Clinical Pocket Companion for

Maternal-Child Nursing Care

Optimizing Outcomes for Mothers, Children, and Families

W0036357

Clinical Pocket Companion for

Maternal-Child Nursing Care

Optimizing Outcomes for Mothers, Children, and Families

Susan L. Ward, PhD, RN
Professor of Nursing
Nebraska Methodist College
Omaha, Nebraska

Shelton M. Hisley, PhD, RNC, WHNP-BC
Assistant Professor of Nursing (Retired)
University of North Carolina at Wilmington
Wilmington, North Carolina

 F.A. Davis Company • Philadelphia

F.A. Davis Company
1915 Arch Street
Philadelphia, PA 19103
www.fadavis.com

Printed in the United States of America

Last digit indicates print number: 10 9 8 7 6 5 4 3 2 1

Publisher, Nursing: Lisa B. Deitch
Developmental Editor: Shirley Kuhn
Director of Content Development: Darlene D. Pedersen
Senior Project Editor: Padraic J. Maroney
Manager of Art and Design: Carolyn O'Brien

As new scientific information becomes available through basic and clinical research, recommended treatments and drug therapies undergo changes. The author(s) and publisher have done everything possible to make this book accurate, up to date, and in accord with accepted standards at the time of publication. The author(s), editors, and publisher are not responsible for errors or omissions or for consequences from application of the book, and make no warranty, expressed or implied, in regard to the contents of the book. Any practice described in this book should be applied by the reader in accordance with professional standards of care used in regard to the unique circumstances that may apply in each situation. The reader is advised always to check product information (package inserts) for changes and new information regarding dose and contraindications before administering any drug. Caution is especially urged when using new or infrequently ordered drugs.

Library of Congress Cataloging-in-Publication Data

Ward, Susan L.
  Clinical pocket companion for Maternal-child nursing care : optimizing outcomes for mothers, children, and families / Susan L. Ward, Shelton M. Hisley.
    p. ; cm.
  Companion for Maternal-child nursing care : optimizing outcomes for mothers, children, and families / Susan L. Ward, Shelton M. Hisley. Philadelphia : F.A. Davis, c2009.
  Includes bibliographical references and index.
  ISBN-13: 978-0-8036-1855-8
  ISBN-10: 0-8036-1855-7
1. Maternity nursing—Handbooks, manuals, etc. 2. Pediatric nursing—Handbooks, manuals, etc. I. Hisley, Shelton M. II. Ward, Susan L. Maternal-child nursing care. III. Title. [DNLM: 1. Maternal-Child Nursing—methods—Handbooks. 2. Cultural Diversity—Handbooks. 3. Evidence-Based Nursing—methods—Handbooks. 4. Holistic Nursing—methods—Handbooks. WY 49 W263c 2010]
  RG951.W369 2010
  618.2'0231—dc22   2009022384

We dedicate the Clinical Pocket Companion to the nurses, students, and faculty who use this book as they provide holistic and culturally sensitive nursing care to mothers, children, and families.

preface

The *Clinical Pocket Companion for Maternal-Child Nursing Care: Optimizing Outcomes for Mothers, Children, and Families* is a handy, concise resource that provides the essential elements for safe, effective nursing practice in maternal and child health. This versatile clinical aid can be beneficial to students and practicing nurses alike. Use it to supplement and reinforce information provided in the parent text during the clinical portion of the course. It also makes a great study guide. As a maternal-child health nurse, you will find it a convenient resource to retrieve important information quickly in a variety of patient settings. Presented in an easy-to-use format, this must-have tool for clinical practice offers students and practicing professional nurses an opportunity to ensure that the care they provide to mothers, children, and families is safe, timely, evidence-based, and culturally sensitive.

The clinical pocket companion is comprised of 32 chapters and is organized in a format that parallels the parent text. The first 14 chapters address ante-, intra-, and post-partal care of the childbearing woman; the final 18 chapters center on the care of infants, children and adolescents.

Pertinent information needed for safe clinical practice is condensed and summarized in a format to facilitate easy retrieval and quick reference. Illustrations enhance and clarify the major concepts presented. Special features focus on the themes of caring, sensitivity, empowerment, holism, spirituality, health promotion, complementary care, and safety.

Each chapter in this clinical pocket companion is organized into the following features:

- Key Terms - Definitions to enhance understanding of key concepts of care
- Focused Assessment - Essential elements of the nursing assessment for specific maternal-child conditions
- Clinical Alerts – Help you to recognize emergent or critical situations
- Diagnostic Tests – Various tests necessary for specific conditions

- Medications – Crucial information about commonly prescribed medications and herbal agents
- Nursing Procedures – Step-by-step instructions to ensure proper technique and positive outcomes
- Ethnocultural Considerations – Emphasize culturally-sensitive care in the clinical setting
- Teaching the Family – Clear teaching guidelines for parents to care for themselves, their infants, and children
- Additional Information for the Clinical Setting – Essential information to facilitate the delivery of safe, effective care in specific circumstances
- Resources – To direct you to various Internet and other sources for additional information

The *Clinical Pocket Companion for Maternal-Child Nursing Care: Optimizing Outcomes for Mothers, Children, and Families* is an easy-to-follow resource designed to help guide your everyday care of patients in the clinical setting. Use it to help you perform an appropriate assessment; formulate a nursing care plan; recognize abnormal findings; teach the mother, child, and family; interpret diagnostic and laboratory data; and provide safe, effective, culturally-sensitive care.

contributors

Deborah Bambini, PhD, WHNP-BC, CNE
Assistant Professor
Grand Valley State University
Grand Rapids, Michigan

Linda Nicholson Grinstead, PhD, RN, CPN, CNE
Professor
Grand Valley State University
Grand Rapids, Michigan

acknowledgments

We thank the editors and production staff of the F.A. Davis Company for their expertise and guidance, especially:

- Lisa Deitch, Publisher, Nursing
- Shirley Kuhn, Special Projects Editor
- Darlene D. Pedersen, Director of Content Development
- Padraic Maroney, Senior Project Editor
- Sam Rondinelli, Assistant Director of Production
- David Orzechowski, Managing Editor
- Julia Reukauf, Marketing Specialist

table of contents

chapter **9**   **The Process of Labor and Birth**   **136**

chapter **10**   **Promoting Patient Comfort During Labor and Birth**   **161**

chapter **11**   **Caring for the Woman Experiencing Complications During Labor and Birth**   **175**

Caring for Women, Families, and Children in Contemporary Society

KEY TERMS

climacteric – Transitional time in a woman's life marked by declining ovarian function and decreased hormone production

dysmenorrhea – Painful menstruation that interferes with daily activities

dysplasia – Abnormal development of tissues or organs

endometriosis – Benign disorder of the reproductive tract characterized by the presence and growth of endometrial tissue outside of the uterus.

hyperprolactinemia – Excessive secretion of prolactin

leiomyoma – Fibroid, a benign smooth muscle uterine tumor

menopause – Permanent cessation of menstrual periods; can only be dated with certainty 1 year after menstruation ceases

mittelschmerz – Abdominal pain in the region of an ovary during ovulation; usually occurs midway through the menstrual cycle

perimenopause – Period of transition of changing ovarian activity before menopause and through the first few years of amenorrhea

prostaglandins – Chemical mediators produced by the tissues and found in many parts of the body; play an important role in menstrual cramps

Infants and Children

FOCUSED ASSESSMENT

Recommended Immunization Schedule for Children

Vaccine ▼ / Age ►	Birth	1 month	2 months	4 months	6 months	12 months	15 months	18 months	19–23 months	2–3 years	4–6 years
Hepatitis B[1]	Hep B	Hep B		see footnote 1	Hep B						
Rotavirus[2]			Rota	Rota	Rota						
Diphtheria, Tetanus, Pertussis[3]			DTaP	DTaP	DTaP	see footnote 3	DTaP				DTaP
Haemophilus influenzae type b[4]			Hib	Hib	Hib[4]	Hib					
Pneumococcal[5]			PCV	PCV	PCV	PCV				PPV	
Inactivated Poliovirus[6]			IPV	IPV	IPV						IPV
Influenza[6]					Influenza (Yearly)						
Measles, Mumps, Rubella[7]						MMR					MMR
Varicella[8]						Varicella					Varicella
Hepatitis A[9]						HepA (2 doses)				HepA Series	
Meningococcal[10]										MCV4	

Range of recommended ages ▭ Certain high-risk groups ▭

Source: Centers for Disease Control and Prevention (2008).

TEACHING THE FAMILY

Nutrition

Guidelines for Infant Feeding	
Infant/Child Age	**Feeding Guidelines**
Birth–1 Month	Breast every 2–3 hours Bottle every 3–4 hours 2–3 oz. per feeding
2–4 Months	Breast or bottle every 3–4 hours 3–4 oz. per feeding
4–6 Months	Breast or bottle 4–6 times per day 4–5 oz. per feeding
6–8 Months	Iron-fortified rice cereal Breast or bottle 4 times per day 6–8 oz. per feeding

Infant/Child Age	Feeding Guidelines
8–10 Months	Finger foods Chopped or mashed foods Sippy cup with formula, breast milk, juice or water Breast or bottle 4 times per day 6–8 oz. per feeding
10–12 Months	Self-feeds with fingers and spoon Most table foods Breast or bottle 4 times per day 6–8 oz. per feeding

Introducing Solid Foods to Infants

Tips for Introducing Solid Foods to Infants
- The infant displays readiness at approximately 6 months of age.
- Assess for developmental cues: ability to sit well with support; disappearance of the extrusion reflex.
- Begin with iron-fortified rice cereal.
- Add vegetables, then fruits.
- Introduce one food at a time; wait 3 to 5 days between new foods.
- Introduce food before formula or breastfeeding; follow each solid food meal with breast milk or formula.

Alert: If the infant is not growing or gaining weight, or if he is unable to suck or swallow or shows any sign of an allergic reaction, promptly seek help from the primary health care provider, nearby clinic, or emergency room.

Additional Information
- Avoid salt, sugar, and additives.
- **Never** prop bottles, put food in bottles, or mix food with formula (choking hazard).
- Offer only small bites of food to prevent choking; when feeding, pay close attention to the infant.

(American Academy of Pediatrics, 2005)

Dental Care

Guidelines for Parents
- Teething typically begins between 4 and 7 months.
- It is normal for an infant to have any number of teeth ranging from no teeth to 8 or more teeth by the first birthday.

- Most children have all 20 primary teeth by the third birthday.
- Signs of teething:
  - Drooling, irritability, desire to chew on objects, crying episodes, disrupted sleep, change in eating patterns
- Interventions for teething discomfort:
  - Give infant a cool wet washcloth to chew on.
  - Place teething rings in the refrigerator for a few minutes before applying.
  - Rub gums with a clean finger.
- Take the infant to the dentist within 6 months of the eruption of the first tooth.
- Cleanse the gums with a damp washcloth or soft toothbrush.
- Do not use toothpaste until the child reaches age 2.

Sleep and Rest

Sleep Requirements			
Age	Hours of Sleep	Additional Naps	Tips
Newborn	15–20	—	"Back to sleep": Always place infant on back for sleep
3 Months	15	—	Put infant to bed drowsy but awake so that he learns to fall asleep on his own.
6 Months	9–14	Two 2-hour naps	
1 Year	9–14	May decrease slightly	
Toddler/ Preschool	14	Usually one nap for 1.5–3 hours	Bedtime resistance often appears. Utilize bedtime rituals.
School Age	10–12 +/–	—	

Prevent Plagiocephaly

- Infant skulls are soft and flexible during the first year of life as the skull enlarges to accommodate the growing brain. During this time, the infant skull can become misshapen or deformed by external pressure. This condition is rarely life threatening, but can cause permanent facial and skull deformities, or in severe cases, the child's vision can be affected.

- Constant pressure on one area of the infant's head can flatten or reshape it. Proper positioning during sleep and waking periods spent in car seats and infant chairs often require the infant to spend considerable time on his back.
- Place the infant on the stomach to play for several times each day. When the infant is very young, place a rolled towel or blanket under his arms for support. This intervention removes pressure from the skull and facilitates the development of strong neck and arm muscles needed for sitting and crawling.
- Place the infant on his side during awake times.
- Alternate the direction the infant faces in the bassinette or crib during sleep times. If the infant's crib is positioned against a wall, alternate the end of the bed where the infant's head is placed to allow her to look out toward the room instead of the less stimulating wall.
- Seek medical advice if a flattened area on the baby's skull does not improve with positioning changes; a customized helmet may be necessary.

Promoting Safety for Infants and Children

Review with parents:

- Car seat guidelines
- Household smoke and carbon monoxide detectors; fire extinguishers
- Storage of medications and cleaning supplies: Install child-safety latches.
- Crib safety: Ensure that bars are less than 2 3/8 inches apart; mattress fits snugly; free from sharp edges and toxic paint.
- Hazards of microwave ovens: Never use to warm infant bottles or food.
- Use of pacifiers: Never place around infant's neck or attach to clothing.
- Proper use of highchairs, strollers, swings, playpens; avoid walkers.
- Infant care basics:
  - Keep one hand on the infant when on a changing table or other high surface.
  - At bath time, test water temperature with wrist, keep both hands on infant.
- Use safety gates at all stairways.

ETHNOCULTURAL CONSIDERATIONS

Infant Feeding

Culture plays an important role in infant feeding. For many new immigrants and members of ethnic minorities, the traditions of their homeland, the consumption of traditional foods, and maintaining traditional food preparations provide comfort in an environment that is new *and* unknown, and is a way of sustaining cultural identity. Some cultural practices include breastfeeding on demand and early introduction of solid foods, whereas others feel that exposure of the breast is indecent and therefore decreases the mother's comfort with breastfeeding. It is imperative for nurses to recognize biases that the Western view of health and nutrition is the only appropriate method to feeding an infant. Nurses need to evaluate the effect of the cultural practices objectively and intervene only if the mother or infant is at risk for harm.

Adolescents

FOCUSED ASSESSMENT

Components of Health Promotion Screening

Screening should include (Michigan Quality Improvement Consortium, 2005a):

- Height, weight, and body mass index (BMI)
- Risk evaluation and counseling:
  - Nutrition, obesity, physical activity, dental health, tobacco use, immunizations, human immunodeficiency virus (HIV) prevention, sexually transmitted diseases prevention and sexual health, sexual abuse, preconception counseling for all women of childbearing age, medication use, and sun exposure
- Safety:
  - Intimate partner violence, seat belt use, use of helmets, firearm safety, and use of smoke and carbon monoxide detectors in the home
- Behavior assessment:
  - Depression, suicide threats, alcohol and drug use, anxiety, stress reduction, risk-taking behaviors and coping skills
  - Consideration of developmental tasks

- Piaget: Thought becomes more abstract
- Erikson: Role experimentation; peer influence
- Freud: Puberty and development of sexuality

TEACHING THE FAMILY

Safety

Discuss the following topics:

- Decision making
- Strategies for conflict resolution
- Reproductive health safety
- Risk-taking behaviors (substance use and abuse, violence, tattooing, body piercing)
- Signs of depression, suicide, eating disorders
- Injury prevention (seatbelt, helmet, other protective wear for sports)

Health Promotion

- Adequate calcium and vitamin D intake
- Adequate sleep, rest, and exercise
- Preparation for the first gynecological visit (ages 13–15); pelvic examination by age 21 or 3 years after the initiation of sexual activity

Adult Health

FOCUSED ASSESSMENT

Preventive Screening Recommendations

Service	19–39 Years	40–64 Years	65 + Years
Aspirin Prophylaxis	Discuss with women post-menopause, men older than 40 years, and younger individuals at increased risk for coronary heart disease.		
Breast Cancer Screening		Annual mammogram for women with risk factors; every 1–2 years for women 50 to 64 years of age with no risk factors	Annual mammogram for women with risk factors; every 1–2 years for women 65 and older with no risk factors

(continued)

Preventive Screening Recommendations (Continued)

Service	19–39 Years	40–64 Years	65 + Years
Cervical Cancer Screening	First Pap smear at age 21 or 3 years after first sexual intercourse, whichever is earlier; every 3 years after 3 consecutive normal results	Every 3 years after 3 consecutive normal results	Pap smear with new sexual partner
***Chlamydia* and Gonorrhea Screening**	All sexually active females, including asymptomatic women age 25 years and younger		
Colon Cancer Screening	All persons 50–79 years of age		
Hypertension Screening	Blood pressure screening every 2 years if <120/80 mm Hg; annual blood pressure screening if 120–139/80–89 mm Hg		
Influenza Vaccine	Annually between October and March for individuals age 50 years and older, those with chronic illnesses, members of the health care team, and others at high risk		
Pneumococcal Vaccine	Immunize individuals at high risk once; re-immunize once after 5 years if at risk for losing immunity.		Immunize at age 65 if not done previously; re-immunize once if first vaccination received >5 years ago and before age 65.
Problem Drinking Screening	Screen for problem drinking among all adults and provide brief counseling.		
Tobacco Cessation Counseling	Assess all adults for tobacco use and provide ongoing cessation services for those who smoke or are at risk for smoking relapse.		
Total Cholesterol and HDL Cholesterol Screening	Fasting fractionated lipid screening for men older than age 34 every 5 years	Fasting fractionated lipid screening for men older than age 34 and for women older than age 44 every 5 years	
Vision Screening			Asymptomatic elderly adults

Sources: American College of Obstetricians and Gynecologists (2007); U.S. Preventive Services Task Force (2007); Institute for Clinical Systems Improvement (2005).

Breast Cancer Risk Factors

- Defects in breast cancer gene 1 (*BRCA1*) or breast cancer gene 2 (*BRCA2*)
- Gender: 100 times more likely to occur in females than in males
- Age: Increasing age, with 50% appearing by age 50
- Personal history of breast cancer in at least one breast
- Family history of breast cancer
- Exposure to radiation
- Excess weight
- Exposure to estrogen: Early onset of menarche, late menopause, or use of hormonal therapy
- Race: Caucasians more likely to develop breast cancer than Hispanics or African Americans
- Smoking
- Exposure to carcinogens
- Excessive use of alcohol
- Diagnosis of precancerous breast changes
- Increased breast density revealed on mammography

(American Cancer Society [ACS], 2006)

Osteoporosis Risk Factors

- Older age, due to decreased estrogen after menopause
- Slender build and small frame
- Low body weight (< 70 kg [150 lbs.])
- Shortened exposure to estrogen, through late menarche or early menopause
- Family history of osteoporosis
- Smoking
- Decreased physical activity or sedentary lifestyle
- Excessive caffeine or alcohol use
- Low calcium and vitamin D intake
- Southeast Asian and Caucasian ethnicity
- Use of corticosteroids, commonly used to treat chronic respiratory disorders and arthritis

DIAGNOSTIC TESTS

Cholesterol and Lipid Screening

Guidelines for Interpreting Lipid Screening Results	
Total Cholesterol	
Below 200 mg/dL:	Desirable
240 mg/dL and above:	High, increased risk of cardiac disease
LDL Cholesterol	
Below 100 mg/dL:	Desirable; target goal for those with cardiac disease or multiple risk factors
100–129 mg/dL:	Elevated; target goal for those with two or more risk factors
130–160 mg/dL:	Borderline high; target goal for those with zero to one risk factor
Above 160 mg/dL:	Significantly elevated
HDL Cholesterol	
Below 40 mg/dL:	Adds a risk factor for cardiac disease
60 mg/dL and above:	Desirable
Triglycerides	
Below 150 mg/dL:	Desirable
200 mg/dL and above:	High

Source: Veterans Health Administration, Department of Defense (2006).

MEDICATIONS

Herbal Remedies for Anxiety and Depression

Herbal remedies for anxiety and depression include kava kava, passionflower, valerian root, gotu kola, and St. John's wort. Although these herbs are believed to reduce anxiety, stress, and muscle tension, the nurse should provide education on the potential side effects of these substances, which include gastrointestinal discomforts, nausea, and dizziness.

ETHNOCULTURAL CONSIDERATIONS

Breast Cancer Screening

There are notable differences in breast cancer screening practices among women of different ethnic backgrounds. Although African American women are at a lower risk for developing breast cancer than Caucasian women are, they are more likely to die from breast cancer due to late diagnosis. According to Husaini et al. (2001), African American women are more likely to have mammogram screening if they are older, married, have a higher level of education, and believe that early detection could lead to a cure. A positive family history of breast cancer and church affiliation have no influence on the incidence of detection.

Asian American and Pacific Islander women have very low rates of breast cancer screening. Factors responsible for the low screening rates include lack of health insurance, low income, and lack of a primary care provider (Kagawa-Singer & Pourat, 2000).

Breast cancer causes a significant number of deaths in Filipino women. In a study by Wu and Bancroft (2006), researchers found that women were more likely to follow recommended screenings if there was support from physicians and family members and if they had insurance. The presence of physical symptoms, family history of breast cancer, and health literacy promote adherence to recommendations.

TEACHING THE FAMILY

Breast Self-Examination (BSE)

1. Visually inspect the breasts in front of a mirror. Assess for color, contour, shape, and size. Assess for dimpling or puckering of the skin; change in nipple direction; and redness, rash, or swelling

2. Repeat the first step with the arms slightly raised above the head.

3. Inspect and palpate the nipple. Gently squeeze the nipple between the thumb and forefinger, looking for discharge. Many women, especially those who have had children, are able to express some discharge by squeezing the nipples. Discharge that is of concern is most often spontaneous (ACS, 2007).

4. Palpate the breast and axillae. Recline on the bed and place a pillow under each shoulder during palpation. Use the left hand to palpate the right breast and the right hand to palpate the left breast. Using the finger pads of the three middle fingers, palpate the entire surface of the breast. Use overlapping dime-sized circular motions and apply three different levels of pressure: light pressure is best to feel the tissue closest to the skin; medium pressure is best to feel a little deeper; and firm pressure is used to feel the tissue closest to the chest and ribs.

5. Move around the breast in an up-and-down pattern, checking the entire breast area until only the ribs are felt.
6. Repeat the entire technique on the other breast (ACS, 2007).

How to Recognize and Cope with Fibrocystic Changes in the Breast

- Palpable thickening in breast tissue, associated with cyclic tenderness, pain
- Common, benign, usually appear during second and third decades of life
- Treat by relieving symptoms (e.g., analgesics, nonsteroidal anti-inflammatory drugs such as ibuprofen), diuretics, use of support bra, avoidance of tobacco and alcohol, application of heat to breasts.

How to Perform Testicular Self-Examination

1. Examine the testicles, one at a time. One should be slightly larger than the other (usually the right one).
2. Feel for lumps and bumps along the front and sides.
3. Using both hands, place your thumbs over the top of each testicle and your index fingers and middle fingers underneath the testicle. Gently roll the testicle, using slight pressure, between your fingers.

4. The epididymis, which carries the sperm, can be felt at the top of the back part of each testicle. It should feel soft and rope-like and be slightly tender to pressure. This is a normal finding.
5. Notify your physician if you notice any swelling, lumps, pains, or changes in color or size of either testicle (The Nemours Foundation, 2007).

ADDITIONAL INFORMATION FOR THE CLINICAL SETTING

Speaking with an Adolescent About Losing Weight

- Discussions about weight loss can be a sensitive issue for many overweight patients, especially during adolescence. Body weight has a dramatic effect on the development of self-image and self-esteem.
- Begin the conversation with expressions of respect that are sensitive to cultural differences related to food choices and eating patterns. Regardless of whether or not the patient is ready to begin a weight control program, she may still benefit from talking openly about healthy eating and exercise.
- Begin with a simple question to determine if the patient is willing to talk about the issue: *"Cindy, can we talk about your weight? What are your thoughts about your weight right now?" "What kind of help would you like from me regarding your weight?"*
- Avoid the use of words that may make patients feel uncomfortable, such as "obese," "obesity," "fat," and "excess fat."
- To determine the degree of readiness to engage in weight control, additional questions can be asked: *"What are your goals concerning your weight?"*

Health Promotion Counseling for Perimenopausal Women

Counsel perimenopausal women about:

- Healthy lifestyle strategies: Smoking cessation, consuming a variety of foods low in saturated fat and cholesterol, limiting salt and alcohol intake, maintaining a healthy weight, and being physically active
- Prevention of osteoporosis: Consuming foods rich in vitamin D and calcium, obtaining moderate exposure to sunlight, engaging in weight-bearing exercises; smoking cessation; and limiting alcohol intake
- Treatment of menopausal symptoms: Alternative therapies; antidepressants; stress reduction; avoidance of spicy foods, alcohol, and caffeine; getting adequate sleep; being physically active; use of selective estrogen receptor modulators (SERMs) for severe symptoms only

Empowering Women to Cope with Symptoms of Menopause

Dietary supplements and herbal therapies have long provided women with alternative treatments to alleviate some of the symptoms associated with menopause (e.g., soy, vitamins, probiotics, and herbs such as black cohosh). Research evidence does not support the ideas that they are efficacious in minimizing menopausal symptoms (Nedrow et al., 2006).

Complementary therapies that are currently being studied for their benefit in diminishing menopausal symptoms include:

- Mind–body therapy
- Energy therapy: Electromagnetic forces, life-force energy
- Manipulative and body-based therapy: Chiropractic, osteopathy, massage
- Traditional Chinese medicine

While there is no current evidence to support their effectiveness in minimizing the symptoms of menopause, these complementary methods are considered to be much safer than herbal and vitamin therapies.

Health Promotion for Older Adults

- Exercise and activity: Improve strength, endurance, flexibility, and balance

- Cognitive functioning
  - Stress management
  - Coping strategies
  - Medical management of physical illnesses
  - Healthy lifestyle choices: good nutrition, moderation of alcohol, elimination of tobacco use
- Functional assessment
- Immunizations
  - Influenza
  - Pneumococcus

REFERENCES

American Academy of Pediatrics. (2005). Policy statement: Breastfeeding and the use of human milk. *Pediatrics, 115*(2), 496–506.

American Cancer Society (ACS). (2006). What are the risk factors for breast cancer? Retrieved from http://www.cancer.org/docroot/CRI/content/CRI_2_4_2X_What_are_the_risk_factors_for_breast_cancer_5.asp?sitearea= (Accessed October 29, 2008).

American Cancer Society (ACS). (2007). How to perform a breast self-exam. Retrieved from http://www.cancer.org/docroot/CRI/content/CRI-2-6x-How-to-perform-a-breast-self-exam-5.asp (Accessed March 4, 2008).

American College of Obstetricians and Gynecologists. (2007). *Women's health care: a resource manual* (3rd ed.). Washington, DC: Author.

Husaini, B.A., Sherkat, D.E., Bragg, R., Levine R., Emerson, J.S., Mentes, C.M., et al. (2001). Predictors of breast cancer screening in a panel study of African American women. *Women and Health, 34*(3), 35–51.

Institute for Clinical Systems Improvement (ICSI). (2005, October). *Preventive services in adults.* Bloomington, MN: Author.

Kagawa-Singer, M., & Pourat, N. (2000). Asian American and Pacific Islander breast and cervical carcinoma screening rates and healthy people 2000 objectives. *Cancer, 89*(3), 696–705.

Michigan Quality Improvement Consortium. (2005a, July). *Adult preventive services (ages 18–49).* Southfield, MI: Author.

Nedrow, A., Miller, J., Walker, M., Nygren, P., Huffman, L.H., & Nelson, H.D. (2006). Complementary and alternative therapies for the management of menopause-related symptoms: A systematic evidence review. *Archives of Internal Medicine, 166*(14), 1453–1465.

Nield, L.S., & Kamat, D.M. (2006). Odd skull shapes: Heads up on diagnosis and therapy, *Consultant for Pediatricians, 5*(11), 701–709.

The Nemours Foundation. (2007). How to perform a testicular self-examination. Retrieved from http://www.kidshealth.org/teen/sexual_health/guys/tse.html (Accessed March 14, 2008).

Veterans Health Administration, Department of Defense. (2006). *VHA/DoD clinical practice guideline for the management of dyslipidemia in primary care.* Washington, DC: Author.

Wu, T.Y., & Bancroft, J. (2006). Filipino American women's perceptions and experiences with breast cancer screening. *Oncology Nursing Forum, 33*(4), E71–E78.

Reproductive Anatomy and Physiology

KEY TERMS

adrenarche – Changes that occur at puberty as a result of increased secretion of adrenocortical hormones

ferning – Palm leaf or arborization pattern found on microscopic examination of a sample of certain fluids such as cervical mucus and amniotic fluid

gonad – Sex gland that produces hormone (ovary and testis)

graafian follicle – Mature ovarian cyst that contains the nearly mature ovum (oocyte); on rupture of the follicle, it is discharged from the ovary (ovulation); the corpus luteum develops within the ruptured graafian follicle

gravid – Pregnant

menarche – The first menstrual period

oocyte – Incompletely developed ovum

oogenesis – Process of oocyte development that results in maturation of human ova

puberty – Biological time frame between childhood and adulthood; during this time the reproductive organs mature and the individual becomes functionally capable of reproduction

sex chromosome – Chromosome associated with the determination of sex: X (female); Y (male)

spinnbarkheit – The formation of a stretchable thread of cervical mucus; occurs at the time of ovulation due to the influence of estrogen

thelarche – Beginning of breast development

FOCUSED ASSESSMENT

Assessment of the reproductive system should start with a general health assessment:

- Chief complaint
- Associated/alleviating factors
- Past medical history
- Family health history
- Social history
- Timeline of development of the secondary sexual characteristics

Female Body Changes Associated with Puberty

Type of Body Change	Body Change	Definition	Average Age Initiated	Average Age Completed
Growth Spurt	Adolescent growth spurt	Height increase 2.4–4.3 inches (6–11 cm) in 1 year	10	11.8
Secondary	Thelarche	Breast budding	9.8	14.6
	Adrenarche	↑ adrenal androgen secretion → axillary and pubic hair	10.5	
Primary	Menarche	First menstrual period	12.8	

FEMALE REPRODUCTIVE SYSTEM

External Structures

Include mons pubis, labia majora, labia minora, clitoris, vestibule of the vagina, urethral (urinary) meatus, Skene's glands, Bartholin's glands, vaginal introitus, hymen, and perineum (Fig. 2-1).

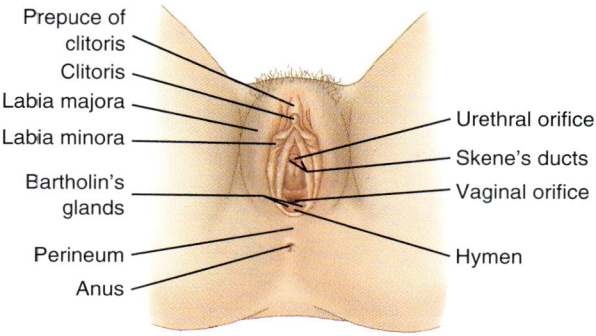

Figure 2-1 Female external genitalia.

The Pelvic Floor
- Muscles include the levator ani and coccygeus.
  o Provide support for internal pelvic structures.

Internal Structures

Include the ovaries, fallopian tubes, uterus, adjacent structures (adnexa), and vagina (Figs. 2-2 and 2-3).

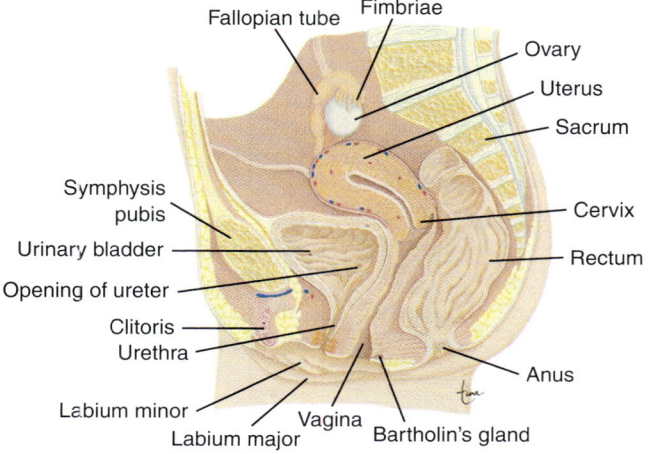

Figure 2-2 Midsagittal view of the female reproductive system.

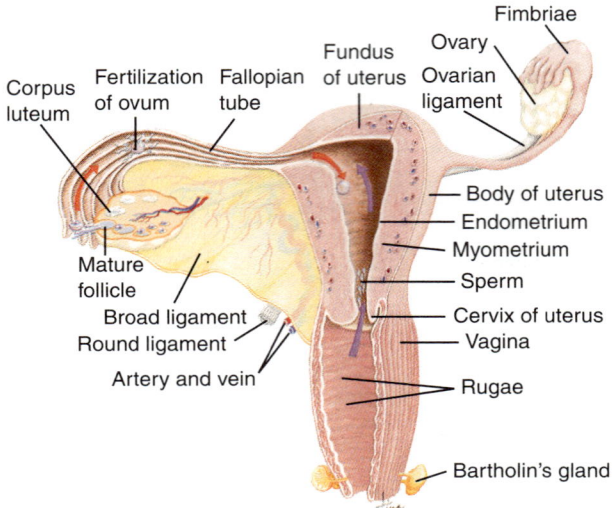

Figure 2-3 The female reproductive system shown in anterior view.

Uterine Anatomy
- Corpus: Upper two thirds of uterine body
- Isthmus: Slight constriction midway between the corpus and the cervix
- Cervix: Lower, narrow end of the uterus, opens into the vagina

Uterine Support Structures
Include the broad, round, cardinal, pubocervical, and uterosacral ligaments (support upper and middle portions of the uterus); and pelvic floor muscles (support lower portion of the uterus).

Bony Pelvis (Fig. 2-4)
- Composed of sacrum, coccyx, and two innominate (hip) bones.
- Includes the "false pelvis" and the "true pelvis."
- True pelvis is divided into inlet, midpelvis, outlet.

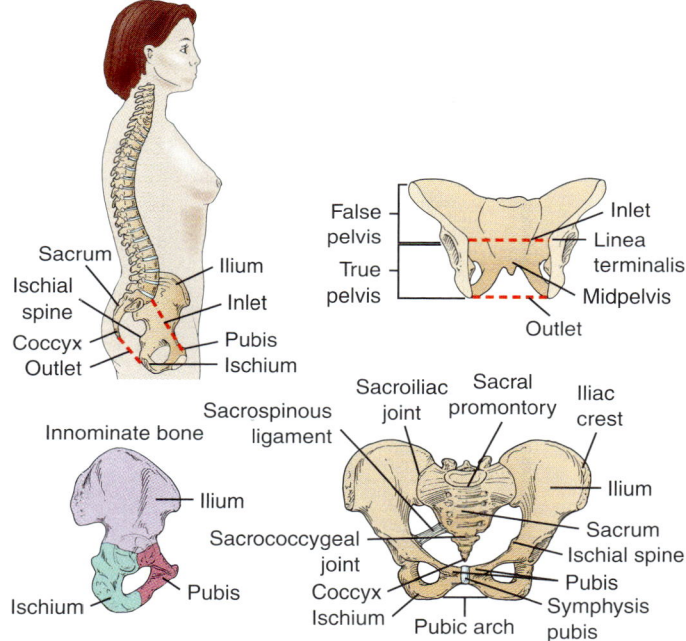

Figure 2-4 The female bony pelvis.

The Breasts

- Considered accessory organs of the reproductive system.
- Consist of glandular, fibrous, and adipose tissue suspended by Cooper's ligaments.
- Primary function is infant nourishment.
- Lactation is triggered by prolactin.
- Parts include nipples, areolae, and Montgomery tubercles.

The Menstrual Cycle and Reproduction

The menstrual cycle is hormonally mediated through events in the hypothalamus, anterior pituitary gland, and ovaries (Fig. 2-5). Interrelationships exist among the levels of hormone secretion, development of the ovarian follicles, and changes in the uterine endometrium (Fig. 2-6).

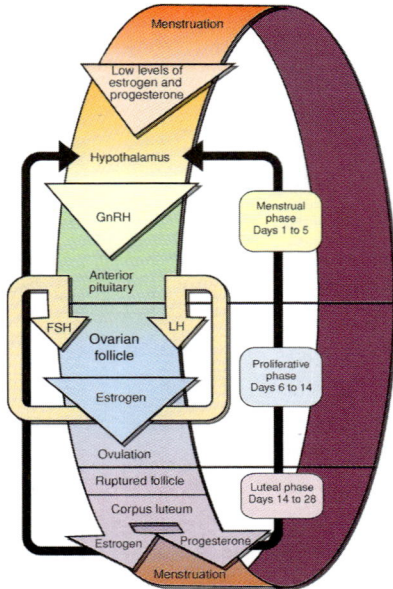

Figure 2-5 Hormonal feedback mechanisms that regulate the female menstrual cycle.

Body Changes Related to the Menstrual Cycle and Ovulation
- Cervical mucus
  - Increased amount: Watery, clear
  - Increased elasticity (spinnbarkheit)
  - Increased ferning
- Physiological changes
  - Increased basal body temperature
  - Mittelschmerz

Natural Cessation of Menses
- Climacteric phase: Decline in ovarian function and loss of estrogen and progesterone production
- Perimenopausal phase: Precedes menopause; characterized by physical/psychological changes related to estrogen depletion
- Menopause (last menstrual period)
- Postmenopausal phase: Time after menopause; estrogen produced by the adrenal glands

Figure 2-6 The female reproductive cycle. Levels of the hormones secreted from the anterior pituitary are shown relative to one another and throughout the cycle. Changes in the ovarian follicle are depicted. The relative thickness of the endometrium is also shown.

MALE REPRODUCTIVE SYSTEM

External Structures

Consist of the perineum, penis, and scrotum (Fig. 2-7).

Internal Structures

Include the testes, epididymis, ducts (vas deferens, ejaculatory duct), urethra, spermatic cords, and accessory glands (seminal vesicles, prostate, bulbourethral glands and urethral glands).

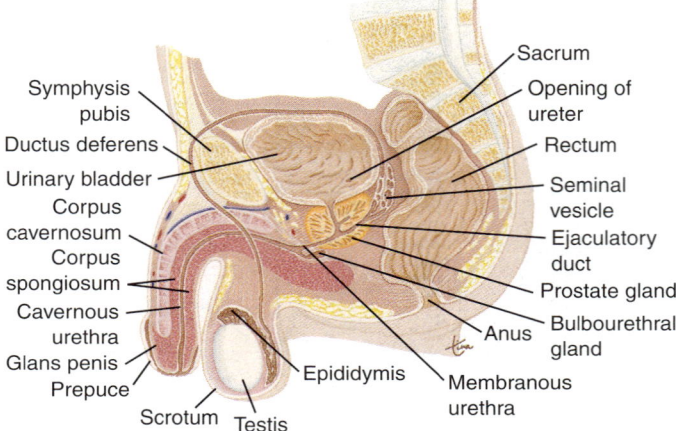

Figure 2-7 The male reproductive system shown in a midsagittal section through the pelvic cavity.

Hormonal Influence

Testosterone is the dominant male hormone.

- At puberty, stimulates enlargement of testes and accessory organs
- Prompts development of the secondary sex characteristics and a linear growth spurt

Human Sexuality and Fertility

KEY TERMS

abortion – Termination of pregnancy before the fetus reaches a viable age, usually less than 20 weeks of gestation or when the fetus weighs less than 500 grams

> **elective a.** Voluntary termination of a pregnancy for other than medical reasons

> **therapeutic a.** Abortion performed when the pregnancy endangers the mother's mental or physical health or when the fetus has a known condition that is incompatible with life

abstinence – Refraining from vaginal intercourse

basal body temperature (BBT) – Lowest body temperature taken immediately on awakening and before arising

bilateral tubal ligation (BTL) – Method of female sterilization in which both fallopian tubes are blocked to prevent conception

contraception – Prevention of conception

dyspareunia – Pain with sexual intercourse

hysterosalpingography – Radiography of the uterus and fallopian tubes after injection of a radiopaque iodine-based dye

infertility – Inability to achieve pregnancy during a year or more of unprotected intercourse

intrauterine device (IUD) – Small plastic device that is inserted into the uterus and left in place for an extended period of time to prevent implantation of a fertilized ovum

menorrhagia – Menstrual bleeding that is excessive in number of days or amount of blood

sterility – Absolute factor prevents reproduction

theoretical effectiveness – Effectiveness in a laboratory setting

toxic shock syndrome (TSS) – Severe, acute disease most often caused by *Staphylococcus aureus*; has also been associated with the use of high-absorbency tampons during menstruation but may complicate any staphylococcal infection

user effectiveness – Number of women who will become pregnant within 1 year of typical use (includes user error)

vasectomy – Male sterilization that involves ligation or the removal of a segment of the vas deferens

zygote – Fertilized ovum that results from the union of an ovum and a sperm

FOCUSED ASSESSMENT

Components of a Reproductive Health History

- General health history: Chronic health problems, tobacco, alcohol and other substance use, medications, herbal supplements
- Menstrual history: Age at onset, frequency, duration, flow, presence of dysmenorrhea or breast tenderness
- Obstetric history: Outcomes of past pregnancies; plans for future pregnancies
- Sexual history and risk assessment: Previous sexually transmitted infections (STIs), dyspareunia, postcoital bleeding, frequency of intercourse (is it consensual?), number of past sexual partners, current partner(s), gender, sexual practices, use of protective devices
- Past contraceptive use: Any difficulties with specific methods

DIAGNOSTIC TESTS

Common Diagnostic Methods Used in the Evaluation of Female Infertility

Type/Name of Test	Role of the Nurse
Prediction of Ovulation Identifies the LH surge (24–36 hours before ovulation) and absence of ovulation. Tests include basal body	Teach the couple how the information helps to determine timing of intercourse to coincide with ovulation. Instruct the woman about recording the BBT and

Type/Name of Test	Role of the Nurse
temperature (BBT), commercial ovulation predictor kits, and assessment of cervical mucus.	assessing the cervical mucus; reinforce directions for using commercial ovulation predictor kits.
Postcoital Test (PCT); Huhner Test Assessment of the quality and quantity of cervical mucus and sperm function at the time of ovulation	Instruct the patient to arrange to come in to the office 6–12 hours after intercourse for evaluation of the cervical mucus.
Ultrasound Examination To evaluate structure of the pelvic organs, identify maturing ovarian follicles and the timing of ovulation	Reassure the patient that sonography uses sound waves, not radiation, to evaluate the pelvic structures. The examination may be conducted transabdominally or transvaginally and specific instructions are given, depending on method.
Hysterosalpingography Radiopaque dye is injected through the cervix, into the uterus and tubes. Evaluates structural integrity of the uterus and tubes.	May experience cramping, referred shoulder pain. Use nonsteroidal anti-inflammatory drugs (NSAIDs) as needed for pain. Report heavy cramping, bleeding, fever or malodorous discharge.
Tests of Endocrine Function Used to evaluate the hypothalamus, pituitary gland and ovaries. Levels of follicle-stimulating hormone (FSH), luteinizing hormone (LH), estrogen, and progesterone are assessed.	Timing of blood tests is very important for accurate interpretation of the results. Explain that FSH and LH stimulate ovulation; and estrogen and progesterone make the endometrium receptive for implantation of the fertilized ovum.
Endometrial Biopsy Involves the removal of a sample of the endometrium with a small pipette attached to suction. Provides information about the effects of progesterone (produced by the corpus luteum after ovulation) on the endometrium.	Teach the patient about the purpose and appropriate timing of the test: it should be performed not earlier than 10–12 days after ovulation (2–3 days before menstruation is expected). Cramping, pelvic discomfort, and vaginal spotting may occur; a mild analgesic (e.g., ibuprofen) may be used to alleviate the discomfort.
Hysteroscopy and Laparoscopy Endoscopic exam of the interior of the uterus and the pelvic organs under general anesthesia. Hysteroscopy may be performed without general anesthesia in the office. Abnormalities such as polyps, myomata (fibroid tumors), and endometrial adhesions are identified.	Explain the purpose of the test and other procedures that may be done at the same time. When general anesthesia is to be used, the patient should take nothing by mouth for several hours before the planned procedure. Advise her that since carbon dioxide gas will be instilled into the abdomen to enhance organ visibility, she may experience postoperative cramping and referred shoulder pain, which can be relieved with a mild analgesic.

Basic Infertility Evaluation and Workup	
Female	**Male**
CBC	Semen analysis: Sperm count should be:
Urinalysis	Volume of 2–6 mL of semen
Pap smear and wet mount	
Serology	>20 million sperm per 1 mL of semen
Luteinizing-hormone-surge	>50% forward moving sperm
ovulation predictor kit	>30% normal sperm
FSH cycle day 3 if >35 years old	
Rh factor, blood grouping	<1 million WBCs/mL of semen
Hysterosalpingography (to reveal	
uterine or tubal obstruction or	
abnormalities)	

MEDICATIONS

Counseling About Medications that Decrease the Effectiveness of Oral Contraceptives

- Take a thorough history.
- Use of certain medications (e.g., Rifadin, Rimactane), isoniazid, barbiturates, and griseofulvin (Fulvicin-U/F, Gris-PEG, Grifulvin V) can decrease effectiveness of oral contraceptives and higher doses of estrogen must be used.
- Vomiting and diarrhea affect the absorption of oral contraceptives; thus patients who experience these symptoms should use a backup method such as condoms.
- Interactions with certain drugs such as acetaminophen, anticoagulants, and some anticonvulsants (e.g., phenytoin sodium, carbamazepine, primidone, topiramate) may reduce the efficacy of oral contraceptives.

TEACHING THE FAMILY

Contraception

Topics to discuss with the patient:

- Use and satisfaction with previous methods
- Lifestyle, ability to manage chosen method
- Indications, contraindications, side effects, efficacy
- Reinforce that no method is 100% effective except abstinence.

Methods of Contraception

Medication-Free Contraception

Method	Description	Teaching
Natural Family Planning (NFP)	Identify fertile time and avoid intercourse during that time.	The only method acceptable to the Roman Catholic Church
Fertility Awareness Methods (FAM)	Identify fertile time and use abstinence or other contraceptive method during that time. Utilizes assessment of BBT, cervical mucus changes, abdominal bloating, and mittelschmerz.	Both NFP and FAM require patients who are very aware of the subtle changes during cycles and who have regular, predictable cycles. Both partners must be motivated to use the method successfully. Stress or illness can affect the timing of the cycle. User effectiveness: 75%
Coitus interruptus	Withdrawal	Ejaculation may occur before full withdrawal. User effectiveness: 71%
Lactational Amenorrhea Method (LAM)	Breastfeeding	Can be effective if breastfeeding exclusively. Some lactating mothers ovulate without menstruating. If exclusively breastfeeding, infant younger than 6 months of age, and no menses since childbirth, user effectiveness approaches 98%.
Abstinence	Refrain from intercourse.	Requires commitment and self-control. User effectiveness: 100%

Barrier Methods of Contraception

With all barrier methods, wash hands before and after use.

Method	Description	Teaching
Diaphragm	Rubber/latex dome-shaped barrier inserted into vagina to cover cervix **CONTRAINDICATIONS:** Latex allergy, predisposition to urinary tract infections (UTIs)	Use spermicide in center and around edges. Place up to 6 hours before intercourse **Must** leave in place 6–24 hours after intercourse. Wash with warm, soapy water. Inspect for holes and tears. *(continued)*

Barrier Methods of Contraception (Continued)

Method	Description	Teaching
		Re-fit with 20% weight change or pregnancy. Provides no protection against STIs. Side effects: UTI, irritation from spermicide User effectiveness: 84%
Cervical Cap	Thimble-shaped latex device fits firmly around cervix **CONTRAINDICATIONS:** History of toxic shock syndrome (TSS), pelvic inflammatory disease (PID), cervical disease, latex allergy	Use spermicide in the cap before placement. Requires dexterity. Provides no protection against STIs. Side effects: Cervical irritation, allergic reaction User effectiveness: 74%
Male Condoms	Placed over erect penis before ANY genital, oral, or anal contact **CONTRAINDICATIONS:** Latex allergy (polyurethane and natural membrane condoms are available but offer no protection against HIV and STIs).	Penis must be erect for placement. Leave space at tip as reservoir. Remove while still erect, grasping at the base and avoiding spillage. Avoid using condoms with the spermicide nonoxynol-9. Side effects: Allergic reaction User effectiveness: 85%
Female Condoms	Polyurethane vaginal sheath with a ring at each end	More expensive than male condom Not latex, so safe for latex allergies Also use spermicides User effectiveness: 75%–82%
Spermicides	Gels, creams, films, and suppositories inserted into vagina to kill sperm before they can ascend **CONTRAINDICATIONS:** Cervicitis	Suppositories and films require 15 minutes to become effective. Provides no protection against STIs. Side effects: Allergic reaction, topical irritation User effectiveness: 71%
Contraceptive Sponge	Round, disposable polyurethane device permeated with spermicide (nonoxynol-9) that fits over cervix	Moisten thoroughly with tap water. Provides protection for up to 24 hours. Must remain in vagina at least 6 hours after intercourse. Provides no protection against STIs. User effectiveness: 84%–87%

Hormonal Methods of Contraception

Combined Hormonal Methods

All combination hormonal contraceptives have both estrogen and progestin, which, in combination, decrease FSH and LH. Progestins also thicken cervical mucus to prevent sperm penetration.

Method	Description	Teaching
Oral Contraceptive Pills (OCPs)	Many different formulations including 21/7 pattern (21 days of hormones, 7 days off); 24/4 pattern; and continuous **CONTRAINDICATIONS:** *Absolute* – smoking and >35 years of age; moderate to severe hypertension (BP 160/100); undiagnosed uterine bleeding; diabetes >20 years duration or with vascular changes; history of pulmonary embolism or deep venous thrombosis (DVT); ischemic heart disease or stroke; severe migraine headaches; known/suspected breast cancer; impaired liver function; pregnancy; major immobilizing surgery within the past month; cholecystitis *Relative:* Hypertension; migraine headaches; epilepsy; obstructive jaundice in pregnancy; gallbladder disease; surgery with prolonged immobilization; sickle cell disease	Must take at the same time every day. Use backup method during first week. Provide no protection against STIs Medications that may interfere: Rifampin, isoniazid, barbiturates, griseofulvin, certain anticonvulsants, anticoagulants, acetaminophen Report ACHES: **A**bdominal pain **C**hest pain **H**eadaches **E**ye problems **S**evere leg pain Side effects: Amenorrhea, nausea, bloating, spotting, breast tenderness, headaches during first 3 months User effectiveness: 95%
Transdermal Patch	Same contraindications as for OCPs	Apply to abdomen, buttock, upper outer arm, upper torso once a week for 3 weeks, then 1 week off for withdrawal bleeding. Rotate sites. Side effects: Same as for OCPs *(continued)*

Combined Hormonal Methods (Continued)		
Method	**Description**	**Teaching**
		In addition: Local irritation User effectiveness: 99%
Vaginal Ring	Same contraindications as for OCPs	Side effects: Same as for OCPs; also vaginal irritation, infection User effectiveness: 98%

Contain only progesterone, which provides contraception by thickening the cervical mucus to prevent sperm penetration and inhibits implantation. The injections and implant also suppress ovulation.

Pills	"Mini pill" Ovulation may occur. **CONTRAINDICATIONS:** Hepatitis; cancer; colitis	Timing of dosage is very important! Side effects: Irregular menses User effectiveness: 92% May be used while breastfeeding No protection against STIs
Injections	Medroxyprogesterone 150 mg IM deltoid or gluteal or 104 mg SQ abdomen or anterior thigh Also suppresses ovulation. Give first injection within 5 days of menses.	Side effects: Irregular bleeding; amenorrhea; weight gain; depression; headache; breast tenderness User effectiveness: 98%–99% No protection against STIs Must return to office/clinic every 3 months for injection
Implant	Subdermal implant inserted on inner side of upper arm. Suppresses ovulation. Implanon is effective for 3 years.	Side effects: Irregular bleeding; amenorrhea; emotional lability; weight gain; headache; depression; dysmenorrhea; acne User effectiveness: Approaches 100% No protection against STIs
Other		
Emergency Postcoital Contraception	"Morning after pill": Estrogen + progestin or progestin-only Take first dose within 72 hours of coitus and second dose 12 hours later.	Side effects: Nausea and vomiting Effectiveness: Estrogen + progestin = 89% of those who would have become pregnant; Progestin only = 95% Provides no protection against STIs.
Intrauterine device (IUD)	Small plastic device inserted into the uterus	Insert during menses.

Other

	Exact mechanism not known but causes sterile inflammatory response that results in a spermicidal intrauterine environment ParaGard (contains copper wire): Replace every 10 years. Mirena (contains progestin): Replace every 5 years; may produce amenorrhea. **CONTRAINDICATIONS:** Pregnancy; current STI; abnormal vaginal bleeding; cancer of genital tract; uterine anomalies or fibroid tumor; allergy to IUD components	Teach the patient to check for presence of "strings" after menses. Side effects: With ParaGard: Menorrhagia; dysmenorrhea. With Mirena: Decreased dysmenorrhea; decreased menorrhagia; amenorrhea Effectiveness: 98%–99% Provides no protection against STIs. Teach **PAINS** warning signs: **P**eriod late **A**bdominal pain, dyspareunia **I**nfection exposure or vaginal discharge **N**ot feeling well, fever/chills **S**tring missing, shorter, or longer
Sterilization	Permanent and irreversible Women: Bilateral tubal ligation (BTL); microinserts Men: Vasectomy	Outpatient or after childbirth (inpatient) Effectiveness: 96.3%–99% Office procedure (microinserts) Not considered complete until 2 negative semen analyses are obtained after procedure. Effectiveness: 99%
Clinical Pregnancy Termination	Elective: Performed at the woman's request Therapeutic: Performed for health reasons Vacuum aspiration: Most commonly used surgical method up to 12 weeks' gestation Dilation and evacuation: Second-trimester procedure	Potential complications: Bleeding, infection Reinforce need for follow-up care. Administer Rh_o (D) immune globulin if indicated (i.e., non sensitized Rh_o D-negative woman). Provide psychosocial support Teach about side effects associated with medications used with medical abortion: Nausea, vomiting, cramping. *(continued)*

Combined Hormonal Methods (Continued)		
Other		
	Medical termination: Can be performed for up to 63 days of gestation. Antimetabolites (e.g., methotrexate), abortifacients (e.g., mifepristone) and medications that induce uterine contractions (e.g., misoprostol) are used.	Teach about signs of complications: Fever 104°F (40°C), abdominal pain, prolonged or heavy bleeding, foul vaginal discharge, no menses within 6 weeks. Teach about contraception.

ETHNOCULTURAL CONSIDERATIONS

Obtaining a Sexual History for Infertility Care

Culturally influenced practices and taboos may create feelings of discomfort for couples when asked specific details of their intimate lives during the infertility care interview. Nurses must be sensitive to these issues and aware of cultural variations. For example, Orthodox Jewish law forbids a couple from engaging in sexual intercourse for 7 days after the menstrual period. This tenet can create an infertility problem if ovulation occurs during the early days after menstruation.

Drugs that Adversely Affect the Female Reproductive System		
Drug Class	**Drug**	**Possible Adverse Reactions**
Androgens	Danazol	Vaginitis, with itching, dryness, burning, or bleeding; amenorrhea
	Fluoxymesterone, methyltestosterone, testosterone	Amenorrhea and other menstrual irregularities; virilization, including clitoral enlargement
Antidepressants	Tricyclic antidepressants	Changed libido, menstrual irregularity
	Selective serotonin reuptake inhibitors	Decreased libido, anorgasmia
Antihypertensives	Clonidine, reserpine	Decreased libido
	Methyldopa	Decreased libido, amenorrhea

Drug Class	Drug	Possible Adverse Reactions
Antipsychotics	Chlorpromazine, perphenazine, prochlorperazine, thioridazine, trifluoperazine, haloperidol	Inhibition of ovulation (chlorpromazine only), menstrual irregularities, amenorrhea, change in libido
Beta Blockers	Atenolol, labetalol hydrochloride, nadolol, propanolol hydrochloride, metoprolol	Decreased libido
Cardiac Glycosides	Digoxin	Changes in cellular layer of vaginal walls in postmenopausal women
Corticosteroids	Dexamethasone, hydrocortisone, prednisone	Amenorrhea and menstrual irregularities
Cytotoxics	Busulfan	Amenorrhea with menopausal symptoms in premenopausal women, ovarian suppression, ovarian fibrosis and atrophy
	Chlorambucil	Amenorrhea
	Cyclophosphamide	Gonadal suppression (possibly irreversible), amenorrhea, ovarian fibrosis
	Methotrexate	Menstrual dysfunction, infertility
	Tamoxifen	Vaginal discharge or bleeding, menstrual irregularities, pruritus vulvae (intense itching of the female external genitalia)
	Thiotepa	Amenorrhea
Estrogens	Conjugated estrogens, esterified estrogens, estradiol, estrone, ethinyl estradiol	Altered menstrual flow, dysmenorrhea, amenorrhea, cervical erosion or abnormal secretions enlargement of uterine fibromas, vaginal candidiasis
	Dienestrol	Vaginal discharge, uterine bleeding with excessive use
Progestins	Medroxyprogesterone acetate, norethindrone, norgestrel, progesterone	Breakthrough bleeding, dysmenorrhea, amenorrhea, cervical erosion, and abnormal secretions

(continued)

Drugs that Adversely Affect the Female Reproductive System (Continued)

Drug Class	Drug	Possible Adverse Reactions
Thyroid Hormones	Levothyroxine sodium thyroid USP, and others	Menstrual irregularities with excessive doses
Miscellaneous	Lithium carbonate	Decreased libido
	L-Tryptophan	Decreased libido
	Spironolactone	Menstrual irregularities, amenorrhea, possible polycystic ovarian syndrome

Source: Dillon, P.M. (2007). *Nursing health assessment. Clinical pocket guide.* Philadelphia: F.A. Davis, pp. 234–235

Selected Medications Used in the Treatment of Infertility

Medication	Actions	Nursing Considerations and Side Effects
Clomiphene Citrate (Clomid)	An antiestrogen that binds with estrogen receptors to trigger FSH and LH release	Contraindicated with hepatic impairment. Patients may experience ovarian enlargement, vasomotor flushes, abdominal distention, nausea and vomiting, breast tenderness, blurred vision, headache, pelvic pain, abnormal uterine bleeding. May cause multiple ovulation.
Bromocriptine Mesylate (Parlodel)	Reduces elevated prolactin secretion by the anterior pituitary, which improves gonadotropin-releasing hormone secretion and normalizes follicle-stimulating hormone and luteinizing hormone release. Ovulation is restored and increased progesterone by the corpus luteum supports early pregnancy.	Patients may experience nausea and vomiting, headache, dizziness, orthostatic hypotension, blurred vision, diarrhea, metallic taste, dry mouth, urticaria, rash.

Medication	Actions	Nursing Considerations and Side Effects
Gonadotropin-releasing Hormone (GnRH) Agonists (GONADORELIN; GOSERELIN [ZOLADEX], LEUPROLIDE [LUPRON], NAFARELIN [SYNAREL])	Stimulates release of pituitary FSH and LH in patients with deficient hypothalamic GnRH secretion. FSH and LH stimulate ovulation (female) and testosterone and spermatogenesis (male).	Advise patients of potential side effects: Headache, depression, nasal irritation (Synarel), vaginal dryness, breast swelling and tenderness, hot flashes, vaginal spotting, decreased libido, and impotence.
GnRH Antagonists (CETRORELIX [CETROTIDE], GANIRELIX [ANTAGON], ABARELIX [PLENAXIS], HISTRELIN [SUPPRELIN])	Reduces the extent of endometriosis; used with medications that stimulate ovulation by suppressing LH and FSH.	Patients are closely monitored for ovarian hyperstimulation (ascites with or without pain, pleural effusion, ruptured ovarian cysts, multiple births), headache, nausea.
Human Chorionic Gonadotropin (hCG) (PROFASI HP, PREGNYL, CHOREX)	Used after failure to respond to therapy with clomiphene citrate; induces ovulation; used in conjunction with gonadotropins (FSH and LH [Pergonal], [Repronex], [Humegon]); ovulation usually occurs within 18 hours. Also stimulates production of progesterone by the corpus luteum.	When used with menotropins, risk for ovarian hyperstimulation, and arterial thromboembolism; other side effects include headache, irritability, restlessness, and depression.
Progesterone (IM, Intravaginal)	Provides luteal phase support—prepares the endometrial lining to promote implantation of the embryo.	Common side effects include nausea, weight gain, and fluid retention.

TEACHING THE FAMILY

Herbs to Avoid When Attempting to Achieve Pregnancy	
Category	**Herb**
Anthraquinone Laxatives	Aloe Buckthorn Cascara sagrada Docks Meadow saffron Senna
Uterine Stimulants	American mandrake Black cohosh Blue cohosh Bloodroot Calamus Cayenne Fennel Feverfew Flax seed Goldenseal Lady's mantle Licorice Make fern Sage Tansy Thuja Thyme Wild cherry Wormwood Mayapple Mistletoe Passion flower Pennyroyal Periwinkle Poke root Rhubarb
Alkaloids/Bitter Principles	Barberry Bloodroot Celandine Cinchona Ephedra Goldenseal

ADDITIONAL INFORMATION FOR THE CLINICAL SETTING

Advanced Reproductive Technologies (ART)

Treatment	Procedure	Indications for Use/Special Considerations	Complications
In Vitro Fertilization (IVF)	Administration of medications to induce ovulation. Oocytes are harvested and mixed with prepared sperm in a culture dish to form embryos. Three or four embryos are placed into the hormonally prepared uterus.	Tubal blockage or damage, endometriosis, cervical mucus abnormalities, male/female immunological infertility, cervical factors, infertility of unknown etiology.	Failure Multiple pregnancy
Intrauterine Insemination (IUI)	Retrieved and prepared sperm are placed into the uterus at the time of natural or induced ovulation.	Seminal deficiencies (e.g., oligospermia [low sperm count]), cervical factors (e.g., inhospitable mucus, stenosis), unexplained infertility	Failure Multiple pregnancy
Gamete Intrafallopian Transfer (GIFT)	Oocytes and sperm are placed in the fallopian tube.	Requires at least one functioning fallopian tube.	Failure Tubal pregnancy Multiple pregnancy
Zygote Intrafallopian Transfer (ZIFT) **Tubal Embryo Transfer (TET)**	After in vitro fertilization, zygotes are placed in one fallopian tube. Placement occurs at the embryo stage.	Requires at least one functioning fallopian tube.	Failure Tubal pregnancy Multiple pregnancy
Intracytoplasmic Sperm Injection (ICSI)	Micromanipulation process for an individual sperm cell which is injected directly into an ovum (in the laboratory)	Absence of the vas deferens; severe male factor (e.g., oligospermia, poor sperm quality)	Failure

(continued)

Advanced Reproductive Technologies (ART) (Continued)

Treatment	Procedure	Indications for Use/Special Considerations	Complications
Cryopreservation	Freezing method	Permits storage of sperm or ovarian tissue or embryos that result from IVF for the future.	Failure

REFERENCE

Dillon, P.M. (2007). *Nursing health assessment. Clinical pocket guide.* Philadelphia: F.A. Davis.

Conception and Development of the Embryo and Fetus

KEY TERMS

amnion – The innermost of the two fetal membranes that form the sac and contain the fetus and the fluid that surrounds it in utero

chorion – Fetal membrane closest to the intrauterine wall; gives rise to the placenta and continues as the outer membrane that surrounds the amnion

chorionic villi – Vascular projections from the chorion, which will form the fetal portion of the placenta

chromosome – A linear strand within the cell nucleus that carries genes; composed of DNA and proteins

dizygotic – Originating from two zygotes (i.e., fraternal twins)

embryo – Conceptus from the fourth day after fertilization until approximately the eighth gestational week

fetus – The developing human, in utero, after completion of the eighth gestational week, until birth

genetics – The study of single genes and their effects

gestation – The period of intrauterine fetal development from conception to birth

karyotype – Photomicrograph of the chromosomes of a single cell; the chromosomes are then arranged in numerical order

monozygotic – Originating from a single fertilized ovum (i.e., identical twins)

mutation – Spontaneous, permanent change in the normal gene structure neural tube defect – A group of congenital structural disorders that result from a failure of the embryonic neural tube to close during development (i.e., cranial fusion disorders: anencephaly, encephalocele; spinal fusion disorders: spina bifida, meningomyelocele, meningocele)

teratogen – Substance that adversely affects normal cellular development in the embryo/fetus

trisomy – Condition in which a chromosome breaks and all or a part of the chromosome is transferred to a different part of the same chromosome or to a different chromosome. Most common trisomies in live newborns: trisomy 18 (Edward syndrome); trisomy 21 (Down syndrome); trisomy 13 (Patau syndrome)

FOCUSED ASSESSMENT

The first prenatal visit should include a careful history to determine factors that may affect the pregnancy:

- Cultural: Health practices and values
- Psychological: Feelings about the pregnancy, preparation, social support, stressors, future plans
- Physical: Past health history, current health issues, menstrual/ovulatory history, structural abnormalities, medications, substance use, tobacco
- Environmental: Exposure to toxins in the home or work place, second-hand smoke, stress

Embryonic and Fetal Growth and Development

Weeks	Weight	Length (crown to rump)	Characteristics	Implications
2 weeks	?	2 mm	Blastocyst implanted in uterus	Adequate secretion of progesterone by corpus luteum crucial to maintain endometrium
4 weeks	0.4 g	4 mm	Embryo is curved, tail prominent. Upper limb buds and otic pits present. Heart prominence evident.	Central nervous system (CNS), organ, and tissue development begins and vulnerable to teratogens.

Weeks	Weight	Length (crown to rump)	Characteristics	Implications
				Folic acid supplement is important.
8 weeks	2 g	3 cm	Head rounded with human characteristics. Unable to determine sex. Intestines still present in umbilical cord. Ovaries and testes distinguishable.	Ends embryonic period and begins fetal period. Organ systems and neuromuscular development remain vulnerable.
12 weeks	19 g	8 cm	Has a human appearance, with disproportionately large head. Eyes fused. Skin pink and delicate. Upper limbs almost reached final length. Intestines in the stomach. Sex distinguishable externally.	Fetus becomes more resistant to damage from teratogens. Able to auscultate heart tones with Doppler ultrasound stethoscope.
16 weeks	100 g	13.5 cm	Scalp hair appears. External ears present. Lower limbs well developed. Arm to leg ratio proportionate. Fetus active.	Maternal serum alpha-fetoprotein (MSAFP) reliable until 22 weeks.
20 weeks	300 g	18.5 cm	Head and body hair (lanugo) present. Vernix covers skin. Quickening felt by the woman.	Ultrasound examination often performed to detect growth abnormalities.
24 weeks	600 g	23 cm	Skin reddish and wrinkled. Some subcutaneous fat present. Some respiratory-like movements. Fingernails present. Lean body.	Fetus now viable.

(Continued)

Embryonic and Fetal Growth and Development (Continued)

Weeks	Weight	Length (crown to rump)	Characteristics	Implications
28 weeks	1100 g	27 cm	Eyes open with eyelashes present. Much hair present. Skin slightly wrinkled; more fat now present.	Gestational diabetes, related to maternal insulin resistance and fetal growth, becomes detectable by glucose tolerance test.
32 weeks	1800 g	31 cm	Skin is smooth. Increase in weight gain more than length. Toenails present. Testes descending.	
36 weeks	2200 g	34 cm	Skin pale, body plump. Body lanugo almost gone. Able to flex arm and form grasp. Umbilicus in center of body. Testes in inguinal canal, scrotum small with few rugae. Some sole creases present.	
40 weeks	3200+ g	40 cm	Skin smooth and pink. Lanugo on upper back and shoulders. Ear lobes formed and firm. Chest prominent and breasts often protrude slightly. Testes with well defined rugae. Labia majora well developed. Creases cover soles of feet.	

MEDICATIONS

Organogenesis occurs from approximately the second until the eighth week of gestation. During this time, the embryo is extremely vulnerable to teratogens.

Teratogen Exposure During Organogenesis	
Teratogen	**Effect**
Fat-soluble Vitamins: Vitamin A Vitamin D deficiency Vitamin E: High doses	Both high and low doses can cause malformations: CNS, microtia, clefts (fissure or elongated opening). Poor fetal growth, neonatal hypocalcemia, rickets, poor tooth enamel May increase risk for bleeding problems.
Alcohol	One of the most potent teratogens known. Safe threshold not established. Associated with fetal alcohol spectrum disorder (FASD) which includes neurological and physical changes.
Tobacco	Small for gestational age (SGA), cleft lip, impaired infant neurobehavior, decreased babbling in infants
Caffeine	Half-life triples during pregnancy. Readily crosses the placenta. CNS stimulant, causing maternal tachycardia and hypertension and affects fetal heart rate and movement; may be associated with preterm labor and intrauterine growth restriction (IUGR) although no clear causation exists.
Cocaine and Crack	Vasoconstriction of uterine vessels Associated with spontaneous abortion, abruptio placentae, stillbirth, IUGR, fetal distress, meconium staining, preterm birth Altered neurological and behavior patterns, neonatal strokes and seizures, congenital genitourinary and limb malformations, intestinal atresia, and heart defects
Opiates	Maternal: Spontaneous abortion, premature rupture of the membranes, preterm labor, increased incidence of STIs, hepatitis, malnutrition Fetal: Death, IUGR, prenatal asphyxia, prematurity, intellectual impairment, neonatal infection
Sedatives	Maternal: Lethargy, drowsiness, CNS depression. Infant: Neonatal withdrawal syndrome, seizures, delayed lung maturity

(continued)

Teratogen Exposure During Organogenesis (Continued)

Teratogen	Effect
Amphetamines	Maternal: Malnutrition, tachycardia, withdrawal symptoms Fetus: IUGR, prematurity, cardiac anomalies, cleft palate, placental abruption Infant: Hypoglycemia, sweating, poor visual tracking, lethargy and difficulty feeding
Marijuana	Maternal: Anemia, low weight gain Fetus: IUGR Infant: Hyperirritability, tremors, photosensitivity, adverse effects on cognitive and language development
Radiation (high levels)	Damage to chromosomes and embryonic cells, stunted fetal growth, mental retardation, deformities, abnormal brain function, cancer that develops later in life
Lead	Spontaneous abortion, fetal anomalies (hemangiomas, lymphangiomas, hydrocele, minor skin abnormalities, undescended testes), preterm birth

FDA Pregnancy Categories

Category	Interpretation
A	Adequate, well-controlled studies in pregnant women have not shown an increased risk of fetal abnormalities.
B	Animal studies have revealed no evidence of harm to the fetus; however, there are no adequate and well-controlled studies in pregnant women. **or** Animal studies have shown an adverse effect, but adequate and well-controlled studies in pregnant women have failed to demonstrate a risk to the fetus.
C	Animal studies have shown an adverse effect and there are no adequate and well-controlled studies in pregnant women. **or** No animal studies have been conducted and there are no adequate and well-controlled studies in pregnant women.
D	Studies (adequate well-controlled or observational) in pregnant women have demonstrated a risk to the fetus. However, the benefits of therapy may outweigh the potential risk. For example, the drug may be acceptable if needed in a life-threatening situation or serious disease for which safer drugs cannot be used or are ineffective.

Category	Interpretation
X	Studies, adequate well-controlled or observational, in animals or pregnant women have demonstrated positive evidence of fetal abnormalities. The use of the product is contraindicated in women who are or may become pregnant.

ETHNOCULTURAL CONSIDERATIONS

Racial and Ethnic Groups with Increased Risk for Diseases Caused by Recessive Genes	
Racial/Ethnic Group	**Disease**
African, Mediterranean, Caribbean, Latin American, or Middle Eastern descent	Hemoglobin gene mutations are more common in persons from these areas. African Americans have an increased incidence of sickle cell anemia. Southeast Asians have a greater likelihood of carrying hemoglobin E, an abnormal hemoglobin.
Mediterranean or Asian origin	These individuals have a higher risk for the hereditary anemia thalassemia.
Jewish ancestry	Individuals with Jewish ancestry have an increased risk for diseases associated with inborn errors of metabolism caused by different enzyme deficiencies (e.g., Tay–Sachs, Canavan, and Gaucher).
Caucasian or northern European descent	The most common disorder found among this population is cystic fibrosis.

TEACHING THE FAMILY

Empowering Through Education

- Teach all women of childbearing age who are capable of becoming pregnant to consume 0.4 mg of folic acid daily to reduce the incidence of neural tube defects.
- Include prenatal screening for maternal drug/substance use as a component of care for all pregnant women.
- Provide pregnant women with information on normal fetal growth and development.
- Display fetal growth charts in visible areas and discuss developmental landmarks throughout gestation to enhance the patient's and family's understanding.

- When appropriate, assemble a team composed of nutritionists, social workers, and home health workers to ensure healthy fetal growth and development.
- Include fathers and other support persons in prenatal education to help optimize the outcome.

TORCH Infections

TORCH infections are a group of maternal infectious diseases that cause harm to the embryo or fetus, especially during the first 12 weeks of gestation when developmental anomalies may occur (Box 4-1). TORCH is an acronym for *t*oxoplasmosis, *o*ther (e.g., hepatitis, syphilis), *r*ubella, *c*ytomegalovirus, and *h*erpes simplex.

Box 4-1 TORCH Infections

Toxoplasmosis
- Associated with consumption of infested, undercooked meat and poor hand washing after handling cat litter.
- If mother acquires toxoplasmosis after conception and passes it to the fetus via the placenta, fetal infection occurs.
- Most infants are asymptomatic at birth, but develop symptoms later.

   Maternal Effects: Flu-like symptoms in the acute phase.
   Fetal/Neonatal Effects: Miscarriage likely in early pregnancy. In neonates, CNS lesions can result in hydrocephaly, microcephaly, chronic retinitis, and seizures; retinochoroiditis may appear in adolescence or adulthood.

Other Infections
- Most commonly includes the hepatitis virus.
- Hepatitis A virus spread by droplets or hands, transmission rare but can occur.
- Hepatitis B virus can be transmitted via placenta, but transmission usually occurs when the infant is exposed to blood and genital secretions during labor and birth.

   Maternal Effects: Fever, malaise, nausea, abdominal discomfort; may be associated with liver failure
   Fetal/Neonatal Effects: Preterm birth, hepatitis infection, intrauterine death

Rubella (German measles)
- Spread by respiratory droplets.
- Obtain signed consent prior to administration of vaccine.

- Vaccine may be safely given to breastfeeding mothers.
- Instruct patients not to become pregnant for 1 month after receiving the immunization.

Maternal Effects: Fever, rash, mild lymphedema

Fetal/Neonatal Effects: Miscarriage, IUGR, cataracts, congenital anomalies, hepatosplenomegaly, hyperbilirubinemia, mental retardation, and death. Other symptoms may develop later. Infants born with congenital rubella are contagious and should be isolated.

Cytomegalovirus (CMV)

- Spread by respiratory droplets, semen, cervical and vaginal secretions, breast milk, placental tissue, urine, feces, and banked blood (nearly 50% of adults in the United States have antibodies for this virus).

Maternal Effects: Asymptomatic illness, cervical discharge, and mononucleosis-like syndrome

Fetal/Neonatal Effects: Fetal death or severe generalized disease with hemolytic anemia and jaundice, hydrocephaly or microcephaly, pneumonitis, hepatosplenomegaly, mental retardation, cerebral palsy, deafness; blood, brain, and liver are most often affected.

Herpes Simplex Virus (HSV)

- HSV II is sexually transmitted.
- Infant usually infected during exposure to lesion in birth canal, most at risk during a primary infection in the mother (50% born vaginally will develop some form of herpes; 60% will die; half of survivors develop problems).

Maternal Effects: Blisters, rash, fever, malaise, nausea, and headache

Fetal/Neonatal Effects: Miscarriage, preterm birth, stillbirth; transplacental infection is rare but can cause skin lesions, IUGR, mental retardation, microcephaly, seizures, and coma.

Communicating with the Family When a Fetal Anomaly Has Been Identified

- When prenatal testing identifies a fetus with a congenital anomaly, families are faced with a flood of emotions and difficult decisions. The nurse plays an important role in providing support and education regarding options available to these couples. A nonjudgmental and caring attitude is vital at this difficult and vulnerable time.

Therapeutic communication is enhanced when the nurse uses statements such as:

- "It's normal to have fear, grief, or even be angry."
- "It's normal to have concerns about your ability to have a normal baby."

- "I am here to answer your questions and listen to your concerns. If I don't know the answers. I will either find and share them or arrange for a colleague to meet with you.

The nurse should avoid using statements such as:

- "You can always have other children."
- "I know how you feel."
- "At least you don't know the baby yet."

ADDITIONAL INFORMATION FOR THE CLINICAL SETTING

Preterm Birth at Less Than 38 Weeks of Gestation

- Nurses must understand fetal growth and development in order to anticipate specific problems when infants are born prematurely.
- An infant born at 28 weeks of gestation has significantly different needs from an infant born at 38 weeks of gestation.

Understanding Abnormalities in Sex Chromosomes

Turner syndrome (monosomy X)

- Most common sex chromosome deviation in females
- Characterized by chromosomal constitution of 45X
- Affected females usually exhibit juvenile external genitalia, undeveloped ovaries, short stature, webbing of the neck, impaired intelligence.

Klinefelter syndrome (trisomy XXY)

- Most common sex chromosome deviation in males
- The extra X chromosome results in poorly developed male secondary sexual characteristics, small testes, infertility, and possible impaired intelligence.

RESOURCES

http://www.ornl.gov/sci/techresources/Human_Genome/publicat/tko/01_foreword.html

http://www.healthypeople.gov/Publications

http://www.nichd.nih.gov/health/topics/preconception_care.cfm

Physiological and Psychosocial Changes During Pregnancy

KEY TERMS

angioma – Tiny, bluish end-arterioles occurring on the neck, thorax, face, and arms; often appear during the second to fifth month of pregnancy and disappear after birth

Chadwick's sign – Bluish purple coloration of the vaginal mucous membrane caused by increased vascularity; visible from approximately the fourth week of pregnancy; a probable sign of pregnancy

chloasma – Increased pigmentation over the cheeks, hairline, brow, and nose of the pregnant woman and in some women taking oral contraceptives; also called the "mask of pregnancy" or "melasma gravidarum"

colostrum – Breast fluid that may be secreted from the second trimester of pregnancy onward; most evident in the first 2 to 3 days after birth and before the onset of true lactation

decidua – The endometrium or lining of the uterus during pregnancy; it is shed after giving birth

diastasis recti abdominis – Separation of the two rectus muscles along the median line of the abdominal wall

epulis gravidarum – Benign red, raised nodules of the gingiva seen in pregnant women

Goodell sign – Softening of the tip of the cervix; a probable sign of pregnancy

leukorrhea – Whitish-yellow discharge from the cervical canal or the vagina; may be normal physiologically or caused by vaginal/endocervical pathology such as infection

linea alba – White line of connective tissue in the middle of the abdomen that extends from the sternum to the mons pubis

linea nigra – Line of darker pigmentation seen in some women during the latter part of pregnancy; appears on middle of the abdomen and extends from the umbilicus to the mons pubis

mean arterial pressure (MAP) – Average of the systolic and the diastolic blood pressures

Montgomery tubercles (glands) – Small, nodular sebaceous glands on and around the areola that provide lubrication for the nipple tissue

operculum – Plug of mucus that fills the cervical canal to protect a pregnancy from outside pathogens

palmar erythema – Rash occurring on the surface of the palms, sometimes seen during pregnancy

pruritis gravidarum – Severe itching during pregnancy

ptyalism – Excessive production of saliva

striae gravidarum – "Stretch marks"—reddish lines on the breasts, abdomen, and thighs caused by stretching of the skin during pregnancy

supine hypotension syndrome (vena caval syndrome) – Fall in blood pressure caused by decreased venous return when the gravid uterus presses on the ascending vena cava when the woman is lying flat on her back; symptoms include dizziness, diaphoresis, nausea and pallor

FOCUSED ASSESSMENT

Physiological Adaptations in Pregnancy

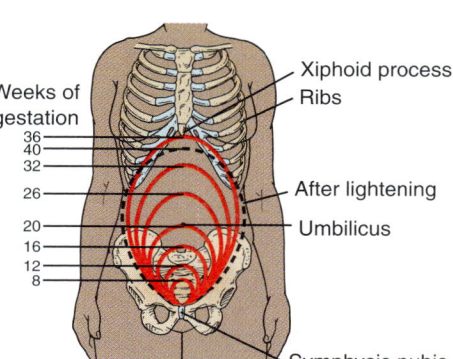

Figure 5-1 Pattern of uterine growth during pregnancy.

Hormones in Pregnancy

Hormone	Action	Effect
Estrogen	Hyperplasia and hypertrophy	Breast tissue enlargement, uterine enlargement, enhanced uterine contractility
Progesterone	Smooth muscle relaxant, vasodilation, inhibits prolactin and oxytocin actions until needed	Slows gastrointestinal (GI) tract to increase absorption of nutrients, relaxes uterus to prevent labor until ready.
Prolactin	Increases 10-fold.	Responsible for initial lactation.
Oxytocin	Causes uterine contractions, stimulates milk ejection.	Labor, "let down" reflex
Prostaglandins	Increase response of the myometrium to the effects of oxytocin.	May contribute to onset of labor, softening of the cervix. Decreased levels may contribute to hypertension and preeclampsia.
Relaxin	Produced by the placenta, softens ligaments.	Lumbar lordosis, change in the center of gravity

Summary of Physiological Adaptations in Pregnancy

Organ/System	Change	Effect
Uterus	Hyperplasia and hypertrophy, hyperemia	Weight increases from 70 g to 1100 g.
Cervix	Hyperemia	Chadwick's sign, operculum, leukorrhea
Vagina and vulva	Hyperemia, elevated glycogen levels, decreased pH	Leukorrhea, increased risk of *Candida albicans*
Ovaries	Luteinizing hormone (LH) causes corpus luteum to produce progesterone for 6–7 weeks.	Corpus luteal cyst may enlarge to golf-ball size, then resolves.
Breasts	Estrogen and progesterone stimulate changes in tissue and mammary gland action.	Early: Enlargement, fullness, tingling, increased sensitivity. Montgomery tubercles enlarge and secrete lubricant, striae develop; colostrum is formed.
Integumentary System	Estrogen, progesterone, melanocyte-stimulating hormones increase. Increased adrenal steroid levels cause connective tissue changes.	Photosensitivity, chloasma, linea nigra, palmar erythema, angiomas. Connective tissue becomes fragile, causing striae.
Neurological System	Unclear	Changes in attention span, concentration, memory, sleep pattern changes
Cardiovascular System	Changes in vascular permeability and vasodilation, relaxation of vascular resistance	Carpal tunnel syndrome, syncope, orthostatic hypotension, vasodilation; allows improved heat dispersion and increases risk for varicose veins, hemorrhoids.
Heart	Hypertrophy, displacement from growing fetus	Exaggerated first and third sounds, systolic murmur
Blood Volume	Increased by 40%–45%	Murmur
Iron	Increased need due to additional oxygen demands	"Physiological anemia of pregnancy" or "pseudoanemia" (normal hemodilution effect related to the plasma volume increase that exceeds the increase in erythrocytes)

Organ/System	Change	Effect
Clotting Factors	Fibrinogen volume increases by 50%.	Increased sedimentation rate, increased factors VII, VIII, IX, and X, leading to a hypercoagulable state
Cardiac Output	Increases by 30%–50%.	Pulse increases, blood pressure drops in second trimester, then returns to normal after 20 weeks; supine hypotension syndrome.
Immune System	Depressed leukocyte function	Increased susceptibility to infection
Respiratory System	Tidal volume increases 30%–40%; estrogen causes hypertrophy and hyperplasia of lung tissue; progesterone causes relaxation of bronchi, bronchioles, alveoli.	Increased oxygen consumption and vital capacity, decreased diaphragmatic movement and increased lateral chest wall movement to compensate for changes
Eyes, Ears, Nose, Throat	Eyes: Corneal thickening, fluid retention, decreased intraocular pressure. Nose: Increased mucus production Throat: Hyperemia	Blurred vision Rhinitis of pregnancy, epistaxis Difficulty swallowing
GI Tract	Increased blood flow, change in mucosa, progesterone slows GI motility, weakens gastroesophageal sphincter, slows bile emptying.	Changes in taste and smell, gingivitis, ptyalism, reflux, pyrosis, nausea/vomiting of pregnancy; hemorrhoids, constipation, pruritis gravidarum
Urinary System	Increased blood flow to kidneys by 30%–50%, pressure on structures by gravid uterus, progesterone relaxes urethra and sphincter musculature	Increased glomerular filtration rate (GFR) and renal tubular reabsorption. Increased excretion, urgency, frequency, nocturia, predisposed to urinary tract infections (UTIs)
Endocrine System		
THYROID	Increased blood flow, hyperplasia from estrogen, elevated levels of triiodothyronine (T_3) and thyroxine (T_4)	Enlarges up to two times, basal metabolic rate (BMR) increases up to 25%.
PARATHYROID	Hyperplasia from estrogen	Calcium demand increases. *(continued)*

Summary of Physiological Adaptations in Pregnancy (Continued)		
Organ/System	**Change**	**Effect**
PANCREAS	Hypertrophy and hyperplasia of insulin-producing beta cells of the islets of Langerhans	Alterations in carbohydrate metabolism
Musculoskeletal System	Hypertrophy of the round ligaments supporting the uterus	"Round ligament pain"
	Abdominal wall weakens. Weight shifts upward and outward.	Diastasis recti
	Symphysis pubis separates, bones of pelvis become loose.	Compensated by lordosis to maintain the center of gravity over the legs. "Pregnancy waddle"

DIAGNOSTIC TESTS

Common Laboratory Values in Pregnancy		
Laboratory Values	**Usual Normal Female Value**	**Normal Value in Pregnancy**
Serum Values		
Hemoglobin (Hgb)	11.7–15.5 g/dL	Decreased by 1.5–2 g/dL Lowest point occurs at 30–34 weeks
Hematocrit (Hct)	38%–44%	Decreased by 4–7%, lowest point at 30–34 weeks
Leukocytes	$4.5–11.0 \times 10^3/mm^3$	Gradual increase of $3.5–10^3/mm^3$
Platelets	$150–400 \times 10^3/mm^3$	Slight decrease
Amylase	30–110 U/L	Increased by 50–100%
Chemistries		
Albumin	3.4–4.8 g/dL	Early decrease by 1 g/dL
Calcium (total)	8.2–10.2 mg/dL	Gradual decrease of 10%
Chloride	97–107 mEq/L	No significant change
Creatinine	0.5–1.1 mg/dL	Early decrease by 0.3 mg/dL
Fibrinogen	200–400 mg/dL	Progressive increase of 1–2 g/L
Glucose (fasting)	65–99 mg/dL	Gradual decrease of 10%
Potassium	3.5–5.0 mEq/L	Gradual decrease of 0.2–0.3 mEq/L
Protein (total)	6.0–8.0 g/dL	Early decrease of 1 g/dL, then stable

Laboratory Values	Usual Normal Female Value	Normal Value in Pregnancy
Sodium	135–145 mEq/L	Early decrease of 2–4 mEq/L then stable
Urea nitrogen	8–20 mg/dL	Decrease in first trimester by 50%
Uric acid	2.3–6.6 mg/dL	First trimester decrease of 33%, rise at term
Urine Chemistries		
Creatinine	11–20 mg/kg per 24 h	No significant change
Protein	10–140 mg per 24 h	Increased by 250–300 mg/day by the 20th week
Creatinine clearance	75–115 mL/min/1.73 m^2	Increased by 40%–50% by the 16th week
Serum Hormones		
Cortisol	8–21 g/dL	Increased by 20 g/dL
Prolactin	3.3–26.7 ng/mL	Gradual increase, 5.3–215.3 ng/mL, peaks at term
T_4 total	5.5–11.0 mcg/dL	5.5–16.0 mcg/dL
T_3 total	70–204 ng/dL	Early sustained increase of up to 50% 116–247 ng/dL (last 4 months of gestation)

Sources: Hacker, Moore, & Gambone (2004); Van Leeuwen, Kranpitz, & Smith, (2006).

ETHNOCULTURAL CONSIDERATIONS

Pregnancy-related Beliefs and Practices

All cultures have beliefs and practices related to the pregnancy and birthing experience. Careful assessment of the patient's beliefs regarding pregnancy and birth is essential to providing culturally sensitive care. The following areas require special attention: the state of pregnancy as a healthy versus a taboo state, nutritional practices such as hot/cold balance, expression of pain during labor, involvement of the father and other family members, over-the-counter remedy or herbal use, and other cultural beliefs.

TEACHING THE FAMILY

Health Education Topics Related to the Physiological Adaptations of Pregnancy			
Topics to Include	**First Trimester**	**Second Trimester**	**Third Trimester**
Physiological Changes of Pregnancy and Related Discomforts	Pain and tingling in breasts Nausea and vomiting (morning sickness) Urinary frequency Fatigue Mood swings	Enlargement of the abdomen Skin pigmentation Striae gravidarum Vascular spiders Constipation Heartburn or gastric reflux Leg cramps Groin pain from round ligament stretching Leukorrhea	Dyspnea Leg and feet cramps Constipation Indigestion, heartburn, gastric reflux Pedal edema Fatigue Vaginal discharge Urinary frequency Braxton Hicks contractions versus true labor
Danger Signs to Report to the Health Care Provider	Vaginal bleeding Abdominal cramping or pain Severe or prolonged vomiting	Vaginal bleeding Burning or painful urination Fever, increased pulse rate Decreased or absent fetal movements Unrelenting nausea and vomiting Abdominal pain or cramping Swelling of face or fingers, headaches, visual disturbances or epigastric pain	Visual disturbances Headache Hand and facial edema Fever Vaginal bleeding Abdominal pain; uterine contractions Premature rupture of the membranes Decreased or absent fetal movements Swelling of face or fingers, headaches, visual disturbances or epigastric pain
General Health Teaching	Schedule of return visits for routine prenatal care General hygiene	Reinforcement and reiteration of previous teaching Comfort measures	Signs and symptoms of labor/preterm labor

Topics to Include	First Trimester	Second Trimester	Third Trimester
	Comfort measures	Anticipatory guidance	When to call the health care provider, when to go to the birthing center or hospital
	Anticipatory guidance	Choices of prenatal education classes	Comfort measures
	Sexual activity and restrictions	Signs and symptoms of preterm labor	Anticipatory guidance
	Physical activities, exercise and rest		Reinforcement and reiteration of previous teaching
	Nutritional guidance		Encouragement to attend a labor and birth class
	Avoidance of alcohol, fetal alcohol effects		
	Effects of smoking, and smoking cessation strategies if indicated.		

Source: Mattson & Smith (2004).

PSYCHOSOCIAL ADAPTATIONS IN PREGNANCY

Health Education Topics Related to the Psychosocial Adaptations to Pregnancy

Topics to Include	First Trimester	Second Trimester	Third Trimester
Psychosocial Changes During Pregnancy	Ambivalence about pregnancy	Active dream and fantasy life	Dislikes being pregnant but loves the child
	Introversion	Concerns with body image	Anxious about childbirth, but sees labor and birth as deliverance
	Passivity and difficulty with decision making	Nesting behaviors	The couple experiments with various mothering or fathering roles
	Sexual and emotional changes	Sexual behavior adjustment	Woman is introspective
	Changing self-image	Expanding to a variety of methods of expressing affection and intimacy	
	Ethical dilemmas of prenatal testing		

Source: Mattson & Smith (2004).

ADDITIONAL INFORMATION FOR THE CLINICAL SETTING

Maternal Tasks of Pregnancy

General Principles	Pregnancy progressively becomes part of the woman's total identity She feels unique because she cannot share her sensory experience with others. Her focus turns inward and she is overly sensitive. She seeks the company of other women and especially pregnant women. Absence of a female support system during pregnancy is a singular index of a high-risk pregnancy.
Acceptance of Pregnancy "Binding-in"	*First trimester.* The woman accepts the idea of pregnancy but not the child. *Second trimester.* With sensation of fetal movement, or "quickening," the woman becomes aware of the child as a separate entity. *Third trimester.* The woman wants the child and is tired of being pregnant.
Acceptance of the Child	*First trimester.* Acceptance of the pregnancy by self and others. *Second trimester.* The family needs to relate to the infant. *Third trimester.* The critical issue is the unconditional acceptance of the child; conditional acceptance may imply rejection by the mother or family members.
Reordering of Relationships, Giving of Self	*First trimester.* Examines what needs to be given up; trade-offs for having the infant May grieve the loss of a carefree life. *Second trimester.* Identifies with the child. *Third trimester.* Has decreased confidence in her ability to become a good mother to her child.
Safe Passage	*First trimester.* Focuses on herself, not on her infant. *Second trimester.* Develops a strong attachment and places great value on her infant. *Third trimester.* Has concern for herself and her infant as a unit, shares a symbiotic relationship. At the seventh month, she is in a state of high vulnerability. She views labor and birth as deliverance and as a hope, not as a threat.

Source: Mattson & Smith (2004).

Developmental Tasks and the Pregnant Adolescent

- Developing a personal value system
- Choosing a vocation or career
- Developing a personal body image and sexuality
- Achieving a stable identity
- Attaining independence from parents

These tasks may be overshadowed by the developmental tasks of pregnancy and create conflicts.

CLINICAL ALERT

Avoiding Supine Hypotension Syndrome

The woman may experience supine hypotension syndrome, or vena caval syndrome (faintness related to bradycardia) if she lies on her back. The pressure from the enlarged uterus exerted on the vena cava decreases the amount of venous return from the lower extremities and causes a marked decrease in blood pressure, with accompanying dizziness, diaphoresis, and pallor (Fig. 5-2). Place the woman on her left side to relieve these symptoms.

Figure 5-2 Supine hypotension, or vena caval syndrome, may occur if the pregnant woman lies on her back. The weight of the gravid uterus causes compression of the vena cava.

REFERENCES

Hacker, N.F., Moore, J.G., & Gambone, J.C. (2004). *Essentials of obstetrics and gynecology* (4th ed.). Philadelphia: W.B. Saunders.

Mattson, S., & Smith, J.E. (2004). *Core curriculum for maternal-newborn nursing.* St. Louis, MO: W.B. Saunders

Van Leeuwen, A.M., Kranpitz, T.R., & Smith, L. (2006). *Davis's comprehensive handbook of laboratory and diagnostic tests with nursing implications* (2nd ed.). Philadelphia: F.A. Davis.

The Prenatal Assessment

KEY TERMS

alpha-fetoprotein (AFP) – Fetal antigen; elevated levels in amniotic fluid are associated with neural tube defects; decreased levels may indicate an increased risk of having an infant with Down syndrome.

MSAFP Maternal serum alpha-fetoprotein

amenorrhea – Absence of menses

ballottement – Passive movement of the unengaged fetus

Braxton Hicks sign – Mild, intermittent uterine contractions

Chadwick's sign – Bluish-purple coloration of the vaginal mucous membrane caused by increased vascularity; visible from approximately the fourth week of pregnancy; a probable sign of pregnancy

diethylstilbestrol (DES) – Synthetic estrogen that was once given to women in early pregnancy to prevent miscarriage. In utero exposure to DES is associated with reproductive tract malformations and vaginal cancer in females and increased rates of infertility in males and females

EDB – Estimated date of birth; also called "estimated date of delivery" (EDD); formerly termed the "estimated date of confinement" (EDC)

engagement – Entry of the presenting part into the maternal pelvis. Fetus is not ballottable.

fetal heart rate (FHR) – Beats per minute (bpm) of the fetal heart; normal range is 110–160 bpm

fetal lie – Position of the fetal spine in relation to the maternal spine: longitudinal (the same as the mother); transverse (fetal spine is horizontal across maternal spine); oblique (fetal spine is at some angle between the longitudinal and the transverse lie).

fundus – Dome-shaped upper portion of the uterus between the points of insertion of the fallopian tubes

Goodell sign – Softening of the tip of the cervix; a probable sign of pregnancy

gravidity – Total number of a woman's pregnancies

Hegar sign – Softening of the lower uterine segment; a probable sign of pregnancy

human chorionic gonadotropin (hCG) – Hormone produced by the chorionic villi; the biologic marker in pregnancy tests

Leopold maneuvers – Four maneuvers to assess the lie, presentation and position of the fetus

LMP – Last menstrual period

multigravida – Woman who has been pregnant two or more times

multipara – Woman who has carried two or more pregnancies to viability, whether they ended in live infants or stillbirths

Naegele's rule – Method for calculating the estimated date of birth: LMP + 7 days – 3 months

nulligravida – Woman who has never experienced a pregnancy

nullipara – Woman who has not yet carried a pregnancy to the point of viability

parity – Number of pregnancies carried to the point of viability, regardless of whether the infant or infants were alive or stillborn

Piskacek sign – Uterine asymmetry with a soft prominence on the implantation site; a probable sign of pregnancy

position (of the fetus) – Location of a fixed reference point on the fetal presenting part in relation to a specific quadrant of the maternal pelvis

presentation – Fetal part that enters the pelvic inlet first and leads through the birth canal during labor. If the head is "presenting," terms used are cephalic, vertex. Other presentations are breech and shoulder

primigravida – Woman who is pregnant for the first time

pseudocyesis – "False pregnancy"; condition in which a woman has the usual signs of pregnancy (e.g., abdominal enlargement, weight gain, cessation of menses, morning sickness) but is not pregnant

quickening – Maternal awareness of the sensation of fetal movement, usually occurs around 17 to 20 weeks of gestation

Rh factor – Inherited antigen present on erythrocytes. The individual who has the factor is known as "positive" (Rh+) for the factor; one who does not have the factor is known as Rh negative (Rh–)

Rh immune globulin (RhIg) – Solution of gamma globulin that contains Rh antibodies

FOCUSED ASSESSMENT

First Visit During the First Trimester

- Comprehensive health history
- Medical history (patient and father of the baby [FOB]; include hospitalizations, chronic and acute illnesses, immunizations, family history)
- Reproductive history
- Menstrual history (age at onset of menses [menarche], frequency, duration, flow)
- Risk exposure (diethylstilbestrol [DES], sexually transmitted infections [STIs], sexual practices)
- Obstetric history: Previous pregnancies (losses, births, preterm labor/birth, preeclampsia, gestational diabetes, perception of the childbearing experience)
- Current pregnancy: Last menstrual period (LMP)–was it "normal?"; any concerns; discomforts; establish the estimated date of birth (EDB)
- Social history (education level, work history, environmental exposure to teratogens, substance use, smoking, alcohol use, occupational hazards)
- Sexual history
- History of intimate partner violence (IPV) (assess every patient)
- Cultural practices (health practices, pregnancy practices, parenting practices, social support)
- Psychological assessment (depression, stress level, coping strategies, developmental stage, adjustment to pregnancy)
- Nutritional assessment (dietary recall, dietary restrictions, prenatal vitamins, folic acid, use of herbal or homeopathic remedies)
- Complete physical assessment: Head-to-toe with clinical pelvimetry, uterine size/fundal height measurement (Fig. 6-1), Pap smear, chlamydia and gonorrhea cultures, fetal heart tones (FHT) if >12 weeks of gestation, body mass index (BMI)
- Patient education

Figure 6-1 Fundal measurement should approximately equal the number of weeks of gestation.

Screening/Diagnostic Tests
- Pap smear
- Chlamydia, gonorrhea
- Complete blood count (CBC: hemoglobin, hematocrit, differential)
- Blood type and rhesus (Rh) factor
- Antibody screen (Kell, Duffy, rubella, varicella, toxoplasmosis, and anti-Rh)
- RDR/VDRL (for syphilis)
- Hepatitis B surface antigen (HbsAB)
- HIV
- Sickle cell screen (women of African, Asian, Middle Eastern descent)
- Urine (protein, ketones, glucose; culture for asymptomatic bacteriuria if indicated)

Assess for Intimate Partner Violence
Developed by the Massachusetts Medical Society (Alpert et al., 1992), "RADAR" is an acronym to guide nurses as they interview patients about relationship violence:

- Routinely screen every patient.
- Ask directly, kindly, and in a nonjudgmental manner.
- Document your findings.
- Assess the patient's safety.
- Review options and provide referrals.

Document Past Pregnancies and Their Outcomes

Pregnancy Classification System	
G	**G**ravida
T	Number of **T**erm pregnancies
P	Number of **P**reterm deliveries
A	Number of **A**bortions, both spontaneous and induced
L	Number of **L**iving children

Assess for Signs of Pregnancy		
Presumptive	**Probable**	**Positive**
Amenorrhea	Abdominal enlargement	Fetal heartbeat
Nausea and vomiting	Hegar sign, Piskacek sign	Visualization of the fetus
Urinary frequency	Goodell sign	Fetal movement palpated by a health care professional
Breast tenderness	Chadwick sign	
Quickening	Braxton Hicks sign	
Skin changes	Positive pregnancy test	
Fatigue	Ballottement	

Calculate the EDB Using Naegele's Rule

Naegele's rule is used to calculate the estimated date of birth (EDB; estimated date of delivery [EDD]).

This calculation is based on the first day of the woman's last normal period.

7 days are added to the LMP and 3 months subtracted and where necessary a year added.

For example, if the woman's LMP was June 8, 2007:

Add 7 days = June 15, 2007

Subtract 3 months = March 15, 2007

Add a year = March 15, 2008   EDB = 3/15/08

(An alternative way is to add 7 days and then add 9 months = year where needed)

Remember to ask the woman about her LMP.
>   Did her period start on the expected date?
>   Was blood loss normal (the same as her usual menstrual blood loss)?
>   Was her period different in any way?

(continued)

Calculate the EDB Using Naegele's Rule (Continued)

Was she using a form of contraception and if so, when was this method discontinued? (Hormonal contraception may delay the return to a normal ovulation pattern).

These questions will help you to determine an accurate date for the woman's last normal menstrual period.

Remember: Some women experience bleeding at the time of implantation, which normally occurs 7 to 9 days after fertilization. Care needs to be taken not to mistakenly use the date of implantation bleeding as the LMP.

Essential Components of Subsequent Prenatal Visits

- Review overall health status (signs/symptoms, discomforts, changes in medications, psychological assessment) and warning signs of pregnancy
- Assess maternal well-being (vital signs, weight, edema, reflexes and clonus if indicated, signs of preterm labor, intimate partner violence)
- Assess fetal well-being (FHTs after week 12) (Fig. 6-2), presence of fetal movements, uterine growth (fundal height measurement), Leopold maneuvers (Figs. 6-3, 6-4, 6-5, and 6-6), and presentation/position (Fig. 6-7)

Figure 6-2 Auscultation of the fetal heart tones with a fetoscope.

Figure 6-3 First Leopold maneuver.

Figure 6-4 Second Leopold maneuver.

Figure 6-5 Third Leopold maneuver.

Figure 6-6 Fourth Leopold maneuver.

Figure 6-7 Assessing fetal presentation/position.

Assessments Specific to Trimester

First Trimester
Every 4 weeks:

- Evaluate weight, blood pressure (BP), urine for glucose, ketones, and protein, fundal height, fetal heart tones (FHTs).
- Evaluate adjustment to pregnancy, nutritional intake, nausea/vomiting, discomforts.

Second Trimester
Every 4 weeks:

- Evaluate weight (normal gain is 1–2 pounds/week), BP, urine for glucose and protein, fundal height, FHTs, fetal movements, perform Leopold maneuvers.
- Nutrition, AFP testing by 20 weeks, general survey ultrasound at 20 weeks.
- Discuss plans for childbirth and prenatal classes.
- Perform preterm labor (PTL) assessment and reinforce teaching about PTL.

Third Trimester

Every 2 weeks from 28 to 32 weeks until 34 weeks, then weekly:

- Evaluate weight (normal gain is 1–2 pounds/week), BP, urine for glucose and protein, fundal height, FHTs, fetal movements, perform Leopold maneuvers.
- At 24–28 weeks perform screen for gestational diabetes, obtain culture for Group B *Streptococcus*.
- Assess for contractions, readiness for childbirth, social support.

Diagnostic Tests	
Test	**Description**
Ultrasound Examination	Routinely performed by many clinicians during the first trimester to confirm dates and to ensure a singleton gestation – may also be obtained later in the pregnancy.
Prenatal Screening*	MSAFP: Screening for open neural tube defects and Down syndrome. Done around 16 weeks of gestation; if indicated, follow-up may include amniocentesis.
Screening for Gestational Diabetes	Offered around 24–28 weeks of gestation Patient drinks solution containing 50 grams of glucose. Blood is drawn 1 hour later; results should be below 140 mg/dL.
Rh Screening	To check for Rh antibodies; if negative, 300 mcg Rh_o immune globulin (RhoGAM) is administered at 28–32 weeks (nonsensitized Rh[D]-negative women).
Hemoglobin/Hematocrit	Usually repeated mid-pregnancy and then as indicated.
Group B *Streptococcus* Screening	Usually offered at 37 weeks of gestation to determine whether antibiotic coverage is needed during labor.

*See Timetable for Prenatal Diagnosis.

Timetable for Prenatal Diagnosis

Test	Significance
Maternal Serum Alpha-fetoprotein Screening (MSAFP)	Sample of maternal blood obtained between 14 and 16 weeks of pregnancy.
	High levels may be indicative of an open neural tube defect, but may also result from incorrect dates, multiple pregnancy or fetal demise.
	Low levels of serum AFP are associated with Down syndrome. The incidence of Down syndrome increases with maternal age to approximately 1 in 100 at age 40 or older.
Triple Test: AFP, human chorionic gonadotropin (hCG) and unconjugated estriol	Levels of hCG are increased when trisomy 21 (Down syndrome) is present.
	A low level of hCG can indicate trisomy 18. The sensitivity of the AFP test in detecting trisomy 21 is increased by 40%–50% when hCG levels are added.

MEDICATIONS

Effects of Recreational Drug Use in Pregnancy

Name	Street Name	Route	Effect	Pregnancy	Newborn
Methamphetamines	Meth Crank	Smoked Snorted	Stimulant	Spontaneous abortion	Withdrawal Tremors
Dextroamphetamine	Speed Ice	Swallowed Injected Inhaled		Prematurity Breastfeeding not recommended	Poor muscle tone ?↑SIDS
Cocaine	Coke	Inhaled Smoked	Stimulant	Spontaneous abortion Placental abruption Preterm birth Breastfeeding not recommended	Birth defects – abnormalities of brain, skull, face, eyes, heart, limbs, intestines, genitals and urinary tract. Neonatal withdrawal Visual disturbances Delay in cognitive and/or learning ability
Ecstasy (methylenedioxymethamphetamine [MDMA]; compound may contain amphetamines and hallucinogens)	E, Adam, Roll, Bean, X and XTC, Clarity, Essence, Stacy, Lover's Speed, Eve	Pill form usually swallowed Crushed and snorted Injected per rectum (known as 'shafting') Smoked	Stimulant Mood enhancer	Spontaneous abortion Placental abruption Preterm birth	Congenital abnormalities: Cleft palate Low birth weight Rats exposed to ecstasy showed memory and learning deficiencies.

(continued)

Effects of Recreational Drug Use in Pregnancy (Continued)

Name	Street Name	Route	Effect	Pregnancy	Newborn
Marijuana, Cannabis	Pot, Weed, Grass, Mary Jane	Ingested, Smoked, Snorted, Injected	Stimulant, Psychedelic, Depressant	Intrauterine growth restriction (IUGR), Preterm birth	Possible link to increased incidence of childhood cancers. Withdrawal symptoms. Decrease in verbal ability and memory, plus lower impulse control
Heroin	Boy, brown, china white, dragon, gear, H, horse, junk, skag, smack	Swallowed	Sedative	Spontaneous abortion, IUGR, Preterm labor/birth, Stillbirth	Neonatal withdrawal syndrome

ETHNOCULTURAL CONSIDERATIONS

Hypertension and Pregnancy

Hypertension is more prevalent in African American and Mexican American cultures, probably due to hereditary factors (Nabel. 2003). It is the most common medical condition affecting pregnancy and may worsen as the pregnancy progresses.

TEACHING THE FAMILY

Strategies to Enhance the Childbearing Year

- Provide education related to stage of pregnancy (i.e., what physical changes to expect or danger signs that need to be reported such as vaginal bleeding or fluid loss, abdominal pain or visual disturbances).
- Encourage attendance in prenatal education classes.
- Encourage tour of facility where patient intends to give birth.
- Educate about care of the newborn (e.g., car seats, male circumcision, immunizations) so that parents can make informed decisions.

ADDITIONAL INFORMATION FOR THE CLINICAL SETTING

Goals that Guide Nursing Care

- To recognize deviations from normal
- To provide individualized, evidence-based care
- To provide culturally appropriate prenatal education designed to meet the patient's learning style and needs
- To empower women to become actively involved in their pregnancy by being informed recipients and shared decision-makers

Procedure 6-1 Obtaining A Mid-Stream Urine Sample

Purpose

A technique for obtaining a clean sample of urine so that it can be examined for bacteria, protein, glucose, and ketones. Findings provide information about the patient's hydration status (e.g., amount, color, specific gravity), infection status (e.g., leukocytes), nutritional status (e.g., ketones), and the status of possible complications such as gestational diabetes (i.e., glucose) or preeclampsia (e.g., protein).

Preparation

1. Complete the information requested on the container label. Include the patient's full name and the date and time of collection of the specimen. If a requisition is needed, note the date and time on the requisition.

2. Explain the procedure to the woman to ensure she understands why a urine sample is requested, the purpose of any tests to be performed, and directions on how to obtain a mid-stream urine sample.

Equipment

- Approved empty sterile container for collection
- Towelette for cleaning in between the labia
- Tissue

Steps

Instruct the patient to do the following:

1. Wash and dry hands thoroughly or use an alcohol-based hand-rub.

2. Remove the container cap and set it on a clean, even surface with the inner surface pointing up. Do not touch the inner surface of the lid or the container.

3. Sit on the toilet seat and separate the labia (vaginal lips) using your nondominant hand. Clean the urogenital area from the front to back with the towelette provided. Wipe for only one stroke and then discard the towelette

Patient cleansing labia

Procedure 6-1 (Continued)

4. Holding the labia apart, begin to pass urine. Allow the beginning urine to go directly into the toilet.

5. Continue to urinate and hold the container under the urine stream. Avoid touching the inside of the container. Remove the container when it is approximately half full.

6. Carefully replace the cap and secure tightly.

7. Wash your hands again after the specimen collection.

Document the procedure.

Patient urinating into specimen cup.

Clinical Alert Pregnant women are at an increased risk for developing urinary tract infections, especially if they are diabetic or have gestational diabetes. Urinary tract infections may also predispose to the onset of preterm labor.

Teach the Patient

Teach the patient to recognize common signs of a urinary tract infection:

- Dysuria: Pain (burning sensation) on urination
- Urinary frequency associated with small amounts of urine
- Hematuria: Blood or red blood cells in the urine

REFERENCES

Alpert, E.J., Freud, K.M., Park, C.C., Patel, J.C., & Sovak, M.A. (1992). *Partner violence: How to recognize and treat victims of abuse.* Massachusetts Medical Society, Waltham, MA.

Nabel, E.G. (2003). Cardiovascular disease. *New England Journal of Medicine, 349*(1), 60–72.

7

Promoting a Healthy Pregnancy

KEY TERMS

anorexia nervosa – Eating disorder marked by weight loss, emaciation, a disturbance in body image, and fear of weight gain

body mass index (BMI) – A method of evaluating the appropriateness of weight for height. Formula for calculating BMI: $BMI = \dfrac{Weight \ (in \ kilograms)}{Height^2 \ (in \ meters)}$

bulimia nervosa – Eating disorder marked by recurrent episodes of binge eating, self-induced vomiting and diarrhea, excessive exercise, strict dieting or fasting, and an exaggerated concern about body shape and weight

intrauterine growth restriction (IUGR) – Undergrowth of the fetus; may be due to deficient nutrient supply, intrauterine infection or associated with a congenital malformation

pica – Consumption of non-nutritive substances or food

small for gestational age (SGA) – Inadequate growth for gestational age

FOCUSED ASSESSMENT

At each prenatal visit: update health history, perform physical examination (as indicated) and conduct appropriate laboratory/ diagnostic testing (see Chapter 6)

DIAGNOSTIC TESTS

Genetic Screening During Pregnancy

Disorder	Population Affected	Pathology	Pregnancy and Newborn Complications
Sickle Cell Disease	African Americans Persons of Mediterranean descent	Autosomal recessive hemolytic disease. Involves an abnormal substitution of an amino acid in the structure of hemoglobin. Red blood cells assume abnormal, sickle shape in response to triggers, including hypoxia, infection, dehydration. Results in inability to oxygenate tissues. Leads to occlusion and rupture of blood vessels.	Spontaneous abortion Preterm labor Intrauterine growth restriction Stillbirth
Tay–Sachs Disease	Ashkenazi Jews Jewish people from Eastern or Central Europe French-Canadians Cajuns	Both parents must carry and pass on the trait to the child.	Infants appear normal at birth, until about 3 to 6 months of age when the neurological system begins to deteriorate. Death occurs between the ages of 2 and 4 years.
Thalassemia	Greeks Italians Southeast Asians Filipinos	Disorder of hemoglobin synthesis Thalassemia minor: person is heterozygous for the trait; experiences fewer symptoms. Thalassemia major: person is homozygous for the trait; experiences more severe symptoms.	Children appear normal at birth. During the first 2 years, children become pale, lethargic, and develop jaundice. Results in enlarged liver, spleen, and heart. Death results from heart failure and infection.

(continued)

Genetic Screening During Pregnancy (Continued)

Disorder	Population Affected	Pathology	Pregnancy and Newborn Complications
Hemophilia	Males are affected. Females are carriers.	Mutation in the gene of coagulation factor VIII. Causes a defect in blood clotting. Leads to frequent bleeding episodes and hemorrhage.	Males can have excessive bleeding when circumcised. Increased incidence of intracranial hemorrhage Easy bruising and bleeding with injuries
Glucose-6-Phosphate Dehydrogenase (G6PD) Deficiency	African Americans Seen mostly in males	Causes drug-induced destruction of red blood cells when taking certain medications (e.g., sulfonamides)	Increased incidence of pathological jaundice or hyperbilirubinemia due to destruction of red blood cells
Cystic Fibrosis	Caucasians	Autosomal recessive genetic disorder Causes exocrine gland dysfunction	Results in chronic obstructive lung disease from thick mucus secretions in the lungs Frequent lung infections occur Causes a deficiency in pancreatic enzymes that prevents normal digestion

MEDICATIONS

Ferrous Sulfate (**fer-**us **sul**-fate)

Pregnancy Category B

Indications Prevention/treatment of iron-deficiency anemia

Actions An essential mineral found in hemoglobin, myoglobin, and many enzymes. Prevents iron deficiency.

Therapeutic Effects Prevents/treats iron deficiency.

Pharmacokinetics
Absorption Therapeutically administered PO iron may be 60% absorbed; absorption is an active and passive transport process.

Contraindications and Precautions
Use cautiously in Peptic ulcer, ulcerative colitis; indiscriminate chronic use may lead to iron overload.
Adverse Reactions and Side Effects Constipation, dark stools, diarrhea, epigastric pain, gastrointestinal bleeding

Route and Dosage (mg elemental iron) 100–200 mg/day (2–3 mg/kg per day) in three divided doses

Nursing Implications
1. Assess nutritional status and dietary history to determine possible cause of anemia and need for patient teaching.
2. Assess bowel function for constipation or diarrhea; notify care provider and use appropriate nursing measures if these symptoms occur.

Data from Deglin, J.H., & Vallerand, A.H. (2009). Davis's drug guide for nurses *(11th ed.). Philadelphia: F.A. Davis.*

ETHNOCULTURAL CONSIDERATIONS

Vitamin D Deficiency

African Americans and other women with dark skin are at the greatest risk for vitamin D deficiency. Women who habitually cover most of their skin with clothing and those who live in northern latitudes with limited exposure to sunlight are also more likely to be deficient in vitamin D.

Anemia During Pregnancy

In the United States, maternal anemia occurs most commonly among adolescents, African American women, and women of lower socioeconomic status.

The Consumption of Non-nutritive Substances

Causes of pica are believed to include nutritional deficiencies, cultural and familial factors, stress, low socioeconomic status, and biochemical disorders. In some cultures, certain non-nutritive food substances are thought to bring health or have positive spiritual effects for those who consume them. Individuals of other cultures believe that the consumption of specific non-nutritive substances plays a role in enhancing fertility or promoting luck within the family.

TEACHING THE FAMILY

Nutrition to Promote a Healthy Pregnancy		
Element	Recommendation During Pregnancy	Comments
Calories	300 kcal/day increase	Focus on healthy eating.
Protein	Moderate increase	Caution regarding undercooked meats, fish high in mercury (shark, swordfish, tilefish, king mackerel).
Water	8–10 8-oz. glasses per day	Four to six glasses should be water; the rest may be other fluids (limit caffeine to <300 mg/day).
Calcium	1000 mg/day	Supplements are important.
Vitamin D	5 mcg	Exposure to sunlight and fortified foods usually adequate. Dark-skinned women are more at risk for deficiency.
Iron	18 mg/day	Starting by 12 weeks of gestation, usually requires supplementation.
Vitamin C	80–85 mg/day	Enhances iron absorption.
Folic Acid	800 mcg/day	Aids in iron absorption; necessary for DNA and RNA production. Deficiency is related to neural tube defects.

Recommended Total Weight Gain During Pregnancy for a Single Birth	
Pre-Pregnancy BMI	**Recommended Total Weight Gain**
Underweight (<19.8)	28–40 lbs.
Normal weight (19.8–26)	25–35 lbs.
Overweight (>26–29)	15–20 lbs.
Obese (>29)	15+ lbs.

Source: National Heart, Lung and Blood Institute (2006).

Iron Supplements

- Teach patients to avoid substances known to decrease iron absorption (bran, tea, coffee, milk, oxylates [found in spinach and Swiss chard], egg yolk) when taking iron supplements.
- Take iron between meals with a beverage other than tea, coffee, or milk.

Vitamin B_{12} Deficiency

- Counsel patients who are vegetarians about the risk for vitamin B_{12} deficiency.
- Associated with the following maternal problems: megaloblastic anemia, glossitis, and neurological deficits
- Infants born to mothers with vitamin B_{12} deficiency are more likely to have megaloblastic anemia and to exhibit neurodevelopmental delays.

Coping with Fatigue

Advise the woman to:

- Get plenty of rest (go to bed earlier, take naps and breaks when possible).
- Cut down on external commitments (e.g., volunteer and social events).
- Eat a healthy, balanced diet; include iron-rich foods and protein; include foods with vitamin C to help with iron absorption.
- Exercise moderately at least 30 minutes each day. Brisk walking is the best exercise for improving alertness and boosting energy levels.

- Avoid food and beverages containing caffeine.
- Drink plenty of fluids.
- Minimize stress.
- Ask for help. One's partner, children, and friends can help, but only if they are aware that help is needed.

Exercise

Advise the woman to:

- Monitor her breathing rate (she should be able to talk comfortably while exercising).
- Protect against overheating.
- Stop when she becomes tired and never exercise to the point of exhaustion.
- Avoid exercises that could cause trauma to the abdomen, rigorous bouncing, arching of the back, or bending beyond 45-degree angle.
- Drink adequate fluids.
- Remember that balance changes as pregnancy progresses.

Complementary Care

- Massage therapy: Increases blood flow to maternal and fetal tissues; enhances relaxation.
- Chiropractic care: Treats lower back pain and headaches related to increased hormone levels.
- Acupuncture and acupressure: Treat many physical ailments during pregnancy without the introduction of medications.
- Relaxation exercises, meditation, and breathing techniques: increase blood flow to maternal and fetal tissues; increase relaxation.
- Light therapy: Enhances mood and treats depression.
- Reflexology: Stimulates nerve pathways to increase blood flow and energy flow to corresponding areas of the body.
- Aromatherapy: Enhances relaxation.

Dealing with Common Discomforts in Pregnancy

Trimester	Common Discomforts	Relief Measures
First	Nausea and vomiting	Consume small, frequent meals, dry crackers. Remain upright after meals. Consider vitamin B_6, acupressure.
	Fatigue	Establish bedtime routine; take naps.
	Urinary frequency and nocturia	Ensure adequate intake; decrease fluid intake 2–3 hours before bedtime. Perform Kegel exercises. Seek help if urine is bloody or if hesitancy or burning during urination is experienced.
	Dyspepsia	Remain upright after eating; consume small, frequent meals; avoid fatty foods and cold liquids.
	Gum hyperplasia and bleeding	Use soft toothbrush and see dentist as recommended.
Second	Dependent edema	Avoid constrictive clothing; elevate legs; use side-lying position when resting.
	Leg varicosities	
	Hyperventilation and shortness of breath	Take slow, steady breaths, raise arms above the head.
	Numbness and tingling of fingers	Wear wrist brace when sleeping.
	Supine hypotensive syndrome	Rest on the side and rise slowly.
	Fatigue	As above
	Urinary frequency	As above
	Dyspepsia	As above
	Flatulence	Avoid gas-forming foods, chewing gum, large meals
	Gum hyperplasia and bleeding	As above
	Leg cramps	Regular exercise, elevate legs, dorsiflex feet, consume adequate calcium and phosphorous
Third	Dependent edema	As above
	Leg varicosities	As above
	Dyspareunia	Try various positions, alternative methods for satisfaction
	Nocturia	As above

(continued)

Dealing with Common Discomforts in Pregnancy (Continued)

Trimester	Common Discomforts	Relief Measures
	Round ligament pain	Warm bath, apply heat, support uterus with pillow or pregnancy girdle
	Supine hypotensive syndrome	As above
All Trimesters	Ptyalism	Small frequent meals, avoid starchy foods, suck on hard candies
	Nasal congestion	Increase fluids, vaporizer, steamy shower
	Back pain	Good body mechanics, physical therapy
	Leukorrhea	Panty liner, cotton underwear
	Constipation	Fluids, fiber, exercise
	Insomnia	Sleep hygiene, proper alignment with pillows

Signs and Symptoms of Danger

Trimester	Warning Sign	Possible Complication(s)
	Severe, persistent nausea and vomiting	Hyperemesis gravidarum Hydatidiform mole
First	Abdominal pain and vaginal bleeding	Spontaneous abortion
	Chills, fever, malaise, anorexia	Infection, e.g., UTI
	Headache, vision changes, elevated blood pressure, edema	Preeclampsia
	Increased vaginal secretions	Vaginitis Premature rupture of the membranes
Second	Regular, persistent contractions or backache	Preterm labor
	Decreased fundal height	IUGR
	Increased fundal height (>2 cm/week)	Hydramnios, multiple gestation, fetal macrosomia
	Decreased fetal movement	Fetus in danger from any of the above
Third	The same as found in the second trimester	As above
	Positive glucose challenge test	Gestational diabetes

Trimester	Warning Sign	Possible Complication(s)
	Painless vaginal bleeding	Placenta previa
	Abdominal pain with or without vaginal bleeding	Abruptio placentae

RESOURCES

American College of Obstetricians and Gynecologists (ACOG)

Association of Women's Health, Obstetrical, and Neonatal Nursing (AWHONN)

USDHHS & U.S. Department of Agriculture

The document "Dietary Guidelines for Americans 2005" is an evidence-based resource guide for professionals and consumers that offers strategies for promoting health and reducing the risk for chronic diseases through diet and physical activity. Dietary guidelines, food composition, the food guide pyramid, dietary supplements, and resource lists are included in the guide (USDHHS & U.S. Department of Agriculture [USDA], 2005) (http://www.nal.usda.gov/fnic/).

REFERENCES

Deglin, J.H., & Vallerand, A.H. (2009). *Davis's drug guide for nurses* (11th ed.). Philadelphia. F.A. Davis.

Obesity and Women's Reproductive Health (2006). National Heart, Lung and Blood Institute. Retrieved from http://www.nhlbi.nih.gov/guidelines/obesity/e_txtbk/ratnl/22111.htm (Accessed December 7, 2008).

Caring for the Woman Experiencing Complications During Pregnancy

KEY TERMS

amniotic infection syndrome – Placental, fetal membrane, and umbilical cord inflammation that occurs after premature rupture of the membranes (PROM)

asymptomatic bacteriuria – Presence of at least 10^5 colony-forming bacteria without symptoms

condylomata acuminata – Genital warts

disseminated intravascular coagulation (DIC) – Hematological disorder characterized by a pathologic form of clotting that is diffuse and consumes large amounts of clotting factors; causes widespread external or internal bleeding or both

ectopic pregnancy – A pregnancy that implants outside of the uterine cavity

erythroblastosis fetalis – Hemolytic disease of the newborn, usually caused by isoimmunization that has resulted from Rh incompatibility or ABO incompatibility

gestational diabetes mellitus (GDM) – Onset of diabetes during pregnancy

glycosylated hemoglobin (Ghb) – Glycohemoglobin (a minor hemoglobin) with glucose attached; Ghb/HbA1c concentration represents the average blood glucose level over the preceding 5 to 6 weeks

Homans' sign – Early sign of deep venous thrombosis in the leg; on dorsiflexion, pain occurs from inflammation of the blood vessel. A negative Homans' sign does not rule out deep vein thrombosis.

hydatidiform mole (molar pregnancy) – Gestational trophoblastic neoplasm, usually results from fertilization of an egg that contains no nucleus

hydramnios (polyhydramnios) – Amniotic fluid in excess of 2.0 liters

hydrops fetalis – Most severe form of fetal hemolytic disorder; may be a sequela to maternal isoimmunization.

isoimmunization – Development of antibodies in a species of animal with antibodies from the same species (e.g., development of anti-Rh antibodies in an Rh-negative mother following exposure to Rh-positive fetal blood)

kernicterus – Bilirubin encephalopathy that involves the deposit of unconjugated bilirubin in brain cells and results in neurological damage or death

ophthalmia neonatorum – Neonatal eye inflammation from *Neisseria gonorrhoeae* that can result in permanent blindness from perforation of the globe of the eye

pregestational diabetes mellitus – Onset of diabetes before pregnancy

premature rupture of the membranes (PROM) – Rupture of the amniotic sac at least 1 hour before the onset of labor at any gestational age

preterm premature rupture of the membranes (PPROM) – Rupture of the membranes before the onset of labor and before 37 completed weeks of gestation

preterm rupture of the membranes – Rupture of the membranes before 37 completed weeks of gestation

salpingectomy – Surgical removal of the fallopian tube

salpingostomy – Surgical opening of a fallopian tube

thyrotoxicosis – Excessive thyroid activity

tocolysis – Use of medications (tocolytics) to inhibit uterine contractions

type 1 diabetes – An absolute insulin deficiency (Expert Committee on the Diagnosis and Classification of Diabetes Mellitus [ECDCDM], 2003)

type 2 diabetes – A combination of insulin resistance and inadequate insulin production (ECDCDM, 2003)

vertical transmission – Transmission of infection occurs antepartally when the virus or bacteria crosses the placenta, intrapartally when it travels (via the bloodstream) from the vagina up into the uterus during labor or following rupture of the membranes, or postpartally through transfer in the breast milk

Bleeding During Pregnancy

FOCUSED ASSESSMENT

The Perinatal Patient at Risk: Causes of Bleeding in Early Pregnancy

Cause	Assessment	Implications	Risk Factors
Implantation	Scant spotting for 1–2 days 1–2 weeks after conception, Painless	Does not affect the pregnancy.	
Abortion: 10%–20% of all pregnancies are "lost."	*Complete:* Complete expulsion of products of conception (POC) before 20 weeks of gestation	Watch for infection, offer counseling.	More than three previous pregnancy losses
	Threatened: Bleeding before 20 weeks of gestation but no cervical dilation	Rest; call if bleeding or cramping increases.	
	Incomplete: Partial expulsion of POC	Dilation and curettage	
	Inevitable: No expulsion of POC yet but bleeding and dilated cervix	Counseling Watch for infection.	
	Missed: Death of embryo or fetus but POC are not expelled		
Ectopic Pregnancy	Abdominal pain, spotting, missed menstrual period	Pregnancy loss, hemorrhage if ruptures, salpingostomy or methotrexate. Counseling	Previous ectopic or other abdominal surgeries, pelvic inflammatory disease (PID), endometriosis
Gestational Trophoblastic Disease	"Molar pregnancy": Bleeding, uterus larger than expected, hyperemesis, preeclampsia, absence of fetal heart tones (FHTs)	Hemorrhage, anemia, shock, choriocarcinoma, not a viable pregnancy Counseling	Maternal age, history of previous molar pregnancy, Clomid

(continued)

The Perinatal Patient at Risk: Causes of Bleeding in Later Pregnancy (Continued)

Cause	Assessment	Implications	Risk Factors
Placenta Previa (Fig. 8-1) Implantation of placenta near or over the cervix	Painless bleeding in second half of pregnancy *Complete*: Placenta covers entire cervix *Partial*: Placenta covers part of the cervix *Marginal*: Placenta encroaches on cervical margin	Vaginal birth not possible with complete placenta previa. Seek immediate care if **any** bleeding or labor. **No vaginal digital exam**	Prior cesarean birth, multiple gestation, smoking, cocaine use, age >35 years, African or Asian ethnicity
Placental Abruption (abruptio placentae) (Fig. 8-2) Premature separation of a normally implanted placenta	Severe abdominal pain, abnormal contractions, increased uterine tone, fetal compromise, third trimester *Concealed*: Bleeding is confined within the uterine cavity, 20% of cases *Revealed*: Vaginal bleeding present	Fetal mortality in 35% of all placental abruptions Maternal mortality 0.5%–5% Actual blood loss is often more than what is visible	Trauma Cocaine use

CLINICAL ALERTS

Early Identification of Maternal Hemorrhage

- The maternal pulse (tachycardia) and/or fetal heart rate (bradycardia or tachycardia) may be the first indicators of maternal instability.
- Blood pressure is a very poor indicator of blood volume deficit.
- Due to the expanded blood volume that normally occurs during pregnancy, the patient may be asymptomatic and exhibit vital signs that remain within normal parameters despite a large amount of blood loss.

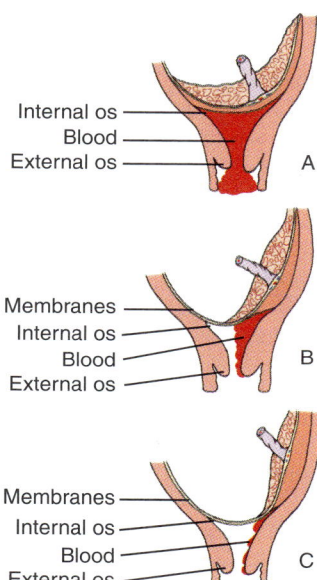

Figure 8-1 Placenta previa. *A*. Complete. *B*. Partial. *C*. Marginal.

Partial separation
(concealed hemorrhage)

Partial separation
(apparent hemorrhage)

Complete separation
(concealed hemorrhage)

Figure 8-2 Abruptio placentae.

Care for the Patient Experiencing an Abruptio Placentae

- Hospitalization
- Intravenous placement with a large-bore catheter (16-gauge)
- Lab work: Includes complete blood count (CBC), coagulation studies (fibrinogen, prothrombin time [PT],

partial thromboplastin time [PTT], platelet count, fibrin degradation products), type and screen for 4 units of blood, Kleihauer-Betke for Rh-negative patients. A "clot test" may be performed: a red top tube of blood is drawn, set aside, and checked for clotting. If a clot does not form within 6 minutes or if it forms and lyses within 30 minutes, a coagulation defect is probably present and the fibrinogen level is <150 mg/dL.

- If birth is not imminent, possibly betamethasone to promote fetal lung maturity
- RhoGAM if indicated
- Continuous evaluation of intake and output
- Continuous electronic fetal monitoring
- Delivery (cesarean or vaginal birth) may be initiated depending on maternal–fetal status
- Continuous maternal–fetal assessment, with ongoing information and emotional support for the patient and her family

DIAGNOSTIC TESTS

With any incidence of bleeding during pregnancy, the following laboratory tests are commonly performed:

- CBC
- Coagulation studies (fibrinogen, PT, PTT, platelet count, fibrin degradation products)
- Type and screen for blood
- Kleihauer–Betke for Rh-negative patients; Rh(D)-negative patients should receive RhoGAM to prevent isoimmunization
- Ultrasound to assess viability of pregnancy, location of placenta, location of conceptus, and to assess for abruption

ETHNOCULTURAL CONSIDERATIONS

Religious Beliefs and Blood Transfusions

Jehovah's Witness prohibits its members from receiving blood products or their derivatives. When bleeding occurs during pregnancy and blood is deemed necessary to save the woman's and/or fetus' life, a very challenging situation exists. Non-blood products may be given but are not always successful. Sometimes a court order is obtained so that blood can be administered to save the life of the woman and/or fetus. Respect the family's beliefs and support them during this very difficult time when the health of both the woman and her fetus as well as their religious beliefs are being challenged.

TEACHING THE FAMILY

Communicating with the Family Who Has Experienced a Perinatal Loss

Approach the family with compassion and sincerity. Expressions of caring are conveyed in the following statements:

- "I understand this is a very difficult time for you and your family, but I want you to know that I am here and willing to listen if you want to talk. You let me know if and when you are ready."
- "It is normal for you to be sad and you will probably feel like this for some time. Losing a baby, no matter how far along in your pregnancy, is very difficult. I can recommend some support groups if you think you might be interested." (If the patient says she does not want the information at this time, continue with) "Please do not hesitate to call us if you change your mind. We can always give you the information."
- "Does your baby have a name?" (refer to the fetus by name instead of "the fetus")

Hypertensive Complications in Pregnancy

Specific Conditions and Implications

Condition	Definition	Implications
Chronic Hypertension (HTN)	HTN present before pregnancy	At increased risk for preeclampsia
Gestational HTN (transient)	HTN appearing after the 20th week of pregnancy without proteinuria	Resolves by 12 weeks postpartum
Preeclampsia	HTN (BP >140/90 mm Hg) with proteinuria appearing after 20 weeks of gestation	Risk for abruption, intrauterine growth restriction (IUGR), fetal demise, disseminated intravascular coagulation (DIC), renal failure, seizure

(continued)

Specific Conditions and Implications (Continued)		
Condition	**Definition**	**Implications**
Hemolysis, **E**levated **L**iver Enzymes, **L**ow **P**latelets (HELLP syndrome)	A complication of preeclampsia that can manifest at any time during pregnancy and the puerperium	Arteriolar vasospasms lead to **h**emolysis, and decreased blood flow to the liver, resulting in tissue ischemia and hemorrhagic necrosis (**e**levated **l**iver enzymes). In response to the endothelial damage caused by the vasospasms, platelets aggregate at the site and a fibrin network is set up, leading to a decrease in the circulating platelets (**l**ow **p**latelets).
Eclampsia	The occurrence of a grand mal seizure	Can occur during pregnancy, labor, or within 72 hours after birth

FOCUSED ASSESSMENT

Risk Factors for Preeclampsia

- Primigravida (6–8 times greater risk)
- Age extremes (<17 years and >35 years)
- Diabetes
- Preexisting hypertension
- Multiple gestation (5 times greater risk)
- Fetal hydrops (10 times greater risk)
- Hydatidiform mole (10 times greater risk)
- Preeclampsia in a previous pregnancy
- Family history
- Obesity
- Immunological factors
- Chronic renal disease
- Rh incompatibility
- African American ethnicity
- Pregnancies that result from donor insemination, oocyte donation, embryo donation (American College of Obstetricians and Gynecologists [ACOG], 2002; Sibai, Dekker, & Kupfermine, 2005)

Assessment Guidelines

Cardiovascular System
- Blood pressure, heart sounds, lung sounds
- Edema

- Early signs or symptoms of pulmonary edema (tachycardia or tachypnea)
- Daily weight taken at the same time of the day and on the same scale
- Skin color, temperature, and turgor
- Capillary refill: May indicate decreased perfusion if >3 seconds

Renal System
- Proteinuria: 24-hour urine sample
- Output of at least 30 mL/hr
- Intake/output measurement

Central Nervous System
- Level of consciousness
- Headache, visual disturbances*
- Hyperreflexia
- Clonus

Hepatic System
- Elevated liver enzymes
- Enlarged liver
- Epigastric pain*

Document the presence or absence of these symptoms.

CLINICAL ALERTS

Facilitating Effective CPR for the Pregnant Patient

Instruct the pregnant patient never to lie on her back. Explain that the weight of the baby exerts pressure on the large blood vessels and impedes blood flow back to the heart. If the pregnant patient experiences a cardiac arrest, this information is essential. CPR is not effective if the fetus remains on the large blood vessels. One nurse must take responsibility to displace the uterus to the left while the cardiac compressions are being performed.

Care of the Pregnant Patient Post Seizure

- Do not attempt to shorten or abolish the initial seizure. Attempts to administer anticonvulsants intravenously without secure venous access can lead to phlebitis and venous thrombosis.
- Prevent maternal injury.

- Maintain adequate oxygenation; administer oxygen via face mask at 10 L/min.
- Minimize the risk of aspiration. Position the patient on her side to facilitate drainage. Ensure suction equipment is ready and working.
- Give adequate magnesium sulfate to control seizures. As soon as possible following the seizure, venous access should be secured with a 4- to 6-gram loading bolus of magnesium sulfate given over 15 to 20 minutes. If the patient seizes after the loading dose, another 2-gram bolus may be given intravenously, over 3 to 5 minutes.
- Correct maternal acidemia. Blood gas analysis allows monitoring of oxygenation and pH status. Respiratory acidemia is possible following a seizure.
- Avoid polytherapy. Maternal respiratory depression, respiratory arrest, or cardiopulmonary arrest is more likely in women who receive polytherapy to arrest a seizure. Remember that anticonvulsants are respiratory depressants and may interact.
- Check the fetus(es) (all must be accounted for). Following a seizure there may be loss of FHR variability and bradycardia on the fetal monitoring tracing.
- Check the patient for ruptured membranes, contractions, and cervical dilation.
- Prepare for birth as indicated.
- Support the patient and her family. This is a very frightening event for them and they need reassurance and need to be kept aware of the plan of care and the well being of their baby (Poole, 2004).

Documentation After a Patient Seizure

- Time and length of seizure
- Associated symptoms
- Vital signs including fetal heart assessment
- Presence or absence of uterine contractions
- Any untoward results such as the rupture of membranes or signs of placental abruption
- Medications that were given. Remember to have the physician write or co-sign any verbal orders that were given during the emergency (Poole, 2004)

Accidental Overdose of Magnesium Sulfate Administration Can Pose a Significant Risk to Both Mother and Newborn

Current Recommendations to Prevent Magnesium Sulfate Accidents

- A standardized unit protocol with standing orders that address the initial bolus and maintenance dose to be administered; how the pump should be programmed; the maintenance IV solutions that will be used and the frequency of the maternal–fetal assessment.
- Administer IV magnesium sulfate (including the initial bolus) only through a controlled infusion device with free-flow protection.
- Use universal standardized dose prepackaged magnesium sulfate.
- Have a second nurse check the initial magnesium sulfate IV bag and pump settings (and every magnesium sulfate IV bag that is added and each subsequent rate change).
- Use a 100-mL (4 g) or 150-mL (6 g) IV piggyback (IVPB) for the initial bolus instead of giving a bolus from the main bag with a rate change on the pump.
- Use color-coded tags on the lines as they go into the pumps and into the IV ports.
- Provide 1:1 nursing care for women in labor who are receiving magnesium sulfate.
- When care is transferred to another nurse, have both nurses together at the bedside review the pump settings for both the magnesium sulfate and mainline IV fluids and review written physician orders for magnesium sulfate infusion orders.
- Implement periodic magnesium sulfate overdose drills with airway management and calcium administration with the physician and nurse team members participating together.
- Maintain the calcium antidote in the patient's room in a locked box.

(Simpson & Knox, 2004).

MEDICATIONS

Magnesium Sulfate (mag-**nee**-zhum **sul**-fate)

Pregnancy Category D

Indications Anticonvulsant in severe eclampsia or preeclampsia. Unlabeled use: Preterm labor.

Actions Plays an important role in neurotransmission and muscular excitability

Therapeutic Effects Resolution of eclampsia

Pharmacokinetics
Absorption IV administration results in complete bioavailability; well absorbed from IM sites.
Distribution Widely distributed. Crosses the placenta and is present in breast milk.
Metabolism and Excretion Excreted primarily by the kidneys
Half-life Unknown

Contraindications and Precautions
Contraindicated in Hypermagnesemia/hypocalcemia/anuria/ heart block/active labor or within 2 hours of labor (unless used for preeclampsia or eclampsia)
Use Cautiously in Any degree of renal insufficiency

Adverse Reactions and Side Effects
Central Nervous System Drowsiness
Respiratory System Decreased respirations
Cardiovascular System Arrhythmias, hypotension, bradycardia
Gastrointestinal System Diarrhea
Dermatological System Flushing, sweating
Metabolic Hypothermia

Interactions Potentiates neuromuscular blocking agents

Route and Dosage
Eclampsia/Preeclampsia Piggyback a solution of 40 g of magnesium sulfate in 1000 mL of lactated Ringer's solution—use an infusion control device (pump) at the ordered rates; loading dose: initial bolus of 4–6 g over 15–30 min; maintenance dose: 1–3 g/hr.
IM: 4–5 g given in each buttock, can be repeated at 4-hour intervals; use Z-track technique

(Note: IM route rarely used because the absorption rate cannot be controlled and injections are painful and may result in tissue necrosis.)

Time/Action Profile for Anticonvulsant Effect
IM: Onset is 60 minutes with peak unknown and duration is 3–4 hours. **IV:** Onset is immediate with peak unknown and duration is 30 minutes.

Nursing Implications
Remember that this is a very potent, high alert drug!
Explain the purpose and side effects of the medication to the patient and her companion.

Explain that she may feel very warm and become flushed and experience nausea and vomiting, visual blurring, and headaches.

Magnesium sulfate must never be abbreviated (i.e., $MgSO_4$ is not acceptable) and requires a written order by the physician for administration.

Always use an infusion pump for administration and run the medication piggyback, not as the main line.

Monitor pulse, blood pressure, respirations, and ECG frequently throughout parenteral administration. Respirations should be at least 16/min before each dose.

Monitor neurologic status before and throughout therapy.

Institute seizure precautions

Keep the room quiet and darkened to decrease the likelihood of triggering seizure activity

Patellar reflexes should be tested before each parenteral dose of magnesium sulfate. If absent, no additional dose should be administered until a positive response returns.

Monitor intake and output. Urine output should be maintained at a level of at least 100 mL/4 hr.

Serum magnesium levels and renal function should be monitored periodically throughout administration of parenteral magnesium sulfate.

Have 10% calcium gluconate available should toxicity occur. Administer 10 mL intravenously over 1–3 minutes until signs and symptoms are reversed.

After delivery, monitor the newborn, for hypotension, hyporeflexia, and respiratory depression.

Data from Deglin, J., & Vallerand, A. (2009). Davis's drug guide for nurses (11th ed.). Philadelphia: F. A. Davis.

Medications Used to Treat Chronic Severe Hypertension in Pregnancy

Agent (trade name)	Class	Dose	Contraindications and Adverse Effects	Breast feeding
Alpha-Methyldopa (Aldomet)	Central alpha-adrenergic inhibitor	Starting dose is 250 mg PO, tid or qid Maximum dosage of 2–4 g/24 hr	Methyldopa hypersensitivity, history of hepatitis, autonomic dysfunction, lethargy, or syncope. Can cause liver damage, fever, Coombs-positive hemolytic anemia.	Safe

(continued)

Medications Used to Treat Severe Hypertension in Pregnancy (Continued)

Agent (trade name)	Class	Dose	Contraindications and Adverse Effects	Breast feeding
Labetalol (Trandate, Normodyne)	Alpha/beta-adrenergic blocker	100–400 mg PO bid–tid (maximum dose 2400 mg a day)	Labetalol hypersensitivity, bradycardia, asthma, heart block, heart failure. Can cause maternal and fetal bradycardia, hypotension, bronchospasm	Safe
Nifedipine (Adalat, Procardia)	Calcium channel blocker	10–30 mg PO tid. Slow release once a day. Maximum of 90 mg/day	Hypersensitivity to calcium channel blockers, persistent dermatologic reactions, congestive heart failure. Can potentiate cardiac depressive effect of magnesium sulfate.	Safe
Furosemide (Lasix)	Loop diuretic	20–80 mg PO, once or twice daily	Hypersensitivity to furosemide, anuria, or depleted blood count. Can cause profound diuresis with water and electrolyte depletions, sensitivity to sunlight exposure, hyperuricemia and gout, exacerbation of SLE, abdominal cramping, diarrhea, tinnitus, dizziness, pancreatitis, and cholestasis.	Safe
Hydrochloro-thiazide (HydroDIURIL)	Loop diuretic	25–50 mg PO daily	Anuria, renal disease, liver disease, SLE, hypersensitivity to hydrochlorothiazide or other sulfonamide derived drugs. Can cause weakness, hypotension, pancreatitis, cholestasis, anemia, allergic reactions, electrolyte disturbance, hyperglycemia, hyperuricemia, dizziness, renal dysfunction.	Risk is remote, but there are concerns about potential thromb-ocytope-nia in infants.

Source: Yankowitz, J. (2004). Pharmacologic treatment of hypertensive disorders during pregnancy. *The Journal of Perinatal & Neonatal Nursing, 18* (3), 230–240. Reproduced with permission.

Medications Used to Acutely Treat Severe Hypertension in Pregnancy		
Agent (Trade Name)	**Class**	**Dosage**
Labetalol hydrochloride (Normodyne, Trandate)	Alpha/beta-adrenergic blocker	IV bolus 20 mg; if no response, double dose and repeat every 15 minutes, up to a cumulative maximum dose of 300 mg.
Hydralazine (Apresoline, Nepresol)	Peripheral/arterial vasodilator	IV bolus 5–10 mg every 15–20 minutes to a maximum dose of 30 mg
Nifedipine (Adalat, Procardia)	Calcium channel blocker	Nifedipine can be given PO in doses of 10 mg repeated every 15 minutes to a maximum of 30 mg.
Sodium Nitroprusside (Nipride, Nitropress)	Vasodilator	0.25 mcg/kg per minute (Increase by 0.25 mcg/kg per minute every 5 minutes to a maximum of 5 mcg/kg per minute.)

Source: Yankowitz, J. (2004). Pharmacologic treatment of hypertension during pregnancy. *The Journal of Perinatal & Neonatal Nursing, 18* (3), 230–240.

TEACHING THE FAMILY

Home Management of the Patient with Pregnancy-induced Hypertension

Before discharge, ascertain that the home environment is conducive to rest and the patient will be able to rest frequently throughout the day. Ensure that the patient can verbalize understanding of the importance of keeping all prenatal appointments and that she must immediately notify her physician or midwife at the first appearance of:

- Blood pressure values greater than those at the time of hospital discharge: MD or CNM should provide parameters.
- Visual changes
- Epigastric pain
- Nausea and vomiting
- Bleeding gums
- Headaches
- Increasing edema, especially of the hands and face
- Decreasing urinary output
- Decreased fetal movement
- "Just not feeling right"

ADDITIONAL INFORMATION FOR THE CLINICAL SETTING

Grading Reflexes and Checking for Clonus

During the assessment, grade maternal reflexes on a 0 to 4+ scale:

4+ Very brisk, hyperactive; often indicative of disease; often associated with clonus

3+ Brisker than average; possibly but not necessarily indicative of disease

2+ Average; normal

1+ Somewhat diminished

0 No response

Clonus is usually noted as "absent" or "present" but it may be rated as:

Mild (2 movements)
Moderate (3–5 movements)
Severe (6 or more movements)

SPASMS: A Memory Enhancer When Caring for a Patient with Preeclampsia

S: Significant blood pressure changes may occur without warning.

P: Proteinuria, a serious sign of renal involvement, is present.

A: Arterioles are affected by vasospasms that result in endothelial damage, leakage of intravascular fluid into the interstitial spaces, and edema.

Figure 8-3 Assessing for clonus.

S: Significant laboratory changes (most notably, liver function tests and platelet count) signal worsening of the disease.

M: Multiple organ systems can be involved, including cardiovascular, hematological, hepatic, renal, and central nervous systems.

S: Symptoms appear after 20 weeks of gestation.

Endocrine Complications in Pregnancy

FOCUSED ASSESSMENT

Diabetes Mellitus

Classification of Diabetes	Characteristics	Implications
Type 1	• Usually diagnosed in persons younger than 30 years of age • Polyuria, polydipsia, weight loss • An abrupt onset that requires emergency medical attention • Approximately 10% of those diagnosed with diabetes	• Requires insulin *Possible sequelae* (dependent on level of glycemic control; HbA_{1c} level used to guide treatment): • 4 times more likely to develop preeclampsia or eclampsia • 5 times increase in perinatal death • 2–3 times increase in congenital malformations and poor fetal growth • Fetal demise
Type 2	• Usually diagnosed in adults older than age 30 • Slow onset with gradual progression of symptoms • Not ketosis prone	Does not always require insulin *Possible sequelae* (dependent on level of glycemic control; HbA_{1c} level used to guide treatment): • 4 times more likely to develop preeclampsia or eclampsia • 5 times increase in perinatal death • 2 to 3 times increase in congenital malformations and poor fetal growth • Fetal demise

(continued)

Diabetes Mellitus (Continued)

Classification of Diabetes	Characteristics	Implications
Gestational	• Develops in the latter half of pregnancy • Symptoms are usually mild and not life threatening • May be treated with either diet or insulin *Risk factors*: • Women older than 25 years of age • Obesity • Insulin resistance • Polycystic ovary syndrome • History of a large-for-gestational age infant, hydramnios, stillbirth, miscarriage, infant with congenital anomalies • Family history of type 2 diabetes • Ethnicity	Increased risk for developing diabetes later in life *Possible sequelae*: (Dependent on level of glycemic control; HbA$_{1c}$ level used to guide treatment): • Fetal demise • Growth abnormalities • Hydramnios • Macrosomia • Newborn hypoglycemia

Other Endocrine Disorders

Disorder	Signs/Symptoms	Tests and Treatment
Hyperthyroidism	Heat intolerance, diaphoresis, fatigue, anxiety, emotional lability, tachycardia, wide pulse pressure, weight loss, goiter, nausea, vomiting, diarrhea, cardiomyopathy	*Tests*: Decreased TSH with increased free T$_4$ *Treatment*: Antithyroid medications (thioamides, propylthiouracil, methimazole), subtotal thyroidectomy, radioactive iodine treatment *Potential effect on pregnancy*: Increased risk of preeclampsia, preterm labor, low birth weight, neonatal mortality
Hypothyroidism	Weight gain, decreased exercise tolerance, constipation, hoarseness, hair loss, brittle nails, dry skin	*Tests*: Increased TSH with normal to low T$_3$ and T$_4$ *Treatment*: Thyroid hormone supplement *Potential effect on pregnancy*: Increased risk of preeclampsia, placental abruption, stillbirth

Disorder	Signs/Symptoms	Tests and Treatment
Hyperemesis Gravidarum	Abnormal condition of pregnancy characterized by protracted, persistent vomiting, weight loss, and fluid and electrolyte imbalance	*Tests:* Electrolytes assessment *Treatment:* Rest; eat small frequent meals of dry, bland foods high in protein; avoid spicy foods; antiemetics; hospitalization if severe for parenteral or enteral feedings.

CLINICAL ALERT

Maternal Diabetes and Preterm Labor

Magnesium sulfate is the drug of choice for diabetic women who experience preterm labor. The use of terbutaline sulfate (Brethine) or antenatal corticosteroids to accelerate fetal lung maturation can cause significant maternal hyperglycemia and precipitate diabetic ketoacidosis (DKA). Follow patients closely in an acute care setting for at least 48 to 72 hours after corticosteroids have been given. An intravenous insulin infusion is usually required and is adjusted on the basis of frequent capillary glucose measurements (Landon, Catalano, & Gabbe, 2002).

DIAGNOSTIC TESTS

The Glucose Challenge Test (Glucola Screening)

- Administer a 50-g oral dose of glucose solution to the woman.
- Take a blood sample 1 hour after the glucose is consumed.
- Follow up with the formal 3-hour oral glucose tolerance test (OGTT) if the patient's 1-hour plasma glucose level is 140 mg/dL or higher.

Oral Glucose Tolerance Test (OGTT)

The 3-hour OGTT requires the fasting patient to ingest 100 g of glucose and have blood drawn at 1-hour intervals. For at least 12 hours before and during the test, the woman should avoid consuming caffeine (it may increase glucose levels) and refrain from smoking. The diagnosis of gestational diabetes mellitus is made when two or more of the threshold values are above the norm. According to the American Diabetes Association (ADA; 2006), normal plasma glucose values are:

Fasting blood sugar	<95 mg/dL
1-hour	<180 mg/dL
2-hour	<155 mg/dL
3-hour	<140 mg/dL

MEDICATIONS

Medications for Nausea and Vomiting of Pregnancy

- Pyridoxine (vitamin B_6, 25–75 mg (orally) per day, used alone or in combination with Doxylamine (Unisom), 25 mg (orally) per day
- Promethazine (Phenergan) 12.5–25 mg (intravenously, intramuscularly, orally, or rectally) every 4 hours
- Dimenhydrinate (Dramamine) 50–100 mg (orally or rectally) every 4–6 hours or 50 mg intravenously (in 50 mL of saline run over 20 minutes) every 4–6 hours
- Metoclopramide (Reglan) 5–10 mg (intravenously, intramuscularly, or orally) every 8 hours

(ACOG, 2004; Cunningham et al., 2005)

ETHNOCULTURAL CONSIDERATIONS

- Gestational diabetes occurs more often in Native Americans, African Americans, Hispanic Americans, Asian Americans, and Pacific Islanders (ADA, 2006).

TEACHING THE FAMILY

Complementary Care for Nausea and Vomiting of Pregnancy

- Ginger, a perennial native to many Asian countries, is effective in treating nausea and vomiting during pregnancy. The antiemetic effect of this root (taken in a dosage of 1 gram per day) is due to its ability to increase gastrointestinal motility. Ginger is available in tablet, capsule, and syrup form. Some concerns about taking ginger during pregnancy have been raised, but to date no significant side effects have been documented.

- Elasticized wristbands (i.e., Sea-Bands®) that use a firm object to place pressure on the Neiguan point (acupressure P6 point) are a nonpharmacological, noninvasive method that may lessen the frequency and severity of nausea and vomiting during pregnancy (Hunter, Sullivan, Young, & Weber, 2007).

ADDITIONAL INFORMATION FOR THE CLINICAL SETTING

Diet and Exercise for the Patient with Gestational Diabetes Mellitus (GDM)

Diet and exercise are important components of care for the woman with GDM. Typically, the patient is placed on a standard diabetic diet that is calculated to include 30 kcal/kg per day, based on a normal preconceptional weight. For the obese woman, the diet may be calculated to include up to 25 kcal/kg per day. On-going nutritional counseling is essential.

Physical activity such as walking and swimming is also important for the woman with GDM. Exercise helps to lower blood glucose levels and may decrease the need for insulin (ADA, 2006).

Planning Care for the Woman with GDM

Although diet and exercise are the mainstays of care for the woman with gestational diabetes mellitus, up to 20% require insulin during pregnancy to maintain euglycemia. If fasting blood glucose levels exceed 105 mg/dL, insulin therapy is initiated (ADA, 2006).

Anticipating Changes in Insulin Needs During Pregnancy

- During the first trimester, maternal blood glucose levels typically decrease and the insulin response to glucose increases. To avoid hypoglycemia, a woman with well-controlled diabetes may need a decreased insulin dosage when she becomes pregnant.

- Maternal insulin resistance begins at about 14 weeks of gestation and increases until it stabilizes during the final weeks of pregnancy.
- During the second and third trimesters, as insulin requirements steadily increase, the insulin dosage must be adjusted to prevent hyperglycemia.

Infections that May Adversely Affect Pregnancy

FOCUSED ASSESSMENT

Various Infections and Their Effects on the Pregnancy

Infection	Signs/Symptoms	Sequelae in Pregnancy	Treatment
Urinary Tract Infection (UTI), Cystitis	Urinary frequency, urgency, dysuria and suprapubic pain	Preterm labor, septic shock, adult respiratory distress syndrome	Anti-infectives for 7–10 days
Pyelonephritis	Flank tenderness, nausea, vomiting, fever and chills together with the symptoms of a lower UTI	If left untreated or inadequately treated, septic shock, adult respiratory distress syndrome and/or preterm labor may result.	Treated aggressively with hospitalization and intravenous antibiotics
Group B *Streptococcus* (GBS)	All women are now screened between 35 and 37 weeks of pregnancy and treated before childbirth.	May cause UTI, chorioamnionitis, or endometritis, preterm labor, neonatal infection	Penicillin-based anti-infective agent
Chlamydia	Vaginal discharge, dysuria, abnormal vaginal bleeding, or asymptomatic	Neonatal infection transmitted during birth (conjunctivitis and pneumonia)	Erythromycin or penicillin-based anti-infectives
Gonorrhea (GC)	Vaginal discharge, dysuria and abnormal vaginal bleeding	Ophthalmia neonatorum, amniotic infection syndrome	Oral or intramuscular cefixime (Suprax) or ceftriaxone (Rocephin)

Infection	Signs/Symptoms	Sequelae in Pregnancy	Treatment
Syphilis	Primary: Chancre Secondary: Palmar rash Tertiary: Neurosyphilis	Delayed treatment or untreated infection results in a range of fetal effects from minor anomalies to preterm birth or fetal death	Penicillin
Human Papillomavirus (HPV) Infection	Genital warts	May be transmitted to fetus transplacentally	Cryotherapy, trichloroacetic acid, dichloroacetic acid, surgical excision
Human Immunodeficiency Virus (HIV) and Acquired Immunodeficiency Syndrome (AIDS)		Vertical transmission to fetus (antepartally, intrapartally); transfer in breast milk (postpartally)	Without identification of HIV-infected women and the aggressive use of preventive therapy, 20%–30% of exposed children will become infected with HIV (CDC, 2006; Landry, 2004; Moran, 2004).
Tuberculosis (TB)	Inflammatory infiltrations in the respiratory tract, the gastrointestinal and genitourinary tracts, bones, joints, nervous system, lymph nodes and skin	The tubercle bacillus can spread to the fetus from the maternal blood by crossing the placenta, and entering the umbilical vein. Bacilli may settle in the fetal liver or the lungs.	Isoniazid (INH), ethambutol, and rifampin

TORCH Diseases

Infection/Agent	Mode of Transmission/ Detection	Maternal Effects	Neonatal Effects	Treatment	Incidence and Prevention	High Risk Potential
Toxoplasmosis Single-celled protozoan parasite *Toxoplasma gondii*	*Transmission:* Transplacental Eating raw meat, especially pork, lamb or venison Touching the hands or mouth after handling undercooked meat containing *T. gondii* Secreted in feces of infected cats Cyst is destroyed with heat. *Detection:* Serological antibody testing IgM specific antibody	Most infections in humans are asymptomatic. However, may include fatigue, muscle pains, and sometimes lymphadenopathy. In the immunocompetent person, toxoplasmosis can be a devastating infection.	Severity varies with gestational age. Congenital infection can occur if a woman develops acute toxoplasmosis during pregnancy (most likely in the third trimester). May have miscarriage if acquired early. Fetal infections are more virulent the earlier the infection is acquired but less frequent. Sequelae include low birth weight, hepatosplenomegaly icterus, anemia, neurological disease, and chorioretinitis.	Pyrimethamine and sulfadiazine may reduce incidence of congenital toxoplasmosis. Treatment of the mother has been shown to reduce the risk of congenital infection. *Pyrimethamine is not recommended for use during the first trimester of pregnancy.*	ACOG does not recommend routine screening except for pregnant women with HIV infection. Incidence varies throughout the world (1–4 infants per 1000 live births). 30% of U.S. women have been exposed. Approximately 40%–50% of U.S. adults have an antibody to this organism. Frequency of seroconversion during pregnancy is ≤5% and approximately 3 in 1000 infants show evidence of congenital infection.	People who consume raw or poorly cooked meat High-risk gestational age is 10–24 weeks. Toxoplasmosis is more common in Western Europe, particularly France.

	IgG seroconversion from negative to positive Most accurate confirmation of active infection is a rise in IgG titer in two appropriately spaced tests.		Clinically significant congenital toxoplasmosis occurs in approximately 1 in 8000 pregnancies.		Incidence of congenital toxoplasmosis infection in the United States is 1 in 1000-8000. More than 60 million people in the United States carry a parasite. Cook meat to a safe temperature. Peel or wash fruits and vegetables.	
Other **HEPATITIS B** **HBV** Incubation usually 60–90 days	*Transmission*: Direct contact with the blood or body fluids of an infected person Sexual Perinatal Percutaneous Transplacental Blood, stool, amniotic fluid, and saliva transmission	The course of the disease is not altered during the pregnancy. Symptoms are seen in only 30%–50% of patients; these include low-grade fever, nausea, anorexia, jaundice, hepatomegaly, malaise, preterm labor, and preterm birth.	Infants infected at birth have a 90% risk of becoming chronically infected with HBV (carrier) and 25% risk of developing significant liver disease—yet if they receive prophylaxis at birth, 95% can be prevented.	Mother: Rest Infant: Vaccine if mother is carrier, infant receives HBIg HBV vaccine is recommended (three doses).	Screen all pregnant women. The incidence of hepatitis B in the United States declined by >60% from 1985 to 1995. Estimated that 1–1.25 million people in the United States are chronically infected with HBV.	High-risk categories: Pregnant women from China, Southeast Asia, Africa, Philippines, and Indonesia Eskimos Prostitutes Homosexuals IV drug users Hemophiliacs

(continued)

TORCH Diseases (Continued)

Infection/Agent	Mode of Transmission/ Detection	Maternal Effects	Neonatal Effects	Treatment	Incidence and Prevention	High Risk Potential
	Shared razors, toothbrushes, towels, and other personal items *Detection:* HBsAg identified 7–14 days after exposure Hepatitis B surface antibody present with HBsAg indicates noninfectious HBcAg, HBeAg, and anti-HBc evaluate stage and progression of the infection	No specific treatment, but may include bedrest and a high-protein, low-fat diet. Mother-to-child transmission of HBV occurs in 10%-20% of women who are seropositive for HBsAg and in 90% of women who are seropositive for both HBsAg and HBcAg. Transmission to the neonate appears to occur as a result of exposure to infected blood and genital secretions during delivery.	Increased risk of transmission to infant if mother is HBeAg-positive (indicating acute infection) Stillbirth Clinical illness is relatively infrequent. Most (90%–95%) of those infected are symptomatic and become chronic hepatitis B carriers. Infants born to women who have hepatitis B infection during pregnancy should be given HBIg within 12 hours of delivery.		Estimated that 300 million people worldwide are chronically infected with HBV. Approximately 8000 acute HBV infections were reported to the CDC. HBV vaccine has been available since 1982. Acute infection occurs in 1–2 per 10,000 pregnancies. Minimize exposure of close physical contact. Heptavax-B (Pregnancy does not contraindicate vaccination.)	Transfusion recipients People with other sexually transmitted diseases or multiple sex partners CDC recommends universal screening of all prenatal patients.

Rubella (3-day German measles) Rubella virus incubation is 2–3 weeks.	*Transmission*: Nasopharyngeal secretions Transplacental *Detection*: Virus isolated from throat Rubella-specific IgM antibodies Hemagglutination-inhibition antibodies Complement-fixing antibodies Rubella antibody titer of 1:8 or more indicates immune status.	Erythematous maculopapular rash on face, neck, arms, and legs lasting 3 days Lymph node enlargement Slight fever, malaise, headache, and arthralgia History of exposure 3 weeks earlier	Overall risk of congenital rubella syndrome is approximately 20% for primary maternal infection in the first trimester. High incidence of congenital abnormalities in newborns whose mother contracted rubella within the first 4 months of pregnancy. Approximately 50% of infants exposed to the virus within 4 weeks of conception will manifest signs of congenital infection. When infection occurs in second 4 week period after conception, approximately 25% of	Women with rubella require no special therapy other than mild analgesics and rest. Infants born with congenital rubella may shed virus for many months and thus be a threat to other infants, as well as to susceptible adults.	Last epidemic in 1965; since introduction of vaccine in late 1960s, rubella has been rare. Absence of rubella antibody indicates susceptibility. Estimated that 6%–25% of women are susceptible. Occurs more commonly in the spring. Vaccinate immediately postpartum and use contraception for a minimum of 1 month after vaccination.

(continued)

TORCH Diseases (Continued)

Infection/Agent	Mode of Transmission/ Detection	Maternal Effects	Neonatal Effects	Treatment	Incidence and Prevention	High Risk Potential
			fetuses will be infected; when infection develops in the third month, approximately 10% of fetuses will be infected. Spectrum anomalies: Deafness (60%–75%) Eye defects (10%–30%) CNS anomalies (10–25%) Cardiac malformation (10%–20%) Risks appear to be almost exclusively associated with women who previously have not been infected with CMV. Even in this case, two thirds of infants will not become infected and only 10%–15% of		Vaccination is contraindicated during pregnancy.	

Cytomegalovirus (CMV)
DNA virus of the herpesvirus group

Transmission: Transmitted horizontally by droplet infection and contact with saliva and urine, vertically from mother to fetus-infant, and as a sexually transmitted infection. Intimate contact with infected secretions (breast milk, cervical mucus, semen, saliva, tears and urine) Transplacental
Detection: Isolation of virus from urine or endocervical secretions

Most infections are asymptomatic, but approximately 15% of adults have a mononucleosis-like syndrome characterized by fever, pharyngitis, lymphadenopathy, and polyarthritis.

the remaining will have symptoms. Infection is most likely to occur with primary maternal infection. The timing of the infection during pregnancy is a major determinant of outcome (first and second trimester being more severely affected). CID includes low birthweight, IUGR, microcephaly. CNS abnormalities, mental and motor retardation, intracranial calcifications, sensorineural deafness, blindness with chorioretinitis, mental retardation, hepatosplenomegaly and jaundice

Mother: Treat symptoms.
Infant: No satisfactory treatment is available.
Isolate the infant.
Approximately 50% of females in the United States have antibodies.
It is estimated that approximately 2% of susceptible pregnant women in the United States acquire primary CMV infection during pregnancy.

.

Maternal immunity to CMV does not prevent recurrence. Found in 0.5%–2.0% of all neonates. Incidence of primary CMV infection in pregnant women in the United States varies from 1% to 3%. Maintain rigorous personal hygiene throughout the pregnancy.

Day care centers are a common source of infection. Prevalence depends on age, sex, SE class, sexual behavior, and occupational or institutional exposure. Serological screening is not recommended by ACOG. Vaccine is experimental.

(continued)

TORCH Diseases (Continued)

Infection/Agent	Mode of Transmission/ Detection	Maternal Effects	Neonatal Effects	Treatment	Incidence and Prevention	High Risk Potential
Herpes Simplex Virus (HSV) Herpes virus type 1 (more common with oral lesions) and type 2 (more common in genital lesions) Incubation is 2–10 days	*Transmission:* Ascending infection Intimate mucocutaneous exposure Transmission is more likely to occur from men to women. Passage through an infected birth canal Transplacental (although rare) if initial infection occurs during pregnancy	Painful genital vesicle lesions Vesicles on the cervix, vagina, or external genitalia area Primary infection is commonly associated with fever, malaise, and myalgia; numbness, tingling, burning, itching, and pain with lesions; lymphadenopathy; and urinary retention.	Rare transplacental transmission have resulted in miscarriage. Mortality of 50%–60% if neonatal exposure is with active primary infection.	Protect neonate from exposure at time of birth. Cultures are obtained when the mother has active lesions. Avoid routine use of scalp electrodes. If lesions are visible, delivery by cesarean section is the current standard of care. Acyclovir has been used near term to suppress viral outbreak.	An estimated 1 million Americans are newly infected with genital HSV annually. Seroprevalence of HSV is approximately 25%. Approximately 1%–2% of pregnancies. 1 in 3000–20,000 live births is at risk for the development of neonatal herpes. Up to 70% of women who give birth to infected infants have no history of genital herpes.	Risk factors include female sex, African-American, or Mexican-American ethnic background, older age, low educational level, poverty, cocaine use, a greater number of lifetime sexual partners, unprotected sex, and having a sexual partner with genital herpes.

Detection:

Tissue culture (swab specimen from vesicles) and immunofluorescent staining of the cell can differentiate HSV-1 from HSV-2. Presence of swelling, redness, and painful lesions

Neurological morbidity such as chorioretinitis, microcephaly, mental retardation, seizures, and apnea

Prophylactic treatment with oral acyclovir may be appropriate in women with frequent recurrent infections in pregnancy.
If symptoms or lesions are present, cesarean delivery should be performed. Avoid genital contact when male partner has penile lesions.
Use condoms.

ACOG = American College of Obstetricians and Gynecologists; Anti-HBc = antibody to hepatitis B core antigen; CDC = Centers for Disease Control and Prevention; CID = cytomegalic inclusion disease; CNS = central nervous system; DNA = deoxyribonucleic acid; HBV = hepatitis B virus; HbsAg = surface antigen to HBC; HbcAg = core antigen to HBV; HbeAg = hepatitis B early antigen; HBIg = hepatitis B immunoglobulin; IgG = immunoglobulin G; IgM = immunoglobulin M; IUGR = intrauterine growth restriction; IV = intravenous.
Source: Moran, B. (2004). Maternal infections. In Mattson, S. & Smith, J. (Eds), *Maternal-child nursing core curriculum.* 3rd ed. Philadelphia: W.B. Saunders. Reproduced with permission.

DIAGNOSTIC TESTS

Caring for the Patient with a UTI: Urine Specimens

- UTI is more likely during pregnancy, when urine becomes more alkaline and vaginal secretions have an increased glycogen level, both of which foster bacterial growth.
- Before collecting a midstream specimen, explain the importance of proper cleansing.
- Obtain a urinalysis and urine culture and sensitivity on all patients with signs of preterm labor.
- Remember that signs and symptoms of UTI commonly are similar to those of normal pregnancy (urgency, frequency).
- Urge the patient to take all prescribed antibiotic(s), even if she feels better before completing the prescription.
- When treatment is complete, expect to retest the patient's urine to confirm the UTI cure.

MEDICATIONS

Antibiotic Use During Pregnancy

- Sulfonamides should not be used near term because they interfere with protein binding of bilirubin.
- Tetracyclines should never be used during pregnancy because they cause retardation of fetal bone growth and staining of fetal teeth.
- Antibiotics that are safe to use during pregnancy include amoxicillin (Amoxil), ampicillin (Marcillin), and cephalosporins (cephalexin [Keflex]).

Immunizations During Pregnancy

- The ideal time for immunizations that prevent disease transmission from mother to fetus is before conception.
- After conception, maternal and fetal benefits of immunization still usually outweigh the theoretical risks of adverse effects.
- The risks of disease exposure and adverse effects on the mother and her fetus must be weighed against the risks, benefits, and efficacy of the vaccine.
- Nurses should educate women about the importance of immunizations and document each patient's immunization status on her permanent medical record.

Special Conditions and Circumstances that May Adversely Affect Pregnancy

Selected Conditions and Their Effects on Pregnancy

Condition	Definition	Implications
Preterm Labor (PTL)	Contractions and cervical dilation before the end of the 37th gestational week. Symptoms can be subtle: backache, pelvic aching, menstrual-like cramps, vaginal discharge, pelvic pressure, urinary frequency, intestinal cramping.	RhoGAM if indicated Preterm birth: >50% survive at 25 weeks, >90% survive at 28–29 weeks. Assess for infection and fetal fibronectins (fFN) (proteins produced by the fetal membranes).
Premature Rupture of Membranes (PROM)	Rupture of membranes before the onset of labor Diagnosed based on history of vaginal discharge and results of Nitrazine and fern tests	Implications depend on gestational age. Monitor for infection.
Multiple Gestation	More than one fetus	Considered a high-risk pregnancy; at risk for PTL, GDM, UTIs, PIH, placenta previa, IUGR, abnormal presentation, cord prolapse
Disseminated Intravascular Coagulopathy (DIC)	Pathological clotting disorder that consumes clotting factors and results in widespread bleeding.	Life-threatening, early detection is crucial. Observe for signs of bleeding, e.g., petechiae, oozing from injection sites, hematuria.
Venous Thromboembolic Diseases	Includes superficial and deep vein thrombophlebitis (DVT), pulmonary embolus (PE), septic pelvic thrombophlebitis, and thrombosis.	Account for 50% obstetric mortality.
Sickle Cell Disease	Recessive genetic disorder resulting in the production of S hemoglobin (HbS) Most commonly affects those of African or Mediterranean descent.	"Sickled" erythrocytes cannot change their shape and are unable to squeeze through the microcirculation, resulting in obstruction, progressive tissue, and organ damage.

(continued)

Selected Conditions and Their Effects on Pregnancy (Continued)

Condition	Definition	Implications
Thalassemia	Defective globin chains damage developing red blood cells	Predominately affects blacks and those of Italian, Greek, Middle-Eastern Indian, Asian, and West Indies descent.
Rho(D) Isoimmunization	Hemolytic disease of the fetus and newborn resulting from maternal production of antibodies against the $Rh_o(D)$ antigens present on the fetal red blood cells.	Fetal RBC deficiency, hyperbilirubinemia, erythroblastosis fetalis, neonatal kernicterus
ABO Isoimmunization	Hemolytic disease in response to ABO incompatibility between mother and fetus. Type O carries no antigens, type A carries A antigen and type B caries B antigen.	Milder reaction than $Rh_o(D)$ incompatibility
Psychiatric Complications	May represent an exacerbation of an ongoing disorder, a resurgence of previously remitted symptoms, or onset of a new illness.	Psychoactive medications cross the placenta; however, the effects of an untreated psychiatric disorder can also affect pregnancy outcome. The risk:benefit ratio must be carefully considered.
Substance Abuse	Frequent drug and/or alcohol use in pregnancy	See Chapter 4.

Other Special Circumstances

Circumstance	Potential Problems and Complications
Antenatal Bedrest	Muscle wasting, failure to gain weight, cardiovascular and psychological difficulties, difficulty regulating blood pressure, dizziness, fainting
Adolescence	Prenatal medical and behavioral risk factors can severely complicate adolescent pregnancy and result in poor birth outcomes, particularly when late or inadequate prenatal care occurs.

Circumstance	Potential Problems and Complications
Older Gravida	Pregnant women older than the age of 35 are more likely to experience obstetrical complications such as placenta previa, abruptio placentae, prolonged labor, cesarean birth, and mortality. The fetus is at a greater risk for low birth weight, macrosomia, chromosomal abnormalities, congenital malformations, and neonatal mortality.
Obese Patient	A pregnant woman is considered **overweight** if she is 20% above ideal weight or has a BMI over 26.1; she is considered **obese** if her weight exceeds 200 pounds, if she is 50% over ideal body weight for height, or if her BMI is above 29. Obesity is associated with a higher incidence of diabetes and hypertension, macrosomia, prolonged labor, shoulder dystocia, and higher cesarean rates. Cesarean delivery is often complicated by excessive operative blood loss, difficult intubations, postoperative wound complications, operative injury, the need for blood transfusions, thromboembolism, and hysterectomy.
Intimate Partner Violence (IPV)	Pregnancy is often a trigger for escalation of violence in a relationship.

FOCUSED ASSESSMENT

Recognizing Thromboembolism

Assess for the following signs and symptoms:

- Pain, tenderness, warmth in the extremity
- Asymmetrical swelling of lower extremities, with a difference of more than 2 cm between the normal and affected leg. (Thigh swelling is especially significant because the risk of pulmonary embolism is associated with femoral or iliac phlebitis.)
- Color change, especially in the left leg
- A palpable cord beneath the tender, painful area
- Positive Homans' sign
- Signs or symptoms of pulmonary embolism: Tachypnea, dyspnea, pleuritic chest pain, atelectatic rales, cough, fever, diaphoresis, tachycardia, hemoptysis, cyanosis, heart gallop or murmur, anxiety, apprehension (Cunningham et al., 2005; McPhedran, 2004)

Screening for Depression During Pregnancy

The U.S. and Canadian Task Forces on Preventive Health Care recommend using the following two "probe questions" to screen women for depression during pregnancy:

- "Over the past 2 weeks, have you felt down, depressed, or helpless?"
- "Over the past 2 weeks, have you felt little interest or pleasure in doing things?"

(Records & Rice, 2007)

CLINICAL ALERTS

Hemodynamic Changes in Pregnancy

A patient with a cardiac disorder is at greatest risk when hemodynamic changes reach their maximum, between the 28th and 32nd weeks of gestation.

Indicators of Decreased Cardiac Output During Labor and Birth

- Decreased or irregular pulse
- Increased respiratory rate
- Dyspnea
- Chest pain
- Abnormal breath sounds (crackles at lung bases)
- Decreased blood pressure
- Decreased urinary output (<30 mL/hr)
- Edema of hands, face, and feet
- Abnormal heart sounds (diastolic murmur at heart's apex)
- Signs or symptoms of air hunger (anxiety)
- Decreased oxygen saturation (<95%)
- Cool, clammy, cyanotic skin
- Increased capillary refill time (>3 seconds)
- EKG changes
- Mental changes (disorientation, fatigue, syncope)

DIAGNOSTIC TESTS

Kleihauer-Betke test: Estimates the number of fetal RBCs in the maternal circulation

Coombs test: Immunological test that is performed on
  newborn's blood at birth and that includes direct and
  indirect Coombs tests
Direct Coombs test: Identifies the presence of maternal
  Rh-positive antibodies in the neonate's blood and
  hemolysis or lysis of RBCs
Indirect Coombs test: Detects Rh-positive antibodies in
  maternal serum

Antepartum Fetal Assessment Tests

Name	Description	Nursing Implications
Chorionic Villus Sampling (CVS)	An invasive procedure in which a thin catheter is inserted vaginally into the intrauterine cavity and a sample of chorionic villus is aspirated from the placenta	Used to obtain a fetal karyotype. Performed between 10 and 12 weeks. The risk of complications with CVS is 1 in 200 and includes infection, fetal loss, rupture of membranes, Rh isoimmunization, and possible fetal limb reduction. After CVS, administer microdose Rh_o(D) immune globulin to the Rh_o(D) negative woman to prevent isoimmunization (Gilbert & Harmon, 2003).
Percutaneous Umbilical Blood Sampling (PUBS)	An invasive procedure in which a needle is inserted through the maternal abdomen and into the fetal umbilical cord	Used to obtain a sample of fetal blood for karyotyping and to test for anemia, isoimmunization, metabolic disorders, and infection. Complications include cord laceration, thromboembolism, preterm labor, premature rupture of the membranes, and infection (Jenkins & Wapner, 2004).
Amniocentesis	An invasive procedure in which amniotic fluid is removed via a needle inserted through the maternal abdomen and into the amniotic sac to obtain a sample of fetal cells	Performed after 12 weeks. May be used to analyze for chromosome abnormalities, fetal lung maturity, infection, the presence of bilirubin in Rh-sensitized pregnancies, amniotic fluid reduction for temporary alleviation of maternal symptoms associated with hydramnios. Complications include rupture of the membranes, preterm labor, infection, fetal injury, and fetal death. If the woman has Rh_o(D)-negative blood, Rh_o(D) immune globulin should be administered after amniocentesis to prevent isoimmunization. *(continued)*

Antepartum Fetal Assessment Tests (Continued)

Name	Description	Nursing Implications
	L/S ratio (Lecithin to sphingomyelin) is determined from amniotic fluid, with a value of 2:1 or more indicating mature fetal lungs.	These proteins are components of surfactant formed by the alveoli beginning around the 22nd week of gestation.
	Phosphatidyl glycerol and desaturated phosphatidylcholine	These two substances are found only in the amniotic fluid once the fetal lungs are mature.
Ultrasonography	Use of high-frequency sound waves to detect differences in tissue density and visualize outlines of structures in the body	Noninvasive and painless. Often performed during the first trimester to confirm the viability and age of the pregnancy; determine the number, size, and location of the gestational sacs; identify uterine abnormalities (and rule out an ectopic pregnancy); and locate the presence of an intrauterine contraceptive device
Kick Counts	A count of the number of times the woman feels the fetus move in a specified time	Many variations have been developed but there are two major methods for performing kick counts: 1. While lying on her side, the woman counts and records 10 distinct movements in a period of up to 2 hours. Once 10 movements have been perceived, the count may be discontinued. 2. The patient counts and records fetal movements for 1 hour three times per week. The count is considered reassuring if it equals or exceeds the woman's previously established baseline.

Name	Description	Nursing Implications
Doppler Ultrasound Blood Flow Studies (umbilical velocimetry)	Used to study blood flow in the umbilical vessels of the fetus, placental circulation, fetal cardiac motion, and maternal uterine circulation by measuring the velocity of red blood cell movement through the uterine and fetal vessels	This noninvasive technology is useful in managing pregnancies at risk because of hypertension, diabetes mellitus, intrauterine growth restriction (IUGR), multiple fetuses, or preterm labor.
Fetal Biophysical Profile (BPP)	A noninvasive "fetal physical examination" that combines electronic fetal heart rate monitoring with ultrasonography to evaluate fetal well-being, producing a more accurate prediction than any single assessment	Comprises five components (Harmon, 2004): 1. Nonstress test 2. Fetal breathing movements (one or more episodes of rhythmic fetal breathing movements for 30 seconds) 3. Fetal movement (three or more discrete body or limb movements) 4. Fetal tone (one or more episodes of extension of a fetal extremity with return to flexion, or opening or closing of a hand) 5. Determination of the amniotic fluid volume (a single vertical pocket of amniotic fluid exceeding 2 cm - provides evidence of adequate amniotic fluid) Each of the five components is assigned a score of 2 (normal or present) or 0 (abnormal). A score of 8–10 is reassuring. *(continued)*

Antepartum Fetal Assessment Tests (Continued)

Name	Description	Nursing Implications
Non-stress Test (NST)	The use of electronic fetal monitoring (EFM) for 20 minutes based on the premise that a normal fetus moves at various intervals and that the central nervous system and myocardium respond to movement, with the response of a healthy fetus demonstrated by an acceleration of the fetal heart rate	Acceptable criteria: The presence of 2 fetal heart rate accelerations of 15 beats per minute that last for 15 seconds each during a 20-minute period (ACOG, 1999)
Acoustic Stimulation/ Vibroacoustic Stimulation	A hand-held instrument such as an artificial larynx (especially designed for this purpose) positioned on the maternal abdomen to produce a low-frequency vibration and a buzzing sound for 1 to 3 seconds	May be used as an adjunct to the NST to elicit an acceleration of the fetal heart rate.
Contraction Stress Test (CST)	Evaluates the fetal heart rate response to uterine contractions, with CSTs evaluated according to the presence or absence of late fetal heart rate decelerations.	A late deceleration, associated with fetal hypoxia, is one that begins at the peak of the contraction and persists after conclusion of the contraction. The test is considered negative (normal) if there is no evidence of late or significant variable decelerations; a positive CST (abnormal) is one in which there are late decelerations after 50% of contractions, even if the frequency is less than three in 10 minutes.
Electronic Fetal Heart Rate Monitoring (EFM)	Use of electronic techniques to give an ongoing assessment of fetal well-being, which can be accomplished by either external or internal means	EFM provides information related to the response of the fetal heart rate in the presence or absence of uterine contractions.

MEDICATIONS

Rho(D) Immune Globulin (arr aych oh **dee** im-**yoon glob**-yoo-lin) (RhoGAM, HypRho-D, BayRho-D, Gamulin Rh, Rhophylac)

Pregnancy Category C

Indications
Administered to Rh-negative women who have been exposed to Rh-positive blood by:

Delivering an $Rh_o(D)$-positive infant
Aborting an $Rh_o(D)$-positive fetus
Having chorionic villus sampling, amniocentesis, or intraabdominal trauma while carrying an $Rh_o(D)$-positive fetus
Having an accidental transfusion of $Rh_o(D)$-positive blood

Action Prevents production of anti-$Rh_o(D)$ antibodies in $Rh_o(D)$-negative patients who were exposed to $Rh_o(D)$-positive blood by suppressing the immune reaction of the $Rh_o(D)$-negative woman to the antigen in the $Rh_o(D)$-positive blood.

Therapeutic Effects Prevents antibody response and subsequently prevents hemolytic disease of the newborn (erythroblastosis fetalis) in future pregnancies of women who have conceived an $Rh_o(D)$-positive fetus. Prevents $Rh_o(D)$ sensitization after a transfusion accident.

Pharmacokinetics
Absorption Well absorbed from IM sites.

Contraindications and Precautions
Contraindicated in $Rh_o(D)$- or Du-positive patients and patients previously sensitized to $Rh_o(D)$ or Du.

Adverse Reactions and Side Effects Pain at IM site

Route and Dosage
One vial *standard* dose (300 mcg) administered intramuscularly:

- At 28 weeks of pregnancy and within 72 hours of delivery
- Within 72 hours after termination of a pregnancy of 13 weeks or more of gestation
- After an accidental transfusion, with dosage calculated based on the volume of blood that was erroneously administered

One vial *microdose* (50 mcg) within 72 hours after chorionic villus sampling (CVS) or termination of a pregnancy of >13 weeks' gestation

Notes:

- More than 300 mcg of RhoGAM may be indicated after a large transplacental hemorrhage or after a mismatched blood transfusion
- Rhophylac can be given IM or IV (prefilled syringes are available).

Nursing Implications

Do not give to infant, to $Rh_o(D)$-positive person, or to $Rh_o(D)$-negative person previously sensitized to the $Rh_o(D)$ antigen. Note: There is no more risk than when given to a woman who is not sensitized – if in doubt, administer $Rh_o(D)$ immune globulin.

Administer into the deltoid muscle.

Give within 3 hours if possible, but may be given up to 72 hours after delivery, miscarriage, abortion, or transfusion.

Explain the purpose of this medication to protect future $Rh_o(D)$-positive infants; before administering, obtain a signed consent form if required by your facility.

Data from Deglin, J., & Vallerand, A. (2009). Davis's drug guide for nurses (11th ed.). Philadelphia: F. A. Davis.

Administer and Document RhoGAM When Clinically Indicated

- Administering and properly documenting $Rh_o(D)$ immune globulin (RhoGAM) is an important nursing action.
- If the mother is Rh-negative and nonsensitized and the baby is Rh-positive:
  - Always check to be sure the patient has received $Rh_o(D)$ immune globulin (RhoGAM), if indicated, before discharge.
  - Make certain that she has received the appropriate dose.
- Patients who have miscarried also must be treated.
- In cases where it is not possible to determine the fetus' or baby's blood type, $Rh_o(D)$ immune globulin (RhoGAM) is still given.
- Question if an order (for $Rh_o(D)$ immune globulin) has not been written.

Safe Administration of Rh₀(D) Immune Globulin (RhoGAM)

- In a RhD-negative woman who is **non**-sensitized, RhoGAM should be given after delivery of an RhD-positive infant. In the United States, the standard dose is 300 mcg and it is given within 72 hours of delivery.
- Educate your patient as to the reason why she is receiving RhoGAM.
- Give your patient documentation that she has received RhoGAM.
- **Never** give RhoGAM to: (1) an Rh(D)-positive woman; (2) a sensitized Rh(D) negative woman; (3) an Rh(D)-negative woman who has given birth to an Rh(D)-negative infant; or (4) the infant or father of the infant.

Recognizing Cardiac Effects of Obstetric Medications

Obstetric medications such as tocolytics and uterine stimulants can have a major impact on circulatory function.

- Terbutaline, administered to suppress premature uterine contractions, may stimulate the heart. Adverse effects may include chest discomfort, dyspnea, irregular pulse, EKG changes, or pulmonary edema. Question the use of this medication in any patient with a cardiac history.
- Prostaglandin is a vasodilator and should not be used in patients with certain cardiac conditions. Oxytocin can cause hypertension and fluid retention and may lead to congestive heart failure.

Nursing Care of the Patient Receiving Tocolytic Therapy

- Explore the woman's understanding of what is taking place.
- Include the woman's partner in all discussions about medications and their effects.
- Provide anticipatory guidance regarding what is likely to happen during medication administration.
- Position the woman on her side for better placental perfusion.
- Explain the side effects and contraindications of the drug.
- Assess blood pressure, pulse, and respirations regularly according to hospital policies (every 15 minutes in many institutions).

- Notify the health care provider if systolic blood pressure is >140 mm Hg or <90 mm Hg.
- Notify the health care provider if diastolic blood pressure is >90 mm Hg or <50 mm Hg.
- Assess for signs of pulmonary edema (chest pain, shortness of breath).
- Assess for the presence of deep tendon reflexes (DTRs).
- Assess output every 1 hour.
- Notify the health care provider if the maternal output is <30 mL/hr.
- Limit intake to 2500 mL/day (90 mL/hr).
- Provide psychosocial support and opportunities for the patient to express anxiety.

(Source: *March of Dimes Nursing Module: Preterm Labor: Prevention and Nursing Management [2004]. Reproduced with permission.*)

Contraindications to the Use of Tocolytics in Preterm Labor

- Significant maternal hypertension (eclampsia, severe preeclampsia, chronic hypertension)
- Antepartum hemorrhage
- Cardiac disease
- Any medical or obstetrical condition that contraindicates the prolongation of pregnancy
- Hypersensitivity to a specific tocolytic agent
- Gestational age >37 weeks
- Advanced cervical dilation
- Fetal demise or lethal anomaly
- Chorioamnionitis
- In utero compromise: Acute—Non-reassuring fetal heart rate pattern; Chronic—Intrauterine growth restriction (IUGR) or substance abuse (Cunningham et al., 2005)

ETHNOCULTURAL CONSIDERATIONS

- RhoGAM is a blood product. Special considerations may be indicated for women who are members of Jehovah's Witness because this medication is made from human plasma.

ADDITIONAL INFORMATION FOR THE CLINICAL SETTING

Various Risk Factors Associated with Preterm Labor and Birth

- History of preterm birth
- Uterine or cervical anomalies
- Multiple gestation
- Hypertension
- Diabetes
- Obesity
- Clotting disorders
- Infection
- Fetal anomalies
- Premature rupture of membranes
- Vaginal bleeding
- Late or no prenatal care
- Illicit drug use
- Smoking
- Alcohol use
- Diethylstilbestrol (DES) exposure
- Intimate partner violence
- Non-Hispanic black race
- Age <17 years or >35 years
- Low socioeconomic status
- Stress
- Long working hours with long periods of standing
- Periodontal disease (ACOG, 2001; Freda and Patterson, 2004)

Considerations When Caring for the Obstetric Trauma Patient

- Maternal stabilization is the initial goal in resuscitation. Resuscitation during pregnancy proceeds as with any other trauma.
- Trauma in pregnancy involves at least two patients (more in the case of multiple gestation).
- The fetal heart rate is often the first vital sign to change. All pregnant trauma patients need continuous fetal monitoring.
- Risk factors predictive of fetal death include ejection during an automobile crash, motorcycle and pedestrian

collisions, abnormal fetal heart rate patterns, maternal tachycardia, and maternal death (Haney, 2004).

RESOURCES

The Association of Women's Health, Obstetric and Neonatal Nurses (AWHONN) (www.awhonn.org), the American College of Obstetricians and Gynecologists (ACOG) (www.ACOG.org), and the American Academy of Pediatrics (AAP) (www.aap.org) have partnered with the March of Dimes (MOD) (www.marchofdimes.com) in a multimillion-dollar research, education, and awareness campaign to address the problem of prematurity. Educating all women of childbearing age about preterm labor is a crucial component of prevention (MOD, 2005).

Sidelines is a national support group for women on bed rest (www.sidelines.org).

The Surgeon General's Call to Action to Prevent Deep Vein Thrombosis and Pulmonary Embolism:
http://www.surgeongeneral.gov/topics/deepvein/calltoaction/call-to-action-on-dvt-2008.pdf.

REFERENCES

American College of Obstetricians and Gynecologists (ACOG). (1999). *Antepartum fetal surveillance* (Practice Bulletin No. 9). Washington, D.C.: Author.

American College of Obstetricians and Gynecologists (ACOG). (2001). *Assessment of risk factors for preterm birth* (Practice Bulletin No. 31). Washington, DC: Author.

American College of Obstetricians and Gynecologists (ACOG). (2002). *Diagnosis and management of preeclampsia and eclampsia* (Practice Bulletin No. 33).

American College of Obstetricians and Gynecologists (ACOG). (2004). *Nausea and vomiting of pregnancy. [miscellaneous]* (Practice Bulletin No. 52).

American Diabetes Association (ADA). (2006). Diagnosis and classification of diabetes mellitus. *Diabetes Care, 29*(Suppl), S543–S548.

Centers for Disease Control and Prevention, Workowski, K., & Berman, S. (2006). Sexually transmitted diseases treatment guidelines 2006. *MMWR Morbidity and Mortality Weekly Report, 51(RR11), 1–23.*

Cunningham, F., Leveno, K., Bloom, S., Hauth, J., Gilstrap, L., & Wenstrom, K. (2005). *Williams obstetrics* (22nd ed.). New York: McGraw-Hill.

Deglin, J., & Vallerand, A. (2009). *Davis's drug guide for nurses* (11th ed.). Philadelphia: F.A. Davis.

Freda, M., & Patterson, E. (2004). In Wieczorek R. (Ed.), *Preterm labor: Prevention and nursing management* (3rd ed.). White Plains, NY: March of Dimes.

Gilbert, E., & Harmon, J. (2003). *Manual of high risk pregnancy and delivery* (3rd ed.). St. Louis, MO: C.V. Mosby.

Haney, S. (2004). Trauma in pregnancy. In S. Mattson & J. Smith (Eds.), *Core curriculum for maternal-child nursing* (3rd ed., pp. 703–726). Philadelphia: W.B. Saunders.

Harmon, C. (2004). Assessment of fetal health. In R. Creasy, R. Resnik & J. Iams (Eds.), *Maternal-fetal medicine: Principles and practice* (5th ed., pp. 357–401). Philadelphia: W.B. Saunders.

Hunter, L.P., Sullivan, C.A., Young, R.E., & Weber, C.E. (2007). Nausea and vomiting of pregnancy: Clinical management. *The American Journal for Nurse Practitioners, 11*(8), 57–67.

Jenkins, T., & Wapner, R. (2004). Prenatal diagnosis of congenital disorders. In R. Creasy, R. Resnik & J. Iams (Eds.), *Maternal-fetal medicine: Principles and practice* (5th ed.). Philadelphia: W.B. Saunders.

Landon, M., Catalano, P., & Gabbe, S. (2002). Diabetes mellitus. In S. Gabbe, J. Niebyl & J. Simpson (Eds.), *Obstetrics: Normal and problem pregnancies* (4th ed., pp. 1081–1116). Philadelphia: Churchill Livingstone.

Landry, M. (2004). Viral infections. In G. Burrow, T. Duffy & J. Copel (Eds.), *Medical complications of pregnancy* (6th ed., pp. 347–374). Philadelphia: W.B. Saunders.

McPhedran, P. (2004). Venous thromboembolism during pregnancy. In G. Burrow, T. Duffy & J. Copel (Eds.), *Medical complications of pregnancy* (6th ed., pp. 87–101). Philadelphia: W.B. Saunders.

Moran, B. (2004). Maternal infections. In S. Mattson & J. Smith (Eds.), *Core curriculum for maternal-newborn nursing* (3rd ed., pp. 592–629). St. Louis, MO: W.B. Saunders

Poole, J. (2004). Hypertensive disorders in pregnancy. In S. Mattson & J. Smith (Eds.), *Core curriculum for maternal-newborn nursing* (3rd ed., pp. 554–591). St. Louis, MO: W.B. Saunders.

Records, K., & Rice, M. (2007). Psychosocial correlates of depression symptoms during the third trimester of pregnancy. *Journal of Obstetric, Gynecologic and Neonatal Nursing, 36*(3), 231–242.

Sibai, B.M., Dekker, G., & Kupfermine, M. (2005). Preeclampsia. *The Lancet. 365*(9461), 785–799.

Simpson, K., & Knox, G.E. (2004). Obstetrical accidents involving intravenous magnesium sulfate: Recommendations to promote patient safety. *The American Journal of Maternal/Child Nursing, 29*(3), 161–171

Yankowitz, J. (2004). Pharmacologic treatment of hypertensive disorders during pregnancy. *The Journal of Perinatal & Neonatal Nursing, 18*(3), 230–240.

The Process of Labor and Birth

KEY TERMS

acceleration – An increase in the fetal heart rate of 15 bpm above the baseline, lasting for at least 15 to 30 seconds.

acrocyanosis – Peripheral cyanosis; a bluish coloration of the hands and feet present in most infants at birth

active phase of labor – Phase in the first stage of labor from 4 to 7 cm of cervical dilation

amniotomy – Artificial rupture of the membranes (AROM)

Apgar score – Numeric expression of the condition of a newborn obtained by assessment at 1 and 5 minutes of age; evaluates five signs of cardiopulmonary adaptation and neuromuscular function

attitude (fetal) – Relationship of the fetal parts to each other in the uterus

baseline fetal heart rate – Average fetal heart rate (FHR) observed between contractions over a ten-minute period

bloody show – Expulsion of blood-tinged mucus plug

bradycardia – Baseline fetal heart rate (FHR) of less than 110 to 120 beats per minute

breech presentation – Presentation in which buttocks or feet are nearest the cervical opening and are born first

cephalic presentation – Fetal head is first into the birth canal

cervical ripening – Softening of the cervix

crowning – Stage of birth when the top of the fetal head is visible at the vaginal introitus as the widest part of the head distends the vulva

deceleration – Any decrease in fetal heart rate below the baseline FHR.

dilation – Stretching and enlargement of the cervix

effacement – Process of shortening and thinning of the cervix

electronic fetal heart rate monitoring (EFM) – Electronic surveillance of the fetal heart rate; may use external or internal methods

false labor – Uterine contractions that do not produce cervical change (dilation or effacement)

first stage of labor – Stage of labor from the onset of regular uterine contractions to full dilation of the cervix

fontanel – Unossified membrane or soft spot that lies between the cranial bones of the skull of a fetus or infant

involution – Reduction in uterine size following birth

latent phase of labor – Phase in the first stage of labor from 0 to 3 cm of cervical dilation

lochia rubra – Bright red vaginal flow that follows birth and lasts 2 to 4 days

long-term variability – Changes in fetal heart rate over a period of time (e.g., 1 minute)

malpresentation – Presentation other than cephalic (e.g., breech, shoulder)

molding – Overlapping or overriding of the fetal cranial bones to accommodate and conform to the bony and soft parts of the mother's birth canal during labor

position – Location of a fixed reference point on the fetal presenting part in relation to a specific quadrant of the maternal pelvis: front, back, or side

second stage of labor – Stage of labor from full dilation of the cervix to the birth of the infant

short-term variability – Beat-to-beat changes in fetal heart rate

station – Level of the presenting fetal part in relation to the maternal ischial spines

tachycardia – Baseline fetal heart rate greater than 160 beats per minute

tachysystole – Greater than 5 contractions in 10 minutes, averaged over a 30-minute window

third stage of labor – Stage of labor from the birth of the infant to the expulsion of the placenta

transition phase of labor – Phase in the first stage of labor from 8 to 10 cm of cervical dilation

uteroplacental insufficiency – Decline in placental function, leading to fetal hypoxia and acidosis

variability – Normal irregularity of fetal cardiac rhythm; fluctuations in the baseline fetal heart rate (FHR) observed on the fetal monitor; absence of variability is non-reassuring

Short-term: beat-to-beat changes in the FHR

Long-term: changes in FHR over a longer period of time (i.e., 1 minute)

FOCUSED ASSESSMENT

The 5 P's of Labor

- Powers: Primary (uterine contractions), secondary (use of maternal abdominal muscles for pushing)
- Passageway: Maternal pelvis and soft tissues
- Passenger: Fetus and fetal membranes (lie, attitude, presentation)
- Passageway/passenger relationship: Engagement, station, position
- Psychosocial influences: Factors other than the physical forces that have an effect on the labor and birth process

Powers

The coordinated efforts of the uterine contractions help to bring about effacement and dilation of the cervix (Fig. 9-1).

Amniotic sac
Amniotic fluid
Internal os
Cavity of cervix
External os

Amniotic fluid
Internal os
External os

A   **B**

Figure 9-1 Cervical effacement and dilation. The membranes are intact. *A*. Before labor. *B*. Early effacement.

Figure 9-1 cont'd *C.* Complete (100%) effacement. The fetal head is well applied to the cervix. *D.* Complete dilation (10 cm).

Assess uterine contractions as follows:

- Frequency: Measured from beginning of one contraction to the beginning of the next contraction
- Duration: Measured from the start of one contraction to the end of the same contraction
- Intensity: Measured by uterine palpation, described as mild, moderate, or strong.

Passageway

The maternal bony pelvis is divided into the inlet, midpelvis, and outlet

Passenger (Figs. 9-2, 9-3, 9-4, 9-5, 9-6, and 9-7)

Figure 9-2 Bones, fontanelles, and sutures of the fetal head. An understanding of the placement and relationships of these structures is essential in making an accurate assessment during the labor process.

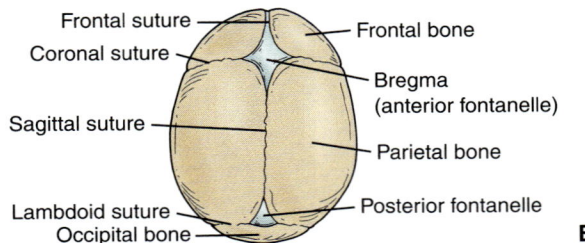

Frontal suture — Frontal bone
Coronal suture — Bregma (anterior fontanelle)
Sagittal suture — Parietal bone
Lambdoid suture — Posterior fontanelle
Occipital bone —

B

Figure 9-2 cont'd

A **B** **C**

Figure 9-3 The fetal lie refers to the relationship of the long axis of the woman to the long axis of the fetus. *A.* Longitudinal lie. *B.* Transverse lie. *C.* Oblique lie.

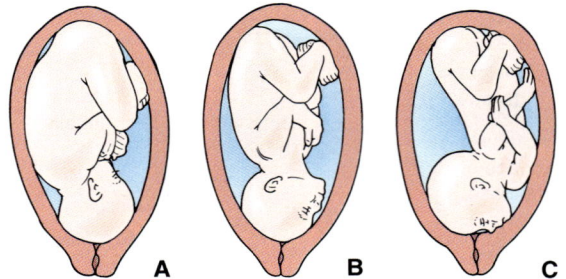

A **B** **C**

Figure 9-4 The fetal attitude describes the relationship of the fetal body parts to one another. *A.* Flexion (vertex). *B.* Moderate flexion (military). *C.* Extension.

Vertex presentation | Military presentation | Brow presentation | Face presentation

Complete flexion | Moderate flexion | Poor flexion (extension) | Full extension

A | B | C | D

Figure 9-5 There are four types of cephalic presentation; the vertex presentation with complete flexion is optimal. Fetal presentation refers to the fetal body part that first enters the maternal pelvis.

A | B | C

Figure 9-6 There are three types of a breech presentation. *A.* Frank. *B.* Complete or full. *C.* Footling breech (single or doubling). Frank breech is the most common variation.

Figure 9-7 Shoulder presentation.

Passage/Passenger Relationship

The relationship between the passageway and the passenger is assessed when determining engagement, station, and the fetal position (Figs. 9-8 and 9-9).

Figure 9-8 The maternal ischial spines represent the narrowest diameter through which the fetus must pass. When the presenting part lies above the ischial spines, it is at a minus station; when the presenting part lies below the ischial spines, it is at a positive station.

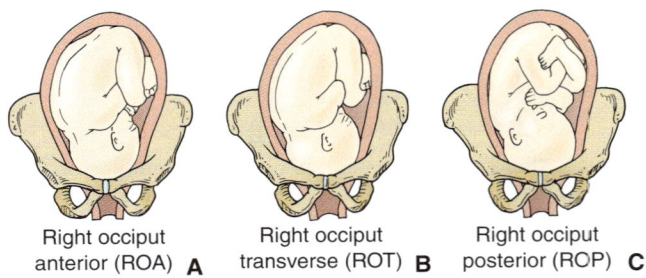

Right occiput anterior (ROA) **A**   Right occiput transverse (ROT) **B**   Right occiput posterior (ROP) **C**

Figure 9-9 Fetal presentations and positions. The presenting part can be right anterior, left anterior, right posterior, and left posterior. These four quadrants designate whether the presenting part is directed toward the front, back, right, or left of the passageway.

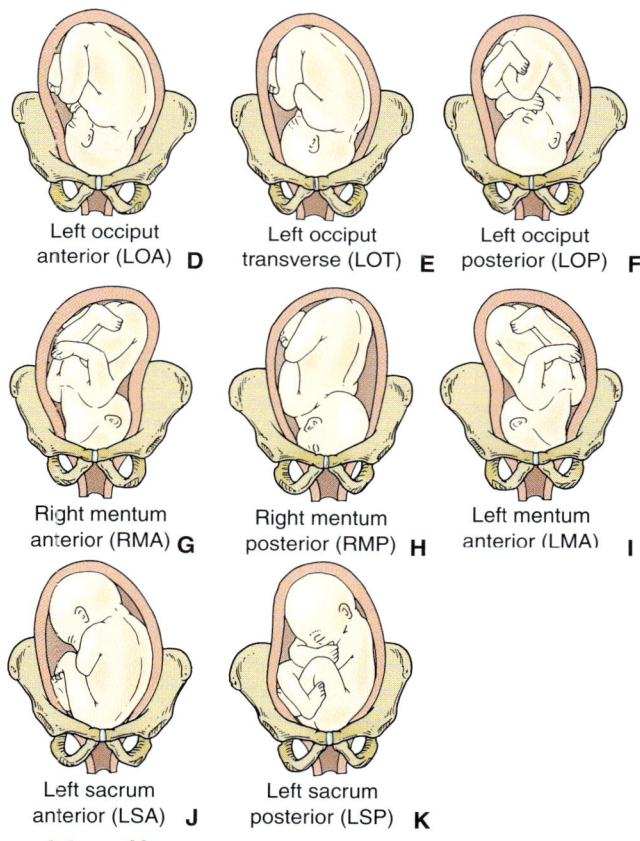

Left occiput anterior (LOA) **D**

Left occiput transverse (LOT) **E**

Left occiput posterior (LOP) **F**

Right mentum anterior (RMA) **G**

Right mentum posterior (RMP) **H**

Left mentum anterior (LMA) **I**

Left sacrum anterior (LSA) **J**

Left sacrum posterior (LSP) **K**

Figure 9-9 cont'd

Psychosocial Influences

Factors that influence the birth experience:

- Readiness for labor and birth
- Level of educational preparedness
- Emotional readiness
- Ethnicity and cultural influences
- Anxiety; fear; fatigue
- Previous experiences with childbirth

Assessment During Labor

Distinguishing True Labor from False Labor	
True Labor	**False Labor**
Contractions at regular intervals	Irregular contractions
Contractions increase in frequency, duration, and intensity.	Usually no increase in frequency, duration, or intensity of contractions.
Pains usually begin in the lower back, radiating to abdomen.	Pains usually occur in abdominal region.
Progressive dilation and effacement of the cervix	No change in the cervix
Activity such as walking usually increased labor pains.	Walking may lessen the pain.

Questions to Ask the Patient Who Calls the Birth Unit

Conduct the telephone assessment by asking the following questions:

"What is your due date?"

"Are your membranes ruptured?" or "Did your water break?" and "Are you having any bleeding or vaginal discharge?"

"Describe your contractions: When did they start? How frequent? How long? How strong?"

"Is the fetus active?"

"What helps to decrease the discomfort?"

"Who is with you?"

Hospital and Birth Center Admission Procedures

Assess the following factors:

- Is this true labor?
- Are the membranes ruptured?
- Is birth imminent?
- Are there any factors that increase risk to the mother and/or fetus?
- What is the gestational age and estimated date of delivery?
- What is the fetal status (FHR and response to contractions; fetal movement)?
- What is the mother's status (physical [vital signs]; psychosocial [coping, supports])?

- What is the contraction status (frequency, duration, intensity)?
- What are the findings from the vaginal exam (cervical dilation, effacement; fetal station, presentation, position)?

Procedure 9-1 Auscultating the Fetal Heart Tones During Labor

Purpose

An auditory method of monitoring the fetal heart tones to assess the fetus. Performed intermittently during labor.

Equipment

- Fetoscope or hand held Doppler ultrasound with gel ("Doppler")
- Disposable wipes

Steps

1. Wash and dry hands and explain procedure and purpose of the examination to the patient

2. Help the patient assume a comfortable position that provides access to the abdomen.

3. Palpate the maternal abdomen using Leopold maneuvers to identify the fetal position to aid in obtaining the location of the fetal heart tones. Note that the fetal heart tones are heard most loudly over the fetal back.

4. Palpate the fundus of the uterus for the presence of uterine contractions. At the end of a uterine contraction place the fetoscope or Doppler over the location of the fetal back. Adjust the fetoscope or Doppler if necessary to obtain a clearly audible fetal heart rate (FHR). Depending on fetal position, the fetal heart sounds may be soft and muffled or loud and clear.

5. Listen for audible fetal heart sounds. Note that two distinctly different sounds can be heard: fetal heart tones that result from blood moving through the placenta and umbilical cord (funic soufflé) and the uterine soufflé, which is the same rate as the maternal pulse.

6. Palpate the maternal radial pulse to ensure that the auscultated fetal heart sounds are at a different rate than the maternal pulse.

(continued)

Procedure 9-1 (Continued)

7. Auscultate the fetal heart sounds for the rate and rhythm. The greatest accuracy for assessment of the fetal heart rate occurs when listening for 1 minute.

   Note: During active labor, 30-second intervals may be more feasible.

8. Count the FHR for 30 to 60 seconds between contractions to determine the baseline rate.

9. Interpret the fetal heart rate: Is the baseline normal between 110 and 160 bpm? Is there tachycardia (baseline >160 bpm) or bradycardia (baseline <110/bpm)? Is the rhythm regular or irregular? Can you note the presence of accelerations or decelerations?

10. Repeat the procedure as indicated according to agency policy.

11. Inform the patient of the findings.

12. Document fetal heart rate according to agency policy.

 Procedure 9-2 Performing the Intrapartal Vaginal Examination

Purpose

Vaginal examination may be performed during the intrapartal period for many reasons including assessment of cervical dilation, effacement and station, position and presentation of the fetus, rupture of the membranes, and prolapse of the umbilical cord.

Equipment

- Sterile examination gloves (clean gloves may be used if the membranes are intact)
- Sterile lubricant
- Antiseptic solution and light source (if required)
- Disposable wipes

Steps

1. Wash and dry your hands. Explain the procedure and purpose of the examination to the patient.

Procedure 9-2 (Continued)

2. Assess for latex allergies.

3. Ensure privacy.

4. Assemble necessary equipment including: clean gloves (if the membranes are intact) or sterile examination gloves (if the membranes are ruptured), sterile lubricant, antiseptic solution (if required).

5. Position the patient in a supine position with a small pillow or towel under her hip to prevent supine hypotension. Instruct the patient to relax and position herself with her thighs flexed and abducted. (Proper positioning facilitates the examination by providing access to the perineum.)

6. Don sterile gloves (clean gloves may be used if the membranes are intact).

7. Inspect the perineum for any redness, irritation or vesicles.

8. Using the nondominant hand, spread the labia majora and continue assessment of the genitalia. Check for discharge including blood or amniotic fluid and lesions. The presence of lesions may be indicative of an infection and possibly preclude a vaginal birth. The presence of amniotic fluid implies that the membranes have ruptured. Bleeding may be a sign of placenta previa.

   Note: Do not perform a vaginal examination if a placenta previa is suspected.

9. Gently insert the lubricated gloved index and third fingers into the vagina in the direction of the posterior wall until they touch the cervix. Stabilize the uterus by placing the nondominant hand on the woman's abdomen.

(continued)

Procedure 9-2 (Continued)

10. Assess the cervix for effacement and the amount of dilation.
11. Assess for intact membranes; if fluid is expressed, test for amniotic fluid.
12. Palpate the presenting part.
13. Assess fetal descent and station by identifying the position of the posterior fontanel.
14. Withdraw the fingers. Assist the patient in wiping her perineum from front to back to remove lubricant or secretions. Help her to resume a comfortable position.
15. Inform the patient of the findings from the examination.
16. Wash hands.
17. Document the procedure on the patient's chart and on the fetal monitor strip (if a fetal monitor is being used). Include the assessment findings and the patient's tolerance of the procedure.

  Procedure 9-3 Assessing for Amniotic Fluid

Purpose

Assessing for the presence of amniotic fluid helps determine whether the membranes have ruptured. There are two tests commonly used to detect amniotic fluid: the Nitrazine tape test and the fern test.

Equipment

- Nitrazine test tape
- Sterile gloves
- Sterile speculum
- Sterile cotton swab and glass slide
- Microscope

Steps

1. Wash and dry hands and explain the procedure and purpose of the examination to the patient, noting what she will experience, and what the results will indicate.

Procedure 9-3 (Continued)

2. Assess for latex allergies.

3. Ask the patient if she has noticed any leakage of fluid from her vagina.

4. Assess for the presence of amniotic fluid before other tests that require the use of lubricant (such as vaginal examination).

5. Don sterile gloves.

6. With one hand, spread the labia to expose the vaginal opening. With the other hand, place a 2-inch (5 cm) piece of Nitrazine tape against the vaginal opening, ensuring contact with enough fluid to wet the tape. Alternately, a sterile cotton-tipped applicator may be used to obtain fluid from the vagina. Touch the applicator to the Nitrazine tape.

7. Remove the tape. Compare the color of the tape with the color guide on the Nitrazine tape container. If the tape turns blue-green, gray or deep blue, amniotic fluid is present. If the tape remains beige, no amniotic fluid has been detected.

   Caution: Blood, *Trichomonas vaginalis*, and other substances may also turn the Nitrazine test strip alkaline or blue.

8. When the Nitrazine test has *not* confirmed the presence of amniotic fluid, the nurse may insert a speculum and sterile cotton swab to collect a sample of fluid from the posterior vagina.

9. Smear the swab on a glass slide and allow it to dry. Then place the glass slide on the microscope. The presence of a ferning pattern confirms the presence of amniotic fluid. The fern test is often indicated if premature rupture of the membranes (PROM) is suspected.

10. Inform the patient of the findings.

11. Document the findings on the admission or labor record.

Characteristics of the First and Second Stages of Labor

	First Stage	Second Stage
Definition	Commences with the onset of regular contractions and ends with full dilation (10 cm) of the cervix	Begins with full dilation of the cervix (10 cm) and ends with the expulsion (birth) of the fetus
Contractions	Latent: 5–10 minutes, may be irregular in frequency, duration 30–40 seconds, mild to moderate strength Active: Regular pattern established (2–5 minutes apart), 40–60 seconds duration and moderate to strong by palpation Transition: 2–3 minutes apart lasting 60–90 seconds duration, strong by palpation.	Contractions continue at a similar rate as during the transition phase: 2–3 minutes apart lasting 60 seconds and strong by palpation.
Dilation	Latent: 0–3 cm Active: 4–7 cm Transition: 8–10 cm	Fully dilated
Physical Discomforts	Latent: Contractions often begin as painful menstrual-like cramps or low backache. Active: Increasing discomfort as contractions become stronger and more regular. May have backache. Transition: Increasing discomfort as contractions are very strong with little time for relaxation in between. As the fetal head descends there may be an increase in rectal pressure and the urge to push.	May have an urge to push that increases as the fetal head descends. Many women prefer to push so that they can use the contractions and work with them. When head is crowning may feel intense pain, burning.
Maternal Behaviors	Latent: Pain often well controlled; various behaviors may be present: excited, talkative, confident, anxious, withdrawn. This stage may be completed at home.	Often during this stage many women get a "second wind" as they see that they are making progress and are embarking on a new (labor) phase.

	First Stage	Second Stage
	Active: Needs to focus more on staying in control and managing the pain; often requires coaching at this stage; quieter and more inwardly focused	Intense concentration with pushing efforts
	Transition: Most intense phase. Often difficult to cope; may experience various emotions; irritable, agitated, hopeless (can't do it); tired (sleeps between contractions)	

Friedman Curve

Figure 9-10 A labor curve assessment tool, often referred to as a "Friedman curve," helps to identify whether a patient's labor is progressing in a normal pattern.

Electronic Fetal Monitoring (EFM)

External Fetal Monitor

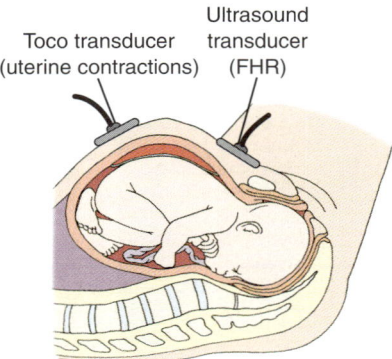

Figure 9-11 The external fetal monitor is composed of a Doppler ultrasound transducer and tocodynamometer that is applied to the maternal abdomen to monitor and display the FHR and contractions.

Internal Fetal Monitor

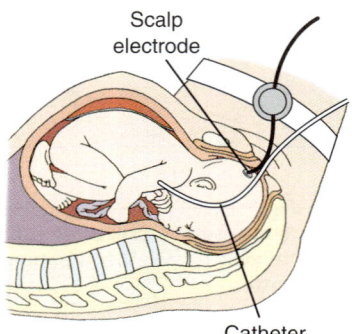

Figure 9-12 The internal fetal monitor is composed of a spiral electrode inserted into the fetal scalp or presenting part. Uterine activity is assessed by an intrauterine pressure catheter (IUPC).

Fetal Heart Rate Patterns

Normal Fetal Heart Rate

Figure 9-13 The normal baseline fetal heart rate at term is 110 to 160 bpm. *Top*: fetal heart rate. *Bottom*: Uterine contractions.

Fetal Heart Rate Accelerations

Figure 9-14 FHR accelerations: often associated with a normal FHR baseline and normal variability.

Early Decelerations

Figure 9-15 Early decelerations: Related to fetal head compression.

Variable Decelerations

Figure 9-16 Variable decelerations: Related to umbilical cord compression.

Late Decelerations

Figure 9-17 Late decelerations: related to uteroplacental insufficiency.

Interpreting Fetal Monitor Tracings

To aid in the interpretation of EFM tracings, the nurse should consider the following parameters:

Uterine Activity

What is the frequency, duration, and intensity of contractions?

Labor Progress

What is the stage of labor?
What is the dilation, effacement, station, presentation and position?

Baseline FHR

What is the baseline FHR?
Is tachycardia or bradycardia present?

Baseline Variability

What is the variability of the FHR (absent, minimal, moderate, marked, or other)?

Periodic Changes in FHR

Are there any FHR changes from the baseline?
Are accelerations present?
Are any decelerations present?
If decelerations are present, are they early, variable, late or prolonged?

Maternal History/Condition

Are there any preexisting conditions that increase the risk for this pregnancy?
Are there any intrapartum high-risk factors (e.g., meconium) that should be noted?

Characteristics of Reassuring and Non-reassuring FHR Patterns by EFM	
Reassuring Patterns	**Non-reassuring Patterns**
Normal baseline FHR (110–160 bpm)	Absence of variability (short-term and long-term)
Presence of short-term and long-term variability	Late decelerations
Presence of accelerations with fetal movement or contractions	Severe variable decelerations
Early decelerations may be noted in active labor.	Prolonged decelerations
	Severe bradycardia or tachycardia
Category I FHR tracing	Category III FHR tracing
Possible category II FHR tracing	Possible Category II FHR tracing

Sources: Macones et al. (2008); Tucker (2004).

Conditions Associated with Fetal Heart Rate Variations	
Tachycardia	**Bradycardia**
Fetal hypoxia	Late hypoxia
Maternal fever	Medications
Maternal medications	Maternal hypotension
Infection	Prolonged umbilical cord compression
Fetal anemia	Bradyarrhythmias
Maternal hyperthyroidism	

PROMOTING EFFECTIVE PUSHING

- Closed-glottis pushing: Encourage the patient to begin pushing at full cervical dilation, regardless of the urge to bear down, by taking a deep breath and holding it for at least 10 seconds while pushing as hard and as long as she is able throughout the contraction.
- Open-glottis pushing: Encourage the patient to hold her breath for only 5 to 6 seconds during pushing and to take several breaths between each bearing down effort. Instruct the woman to exhale throughout the bearing down attempts.

Characteristics of the Third and Fourth Stages of Labor		
	Third Stage	**Fourth Stage**
Description	Begins with the birth of the infant and ends with the delivery of the placenta. Usually 5–10 minutes, may take up to 30 minutes.	A time of physiological adaptation that begins after delivery of the placenta and lasts 1–2 hours.
Contractions	Uterus should be firmly contracted.	Uterus should be firmly contracted.
Assessment	Uterus becomes globelike. Uterus rises upward. Umbilical cord descends further. Gush of blood as placenta detaches.	Uterus remains firmly contracted. Lochia rubra, blood red flow with occasional small clots. Vital signs return to prelabor values.
Physical Discomforts	Discomfort or cramping as the placenta is expelled.	Some women experience perineal discomfort usually related to trauma from the episiotomy or tearing, or hemorrhoids.

	Third Stage	Fourth Stage
Maternal Behaviors	Focus on infant well-being Crying common	Excited, tired Bonding and attachment with infant
	Expressions of relief Culturally influenced	Initiation of breastfeeding Culturally influenced

CLINICAL ALERTS

Preventing Supine Hypotension

Much of the fetal assessment involves the maternal abdomen. To avoid supine hypotension, do not position the patient flat on her back. Slightly elevate the head of the bed or place a wedge under the patient's hip to prevent compression of the maternal vena cava caused by the gravid uterus.

Fourth Stage Risk Signs

The following risk signs that may occur during the fourth stage of labor are associated with hemorrhage and must be reported immediately: hypotension, tachycardia, excessive bleeding, or a boggy, non contracting uterus. If the uterus is boggy, the nurse must immediately initiate fundal massage and continue until the uterus becomes firm.

MEDICATIONS

Oxytocin (ox-i-**toe**-sin)

Pitocin, Syntocinon

Pregnancy Category B

Indications Induction of labor at term. Facilitation of uterine contractions at term. Control of postpartum bleeding after expulsion of placenta.

Actions Stimulates uterine smooth muscle producing uterine contractions similar to those in spontaneous labor (administered IV). Stimulates mammary gland smooth muscle facilitating lactation (administered intranasally). Has vasopressor and diuretic effects.

Therapeutic Effects Induces labor. Reduces postpartum bleeding. Induces breast milk letdown.

Pharmacokinetics

Absorption Well absorbed from the nasal mucosa when administered intranasally.

Distribution Through extracellular fluid. Small amounts reach the fetal circulation.

Metabolism Metabolized rapidly in kidneys and liver.

Excretion Small amounts excreted in urine, half-life 3–9 minutes

Contraindications and Precautions

Contraindicated in Cephalopelvic disproportion or deliveries that require conversion (e.g., transverse lie).

Use with caution in First and second stage of labor.

Adverse Reactions and Side Effects Maternal adverse reactions are associated with IV use only. Painful contractions and increased uterine motility most common. May contribute to maternal coma, seizures, hypotension. May contribute to fetal asphyxia or arrhythmias.

Route and Dosage May be added to IV for labor induction or given IV or IM to control postpartum bleeding (do not administer IM and IV routes simultaneously). Intranasal spray is administered 2 to 3 minutes before planned breastfeeding.

Nursing Implications Fetal maturity, presentation, and maternal pelvic adequacy should be assessed prior to administration to induce labor. Monitor contractions, resting uterine tone, and fetal heart rate frequently. Monitor the uterus for firmness and early detection of bogginess. Monitor lochia for signs of excessive bleeding.

Data from Deglin, J.H., & Vallerand, A.H. (2009). Davis's drug guide for nurses (11th ed.). Philadelphia: F.A. Davis.

The Apgar Scoring System

Physiological Parameter	Score 0	Score 1	Score 2
Heart Rate	Absent	Slow: Below 100	Above 100
Respiratory Effort	Absent	Slow: Irregular, weak cry	Good; strong cry
Muscle Tone	Flaccid	Some flexion of extremities	Well flexed
Reflex Irritability	No response	Grimace	Vigorous cry
Color	Blue, pale	Pink body, blue extremities	Completely pink

Range of Apgar Score: From 0 to 10

A score of 8–10 reflects a newborn in good condition who usually requires only nasopharyngeal suctioning. A score of <8 may warrant further resuscitation measures.

ETHNOCULTURAL CONSIDERATIONS

Assessing Cultural Influences on the Laboring Patient

To provide culturally sensitive care to the laboring patient, the nurse should consider:

- The patient's and family's level of comfort with the nurse's "language" and whether an interpreter is needed
- Who the designated birth support person is and the extent of this person's role
- The patient's level of comfort with touch
- If any special rituals or practices will be used during the childbirth experience

TEACHING THE FAMILY

Providing Patient Guidelines for Reporting to the Birthing Center

Questions to Ask the Patient	Guidelines for Admission
Describe your contractions: frequency, duration, and intensity.	Primigravida: Contractions are regular, occur about every 5 minutes for at least 1 hour. Multipara: Contractions are regular, occur about every 10 minutes for at least 1 hour.
Have your membranes ruptured?	*Any* gush of fluid needs to be evaluated, even if there are no contractions.
Is there any vaginal bleeding?	The mucous plug or "bloody show" is usually pink or dark red. Any bright red bleeding requires immediate evaluation.
Has there been a decrease in the movement of the baby?	Any decrease in fetal movement signals the need to report to the birthing center.
Has there been any change in your health?	Any cause for worry or anxiety in the pregnant woman needs to be explored by the nurse and may lead to admission.

ADDITIONAL INFORMATION FOR THE CLINICAL SETTING

Determining and Documenting Fetal Position

During the assessment, the nurse determines that the fetal occiput is in the right anterior quadrant of the maternal pelvis. The position is correctly documented as ROA. If the fetus were presenting in the frank breech position with the buttocks positioned to the left maternal posterior quadrant, the position would be correctly documented as LSP (left sacral posterior).

RESOURCES

National Certification Corporation monograph (2006). *Applying NICHD terminology and other factors to electronic fetal monitor interpretation.* Retrieved on February 14, 2008 from http://www.nccnet.org/public/files/NICHDMonograph.pdf.

REFERENCES

Deglin, J.H. & Vallerand, A.H. (2009). *Davis's drug guide for nurses* (11th ed.). Philadelphia: F.A. Davis.

Macones, G.A., Hankins, G.D., Spong, C.Y., Hauth, J., & Moore, T. (2008). The 2008 National Institute of Child Health and Human Development Research Workshop Report on Electronic Fetal Heart Rate Monitoring. *Journal of Obstetric, Gynecologic, & Neonatal Nursing, 37*(5), 510–515.

Tucker, S.M. (2004). *Pocket guide to fetal monitoring and assessment* (5th ed.). St Louis, MO: C.V. Mosby.

Promoting Patient Comfort During Labor and Birth

KEY TERMS

acupressure – Massage technique applied to specific points along the body's energy pathways (meridians); also called "Chinese massage"

acupuncture – A form of treatment that involves the insertion of fine, stainless steel needles into specific points along the energy pathways to correct, enhance, and rebalance the flow of body energy

aromatherapy – The use of essential oils whose aroma is believed to have a therapeutic effect in treating illness and promoting health and well-being

autologous epidural blood patch – The administration of 10 to 20 mL of the patient's blood into the lumbar epidural space to form a clot in the hole in the dura mater around the spinal cord. The clot effectively seals the area from further cerebrospinal fluid (CSF) leakage.

analgesia – Relief, to some degree, from pain without loss of consciousness

anesthesia – the partial or complete loss of sensation with or without the loss of consciousness

biofeedback – Treatment method that uses monitors to provide patients with physiological information of which they are normally unaware. Practice during the prenatal period enhances the woman's body awareness and ability to recognize her responses to stimuli. She can then use various strategies (e.g., focal points, breathing techniques) during labor to control her response to uncomfortable stimuli.

cleansing breath – A slow, deep breath taken in through the nose and out through the mouth

effleurage – Gentle stroking technique performed in rhythm with uterine contractions

epidural anesthesia and analgesia block – Regional anesthesia produced by injection of a local anesthetic into the epidural space between L4 and L5

general anesthesia – Induced unconsciousness

hydrotherapy – Water therapy; the use of water to promote comfort and relaxation

hypnotherapy – Technique used to enable an individual to achieve a state of heightened awareness and focused concentration to alter the perception of pain

intrathecal analgesia – Injection of opioids into the subarachnoid space

postdural puncture headache – A complication following spinal anesthesia block; occurs from leakage of cerebrospinal fluid (CSF) from the puncture site in the dura mater

referred pain – During labor, pain that originates from the uterus and radiates to the abdominal wall, lumbosacral area, iliac crests, gluteus maximus, and down the thighs

regional anesthesia – Temporary and reversible loss of sensation

somatic pain – Perineal discomfort that results from stretching and distention of the perineal tissues

sympathetic blockade – Decreased cardiac output that results from vasodilation with pooling of blood in the lower extremities after the administration of an epidural anesthetic

transcutaneous electrical nerve stimulation (TENS) – Delivery of an electric current through electrodes applied to the skin over the painful region of a peripheral nerve

visceral pain – A slow, deep, diffuse pain, the predominant discomfort during the first stage of labor. Usually located over the lower abdomen, and radiates to the lumbar area and thighs. Related to cervical dilation and effacement, distention of the lower uterine segment, and uterine ischemia.

FOCUSED ASSESSMENT

Types of Pain During Labor and Birth

- Visceral pain
- Referred pain
- Somatic pain

Factors that Affect the Experience of Pain		
Physical	**Physiological**	**Psychological**
Labor intensity	History of dysmenorrhea	Anxiety
Cervical readiness	Maternal position	Fear
Fetal position	Maternal control	Previous experience
Pelvic dimensions	Fetal size	Support system
Fatigue		Childbirth preparation
Medical interventions		

Assessing Pain During Labor

- Using appropriate pain assessment tools, conduct an initial assessment and continuously evaluate the patient and address her needs for comfort measures.
- Develop an individualized plan of care that includes pain relief interventions acceptable to the patient.

Recognizing the Anxiety–Tissue Anoxia–Pain Connection

- Pain triggers the body's general stress response.
- The release of epinephrine causes peripheral and uterine vasoconstriction and results in tissue anoxia and increased pain.
- Decrease the patient's anxiety by assisting with relaxation techniques to reduce anxiety; administer antianxiety medications as needed to reduce vasoconstriction and pain.

Other Maternal–Fetal Assessments During the Intrapartal Period

- Assess for risk factors: Bleeding, infection, ruptured membranes, fetal presentation, prolapsed cord,

precipitous labor, meconinum-stained amniotic fluid, postmaturity, prematurity, or fetal heart rate irregularities.
- Assess maternal vital signs per facility protocol.
- Assess the patient's anxiety level, coping mechanisms, and labor support.
- Assess the progress of labor.
- Assess the fetal heart rate, lie, and presentation.
- Assess the maternal and fetal responses to each comfort measure.
- Carefully document all findings.

Nonpharmacological Pain Relief Measures for Labor

- Position of comfort (e.g., movement, slow dancing, squatting bar, hands/knees, birth ball, kneeling)
- Breathing techniques
- Music
- Relaxation techniques
- Guided imagery
- Massage, touch, effleurage
- Hydrotherapy
- Hypnotherapy
- Aromatherapy
- Heat/cold application
- Biofeedback
- Acupressure and acupuncture
- Transcutaneous electrical nerve stimulation

CLINICAL ALERTS

Flumazenil to Reverse the Effects of Benzodiazepine Sedatives

Flumazenil (Romazicon) is an intravenously administered medication that reverses the effects of benzodiazepine sedatives. Ensure that flumazenil is readily available in any childbirth setting where benzodiazepines are used.

Combining Butorphanol with Other CNS Depressants

Butorphanol (Stadol) is associated with respiratory depression in both the mother and fetus. When administering butorphanol with other central nervous system (CNS) depressants (e.g., hypnotic agents, phenothiazines, sedatives, other tranquilizers, and general anesthetics), closely monitor the patient's respiratory and cardiac status for signs of respiratory depression. Ongoing observation of the maternal level of consciousness, vital signs, and pulse oximetry, and continuous electronic fetal heart rate monitoring is recommended. Naloxone (Narcan), the specific antagonist for this medication, should be readily available to reverse the drug effects if needed.

Complications Associated with Spinal Anesthesia Block

- Maternal hypotension (before administration, assess fluid balance, administer intravenous fluids; after administration, assess and document pulse, blood pressure, respirations and fetal heart tones (FHTs) every 5 to 10 minutes).
- Decreased placental perfusion
- Ineffective breathing pattern
- Sympathetic blockade
- Postdural puncture headache

Severe Maternal Hypotension and Decreased Placental Perfusion

In the event of severe maternal hypotension, the nurse takes the following actions:

1. Place the patient in a lateral position or use a wedge under the hip to displace the uterus; elevate the legs.
2. Maintain or increase the IV infusion rate, according to institutional protocol.
3. Administer oxygen by face mask at 10 to 12 L/min, or according to institutional protocol.
4. Alert the primary care provider, anesthesiologist or nurse anesthetist.
5. Administer an IV vasopressor (e.g., ephedrine 5 to 10 mg) according to institutional protocol, if the above measures are ineffective.
6. Remain calm, offer reassurance, and continue to assess maternal blood pressure and fetal heart rate (FHR) every 5 minutes until stable or per order from the primary care provider.

Postdural Puncture Headache

- Develops within 48 hours after the puncture.
- Typically intensified when the patient assumes an upright position.
- Relieved when the patient assumes a supine position.
- Accompanying symptoms include auditory (tinnitus) and visual (blurred vision, photophobia) problems.
- Interventions include oral analgesics, bed rest in a darkened room, caffeine, hydration, and autologous epidural blood patch.

MEDICATIONS

General Guidelines

- Ensure that the woman understands the alternative methods of pain relief that are available in the birth facility. When indicated, ask the primary care provider for further details or clarification.
- Explain that nonpharmacological measures promote relaxation and potentiate the effects of analgesic agents.
- Obtain informed consent for interventions after fully explaining advantages and disadvantages. The patient must agree with the plan of care as it is described to her; the patient's consent must be given freely without coercion or manipulation from her health care provider (Lowe, 2004).
- Initiate pain control before the pain intensifies to the point that catecholamines are released and the labor is prolonged.

Types of Medications Used During Labor and Birth

- Sedatives and antiemetics: Used during early latent phase and to augment analgesics
- Barbiturates: Produce mild sedation; rarely used in labor because of undesirable effects (i.e., maternal and neonatal respiratory and vasomotor depression)
- Benzodiazepines: Used to treat anxiety
- H_1-Receptor antagonists: Used for sedation and antiemetic effects

- Systemic analgesia: Provides central analgesia to patient and fetus (opioid agonists, opioid agonist–antagonists)
- Nerve block analgesia and anesthesia (regional analgesia, regional anesthesia)

Pharmacological Interventions for Intrapartal Pain Control According to Stage of Labor

First Stage of Labor
Systemic Analgesia
- Opioid agonists, e.g., hydromorphone hydrochloride (Dilaudid), meperidine (Demerol), fentanyl citrate (Sublimaze), sufentanil citrate (Sufenta)
- Opioid agonist–antagonists, e.g., butorphanol (Stadol); nalbuphine (Nubain)

Nerve Block Analgesia
- Epidural
- Combined spinal–epidural

Second Stage of Labor
Nerve Block Analgesia and Anesthesia (Fig. 10-1)
- Local infiltration
- Pudendal block
- Spinal block
- Epidural block
- Combined spinal–epidural

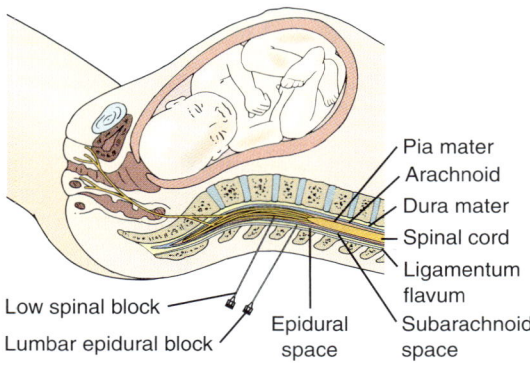

Figure 10-1 The spinal canal: Injection sites for regional anesthesia.

Opioid Agonist Analgesics

Opioid-Agonist Analgesic	Route and Dosage	Nursing Considerations
Hydromorphone Hydrochloride (Dilaudid)	IV: 1 mg q–3hr prn IM: 1–2 mg q3–6hr prn	Monitor vital signs, FHR pattern, and uterine activity before and during administration; observe for maternal respiratory depression; encourage voiding q2hr, palpate for bladder distention; if birth occurs within 1–4 hours after administration, observe the neonate for respiratory depression.
Meperidine hydrochloride (Demerol)	IV: 25 mg q1–3hr prn IM: 50–100 mg q1–3hr prn	
Fentanyl Citrate (Sublimaze)	IV: 25–50 mg; 1–2 mg with 0.125% bupivacaine at rate of 8–10 mL/hr epidurally	
Sufentanil Citrate (Sufenta)	IV: 1 mg with 0.125% bupivacaine at a rate of 10 mL/hr	

Safety Measures for Women Who Receive Opioid Analgesics
- Administer cautiously to women with respiratory or cardiovascular disorders, as opioid analgesics may cause bradycardia/tachycardia, hypotension, and respiratory depression (Lehne, 2006).
- Assist with ambulation and observe for adverse effects because patients may experience sedation and dizziness after administration.

Pharmacological Interventions for Intrapartal Pain Control According to Birth Method

Vaginal Birth
- Local infiltration anesthesia
- Pudendal block
- Epidural block analgesia/anesthesia
- Spinal block anesthesia
- Combined spinal–epidural analgesia/anesthesia

Cesarean Birth
- Spinal block anesthesia
- Epidural block anesthesia
- General anesthesia

Commonly Used Regional Blocks for Labor and Birth

Type of Block; Areas Affected	When Used During Labor and Birth	Nursing Implications
Local Perineal Infiltration **AFFECTED AREA:** Perineum	Immediately before birth for episiotomy; after birth for repair of lacerations	Assess the patient's knowledge and understanding; provide information as needed. Observe the perineum for bruising or discoloration during the recovery period.
Pudendal Nerve Block **AFFECTED AREAS:** Perineum and lower vagina	Late in the second stage for episiotomy, forceps or vacuum extraction; during third stage for repair of episiotomy or lacerations	Assess the patient's level of knowledge and understanding; provide additional information as needed.
Spinal Anesthesia Block **AFFECTED AREAS:** Uterus, cervix, vagina, and perineum	First stage for both elective and emergent cesarean births; low spinal anesthesia block may be used for vaginal birth—not suitable for labor	Assess the patient's level of knowledge and understanding; provide additional information as needed. Monitor maternal vital signs and FHR status.
Lumbar Epidural Block **AFFECTED AREAS:** Uterus, cervix, vagina, and perineum	First and second stages	Assess the patient's level of knowledge and understanding; provide additional information as needed. Monitor maternal blood pressure—the major side effect is hypotension. Provide ongoing support.
Combined Spinal–Epidural **AFFECTED AREAS:** Uterus, cervix, vagina, and perineum	Spinal analgesia may be administered during the latent phase for pain relief. Epidural is given when active labor begins	Assess the patient's level of knowledge and understanding; provide additional information as needed. Monitor maternal vital signs and FHR status. Provide ongoing support.

Procedure 10-1 Assisting with the Administration of Spinal Anesthesia

Purpose

To facilitate safe, effective care during conduction of spinal anesthesia

Equipment

- Blood pressure cuff
- Stethoscope
- Fetal monitor

Steps

1. Wash and dry hands and explain procedure and purpose to the patient.
2. Assist the patient to a sitting position on the edge of the bed or operating table (as directed by the nurse anesthetist or anesthesiologist).
3. Provide support, promote comfort, and limit motion during the procedure.
4. Check the intravenous infusion for patency.
5. Assist the patient to lie down on her back after anesthesia administration (as directed by the nurse anesthetist or anesthesiologist).
6. Place a pillow under her head and a wedge under her right hip.
7. Monitor the pulse, blood pressure, and respirations every 1–2 minutes for the first 10 minutes, then every 5–10 minutes. Use electronic monitor to continuously monitor the FHR.
8. Document the procedure.

Nursing Consideration

The nurse informs the nurse anesthetist or anesthesiologist when a contraction is beginning so that the anesthetic will not be administered during a contraction.

Contraindications to Spinal/Epidural Block Anesthesia

- Maternal refusal
- Local or systemic infection
- Coagulation disorders

- Actual or anticipated maternal hemorrhage
- Allergy to specific anesthetic agents
- Lack of trained staff available (Cunningham et al., 2005)

Nursing Actions After Administration of Epidural and Intrathecal Opioids

- Monitor and record patient's respiratory rate every hour for 24 hours (or per institutional protocol) after administration of epidural or intrathecal opioids.
- Administer naloxone (Narcan) if the maternal respiratory rate decreases to <10 breaths per minute or if the maternal oxygen saturation rate decreases to <89%; administer oxygen by face mask and notify the anesthesiologist.

Epidural Block and Second Stage Labor

- The patient who has received an epidural block may need assistance with pushing owing to an inability to feel contractions or experience the urge to push. She may need someone to hold or control her legs in order to push.
- After the birth, ensure that full sensation has returned and the patient can control her legs before permitting ambulation (depending on drug and dose, it may take several hours).

Shiver Response After Epidural Block Administration

- If the patient exhibits a shiver response after administration of an epidural block, apply warm blankets and offer reassurance.

ETHNOCULTURAL CONSIDERATIONS

Realities of the Cultural Model

Cultural models of health care frequently stereotype women who share the same cultural heritage. In so doing, they may immobilize health providers who seek to change unfavorable health care situations in the name of protection of the cultural heritage (Meleis, 2003).

Recognizing Cultural Influences on the Experience of Pain

Culture strongly influences how one perceives and copes with pain. Women from certain cultures seek pain relief through prayer; others rely on herbal remedies, the application of cold or warmth, acupuncture, the "laying on of hands," and therapeutic massage. Assessment of cultural beliefs and practices, questions to identify specific needs, and encouragement and support to use safe interventions is key in providing culturally sensitive care that empowers the patient to maintain her sense of control over her labor and childbirth experience.

TEACHING THE FAMILY

Discharge Instructions After Autologous Epidural Blood Patch

- Maintain bedrest for 24 to 48 hours.
- Apply cold packs to the area as needed for pain relief.
- Increase oral fluids.
- Avoid the use of analgesics that affect platelet aggregation (e.g., nonsteroidal anti-inflammatory drugs) for 2 days.
- Observe for signs of infection at the site.
- Observe for signs of neurological complications (pain, numbness, tingling in the legs, difficulty with ambulation).

ADDITIONAL INFORMATION FOR THE CLINICAL SETTING

Environmental Strategies to Enhance Comfort During Labor

- Provide privacy, comfort, and a sense of security.
- Allow the patient to regulate the amount of noise, light, and temperature to foster relaxation and a sense of control.
- Keep medical equipment from the patient's view unless it needs to be used.

Precautions When Using Aromatherapy

Never apply essential oils to the skin in a full-strength form. Instead, dilute the oil(s) before application and caution patients that not all aromatherapy oils are safe to use during pregnancy.

Breathing Techniques for Labor and Childbirth
Slow-paced Breathing Pattern
- Use in early labor.
- Cleansing breath at the beginning of the contraction.
- Slowly breathe in through the mouth while the coach counts "one, two, three, four" and slowly breathe out as the coach counts "one, two, three, four."
- Rate = 6 to 8 breaths/min

Modified-paced Breathing Pattern
- Use as contractions increase in frequency and intensity.
- Shallower than slow-paced breathing pattern and faster rate.
- Rate = 32 to 40 breaths/min
- Cleansing breath at the beginning of the contraction.
- Inhale slowly; exhale at a faster pace.
- End with a cleansing breath.
- Requires more concentration.

Pattern-paced Breathing Pattern
- Use during the transition phase of labor.
- Cleansing breath at the beginning of the contraction.
- 3:1 pattern of breathing in and out 2 times, then breathe in and blow out; repeat throughout the contraction.
- End with a cleansing breath.

Assisting the Laboring Patient to Remain Focused During Contractions

Offer words of support and encouragement with statements such as:

- "You're doing a great job!"
- "You're almost there!"
- "I can see your baby's head - reach down and feel it!"
- "You can do it!"

Recognizing and Managing Hyperventilation

- Alert the patient and her support person to symptoms of respiratory alkalosis (light-headedness, dizziness, tingling of the fingers, or circumoral numbness)

- Instruct the patient to breathe into a paper bag held tightly around her mouth and nose. If a bag is not available, instruct her to breathe into her cupped hands.

Using Heat and Cold for Pain Relief During Labor

- Application of heat or cold over anesthetized body areas can cause tissue damage.
- Use hot and cold packs only after one to two layers of cloth have been placed between the pack and the patient's skin (Simkin & Bolding, 2004).

RESOURCES

American College of Obstetricians and Gynecologists: http://www.acog.org/index.cfm

Association of Women's Health, Obstetrical, and Neonatal Nursing (AWHONN): http://www.awhonn.org/awhonn/

Childbirth Connection: http://www.childbirthconnection.org/

Lamaze International: http://www.lamaze.org/

REFERENCES

Cunningham, F., Leveno, K., Bloom, S., Hauth, J., Gilstrap, L., & Wenstrom, K. (2005). *Williams' obstetrics* (22nd ed.). New York: McGraw-Hill.

Lehne, R. (2006). *Pharmacology for nursing care* (6th ed.). Philadelphia: W.B. Saunders.

Lowe, N. (2004). Context and process of informed consent for pharmacologic strategies in labor pain care. *Journal of Midwifery & Women's Health, 49*(3), 250–259.

Meleis, A. (2003). Theoretical considerations of health care for immigrant and minority women. In P. St. Hill, J.G. Lipson, & A.I. Meleis (Eds.), *Caring for women cross-culturally* (pp. 1–10). Philadelphia: F.A. Davis.

Simkin, P., & Bolding, A. (2004). Update on nonpharmacologic approaches to relieve labor pain and prevent suffering. *Journal of Midwifery & Women's Health, 49*(6), 489–504.

Caring for the Woman Experiencing Complications During Labor and Birth

KEY TERMS

amnioinfusion – The instillation of warmed normal saline or lactated Ringer's solution into the uterus via a sterile intrauterine catheter. Performed in an attempt to increase the fluid around the umbilical cord and prevent compression during contractions. Also used to dilute and help wash out thick meconium to avoid neonatal meconium aspiration syndrome.

amniotic fluid embolism (AFE) – Embolism that results from amniotic fluid entering the maternal circulation during labor and birth and after rupture of the membranes; may cause maternal death if it is a pulmonary embolism

artificial rupture of membranes (AROM) – Rupture of the membranes using a plastic device (Amnihook) or surgical clamp

augmentation of labor – The use of chemical modalities to stimulate uterine contractions after labor has begun spontaneously but is not progressing satisfactorily

Bishop score – A rating system to evaluate cervical inducibility; a higher score is associated with a greater likelihood for successful labor induction

cephalopelvic disproportion (CPD) – Condition in which the fetal head is of a shape, size, or position that prohibits it from passing through the maternal pelvis; may also be caused by maternal pelvic problems

cesarean birth – Birth of a fetus through an incision in the maternal abdominal wall and uterus

dystocia – A long, difficult, or abnormal labor and birth

forceps – Instrument consisting of cephalic-curved blades similar to the shape of the fetal head; used during birth to protect the fetal head and to apply traction to assist the birth

hypertonic labor contractions – Uterine contractions that are uncoordinated, frequent, and often painful but are ineffective in producing cervical effacement and dilation

hypotonic labor contractions – Uterine contractions that are weak and ineffective; this labor pattern usually occurs during the active phase of labor

induction of labor – The use of chemical or mechanical modalities to initiate uterine contractions before their spontaneous onset to bring about childbirth.

intrauterine resuscitation – Interventions initiated when a nonreassuring fetal heart rate pattern is noted; directed at improving uterine and intervillous space blood flow and cardiac output

macrosomia – Large body size; fetal birth weight above the 90th percentile on an intrauterine growth chart for that gestational age; often seen in neonates of diabetic or prediabetic mothers

meconium – First stools of the infant; characteristically viscid, dark greenish brown, sticky, sterile, and odorless

meconium stained amniotic fluid – In response to hypoxia, fetal intestinal activity increases and the anal sphincter relaxes, resulting in the passage of meconium into the amniotic fluid. Normally seen in breech presentations

nuchal cord – Encircling of the fetal neck by one or more loops of the umbilical cord

oligohydramnios – Less than 300 mL of amniotic fluid

pelvic dystocia – Occurs when contractures of the pelvic diameters reduce the capacity of the bony pelvis: the midpelvis; the outlet; or any combination of these planes

postdate pregnancy – A pregnancy that has gone past the estimated date of birth

postterm pregnancy – A pregnancy that extends beyond 294 days or 42 weeks past the first day of the last normal menstrual period

precipitate (precipitous) labor – Rapid or sudden labor that lasts less than 3 hours from the beginning of contractions to birth

spontaneous rupture of membranes (SROM) – Rupture of the membranes by natural means

shoulder dystocia – Occurs when the fetal head is born but the anterior shoulder cannot pass under the maternal pubic arch

soft tissue dystocia – Occurs when the birth passage is obstructed by an anatomic abnormality other than that involving the maternal bony pelvis

trial of labor (TOL) – Observation period to determine if a woman in labor is likely to successfully progress to a vaginal birth

umbilical cord prolapse – Protrusion of the umbilical cord in advance of the presenting part

vacuum-assisted birth (also termed vacuum extraction) – Birth involving the attachment of a vacuum cup to the fetal head and using negative pressure to assist in the birth of the fetus

vaginal birth after cesarean (VBAC) – Giving birth vaginally after a previous cesarean birth

version – Act of turning the fetus in the uterus from one presentation to another

    external cephalic v. – Turning the fetus to a vertex position by externally exerting pressure on the fetus through the maternal abdomen

FOCUSED ASSESSMENT

Uterine Contraction Patterns (Fig. 11-1)

- **A** – Normal uterine contraction pattern (brings about cervical effacement and dilation)
- **B** – Hypertonic uterine contraction pattern (uncoordinated, frequent, painful)
- **C** – Hypotonic uterine contraction pattern (weak, ineffective)

Figure 11-1 Uterine contraction patterns. *A.* Normal uterine contraction pattern. *B.* Hypertonic uterine contraction pattern. *C.* Hypotonic uterine contraction pattern.

Factors Associated with Increased Risk for Hypertonic Labor Contractions

- Increased maternal catecholamine release (e.g., epinephrine, norepinephrine)
- Maternal anxiety (primiparous labor, fear of loss of control, history of sexual abuse, lack of support, cultural differences)
- Fetal occiput–posterior malposition

Factors Associated with Increased Risk for Hypotonic Labor Contractions

- Fetal macrosomia
- Multiple gestation
- Hydramnios
- Maternal obesity unaccompanied by diabetes
- Pharmacological agents used for pain relief

Factors Associated with an Increased Risk for Uterine Dystocia

- Uterine abnormalities, such as congenital malformations and overdistention (e.g., hydramnios, macrosomia, multiple gestation)

- Fetal malpresentation or malposition
- Cephalopelvic disproportion (CPD)
- Maternal body build (>30 lbs. [13.6 kg] overweight, short stature)
- Uterine overstimulation with oxytocin
- Inappropriate timing of administration of analgesic/anesthetic agents
- Maternal fear, fatigue, dehydration, electrolyte imbalance (Gilbert, 2006)

How to Recognize Indicators of Dystocia

- Lack of progress in rate of cervical dilation, fetal descent, and expulsion
- Alteration in the pattern of normal uterine contractions

Assessment of the Patient Undergoing an Amniotomy

- Assess maternal understanding of the procedure.
- Assess vital signs, cervical effacement and dilation, station, fetal heart rate (FHR), and contractions.
- Ensure equipment is assembled (hip pad, padded bedpan, sterile gloves, lubricant, Amnihook, or Allis clamp; Fig. 11-2).
- Place the hip pad under the buttocks and position the padded bedpan to elevate hips.
- Assess the FHR immediately before and after artificial rupture of membranes (AROM).
  - Transient fetal tachycardia is common.
  - Bradycardia or variable decelerations may indicate cord compression or prolapse.
- Assess color, odor, consistency, clarity, and amount of amniotic fluid.
- Assess for signs of maternal infection.
  - Take temperature at least every 2 hours.
  - Assess for chills, uterine tenderness, foul-smelling vaginal discharge, fetal tachycardia.

Amniotic
membrane

Figure 11-2 An Amnihook is used to rupture the membranes.

Assessing Cervical Inducibility with the Bishop Score				
Score	**0**	**1**	**2**	**3**
Dilation (cm)	0	1–2	3–4	≥5
Effacement (%)	0–30	40–50	60–70	≥80
Station (cm)	–3	–2	–1	+1, +2
Cervical Consistency	Firm	Medium	Soft	
Cervix Position	Posterior	Midposition	Anterior	

Source: Cunningham et al. (2005).

Assessment and Documentation During Oxytocin Administration

- Patient's vital signs (blood pressure, pulse, and respirations every 30 to 60 minutes and with every increment in medication dose)
- FHR (via electronic monitoring)
- Frequency, duration, and strength of contractions (note contraction pattern and uterine resting tone every 15 minutes and with every increment in medication dose during first stage; then monitor every 5 minutes during second stage).
- Cervical effacement and dilatation
- Fetal station and lie
- Rate of oxytocin infusion
- Intake and urine output (limit IV intake to 1000 mL/8 hr; output should be 120 mL or more every 4 hours)

- Any untoward effect of the medication administration (nausea, vomiting, headache, hypotension)
- Psychological response of the patient

(American College of Obstetricians [ACOG], 1999; Gilbert, 2006; Simpson, 2005)

CLINICAL ALERTS

Contraindications to the Use of Oxytocin to Stimulate Labor

- Vasa previa or complete placenta previa
- Transverse fetal lie
- Umbilical cord prolapse
- Previous transfundal uterine surgery

Conditions that Necessitate Special Precaution During Oxytocin Administration

- Breech presentation
- Multifetal pregnancy
- Presenting part above the pelvic inlet
- Severe hypertension
- Maternal heart disease
- Polyhydramnios
- One or more previous low-transverse cesarean deliveries (ACOG, 1999)

MEDICATIONS

Administering Oxytocin

1. Obtain written order for oxytocin for labor induction or augmentation from patient's primary health care provider.
2. Explain procedure and assess the patient's level of understanding.
3. Assist the patient to a side-lying or upright position.
4. Assess the patient and fetus and document the findings.
5. Prepare the primary IV solution and administer with a pump delivery system according to the prescribed orders.

6. Connect the piggyback solution with the medication to the intravenous infusion at the port nearest the point of venous insertion, and administer as ordered.
7. Perform ongoing maternal-fetal assessments according to institutional protocol.
8. Document:
   - Medication name and amount
   - Times of beginning infusion and any dose changes
   - Maternal–fetal reactions (FHR and pattern, maternal vital signs, pattern and progress of labor, and nursing interventions and maternal response)
   - Notification of primary health care provider of any change

Cervical Ripening Agents

Medication	Action	Adverse Effects	Dosage
Prostaglandin E$_1$ Misoprostol (Cytotec)	Induces labor contractions.	Diarrhea, abdominal pain, headaches, fever, tachysystole, uterine hyperstimulation	Intravaginally: 25 mcg; repeat every 4–6 hours until Bishop score equals 8 or greater
Prostaglandin E$_2$ Dinoprostone (Cervidil Insert, Prepidil Gel)	Promotes initiation of cervical ripening. May stimulate labor contractions.	Uterine hyperstimulation, fever, back pain, headache, nausea and vomiting, diarrhea, hypotension, tachysystole *Adverse effects are more common with intracervical administration.*	Cervidil insert: (10 mg dinoprostone gradually released over 12 hours). Remove after 12 hours or at labor onset. Keep insert frozen until ready to use. Prepidil Gel: (2.5-mL syringe containing 0.5 mg of dinoprostone). Repeat gel insertion in 6 hours as needed (maximum = 1.5 mg or 3 doses/24 hr). Allow the gel to reach room temperature before administration; do not heat. Continue administration until

Medication	Action	Adverse Effects	Dosage
			the maximum dose is reached, or uterine contractions are established (3/10 min) or the Bishop score equals 8 or greater or adverse reactions occur.

ETHNOCULTURAL CONSIDERATIONS

Communication Difficulties During Labor

Nurses need to be sensitive to cultural differences among women experiencing hypertonic labor, a pattern characterized by strong, painful contractions that do not produce cervical effacement and dilation. Maternal anxiety, related to factors such as fear of pain, loss of control, lack of support, and cultural differences, produces high levels of catecholamines, which can result in poor uterine contractility. Women who are unable to speak or understand the English language may have difficulty communicating their feelings. A therapeutic environment that fosters trust, comfort, relaxation, and rest, along with other measures such as hydration and sedation, help to reduce the irritability of the uterus and diminish the ineffective contractions.

Trends in Preterm Labor and Birth

Black women are at a higher risk for preterm birth than are Caucasian women. When preterm birth rates of married, educated women are compared with those of matched Caucasian women, a disparity continues to be noted among the Black women. The increase in cases of preterm labor results in a greater percentage of infant mortality in the Black population (Moore, 2003).

Minority Women and Level of Care Received

The Institute of Medicine (2003) reported that members of minorities do not receive the same level of quality care as do white Americans. A nurse working in the birth unit needs to be attentive to this problem. It is incumbent upon all nurses to advocate for patients any time there appears to be an ethnic bias in treatment. The nurse also must be aware of any personal prejudices that could affect care. In institutions that serve minority populations, it is essential that all hospital staff members undergo frequent in-service educational offerings that focus on heightening cultural sensitivity.

Cultural Aspects of Loss

Reactions to perinatal death vary among cultures. Tears and emotional outbursts are common to some cultures; others are quiet and introspective. The Hispanic culture that includes Mexicans, Puerto Ricans, and Cubans views children as their future. The loss of a child denies that future. Hispanic individuals tend to welcome touch from others and expect health care professionals to respect their need for extended family during this time frame (Gilbert, 2006).

TEACHING THE FAMILY

Preparing the Patient for an Amniotomy

- Ensure that the patient understands the procedure and the reason for it.
- Explain that the membrane rupture is painless for her and the fetus, but that she may feel some discomfort when the instrument is inserted.

Exploring Concerns of the Patient Experiencing Preterm Labor

- Use active listening; remain nearby; provide ongoing information.
- Encourage the patient to participate in decision making.
- Teach the patient and her partner about the process of labor and how they can support and help one another throughout the labor and birth experience.

Educating the Patient About Cervical Ripening Agents

- Assess knowledge of the medication.
- Explain the purpose of the medication and its side effects.

- Discuss comfort options to offset the side effects of the medication.
- Instruct the patient to void before insertion of the medication.
- Instruct the patient to maintain a supine position with a lateral tilt or side-lying position for 30 to 40 minutes after insertion of the medication.

(Deglin & Vallerand, 2009; Turkoski, Lance, & Bonfiglio, 2004)

ADDITIONAL INFORMATION FOR THE CLINICAL SETTING

Assisting with a Precipitous Birth

- Request a translator to interpret for patients unable to speak or understand English.
- Assist the laboring woman to breathe through each contraction to prevent pushing.
- Provide continuous emotional support.
- Provide perineal support with warm cloths.
- Frequently monitor the maternal and fetal vital signs and immediately report any abnormal findings to the physician or certified nurse midwife.
- After birth, carefully monitor the patient for signs of hemorrhage; assess for trauma to the perineum.
- Assess the neonate for evidence of trauma and report and document all findings.

Nursing Actions During a Trial of Labor (TOL)

Nursing responsibilities during a TOL include assessment of maternal vital signs and FHR and pattern. If complications arise, the nurse notifies the primary health care provider, and evaluates and documents the maternal–fetal responses to the interventions. Offering support and encouragement to the woman and her labor partner and ongoing information about labor progress are essential components of care.

Nursing Actions When a Non-reassuring FHR Pattern Is Detected

- Provide information to the patient; assist her to a lateral position.

- Encourage relaxation and mental imagery to reduce anxiety.
- Assess for and correct maternal hypotension by elevating the legs.
- Increase the rate of the maintenance IV fluids.
- Assess for hyperstimulation by palpating the uterus.
- Discontinue oxytocin if infusing.
- Administer oxygen at 8 to 10 L/min by mask.
- Consider internal monitoring to obtain more accurate fetal/uterine assessments.
- Apply fetal scalp or acoustic stimulation.
- Assist with fetal oxygen saturation monitoring if ordered.
- Assist with birth (cesarean or vaginal-assisted) if a non reassuring FHR pattern cannot be corrected.

Communicating Effectively When a Non-reassuring FHR Pattern Is Detected by Electronic Monitoring

When electronic monitoring reveals a non-reassuring FHR pattern, the nurse needs to maintain a calming presence and offer factual, simple explanations for all actions. For example, the nurse may say:

"We are concerned about your baby's heart rate pattern."
"I am going to change your position to your side to increase oxygen flow to your baby."
"I am also going to place this oxygen mask on your face to increase the oxygen flow to you and to your baby, and increase your IV rate."
"Do you have any questions?"
"I am here to help in any way and I will stay here with you. Please let me know what concerns you have."

Assisting with Intrauterine Resuscitation

Nursing priorities:

1. Open the maternal and fetal vascular systems.
2. Increase the blood volume.
3. Optimize oxygenation of the circulating blood volume.

These interventions are accomplished by:

- Changing the maternal position
- Increasing the rate of the primary IV
- Providing oxygen by face mask

Caring for a Patient Undergoing Amnioinfusion

1. Assess the patient's response to the fluid infusion.
2. Continually monitor the frequency and intensity of uterine contractions.
3. Stop the infusion if the following signs and symptoms are noted: Maternal shortness of breath, an over-distended uterus, hypotension, or tachycardia.

Recognizing and Responding to Problems During Labor Induction with Oxytocin

During induction of labor with oxytocin, be alert to signs indicative of complications: uterine hyperstimulation, nonreassuring fetal heart rate pattern, and suspected uterine rupture. Immediate emergency measures include discontinuing the oxytocin per institutional protocol; positioning the patient on her side; increasing the primary IV rate up to 200 mL/hr (unless there is evidence of water intoxication—in this situation, the rate is decreased to one that keeps the vein open); administering oxygen by face mask at 8 to 10 L/min or per physician order or institutional protocol.

Alternative Measures for the Induction of Labor

Herbal Remedies

Black haw, primrose oil, black and blue cohosh, chamomile, and red raspberry leaves are medicinal agents with some properties similar to those of oxytocin. Although used as labor inducers in some cultures, there is a lack of scientific research and validation of their effectiveness.

Nonherbal Methods

Nonherbal methods include acupuncture, the ingestion of a laxative (e.g., castor oil), and the stripping of membranes.

Assisting with External Cephalic Version (ECV): Nursing Responsibilities (Fig. 11-3)

1. Obtain consent.	The physician is responsible for explaining the procedure.
2. Assess for contraindications to a version.	Contraindications include previous cesarean birth, uterine anomalies, CPD, placenta previa, multifetal gestation, oligohydramnios
3. Provide teaching regarding the procedure.	Before the version, ultrasonography, non-stress testing, and/or electronic FHR monitoring is performed. The ECV may not be successful; complications include rupture of the membranes, fetal bradycardia, discomfort, and the potential for cesarean birth if maternal or fetal compromise occurs.
4. Administer medications if ordered.	Tocolytic agents (e.g., magnesium sulfate, terbutaline) may be ordered.
5. Maintain constant maternal and fetal surveillance.	Assess for fetal or maternal compromise.
6. Administer Rh immune globulin if the patient is Rh-negative	Manipulation may cause fetal–maternal bleeding.

Intravenous tocolytic drug

A   B

Figure 11-3 External cephalic version is a maneuver performed through the maternal abdominal wall in an attempt to change the fetal position from a breech to a cephalic presentation.

Breech Presentation and the Presence of Meconium in the Amniotic Fluid

When the fetus is in a breech presentation, the presence of meconium in the amniotic fluid may not be indicative of fetal distress. Pressure exerted on the fetal abdomen during the birth process may cause the passage of meconium. It is important to assess the FHR and pattern to ensure there are changes indicative of fetal hypoxia. When the fetus is in a breech position, the FHR is best auscultated at or above the maternal umbilicus.

Intrapartal Neonatal Suctioning and Meconium-Stained Amniotic Fluid

The nasopharynx and oropharynx of the neonate born in the presence of meconium-stained amniotic fluid are often suctioned before the first breath to reduce the incidence and severity of meconium aspiration syndrome (MAS). However, because research does not support the efficacy of routine intrapartum suctioning to prevent MAS, this practice is no longer recommended (Vain et al., 2004).

Actions to Reduce the Risk of Umbilical Cord Prolapse

When SROM occurs, maintain the patient on bed rest until the fetal presenting part is engaged. AROM should not be attempted until engagement has occurred. To rule out umbilical cord prolapse, assess the fetal heart sounds immediately after spontaneous or artificial rupture of the membranes.

Nursing Actions After Prolapse of the Umbilical Cord (Fig. 11-4)

1. Call for assistance; notify the primary health care provider.
2. Using the gloved examining hand, insert two fingers into the vagina to the cervix. Place one finger on either side of the cord or both fingers to one side and quickly exert upward pressure against the presenting part to relieve compression of the cord.
3. Assist the woman into an extreme Trendelenburg, modified Sims, or knee–chest position.

4. If the cord is protruding from the vagina, wrap it loosely in a sterile towel saturated with a warmed, sterile normal saline solution.

5. Administer oxygen at 10 L/min by facemask.

6. Increase the IV fluids; administer a tocolytic agent as ordered.

7. Continuously monitor the FHR by internal fetal scalp electrode if possible.

8. Provide information and support to the patient and her birth partner.

9. Prepare for an immediate vaginal birth if the cervix is fully dilated or for cesarean birth if it is not.

Figure 11-4 Interventions to relieve pressure on a prolapsed umbilical cord until birth can be effected. *A.* A gloved hand is placed in the vagina to lift the presenting part off the cord. *B.* The knee–chest position uses gravity to shift the fetus out of the maternal pelvis. *C.* The maternal hips are elevated with two pillows; this intervention is often combined with a Trendelenburg position.

Actions When Attending a Forceps-Assisted Birth

- Assess and record the FHR and pattern before the forceps application (there is a danger of compression of the cord between the fetal head and the forceps blade; cord compression causes a decrease in the FHR) (Fig. 11-5).
- Assess and record the FHR and pattern again *immediately* after the forceps application

Simpson forceps (outlet)

Tucker-McLean forceps (outlet)

Piper forceps (aftercoming head in breech)

Direction of gentle traction for outlet forceps delivery

Figure 11-5 Forceps are instruments with curved blades that are used to facilitate birth of the fetal head.

Nursing Responsibilities Associated with a Vacuum-Assisted Birth (Fig. 11-6)

- Management of patient care.
- Control the vacuum gun and pressure while the physician applies the vacuum apparatus to the fetal head.
- Thoroughly document the sequence of events.
- Communicate progress or lack of progress to all members of the perinatal team.
- Assess maternal and fetal status and advocate for cesarean birth if maternal exhaustion and/or failure of descent indicates that the vacuum assistance is not effective.
- Be aware that after an assisted birth, the nurse who assesses the neonate is also liable with regard to the documentation of vital signs and the neonatal assessment (Mahlmeister, 2005).

Nursing Actions When Birth Is Complicated by Shoulder Dystocia

- Assist the patient in assuming the position ordered by the physician.
- Assist the physician with maneuvers (e.g., suprapubic pressure; McRoberts maneuver) to facilitate birth (Fig. 11-7).
- Document all procedures.
- Provide instruction to the patient to facilitate cooperation and understanding.

A   B

Figure 11-6 Vacuum extraction also facilitates the delivery of the fetal head and is associated with fewer lacerations of the maternal birth canal. *A.* Vacuum extractor is applied with a downward and outward traction. *B.* A caput succedaneum, or chignon, is formed from the suction cup.

- After birth, closely observe the mother for signs of hemorrhage and soft tissue trauma of the birth canal.
- Assess the neonate for birth asphyxia, fracture of the clavicle or humerus, and/or brachial plexus injuries

Figure 11-7 Methods to relieve shoulder dystocia. *A.* Pressure is applied immediately above the maternal symphysis pubis to push the fetal anterior shoulder downward. *B.* McRoberts maneuver. The woman's thighs are sharply flexed on her abdomen to straighten the pelvic curve. *C.* Angle of pelvis before maneuver. *D.* Angle of pelvis after maneuver.

Understanding Types of Uterine Rupture

Type	Description	Symptoms
Complete Rupture	Extends through the endometrium, myometrium, and peritoneum.	Sudden, severe, abdominal pain during a contraction followed by cessation of the pain and contractions with bleeding into the abdominal cavity and possibly into the vagina.
Incomplete Rupture	Extends into the peritoneum but not into the peritoneal cavity or broad ligament.	Bleeding is usually internal and the woman may be asymptomatic (a "silent" rupture) or complain of localized tenderness and aching pain over the lower uterine segment.

Umbilical Cord and Placental Variations

Variation	Description	Implications
Velamentous Insertion of Cord	The fetal vessels separate at the distal end of the cord and insert into the placenta at a distance away from the margin.	Vessels are not protected by Wharton's jelly and are subject to rupture and/or thrombosis. Most common with placenta previa and multiple pregnancies.
Vasa Previa	The umbilical cord is implanted into the fetal membranes rather than the placenta; the vessels cover the cervical os and precede the fetus.	Hemorrhage
Circumvallate Placenta	A ring composed of a double fold of amnion and chorion forms near the fetal surface.	Associated with antepartum hemorrhage, preterm birth, and fetal malformations.
Succenturiate Placenta	Placenta contains one or two separate lobes, each with its own circulation.	After childbirth, one of the separate lobes may be retained in the uterus and impede contractions, resulting in severe maternal hemorrhage. The remaining lobes must be manually removed from the uterus to prevent hemorrhage.
Battledore Placenta	The umbilical cord is implanted near the margin of the placenta.	Associated with fetal hemorrhage, especially after marginal separation of the placenta
Placenta Accreta	A slight penetration of the myometrium by the trophoblast.	Hemorrhage
Placenta Increta	A deep placental penetration of the myometrium.	Hemorrhage and possible hysterectomy
Placenta Percreta	Perforation of the uterus by the placenta.	Hemorrhage, hysterectomy

Disseminated Intravascular Coagulation (DIC)

Be alert for maternal clinical signs indicative of DIC:

- Bleeding from multiple sites: intravenous access site, venipuncture site, site of urinary catheter insertion

- Spontaneous bleeding from the gums and nose
- Widespread petechiae and bruising
- Gastrointestinal bleeding
- Tachycardia
- Diaphoresis

Care of the Patient Experiencing an Intrapartal Hemorrhage

Assessment	Plan	Intervention	Evaluation
Vital Signs	Establish maternal stability.	Take every 5 minutes if unstable, or every 15 minutes if stable. Use pulse oximetry. Auscultate respirations.	Vital signs are within normal range. Pulse is between 60 and 120 beats per minute. Respirations are between 14 and 26 breaths per minute. Temperature is <100.4°F (38°C); BP is >90/60 mm Hg.
Bleeding	Resolve hemorrhage. Prevent shock.	Start two large-bore IV sites. Infuse normal saline and lactated Ringer's solution. Estimate blood loss. 1 g = 1 mL for replacement Infuse blood products as necessary. Monitor circulatory volume using central venous pressure (CVP)/Swan-Ganz catheter as needed for extreme bleeding.	Bleeding is minimized. Homeostasis is established.

(continued)

Care of the Patient Experiencing an Intrapartal Hemorrhage (Continued)

Assessment	Plan	Intervention	Evaluation
		Send blood sample to lab for analysis of gases. Document blood loss.	
Intake/Output	Prevent volume depletion.	Insert in-dwelling urinary catheter. Measure and record output every hour. Measure and record input every hour.	Urine output will be >30 mL/hr.
Fetal Status	Prevent fetal injury.	Continuous electronic fetal monitoring	Fetal heart rate tracings remain between 120 and 160 bpm. There is no evidence of abnormal tracings.
Emotional Response	Assist the patient to cope with the condition.	Educate the patient regarding all procedures. Inform the patient of her status throughout the bleeding crisis. Provide relaxation and breathing techniques. Provide spiritual support as necessary.	The patient verbalizes an understanding of her condition. The patient's face displays no grimace. The muscles remain relaxed.
Pain	Reduce pain.	Provide relaxation and breathing techniques. Use guided imagery.	The patient reports pain on a rating scale of 1–10 as between 3 and 5.

Assessment	Plan	Intervention	Evaluation
		Offer massage. Monitor contractions. Offer limited pain medication as ordered.	

Sources: MacMullen, Dulski, & Meagher (2005); Curran (2003); Mandeville & Troiano (1999).

Nursing Actions When Amniotic Fluid Embolism (AFE) Develops

Immediately perform the following actions:

- Administer oxygen by facemask or cannula at a rate of 8 to 10 L/min; or resuscitation bag to deliver 100% oxygen.
- Prepare for intubation and mechanical ventilation.
- Initiate or assist with cardiopulmonary resuscitation (CPR). Position the pregnant patient in a 30-degree lateral tilt to displace the uterus.
- Administer intravenous fluids and blood (e.g., packed cells; fresh frozen plasma).
- Insert indwelling urinary catheter; measure hourly urine output.
- Continuously monitor maternal–fetal status.
- Prepare for emergency birth once the patient is stable.
- Provide ongoing information and emotional support to the patient and her family.

Risks Associated with Multiple Gestations

- Antepartal complications: Hypertension of pregnancy, anemia, gestational diabetes
- Intrapartal complications: Hemorrhage (related to atony from uterine overdistention); abruptio placentae, multiple or adherent placentas, abnormal fetal presentation(s), fetal distress (related to cord prolapse and the onset of placental separation after the birth of the first fetus)
- Fetal/newborn complications: primarily related to problems associated with low-birth-weight infants due to preterm birth and intrauterine growth restriction

Medical Indications for Elective Preterm Birth in Women with Diabetes

- Poor metabolic control
- Worsening hypertensive disorder
- Fetal macrosomia or fetal growth restriction (ACOG, 2001; Cunningham et al., 2005)

Postpartal Complications in Diabetic Women

Increased risk for:

- Preeclampsia/eclampsia
- Hemorrhage (more likely following uterine overdistention [e.g., hydramnios, macrosomia])
- Infection (e.g., endometritis)

Intrapartal Nursing Care for Patients with Preeclampsia

Blood Pressure

- Check every 4 hours (or more frequently according to physician orders or institutional protocol).
- Use the same arm at each assessment.
- Encourage a side-lying position to enhance uterine perfusion.
- Record all data.
- Notify the physician of an increase in blood pressure.

Medication Administration

- Administer as ordered and evaluate its effect.
- Adhere to hospital protocol for magnesium sulfate infusion.
- Monitor maternal vital signs, FHR, urine output, deep tendon reflexes (DTRs), IV flow rate, and serum magnesium levels.
- Assess for magnesium sulfate toxicity (e.g., depressed respirations, hyporeflexia, sudden onset of hypotension, oliguria, indicators of fetal compromise).
- Administer calcium gluconate (the antidote for magnesium sulfate toxicity) for respirations below 12/min and discontinue the magnesium sulfate infusion.

Renal Balance

- Assess edema on a scale of 1 to 4 (4 is generalized massive edema that includes the face, abdomen, and sacrum).

- Assess and record urinary output. An indwelling urinary catheter may be inserted to measure urinary output more accurately. A urine output <30 mL/hr is indicative of oliguria and the physician must be notified.
- Assess urine for protein every 4 hours. A dipstick reading >2+ is indicative of a worsening condition.

Neurological Status
- Assess DTRs every 4 hours (or more frequently) on a scale of 1 to 4. Reflexes >2+ are a sign of worsening status.
- If dorsiflexion of the foot produces clonus (convulsive spasm), the maternal condition is deteriorating.

Pulmonary
- Auscultate the lungs every 4 hours (or more frequently).
- Assess for dyspnea, crackles, and diminished breath sounds (may be indicative of pulmonary edema).
- Assess the respiratory rate every 4 hours (or more frequently).
- Patients who are receiving magnesium sulfate require more frequent respiratory assessments because a respiratory rate below 12 is an indicator of magnesium toxicity.
- Hemoglobin oxygen saturation can be assessed with a pulse oximeter.

Psychological Status
- Assess for indicators of anxiety and fear.
- Provide information to the patient and family about the treatment protocols and status of the maternal-fetal conditions.
- Assess the patient's and family's level of understanding and provide updates when indicated.

Advancing Symptoms
Headaches, blurred vision, severe right upper quadrant epigastric pain, and restlessness are all indicators of impending eclampsia. Prepare for immediate delivery.

Seizures
Protect the patient. Keep the airway patent: turn the head to one side and place a pillow or folded linen under one shoulder or back. Call for assistance. Ensure that the side rails have been raised. Observe and document all seizure activity. Notify the physician and prepare for delivery. Administer oxygen.

Fetal Status

Monitor the fetal heart rate every 4 hours or more frequently as indicated. Assess fetal movements. Notify the physician if indicators of fetal compromise are noted.

Factors that May Necessitate Immediate Intervention to Facilitate Birth in Patients with Hypertensive Disorders

- Uncontrolled severe hypertension
- Eclampsia
- Persistent oliguria (<500 mL/24 hr)
- Abruptio placentae
- Platelet count <100,000/mm^3
- Elevated liver enzyme levels with epigastric pain or right upper quadrant tenderness
- Pulmonary edema
- Persistent severe headache or visual changes
- Spontaneous labor
- Fetal death
- Rupture of the membranes
- Gestational age <34 weeks (an observational period may be initially attempted as a conservative management approach)
- Evidence of fetal compromise

Supporting the Mother Whose Newborn Has Died

When caring for the mother whose infant has died, the nurse conveys compassion by simply being available. Often, the mother finds comfort in talking about the birth experience, her infant, and how she will cope with her loss. The nurse can gain insights into the mother's support systems by asking the following questions:

"What are you most worried or fearful about?
"How supportive is the baby's father and your family or friends?
"What coping techniques have been helpful for you in the past?" (Gilbert, 2006)

REFERENCES

American College of Obstetricians and Gynecologists (ACOG). (1999). *Induction of labor.* ACOG Practice Bulletin No. 10. Washington, DC: Author.

American College of Obstetricians and Gynecologists (ACOG). (2001). *Gestational diabetes.* ACOG Practice Bulletin Number 30. Washington, DC: Author.

Cunningham, F., Leveno, K., Bloom, S., Hauth, J., Gilstrap, L., & Wenstrom, K. (2005). *Williams' obstetrics* (22nd ed.). New York: McGraw-Hill.

Curran, C. (2003). Intrapartum emergencies. *Journal of Obstetric, Gynecologic, and Neonatal Nursing, 32*(6), 802–813.

Deglin, J.H., & Vallerand, A.H. (2009). *Davis's drug guide for nurses* (11th ed.). Philadelphia: F.A. Davis.

Gilbert, E.S. (2006). *Manual of high risk pregnancy and delivery.* St. Louis, MO: C.V. Mosby.

Institute of Medicine. (2003). *The future of the public's health in the 21st century.* Washington, DC: National Academy Press.

MacMullen, N., Dulski, L., & Meagher, B. (2005). RED ALERT: Perinatal hemorrhage. *The American Journal of Maternal Child Health, 30*(1), 46–51.

Mahlmeister, L. (2005). Nursing responsibilities in preventing, preparing for and managing epidural emergencies. *Journal of Perinatal and Neonatal Nursing, 17*(1), 19–34.

Mandeville, L., & Troiano, N. (1999). *High-risk and critical care: Intrapartum nursing* (2nd ed.). Philadelphia: Lippincott.

Moore, M. (2003). Preterm labor and birth: What have we learned in the past two decades? *Journal of Obstetric Gynecological and Neonatal Nursing, 32,* 638–649.

Simpson, K. (2005). The context and clinical evidence for common nursing practices during labor. *MCN American Journal of Maternal/Child Nursing, 30*(6), 356–363.

Turkoski, B.B., Lance, B.R., & Bonfiglio, M.F. (2004). *Lexi comp's drug information for nursing: Including assessment, administration, monitoring guidelines, and patient education* (6th ed.). Hudson, OH: Lexi-Comp.

Vain, N., Szyld, E., Prudent, L., Wiswell, T., Aguilar, A., & Vivas, N. (2004). Oropharyngeal and nasopharyngeal suctioning of meconium-stained neonates before delivery of their shoulders: Multicentre, randomized, controlled trial. *Lancet, 364*(9434), 597–602.

12

Caring for the Postpartal Woman and Her Family

KEY TERMS

afterpains (afterbirth pains) – Painful intermittent uterine contractions that occur for approximately 2 to 3 days, during the process of uterine involution.

couplet care – Situation when one nurse, who has been educated in both mother and infant care, serves as the primary nurse for the mother and the infant, even when the infant is kept in the nursery. Also known as "mother–baby care"

engorgement – Distention or vascular congestion

   breast e. Excessive swelling of the breast and areola brought about by an increase in blood and lymph supply to the breast, which precedes lactation. Typically occurs between the 3rd and 5th postpartum day and lasts about 24 hours.

involution – Reduction in uterine size after birth

lactogenesis – Process by which the breasts secrete milk

latch-on – Proper attachment of the infant to the breast for feeding

"let-down" reflex – Release of milk from the breast, caused by the contraction of the myoepithelial cells within the milk glands in response to oxytocin. Also termed "milk ejection reflex"

lochia – Vaginal discharge during the postpartal period; consists of blood, tissue, and mucus

   l. alba Thin, yellowish-white vaginal discharge that follows lochia serosa on approximately the tenth day after birth

   l. rubra Bright red vaginal flow that follows birth and lasts 2 to 4 days

l. serosa Serous, pinkish-brown thin vaginal discharge that follows lochia rubra until about the 10th day after birth

maternal blues/baby blues/postpartum blues – Feelings that include sadness, forgetfulness, tearfulness and mood swings; usually begin 2 to 3 days after giving birth and disappear within 1 to 2 weeks

nipple confusion – Difficulty experienced by some infants when attempting proper latch-on to the breast; occurs after the breastfed infant is given supplemental feedings with a bottle

parturition – The act of giving birth

puerperium – Period that begins after the third stage of labor and lasts until uterine involution is complete, usually 3 to 6 weeks; also known as the "fourth trimester"

sitz bath – Application of moist heat to the perineum; may be accomplished by sitting in a tub or basin filled with warm water

subinvolution – Failure of a part (e.g., the uterus) to return to its normal size and condition after enlargement from a functional activity (e.g., pregnancy)

FOCUSED ASSESSMENT

Assessment of Vital Signs During the Early Puerperium		
Parameter	**Frequency**	**Expected Findings**
Temperature		May increase up to 100.4°F (38°C) during first 24 hours due to exertion and dehydration.
Heart Rate	All vital signs are assessed q15min × 4; q30min×2hr; qhr × 1; then q8hr	Bradycardia (50–70 bpm) is common for the first 6–10 days.
Blood Pressure		Compare with pre-pregnancy norms. Orthostatic hypotension is common.
Respirations		Should remain in a normal range.

BUBBLE-HE: Essential Components of a Postpartum Assessment

Letter	Assess	Assessment Includes
B	Breasts	Inspection of nipples: Everted, flat, inverted? Breast tissue: Soft, filling, firm? Temperature and color: Warm, pink, cool, red streaked?
U	Uterus	Location (midline or deviated to right or left side) and tone (firm, firm with massage, boggy)
B	Bladder	Last time the patient emptied her bladder (spontaneously or via catheter)? Palpable or nonpalpable? Color, odor, and amount of urine?
B	Bowels	Date/time of last bowel movement; presence of flatus and hunger (unless the colon was manipulated, do not need to auscultate for bowel sounds)
L	Lochia	Color, amount, presence of clots, any free flow?
(I) E	(Incision) Episiotomy	Type as well as other tissue trauma (lacerations, etc.) Assess using REEDA (redness, edema, ecchymosis, drainage/discharge, approximation of episiotomy, if present)
L/H	Legs (Homans' sign)	Pain, varicosities, warmth or discoloration in calves; presence of pedal pulses; sensation and movement (after cesarean birth)
E	Emotions	Affect, patient–family interaction, effects of exhaustion
(B)	Bonding	Interaction with infant—"taking in" phase: Presence of finger tipping, gazing, enfolding, calling infant by name, identifying unique characteristics

Performing the Uterine Assessment

- Assist the patient to a supine position.
- Observe the abdomen for contour to detect distention, striae, or diastasis (separation).
- Place one hand immediately above the symphysis pubis to stabilize the uterus.
- Place the other hand at the level of the umbilicus.
- Press inward and downward with the hand positioned on the umbilicus until the fundus is located.

- Note and document the findings: the fundus should feel like a firm, globular mass located at or slightly above the umbilicus (first hour after birth; Fig. 12-1).
- Uterus descends in the pelvis at a rate of about 1 cm/day (one fingerbreadth; Fig. 12-2).

Figure 12-1 To palpate the uterus, the upper hand is cupped over the fundus; the lower hand stabilizes the uterus at the symphysis pubis.

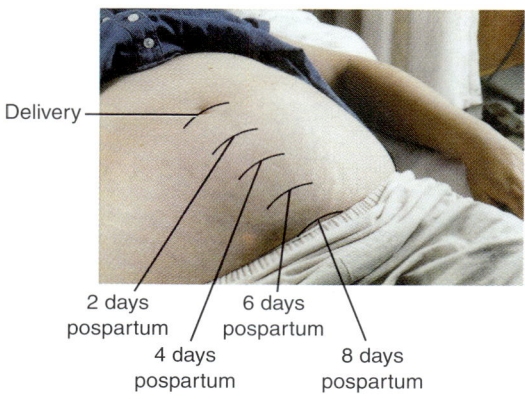

Figure 12-2 Fundal heights postpartum.

Assessment and Documentation of Uterine Involution

Time	Location of Fundus	Documentation
Immediately after birth	Midline, midway between umbilicus and symphysis pubis	
1–2 hours	At the level of the umbilicus	at U (umbilicus)
12 hours	1 cm above umbilicus (1 fingerbreadth)	U+1
24 hours	1 cm below umbilicus	U–1
2 days	2 cm below umbilicus (2 fingerbreadths)	U–2
3 days	3 cm below umbilicus (3 fingerbreadths)	U–3
7 days	Palpable at the symphysis pubis	
10 days	Not palpable	

Assessment and Documentation of Lochia Flow

- Pattern of lochia flow progresses from lochia rubra to serosa to alba; should not reverse.
- Lochia should contain no large clots.
- Lochia odor is similar to that of menstrual blood.
- Document lochia in amounts described as scant, small, moderate, heavy (Fig. 12-3).
- Always include the time factor associated with the flow of lochia.

Scant: Blood only on tissue when wiped or 1- to 2-inch stain

Light: 4-inch or less stain

Moderate: Less than 6-inch stain

Heavy: Saturated pad

Figure 12-3 Assessment of lochia flow in 1 hour.

ASSESSMENT AND CARE OF THE PERINEUM

The REEDA Acronym to Guide the Perineal Assessment					
Points	Redness	Edema	Ecchymosis	Discharge	Approximation
0	None	None	None	None	Closed
1	Within 0.25 cm of incision bilaterally	Less than 1 cm from incision	1–2 cm from incision	Serum	Skin separation 3 mm or less
2	Within 0.5 cm of incision bilaterally	1–2 cm from incision	0.25–1 cm bilaterally or 0.5–2 cm unilaterally	Serosanguineous	Skin and subcutaneous fat separated
3	Beyond 0.5 cm of incision bilaterally	Greater than 2 cm from incision	Greater that 1 cm bilaterally or 2 cm unilaterally	Bloody, purulent	Skin, subcutaneous fat, and fascial separation

Providing Early Episiotomy Care

1. Apply an ice bag or commercial cold pack, wrapped in a cover, to the perineum during the first 24 hours. Application of cold provides local anesthesia and promotes vasoconstriction while reducing edema and the incidence of peripheral bleeding.

2. After 24 hours, encourage the use of moist heat (sitz bath) between 100° and 105°F for 20 minutes three to four times/day. The sitz bath increases circulation to the perineum, enhances blood flow to the tissues, reduces edema, and promotes healing.

3. Dry heat, in the form of a commercial perineal "hot pack," may also be used. Women should be cautioned to apply a washcloth or gauze square between the hot pack and their skin to prevent a potential burn.

Assessment and Interventions for the Urinary System

Patient's Signs and Symptoms	Nursing Interventions
Location of fundus above the baseline level	Promote voiding: Provide privacy; turn on the lavatory faucet.
Fundus displaced from midline	Promote hydration.
Bulge of bladder above the symphysis pubis	Promote ambulation.
Frequent voiding of <150 mL of urine; urinary output disproportionate to fluid intake Bladder discomfort	Administer an analgesic before voiding, as prescribed. Place ice on the perineum to reduce swelling and pain. Encourage the use of a sitz bath.

Special Considerations for Assessment and Care After a Cesarean Birth

In addition to the BUBBLE-HE assessment:

- Facilitate bonding (recovery from anesthesia and incision pain may inhibit maternal–newborn bonding).
- Assess REEDA as well as warmth, redness, and tenderness around the incision.
- Monitor anesthesia recovery.
- Facilitate pulmonary exercises.
- Prevent deep venous thrombosis (DVT)—with leg exercises (flexion and extension of the knee) and application of compression boots as ordered by the physician.

PROMOTION OF INFANT NOURISHMENT

Assessing for Infant Feeding-Readiness

The infant demonstrates readiness for feeding when she:

- Begins to stir.
- Bobs the head against the mattress or mother's neck/shoulder.
- Makes hand-to-mouth or hand-to-hand movements.
- Exhibits sucking or licking.
- Exhibits rooting.
- Demonstrates increased activity; arms and legs flexed; hands positioned in a fist.

Assessing for Milk Let-down

Cues that indicate that the milk let-down reflex has occurred:

- The mother reports a tingling sensation in the nipples (not always present).
- The infant's quick, shallow sucking pattern transitions to a slower, more drawing pattern.
- The infant exhibits audible swallowing.
- The mother reports uterine cramping; increased lochia may be present.
- The mother states she feels extremely relaxed during the feeding.
- The opposite breast may leak milk.

Assessing Infant Weight Gain During the Early Days of Life

- Expected loss: Up to 5% of birth weight
- Greater than 7% weight loss indicates need for closer assessment/evaluation

Assessing Maternal–Infant Attachment

Assess for the following indicators:

Does the mother show eagerness to feed and care for her infant?

What is her response when the baby cries?

Does she make eye contact when holding and feeding her baby?

CLINICAL ALERTS

Proper Technique for Uterine Palpation

Never palpate the uterus without supporting the lower uterine segment. Failure to do so may result in uterine inversion and hemorrhage.

Assessing for a Hematoma After an Episiotomy

- Look for discoloration of the perineum.
- Listen for the patient's complaints or expression of severe perineal pain.
- Observe for edema of the area.
- Listen for the patient's expression of a need to defecate (the hematoma may cause rectal pressure).
- Don sterile gloves; gently palpate the area and observe for the patient's degree of sensitivity to the area by touch.
- Call the physician or nurse-midwife to report the findings immediately if hematoma is present. The bleeding that has produced the hematoma must be promptly identified and halted.

Teaching the Patient to Avoid the Knee–Chest Position

Teach the patient to avoid a knee–chest position until at least the third postpartal week. This position causes the vagina to open. Since the cervical os is still open to some extent, there is a danger that air can enter the vagina, pass into the cervix and enter the open blood sinuses inside the uterus. Entry of air into the circulatory system can cause an air embolus.

MEDICATIONS

Commonly Used Medications in the Postpartum Period			
Classification	**Medication**	**Dose and Safety of Use in Breastfeeding Mothers**	**Indication for Use During the Postpartum Period**
Stool Softener	Docusate sodium (Colace)	50–500 mg by mouth daily until bowel movements are normal Not contraindicated in breastfeeding mother	Used in the treatment of constipation

Classification	Medication	Dose and Safety of Use in Breastfeeding Mothers	Indication for Use During the Postpartum Period
Stool Softener	Bisacodyl (Dulcolax)	10–30 mg by mouth until bowel movements are normal Not contraindicated in breastfeeding mother	Used in the treatment of constipation
Topical Anesthetic	Lidocaine spray	Apply spray to the perineal area after sitz bath or perineum care. Not contraindicated in breastfeeding mother	Used on the skin to relieve pain and itching
Hemorrhoid Care	Witch hazel (Tucks)	Apply to the perineal area after sitz bath or perineum care. Not contraindicated in breastfeeding mother.	Used on the skin to relieve the itching, burning, and irritation associated with hemorrhoids
Nonsteroidal Anti-inflammatory Drugs (NSAIDs)	Ibuprofen (Motrin)	400 mg by mouth every 4–6 hours as needed for pain Not contraindicated in breastfeeding mother	Used for the treatment of mild to moderate pain
Opioid Analgesics	Propoxyphene napsylate and acetaminophen (Darvocet)	Take one tablet by mouth every 4 hours as needed for pain. Not contraindicated in breastfeeding mother	Used for the treatment of moderate to severe pain
Opioid Analgesics	Oxycodone and acetaminophen (Percocet)	Take one to two tablets every 4–6 hours as needed for pain. Not contraindicated in breastfeeding mother	Used for the treatment of moderate to severe pain

Breastfeeding and Afterpains

Analgesics such as ibuprofen (Advil, Motrin) or naproxen (Aleve, Anaprox) are frequently administered to lessen the discomforts of afterpains. Breastfeeding women should take pain medication approximately 30 minutes before nursing the baby to achieve maximum pain relief and to minimize the amount of medication that is transferred in the breast milk.

MEDICATIONS

Methylergonovine (meth-ill-er-goe-**noe**-veen); Methergine

Pregnancy Category C

Indications Prevention and treatment of postpartum and postabortion hemorrhage caused by uterine atony or subinvolution

Actions Directly stimulates uterine and vascular smooth muscle

Therapeutic Effects Uterine contraction

Pharmacokinetics
Absorption Well absorbed following oral or IM administration
Onset of Action Oral: 5 to 10 minutes; IM: 2 to 5 minutes; IV: Immediately
Distribution Oral: 3 hours; IM: 3 hours; IV: 45 minutes. Enters breast milk in small quantities
Metabolism and Excretion Probably metabolized by the liver
Half-life: 30–120 minutes

Contraindications and Precautions
Contraindicated in Hypersensitivity. Should not be used to induce labor.
Use cautiously in Hypertensive or eclamptic patients (more susceptible to hypertensive and arrhythmogenic side effects); severe hepatic or renal disease; sepsis
Exercise extreme caution in Third stage of labor

Adverse Reactions and Side Effects
CNS Dizziness, headache
Eye, ear, nose, throat Tinnitus
Respiratory Dyspnea
Cardiovascular Hypotension, arrhythmias, chest pain, hypertension, palpitations
Gastrointestinal Nausea, vomiting

Genitourinary Cramps
Dermatological Diaphoresis

Route and Dosage
PO: 200–400 mcg (0.4–0.6 mg) q6–12hr for 2–7 days
IM: IV: 200 mcg (0.2 mg) after delivery of fetal anterior shoulder, after delivery of the placenta, or during the puerperium; may be repeated as required at intervals of 2–4 hours up to 5 doses

Nursing Implications
1. Physical assessment: Monitor blood pressure, heart rate and uterine response frequently during medication administration. Notify the primary health care provider if uterine relaxation becomes prolonged or if character of vaginal bleeding changes.
2. Assess for signs of ergotism (cold, numb fingers and toes, chest pain, nausea, vomiting, headache, muscle pain, weakness)

Data from Deglin, J.H., & Vallerand, A.H. (2009). Davis's drug guide for nurses (11th ed.) Philadelphia: F.A. Davis.

 Procedure 12-1 Preparing a Sitz Bath

Purpose
To facilitate healing through the application of moist heat.

Equipment
- Sitz bath tub/toilet insert with water receptacle
- Medications to be added to water or saline, as ordered
- Towels for drying the perineal area after the treatment
- Clean perineal pad to be applied after the treatment

Steps

1. Explain the procedure to the patient to ensure she understands that a sitz bath is a method for applying moist heat to the perineum to facilitate healing and comfort.
2. Wash your hands, identify the patient, and explain the procedure.

(continued)

Procedure 12-1 (Continued)

3. Assess the patient to confirm that she is able to ambulate to the bathroom.

4. Assemble equipment and ensure that all equipment is clean.

5. Raise the toilet seat in the patient's bathroom.

6. Insert the sitz bath apparatus into the toilet. The overflow opening should be directed toward the back of the toilet.

7. Fill the collecting bag with water or saline, as directed, at the appropriate temperature (105°F [41°C]).

8. Test the water temperature. It should feel comfortably warm on the wrist.

9. If prescribed, add medications to the solution.

10. Hang the bag overhead to allow a steady stream of water to flow from the bag, through the tubing, and into the reservoir.

11. Assist the ambulating patient to the bathroom. Help with removal of the perineal pad from front to back. Assist the patient to sit in the basin.

12. Instruct the patient to use the tubing clamp to regulate the flow of water. Ensure that the patient is adequately covered with a robe or blankets to prevent chilling.

13. Verify that the call bell is within reach and provide for privacy.

14. Encourage the patient to remain in the sitz bath for approximately 20 minutes.

15. Provide assistance with drying the perineal area and applying a clean perineal pad by grasping the pad by the ends or bottom side.

Procedure 12-1 (Continued)

16. Assist the patient back to the room.

17. Assess the patient's response to the procedure. Reinforce teaching about continued perineal care at home.

18. Document procedure and patient's response.

Clinical Alert The warm environment associated with a sitz bath may cause the patient to feel light-headed or dizzy. It is important to monitor the patient frequently throughout the intervention to ensure safety and tolerance.

Teach the Patient

1. The benefits of using the sitz bath, which include enhanced hygiene, comfort, and improved circulation

2. To use the sitz bath as often as recommended— usually three to four times per day or as needed for discomfort

3. To contact the nursing staff immediately if she becomes light-headed or dizzy

4. To check the temperature of the solution before use. Applying water or solution that is too warm may result in local trauma or burns to the area

Note

If the patient prefers to prepare a sitz bath in the tub at home, she should be instructed not to use the same water for bathing. Instead, fresh water should be drawn for washing to diminish the potential for infection.

Caution

The nurse must check the temperature of the water before administration of the sitz bath to ensure that it is not too warm.

ETHNOCULTURAL CONSIDERATIONS

Pregnancy-Related Skin Changes in the Puerperium

Although abdominal stretch marks (striae gravidarum) appear more pronounced immediately after childbirth, they tend to fade over the following 6 months. In Caucasian women, striae become pale and white in color; in African American women, they will appear as a slightly darker pigment.

Cultural Influences and Interventions for Breastfeeding Discomfort

Many non-Western cultures such as Asian, Latin, and African cultures embrace a hot and cold "humoral theory." Breastfeeding mothers from these cultures may choose not to use a cold modality for the relief of breast engorgement or discomfort. Although the nurse may explain the clinical rationale for applying ice packs to the breasts, the patient is culturally bound to adhere to her beliefs. Nurses must remain sensitive to culturally influenced customs and allow patients to use relief measures that do not conflict with their personal beliefs.

TEACHING THE FAMILY

Perineal Care

To enhance the patient's understanding about proper perineal care, provide the following instructions:

- Fill the squeeze/peri bottle with warm tap water (comfortable to your wrist).
- Sit on the toilet with the bottle positioned between your legs. Aim the bottle opening at your perineum and spray so that the water moves from front to back. Do not separate the labia and do not spray the water into your vagina. Empty the entire bottle over the perineum (takes about 2 minutes).
- Gently pat the area dry with toilet paper or cotton wipes. Move from front to back. Use each wipe once and drop into toilet.
- Grasp the bottom side or ends of a clean perineal pad and apply it from front to back.

Pain Relief Measures

- Suggest nonpharmacological methods for pain relief such as imagery, therapeutic touch, relaxation, distraction, and interaction with the infant.
- Provide pain relief by administering prescribed agents such as ibuprofen, propoxyphene napsylate/acetaminophen (Darvocet-N), or oxycodone/acetaminophen (Percocet).
- Suggest over-the-counter medications and alternative therapies such as tea tree oil for self-care after hospital discharge.

- Teach the patient that medications such as acetaminophen or ibuprofen may be equally as effective as narcotic analgesics.
- Reassure the patient that the pain and discomfort should not persist beyond 5 to 7 days, and that because the episiotomy sutures are made of an absorbable material, they will not need to be removed.
  - Instruct breastfeeding mothers to wash the nipples with warm water.
  - Avoid soaps because they have a drying effect and cause cracked nipples.
  - Avoid breast creams because they block the natural oil secreted by the Montgomery tubercles and may contain alcohol.
  - Avoid creams or oils that contain vitamin E because the infant may absorb toxic amounts of the fat-soluble vitamin.

Storage of Breast Milk

Freshly pumped breast milk can be safely stored:

- At room temperature for 4 hours
- Refrigerated at 34 to 39° F (0°C) for 5 to 7 days after collection
- Frozen at 0°F (–19°C) for 6 to 12 months (Lawrence & Lawrence, 2005)

Manual (Hand) and Electric Expression of Breast Milk

- Sometimes necessary due to medical complications or occupational reasons
- Frequent expression of breast milk during the early postpartum period helps to establish and increase the milk supply for later breastfeeding needs
- Once lactation is established, the mother may express milk either manually or with an electric breast pump, whichever method is most convenient

Preventing Infant Nipple Confusion

- The infant exhibits difficulty with latch-on.
- Teach parents to avoid bottles until breast feeding is well established (3 to 4 weeks).

Preparing Infant Formula

Provide the following safety instructions to parents who plan to formula feed their infant:

- Wash hands before beginning to prepare formula and after any interruptions.
- Always shake and wash tops of liquid formula cans before opening.
- Reconstitute the formula according to the manufacturer's recommendations.
- Store the ready-to-feed formula according to the manufacturer's recommendations.
- Shake the bottle well before feeding.
- Discard any formula that the infant does not drink.
- Wash thoroughly and sterilize all equipment used to prepare the infant formula and use a bottle and nipple brush to remove milk residue.
- Replace the nipples regularly.

Helping Older Siblings Adjust to the New Baby

- Talk with the child(ren) about their feelings regarding the new baby. Listen and validate their feelings.
- Teach the older sibling how to play with the new baby; encourage gentleness.
- Help develop the child's self-esteem by giving him/her special jobs (e.g., bringing the diaper when you are changing the baby). Praise each contribution.
- Praise age-appropriate behaviors and do not criticize regressive behaviors.
- Set aside time to be alone with the older sibling and remind him that he is loved very much.

Warning Signs Indicative of Poor Sibling Adjustment
Professional help may be needed if the child:

- Continually avoids or ignores the baby
- Shows the baby no affection
- Is consistently angry, taunting, or demonstrating aggressive behavior toward the baby or other family members
- Experiences nightmares and sleeping difficulties (International Childbirth Education Association [ICEA], 2003)

Maternal Mood Changes During the Postpartal Period

Teach the mother and her partner that:

- Emotional changes (e.g., sadness, weepiness) often appear on the second or third postpartal day
- "Mood swings" and periods of unexpected crying or anxiety occur in 70%–80% of postpartal women
- The health care provider should be contacted if the following symptoms persist for more than 2 weeks:
  - Crying excessively
  - Significant changes in appetite
  - Feeling helpless
  - Experiencing extreme worry, concern
  - Difficulty sleeping or wanting to sleep all of the time
  - Inability to care for self or for the baby
  - Experiencing panic attack(s)
  - Experiencing a fear of harming self or the baby

ADDITIONAL INFORMATION FOR THE CLINICAL SETTING

Actions to Protect the Infant from Abduction

- Educate personnel, parents, and significant others about various measures that have been implemented to protect the safety of the infant.
- During infant transport from the nursery to the mother's room, all staff must follow the hospital's protocol. In most facilities:
  - Infants may be transported only in a bassinet.
  - Parents are prohibited from carrying the infant in the halls.
  - When identification bracelets are used, they are matched before giving the infant to the mother.
- Instruct mothers to release the infant only to properly identified hospital personnel.
- Ensure that admission photographs and footprints, most likely taken after birth, are affixed to the permanent record
- Follow institutional protocol for infants that have a similar or same last name: frequently, the infants' cribs

and charts indicate the mother's first name, and bear a label that designates a "NAME ALERT."

- Follow institutional protocol for multiple births: the infants' cribs may be labeled with the infant's name followed by a letter of the alphabet (i.e., A, B, C, or D).
- Ensure that all hospital personnel follow institutional identification protocol: prominently displayed photo identification when working in the maternal–child unit; freedom to question any suspicious activity or individuals who are present on the maternal–child unit.
- Ensure that all visitors follow institutional identification protocol: prominently displayed identification badges while on the maternal–child unit.

Postpartum Discharge Teaching: Danger Signs to Report

Alert patients to signs and symptoms to report to the health care provider. Ensure that the patient is given written information and knows how to reach her care provider. She should immediately report any of the following:

- Temperature >100.4°F (38.0°C), chills, or flu-like symptoms
- Abdominal incision that is red, tender to touch, or painful, or if edges of the incision have separated.
- Difficulty initiating urination, urinary frequency, or painful urination
- Increased vaginal bleeding with or without clots, or foul-smelling vaginal discharge
- Persistent pain or marked swelling at the site of a perineal laceration or episiotomy
- Swelling or masses in the breasts; red streaks; shooting pain in the breasts; or cracked, bleeding nipples.
- Swelling, warmth, tenderness, or painful areas in the legs
- Blurred vision or persistent headache that is not relieved by pain medication
- Overwhelming feelings of sadness or an inability to care for self or the baby

RESOURCES

American Academy of Pediatrics (AAP):
http://www.aap.org/healthtopics/breastfeeding.cfm

American College of Obstetricians and Gynecologists (ACOG):
http://www.acog.org/navbar/current/publications.cfm

Association of Women's Health, Obstetric and Neonatal Nurses
(AWHONN): http://awhonn.org/awhonn/

International Childbirth Education Association (ICEA):
http://icea.org/

Lactation Education Resources: http://www.leron-line.com/

La Leche League International:
http://www.lalecheleague.org/philosophy.html

REFERENCES

Deglin, J.H., & Vallerand, A.H. (2009). *Davis's drug guide for nurses* (11th ed.). Philadelphia: F.A. Davis.

International Childbirth Education Association (ICEA). (2003). *Siblings and the new baby.* (Brochure). Minneapolis, MN: Author.

Lawrence, R., & Lawrence, R. (2005). *Breastfeeding: A guide for the medical profession* (6th ed.). Philadelphia: Elsevier Mosby.

13

Caring for the Woman Experiencing Complications During the Postpartal Period

KEY TERMS

endometritis – Postpartum uterine infection

hematoma – Collection of blood in tissue; results from damage to a blood vessel

Homans' sign – Early sign of deep venous thrombosis in the leg – upon dorsiflexion, pain occurs from inflammation of the blood vessel. A negative Homans' sign does not rule out deep venous thrombosis.

magnetic resonance imaging (MRI) – Diagnostic test that uses electromagnetic energy to provide images of the heart, large blood vessels, brain, and soft tissues. In obstetrics, may be used to evaluate fetal structures, the placenta, and amniotic fluid volume.

mastitis – Infection in a breast; typically characterized by redness and tenderness in the affected breast along with influenza-like symptoms

postpartum – Occurring after birth (mother)

> **p. depression** Symptoms including depressed mood or decreased interest in previously enjoyable activities, occurring within 6 months after giving birth and lasting longer than postpartum blues.

> **p. hemorrhage** Excessive bleeding after childbirth; traditionally defined as a blood loss greater than 500 mL after a vaginal birth and 1000 mL or more after a cesarean birth.

p. psychosis Rare, severe form of mental illness; symptoms begin as postpartum blues or depression. However, distinguishing signs of psychosis, including hallucinations, delusions, agitation, confusion, and suicidal and homicidal thoughts can occur.

thrombophlebitis – Obstruction of a vein with secondary clot formation

thrombosis – Formation or presence of a blood clot within the vascular system

FOCUSED ASSESSMENT

Postpartum Hemorrhage (PPH)

Early hemorrhage: Occurs within first 24 hours after birth
Late hemorrhage: Occurs more than 24 hours after birth but <6 weeks postpartum

Early Postpartum Hemorrhage

Acronyms for Causes of Early Postpartum Hemorrhage	
"LARRY" (common causes of PPH)	**"4 T's" (factors associated with PPH)**
L: Lacerations	**T:** Tone (uterine)
A: Atony	**T:** Trauma (genital tract)
R: Retained placental tissue	**T:** Tissue (retained placenta)
R: Ruptured uterus	**T:** Thrombin (maternal coagulation disorders)
Y: "You pulled too hard on the cord!"	

Using a Standardized Assessment for Blood Loss After Childbirth
- Scant: Peripad blood stain <2 inches (<10 mL) within 1 hour
- Small: Peripad blood stain >2 inches, >4 inches (10–25 mL) within 1 hour
- Moderate: Peripad blood stain >4 inches but <6 inches (25–50 mL) within 1 hour
- Large: Peripad blood stain >6 inches to saturated peripad (50–80 mL) within 1 hour (Lugenbiehl et al., 1990)

Characteristics that Point to the Source of Postpartal Bleeding

Source	Color	Uterus
Uterine Atony	Dark red with clots	Soft/boggy
Retained Placenta	Dark red with clots	Soft/boggy
Lacerations of Cervix or Vagina	Bright red	Firm, contracted

Risk Factors for Uterine Atony

Uterine overdistention
  Large baby
  Multiple gestation
  Hydramnios
Bladder distention
Prolonged first and/or second stage labor
Precipitous labor

Labor induction/augmentation with
  Pitocin
Tocolytic therapy (especially with
  magnesium sulfate)
High parity
Retained placental fragments
Halogenated anesthetic agents
Prolonged/mismanaged third stage
  of labor

If hemorrhage results from uterine atony, perform continual fundal massage with lower uterine segment support.

Procedure 13-1 Performing Fundal Massage

Purpose

Fundal massage is used as an emergency measure to contract the uterus that is soft and boggy due to atony. It is performed to promote uterine tone and consistency and minimize the risk of hemorrhage. Uterine atony may result from prolonged labor, rapid or precipitous labor and birth, high parity, medications during labor (i.e., oxytocin, magnesium sulfate, inhalation anesthesia), intra-amniotic infection, operative delivery, and uterine overdistention from multiple gestation, hydramnios, or macrosomia.

Equipment

- Clean examination gloves
- Disposable cleansing wipes
- Two clean peripads

Procedure 13-1 (Continued)

Preexamination Preparation

1. Wash and dry hands; explain the procedure and its purpose to the patient. Ensure privacy.
2. Assemble necessary equipment, including clean examination gloves, disposable cleansing wipes, and clean peripads.
3. Ask the patient to void, unless fundal massage must be performed immediately due to excessive bleeding
4. Assist the woman to a supine position with the knees flexed and the feet placed together.

Steps

1. Don gloves, remove the peripad, and inspect the perineum. Observe the character and amount of drainage on the pad and the presence of clots. Apply a clean peripad.
2. Place one hand on the abdomen, just above the symphysis pubis.
3. Place the other hand around the top of the fundus.
4. With the lower hand maintained in a stable position, rotate the upper hand and massage the uterus until it is firm. Avoid overmassaging the uterus. Massaging a firm uterus may result in muscle fatigue and uterine relaxation. Overly aggressive fundal massage may result in uterine prolapse.

(continued)

Procedure 13-1 (Continued)

5. Once the uterus has become firm, *gently* press the fundus between the hands. Apply a slight downward pressure against the lower hand.

6. Observe the perineum for the passage of clots and the amount of bleeding.

7. Once the uterus remains firm, cleanse the perineum and apply a clean peripad. Dispose of the soiled gloves and pads according to institutional policy.

8. Document the findings. Continue to assess the fundus and vaginal drainage according to institutional protocol. Alert the physician or nurse midwife if the fundus does not remain contracted or if bleeding persists.

Risk Factors for Postpartum Hemorrhage from Tissue Trauma

- Rapid second stage labor
- Rapid/precipitous labor (<3 hours from onset to birth)
- Operative vaginal deliveries (forceps, vacuum extraction)
- Fetal manipulation (extrauterine or intrauterine version, corkscrew maneuver for shoulder dystocia [corkscrew maneuver: a progressive 180 degree manual rotation of the baby's posterior shoulder to release the impacted anterior shoulder])
- Large episiotomy, including extension
- Large infant
- Cesarean birth
- Uterine rupture (increased incidence with previous uterine surgery, tetanic contractions, labor stimulation, versions, placental attachment abnormalities)

Source: Cunningham et al. (2005).

CLINICAL ALERTS

Postpartal Blood Loss and Vital Signs

In the presence of a firm uterus, continuous vaginal bleeding in a slow but steady trickle, with or without clots, can result in significant blood loss. Normal physiological adaptations in pregnancy mean that a large loss of blood can occur before changes in vital signs (decreased blood pressure and increased pulse) are evident. The usual signs of shock (restlessness, anxiety, pallor, cool, clammy skin, increased pulse, tachypnea, shaking, decreased blood pressure) may not be evident until 30% to 40% of the patient's total circulating blood volume has been lost. A decrease in the mean arterial pressure (MAP) measurement may be the first indicator of hypovolemia. The lack of objective signs and symptoms may lead to a delay in treatment.

Postpartal Blood Loss and the Behavioral Assessment

Assess the patient for:

- Restlessness
- Level of consciousness
- Vague complaints
- Level of pain

Immediate Intervention for Uterine Atony

As soon as excessive blood loss is noted, begin fundal massage. Support the lower uterine segment by placing a hand in a slight "C" position just above the symphysis pubis. Do not express clots if the uterus does not become firm with massage. The clots may protect the patient from an even greater blood loss.

Lacerations of the Cervix or Vaginal Canal

Lacerations are usually internal and are not visible when the nurse examines the perineum. Identifying either a vaginal wall or cervical laceration usually requires that the physician or midwife examine the patient while she is in the lithotomy position. Often the physician locates and repairs a laceration before the patient's transfer to the postpartum unit.

Hematoma

- May cause excessive blood loss and severe discomfort and tenderness
- Occurs most frequently in the vulva; also occurs in the vagina and retroperitoneal area (Figs. 13-1 and 13-2).
- Risk factors
  - Genital tract lacerations

- Episiotomy
- Operative vaginal delivery
- Difficult or prolonged second stage of labor
- Nulliparity
- Examination may reveal discoloration, bulging of tissue at hematoma site
- Treatment: ice (first 24 hours); sitz baths (after 24 hours); analgesics; may require incision and drainage (if larger than 5 cm)

Late Postpartum Hemorrhage

- Causes
  - Retained placental fragments
  - Subinvolution
  - Uterine infection

Figure 13-1 Vulvar hematoma.

Figure 13-2 Vaginal wall hematoma.

- Treatment
  - Ergonovine medication (Ergotrate; methergine)
  - Antibiotics
  - Dilation and curettage

Postpartum Infection

May involve:

- Endometrium (endometritis)
- Operative wound (cesarean incision; episiotomy)
- Urinary tract
- Breasts (mastitis) (Fig. 13-3)
- Septic pelvic thrombophlebitis

Figure 13-3 Mastitis.

Postpartum Infection: Endometritis

Type of Infection	Risk Factors	Onset	Signs and Symptoms	Causative Organisms	Diagnosis Based on	Collaborative Treatment	Prognosis and Complications
Endometritis (inflammation and infection of the inner lining of the uterus) Incidence: Vaginal birth: 1%–3% and cesarean birth 10%–20% (Kennedy, 2005)	Cesarean birth Prolonged rupture of the membranes, multiple vaginal examinations, internal electronic fetal heart rate (FHR) monitoring, low socio-economic status, poor nutrition, young age, diabetes, prior genital infection, lapse in aseptic technique, anemia, smoking, nulliparity, operative vaginal delivery, poor postpartum perineal care	2–4 days following childbirth	Prolonged fever ≥100.4°F (38°C), foul smelling lochia, uterine or abdominal tenderness, chills, poor appetite, malaise, increased pulse rate, cramping pain, increased WBC count (above 20–30,000)	Normal vaginal flora and enteric bacteria	Clinical signs and symptoms Vaginal and bimanual examination Laboratory test results: Culture of lochia; elevated WBC count (Must also rule out urinary tract infection.)	1. MD/CNM: Order antibiotics. 2. Treat symptoms: a. Rest b. Antipyretics c. Increase fluid intake. d. Encourage high-protein, high-vitamin C foods. e. Promote uterine drainage via ambulation and Fowler's position. f. Instruct in perineal care. 3. Explain treatments to patient/family.	90%–95% improvement within 48–72 hours after treatment. May be discharged on oral antibiotics. *Complication:* Extension of infections via lymphatic system to connective tissues (pelvic infection) Dehiscence of cesarean section incision or episiotomy Peritonitis

4. Home antibiotic therapy may need to be arranged with follow-up by a home care nurse.
5. Promote infant attachment.

Sources: The American Academy of Pediatrics (AAP) & The American College of Obstetricians and Gynecologists (ACOG), 2007; Cunningham et al. (2005); Gibbs, Sweet, & Duff (2004); Kennedy (2007).

Postpartum Infection: Wound Infections

Type of Infection	Risk Factors	Onset	Signs and Symptoms for ALL	Causative Organisms	Diagnosis Based on	Collaborative Treatment	Prognosis and Complications
Wound Infections *Perineal* Incidence: 0.35%–10% *Cesarean incision* Incidence: 3%–5%	Endometritis (infected lochia), poor hygiene, fecal contamination, hematoma ALL wound infections: obesity, diabetes, hypertension, immunosuppression, malnutrition, anemia, hemorrhage, prolonged labor, chorioamnionitis prolonged rupture of membranes, hematoma	Early: 48 hours Late: 6–8 days	Pain, foul-smelling discharge, edema, low-grade fever Sudden chills, high fever, abdominal tenderness, erythema, edema, warmth of incision, drainage from the incision	Polymicrobial, normal vaginal flora *Staphylococcus aureus,* aerobic streptococci, aerobic and anaerobic bacilli	Clinical signs and symptoms, subjective complaints Clinical signs and symptoms, along with a poor response to antibiotics given for endometritis. Laboratory test results: elevated white blood cell (WBC) count	1. Antibiotics per order 2. May require incision and drainage with placement of drain to facilitate healing by secondary intention.* If packing has been placed in the wound to keep it open and maintain drainage, alert the patient to exercise caution when changing her perineal pads to avoid dislodging the packing. 3. Perineal: Sitz baths; instruct in perineal care	Improvement usually within 24–48 hours; may require long-term antibiotic therapy **Complications** Necrotizing fasciitis, abscess, wound dehiscence

4. Cesarean: Wet to dry dressing changes 3+ times/day
5. Pain medication per order (usually nonsteroidal anti-inflammatory drugs [NSAIDs])
6. Instructions to patient and family about wound care
7. Possible referral for home health or community health nurse visits

*Secondary intention: Healing from the inside of the wound out to the skin.

Sources: Cunningham et al. (2005); Franzblau & Witt (2006); Gibbs, Sweet, & Duff (2004); Kennedy (2007).

Postpartum Infection: Urinary Tract Infections (UTI)

Type of Infection	Risk Factors	Onset	Signs and Symptoms	Causative Organisms	Diagnosis Based on	Collaborative Treatment	Prognosis and Complications
Urinary Tract Infections Incidence: 2%–4%	Catheterization, multiple vaginal exams, poor postpartum hygiene, genital tract trauma, epidural anesthesia, cesarean birth, premature rupture of the membranes, poor nutritional status, history of UTIs during pregnancy, diabetes, decreased bladder sensation after birth	Any time during pregnancy or after birth	May have none. Dysuria (painful urination), frequency, burning on urination, difficulty voiding and/or retention, costovertebral angle tenderness (CVAT), back or suprapubic pain, hematuria (blood in the urine); fever, fatigue, nausea, vomiting	Most common: *Escherichia coli* (60%–90% of all UTIs); *Proteus mirabilis, Klebsiella pneumoniae,* group B hemolytic streptococcus, *Staphylococcus saprophyticus*	Clinical signs and symptoms Laboratory test results: urine culture & sensitivity, presence of leukocytes and blood on urine dipstick	1. Antibiotics per order (usually sulfonamides, aminopenicillins, anti-infectives, nitrofurantoin, or cephalosporins × 3 to 10 days depending on symptoms). Teach importance of taking all medication. 2. Encourage increased fluid intake, including cranberry juice. 3. Encourage rest. 4. Instruct in perineal care.	Improvement within 48–72 hours after initiation of antibiotic therapy Can reoccur with bacteremia and scarring of the kidney followed by hypertension and kidney damage.

5. Instruct in monitoring temperature, bladder function, normal appearance of urine.
6. Instruct in/administer antipyretics, antispasmodics, analgesics, and antiemetics.
7. Educate the patient to avoid recurrence:
   - When intercourse resumes, void following
   - Clean from front to back

Data from Cunningham et al. (2005); Franzblau & Witt (2006); Kennedy (2007).

Postpartum Infection: Mastitis

Type of Infection	Risk Factors	Onset	Signs and Symptoms	Causative Organisms	Diagnosis Based on	Collaborative Treatment	Prognosis and Complications
Mastitis	Milk stasis, plugged milk duct, infrequent breastfeeding, fatigue, nipple trauma, primiparity	3–4 weeks postpartum	Warm, tender, hardened area on breast (usually only one), enlarged axillary lymph nodes, fever (up to 102°F 38.9°C]), chills, generalized aching, headache, malaise	Most common: *Staphylococcus. aureus*; also: *Haemophilus parainfluenzae* (from infant's mouth and nose), *Candida albicans*, *Streptococcus viridans*	Clinical signs and symptoms Laboratory test results: culture of breast milk	1. Notify the MD/CNM. 2. Initiate antibiotics. 3. Continue breastfeeding or manual/electrical expression of milk to maintain lactation. May be instructed to discard the milk. 4. Promote rest. 5. Increase fluid intake. 6. Pump breast after infant feeding to ensure breast is empty. 7. Apply warm compress or ice to breast for comfort. 8. Administer antipyretics	Improvement within 24–48 hours after initiation of antibiotics *Complication:* Breast abscess If breast abscess occurs: Must discontinue breastfeeding on the affected side—may lead to decreased maternal–infant attachment, low self-esteem and feelings of disappointment and guilt.

9. Instruct in high-protein, high-vitamin C diet.
10. Educate regarding hygiene and prevention of future recurrence.
11. Assess the infant's mouth for signs of thrush (oral *Candida*), an overgrowth of fungal organisms related to the mother's antibiotic therapy.

Sources: Lawrence & Lawrence (2005); Mass (2004).

Postpartum Infection: Septic Pelvic Thrombophlebitis

Type of Infection	Risk Factors	Onset	Signs and Symptoms	Causative Organisms	Diagnosis Based on	Collaborative Treatment	Prognosis and Complications
Septic Pelvic Thrombophlebitis	Cesarean birth, genital tract lacerations, history of varicosities, immobility, operative vaginal delivery, prolonged labor, multiple vaginal exams	48 hours to 4–6 weeks post partum	Fever ≥ 102.2°F (39°C) with spikes after initiation of antibiotic therapy, abdominal and/or back pain, chills, increased pulse (resting tachycardia), few or absent bowel sounds	Normal vaginal flora and enteric bacteria—is usually an extension of endometritis	Clinical signs and symptoms. Pelvic CT or MRI to confirm the clinical picture. Laboratory test results: CBC; coagulation profile; blood chemistries	1. MD/CNM: prescribe antibiotics. 2. Add heparin therapy to increase APTT (activated partial thromboplastin time) to 1.5–2 times the normal value. 3. Rest in Fowler's position. 4. High-protein, high-vitamin C diet 5. Increased fluids 6. Comfort measures: Pain medications, antipyretics 7. Complementary therapies: Heat, cold, relaxation, music, touch, etc. 8. Explain treatments. 9. Promote infant attachment.	Improvement usually within 48–72 hours of heparin initiation; may need to continue anticoagulant therapy for 6 months (7–10 days of heparin) followed by warfarin (Coumadin) *Complication*: Pulmonary embolism Possible decreased infant attachment; prolonged hospitalization

Sources: Cunningham et al. (2005); Franzblau & Witt (2006); Gibbs, Sweet, & Duff (2004).

Thrombophlebitis and Thrombosis

- Inflammation of the venous circulation and blood clot formation.
- Typically occurs in the lower extremities.
- Related to venous stasis and hypercoagulation associated with pregnancy.
- Early ambulation is key in prevention.
- Risk factors:
  - Smoking
  - Obesity
  - Age >35 years
  - Pregnancy-related complications (e.g., preeclampsia)
  - Immobility
  - Grand multiparity
  - Operative childbirth
  - Hemorrhage
  - Sepsis
  - Chronic health problems (e.g., inflammatory bowel disease, lupus erythematosus, varicose veins, factor V Leiden mutation)
  - History of DVT
- Symptoms may include tenderness, edema, redness, localized heat, decreased peripheral pulse, palpable cord, change in skin color, positive Homans' sign.
- Diagnosis with venous duplex ultrasonography (real-time imaging and Doppler flow studies); magnetic resonance imaging (MRI).
- Management:
  - Bedrest
  - Anticoagulation therapy (heparin; warfarin)
  - Analgesics
  - Elevation of affected extremity
  - Elastic support to affected leg
  - Increased fluid intake
  - Local application of moist, warm packs
- Nursing considerations:
  - Assess for bleeding.
  - Assess circulation to affected extremity.
  - Measure and document circumference to affected extremity.
  - Provide discharge teaching (e.g., medication side effects; avoidance of salicylic acid).

Recognizing Signs and Symptoms Indicative of DVT

Additional signs and symptoms that may be associated with DVT include elevated temperature, cough, tachycardia, hemoptysis, pleuritic chest pain and increasing apprehension. The presence of dyspnea and tachypnea may signal pulmonary embolism. Pulmonary embolism is a complication of DVT that occurs when part of a blood clot breaks away and travels to the pulmonary artery, where it occludes the vessel and obstructs blood flow to the lungs.

Clinical Alert

Avoid Extremity Massage When DVT Is Suspected

If DVT is present or suspected, it is essential to refrain from massaging the affected area. This action could loosen the clot and result in a pulmonary or cerebral embolism.

Postpartum Psychosocial Complications

May include:

- Postpartum blues (within first 2 weeks after childbirth; common; self-limiting)
- Postpartum depression (occurs in 8% to 15% of women; onset within the first year after childbirth; treated with psychotherapy, medications, and complementary therapies)
- Postpartum psychosis (rare, characterized by hallucinations, delusions, agitation, confusion, suicidal/homicidal thoughts, loss of touch with reality)

Signs and Symptoms of Postpartum Depression

Decreased appetite	Excessive fears about the infant's health/safety
Insomnia or fragmented sleep	Hopelessness
Fatigue	Negativity
Inability to concentrate	Complaints about "loss of self" and a
Confusion	"sense of loneliness" (Clemmens
Withdrawal	et al., 2004)
Decreased self-esteem	Guilt
Suicidal thoughts	Decreased interest and functioning in
Infant neglect or abuse	both self and infant care

Data from Beck, Records, & Rice (2006); Clemmens, Driscoll, & Beck (2004); Franzblau (2006); Logsdon et al. (2005); Stoops & Mann (2004).

Recognizing Behavioral Cues that Signal Postpartum Psychosis

- Hyperactivity
- Agitation
- Confusion
- Suspiciousness
- Excessive complaints

DIAGNOSTIC TESTS

Tests to Help Identify a Postpartum Infection

- Complete blood count (CBC) with differential
- Blood cultures if sepsis is suspected
- Urinalysis with culture and sensitivity
- Cervical, uterine or wound culture as needed

Laboratory Findings with Disseminated Intravascular Coagulation (DIC)

- Low hemoglobin
- Low hematocrit
- Low platelets
- Elevated fibrin split/degradation products
- Low fibrinogen

MEDICATIONS

Medications and Nursing Considerations for Postpartum Hemorrhage

Name	Action	Dosage/Route	Contraindications	Nursing Considerations
Oxytocin (Pitocin)	Stimulates uterine smooth muscle and produces contractions similar to those that occur during spontaneous labor.	10 units IM if no IV access; 10–40 units in 1000 cc crystalloid IV fluid (lactated Ringer's or normal saline)	Hypersensitivity	Monitor uterine response. DO NOT administer a bolus of undiluted oxytocin, as it can cause hypotension and cardiac arrhythmias. Consider administration of pain medication for uterine cramping.
Methylergonovine (Methergine)	Causes uterine contractions by stimulating uterine and vascular smooth muscles.	0.1–0.2 mg IM followed by 0.2 mg PO q4–6hr × 24 hours	Hypersensitivity History of, or current elevation of blood pressure	Keep refrigerated. DO NOT add it to IV solutions or mix in a syringe with other medications.
Carboprost* (Hemabate)	Stimulates contractions of the myometrium.	250 mcg IM or directly into the uterus (by MD or CNM); may repeat dosage	Asthma or glaucoma	Do not administer if patient demonstrates shock, as it will not be well absorbed. Keep refrigerated. This medication is VERY expensive.

| Misoprostol (Cytotec) | Acts as a prostaglandin analogue; stimulates powerful contractions of the myometrium. | 400–1000 mcg rectally | Hypersensitivity to prostaglandins | Stable at room temperature Rectal absorption is likely slower than IV medication. Monitor uterine response. Note: Misoprostol is neither marketed by its manufacturer for obstetrical use nor approved by the FDA for obstetrical use although its effectiveness in abating postpartum hemorrhage is now generally accepted. |

*Eighty to ninety percent effective in stopping postpartum hemorrhage when unresponsive to Pitocin or Methergine (Smith & Brennen, 2006).

Sources: Adams, Josephson, & Holland (2005); Cunningham et al., (2005); Smith & Brennan (2006); Tucker (2004); Walters & Wing (2007).

MEDICATIONS

Herbal Medication: Echinacea Purpurea (Ek-i-**neigh**-sha)

Pregnancy Category Injectable form not recommended during pregnancy

Indications Treatment of wounds, injuries, enlarged lymph nodes; prevent and reduce symptoms and duration of common cold and bacterial infections of the upper respiratory tract; used by Native Americans to treat burns and insect and rattlesnake bites

Actions Boosts the immune system by increasing phagocytosis of the WBCs and by inhibiting the bacterial enzyme, hyaluronidase; also stimulates the production of interleukin and interferon; exerts an anti-inflammatory action

Therapeutic Effects Used by proponents to both prevent and treat infections; juice from leaves used as a supportive treatment for vaginal yeast infections; approved in Germany for treatment of the common cold and influenza

Contraindications and Precautions Herb–drug interactions with amiodarone, anabolic steroids, ketoconazole, methotrexate (possible increased hepatic toxicity)

Possible exacerbation of autoimmune diseases (rheumatoid arthritis, lupus, multiple sclerosis, etc.) because of its immune system stimulation properties (no clinical evidence to support)

Is a member of the daisy family: Possible cross-over allergic reaction

Adverse Reactions and Effects No toxicity noted with even extremely high doses of oral *Echinacea*; the most common side effects from oral form are gastrointestinal symptoms and increased urination. INJECTIONS: Side effects are short-term nausea, vomiting, shivering, headache, fever

Route and Dosage Tincture, oral, injection (dosage individualized)

Nursing Implications
1. Be sure to ask every patient if she uses herbal remedies.
2. Instruct the patient that daily dosages of *Echinacea* in an attempt to prevent infections may decrease the immunostimulating effects of this herb.
3. Because the U.S. Food and Drug Administration (FDA) has not approved herbal treatments/remedies, encourage

the patient to be sure that she uses a reputable form of the herb to ensure its quality (Adams, Josephson, & Holland, 2005; Deglin & Vallerand, 2009; Lincoln & Kleiner, 2004).

Warfarin (**war**-fa-rin), Coumadin

Pregnancy Category X

Indications Prevention of thrombosis (clot) formation

Actions Inhibits the hepatic synthesis of coagulation factors II, VII, IX, and X; inhibits the action of vitamin K

Therapeutic Effects Used in patients who are at high risk for development of or who have a history of deep vein thrombosis or other thrombophilia (love of clot formation) conditions

Pharmacokinetics 99% binds to plasma proteins, thereby delaying the effects of warfarin

Route and Dosage Orally; dosage adjusted on the basis of international normalized ratio (INR) results (range is 2.5–15 mg daily)

Contraindications and Precautions

Drug–drug interactions occur with NSAIDs, diuretics, antidepressants, steroids, some antibiotics, vaccines, and vitamin K. Concurrent use with NSAIDs may increase the risk of bleeding.

Herbal supplements such as garlic, ginger, and feverfew may increase the risk of bleeding.

Arnica may increase the anticoagulant effect of warfarin.

Even after the drug is discontinued, its effects may continue for up to 10 days.

Warfarin dosage must be individualized on the basis of prothrombin time results. The INR is now used for dosage adjustments. A normal INR is 2.0–3.5.

Adverse Reactions and Effects Overdosage leads to excessive blood loss that may appear via gastrointestinal bleeding, bleeding from the gums, nosebleeds, petechiae, excessive bruising, etc. The patient begins with heparin therapy for anticoagulation and transitions to warfarin. Because normal clotting factors circulate in the patient's blood stream routinely, several days of both heparin and warfarin therapy may be required for the anti-coagulant effect.

Nursing Implications

1. This drug is dangerous. The patient and family must receive detailed information regarding follow-up care and drug–drug, drug–herb, and food–drug interactions.
2. Instruct the patient to notify the doctor of excessive bruising, to take warfarin at the same time each day, and to avoid activities that could result in a bleeding injury.
3. Be sure the patient receives instructions on foods to minimize/avoid. (Involve the dietitian.)

Data from Deglin, J.H., & Vallerand, A.H. (2009). Davis's Drug Guide for Nurses (11th ed.). Philadelphia: F.A. Davis.

Medications Used to Treat Postpartum Depression		
Selective Serotonin Reuptake Inhibitors (SSRIs)	**Serotonin–Norepinephrine Reuptake Inhibitors (SNRIs)**	**Tricyclics Pamelor (Nortriptyline)**
Fluoxetine (Prozac) Paroxetine (Paxil) Sertraline (Zoloft)	Venlafaxine (Effexor) Duloxetine (Cymbalta)	Imipramine (Tofranil) Doxepin (Sinequan)

TEACHING THE FAMILY

Educating Patients About Risk Factors for Puerperal Infection

- Alert the patient about antepartum or intrapartum events that are risk factors for postpartum infection.
- Alert the family to the importance of promptly notifying the health care provider if symptoms (e.g., low abdominal tenderness; fever; red vaginal drainage beyond 1 week; foul smelling vaginal drainage) occur.
- Inform the family about arrangements for a community health nurse visit after hospital discharge.

Educating Patients About the Prevention of Infection

Teach the patient to:

- Thoroughly wash her hands before and after using the toilet, when changing peripads, changing the baby's diaper, etc. Hand washing with friction removes infection-causing microorganisms.

- Use a squeeze bottle with warm water to cleanse the perineum, then pat the perineum dry, and remove and replace peripads from front to back. Front to back patting and pad removal/application prevents bringing rectal organisms forward to the perineum and vagina.

- Drink extra fluids (eight 8-ounce glasses of water) to increase urine production. The increased blood flow and urine production will decrease the stagnation of microorganisms in the urinary tract.

- Gently wash incisions with soap and water. Be sure to dry the incision completely. If necessary, use a hair dryer set on low heat to ensure that the incision is dry. A dry incision is less likely than a wet one to promote bacterial growth.

- Feed the infant every 2–3 hours and alternate feeding positions if breastfeeding. Be sure that the baby gets as much of the nipple and areola in his mouth as possible. These actions reduce the likelihood of injury to the nipple.

- Properly care for the nipples. For a breast infection to occur, a cracked or blistered nipple is necessary. Use lanolin, vitamin E, cod liver oil, or express breast milk and rub any of these into the nipple to help reduce soreness and to protect the nipple from trauma.

- Consider alternative therapies to boost the immune system (e.g., *Echinacea*)

- Notify the health care provider if pain, redness, or swelling at the site of any incision develop.

- Notify the health care provider if a fever of 100.4°F (38°C) or greater develops. (If breastfeeding, a temperature elevation to 100.4°F [38°C] may occur when the milk production begins) (Lincoln & Kleiner, 2004).

Teaching Patients About Aspirin and Anticoagulants

- Caution patients to avoid medications that contain aspirin (salicylic acid) because it prevents blood clotting and increases the risk of bleeding.

ADDITIONAL INFORMATION FOR THE CLINICAL SETTING

Nursing Actions for the Patient Experiencing Hemorrhage

- Monitor and record intake and output (indwelling urinary catheter).
- Weigh pads, linens, and other bloody items on a gram scale.
- Administer oxygen at 10 to 12 L/min according to institutional protocol.
- Obtain appropriate lab studies (e.g., complete blood count; prothrombin time; partial thromboplastin time; fibrinogen degradation products).
- Type and cross-match for replacement blood.
- Assess for indicators of disseminated intravascular coagulation (DIC).

Alternative Therapies for Postpartum Depression

- Hypnosis: Enhances relaxation and an ability to focus on daily tasks.
- Exercise: Increases levels of neurotransmitters that communicate with brain cells to increase feelings of euphoria.
- St. John's wort (*Hypericum perforatum*): Believed to bind with neuroreceptors in the brain to prevent a response to the "depression" neurotransmitters (Lincoln & Kleiner, 2004). Do not use in combination with SSRI antidepressants.
- Biofeedback: Promotes relaxation and decreases anxiety.
- Meditation: Helps the woman to focus on "being rather than doing," thereby relieving stress and tension.
- Humor: Has been shown to decrease anxiety, fear, tension, anger, and frustration and to stimulate the immune system.
- Acupuncture, aromatherapy, and massage: Additional complementary therapies that may also be beneficial.

RESOURCES

Centers for Disease Control and Injury (CDC), National Center for Injury Prevention and Control: http://www.cdc.gov/ncipc/

Family Violence Prevention Fund: www.endabuse.org

LaLeche League International: http://www.lalecheleague.org/philosophy.html

National Center for Complementary and Alternative Medicine (NCCAM): http://info@nccam.nih.gov/

The National Women's Health Information Center: http://www.forwoman.gov/faq/depression-pregnancy.cfm

REFERENCES

Adams, M.P., Josephson, D.L., & Holland, L.N. (2005). *Pharmacology for nurses: A pathophysiologic approach.* Upper Saddle River, NJ: Pearson Education.

American Academy of Pediatrics (AAP) & The American College of Obstetricians and Gynecologists (ACOG). (6th ed.) (2007). *Guidelines for perinatal care.* Washington, DC: Author.

Beck, C.T., Records, K., & Rice, M. (2006). Further development of the Postpartum Depression Predictors Inventory-Revised. *Journal of Obstetric, Gynecologic, & Neonatal Nursing, 35*(6), 735–745.

Clemmens, D., Driscoll, J.W., & Beck, C.T. (2004). Postpartum depression as profiled through the postpartum depression screening scale. *The American Journal of Maternal/Child Nursing, 29*(3), 180–185.

Cunningham, F., Leveno, K., Bloom, S., Hauth, J., Gilstrap, L., & Wenstrom, K.D. (2005). *Williams obstetrics* (22nd ed.). New York: McGraw-Hill.

Deglin, J.H., & Vallerand, A.H. (2009). *Davis's Drug Guide for Nurses* (11th ed.). Philadelphia: F.A. Davis.

Franzblau, N., & Witt, K. (June 26, 2006). Normal and abnormal puerperium. Retrieved from http://www.emedicine.com/med/topic3240.htm (Accessed April 18, 2009).

Gibbs, R., Sweet, R., & Duff, P. (2004). Maternal and fetal infectious disorders. In R. Creasy, R. Reznik, & J. Iams (eds.), *Maternal-fetal medicine: Principles and practice* (5th ed., pp. 955–986). Philadelphia: W.B. Saunders.

Kennedy, E. (August 8, 2007). Pregnancy, postpartum infections. Retrieved from http://www.emedicine.com/emerg/topic482.htm (Accessed April 18, 2009).

Lawrence, R., & Lawrence, R. (2005). *Breastfeeding: A guide for the medical profession* (6th ed.). Philadelphia: C.V. Mosby.

Lincoln, V., & Kleiner, K. (2004). Holistic health: Complementary thera-peutic disciplines and remedies. In M. Condon (Ed). *Women's health: An integrated approach to wellness and illness* (pp. 195–225). Upper Saddle River, NJ: Pearson Education.

Logsdon, M.C., Birkimer, J.C., Simpson, T., & Looney, S. (2005). Postpar-tum depression and social support in adolescents. *Journal of Obstetric, Gynecologic & Neonatal Nursing, 34*(1), 46–54.

Luegenbiehl, D.L., Brophy, G., Artigue, G., Phillips, K., & Flack, R. (1990). Standardized assessment of blood loss. *MCN: American Journal of Maternal-Child Nursing,* 15(4), 241–244.

Mass, S. (2004). Breast pain: Engorgement, nipple pain, and mastitis. *Clini-cal Obstetrics and Gynecology, 47*(3), 676–682.

Smith, J.R. & Brennan, B. (June 13, 2006). Postpartum hemorrhage. Retrieved from http://emedicine.com (Accessed April 18, 2009).

Stoops, J., & Mann, N. (2004). Psychological/emotional wellness and illness. In M. Condon (Ed). *Women's health: An integrated approach to wellness and illness* (pp. 538–556). Upper Saddle River, NJ: Pearson Education.

Tucker, M.E. (2004). Treat before hypotension occurs: Avoiding hysterec-tomy for postpartum hemorrhage. *OB GYN News, 39*(11), 22–23.

Walters, K.C., & Wing, D.A. (2007). Misoprostol and postpartum hemor-rhage. *The Female Patient, 32*(7), 53–60.

Physiological Transition of the Newborn

KEY TERMS

acrocyanosis – Peripheral cyanosis; bluish coloration of the hands and feet present in most infants at birth

apnea – Temporary cessation of breathing that lasts more than 20 seconds, associated with generalized cyanosis

bilirubin – Yellow-orange pigment that is a breakdown product of hemoglobin

brown adipose tissue (BAT) – Unique neonatal heat source that is capable of greater thermogenic activity than ordinary fat. Deposits are located around the adrenal glands, kidneys, neck, between the scapulas and behind the sternum. Also termed "brown fat."

hyperbilirubinemia – Elevation of unconjugated serum bilirubin concentrations

icteric – Yellow discoloration of the body tissues (skin, sclera, oral mucous membranes) caused by the deposit of bile pigments (unconjugated bilirubin); jaundice

immunity – Protection from diseases, especially infectious diseases

> **acquired i.** Immunity that results either from exposure to an antigen (response to the infection) or from the passive injection of immunoglobulins
>
> **active i.** Immunity that develops in response to actual infection or vaccination
>
> **natural i.** Immunity that is genetically determined in a specific species; the first line of defense
>
> **passive i.** Immunity that is acquired by the introduction of preformed antibodies into an unprotected individual

(e.g., maternal antibodies that pass to the fetus through the placenta)

insensible water loss (IWL) – Evaporative water loss that occurs mainly through the skin and respiratory tract

jaundice – Yellow discoloration of the body tissues (skin, sclera, oral mucous membranes) caused by the deposit of bile pigments (unconjugated bilirubin); icterus

kangaroo care – Skin-to-skin infant care; provides warmth to the infant

kernicterus – Bilirubin encephalopathy that involves the deposit of unconjugated bilirubin in brain cells. Results in neurological damage or death.

neutral thermal environment (NTE) – Range of temperature in which the newborn's body temperature can be maintained (at least 36.5°C) with minimal metabolic demands and oxygen consumption

nonshivering thermogenesis – Infant's method of producing heat from brown adipose tissue by increasing the metabolic rate

periodic breathing – Sporadic episodes of cessation of respirations for periods of 5 to 15 seconds, not associated with cyanosis

polycythemia – Increased number of erythrocytes per volume of blood

respiratory distress syndrome (RDS) – Developmental disorder that results from decreased pulmonary gas exchange leading to carbon dioxide retention (increased arterial Pco_2). In the neonate, most commonly associated with prematurity, perinatal asphyxia, and maternal diabetes mellitus. Also known as hyaline membrane disease.

surfactant – Phosphoprotein necessary for normal respiratory function; prevents alveolar collapse and permits reexpansion after exhalation

thermogenesis – Production of heat

FOCUSED ASSESSMENT

Adaptation of the Respiratory System

Initiation of the neonate's first breath influenced by:

- Internal stimuli
  - Chemical factors (hypercarbia, acidosis, hypoxia)

- External stimuli
  - Sensory factors (tactile, visual, auditory)
  - Thermal factors (cool air)
  - Mechanical factors (chest compression – "thoracic squeeze") (Fig. 14-1)

Factors that interfere with initiation and maintenance of respirations include:

- Prematurity
- Birth asphyxia
- Trauma
- Maternal medications
- Mode of birth

Recognizing Normal Neonatal Lung Sounds During Early Auscultation

The neonate's lung sounds may sound moist during early auscultation, but should become clear within the following 24 hours as the lung fluid is gradually absorbed into the lymphatic and circulatory systems.

Figure 14-1 Internal and external factors involved in the initiation of respirations.

Cardiopulmonary Transitions

Conversion from fetal to newborn circulation: normal sequence of events (Fig. 14-2):

1. Air enters lungs, leading to increased Po_2 in the alveoli.
2. Relaxation of the pulmonary artery leads to decreased pulmonary vascular resistance.
3. Increased pulmonary blood flow leads to conversion to newborn circulation.

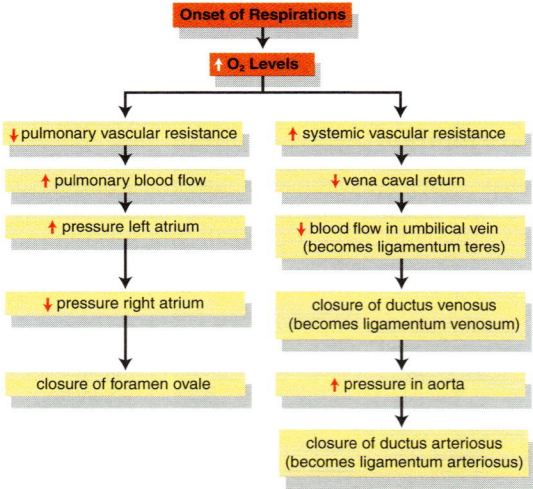

Figure 14-2 Major events that occur during the transition from fetal to neonatal circulation include closure of the foramen ovale, the ductus arteriosus, and the ductus venosus.

Structural Changes in Circulation After Birth		
Fetus	**Neonate**	**Mechanism**
Umbilical vein	Ligamentum teres	Constricts after placental separation.
Ductus venosus	Ligamentum venosum	Once the umbilical cord is clamped, cessation of umbilical venous blood return, along with mechanical pressure changes, lead to closure of the ductus venosus. Closure of the bypass route forces enhanced blood flow to the liver. Closure usually occurs by the end of the first week.

Fetus	Neonate	Mechanism
Foramen ovale	Closed atrial septum	Blood flow increases to the pulmonary veins, leading to increased left atrial pressure, which causes the foramen ovale flap to close. Fibrin and cells seal the shunt; it is physiologically closed by 1 month of age.
Ductus arteriosus	Ligamentum arteriosum	The pathway for most of the fetal blood due to the high pulmonary vascular resistance. Once the umbilical cord is clamped, placental blood flow ceases, and systemic blood pressure and vascular resistance increase. As the lungs oxygenate the blood, the increased Pao$_2$ stimulates the closure of the ductus arteriosus. Occurs within the first 72 hours of life.
Umbilical artery	Superior vesical (bladder) artery Lateral vesicoumbilical ligaments	Constricts after placental separation.

Thermogenic Adaptation

Mechanisms for Neonatal Heat Loss

Mechanism	Description	Nursing Actions
Evaporation	Heat loss when water is converted into a vapor.	Thoroughly dry the neonate immediately after birth, remove wet blankets, place hat on the head.
Conduction	Heat loss to a cooler surface by direct skin contact.	Place the infant on a pre-warmed radiant warmer, use warmed blankets, cover the scales with blankets before weighing, and avoid the use of cold instruments. The newborn can also be placed skin to skin with the mother to facilitate body warming and bonding (kangaroo care).
Convection	Heat loss from the warm body surface to the cooler air currents.	Prevent drafts in the birth area; place the newborn away from doors or windows; keep the neonate warmly clothed and possibly swaddled to prevent cooling from air currents.
Radiation	The transfer of heat between objects that are not in direct contact with one other (e.g., the walls of the nursery or the incubator)	Have a prewarmed radiant warmer present at the birth; avoid placing the crib or incubator by a cold window; and keep cold objects well away from the neonate.

Factors Related to Cold Stress
- Large body area in relation to body mass
- Limited subcutaneous fat
- Limited ability to shiver
- The skin is thin and the blood vessels are close to the body surface

Hematopoietic Adaptation

Changes in Hematopoietic Components	
Component	Change
Blood Volume	Approximately one half of the fetal blood volume is transferred from the placenta to the neonate by the end of the first minute of life.
Erythrocytes and Hemoglobin	Fetal RBCs have a shorter lifespan (90 days) than do adult RBCs, but carry 20%–50% more oxygen. The faster deterioration of fetal RBCs may cause physiological anemia of infancy and lead to higher bilirubin levels.
Platelets	Lack of vitamin K at birth places the neonate at risk for a blood clotting deficiency during the first few days of life.

Hepatic Adaptation

The liver is responsible for regulation of blood glucose, iron storage, bilirubin conjugation, and coagulation of the blood.

Risk Factors for Hypoglycemia in the Neonate
- Prematurity
- Postmaturity
- Intrauterine growth restriction (IUGR)
- Large or small for gestational age (LGA or SGA)
- Asphyxia
- Difficult transition at birth
- Cold stress
- Maternal diabetes
- Maternal intake of ritodrine (Yutopar) or terbutaline (Brethine)
- Infection

Conjugation of Bilirubin

1. Bilirubin is produced from hemolysis of erythrocytes (RBCs).

2. Reticuloendothelial system: Removes aging RBCs; converts hemoglobin to unconjugated bilirubin.
3. Bilirubin is transported via blood albumin to the liver.
4. In the liver, bilirubin is conjugated with glucuronic acid.
5. Resulting conjugated (direct) bilirubin is excreted into the common duct and duodenum.
6. Direct bilirubin is excreted in stools and urine (Fig. 14-3).

Factors that May Influence Bilirubin Levels in the Neonate

- Cultural background: Chinese, Japanese, Korean, and Native American neonates exhibit higher bilirubin levels than do European and American Caucasian neonates. The elevated levels of bilirubin persist for a longer period of time and cause no apparent adverse effects.
- Perinatal events (i.e., delayed cord cutting, breech presentation, the use of Pitocin)
- Prematurity
- Maternal diabetes

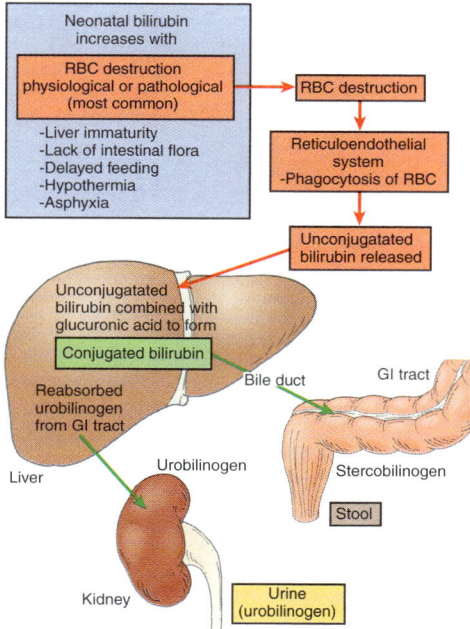

Figure 14-3 Physiological pathway for the excretion of bilirubin.

- Excess bilirubin production (e.g., hemolytic diseases such as Rh isoimmunization and ABO incompatibility; sepsis; metabolic disorders)
- Delayed feedings
- Liver immaturity (i.e., prematurity; glucose-6-phosphate dehydrogenase deficiency)
- Birth trauma
- Family history of jaundice or a previous child with jaundice
- Neonatal complications (i.e., asphyxia neonatorum, cold stress, hypoglycemia) (MacDonald, Mullett, & Seshia, 2005; Wong et al., 2006)

Types of Jaundice

Type	Definition	Comments
Physiological Jaundice (nonhemolytic)	Yellow tinge to skin and mucous membranes related to increased serum levels of unconjugated bilirubin	**Occurs in >60% term and >80% preterm newborns.** Typically occurs 24–48 hours after birth. Peaks between 5 and 7 days.
Pathological Jaundice (non-physiological jaundice)	Jaundice is usually noticeable within the first 24 hours of life. Caused by an abnormal condition such as Rh or ABO incompatibility. Results in bilirubin toxicity (i.e., kernicterus).	Total serum bilirubin (TSB) concentration increases by 5 mg/dL per day. Occurs within the first 24 hours of life. TSB >12.9 mg/dL in a term infant TSB >15 mg/dL in a preterm infant
Breastfeeding Jaundice (early onset)	Occurs between the 2nd and 4th days of life, peaks at 72 hours of life. Occurs when there is a decreased intake of breast milk and a decreased passage of meconium.	TSB peaks at 15–19 mg/dL by 72 hours of life. Believed to be associated with poor feeding practices, not related to the composition of the breast milk. Primary therapy centers on early and frequent feedings and avoidance of formula and glucose supplementation (Hertz, 2005).
Breast Milk Jaundice (late onset)	Typically occurs in the full term infant after the fifth day of life; peaks around day 10.	Infant thrives, stools appropriately, and gains weight. No evidence of hemolysis. Gradually declines over a few weeks.

Gastrointestinal Adaptation

- Bowel sounds are present within the first 15 to 30 minutes of life.
- First stool occurs within 8 to 24 hours of life (meconium).
- Stools may occur up to 10 times per day.
- Cardiac sphincter immature; regurgitation may occur after feedings.

Genitourinary Adaptation

Kidney Function

- The nephrons are fully functional by 34 to 36 weeks of gestation.
- The glomerular filtration rate is lower than that of the adult.
- There is a limited capacity for the reabsorption of HCO_3^- and H^+.
- Initially unable to dispose of fluid rapidly or to concentrate urine.
- Most newborns void immediately after birth; some may not void for up to 24 hours.

Immunological Adaptation

Recognizing and Preventing Newborn Infections	
Signs and Symptoms of Infection	**Nursing Interventions**
Subtle behavior changes Poor feeding patterns Respiratory distress Hypothermia	Maintain skin integrity. Assess for potential risk factors (e.g., maternal group B *Streptococcus* exposure). Assess all breaks in skin integrity (e.g., circumcision site, heel sticks, umbilical stump). Provide parents with thorough discharge instructions regarding infant hygiene, proper skin care, awareness of signs and symptoms of infection.

Psychosocial Adaptation

Early Stages of Activity	
Period	**Description**
First Period of Reactivity	First period of active, alert wakefulness displayed immediately after birth Rapid heart rate and respirations Increased muscle tone and activity Decreased body temperature Absent bowel sounds May last from 30 minutes to 2 hours Excellent time to initiate breastfeeding
Period of Inactivity and Sleep	Follows the first period of reactivity Decreased muscle activity Difficult to awaken Heart rate and respirations return to a normal range May last up to 4 hours
Second Period of Reactivity	Newborn becomes alert once again. Most infants show signs for feeding readiness. Infant becomes more responsive to stimulation. Lability in heart rate and respirations is common. Bowel sounds are usually present.

Newborn Behavioral States	
Sleep States	Sleep occurs in intervals of approximately 50 minutes.
Deep/Quiet	45% of sleep is "quiet" sleep.
Rapid Eye Movement (REM)	Approximately one half of the infant's total sleep is "active" (REM) sleep.
Alert States	
Drowsy/Semidozing	Open or closed eyes, fluttering eyelids; semidozing appearance; and slow, regular movement of the extremities. There is a delayed response to external stimuli.
Wide Awake	The infant is alert and follows and fixates on attractive objects, faces, or auditory stimuli. There is minimal motor activity and a delayed response to external stimuli.

Alert States	
Active Awake	The eyes are open; motor activity is intense, and the infant displays thrusting movements of the extremities. Environmental stimuli increase the motor activity.
Crying	Jerky movements accompany intense crying. Crying often serves as a distraction from unpleasant stimuli such as hunger and pain; it allows the infant to discharge energy and elicits a helpful response from the parents.

CLINICAL ALERT

Recognizing Hypoglycemia in the Neonate

When assessing the neonate during the transitional period, be alert to signs and symptoms of hypoglycemia: jitteriness; diaphoresis; poor muscle tone; poor sucking reflex; temperature instability (low temperature); respiratory distress; tachycardia; dyspnea; apnea; high-pitched cry; irritability; lethargy; and seizures or coma. Awareness of prenatal and perinatal risk factors that may predispose to postnatal hypoglycemia is essential as the infant may be asymptomatic.

DIAGNOSTIC TESTS

Laboratory Values for the Normal Term Neonate – Blood	
Blood Component	**Normal Range**
Albumin	3.6–5.4 g/dL
Amylase	0–1000 IU/hr
Bicarbonate	20–26 mmol/L
Bilirubin, direct	<0.5 mg/dL
Bilirubin, total	<2.8 mg/dL (cord blood)
0–1 days	2.6 mg/dL (peripheral blood)
1–2 days	6–7 mg/dL (peripheral blood)
3–5 days	4–6 mg/dL (peripheral blood)
Bleeding time	2 Minutes

(continued)

Laboratory Values for the Normal Term Neonate – Blood (Continued)

Blood Component	Normal Range
Arterial blood gases	
pH	7.35–7.45
$Paco_2$	35–45 mm Hg
Pao_2	50–90 mm Hg
Venous blood gases	
pH	7.35–7.45
$Paco_2$	41–51 mm Hg
Pao_2	20–49 mm Hg
Calcium, ionized	2.5–5 mg/dL
Calcium, total	7–12 mg/dL
Glucose	30–125 mg/dL
Hematocrit	48%–64%
	53% (cord blood)
Hemoglobin	17–18.4 g/dL
	16.8 g/dL (cord blood)
Platelets	$150,000 – 300,000/mm^3$
Immunoglobulins, total	660–1439 mg/dL
Iron	100–250 mcg/dL
Red blood cell count	$4,800,000–7,100,000/mm^3$
White blood cell count	$9000–30,000/mm^3$

Sources: Nettina (2007); Pagana & Pagana (2006).

Laboratory Values for the Normal Term Neonate – Urine

Urine Component	Normal Range
Casts, WBC	Normal to be present for the first 2–4 days
Osmolality (maximum concentration ability)	800 mOsmol/L
(Maximum diluting ability)	25–30 mOsmol/L
pH	4.5–8.0
Phenylketonuria	No color changes
Specific gravity	1.002–1.010
Protein	May be present during first 2–4 days
Glucose	Negative
Blood	Negative
Leukocytes	Negative

Sources: Cloherty, Eichenwald, & Stark (2004); Nettina (2007).

MEDICATIONS

Betamethasone (bay-ta-**meth**-a-sone), **Dexamethasone** (dex-a-**meth**-a-sone)

Pregnancy Category C

Indications To prevent or reduce the severity of respiratory distress syndrome in preterm infants between 24 and 34 weeks of gestation (unlabeled use)

Action Stimulates fetal lung maturation by promoting the release of enzymes that induce the production or release of lung surfactant.

Classification(s)
Therapeutic Stimulates fetal lung maturation
Pharmacological Glucocorticoids (corticosteroids)

Pharmacokinetics
Absorption Preferred method of absorption is via injection
Distribution Crosses the placenta; enters the breast milk
Metabolism and Excretion Metabolized in the liver and excreted by the kidneys
Half-life 6.5 hours

Contraindications and Precautions Contraindicated in women in whom there is a medical indication for delivery (i.e., severe pregnancy induced hypertension [PIH], cord prolapse, chorioamnionitis, abruptio placentae) and in women with systemic fungal infection.

Adverse Reactions and Side Effects Seizures, headache, vertigo, hypertension, increased perspiration, petechiae, ecchymoses, and facial erythema, maternal infection, pulmonary edema (if administered with beta-adrenergic medications). May worsen certain maternal conditions such as diabetes and hypertension.

Route and Dosage 12 mg IM q24hr × 2 doses

Nursing Implications
1. Inform the woman of the benefit of medication and the need to administer to prevent respiratory distress syndrome in her preterm infant.
2. Teach the woman the signs and symptoms of pulmonary edema; assess lung sounds.
3. Shake the suspension well; prolonged exposure to heat and light must be avoided.

4. Administer the medication into a large muscle; avoid the deltoid to prevent local atrophy.
5. Vital signs must be monitored frequently and fetal monitoring should be performed according to institution policy.
6. Accurate intake and output must be monitored and recorded.
7. Monitor blood sugars if the woman is diabetic or at risk for diabetes.
8. Do not administer if the woman has an infection

NOTE: The FDA has not approved the medication for this use.

Data from Deglin & Vallerand (2009); Hayes, Kee, & McCuistion (2006).

ETHNOCULTURAL CONSIDERATIONS

Neonatal Jaundice and RBC Enzyme Defects

Jaundice occurs with greater frequency in infants of Chinese, Japanese, Korean, Native American, and Greek descent. In these populations there is an increased incidence of red blood cell enzyme defects, including glucose-6-phosphate dehydrogenase (G6PD) deficiency and pyruvate kinase deficiency. It occurs most frequently in Mediterranean, Middle-Eastern, Southeast Asian, and African infants. Pyruvate kinase deficiency is the next most common enzyme deficiency. Affected infants typically display symptoms of jaundice, anemia and reticulocytosis (MacDonald, Mullett, & Seshia, 2005).

ADDITIONAL INFORMATION FOR THE CLINICAL SETTING

Facilitating Newborn Transition in a Non-hospital Setting

When assisting with an unexpected birth in a non-hospital setting:

- Evaluate the mother before childbirth if possible.
- Manipulate the environment to facilitate immediate care for the neonate.
- Remain alert to signs of transitional difficulties.
- Ensure effective respirations.

- Facilitate a neutral thermal environment.
- Establish safe transport to the hospital for the mother and newborn.
- Manage maternal–neonatal care until the transport team arrives.

Preventing Cold Stress in the Newborn

During nonshivering thermogenesis, the newborn metabolizes brown fat. This process increases the metabolic rate, oxygen consumption, and risk for metabolic acidosis. Decreased oxygen causes peripheral vasoconstriction and increases the likelihood of respiratory distress. Peripheral vasoconstriction can lead to increased pulmonary vascular resistance, and a return to fetal circulation as a compensatory mechanism.

Assessing Neonatal Blood Glucose

Capillary blood obtained from the neonate's heel is commonly used to assess blood glucose. When available, a heel warmer is used to increase blood flow to the sample site. Cleanse the area with a sterile alcohol pad. Gently puncture the heel, taking care to avoid the middle area, where there is a risk for nerve damage or puncture of the plantar artery. Place a large drop of blood on the test strip. Apply a sterile bandage to apply pressure on the sample site.

REFERENCES

Cloherty, J., Eichenwald, E., & Stark, A. (2004). *Manual of neonatal care* (5th ed.). Philadelphia: Lippincott Williams & Wilkins.

Deglin, J.H., & Vallerand, A.H. (2009). *Davis's drug guide for nurses* (11th ed.). Philadelphia: F.A. Davis.

Hayes, E., Kee, J., & McCuistion, L. (2006). *Pharmacology, a nursing process approach* (5th ed.). St. Louis, MO: W.B. Saunders/Elsevier.

Hertz, D. (2005). *Care of the newborn: A handbook for primary care.* Philadelphia: Lippincott.

MacDonald, M., Mullett, M., & Seshia, M. (2005). *Avery's neonatology, pathophysiology & management of the newborn* (6th ed.). Philadelphia: Lippincott Williams & Wilkins.

Nettina, S. (2007). *Lippincott manual of nursing practice.* Philadelphia: Lippincott Williams & Wilkins.

Pagana, K., & Pagana, T. (2006). *Mosby's manual of diagnostic and laboratory tests* (3rd ed.). St. Louis, MO: C.V. Mosby.

Wong, R., DeSandre, G., Sibley, E., & Stevenson, D. (2006). Neonatal jaundice and liver disease. In R. Martin, A. Fanaroff, & M. Walsh (Eds.), *Fanaroff and Martin's neonatal-perinatal medicine: Diseases of the fetus and infant* (8th ed., pp. 578–586). Philadelphia: C.V. Mosby.

Caring for the Normal Newborn

KEY TERMS

caput – Occiput of the fetal head appearing at the vaginal introitus preceding birth of the head

  c. succedaneum Swelling of the tissue over the presenting part of the fetal head; caused by pressure during labor

cephalhematoma – Extravasation of blood from ruptured vessels between a skull bone and its external covering (the periosteum). The hemorrhage does not cross the suture lines; swelling is limited by the margins of the cranial bone affected.

circumcision – Surgical procedure in which the prepuce (epithelial layer covering the penis; foreskin) is separated from the glans penis and excised

developmental dysplasia of the hip (DDH) – Abnormal development of the hip joint, resulting in instability of the hip causing one or both of the femoral heads to be displaced from the acetabulum

erythema toxicum – Transient pink papular rash in the neonate. Cause is unknown and it may persist up to 1 month of life. Also called "erythema neonatorum."

hypospadias – Anomalous positioning of the urinary meatus on the undersurface of the penis or close to or just inside the vagina

imperforate anus – Congenital absence of an opening in the anal ring

meningocele – Congenital hernia in which the meninges protrude through a defect in the skull or spinal column

microcephaly – Congenital anomaly characterized by abnormal smallness of the head in relation to the rest of the body; underdevelopment of the brain and mental retardation

molding – Overlapping or overriding of the fetal cranial bones to accommodate and conform to the bony and soft parts of the mother's birth canal during labor

myelomeningocele – Hernia of the spinal cord and meninges through the posterior vertebral column; results from failure of the neural tube to close during embryonic development

necrotizing enterocolitis (NEC) – Acute inflammatory bowel disorder that occurs primarily in preterm or low-birthweight infants. Occurs when bowel ischemia results in destruction of the intestinal mucosa; may lead to perforation and peritonitis.

nevus – Natural blemish or mark, a congenital deposit of pigmentation in the skin; mole

> **n. flammeus** "port wine stain"; a nonelevated capillary angioma located directly below the epidermis

> **n. vasculosus (strawberry hemangioma)** Elevated lesion of immature capillaries and endothelial cells – slowly regresses over a period of years

omphalitis – Inflammation of the umbilical stump, characterized by redness, edema, and purulent exudate in severe infections

ophthalmia neonatorum – Neonatal eye infection usually resulting from gonorrheal or other infection contracted during passage through the vagina at the time of birth

plethora – Deep purplish-red coloration of a newborn caused by an increased number of circulating red blood cells

simian crease – Single, straight crease that appears in the middle of the palm on one or both hands. May be present in a variety of developmental abnormalities including Down syndrome, Turner's syndrome and Klinefelter's syndrome

telangiectasia – Permanent dilation of groups of superficial capillaries and venules

telangiectatic nevus – "Stork bite"; "angel kiss." Small, red, localized area of capillary dilation frequently seen in neonates; may occur on the nape of the neck, eyebrows, eyelids, nose or upper lip

tetralogy of Fallot – Congenital heart defect that involves four distinct cardiac anomalies: transposition of the aorta and pulmonary artery; right ventricular hypertrophy; pulmonary stenosis; and ventricular septal defect

Wharton's jelly – Specialized white, gelatinous connective tissue that surrounds the umbilical vessels within the cord

FOCUSED ASSESSMENT

The Immediate Neonatal Assessment

- Follow universal precautions.
- Suction oral, pharyngeal, or endotracheal area according to policy (see Procedure 15-1).
- Place the infant on the mother's abdomen, if stable, or under a pre-warmed radiant warmer (unclothed).
- Dry the infant vigorously with warmed blankets (also stimulates respiratory effort).
- Place a cap on the infant's head.
- Observe the respiratory effort, color, and muscle tone.
- Assess the heart rate: May be done by palpating the base of the umbilical stump.
- Lightly flick the soles of the feet to prompt crying, if necessary.
- Document 1-minute and 5-minute Apgar scores.

 Procedure 15-1 Suctioning the Infant's Oral and Nasal Passages

Purpose
To clear secretions from the oral and nasal passages

Equipment
- One bulb syringe
- Tissue

Steps for Oral Suctioning
1. Assess the infant for oral secretions.
2. Position the infant's head to the side or downward if he is vomiting or gagging.
3. Compress the bulb syringe.
4. Insert the bulb syringe approximately 1 inch into one side of the infant's cheek.
   Avoid contact with the roof of the mouth and the back of the throat.

Procedure 15-1 (Continued)

5. Gently release compression of the bulb syringe and allow it to fill with oral secretions.
6. Gently remove the bulb syringe; expel drainage into a tissue.
7. Repeat the process on the other side of the infant's cheek.
8. Repeat as needed.
9. Document procedure.

Steps for Nasal Suctioning

1. Assess the infant for nasal congestion.
2. Position the infant's head to the side or downward if he is vomiting or gagging.
3. Compress the bulb syringe.
4. Insert the bulb syringe into the tip of the infant's nostril. Avoid obstructing the nasal passageway.
5. Gently release the compression of bulb syringe to allow it to fill with mucus or nasal drainage.
6. Gently remove the bulb syringe; expel drainage into a tissue.
7. Repeat as needed.
8. Document the procedure.

Normal Neonatal Parameters at Birth	
Parameter	**Normal Finding**
Respirations	Rate 30–60 breaths/min, irregular with no retractions or grunting
Apical pulse	Rate 120–160 beats/min
Temperature	97.8°F (36.5°C)
Skin color	Pink body, blue extremities
Umbilical cord	Contains two arteries and one vein
Gestational age	Full term: >37 completed weeks (should be 38–42 weeks to remain with parents for an extended time period)

The Later Neonatal Assessment

Vital Signs

Recognizing Normal Newborn Vital Signs			
Temperature	**Pulse**	**Respirations**	**Blood Pressure**
Normal 97.7°–99.4°F (36.5°–37.0°C) Axillary 97.5°–99°F (36.5°–37.2°C)	120–160 beats per minute (bpm) (count pulse rate for 1 full minute) During sleep the pulse rate can be as low as 80 bpm. During crying the pulse rate can be as high as 180 bpm.	30–60 respirations per minute (count respiratory rate for 1 full minute) Abdominal breathing is normal. Periodic breathing is considered normal; is classified as short pauses in the breathing of the newborn that last approximately 3 seconds. Apneic episodes are significant if they last more than 15–20 seconds; they may be accompanied by abrupt pallor, hypotonia, cyanosis, and bradycardia. Apnea must be differentiated from periodic breathing, which is normal in the newborn. *Caution*: Withhold the oral feeding if the respiratory rate is >60 respirations per minute.	Systolic: 60–80 mm Hg; diastolic: 40–50 mm Hg at birth Systolic: 95–100 mm Hg; diastolic: slight increase at 10 days of age

Importance of Temperature Assessment

If the newborn's temperature drops to 97.5°F (36.4°C) or below, immediately initiate temperature stabilization measures such as skin-to-skin contact by placing the infant directly on the mother's unclothed arms, chest, or abdomen or move him to a radiant warmer. Once the newborn's temperature reaches 98.6°F (37.0°C) or above, dress him in a T-shirt and hat and cover him with two or three blankets.

Assessment of the Neonate: A Systems Approach

Level of Reactivity Responsiveness, symmetrical movement, sleep pattern

Overall Size and Symmetry

Measurements Weight, length, head, chest, and abdominal circumference

- Average weight is 3400 grams; range is 2500 to 4300 grams.
  - Place a cover on the scale to prevent cross-infection (Fig. 15-1).
  - Protect the infant against heat loss.
  - Remain with the infant.
- Average length is 45 to 55 cm (18–22 in.) (See Procedure 15-2.)
- Average head circumference (frontal–occipital circumference) is 33 to 38 cm (13–15 in.).
  - Place the tape measure immediately above the eyebrows and pinna of the ears (Fig. 15-2).
  - Wrap the tape measure around to the occipital prominence at the back of the head.
  - Measure three times; record the largest finding.

Figure 15-1 Weighing the infant.

Figure 15-2 Measuring the head circumference.

- Average chest circumference is 30.5 to 33 cm (12–13 in.).
  - Place the tape measure on the nipple line (Fig. 15-3).
  - Wrap the tape measure around the entire thoracic area.
- The abdominal circumference should approximate the chest circumference.
  - Place the tape measure directly above the umbilicus (Fig. 15-4).
  - Wrap the tape measure around the infant's body.

Skin, Scalp, Body Hair, Nails Assess color, texture, distribution, disruptions, eruptions, birthmarks

Head Assess size, symmetry, suture lines, placement and condition of the eyes, nose, mouth, and ears, patency of both nares, integrity of the anterior and posterior fontanels, and the presence of a caput succedaneum or cephalhematoma

Respiratory System Assess symmetry in the movement of the chest, placement and size of the breast tissue, the respiratory rate and effort, and the presence of retractions or grunting

Cardiovascular System Palpate the point of maximum impulse (PMI), the heart rate, capillary refill, femoral pulses, brachial pulses; auscultate for murmurs or extra heart sounds

Figure 15-3 Measuring the chest circumference.

Figure 15-4 Measuring the abdominal circumference.

Gastrointestinal System Inspect the abdominal shape and the umbilical cord; auscultate bowel sounds, palpate and note structures; assess for the presence of a hernia

Genitourinary System: Assess patency of the anus, elicit the anal wink reflex, note passing of stool.

Males: Examine the scrotum and palpate for the presence of both testes; note location of urinary meatus; palpate the penis; note the presence of smegma.

Females: Examine the labia; note any discharge.

Musculoskeletal System Inspect extremities for differences in length or size, the number of digits, muscle tone and symmetry in movement; palpate the clavicles and hips for crepitus, perform passage range of motion on the remaining joints; assess rotation of the neck; assess for developmental dysplasia of the hip

Neurological System Assess reflexes, especially the gag reflex, Babinski, Moro, and Galant reflexes; assess integrity of the spine.

 Procedure 15-2 Measuring the Newborn's Length

Purpose

To establish and document the newborn's length

Equipment

- Standard paper tape measure

Steps

1. Place the infant on a paper-covered flat surface.
2. Fully extend the infant's body by holding the head midline.
3. Gently grasp the knees and place them together.
4. Push down gently on the knees until they are fully extended and flat against the table surface.
5. Measure the crown-to-heel recumbent length by placing the paper tape measure beside the infant with the 0 end of the tape at the top of the head. Keep the infant's body in alignment and carefully extend one leg. Ensure that the tape measure remains straight.

(continued)

Procedure 15-2 (Continued)

As an alternate measurement method, make a slash mark with a pen at the end points by the top of the infant's head and the heels of the foot. While providing continuous support, gently roll the infant to the side and measure between the two points with a paper tape measure that has increments designated in tenths.

6. Document the procedure and record the measurement.

Gestational Age Assessment (Fig. 15-5)
- Performed within the first 12 hours of life.
- Includes neuromuscular maturity and physical maturity components.
- Scores from each component are added together.
- Combined scores are mathematically extrapolated onto the maturity rating scale to determine the infant's gestational age by examination.
- Identifies the decreased levels of muscle and joint flexibility characteristic of the premature infant, and the mature term infant's ability to return to the original position after movement.
- The infant's maturity scoring does not directly translate to the gestational age in weeks (Ballard et al., 1991).

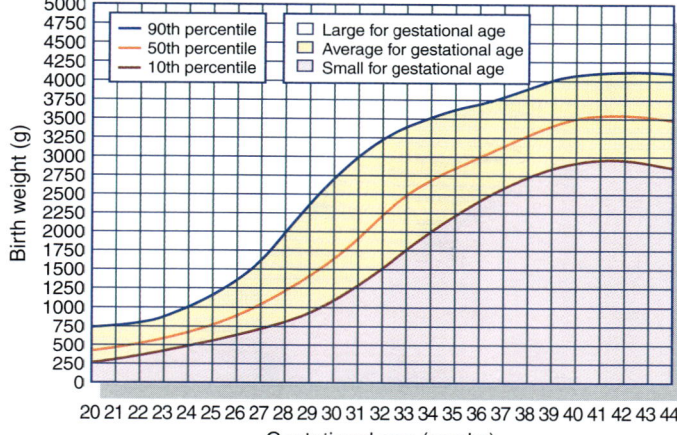

Figure 15-5 Gestational age assessment.

Procedure 15-3 Performing the Barlow–Ortolani Maneuver

Purpose

To assess for developmental dysplasia of the hips

Steps

1. Place the infant supine on a flat surface.
2. Place your thumbs on the infant's inner thighs and your fingers on the outside of the greater trochanters of the hips.

(continued)

Procedure 15-2 (Continued)

3. Flex the infant's knees and move the legs inward until your fingers touch.

4. Using gentle but firm pressure, rotate the hips outward so that the knees touch the flat surface. No clicking or crepitus should be detected. The presence of clicking or crepitus indicates joint instability.

5. Document the procedure.

Newborn Reflexes

Reflex	Indicator/Method for Assessment
Palmar Grasp	The infant curls his fingers around an object.
Toe or Plantar Grasp	The infant curls his toes around an object that has been placed at the sole of the foot.
Rooting and Sucking Reflexes 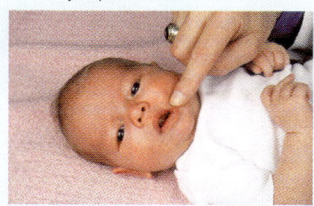	Stroke the infant's cheek and watch him turn toward the finger, open his mouth, and suck on an object placed in his mouth.
Extrusion Reflex	Touch the tip of the infant's tongue and the tongue will protrude outward.

(continued)

Newborn Reflexes (Continued)

Reflex	Indicator/Method for Assessment
Stepping Reflex	Hold the infant in an upright position with the legs flexed. The soles of the feet are lightly brushed against a flat surface. In response to the stimulation, the infant lifts his feet and then places them back down in a stepwise pattern that imitates walking.
Tonic Neck or Fencing Reflex	Observe the infant, in a supine position, extend his arm and leg on the side to which his head and jaw is turned while flexing his arm and leg on the opposite side.
Glabellar Reflex	Tap on infant's forehead and observe him blink for the first few taps.
Babinski Reflex	Lightly stroke the plantar surface of the foot from the heel toward the toes. The infant responds to this stimulation by first incurving the toes, then uncurling and stretching them out.

Reflex	Indicator/Method for Assessment

Moro Reflex

Observe the infant's head as it is lifted while the nurse mimics a release and watches for extension of both arms along with flexion of the legs.

Magnet Reflex

With the infant in a supine position, flex the leg and apply pressure to the soles of the feet. Observe the infant extend his legs against the pressure.

Galant Reflex or Trunk Incurvation Reflex

Hold or support the infant in a prone position. Stroke one side of the vertebral column. Observe the infant respond to this stimulus by moving his buttocks in a curving motion toward the side that is being stroked.

Crawling Reflex

Place the infant on his abdomen; observe his attempts to crawl.

(continued)

Newborn Reflexes (Continued)

Reflex	Indicator/Method for Assessment
Crossed Extension	With the infant in a supine position, stimulate one foot; observe flexion, adduction, and then extension of the opposite leg.

Common Skin Findings in the Neonate

Finding/Condition	Description
Acrocyanosis	The bluish coloring of the hands and feet that results from vasomotor insufficiency and poor peripheral perfusion
Birthmarks	Distinct areas of color that may be red, tan, brown, white or red. Their appearance varies but generally these lesions are small and flat.
Blue Nevus	Appears as a distinct blue or blue-black birthmark often found on the buttocks, hands and feet, usually ≤1 cm in size.
Brown Nevi	Brown skin marks, or birth marks whose color can vary from brown to deep black
Café-au-lait	Flat, tan spots that are quite common and insignificant unless the infant exhibits six or more marks that are >1 cm in diameter
Coloboma	A disruption in the iris; appears as a keyhole in the circle of the iris and pupil and will affect vision in that eye.
Epstein's Pearls	Whitish hardened nodules found along the newborn's gum margins and at the junction of the soft and hard palates; disappear within a few weeks
Erythema Toxicum	Transient pink papular rash in the neonate. Cause is unknown and it may persist up to one month of life. Also called "erythema neonatorum."
Hypopigmentation	Diminished pigment in the tissue

Finding/Condition	Description
Jaundice	Yellow discoloration of the body tissues (skin, sclera, oral mucous membranes) caused by the deposit of bile pigments (unconjugated bilirubin); icterus
Milia	Small white papules or sebaceous cysts that may be present on the newborn's forehead, nose, cheeks and chin
Mongolian Spots	Gray, dark blue, or purple non-elevated pigmented area most often located on the back and buttocks in some neonates, especially those of nonwhite ethnicity
Nevus Flammeus	Often referred to as a "port wine stain," a capillary angioma located directly below the epidermis; a non-elevated, red to purple network of dense capillaries that varies in size, shape, and location, although it commonly appears on the face. It does not blanch on pressure, disappear, or grow in size.
Nevus Vasculosus	"Strawberry mark," a red, raised capillary hemangioma that can occur anywhere on the neonate's body. This birthmark usually has sharp borders and a rough surface that resembles a strawberry.
Periauricular Papillomas	Skin tags around the ear
Plethora	Deep purplish-red coloration of a newborn caused by an increased number of circulating red blood cells
Pustular Melanosis	A condition in which small pustules are formed before birth
Sturge–Weber Syndrome	A clinical condition involving the fifth cranial nerve; may be present when a nevus flammeus is accompanied by convulsions or other indicators of neurological problems.
Telangiectatic Nevus	"Stork bite"; "angel kiss": Small, red, localized area of capillary dilation frequently seen in neonates; may occur on the nape of the neck, eyebrows, eyelids, nose, or upper lip.
Torticollis	A deviation of the neck to one side caused by a spasmodic contraction of neck muscles. In the neonate, a torticollis is apparent when the head is positioned on one side while the chin points to the opposite side.

Obtaining an Accurate Assessment of the Infant's True Skin Color

- Use a variety of light sources (helps ascertain the "true" color).
- Examine the infant's entire skin surface.
- Carefully inspect the palms, soles of the feet, lips, and areas behind the ears.
- Gently palpate bony prominences (nose, sternum, sacrum, wrists, ankles):
  - Apply slight pressure for 1 second ("blanching").

- Observe for true skin color, reflective of the infant's ethnic heritage.
- Record true skin color; yellow is indicative of jaundice; white is indicative of pallor.

Understanding Classifications for Newborn Weight

Large for gestational age (LGA): Weight is above the 90th percentile at any week.

Appropriate for gestational age (AGA): Weight falls between the 10th and 90th percentiles for the infant's age.

Small for gestational age (SGA): Weight falls below the 10th percentile for the infant's age.

CLINICAL ALERTS

Safe Suctioning

Always suction the mouth before suctioning the nares because fluids and secretions that could obstruct the respiratory tract may be present in the mouth or the nares or both. Placing the syringe in the nares first may trigger an inspiratory gasp, causing the infant to pull mucus further into the respiratory tract.

Timely Recognition of Tachypnea

An increasing respiratory rate is often the first sign of respiratory comprise or obstruction. If this occurs, initiate and maintain effective ventilation.

Recognizing Immediate Neonatal Respiratory Distress

- During the neonatal assessment, the nurse is alert to the following signs and symptoms that are indicative of respiratory distress. If any of these symptoms are present, notify the physician immediately.
- Generalized cyanosis
- Tachycardia (heart rate >160 beats/min)
- Tachypnea (respiratory rate >70 breaths/min)
- Rib retractions
- Expiratory grunting
- Flaring nostrils

Safe Positions to Prevent Sudden Infant Death Syndrome (SIDS)

- Place all newborns on their backs to sleep.
- When using a side-lying position, place the infant's dependent arm forward to lessen the likelihood that the infant will roll into a prone position.

Recognizing an Ophthalmic Emergency in the Infant

Absence of the red reflex indicates an interference with the transmission of light to the retina. This is an ophthalmic emergency that requires immediate medical attention, as optic nerve suppression from obstructed light pathways may result in permanent blindness.

Recognizing Acute Abdomen in the Neonate

The following symptoms may indicate an acute abdomen:

- Rigid, board-like abdomen
- Inability to palpate abdominal organs
- Indicators of pain (continuous crying, facial changes, gross motor movements)

Scrotal Auscultation

If bowel sounds are present in the scrotum, immediately notify the physician. This is a medical emergency.

Protecting the Infant from the Sun

Advise parents to check with their health care provider about use of sunscreen products, as many do not recommend sunscreens until the infant is at least 6 months of age.

DIAGNOSTIC TESTS

Mandatory Newborn Metabolic Screening

- Mandatory in the United States to screen for inborn errors of metabolism (e.g., phenylketonuria (PKU), galactosemia, hemoglobinopathy, hypothyroidism)

- Serum sample obtained from a heel stick
- Performed 24 hours to 7 days after birth

MEDICATIONS

Eye Prophylaxis to Prevent Ophthalmia Neonatorum

- The Centers for Disease Control and Prevention (CDC) recommends that the medication (e.g., erythromycin, tetracycline, silver nitrate) be administered as soon as possible after birth.
- Some birth facilities delay neonatal eye prophylaxis up to an hour to allow eye contact to facilitate parent–infant bonding. If instillation is delayed, the facility should have a monitoring system in place to ensure that all infants receive the prophylaxis (CDC, Workowski & Berman, 2006).

Erythromycin (eh-rith-roe-**mye**-sin), Ilotycin

Pregnancy Category B
Indications
Infants Prophylaxis of ophthalmia neonatorum

Actions Suppresses protein synthesis at the level of the 50S ribosome

Therapeutic Effects Bacteriostatic action against susceptible bacteria spectrum: Streptococci, staphylococci, gram-positive bacilli

Pharmacokinetics
Absorption Minimal absorption may follow topical or ophthalmic use.

Contraindications and Precautions
Contraindicated in Hypersensitivity

Adverse Reactions and Side Effects Irritation

Route and Dosage Apply a thin strip to each eye as a single dose.

Nursing Implications
1. Inform the parents of medication administration.
2. Prepare to administer the eye ointment to the infant 1 hour after birth.

3. Apply a thin strip to each eye as a single dose.
4. Start at the inner canthus and move to the outer canthus.
5. Dab excess medication off gently, do not wash away the medicine.

Data from Deglin, J., & Vallerand, A. (2009). Davis's drug guide for nurses (11th ed.). Philadelphia: F.A. Davis.

AquaMEPHYTON Phytonadione (fye-toe-**na**-dye-one)

AquaMEPHYTON, Mephyton, Vitamin K

Classifications
Therapeutic Antidotes, vitamins
Pharmacological Fat-soluble vitamins

Pregnancy Category UK

Indications
Prevention and treatment of hypoprothrombinemia, which may be associated with excessive doses of oral anticoagulants, salicylates, certain anti-infective agents, nutritional deficiencies, and prolonged total parenteral nutrition. Prevention of hemorrhagic disease of the newborn.

Action
Required for hepatic synthesis of blood coagulation factors II (prothrombin), VII, IX, and X.
Therapeutic Effects Prevention of bleeding due to hypoprothrombinemia.

Pharmacokinetics
Absorption Well absorbed after oral, IM, or subcutaneous administration
Distribution Crosses the placenta; does not enter breast milk
Metabolism and Excretion Rapidly metabolized in the liver
Half-life Unknown

Contraindications and Precautions
Contraindicated in Hypersensitivity, hypersensitivity or intolerance to benzyl alcohol (injection only)
Use Cautiously in Impaired liver function.
Exercise Extreme Caution in Severe life-threatening reactions have occurred after IV administration; use other routes unless IV is justified.

Adverse Reactions and Side Effects

Gastrointestinal Gastric upset, unusual taste
Dermatological Flushing, rash, urticaria
Hematological Hemolytic anemia
Local Erythema, pain at injection site, swelling
Miscellaneous Allergic reactions, hyperbilirubinemia (large doses in very premature infants), kernicterus.

Route and Dosage IV use of phytonadione should be reserved for emergencies.

Prevention of hemorrhagic disease of the newborn:

IM (Neonates): 0.5–1 mg, given within 1 hour of birth. May be repeated in 2–3 weeks if the mother received previous anticonvulsant/anticoagulant/anti-infective/antitubercular therapy. 1–5 mg may be given IM to the mother 12–24 hours before delivery.

Nursing Implications

- Inform the parents of medication administration.
- Prepare to administer the injection to the infant 1 hour after birth.
- Administer IM injection into the anterolateral muscle of the newborn's thigh.
- Report any symptoms of unusual bleeding or bruising (bleeding gums, nose bleed, black, tarry stools, hematuria, bleeding from the base of the umbilical cord or other open wounds)
- A decrease in hemoglobin and hematocrit levels or any bleeding may indicate that the desired effects of the medicine have not been achieved and that more vitamin K may be necessary. Call the physician for further instruction.

Data from Deglin, J., & Vallerand, A. (2009). Davis's drug guide for nurses (11th ed.). Philadelphia: F.A. Davis.

Hepatitis B Vaccine (Recombivax HB, Enerix-B)

- Series of three doses, beginning at birth
- Recommended for all infants
- Parental consent required
- Administered into the vastus lateralis muscle
- Repeat doses at 1 and 6 months of age

ETHNOCULTURAL CONSIDERATIONS

Accepting Customs and Traditions

Valued health beliefs from various ethnic backgrounds frequently extend to the area of infant care. For example, some Asians, Hispanics, Eastern Europeans and Native Americans delay the initiation of breastfeeding because of the belief that colostrum is "bad" (D'Avanzo & Geissler, 2003; Dillon, 2007). Be respectful and accepting of cultural beliefs such as these.

TEACHING THE FAMILY

Proper Bulb Suctioning

- Ensure that parents understand the proper technique for use and care of the bulb syringe; ask for a return demonstration.
- Compress the bulb syringe first, then insert it into the infant's nostril or mouth; if the bulb syringe is inserted and then compressed, secretions may be forced further back into the nose or throat and cause obstruction.
- Position the infant's head to the side or downward if he is vomiting or gagging.
- Always wash the bulb syringe in warm, soapy water each day and after each use.
- Store the bulb syringe at the infant's bedside.

How to Recognize Breathing Difficulties

Teach parents the signs of breathing difficulties in their infant:

- Above normal respirations
- Prolonged (>15 seconds) periods of breath holding
- Sucking-in and see-saw movements around the rib cage
- Nasal flaring
- Grunting

Umbilical Cord Care

- Teach parents about the cord's normal appearance and when to expect complete cord detachment.

- Show parents how to fold and position the diaper below the cord stump; emphasize the need to keep the area free from urine and wetness during bathing.
- Alert parents to potential danger signs such as bleeding or a foul odor.

Basics of Newborn Care

Topic	Essential Instructions
Bathing	Use a warm area that is free from drafts. Use only warm water for the first few days of life. Sponge bathe until the umbilical stump falls off (approximately 2 weeks). Use unscented products. There is no need to bathe every day.
Clothing	At home, dress as other family members, appropriate for temperature and season. Protect from wind or drafts and sun.
Diapering	Wash cloth diapers separately from other clothing. Infants may develop rash from perfumes in disposable diapers; if so, try another brand. Contact a health care professional if the rash persists.
Circumcision	Use petroleum gauze dressing for 1-2 days to prevent the diaper from adhering to the surgical site (unless a Plastibell is used). Cleanse with water only until healed.

How to Care for the Infant/Child Who Has Not Been Circumcised

Teach the parents:

- Keep the uncircumcised penis clean by gently washing the genital area while bathing. No special cleansing (e.g., with cotton swabs or antiseptics) is necessary.
- The foreskin usually does not fully retract for several years and should not be forced.
- When the foreskin fully retracts (4–5 years of age), teach your son to clean his foreskin by gently pulling it back away from the head of the penis and then rinsing the head of the penis and inside fold of the foreskin with soap and warm water every day. After washing, the foreskin should be pulled back over the head of the penis.

Safe Car Seat Use

- Ensure that the car seat meets federal guidelines; look for a label on the seat tag or packaging box that confirms this; guidelines are also available at the American Academy of Pediatrics Web site (www.AAP.org).
- Follow car seat instructions when installing the car seat.
- Car seats for initial hospital dismissal may be obtained through various community resources (e.g., hospital or birthing center, American Red Cross, local health and safety council, State Department of Health).
- Dress the infant in clothing that facilitates ease of positioning and strap placement.
- Provide infant head support: Use a commercially made product or place a rolled-up receiving blanket around the head and neck area.
- To prevent burns and overheating in warm weather, check the temperature of the car seat by touching the surface.
- Trained professionals may be available to perform safety checks to help parents with proper car seat use. New cars are required to be equipped with tethers and lower anchors to ensure safe car seat installation and use.

How to Plan for and Assess Child Care Arrangements

Encourage the family to:

- Communicate their needs and express their concerns about child care.
- Interview the facility director along with other individuals who may be involved in the child's care.
- Evaluate the educational programs related to qualification of teachers and structure of the learning environment (structured or unstructured).
- Investigate the provision of meals, nutrition, and related sanitation.
- Visit the child care facility on a few occasions, announced and unannounced.
- Identify practical aspects of child care such as location, hours of operation, fee requirements and payment schedule, child to worker ratio, environmental safety, indoor and outdoor space, sick day policies, and availability of care during a holiday or inclement weather.

- Evaluate the infection control and injury prevention measures.
- Gain broader information about the facility related to breast feeding, discipline, nurturing, diapering/toileting, stimulating growth and development, play, nap/rest time, and field trips.
- Discover state regulations and read the care facility's policies and related public records.
- Become familiar with early childhood programs that offer voluntary accreditation such as the National Academy of Early Childhood Programs.

ADDITIONAL INFORMATION FOR THE CLINICAL SETTING

Documenting Appropriate Birth Information

- Exact time of birth
- Status of infant's respirations (spontaneous or assisted)
- 1- and 5-minute Apgar scores
- Birth weight in pounds and kilograms
- Axillary temperature
- Number of vessels in the umbilical cord
- Type and amount of medication instilled for eye prophylaxis
- Injection sites for vitamin K and hepatitis B vaccine administration
- Findings from the general physical assessment
- Observations of voiding or stooling
- All laboratory testing obtained, such as blood glucose or cultures
- Legally register the neonate with the State Bureau of Vital Statistics (mother's name, father's name [if the mother gives permission], date, time, place of birth)

Fostering Family Attachment

- Provide time in the first few hours after birth for privacy and time for the new family to get to know one another.
- After birth, delay any procedures that are not immediately necessary such as measurements and other admission procedures, to allow the family adequate time alone.

- Encourage early breast-feeding by providing proper education and support.
- Teach parents about infant behavioral cues for feeding (rooting, sucking on their fingers or fist, increasing motor activity or crying) and how to respond to them.
- Help parents understand that crying is the infant's way of communicating, and all newborns have distinguishable cries for hunger, pain, tiredness, fussiness, or getting attention.
- Teach parents that newborns have a built-in capacity to console themselves and do so by sucking, motion, and distraction.
- Help parents to recognize the joys and frustrations that go along with ongoing parenting. Assure them that it takes time to feel comfortable in meeting their newborn's unique needs.
- Introduce the concept of anticipatory guidance to help prepare parents for important developmental milestones that will occur.
- Encourage the parents to invite siblings and other family members to visit for short periods of time to share the joy and to provide support.
- Provide consistent nurses throughout the hospital or birthing center stay.

RESOURCES

Centers for Disease Control and Prevention (CDC). National Center for Health Statistics. (2007). *National Health and Nutrition Examination Survey*. Available at:
http://www.cdc.gov/nchs/about/major/nhanes/growthcharts/charts.htm

National Newborn Screening and Genetic and Resource Center: *National newborn screening status report*. Available at:
http://genes-r-us.uthscsa.edu/nbsdisorders.pdf

Recommended Childhood and Adolescent Immunizations Schedule - United States (2007). Approved by the Advisory Committee on Immunization Practices (www.cdc.gov/nip/acip), the American Academy of Pediatrics (www.aap.org), and the American Academy of Family Physicians (www.aafp.org). Available at: http://www.cdc.gov/vaccines/recs/acip/default.htm

U.S. Preventive Services Task Force (USPSTF) (2001). *Screening for newborn hearing. Recommendation statement*. Available at: www.ahrq.gov/clinic/uspstf/uspsnbhr.htm

REFERENCES

Ballard, J.L., Khoury, J.C., Wedig, K., Wang, L., Eilers-Waisman, B.L., & Lipp, R. (1991). New Ballard score, expanded to include extremely premature infants. *Journal of Pediatrics, 119*, 417–423.

Centers for Disease Control and Prevention (CDC), Workowski K., & Bergman, S. (2006). Sexually transmitted disease treatment guidelines, 2006. *MMWR Morbidity and Mortality Weekly Report, 55*(RR-11), 1–94.

D'Avanzo, C., & Geissler, E. (2003). *Pocket guide to cultural assessment* (3rd ed.). St. Louis, MO: C.V. Mosby.

Deglin, J., & Vallerand, A. (2009). *Davis's drug guide for nurses* (11th ed.). Philadelphia: F.A. Davis.

Dillon, P.M. (2007). *Nursing health assessment: A critical thinking, case studies approach* (2nd ed.). Philadelphia: F.A. Davis.

Caring for the Newborn at Risk

KEY TERMS

preterm – An infant born before 37 completed weeks of gestation

term newborn – Live infant born between weeks 38 and 42 of completed gestation

postterm – An infant born after week 42 of completed gestation

FOCUSED ASSESSMENT

- Lung maturity: Fetal lung maturity develops in utero progressively until term. Fetal lung is determined via the lecithin/sphingomyelin (L/S) ratio and phosphatidyl glycerol (PG) values, which are essential in promoting oxygenation of the lung alveoli.
- Circulatory maturity: Fetal circulation functions in utero to oxygenate the organs needed for intrauterine growth.
- Neurological maturity: The neurological system, including the central and peripheral nervous systems and the parasympathetic and sympathetic nervous systems, is underdeveloped at birth. The preterm newborn is at an increased risk resulting in the inability to cope with the extrauterine stimuli at birth.

Viability Related to Newborns Classified According to Gestational Age (GA)

- Viable: Newborns whom all neonatal clinicians agree should be treated (gestational age [GA] greater than or equal to 25 weeks)

- Nonviable: Newborns whom nearly all neonatal clinicians agree should not be treated (GA less than or equal to 22 weeks)
- Viability uncertain: Newborns for whom the need for resuscitation or treatment (GA 23–24 weeks) is debated and discussed by clinicians, often with disagreement (Taeusch, Ballard, & Gleason, 2005).

Newborn Classification by Birth Weight and Gestational Age

Birth weight is compared to gestational age for a more accurate assessment of risk factors and specific growth patterns

- Small for gestational age (SGA): Weight below the 10th percentile for gestational age
- Average for gestational age (AGA): Weight between the 10th and 90th percentile for gestation age
- Large for gestational age (LGA): Weight above the 90th percentile for gestational age

Signs of Cold Stress

- Poor feeding
- Lethargy
- Central cyanosis or pallor
- Respiratory distress
- Bradycardia (Klaus & Fanaroff, 2005)

Temperature

- Normal skin temperature: 97–98°F (36.2–36.8°C)
- Normal axillary temperature: 97.7–99.5°F (36.5–37.5°C)
- Normal rectal temperature: 97.9–100.4°F (36.6–38°C)

Pain

High-risk newborns undergo numerous life-saving interventions, many of which produce pain. Pain should be assessed during both procedural and routine care. The Premature Infant Pain Profile is commonly used for pain assessment in the NICU (Fig. 16-1).

	0	1	2	3
GA	>/= 36 Wks	32–36 6/7 Wks	28–31 6/7 Wks	</= 28 Wks
Behavioral state	Active/awake	Quiet/awake	Active/sleep	Quiet/sleep
HR	0–4 beats/minute Inc	5–14 beats/minute Inc	15–24 beats/minute Inc	25 beats or > Inc
O2 Sats	0–2.4% Decrease	2.5–4.9% Decrease	5–7.4% Decrease	7.5% or Decrease
Brow bulge	None	Minimum	Moderate	Maximum
Eye squeeze	None	Minimum	Moderate	Maximum
Nasolabial furrow	None	Minimum	Moderate	Maximum

Figure 16-1 Premature infant profile.

Relationship Between pH and Concentration of Arterial Blood Gases

	pH	pco$_2$	pao$_2$	pHCO$_3$
	Measures blood acidity	Partial pressure of carbon dioxide in blood	Partial pressure of oxygen in blood	Partial pressure of bicarbonate (alkaline or base) in blood
Normal Neonatal Values	pH = 7.25–7.45	pco$_2$ = 35–40 mm Hg	pao$_2$ = 50–80 mm Hg	pHCO$_3^-$ = 20–22 mEq/L
Respiratory Acidosis (due to poor ventilation)	↓pH	↑pco$_2$	WNL	WNL
Metabolic Acidosis (anaerobic metabolism from hypoxia, diarrhea, or kidney disease)	↓pH	WNL	WNL	↑pHCO$_3^-$
Respiratory Alkalosis (hyperventilation)	↑pH	↓pco$_2$	↑pao$_2$	WNL
Metabolic Acidosis (vomiting, diarrhea, hypocalcemia)	↑pH	WNL	WNL	↑pHCO$_3^-$

WNL = within normal limits.
Adapted from Noerr, B. (2000). Neonatal respiratory disease and management strategies, May 18, Hershey, PA. A continuing education service of Penn State's College of Medicine at the Milton S. Hershey Medical Center.

Assessment of the Preterm Infant

Skin	Head	Chest	Cardiac	Abdomen	Musculoskeletal	Genitalia	Neurological/Sensory
Skin tags	Irregular shaped head, molding after delivery, caput succedaneum cephalhematoma	Funnel or pigeon chest	Apical heart rate is assessed for a full minute.	Cord does not have two arteries and one vein.	No flexion of extremities resulting in increased susceptibility to heat loss and skin breakdown	Male scrotum has no rugae and the testes are often undescended.	Marked head lag in all positions
Translucent	Large anterior and posterior fontanels present. Fused sutures. Bulging or depressed fontanels	Supernumerary nipples or nipples are flat on the chest wall	The heart rate may normally be above 160 bpm but it should not be above 180 bpm.	Palpate for masses.	Assess for fractures or developmental hip dysplasia or fractured clavicle.	Female clitoris is often prominent and not covered by the labia minora. The labia majora is also small.	Consistent caregivers read the cues and notice subtle changes.
Lanugo covering the shoulders, back, thighs, forehead and ears	Ear pinnas are flat and readily fold upon themselves	Ribs are visible.	Heart auscultation is done in the second and fourth right and left intercostal spaces as well as the apex and axillae area	Auscultate bowel sounds.		Inguinal hernias are common.	Sucking and gagging reflexes are often absent until 32–34 weeks of gestation.

Little subcutaneous fat	Eyes are fused before 24 weeks of gestation.	Grunting, nasal flaring, or retractions (subcostal, sternal or suprasternal) are signs of respiratory distress.	Auscultation of heart sounds should be done routinely to detect murmurs that may or may not be innocent	Abdominal circumference is measured to assess for distention that may indicate necrotizing enterocolitis (NEC).	Female absence of vaginal or male urethral opening covered by prepuce	Moro reflex may be absent to weak.
Fragile and easily injured	Nose flattened or bruised Nasal patency Low placement of ears	Auscultate anterior, posterior, and at the sides of the chest	Blood pressure readings are taken on all four extremities to determine any wide variations that may be indicative of a ductal defect.		Meconium found in the vaginal opening	Any signs or symptoms of increased intracranial may be related to cerebral insults.
Mottled related to poor peripheral perfusion	Facial anomalies	Auscultate respiratory rate for a full minute.	Persistent central cyanosis	Enlarged liver or spleen	Ambiguous genitalia	Hypotonia or hypertonia
Prominent veins		Respiratory rate is between 60 and 80 respirations per minute.	Displacement of apex		Bladder exstrophy	Twitches, jittery, myoclonic jerks

(continued)

Assessment of the Preterm Infant (Continued)

Skin	Head	Chest	Cardiac	Abdomen	Musculoskeletal	Genitalia	Neurological/Sensory
Covered in vernix		Respiratory rates above 80 breaths per minute are not within normal limits.	Cardiomegaly				Eye lids edematous, drainage present, minimal reactivity to light, congenital cataracts, absence of red reflex, inability to follow object or bright light
Pale (pallor) related to anemia from blood loss		Asymmetrical chest movement may suggest respiratory conditions such as pneumothorax or diaphragmatic hernia.					Eyes have nystagmus, or strabismus, or ruptured capillaries.
Congenital strawberry hemangiomas		Excessive secretions will affect the oxygen intake.					

Diaper rash is common and related to the increase in irritation of the stool when the newborn is on antibiotics and the fragility of the skin

Soles of the feet are smooth.

Figure 16-2 Laboratory evaluation of the jaundiced infant of 35 or more weeks' gestation.

Jaundice

Jaundice is diagnosed in term infants with a serum bilirubin level greater than 12.9 mg/dL and in preterm infants with a serum bilirubin >15 mg/dL. If jaundice appears, a bilirubin level to determine the bilirubin factor is plotted on the bilirubin graph in relation to hours of age (American Academy of Pediatrics [AAP], 2004) (Fig. 16-2).

Neonatal Abstinence Syndrome (NAS)

The following are signs and symptoms of withdrawal or neonatal abstinence syndrome (NAS) to determine if a newborn is an infant of a drug-abusing mother (IDAM):

- Irritability
- Tremors
- Wakefulness
- Uncoordinated feeding pattern
- Loose stools
- Yawning or hiccups
- Poor weight gain
- Hypertonia
- Seizures
- Exaggerated rooting reflex
- Regurgitation and vomiting
- Tachypnea or apnea
- Sneezing and stuffy nose
- Lacrimation

CLINICAL ALERTS

Fractured Clavicle

- The T-shirt is sometimes pinned so that the arm is in a flexed position to produce a loose splint.
- The affected arm is pinned to the opposite shoulder by the hand cuff of the newborn T-shirt.
- Pain management may be needed if the newborn appears uncomfortable.
- Keep the newborn off the injured side to decrease pain and promote alignment.

Microcephaly

- It is critical to maintain accurate and consistent head measurements by plotting them on the growth chart and monitoring the newborn for neurological symptoms.

Taking the Newborn's Blood Pressure

Attempt to take the blood pressure while the newborn is sleeping or use a pacifier to quiet the newborn for the procedure.

Aspiration

Never feed newborns with greater than 60 respirations/minute orally because they have an increased risk of aspiration pneumonia.

Calculating Standard Newborn Formulas

To maintain adequate growth, newborns need a caloric intake of 100 to 120 kcal/kg per day and a fluid intake of 150 to 180 mL/kg per day (Gomella, 1999).

$$\text{kcal/kg per day} = \frac{\text{kcal/mL} \times \text{total mL of formula}}{\text{weight}}$$

DIAGNOSTIC TESTS

Hypoglycemia and Hyperglycemia

- Hypoglycemia is diagnosed when glucose levels fall below 60 mg/dL. The newborn may also start building up ketones.

- Hyperglycemia is rarer than hypoglycemia but is still significant. A blood glucose level above 150 mg/dL is considered hyperglycemia and can cause dehydration and weight loss. Severe hyperglycemia may also cause cerebral hemorrhage (Treusch et al., 2005).

Hemoglobin and Hematocrit Levels

- Closely monitor hemoglobin, hematocrit, and bilirubin levels.
- Exchange transfusions may be ordered for hematocrits greater than 65% in the first 24 hours of life to prevent neurological deficits.
- Exact hematocrit values at which complications will occur are difficult to determine because different newborns become symptomatic at different levels.
- Monitor questionable hematocrit levels by venous blood because capillary hematocrits are less exact.
- Assess the newborn for neurological symptoms such as high pitched cry, feeding problems, irritability, and apnea.
- Test urine for blood and macroscopic analysis (Klaus & Fanaroff, 2005).

Normal Newborn Blood Counts

Value	28 Weeks' Gestation	34 Weeks' Gestation	Term
Hemoglobin (g/dL)	14.5	15	16.8
Hematocrit (%)	45	47	53
Red blood cells (mm³)	4	4.4	5.25
MCV (μm³)	120	118	107
MCH (pg)	40	38	34
MCHC (%)	31	32	31.7
Reticulocytes (%)	5–10	3–10	3–7
Platelets (1000/mm³)			290

Source: Klaus & Faranoff (2005).

Radiology

The radiographs of respiratory distress syndrome (RDS) show a reticulogranular pattern that looks like "ground glass," possible atelectasis that looks like white correction fluid, and obscure heart borders (Noerr, 2000).

Differential White Blood Cell Count

The formula for a total neutrophil ratio (I/T ratio) is bands divided by segs + bands:

$$\frac{\text{bands}}{\text{segs} + \text{bands}}$$

For example:

$$\frac{7 \text{ bands}}{54 + 7} = 0.11 \text{ shift}$$

This is a less than 0.3 shift and is not indicative of an infection.

White Blood Cell Count for a 1-Week-Old Newborn		
	<1500 g	1500–2500 g
Total WBC count	16.8 ($\times$ 10³/mm³)	13.0 ($\times$ 10³/mm³)
Segmented	54	55
Unsegmented	7	8
Eosinophils	2	2
Basophils	1	1
Monocytes	6	5
Lymphocytes	30	29

Source: Klaus & Faranoff (2005).

MEDICATIONS

In high-risk infants, after an airway has been established, the administration of synthetic surfactant within 15 to 30 minutes of the birth is required. Newborns larger than 1000 g benefit from surfactant therapy at any time during the first 2 to 6 hours of life.

Beractant (Survanta)

Classifications Sterile nonpyrogenic pulmonary surfactant.

Indications Lowers minimum surface tension and increases pulmonary compliance and oxygenation in preterm newborns. Prevents and treats respiratory distress syndrome.

Action Lowers surface tension at the alveolar level.

Storage Refrigerate and protect from light.

Pharmacokinetics
Absorption Absorbed only in lungs.
Distribution Is not absorbed systemically.

Contraindications and Precautions Monitor heart rate and respiration.

Adverse Reactions and Side Effects Transient bradycardia, oxygen desaturation, possible increased nosocomial infections.

Route and Dosage Intratracheal 4 mL/kg q6hr × 4 (maximum of 4 doses in first 48 hours)

Nursing Implications
1. Give within 15 minutes of birth to premature newborns.
2. Perform naso-oral suction before administration.
3. Warm the vial 20 minutes to room temperature or 8 minutes by hand.
4. Do not suction for 1 hour after administration.
5. Discard vial after use; do not re-refrigerate once it is warmed.

Data from RxList (2008).

Drugs that Can Cause Withdrawal Symptoms in Newborns		
Opiates	**Barbiturates**	**Others**
Codeine	Butabarbital	Alcohol
Heroin	Phenobarbital	Amphetamine
Meperidine	Secobarbital	Chlordiazepoxide
Methadone		Clomipramine
Morphine		Cocaine
Pentazocine		Desmethylimipramine
Propoxyphene		Diazepam
		Diphenhydramine
		Ethchlorvynol
		Fluphenazine
		Glutethimide
		Hydroxyzine
		Imipramine
		Meprobamate
		Phencyclidine

Source: Gomella (1999).

Medications Used to Treat Infant of a Drug-abusing Mother (IDAM)

- Paregoric (camphorated tincture of opium)
- Phenobarbital (Luminal)

- Clonidine (Catapres)
- Chlorpromazine (Thorazine)
- Diazepam (Valium)

Naloxone (Narcan) in a Newborn with Neonatal Abstinence Syndrome

Do not use Naloxone (Narcan) if the mother is a suspected drug abuser. It may increase the severity of drug withdrawal.

ETHNOCULTURAL CONSIDERATIONS

Racial Disparities in Preterm Deliveries

- White and Asian women: 10.7%
- Hispanic women: 11.4%
- African American women: 17.6% (Cuevas et al., 2005)

Recording Weights

Record the newborn's weight in units corresponding to the parents' culture:

- North American: pounds
- European and Asian: kilograms

TEACHING THE FAMILY

Communicating to Parents About Cleft Lip and Palate Repair

- Provide parents emotional support related to their newborn's cleft lip and palate repair.
- Refer parents to Web sites that contain valuable information (see Resources at end of chapter).

Orienting Family Members to the Neonatal Unit

Orient parents to the neonatal intensive care units' (NICU) environment and policies and procedures and Health Insurance Portability and Accountability Act of 1996 [HIPAA] regulations.

- Assign one primary care nurse as the main contact for the parents.

- Explain the rationale for policies and procedures.
- Listen to the parent's expectations of their role in the NICU.
- Explain the integration of caretaking roles between parents and staff.
- Use a white board at the newborn's bed to relay messages back and forth.
- Encourage parents to call the NICU and inquire about their newborn 24/7.
- Encourage parents to bring in the newborn's personal clothes when the newborn can be dressed.
- Encourage parents to verbalize if there is dissatisfaction with newborn's care. Try to incorporate parent's suggestions into care when possible.

ADDITIONAL INFORMATION FOR THE CLINICAL SETTING

Weaning the Newborn from the Incubator

- When the newborn is being "weaned" from the servo (skin) mode of the incubator the temperature is decreased gradually every few hours while the body temperature is checked.
- When the newborn can maintain his temperature above 97.7°F (36.5°C) axillary, switch to air mode and dress the newborn.
- Closely observe the newborn's temperature, weight gain, and behavioral status during the weaning process.

Hypoglycemia in the Newborn

The nurse must understand the dynamics of hypoglycemia and remember that not all newborns are symptomatic:

- Monitor glucose levels carefully in SGA newborns. Glucose testing is often performed via heelstick (capillary blood sampling). A heelstick is done by pricking the heel and scooping the dripping heel blood into the appropriate neonatal laboratory tubes. Approximately 1 mL of blood is required for testing.
- Optimal glucose levels are 70 to 100 mg/dL, as they are in adults. The lowest clinically acceptable level is 60 mg/dL.

At a level of 40 mg/dL the newborn may become symptomatic.

- Many NICUs have protocols requiring blood glucose levels at specific intervals for SGA newborns (e.g., at birth, 1, 2, 4, and 8 hours of age; Klaus & Faranoff, 2005). Some NICUs repeat glucose levels at 12 and 24 hours of age.
- For newborns on IV therapy, since a basic component of the parenteral fluid is glucose, nurseries maintain routine blood glucose checks. IV therapy consists of providing glucose at a rate of 4 to 8 mg/kg per minute.
- If a stable newborn is found to be hypoglycemic on routine blood glucose check, start enteral feedings immediately. Recheck the glucose level 30 minutes after feeding.

Transient Tachypnea of the Newborn

The nurse must perform an accurate assessment of the respiratory system because immediately after birth or into the transitional period (within 1–2 hours) the neonate's respiratory rate should be **below 60** breaths/min with **no** retractions, nasal flaring, or grunting and a peripheral pulse oximeter reading of >92%. If any of these parameters are not met immediately after birth or in the transition period, immediate attention and supplemental oxygen are warranted.

Caring for the Infant with Jaundice

- Shield the newborn's eyes with an opaque mask during phototherapy. Remove the mask during feedings so the infant can receive visual stimulation.
- Assess the newborn's eyes every 4 hours for discharge or corneal irritation.
- Cover the infant's genital area.
- Keep the newborn warm during phototherapy. The infant is susceptible to hypothermia due to skin exposure and his temperature needs to be monitored closely.
- Provide proper nutrition to ensure the clearance of the bilirubin. Encourage the mother to feed the child as often as every 2 hours.
- Explain treatment measures to parents to help decrease their anxiety.

- Instruct parents to report any changes in the infant's condition such as an increase in jaundice, poor feeding, lethargy, or vomiting.

Retinopathy of Prematurity

Because retinopathy of prematurity (ROP) may be a complication of oxygen therapy, the nurse must maintain the lowest level of oxygen possible to maintain the pulse oximeter reading above 92%.

Extracorporeal Membrane Oxygenation

- Extracorporeal membrane oxygenation (ECMO) is used for newborns who are not responding to conventional or high-frequency ventilation.
- ECMO has only an 80% success rate and it is used as a last resort for respiratory support.
- Delivering ECMO is complicated, and it is a heart and lung bypass procedure used mainly for newborns with meconium aspiration pneumonia, neonatal pneumonia, and congenital diaphragmatic hernias.
- Newborns less than 34 weeks' gestation or 2000 g are not candidates owing to the need for heparinization of the blood, which can cause a cerebral hemorrhage in small or preterm newborns.
- ECMO is accomplished by inserting a catheter into the right internal jugular vein that extends into the right atrium and another catheter inserted into the right carotid artery into the aorta arch. The system drains venous blood and replaces arterial blood with oxygenated packed red blood cells, platelets, and fresh frozen plasma.
- The procedure is expensive, work intensive, and carries a multitude of complications.
- ECMO is available only at select Level III neonatal centers (Taeusch et al., 2005).

Necrotizing Enterocolitis

- Measure and record frequent abdominal circumferences.
- Auscultate bowel sounds before every feeding, and observe the abdomen for distention (observable loops or shiny skin indicating distention).

- Before a feeding, check for aspirates at each feed for undigested formula or breast milk. If excessive (20%) undigested breast milk or formula is found, follow the hospital's protocol, which may suggest that the next feeding be held and the primary care practitioner notified.
- Record all bowel movements (amount, consistency, and frequency).
- Hematest of stools may be needed to detect occult (nonvisible) fecal blood.

Most Common Causes of Neonatal Sepsis According to Onset of Symptoms

Neonatal sepsis is a systemic infection and can be due to any number of causes.

Early Onset and Late Onset	Nosocomial Onset
Group B *Streptococcus* (GBS)	*Staphylococcus epidermidis*
Listeria monocytogenes	*Pseudomonas*
Staphylcoccus	*Klebsiella*
Streptococcus	*Serratia*
Haemophilus influenzae	*Proteus*

 Procedure 16-1 Taking a Newborn's Blood Pressure

Purpose
Blood pressure is the pressure of blood as it is forced against the arterial walls during a cardiac contraction and is an indicator of a newborn's state of health.

Equipment
- Appropriate size cuff
- Blood pressure (B/P) machine
- Method to record results

Steps
1. Choose the appropriate size cuff by measuring the midpoint of the limb.
2. Do not use an extremity that has an IV.
3. Do not apply to broken skin areas.
4. Do not extend the cuff over a joint.

(continued)

Procedure 16-1 (Continued)

5. Inspect the cuff for intactness and decompress it to ensure it is not leaking.
6. If the cuff has an arterial mark, palpate the artery and line up the mark.
7. Wrap cuff snugly.
8. Connect the cuff to the air hose.
9. Start the blood pressure device.
10. Remove the cuff and inspect the skin (Stebor, 2005).
11. Document the procedure.

Clinical Alert Attempt to take blood pressures while the newborn is sleeping or use a pacifier to quiet the newborn for the procedure.

Note

The blood pressure is usually slightly higher in the legs.

Caution: A wide pulse pressure may indicate: Arteriovenous malformation, truncus arteriosus, or patent ductus arteriosus (PDA). A narrowed pulse pressure may indicate: peripheral vasoconstriction and cardiac failure. A systolic pressure in the arms that is 20 mm Hg or higher may indicate aortic coarctation.

Teach Parents

The nurse can teach the parents that the blood pressure is an indicator of the newborn's state of health.

Developmental Care

Providing an environment for optimal growth is the primary philosophy of developmental care. Developmental care assists in modulating the preterm newborn's behavioral states. Some of the environmental issues that can be controlled by the nurse in order to promote developmental growth include:

- Decrease noise level.
- Keep lighting subdued, and use light–dark cycles.
- Promote non-nutritive sucking.
- Provide cluster care (1–3 hours of undisturbed time between vital signs, feedings, and treatments).
- Include parents in discharge planning.

- Encourage nesting (a concept in which the linen is used to safely contain the newborn in a flexed position).

Acquainting Parents with the NICU

Explain to parents that HIPAA [Health Insurance Portability and Accountability Act of 1996 from the U.S. Department of Health and Human Services (HHS)] is taken seriously within the unit:

- Parents may be asked to step out of the unit during medical rounds, nursing report times, and possibly in emergencies to protect the privacy of all newborns.
- Phone inquiries can be done by the parents only after they identify themselves by the infant's medical record or bracelet number and they have signed a consent permitting nursing and medical personnel to discuss information on the phone with them.
- Nurses and physicians will not answer questions regarding the condition of other newborns in the unit.
- Pictures of their own newborn are allowed but they cannot photograph other newborns in the unit.

The Transport Team

The S.T.A.B.L.E. Program is designed to assist health care professionals in the postresuscitation/pretransport phase of neonatal care. It is an acronym for aspects critical to stabilization of the high-risk newborn.

S Sugar
T Temperature
A Airway
B Blood pressure
L Lab work
E Emotional support (S.T.A.B.L.E., 2006).

Endotracheal Tube (ET Tube) Size According to the Newborn's Weight and Gestational Age		
500–1000 g	<28 weeks' gestation	2.5 mm internal diameter
1000–2000 g	28–34 weeks' gestation	3.0 mm internal diameter
2000–3000 g	34–38 weeks' gestation	3.5 mm internal diameter
>3000 g	>38 weeks' gestation	3.5–4.0 mm internal diameter

Source: American Academy of Pediatrics (2000).

Types of Mechanical Ventilation Used for the Newborn

Conventional Ventilation	Conventional ventilators are set at rate of 20–60 (usually 30) breaths/min. The inspiratory time is 3-5 seconds and the peak inspiration pressure is set at 12–20 cm H_2O based on tidal volume. The flow rate is set at 6–8 L/min and they can be set to work on a timed cycle or volume cycled. Ventilators can also be patient triggered, whereby the newborn can take a spontaneous breath in between timed ventilations.
High-frequency Ventilation (HFV)	This machine uses small tidal volumes at rapid frequency (60–150 breaths/min) to decrease dead space. This is used when lower volumes would be less stressful for the neonate's respiratory system.
High-frequency Jet Ventilation (HFJV)	This method is used to limit air leaks that are problematic with atelectasis. It delivers very minute volumes at high frequency (60–600 breaths/min).
High-frequency Oscillatory Ventilation (HFOV)	This method also increases frequency to decrease volume and minimize pressure to the newborn lung. These machines are set at 300–3000 breaths/min.
Liquid Ventilation	Uses fluorocarbons, which absorb respiratory gases even better than blood. It has a low surface tension and is easily eliminated by vaporization. To date there have been no clinical trials using liquid ventilation in the newborn population (Taeusch et al., 2005).
Nitric Oxide	Used to reduce pulmonary hypertension.

RESOURCES

Parent information on discharge topics:
http://www.advanceinneonatalcare.org

Cleft Lip and Palate Association: http://www.clapa.com/

American Society of Plastic Surgeons:
http://www.plasticsurgery.org/public_education/procedures/CleftLipPalate.cfm

March of Dimes: http://www.marchofdimes.com/pnhec/4439.asp

S.T.A.B.L.E. Program: http://www.stableprogram.org/addinfo.html

National Association of Neonatal Nurses: http://www.nann.org

Cleft lip and palate information: http://www.rxlist.com/

Wide Smiles: http://www.widesmiles.org/

REFERENCES

American Academy of Pediatrics (AAP), Clinical Practice Guidelines. (2004). Management of Hyperbilirubinemia in the Newborn Infant 35 or More Weeks of Gestation, Subcommittee on Hyperbilirubinemia. *Pediatrics, 114*(1), 297–316.

Cuevas, K., Silver, D., Brooten, D., Younglut, J., & Bobo, C. (2005). The cost of prematurity: hospital charges at birth and frequency of rehospitalizations and acute care visits over the first year of life. *AJN 105*(7), 56–64.

Gomella, T. (1999). *Neonatology*. Stamford, CT: Appleton & Lange.

Klaus, M., & Fanaroff, A. (2005). *Care of the high-risk neonate* (5th ed.). Philadelphia: W.B. Saunders.

Noerr, B. (2000). Neonatal respiratory disease and management strategies, May 18. Hershey, PA. A continuing education service of Penn State's College of Medicine at the Milton S. Hershey Medical Center.

S.T.A.B.L.E. Program (2006). Retrieved from http://www.stableprogram.org/addinfo.html (Accessed April 3, 2009).

Stebor, A.D. (2005). Basic principles of noninvasive blood pressure measurement in infants. *Advances in Neonatal Care: Official Journal of the National Association of Neonatal Nurses, 5*(5), 252–261.

Taeusch, H., Ballard, R., & Gleason, C. (2005). *Avery's diseases of the newborn.* (8th ed.) Philadelphia: Elsevier Saunders.

*Caring for
the Developing Child*

KEY TERMS

age groups

Newborn: birth to 1 month

Infant: 1 month to 1 year

Toddler: 1 to 3 years

Early childhood/preschool: 3 to 6 years

School-age: 6 to 12 years

Adolescence: 12 to 19 years

FOCUSED ASSESSMENT

Principles of Childhood Growth and Development

- It is important for the pediatric nurse to have a working knowledge of growth and development in order to tailor care to the specific needs of the child and help the family understand the normal limits of behavior and development.
- *Nature* describes the traits inherent in the infant: biologically imposed idiosyncratic factors that create what and how each person "is."
- *Nurture* refers to the influence of external events such as parenting received, culture, or the "times" in which a child lives. Both are intrinsically influential.
- Each child moves at her own pace and in her own way. One child may move quickly through physical tasks, only to be slower with words.

- Growth refers to the continuous adjustment in the size of the child, internally and externally.
- Development refers to the ongoing process of adapting throughout the lifespan.
- Growth and development is a continuous process from conception to death.
- Development advances in an orderly sequence and each child progresses through the predictable stages within a predictable timeframe.
- Development proceeds in a cephalocaudal direction from head to tail (top to bottom).
- Development proceeds proximodistally, meaning from near to far and midline to periphery.
- Development proceeds from gross motor skills (e.g., walking, jumping, riding a bike) to fine motor skills (using utensils, coloring, cutting with scissors).
- Growth and development can be discussed in terms of theoretical approaches as well as developmental domains. A theoretical approach explains, describes, and predicts the various aspects of growth and development. A developmental domain refers to a way of understanding the total child in relation to the mind, body, and spirit. Understanding both the theoretical and developmental aspects is important because each contributes to a broader understanding about the child.

CLINICAL ALERTS

Reflexes

It is imperative to note important infant reflexes:

- Rooting: The infant's head turns and she begins to suck when her cheek or lower lip is stroked
- Sucking: Motion of lips, mouth, and tongue allowing the infant to take in sustenance
- Moro: Startle response when the infant is surprised
- Grasping: When palm of hands or soles of feet are stroked
- Babinski: Turning in of foot and spreading out of toes when sole of foot is stroked

Privacy

Guard the privacy of a school-age and adolescent child. Be aware of self-conscious behavior related to physical changes in the body that are occurring. Pay attention to other issues affecting the child and family such as menstruation, development of secondary sexual characteristics, hormonal imbalances, mood swings, family dynamics, social needs and other specific areas identified by the child and family.

ETHNOCULTURAL CONSIDERATIONS

Attachment

Infants from various cultures bond with parents and caregivers in the manner appropriate to their culture. Some cultures are more comfortable with physical touch and others with verbal exchange. Infants respond based on the cultural norms.

Puberty

African American girls tend to develop secondary sexual characteristics and begin menses somewhat earlier than Caucasian girls do.

TEACHING THE FAMILY

Introducing Solid Foods

- The infant is ready for the introduction of solid foods at approximately 6 months of age. To help determine if the infant is ready for solid foods, look for developmental cues such as the ability to sit well with support and the decrease or disappearance of extrusion reflex. The infant may also watch very intently as you eat, and may seem hungry between bottles or breastfeeding.
- Iron-fortified rice cereal is recommended as the infant's first solid food because it is the least allergenic of the grains, and the iron helps the infant replenish the iron stores received in utero. Mix the rice with formula, breast milk, or boiled and cooled water until it is soupy. As the infant adjusts to solids, you can increase the consistency of the cereal.

- When the infant is eating about 4 tablespoons of cereal twice per day, you can begin introducing vegetables and fruits. Starting with vegetables may help to increase acceptance by an infant not yet exposed to the sweet taste of fruits.
- Introduce one food at a time, waiting 3 to 5 days between new foods so you will be able to identify any reactions to particular foods.
- Introduce food before formula or breastfeeding when the infant is hungry, and then follow each solid food meal with a bottle or breast.
- If the infant is not growing or gaining weight, cannot suck or swallow, or shows any sign of allergic reaction it is important to seek help from the primary health care provider, nearby clinic, or emergency room if the problem is urgent.
- Keep salt, sugar, and additives to a minimum or avoid them altogether. If you make your own baby food, do not add salt or sugar.
- To prevent aspiration, **never** put solid food in bottles or mix with formula.
- Pay close attention while feeding and keep bites small to prevent choking

When Parents Inquire About the Development of Their Child

- Each child does not always reach the appropriate developmental stage based on chronological age alone.
- Certain events or variables, such as illness, may stunt the child's attempts to advance developmentally.
- Certain events or variables may move the child toward maturity.
- The child must successfully complete one stage before advancing to the next.

Anticipatory Guidance

Provide caregivers with information of what to expect with the child's next developmental phase (e.g., discipline, nutrition, safety, schooling, elimination, immunizations, and play).

Discipline

- Discipline teaches the child socialization and safety.
- Discipline corrects, molds, or enhances mental capacities and moral character.
- Early forms of discipline take place when the caregiver molds and structures the infant's daily routines and responds to the infant's needs.
- Parents often learn how to discipline from their own experiences as children.
- Teach parents what to expect at each of the developmental stages and how to recognize appropriate strategies for teaching and limit-setting.

Discipline Strategies

Distraction: Providing a toy or activity to divert the child's attention.

Time-out: Moving the child to a "cooling-off" place where the child can calm down or redirect. This can be a predetermined chair, step, or space that is associated with calming down.

Removal of privileges: Withholding a favorite toy or refusing to show a favorite video until the child's behavior is appropriate.

Verbal reprimands: Spoken warnings or disapprovals without berating the child or judging the child as "bad."

Corporal punishment (not recommended): e.g., spanking, swatting, grabbing.

ADDITIONAL INFORMATION FOR THE CLINICAL SETTING

Newborn and Infant

- The newborn or neonatal period of development refers to the first 4 weeks of life.
- The infant period of development encompasses the development from 1 to 12 months of life. This period of development continues to be a time of intense change in all aspects of development.
- Sensory development (the infant uses the five senses to explore and to learn about the world).
- Touch is extremely important and is the first sense to develop. The ability to feel objects, textures, and other people opens up the newborn's world of learning.

- The infant responds to smells within the first few days and has an innate preference for sweet tastes.
- Hearing is well developed at birth. A newborn can immediately recognize the difference between male and female voices and will generally turn toward the female voice.
- Vision is the least developed of the senses at birth. Newborns are fascinated with faces and with designs or objects that resemble faces. They may also demonstrate the beginnings of eye–hand coordination.
- Gross motor skills (the ability to use large muscles for movement) are the first to develop in the newborn and infant.
- Fine motor skills (the use of muscles to accomplish minute tasks such as pinching or picking up food) build on the gross motor skills.
- The infant must achieve three major tasks during this phase of development (separation, object permanence, mental representation)
- Infants initially communicate through cries (a universal language) that indicate physical discomfort or loneliness.

Infant Temperament

- Temperament refers to the characteristics present at birth that govern the way in which an infant responds to her surroundings. Understanding an infant's temperament is essential in her care to help both the parent and infant adapt to these experiences.
- Based on the work by Thomas, Chess, and Brich (1956), the following descriptors can be used to help recognize the infant's unique personality:
  - Regularity: Regularity refers to the need for reliability in sleeping, eating, and bowel habits. A child who is "easy" is one who can adapt to relatively flexible schedules. A child who is "difficult" has trouble when the schedule has been disrupted.
  - Reaction to new people and situations: The easy child responds easily to new people in her environment. Another child may stand back or withdraw when something or someone new is present.
  - Adaptability to change: This trait refers to a child's willingness to change routine. An easy child makes transitions with little or no discomfort. A slow-to-adapt child will become distressed with even the smallest changes, for instance, taking a different route home from school.

- Sensory sensitivity: An easy child with lower sensitivity appears much less meticulous or disturbed by her senses. A difficult child with high sensitivity may react strongly when exposed to sensory stimuli. The child may chafe against certain textures, tastes, smells, or sounds.
- Emotional intensity: An easy child may show little or no response to a situation. An intense child reacts dramatically and profoundly, whether that reaction is loud or withdrawn.
- Level of persistence: This trait refers to the child's willingness to stay engaged regardless of setbacks. A persistent child has difficulty giving up until the goal is reached. A less persistent child may be more flexible and give up easier.
- Activity level: An easy child is less frenetic with activity. A difficult child has difficulty with inactivity, preferring to always be on the move.
- Distractibility: The distractible child has difficulty concentrating on tasks in which he is not immersed. This is not the same as attention deficit disorder (ADD). A less distractible child is able to stay with a task longer.
- Mood: An easy child tends to see the world in a more positive way. A difficult child reacts more negatively.

Toddler (1 to 3 years)

- As the physical growth rate slows, the toddler develops skills (physical, cognitive, and emotional) that help her become more independent.
- As the toddler develops mobility, he is in a wonderful position to start exploring how things work and his senses become more refined.
- The toddler uses newly acquired gross motor skills.
- Tantrums are the toddler's way of working things out internally and are normal for the toddler. It may be possible to anticipate when tantrums are most apt to occur. For instance, when the toddler is tired, hungry, or overwhelmed by new situations, reserves are low; therefore, he may be more likely to explode or "melt down."
- If tantrums can be anticipated, they may be avoided or minimized.

- Finding a way for a tired toddler to rest or feeding a hungry child will do wonders in decreasing her frustration level.
- When the child is wailing and thrashing, but not doing any harm, the toddler should be ignored. Often this is not possible, and it may be necessary for a parent to intervene quickly and decisively to remove the child to a quieter or safer place.
- Some children respond to soothing touch, others can be distracted, and still others may need to continue the tantrum under the watchful eye of a parent.
- The goal is for the child to feel (and be) safe without being reinforced (positively or negatively) for having a tantrum.

Early Childhood (Preschooler; 3 to 6 years)

- The preschooler is much more agile; he can climb stairs using alternating feet and is able to ride his tricycle.
- As the brain becomes more developed the preschooler is better able to pick things up with the fingers.
- The preschooler engages in magical thinking.
- The preschooler has increased ability to verbalize; vocabulary has increased, from 1500 to 2000 words between the ages 3 and 5.
- Tantrums generally begin to subside.
- The preschooler is still egocentric (focused only on his own sense of things) and therefore is limited socially.
- It is a time of exploration of new skills and figuring out how to get and do things for oneself.

School-Age Child (6 to 12 years)

- There are many variations in size and shape of children in this period. These variations are influenced not only by familial and cultural genetics, but also by environmental factors such as diet and exercise.
- Sexual development begins.
- The school-age child is more able than the younger child to think logically.
- The school-age child builds on experience and begins to recognize consequences of actions.
- The school-age child is more able to determine what is important to remember and what is not.

- Language improves considerably; the child uses words more accurately and is able to elaborate on concepts that she wants to get across.
- The school-age child has a more definite sense of self-esteem or competence based on the ability or lack of ability to perform.
- Best friends tend to be of the same gender, although mixed-gender groups of school-age children become common as they reach the preteen and early teen years.

Adolescence (12 to 19 years)

- Adolescence technically begins with the onset of puberty when the pituitary gland relays messages to the sex glands to manufacture hormones necessary for reproduction.
- It is a period of great growth.
- The adolescent thinks abstractly and uses logic to solve problems and to test out hypotheses.
- Three major tasks must be confronted: choose an occupation or course of study, subscribe to a set of values, and develop a satisfactory sexual identity.

The Adolescent and the Informed Consent Process

- An informed consent is a way to elicit permission that is given freely that protects a person's right to autonomy and self-determination. Informed consent is given when the person understands the usual procedures and their rationales and associated risks.
- A legal parent or guardian customarily gives informed consent on behalf of the child.
- As children gain critical thinking skills they can become more active in the consent process.
- Depending on state law, people 18 to 21 years of age can give legal informed consent in the following situations: when they are minor parents of a child patient, when they are between 16 and 18 years of age seeking birth control, counseling or help for substance abuse, or when they are self-supporting (emancipated).
- In many states, a pregnant teen is considered emancipated.
- The physician is ultimately responsible for explaining the procedure and related risks while the nurse's role is to

serve as a witness to the parents' signature for the child or an emancipated adolescent's signature

- The nurse has a responsibility to notify the physician if the parent (or legal guardian) does not understand the procedure or related risks.
- This is a time of great questioning and consternation as the adolescent learns that it is possible for several views of morality to exist.

Helping the Teen Make Healthy Decisions

- Listen: Pay close attention not only to what the adolescent is saying, but also to his nonverbal cues. Try to understand his view of the world and the situation. Stay open minded when listening to the teen's views.
- Discuss without judging: The nurse can share his understanding of the issues and his perspectives while respecting those of the teenager.
- Encourage critical thought: Allow the teenager to explore and further develop his options.

RESOURCES

American Academy of Pediatrics. Topics on children and adolescents. http://www.aap.org

REFERENCE

Thomas, A., Chess, S., & Birch, H.G. (1968). *Temperament and behavior disorders in children*. New York: New York University Press.

18

*Caring for the Child
in the Hospital
and in the Community*

KEY TERMS

acute pain – Pain that occurs 24 to 48 hours after trauma and surgery; severe pain that gradually subsides over time

chronic pain – Pain that lasts more than 3 months

informed consent – Involves providing the patient with the necessary knowledge to make a decision regarding health; implies that the person understands the benefits and risks of treatment or the refusal of treatment

FOCUSED ASSESSMENT

Gathering the Child's Health History

Use the mnemonics Old Cat and SODA to gather a child's health history (Bickley & Szilagyi, 2007, p. 31).

Old Cat

Onset: "When did the child become ill?"
Location: "Where is the pain?"
Duration: "How long does the pain last?"
Character: "Can you tell me on a scale of 1 to 10 how bad it is?" Or, for a younger child, ask the parents, "How much pain do you think the child is experiencing?"
Aggravating/Alleviating: "What has made the pain better or worse?"
Timing: "When does the pain start/stop?"

SODA

Sleep: "How has your child been sleeping?"

Output: "How many times per day do you _____?" (Use the expression the family has adopted to convey urine/stool output.) Or, for the younger child ask, "How many wet diapers has he had today?"

Diet: "How much fluid has your child taken in today?" "Has the illness affected the child's appetite or diet?"

Activity: "Has the child's activity level changed since he has been ill?"

Comprehensive Health History

Family Medical and Social History

- Ages and cause of death of any deceased parents, grandparents, and siblings
- Chronic illnesses experienced by family members
- Inherited diseases
- Parents' professions, religious affiliations or spiritual beliefs, and family activities
- For the older child, interviewed without the presence of the parent, the social history must also include information regarding grade level, friendships, drug or alcohol use, smoking, sexual activity, and safe sex practices

Past Medical History

- History of the pregnancy
- Labor and delivery
- Health of the baby at birth (birth weight and APGAR scores, difficulties with feeding, breathing, jaundice, or other medical problems in the early neonatal period)
- Acute illness(es)
- Chronic illness(es)
- Medication(s)
- Herbal product(s) and home remedy(ies)
- Review all encounter form(s) and determine the reason for the visit(s), resultant medical diagnose(es), and outcome(s) of previous treatment(s)
- Immunizations
- Patterns of daily activities: sleep, nutrition, play (activities and schoolwork)

Developmental Milestones

Age	Gross Motor	Fine Motor	Sensory/Language/Play
Newborn Birth–1 Month	Reflexes present Absence of head control, but can momentarily hold the head in midline Hand lag when the newborn is pulled from a lying to a sitting position Assumes flexed position When supine assumes tonic neck flex position Kicks legs and waves arms Rounded back when sitting Rolls over accidentally	Hands predominately closed Strong grasp reflex	Touch: First sense to develop Smell: Recognizes mother and has a taste preference for sweets Hearing well developed; Becomes quiet when hears a familiar voice Limited visual acuity 20/100, fascinated with faces, follows moving objects, contrasting colors (black and white) Language: Cries and smiles during sleep Play: Interaction with parents and caregivers
Infant 1–2 Months	Less head lag when pulled to sitting position When prone can slightly lift head off of floor Improved head control, turns and lifts head from side to side when prone	Hold hands open Grasp reflex absent Call pull at clothes and blanket, bats at objects	When supine follows dangling toys Visually searches for sounds Turns head to sound Language: Coos, has social smile Play: Interaction with parents and caregivers, through gross and fine motor skills and senses

Infant 3–6 Months

Can hold head more erect when sitting, still some babbling, by 6 months sturdy head control

Only slight head lag, by 6 months no head lag

Raises head to 45 degrees to 90 degrees off of floor

In sitting position (tripod) back is straight and balances head well, sits alone by 8 months

When held in a standing position can bear some weight, by 8 months readily bears weight

Rolls from back to side and then abdomen to back

When supine puts feet to mouth

Begins to creep on hands and knees

Plays with toes

Clutches own hands, inspects and plays with hands

Pulls blanket over face

Rakes objects

Grasps objects with both hands (palmer grasp)

Shakes rattle and holds bottle

Eventually able to put objects in container and bang them together

Carries objects to mouth

Transfers objects from hand to hand

Reaches and bangs toys on table

Likes mirror images

Follows object 180 degrees

Good vision

Locates sound by turning head

Beginning eye–hand coordination

Pursues dropped object visually

Sees small objects

Responds to name

Language: Coos and babbles

Play: Interaction with parents and caregivers, through gross and fine motor skills and senses

Infant 9–12 Months

Creeps on hands and knees

Pulls self to standing position

Stands while holding onto furniture and begins to cruise

Stands alone

Changes from prone to sitting position

Can reach backwards while sitting

Can sit down from standing position alone

Begins to walk holding hand and then independently, takes first step

Uses pincer grasp

Hand dominance evident

Releases and rescues an object

When sitting, purposely reaches around back to retrieve object

Can randomly turn pages in a book

Can make a simple mark on paper

Waves bye-bye and plays pat-a-cake

Begins to feed self finger foods

Increasing depth perception

Moves toward sound

Thoroughly explores and experiences objects

Points to simple objects

Language: Says "mama" and "dada"

Play: Plays alone, continues interaction with parents and caregivers, through gross and fine motor skills and senses

(continued)

Age	Gross Motor	Fine Motor	Sensory/Language/Play
Toddler 1–3 Years	Stands without support Walks independently Creeps upstairs Pulls toys while walking Runs with wide stance Jumps in place with both feet Climbs Begins to stand on one foot momentarily Can walk up and down stairs with alternate feet	Holds a pencil or a large crayon Makes artwork that is more representative of the object Copies a circle Knows colors Feeds self with a spoon and drinks from a cup Constantly throws objects on floor Builds tower of 3-4 cubes eventually building tower of 7-8 cubes Screws/unscrews Turns pages in a book one page at a time Turns knobs Removes shoes and socks, learns to undress self	Well developed vision Can identify geometric objects Intense interest in book's pictures Distinguishes food preferences based on senses Language: Single words and simple phrases, "I do," "Want drink." By 15 months knows 15 words Play: Play along side another child
Early Childhood (preschooler) 3–6 Years	Dress self Throws and catches ball Pedals tricycle Kicks ball forward Stands on one foot for 5–10 seconds Skips and hops on one foot Walks down steps with alternate feet Jumps from bottom step Balances on alternate feet with eyes closed	Moves around in more balanced fashion Builds a tower or 9–10 cubes Draws stick figure with 6 parts Uses scissors to cut outline of picture Copies and traces geometric patterns Ties shoe laces Uses fork, spoon, and knife with supervision Colors, prints letters Mostly independent toilet training	Well developed senses Preferences based on the use of senses Language: Vocabulary has increased from 1500 to 2000 words, eventually speaks in complete sentences Play: Plays with peers, make believe, dramatic play

| School-age 6–12 Years | Gradual increase in dexterity and becomes limber
Improves coordination and balance, rhythm
Climbs, bikes, skips, jumps rope, swings
Learns to swim, dance, do somersaults and skate | Good eye–hand coordination
Balance improves
Can sew, draw, makes arts and crafts, build models, play video games
Prints and writes
Likes activities that promote dexterity such as playing a musical instrument | 20/20 Visual acuity
Color discrimination fully developed
Mature sense of smell
Hearing deficits may be discovered as language develops
Language: Accelerated, vocabulary expands to 8000–15,000 words
Play: Play with peers, solitary activities and active play (e.g., dance, karate) |
| Adolescence 12–19 Years | Begin to develop endurance
Speed and coordination
Focuses skills on interest area | Manipulates complicated objects
High skill level playing video games and computer
Good finger dexterity for writing and other intricate tasks
Precise eye–hand coordination | Increased concentration so can follow complicated instructions
Senses tied into body image
Develops adult preferences based on senses
Language: Continues to develop and refine with increased vocabulary up to 50,000 words; improved communication skills
Play: Peer groups, team sports, solitary time, school or community activities, dating |

Review of Systems

- General: Usual weight, change in weight, weakness, fatigue, fever, or allergies
- Skin: Rashes, pruritus, turgor, changes in color, indications of injury, acne, changes in nails or hair
- Head, eyes, ears, nose, throat (HEENT): Injury to head, headaches, dizziness; eye infections, itching or watering eyes, behaviors indicating change in visual acuity, use of glasses, date of last eye exam; ear infections, behaviors indicating change in hearing; nose bleeds, colds, hay fever, sinus infections; sore throats, tonsils, dentition, caries
- Neck: Neck pain, enlarged lymph glands, neck range of motion
- Chest: Respiratory infections, asthma, chronic cough, wheezing, shortness of breath, breast changes
- Cardiovascular: Heart murmur, anemia, palpitations, date of last blood work
- Gastrointestinal: Regurgitation, vomiting, changes in bowel habits, constipation, diarrhea, food intolerance, abdominal pain, changes in appetite or eating pattern
- Genitourinary: *General*—dysuria, urgency, odor to urine, date of last urinalysis; signs of puberty, urethral or vaginal discharge, presence of lesions, sexual habits, contraceptive use, and symptoms or history of sexually transmitted infections; *males*—changes in groin/scrotum/glans, presence of circumcision; *females*—menarche, date of last menstrual period, dysmenorrhea, and date of last Pap smear (if appropriate)
- Musculoskeletal: Injuries, fractures, weakness, clumsiness, gait, muscle pains
- Neurological: Seizures, tics, psychiatric diseases, anxiety, depression
- Endocrine: History or symptoms of thyroid disease or diabetes or diseases that affect normal growth

Health Assessment

Anthropometric Measurements
- Length
- Weight
- Body mass index (BMI)
  - Calculate by measuring the weight in kilograms and the height in meters squared

- Help the family calculate their child's BMI by accessing the Centers for Disease Control and Prevention (CDC) Web site. This Web site has a BMI Percentile Calculator for the Child and the Teen: http://apps.nccd.cdc.gov/dnpabmi/Calculator.aspx
- Access growth charts from the National Center for Health Statistics (NCHS) are available at http://www.cdc.gov/nchs/about/major/nhanes/growthcharts/charts.htm
- Head circumference (Fig. 18-1)
- Skinfold thickness

Figure 18-1 Measuring head circumference.

Vital Signs

Expected Temperatures in Children		
Age	**Degrees Fahrenheit (°F)**	**Degrees Centigrade (°C)**
2 months	99.4	37.5
4 months	99.5	37.5
1 year	99.7	37.7
2 years	99.0	37.2
4 years	98.6	37.0
6 years	98.3	36.8
8 years	98.1	36.7
10 years	98.0	36.7
12 years	97.8	36.6

Centigrade to Fahrenheit Temperature Conversions

$°F = (°C \times 9/5) + 32$, or $(°C \times 1.8) + 32$
$°C = (°F - 32) \times 5/9$, or $(°F - 32) \times 0.55$

°C	°F
35.0	95.0
35.2	95.4
35.4	95.7
35.6	96.1
35.8	96.4
36.0	96.8
36.2	97.2
36.4	97.5
36.6	97.9
36.8	98.2
37.0	**98.6**
37.2	99.0
37.4	99.3
37.6	99.7
37.8	100.0
38.0	100.4
38.2	100.8
38.4	101.1
38.6	101.5
38.8	101.8
39.0	102.2
39.2	102.6
39.4	102.9
39.6	103.3
39.8	103.6
40.0	104.0
40.2	104.4
40.4	104.7
40.6	105.1
40.8	105.4

Average Range for Pediatric Vital Signs

Age Group	Heart Rate (beats/min)	Respiration Rate (breaths/min)	Blood Pressure Systolic	Blood Pressure Diastolic
Infant	80–150	25–55	65–100	45–65
Toddler	70–110	20–30	90–105	55–70
Preschooler	65–110	20–25	95–110	60–75
School-age Child	60–95	14–22	100–120	60–75
Adolescent	55–85	12–18	110–125	65–85

Physical Assessment

General Impression

As the nurse meets the child and the parents and engages in conversation with them, an impression begins to take form. This subjective feeling about the child encompasses many areas of assessment.

- How does the child react to questions?
- What is the child's speech like?
- Is the child quiet, pleasant, talkative, uninterested, or angry?
- For the younger child: Does the child listen to parents, interact in a meaningful way, or engage in age-appropriate behavior?
- Is the child clean and appropriately dressed for the season?
- Observe body size, skin color, eyes, and the condition of the hair for evidence of a good overall nutritional state.

Skin

- Assess the skin for color, turgor, and lesions.
- Skin color reflects ethnicity, diet, disease, and injury.
- Assess for evidence of dehydration by grasping a small area of skin and pulling up. Once released, the skin should quickly return to its normal position.
- Inspect the texture of the hair and the condition of the scalp, palms, and nails. Normal nails are pink and convex, with white edges extending over the end of the fingers.
- Examine the palms for the normal flexion creases.

Head

- Observe the head for symmetry and shape.
- Palpate the skull to evaluate fontanels, sutures, contusions, or other swellings.
- The posterior fontanel closes within 1 to 3 months after birth, while the diamond-shaped anterior fontanel remains open until 12 to 18 months of age. The anterior fontanel is the most significant fontanel for evaluation (Fig. 18-2).
- Examine the face for general appearance and compare features with those of the parents.

Figure 18-2 Anterior and posterior fontanels.

Neck

- Palpate the lymph nodes of the head and neck systematically, starting at the preauricular area, proceeding to the postauricular area, and then to the occipital nodes (Fig. 18-3).
- Palpate the trachea for midline placement and masses. A lateral deviation of the trachea may be due to a mass or a collapsed lung.
- Examine the thyroid gland for enlargement, nodules, and goiters.

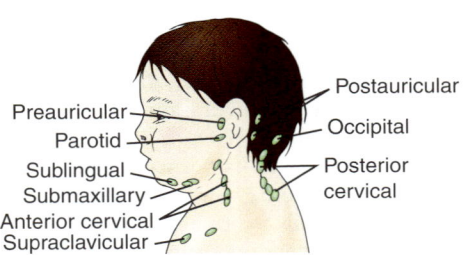

Figure 18-3 Lymph nodes of the head and neck.

Eyes

- Observe the eyes to assess symmetry, shape, and placement in relation to the nose.
- Assess for symmetry and size of the pupils and their response to light.
- Observe the conjunctiva and lids for conjunctivitis, styes, or chalazia.
- Inspect the color of the sclera.
- Note erythema, swelling, or discharge from the eyes.

Ears

- Examine the external ears for size, shape, placement, pain, and presence of drainage from the ear canal.
- Examine the tympanic membrane for the presence of normal anatomic landmarks (Fig. 18-4).
- The pinna of the ear should be above the imaginary horizontal line drawn from the medial and lateral canthi toward the occiput.
- Low-set ears may indicate a congenital anomaly such as Down syndrome.
- To assess for pain, move the pinna of the ear up and down.
- Check for purulent drainage. This may indicate a foreign body in the external ear canal or a ruptured tympanic membrane.
- Immediately report any clear drainage from the ear, particularly after head trauma or with cranial infections. This fluid may indicate a cerebrospinal fluid leak.

Figure 18-4 Tympanic membrane landmarks.

Nose/Sinuses

- Inspect the nasal mucosa for color and inflammation. Pale, boggy mucosa is a typical finding in a child with allergic rhinitis.
- Purulent discharge from the nose may indicate a viral or bacterial condition.
- Purulent discharge occurring in one nostril is suggestive of a foreign object in the other nostril.
- Inspect the septum for the midline position.
- Palpate maxillary sinuses for tenderness, using the thumbs of both hands and holding the child's head.

Throat/Mouth

- Eliciting the sound *eeehh* flattens the tongue better than the sound *aaahh* and visualization of the posterior pharynx is possible without the use of the tongue blade.
- Assess the palate, uvula, tonsils, and mucous membranes for color, exudate, and odor.
- Observe the lips for shape, symmetry, color, dryness, fissures at the corners of the mouth indicative of vitamin B_2 (riboflavin) deficiency, and clefts.
- Inspect teeth for number present, condition, color, alignment, and caries.
- Inspect the color and condition of gingival tissue. The gingival tissue should be the same color as the surrounding mucous membranes and should not be hypertrophied or show evidence of bleeding.

Chest

- Inspect the chest for size, shape, symmetry, respiratory effort, and breast development in infants. The anteroposterior diameter is fairly equal to the lateral diameter. By 2 years of age, the lateral diameter is greater than the anteroposterior diameter. Equal anteroposterior and lateral diameter after the age of 2 years may indicate chronic lung disease.
- A chest that is larger on the left than on the right may indicate an enlarged heart or a collapsed right lung.
- Pectus carinatum is a protrusion of the sternum.
- Pectus excavatum is a depression of the lower portion of the sternum.
- Retractions may also be seen in the suprasternal, substernal, subcostal, and suprasternal notch regions.

- Lung sounds are best auscultated with the child in a sitting position.
- Using a stethoscope with an appropriately sized pediatric diaphragm, auscultate the five lobes of the lungs, anteriorly and posteriorly, beginning with the apices and then moving side to side to compare bilateral lung sounds.
- Direct observation of breathing can also indicate inadequate oxygenation.
- The child's posture can be indicative of adequate or inadequate oxygenation. The child in respiratory distress sits in a tripod position sitting upright, leaning forward on outstretched arms with the jaw thrust forward. This particular position helps maximize opening up the airway and use of accessory muscles of respiration.
- Normal breath sounds are classified as bronchial (crackles), bronchovesicular (wheezes), or vesicular (rhonchi). Bronchial breath sounds are loud, high-pitched, and heard only over the trachea. The inspiratory and expiratory sounds are equal in length. Bronchovesicular breath sounds are of intermediate intensity and pitch, with equal inspiratory and expiratory phases.

Cardiac

- The chest is inspected for symmetry and pulsations and all peripheral pulses are palpated
- The nurse begins palpation with the carotid pulse, noting any distended neck veins, and continues with the brachial and radial pulses.
- Capillary refill is assessed as well as changes in the fingernails, e.g., clubbing of the fingers is noted.
- Peripheral edema and cyanosis are assessed during palpation of the femoral, popliteal, posterior tibial, and dorsalis pedis pulses.

Cardiac Assessment Techniques

Assessment Technique	What to Look for	Normal Findings	Abnormal Findings	Rationale
Inspection	Skin color, shape, and symmetry of chest, clubbing	Pink, symmetrical chest	Pallor, cyanosis, asymmetry of chest shape and movement, hyperdynamic precordium	Poor cardiac output. Deoxygenated circulating blood, ventricular failure or hypertrophy, tachycardia
Palpation	Skin and body temperature, moisture, chest movement, point of maximal impulse (PMI)	Warm, dry, symmetrical movement. PMI at 4th or 5th intercostal space at midclavicular line	Cold extremities, dry flaky skin, diaphoresis. Thrills or heaves	Poor circulation, heart failure, ventricular hypertrophy
Percussion	Heart shape and size	Normal size and shape for age and weight	Enlarged heart, axis deviation	Heart failure and hypertrophy
Auscultation	Murmurs, other sounds	No murmurs, innocent murmurs. Quiet precordium	Murmurs, clicks, rub, snaps.	Structural defects, increased workload of heart and volume overload

© Judith M. Marshall (2006).

- The point of maximal impulse (PMI), or area of most intense pulsation, and the point of apical impulse, or the impulse corresponding to the apex of the heart, are usually located in the same area of the chest.
- To assess for the first heart sound (S_1— the *lub* sound), begin at the fourth or fifth *left* intercostal space at the midclavicular line. The first heart sound reflects the closure of the mitral and tricuspid valves and signifies the beginning of ventricular contraction or systole.
- The second heart sound (S_2—the *dub* sound) reflects the closure of the pulmonary and aortic valves and signifies the beginning of atrial contraction or diastole. You hear *lub dub*.
- Murmurs are attributed to turbulent blood flow within the vessels. Assess for intensity, location, radiation, timing, and quality.

Abdominal

- Inspect the abdomen and its contour, which may be flat, round, protuberant, or scaphoid (shaped like a boat).
- Visible peristalsis may be noted in a thin child, and should be documented and reported.
- Inspect the umbilicus and inguinal areas for bulging. Note any scars, rashes, and lesions or piercings.
- The abdomen is divided into four quadrants: right upper quadrant (RUQ), left upper quadrant (LUQ), right lower quadrant (RLQ), and left lower quadrant (LLQ) (Fig. 18-5).
- Listen for up to 1 minute before determining the absence of bowel sounds in any one quadrant.
- After inspection, auscultate the abdomen in all four quadrants to assess for bowel motility. These high-pitched sounds occur every 5 to 10 seconds. Allow enough time to adequately assess frequency and character of the bowel sounds.
- Palpate the abdomen last so as not to disrupt bowel sounds. Palpation is divided into light palpation and deep palpation. Light palpation assists in identifying abdominal tenderness; these areas should be palpated last. Deep palpation is useful when assessing for masses in the liver, kidneys, spleen, inguinal and lymph nodes.
- Throughout the abdominal assessment, observe for changes in facial expression, guarding, and tensing of the abdominal muscles.

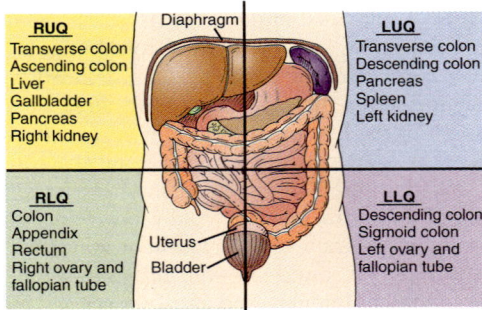

RUQ	Diaphragm	**LUQ**
Transverse colon Ascending colon Liver Gallbladder Pancreas Right kidney		Transverse colon Descending colon Pancreas Spleen Left kidney
RLQ Colon Appendix Rectum Right ovary and fallopian tube	Uterus Bladder	**LLQ** Descending colon Sigmoid colon Left ovary and fallopian tube

Figure 18-5 Abdomen divided into quadrants and organs in each quadrant.

Genitourinary and Perineal

- Assess boys and girls for Tanner staging of hair growth, evidence of normal development for the age of the child, signs of sexual abuse, and precocious puberty.

Tanner Staging of Development of Secondary Sex Characteristics

Sex Characteristics	Scoring				
	1	2	3	4	5
Breast Development in Females	Slight to no elevation of papilla	Breast buds appear; areolar widening with slight elevation	Entire breast enlarged with no protrusion of the papilla or nipple	Enlargement of the entire breast with formation of secondary mound of areola and papilla	Mature breast with protrusion of nipple only. No protrusion of the papilla
Pubic Hair Development in Females	None	Sparse, lightly pigmented, straight along border of labia	Darker and increasing amount on labia and pubis. Distribution in typical female inverted triangle	Coarse, thicker, curly. Increasing amount, less than adult.	Adult female triangle with extension of hair onto medial thighs
Pubic Hair and Genital Development in Males	No pubic hair. Preadolescent genitalia	Scant, long, slightly pigmented pubic hair. Slight enlargement of scrotum and testes; scrotum reddens and becomes more textured	Pubic hair darker, starting to curl and extends across pubis. Scrotum and testes continue to enlarge. Penis becomes longer and slightly wider.	Pubic hair is coarse, curly, less quantity than adult. Scrotum is darker; penis increases in length and breadth. Glans is broader.	Adult distribution of pubic hair with extension to medial thighs; genitalia adult in size and shape

Adapted from Tanner, J.M. (1962). *Growth at adolescence* (2nd ed.). Oxford: Blackwell.

- The anus is not routinely examined in children unless indicated due to abdominal, bowel, rectal, or stool abnormalities.

Musculoskeletal

- Perform the musculoskeletal exam while observing the child for range of motion, symmetry of movement, general alignment, and any deformities.
- Palpate each joint for range of motion and the presence of erythema or swelling.
- Assess the muscles for strength of movement.
- To test upper extremity strength, ask the child to hold both arms out to the sides and then out to the front. Ask the child to hold these positions as you apply downward pressure to both arms.
- Assess the symmetry of strength in both hands by having the child squeeze your index fingers.
- Test the strength of the legs by asking the child to lie supine and raise his legs while you apply downward pressure on the legs.
- Screen for scoliosis by age 14. A scoliometer can be used to assess for the condition as well as noting if the back appears straight and the hips are even.

Neurological

- Assess mental status by observing the infant's interaction with the parents, or by asking the older child to answer questions and listening for clear speech in the responses.
- Assess motor functioning during the skeletal examination. Ask the child to hop, skip, or jump to assess symmetry of movement.
- Sensory testing is done if there is a question regarding sensory functioning.
- Check cerebellar function by observing the child's posture and gait or by using the finger-to-nose test.
- Use the Romberg test to assess cerebellar functioning; the child stands with eyes closed and arms outstretched and is assessed for the ability to stand without swaying.
- Assess for persistence of primitive reflexes, which normally disappear during infancy (e.g., Babinski, Moro), palmar, plantar, and tonic neck reflexes are a few that are seen in the neonate but that disappear over time. Persistence of these reflexes may indicate cerebral dysfunction.

- Check deep-tendon reflexes (DTRs) with the reflex hammer. DTRs are difficult to elicit in some children and a distraction may be needed while testing reflexes.
- Cranial nerve assessment is an integral part of the physical examination and may be completed throughout the exam or as a separate part of the exam.

Cranial Nerve Testing

Cranial Nerve (CN)	How to Test
I. Olfactory	Ask the child to close both eyes and have the child identify smells. Rarely done during a routine examination.
II. Optic	Perform vision screen for test of visual acuity and color vision, test for peripheral vision, and examine the optic disc with the ophthalmoscope.
III. Oculomotor	Ask the child to follow an object through the six cardinal positions of gaze. Assess for papillary response and drooping of upper lids.
IV. Trochlear	CN III, IV, and VI are tested together.
V. Trigeminal	Observe the child chewing on a cracker. With eyes closed, gently stroke different areas of the face with a cotton ball to assess sensory function.
VI. Abducens	CN III, IV, and VI are tested together.
VII. Facial	Observe the child's facial expressions during the interview and exam. May need to ask child to frown and then smile.
VIII. Acoustic	Cause a loud sound and assess if child turns toward the sound.
IX. Glossopharyngeal	Stimulate gag reflex.
X. Vagus	Assess the uvula in midline. Assess the ability to swallow by asking child to do so.
XI. Accessory	While providing resistance, ask the child to shrug his shoulders and turn his head side to side.
XII. Hypoglossal	Observe infant sucking on a bottle. Ask the child to stick out the tongue. Listen for clarity of speech.

Feeding

- Basic knowledge of nutritional requirements is essential when working with children.
- Formula-fed infants require no more than 24 to 32 ounces of iron-fortified formula daily.
- Assess the older child, by taking a diet history and asking about routines at mealtimes.
- Children are often prescribed an "as tolerated" diet and they are able to select foods that appeal to them.
- Encourage the intake of wholesome and nutritious foods and snacks.
- Foods ingested are also important for their fluid content (e.g., gelatin and ice pops).
- Encourage parents to bring in favorite foods from home.
- Cultural preferences may make a difference in whether or not a child eats while hospitalized.
- Evaluate if foods and caloric intake are appropriate for age and developmental level.

Average Daily Caloric Requirements for Children	
Age	**Daily caloric requirements**
0–1 month	100–110 kcal/kg per day
2–4 months	90–100 kcal/kg per day
5–60 months	70–90 kcal/kg per day
>5 years	1500 kcal for first 20 kg + 25 kcal for each additional kg/day

Source: Hay W.W. Jr. et al. (2005). *Current pediatric diagnosis & treatment* (19th ed). New York: Lange Medical Books/McGraw-Hill.

Measuring Intake and Output
Calculation of Daily Maintenance Fluid Requirements

- The surface area method is the most common and used for children weighing more than 22 lbs. (10 kg): 1500 to 2000 mL/m² per day.

- Daily maintenance fluid requirements:

Calculation of Daily Maintenance Fluid Requirements	
Child's Weight	**Daily Maintenance Fluid Requirement**
0–10 kg (0–22 lbs.)	100 mL/kg of body weight
11–20 kg (24.2–44 lbs.)	1000 mL + 50 mL/kg for each kg >10
>20 kg (>44 lbs.)	1500 mL + 20 mL/kg for each kg >20
Example: A child weighs 48 kg. For the first 20 kg the child needs 1500 mL. For the next 28 kg the child needs 20 mL/kg. So, 500 mL + (28 kg × 20 mL) = 1500 mL + 560 mL = 2060 mL/day.	

- Normal urinary output is 1 to 2 mL/kg per hour.

Pain

- Remember that *"pain is whatever the child says it is."*
- Mild pain is a slight discomfort and is managed with minor analgesics along with comfort measures or distraction.
- Moderate pain may be relieved by using distraction and in conjunction with regularly timed analgesic administration, including milder opioids such as codeine in varying combinations of acetaminophen (Children's Tylenol).
- Severe pain causes pallor, sweating, piloerection (elevation of the hair above the skin), dilated pupils, increased respiration and blood pressure, and muscle tension. Management of severe pain, often associated with surgical interventions, is usually managed with strong analgesics such as morphine (Astramorph).
- Pain may be either acute or chronic. Acute pain occurs 24 to 48 hours after trauma or surgery. It is initially experienced as severe pain, and gradually subsides over time. Chronic pain in children is any pain lasting more than 3 months. It can result in fear of reinjury, anorexia, weight loss, changes in sleep patterns, guarded movements, a rigid facial expression, and diminishment of the child's joy of living.

Characteristics of Acute and Chronic Pain

Acute Pain	Chronic Pain	Chronic Cancer Pain
Identifiable cause	Cause difficult to determine	Usually identifiable cause
Short duration	Lasts longer than 3 months	Duration varies
Sudden onset	Begins gradually and persists	Onset varies
Well defined	May or may not be well defined	May or may not be well defined
Limited	Unlimited	Unlimited
Decreases with healing	Persists beyond healing time	May persist beyond healing
Reversible	Exhausting and useless	Exhausting and useless
Objective signs and symptoms	Objective signs absent	Objective signs absent
Anxiety	Depression and fatigue	Depression, fatigue, and anxiety

Source: Otto, S. E. *Oncology nursing*. St. Louis: C.V. Mosby, 1991. Reprinted in *Mosby's medical, nursing and allied dictionary* (4th ed.), p. 1144.

Several statistically reliable pain scales are available for use with children of different ages and stages of cognitive development. The most commonly used pain scales are the numeric scale, the Wong Faces Scale, and the FLACC pain scale (Fig. 18-6).

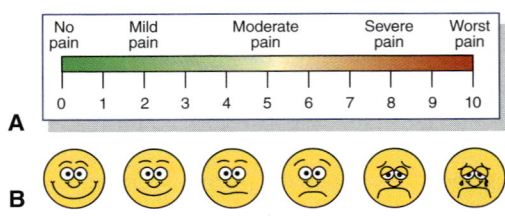

Figure 18-6 Pain scales. *A.* Numeric pain scale (about 12 years or older). *B.* Wong-Baker Faces pain scale (preschool through school-age).

FLACC Pain Scale

	Scoring		
Categories	**0**	**1**	**2**
Face	No particular expression or smile; disinterested	Occasional grimace or frown; withdrawn	Frequent to constant frown, clenched jaw, quivering chin
Legs	Normal position or relaxed	Uneasy, restless, tense	Kicking, or legs drawn up
Activity	Lying quietly, normal position, moves easily	Squirming, shifting back and forth, tense	Arched, rigid, or jerking
Cry	No cry (awake or asleep)	Moans or whimpers, occasional complaint	Crying steadily, screams or sobs, frequent complaints
Consolability	Content, relaxed	Reassured by occasional touching, hugging, or talking to. Distractible.	Difficult to console or comfort.

Each of the five categories—(F) Face; (L) Legs; (A) Activity; (C) Cry; (C) Consolability—is scored from 0 to 2, which results in a total score between 0 and 10

CLINICAL ALERTS

Important Respiratory Signals

Normal breath sounds are equal bilaterally in intensity, rhythm, and pitch. The following respiratory signals may indicate the presence of a respiratory condition in a child:

- Noisy breathing or snoring (air passing through a narrowed upper airway) may indicate nasal polyps, foreign body obstruction, choanal obstruction, hypertrophied adenoid tissue, or obesity.
- Grunting is caused by the glottis closing at the end of expiration and may suggest respiratory distress or pneumonia.
- Nasal flaring (intermittent outward movement of the nostrils) occurs on inspiration and is a form of accessory muscle use found in a variety of conditions such as respiratory distress syndrome (RDS) (Venes, 2005).

- Coughing (a forceful expiratory effort) is a normal process that clears the throat, but can indicate an infection, asthma, lung disease, or sinusitis.
- Stridor (a high-pitched, harsh sound occurring during inspiration) results from air moving through a narrowed trachea and larynx and can indicate croup (Venes, 2005).
- Wheezing (a musical noise) results from air moving through mucus or fluids in a narrowed lower airway that is associated with asthma.
- Hoarseness is a rough quality in the child's voice and can mean that the airway is inflamed.
- Crackles is a fine, high-pitched sound lung heard on inspiration or expiration produced by air passing over retained airway secretions or the sudden opening of collapsed airways found in several respiratory conditions (Venes, 2005).
- Rhonchi is a low-pitched wheezing, snoring, or squeaking sound indicating a partial airway obstruction. Mucus or other secretions in the airway, bronchial hyperreactivity, or tumors that occlude respiratory passages can cause the airway obstruction (Venes, 2005).
- Color changes in the skin (pallor, mottling and cyanosis) are significant respiratory signals and usually indicate cardiac involvement.
- Chest pain is caused by alteration in chest structures, nonpulmonary involvement, or a variety of respiratory conditions
- Clubbing (excessive growth of the soft tissues at the ends of the fingers or toes) is usually associated with chronic hypoxia and pulmonary disease.

Safety Measures

Keeping Children Safe in the Home or Hospital

- Parents must imagine how a child thinks. Suggest that parents get down on the floor in their home to see what their child sees (e.g., electrical plugs and outlets, tablecloths ready to be pulled, hot coffee mugs or tea saucers perched on the edge of the coffee table).
- In the hospital, store toxic and nontoxic materials in a locked utility room, on the top shelf of a cabinet, or in another location where children do not have ready access. Keep utility rooms, kitchens, medication carts, treatment rooms, and supply rooms locked. Lock play areas unless the child is accompanied by an adult.

Handwashing

- Wearing gloves does not replace the need for handwashing. Gloves may have small defects that allow the hands to become contaminated during removal of the gloves. Handwashing is essential if the caregiver touches any item in the child's room, as objects may have been touched by the child and are considered contaminated.

Risk of Infection

- With any procedure where the skin barrier is compromised, adhere to sterile techniques for dressing changes over IV sites and to monitor for signs and symptoms of infection (change in temperature, erythema, edema, pain at IV site, tenderness on palpation).

Gastrostomy Tubes

- A gastrostomy tube may move into the duodenum and cause an obstruction as it occludes the pyloric sphincter. Mark the tube with indelible ink to make it easy to observe for migration. Report any vomiting, abdominal distention, or evidence of bile drainage as aspirate.

Naloxone (Narcan)

- When giving morphine sulfate, be sure to have the opioid antagonist naloxone (Narcan) available. Narcan completely blocks the respiratory depression caused by the opioids, including central nervous system (CNS) effects. The dose for children is 5-10 mcg/kg (0.01 mg/kg) (Deglin & Vallerand, 2009).

DIAGNOSTIC TESTS

Body Mass Index (BMI)

- A BMI-for-age plotted below the 5th percentile indicates that a child is underweight; a BMI-for-age between the 5th and 85th percentile is considered a healthy weight; a child with a BMI-for-age between the 85th and 95th percentile are considered at risk for obesity; and those with a BMI-for-age greater than 95% are considered obese.

Eye Assessment Tools

- Visual screening for children can begin at the age of 2 $\frac{1}{2}$ years. Various charts are available to assist in the assessment of visual acuity.
- Visual acuity for each eye is assessed by occluding the contralateral eye with a plastic paddle.
- With all charts the objects, letters and numbers decrease in size. The Allen chart requires the child to identify common objects; the "tumbling E" requires the child to identify in which direction each E is facing; and the Snellen charts require the child to identify letters or numbers (Fig. 18-7).
- A common method for assessing ocular alignment is the Hirschberg corneal light reflex test, in which a light is shone directly into the child's eyes and note is taken of the position of the corneal light reflection in both eyes. The reflection should fall in the same location on the cornea of each eye.
- The second screening test is the cover–uncover test, in which the child is asked to focus on a distant object across the room. Cover the first eye while watching the second eye for any movement. Remove the cover and observe for any movement. If no movement is detected, ocular alignment is intact. Repeat the examination on the opposite eye.

A   **B**

Figure 18-7 Eye charts used to assess vision.

- Test the red reflex by viewing the pupil through an ophthalmoscope from a distance of ten inches. If the pupil appears red, the finding is normal. A white retinal reflex may indicate cataracts, retinoblastoma, or chorioretinitis.
- Children should be screened at least once during the school-age years for the ability to discriminate between red, yellow, and green. A common method for detecting color blindness is the use of the Ishihara pseudochromatic charts. The inability to identify the numbers indicates color blindness.

Hearing Screening Techniques

- Hearing screening should be done before any injections, vaccines, or laboratory work. Assess for frequency (pitch) and the decibel level (loudness). Frequency is defined as the number of vibrations a sound creates per second. As the frequency increases, the pitch of the sound also increases. The frequency range is 250 to 6000. For a normal finding, the child should hear at all frequencies at the 20-decibel range.
- Conditioned play audiometry (CPA) is a common test for children older than 3 years. Engage the child in a play-oriented activity (e.g., placing a colorful block in a box each time a sound is heard). The child is subjected to sounds of different frequencies that a child with normal hearing could hear.
- A conventional audiogram assesses hearing acuity by asking the child to raise his hand or press a button each time a sound is heard. The child must be able to understand the language spoken, be able to follow directions, pay attention, and wait to listen to the sounds.
- Use tympanometry to assess the status of the middle ear. Places a probe into the ear canal. The amount of sound that is reflected by the tympanic membrane is measured along with the pressure in the canal. The tympanogram delineates the movement of the eardrum as stiffness, floppiness, or normal eardrum movement.
- The Weber test involves striking the tines of the tuning fork and immediately placing the handle of the tuning fork midline on top of the child's head. Ask the child in which ear he hears the sound best. If hearing is normal, sound is heard equally in both ears. Sound heard in one ear better than the other indicates a conductive hearing loss.

- Use the Rinne test to assess air and bone conduction of sound. Bone conduction is tested by placing the handle of the vibrating tuning fork on the mastoid process behind the ear. The child informs the nurse when he no longer can hear the sound of the vibrating tuning fork and the nurse immediately moves the tines forward to within 1 to 2 inches of the auditory meatus. The child should hear the air-conducted sound of the vibrating tines twice as long as he heard the bone-conducted sound.

Analysis of Cerebrospinal Fluid (CSF)

- With the lumbar puncture, a needle is inserted into the subarachnoid space at the level of L4 or L5 to withdraw CSF for analysis. CSF samples are sent for culture, glucose, red blood cell (RBC) and white blood cell (WBC) count, and protein.
- Normal values for total WBC and differential in adult males and females are:
  - Total WBC: 4500 to 10,000
  - Bands or stabs: 3% to 5%
  - Granulocytes (or polymorphonuclears)
    - Neutrophils (or segs): 50% to 70% relative value (2500–7000 absolute value)
    - Eosinophils: 1% to 3% relative value (100–300 absolute value)
    - Basophils: 0.4% to 1% relative value (40–100 absolute value)
  - Agranulocytes (or mononuclears)
    - Lymphocytes: 25% to 35% relative value (1700–3500 absolute value)
    - Monocytes: 4% to 6% relative value (200–600 absolute value)

Analysis of Cerebrospinal Fluid					
	Pressure (mm Hg)	Protein (mg/dL)	RBCs	Glucose (mg/dL)	WBCs (%)
Infant	<200	20–170	None	34–119	0–30
Child	<200	5–40	None	60–80	0–20

MEDICATIONS

Pain Management with Acetaminophen

Acetaminophen is an over-the-counter medication that is used for mild to moderate pain and fever control in children. Acetaminophen comes as a liquid in drop or elixir form; as a tablet in the form of chewable tablets, swallowable caplets, and capsules; and as a suppository. Acetaminophen is the generic name for Tylenol, Panadol, Tempra, Liquiprin, in drop form; Paracetamol, St. Joseph Aspirin-Free Chewable, and Chewable Anacin 3 in tablet form; and Fever-all in suppository form.

How to Determine the Recommended Dose of Medication Based on the Child's Age and Weight

	3 mo	4–11 mo	12–23 mo	2–3 yr	4–5 yr	6–8 yr	9–10 yr	11 yr	12 yr
Weight (lbs.)	6–11	12–17	18–23	24–35	36–47	48–59	60–71	72–95	>96
Dose (mg)	40	80	120	160	240	320	400	480	650
Liquids									
Drops (1 dropper = 80 mg/ 0.8 mL)	½	1	1–1½	2	—	—	—	—	—
Elixir/ suspension 160 mg/5 mL (1 tsp)	—	½ tsp	¾ tsp	1 tsp	1½ tsp	2 tsp	2½ tsp	3 tsp	—
Tablets									
Chewable 80 mg/tab	—	—	—	2	3	4	—	—	—
Swallowable 160 mg/tab	—	—	—	1	1½	2	2½	3	4
Capsules 80 mg	—	—	—	2	3	4	—	—	—
Capsules 160 mg	—	—	—	1	—	2	—	3	4

Suppository									
Infant strength 80 mg	$1/2$	1	—	—	—	—	—	—	—
Child strength 120 mg	—	$1/2$	1	1	2	—	—	—	—
Junior strength 325 mg	—	—	—	—	—	1	1	$1\ 1/2$	2

- Age-appropriate doses can be repeated every 4 to 6 hours according to instructions on the label and the recommendation of your health care provider.
- Do not exceed five doses in 24 hours.
- There are few side effects associated with acetaminophen when the appropriate dose for age and weight are followed.
- Gastrointestinal (stomach) upset can occur in some people. If this occurs, food or milk may be given to reduce the stomach upset.
- Signs of an allergic reaction may include fever and rash and should be reported to your health care provider if suspected.
- Signs of toxicity (overdose of the medication) that require immediate reporting to your health care provider include paleness, bluish discoloration of the skin or nails, weakness, irregular or rapid heart beat, shortness of breath, unexplained bleeding or bruising, sore throat, fatigue, headache or dizziness, and nausea or vomiting.
- Signs of chronic poisoning or overdose include abdominal pain, yellow skin and eyes, dark urine, itchy skin, and clay-colored bowel movements.

Essential Information

Acetaminophen is also found in other medications, such as cold and flu preparations. To prevent accidental overdose, check with your pharmacist or health care provider to ensure that your child is not receiving too much medication if you are using a combination of over-the-counter preparations that contain acetaminophen.

Commonly Used Herbal Preparations

Herb	Use	Concerns
Aloe Vera	Minor skin wounds and irritations.	No known side effects for topical applications.
Bilberry	The tea form is used for the treatment of diarrhea.	Can affect clotting time by decreasing platelet aggregation.
Cayenne Pepper	Relief of pain associated with tonsillitis (capsule form) and sore muscles (ointment).	Ointment may cause burning sensation when used topically.
Chamomile	Pain associated with colic, teething and stomach aches.	Hypersensitivity reaction. Contraindicated in those allergic to daisies, marigolds or ragweed.
Echinacea	Symptoms of the common cold and mild infections.	Do not use for autoimmune disorders, diabetes, AIDS, HIV. Use for short-term illnesses only.
Fennel	Colic, stomach spasms and cough associated with respiratory infections.	May have a laxative effect.
Feverfew	Migraines	Not safe for children younger than 2 years of age. Administration of nonsteroidal anti-inflammatory drugs (NSAIDs) inhibits the effect of feverfew.
Licorice	The oral form treats cough; the topical form is used in the treatment of eczema.	Safe for children if taken for short-term illness. Contraindicated in diabetes, hypertension, and liver and kidney disease.
Nettle	Asthma and allergy symptoms	May increase blood sugar.
St John's Wort	Mild depression	May cause photosensitivity; many herb–drug interactions
Tea Tree Oil	The topical form is used as an antibacterial	Use restricted to topical application.
Valerian	Mild to moderate insomnia	May potentiate sedative effects of barbiturates, anesthetics, and CNS depressants. May cause GI upset

Source: Bascom (2002).

Ibuprofen (Children's Advil)

- A common nonsteroidal anti-inflammatory drug (NSAID) given to children as a fever-reducing measure
- Given every 6 hours and may be an advantage when rest is crucial or when administering medications to the child is a challenging task.
- Dyspepsia and nausea are common side effects.
- Can be given (chewable tablet, caplet, or liquid) with food or after meals if gastrointestinal (GI) upset occurs.
- Monitor the child for GI bleeding.
- Dosing for ibuprofen is dependent on the temperature of the child. A fever below 102.6°F (39.2°C) warrants a dose of 5 mg/kg of body weight.
- Increase the dose to 10 mg/kg of body weight, if a child's temperature is over 102.6°F (39.2°C).
- Assess the efficacy of antipyretic medication by retaking the child's temperature one hour after administration.

Morphine Sulfate (Astramorph)

- Morphine sulfate (Astramorph) is an opioid analgesic that is frequently used for children with chronic pain.
- Administer PO, IV, IM, epidurally, or via a patient-controlled analgesia (PCA) pump. For children weighing less than 50 kg the dose is:

0.3 mg/kg PO every 3 to 4 hours, or 0.1 mg/kg IV or IM every 3 to 4 hours (Deglin & Vallerand, 2009).

ETHNOCULTURAL CONSIDERATIONS

Stereotyping

Avoid stereotyping an individual or family based on a specific racial or cultural background, or assuming that all members of a particular culture subscribe to the traditions, beliefs, and customs associated with that culture. Length of time in the country, level of education, level of acculturation, and economic status affect the degree to which the culture shapes the parent's approach to health care (Salimbene, 2005).

Skin Assessment

The sclera is white in light-skinned individuals. It is normal for the sclera to be slightly yellow with small black marks in darker-skinned individuals.

Lead Exposure in Folk Medicines

Folk medicines used by Indian, Middle Eastern, West Asian, and Hispanic cultures may contain high levels of lead. Inquire as to the use of greta, azarcon (coral, *luiga*, *maria luisa*, or *rueda*), ghasard, or ba-baw-san.

TEACHING THE FAMILY

Caring for the Child with a Disability

- Maintain a respectful attitude toward the parents and the child.
- Listen carefully to the parents' concerns. They know their child best.
- Evaluate how social and health care agencies can assist the parents and the child to manage the disability (financial, medical, community services).
- Assess the child's skills for coping with pain or fatigue
- Evaluate the need for respite care and reliable community resource providers.

Using Cotton Swabs

Instruct parents to use cotton swabs to clean only the external ear (not the ear canal) to avoid pushing cerumen into the canal, where it cannot be removed by the mechanical action of the tiny ear hairs. Cerumen dries, hardens, and becomes difficult to remove over time. Impacted cerumen in the ear canal may lead to hearing deficits.

Decreasing Exposure to Lead

- Encourage parents to contact the water authority to determine the lead content in the water. The EPA states that 15 parts per billion is acceptable.

- If mixing formula from powder or concentrate, advise parents to flush water from the system by running the tap for 1 to 2 minutes before using the water. Most of the lead comes from the corrosion of older pipes that leak into the water supply after sitting in the pipes for several hours.

Preparing Children for Procedures

Infant
- Describe the procedure to the parents; explain what will happen and how long it will take.
- Encourage the parents to stop you at any point if they have a question.
- Remind parents that infants often cry for reasons other than discomfort, but be honest about any discomfort the infant may experience with the procedure.
- Identify what restraints may be used and provide an explanation as to why they are needed. Allow parents to decide whether they would like to be present for the procedure. Parents may prefer to leave the room and return immediately after the procedure to comfort their child.

Toddler
- Describe the procedure to the parents, explaining what will happen and how long it will take.
- Use play to demonstrate the procedure to the toddler. Encourage him to demonstrate/practice with a doll or teddy bear.
- Use simple, concrete language to describe the procedure and how it might feel to the toddler.
- Limit preparation to 5 to 10 minutes due to the shorter attention span of the toddler.
- Identify the restraints that may be used and give an explanation as to why they are needed. Allow parents to decide whether they would like to be present for the procedure. Parents may prefer to leave the room and return immediately after the procedure to comfort their child.

Preschooler
- Explain the procedure in terminology the child can understand.

- Begin preparation immediately before the procedure so the child does not worry for hours or days.
- Use play to demonstrate the procedure to the child; encourage her to demonstrate/practice with a doll or teddy bear.
- Set limits for the child so she is aware of expectations (e.g., tell her she can yell and scream as much as she wants, but must hold very still).
- Give legitimate choices to the child whenever possible.
- Allow parents to decide whether they would like to be present for the procedure. Parents may prefer to leave the room and return immediately following the procedure to comfort their child.
- Use distraction techniques such as deep breathing, singing, or squeezing a parent's or nurse's hand.

School-age Child

- Explain the procedure in terminology that the child can understand. Children in this stage of development have a good concept of time, so preparation can begin in advance of the procedure.
- For the younger school-age child, use play to demonstrate the procedure and if possible have the child demonstrate on and practice positioning with a doll or teddy bear. Allow the child to touch and explore equipment to be used in the procedure, and involve the child in simple tasks during the procedure when possible. Set limits for the child so she is aware of expectations (e.g., tell her she can yell and scream as much as she wants, but must hold very still). Give legitimate choices to the child whenever possible.
- Allow parents and the child to decide together whether parents will be present for the procedure. Some school-age children may be modest about exposing body parts in front of family members.
- Teach the child techniques such as deep breathing, counting, reciting a silly rhyme, or anything else that might help distract and relax the child during the procedure.

Adolescent

- Describe the procedure, explaining exactly what will happen and how long it will take.
- Encourage the adolescent to stop you at any point if she has a question.

- Be honest. Describe potential risks and pain associated with the procedure, but do not dwell on it.
- Allow the adolescent to take as active a role as possible in the procedure. Practicing positioning or demonstrating the equipment prior to the procedure helps give the adolescent a sense of control.
- Provide a peer video of the procedure if possible.
- Allow the adolescent to make decisions such as when the procedure should take place, if possible.
- Offer tips for distraction such as deep breathing, relaxation, counting, or squeezing an object or parent's hand.

Insurance for Children

- Teach the family how to obtain health insurance for their child.
- Encourage the family to call 1-877 KIDS NOW (1-877-543-7669) or go to your state's program: http://www.insurekidsnow.gov/states.asp
- Children who are eligible for Medicaid cannot enroll in the state program because Medicaid provides comprehensive health benefits.

Promoting Resiliency

- Express love and gratitude.
- Foster competency and positive attitudes.
- Nurture positive emotions.
- Encourage helping others.
- Teach peace-building skills.
- Reinforce positive behaviors.
- Reduce stress.

ADDITIONAL INFORMATION FOR THE CLINICAL SETTING

Use of Herbal Products

- The use of herbal products and home remedies is common (Lanski et al., 2003), but often parents do not divulge herbal product use for their children in encounters with health care providers.

- Ask about the use of herbal products to avoid inadvertent drug interactions.

Key Actions in Caring for the Child Confined to Bed

- Keep skin clean and dry.
- Assess nutritional status for adequate protein.
- Use the draw sheet for position changes.
- Assess skin for irritated areas.
- Assess for pressure ulcers by looking for the "red flush" (the first sign of tissue compromise and ischemia).

Encouraging Adequate Intake

- Offer small portions at frequent intervals.
- Host a "tea party" using medicine cups filled with the child's favorite drink.
- Make food into fun shapes (trace a smile face with mayonnaise on a sandwich, use a cookie cutter to make different shapes for sandwiches).
- Offer incentives of more time doing a favored activity.
- To provide autonomy, offer two choices (e.g., a straw or a colored cup).

Spiritual Care

Comfort may be found in dialogue with a priest, monk, chaplain, deacon, rabbi, imam, or other trusted person with a religious affiliation. At times when parents ask "why is this happening to my child?" it may be beneficial for the nurse to arrange a meeting to discuss the parents concerns and issues.

Before, During, and After a Procedure

Before

- Think through the procedure in advance and anticipate problems.
- Gather all equipment and check to make sure it functions properly.
- Establish trust. Get to know the child first.
- Through the use of play, allow the child to "perform" the procedure on her doll, teddy bear, or other appropriate surrogate.

- Offer a coping strategy such as guided imagery or relaxation breathing.
- Give the child realistic choices.
- Be sure informed consent is signed.
- Wash hands.
- Let the child know that it is "OK" to cry.

During

- Whenever possible, schedule all treatments away from the child's bed or "safe area."
- Expect the child to do well.
- Talk to the child and ask how he is doing.
- Keep the child informed as to the progress of the procedure.
- Use distraction techniques such as pop-up picture books, bubbles, "shutting off the pain switch," or other techniques that have been practiced before the procedure.
- When appropriate, give the child some control by allowing him to make some of the decisions.
- Encourage the parent to provide comfort to the child, if the parent is able. Sometimes a parent's presence at the procedure may not be beneficial for the child.

After

- Praise the child for completing the procedure.
- Provide an opportunity for the child to verbalize feelings.
- If the parents were not involved in the procedure, comment on a positive aspect involving the child during the procedure (e.g., "Jill was able to help out and keep still when she was asked to do so! She did a great job!").
- Give a reward (stickers, small toy, previously agreed-upon reward negotiated with parents).
- Document the child's response to procedure and outcomes.

Using Developmentally Appropriate Words

- For children with beginning language skills, use simple terms that are familiar to the child, such as "go potty," "owie," and "boo boo."
- For the concrete thinker who takes what is said literally, do not use words that may frighten the child: "*dye* in your vein," "*shot* in the arm," "*cut* out the tonsils," and "*take* your temperature."

- Instead use "*special medicine* in your vein," "*special medicine* in your arm," "*make* your tonsils *better*," "*check* to see if your temperature *is working*."
- Be honest and patients will learn to trust you.

Obtain Written Consent Before a Procedure

- Obtain informed consent before a procedure is performed.
- It is the physician's responsibility to explain the procedure and the risks and benefits of treatment.
- Alternatives to the prescribed treatment should be discussed.
- When signed by the emancipated minor or parent, an informed consent is a legal document denoting that the emancipated minor or parent understands the nature of the procedure, risks, and benefits.
- The nurse is a witness to the signature.

Procedure 18-1 Guidelines for Inserting an Oro- or Nasogastric Tube

Purpose

To maintain the child's nutrition using a feeding tube that is passed through the mouth or nares and into the stomach

Equipment

- Oro- or nasogastric tube
- Tap water or a water soluble lubricant
- Syringe
- pH indicator paper

Steps

1. Wash hands and don gloves.
2. Determine tube length required by measuring from the nose to the earlobe and to the midway point between the end of the xiphoid process and the umbilicus.
3. Note the measurement by finding the manufacturer's black mark on the appropriately sized feeding tube.

(continued)

Procedure 18-1 (Continued)

4. Lubricate the tube with tap water or a water-soluble lubricant. Follow the manufacturer's guidelines. Using the dominate hand gently direct the tube toward the back of the throat. If using the nose, direct toward the occiput.

5. Aspirate stomach contents.

6. Check for proper placement using the method following the institution's policy:

   - Use pH indicator paper for assessment of gastric aspirate.

   - Inject a small amount of air into the tube while auscultating over the stomach; the nurse should hear a "swoosh" as the air enters the stomach.

   - Obtain an X-ray film to verify placement. This method is not practical for every feeding, but is often used after initial placement of the oro- or nasogastric feeding tube when used for continuous feeding.

7. Document the procedure.

Clinical Alert There are some risks with an oro- or nasogastric tube. The liquid from the feeding or medication may enter the lungs and possibility cause pneumonia. In addition, the feeding tubes may cause the child discomfort. The tube can also become plugged, causing pain, nausea, or vomiting.

Teach Parents

It is important to teach parents about artificial nutrition and hydration as well as the function of the oro- or nasogastric tube. Parents can be encouraged to report displacement of the tube, noted distress in the child and tube placement if necessary.

Psychosocial Needs of the Infant Receiving Gavage Feedings

- Place the infant comfortably in the mother's arms with the head elevated.
- Provide the infant with a pacifier to help simulate an actual feeding.

- Nonnutritive sucking has been shown to increase weight gain and decrease crying, and allow for the normal muscular development of the mouth and tongue.

Care of the Child in Restraints

- Remove restraints every 2 hours to assess skin and provide range of motion (ROM) exercises to the affected extremity.
- Provide supervised time with restraints off, if appropriate, to allow the child to engage in activities of daily living (toileting, feeding, reading a book, watching TV, etc.).
- Encourage games and activities that promote growth and development.
- Reapply restraints.
- Document condition of skin, nursing care given with restraints off, removal, and reapplication of restraints.
- Teach parents how to remove and reapply restraints.

Myths About Pain Management

- Children don't feel pain with the same intensity as adults.
- Neonates do not feel pain because their nervous systems are not mature.
- Children cannot tell where they hurt.
- Children will tell you if they are really having pain.
- Children become accustomed to pain.
- Narcotic analgesics are dangerous for children because they will become addicted or go into respiratory distress.
- If children can be distracted, they are not in pain.
- If children say they are in pain, but don't look in pain, they don't need to be medicated.
- Being in pain for only a little while isn't that bad.
- After children have undergone surgery, they should not be given analgesia until they can vocalize pain, because they received enough anesthetic to "cover" their pain.
- The best way to give analgesics is intramuscularly.
- Children with neurological impairments do not feel pain as much as other children.
- Children, especially boys, should learn to tolerate pain; they will make better, stronger adults.

Pain Management Strategies

Age (Guideline only)	Reactions	Concerns/ Distraction	Environment	Involvement	Parental Preparation	Positions	Post Procedure Comforting
Infant/Toddler (0–3 years)	Separation anxiety Protest Despair Denial	Pacifier Swaddling Rocking Eye contact Music Picture books	Controlled lighting and noise Use treatment room	Encourage parental presence, provide guidance, comfort/cuddle baby during procedure.	Prepare parent: offer explanations of what they will see and hear. Develop a plan "who will do what"	Swaddle Cuddle	Soothe Swaddle Hold and rock Soft music Soothing voice
Preschool (3–6 years)	Separation anxiety Concerns with body image Develops fantasies with illness and treatment Battle for control	Distraction kit Deep breathing Bubble blowing Counting Singing	Use treatment room Music Controlled lighting and noise	Encourage parental presence and provide guidance in encouraging participation during strategies.	Medical play with relevant medical equipment and participation Pre-procedural teaching Reassurance of what child is to expect (focus on senses)	Lap Parent or staff may support patient or have other close physical contact.	Praise and reward stickers Medical play Play Stories
School-age (6–11 years)	Has questions regarding body and illness	Deep breathing Hand squeezing Riddles/trivia Pretend games	Use treatment room Music Controlled lighting and noise	Encourage parental presence and provide guidance	Simple medical terms to describe what will happen	Lap	Praise, reward stickers Play, medical play

Age	Developmental Concerns	Distraction Techniques	Environment	Parental Involvement	Interventions	Positioning/Choices	Evaluation
	Concerns of helplessness, passivity, and dependency; Tend to be phobic and develop fears; Anger	Talking; Distraction kit		Encourage parents to be part of the team.	Allow appropriate play with medical equipment. Explain reasons for various components of tests and allow appropriate participation by patient.	Parent may support patient or have other close physical contact. Present patient with choices.	Stories; Evaluate procedures and discuss suggestions for next time.
Teens (12 years and older)	Illness interferes with struggle for independence; Illness is a major threat to developing self-image; Very threatened by helplessness and loss of privacy; Denial, withdrawal, anger, hostility, disappointment	Imagery; Walkman; Deep breathing; Hand squeezing; Talking; Jokes; Distraction kit	Use treatment room; Music; Controlled lighting and noise	Ask permission of patient for parental involvement. Encourage parents to be part of the team.	Clarify misconception and initiate discussions about the past experiences with procedures. Allow appropriate participation by patient. Pre-procedural teaching utilizing medical play	Present patient with choices. Plan positioning with teen	Praise, reward stickers; Play, medical play; Stories; Evaluate procedures and discuss suggestions for next time.

Distraction

A distraction kit is a set of materials that help divert the child's attention to a more pleasant experience than the painful experience.

- Appropriate for any age
- Use before, during, and after procedure
- Other suggestions: Hold someone's hand really tight, say 'ouch' really loud, count to 10 or count backwards, sing a song, pretend to be somewhere else.

Environment

- Use designated treatment rooms when possible.
- The child's inpatient room should be kept as a "safe area" whenever possible.
- Ensure lighting is sufficiently bright and focused on safety, without glare.

Preparations

- Relieve parental anxiety so they can help prepare and reassure the child/youth. Provide an explanation of what they will see and hear.
- Relieve patient anxiety. Use simple explanations that are developmentally appropriate to explain how, why, where, and when

(Stollery Children's Hospital, Edmonton, Alberta, Canada).

RESOURCES

U.S. Department of Health and Human Services. Insure Kids Now! http://www.insurekidsnow.gov/questions.asp#why1

Child immunization schedules: http://www.cdc.gov/vaccines

Denver II Developmental Screening Test:
http://www.denverii.com/DenverII.html

Food Guide Pyramid for Young Children:
http://www.mypyradmid.gov/kids/index.html

Lead Poisoning:
http://www.cdc.gov/nceh/lead/publications/books/plpyc/chapter3.htm#top

Insurance for children: http://www.insurekidsnow.gov/states.asp

REFERENCES

Bascom, A. (2002). *Incorporating herbal medicine into clinical practice.* Philadelphia: F.A. Davis.

Bickley, L.S., & Szilagyi, P.G. (2007). *Bates' guide to physical examination and history taking* (9th ed). Philadelphia: Lippincott Williams & Wilkins.

Deglin, J.H.L., & Vallerand, A.P. (2009). *Davis's drug guide for nurses* (11th ed). Philadelphia: F.A. Davis.

Karch, A. (2009). *Lippincott's nursing drug guide.* Philadelphia: Lippincott Williams & Wilkins.

Lanski, S.L., Greenwald, M., Perkins, A., & Simon, H.K. (2003). Herbal therapy use in a pediatric emergency department population: Expect the unexpected. *Pediatrics, 111*(5), 981–986.

Otto, S.E. (1991). *Oncology nursing.* St. Louis: C.V. Mosby. Reprinted in *Mosby's medical, nursing, and allied dictionary* (4th ed.), p. 1144.

Salimbene, S. (2005). *What language does your patient hurt in?* St. Paul, MN: EMCParadigm.

Stollery Children's Hospital, 8440-112 Street, Edmonton, Alberta, Canada

Venes, D. (Ed.). (2005). *Taber's cyclopedic medical dictionary* (20th ed.). Philadelphia: F.A. Davis.

19

Caring for the Family Across Care Settings

KEY TERMS

despair – Phase of separation experienced by a hospitalized child in which he seems to withdraw from the environment and becomes very apathetic

detachment – Final phase of separation experienced by a hospitalized child when he has begun to internalize the stressor and seems outwardly happy, although the stressor is still present

health screening – To test or examine children for the presence of a disease, illness, chronic condition, developmental delay, or mental health issue

health surveillance – Continuous observation related to tracking health conditions and risk behaviors

protest – Phase of separation experienced by a hospitalized child that begins when he realizes his parents are leaving or that he is separated, even if for a brief period, from his parents

therapeutic play – The use of play as therapy to help children who have had or will have a stressful experience decrease their fear and anxiety of the experience

FOCUSED ASSESSMENT

Developing a Plan of Care

Ask parents the following questions:

- What are your child's daily routines related to eating, elimination, sleeping, bathing, and play?

- Who are the important people in your child's life?
- Does your child have a favorite toy or attachment object?
- What has your child been told about hospitalization?
- Does your child have any fears that the staff should know about?
- Have there been any recent changes or problems in your child's life?
- How does your child usually react to pain or when frightened?

Include the Parents in the Plan of Care When Their Child Is Admitted to the Hospital

- Request information about the child's personal routine and schedule at home.
- Inquire about previous hospitalizations.
- Ask about the child's anxieties and fears.
- Encourage the parent's presence, involvement, and participation in caring for the child.
- Recognize the parent's concerns, including possible guilt, fear, or other anxieties about the child's hospitalization.
- Provide positive reinforcement for the family to alleviate as much stress as possible.

The Nurse's Role in Health Screening and Surveillance

- Pay attention to voiced parental concerns.
- Ask questions about the child's growth and development.
- Observe the child's mental, physical, and spiritual state (not just a diagnosed condition).
- Note any risk factors that may be present.
- Document specific observations and findings.
- Provide community resources and make appropriate referrals.
- Track disease incidence and demographics of illnesses.
- Implement policies that may prevent further spread of diseases.
- Initiate follow-up care for any concerns and conditions.

CLINICAL ALERT

Common Problems of Critical Illness

Common problems of critical illness are shock, acute respiratory failure, chronic respiratory failure, infection, sepsis, renal failure, neurological conditions, bleeding and clotting disorders, and multiorgan dysfunction.

TEACHING THE FAMILY

Teaching Tips for Families

Ask the family to bring a list of questions or concerns to discuss when visiting the primary care physician's office:

- Bring a list of any allergies that the child has, as well as medications the child is currently taking.
- Be ready to share information as to how the child is growing and changing. Keep track of the child's developmental progress.
- Inquire about resources including community organizations that may provide assistance.
- Request to meet the health care team members who will be working the child (a nurse, a referral coordinator, and a medical assistant).

Caring for the Child at Home After Minor Surgery

Teach parents how to care for their child at home after minor surgery. Explain:

- How to take the child's axillary temperature.
- How to assess the child's level of consciousness.
- When to begin giving the child liquids based on type of surgery, prescribed diet, and age.
- When to offer solid food based on type of surgery, prescribed diet, and age.
- What type of activity is expected or should be encouraged.
- The actions and side effects of medications.
- The signs and symptoms of infection.
- The signs of poor airway exchange.

- How to use assistive devices and medical equipment and perform home treatments.
- How to contact a nurse, pharmacist, health care professorial, or community agency.
- When to call the doctor.

Follow-up Care

- Inform the family of the following: Rehabilitation services are generally provided in a hospital or community center where the child can begin to recuperate and receive physical, occupational, audiology, or speech assessment and therapy.
- Other health care professionals will assist the child in working toward the achievement of optimal function and the relief of pain.
- The ultimate goal is to assist the child's physical recovery and reentry into the community, home, and school.
- A social worker may also be involved in the child's care to assess the capacities of the family's ability to cope with the impact of the condition and situation.
- A social worker can also offer a broad range of community services and may serve as emotional support to referrals for community resources.

ADDITIONAL INFORMATION FOR THE CLINICAL SETTING

Outcomes of a Medical Home and Coordinated Care

Children with special needs receive coordinated ongoing comprehensive care within a medical home (provides comprehensive primary care services on an ongoing basis, in a manner encouraging a positive relationship with the child, family, and the health care team) based on these outcomes:

- Families of children with special health care needs have adequate private and/or public insurance to pay for the services needed.
- Children are screened early and continuously for special health care needs and will have increased wellness.
- Services for children with special health care needs are organized in a manner that fosters trust, considers the

family's cultural and religious beliefs, and builds support for the child and family.

- Families of children with special needs will partner in decision making at all levels, and will be satisfied with the services they receive.
- All youth with special needs receive the services necessary to make appropriate transitions to adult health care, work, and independence.
- Families will have increased satisfaction with their health care.

Benefits of a Medical Home

- A child regularly sees the same primary care physician and staff.
- There is coordination of care for the child.
- There is an open exchange of information in an honest and respectful manner.
- There is support for finding resources and information related to all stages of growth and development and medical conditions.
- The family is connected to information and family support organizations.
- The medical home partnership promotes health and quality of life as the child grows and develops.

Primary Health Care Provider or Clinic Setting

- A private medical office or clinic
- Provision of health information
- Discussions about how to take care of the child at home
- Comprehensive and safe nursing care
- Education about child's condition
- Recommendations for additional community resources
- Reasonable cost of care and continuity of care (child remains in the care of the family)

The Hospitalized Child

- Hospitalization is required when the child becomes ill.
- It may be a new experience wherein both the child and family are exposed to an unfamiliar medical environment.

- Children are more vulnerable to the stress of hospitalization because they do not have a full range of coping mechanisms.
- The child and family are also introduced to an entirely new group of people
  - Children's hospital: Specialty pediatric hospital that is specially designed and managed specifically for children
  - Day hospital: Specialized hospital that serves children who require medical treatments
  - Ambulatory surgery center: Surgical center is where children receive minimal surgical treatment, recover from the procedure, and are discharged soon after the surgery

Stages of Separation with a Hospitalized Child

- Protest phase: The child realizes parents are leaving and could cry, cling, and act aggressively.
- Despair phase: The child seems to withdraw and becomes apathetic.
- Detachment phase: The child represses pain at the sense of loss and shows disinterest on parent's return.

Ways to Decrease the Stress of Hospitalization

- Rooming-in is when parents stay in the room both during the day and through the night
- Encourage child to do the following:
  - Bring something from home.
  - Draw a picture that can be hung up.
  - Watch a movie or select a game.

Therapeutic play is the use of play as therapy to help children who have had or will have a stressful experience. Therapeutic play may decrease the child's fear and anxiety. It also may help to correct misconceptions the child may have about being in the hospital. There are two types of play techniques:

- Directed therapeutic play is guided by an adult who facilitates the play, including determination of the goals.
- In nondirected therapeutic play, the child is in control of the activity, although an adult may select the materials.

Guided imagery is a relaxation technique that aims to ease stress and to promote a sense of peace and harmony during a difficult time.

- Guided imagery can be used by persons of all ages.
- Guided imagery encompasses the power of the mind, to help heal the body, while maintaining a relaxed state including all of the body's senses (touch, smell, sound, sight and visual) (Tusek, 2008).

Role modeling refers to a process by which the child learns certain behaviors by observing the behavior of others. Role models can also come from videotapes, movies, or even their peers. Role models who are similar in age, sex, race, and attitudes are more likely to be imitated as well as models who have a caring demeanor (Watson, 1996). For example, a child might view a video about another child and his or her experience preparing for hospitalization and surgery. Viewing how the child in the video prepares for surgery may help the child who is facing surgery to find ways to cope with the anxiety and stress of the procedure.

Assist Parents in Adapting to the Child's Hospitalization

- Involve the parents.
- Assess home routines, preferences, and developmental and special needs.
- Allow parents to tell their story.
- Promote trust.
- Give prompt attention to the child's needs.
- Allow the parents to participate in care.
- Give positive reinforcement.
- Conduct ongoing evaluation.

Nursing Interventions to Help Parents Cope with a Child's Hospitalization

- Encourage parents to visit the hospital to see where the child will be staying.
- Encourage constant and open communication with the health care team.
- Encourage visitation of parents, friends, and family members.

- Perform ongoing assessment to ensure that the nurse fully understands any changes in the child's plan of care.
- Observe for the need for crisis intervention, should the child's condition deteriorate or change.
- Encourage the parents to participate in the child's care, while being supportive of the child and family.

Twenty-Four-Hour Observation Unit

- Short-stay hospitalization experience.
- Sudden illness; most likely will recover quickly.
- Nurse provides acute nursing care.
- Quickly begins to prepare the child and family for discharge.

Ambulatory Surgery Center

- Surgical treatment is minimal.
- The child recovers from the procedure and then is discharged home soon after the surgery.
- Minimizes separation between the child and family (emotionally less stressful).
- Teaches the family about the surgery and ways to care for the child at home.

Critical Care Unit

- The child is admitted to the critical care unit through the emergency department or operating room, or transferred from a medical-surgical floor.
- After delivery, a newborn who requires intensive care is transferred to a neonatal intensive care unit.
- Other types of critical care units include cardiac, surgical, or psychiatric critical care units.
- The child is extremely ill and receives specialized care, medication, intravenous fluid, respiratory, or ventilator support.

Emergency Department

- Used for quick treatment for children who have become suddenly ill or experienced a severe injury
- Open 24 hours/day, 7 days/week
- Rapid screening or triage assessment

- Several areas of treatment
- Patient may be admitted to the hospital from emergency department

Community Settings

- The majority of a child's health care is provided in a community setting today.
- Community settings are on the front line of prevention and early detection.
- These settings may be located in neighborhood clinics, schools, shopping malls, or health care centers.

RESOURCES

Maternal and Child Health Bureau:
http://www.mchb.hrsa.gov/programs/

The National Center for medical home initiatives for children with special needs: http://www.mchb.hrsa.gov/programs/

The National Center for medical home initiatives for children with special needs: http://www.medicalhomeinfo.org/

Guided imagery: http://www.guidedimageryinc.com/guided.html

National Association of School Nurses: http://www.nasn.org/

Web MD, 2008: http://www.webmd.com

REFERENCES

Tusek, D. (2008). What is guided imagery? Retrieved from http://www.guidedimageryinc.com/guided.html (Accessed April 4, 2009).
Watson, J. (1996). Watson's theory of transpersonal caring. In P.H. Walker & B. Neuman (Eds.). *Blueprint for use of nursing models: Education, research, practice, and administration* (pp. 141–184). New York: National League for Nursing Press.

Caring for the Child with a Psychosocial or Cognitive Condition

KEY TERMS

developmental psychopathology – A discipline that evolved from the contribution of multiple fields of study with the goal to provide understanding between psychopathology and normal adaptation

encopresis – Repeated passage of feces into inappropriate places (e.g., clothing or floor)

enuresis – Occurrence of wetting clothing or the bed at least two times per week for at least 3 months, or that causes significant embarrassment or restriction of activities for the child

obesogenic – Role that environment plays in the development of obesity

FOCUSED ASSESSMENT

Assessing the Child for Posttraumatic Stress Disorder (PTSD)

After a trauma, a child with posttraumatic stress disorder (PTSD) exhibits symptoms within each of the following sets of reactions:

- Reexperiencing the trauma, perhaps in the form of a flashback (intense "remembering" of the event while feeling as if it were happening at the present moment), or nightmares, or sensations

- Avoidance of anything that could trigger the memories, through dissociation (a sense of being detached emotionally, mentally, and perhaps even physically) or avoiding places or events reminiscent of the trauma
- Physiological symptoms of anxious arousal (insomnia, startle response, sense of panic) (Commission on Adolescent Anxiety Disorders, 2005).

Assessing the Child for Bipolar Disorder (BPD)

As bipolar disorder (BPD) is a combination of major depression and mania, the nurse must be aware of symptoms of depression.

Manic and Depressive Symptoms	
Mania	**Depression**
Severe changes in mood—either extremely irritable or overly silly and elated	Persistent sad or irritable mood
Overly inflated self-esteem; grandiosity	Loss of interest in activities once enjoyed
Increased energy	Significant change in appetite or body weight
Decreased need for sleep—able to go with very little or no sleep for days without tiring	Difficulty sleeping or oversleeping
	Physical agitation or slowing
	Loss of energy
Increased talking—talks too much, too fast; changes topics too quickly; cannot be interrupted	Feelings of worthlessness or inappropriate guilt
	Difficulty concentrating
Distractibility—attention moves constantly from one thing to the next	Recurrent thoughts of death or suicide
Hypersexuality—increased sexual thoughts, feelings, or behaviors; use of explicit sexual language	
Increased goal-directed activity or physical agitation	
Disregard of risk – excessive involvement in risky behaviors or activities	

Source: National Institute of Mental Health (2000). Child & adolescent bipolar disorder: An update from the National Institute of Mental Health. NIH Publication No. 00-4778.

Assessing the Child for Suicide

The nurse should suspect suicide potential when faced with any of the following:

- Symptoms of depression or other mental illness
- Alienation or withdrawal from friendships or relationships
- Personality changes
- Decline in schoolwork
- Giving away personal possessions that were once prized

- Preoccupation with death in writing or drawings
- References to dying or to no longer being around
- Access to a method of suicide (e.g., medications, weapons)

Continued Assessment for Suicide

The nurse must ask the child about suicidal thoughts or behaviors. Examples of questions that the nurse might ask include:

"Have you thought about doing something to hurt yourself or take your life?"

"Do you ever wish you were not alive?"

"What would you do if you were to hurt yourself?"

Assessing the Child for Failure to Thrive

During a nursing assessment, the nurse can discern:

- How does the caretaker interact with the child?
- Are there signs of abuse or neglect?
- Does the caretaker understand appropriate feeding amounts and routines?
- Does the caretaker mistakenly believe that a healthy adult diet (i.e., lower fat) is also healthy for an infant?

Assessing the Child for Attention-Deficit/ Hyperactivity Disorder (ADHD)

Developmentally inappropriate or maladaptive symptoms consist of either inattentive symptoms, hyperactive or impulsive symptoms, or a combination

Symptoms of ADHD	
Inattention	**Hyperactivity or Impulsivity**
Distractibility	Excessive energy and activity
Inability to complete projects	Restlessness
Easily bored	Overactivity
Disorganized	Inability to sit still or stay in one place for long
Inattentiveness	Excessive talking
Avoidance of detailed tasks	Poor boundaries—interrupts or intrudes
Forgetfulness	Difficulty delaying

Assessing the Child for Maltreatment of Children

Type of Abuse	Tactics of Abuse	Possible Signs and Symptoms in the Child
Physical: Bodily injury caused by intentional or unintentional physical aggression.	Beating, hitting, slapping, poisoning, kicking, pinching, biting, choking, pulling hair, burning Excessive corporal punishment Shaken baby syndrome Munchausen by proxy	Suspicious bruises, welts, or burns Unexplained fractures or dislocations New and healing or healed lacerations or abrasions Wariness of adults or caregivers Fearful of going home Acting out with aggression Retinal hemorrhages CNS injury Prolonged or recurrent illnesses or injuries that cannot be explained
Sexual: Sexual acts between an adult and a child.	Penetration, incest, rape, Violations of bodily privacy Exposing children to adult sexuality Commercial exploitation Sexual exploitation (prostitution or pornography)	Inappropriate or precocious interest in or knowledge of sexuality Poor peer relationships Sudden changes in behavior Running away from home Substance abuse Declining school performance Suicide attempts
Emotional: Attitude, behavior, or failure to act that interferes with a child's mental health or social development	Intimidation, belittling, shaming, lack of affection and warmth, habitual blaming, ignoring or rejection, extreme punishment, exposure to violence, child exploitation, child abduction	Apathy, depression Hostility Difficulty concentrating
Neglect: Pattern of failing to meet basic needs	Physical, educational, emotional	Clothing unsuited to the weather Poor hygiene Hunger Lack of supervision

Evaluating the Child for Substance Abuse

Two common ways of evaluating for substance abuse are CRAFFT and CAGE.

CRAFFT	CAGE
Have you ever ridden in a **C**ar driven by someone (including yourself) who was high or had been using alcohol or drugs?	Have you ever felt like **C**utting down on your drinking?
Do you ever use alcohol or drugs to **R**elax, feel better about yourself, or fit in?	Have people made you **A**ngry by talking about your drinking?
Do you ever use alcohol or drugs while you are by yourself **A**lone?	Have you ever felt **G**uilty about your drinking?
Do you ever **F**orget things you did while using alcohol or drugs?	Do you ever need a drink first thing in the morning to have enough **E**nergy or to feel ready for the day?
Do your **F**amily or **F**riends ever tell you that you should cut down on your drinking or drug use?	Scoring: 2 or more positive answers = an alcohol problem.
Have you ever gotten into **T**rouble while you were using alcohol or drugs?	*Note: This tool is used with individuals 16 and older.*
Scoring: 2 or more positive items indicate the need for further assessment.	

Source: Reprinted from Center for Adolescent Substance Abuse Research at Children's Hospital, Boston.

Source: Ewing, J.A. (1984). Detecting alcoholism: The CAGE questionnaire. Public domain.

Assessing the Child for Sleep Disorders

Sleep disorders can be diagnosed based on a positive answer by the caregiver to one or more of these questions:

- Is it hard for your child to fall asleep?
- Is it hard for your child to stay asleep though the night?
- Does your child wake up feeling tired?
- Is your child sleepy during the day?

CLINICAL ALERTS

Suicidal Behavior Related to Antidepressant Therapy

The Food and Drug Administration (FDA) requested that pharmaceutical companies manufacturing selective serotonin reuptake inhibitors (SSRIs) add a "black box" warning to the packaging because of an apparent rise in suicide in children and adolescents recently prescribed an SSRI for depression. Several factors have been proposed to explain the occurrence of suicide ideation in children treated with these medications:

- The prescription may be an inadequate dose and therefore the depression is not treated.
- An energizing phenomenon, which describes a situation in which the depressive symptoms related to energy decrease before the mood symptoms, may occur, thus making it more possible for the depressed individual to have the energy to attempt suicide.
- The emergence of an activation syndrome may be related to a toxic reaction to the medication.
- Motor restlessness related to akathisia (motor restlessness that may appear as a side effect of antipsychotic medication)
- The shift from depression to mania in a not-yet-diagnosed bipolar child may occur
- Idiosyncratic reactions (perhaps related to gene-drug reactions) may occur

(Goodman, Murphy, & Storch, 2007).

Attachment Therapies to Avoid

Because there have been child deaths related to the following treatments, they should be avoided:

- Holding therapy
- Rage reduction
- Rebirth

(Barth et al., 2005; Stafford & Zeanah, 2006).

Anorexia Nervosa

Anorexia nervosa can become a life-threatening problem or cause death because the severe weight loss can result in electrolyte imbalance and hemodynamic instability.

MEDICATIONS

Somatic Therapies for Depression

Serotonin Selective Reuptake Inhibitors (SSRIs)

- Open-label studies suggest that fluoxetine (Prozac) is an effective medication in the treatment of pediatric major depression and dysthymia in patients with and without co-occurring mental health disorders (Findling et al., 2004).
- This type of medication has been used in children as young as 8 years of age (National Institute of Mental Health [NIMH], 2001).
- Other SSRIs are used off-label (i.e., use other than specifically approved for by the Food & Drug Administration [FDA]) such as sertraline (Zoloft), paroxetine (Paxil), citalopram (Celexa), escitalopram (Lexipro), or fluvoxamine (Luvox) have also been prescribed by some clinicians (NIMH, 2001).
- Recent evidence that SSRIs can contribute to suicidal ideation in adolescents and children have left many parents and physicians wary of using medication to treat depression in young people.

Valproate (Depakote)

- The nurse needs to be aware that most medications used for the treatment of bipolar disorder have not been studied specifically with children.
- Lithium carbonate (Eskalith, Lithobid) has been the most common treatment. It is a mood stabilizer that calms the manic symptoms.

Pharmacological Treatments for Psychological Difficulties		
Category	**Medications**	**Uses**
Antianxiety	Beta blockers Propanolol (Inderal) Alpha blockers Clonidine (Catapres)	Anxiety
Antidepressants	**SSRIs** Fluoxetine (Prozac) Sertraline (Zoloft) Paroxetine (Paxil) Citalopram (Celexa) Escitalopram (Lexapro) Fluvoxamine (Luvox)	Depression Anxiety Obsessive–compulsive disorder (OCD) Selective mutism

Category	Medications	Uses
	Tricyclics Imipramine (Tofranil) Clomipramine (Anafranil) **Other** Bupropion (Wellbutrin) Venlafaxine	Enuresis Autism
Mood Stabilizer	Lithium carbonate (Lithobid, Lithane, or Eskalith)	Bipolar disorder (BPD) Mania Oppositional defiant disorder (ODD) Attention-deficit/hyperactivity disorder (ADHD)
Anticonvulsants	Valproate (Depakote)	Bipolar disorder (BPD) Mania
Antipsychotics	Traditional: Haloperidol (Haldol) Atypical: Risperidone (Risperdal) Olanzapine (Zyprexa) Quetiapine (Seroquel) Ziprasidone (Geodon) Aripiprazole (Abilify)	Autism Psychosis Tourette's syndrome Behavioral problems related to other psychiatric disorders (oppositional conduct disorder), Attention-deficit/hyperactivity disorder (ADHD), and developmental disabilities
Stimulants	Methylphenidate (Ritalin and Concerta) Dextroamphetamine (Dexedrine and Adderall)	Attention-deficit/hyperactivity disorder (ADHD)
Nonstimulants	Atomoxetine (Strattera)	Attention-deficit/hyperactivity disorder (ADHD)

Enuresis

- Early pharmacological treatments included the use of the tricyclic antidepressant imipramine (Tofranil).
- It is important to note that other tricyclics do not stop bedwetting.
- DDAVP (desmopressin), a vasopressin analogue, has been shown to work to decrease nighttime enuresis. It is administered either nasally or orally.

ETHNOCULTURAL CONSIDERATIONS

Promoting Understanding of Culture in Diverse Families

- Nurses working with children and families of various diverse and socioeconomic backgrounds must take an approach of listening, providing as much positive feedback as possible for what families are doing well, and keep resilience-promoting strategies in mind.
- Using anticipatory guidance, nurses working with children and their families might be most effective suggesting alternative ways of handling a specific cognitive or psychosocial-related concern.

Differences in Incidence of Childhood Obesity

Despite the fact that African American and Latino children and adolescents have higher prevalence rates of obesity compared to white children and adolescents, researchers have found that:

- African American and Latino children receive much less attention related to obesity. African American and Latino are also more likely to develop obesity related problems, such as type 2 diabetes (Caprio, 2006).
- Children of low-income families also experience higher levels of obesity. Access to high-quality, low-fat foods is limited, as is often the education of the parents in providing such foods. Lower-income families often have less access to educational programs on weight management that more privileged families may have (Kumanyika & Grier, 2006).
- Nurses, especially nurses of African American and Latino backgrounds, can help eliminate these disparities by becoming involved or taking leadership roles in programs that identify and involve these youngsters and their families in interventions.

TEACHING THE FAMILY

Therapeutic Parenting Techniques

The nurse can teach the family and the child, as well as model the following therapeutic parenting techniques (Child and Adolescent Bipolar Foundation [CABF, 2008]).

- Practice and teach the child relaxation techniques.
- Use firm restraint to help the child contain rages.
- Prioritize battles and let go of less important matters.
- Reduce stress in the home.
- Use good listening and communication skills.
- Use music, sound, lighting, water, and massage to assist the child with waking, falling asleep, and relaxation.
- Become an advocate for stress reduction and other accommodations at school.
- Help the child anticipate and avoid, or prepare for stressful situations by developing coping strategies beforehand.
- Engage the child's creativity through activities that express and channel gifts and strengths.
- Provide routines, structure, and freedom within limits.
- Remove objects from the home (or lock them in a safe place) that could be used to harm self or others during a rage, especially guns.
- Keep medications in a locked cabinet or box.

Maltreatment

- Educate parents about what to expect from parenthood and from child rearing.
- Help parents develop resources for support such as babysitters, family members, community sites, and health care resources that may help them find ways to cope with parenting.
- Provide parents with information regarding "normal" stages of growth.
- Discuss with parents ways to discipline the child that does not involve physical or verbal aggression.
- Educate children and adolescents about the body and personal boundaries.

Sleep Hygiene

- Provide a quiet, dark, and comfortable environment or bedroom.
- Set a strict bedtime and awake routine that remains consistent on a daily basis.
- Avoid long daytime naps.
- Allow a long space of time between daytime nap and bedtime.

- Provide a healthy snack before bedtime so the child is not hungry.
- Avoid substances such as caffeine, chocolate, medication containing alcohol, and other foods/beverages that are stimulating to children.
- Cut down on fluids before bedtime so that a full bladder or wetness does not interrupt sleep.
- Avoid a high level of activity and television viewing before bedtime and replace it with quiet activities (e.g., reading books).
- Encourage children to fall asleep without a caregiver in the room (Sheldon, 2005).

Toilet Training

Indications to begin toilet training (American Academy of Family Physicians, 2006; Child Welfare Information Gateway, 2007):

- When the child indicates his diaper is soiled or wet or when he indicates he wants to use the toilet (generally 18 to 24 months, but could be 2 1/2 to 3 years)
- When parents can devote about 3 months of time to offer lessons and encouragement
- When the child shows interest in other people using the bathroom or interest in wearing underwear

ADDITIONAL INFORMATION FOR THE CLINICAL SETTING

Mindful Breathing

The pediatric nurse can teach deep breathing to avoid or help with an anxious episode:

- Consciously direct your attention to your breathing.
- Breathe in slowly, paying attention as the air enters your nose or mouth and fills your lungs.
- Breathe out slowly, paying attention as the air leaves your body.
- Allow your mind to follow your breath in and out.
- Imagine yourself in a rubber raft riding the gentle waves of your breath.

Understanding Autism Spectrum Disorder

Developmental disorders have subtle signs and may be easily missed.

The "First Signs" program uses the acronym Autism A.L.A.R.M. to highlight important clinical guidelines (Wiseman, 2006):

Listen to parents:

- Early signs of autism are often present before 18 months.
- Parents usually do have concerns that something is wrong.
- Parents generally do give accurate and quality information.
- When parents do not spontaneously raise concerns, ask if they have any.

Act early:

- Make screening and surveillance an important part of your practice.
- Know the subtle differences between typical and atypical development.
- Learn to recognize red flags.
- Improve the quality of life for children and their families through early and appropriate intervention.

Refer:

- To early intervention or a local school program (do not wait for a diagnosis).
- To an autism specialist, or team of specialists, immediately for a definitive diagnosis.
- To audiology department to rule out a hearing impairment.
- To local community resources for help and family support.

Monitor:

- Schedule a follow-up appointment to discuss concerns more thoroughly.
- Look for other features known to be associated with autism.
- Educate parents and provide them with up-to-date information.
- Advocate for families with local early intervention programs, schools, respite care agencies, and insurance companies.

- Continue surveillance and watch for additional or late signs of autism and/or other developmental disorders.

Youth Violence: Fact Sheet

The Youth Violence: Fact Sheet (http://www.cdc.gov/ncipc/factsheets/yvfacts.htm) offers a comprehensive resource about the problem of violence (compiled and referenced from research and refereed articles). The nurse can access this information to be used as an educational tool when talking to youth and families about violence. Examples of fact sheet topics are the following:

- Occurrence
- Consequences
- Groups at Risk
- Risk Factors
- Individual Risk Factors
- Family Risk Factors
- Peer/School Risk Factors
- Community Risk Factors
- Protective Factors
- Individual Protective Factors
- Family Protective Factors
- Peer/School Protective Factors

Child Abuse

- All states in the United States have mandatory reporting guidelines for cases of child abuse; the national hotline in the United States is 1-800-4-A-Child.
- All allegations must first be investigated before confirmed.
- After documented confirmation, the child is placed in an environment safe and free of abuse.

Prevention of Childhood Obesity in Schools

- Ensure that the school provide healthy meals and replace soda machines with water.
- Encourage improved physical activity.
- Provide education about nutrition, physical activity, and acceptable weight.
- Provide health education to promote healthy eating, physical activity, and well-being.
- Research and advocate for changes in school policy.

RESOURCES

de Benedictis T, Jaffe-Gill E, & Segal J. (2007). Child abuse: Types, signs, symptoms, causes and help.
http://www.helpguide.org/mental/child

Child & Adolescent Bipolar Foundation: http://www.bpkids.org

Could it be autism? http://www.firstsigns.org

Office of Science Policy National Institute of Health:
http://www.science.education.nih.gov

The Youth Violence: Fact Sheet:
http://www.cdc.gov/ncipc/factsheets/yvfacts.htm

REFERENCES

American Academy of Family Physicians (AAFP). (updated 2006). Toilet training your child. Retrieved from http://familydoctor.org/online/famdocen/home/children/parents/toilet/179 (Accessed April 4, 2009).

Barth, R.P., Crea, T.M., John, K., Thoburn, J., & Quinton, D. (2005). Beyond attachment theory and therapy: Towards sensitive and evidence-based interventions with foster and adoptive families in distress. *Child and Family Social Work*, *10*(4), 257–268.

Caprio, S. (2006). Treating child obesity and associated medical conditions. *The Future of Children*, *16*(1), 209–224. Retrieved from www.futureofchildren.org (Accessed April 4, 2009).

Child and Adolescent Bipolar Foundation. Retrieved from http://www.bpkids.org/site/PageServer (Accessed April 4, 2009).

Child Welfare Information Gateway (2007). Surviving toilet training. Retrieved from http://www.childwelfare.gov/preventing/supporting/resources/toilettraining.cfm (Accessed April 4, 2009).

Commission on Adolescent Anxiety Disorders. (2005). Anxiety disorders. In D.L. Evans, E.B. Foa, R.E. Gur, H. Hendin, C.P. O'Brien, M.E.P. Seligman, & B.T. Walsh (Eds.). *Treating and preventing adolescent mental health disorders: What we know and don't know: A research agenda for improving the mental health of our youth* (pp. 162–253). New York: Oxford University Press.

Ewing, J.A. (1984). Detecting alcoholism: the CAGE questionnaire. *JAMA*, *252*(14), 1905–1907.

Findling, R.L., Feeny, N.C., Stansbrey, R.J., Delporto-Bedoya, D., & Demeter, C. (2004). Special articles: Treatment of mood disorders in children and adolescents: Somatic treatment for depressive illnesses in children and adolescents. *Psychiatric Clinics of North America*, *27*(1), 113–137.

Goodman, W.K., Murphy, T.K., & Storch, E.A. (2007). Risk of adverse behavioral effects with pediatric use of antidepressants [Electronic version]. *Psychopharmacology*, *191*(87), 87–96.

Kumanyika, S., & Grier, S. (2006). Targeting interventions for ethnic minority and low-income populations. *The Future of Children, 16*(1), 187–207.

National Institute of Mental Health (NIMH). (2000). Child & adolescent bipolar disorder: An update from the National Institute of Mental Health. (NIH Publication No. 00–4778). Retrieved from http://www.nimh.nih.gov/publicat/index.cfm (Accessed April 4, 2009)

National Institute of Mental Health (NIMH). (2001). Blueprint for change: Research on child and adolescent mental health: Report of the National Advisory Mental Health Council's Workgroup on Child and Adolescent Mental Health Development and Deployment. Washington, DC: Office of Communications and Public Liaison (ERIC Document Reproduction Service No. ED462650).

Sheldon, S H. (2005). Introduction to pediatric sleep medicine. In S.H. Sheldon, R. Ferber, & M.H. Kryger (Eds.). *Principles and practice of pediatric sleep medicine* (pp. 1–16). Philadelphia: Elsevier Saunders.

Stafford, B.S., & Zeanah, C.H. (2006). Attachment disorders. In J.L. Luby (Ed.). *Handbook of preschool mental health: Development, disorders, and treatment* (pp. 231–251). New York: Guilford Press.

Vieth, V., Bottoms, B.L., & Perona, A. (2006). *Ending child abuse: New efforts in prevention, investigation, and training.* Binghamton, NY: The Haworth Maltreatment & Trauma Press.

Wiseman, N.D. (2006). *Could it be autism? A parent's guide to the first signs and next steps.* New York: Broadway Books.

Caring for the Child with a Respiratory Condition

KEY TERMS

retractions – Drawing back of the chest wall with inspiration; seen when the accessory muscles are used for breathing. Common sites for retractions include suprasternal, supraclavicular, intercostal, subcostal, and substernal (Ball & Binder, 2006).

status asthmaticus – Persistent and intractable asthma where the child does not respond to therapy and a medical emergency ensues

FOCUSED ASSESSMENT

Nursing Assessment

The nurse must use a complete nursing assessment to assess the child's respiratory condition:

- Watch for subtle changes in the child's color, respiration, behavior, heart rate, and general health.
- Subtle changes can occur before they can be recognized by technological methods.
- Use innate instincts when caring for the child; if the nurse senses impending crisis it is important to pay attention to this instinct and act accordingly (getting emergency equipment ready).
- Remember that children have an uncanny ability to compensate. When a child is no longer able to compensate, he or she "crashes" and may then have a poor probability of recovery.

Pediatric Respiratory Emergencies

Assessment	Critical	Unstable	Potentially Unstable	Stable
Airway	Completely or severely obstructed	Partially obstructed, excessive secretions or blood	Open with secretions	Open
Breathing Rate	May be slow, absent, or very fast with periods of slowing	Increased	Occasionally increased	Normal
Breathing Effort	Absent or greatly increased with periods of weakness	Increased	Normal	Normal
Breath Sounds	Grunting, faint, or absent	Wheezing or stridor, decreased breath sounds	Normal or slight wheezing	Normal
Skin Color	Pale, mottled, or blue	Pink or pale	Pink	Pink
Inspection	Normal, decreased, or absent chest movement	Normal or decreased chest movement	Runny nose, red eyes, fever	Runny nose
Actions	Immediately open airway, suction, give high concentration oxygen with assisted ventilation, and transport	Move at moderate pace; give high concentration oxygen; prepare for transport; reassess frequently	Move at moderate pace; help into position of comfort; give high concentration oxygen; prepare for transport	Begin focused history and physical exam

Based on CUPS Assessment table in Sanddal, N., et al. (1997). *Critical trauma care by the basic EMT* (4th ed.). Bozeman, MT: Critical Illness and Trauma Foundation.

Classification of Asthma Severity

Criteria for Classification of Asthma Severity in Children 0–4 Years of Age				
Severity	**Day Symptoms**	**Night Awakenings**	**SABA Use***	**Limit to Activity**
Intermittent	≤2 days/week	None	≤2 times/week	None
Mild Persistent	3–6 days/week	1–2X/month	>2 days/week	**Minor**
Moderate, Persistent	Daily	3–4X/month	Daily	Some
Severe, Persistent	Several X/day	>1X/week	Several X/day	Extreme

*Short-acting beta 2 agonists (SABA) such as albuterol use does not include prevention of exercise induced bronchospasm (EIB).
The U.S. Department of Health and Human Services 2007, the National Asthma Education and Prevention Program. Expert panel report 3: Guidelines for the diagnosis and management of asthma.

CLINICAL ALERTS

Respiratory Rate Exceeding 60 Breaths/Minute

A respiratory rate that exceeds 60 breaths/min is dangerous! At this high rate, sufficient oxygen does not reach the alveoli for adequate gas exchange. **Never** feed an infant or child orally if the respiratory rate exceeds 60 breaths/min because of potential aspiration.

Retractions

- Retractions are a drawing back of the chest wall with inspiration and are seen when the accessory muscles are used for breathing.
- Common sites for retractions include suprasternal, supraclavicular, intercostal, subcostal, and substernal.

The Mother's Obstetrical History

- If the nurse caring for a newborn observes the infant to be drooling excessively and/or having persistent choking spells and color change with feedings, it is important for the nurse to check the mother's obstetrical history.

- These symptoms are highly suspicious of esophageal atresia and tracheoesophageal fistula.
- If there is history of polyhydramnios, the nurse must immediately report the observed symptoms to the baby's pediatrician.

Suctioning

- Preoperatively, nasogastric, or orogastric tube placement for suctioning must be done extremely carefully and gently, and progression stopped immediately if any resistance is met to avoid perforating the esophageal tissue of an infant with an anomaly.
- Postoperative oral or nasal suctioning of the infant with esophageal atresia (EA), tracheoesophageal fistula (TEF), or congenital diaphragmatic hernia (CDH) must be done extremely carefully to avoid disruption of the repairs. Ensure that the tube is not inserted any further than the distance from the nares to the ear lobe.

Assisted Mechanical Ventilation

Neonates with severe respiratory distress syndrome (RDS) and those with complications require assisted mechanical ventilation.

Signs of Bleeding After Tonsillectomy

Continuous swallowing is indicative of bleeding. Additional signs to be observed are restlessness, increased pulse rate, and pallor (late symptom).

Rupture of the Tympanic Membrane

Rupture of the tympanic membrane brings immediate pain relief, a gradual decrease in temperature, and the presence of a purulent discharge in the external auditory canal. However, rupture of the tympanic membrane may lead to scarring and hearing loss.

DIAGNOSTIC TESTS

Common Diagnostic Tests

Test	Indications	Preparation	Post-test Care
Bronchoscopy Insertion of a rigid or flexible fiberoptic bronchoscope to evaluate lungs, larynx, vocal cords, trachea, bronchi	Recurrent and persistent pneumonia or atelectasis, unexplained and persistent wheezes, presence of a foreign body, hemoptysis, congenital anomalies, and unexplained interstitial conditions	Explain procedure: IV inserted to infuse anesthetics and analgesics, general anesthetic in most cases, NPO 6 hours. Written and informed consent required.	Monitor vital signs. Explain that the patient may have sore throat or hoarseness. Observe for hemoptysis, difficulty breathing, cough, pain, absent breath sounds over affected area. Evaluate for symptoms of pneumothorax: dyspnea, tachypnea, anxiety, decreased breath sounds, restlessness.
Chest X-ray Radiologic study to identify and detect abnormalities in size, structure, and shape of bony structures and tissues.	Pneumonia, bronchitis, pleural effusion, atelectasis, tuberculosis, pneumothorax, tumors, presence of foreign body	Explain procedure. Record date of last menstrual period and determine the possibility of pregnancy.	
Computed Tomography (CT) Noninvasive cross-sectional and three dimensional study of internal structure of thorax	Mediastinal and pleural effusions, suspected bronchiectasis.	Explain the procedure: IV may be inserted for infusion of contrast medium or sedatives. The patient may experience a feeling of warmth and a salty or metallic taste if contrast medium is given. Fluids may be restricted before the test. Remove jewelry and metallic objects. Written and informed consent is required.	If contrast is used, observe for delayed allergic reactions such as rash, urticaria, tachycardia, nausea, or vomiting.
Lung Biopsy (surgical) Removal of living tissue from lungs for diagnostic purposes	Inflammatory diseases, infections	Explain the procedure: IV line will be inserted, NPO 6 hours. Record date of last menstrual period and determine possibility of pregnancy. Written and informed consent is required.	Monitor vital signs according to agency protocol. Observe the biopsy site for bleeding. Observe patient for hemoptysis, difficulty breathing, cough, pain, or absent

Test	Indications	Preparation	Post-test Care
			breath sounds over the affected area. Monitor chest tube patency and drainage after a thoracotomy.
Pulmonary Function Studies Tests measuring the volume, pattern, and rates of airflow of lungs	Differentiate between restrictive and obstructive conditions. Determine progression of disease. Determine responsiveness to respiratory therapies.	Explain the procedure. Obtain height and weight data. No smoking for 4 hours before procedure.	
Sweat Chloride Noninvasive study to assist in diagnosis of cystic fibrosis	Screen for suspected cystic fibrosis.	Explain that sweat is collected on filter paper disks by introducing a small electrical current to the skin which may result in a stinging sensation.	Observe site for unusual color, sensation, or discomfort.

Adapted from Van Leeuwen, A.M., Kranpitz, T.R., & Smith, L. (2006). *Davis's comprehensive handbook of laboratory and diagnostic tests with nursing implications.* Philadelphia: F.A. Davis.

Pulmonary Function Tests

Category	Test	Definition
Slow Vital Capacity Tests	Tidal volume (TV)	The amount of air inhaled and exhaled during normal respiration
	Inspiratory capacity (IC)	The maximum amount of air inhaled after the end of tidal volume expiration during normal respiration
	Expiratory reserve volume (ERV)	The maximum amount of air exhaled after the end of tidal volume expiration during normal respiration
	Inspiratory reserve volume (IRV)	The maximum amount of air inhaled after the end of tidal volume inspiration during normal respiration

(continued)

Pulmonary Function Tests (Continued)

Category	Test	Definition
	Vital capacity (VC)	The maximum amount of air exhaled following a maximal inhalation (VC = ERV + IC)
Lung Volume Studies	Residual volume (RV)	The amount of air that remains in the lungs after maximal exhalation
	Functional residual capacity (FRC)	The amount of air left in the lungs after normal exhalation (FRC = ERV + RV)
	Total lung capacity (TLC)	The total amount of air in the lungs at maximal inhalation (TLC = V + RV or TLC = FRC + IC)
Lung Volumes and Capacity	Forced vital capacity (FVC)	The maximum amount of air that can be exhaled as hard, fast, and long as possible after a maximum inhalation
	Forced inspiratory volume (FIV)	The maximum amount of air that can be inhaled after a maximum exhalation

Normal Values for Arterial Blood Gases

Component	Definition	Normal Values	Interpretation
pH	Acid–base status of the body	Preterms: 7.3–7.4 Full term: 7.3–7.4 Children 7.35–7.45	Acidosis <7.35 Alkalosis >7.45
Paco$_2$	Pressure exerted by CO_2 in blood	Newborn: 30–40 mm Hg Infant: 30–41 mm Hg Children: 35–45 mm Hg	Acidosis >45 mm Hg Alkalosis <35 mm Hg
HCO$_3$$^-$	Buffering effect of acid in blood	Children >7 yr 20–22 mEq/L	Acidosis: 22 mEq/L Alkalosis: 26 mEq/L
Base Excess	Status of bases in blood	Newborn: −10 to −2 mEq/L Infant: −7 to −1 mEq/L Children: −4 to +2 mEq/L Thereafter: −3 to +3 mEq/L A positive or negative number indicate increasing or decreasing range of bicarbonate ion concentration	Acidosis more + Alkalosis more −

Component	Definition	Normal Values	Interpretation
Pao_2	Pressure exerted by dissolved O_2 in blood	Newborn: 60–90 mm Hg Infant: 80–100 mm Hg Children: 80–100 mm Hg	Acidosis: <80 mm Hg Alkalosis: >100 mm Hg

Sputum Culture and Sensitivity

To be able to establish the causative organism and most effective antibiotic a culture and sensitivity test of the sputum is done.

- A specimen may be obtained by a direct throat swab immediately after coughing.
- In some cases, a sterile catheter may be inserted directly into the trachea through the endotracheal tube or during direct laryngoscopy.
- An early morning fasting specimen obtained by gastric aspiration may also be obtained.

Tuberculin Skin Test (TST)

The tuberculin skin test (TST) is an exact indicator of whether a child has been infected with the tubercle bacillus.

- Inject a measured amount of the intermediate strength of 5 tuberculin units of tuberculin purified protein derivative (PPD) intradermally to form a small wheal in the forearm.
- In 48 to 72 hours, a positive reaction is marked by an area of red induration (an area of hardened tissue).
- Reactions greater than 10 mm in size are considered positive in non-immunocompromised patients.

MEDICATIONS

Erythromycin (eh-rith-roe-**mye**-sin)

Indications IV, PO: Infections caused by susceptible organisms including upper and lower respiratory tract infections and otitis media.

Action Suppresses protein synthesis at the level of the 50S ribosome.

Therapeutic Effects Bacteriostatic action against susceptible bacterial spectrum: streptococci, staphylococci, gram-positive bacilli.

Pharmacokinetics
Absorption Variable absorption from the duodenum after oral administration.

Contraindications and Precautions
Contraindicated in Hypersensitivity

Adverse Reactions and Side Effects Irritation

Route and Dosage Children **PO:** 30–50 mg/kg divided doses q6–8hr Neonates **PO:** 20–50 mg/kg per day divided q6–12hr.

Nursing Implications Inform parents of medication administration.

Prepare to administer around the clock. Use a calibrated measuring device for liquid preparations. Do not crush or chew delayed–release capsules or tablets; swallow whole.

> *Data from Deglin, J., & Vallerand, A. (2009). Davis's drug guide for nurses (11th ed.), pp. 498–501. Philadelphia: F.A. Davis.*

Oseltamivir (o-sel-**tam**-i-vir) (Tamiflu)

Pregnancy Category C

Indications Uncomplicated acute illness due to influenza infection in adults and children older than 1 year of age who have symptoms for ≤2 days. Prevention of influenza in patients ≥13 years of age.

Actions Inhibits the enzyme neuraminidase, which may alter virus particle aggregation and release.

Therapeutic Effects Reduced duration of flu related symptoms

Pharmacokinetics
Absorption Rapidly absorbed from the GI tract and converted by the liver to the active form, oseltamivir carboxylate; 75% reaches the systemic circulation as the active drug.

Contraindications and Precautions
Contraindicated in Hypersensitivity and children <1 year old

Adverse Reactions and Side Effects
CNS Insomnia, vertigo
Respiratory Bronchitis

Gastrointestinal Nausea, vomiting

Route and Dosage PO: Children >40 kg: 75 mg twice daily for 5 days. Children 23–40 kg: 60 mg twice daily. Children 15–23 kg: 45 mg twice daily. Children ≤15 kg and 1 year or older: 30 mg twice daily.

Nursing Implications Monitor influenza symptoms. Additional supportive treatment may be indicated to treat symptoms. Treatment should be started as soon as possible at the first sign of flu symptoms. Administer with food or milk to minimize GI irritation. Drug should be used within 10 days of the infection. Caution patients/parents that Tamiflu should not be shared with anyone even if they have the same symptoms.

According to immunization guidelines, Tamiflu is not a substitute for flu shots. Advise patient to consult a health care professional before taking any medications concurrently with Tamiflu.

Data from Deglin, J., & Vallerand, A. (2009). Davis's drug guide for nurses (11th ed.), pp. 916–917. Philadelphia: F.A. Davis.

Albuterol (al-**byoo**-ter-ole) (Ventolin, Salbutamol)

Indications Control and prevent reversible airway obstruction caused by asthma or COPD Inhalant: Used as a quick relief agent for acute bronchospasm. **PO:** Used as a long-term control agent in patients with chronic/persistent bronchospasm.

Actions Binds to beta adrenergic receptors in airway smooth muscle.

Therapeutic Effects Bronchodilatation

Pharmacokinetics
Absorption Well absorbed after oral administration but rapidly undergoes extensive metabolism.

Contraindications and Precautions
Contraindicated in Hypersensitivity to adrenergic amines and to fluorocarbons (some inhalers).

Adverse Reactions and Side Effects Nervousness, restlessness, tremors, chest pains, palpitations.

Route and Dosage PO: Children 2–6 years: 0.1 mg/kg 3 times daily, not to exceed 2 mg 3 times daily initially; children 6–12 years: 2 mg 3–4 times daily or 0.3–0.6 mg/kg/day not to exceed 8 mg/day; children older than 12 years: 2–4 mg 3–4 times daily not to exceed 32 mg/day. **Inhalant:** Children older than 4 years – via metered-dose inhaler 2 inhalations every 4–6 hours. For acute asthma exacerbations: 4–8 puffs every 20 min for 3 doses, then every 1–4 hours; children older than 12 years: via nebulization or intermittent positive pressure breathing (IPPB): 2.5–5 mg every 20 minutes for 3 doses then 2.5–10 mg every 1–4 hours. PRN; children 2–12 years: via nebulization or IPPB: 0.15 mg/kg per dose (minimum dose 2.5 mg) every 20 minutes for three doses, then 0.15–0.3 mg/kg (not to exceed 10 mg) every 1–4 hours PRN or 1.25 mg 3–4 times daily for children 10–15 kg or 2.5 mg 3–4 times daily for children weighing more than 15 kg; children older than 4 years via Rota inhaler inhalation device: 200 mcg (as Ventolin Rotacaps) every 4–6 hours (up to 400 mcg every 4–6 hours).

Nursing Implications Assess lung sounds and vital signs before administration and during peak of medication. Note the amount, color, and characteristics of the sputum produced. Monitor pulmonary function test (PFT) periodically. If wheezing occurs, withhold medications and notify the physician immediately.

Data from Deglin, J., & Vallerand, A. (2009). Davis's drug guide for nurses (11th ed.), pp. 120–122. Philadelphia: F.A. Davis

ETHNOCULTURAL CONSIDERATIONS

Asthma

- In the United States, the poor, especially of black or Hispanic background, experience disproportionally high rates of both asthma and morbidity (Castro et al., 2001; Mannino et al., 2002).
- There is great worldwide variability in prevalence with industrialized areas having consistently high rates.

TEACHING THE FAMILY

Esophageal Atresia with or without Tracheoesophageal Fistula

- Teach parents proper sterile technique of suctioning and how to handle the equipment appropriately.
- Ensure that all emergency calling numbers are written down so emergency care can be provided in a serious situation.
- Ensure that parents know how to identify respiratory distress.
- Ensure that parents know feeding techniques for a gastrostomy tube and how to handle tube plugging and dislodging.
- Instruct parents in performing CPR before the child goes home.
- Encourage parents to use different toys and games to promote stimulation during regular care.
- Mobilization can be as simple as holding or rocking while action play can be games, toy figures, or crafts.
- Involve other siblings in adapting the young child with EA or TEF.
- Ensure the family knows how to operate equipment and knows proper maintenance of the equipment used at home.

Caring for the Child with Cystic Fibrosis at Home

- Teach the family about the nature of the disease and prepare them to manage day-to-day minor complaints.
- Assist in arranging for the portable suction machine and about the proper suctioning technique at home.
- Instruct the parents to perform respiratory therapy before meals because chest physiotherapy may induce vomiting of the thick tenacious mucus.
- Teach the parents different techniques for chest physiotherapy and postural drainage and about coughing exercises based on their child's age. The child needs to be suctioned followed by chest physiotherapy and inhalation to liquefy the thick secretions.
- Teach the family about the preferred meal plans, high-calorie diet, and mixing pancreatic enzymes with meals.

- Instruct the family to monitor the child's weight to ensure proper growth patterns.
- Teach the family how to administer medications properly.
- Inform the family how to access community resources and how to contact their home health nurse.

Avoiding Sinusitis

- Use an oral decongestant or a nasal spray decongestant when initial signs and symptoms appear.
- Have the child gently blow his nose, blocking one nostril while blowing through the other.
- Ensure the child drinks plenty of fluids to keep nasal discharge thin.
- Apply warm compresses or heating pad on low heat over the inflamed area.
- Use a cool mist humidifier.
- Avoid air travel. If it cannot be avoided, use a nasal spray decongestant before "take off" to help prevent blockage of the sinuses, allowing mucus secretions to drain.
- Avoid contact with main allergens.
- Use air conditioning to ensure even room temperature.
- Use electrostatic filters attached to heating and air con-ditioning systems to help remove allergens (American Academy of Otolaryngology, Head and Neck Surgery, 2008).

Home Discharge Instructions After a Tonsillectomy

- Keep the child away from highly seasoned food and "sharp" foods (nacho chips) for a period of 2 weeks. The postsurgical scab is most likely to be dislodged at the 8–12-day period.
- Ensure the child avoids gargling and vigorous tooth brushing.
- Instruct the child to avoid coughing or clearing the throat.
- Limit activities that may result in bleeding.

Preventing External Otitis Media

- Advise children to limit their stay in the water to less than an hour. Ears should be completely dry before entering the water again.

- Shaking the head and judicious use of the corner of a towel or small tuft of cotton can remove most excess water.
- To keep the ear dry, the parent can pull the auricle up and out to straighten the canal, then use a conventional hair dryer set on low or no heat held at a distance of 18 to 24 inches for 30 seconds, three times a day.
- Earplugs may be recommended.
- Advise against swimming in dirty water and in public swimming pools that do not maintain good control of the chlorine and pH pool testing and treatment.

Salicylates (Aspirin)

- Avoid giving salicylates (aspirin) because of the possibility of Reye syndrome.
- Watch for symptoms (nausea, vomiting, lethargy, and indifference). In severe cases there may be irrational behavior, delirium, and rapid breathing.

The Heimlich Maneuver

Conscious Child Older Than 1 Year of Age

1. Give five blows to the child's back with the heel of your hand with the child sitting, kneeling, lying.
2. If the obstruction persists, go behind the child and pass your arms around the child's body; form a fist with one hand immediately below the child's sternum. Place the other hand over the fist and pull upwards into the abdomen. Repeat five times.

3. Check the child's mouth for any obvious obstruction that can be removed.
4. If necessary, repeat the sequence and ask for help to call 911 or rush to the nearest hospital.

Heimlich Maneuver on an Infant

1. Lay the infant on your arm or thigh with the infant's head down.
2. Give five blows to the infant's back using the heel of your hand.

3. If the airway obstruction continues, turn the infant over with the head down and give five chest thrusts using two fingers at a distance of 1 fingerbreadth below the nipple level in midline.

4. Check the infant's mouth for any obvious obstructions that can be removed.
5. If necessary, repeat the sequence and ask for help to call 911 or rush to the nearest hospital (The AHA Subcommittee on Pediatric Resuscitation, 2006. http://pediatrics. appublications.org/cgi/content/full/117/5/e989).

Peak Flow Meter

 Procedure 21-1 Using a Peak Flow Meter

Purpose

The purpose of a peak flow meter is to keep track of the results and help the parents and child learn about asthma. Keeping a daily record may also help determine if the child's asthma is getting worse.

Equipment

- Peak flow meter
- Peak flow record

Procedure 21-1 (Continued)

Steps

1. Before each use, make sure the sliding marker or arrow on the peak flow meter is at the bottom of the numbered scale (zero or the lowest number on the scale).

2. Instruct the child to stand up straight and to remove gum or any food from the mouth.

3. Instruct the child to take a deep breath and to put the mouthpiece of the peak flow meter into the mouth. Close the lips tightly around the mouthpiece. Be sure to keep the tongue away from the mouthpiece.

4. Instruct the child to take in one breath and to then blow out as hard and as quickly as possible. Blow a "fast and hard blast" rather than "slowly blowing" until all of the air is emptied from the lungs.

5. Teach the parents that the force of the air coming out of the lungs causes the marker to move along the numbered scale. Record the number where the marker landed on a peak flow record.

6. Repeat the entire routine three times (if the routine is done correctly the numbers from all three tries are very close together).

7. Record the highest reading. Do not calculate an average.

8. Measure the peak flow rate at the same time each day. A good time to measure the peak flow rate is between 7 and 9 A.M. and between 6 and 8 P.M. Note: It may be a good idea to measure the peak flow rate before or after using asthma medicine.

9. Keep a chart of the peak flow rates on a peak flow record.

Clinical Alert A peak flow meter package usually contains a peak flow record when the peak flow readings are recorded regularly.

Teach Parents

Teach parents about the child's personal best. The "personal best" peak flow is determined when the child is symptom free. It is important for the child, parents,

(continued)

Procedure 21-1 (Continued)

and the physician to discuss what is considered "normal." Remind parents of the need to discuss the readings with the physician.

Spacers

The nurse understands that for children less than 5 years of age, a spacer or a valved holding chamber (VHC) is recommended which is attached to the MDI. A spacer may deliver the medication to the child's lungs better than an inhaler alone and may be easier for the child to use than an MDI alone. In addition, for ease of delivery, child sized masks are available that fit the VHC. With this device there is more medication deposited in the lungs and less systemic side effects. After VHC use the nurse can have the child follow with mouth washing and spitting to decrease swallowing medication and side effect including, in the case of inhaled corticosteroids (ICS), prevention of oral *Candidiasis* (U.S. Department of Health and Human Services, 2007).

Asthma Action Plan

The Asthma Action Plan is an educational tool used for communication between the health care provider and the patient, with their family and caregivers, to properly manage asthma and respond to asthma episodes. Found at http://www.lungusa.org

- Ensure it is completed by the child's primary care provider.
- It includes the symptoms and management for each color zone including peak flow measurements appropriate for each color zone.
- Provide adequate instructions on how to use, interpret, and complete the form.

ADDITIONAL INFORMATION FOR THE CLINICAL SETTING

Assessing Respiratory Status

- Assess the infant's respiratory status including increasing respiratory rate and decreasing oxygenation. The child who has a severe case of bronchopulmonary dysplasia (BPD) may need recurrent hospitalization; therefore, the nurse must be able to provide emotional support to parents during these crucial moments.

Preventing Respiratory Illnesses in Patients with BPD

- Instruct all visitors to wash their hands before touching the neonate. The nurse should politely ask visitors with current respiratory infections to leave the room, explaining that the infant is at an increased risk for infection.

Promoting Respiratory Function

- To ensure respiratory function, a multidisciplinary approach should be taken. A physician, nurse, respiratory therapist, social worker, dietitian, and psychologist are the important professionals in the management of a child with cystic fibrosis (CF).

Nutrition

- The best outcome for a child with CF is a well-balanced, high-protein, high-caloric diet. Pancreatic insufficiency results in malabsorption of fat-soluble vitamins (vitamins A, D, E, K). Daily vitamin supplementation is recommended. The nurse can also work closely with the family to prevent infection as well as optimize nutrition and growth of a child.

Acute Epiglottitis or Supraglottitis; a Medical Emergency

Acute epiglottitis or supraglottitis is a sudden, potentially lethal condition characterized by high fever, sore throat, dyspnea, and rapidly progressing respiratory obstruction. It is considered a serious obstructive inflammatory condition and a medical emergency that requires immediate attention.

- The child goes to bed asymptomatic and awakens with complaints of sore throat and pain on swelling accompanied by a febrile state.

- The child typically assumes the tripod position: leaning forward and sitting upright with chin thrust, mouth open while bracing on the arms, and tongue protruding with drooling of saliva.
- The child is irritable and restless with a thick and muffled voice and there is a froglike croaking sound on inspiration.
- Suprasternal and substernal retractions may be visible.
- The child breathes slowly, the throat is red and inflamed, and there is a distinctive large, cherry red edematous epiglottis.
- The nurse must never assess the child's throat with a tongue blade unless a respiratory therapist or medical doctor is present.

Preventing RSV

- RSV immunoglobulin (RSV-IGIV), an intravenous preparation of immunoglobulin G that provides neutralizing antibodies against RSV, may be given just before the start of the RSV season to prevent RSV.

What to Do in Cases of an Acute Asthma Attack

An asthma attack may occur anytime and anywhere. It may happen in the home, at a school, in a mall, or in a park. To guide parents, teachers, and people who work in places where children go, the nurse can provide the following tips:

Teachers and school administrators should be familiar with the health history of the child. It is important to coordinate care and share information with the school health nurse. The nurse should also know the school district's rules and regulations regarding carrying asthma medications to school, including where the medications are to be kept and how to use the medications. In coordination with the child's physician and parents the nurse can fill out an emergency asthma action plan, including the child's triggers. The nurse needs to post emergency phone numbers in case of an attack. In addition, the nurse must know the child's peak flow readings, the child's personal best, and when the child runs into trouble. The nurse can also educate the teachers and other personnel who come in contact with the child.

Parents should be sure to carry the child's quick relief medications. It is helpful if the school-age child carry it too, along with the instructions about how the medication is used.

Nurses can give information on environmental control and creating an allergen-free environment. In addition, through community health education, the nurse can emphasize that when child exhibiting difficulty breathing, wheezing, and coughing, it is important to be calm and reassure the child. It is important to find out if the child's medicine is available; if not, call 911.

Personnel in parks, mall, and play areas should be briefed about possible pediatric emergencies including management in an emergency situation.

RESOURCES

American Academy of Family Physicians. (2005). Asthma action plan. http://www.familydoctor.org/online/famdocen/home.html

American Lung Association: http://www.lungusa.org

Cystic Fibrosis Foundation: http://www.cff.org

REFERENCES

American Academy of Otolaryngology, head and neck surgery (2008). Retrieved from: http://entmd.org/healthinfo/sinus/sinusitis.cfm (Accessed June 20, 2008).

Castro, M., Schechtman, K., Halstead, J., & Bloomberg, G. (2001). Risk factors for asthma morbidity and mortality in a large metropolitan city. *Journal of Asthma, 38*(8), 625–635.

Deglin, J. & Vallerand, A. (2009). *Davis's drug guide for nurses* (11th ed.). Philadelphia: F.A. Davis.

Mannino, D.M., Homa, D.M., Akinbami, L.J., Moorman, J.E., Gwynn, C., & Redd, S.C. (2002). Surveillance for asthma—United States, 1980–1999. *MMWR. Surveillance Summaries: Morbidity and Mortality Weekly Report. Surveillance Summaries / CDC. 51*(1), 1–13.

U.S. Department of Health and Human Services. (2007). National asthma education and prevention program. Expert panel report 3: Guidelines for the diagnosis and management of asthma. Full report 2007. NIH Publication No. 07-4051. Bethesda, MD: NHLBI Health Information Center. Retrieved from http://www.nhlbi.nih.gov/guidelines/asthma/asthgdln.htm (Accessed July 8, 2008).

Venes, D. (Ed.). (2005). *Taber's cyclopedic medical dictionary* (20th ed.). Philadelphia: F.A. Davis.

Caring for the Child with a Gastrointestinal Condition

KEY TERMS

biliary atresia – Extrahepatic biliary atresia (EHBA), an idiopathic, progressive, inflammatory process that causes both intrahepatic and extrahepatic bile duct fibrosis and obstruction

constipation – Difficult or infrequent passage of hard stool, which is often associated with straining, abdominal pain, or withholding behaviors

encopresis – Stool incontinence beyond the age when children should normally be able to control their bowels, which is usually after the age of 4 years

intussusception – Condition that occurs when a proximal section of the intestine and the mesentery (the peritoneal fold that encircles the small intestine and connects it to the posterior abdominal wall) "telescopes" into a distal section of the intestine

irritable bowel syndrome (IBS) – A functional disorder that is commonly cause of recurrent abdominal pain in children

lactose intolerance – Inability to digest milk and some dairy products, which leads to symptoms of bloating, cramping, and diarrhea

nissen fundoplication – Wrapping the gastric cardia with adjacent portions of the gastric fundus

omphalitis – Infection of the umbilical stump; occurs once the umbilicus is colonized with streptococci, staphylococci, or gram-negative organisms, which may cause a local infection

probiotics – Food preparations containing microorganism, such as *Lactobacillus*; can improve lactose intolerance when live cultures are fermented in dairy products

FOCUSED ASSESSMENT

Classic Symptomatic Triad for Intussusception

- Paroxysmal, episodic abdominal pain with vomiting every 5–30 minutes.
- Screaming with drawing up of the legs with periods of calm, sleeping, or lethargy between episodes.
- Stool, possible diarrhea in nature, with blood (currant jelly) (Petersen-Smith, 2004, p. 862).

Appendicitis Physical Examination

- The child diagnosed with appendicitis experiences a progression of symptoms, with no single test providing overall confirmation of the diagnosis.
- Laboratory findings may demonstrate an elevated white blood cell (WBC) count.
  - An elevated WBC count does not distinguish simple appendicitis from perforated appendicitis.
  - Children with appendicitis may also have a normal WBC count (Burd & Whalen, 2001).
- An abdominal radiograph may reveal fecal matter, or some other obstruction, although this rarely confirms the diagnosis.
- If there is uncertainty in young children, ultrasound and computed tomography (CT) scan may help differentiate abdominal pain from other causes, although the usefulness is variable (Mow, 2005).

Appendicitis	
Signs and Symptoms	**Reaction**
Rebound Tenderness	Presence of involuntary guarding, rebound tenderness with pain over McBurney's point, which is located 1.5–2 inches in from the right anterior superior iliac crest on a line toward the umbilicus and is best elicited on palpation
Heel-drop Jarring Test	Stand on toes for 15 seconds, then drops on heels; inability to stand straight or climb stairs; winces when getting off examination table.

(continued)

Appendicitis (Continued)

Signs and Symptoms	Reaction
Psoas Sign	Abdominal pain with right hip flexion against resistance
Obturator Sign	Pain on passive internal rotation of the flexed right thigh
Rovsing Sign	Deep pressure in lower left quadrant elicits pain with a sudden release (Petersen-Smith, 2004).

Comparison of Hepatitis A (HAV), Hepatitis B (HBV), and Hepatitis C (HCV)

Clinical Features	HAV	HBV	HCV
Onset	Usually rapid, acute	More insidious	Usually insidious
Fever	Common and early	Less frequent	Less frequent
Anorexia	Common	Mild to moderate	Mild to moderate
Nausea and Vomiting	Common	Sometimes	Mild to moderate
Rash	Rare	Common	Sometimes
Arthralgia	Rare	Common	Rare
Pruritus	Rare	Sometimes	Sometimes
Jaundice	Present	Present	Present

Sources: Diagneau (2007) and Sokol & Narkewicz (2007).

CLINICAL ALERTS

Abdominal Pain in Children

- In children, abdominal pain can be referred from an extra-abdominal source (e.g., pneumonia, urinary tract infection, or testicular torsion) or it can be associated with a systematic disease.
- Abdominal pain is a common complaint in ill children and can be found in conditions such as streptococcal pharyngitis, lower lobe pneumonia, sickle cell disease, cystic fibrosis, or in other conditions (Duderstadt, 2006).
- A child's abdominal pain experience is usually limited and the child may be unable to accurately describe or pinpoint the location or sensation.

Vomiting

- Projectile vomiting is the classic and most common symptom of hypertrophic pyloric stenosis.

Signs of Perforation and Peritonitis

- The nurse is responsible for monitoring the infant for signs of perforation (a hole), peritonitis (inflammation of the abdominal cavity), or shock in addition to evidence of increased pain. The nurse also monitors and records the child's stools. The nurse understands that the spontaneous passing of a stool may indicate a resolution of the obstruction.
- Perforation: Acute pain, beginning over the perforated area and spreading over the abdomen; abdomen may become rigid; nausea; vomiting; tachycardia; fevers; chills; sweats; confusion; decreased urinary output (Venes, 2005).
- Peritonitis: Moderate or mild abdominal pain that worsens with movement; fever; change in bowel habits; malaise; nausea; loss of appetite; fever; hypothermia; distended abdomen with decreased bowel sounds (Venes, 2005).

Shock

- Signs of shock include tachycardia, tachypnea, hypotension, and cool, clammy, or cyanotic skin (Venes, 2005).

Irritable Bowel Syndrome (IBS)

- Symptoms of IBS include fever, severe abdominal pain and/or vomiting blood require immediate attention; surgical evaluation and/or intervention may be necessary.

Appendicitis

- Children with suspected appendicitis who respond with a "yes" to being hungry most likely do not have appendicitis because in most cases the child does not feel like eating (Potts, 2002).

Constipation

- Most children who are constipated usually have some abdominal pain due to cramping.
- If the onset of constipation and severe abdominal pain is acute and/or accompanied by fever, vomiting, or other symptoms, the child must be evaluated for a bowel obstruction.

Probiotics

- Concern regarding the potential for decreased bone mineral density and osteoporosis in children and adolescents with lactose intolerance reinforces the recommendations for the ingestion of small amounts of dairy products with meals.
- Probiotics (food preparations containing microorganism) such as *Lactobacillus* can improve lactose intolerance when live cultures are fermented in dairy products.
- *Lactobacillus* is a non-pathogenic bacterium that produces lactic acid from carbohydrates. The active culture in yogurt provides a source of calcium for persons with lactose intolerance in addition to producing some of the lactose enzyme required for proper digestions.

Complications of a Central Venous Line

Observe infusion site at least every 4 hours for the following complications (Venes, 2005):

- Infiltration
- Thrombophlebitis
- Fluid or electrolyte overload
- Air embolism

DIAGNOSTIC TESTS

- Diagnosis of hypertrophic pyloric stenosis can be made by palpating the pyloric mass. The mass is olive-shaped, movable, firm, and best palpated from the left side and located above and to the right of the umbilicus in the mid-epigastrium (the superior central portion of the abdomen) beneath the liver edge (Bishop, 2006).

- An abdominal x-ray film may show an enlarged stomach with diminished or absent gas in the intestine (Bishop, 2006).
- Examination of the pylorus on ultrasound shows elongation and thickening of the pylorus, which may be confirmed by a barium upper GI series.
- Confirmation by an upper GI series demonstrates a "string sign," which is caused by the barium passing through narrowed pylorus (Bishop, 2006).

Ultrasound

A diagnosis is often made after the history and physical examination. The diagnosis can be established 60% to 80% of the time by an experienced examiner. For example, if the diagnosis of hypertrophic pyloric stenosis is inconclusive, an ultrasound can be used to demonstrate an elongated muscular mass surrounding a long pyloric canal. Ultrasound confirms the diagnosis of hypertrophic pyloric stenosis.

Intussusception

- A flat-plate x-ray film in the child can appear normal early in the course of the disorder. However, an abdominal "ultrasound establishes the diagnosis in 90% of the cases" (Petersen-Smith, 2004, p. 862).

Laboratory Findings for Ulcerative Colitis

Laboratory findings for ulcerative colitis may include elevated sedimentation rate, microcytic anemia, and elevated white blood cell count with left shift, antineutrophil cytoplasmic antibodies (ANA) present in 80% (Petersen-Smith, 2004).

Conditions, Laboratory Tests, and Their Implications

Condition	Laboratory Tests	Implication
Cyclic Vomiting Syndrome	Complete blood count (CBC) with differential, electrolytes, glucose, liver function tests, metabolic screening, urinalysis, urine culture, urine organic acids	Rule out other conditions

(continued)

Conditions, Laboratory Tests, and Their Implications (Continued)

Condition	Laboratory Tests	Implication
Crohn's Disease	CBC with differential, serum iron, total iron-binding capacity, serum albumin, sedimentation rate, C-reactive protein	Inflammation, malnutrition
Ulcerative Colitis	CBC with differential, sedimentation rate	Inflammation, malnutrition
Short Bowel Syndrome	Electrolytes	Diarrhea, malnutrition, dehydration
Biliary Atresia	CBC, electrolytes, bilirubin, liver enzymes, TORCH titer, urine cytomegalovirus, sweat test	For diagnosis and to rule out other conditions

Tests, Purpose, and Condition

Test	Purpose	Condition
Anorectal Manometry	Measures pressure of the internal and anal sphincters	Hirschsprung disease
Barium Enema	Allows visualization of bowel; may reduce intussusception	Intussusception, Hirschsprung disease
Barium Swallow	Allows visualization of upper gastrointestinal tract	Post swallowing reflux
Intraesophageal pH Monitoring Study	Records presence of acid reflux	Gastroesophageal disease
Intravenous Pyelogram	Provides information about structure and function of the kidney, ureters, and bladder	Anorectal malformations
Liver Biopsy	Establishes degree of disease	Hepatitis
Radionuclide or Meckel Scan	Creates images of body parts through injection and detection of radioactive isotopes	Meckel diverticulum
Ultrasound	Outlines shape of tissues and organs	Anorectal malformations; hypertrophic pyloric stenosis; intussusception; appendicitis
Voiding Cystogram	Allows visualization of bladder and urethra	Urinary tract defects associated with anorectal malformations

Chronic Diarrhea

- Chronic diarrhea is defined as "one or more liquid to semiliquid stools passed per day for 14 days or longer" (Petersen-Smith, 2004, p. 878).
- Diagnostic assessment may include stool for culture and sensitivity, ova and parasites.

 Procedure 22-1 Stool for Culture and Sensitivity and Ova and Parasites

Purpose

Collecting stool for culture and sensitivity and ova and parasites is used to detect the presence of bacterial overgrowth; to confirm bacterial gastroenteritis; and to assess sensitivity of specific antimicrobials.

Equipment

- Gloves
- Patient identification label
- Sterile culture tube and cotton swab to collect specimen
- Biohazard container

Steps

1. Don gloves.
2. Using the sterile cotton swab collect (scrape) a fresh, warm specimen of stool from the diaper or stool receptacle and place it into the sterile culture tube.
3. Label both the sterile culture tube and the biohazard bag with the patient's identification information.
4. Place the sterile culture tube into the biohazard bag.
5. Deliver the fresh specimen of stool to the laboratory promptly after collection.
6. Document the procedure.

Clinical Alert

- Avoid external contamination of stool and deliver to laboratory promptly.
- Provide samples from several areas of the stool to assure that organisms are isolated. Failure to do so may yield a false-negative result.
- Inform the lab of antimicrobial or antiamebic therapy within 10 days as it may yield false-negative results.

(continued)

Procedure 22-1 (Continued)

- Medications such as antacids, antibiotics, antidiarrheals, iron, and castor oil may interfere with analysis.

Teach Parents

Teach the parents that a stool for culture and sensitivity is used to detect the presence of bacterial overgrowth; confirm bacterial gastroenteritis; and to assess sensitivity of specific antimicrobials.

Teach parents that a stool for ova and parasites (O & P is used to aid in diagnosis of parasites or their eggs).

Source: Schnell, Van Leeuwen, & Kranpitz (2003).

MEDICATIONS

Medications for Gastrointestinal Conditions

Category	Examples	Treatment of
Antiemetics	Promethazine Ondansetron Trimethobenzamide	Cyclic vomiting syndrome
Antispasmodics	Atropine Hyoscyamine Scopolamine	Irritable bowel syndrome
Laxatives	Milk of magnesia Polyethylene glycol	Constipation
Prokinetics	Metoclopramide	Cyclic vomiting syndrome Gastroesophageal reflux
Proton Pump Inhibitors	Lansoprazole Omeprazole	Gastroesophageal reflux

Steroid Side Effects

In gastrointestinal disorders steroids can help with inflammation. However there are side effects the nurse needs to be aware of:

- Cardiovascular: Edema, hypertension, congestive heart failure
- Central nervous system: Vertigo, seizures, psychoses, headache

- Dermatologic: Acne, skin atrophy, impaired wound healing, petechiae, bruising
- Endocrine and metabolic: Cushing's syndrome, growth suppression, glucose intolerance, sodium and water retention
- Gastrointestinal: Peptic ulcer, nausea, vomiting
- Genitourinary: Menstrual irregularities
- Neuromuscular and skeletal: Muscle weakness, osteoporosis, fractures
- Ocular: Cataracts, elevated intraocular pressure, glaucoma (Deglin & Vallerand, 2009).

Medications Used for Vomiting

- A combination of medications is used for sedation and the relief of pain and nausea and vomiting, which may include a combination of diphenhydramine (Benadryl), lorazepam (Ativan), promethazine (Phenergan), and meperidine (Demerol).
- Metoclopramide (Reglan) is a prokinetic agent that accelerates gastric emptying.
- Migraine relief includes sumatriptan (Imitrex) for acute episodes; amitriptyline (Elavil), cyproheptadine (Periactin), phenobarbital (Luminal), propranolol (Inderal) for prophylaxis; and ethinyl estradiol (Loestrin) for menstrual pain relief.
- Erythromycin (E-Mycin, E.E.S., EryPed) as a prokinetic is not used much in children secondary to the gastric effects and questionable efficacy.

ETHNOCULTURAL CONSIDERATIONS

Occurrence of Hypertrophic Pyloric Stenosis

- Hypertrophic pyloric stenosis occurs in approximately 6–8 of 1000 live births in the United States (Bishop, 2006).
- The incidence of pyloric stenosis is more common in the Caucasian population compared to 1.8 per 1000 live births in the Hispanic population and 0.7 in the African American population (Letton, 2001).

- Males, especially firstborns, are affected two to four times more often than females are, and there may be a positive family history (Letton, 2001).

Colic

- Chamomile, vervain, licorice, fennel, and balm mint have antispasmodic properties that are found in herbal teas and are used as a remedy for colic in Israel.

Occurrence of Lactose Intolerance

- Asians, southern Europeans, Arabs, Israelis, and African-Americans experience a high incidence of primary lactase deficiency.

Occurrence of Celiac Disease

- Celiac disease primarily affects people of northern European descent. The average incidence of celiac disease in Europe is 1 per 1000 live births with a ratio of 1 per 250 in Sweden to 1 per 4000 in Denmark (Potts, 2002).

TEACHING THE FAMILY

Inguinal Hernia

- If the child has an inguinal hernia, tell the parents that the surgery will repair the defect caused by the hernia.
- Recovery for an inguinal hernia is usually rapid and the child will return home the same day as the surgery.
- After surgery, the nurse can inform the parents that the child's vital signs are monitored frequently and that the child's position will be changed often to avoid undue stress on the surgical area.
- Postoperative care includes keeping the wound clean and dry and managing the child's pain.
- For a child who is not toilet trained, changing diapers as soon as possible is important to prevent wound irritation and infection.

- Discharge instructions include informing the parents on wound care and the importance of keeping the surgical site clean and dry.
- The nurse can also tell the parents that the child can resume normal activity within 4–6 weeks and that they may be given a prescription for stool softeners for the child to prevent straining during defecation (Venes, 2005).

Irritable Bowel Syndrome (IBS)

- Explain to the family that stress can trigger the symptoms of IBS (school, family circumstances).
- Instruct parents and children to keep a food diary to determine the triggers that cause flares of IBS.
- Family counseling may be recommended.

Dealing with Food Jags with Young Children

- Reassure the parents that food jags are normal and that these tendencies will pass. Stress that a little patience will keep both parents and child from further gastrointestinal upsets.
- Suggest that the parents not force the child to eat foods he is not interested in but to provide a variety of nutritious foods during meals and for between-meal snacks in the amount appropriate for the child's age.
- Inform the family about treatments and when they need to seek additional help.

Management Strategies for Infantile Colic (Petersen-Smith, 2004)

- Support parents and assure them the child is in good health.
- Reinforce parents' efforts to comfort the child.
- Instruct parents on strategies to calm infant (swaddling, decreasing environmental stimulation, rocking).
- Assess feeding techniques and instruct as needed.
- Provide an opportunity for parents to express frustrations

Preventing Spread of Rotavirus

Rotavirus	Incidence	Protecting Children	Dehydration Secondary to Gastroenteritis
Viral gastroenteritis causes approximately 80% of all cases of diarrhea in children younger than 1 year of age. Accounts for approximately one third of hospitalizations of children in industrialized countries. By 5 years of age, nearly every child will have had at least one episode of rotavirus-induced illness. Primary transmission of this virus is via the fecal–oral route. Virus is very hearty and stable on surfaces for long periods of time, increasing the risk for transmission through contaminated surfaces or food. The virus has been found in the respiratory tract of infected individuals, raising concern for transmission via infectious secretions.	Does not vary between industrialized and developing countries. Has not been shown to decrease with increased sanitation in developing nations. The incubation period for rotavirus is 1–3 days followed by fever, vomiting, diarrhea, and abdominal pain. Vomiting and diarrhea may be severe enough and require intervention to prevent dehydration. A primary factor in survival of rotaviral induced gastroenteritis is access to adequate medical care. Therapy primarily consists of oral rehydration.	The immunization schedule for ages 0–6 years of age now currently includes a recommendation for a three-dose series of the rotavirus vaccine (Rota). First dose is recommended between 6 and 12 weeks of age with the initial dose not to be started later than age 12 weeks (American Academy of Pediatrics, 2006).	Rotaviral gastroenteritis is self-limiting disease. Deaths due to dehydration. Early signs of dehydration require medical treatment: • Decreased number wet diapers • Sunken fontanel and eyes • Listlessness • Cool, pale skin Families should be given specific instructions regarding oral intake goals during treatment for rotavirus and instructed to return for follow up if a child is unable to meet the goals or the appearance of any of the above symptoms of dehydration.

Complementary Care for Diarrhea

- Products containing *Lactobacillus acidophilus*, such as yogurt, can be used to decrease the incidence of rotavirus diarrhea in infants 5–24 months of age (Blosser, 2004).
- *Lactobacillus* is a nonpathogenic bacterium that produces lactic acid from carbohydrates and is normally found in milk, feces of infants fed by bottle, and adults.
- The addition of *Lactobacillus acidophilus* to the diet changes the bacterial flora of the GI tract, hence treating the overgrowth of pathogenic or diarrhea-causing organisms in the GI tract.

Common Causes of Vomiting	
Origin	**Cause**
Upper GI	Gastritis
	Esophagitis
	Pyloric stenosis
Small Intestine	Intestinal malrotation with volvulus
Colon	Hirschsprung's disease
	Intussusception
	Fecal impaction
Liver or Pancreas	Hepatobiliary dysfunction
Infections	Bacterial enteritis
	Otitis media
	Urinary track infection
	Viral gastroenteritis
	Hepatitis
	Sepsis
Neurological	Hydrocephalus
	Brain tumor
	Migraine headache
	Head trauma
	Congenital malformation
Other	Cow's milk protein allergy
	Maternal drug exposure and withdrawal
	Toxic ingestion
	Appendicitis
	Inborn error of metabolism
	Pneumonia
	Drug or alcohol ingestion
	Eating disorders
	Pregnancy

Short Bowel Syndrome

- The major symptoms of short bowel syndrome are diarrhea, malabsorption, malnutrition, and dehydration.
- Electrolyte imbalance is abnormal and usually secondary to diarrhea and malabsorption.

Hepatitis Viruses					
	HAV	**HBV**	**HCV**	**HDV**	**HEV**
Type of Virus	Enterovirus	Hepadnavirus	Flavivirus	Incomplete	Calicivirus
Transmission	Fecal–oral	Parenteral, sexual, vertical	Parenteral, sexual, vertical	Parenteral, sexual	Fecal–oral
Incubation Period	15–40 days	50–150 days	30–150 days	20–90 days	14–65 days
Diagnostic Tests	Anti-HAV IgM	HBsAg, anti-HBc IgM	Anti-HCV, PCR–RNA test	Anti-HDV	Anti-HEV
Mortality Rate	0.1–0.2%	0.5–2%	1–2%	2–20%	1–2% (20% in pregnant women)
Carrier State	No	Yes	Yes	Yes	No
Vaccine Available	Yes	Yes	No	Yes (HBV)	No
Treatment	None	Interferon-α, nucleoside analogues (lamivudine, tenofovir, adefovir, entecavir)	Interferon-α, (pegylated interferon in adults) plus ribavirin	Treatment for HBV	None

Source: Sokol & Narkewicz (2007).

Comparison of Hepatitis A (HAV), Hepatitis B (HBV), and Hepatitis C (HCV)

HAV	HBV	HCV
Usually rapid, acute	More insidious	Usually insidious
Common and early	Less frequent	Less frequent
Common	Mild to moderate	Mild to moderate
Common	Sometimes present	Mild to moderate
Rare	Common	Sometimes present
Rare	Common	Rare
Rare	Sometimes present	Sometimes present
Present	Present	Present

Sources: Diagneau (2007); Sokol & Narkewicz (2007).

Injuries Caused by Abdominal Trauma

Organ	Incidence and Description	Management
Abdomen	Approximately 8% of pediatric trauma Risk of blunt trauma injuries increased because of relative size and close proximity of organs Penetrating trauma accounts for <10% or pediatric abdominal trauma Gunshot wounds involve multiple organs in 80% of the cases	Serial examination is primary in decisions regarding surgical interventions Surgical intervention may be required if vital signs are persistently unstable along with aggressive fluid replacement. Laparoscopy may be indicated with peritoneal irritation and abdominal wall discoloration. CT is valuable for assessing intra-abdominal trauma.
Spleen	Most frequently injured abdominal organ in children Positive Kehr sign (pressure on the left upper quadrant eliciting left shoulder pain) related to diaphragmatic irritation from ruptured spleen Spleen injury suspected with left upper quadrant abrasions or tenderness Splenic injury may include capsular tear to a complete rupture	CT scan can be used to grade splenic injury. Treatment of choice is nonoperative management. Surgery is indicated for blood loss greater than 40 mL/kg or transfused blood in 24–36 hours or evidence of hemodynamic instability. With splenectomy penicillin prophylaxis is recommended *(continued)*

Injuries Caused by Abdominal Trauma (Continued)

Organ	Incidence and Description	Management
Liver	Accounts for 40% of all deaths associated with blunt abdominal trauma in children Right lobe injuries are more common Diagnosis based on Kehr sign (pressure on the right upper quadrant eliciting right shoulder pain) Severe hemorrhage is more common with injury to the liver than to other abdominal organs	Conservative management is recommended with ongoing monitoring of blood loss, hepatic function, and liver structure with serial CR scans or ultrasound. Operative management is reserved for life-threatening situations.
Pancreas and Duodenum	Less common in children than adults Seen in bicycle handlebar injuries, motor vehicle crashes, and nonaccidental trauma Diagnosis difficult unless obvious injury to overlying structures Diffuse abdominal tenderness, pain, and vomiting accompanied by elevation of amylase and lipase may be indicative of injury although often do not occur for several days after injury Duodenal injuries include hematomas and perforation Perforations are difficult to diagnose	Management includes nasogastric suction and parenteral nutrition. Nonoperative management is appropriate for contusions. Surgical interventions may be required with distal transection. Perforation is not always obvious on a CT scan.
Intestinal	Injury occurs less often than in solid intra-abdominal organs. Risk varies with the amount of intestinal contents, i.e., a full bowel is likely to shear more easily than an empty bowel. Lap belt or seatbelt in a motor vehicle crash results in a sudden deceleration and increase in intraluminal pressure and can lead to perforation.	Presence of a contusion over the seatbelt area and abdomen or back pain indicates a need to pursue the diagnosis of intestinal injury. Pneumoperitoneum in association with intestinal perforation occurs in about 20% of patients

Source: Marcdante (2006).

RESOURCES

American Academy of Pediatrics: http://www.aap.org

Celiac Sprue Association: http://www.csaceliacs.org

Crohn's and Colitis Foundation of America: http://ccfa.org

Food and Nutrition Information Center:
http://www.nal.usda.gov/fnic/

My Pyramid.gov: http://www.mypyramid.gov

United States Department of Agriculture Healthy Food
Guidelines: http://www.mypyramid.gov

REFERENCES

Bishop, W.F. (2006). The digestive system. In R.M. Kliegman, K.J. Marcdante, H.B. Jenson, & R.E. Behrman (Eds.). *Nelson essential of pediatrics* (5th ed., pp. 579–624). St. Louis: Elsevier.

Blosser, C.G. (2004). Complementary medicine. In C.E. Burns, A.M. Dunn, M.A. Brady, N.B. Starr, & C.G. Blosser (Eds.). *Pediatric primary care: A handbook for nurse practitioners* (3rd ed., pp. 1211–1248). St. Louis: Elsevier.

Burd, R.S., & Whalen, T.V. (2001). Evaluation of the child with suspected appendicitis. *Pediatric Annals, 30*(12), 721–725.

Daigneau, C.V. (2007). The child with gastrointestinal dysfunction. In M.J. Hockenberry & D. Wilson (Eds.). *Wong's nursing care of infants and children* (8th ed, pp. 1387–1435). St. Louis: Elsevier.

Deglin, J. & Vallerand, A. (2009). *Davis's drug guide for nurses* (11th ed.). Philadelphia: F.A. Davis.

Duderstadt, K.G. (2006). *Pediatric physical examination: An illustrated handbook.* St. Louis: Elsevier.

Letton, R.W. (2001). Pyloric stenosis. *Pediatric Annals, 3*(12), 745–750.

Marcdante, K.J. (2006). The acutely ill or injured child. In R.M. Kliegman, K.J. Marcdante, H.B. Jenson, & R.E. Behrman (Eds.). *Nelson essentials of pediatrics* (5th ed, pp. 179–216). St. Louis: Elsevier.

Mow, W. (2005). Disorders of the intestine. In L.M. Osborn, T.G. DeWitt, L.R. First, & J.A. Zenel (Eds.). *Pediatrics* (pp. 670–677). St. Louis: Elsevier.

Petersen-Smith, A.M. (2004). Gastrointestinal disorders. In C.E. Burns, A.M. Dunn, M.A. Brady, N.B. Starr, & C.G. Blosser (Eds.). *Pediatric primary care: A handbook for nurse practitioners* (3rd ed, pp. 839–884). St. Louis: Elsevier.

Potts, N. (2002). Gastrointestinal alterations. In N.L. Potts & B.L. Mandleco (Eds.). *Pediatric nursing: Caring for children and their families* (pp. 653–696). Clifton Park, NY: Delmar-Thomson Learning

Schnell, Z.B., Van Leeuwen, A.M., & Kranpitz, T.R. (2003). *Davis's comprehensive handbook of laboratory and diagnostic tests with nursing implications.* Philadelphia: F.A. Davis.

Sokol, R.J., & Narkewicz, M.R. (2007). Liver and pancreas. In W.W. Hay, M.J. Levin, J.M. Sondheimer, & R.R. Deterding (Eds.). *Current diagnosis & treatment in pediatrics* (18th ed, pp. 638–683). New York: Lange Medical Books/McGraw-Hill.

Venes, D. (Ed.). (2005). *Tabers cyclopedic medical dictionary.* Philadelphia: F.A. Davis.

Caring for the Child with an Immunological or Infectious Condition

KEY TERMS

allogeneic cell transplantation – Cell donation from a donor (family member) who has a compatible human leukocyte antigen

anaphylaxis – Immediate hypersensitivity reaction to an excessive release of chemical mediators affecting the entire body; a medical emergency

autoimmune disorder – Immune response against one of the body's own tissues or cells

autologous transplant – The child's own cells are taken, stored, and reinfused after the child has received chemotherapy

immune response – Defends the body against microorganisms, parasites, and foreign cells such as cancer cells and transplanted cells; key to a normal immune response is the body's ability to recognize foreign substances as non-self and then to mobilize defenses and attack the invaders

isogeneic transplantation – Cells are taken from an identical twin

pathogenicity – Percentage of children exposed to the pathogen who will eventually develop the disease

virulence – The severity of the health problems caused by the agent

FOCUSED ASSESSMENT

Anaphylaxis

Signs and symptoms of anaphylaxis develop suddenly and require prompt recognition and treatment.

- Wheezing
- Tachycardia
- Hypotension
- Cyanosis
- Alteration in level of consciousness
- Nasal congestion
- Facial edema
- Anxiety
- Hives
- Urticaria
- Nausea and vomiting
- Abdominal pain
- Laryngospasm
- A sense of impending doom
- Vascular collapse and cardiac arrest

Key Components of Physical Assessment for the Child with an Infectious Disease

Vital Signs

- Temperature (see Chapter 18, Expected Temperatures in Children)
- Heart rate
- Respiratory rate
- Blood pressure

Average Range for Pediatric Vital Signs

Age Group	Heart Rate	Respiration Rate	Blood Pressure Systolic	Blood Pressure Diastolic
Infant	80–150	25–55	65–100	45–65
Toddler	70–110	20–30	90–105	55–70
Preschooler	65–110	20–25	95–110	60–75
School-age	60–95	14–22	100–120	60–75
Adolescent	55–85	12–18	110–125	65–85

- Pain (the most commonly used pain scales are the numeric scale, the Wong Faces Scale, and the FLACC pain scale)

Respiratory Assessment
- Upper respiratory infection symptoms
- Breath sounds
- Work of breathing
- Pulse oximeter reading
- Skin/mucous membrane color
- Secretions; color, character, amount

Neurological Assessment
- Febrile seizures
- Early identification of neurological complications
- Level of consciousness (the pediatric Glasgcow Coma Scale consists of three components of assessment: eye opening, verbal response, and motor response)

Gastrointestinal Assessment
- Fluid intake
- Presence of vomiting or diarrhea

Skin
- Presence of rash, pruritus, lesions

CLINICAL ALERTS

Increased Risk for Infection

Something as simple and common as irritation from diaper rash, but also as a potential portal of entry for microorganisms.

Administration of Steroids

- Never stop steroids abruptly due to adrenal insufficiency (the greatest risks come from sudden withdrawal).
- Clinical manifestations of adrenal insufficiency include hypotension, weight loss, weakness, nausea, vomiting, anorexia, lethargy, confusion, and restlessness.
- Educate parents about the proper use of steroids; must be taken as directed.
- Slowly taper the use of steroids when it is time to discontinue use.

Systemic Lupus Erythematosus (SLE)

- Assess for signs and symptoms to ensure prompt recognition of an exacerbation (prevention is the most important component of nursing care).
- Emphasize the importance of rest and adequate nutrition to maximize immune system function.
- Facial rash, fatigue, and arthritic changes may put the child at risk for depression and altered body image.
- Refer family to support group to help adjust to life with SLE.

Reye Syndrome Risk with Use of Aspirin

- Administration of salicylates (aspirin) to children with acute viral illness is linked to Reye syndrome.
- Educate parents regarding use of aspirin-free medications (Alka-Seltzer, Anacin, Ascriptin, Bayer Arthritis Pain and Aspirin preparations, Doan's, Dristan, Ecotrin, Excedrin, Kaopectate, Pamprin, Pepto-Bismol, Sine-Off Sinus Medicine, St. Joseph Adult Aspirin, Vanquish).
- The National Reye Syndrome Foundation can be accessed at www.reyessyndrome.org/

Preventing Cytomegalovirus (CMV) Infection in Immunocompromised Children

Cytomegalovirus (CMV) infection is a source of significant morbidity and mortality in immunocompromised children.

- Good hand washing is the best preventive measure.
- Disposable gloves should be worn when handling linen or underclothes soiled with feces or urine.
- CMV-negative blood should be provided to immunocompromised children.

Adverse Effects of Immunizations

- Local effects: Mild, occur most frequently. Symptoms include soreness, redness, and pain at the site of injection. Manage with heat or ice to the site.
- Systemic effects: Less frequent; fever and mild irritability. Manage the effects with acetaminophen (Children's Tylenol) administered before immunization; continuing every 4 hours as needed for 24 hours.

- Allergic reaction: Rare but serious. Seek immediate medical assistance if the child exhibits the following symptoms: high fever; altered mental status (excessive irritability, lethargy, nonresponsiveness, seizures); increased difficulty breathing; hoarseness or wheezing when breathing; hives, pale, cool skin.

Postexposure Treatment for Rabies

- Exercising caution with unknown animals is essential.
- Most exposures to rabies occur through bites of wild animals that allow contaminated saliva to enter the bite wound.
- If an animal has injured a child, the parents must contact their health care provider immediately!

Clusters of Human H5N1 Cases

- Clusters of human H5N1 cases ranging from 2 to 8 cases per cluster have been identified in most countries that have reported H5N1 cases.
- Nearly all of the cluster cases have occurred among blood relatives living in the same household.
- Most people in these clusters have been infected with H5N1 virus through direct contact with sick or dead poultry or wild birds.
- Limited human-to-human transmission of H5N1 virus cannot be excluded in some clusters.
- CDC Web site: http://www.cdc.gov/flu/avian/outbreaks/current.htm

DIAGNOSTIC TESTS

Human Immunodeficiency Virus (HIV) Testing

There are two primary methods for confirming the diagnosis of Human immunodeficiency virus (HIV):

- Enzyme-linked immunosorbent assay (ELISA): A test that identifies the presence of HIV antibodies and is performed within 48 hours after birth. The use of ELISA is ineffective in children younger than 18 months due to the presence of maternal antibodies.

- Polymerase chain reaction (PCR): A test that identifies the proviral DNA, specific to HIV. The PCR is more expensive but has greater sensitivity. PCR has a greater number of false-positive results.

Blood Culture

A simple blood culture can detect bacteria or fungi in the blood. To test for an infection in the blood:

- A phlebotomist will draw a sample of blood from a vein.
- In the laboratory, the blood sample will be mixed with substances that promote the growth of bacteria or fungi.
- In most cases, bacteria can be detected in the blood culture within 2 to 3 days. Some types of blood infections can take 10 days or longer and fungal infections in the blood can take up to 30 days for results.
- A normal blood culture (negative) result will report that no bacterium or fungus has been found in the blood.
- An abnormal result (positive) will report that a bacterium or fungus has been found in the blood.

Identification of an Infectious Disease

- Complete blood count (CBC) with differential
- Urinalysis (UA)
- Spinal fluid analysis
- Cultures from fluids, secretions, drainage
- Pulse oximetry
- Chest x-ray exam
- Computerized tomography (CT)

MEDICATIONS

Trimethoprim-Sulfamethoxazole (TMP-SMZ) (Bactrim or Septra) (trye-**meth**-oh-prim/sul-fa-meth-**ox**-a-zole)

Indications Prevention of *Pneumocystis carinii* pneumonia (PCP). Prevention of bacterial infections in an immunosuppressed child.

Actions The combination inhibits the metabolism of folic acid in bacteria at two different points.

Therapeutic Effects Bactericidal action against susceptible bacteria.

Pharmacokinetics
Absorption Well absorbed from the GI tract.

Contraindications and Precautions
Contraindicated in Hypersensitivity to sulfonamides or trimethoprim, megaloblastic anemia secondary to folate deficiency, severe renal impairment, and children <2 months of age.

Adverse Reactions and Side Effects Hepatic necrosis, nausea, vomiting, diarrhea, toxic epidermal necrolysis, Stevens-Johnson syndrome, erythema multiforme, rashes, agranulocytosis, aplastic anemia, and phlebitis with IV insertion.

Route and Dosage PCP prevention: **PO** (children): 75 mg/m³ TMP/325 mg/m³ SMZ q12hr on 3 consecutive days/week. Not to exceed 320 mg TMP/1600 mg/SMZ per day.

Nursing Implications
1. Assess the child for infection. Advise the family to notify the health care provider for any signs of infection.
2. Assess for allergy to sulfonamides.
3. Monitor lab values periodically throughout therapy. TMP-SMZ may produce elevated serum bilirubin, creatinine, and alkaline phosphatase.

Data from Deglin, J., & Vallerand, A. (2009). Davis's drug guide for nurses (11th ed.), pp. 1205–1207. Philadelphia: F.A. Davis.

Methylprednisolone (A-Methapred) (meth-ill-pred-**niss**-oh-lone)

Indications Anti-inflammatory or immunosuppressant agent

Actions Suppress inflammation and the normal immune response.

Therapeutic Effects Suppression of inflammation and modification of the normal immune response.

Pharmacokinetics
Absorption Well absorbed after oral administration.

Contraindications and Precautions
Contraindicated in Acute untreated infections.

Cautions Chronic use in children will result in decreased growth. During stress (surgery, infections) supplemental doses may be needed.

Adverse Reactions and Side Effects Peptic ulceration, anorexia, nausea, acne, decreased wound healing, hirsutism, petechiae and bruising, muscle wasting, osteoporosis, cushinoid appearance, and thromboembolism.

Route and Dosage PO (children): 0.417 mg/kg–1.67 mg/kg (12.5–50 mg/m²) per day in 3–4 divided doses. Rectal (children): 0.5–1 mg/kg (15–30 mg/m²) daily or every other day for at least 1 week. **IV, IM** (children): 139–835 mcg/kg (4.16–25 mg/m²) every 12–24 hours.

Nursing Implications

1. Assess for signs and symptoms of adrenal insufficiency (hypotension, weight loss, weakness, nausea, vomiting, anorexia, lethargy, confusion, restlessness).
2. Monitor fluid status, daily weights.
3. Monitor electrolytes and glucose levels.
4. Administer oral medications with food.
5. Instruct family regarding need to take medications as ordered due to risk of adrenal insufficiency with sudden withdraw of medication.
6. Instruct family regarding possibility of immunosuppression, need to avoid ill contacts and report possible infections to health care provider immediately.
7. Instruct family to inform health care provider promptly for severe abdominal pain, tarry stools, increased bruising, non healing sores, sudden weight gain, or behavior changes.
8. Immunizations should be discussed with health care provider on an individual basis.

Data from Deglin, J., & Vallerand, A. (2009). Davis's drug guide for nurses (11th ed.), pp. 350–367. Philadelphia: F.A. Davis.

Epinephrine (Adrenaline) (e-pi-**nef**-rin)

Indications IV: Management of severe allergic reactions

Actions Inhibits the release of mediators of immediate hypersensitivity reactions from mast cells.

Therapeutic Effects Maintenance of heart rate and blood pressure.

Pharmacokinetics
Absorption Well absorbed.

Contraindications and Precautions
Contraindicated in Hypersensitivity.

Adverse Reactions and Side Effects
CNS Nervousness, restlessness, tremor.
Cardiovascular Arrhythmias, hypertension, tachycardia.

Route and Dosage
IV (severe anaphylaxis): 0.1–0.25 mg q5–15 minutes; may be followed by a 1–4 mcg/min continuous infusion (may be increased up to 1.5 mcg/kg per minute)

Nursing Implications
1. Assess volume status. Hypovolemia should be corrected prior to administration of IV epinephrine.
2. Monitor blood pressure, perfusion, ECG, respiratory rate, and urine output during administration.
3. Assess for hypersensitivity reaction: Rash, urticaria, swelling of face, lips, eyelids.
4. IV administration: Administer at a dilution of 1:10,000; this may be prepared through dilution of 1 mg of 1:1000 solution in at least 10 mL of 0.9% NaCl.

Administer each 1 mg of 1:10,000 solution over at least 1 minute.

Data from Deglin, J., & Vallerand, A. (2009). Davis's drug guide for nurses (11th ed.), pp. 480–484. Philadelphia: F.A. Davis.

Diphenhydramine (Benadryl) (dye-fen-**hye**-dra-meen)

Indications Relief of allergic symptoms caused by histamine release including: anaphylaxis, allergic rhinitis, allergic dermatoses. Relief of pruritis.

Actions Antagonizes the effects of histamine at H_1-receptor sites. Significant CNS depressant and anticholinergic properties.

Therapeutic Effects Decreased symptoms of histamine excess (sneezing, rhinorrhea, nasal and ocular pruritus, ocular tearing and redness, urticaria)

Pharmacokinetics
Absorption Well absorbed after oral or IM administration

Contraindications and Precautions
Contraindicated in Hypersensitivity.

Adverse Reactions and Side Effects
Drowsiness, paradoxical excitation (more common in children). Anorexia, dry mouth.

Route and Dosage
PO (children 6–12 years): 12.5–25 mg q4–6hr. **PO** (children 2–6 years): 6.25–12.5 mg q4–6hr. **IM/IV** (children): 1.25 mg/kg 4 times/day. Not to exceed 300 mg/day.

Nursing Implications
1. Provide child and family education regarding medication, caution not to exceed recommended dose.
2. Inform parents that medication may cause drowsiness or excitability in the child.
3. Provide education regarding common side effect of dry mouth. Management strategies include frequent mouth care and oral rinses.

Data from Deglin, J., & Vallerand, A. (2009). Davis's drug guide for nurses (11th ed.), pp. 424–426. Philadelphia: F.A. Davis.

Ganciclovir (Cytovene) (gan-**sye**-kloe-vir)

Indications
Treatment of CMV retinitis in the immunocompromised child.

Prevention of CMV infection in the transplant child at risk

Actions
CMV converts ganciclovir to its active form inside host cell, where it inhibits viral DNA polymerase.

Therapeutic Effects
Antiviral effect directed against CMV-infected cells.

Pharmacokinetics
Absorption 5% to 9% absorbed with oral administration. IV administration results in complete bioavailability.

Contraindications and Precautions
Contraindicated in Hypersensitivity to ganciclovir or acyclovir

Adverse Reactions and Side Effects
Seizures, headache, malaise, drowsiness, ataxia
GI bleeding, nausea, vomiting, increased liver enzymes.
Neutropenia, thrombocytopenia, anemia.
Hypotension, hypertension
Renal toxicity

Route and Dosage Pediatric doses not established. **IV** (Adults): Induction 5 mg/kg q12hr for 14–21 days. Maintenance: 5 mg/kg per day or 6 mg/kg for 5 days/week; may increase to q12hr. **PO** (Adults): Maintenance: 1000 mg 3 times/day or 500 mg 6 times/day.

Nursing Implications

1. Pediatric dose not established.
2. Increased risk of bone marrow depression when used with antineoplastics or zidovudine
3. Assess the child during treatment for signs of infection, bleeding, or development of CMV retinitis.
4. Administer IV at slow rate, using in-line filter.
5. Advise the child/family to notify the health care provider for any signs of bleeding.

Data from Deglin, J., & Vallerand, A. (2009). Davis's drug guide for nurses (11th ed.), pp. 594–596. Philadelphia: F.A. Davis.

Amphotericin B (Amphocin) (am-foe-**ter**-i-sin)

Indications Treatment of active, progressive, potentially fatal fungal infections

Actions Binds to fungal cell membrane, allowing leakage of cellular contents

Therapeutic Effects Fungistatic action

Pharmacokinetics
Absorption Not absorbed orally.

Contraindications and Precautions
Contraindicated in Hypersensitivity

Adverse Reactions and Side Effects Headache, hypotension, diarrhea, nausea, vomiting, nephrotoxicity, hypokalemia, chills, fever, and hypersensitivity reactions

Route and Dosage Specific dosage and duration of therapy depend on infection being treated.
Amphotericin Deoxycholate IV (children): 0.25 mg/kg infused initially; increase by 0.25 mg/kg every other day to a maximum of 1 mg/kg per day.
Amphotericin B Cholesteryl Sulfate IV (children): 3–4 mg/kg per day
Amphotericin B Lipid Complex IV (children): 5 mg/kg per day.
Amphotericin B Liposome IV (children): 3–5 mg/kg q24hr

Nursing Implications

1. Premedication with antipyretics, corticosteroids, antihistamines, and antiemetics may reduce incidence of fever, chills, headache, nausea, or vomiting.
2. Monitor VS and above noted symptoms every 15–30 minutes during test dose and every 30 minutes for 2–4 hours after the test dose.
3. Monitor VS and above symptoms closely for first 1–2 hours of each subsequent dose.
4. Monitor for thrombophlebitis because the drug is highly irritating to tissues.
5. Monitor CBC and platelet counts weekly, BUN and serum creatinine every other day while increasing dose, then twice weekly. Monitor potassium and magnesium levels biweekly.
6. Ensure resuscitation equipment readily available before administration.

Data from Deglin, J., & Vallerand, A. (2009). Davis's drug guide for nurses (11th ed.), pp. 160–164. Philadelphia: F.A. Davis.

Vaccines

- Vaccine schedules may be obtained through the Centers for Disease Control and Prevention (CDC) Web site: http://www.cdc.gov/vaccines/recs/schedules/
- Vaccine Information Statements (in many languages) may be accessed at www.cdc.gov/nip or www.immunize.org

Type	Definition	Example
Inactivated	Disease-causing microbe is killed but is still capable of inducing the body to produce antibodies.	Inactivated poliovirus vaccine (IPV; injection)
Live (attenuated)	Disease-causing organism is not killed but under special conditions is designed to decrease virulence.	Measles vaccine (injection)
Toxoid	Inactivated form effective in producing an immune response geared toward a toxin-producing organism.	Tetanus toxoid (injection)

(continued)

Type	Definition	Example
Subunit	Portion of the virus or bacterium is used to produce the desired immunological response without the undesirable effects that are seen with some of the other surface antigens.	*Bordetella pertussis* vaccine included in the acellular DPT (injection)
Polysaccharide	Made from portions of the polysaccharides capsule and are effective in producing immunity in children older than the age of 2 years. At exposure the polysaccharide capsule does not elicit a T-cell response, the duration of immunity is variable and not life long.	Pneumovax (injection)
Conjugate	Links a recognizable antigen with the "hidden" bacterial antigen thereby enabling the immature immune system to identify the bacteria as non-self and respond.	*Haemophilus influenzae* type b (Hib; injection)
Recombinant	Inserts genes for production of the antigens desired into a low-virulent vector using genetic engineering.	Hepatitis B virus (HBV; injection)

TEACHING THE FAMILY

Anaphylaxis Reaction

- For children who have experienced an anaphylactic reaction the nurse must provide follow-up care to families to prevent recurrences.
- If the child has allergies that cannot be completely eliminated, a follow-up referral to an allergist for desensitization treatments or a self-administration epinephrine prescription, such as an EpiPen.
- It is important that parents are taught to recognize early indicators of anaphylaxis and are confident in their ability to act quickly on this assessment.

Immunizations

1. Discuss the immunization's purpose as well as the administration and potential side effects.
2. Give parents educational materials.
3. Tell parents about immunization clinics in nontraditional settings such as churches, synagogues, mosques, community centers, or shopping malls.
4. Provide opportunities and encourage parents to communicate their concerns about immunizations.
5. Encourage parents to investigate immunizations using reputable Web sites and other resources such as education pamphlets.
6. Assist the parents in understanding how to keep track of immunizations and when the next immunizations are due.
7. Assist parents in investigating funding resources for immunizations (this is a possible barrier to immunization for many families).

Use of Insect Repellants

Instruct parents to apply insect repellant to clothing and not to the child's skin to decrease the chance of systemic absorption of a potentially harmful substance.

Avian Flu Preparation

1. Discuss the differences between seasonal flu and pandemic flu.
2. Describe actions being taken by the health care community to monitor and prepare for the pandemic and encourage families to take an active role.
3. Assist families to establish their own plan for care in the event of a pandemic including:
   - Storage of a 2-week supply of food and water for the family
   - Maintenance of a supply of needed medications.
   - Maintenance of a supply of over-the-counter medications needed to treat symptoms of flu.
   - Establish a plan for family members living alone.
4. Encourage families to become involved with community groups to help prepare and plan for the pandemic.

5. Reinforce basic infection control techniques to limit the spread of influenza.
6. Provide families with links to CDC resources with preparation checklists. Encourage them to utilize the checklists to assist in preparation.

ADDITIONAL INFORMATION FOR THE CLINICAL SETTING

Complementary care: Nonpharmacological adjuncts to pain management:

- Guided imagery
- Hypnosis
- Prayer
- Meditation
- Music
- Aromatherapy
- Proper preparation (e.g., show diagrams, allow handling of equipment, introduce to child to personnel, visit special rooms where the child may go after the procedure)
- Distraction (e.g., blowing bubbles, singing songs, reading a book, playing with a favorite toy)
- Relaxation (guided imagery or hypnosis, easy-to-read relaxation books)

Systemic Lupus Erythematosus (SLE) Resources

The nurse can encourage an adolescent recently diagnosed with systemic lupus erythematosus (SLE) to contact a local support group. In addition, several good resources are available online through the organizations located at the following Web sites:

- Lupus Foundation of America
  http://www.lupus.org/
- National Institute of Arthritis and Musculoskeletal and Skin Disorders
  http://www.niams.nih.gov
- SLE Foundation, Inc.
  http://www.lupusny.org/
- Association of Rheumatology Health Professionals, American College of Rheumatology
  http://www.rheumatology.org/

- Arthritis Foundation
  http://www.arthritis.org/

Nursing Care for Anaphylaxis

- Perform cardiopulmonary resuscitation.
- Activate the emergency system.
- Ensure adequate airway: endotracheal intubation or oxygen.
- Administer epinephrine (adrenaline).
- Place a tourniquet proximal to the site of injection or insect sting.
- Keep the child lying flat, warm, and with feet slightly elevated.
- Administer corticosteroids and antihistamines.
- Determine the cause of the attack.

Communicable Diseases in Childhood

See Table 26–1 in Chapter 26 of Ward, S. & Hisley, S. (2009). *Maternal child nursing care: Optimizing outcomes for mothers, children & families*. Philadelphia: F.A. Davis.

Common Fungal Infections

Fungal Infection	Location	Treatment	Parent Information
Tinea Capitis (ringworm)	Begins as an infection of a single hair follicle but spreads rapidly in a circular pattern and produces a one inch in diameter lesion. The circular pattern becomes filled with dirty-appearing scales and the hairs involved break off.	Oral griseofulvin (Fulvicin)	**1.** Adolescents warned not to use alcohol due to tachycardia. **2.** Children do not need to be kept home from school. **3.** Family members must not share towels or combs.

(continued)

Common Fungal Infections (Continued)

Fungal Infection	Location	Treatment	Parent Information
Tinea Pedis (Athlete's Foot)	Skin lesions between the toes and on the plantar surface of the foot	Liquid preparations of clotrimazole (Lotrimin)	1. Antiseptic foot baths 2. Do not let others share personal items such as foot wear, towels, clothes, or sports equipment. 3. Wear thongs or swim shoes in public showers and stocking/shoes in locker rooms.
Tinea Cruris (jock itch)	Found on the inner aspects of thighs and scrotum	Liquid or powder preparations of clotrimazole (Lotrimin)	1. Shower or bathe frequently if necessary. 2. Dry scrotal area thoroughly when damp. 3. Wear cotton underwear 4. Do not let others share personal items such as foot wear, towels, clothes, or sports equipment.
Tinea Corporis (epidermal layer of the skin)	Fungal infection of the epidermal layer of the skin that has a circular lesion with a clear center and scaly inflammation	Topical clotrimazole (Lotrimin)	1. Do not let others share personal items such as foot wear, towels, clothes, or sports equipment.

The Role of the Nurse in Immunizations

The primary nursing goal is up-to-date immunizations for all children based on their particular health status. The pediatric nurse has several roles in the area of immunization:

- Address family concerns regarding immunizations.
- Organize and carry out vaccination programs and distributing accurate and timely information regarding childhood immunizations.

- Use the current immunization schedule and recognize that the complicated schedule may pose some challenges for parents.
- Ensure that the parent has a vaccine information sheet (VIS) that records the immunizations.
- Remind parents when the next immunizations are due.
- Stay abreast of current information and discuss the parents' concerns.
- Contact and immunize high-risk unimmunized children such as children who are homeless, immigrant, refugee, home schooled, frequently mobile, or who have chronic or life-threatening illnesses.
- Report adverse effects of the vaccine.

Legal Considerations in Immunization Education

The National Childhood Vaccine Injury Act of 1986 provides that parents or legal representatives of children receiving immunizations must be given a VIS developed by the Centers for Disease Control and Prevention (CDC) before immunization. The purpose of the VIS is to ensure uniform education regarding vaccines. The VIS must be used with the following vaccinations: DTaP, Td, MMR, polio, hepatitis B, Hib, varicella, and pneumococcal conjugate.

- Provide the parent or legal guardian with the appropriate VIS before immunization.
- Record on the medical record the date that the VIS was given, the date of publication for the VIS, the name, address, and title of the person giving the vaccine, the date of administration of vaccine, the manufacturer of the vaccine, and the vaccine lot number.
- The VIS must not be altered in any way.
- VIS forms (in many languages) may be accessed through the web at www.cdc.gov/nip or www.immunize.org
- Hardcopies may be ordered through the CDC website at www.cdc.gov/nip/publications
- Individual state health departments with camera-ready copies can be obtained.
- Additional resources and additional education provided to the parent must also be recorded.

Note: Additional VIS sheets are available for use with other common childhood vaccines.

Identifying Contraindications to Immunizations

Only one universal contraindication exists to all vaccines:

- Previous severe allergic reaction (anaphylaxis) to the vaccine or its component of vaccine.

Individual vaccines carry additional contraindications:

- DTaP: Progressive neurological disease, i.e., infantile spasms, encephalopathy
- MMR: Pregnancy, severe immunodeficiency

Circumstances requiring postponement of vaccine administration include:

- Moderate to severe illness.
- Administration of immunoglobulin within last 3 to 11 months (precise period depends on specific immunoglobulin).

Note: Individual vaccines may have additional contraindications and precautions. Safe administration of vaccines requires the nurse to screen for contraindications and precautions prior to administration.

RESOURCES

Lupus Foundation of America: http://www.lupus.org/

National Institute of Arthritis and Musculoskeletal and Skin Disorders: http://www.niams.nih.gov

SLE Foundation, Inc.: http://www.lupusny.org/

Association of Rheumatology Health Professionals, American College of Rheumatology: http://www.rheumatology.org/

Arthritis Foundation: http://www.arthritis.org/

Planning Checklists: http://www.pandemicflu.gov/plan/checklists.html

REFERENCE

Deglin, J., Vallerand, A. (2009). *Davis's drug guide for nurses* (11th ed.). Philadelphia: F.A. Davis.

Caring for the Child with a Cardiovascular Condition

KEY TERMS

cardiac output – Amount of blood discharged from the left or right ventricle per minute (Venes, 2005); the product of stroke volume (SV) and heart rate (HR)

stroke volume – Amount of blood ejected by the left ventricle with each heartbeat (Venes, 2005); the product of preload, after-load and contractility (inotropy).

FOCUSED ASSESSMENT

Syndromes Associated with Cardiac Disease

Syndrome/Disease/ Chromosomal Aberrations	Cardiac Defect/Condition	Other Physical Findings
Down Syndrome	Atrioventricular canal defect (AVC), ventricular septal defect (VSD)	Down facies, developmental delay
Noonan Syndrome	Pulmonic valve stenosis, left ventricular hypertrophy (LVH)	Elfin facies, pectus deformity, joint laxity, undescended testes, spine abnormalities, hypotonia, seizures
Williams Syndrome	Supravalvular aortic stenosis, pulmonary artery (PA) stenosis	William's facies: small upturned nose, long philtrum (upper lip length), wide mouth, full lips, small chin, and puffiness around the eyes; hypercalcemia, dental abnormalities, renal problems, sensitive hearing, hypotonia, joint laxity, overly friendly personality
DiGeorge or Velo-cardio-facial Chromosome	Interrupted aortic arch, truncus arteriosus, ventricular septal defect (VSD), patent ductus arteriosus (PDA), tetralogy of Fallot (TOF)	Decreased immune response, low set ears, palate problems, hypoparathyroidism, hypocalcemia
Duchenne Muscular Dystrophy	Cardiomyopathy	Generalized weakness and muscle wasting first affecting the muscles of the hips, pelvic area, thighs, and shoulders; calves often enlarged
Marfan Syndrome	Aortic aneurysm, aortic and/or mitral regurgitation	Arms disproportionately long, tall and thin with laxity of joints, dislocation of lenses, spinal problems, stretch marks, hernia, pectus abnormalities, and restrictive lung disease

Syndrome	Cardiac defects	Other features
Trisomy 18	Ventricular septal defect (VSD), patent ductus arteriosus (PDA), pulmonic stenosis or pulmonic valve stenosis (PS or PVS)	Multiple joint contractures, spina bifida, hearing loss, radial aplasia (underdevelopment or missing radial bone of forearm), cleft lip, birth defects of the eye
Trisomy 13	Ventricular septal defect (VSD), patent ductus arteriosus (PDA), dextrocardia	Omphalocele, holoprosencephaly (an anatomic defect of the brain involving failure of the forebrain to divide properly), kidney defects, skin defects of the scalp
CHARGE	Tetralogy of Fallot (TOF), truncus arteriosus, vascular ring, interrupted aortic arch	Coloboma of the eye, *Heart* defects, *Atresia* of the choanae, *Retardation* of *Growth* and development, and *Ear* abnormalities and deafness
Fetal Alcohol Syndrome	Ventricular septal defect (VSD), patent ductus arteriosus (PDA), atrial septal defect (ASD), Tetralogy of Fallot (TOF)	Growth deficiencies, skeletal deformities, facial abnormalities, organ deformities: genital malformations; kidney and urinary defects, central nervous system handicaps
VATER (VACTERLS)	Ventricular septal defect (VSD)	*Vertebral* anomalies, vascular anomalies, *Anal* atresia, *Cardiac* anomalies, *Tracheoesophageal* (T-E) fistula, *Esophageal* atresia, *Renal* anomalies, radial dysplasia, *Limb* anomalies, Single umbilical artery
Turner Syndrome	Coarctation of the aorta (CoA), atrial septal defect (ASD), aortic stenosis or aortic valve stenosis (AS or AVS)	Kidney problems, high blood pressure, overweight, hearing difficulties, diabetes, cataracts, thyroid problems, lack of sexual development, a "webbed" neck, a low hairline at the back of the neck, drooping of the eyelids, dysmorphic, low-set ears, abnormal bone development, multiple moles

CLINICAL ALERTS

Renal Failure

Renal failure is considered when the output is less than 1 mL/kg per hour along with an elevation in serum creatinine and blood urea nitrogen.

- Monitor blood lab values for postoperative bleeding and post-pump electrolyte imbalances.
- Suction secretions.
- Maintain chest tubes that remove secretions and reexpand the lungs. Check drainage for quantity and color.

Postoperative Hemorrhage

Postoperative hemorrhage is considered when there is excessive chest tube drainage greater than 5–10 mL/kg in 1 hour or more than 3 mL/kg per hour in 3 consecutive hours.

- Assess for complications (e.g., cardiac, neurological, pulmonary, or hematological changes; infection; and delayed growth and development).
- Consider the child's level of development in order to provide developmentally appropriate care.
- Ensure rest, which is essential to promote healing and decrease the work load of the heart.
- Manage pain via comfort measures and the administration of medication.
- Group nursing care to avoid imposing unnecessary fatigue and weakness.
- Provide emotional support and information about home care.

Survival

- With any congenital defect, as long as there is mixing of oxygenated and deoxygenated blood, the child survives. A more definitive surgery such as a Fontan procedure is performed at a later date to correct the condition.

Tetralogy of Fallot

- The hallmark sign of Tetralogy of Fallot is cyanosis with crying or playing, which is relieved by squatting or drawing up the legs. These episodes are called "TET" spells: cyanotic events exacerbated by excitement and crying, then relieved by a decrease in pulmonary vascular resistance.

Kawasaki Disease

If the child has five out of six of the following signs, the diagnosis is Kawasaki disease:

- Persistent fever (5 days or more, spiking to 104°F [40°C])
- Skin rash
- Cervical lymphadenopathy, typically unilateral, greater than 1.5 mm in diameter
- Edema and erythema of hands and feet with eventual peeling of skin
- Irritation and inflammation of the mouth with "strawberry tongue," erythema, and cracking lips
- Conjunctivitis without exudate

Thrombus Formation

- Children with aneurysm formation as a result of Kawasaki disease require long-term follow-up for continued assessment related to other vascular changes such as stenosis or tortuosity (twisting) (AHA, 2004; Park, 2003).
- Occasionally, cardiac catheterization is indicated to diagnose aneurysm formation.
- Thrombotic agents such as streptokinase (Streptase), urokinase (Abbokinase), and alteplase (tPA or Activase) have been used with some success in thrombus formation.
- Long-term use of anticoagulants such as warfarin. (Coumadin) or clopidogrel (Plavix) may be used to prevent thrombus formation in the engorged or aneurysmal vessels.

Blood Pressure Post-Catheterization

- The child's blood pressure should remain within normal limits.
- Watch the pulse pressure (the difference between the systolic and diastolic BP; normal is <40 mm Hg).

Complications of Cardiac Transplantation

The four main complications of cardiac transplantation are:

- Rejection
- Infection
- Posttransplant lymphoproliferative disorder (PTLD)
- Transplant coronary artery disease (TCAD)

Postoperative Vital Signs

- Record vital signs every 15 minutes for the first few hours, then every 30 minutes, then once an hour until the child is stable.
- Adjust frequency based on stability of the patient.
- Document and report to the physician even the most subtle change in vital signs.

DIAGNOSTIC TESTS

Cholesterol Levels in Children			
	Desirable	**Borderline**	**Associated with Higher Risk**
Total Cholesterol	Less than 170 mg/dL	170–199	200 or more
LDL Cholesterol	Less than 110 mg/dL	110–129	130 or more

Tilt Test

The tilt test is used to diagnose neurally mediated syncope (NMS).

1. Place the child in a supine position on a table equipped with a foot board that may be tilted to an upright position between 45 to 90 degrees.
2. After a short time, tilt the table to a full 90-degree angle, standing the child upright.
3. If there is a remarkable drop in BP or HR and the child experiences syncope or presyncope, the tilt test is positive.
4. If the child does not exhibit any symptoms, lay the table flat again and administer isoproterenol (Isuprel) to stimulate a fast heart rate. Tilt the table again to elicit syncopal response or a drop in the blood pressure. If there is

no response in change in vital signs, the test is considered negative and other causative factors are evaluated.

Electrocardiogram

- An ECG or EKG is a graphic display of electrical activity produced by changes in the intracellular charge of the cardiac muscles.
- The components of an ECG or EKG are marked with the letters PQRST (Fig. 24-1)

Invasive Tests

Cardiac Catheterization
- Determines the pressures in heart and radiographic picture of heart anatomy.
- Interventional catheterization is a corrective procedure.
- Post-catheterization (monitor: pressure dressing in the groin, heart rate, respirations, and blood pressure).

Angiography
- Visualizes the structures and function of the ventricles, vessels, and valves; size and location of septal defects; directs medical treatment.

Biopsy
- Routine biopsies to assess for cardiac transplant rejection

Closure Devices
- Close simple intracardiac communications or shunts

Opening Devices
- Angioplasty or valvuloplasty
- Opens narrow vessels or valves

Figure 24-1 Components of electrocardiogram are PQRST.

Balloon Atrial Septostomy

- Emergent palliative procedure necessary to keep the child alive

Laboratory Values

- Lab values are unstable and require close monitoring.
- Electrolyte measurement (especially potassium) is the most critical lab test during the postoperative period because the cardiac bypass machine homolyses the cells, which creates a high concentration of extracellular potassium.
- Hemoglobin and hematocrit tests are required to check for bleeding and coagulation factors.
- Assess arterial blood gasses frequently to determine the concentrations of gases such as carbon dioxide and oxygen.

MEDICATIONS

Carvedilol (kar-**ve**-dil-ole)

Brand Name Coreg (co-rĕg)

Generic name Carvedilol

Classification(s) β-Adrenoreceptor blocker, α-adrenergic

Pregnancy Category C

Indications Coreg is indicated for the treatment of mild to severe heart failure of ischemic or cardiomyopathic origin.

Actions Beta blockade, slows tachycardia, vasodilation, decreases peripheral vascular resistance, decreases renal vascular resistance, reduces plasma renin levels, increases atrial natriuretic peptide levels

Therapeutic Effects Increase stroke volume, decrease blood pressure and improve renal flow, decrease heart rate.

Pharmacokinetics
Bioavailability 25–35%.
Onset of Effect 1–2 hours
Half-life 7–10 hours

Contraindications and Precautions Monitor for possible deterioration of CHF, liver injury, bronchospastic disease, thyrotoxicosis.

Adverse Reactions and Side Effects Chest pain, dizziness, hyperglycemia, bradycardia, nausea.

Route and Dosage
Oral: 0.07 mg/kg per dose
Maximum dose: 0.5 mg/kg
Once or twice daily dosing
Reduce dose for bradycardia <55 beats/min

Nursing Implications
1. Initiate with low dose and titrate up as tolerated.
2. Monitor blood pressure for 1 hour after initial dosing.
3. Monitor blood pressure, pulse and ECG frequently.
4. Take with food.

Data from Deglin, J., & Vallerand, A. (2009). Davis's drug guide for nurses (11th ed.), pp. 271–273. Philadelphia: F.A. Davis.

Idiopathic Primary Pulmonary Arterial Hypertension (IPAH)

- Prostacyclin (Flolan) dilates blood vessels and decreases pulmonary vascular resistance.
- Inhaled nitric oxide relaxes pulmonary (not systemic) vessels.
- Sildenafil (Revatio) decreases pulmonary artery pressures.
- Bosentan (Tracleer) blocks hormone that causes vasoconstriction.

ETHNOCULTURAL CONSIDERATIONS

Hypertension

- Hypertension has a higher incidence among black children than in other ethnic groups.
- Educate the child and family about the condition.
- Promote a reasonable sodium intake.
- Teach the family how to reduce the saturated fat and cholesterol in the child's diet.

TEACHING THE FAMILY

Hypercholesterolemia–Hyperlipidemia

- Treatment includes diet modification, exercise, and medication.
- Recommend balanced diet per day (less than 10% of total calories from saturated fatty acids, 30% or less total calories from fat, less than 300 mg of cholesterol).
- Pharmacological treatment is recommended for children over 10 years of age whose LDL is greater than 190 mg/dL.
- Recommend testing children 2 years old or older if the following factors apply:

At least one parent with high cholesterol (240 mg/dL or greater), family history of early heart disease such as a male parent or grandparent with Congenital Heart Disease (CHD) before age 55, or a female parent or grandparent with CHD before age 65, diabetes, obesity, immunosuppressant drug use (AHA, 2005).

Neurally Mediated Syncope (NMS)

- Inform the family of a teen of driving age who has syncope that he must be syncope free for 6 months in some states before he can drive again.

Pacemakers

- Permanent pacemakers may be placed in the abdomen in younger children and in the subclavicular area in older children.
- Pacemakers must be protected (consideration must be taken with children who are athletic).
- Pacemakers must be replaced every 5 to 10 years.
- Use of a pacemaker is controversial for vaso-vagal syncope.
- Pacemaker placement is not recommended for neutrally mediated syncope.

Caring for the Child with a Cardiac Condition

- A home health nurse may evaluate the child at intervals to see if help at home is needed and if a parent needs to take vital signs at night.

- The family must receive crucial information related to the timing and the routine of medication administration.
- Teach the family that one of the most important aspects of medication administration is proper dosing. Many medications are given in a liquid form. The medication dosing should always be in milliliters (mL) or cubic centimeters (cc) and not tsp or other household measures.
- Educate the family about the disease; there are many resources in print and on the Internet. Ensure that the most up-to-date information is provided.
- Educate the family that it is necessary for a team approach in treating the cardiac disease.

ADDITIONAL INFORMATION FOR THE CLINICAL SETTING

- The heart consists of four chambers, two reservoirs (atria) and two pumping chambers (ventricles; Fig. 24-2).
- There are four valves in the heart. Two are atrioventricular (AV) valves connecting the atria and ventricles (Fig. 24-3).
- There are major vessels that lead to and from the heart (Fig. 24-4).
- The vena cava carries the blood from body tissues to the right atrium.
- The superior vena cava lies above the heart and carries blood from the head, arms, and upper body.
- The inferior vena cava lies below the heart and carries blood from the legs, abdominal organs, and lower part of the body.

Figure 24-2 Chambers of the heart.

Figure 24-3 Valves of the heart.

- The pulmonary artery is the only named artery in the body that carries deoxygenated blood. It is called an artery because it carries blood away from the heart, but since it arises from the right ventricle, it carries deoxygenated blood. It carries this blood to the pulmonary capillary bed, where it interfaces with the alveoli in the lungs and "picks up" oxygen. From the lungs, the blood returns to the heart through the pulmonary veins into the left atrium (the only veins that carry oxygenated blood). The blood leaves the left ventricle through the aortic valve, through the aorta and out to the body.
- Venous system, venae cavae, right atrium tricuspid valve, right ventricle, pulmonic valve, pulmonary artery, and lungs pick up O_2. The pulmonary veins, left atrium, mitral valve, left ventricle, aortic valve, aorta, and arteriole system delivers O_2 via the blood to the cells of the body (Fig. 24-5).

Figure 24-4 Vessels of the heart.

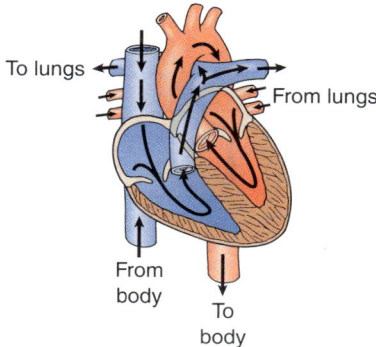

Figure 24-5 Normal blood flow.

- An atrial septal defect (ASD) results when the two septae fail to form properly (Fig. 24-6).
- A ventricular septal defect (VSD) is the most common congenital heart defect. The septum can have a single opening or be fraught with multiple defects (Fig. 24-7).

Figure 24-6 Atrial septal defect.

Figure 24-7 Ventricular septal defect.

- An atrioventricular canal defect (AVC) is somewhat of a combination of an ASD and VSD. However, it is much more than that, as it involves the valves. In its simplest definition, an AVC is a large hole in the center of the heart (Fig. 24-8).
- A patent ductus arteriosus is probably the simplest form of vessel defect. Remember that the ductus arteriosus is a normal structure during fetal life. In utero, the pulmonary resistance is high because the lungs are filled with fluid and not air. The blood is oxygenated through the placenta by the umbilical vein. Instead of the blood moving from the pulmonary artery (PA) to the lungs, the ductus is a pop-off valve for the large volume of fluid. As the blood flow follows the "path of least resistance," the blood moves through the ductus, into the aorta, and out to the body tissues. Directly after birth and the baby's first breaths, the pulmonary resistance starts to drop and the blood flows from the PA into the lungs. Since there is decreased flow through the PDA, the duct starts to close. Changes in prostaglandin level assist the closure as well. In 8 to 10% of the population, the PDA remains open (Fig. 24-9).
- Pulmonic stenosis or pulmonic valve stenosis (PS or PVS) is a malformation of the pulmonary artery or pulmonic valve. The narrowing of the valve causes an increased workload on the right ventricle which in turn leads to congestive heart failure (CHF) (Fig. 24–10).
- Pulmonary atresia is absence of the pulmonary valve, pulmonary artery, or both (Fig. 24-11).

Figure 24-8 Atrioventricular canal defect.

Figure 24-9 Patent ductus arteriosus.

Figure 24-10 Pulmonary stenosis.

Figure 24-11 Pulmonary atresia.

- Aortic stenosis or aortic valve stenosis (AS or AVS) is a malformation and narrowing in the aorta or around the aortic valve. A narrowing in this area causes an increased workload on the left ventricle and eventually leads to hypertrophy (increase in size) and heart failure (Fig. 24-12).

Figure 24-12 Aortic stenosis.

- Coarctation of the aorta (CoA) is a narrowing or stricture of the descending aorta distal to the carotid arteries. The coarctation is classified by its location: preductal, ductal, or postductal (Fig. 24-13).
- Tricuspid atresia (TA) occurs when there is an error of the formation of the tricuspid valve. As a single defect, this condition is incompatible with life, as no blood from the right atrium (RA) reaches the right ventricle (RV) and thus the right ventricular outflow tract (RVOT) leading to the PA and the lungs. For this reason, most children born with TA also have comorbidity with a septal defect such as ASD or VSD as well as a PDA. The deoxygenated blood must reach the pulmonary bed to sustain life (Fig. 24-14).
- Epstein's malformation occurs when the tricuspid valve is displaced into the right ventricle (Fig. 24-15).

Figure 24-13 Coarctation of the aorta.

Figure 24-14 Tricuspid atresia.

Figure 24-15 Epstein's malformation.

- Total anomalous pulmonary venous return (TAPVR) is a condition in which the pulmonary blood flow returns to the heart through the right atrium rather than the left (Fig. 24-16).
- Transposition of the great arteries or vessels (TGA or TGV) occurs in utero when the signals cross and instead of twisting there is simply a septation and the aorta arises from the right side of the heart and the pulmonary artery arises from the left (Fig. 24-17).
- In truncus arteriosus, the trunk has not twisted or septated. There are multiple variations of the condition, classed I to IV, but the general physiology is that the aorta and pulmonary arteries (PAs) are combined, with full mixing of blood. Sometimes the PAs arise from the aorta, either ascending or descending (Fig. 24-18).

Figure 24-16 Total anomalous venous return.

Figure 24-17 Transposition of the great vessels.

Figure 24-18 Truncus arteriosus.

- In tetralogy of Fallot, there are always four associated conditions: VSD, overriding aorta, hypertrophic RV, and pulmonary stenosis or atresia (Fig. 24-19).
- Hypoplastic left heart syndrome is a defect in which the left ventricle is extremely small or hypoplastic and unable to maintain an adequate cardiac output (Fig. 24-20).

Figure 24-19 Tetralogy of Fallot.

Figure 24-20 Hypoplastic left heart syndrome.

- Long Q-T syndrome (LQTS) is an electrophysiological condition predisposing the child to fatal arrhythmias such as ventricular tachycardia (VT), torsade de pointes, and ventricular fibrillation (Fig. 24-21).
- Narrow vessels or valves may be opened or dilated with a balloon angioplasty or valvuloplasty as an initial treatment or a stent may be placed in a vessel as a long-term treatment. This treatment is performed during a cardiac catheterization procedure. A special catheter with a balloon (similar to a Foley balloon) catheter is passed into the heart and into the narrow vessel. The balloon is then inflated, causing the stenotic area to expand (Fig. 24-22).

Figure 24-21 Long QT syndrome.

Figure 24-22 Balloon angioplasty with stent.

Postoperative Management

Provide immediate postoperative care in the intensive care unit:

- Record the vital signs frequently until the child is stable.
- Maintain "lines" (there may be several):
  - A peripheral IV line is used to administer fluid and medications.
  - A central venous pressure line (CVP) is inserted in a large vessel in the neck and is used to measure central venous pressure.
  - Intracardiac lines are inserted in the right atrium, left atrium, and pulmonary artery and are used to measure the pressures inside the cardiac chambers that provide essential information about cardiac output, blood volume, pulmonary pressures, ventricular function, and drug therapy response.

- Assess and maintain respiratory status. Respiratory assessment is done frequently.
- Provide oxygen via mechanical ventilation.
- Monitor fluid status. Accurately measure the intake and output of all fluids.
- Assess for signs and symptoms of infection.

A Way to Remember Cyanotic Defects

- All defects starting with a "T" are cyanotic defects.

Valve Replacement

- Replace every 5 years if originally replaced in infancy or childhood.
- If replaced in adolescence, replace approximately every 10 years.

Electrocardiogram

The abbreviations ECG/EKG are used interchangeably. (The K indicates the German spelling of cardiac.)

- An electrocardiogram (ECG) is a graphic display of electrical activity produced by changes in the intracellular charge of the cardiac muscles.
- An isoelectric line is the imaginary baseline of the ECG/EKG. One measurement in reading ECGs is how far the wave is from the baseline.
- A lead refers to the actual recording.
- The electrode is the device that is placed on the chest where the lead wire is attached.
- It typically takes two electrodes to make one lead.
- The electrical activity in the heart can then be graphed and evaluated.

Caring for the Child with a Cardiac Condition in a Clinic

- Monitor vital signs (heart rate, blood pressure, respiratory rate).
- Monitor the oxygen saturation of the patient's blood using a pulse oximeter (acceptable normal ranges are from 95 to 100% however, some children normally have a value as low as 85%. The nurse should confirm the range of normal oximeter readings with the practitioner).

- Review medications and discuss changes with the caregiver.
- Verify all medications and provide necessary instruction.
- Ensure that the family has enough medication refills. If there are any changes in medication or adjustments in dosages, document it in the child's record.
- Medications are frequently altered due to growth (weight) of the child.
- Laboratory tests may be required.
- Children requiring warfarin (Coumadin) to prevent thrombus must have the pro-time and international normalized ratio checked routinely. The ratio is checked frequently when this drug is first initiated, then every 4 weeks to 3 months after it is stabilized. Note any changes made to the dosage.
- Electrogram monitoring in the clinic usually includes a 12-lead ECG to identify potential or existing arrhythmias, chamber size, and strain on the heart muscle.
- Often the Holter monitor or event recorders are applied in the clinic.
- Other recording devices may be distributed to parents for home use (e.g., apnea monitors, pulse oximeters).

 Procedure 24-1 Taking a Blood Pressure Reading

Purpose

Taking the blood pressure is an indicator of the child's state of health. Blood pressure is the pressure of blood as it is forced against the arterial walls during a cardiac contraction.

Equipment

- Blood pressure cuff (**sphygmometer**) Stethoscope (Venes, 2005)

Steps

1. Measure the child's bare limb to determine the appropriate size cuff.
2. Have the child sit comfortably without dangling feet.
3. Encourage the child to be quiet and relaxed before taking the BP.
4. Apply the cuff to the arm.

Procedure 24-1 (Continued)

5. Palpate the brachial pulse just below and slightly medial to the antecubital area.
6. Rapidly inflate the cuff to about 30 mm Hg about the level at which the pulse disappears.
7. Slowly open the valve and watch the mercury drop.
8. Continue deflating the cuff, noting the point at which the pulse disappears or becomes muffled (fourth Korotkoff sound).
9. Document the procedure.

Clinical Alert Sometimes blood pressure is taken over clothing with the thought that children may become more afraid if asked to put on a gown. This practice will result in an inaccurate measurement of BP. In addition, the BP should not be taken in the same arm where an IV is placed.

Teach Parents

Teaching parents about the importance of taking the child's blood pressure as it is a physical sign concerning functions essential to life (Venes, 2005).

Subacute Bacterial Endocarditis (SBE)

- Subacute bacterial endocarditis (SBE) occurs subsequent to a bacterial infection or introduction of an infective agent into the child's blood stream.
- The infection may be caused by an invasive procedure such as surgery, urological procedures, or most often dental cleaning.
- Initially, vague symptoms may include a low-grade fever, malaise, loss of appetite, and muscle aches. A high fever, chills, sweating, stiff joints, or back pain can indicate that acute illness has occurred.
- As the condition worsens, symptoms of heart failure occur (Venes, 2005).
- Blood cultures to identify bacteria or fungi in the bloodstream may detect endocarditis.

The guidelines for administration and dosage of prophylactic antibiotics are determined by the American Dental Association

(ADA) and the American Heart Association (AHA). Guidelines for prescribing prophylaxis treatment were updated in April 2007:

- Patients with a prosthetic cardiac valve
- Patients who previously had endocarditis
- Patients with congenital heart disease only in the following categories:
  - Unrepaired cyanotic congenital heart disease, including those with palliative shunts and conduits
  - Completely repaired congenital heart disease with prosthetic material or device, whether placed by surgery or catheter intervention, during the first 6 months after the procedure
  - Repaired congenital heart disease with residual defects at the site or adjacent to the site of a prosthetic patch or prosthetic device (which inhibit endothelialization)
- Cardiac transplantation recipients with cardiac valvular disease
- If valve destruction occurs, the valve may need to be repaired or replaced

Sinus Arrhythmias

A normal irregular rhythm in which the rhythm varies with respiration is called sinus arrhythmia. Sinus arrhythmia has no adverse effect on the cardiac output.

- The heart rate increases with inspiration (Remember: "Inspiration" and "Increase" both start with an "I").
- The heart rate decreases with expiration.

Typical Post-Cardiac Catheterization Medical Orders

1. Admit to postsurgical observation unit.
2. Check vital signs (q15min × 4, then q1hr × 2, then q2hr × 2, then q4hr).
3. Check peripheral pulses with vital signs (especially on affected extremity).
4. Keep O_2 saturation above (95–100%) or _____.
5. Call house officer for HR > _____, BP > _____ (age and baseline dependent) and temperature >_____.
6. Give acetaminophen (Children's Tylenol) for pain (based on weight).

7. Keep the child flat in bed for 6 hours.
8. Check pressure dressing with Vital Signs for bleeding.
9. Call the medical doctor or house officer for complaints of abdominal pain or urine output. < _____ or no urine output.
10. Increase diet as tolerated.
11. Give _____antiemetic for nausea.

Note: The blank lines indicate the physician's particular medical order.

Administering Medication Properly

- It is crucial for the nurse to understand the desired and undesired effects of the child's medication.
- Before giving any medication, the nurse must check the proper dosage (with calculations) and route.
- At times, medications are given in very small amounts and an error in decimal placement can mean a fatal overdose or other detrimental effects.
- Be sure to use the 5 rights of medication administration.

Waking the Child during the Night for Vital Signs

- The best outcome for a child with a cardiac condition is proper healing along with adequate growth and development.
- Assess if the child needs to be awakened during the night for vital signs or can be allowed to sleep.

RESOURCES

American Heart Association: http://www.americanheart.org

Children's Heart Society: http://www.childrensheart.org

Congenital Heart Information Network: http://www.tchin.org

Cardiomyopathy: http://www.cardiomyopathy.org

Heart Rhythm Society: http://www.hrsonline.org

Kawasaki Disease: http://www.kdfoundation.org

Long QT Syndrome: http://www.long-qt-syndrome.com

March of Dimes: http://www.marchofdimes.com

Pectus: http://www.pectusinfo.com

Sudden Arrhythmia Death Syndrome (SADS) Foundation:
http://www.sads.org

REFERENCES

American Heart Association. (2004). Scientific statement: Diagnosis, treatment, and long-term management of Kawasaki disease. *Circulation, 110,* 2747–2771.

American Heart Association (AHA). (2005). Scientific Statement: Dietary recommendations for children and adolescents. *Circulation, 112,* 2061–2075.

Deglin, J., & Vallerand, A. (2009). *Davis's drug guide for nurses* (11th ed.). Philadelphia: F. A. Davis.

Park, M. (2003). *The pediatric cardiology handbook* (3rd ed). St. Louis: C.V. Mosby.

Venes, D. (Ed.). (2005). *Taber's cyclopedic medical dictionary* (20th ed.). Philadelphia: F.A. Davis.

Caring for the Child with an Endocrinological or Metabolic Condition

KEY TERMS

kussmaul breaths – Very deep and laborious breaths; in an attempt to correct metabolic acidosis, the respiratory system works hard to "blow off" excess carbon dioxide

FOCUSED ASSESSMENT

Proper Growth Assessment

- Plot the child's height and weight accurately at each outpatient visit on the appropriate growth chart.
- If the child is of short stature (below the 3rd or 5th percentile) and is not chartable on the usual chart or has Down syndrome, go to the Centers for Disease Control and Prevention (CDC) Web site to access the most appropriate chart, located at http://www.cdc.gov/nchs/about/major/nhanes/growthcharts/charts.htm.
- Be sure to use the same growth chart at each visit.
- Weigh an infant completely undressed (including diaper) and children in underwear only.

Signs and Symptoms of Diabetes Insipidus	
Infant	**Child**
Irritability	Excessive thirst (polydipsia)
Poor feeding (despite vigorous suck)	Excessive urine production (polyuria)
Failure to grow/thrive	Enuresis (nocturnal bed wetting)
Vomiting	
Constipation	
High fevers	

Signs and Symptoms of Acute Adrenocortical Insufficiency (Adrenal Crisis)

- Weakness, feeling tired, nausea, vomiting, loss of appetite, weight loss, low blood pressure, abdominal pain, fever, confusion, or coma

Assessing for Hyperreflexia of Muscles

- Tap on the facial nerve.
- Facial muscle spasm (Chvostek sign) confirms that the child has muscle pain, cramps, and probably twitches.
- These muscle manifestations may progress to numbness and tingling of the hands and feet as well as stiffness.
- Remember that infants and small children cannot express these manifestations and therefore may cry to communicate their pain.

Signs and Symptoms of Cushing's Syndrome

- Common signs and symptoms of Cushing's syndrome include weight gain, especially, pendulous abdomen; fatigue; muscle wasting and weakness, thin extremities; round "moon" face; facial flushing; fatty pad between shoulders (buffalo hump); and pink or purple stretch marks (striae) on abdominal skin, thighs, breasts, and arms.
- The child's skin is thin and fragile with little subcutaneous tissue, causing easy bruising; slow healing of cuts, insect bites, and infections due to a lessened inflammatory response.

- The child may exhibit depression, anxiety and irritability, euphoria, and frank psychoses; irregular or absent menstrual periods in females; and erectile dysfunction in adolescent males.
- Hyperglycemia may eventually lead to latent or overt diabetes, high blood pressure, or arteriosclerosis.
- Owing to the excess production of androgens, signs and symptoms related to secondary sexual characteristics can also be seen.

Signs and Symptoms of Diabetes Mellitus Type 1

- Excessive urination, in volume and frequency (polyuria)
- Loss of bladder control in children after they had already been trained, especially at night
- Excessive intake of water and/or food (polydipsia and/or polyphagia)
- Unintended weight loss over several days and tendency to be thin
- High glucose levels in the blood and urine (hyperglycemia and glycosuria)
- Nausea and vomiting, abdominal pain or discomfort
- Weakness and excessive fatigue
- Increased susceptibility to infection, especially urinary tract, respiratory, and skin infections
- Dehydration
- Blurred vision
- Irritability, restlessness, apathy

Signs and Symptoms of Diabetes Mellitus Type 2

- High blood glucose levels
- Sometimes mimic type 1 diabetes

Signs and Symptoms of Diabetic Ketoacidosis (DKA)

- Toddlers: Classic manifestations often absent
- Altered mental status, tachycardia, tachypnea, Kussmaul respirations, normal or low blood pressure, poor perfusion, lethargy and weakness, fever, acetone breath

CLINICAL ALERTS

Exogenous Hormones

- Alert parents of the dangers of hidden toxins in everyday products that can harm their children.
- Make parents aware of "endocrine disruptors".
- Refer parents to this Web site: http://www.mindfully.org/Pesticide/EDs-PWG-16jun01.htm.

Dehydration

- Dehydration can be seen in all cases, causing the infant/child to be irritable with many other manifestations: dry mucous membranes, decreased skin turgor (tenting of abdominal skin in infant), decreased tears when crying, sunken fontanel, and tachycardia.
- If dehydration is severe, the child's pulse may be thready and very rapid.
- Hypotension may be present and could lead to hypovolemic shock.

Hyponatremia

- Thoroughly and accurately track intake, output, and daily weights of the child.
- Hyponatremia (low serum sodium of less than 125 mEq/L) may cause seizures in the child with syndrome of inappropriate antidiuretic hormone secretion (SIADH).
- Keeping the serum sodium level as near as normal is the goal of treatment.

Thyroid Storm

- A rare and potentially fatal complication of hyperthyroidism
- Occurs in patients with untreated or partially treated thyrotoxicosis (a term often used interchangeably for hyperthyroidism) who experience a precipitating event such as surgery, infection, or trauma
- Must be recognized and treated on signs and symptoms alone, as laboratory confirmation often cannot be obtained in a timely manner

- Patients typically appear markedly hypermetabolic with high fevers, tachycardia, nausea and vomiting, tremulousness, agitation, and psychosis if untreated.
- Late in the progression of the disease (hyperthyroidism), patients may become stuporous or comatose with hypotension.

Symptoms of an Addisonian Crisis

- Sudden penetrating pain in the lower back, abdomen, or legs, severe vomiting and diarrhea, dehydration, low blood pressure, and a loss of consciousness
- If left untreated, a child with Addison's disease in crisis can die (NIH, 2004).

Cortisone Insufficiency

- Be aware of the signs and symptoms observed before an adrenal crisis (headache, dizziness, and nausea) or vomiting (stomachache) or wobbly knees.
- By the time the child exhibits extreme weakness and mental confusion, the adrenal crisis will be eminent.

Diabetic Ketoacidosis (DKA)

- Infection is the most frequent cause of DKA, particularly in known diabetics.
- Aggressive evaluation for infection is necessary.
- Empiric antibiotic therapy should strongly be considered until culture results return.
- Other patient-related issues may be the cause (noncompliance with insulin regimens, thelarche, adrenarche, menarche, caregiver's lack of competence, insulin pump failure).

DIAGNOSTIC TESTS

Diagnosis of Diabetes Insipidus

Water Deprivation Test

1. Monitor the patient's vital signs every hour if necessary and watch for fever and hypotension.

2. Collect urine and blood samples early in the day and test for osmolarity and electrolytes.
3. Deprive the child of water until significant dehydration occurs.
4. Weigh child every 2 hours until 2% to 5% of body weight is lost.
5. Monitor urine specific gravity hourly; stop when specific gravity is 1.014 or higher.
6. Complete test within 4 hours for an infant and 7 hours for a child.

Serum Levels

Diagnosis of diabetes insipidus is confirmed when the following values are found:

- High urine osmolarity (greater than 1200 Osmol/kg)
- High urine specific gravity (greater than 1.030)
- Low serum osmolarity (less than 275 mOsm/kg)
- Low serum sodium (less than 125 mEq/L)

Potassium Depletion

- Treatments for adrenal crisis cause potassium depletion; must closely watch the child's lab values.
- Watch for warning signs of hyperkalemia and hypokalemia (apnea, cardiac arrhythmias, paralysis, poor muscle control, weakness).

Hyperaldosteronism

- Blood chemistry studies indicate decreased potassium level, increased aldosterone level, and decreased renin activity.
- Urinalysis reveals an elevated aldosterone level.
- CAT scan of abdomen reveals an adrenal mass.
- EKG shows abnormalities.

Equivalent of A1C Level and Blood Glucose Level

Hemoglobin A1C Levels (mean %)		Mean Blood Glucose Level (mg/dL)
Normal	4	60
	4.5	
	5	90
	5.5	
	6	120
Slightly Elevated	6.5	
	7	150
	7.5	
	8	180
Elevated	8.5	
	9	210
	9.5	
	10	240
Severely Elevated	10.5	
	11	270
	11.5	
	12	300
	12.5	
	13	330
	13.5	
	14	360

Modified from the American Diabetes Association (2005). Standards of medical care in diabetes: Clinical practice recommendations. *Diabetes Care 28 (Suppl)*, S4–S36.

Plasma Blood Glucose and Hemoglobin A1C Goals for Type 1 Diabetes by Age Group

Age Group (years)	Plasma Blood Glucose Goal Range (mg/dL)		Hemoglobin A1C (%)	Rationale
	Morning Before Meals	Bedtime/ Overnight		
Toddlers and Preschoolers (0–6 years)	100–180	110–200	< 8.5% (but > 7.5%)	High risk/ vulnerability to hypoglycemia
School-age (6–12 years)	90–180	100–180	< 8%	Risk of hypoglycemia and low risk of complications before puberty

(continued)

Plasma Blood Glucose and Hemoglobin A1C Goals for Type 1 Diabetes by Age Group (Continued)				
Age Group (years)	**Plasma Blood Glucose Goal Range (mg/dL)**		**Hemoglobin A1C (%)**	**Rationale**
	Morning Before Meals	**Bedtime/ Overnight**		
Adolescents and Young Adults (13–19 years)	90–130	90–150	< 7.5%	Risk for severe hypoglycemia Developmental and psychological issues Lower goal of < 7.0% is reasonable if it can be achieved without excessive hypoglycemia

Modified from the American Diabetes Association (2007). Standards of medical care in diabetes – 2007. *Diabetes Care 30 (Suppl), S4–S41.*

MEDICATIONS

Desmopressin (DDAVP)

- Desmopressin (DDAVP) is a synthetic vasopressin analogue

Accurate Administration of Intranasal Medication Doses
- Instruct the child to blow his nose before medication is given.
- Administer intranasal DDAVP through a rhinal tube.
- Position the child on the side the medication is given to enhance absorption of the medication.
- Provide parents with clear instructions and refer them to the Family Resource Center Library (www.childrensmn.org) for patient family education materials.

Administration of Hormone Tablets

- Teach parents proper administration of the medication.
- Pills can be crushed in a spoon, dissolved with a small amount of water or other liquid immediately before

administration, and administered to the child with a syringe, dropper, or nipple.

- Toddlers can be allowed to readily chew the tablets (Postellon, 2006).
- Do not mix in a full bottle of formula (to avoid ruining the taste of the infant's sole source of nutrition).

Side Effects of Antithyroid Medications

Mild Effects	Severe Effects (can be *Fatal*)
Skin rash	Agranulocytosis (sore throat, high fever)
Mild leukopenia	Lupus-like syndrome
Loss of taste	Hepatitis
Arthralgia	Hepatic failure
Loss/abnormal hair pigmentation	Glomerulonephritis

Accurate Administration of Intravenous Calcium

- Check the IV site for accurate placement as infiltration of the intravenous calcium supplements cause extravasation and sloughing of the tissue around the site.
- Intravenous calcium supplements must be properly calculated, diluted, and administered strictly according to hospital's standards of care and protocols.

Steroid Administration

- Never stop steroid administration abruptly (can cause an adrenal crisis).
- Slowly wean according to the physician's orders.

Insulin Dosage and Frequency

- Dosage is based on the individual needs of the patient (common dosage for an adolescent is 1.0 to 1.7 units/kg per day; common dosage for a child is 0.75 to 1.0 units/kg per day).
- If treatment calls for two doses, usually 60% to 75% of the insulin is given before breakfast and the remainder is given with dinner.

Insulin Types and Peak Effects

Insulin Name	Insulin Type	Begins to Work	Peak Effect	Used Up
Humalog/ NovoLog	Short-acting	10–15 minutes	30–90 minutes	4 hours
Regular	Short-acting	30–60 minutes	2–4 hours	6–9 hours
NPH	Intermediate acting	1–2 hours	3–8 hours	12–15 hours
Ultralente	Intermediate acting	2–4 hours	6–14 hours	18–20 hours
Lantus	Long-acting	1–2 hours	2–22 hours	24 hours

Insulin "Cocktails"

Insulin Name	Insulin Type	Begins to Work	Peak Effect	Used Up
Lente	Premixed	1–2 hours	3–14 hours	18–20 hours
70/30 NPH/Regular	Premixed	30–60 minutes	3–8 hours	12–15 hours
75/25 NPH/Humalog	Premixed	10–15 minutes	30 minutes– 8 hours	12–15 hours

ETHNOCULTURAL CONSIDERATIONS

Shock in Dark-Complexioned Children

- When assessing for shock in children with a dark complexion look at the palms of the hands, feet, and lips to ascertain color changes.

Type 2 Diabetes

- Type 2 diabetes in children is often associated with ethnic background (African American, Hispanic, Asian, or American Indian), obesity (85% at diagnosis), and a family history of type 2 diabetes (74%–100%) as well as with insulin resistance.

TEACHING THE FAMILY

Hydrocortisone (A-Hydrocort) Administration

- Medication must be used as prescribed.
- Always have the injectable hydrocortisone available at home, school, and wherever the child travels.
- Keep an emergency kit on hand at all times with a cortisol supply. Administer to the child during acute illness, vomiting, diarrhea, or during stressful circumstances. When oral dose cannot be tolerated, injectable dose must be readily available.
- Administer the medication on time because this follows the child's body's normal cortisol release patterns (Wilson, 2006).

 Procedure 25-1 Teaching Parents How to Inject Insulin

Purpose

To teach parents how to inject insulin

Equipment

- Insulin bottle from refrigerator (remove up to one hour before injection to allow it to warm to room temperature)
- Appropriate syringe (U-30, U-50, or U-100)
- Alcohol wipes
- Container for the dirty, used syringe

Steps

1. Check the expiration date on the insulin bottle.
2. Wash hands.
3. Clean rubber stopper on insulin bottle with alcohol wipe.
4. Remove the syringe cap and pull air into the syringe line up the end of the black plunger to the exact amount the insulin dose will be.
5. Put the syringe needle through the bottle rubber top and push syringe plunger so that all the air goes from the syringe into the bottle.

(continued)

Procedure 25-1 (Continued)

6. Turn the insulin bottle upside down and pull the syringe plunger so that the insulin enters the syringe until the top of the black plunger exactly lines up with the dose of insulin to be given.

7. Remove every air bubble, always checking that the dose is exact.

8. Choose (or let the child choose) the site of the injection.

9. Clean the injection site with an alcohol swab.

10. Pinch up the skin slightly and gently, with the syringe at a 90-degree angle (perpendicular) to the skin, with a dart-like motion, insert the needle into the skin, release the skin.

11. Slowly inject the dose of insulin.

12. Discard the used syringe in a hard, rigid container with a tight-fitting lid.

13. Document the procedure.

Clinical Alert The nurse teaches the parents to evaluate the child for the signs and symptoms of either hypo- or hyperglycemia. In understandable terms explain these signs and symptoms to the parents so they can watch for them at home.

Hypoglycemia (*LOW* Blood Sugar)	Hyperglycemia (*HIGH* Blood Sugar)
Cold, pale skin (cold sweat)	Increased thirst, even if consuming a large amount of liquids
Shakiness/hand tremors	Loss of appetite, nausea/vomiting
Sudden hunger (crave salt/sweet)	Weakness, stomach pains/aches
Emotional outbursts (personality changes)	Heavy, labored breathing
Drowsiness/extremely tired	Fatigue, tired often sleepy
Pounding heartbeat/ palpitations	Large amounts of sugar in urine
Nervousness/dizziness	Ketones in urine
Anxiety/irritability	Frequent urination

Procedure 25-1 (Continued)

Headache, mental confusion, difficulty concentrating

Blurred/double vision

Numbness or tingling of lips/mouth

Poor coordination/ staggering, unable to walk

Slurred or slow speech

Dilated, enlarged pupils

Fainting (needs emergency treatment *NOW*)

Teach Parents

If the child expresses that the injection is painful, the following measures can be taken to decrease the pain:

Inject only room-temperature insulin.

Clear even the tiniest air bubbles from the syringe.

Allow the alcohol to dry completely.

Tell the child to relax muscles in the area of injection (the more tense the muscles during injection, the more painful the procedure).

Using the syringe like a dart, pierce the skin quickly.

Do not change the needle direction during insertion or withdrawal.

Never reuse needles/syringes.

Rotate sites with *each* injection (giving the insulin in the *same* place twice in one day can cause unnecessary discomfort for the child and undue stress on the tissue).

Document exactly where each injection was given so as to avoid the same place more than once a day.

Create and keep a Diabetes Management Notebook with the plan and a place to record daily Blood Sugar values as well as doses of insulin administered including injection site.

Dealing with a Hypoglycemic Crises

- Recognize the signs of hypoglycemia (skin pale and sweaty, dizzy, shaky, tremors, confused, irritable, numb on lips or mouth, altered mental status).
- Check blood glucose level.
- If the blood glucose level is less than 70 mg/dL, rapidly give one of the following sources of carbohydrates (about 10–15 grams each), the right amount to treat hypoglycemia:
  - 1/2 to 3/4 cup of orange or grape juice (a juice box is good when you're away from home)
  - 2 glucose tablets or 2 doses of glucose gel
  - 2 to 4 pieces hard candy
  - 5 gumdrops
  - 1 to 2 tablespoons of honey
  - 1 small box of raisins
  - 6 oz. regular (not diet) soda (about half a can)
  - 2 tablespoons of cake icing
- Recheck blood glucose in 15 minutes, if reading is still below <70 mg/dL, then give another glass of juice, etc.
- Recheck blood glucose again after another 15 minutes.
- When blood glucose returns to at least 80 mg/dL, give a more substantial snack that is not sugar concentrated (i.e., cheese and crackers, bread and peanut butter) if the next meal is more than 30 minutes away or if a physical activity/exercise is planned.
- If the child is unconscious, give glucagon subcutaneously or intramuscularly (American Diabetes Association [ADA], 2007a).

Educating Different Groups on Diabetes

Content Topics	Parent	Child	Adolescent
Disease Process	Include type of diabetes, treatment options, and benefits of a healthy lifestyle.	Explain the disease simply. Begin to teach self-care. Include in treatment plan.	Talk to as an adult. Expect self-care, but with limitations.
Nutritional Guidelines	Address breastfeeding. Erratic eating habits How to read labels	Provide instruction on how to make appropriate food choices (restaurant). Discuss ways to change food behavior habits (fast food).	

Content Topics	Parent	Child	Adolescent
	Family goes grocery shopping. Controversy of artificial sweeteners	Provide guidelines for meal and snack planning. Address after-school and party eating habits. Discuss coordination of school, activities, and meals.	
Activities	Explain how activity and glucose level interact. Younger children have a high energy level. Incorporate walking into family outings.	Limit sitting in front of TV or computer. Play outside. Join a sport or activity. Walk to a friend's house if possible.	Explain how exercise increases glucose use. Decrease sedentary (computer) time. Exercise every day, not just on weekends. Increase time, amount, and frequency of activity.
Medications	Understand the medication to be given. Discuss dose, frequency, action, adverse reactions. Insulin storage, dose, adminis- tration technique if appropriate. Choose medication schedule to fit the family's lifestyle.	Needs supervision at all times. Plans medications around normal schedule. Provide for lunch time dose if needed (talk to school RN, teacher)	Educate on self-treatment Adapting to hectic high school schedule Treat to target blood glucose. Monitor patterns in blood glucose to improve control.
Complications Acute Chronic	Discuss signs/ symptoms of hypo/ hyperglycemia. Discuss DKA emergency procedures and when to go to the ER. Explain the risk of long-term uncontrolled diabetes and effect on neurological and vascular systems.	Begins to understand hyper/ hypoglycemia. Recognizes patterns. Links causes to high and low blood sugar. Understands consequences of actions.	Identify cause and effect of hyper/ hypoglycemia. Instruct on how to prevent high and low blood sugar levels. Discuss driving precautions. Explain effect of long-term, uncontrolled diabetes on neurological and vascular systems.

(continued)

Educating Different Groups on Diabetes (Continued)

Content Topics	Parent	Child	Adolescent
Outcome Criteria	Family lifestyle changes Discuss goals that can be met. Boost confidence in technical skills. Management of child during illness Understand blood glucose readings and hemoglobin A1C results.	Work toward independence. Learn technical skills; expect frustrations. Emotional immaturity	Goals should be realistic and attainable Problem solving each day How to manage heat, sun, dehydration
Psychosocial Adjustments	Avoid giving too much responsibility too soon. Identify friends at whose homes the child could spend the night. (friends know child's care routine.) Notify teachers, principal of child's health needs. Adaptation of family life to incorporate care without stress. Stress reduction Parental relief (who could stay overnight with family so parents can "get away")	Blood glucose testing before meals at friends, in restaurant, at school (in public) Learn weight control. Manage overnight stays. Promote healthy habits amid unhealthy environments.	Body image and weight concerns Puberty and effect of hormonal changes Learn to prevent complications. Prevent DKA. Modify high-risk behaviors. Diabetes and dating, sex, and conception Peer pressure Alcohol, tobacco, drugs

Source: Atkinson, A., & Radjenovic, D. (2006).

ADDITIONAL INFORMATION FOR THE CLINICAL SETTING

Weighing Children

Weigh an infant completely undressed (including diaper) and children in underwear only.

Daily Weights to Ensure Accurate Medication Doses

- Use metric system (kilograms) daily to ensure medication dosages are accurately calculated and administered.
- Recalculate medication dosages with every weight variance.
- Notify the physician if the dose ordered is inaccurate based on the current weight.

Helping Children Express Themselves About Growth Hormone Treatments

- Be honest about growth hormone treatments.
- Refer families to the Magic Foundation Web site (see Resources) for online videos.
- Help the child respond to the following questions:
  "How do you feel?"
  "What do you tell your friends about the GH medication?"
  "How have you changed since the GH treatments began?"
  "What advice do you have for other children beginning GH treatment?"

Action of Diuretics on the Kidney

Diuretics impede the sodium chloride reabsorption that occurs in the distal tubule of the kidney. This reduces the loss of free water and increases the concentration of the child's urine. Reduction in urine volume derives from a concomitant action on the proximal tubule, which causes reabsorption of sodium chloride from the glomerular filtrate, thus drawing additional water along. This results in both a smaller volume and a higher concentration of the urine (Chan & Roth, 2006).

Switching from Milk-Based Formula to Soy-Based Formula

- Soy-based formula may cause a decrease in absorption of levothyroxine (Synthroid).
- When an infant is switched from a milk-based formula to a soy-based formula, the dose of thyroid hormone may need to increase to maintain a euthyroid status (Postellon, 2006).

Proper Nutrition for Hypoparathyroidism

The following supplements have been used clinically and may be valuable adjuncts in the treatment of hypoparathyroidism:

- Calcium, if dietary intake is not adequate.
- Magnesium, which aids in the absorption of calcium; also, often low levels of magnesium are present in the case of hypoparathyroidism.
- Boron, which enhances the absorption of calcium.
- Vitamin K, produced by bacteria in the intestines or obtained through the diet (e.g., dark leafy greens) is important for the uptake of calcium by cells throughout the body.
- Foods rich in calcium include almonds, legumes, dark leafy greens, blackstrap molasses, oats, sardines, tahini, prunes, apricots, and sea vegetables.
- Calcium and vitamin D are thought to be best absorbed in an acidic environment (e.g., lemon juice may be added to salad to facilitate calcium absorption).
- Limit carbonated beverages, as they are high in phosphates and may reduce calcium absorption; dairy may diminish calcium absorption for similar reasons.
- Avoid caffeine (such as in coffee, black tea, colas, and chocolate); it can lead to calcium loss through the urine (A.D.A.M., 2006).

Adrenal Crisis

- Adrenal crisis is a life-threatening condition caused by the anterior pituitary gland not making enough adrenocorticotropic hormone (ACTH). Without ACTH, the adrenal gland cannot regulate bodily functions.
- Never stop steroids abruptly. Abrupt withdrawal can cause an adrenal crisis.
- Parents must seek emergency medical care immediately if there is suspicion of adrenal crisis.

Pheochromocytoma

- Perform frequent assessments.
- Never touch or manipulate an adrenal tumor. Palpation can cause further release of catecholamines, increasing the likelihood of a severe hypertensive crisis. This can cause potentially harmful tachyarrhythmias.

Clinical Comparison of Hypoglycemia and Hyperglycemia

Clinical Condition due to	Manifestations	Critical Nursing Actions
Hypoglycemia Too much insulin for amount of food eaten Injected insulin into muscle Too much activity for insulin dose Too much time between meals Too few carbohydrates eaten Illness or stress	Rapid onset Irritable Nervous Shaky feeling, tremors Difficult to concentrate Difficult to speak Behavior change Confused Repeats over and over Unconscious Seizure Tachycardia Shallow breathing Pale, sweaty Hungry Headache Dizzy Vision blurry or double Photophobic Numbness of mouth or lips	Give 15 grams of carbohydrates ($^1/_2$ glass orange juice). Recheck blood glucose in 15 minutes. If blood glucose level is <70 mg/dL give another 15 grams of carbohydrates. Recheck again in another 15 minutes. If unconscious, give IM glucagon.
Hyperglycemia Too little insulin for the food eaten Illness or stress Too many carbohydrates eaten Meals too close together Too many snacks Insulin given just under skin Too little activity	Gradual onset Lethargic Sleepy Slow response Confused Breathes deeply and rapidly Skin flushed and dry Mucous membranes dry Thirsty, hungry, dehydrated Weak, tired, headache Abdomen hurts Nausea and vomiting Vision blurry Shock	Give additional insulin at the usual injection time. Use sliding scale doses for specific level of blood glucose. Increase fluids. If ketone levels are elevated, give an extra insulin injection.

RESOURCES

Audio and visual injection techniques:
http://www.bddiabetes.com/us/main.aspx?cat=1&id=258

Growth charts: http://www.cdc.gov/growthcharts

Growth charts: www.growthcharts.com

Human Growth Foundation: http://www.hgfound.orgParenting:
http://www.primalspirit.com/ps3_1lyn-piluso.htm

Magic Foundation: http://www.magicfoundation.org/www

Short Stature Foundation:
http://www.kumc.edu/gec/support/dwarfism.html

REFERENCES

A.D.A.M. (2006). *Alternative medicine.* Retrieved from http://www.adam.com/ (Accessed July 15, 2008).

Atkinson, A., & Radjenovic, D. (2006). Meeting quality standards for self-management education in pediatric Type 2 diabetes. *Diabetes Care,* 40–46.

American Diabetes Association (ADA). (2007a). Nutrition recommendations and interventions for diabetes. *Diabetes Care,* S48–S65.

American Diabetes Association (ADA). (2007b). Standards of medical care in diabetes—2007. *Diabetes Care,* S4–S41.

Chan, J.C., & Roth, K.S. (2006, July 26). Diabetes insipidus. Retrieved from http://www.emedicine.com/ped/topic580.htm (Accessed November 20, 2008).

NIH Publication No. 04–3054 (2004, June). Addison's disease. Retrieved from http://www.endocrine.niddle.nih.gov/pubs/Addison/Addison.htm (Accessed April 13, 2009).

Postellon, D. (2006, August 23). EMedicine: Congenital hypothyroidism Retrieved from http://www.emedicine.com/ (Accessed November 20, 2008).

Wilson, T.A. (2006, November 17). EMedicine: Congenital adrenal hyperplasia. Retrieved from http://www.emedicine.com/ (Accessed November 20, 2008).

Caring for the Child with a Neurological or Sensory Condition

KEY TERMS

color blindness – An X-linked recessive inheritable color vision deficiency that causes loss of accurate color perception

encephalopathy – Generalized brain dysfunction marked by varying degrees of impairment of speech, cognition, orientation, and arousal, as well as trauma (Venes, 2005).

intracranial pressure (ICP) – Pressure of the cerebrospinal fluid in the subarachnoid space between the skull and the brain

meningocele – Protruding sac located on the cervical, thoracic, or lumbar spine at the level of the defect with a thin layer of muscle and skin usually covering the lesion

nystagmus – Rapid irregular involuntary eye movement caused by a disorder of the central nervous system which may be congenital or acquired

papilledema – Mass of blown-out blood vessels located around the optic nerve; an important sign of increased intracranial pressure (ICP)

strabismus – Condition of nonparallelism in the different fields of gaze causing visual lines to cross even when focused on the same object

tympanogram – Radiographic examination of the eustachian tubes and middle ear after introduction of a contrast medium (Venes, 2005).

FOCUSED ASSESSMENT

States of Consciousness Technique and Patient Response

State	Technique	Response
Alertness	Speak in a normal tone of voice.	Answers appropriately while opening his eyes and responding fully.
Lethargy	Speak in a loud voice.	Opens eyes, appears drowsy, answers questions appropriately but falls asleep easily.
Obtundation	Shake gently to arouse.	Opens eyes and looks at the stimuli, appears slightly confused; alertness and interest in surroundings decreased.
Stupor	Use a painful stimulus.	Responds only to painful stimuli; verbal responses slow or absent; ceases to respond to painful stimuli.
Coma	Apply repeated painful stimuli.	No response to internal or external stimuli, remains in unaroused state with eyes closed

Source: Bickley & Szilagi (2003).

Pediatric Glasgow Coma Scale (GCS)

- Monitor the child's neurological status by assessing his level of consciousness with the GCS (Fig. 26-1).

Pediatric Glasgow Coma Scale

Score for Infant/Nonverbal Child			Verbal Child	
Eye Opening	4	Spontaneously	Spontaneously	
	3	To speech	To verbal command	
	2	To pain	To pain	
	1	No response	No response	
Best Motor Response	6	Normal spontaneous movement	Obeys command	
	5	Withdraws to touch	Localizes pain	
	4	Withdraws to pain	Flexion withdrawal	
	3	Abnormal flexion	Abnormal flexion	
	2	Extension (decerebrate)	Extension (decerebrate)	
	1	No response	No response	
			2–5 years	>5 years
Best Verbal Response	5	Cries appropriately, coos	Appropriate words	Oriented
	4	Irritable crying	Inappropriate words	Confused
	3	Inappropriate screaming/ crying	Screams	Inappropriate
	2	Grunts	Grunts	Garbled
	1	No response	No response	No response

Adapted from Marcoux, K. (2005).

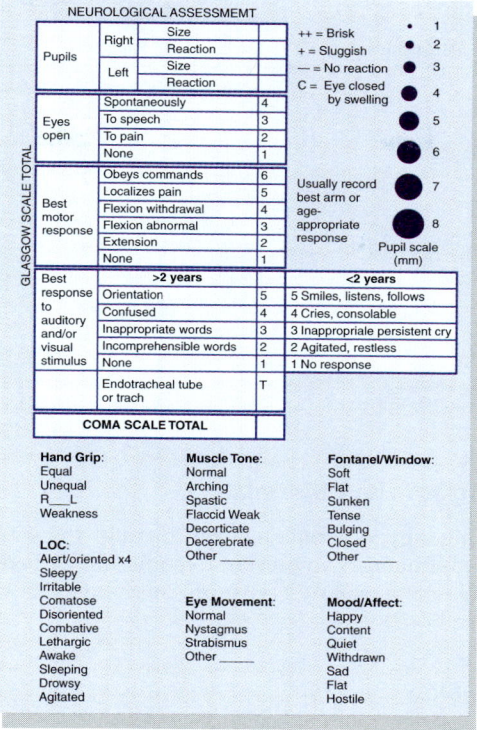

Figure 26-1 Pediatric Glasgow Coma Scale.

Assigning a Numeric Value for Level of Response with Modified GCS

- Assign a value to each level of response (1–5); highest score is 15 (unaltered state of consciousness).
- 8 or below: Coma
- 3: Deep coma
- Coma scale scores may fluctuate if a change in neurological state occurs (e.g., cerebral ischemia, administration of paralytics and sedatives, regaining of consciousness).

Signs and Symptoms of Increased Intracranial Pressure in Infants

Early Signs and Symptoms	Late Signs and Symptoms
Headache	Further decrease in level of consciousness (LOC)
Emesis	Bulging fontanels (infant)
Change in LOC	Decreasing spontaneous movements
Decrease in GCS score	Posturing
Irritability	Papilledema
Sunsetting eyes	Pupil dilation with decreased or no response to light
Decreased eye contact (infant)	Increased blood pressure
Pupil dysfunction	Irregular respirations
Cranial nerve dysfunction	Cushing's triad (late, ominous sign)
Seizures	

Adapted from Marcoux, K. (2005). Management of increased intracranial pressure in the ill child with an acute neurological injury. *AACN Advanced Critical Care, 16*(2), 212–231.

Assessing for Hypothermia

When using a hypothermia blanket, monitor the patient's temperature continuously to prevent hypothermia (a body temperature below 95°F or 35°C). Hypothermia causes shivering and an increase in ICP.

Kernig's Sign

Classic finding on examination for a child suspected of meningitis include a positive Kernig's or Brudzinski sign (Behrman, Kleigman, & Jenson, 2004).

- Place child in the supine position with hips flexed.
- When the lower leg is raised to straighten it, the child cries out or resists the leg extension.
- It is an abnormal finding if the child experiences pain behind the knee when it is fully extended.
- Bilateral increased resistance and pain upon extension of the knee is a positive Kernig sign and may indicate meningeal irritation.

Brudzinski Sign

- Lie the child flat.
- Attempt to raise the child's head toward her chest and place the chin on the chest.

- If there is pain or resistance, the child will immediately flex the hip and knee, which indicates meningeal inflammation may be present (Bickley & Szilagyi, 2003).

Reye Syndrome

There are several stages of Reye syndrome. The child may progress through all of the stages or stop at any stage if treatment is effective (McCance & Huether, 2002).

The Stages of Reye Syndrome

Stage I: Lethargy, vomiting, drowsiness, liver dysfunction
Stage II: Disorientation, combativeness, aggressiveness, delirium, hyperactive reflexes, hyperventilation, shallow breathing, stupor, liver dysfunction
Stage III: Obtundation, coma, decorticate posturing hyperventilation
Stage IV: Deepening coma, large fixed pupils, decerebrate posturing, loss of focular reflexes, liver dysfunction
Stage V: Loss of deep tendon reflexes, seizures, flaccidity, respiratory arrest, usually no liver dysfunction

Head Circumference Measurement	
Birth to 3 months (average head size at birth is 33–38 cm, 12–14 inches)	Head circumference increases 2 cm/month (0.75 inch)
4–6 months (average head size at 6 months is 43 cm, 17 inches)	Head circumference increases 1 cm/month (0.4 inch); average head size at 6 months is 43 cm (17 inches)
6–12 months (average head size at 1 year is 46 cm, 18 inches) By one year of age the child's head size has increased by 33%	Head circumference increases 0.5 cm/month (0.2 inch); average head size at 1 year is 46 cm (18 inches)

Near Drowning (Submersion Injuries)

- A submersion injury occurs when the child is submerged in water tries to breathe and aspirates water (wet drowning) or has a laryngospasm without aspiration (dry drowning).
- The most significant contributing factors to morbidity and mortality are hypoxemia with decreasing oxygen delivery to vital tissues.

- Central nervous system (CNS) damage may occur during the incident (primary injury) or may result from ongoing pulmonary injury, injury due to reperfusion, or multiorgan dysfunction (secondary injury).
- Early resuscitation is associated with an improved prognosis.
- Clinicians use an Orlowski scale to predict the likelihood of neurologically intact survival (Verive, 2006).

Orlowski Scale

Each item listed below is assigned one point. If a child has a score of 2 or less, there is a 90% likelihood of a complete recovery. If a child has a score of 3 or more, there is a 5% chance of survival (Verive, 2006).

- Three years of age or older
- Submersion time greater than 5 minutes
- No resuscitation efforts for more than 10 minutes after rescue
- Comatose on admission to the emergency room
- Arterial pH <7.10

Shaken Baby Syndrome

- Shaken baby syndrome results from major rotational forces and angular deceleration encountered when an infant is shaken forcefully (intentional or unintentional).
- Most victims are younger than 6 months of age and the source of the abuse is usually the father or a male acquaintance of the mother.
- The prognosis for an infant depends on the severity of the injury and response to medical therapy.
- A child may experience neuromotor impairment, visual impairment, and developmental delays.

Signs and Symptoms
- Seizure activity
- Apnea
- Bulging or full fontanelles
- Coma
- Hemorrhage
- Bradycardia
- Complete cardiovascular collapse

Symptoms Exhibited in Less Severe Shaken Baby Syndrome Cases

- Vomiting
- Hypothermia
- Poor feeding
- Failure to thrive
- Increased sleeping
- Lethargy
- Irritability
- Difficulty arousing
- The hallmark of shaken baby syndrome is an absence of external trauma to the head, face, and neck of an infant along with massive intracranial or intraocular pressure.

Hirschberg Asymmetrical Corneal Light Reflex Test

- Hold a penlight or flashlight in front of the child's face. Note the light reflection on the cornea in both eyes.
- Negative corneal light reflex exam (and normal muscle alignment) is when there is symmetrical placement on both eyes at the same time and in the same location on each eye.
- A positive asymmetrical corneal light reflex test (suggestive of strabismus) is when the light falls slightly medially to the center of the pupil on the iris. If this occurs, perform a cover test.

CLINICAL ALERTS

Monroe–Kellie Hypothesis

- The pressure–volume relationship between the blood, intracranial pressure (ICP), volume of cerebrospinal fluid (CSF), and brain tissue and cerebral perfusion pressure is the Monroe–Kellie hypothesis or Monroe–Kellie doctrine.
- This hypothesis states that if one of the components increases, the other components must compress (LeJune & Howard-Fain, 2002).
- The body tries to compensate by an increase in cerebrospinal fluid absorption, by a decrease in CSF production, by a reduction in blood volume or by a decrease in brain mass.
- When compression is exhausted, the intracranial pressure will rise.

- As a result of increased ICP, blood flow and oxygen delivery may be compromised.
- When blood flow and oxygen decrease, secondary brain injury occurs (Marcoux, 2005).

Patient Safety

When a child has increased ICP never place her head lower than her body. This position significantly increases the pressure more.

Seizure Precautions

- Maintain airway patency.
- Maintain a safe environment
- Do not place anything in the child's mouth during a seizure. A loose tooth may be aspirated or knocked out.
- Monitor oxygenation. Ensure the child's color remains pink; the pulse oximeter should read 95% or greater and the heart rate should be normal or slightly raised.
- Administer intravenous medications during a seizure slowly to reduce the risk of side effects such as respiratory or circulatory failure.
- Raise and pad the side rails of the crib or bed to protect the child from harm.
- Recommend that a helmet be worn to protect his head.
- Encourage the use of a medical identification bracelet at all times.

Cricoid Pressure

With neurological injuries apply cricoid pressure or empty the stomach contents with a nasogastric tube to avoid vomiting during intubation (Orlowski & Szpilman, 2001).

Autonomic Dysreflexia

- Autonomic dysreflexia is a stress syndrome caused by massive amounts of stimuli overloading the autonomic system, resulting in hyperactive sympathetic stimulation.
- Autonomic dysreflexia leads to extreme anxiety, headache, visual and auditory sensation changes, nausea, seizures, hypertension, peripheral vascular dilation or flushing, and bradycardia.

- Immediate management of hypertension and cardiac, and neurological complications is required.

DIAGNOSTIC TESTS

Determining Increased Intracranial Pressure (ICP)

- Magnetic resonance imaging (MRI) or computerized tomography (CT) is used to determine etiology and severity of increased ICP.
- Avoid computed tomography (CT) contrast in the presence of intracranial bleeding.
- Monitor ICP by inserting an intracranial catheter.

Brain Abscess

- Serum laboratory studies may be ordered (CBC, blood cultures, C-reactive protein).
- Usually moderate leukocytosis and elevated erythrocyte rate and C-reactive protein level occur.
- If the abscess is aspirated, culture the specimen to identify causative microorganism (Brook, 2004).

Hydrocephalus

- Use CT, MRI, and ultrasound to diagnose hydrocephalus.
- Cisternogram may be used to evaluate CSF flow dynamics in brain and spinal cord. This procedure reveals CSF concentration, leakage, obstruction, and pressure.

Audiologic Testing

One or several procedures may be used. The otoacoustic emissions test (OAE) and auditory brain stem evoked response (ABER) determine the degree of hearing loss.

MEDICATIONS

Phenytoin (Dilantin)

- Phenytoin (Dilantin) may cause gingival hyperplasia.
- The nurse observes for swelling and bleeding of the child's gums and provides good dental hygiene.

- Parents need to be taught the necessity of performing proper hygiene.

Mannitol (man-i-tol) (Osmitrol)

Classification(s) Osmotic Diuretic, Diagnostic Agent

Indications Reduction of intracranial pressure and treatment of cerebral edema

Action Increases the osmolarity of the glomerular filtrate, preventing the reabsorption of water and resulting in a loss of sodium chloride and water

Contraindications Use cautiously with dehydration, pulmonary congestion, renal disease and active intracranial bleeding (except during craniotomy)

Incompatibilities Do not add to blood products.

Adverse Reactions and Side Effects Seizures, hypotension, tachycardia, skin necrosis with infiltration, hyponatremia, diuresis, and urticaria

Route and Dosage Dosage for children <12 years of age not established

Nursing Implications
1. Do not administer electrolyte-free mannitol with blood products. If blood is administered, add at least 20 mEq of NaCl to each liter of mannitol.
2. Do not expose mannitol to low temperatures. If crystallization occurs, warm the bottle in a hot water bath and cool the medication to body temperature before administering.
3. Monitor serum electrolytes throughout therapy.

Data from Deglin, J., & Vallerand, A. (2009). Davis's drug guide for nurses (11th ed.), pp. 770–771. Philadelphia: F.A. Davis.

Seizure Medications

Type of Seizure	Medication	Dose Range	Adverse Reactions	Nursing Care
Partial Complex (Psychomotor)	Carbamazepine (Tegretol)	10–30 mg/kg per day in divided doses. Increase until best response is achieved.	Drowsiness, nausea, liver changes, increased appetite	Give with food but not milk.
	Valproic acid (Depakene)	0.1–0.2 mg/kg per day in two or three divided doses per day	Confusion, ataxia, nystagmus, nausea, gingival hyperplasia, bleeding disorders	Always give with food and monitor serum drug levels. Teach parents about oral hygiene and wear a medical alert tag. Teach parents to watch for adverse effects indicating toxicity.
	Phenytoin (Dilantin)	5 mg/kg per day in two to three divided doses	May cause dizziness, drowsiness, or physical incoordination. Avoid abrupt discontinuation of use. Daily multivitamin is recommended while on this medication.	Give with water, juice, or milk.
	Phenobarbital (Luminal)	Infants: 5–6 mg/kg per day in one or two divided doses		

Type of Seizure	Medication	Dose Range	Adverse Reactions	Nursing Care
	Fosphenytoin (Cerebyx)	Children 1–6 years: 6–8 mg/kg per day in one or two divided doses Loading dose of 10–20 mg/kg. Then 4–6 mg/kg per day		
Generalized Tonic–Clonic	Valproic acid (Depakene) and carba-mazepine (Tegretol) Phenytoin (Dilantin) Phenobarbital Ketogenic diet high in fat and low in protein and carbohydrates	May be an inexpensive medication. Causes a high level of ketones which decrease myoclonic or tonic–clonic seizure activity.	Monitor for sleepiness, hyperactivity, drowsiness, and school performance changes. Nausea, vomiting, headache, drowsiness, dizziness	This diet is hard to maintain for a long period of time because of the lack of food variety and difficulty of food preparation and parental involvement.
Absence (Petit Mal)	Ethosuximide (Zarontin) or Valproic acid	3–8 mg/kg per day		Avoid antacids.
Partial Simple	Topiramate (Topamax)	1–3 mg/kg per day	Weight loss, dizziness, diarrhea, cognitive dysfunction	Avoid antidepressants and antacids.

Community Education about DEET (N,N-diethyl-m-toluamide)

- Educate the community about DEET. Insect repellents containing DEET (N,N-diethyl-m-toluamide, also known as N,N-diethyl-3-methylbenzamide) with a concentration of 10% appear to be as safe as products with a concentration of 30% when used according to the directions on the product labels.
- The American Academy of Pediatrics recommends that repellents with DEET should not be used on infants younger than 2 months old.

Antimicrobial Therapy Used in Brain Abscesses

- Meningitis: Neonates: Cefotaxime+ampicillin; infants and children: ceftriaxone or cefotaxime+vancomycin
- Cyanotic congenital heart disease: Ampicillin+ chloramphenicol, or ceftriaxone+metronidazole, or ampicillin-sulbactam
- Otitis or sinusitis: Ampicillin+chloramphenicol, ceftriaxone+metronidazole or ampicillin-sulbactam
- Ventriculoperitoneal shunt or trauma: Vancomycin+antipseudomonal cephalosporin (i.e., cefepime or ceftazidime)
- Immunocompromised: Vancomycin+ceftazidime +metronidazole. If no response within 7 days, Amphotericin B should be added
- Endocarditis: prostatic valve: Vancomycin+gentamicin or ceftazidime; natural valve: ampicillin or an aminoglycoside or penicillin+ceftriaxone

Medications Containing Acetylsalicylic Acid

Non-prescription	Prescription	Topical
Alka-Seltzer	Darvon	Acne cleaners
Excedrin	Norgesic	Acne creams
Pepto-Bismol	Robaxisal	Astringents
Anacin	Talwin	Facial masks
Kaopectate	Butalbital	Wart removers
Pamprin	Percodan	Dandruff shampoos
	Roxiprin	Muscle pain relief creams
	Lortab	Wintergreen scented oils
	Propoxyphene	Arthritis pain rubs
	Soma	Facial scrubs
		Sport strength sun block

ETHNOCULTURAL CONSIDERATIONS

Head Circumference in Infants of Asian Heritage

- Infants of Asian heritage generally have smaller head circumferences than Caucasian infants.
- When Asian infants are measured, the measurement obtained may indicate the infant is SGA; this may in fact not be true.
- The infant may be considered to be at risk for medical diseases and complications based on the data, which may be based on inaccurate conclusions.

TEACHING THE FAMILY

General Instructions

- Provide the family with specific instructions for care if the child will be cared for at home.
- Communicate information about bathing, feeding, medical equipment, tracheostomy suctioning, gastrostomy tubes, urinary catheterization, positioning, and range-of-motion exercises.
- Stress the importance of performing these procedures correctly.
- To validate parental understanding, require parents to demonstrate the tasks. Parents may appear reluctant and fearful.
- Remain supportive and patient as parents learn new skills.

Reye Syndrome

- Instruct parents not to administer any product containing acetylsalicylic acid (aspirin) to a child younger than the age of 19 because of the risk of Reye syndrome.

Ventricular Shunts

- Continuous monitoring and assessment is essential because hydrocephalus is a lifelong disorder.
- Recognize complications: Increased ICP and shunt malfunction (kinking, plugging within the ventricle from tissue, or exudate or obstruction at the distal end from thrombosis or displacement of tubing due to growth).
- Observe for signs of infection: Nausea and vomiting, headache, change in customary behavior, lethargy, unresponsiveness, elevated temperature.
- Instruct parents that the child cannot participate in contact sports.
- Emphasize the importance of safe transport and positioning during transport.

Language Disorder

- Encourage caregivers to help the children how to say speech sounds correctly, improve language comprehension, and develop conversational skills.

- Inform caregivers that the disorder may impact the child's educational and social interactions.
- Advise the family about how to find a speech pathologist in the community

ADDITIONAL INFORMATION FOR THE CLINICAL SETTING

Benefits of Massage

- Helps promote a sense of well-being and enhances self-esteem while benefiting the immune and circulatory systems.
- The resulting sense of well-being decreases the amounts of the circulating stress hormones cortisol and norepinephrine that may weaken the immune system.
- Decreased anxiety and tension allows people to feel more serene and enhances their ability to cope with life stressors.
- Different massage techniques have been integrated into various complementary therapies.
  - Gentle massage or stroking releases endorphins (the body's natural pain killers) and a feeling of comfort is experienced.
  - Stronger, more vigorous massage helps to stretch tense and uncomfortable muscles, leading to improved mobility and flexibility.
- Aids in relaxation by affecting the body system that controls blood pressure, digestion, and respiration.
- The stimulation of circulation improves the supply of oxygen and nutrients to the body's tissues and enhances skin tone.
- Stimulation of the lymphatic system improves the body's ability to eliminate lactic acid and other chemical wastes that cause muscle stiffness and pain (Woodham & Peters, 2006).

Cushing's Triad

- A child with significantly increased intracranial pressure may exhibit Cushing's triad. Symptoms of Cushing's triad

are hypertension (with widening pulse pressure), bradycardia, and an irregular respiratory pattern.
- Cushing's triad is usually indicative of impending herniation (the displacement of the foramen magnum) (Venes, 2005)

Intravenous Fluids

- Avoid hypotonic intravenous fluids (i.e., D5W) because they cross the blood–brain barrier, resulting in increased cerebral edema and ICP.

Intracranial Pressure Monitoring

- To monitor ICP accurately, a pressure line may be inserted. Several types of monitoring devices are available, including intracranial bolts, intraventricular catheters, and intraparenchymal fiber optic catheters.
- ICP monitoring is indicated for the child who has a Glasgow Coma Scale (GSC) score of less than 8, exhibits signs of increasing ICP, is status post major neurosurgical procedures, or has a high probability of having increased ICP.
- The best outcome for ICP monitoring is to maintain cerebral perfusion pressure between 50 and 70 mm Hg, maintain ICP at <20 mm Hg, and detect occurrences such as herniation or bleeding (Marcoux, 2005).

Signs and Symptoms of Seizures

Type of Seizures	Brain Location/Cause	Signs and Symptoms
Partial (focal)	Localized to one area	One area affected: Hands, lips, wrist, arms face. Impaired loss of consciousness at onset.
Partial Complex (psychomotor)	Temporal lobe	Loss of consciousness and loss of awareness or surrounding. Change in behavior: Lip smacking, picking, inappropriate mannerisms, confusion follows the seizure. *(continued)*

Signs and Symptoms of Seizures (Continued)

Type of Seizures	Brain Location/Cause	Signs and Symptoms
Partial Simple		Lasts 5 minutes, child only remembers the aura. Automatisms are noted. No loss of consciousness or awareness. Motor signs are isolated to one area of the body and then spread to the rest of the body. May experience senses such as buzzing sounds, tingling, flashing lights, anxiety, fear or anger.
Generalized Tonic–Clonic	Genetic predisposition or brain injury secondary to anoxia.	Partial simple and complex seizures evolve to generalized seizures. Aura is experienced followed by loss of consciousness and tone. Patient falls to the floor with tonic clonic muscle contractions. Patient is postictal and confused after the seizure is over. Loss of urine may occur.
Atonic: Loss of muscle tone, drop attacks. Absence (petitmal) Tonic Myoclonic Clonic Myoclonic and Akinetic	Metabolic etiology	Sudden drop to the floor due to loss of motor muscle tone. Seen in children 2–4 years of age. No loss of consciousness but experiences loss of awareness. Nonconvulsive. Periods of staring or minor movements lasting seconds. May occur several times a day, interferes with learning and school work. Stiffening of the body that is sustained, involving all four extremities. Single or multiple jerks or flexion of limbs. Intermittent rhythmic jerking, one to three per second, may start in one body location and move or migrate to another location. Complete or total lack of movement

Source: Fox (2002).

Nursing Care for the Child Having a Seizure

1. Call for help (in a hospital setting use the designated emergency number; in the community setting, call 911).
2. Maintain safe environment and a patent airway. If the airway is occluded, open the airway with a jaw thrust maneuver. Administer oxygen if needed and available. Do not put anything in the mouth. If the situation warrants emergency medical care, qualified health care personnel can insert an appropriate sized oral airway.
3. Place the child on his side to prevent aspiration of secretions.
4. Loosen restrictive clothing to ensure adequate circulation to essential body organs.
5. Administer medications such as diazepam (Valium), lorazepam (Ativan), or fosphenytoin (Cerebryx) as ordered by the physician. An exception is in the neonate where these medications become toxic due to immature liver function.
6. Continue to monitor respiratory status and circulatory status throughout the seizure.
7. When the seizure is over, place the child in the recovery position or the left lateral recumbent position.
8. Inform the child that he or she has just had a seizure. Tell the family that the child may still be confused and disoriented for a short time.
9. Stay with the child (support is essential because a seizure can be frightening to both the child and family).
10. Document important details about the seizure (e.g., time and duration of seizure, antecedent activity or event, type or description of the seizure, assessment data, care measures provided such as positioning, oxygen, suctioning, mechanical ventilation or CPR, medication administration, physician notification or presence at the child's side, and response to seizure such as condition and disposition of the child after the seizure).

Complications from Encephalitis

- The complications may include motor or cognitive deficits, seizure disorders, hearing or vision loss, memory loss, and paralysis (Wisniewski, 2003).

- If a child has permanent or lingering problems, the treatment plan for them may be multidisciplinary.
- This multidisciplinary approach optimizes the child's recovery and maximizes skills necessary for life.

Liver Biopsy

- Monitor bleeding after a liver biopsy because child is predisposed to bleeding as the liver is highly vascular.
- After the biopsy, the physician places a dressing to splint the puncture site. Lie the child on the right side for 2 hours (Lewis et al., 2007).

Preventing Injury of the Sac (Spina Bifida)

- Use sterile technique to cover the defect as quickly as possible with a sterile, non-adherent dressing that is moistened with sterile saline to maintain moisture and prevent drying.
- Change dressing every 2 to 4 hours or as prescribed or when soiled.

Rectal Temperature

Do not obtain a rectal temperature of a child with spina bifida because rectal irritation and rectal prolapse may occur.

Ventricular Shunts

- A shunt may be placed to drain excessive intracranial CSF.
- Ventricular shunts have greatly improved the quality of life for children with hydrocephalus.
- A ventricular shunt consists of several parts including a proximal catheter that enters the lateral ventricle, a one-way valve that is set at a desired pressure to prevent CSF being drained too fast due to gravity, a small reservoir, and a distal catheter that terminates in the peritoneal cavity or alternate drainage site.
- The peritoneal cavity is the preferred site for placement of the distal catheter because of easy accessibility and decreased risk of complications.
- When the catheter is placed in the peritoneum, the shunt is called a ventriculoperitoneal shunt.

Measuring Head Circumference

 Procedure 26-1 Measuring Head Circumference

Purpose

Measuring head circumference is an important component of evaluation of a child's growth as well as his health status.

Equipment

- Flexible nonstretchable tape measure
- Child's chart

Steps

1. Obtain a flexible nonstretchable tape measure (preferably one in which one end inserts into the other end).
2. Allow the parent to hold the child in his or her arms or lap.
3. Remove braids, barrettes, or other hair decorations.
4. Place the tape measure over the most prominent part of the occiput (back of the head) and just above the supraorbital ridges (above the eyebrows).
5. Pull the tape measure snugly to compress the hair and underlying tissues.
6. Read the measurement to the nearest 0.1 cm or 1/8 inch.
7. Document the measurement on the chart.

Clinical Alert If an abnormal circumference is found based on the child's age, reposition the tape and measure the head circumference again. The new measurement should agree with the first measurement within 0.2 cm or 1/4 inch.

Teach Parents

To help ensure an accurate head circumference measurement, teach the parents how to hold the child firmly while offering verbal comfort and encouragement.

Intravenous Therapy

- If shunt surgery is anticipated, the nurse should not use scalp veins for intravenous therapy because the IV may be located near the surgical site.

Basal Skull Fracture

- Do not insert a nasogastric tube if a basal skull fracture is suspected because the tube may enter the brain through fracture.
- Insert an orogastric tube if needed (Brettler, 2004).

Common Acute Eye Disorders

Eye Disorder	Cause/Organism	Signs and Symptoms	Treatment
Conjunctivitis	An inflammation of the conjunctiva	Excessive tearing, erythematous, edema and with clear, watery, yellow or green drainage and eyelid crusting	Apply warm soaks to remove crusting, use good hand hygiene and apply cool compresses to edematous eyes.
Neonatal Conjunctivitis–Ophthalmia Neonatorium	Chemical irritation caused by maternal sexually transmitted diseases acquired at birth such as *Chlamydia, gonorrhea,* herpes.	Purulent drainage either white or yellowish.	Prophylactic antibiotic ointment is used in all neonates. Lack of treatment can cause eye damage.
Sty	A localized inflammatory swelling of one or more of the glands of the eyelid.	Painful, erythematous lesion on the lid margin. Slight edema, some lymph node tenderness or induration.	Apply warm moist compresses with an antibiotic ointment. Good hand hygiene is necessary.
Chalazion	Granuloma of the meibomian gland on the eyelid.	Hard, small nodule on either eye lid may be painful.	Apply warm moist compresses and massage, antibiotic ointment, may resolve the condition spontaneously.

Continued

Common Acute Eye Disorders (Continued)

Eye Disorder	Cause/Organism	Signs and Symptoms	Treatment
Blepharitis Marginalis	Staphylococcal infection of the lid margin.	Erythematous eyelid margin with crusted eye drainage.	Apply an antibiotic ointment to the lower affected eye lid. Apply warm moist compresses to remove crusting drainage.
Keratitis	Inflammation and infection of the corneal layers due to bacterial, viral, fungal, or foreign body infiltration.	Very painful, excessive tearing, photophobia, and erythema.	An ophthalmologist must examine the cornea to monitor or treat potential scarring and prevent loss of vision.
Periorbital Cellulitis	Inflammation of the subcutaneous tissues and skin about the eye may be bacterial or viral.	Edema, pain, erythema in the skin and orbital folds of the affected eye.	Use intravenous antibiotic therapy for 7 days.
Blocked Tear Duct (Dacryostenosis/ Dacryocystitis)	Obstruction of the nasolacrimal tear duct causing inflammation or cystitis.	Tearing, yellow drainage, crusting, small bump in the inner canthus of the affected eye. Usually unilateral, may be painful.	Apply warm compresses and gentle massage of the lacrimal sac with the forefinger milking any exudates toward the nose.

Chemical Burns

- Prompt assessment is essential.
- Monitor for signs of infection, hemorrhage, and increased intraocular pressure (IOP). Provide emotional and social support for the child and family.
- Follow-up care for evaluation of the cornea for scarring and IOP testing to determine post inflammatory response is necessary.
- Patching and administering eye medication may be required at home.
- School and normal activities are allowed after physician consultation.

Communicating with the Hearing Impaired Child

- Recognize behavioral cues suggestive of hearing loss.
- Obtain the child's attention before speaking.
- Face the child when speaking.
- Position yourself at the child's eye level.
- Speak slowly and loudly.
- Modify the environment; unnecessary noises should be reduced.
- Offer emotional support: a child with a hearing loss may face a potential stigma associated with his communication difficulty.

RESOURCES

American Academy of Pediatrics:
http://www.bt.cdc.gov/cdclinkdisclaimer.asp?a_gotolink=http://www.aap.org/family/wnv-jun03.htm

About Pediatrics.com:
http://pediatrics.about.com/cs/conditions/a/hydrocephalus_2.htm

About Pediatrics.com:
http://pediatrics.about.com/cs/conditions/a/hydrocephalus2.htm About Pediatrics.com

About Pediatrics.com:
http://pediatrics.about.com/cs/weeklyquestion/a/032002_ask.htm

American Foundation for the Blind Information Center:
http://www.afb.org

American Society for Deaf Children: http://www.deafchildren.org

American Speech-Language-Hearing Association:
http://www.asha.org

Alexander Graham Bell Association for the Deaf and Hard of Hearing: http://www.agbell.org

Colored blindness:
http://www.nlm.nih.gov/medlineplus/colorblindness.html

American Deafness and Rehabilitation Association:
http://www.adara.org

Centers for Disease Control and Prevention:
http://www.cdc.gov/ncbddd/autism/actearly

Epilepsy Foundation: http://www.epilepsyfoundation.org

Individuals with Disability Education Act of 2004 (IDEA): http://idea.ed.gov

March of Dimes: http://www.marchofdimes.com

Meningitis Foundation of America: http://www.musa.org

National Association of Neonatal Nurses: http://www.NANN.org

National Eye Institute: http://www.nei.nih.gov

National Headache Foundation: http://www.headaches.org

National Institute on Deafness and other Communication Disorders: http://www.nidcd.nih.gov/health/statistics/hearing.asa

Normal Growth of Young Children: http://pediatrics.about.com/cs/weeklyquestion/a/032002_ask.htm

National Institutes on Disability and Rehabilitation Research: http://www.ed.gov/about/contact/gen/index.htmo?src_1n

National Institute of Neurological Disorders and Stroke: http://www.ninds.nih.gov

National Reye's Syndrome, Inc.: http://www.reyessyndrome.org

National Spinal Cord Injury Association: http://www.spinalcord.org

Spina Bifida Association of America: http://www.sbaa.org

US Department of Health and Human Services: Health Resources and Services Administration Maternal and Child Health Bureau: http://depts.washington.edu/growth/module5/text/page5a.htm

REFERENCES

Behrman, R., Kleigman, R., & Jenson, H. (2004). *Nelson textbook of pediatrics* (16th ed.). Philadelphia: W.B. Saunders.

Bickley, L., & Szilagyi, P. (2003). *Bate's guide to physical examination and history taking* (8th ed.). Philadelphia: Lippincott Williams & Wilkins.

Brettler, S. (2004). Trauma nursing: Traumatic brain injury. Retrieved from http://www.rnweb.com/rnweb/article/articleDetail.jsp?id=110100 (Accessed July 22, 2008).

Brook, I. (2004). Microbiology and management of brain abscess in children. *Journal of Pediatric Neurology*, 2(3), 125–130.

Deglin, J., & Vallerand, A. (2009). *Davis's drug guide for nurses* (11th ed.). Philadelphia: F.A. Davis.

Fox, J.A. (2002). *Primary health care of infants, children and adolescents.* St Louis, MO: C.V. Mosby.

LeJune, M., & Howard-Fain, T. (2002). Caring for patients with increased intracranial pressure. *Nursing, 32*(11), 1–5.

Lewis, S., Heitkemper, M., Dirksen, S., O'Brien, P., & Bucher, L. (2007). *Medical-surgical nursing: Assessment and management of clinical problems.* St. Louis, MO: Mosby Elsevier.

Marcoux, K. (2005). Management of increased intracranial pressure in the ill child with an acute neurological injury. *AACN Advanced Critical Care, 16*(2), 212–231. Retrieved from http://www.nursingcenter.com/library/JournalArticle. asp? Article_ID=594176 (Accessed January 4, 2007).

McCance, K., & Huether, S. (2002). *Pathophysiology: The biologic basis for disease in adults and children* (4th ed.). St. Louis, MO: C.V. Mosby.

Orlowski, J.P., & Szpilman, D. (2001). Drowning: Rescue, resuscitation, and reanimation. *Pediatric Clinics of North America, 48*(3), 627–646.

Venes, D. (Ed.). (2005). *Taber's cyclopedic medical dictionary.* Philadelphia: F.A. Davis.

Verive, M. (2006). Near drowning. Retrieved from www.emedicine.com/ped/ topic/2570.htm (Accessed November 23, 2008).

Wisniewski, A. (2003). Closing in on clues to encephalitis. *Nursing, 33*(4), 70–71.

Woodham, A., & Peters, D. (2006). Healing massage. *Saturday Evening Post,* May/June, 2006.

Caring for the Child with a Musculoskeletal Condition

KEY TERMS

cast syndrome – Results when a child is placed in a spica cast and a portion of the duodenum is compressed between the superior mesenteric artery and the aorta, causing vomiting, abdominal distention, and bowel obstruction

closed reduction – Treatment of bone fractures by placing the bones in their proper position without surgery (Venes, 2005)

compartment syndrome – Caused by an accumulation of fluid in the fascia; increases the pressure on the muscles, blood vessels, and nerve tissue that the fascia surrounds; too much pressure can cause tissue ischemia, nerve damage, and necrosis

open reduction – Treatment of bone fractures by the use of surgery to place the bones in their proper position (Venes, 2005)

FOCUSED ASSESSMENT

Performing the Neurovascular Assessment

Neurovascular status must be assessed carefully and every 1 to 2 hours for the first 48 hours and then every 4 hours after that if there is no compromise in circulation.

Pain

- Does the child complain of pain in the affected limb?
- Is it relieved by narcotic medication?

- Does it become worse when fingers or toes are flexed? If yes, notify the physician immediately (compartment syndrome).

Sensation
- Can the child feel touch on the extremity?
- Is two-point discrimination decreased? If yes, notify the physician immediately (compartment syndrome).

Motion
- Can the child move fingers or toes?
- Lack of movement may indicate nerve damage.

Temperature
- Does the affected limb feel warm?
- Does it feel cool? A cool extremity may change to feeling warm if a blanket is placed over it and the extremity is elevated. If the extremity is still cool after these interventions, there is poor circulation.

Capillary Refill Time (CRT)

Apply brief pressure to the nail bed and note how quickly pink color returns to the nail bed (normal, <3 seconds; circulation is poor if >3 seconds) (Fig. 27-1).

Color
- Note the color of the affected limb. Compare that color to the color of the unaffected limb. Pink is the norm.
- If the color is paler than in the unaffected limb, circulation is poor.

Figure 27-1 Assessing capillary refill time.

Pulses

- Check pulses distal to the injury or cast.
- If the pulse is difficult to locate, assess the area with a Doppler and mark the spot with an 'X'. If the cast covers the foot or hand, this may not be possible to assess.

Slipped Capital Femoral Epiphysis

Stage

- Preslip: The child complains of weakness in the leg. There is pain in knee or hip when standing or walking for long periods of time.
- Acute slip: The child falls and then reports hip pain.
- Chronic slip: The femoral head gradually slips off the femoral neck and then remodels for the incorrect position.
- Acute to chronic slip: Slow progressive slip that becomes more displaced.

Severity

- Grade I (preslip): Widening of the physis without any displacement of the epiphysis.
- Grade II (minimal slip): A one third displacement of the femoral head from the femoral neck.
- Grade III (moderate slip): More than one third but less than one half displacement of the femoral head from the femoral neck.
- Grade IV (severe slip): More than one half displacement of the femoral head from the femoral neck.

Classification of Fractures

- Classification of fractures is based on the location and description of the fracture.
- The location is where the fracture occurs along the shaft of the bone. Fractures are described in terms of the amount of injury.
- Closed fracture: No break in the skin.
- Open fracture: Bone has penetrated through the skin (type I, II, or III, based on the degree, severity of soft tissue damage, size of the wound, and amount of contamination), potential for infection is greatest with an open fracture.

Epiphyseal

- Type I: Separation of epiphysis; may be mistaken for a sprain; does not affect growth.
- Type II: Fracture separation of the epiphysis; circulation is intact; does not usually affect growth.
- Type III: Fracture through the epiphysis into the joint, does not usually affect growth if reduced properly.
- Type IV: Fracture through epiphysis into the joint and the metaphysis; open reduction and internal fixation necessary; can prevent growth disturbance.
- Type V: Rare occurrence; crush injury to epiphyseal plate; results in premature closure of epiphyseal plate and growth arrest.

Classification by Breaks

Transverse
Line crosses the shaft at a 90-degree angle.

Spiral
A diagonal line coils around the bone. Caused by a twisting force.

Oblique
A diagonal line across the bone.

Greenstick
Bone is bent, but not broken.
More common in children.

Comminuted
Three of more fractured fragments.

Compression
Bone becomes wider and more flat.
Usually seen in the spine.

Sprains

First Degree

- Mild; ligament is stretched and the affected joint is stable.
- Minimal pain, swelling, ecchymosis.
- Full range of motion and weight bearing.

Second Degree

- Moderate; ligament is partially torn and joint laxity is present.
- Moderate pain, swelling, and ecchymosis.
- Motion is slightly limited and painful.
- Mild joint laxity with tenderness over the joint.
- The patient may be unable to bear weight.

Third Degree

- Severe; ligament is completely torn and the joint is unstable.
- Significant swelling and severe ecchymosis occur within the first 30 minutes.
- Severe pain over the joint makes examination difficult.
- Cannot bear weight or otherwise use the extremity.

Gower Maneuver

- A child with muscular dystrophy uses the Gower maneuver to rise from the floor.
- The child moves to a kneeling position with hands on the floor to stabilize himself.
- With hands on the floor, he rises to his feet.
- The child uses his hands to walk up his legs until he reaches a standing position.

Scoliosis

- Scoliosis is a nonpainful lateral curvature of the spine and is the most common spinal deformity in children. The spine either curves laterally in only one direction ("C" curve) or in two opposite directions ("S" curve).
- The child is asked to bend at the waist with arms hanging loosely (Adam's position or bend over test) to determine scoliosis (Fig. 27-2).

Figure 27-2 By doing the Adam's test or bend over test, scoliosis is obvious.

CLINICAL ALERTS

Complication of the Child with a Fracture: Compartment Syndrome

- Complications can occur when a child is immobilized in a cast. The major complication that can occur is compartment syndrome, which is caused by an accumulation of fluid in the fascia.
- The classic sign of compartment syndrome is unrelenting pain that is unrelieved by narcotics.
- Notify the physician immediately.
- The best treatment of compartment syndrome is prevention. Prevention is achieved by elevating the extremity to prevent excessive swelling and frequent neurovascular checks.

Osteomyelitis

- Osteomyelitis is an inflammation of bone and marrow, usually caused by infection.
- Acute osteomyelitis is a serious complication that may be caused by open fracture, penetration of the skin by a contaminated object, a septic joint, infected wound, bacterial infection from somewhere else in body (like

dental caries), blunt trauma, premature babies and infants with birth complications the first year of life.

- All types of osteomyelitis require immediate treatment (broad-spectrum antibiotics after blood cultures are drawn).
- Evaluate the child's response to the antibiotic therapy about 2 or 3 days after the initial dose.
- If the child demonstrates a response to the intravenous antibiotic therapy at this point, more blood cultures are drawn, intravenous antibiotics are stopped, and the child continues therapy on oral antibiotics for 4 to 8 weeks at home.
- If the child demonstrates poor response to the intravenous antibiotic therapy, antibiotic therapy is continued for a much longer time period.

Chronic Osteomyelitis

- Chronic osteomyelitis is uncommon and occurs when bone tissue dies as a result of the lost blood supply.
- Children with chronic osteomyelitis have had symptoms for longer than 3 weeks and there is a history of prior bone infection within weeks or months after surgery or trauma.
- The treatment for chronic osteomyelitis is prolonged, painful, and frustrating for the child and family. For the first few days of hospitalization, the affected limb is placed in a splint. Oral analgesics, including acetaminophen (Children's Tylenol), ibuprofen (Children's Motrin), or narcotic analgesics such as acetaminophen with codeine (Percocet) can be used to manage pain.
- Make the child as comfortable as possible.
- Monitor intravenous site for infiltration because the antibiotics used to treat osteomyelitis are caustic to the veins. A peripherally inserted central catheter (PICC) or tunneled central line is placed if intravenous therapy continues for more than 2 to 3 days.
- Use diversional activities while activity is limited.

DIAGNOSTIC TESTS

Orthopedic Imaging Tests

Diagnostic Imaging Test	Benefits	Limitations
Radiograph	Easily available Visualizes fractures well No sedation needed Inexpensive	Two-dimensional Does not visualize soft tissue such as cartilage. Patient must be positioned properly. Radiation exposure
Fluoroscopy	Guides many orthopedic procedures Can be used with contrast Real-time radiography Inexpensive	Radiation exposure
Arthrography	Provides visualization of joints Three-dimensional view	Risk of reaction to contrast Depends on the skill of the radiographer Radiation exposure
Computed Tomography (CT scan)	Cross-sectional view of anatomy More clear than radiographs Software programs can show reconstruction Can use contrast	Expensive May require sedation Risk of reaction to contrast
Bone Scan (nuclear medicine)	Excellent at finding changes in bone as a result of infection, trauma, or tumor	Takes 4 hours Not always available on emergency basis Cannot distinguish benign from malignant tumors Radiation exposure to entire body IV access required
Ultrasound	Easily available No radiation No sedation needed Good for visualizing soft tissue masses and cysts Painless Inexpensive	Limited use Depends on the skill of the radiographer
Magnetic Resonance Imaging (MRI)	Visualizes hard and soft tissue and bone marrow No radiation	Not readily available No metal Sedation may be needed Need experienced radiologist to read MRI

Blood and Body Fluid Analysis for the Child with Alterations in Musculoskeletal Conditions

Diagnostic Test	Function of the Test	Indications	Normal Values
Complete Blood Count (CBC)	Blood sample that evaluates many components.	Lower platelet count indicates a bleeding disorder. Greater WBC count indicates a bacterial infection or septic arthritis.	Platelets: 150,000–400,000/μL WBCs: 4500–10,000/μL
CBC Differential	Breaks down WBCs into various types (five total). Numbers indicate a percentage of total WBCs. Gives an indication of the type of infection.	↑Monocytes indicate a long-term infectious process. ↑Lymphocytes indicate an increase in viral illness. ↑Eosinophils indicate an allergic or parasitic condition. ↑Basophils indicate a chronic inflammatory condition. ↑Neutrophils (Polys) -Bands are immature neutrophils. -Segs are mature neutrophils. An increase in the band neutrophils suggest a severe bacterial infection such as sepsis.	0% for bands and 31%–57% for segs Presence of bands is highly indicative of a bacterial infection.

Diagnostic Test	Function of the Test	Indications	Normal Values
C-Reactive Protein (CRP)	Measures a protein in blood that is released when an infection is present.	>0.9 indicates an infection or septic arthritis.	<1.0 mg/dL
Calcium and Phosphate	Measures the amount of these minerals.	Low levels may indicate rickets.	Calcium: 8.5–11 mg/dL Phosphorus: 3.0–4.5 mg/dL
Rheumatoid Factor (Rh factor)	Measures the body's autoimmune response to an antigen.	If positive, may indicate juvenile arthritis. Not all children with juvenile arthritis have a positive Rh factor.	Negative
Erythrocyte Sedimentation Rate (ESR)	Measures the speed at which RBCs settle out in solution.	Elevated indicates septic arthritis; may also indicate infection.	0–10 mm/hr
Blood Cultures	Measures whether organisms grow out in the laboratory.	Can identify an organism causing infection; 40% of children with septic arthritis have a positive blood culture.	No growth
Bone Biopsies	Diagnose tumor or infection of the bone.	Osteomyelitis Bone tumor	Normal bone cells
Fluid Aspiration from Joints	Diagnose an infection of the joint or drain fluid from a joint to relieve pressure.	Drainage is purulent. Culture of fluid is positive.	Clear fluid No growth from culture

MEDICATIONS

Medications for Juvenile Arthritis (JA)

- Use approved nonsteroidal anti-inflammatory drugs (NSAIDs): Ibuprofen (Children's Advil), naproxen (Aleve), tolmetin (Tolectin), and choline magnesium trisalicylate (Trilisate), indomethacin (Indocin), and diclofenac (Cataflam). An NSAID is selected based on dosing schedule, patient preference, or medication taste because there is a lack of agreement on the best NSAID for patients with Juvenile Arthritis (JA).
- Common disease-modifying antirheumatic drugs (an agent that prevents or relieves rheumatism) (DMARDs): medications are methotrexate (Rheumatrex) (most commonly prescribed), cyclophosphamide (Cytoxan), sulfasalazine (Azulfidine) and infliximab (Remicade). It is effective in polyarticular JA and has been used for the past 10 years. The most common side effect of methotrexate (Rheumatrex) is gastrointestinal symptoms.
- New drugs potentially available for use with juvenile arthritis are leflunomide (Arava) and etanercept (Enbrel). Leflunomide is an immunosuppressant. Side effects are diarrhea, elevated liver enzymes, alopecia, and rash. It has been approved for use in patients with adult rheumatoid arthritis (RA), but has not yet been approved for use with children. There is a teratogenic potential that would be of concern with children, particularly adolescent girls. Etanercept (Enbrel) reduces the signs and symptoms of moderately severe to severe polyarticular juvenile arthritis. It is a potent inhibitor of tumor necrosis factor (TNF), which is a key proinflammatory cytokine found in the synovial tissue of patients with JA (Ilowite, 2002).
- Infliximab (Remicade) is another TNF-neutralizing agent. Efficacy data are limited for use of this medication.
- Prednisone (Deltasone) and other corticosteroids are very potent and should be administered at the lowest possible dose and for the shortest possible period of time. Side effects such as Cushing syndrome, osteoporosis, increased risk of infection, glucose intolerance, cataracts, and growth retardation can occur.

Neuromuscular Blocking Agent

When caring for a child treated with a neuromuscular blocking agent, remember:

- The child has total paralysis, including respiratory function.
- The child is not able to communicate.
- The child is anxious.
- The child is aware of all activity around him or her.

The nurse can:

- Anticipate the child's needs.
- Explain all procedures.
- Never leave the child alone.
- Reduce the child's anxiety (e.g., use a calm and reassuring manner, support her fear, encourage parents to stay with the child).
- Medicate with an anxiolytic (antianxiety agent).

Medications Used in Tetanus (Lockjaw)

Medications are used to alleviate the muscle spasms and seizures.

- Diazepam (Valium) is the drug of choice to control seizures.
- Lorazepam (Ativan) is an anticonvulsant. It may cause respiratory depression, especially when used in combination with other sedatives. Onset of action is 1 to 5 minutes intravenously, 30 to 60 minutes intramuscularly and 20 to 30 minutes orally, with a duration of action of 6 to 8 hours.
- Intrathecal baclofen (Lioresal) is a centrally reacting skeletal muscle relaxant. Avoid abrupt withdrawal. Administer oral doses with food or milk. Use with caution in children with a seizure disorder or impaired renal function (Robertson & Shilkofski, 2005).
- Dantrolene sodium (Dantrium) is a skeletal muscle relaxant. Use caution when administering to a child with cardiac or pulmonary impairment. Avoid unnecessary exposure to light. Do not allow it to extravasate into the surrounding tissue. Discontinue if benefits are not evident in 45 days (Robertson & Shilkofski, 2005).
- Midazolam (Versed) may be effective, but is contraindicated in patients with narrow-angle glaucoma and shock because

it causes respiratory depression, hypotension, and bradycardia. Cardiovascular monitoring is necessary. Reduce doses when given in combination with narcotics or in patients with respiratory compromise. Serum concentrations may be increased by cimetidine (Tagamet), erythromycin, itraconazole, ketoconazole, and protease inhibitors. Sedative effects may be antagonized by theophylline. The effects of the medication can be reversed with flumazenil (Romazicon) (Robertson & Shilkofski, 2005).

- Use neuromuscular blocking agents when the child is suffering severe unresponsive tetanus. The following are two nondepolarizing neuromuscular blocking agents:

Rocuronium (Zemuron) may cause hypertension, hypotension, tachycardia, and bronchospasm. There is a risk of increased neuromuscular blockade when administered in conjunction with aminoglycosides, clindamycin, tetracycline, magnesium sulfate, quinine, quinidine, succinylcholine, and inhalation anesthetics. There is a risk of a reduction in neuromuscular blocking effects when used in conjunction with carbamazepine, phenytoin, azathioprine, and theophylline. Peak effects occur in 0.5 to 1 minute. Duration is 30 to 40 minutes (Robertson & Shilkofski, 2005).

- Vecuronium bromide (Norcuron) may cause arrhythmias, rash, and bronchospasm. Use with caution in patients with renal or hepatic failure and neuromuscular disease. Infants from 7 weeks to 1 year of age are more sensitive to the medication and may have a longer recovery period. Children from 1 to 10 years may need higher and more frequent doses. Potency can be increased with administration of enflurane, isoflurane, aminoglycosides, magnesium salts, tetracyclines, bacitracin, and clindamycin. Neostigmine, pyridostigmine and edrophonium are antidotes. Onset is 1 to 3 minutes. Duration is 30-90 minutes (Robertson & Shilkofski, 2005).

ETHNOCULTURAL CONSIDERATIONS

Caring for a Hispanic Child

Hispanics have the following beliefs and they must be respected:

- "Mal ojo" or Evil Eye is an illness that affects a child when someone with special powers looks at or admires the child

but does not touch the child. Touching a Hispanic child when making an admiring statement is important.
- Curanderos and curanderas treat a child through touch and prayer and have the child wear special amulets or charms to protect her.
- Saints help sick children and parents place holy pictures around the sick child.

TEACHING THE FAMILY

Instructions for Caregivers of a Child Who Is Casted for Clubfoot

- Call the physician if the child has a fever, infection, cast syndrome, or unrelieved pain.
- Take the child to the health care professional if the cast becomes loose, soft, or cracked.
- Perform good hygiene to prevent skin breakdown.
- Stimulate the child's development by reading and playing.
- Provide reassurance that when the cast is removed the child will quickly return to the expected developmental level.
- Encourage compliance with follow-up because there is potential for recurrence. Make first follow-up appointment with the parents for the child before the child is discharged.

Osteogenesis Imperfecta

Teach parents to:

- Watch for signs of a fracture (irritability, fever, refusal to eat).
- With an older child, watch for pain, swelling, and possible deformity at the site.

ADDITIONAL INFORMATION FOR THE CLINICAL SETTING

Preventing Cast Syndrome

- Reposition the child frequently.
- Encourage fluids and increased fiber in the child's diet.
- Cut a "belly hole" or a window to allow for abdominal expansion.

Procedure 27-1 Petaling a Cast

Purpose

The purpose of petaling a cast is to promote good hygiene by protecting the proximal edges of the long leg casts and the perineal area of the hip-spica casts from soiling.

Equipment

- Moleskin
- 1-inch waterproof adhesive tape
- Plastic bag to place adhesive tape on
- Scissors

Steps

1. Use scissors to cut 1-inch wide by 1 1/2 to 2 inches long strips of moleskin.

2. Use scissors to cut 1-inch wide strips of waterproof adhesive tape.

   The length of the waterproof adhesive tape should be about 1 1/2 to 2 inches long.

3. The edge on one end of both the moleskin and waterproof adhesive tape must be rounded.

4. Place strips of the 1-inch waterproof adhesive tape on the plastic bags.

5. Apply the first strip of waterproof adhesive tape to any edge of the cast that is likely to become soiled by urine or stool. Place the rounded ends of the moleskin and adhesive tape over the cast edge to the outside.

6. Tuck the straight (unrounded) end inside the cast.

Procedure 27-1 (Continued)

7. With your forefinger, gently ensure that the inside end is flat and not sticking to the child's skin.

8. Repeat the procedure, overlapping each additional strip, until all rough edges are completely covered.

9. Begin the same procedure with the moleskin to edges of the cast that are not likely to become soiled by urine and stool.

10. Document the procedure.

Clinical Alert It is a good idea to petal the edges of the cast that are likely to be soiled by urine and feces on the first postoperative day and preferably before the Foley catheter is removed.

Teach Parents

The nurse can teach the parents that diapering needs to be modified. To achieve this, a small diaper or peripad is placed in the perineal area with all edges of the cast outside this small diaper. Then a larger diaper is placed outside the smaller diaper and taped in the normal fashion. The nurse needs to ensure that the perineal edges of the cast remain outside of the diaper.

Skin Traction

Skin traction is used for an extremity with a type of strapping material applied to the limb. It is used for short periods of time.

Russell's Traction

- Used when the child weighs more than 26.4 lbs. (12 kg).
- Most often used to stabilize femur fractures until a callus forms or with Legg–Calve–Perthes disease.
- The child lies supine with hip flexed and abducted.
- There are two lines of pull in Russell's traction and the hips need to remain in alignment (Fig. 27-3).
- Secure a trapeze on a cross-bar above the bed to assist with repositioning and maintaining upper body strength.
- A sling is placed under the knee. Assess placement of the sling frequently.
- Increase countertraction with the foot of the bed elevated and the head of the bed flat.

Figure 27-3 Russell's traction.

Skeletal Traction

Skeletal traction is used for long periods of time until the bone is ready for casting or open reduction (surgery to place the bones in their proper position).

- Crutchfield tongs: Used to treat cervical and thoracic fractures; tongs are placed into the skull (Fig. 27-4).
- 90/90 femoral traction: Most commonly used to treat femur fractures and complicated femur fractures (Fig. 27-5).
- Dunlop traction: Used to treat supracondylar fractures of humerus (Fig. 27-6).

Figure 27-4 Crutchfield tongs.

Figure 27-5 90/90 femoral traction.

Figure 27-6 Dunlop traction.

Preventing Pneumonia

- Include assessment and methods to increase lung expansion.
- Initiate incentive spirometry in school-age and adolescent children.
- In younger children who cannot comprehend the concept of spirometry, encourage the same concept through other means (e.g., blowing bubbles or a party favor).

Talipes Equinovarus (Clubfoot)

When caring for an infant just delivered with clubfoot, the nurse can ask questions such as:

- "How are you feeling at this time?"
- "Do you know what this condition is called?"
- "Do you know anything about clubfoot?"
- "Can I stay with you to offer support while you hold the baby?"
- "After you rest we can talk more about the baby's condition."

Legg–Calve–Perthes Disease

There are four stages of Legg–Calve–Perthes Disease (LCPD):

- Aseptic necrosis (flattening of femoral head): Lasts several weeks, is characterized by synovitis and a decrease in ossification in the nucleus of the femoral head secondary to ischemia.
- Revascularization: Lasts 6 to 12 months, is characterized by increased joint space, increased cartilage thickness, and a decrease in size and density of femoral head.

- New bone formation: Lasts 1 to 2 years, is characterized by collapse and superolateral displaced head, and avascular bone is reabsorbed.
- Regenerative phase: Reconstitution of femoral head with remodeling and final healing.

Visiting Nurse's Responsibilities with a Child with Legg–Calve–Perthes Disease

- Assess the family's support systems in their own environment.
- Ensure that the family is able to provide the care needed.
- Ensure compliance with the use of the conservative devices.
- Ensure the non–weight-bearing status of the child.
- Assess the knowledge of the parents and child about ongoing care.
- Encourage the use of creative quiet activities and hobbies.
- Ask the family about follow-up care with the physician.

Caring for a Child with a Fracture in a Cast

- Elevate the casted extremity on pillows for at least the first 24 hours.
- Avoid indenting the cast.
- Observe the extremity for swelling and discoloration.
- Observe the extremity for sensation and movement.
- Call the health care professional if abnormalities are noted.
- Follow activity restrictions.
- Do not allow the affected limb to hang down for any length of time.
- Prevent the child from putting anything inside the cast.
- Keep a clear path for ambulation.
- Ensure the child uses crutches appropriately.
- Encourage rest.
- Encourage quiet activities.
- Instruct the child to move joints above and below cast.

Soft Tissue Injuries

Immediately after the initial injury, use the RICE acronym:

R: Rest the injured extremity prevents further injury and allows the ligament to heal.

I: Ice for the first 48 hours; keep ice packs in place for 15-minute intervals to decrease swelling.

C: Compression; apply an ace wrap or some other method to apply pressure to the affected joint to help reduce swelling of the joint.

E: Elevation and early motion of the affected joint; elevation reduces swelling and early motion of the affected joint helps keep the full range of motion of the joint.

Log Rolling

- Use log rolling to turn the child in Crutchfield tongs or after a spinal fusion.
- Two or more nurses turn the patient in complete unison.
- Turn head, shoulders, hips, and legs as one unit, keeping the back in a straight line (Fig. 27-7).

Tetanus (Lockjaw)

Signs and Symptoms

- Progressive stiffness and tenderness of the muscles in the neck and jaw
- Trismus (difficulty opening the mouth)
- Risus sardonicus (a peculiar grin)
- Opisthotonus posturing
- Laryngospasm of the respiratory muscles
- Tetanus prophylaxis through immunization is the key to preventing tetanus

Figure 27-7 Logrolling technique.

Nursing Care

- Tetanus immune globulin (TIG) and antibiotics
- Closely monitored and respiratory support
- Fluids and electrolytes as well as caloric intake monitored
- Nasogastric (NG) feedings or Total Parental Nutrition (TPN)
- Endotracheal (ET) intubation (laryngospasms)
- Eliminate stimulation
- Frequent neurological assessments
- O_2 saturation and blood gases
- Oropharyngeal suctioning
- Medications
- Hydration and nutrition
- Collaboration

RESOURCES

Arthritis Foundation: http://www.arthritis.org

Muscular Dystrophy Association: http://www.mdausa.org

Osteogenesis Imperfecta Foundation: http://www.oif.org

REFERENCES

Ilowite, N. (2002). Current treatment of juvenile rheumatoid arthritis. *Pediatrics, 109*, 109–115.

Robertson, J., & Shilkofski, N. (2005). *Harriet Lane handbook: A manual for pediatric house officers,* 17th ed. St. Louis, MO: C.V. Mosby.

Venes, D. (Ed.). (2005). *Taber's cyclopedic medical dictionary* (20th ed.). Philadelphia: F.A. Davis.

Caring for the Child with an Integumentary Condition

KEY TERMS

dermis – Layer of skin containing the nerves, muscles, connective tissue, sebaceous and sweat glands, blood vessels, and lymph channels

epidermis – Layer of skin that serves as the outlet for the sweat glands and through which the hair follicles protrude

FOCUSED ASSESSMENT

Common Skin Lesions and Associated Conditions

Lesion Name	Description	Examples
Macule	Flat, circumscribed area that has color change and is <1 cm in diameter	Freckles Flat moles Petechiae Measles Scarlet fever
Papule	Raised, circumscribed area <1 cm diameter	Warts Moles Lichen planus Scabies
Patch	Macule that is flat, nonpalpable, of irregular shape, and >1 cm diameter	Port-wine stains Café-au-lait spots
Nodule	Raised, firm, circumscribed (deeper than a papule) 1–2 cm diameter	Lipomas Erythema nodosum
Tumor	Raised and solid. May be clear, deep in the dermis, <2 cm in diameter.	Lipoma Hemangiomas Neoplasms Benign tumors
Vesicle	Raised, circumscribed, superficial, filled with serous fluid, <1 cm in diameter	Varicella Herpes zoster (shingles)
Pustule	Raised, superficial-like vesicle, but fluid is purulent	Impetigo Acne

Lesion Name	Description	Examples
Bulla	Vesicle >1 cm in diameter	Blister
Wheal	Raised, irregular shape, cutaneous swelling, solid. Diameter is variable (usually transient)	Urticaria Insect bites Allergic reaction
Crust	Dried body fluid on the skin surface: serum, pus, or blood	Disease where the skin weeps: eczema, impetigo, seborrhea
Scales	Raised cluster of keratinized cells, irregular, diameter is variable, can be thick or thin, dry or oily	Seborrheic dermatitis Dry skin Skin flaking after allergic reaction
Lichenification	Rough, thickened epidermal area often in the flexor surface of extremity	Chronic dermatitis
Scar	Fibrous tissue, thin or thick, coloration may be lighter or darker than surrounding skin	Healing wound of any etiology
Keloid	Fibrous tissue (scar) of irregular shape, raised and grown beyond the boundary of the original wound	Postoperative wound healing (more common in persons of color)

(continued)

Common Skin Lesions and Associated Conditions (Continued)

Lesion Name	Description	Examples
Fissure	Linear crack in the epidermis may be deeper, moist or dry	Athlete's foot Cracks at the corner the mouth or anus
Erosion	Depressed, moist, loss of part of the epidermis	After rupture of vesicle or bulla, e.g., varicella
Ulcer	Concave, moist, loss of epidermis and dermis	Ulceration: stasis, decubitus

Adapted from Potter & Perry (2004).

Questions for Assessing Acne in an Adolescent

- When did your acne begin?
- What types of cleaning products, makeup, or moisturizers and hair care products are you currently using?
- Can you tell me what medications you are taking? Please include over-the-counter and natural products.
- What type of foods do you eat?
- Have you noticed any foods, activities, or environmental factors that affect your acne?
- Do you notice a change in your acne related to your menses? (female patients)
- What other dermatological problems have you had recently or in the past?
- Can you tell me how you feel about having acne?

Ringworm

The most common ringworm infections are as follows:

- Tinea capitis: Involves the hair of the scalp, usually seen in prepubertal children between the ages of 1 and 10 years.

- Tinea corporis: Involves the skin of the body, except the scalp, groin, hands, and feet; seen in children and adolescents.
- Tinea cruris: Known as "jock itch"; involves the inner thighs, inguinal creases, or perineal area (rare before adolescence).
- Tinea pedi: Athlete's foot, involves the kinesthetic webbed areas of the toes and feet; seen in children and adolescents.

Assessing for a Systemic Allergic Response

The nurse must recognize the key assessments in a systemic allergic response.

- Assess for edema or laryngospasms in the airway, which has the potential to cause blockage.
- Assess for cyanosis and listen for audible sounds of upper airway respiratory distress such as wheezing or stridor.
- Assess the vital signs, specifically hypotension.

Lyme Disease Presents in Three Stages

- In the first stage, days to weeks after the tick bite, the child has a mild local rash. The rash from Lyme disease may occur as a bull's-eye rash or as disseminated erythematous (red) rash and erythema migrans (bulls-eye rash) (CDC, 2005b).
- Other symptoms include headache, nuchal rigidity (stiff neck), and joint and muscle pain.
- In the second stage, the disease may last from a few days to up to 10 months after the tick bite. During stage 2, the infection spreads through the blood and the child may exhibit signs of arthritis (especially in the knees), arthralgia (muscle pain), cardiac dysrhythmias, lymphadenopathy, pericarditis, or meningoencephalitis.
- In the third stage, lasting from weeks to years after the tick bite (chronic stage), the child develops mild to severe arthritis. Neurological symptoms that occur in stage 3 include cranial nerve palsy, depression, meningitis, neuropathy, radiculopathy, and encephalopathy.

Questions for Gathering Important Information About Burns

- What was the offending agent?
- When did this burn occur?
- Who was present or witnessed the injury?
- What first aid was given?
- How did the burn feel when it first occurred?
- How does the burn feel now?
- Has the child had any like accidents or injuries before?
- What other medical history is important?

Classifying Hypothermia		
Classification	**Body Temperature**	**Clinical Signs and Symptoms**
Mild	90°–95°F (32.2°–35°C)	Shivering, rapid heart rate, rapid respiratory rate, vasoconstriction, increased urine output As temperature decreases, the child displays apathy, lethargy, and impaired judgment
Moderate	82.4°–90°F (28°–32.3°C)	Decreased heart rate, decreased respiratory rate, hypotension, loss of consciousness, decreased pupillary response
Severe	<82.4°F (<28°C)	Apnea, asystole, coma It may not be possible to readily differentiate between severe hypothermia and death

Source: McCullough, L., & Arora, S. (2004).

CLINICAL ALERTS

Group A *Streptococcus*

Group A *Streptococcus* can cause necrotizing fasciitis (flesh-eating bacteria). Be alert to the following clinical manifestations of necrotizing fasciitis:

- Bruising
- Crepitus
- Bullae filled with bluish/purple colored fluid over the induration (Lipsky, 2003).

Stevens–Johnson Syndrome (Erythema Multiforme)

Stevens-Johnson syndrome (also known as erythema multiforme) is a serious reaction that may be fatal (Knowles, Shapiro, & Shear, 2003; Venes, 2005).

- Stevens–Johnson syndrome is the leading cause of severe allergic response to a medication.
- This condition begins with a nonspecific upper respiratory system infection; however, the defining signs of this condition are bullae that appear on the lips, mouth, eyes, and genitalia, often in a target-like pattern.
- It is essential to eliminate the causative agent.
- Treat the skin lesions using aseptic technique along with an air- or fluid-filled bed, nutritional support, IV fluids, and pain management.
- Antibiotics can be given for secondary infections and an ophthalmologist should be contacted to assess for lesions in the eyes.
- As the fluid-filled lesions erupt and slough off internally and externally it is vital to ensure a patent airway. This may progress to the necessity of intubation and mechanical ventilation.
- As these lesions rupture large amounts of body surface area may become exposed. The child may experience large fluid losses and should be treated similarly to a burn patient.

A Severe Reaction to a Bite

A child who has had a severe reaction to bees or wasps should wear a medical alert bracelet or necklace and carry an EpiPen (epinephrine) or EpiPen Jr.

Material Safety Data Sheets

To protect personal and patient safety the nurse must:

- Know where to find material safety data sheets (MSDS) in your facility.
- Know your facility's special telephone hotline for MSDS information (usually in case of chemical exposure).
- Know the telephone number of the local poison control center, where you can receive accurate telephone advice and faxed information on management of spilled chemicals or ingested substances.

Hypothermia

- Hypothermia in children may have a metabolic or neurological etiology.
- The cause of hypothermia must be investigated when no environmental explanation is appropriate.
- Wet clothes increase the risk and should be removed as soon as possible and replaced with dry clothes.

DIAGNOSTIC TESTS

Monitoring Isotretinoin Therapy

- Approval for continued isotretinoin (Accutane) therapy depends on the patient's willingness to comply with pregnancy testing (girls) and blood testing of liver enzymes (both girls and boys).
- Liver enzymes must be tested once a month to ensure that liver damage is not occurring from the isotretinoin (Accutane).
- Teens are particularly difficult to manage because of their developmental age. They may feel invincible and may be less likely to comply with treatment unless they see a quick and direct improvement in their acne.

Procedure 28-1 Obtaining a Fungal Culture

Purpose
To test for the presence of fungi and, if found, to identify the type.

Equipment
- Gloves
- Tongue blade
- Sterile cotton swab
- Sterile test tube

Steps
1. Explain the procedure to the child in age-appropriate terms.
2. Gather all supplies.
3. Using aseptic technique, place a sterile cotton swab against a plaque.
4. Vigorously rub the plaque with the cotton swab.

5. Place the swab into a covered, sterile test tube provided by the laboratory and place in a biohazard bag.

6. Have the specimen transported to the lab within 15–30 minutes to ensure accurate test results.

7. Monitor the child's oral mucosa for bleeding, which may result from attempting to remove the oral thrush (Elewski, 2002).

8. Explain to parents that final culture results will not be available for 48 to 72 hours, although preliminary results may be available sooner.

9. Document the procedure.

Clinical Alert The nurse must remember that attempting to remove the oral thrush can cause the lining of the oral mucosa to bleed.

Teach Parents

The final culture is not available for 48–72 hours; preliminary culture results may be available sooner.

Laboratory Results in Rocky Mountain Spotted Fever

Expect elevated white blood cells (WBCs), thrombocytopenia (low platelets), hyponatremia (decreased sodium in the blood), and elevated liver enzymes (CDC, 2005a). The child's WBCs will likely remain low in the early stage and rise to slightly abnormal in later stages.

WBCs: 5,000–10,000/mm³ (later stage: 10,000–12,000/mm³)
Platelets: 150,000–400,000/mm³ (thrombocytopenia: <150,000/mm³)
Sodium: 136–145 mEq/L (hyponatremia: <136 mEq/L)
Bilirubin (total): 0.3–1.0 mg/dL (hyperbilirubinemia: >1.0 mg/dL)
Urine testing may reveal red blood cells and protein (Gandhi, 2005).

MEDICATIONS

Tetracycline (Sumycin)

- Tetracycline (Sumycin) will autofluorescence in the presence of ultraviolet light, thus making the person noticeably "glow" in environments that are lit by black lights.

- Tetracycline (Sumycin) can also darken the teeth in children younger than the age of 8 years and should not be used in this age group.

Isotretinoin (Accutane)

- Isotretinoin (Accutane) causes severe birth defects.
- Women must not take this medication if there is any chance of becoming pregnant because of the risk of birth defects. It is important to discuss this with adolescents if pregnancy is a possibility.
- Pregnancy tests must be performed before treatment with this medication, monthly during treatment, and 1 month after the cessation of treatment.
- In addition, women must use two forms of birth control if considering this treatment.
- Visit iPLEDGE: Committed to Pregnancy Prevention program at http://www.ipledgeprogram.com/ to view the information appropriate for clients undergoing isotretinoin (Accutane) treatment.
- Other side effects include hypercholesteremia, drying of the mucous membranes, decrease in night vision, headaches, depression, and liver damage.

Benzathine Penicillin G (**ben**-za-**theen** pen-i-**sill**-in **gee**) Bicillin L-A

Pregnancy Category B

Indications Treatment of a wide variety of infections: pharyngeal/tonsil/skin.

Prophylaxis for rheumatic fever

Actions Binds to bacterial cell wall, resulting in cell death.

Therapeutic Effects Bacteriostatic action against susceptible bacterial spectrum: Streptococci, staphylococci, and some gram-negative organisms

Pharmacokinetics
Absorption IM delayed and prolonged to sustain therapeutic blood levels.

Contraindications and Precautions Contraindicated in hypersensitivity

Adverse Reactions and Side Effects
Pain at injection site.

GI Diarrhea, epigastric distress, nausea/vomiting
Endocrine Rash
Respiratory Anaphylaxis

Route and Dosage
IM: Children >27 kg, 900–1.2 million units (single dose). **IM:** Children <27 kg, 300,000–600,000 units (single dose)

Nursing Implications
Assess for history of hypersensitivity.
Observe the patient for signs of anaphylaxis for a minimum of 15 minutes after injection.
Reconstitute with D_5W or 0.9% NaCl.
Administer deep into a well-developed muscle mass.

Data from Deglin, J., & Vallerand, A. (2009). Davis's drug guide for nurses (11th ed.), pp. 958–961. Philadelphia: F.A. Davis.

Ibuprofen (eye-byoo-**proe**-fen) Children's Advil/Motrin

Pregnancy Category B (first trimester)

Indications Mild to moderate pain. Inflammation

Actions Inhibits prostaglandin synthesis.

Therapeutic Effects Antipyretic, analgesic, nonsteroidal anti-inflammatory, antirheumatic

Pharmacokinetics
Absorption Well absorbed from the GI tract

Contraindications and Precautions Contraindicated in hypersensitivity. Cross-sensitivity with other nonsteroidal anti-inflammatory drugs (NSAIDs) and aspirin

Adverse Reactions and Side Effects Headache, constipation, nausea/vomiting

Route and Dosage
PO: Children 6 months–12 years: 20–40 mg/kg/day in 3–4 divided doses/day (every 6–8 hours).

Nursing Implications
Assess for history of sensitivity.
Assess pain and monitor temperature (if given as an antipyretic).
Ibuprofen may cause anticoagulation effects.

Data from Deglin, J., & Vallerand, A. (2009). Davis's drug guide for nurses (11th ed.), pp. 654–656. Philadelphia: F.A. Davis.

Topical Treatments

Classification	Names	Precautions
Anesthetics	Benzocaine (Americaine) Lidocaine and prilocaine (EMLA)	Allergy Do not use over wounds. Do not use over large areas; avoid the eyes.
Antibacterial	Bacitracin and polymyxin B (AK-Poly-Bac) Neomycin (Myciguent) Mupirocin (Bactroban)	Allergy Existing infection (for prevention of infection) Antibiotic resistance Use for only minor cuts/scrapes/burns.
Antifungal	Clotrimazole (Lotrimin) Ketoconazole (Nizoral) Miconazole (Aloe Vesta) Nystatin (Mycostatin)	Cautious use in nail and scalp infections
Anti-itch	Diphenhydramine (Benadryl)	Allergy Photosensitivity
Emollients	White petrolatum jelly Mineral oil Lanolin Glycerin	Allergy Choose fragrance-free products.
Steroids	Varying strengths Strongest: Group I: betamethasone (Diprolene) Group II: Desoximetasone (Decadron) Group III: Triamcinolone 0.5% (Kenalog) Group IV: Fluocinolone (Lidex) Group V: Hydrocortisone 0.2% (A-Hydrocort) Group VI: Desonide (Tridesilon) Group VII: Hydrocortisone 1% (A-Hydrocort)	Allergy Repeated use in the same area of the skin will cause thinning of the skin May inhibit the skin's ability to fight infection. Should be used in the lowest strength on the thin skin of the face and genitalia. Avoid the eye area: places the client at risk for glaucoma or cataract formation.

Data from Deglin, J., & Vallerand, A. (2009). *Davis's drug guide for nurses* (11th ed.). Philadelphia: F.A. Davis.

Topical Agents

- Topical agents that promote healing are frequently used for rashes: cow udder balm (bag balm), green tea extract, vitamin E preparations, aloe vera, milk, calamine, and colloidal oatmeal (Beltrani, 2002).

ETHNOCULTURAL CONSIDERATIONS

Vulnerable Populations

African Americans and Native Americans (CDC, 2006) and persons living in rural areas (Ahrens, 2001) are most vulnerable to fire-related injuries and death.

Pressure Ulcers

In children with dark pigmented skin, blanching may look red or purple.

TEACHING THE FAMILY

Impetigo

For a child with impetigo, teach the child and family the following:

- Wash your hands thoroughly and often.
- Do not scratch the lesions.

Cellulitis

- Teach the caregiver the following: Administer all antibiotics as ordered, even if the skin improves before completing the antibiotic course, because failure to finish the antibiotic may lead to recurrence of the infection.
- Use warm, moist packs to relieve discomfort as needed. Cool, moist packs are also acceptable if they relieve discomfort.
- Administer an analgesic, such as ibuprofen (Children's Advil) or acetaminophen (Children's Tylenol), if needed for comfort.
- If the infection is in a limb, elevate the limb to reduce swelling and increase comfort.
- Contact the physician if redness or edema worsens, if the child's pain increases, or if temperature remains above 101.5°F (38.6°C) for 48 hours after starting the antibiotic.

(Thomson Micromedex, 2006)

Herpes Simples Virus (HSV-1)

To decrease transmission of the virus and prevent future outbreaks, teach the child to do the following:

- Keep his hands away from his face.
- Wash his hands thoroughly. (To ensure that a young child washes for the proper amount of time, teach him to sing the alphabet song while washing.)
- Decrease stress.
- Avoid prolonged sun exposure.
- Use a moisturizing sunscreen on the lips during summer months.

(Hurtado, 2005)

Lice (Pediculosis)

Teach caregivers the following:

- To detect lice, examine the child's head under good lighting. Pay particular attention to areas behind the ears and at the nape of the neck.
- To treat lice, use an over-the-counter shampoo that contains permethrin (for an infant or young child) or lindane (for an older child).
- Wash the child's hair according to the instructions on the product.
- After shampoo is rinsed from the hair, remove nits by backcombing with a fine-tooth comb. Nits are easier to remove when the hair is damp.
- If the child cannot tolerate the medicated shampoo, an asphyxiant such as petrolatum or food oil (e.g., olive oil) may be used (Wiederkehr & Schwartz, 2003).
- Nits on eyelashes may be removed by applying petrolatum to the eyelashes twice daily for 8 days.
- Clean the home thoroughly (dust, vacuum, scrub), wash clothing and bedding, and wipe hats, bicycle helmet, and toys.
- If a soft or cloth toy is not washable, it must be placed in a sealed plastic bag away from family members' rooms for 14 days.
- All bed linens should be laundered in hot water and dried in a dryer.
- Pillows used by the child should be thrown away.
- Anti-lice spray can be used for furniture and other environmental objects that are not disposable.

- Hair-care items can be boiled (hot water above 140°F) or soaked in anti-lice shampoo and should never be shared.
- The child should stay home from school until lice-free, in keeping with the school's anti-lice policy. The child may need to be checked by the school nurse or day care provider before returning.
- The child should be rechecked for lice in 7 to 10 days if the itching resumes, if itching disrupts the child's sleep, or if the condition fails to clear after 1 week of treatment.
- More information is available from the National Pediculosis Association at http://www.headlice.org

Animal Bite Prevention

Teach children and families the following:

- Never leave a child alone with an animal.
- Never put your face close to an animal.
- Never tease or overexcite an animal.
- Avoid dogs and other animals that you do not know.
- Ask the owner's permission before touching or petting an animal.
- Play with animals only under adult supervision.
- Report strange animal behavior, even if you know the animal.
- Do not disturb animals that are eating, sleeping, or feeding their young.
- Spay or neuter pets to reduce aggression.
- Stay away from wild animals.
- Do not run away from an aggressive animal; instead, lie down in a ball, protect your face, and stay quiet.

(National Center for Injury Prevention and Control, 2008)

Burn Prevention

Teach parents the following:

- Set the home water heater no higher than 120°F to prevent scald injuries.
- When cooking, turn pot handles inward so children cannot reach them.
- Make sure electrical cords from cooking appliances are not dangling within the child's reach.

Managing Minor Burns

Teach parents and caregivers the following:

- Remove any clothing that is hot or has been in contact with an offending chemical.
- Cool a burn immediately using gauze or a clean cloth soaked in cool (54°F) saline solution or water.
- Do not put ice on a burn.
- Wash a wound with mild soap, and rinse well with water.
- Bacitracin (Baciguent) may be used topically to prevent infection. For moderate or major burns, the child will receive a different type of anti-infective and a tetanus booster.
- Cover the burn with gauze to prevent infection, decrease pain, and absorb drainage.
- Give acetaminophen (Children's Tylenol) or ibuprofen (Children's Advil) to decrease pain. If pain disrupts the child's sleep, play, or mood, give the medication on a schedule (Morgan, Bledsoe, & Barker, 2000).

Frostbite

Teach parents and caregivers the following:

- Place the child in a warm area, remove all wet and cold clothing, and replace with warm ones.
- If frostbite is in the hands or feet, they are immersed in warm tap water (100°F) for up to one half hour (McCullough & Arora, 2004).
- Check the water temperature frequently, as the body part cools the tub of water.
- Do not run warm water directly from the tap over the area, as tap water can change in temperature rapidly based on use by other household members. The water must also be monitored closely so a secondary burn does not occur in the process of rewarming.
- Do not rewarm the frozen part with massage or dry heat (McCullough & Arora, 2004).
- After rewarming is complete, the extremity is wrapped in a soft cloth and the child can be encouraged to rest.
- If no subsequent problems arise, the child can remove the soft cloth and return to inside activities.
- If parents suspect continued problems the heath care provider is called.

ADDITIONAL INFORMATION FOR THE CLINICAL SETTING

Infant Skin and Temperature

An infant's skin is very thin and contains very little subcutaneous fat. Temperature regulation becomes an important issue, as the infant tends to lose heat rapidly.

- Do not to leave an infant uncovered and exposed for a prolonged time.

Superficial Wound Management

- Superficial wounds are often closed with tissue adhesives (DERMABOND) that work like glue.

Cleansing an Adolescent's Face and Treating Acne

Follow these steps, giving the adolescent as much autonomy as possible in cleansing and treating the area:

1. Wash hands thoroughly.
2. Use a warm, moist cloth and antibacterial soap to soak and soften the crusting.
3. Gently wipe away as much crusting as possible.
4. Apply the prescribed topical antibiotic ointment using a cotton swab or a gloved finger.
5. Apply water-soluble moisturizer.
6. Wash hands thoroughly.

Family Compliance

- The best outcome for a child receiving an antibiotic is for the family to be adherent and administer the entire medication as prescribed.
- If the family has a history of nonadherence to a medical plan, or if the child cannot take the medication as prescribed, the nurse must notify the healthcare provider immediately. The healthcare provider may then choose to order a single dose of intramuscular penicillin instead of the oral medication.
- Using a topical anesthetic such as EMLA (lidocaine/prilocaine) at the injection site at least an hour before the injection can help decrease the pain.

Human Papillomavirus: Warts

Type of Wart	Treatment	Description
Common Wart (verruca vulgaris)	Topical keratolytic acids (OTC)	Applied by dropper or cotton swab. Place thick liquid directly on top of the wart, taking care to keep the highly acidic fluid off the surrounding skin. The wart will peel away in layers as the acid kills the superficial layers, one at a time.
	Liquid nitrogen cryosurgery	Application of liquid nitrogen to the wart by a practitioner is a common method of removal. It is mildly painful but efficient. The practitioner directs a narrow flow of liquid nitrogen to the wart, freezing and therefore killing the wart tissue.
Flat Wart (verruca plana)	Topical tretinoin cream (prescription)	Treatment is applied in a thin coating via a gloved finger.
Plantar Wart (verruca plantaris)	Topical keratolytic acids	Applied by dropper or cotton swab. Place thick liquid directly on top of the wart, taking care to keep the highly acidic fluid off the surrounding skin.
	Liquid nitrogen cryosurgery (with paring and topical chemodestruction to enhance effectiveness).	Application of liquid nitrogen to the wart by a practitioner is a common method of removal. It is mildly painful but efficient. The practitioner directs a narrow flow of liquid nitrogen to the wart, freezing and therefore killing the wart tissue.

Source: Krusinski, P.A., & Flowers, F.P. (2000).

How to Tell Oral Thrush from Formula or Breast Milk on the Tongue of the Infant

Gently scrape the white film on the infant's tongue with a tongue blade. If it comes off, it is formula or breast milk. If it does not come off, it is thrush.

Preventing Atopic Dermatitis Secondary Infection

- Use good hygiene.
- Follow prescribed treatment protocols.

- Maintain skin hydration.
- Assess rash frequently.

Removing a Tick

1. Clean the skin with a topical antiseptic.
2. Don gloves.
3. Using tweezers, grasp the tick firmly, as close to the skin as possible.
4. Pull the tick out with a firm, steady motion. Do not twist the tick.
5. Clean the skin again with a topical antiseptic.
6. Seal the tick in a bag, write the date on the bag, and place it in the freezer in case the tick needs to be tested for disease.

Classifying Burns

Determine the extent of the burn by calculating the total body surface area (TBSA). TBSA can be determined by using several methods:

- Lund and Browder Chart or the Burn Calculations Rule of 9's (Fig. 28-1)
- Categorized according to severity

PERCENTAGES IN A CHILD

Figure 28-1 Rule of 9's.

Classification of Burn Severity

Classification	Characteristics	Treatment
Mild	First or second degree, <10% body surface area (BSA) Third degree, <2% BSA No area of face, feet, hands, genitals burned	Can be treated on an outpatient basis.
Moderate	Second degree, 10%–20% BSA Third degree, <10% BSA	Can be treated in a burn unit or general hospital.
Severe	Second degree, >20% BSA Third degree, >10% BSA Burns on hands, feet, and genitals that may lead to functional impairment Smoke inhalation is present	Should be treated in a specialized burn center.

Sources: American Burn Association (2006); and Perry, C. (2003).

Criteria for Transfer to a Burn Center

- Partial-thickness burn over greater than 10% of body surface area (BSA)
- Burn involving face, hands, feet, or genitals
- Third-degree burn
- Electrical burn, including lightning injury
- Chemical burn
- Inhalation burn
- Burn injury in a person with a preexisting condition that could prolong the recovery period
- Burn injury in a person with coexisting trauma (e.g., fracture) when the burn poses a greater risk of morbidity or mortality than the trauma.
- The patient is a child in a facility without qualified personnel or equipment to care for a child.
- The patient needs special emotional, social, or long-term burn rehabilitation

(American Burn Association, 2006)

Overall Goals of Burn Treatment

The best outcome for a burned child considers the following interventions.

Burn Assessment

- The initial nursing assessment includes emergency care related to airway, breathing, and circulation (ABCs).
- After the ABCs are addressed and the child is being safely transported to an emergency room, the nurse or emergency medical technician (EMT) removes all clothing and jewelry to decrease continued burning at any site.
- Once the child is in a hospital, burn wounds are decontaminated and assessed for depth, surface area, and severity. The depth of the wounds is measured in millimeters or centimeters, circumference measurements are also necessary to provide a full clinical picture.
- The surface of the burn wound is assessed for color, blanching, desiccation (dryness), turgor/elasticity, blisters, or sloughed blisters.
- TBSA and all other skin assessments are taken into consideration to help classify the burn.

Fluid Resuscitation

- Children with burns greater than 15% of BSA require intravenous fluid resuscitation to maintain adequate perfusion.
- The IV fluid of choice is lactated Ringer's solution (Behrman, Kliegman, & Jenson, 2004).
- The Parkland formula is one means of determining the fluid needs of the child with a burn injury (Bollero et al., 2000). See page 568.
- Effectiveness of fluid resuscitation is monitored by adequate urine output. Normal urine output for children is 1 to 2 mL/kg per hour. If adequate urine output is not achieved, additional fluid resuscitation may be required.

Adequate Nutrition

- The caloric requirement for a patient with a >30% burn is 2000 to 2200 calories/day.
- In major burns enteral nutrition is necessary to keep up with the increased energy demand of the body, secondary to the stress response (Rimdeika et al., 2006).
- Enteral feeding is often initiated within 6 hours of the burn injury to support the child's increased needs.

Pain Management

- Initially morphine sulfate (Duramorph) is most commonly used for pain.

- The use of anxiolytics such as midazolam (Versed) or lorazepam (Ativan) is helpful
- Nonpharmacological interventions are also used

Meticulous Wound Care
- Wounds are initially decontaminated.
- Subsequent burn wound care includes cleansing the wound with a special solution or débridement.
- After cleansing, antibiotic ointment is applied and the wound is then re-dressed.
- Wounds can also be cleansed in a tub or a whirlpool, allowing the movement of the water to soften skin, and gently removing some loose dead skin.
- Escharotomy may be required if circulation or perfusion is impeded.
- Silvadene™ is the most commonly used burn cream to both prevent and treat burn infection.

Burn Recovery
- Burn injuries for children are managed by phases of recuperation as well as the type and severity of burns.
- The acute, or early phase, is from the time of the initial assault until wound closure.
- The second phase, recovery, is from the time of wound closure until scar maturation, which could be as long as 16 months (Selvaggi et al., 2005).
- For some children burn recovery may last a lifetime.

The Parkland Formula for Fluid Resuscitation

Fluid (milliliters) for first 24 hours: $4 \times$ patient's weight in kg $\times$ %TBSA

- Give half of the resulting IVF volume over the first 8 hours.
- Give the remaining half at an even rate over the next 16 hours.

  Example: A child weighing 50 kg (110 lbs.) with a 20% TBSA burn
  4 ml $\times$ 50 kg $\times$ 20% TBSA = 4000 mL.
  First 8 hours, IVF = 2000 mL/8 hr = 250 mL/hr
  Next 16 hours, IVF = 2000 mL/16 hr = 125 mL/hr
  IVF = intravenous fluid; TBSA = total body surface area

(Behrman, Kliegman, & Jenson, 2004)

Using Distraction During Dressing Changes

- Use distraction techniques to reduce pain and anxiety based on the patient's age and developmental stage.
- Examples of distraction include singing, counting, watching television, focusing on a picture, talking about familiar events or places, playing a game, or blowing a pinwheel or bubbles.
- If the child is anxious or has severe pain, medication may be required before dressing changes.
- Praise the child when the dressing change is complete, focusing on all of the positive behaviors the child displayed.

Hypothermia

- Hypothermia is secondary to cold air exposure, wet clothes, and immersion in water.
- Hypothermia is a condition in which the child's core body temperature falls below 95°F (35°C).
- Hypothermia is a life-threatening emergency.

Types of Heat Loss	
Radiation	Heat loss from the head and areas with less subcutaneous fat and thin skin, e.g., prematurity of the newborn. This is the most rapid method of heat loss and accounts for at least 50% of heat loss
Conduction	Transfer of heat away for the body by direct contact with a cooler surface, e.g., wet clothing or immersion
Convection	Transfer of heat away from the body by the movement of air over the skin surface, e.g., wind and drafts
Evaporation	Transfer of heat away from the body, e.g., skin moisture turned to vapor as it is dried by the movement of air
Respiration	Expiration of heat from the lungs, e.g., cold and windy weather

Pressure Ulcers

Pressure ulcers are the result of compression on one or more areas of the body for an extended period. Pressure ulcers occur when children and infants:

- Have decreased mobility.
- Have motor delays and cannot easily move their head or extremities.

- Have paralysis or other forms of limited mobility.
- Use mobility devices such as crutches, walkers, and wheelchairs.
- Have casts.
- Are malnourished.
- Have infections or anemia.
- Are bed bound for any period of time.
- Have decreased sensation to pressure or pain.

The four stages of ulcer formation can assist the nurse through skin assessment (Fig. 28-2).

Signs of Pressure Ulcer Formation
- The earliest sign of skin damage is a reddened area on the skin that does not disappear within 30 minutes of removing the cause of the pressure or irritant.
- The skin can appear to have an abrasion and look raw or rubbed.
- Further damage extends through the dermis forming the ulcer.

Nursing Care Related to Pressure Ulcer Formation
- Carefully inspect the child's skin at least three times a day, noting the color of the affected area, signs of infection, character of the skin lesion, wound edges, and drainage; measure the diameter; and determine the depth of the pressure ulcer.
- Address anemia by providing a diet high in iron.

Figure 28-2 Stages of ulcer formation. *A.* Stage 1. *B.* Stage 2. *C.* Stage 3. *D.* Stage 4.

- Keep bed clothing straight and wrinkle-free to decrease areas of pressure.
- Use air, water, or gel mattresses and pads.
- Keep the child's skin both clean and dry.
- Keep the child off the affected area as much as possible.
- Stage 1 and 2 pressure ulcers are cleansed and allowed to dry.
- For stage 3: use hydrophilic gels or hydrocolloidal dressings for the ulcer.
- For stage 4 ulcers, surgical débridement and closure may be the treatment of choice.

Prevention of Pressure Ulcers

- Routinely move and shift the weight of the child off bony prominences on a regular basis.
- Move a child who is confined to bed at least every 2 hours.
- A child who is in a sitting position (e.g., in a wheelchair) should shift his weight every 15 minutes.
- If the child wears braces, inspect the skin for redness or irritation at least once a day. If any redness is noted, the nurse must not reapply the brace and notify the physician immediately.

RESOURCES

Braden Scale: http://www.bradenscale.com

iPLEDGE: Committed to Pregnancy Prevention: http://www.ipledgeprogram.com

National Pediculosis Association: http://www.headlice.org

Phoenix Society for Burn Survivors: http://www.phoenix-society.org

REFERENCES

Ahrens, M. (2001). The U.S. fire problem overview report: Leading causes and other patterns and trends [Electronic Version]. Quincy, MA: National Fire Protection Association.

American Burn Association (2006). National burn repository: 2005 report. Retrieved from http://www.ameriburn.org/NBR2005.pdf (Accessed July 27, 2008).

Behrman, R.E., Kliegman, R.M., & Jenson, H.B. (2004). *Nelson's textbook of pediatrics* (17th ed.). Philadelphia: W. B. Saunders.

Beltrani, V.S. (2002). An overview of chronic urticaria. *Clinical Reviews in Allergy and Immunology*, 23, 147–170.

Bollero, D., Stella, M., Calcagni, M., Guglielmotti, E., & Magliacani, G. (2000). Does inhalation injury really change fluid resuscitation needs? A retrospective analysis. *Annals of Burns and Fire Disasters*. 13, 198–200.

Centers for Disease Control and Prevention (CDC). (2005a, May). Rocky Mountain spotted fever. Retrieved from http://www.cdc.gov/ncidod/dvrd/rmsf/Epidemiology.htm (Accessed July 27, 2008).

Centers for Disease Control and Prevention (CDC). (2005b, October 7). Lyme disease prevention and control. Retrieved from http://www.cdc.gov/ncidod/dvbid/lyme/ld_prevent.htm (Accessed July 27, 2008).

Centers for Disease Control and Prevention (CDC). (2006, July 6). Mass casualties: Burns. Retrieved from http://www.bt.cdc.gov/masscasulties/burns.asp (Accessed July 27, 2008).

Deglin, J., & Vallerand, A. (2009). *Davis's drug guide for nurses*. (11th ed.). Philadelphia: F.A. Davis.

Elewski, B.E. (2002, January 24). Common fungal infections of the skin. Retrieved from http://merck.micromedex.com/index.asp?page=bpm_brief&article_id=CPM02DE405&hilight=candida|albicans (Accessed February 16, 2006).

Gandhi, M. (2005, June). Rocky mountain spotted fever. Retrieved from http://www.nlm.nih.gov/medlineplus/ency/article/000654.htm (Accessed July 27, 2008).

Hurtado, R. (2005). Herpes simplex. Retrieved from http://www.nlm.nih.gov/medlineplus/ency/article/001324.htm (Accessed July 28, 2008).

Knowles, S.R., Shapiro, L.E., & Shear, N.H. (2003, July). Cutaneous drug reactions. Retrieved from http://merck.micromedex.com/index.asp?page=bpm_brief&article_id=BPM01DE15&hilight=drug|reactions (Accessed February 27, 2006).

Krusinski, P.A., & Flowers, F.P. (2000, March). Common viral infection of the skin. Retrieved from http://merck.micromedex.com/index.asp?page=bpm_brief&article_id=CPM02DE404&hilight=herpesvirus (Accessed July 29, 2008).

Lipsky, B.A. (2003, July 1). Cellulitis, erysipelas, and necrotizing soft-tissue infections. Retrieved from http://merck.micromedex.com/index.asp?page=bpm_brief&article_id=BPM01ID08&hilight=cellulitis (Accessed February 25, 2006).

McCullough, L., & Arora, S. (2004). Diagnosis and treatment of hypothermia [Electronic Version]. *American Family Physician, 70*(12), 2325–2332.

Morgan, E.D., Bledsoe, S.C., & Barker, J. (2000). Ambulatory management of burns [Electronic Version]. *American Family Physician, 62*(9), 2015–2026.

National Center for Injury Prevention and Control. (2008). National dog bite prevention week. Retrieved from http://www.cdc.gov/ncipc/duip/biteprevention.htm (Accessed July 27, 2008).

Perry, C. (2003). Thermal injuries. In P.A. Maloney-Harmon & S.J. Czerwinski (Eds), *Nursing care of the pediatric trauma patient* (pp. 277–294). St. Louis, MO: W.B. Saunders.

Potter, P.A., & Perry, A.G. (2004). *Fundamentals of nursing* (6th ed.). St. Louis, MO: C. V. Mosby.

Rimdeika, R., Gudaviciene, D., Adamonis, K., Barauskas, G., Pavalkis, D., & Endzinas, Z. (2006). The effectiveness of caloric value of enteral nutrition in patients with major burns. *Burns: Journal of the International Society for Burn Injuries, 32*(1), 83–86.

Selvaggi, G., Monstrey, S., Van Landuyt, K., Hamdi, M., & Blondeel, P. (2005). Rehabilitation of burn injured patients following lightning and electrical trauma [Electronic Version]. *NeuroRehabilitation, 20*, 35–42.

Thomson Micromedex (2006). Micromedex healthcare series. Retrieved from http://www.thomsonhc.com/hcs/librarian/ND_PR/Main/SBK/2/PFPUI/LQ4m3Y21lSzztq/ND_PG/PRIH/CS/57CE9B/ND_T/HCS/ND_P/Main/DUPLICATIONSHIELDSYNC/85BB5A/ND_B/HCS/PFActionId/hcs.common.RetrieveDocumentCommon/DocId/1746/ContentSetId/31#pharmacokineticsSection (Accessed June 5, 2006).

Venes, D. (Ed.). (2005). *Taber's cyclopedic medical dictionary* (20th ed.). Philadelphia: F.A. Davis.

Wiederkehr, M., & Schwartz, R.A. (2003, October). Lice, scabies, and bedbugs. Retrieved from http://merck.micromedex.com/index.asp?page=bpm_brief&article_id=BPM01DE11&hilight=lice (Accessed March 18, 2006).

Caring for the Child with a Renal, Urinary Tract, or Reproductive Condition

KEY TERMS

urinary tract infection (UTI) – An acquired infection of the urinary system caused by bacteria, virus, or fungus (Hogan & White, 2003)

pyelonephritis – An infection in the renal pelvis that causes renal scarring and, with repeated infections, hypertension or end-stage renal disease

FOCUSED ASSESSMENT

Fluid Deficit

- A fluid deficit occurs when fluids are lost through diaphoresis, vomiting, diarrhea or hemorrhage.
- To determine normal values use calculation of daily maintenance fluid requirements. See page 581.

Fluid Deficit

Causes	Signs and Symptoms	Nursing Care
Diminished fluid intake Diaphoresis Vomiting Diarrhea Nasogastric suction Fever Hemorrhage	Dry skin Sticky mucous membranes Poor skin turgor Thirst Poor perfusion Decreased urinary output Weight loss Fatigue Tachycardia Tachypnea Decreased blood pressure High urine specific gravity High hematocrit	Determine the underlying cause. Replace fluids. Replace electrolytes. Provide oral hydration. Provide IV hydration. Measure intake and output. Monitor vital signs. Monitor laboratory values.

Fluid Excess

- A fluid overload occurs from conditions that create impaired fluid excretion, such as kidney disease or congestive heart failure. Fluid overload also can occur due to excessive administration of intravenous fluids (Venes, 2005).
- To determine normal values use calculation of daily maintenance fluid requirements. See page 581.

Fluid Excess

Causes	Signs and Symptoms	Nursing Care
Excessive oral/IV intake Hypotonic fluid overload Kidney disease	Pulmonary edema (crackles) Weight gain (fluid retention) Lethargy Decreased level of consciousness Slow, bounding pulse Low urine specific gravity Decreased hematocrit	Determine the underlying cause. Decrease fluid intake. Administer diuretics. Monitor vital signs. Monitor laboratory values (electrolytes).

Vesicoureteral Reflux (VUR) and Urinary Tract Infection (UTI)

- Be aware that infants and small children cannot express urinary discomfort easily.
- Observe for discomfort during voiding or straining to void, dribbling of urine, and starting and stopping of the stream.
- Fever of unknown origin and irritability may suggest UTI, especially in nonverbal children.
- Take extreme care to obtain a reliable clean-catch urine specimen by helping older children collect the sample and properly handling a bagged specimen in younger children.
- Explain the urinary system to children old enough to understand it through the use of drawings, models, or dolls (Montagnino & Currier, 2005).

Hemolytic Uremic Syndrome

- Assess the child for abdominal symptoms, such as diffuse abdominal pain, intussusception (telescoping of the bowel), nausea, vomiting, diarrhea, and fever. These symptoms may occur up to 1 week after exposure to the *E. coli* 0157.H7 toxin (Razzaq, 2006).
- Look for evidence of bleeding related to thrombocytopenia.
- Observe for petechiae, epistaxis (nosebleed), prolonged bleeding at venipuncture sites, and ecchymoses.
- Because of the increased risk for neurological sequelae, look for evidence of increased intracranial pressure (ICP), including altered level of consciousness and seizures.

Accurate Weight Measurement

- It is critical that children be weighed properly and their weights monitored carefully. An inaccurate weight recorded in a computer charting system can cause life-threatening harm for the patient.
- Weights are commonly ordered every 12–24 hours in children and must be done at the same time of day.

Glomerular Disease

Glomerular disease (glomerulonephritis) can be due to primary kidney disease or secondary multisystem diseases that cause damage to the glomerulus.

Poststreptococcal Glomerulonephritis

- A beta-hemolytic streptococcus is the cause of postinfectious glomerulonephritis.
- Gross hematuria, either tea- or coffee-colored urine, develops, accompanied at times by edema, which may be seen in the periorbital region (around the eye orbits).
- If the symptoms become more severe, the child may develop hypertension and headache.
- Severe disease causes significant proteinuria and possibly even ascites, due to fluid shifting (Lum, 2007).

Signs and Symptoms of Renal Trauma

- Localized flank tenderness
- Hematoma
- A palpable mass
- There also can be other symptoms related to abdominal injury such as tenderness, peritonitis, paralytic ileus, and resulting hypovolemic shock.

Signs and Symptoms of Acute Renal Failure

- Rash
- Bloody diarrhea
- Pallor
- Vomiting and diarrhea
- Abdominal pain
- Hemorrhage
- Shock
- Anuria or polyuria
- Other life-threatening signs and symptoms include gastrointestinal bleeding, hypertension, anemia, neurological symptoms, as well as the skin becoming ecchymotic.

History Information in Chronic Renal Failure

- Look for malaise, poor appetite, vomiting, bone pain, headache (if hypertensive), and polyuria.
- Listen for these problems in the patient's history: perinatal complications, oligohydramnios, recurrent UTIs, and enuresis.
- Stay alert for evidence of renal disease and hearing impairment in the patient's family history (Schwartz, 2005, p. 712).

Physical Examination Findings Correlated with Underlying Pathophysiological Mechanisms for Chronic Renal Failure

Organ System	Physical Findings	Correlation with Pathophysiological Mechanisms
Skeletal	Osteitis fibrosa (bone inflammation with fibrous degeneration) Bone demineralization (principally subperiosteal loss of cortical bone in the fibers, lateral ends of the clavicles, and lamina dura of the teeth) Spontaneous fractures, bone pain; osteomalacia (rickets or rachitic changes) with end-stage renal failure Edema Absent patella	Bone resorption associated with hyperparathyroidism, vitamin D deficiency, and demineralization Lowered calcium and raised phosphate levels
Cardiopulmonary	Hypertension, pericarditis with fever, chest pain, and pericardial friction rub, pulmonary edema, Kussmaul respirations Flow murmur Gallop Rub	Extracellular volume expansion as cause of hypertension Hypersecretion of renin also associated with hypertension Fluid overload associated with pulmonary edema and acidosis leading to Kussmaul respirations
Neurological	Encephalopathy (fatigue, loss of attention, difficulty problem solving) Peripheral neuropathy (pain and burning in the legs and feet, loss of vibration sense and deep tendon reflexes)	Uremic toxins associated with end-stage renal disease

Organ System	Physical Findings	Correlation with Pathophysiological Mechanisms
	Loss of motor coordination, twitching, fasciculations, stupor, and coma with advanced uremia Hypotonia Irritability	
Endocrine and Reproductive	Retarded growth in children (short stature) Osteomalacia High incidence of goiter Sexual dysfunction: menorrhagia, amenorrhea, infertility, and decreased libido in women; decreased testosterone levels, infertility, and decreased libido in men	Decreased growth hormone Elevated parathyroid hormone Decreased thyroid hormone Elevated hormones: luteinizing hormone (LH), follicle-stimulating hormone (FSH), prolactin, and LH-releasing hormone; decreased testosterone, estrogen, and progesterone
Hematological	Anemia, usually normochromic normocytic; platelet disorders with prolonged bleeding times (increase in bleeding gums)	Reduced erythropoietin secretion associated with loss of renal mass, leading to reduced red cell production in the bone marrow; uremic toxins associated with shortened red cell survival
Gastrointestinal	Anorexia, nausea, vomiting Mouth ulcers, stomatitis, ruinous breath (uremic fetor), hiccups, peptic ulcers, gastrointestinal bleeding, and pancreatitis associated with end-stage renal failure	Retention of urea, metabolic acids, and other metabolic waste products, including methylguanidine
Integumentary	Abnormal pigmentation and pruritus	Retention of urochromes, contributing to sallow, yellow color High plasma calcium levels associated with pruritus
Immunological	Increased risk of infection that can cause death Decreased response to vaccination	Suppression of cell-mediated immunity Reduction in number and function of lymphocytes Diminished phagocytosis. *(continued)*

Physical Examination Findings Correlated with Underlying Pathophysiological Mechanisms for Chronic Renal Failure (Continued)		
Organ System	**Physical Findings**	**Correlation with Pathophysiological Mechanisms**
HEENT	Retinal changes Preauricular pits Hearing deficit	Uremic toxins
Abdomen	Palpable kidneys Suprapubic mass	

Varicocele

- Expect scrotal veins to distend when the patient stands and to decrease in visibility when the patient is supine.
- Look for accentuation of the veins with Valsalva maneuver.
- Be aware that testes are often smaller in varicocele.

Signs and Symptoms of Testicular Torsion

- The torsed testicle may be lying horizontally or appear higher in the scrotal sack than the opposite testicle.
- Although most commonly, the situation is unilateral, it may be bilateral. Scrotal edema is usually present within 12 hours.
- Especially in the neonate, the torsed testicle may feel quite hard.
- One way to differentiate the diagnosis of testicular torsion is to attempt to elicit the cremasteric reflex, which is normally absent on the torsion side.
- Prehn's sign, which is relief of pain from elevating the testicle, is also usually absent in torsion (Cole & Vogler, 2004).

CLINICAL ALERTS

Calculation of Daily Maintenance Fluid Requirements

Fluid balance means that the liquid in the body is regulated in such a way to maintain homeostasis (a state of equilibrium). The body's intake and output of fluid in a 24-hour period is approximately the same. Fluid balance is measured by daily discrepancies in body weight and by monitoring fluid intake and output. There are two methods of fluid maintenance:

- The surface area method is the most common and used for children >22 lbs. (10 kg): 1500 to 2000 mL/m² per day.

Daily Maintenance Fluid Requirements	
Child's Weight	**Daily Maintenance Fluid Requirement**
0–10 kg (0–22 lbs.)	100 mL/kg of body weight
11–20 kg (24.2–44 lbs.)	1000 mL + 50 mL/kg for each kg >10
>20 kg (>44 lbs.)	1500 mL + 20 mL/kg for each kg >20

Note: The method used to measure normal urinary output is 1–2 mL/kg per hour.

Types of Dehydration

Depending on the cause of the fluid loss, a child will lose water and electrolytes.

- *Isotonic* dehydration occurs when electrolyte and water deficits are present in balanced proportions (sodium and water are lost in equal amounts). Serum sodium remains in normal limits 130 to 150 mEq/L. This is the most common type of dehydration. Hypovolemic shock is the greatest concern.
- *Hypotonic* dehydration occurs when the electrolyte deficit exceeds the water deficit. Serum sodium concentration is <130 mEq/L. Physical signs are more severe with smaller fluid losses.
- *Hypertonic* dehydration is the most dangerous type and occurs when water loss is in excess of electrolyte loss. Sodium serum concentration is >150 mEq/L. Seizures are likely to occur.

Pathophysiology of Dehydration

Reasons for Dehydration
- Fever
- Vomiting
- Diarrhea
- Diaphoresis
- Hemorrhage
- Burns

- Trauma
- Diminished fluid intake

Possible Results of Dehydration
- Rapid and sudden extracellular fluid loss
  - Electrolyte imbalance
  - Intracellular fluid loss
  - Cellular dysfunction
- Hypovolemic shock (tachycardia, tachypnea, hypotension, cool, clammy, or cyanotic skin, decreased urine output)
  - Death

Sources of *E. coli* 0147.H7

- Undercooked ground beef is a primary source of *E. coli* 0147.H7, which can cause hemolytic uremic syndrome. Meat should be cooked until it reaches an internal temperature of 160°F and is no longer pink.
- *E. coli* outbreaks have originated in fast-food and other restaurants and have been linked to nonpasteurized cider, milk, juice, alfalfa sprouts, strawberries, and most recently, raw spinach.

Hematuria

- Hematuria usually is considered the cardinal marker of renal injury.
- Any degree of hematuria suggests underlying renal injury or anomaly.
- Hematuria out of proportion to the mechanisms of injury suggests a congenital anomaly or neoplasm.

Signs of Kidney Transplant Rejection

- Hypertension
- Decreased urinary output
- Fever
- Weight gain
- Edema
- Graft site pain
- Increasing BUN and creatinine levels

(Kenner et al., 2007).

DIAGNOSTIC TESTS

Sodium (Na⁺) Deficit (Hyponatremia; Serum Sodium Concentration <130 mEq/L)

Causes	Signs and Symptoms	Nursing Care
Decreased sodium intake Excessive sweating Fever Malnutrition Vomiting Diarrhea Nasogastric suction Diabetic ketoacidosis Kidney disease	Dehydration Nausea Weakness Lethargy Abdominal cramping Dizziness Weak pulse Decreased blood pressure	Determine the underlying cause. Administer IV fluids with the appropriate amount of sodium added. Monitor laboratory values (electrolytes).

Sodium (Na⁺) Excess (Hypernatremia; Serum Sodium Concentration ≥150 mEq/L)

Causes	Signs and Symptoms	Nursing Care
Excessive salt intake Fever High insensible water loss Diabetes insipidus Hyperglycemia Kidney disease	Oliguria Nausea Vomiting Muscle twitching Lethargy	Determine the underlying cause. Monitor neurological status. Monitor laboratory values (electrolytes).

Potassium (K⁺) Deficit (Hypokalemia; Serum Potassium Concentration ≤3.5 mEq/L)

Causes	Signs and Symptoms	Nursing Care
Diuresis Starvation IV fluid without potassium added Diarrhea Vomiting Nasogastric suction Administration of diuretics or corticosteroids Burns that are healing Alkalosis	Muscle weakness Muscle cramping and stiffness Hypotension Hyporeflexia Cardiac arrhythmias (tachycardia or bradycardia) Fatigue Drowsiness	Determine the underlying cause. Monitor vital signs. Offer high-potassium foods. Administer oral potassium supplements (assess for adequate output before administration). Administer IV potassium slowly. Obtain ECG (for IV potassium bolus). Monitor laboratory values (electrolytes). Evaluate acid–base status.

Potassium (K⁺) Excess (Hyperkalemia; Serum Potassium Concentration ≥5.5 mEq/L)

Causes	Signs and Symptoms	Nursing Care
Increased intake of potassium	Muscle twitching	Determine the underlying
Severe dehydration	Muscle weakness	cause.
Rapid administration of IV	Flaccid paralysis	Monitor vital signs.
potassium chloride	Hyperreflexia	Obtain ECG.
Potassium sparing diuretics	Oliguria	Administer IV fluids as
Burns	Apnea (respiratory arrest)	ordered.
Kidney disease (failure)	Bradycardia	Administer IV insulin to
Adrenal insufficiency	Ventricular fibrillation	facilitate potassium
(Addison disease)	(cardiac arrest)	moving into cells (if
Metabolic acidosis		ordered).
		Monitor laboratory values
		(electrolytes).
		Evaluate acid–base status.

Calcium (Ca²⁺) Deficit (Hypocalcemia; Serum Calcium Concentration <8.8 mEq/L)

Causes	Signs and Symptoms	Nursing Care
Inadequate dietary intake	Tetany	Determine the underlying
Vitamin D deficiency	Convulsions	cause.
Feeding cow's milk to infants	Neuromuscular irritability	Administer oral calcium
Advanced adrenal insufficiency	Hypotension	supplement as prescribed.
	Tingling (nose, ears, toes	Administer IV calcium
	and fingertips)	slowly and monitor IV site
	Cardiac arrest	(irritation).
		Monitor laboratory values
		(serum calcium and
		potassium levels).

Calcium (Ca²⁺) Excess (Hypercalcemia; Serum Calcium Concentration >10.8 mEq/L)

Causes	Signs and Symptoms	Nursing Care
Excessive vitamin D intake	Weakness	Determine the underlying
Acidosis	Fatigue	cause.
Immobilization (prolonged	Constipation	Obtain ECG.
periods of time)	Anorexia	Monitor laboratory values
Increased bone catabolism	Nausea	(electrolytes).
Hyperthyroidism	Vomiting	
Kidney disease	Thirst	
	Bradycardia (cardiac arrest)	

Determining Problems with the Urinary Tract

- The renal ultrasound depicts the ureters but does not discern if there is an infection.
- A voiding cystourethrogram (VCUG) depicts urethral and bladder anatomy.
- An intravenous pyelogram (IVP) assists with identifying the size, shape, and position of the urinary system as well as elimination function by noting length of time for passage of contrast material through the kidneys.
- Nuclear cystography visualizes the bladder and is good for detecting VUR.
- Nuclear cortical scanning detects tubular damage and scarring

(Egland & Egland, 2006; Pagana & Pagana, 2003).

Voiding Cystourethrograms (VCUG)

Gradations of VUR are provided in the International Reflux Grading System, with a range from Grade I to Grade V (Fig. 29-1).

Grade I	Urine backs up into the ureter only, and the renal pelvis appears healthy, with sharp calyces.
Grade II	Urine backs up into the ureter, renal pelvis, and calyces. The renal pelvis appears healthy and has sharp calyces.
Grade III	Urine backs up into the ureter and collecting system. The ureter and pelvis appear mildly dilated, and the calyces are mildly blunted.
Grade IV	Urine backs up into the ureter and collecting system. The ureter and pelvis appear moderately dilated, and the calyces are moderately blunted.
Grade V	Urine backs up into the ureter and collecting system. The pelvis severely dilates, the ureter appears tortuous, and the calyces are severely blunted.

Source: Cendron & Benedict (2006, p. 1).

I II III IV V

Figure 29-1 Gradations of VUR are found in the International Reflux Grading System, ranging from Grade I to Grade V.

Procedure 29-1 Urine Collection

Purpose

The purpose of collecting a urine specimen is to screen for early signs of disease

Equipment

Packaged urine culture set (usually contains three iodine or antiseptic towelettes and a sterile plastic collection container)

Steps

1. Wipe (or have the child wipe) the labia or penis with the three iodine or antiseptic solution towelettes. The customary procedure is to wipe the area three times.

   - In males, wipe the urethral tip three times in a circular fashion, once with each wipe.

   - In females, holding the labia open to expose the urethra, wipe the right side top to bottom and discard the wipe. Repeat on the left side, discarding the wipe. Finally, wipe top to bottom over the central area and the urethral meatus and discard that wipe.

2. Ask the child to start urinating into the toilet, bedpan, or urinal, and then to stop urinating.

3. Position the sterile urine container so that it catches about 3 to 4 ounces of "mid-stream" urine, which needs to be about 3–4 oz. of urine.

4. Remove the container and cap it, taking care not to contaminate the inner container with your gloved hands.

5. Allow the child to finish voiding into the toilet, bedpan, or urinal.

6. Do not keep the urine sample at room temperature any longer than 10 minutes, unless it is directly in transport to the laboratory. If the specimen cannot be sent to the laboratory immediately, it is necessary to refrigerate it in a plastic specimen bag.

7. Note the time and date of urine collection on the container label and in the patient's chart. The container label should also contain the patient's name and other identifying information, such as identification number.

Procedure 29-1 (Continued)

8. If the patient's parents will be responsible for collecting urine at home, instruct them in sterile collection and proper storage of the specimen.
9. Document the procedure.

Clinical Alert Do not keep a urine culture at room temperature any longer than 10 minutes, unless it is directly in transport to the laboratory. If the specimen cannot be sent to the laboratory immediately, it is necessary to refrigerate it in a plastic specimen bag to prevent the overgrowth of organisms that interfere with the interpretation of the culture and sensitivity to specific antibiotics. The specimen is plated on a nutrient medium and bacteria that are present are allowed to grow and then are counted. Usually, different antibiotic discs are placed on the inoculated medium to show which ones decrease the colony counts (sensitivity).

Teach Parents:

Parents may be responsible for collecting urine cultures of their children at home or in the medical office, so they must be instructed on the sterile techniques of handling the specimen. If the specimen is collected at home, it may need to be refrigerated before bringing it to the laboratory.

Urine Dipstick Test

To perform an accurate urine dipstick test, obtain proper quantities of urine to dip the sticks into, and then wait the appropriate amount of time to test each specimen (Fig. 29-2).

Figure 29-2 Nurses should be able to perform an accurate dipstick test.

Normal Urinalysis Values

Urinalysis Component	Normal Values
Appearance	Clear
Color	Amber yellow
Odor	Aromatic
pH	4.6–8.0 (average 6.0)
Osmolarity	50–1,400 mOsm/L
Protein	None or up to 8 mg/dL
	50–80 mg/24 hr (at rest)
	<250 mg/24 hr (exercise)
Specific gravity	Adult: 1.005–1.030 (usually 1.010–1.025)
	Elderly: values decrease with age
	Newborn: 1.001–1.020
Leukocyte esterase	Negative
Nitrites	Negative
Ketones	Negative
Crystals	Negative
Casts	None present
Glucose	Brand new specimen: Negative
	24-hour specimen: 50–300 mg/day or 0.3–1.7 mmol/day (SI units)
White blood cells (WBCs)	0–4 per low-power field
WBC casts	Negative
Red blood cells (RBCs)	Up to 2
RBC casts	None

Common Urinalysis Findings of Acute Renal Failure

Findings	Interpretation
Sediment	Intrinsic kidney failure
Color	"Dirty" brown: Intrinsic renal failure Reddish brown: Acute glomerulonephritis Bilious tinge: Mixed hepatic and renal failure
Proteinuria	Glomerulonephritis Interstitial nephritis Toxic and infectious causes
Casts	Red blood cells: Glomerulonephritis or vasculitis White blood cells: Interstitial nephritis Granular: Glomerulonephritis Uric acid crystals: Tumor lysis syndrome Calcium oxalate crystals: Ethylene glycol ingestion Acetaminophen (Tylenol) crystals: Acetaminophen toxicity acute

Renal Tubular Function

The fractional excretion of sodium (FE_{NA}) is an index of renal tubular function.

FE_{NA} = ([U_{NA}/P_{NA}]/Ucreat/Pcreat) × 100 (Schwartz, 2005, p. 711).

- An FE_{NA} greater than 2 is correlated with acute interstitial nephritis or acute tubular necrosis.
- An FE_{NA} less than 1 is correlated with hemolytic uremic syndrome, acute glomerulonephritis, or prerenal causes.

Laboratory Differential Diagnosis of Acute Renal Failure

	Prerenal		Intrarenal		Postrenal
	Child	Neonate	Child	Neonate	
Urine Na⁺ (mEq/L)	<20	<20–30	>40	>40	Variable, may be >40
FEna* (%) Should not be obtained after a diuretic is given as renders the test inaccurate	<1	<2–5	>2	>2.5	Variable, may be >2

(continued)

Laboratory Differential Diagnosis of Acute Renal Failure (Continued)

	Prerenal		Intrarenal		Postrenal
	Child	**Neonate**	**Child**	**Neonate**	
Urine Osmolality (mOsmol/L)	>500	>300–500	>300	>300	Variable, may be <300
Serum BUN-to-Creatinine Ratio	>20	≥10	>10	>10	Variable, may be >20
Urinalysis	Normal		RBCs, WBCs, casts, proteinuria		Variable to normal, possible crystals
Comments	History: Diarrhea, vomiting, hemorrhage, diuretic Physical: Volume depletion		History: Hypotension, anoxia, exposure to nephrotoxins Physical: Hypertension, edema		History: Poor urine stream and output Physical: Flank mass, distended bladder

*Fractional excretion of sodium = [(urine sodium/plasma sodium) + (urine creatinine/plasma creatinine)] × 100.
RBCs, red blood cells; WBCs, white blood cells.
Source: Kliegman et al. (2006, p. 761).

Diagnostic Tools Determining Reason for Amenorrhea

- Genetic testing may be required to determine disorders such as Turner's syndrome.
- Pelvic ultrasound or transvaginal (ultrasound wand in the vaginal canal) is used to test for pregnancy, ovarian cysts, and other gynecological abnormalities. Patients normally are required to drink four 8-ounce glasses of water 1 hour before a pelvic ultrasound to elevate the bladder in order to view the pelvic organs.

Laboratory Tests for Amenorrhea

Urine Pregnancy Test	Widely available over the counter, but more sensitive tests are available in clinical facilities.
Serum Pregnancy Test	Qualitative and quantitative tests show positive pregnancy and approximate duration of pregnancy, respectively. More accurate than urine pregnancy tests, and detect pregnancy earlier.

Thyroid-stimulating Hormone (TSH) Level	A general test for hypothyroidism and hyperthyroidism. May be accompanied by test of free thyroxine test to specify the disorder more clearly
Prolactin Level	Elevated in hyperprolactinemia, which may be seen with hypothyroidism or with a benign pituitary adenoma. Prolactin is a hormone produced in the pituitary gland and associated with breast-feeding.
Follicle-stimulating Hormone (FSH) Level	May be decreased in polycystic ovary syndrome (PCOS).
Luteinizing Hormone (LH) Level	May be increased in PCOS.
Testosterone Level	May be increased in PCOS, along with dehydroepiandrosterone (DHEA) level.

Tests for Testicular Torsion

- Doppler ultrasonography is the preferred diagnostic test and should be ordered immediately.
- The test can differentiate between ischemia; inflammation, such as that seen in orchitis (inflammation of a testis); and epididymitis (inflammation of the epididymis), often seen with gonorrhea.
- In possible false-negative results, a technetium scintigraphy test will show definitive testicular torsion (Ringdahl & Teague, 2006).
- The testicle may be enlarged and may have decreased or absent blood flow.

MEDICATIONS

Broad-Spectrum Antibiotics

- Stress to the parents the need for the child to complete the prescribed amount and to maintain adequate intake of fluids.
- For those children taking prophylactic low-dose antibiotics, taking the medication at night allows the drug more time in the bladder.
- Children who receive broad-spectrum antibiotics that are likely to alter GI and periurethral flora are at increased risk for UTI because these drugs disturb the natural defense against colonization by pathogenic bacteria (Hellerstein, 2007, p.4).

Common Anti-Infectives, Side Effects, and Nursing Interventions

Generic Drug Name Trade name	Side Effects	Nursing Interventions and Patient Teaching
Ampicillin (IV) *Marcillin*	Nausea, vomiting, diarrhea, Rash	Hold and notify MD if rash or diarrhea. With prolonged therapy periodically monitor renal, hepatic and hematological lab work.
Cefixime (PO) *Suprax*	Serious side effects: Stevens–Johnson syndrome, nephrotoxicity, blood dyscrasias Superinfections (can occur with any antibiotic)	Monitor BUN, serum creatinine, and input & output (I & O). Teach how to recognize superinfection, e.g., furry tongue, perineal itching. Tell the patient to take with yogurt/buttermilk to decrease superinfection by maintaining intestinal flora.
Cefotaxime (IV) *Claforan*	Mild diarrhea, mild abdominal cramping	Monitor fluid intake.
Ceftriaxone (IV) *Rocephin*	Serious side effect: Antibiotic-associated colitis manifested as severe abdominal pain, tenderness, fever, and diarrhea that is severe and watery	Assess bowel pattern or pain. Monitor I & O.
Cephalexin (PO) *Biocef, Keflex*	Serious side effects: Antibiotic-associated colitis and other superinfections, nephrotoxicity with preexisiting renal disease, angioedema, bronchospasm, and anaphylaxis (especially if allergies to penicillin or cephalosporins)	Monitor I & O for nephrotoxicity. Assess bowel activity, stool consistency, and increasing GI effects. Advise taking with food or milk if mild GI upset occurs. Assess mucous membranes and tongue for white patches.
Ciprofloxacin (PO) *Cipro*	Many IV incompatibilities Serious side effects: superinfection, nephrotoxicity, cardiac arrest, cerebral thrombosis Arthropathy may occur in children younger than 18 years.	Monitor I & O; assure that appropriate fluid intake maintained. Caution regarding sun exposure affecting eyes, skin.

Generic Drug Name Trade name	Side Effects	Nursing Interventions and Patient Teaching
		If patient wears contact lenses, remove if taking ophthalmic solution or ointment.
Gentamicin (IV) *Garamycin*	Serious side effects: Ototoxicity, nephrotoxicity	Monitor urinalysis. Therapeutic peak 5-10 mcg/mL and trough is 2 mcg/mL. The family should notify physician of any balance, hearing, urinary, or vision problems even after drug is completed.
Nitrofurantoin (PO) *Macrodantin, Furadantin*	Serious side effects: Stevens–Johnson syndrome, liver toxicity, peripheral neuropathy, impairment of pulmonary function	Monitor for peripheral neuropathy, e.g., numbness and/or tingling of extremities. Monitor for liver toxicity signs and symptoms. Monitor respiratory system and chest pain, cough, or difficulty with respirations.
Sulfamethoxazole/ Trimethoprim (PO) *Bactrim, Septra, Generic*	Serious side effects: Fatalities secondary to Stevens-Johnson syndrome, toxic epidermal necrolysis, fulminant hepatic necrosis and other blood dyscrasias, such as agranulocytosis, aplastic anemia	Contraindicated in children younger than 2 months of age; kernicterus may result if used with newborns. Monitor I & O; assess skin for pallor, purpura, and rash or overt signs of bleeding, swelling. Monitor hematology and liver and renal function lab results. Tell the family to report new symptoms, e.g., bruising, fever, sore throat, or other skin reactions.

Medications Used to Treat Complications of Acute Renal Failure

Medication	Action/Indication	Nursing Implications
Hyperkalemia		
Kayexalate	Exchanges sodium for potassium.	May require up to 4 hours to take effect.
Calcium gluconate 10%	Counteracts potassium-induced increased myocardial irritability.	Monitor for ECG changes. Intravenous infiltration may result in tissue necrosis.
Albuterol	Shifts potassium to the cells.	Give by inhalation.
Metabolic Acidosis		
Sodium bicarbonate or sodium citrate	Helps correct metabolic acidosis by exchanging hydrogen for potassium.	Do not mix with calcium. Complications include fluid overload, hypertension, and tetany.
Hypocalcemia		
Calcium gluconate 10%	Used in the presence of tetany; provides ionized calcium to restore nervous tissue function to control serum phosphorus.	Administer slowly to prevent bradycardia. Monitor for ECG changes.
Malignant Hypertension (B/P>95% for age)		
Sodium nitroprusside, nitroglycerin	Relaxes smooth muscle in peripheral arterioles.	Administer by continuous intravenous infusion; fall in blood pressure is seen within 10–20 minutes.

Medications Commonly Used for Children with Chronic Renal Failure

Medication	Action or Indication	Nursing Considerations
Vitamin and mineral supplement (Nephrocaps)	Adds vitamins and minerals missing from heavily restricted diet.	Only prescribed vitamins should be used; over-the-counter brands may contain elements that are harmful.
Phosphate binding agents: Calcium carbonate (Tums), calcium acetate (PhosLo), or sevelamer hydrochloride (Renagel)	Reduce absorption of phosphorus from the intestines.	Ensure that phosphate binding agent is aluminum free.

Medication	Action or Indication	Nursing Considerations
Calcitriol (Rocaltrol)	Replaces the calcitriol that kidneys are no longer producing to keep calcium balance normal.	Monitor serum calcium level. Ensure that calcium supplement is provided.
Epoetin alfa (Epogen, Procrit)	Stimulates bone marrow to produce red blood cells; treats anemia due to chronic renal failure (CRF).	Given by IV or subcutaneous injection. Monitor blood pressure as hypertension is an adverse effect. Monitor hematocrit and serum ferritin level according to facility guidelines.
Iron supplementation	Treats iron deficiency when epoetin alfa is prescribed.	May be administered orally or IV during hemodialysis.
Growth hormone (rhGH)	Used to stimulate growth in children with CRF.	Record accurate height measurements at regular intervals.
Antihypertensive agents: Angiotensin-converting enzyme (ACE) inhibitor (enalapril, lisinopril) Loop diuretics	Used with proteinuric kidney disease as it slows the progression to end-stage renal disease Used when volume overload is present.	Monitor renal function and electrolyte balance.

Medications Used for Enuresis

- Desmopressin (DDAVP) is a synthetic analogue of the antidiuretic hormone (ADH). This medication, administered orally or via a nasal spray, acts to lower nocturnal urinary production. The spray is given intranasally at doses of 1 to 40 mcg (1 to 4 sprays) each night, beginning with the lowest effective dose. If given orally, desmopressin (DDAVP) is available in 0.2 mg tablets given in dosages of 0.2 mg to 0.6 mg per night. Success rates range from 10% to 65%, but unfortunately, relapse rates are high, at 80%, when the drug is discontinued. Although there is a slight risk of water intoxication, the drug overall appears safe and efficacious (National Guidelines Clearinghouse, 2004).

- Imipramine (Tofranil) has been used for enuresis. Imipramine (Tofranil) may be used in a bedtime dose of 1 to 2.5 mg/kg with up to 60% effectiveness. As imipramine (Tofranil) is a tricyclic antidepressant, it is subject to risk of cardiac arrhythmia and therefore pretreatment EKG is required (National Guidelines Clearinghouse, 2004).

Topical Antifungal Medications for Candida vulvovaginalis				
Medication	**Pregnancy Category**	**Mechanism**	**Absorption**	**Use**
Miconazole (Monistat products)	C	Damages fungal cell wall membrane, which causes nutrients to leak.	Small amount through the vagina	Apply topically, very sparingly, to external vagina once or twice daily in adolescents; may be applied with vaginal applicator in adolescents.
Nystatin (Mycostatin products)	B	Binds to sterols in fungal cell membrane, changing wall permeability	Not absorbed through mucous membranes, therefore safer for children	Gently massage cream or ointment into skin two to four times daily.
Clotrimazole (Lotrimin, Mycelex products)	B (topical)	Binds to phospholipids in cell membrane, causing cell wall permeability and loss of cell contents	Negligible through intact skin topically; 3% to 10% absorption when applied intravaginally	In children older than age 3, apply vaginal cream (Mycelex) 2% bid to external vagina. In children older than age 12 and adults, vaginal applicator may be used for cream.

Source: Taketomo, Hodding, & Kraus (2007).

ETHNOCULTURAL CONSIDERATIONS

Kidney Failure

"African Americans constitute about 32 percent of all patients treated for kidney failure in the United States, but only about 13 percent of the overall U.S. population. Anyone with high blood pressure, diabetes, or a family history of kidney disease is at risk and should have his or her kidney function tested" (Former U.S. Surgeon General Dr. Joycelyn Elders).

Enuresis

Toileting patterns and expectations vary among different cultural and ethnic groups. Enuresis may be considered more problematic for some people than for others, and expectations of bladder and bowel control vary among parents, teachers, health care professionals, and daycare providers.

TEACHING THE FAMILY

Arteriovenous (AV) Fistulas

- Teach the child (and family) with a new AV fistula to wash the access site with soap and water each day and always before dialysis.
- Instruct the child not to scratch the area or pick at scabs.
- Tell the child and family to check the area daily for signs of infection, including warmth and redness.
- Teach them to check for blood flow in the area daily by showing them the vibration (thrill) that should be present over the access site. Tell the child and family to notify a health care provider at the dialysis center if this vibration changes or stops.
- Urge the child to avoid traumatizing the arm with the access site, including by not wearing tight clothes or jewelry, carrying heavy objects, or sleeping on the arm.
- Instruct the child and family to remind all health care providers not to take blood or blood pressure measurements using that arm.
- Tell the child and family that needle sites should be rotated.
- Tell the child and family to apply gentle pressure to stop bleeding when the needle is removed. Also explain that gentle pressure should be applied if bleeding resumes later. A health care provider should be called if bleeding is excessive or does not stop within 30 minutes.

Vulvovaginitis

- Suggest tub baths with clear, warm water once to twice daily for 10 to 15 minutes, followed by washing with a bland soap such as unscented Dove, Basis, Aveeno, or Neutrogena. The soap should not be applied to the vulvar area, and the vulva should never be scrubbed.

- Discourage shampooing the hair in the bathtub to keep the vulva from being exposed to shampoo chemicals. Showering is a better option.
- Instruct the patient to gently pat the vulvar area dry after bathing.
- Sleeper pajamas are not recommended due to their occlusive nature.
- Underwear should be all cotton for greater ventilation, and they should be washed in mild, unscented detergent without bleach.
- Some health care providers recommend applying a small amount of A+D ointment, Vaseline, or Desitin ointment to protect the vulvar skin. Loose-fitting clothing is ideal, especially in warm weather.
- Persistent discharge is occasionally treated with certain oral or topical antibiotics.
- Pinworms may cause recurrent vulvovaginitis; it may be necessary to instruct parents to inspect their child's anal area at night with a flashlight or apply a small piece of cellophane tape over the anal area to catch the pinworms or their eggs (Emans, 2005).

Vaginal Candidiasis

Instruct the patient in the following:

- Wear cotton underwear to allow better ventilation.
- Avoid wearing wet clothing, such as bathing suits, for long periods.
- Avoid taking bubble baths and using perfumes or powder near the vaginal area.
- In menstruating females, avoid scented sanitary pads or tampons.
- Avoid excessive sugars and simple carbohydrates in the diet.
- Eat yogurt, which contains natural lactobacilli, to maintain normal bacterial balance in the GI tract, keeping yeast in check.

Causes of Secondary Amenorrhea

Review with the patient these possible causes of secondary amenorrhea:

- Pregnancy
- Corpus luteum cyst

- Lactation
- Menopause (premature or normal)
- Hypothyroidism or hyperthyroidism
- Chemotherapy
- Polycystic ovarian syndrome (PCOS)
- Diabetes mellitus
- Stress
- Excessive exercise
- Weight loss

(Herban, Hill, & Sullivan, 2004)

Cryptorchidism

- Teach patients and caregivers that human chorionic gonadotropin may cause penile growth, increased pigmentation, and pubic hair.
- Urge them to talk about any anxieties raised by the risk of testicular cancer and decreased fertility.

Gynecomastia

- Teach the patient and parents that gynecomastia is usually a temporary condition.
- If obesity is an issue, work with the patient and family members to establish an age-appropriate dietary plan. Referral to a nutritionist may be useful.
- Explain to the family and patient that certain blood tests may be used to eliminate any risk of pathological causes of the gynecomastia.
- Discuss ways the child can respond to hurtful comments from other children.

ADDITIONAL INFORMATION FOR THE CLINICAL SETTING

Fluid and Electrolyte Balance Nursing Interventions

- Obtain daily weights (same scale, same time and wearing the same clothing, infants are weighed naked and oftentimes older children only have on their underwear).
- Measure intake and output (weigh diapers to assess output). Assess hydration status which includes assessing for presence of tears, skin turgor, anterior fontanel (up to 18 months), sticky mucous membranes, sunken eyeballs,

urine and stool output, weight loss, tachycardia, tachypnea, decreased blood pressure, temperature and thirst.

- Laboratory tests include specific gravity, hematocrit, blood urea nitrogen (BUN), creatinine, Na^+, K^+, and Ca^{2+}.
- Assess type of acid–base disturbance (metabolic acidosis, metabolic alkalosis, or respiratory acidosis).
- Administer oral clear liquids as ordered (1 to 2 oz. every hour).
- Start an IV for fluid and electrolyte replacement as ordered.
- Before administering intravenous potassium (K^+), ensure the child has voided.
- Cleanse the perineal area and apply protective topical ointment.
- Encourage parents to be involved in the care of the child.
- Educate parents about signs and symptoms of dehydration, rehydration, and when to call the doctor.
- Encourage parents to be compliant with follow-up appointments.

Causes of UTI

- Bacterium, virus, or fungus
- Structural anomalies, catheterization, urinary tract instrumentation, and sexual activity (Lum, 2007; Wise & Cardinal-Busse, 2007).
- Boys are affected more than girls owing to a higher rate of congenital abnormalities (Lippincott Williams & Wilkins, 2004).
- Starting at 6 months, girls are at greater risk until school age and then again when they enter adolescence, owing to the proximity of the anus with fecal flora that are available to colonize easily within the urethra.
- Sexually active adolescent girls. The causative agent is *Chlamydia*.
- UTIs are also more common in uncircumcised males (Elder, 2004).
- Conditions associated with chronic perineal irritation such as poor hygiene, bubble baths, soaps, pinworms, or perineal trauma that experienced cyclists, dirt bikers, or equestrians may experience are important associations to consider in predisposing the individual to UTIs.

- Conditions such as constipation, neurogenic bladder, and voiding dysfunction, or a history of abnormal voiding patterns are potential underlying etiological factors.
- Fungus, particularly *Candida* (yeast) species in immunocompromised children (Kennedy, 2003).
- A child with a UTI may also have an anatomical abnormality called vesicoureteral

Hematuria

- The main sign of hematuria is blood in the urine.
- The color of the urine may be significant; tea-colored or brownish urine, especially if it contains protein and casts

Causes of Acute Renal Failure	
Prerenal, Hypovolemic, Hypotension	Dehydration Septic shock Heart failure Hemorrhage Burns Peritonitis Ascites Cirrhosis
Intrinsic, Intrarenal, Parenchymal	Acute tubular necrosis (nephrotoxins [drugs], reversible if caught early) Acute cortical necrosis (not reversible) Glomerulonephritis Interstitial nephritis Renal vein thrombosis Arterial thromboembolus (umbilical artery catheter) Disseminated intravascular coagulation Immune mediated (scleroderma) Hemoglobinuria, myoglobinuria (pigmented)
Postrenal (Obstruction)	Urethral obstruction (stricture, posterior urethral valves, diverticulum) Ureterocele Extrinsic tumor compressing bladder outlet Extrinsic urinary tract tumors Tumor lysis syndrome

Source: Kliegman et al. (2006, p. 760).

Signs and Symptoms of Electrolyte Imbalances in Acute Renal Failure

Electrolyte Imbalance	Clinical Manifestations	Clinical Treatment
Hyperkalemia (>6.0 mEq/L) Results from inability to adequately excrete potassium derived from diet and catabolized cells. In metabolic acidosis, there is also movement of potassium from intracellular fluid to extracellular fluid	Peaked T waves, widening of QRS on ECG Dysrhythmias: ventricular dysrhythmias, heart block, ventricular fibrillation, cardiac arrest Diarrhea Muscle weakness	Elimination of all intake of potassium (dietary, parenteral, or TPN) Administration of alkalinizing agents Kayexalate orally or in retention enema when K^+>7.0 mEq/L Other drugs may be ordered by physician, including calcium gluconate 10% solution, sodium bicarbonate, and regular insulin when K^+>7.0 mEq/L Dialysis if other methods to reduce the potassium level are ineffective
Hyponatremia In the acute oliguric phase, hyponatremia is related to the accumulation of fluid in excess of solute.	Change in level of consciousness Muscle cramps Anorexia Abdominal reflexes, depressed deep tendon reflexes Cheyne–Stokes respirations Seizures	Electrolyte replacement, sodium bicarbonate Dialysis to correct severe electrolyte disturbance
Hypocalcemia Phosphate retention (hyperphosphatemia) depresses the serum calcium concentration. Calcium is deposited in injured cells. Hyperkalemia and metabolic acidosis may mask the common clinical manifestations of severe hypocalcemia.	Muscle tingling Changes in muscle tone Seizures Muscle cramps and twitching Positive Chvostek sign (contraction of facial muscles after tapping facial nerve just anterior to parotid gland)	Calcium gluconate Low-phosphorus diet Phosphate binders, e.g., Tums tablets, calcium acetate and sevelamer. (Aluminum-based binders not utilized to prevent possible aluminum toxicity.) Calcium IV not given except for tetany to prevent calcium salt deposition into tissues) Dialysis to correct severe electrolyte disturbance

Complications of Acute Renal Failure

System	Complications
Metabolic	Hyperkalemia Metabolic acidosis Hyponatremia Hypocalcemia Hyperphosphatemia Hypermagnesemia Hyperuricemia
Cardiovascular	Pulmonary edema Arrhythmias Pericarditis Pericardial effusion Pulmonary embolism Hypertension Myocardial infarction
Gastrointestinal	Nausea Vomiting Malnutrition Gastrointestinal hemorrhage
Neurological	Neuromuscular irritability Asterixis (flapping tremor) Seizures Mental status change
Hematological	Anemia Bleeding
Infectious	Pneumonia Septicemia UTI
Other	Hiccups Increased parathyroid hormone level Low total triiodothyronine level Low thyroxine level Normal free thyroxine level

Four Stages of Chronic Renal Failure According to Glomerular Filtration Rate (GFR)

Percentage of Reduction of GFR	Stage of Renal Failure	GFR as Applied to Children Age 2 and Older*
35%–55% of normal	1. Reduced renal reserve	90 or higher
25%–35% of normal	2. Renal insufficiency	60–89
20%–25% of normal	3. Renal failure	30–59
<20% of normal	4. End-stage renal disease (ESRD)	15–29*

*If GFR <15, dialysis is needed.

Dialysis in Pediatric Nursing

Dialysis is a life-extending procedure for children with severe renal compromise. Dialysis may be done through the peritoneal wall (peritoneal dialysis) or through cleansing the blood by using a dialysis machine (hemodialysis).

Peritoneal Dialysis
- Utilizes the peritoneal membrane (abdominal lining) to filter blood and purify it.
- A dialysis solution composed of dextrose sugar and other minerals in water is inserted into the child's abdomen through an abdominal catheter.
- Through an osmotic process, the dialysis solution draws toxins, excess water, and waste chemicals from the blood into the dialysis solution.
- Then it is drained through an abdominal tube out of the abdomen. The amount of time the dialysis solution is in the abdomen is termed the dwell time, and the entire process of filling and emptying the abdomen is termed an exchange, which normally lasts 30 to 40 minutes.
- There are two essential types of peritoneal dialysis: continuous ambulatory peritoneal dialysis (CAPD) and continuous cycling peritoneal dialysis (CCPD).
- Nurses monitor the abdominal catheter sites for signs of infection or malfunctioning equipment and make certain that the returning dialysate solution remains clear.

Hemodialysis
- The child's blood is moved through a filter called a dialyzer, which is part of a complex machine.
- Extra water, extra salt, and toxic waste products are removed, while the blood pressure and electrolytes such as potassium, calcium, sodium, and bicarbonate are kept in balance.
- A special port is placed in the child, usually in the wrist, for vascular access. Through this port, the blood is removed through tubing into the dialyzer, cleansed, and then returned through a different set of tubes back to the child's body.
- Three types of ports are used: Arteriovenous (AV) fistulas, AV grafts, and venous catheters.
- It is imperative for pediatric nurses to teach the patient and parents or guardians how to keep the AV fistula, AV graft, or venous catheter safe and clean.

Dysfunctional Voiding

Dysfunctional elimination syndrome (DES), also called voiding dysfunction, is an abnormal but common pediatric elimination pattern associated with bladder and bowel withholding and incontinence. There are numerous types of voiding disorders:

- Urge incontinence
- Lazy bladder syndrome
- Giggle incontinence
- Bladder-sphincter dyssynergia
- Vaginal voiding

Alternative Treatments for Enuresis

- Hypnotherapy: Four to six sessions of hypnotherapy can train a child to awaken when his or her bladder feels full.
- Psychological evaluation: Although not every child with enuresis has psychological problems, there is an increased incidence of psychological issues in secondary enuresis, including parental divorce, school trauma, hospitalization, and sexual abuse (Practice Parameter for the Assessment and Treatment of Children and Adolescents With Enuresis http://www.aacap.org/galleries/PracticeParameters/Enuresis.pdf).
  - Also, psychological counseling is vital. Associated psychological and educational problems include learning disabilities, attention–deficit/hyperactivity disorder (ADHD), low motivation, sensory problems, and family issues. Parents and other family members may need assistance in dealing with these issues.
- Acupressure or massage therapy: These may be useful in some cases of neurologically induced enuresis.
- Homeopathic remedies: These should be provided by a licensed homeopathic provider.
  - Promote adequate hydration by ensuring that the child is hydrated with 8 ounces of water with each meal and then encouraged to void every 2 hours.
- Behavioral management and biofeedback
  - Voiding charts and diaries may help in tracking behavior and recording successes.
  - Biofeedback training helps the patient gain control over bladder muscles and relaxes the external sphincter. Children wear electromyogram (EMG) patches near the perineum or abdomen to assist in training.

Exstrophy of the Bladder

- Exstrophy of the bladder is a congenital defect where the anterior surface of the bladder is open on the abdominal wall. The defect has a variety of degrees of severity.
- Ultrasound is the tool used to diagnose exstrophy of the bladder.
- Surgery is necessary within the first 48 hours of the infant's life.
- The area must be kept clean because urine on the skin can cause irritation.
- Diapers should be loose-fitted and changed frequently.
- The exposed bladder may be covered with Vaseline gauze (Stein, 2007).

Cryptorchidism

- Cryptorchidism is defined as absent, undescended, or ectopic testicles.
- Gentle compression of the inguinal canals should reveal a palpable nodule in undescended testicles (Fig. 29-3).
- The surgical repair is termed orchiopexy and is usually done between ages 1 and 2.
- Instruct the caregiver to have the child wear loose clothing to increase comfort; use appropriate analgesics as ordered, including acetaminophen (Children's Tylenol); observe for erythema, purulent discharge, fever, and increased pain at the incision site as potentially indicative of infection.
- Instruct the caregiver to change diapers more frequently and to avoid having the older child engage in any sports or straddle riding toys that might injure the surgical site (Kenner et al., 2007).

Above the groin
In the groin area
Close to top of scrotum
Normal scrotal

Figure 29-3 An undescended testis is palpable in various areas and needs to be surgically corrected.

Hypospadias and Epispadias

- Hypospadias and epispadias are genetic congenital conditions, which imply an abnormal positioning of the urethral meatus in boys.
- In hypospadias, the meatus is inferior to its usual position.
- In epispadias, the meatus is superior to its usual position and a surgical correction with possible penile urethral lengthening may be necessary (Montagnino & Currier, 2005).
- Recognize that parents of these children may be deficient in knowledge about the defects and their repair.
- Assess the parents' feelings about having a child with a congenital defect (Kenner et al., 2007).

Ambiguous Genitalia

- External reproductive organs that are not easily identified as male or female (Venes, 2005).
- The nurse may assist the patient's family by suggesting endocrinology and genetic referrals.
- Some patients with ambiguous genitalia become surgical candidates (Gray & Campbell, 2002).

RESOURCES

American Academy of Child and Adolescent Psychiatry: http://www.aacap.org

Bedwetting Store: http://www.bedwettingstore.com

National Guideline Clearinghouse: http://www.guideline.gov

National Kidney Foundation: http://www.kidney.org

REFERENCES

Cendron, M., & Benedict, J. (2006). Vesicoureteral reflux. Retrieved from http://www.emedicine.com/med/topic2838 (Accessed April 24, 2009).

Cole, F.L., & Volger, R. (2004). The acute, nontraumatic scrotum: Assessment, diagnosis, and management. *Journal of the American Academy of Nurse Practitioners, 16*(2), 50–56.

Davis' Drug Guide for Nurses (2009). Imipramine. Retrieved from http://www.drugguide.com/monograph_library/psychotropic_drugs/imipramine.htm (Accessed April 24, 2009).

Elder, J. (2004). Urinary tract infections. In R.E. Behrman, R.M. Kleigman, & H.B. Jenson. *Nelson's textbook of pediatrics* (17th ed., pp. 1785–1789). Philadelphia: W.B. Saunders.

Emans, S.J. (2005). Vulvovaginal problems in the prepubertal child. In S.J. Emans, M.R. Laufer, & D.P. Goldstein (Eds.). *Pediatric & adolescent gynecology* (5th ed.). Philadelphia: Lippincott Willliams & Wilkins.

Egland, A. & Egland T. (2006). Pediatrics, urinary tract infections and pyelonephritis. Retrieved from http://www.emedicine.com/emer/topic 769.htm (Accessed April 24, 2009).

Gray, M., & Campbell, F. (2002). Urinary system. In J.A. Fox (Ed.). *Primary health care of infants, children, & adolescents* (2nd ed., pp. 670–693). St. Louis, MO: Mosby.

Hellerstein, S. (2007). Urinary tract infection. Retrieved from http:// www.emedicine.com/ped/topic2366.htm (Accessed April 24, 2009).

Herban Hill, N., & Sullivan, L.M. (2004). *Management guidelines for nurse practitioners working with children and adolescents* (2nd ed.). Philadelphia: F.A. Davis.

Hogan, M. & White, J. (2003). *Child health nursing: Reviews & rationales.* Upper Saddle River, NJ: PrenticeHall.

Kennedy, T. (2003). Urinary tract infection. In C. Rudolph & A. Rudolph (Eds.). *Rudolph's pediatrics* (21st ed., pp. 1667–1671). Chicago: McGraw-Hill.

Kenner, C., Moran, M., Zebold, K.F., Keating, B.J., & Amlung, S.R. (2007). Genitourinary alterations. In N.L. Potts & B.L. Mandleco (Eds.). *Pediatric nursing: Caring for children and their families* (2nd ed., pp. 623–659). Clifton Park, NY: Thompson Delmar.

Kliegman, R., Marcdante, K., Jenson, J. & Behrman, R. (2006). *Nelson essentials of pediatrics.* Philadelphia: Elsevier Saunders.

Lippincott Williams & Wilkins. (2004). *Straight A's in pediatric nursing.* Philadelphia: Lippincott Williams & Wilkins.

Lum, G.M. (2007). Kidney & urinary tract. In W.W. Hay, Jr., M.J. Levin, J.M. Sondheimer, & R. R. Deterding (Eds.). *Current pediatric diagnosis & treatment.* (18th ed). New York: Lange Medical Books/McGraw-Hill.

Montagnino, B., & Currier, H. (2005). The child with genitourinary dysfunction. In M.J. Hockenberry, D. Wilson, & M.L. Winkelstein (Eds.). *Wong's essentials of pediatric nursing* (7th ed., pp. 984–1010). St. Louis, MO: Mosby.

National Guideline Clearinghouse. (2004). Practice parameter for the assessment and treatment of children and adolescents with enuresis. Retrieved from http://www.guideline.gov (Accessed April 24, 2009).

Pagana, K., & Pagana, T. (2003). *Mosby's diagnostic and laboratory test reference.* Philadelphia: Mosby.

PDRhealth. (2007). Tofranil. Retrieved from http://www.pdrhealth.com/ drug_info/rxdrugprofiles/drugs/tof1448.shtml (Accessed April 24, 2009).

Razzaq, S. (2006). Hemolytic uremic syndrome: An emerging risk. *American Family Physician, 74*(6), 991–996.

Ringdahl, E., & Teague, L. (2006). Testicular torsion. *American Family Physician, 74*(10), 1739–1744.

Schwartz, M.W. (2005). *The 5 minute pediatric consult.* Philadelphia: Lippincott Williams & Wilkins.

Stein, A.M. (Ed.). (2007). *Nursing review series: Pediatric nursing.* Clifton Park, NY: Thomson Delmar Learning.

Taketomo, C.K., Hodding, J.H., & Kraus, D.M. (2007). *Pediatric dosage handbook*. Hudson, OH: Lexi-Comp.

Venes, D. (Ed.). (2005). *Taber's cyclopedic medical dictionary* (20th ed.). Philadelphia: F.A. Davis.

Wise, B. & Cardinal-Busse, B. (2007). Common illness of the reproductive and urologic systems. In N. Ryan-Wenger (Ed.). *Core curriculum for primary care pediatric nurse practitioners*. St. Louis, MO: Mosby.

Caring for the Child with a Hematological Condition

KEY TERMS

allogeneic transplant – A transplant in which the recipient's human leukocyte antigens (HLA) are matched to a compatible donor, usually a sibling

autologous transplant – A transplant in which the ill child is her own donor of stem cells

febrile reaction – A fever greater than 1.8 degrees Fahrenheit from the baseline temperature

hemarthrosis – Bloody effusion within a joint and soft tissue bleeding (Sevier, 2005)

neutropenia – When an absolute neutrophil count is <1000/µL in infants <1 year of age and 1500/µL for those older than 1 year of age

pancytopenia – Reduction in all cellular elements of the blood caused by bone marrow hematopoiesis failure (Hillman, Ault, & Rinder, 2005)

plasmapheresis – Removal of plasma containing harmful components such as circulating complexes, antibodies (IgM, IgG), cholesterol

syngeneic transplant – A transplant in which the donor of the bone marrow is an identical sibling

FOCUSED ASSESSMENT

Anemia

Signs and Symptoms
- Mild anemia, may be asymptomatic and not diagnosed until blood tests are completed. Initial signs include fatigue, shortness of breath, headache, difficulty concentrating, dizziness, and pale skin.
- Moderate to severe anemia: Irritability, fatigue, delayed motor development, tachycardia, shortness of breath, decreased activity level, pale, listless, systolic heart murmur, hepatomegly, congestive heart failure.

Iron-Deficiency Anemia

Signs and Symptoms
- Asymptomatic (mild anemia)
- Decreased hemoglobin (Hgb) and hematocrit (Hct)
- Irritability, fatigue, delayed motor development, shortness of breath, decreased activity level, and pallor
- Remember that it is possible for an overweight child to be diagnosed with iron-deficiency anemia

Epistaxis

Signs and Symptoms
- Bleeding from the nose

Sickle Cell Disease (SCD)

Signs and Symptoms
- Result of vaso-occlusion
- Weakness
- Pallor
- Fatigue
- Tissue hypoxia
- Jaundice
- Pain

Beta-Thalassemia

Signs and Symptoms
- Enlarged liver and spleen
- Mild jaundice

- Growth retardation
- Moderate to severe anemia
- Bony deformities
- Increased susceptibility to infection

Hereditary Spherocytosis (HS)

Signs and Symptoms
- Hyperbilirubinemia
- Splenomegaly
- Negative Comb's test

Hemophilia

Signs and Symptoms
- Present with bleeding or known family history of bleeding disorders
- Hemarthrosis

von Willebrand's Disease

Signs and Symptoms
- Epistaxis
- Bleeding from the oral cavity
- Menorrhagia
- Easy bruising

Idiopathic (Immune) Thrombocytopenia Purpura (ITP)

Signs and Symptoms
- Detected after a recent viral infection
- Petechiae
- Bruising
- Mucocutaneous bleeding
- Epistaxis
- Menorrhagia (adolescent)

Disseminated Intravascular Coagulation (DIC)

Signs and Symptoms
- Excessive bleeding from orifices
- Petechia, purpura, and hypotension
- Multiorgan failure

Aplastic Anemia

Signs and Symptoms
- Pancytopenia
- Anemia, pallor, dizziness, and fatigue
- Petechia, epistaxis
- Increased susceptibility to infections and oral ulcerations

Neutropenia

- The nursing plan of care for children with neutropenia is based on the severity of neutropenia.
- Absolute neutrophil count (ANC) is a measure of the number of neutrophil granulocytes present in the blood.
- Calculation of the absolute neutrophil count (ANC) is the total number of white blood cells multiplied by the percentage of neutrophils (segs and bands). See page 647.
- The National Cancer Institute neutropenia grading system classifies slight neutropenia as grade 1 with ANC of less than 2000, minimal neutropenia grade 2 with ANC of <1500, and moderate neutropenia grade 3 with ANC less than 1000. The most severe neutropenia is grade 4 with an ANC of <500.

Signs and Symptoms
- Lymphadenopathy
- Organomegaly
- Pallor
- Bruising
- Petechia

Thrombosis

Risk Factors
- Prolonged immobility
- Disease states, obesity, medications, hereditary factors
- Major surgery or trauma

Signs and Symptoms
- Lungs: Shortness of breath, lightheaded, and increased heart rate
- Kidney: Blood in the urine
- Skin: Hemorrhagic spots
- Artery or extremity: Cold, pale, blue, and absent pulse

Complications
- Stroke
- Deep vein thrombosis
- Pulmonary emboli

CLINICAL ALERTS

Screening Guidelines

- According to the recommendations in the American Academy of Pediatrics screening guidelines, hemoglobin and hematocrit should be evaluated once during infancy (6–9 months of age), early childhood (1–5 years of age), late childhood (5–12 years of age), and adolescence (14–20 years of age).
- Identifies children who may benefit from treatment for anemia.

Iron-Deficiency Anemia

- Iron-deficiency anemia is defined as a microcytic, hypochromic anemia caused by an inadequate supply of iron (Nathan et al., 2003).
- Iron-deficiency anemia is more common in infants. Premature infants are at high risk due to their decreased fetal iron supply (Nathan et al., 2003).
- Be vigilant for overweight infants who may have iron deficiency anemia because of excessive milk ingestion, known as "milk baby." These infants will be chunky, pale, with a "porcelain like" appearance. Other clinical features of these "milk babies" include poor muscle development as well as being susceptible to infections.

A Child Who Is Asplenic

- Seek immediate medical attention if a child has a temperature greater than 101.5°F (38.6°C). The child needs blood cultures and broad-spectrum antibiotics to prevent sepsis.
- There is an inability to filter certain encapsulated bacteria, which causes a low-grade bacterial infection or serious sepsis.

- Ensure that parents know that is critical for children to receive the pneumococcal and *H. influenzae* type b vaccine and other routine vaccinations.

Accumulation of Iron (Hemosiderosis)

- Chronic blood transfusion therapy may cause iron to accumulate in tissues and organs that the body cannot eliminate. Treatment is necessary to prevent toxic levels of iron in the body, which may result in death.
- Chelating agents are used to remove iron from the body through excretion of urine and stool. The main chelating agent is deferoxamine B (Desferal) (Lo & Singer, 2002). This drug is rapidly excreted in the urine; therefore it must be administered intravenously or subcutaneously over 8 to 10 hours, usually at bedtime, at least 5 days a week.
- Teach parents and older children how to insert the butterfly catheter and administer the drug via an infusion pump at home without difficulty.
- Monitoring iron levels is indicated for patients on chelation therapy to evaluate compliance and effectiveness of treatment.
- Evaluate patients at risk for hemosiderosis for long-term complications. Complications that may occur are a result of iron deposits that may damage vital organs causing hearing loss, diabetes, organ failure, and ultimately death.

Administration of Intravenous Anti-D Antibody

- Is the newest treatment for acute ITP patients who are Rh+.
- Common side effects: Transient hemolytic anemia that often resolves as the IgG disperses, fever, chills, and headache after infusion.
- Closely monitor vital signs.

Intracranial Bleeding

- Intracranial bleeding is the most serious complication in idiopathic (immune) thrombocytopenia purpura (ITP).
- Alert caregivers to report any changes in level of consciousness or behavior, severe headaches, vision

changes, ataxia, slurred speech, weakness or numbness, severe vomiting not associated with nausea.

Anaphylactic Reaction in Children Who Receive Antithymocyte Globulin (ATG)

- A severe anaphylactic reaction could occur (signs and symptoms include hypotension, tachycardia, shortness of breath, chest pain).
- Administer a test dose to check for allergic reaction, but be aware that an allergic reaction could occur beyond the test dose.
- If there is an allergic reaction, ATG may still be used following a desensitizing process and/or administration of pre-medications such as antihistamine and steroids.

Blood Transfusion Safety Measure

- To prevent a fatality, ensure a child receiving a transfusion is wearing a blood identification bracelet. The blood to be given must match identifying numbers on the bracelet.

The Administration Process for Blood Products

Pretransfusion

- Do not call for the product until it is needed.
- Verify the physician's orders including the appropriate product and volume to be infused. For packed red blood cell infusions appropriate volume is 10 to 13 mL/kg. Check with the institutional policies and procedures. The transfusion must be started within 30 minutes after the blood has left the blood bank.
- The maximum time for the infusion is 4 hours, which includes the first 30 minutes. Transfusion needs to start immediately due to the risk of bacterial contamination and cell lysis. Most blood banks will not accept blood back after 30 minutes.
- Follow institutional policy for obtaining, verifying, and transporting blood products obtained from the blood bank.
- Complete the appropriate forms and ensure accurate patient identification.
- Indicate product type and check for any special orders such as CMV safe, irradiated.

- Always check to see if any premedications were ordered before administration.
- Use PPE (personal protective equipment). Wear goggles and gloves.
- All blood products must be checked at the patient's bedside by two appropriate health care team members as per your institution's policy.
- Remember the two patient identifiers: Matching the numbers on the blood product and blood identification bracelet.

Initiation of the Transfusion
- Obtain baseline vital signs.
- Start the infusion slowly for the first 15 minutes.
- Designate a nurse to remain with the patient for the first 15 minutes of transfusion in the event of an adverse reaction.

During the Transfusion
- Do not infuse any other solutions simultaneously with blood through the same intravenous line; the only exception to this is normal saline (AABB Guidelines, 2004).
- Never add any medications to blood.
- Monitor vital signs per the institution's policy and procedures.
- All identification information that is attached to the blood product must remain attached until the transfusion is completed.
- Monitor for signs and symptoms of adverse reactions.

Posttransfusion
- Save the transfusion bag for at least 1 hour after the transfusion has ended.
- Complete the blood slip per the institution's policy.
- As per the American Association of Blood Bank (AABB). guidelines, include the following information on the child's medical record: Transfusion order, type of blood product, donor unit number, date and time of transfusion, pre and post vital signs, volume infused, required signatures, and any transfusion adverse events.
- Place the chart copy and blood bank copy of the blood slip in an appropriate area and keep on file as per policy and procedure.

Transfusion-Related Acute Lung Injury

- Transfusion-related acute lung injury (TRALI) occurs when there is an antigen–antibody reaction.
- The child who is experiencing TRALI may develop respiratory distress such as shortness of breath, hypoxia, hypotension, fever, and abnormal breath sounds.
- The reaction typically occurs within 1 to 2 hours after the transfusion has started and full-blown acute respiratory distress may occur within 6 hours (Knippen, 2006).
- Based on the severity of symptoms, respiratory support with a ventilator may be indicated. For mild cases of TRALI, supportive care is indicated.
- If this complication is suspected, it is reportable to the FDA (U.S. Food and Drug Administration, 2002).

DIAGNOSTIC TESTS

Hemoglobin and Hematocrit (Hgb & Hct)

- Complete blood count (CBC) and reticulocyte count are obtained to evaluate the hemoglobin and hematocrit.
- Anemia exists when the hemoglobin content is less than required to meet the oxygen demands of the body.
- Hemoglobin level is measured as the amount of hemoglobin per deciliter of whole blood. The average hemoglobin in the blood varies based on the age and gender of the individual. Normal Hemoglobin (Hgb; g/dL) lab values for children are:
  - Newborn: 12.7–18.6 g/dL
  - 2 Months: 9.0–14.0 g/dL
  - 2 Years: 10.5–12.7 g/dL
  - 6–12 Years: 11.2–14.8 g/dL
  - 12–18 Years: 10.7–15.7 g/dL
- The hematocrit is the percentage of whole blood that is composed of RBCs. The hematocrit measures both the number and size of the RBCs and is approximately three times greater than the hemoglobin value. The hematocrit indirectly measures the hemoglobin. The average hematocrit value is between 35% and 45% (Gilbert-Barness & Barness, 2003).

Complete Blood Count, Reticulocyte, and Peripheral Smear Lab Values for Children

- When evaluating for the presence of anemia, initial laboratory tests should include complete blood count (CBC) and a reticulocyte count. The CBC includes hemoglobin, hematocrit, red blood cell (RBC) indices, platelet count, white blood cell (WBC) count with a differential, and a peripheral smear to examine the morphology of the RBCs.
- For the patient with suspected anemia, the peripheral blood smear is imperative to confirm the appropriate diagnosis (Gilbert-Barness & Barness, 2003).

Normal Lab Values According to Age					
	Newborn	2 Months	2 Years	6–12 Years	12–18 Years
Red Blood Cell (RBC) Count	4.1–5.74	2.7–4.9	3.9–5.03	4.93–5.3	3.7–5.5
Hemoglobin (Hgb) (g/dL)	12.7–18.6	9.0–14.0	10.5–12.7	11.2–14.8	10.7–15.7
Hematocrit (Hct) (%)	37.4–56.1	28.0–42.0	31.7–37.7	34.0–43.9	33.0–46.2
White Blood Cell (WBC) Count	6.8–14.3	5.0–19.5	5.3–11.5	4.5–10.1	4.4–10.2
Platelets 10³/mm³(µL)	164–586	164–586	206–459	189–403	175–345

Normal White Blood Cell Differential Count According to Age

Age/White Blood Cell Component	Function	Newborn	2 Months	2 Years	6–12 Years	12–18 Years
Neutrophils (%)	Phagocytosis	19–49	15–35	13–33	32–54	34–64
Eosinophils (%)	Allergic reactions	0–4	0–3	0–3	0–3	0–3
Basophils (%)	Inflammatory reactions	0–1	0–1	0–1	0–1	0–1
Lymphocytes (%; B cells and T cells)	Humoral immunity (B cell) and cellular immunity (T cell)	38–46	42–72	46–76	27–57	25–45
Monocytes (%; macrophages)	Phagocytosis and antigen processing	0–9	0–6	0–5	0–5	0–5

Red Cell Lab Values for Children

Test	Reference Range	Comments
Mean Corpuscular Volume (MCV)	79–95 µm³	Average size of a single RBC, expressed as cubic microns (µm³)
Mean Corpuscular Hemoglobin (MCH)	25–33 pg/cell	Average weight of the Hgb within a RBC, expressed in picograms (pg)
Mean Cell Hemoglobin Concentration (MCHC)	31%–37% Hgb [g]/dl RBC	Average concentration of Hgb in each RBC
Reticulocyte Count	0.5%–1.5%	Measure of the production of mature RBCs by the bone marrow
Peripheral Smear	Size, shape, and structure of the RBCs, as well as an estimate of the amount of Hgb in the RBCs	Can indicate variations in size and shape of RBCs: microcytic, macrocytic, or normocytic

Evaluating a CBC		
Blood Elements	**Increase**	**Decrease**
RBC (Hgb/Hct)	Polycythemia	Anemia
WBC	Leukocytosis	Leukopenia
Platelets	Thrombocytosis	Thrombocytopenia

Epistaxis Diagnostic Workup: Laboratory Tests to Diagnose Bleeding Disorder		
Test	**Range**	**Significance**
Prothrombin Time (PT)	11–14 seconds	Measures the extrinsic pathway for bleeding, requires fibrinogen, prothrombin, and factors V, VII, and X. Prolonged times may indicate deficiencies of vitamin K liver factors, malabsorption, and liver disease.
Partial Thromboplastin Time (PTT)	25–38 seconds	Measures the intrinsic pathway for bleeding, requires factors V, VIII, IX, X, XI, and XII and fibrinogen and prothrombin. Prolonged times may indicate a bleeding disorder.

Source: H llman, Ault, & Rinder (2005).

Further Testing for Infants Suspected of Having Sickle Cell Disease

- If sickle cell disease is suspected, infants will need further testing, such as a hemoglobin electrophoresis (Fixler & Styles, 2002).
- A hemoglobin electrophoresis is a more specific blood test that identifies sickle cell disease versus sickle cell trait in a child (Gilbert-Barness & Barness, 2003).

Procedure 30-1 Obtaining a Fecal Occult Blood Test Sample

Purpose

A fecal occult blood test (FOBT) is performed to detect hidden (occult) blood in the stool.

Equipment

- Hematest cards
- Gloves
- Sterile tongue blade
- Chemical reagent

Steps

1. Wash hands and don gloves.
2. Verify the identity of the patient.
3. Check the manufacturer's instructions for specific Hematest cards.
4. Keep the Hematest cards at room temperature.
5. Use a sterile tongue blade to remove a sample of stool from the diaper.
6. Place a smear of stool on both windows of the Hematest card as indicated on the instructions.
7. Cover the windows with the paper flaps and wait the correct amount of time before reading the results.
8. Apply the recommended drops of developing solution to the Hematest card.
9. Read the back flap of the sample card within the recommended time of application of developing solution.
10. The Hematest card should change color to indicate the test results.
11. Document the procedure.

Clinical Alert When the nurse records the results, it is important to notify the health care provider of any abnormal findings. In addition, the nurse should check the expiration date on the developing solution.

Teach Parents

It is important to teach the parents the rationale for the test.

Type and Screen and Type and Crossmatch

The best outcome exists for the child when the nurse understands the difference between the type and screen and type and crossmatch.

Type and Screen
- Obtained in anticipation that a child may need blood.
- ABO group and Rh type of patient identified.
- Does not remove blood from inventory.

Type and Crossmatch
- Obtained if almost certain the child will require blood.
- ABO/Rh compatible donor red cells combined.
- Crossmatch is good for 72 hours (Hillman et al., 2005).

Understanding Blood Type

- When the clinical criterion is met, the nurse may proceed and obtain the product to be infused from the institution's blood bank or pharmacy. Understand that blood type is essential information for the nurse.

Blood Type	Can GIVE to:	TAKE from:
A+	A+	A+, A–, O–
A–	A+, A–	A–, O–
B+	B+	B+, B–, O+, O–
B–	B+, B–	B–, O–
AB+	AB+	All types
AB–	AB–	A–, B–, AB–, O–
O+	A+, B+, AB+, O+	O+, O–
O–	All types	O–

MEDICATIONS

Ketorolac (Toradol)

Generic Name Ketorolac (Kee-**toe**-role-ak)

Pregnancy Category C (D if used in the 3rd trimester)

Indications Short-term (≤5 days) management of moderate to severe pain, including post operative pain.

Actions Inhibits prostaglandin synthesis by decreasing activity of the enzyme, cyclooxygenase, which results in a decrease of prostaglandin precursors.

Therapeutic Effects Pain relief

Pharmacokinetics
Oral Well absorbed; 100%
IM/IV Rapid and complete

Contraindications and Precautions
Contraindicated in Hypersensitivity to Toradol, aspirin, or other NSAIDs
Patients with peptic ulcer disease or anyone with bleeding tendencies

Adverse Reactions and Side Effects Dizziness, headache, rash, diarrhea, GI pain, bleeding, prolonged bleeding times, anaphylaxis, hypersensitivity reactions.

Route and Dosage Ketorolac injection is approved for use in pediatric patients only as a single IM or IV dose in children 2–16 years of age; the use of ketorolac injection in children <2 years of age, the use of multiple doses of the injection in children <16 years of age, and the use of the tablets in children <16 years of age are outside of product labeling; ophthalmic solutions are approved for use in children ≥3 years of age.
Single-dose treatment: Manufacturer's recommendations:
IM: 1 mg/kg as a single dose; maximum dose: 30 mg
IV: 0.5 mg/kg as a single dose; maximum dose: 15 mg

Nursing Implications
Teach the patient and parents medication administration.
Do not exceed 5 days of total use.
Avoid alcohol.
May cause drowsiness and impair the ability to perform activities requiring mental alertness.

Additional Information 30 mg of Toradol provides analgesia comparable to 12 mg of morphine or 100 mg of meperidine.

Data from Deglin, J., & Vallerand, A. (2009). Davis's drug guide for nurses (11th ed.), pp. 716–718. Philadelphia: F. A. Davis.

Pneumococcal and *Haemophilus influenzae* Type b (Hib) Vaccine

- Children with hereditary spherocytosis (HS) should receive the pneumococcal and *Haemophilus influenzae* type b (Hib) vaccine before the splenectomy to prevent life-threatening bacterial infections.
- Children should also be given prophylactic penicillin to prevent fatal infections.

Proper Replacement Factors

- Now recombinant factor products are the main treatment of hemophilia patients (Sevier, 2005).

Hematopoietic Growth Factors

- Hematopoietic growth factor is granulocyte colony stimulating factor (GCSF), also known as Neupogen.
- GCSF stimulates the WBC lines.
- Growth factors for the WBCs are given to prevent profound neutropenia and prevent the patient from being susceptible to life threatening infections.
- Given by subcutaneous injection once a day by child's caregiver.
- Possible side effects: Fever, bone pain, headache, local reaction at injection site.

ETHNOCULTURAL CONSIDERATIONS

Sickle Cell Disease

- Most prominent in children of African American or Mediterranean descent
- May also be seen in Hispanics, Caucasians, and Italians

Jehovah Witness

- It is against this faith to receive blood and blood products, including self-donation.
- All alternatives should be explored to respect these beliefs.
- If the child is in a life-threatening situation, the courts may be called in to make a decision.

TEACHING THE FAMILY

Nutritional Counseling for the Prevention of Iron-Deficiency Anemia

- Feed the infant breast milk or commercial infant formula for the first 12 months of life.
- Use iron-fortified cereal from 6 to 12 months of age.
- Do not feed the infant cow's milk before 12 months of age (for infants 12 months and older limit the amount of cow's milk to 18 to 24 ounces per day).
- Once solids are introduced, offering the bottle before the feeding helps prevent iron deficiency.
- It is important for adolescents on a vegetarian diet or weight reduction diet to understand proper dietary alternatives to prevent iron-deficiency anemia.
- Dietary alternatives such as red meats, beans, whole grains, nuts, and iron-fortified cereals are good sources of iron.

Education About Oral Iron

- Educating parents on the proper administration of oral iron is a vital nursing responsibility.
- The iron supplement needs to be taken between meals because absorption is improved in an acidic environment.
- Administering iron with a glass of orange juice may also enhance absorption.
- Iron supplements should not be taken with tea because they may adversely affect the absorption process.
- Inform parents that liquid iron preparations may stain teeth so it is important to administer the medication with a dropper or drink it through a straw. Encourage the child to rinse his or her mouth after taking this liquid medication.

- Make parents aware that iron can be constipating and it is necessary to increase the fiber and water intake to prevent this possible complication.
- Possible side effects of iron therapy include gastric upset, nausea, vomiting, and constipation. Black tarry stools are a common finding and are normal for children taking iron supplements.
- Encourage parents to keep no more than a 1-month supply in the home and to store it out of reach of small children because ingestion of excessive quantities may be toxic or even fatal.

Education About Sickle Cell Disease

- Ensure that families know signs and symptoms of sickle cell crisis so they can report them to health care provider.
- Educate the family about the goals of ongoing care including the prevention of complications such as infections, hypoxemia and vaso-occlusive crisis.
- Avoid strenuous activities that may precipitate hypoxia.
- Maintain rest and adequate hydration to avoid sickle cell crisis.
- Adhere to prophylactic penicillin as prescribed to prevent sepsis.
- Use supplemental folic acid to assist with red blood cell production.
- Instruct a patient who experiences a mild sickle cell crisis at home to stop what she is doing, rest, drink fluids, and take prescribed pain medication. If there is no improvement, tell her to seek help from health care provider or go to nearest emergency facility for treatment.
- Advise parents about genetic screening and counseling.

The Child with Hemophilia

- Instruct families on what signs and symptoms require prompt medical attention. Most importantly, any trauma to the head or a change in the level of consciousness is a medical emergency.
- Teach the family about the factor replacement products; including how to obtain the products.
- Teach parents how to administer prophylactic dose of factor replacement at home.

- Ensure that the family is aware that safety is of utmost importance. Injury prevention should be reviewed at all stages of development as risk factors change based on the child's age. Contact sports are highly discouraged. The child should be fitted for a safety helmet to prevent head injury when bike riding.
- Communicate to the family that an interdisciplinary team reviews home environmental factors that can affect the treatment plan.
- Inform the family that for children who have experienced bleeding into the joints, physical therapy may be necessary to preserve and maintain functional status.
- Encourage the child to wear a medical alert bracelet in the event that a medical emergency occurs outside the home.
- Reinforce to the family that genetic counseling is recommended because hemophilia is an inherited disorder (Lea & Williams, 2002).
- Collaboration with the social worker is essential to assist with insurance issues, obtaining medications and supplies, rehabilitation services, home nursing, and other concerns. The social worker is also available for emotional/psychosocial support.
- Numerous resources are available at comprehensive hemophilia centers and also online by the National Hemophilia Foundation at www.hemophilia.org.

Diagnosing Idiopathic (Immune) Thrombocytopenia Purpura

- The following tests are required to confirm the diagnosis of ITP: CBC, peripheral smear examination, coagulation analysis, bone marrow aspirate if steroid therapy is implemented or to rule out an underlying malignancy.
- CBC usually shows isolated and severe thrombocytopenia, usually a platelet count of less than 20,000.
- Peripheral smear is often normal with the exception of thrombocytopenia with normal to large-sized platelets (Di Paola & Buchanan, 2002).

The Neutropenic Child

Teach families and children with neutropenia the following measures to reduce the incidence of infection:

- Always keep routine visits.
- Be aware of the signs and symptoms of infections such as fever (>101.5°F [38.6°C]).
- Avoid large crowds or anyone who may be sick with a cold, flu, etc.
- Keep the child's body clean by bathing every day, brushing teeth after meals and before bedtime.
- Avoid hot tubs.
- Always wash the child's hands before eating or touching the face, eyes, nose, mouth, etc.
- Avoid constipation and straining to have a bowel movement by drinking 2 quarts of fluid each day, exercising, and using a stool softener.
- Avoid putting anything in the child's rectum, including thermometers and suppositories.
- Avoid exposure to fresh flowers or live plants.
- Avoid exposure to stool droppings from pets and cleaning bird cages as well as cleaning cat litter boxes.
- Do not share bath towels or drinking glasses with others, including family members.
- Avoid eating the following items:
  - Raw milk or milk products; any milk product that has not been pasteurized, including cheese and yogurt made from unpasteurized milk
  - Raw or uncooked meat, fish, chicken, eggs, tofu
  - Any food that contains mold, for example, blue cheese
  - Raw honey (honey that has not been pasteurized)
  - Uncooked fresh fruit or vegetables
  - Any outdated foods or foods left at room temperature for more than 2 hours
- Adolescents should not use tampons, vaginal suppositories, or douche.
- Adolescents should avoid manicures, pedicures, acrylic nails, or nail tips.
- Adolescents should use an electric shaver instead of a razor.

ADDITIONAL INFORMATION FOR THE CLINICAL SETTING

Nursing Care for Iron-Deficiency Anemia

- Arrange for nutritional counseling and provide assistance in obtaining the recommended iron-fortified formula.
- Administer oral iron supplements.

Controlling Epistaxis (Nosebleeds)

1. Wear gloves and place child in a sitting position, leaning forward.
2. Apply direct pressure to anterior nasal septum for 10 to 15 minutes.
3. Remind the child to breathe through his mouth to avoid becoming anxious.
4. Apply ice to the nose area.
5. Monitor vital signs if there is a large amount of blood loss.
6. If severe nose bleeding persists beyond 10 to 15 minutes, begin nasal packing and apply topical adrenaline (epinephrine).
7. When infection is present, antibiotics may be ordered (Kucik & Clenney, 2005).
8. Keep child and family calm by providing support and reassurance.
9. Ensure family can demonstrate first aid measures necessary to control epistaxis.

Nonpharmacological Pain Interventions

- Distraction
- Guided imagery
- Relaxation techniques
- Music therapy
- Comfort care
- Cutaneous stimulation
- Play therapy

Idiopathic (Immune) Thrombocytopenia Purpura (ITP) Management

- Platelet count >20,000, asymptomatic; does not require treatment and platelet counts should be monitored.

- Platelet count <20,000, bruises, petechia, no bleeding; treat with steroid, immune gamma globulin (IVIG) or Anti-D antibody (WinRho).
- Platelet count <20,000, bleeding; hospitalization with close observation and a 2- to 3-day course of immune gamma globulin (IVIG).

Understand Institutional Guidelines Related to Intravenous Immune Gamma Globulin (IVIG)

- Understand that intravenous immune gamma globulin (IVIG) is a blood product and blood product consent may be necessary based on institutional guidelines.
- Administration of this product requires frequent measurement of vital signs to monitor for possible side effects.
- Side effects may include fever, chills, hypotension, nausea, and headache.
- It is important for the nurse to check product-specific information for administration guidelines (Di Paola & Buchanan, 2002).

Supportive Care for Patients with Aplastic Anemia

- Provide transfusions of red blood cells and platelets.
- Use transfusions cautiously to prevent development of antibodies and possible graft versus host disease.
- Antibiotics are given to treat infections but generally not recommended prophylactically.

Obtain Transfusion Consent

- Transfusion consent must be obtained before the transfusion of all blood products.
- Transfusion consent must include the description of the procedure for transfusion, risks/benefits, treatment alternatives, and appropriate signatures including the health care provider, signature of patient if 18 years or older, or signature of parent or other legal representative and witness (AABB, 2004).
- Provide the opportunity for the family to ask questions.
- The family has the right to revoke the consent if they wish.

Transfusion Products

Transfusion Product	Indications	Critical Nursing Actions
Red Blood Cells	Hemoglobin <8 grams on a stable patient with a chronic anemia Hypovolemia due to acute blood loss Evidence of impending heart failure secondary to severe anemia Patients on hypertransfusion regimen for sickle cell disease and history of: • Cerebral vascular accident • Splenic sequestration • Acute chest syndrome • Recurrent priapism • Preoperative preparation for surgery with general anesthesia • Hypoxia Children requiring increased oxygen carrying capacity (i.e., complex congenital heart, intracardiac shunting, severe pulmonary disease—acute respiratory distress syndrome [ARDS]): • Shock states (decreased blood pressure, increased peripheral vasoconstriction, pallor, cyanosis, diaphoresis, clamminess, mottled skin, increased oxygen requirement, decreased urinary output) • Cardiac failure • Respiratory failure requiring significant ventilatory support • Postoperative anemia	Observe for clinical signs and symptoms of anemia: Fatigue Syncope Pallor Tachycardia Diaphoretic Shortness of breath Inability to perform activities of daily living Don appropriate PPE (personal protective equipment) for all blood product transfusions. Monitor vital signs per hospital policy and procedure. Monitor hemoglobin and hematocrit Observe for adverse reactions. Store blood in a designated blood refrigerator. Generally 10-15 ml/kg of packed red blood cells are transfused (Khilnani, 2005).
Autologous Blood (Self-donated blood product)	For general scheduled surgical procedures in which there is clinical indications that a blood transfusion may be necessary during the intraoperative or postoperative period, the patient may elect to self-donate. Check with blood bank facilities for time criteria for this type of donation. For general surgical procedures, the recommended hemoglobin is 10 grams or greater and for orthopedic surgery, the recommendation is hemoglobin of 11.5 grams or greater.	Verify with the parent that self-donation has occurred. Patient identification and administration process is the same as with all other blood products.

Transfusion Product	Indications	Critical Nursing Actions
Whole Blood or Packed Red Blood Cells (PRBCs) Reconstituted with Fresh Frozen Plasma (FFP)	Hypovolemia due to acute blood loss non-responsive to crystalloids • Hct <35% • Hypovolemia due to acute massive blood loss (i.e., major trauma) • History of blood loss at delivery or large amount of blood drawn for lab studies (10% blood volume) • Cardiac patients Hct <40% (structural heart disease, cyanosis, or CHF) • Drop in Hgb to below 10 grams intraoperatively • Exchange transfusion	Same nursing actions applicable to red blood cell infusions In major trauma situations, may transfuse patient with O negative blood, the universal donor. Use blood warmer and rapid infuser if available.
Platelets	Platelet count <20,000 Active bleeding with symptoms of DIC or other significant coagulopathies Platelet count <50,000 with planned invasive procedure (i.e., surgical procedure, central line insertion, does not include drawing blood or intramuscular injection of intravenous catheter insertion) Prevention or treatment of bleeding due to thrombocytopenia (secondary to chemotherapy, radiation or bone marrow failure) Treatment of patients with severe thrombocytopenia secondary to increased platelet destruction or immune thrombocytopenia associated with complication of severe trauma Massive transfusion with platelet dilution.	Know normal platelet count (150,000 to 400,000). Obtain CBC. Assess bruising, petechiae, and bleeding.
Fresh Frozen Plasma (FFP)	Replacement for deficiency of factors II, V, VII, IX, X, XII, protein C, or protein S. Bleeding, invasive procedure, or surgery with documented plasma clotting protein deficiency (i.e., liver failure, DIC, or septic shock) Prolonged PT and/or PTT without bleeding.	Notify the blood bank to thaw FFP, product must be used within 6 hours of thawing. Don appropriate PPE for all blood product transfusions. Monitor vital signs per hospital policy and procedure.

(continued)

Transfusion Products (Continued)

Transfusion Product	Indications	Critical Nursing Actions
	Significant intraoperative bleeding (>10% blood volume/hr) in excess of normally anticipated blood loss that is at high risk of clotting-factor deficiency Massive transfusion Therapeutic plasma exchanges Warfarin anticoagulant overdose	Monitor coagulation studies. During FFP infusions, observe for adverse reactions.
Cryoprecipitate	Fibrinogen levels <150 mg/dL with active bleeding Bleeding or prophylaxis in von Willebrand's disease or in factor VIII (hemophilia A) deficiency unresponsive to or unsuitable for DDAVP or factor VII concentrates Replacement therapy, bleeding, or invasive procedure in patients with factor XIII deficiency Patients with active intraoperative hemorrhage in excess of normally anticipated blood loss that are at risk of clotting factor deficiency	Assess for signs and symptoms of bleeding. Don appropriate PPE (personal protective equipment) for all blood product transfusions. Monitor vital signs per hospital policy and procedure. Monitor coagulation studies. During cryoprecipitate infusions, observe for adverse reactions.
Granulocytes (White Cell Transfusion)	Bacterial or fungal sepsis (proven or strongly suspected) unresponsive to antimicrobial therapy Infection (proven or strongly suspected) unresponsive to antimicrobial therapy	Type and crossmatch required for all WBC transfusions. Premedications may be ordered, such as antihistamines or acetaminophen.
Factor VII	Factor VII deficiency Factor VIII inhibitors Factor IX inhibitors Idiopathic uncontrolled bleeding	Assess for signs and symptoms of bleeding. Don appropriate PPE for all blood products, even recombinant. Monitor coagulation studies. If undiluted, dilute vial with indicated amount of sterile water and administer intravenously as per manufacturer's guidelines.

Transfusion Product	Indications	Critical Nursing Actions
Factor VIII Concentrate	Hemophilia A (factor VIII deficiency). Patient with factor VIII inhibitors Patients with von Willebrand's disease	Assess for signs and symptoms of bleeding. Don appropriate PPE for all blood products. Monitor coagulation studies. Check product to see if refrigeration necessary. Record expiration date and lot number of product.
Factor IX Concentrate (Prothrombin Complex)	Hemophilia B Hemophilia A with factor VIII inhibitors Patients with congenital deficiency of prothrombin, factor VII, and factor X	Assess for signs and symptoms of bleeding. Don appropriate PPE for all blood products. Monitor coagulation studies. Record expiration date and lot number of product.
Intravenous Immunoglobulin (IVIG)	Congenital or acquired antibody deficiency Immunological disorders such as idiopathic thrombocytopenia (ITP), Kawasaki disease Posttransplant patients used prophylactically; newborns with severe bacterial infections	Don appropriate PPE (for all IVIG infusions). Monitor vital signs per hospital policy and procedure. Start infusion slowly and increase rate/titrate per physician orders. During IVIG infusion, observe for adverse reactions such as fever, chills, and headache. Product is obtained from the pharmacy. Record the expiration date and lot number of the product.

The Administration of Blood

- Strict observance to the institutional policy regarding the administration of blood products cannot be stressed enough.
- The accuracy of patient verification is a critical nursing action that can help prevent a transfusion reaction.

Transfusion Reactions

- Most transfusion reactions occur during the initiation of a transfusion, but a reaction can occur at any time during this process (AABB, 2004).

- These reactions can vary from a mild reaction, such as mild fever, to the most severe complication of death.
- Children who have received multiple transfusions are at higher risk for developing a transfusion reaction (Knippen, 2006).

Febrile Reaction

- The most common blood transfusion reaction is a nonhemolytic febrile reaction in which the child develops a fever >1.8°F from the baseline temperature.
- Occurs on initiation of the transfusion, but have been known to occur up to 12 hours posttransfusion.
- Signs and symptoms: Fever and chills, which then may progress to more serious complications such as tachycardia, tachypnea, and hypotension.
- Nursing care: Premedication with acetaminophen (Children's Tylenol) can sometimes prevent this type of reaction. Monitoring the child's temperature to recognize febrile reactions early and prevent progression. Stop the transfusion, monitor vital signs closely, and notify the physician.

Allergic Reaction

- A nonhemolytic reaction that occurs during a transfusion in which the child has had a previous exposure to a particular allergen in the blood product.
- Signs and symptoms: Rash, hives, pruritus, swelling of the lips, wheezing, and anxiety.
- Nursing care: Stop the transfusion immediately, monitor vital signs closely, and notify physician. The administration of an antihistamine such as diphenhydramine (Benadryl) resolves an allergic response.

Bacterial Contamination

- Occurs during the initiation of the infusion.
- Guidelines from the AABB (2004) require strict adherence to the completion of all transfusions in 4 hours or less to prevent this from happening.
- Signs and symptoms: Shaking chills, fever, vomiting, diffuse erythema, and the onset of hypotension that may progress to shock. In severe cases hemoglobinuria, actual renal failure, and DIC may develop.
- Nursing care: Stop the transfusion immediately, monitor vital signs closely, start a normal saline infusion, notify the physician, and prepare emergency care (support

oxygenation and ventilation, antibiotics, and vasopressors may be ordered). Nursing responsibilities also include obtaining blood samples for culture and sensitivity and sending the blood product with tubing to the blood bank also to be cultured.

Circulatory Overload
- This reaction is rare and occurs when the infusion is given too rapidly or an excessive quantity of blood is given.
- Signs and symptoms: Dry cough, dyspnea, rales, distended neck veins, hypertension/hypotension, bradycardia/ tachycardia, clammy skin, and cyanosis of the extremities.
- Nursing care: Accurate verification of physician orders, double-checking the volume to be infused, and the use of an intravenous pump. If any of the signs and symptoms are identified, the nurse must immediately stop the transfusion, monitor vital signs closely, place the child upright with feet in a dependent position to increase venous resistance, notify physician, and prepare emergency care (support oxygenation and ventilation as well as diuretics may be ordered).

Acute Hemolytic Transfusion Reaction
- This reaction is rare but it is the most severe type of reaction. It occurs when the donor RBCs and the recipient plasma are incompatible, and there is an ABO mismatch. Acute hemolytic transfusion reactions occur upon initiation after exposure to a small amount of blood (Hillman et al., 2005).
- Signs and symptoms: Fever, shaking chills, pain at the intravenous site, tightness of the chest, difficulties breathing, impending sense of doom, pallor, jaundice, nausea/vomiting, red or black urine, flank pain, and progressive signs of shock such as tachycardia and hypotension.
- Nursing care: Stop the transfusion, monitor vital signs closely, start a normal saline infusion, verify patient identification, notify the physician, and prepare emergency care (support oxygenation and ventilation, antihistamines, fluids, diuretics, and vasopressors may be ordered). Other nursing responsibilities include obtaining blood and urine samples and sending them to the laboratory to analyze for the presence of hemoglobin, which indicates intravascular hemolysis. Insert a urinary catheter to monitor the child's output more accurately.

Complications of Apheresis

Complication	Critical Nursing Actions
Hypocalcemia	Obtain ionized calcium levels before treatment. Correct all abnormal levels before initiating treatment. For apheresis lasting longer than 1 hour in length, monitor ionized calcium levels every hour until the end of the procedure. Consider calcium drip if needed: ● Calcium chloride: 20–25 mg/kg per dose used for acute hypocalcemia ● Calcium gluconate: 100–500 mg/kg per day (Robertson & Shilkofski, 2005)
Hypotension	Hypotension may occur with onset of treatment. Be sure to have fluid readily available at bedside. Patients receiving inotropic support may need an increase in the rate of administration.
Risk for Bleeding	Prothrombin time (PT), partial thromboplastin time (PTT), fibrinogen level, platelet count, Hct, and activated clotting time (ACT) are measured before and after apheresis. Measure ACT at the bedside at regular intervals, and adjust citrate and/or heparin doses accordingly. Platelet or other blood products such as clotting factors may be required during the procedure.
Hypothermia	Hypothermia may result from the blood being circulated in the extracorporeal circuit outside the body. Use a blood warmer on the pheresis machine. Monitor frequent temperatures to avoid hypothermia. Assess the patient for other signs of hypothermia (e.g., bradycardia and shivering). Keep the child warm with blankets and/or an external warmer. Increase ambient room temperature.
Transfusion Reaction	Use leukodepleted blood. Monitor for transfusion reactions from the replacement products. Follow the transfusion reaction protocol if this occurs. Consider administration of an antihistamine for patients receiving multiple treatments.
Infection	Maintain strict sterile technique with all intravenous lines.
Air Embolism	Monitor tubing and connection sites. Check that all are secured properly.
Thrombus	Obtain platelet count before catheter placement and be aware when possible transfusion of platelets are necessary. Flush vigorously with adequate volumes of normal saline as per institution's policy.

RESOURCES

American Sickle Cell Anemia Association: http://www.ascaa.org

Aplastic Anemia and MDS International Foundation: http://www.aamds.org

National Hemophilia Foundation: http://www.hemophilia.org

National Marrow Donor Program: http://www.marrow.org

Sickle Cell Anemia Association: http://www.sicklecelldisease.org

REFERENCES

American Association of Blood Banks (AABB) Guidelines. (2004). Bethesda, MD: AABB Press.

Deglin, J., & Vallerand, A. (2009). *Davis's drug guide for nurses* (11th ed.). Philadelphia: F.A. Davis.

Di Paola, J., & Buchanan, G.R. (2002). Immune thrombocytopenic purpura. *Pediatric Clinics of North America, 49,* 911–928.

FDA Patient safety news. October 2004.

Fixler, J., & Styles, L. (2002). Sickle cell disease. *Pediatric Clinics of North America, 49,* 1193–1210.

Gilbert-Barness, E., & Barness, L. (2003). *Clinical use of pediatric diagnostic tests.* Philadelphia: Lippincott Williams & Wilkins.

Hillman, R.S., Ault, K.A., & Rinder, H.M. (2005). *Hematology in clinical practice: a guide to diagnosis and management.* New York: McGraw-Hill.

Knipper, M. (2006). Transfusion-related acute lung injury. *AJN, 106*(6), 61–64.

Khilnani, P. (2005). *Practical approach to pediatric intensive care.* New York: Oxford University Press.

Kucik, C.J., & Clenney, T. (2005). Management of epistaxis. *American Family Physician. 71*(2), 305–311.

Lea, D., & Williams, J. (2002). Genetic testing and screening, use them as part of routine nursing practice. *American Journal of Nursing, 102*(7), 36–43.

Lo, L., & Singer, S. (2002). Thalassemia: Current approach to an old disease. *Pediatric Clinics of North America, 49,* 1165–1191.

Nathan, D.G., Orkin, S.H., Ginsburg, D., & Look, A.T. (2003). *Nathan and Oski's hematology of infancy and childhood* (6th ed.). Philadelphia: W.B. Saunders.

Robertson, J., & Shilkofski, N. (2005). *The Harriet Lane handbook* (17th ed.). Philadelphia: Elsevier Mosby.

Sevier, N. (2005). Inherited coagulation factor abnormalities: A pediatric review. *Journal of Pediatric Oncology Nursing, 22*(3), 137–144.

U.S. Food and Drug Administration. (2002). Current good manufacturing practice for blood and blood components: Adverse reaction file. Title 21 part 606.170(b).

Caring for the Child with Cancer

KEY TERMS

mucositis – A diffuse inflammation of the mucosa of the mouth, a change in the integrity of the mucous membranes characterized by soreness, redness, and swelling; lesions on the mucous membranes allow bacteria to attach themselves to the affected areas and are a source of localized and systemic infection

FOCUSED ASSESSMENT

Acute Lymphocytic Leukemia (ALL)

Signs and Symptoms
- Fever, fatigue, lethargy, anemia, pale skin, anorexia, bone or joint pain
- Increased white blood cell (WBC) count

Acute Myelogenous Leukemia (AML)

Signs and Symptoms
- Symptoms resembling the flu, anemia, pallor, fatigue, bone pain, fever, headache or dizziness, petechiae, easy bruising, nosebleeds, or bleeding gums
- Increased WBC count

Chronic Myelogenous Leukemia (CML)

Signs and Symptoms
- Fever, fatigue, weight loss, anorexia
- Increased WBC count and splenomegaly

Brain Tumors

Signs and Symptoms
- Depends on the tumor location, tumor type, and the age of the child
- Obstruction of cerebrospinal fluid (CSF) drainage leading to increased intracranial pressure (ICP)

Neurological Assessment
- Tumors of the brain or CNS are the second most common cancer in children after leukemia.
- Virtually all childhood brain tumors are primary tumors, meaning that they originate in the brain.

Performing the Neurological Exam
- The main focus of a physical assessment of a child with a brain tumor should be the neurological exam.
- A patient's baseline assessment is important to detect any subtle changes.
- The exam includes vital signs; pupil size, equality, and response to light; level of consciousness; strength and equality of grip of hands; and movement of the legs.
- Head circumference and the assessment of the anterior fontanel is also important in assessing an infant's intracranial pressure.
- Parents may first notice behavioral changes.
- The neurological exam can change rapidly.
- Timely responses to neurological changes are of vital importance for the child with a brain tumor.

Neuroblastoma

Signs and Symptoms
- Wide variety depending on site of primary tumor
- On palpation tumor crosses midline; hard painless mass in neck or abdomen

Wilms' Tumor (Nephroblastoma)

Signs and Symptoms
- Painless abdominal mass in one or both kidneys (seldom crosses midline)

Palpitation of the Abdomen in a Child with Wilms' Tumor

- Once a child has been diagnosed with Wilms' tumor, never palpate the abdomen or allow anyone else to do so.
- Palpating this kind of encapsulated tumor can cause it to rupture or lead to further metastasis.
- Place a warning sign on the child's hospital room door that says, "No abdominal palpation."

Rhabdomyosarcoma

Signs and Symptoms

- Depends on location of primary tumor and metastasis (head and neck, nasopharynx, genitourinary, extremities skeletal or smooth muscle perianal regions)

Retinoblastoma

Signs and Symptoms

- Leukocoria, strabismus, red painful eyes (blindness is a late sign)

Osteosarcoma

Signs and Symptoms

- Pain and swelling
- Limp
- Dull aching pain
- Palpation at site, tenderness, swelling, warmth, and erythema

Ewing's Sarcoma

Signs and Symptoms

- Pain or tenderness and swelling at the site of the tumor (chest wall tumor causes respiratory distress)

Hodgkin's Disease (HD)

Signs and Symptoms

- Painless, firm, cervical, or supraclavicular lymphadenopathy

Non-Hodgkin's Lymphoma (NHL)
Signs and Symptoms
- Pain or swelling (abdomen, chest and head/neck)

Liver Cancer

- Hepatoblastoma or Hepatocellular carcinoma
Signs and Symptoms
- The first sign is a mass in the abdomen (upper right side).
- Abdominal fullness, pain, vomiting, diarrhea, fever, abnormal weight loss, jaundice, or general itching

Medical Emergencies

Hemorrhagic Cystitis
Signs and Symptoms
- Bloody or painful urination

Tumor Lysis Syndrome
Signs and Symptoms
- Lethargy, nausea and vomiting, oliguria, flank pain, pruritus, tetany, and altered level of consciousness
- Renal failure can also occur.

Septic Shock
Signs and Symptoms
- Confusion, fever, tachypnea, decreased urinary output, and cold, clammy skin.
- Note: Decreased blood pressure is a late sign.
- Laboratory studies reveal acidosis and sometimes renal failure.

The Psychological Impact of Pediatric Cancer
Signs and Symptoms
- Shock, denial, confusion, fear, blame, and loss of control.

CLINICAL ALERTS

Brain Tumors

- First the tumor is staged.
- Tumor tissue is needed for the pathologist to determine the histological diagnosis so that proper treatment can be determined.

- Treatment may include surgical resection, radiation therapy, chemotherapy, or a combination of these.

Surgical Resection

- The extent of surgical resection (cutting off) of the tumor correlates with the prognosis.
- Radical resections are particularly important in children younger than 2 years of age because cranial radiation can be deferred in these patients.
- Because many brain tumors infiltrate into surrounding normal brain, complete resection often is not possible.

Discarding Chemotherapy Drugs

- When handling equipment or material that has contained chemotherapy drugs, discard it in a designated container that is properly labeled.
- Chemotherapy drugs are considered hazardous waste material.

Radiation

Radiation therapy is using ionizing radiation to break apart the bonds within a cell, damaging it and causing it to die. Address the radiation side effects:

- Nausea
- Alopecia
- Fatigue and malaise
- Low WBC count
- Skin desquamation
- Mucous membrane inflammation and irritation

Extravasation

- Chemotherapeutic drugs must be handled carefully to avoid extravasation (accidental leakage of drug into the subcutaneous tissues surrounding the injection site/IV site). This is caused by known vesicants or a chemotherapy agent that can produce a blister or tissue destruction.
- It is important to handle chemotherapy agents safely

- For central lines, it is important to make sure there is a blood return in the line to ensure patency before administering any chemotherapeutic agents by this route.
- Monitor closely the intravenous (IV) site.
- Before administering a known "vesicant," a chemotherapy agent that can result in tissue necroses and even potentially the loss of a limb, make sure the peripheral IV or central line is patent.
- It is important to flush the IV site and check a return blood flow.
- The nurse infusing these agents be specially trained and certified in the administration of chemotherapy agents. Through this training, the nurse learns that vigilant monitoring is paramount.

Medical Emergencies

Septic Shock

Septic shock response can occur immediately or up to 48 to 72 hours later.

Other Emergencies

- Superior vena cava syndrome: Obstruction or thrombus in the superior vena cava
- Superior mediastinum syndrome: Tracheal compression
- Pericardial effusion: Fluid in the pericardial cavity, between the visceral and the parietal pericardium. This condition may produce symptoms of cardiac tamponade, such as difficulty in breathing (Venes, 2005).
- Pleural effusion: Fluid in the thoracic cavity between the visceral and parietal pleura. It may be seen on a chest radiograph if the fluid exceeds 300 mL (Venes, 2005).
- Abdominal emergencies: Esophagitis, gastric hemorrhage, perirectal abscess, hemorrhagic pancreatitis, massive acute hepatomegaly, bowel obstruction.
- Neurological conditions: Stroke, seizure, spinal cord compression.
- Shock: Hypovolemic, cardiogenic, distributive.
- Hyperleukocytosis: WBC count >100,000 mm^3.

DIAGNOSTIC TESTS

Staging

- Staging describes the severity of the patient's cancer. It classifies tumors in relation to the degree of differentiation, possibility of responding to therapy, and prognosis (Venes, 2005).
- Stage 0 indicates early cancer that is present only in the layer of cells in which it began.
- Stages I, II, and III indicate more extensive disease, greater tumor size, and/or spread of the cancer to nearby lymph nodes or adjacent organs.
- Stage IV indicates that the cancer has spread to another organ(s).

Lumbar Puncture

- A lumbar puncture (LP), or "spinal tap," is the insertion of a needle into the subarachnoid space of the lumbar spinal cord to remove a sample of CSF to test for infection.
- Insert the needle with a stylet into the interspace between the third and fourth lumbar vertebrae under strict sterile technique (Fig. 31-1).
- It is used to introduce chemotherapeutic agents into the CSF space in cancer patients.

Neutropenia

- Neutropenic children have few WBCs and often do not show signs of infection, such as swelling, redness, or drainage.

Figure 31-1 Lumbar puncture.

- The only sign may be fever.
- A fever in an oncology patient is 101.2°F (38.5°C) in a 24-hour period or 100.4°F (38.0°C) three times in a 24-hour period.
- A severe neutropenic patient has an absolute neutrophil count (ANC) of <500.
- An ANC of 500 to 1000 is considered moderately neutropenic
- ANC >1000 is considered mildly neutropenic.
- When a child undergoing chemotherapy develops a fever, it is considered an emergency.

Calculating the Absolute Neutrophil Count (ANC)
Formula:
ANC = (WBC × 10) × (Bands + Neutrophils)
Example: If WBC = 8.8, neutrophils = 82, bands = 5
ANC = (8.8 × 10) × (82 + 5)
ANC = (88) × (87)
ANC = 7656

Liver Cancer

- Both hepatoblastoma and hepatocellular carcinoma can produce a protein called alpha-fetoprotein (AFP), which can be detected in the blood via a simple blood test.
- If AFP levels fall, it indicates that treatment is working. If AFP levels rise, it means the tumor is not responding.

 Procedure 31-1 Checking Urine Specific Gravity

Purpose
The purpose of checking the specific gravity of urine is to measure the concentration of the particles in the urine.

Equipment
- Refractometer
- 3- or 5-mL syringe (needleless)

Steps
1. Have the child urinate into a urine collection receptacle.
2. Using a 3- or 5-mL syringe, draw up 0.5 mL of urine into the syringe

(continued)

Procedure 31-1 (Continued)

3. Place the syringe into a universal precaution container.

4. Take the urine specimen to the testing area.

5. Open the refractometer.

6. Place one drop of urine in the center of the square opening.

7. Close the lid.

8. Look through the focused eyepiece to see the horizontal line clearly.

9. Note where the blue horizontal line crosses the markings (see picture below).

10. Document the procedure.

Clinical Alert If the institution does not have a refractometer, it is acceptable to use a urine dipstick, with the realization that this is not as detailed. The specific gravity markings on a urine dipstick are in increments of 0.005. On a refractometer, the markings are in increments of 0.001.

Teach Parents

The nurse can teach the parents about the purpose of a specific gravity measurement.

Checking Urine Specific Gravity

- Check urine specific gravity for patients receiving cytoxan, ifosfamide, cisplatin, high-dose carboplatin, high-dose methotrexate.
- Specific gravity must be less than or equal to 1.010 before the start of chemotherapy and then for at least 24 hours after its completion.

- If at any time the specific gravity rises above 1.010, the patient should receive a fluid bolus (extra fluid). DO NOT turn off the main IV. The bolus is in addition to the main intravenous fluid (IVF).
- If giving more than two or three fluid boluses, notify the oncologist on call.

Urine pH

- Monitor when the patient is receiving methotrexate (Amethopterin).
- Urine pH must be higher than 7.0 before starting methotrexate, and must be maintained at that level until the methotrexate serum blood level is <0.1 mg/dL.
- Before receiving high-dose methotrexate, patients are hydrated with IVF of D5^1/$_4$ with 40 mEq/L of $NaHCO_3$. The $NaHCO_3$ is needed to keep the urine alkalinized.

Bone Marrow Biopsy

Pretest

- Obtain a written, informed and signed consent for the procedure.
- Review the procedure with the child and parents. Explain that the child will receive topical anesthetic (EMLA) and/or pain medication before the procedure.
- If receiving conscious sedation, review the institution's policy on restriction of food and fluids.
- If parents choose to be present, explain how they might assist their child through diversionary activities, breathing techniques, and verbal support.

Intratest

- Depending on age, have the patient void before the procedure.
- Identify the patient.
- Take the patient to the treatment room.
- Assist the child to the desired position depending on the site to be used:
  - Proximal tibia (supine with pillow beneath knee)
  - Vertebral bodies (on side with head and knees tucked)
  - Posterior iliac crest (prone)
  - Anterior iliac crest or sternum (supine)
- Restrain as necessary with two adults.

- Record baseline vital signs and continue to monitor during procedure. If receiving conscious sedation, pulse and oxygen saturation monitoring are also necessary.

Posttest

- Apply pressure dressing if child's platelet count is 50,000 or less.
- Monitor vital signs and neurologic status for at least 1 hour or until child returns to a premedicated state.
- Observe site for bleeding, inflammation, or hematoma.
- Administer antiemetic and analgesic medications as needed.
- Instruct patient/family to report any redness, edema, bleeding, or pain at the site. Instruct patient/family to report chills or fever and to keep the site clean and change dressing as needed.

(Adapted from Van Leeuwen, A.M., Kranpitz, T.R., & Smith, L. (2006). *Davis's comprehensive handbook of laboratory and diagnostic tests with nursing implications.* Philadelphia: F.A. Davis, pp. 209–211.)

Bone Scan

Pretest

- Obtain a written, informed, and signed consent for the procedure.
- Explain the procedure to the child and family.
- Inform child and family that the technologist will administer an intravenous injection of an isotope and they will need to return 1 to 3 hours later for the scan.
- After the injection, encourage child to increase fluid intake and continue normal physical activity.

Intratest

- Confirm the child's identity.
- Ask the child to remove any jewelry, watches, and other metallic objects.
- Depending on the age of the child, ask the child to void.
- If the child is unable to lie still, sedation is necessary.
- Place the child supine with foam wedges to help maintain position and immobilization while multiple images are obtained.

Posttest

- If the child is sedated, monitor vital signs and neurologic status for at least 1 hour or until child returns to a premedicated state.
- Encourage increased fluid intake.
- Check the injection site for bleeding, redness, or hematoma (Van Leeuwen, 2006).

Lumbar Puncture

Pretest

- Obtain a written, informed, and signed consent for the procedure.
- Review the procedure with the child and parents. Explain that the child will receive topical anesthetic (EMLA) before the procedure.
- If parents choose to be present, explain how they might assist their child through diversionary activities, breathing techniques, and verbal support.

Intratest

- Confirm the child's identity.
- Take to treatment room.
- Obtain baseline vital signs and continue to monitor during procedure, particularly for signs of respiratory compromise due to positioning of the child. For infants, pulse and oxygen saturation monitoring may be required.
- Have emergency equipment readily available.
- Position and restrain the child in the knee chest position at the side of the examination table in order to best expose the L3–L4 site or the L4–L5 site. For older children the sitting position with neck and chest bent to the knees is an alternative.
- Instruct the child to breathe normally and to avoid unnecessary movement while vials of CSF are obtained.

Posttest

- Apply an adhesive dressing to the site.
- Observe site for bleeding, CSF leakage, or hematoma.
- Monitor vital signs and neurological status and compare to baseline values.

- The child should lie flat for at least 1 hour or according to the health care provider's instructions (Van Leeuwen, 2006).

Lymphangiogram

Pretest
- Obtain a written, informed, and signed consent for the procedure.
- Review the procedure with child and parents.
- Ask the child to remove any jewelry, watches, or other metallic objects before going to the radiology department.
- Ask the child and family if the child has an allergy to iodine or shellfish.

Intratest
- Confirm the child's identity.
- Have emergency equipment readily available.
- Obtain baseline vital signs and assess neurological status.
- Encourage the child to remain still throughout the procedure.
- Explain that a local anesthetic is injected before the injection of the contrast medium into the area between the first three toes of the foot or the web of skin between the fingers.
- Remind the child that he will need to inhale deeply and hold his breath while the x-ray images are taken.
- Monitor the child for complications related to the contrast medium (e.g., allergic reaction, anaphylaxis, bronchospasm).

Posttest
- Monitor vital signs and neurological status every 15 minutes and compare with baseline values.
- Observe the site for bleeding, inflammation, and hematoma and monitor for signs of infection.
- Observe for delayed allergic reaction or pulmonary embolus (shortness of breath, increased heart rate, pleuritic pain, hypotension, low-grade fever, and cyanosis) (Van Leeuwen, 2006).

MEDICATIONS

Chemotherapeutic Agents and Common Drugs Used with Cancer Patients

Agent	Indications	Route	Side Effects
Asparaginase (Elspar, Kidrolase) Classification: Antineoplastic Pharmacological action: Enzyme	Acute lymphoblastic leukemia (ALL)	IM, IV	Seizures, hyperglycemia Nausea/vomiting, rashes, coagulation abnormalities, hepatotoxic, pancreatitis, anaphylaxis (have emergency medications available)
Bleomycin (Blenoxane) Classification: Antineoplastic Pharmacological: Antitumor antibiotics	Hodgkin's disease Osteosarcoma Testicular embryonal cell carcinoma	IM, IV, SQ	Pulmonary fibrosis Pneumonitis, hypotension, nausea/vomiting, anorexia, hyperpigmentation, rashes, anaphylaxis (fever, chills)
Carboplatin **(Paraplatin, Paraplatin AQ)** Classification: Antineoplastic Pharmacological: Alkylating agent	Brain tumors Soft tissue sarcoma Osteosarcoma Retinoblastoma Neuroblastoma	IV	Ototoxicity, nausea/vomiting, constipation, diarrhea, stomatitis, renal and liver toxicity, hypocalcemia, hypokalemia, hyponatremia, hypomagnesemia Anaphylactic-like reactions

(continued)

Chemotherapeutic Agents and Common Drugs Used with Cancer Patients (Continued)

Agent	Indications	Route	Side Effects
Corticosteroid (Dexamethasone, Decadron, Hydrocortisone, Prednisone) Classification: Corticosteroid Pharmacological: Systemic corticosteroids, anti-inflammatory	ALL Non-Hodgkin's lymphoma HD Cerebral edema	PO, IV, IT	Immunosuppression Weight gain, hypertension, anorexia, nausea/vomiting, acne, delayed wound healing, hirsutism, petechiae, osteoporosis, growth delay Cushinoid appearance
Cyclophosphamide (Cytoxan, Neosar, Procytox) Classification: Antineoplastic, Immunosuppressant Pharmacological: Alkylating agent	NHL HD ALL Neuroblastoma Wilms' tumor Bone and soft tissue sarcoma Retinoblastoma	PO, IV	Myelosuppression Nausea, vomiting, anorexia, diarrhea, pulmonary and myocardial fibrosis, hemorrhagic cystitis, leukopenia, hematuria, alopecia, sterility, SIADH May cause second neoplasm
Daunorubicin (Daunomycin, Cerubidine) Classification: Antineoplastic Pharmacological: Anthracyclines	ALL AML Osteosarcoma Soft tissue sarcoma	IV	Blistering, myelosuppression, cardiotoxic: arrhythmias, acute cardiac myopathy-delayed Nausea/vomiting, stomatitis, potentiation of radiation, alopecia, rash, hyperpigmentation of nails

Doxorubicin
(Adriamycin, Adria, DOX, Rubex)
Classification: Antineoplastic
Pharmacological: Anthracyclines

ALL
AML
Osteosarcoma
Soft tissue sarcoma
Neuroblastoma

IV

Blistering, nausea/vomiting, stomatitis, esophagitis, diarrhea, red urine, anemia, hypersensitivity reaction, sterility. Cardiotoxic: arrhythmias, acute cardiomyopathy—delayed, potentiation of radiation, hyperpigmentation of nails, seizures, hypertension, edema, diarrhea, cough, shortness of breath, rash, thrombotic events

Epoetin/Erythropoietin
(Epogen, EPO, Procrit)
Classification: Biological Response Modifier
Pharmacological: Hormone

Anemia

IV, SQ

Pulmonary edema, CHF, MI, hypotension, nausea/vomiting, anaphylaxis

Etoposide
(VP-16, VePesid)
Classification: Antineoplastic
Pharmacological: Podophyllotoxin derivative

AML, ALL
NHL
HD
Bone and soft tissue sarcoma
Wilms' tumor
Brain tumor
Neuroblastoma
Retinoblastoma

IV

Excessive leukocytosis, pain and redness at subcutaneous site.

Filgrastim (GCSF—granulocyte colony stimulating factor)
(Neupogen)
Classification: colony-stimulating factor
Pharmacological: Hematopoietic progenitor mobilizer

Recovery drug for neutropenia

IV, SQ

Medullary bone pain

(continued)

Chemotherapeutic Agents and Common Drugs Used with Cancer Patients (Continued)

Agent	Indications	Route	Side Effects
Fluorouracil (5-FU, Adrucil) Classification: Antineoplastic Pharmacological: Antimetabolite	Brain tumors Germ cell tumors Osteosarcoma Soft tissue sarcoma NHL ALL	IV	Myelosuppression, nausea/vomiting (mild), mucositis (severe), hyperpigmentation of nails, nail loss, dermatitis, phototoxicity, myelosuppression, diarrhea, neurotoxicity (encephalopathy, hallucinations), hepatoxicity, hemorrhagic cystitis, alopecia, sterility, may cause second neoplasm
Ifosfamide (Ifex) Classification: Antineoplastic Pharmacological: Alkylating agent	Stops methotrexate from harming the cells when given in high doses	IV	Allergic reactions: rash, urticaria, wheezing
Leucovorin (Citrovorum factor, folinic acid, Wellcovorin) Classification: Antidote (for methotrexate), vitamins Pharmacological: Folic acid analog	Recovery drug to prevent hemorrhagic cystitis from ifosfamide and cyclophosphamide	IV, PO	*Dose dependent on methotrexate level *Given 24 hrs after first methotrexate level has begun
Mesna (Mesnex, Uromitexan) Classification: Antidote Pharmacological: Ifosfamide detoxifying agent	Prevention of ifosfamide-induced hemorrhagic cystitis	IV, PO, IM, IT	Dizziness, drowsiness, headache, anorexia, diarrhea, nausea/vomiting, unpleasant taste, flushing, flu-like symptoms

Methotrexate (MTX, Amethopterin) Classification: Antineoplastic Immunosuppressant Pharmacological: Antimetabolite	ALL Osteosarcoma NHL	IV	Myelosuppression, nausea/vomiting/stomatitis, alopecia, hepatotoxicity, neurotoxicity, photosensitivity, rash, pulmonary fibrosis, aplastic anemia
Ondansetron (Zofran) Classification: Antiemetic Pharmacological: 5-HT$_3$ antagonist	Prevention of nausea/vomiting association with chemotherapy	IV, PO	Headache, diarrhea, constipation, dry mouth, extrapyramidal reactions
PEG-L-asparaginase (pegaspargase) (Oncaspar) Classification: Antineoplastic Pharmacological: Enzymes	ALL HD	IM, IV	Seizures, pancreatitis, lip edema, headache, nausea/vomiting, diarrhea, DIC, hemolytic anemia, pancytopenia, chills, night sweats
Vincristine (Oncovorin, Vincasar PFS) Classification: Antineoplastic Pharmacological: Vinca alkaloids	Wilms' tumor Ewing's sarcoma Brain tumor	IV	Altered LOC, blistering, peripheral neuropathy, alopecia, constipation, SIADH, seizure, nausea/vomiting

IV = intravenous; IM = intramuscular; SQ = subcutaneous; PO = by mouth; IT = intrathecal.
Data from Deglin, J., & Vallerand, A. (2009). *Davis's drug guide for nurses* (11th ed.). Philadelphia: F.A. Davis.

Topical Anesthetics

- Use topical anesthetics when possible for procedure-related pain such as EMLA (Astra Zeneca) cream, which is a lidocaine/prilocaine 1:1 mixture.
- The nurse applies a thin coating of ointment to the projected insertion site(s) and covers the site(s) with a hydrocolloid dressing (such as DuoDERM).
- It is important to keep the cream on for at least 1 hour (sometimes longer) before the procedure (Bryant, 2003).

Common Antiemetics

Odansetron (Zofran)

- 0.15 mg/kg every 8 hours
- Duration
  - IV: 24 hours
  - PO: 8 hours
  - Not as effective as a prn
  - Not as effective if vomiting has begun
  - While the child is receiving chemotherapy, give 30 minutes before chemotherapy, then every 6 to 8 hours for 24 hours

Diphenhydramine (Benadryl)

- 1 mg/kg per dose every 6 hours
- PO/IV immediate onset
- Duration 4 to 7 hours
- Side effects: Sedation, dry mouth, blurred vision

Lorazepam (Ativan)

- IV: 0.4 mg/kg per dose every 6 hours
- IV duration: 4–6 hours
- Often used for anticipatory nausea/vomiting
- Side effects: Sedation, euphoria

Agents Known to Cause Extravasation

- TPN and other hyperosmolar fluids
- Dilantin
- Chemotherapeutic agents (doxorubicin, daunorubicin, mitomycin C, vincristine, vinblastine, VP-16, dacarbazine)

ETHNOCULTURAL CONSIDERATIONS

Caring for a Hispanic Child with Cancer

- Respect the family's values and incorporate their folk practices when possible.
- Provide written instruction for the child and parents in Spanish so they understand the plan of treatment.
- Do a thorough pain assessment and do not rely on verbal or observational cues, as Hispanics are known to be stoic and not express pain.
- Explore the parents' or caregivers' beliefs as well as the child's beliefs so that optimal pain control can be achieved.

TEACHING THE FAMILY

Suggestions for Nutrition

- Offer suggestions to the family to help the child maintain good nutrition.
- Encourage the family to plan a diet that includes foods from all four food groups.
- Refer to the nutritionist if necessary.

Nausea/Vomiting

- Offer plain, bland foods such as cereal, canned or fresh fruit, rice, pasta, toast, mashed potatoes, soup, crackers, or plain meat.
- Avoid spicy, heavy, or fatty foods.
- If food smells bother the child, choose cold or room-temperature foods; use a cup with a lid.
- Do not offer solid food and liquid at the same time, as this can induce nausea by making the child feel too full; give liquids 30 to 60 minutes after solid food.

Diarrhea

- Offer plenty of liquids.
- Suggest eating bananas, rice, applesauce, toast, and tea.
- Suggest cutting back on fiber in the diet.

Constipation

- Provide extra liquids; offer beverages that contain caffeine, like coffee, tea, and cola.
- Increase fiber in the diet.
- Encourage the child to increase activity level.

Poor Appetite

- Offer small amounts of food four or more times a day.
- Offer liquids between meals.
- Make every bite count by offering "power-packed foods."
- Start with small portions, and then gradually increase them.
- Allow the child to have foods and beverages that he or she especially likes.

Sore Throat and Mouth

- Offer soft foods such as pudding, Jell-O®, macaroni and cheese, applesauce, bananas, ice cream, Italian ice, popsicles.
- Avoid acidic foods like oranges and tomatoes, spicy foods, or foods that require a lot of chewing.
- Encourage good oral hygiene.

Heartburn or Reflux

- Do not give the child high-fat, spicy foods, caffeine, citrus juices, cinnamon, peppermint, or pepper.
- Keep the child upright for at least 1 hour after eating.

Difficulty Chewing or Swallowing/Dry Mouth

- Give the child soft, moist foods.
- Encourage sips of liquids while eating.
- Avoid hard foods that require a lot of chewing.
- Cut the food into small pieces.
- Use extra butter, sauces, or gravies.
- Offer hard candy to suck on.

Belching, Intestinal Gas, or Cramps

- Avoid gas-forming foods such as cabbage, broccoli, cauliflower, cucumbers, beans, and carbonated beverages.

- Encourage the child to eat or drink slowly.
- Do not allow the child to chew gum.

(Steen & Mirro, 2000).

Recognizing Signs and Symptoms of Infection

If any of these signs and symptoms or a combination of them occur, report them to the physician immediately.

- Fever
- Decrease in temperature
- Runny nose (or other respiratory illness)
- Sore throat
- Childhood disease such as chickenpox
- Lethargy
- Pale or ashen color
- Chills
- Diaphoresis
- Poor appetite
- Poor fluid intake
- Nausea, vomiting, or diarrhea
- Decreased urination
- Foul smelling urine, or pain or burning upon urination

ADDITIONAL INFORMATION FOR THE CLINICAL SETTING

Factors Predisposing to Childhood Leukemia

Genetic Conditions	Environmental Factors
Down syndrome	Ionizing radiation
Fanconi syndrome	Drugs
Bloom syndrome	Alkylating agents
Shwachman syndrome	Nitrosourea
Klinefelter syndrome	Epipodophyllotoxin
Turner syndrome	Benzene exposure
Neurofibromatosis	Advanced maternal age
Li–Fraumeni syndrome	
Severe combined immune deficiency	

Visualization and Distraction

- Use visualization and distraction to help avoid anxiety before a procedure (e.g., imagine a trip to his favorite place).

- Have the child close his or her eyes while the nurse plays tour guide.
- Ask the child questions about the favorite place and encourage the child to be part of the story or trip.
- Use distraction depending on the child's developmental level (e.g., blowing bubbles, reading a story).

Bone Marrow Transplant

- This is the treatment option for children who have a second remission after relapse.
- The child is given high doses of chemotherapy and/or radiation to eradicate disease or cancer and then the patient is rescued with a source of stem cells that allows for recovery of healthy bone marrow.
- There are two basic types of bone marrow transplants: Autologous and allogeneic. In an autologous transplant, the patient's own peripheral blood or bone marrow is given back. An allogeneic transplant can be from a matched sibling, a relative, or an unrelated donor accessed through the National Marrow Donor Program.

When a Child Is Diagnosed with a Brain Tumor

- The family or the child does not understand the exact nature or future implications of a brain tumor.
- Treat the child as normally as possible.
- It is acceptable to communicate with the child and family while the child plays.
- Support the parents or caregivers and allow them time to "absorb" the diagnosis.

Things to say to the family:

- "It is important for you to verbalize and express your feelings."
- "You may find it helpful to talk with others who have had the same experience as you. I have contact information for a support group. Would you like me to make a call for you?"
- "I know this is a very difficult time for you. Let's take this a day at a time and make your child's daily routine as normal as possible.

Venous Access Devices

Name	Description	Advantage	Nursing Care
Central Implanted Ports such as Infus-a-port, Mediport, Port-a-cath, or Norport	A saucer-shaped plastic device with a self-sealing injection port that can be accessed from the top or side. Requires placement in operating room.	Decreased risk of infection Placed under the skin; reducing the chance of becoming dislodged or pulled out Limited noticeably (small bump under the skin) Patency is maintained by administering heparin after access Little maintenance or care: child can participate in regular activities	Cleanse skin with warm water and soap before use. Administer topical anesthetic such as EMLA (lidocaine and prilocaine) before accessing the port. Use a Huber needle to access the port. Observe the child during medication administration for dislodgment of the needle. When treatment complete the port must be surgically removed.
Central Groshong Catheter	A silicone, flexible and clear catheter. At the proximal end, there is a closed-tip two-way valve. Requires placement in operating room.	Easy for self-administered medications and fluids No heparin required No clamping needed due to two-way valve Minimal backflow Decrease possibility of air embolism	Weekly irrigation with normal saline Parents can learn catheter care (site must be kept clean and dry). Teaching includes: (1) strenuous activity and water sports are restricted and (2) safety as the catheter protrudes from body and may be pulled out. Offer support based on body image disturbance *(continued)*

Venous Access Device (Continued)			
Name	**Description**	**Advantage**	**Nursing Care**
Central Tunneled Catheter such as Broviac or Hickman	An open-ended silicone, flexible, radiopaque catheter. Requires placement in operating room	Easy for self-administered medications and fluids Decrease risk of infection	Daily heparin flushes Parents can learn catheter care (site must be kept clean and dry) When not in use must be clamped Teaching includes; (1) strenuous activity and water sports are restricted (2) safety as the catheter protrudes from body and may be pulled out
Peripherally Inserted Central Catheters	Catheter made of silastic or polyurethane material Single- or double-lumen available Inserted into antecubital fossa passing through the cephalic or basilic vein entering the superior vena cava	Does not require placement in operating room. Pediatric nurse practitioners can insert the line using a small lumen needle Decrease risk of infection	Flushed with saline using 5 to 10-mL syringe Not suitable for rapid fluid replacement (small lumen needle) Sometimes can be difficult to remove because of resistance

Insertion of Central Venous Catheters

- The insertion of central venous catheters is one of the most frequent surgical procedures performed (Fig. 31-2).
- Long-term central venous access devices make it safer to administer chemotherapy and total parenteral nutrition; also used to administer antibiotics and to obtain blood specimens (Alcoser & Rodgers, 2003).

Figure 31-2 The insertion of a central venous catheter helps in administering chemotherapy and is one of the most frequent surgical procedures performed on children with cancer.

Nursing Care of Children with Cancer

- Children with cancer still want to be loved and treated like other children.
- Encourage these children to play and be involved in self-care activities as their condition allows.
- Encourage them to talk about their dreams, feelings, and fears.

Negative Effects of Chemotherapy

- Chemotherapy is toxic to the body because it kills not only cancer cells but healthy cells as well.
- As soon as chemotherapy is administered the nurse ensures that the child is also well hydrated so that the chemotherapeutic agent (or toxin) is flushed out of the system.
- Measure specific gravity of the urine to ensure proper hydration.
- The urine specific gravity should be 1.012 or below. If it rises above this, IV fluid boluses are required.

Loss of Hair (Alopecia)

- Explain that hair will probably start to fall out 10 days to 2 weeks after chemotherapy begins and that it may fall out in sections.

- Assure the child that once the chemotherapy has been completed, his or her hair will grow back.
- Emphasize that just because his or her hair falls out, it does not change the person the child is inside (just looks a little different for a short time).
- Suggest arranging for a first "cool hat" purchase before the child leaves the hospital.

Safe Handling of Chemotherapeutic Agents

- Use disposable gloves and gowns when handling or preparing chemotherapy medications to prevent contact with medication.
- Use aseptic technique when administering medications.
- Prepare drugs in a well ventilated room.
- Dispose all medications, contaminated needles, syringes, intravenous tubing, gloves, and gowns in an appropriate leak-proof, puncture-resistant container (Alcoser & Rodgers, 2003).

Neutropenic Patient Admitted to a Pediatric Unit

- Place the child in a private room by him- or herself for the best outcome.
- If a private room is not available, assigning the child to a room with a noninfectious child such as a fractured femur is acceptable.

Nutrition

- Maintain good nutrition.
- Assess for poor nutrition.
- Assess side effects of chemotherapy and recommend foods accordingly.
- Maintain the immune system.
- Try simple care measures first (enteral feedings or TPN may be the only option).
- Communicate to the parents that their child may eventually be able to eat independently again.

Infection

- Monitor for systemic and localized signs of infection every 2 to 4 hours.
- Take temperature every 4 hours.
- Report a single temperature >101.20°F (38.50°C) in a 24-hour period or 100.40°F (38.00°C) three times in a 24-hour period.
- Provide meticulous skin care and use good hand washing (instruct visitors).

- Use universal precautions and designated isolation precautions.
- Monitor and report lab values.
- Teach family about the principles of prophylactic antibiotics and signs and symptoms of infection.

Radiation Side Effects
- Nausea
- Alopecia
- Fatigue and malaise
- Low WBC count
- Skin desquamation
- Mucous membrane inflammation and irritation

Surgery
Surgery is used as an adjunct to both chemotherapy and radiation.

- It also has an important role in the diagnosis of a tumor via biopsy.

The biopsy is obtained through a fine-needle aspiration or an open biopsy procedure.

Pain Control
- Pain medications combined with adequate rest and sleep, massage, heat, distraction, and social support
- Topical anesthetics

Psychological Support
- Provide holistic nursing care.
- Encourage parents or another support person to stay with the child 24 hours a day.
- Involve the child-life specialist.
- Be present and listen.
- Provide family with community resources, reliable internet sources, or information about support groups.

Negative Effects of Chemotherapy
- Nausea and vomiting (administer antiemetics)
- Alopecia (address body image)
- Extravasation (prevent accidental leakage of drugs)
- Mucositis (keep oral cavity clean)
- Diarrhea (skin care, diet, and medication)
- Constipation (diet, activity, and medication)
- Anemia (signs and symptoms, diet, vitamin, RBC transfusion, administer hematopoietic growth factors)

- Thrombocytopenia (platelet transfusion)
- Neutropenia (assess fever, blood cultures, and administer antibiotics)

Medical Emergencies

Hemorrhagic Cystitis
- Maintain hydration.
- Test urine for blood, pH and specific gravity (see Procedure 31-1).
- If urine is positive for blood, notify the physician immediately.
- Monitor intake and output.
- Obtain daily BUN and creatinine levels.
- Administer MESNA (Mesnex, Uromitexan)

Tumor Lysis Syndrome
- Keep urine alkalinized.
- Maintain a low-phosphate diet.
- Administer allopurinol (Aloprim).
- Maintain adequate hydration.
- Monitor electrolytes.
- Obtain BUN and creatinine levels.
- Dialysis or exchange transfusions may be necessary.

Septic Shock
- When a neutropenic child is given antibiotics; take vital signs every 10 to 15 minutes during the antibiotic administration to recognize signs of septic shock.
- Administer large amounts of an isotonic fluid (normal saline).
- Check peripheral pulses and capillary refill to monitor perfusion.
- Use the ABCs and other emergent care measures:
  - Airway
  - Breathing
  - Circulation
  - Fluid resuscitation
  - Evaluation of etiology (CBC, electrolytes, DIC panel, blood cultures, liver and renal functions)
  - Blood products
  - Antibiotics
  - Vasopressors

Psychological Aspects

- Suggest support.
- Encourage adequate rest and nutrition for parents.
- Be honest.
- Use a multidisciplinary approach.
- Tailor information to developmental stage.
- Keep lines of communication open.
- Offer spiritual care.
- Help the child and his family express feelings.

Handling Siblings of an Ill Child

- While children with cancer are undergoing many stressful events, do not forget about their siblings (visiting a sick sibling is stressful for both sides).
- Help make the sibling's day special by telling her a story, or by giving her a sticker or a coloring book and crayons.
- Encourage the ill child to color a picture for his or her sibling and hang it in the room.
- A sincere demeanor and common pleasantries such as saying hello or calling the sibling by their name can make the visit special and less stressful.

RESOURCES

Association of Pediatric Hematology/Oncology Nurses:
http://www.apon.org

American Cancer Society (for children):
http://www.cancer.org/docroot/CRI/CRI_2_6x_Children_and_Cancer.asp

Candlelighters Childhood Cancer Foundation:
http://www.candlelighters.org

The Leukemia and Lymphoma Society: http://www.leukemia.org

REFERENCES

Alcoser, P., & Rodgers, C. (2003). Treatment strategies in childhood cancer. *Journal of Pediatric Nursing, 18*(2), 103–112.

Bryant, R. (2003). Managing side effects of childhood cancer treatments. *Journal of Pediatric Nursing, 18*(2), 113–125.

Deglin, J., & Vallerand, A. (2009). *Davis's drug guide for nurses* (11th ed.). Philadelphia: F.A. Davis.

Steen, G., & Mirro, M (2000). *Childhood cancer. A handbook from St. Jude Children's Research Hospital.* Cambridge, MA: Perseus.

Van Leeuwen, A.M., Kranpitz, T.R., & Smith, L. (2006). *Davis's comprehensive handbook of laboratory and diagnostic tests with nursing implications.* Philadelphia: F.A. Davis

Venes, D. (2005). *Taber's cyclopedic medical dictionary* (20th ed.). Philadelphia: F.A. Davis.

Caring for the Child with a Chronic Condition or the Dying Child

KEY TERMS

caregiver burden – Unrelenting pressure and anxiety in providing daily care to a child with disabilities while meeting other family needs; can be a major source of stress

chronic sorrow – Period of episodic grieving interspersed with periods of denial

end-of-life care – A holistic approach to care that includes physical, emotional, social, and spiritual interventions, and complementary care during the final 6 months of life

general growth failure – Growth that is slower than normal and the height and weight is in a lower percentile on the growth charts than those of children the same age

hospice care – A program that focuses on quality of life for dying persons; method of treating a serious illness when cure or meaningful improvement is no longer possible and end-of-life care describes a certain time frame where care is given during the final 6 months of life

palliative care – Type of care that the child receives at the end of life after it becomes obvious that no cure is possible; emphasizes physical, emotional, and spiritual care of the child and family

pathological grief – Deviation from a healthy or normal grief where intense grief feelings or a dysfunctional personality may easily bring about such behaviors as violence, addictions, or poor decision making

regression – An abnormal return to an earlier reaction, characterized by emotions or behaviors that are inappropriate for the current age and may include the loss of recently acquired skills (Venes, 2005)

respite care – Short-term care offered to families living with a child who has a chronic condition; the main goal is to provide temporary relief for family members from the burden and stress of sustained care giving (Venes, 2005)

technology dependent – Reliance on some type of medical device to compensate for the loss of normal use of a vital body function

FOCUSED ASSESSMENT

- Use either the numeric scale, the Wong faces scale, or the FLACC pain scale to determine a child's level of pain. See Chapter 18.

Impact of the Chronic Condition on the Infant

- Bonding process
- Pain
- Changes in diet and sleep may alter growth and development

Impact of the Chronic Condition on the Toddler

- Unable to achieve autonomy
- Pain, anxiety, and separation from parents
- Sensitive to bodily harm
- Hindered gross and fine motor development
- Stress and regression present

Impact of the Chronic Condition on the Preschooler

- Feels he or she is being punished for wrongdoing
- Reacts aggressively
- Regresses
- Withdraws from others
- Difficulty sleeping (fears falling asleep)

Impact of the Chronic Condition on the School-age Child

- Altered autonomy and peer relationships
- Interrupts independence
- Refuses to comply with treatments or to follow a special diet
- Cannot completely comprehend all information (reluctant to answer questions)
- May understand significance of illness and lifelong consequences

Impact of the Chronic Condition on the Adolescent

- There may be a dilemma where to place the adolescent; in a pediatric ward or on an adult floor?
- In spite of trying to achieve independence, dependence on caregivers may occur
- Lack of privacy
- Maladaptive coping behaviors
- Refuses treatments
- Easily overwhelmed and may show regression
- Worries about condition, self-esteem, identity, and family

Impact of the Chronic Condition on the Sibling

- May have decreased self-esteem
- May receive less attention and support from parents
- May have mood swings and lack understanding about the condition
- May display a negative attitude toward the ill sibling
- May have feelings of jealousy, embarrassment, resentment, loneliness, and isolation
- May think that he or she caused the condition or might acquire the condition too

Handling a Sibling Who Is Acting Out

Best outcome: The sibling has time to regain control and can express feelings. Some examples are below:

- "You seem very angry today." (reflection)
- "It is all right to be angry at your sister's condition and about the situation." (validating the sibling's feelings)

- "It must be difficult for you to have your sister in the hospital." (empathizing and understanding)
- The nurse can then help the sibling find a positive outlet for the anger such as art therapy (channeling).
- Encourage the sibling to tell an adult when the anger returns (providing an outlet).

Children Living with Chronic Conditions

Children living with a chronic condition experience one or more of these symptoms (Judson, 2004):

- Limitation in bodily functions appropriate for age and development
- Disfigurement
- Dependency on medical technology
- Dependency on medication or special diet to ensure normal functioning or control of the condition
- Ongoing need for medical care or related services compared to other children the same age
- Special ongoing treatments at home or at school

Emotional Responses to a Chronic Condition

- Disruption of family equilibrium
- Feelings of shock, chaos, anger, fear, disbelief, anxiety, pain, and stress ("emotional roller coaster")

Perceptions of Death

Infant
- Based on the degree of discomfort and the reactions of the parents and others in the environment

Toddler
- Has difficulty with separation from parents and/or disruption in routine

Preschooler
- Magical thinkers: Illness or injury may be viewed as punishment for bad behaviors
- Concrete thinkers: Death should not be described as "going to sleep."

School-age
- Understanding is not precise until the child can understand the concept of time
- After age 8 or 9 children understand the permanence of death.

Adolescent
- Adult level of understanding and fear of dependence on others
- Difficulty accepting death as reality and often think that death can be defied

Recognition of Physical Signs of Impending Death

- Loss of sensation
- Loss of the body's ability to maintain thermoregulation: skin may feel cool
- Loss of bowel and bladder function
- Loss of awareness or consciousness and slurring of speech
- Alteration in respiratory status
- Cheyne–Stokes respirations (a waxing and waning in the depth of respirations with regular periods of apnea)
- Noisy chest or respirations with the accumulation of fluid in the lungs or in the posterior pharynx
- Decreased, weak, or slow pulse rate and drop in blood pressure

Somatic Grief Response

- Somatic distress that includes feelings of tightness in the throat or chest, sighing
- Weakness or shortness of breath
- Preoccupation with the image of the deceased (e.g., hearing or seeing the person who died)
- Inability to focus on anything other than the loved one who died
- Emotionally distancing self from others
- Feelings of guilt
- Feeling responsible for the loved one's death
- Searching for what could have been done differently, thinking in terms of "if only I had done..."
- Hostile reactions that include feelings and expressions of anger
- Inability to complete daily tasks

Subtle Indicators of Grief

These subtle signs are warning signs and may not necessarily indicate a severe problem. It is the intensity and duration of these behaviors that are the deciding factors indicating the need for professional help.

- Absence of grief, such as showing little or no emotion
- Persistent blame or guilt
- Anxiety
- Aggressive and destructive outburst
- Depression and suicidal thoughts or actions
- Unwillingness to speak about the deceased
- Expressing only positive or only negative feelings about the deceased
- Prolonged dysfunction in school
- Always assuming a caregiver role
- Stealing or other illegal acts
- Signs of addictive behavior: drugs, food, certain activities

Paying Attention to Personal Needs

The nurse can pay attention to personal needs by asking:

- How do I feel?
- Am I comfortable caring for a child who is dying?
- Can I cope with the needs of the family as well?
- Am I becoming overwhelmed or attached when caring for this child and family?
- If the nurse feels uncomfortable with any of these questions, it is time for reflection and self-care.
- Determine if the situation becomes too great to bear.

CLINICAL ALERTS

Principles of Pain Medication Administration

- Administer pain medications orally for as long as possible.
- Alternative routes for pain medication administration include intravenous, subcutaneous, transcutaneous, transmucosal, rectal, nasal, epidural, and intrathecal.
- The enteral route (or through a gastrostomy tube) is the preferred route for children in the dying process.

- Adjuvants (drugs added to a prescription to hasten or increase the action of a principal ingredient in the medication) must be considered. They are medications not used as the principal pain medication but offer analgesia in certain situations, including anticonvulsants, antidepressants, or muscle relaxants (Hain et al., 2004).

MEDICATIONS

- Pain management includes medication and other traditional nursing comfort measures (e.g., clean sheets, good hygiene measures, oral care, and skin care).
- Answer questions about treatment, procedures, and medications honestly and at a level the child can understand.
- General growth failure means that the child grows more slowly than normal and that the height and weight are in a lower percentile on the growth charts than for children of the same age. It may result from the condition itself or from related treatments and medications.
- A large proportion of children taking herbal medications are also taking over-the-counter medications.

ETHNOCULTURAL CONSIDERATIONS

Cultural Practices

- The nurse must be knowledgeable about the cultural practices of the child and family.
- Include the right support person to facilitate the cultural care of the dying child.
- By including cultural rituals or customs, nursing care can provide comfort during the death process for the child and family.
- Special ceremonies or rites may be requested by the family and should be accommodated whenever possible.
- Other cultural care measures may include use of spiritual texts and symbols, using prayer or meditation, chanting, offering music, lighting a candle, listening in silence, being present in the moment, or including other methods of care as deemed appropriate by the culture.

Hispanic Culture and Grieving

- Hispanics are predominantly of the Roman Catholic faith tradition and have a close extended family network within the social structure. A child who dies is viewed as an angel who has returned to heaven. This belief brings comfort to the parents and the extended family, particularly the grandparents, and allows them to move on through the grieving process.
- To honor the deceased child, pictures are displayed in the home as a tribute, keeping the memory alive.
- Outward expressions of happiness (parties, celebrations, music in the house) are discouraged for usually a year.
- In some instances, the relatives wear black clothing to signify that they remember the loved one.
- If these traditions are not observed, there may be criticism from others and criticism is of the utmost concern to the family.

TEACHING THE FAMILY

The Sibling Needs to Say Good-Bye

- Visits from siblings are important and should be encouraged.
- Parents often try to protect the dying child by limiting visitation.
- Encourage siblings to write letters or draw pictures for the dying child as a way of saying good-bye.
- Siblings need to be included in the grieving process and to have the opportunity to say good-bye.
- The child who has been included in the death and mourning process with the family is able to let go in a healthy way (Kübler-Ross, 1983).

ADDITIONAL INFORMATION FOR THE CLINICAL SETTING

Other Terms Associated with a Chronic Condition

- Disability is similar to a chronic condition in that it also refers to the limitations that prevent or interfere with a child's ability to perform daily activities.

- Handicap is the inability to carry out tasks or access certain aspects of the environment due to one or more impairments. The terms "activity limitation" or "participation restriction" are preferred by many specialists in physical, occupational, and speech therapy as well as those in related fields (Venes, 2005).

Understanding the Type of Technological Equipment Required

Technology dependent children are grouped according to the type of equipment required. According to a United States Congress report, the groups are designated from the most complex equipment to the least complex equipment required:

- Group 1: Children who require a ventilator.
- Group 2: Children who require devices for total parenteral nutrition.
- Group 3: Children who have a daily dependence on some other device for respiratory or nutritional support (e.g., tracheostomy, oxygen support, tube feeding).
- Group 4: Children who require an apnea monitor, peritoneal dialysis, hemodialysis or other devices, such as catheters and colostomy bags.
- The infants and children who fall into groups 1 and 3 are further defined as needing high-technology care; medically fragile (Judson, 2004).

Impact of a Chronic Condition

- Creates a threat of the unknown, loss of control, and has long-term effects.
- Frequent hospitalizations or clinic visits may be needed.
- Disrupts normal home routines.
- Demands are placed on the caregiver.
- Parents may become controlling and overprotective.
- The child may have to cope with unfamiliar people, places, and medical treatments.
- The family may be overwhelmed and experience social, financial, and psychological strain.

Nursing Care of the Infant with a Chronic Condition

- Rock, hold, comfort, and use a soothing voice.
- Provide visual and auditory stimulation.

- Use group nursing care measures and protect nap time.
- Maintain the crib as a safe place.
- Encourage parents to hold the infant.
- Encourage siblings to visit.

Nursing Care of the Toddler with a Chronic Condition

- Maintain the bond between parents and child.
- Promote realistic developmental skills.
- Do not react negatively to regression.
- Praise the child for attempts at self-care.
- Instruct the parents on realistic methods of discipline.
- Manage pain.
- Maintain the home routine as much as possible.
- Allow the child to express his or her feelings through play.

Regression
- An abnormal return to an earlier reaction, characterized by emotions or behaviors that are inappropriate for the current age and may include the loss of recently acquired skills (Venes, 2005).
- Can be both physical and emotional.

Nursing Care of the Preschooler with a Chronic Condition

- Provide the opportunity to express fears and frustrations.
- Tell stories and read books.
- Allow the preschooler to use dramatic play.
- Ask the child-life specialist for assistance.
- Maintain a normal home schedule as much as possible and enforce consistent limits.
- Reassure the child that nothing he or she did caused the illness.
- Be honest when explaining and preparing the child for procedures.
- Understand the child's limited concept of time.

Nursing Care of the School-age Child with a Chronic Condition

- Maintain pain management.
- Reassure that personal behavior has not caused the illness.
- Answer questions at a level the child can understand.

- Use play as an outlet (unstructured).
- Include peers as much as possible.
- Communicate to family about nonverbal cues.
- Maintain open and honest dialogue.

Nursing Care of an Adolescent with a Chronic Condition

- Provide solitary time.
- Give realistic choices.
- Include the adolescent in medically related matters when possible.
- Use peer support and interaction.
- May expand networks to include support groups and community programming.

Nursing Care of a Sibling of a Child with a Chronic Condition

- Instruct parents to maintain familiar home routines as much as possible.
- Include the sibling in simple care.
- Provide information about the ill child.

Child Life Specialist

- Whenever a child is diagnosed with a chronic condition, it is important to involve the child life specialist.
- The child life specialist is an expert in child development and therapeutic play and can assist in diversion activities during procedures, arrange for therapeutic play, or simply let the child take time to play.

Caregiver Burden

- Caregiver burden, as described by Kuster et al. (2004), is the unrelenting pressure and anxiety in providing daily care to a child with disabilities while meeting other family needs and can be a major source of stress.

Respite Care

- Respite care is short-term care offered to families living with a child who has a chronic condition.

- The main goal of respite care is to provide relief for family members of the burden and stress of sustained care giving (Venes, 2005).
- Parents can also use respite care in situations in which someone besides them can accompany the child to a doctor's appointment.
- The availability of respite care varies in every community (Orloff et al., 2004).
- It is important to note that respite care is not always paid for by private insurance. Sometimes state agencies or national programs can reimburse the family for respite care.

Talking About the Chronic Condition

- When talking about the child's chronic condition with the family, the nurse must be sure to use the child's name and personalize the discussion.
- It is important that the nurse avoid labeling the child by, for example, saying "CF kids." Instead, the nurse can say, "Timmy will need ongoing care for his cystic fibrosis."
- This kind of communication places the emphasis on the child and not on the condition.
- It is also important to listen to the family so that home routines can be continued during hospitalization.

Establishing Trust with the Family

Godshall (2003) suggests that the nurse take the following actions when establishing trust:

- Consider the needs of the entire family; do not forget the siblings.
- Familiarize yourself with the child's condition and know about the disease process.
- Be open and honest.
- Show the family that the burden of care is understood. Burden of care includes the combination of physical, psychological, social, and financial burdens the family may face.
- Take time to listen to the child and to the caregiver.
- Include parents in the plan of care. Some parents like to participate in the child's care while the child is hospitalized. It is also important to maintain home rituals as much as possible while the child is hospitalized.

- Treat each child as an individual. It is essential that the nurse not label the child according to the disease process.
- Allow the child to make decisions about the care when possible. Decision making is especially important for the adolescent.
- Maintain confidentiality.
- Do not prematurely judge the parents. Some parents cannot stay with the child in the hospital because of personal needs and responsibilities.
- Arrange for continuity of nursing care.
- Assess the family's support systems and resources.

The Dying Child

Do Not Resuscitate

- A Do Not Resuscitate (DNR) request means withholding life-sustaining treatment and requires that no attempt be made to revive a child who has clinically died.
- Withholding life-sustaining medical treatment includes decisions to withhold, withdraw, or limit medical treatment.
- Some medical ethicists feel that there is no difference between withholding and withdrawing treatment if the treatment is no longer beneficial to the child. When making recommendations to withhold, withdraw, or limit medical treatment, the benefits of treatment must be weighed against the burden of continuing treatment for the child.
- A DNR order means that no lifesaving measures will be initiated in the event of cardiac or respiratory arrest.
- This decision also can mean removing medical equipment such as a ventilator or monitor, dialysis machine, feeding tube used for artificial nutrition, and intravenous fluids for hydration. Aggressive treatments such as chemotherapy or radiation therapy are also terminated.
- Wiegand (2006) states that the child and family participating in the process of withdrawal of life-sustaining therapy need consistency among health care providers and the delivery of consistent messages.
- All members of the interdisciplinary team need to communicate effectively with each other so that families receive ongoing and reliable information.

Before the Child Dies
- Complete the institution's checklist to ensure policies and procedures are followed.
- Contact the bereavement team.
- Create a file and include community resources.
- Make a follow-up ledger and phone call.

Facilitators and Barriers to Providing a "Good Death" Experience in the ICU	
Facilitators	**Barriers**
Make environment changes to facilitate dying with dignity.	Staffing patterns and nursing shortage
Communicate challenges.	Treatments based on medical regimens rather than on child and family needs
Manage pain and discomfort.	
Follow child's and family's wishes for end-of-life care.	
Promote early cessation of treatments if requested.	
Eliminate aggressive treatments, especially when the treatments are futile.	
Ensure effective communication among the total health care team.	

Source: Beckstrand, Callister, & Kirchoff (2006).

Care of the Dying Child
- Care of the dying child includes holistic nursing interventions that address the physical, emotional, and spiritual aspects:
  - Palliative care: Follows a medical model
  - Hospice care: Holistic approach; focuses on quality of life
  - End-of-life care: End of life is about 6 months away; the objective is peaceful death without pain
- Shift from the curative technological approach to providing care that enables the child to move toward death accessing own inner resources for healing.
- Help the child restore mental, physical, and spiritual balance to attain peace at the time of death.
- Be present.
- Use touch.
- Give the family choices.
- Assess the situation and determine the proper environment.

Complementary and Alternative Medicine

- Complementary and alternative medicine (CAM) has become increasingly popular in palliative care (e.g., relaxation, aromatherapy, acupuncture, or other therapies performed by a licensed practitioner). Other therapies, including dietary supplements and herbal remedies, are unregulated.
- The frequency and type of CAM are dependent on the child's condition and prognosis.
- Spiritual blessings and prayers may be beneficial to various types of chronic illnesses

Advantages of CAM

- Easy to understand
- Familiar methods
- Many are noninvasive
- Many have fewer side effects compared to medical treatments
- Help improve the overall quality of life
- Help maintain current state of health
- More holistic and in balance with nature (Suzuki, 2004)

Disadvantages of CAM

- Some treatments are complex
- They have not undergone adequate testing of effectiveness
- Many herbal preparations and remedies lack FDA approval
- Many are not covered by third-party reimbursement

The Hospice Approach

- Family-centered care is essential.
- A comprehensive, holistic approach can meet the child's physical, emotional, social, and spiritual needs.
- Effective symptom control and pain management are paramount.
- Care is provided by an interdisciplinary team.
- The child can be cared for at home or in a homelike environment.
- Coordination and continuity of care is a priority.
- In addition to regularly scheduled home care visits, services are available on a 24-hour, 7 days-a-week, on-call basis.
- The focus of care is on improving the quality of remaining life; that is, on palliative, not curative, measures.

- Bereavement follow-up services are offered to family members in the year after the death of the loved one (Lattanzi-Licht & Connor, 1995).

Children's Hospice International, 2005

- Children's Hospice International, 2005 states that it is important to give clear answers to children who are dying. Evasive answers may confuse the child.
- The child may be at a developmental level at which he or she may take conversations literally. When talking to the child, it is important to remember:
  - Do not tell the child that death is sleeping peacefully. The child may fear going to sleep.
  - Do not tell the child abstract concepts like, "It is God's will" or "You are such a good boy that God wants you to be with him." He or she may start to misbehave so as not to die.
- Approach the child with compassion, honesty, support, and love (Children's Hospice International, 2005).

Critical Nursing Actions: Holistic Care for the Dying Child

Comfort Measures	Emotional Support	Spiritual Interventions	Complementary Care
Pain management Good hygiene Repositioning Nutrition and diet management Physical or occupational therapy Help the family create new rituals when the old ones no longer work due to the disease process.	Active listening and showing empathy Distraction Encourage positive coping. Encourage verbalization and ventilation of feelings. Psychotherapy referral Suggest support groups. Discuss topics about grief, loss, isolation, fear, guilt, and relationships. Discuss concerns about life after the child's death that relate to family, friends, and others.	Offering presence Meditation Music Prayer Read from spiritual text or poetry Allow for sacrament. Contact the family's religious or spiritual community. Discuss God/Higher Power or spiritual source.	Art therapy Energy-based therapy (healing touch, therapeutic touch, Reiki) Relaxation Guided imagery Acupuncture Reasonable exercise Aromatherapy

National Cancer Institute

- The National Cancer Institute (NCI) has resources available by calling the Cancer Information Service (CIS) Toll-free: 1-800-4-CANCER (1-800-422-6237) TTY (for deaf and hard of hearing callers): 1-800-332-8615.
- The NCI's Web sites are located at http://www.cancer. gov or http://www.cancer.gov/cancer_information/coping/ (click on the title under "End-of-Life Issues"). Cancer information specialists offer online assistance through the *LiveHelp* link on the NCI's Web site.

Fact Sheets

- The NCI fact sheet about hospice care includes contact information for hospice organizations.
- The NCI Advance Directives fact sheet discusses a patient's rights regarding medical treatment.
- The NCI fact sheet on Home Care for Cancer Patients provides information and resources related to home care services.
- The NCI booklet "Advanced Cancer: Living Each Day" provides support to cancer patients, families, and friends.

After the Child Dies

- Prepare the family about the child's appearance and description of the death.
- Offer the family the choice of seeing the child alone or with the nurse.

Handling the Child's Belongings

- Treat the child's belongings with respect and package in a special container instead of a plain plastic bag.
- Show sensitivity as these are the child's final possessions.

Grief

- Grief is a normal and appropriate emotional response to loss.
- Grief is unique to every individual and there is no timetable in which grief is complete.
- The stages of grief may come and go.
- Feelings of grief can return when least expected.
- Parents may not realize that grief begins the moment the child's diagnosis is communicated (Steen & Mirro, 2000).

Helping the Family Understand the Situation

- Listen empathetically and encourage the family to take the situation one day or one moment at a time.
- Help the family understand that there will be "good days" and inevitably "bad days."
- Give the family hope that over time the emotional pain may dissipate and that they can better come to terms with the experience of their child's death.

Coping Patterns

- Recognize exhibited coping patterns and find ways to support family:
  - Listen, sit silently, refer to pastoral care, offer spiritual care.
  - In case of destructive behavior to self or others call the physician or professional counselor.
  - Do not alter the coping pattern completely.

Pathological Grief

- Subtle indicators
- Suicidal or homicidal ideation
- Violent behavior
- Grief influenced by drugs and alcohol
- Extreme denial

Saying Good-bye

- Saying good-bye should not be rushed.
- Include siblings in the grieving process, encourage them to visit, and give them the opportunity to say good-bye.
- Call the child by his or her name.
- What to say to parents and family:
  - "I'm sorry"
  - "This must be terribly hard for you"
  - "Is there anyone I can call for you?"
  - "Would you like me to stay with you for a while?"

Caring for the Sibling of a Dying Child

- Listen and help the sibling express his or her feelings.
- Model to the family about how to acknowledge the sibling's presence during this difficult time (initiate a

simple conversation, turn on cartoons, offer a drink or snack, or show the sibling how to touch the dying child).
- Explain the situation to the sibling and relate appropriate information in terms understandable for the sibling's age.
- Help the sibling understand that he or she is not responsible for the death.
- Contact a child life specialist who can assist the sibling with art therapy.
- Encourage simple ways to be involved in the care such as making a final gift for the sibling to keep at the bedside.

RESOURCES

Compassionate Friends: http://www.compassionatefriends.org

National Cancer Institute: http://www.cancer.gov

End-of-Life Issues": http://www.cancer.gov/cancer_information/coping/

REFERENCES

Beckstrand, R.L., Callister, L.C., & Kirchhoff, K.T. (2006). Providing a "good death": Critical care nurses suggestions for improving end-life-care. *American Journal of Critical Care, 15*(1), 38–45.

Children's Hospice International (2005). Retrieved from http://www.chionline.org/resources (Accessed August 22, 2008).

Godshall, M. (2003). Caring for the families of chronically ill kids. *RN, 66*(2), 30–35.

Hain, R., Weinsten, S., Oleske, J., Orloff, S.F., & Cohen, S. (2004). Holistic management of symptoms. In B.S. Carter & M. Levetown (Eds.). *Palliative care for infants, children, and adolescents: A practical handbook* (pp. 163–195). Baltimore: The Johns Hopkins University Press.

Judson, L. (2004). Protective care: mothering a child dependent on parenteral nutrition. *Journal of Family Nursing, 10*(1), 93–120.

Kübler-Ross, E. (1983). *On children and death.* New York: Macmillan.

Kuster, P.A., Badr, L.K., Chang, B.L., Wuerker, A.K., & Benjamin, A.E. (2004). Factors influencing health promoting activities of mothers caring for ventilator assisted children. *Journal of Pediatric Nursing, 19*(4), 276–287.

Lattanzi-Licht, M., & Connor, S. (1995). Care of the dying: The hospice approach. In H. Wass & R.A. Neimeyer (Eds.). *Dying: Facing the facts.* Washington, DC: Taylor and Francis.

Orloff, S., Quance, K., Perszyk, S., Flowers, W., & Veale, E. (2004). Psychosocial and spiritual needs of the child and family. In K.M. Foley, B.S. Carter, & M. Levetown (Eds.). *Palliative care for infants, children, and adolescents* (pp. 141–162). Baltimore: The Johns Hopkins University Press

Suzuki, N. (2004). Complementary and alternative medicine: A Japanese perspective. *Evidenced-based Complementary and Alternative Care, 1*(2), 113–118.

Steen, G., & Mirro, M. (2000). *Childhood cancer. A handbook from St. Jude Children's Research Hospital*. Cambridge, MA: Perseus.

Venes, D. (Ed.). (2005). *Tabers cyclopedic medical dictionary*. Philadelphia: F.A. Davis.

Wiegand, D. (2006). Withdrawal of life-sustaining therapy after sudden, unexpected life-threatening illness or injury: Interactions between patients' families, healthcare providers, and the healthcare system. *Journal of Critical Care, 15*(2), 178–187.

PHOTO AND ILLUSTRATION CREDITS

Chapter 1

First figure. Centers for Disease Control and Prevention, 2008.

Visual breast inspection. Dillon, P. (2007). *Nursing health assessment: A critical thinking, case studies approach* (2nd ed., p. 544). Philadelphia: F.A. Davis.

Arms raised overhead. Dillon, P. (2007). *Nursing health assessment: A critical thinking, case studies approach* (2nd ed., p. 544). Philadelphia: F.A. Davis.

Nipple assessment. Dillon, P. (2007). *Nursing health assessment: A critical thinking, case studies approach* (2nd ed., p. 550). Philadelphia: F.A. Davis.

Breast palpation. Dillon, P. (2007). *Nursing health assessment: A critical thinking, case studies approach* (2nd ed., p. 550). Philadelphia: F.A. Davis.

Testicular self-examination. Williams, L., & Hopper, P. (2007). *Understanding medical surgical nursing* (3rd ed., p. 896). Philadelphia: F.A. Davis.

Chapter 2

Figure 2-1 Dillon, P. (2007). *Nursing health assessment: A critical thinking, case studies approach* (2nd ed., p. 612). Philadelphia: F.A. Davis.

Figure 2-2 Scanlon, V., & Sanders, T. (2007). *Essentials of anatomy and physiology* (5th ed., p. 463). Philadelphia: F.A. Davis.

Figure 2-3 Scanlon, V., & Sanders, T. (2007). *Essentials of anatomy and physiology* (5th ed., p. 464). Philadelphia: F.A. Davis.

Figure 2-5 Dillon, P. (2007). *Nursing health assessment: A critical thinking, case studies approach* (2nd ed., p. 613). Philadelphia: F.A. Davis.

Figure 2-7 Scanlon, V., & Sanders, T. (2007). *Essentials of anatomy and physiology* (5th ed., p. 459). Philadelphia: F.A. Davis.

Chapter 6

Figure 6-1 Dillon, P. (2007). *Nursing health assessment: A critical thinking, case studies approach* (2nd ed., p. 836). Philadelphia: F.A. Davis.

Figure 6-2 Dillon, P. (2007). *Nursing health assessment: A critical thinking, case studies approach* (2nd ed., p. 837). Philadelphia: F.A. Davis.

Figure 6-3 Dillon, P. (2007). *Nursing health assessment: A critical thinking, case studies approach* (2nd ed., p. 838). Philadelphia: F.A. Davis.

Figure 6-4 Dillon, P. (2007). *Nursing health assessment: A critical thinking, case studies approach* (2nd ed., p. 838). Philadelphia: F.A. Davis.

Figure 6-5 Dillon, P. (2007). *Nursing health assessment: A critical thinking, case studies approach* (2nd ed., p. 838). Philadelphia: F.A. Davis.

Figure 6-6 Dillon, P. (2007). *Nursing health assessment: A critical thinking, case studies approach* (2nd ed., p. 838). Philadelphia: F.A. Davis.

Figure 6-7. Dillon, P. (2007). *Nursing health assessment: A critical thinking, case studies approach* (2nd ed., p. 838). Philadelphia: F.A. Davis.

Chapter 8

Figure 8-1 Holloway, B., Moredich, C., & Aduddell, K. (2006). *OB peds women's health notes: Nurse's clinical pocket guide,* p. 43, Philadelphia: F.A. Davis.

Figure 8-2 Holloway, B., Moredich, C., & Aduddell, K. (2006). *OB peds women's health notes: Nurse's clinical pocket guide,* p. 45, Philadelphia: F.A. Davis.

Figure 8-3 Dillon, P. (2007). *Nursing health assessment: A critical thinking, case studies approach* (2nd ed., p. 785). Philadelphia: F.A. Davis.

Chapter 9

Figure 9-8 Holloway, B., Moredich, C., & Aduddell, K. (2006). *OB peds women's health notes: Nurse's clinical pocket guide* (p. 53). Philadelphia: F.A. Davis.

Figure 9-11 Holloway, B., Moredich, C., & Aduddell, K. (2006). *OB peds women's health notes: Nurse's clinical pocket guide* (p. 55). Philadelphia: F.A. Davis.

Figure 9-12 Holloway, B., Moredich, C., & Aduddell, K. (2006). *OB peds women's health notes: Nurse's clinical pocket guide* (p. 56). Philadelphia: F.A. Davis.

Figure 9-13 Holloway, B., Moredich, C., & Aduddell, K. (2006). *OB peds women's health notes: Nurse's clinical pocket guide* (p. 57). Philadelphia: F.A. Davis.

Figure 9-14 Holloway, B., Moredich, C., & Aduddell, K. (2006). *OB peds women's health notes: Nurse's clinical pocket guide* (p. 59). Philadelphia: F.A. Davis.

Figure 9-15 Holloway, B., Moredich, C., & Aduddell, K. (2006). *OB peds women's health notes: Nurse's clinical pocket guide* (p. 60). Philadelphia: F.A. Davis.

Figure 9-16 Holloway, B., Moredich, C., & Aduddell, K. (2006). *OB peds women's health notes: Nurse's clinical pocket guide* (p. 60). Philadelphia: F.A. Davis.

Figure 9-17 Holloway, B., Moredich, C., & Aduddell, K. (2006). *OB peds women's health notes: Nurse's clinical pocket guide* (p. 60). Philadelphia: F.A. Davis.

Chapter 12

Figure 12-1 Holloway, B., Moredich, C., & Aduddell, K. (2006). *OB peds women's health notes: Nurse's clinical pocket guide* (p. 83). Philadelphia: F.A. Davis.

Figure 12-2 Dillon, P. (2007). *Nursing health assessment: A critical thinking, case studies approach* (2nd ed., p. 844). Philadelphia: F.A. Davis.

Chapter 13

Figure in Procedure 13-1. Holloway, B., Moredich, C., & Aduddell, K. (2006). *OB peds women's health notes: Nurse's clinical pocket guide* (p. 83). Philadelphia: F.A. Davis.

Chapter 15

Figure 15-1 Dillon, P. (2007). *Nursing health assessment: A critical thinking, case studies approach* (2nd ed., p. 857). Philadelphia: F.A. Davis.

Figure 15-2 Dillon, P. (2007). *Nursing health assessment: A critical thinking, case studies approach* (2nd ed., p. 856). Philadelphia: F.A. Davis.

Figure 15-3 Dillon, P. (2007). *Nursing health assessment: A critical thinking, case studies approach* (2nd ed., p. 856). Philadelphia: F.A. Davis.

Figure 15-4 Dillon, P. (2007). *Nursing health assessment: A critical thinking, case studies approach* (2nd ed., p. 857). Philadelphia: F.A. Davis.

Figure 15-5 Courtesy of Mead Johnson Nutritionals.

Procedure 15-2 Dillon, P. (2007). *Nursing health assessment: A critical thinking, case studies approach* (2nd ed., p. 857). Philadelphia: F.A. Davis.

Procedure 15-3, first photo. Dillon, P. (2007). *Nursing health assessment: A critical thinking, case studies approach* (2nd ed., p. 866). Philadelphia: F.A. Davis.

Procedure 15-3, second photo. Dillon, P. (2007). *Nursing health assessment: A critical thinking, case studies approach* (2nd ed., p. 866). Philadelphia: F.A. Davis.

Procedure 15-3, third photo. Dillon, P. (2007). *Nursing health assessment: A critical thinking, case studies approach* (2nd ed., p. 866). Philadelphia: F.A. Davis.

Palmar grasp. Dillon, P. (2007). *Nursing health assessment: A critical thinking, case studies approach* (2nd ed., p. 869). Philadelphia: F.A. Davis.

Toe or plantar grasp. Dillon, P. (2007). *Nursing health assessment: A critical thinking, case studies approach* (2nd ed., p. 869). Philadelphia: F.A. Davis.

Rooting and sucking reflexes. Dillon, P. (2007). *Nursing health assessment: A critical thinking, case studies approach* (2nd ed., p. 871). Philadelphia: F.A. Davis.

Extrusion reflex. Dillon, P. (2007). *Nursing health assessment: A critical thinking, case studies approach* (2nd ed., p. 871). Philadelphia: F.A. Davis.

Stepping reflex. Dillon, P. (2007). *Nursing health assessment: A critical thinking, case studies approach* (2nd ed., p. 870). Philadelphia: F.A. Davis.

Tonic neck or fencing reflex. Dillon, P. (2007). *Nursing health assessment: A critical thinking, case studies approach* (2nd ed., p. 868). Philadelphia: F.A. Davis.

Glabellar reflex. Dillon, P. (2007). *Nursing health assessment: A critical thinking, case studies approach* (2nd ed., p. 872). Philadelphia: F.A. Davis.

Babinski reflex. Dillon, P. (2007). *Nursing health assessment: A critical thinking, case studies approach* (2nd ed., p. 872). Philadelphia: F.A. Davis.

Moro reflex. Dillon, P. (2007). *Nursing health assessment: A critical thinking, case studies approach* (2nd ed., p. 868). Philadelphia: F.A. Davis.

Magnet reflex. Dillon, P. (2007). *Nursing health assessment: A critical thinking, case studies approach* (2nd ed., p. 873). Philadelphia: F.A. Davis.

Galant reflex. Dillon, P. (2007). *Nursing health assessment: A critical thinking, case studies approach* (2nd ed., p. 873). Philadelphia: F.A. Davis.

Crawling reflex. Dillon, P. (2007). *Nursing health assessment: A critical thinking, case studies approach* (2nd ed., p. 872). Philadelphia: F.A. Davis.

Crossed extension. Dillon, P. (2007). *Nursing health assessment: A critical thinking, case studies approach* (2nd ed., p. 872). Philadelphia: F.A. Davis.

Chapter 16

Figure 16-1 Stevens, B., Johnston, C., Petryshen, P., & Taddio, A. (1996). Premature infant pain profile: Development and initial validation. *Clinical Journal of Pain, 12*(1), 13–22.

Chapter 18

Figure 18-1 Dillon, P. (2007). *Nursing health assessment: A critical thinking, case studies approach* (2nd ed., p. 856). Philadelphia: F.A. Davis.

Figure 18-6B *Wong's essentials of pediatric nursing* (6th ed). St. Louis: Mosby. Copyright by Mosby, Inc. Reprinted with permission.

Figure 18-7 Wilkinson, J.M., & Van Leuven, K. (2007). *Fundamentals of nursing: Theory, concepts & application,* Vol. 2 (p. 254). Philadelphia: F.A. Davis.

Chapter 21

Heimlich maneuver, chest thrusts. Hopkins, T., & Myers, E. (2007). *Medical surgical notes* (2nd ed., p. 168). Philadelphia: F.A. Davis.

Heimlich maneuver, back blows. Hopkins, T., & Myers, E. (2007). *Medical surgical notes* (2nd ed., p. 168). Philadelphia: F.A. Davis.

Chapter 26

Figure 26-1 Teasdale, G., & Jennettt, B. (1974). Assessment of coma and impaired consciousness. A practical scale. *The Lancet, 13*,2(7872), 81–84.

Chapter 27

Figure 27-2 Dillon, P. (2007). *Nursing health assessment: A critical thinking, case studies approach* (2nd ed., p. 708). Philadelphia: F.A. Davis.

Assessment Tools: Transverse break. Williams, L., & Hopper, P. (2007). *Understanding medical surgical nursing* (3rd ed., p. 995). Philadelphia: F.A. Davis.

Assessment Tools: Spiral break. Williams, L., & Hopper, P. (2007). *Understanding medical surgical nursing* (3rd ed., p. 995). Philadelphia: F.A. Davis.

Assessment Tools: Oblique break. Williams, L., & Hopper, P. (2007). *Understanding medical surgical nursing* (3rd ed., p. 995). Philadelphia: F.A. Davis.

Assessment Tools: Greenstick break. Williams, L., & Hopper, P. (2007). *Understanding medical surgical nursing* (3rd ed., p. 995). Philadelphia: F.A. Davis.

Assessment Tools: Comminuted break. Williams, L., & Hopper, P. (2007). *Understanding medical surgical nursing* (3rd ed., p. 995). Philadelphia: F.A. Davis.

Chapter 28

Figure 28-1 Venes, D. (2005). *Taber's cyclopedic medical dictionary* (20th ed., p. 1931). Philadelphia: F.A. Davis.

Figure 28-2 Dillon, P. (2007). *Nursing health assessment: A critical thinking, case studies approach* (2nd ed., p. 239). Philadelphia: F.A. Davis.

Macules. Dillon, P. (2007). *Nursing health assessment: A critical thinking, case studies approach* (2nd ed., p. 231). Philadelphia: F.A. Davis.

Papule. Dillon, P. (2007). *Nursing health assessment: A critical thinking, case studies approach* (2nd ed., p. 233). Philadelphia: F.A. Davis.

Patches. Dillon, P. (2007). *Nursing health assessment: A critical thinking, case studies approach* (2nd ed., p. 233). Philadelphia: F.A. Davis.

Tumor. Dillon, P. (2007). *Nursing health assessment: A critical thinking, case studies approach* (2nd ed., p. 234). Philadelphia: F.A. Davis.

Vesicles. Courtesy of Centers for Disease Control and Prevention.

Pustules. Courtesy of Centers for Disease Control and Prevention.

Bullae. Courtesy of Centers for Disease Control and Prevention.

Wheals. Courtesy of Centers for Disease Control and Prevention.

Crust. Courtesy of Centers for Disease Control and Prevention.

Scales. Courtesy of Centers for Disease Control and Prevention.

Licherification. Courtesy of Centers for Disease Control and Prevention.

Keloids. Dillon, P. (2007). *Nursing health assessment: A critical thinking, case studies approach* (2nd ed., p. 237). Philadelphia: F.A. Davis.

Fissure. Dillon, P. (2007). *Nursing health assessment: A critical thinking, case studies approach* (2nd ed., p. 238). Philadelphia: F.A. Davis.

Ulcer. Dillon, P. (2007). *Nursing health assessment: A critical thinking, case studies approach* (2nd ed., p. 238). Philadelphia: F.A. Davis.

Index

Note: Page numbers followed by f refer to figures.

Psychopathology, developmental, 381
Psychosis, postpartal, 223, 240–241
Ptyalism, 52
  in pregnancy, 86
Puberty, 17, 18
  ethnocultural considerations in, 316
Pubic hair, 341
Pudendal nerve block, 169
Puerperium. *See* Postpartum period
  (puerperium)
Pulmonary artery, 464, 464f
Pulmonary atresia, 466, 467f
Pulmonary function testing
  in children, 401–402
  peak flow meter for, 410–412
Pulmonary vein, 464, 464f
Pulmonic stenosis, 466
Pulmonic valve stenosis, 466, 467f
Pulses
  in musculoskeletal injury, 527
  neonatal, 269, 270
  pediatric, 337
Pushing, in labor, 156
Pustule, 548
Pyelogram, intravenous, 422
Pyelonephritis, 574
Pyloric stenosis, hypertrophic,
  420–421, 425–426
Pyridoxine, in pregnancy-related
  nausea and vomiting, 108
Pyruvate kinase deficiency, 264

Q
Quickening, 64

R
Rabies, 438
RADAR, for intimate partner violence
  screening, 66
Radiation, heat, 255, 569
Radiation therapy, 644, 667
  teratogenicity of, 46
Radiography, 533
Radiology, in preterm infant, 302
Radionuclide scan, 422
Rage reduction therapy, 386
Rebirth therapy, 386
Rebound tenderness, 417
Red blood cells
  neonatal, 262
  pediatric, 619, 620
  preterm infant, 302
  urinary, 588, 590

Red reflex, 283, 351
Referred pain, 162
Reflex(es)
  Babinski, 278, 315
    in children, 342–343
  corneal, 350, 505
  crawling, 279
  crossed extension, 280
  extrusion, 277
  fencing, 278
  Galant, 279
  glabellar, 278
  grasping, 315
  magnet, 279
  Moro, 279, 315
  neonatal, 277–280
  palmar grasp, 277, 315
  plantar grasp, 277, 315
  in preeclampsia, 199
  in pregnancy, 104, 104f
  red, 283, 351
  rooting, 277, 315
  stepping, 278
  sucking, 277, 315
  toe grasp, 277
  tonic neck, 278
  trunk incurvation, 279
Reflexology, in pregnancy, 84
Regression, 672, 680
Relaxation exercise, in pregnancy, 84
Relaxin, in pregnancy, 53
Renal failure, in children, 456
Renal tubular function, 589
Reproductive health history, 26
Reproductive system
  in chronic renal failure, 579
  female, 18–23, 19f, 20f
    drug effects on, 34–36
    external structures of, 18–19, 19f
    focused assessment of, 18
    health history for, 26
    internal structures of, 19–20, 19f,
      20f
    menstrual cycle and, 21–23, 22f, 23f
  male, 23–24, 24f
Residual volume, 402
Resiliency, in children, 362
Respiration
  Cheyne-Stokes, 675
  heat loss with, 569
  pediatric, 347–348
Respiratory distress
  neonatal, 282
  pediatric, 337

Welcome
to the rewarding world of maternity and pediatric nursing!

Master all of the need-to-know information!

A thematic organization reflects the state-of-the-art in nursing today.
- Holistic Care
- Critical Thinking
- Validating Practice
- Tools of Care

Understand how to apply it in clinical!

A unique emphasis supports care in traditional and community settings.
- Optimizing Outcomes
- Research
- Evidence-based Practice
- Compassionate Care

Use the wealth of resources to make learning and studying easier!
- A feature-rich textbook
- BONUS! An interactive Electronic Study Guide on CD-ROM
- BONUS! Web-based tools on *DavisPlus*
- More!

From *class* to *clinical* through

Holistic Care

Nursing Insight Boxes—Step into a variety of nursing roles with helpful hints from experienced nurses that show you how to apply what you're learning.

What to Say Boxes—Learn what to say to your patients and how to ask questions in all types of situations.

An Inspirational Quotation or Story

Collaboration in Caring

Ethnocultural Considerations

Complementary and Alternative Care Modalities

Across Care Settings

Nursing Insight— *Gastroesophageal reflux*

Frequent use of an infant seat for positioning should be avoided as it reduces truncal tone in infants and increases intraabdominal pressure, which can promote reflux. (Potts, 2002)

"What to say" — *When planning the adolescent mother's hospital discharge*

The adolescent mother has unique needs for discharge planning. The nurse can best explore the young patient's immediate plans for herself and the baby by initiating dialog in a supportive, nonthreatening environment. Examples of appropriate questions that the nurse may ask include the following:

"Do you have someone available to offer you help and/or support?"

"Do you feel a sense of closeness or attachment to your baby?"

"After you leave the hospital, will anyone be helping you to care for your baby?"

"Will anyone be taking care of the baby so that you can go back to school?"

"Where will you take the baby for follow-up care?"

Family Teaching Guidelines— Helping Older Siblings Adjust to the New Baby

Nurses can be instrumental in arming parents with strategies to help their children accept and adjust to a new infant. The following tips may be useful:

- Talk with the child(ren) about their feelings regarding the new baby. Listen and validate their feelings.
- Teach the older sibling how to play with the new baby; encourage gentleness.
- Help develop the child's self-esteem by giving him/her special jobs, for example, bringing the diaper when you are changing the baby. Praise each contribution.
- Praise age-appropriate behaviors and do not criticize regressive behaviors.
- Set aside a special time each day for the older child for you to be alone with him/her, remind the child that he/she is loved very much.

TOPIC: Warning signs indicative of poor sibling adjustment

Professional help may be needed when the child:

- Continually avoids or ignores the baby
- Shows the baby no affection
- Is consistently angry, taunting or demonstrating aggressive behavior towards the baby or other family members
- Experiences nightmares and sleeping difficulties

Adapted from International Childbirth Education Association (ICEA), 2003. *Siblings and the new baby.*

Family Teaching Guidelines—Review what and how to teach family members to care for themselves and their families.

Nursing Care Plans—Study the care plans to learn how to apply the chapter content to clinical practice and develop care plans for your own patients.

Nursing Care Plan Acute Pain/Discomfort in the Postpartal Patient

Nursing Diagnosis: Acute Pain related to tissue damage secondary to childbirth

Measurable Short-Term Goal: The patient will report decreased pain to a level that is acceptable to her.

Measurable Long-Term Goal: The patient will report minimal or no pain upon discharge from hospitalization.

NOC Outcomes:
Pain Level (2102) Severity of observed or reported pain
Pain control (1605) Personal actions to control pain

NIC Interventions:
Pain Management (1400)
Analgesic Administration (2210)
Heat/Cold Application (1380)

Nursing Interventions:

1. Perform routine, comprehensive pain assessments to include: onset, location, intensity, quality, characteristics, and aggravating and alleviating factors of the discomfort. Note verbal and nonverbal indications of discomfort.

    RATIONALE: Routine, comprehensive pain assessments enable the nurse to provide interventions in a timely manner to enhance effectiveness of medications and ensures early identification of complications resulting in painful stimuli.

2. Ask the patient to rate her pain on a standard 0 to 10 pain scale before and after interventions and to identify her own acceptable comfort level on the scale.

    RATIONALE: Use of a consistent pain scale provides objective measurement of the patient's perception of pain, the effectiveness of interventions, and the acceptable comfort level for the individual.

3. Identify cultural or personal beliefs about the experience of pain and the use of pain interventions, including prescribed medications.

    RATIONALE: Expression of pain and use pain relief interventions may vary according to culture and personal beliefs. Patients may prefer a stoic response to pain or fear becoming addicted to narcotics.

4. Pr... ...al, no... ...ntal information regarding pain interventions that are availabl... ...

NCLEX to *practice...*

  Critical Thinking

Case Studies—Apply your knowledge to actual practice situations.

Clinical Alerts—Recognize the emergent or critical situations you'll encounter in practice.

Critical Nursing Actions—See how to apply important clinical concepts to real-life situations.

NCLEX-Style Review Questions—Answer the end-of-chapter review questions to make sure you understand what you've just read.

Concept Maps—Study the visual summaries of the most important concepts presented in the chapter. Great for review, too.

Validating Practice

Optimizing Outcomes—See how to establish the course of action that achieves the best possible outcomes for your patients.

Moving Toward Evidence-Based Practice Boxes—Read about the current research relevant to the topic under discussion and answer the critical thinking questions to see how this research affects practice.

Where Research and Practice Meet—Understand the 'big picture' through the link between research and practice.

Be Sure To...—Be aware of the importance of legal issues and liabilities and be able to quickly analyze potential problems.

Now You Can!—Make sure you comprehend and can apply the material as you progress through each chapter.

Optimizing Outcomes— Assessing for milk let-down

The nurse assesses for cues that indicate that the milk let-down reflex has occurred:

- The mother reports a tingling sensation in the nipples (not always present).
- The infant's quick, shallow sucking pattern transitions to a slower, more drawing pattern.
- The infant exhibits audible swallowing.
- The mother reports uterine cramping; increased lochia may be present.
- The mother states she feels extremely relaxed during the feeding.
- The oppos

moving toward evidence-based practice — Probiotic Use in Antibiotic-Associated Diarrhea Prevention

Johnston, B.C., Supina, A.L., & Vohra, S. (2006). Probiotics for pediatric antibiotic-associated diarrhea: A meta-analysis of randomized placebo-controlled trials. *CMAJ, 175*(4), 1–14.

The purpose of this study was to assess the efficacy of probiotics in the prevention of antibiotic-associated diarrhea in children. Adverse events associated with coadministration of probiotics and antibiotics were also explored. The incidence of antibiotic-associated diarrhea in children who received broad-spectrum antibiotics was reported as 11% to 62%. A systematic review of probiotic trials was completed. The analysis included six pediatric trials with a total of 707 patients. A significant reduction in the incidence of antibiotic-associated diarrhea in children was reported in all studies. Four of the six studies reported use of *Lactobacillus GG, L. sporogenes,* or *Saccharomyces boulardii* and showed evidence of preventive effects with no reported adverse

events. None of the studies provided a definition for adverse events although four reported minor events to include rash, gas, vomiting, increased phlegm, and chest pain. Overall findings indicated that the treatment of six patients should prevent one case of diarrhea.

1. Based on the findings from this study, are probiotics effective in the treatment and prevention of antibiotic associated diarrhea?
2. How is this information useful to clinical nursing practice?

Suggested Response
the Electronic Study

where research and practice meet: Crohn's disease

Research exploring the use of an enteric-coated fish oil preparation in adult Crohn's disease patients found that those who received the fish-oil preparation were less likely to have relapses than patients who received placebos. Fish oil has been found to not only have ...atory actions but also to increase the absorption of ...resulting in improved nutrition (Hockenberry & Wilson

...care includes the administration of medication and nutri-...agement, emotional support, and community referral ...). The focus of care during periods of remission involves ...compliance. As symptoms resolve, the child may resist ...ications. The adolescent with Crohn's disease presents ...enges in the treatment of his or her disease. Adolescents ...ral desire to be "normal" and to be like their peers. This ...e adolescent to resist taking prescribed medications that ...us side effects, such as those experienced with pro-...of steroids.

Be sure to— Obtain consent for genetic testing

In the case of genetic testing of children the risks and benefits of testing should be discussed with the child as appropriate for their level of development. Most testing requires only a blood sample with little physical risk, although there can be psychological risks to the child that include decreased self-worth anxiety, and disruption of family bonds (Chasson, Gutt, & Ihlenfeld, 2002). The best interest of the child should be the primary consideration when genetic testing is ordered with counseling provided before the testing. Where possible both parents and the child should provide info...

Now Can You— Promote self-care for the puerperium?

1. Outline postpartal teaching guidelines that include information about self- assessment of the fundus, lochia, hygiene, incisional site, body temperature, and elimination?
2. Demonstrate appropriate exercises for the postpartal patient?
3. Identify at least six symptoms indicative of poor emotional adjustment that, if present for more than 2 weeks, should be reported to the healthcare provider?

Tools for Care

Procedure Boxes—Follow the step-by-step instructions for performing common procedures and review the documentation examples.

A & P Review

Labs Boxes

Medication Boxes

Assessment Tools

Diagnostic Tools

Procedure 25-1 Collecting Stool for Culture and Sensitivity and Ova and Parasites

Purpose
Collecting stool for culture and sensitivity and ova and parasites is used to detect the presence of bacterial overgrowth; to confirm bacterial gastroenteritis; and to assess sensitivity of specific antimicrobials.

Equipment
- Gloves
- Patient identification label
- Sterile culture tube and cotton swab to collect specimen
- Biohazard container

Steps
1. Don gloves.
   RATIONALE: *Prevents the spread of bacteria.*
2. Using the sterile cotton swab collect (scrape) a fresh, warm specimen of stool from the diaper or stool receptacle and place it into the sterile culture tube.
3. Label both the sterile culture tube and the biohazard bag with the patient's identification information.
   RATIONALE: *Accurate labeling is essential for correct patient identification.*
4. Place the sterile culture tube into the biohazard bag
   RATIONALE: *To ensure that the properly identified specimen is safely transported to the laboratory.*
5. Deliver the fresh specimen of stool to the laboratory promptly after collection.
   ...f the specimen may

Clinical Alert
- Avoid external contamination of stool and deliver to laboratory promptly.
- Provide samples from several areas of the stool to ensure that organisms are isolated. Failure to do so may yield a false-negative result.
- Inform the lab of antimicrobial or antiamebic therapy within 10 days as it may yield false-negative results.
- Medications such as antacids, antibiotics, antidiarrheals, iron, and castor oil may interfere with analysis

Teach Parents
Teach the parents that a stool for culture and sensitivity is used to detect the presence of bacterial overgrowth; confirm bacterial gastroenteritis; and to assess sensitivity of specific antimicrobials.

Teach parents that a stool for ova and parasites (O & P is used to aid in diagnosis of parasites or their eggs).

Documentation
10/12/10 0900 Stool for culture and sensitivity and ova and parasites collected from the diaper, labeled, placed in biohazard bag and sent to laboratory via laboratory collection personnel.

N. Kramer, RN

Source: Schnell, Van Leeuwen, & Kranpitz (2003).

The ideal companions to the text!

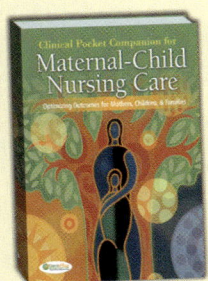

Clinical Pocket Companion for Maternal-Child Nursing

Susan L. Ward, PhD, RN
Shelton M. Hisley, PhD, RNC, WHNP

This handy pocket reference helps you provide safe, effective, and compassionate care in clinical. Full-color images of nursing skills and procedures as well as tools and charts make bedside reference quick and easy.

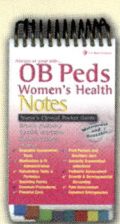

Holloway, Moredich & Aduddell
OB Peds Women's Health Notes Nurse's Clinical Pocket Guide

This handy, spiral-bound reference puts the key clinical information you need to care for obstetric, gynecologic, and pediatric client in your pocket. Organized for fast access, its waterproof, reusable pages wipe clean with alcohol.

Deglin • Vallerand
Davis's Drug Guide for Nurses, 11th Edition

This **Drug Guide** has it all! The Resource Kit CD-ROM includes FREE PDA access to 400 complete drug monographs and DrugGuide.com will keep you current throughout the year with monthly updates. Plus, only in **Davis's Drug Guide** will you find unique coverage of maternity and pediatrics.

Resources for students online at Davis*Plus*.
Visit www.fadavis.com

The perfect review books!

Davis's SUCCESS SERIES

Course review now. NCLEX®-prep later.

✓ Thousands of questions, most at application and analysis levels. (Alternate format, too!)
✓ Comprehensive rationales for correct and incorrect answers.
✓ Test-taking tips for most questions.

DeSevo
Maternity/Newborn Success
A Course Review Applying Critical Thinking to Test Taking

Richardson
Pediatric Success
A Course Review Applying Critical Thinking to Test Taking

Taber's brings meanings to life!

NEW Edition!
Taber's Cyclopedic Medical Dictionary, 21st Edition

Bring meanings to life! With over 60,000 terms, 1,100 images (300 on the bonus DVD,) and so much more!

Visit www.fadavis.com for a complete description of all that's new, including information on one free year of **Taber's Online** powered by Unbound Medicine® and one free year of **Taber's Mobile** powered by Skyscape®.

NEW Edition!

Van Leeuwen • Poelhuis-Leth
Davis's Comprehensive Handbook of Laboratory and Diagnostic Tests with Nursing Implications, 3rd Edition

This easy-to-read, nursing-focused reference provides you with all of the information you need to know before, during, and after each test. Plus, it delivers more maternity and pediatric information throughout each **monograph,** and the online **Student Workbook.**

Resources for students online at Davis*Plus*.
Visit www.fadavis.com

Superb tools make *learning* and *studying* easier!

Maternal-Child Nursing Care

Optimizing Outcomes for Mothers, Children, and Families

Susan L. Ward, PhD, RN

Professor of Nursing
Nebraska Methodist College
Omaha, Nebraska

Shelton M. Hisley, PhD, RNC, WHNP-BC

Assistant Professor of Nursing (Retired)
University of North Carolina at Wilmington
Wilmington, North Carolina

F.A. Davis Company · Philadelphia

F.A. Davis Company
1915 Arch Street
Philadelphia, PA 19103
www.fadavis.com

Printed in the United States of America

Last digit indicates print number: 10 9 8 7 6 5 4

Publisher, Nursing: Lisa Deitch
Developmental Editor: Shirley Kuhn
Content Development Manager: Darlene Pedersen
Senior Project Editor: Padraic Maroney
Manager of Art and Design: Carolyn O'Brien
Cover Illustration: Jose Ortega

As new scientific information becomes available through basic and clinical research, recommended treatments and drug therapies undergo changes. The author(s) and publisher have done everything possible to make this book accurate, up to date, and in accord with accepted standards at the time of publication. The author(s), editors, and publisher are not responsible for errors or omissions or for consequences from application of the book, and make no warranty, expressed or implied, in regard to the contents of the book. Any practice described in this book should be applied by the reader in accordance with professional standards of care used in regard to the unique circumstances that may apply in each situation. The reader is advised always to check product information (package inserts) for changes and new information regarding dose and contraindications before administering any drug. Caution is especially urged when using new or infrequently ordered drugs.

Library of Congress Cataloging-in-Publication Data

Ward, Susan L.
Maternal-child nursing care: optimizing outcomes for mothers, children, and families / Susan L. Ward, Shelton M. Hisley.
    p. ; cm.
    Includes bibliographical references and index.
    ISBN-13: 978-0-8036-2813-7 (alk. paper)
    ISBN-10: 0-8036-2813-7 (alk. paper)
1.   Maternity nursing--Textbooks. I. Hisley, Shelton M. II. Title.
    [DNLM: 1.   Maternal-Child Nursing--methods. 2.   Cultural Diversity. 3.   Evidence-Based Nursing--methods. 4.   Holistic Nursing--methods. WY 157.3 W263m 2009]
RG951.W37 2009
618.2'0231--dc22   2008051815

In loving memory of my mother, Betty A. Tighe, who always said "it's possible".
With great love and appreciation to my family, particularly to my intelligent
children Kathleen, Frank, and William.
To my co-author, Shelton Hisley, who has amazing fortitude. To faculty,
administration, and staff at Nebraska Methodist College.
To the skilled and caring nurses at Children's Memorial and Methodist Hospitals.
To my dear friend, Jeanne Snowden.

Susan Ward

To my husband, Jack, whose love and encouragement, especially during the dark
days of my cancer diagnosis and treatment, kept me aloft and convinced that I could
achieve this goal.
To my parents, Barbara and Hubert McLendon, for a lifetime of love and support.
Also to Susan, my co-author and friend, for whom I hold the greatest admiration
and respect.

Shelton Hisley

Maternal–Child Nursing Care: Optimizing Outcomes for Mothers, Children, and Families springs from our passionate commitment to providing the best nursing care possible to mothers and children and our desire to inspire others to make that same commitment. In this all-inclusive source, we provide students with current, comprehensive information about maternal–child nursing in creative, dynamic ways and in a concise, accessible format. Building upon theoretical foundations in basic nursing care, communication skills, and principles of health promotion, the text challenges students to optimize outcomes for their maternal and pediatric patients using critical thinking as they care for them in the hospital and community environments. We focus on aesthetics, cultural sensitivity, and a caring approach. The textbook also serves as an excellent resource for practicing nurses who work with women, children, and families in a variety of settings. We believe that combining essential information about the two specialties into a single textbook supports good educational practice while being economically practical.

Philosophy

The primary objective of this textbook is to identify the myriad of options for holistic, evidence-based practice in maternal and child nursing care in this new millennium, based on a philosophy of physiological and developmental normalcy and stressing safety and optimization of outcomes for mother and child. In addition to comprehensive coverage of maternal and child nursing care in traditional settings, essential elements for providing cost-effective, high-quality, innovative nursing care in community settings are presented. Discussion of health care delivery in community settings is crucial in contemporary nursing education and reflects the present trend for women, families, and children to obtain health care in the diverse settings in which they live, grow, play, work, or go to school.

This book is built upon a framework that views the delivery of nursing care as a continuum spanning the traditional hospital in-patient environment to the community setting. Students are presented with information essential to providing appropriate, culturally sensitive nursing care to women, families, and children. A variety of creative learning aids are used to assist students in subject mastery and prompt the delivery of care that appropriately addresses contemporary needs while incorporating innovative approaches that integrate provider–patient partnerships and alliances with coalitions that serve women, families, and children across the lifespan. Because the traditional hospital experience constitutes an important component of nursing education, content on hospital-based nursing care for women, families, and children examines acute, traumatic, chronic, and terminal conditions. Likewise, content that addresses community-based nursing care for women, families, and children explores strategies and resources for the provision of appropriate care in many different outpatient settings. With this text, students learn that community-based care can take place in a variety of ways at any time and in any place. It is our hope that the users of this textbook will acquire the essential knowledge for professional nursing practice in the specialties of maternal and child nursing and that they will gain insights about providing nursing care in a myriad of settings and with diverse populations.

Organization

Each chapter opens with a culturally or spiritually oriented story, literary piece, caring element, or quotation that creatively expresses various dimensions of aesthetics in nursing. Because contemporary nursing is a dynamic profession with a rich past, present, and future, we emphasize and promote the importance of innovative, state-of-the art technology balanced with compassionate, humanistic care. "Learning Targets" offer a guided approach to chapter content and provide a gauge for assessing outcomes.

Chapter introductions provide a preview of content and assist students in identifying essential information and major concepts. Key words appear in boldface print accompanied by brief definitions in the text and are grouped in the glossary for easy, quick reference on the Electronic Study Guide. Color illustrations and photos provide visual cues to enhance understanding. These features facilitate students' learning and promote an understanding of the relationship between classroom or textbook information and the delivery of nursing care in the clinical setting.

A short review of anatomy, physiology, and pathophysiology is provided in applicable chapters to foster understanding of new applications of concepts previously learned. Eye-catching display boxes draw students' attention to essential information about medications, critical nursing actions, nursing procedures, related research studies, assessment tools, diagnostic modalities, safety issues, therapeutic communication strategies, and family teaching guidelines.

Each chapter concludes with a concept map that visually summarizes the relationships among the most important concepts presented. The map reinforces students' learning, promotes mastery of information, and assists students in critical analysis. It is a useful tool for confirming that students have identified the essential chapter elements and for applying classroom information to the clinical setting.

A number of strategies designed to prompt and enhance critical thinking weave through the text. Case studies, nursing care plans, NCLEX-style review questions, and exercises in clinical decision-making assist students in mastering content and in integrating new information. These creative learning activities help students to assimilate and internalize information as they build upon previously learned nursing knowledge and prepare to apply newly introduced concepts in various maternal–child clinical practice areas.

Themes and Key Features

The overarching theme of this comprehensive maternal–child resource focuses on how to provide contemporary nursing care to women, families, and children in the community as well as in the traditional hospital setting. In service to that goal are the broad themes of holistic care, critical thinking, validating practice, and tools for care. We use the following key features throughout the chapters to creatively illustrate and emphasize information essential for the delivery of safe, effective nursing care to diverse populations across care settings, thus ensuring an educational experience rich with critical thinking activities and clinical application opportunities.

HOLISTIC CARE

- Each chapter begins with a culturally or spiritually oriented story, literary piece, caring element or quotation that creatively expresses aesthetics in nursing.
- "Nursing Insight" boxes show students how experienced nurses use their five senses to gain a deeper understanding about the clinical situation or the patient's condition.
- "Collaboration in Caring" provides guidelines for working with other health care professionals to care for patients and families in in-patient and community-based environments.
- "Ethnocultural Considerations" emphasize cultural humility in both the hospital and community settings.
- "What to Say" helps students develop and enhance their communication skills by providing verbatim examples or helpful hints.
- Nursing Care Plans incorporating NANDA, NOC, and NIC terminology relate classroom and textbook knowledge to clinical practice, while evidence-based rationales for interventions show how research supports practice.
- "Complementary Care" shows students the wide range of complementary options available for integration with conventional approaches to provide safe, timely, and compassionate care.
- "Across Care Settings" foster students' responsiveness to trends in health care by highlighting holistic health care in acute care and community-based settings in which children and families live, grow, play, work, or go to school. Sensitivity to diverse patient populations is also underscored.
- "Family Teaching Guidelines" help students teach families essential components about caring for themselves and their children and are offered both in English (in the text and on the Electronic Study Guide) and Spanish (on the Electronic Study Guide).

CRITICAL THINKING

- "Learning Targets" offer a guided approach to chapter content and provide a gauge for assessing outcomes.
- Key words appear in boldface type accompanied by brief definitions. Key words are also stored in the glossary for easy, quick reference on the Electronic Study Guide and DavisPlus.
- "Case Studies" facilitate students' practice in the assimilation of content from various chapters into actual patient situations. As students work through the various case studies, they are challenged to apply critical thinking and practice clinical decision-making.
- Nursing Diagnoses foster the development of new nursing knowledge where diagnoses are developed based on information obtained during a nursing assessment. A standardized statement about the health of a patient is created for the purpose of providing nursing care. The nursing diagnoses portray patients' responses to their condition where the nurse can address the problems independently.
- "Clinical Alerts" help students recognize emergent or critical situations and relate classroom or textbook information as they deliver safe, effective nursing care in the hospital and community-based environments.
- "Critical Nursing Actions" prompt students to assimilate and internalize information as they prepare to apply important concepts in the clinical area.
- NCLEX-style review questions located at the end of each chapter prompt and enhance critical thinking and help to prepare students for licensure examination.
- Concept Maps visually summarize the relationships among the most important concepts presented in every chapter. The concept map can be used by students to think critically, to review, and to more clearly see the application of classroom information to the clinical setting.

VALIDATING PRACTICE

- "Moving Toward Evidence-Based Practice" highlights current relevant research and encourages students to incorporate evidence-based findings into their everyday practice.
- "Optimizing Outcomes" enhance critical thinking skills for clinical application and help establish the best possible outcomes and how to obtain them.
- "Where Research and Practice Meet" focus on investigative initiatives that may impact practice in the future, underscoring the value of clinical inquiry in ensuring positive outcomes for patients and their families.
- "Be Sure To…" alert new nurses to important legal issues that impact the clinical environment and help them recognize how to critically analyze potentially litigious situations.
- "Now Can You?" prepares students to assimilate and internalize information presented throughout the chapter and serve as a mini check to ensure mastery of material before proceeding to the next section.
- "Summary Points" bring together the information students should be most careful to comprehend from the chapter.
- References provide current citations that validate practice and support the chapter content.

TOOLS FOR CARE

- "A & P Review" of chapter-specific anatomy, physiology, and pathophysiology foster understanding of new applications of previously learned concepts.
- "Labs" boxes present crucial information about laboratory testing and its relationship to the patient's overall health status.

- Procedures provide step-by-step instructions for performing common procedures in maternal–child nursing and the rationales for why things are done a particular way. Each procedure includes an example of documentation to emphasize the critical nature of proper, accurate documentation.
- "Medication" boxes present crucial information about commonly prescribed medications and help students in their care of mothers, children, and families.
- "Assessment Tools" facilitate understanding of clinical evaluation and help students make the connection between classroom or textbook knowledge and the clinical setting.
- "Diagnostic Tools" present crucial information about common diagnostic measures and their relationship to various disease entities.

Teaching Ancillaries and Other Related Products

INSTRUCTOR'S RESOURCE DISK

The components on the Instructor's Resource Disk seamlessly guide faculty through the content and offer innovative strategies for creatively supplementing the text. This complete and easy-to-use collection of teaching aids for maternal–child content includes the following components.

Instructor's Guide

The course syllabus includes a proposed class schedule for a traditional 15-week semester and for an accelerated 8-week semester along with reading assignments and testing content. The syllabi provide a guide for using the text in the most efficient way.

"Teaching Plans" provide a user-friendly lesson plan for each chapter whether teaching in separate or combined courses. The Teaching Plans integrate teaching tips, PowerPoint presentations, and suggested students assignments.

"Tips for Teaching a Combined Maternal–Child Course" offer suggestions about how to effectively teach these two specialties in one course.

Case Studies

The case studies provided to the instructor are more extensive and detailed than those provided in the text or on the Electronic Study Guide so they can be used for testing as well as post-conference discussions. Answers to the case studies are provided to promote and enhance critical thinking skills and facilitate the application of theoretical concepts into the clinical setting.

Concept Maps

Concept maps are constructed to underscore the relationships among the essential concepts in each chapter. They prompt critical thinking and may be used as a guide for students assigned to create additional maps about other important theoretical elements.

Electronic Test Bank

The electronic test bank is a collection of NCLEX-style questions and rationales to enable students to identify areas of strength and weakness and prepare for course tests and the national licensure examination.

PowerPoint Presentations

A collection of slides is provided that form the basis for a lecture for each chapter, which can be modified based on the instructor's preferences.

Media Ancillary

Electronic files of the images from the text are included for use in the classroom, as are audio selections of heart sounds.

ELECTRONIC STUDY GUIDE

A complimentary electronic study guide is included with the text. This is intended to assist and enhance students' learning and offers creative ways to supplement and reinforce the textbook information. It contains the following:

Interactive Exercises

These provide a creative and enjoyable way to enhance students' learning and include:

- Don't Tip the Scale
- Quiz Show
- Critical Thinking
- Drag and Drop Bucket
- Fill-in-the-Blank Clue

Case Studies

Thirty-one relevant case studies from selected chapters facilitate students' practice in the assimilation of content from various chapters into actual patient situations.

Nursing Care Plans

All care plans from the textbook are provided and are printable. There are also twelve expanded care plans that are not included in the text (six for Obstetrics and six for Pediatrics) to provide in-depth information and guidance for planning and providing care to maternity and pediatric patients with commonly encountered normal and pathological conditions.

Family Teaching Guidelines

English and Spanish versions of the Family Teaching Guidelines from the text, as well as additional ones unique to the Electronic Study Guide, can be personalized and printed and used in actual patient care situations.

NCLEX-style Review Questions

A collection of NCLEX-style questions and rationales can help students identify areas of strength and weakness, and prepare for course tests and the national licensure examination.

Sound Collection

Heart sounds depicting various normal and abnormal heart sounds are included to help students recognize when there is a problem.

Podcasts

Podcasts directs students to key chapter concepts and reinforces essential information.

Concept Maps

For students' convenience, all concept maps from the text are included on the Electronic Study Guide.

Clinical Pathways

Clinical pathways display patient goals and corresponding sequence nursing actions to achieve those goals.

DavisPlus Website

In addition to all the Web-suitable content from the Instructor's Resource Disk and the Electronic Study Guide (instructor materials are password protected; students' materials are not), the Web site contains Internet links related to specific content areas presented throughout the book; links to useful Web sites, links to the F.A. Davis Web site and product page, and bonus material, including interactive exercises for pediatric dosage calculations.

CLINICAL POCKET COMPANION TO MATERNAL–CHILD NURSING

The separate, for-sale *Clinical Pocket Companion* contains critical information to facilitate the delivery of safe, effective, compassionate care in maternity and pediatric clinical settings. Information is extracted from the core text and is presented in easy-to-access formats. In addition to nursing skills and procedures, nursing tools and charts, and color illustrations from the parent text, each chapter in the *Clinical Pocket Companion* covers:

- Key Terms
- Focused Assessments
- Clinical Alerts
- Diagnostic Tests
- Medications
- Ethnocultural Considerations
- Teaching the Family
- Additional Information for the Clinical Setting
- Resources

Thank you for choosing *Maternal–Child Nursing Care: Optimizing Outcomes for Mothers, Children, and Families.* It is our sincere hope that this textbook and ancillary package will provide you with the tools needed to convey the essentials of care for the childbearing/child-rearing family.

We believe that providers of contemporary nursing education are challenged to present timely, evidence-based information grounded in a framework of holistic, compassionate care. We appreciate that you will bring your own unique approach as you guide students toward providing competent, sensitive care for mothers, children, and families. We share your passion for maternal–child nursing and hope that this learning package may be instrumental in sparking this same passion in others.

Susan L. Ward

Shelton M. Hisley

Acknowledgments

Dedicated Participants

It has taken a village of professionals to bring this project to fruition, and we thank the editors and production staff of the F.A. Davis Company for their expertise and guidance, especially:

- Lisa Deitch, Publisher, Nursing
- Shirley Kuhn, Special Projects Editor
- Darlene Pedersen, Director of Content Development
- Padraic Maroney, Senior Project Editor
- Doris Wray, Executive Editorial Coordinator
- Sam Rondinelli, Assistant Director of Production
- David Orzechowski, Managing Editor
- Julia Reukauf, Marketing Specialist

We are indebted to the following for helping us shoot and collect the photographs used in the text:

Billings Photography, Omaha, Nebraska
Children's Memorial Hospital, Omaha, Nebraska
Methodist Health System, Birth Services, Omaha, Nebraska
Nebraska Methodist College, Omaha, Nebraska
Betsy Toole Media Production Services, St. Luke's Hospital & Health Network, Bethlehem, Pennsylvania
Miami Children's Hospital, The Mary Ann Knight International Institute of Pediatrics, Founded as Variety Children's Hospital, Miami, Florida
Chandra Vig, Ann Harms, and Susan Ward's nursing students, family members, and friends

Many thanks to the following people who helped us supply sketches for the professional illustrator to create many of the line drawings in the text: John C. Hisley, MD, William R. Ward, and Matthew T. Blaszko.

Many colleagues and friends assisted the chapter contributors through mentoring, editing and offering content expertise. A special thank you goes to the following individuals:

Tem Adair, BS (and other Methodist College Library Staff)
Rita Atwell, MS, CRNP
Joanna E. Cain, BSN, RN
Kathy Cassandra, RN, MS
Megan Connelly, MSN, APRN, CCRN, CPNP-AC
Carolyn Gilmore, BSN
Kayli A. Hall, BS, MEd
Christine A. Hamilton, DHSc, RRT, AE-C
Patricia Harris, MS, CRNP-PMH
Sue Hinds, RN, MSN, CPN
Nancy Koster, MS, APN
Melissa Lanza, RN, MS, APRN-BC
Kerry Lazewski, MS, PNP
Casey O'Brien, BSN
Barbara Paliughi, RN, BSN
Ellen Reyerson, MS, NP
Judith Rocchiccioli, PhD, RN
Sherrie Rodgers, MS, PNP
Kathleen A. Ward, BA, JD
Frankie J. Ward, BA, MSc
Cathy Webb, RN, MA
Joyce Weisshar, MS, CNS
Renee Zubay Fife, RN, MSN

Contributors

Sharon Akes-Caves, RN, MS, MSN
Corporate Nursing Education Program and Interim ADN
    Program Director
Prima Medical Institute
Mesa, Arizona
    Chapter 1

Jan Andrews, RNC, PhD, WHNP
Professor and Associate Dean of Nursing and Health
    Sciences
Macon State College
Macon, Georgia
    Chapter 6

Kimberly Attwood, PhD(c), MSN, CRNP, APRN, BC, NP-C
Assistant Professor of Nursing
DeSales University
Center Valley, Pennsylvania
    Chapter 15

Deborah Bambini, PhD, WHNP-BC, CNE
Assistant Professor
Grand Valley State University
Grand Rapids, Michigan
    Clinical Pocket Companion

Sharon Bator, RN, MSN, PNP, CPE, PhD Student
Assistant Professor of Nursing
Southern University School of Nursing
Baton Rouge, Louisiana
    Chapter 32

Bridget Bailey, RN, MSN
Associate Professor
Iowa Lakes Community College
Emmetsburg, Iowa
    Chapter 22

Diane M. Bligh, MS, RN
Associate Professor, Nursing
Front Range Community College
Westminster, Colorado
    Concept Maps in all Chapters and Ancillaries

Michelle Lynn Burke, MSN, ARNP, CPN, CPON
Clinical Specialist
Department of Hematology Oncology
Miami Children's Hospital
Miami, Florida
    Chapter 33

Irma Bustamante-Gavino, PhD, RN
Associate Professor
The Aga Khan University School of Nursing
Karachi, Pakistan
    Chapter 24

Marsha Cannon, MSN, RN
Associate Professor
University of West Alabama

Livingston, Alabama
    Chapter 29

Patricia M. Connors, RNC, MS, WHNP
Perinatal Clinical Nurse Specialist
Massachusetts General Hospital
Boston, Massachusetts
    Chapter 11

Sherrill Anne Conroy, D Phil, Med, BN, RN
Assistant Professor
University of Alberta
Edmonton, Alberta, Canada
    Chapter 21

Janine L. Dailey, RN, MSN
Instructor
Nebraska Methodist College
Omaha, Nebraska
    Clinical Pathways in Ancillaries

Wendy A. Darby, PhD, CRNP
Associate Professor, Family Nurse Practitioner
University of North Alabama
Florence, Alabama
    Case Studies for Pediatric Chapters in Ancillaries

Michele D'Arcy-Evans, CNM, PhD
Professor
Lewis-Clark State College
Lewiston, Idaho
    Chapter 9

Jacqueline Maria Dias, RN, RM, MEd
Assistant Professor
The Aga Khan University School of Nursing
Karachi, Pakistan
    Chapter 24

Elizabeth Fahrenholtz, APRN, MSN
Assistant Professor
Creighton University
Hastings, Nebraska
    Chapter 5

Brian G. Fonnesbeck, RN, BSN, MN
Associate Professor
Lewis-Clark State College
Lewiston, Idaho
    Chapter 3

Marcia L. Gasper, EdD, RNC
Associate Professor of Nursing
East Stroudsburg University
East Stroudsburg, Pennsylvania
    Interactive Exercises

Maryann Godshall, MSN, CPN
Assistant Professor of Nursing
DeSales University

Center Valley, Pennsylvania
Chapters 31, 34 and 35

Jacqueline L. Gonzalez, ARNP, MSN, FAAN, CNAA-BC
Senior Vice President/Chief Nursing Officer
Miami Children's Hospital
Miami, Florida
Chapter 22

Linda Nicholson Grinstead, PhD, RN, CPN, CNE
Professor
Grand Valley State University
Grand Rapids, Michigan
Clinical Pocket Companion

Ann M. Harms, RN, MSN, CS
Assistant Professor
Creighton University School of Nursing
Hastings-Mary Lanning Campus
Hastings, Nebraska
Chapters 20 and 23

Dawn Hawthorne, MSN, RN, CCRN, IBCLC
Family Educator and Lactation Consultant
Joe DiMaggio Children's Hospital at Memorial
   Hospital
Hollywood, Florida
Chapter 15

Mary A. Helming, PhD, APRN, FNP-BC, AHN-BC
Associate Professor of Nursing and FNP Track
   Coordinator
Quinnipiac University
Hamden, Connecticut
Chapter 32

Shelton M. Hisley, PhD, RNC, WHNP-BC
Assistant Professor of Nursing (Retired)
University of North Carolina at Wilmington
Wilmington, North Carolina
Chapter 18

Jodi L. Jenson, RN, MSN
Assistant Professor
Nebraska Methodist College
Omaha, Nebraska
PowerPoints for Pediatric Chapters in Ancillaries

Helen W. Jones, RN, APN, C., PhD
Chairperson of Health Science Education
Raritan Valley Community College
Somerville, New Jersey
PowerPoints for Maternity Chapters in Ancillaries

Marcia Jones, RN, N.D.
Assistant Professor of Nursing
Bronx Community College
Bronx, New York
*Case Studies and Family Teaching Guidelines for Maternity
   Chapters in Ancillaries*

Esperanza Villanueva Joyce, EdD, CNS, RN
Associate Dean for Academics
University of Texas at El Paso
El Paso, Texas
Spanish Translations of Family Teaching Guidelines

Kathy Jo Bertelsen Keever, RNC, CNM, MS
Associate Professor of Nursing
Women's Health
Anne Arundel Community College
Arnold, Maryland
Chapter 8

Patricia A. Kiladis, MS, RN
Director of Undergraduate Nursing Program
Northeastern University
Boston, Massachusetts
Chapter 14

Cynthia Kildare, RN, MSN, APRN-CNS
Nurse Specialist
University of Nebraska Medical Center, College of
   Nursing
Lincoln, Nebraska
Chapter 31

Nancy Kramer, EdD, CPNP, CNE, ARNP
Associate Dean, Head of the Division of Nursing, Professor
Allen College
Waterloo, Iowa
*Chapter 25, Evidence-Based Practice Features for all
   Chapters, and Family Teaching Guidelines for Pediatric
   Chapters in Ancillaries*

Marilee LeBon, BA
Developmental Editor/Writer
Mountaintop, Pennsylvania
NCLEX-style Questions for Pediatrics in Ancillaries

Karla Luxner, DNP, RNC
Assistant Professor of Nursing
Milikin University
Decatur, Illinois
Nursing Care Plans in all Chapters and Ancillaries

Judith M. Marshall, MS, APRN
Family Nurse Practitioner
Children's Memorial Hospital
Chicago, Illinois
Chapter 27

Betsy B. McCune, MSN, RNC
OB Clinical Nurse Specialist
Borgess Medical Center
Kalamazoo, Michigan
Chapter16

Karen McQueen, RN, MA(N), PhD
Assistant Professor
Lakehead University School of Nursing
Thunder Bay, Ontario, Canada
Chapter 12

Deborah Naccarini, RN, MSN
Assistant Professor Nursing
Carroll Community College
Westminster, Maryland
Chapter 21

Margaret A. O'Connor, RN, MS
Assistant Clinical Professor
Lawrence Memorial/Regis College Nursing Program
Medford, Massachusetts
Chapter 30

Nicole K. Olshanski, MSN, RN
Instructor of Nursing
University of Pittsburgh School of Nursing
Pittsburgh, Pennsylvania
  Chapter 13

Helen Papas-Kavalis, RNC, MA Nursing
Bronx Community College
Bronx, New York
  *NCLEX-style Questions as Review Questions in
    Pediatric Chapters*

Karen Joy Poole, RN, BScN, ME, MA
Director and Associate Professor
Lakehead University
Thunder Bay, Ontario, Canada
  Chapter 12

Karen L. Pulcher, MSN, BSN, ARNP, BC
Assistant Professor of Nursing
University of Central Missouri
Lee's Summit, Missouri
  Chapter 29

Fatima Ramos-Marcuse, PhD, APRN, BC
Adjunct Assistant Professor and Psychotherapist
University of Maryland School of Nursing
Baltimore, Maryland
  Chapter 23

Nancy Redfern-Vance, PhD, MN, CNM
Associate Professor
Valdosta State University
Valdosta, Georgia
  Chapter 2

Sarah Roland
Associate Degree Nursing Instructor
Central Carolina Technical College
Sumter, South Carolina
  Teaching Plans for Pediatric Chapters in Ancillaries

Maria A. Rosen, RN, PNP, PhD
Program Director
Becker College
Worcester, Massachusetts
  Chapter 21

Melodie Rowbotham, PhD, RN
Assistant Professor
Southern Illinois University School of Nursing
Edwardsville, Illinois
  Teaching Plans for Maternity Chapters in Ancillaries

Deborah Salani, ARNP, MSN, CPON
Director of the Emergency Department
Miami Children's Hospital
Miami, Florida
  Chapter 33

Jacoline Sommer, RN, RM, BScN
Senior Instructor
The Aga Khan University School of Nursing
Karachi, Pakistan
  Chapter 24

Deborah Stiffler, PhD, RN, CNM
Assistant Professor
Coordinator, Women's Health Nurse Practitioner Major
Indiana University School of Nursing
Indianapolis, Indiana
  Chapter 10

Angela S. Taylor, PhD, RN, BC
Director of Nursing Program and Associate Professor
Department of Nursing, School of Health Sciences and
    Human Performance
Lynchburg College
Lynchburg, Virginia
  Chapters 4 and 10

Dawn Michele Teeple, RN, BSN, MS, CCE
Assistant Professor
Anne Arundel Community College
Arnold, Maryland
  Chapter 17

Joan Nalani Thompson, NNP, MSN, RNC
Assistant Professor
University of Hawaii at Hilo
Hilo, Hawaii
  Chapter 7

Wendy Thomson, EdD(c), MSN, BSBA, RN, IBCLC
Assistant Professor and Technology Coordinator
Nursing Department
Nova Southeastern University
Fort Lauderdale, Florida
  Chapter 15

Kelly Tobar, RN, EdD
Associate Professor
California State University Sacramento
Sacramento, California
  Chapter 26

Chandra Vig, BSN
Curriculum Developer
Bow Valley College
Calgary, Alberta, Canada
  Chapter 20

Susan L. Ward, PhD, RN
Professor of Nursing
Nebraska Methodist College
Omaha, Nebraska
  Chapter 18

Nancy Watts, RN, MN, PNC (C)
Clinical Nurse Specialist
London Health Sciences Centre
London, Ontario, Canada
  *Maternity NCLEX-style Questions for Text, Electronic
    Study Guide, and Instructors Materials*

Ruth A. Wittmann-Price, D.N.Sc., RN, CNS, CNE
Assistant Professor
Drexel University College of Nursing and Health
    Professions
Philadelphia, Pennsylvania
  Chapter 19

Roseann Mary Zahara-Such, APRN, BC, MSN, CCNS
Assistant Clinical Professor of Nursing
Purdue University
Hammond, Indiana
    Chapter 28

Kelly K. Zinn, MSN, RN
Assistant Professor
Nebraska Methodist College
Omaha, Nebraska
    Coordinator for certain Ancillary Components

Reviewers

Marie Adorno, APRNC, MN
Assistant Professor of Nursing
Our Lady of Holy Cross College
New Orleans, Louisiana

Rebecca L. Alleen, RN, MNA
Assistant Professor
Clarkson College
Omaha, Nebraska

Anita Dupre Althans, RNC, BSN, MSN
Assistant Professor of Nursing
Our Lady of Holy Cross College
New Orleans, Louisiana

Elaine Andolina, BS, MS
Director of Admissions, School of
    Nursing
University of Rochester
Rochester, New York

Bridget Bailey, RN, MSN
Nursing Instructor
Iowa Lakes Community College
Emmetsburg, Iowa

Margaret Batson, RN, MSN
Nursing Instructor
San Joaquin Delta College
Stockton, California

Samantha H. Bishop, MN, RN, CPNP
Assistant Professor of Nursing
Gordon College
Barnesville, Georgia

Linda Boostrom, RN, MSN
Instructor of Nursing Program
Henderson Community College
Henderson, Kentucky

Susan J. Brillhart, MSN, APRN, BC, PNP
Assistant Professor of Nursing
Borough of Manhattan Community
    College
New York, New York

Linda A. Browne, MSN, RN
Program Director/Instructor
Southwest Georgia Technical College
Thomasville, Georgia

Tammy Bryant, RN, BSN
Program Director
Southwest Georgia Technical College
Thomasville, Georgia

Gloria Haile Coats, RN, MSN
Professor of Nursing
Modesto Junior College
Modesto, California

Jami-Sue Coleman, MS, RN
Nursing Instructor
Western Nevada Community College
Carson City, Nevada

Meghan Connelly, MSN, APRN,
CCRN, CPNP-AC
CNS/NP
Children's Hospital
Omaha, Nebraska

Susan Craig, RN, MSN
Faculty
Butte Community College
Oroville, California

Robin Culbertson, RN, MSN, EdS
Nursing Instructor
Okaloosa Applied Technology Center
Fort Walton Beach, Florida

Lori DuCharme, RN, BSN, MS
Nursing Faculty
Front Range Community College
Westminster, Colorado

Susan Ellison, MSN, RNC
Senior Instructor
The Charles E. Gregory School of
    Nursing
Perth Amboy, New Jersey

Marie Esch-Radtke, MN, RN
Nursing Faculty
Highline Community College
Des Moines, Washington

Polly D. Fehler, RN, BSN, MSN
Instructor of Nursing
Tri-County Technical College
Pendleton, South Carolina

Denise M. Fitzpatrick, RNC, MSN
Instructor/Course Coordinator
Dixon School of Nursing
Willow Grove, Pennsylvania

L. Sue Gabriel, MSN, MFS, RN, SANE
Assistant Professor
Bryan LGH College of Health Sciences
Lincoln, Nebraska

Marilyn Johnessee Greer, RN, MS
Associate Professor of Nursing
Rockford College
Rockford, Illinois

Kristin J. Hanak, MS, RN, PNP
Nursing Faculty
Front Range Community College
Westminster, Colorado

Donna Healy, MS, RN
Associate Professor of Nursing
Adirondack Community College
Queensbury, New York

Debra L. Hyde, RN, MSN, CNS
Faculty
Aultman College of Nursing and
    Health Sciences
Canton, Ohio

Paula Karnick, PhD, ANP-C, CPNP
Associate Professor
North Park University
Chicago, Illinois

Mary Beth Kempf, BSN, RNC, MSN, OB
Associate Degree Nursing Instructor
Northeast Wisconsin Technical
    College
Green Bay, Wisconsin

Cynthia A. Kildare, RN, MSN,
APRN-BC
Assistant Professor
Bryan LGH College of Health
    Sciences
Lincoln, Nebraska

Karen M. Knowles, RN, MS
Faculty/Specialty Chairperson
Crouse Hospital School of Nursing
Syracuse, New York

Kathleen Nadler Krov, RN, CNM,
MSN, FACCE
Assistant Professor
Raritan Valley Community College
Somerville, New Jersey

Barbara Leser, PhD, RN, RM
Doctor
Northwest Nazarene University
Nampa, Idaho

Randee L. Masciola, RN, MS, CNP
Clinical Instructor and Women's
    Health Nurse Practitioner
Ohio State University
Columbus, Ohio

Kathleen Matta, MSN, CNS, IBCLC
Visiting Faculty
University of New Mexico
Albuquerque, New Mexico

Sheila Matye, MSN, RNC
Adjunct Assistant Professor
Montana State University
Great Falls, Montana

Trilla Mays, RN, MSN
Nursing Instructor
Midlands Technical College
Columbia, South Carolina

Barbara McClaskey, PhD, MN,
RNC, ARNP
Professor, Department of Nursing
Pittsburg State University
Pittsburg, Kansas

Michelle Michitsch, RN, MS, CPNP-PC
Adjunct Nursing Professor
Borough of Manhattan Community
    College
New York, New York

Nancy Miller, MSN, RNC, CCM
Nursing Professor
Keiser University
Fort Lauderdale, Florida

Georgia Moore, PhD, MSNed, RN-BC
Consultant/Online educator
Louisville, Kentucky

Julie Moore, RNC, MSN, MPH, WHNP
Associate Professor of Nursing
Hawaii Community College
Hilo, Hawaii

Cindy Morgan, CNM
Instructor
University of Tennessee at
    Chattanooga
Chattanooga, Tennessee

Deborah Naccarini, RN, MSN, FNP
Assistant Professor
Carroll Community College
Westminster, Maryland

Debbie Ocedek, RN, BSN, MSN
Professor of Nursing
Mott Community College
Flint, Michigan

Donna Paulsen, RN, MSN
Nursing Faculty
North Carolina Agricultural and
    Technical State University
Greensboro, North Carolina

Melissa A. Popovich, RN, MSN
Clinical Faculty
Ohio State College of Nursing
Columbus, Ohio

Karen L. Pulcher, ARNP/CPNP,
MSN, RN
Assistant Professor in Nursing
University of Central Missouri
Lee's Summit, Missouri

Jacquelyn Reid, MSN, EdD, CNM, CNE
Associate Professor
Indiana University Southeast
New Albany, Indiana

Jean Rodgers, RN, BSN, MN
Nursing Faculty
Hesston College
Hesston, Kansas

Kathryn Rudd, RNC, MSN
Clinical Educator
MetroHealth Medical Center
Cleveland, Ohio

Christine L. Sayre, MSN, RN
Auxiliary Faculty
Ohio State University
Columbus, Ohio

Gwenneth C. Simmonds, PhDc, CNM,
MSN, RN
Clinical Instructor
Ohio State University
Columbus, Ohio

Lisa H. Simmons, RN, MSN
Instructor and Coordinator Child
    Health Nursing
University of South Carolina Aiken
Aiken, South Carolina

Cordia A. Starling, BSN, MS, EdD
Division Chair of Nursing
Dalton State University
Dalton, Georgia

Nora F. Steele, DNS, RNC, PNP
Professor
Charity/Delgado Community College
New Orleans, Louisiana

Suzan Stewart, RN, BS
Lab Coordinator
Community College of Denver
Denver, Colorado

Deborah Terrell, RN, MSN, APN, DNSc
Associate Professor
Harry S. Truman College
Chicago, Illinois

Barbara Tewell, RNC, BSN
Perinatal Staff Nurse
Naval Medical Center
San Diego, California

Donna J. Gryctz Thomas, RN,
BSN, MSN
Assistant Professor of Nursing
Kent State University
New Philadelphia, Ohio

Joan Thompson, NNP, MSN, RNC
Assistant Professor
University of Hawaii at Hilo
Hilo, Hawaii

Pat Twedt, RN, MS, Med, MS
Associate Professor of Nursing
Dakota Wesleyan University
Mitchell, South Dakota

Becky C. Vicknair, RNBS, APRN,
MSN, PNP
Pediatric Instructor
Delgado/Charity School of Nursing
New Orleans, Louisiana

Sherry Warner, RN
Nursing Instructor
Fulton-Montgomery Community
    College
Johnstown, New York

Maribeth Wilson, MSN, MSPH
Nursing Faculty
Keiser University
Tallahassee, Florida

Jennifer J. Woods, RN, MSN
Instructor
Delgado/Charity School of Nursing
New Orleans, Louisiana

Detailed Table of Contents

unit three
The Prenatal Journey   191

chapter 8

Physiological and Psychosocial Changes During Pregnancy   193

chapter 7

Conception and Development of the Embryo and Fetus   164

chapter 9

The Prenatal Assessment   215

chapter 10

Promoting a Healthy Pregnancy   256

chapter 11

Caring for the Woman Experiencing Complications During Pregnancy   291

unit four
The Birth Experience   353

chapter 12
The Process of Labor and Birth   355

unit five
Care of the New Family   467

chapter 15

Caring for the Postpartal Woman and Her Family   469

chapter 16

Caring for the Woman Experiencing Complications During the Postpartal Period   511

chapter 17

Physiological Transition of the Newborn   541

chapter 18

Caring for the Normal Newborn   563

chapter 19

Caring for the Newborn at Risk   603

unit six
Caring for the Child and Family 639

chapter 20
Caring for the Developing Child 641

chapter 21
Caring for the Child in the Hospital and in the Community 664

chapter 32

Caring for the Child with a Renal, Urinary Tract, or Reproductive Condition   1033

chapter 33

Caring for the Child with a Hematological Condition   1071

chapter 34

Caring for the Child with Cancer   1104

Special Features

Case Studies

Clinical Alerts

Collaboration in Caring

Complementary Care

Diagnostic Tools

Ethnocultural Considerations

Family Teaching Guidelines

Labs

Medications

Moving Toward Evidence-Based Practice

Now Can You

Nursing Care Plans

Nursing Diagnoses

Nursing Insights

Optimizing Outcomes

Procedures

What to Say

Where Research and Practice Meet

one
two
three
four
five
six
seven

Foundations in Maternal, Family, and Child Care

Traditional and Community Nursing Care for Women, Families, and Children

As a Family-Centered Nurse

Learn of the essence of family-centered nursing,
while you walk with a worried family
until you wear side-by-side paths in the carpet;
Suffer the emotions of a troubled family
When they soar in their hope for healing and recovery;
Stay through the darkest hour of a mother, father, sister or brother,
as they silently cry for a member's pain;
Experience the failure, disappointment and challenges
presented with each health care encounter;
Never cease to be amazed at the resilience
of a family's strength, spirit and protective value.

—S. Caves

LEARNING TARGETS *At the completion of this chapter, the student will be able to:*

◆ Explore the impacts of ethnocentrism, ethnopluralism, paternalism, the medical model, and consumerism on nursing.

◆ Compare the roles of nurses, families, and patients in various health care settings.

◆ Discuss theories of caring and holism as they apply to the nursing care of women, families, and children.

◆ Clarify nursing responsibilities using NANDA, NIC, and NOC taxonomy related to diagnosis, management, and outcome evaluation of family-centered medical and nursing problems.

◆ Summarize the importance of cultural competency in fulfilling the role of nurse teacher.

◆ Evaluate the nurse's role in promoting self-healing.

◆ Discuss how responsibility and professional accountability are enhanced by evidence-based knowledge.

◆ Contrast the focus of the advanced practice nurse with that of the professional registered nurse.

---

 moving toward evidence-based practice Concept Maps and Learning-Style Preference

Kostovich, C.T., Poradzisz, M., Wood, K., & O'Brien, K.L. (2007). Learning style preference and student aptitude for concept maps. *Journal of Nursing Education, 46*(5), 225–231.

The purpose of this study was to describe the relationship between nursing students' learning-style preferences and aptitude for concept mapping. A correlational, descriptive study conducted at a private Midwestern university included 120 students enrolled in an adult medical–nursing course taken in the junior year. The students completed the Kolb's Learning Style Survey (LSS) and a Concept May Survey, instruments developed by the researchers. The LSS consists of several phases and is designed to determine preference for learning experiences, i.e., concrete, active experimentation, abstract conceptualization,

continued

and reflective observation. The Concept Map Survey consisted of nine open-ended questions related to preference for creating concept maps.

The students were also given a concept map assignment, which included both written and verbal instructions since the majority of the students had not created a concept map before this class. Concept maps were graded using a rubric. As the course was co-taught, each faculty member corrected one half of the concept maps using the same criteria. The interrater reliability was reported as moderately low. Final course grades and concept map grades correlated weakly ($R = 0.37$, $p < 0.01$). A one-way analysis of variance (ANOVA) was performed to assess the influence of learning preference on concept map grades. The researchers reported that although "students in the abstract conceptualization group had higher mean concept map grades than did students with other learning preferences, the difference was not significantly higher." Students were also asked whether they preferred concept maps or case studies as a learning tool. The researchers reported that nearly twice as many students in the abstract learning preference group preferred the use of concept maps. The researchers concluded that learning style preference does not impact students' abilities to use concept maps as a learning tool, and hence they can be used for all learning style categories.

1. Based on the information provided in the synopsis of this study, do you believe that sufficient evidence exists to require students to use strategies that are not consistent with their learning style preference in order to develop a range of problem-solving skills?
2. How is this information useful to clinical nursing practice?

See Suggested Responses for Moving Toward Evidence-Based Practice on the Electronic Study Guide or DavisPlus.

Introduction

Most nurses and students have personal understandings of what it means to be a nurse caring for women, families, and children—the field of family and child nursing. They may have even developed a broad range of strategies, knowledge, values, and competencies to use when caring for women, families, and children. Nurses conversely may approach family and child nursing no differently than they would if providing care for any other patient. Realizing how the nurse, the patient, other health care providers, and outside forces of influence have framed family and child nursing through the last century provides the nurse with insights into the level and outcome of care historically and currently received and given to families and children.

There is a fairly consistent view of how family and child patients are defined, from one of three family and children perspectives: as an individual affected by some health event; the family unit involved in that event; and the whole of supporting mind-body-spirit, culture, and community affected by the experience (Harmon Hanson, Gedaly-Duff, & Kaakinen, 2005). Nurses as well as families are being challenged by ever-increasing numbers of health care and societal changes to adapt and expand these perspectives on family and child health.

The traditional hospital that served as the center of care for families and children has been replaced by a myriad of community-based settings. With this change in setting, often the thrust of power has shifted from the traditional nursing and medical models to one of family-centered decision making.

Becoming a part of this care experience, engaging in the patient's lived experience throughout its entirety instead of functioning as a part of the process by doing "for" the patient, is one of the emerging roles for the family and child nurse. Using this engaging transpersonal approach to understanding the experience of the patient's entire mind-body-and-soul during times of health threats may offer one of the most fulfilling roles for the nurse, and one of the first experiences of empowered caring for the patient. This return to the development of a therapeutic nurse–patient relationship through communication and the artistry of nursing provides the nurse the opportunity to experience the ultimate caring component of nursing for which the profession is known.

This chapter begins with an historical overview of nursing, family and child health care, and the influences that have shaped and driven some of the changes toward a more contemporary approach to family and child nursing. It discusses the many professional roles of the family and child nurse, how they have changed over time, and where the future will take them, irrespective of the type of care setting. The focus of the chapter is on the art of caring and its centrality to the family and child nurse experience.

Traditional Nursing Care

Taking a look at the traditional role of nursing in the care of families and children helps identify the significance of both positive and unfavorable changes that have occurred during the past century and framed current standards of care.

HISTORICAL PERSPECTIVE

Physicians, the general public, and the nursing profession historically viewed health as the absence of disease and the presence of optimal functioning. Illness was seen as pathological and something of which the health care provider worked to rid, heal, or cure the patient. This curative approach commonly was referred to as the **medical model**. It often entailed a paternalistic, one-way channel of communication between the powerfully dominant and more knowledgeable health care provider and the submissive and uneducated patient or family. The power base for all decisions rested with the medical or, infrequently, the nurse provider who together often took an objective, detached biomedical approach (Gordon & Nelson, 2005).

Over the previous quarter century, a number of influences have affected how family and child health and nursing care are now defined in the 21st century (Fig. 1-1). The infusion of multiple cultures and beliefs about health care systems, along with exponential growth in scientific and technological capabilities, have been major forces in shaping the structure and delivery of nursing care. In addition, increased consumer access to health-related information via the Internet, mass media, and other sources that may or may not be accurate, the unprecedented rise in health care costs, and increasing imposition of cumbersome regulations have also contributed to change.

🌀 **Now Can You—** **Discuss elements of contemporary nursing and health care for families and children?**

1. Identify a major force that accounts for the present-day shift toward family-centered decision making in health matters?
2. Describe a nursing approach that fosters empowered caring for the patient?
3. Name four factors that have shaped contemporary family and child health and nursing care?

The growth of **ethnopluralism** (diverse cultures) daily impacts health care systems and providers. Often each culture comes with its own beliefs, values, and practices about health and illness. The United States Department of Commerce, Bureau of the Census, projects that within the next 10 to 12 years, only one-half of the U.S. population will be of Euro-Caucasian descent, although the medical model formed and that continues to be supported is based on this group (U.S. Census Bureau, 2008). The population of other ethnicities and cultures will double and triple in that time, rapidly making up the other half of the U.S. population and bringing to the forefront their beliefs, values, and health practices.

During the past century the values, beliefs, and practices of the predominantly Euro-Caucasian male health care provider system drove health care decisions, interactions, and treatments based on the belief that these were unquestioningly in everyone's best interest and by far superior to all others: a belief referred to as **ethnocentrism** (Leininger & McFarland, 2002).

In a culture changing as rapidly as is that of the United States today, ethnocentrism can critically compromise effective health care. One of the predominant problems with a health care system founded on ethnocentrism, paternalism, and the medical model is the system's closed-mindedness and prejudice toward other solutions and viewpoints of health. It is this viewpoint that often alienates people in need of health care and deters them from seeking or accepting help.

HEALTH–WELLNESS CONTINUUM

For decades, the goal of nursing has been to move the patient toward well-being and away from disease and pathology. The aim of the nurse–patient relationship was to facilitate the attainment of that goal. The relationship process had a beginning (illness), middle (treatment), and end (wellness). This prominent emphasis on treating illness defined the scope of the nurse's practice, or the **nursing process:** assess for signs of illness, diagnose alterations in health, determine interventions to restore health, conceptualize a targeted health outcome moving away from illness, and evaluate the treatment plan for nurse-determined modifications (Fig. 1-2).

In nursing there has recently been a shift in this health–wellness continuum and process. The emphasis is changing from a linear beginning-to-end, illness-to-wellness process. No longer is the predominant nursing perspective to return the patient from illness (beginning) to a prior disease-free state (end) but toward a shared experience of transcending or controlling the health threat and changing it into one of purposeful meaning (LeVasseur, 2002). The nurse–patient relationship now is a circular or spiral process formed to motivate the patient or family toward promotion, maintenance, and restoration of health; health potential; prevention of illness; and self-care (Fig. 1-3).

✳️ *Ethnocultural Considerations—* **Perceptions of desired health and health outcomes**

Based on personal beliefs, values, and practices, an ever-increasing culturally diverse population has many differing definitions of health and the outcomes desired during health-seeking encounters.

Figure 1-1 Evolution of family and child health nursing model.

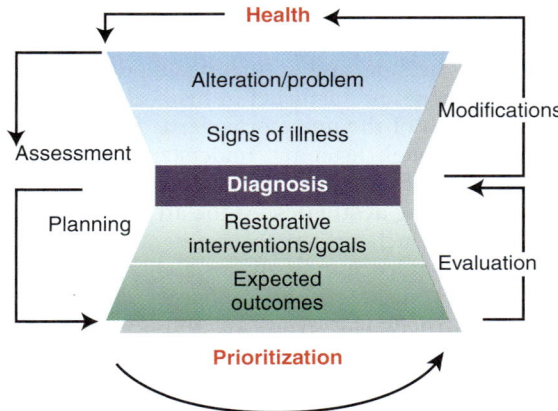

Figure 1-2 Traditional nursing process.

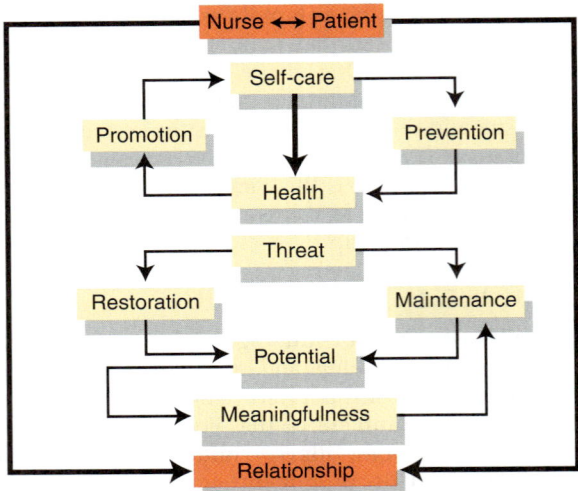

Figure 1-3 Health promotion nursing process.

Through health promotion, the nurse helps the woman, child, or family understand health risk factors and adopt lifestyle changes that foster health maintenance, prevent health threats through early detection and recognition, and explore options for health restoration.

 Across Care Settings: **Health protection for families**

With increasing international travel comes also the transport of illness vectors previously unknown in certain locales. Providing information about ways to protect children and families from these new sources of illness and injury through the use of individual instruction, educational videos, and use of the mass media can help the family maintain confidence in their ability to protect themselves from new threats.

This form of nursing entails a shared connectedness between patient and nurse. The goal is to experience the illness or health threat in the same way the patient perceives it. The nurse moves with the patient beyond the illness through the patient's own inner healing process to a patient-defined state of coping, harmony, wholeness **(holism)**, and unity with the illness and healing outcome; and hope, purpose, meaning **(spirituality)**, and health potential beyond the illness toward healing. The power base for this healing and future health decisions rests within the patient and his belief in his health potential.

The approach of the nurse provider is to form a caring relationship through listening, understanding, experiencing, presencing, facilitating, valuing, and using nursing aesthetics. **Nursing aesthetics,** or the art of nursing, is the low-tech, high-touch artistry of caring that strengthens the patient's confidence in her or his ability to manage the healing process, make change, or master the threatening health event (Stichler & Weiss, 2001). It is the way the nurse and patient help each other find meaning in the experience. It is a transformative, spiral process with a beginning (a threat), middle (relational building of trust and connection), and future (experiencing new possibilities for health change and outcomes) (Rhea, 2000).

Some nursing interventions that fall under this art of aesthetics include imagery, music therapy, and touch (Ward, 2002). Guiding the family or child's imagination **(guided imagery)** to visualize repeatedly a positive outcome has been demonstrated to enhance healthy outcomes. Music therapy helps bond the mind–body–spirit components of health and is especially successful with children. Touch and speech patterns of the nurse have descriptively been shown to soothe, calm, and encourage patients toward the health outcome of their choosing. One only needs to watch a caregiver stroke, rock, and sing to a sick child to know that this form of the nursing art works.

 Across Care Settings: **Teaching simple strategies for stress relief**

Most have heard of the beneficial effects of slow, deep, deliberate abdominal breathing patterns on the stress, anxiety, and pain associated with labor and birth. Nurses can teach these simple techniques to patients who anticipate stress, anxiety, or pain in any care setting.

 Ethnocultural Considerations— **Use of imagery, chanting, and afterlife encounters**

One often thinks of imagery as a collection of nurse-initiated instructions given to the patient. To the woman undergoing treatment for cancer, the nurse may suggest: "Imagine all of the cancer cells flowing up through your body, gathering all of the bad cells with them, and finally bursting into an explosion of color and sparkles like an explosion of fireworks from your body. Out into the atmosphere they go, floating higher and higher as they disintegrate into outer space." But, have nurses considered the healing power connected with objects used by some non-European Caucasian cultures? For example, the healing feather used by Native Americans, or the "seeing" of spirits practiced in Asian cultures, the casting of spells performed in the Caribbean Island culture, and the prayer beads used in Middle Eastern cultures. The healing effects of music and speech patterns have been well documented. But do health professionals consider of equal value the healing value of chanting by the Native American, or the wails of sorrow of the Central and Eastern European culture? One's awareness of various cultural practices is important. Even more important to their healing powers is the nurse's sensitivity and incorporation of them into a shared perspective of healing with the patient and family.

While the family or child relates stories of a lived experience, maintaining en-face eye contact, symbolically enfolding them through proximity, and staying focused solely on them acknowledges their worthiness. Imaginatively being in the patient's experience, reflectively sharing that experience through the use of body language, and avoiding demonstrations of disappointment and frustration gives the nurse a shared point of reference from which to help the family and child create meaning out of a threatening health experience (Fig. 1-4).

CHANGING DEMANDS AND DEMOGRAPHICS

This nursing approach of **engaging transpersonal care** has evolved from the simple nursing basics of providing treatment-driven, high-technology-centered care. It is an opportunity for the family–child nurse to utilize the nursing process in a new way. The nurse assesses the patient and family's confidence to address and manage the health threat, diagnoses the health alteration from the patient's viewpoint, conceptualizes the outcome as the patient and family envision it, and supports the patient in his or her chosen changes directed at restoring health or transcending the threat. Finally, the nurse evaluates the ongoing maintenance of health as it is lived by the patient and family.

Over the last half century, public trust in health care providers has continually declined. Some surveys have noted that the public trusts health care providers only slightly more than they do the Internal Revenue Service and the tobacco industry (Ford & Fottler, 2000). According to data from the National Coalition on Health Care (2006), much of this is likely due to health care providers' minimal awareness of consumer preferences and desire for personal control. Starting in the 1960s, health care seekers became increasingly critical of health care providers.

Family–child nursing responded to this call for consumer advocacy (consumerism) by supporting the consumer demand for a shift in the thrust of decision-making power. Other strategies included advocating for the provision of health care in facilities outside of the standard hospital setting (accessibility) and by providing family-centered approaches to care that emphasized health promotion and education. During the next half-century, other societal changes occurred that continued to alter health care delivery.

Figure 1-4 Nursing aesthetics that strengthen confidence in mastering a health threat.

 Across Care Settings: Family-centered care

The need for family members to feel significant and competent to care for their loved ones is universal, and should not be affected by the setting in which care is provided. Being friendly, encouraging family participation, and modeling of care are techniques that accomplish this goal in any setting.

Family structures (who the members are), functions (the roles members play), and definition of the family (a group of people sharing interpersonal bonds, tasks, and activities) have changed during the last half-century. Dyad families can comprise two cohabitating companions or spouses; traditional nuclear families of husband, wife, and children; extended multigenerational families; communal families of shared religious or social beliefs and values; blended families from separate prior marriages; families of same-sex unions; foster families; and adoptive families (see Chapter 3).

Social and technological advances of the past half-century have changed family structure, function, and definition. With the increasing acceptance and technologically available birth control options made available to families since the 1970s, family size has also changed. The sexual revolution of the 1960s resulted in an increase in the number of single-parent families. The feminist movement of the 1970s sent ever-growing numbers of mothers outside the home into a second work environment. As the workforce increased, industries flourished, cities grew, and families became more mobile in search of better lives for themselves, often leaving behind the extended multigenerational family they had learned to depend upon.

In the family's search for a better life, family health consciousness increased, as did usage of health care services and costs. The changes had implications for the way nursing delivered care and families sought it. Smaller families, single-parent families, families dispersed in search of better lives, and dual-income families meant fewer support persons present during family illnesses and crises. As a result, the role of the nurse inevitably changed from a focus on carrying out medical orders to a fuller scope of providing family support services.

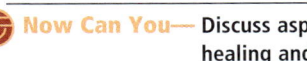 **Now Can You—** Discuss aspects of cultural practices for healing and comfort, transpersonal care, and components of the family unit?

1. Explain why nurses should develop awareness and understanding of cultural practices intended to foster comfort and promote healing?
2. Discuss a nursing approach that incorporates engaging transpersonal care?
3. Differentiate among family, family structures, and family functions?

PROFESSIONAL NURSING ROLES

Since the time of Florence Nightingale, nurses have played a role that involved clinical interventions, patient and family education, empathetic support, development of therapeutic relationships, and unique opportunities to make a difference in the lives of families during illness.

Nursing's domain in the earlier times consisted of being a provider of care and a teacher. As a provider of care, the nurse would change elements of the patient's environment through hygienic measures, nourishment, and comfort to enable the best opportunity for recovery. As a teacher, the nurse would prepare the patient for procedures, surgery, and the uncertainties of hospitalization.

Even in the 1860s, nurses saw their patient responsibilities not only for the individual for whom they ministered but also for the living conditions of the individual's family. The most frequent cause of illness and death during these years was infectious diseases. The nursing emphasis on sanitation, nutrition, and family education played a key role in the decline in deaths well into the 1950s when antibiotic drugs and scientific treatments became widely available.

Until the late 20th century, nurses continued to be seen as passive, deferential, and compliant advocates to paternalistic physicians. Nurses still practiced from the male dominated, ethnocentric, patriarchal medical model of the professional nurse. In 1963, the nursing process began to change that.

The **nursing process** was developed as a framework of systematic problem solving and actions to be used by nurses in identifying, preventing, or treating the individual health needs of patients. The nursing process was problem oriented, goal directed, and involved critical thinking and decision making. Clear differentiations were made between nursing and medical diagnoses, interventions, and outcomes. Ten years later, the North American Nursing Diagnosis Association (NANDA) developed a list of standardized nursing diagnoses used by the nurse through individualized patient care plans to express to other caregivers the findings of the nurse's assessment, diagnosis, and plans of action (Johnson et al., 2006). An example of the use of the NANDA-I Diagnosis to formulate a nursing care plan for a child with culturally different verbal communication is presented in Box 1-1.

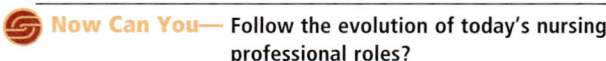 **Now Can You**— Follow the evolution of today's nursing professional roles?

1. Explain the central focus of the nurse as a provider of care and teacher before the 1950s?
2. Describe how the introduction of the nursing process as a systematic framework changed the nurse's professional role?

Contemporary Nursing Care

As families became more prosperous in the late 20th century, they also became more conscious of health promotion and advanced health technology. They demanded more knowledge about how to stay healthy, prevent common illnesses, and use technology to detect and treat early signs of health alterations. With this increased demand on the health care system came increasing costs. In response to increased health care costs, health care systems, and third-party payers focused on monitoring, controlling, and curtailing expenditures. As the costs for health care rose, the resultant changes impacted family and child health, and nursing's professional role.

Hospitals and third-party payers responded to increasing costs in a number of ways that included managed care systems and the development of alternative settings for health care delivery. In addition, greater emphasis was placed on patient and family accountability and responsibility for their own health promotion and disease prevention. This approach shifted the thrust of decision making power to the consumer. Other measures included a redefining of nursing functions, work loads, and methods for care delivery.

CURRENT HEALTH CARE SETTINGS

Cost containment, tightened reimbursement for services, and advanced technology have become important determinants of the current settings in which health care is received. Patients are being discharged earlier from acute care hospitals. Care is being provided in the home by family members using highly technical equipment. Many conditions that previously required acute care hospital stays are now being treated in ambulatory settings and the community-based health care service sector is almost limitless. Hospitals, homes, and community service centers have become interdependent providers in the ever-expanding health care arena.

Regional and specialized acute care hospitals for women, families, and children have undergone a multitude of changes since their inception in the late 1950s. Liberalized family, sibling, and children visiting; 24-hour family partnering with caregivers; policies; and procedures based on theories of child and family growth and development; and a heightened level of acuity in these acute care settings have had both beneficial and challenging effects on nurses, families, and children. A strong knowledge base in the care of families and children, highly developed critical thinking skills, expertise with advanced technology, and dedication to evidence-based practice are stringent requirements for nurses caring for families and children in all settings.

When referred to these modern, highly technologically advanced facilities, family members are often separated by great distances from children and other support persons. Emotions of separation, anxiety, abandonment, fear, and guilt compound already tenuous physical conditions. The accessibility to follow-up care in these comprehensive settings is frequently made difficult by time, distance, and coordination of return visits to multiple providers of segmented and specialized care.

Even with the heightened acuity of patients in acute and tertiary care hospitals, the length of stay in the settings continues to decrease. With these decreasing hospital stays, alternative settings were created for what once was considered "inpatient care."

At the other end of the health provider environment, from the specialized tertiary and acute care hospitals, are the acute care 24-hour observation unit, freestanding short stay, and urgent care centers. The facilities are less costly than acute care settings, in part because they minimize the high cost of advanced technology in specialized hospitals. These settings present their own challenges for the nurse, family, and patient. Assessment, risk identification, counseling, and teaching must all be accomplished

---

Box 1-1 Use of NANDA-I Diagnosis to Formulate a Nursing Care Plan

 Care Plan for the Patient with Culturally Different Verbal Communication

Patient and Family Data: Extended three-generational family comes to the health care provider with a complaint of weakness and loss of appetite in a 3-year-old family member. The family has arrived from a Middle Eastern country within the previous 2 weeks; they do not speak English and converse among themselves loudly and with much gesturing.

NANDA Nursing Diagnosis: Impaired Verbal Communication related to patient-care provider cultural and language difference

Measurable Short-term Goal: The family will have an opportunity through appropriate interpretation resources to share and interpret information regarding the well-being of the child.

Measurable Long-term Goal: The family will express concerns, needs, wants, ideas, questions, and understanding about immediate and long-term home care of the child.

NOC Outcome:
Communication (0902): Reception, interpretation, and expression of spoken, written, and nonverbal messages

NIC Interventions:
Active Listening (4920)
Culture Brokerage (7330)

Nursing Interventions:

1. Assess contributing cultural and language factors that may impede simple communication.

   RATIONALE: A shared understanding of culture and language is necessary for communication to take place.

2. Evaluate extent and level of impairment.

   RATIONALE: Misunderstandings of intent and content are heightened with increased levels of communication disparity.

3. Establish a therapeutic relationship by listening carefully.

   RATIONALE: Communication is enhanced when intent of trust and understanding is established.

4. Assist the family and patient to establish means of communication via an interpreter.

   RATIONALE: Law mandates that interpretation services be made available for accurate and precise basic understanding of medical terminology and care provided.

5. Validate the meaning of nonverbal and verbal communication.

   RATIONALE: Words and gestures can easily be misinterpreted, and affect the delivery and reception of important concepts.

Documentation Focus:

1. Assessment of pertinent patient physical, psychological, and cultural concerns

2. Description and meaning of nonverbal cues as related by interpreter

3. Type of interpreter services utilized

4. Teaching and explanations communicated

5. Level of outcome (NOC) completion/accomplishment

6. Discharge needs, referrals, and stated family/patient understanding

---

NIC = Nursing Interventions Classification; NOC = Nursing Outcomes Classification.
Adapted from Doenges, M.E., Moorhouse, M.F., Murr, A.C., & Murr, A.G. (2006). *Nursing care plans: Guidelines for individualizing client care across the life span.* Philadelphia: F.A. Davis.

---

in a crucially compressed time. The nurse in these settings may be responsible for direction of unlicensed assistive personnel who may not have the highly developed expertise needed to recognize subtle physiological changes in a patient's condition before discharge. Follow-up procedures that once were performed and monitored by nurses in the acute care setting now must be taught to the patient and family as they prepare for a rapid return to their home.

 Collaboration in Caring— *Preparing the family for community-based care*

The nurse can prepare the patient and family for care outside of the acute setting by:
- Discussing the feasibility of using specialized equipment in the home
- Encouraging the patient and family to investigate health insurance coverage for home care

- Suggesting the parents of a young patient contact school officials before a child returns after an illness
- Evaluating the family's transportation needs for follow-up care
- Discerning when an interaction in the acute care setting is conducive to teaching and learning

Since the early 1990s, there has been a dramatic increase in home- and community-based nursing care. Home- and community-based nursing care is provided in settings such as adult and child day-care centers; public and private schools; churches and religious body parishes; penal systems; health- and disease-related camps; foster homes and homeless shelters; physicians' offices; public health systems; and nurse-managed care centers (Fig. 1-5). Nurses in these settings often experience different degrees of professional independence and accountability, yet still need to possess expert skills as providers of clinical interventions, health history interviewers, culturally competent teachers, coordinators of extended care services, managers of allied health colleagues, supporters of family functionality, and advocates for family-centered care.

 Now Can You— Recognize the changes created by family-centered care for professional nursing in acute care settings?

1. List at least four characteristics of acute care hospitalization that have changed since the introduction of family-centered care?
2. Identify at least five community-based care settings in which the nurse may practice family-centered care?
3. Compare and contrast the role of the professional nurse in acute and specialized care hospitals and alternative care settings?

FAMILY-CENTERED CARE

Acute care providers have made strides toward keeping family members informed of hospital procedures and processes affecting their loved ones, and the patient outcomes expected. Acute care settings still, however, are major sources of family disruption during times of stress and illness. Placing family relationships, their coping mechanisms, values,

priorities, and perceptions at the center of a patient's health care needs is the essence of **family-centered care (FCC).**

Family-centered care requires sensitivity to the beliefs, values, and customs of each family member and those of their supporting culture or community. The role of the family-centered nurse is to facilitate and assist the family in making informed choices toward the outcome the patient and family desire. Family-centered care necessitates that the nurse relinquish an authoritarian role that tells the family what is best for them while the nurse does things to and for them. The nurse becomes a human just like all other members of the family, each with their special abilities to support the patient. The center of power shifts from the one with the most clinical knowledge to the whole of the group's knowledge.

This is a large shift for the nurse educated under traditional Euro-Caucasian theories of nursing care. The global nature of health care as a multiethnic (ethnopluralitic), multicultural composite of health-seeking people requires an ever-growing sensitivity on the part of the nurse. Consideration of the family's cultural influences allows the nurse to take a more in-depth approach to health assessment and outcome-directed interventions. For example, the proximity and quality of the family's support systems; religious and spiritual beliefs; customs and traditions, especially as they relate to health, illness, and healing; micro-living environment of the home; and macro-living environment of the neighborhood all must be incorporated into the plan of care. Other elements to be considered include financial resources, including willingness to ask for and accept additional resources; significant historical events, especially crises, losses, and new beginnings; and the members' communication patterns and verbal abilities, coping strategies, and problem-solving techniques.

One format used for assessing the health of a family is the community health map (Falk-Rafael, 2004). With this tool, the nurse assesses the family structure, function, and support networks. The map provides a diagram of significant data and helps the nurse focus on the family as it interacts with the social systems within and around them (Fig. 1-6). Actively including the family members in the development of the community health map provides the nurse insights into the family's health experience and fosters the nurse–family alliance. The nurse should remember that the focus is on family health, past successes, and current strengths, not on family problems.

Learning, recognizing, and comprehending that these cultural factors are what shape a family's perception of their health and health-related events is known in nursing as **cultural sensitivity**. The nurse does not need to seek congruency between these factors, values, traditions, and beliefs and his or her own. The nurse does, however, need to recognize that how the patient and family comprehend and respond to a particular health event is shaped by these factors, values, and beliefs.

In order to use **cultural competence** as a nursing assessment tool, the nurse must be open and receptive to gaining awareness and respect of these cultural influences. Nursing interventions that are based on a solid knowledge of these values and practices have been demonstrated to achieve much higher levels of successful outcomes for families and patients (Locsin, 2002). Listening to the cultural voices and experiences of family and patients

Figure 1-5 The nurse is instrumental in providing family-centered care in the community setting.

Structural Family Assessment	**Developmental Family Assessment**	**Functional Family Assessment**
• Number males/females	• Parent's family of origin	• Socio-economic systems in place
• Marriage status	• Emotional reactions to changes	• Physical problems and strengths of patient
• Number/order children	• Spiritual beliefs	• Family strengths and weaknesses in shared caregiving
• Family members loss/death	• Recent life changes	• Who identifies and problem solves what issues
• Significant contacts and strength of relationship (work, church, medical, school, friends, extended family, clubs/organizational participation)	• Degree of family stability	• Parental discipline habits
	• Recent or expected shifts in family structure/relationships	• Perceptions of health, control over health, strengths, and weaknesses
• Ethnicity	• Affectional bonds	• Health priorities (individual and shared)
• Religion	• Feelings about family roles	• Health values (individual and shared)
• Socio-economic status/environment	• Childcare-work-relaxation balance	• Cultural values (individual and shared)
• Culture	• Alone time balance	• Spiritual values (individual and shared)
• Health problems	• Hopes for future	• Goals for a fulfilling life
• Living difficulties	• View of extended family	• Permeability of family boundaries — who is allowed into inner circle and for what function
	• Previous health crises	• Willingness to accept help
	• Method of coping with crises	• Communication styles, patterns
		• Use of power, by whom, when
		• Emotional closeness

Figure 1-6 Community health map.

affirms their value and is critically important to unifying the nurse–patient relationship as it motivates the patient toward positive health-promoting activities.

Across Care Settings: Ensuring cultural sensitivity and reliable information

In all care settings, nurses should use the services of professionals who can interpret word meanings correctly. Relying on family members often results in literal translation of words and omission of information—problems that create confusion and misunderstanding. In settings where professional interpreters are not available, the use of services like AT&T, Roget's International Thesaurus, or handheld personal information devices can be useful alternatives.

Delivering nursing care that is sensitive to and understands cultural differences, whether in knowledge, values, beliefs, or role expectations, should help the nurse evolve into a culturally competent professional who makes assessments and plans interventions from a holistic framework. Framing one's nursing assessment, intervention, outcome expectation, and evaluation with a holistic perspective gives the nurse a better assurance that no significant physiological, psychological, cultural, spiritual, or social component is excluded.

Ethnocultural Considerations— Cultural prescriptions and proscriptions for women and children

Cultural prescriptions are folk beliefs, practices, and values of a group that tell women and children what they should do—what their respective roles should be.

Cultural proscriptions are folk beliefs, practices, and values of a group that tell women and children what they should not do—what is "not" incorporated in their respective roles. When assessing cultural prescriptions and proscriptions, it is helpful to consider elements such as clothing, exercise, sexual participation, disciplinary efforts, dietary habits, family roles and relationships, verbal and nonverbal communication, cleanliness, illness remedies, and displays of emotion.

In some cultures, women and children do not have the permission, the decision-making power, or the means to access the American health care system. Legal barriers, language differences that restrict access to medical care and lack of diversity in the health care workforce are some of the obstacles that may prevent immigrant minorities from accessing care. In addition to the barrier(s) that culture may place on accessibility of modern health care for women and children, in many situations, health care providers are not available in the areas where culturally bound groups reside. The real or perceived lack of accessibility, affordability, and availability of health care services to growing numbers of individuals leaves the provision of health care delivery to the family, especially in multicultural societies. In these situations, nurses must help family members identify needs, strengths, resources, coping mechanisms, and desired outcomes. The functions of the nurse and family are intertwined and require collaborative planning, delegation, coordination, and provision of care (Goldberg, Hayes, & Huntley, 2004).

COMBINING MODERN TECHNOLOGY WITH THE CARING TOUCH

In settings where modern health care may not be accessible, affordable, and available or is culturally restricted, **complementary and alternative health care/medicine (CAM)** methods often are used. The focus of these low-tech high-touch noninvasive, nonintrusive, nontraditional interventions is the support of the family and child's whole mind, body, energy, environment, and spiritual healing. The nurse approaches this healing methodology from a holistic philosophy of caring, aimed toward a goal of patient-centered autonomy and a patient-defined sense of well-being.

In 1998 an Advanced Practice Nurse (APN) established a "Nurses' Tool Box" of CAM nursing interventions found to be effective in establishing patient and family autonomy; relieving various illness symptoms, controlling pain, improving immune function, decreasing anxiety and depression, improving circulation, excreting toxins, and enhancing healing (Ward, 2002). CAM interventions range from guided imagery, aromatherapy, imagining, creating art and writing; prayer, chanting, meditation, and channeling; therapeutic touch, stroking, and cuddling; acupressure, tai chi, magnetic forces and massage; music, singing, tonal vibrations, and various water therapies; to storytelling, joking and humor (Helms, 2006) (Fig. 1-7).

It is estimated that Americans spent more than 27 billion dollars on CAM in 2005. This statistic reflects the level of consumer interest and demand for low-tech medical and nursing interventions, and self-directed healing (Lucey, 2006). The nurse must be aware that not all CAM interventions are noninvasive, nonintrusive, or free from side effects and negative consequences. CAM also involves the use of nutritional and herbal supplements, diet adjustments and fasting, chiropractic and body manipulation, and the use of drugs that have not been fully tested for safety and efficacy. Today, much confusion about CAM remains in both the consumer and health provider sectors (Box 1-2).

 Collaboration in Caring— *Supporting the family that uses CAM*

The nurse can provide support to the patient or family that uses CAM by:
- Investigating what they think caused a health event and how they have been able to avoid it in the past
- Encouraging them to seek all approaches of healing that are evidence-based, including both traditional and alternative medicine
- Respecting the participation of a family-chosen folk healer
- Acknowledging the patient's/family's religious and spiritual beliefs
- Reflecting on and understanding personal beliefs and recognizing when they may be in conflict with those of the patient
- Avoiding judgment

The family-centered nurse has a responsibility to advocate for the patient and family who choose to use CAM; to assess for and educate about the implications, contraindications, and benefits of CAM to the family and patient; and to promote health practices that have been proven safe and effective in restoring well-being, whether via conventional treatments or CAM. The nurse must recognize that health can be achieved through various means, both high-tech and high-touch, and that individual well-being is most optimally accomplished when care is directed by concerns expressed, interventions chosen, and outcomes defined by the patient. It is easy to understand why the nurse–patient relationship and a focus on the patient as a whole being (mind, body, energy, environment, and spirit) are key to the success of CAM healing.

Also key to a healthy outcome when using CAM therapy, as with all nursing interventions, is the responsibility to encourage evidence-based decision making. This method of **evidence-based practice** is built on the premise that interventions need to be questioned, examined, and confirmed or refuted in their ability to support healthy outcomes. The nurse using evidence-based practice searches computer databases and current literature for reports that evaluate the safety, quality, and credibility of particular interventions. These searches produce reports from rigorous research studies, textbook and journal readings, stated expert opinions, and best practices resulting from quality improvement activities. It is the nurse's responsibility to use the best evidence available and make decisions accordingly, especially when working with practices such as CAM that are viewed by many as mythical, magical, and nontraditional.

Another source of evidence-based guidelines available to the nurse is the standards of care/practice developed by nursing professional organizations such as the American Nurses Association (ANA); Society of Pediatric Nurses (SPN); National Association of Neonatal Nurses (NANN); National Association of Pediatric Nurse Associates and Practitioners (NAPNAP) and Association of Women's Health, Obstetric, and Neonatal Nurses (AWHONN) (ANA, 2008; AWHONN, 2008). These published guidelines promote consistency and quality in nursing care and outcomes. Because of the time it takes to search and retrieve evidence-based knowledge, these guidelines provide the nurse a reliable source of high-quality interventions on which to base practice.

Figure 1-7 Storytelling, joking, and humor are therapeutic complementary and alternative medicine interventions.

Box 1-2 Confusion about CAM Through the Ages

A HISTORY OF MEDICINE
(Author unknown)

2000 B.C.	"Here, eat this root."
1000 A.D.	"That root is heathen. Say this prayer."
1850 A.D.	"That prayer is superstitious. Drink this potion."
1940 A.D.	"That potion is snake oil. Swallow this pill."
1985 A.D.	"That pill is ineffective. Take this antibiotic."
2000 A.D.	"That antibiotic doesn't work anymore. Here, eat this root."

Source: Helms, J.E. (2006). Complementary and alternative therapies: A new frontier for nursing education? *Journal of Nursing Education, 45*(3), 117.

Now Can You— Discuss the community health map, aspects of complementary and alternative health healing, and evidence-based practice?

1. Discuss the value of a community health map as a nursing assessment tool?
2. Identify at least five ways that nurses can offer support for the patient/family who uses CAM?
3. Explain what is meant by evidence-based practice?

PROFESSIONAL NURSING ROLES

Ever since Florence Nightingale's time, helping patients and families gain understanding into their health practices has been integral to the profession of nursing (Nightingale, 1859). The role of the nurse as patient and family teacher has been sustained over the years as a foundation of the profession and continues to be reinforced through professional standards of care/practice. The professional nurse teaches the patient and family by helping them gain knowledge and skills about the health risk affecting them, and of behaviors that can assist in accomplishing the health outcome they desire. There is a sharing of knowledge, and through that knowledge a gathering of strength that can be directed toward the health condition.

The nurse, patient, and family combine their strengths, through collaboration, to describe what the health issue is and means in their lives, and what interventions and decisions are possible and preferable. This collaboration results from, and becomes an act of, mutual respect for each other's values, abilities, expectations, and experiences with the health event and life (Rhea, 2000). Collaboration with the patient and family about health education needs pulls the nurse away from the traditional "banking" concept of patient teaching and learning in which facts, skills, and knowledge are offered by the nurse and deposited for storage in the patient's vault (Freire as cited in Sanford, 2000, p. 6).

Collaboration requires two-way dialogue and sharing between the patient and nurse of both personal and health-related problems and solutions. Each participant is an equal possessor of knowledge and shares the power of determining what is to be learned. Each has a desire to learn more from and about the other. Participants become personally engaged and share a deeper level of understanding of each other, the health risk as each perceives it, and the available and chosen interventions to explore in collaboration.

The nurse still holds responsibility as the provider of care to implement the chosen interventions, or to accept accountability for their delivery. Even though family-centered care encourages patient and family involvement in therapy delivery, it is still expected that the nurse will be actively involved and skilled in the provision of health assessment, treatment, care, and follow-up evaluation. The nurse plays a vital role in collaborative care across a range of settings, especially in the follow-up evaluation and ongoing treatment. It is the nurse's task to collaborate with the discharge planner, child's teacher, physician, physical or speech therapist, dietitian, and community services worker to develop with the family the best plan of care for the desired long-range health outcome.

 Now Can You— Describe the role of the nurse as a teacher, collaborator, and provider?

1. Explain how the nurse functions in the role of patient/family teacher?
2. Discuss aspects of therapeutic nurse–patient collaboration?
3. Describe the need for accountability on the part of the nurse as a provider of care?

The nursing process is the foundation for the professional role as collaborator and provider of care and guides the nurse in helping the patient and family choose appropriate interventions, and in quantifying and evaluating the chosen outcome goal. By using the NANDA International **Nursing Outcomes Classification (NOC)** and **Nursing Interventions Classification (NIC)**, the nurse is able to evaluate more clearly associations between interventions and outcomes (Johnson et al., 2006). Using these standards also helps nursing students and novice professionals develop the intellectually and technically complex competencies required to link assessment cues accurately with outcomes and interventions (Lunney, 2006).

Nursing interventions are more than the actions nurses take to help patients and families toward their desired outcome. One NIC may entail up to 30 actions or activities the nurse and family selectively choose from in order to individualize the intervention to the specific health condition as it is perceived at that moment (Johnson et al., 2006). The NIC also involves the evidence-based practices and critical thinking processes the nurse undertakes when judging for appropriateness and feasibility of activities chosen to reach resolution of the health problem and achieve desired outcomes.

Nursing interventions must be appropriate for both the selected nursing outcomes and diagnoses. They require comprehensive, preliminary assessment of patient and family strengths and health concerns; acceptability to the patient and family of the chosen interventions; and the nurse's and family's capabilities to fulfill or coordinate with other health care providers, both professional and familial, the chosen health outcomes.

Before nursing interventions are selected, appropriate, feasible, and family-agreed-upon outcomes must be clearly identified. The chosen NOCs help the nurse identify, prioritize, and differentiate the critical from the sometimes exhaustive list of other relevant interventions and actions. Just as nursing interventions are more than the sum of outcome-directed actions, outcomes are more than the ultimate, end goal of the health state. Outcomes are dynamic and demand frequent measurement of the responsiveness of the chosen interventions. Outcomes should be evaluated for continuing meaningfulness, both physiologically and personally; for direction and purpose, whether health restoration, maintenance, promotion or threat prevention; and for consistency with the culturally lived experience of the patient and family.

The Caring Art and Science of Nursing

Just as a family's culture is their centering foundation in times of health and illness, caring is the centering foundation of nursing. "Caring transcends language, customs, and cultural differences... it is universal" (Watson as cited in Rexroth & Davidhizar, 2003, p. 298). It "defines the characteristics and parameters of practice" (Falk-Rafael, 2005, p. 38). The National League for Nursing Accrediting Commission (NLNAC) supports caring as a vital core value of nursing (NLNAC, 2005). Caring often leads to new outcomes, ways of being, and experiencing life for a patient and family (Watson, 2002).

"Many circumstances in contemporary society have made caring more difficult now than in the past" (Rosalynn Carter as cited in Cluff & Binstock, 2001, p. 15). Advanced technology, the rapid pace of health care, and a focus on the legal ramifications of one's professional actions have placed great demands on the time and support a nurse can offer a patient and family. Understanding the many dimensions of caring one brings to, and gets from, the patient encounter is essential to the nurse's ability to recognize the pain, suffering, and vulnerability that patients experience.

THEORIES THAT FRAME CARING AS THE CORE OF NURSING

Florence Nightingale's model of nursing encouraged a focus on the spiritual, physical/environmental, emotional, mental, and social needs of the patient and is known as a holistic view of the patient (Nightingale, 1859). She described the base of nursing activities as observation, experience, knowledge of sanitation, nutrition, caring, and compassion; and the focus of nursing as the patient rather than the illness (Nightingale, 1859). Nightingale viewed all people as equal in their abilities to attain health. In addition to her emphasis on improving the patient's environment, she encouraged the use of imagination and retelling of pleasant life events as appropriate healing interventions to help restore the patient to the best possible condition so that natural healing could occur (Nightingale, 1859).

Watson and Leininger are two modern-day theorists known for their inclusion of caring as a core of nursing. The commonalities between these two theorists are especially important in understanding how to incorporate caring as a recognized nursing intervention with a measurable outcome.

In her *Theory of Human Caring*, **Jean Watson** contends that caring as a nurse demands that attention be given not only to the body but also to the soul and spiritual dimension of the patient and family (Watson, 2005). She defines the soul as the ideal self of an individual, and notes that the individual is constantly striving to achieve that ideal self by creating harmony among the body, mind, and spirit; between the ideal self (referred to as 'I') and the current self as living the experience (referred to as "me") (Watson, 2005). The state of health is related to the congruence between I and me, and the effect that the differences in I and me is having on the body, mind, and spirit (Watson, 2005).

By participating in transpersonal therapeutic relational nurse–patient communication in which each participant gives and gains equally and learns to identify with the other, the nurse and patient demonstrate mutual caring, recognize the other as more than an object, and move the patient toward a desired state (Watson, 2005). This caring by the nurse begins with the feelings elicited and responses demonstrated toward the patient's condition, allowing or encouraging the patient to also release feelings and thoughts about the condition and self (Watson, 2005). The focus of the encounters, referred to by Watson as caring occasions, is on "caring, healing and wholeness, rather than on disease, illness and pathology" (Watson, 2005).

The goals of the nurse–patient transpersonal therapeutic relational communication are to find meaning and develop a wholeness in the body–mind–spirit; assist the patient in transcending beyond the current health state toward his or her ideal; give meaning to the patient's being; and "release some of the disharmony, the blocked energy that interferes with the natural healing processes; thus the nurse helps another through this process to access the healer within, in the fullest sense Nightingale's view of nursing" (Watson, 2005, p. 89).

Madeleine Leininger also believes that caring is the core value of nursing. "Caring is essential for curing, but curing is not essential for caring" (Leininger as cited in Jeffreys, 2006, p. 37). Her *Theory of Transcultural Care Diversity and Universality* sees caring and culture as embedded with each other. You cannot have one without the other.

Caring necessitates understanding of the patient's cultural beliefs, values, methods of providing or showing caring, causes of illness and how it is viewed, and how wellness is achieved. This level of understanding only comes through a trusting relationship. Developing that trusting relationship is an ongoing process. When the nurse takes the time to clarify the patient's health beliefs and practices, reflect on one's own health values and actions, and validate through an unprejudiced and unbiased eye (avoiding judgment of what seems logical, sensible, or reasonable), the strengths and weaknesses of each, a caring relationship is established.

 Now Can You— **Compare and contrast the caring base of nursing as described by Nightingale, Watson, and Leininger?**

1. Describe Nightingale's focus of nursing?
2. List three of Watson's goals for a caring, therapeutic nurse–patient relational communication?
3. Discuss Leininger's advice for a nurse who wishes to develop a caring nurse–patient relationship?

ESSENTIAL CHARACTERISTICS OF CARING

Trust, built through an interactional relationship in which the nurse is cognizant of both personal and the patient's feelings and meaning of the health experience, is an essential characteristic of caring. It can involve such concrete actions as listening and observing for cues as to what the health event means to the patient, and what the patient views as her needs, how they should be met, and what the desired outcome should be. It is the aesthetic engagement, or art of nursing, that is defined as caring (see Fig. 1-4).

Caring provides a sense of empowerment (some believe caring is the opposite of power), capability, inner peace, and self-determination. It requires an understanding of one's own beliefs, prejudices, and values so that those of the patient can be addressed with respect and dignity (Davis, 2005).

A study of patients in an intensive care unit (Rosenthal as cited in Rexroth & Davidhizar, 2003, p. 301) helped divide caring characteristics into instrumental behaviors of caring and expressive behaviors of caring, or technical and non-technical components. It is important to know that nursing behavior that is considered caring first depends on clinical competence and technical expertise. "Without knowledge, caring is just a matter of good intentions" (Mayeroff as cited in Falk-Rafael, 1998, p. 41). It was found that where the patient perceived himself to be on the health-wellness continuum, or how critically ill, played a big role in the value he placed on the instrumental versus expressive caring behavior of the nurse (Meyeroff as cited in Falk-Rafael, 1998, p. 41) (Fig. 1-8).

🌸 Collaboration in Caring— *Enhancing family and patient coping*

The nurse caring for a patient in an intensive care unit can facilitate coping by:
* Encouraging family presence, interaction, and touching
* Encouraging the family to adhere to home/daily routines as much as possible
* Including the family in the plan of care; offering choices when possible
* Encouraging discussion of family fears and anxieties
* Offering to contact a spiritual leader or healer
* Encouraging the family to place familiar and comforting articles nearby

In a 2005 study on the components of caring as described by patients, expressive behaviors such as smiling, gentleness in touch, praising the patient for her efforts, and making the patient feel important were consistently classified as elements of caring (Davis, 2005). Communication was identified as another essential element. Communication with the patient and family that they mattered to the nurse personally; about the patient's hopefulness for the future and awareness of a higher source of healing; and with the physician that things were going well or not going well as defined mutually by the patient and caregiver were all recognized as supportive, caring ways of conveying concern, interest and compassion (Cluff & Binstock, 2001).

In addition to instrumental and expressive characteristics of caring, a spiritual component was reported by patients. Spiritual caring, however, did not necessarily equate with attention to one's religion, rituals, or beliefs. Rather, **spirituality** addressed the meaning of life, including the present as being experienced, the past, and the future. It entailed learning about a patient's and one's own perceived weaknesses, vulnerabilities, and mortality, and where the power lies to transcend or accept them (Kelly, 2004). Again, many of the same expressive characteristics were found when describing nurses who addressed spiritual caring (touching, listening, respecting, trusting, and humor). It is important to note that more than 80% of the patients questioned about caring stated they did not expect the nurse to address their spiritual needs, although they would have liked it (Davis, 2005).

Tolstoy said that "the essence of caring is the need to have one's position grasped." (Cluff & Binstock, 2001, p. 47) Caring's "unifying essence, however, is concern for and responsiveness to the needs and worth of the person receiving it....How often do I turn my focus from my performance to the needs of the patient?" (Cluff & Binstock, 2001, p. 1).

🌀 Now Can You— **Define the essential characteristics of caring?**

1. List three nursing actions designed to build trust?
2. Discuss the importance of instrumental, expressive, and spiritual behaviors of caring?
3. Identify three ways that communication is translated into caring behavior?

PROFESSIONAL NURSING ROLES

Provider of Care

As a provider of care, the nurse expertly includes caring behaviors that address all the physical, psychosocial, and spiritual needs of the patient and family. Through careful assessment of all three categories of needs, diagnosis of the patient's response to the health event, planning of interventions that promote the patient's strengths and follow-up, and evaluation of the patient's transition and potential for a new health state, the nurse can accomplish the most effective, efficient, and desirable outcome.

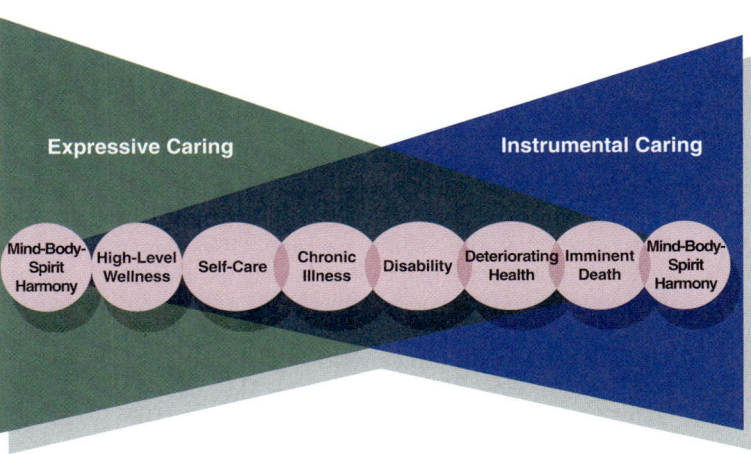

Figure 1-8 Health–illness continuum and the patient's need for caring behaviors.

One of the major responsibilities of the nurse as a provider of care is to stay current and competent in the operation of technical procedures and monitoring equipment. This professional responsibility requires knowledge of not only how to perform the procedures and operate the equipment, but also an understanding of why the procedure and equipment are necessary.

It means the nurse is not only responsible for safely executing the procedure, but also accountable for recognizing and interpreting the data gathered during the procedure and from the equipment read-outs. This level of responsibility and accountability evolves from an ongoing development of critical, analytical thinking on the part of the nurse.

Critical Thinker

Critical thinking is the "precise, disciplined thinking that promotes accuracy and depth of data collection and seeks to clearly identify the problems, issues, and risks at hand" (Alfaro-LeFevre, 2004, p. 61). Much of what it entails comes from experience, knowledge seeking, practiced hands-on work, and contextual discernment. Much of critical thinking is also built on inner personal skills, including: ability and willingness to self-reflect on values and beliefs, open-mindedness to diverse and unique perspectives, persistence in seeking the most reasonable answer, comfort and confidence with calculated risk-taking, and devotion to listening with a passion for true comprehension and understanding (Alfaro-LaFevre, 2004). The overriding purpose of critical thinking always is to make the best clinical judgment possible.

 Now Can You— Describe why critical thinking is key to the successful clinical practice of nursing?

1. Define critical thinking?
2. Name four avenues for developing successful analytical critical thinking?
3. Discuss the personal skills that help build critical thinking analysis?

Effective Communicator

Good listening and communication skills are essential to the nurse, especially when providing care for children and families. Often the nurse receives key information through subtle tones of voice and snippets of dialogue with a child or parent. Listening carefully allows the nurse to evaluate the level of language development of a child and to effectively use words that can be understood. It also offers the nurse an opportunity to view how the family communicates with each member, often delineating the family roles and structure. Listening to communication patterns can clue the nurse to components of the patient's value system and cultural approaches. For example, some cultures consider it rude to offer an immediate response when asked a question. Silence signifies that the receiver values the question and the person, and is giving it serious consideration. Some cultures communicate through storytelling; "Remember when Aunt Margie was in the hospital and…" The nurse can use this insight to help tailor much of the interactions that will take place during the

health event encounter. Listening to the family communicate can provide insight into the most favorable method of interacting.

The nurse often has the potential to role model for the child, and even the parent, effective ways of verbally expressing ideas, thoughts, and feelings. One way of role modeling appropriate expressive language is by the use of reflective listening and rephrasing. A parent who tells a 3-year-old, "Now be a good boy and stop crying. Big boys don't cry," might benefit from the nurse rephrasing the statement for her by saying, "Mommy knows your head hurts, and it's all right to cry. You did such a good job helping the nurse see how warm your body was."

Tone and quality of voice sometimes communicate more than the actual words themselves. This is especially true with infants and toddlers. All audible sounds convey meaning, even when the tone is incongruent with the word. Caution should be taken when using a stern tone to express endearments like, "Get over here so I can put some love on you." The young child is more likely to hear the stern tone of the voice than he or she is to hear the loving words. Touch, eye contact, and body language are also key components of communication the nurse must recognize as having the potential for enhancing or impeding a healthy outcome.

 ### *Ethnocultural Considerations*— Patterning effective communication styles

Most of us have seen the way an infant responds to the pace of our speech. Talk slowly, and the infant's body movements become slower to match the pace of the spoken words. Talk very quickly, and the infant becomes very active with her movements. To communicate effectively with various cultures, nurses need to become aware of the pacing of their speech. The pacing of the spoken word for people from the southern United States is often slow and drawn out, commonly called a "Southern drawl," while the spoken word of the person from New York City is often rapid and clipped, commonly called "rapid-fire chatter." Responding to a Southerner with rapid-fire answers, or to a New Yorker with slow, drawn out responses, may be perceived as rude. Listening to the speech pattern of the patient can allow the nurse to match that pattern when communicating with her.

Listening, touching, establishing eye contact, patterning, and paying attention to body language are all essential components of effective communication. The vital distinguishing factors of therapeutic communication, however, are that it is purposeful, goal driven, and focused on the outcome. Therapeutic communication should most often start with an introduction of the nurse, by name and role. This helps differentiate the purpose of therapeutic communication from that of social interaction. Maintaining focus of the communication on the outcome desired (i.e., meeting the patient's needs) helps not only in the nurse's time management but also in identifying data that is important from that which may be interesting but not necessary for a healthy outcome.

Teacher

The nurse's professional role as a teacher relies heavily on effective therapeutic communication. In order to meet the patient's desired health outcome, in addition to caring and competent nursing care, the patient needs information and education. Teaching what to expect regarding a procedure, surgery, or hospitalization; how to prevent complications, injuries, or illnesses; preparation toward discharge, continuing and self-care efforts; guidance in nutrition, safety and general wellness behaviors; and identification and avoidance of high-risk behaviors are all professional obligations of the nurse (DHHS, 2000). With patient encounters sometimes controlled by the clock, opportunities for effective teaching must be expertly recognized, planned, and executed.

Using multiple communication approaches can facilitate the nurse's health education encounter with the patient and family. Because children are introduced to television, animated computer games, and interactive learning early in their development, simple talking to them may not achieve the effect the nurse desires. Just as health assessment is a key role for the nurse when providing care, so is learning assessment. Finding out the desired educational outcome of the patient, her preferred learning style, and the most effective methods of delivery are fundamental to the nurse's role as a health teacher.

It is especially important to allow additional time for questions and answers. Most have experienced a precocious 3-year-old child's persistent and repeated use of the word "Why?", and the adolescent's ongoing "Yeah, but what if?" The nurse must feel comfortable in permitting the child all the time necessary to have these questions, no matter how seemingly insignificant, answered. Not only does it provide an avenue for teaching and learning, but it also demonstrates to the child and parent that the child is important to the nurse. Taking the time to exhaust all the questions helps establish and enhance therapeutic nurse–patient communication. Keep answers and explanations simple until asked for more elaboration.

Optimizing Outcomes— Identifying patient expected learning outcomes

Best Outcome: The nurse establishes the targeted learning outcome by talking and negotiating with the patient and family about what is most important. For example, an 8-year-old child learning how to control his asthma may be more interested in the mechanics of the use of the inhaler, while a 13-year-old might want to know how long he can wait to use his inhaler when he first experiences difficulty breathing (wanting to avoid at all costs the appearance of being different from the other children). Finding out what the child or adult wants to learn increases the success of changed behavior through new knowledge—always the underlying goal of teaching.

Mutually establishing the patient desired learning outcome is important to the success of the teaching encounter. Discussion of outcomes is futile if the patient is not ready to learn. Assessing readiness to learn is critical to the outcome of teaching. If there are basic needs yet unmet, such as physical hunger, safety or pain; psychological anxiety, fear, or guilt; and spiritual rituals, fears, and traditions, then learning is likely to be less effective. After ensuring that basic needs are met, the nurse can then assess for the patient's readiness to learn while taking into consideration the language development; current level of knowledge and experience with the topic; growth and development stage of life and capabilities; psychomotor, cognitive, and emotional skills; cultural rituals, beliefs, and values; and the learning environment.

In addition to setting mutually understood learning outcomes and assessing the readiness of the learner, there are some other key principles the nurse needs to be cognizant of when performing health teaching. Praise and positive feedback foster feelings of competence and motivation to learn more. The nurse is the ultimate role model for health teaching. Actions are remembered and patterned much more easily and create a more lasting effect than words. It is important to remember that along with the topic that the child, his family and the nurse have chosen, growth and development learning tasks are also underway, so the teaching should be planned as not to overwhelm the child. Topics should be taught in a manner that moves from the simple to the complex, with the recognition that follow-up teaching may need to be delivered in another setting at a later date.

Collaborator

The nurse plays a key role as a collaborator and coordinator of health teaching, especially when it must occur and be reinforced across multiple care settings and with multiple caregivers. Continuity of care involves not only addressing the continuing physical, emotional, and spiritual needs of the patient, but also the learning needs. Planning, implementing, and evaluating a teaching plan should involve members of multiple health disciplines: dietitians, community health nurses, social workers, home health aides, discharge planners, respiratory therapists, criminal justice workers, school teachers, pharmacists, physical therapists, ministers, respite providers, physicians, clinical nurse specialists, nurse practitioners, and family supporters.

In today's managed care health environment where patients are being pushed farther and farther away from the acute care setting, it is unreasonable to expect the patient's learning needs to be assessed, met, and adequately evaluated all during the brief initial nurse–patient encounter. Coordinating and collaborating about the learning needs of the patient with health care providers present during the provision of continuing care beyond the initial encounter are critical to a successful outcome.

Now Can You— Discuss three professional nursing roles that rely heavily on therapeutic communication?

1. Explain why listening skills are important to the nurse's role as provider of care?
2. Discuss five areas of readiness to learn that the nurse must assess before teaching begins?
3. Clarify the professional nursing role of collaborator as it relates to patient teaching and learning?

Advocate

When coordinating care for the patient who is receiving services from multiple providers, the nurse may be called upon to speak on the patient's behalf. As the number of providers increases, the potential for patient confusion and disillusionment also increases. Making certain that the patient's wishes, needs, plans, decisions, resources, and expected outcomes are recognized and guiding the provision of care is a vital role for the nurse. In this role as advocate, the nurse can promote patient- and family-centered care, all the while ensuring that the patient's and family's vision of health and healing remain the ultimate goal.

As an advocate for the patient and family, however, the nurse must take caution to avoid influencing the care from a personal values perspective rather than from that of the patient and family. Self-reflection of one's own values, beliefs, perceptions, and moral standards can help the nurse minimize the imposition of health-related decisions driven by personal values rather than the values of the patient and family. Advocacy should always provide the patient more control, power, and self-determination of the outcome of the health experience (Falk-Rafael, 2005). There should be clear agreement concerning when the patient wants, or needs, the nurse to speak for him or her. A well-established transpersonal relationship can foster this level of understanding and agreement.

Advocating for patients through group organizations (political, social and professional; local, state-wide, national and international) can also have an important impact on health care. Finding solutions to broad-based health problems and disparities among groups of people, such as children, women, and the poor, can be accomplished through nurses' political and social advocacy on their behalf.

The percentage of children living in poverty has remained between 17% and 20% for the past two decades (Forum on Child and Family Statistics [FCFS], 2005). Economic security has been identified as a key indicator of well-being and health (FCFS, 2005). Poverty affects the child and family's ability to access health care, educational opportunities, housing, transportation, health prevention measures, adequate nutrition, and continuity of care (FCFS, 2005).

Impoverished children are at higher risk for a number of health threats including obesity, violence, asthma, lead poisoning, teen pregnancy, and mental disorders (Velsor-Friedrich, 2000). Nurses have the ability, opportunity, and ethical responsibility to advocate for this group of vulnerable individuals. Nurses can use their image, knowledge, and numbers to advocate for change in these and other health disparities that exist between the economically secure and the impoverished.

🌼 Collaboration in Caring— *Helping impoverished families*

The nurse can be instrumental in helping impoverished families by:
- Providing the telephone number/contact information for federal food stamps; reduced-fee community health clinics, dental and mental health programs; Women, Infants and Children Special Supplemental Food Programs (WIC); State Children's Health Insurance Program (SCHIP); State Medicaid: HeadStart; Lion's Eyeglass Services
- Helping the patient investigate reduced-fee pharmaceutical options
- Connecting the family with Big Brother and Sister programs for family respite

EVIDENCE-BASED PRACTICE

The link between poverty as a risk factor and the health outcomes of obesity, violence, asthma, lead poisoning, teen pregnancy, and mental disorders has been demonstrated through epidemiologic, controlled quantitative, and qualitative studies and nursing research (FCFS, 2005). Nurses and others interested in improving the health of these vulnerable groups have taken research findings and developed **evidence-based practices (EBPs)** that promote, prevent, and protect health behaviors in vulnerable populations.

This scientific literature helps nurses not only stay current in their technical clinical abilities, but also in their choice of the most effective interventions. Professional organizations such as AWHONN, SPN, ANA, NAPNAP, and NANN have developed evidence-based clinical practice guidelines (CPGs) for the safest, most consistent, and effective provision of family-centered nursing care. Not only are these evidence-based practice guidelines beneficial to the individual nurse's practice, but they can also be used by the nurse to advocate for change in the ritualistic, unverified, rules-oriented, and opinion laced traditions (i.e., accustomed practice) of institutional nursing. With an ever-increasing level of patient knowledge and health-seeking sophistication, the demand for higher level nursing knowledge quickly becomes evident (Catalano, 2006).

Evidence-based guidelines are available for a number of interventions including newborn bathing, use of adhesives on premature newborns, positioning and snuggling of premature newborns, childhood asthma management, HIV/AIDS treatment, childhood cancer treatments, hypertension management, pregnancy weight gain, play therapy, and family-centered care (National Guideline Clearinghouse, 2006). The nurse must be diligent in seeking out these evidence-based guidelines so that excellence in practice can always be achieved, measured, and held up for scrutiny. However, as one nurse researcher (Schultz, 2005) cautions, nurses must be careful to remember that evidence-based practice is not "best practice" until it combines the investigational guidelines and scientifically sound interventions with clinical expertise and the patient's values and preferences.

Accessing a wide variety of evidence-based information is important when evaluating the quality of data to be used in one's nursing practice (Box 1-3). Examples of three sources of peer-reviewed, critically evaluated research summaries and reports available to the nurse for use in assessing research studies are The Cochrane Database of Systematic Reviews Library, the Agency for Healthcare Research and Quality (AHRQ), and MEDLINE.

Questioning nursing practice, collecting relevant evidence to support or change practice, and evaluating the best data for the desired patient outcome help provide the best care. As more responsibility and accountability for practice and patient outcome are shifted to the

Box 1-3 Evaluating Evidence-Based Data

- Ensure data have been reviewed by at least two or three experts in an area when using information from a journal or Web site.
- Check the author's and publisher's credentials.
- Evaluate for prejudice, bias, or vested interest of author.
- Check timeliness of data.
- Check for balance between explanatory graphs and text.
- Ensure consistency across populations, settings, and time.

Source: Catalano, J.T. (2006). *Nursing now: Today's issues, tomorrow's trends* (4th ed., pp 547-550). Philadelphia: F.A. Davis.

individual nurse, the role of the nurse will continue to change. Advancing nurses' accountability for the quality of care provided also advances autonomy of practice.

The advanced practice nurse (APN) enjoys the highest level of autonomy because of additional education, occasionally through certification but most often through a master's level of post-secondary education. There are various advanced practice nursing roles, including certified nurse midwife (CNM), family nurse practitioner (FNP), clinical nurse specialist (CNS), pediatric nurse practitioner (PNP), and certified nurse anesthetist (CRNA).

 Across Care Settings: **Practice possibilities for advanced practice nursing**

The Advanced Practice Nurse can practice in all types of health care settings: nurse-owned and -run clinics, nursing homes, rehabilitation centers, hospitals, physician offices, sports health centers, surgical centers, student health centers, birthing centers, private outpatient practice, community health centers, primary and secondary schools, research centers, private consultation, academia, military fields, and state and federal legislature.

APNs make independent clinical judgments and provide primary care to individuals and groups of patients. Of the 2,909,467 licensed registered nurses living and working in 2004 in the United States, 4.8% were prepared to practice as nurse practitioners (NPs), 2.5% as clinical nurse specialists, 1.1% as nurse anesthetists, 0.5% as nurse midwives, and fewer than 0.5% as neonatal nurse practitioners (NNPs) (Health Resources and Services Administration, 2004).

The University of Pennsylvania conducted a 1-year study (Kennedy, 2004) to evaluate the effect of APN versus traditional hospital-based care on death, re-hospitalization, complications, and cost for elderly patients with congestive heart failure health problems. There was a 13.7% lower death and re-hospitalization rate, an average of 110 days longer period of time without complications, and a savings of $4,845.00 for patients cared for by APNs. Although not statistically linked, it was hypothesized that the difference resulted from the holistic mind–body–soul perspective taken by the APNs in their approach to patient care; the more patient-friendly atmosphere of a primary, non-acute care setting; and a focus on health prevention, promotion, and protection.

 Now Can You— Discuss evidence-based practice and contrast the focus of the advanced practice nurse with that of the professional registered nurse?

1. Describe the difference(s) between "best practice" and "evidence-based practice"?
2. Explain six key elements to look for when evaluating the quality of evidence-based data found in journals or on Web sites?
3. Compare and contrast the licensed Registered Nurse and the Advanced Practice Nurse's role and preparation?

THE NURSING PROCESS

Evidence-based practice constantly questions the status quo and focuses on the outcome rather than the process of treatment. It helps to take the nursing process to the next level, from treating illness to predicting and preventing health problems, complications, and risks (Alfaro-LeFevre, 2004). A nurse using the traditional nursing process of assess, diagnose, plan, implement, and evaluate most likely uses some form of a body systems approach to data collection, focused primarily on medical systems health problems. A nurse practicing from an evidence-based focus assesses for health risk factors; patient and family strengths and self-worth; learning needs; family role and relationship patterns; values, cultural beliefs and spiritual health; and patient perception of or response to the risk or problem, in addition to the medical body systems assessment (Alfaro-LaFevre, 2004).

The evidence-based nurse diagnoses not only health problems but is also able to predict potential problems based on knowledge of prior research. That evidence-based knowledge includes awareness of signs, symptoms, and related health factors of potential problems as well as a grounded understanding of their etiology. The use of a concept map, clinical pathway, or care map can aid the nurse in this awareness of relationships. The maps also help in prioritizing diagnoses.

The concept map is a five-step process, just as the traditional nursing process is. It is built on the nursing process and is especially helpful in the analysis of relationships of data to the health problem and the development of critical thinking.

Although there are different ways to create a concept map, a format that is often used parallels the steps in the traditional nursing process. First, assessment data is gathered. In Step 2 of the map, the nurse analyses the data to determine the patient's key medical and nursing problems. The medical diagnosis occupies the center of the map. The nursing diagnoses are those problems or responses the medical diagnosis has caused for the patient.

When creating a concept map, one begins by drawing a skeleton diagram with the medical diagnosis placed in the center and the nursing diagnoses, patient responses, or general impressions of health threats surrounding the medical diagnosis (Fig. 1-9). At this point in the map development, potential problems are yet to be addressed. The initial focus is on problems that are currently major issues in maintaining wellness.

Figure 1-9 Concept map construction begins with gathering and analyzing assessment data.

After the initial diagram is constructed, depicting what is believed to be the key problems, it is then time to investigate the medical diagnosis and gain knowledge of the treatment options. A review of assessment and evidence-based information on the following patient areas guide the nurse in the next step of the map:

• Growth and development tasks
• Past medical history
• Current laboratory values
• Medication taken and likely to be ordered
• Allergies
• Pain rating
• Diet and fluid intake, needs, and preferences
• Recent elimination patterns
• Usual activity rituals and current limitations

Step 2 in developing the concept map is to categorize the assessment data gathered under one or more of the identified patient problem areas (Fig. 1-10). Then the nurse describes the essential ongoing assessment data that

signifies improvement or deterioration in the health status of the primary medical diagnosis (Fig. 1-11). Step 3 of the map involves analyzing the relationships among, and prioritizing the patient responses that led to the nursing diagnoses. The problem or diagnosis with the most supporting data is usually the most important (Fig. 1-12).

Step 4 of the concept map requires the nurse, along with the patient and family, to develop the beneficial goals and outcomes they hope to attain. This step corresponds to the planning phase of the nursing process. The outcomes are what drive the selection of interventions to be initiated by the nurse, patient, and family and other caregivers. They should describe the assessment data that determines if there has been successful progress toward achieving them. The outcomes should address clinical health (the medical diagnosis, signs and symptoms), functional health (mind–spirit–emotions), quality of life (as defined by the patient), health risk reduction, health protection, health promotion, therapeutic relationships, and personal satisfaction (Alfaro-LeFevre, 2004). "Simply put, determining expected outcomes requires you to reverse the problem (state what happens when the person doesn't have the problem)" (Alfaro-LeFevre, 2004, p. 173).

Whether the nurse uses Maslow's hierarchy of needs or a professional theorist to determine the priority status of outcomes and interventions, it is important to recognize that the context or circumstances in which the health problem is occurring plays a key role in the prioritization and implementation. When the above mentioned steps are completed, it becomes much easier to choose interventions that are achievable within the time and environmental constraints of the health event; build upon the strengths of the patient and family; and increase the likelihood that they will be carried out by all those providing care.

Step 5 of the map is the evaluation of the patient's response to the health event, interventions, and progress toward the outcome goals. Evaluation is not a one-time nursing responsibility, but an ongoing process. The nurse is looking for a pattern of patient responses to the health event that should guide ongoing reassessment, planning,

Figure 1-10 Categorizing the assessment data.

Figure 1-11 Identifying essential assessment data to evaluate the health status.

Figure 1-12 Analyzing relationships and prioritizing patient responses.

and provision of safe and effective care. Concept mapping helps the nurse develop disciplined, critical thinking that promotes accuracy, depth of data collection, early identification of risks, realistic goals, and a broader understanding of patient health problems (Alfaro-LeFevre, 2004).

 Collaboration in Caring— *Promoting optimal care for the family*

The nurse can manage the care of the family best by:
- Establishing therapeutic communication with the patient and family
- Developing relationship-centered, patient-focused encounters
- Discussing the concept map with other caregivers
- Designating discharge planning needs and personnel in the concept map
- Consulting with the case manager when evaluating the concept map outcomes
- Investigating evidence-based practice from all health care disciplines (i.e., medicine, nursing, pharmacology, respiratory therapy, primary school education, criminal justice, and social sciences)

summary points

◆ Contemporary family and child health care nursing has shifted to a framework that emphasizes health promotion, protection, prevention, maintenance, and caring.

◆ Modern family-centered nursing applies a circular or spiral process that builds a nurse–patient–family connectedness by mutually identifying health threats, potentials, and meaningfulness for the family.

◆ Nursing aesthetics is the low-tech, high-touch component of providing health care, and the centering, caring foundation of nursing.

◆ The use of a community health map can help the nurse assess the family's support systems, strengths, and coping mechanisms.

◆ Today, health care may be provided in the acute care hospital, tertiary research center, free standing short stay unit, community health center, school, nurse-managed center, and private home. Different settings require increased independence, accountability, and expertise from the nurse.

◆ The essence of family-centered care is the placement of family relationships, coping mechanisms, values, priorities, and perceptions at the center of the health event.

◆ A holistic view of the patient and family includes the spiritual, physical, emotional, mental, social, and cultural indicators of patient health.

◆ Concept mapping helps the nurse develop critical thinking that promotes accuracy, depth of data collection, early identification of risks, realistic patient centered goals, and a broader understanding of patient health problems.

◆ When coordinating care for the patient and family who are receiving services from multiple providers, the nurse must advocate for the patient's wishes, needs, plans, decisions, resources and expected outcomes, and ensure that they are recognized and are the guiding force in the provision of care.

review questions

Multiple Choice

1. The new nurse explains to the clinic nurse that the nursing process currently being taught has an emphasis on:
   A. Health promotion
   B. Disease and illness
   C. Linear progression of the illness
   D. Assessment for signs and symptoms of disease

2. As a vital part of family-centered care, the clinic nurse works with the patient and family to discover what the health issue is and what interventions are preferable in a process of:
   A. Collaboration
   B. Assessment
   C. Development
   D. Knowledge

Fill-in-the-Blank

3. The clinic nurse collaborates with other multi-disciplinary members to provide care to a 60-year-old woman with uterine cancer who is anticipating a hysterectomy. The patient's care includes _____ and _____ needs as well as _____ needs.

4. The clinic nurse knows that the patient's _____ and preferences as well as the nurse's clinical expertise combined with the use of national guidelines is described as _____ practice.

5. The clinic nurse demonstrates for the new nurse strategies that are helpful to children in a crisis. The nurse maintains _____ eye contact, stays _____ on the children and _____ shares their experiences.

6. The clinic nurse understands that increased _____ has led to many patients and families having an increased focus on health _____ and _____.

7. The clinic nurse demonstrates elements of spiritual caring by learning about a patient's _____ or _____.

True/False

8. The nurse who is able to share the patient's perception of a health threat, and support the patient's changes in order to cope and understand their outcomes is part of a process of engaging transpersonal care.

9. The nurse collaborates with a family on outcomes that are realistic and culturally appropriate prior to the development of any interventions.

10. The clinic nurse defines critical thinking as promotion of an accurate and strong data collection that clearly identifies problems, issues and risks for a patient.

See Answers to End of Chapter Review Questions on the Electronic Study Guide or DavisPlus.

REFERENCES

Alfaro-LeFevre, R. (2004). *Critical thinking and clinical judgment: a practical approach* (3rd ed.). St. Louis, MO: Saunders Elsevier.

American Nurses Association (ANA). (2008). Retrieved from http://www.nursingworld.org/MainMenuCategories/HealthcareandPolicy-Issues/ANAPositionStatements.htm (Accessed February 27, 2008).

Association of Women's Health, Obstetric, and Neonatal Nurses (AWHONN). (2008). Retrieved from http://awhonn.org/awhonn/content.do?name=05_HealthPolicyLegislation/5H_PositionStatements.htm (Accessed February 27, 2008).

Bulechek, G., Butcher, H.M., & Dochterman, J. (2008). *Nursing interventions classification (NIC)* (5th ed.). St. Louis, MO: C.V. Mosby.

Catalano, J.T. (2006). *Nursing now! Today's issues, tomorrow's trends* (4th ed.). Philadelphia: F.A. Davis.

Cluff, L.E., & Binstock, R.H. (2001). *The lost art of caring: a challenge to health professionals, families, communities, and society.* Baltimore: The Johns Hopkins University Press.

Davis, L.A. (2005). A phenomenological study of patient expectations concerning nursing care. *Holistic Nursing Practice, 19*(3), 126–133.

Department of Health & Human Services (DHHS). (2000). *Healthy people 2010.* Washington, DC: Author.

Doenges, M.E., Moorhouse, M.F., Murr, A.C., & Murr, A.G. (2006). *Nursing care plans: Guidelines for individualizing client care across the life span.* Philadelphia: F.A. Davis.

Falk-Rafael, A. (2005). Advancing nursing theory through theory-guided practice: the emergence of a critical caring perspective. *Advances in Nursing Science, 28*(1), 38–49.

Ford, R.C., & Fottler, M.D. (2000). Creating customer-focused health care organizations. *Health Care Management Review, 25*(4), 18–33.

Forum on Child and Family Statistics (FCFS). (2005). America's children: key national indicators of well-being. Retrieved from http://www.childstats.gov (Accessed February 26, 2008).

Freire, P. (1997). Pedagogy of the oppressed. Cited in Sanford, R.C. Caring through relation and dialogue: A nursing perspective for patient education (healing and caring). *Advances in Nursing Science, 22*(3), 1–15.

Goldberg, J., Hayes, W., & Huntley, J. (2004, November). Understanding Health Disparities. *Health Policy Institute of Ohio,* 13.

Gordon, S., & Nelson, S. (2005). An end to angels. *American Journal of Nursing, 105*(5), 62–69.

Harmon Hanson, S.M., Gedaly-Duff, V., & Kaakinen, J.R. (2005). *Family health care nursing: theory, practice, and research* (3rd ed.). Philadelphia: F.A. Davis.

Health Resources & Services Administration (HRSA). (2004). The registered nurse population: National sample survey of registered nurses. Retrieved from http://www.bhpr.hrsa.gov/healthworkforce/reports/rnsurvey (Accessed February 24, 2008).

Helms, J.E. (2006). Complementary and alternative therapies: A new frontier for nursing education? *Journal of Nursing Education, 45*(3), 117–123.

Jeffreys, M. (2006). Cultural competence in clinical practice. *NSNA Imprint, 53*(2), 36–41.

Johnson, M., Bulechek, G., Butcher, H., McCloskey Dochterman, J., Maas, M., Moorhead, S., & Swanson, E. (2006). *NANDA, NOC, and NIC Linkages: nursing diagnoses, outcomes, & interventions* (2nd ed.). St. Louis, MO: Mosby Elsevier.

Kelly, J. (2004). Spirituality as a coping mechanism. *Dimensions in Critical Care Nursing, 23*(4), 162–168.

Kennedy, M. (2004). APN's: improved outcomes at lower costs. *American Journal of Nursing, 104*(9), 19.

Leininger, M., & McFarland, M.R. (2002). *Transcultural nursing: Concepts, theories, research & practice* (3rd ed.). New York: McGraw-Hill.

LeVasseur, J.P. (2002). A phenomenological study of the art of nursing: experiencing the turn. *Advances in Nursing Science, 24*(4), 14–26.

Locsin, R.C. (2002). Culture perspectives. *Holistic Nursing Practice, 17*(1), ix–xii.

Lucey, J.F. (2006). When trust in doctors erode, other treatments fill the void. *Pediatrics, 117*(4), 1242.

Lunney, M. (2006). Helping nurses use NANDA, NOC, and NIC: Novice to expert. *Journal of Nursing Administration, 36*(3), 118–125.

Mayeroff, M. (1971). *On caring*. New York: Harper Perennial. Cited in Falk-Rafael, A.R. (1998). Nurses who run with the wolves: The power and caring dialectic revisited. *Advances in Nursing Science, 21*(1), 29–42.

Moorehead, S., Johnson, M., Mass, M., & Swanson, E. (2008) *Nursing outcomes classification (NOC)* (4th ed.). St. Louis, MO: C.V. Mosby.

National Coalition on Health Care (2006). The impact of rising economic costs on the economy. Retrieved from http://www.nchc.gov (Accessed April 20, 2006).

National Guideline Clearinghouse (2008). http://www.guideline.gov (Accessed February 24, 2008).

National League for Nursing Accrediting Commission (2005). *Accreditation manual with interpretive guidelines by program type for post secondary and higher degree programs in nursing*. New York: Author.

Nightingale, F. (1859). *Notes on nursing*. Philadelphia: Lippincott Williams & Wilkins.

Rexroth, R., & Davidhizar, R. (2003). Caring: Utilizing the Watson theory to transcend culture. *The Health Care Manager, 22*(4), 295–304.

Rhea, S.C. (2000). Caring through relation and dialogue: A nursing perspective for patient education. *Advances in Nursing Science, 22*(3), 1–15.

Schultz, A. (2005). Clinical scholar mentorship model. *Excellence in Nursing Knowledge,* Feb. http://www.nursingknowledge.org (Accessed February 24, 2008).

Stichler, J.F., & Weiss, M.E. (2001). Through the eye of the beholder: Multiple perspectives on quality in women's health care. *Journal of Nursing Care Quality, 15*(3), 59–74.

U.S. Census Bureau (2008). The 2008 statistical abstract: The national data book. Retrieved from http://www.census.gov/compendia/statab (Accessed February 27, 2008).

Velsor-Friedrich, B. (2000). *Healthy People 2000/2010*: Healthy appraisal of the nation and future objectives. *Journal of Pediatric Nursing, 15*(1), 54–59.

Ward, S.L. (2002). Ask the expert: Balancing high-tech nursing with holistic healing. *Journal for Specialists in Pediatric Nursing, 7*(2), 81–84.

Watson, J. (2002). *Nursing: Human science and human care, a theory of nursing.* New York: National League for Nursing.

Watson, J. (2005). Theory of human caring. Retrieved from http://hschealth.uchsc.edu/son/faculty/caring.htm (Accessed February 27, 2008).

SUGGESTED RESOURCES

Agency for Health Care Policy and Research: Evidence-based Practice: http://www.ahrq.gov/clinic/epcix.htm

American Academy of Pediatrics: http://www.aap.org

American Association of Birth Centers: http://www.birthcenters.org

American College of Nurse Midwives: http://www.acnm.org

American College of Obstetricians and Gynecologists: http://www.acog.org

American Holistic Nurses' Association: http://www.ahna.org

American Medical Association Compendium of Cultural Competence Initiatives in Health care: http://www.kff.org/uninsured/loader.cfm?url=/commonspot/security/getfile.cfm

American Nurses Association: http://www.nursingworld.org

Assessing Cultural Competence in Health Care: Recommendations for National Association of Maternal and Child Health Programs: http://amchp.org

Center for Cross-Cultural Health: http://www.crosshealth.com

Childbirth Connection: http://www.childbirthconnection.org/

Diversity Rx: http://www.diversityrx.org

Federal Interagency Forum on Child and Family Statistics: http://www.childstats.gov

Georgetown University: National Center for Cultural Competence: http://www11.georgetown.edu/research/gucchd/foundations/frameworks.html

Healthy Mothers, Healthy Babies Coalition: http://www.hmhb.org

Institute for Women's Policy Research: http://www.iwpr.org

International Confederation of Midwives: http://www.internationalmidwives.org/

International Council of Nurses: http://www.icn.ch

NANDA International: http://www.nanda.org

National Association of Pediatric Nurse Practitioners: http://www.napnap.org

National Center for Cultural Competence: http://www.11.georgetown.edu/research/gucchd/nccc/

National Guideline Clearinghouse: http://www.guideline.gov

National Institute of Nursing Research: http://www.nih.gov/ninr

National League for Nursing: http://www.nln.org

National Library of Medicine – National Institutes of Health: http://www.nlm.nih.gov/

National Perinatal Association: http://www.nationalperinatal.org

National Resource Center for Family Centered Practice: http://www.uiowa.edu/~nrcfcp/

Survey on Women's Health in the United States: http://www.kff.org/womenshealth/

The Association of Women's Health, Obstetric, and Neonatal Nurses: http://awhonn.org

The Cochrane Database of Systematic Reviews Library: http://www.cochrane.org

The National Institute of Medicine: http://www.ncbi.nlm.nih.gov

The National Multicultural Institute: http://www.nmci.org

Urban Institute: National Survey of America's Families: http://www.urban.org/center/

U.S. Department of Health and Human Services, Health Resources and Services Administration (HRSA), Maternal and Child Health Bureau: http://www.mchb.hrsa.gov/

 DavisPlus DavisPlus.fadavis.com   **For more information, go to http://davisplus.fadavis.com/**

CONCEPT MAP

Nursing Care: Women, Families, and Children

Traditional Nursing Care

Contemporary Nursing Care

Caring: The centering foundation of nursing

Historic Nursing Approach:
- Health = absence of disease
- Medical model
  - Rid, heal, cure
  - Paternalistic
- Submissive patient
- Ethnocentrism
- Treatment-driven care

Theories of Caring:
- Nightingale
- Leininger
- Watson

Characteristics:
- Establish trust
- Recognize patient feelings/perception of illness
- Expressive behavior → touch
- Communication
- Technical skill/ knowledgeable
- Spiritual awareness

Family Centered Care:
- Sensitivity to culture, beliefs/values of family and community
- Collaborative versus authoritarian role
- Recognize knowledge of family group
- In-depth assessment of family → use of Community Health Map

Forces of Change:
- Consumerism
- Change in family structure/ accessibility
- Increase in health consciousness
- Social/technical advances
- Increased patient/family accountability
- Ethnopluralism

Nursing Roles:
- Provider
  - Use up-to-date, evidence-based interventions
  - Form a caring relationship
  - Implement the art of nursing aesthetics → imagery, music therapy, art
- Collaborator across care settings
- Implement nursing process using NIC/NOC
- Critical thinker
- Communicator
- Patient Advocate
  - Support decision making power
  - Increase access to health care
  - Emphasize education
  - Increase family-centered approaches
- Patient/family teacher

Home & Community-Based Care:
- Independent practice
- Expert skill in:
  - Health history
  - Cultural competence
  - Coordinating extended care
- Manage other health care workers
- Advocate for family-centered care
- Advocate for patients using CAM

A New Nursing View:
- Transcend/control health threat
- Motivate toward health promotion, prevention, maintenance
- Self-care
- Shared connection
- Patient-defined wholeness
- Engaged, transpersonal care

24-Hour Observation/Urgent Care:
- Manage time to:
  - Assess, ID those at risk, counsel, teach
  - Direct unlicensed personnel
  - Teach follow-up procedures to family

Specialized Acute Care:
- Strong knowledge base → care of the family/child
- Critical thinking
  - Technological expertise
  - Evidence-based

Collaboration In Caring:
- Prepare the family for community-based care
- Support CAM use; respect family healer; reflect on personal beliefs
- Enhance family/patient coping

Across Care Settings:
- Teach families who travel about protection against illness vectors
- Encourage family participation in care across all settings
- Use professional translator when possible

Ethnocultural Considerations:
- Health care beliefs and desired outcomes vary among cultures
- Use of imagery/music → based on cultural definition of said therapies
- Include cultural prescriptions/proscriptions
- Match pace of speech to the patient's speech pattern

Now Can You:
- Identify a major force that accounts for the present-day shift toward family-centered decision making in health matters
- Define present-day trends in nursing focus related to the health-wellness continuum
- Discuss a nursing approach that incorporates engaging transpersonal care
- Explain what is meant by evidence-based practice
- Identify how the nursing process has changed the professional role of the nurse
- Identify the essential characteristics of caring

Contemporary Issues in Women's, Families', and Children's Health Care

 In these days of investigation and statistics, where results are described with microscopic exactness and tabulated with mathematical accuracy, we seem to think figures will do instead of facts, and calculation instead of action. We remember the policeman who watched his burglar enter the house, and waited to make quite sure whether he was going to commit robbery with violence or without, before interfering with his operations. So as we read such an account as this we seem to be watching, not robbery, but murder going on, and to be waiting for the rates of mortality to go up before we interfere; we wait to see how many of the children playing round the houses shall be stricken down. We wait to see whether the filth will really trickle into the well, and whether the foul water really will poison the family, and how many will die of it. And then, when enough have died, we think it time to spend some money and some trouble to stop the murders going further, and we enter the results of our "masterly inactivity" neatly in tables; but we do not analyse and tabulate the saddened lives of those who remain, and the desolate homes in our "sanitary districts."

—Florence Nightingale, writing on rural hygiene

LEARNING TARGETS *At the completion of this chapter, the student will be able to:*

◆ Describe a multilevel approach for prevention and intervention in addressing contemporary health care issues.

◆ Discuss the major purpose and goals of *Healthy People 2010* and their relevance to nurses.

◆ Explain social, political, economic, and cultural trends that affect the health status of women, children, and families.

◆ Compare morbidity and mortality statistics between different populations and age groups of women, children, and families.

◆ Evaluate current gaps in health care delivery systems that impact women's, children's, and families' health.

◆ Discuss examples of major barriers to accessing health care in the United States.

◆ Apply four bioethics principles to analyze ethical issues in maternal–child and family health.

◆ Describe trends in integrative health care as it is used with women, children, and families.

◆ Identify examples of public policies and programs that have benefited childbearing families.

◆ Describe vulnerable populations in the United States and the nurse's role in advocating for neglected and stigmatized persons.

◆ Discuss some potential concerns that a nurse of the future might face and what skills will be needed.

moving toward evidence-based practice Reducing Health Disparity

Shoultz, J., Fongwa, M., Tanner, B., Noone, J., & Phillion, N. (2005). Reducing health disparities by improving quality of care: Lessons learned from culturally diverse women. *Journal of Nursing Care Quality, 21*(1), 86–92.

The purpose of this study was to view culturally diverse women's perspectives on health care services as a framework for improving the quality of health care using Fongwa's Quality of Care Model. The study design was based on an analysis of existing data from 15 focus groups that consisted of participants from 5 different cultural subgroups. Findings from three previous studies completed by the researchers were applied to Fongwa's Model. The model was selected for its usefulness in identifying ways to improve the health care system and enhance quality of care from the perspective of diverse cultures. The original studies were conducted to gain women's perspectives on alcohol and drug use, smoking cessation, and domestic violence. Themes that emerged from these studies were reflective of the women's perceptions of the care they received. The findings led the researchers to reframe their focus for the improvement of health care by exploring three common aspects: patient/client/consumer, provider, and setting.

From the patient/client/consumer perspective, women identified that they wanted to include their partners in health promotion activities. They also requested that education on domestic violence be integrated into a variety of community activities. The participants believed that this approach would allow them to access the information without fear that the perpetrator of violence would be suspicious of their activities. The women further stated that they preferred a female provider of their own ethnicity or one who understood their values and beliefs. They felt it would be easier to discuss difficult topics with such a provider.

The study participants reported that their providers frequently appeared rushed and overly busy, which was perceived as a barrier to receiving quality care. They believed that in order to develop a trusting professional relationship, it was important for the provider to take time and listen, remain nonjudgmental, and ensure confidentiality. They felt that any care given should be modified to fit the specific needs of the individual.

The women preferred that the clinical environment include brochures and flyers written in appropriate languages. In their view, these actions would help to create an environment responsive to the participants' needs, and supportive of their making changes to improve health.

The researchers concluded that encouraging women's input, listening to their needs and modifying the system based on their suggestions would encourage the women to recognize their power in improving their own health and the health care system in general.

1. Based on the study do you believe that sufficient evidence exists to generalize these findings to all culturally diverse populations?
2. How is this information useful to clinical nursing practice?

See Suggested Responses for Moving Toward Evidence-Based Practice on the Electronic Study Guide or DavisPlus.

Introduction

This chapter examines contemporary trends in women's, children's, and families' health care from a holistic, action-oriented perspective. Emphasis is on the professional nurse's role as change agent using the intervention wheel model and *Healthy People 2010* as guides for improvement. Biostatistical data are used to assess the current status of women, children, and family health, highlighting health inequities, vulnerable populations, and gaps in health care access and delivery. Societal trends and issues are examined from political, social, economic, and cultural perspectives, illustrating how these important dimensions become determinants of health. An overview of legal, ethical, and social justice is presented, with the nurse as a key player in transforming and maintaining a more effective health care system in the future.

Framework: The Public Health Intervention Model

Nurses have always been tenacious in their responsiveness to the rapidly changing health and societal landscape, and are well situated to address contemporary family health issues. This is an era of unprecedented change in health care. Some of these fast-paced trends include rapid technological advances, escalating health care costs, managed care, demands for increased accountability for public agencies, and terrorism threats. Modern nurses maintain a readiness to address new and resurfacing health-related issues, illnesses, or disaster management responsibilities. Nurses frequently serve as catalysts to help coordinate societal, community, and individual efforts to help achieve health and wellness goals.

It is useful to have a framework when thinking critically about the complex topics encountered in family health. The Intervention Wheel, formerly known as Minnesota's "public health intervention model," is particularly well suited for examining health issues with an action-oriented, holistic lens. The lens used to view the intervention model is population-based, meaning that epidemiology of the population's health status as a whole is assessed (Keller, Strohschein, Schaffer, & Lia-Hoagberg, 2004b) (Fig. 2-1).

The model is an inclusive framework and was developed, refined, and extensively critiqued by more than 200 nurses throughout the country (Keller et al., 2004a). It encompasses three levels at which interventions can be initiated, from the micro-level of the individual to the

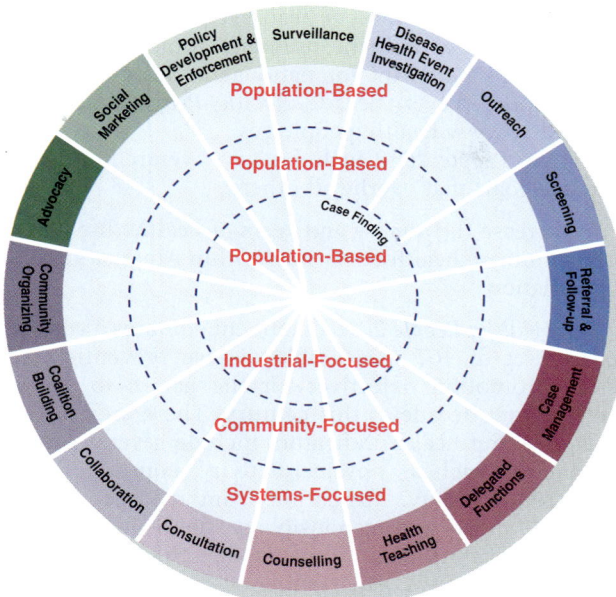

Figure 2-1 The Public Health Intervention Model.

macro-level environment. Interventions are targeted toward individuals/families, communities, and larger institutional and societal systems. Thus, broad determinants of health such as environment, employment, insurance, class, race, social support, access to health services, genetic endowment, and personal histories can be integrated, making health care interventions more comprehensive and effective.

In short, the public health intervention model is population-based, defines levels of practice, and has a comprehensive prevention focus. There are 17 categories of intervention tactics outlined in the model: social marketing, advocacy, policy development, surveillance, disease investigation, outreach, screening, case finding, referral, case management, delegated functions, health teaching, counseling, consultation, collaboration, coalition building, and community organizing (Keller et al., 2004b).

HOW THE INTERVENTION WHEEL WORKS

The issue of childhood obesity provides a good example for demonstrating how the Minnesota public health intervention model can be used to confront a contemporary health problem. Approaches that are currently being used to address the problem of childhood obesity range from those at the micro-level to the macro-level spheres of practice.

Childhood obesity has traditionally been framed as an issue of personal or parental responsibility. Viewing childhood obesity as merely a personal responsibility excuses society's responsibility and limits shared solutions. Nurses need to broaden their scope to examine health processes more globally. For example, nurses need to ensure that social, political, and structural conditions are addressed so that it is possible for people to achieve health.

There are many interesting and promising strategies for addressing childhood obesity. Some urban areas are proactively collaborating to redesign their communities. One

intervention is to build community sidewalks, establishing a more inviting environment for children to bicycle or walk to school. Communities have formed coalitions that advocate for neighborhood safety, so that walking, biking, and running can be safe. Some have looked at the strategic geographical proximity of fast food restaurants to schools, and have brought those observations to public consciousness. Fast food restaurants are clustered three to four times more often within walking distances of schools (Austin et al., 2005). This deliberate geographical placement exposes America's children to poor quality food that is frequently inadequate for health promotion.

Other strategies are targeted at schools, such as altering choices in school vending machines and cafeterias to include healthy alternatives to junk food. Some schools have already done so on their own. Others are advocating interventions at the state and federal levels, such as bringing back physical education courses in schools where they have been eliminated.

Currently, only 8% of U.S. public schools require daily physical education. Some schools collaborate with community health programs and screen for body mass index (BMI) and refer overweight children for early intervention and follow-up. Several schools have implemented the *Planet Health* program, developed by The Harvard School of Public Health. The *Planet Health* curriculum is intertwined with existing lessons already being taught in middle schools, such as science, math, and English. Students who participated in the pilot *Planet Health* interdisciplinary studies increased their fruit and vegetable intake, decreased their television viewing time, and lowered their BMI (Gortmaker et al., 1999).

Television presents another avenue for targeting obesity in children. Television is used more as an electronic babysitter than ever before. According to a 2006 Kaiser Foundation study, children younger than 6 years of age average 2 hours of media viewing per day (Kunkel et al., 2004). It is "used by parents to help manage busy schedules, keep the peace, and facilitate family routines such as eating, relaxing, and falling asleep" (Rideout & Hamel, 2006). Television viewing contributes to childhood obesity because it fosters physical inactivity as well as exposes children to a bombardment of junk food advertising (Fig. 2-2).

The American Psychological Association has a task force that researches television advertising that is specifically aimed at children. The task force has learned that children younger than the age of 8 do not yet have the experience and knowledge to critically evaluate advertising messages, and they tend to accept advertising as factual. American children view an average of 40,000 television ads per year (Kunkel, 2001). Many messages are aimed at marketing unhealthy foods to children, and are aired strategically at times when children are most likely to watch. One study demonstrated an average of 11 food commercials per hour during children's Saturday morning cartoons (Kunkel, 2001). Therefore, an average child is exposed to approximately one food commercial every five minutes. Advertising strategies for snacks, sugared cereals, soft drinks, and fast food contribute to the epidemic of childhood obesity, and the task force is urging policymakers to better protect young children from this exposure (Kunkel et al., 2004).

Figure 2-2 Typical American child fixed on the television set while snacking on popcorn.

There are initiatives at the federal level to address the childhood obesity problem as well. For example, the U.S. Food and Drug Administration (FDA) recommends strengthening food labeling in grocery stores as well as in restaurants. In some cases, consultation with restaurants is resulting in healthier portion sizes and the offering of lower fat options. The Centers for Disease Control (CDC) is using a multicultural social marketing technique to spread the word nationally about exercise benefits to children.

The public health intervention model gives an integrated view because it includes both the local and the more global system realms. The use of this model guides health professionals toward enhancing the capacity of all segments of society to move toward health and wellness. For nurses, it is becoming increasingly clear that the traditional approach to "caring" must be broadened beyond the individual patient, and instead become oriented toward the public's health in order to effect real change in health outcomes. Intervention programs must be multitiered and oriented toward the broader social context because this is where most patients are located.

Now Can You— Discuss the public health intervention model?

1. Describe the three levels of intervention in the public health intervention model?
2. Apply the intervention model to the health problem of childhood obesity?
3. Discuss why the public health intervention model provides an integrated view of health and wellness?

Healthy People 2010: A Blueprint for Action

Healthy People 2010 is the guide that defines health priorities for the United States. It is the nation's compass that points to specific focus areas that will guide progress toward the ultimate goal of optimal health for all Americans. The *Healthy People 2010* blueprint for action is coordinated by the Office of Disease Prevention and Health Promotion in the U.S. Department of Health and Human Services. Prominent health scientists, both inside and outside of government, use population-based studies to create this blueprint for national health goals which are renegotiated every decade. *Healthy People 2010* can be accessed at www.healthypeople.gov.

Healthy People 2010 includes two overarching health outcome goals that overlie all others:

- To increase the quality and years of healthy life
- To eliminate health disparities within America's population

The *Healthy People 2010* document contains a comprehensive set of 467 measurable disease prevention and health promotion objectives for the nation to achieve over the first decade of this century. There are 28 focus areas. Leading health indicators include several prevention factors such as physical activity, control of overweight and obesity, abstention from tobacco use and substance abuse, and responsible sexual behavior. Other leading indicators include mental health, prevention of injury and violence, environmental quality, immunization, and access to health care.

Ideally, the best method to address health priorities is through the early prevention of health problems. There are three levels of prevention. The most desirable level is **primary prevention**, which encompasses health promotion as well as activities specifically meant to prevent disease from occurring. **Secondary prevention** refers to early identification and prompt treatment of a health problem before it has an opportunity to spread or become more serious. Finally, **tertiary prevention** is intended to restore health to the highest functioning state possible. These three levels of prevention may be applied to a child's day-care setting. Primary prevention would involve teaching children and workers proper hand hygiene to prevent illness. Secondary prevention would encompass screening and isolating children who develop signs and symptoms of infection to prevent its spread. Tertiary prevention would involve strategies such as keeping the child at home, administering fluids, encouraging rest, and administering antibiotics if indicated, until the child is once again restored to health. This focus on prevention has the potential to make an enormous difference in family health status.

Current health indicators demonstrate that Americans today are healthier than they have ever been, with a steady upward trend to an average life expectancy of 77.3 years. Dreaded diseases that struck terror in families 100 years ago such as plague, polio, tetanus, and whooping cough (pertussis) are under control even though new health problems continually threaten to surface. Although heart disease remains the leading cause of death in the United States, rates have plummeted in recent years, most likely due to the present emphasis on healthy lifestyles and the availability of cholesterol-lowering medications.

However, there is no room for complacency regarding the present state of the nation's health. Despite some positive trends, the United States lags behind other industrialized countries. The World Health Organization ranks the United States as 37th in health system status, even though health spending per capita in the United States exceeds that of all other countries. Remarkably, health spending consumes one-seventh of the United States' gross national budget.

Despite large health care expenditures, health care and other resources are unevenly distributed in the United States. Persistent health disparities remain disturbing. An African American baby, for example. is more than twice as likely to be low birth weight and two and one-half times more likely to die during the first year of life than a European American baby. Sudden infant death syndrome (SIDS) is more than three times higher in American Indian and Alaska native babies than in European American babies. Additional information about health disparities can be accessed at the Centers for Disease Control's Web site, http://www.cdc.gov/.

 Now Can You— **Relate the value of having national** ***Healthy People 2010* goals to align health care improvement efforts?**

1. Discuss the two overarching goals of *Healthy People 2010*?
2. Define the three levels of prevention and give an example of each?
3. Describe prevention measures that have made a difference in reducing heart disease, the leading cause of death in the United States?

Overview of Selected Societal Trends

What is meant by the term "health"? Is health merely the absence of illness? If nurses are to effect improvements in national health status, a more comprehensive definition of health is needed. A holistic definition would include more than the physical body and instead extend into the interconnected mental, social, and spiritual realms. Health would encompass energy levels, balance, and resiliency. The World Health Organization defines health as a state of complete physical, mental, and social well-being and not merely the absence of disease or infirmity. Purnell and Paulanka (2003) expand this definition by describing health as a state of wellness that includes physical, mental, and spiritual states and is defined by individuals within their ethnocultural group.

Health as a concept may be self-defined, but to examine a population's health, one is limited to using health status indicators that can be directly measured. The health of a nation is measured by collecting statistical data and making inferences. **Epidemiology** is the statistical analysis of the distribution and determinants of disease in populations over time. **Mortality** (death) and **morbidity** (illness) rates are examined for trends. For example, epidemiological studies of heart disease reveal how many people develop heart disease, what type of heart disease they have, and what factors are associated with heart disease, such as smoking, obesity, diet, hyperlipidemia, working hazards, family dynamics, and other environmental factors. Mortality rates provide information about where nursing efforts should be focused. Morbidity rates identify populations where the illness occurs most frequently.

There have been many achievements that translate to measurable improvements in health status indicators. Yet the nation still has a long way to go. According to the United Nations 2006 Human Development Index, the United States ranks 38th in the world in life expectancy,

lagging behind countries with half the national income per capita and with a fraction of the expenditure on medical care. Certain national health problems, including acquired human immunodeficiency virus (AIDS), drug abuse, family violence, and homelessness continue to signal special cause for concern. More than 3 million people will experience homelessness in a given year and families with children comprise 33% of the homeless population. In addition, more than 38 million individuals living in the United States have experienced what has been termed "food insecurity" (Los Angeles Homeless Services Coalition [LAHSC], 2007).

To understand better the myriad of issues that impact the nation's health, it is helpful to consider some of the major trends that exert an influence on health status. These include the aging population, ethnic diversity, health care disparities, childbirth trends, and patterns of physical fitness.

 Now Can You— **Discuss why analysis of statistical health data in the United States is useful?**

1. Define the term epidemiology and describe how analysis of epidemiological data may guide public health interventions?
2. Discuss why mortality/morbidity biostatistics about disease and illness are useful?
3. Describe three health problems in the United States today that are of particular concern?

AGING POPULATION WITH MORE CHRONIC ILLNESSES

The population of persons ages 65 and older (one in eight in the United States) is growing steadily. This trend is attributed to the present increase in life expectancy and is expected to continue as the baby boom generation ages. It is predicted that by 2030, one in five persons will be elderly (U.S. Census Bureau, 2006). With the increased length of life comes more chronic illnesses, such as strokes, diabetes, arthritis, and Alzheimer's disease. Management of chronic illnesses presents a major challenge to health care systems that is expected to continue well into the years ahead.

INCREASED RACIAL AND ETHNIC DIVERSITY

The composition of the U.S. population is rapidly changing, and racial and ethnic diversity (difference) is greater than ever before. The historically designated U.S. minority populations can be classified as Hispanic, Black/African American, Asian, and Native American. The percentage of minority populations increased from 16% in 1970, to 27% in 2006, and it is projected to rise to 50% of the population by 2050, if current trends continue. As the population becomes more diverse, delivering culturally competent care becomes crucial for nurses. The delivery of health care within a culturally appropriate framework will help patients to feel better satisfied with their care and empower nurses to contribute more actively to the healing process.

Everyone, regardless of his or her professional status, is interested in the concept of racial and ethnic diversity. However, a most important point to remember is that racial and ethnic categories (Hispanic, Black/African American, Asian, European American, and Native American) are constructed by social systems (i.e., people) and their differences are based on visible physical characteristics. In scientific terms, these differences are phenotypic genetic expressions. There is no known biological basis for what society calls "race." Scientists have noted that there is more diversity within each of these artificial categories than there is between them. Migration, intermarriage, and genetic modifications have served to form one race, the human race. Despite the fact that "race" cannot be supported by scientists as a biological concept, as a social concept (i.e., how persons see one other and label one other) it is still very real.

DISPARITIES IN HEALTH CARE

Health disparities can be viewed as the extra burden carried by certain racial, ethnic, gender, and age groups for different health problems. Statistics indicate that the risk of death for women of color, for example, is nearly four times higher than it is for Caucasian women. More than half of 45- to 64-year-old African American women have hypertension, an incidence that is twice the rate for European Americans. Although Hispanic and African American women have a lower incidence of breast cancer than European Americans, they experience greater mortality from this disease. For reasons that include gender bias and difficulty establishing a correct diagnosis, a woman who presents to the hospital with symptoms of a heart problem is less likely than a man to receive a heart catheterization or to be given certain heart medications. The same scenario applies to Hispanics and African Americans of both genders.

Access to health care is disproportionate among different population groups. The status of one's health insurance remains the greatest factor that determines access. Insurance status is also the largest predictor of the quality of the health care that one receives. Yet insurance status alone cannot explain racial and ethnic disparities. Disparities exist even when clinical factors, such as comorbidities, age, stage of disease presentation, and severity of disease, are taken into account (Issacs & Schroeder, 2004).

Many other factors, such as the role of discrimination and stereotyping in health care settings, must also be considered when health disparities are analyzed. Nurses have long considered themselves to be "caring professionals." However, nurses are not immune from societal beliefs and values that result in discrimination and stereotyping of different populations. Nurses must continually remain vigilant for signs of these attitudes in themselves, and in turn, develop an awareness of how they influence their nursing practice. To heighten awareness of these issues, the Institute of Medicine published *Unequal Treatment: Confronting Racial and Ethnic Disparities in Health Care* in 2002. This compilation of studies clearly demonstrated that racism does indeed exist in medicine—and nursing is no exception.

Racism can be defined as the assumption that one's "race" is superior to others', resulting in unfair and harmful treatment. Racism can include attitudes and behaviors, it can be overt or covert, and it can exist at the individual and the institutional levels. Porter and Barbee (2004)

reviewed nursing research from the 1970s to the present. One study examined by these authors was an investigation by McDonald in 1994, which retrospectively explored pain medication administration after uncomplicated appendectomies. Record reviews revealed that "there were large and unexplainable differences in total doses that were received by Asian, Black and Hispanic Americans compared to White patients" (Porter & Barbee, 2004, p. 21). These findings provided a clear example of how nurses' beliefs and values influenced their clinical practice.

 Now Can You— Discuss health inequities and limited access to health care?

1. Identify both the age and racial/ethnic diversity trend of the U.S. population and discuss what that means in terms of nursing and health care provision?
2. Describe the greatest factor that limits access to health care?
3. Explain the roles that discrimination, stereotypes, and racism play in perpetuating health inequities?

CHILDBIRTH TRENDS

Today, many women are choosing to delay childbirth, and this trend is believed to be due to the desire to complete education and to securely establish careers, relationships, and finances. In 1970, the average age for a woman to have her first baby was 23.4 years; in 2001, the average age had risen to 27.6 years. In 1970, 9% of first-time mothers were older than age 30; by 2001 that proportion had risen to 34%. Because fertility decreases with age, some couples may miss the opportunity to have children altogether. Other related trends in society include children leaving home later and forming unions such as marriage at an older age.

In addition, more women are electing to give birth by cesarean section even when there is no medical reason for doing so. Patient-choice cesarean births in 2001 accounted for 1.87% of births. However, by 2003, this figure had risen to 2.55%, representing an increase of 36.6% in only 2 years (Wax, Cartin, Pinette, & Blacksone, 2004). Much controversy continues to surround this trend, since a cesarean birth is major abdominal surgery with all of the accompanying risks.

PATTERNS OF PHYSICAL FITNESS

Physical inactivity and its consequences are becoming a significant health problem for families in the United States. According to the Centers for Disease Control and Prevention ([CDC], 2005), only 13% of American women "engage in the recommended physical activity sufficient to reduce the risk of cardiovascular disease and other chronic debilitating diseases" (Peterson, Yates, Atwood, & Hertzog, 2005, p. 94). Research by the American Heart Association has shown that physically active women have a 60% to 75% lower risk of cardiovascular disease than inactive women (Peterson et al., 2005).

Obesity has made a steady climb upward. More than half of all Americans are overweight or obese (Ogden et al., 2006). It makes sense that increasing physical activity and reducing obesity are underscored in *Healthy People*

2010 as a primary means for reaching the nation's major health outcome goal: increasing the quality and years of healthy life.

THE INTERSECTION OF RACE, CLASS, AND HEALTH

While great strides have been made in family health, the progress achieved is not universal. The gap is widening between persons in lower and upper socioeconomic classes. "Upper class" in this context refers to those who live in contented neighborhoods, have a quality education, and bring home adequate wages. Persons from the lower classes, many of whom are African American, Hispanic, or Native American, live shorter and less healthy lives. Eighteen percent of all children in the United States currently live in poverty (U.S. Census Bureau, 2006).

It is important for nurses to work toward eliminating discrimination and racism, but if they are to make a difference in rates of illness and premature death, it is also important to work toward improving socioeconomic opportunities for all Americans (Isaacs & Schroeder, 2004). All too often, life and health choices are limited by socioeconomic status. The vision of the "American dream" and the ideology of "personal choice" obscure the fact that there are enormous constraints and limited choices that accompany poverty. A hungry and desperate person loses the capacity to choose.

 Now Can You— **Identify certain population trends that relate to health?**

1. Discuss U.S. fertility trends and trends toward surgical birth and what it means for women's health?
2. Discuss the trend toward inactivity in the United States and describe what consequences might be seen in the future health care status of Americans as a result?
3. Describe the role poverty plays in increasing health care disparities?

The Current Health Status of the Nation

INFANTS AND YOUNG CHILDREN

The plummeting rates of infant mortality in the past century allowed health care professionals to move forward beyond infant survival and focus on prevention and early intervention with children's health. Ideally, health prevention strategies targeting children's health would begin as early as preconception. It has been learned, for example, that folic acid supplementation helps to prevent certain birth defects. A fetus' exposure to harm could potentially be prevented if a woman were counseled *before* pregnancy about the harmful effects of alcohol, tobacco, toxoplasma, and other **teratogens** (substances that adversely affect normal cellular development in the embryo/fetus). The fetal neurological system, especially the brain, is extremely vulnerable to even small amounts of potentially toxic substances.

Early intervention is especially important when it comes to growth and developmental delays. There is a well established link between developmental delays and learning difficulties (Shonkoff & Phillips, 2000). Once children reach school age, interventions are less likely to be effective if they have already begun to fail academically or socially. Today, a number of infant and child development screening tools have been developed and refined. Unfortunately, however, close to one-third of developmental or behavioral disorders are not detected until children begin to attend school (Glascoe, 2000; Tebruegge, Nandini, & Ritchie, 2004).

The leading causes of death by age groups are revealing and offer clues about how to prioritize nursing interventions. SIDS is the leading cause of death among infants between the ages of 1 and 12 months. Accidents, or unintentional injuries, constitute the leading cause of death in children older than 1 year of age, which suggests that more community education and effort are needed to address child safety hazards. Although the incidence varies by age group, congenital malformations and malignant neoplasms shift between the second and fourth place for the leading cause of death in children.

Violence also takes a harsh toll on America's children. Homicidal assaults are the third leading cause of death of children in the 1- to 4-year-old age group, and also in the 15- to 19-year-old age group. Suicide is the third leading cause of death in teenagers and young adults, ages 15 to 24; it is the sixth leading cause of death among children ages 5 to 14. Family violence, child maltreatment, and violence in schools such as bullying are also issues of great concern.

Anthropologists such as Sanday (1994) note that in American culture, "inter-personal violence has become a national pastime" (p. 2). The most watched television shows of 2005, *Law and Order* and *CSI*, were routinely based on violent acts. It is estimated that the average child will witness 9000 media murders by the time he or she finishes elementary school (Kunkel, 2001).

Violent video games are a more recent trend and research is still sparse regarding their effects on children. A study by Anderson and Dill (2000) suggests that they may be even more harmful because they are interactive and the aggressor is the one glorified and with whom the player identifies.

There are other potentially preventable children's health issues. Lead exposure provides another example where early intervention and teaching can have a positive impact on children's health. Exposure to lead can occur from contact with lead-based paint in older homes; contaminated soil; a parent's occupation; certain vinyl mini-blinds; various folk remedies; living close to major highways; and from contact with imported pottery, jewelry or cosmetics. The American Academy of Pediatrics (AAP) recommends that all children between the ages of 1 and 2 years receive testing for lead exposure, since 25% of homes presently occupied by children younger than the age of 6 have known lead contamination. Lead exposure has been linked to a number of medical and developmental problems, including anemia, seizures, and mental retardation.

A trend not well understood is the alarming increase in childhood asthma, a condition that constitutes the most common cause of time missed from school. Asthma and allergies account for the loss of an estimated 2 million school days per year. In fact, the number one reason for pediatric emergency room visits due to chronic illness is for asthma-related problems.

Other trends in children's health status include a significant rise in the diagnoses of attention-deficit/hyperactivity disorder (ADHD) and developmental delays due to autism. Children with ADHD are typically fidgety, act without thinking, and have difficulty focusing. ADHD now affects 4% to 8% of all school-age children (Glascoe, 2000). Autism is the third most common type of developmental delay in the United States. An autistic child presents as a solitary child and notably lacks social responsiveness to others. Autism affects language, which is absent, abnormal, or delayed. Autistic children may demonstrate a strong resistance to change and show an abnormal attachment to objects. The prevalence of this disorder is difficult to gauge, since autism is not an easily accepted diagnosis, but it is estimated that it affects approximately 6 out of every 1000 children (Charles, 2006).

One way to visualize children's health is to view it as an obstacle course. The fortunate child is one who was desired and planned for before conception and who has parents with a good genetic profile, adequate resources, and who harbor no chronic illnesses. The fortunate child's mother would have healthy eating habits; maintain her ideal body weight; access early and regular prenatal care; and abstain from the use of alcohol, tobacco, and other harmful substances. The child who does well through fetal life must then encounter birth and avoid major complications such as prematurity or aspiration pneumonia.

Following birth, the child must encounter the hurdles of the first year of life to avoid becoming an infant mortality statistic. She has to dodge SIDS and shaken baby syndrome, and needs to be taken to health care providers for the hectic schedule of immunizations needed to prevent major childhood diseases. She must be fed and stimulated enough to grow physically, psychologically, socially, and emotionally. The child whose mother breastfeeds her gains an added bonus of immunities.

As the child matures, there are more obstacles to confront. The child who attends day care faces a significantly higher risk of infections. The tendency toward obesity and all the tempting fast food commercials on television offer additional stumbling blocks. She has to dodge all kinds of accidents that cause unintentional injury, tackle each developmental milestone, and land solidly in the "normal" grid of childhood growth charts. Ideally, she will not develop asthma, autism, or ADHD. She will hope to avoid the stumbling blocks of sexual abuse, or coping with poverty, and poor housing in unsafe neighborhoods. While parents work, the child's day-care environment may be laden with communicable childhood illnesses to be avoided. School-age children need to dodge being one of the 16% who are bullied (Volk, Craig, Boyce, & King, 2006). The obstacle course continues to pose challenges throughout childhood, and when adolescence arrives, the child again faces new foothills and crags.

Adolescents

Adolescents represent a population group with a set of issues uniquely their own. With regard to health care, adolescents are most often at risk for falling through the cracks. The adolescent must confront issues of self-esteem along with demands to meet a cultural ideal, while at the same time deal with pressure to conform to gain peer acceptance. The adolescent may have to cope with changes in appearance such as acne and awkwardness. Reproductive issues also arise. Girls must bridge the experience of menses, while boys encounter embarrassing erections and emissions. Issues such as sexuality, teen pregnancy, and sexually transmitted infections may pose further stumbling blocks. Alcohol, tobacco, and drug use as well as bullies, gangs, and school violence may force more hurdles in the envisioned obstacle course for the child to seek a full and healthy life.

One way nurses can make a difference is by learning and teaching others how to listen to children respectfully and value their experiences. Nursing can be called a "narrative profession" since patients present first and foremost with their narratives of symptoms and illness. Children do so as well but it takes patience to really listen.

 Nursing Insight— *Listening to our youngest patients*

Children tell us that we do not respect their expertise. The child who lives with an illness day by day holds the greatest insight into what it is to experience that illness. They come to know what the illness feels like, what treatments are necessary, what works, and what doesn't. They often develop quite sophisticated knowledge about their medications and treatment. The difficulty is that we do not give this knowledge and experience the same value as that held by the adults around them. Children also tell us that we do not give them uninterrupted time to tell their story their way. Children, with their varying cognitive and communication abilities, need time to explain their illness experience and time to respond to our questioning. Sometimes, through adult eyes, their way of telling us seems long and convoluted, and we therefore cannot resist the temptation of jumping in or interpreting what we think they are trying to say. Long story-telling does not fit well in the busy world of practice (Dickinson, 2006).

Two of the priority goals for children in *Healthy People 2010* address childhood vaccinations. One goal is to achieve and maintain effective vaccination coverage levels for universally recommended vaccines to 90% of children from 19 to 35 months of age and increase routine vaccination coverage for adolescents. The second goal is to reduce vaccine preventable diseases as follows: (1) measles, mumps, and rubella to zero cases and (2) pertussis in children younger than 7 years to no more than 2000 cases per year (CDC, 2005).

 Now Can You— Describe nursing actions that can serve to improve the current status of children's health in the United States?

1. Describe two benefits of preconceptual health guidance and early intervention?
2. Discuss major causes of child mortality and describe nursing interventions that can make a difference?
3. Compare and contrast communication strategies for children with those of adults?

FAMILIES

Today's world is full of complex, overlapping conditions and trends that influence the health of American families. Families are often the core unit where health habits are first formed. One of nursing's most important roles is to foster the health capacity of families, whether those families are blood-related or are families of choice.

Families do not exist in a vacuum, but are situated within communities and regions that often have unique social and physical characteristics. Surrounding environmental hazards affect family health. Natural disasters such as earthquakes, hurricanes, tornadoes, floods, and fires have favorite regional targets. Such disasters cause more damage when they strike high-population areas. Communities with high poverty rates are more likely to have older, run-down homes with more asthma-producing sources, such as mold, lead, and pests. Poorer neighborhoods are more likely to be closer to highways and regional waste sites.

Access to health insurance is an enormous factor that affects the health status of families in what is considered the richest country in the world. There is an ever increasing number of uninsured and underinsured citizens in the United States. More than 45 million Americans were uninsured at last count in 2004 (U.S. Department of Health and Human Services [DHHS], 2005b). One concerning trend is the erosion of employer-provided insurance. Today's employees are no longer guaranteed health insurance coverage through their jobs. According to the National Coalition on Health Care (2007), employer-sponsored health insurance fell 5 percentage points between 2000 and 2004, from 66% to 61%.

A recent study conducted by investigators at Harvard University found that illness and medical bills constitute the leading cause of personal bankruptcy and affect approximately 2 million Americans each year (Warren, 2005). Those with health insurance coverage frequently have gaps in coverage that can lead to missed appointments or the inability to fill a needed prescription. Health care problems among children extend beyond the millions who are uninsured, because for each of those children is another who misses a doctor's appointment or filled prescription due to coverage gaps in their parents' plans. Researchers suggest there are many more children in the nation receiving inadequate health care than are reflected in the uninsured figures. Persons without health insurance have limited access to health care and are left vulnerable to the effects of illness, both physical and financial. One of the more ambitious goals of *Healthy People 2010* is to increase to 100% the proportion of persons with health insurance.

WOMEN

The leading cause of death for women in the United States in 2005 was heart disease, which accounted for 28.6% of all female deaths. Cancer represented the second leading cause at 21.6%, followed by cerebral vascular disease (stroke) as third, which accounted for 8.0%.

There is plenty of room for improvement in health behaviors that are precursors to heart disease. According to the 2002 CDC's Behavior Risk Factor Surveillance System (BRFSS), two-thirds of women in the 25- to 65-year-old age group do not get the recommended 30 minutes of daily physical activity. One in five adult women smoke tobacco. With regard to nutrition, 72% of women do not get the recommended five or more servings of vegetables and fruits per day. There are also deficiencies in calcium and folic acid intake, nutrients important to women's health. Folic acid is a B vitamin that is linked to prevention of certain birth defects. Calcium is important to bone health. Lack of calcium contributes to osteoporosis, which makes a person susceptible to fractures, which can lead to disability and death (U.S. DHHS, 2005a).

Perinatal Health

In the area of perinatal health, national statistics reveal that over the past 20 years, there has been no decline in the number of pregnancy-associated deaths. According to the CDC (2005), two to three women in the United States die from pregnancy complications each day. Studies show that at least one-half of pregnancy-related deaths could be prevented. One reason for the recent escalation in high-risk pregnancies is related to pregnancies that occur in women with preexisting chronic conditions. Complications before childbirth account for more than 2 million hospital days of care and more than $1 billion spent each year in this country. In actuality, this number would be even higher if it also included complications that occur during and after childbirth.

Several years ago, health care professionals in Florida developed a program to address these issues at the state-wide level. Florida's Pregnancy Associated Mortality Reviews (PAMR) is a best practices example of how nurses initiated a plan to mobilize an entire state to work on improving pregnancy outcomes and reducing maternal mortality. PAMR started in 1996 in response to a cluster of maternal deaths noted in one particular county. Nurses organized an interdisciplinary team with wide representation, consisting of nurses, nurse-midwives, obstetricians, fetal-medicine specialists, family physicians, emergency medical services personnel, medical examiners, pediatricians, social workers, researchers from colleges of public health, and insurance payers. Using all available sources of data (i.e., physician office and hospital records, EMS records, autopsy reports), a nurse abstractor compiles the cases and sends them to each team member for review. The interdisciplinary team then meets, reviews each case, and collectively develops solutions for the identified problems. Confidentiality is key to the entire process. No providers' names are ever used and if team members recognize case details, they do not reveal that information. Contracts of confidentiality are signed at each quarterly session. To date, several important gaps in care have been discovered and recommendations and changes were made based on team findings. In addition, trends in pregnancy-associated deaths have been identified, leading to enhanced services and innovative approaches in caring for pregnant women.

Four million women give birth each year in the United States. Interestingly, in this day where there are more contraceptive methods than ever before, at least one-half of all pregnancies are unintended or mistimed. Another *Healthy People 2010* goal is to reduce unintended pregnancies to 30% or lower by 2010. Currently, there are some positive trends in perinatal health. For example, women are starting their prenatal care earlier. In the latest CDC Behavioral Risk data (2004), 83.9% of women initiated prenatal care during the first trimester. Smoking during pregnancy decreased from 20% in 1989 to less than 11% in 2003. Also, today, there is more published information about proper nutrition, folic acid, and healthy lifestyles than ever before.

There is evidence that contemporary health care systems are more cognizant of women's needs. Children maneuvering giant balloons as they eagerly bounce down the postpartum hall en route to visit their mothers and newborn siblings is a welcome and familiar sight. There is more understanding in research circles about the differences in the health care needs of women and men. Women are being empowered more in health care settings, enabling them, in turn, to make better health care decisions for their families.

 Now Can You— **Discuss elements of the current health status of American families and women?**

1. Discuss how recent national trends have affected families' access to health insurance?
2. Identify the three leading causes of death in women in the United States?
3. Describe a statewide model developed by nurses to improve pregnancy outcomes and reduce maternal mortality?

Politics, Socioeconomics, and Culture: Contemporary Influences and Trends

To facilitate understanding of present-day health care issues, it is helpful to consider political, socioeconomic, and cultural influences and trends. Family health issues are shaped, in part, by other elements as well. These elements include historical factors, family features, and biological and ecological influences. All of these factors intermingle and intersect with personal life experiences to comprise a health issue.

POLITICAL INFLUENCES AND TRENDS

Health policy decisions always involve choices, and whenever there are choices to be made, values and the potential for values conflicts are involved. One of the most polarizing political debates in modern times concerns the issue of abortion. Throughout the years since the passage of *Roe vs. Wade*, "abortion has kept its grip on the American imagination…dividing the body politic on issues of control of women's bodies, rights to privacy, fetal viability, and broader concerns over the moral shape of our country…" (Ginsburg, 1998, p. ix).

How and where a nation spends money has a major influence on the overall health of the population. National economic policies often dictate who has access to health care and who will be able to obtain medications. Policies related to social income programs such as Social Security and welfare assistance significantly affect the health of populations. Transportation issues and housing policies are critical as well. Education policies, such as the removal of physical education requirements from schools, have far-reaching and long-lasting effects on the health of children.

Health Care Delivery

Changes in health care delivery are omnipresent. The current health care delivery system is less of a system than it is a collection of entities. Health care today is corporate, and thus is more market driven than based on the common good or the actual needs of populations. Care is increasingly centralized into major medical centers. Small hospitals are closing due to an inability to remain solvent. Managed care is the rule rather than the exception, and is expanding as more and more health care providers and institutions are pressured into joining networks for health care delivery. Many of the provider networks operate on capitation, where they negotiate and are paid a set amount in order to provide complete health care for a certain number of clients.

Quality of health care and consumer satisfaction are the drivers of health care, just as in the retail industries. National databases regarding quality of care and specific conditions are only now beginning to be organized. Although a dearth of information is available on the quality of health care in the United States, this is changing as the focus on accountability in government and institutions moves to the forefront. The trend toward increased media attention concerning health care errors represents a vivid example of a growing demand for accountability. Workplace satisfaction and nursing shortages are issues that need to be addressed as well.

Public Policies and Programs

There are several public policies and programs that make a difference in women's, children's, and families' health. One highly influential program is the Women, Infants, and Children (WIC) program. WIC targets pregnant women, infants, and children, age 5 or younger, who are nutritionally at risk and provides supplemental nutritious foods and nutrition counseling and education. WIC serves low-income families as well as any pregnant woman who has particular nutrition challenges such as diabetes or anemia. Forty-five percent of infants born in the United States participate in the WIC program. Another nutrition program, The National School Lunch/Breakfast program, provides free or reduced-price meals to children from low-income families.

Medicaid, legislated through Title XIX of the Social Security Act, is a major publicly funded program that helps to boost the health status of women, children, and families. Funding for Medicaid is shared between federal and state governing bodies. Medicaid offers medical assistance after specific sets of complex eligibility criteria have been met. The Medicaid program is the largest safety net source of funding for health care services for the poorest populations in the United States.

The Newborn and Mothers Health Protection Act was passed in 1996. This legislation ensures that mothers and their newborn infants can remain in the hospital for at least 48 hours after a vaginal birth, or 96 hours following a cesarean birth. Another influential source of legislation for families is the Family and Medical Leave Act (FMLA) of 1993. This law permits American workers to take up to 12 weeks of unpaid leave per year from their jobs for recovery from serious illness or to provide care for a sick family member.

SOCIOECONOMIC INFLUENCES AND TRENDS

The most egregious effects of inequality in the United States are seen on the streets of the inner cities among persons with little hope for the future. The more subtle but far-reaching effects are seen in workers with insecure jobs. These are persons who rightly fear that major illness would result in personal catastrophe. Many single mothers report that they are merely one sick child away from losing their jobs and entire paychecks (Edin & Lein, 1997; Redfern-Vance, 2000).

In addition, there are the elderly who must expend nearly all of their resources before they can accept public funding for needed long-term care. For the elderly, the cost of medications can add up at the same rapid rate as do the chronic health conditions associated with the aging process. There are also those who may be classified in a low- or a high-income group, may be young or may be elderly, may be living in a busy metropolis, in suburbia, or in a lonesome rural area, and yet maintaining lives that offer little opportunity for control or meaningful social participation. Certainly these inequalities are, in part, inequalities in income. However, more than an inequality of income is at issue. In a fundamental sense, these inequalities are reflective of a society that works well for those at the top, and far less well for everyone else.

The Increasing Rate of Poverty

Most persons consider items like adequate food, housing, clothing, heat, electricity, telephone service, and essential health care as necessities rather than luxuries. This is not true for everyone. Overall, 12.7% of Americans were living in poverty in the United States in 2004. The number has risen each year since 2000 (U.S. Census Bureau, 2006). Economic changes, racial inequality, suburban movement, manmade and natural disasters, and industrialization all contribute to poverty circumstances.

The Feminization of Poverty

Women are the most impoverished demographic group in American society (Edin & Lean, 1997). In 2005, 56% of persons older than age 18 living in poverty were women. Single mothers with their children constitute 82% of the poverty population. More than 60% of U.S. women with children younger than the age of 2 now work outside the home (U.S. Census Bureau, 2000).

In 2000, one-fifth of all U.S. children were living in poverty. Between 2000 and 2003, the number and percentage of single mothers living in poverty increased while the percentage of single mothers with jobs fell. At the same time, poverty among children rose, and the number of children living below half of the poverty line (about $620 a month in 2003 for a single mother with two children) increased by nearly 1 million. These structural features of U.S. society have contributed to what has been coined as the "feminization of poverty."

Single mothers face oppressive barriers to achieve the "economic self-sufficiency," now legislatively prescribed for them, commonly referred to as "welfare to work." The essence of the new legislation, entitled Temporary Assistance for Needy Families (TANF), is that work now becomes compulsory and lifetime limits are imposed.

TANF replaces the former public assistance program that was known as Aid to Families with Dependent Children (AFDC). There is a maximum period that a person is allowed to receive public assistance at one time, and a lifetime limit. The mandates apply to pregnant women as well as those with infants older than the age of 3 months.

The Wage Gap

Gender inequity persists and the ratio of full-time working women's weekly earnings to those of men was 77 cents to the men's dollar in 2004. Proportionately, more families are being supported by women today than ever before. Three out of five U.S. families were headed by women and 22% of all children in the United States lived in mother-only families in 1990, an increase of 11% since 1970 (U.S. Census Bureau, 2006).

 Now Can You— Discuss aspects of political and socioeconomic influences that impact the nation's health?

1. Identify and discuss three socioeconomic trends that have a negative impact on the health of persons living in the United States?
2. Describe two public programs intended to improve the health of American women, children, and families?
3. Describe what is meant by the phrase "the feminization of poverty"?

Communications and the Digital Divide

One of the factors promoting patient empowerment is the ready access to health care information over the Internet. Fox (2006), reporting on the Internet and health, found that "looking specifically at online discussion groups devoted to health and well-being, the audience is also stable—about half of internet users helped someone else through an illness in the past two years; one in five internet users dealt with their own illness during that time" (p. 5).

In modern society, however, there exists what has been termed the "digital divide" (Wagner, Bundorf, Singer, & Baker, 2005). Families with discretionary income and with some formal education are more likely to access health information and educational resources from the worldwide Web. Those with less income, in particular those from racial and ethnic minority backgrounds, are less likely to have access to electronic materials. In addition, there is what is called the "gray gap," referring to seniors who do not use Internet technology. Approximately 68% of Americans reported ready access to the Internet in 2005. In families with incomes of $75,000, 95% of children have a computer at home. One out of five Americans claims they have never used the Internet or e-mail. Again, the "digital divide" separates and discriminates against the poor or elderly who do not have access to computers or who have not learned computer skills (U.S. Census Bureau, 2007).

Vulnerable Populations

Bellah, Madsen, Sullivan, Swiler, and Tipton (1991), who conducted a landmark study of mainstream American culture, articulated a problem described as "excessive individualism." The cultural norm of individualism focuses attention away from critical societal issues such as the ever-increasing gap between the "haves" and the "have-nots," as evidenced by the alarming rise in homelessness, hunger, and violence. The dark side of individualistic thinking advocates a policy of "choosing and creating your own reality" which then leads to "blaming the victim" and ignoring the social context, where "choices" are not, and have never, been equal. As a society, it behooves Americans to focus on a shared vision and goals, such as those afforded to us by the *Healthy People 2010* initiative. To do so, it is important to consider the vulnerable populations in the United States. As Aday (2001) notes, "as members of human families and communities, we are all potentially vulnerable" (p. 53). Vulnerability encompasses threats to physical and psychological health, as well as vulnerable social circumstances and stages within the life course.

HOMELESSNESS. Homelessness is rising among all populations, but most noticeably for families. There is an increase in families at the extreme poverty level (about $17,000 for a family of three in 2007). Income levels such as this are woefully inadequate to maintain a household. The increase in homelessness has resulted in more and more entire families who regularly visit homeless shelters and soup kitchens across the country. In New York City, 73% of the shelter population comprises children and their parents. The random collection of community shelters and free food kitchens that have proliferated throughout the United States during the past several years have had a difficult time keeping up with the needs. It has not helped that recent policy changes have resulted in the elimination of several programs that previously served as safety nets for health care and housing subsidies. Persons displaced as a result of wars and disasters have also added to the number of those desperately seeking assistance.

For homeless persons and families, health is a momentous challenge. The poverty, stigma, poor nutrition, and increased susceptibility to violence and mental illness all take their toll. Access to health care is a problem due to lack of transportation and finances, so that hospital emergency rooms are often the only option for medical attention. It is difficult to obtain accurate numbers on the homeless population but the Partnership for the Homeless estimates that currently there are about 2 million homeless persons in the United States, with 8105 homeless families in New York City alone.

✿ Nursing Insight— *Putting Homelessness into Proper Perspective*

To enhance understanding of the magnitude of the problem of homelessness in the United States, it is useful to consider the following statistics. These figures relate to families who were sleeping in Department of Homeless Services (DHS) city shelters in New York City during 1 month in 2005:

- 8105 families
- 13,062 children
- 11,854 adults
- Average family size: 3.18
- Average length of stay: 361 days
- 32.3% remain in shelters more than 1 year
  Source: http://www.partnershipforthehomeless.org/

UNDOCUMENTED IMMIGRANTS AND REFUGEES. Undocumented persons who enter the United States illegally in order to work constitute another highly vulnerable population. Many persons are from Mexico or Central America and are drawn to the United States for economic reasons or to escape political conflicts. Undocumented persons are willing to work in what are considered the lowest paid and least desirable occupations in the United States. They generally have no job security, health care access, or decent housing. Most face language barriers as well. Without financial resources, hospital and health clinic doors are generally closed to them. In addition, this population is experiencing mounting resentment from a public that is leaning more and more toward isolationism since the World Trade Center attack (Goldman, Smith, & Sood, 2006).

PERSONS RESIDING IN RURAL AREAS. Persons living in rural neighborhoods are less likely to have access to quality health care. Primary care providers are increasingly reluctant to locate in rural areas. Many small, rural hospitals have been forced to close because of centralization of intensive care services.

ABUSED AND NEGLECTED CHILDREN. The National Child Abuse and Neglect Data System (NCANDS) is the federal reporting system that analyzes data on child abuse that are collected on an annual basis. In 2006, NCANDS reported that the information obtained in the 2004 count included 3 million cases of reported child abuse. Child abuse can take many forms. The most common is child neglect, which can mean withholding food, clothing, shelter, love, supervision, or medical attention. Physical and child sexual abuse are other types and it is not uncommon for all three forms of abuse and neglect to overlap. According to the American Academy of Pediatrics, study estimates predict that one out of four girls and one out of eight boys will be inappropriately touched sexually by the time they turn 18 (Kellogg and the Committee on Child Abuse and Neglect, 2005).

NCANDS reports that three children die of child abuse in the home each day (U.S. DHHS, 2007). Fewer than 1% of children are abused by strangers. Children are most commonly abused by someone they know. In 79% of cases, the perpetrator is a parent. Child abuse can set up a perpetuating cycle of suffering and more violence later in life, potentially reaching into future generations.

Nurses have a legal obligation to report any observed known or suspected child abuse to child protective services. Thus, it is critical for nurses to learn to assess the signs and symptoms of child abuse (see Chapter 23).

VICTIMS OF SEXUAL VIOLENCE. Historical beliefs and attitudes toward women continue to influence women's lives and health. In the past, women were viewed as physically and psychologically inferior to men. They were denied rights and privileges routinely granted to men, such as owning property and voting.

Sexual violence haunts the lives of all women, both with its frequency and its impact. In a U.S. Department of Justice, Office of Justice Programs, National Violence Against Women Survey (NVAWS), nearly one out of five to six women report having been raped (Tjaden & Thoennes, 2000). Some have called the United States a "rape-prone" society (Buchwald, Fletcher, & Roth, 1995).

Sexual violence is linked with deleterious long-term psychological, social, and physical effects such as substance abuse, major depression, gynecological disorders, and others (Koss & Harvey, 1991; Wolfe, 1996). Unwanted sexual attention also devalues women and takes a toll on their health. Lewd sexual comments, cat calls, whistling, and intrusive looks are demeaning actions that negatively affect women's health (Esacove, 1998).

VICTIMS OF INTIMATE PARTNER VIOLENCE. It is difficult to obtain accurate numbers about intimate partner violence (IPV) because of varying definitions and widespread underreporting. The National Violence Against Women Survey (National Institute of Justice and the Centers for Disease Control and Prevention) revealed that nearly 5.3 million incidents of IPV occur each year among U.S. women ages 18 and older, and 3.2 million IPV incidents occur among men. The majority of reported assaults did not result in serious injury and consisted of pushing, grabbing, shoving, slapping, and hitting (Tjaden & Thoennes, 2000a).

Research suggests that nurses in clinical settings are still reluctant to question patients about intimate partner violence. Nurses need to routinely ask the violence screening questions and offer to help abused patients develop a safety plan. It is important for nurses to know that the most dangerous times for abused women are during pregnancy and when a woman tries to leave her partner.

GAY/LESBIAN/TRANSGENDERED INDIVIDUALS. Studies repeatedly demonstrate that access to sensitive health care for gay, lesbian, and gender transitioning patients is extremely limited. Stigma and prejudice continue to prevail in attitudes toward those living an "other than heterosexual" lifestyle (see Chapter 6 for further discussion about specific health issues among this population).

INCARCERATED WOMEN. An invisible population of marginalized women exists within the hidden pockets of the richest country in the world. One hears very little about incarcerated women, yet they currently inhabit U.S. jails and prisons in ever increasing numbers, with a sixfold increase during the past 20 years (Braithwaite, Arriola, & Newkirk, 2006). The growth rate of women prisoners has now bypassed the growth rate of male prisoners, and at present, women constitute 10% of the total inmate population (Hufft, 2004). In this country, which has the highest incarceration rate in the world, there are approximately 1 million women behind bars.

As a population, incarcerated women are not healthy. They tend to have a myriad of health problems, particularly illnesses that stem from the stresses of poverty, physical and sexual abuse, addiction, and motherhood. Imprisoned women frequently do not have access to the benefits of health education. Mental health issues abound in this vulnerable population as well.

More than 70% of incarcerated women are mothers. This is an issue that greatly impacts the health of families. Approximately 1.3 million minor children have no mother to care for them on a daily basis. Inevitably, children are affected by the abrupt changes commonly associated with incarceration of a parent. They may experience a sudden change in caretaking arrangements, social stigma, the potential for abandonment, and the loss of family support and financial resources.

The Girl Scouts of America organization has developed a unique program for girls who are separated from their mothers because of incarceration (Hufft, 2004). Called "Girl Scouts Behind Bars," this program is similar to regular scouting programs and has the same goals of self-esteem building and incremental accomplishments. It includes prison visitation between mothers and daughters, and especially targets social risks for which these young women are more vulnerable. The program also attempts to help incarcerated women hone their parenting skills. Forensic psychiatric nurses play an important consulting role in this national program, now operational in 13 states.

A nurse who is able to deliver culturally competent care to incarcerated populations quickly becomes cognizant of the challenges as well as the importance of raising standards and improving the present system. Work performed with this vulnerable population is significant far beyond the prison walls. Nearly 95% of prisoners will eventually be released into communities where they will likely face poverty, stigma, unemployment, and deficiencies in health care.

PERSONS WHO ARE SUBSTANCE ABUSERS. Substance abuse is a major health issue for families. Unfortunately, children are often the ones who suffer the most. Children in families with substance use problems are likely to be abused and neglected. These same children are also more likely to become substance users themselves. See Chapters 11 and 23 for further information.

 Now Can You— **Identify vulnerable populations of women, children, and families that exist in the United States today?**

1. Identify and describe four vulnerable populations in the U.S.?
2. Describe the population group at present experiencing the largest rise in homelessness?
3. Explain why undocumented immigrants are considered a vulnerable population?

PERSONAL AND CULTURAL INFLUENCES AND TRENDS

The world of today has dramatically changed from the era when telephones, televisions, and airplanes were giant novelties. Now nursing students "text message" friends on their cell phones in real time. The population relies on mass media for news and entertainment and the electronic gaming industry is thriving. Even dating relationships have changed. According to the U.S. Census Bureau, of the 44% of American adults who are single, 40% have tried online dating (Madden & Lenhart, 2006). The global education businesses that use e-learning are estimated to climb to a worth of $212 billion by the year 2010.

Other cultural changes include an increase in language barriers and cultural differences within the U.S. population. There is also a cultural component to many health issues. For example, the dramatic rise in eating disorders demonstrates how present-day popular culture can strongly influence health. Media images of so-called "perfection" flood the media, yet these images rarely represent healthy role models.

Self-Care and Patient Involvement

Autonomy and social participation have important influences on health status. Trends that present themselves in the health care arena include a focus on more consumer involvement and self-care tactics. Today there is an abundance of self-help groups, many of which are modeled along the lines of Alcoholics Anonymous, with varying purposes. For example, there are groups for tobacco dependency, "co-dependency" (CODA), drug addictions (Narcotics Anonymous), eating disorders (Overeater's Anonymous), and for families of addicts (Al-Anon and Alateen). In addition, there are self-help groups for nearly every medical ailment or illness imaginable. Some communities offer peer visitation programs whereby a person with the same illness or condition shares personal experiences with the newly diagnosed patient to help him or her understand what to expect in the days ahead.

In many situations, increased patient autonomy has resulted in more of a partnership model for the nurse. The nurse's role becomes increasingly one of facilitator and "cultural broker" to help the patient negotiate mutually acceptable plans of care. In obstetrics, it has meant that traditional childbirth practices of the past are increasingly challenged to become more personalized and family-centered. In pediatrics, it has meant that parents are encouraged to remain in their everyday roles as the primary support persons for their children.

The trend toward early discharge from hospitals has resulted in sicker patients in hospitals. Early discharge trends have also led to the blossoming of home health organizations. It is estimated that within the next few years, 70% of nursing care will be administered in the home setting. Literature has indicated that community-based care will be essential to nursing in the 21st century.

Complementary and Alternative Therapies

There is a growing trend toward the use of complementary and alternative medicine (CAM) therapies. The majority of persons in the United States now use some sort of CAM therapy, but many are reluctant to disclose that information to traditional medical personnel. There is sometimes the perception that nurses and physicians, since most are trained using the biomedical model, may not approve of the use of CAM. It is important for health care providers to have a working knowledge of CAM and try to integrate the two types of medicine. In this way, the patient obtains the benefit of each. Integrating CAM with conventional health care is called "integrative health care." Ideally, the nurse can thread integrative health care with the practice of conventional maternal child nursing for the maximum benefit of the patient.

One common lay perspective that is difficult to counter is the belief that because something is marketed as "natural," it means that it is harmless or without side effects. There have been publicized incidences of children being given unsafe treatments that resulted in harm or death. Mantle (2005) notes that the Children's Act of 1989 states: the "interests of the child are paramount. This includes the child's physical welfare and anything relevant to this, including nutrition and access to appropriate medical care" (p. 24).

 Complementary Care: *Blogging as Therapy*

Some health programs recommend "blogging" to facilitate healing when faced with serious diseases. Patients write daily about their experiences in diary format on the Internet. Blogs are a recording of personal experience, a participatory form of self-expression. Blogs help the creativity of individuals to surface and can be comforting during health crises. Blogs bypass editors and publishers and can be produced at the person's own pace. A strong sense of community can grow from blogging for health, and it is free of charge for those with computers and Internet access.

 Now Can You—Discuss personal and cultural trends that may impact an individual's health status?

1. Discuss some of the effects of self-care and autonomy on a person's health status?
2. Explain what is meant by the term "integrative health care"?
3. Discuss why blogging may be viewed as a complementary care method?

Health Care for the Nation

Recent years have brought an exponential growth of information and knowledge in all areas, especially in the field of health care. It is estimated that the total amount of information doubles every 6 years. Knowledge becomes obsolete at a rapid pace. Learning how to access current and accurate knowledge is critical for all health care providers. The implementation of community-based programs that are responsive to population needs for health promotion, education, and screening is an important nursing strategy to help meet many of the national goals of the *Healthy People 2010* initiative.

 Across Care Settings: Serving the community through parish nursing

Parish nursing, also known as faith community nursing, congregational nursing, or church nursing, is a phenomenon born from the marriage of nursing to the healing ministry of churches and religion. A **parish nurse** is a registered nurse who ministers to a church community, and honors the connection between faith, health, and well-being. The parish nurse has a holistic approach that recognizes the spiritual domain as an essential component of health. The parish nurse usually focuses on health promotion, health education, and prevention of illness. To achieve this goal, the parish nurse might conduct regular health seminars, perform health screening assessments, organize health support groups, or serve as a link from the parishioner to health resources in the community. Smaller congregations sometimes share a parish nurse with other congregations, while large congregations may hire a full-time nurse to serve their church community.

There is also a growing trend toward the use of "high-tech" medical care. Remarkable advances in technology have fostered the development of new strategies for delivering health services across care settings. The United States leads the world in its investment in biomedical technology, and owns 85% of the intellectual property associated with biotechnology. Telemedicine/home telecare provides one example of an innovative approach that has become increasingly available during the past decade.

DELIVERY SYSTEMS

Telemedicine

Telemedicine, whereby specialists can be remotely based and still assess and counsel patients, is another growing trend in health care delivery systems. Digital photos can be sent by the Internet from the patient's location to the specialist, at substantial cost savings. For example, in sexual assault crisis centers, a nurse practitioner can capture a colposcopy image and have ready access to a consultant through telecommunications technology. Wireless technology has progressed to the point where remote telemetry is possible. Wireless sensors are capable of detecting changes in blood pressure, or respiratory rate and sending alerts. It is possible to monitor medication adherence, and when a pill is missed an alert can be sent to the patient's pharmacist or provider. Webcams can be used to assess patients who have disabilities or live in remote areas. As the aging population increasingly grows, so do chronic health disabilities. Because the majority of health care providers remain concentrated in metropolitan areas, this type of technology may help bridge the gap, especially for those in remote or rural locations.

Telemedicine technology can be used for access to medical interpreters, desperately needed in many areas with multiethnic populations. It can also be used for home surveillance of elderly persons. Eighty percent of elderly persons who need help with their activities of daily living are cared for by family members, most of whom work. It is now possible to turn on a webcam at work to "look in" on a grandparent who is at home alone. In some areas, pediatric remote home monitoring services are offered to reach underserved children who have asthma.

CHALLENGES FOR NURSES IN CONTEMPORARY SOCIETY

An Ethical Framework for Professional Practice

Nurses are intimately drawn into daily encounters with other humans, and as a result often face difficult legal and ethical concerns. The Patient's Bill of Rights, informed consent, confidentiality, pain relief, and end of life care are examples of ethical concerns.

There are four basic principles that are commonly used to help solve ethical dilemmas. Those principles are beneficence, nonmaleficence, respect for autonomy, and justice or fairness. **Beneficence** means acting for the patient's benefit. **Nonmaleficence** is known best by the saying that is credited to Hippocrates, "First, do no harm" or *"Primum non nocere"* in Latin. **Respect for autonomy** means that patients have a right to make decisions about themselves as well as the right to have the information that is needed to make certain decisions. **Justice** or **fairness**

means that all patients should be treated equally. Discrimination should not occur based on social or economic status or type of illness.

The problem is that it is not unusual for those principles to be in conflict. Consider, for example, the Jehovah's Witness mother who refuses to accept blood, even if it means the death of herself or her child. Beneficence and respect for autonomy are clearly in conflict. Jonson, Siegler, and Winslade (2002) suggest that beyond the four principles, ethics must consider contextual data to be more useful in the complex medical world that nurses work in today. These authors developed a clinical pocket guide to help clinicians analyze case circumstances in context (Table 2-1).

 Collaboration in Caring— *Providing a nursing perspective for resolving ethical dilemmas*

Many health care settings have bioethics committees who confront the more difficult ethical problems. Nurses are often asked to sit on these types of interdisciplinary committees that usually include clergy, attorneys, social workers, physicians, and ethics consultants.

IMPLICATIONS OF THE HEALTH INSURANCE PORTABILITY AND ACCOUNTABILITY ACT (HIPAA). The Health Insurance Portability and Accountability Act (HIPAA) is a law that was passed in 1996. It has several components, including procedural mandates designed to protect the privacy of an individual's health information. The portability component ensures that a person moving from one health plan to another will be able to continue his or her insurance coverage. Expanded federal sanctions attached to health care fraud are also included in the HIPAA law.

HIPAA resulted in a flurry of health care system-wide modifications. Many office settings were required to reorganize their sign-in procedures. Others had to rebuild patient interviewing spaces, install expensive computer safeguarding mechanisms, supply units with paper shredders, and extend continuous training to employees. With this law, patients clearly have the right to protected health information (PHI). The consequences for breaking a HIPAA law can be both civil and criminal charges. Substantial fines and imprisonment can be imposed if a patient's health information is knowingly disclosed.

Since nurses frequently have ready access to confidential patient data, extreme vigilance is required. Addresses, telephone numbers, occupations, and e-mail addresses need to be protected, along with the patient's medical history, diagnosis, and condition. Nurses must be particularly cautious with conversations that take place in public places such as elevators and lunchrooms. Communication needs to be limited to only those who *need* to know the specific information in order to provide care for the patient.

THE HUMAN GENOME PROJECT. The Human Genome Project (HGP) was a 13-year project completed by the U.S. Department of Energy and the National Institutes of Health. In 2003, the project produced the first draft of a

Table 2-1 Ethics Guide for Clinical Practice

Medical Indications

The Principles of Beneficence and Nonmaleficence

1. What is the patient's medical problem? history? diagnosis? prognosis?
2. Is the problem acute? chronic? critical? emergent? reversible?
3. What are the goals of treatment?
4. What are the probabilities of success?
5. What are the plans in case of therapeutic failure?
6. In sum, how can this patient be benefited by medical and nursing care, and how can harm be avoided?

Patient Preferences

The Principle of Respect for Autonomy

1. Is the patient mentally capable and legally competent? Is there evidence of incapacity?
2. If competent, what is the patient stating about preferences for treatment?
3. Has the patient been informed of benefits and risks, understood this information, and given consent?
4. If incapacitated, who is the appropriate surrogate? Is the surrogate using appropriate standards for decision-making?
5. Has the patient expressed prior preferences, e.g., Advance Directives?
6. Is the patient unwilling or unable to cooperate with medical treatment? If so, why?
7. In sum, is the patient's right to choose being respected to the extent possible in ethics and law?

Quality of Life

The Principles of Beneficence and Nonmaleficence and Respect for Autonomy

1. What are the prospects, with or without treatment, for a return to normal life?
2. What physical, mental, and social deficits is the patient likely to experience if treatment succeeds?
3. Are there biases that might prejudice the provider's evaluation of the patient's quality of life?
4. Is the patient's present or future condition such that his or her continued life might be judged undesirable?
5. Is there any plan and rationale to forgo treatment?
6. Are there plans for comfort and palliative care?

Contextual Features

The Principles of Loyalty and Fairness

1. Are there family issues that might influence treatment decisions?
2. Are there provider (physicians and nurses) issues that might influence treatment decisions?
3. Are there financial and economic factors?
4. Are there religious or cultural factors?
5. Are there limits on confidentiality?
6. Are there problems of allocation of resources?
7. How does the law affect treatment decisions?
8. Is clinical research or teaching involved?
9. Is there any conflict of interest on the part of the providers or the institution?

Source: Jonson, A.R., Siegler, M., & Winslade, W.J. (2002). *Clinical ethics: A practical approach to ethical decisions in clinical medicine* (5th ed.). New York: McGraw-Hill.

map that identified the estimated 20,000 to 25,000 genes in human DNA. More than 3 billion sequences of human DNA base pairs were revealed. The base pairs are the chemical building blocks (A, T, C, and G) that are contained in the long, twisted chains that make up the DNA of the 24 different human chromosomes. It is the DNA that provides the gene with detailed instructions about how to manage all the processes within the human body. In May 2006, Human Genome Project (HGP) researchers filled in gaps from the first draft and completed the DNA sequence for the last of the 24 human chromosomes.

Knowledge gained from the Human Genome Project offers great potential in health care. It also brings to the surface some difficult ethical issues. For example, who will control genetic information? Commercialization has already begun in the areas of genetic testing and exploration of the promise of gene therapy, including more targeted medications. Yet social consequences have not been fully resolved. If sophisticated genetic testing is available, how will privacy be maintained? What will be the psychological impact of having genetic information, especially if

it is thought to be predictive of a genetically related illness or condition? Could the information potentially jeopardize insurance coverage for an entire family? Technologies developed for more sophisticated fetal testing will invariably lead to more controversy regarding reproductive rights. The ethical, legal, and social issues associated with the Human Genome Project were built in as part of the scientific study, and many have called the project the "world's largest bioethics program."

The American Nurses Association (ANA) proactively produced a thoughtful position statement on cloning in preparation for future ethics challenges. In their statement, the ANA emphasizes that nurses "…must be able to participate actively in the public debate about the possibility of cloning human beings by means of blastomere splitting or somatic cell nuclear transplantation. It is likely that there will be attempts to clone human beings in the near future and nurses must be able to speak to the ethical implications of such developments and point out possible advantages and disadvantages for the human species" (ANA, June 2000, p. 1, see Chapter 7).

Nursing Insight— *Professional responsibilities and genetics research*

The possibility of using cloning techniques to create human embryos and possibly human beings raises profound ethical, social, and health concerns. It is crucial that nurses understand the science of cloning techniques and appreciate the implications of related developments in germ line gene therapy and stem cell research.

 Now Can You— Discuss aspects of an ethical framework for nursing practice?

1. Describe the four basic principles involved in resolving ethical dilemmas?
2. Define HIPAA and give two examples of a breach of this legislation?
3. Discuss implications of the Human Genome Project for professional nursing practice?

Current Trends in Clinical Practice

Innovative approaches in health care delivery systems coupled with technological advances in patient management have prompted the emergence of new trends in nursing. Increased complexities in modern-day patient care are evident. Programmable electronic pumps that deliver specific rates of fluid and medications have replaced tedious bedside calculations of intravenous drips. "Paperless" (computerized) charting is quickly becoming the norm, replacing the alternating black and red inked pens that separated night shift from the day. Also gone are the large vats of medications that once lined the shelves of medicine rooms. Today, medications are dispensed in individually dosed packages stored in locked robotic machines that require computerized entry.

The aging of the population has created a shift in focus from acute to chronic care. Nurses in every specialty area are challenged to manage a rapidly expanding evidence base to guide their clinical practice. The global community, evident in patient populations, has underscored the need for collaboration and the use of "interdisciplinary" models to manage care.

Nurses are involved in cutting-edge approaches to health care delivery to patients in a variety of settings. Nursing resources and expertise have helped to develop cost-effective, innovative programs. For example, children with asthma can now be monitored in their own homes for blood pressure, pulse rate, temperature, blood oxygenation, and breathing rate. The results, quickly relayed by conventional phone lines to a secure server, are sent to health centers where nurses can assess and manage the patient who remains comfortable in the home environment.

In the area of maternal health care, a perinatal nursing service may be prescribed for women at risk for preterm labor. The service provides daily contact with a perinatal nurse and the use of an electronic device for conducting home monitoring to detect uterine contractions. Telecare is also used to monitor wound healing in medical-surgical patients. An inexpensive digital camera attached to a computer allows specialists to view the various stages of wound healing, make clinical assessments, and provide patient consultation.

The use of telemedicine has great potential for reducing the need for hospital admissions and frequent office visits. Some nurses resist home telecare, fearful that "high-touch" care is being replaced by "high-tech" care. However, home telecare, when creatively and appropriately used, can serve to administer personalized patient care and communication, result in better outcomes, and increase patient satisfaction. The increased application of technology ensures that nurses' caring presence in the virtual world will continue to expand. Despite the movement into "high technology," nurses must remain cognizant of the need to provide "human-centered," holistic care. Holism is a philosophy of care that is built upon a framework that values the human relationship and focuses on meeting the physical, emotional, spiritual, and social needs of the person.

To practice holistic nursing is to blend technology with healing while providing care that encompasses the interrelated relationships between the patient, the patient's family and other support persons, the provider(s), and the community.

Nursing Insight— *A holistic approach to care*

The practice of holistic nursing encompasses approaches and interventions that address the needs of the whole person: mind, body, and spirit. Florence Nightingale recognized the value of caring for the whole person and encouraged the use of touch, light, aromatics, empathetic listening, music, quiet reflection, and other methods to empower the individual's ability to draw upon inner strengths to promote healing (American Holistic Nurses' Association, 2005).

NANDA-I Nursing Diagnoses for Holistic Nursing

NANDA-I Classification of Nursing Diagnoses, Nursing Interventions Classification (NIC) and Nursing Outcomes Classification (NOC) were described in Chapter 1 as classifications systems used to name nursing interventions. Examples of how holistic nursing and complementary therapies fit nicely into nursing taxonomies for documenting care are presented in Table 2-2.

 Now Can You— Discuss current trends in clinical nursing practice?

1. Provide two examples of ways that home telecare can improve patient outcomes?
2. Explain how nurses can provide sensitive, personalized care that enhances the "high-tech" methods used?
3. Describe what is meant by holistic care?

CONTEMPORARY ISSUES AND NURSING ROLES

The scope and complexity of current health problems continue to present formidable challenges for nurses. There is no room for complacency in nursing's future. Nurses will inevitably need to struggle to keep up with the exponential growth of information, evidence-based

Table 2-2 Selected Nursing Diagnoses and Nursing Interventions: Possible Pairings of Nursing Concerns and Complementary/Alternative Interventions

Impaired Comfort	Acupressure, therapeutic touch	To decrease perceived pain
Disturbed Sleep Pattern	Massage	To promote relaxation, rest
Social Isolation	Pet therapy	To provide affection
Impaired Coping	Humor	To facilitate appreciation of that which is funny, to relieve tensions
Hopelessness	Hope instillation	To promote a positive sense of the future
Spiritual Distress	Spiritual support	To facilitate a sense of inner peace
Spiritual Well-Being	Spiritual growth facilitation	To support growth/ reflection/reexamination of values
Anxiety or Fear	Guided imagery, relaxation therapy, biofeedback, calming techniques	To reduce sense of anxiety
Impaired Communication	Art therapy	To facilitate expression

Source: Frisch, N. (May 31, 2001). Nursing as a context for alternative/ complementary modalities. *Online Journal of Issues in Nursing, 6*(2), Manuscript 2. Available online: http://www.nursingworld.org/ojin/topic15/ tpc15_2.htm

knowledge, and technological advances. Nurses are likely to deal with ethics questions that have never been faced before. The growth and diversity of the population will require more cultural sensitivity than ever before. The continual threat of chronic diseases demands creative, holistic approaches. Infectious disease threats will continue to challenge health care resources at the national and international levels. Terrible natural and manmade disasters will tax the nation's systems to their fullest extent. All citizens will feel the effects of HIV-AIDS as the disease trends toward women and children.

Nurses must extend their caring work beyond individual patients and families to communities, sociopolitical systems, and national and global health arenas if they are to have a significant impact on health promotion. Major disparities in health outcomes between families and children from racial and ethnic backgrounds and those of European American backgrounds must be confronted. Nurses have serious work to do to empower the many Americans who are without adequate health care coverage and access to services.

Broad-based efforts are needed to work through societal, economic, and cultural issues. Nursing's passion for evidence-based solutions must continue and remain focused on conditions that determine the health of individuals and populations. The *Healthy People 2010* national initiative is a step in the right direction. States, communities, and national organizations have rallied behind the priorities, goals, and objectives set in *Healthy People 2010* and have used it to guide their own health planning efforts.

A caring, holistic nurse is one who endeavors to develop and apply critical thinking skills to bring about changes, not only to bedside nursing of the individual, but to social justice issues that are determinants of health. Nurses have continually been ranked as the top professionals in the public trust in Gallup's annual Honesty and Ethics Poll since they were added to the list in 1999. The only exception occurred in the year after the World Trade Center attacks, when firefighters were ranked number one. As a profession, nursing's challenge is to step up and claim that popular power with the public and use it to be a dynamic force in transforming family and community health systems.

summary points

◆ There is much work to be done and health care challenges can best be faced by using multitiered, holistic approaches such as those articulated in the Intervention Wheel model.

◆ *Healthy People 2010*'s visionary blueprint prioritizes national goals for health so that health promotion efforts can be focused and aligned.

◆ A priority goal of *Healthy People 2010* centers on resolving health inequities in the United States.

◆ An overview of societal trends reveals where present and future health problems are arising and where efforts should be concentrated.

◆ Technological trends such as the Internet, telemedicine, and genetics research highly influence health issues.

◆ Cultural trends must be used to guide the designing of effective, culturally acceptable health interventions and programs.

◆ Nurses need to be vigilant and confront the negative effects of racism and prejudice in all health care settings.

◆ Nurses need to be familiar with health policy and programs of assistance so that patients can be referred to needed resources whenever possible.

◆ There are numerous vulnerable populations in the United States and the "common good" ethic needs to be rediscovered.

◆ The nurse of the future will face unprecedented ethical challenges that can be analyzed using a systematic framework like the one described by Jonson and colleagues.

review questions

Multiple Choice

1. The clinic nurse is providing information to Tracy and her 5-year-old child who has just been diagnosed with rubella. The nurse encourages rest, acetaminophen (Children's Tylenol), and increased fluids. This intervention is an example of:
   A. Primary health prevention
   B. Secondary health prevention
   C. Tertiary health prevention
   D. Mandatory health care

2. The clinic nurse is aware that a specific health concern for African American women in the population between 45 and 64 years of age is:
A. Stroke
B. Breast cancer
C. Hypertension
D. Motor vehicle collisions

3. The clinic nurse understands that nonmaleficence is a concept used in ethical decision making. It means:
A. First do no harm
B. Acting on the patient's behalf
C. Patients have a right to information
D. Patients should be treated equally

True/False

4. The perinatal nurse is aware of the Intervention Wheel and its potential for nurses working with community leaders to examine health issues more holistically.

5. Nurses who are taking a more proactive approach to childhood obesity would support the Food and Drug Administration (FDA) program to increase food labeling and decrease portion sizes in restaurants.

6. The clinic nurse is aware that with telemedicine, photos may be sent to the clinic doctors from remote sites and diabetics may send their "logs" for review before their appointments.

Fill-in-the-Blank

7. The clinic nurse is aware of the *Healthy People 2010* report and its identification of health _____ for the nation.

8. The public health nurse understands that when studying effects of diseases, it is the _____ rate that should be the focus of attention.

9. The pediatric nurse is aware that "race" as a concept is best defined as how persons _____ one another and _____ one another.

10. The clinic nurse is aware of the effects of poverty on the families seen in the clinic as the poverty rate has _____ yearly since the year 2000. At present, the most impoverished group is _____.

See Answers to End of Chapter Review Questions on the Electronic Study Guide or DavisPlus.

REFERENCES

Aday, L.A. (2001). *At risk in America: The health and health care needs of vulnerable populations in the United States* (2nd ed.). San Francisco: John Wiley & Sons, Inc.

American Holistic Nurses' Association (AHNA). (2005). About AHNA. Flagstaff, AZ: Author. www.ahna.org/about/about.html (Accessed March 21, 2007).

American Nurses Association (ANA). (2000). http://www.nursingworld.org/readroom/position/ethics/Etclone.htm (Accessed March 17, 2007).

American Nurses Association (ANA) Council of Cultural Diversity in Nursing Practice. (1991, October). ANA Ethics and Human Rights Position Statement.

American Nurses Association (ANA) Council. (2000, June). Human cloning by means of blastomere splitting and nuclear transplantation. ANA Ethics and Human Rights Position Statement.

Anderson, C.A., & Dill, K.E. (2000). Video games and aggressive thoughts, feelings, and behavior in the laboratory and in life. *Journal of Personality and Social Psychology, 78*(4), 772–790.

Annie E. Casey Foundation—Kids Count data. Retrieved from http://www.aecf.org/cgi-bin/aeccensus.cgi?action=profileresults&area=00N (Accessed May 28, 2007).

Austin, S.B., Melly, J., Sanchez, B.N., Patel, A., Buka, S., & Gortmaker, S.L. (2005). Clustering of fast food restaurants around schools: A novel application of spatial statistics to the study of food environments. *American Journal of Public Health, 95*(9), 1575–1581.

Bellah, R., Madsen, R., Sullivan, W., Swidler, A., & Tipton, S. (1991). *The good society.* New York: Vintage Books.

Braithwaite, R.L., Arriola, K.J., & Newkirk, C. (2006). *Health issues among incarcerated women.* Piscataway, NJ: Rutgers University Press

Buchwald, E., Fletcher, P., & Roth, M. (1995). *Transforming a rape culture.* Minneapolis, MN: Milkweed Editions

Bulechek, G., Butcher, H.M., & Dochterman, J. (2008). *Nursing interventions classification (NIC)* (5th ed.). St. Louis, MO: C.V. Mosby.

Centers for Disease Control and Prevention (CDC). (2005). Trends in leisure-time physical inactivity by age, sex, and race/ethnicity—United States, 1994–2004. *MMWR: Morbidity and Mortality Weekly Recommendations and Reports, 54*(39), 991.

Charles, J.M. (2006). Autism spectrum disorders: An introduction and review of prevalence data. *Journal of the South Carolina Medical Association, 102*(8), 267–270.

Dickinson, A.R. (2006, May). 'We are just kids': Children within healthcare relationships. *Contemporary Nurse, 21*(2), Retrieved from http://www.contemporarynurse.com/18.1/18-1p3.php (Accessed January 13, 2007).

Edin, K., & Lein, L. (1997). *Making ends meet: How single mothers survive welfare and low-wage work.* New York: Russell Sage Foundation.

Esacove, A.W. (1998). A diminishing of self: Women's experiences of unwanted sexual attention. *Health Care for Women International, 19,* 181-192.

Fox, S. (2006). Demographics, degrees of Internet access, and health. Presented June 19–20 at: Identifying and disseminating best practices for health eCommunities, Chapel Hill, NC : http://www.pewinternet.org/ppt/Fox_UNC_June_2006.pdf (Accessed March 19, 2007).

Ginsburg, F.D. (1998). *Contested lives: The abortion debate in an American community.* Berkeley, CA: University of California Press.

Glascoe, F.P. (2000). Detecting and addressing developmental and behavioural problems in primary care. *Pediatric Nursing, 26*(3), 251–266.

Goldman, D.P., Smith, J.P., & Sood, N. (2006, November–December). Immigrants and the cost of medical care: Immigrants use disproportionately less medical care than their representation in the U.S. population would indicate. *Health Affairs, 25*(6), 1700–1711.

Gortmaker, S.L., Peterson, K.E., Wiecha, J.L., Sobol, A.M., Dixit S., Fox, M.K., & Laird, N. (1999). Reducing obesity via a school-based interdisciplinary intervention among youth: Planet Health. *Archives of Pediatric Adolescent Medicine, 153*(4), 409–418.

Hufft, A.G. (2004, March/April). Supporting psychosocial adaptation for the pregnant adolescent in corrections. *MCN, American Journal of Maternal Child Nursing, 29*(2), 122-127.

Isaacs, S.L., & Schroeder, S.A. (2004, September 9). Class—the ignored determinant of the nation's health. *The New England Journal of Medicine, 351*(11), 1137–1142.

Johnson, M., Bulechek, G., Butcher, H., McCloskey Dochterman, J., Maas, M., Moorhead, S., & Swanson, E. (2006). *NANDA, NOC, and NIC Linkages: nursing diagnoses, outcomes, & interventions* (2nd ed.). St. Louis, MO: Mosby Elsevier.

Jonson, A.R., Siegler, M., & Winslade, W.J. (2002). *Clinical ethics: A practical approach to ethical decisions in clinical medicine* (5th ed.). New York: McGraw-Hill.

Kaiser Family Foundation. (2006). New study shows how kids' media use helps parents cope. Available at http://www.kff.org/entmedia/entmedia052406nr.cfm (Accessed March 17, 2007).

Keller, L.O., Strohschein, S., Schaffer, M.A., & Lia-Hoagberg, B. (2004a). Population-based public health interventions: Innovations in practice, teaching, and management, part II. *Public Health Nursing, 21*(5), 469–487.

Keller, L.O., Strohschein, S., Schaffer, M.A., & Lia-Hoagberg, B. (2004b). Population-based public health interventions: Practice-based and evidence supported, part I. *Public Health Nursing, 21*(5), 453–468.

Kellogg, N., and the Committee on Child Abuse and Neglect (2005). American Academy of Pediatrics Clinical Report. The evaluation of sexual abuse in children. *Pediatrics, 116,* 506–512.

Koss, M.P., & Harvey, M.R. (1991). *The rape victim: Clinical and community interventions.* Newbury Park, CA: Sage Publications.

Kunkel, D. (2001). Children and television advertising. In D. Singer, & J. Singer (Eds.), *Handbook of children and the media.* Thousand Oaks, CA: Sage Publications.

Kunkel, D., Wilcox, B., Cantor, J., Palmer, E., Linn, S., & Dowrick, P. (2004). Report of the APA task force on advertising and children, Section: Psychological issues in the increasing commercialization of children. Retrieved from http://www.apa.org/releases/childrenads.pdf (Accessed September 12, 2007).

Los Angeles Homeless Services Coalition (LAHSC). (2007). United States homeless statistics. Retrieved from http://www.lahsc.org/wordpress/educate/statistics/united-states-homeless-statistics/ (Accessed February 29, 2008).

Madden, M., & Lenhart, A. (2006). *Online Dating.* PEW Internet & American Life Project. Washington, DC.

Mantle, F. (2005). Complementary medicine and children. *Primary Health Care, 15*(8), 23–25.

Moorehead, S., Johnson, M., Mass, M., & Swanson, E. (2008) *Nursing outcomes classification (NOC)* (4th ed.). St. Louis, MO: C.V. Mosby.

NANDA International. http://www.nanda.org

National Center for Health Statistics (NCHS). (2005). Health, United States, 2005 with chartbook on trends in the health of Americans. Hyattsville, MD.

National Child Abuse and Neglect Data System (NCANDS). http://www.ndacan.cornell.edu/NDACAN/AboutNDACAN.html (Accessed May 28, 2007).

National Coalition on Health Care (NCHC). (2007). Health insurance cost. Retrieved from http://www.nchc.org/facts/cost.shtml (Accessed March 21, 2007).

Ogden, C.L., Carroll, M.D., Curtin, L.R., McDowell, M.A., Tabak, C.J., & Flegal, K.M. (2006). Prevalence of overweight and obesity in the United States, 1999–2004. *JAMA 295*, 1549–1555.

The Partnership for the Homeless. (2005). The cycle of homelessness. Retrieved from http://www.partnershipforthehomeless.org/ (Accessed March 17, 2007).

PBS, *Frozen Angels.* Retrieved from http://www.pbs.org/independentlens/frozenangels/makingbabies.html (Accessed June 8, 2007).

Peterson, J., Yates, B., Atwood, J., & Hertzog, M. (2005). Effects of a physical activity intervention for women. *Western Journal of Nursing Research, 27*(1), 93–110.

Porter, C.P., & Barbee, E. (2004). Race and racism in nursing research: Past, present and future. In J.J. Fitzpatrick, A.M. Villarruel, & C.P. Porter (Eds.), *Annual review of nursing research* (Vol. 22). New York: Springer Publishing.

Purnell, L.D., & Paulanka, B.J. (2008). *Transcultural health care: A culturally competent* approach (3rd ed.) Philadelphia: F.A. Davis.

Redfern-Vance, N. (2000). "Can't win for losin'": The impact of WAGES on single mothers with young children in a North Tampa Community. *Practicing Anthropology, 22*(1), 12–19.

Rideout, V., & Hamel, E. (2006, May). The media family: Electronic media in the lives of infants, toddlers, preschoolers, and their parents. Menlo Park, CA: The Henry K. Kaiser Family Foundation. Retrieved from http://www.kff.org/entmedia/upload/7500.pdf (Accessed February 2, 2007).

Sanday, P.R. (1994). Trapped in a metaphor. *Institute for Criminal Justice Ethics, 13*(2), 32–39.

Shonkoff, J.P., & Phillips, D.A. (2000). Executive summary. In J.P. Shonkoff & D.A. Phillips (Eds.), *From neurons to neighborhoods. The science of early childhood development.* Washington, DC: National Academy Press.

Spencer, N. (1999). Health of children—Causal pathways from macro to micro environment, *Health Ecology*, 175–192.

Tebruegge, M., Nandini, V., & Ritchie, J. (2004). Does routine child health surveillance contribute to the early detection of children with pervasive developmental disorders? An epidemiological study in Kent, U.K. *BMC Pediatrics, 3*(4), 4.

Tjaden, P., & Thoennes, N. (2000). Full Report of the Prevalence, Incidence, and Consequences of Intimate Partner Violence Against Women: Findings from the National Violence Against Women Survey. Report for grant 93-IJ-CX-0012, funded by the National Institute of Justice and the Centers for Disease Control and Prevention. Washington, DC: NIJ

U.S. Census Bureau. (2007). Internet access and usage and online service usage. Retrieved from http:///www.census.gov/compendia/statab/tables (Accessed August 14, 2007).

U.S. Department of Health and Human Services (DHHS), Health Resources and Services Administration (2005a). *Women's health USA 2005.* Rockville, MD: Author.

U.S. Department of Health and Human Services (DHHS), Office of the Assistant Secretary for Planning and Evaluation. (2005b). Overview of the Uninsured in the United States: An analysis of the 2005 Current Population Survey. Rockville, MD: Author. Retrieved from http://aspe.hhs.gov/health/reports/05/uninsured-cps/ (Accessed May 17, 2007).

U.S. Department of Health and Human Services (DHHS), Administration on Children, Youth and Families. (2007). *Child Maltreatment 2005.* Washington, DC: U.S. Government Printing Office.

Volk, A., Craig, W., Boyce, W., & King, M. (2006). Adolescent risk correlates of bullying and different types of victimization. *International Journal of Adolescent Medical Health, 18*(4), 575–586.

Wagner, T.H., & Bundorf, M.K., Singer, S.J., & Baker, L.C. (2005, April). Free internet access, the digital divide, and health information. *Medical Care, 43*(4), 415–420.

Warren, E. (2005, February 9). Sick and broke. Washington Post.com. Retrieved from http://www.washingtonpost.com/wp-dyn/articles/A9447-2005Feb8.html (Accessed May 5, 2007).

Wax, J.R., Cartin, A., Pinette, M.G., & Blacksone, J. (2004). Patient choice cesarean: An evidence–based review. *Obstetrics & Gynecological Survey, 59*(8), 601–616.

Wolfe, J. (1993). Female military veterans and traumatic stress. *PTSD Research Quarterly, 4*(1), 1–7.

 For more information, go to http://davisplus.fadavis.com/

CONCEPT MAP

Societal Health Trends

Contemporary Issues In Women's, Families', and Children's Health Care

Factors/Trends Influencing Health Issues

- US: 27th in life expectancy
- Major national health problems:
  - AIDS; homelessness: drug abuse; domestic violence
- Increased need for chronic illness management in the aged
- Increasing need for delivering culturally competent health care
- Disparities in HC: access; treatment; role discrimination
- Childbirth trends: increased maternal age at birth; more elective C-sections
- Physical inactivity/obesity
- "Class" gap = shorter, less healthy lives for "lower" class

Politics:
- How & where $$$ is spent
- How health care is delivered
- Public programs/policies

Socioeconomics:
- Poverty rates: women most impoverished
- Male-female wage-gap
- Digital divide: have/have not
- Increasing vulnerable populations

Personal/cultural trends:
- Increased use of technology
- Cultural/language barriers
- Degree of patient autonomy/self-care
- Trend toward early discharges
- Increased use of CAM therapies

Current Health Status/ Health Issues

Infants/Children:
- Infant mortality rate falling
- Leading causes of death:
  - SIDS; accidents/violence; malignant neoplasms; homicidal assaults; suicide
- Health issues/trends
  - Obesity/Type II diabetes
  - Lead exposure
  - Asthma
  - Rise in ADHD/autism
  - Self-image issues
  - Sexuality/pregnancy
  - Substance abuse

Families:
- Environmental hazards
- Natural disasters
- Poverty-related concerns asthma & waste sources
- Increased rates of uninsured/under-insured

Women:
- Causes of death: heart disease, cancer, stroke
- Nutritional deficits
- Lack of exercise
- Increased smoking
- No decline in # of pregnancy-associated deaths in 20 years
- 1/2 of all pregnancies unintended/unwanted

Nursing Insight:
- Critical to listen to young patients' illness stories
- Develop awareness of relevant statistics
- Understand implications of genetic research
- Holistic nursing = addressing needs of mind/body/spirit

Intervention Wheel

Guided by

Professional Nursing Role: Change Agent

Guided by

Healthy People 2010

- Assesses epidemiology of population's health
- Uses broad determinants of health
- Encompasses three intervention "levels" and 17 intervention categories
- Comprehensive focus on prevention

- Know how to access current/accurate knowledge
- Implement community-based programs for screening/prevention/education
- Be aware of alternative HC delivery systems & nursing role
- Develop an ethical framework for practice

- US Dept. HHS
- Blueprint for national health goals
  - Increase quality/years of healthy life
  - Eliminate health disparities within the US population
- 28 focus areas
- 467 disease prevention/health promotion objectives

Complementary Care:
- Blogging to facilitate healing: promote sense of community

? Now Can You:
- Discuss the Intervention Wheel and Healthy People 2010 goals
- Identify population trends that relate to health, including identifying vulnerable populations
- Describe nursing actions that improve children's health in the US
- Discuss influences that impact the nation's health

Collaboration In Caring:
- Bioethical committees

Across Care Settings:
- Parish nurse serving the church community

The Evolving Family

 Question of Family

What is a family but a collection of beings dwelling together?
But it is more than that
One person might see a refuge from the storms of society...
Another, a prison to prevent help from the outside world.
It can be both and more.
We draw our first breath in the presence of our family and hopefully
... we are held in family's arms when we sigh our last.
We learn all that is good in its caring boundaries or keep secrets of terror locked in its heart.
The difference between knowing love and trust and learning never to love or trust is in what passes between members of the family and what is passed on through members to their families.
What have you learned from your family?
What will you pass to your family?

— Brian Fonnesbeck, 2006

LEARNING TARGETS *At the completion of this chapter, the student will be able to:*

◆ Identify different structures of the modern American family.

◆ Describe theoretical concepts that apply to the family.

◆ Assess the family using selected family assessment tools during an interview.

◆ Apply specific family nursing diagnoses and interventions to the family.

◆ Discuss special family problems that often require nursing intervention.

◆ Compare various family cultural characteristics that may impact nursing care.

◆ Expand patient care to include and involve the family in every nursing setting.

---

 moving toward evidence-based practice: Parenting Concepts Among Culturally Diverse Cultures

McEvoy, M., Lee, C., O'Neill, A., Groisman, A., Roberts-Butelman, K., Dinghra, K., & Porder, K. (2005). Are there universal parenting concepts among culturally diverse families in an inner-city pediatric clinic? *Journal of Pediatric Nursing, 19*(3), 142–150.

The purpose of this study was to examine universal concepts in parenting philosophies and practices, which are in common across multiple cultures. The researchers used a grounded theory approach with ethnographic interviews of 46 English-speaking families representing 27 countries. All participants were from families of well children in an inner city hospital clinic in the Bronx, New York. The children's ages ranged from 7 days to 15 years of age. The researchers stated that New York City has

long established immigrant neighborhoods, tolerance, and plentiful jobs, factors that have been instrumental in attracting diverse cultures during the past century.

Interviews were completed using a question guide composed of open-ended questions, which were developed by the research team. The purpose of the questions was to elicit stories or examples from parents regarding the everyday care of their children. From transcribed interviews, 22 thematic categories

(continued)

moving toward evidence based practice (continued)

were identified, which were condensed into 11 common themes. The themes were subdivided into three broad headings: parenting philosophies; influence of American culture and perceived opportunities for children; and parenting practices. Similarities were identified among families in all categories.

Findings from the study indicated that a sense of community, family, and spirituality or religion was strong among all cultures, as was the importance of teaching values, respect, and the need for strict discipline. Television was considered to be an educational influence and parents believed that opportunities existed for jobs and higher education for their children. Parents expressed concern for child safety when playing alone outside and mistrusted nonfamily babysitters. Parents also indicated a preference for medical treatment rather than home remedies during episodes of acute illness. They expressed concern regarding the desire for preserving individual cultural heritage versus becoming assimilated into American society.

1. Based on this research, do you believe that sufficient evidence exists to generalize the study findings to all culturally diverse populations?
2. How useful is this information to clinical nursing practice?

See Suggested Responses for Moving Toward Evidence-Based Practice on the Electronic Study Guide or DavisPlus.

Introduction

This chapter addresses the assessment of families and highlights interventions for families encountered in a variety of nursing settings. Viewed through the lens of the media, actual and perceived changes that have taken place in the American family since the 1940s are explored. Modern-day family structures and challenges are described and various theories from psychology, sociology, and nursing are presented to provide a reference point for family assessments and interventions. A nursing diagnosis is presented and described in detail to illustrate the possible goals, interventions, and evaluation criteria that could be used with a family that is experiencing problems with daily functioning.

Concepts such as developmental and group stages of the family, communication, roles and relationships, and special need families are presented to assist with the planning and implementation of family centered care. Cultural characteristics and comparisons of American family orientation with families from various ethnic backgrounds provide the nurse with a starting point for the delivery of culturally sensitive care for American and international families.

The Evolving Family

VIEWING THE FAMILY IN A NURSING CONTEXT

A nurse hears in report, "…that family is starting to get to me. They have a million questions and want to be involved in any decisions that are made related to the patient." Another nurse asks, "Why is this patient still a full-code status? Someone needs to clue the family in on what the actual prognosis is. They are grasping at straws!" Another's comments: "I had to ask the boyfriend to leave again…the family does not want him around their daughter any more."

The preceding statements reflect an often-prevailing narrow point of view related to families and their involvement in nursing care. The literature describes the ideal nursing approach as one that views the entire family as the recipient of care, rather than only the individual patient (Harmon Hanson, Gedaly-Duff, & Rowe, 2005). In most practice settings, under the best circumstances, the family is seen as contextual background for the patient, and, under the worst, the family represents a pesky interference or additional stressor in the patient's hospitalization and treatment. Nurses should lead the team of health professionals who welcome and embrace the involvement of families in every care setting. In most situations, the family represents a rich source of information and support for the patient. An important role for nursing involves tailoring each plan of care to include the family in interventions that will assist the patient's reintegration back into the family unit following discharge.

THE *HEALTHY PEOPLE 2010* NATIONAL INITIATIVE

The family is the starting point for societal changes needed to ensure the health of families in the future. The national initiative *Healthy People 2010* outlines objectives and indicators that provide the basis for interventions, education, and policy on improving health in this decade. All of the indicators encompassed in this important national health initiative have an impact on the family, such as physical activity, overweight and obesity, tobacco use, substance abuse, responsible sexual behavior, mental health, injury and violence, environmental quality, immunization, and access to health care (USDHHS, 2000). Target areas concerning social policy and access to health care for families are underscored in the charge to "… reduce the proportion of families that experience difficulties or delays in obtaining health care or do not receive needed care for one or more family members" (Hitchcock, Schubert, & Thomas, 2003, p. 435).

Families Today

The family is widely defined by many different sources reflective of the social, biological, and legal domains (Friedman, Bowden, & Jones, 2003; Harmon Hanson et al., 2005). Various definitions describe members who comprise the family, their interdependence, and methods of interaction. A **family** consists of two or more members who self-identify as a "family" and interact and depend on one another socially, emotionally, and financially (Harmon Hanson, 2005). Most often, family structure involves either the **family of origin** (the family that reared the individual) or the **family of choice** (the family adopted through marriage or cohabitation). A single person belongs to a family of origin, but may choose not to become a member of a family of choice. A single individual cannot constitute a family. Instead, most definitions of family include a prerequisite of at least one other person who is self-defined as being a part of the family (Harmon Hanson et al., 2005; Friedman et al., 2003; Wright & Leahey, 2005).

 Nursing Insight— *Differentiating among various family configurations*

In contemporary society, the traditional **nuclear family**, which consists of a male partner, female partner and their children, actually represents only a small number of families. Other family members, termed **extended family**, may also live in the same household. According to the Urban Institute, there are five categories of families (Wherry & Finegold, 2004):

1. The **married-parent family** includes biological or adoptive parents. This family structure accounts for approximately 64% of American families. It describes 69% of Caucasian, 55% of Hispanic, and 26.6% of African American families (Wherry & Finegold, 2004).
2. The **single-parent family** consists of an unmarried biological or adoptive parent who may or may not be living with other adults (Wherry & Finegold, 2004). The **homosexual family** (lesbian and gay) consists of same-sex partners who live together with or without children. This family structure may also consist of single gay or lesbian parents or multiple parenting figures (Friedman et al., 2003).
3. The **married-blended family**, formed as a result of death or divorce, consists of unrelated family members who join together to form a new household.
4. The **cohabiting-parent family** describes one in which children live with two unmarried biological parents or two adoptive parents.
5. The **no-parent family** is one in which children live independently in foster or kinship care, such as living with a grandparent or aunt.

 Ethnocultural Considerations— **Patterns of family structure**

Patterns of family structure tend to be culturally influenced. For example, Hispanic children are more than twice as likely as African American children to live in cohabiting-parent families and they are approximately four times as likely as Caucasian children to live in this type of family configuration (Wherry & Finegold, 2004).

THE CHANGING FAMILY AS REFLECTED IN THE MEDIA

Family changes and adaptations from the Cro-Magnon era to the present day have been well researched and documented, but it is useful to examine the more recent changes that have taken place over the past 20 to 40 years. During this time, family structure and roles have changed rapidly and at present seem to be in a state of flux. As American families transition and evolve, television and theater often provide useful insights into the predominant family themes of the time.

For example, in the 1950s and 1960s, a nuclear family was presented with little emphasis on the extended family. Programs such as *Ozzie and Harriet*, *Leave It to Beaver*, *The Dick Van Dyke Show*, and *Father Knows Best* portrayed the typical family as one that included the mother and father along with one to three children. Family roles typically portrayed a father-dominated household and a homemaker mother who would occasionally flex her decision-making authority when the father's advice did not work. Issues were generally simple and resolvable with an occasional foray into societal issues such as racism or mental health. When problems such as alcoholism were presented, they tended to be in the context of an outsider who temporarily touched the family and then left. Rarely was there depiction of a serious internal family mental health problem. Instead, scenarios involved events such as girlfriend–boyfriend situational crises or friend-related peer pressure. Occasional variations in family structure were offered in weekly programs such as *Bonanza*, *Family Affair*, and *My Three Sons* that portrayed households run by males who received assistance from a housekeeper or relative.

Programming during the 1960s and early 1970s reflected a growing trend toward themes that included blended families with shows such as *The Brady Bunch*. These weekly programs tended to present upper income families with housekeepers and stay-at-home mothers who deferred major decisions to the father. Widowhood, as opposed to divorce, usually constituted the reason for remarrying, and this situation neatly sidestepped the unpleasantness of a broken home resulting from divorce.

Family issues continued to relate primarily to difficulties associated with school and dating. Major breakthroughs were achieved with *All in the Family*, *The Jeffersons*, *What's Happening*, and other sit-coms in the 1970s that dealt with the turbulent issues of civil rights and sex equality and changing views on race and gender.

During this time, there were also shows that began to present selected variations of family. For example, *The Mary Tyler Moore Show* centered on a career woman whose close work relationships served as a central component of family. *Gilligan's Island* presented family-like associations that dealt with work or survival issues as a team and shared support and platonic love and loyalty that would have normally been received from a family. The 1990s to 2000s version of this theme was expanded in *Friends* and *Seinfeld*, programs that introduced the idea that people could remain single longer without the expectation that a family was defined by marriage and procreation. This trend is again reflected in more recent programs such as *Grey's Anatomy*, where unrelated individuals form a family with "ties" that sometimes are actually stronger than those with their biological relatives who may not always "be there" for them.

Television programs during the 1980s and 1990s also began to address variations in social class and politics with shows such as *Family Ties*, which explored social issues such as premarital sex, dealing with the death of friends, and Alzheimer's disease. Interestingly, the episodes did not always present a clean resolution of an issue but instead focused on the importance of family closeness and support in dealing with the problem within the context of battling political views. *The Cosby Show* depicted a African American upper middle-class family in which both parents were white-collar professionals.

The 1990s brought increased awareness of the challenges facing families dealing with poverty, alcoholism, and abuse within their own ranks rather than as a problem that occurred only outside of the family. *Grace Under Fire* presented a single head of household who was a recovering alcoholic. *Roseanne* revolved around a matriarchal family structure in a lower economic setting where both parents had to work to make ends meet. One particular episode in this series dealt with how to write a check in a way that delayed cashing (and subsequently, "bouncing") it, to allow extra time for sufficient funds to be deposited into the account.

Television sitcoms in the new millennium continue to reflect trends consistent with societal changes. Family structures such as the binuclear arrangement (two intact nuclear families sharing a home), and the divorced family living with a brother and sharing responsibility for rearing a son (*Two and a Half Men*) are examples of alternate family themes that have emerged in recent times. Programs such as these may be preparing the way for shows that depict same-sex unions with or without children.

Also reflective of contemporary society is the trend of sitcoms that feature extended family members such as the live-in father in *King of Queens* and the very intrusive parents in *Everybody Loves Raymond*. The success of the movie *My Big Fat Greek Wedding* opened the door for depicting ethnic families that were keeping their own values and beliefs separate from those of the prevailing culture. Hispanic, Jewish, Asian, and other ethnic groups have revealed their differences in humorous but culturally sensitive ways. The media, however, generally provides only a superficial representation of the varied and complex challenges faced by the modern-day family.

 Collaboration in Caring— *Five functions of the family*

1. Physical Needs: Meets the primary basic needs such as food, water, clothing, and shelter.
2. Economic Needs: Access to enough financial resources to adequately meet the family's needs and wishes.
3. Reproductive Needs: Ways that add new life to the family unit and maintain a healthy sexual relationship between parents.
4. Affective and Coping Needs: Strategies to deal with everyday stresses of life and encourage a nurturing environment.
5. Socialization Needs: Processes whereby families acquire the skills, knowledge, attitudes, and values necessary for performing their social roles.

STRESSORS ON FAMILIES TODAY

Health Care

Today's families face varied and complex challenges. Baby boomers are aging and entering retirement. This shift in the contemporary workforce leaves openings and shortages in critical areas such as education and health care and at the same time adds increased demands on a health care system already burdened with an aging population. For many, insurance coverage changes and often becomes more expensive as retirees transition from employment insurance to retirement insurance options such as Medicare and Social Security. In many instances, families have no options for insurance because of part-time work or unemployment.

At present, more than 45 million families in the United States are uninsured (U.S. Department of Health and Human Services [DHHS], 2005b) and as many as 13.5 million individuals have been homeless at some point during their lifetime (Harmon Hanson et al., 2005). All too frequently, families are counted among these staggering statistics. Health issues among homeless families and individuals are numerous and usually result from a lack of preventive care and a lack of resources in general. For example, in addition to the problems associated with extreme poverty, homeless women are at an increased risk for illness and injury and many have been victims of rape, assault, and domestic abuse (American College of Obstetricians and Gynecologists [ACOG], 2005).

The rural homeless are more likely to be families who are living with other families or migrant workers who live in vehicles and follow crop harvesting. Access to health care and discrimination in health care practices are major problems for this population. At present, there are approximately 3 million migrant and seasonal farm workers in the United States, and of these, 21% are women. Although the workers represent a number of ethnic and cultural groups, 75% were born in Mexico, 81% speak Spanish, their average age is 33, and the majority have not been educated beyond the seventh grade (U.S. Department of Labor National Agricultural Workers Survey, 2005). As the nation becomes more culturally diverse, there is a growing imperative to eliminate racial and ethnic health care disparities by providing ready access to quality care for diverse populations (Weissman et al., 2005).

 Nursing Insight— *Health care resources for women without U.S. citizenship*

Approximately 26% of women who do not have U.S. citizenship lack a regular health care provider and 45.5% have no health insurance coverage. Their access to health care is further compromised by policies that restrict Medicaid eligibility for this population (Kaiser Commission, 2003a). In a study that compared the health care costs of immigrants to those of U.S. citizens, it was found that total health care expenditures for immigrant adults and children were significantly lower than those of U.S.-born citizens (Mohanty et al., 2005).

Mental Illness

Other problems that arise from both internal and external causes also impact families. In any given year, an estimated 57 million individuals and their families deal with mental illness (U.S. Census Bureau, 2005). Affected families not only face dealing with a potentially chronic illness that continues to be stigmatized by society, but they also must grapple with paying for treatment of a diagnosis that is largely exempt from insurance coverage. Challenges that come from external forces outside of the family system include environmental assaults such as catastrophic weather, forest fires, and earthquakes. An entire region of families continues to be affected by problems that follow in the aftermath of hurricanes, fires, and floods.

Nursing Insight— Recognizing the relationship between family stressors and poor health outcomes

Families may have multiple stressors that increase their vulnerability to poor health outcomes. Problems such as substance abuse, mental illness, domestic violence, and limited access to medical care due to unemployment, loss of medical insurance, or inadequate insurance coverage can affect families across all strata of society.

Societal Pressures

The family also faces societal pressures. The incidence of violent crimes has decreased in major urban areas, but suicide among children and adolescents continues to represent an important societal issue. The number of families currently affected by AIDS is increasing at a startling rate. Women and children, a vulnerable population due to barriers associated with access to health care, constitute the fastest growing segment of the population to contract HIV. Public education is in a state of crisis as demands increase on teachers who are confronted with diminishing resources.

These and many other issues continue to challenge families. Meanwhile, family structure and roles are undergoing changes that frequently increase the potential for further family problems. Present trends show a diminishing number of nuclear family households. The traditional family structure is being replaced by one that includes a single head of household, most frequently a divorced or abandoned mother. The number of unmarried mothers continues to increase. Statistics reflect the current trend: the percentage of children living with two married parents decreased from 85% in 1970 to 68% in 2004. A divorced or single woman is usually the head of household in those families, although recently there has been an increase in single male head of household families from 1% to 5% (Child Trends Data Bank, 2006). In other situations, the head of household is homosexual or sharing a home with a same-sex partner.

These trends reflect increasing opportunities for alternative forms of parenthood within contemporary American society. The nontraditional parenting arrangements result from more liberal social mores as well as the technological and medical advances that now offer the possibility of parenthood to single men and women (Greenfield, 2005). Homosexuality and same-sex partnerships/marriages and their effects on the family raise political, social, and religious issues that have increasingly found their way into present-day discussions. Although the far-reaching impact of same-sex relationships on family structure and function has not been adequately studied, areas that frequently must be addressed concern child custody, legal consent, power of attorney, and confidentiality. The following case study provides an example of some of the issues and questions that may need to be addressed by the family and the patient's care providers.

❝ **What to say** ❞ *— Effective tools for families*

Covey (2006) discusses effective tools that may enhance family performance. The nurse can communicate these principles to families that may promote healthy family functioning.

- Be proactive: Become an agent of change in the family.
- Begin with the end in mind: Develop a family mission statement.
- Put first things first: Make the family a priority in a turbulent world.
- Think "win–win": Move from me to we.
- Seek first to understand then be understood: Solve family problems through empathetic communication.
- Synergize: Build family unity through celebrating differences.
- Sharpen the saw: Renew family spirit through traditions.

 case study The Family with Same-Sex Partners

Julia, a 37-year old comatose woman, is dying of ovarian cancer. She is on life support in the hospital. The family, which includes ex-husband, Dan, and two children—John, age 12 and Tami, age 14—has gathered in the visitors' lounge. Cindy, Julia's life partner, is also present in the lounge. The family is discussing whether to extend Julia's present level of care or to begin to wean her from life support. Although Julia has a living will, there is concern and conflict among the family members and Cindy regarding how and when the will should be honored. Dan questions the appropriateness of Cindy's being in attendance for the discussion.

1. What would the nurse need to know to help the family problem-solve in this situation?

2. What resources are available to the family and the nursing staff to help clarify these issues?

◆ See Suggested Answers to Case Studies in text on the Electronic Study Guide or DavisPlus.

The **skip generation**, an arrangement in which the grandparents rear grandchildren with or without the parents' help, describes another present-day variation in family structure. In 1994, 16% of preschool children of working parents were cared for by a grandparent. Today, 2.4 million grandparents assume primary responsibility for more than 6 million children and many of these households do not have the children's parents living in the home with them (AARP, 2006).

 Now Can You— Discuss contemporary family changes and stressors?

1. Define family and identify five family categories?
2. Identify three changes in family structure that have been highlighted in the media?
3. Identify five stressors faced by the American family today?

Family Theories and Models

Development of a specialized body of knowledge provides the foundation for a profession. While nursing theories and models are essential in defining nursing and nursing practice, theories from other disciplines are important in providing insights into other dimensions of health and human behavior. For example, family theory, which draws from a number of related disciplines (Harmon Hanson et al., 2005), helps to guide assessment and intervention within a holistic framework that views the entire family as client. The following discussion presents several theoretical models representing a cross section of useful concepts to assist in the nursing assessment and to facilitate a creative application to various family interactions.

FAMILY SYSTEMS THEORY

A systems approach to understanding the family centers on the recognition that changes that occur in one member affect the entire family. The family systems theory, which views persons as "open systems," has at its central theme: "The sum of the parts is greater than the whole" (Harmon Hanson et al., 2005). According to this theory, the family shares a unique identity that is far more complex than that of its collective members. The family is dynamic, constantly adjusting to information that filters in from the surrounding environment and from within the family.

 Nursing Insight— *Clinical application of the family systems theory*

When working with families, the nurse uses the family systems theory to "view the family as a unit and focus on observing the interaction among family members rather than studying family members individually" (Wright & Leahey, 2005).

The following situation helps to illustrate application of the family systems theory: An addicted member receives help for the addiction and then returns to the family system. The changes in the recovering family member have a significant impact on how the entire family acts and reacts. A new system of communication is established. In the new system, the family members communicate assertively and supportively with each other and no longer adhere to the former framework of denial that a problem exists and secret keeping. The nurse working with the family recognizes that teaching and referrals to appropriate community resources are most likely be needed to facilitate the family's healthy adjustment to the changes.

Boundaries

Another concept inherent in family systems theory concerns boundaries. Each system contains a boundary that affects how the outside world is allowed to interact with the family members. Stated another way, boundaries identify the family's control of how the family system interacts with the outside world. A family whose children obtain food and shelter by begging from the neighbors demonstrates a problem with boundaries that are too permeable. Permeability refers to the degree that information and interchange are allowed to flow between systems. An ideal system is one that is semipermeable. In a semipermeable system, the boundaries are secure enough to keep the family intact, but still allow for free interchange with the outside world. In this situation, the family system readily interacts with outside systems. A healthy family has a semipermeable boundary that allows and encourages interaction with outside agencies such as work, school, church, and family, and friends.

A closed boundary serves to keep family secrets inside and therapeutic interventions outside. Closed boundaries often occur in families with issues of addiction or abuse.

Families of alcoholics soon learn not to disclose information about their problems to outsiders. Conversely, a family that is so lacking in structure that it allows an uninterrupted free flow of information/intervention to and from outsiders can be said to have an open boundary or no boundary at all. For example, an open boundary exists with a family whose children are so neglected that they rely on friends or neighbors to feed them.

 Nursing Insight— *Recognizing the childbearing family's boundary permeability*

The extent to which the **suprasystem** (the broad system that surrounds the family unit, such as the cultural community) influences the childbearing family's participation in activities such as childbirth education, prenatal care, and infant care is dependent upon the family's boundary permeability.

Subsystems

Family systems are further divided into subsystems. A family of four may constitute the "main" system. The mother and father represent a subsystem that has a permanent or temporary relationship that is a part of, yet separate from, the main family system. Children often form alliances with other siblings or with one parent. A subsystem can develop when a sibling marries or cohabits with another individual who is temporarily or permanently accepted into the family. Subsystems are necessary parts of family functioning, especially in health crisis situations when families must make decisions for sick or disabled members, or when new dependent members join the family. For example, the birth of a baby introduces a new member who becomes part of the family system, but is also a subsystem with the mother or father or other family caregiver(s).

 Ethnocultural Considerations— **Boundaries and receptivity to information**

Families that have recently immigrated to this country may be receptive to health information only from extended family members or from persons within their cultural community.

Balance and Homeostasis

The family system continually strives to return to balance or achieve homeostasis after a crisis. When a family member is sick or injured, or when an emergency arises that requires a reorganization of the family (i.e., an evacuation during a storm), the family quickly attempts to return to former routines and rules as a way of reestablishing homeostasis. At certain times the family is unable to return to former normalcy and instead must adjust or form adaptive behaviors. For example, the family may learn to work with a wheelchair and other adaptive devices when a member suffers a stroke or spinal cord injury. Over time, adaptations become the norm for the family.

Maladaptive behaviors are an alternate adaptation that involves the use of unhealthy or abnormal behaviors to adapt to a family crisis. Enabling and codependency are common maladaptive behaviors that are often adopted by an addictive family (Townsend, 2005). Enabling involves making excuses or obtaining substances for the addictive family member. Codependency is a maladaptive behavior in which the nonaddicted family member joins the addicted member in the use of alcohol or other substances as a way of interacting or communicating.

FAMILY DEVELOPMENTAL STAGES AND THEORY

Developmental theory (Friedman et al., 2003; Harmon Hanson et al., 2005) has at its core the idea that every life moves through developmental stages with tasks that need to be accomplished before moving on to the next stage. Duvall identifies eight family stages: beginning, childbearing, preschool children, school-age, teenagers, launching, middle-aged, and retirement (Friedman et al., 2003). Each stage is accompanied by specific tasks that are performed to assist with the physical and emotional development of the family members in that particular stage.

When working with families, the nurse should identify what stage(s) the family is in and assess how well the needs for that particular stage are being met. Learning, attachment, and grieving represent specific tasks that are affected by the developmental stage. Teaching needs and nursing interventions are structured and implemented according to the developmental stages of the family and its members. Although the stages follow one another in a linear progression, some families may simultaneously be in more than one stage or they may revert to previous stages (Wilkinson & Van Leuven, 2007).

Beginning Families

Beginning families are those that have just been formed through marriage or that self-identify as family, as in the case of common-law unions. The beginning family identifies shared goals that may include career paths, home-building, and planning for children. Creating shared time together in order to build the relationship constitutes a central developmental task for all families and this special together time traditionally is initiated during the honeymoon period. Combined households and property are common features of all families. One of the limitations of Duvall's theory concerns its application with the childless family. If the family has no children, many of the developmental stages are not applicable until the couple reaches middle age and beyond. If the family does have a child, the family developmental stage parallels the age of the child. When more than one child is present, the family is usually in more than one developmental stage.

Childbearing Stage

The childbearing developmental stage begins with conception. Early tasks during this stage include seeking prenatal care and planning for space for the child. If there are other children already in the home, the family begins to prepare and socialize the other children into a sibling role. Ideally, the family involves the children in decision making related to preparation for the expected baby. For example, siblings can help to choose paint colors for the baby's room or offer advice regarding toys or clothes to select for the baby. When the baby is born, the family must adapt its routines to include the various tasks associated with feeding and caring for the baby. Family teaching needs may include dealing with sleep pattern disturbances related to feeding and changing diapers through the night. Along with strategies for successfully coping with these adjustments, the nurse can offer support and reassurance. The nurse assesses the family's readiness and openness to learn and receive help (an open boundary) and, according to specific needs, may provide additional information concerning nutrition, the importance of well-baby visits, car seats, immunization schedules and infant crib monitors.

> ### Optimizing Outcomes— Applying developmental theory when caring for the childbearing family
>
> An understanding of the normal phases of the life cycle helps the nurse to provide anticipatory guidance for the childbearing family. Strategies to bolster the young child's sense of security when a newborn is brought home may divert a potential family crisis.

Preschool Stage

The preschool developmental stage includes toddlerhood and attending kindergarten. During this stage, the child has learned to walk and actively explore her world, which encompasses siblings and other family members and friends. At this time, families need information about the prevention of injuries and interventions for accidents that usually result from the child's increased motor abilities coupled with less-developed judgment and coordination. The nurse should be alert for signs of abuse or neglect during this stage. Points of contact that allow the nurse to assess developmental progress occur during well-child checks, immunization appointments and office or hospital visits for the child or other family members.

School-Age and Adolescent/Teenage Stages

The school-age and adolescent/teenage developmental stages provide the optimal opportunity for teaching about drugs, sex, and health promotion. Personal values are shaped and clarified and ethical development occurs during this time. Surveys have shown that nurses are included among the top ten trusted people sought by school-aged children to discuss issues important to them.

Launching, Middle Age, and Retirement Stages

The launching, middle-age, and retirement developmental stages bring the family full-circle back to the early issues of self and couple-building with less emphasis on children (if successfully launched) and more involvement in community and hobby-related interests. The young adult who is not successfully launched from the childhood home presents a complication of incomplete launching. This situation may represent a temporary arrangement necessary for continuing education or it may provide a convenient and economical "non-action" by the son or daughter until ties with others have been established. The nurse's role in this situation is to assess whether the living arrangement creates a problem (e.g., anger, frustration, and delay in meeting goals) for either the parents or the child. Interventions may include strategies to improve communication between the parents and the child and/or community referrals for assistance with goal setting and vocational training.

STRUCTURAL–FUNCTIONAL THEORY

Structural–functional theory focuses on the functioning of the family and the roles assumed by each family member to promote family function. Necessary roles include provider, housekeeper, child caregiver, socializer, sexual partner, therapist, recreational organizer, and kinship member. Although a family member often assumes more than one role, some roles may be exclusive to only one identified member. This arrangement takes on added significance concerning the family's ability to move forward when a member is unable to fulfill his or her exclusive role (Friedman et al., 2003; Harmon Hanson et al., 2005; Wright & Leahey, 2005). According to structural–functional theory, if any of the roles are not managed by one or more members of the family, problems such as disorganization, deficits in hygiene, isolation, and other negative situations will emerge that may require a nurse's intervention to help the family return to balance (Harmon Hanson et al., 2005).

Provider Role

The provider role is the money-earner or the resource gatherer. One or more family members pay the bills and distribute resources to other family members for clothing, food, and recreation. If the provider is sick or hospitalized, the family identifies an alternate provider to temporarily meet that need or identify other resources such as savings, insurance, or public assistance in order to pay bills.

Housekeeper

During recent years, the housekeeper role has evolved from the traditional stay-at-home mother as increasing numbers of women are engaged in full-time employment outside of the home. Housekeeping involves not only the physical cleaning and maintenance of the family environment but also the organization of family duties to maintain a stable, healthy living situation for the family.

Child-Caregiver

The child-caregiver role is assumed by the person (usually the mother) who is designated as the primary care provider for the children. This role is performed by a designated member such as the mother, father, grandmother, or uncle, depending on the family structure. Someone (i.e., childcare facility, babysitter) is responsible to ensure that the children are supervised and cared for even when the primary child-caregiver is away from home.

Socializer and Recreational Organizer

The socializer and recreational organizer roles may not be as consciously directed as the previous roles, but they encompass how the family interacts with others. Initially, the parents or guardians may arrange interactions for the children through family and friend gatherings, trips, and activities. Eventually, most members begin to organize their own social events through personal friendship choices and preferred activities outside the home. Socialization is taught by the family and may be a role that is shared equally among family members unless a problem occurs. Family trips, holidays, and birthdays are important events that teach family patterns that children will later use to help them develop their own family's social and recreational roles.

Sexual Partner

The sexual partner role should exist between the parental units. Variations exist in different family structures. In every structure, children should have education and role modeling on how to interact in socially and sexually appropriate ways. Healthy family interactions constitute the first defense against abuse and violence.

Therapist

The therapist role is assumed when one family member expresses concern for another's health or emotional well-being. For example, concern about the husband's blood pressure prompts the wife to make a doctor's appointment for him. The therapist role can also involve active listening and other expressions of caring as family members help one other through a loss or a crisis.

Kinship

The family member who organizes family reunions, corresponds with friends, sends birthday and holiday greetings, and reminds children to write thank-you notes assumes the kinship role. The wife most often assumes this role and is charged with the responsibility of remembering important dates for her spouse's family as well as for her own.

 Optimizing Outcomes— Applying the structural–functional theory

Structural–functional theories view the family as a social system and focus on outcomes, not process. Nurses can use structural–functional theory to assess how well the family functions internally among family members and externally with outside systems.

COMMUNICATION THEORY

Communication theory asserts that emotional problems result from the way people interact with each other in the context of the family (Harmon Hanson et al., 2005). Healthy families have clear rules such as "we don't interrupt each other when speaking" or "we don't yell at each other." Communication is clear and congruent and nonverbal cues match what is being said. Unhealthy families give mixed or double-binding messages, which are statements accompanied by nonverbal expressions that are inconsistent and incongruent with the verbal message. Healthy families communicate love and support clearly and often. Verbal communication is matched by nonverbal communication (such as hugs, voice tone, and eye-contact) that supports the intended message. Families check with each other to make sure the intended meaning is understood. For example, a parent explains; "I am setting a curfew because I care about you and want you to be safe. Does that make sense to you?" The parent then encourages discussion to ensure clarity and understanding of the purpose of curfew.

💮 *Nursing Insight*— *Family communication patterns*

Patterns of family communication reveal much about family functioning. In addition to providing information about "who is saying what and to whom," they also convey information about the structure and functions of family relationships in relation to the power base, decision-making processes, affection, trust, and coalitions. Dysfunctional communication inhibits healthy nurturing and diminishes personal feelings of self-esteem and self-worth.

The nurse or family therapist assesses a repeating negative pattern such as excessive drinking to determine if it has been replaced instead by an assertive yet supportive and positive communication. For example, a wife complains to the nurse that her husband drinks more whenever they have an argument about their children. The husband notes that his wife complains to him about the children whenever he tries to relax by drinking. The nurse educates the family that interventions regarding either the arguing or the drinking could help to break the pattern of negative communication and refers them to a support group or a counselor to learn new patterns.

GROUP THEORY

Group theory can be applied to the family as a group. Norms (rules of conduct), roles, goals, and power structure are inherent family concepts along with the division of household chores, expectations of completed homework, and curfew enforcement. According to group theory, stages of groups (forming, storming, norming, performing, and adjourning/terminating) explain expected behaviors that occur in any given stage (Clark, 2003; Johnson & Johnson, 2003).

Forming describes the beginning phase of the group. In families, the forming stage usually occurs through marriage or cohabitation. Storming, the next stage, is the disordered time of confusion or chaos when two or more distinct personalities discover their differences. Norming describes how groups (or families) adjust to individual members by applying rules and procedures that the members agree to obey. Performing is the ideal stage in which the group (i.e., the family) accomplishes their goals and produces results. In the family, desirable results would include good citizenship, education and health of its members, and active contribution to society. Adjourning/terminating represents the final stage in a group when it has accomplished its goals and disbands to possibly form a different group. Families experience this stage when members die, divorce, or leave the family to begin their own families.

Since families represent long-term relationships anchored in the performing stage of meeting goals and taking care of one another, the stages tend to be more stable than with groups. Forming occurs when a child is brought into the family by birth or by adoption. Storming describes the emotional clashes that occur during times of transition (i.e., an adolescent testing the rules) or crisis (i.e., adjusting to a move or job change). Norming generally occurs when parental rules are imposed. For example, family norming may involve teaching the children to talk more softly inside the house than when playing in the yard. Performing occurs as each family member performs specific duties to accomplish the daily tasks of life. Adjourning or termination may follow a death in the family, or it can also follow the launching of a high school graduate into college. The healthy family adjusts for the loss and resets roles and norms to fit the new family structure.

BOWEN'S FAMILY SYSTEMS THEORY

Family systems theory, based on Bowen's concepts, is useful when identifying family problems or challenges that are rooted in family processes such as communication, connecting between members, and teaching values (Harmon Hanson et al., 2005). The nuclear family emotional system describes the pattern of adaptive/maladaptive emotional expression that exists as a theme in the family. According to this theory, one family could be characterized as stoic or cold in their interactions with others, while another is described as emotional and highly reactive to situations and circumstances.

According to family systems theory, differentiation of self is demonstrated when a family member breaks away from the learned emotional system and instead expresses emotions that differ from the learned family pattern. For example, a father whose family of origin is nondemonstrative of love and caring may openly hug and kiss his spouse and children and verbally express his love for them. In an emotional cut-off, a family member has separated from the original family pattern in a dramatic and sometimes permanent way. This may occur when a family member who was reared in a dysfunctional family chooses not to perpetuate the learned pattern of alcoholism or abuse.

Family systems theory also views birth order as a predictor of certain patterns of behavior that may be desirable or conflicting, depending on the birth order of the chosen mate. A firstborn child with behaviors related to high responsibility and control may clash with a spouse who is also a firstborn. The "baby of the family" (youngest sibling) may seek out a spouse who was a firstborn to serve as a caretaker.

With the family systems approach, most interactions take place in the form of a duo or dyad. Triangulation occurs when the dyad diverts attention away from its own conflict by focusing on a third person such as the child, teacher of the problem child, or police officer who comes into a domestic disturbance. Police, nurses, and counselors have often taken the displaced anger of a couple they are trying to help and have instead unwittingly become the third part of a triangle.

The multigenerational transmission process describes how one learns or transmits family emotional systems across generations. Watching grandparents express affection teaches patterns to grandchildren who will model similar behaviors to their children (unless self-differentiation or an emotional cut-off changes the pattern). Family projection process is how and what children are taught. Societal regression describes patterns of the family projection process that exist in cultures as part of a dominant theme. For example, in the United States, independence and individuality are recognized as desirable qualities and thus are replicated throughout family culture. This is in contrast with some Asian cultures that value interdependence and the importance of being a part of a group.

NURSING THEORIES

Nursing theories define the family–nurse relationship in various ways. Nightingale viewed family as a support system for the primary patient. King described interactions that result in a shared or mutual transaction (similar to the nursing care plan). Roy placed family in the context of the adaptive system of the client. Neuman viewed families as systems and subsystems. According to this framework, the family can become the self-care agent of a patient who is unable to meet her own needs. Rogers described the family as an open system that interacts through the exchange of matter and energy (George, 2002).

Many nursing theorists and practitioners blend theories, which then become "integrated" nursing theories. Friedman et al. (2003) merged concepts from general systems theory and structural functional theory to form an assessment model. Harmon Hansen and colleagues (2005) used the family assessment intervention model with the Family Systems Stressor-Strength Inventory to apply Neuman's theory in a quantitative measurement tool for assessing families. The Calgary Family Assessment Model (Wright & Leahey, 2005) draws on postmodernism, systems theory, cybernetics, communication theory, change theory, and biology of cognition to form a multidimensional assessment model for family nursing care.

The theories described in this chapter have been selected for their clarity and applicability to a variety of family structures and situations. Many theories from nursing and related disciplines have utility in a range of family settings and can be successfully applied to guide and direct nursing care. Familiarization with a variety of theories allows for selection of the theory or theories that best fits the family nursing assessment and interventions. Nursing is both an art and a science. The science component involves the research of concepts and development of theories to describe phenomena. The art of nursing is the application of theory or theories to a specific family interaction.

 Now Can You— **Discuss family theory for nursing practice?**

1. Identify at least four types of theories used in family nursing?
2. Name three components of Bowen's Family Systems Theory?
3. Discuss a theory that describes stages experienced by the family during the life span of the children?

FAMILY ASSESSMENT

Theories are useful for helping to explain and categorize behaviors of individuals and families. The next logical step, applying theory to the assessment of families, provides information from which to base interventions to either improve or correct the family's health. The nurse is sensitive to family needs and is in a unique position to interact with the family during the assessment process.

THE NURSING ROLE IN FAMILY ASSESSMENT

It is difficult to fit modern American families into any particular mold. Variations in size and structure and parenting style, along with religious, cultural, and socioeconomic orientation all affect how the family deals with economic, educational, social, and health care issues. To guide the delivery of appropriate care to the family unit, it is helpful to examine the nurse's role in assessment and intervention and explore some of the major factors that influence family structure. During the assessment interview, the nurse addresses important concepts including family size and structure; parenting style; and religious, cultural, and socioeconomic orientation.

Family Size and Structure

Family size has generally decreased since the founding of the country when large families ensured more workers for the family business. As recently as one generation ago, families consisting of more than six members were more reflective of the norm than today's families that average two and a half children. Birth rates have declined in Caucasian families while remaining the same in some ethnic cultures. It has been predicted that by the year 2020, the "minority" family will represent 51% of the total American population.

Family structure is becoming increasingly different from the traditional two-parent, two-child nuclear family portrayed during the 1950s. Single-parent (mother or father head of household), binuclear (two families living together), skip-generation (grandparents rearing grandchildren), and extended family (grandparents or other relatives living with the nuclear family) are all represented in the American family of today.

Parenting Style

Parenting style is the manner in which knowledge and values first observed and ingrained during one's own upbringing and other observed experiences are then used in rearing one's own children. Parenting style includes discipline, communication, and distribution of power. Blue collar or working class families tend to view corporal punishment (usually in the form of spanking) as the normal approach to discipline. Conversely, white-collar (professional class) families favor disciplinary measures that include times-out, positive reinforcement, and other nonphysical methods. Three distinct styles of parenting have been identified:

- **Authoritarian** or **dictatorial:** Enforces absolute rule; parents enforce rules and strict expectations of each family member; children have little say in decision making and punishment follows any deviation from the established rules; punishment is not necessarily corporal but often includes withdrawal of approval; children from this style of parenting tend to be shy, sensitive, conforming, submissive, loyal, and honest.
- **Laissez-faire** or **permissive:** Allows the children control over their environment and subsequent behavior with less input from the parents; few rules to follow; children are able to make their own decisions; punishment is inconsistent when used; children from this family tend to be disrespectful, aggressive, and disobedient, possibly growing up to be irresponsible members of the community.
- **Authoritative** or **democratic:** Parents have a combination of characteristics from both the authoritarian and laissez-faire parenting styles; parents find a common ground between enforcing rules and allowing some freedom for their children to participate in decisions; parents are firm, set realistic standards and punishment centers on assisting the child develop an inner consciousness about behavior; produces children who are assertive, self-reliant, and highly interactive with high self-esteem (Wilson, Hockenberry-Eaton, Winkelstein, & Schwartz, 2001). Although each type of parenting style has benefits and drawbacks, authoritative parenting tends to meet the child's needs better than the other styles.

The nurse recognizes that disciplining children is an important concept for parents to understand. Discipline is training the child to meet a pattern of behavior with the intention of instilling good moral judgment, achieving competence and maintaining self-control, promoting self-direction, and learning to respect others. Consistency with rule setting is a key concept that parents must understand. A reliable and steady discipline approach by parents reinforces to the child that their misbehavior will be corrected. Often, redirecting the child away from the behavior to alternative activity can be an effective way to discipline. With older children, reasoning or explaining to the child why the behavior is unacceptable may also be useful. The nurse can help parents understand that positive and effective child-rearing practices can be straightforward and firm without being negative or abusive.

During the family parenting-style assessment, the nurse observes for indicators of neglect or physical abuse, but otherwise supports consistent and predictable consequences and rewards appropriate to the age of the child. Parents should be given information about disciplining consistently and without anger. When indicated, parents can be referred to parenting courses or support groups.

Religious, Cultural, and Socioeconomic Orientation

Religious orientation has varying effects on families. The majority of Americans claim some affiliation with a church or spiritual group, but fewer than 30% actually attend a spiritual institution on a regular basis (McIntosh, 2004). Values that tend to be rooted in religious beliefs include practices concerning the observation of holidays and beliefs toward abortion, birth control, marriage, and advance directives (legal documentation that directs that "no heroic" measures be taken to extend life).

Religion also influences attitudes toward alternate lifestyle choices such as homosexuality and sexual abstinence and other moral choices such as euthanasia or suicide. Religious beliefs can provide comfort and a sense of peace to believers in times of sickness or grieving. Religion-based movements such as the "Promise-Keepers" and the "Million Man March" were created, in part, as a positive force to encourage men to become more responsible fathers and husbands.

The nurse assesses the family's religious or spiritual affiliation and, when indicated, assists in contacting the appropriate spiritual advisor or clergy member. Hospitals provide clergy and chaplain services for a variety of needs and occasions. The nurse avoids imposing personal beliefs and values on the family, but instead helps them obtain the resources necessary to help them to regain balance in crisis situations.

Cultural orientation includes family communication styles, structure of family, health beliefs, and power distribution. The nurse assesses family cultural affiliation and avoids generalities or stereotypes by validating all cultural information with the family.

✸ Ethnocultural Considerations— When assessing families

It is important for the nurse to be aware of ethnocultural variations that may exist in family structure and communication styles. Many cultures emphasize the extended family to a much greater extent than the American nuclear family. Often, grandparents as well as aunts, uncles, and cousins may be considered a part of the primary family. In some Native American tribes, a sister or aunt or grandparent may be the primary caretaker of the family and this individual needs to be included in health planning and teaching. Certain cultures give preference to the matriarch while others are more male-dominated. In some Hispanic cultures, the adult son makes health care decisions for the family. Nonverbal forms of communication can vary widely across cultures. There may be differences in eye contact, the practice of formal and informal touch, the level and tone of voice, and how respect is shown. A nod by individuals in some Pacific Rim countries may be an indicator of respect but does not necessarily convey an understanding of the nursing instructions given. Although a family member translator may be comforting to the family, this situation is not reflective of best practice methods, especially for informed consent purposes. Instead, a non-family professional translator should be used (Ehrlich, McCloskey, & Daly, 2004; Wilkinson & Van Leuven, 2007).

Socioeconomic status impacts the family's ability to access and pay for health care and other services. The nurse assists with referrals to social workers or other community experts to secure resources appropriate to the family's needs. Available resources include state and government supplemental programs, insurance sources, loans and grants, and church or community programs that aid families through catastrophic losses such as fire or health crises.

Historically recognized as important advocates for the family, nurses lead efforts to change or adjust laws and legislation to assist and empower families in areas such as child care, elder care, work leave for births or care of sick family members, tax breaks for dependents including elderly members, assistance with health care costs, and public service education for health care choices. Legislation concerning helmets, seat belts, and child safety seats illustrates several government interventions designed to foster and enhance the well-being of families and individuals. Policies concerning stem-cell research, same-sex marriage, property laws, pro-choice rights, and minimum wages are but a few examples of the government's far-reaching impact on the family.

TOOLS TO FACILITATE THE FAMILY ASSESSMENT

Qualitative and Quantitative Surveys

For most hospital settings, assessment of the family is limited to gathering a history, usually during admission, related to the patient's illness. However, in a family nursing approach that encompasses care of the entire family, more thorough formats for family assessment are used. Friedman et al. (2003), Harmon Hanson et al. (2005), Wright and Leahey (2005), and others have developed family nursing assessment forms to provide either a qualitative or a quantitative view of the family. A variety of assessment tools are available and those frequently used include surveys, genograms, ecomaps, and strengths and problems lists.

Qualitative tools assess the description and depth of family experiences. **Quantitative** tools measure the frequency with which behaviors or situations exist. Most survey tools emphasize either the qualitative or quantitative dimensions of family, but usually contain elements of both. Friedman et al. (2003) have developed both a long form and a short form to qualitatively assess the roles and structure of the family and its members. Harmon Hanson et al. (2005)

utilize the Family Systems Stressors-Strength Inventory, an instrument that elicits a numbered ranking of each family member's perception of the severity of stressors in selected categories. Wright and Leahey (2000) use the Calgary Family Assessment Model (CFAM) and combine this tool with the Calgary Family Intervention Model (CFIM) to provide a complete assessment and treatment map.

Before implementation of the selected assessment tool, agreements and sometimes written consents are obtained that relate to the confidentiality of the information sought, how it will be used, and what treatment options and referrals may be recommended. Before the assessment, it is important for the family to understand that the nurse is legally bound to mandatory reporting obligations in cases of abuse or violence, and also that member safety remains a priority above all other interventions. Following these disclosures, or "ground rules," the family may choose to end the therapeutic relationship with the nurse before any information is shared.

Genogram and Ecomap

Family assessment usually begins with a simple diagram (of the family history) in the form of a **genogram** (Fig. 3-1). A genogram is a set of symbols that is used to illustrate the present family structure and compare generations within the same family. The genogram may be used to highlight generational influences of behaviors, illnesses, vocational information, or any other pertinent information that provides a larger picture of patterns that exert influence on the family's current situation. Dates of births, divorces, deaths, stillbirths, and other pertinent elements of family information are represented. A key to guide interpretation of the various symbols is included on the form. Depending on the situation, the nurse either assists the family in drawing the genogram or instructs them in producing a genogram that will be reviewed during the next assessment visit. To make the information more meaningful to the assessor, the genogram should include at least three family generations.

The nurse also helps the family create an ecomap. An ecomap is a tool that displays the various outside systems used by the family. An ecomap illustrates the relationship between the family as a whole system and the various systems with which the family most often interacts, including school, job, church, and other institutions (Fig. 3-2).

To create a family ecomap, the nurse inquires about schools, health care agencies, employment, church, and other outside systems with which the family has routine interaction. Families may have closed boundaries with some systems and maintain open boundaries with others. For example, the parents may conduct home schooling yet contract with the public schools to provide their children with opportunities for extracurricular involvement. During the family assessment, the nurse looks for balance and self-regulation in the family system.

Strengths and Problems Lists

Early in the assessment process, the nurse asks the family to list their strengths (strengths list). The strengths list gives the family an opportunity to express the positive characteristics, or attributes, of their family as a whole and strengths that each member brings to the constellation. The family also creates a problems list, which identifies the difficult or negative characteristics. The family and the nurse collaboratively create both lists. The nurse can

provide input based on observations related to the family's strengths and weaknesses, but should not take over this process. In the therapeutic situation, the family must assume ownership of all identified strengths and problems so that they can participate fully during the assessment and treatment phases of the nursing intervention. The nurse helps the family focus on major issues or problems that will form the starting point of intervention.

Next, the family makes a commitment with the nurse and appropriate referral agencies to participate in the mutually agreed upon interventions. Depending on the situation, the family may be assisted in completion of the assessment tools or the tools may be given to each member to complete and return at a later date. Usually, more tools are completed when the family is assisted with this task in the nurse's presence.

The nurse compiles and summarizes the information provided and discusses the results with the family. The initial assessment, which utilizes the selected assessment

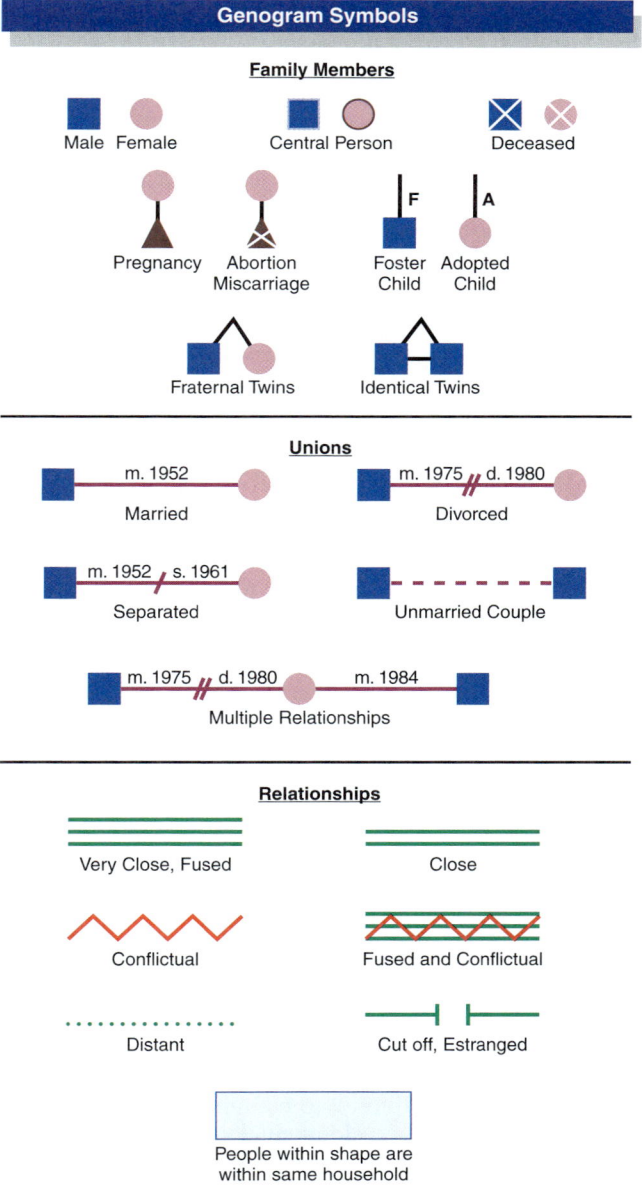

Figure 3-1 Example of a genogram template.

Our "Identified Family" consists of Helen, Chris, Molly and Brett.
They all live in the same household.

Helen married Brett and Molly's father George in 1987.

George, a Civil Service worker, was abusive and the couple divorced in 1994.
Not much is known about George's family and there is little contact with Helen.

George and Brett continue to be close and have weekly visits.

Brett was born in 1987 and is currently troubled, running away often to his father George's house.

Helen had a miscarriage in 1991.

Molly was born in 1993.

Helen and Chris married in 1996 and are currently expecting their first child together.

Helen is a Dental Hygienist and Chris is an Engineer.

Helen's Background:
Helen's parents Herman and Joyce were married in 1959 until Herman's death in 1989.

Herman was an alcoholic.

Helen was closer to her father than to her mother.

Joyce is very active in her local community.

Helen has brothers who are identical twins, Jason and Jared. They are very close.

Chris' Background:
Chris' parents Sirus and Mary were married in 1961, but have been separated since 1999.

Sirus has health difficulties due to diabetes and relies often on Chris to help him.

Chris' sister Anna is in a relationship with Donna, which has distanced her from their mother Mary.

Chris is close to Anna.

Figure 3-1 cont'd Example of a genogram template.

tools and surveys, is frequently completed within an hour and is then followed by daily or weekly conferences, depending on the setting and the time available. The follow-up conference provides an opportunity to review the assessment information and to identify progress made toward achieving the goals. During these conferences, the nurse and family agree upon priority issues and begin to formulate a treatment plan.

Many of the following components of the family assessment were introduced earlier in the discussion of theories. They are included in the discussion that follows to demonstrate types of information that can be obtained during assessments conducted via observation, direct questioning, or through the administration of various assessment tools and surveys. Components of family assessment include but are not limited to communication, roles and relationships, family developmental stages, rituals, family building activities, triangulation, and other concepts from selected theories.

COMPONENTS OF THE FAMILY ASSESSMENT

Assessment of Communication Patterns

Communication is how the family exchanges information, values, and emotional connection. The nurse assesses the type, frequency, and direction of communication among the family members. For example, the nurse seeks answers to questions such as: "What is the nature of the interpersonal messages—supportive or attacking?"; "What emotional content is expressed?"; "Who is sending and receiving the messages?"; and, "Are there any patterns of dominance or powerlessness?". In some situations, one family member may dominate the responses to the assessment. The nurse assesses whether the entire family agrees with the information presented or if one member's point of view is ignored or suppressed. A family with addiction issues may present information cautiously and censure members who give information that indicates a problem.

Key to Ecomap

Circles represent systems that
interact with Smythe Family

Dotted line indicates strained
relationship

Figure 3-2 Example of an ecomap.

The nurse looks for themes of emotional connectedness or isolation among the family members. There may also be clues that indicate the presence of family violence or neglect. In their interactions, the healthy family conveys a sense of connection and an appreciation of the family unit and of its individual members. The healthy family is open with problem identification and exploring coping patterns. There may also be clues that indicate the presence of family violence or neglect. Conversely, the unhealthy family tends to control or hide information or block access (of information) from other family members. The nurse should always conduct follow-up interviews with family members who were absent or not accessible during the initial interview.

Optimizing Outcomes— **During assessment of family communication patterns**

During the family interview, the nurse should be cautious not to rely solely on information provided by family members. Often, dysfunctional communication patterns are suppressed as members attempt to present themselves most favorably. It is important to observe verbal and non-verbal communication with and *among* family members.

ASSESSMENT OF ROLES AND RELATIONSHIPS

Roles and relationships are the job descriptions and connections of the individual family members. One or more family members assumes the responsibility of earning or obtaining money and resources, paying bills, providing meals, cleaning the living space, transporting family members, choosing entertainment and recreation activities, and promoting health and emotional security. The nurse assesses (through observation and/or application of assessment tools/surveys) for the delegation of tasks that meet the family needs on a daily basis. Certain roles clearly fall in the domain of specific family members, such as the parent who pays the bills.

Other roles may be more fluid, like the mother or older sister with a driver's license who takes turns transporting the younger child to soccer practice. Relationships are usually clearly delineated: father, mother, brother, and sister. Relationships may also be self-declared or assigned. Examples of these types of relationships include brothers or cousins who are best friends or an oldest sibling who becomes the "boss" of younger siblings while the parents are away. Some roles and relationships are blended together: the mother who is also the nurturer; the father who is also the enforcer of rules. Roles and relationships should have an observable outcome on the family home/household.

Nursing Insight— *Family roles, cultural influences, and maternity care*

When working with the childbearing family, nurses need to be aware that social class and cultural norms frequently affect the roles of various family members. The male's likelihood to participate in the childbearing experience, for example, is culturally influenced. Traditional Mexican and Arab families may view pregnancy and birth as events that are strictly "female affairs."

The nurse assesses the effectiveness of family roles by observing the condition of the house and living conditions (by conducting a home visit, if possible, or by obtaining the information during the interview), the clothing and personal hygiene of the family members, and gathers other information to determine if family members are carrying out individual role assignments. There is much variation on how different family members meet their role requirements. For example, a single mother may need to seek public assistance in order to fulfill the provider role and obtain essential resources for her family. This process involves contacting various agencies, completing lengthy forms, waiting in lines, and engaging in other activities that can sometimes take as much time as working at a job to meet the family's needs. Fulfilling roles also encompasses the completion of tasks appropriate to each member's and the family's stage of development.

ASSESSMENT OF THE FAMILY DEVELOPMENTAL STAGE

The **Family Developmental Stage** (Friedman et al., 2003; Harmon Hanson et al., 2005; Wright & Leahey, 2005) is the time in the family's life span that is focused on a particular age of a child or a specific family situation. This stage is assessed by means of the interview, the application of tools and surveys, and during observation of the family. At any given time, most families exist in simultaneous stages. They may be launching a high school graduate off to work or college and still have an infant (their child or grandchild) in the home. The family must accomplish a specific set of tasks for each stage. An infant requires feeding and changing and napping and nurturing throughout the day. The high school graduate most likely needs assistance and support whether planning for college or making career choices. An extended living situation at home may be needed while a family member is in transition. The nurse assesses (by the observation of the presence or absence of resources and material goods such as clothing, food, and furniture appropriate to the family stage) that the family is successfully meeting the tasks for each stage or that they are obtaining appropriate assistance from outside resources (e.g., a student loan) to help meet their needs.

ASSESSMENT OF FAMILY RITUALS

Family rituals consist of routines or activities that the family performs and teaches its members as a part of continuity and stability. Rituals encompass meal and bedtime routines, greeting and dismissing behaviors (a kiss goodbye or good night; a hello or a good-morning shout across the room), and observation of celebrations or terminations (birthdays or funerals). The nurse assesses (through observation and direct inquiry, or as guided by the assessment survey) for family member agreement on how important days are observed or if they are acknowledged at all. For example, birthday celebrations may be elaborate, informal, or summarily dismissed. Holiday presents may be opened before or during the holiday or not exchanged at all. Families may always or never share meals together.

 Nursing Insight— *Family-building activities, rules, mottos, and beliefs*

Family-building activities are an extension of rituals that center on recreation and leisure, such as family trips and vacations. Although a best friend may be invited to participate in some family events, a healthy family generally designates special "together time" that isn't open to non-family members. Family rules, mottos, and beliefs are the ways the family views itself and describes itself to others. "We always finish what we start" or "We stick together through thick and thin" are oft-used sayings that a family may identify with, whether or not they are consistent in holding to those beliefs. As a component of the assessment, the nurse can ask for three or four sayings or beliefs that the family feels are important in maintaining their family system. The nurse then asks for examples of responses to situations that illustrate or confirm this belief.

ASSESSMENT FOR TRIANGULATION

Triangulation, assessed through family observation, occurs when two family members focus on or team up against a third family member to compensate for friction between the two members (Bowen, 1978; Harmon Hanson et al., 2005). Triangulation balances the family in a manner similar to how a furniture builder adds a third leg to balance a two-legged stool. The family reaches out or even attacks a third member or outside person as a way to decrease tension between two members and to obtain balance. For example, rather than blame one another for the child's asthma symptoms, the parents instead focus on seeking outside medical help for the condition. This scenario illustrates a positive use of triangulation.

Conversely, tobacco-using parents who focus on their child's asthma symptoms while ignoring their own tobacco addiction (and the unhealthy environment that accompanies it) illustrate a potentially negative triangulation. Two brothers who team up against the policeman called to break up their drunken dispute is an example of triangulating with an outside source. Family therapists are particularly vulnerable to triangulation when working with families, and they must learn to recognize when triangulation is being negatively used and teach families other strategies for maintaining stability.

ASSESSMENT FOR THE PRESENCE OF DYADS AND OTHER SUBSYSTEMS

A dyad (Bowen, 1978; Harmon Hanson et al., 2005) is a structure in which two family members form a bond to become a subsystem of the greater family system. Within a family of four, existing dyads generally include the husband–wife dyad, father–son dyad, brother–sister dyad, or other combinations. The dyad may be a natural alliance for the purposes of intimacy or play or related activities. Dyads may form as siblings team up against a perceived unfair parental rule. The nurse observes for the presence of dyads, and notes whether or not they are self-identified, and whether a positive or negative impact on the family is known or acknowledged.

❝ **What to say** ❞ — *Specific questions to ask during the family assessment*

To elicit family identifying data, the nurse may ask:

"Who in your family lives in your home?"

"What other family members live elsewhere?"

"What are the sources of income or other resources for your family?"

Questions to determine the family's developmental stage can include:

"What are the ages of the children in family?"

"What jobs or tasks take up the most time in providing care for the children?" Environmental data includes information about the neighborhood of residence and local resources such as stores, schools, hospitals, and entertainment centers. Other questions are intended to elicit information concerning family structure ("Who makes decisions?"), function ("How is emotion and affection shown?"), and health care ("What health appointments are made and by whom?") (Friedman et al., 2003).

Once all pertinent information has been obtained and documented, the nurse elicits the family's assistance in prioritizing the most pressing and problematic issues. These issues are then addressed in the family treatment plan that forms the basis for all family-centered interventions. Depending on the specific situation, nursing interventions for families most often include referrals, education, and counseling.

 Optimizing Outcomes— **With nursing interventions for families**

Referrals may be made to support groups (i.e., Alcoholics Anonymous, Al-Anon, Gamblers Anonymous), physicians, social services, and mental health agencies. Education may center on the use of prescribed medications and therapies, nutrition, and family health promotion. When indicated, licensed professional counselors, nurse practitioners, psychologists, and family therapists provide in-depth family counseling.

Now Can You— Apply tools and concepts to assess a family?

1. Describe two tools used to diagram family structure and function?
2. Discuss at least five concepts that can be assessed in the family?
3. Explain the nurse's role in the assessment of the family?

Family-Centered Care

After the assessment process has been completed, the nurse selects all applicable nursing diagnoses and formulates the family care plan. The family's assistance is elicited to ensure that they are in agreement with the identified diagnoses. The nurse guides the family in writing mutually agreed-upon goals that they will work on together. Diagnoses may be psychosocial, physiological, or both and they may be focused on the individual or on the family (Box 3-1).

In the following discussion the nursing diagnosis "Altered Family Processes" is presented and described in detail to illustrate the possible goals, interventions, and evaluation criteria that could be appropriate for families experiencing problems in their day-to-day functioning.

NURSING DIAGNOSIS: ALTERED FAMILY PROCESSES

This nursing diagnosis describes a family that experiences problems in their everyday functioning. Problems often center on communication issues or difficulties with member role fulfillment. In these situations, the family is in need of education and/or intervention to help them return to normal daily functioning. As an example, a family with an infant may not be communicating about sharing the

---

Box 3-1 Examples of Family Nursing Diagnoses

Any NANDA diagnosis may be appropriate for describing an individual family member's health status. A family diagnosis is intended to describe the health status of the family as a whole. Examples of family diagnoses include the following:

Caregiver Role Strain (actual and risk for)
Dysfunctional Family Processes: Alcoholism
Family Coping: Compromised
Family Coping: Disabled
Impaired Parenting (actual and risk for)
Ineffective Family Therapeutic Regimen Management
Readiness for Enhanced Family Coping
Readiness for Enhanced Parenting
Risk for Parent-Infant-Child Attachment
Social Isolation
Spiritual Distress

NOC outcomes specifically for families as units are included in the NOC domain "Family Health." This category includes the following classes: Family Caregiver Status, Family Member Health Status, Family Well-Being and Parenting. Outcomes from other domains may also apply. *NIC interventions* for families as units are included in the NIC domain "Family." This category includes the following classes: Childbearing Care, Childrearing Care and Life-Span Care.
Sources: Carpenito-Moyet (2006); Wilkinson & Van Leuven (2007).

---

new roles brought about by the baby's arrival. The mother feels resentful that the father is not helping more; the father senses the resentment but doesn't recognize what is wrong. The nurse identifies clues to tension in the relationship during well-baby check-ups or perhaps even prior to discharge from the hospital.

GOAL: RETAIN/MAINTAIN OPEN LINES OF COMMUNICATION. The family will discuss feelings openly and nonjudgmentally with each other using "I feel" statements (Clark, 2003) and avoiding defensive communication techniques (Johnson & Johnson, 2003). All members will negotiate what it is they would want for the other member to understand about their feelings and needs.

GOAL: ADAPT TO CHANGES IN FAMILY PROCESS/SITUATION BY SHARING RESPONSIBILITIES. To meet this goal, various family roles need to be adjusted. For example, having an older sister help babysit the infant in order to give the mother more time for rest represents a family adaptation necessitated by a change in the home situation. After the birth of a baby, the father may need to take family leave so that he can share in child care. In another family, the mother-in-law may be asked to assume a more active role in assisting with newborn or child care.

GOAL: RESPECT THE INDIVIDUALITY OF EACH MEMBER'S ACTIONS. The family may need to allow a member to isolate from an event until he or she is able to handle the situation with the rest of the family. For example, it is developmentally appropriate for a teenager to want to continue with contact from friends while the family is experiencing a situational crisis.

GOAL: PARTICIPATE IN THE CARE OF INDIVIDUALS. The family needs to prioritize care for its sick or disabled members over lesser psychosocial needs such as having friends over for the school-aged children. All needs should be addressed eventually, but safety and physiological needs should be addressed first.

GOAL: SEEK/ACCEPT RESOURCES AS NEEDED. As a system, the family opens its boundaries to appropriate outside sources (i.e., the pediatrician, internist, and social worker or community health department) as needed to help provide appropriate health care for its members. Families with issues such as domestic violence often have difficulty trusting another system due to the fear of legal intervention. The family may have difficulty accepting help if they do not perceive or acknowledge the problem. The nurse may use a number of interventions to help the family obtain their goals under this nursing diagnosis.

The following are examples of applicable nursing interventions.

INTERVENTION: IDENTIFY FAMILY DYSFUNCTION AND THE FAMILY'S AWARENESS OF THE PROBLEM(S). As part of an ongoing collaborative process with the family, the nurse adds entries to the problem list as needed to keep the list current and applicable. The problem list is then reviewed during each nursing visit. For example, the nurse may recognize that the family does not use proper car safety seats for the younger children. Throughout the collaborative process, as problems are identified by a family member, the nurse assesses other members' understanding and willingness to participate in the proposed solutions.

INTERVENTION: GUIDE THE FAMILY THROUGH MEDICAL ADMIS-SIONS/INTERVENTIONS. The nurse acts as the liaison with family member hospitalizations and other referrals. In this role, the nurse provides information about medical procedures, coordinates care with various community resources and helps to clarify medical explanations to the family when one of the members receives medical assistance.

INTERVENTION: ASSESS THE IMPACT OF IDENTIFIED PROBLEMS ON THE STABILITY AND FUNCTIONING OF THE FAMILY. The nurse identifies roles or functions that are neglected by the family and helps the family adjust as they struggle to meet the health needs of members.

INTERVENTION: LISTEN ATTENTIVELY TO ALL MEMBERS. The nurse helps the family to identify the meaning of the dysfunction and assists the family in improving communication among its members.

INTERVENTION: SCHEDULE FAMILY CONFERENCES. Family conferences give all members an opportunity to express themselves and share in the family situation. This strategy is particularly important in an emergency hospitalization when the family members are not all initially involved in the decision making concerning treatments received. For example, a sister who arrives late from out of town may not initially understand the decision to withhold treatment in respect to advance directives.

INTERVENTION: IDENTIFY, REFER, AND INFORM THE FAMILY OF AVAILABLE RESOURCES. After hospitalization of a family member, the nurse may identify a social worker to assist with discharge plans and payment issues. In another situation, the nurse may serve as an advocate to help the family receive rehabilitative care for a member with a head injury.

INTERVENTION: DISCUSS ROLE CHANGES AND THEIR IMPACT ON FAMILY MEMBERS. A family situation may involve a sister caring for a parent with Alzheimer's disease who needs support and respite care to meet her own needs and those of her children. The nurse has the objectivity to identify the sister's needs and facilitate her communication of these needs to other family members.

Periodically, the nurse and family assess the extent to which the goals have been accomplished and the effectiveness of the nursing interventions. Adjustments in goals and interventions are made when necessary.

Evaluation

Expected outcomes may include the following:

- Effective communication takes place among family members in an assertive and nonthreatening manner that allows members' needs to be expressed and met.
- Family tasks and roles are appropriately distributed so that students attend school and employed members go to work, medical appointments are made and kept; and food and shelter is adequately provided.

Many other nursing diagnoses are applicable for the family experiencing health or social problems. For example, Family Coping: Potential for Growth is particularly useful for the family that is not experiencing health or social crisis, but can still benefit from nursing education for improvement in selected areas.

 Now Can You— **Apply family nursing diagnoses to a family?**

1. Identify two family nursing diagnoses that may be applied to a variety of situations?
2. List three goals for each nursing diagnosis identified?
3. List three nursing interventions for each nursing diagnosis identified?

Families with Special Needs

Sometimes families are in special need of nursing intervention due to situational or developmental crises that go beyond the family's internal resources. Situational crises include environmental disasters such as floods, hurricanes, or fires. The loss of a home, job, family member, or close friend are all unexpected and unplanned for events that initially send the family into a state of chaos and often require outside help for the process of reorganization. Developmental crises occur as part of expected growth events that can take place during any developmental stage of the family or its individual members. Toddlerhood and adolescence are examples of two developmental stages that often disrupt family balance if no preparations were made in anticipation of the changing needs of the child and young teen.

Whether related to developmental stages or situational changes, certain events often require some level of intervention to help restore the family's balance and function, such as hospitalization, chronic mental illness (i.e., Alzheimer's disease, attention deficit disorder, autism, schizophrenia), substance abuse, sexual or physical abuse, posttraumatic stress disorder, chronic illness, and loss of a family member.

HOSPITALIZATION

The hospitalization of a family member often triggers a crisis that requires assistance and interventions from various outside sources. The scope of the family's needs is related to their resources, level of adaptability, and prior experience. In most situations, intervention includes treatment and education provided by the physician, care and additional education provided by the nurse, and discharge planning with community support arranged by designated hospital staff. Depending on the circumstance, the chaplain, social worker, community health nurse, and rehabilitation professional may all be members of the health care team that assists in the transition from the hospital to the home or community facility. At times, the nurse is responsible for identifying and coordinating these resources to facilitate the patient's and family's transition and may involve various other interventions.

CHRONIC MENTAL ILLNESS

A family with a member who has a chronic mental illness such as schizophrenia or bipolar disorder is a lifelong partner with the mental health system. This partnership can be therapeutic or antagonistic, depending on the resources available, the family's history in using these resources, and the amount of continuity that exists between the professionals and the families as they work together. The nurse's role is that of mediator/facilitator between the family system and the mental health system.

Establishing a diagnosis serves as the beginning point in helping the family to proceed with care for their family member. This task can be accomplished with the assistance of outpatient experts such as psychiatrists, social workers, psychologists, and advanced practice nursing specialists. Diagnostic work-ups are usually conducted as a team approach and most often involve an initial hospitalization for patient stabilization and medication. The family should be educated about prescribed medications, their side effects and planned treatments, and provided with information about financial resources such as Medicaid, Social Security, vocational rehabilitation, and other resources. The family is also in need of information and guidance concerning voluntary and involuntary commitment, guardianship, and other legal issues that often emerge as the illness progresses.

In many cases, problems with treatment are related to noncompliance or taking medications improperly (i.e., skipping doses or combining them with other substances). Sometimes the family assumes responsibility for the administration of medications for the family member. Another issue that often arises concerns an inability to pay for the medication. The nurse assists the family and/or family member in securing financial resources.

An important problem that should be addressed with families that have a mentally disabled member concerns social isolation. Social isolation is a situation that occurs when the ill family member is afraid or does not have the energy to participate in activities without continued prompting and encouragement by the family. Another potential problem involves nutritional deficit due to paranoia about harmful substances in the food or changes in eating habits related to depression. Certain medications are associated with weight gain, a problem that can lead to other health issues. Mental illness can also affect sleeping and rest patterns, and this problem is often associated with bipolar disease.

Special attention must be paid to the patient's suicidal potential and risk for harm to others. The nurse teaches the family to be especially vigilant when the patient is recovering from an immobilizing depression, an especially vulnerable time associated with newfound energy to carry out a plan. The person suffering from depression, bipolar disorder, or schizophrenia is also at risk when the normal impulse control becomes affected by influences such as drug or alcohol abuse or the rapid cycling associated with bipolar disorder. An important nursing role involves teaching the family techniques to assess for deficits, strategies for intervention, and recognizing when to call for assistance. Extended family should be recruited to help prevent caregiver strain by being available to help with the family member or offer respite care. Caregiver strain occurs when the main caregiver becomes overwhelmed and feels "under helped" in regard to the tasks concerned with the care of the family member. In this situation, mounting bitterness and withdrawal from other family members may cause caregivers to push away any potential helpers. Respite care occurs when someone else assumes the care of the sick family member in order to give the caregiver time off to rest.

 case study The Family of a Young Adult with Schizophrenia

Ricky, age 24, was diagnosed with schizophrenia at the age of 16. His symptoms include paranoia, auditory hallucinations (hearing voices), and social isolation. He has been hospitalized several times over the years but his symptoms are currently stable on a newer antipsychotic medication. The family is willing for him to be discharged from the state hospital where he had been receiving treatment and come back home to live with them.

1. What information would the family require to be able to properly care for Ricky at home?

2. What are some of the resources the nurse should provide to help Ricky and his family cope with his illness?

◆ See Suggested Answers to Case Studies in text on the Electronic Study Guide or DavisPlus.

SUBSTANCE ABUSE

Substance abuse negatively affects the family system. Family functions frequently become reorganized to sustain and cover up the addiction. If a parent is the substance abuser, parental roles are shifted to the other parent or to a child to provide meals, wash clothes, get the children to school, and call in sick for the affected parent. This process, termed enabling, is necessary in order for the addicted member to appear to be functioning normally. Sometimes another member of the family is so closely enmeshed with the affected member's addiction that he or she becomes codependent (Townsend, 2005). Although the codependent member may not be abusing substances with the addict, he or she is equally impaired through the continued cooperation in the addiction.

Often the remaining family members assume roles that help the addiction to continue. One child, usually the oldest, takes on the learned role of responsible child. This responsible child, who is either self-selected or is family assigned by default, takes over for the mother if she is drinking with the alcoholic partner or engaging in other enabling behaviors that make her unavailable to the family, and makes sure the younger children are being cared for. The responsible child makes lunches, gets the siblings off to school and extracurricular activities, and may even help with paying the bills. The hero is another role that may evolve in children of families with an impaired member. The child in a hero role serves as the family standard-bearer, ready to proclaim that the family cannot really be impaired if it produced such a star. The hero is academically successful and excels in sports and other extracurricular activities.

Two additional roles that may be found in the substance- or alcohol-impaired family are the scapegoat and the lost child. The scapegoat is the opposite of the hero. The scapegoat fails at school and social activities and may have run-ins with the law for vandalism or shoplifting or fighting at school. The family presents the scapegoat to the world with the message: "Look at what we have to endure! No wonder we have a difficult life!" The hero and the scapegoat are actually diversions for what is really happening to the family due to substance abuse. The lost child is a symptom of a family that is too chaotic to meet the needs of the child or notice the child at all. The lost child keeps a low profile at home and school and does not usually fail but also does not particularly stand out in anything, either.

Along with the family roles are family rules that are implicitly followed by all members, such as: "Don't talk and don't feel." Family members know not to discuss family problems with outsiders such as teachers, nurses, or even friends. Secrets are the hallmark of addictive families both for social and legal reasons. Family members also learn not to feel the disappointment or anger or sadness that the addiction causes them. Parents do not make it to the children's games or teacher conferences, or even to major events such as graduation. The children deny that the parent's lack of involvement impacts their feelings. If changes do not take place in these types of family systems, there is a great likelihood that the children will be socially and personally impaired and a high percentage turns to substance abuse themselves (Townsend, 2005).

The nurse and the family with substance abuse/alcohol abuse must assess the amount, type, and length of time the addiction has been a part of the family. If the main substance abuser is actively engaged in treatment, the family should be referred to therapy or support groups such as Al-Anon that can help them to identify and change their own behaviors, wants, and needs apart from those of the alcoholic. If treatment is not obtained for the affected member, the nurse should refer family members to organizations such as Alcoholics Anonymous or to legal agencies that can identify options for getting the member into treatment or strategies for keeping the family safe from the member.

 case study The Family Members of an Alcoholic

A 9-year-old boy has been sent home from school several times for fighting. The father has a history of scrapes with the law related to public drunkenness and bar fights. The mother tells the school nurse that the father has been laid off at work and has a lot of issues on his mind to work through. She further states that the boy has been nothing but trouble and is an embarrassment to the family, unlike his sister, who is a junior high cheerleader and "straight A" student.

1. What roles are being played in this family?

2. What is the purpose of these roles?

3. What interventions would the nurse bring to this family?

◆ See Suggested Answers to Case Studies in text on the Electronic Study Guide or DavisPlus.

SEXUAL OR PHYSICAL ABUSE

Sexual or physical abuse in the family is similar to substance abuse in how it affects the family system. In general, this problem can exist only in a family system that keeps secrets and creates specific roles that allow its continuance. When an incestuous father/child sexual relationship occurs, the mother or marital partner has taken on the role of either ignoring or covering up the abuse. In some situations, the mother feels threatened and acts as a sexual competitor (against the daughter) for the husband's affection. In many cases, one person is singled out for the physical or sexual abuse. Other family members have a relatively normal relationship with the abuser and with one other. If the abused member is removed from the family, there may be a transfer of the behavior to another member.

In all situations, the nurse is legally obligated to report the abuse to the proper investigating agency. However, the nurse is not responsible for investigating or intervening with the family once the report has been made. When unsure, the nurse can verify suspicions of abuse with other treatment team members, but once the suspicions are confirmed, either the nurse, nursing supervisor, or treatment team leader is mandated to report the abuse. The nurse then makes a therapeutic alliance with the family unit (probably without the abuser) to help return them to normal roles and relationships. The nurse must remain vigilant for signs of continued abuse or violence with the remaining members or with the primary abuser if he (or she) is returned to the family.

 case study Elder Abuse in the Family

The nurse is conducting a home visit with an 85-year-old mother who is being cared for by her adult daughter. The daughter exhibits an attitude of detachment toward her mother. A general assessment of the elderly patient is remarkable for strong body odor, stained clothes, and an overall disheveled appearance. The mother is alert but hesitant to talk with the nurse and evasive with her answers. The daughter appears to be impatient and explains that she needs to go shopping.

1. What other assessment information would be needed to verify whether or not the patient was being neglected?

2. What steps should be taken if abuse or neglect is suspected?

◆ See Suggested Answers to Case Studies in text on the Electronic Study Guide or DavisPlus.

POSTTRAUMATIC STRESS DISORDER

Posttraumatic stress disorder (PTSD) is a condition that results from experiencing a catastrophic event such as rape, battering, accident, mugging, or war. The survivor or survivors of the traumatic event may experience nightmares and flashbacks (vivid re-experiencing of events while awake) and frequently develop a detached view of life. Involved families "lose" an active participant in their lives while the family member with PTSD vacillates between apathy and extreme vigilance and overprotectiveness. The affected family member may also turn to substance abuse in an attempt to dull the memories associated with the event.

An entire family may experience PTSD after a shared event such as surviving a flood or tornado that destroyed everything and left them homeless. Often, symptoms do not appear for days or weeks following the event. The delay may result from the initial gestures of support provided by the family and the community. The nurse assesses for symptoms of PTSD during the interview, with questions focused on sleep disturbances or flashbacks of the traumatic event and the individual's inability to participate fully in the family's life. When identified, the family member(s) is referred for appropriate intervention. Alternately, the nurse may elicit the assistance of an expert trained in Critical Incident Stress Debriefing or who has experience with other proven techniques for treating survivors. Support groups are usually therapeutic in helping both the victim and the family ease the affected member back into their world.

CHRONIC PHYSICAL ILLNESS

Asthma, diabetes, and Crohn's disease are often viewed as medical conditions that are affected by psychological factors (Kneisl, Wilson, & Trigoboff, 2004) because of the strong emotionality involved. Although emotions do not cause these illnesses, they may exacerbate the symptoms by decreasing the family member's compliance with the treatment or by increasing the anxiety related to the symptoms. Families need to be educated about various aspects of daily care for members who experience chronic illness. For example, the nurse may teach about monitoring the diabetic family member's blood glucose analysis or self-administration of insulin or how to assist the asthmatic with inhalation therapy.

In some situations, a teenager may not fully accept his illness and choose not to take prescribed medications. This behavior often stems from a need to prove to self or others that he does not truly need the medications or treatment. An older adult living in the home may not fully understand the temporal demands associated with a medication schedule and may require additional teaching and close monitoring, especially if the medications have recently been changed. The nurse helps the family transition from dependence on the health care worker to family member independence, although, depending on the circumstances, some supervision by the family may always be necessary. The family benefits through an ongoing partnership with a provider or clinic that enables them to receive progress reports, treatment updates, and needed medications. The nurse facilitates family empowerment by helping them to get the information necessary to provide continued support and treatment of their family member. To learn more about caring for the family with chronic physical illness, see Chapter 35.

 case study The Family of a Diabetic Teen

Shelley is a 15-year-old with type 1 diabetes mellitus who presents periodically to the emergency department with a blood sugar level of greater than 300 mg/dL. The family states she has been snacking on foods not on her diet, is sporadic with her blood sugar testing, and inconsistent in the management of her sliding scale method of insulin administration. The nurse's conversation with Shelley reveals that Shelley is resentful of her illness and angry that she has to do things that "the other girls do not have to do."

1. In view of Shelley's developmental stage, what information should the nurse give to Shelley and her family regarding diabetes?

2. How would the information be presented differently if Shelley were 6 years old?

◆ See Suggested Answers to Case Studies in text on the Electronic Study Guide or DavisPlus.

DEATH OF A FAMILY MEMBER

The nurse is often the first point-of-contact when a family member has died in the hospital or at home if home nursing was involved in the member's care. The particular developmental stage affects the way in which each family member grieves. While the length of time that elapses between the stages of grief and the manifestations of grief vary, all family members grieve in some manner. Stages of grieving have been described by a number of theorists; several are presented in

Table 3-1 The Grieving Process as Described by Various Theorists				
Kubler-Ross' Stages of Grieving	**Rodebaugh's Stages of Grieving**	**Harvey's Phases of Grieving**	**Epperson's Phases of Grieving**	**Rando's Reactions of Bereaved Parents**
Denial (shock and disbelief)	Reeling (stunned disbelief)	Shock, Outcry, and Denial (external response to loss)	High Anxiety (physical response to emotional upheaval)	Avoidance (confusion and dazed state, avoidance of reality of loss)
Anger (toward God, relatives, the health care system)	Feelings (emotionally experiencing the loss)	Intrusion of thoughts, distractions, and obsessive reviewing of the loss (internal response, isolation)	Denial (protective psychological reaction)	Confrontation (intense emotions, anger, sadness, feeling the loss)
Bargaining (trying to attain more time, delaying acceptance of the loss)	Dealing (taking care of details, taking care of others)	Confiding in others to emote and cognitively restructure (integration of internal thoughts and external actions to move on)	Anger (directed inwardly, toward another family member, or toward others)	Reestablishment (intensity declines, and the parents resume their lives)
Acceptance (readiness to move forward with newfound meaning or purpose in one's own life)	Healing (recovering and reentering life)		Remorse (feelings of guilt and sorrow)	
			Grief (overwhelming sadness)	
			Reconciliation (adaptation to existing circumstances)	

Table 3-1. The nurse provides time and space (family visiting room, chapel, or the patient's room) for the family to gather. The nurse also inquires about the family's preferences concerning participation in preparation activities before the arrival of the mortuary representatives. Some cultures and religions wish to ritually bathe and dress the body.

The family must also decide which members should be involved in the various tasks and this decision is affected by the age or developmental level of the child or adult. For example, a developmentally challenged adult may need the same approach as a younger child. In most situations, viewing the deceased (after equipment such as tubes and drainage bags have been removed) helps family members of all ages accept that death has occurred. They can then begin the grieving process.

The nurse participates in the accepting/searching for answers stage that often occurs early during grieving by providing answers regarding the illness or procedures or treatments that were involved. As appropriate, the nurse may seek assistance from the physician, other members of the health care team, or from other resources. The family's minister or hospital chaplain may be asked to offer spiritual support, provide counseling, and address concerns. The nurse may wish to participate in prayer led by the family's clergy or hospital chaplaincy. Providing a presence and remaining with the family as long as possible are often the best nursing approaches for the family that has experienced a loss. The nurse may also have an opportunity to advise family friends that a critical time for them to be available to the family is around the third or fourth week after the funeral, when the family is left to deal with the full impact of the loss (Wilkinson & Van Leuven, 2007).

🌼 *Across Care Settings:* Family care in inpatient, outpatient, and hospice settings

In hospital inpatient units, families should be oriented to visiting hours, waiting rooms, meals, and overnight accommodations. Nurses reinforce patient admission data such as advance directives and organ donation policies and encourage an open discussion between the patient and family to prevent confusion regarding who would act as the patient's agent to make decisions in the event of incapacity or death. Families often need assistance with medical information, billing information, and admission and discharge information. In pediatrics units, families should be alerted to policies concerning staying with their sick child and assistance should be offered in making arrangements for the care of other children. In long-term inpatient settings, families rely on visits, telephone calls, mail, and e-mail to stay in touch with members. In outpatient units, nurses can educate the family about strategies to enhance patient recovery, reinforce discharge instructions, and provide written information about follow-up visits.

In home health and hospice settings, the nurse assists the family in reaching a comfortable balance between direct involvement in the family member's care and respite time for family building activities with other members. Demystifying medical procedures such as medication administration, catheterization, and tube feeding empowers the family to decide what they can do and how and when to seek assistance from the nurse and other care staff.

 Now Can You— Identify and plan care for special problems and issues faced by the American family?

1. List eight special problems that may be experienced by families?
2. Identify various nursing roles and interventions appropriate for these families?
3. Describe the nurse's role when abuse is suspected?

Family Cultural Characteristics

An understanding of the prevailing concepts of acculturation, assimilation identity, time, connectedness, communication, and social class facilitates the nursing assessment and guides the application of interventions within different cultural frameworks. To enhance understanding of the concepts, it is helpful to examine characteristics of the "typical" American family. General comparisons with selected cultural groups provide the nurse with a staring point for understanding and interacting with families in a culturally appropriate way.

ACCULTURATION AND ASSIMILATION

The American family exhibits many variations owing to its unique blending with other cultures. The rich cultural heritage that has evolved from the mixing of various ethnic groups that comprise the American family constitutes the hallmark of this relatively new culture. **Acculturation** describes the changes in one's cultural pattern to match those of the host society (Spector, 2004). The changes occur within one group or among several groups when individuals from different cultures come into contact with one another. Certain characteristics of the primary culture may be retained while other practices of the dominant cultural society are adopted. For example, culturally influenced customs and traditions such as food choice and preparation, language patterns, and health practices are usually retained for long periods of time. **Assimilation** is the process in which the family loses its unique cultural identity and identifies instead with the prevailing or dominant culture (Spector, 2004).

IDENTITY

The identity (how the family views itself) of the American family is related to whether or not the family aligns itself with a particular ethnic group (e.g., Italian American, Irish American) or instead only sees itself as "American." Identifying with a particular ethnic group usually involves adopting that group's world view or approach to life. Anglo-Americans, for example, view themselves as independent individuals often separate from families (Friedman, 2003). Other cultures (i.e., Hispanic, Asian, and Pacific Islander) consider individuals in the context of family members and place less of an emphasis on who they are as individuals (Wilkinson & Van Leuven, 2007).

The American family may influence a member's choice of occupation, but usually to a lesser degree than that found in some cultures. For example, in earlier times, the English names of "Butcher" and "Baker" reflected a family occupation and set of expectations. In general, an American child is free to choose a career based on personal preferences and talents that have been developed in outside systems such as school, church, or extra-curricular activities rather than one exclusively imposed by the family.

Time orientation is a concept that refers to whether or not the family views itself to be strongly connected to previous generations. The American family tends to be focused on the present and future much more so than many cultures. This current-future time orientation may be related to the relative newness of America as a country, as compared to an ancient civilization such as China. In the American family, the individual is expected to be punctual and conform to deadlines at school and work. Making future plans by saving money or pursuing higher education is also valued. Many industrialized countries share a present and future time orientation, while other countries value a slower pace with greater emphasis on the connection to the past in terms of ancestors and traditional beliefs (Friedman et al., 2003; Townsend, 2005).

CONNECTEDNESS

Connectedness is a concept that emphasizes who the family identifies with and relates to as family members. The generality that American families are often organized into smaller nuclear families that consist of one or two parents and children is being replaced by the fact that only 52% of American families presently fit that pattern (Friedman et al., 2003). Some American families and many other cultures highly value and place great importance on the inclusion of grandparents, aunts, uncles, and cousins in their family circle. That level of extended connectedness may also include the community, especially if other members of the same ethnic group live in the neighborhood. In some American families, members spend more time commuting to outside interests than engaging in neighborhood and home-based family activities.

COMMUNICATION PATTERNS

Patterns of communication vary according to ethnic group. Cultural customs often guide selection of the family member who will be designated as the primary historian in a health care interview. American families tend to be more fluid and open in designating which member speaks to outsiders, although legal contracts most often favor the parents. Other cultures (i.e., Hispanic families from Mexico) may be more patriarchal (male dominant) or matriarchal (female dominant) and the caregiver role may rely heavily on a grandparent or aunt rather than the parents. The designated caregiver is usually the communicator in the health care setting. When planning interventions, it is important to consider the cultural role of the family member who makes the primary decisions (Wilkinson & Van Leuven, 2007).

 Nursing Insight— *Culture, communication, and emotional expression*

Culture is the essence of what defines us as people. Gaining an understanding of culture gives insights into family patterns of human interaction as well as expressions of emotion (Munoz & Luckmann, 2005).

The American family member is more likely to speak on her own behalf in public situations such as in schools and health care settings and is encouraged (within legal limits) to do so. Language other than American English often contains built-in formal and informal variations of words intended to convey respect to parents and elders, who frequently serve as spokespersons in settings such as hospitals and physicians' offices.

SOCIOECONOMIC CLASS

Social class refers to occupation and economic status. In America, status is related to social and economic variables, and mobility between the different classes is more fluid than in some countries. Religious and political influences significantly influence how the family interacts and responds to outside systems such as schools and community health programs. For example, some religious groups advocate home, rather than public schooling; political and religious orientation often shapes family beliefs about abortion or birth control. Other values are influenced by the prevailing societal view. For example, the contemporary American family tends to value its members according to the individual's line of work and educational achievements rather than the family's identity (Harmon Hanson et al., 2005).

HOLISTIC NURSING ENCOMPASSES A CULTURALLY SENSITIVE FAMILY APPROACH

Family assessment is integral to the delivery of competent, appropriate, holistic care. For most nurses, developing a knowledge base that is sensitive to the cultural variations of structure and function in the American family presents a personal challenge. Awareness of personal perceptions and values that may negatively impact therapeutic interactions with families is a professional responsibility. Nurses at every level of preparation and throughout their professional careers must engage in an ongoing process of developing and refining attitudes and behaviors that will promote culturally competent care (Taylor, 2005). The professional nurse grows in cultural competence by seeking more knowledge through review of literature and evidence-based practice, attendance at cultural seminars, and exposure to other cultures in a variety of settings. The more we learn about other cultures, the more we learn about ourselves as nurses and as human beings.

 Now Can You— **Recognize cultural differences that may impact the nursing assessment and interventions with the family?**

1. Identify "typical" characteristics of the American family related to time and goal orientation?
2. Explain how culture influences the family's degree of connectedness and patterns of communication in the health care setting?
3. Describe adjustments the nurse may make to heighten cultural awareness and enhance a culturally appropriate family assessment and intervention?

summary points

◆ The competent nurse views the family as a focus of care, not as an inconvenient intrusion into the nursing routine.

◆ While family structure has undergone dramatic changes over the past 60 years, the importance of family has not diminished.

◆ Family theories and models give the nurse a reference point from which to analyze the information obtained from a family assessment.

◆ The nursing process is applicable and appropriate to guide nursing interventions with the family.

◆ The family nurse possesses an understanding of the norms related to roles, relationships, developmental stages, and family functioning, and uses this information to guide the family assessment and plan appropriate interventions.

◆ The nurse recognizes special needs that affect family functioning and applies strategies to assist the family in the fulfillment of healthy roles and relationships.

◆ Culture is the context by which family behavior is understood.

◆ Working with families in the home and in community health care settings is a challenging and rewarding aspect of nursing.

review questions

Multiple Choice

1. The clinic nurse is taking a history from Karen and her common-law husband, Dave. The best description of this type of relationship is that of a:
   A. Family
   B. Family of origin
   C. Family of choice
   D. Extended family

2. The obstetrical nurse who understands the systems theory of family interaction is aware that an integral part of the nursing role is to facilitate the development of a bond between the:
   A. New subsystem of mother/infant and the father
   B. Subsystem of mother/father and new infant
   C. Subsystem of mother/father/infant and extended family
   D. New subsystem of mother/infant and significant others

3. The pediatric nurse who understands the developmental theory of families would provide information to families with preschool children on:
   A. Injury prevention and immunization
   B. Sibling rivalry
   C. Sleep–wake patterns
   D. Couple building and family adjustment

4. The clinic nurse is providing assistance to the Macy family who has just lost their son in a tragic motor vehicle collision. Future planning would include counseling the Macys that one of the most critical times in their grieving occurs when they will need to deal with the full impact of their loss. This usually takes place in the:
   A. First two weeks
   B. Third to fourth week
   C. Fifth to sixth week
   D. Eighth to tenth week

True/False

5. The clinic nurse is aware that in the 1990s, the media began to depict family challenges such as poverty and substance abuse.

6. The nurse who understands communication theory is aware that emotional problems surface with the interactions that occur within the family.

Fill-in-the-Blank

7. The pediatric nurse recognizes that the most ideal way to describe a patient/family's involvement in a patient's care provision is that the entire family is the _____ of care.

8. The perinatal nurse understands that the process of passing values and cultural heritage between generations is described as the _____ _____ process.

9. The clinic nurse talks to a family who has come in to describe their situation after a fire in their home yesterday. This type of crisis would be described as a _____ crisis that would require the nurse's _____ to locate helpful community resources.

10. The clinic nurse understands that awareness of any form of _____ in a family involves a legal obligation to report it. However, the nurse is not required to _____ or _____ once the report has been made.

See Answers to End of Chapter Review Questions on the Electronic Study Guide or DavisPlus.

REFERENCES

American Association of Retired Persons. (2006, October). October 2006 Fact Sheet. Retrieved from http://www.gicvlocalsupport.org/pages/statefact sheets.cfm (Accessed May 22, 2007).

American College of Obstetricians and Gynecologists (ACOG). (2005). Health care for homeless women. ACOG Committee Opinion No. 312. *Obstetrics and Gynecology, 106,* 429–434.

Bowen, M. (1978). *Family therapy in clinical practice.* New York: Jason Aronson.

Bulechek, G., Butcher, H.M., & Dochterman, J. (2008). *Nursing interventions classification (NIC)* (5th ed.). St. Louis, MO: C.V. Mosby.

Carpenito-Moyet, L. (2006). *Handbook of nursing diagnosis.* Philadelphia: Lippincott, Williams, & Wilkins

Child Trends DataBank. (2006). Family structure and living arrangements. Retrieved from www.childtrendsdatabank.org/ (Accessed February 27, 2008).

Clark, C. (2003). *Group leadership skills.* New York: Springer.

Covey, S.R. (2006). *The 7 habits of highly effective families.* New Delhi: B. Jain Publishers.

Ehrlich, R., McCloskey, E., & Daly, J. (2004). *Patient care in radiography.* St.Louis, MO: C.V. Mosby.

Federal Interagency Forum on Children and Family Statistics. (2007). America's children in brief: Key national indicators of well-being, 2007. Retrieved from www.childstats.gov (Accessed February 27, 2008).

Friedman, M., Bowden, V., & Jones, E. (2003). *Family nursing: Research, theory, and practice.* Upper Saddle River, NJ: Prentice-Hall.

George, J.B. (2002). *Nursing theories: The base for professional nursing practice* (5th ed.). Upper Saddle River, NJ: Prentice-Hall.

Greenfield, D. (2005). Reproduction in same sex couples: Quality of parenting and child development. *Current Opinion in Obstetrics and Gynecology, 17*(3), 308–312.

Harmon Hanson, S., Gedaly-Duff, V., & Rowe, J.K. (2005). *Family health care nursing: Theory, practice, & research* (3rd ed.). Philadelphia: F.A. Davis.

Hitchcock, J., Schubert, P., & Thomas, S. (2003). *Community health nursing: Caring in action.* Clifton Park, NY: Thomson–Delmar Learning.

Johnson, D., & Johnson, F. (2003). *Joining together: Group theory and group skills.* Boston: Allyn and Bacon.

Johnson, M., Bulechek, G., Butcher, H., McCloskey Dochterman, J., Maas, M., Moorhead, S., & Swanson, E. (2006). *NANDA, NOC, and NIC Linkages: nursing diagnoses, outcomes, & interventions* (2nd ed.). St. Louis, MO: Mosby Elsevier.

Kaiser Commission on Medicaid and the Uninsured. (2003a). The uninsured in rural America. Retrieved from www.kff.org/uninsured/upload/The-Uninsured—in-Rural-America-Update-PDF.pdf (Accessed February 27, 2008).

Kneisl, C., Wilson, H., & Trigoboff, E. (2004). *Contemporary psychiatric-mental health nursing.* Upper Saddle River, NJ: Pearson-Prentice–Hall.

McIntosh, G. (2004). *One church four generations.* Grand Rapids, MI: Baker Books

Mohanty, S., Woolhandler, S.L., Himmelstein, D., Pati, S., Carrasquillo, O., & Bor, D. (2005). Health care expenditures of immigrants in the United States: A nationally representative analysis. *American Journal of Public Health, 95*(8), 1431–1438.

Moorehead, S., Johnson, M., Mass, M., & Swanson, E. (2008) *Nursing outcomes classification (NOC)* (4th ed.). St. Louis, MO: C.V. Mosby.

Munoz, C., & Luckmann, J. (2005). *Transcultural communication in nursing* (2nd ed.). Clinton Park, NY: Thompson Delmar Learning.

NANDA International. http://www.nanda.org

Spector, R. (2004). *Cultural diversity in health and illness* (6th ed.). Upper Saddle River, NJ: Prentice-Hall.

Taylor, R. (2005). Addressing barriers to cultural competence. *Journal for Nurses in Staff Development, 21*(4), 135–142.

Townsend, M. (2005). *Essentials of psychiatric mental health nursing* (5th ed.). Philadelphia: F.A. Davis.

U.S. Census Bureau Population Estimates by Demographic Characteristics. Table 2: Annual Estimates of the Population by Selected Age Groups and Sex for the United States: April 1, 2000 to July 1, 2004 (NC-EST 2004-02). Source: Population Division, U.S. Census Bureau Release Date: June 9, 2005. http://www.census.gov/popest/national/asrh/ (Accessed September 14, 2008).

U.S. Department of Health and Human Services (USDHHS). (2000). *Healthy people 2010: Understanding and improving health.* Washington, DC: Author, Government Printing Office.

U.S. Department of Health and Human Services (USDHHS). (2005a). Health Resources and Services Administration. Women's Health USA 2005. Retrieved from www.hrsa.gov/womenshealth (Accessed May 15, 2007).

U.S. Department of Health and Human Services (DHHS), Office of the Assistant Secretary for Planning and Evaluation. (2005b). Overview of the uninsured in the United States: An analysis of the 2005 Current Population Survey. Rockville, MD: Author. Retrieved from http://aspe.hhs.gov/health/reports/05/uninsured-cps/ (Accessed May 17, 2007).

U.S. Department of Labor, Office of the Assistant Secretary for Policy, Office of Programmatic Policy. (2005). Findings from the National Agricultural Workers Survey (NAWS) 2001-2002. A demographic and employment profile of United States farm workers. Washington, DC: Author, Office of the Assistant Secretary for Policy, Office of Programmatic Policy, Research Report No. 9. March 2005. Retrieved from www.doleta.gov/agworker/naws.cfm (Accessed February 27, 2008).

Weissman, J., Betaqncourt, J., Campbell, E., Park, E., Kim, M., Clarridge, B., et al. (2005). Resident physician's preparedness to provide crosscultural care. *JAMA, 294*(9), 1058–1067.

Wherry, L., & Finegold, K. (2004). Marriage promotion and the living arrangements of black, Hispanic and white children. The Urban Institute. Retrieved from www.urban.org/url.cfm?ID=311064 (Accessed May 15, 2007).

Wilkinson, J.M., & Van Leuven, K. (2007). *Fundamentals of nursing: Theory, concepts & applications.* Philadelphia: F.A. Davis.

Wilson, D., Hockenberry-Eaton, M., Winkelstein, M.L., & Schwartz, M. (2001). *Wong's Essentials of Pediatric Nursing.* St. Louis: C.V. Mosby.

Wright, L., & Leahey, M. (2005). *Nurse and families.* (4th ed.) Philadelphia: F.A. Davis.

 For more information, go to http://davisplus.fadavis.com/

CONCEPT MAP

The Evolving Family

Family Theories/Models: guide holistic nursing care
- Family systems theory
- Family developmental stages and theory
- Structural-functional theory
- Communication theory
- Group theory
- Bowen's Family Systems theory
- Nursing theories: Florence Nightingale; King, Roy; Neuman; Friedman; Hansen: Calgary Family model

Family stressors:
- Health care access
- Insurance/lack of
- Homelessness
- Catastrophic events
- Societal pressures:
  - Crime, suicide, AIDS
- Changing family structure
- "Skip" generation responsibilities

Family with special needs:
- In situational crises
  - Disasters, losses
- Developmental crises
  - e.g., adolescence
- Hospitalization
- Chronic mental illness
- Substance abuse
- Physical/sexual abuse
- PTSD
- Chronic physical illness
- Death of a member

Family cultural characteristics:
- Acculturation and assimilation
- Identity
- Time orientation
- Connectedness
- Communication
- Social class

Contemporary Family Categories
- No-parent
- Cohabiting-parent
- Married blended
- Single parent
- Married parent
- Nuclear and Extended

Family **Patient**

Family of origin

- Two or more members
- Self-identify as family
- Interact/depend on each other: socially, emotionally, financially

Family of choice

Assessment Tools: Family Assessment
- Friedman's qualitative tool
- Family Systems Stressors-Strengths Inventory
- Calgary Family Assessment Model
- Genogram & Ecomap

Nursing assessment of families; concepts; components; factors that influence structure:
- Family size: roles and relationships
- Parenting styles
- Communication styles/patterns
- Religious orientation/beliefs/affiliation
- Ethnicity/culture
- Socioeconomic status
- Developmental stage of the family
- Family rituals/rules/mottos/beliefs
- Family-building activities
- Family dyads/subsystems
- Triangulation within the family

Potential Nursing Interventions: Family Centered Care
Dx: Altered Family Processes
- Identify family dysfunction/family's awareness
- Guide family through medical admissions/interventions
- Assess impact of problems on family stability/functioning
- Listen attentively to all members
- Schedule family conferences
- Identify resources and refer
- Discuss role changes and impact on family members
Evaluation: Outcomes may include effective family communication patterns; appropriate distribution of family tasks and roles

Now Can You:
- Discuss contemporary family changes/stressors
- Discuss family theory for nursing practice
- Apply family nursing diagnoses to a family
- Identify families with special needs/distinct cultures

Caring for Women, Families, and Children in Contemporary Society

 The secret of health for both mind and body is not to mourn for the past, not to worry about the future, or not to anticipate troubles, but to live the present moment wisely and earnestly.

—The Buddha

LEARNING TARGETS *At the completion of this chapter, the student will be able to:*

◆ Determine appropriate timing for health screening examinations based on national recommendations.

◆ Discuss health promotion and disease prevention strategies related to infants and children, including nutrition, dental care, safety, activity, immunizations, and sexuality.

◆ Discuss health promotion and disease prevention strategies related to adolescents, including nutrition, dental care, safety, health promotion screening, sexual behavior, and menstrual disorders.

◆ Discuss health promotion and disease prevention strategies related to young adults, including safety, health promotion screening, and gynecological disorders.

◆ Discuss health promotion and disease prevention strategies related to middle-aged adults, including health promotion screening, perimenopause, menopause, and gynecological disorders.

◆ Discuss health promotion and disease prevention strategies related to older adults, including health promotion screening, gynecological disorders, prostate cancer, and mental and emotional health.

---

moving toward evidence-based practice Eating and Activity Habits of Adolescents

Sweeney, N.M., Glaser, D., & Tedeschi, C. (2007). The eating and physical activity habits of inner-city adolescents. *Journal of Pediatric Health Care, 21*(1), 13–21.

The purpose of this study was to analyze the body mass index (BMI) percentile and eating and physical activity habits of adolescents in relation to gender, ethnicity, country of birth, and household type. An additional purpose was to evaluate diet and activity analysis software for use by practitioners and clients.

A convenience sample of 74 participants included 9th-grade students enrolled in physical education classes, Jr. ROTC, and cooking classes. The age range of the participants was from 14 to 18 years and 53% were females. Sixty percent were Hispanic; 22% were Asian, Pacific Islanders or Philippino; 16% were African American or African; and 3% were Caucasian. Sixty percent of the participants were U.S. born and 65% were from two-parent households. Twenty percent lived with a single mother, 11% lived with a single father, and 4% lived with other relatives.

For study purposes, a 24-hour recall form was developed to obtain information related to eating and physical activity habits. Questions focused on the number of hours of sleep and awake time, participation in sports or exercise, time spent doing homework and engaged in other school-related activities, and time spent watching TV and engaging in tobacco use (smoking). Private interviews were conducted to ensure accuracy of the information provided, and each participant's height and weight were recorded at this time.

Participants were assisted in developing a personal profile on the MyPyramidTracker program available online through the U.S. Department of Agriculture (2005). Each participant's age, gender, height and weight, and 24-hour recall data were entered into the program. Exercise and eating habits in relation

(continued)

to personal characteristics were analyzed and each participant received a report that included the percentage of each food group consumed, a comparison of the food consumed, and established dietary recommendations, the overall intake of calories and nutrients and the total number of calories expended during participation in physical activity.

Data from the MyPyramidTracker program were coded and imported into SPSS (Statistical Package for the Social Sciences). Parametric and nonparametric methods were used to test the associations and between group comparisons.

- Fifty-four percent of the participants were considered to be at a healthy weight; 22% were at risk for overweight or (already) overweight according to the MyPyramidTracker statistical analysis. Of the "at risk for" or "already" overweight group, 50% were Hispanic and 41% were African Americans.

The following findings were related to eating habits: 62% of the participants ate before coming to school, 35% ate between 7:30 A.M. and lunchtime, 77% ate at lunch time, and 97% ate during the time interval between returning home from school and bedtime.

- Boys tended to eat more often and before coming to school.
- Foreign-born students were less likely to eat during all four periods.
- African Americans were less likely than Hispanics and Asians to eat during the periods before lunchtime.

The participants' total caloric and nutrient intake was also examined. Forty-five percent consumed more calories than the recommended daily allowance (RDA). In addition,

- 92% consumed more than the RDA for carbohydrates.
- 68% consumed more than the RDA for sodium.
- 23% consumed more than the RDA for cholesterol.
- 89% consumed less than the RDA for fiber.
- 69% consumed less than the RDA for calcium.
- 16% consumed less than the RDA for protein.

Girls consumed more calories and fiber; boys consumed more nutrients. Hispanic participants consumed more calories, calcium, and sodium. Asians and African American participants tended to include more protein, carbohydrates, and cholesterol in their diets although none of the differences among the ethnic groups were significant.

When addressing the purpose of the study, analyzing the BMI percentile and physical activity habits of adolescents, the results showed:

- The average BMI scores were higher in Hispanics and African American participants. Of the total group of participants, females, Hispanics, foreign-born, and those residing in a home with a single-parent mother had the highest mean BMI percentiles, consumed the least healthy diets and engaged in the least amount of physical activity.
- Seventy-three percent of the participants engaged in sports or exercise. Students born in the United States were more likely to engage in physical activity than were foreign-born students. African Americans were the ethnic group least likely to participate in sports or exercise although the differences were not significant. The difference was significant for the participation of boys over girls in sports.

When addressing the additional purpose of the study, evaluating diet and activity analysis software for use by practitioners and clients, the results showed:

- The MyPyramidTracker software was determined to be suitable for use by adolescents for tracking nutrition, diet, and activity habits.

1. What may be considered as limitations to this study?
2. How is this information useful to clinical nursing practice?

See Suggested Responses for Moving Toward Evidence-Based Practice on the Electronic Study Guide or DavisPlus.

Introduction

This chapter focuses on health promotion and disease prevention across the life span. Health promotion refers to the advancement of health to the highest degree possible for an individual. Disease prevention focuses on the implementation of strategies to reduce the incidence of disease or the development of comorbid illnesses in individuals with existing diseases. Health promotion has become a focus of health care since the advent of managed care. *Healthy People 2000* identified areas of priority for people of all ages regarding health promotion, which have been updated in *Healthy People 2010*, and include physical activity, control of overweight and obesity, responsible sexual behavior, and immunization (U.S. Department of Health and Human Services [USDHHS], 2000).

Health assessment and health promotion screening are perhaps the most important aspects related to promotion of health and prevention of disease. For women, this includes breast cancer screening and pelvic examinations on a recommended basis. For men, it is important to encourage screening for testicular and prostate cancer. Colon and rectal cancer screening should be routinely performed on all adults.

Nurses are perfectly situated to provide anticipatory guidance in areas of health promotion, thereby making accurate information available to family members. With all of the health information currently available in popular magazines, television programming, advertisements, and the Internet, patients do not always have the backgrounds to separate accurate information and practices from propaganda. A solid foundation in anatomy, physiology, sociology, and psychology, along with knowledge of current health promotion research, enables nurses to provide accurate patient information in the areas of nutrition, physical activity, stress management, and safer sexual practices.

Nurses assume many roles when caring for families. Theory-driven knowledge, experiential understanding, and evidence-based clinical practice are essential tools that enable nurses to teach patients at a variety of age and developmental levels. In the areas of infant and child health, major health promotion concerns include nutrition, safety, activity and play, and immunizations.

Adolescents can be considered to be relatively healthy individuals. As such, health promotion for this age group is often ignored. Because peer relationships constitute an important component of adolescent development, peer pressure can precipitate high-risk behaviors that may lead to health complications and the early initiation of chronic illnesses. Nurses play a vital role in the education of adolescents in health care settings and in the community. A holistic approach is tremendously beneficial with this patient population. Teaching healthy practices regarding nutrition, safety, health screening, and safe sexual practices and sexual health can provide avenues for improvement in health practices that can last a lifetime.

During young adulthood, there continue to be health concerns related to nutrition and safety. However, the primary focus of health promotion for this population shifts to reproductive concerns, as this is the time when many patients are engaging in more mature relationships, marriage, and childbearing. For women, gynecological disorders, including infertility, may be diagnosed, requiring additional education for maintaining health and preventing complications.

Health screening is essential for patients in middle adulthood. For this age group, health promotion screening includes mammography, colonoscopy, cholesterol and lipid screening, and osteoporosis screening. While gynecological disorders are still a major health concern for women, reproductive health begins to concentrate on the period preceding menopause, known as perimenopause, with interest targeted on the physiological and psychological changes that occur, the hormone replacement debate, and the use of alternative therapies for symptom relief.

Older adults experience physical and psychological changes due to the aging process. These changes shift health promotion concerns for older adults, including concerns related to sexual functioning, exercise and activity, and cognitive functioning. Gynecological topics that nurses should address for women include menopause, osteoporosis, cancer, and pelvic floor dysfunction.

Health Promotion Screening

Health screening is essential for all family members. Recommendations for examinations, laboratory, and diagnostic tests have been developed by diverse professional and community agencies. Guidelines for addressing high-priority services through preventive screening delivery (Institute for Clinical Systems Improvement, 2005) have been developed and are presented in Table 4-1.

HEALTH SCREENING SCHEDULE

The health maintenance examination (HME) (Michigan Quality Improvement Consortium, 2005a, 2005b) is one of the primary components of health promotion screening. Screening should begin in adolescence and should cover a diversity of health promotion topics (Box 4-1). According to these guidelines, adolescents and young adults 18 to 49 years of age should have one HME every 1 to 5 years according to their risk status. Adults 50 to 64 years of age should have one HME every 1 to 3 years based on their risk status, and older adults 65 years of age and older should have one HME at least every 2 years regardless of risk status.

Infant and Child Health

Health promotion and anticipatory guidance are particularly important in infant and child health. Parents need to have an understanding of nutritional needs, including selection of healthy snacks. Proper dental care is also important in maintaining a child's health. Since infants and children are developing cognitively and physically during this time, there are specific considerations that must be given to safety needs. Immunizations provide protection from and prevention of disease and selection of appropriate toys encourages developmental play that meets safety requirements and facilitates development of social roles. Sexual development and sexual education promote healthy sexual behavior in later years.

NUTRITIONAL GUIDANCE

Infant Feeding

The first decision that parents make regarding infant nutrition is the decision to breastfeed or bottle feed their newborn. Although the composition of infant formula is similar to that of breast milk, and many babies thrive on proprietary formula, breast milk is still considered to be the best option for optimal health promotion and disease prevention in the newborn. One of the primary benefits of breastfeeding is the decreased incidence of bacterial and viral infections as a result of passive immunity, acquired via the transfer of maternal antibodies. According to the U.S. Department of Health and Human Services' Office on Women's Health (2005), breastfed infants are less likely to develop allergies, gastrointestinal tract diseases, respiratory tract diseases, ear infections, and childhood obesity. They also have fewer systemic bacterial infections, urinary tract infections, and bacterial and viral infections of the respiratory tract.

Since an infant's immune system does not become fully mature until 2 years of age, the maternal transfer of antibodies and immune factors enhances development of the immune system and facilitates the neonate's immune system response. The longer the time that an infant is breastfed, the stronger the protection against infection and the earlier the maturation of the infant's immune system. In addition, some studies have indicated that breastfed infants experience lower rates of diabetes, lymphoma, leukemia, Hodgkin's disease, and sudden infant death syndrome (SIDS) (American Academy of Pediatrics [AAP], 2005).

Table 4-1 Preventive Services Delivery Schedule: High-Priority Services			
Service	**19–39 Years**	**40–64 Years**	**65+ Years**
Aspirin Prophylaxis	Discuss with women post-menopause, men over age 40, and younger individuals at increased risk for coronary heart disease		
Breast Cancer Screening		Annual mammogram for women with risk factors; every 1–2 years for women 50 to 64 years of age with no risk factors	Annual mammogram for women with risk factors; every 1–2 years for women 65 and older with no risk factors
Cervical Cancer Screening	First Pap smear at age 21 or 3 years after first sexual intercourse, whichever is earlier; every 3 years after 3 consecutive normal results	Every 3 years after 3 consecutive normal results	Pap smear with new sexual partner
***Chlamydia* and Gonorrhea Screening**	All sexually active females, including asymptomatic women aged 25 years and younger		
Colon Cancer Screening		All persons 50–79 years of age	
Hypertension Screening	Blood pressure screening every 2 years if less than 120/80 mm Hg; annual blood pressure screening if 120–139/80–89 mm Hg		
Influenza Vaccine	Annually between October and March for individuals aged 50 and above, those with chronic illnesses, members of the health care team, and others at high risk		
Pneumococcal Vaccine	Immunize individuals at high risk once; re-immunize once after 5 years if at risk for losing immunity		Immunize at age 65 if not done previously; re-immunize once if first vaccination received greater than 5 years ago and before age 65
Problem Drinking Screening	Screen for problem drinking among all adults and provide brief counseling		
Tobacco Cessation Counseling	Assess all adults for tobacco use and provide ongoing cessation services for those who smoke or are at risk for smoking relapse		
Total Cholesterol and HDL Cholesterol Screening	Fasting fractionated lipid screening for men older than age 34 every 5 years	Fasting fractionated lipid screening for men older than age 34 and for women older than age 44 every 5 years	
Vision Screening			Asymptomatic elderly adults

Sources: American College of Obstetricians and Gynecologists (2007); U.S. Preventive Services Task Force (2007); Institute for Clinical Systems Improvement (ICSI, 2005).

Box 4-1 Components of Health Promotion Screening

Beginning in adolescence, screening should include:

- Height, weight, and body mass index (BMI)
- Risk evaluation and counseling: Nutrition, obesity, physical activity, dental health, tobacco use, immunizations, human immunodeficiency virus (HIV) prevention, sexually transmitted diseases prevention and sexual health, sexual abuse, preconception counseling for all women of childbearing age, medication use, and sun exposure
- Safety: Domestic violence, seat belt use, use of helmets, firearm safety, and use of smoke and carbon dioxide detectors in the home
- Behavior assessment: Depression, suicide threats, alcohol and drug use, anxiety, stress reduction, and coping skills

Data from Michigan Quality Improvement Consortium. (2005, July). *Adult preventive services (ages 18–49)*. Southfield, MI: Author.

Human breast milk contains more carbohydrates, less protein, and less casein than cow's milk or infant formulas. This difference in chemical composition facilitates digestion of breast milk and enables the infant to more readily utilize the nutrients provided. At 1 year of age, breastfed infants are leaner than their formula-fed counterparts. In addition, breastfed infants tend to gain less weight during childhood, a factor that may lead to reduced overweight and obesity in later life.

While breastfeeding and breast milk are associated with many benefits, commercially prepared formula, based on cow's milk, also provides the essential nutrients for infant growth and development. Soy-based formulas are available for infants who have an intolerance to formulas based on cow's milk. Sucrose and corn syrup, the carbohydrates in soy formulas, tend to be more easily digested than lactose, the carbohydrate in cow's milk-based formula. However, cow's milk formulas provide a better source of protein than the soy formulas. Hydrolyzed-protein formulas are also available for infants with intolerance to cow's milk-based formula. Because the protein has already been broken down, the likelihood of an allergic response is diminished.

Whole milk should be introduced into the infant's diet at 1 year of age. By this time, the infant's digestive system has developed enough to provide the enzymes necessary for appropriate absorption and use. The use of whole milk is important in ensuring that the child receives enough fat and calories to meet nutritional and developmental needs (Table 4-2).

Table 4-2	Infant Feeding Patterns
Birth–1 month	Breast every 2–3 hours
	Bottle every 3–4 hours
	2–3 oz. per feeding
2–4 months	Breast or bottle every 3–4 hours
	3–4 oz. per feeding
4–6 months	Breast or bottle 4–6 times per day
	4-5 oz. per feeding
6–8 months	Iron-fortified rice cereal
	Breast or bottle 4 times per day
	6–8 oz. per feeding
8–10 months	Finger foods
	Chopped or mashed foods
	Sippy cup with formula, breast milk, juice, or water
	Breast or bottle 4 times per day
	6–8 oz. per feeding
10–12 months	Self-feeds with fingers and spoon
	Most table foods are allowed
	Breast or bottle 4 times per day
	6–8 oz. per feeding

 ### *Ethnocultural Considerations*— **Infant feeding**

Culture plays an important role in infant feeding. For many new immigrants and members of ethnic minorities, the traditions of their homeland, the consumption of traditional foods, and maintaining traditional food preparations provide comfort in an environment that is new and unknown, and is a way of sustaining cultural identity. Some cultural practices include breastfeeding on demand and early introduction of solid foods, where others feel that exposure of the breast is indecent–a view that decreases the mother's comfort with breastfeeding. It is imperative for nurses to recognize biases that the Western view of health and nutrition is the only appropriate method to feeding an infant. Nurses need to evaluate the effect of the cultural practices objectively and intervene only if the mother or baby is at risk for harm.

Introduction of Solid Foods

As a child moves from infancy to toddlerhood, parents should introduce solid foods into the diet, including finger foods. The foods that should be introduced are based on the developmental stage and nutritional need. Solid food should not be introduced until the infant is at least 4 months of age since the digestive tract is still developing until this point. In addition, solid food should not be put in an infant's bottle. Instead, the child needs to learn that food is to be eaten and taken from a spoon.

Between 4 and 6 months of age, infants begin to exhibit signs of readiness for the introduction of solid foods. These signs include the ability to hold up the head, sit in a high chair, and move the tongue around the mouth without pushing food out of the mouth (as the extrusion reflex disappears). In addition, the infant should be teething, gaining weight (should be doubled from the birth weight), and remain hungry after 8 to 10 breastfeedings or after consuming 40 ounces of formula per day. The first solid food offered to the infant should consist of an iron-fortified rice cereal prepared by mixing one teaspoon of cereal with 4 to 5 teaspoons of breast milk or formula. Over the following weeks, the cereal mixture consistency should be thickened, and the amount gradually increased to 1 tablespoon of cereal per day. New cereals, such as those containing oats and barley, may be added, but parents should wait at least 1 week before adding each new food in order to identify signs of potential allergy.

Between the ages of 6 and 8 months, the infant's cereal intake should increase to 3 to 9 tablespoons per serving, given two to three times per day. In addition, parents should introduce pureed or strained fruits, such as bananas, pears, apples, and peaches, into the diet, beginning with 1 teaspoon and increasing to one-fourth to one-half cup in two to three feedings. At 1-week intervals, pureed or strained vegetables such as carrots, squash, sweet potatoes, avocado, green beans, and peas should also be introduced in the same form as the fruit.

Finger foods can be introduced once the infant reaches 8 to 12 months of age. Signs of readiness for finger foods include the ability to pick up objects with the thumb and forefinger (known as development of the pincer grasp), the ability to transfer items from one hand to the other, and the tendency to put everything into the mouth. Examples of appropriate finger foods include small pieces of lightly toasted bagels, small pieces of ripe bananas, well-cooked spiral pasta, teething crackers, and low-sugar "O"-shaped cereal. During this age, mixed cereals may also be introduced, along with small amounts of yogurt and cottage cheese, small amounts of protein (e.g., egg yolk, pureed meats and poultry, mashed beans with soft skins), and apple and pear juice. Citrus juices should not be introduced, as the digestive system has not developed enough to utilize the nutrients.

From 1 year to 18 months of age, the toddler should begin to use a spoon and eat some of the same foods (mashed or chopped into bite-size pieces) as the older family members. Whole milk, eggs, full-fat yogurt, and cottage cheese, and citrus juices can be introduced at this time. New vegetables, such as broccoli and cauliflower can also be introduced.

New foods are then introduced over the next 18 months as the infant begins to feed himself more and make his own choices. Fruit, cut up into bite-size pieces, and diced vegetables may be added to the diet. As the toddler develops his own taste, combination foods such as macaroni and cheese and spaghetti may also be introduced.

Family Teaching Guidelines...
Introducing Solid Foods to Infants

The baby is ready for the introduction of solid foods at approximately 6 months of age. To help determine if the baby is ready for solid foods, look for developmental cues such as the ability to sit well with support and the decrease or disappearance of the extrusion reflex. The baby may watch very intently as you eat, and may seem hungry between bottles or breastfeeding.

◆ Iron-fortified rice cereal is recommended as baby's first solid food for a couple of reasons. Rice is the least allergenic of the grains and the iron helps the baby replenish the iron needed for growth and development. When introducing the rice cereal to the baby, you can mix it with formula, breast milk, or boiled and cooled water until it is very soupy. As the baby becomes accustomed to solid foods, the consistency of the cereal can be gradually adjusted to create a less soupy texture.

◆ When the baby is eating about 4 tablespoons of cereal twice a day, introduce vegetables and fruits. It is recommended to start with vegetables and then expose the baby to the sweet taste of fruits, as babies are typically more accepting of the sweet tastes.

◆ Introduce one food at a time, waiting 3–5 days between new foods so you will be able to identify any reactions to particular foods.

◆ Introduce food before formula or breastfeeding when the infant is hungry, and follow each solid food meal with breast milk or formula.

Seeking Additional Help:

◆ If the infant is not growing or gaining weight, if he is unable to suck or swallow or shows any signs of an allergic reaction, it is important to promptly seek help from the primary health care provider, nearby clinic, or emergency room.

Essential Information:

◆ Keep salt, sugar, and additives to a minimum or avoid them altogether. If you make your baby's food, do not add salt or sugar.

◆ **Never** put food in bottles or mix food with formula because it can cause choking.

◆ Offer only small bites of food to prevent choking and pay close attention to your baby when feeding.

Data from American Academy of Pediatrics. (2005). Policy statement: Breastfeeding and the use of human milk. *Pediatrics*, *115*(2), 496–506.

Now Can You— Discuss infant and child nutrition?

1. Discuss the benefits of breastfeeding when compared to bottle feeding?
2. Describe the recommended process for introducing solid foods into an infant's diet?
3. Identify at least four safe, nutritious finger foods for infants and toddlers?

Childhood Nutrition

Once the child reaches 3 years of age, parents should be introduced to the Food Pyramid for Kids (U.S. Department of Agriculture, 2005). As with the Food Pyramid developed for adults, the servings per day are calculated based on weight and activity. Specific suggestions are included, such as limiting the intake of juice, ensuring that all juices are 100% natural, and incorporating whole grains to comprise half of the daily grain intake (Fig. 4-1).

Snacks for children are often the most difficult aspect of planning meals. Parents need to be taught that snacks should be nutritious, and that any food item that is appropriate for a meal is appropriate for a snack. Children typically need to eat every 3 to 4 hours to maintain energy needs. Thus, parents must consider portion sizes when providing snacks for their children. Nutritious snacks include grain products, fruit and vegetable juices, fresh fruits and vegetables, dried fruit, nuts, and seeds (Box 4-2).

DENTAL CARE

Teething typically begins between 4 and 7 months of age. The first teeth to erupt are usually the bottom central incisors followed by the upper central and lateral incisors. The next to erupt are the bottom lateral incisors followed by the first molars. An infant may have any range from no teeth to eight or more teeth by her first birthday. Most children will have all 20 of their primary teeth by their third birthday.

Signs of teething include increased drooling, irritability, desire to chew on objects, crying episodes and disrupted sleeping, and eating patterns. Caregivers can be encouraged to give teething infants a cool wet washcloth, teething rings that have been cooled in the refrigerator, or a clean finger rubbed on the gums to help ease the discomfort.

The American Dental Association (ADA) recommends that a dentist examine a child within 6 months of the eruption of the first tooth and no later than the first birthday. Daily dental care can begin even before the first tooth emerges. Gums can be gently wiped with a damp washcloth or gauze, and when the first tooth emerges, a soft toothbrush and water can be used. Toothpaste cannot be used until age two.

SLEEP AND REST

Newborns sleep approximately 15 to 20 hours per day in 2- to 3-hour increments. By 3 months of age, infants sleep approximately 15 hours in a 24-hour period. At 6 months, the infant may have two naps of 2 hours each during the day and sleep 9 to 14 hours per night. From 9 months to 1 year, the length of naps may decrease slightly, with nighttime sleep remaining in the 9- to 14-hour range.

Infants are not born knowing how to put themselves to sleep. To help the infant learn to fall asleep on his own, caregivers can put the infant to bed drowsy but awake, rather than breastfeeding or rocking the infant to sleep. By training the infant to fall asleep independently, if he wakens in the night, he is more likely to self-soothe back to sleep.

Dr. T. Berry Brazelton describes six states of behavior in the newborn: quiet sleep, active sleep, drowsiness, quite alert, active awake, and crying. These states include body activity, eye movements, facial movements, breathing patterns, and response to external and internal stimuli. The nurse can provide anticipatory guidance by educating

Figure 4-1 MyPyramid for Kids.

caregivers about how to recognize these states in the newborn. Often caregivers think the infant is waking, when the infant is actually in a period of active sleep and if left for a few minutes, he will settle back into a quiet sleep state.

In 1992, the American Academy of Pediatrics recommended that infants be placed on their backs to sleep to reduce the risk of sudden infant death syndrome (SIDS). According to the Centers for Disease Control and Prevention (CDC), SIDS rates have declined up to 50% in recent years. Premature infants and infants with certain illnesses may be required to sleep in a prone or side-lying position.

Toddlers and preschoolers require the same amount of sleep per day as do infants. Toddlers and preschoolers sleep approximately 14 hours in a 24-hour period, 11 of those hours at night. One 1.5- to 3-hour afternoon nap provides the additional needed rest. Bedtime resistance is likely to appear in this developmental stage. The nurse can provide anticipatory guidance by recommending sleep strategies for caregivers to implement with toddlers.

School-age children require about 10 to 12 hours of sleep per night. Depending on activity level, some children may require a little more or a little less. The nurse can educate the caregiver to assess their child's mood, temperament, and energy levels throughout the day to determine if the amount of sleep they are getting is sufficient.

Box 4-2 Snacks for Children

- Grain products
  - Bread products: Yeast breads and quick breads, made from whole wheat, rye, oatmeal, mixed grains, and bran; rye crisps; whole-grain crackers. Serve with crackers and cheese, peanut butter, or milk.
  - Cereals: Dry cereals with less than 5 grams of sugar. Serve with milk. Add dried fruits.
  - Popcorn: Top with grated cheese instead of butter and salt.
  - Cookies: Use whole-wheat flour for baking. Try oatmeal or peanut butter cookies. Serve with milk.
- Beverages: Fruit juices and vegetable juices. Serve milk with breads, cereals, and cookies. Blend fruit with milk in a blender.
- Vegetables: Cut up raw vegetables. Serve with peanut butter, cheese, or milk. Include broccoli, carrots, celery, green beans, zucchini, and others.
- Fresh fruit: Serve with peanut butter, yogurt, or milk. Include apples, bananas, grapes, melons, oranges, and peaches.
- Nuts and seeds: Include almonds, cashews, and peanuts.

Family Teaching Guidelines...
Preventing Plagiocephaly

- Infant skulls are soft and flexible during the first year of life as the skull enlarges to accommodate the growing brain. During this time, the infant skull can become misshapen or deformed by external pressure. This condition is rarely life threatening, but can cause permanent facial and skull deformities, or in severe cases, the child's vision can be affected.

- Constant pressure on one area of the infant's head can flatten or reshape it. The Back to Sleep campaign initiated by the American Academy of Pediatrics has had the unintended effect of increasing the incidence of plagiocephaly. Proper positioning during sleep and waking periods spent in car seats and baby chairs often require the infant to spend considerable time on his or her back.

- Place the baby on the stomach to play for several times each day. When the baby is very young, placing a rolled towel or blanket under his arms for support helps the infant to be more comfortable. This intervention removes pressure from the skull and facilitates the development of strong neck and arm muscles needed for sitting and crawling.

- Alternating the direction the baby faces in the bassinet or crib during sleep times is also helpful. If the baby's crib is positioned against a wall, alternating the end of the bed where the baby's head is placed allows her to look out toward the room rather than at the less stimulating wall.

SEEKING ADDITIONAL HELP

- If you notice a flattened area on the baby's skull that does not seem to be improving with positioning changes, you should talk with the physician. The baby may need to be fitted with a customized helmet that is worn for 23 hours a day. This helmet is designed to prevent the baby's head from assuming one position, and allows the skull to expand into the flattened area.

ESSENTIAL INFORMATION

- The baby may also be placed on his side while he is awake. The mother can lie on her side, face the baby, and both parties can entertain each other with toys and facial expressions. It is a wonderful way to bond with the baby. Newborn babies love to look at their parents' faces, so this is a very enjoyable activity for them.

Data from American Academy of Pediatrics (1992).

SAFETY

Infants and children are at particular risk for accidents and injuries as a result of their cognitive and physical development during these years. Parents need to be taught how to prevent injuries and accidents, as well as how to prepare for risk-taking behaviors that may arise in late childhood. These risk-taking behaviors may include experimenting with substance use and sexual activity.

Injury Prevention

One of the best methods for prevention of injury to infants and children is for parents to prepare and keep their homes safe. This process, ideally begun before the infant is brought home from the hospital, should be re-evaluated and modified as the child moves through each developmental stage. Smoke and carbon monoxide detectors should be installed throughout the home. Medications and chemicals should be moved to a high shelf, placed in a sealed area, or stored in a cupboard equipped with child safety locks. A fire extinguisher should be readily available on every floor in the home and an additional unit placed in the kitchen. A fire escape route should be planned.

An appropriate car seat should be obtained in anticipation of bringing the new infant home from the hospital. Proper use of a car seat, which has been shown to reduce the chance of injury by 70% and the chance of death by 90%, includes placing the unit in a backward-facing direction in the back seat.

When the infant is brought home from the hospital, new areas of concern must be considered. Crib safety is one of these. Parents should be cautioned about buying older (made prior to 1989) models of cribs, as they do not meet current safety standards. The distance between the slats of the crib railings should be less than 2 3/8 inches to prevent head entrapment and potential strangulation. There should be no sharp edges, and the crib mattress should fit snugly with the end panels extending below the mattress to prevent suffocation. Bumper pads should be used to pad the crib; these should be removed once the infant is able to stand. The furniture paint should be non-toxic and all furniture in the infant's nursery should be positioned to avoid windows, curtains, blinds, lamps, electrical cords, outlets, and appliances.

With regard to infant feeding and safety, teach parents to warm bottles slowly, never to use a microwave oven to heat breast milk or formula, and never prop a bottle in the infant's mouth, as this practice creates a choking hazard. Remind parents to keep all hot liquids and foods away from the baby and to place them well away from the edges of tables and counter tops. If a pacifier is used, one with shields large enough to prevent placement of the entire pacifier in the mouth should be selected, and the pacifier should be frequently inspected for breakage or cracks. Never place the pacifier on a cord around the infants' neck or attached to the infant's clothes with a clip or cord.

At 3 months of age, infants begin to roll over from stomach to back and to turn toward loud sounds. These activities can pose a safety hazard related to the changing tables used for changing diapers. Teach parents to keep one hand on the infant at all times and never to leave the infant alone on the table. Powders, oils, and lotions should be used cautiously to prevent poisoning or illness if swallowed. To prevent aspiration, powders should never be shaken close to the infant's face. Current recommendations for powder use include having the parents first place the powder in their hands and then rub it onto the infant.

Since serious falls and injuries can occur with the use of high chairs, playpens, strollers, and swings, these items should be used only under supervision of an adult. Playpens should not be used in place of cribs in order to prevent injury from suffocation that can occur while the infant is asleep. The use of walkers is not recommended, as serious brain injury, fractures, and concussions have resulted from accidents that involve the walker tipping over or falling down a staircase. Also, the development of gross motor skills may be hindered with walker use, as babies who use them learn to walk on the tips of the toes.

Play time and bath time are associated with potential hazards as well. Risks of accidental choking and suffocation are significant for children younger than the age of 6 months who tend to place small objects in their mouths as their cognitive and fine motor skills are developing. Parents must ensure that crib gyms and mobiles are placed at an appropriate height, toys and stuffed animals have no removable parts or sharp edges, and pull toys do not have long cords. Bath safety includes ensuring that the water temperature is below 120°F. Teach parents to test the water temperature before placing the child in the bath and to use bath mats or towels to prevent slipping. During the bath, the parent should keep both hands positioned securely on the infant, while using one hand to constantly hold the infant and the other hand to wash the infant.

By 14 months of age, the child has developed the skills necessary for walking; the majority of children walk well by this time. Once the child begins to crawl, creep, and walk, additional environmental safety hazards are present. Kitchen and bathroom cabinets should be equipped with firm latches or locks to prevent injury from medications, poisonous chemicals, and sharp implements. Stove guards should be placed over knobs and burners to prevent accidental injury from burns. Remind parents to turn all pot handles away from the front of the stove and to install locks or latches on appliance doors to prevent entrapment and suffocation.

Stairs and windows present safety hazards related to falls. Safety gates at the tops and bottoms of staircases should be used at all times; accordion gates are not recommended. Railings on steps, decks, and balconies should be covered with netting to prevent children from getting trapped between the posts or falling. Safety guards can be placed on windows to prevent them from opening more than 4 inches; however, these should not be used on windows designated for fire escape. Furniture should not be placed near windows as children can climb on the furniture and fall through the windows. Poisoning accidents can occur through the ingestion of harmful plants or peeling paint chips, particularly in homes built before 1978 that contain lead-based paint.

 Now Can You— **Discuss strategies to ensure infant and toddler safety?**

1. Describe methods for ensuring crib safety?
2. Identify ways to promote bath safety?
3. Discuss strategies for making stairways and window areas safe?

By 24 months of age, cognitive skills have developed that allow the toddler to begin logical reasoning. During this time, play activities pose the greatest risk of injury. While playing indoors, children should not be allowed to run or jump, and the kitchen and bathroom should be off limits. Refrigerators and freezers should be locked, and closets, attics, and basements should be sealed to prevent accidental injuries. Outside safety includes having a

fenced-in yard with a locked gate and ensuring that all playground equipment is installed securely. A soft surface should be placed under playground areas to provide cushioning for falls. All yard equipment should be safely stored away from children.

Water safety is also important. Swimming in pools, lakes, and rivers should take place only under adult supervision, and children should not be allowed to dive or jump into water less than 12 feet in depth. Chemicals used in pools and hot tubs are poisonous and should be kept out of the reach of children. If possible, a separate fence should be placed around the pool, equipped with a safety alarm system to alert parents when children are near the water.

Risk-taking Behaviors

Children engage in risk-taking behaviors as a normal progression through cognitive development. Risk-taking enables children to develop skills and self-confidence as well as to understand their strengths and limitations. Through risk-taking behavior, children learn boundaries and develop an awareness of the outside world.

TESTING LIMITS. Risk-taking actually begins in infancy, as infants explore their worlds, place objects in their mouths, and learn to identify parental facial expressions and gestures. Once the child begins to walk, limit-testing heightens through activities such as climbing, reaching, and balancing. Parents who allow the child's exploration send a message that when performed in appropriate situations, a certain degree of risk-taking is necessary for development. Conversely, parents who do not allow exploration convey the message that experimentation is undesirable and should not be done. Close to age 2, when the child enters the developmental stage of *autonomy versus shame and doubt*, risk-taking may present itself in the form of saying "no" to parents.

Preschoolers may engage in risk-taking behaviors as a result of their physical development. As gross motor skills develop, their physical abilities exceed their ability to logically reason the danger associated with their activities. Parents need to monitor their children's activities, while allowing them to maintain a sense of control. In so doing, the parent helps the child to develop the confidence needed to try something new or difficult in the future and facilitates the child's successful mastery of the developmental task associated with *initiative versus guilt*.

School-age children's risk-taking behavior, as opposed to the preschoolers' behavior, is more closely related to cognitive rather than physical development. At this time, the child has moved into the stage of *industry versus inferiority* and is developing a sense of self-esteem. Risk-taking allows the school-age child to experience heightened feelings of self-worth following success and to learn to evaluate mistakes and develop alternative strategies for the future when they meet with failure. See Chapter 20 for more information on developmental stages.

PLAY

Play enables children to explore their world, express their thoughts and feelings, and meet and solve problems. The foundation for play begins immediately after birth. The infant reflexively grasps objects or moves extremities and through this, discovers enjoyment of the sounds, tastes, textures, and smells. These discoveries gradually lead the infant to perform such activities purposefully. Playing with an infant begins with engaging all of the senses. Infants enjoy looking at faces, black-and-white objects, hearing voices, and sucking on hands in the reflexive play stage. It is important for caregivers to play with their babies, as much of an infant's learning occurs through play. For the first few months, the caregiver must play with the baby during quiet alert periods. This is the best learning time for a young infant. As the baby grows and abilities and mobility increase, the infant plays for longer periods and becomes adept at expressing feelings. Signs of boredom or lack of interest become more obvious, at which point the caregiver can switch to a new game.

As physical coordination and sensory ability increase rapidly, the infant is able to examine objects more closely. By looking, touching, and placing objects in the mouth, the infant discovers different textures, tastes, and colors. As the infant develops, he learns cause and effect. For example, when an infant shakes the rattle, it makes a pleasant sound. This recognition of cause and effect encourages the infant to repeat activities to achieve the desired result.

As the infant approaches the 1-year mark, the play environment increases dramatically as the infant learns to crawl and walk. In addition, the ability to communicate increases steadily as the infant reaches 12 months. At this time, the infant can point to objects, voice frustrations at having toys taken away, and use body language and sounds in an attempt to express emotions. Play in childhood is based on cognitive as well as physical development. While there are five types of developmental play in which older children can participate, children must progress from the lower levels to the higher levels. In order to meet the developmental needs of each stage of play as the child grows and matures, specific activities, toys, and games should be introduced (Table 4-3).

- Solitary play (type 1): The child plays alone, without regard for those around him.
- Onlooker play (type 2): The child observes the other children around him as he plays alone; may alter own play activities based on what he sees the others doing or may be content to continue in his play while simply talking with the other children; play activities are different (e.g., one child may be bouncing a ball while another is playing with jacks).
- Parallel play (type 3): Children play with the same materials and items, but they do not yet play together.
- Associative play (type 4): The peer group is developed to the extent that children play together, but in a loosely organized manner.
- Cooperative play (type 5): Children assume designated roles in the games, have goals for the games, and rely on one another for the game to continue and progress.

Now Can You— **Provide developmentally appropriate play activities for school-age children?**

1. Identify the five types of play?
2. Describe the developmental tasks associated with each type of play?
3. Identify play activities that are appropriate for each type of play?

IMMUNIZATIONS

Immunizations are the child's first and best defense against several diseases that can be fatal or cause serious disability. Since the child's immune system is immature, the administration of vaccines enables the child to develop antibodies against specific potential organisms. The CDC (2006b) has developed a recommended schedule to enable health care practitioners and parents to ensure that early and appropriately timed immunization is in place (Fig. 4-2).

SEXUALITY

It is never too early to begin sexual education with children. Correct information enhances appropriate decision-making regarding sexual behavior in the later years. The infant is aware of the differences in touch in certain parts of the body and is capable of deriving comfort and pleasure from touch. Male babies have erections and female babies experience vaginal lubrication. Infants can experience orgasm as early as 4 or 5 months of age. Sexuality at these young ages is an expression of exploration and comfort.

As early as 18 months of age, toddlers begin to explore their bodies and express concerns and questions about their bodies. Parents should teach their children the proper names for sex organs and allow masturbation, in a private manner, as children begin normal body exploration. By age 4, children can be taught that males and females have different sexual organs. While sexual exploration with other children is normal developmentally, the parents should set limits and discourage it if seen. During the preschool years, the question of where babies come from usually arises. It is best if parents are direct and honest and provide a simple and straightforward answer that babies come from inside the mother. School-age children, who tend to associate and play more with children of their same gender, are still attempting to learn the difference between the sexes. At this time, parents must continue to provide truthful, direct information and encourage questions to prevent their children from receiving incorrect information from friends.

During the years between 8 and 11, children begin to focus on their own development and contrast it with that of their friends. Reassurance from parents decreases anxiety and helps children to realize that they are in the normal range of development. At this time, parents should begin to educate their children about the names and functions of the male and female sexual organs, puberty, the menstrual cycle, sexual intercourse, pregnancy, pregnancy prevention, same-sex relationships, masturbation, and the spread of sexually transmitted infections. They should also encourage dialogue about personal expectations and values regarding sexual activity.

ADOLESCENT HEALTH

Adolescents are in a vulnerable life stage as they are between the states of childhood and adulthood and are experiencing significant physical and emotional growth. A number of developmental tasks are associated with this period (Box 4-3). The most important changes that occur between the ages of 11 and 18 are sexual developmental changes. The influx of sexual hormones, combined with the growth of primary and secondary sexual characteristics

Table 4-3 Play Activities for Children

Developmental Age	Type of Play	Purpose of Play	Activities
Infant	• Solitary play (type 1): The child plays alone, without regard for those around him.	To stimulate sensorimotor development with simple imitative games	• Patty cake • Peek-a-boo • Itsy-bitsy spider • Finger painting • Ball rolling • Songs • High chair fishing
Toddler	• Parallel play (type 3): Children play with the same materials and items, but they do not yet play together	To help children make the transition from solitary play to associative play by stimulating sensorimotor and psychosocial development	• Matching games • Simple puzzles • Blowing bubbles • Bean bag toss • Catching fireflies • Ring around the Rosy • London Bridge • Duck-duck goose • Hide and seek • Coloring • Drawing
Preschooler	• Associative play (type 4): The peer group is developed to the extent that children play together, but in a loosely organized manner.	To help children learn how to share, play in small groups and to learn simple games with rules, concepts of language, and social rules	• Memory • Chutes and Ladders • Candyland • Hokey Pokey • Hot Letters • Alphabet games • Color games • Checkers
School-age	• Cooperative play (type 5): Children assume designated roles in the games, have goals for the games, and rely on one another for the game to continue and progress.	To teach children how to bargain, cooperate, and compromise in order to develop logical reasoning, which increases social skills	• Baseball • Soccer • Gymnastics • Swimming • Dodge ball • Board games • Simple card games • Computer games • Video games • Puzzles • Crosswords • Word search puzzles
Adolescent	• Cooperative play (type 5): Children assume designated roles in the games, have goals for the games, and rely on one another for the game to continue and progress.	To teach children how to bargain, cooperate, and compromise in order to develop logical reasoning, which increases social skills	• Video games • Computer games • Board games • Card games • Team sports • Charades

Vaccine ▼ Age ▶	Birth	1 month	2 months	4 months	6 months	12 months	15 months	18 months	19–23 months	2–3 years	4–6 years
Hepatitis B[1]	Hep B	Hep B		see footnote 1		Hep B					
Rotavirus[2]			Rota	Rota	Rota						
Diphtheria, Tetanus, Pertussis[3]			DTaP	DTaP	DTaP	see footnote 3	DTaP				DTaP
Haemophilus influenzae type b[4]			Hib	Hib	*Hib*[4]	Hib					
Pneumococcal[5]			PCV	PCV	PCV	PCV					PPV
Inactivated Poliovirus			IPV	IPV		IPV					IPV
Influenza[6]							Influenza (Yearly)				
Measles, Mumps, Rubella[7]						MMR					MMR
Varicella[8]						Varicella					Varicella
Hepatitis A[9]						HepA (2 doses)				HepA Series	
Meningococcal[10]										MCV4	

Range of recommended ages	Certain high-risk groups

Figure 4-2 Recommended immunization schedule for children (CDC, 2006b).

Box 4-3 Developmental Tasks of Adolescence

- Formal Operational Thought: Piaget's Theory of Cognitive Development indicates that adolescents' thought becomes more abstract. They develop the ability to logically reason, generating hypotheses and potential consequences of action.
- Learning Identity: Erikson's Theory of Psychosocial Development suggests that the adolescent experiments with different roles in an attempt to identify the role with which he or she is most comfortable. The adolescent, through achievement, becomes more confident in his abilities and gradually develops a set of ideals with which he can identify. As the adolescent experiments with different societal roles, peer influences play an increasingly important role in development.
- Sexual Identity: Freud's Theory of Psychosexual Development proposes that, as adolescents enter puberty, instinctual impulses create stress and uncertainty. As the adolescent develops a sense of sexuality, the stress is decreased, and balance is restored, allowing the adolescent to engage in healthy sexual relationships.

and the focus on peer relationships, place adolescents at increased risk of injury and disease. During this developmental period, special attention needs to be placed on nutrition, safety, sexual health promotion, and prevention of illness.

NUTRITION

Diet and nutrition are especially important for facilitating optimal growth and development during adolescence. Adequate nutritional intake is essential to accommodate the growth spurt that occurs during this time. Adolescents gain approximately 25% of their adult height and 50% of their adult weight throughout this time period. In addition to the nutritional needs to promote growth and development, adolescents are tasked with developing a positive body image and a personal identity. When conflicts exist, adolescents are at increased risk for eating disorders, which can lead to overweight, underweight, hypertension, and diabetes mellitus.

Obesity in Adolescence

During adolescence, it is common for the appetite to increase. In addition, adipose cells develop rapidly, leading to an increased potential for adipose tissue development and overweight. This growth is dependent on both nutritional and environmental factors. It is essential to balance the energy intake and output in the adipose cells to prevent the growth of larger adipose cells, which can lead to obesity. Overweight and obesity result from a decreased ability to release fat during periods of energy expenditure.

The effects of heredity and environment should be considered as contributing factors in adolescent obesity. A child born to two obese parents has a 75% chance of being obese. A child born to parents where only one is obese has a 25% chance of being obese. However, the influence of heredity must be considered in the context of the adolescent's environment. Psychological, social, and health factors collectively shape the adolescent's environment and its impact on nutritional health.

PSYCHOLOGICAL FACTORS. Perhaps the factor that has the greatest psychological effect on body image and nutritional health is the media. Television and advertising both encourage and condone the eating of high-fat, high-carbohydrate foods, using thin, attractive people in the commercials. In addition, the mere fact that adolescents spend approximately 3 to 4 hours each day watching television adds to the problem of obesity, as television viewing is a sedentary activity.

The impact of the media on the developing adolescent's body image is crucial. Body image is affected by physical characteristics, body-related experiences, social response to appearance, and social value placed on body characteristics. Each of these factors has an effect on personality development, and is influenced by individual responses. Many times, these factors combine to create a focus on excessive dieting and scale-weighing behaviors. In addition, there is a relationship between impaired body image in adolescents and depression.

SOCIAL FACTORS. Social factors such as the influence of family and peers interact with the psychological factors that impact adolescent obesity. In many families, eating and mealtime behaviors are instituted at an early age. Little time may be spent on meal preparation, and time spent with family members while eating may be nonexistent. As the dual-income family has become the norm in modern society, fast food and eating "on the go" has also become the norm. Eating patterns that lead to adolescent obesity may include the regular consumption of high-calorie, low-nutrient-dense foods, a lack of understanding about nutrition, a lack of structure and sociability in eating patterns, a tendency to eat late in the evening, binge eating when hungry or bored, and the habit of eating rapidly.

Adolescence is also a time when peer relationships become extremely important in the development of a personal identity. Adolescents frequently congregate and socialize in areas where food is consumed, such as fast food restaurants, pizza parlors, and at parties. For many, eating becomes a social event in and of itself. In these settings, peer pressure may influence the healthy eaters to consume high-fat, high-caloric food in order to fit in with the majority. Over time, many adolescents become conditioned to eat poorly and to elude structure in their eating behaviors.

One's level of physical activity is associated with weight, and a sedentary lifestyle constitutes a significant factor in obesity. When adolescents are not with their peers, they are often engaging in sedentary activities, such as watching television, using the computer, talking on the telephone, and text messaging. Without energy expenditure, the excess in calorie consumption increases the number of adipose cells and leads to further weight gain.

MEDICAL FACTORS. The psychological and social factors may predispose to an increased risk for disease related to overeating and obesity. Depression is one of the most common disorders associated with adolescent obesity. While attempting to fit into the peer group by engaging in unhealthy eating behaviors, adolescents are meanwhile being bombarded with media images of thin, attractive individuals overeating and societal messages that obesity is unattractive and shameful. There is an unspoken viewpoint that obese individuals are overindulgent and lack self-control. These influences negatively impact the adolescent's body image and self-esteem, and create a risk for depression, feelings of social isolation, rejection, failure, and thoughts of suicide.

Obesity in adolescence leads to medical problems, including cardiovascular disease, type 2 diabetes mellitus, kidney disease, gallbladder disease, liver disease, and orthopedic problems. Hypercholesterolemia and hyperlipidemia increase the workload on the heart, resulting in hypertension. These disorders, when combined with

hyperinsulinemia, result in insulin resistance syndrome. Insulin resistance is highly associated with the development of type 2 diabetes mellitus, long thought to be an adult disease. Over the past 10 years, however, there has been an increased incidence of type 2 diabetes mellitus developing in childhood and adolescence (Menon, Burgis, & Bacon, 2007).

For the adolescent female, insulin resistance and obesity may affect reproductive and gynecological health. Insulin resistance causes an increase in circulating insulin, and stimulates an increase in the production of androgens. Increased androgens, combined with the increased levels of circulating insulin, have been reported to trigger polycystic ovarian syndrome (PCOS) (Dunaif, 2006). PCOS is associated with anovulation, and is manifested by dysmenorrhea, hirsutism, and acne. Insufficient progesterone production results in infertility and an increased risk of endometrial cancer.

"What to say" — *When talking with an adolescent about losing weight*

Discussions about weight loss can be a sensitive issue for many overweight patients. During adolescence, body weight has a dramatic effect on the development of self-image and self-esteem and can be an even more sensitive issue for discussion. An important strategy in discussions about weight and weight loss with adolescents is to begin the conversation with expressions of respect that are sensitive to cultural differences related to food choices and eating patterns. Regardless of whether or not the patient is ready to begin a weight control program, she may still benefit from talking openly about healthy eating and exercise. To open the conversation, the nurse can begin with a simple question to determine if the patient is willing to talk about the issue:

"Cindy, can we talk about your weight? What are your thoughts about your weight right now?"

To determine the degree of readiness to engage in weight control, additional questions can be asked:

"What are your goals concerning your weight?"

"What kind of help would you like from me regarding your weight?"

Nurses should avoid the use of words that may make patients feel uncomfortable, such as "obese," "obesity," "fat," and "excess fat."

Eating Disorders

In addition to overweight and obesity associated with overeating, other eating disorders such as anorexia nervosa and bulimia nervosa may develop during adolescence. These two eating disorders adversely affect nutrition and the overall health status and impact growth and development. The underlying issue associated with eating disorders concerns the improper use of food: eating too little, eating too much, or eating too much and purging in an attempt to rid the body of excessive calories.

Eating disorders are rooted in issues related to body image development. The core of the problem involves a distortion in body image and a delay in achieving progress toward a healthy, adult body image. In essence, adolescents with severe eating disorders are struggling with another developmental task, that of autonomy. They tend to have an unrealistic view of themselves, and depend on social opinions and judgments, as evidenced by their preoccupation with food, dieting, and exercise patterns.

ANOREXIA NERVOSA. **Anorexia nervosa** is a chronic eating disorder that stems from a distorted body image. This condition develops as a result of obesity or a perception of obesity that creates an obsession with weight loss and a denial of hunger. The fear of gaining weight, combined with a low self-esteem, creates a life-threatening disorder that can, if not properly treated, lead to serious medical complications and death. Individuals with anorexia nervosa undertake strict and severe diets and engage in rigorous excessive exercise in order to maintain an unrealistic body weight. Psychological traits associated with anorexia nervosa include perfectionism, obsessive–compulsive behavior, social isolation, a focus on high achievement without satisfaction, and depression (Menon et al., 2007).

Due to a pervasive malnutrition that affects all organ systems, symptoms include weakness, dizziness, excessive weight loss, intolerance to cold, bradycardia, hypotension, bone loss with consequent fractures, constipation from dehydration, and the development of lanugo. The continued restriction of calories suppresses the hypothalamic–pituitary–adrenal axis, and results in decreased production of cortisol and growth hormone. In females, luteinizing hormone and follicle-stimulating hormone are suppressed, resulting in a decreased production of estrogen. Decreased estrogen levels are associated with anovulation, amenorrhea, loss of secondary sex characteristics, and infertility. Over time, inadequate nutrition results in blood and electrolyte abnormalities, which may lead to death.

BULIMIA NERVOSA. **Bulimia nervosa** is a syndrome that consists of a cycle of binge eating and purging. Binge eating entails eating large amounts of food at least 2 days per week for at least 3 months. When this behavior is combined with extreme measures to rid the body of the excess food, a cycle ensues. Adolescents with bulimia may use laxatives, diuretics, or emetics to rid the body of excess calories (purging behavior), or they may engage in excessive exercise or fasting (nonpurging behavior). These behaviors are performed in an effort to alleviate the guilt associated with overeating; as the guilt feelings pass, the tension returns, and the binging behavior begins once again.

Adolescents with bulimia nervosa typically maintain a normal weight, although psychological factors associated with bulimia include poor impulse control, low self-esteem, depression, and anxiety disorder. In addition, comorbid behaviors such as alcohol and substance abuse, unprotected sexual activity, self-mutilation, and suicide attempts may be present. Similar to anorexia, bulimia is an eating disorder that is usually associated with some degree of depression.

Physically, the adolescent with bulimia nervosa may present with symptoms related to forced excessive vomiting: cracked and damaged lips, tooth damage, callused fingers and hands, and broken blood vessels in the face. Symptoms that may not be physically noticeable include throat irritation, esophageal inflammation, and parotitis from vomiting, as well as rectal bleeding from overuse of laxatives. While life-threatening conditions are less common in adolescents with bulimia than in adolescents with anorexia, they may still be at risk for dehydration, electrolyte imbalances, ruptures in the gastrointestinal tract, kidney disease, and cardiac arrhythmias.

DENTAL CARE. For adolescents, twice yearly dental visits for checkups and cleaning are required. It is common for adolescents to have dental work performed to correct tooth malformations. Obvious dental correction can create body image problems, particularly if wearing braces or a headgear is required. Education regarding the proper care of teeth with dental appliances must be received at the dentist's office and reinforced by caregivers at home.

SLEEP AND REST

Adolescents are commonly chronically sleep deprived as activities, schoolwork, and after-school jobs keep them up later at night. Often the adolescent sleeps extensively on weekends to make up for the deficiency during the week, but this is generally more detrimental as the body has difficulty adapting to irregular sleeping patterns. Sleep deprivation can impair memory and inhibit creativity, making it difficult for sleep-deprived adolescents to learn.

The nurse can encourage caregivers and adolescents to keep evening activities to a manageable level that allows for some quiet time before bed and an appropriate bedtime. Involving the adolescent in the decision-making process regarding which activities to reduce or eliminate will help the teen comply with the limits set. In addition, if the adolescent adheres to a similar bedtime and wake time on the weekends as during the week, excessive fatigue can be controlled.

SAFETY

Since adolescents are still developing formal thought operations, they may not have the cognitive abilities to make appropriate decisions regarding safety. Their decisions are likely to result in accidents and injuries and risk-taking behaviors for which adults may not be at risk. However, the accidents and injuries most common in adolescents differ from those in infancy and childhood. In addition, adolescents must be taught information related to safe sexual practices, substance use and abuse, violence, and suicide prevention.

Accidents and Injuries

The three leading causes of death in adolescents are motor vehicle accidents, homicide, and suicide, respectively. The risk for motor vehicle accidents is greater among adolescents than for any other age group, with more than 5000 adolescents between the ages of 16 and 19 dying from injuries related to crashes (Insurance Institute for Highway Safety, 2005). For male adolescents, the risk is two times higher than that of female adolescents. Risk factors for these statistics include the inability to assess hazardous situations while driving, speeding, driving under the influence of drugs or alcohol, and a low compliance with seat belt use.

In relation to homicides, approximately one-third of all homicides in the United States occur among adolescents. Individual factors related to this level of violence in adolescence include a history of abuse and the observation of violent acts at home. Certain familial characteristics have also been linked to adolescent homicide: distant, passive, or absent fathers; dominant, overprotective, and sexually inappropriate mothers; violence between family members; turmoil in the home setting; and feelings of distrust among the children in the home. Health care providers need to be aware of protective factors that have been identified in order to provide health care teaching to adolescents and empower them with strategies to reduce their risk. Education, spiritual support, improved economic conditions, conflict resolution skills, and reduced use of drugs and alcohol are areas of education focus and patient advocacy that can be addressed by health care providers. Finally, since access to guns impacts the adolescent homicide rate, implementation of gun safety classes is another appropriate area for intervention.

Suicide is the third leading cause of death in adolescents, and, as such, needs to be understood and addressed by health care providers. As a result of their developing personality and peer and family pressures, adolescents may become easily overwhelmed and anxious and look to suicide as an answer to their distress. Although female adolescents are more likely to engage in suicide attempts, males are more likely to complete them, and account for approximately 85% of all suicides, while females account for 15%. Adolescent Native Americans and Alaskan Natives have the highest rates of suicide; African Americans, Hispanics, and Asians have the lowest rates of suicide (Menon et al., 2007).

Common symptoms of suicidal ideation that can be addressed by health care providers include the following: reports of crying frequently, fatigue and insomnia; feelings of isolation; and changes in body weight. Adolescents may exhibit additional symptoms, such as behavior problems, violence, sexual promiscuity, a drop in academic performance, and school absence. Nurses who are aware of any of these symptoms should ask if the adolescent has plans to commit suicide, the means to commit suicide, and if there have been any previous attempts at suicide. Adolescents who are determined to be at low risk for suicide should be referred to a mental health professional; those determined to be at high risk for suicide should be immediately evaluated by a mental health professional.

Risk-taking Behaviors

As in childhood, it is normal for adolescents to engage in risk-taking behavior. Taking healthy risks provides an avenue for discovering and developing one's own identity. Parents need to be taught that they can facilitate healthy risk-taking through talking with their adolescent openly and honestly and helping their child to understand the consequences of healthy versus non-healthy risk-taking behaviors. Ongoing dialogue provides an opportunity to explore alternative actions and sharing a personal history of past risk-taking behaviors conveys the message that making mistakes is not a fatal act.

Health care providers and parents can assist adolescents in finding alternative behaviors to provide outlets for identity development through providing them with challenges that create risk while promoting healthy decision making (Box 4-4).

Injury Prevention

Unhealthy risk-taking often leads to injuries for adolescents, and the most common injuries are related to motor vehicles, bicycles, firearms, and water. Nurses and parents can provide valuable teaching to adolescents and empower them to take necessary precautions to avoid injury. One of the most important ways in which parents can affect adolescent safety is to set a good example and be a positive role model.

DRIVING SAFELY. Since motor vehicle accidents occur so commonly and cause such significant injury, there needs to be a strong focus on injury prevention for this activity. Recommendations for parents to ensure safe driving include establishing limits, such as the number of passengers and restriction to daytime driving, enforcing penalties for unsafe driving practices, adult supervision of adolescents while driving, ensuring mechanical safety, and mandating the use of seat belts.

BICYCLE SAFETY. Another common area of injury in adolescence, and one that is not often discussed includes activities that involve bicycles, in-line skating, and skateboarding. Head injuries related to these activities are quite common in this age group. Approximately 50% of young adolescents hospitalized for a bicycle-related injury have some degree of brain injury. Behaviors that cause the majority of the injuries include riding into a street without yielding or stopping, swerving into traffic, and riding against the flow of traffic.

Box 4-4 Healthy Risk Alternatives for Adolescents

- Physical activities
  - Team sports
  - Horseback riding
  - Camping
  - Rock climbing (with supervision)
  - White water rafting (with supervision)
- Creative activities
  - Joining a band
  - Acting in a play
  - Photography
  - Dance
  - Producing a video
- Developing relationships
  - Talking openly about sex and relationships
  - Volunteering in the community
  - Participating in a student exchange program
- Learning responsibility
  - Getting a part-time job
  - Tutoring

Consistent use of a helmet is one of the best preventive strategies. It is essential that the helmet fit properly—it should not move around when the straps are fastened—and the straps should remain fastened when in use. When worn and used correctly, helmets can reduce the risk of a head injury by 85% and the risk of brain damage by 88%. All helmets should meet the standards established by the American National Standards Institute, the American Society for Testing and Materials, and the United States Consumer Product Safety Commission.

FIREARM SAFETY. Curiosity and impulse control remain important factors in firearm-related injuries and deaths among adolescents. Parents should consider the risks associated with storing a firearm in the home. In this age group, ready access to a firearm is the most frequent cause of the experimentation. If parents choose to keep a firearm in the home for protection or for hunting, it should be safely stored in a locked cabinet and all ammunition placed in a separate, locked location. A firearm safety class should be mandatory for adolescents who engage in the sport of hunting with parents or peers.

WATER SAFETY. Adolescents, who are in the process of developing formal operational thought, have an increased risk of drowning when swimming due to an overestimation of ability and skill, a lack of awareness of water depth and currents, and the use of alcohol and drugs. Safety measures include insisting that adolescents do not swim alone and teaching them never to dive into shallow water, above-ground pools, or the shallow end of an in-ground pool. In addition, adolescents riding in a boat should be required to wear personal flotation devices that are securely fastened. Parents and health care providers should routinely incorporate safety education into discussions with adolescents.

⊛ **Now Can You**— Provide safety education to adolescents?

1. Identify the three leading causes of death in adolescents?
2. Discuss methods for improving driving safety?
3. Identify the best method of preventing injury related to bicycle riding?
4. Describe methods to facilitate firearm safety?

REPRODUCTIVE HEALTH SAFETY Safety with regard to reproductive health can be positively impacted through proper, sensitive, and honest education on topics related to sexual activity. While the majority of parents indicate that they believe education on issues of sexual health should be taught in the family, most also agree that they do not feel prepared to do so alone. Many schools have subsequently incorporated education on sexuality into curricula in an effort to facilitate transfer of factual information.

Developmentally, adolescence is characterized by attempts to develop a personal identity, which includes sexual and gender identity. Young people are bombarded with sexual images from music, television, advertisements, and movies on a daily basis. Providing adolescents with correct information on issues of sexuality helps to empower them to make healthy decisions regarding their own sexual behavior. Whether taught by parents, health care providers, or classroom educators, educational content should

include human development, reproductive anatomy and physiology, relationships, personal coping skills and decision-making, sexual behavior, contraceptive use, condom use, sexual health, and gender role development.

It is also important that the information provided is appropriate to the age and sexual experience of the adolescent. For those who have not engaged in sexual intercourse, an approach that focuses on abstinence as the only absolute way to avoid pregnancy and sexually transmitted infections may be appropriate. Education that focuses on the avoidance of unprotected sex by the use of a condom with every sexual encounter may be an appropriate approach for adolescents who have begun to have sexual intercourse. Life-building skills that are necessary for adolescents, and which may facilitate appropriate decision-making, include negotiation skills, values clarification, goal setting, and interpersonal communication.

SUBSTANCE ABUSE. Experimentation and risk-taking behavior as a means of self-discovery and identity development are common during adolescence. Often this experimentation involves the use of drugs and alcohol. The reasons that adolescents give for trying drugs and alcohol include: to satisfy curiosity, to achieve a feeling of well-being while under the influence, to reduce stress, and to fit in with peers. Adolescents who are at an increased risk for developing dependency are those with low self-esteem, a family history of substance abuse, depression, and those who do not feel accepted by their peers.

Alcohol and marijuana are the most common drugs used by adolescents. On average, alcohol use begins at age 12 and marijuana use at age 14. Adolescent substance use is associated with school failure, an increased risk for accidents, violence, suicide, and unplanned and unsafe sexual activity.

There are many warning signs to alert parents to adolescent substance abuse. Physical signs include fatigue, red and glazed eyes, chronic cough, and health complaints. Emotional signs include personality changes, sudden mood swings, irritability, poor judgment and decision making, depression, and lack of interest in things that were of previous interest. As the substance abuse continues, adolescents may demonstrate a negative attitude, withdraw from the family or from previous friends, and become increasingly argumentative and secretive. Academic performance often drops and school officials report problems with truancy and discipline.

Parents need to be informed about the types of drugs that adolescents may use as well as the possible adverse consequences associated with each. Early and ongoing parent-adolescent education, open communication, appropriate role modeling and the early recognition of developing problems are the best strategies for prompt identification and interventions for substance use.

VIOLENCE AND ABUSE. Negative consequences are also seen in the rising degree of violence and abuse in the adolescent population. In a nationwide survey of high school students, 33% reported being involved in a physical fight one or more times in the preceding year, while 17% reported carrying a weapon one or more days in the preceding month (Centers for Disease Control and Prevention, 2004). It is estimated that 30% of all middle school students encounter some type of bullying, either as the bully, as a victim of the bully, or both.

Violence is a learned behavior. Adolescents learn to solve problems through violence by watching parents, teachers, and others in the community and in the media and by role modeling their behavior. In order to engage in problem-solving behavior without violence, adolescents need to be taught how to assess the conflict, see the other person's point of view, and then redefine the conflict so that they and the others involved can negotiate to a decision without violence.

Parents need to allow the adolescent to develop social relationships outside of the family in order to mature and define their identity. At the same time, they need to continue to set limits to adolescent behavior, maintain open and honest communication on problem-solving, and allow the adolescent to evaluate options to conflict resolution in passive, yet assertive ways.

Successful conflict resolution strategies enable the adolescent to remain calm in a potentially violent situation and to understand that the aggressor is attempting to resolve the conflict in ways that are understood by him. If communication and respect are not facilitating conflict resolution, the adolescent should be taught to remove himself from the potentially dangerous situation.

 ***Ethnocultural Considerations—* Exploring differences in ethnicity and race in adolescent violence**

- African Americans, Native Americans, and Hispanics are more likely to be victims or the persons responsible for fatal violence than Asians or Caucasians.
- These differences are more pronounced in adolescent aggression resulting in homicide than adolescent aggression not resulting in homicide.
- African Americans, Native Americans, and Hispanics are arrested more often for acts of interpersonal violence than Asians or Caucasians.
- Hispanic adolescent males are more likely to be victims of homicide than African Americans or Caucasians.
- African Americans account for the majority of all adolescents known to have committed murder.

Source: Center for the Study and Prevention of Violence (2004). *CSPV fact sheet: Ethnicity, race, class and adolescent violence.* Boulder, CO: Author.

Adolescents are particularly vulnerable to violence and abuse in dating relationships as well. Parents should be encouraged to discuss these issues openly before dating begins in order to prevent this type of abuse from occurring. Dating provides an opportunity to develop healthy love relationships that are built on mutual respect and trust. Similar to abusive situations, relationships can become coercive and escalate to physical abuse at a later time. Indicators of a coercive relationship include:

- Telling a partner what to wear
- Telling a partner where she is allowed to go
- Telling a partner who she can be friends with or talk to
- Making a partner do something she does not want to do

- Destroying the partner's personal property
- Threatening to hurt oneself if the partner breaks up with him
- Repeatedly contacting the partner after a break-up

Indications of abuse, which may be directed toward the male or female partner, can include rude and swearing talk, forcing sexual activity against the partner's will, humiliating one's partner in front of other people, and hitting or hurting one's partner in any way. If any of these behaviors are known by parents, it is the parents' responsibility to intervene, even to the point of legal action. Through interaction and communication, parents can have a lasting effect on helping their adolescent to develop future healthy relationships with others.

TATTOOING AND BODY PIERCING. Tattooing and body piercing are examples of adolescent risk-taking behavior (Roberts & Ryan, 2002; Stephens, 2003), and are associated with other high-risk activities, including smoking, alcohol use, use of smokeless tobacco, and riding in a vehicle driven by another individual who has been drinking. Health risks associated with tattooing and body piercing may be infectious or noninfectious.

Infectious health risks include viral, bacterial, and fungal diseases, most commonly infections caused by viruses and bacteria. The most common infections associated with tattooing and body piercing include hepatitis, human immunodeficiency virus (HIV), and human papilloma virus (HPV). Bacterial infections may be caused by *Staphylococcus*, *Streptococcus*, *Pseudomonas*, *Clostridium*, and *Mycobacterium* (Drifmeyer & Batis, 2007). These organisms have the potential to cause lifelong infection with adverse effects on various body systems or the progression to other diseases, such as cancer and tuberculosis. Allergic or hypersensitivity reactions are the most common noninfectious responses to tattooing and body piercing. Although these reactions may be transient, they can lead to the development of more serious lesions that require surgical intervention.

HEALTH PROMOTION

Although the majority of adolescents have not yet become sexually active, it is important that health care providers promote activities to prevent health problems from developing as they mature. Adolescents can be taught to perform breast self-examination (BSE) early in their development and to engage in activities to promote optimal bone health. Once adolescents become sexually active, they should be encouraged to have regular gynecological examinations.

Prevention of Osteoporosis

While adolescents are not at high risk for the development of **osteoporosis** (a condition characterized by loss of bone mass throughout the skeleton), it is essential that steps be taken at this early age to decrease the risk later in life. Strategies that are appropriate for adolescents include maintaining an adequate intake of calcium and vitamin D and engaging in regular exercise. Adolescents are at an increased risk for unhealthy eating behaviors that result in a calcium intake that falls far short of the amount needed for bone strengthening. Thus, nutritional intake during the adolescent years becomes even more important. In addition, adequate amounts of vitamin D are necessary to facilitate the absorption of calcium. Regular exercise helps the adolescent to achieve peak bone density levels. Weight-bearing exercises, including walking, dancing, sports, and hiking, are the best activities for young people to develop strong muscles and bones.

Gynecological Examinations

Another aspect of developing health practices that continues into later years is the initiation of gynecological examinations during adolescence. It is important for parents and adolescents to understand that the first visit may not necessarily include an internal pelvic examination and collection of specimens.

The first visit, which should occur between the ages of 13 and 15, should be used as an introduction to reproductive health care. The health care provider should discuss issues of sexuality with the adolescent to help prepare her for making appropriate decisions. Information and reassurance can be provided regarding normal development and education on sexually transmitted infections and sexual behavior can empower the adolescent for informed sexual decision making.

The first pelvic examination should be performed at age 21 or 3 years after the initiation of sexual activity, whichever comes first. Other reasons for pelvic examination include unexplained pain in the lower abdomen or pelvic region; vaginal discharge that causes itching, burning, or has an odor; delayed menstruation; prolonged menstruation lasting more than 10 days; dysmenorrhea; and missed periods.

PELVIC EXAMINATION. The frequency of pelvic examinations varies based on age. Females should have pelvic examinations once they become sexually active. Women ages 20 to 40 should undergo a pelvic examination at least every 3 years or annually if high risk. "High risk" includes those with abnormal findings on previous examinations, the presence of a sexually transmitted infection, sexual activity before age 18, multiple sexual partners, or abnor-

Figure 4-4 Using the thumb and index finger to separate the labia to assess the external genital structures.

mal spotting or bleeding. After the age of 40, pelvic examinations should be performed every 1 to 3 years, based on personal risk factors and history (Institute for Clinical Systems Improvement, 2005).

The nurse assists the patient with relaxation techniques before the pelvic examination, performed in a lithotomy position, is initiated. Anxiety is common, especially in women with a history of sexual abuse or assault. Deep breathing, a helpful relaxation strategy, is easy to perform. The patient is encouraged to take slow, deep breaths, in through the nose and out through the mouth. She should be observed for signs of hyperventilation and instructed to slow down her breathing if necessary. Visual imagery is another useful relaxation technique. Many health care providers place engaging pictures on the ceiling for the recumbent patient to view. Some women relax with conversation. Others prefer to quietly concentrate on deep breathing and visualization. It is important to ask the patient whether or not she prefers to talk during the examination.

EXTERNAL INSPECTION. The skin, including the labia majora, is inspected for color, bruising, erythema, lesions, and hair distribution (Fig. 4-3). Using a gloved hand, the examiner gently spreads the labia to assess the external genital structures (Fig. 4-4). The clitoris, labia minora, urethral opening, and vaginal opening are inspected for inflammation, lesions, and lumps. Bartholin's glands, which secrete fluid for lubrication, are palpated using the index finger and thumb, and are assessed for edema, pain, and discharge. The vaginal orifice is opened slightly, and the patient is asked to squeeze the vaginal muscles. This technique allows the examiner to inspect for cystocele, rectocele, uterine prolapse, and incontinence.

VULVAR SELF-EXAMINATION. Nurses can play a vital role in the early detection and treatment of vulvar and vaginal cancer by teaching patients about monthly self-examination. Routine self-examination frequently allows for the early identification and evaluation of abnormalities.

INTERNAL INSPECTION. The examiner uses a speculum for the internal inspection (Fig. 4-5). The speculum should be warmed or maintained at room temperature and moistened with water to avoid damage to cells that are collected for cytological analysis. Depending on the situation, specimens may be collected for cervical cancer screening (Papanicolaou test), gonorrhea, chlamydia, trichomoniasis, bacterial vaginosis, candidiasis, group B *Streptococcus*, and herpes

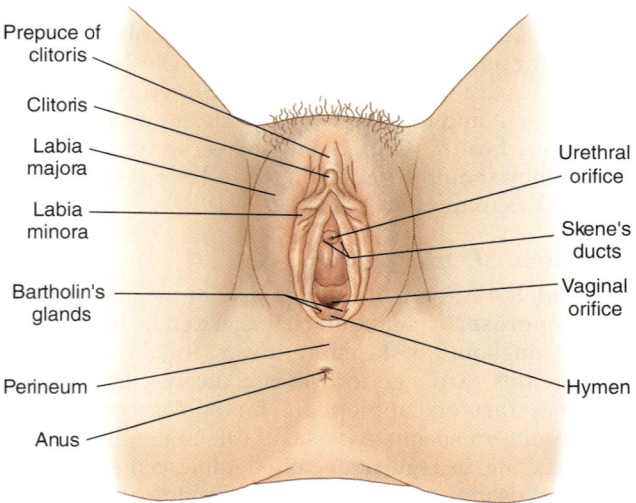

Prepuce of clitoris

Clitoris

Labia majora

Labia minora

Bartholin's glands

Perineum

Anus

Urethral orifice

Skene's ducts

Vaginal orifice

Hymen

Figure 4-3 Female external genitalia.

Family Teaching Guidelines...
Performing Vulvar Self-Examination

To prepare for vulvar self-examination, the woman places a flashlight and mirror within easy reach. She washes her hands, removes clothing from the waist down and sits comfortably on the floor or bed, with a pillow support behind her back. The following steps should then be performed:

1. While bending her knees, she leans backward and allows her knees to fall slightly apart to expose the genital area. The mirror and flashlight should be positioned for optimal visualization.
2. External inspection of the genital area includes visualizing the labia, the clitoris, the urethral meatus, the vaginal opening, and the anal opening.
3. Using her fingers, the woman should gently spread the labia and inspect the vaginal vault. The vaginal walls should be pink and contain small folds or ridges, called rugae.
4. The vaginal discharge should be evaluated at this time as well. Normal vaginal discharge is clear to cloudy and white, with a slightly acidic odor; it may be thick or thin, depending on the timing of the examination with regard to the menstrual cycle.
5. Findings that need to be reported to the health care provider include the presence of sores or growths on the labia or vaginal walls, an unpleasant odor to the vaginal discharge, and tissue redness. Sores, redness, abnormal growths, malodorous or excessive vaginal discharge, and itching may indicate irritation or infection.

Source: Vulval Pain Society (2005). *How to perform a vulval self-exam*. Retrieved from http://www.vulvalpainsociety.org/html/selfexam.htm

simplex virus. The specimens for cervical cancer screening must be obtained first to avoid cell damage during the collection of additional specimens. Common sexually transmitted infections (STIs), symptoms, and methods of diagnosis are presented in Table 4-4 (CDC, 2006c). (See Chapters 9, 11, and 19 for further discussion.)

Once the speculum is inserted, the blades are opened fully to allow complete visualization of the cervix and cervical os (Fig. 4-6). The cervix should be pink, smooth, and absent of lesions or lacerations. It should be midline with no lateral displacement. The cervical os is rounded in nulliparous women and slit-shaped in multiparous women. Secretions in the cervical area may appear thin and watery

Figure 4-5 Inserting the speculum.

or thick and stringy, depending on the day of the menstrual cycle. The secretions should be clear to opaque and have no foul odor. Around the time of ovulation, the cervical secretions are more profuse, slippery, and stretchy to facilitate sperm transport through the cervical mucus. Once the specimens have been collected, the speculum is slowly removed and the vaginal vault is inspected for color and the presence of inflammation, edema, bleeding, and discharge. (See Chapter 9 for further discussion.)

PAPANICOLAOU TEST. The Papanicolaou test (Pap smear) is the microscopic examination of cells taken from the cervical area by various techniques. It is the most reliable method used to screen the patient for preinvasive cervical cancer. The U.S. Preventive Services Task Force (USPSTF) and the American Cancer Society (ACS) recommend that Pap tests should begin approximately 3 years after a woman becomes sexually active but not later than age 21. Yearly screening is recommended to age 30 (with the conventional Pap test; every 2 years with liquid-based Pap tests). After age 30 and three negative Pap tests, screening may be performed every 2 to 3 years, in consultation with the health care provider. Women ages 65 to 70 who have had no abnormal tests in the previous 10 years may choose to stop Pap screenings (ACS, 2006a; USPSTF, 2005). Women in high risk categories should have more frequent Pap tests.

The Papanicolaou test should not be performed if the woman is menstruating or has an infection. The best time to collect the specimen is at mid-cycle to ensure the absence of menstrual blood, which may distort results. The nurse should confirm that the woman has not had intercourse or douched within the 24 hours preceding the test. Using a spatula or an endocervical sampling device, cells are scraped from the cervical os and from around the cervical opening. With one cytological preparatory technique, the sample is smeared onto a slide, sprayed immediately with a fixative solution, and allowed to dry. With another method (e.g., the ThinPrep Pap Test), the specimen is placed directly into a prepared vial of preservative. Regardless of the method used, the sample is labeled and sent to a laboratory for cytological examination.

BIMANUAL PALPATION. The examiner lubricates the first and second (gloved) fingers with water-soluble lubricant. The vaginal canal is palpated for the presence of tenderness, lesions, and nodules (Fig. 4-7). The cervix is palpated for position, consistency, contour, and mobility. It should be soft and movable without tenderness. The uterus is palpated to determine if it is in a midposition, or retroverted or anteverted (Fig. 4-8). It should be soft, movable, and nontender. The uterine fundus (upper area above the openings of the fallopian tubes) should be rounded. The examiner then palpates the adnexa to assess for masses or tenderness. The ovaries may or not be palpable. If palpable, they should be mobile, smooth, and firm. Ovarian palpation may cause some slight discomfort (Fig. 4-9). Structures on each side of the uterus are palpated. As the examiner's fingers are removed, the patient is asked to tighten her vaginal muscles to facilitate assessment of pubococcygeal muscle strength. This component of the examination provides an opportune time to teach about Kegel exercises. (See Chapter 9 for further discussion.)

Table 4-4 Summary of Common Sexually Transmitted Infections

Infection	Symptoms (May Be Asymptomatic)	Detection
Gonorrhea	Yellow-green vaginal discharge	Endocervical culture
	Dyspareunia	Urine test
	Abdominal pain	
	Dysuria	
Chlamydia	Mucopurulent discharge	Endocervical culture
	Postcoital bleeding	Urine test
	Dyspareunia	
	Abdominal pain	
	Dysuria	
Trichomoniasis	Frothy malodorous vaginal discharge	Saline wet mount of vaginal discharge viewed under microscope
	Dyspareunia	
	Vaginal itching/irritation	
	Dysuria	
Hepatitis	Fatigue	Serological testing
	Dark urine	
	Clay-colored stool	
	Jaundice/abdominal pain	
Human papilloma virus (HPV)	Many subtypes exist, some associated with cervical dysplasia	Pap smear report Colposcopy/biopsy
	Visible wartlike growths in genital area associated with subtypes 6, 11	
Syphilis	**Primary**	**Serological testing**
	Chancre (painless raised ulcer)	Nontreponemal (RPR, VDRL)
	Secondary	• Reported quantitatively (titers)
	Skin rash, lymphadenopathy	• Fourfold change in titers clinically significant
	Latent	• Effective treatment will result in falling titers
	Lacking clinical manifestations	• False-positive possible; verify with treponemal test
	Tertiary	Treponemal (FTA-ABS)
	Cardiac, ophthalmic, auditory involvement	• Reported as positive or negative
HIV	Fever	Serological testing (Pretest and posttest counseling with informed consent required)
	Malaise	
	Lymphadenopathy	Positive screen must be confirmed by more specific test (Western blot)
	Skin rash	
Herpes simplex virus (HSV)	Painful, recurrent vesicular lesions	Viral culture with DNA probe
	Fever, malaise	
	Enlarged lymph nodes	

Source: Holloway, B.W., Moredich, C., & Aduddell, K. (2006). *OB peds women's health notes: Nurse's clinical pocket guide*. Philadelphia: F.A. Davis.

RECTOVAGINAL PALPATION. The examiner changes gloves before this component of the examination. Following application of a water-based lubricant, the examiner inserts the index finger into the vagina and the middle finger into the rectum. To facilitate insertion and assessment of muscle strength, the patient is asked to bear down during the insertion. The procedures of the bimanual palpation are repeated, allowing the examiner to palpate the rectovaginal wall, the posterior side of the uterus, and the area behind the adnexa. Palpation should reveal no tenderness or the presence of fissures or masses along the rectovaginal wall. The uterus and adnexa should be nontender, soft, movable and absent of masses (Figs. 4-10, 4-11, and 4-12).

Figure 4-6 Opening the speculum.

Figure 4-7 The vaginal canal is palpated for the presence of tenderness, lesions and nodules.

Figure 4-8 Palpating the uterus.

Figure 4-9 Palpating the ovaries.

Figure 4-10 Inserting fingers for rectovaginal exam.

Figure 4-11 Performing rectovaginal exam.

Figure 4-12 Proper position of hands.

 Now Can You— Discuss the pelvic examination process?

1. Discuss patient preparation for the procedure?
2. Identify the structures that are examined during the external assessment?
3. Identify the specimens collected during the internal inspection and explain their importance?
4. List the structures that are evaluated during the bimanual palpation?

MENSTRUAL DISORDERS

Various menstrual disorders may occur during adolescence. The most common conditions are menstrual cramps, **dysmenorrhea** (painful menstruation that interferes with daily activities), and premenstrual syndrome (PMS). Painful cramping in the uterus during menstruation occurs from myometrial contractions induced by prostaglandins during the second phase of the menstrual cycle. **Prostaglandins** are chemical mediators that cause pain as part of the inflammatory response; during menstruation, the cramps are frequently accompanied by back pain and headache. Peaking levels of prostaglandins cause the symptoms to begin a day or two before the beginning of menstrual flow and continue until about the second or third day of menstrual flow.

Dysmenorrhea is painful menstruation that affects a woman's ability to perform daily activities for 2 or more days each month. Health care teaching for females experiencing dysmenorrhea should be holistic in nature and include relaxation and breathing techniques, the use of heat to reduce uterine contractions and increase blood flow to the uterine tissues, exercise or rest, and the use of nonsteroidal anti-inflammatory drugs to inhibit the synthesis of prostaglandin. For some women, dysmenorrhea is symptomatic of other conditions, including pelvic inflammatory disease and endometriosis. Severe pain and dysmenorrhea that disrupts a women's life should be evaluated by a health care provider.

Premenstrual syndrome (PMS) is another commonly occurring disorder associated with menstruation that affects adolescents. Approximately 85% of all females experience some degree of symptoms related to PMS. Symptoms range from irritability and mood changes to fluid retention, heart palpitations, and visual disturbances. While the most common cause of PMS is the normal fluctuation of estrogen and progesterone during the menstrual cycle, other factors may be associated with PMS symptoms as well. For example, some PMS symptoms may result from the following: an imbalance in the levels of estrogen and progesterone; **hyperprolactinemia** (an excessive secretion of prolactin, the hormone responsible for stimulation of breast development); alterations in carbohydrate metabolism and hypoglycemia; and an excessive production of aldosterone resulting in sodium and water retention.

Recommendations for reducing the severity of the symptoms associated with PMS include the incorporation of simple lifestyle changes. Adolescents should be encouraged to exercise three to five times a week, eat a well-balanced diet, and get adequate sleep and rest. Dietary changes include increasing the daily intake of whole grains, vegetables, and fruits, while decreasing the intake of salt, sugar, and caffeine.

For more problematic symptoms, treatment may include the use of diuretics to reduce fluid retention, the administration of nonsteroidal anti-inflammatory drugs to inhibit synthesis of prostaglandins and provide pain relief, oral contraceptives to inhibit ovulation, central nervous depressants to promote relaxation, antidepressants, and vitamin supplements.

YOUNG ADULTHOOD HEALTH

Formal operational thought is completed as individuals move from adolescence into young adulthood (ages 19 to 34). The developmental stage during this time period is *intimacy versus isolation*. The individual no longer views the family as the primary source of identity and developmental tasks center on making a personal commitment to

another individual as a partner or spouse. With the increased independence associated with young adulthood and the concomitant increase in age, new challenges to health promotion and disease prevention arise. During young adulthood there is a focus on safety, sexual health, reproductive health promotion that includes monthly breast self-examination and yearly clinical breast examinations, and awareness of potential gynecological disorders common to this age group.

SAFETY

As young adults attempt to engage in dating relationships, the safety risks associated with substance use, sexual practices, and intimate partner violence become more evident. It is during this time, when young adults are developing relationships with members of the opposite or same sex in intimate ways, that nurses can provide education and counseling and empower women to care for themselves in healthy ways.

Substance Use

Once young adults reach the age of 21, they can legally purchase and consume alcoholic beverages. This "rite of passage" places them at an increased risk for problems associated with alcohol use. The newly gained independence that comes as the young adult moves out of the parent's home, combined with the social acceptance of drinking during this time, may coincide to place the young adult in situations where excessive and binge drinking can be common and frequent. Although formal operational thought has been developed by this age, the brain continues to mature during young adulthood. Heavy or binge drinking during this time of brain development and independent decision-making may cause serious health risks as well as risks to social growth.

In addition to alcohol consumption, young adults continue to be at risk for the use of illicit drugs. Peak use, similar to that of alcohol, occurs during the early 20s, declines in the late 20s, and tends to come to an end around age 30. The most reliable theory related to illicit substance use focuses on role development during young adulthood, specifically with regard to role normalization and role compatibility. As young adults take on more adult roles associated with employment, marriage, and parenting, the use of illicit drugs may decrease as performance is altered or the person is unable to meet role expectations. Similarly, when the adult roles are seen as being incompatible with illicit drug use and non-normative behavior, substance use declines.

SEXUAL HEALTH. While increased alcohol consumption and illicit drug use are associated with greater degrees of sexual freedom and loss of sexual inhibition, young adults are faced with sexual decision making regardless of substance use. Both males and females tend to have their sexual peak, with regard to interest, desire, ability, and performance in the mid- to late-20s, with sexual interest and ability beginning to decrease during the 30s. This is particularly true of males, as testosterone production and ejaculation decline later during young adulthood.

With regard to safe sex practices during young adulthood, it is essential for nurses to educate women regarding the anatomy and physiology of their bodies in an effort to facilitate an understanding of the heightened risk of susceptibility to sexually transmitted infections. Physiological factors that predispose women to increased susceptibility include an increased genital mucosal surface area, retention of semen in the vagina for several hours following intercourse, and the pH of the vagina. During menstruation, women are more vulnerable to infection as the pH of the vagina becomes more alkaline, thereby becoming more hospitable to viral and bacterial transmission and growth.

During young adulthood, abstinence remains the only safe method for protection against sexually transmitted infections. However, as young adults begin to experiment with sexual activity, nurses must continue to educate them on the proper use of condoms, including the use of a water-based lubricant to prevent tears in the mucosa, use of a barrier during oral sex, and protection and cleaning of sexual toys that may be used. While some nurses may find these topics difficult to approach and discuss openly, it is only through open communication that young adults are likely to incorporate safe practices into their development and experimentation.

HEALTH PROMOTION

Health practices, both positive and negative, that were initiated during adolescence will likely continue into young adulthood. During this time, dietary and exercise behaviors are more likely to either protect from or increase the risk of developing obesity, hypertension, type 2 diabetes mellitus, and cardiovascular disease. Specifically, the chronic illnesses that are more likely to emerge during young adulthood include cancer, cardiovascular disease, type 2 diabetes mellitus, and autoimmune diseases such as lupus erythematosus and multiple sclerosis.

For women, stress-related disorders become more apparent during this time. Stress can trigger behaviors such as overindulgence in comfort foods, alcohol abuse, and the use of marijuana and other drugs to reduce tension. It is encouraging that women in young adulthood are more likely to experiment with alternative therapies to relieve stress. Herbal methods, homeopathic remedies, spiritual approaches, music and dance, and art therapy may be used. Nurses need to understand and support these positive, alternative methods for stress reduction to promote a holistic approach to health and wellness.

🌸 Complementary Care: *Anxiety and depression*

Herbal remedies for anxiety and depression include the use of kava kava, passionflower, valerian root, gotu kola, and St. John's wort. While these herbs are believed to reduce anxiety, stress, and muscle tension, the nurse should provide education on the potential side effects of these substances, which include gastrointestinal discomforts, nausea, and dizziness.

TESTICULAR CANCER SCREENING. Although considered rare, testicular cancer is the most common cancer found in young men 20 to 34 years of age. It is the second most common cancer in men 35 to 39 years of age, and the third most common cancer in men between the ages of 15 and 19. Risk factors for testicular cancer include a positive family history and a personal history of undescended testes; congenital gonadal dysgenesis; and Klinefelter's syndrome, a sex-linked genetic disorder. Interestingly, the majority of testicular tumors are discovered during self-examination. The National Cancer Institute (2006) does not recommend routine screening, other than clinical palpation, for testicular cancer since treatment is effective at each state of diagnosis. However, all males should be taught to palpate the testes for abnormal lumps and masses on a regular basis.

Family Teaching Guidelines...
Testicular Self-examination

The best time to perform a testicular self-examination is during or immediately following a hot shower or bath since the scrotum is more relaxed at this time. The following steps should be performed, examining one testicle at a time:

1. Examine the testicles. One should be slightly larger than the other, usually the right testicle.
2. Feel for lumps and bumps along the front and sides.
3. Using both hands, place your thumbs over the top of the testicle and your index fingers and middle fingers underneath the testicle. Gently roll the testicle, using slight pressure, between your fingers (Fig. 4-13).
4. The epididymis, which carries the sperm, can be felt at the top of the back part of each testicle. It should feel soft and rope-like and be slightly tender to pressure. This is a normal finding.
5. Notify your doctor if you notice any swelling, lumps, pain, or changes in color or size of either testicle.

Source: The Nemours Foundation (2007). *How to perform a testicular self-examination*. Retrieved from http://www.kidshealth.org/teen/sexual_health/guys/tse.html

Figure 4-13 Testicular self-examination.

GYNECOLOGICAL DISORDERS. Along with specific medical problems, certain gynecological disorders are more common during young adulthood as well. Endometriosis, cervical cancer, breast cancer, and urinary tract infections are more likely to occur during this time. Also, since young adulthood marks the time when most women try to begin a family, problems associated with infertility may be discovered at this time as well.

ENDOMETRIOSIS. Endometriosis, a benign disorder of the reproductive tract, is characterized by the presence and growth of endometrial tissue outside of the uterus. Women ages 30 to 40 are most likely to develop endometriosis. Endometrial tissue may implant on the fallopian tubes, ovaries, and the tissues surrounding and lining the pelvis. The endometrial tissue responds to hormonal influences during the secretory and proliferative stages of the menstrual cycle, where it grows and thickens, in a similar fashion to the endometrial tissue lining the uterus. However, during the ischemic and menstrual phases of the cycle, the misplaced endometrial tissue breaks down and bleeds into the surrounding tissue, causing inflammation. The blood becomes trapped in the surrounding tissues causing the development of blood-containing cysts. Recurring inflammation in the areas outside of the uterus eventually result in scarring, fibrosis, and the development of adhesions, scar tissue that binds the organs together causing increased abdominal pain and a risk of infertility.

Abdominal pain of varying intensity is the most common symptom associated with endometriosis. However, the degree of pain associated with endometriosis is not a reliable indicator of the extent of the disorder. Other symptoms may include pain during ovulation (**mittelschmerz**), heavy bleeding during menstruation, and episodes of diarrhea and constipation, which may be mistaken for irritable bowel syndrome. Women may also experience dyspareunia or pain during defecation.

Although the etiology of endometriosis is unknown, the most commonly held theory is "retrograde menstruation." During menstruation, endometrial tissue is refluxed through the fallopian tubes and out into the peritoneal cavity where it implants on the ovaries and surrounding organs. While 90% of all women experience retrograde menstruation, only about 5% to 10% develop endometriosis, indicating a possible difference in immune function, genetic predisposition, or environmental influence.

The diagnosis of endometriosis may be made by pelvic examination although it is often impossible to palpate small areas of localized endometrial tissue. A vaginal ultrasound may be performed to provide imaging of the displaced endometrial tissue or cyst. The physician may also perform a laparoscopy to visualize the abdominal organs and locate signs of abnormally located endometrial tissue. Laparoscopy provides information concerning the location, size, extent of disease, and the presence of scars and adhesions.

Medical management includes pain control, the use of hormonal therapy to shrink the abnormal tissue, and, at times, surgery to remove the abnormal tissue. The pain associated with tissue inflammation may be managed with nonsteroidal anti-inflammatory drugs, such as ibuprofen, to inhibit the synthesis of prostaglandin and reduce the inflammation. If conservative treatment is not helpful, supplemental hormonal therapy may be introduced, with the goal of stabilizing the release of estrogen and progesterone to decrease tissue swelling and bleeding.

When pregnancy is not an immediate goal, oral contraceptives with a low estrogen to progestin ratio may be used to inhibit the production of hormones and suppress ovulation. Gonadotropin-releasing hormone (Gn-RH) agonists and antagonists, such as leuprolide (Lupron) or nafarelin (Synarel), suppress the secretion of pituitary gonadotropins, decrease the release of follicle-stimulating hormone (FSH) and luteinizing hormone (LH), and diminish ovarian function. Danazol (Danocrine), another medication that suppresses the release of FSH and LH, may be used. However, the side effects of acne and facial hair growth make danazol a less commonly prescribed medication. Medroxyprogesterone (Depo-Provera) is an injectable medication used to reduce the growth of the endometrial tissue, but its undesired side effects include weight gain and depression. Newer pharmacological modalities utilize aromatase inhibitors, including anastrozole (Arimidex), exemestane (Aromasin), and letrozole (Femara), chemicals that block the conversion of androgens to estrogen and suppress the production of estrogen from the abnormal endometrial tissue, thereby decreasing tissue growth.

When pharmacological approaches are not successful, or when pregnancy is desired, the endometrial tissue growths, scar tissue, and adhesions can be removed surgically through laparoscopy. When endometriosis is severe, however, radical surgery that includes removal of the uterus, fallopian tubes, and ovaries (bilateral salpingo-ööphorectomy) may be indicated.

CERVICAL CANCER. Cervical cancer develops gradually as cells change their growth pattern. Pre-cancerous cellular changes, called **dysplasia**, may eventually become cancerous. There are two types of cervical cancer: squamous cell carcinoma and adenocarcinoma. Approximately 80% to 90% of all cervical cancers are squamous cell carcinomas that cover the surface of the cervix.

While not all cervical dysplasia develops into carcinoma, screening and treatment of cervical dysplasia significantly reduces the chances that carcinoma will develop. This fact lends credence to the recommendation that screening through Papanicolaou testing be performed on all young adults. Furthermore, 50% of all women diagnosed with cervical cancer are diagnosed during the ages of young adulthood.

The primary risk factor for cervical cancer is human papilloma virus (HPV) infection. There is a strong correlation between infection with the high-risk types of HPV and the development of cervical cancer. Seventy percent of cervical cancers are caused by HPV-16 or HPV-18. Other types of HPV are associated with the development of **papillomas**, which are benign growths found primarily in the genital and anal regions. While there is no treatment for HPV, a new vaccine, Quadrivalent Human Papillomavirus (Types 6, 11, 16, 18) Recombinant Vaccine (Gardasil), has recently been marketed and is targeted for adolescent and young adult women. This vaccine is recommended for girls and women ages 9 through 26 years to protect against the development of cervical cancer; abnormal lesions of the cervix, vulva, and vagina; and genital papillomas (Merck & Co., Inc., 2006). It is important for nurses to remind patients receiving the vaccine to continue to have routine cervical cancer screenings.

The vaccine is given in three doses: the second dose is administered 2 months after the first dose, and the third dose is administered 6 months after the first dose.

Medical management is determined by biopsy and staging of the cancer. Following identification of an abnormal Pap smear, **colposcopy** (use of a stereoscopic binocular microscope to examine the cervix under magnification) is usually performed. An acetic acid solution applied to the cervix enhances visualization of the epithelium and helps to identify areas for biopsy. Cervical biopsies are then obtained and pathologically examined for the presence and extent of cancer. Several outpatient biopsy methods are available. The endocervical curettage (ECC) is an effective diagnostic method in about 90% of cases. The **cone biopsy** involves removal of a cone- or cylinder-shaped sample of tissue. **Loop electrosurgical excision procedure** (LEEP) is a newer method for cervical biopsy and the removal of abnormal cells. With this procedure, an electrically charged wire loop is inserted through a speculum and a thin layer of cells is removed from the cervix. The LEEP technique provides excision and cautery with minimal tissue damage. Patients should be instructed that vaginal drainage is normal and expected following the procedure and may last up to 3 weeks. The patient should refrain from using tampons or having sexual intercourse for the following 4 weeks to minimize the risk of infection. Nonsteroidal anti-inflammatory medications may be taken to reduce the mild cramping that may occur following the procedure.

Following the biopsy, further and more extensive treatment may be required if the cancer has spread to other areas of the cervix or beyond the cervix. The three primary methods of cervical cancer treatment include surgery, radiation, and chemotherapy. It is not uncommon for a combination of two treatment methods to be used.

---

 case study Young Adult with Cervical Dysplasia

Vanessa, a 32-year-old woman, visits the women's health clinic in a small, rural community. She requests a gynecological examination, and states this is her first exam in 3 years. Vanessa has recently married and engages in normal sexual activity with her husband. Her medical history is positive for asthma, and she takes one Singular 10 mg tablet at bedtime and Flovent two puffs twice daily. Her Pap test reveals cervical dysplasia, and the physician recommends a LEEP procedure, with follow-up Pap tests every 3 months for 1 year.

1. Review the preceding information. List as many potential patient problems or risks as you can identify; prioritize your list.

2. Write a nursing diagnosis for each problem.

3. Develop a care plan for the top three nursing diagnoses. Include: (a) goals for the patient, (b) nursing interventions, (c) rationale(s) for each nursing intervention, and (d) how you would evaluate whether or not each goal was met.

   Did you include *Deficient knowledge* or patient teaching in your care plan? Be sure to include the overall goal of your teaching, teaching strategies, content to be taught, and how you will evaluate patient learning.

◆ See Suggested Answers to Case Studies in the text on the Electronic Study Guide or DavisPlus.

URINARY TRACT INFECTIONS. Urinary tract infections (UTIs) can be very serious in young adults and may lead to major problems if not diagnosed or treated. Infections of the urinary tract are the second most common type of infection in adults, and young adults are more susceptible due, in most instances, to increased sexual activity during this time. Women tend to be more vulnerable than men because the short urethral length and the proximity of the urethral meatus to the anus allow for the easy ascension of bacteria. However, urinary tract infections in men can be more serious than in women. The majority of UTIs are caused by the microorganism *Escherichia coli* (*E. coli*), which is normally found in the colon. Once introduced into the urethra, the bacteria colonizes, causing urethritis. As the bacteria multiply and migrate into the bladder, cystitis develops. Left untreated, the infection can spread up the ureters and into the kidneys, causing pyelonephritis.

Symptoms of urinary tract infections include burning, urinary frequency, and urgency during urination, and a strong sensation of the need to void followed by passage of only a small amount of urine. Women often report a sensation of fullness noted above the symphysis pubis; in men, infection triggers a sensation of rectal fullness. Other clinical manifestations of infection include fever, general malaise and fatigue, elevated white blood cell count, and chills. The urine may appear cloudy due to the presence of white blood cells.

Medical management centers on the use of antibiotics. Trimethoprim/sulfamethoxazole (Bactrim, Septra) are the medications most commonly prescribed. Depending on the strain of bacteria and results from culture and sensitivity testing, other agents such as amoxicillin (Amoxil, Trimox) and ampicillin (Omnipen) may be used. Nitrofurantoin (Macrodantin) or ciproflaxin (Cipro) may be prescribed for more complicated infections.

Patient education should focus on the prevention of urinary tract infections. Everyone should drink adequate water each day and urinate when the urge is felt. Following urination and defecation, women should wipe from front to back to prevent bacteria from entering the urethra from the colon, and encouraged to take showers instead of tub baths. Bath oils, perfume, and bubble baths should be avoided if tub baths are taken. Feminine hygiene sprays and scented douches should be avoided to prevent irritation, and cotton underwear should be worn to decrease perineal moistness and warmth that can enhance the growth of bacteria.

MIDDLE ADULTHOOD HEALTH

As the young adult matures into middle age, which includes ages 40 to 64, there is a decrease in the risk for some health problems and an increased risk for others. It is during this age group that mammography screenings should begin, along with colonoscopies, cholesterol and lipid screening, and osteoporosis screening. Most women begin to experience symptoms of perimenopause during middle age and need to make decisions on managing these symptoms. Certain gynecological disorders become more common during middle age, including fibroid tumors, ovarian cysts, ovarian cancer, and endometrial cancer.

HEALTH PROMOTION SCREENING

Health promotion screenings can be of great benefit to people in middle age as there are a variety of diseases that become more prevalent during this time. Breast cancer is the leading cause of death in women between the ages of 40 and 55. Breast cancer is the second leading cause of cancer death in U.S. women (American Cancer Society, 2006a), and there is a one in eight chance that a woman will develop breast cancer at some time during her lifetime.

The promotion of breast health encompasses several areas, including cancer screening, optimal nutrition, and physical activity. It is important for nurses to educate women throughout the life span about strategies for promoting breast health. Personal awareness of the normal appearance and feel of the breasts constitutes an essential first step in promoting and maintaining breast health (Box 4-5).

Box 4–5 Knowing and Understanding Your Breasts

- As you age, your breasts experience loss of milk glands and shrinkage of collagen. This causes an increase in the fat tissue and loosening of the breast tissue. Instead of getting larger with the increase in fat tissue, however, the breast tissue begins to sag, causing the breasts to drop.
- Breast tissue weighs less than most people think: an A-cup weighs 1/4 lb, a B-cup weighs 1/2 lb, a C-cup weighs 3/4 lb, and a D-cup weighs about 1 lb.
- The skin covering the breasts stretches as you grow, causing the skin to become thinner than the skin on other parts of the body.
- It is not uncommon for women to have some degree of hair surrounding their nipples. The darker the skin, the more hair there is likely to be.
- A woman's nipples may be different sizes and may be located in slightly different locations on each breast. This may cause the nipples to point in different directions, which is considered a normal finding.
- Fluctuating hormone levels during the monthly cycle cause changes in breast tissue. Following menstruation, when hormone levels are at their lowest, the breast tissue is smooth and nontender. As estrogen levels increase mid-cycle, breasts may become more sensitive. Also, just before menstruation, when progesterone is elevated, the breasts become swollen and tender, with palpable nodules.
- The health care provider should perform clinical breast examinations one week following menstruation, when the breast tissue is nontender and smooth.
- Breast implants still pose health risks, including deflation, leakage, and wrinkling. In addition, capsular contraction can occur, causing the scar tissue surrounding the implant to tighten and the breast to become hard.
- The area between the breasts has several oil and sweat glands, creating an atmosphere conducive to the growth of bacteria.
- Sleeping on your side, with a pillow to support your breasts, provides the best position for maintaining breast shape and contour over time.
- Regular exercise can strengthen the pectoral muscles, reducing sagging over time and creating a natural lift.
- It is not uncommon to have a third nipple, stemming from breast buds that form during early fetal development. These extra nipples, however, rarely contain milk glands.
- Pregnancy darkens the color of the nipple, which is an enhancement for the breastfeeding baby. This darker color does not disappear after pregnancy.
- The left breast is usually larger then the right breast.
- Breasts do not reach their full size until the early 20s.

Optimizing Outcomes— Teaching about fibrocystic breast changes

When teaching women about breast self-examination, nurses can include information about **fibrocystic changes**, palpable thickening in the breasts often associated with pain and tenderness that fluctuates with the menstrual cycle. Fibrocystic changes are common, benign, and tend to appear during the second and third decades of life. Treatment for the condition, which may be related to an imbalance in estrogen and progesterone, centers on relief of symptoms and may include analgesics, nonsteroidal anti-inflammatory drugs (e.g., ibuprofen), diuretics, use of a supportive bra, avoidance of tobacco and alcohol and the application of heat to the breasts.

Breast self-examination (BSE), clinical breast exams, and **mammography** (x-ray filming of the breasts) can assist in early detection and early treatment. The initiation and frequency of mammography depends on the woman's age and risk factors. Magnetic resonance imaging (MRI) appears to be more sensitive in detecting tumors in women with an inherited susceptibility to breast cancer, and recent findings suggest that this diagnostic method can detect cancer in the contralateral breast that was missed by mammography in women with recently diagnosed breast cancer (Lehman et al., 2007).

While breast cancer is more common in women, colon cancer is the fourth most common cancer in both men and women. In addition, risk for heart disease related to elevated cholesterol and lipids increases in both genders during middle age. Osteoporosis, which may also occur in men, becomes more common and debilitating in women in the latter years of middle age, as they move from perimenopause into menopause.

Ethnocultural Considerations— Breast cancer screening

There are notable differences in breast cancer screening practices among women of different ethnic backgrounds. Although African American women are at a lower risk for developing breast cancer than Caucasian women, they are more likely to die from breast cancer due to late diagnosis. According to Husaini et al. (2001), African American women are more likely to have mammogram screening if they are older, married, have a higher level of education, and believe that early detection could lead to a cure. A positive family history of breast cancer and church affiliation have no influence on the incidence of detection.

Asian American and Pacific Islander women have very low rates of breast cancer screening. Factors responsible for the low screening rates include lack of health insurance, low income, and lack of a primary care provider (Kagawa-Singer & Pourat, 2000).

Breast cancer causes a significant number of deaths in Filipino women. In a study by Wu and Bancroft (2006), researchers found that women were more likely to follow recommended screenings if there is support from physicians and family members, and if they had insurance. In addition, the presence of physical symptoms, family history of breast cancer, and health literacy promote adherence to recommendations.

Breast Self-examination

Familiarization with one's breasts facilitates the early detection of problems and allows for prompt evaluation. Breast self-examination (BSE) is a way for women to learn how their breasts normally feel. Routinely performing BSE is an approach that focuses on the importance of self-awareness and helps women to notice changes in breast tissue (ACS, 2003).

Family Teaching Guidelines...
Breast Self-Examination

1. Visually inspect the breasts in front of a mirror. Assess for color, contour, shape, and size. Assess for dimpling or puckering of the skin; change in nipple direction; and redness, rash, or swelling.

2. Repeat first step with the arms slightly raised above the head.

3. Inspect and palpate the nipple. Gently squeeze the nipple between the thumb and forefinger, looking for discharge. Many women, especially those who have had children, are able to express some discharge by squeezing the nipples. Discharge that is of concern is most often spontaneous (ACS, 2007).

4. Palpate the breast and axillae. Recline on the bed and place a pillow under each shoulder during palpation. Use the left hand to palpate the right breast, and the right hand to palpate the left breast. Using the finger pads of the three middle fingers, palpate the entire surface of the breast. Use overlapping dime-sized circular motions and apply three different levels of pressure: *light pressure* is best to feel the tissue closest to the skin; *medium pressure* is best to feel a little deeper; and *firm pressure* is used to feel the tissue closest to the chest and ribs.

5. Repeat step 4 while standing or sitting. Many women find step 5 easier to complete if the skin is wet, and complete this step while in the shower. Move around the breast in an up and down pattern, checking the entire breast area until only the ribs are felt; repeat the entire technique on the opposite breast (ACS, 2007).

Clinical Breast Examination

All women should have a clinical breast examination performed at recommended intervals by a skilled health care provider. The clinical breast exam should be performed every 3 years for women aged 18 to 39, every 1 to 2 years for women aged 40 to 49, and annually for women age 50 and over (Michigan Quality Improvement Consortium, 2005a, 2005b).

Mammography

A mammography examination is used to aid in the early diagnosis of breast cancer. The examination, which requires exposure to small doses of ionizing radiation, allows for identification of small breast tissue abnormalities that may require further investigation. Two enhancements have been made to traditional mammography: digital mammography and computer-aided detection (CAD). Digital mammography, also called full-field digital mammography (FFDM), converts the x-rays to electrical signals, similar to those found in digital cameras. These signals produce images that can be viewed on a computer screen or printed on special film. The images are stored for future comparison. Preliminary results from a clinical study sponsored by the National Cancer Institute indicate that digital mammography provides improved screening for women determined to be at high risk for developing breast cancer (Pisano et al., 2005). This latest technology is enhanced with the use of computer software that highlights areas of increased density, masses, and calcifications.

Lifestyle Choices and Breast Health

Lifestyle choices, including moderate alcohol consumption, weight maintenance, and avoidance of smoking can affect breast health as well. Alcohol consumption is known to be associated with an increased risk of breast cancer. The American Cancer Society (2006b) recommends limiting alcohol intake to one drink per day. The risk of breast cancer is increased 1.5 times in women who consume two to five drinks per day.

Routine exercise, which helps to maintain a healthy weight, is associated with a decreased risk of breast cancer. Maintenance of a healthy weight is recommended for optimum breast health. Obesity is associated with an increased risk of breast cancer, particularly in postmenopausal women. Following menopause, estrogen is produced in the fat cells. In combination with dietary fat, estrogen significantly increases the likelihood of breast cancer development. Smoking is associated with an increased risk of breast cancer, lung cancer and heart disease in women (National Women's Health Resource Centers, Inc., 2006).

BREAST CANCER. While the majority of lumps found in the breast and axillary tissue are not cancerous, discovery of a mass remains the most common sign of breast cancer. Other signs of breast cancer include a clear or bloody discharge from the nipple, retraction or indentation of the nipple, dimpling of the breast tissue, and change in the size or contour of the breast. While the exact etiology of breast cancer remains unclear, there are factors that place a woman at greater risk for developing breast cancer (Box 4-6).

Box 4-6 Risk Factors Associated with Breast Cancer

- Defects in breast cancer gene 1 (*BRCA1*) or breast cancer gene 2 (*BRCA2*)
- Gender: 100 times more likely to occur in females than in males
- Age: Increasing age, with 50% appearing by age 50
- Personal history of breast cancer in at least one breast
- Family history of breast cancer
- Exposure to radiation
- Excess weight
- Exposure to estrogen: early onset of menarche, late menopause, or use of hormonal therapy
- Race: Caucasians more likely to develop breast cancer than Hispanics or African-Americans
- Smoking
- Exposure to carcinogens
- Excessive use of alcohol
- Diagnosis of precancerous breast changes
- Increased breast density revealed on mammography

Source: American Cancer Society (2006).

 Now Can You— Discuss ways to enhance breast health?

1. Identify the steps for performing breast self-examination?
2. Discuss recommendations regarding clinical breast examination and mammography?
3. Discuss risk factors associated with breast cancer?
4. Identify lifestyle choices that decrease the risk of developing breast cancer?

 Optimizing Outcomes— Screening for breast cancer

Best outcome: Monthly breast-self examination, clinical breast examinations, and routine mammography allow health care practitioners to detect potentially cancerous tumors at the earliest stage possible. This multipronged screening approach facilitates early diagnosis and early treatment, providing the best outcome possible (National Comprehensive Cancer Network, 2006).

When breast self-examination, clinical breast examination, mammography, and MRI detect possible cancerous tumors in the breast or axillae, a biopsy procedure is performed to determine if cancer is indeed present. One type of biopsy procedure is the fine-needle biopsy, which is the simplest method. A thin, hollow needle is used to withdraw cells for histological analysis. Core needle biopsy may be performed to withdraw multiple (e.g., up to 15) tissue samples. This procedure is used when tissues, instead of cells, are necessary for diagnosis. A stereotactic procedure may be used for a nonpalpable lump that is detected by mammography. In this procedure, mammography is used as a placement guide for the core needle biopsy. In the unusual instance when a lump cannot be evaluated via a stereotactic procedure, the physician may use mammography to guide insertion of a thin wire into the breast lump. This procedure usually precedes a surgical biopsy and is used for localization of the problem area. Surgical biopsy, which involves removal of a part or all of a breast lump for analysis, is the most accurate method of breast biopsy.

Medical management of breast cancer is complicated and may require a multi-treatment approach, including surgery and adjunctive treatment, such as radiation, chemotherapy, and hormone therapy. The simplest surgical treatment option is a lumpectomy: the lump and an area of surrounding normal tissue are removed. The lumpectomy is usually followed by radiation treatment to remove any remaining cancerous cells. A partial or segmental mastectomy involves removal of the tumor, the surrounding breast tissue, a portion of the lining of the chest wall, and some of the axillary lymph nodes. This procedure is usually followed with radiation therapy as well. A simple mastectomy involves the removal of all of the breast tissue along with the area surrounding the nipple and areola. Radiation, chemotherapy, or hormone therapy may follow this surgical procedure. In a modified radical mastectomy, the entire breast and several axillary lymph nodes are removed, leaving the chest wall intact. While this procedure makes breast reconstruction easier for the patient, complications including lymphadenopathy and paresthesia are more likely to occur.

Many women choose to undergo breast reconstruction after a mastectomy. This surgical option, performed by a plastic surgeon, is a personal decision that requires considerable individualized counseling and education. Since the reconstruction can be performed at the same time as the mastectomy, it is important to consider the options early. Breast reconstruction methods include use of a synthetic breast implant or reconstruction using one's own tissue. Synthetic implants typically are composed of a silicone shell filled with a saline solution. A tissue expander may be needed to cover the implant. To accomplish tissue expansion, an empty implant shell is placed under the skin and muscles and gradually filled with the saline solution over several months. Once the skin is stretched sufficiently, the expander is removed and replaced with a permanent implant. Recovery usually takes several weeks.

Women who choose to undergo breast reconstruction using their own tissue may have a transverse rectus abdominis myocutaneous (TRAM) flap procedure. The breast is reconstructed using fat and muscle tissue taken from the abdomen, back, and buttocks. Recovery following the procedure usually takes 6 to 8 weeks, and there is an increased risk of infection and tissue necrosis. Deep inferior epigastric perforator (DIEP) reconstruction is a slightly less complicated surgical procedure. This method is similar to the TRAM flap procedure, but the abdominal muscles are left intact. The DIEP procedure is associated with fewer complications and less postoperative pain. Following reconstruction of the breast tissue, the surgeon can reconstruct the nipple and areola using tissue from other areas of the body. A small mound is constructed to resemble a nipple, and tattooing may be used to create an areola; the areola may also be created by using a skin graft and slightly raising the skin, then tattooing the skin graft.

Adjuvant therapies may include radiation therapy, chemotherapy, or hormone therapy. Radiation is usually begun 3 to 4 weeks after surgery, and treatments are given 5 days per week for 5 to 6 weeks. Chemotherapy that includes a combination of two or more drugs may also be prescribed. Chemotherapeutics may be administered orally or intravenously, and usually require four to eight treatments over 3 to 6 months. Hormone therapy is most commonly used to treat advanced metastatic cancer or as an adjuvant treatment to prevent recurrence of cancer. Normally, estrogen and progesterone bind to receptor sites in the breast tissue and encourage growth of cancerous cells. Prescribed hormone medications bind to the sites instead, and prevent estrogen from reaching them. Medications used in hormone treatment include tamoxifen (Nolvadex), a selective estrogen receptor modulator (SERM), and aromatase inhibitors, which block the conversion of androgens into estrogen.

Colon Cancer Screening

A colonoscopy is the best method for identifying possible colon and rectal cancer. Since more than 90% of colon and rectal cancers are diagnosed after the age of 50, recommendations suggest having a colonoscopy at this age. Other tests that can be helpful in screening for colon cancer include:

- Fecal occult blood test (small amounts of blood can be detected in the stool)
- Sigmoidoscopy (detects polyps and cancer inside the rectum)

- Lower colon double-contrast barium enema (x-ray films are taken of the colon and rectum)
- Digital rectal exam (usually included as part of a routine physical exam)

A colonoscopy is an examination that involves insertion of a colonoscope (a thin catheter with a light and lens) into the rectum to allow the physician to visualize and photograph the tissues and, when indicated, remove specimens for pathological examination. Preparation for the procedure usually includes a clear liquid diet for 1 to 3 days before the examination and administration of a laxative or enema on the evening prior to the procedure. Patients who take anticoagulants, nonsteroidal anti-inflammatory drugs, or oral antidiabetic agents are instructed when to withhold their medications in preparation for the procedure.

Colonoscopy is performed under conscious sedation. The patient is placed on the left side and given an analgesic and a sedative. Once the patient is relaxed and the colonoscope is inserted into the rectum, the patient is asked to change positions several times to enhance visualization of the colon. Abnormal growths or tissue are removed for laboratory analysis. The procedure usually takes about 30 to 60 minutes and the patient may experience mild cramping and slight bleeding afterwards.

Cholesterol and Lipid Screening

Cholesterol is essential for cell membranes, synthesis of bile acids, and synthesis of steroid hormones. Included in the cholesterol are chylomicrons, very low density lipids (VLDLs), low-density lipids (LDLs), and high-density lipids (HDLs). **Chylomicrons** are lipoproteins that are present shortly after eating, then disappear within a couple of hours following a meal. HDLs are considered to exert a positive influence on prevention of heart disease: they carry cholesterol to the liver for excretion in the bile. Conversely, LDLs carry cholesterol into the bloodstream. Comparison of results with normal values provides the nurse with information to evaluate cardiac disease risk and provide patient education on healthy eating behaviors (Box 4-7).

THE CLIMACTERIC, MENOPAUSE, PERIMENOPAUSE, AND POSTMENOPAUSE

The **climacteric** is a transitional time in a woman's life marked by declining ovarian function and decreased hormone production. The climacteric begins at the onset of ovarian decline and ends with the cessation of postmenopausal symptoms. **Menopause**, a term derived from Latin *mensis* for month and Greek *pausis*, meaning to cease, refers to the last menstrual period and can be dated with certainty only 1 year after menstruation ceases. The average age at menopause in the United States is 51.4 years; the normal age at menopause ranges from 35 to 60 years.

Perimenopause is the period of time preceding menopause, usually between 2 and 8 years before menopause. The age at onset of perimenopause ranges from 39 to 51 years (Speroff & Fritz, 2005). Although perimenopause may last as few as 2 or as many as 10 years, on average, it lasts 4 years. During this time of transition, levels of estrogen and progesterone increase and decrease at uneven intervals, causing the menstrual cycle to become longer, shorter, and eventually absent. Ovulation is sporadic.

Box 4-7 Lipid Screening Results

GUIDELINES FOR INTERPRETING LIPID SCREENING RESULTS

Total Cholesterol

Below 200 mg/dL:	Desirable
240 mg/dL and above:	High, increased risk of cardiac disease

LDL Cholesterol

Below 100 mg/dL:	Desirable; target goal for those with cardiac disease or multiple risk factors
100–129 mg/dL:	Elevated; target goal for those with two or more risk factors
130–160 mg/dL:	Borderline high; target goal for those with zero to one risk factor
Above 160 mg/dL:	Significantly elevated

HDL Cholesterol

Below 40 mg/dL:	Adds a risk factor for cardiac disease
60 mg/dL and above:	Desirable

Triglycerides

Below 150 mg/dL:	Desirable
200 mg/dL and above:	High

Source: Veterans Health Administration, Department of Defense (2006). *VHA/DoD clinical practice guideline for the management of dyslipidemia in primary care.* Washington, DC: Author.

Symptoms of perimenopause, including irregular menses, hot flashes, vaginal dryness, dyspareunia, and mood changes are associated with the fluctuation and decline in hormone levels.

During **postmenopause**, the time after menopause, estrogen is produced solely by the adrenal glands; the ovaries are no longer involved in estrogen production.

While there is no specific treatment for perimenopause, use of oral contraceptives may help to regulate menstrual periods and alleviate hot flashes and vaginal dryness. **Hormone replacement therapy** (HRT), provided as estrogen only or a combination of estrogen and progestin, is usually a consideration at this time. Estrogen-only HRT increases the risk of endometrial cancer and breast cancer. Estrogen–progestin therapy increases the risk of cardiovascular disease, stroke, and deep vein thrombosis by decreasing protective factors. In a recent position statement, the North American Menopause Society (NAMS) suggests that estrogen therapy (for women who have had hysterectomies) or the combination of estrogen and progesterone therapy offers the greatest benefit and smallest risk to women who are within 10 years of menopause (NAMS, 2007). (See Chapter 5 for further discussion.)

 Be sure to— Provide patients with accurate information on menopausal hormone therapy

In 2002, the National Heart, Lung and Blood Institute of the National Institutes of Health halted a major landmark study, called the Women's Health Initiative. The study was intended to evaluate the risks and benefits of **menopausal hormonal therapy** (MRT). The study was immediately stopped when results indicated an increased risk of breast cancer and a lack of overall benefit for the relief of menopausal symptoms with the use of estrogen and pro-

gestin, known as hormonal replacement therapy (HRT) (Writing Group for the Women's Health Initiative Investigators, 2002). The findings also indicated an increased risk of heart attack, stroke, and blood clots; a reduced risk of colorectal cancer; fewer fractures; and no improvement in cognitive function.

The study component designed to investigate the use of **estrogen-only replacement therapy** (ERT) was allowed to continue. The findings from this branch of the study revealed no difference in the risk for heart attack or colorectal cancer; an increased risk of stroke and blood clots; an uncertain effect on breast cancer risk; and a reduced risk of fractures (The Women's Health Initiative Steering Committee, 2004).

Given the findings of this 15-year study, nurses should focus perimenopausal counseling on:

- Healthy lifestyle changes: Smoking cessation, consuming a variety of foods low in saturated fat and cholesterol, limiting salt and alcohol intake, maintaining a healthy weight, and being physically active
- Prevention of osteoporosis: consuming foods rich in vitamin D and calcium, obtaining moderate exposure to sunlight, engaging in weight-bearing exercises; smoking cessation; and limiting alcohol intake
- Treatment of menopausal symptoms: alternative therapies; antidepressants; stress reduction; avoidance of spicy foods, alcohol, and caffeine; getting adequate sleep; being physically active; and the use of selective estrogen receptor modulators (SERMs) for severe symptoms only

 Complementary Care: *Managing the symptoms of menopause*

Dietary supplements and herbal therapies have long provided women with alternative treatments to alleviate some of the symptoms associated with menopause. These biologically based therapies include soy, vitamins, probiotics, and herbs such as black cohosh. However, research evidence does not support the ideas that they are efficacious in minimizing menopausal symptoms (Nedrow et al., 2006).

Complementary therapies that are currently being studied for their benefit in diminishing menopausal symptoms include:

- Mind–body therapy
- Energy therapy: Electromagnetic forces, life-force energy
- Manipulative and body-based therapy: Chiropractic, osteopathy, massage
- Traditional Chinese medicine

While there is no current evidence to support their effectiveness in minimizing the symptoms of menopause, these complementary methods are considered to be much safer than herbal and vitamin therapies.

Nursing Insight— *Framing menopause as a celebration of midlife*

Once considered by many to be a sign of "old age," menopause has come to be viewed as a natural passage in a maturing woman's life. Through education and support, nurses can help empower women to embrace menopause and midlife as a liberating time that brings freedom from the worry of an unplanned pregnancy; an end to childrearing responsibilities; and an opportunity to focus on hobbies, career, interpersonal relationships, and self-discovery.

GYNECOLOGICAL DISORDERS

During middle age, there is an increased incidence of certain gynecological disorders due to hormonal and environmental influences. Leiomyomas are present in about 20% of women during this age period. Ovarian cysts, which may occur at any age, are most common during the childbearing years up to the time of menopause. Endometrial cancer is the most common malignancy of the reproductive system. Ovarian cancer, the second most frequently occurring reproductive cancer in females, is the most common cause of death of all of the reproductive cancers due to its rapid growth and nonspecific symptomatology. Endometrial cancer is slow-growing and when detected at a localized stage, the survival rate is much greater than with ovarian cancer (ACS, 2006a).

Leiomyomas

Leiomyomas, or uterine fibroid tumors, are benign growths that arise from the smooth muscle in the uterus. They occur most often after age 50 and are more common in African American women and in women who have never been pregnant. While the exact cause is unknown, their growth is dependent on estrogen. Leiomyomas begin as small masses of tissue that spread into and throughout the myometrium. They rarely become malignant and shrink after menopause when levels of the ovarian hormones have declined.

Leiomyomas are often asymptomatic and may not be detected until there is evidence of infertility. Symptoms, if present, may include a sensation of fullness or pressure in the lower abdomen, increased pain and cramping with menstrual periods, abdominal distention, urinary frequency, or heavy menses. Uterine tumors may be identified during a pelvic examination through palpation of the uterus. A transvaginal ultrasound may be performed to confirm the diagnosis. If cancer is suspected, a laparoscopy may be indicated.

Medical management may include the use of nonsteroidal anti-inflammatory drugs for dysmenorrhea. Oral contraceptives may be prescribed to control heavy periods and decrease tumor growth. Leuprolide (Lupron), a medication that suppresses the production of estrogen and progesterone, may be used to shrink leiomyomas although patients may complain of menopausal symptoms such as vaginal dryness, hot flashes, and mood changes.

If the fibroid tumors are growing inside the uterus, a hysteroscopic uterine **ablation** (vaporization of tissue) may be performed under local or general anesthesia. In this procedure, a hysteroscope, a small camera, and surgical instruments are inserted through the vagina and into the uterus. After the procedure, scarring and adhesions that interfere with fertility may form in the uterine cavity. **Myomectomy** (removal of the fibroid tumor) is an alternative surgical treatment that may be performed for women who wish to preserve their fertility. Myomectomy can be done through an abdominal incision, or through a laparoscopic or vaginal (hysteroscopic) approach.

Ovarian Cysts

Ovarian cysts are benign fluid-filled sacs that develop on the ovaries and cause pain and, at times, bleeding. The most common type of ovarian cyst is a functional, or "simple" cyst in which fluid is contained within a thin wall inside the ovary. Functional ovarian cysts result when the ovarian follicle fails to rupture and release an oocyte. Instead, the fluid remains in the follicle and develops into a cyst. This type of cyst occurs most often during a woman's childbearing years and disappears without treatment.

There are, however, other types of ovarian cysts. A follicular cyst develops when ovulation does not occur or when an immature follicle does not reabsorb fluid following ovulation. Follicular cysts are usually asymptomatic and shrink after two or three menstrual cycles. However, rupture of the cyst causes severe pelvic pain.

A corpus luteum cyst occurs after ovulation. Under normal circumstances, if fertilization does not occur, the corpus luteum shrinks and disappears. When the corpus luteum persists, it can become filled with fluid or blood and remain on the ovary. Symptoms associated with a corpus luteum cyst include abdominal pain, ovarian tenderness, and delayed or irregular menses. If bleeding occurs within the cyst, it is known as a hemorrhagic cyst. Rupture can cause an intraperitoneal hemorrhage. Corpus luteum cysts typically resolve spontaneously within one or two menstrual cycles.

A dermoid cyst is a germ cell tumor that usually affects women at an earlier age. This type of ovarian cyst may grow to 6 inches in diameter, and can contain fat, teeth, bone, hair, and cartilage. Dermoid cysts can develop bilaterally and may cause lower abdominal pain or complications related to torsion. Surgical removal is the usual treatment.

Endometrioid cysts result from the growth of endometrial tissue in the ovaries. They are often filled with dark blood and may cause chronic pelvic pain. Treatment involves removal to prevent rupture and the development of a hemoperitoneum.

Ovarian Cancer

Cancer of the ovary is the second most frequently occurring reproductive cancer and causes more deaths than any other genital tract cancer (ACS, 2006a). While the cause is unknown, there are identified risk factors, including nulliparity, pregnancy later in life, presence of *BRCA1* and *BRCA2* genes, a personal history of breast cancer, and a family history of breast or ovarian cancer. Associative causes include the use of fertility medications, exposure to asbestos, genital exposure to talc, a high-fat diet, and childhood mumps infection. Older women are at increased risk as compared to younger women. Approximately two-thirds of the deaths associated with ovarian cancer occur in women who are age 55 and older, while approximately 25% occur in women between the ages of 35 and 54. Pregnancy and oral contraceptive use provide some protection against ovarian cancer, and the use of postmenopausal estrogen may increase the risk (ACS, 2006a).

Symptoms are usually vague and nonspecific, and include pelvic fullness, lower abdominal pain, weight gain, irregular menstrual cycles, back pain, abdominal distention and increased abdominal girth (related to ovarian enlargement or ascites), urinary urgency, urinary frequency, indigestion, lack of appetite, feeling full after eating only a little bit and bloating (Goff et al., 2007). Since ovarian cancer is a rapidly growing neoplasm, the diagnosis is usually not made until the cancer has metastasized, giving rise to the nickname for ovarian cancer as "the silent killer."

The diagnosis is made via transvaginal ultrasonography, CA-125 antigen (a tumor-associated antigen) testing, or laparotomy. The preferred treatment for ovarian cancer is surgical removal, and usually requires a hysterectomy with bilateral salpingo-ööphorectomy. After surgery, chemotherapy is used to treat any remaining cancer. Radiation therapy may be used as a palliative measure although it is not typically used as a treatment option for ovarian cancer.

Older Adulthood Health

As individuals move into the later stages of life, physiological changes as well as psychological changes alter their health and increase their risk of disease. During these years, health promotion and disease prevention is imperative in order to maintain quality of life and encourage empowerment in managing health and daily activities. Health care management focuses on gynecological health and mental and emotional health.

HEALTH PROMOTION

Health promotion is complex and challenging in older adults as they are experiencing changes in sexual functioning, exercise and activity, cognition, and function. Many considerations must be incorporated into patient education during older age.

Sexual Functioning

Intimacy and sexual activity during the later years remain important in fulfilling relationships that can positively affect one's physical and emotional health. However, physical and psychological changes that occur in the body can affect intimacy as one ages. Testosterone, the hormone that regulates the sex drive, does not decrease significantly as one ages. Instead, other changes exert a more immediate impact on intimacy and sexual functioning.

For women, the most significant change is the decrease in estrogen that accompanies menopause. Low levels of estrogen are associated with decreased vaginal lubrication and a slowed response to sexual stimulation. In addition, the vaginal tissue loses elasticity, resulting in increased dryness and dyspareunia. Prolonged foreplay and use of a water-soluble lubricant or an estrogen cream that can be applied directly to the vagina can facilitate lubrication and help in maintaining elasticity.

For men, it may take longer to achieve an erection. Once achieved, the erection may not be as firm or last as long as in previous years. To help with this problem, the health care provider can make recommendations including medications, a penile vacuum pump, or vascular surgery.

For both genders, changes in physical appearance can adversely affect one's emotional ability to develop an intimate relationship with another. The presence of gray hair, wrinkles, and increased body fat may cause the older adult to feel less attractive and experience a reduced libido. Talking to one's partner about these feelings and emotions can stimulate intimacy and help the couple connect on a more comfortable level with one other.

For those who are single, it is imperative that health providers address sexually transmitted infections and safe sex practices. About 20% of all adults with HIV infection are older adults, and the risk increases for women due to the increased dryness and loss of elasticity of the vaginal mucosa. Barriers should be used for sexual intercourse as well as for oral sex for all sexually active adults.

Exercise and Activity

Maintaining exercise and activity during the later years can improve an adult's strength, balance, flexibility, and endurance, which can combine for healthier living and increased independence. Strength exercises build muscles, increase metabolism, and help with maintaining healthy body weight and blood sugar levels. Exercises that can be performed safely by older adults to help in strength building include arm raises, bicep curls, triceps extensions, and knee flexion. Balance exercises help adults to build leg muscles, which can help to prevent falls. Included in the balance exercises are side leg raises, hip flexion, and hip extension. Stretching exercises improve movement and allow one to be more physically active during the later years. Included in the stretching exercises are triceps stretches and double hip rotations. Endurance exercises include cardiovascular exercises that increase the heart rate and respiratory rate and help to build up endurance gradually. The activities can include any activity that builds cardiovascular health in this way, from walking to jogging to swimming and biking. Older adults who have not engaged in endurance exercises should begin slowly, with only about 5 minutes of activity per day.

Cognitive Functioning

While cognition includes memory and knowledge, there are other factors incorporated into cognitive ability. Cognition is a combination of acquiring knowledge, perceiving events that surround us, using language, making decisions, using judgment, and executing motor skills. As cognitive changes occur due to the aging process, older adults begin to notice changes in memory and the ability to execute normal daily functions.

Most of the decline seen in cognitive functioning due to the aging process is irreversible. However, there are some factors that can slow the decline. Stress management and coping strategies can lessen depression and increase concentration and memory. Medical management of physical illnesses can control renal disease, liver disease, endocrine disorders, and electrolyte imbalances that can contribute to diminishing cognitive functioning. Good nutritional intake, including folate, riboflavin, and thiamine can improve cognition. Finally, moderation or elimination of alcohol use can reduce cognitive impairment.

A simple cognitive assessment that can be performed on all adults includes the use of clock drawing, box copying, and narrative writing to describe a pictured scene. These activities allow the health care provider to gather information regarding cognitive function in a relatively quick fashion. A Mini-Mental Status Examination can be performed to provide a better gauge of cognitive difficulty. The specific components in the Mini-Mental Status Examination are time orientation, place orientation, registration of three words, serial 7's as a test of attention and calculation, recall of three words, naming, repetition, comprehension, reading, writing, and drawing (Tufts New England Medical Center, 2007).

Functional Ability

Functional ability may also decrease with aging, especially if the older adult has any disability or does not engage in physical activity and exercise. When assessing functional ability, it is important to consider how a person manages her day-to-day activities, the impact of any disease on the daily activities, and the overall quality of life being experienced by the individual. To gain this information, the health care provider should perform a functional assessment.

The functional assessment needs to incorporate physical, social, psychological, demographic, financial, and legal issues. Questions asked should be designed to provide answers regarding self-concept and self-esteem, occupation, activity and exercise, sleep and rest, nutrition and elimination, interpersonal relationships and resources, coping and stress management, and environmental hazards.

 ### Across Care Settings: Optimizing senior health

Older adults should be encouraged to become more involved in activities that can improve health, endurance, and the enjoyment of life. Whether the individual is at home, in the workplace, in the community, or residing in a senior living environment, regular activity needs to be promoted. Physical activities may include walking, exercise classes, strength training, or swimming. In addition, cognitive functioning can be improved through conversation, puzzles, board games, and card games. Many communities have organizations that provide activities to promote healthy living for seniors, and nurses can play an integral role in encouraging and providing information on available resources.

Immunizations

Recommended immunizations for the older adult focus on disease prevention related to highly communicable illnesses (CDC, 2006a). An influenza vaccination should be administered annually to prevent infection from influenza, and this is particularly important in older adults with chronic respiratory and cardiac diseases. Other older adults at high risk for infection are those who reside in assisted living or long-term care facilities. The pneumococcal vaccine, which provides protection against pneumococcal pneumonia, should be administered to all adults around the age of 65. Individuals at higher risk for infection and complications related to infection are those who reside in assisted living or long-term care facilities as well as older adults with chronic respiratory, cardiac, renal, and hepatic disease.

COMMON HEALTH PROBLEMS IN WOMEN

Health problems that frequently develop in women during older age include osteoporosis, endometrial cancer, and pelvic floor dysfunction. Medical management of each of these disorders can prolong life and, in many cases, provide for a healthier ability to engage in daily activities.

Osteoporosis

As individuals age, there is a progressive decrease in bone density. **Osteoporosis** is a generalized, metabolic disease characterized by decreased bone mass and an increased incidence of bone fractures. Although osteoporosis occurs primarily in older women, it can also occur in older men, in persons with decreased levels of calcium and phosphorus, and in conjunction with increased corticosteroid release or administration. The most common problem associated with osteoporosis is the increased risk of bone fracture, primarily in the spine, hip, or wrist. While normal changes in bone density occur with aging, there are a number of risk factors that are associated with the development of osteoporosis (Box 4-8).

SCREENING. Screening for osteoporosis through measurement of bone density should begin for all women at age 65, and initiated between ages 60 and 64 for women at increased risk for developing osteoporosis.

A variety of tests are available for osteoporosis screening. Dual-energy x-ray absorptiometry (DXA), measured at the femoral head of the hip, spine, and wrist, is the best indicator of an increased risk for hip fracture, although measurements at different areas can be used to determine the presence and degree of osteoporosis. Peripheral sites can also be used for screening purposes, through quantitative ultrasonography, radiographic absorptiometry, single-energy x-ray absorptiometry, peripheral dual-energy x-ray absorptiometry, and peripheral quantitative computed tomograpy (Nelson, Helfand, Woolf, & Allan, 2002).

Medical management of osteoporosis is usually pharmacological, and focuses on the goals of preventing increased bone density loss and, if possible, increasing bone density over time. Bisphosphonates, the most common group of medications used, inhibit osteoclast activity,

---

Box 4-8 Risk Factors for Developing Osteoporosis

Risk factors for developing osteoporosis include:

- Age, due to decreased estrogen following menopause
- Slender build and small frame
- Low body weight (<150 lb [70 kg])
- Shortened exposure to estrogen, through late menarche or early menopause
- Family history of osteoporosis
- Smoking
- Decreased physical activity or sedentary lifestyle
- Excessive caffeine or alcohol use
- Low calcium and vitamin D intake
- Southeast Asian and Caucasian ethnicity
- Use of corticosteroids, commonly used to treat chronic respiratory disorders and arthritis

preserve bone mass, and increase bone density. The most common bisphosphonates are alendronate (Fosamax), ibandronate (Boniva), and risedronate (Actonel), which can be taken on a weekly or monthly basis. Raloxifene, a selective estrogen receptor modulator, can also be used for women with osteoporosis since this medication reduces loss of bone density without increasing the risk of breast or endometrial cancer.

Prevention is the best strategy for reducing the risk of fractures associated with osteoporosis. Health-promoting activities that facilitate prevention include adequate amounts of calcium and vitamin D, moderate exposure to sunlight, strength training exercises, endurance exercises, adding soy, which contains plant estrogens, to the diet, cessation of smoking and the avoidance of excess caffeine and alcohol.

Pelvic Floor Dysfunction

The pelvic muscles atrophy after menopause, becoming weak and unable to adequately support the pelvic structures and organs. As the pelvic organs shift position, they begin to press against the vagina, resulting in prolapse, usually of the vagina or bladder. The most common cause of pelvic muscle weakness results from damage to the muscles during vaginal birth, particularly if the baby was large or if the labor was difficult. Other factors related to weakening of the pelvic floor include obesity, chronic cough, chronic constipation, and strenuous exercise. A prolapse can result in pain during intercourse and urinary incontinence. In severe cases, the vagina may prolapse and protrude through the vaginal orifice.

Different types of prolapse can occur, depending upon the muscles and organs that are affected. A **cystocele** results when the bladder herniates into the vagina. Symptoms include difficulty in voiding, incontinence, and dyspareunia. A **rectocele** occurs when the muscles behind the vagina are damaged, allowing the rectum to press into the vagina. When the muscle damage occurs in a higher location in the colon, it is referred to as an **enterocele**. Symptoms associated with both of these types of prolapse include constipation, difficulty in completing a bowel movement, and dyspareunia. Uterine and vaginal vault prolapses occur when the uterus and cervix press downward, resulting in a sensation of pressure in the abdomen and vagina, dyspareunia, and back pain.

Exercise can strengthen the muscles; however, muscle damage cannot be reversed. Surgery is the primary treatment for pelvic prolapse; the timing of the surgery depends upon the woman's symptoms and their effect on her daily activities.

Some symptoms can be medically managed until surgery is appropriate. Many treatment options are available for urinary incontinence, especially if it is not accompanied by a cystocele. Exercises to strengthen the pelvic muscles, including Kegel exercises, can be beneficial in decreasing the incidence of urinary incontinence (see Chapter 10 for more information). Vaginal cones, which may also be vaginal weights, can be used to strengthen the vaginal muscles as well. These tampon-shaped cones are inserted into the vagina, beginning with the lightest weight. Once inserted, the patient should contract the pelvic muscles in an effort to keep the cone in place for minutes. As the muscles strengthen, the patient then transitions, one at a time, to the next heaviest cone. It is helpful to use the cone while doing Kegel exercises as well. As the pelvic muscles strengthen, patients can use the cones while engaging in exercise.

Electrical stimulation during Kegel exercises stimulates and contracts the pelvic muscles in a manner similar to the Kegels. This approach, conducted in the health care practitioner's office, may be helpful for women who have difficulty contracting the pelvic muscles voluntarily. With biofeedback, the patient is taught to voluntarily control the pelvic muscles and bladder. With an electrode attached to the skin, biofeedback machines measure the electrical signals elicited when the pelvic muscles and urinary sphincter are contracted. Through the visual cues from the graph shown on the monitor, patients can learn to control these muscles voluntarily.

Some women choose to use a **pessary**, which is a device inserted into the vagina to support the prolapsed bladder or uterus. This device must be fitted by a health care practitioner, and needs to be removed and cleaned regularly with soap and water to reduce the risk of infection.

Pharmacological management of incontinence is aimed at relaxing the involuntary contractions that occur in the bladder. For overactive bladder, common medications include tolterodine (Detrol), oxybutynin (Ditropan), and imipramine (Tofranil). Common side effects associated with these medications include dry mouth, nausea, dizziness, drowsiness, and constipation. For **urinary stress incontinence** (USI), in which there is an involuntary loss of urine during sneezing, coughing, or laughing, the goal of treatment is to increase muscle tone in the urinary sphincter. Postmenopausal women may choose to use estrogen replacement therapy following careful consideration of the risks and benefits. For weak or underactive bladder problems, bethanechol (Urecholine) is the usual medication of choice.

Surgical interventions include laparoscopic or abdominal procedures to support the bladder and urethra in the correct anatomical position or methods to tighten the sphincter muscles. In one type of procedure, the surgeon sutures the vaginal wall to the tissue near the pubic bone. Another involves the creation of a sling using synthetic material or tissue taken from the abdomen or from beneath the thigh. The sling is then positioned beneath the urethra to provide support and prevent urine leakage. A newer procedure uses a mesh-like tape, called tension free transvaginal tape (TVT), which is surgically inserted through the vagina and positioned to support the neck of the urethra and the bladder. This procedure is performed under local anesthesia and intravenous sedation. A final procedure involves injections of collagen or silicone into the lining of the urethra. The injected substance increases the bulk of the surrounding tissues, allowing the urethra to close tightly and prevent leakage of urine. This technique usually requires two to three injections before symptom improvement is noticed.

Following either type of surgical repair, the patient should not engage in exercise for 2 weeks and avoid lifting objects weighing more than 10 pounds for 3 months after the surgery. At that time, exercises to protect and strengthen the pelvic muscles are initiated.

Endometrial Cancer

Endometrial cancer occurs most often in women between the ages of 60 and 70, and is the most common malignancy of the reproductive system. Endometrial cancer is slow growing and most women are symptomatic in the early stages, factors that lead to early diagnosis and, frequently, successful treatment. For postmenopausal women, the cardinal symptom is vaginal bleeding; perimenopausal women may have heavy or prolonged menstruation or spotting or bleeding between menses. Other symptoms for all women with endometrial cancer include pelvic pain, dyspareunia, and/or weight loss.

An increased estrogen level, which stimulates growth of the endometrium during the menstrual cycle, is the most common cause of endometrial cancer. However, several additional risk factors have been identified: early age of menarche (before the age of 12), combined with late menopause; nulliparity; irregular ovulation, which may result from obesity or polycystic ovarian syndrome; a high-fat diet, which increases the levels of circulating estrogen; diabetes (a condition closely related to obesity and a high-fat dietary intake); estrogen-only replacement therapy; ovarian tumors that produce estrogen; age greater than 40 years; a personal history of breast cancer or ovarian cancer; breast cancer treatment with tamoxifen; Caucasian race; and hereditary nonpolyposis colorectal cancer (HNPCC), a specific type caused by a gene that inhibits DNA repair.

The diagnosis is made by histologic examination. Most often, tissue is obtained by endometrial biopsy, an outpatient procedure performed using local anesthesia. A suction-type curette is used to remove the tissue for laboratory analysis. Dilatation and curettage (D and C), a surgical procedure performed under general anesthesia, may also be used to obtain endometrial tissue for sampling. If endometrial cancer is present, staging, which may include chest radiography, abdominal CT scan, and serum testing for the presence of cancer antigen 125 (CA 125, released by some endometrial and ovarian cancers), is done to determine the degree of metastasis.

Hysterectomy (surgical removal of the uterus) is the most common treatment for endometrial cancer. In most cases, a bilateral salpingo-ööphorectomy is also performed, along with removal of local lymph nodes. If metastasis has occurred, adjunctive treatment may be needed. Radiation therapy may be recommended if the cancer has metastasized or if there is a high risk for recurrence. Hormone therapy involving synthetic progestin may be used for those premenopausal patients or for those who wish to preserve fertility. Chemotherapy may also be used to reduce the tumor size or prevent recurrence.

PROSTATE CANCER SCREENING

Prostate cancer is the most common cancer diagnosed in men. Risk factors include a positive family history, environmental exposure to carcinogens, hormonal influences, especially elevated levels of androgens, and advancing age. Currently, prostate cancer in the leading cause of cancer in men, regardless of race. Benign hypertrophy of the prostate (BPH) is associated with prostate cancer. However, there is no evidence that a causative link exists. While BPH does not usually cause symptoms in men before the age of 40, more than 50% of men in their 60s and 90% of men in their 70s and 80s have some symptoms of BPH, including difficulty voiding, dribbling, and urinary retention.

Prostate screening should be initiated at age 50. Two screening tests are used to determine the need for prostate biopsy: the digital rectal examination (DRE) and the serum prostate specific antigen (PSA). To perform a DRE, the examiner inserts a gloved and lubricated finger into the rectum and carefully palpates the prostate gland. The examination is considered normal when palpation reveals a prostate that is smooth, absent of nodules, and of normal size and shape.

When the DRE is determined to be normal, there may be other findings (i.e., changes in the texture of the prostate over time or the presence of cysts that cannot be differentiated from a tumor) that signal a need for further screening. If the DRE reveals the presence of enlargement, nodules or an abnormal glandular shape, a blood test measuring the serum tumor marker prostate-specific antigen (PSA) is obtained. The total PSA and free PSA ratio are used to determine the risk of prostate cancer in men whose total PSA is greater than 4 ng/mL. A total PSA between 4 and 10 ng/mL indicates a 25% risk of prostate cancer; a total PSA greater than 10 ng/mL indicates a 67% risk of prostate cancer. Men whose total PSA is greater than 4 ng/mL benefit from the inclusion of a free PSA test, which is the ratio of free-circulating PSA and total PSA. Men who have a free PSA of 20% or less should have a prostate biopsy performed to determine if cancer is present.

A prostate biopsy is typically performed with the assistance of transrectal ultrasonography. During the procedure, an ultrasound probe is inserted into the rectum and ultrasonographic pictures are transmitted for viewing. This procedure allows the physician to determine the size and shape of the prostate and location of abnormal growths. A fine needle is then inserted into the gland and several samples of prostate tissue are removed for pathological examination.

Preparation for Prostate Biopsy

Patients are provided with the necessary information for biopsy preparation at least 2 weeks before the procedure. Although men who have a history of cardiac valvular disease must receive antibiotic prophylaxis before the procedure, many physicians prescribe prophylactic antibiotic therapy for all patients prior to the procedure to decrease the incidence of postprocedure infection. Patients who are taking coagulation-modifier agents or anti-inflammatory agents are instructed to discontinue the use of these medications 7 to 10 days before the procedure, and blood tests, including prothrombin time (PT) and international normalized ratio (INR), are performed before the procedure on the day of the biopsy to determine if bleeding times are normal. The patient is also instructed to administer an enema for bowel cleansing the day before the scheduled procedure.

After the procedure, the patient is instructed to refrain from taking coagulation-modifier agents and anti-inflammatory agents for 3 days, and to drink plenty of water. A sitz bath or warm soak is recommended for rectal tenderness. Antibiotics are prescribed for all postprocedure patients to prevent infection.

MENTAL AND EMOTIONAL HEALTH

Some older adults may experience declines in health and cognitive ability, which can lead to behavioral and emotional problems and physical complaints. Signs of altered mental and emotional health may begin with subtle changes in personality or with dramatic alterations that require immediate intervention from a health care professional. Symptoms that require immediate intervention include hallucinations, paranoia, incoherent thinking or language, extreme lack of motivation or flat affect, and expression of suicidal thoughts or actions. Less serious symptoms that also require intervention include changes in sleeping or eating patterns, loss of interest in activities, neglect of grooming and personal hygiene, changes in sexual habits, and refusal to take prescribed medications.

Treatment for alterations in mental and emotional health requires a collaborative approach. Psychologists and neurologists may be involved in initial testing and diagnosis, while psychiatrists and nurses become an integral part of the treatment and management team. Pharmacists are an important part of the team as they have specialized knowledge in drugs and drug interactions. Psychologists provide psychotherapy treatment and counseling for the patient and the family. Social workers are essential in coordinating care with regard to medical care, benefits, and housing. Occupational therapists are experts that evaluate and restructure a person's physical environment as well as provide mental activities to enhance independent functioning. Community health nurses visit the home to assess the patient and family and to gauge understanding and acceptance of the treatment plan.

 Collaboration in Caring— *Culturally sensitive community approaches to enhanced health care for older citizens*

Organizations, groups, and health care facilities recognize the importance of culturally sensitive approaches to meet the health needs of older citizens. Information gained from these collaborative endeavors benefits diverse communities by generating new knowledge and understanding and by providing insights for further investigation. Examples of successful projects include the following:

- The National Asian Pacific Center on Aging (NAPCA) organized community forums to share assessment results with participants. Three translators were available throughout the forums. Working groups were then developed to implement interventions to meet the identified needs.
- An advisory committee was used to evaluate the methodology and language used for a breast cancer study in Vietnamese women conducted by the University of California at San Francisco. Vietnamese women were hired to conduct the interventions in the study to improve accuracy of the results.
- The American Society on Aging conducted a study to determine the drinking habits of elders in the Chinese community. The written survey was translated into Chinese, and included alcoholic beverages specific to that culture, including plum wine. The researchers were able to acquire more accurate results by using culturally appropriate content (American Society on Aging, 2006).

Advancing age raises issues related to death and dying for most individuals. As they age, individuals may lose a spouse, family member, or close friend, which can significantly alter their living situation and their emotional health. As with persons of any age, the patient needs to be encouraged to grieve. However, it is essential for the nurse to be sensitive to the specific issues that frequently arise following the loss of the loved one: fear about living arrangements; preoccupation with one's own death; agitation and an inability to perform daily activities; and an overwhelming sadness or withdrawal. Counseling, support groups, and antidepressant medications are often beneficial for individuals who are experiencing difficulty with coping.

Another issue related to emotional and mental health concerns the older person's ability to remain connected to other people. Declines in health, physical mobility, and cognitive function may contribute to problems of isolation for the older adult. Family members should be encouraged to maintain frequent contact and engage the elderly in a variety of social activities to keep their loved ones involved in life and socially connected. Many community health agencies or elder day care facilities offer programs with supervised stimulation for adults experiencing difficulty in these areas. Respite care, which allows family members an opportunity for time away from the care-giving situation, may also be beneficial.

summary points

- Health promotion screening can provide early detection and treatment of health disorders, including reproductive cancers, hyperlipidemia, osteoporosis, and gynecological disorders
- Nurses play a key role in collaborative care for all patients, at each stage of the life span, from infancy to older age
- A holistic approach to health promotion includes focusing on nutrition, dental care, safety, injury prevention, screening for early diagnosis and treatment, and other strategies to facilitate healthy development
- Cultural and ethnic differences must be taken into consideration when providing anticipatory guidance and health promotion education to patients

review questions

Multiple Choice

1. The outpatient clinic nurse correctly makes a recommendation that Henry, a 65-year-old patient, schedule a health maintenance examination every:
   A. Year
   B. 2 years
   C. 3 years
   D. 5 years

2. The pediatric clinic nurse correctly identifies the most appropriate milk to introduce to the child at 1 year of age as:
   A. Whole milk
   B. 1% milk
   C. 2% milk
   D. Skim milk

3. The clinic nurse teaches new parents that the most normal time for children to ask about "where babies come from" is approximately:
A. 2 to 3 years of age
B. 3 to 5 years of age
C. 5 to 7 years of age
D. 7 to 9 years of age

4. The clinic nurse assesses Tom's risk for obesity by reviewing his parent's health records. Both of his parents have a BMI (body mass index) of 32. This finding gives Tom a risk of obesity of:
A. 25%
B. 50%
C. 75%
D. 90%

Select All that Apply

5. The clinic nurse teaches the new mother about feeding readiness that she may see in her infant:
A. Reaching 4 to 6 months of age
B. A doubling of the infant's birth weight
C. An ability to hold up the head
D. Hunger after five or six breastfeeds per day or 30 ounces of formula

6. Julie, a mother of a 9-month old infant, asks about appropriate finger foods for her baby. The clinic nurse could suggest:
A. Small pieces of ripe banana
B. Teething crackers
C. Cooked spiral pasta
D. Bite-size orange sections

7. The clinic nurse recognizes that adolescents have an increased risk of injury and disease due to:
A. The importance placed on peer relationships
B. An increased level of sex hormones
C. A developmental need to learn to trust
D. The natural development of primary sexual characteristics

Fill-in-the-Blank

8. The clinic nurse is aware that water safety is an important health promotion topic to discuss with adolescents and their parents. Teens have an increased risk of drowning due to an overestimation of their _____ and _____ in the water.

9. The clinic nurse is aware that the greatest effect on _____ _____ is the media. Teens watch approximately 3 to 4 hours of television a day which increases the likelihood for decreased exercise and adds to their risk for _____ .

10. As a component of health promotion, the clinic nurse screens all overweight teens in the clinic for _____ because of their increased risk for this condition.

See Answers to End of Chapter Review Questions on the Electronic Study Guide or DavisPlus.

REFERENCES

American Academy of Pediatrics (AAP). (2005). Policy statement: Breastfeeding and the use of human milk. *Pediatrics, 115*(2), 496–506.

American Cancer Society (ACS). (2003). Role of breast self-examination changes in guidelines: Focus on awareness rather than detection. Retrieved from http://www.cancer.org/docroot/NWS/content/NWS_1_1x_Role_Of_Breast_Self-Examination_Changes_In_Guidelines.asp (Accessed March 4, 2008).

American Cancer Society (ACS). (2006a). *Cancer facts and figures 2006.* New York: Author.

American Cancer Society (ACS). (2006b). What are the risk factors for breast cancer? Retrieved from http://www.cancer.org/docroot/CRI/content/CRI_2_4_2X_What_are_the_risk_factors_for_breast_cancer_5.asp?sitearea= (Accessed October 29, 2006).

American Cancer Society (ACS). (2007). How to perform a breast self-exam. Retrieved from http://www.cancer.org/docroot/CRI/content/CRI-2-6x-How-to-perform-a-breast-self-exam-5.asp (Accessed March 4, 2008).

American College of Obstetricians and Gynecologists. (2007). *Women's health care: a resource manual.* (3rd ed.). Washington, DC: Author.

American Society on Aging. (2006). Conducting culturally appropriate needs assessments. In Blueprint for health promotion: Foundation module. Retrieved from http://www.asaging.org/cdc/module1/phase1/phase1_3cbis2.cfm (Accessed March 14, 2007).

Bulechek, G., Butcher, H.M., & Dochterman, J. (2008). *Nursing interventions classification (NIC)* (5th ed.). St. Louis, MO: C.V. Mosby.

Center for the Study and Prevention of Violence (2004). *CSPV fact sheet: Ethnicity, race, class and adolescent violence.* Boulder, CO: Author.

Centers for Disease Control and Prevention. (CDC). (2004). Youth risk behavior surveillance—United States, 2003. *Morbidity and Mortality Review 53*(SS02), 1–96.

Centers for Disease Control and Prevention. (CDC). (2006a). Recommended adult immunization schedule, United States, October 2006–September 2007. *Morbidity and Mortality Weekly Report, 55*(40), Q1–Q4.

Centers for Disease Control and Prevention (CDC). (2006b). Recommended immunization schedules for persons aged 0–18 years—United States, 2007. *Morbidity and Mortality Weekly Report, 55*(51 & 52), Q1–Q4.

Centers for Disease Control and Prevention (CDC). (2006c). Sexually transmitted diseases treatment guidelines. Retrieved from www.cdc.gov/std (Accessed June 5, 2007).

Drifmeyer, E., & Batis, K. (2007). Breast abscess after nipple piercing. *Consultant* (April), 481–482.

Dunaif, A. (2006). Insulin resistance in women with polycystic ovarian syndrome. *Fertility and Sterility, 86*(Suppl. 1), S13–S14.

Goff, B.A., Matthews, B.J., Larson, E.H., Andrilla, C.H., Wynn, M.W., Lishner, D.M., & Baldwin, L.M. (2007). Predictors of comprehensive surgical treatment in patients with ovarian cancer. *Cancer, 109*(10), 221–227.

Husaini, B.A., Sherkat, D.E., Bragg, R., Levine R., Emerson, J.S., Mentes, C.M., et al. (2001). Predictors of breast cancer screening in a panel study of African American women. *Women and Health, 34*(3), 35–51.

Institute for Clinical Systems Improvement (ICSI). (2005, October). *Preventive services in adults.* Bloomington, MN: Author.

Insurance Institute for Highway Safety (IIHS). (2005). *Fatality facts: Teenagers 2003.* Arlington, VA: Author.

Johnson, M., Bulechek, G., Butcher, H., McCloskey Dochterman, J., Maas, M., Moorhead, S., & Swanson, E. (2006). *NANDA, NOC, and NIC Linkages: nursing diagnoses, outcomes, & interventions* (2nd ed.). St. Louis, MO: Mosby Elsevier.

Kagawa-Singer, M., & Pourat, N. (2000). Asian American and Pacific Islander breast and cervical carcinoma screening rates and healthy people 2000 objectives. *Cancer, 89*(3), 696–705.

Lehman, C.D., Gastonis, C., Kuhl, C., Hendrick, R.E., Pisano, E.D., Hanna, L., Peacock, S., et al. (2007). MRI evaluation of the contralateral breast in women with recently diagnosed breast cancer. *The New England Journal of Medicine, 356*(13), 1295–1303.

Menon, S., Burgis, J., & Bacon, J. (2007). The college-aged examination: A comprehensive approach to preventive medicine. *The Female Patient, 32*(7), 32–36.

Merck & Co., Inc. (2006). *USPPI Patient Information about Gardasil®.* Whitehouse Station, NJ : Author.

Michigan Quality Improvement Consortium. (2005, July). *Adult preventive services (ages 18–49).* Southfield, MI: Author.

Michigan Quality Improvement Consortium. (2005, July). *Adult preventive services (ages 50–65+).* Southfield, MI: Author.

Moorehead, S., Johnson, M., Mass, M., & Swanson, E. (2008) *Nursing outcomes classification (NOC)* (4th ed.). St. Louis, MO: C.V. Mosby.

National Cancer Institute (2006, July 21). *Testicular Cancer (PDQ®): Screening.* Retrieved from http://www.cancer.gov/cancertopics/ pdq/ screening/testicular/HealthProfessional (Accessed October 30, 2006).

National Comprehensive Cancer Network. (2006, October 1). Your breast cancer survival guide. Retrieved from http://www.nccn.org/about/ publications/pdf/Your_Breast_Cancer_SURVIVAL_Guide.pdf (Accessed March 14, 2007).

National Women's Health Resource Centers, Inc. (2006, September 20). *Take 10 for breast cancer awareness.* Retrieved from http://www. healthywomen.org/breastcancer2006/pg1.html (Accessed October 29, 2006).

Nedrow, A., Miller, J., Walker, M., Nygren, P., Huffman, L.H., & Nelson, H.D. (2006). Complementary and alternative therapies for the management of menopause-related symptoms: A systematic evidence review. *Archives of Internal Medicine, 166*(14), 1453–1465.

Nelson, H.D., Helfand, M., Woolf, S.H., & Allan, J.D. (2002). Screening for postmenopausal osteoporosis: A review of the evidence for the US Preventive Services Task Force. *Annals of Internal Medicine, 137,* 529–541.

Pisano, E., Gatsonis, C., Hendrick, E., Yaffe, M., Baum, J., Acharyya, S., et al. (2005). Diagnostic performance of digital versus film mammography for breast cancer screening: The results of the American College of Radiology Imaging Network (ACRIN) digital mammographic imaging screening trial (DMIST). *The New England Journal of Medicine, 353*(17), 1773–1783.

Roberts, T.A., & Ryan, S.A. (2002). Tattooing and high-risk behavior in adolescents. *Pediatrics, 110*(6), 1058–1063.

Speroff, L., & Ritz, M. (2005). *Clinical gynecologic endocrinology and infertility* (7th ed.). Philadelphia: Lippincott Williams & Wilkins.

Stephen, M.B. (2003). Behavioral risks associated with tattooing. *Family Medicine, 35*(1), 52–54.

The Nemours Foundation. (2007). *How to perform a testicular self-examination.* Retrieved from http://www.kidshealth.org/teen/sexual_ health/guys/tse.html (Accessed March 14, 2007).

The North American Menopause Society (NAMS). (2007). Position Statement: Estrogen and Progestogen use in peri and post menopausal women: March 2007 position statement of the North American Menopause Society. *Menopause: The Journal of the North American Menopause Society, 14*(2), 168–182.

The Women's Health Initiative Steering Committee (2004). Effects of conjugated equine estrogen in postmenopausal women with hysterectomy. *Journal of the American Medical Association, 291*(14), 1701–1712.

Tufts New England Medical Center (2007). *The Mini Mental State Examination.* Retrieved from http://www.nemc.org/psych/mmse.asp (Accessed May 27, 2007).

U.S. Department of Agriculture (USDA), Food and Nutrition Service (2005). *MyPyramid for kids.* Washington, DC: U.S. Government Printing Office.

U.S. Department of Agriculture (USDA). (2005). MyPyramid-Tracker. [Computer software]. Retrieved from http: www. mypyramidtrackergov (Accessed May 5, 2007).

U.S. Department of Health and Human Services (USDHHS). (2000). *Healthy People 2010: Understanding and Improving Health.* Washington, DC: U.S. Government Printing Office.

U.S. Department of Health and Human Services (USDHHS), Office on Women's Health. (2005, October). *Benefits of breastfeeding.* Retrieved from http://www.4woman.gove/Breastfeeding/index.cfm?page=227 (Accessed February 11, 2007).

U.S. Preventive Services Task Force (USPTF). (2005). *The guide to clinical preventive services 2005. Screening for cervical cancer.* AHRQ Publication No. 05-0570, June 2005. Rockville, MD: Agency for Healthcare Research and Quality.

U.S. Preventive Services Task Force (USPSTF). (2007). *The guide to clinical preventive services 2007: Recommendations of the U.S. Preventive Services Task Force.* AHRQ Publication No. 07-05100, September 2007, Rockville MD. Available at http://www.ahrq.gov/

Veterans Health Administration, Department of Defense. (2006). *VHA/ DoD clinical practice guideline for the management of dyslipidemia in primary care.* Washington, DC: Author.

Vulval Pain Society. (2005). *How to perform a vulval self-exam.* Retrieved from http://www.vulvalpainsociety.org/html/selfexam.htm (Accessed March 15, 2007).

Writing Group for the Women's Health Initiative Investigators (2002). Risks and benefits of estrogen plus progestin in health postmenopausal women: Principal results from the Women's Health Initiative randomized controlled trial. *JAMA, 288*(3), 321–333.

Wu, T.Y., & Bancroft, J. (2006). Filipino American women's perceptions and experiences with breast cancer screening. *Oncology Nursing Forum, 33*(4), E71–E78.

 For more information, go to http://davisplus.fadavis.com/

CONCEPT MAP

Caring for Women, Families, and Children in Contemporary Society

Health Promotion / Disease Prevention

Infant/Child Health
Nutrition:
- Feeding: bottle vs. breast
- Solid food introduction based on developmental stage
- For >3 yrs: use food pyramid guide

Dental:
- Daily dental care

Sleep/Rest:
- Nighttime rest and naps based on developmental level

Safety:
- Home safety for injury prevention
- Control environment: crib, car, toys
- Risk-taking behavior: testing limits; sexual exploration

Activity:
- 5 types of developmental play with specific toys/games

Immunizations:
- CDC recommendations

Sexuality:
- Child perception based on developmental level

Adolescent Health
Nutrition:
- To facilitate optimal growth/development
- Risk factors for obesity: psychological/societal/medical
- Risk for eating disorders: anorexia/bulimia

Dental:
- Checkup and cleaning twice yearly

Sleep/Rest:
- May need to decrease extracurricular activities

Safety:
- Accidents/injuries; MVA, homicides, suicides
- Risk-taking behaviors; developing own identity
- Injuries: MV, bikes, firearms, water
- Substance abuse: ETOH, drugs
- Violence/abuse
- Tattooing and piercing
- Reproductive health

Health Promotion:
- Begin osteoporosis prevention
- Gynecological exams: introduction to reproductive health care
- Pap tests; pelvic exams; BSE; TSE
- Manage menstrual disorders: dysmenorrhea; PMS

What To Say:
- Speak with respect when discussing weight issues with adolescent

Ethnocultural Considerations:
- Adolescent violence
- Breast cancer screening practices

Family Teaching Guidelines:
- Performing vulvar self-exam
- Performing TSE

Young Adult Health
Safety:
- Substance use: ETOH, illicit drugs
- Safe sex

Health Promotion:
- Positive lifestyle choices to decrease risk of chronic illness
- Stress management
- Testicular cancer screening

Gynecological disorders:
- Endometriosis
- Cervical & breast cancer
- Urinary tract infections

Middle Adult Health
Health Promotion:
- Screenings: BSE; mammogram; clinical breast exam; colon cancer screening; cholesterol/lipids
- Lifestyle choices: ETOH, weight, smoking

Issues with menopause:
- Climacteric; peri/postmenopause
  - cessation of ovulation/menstruation
  - distressing symptoms
- HRT decisions

Gynecological disorders:
- Leiomyomas
- Ovarian cysts/ovarian cancer

Older Adult Health
Health Promotion:
- Sexual functioning; physical/psychological changes affect intimacy
- Still at risk for STI/HIV
- Exercise: balance, flexibility, endurance
- Cognitive functioning: stress management/coping strategies; manage physical illnesses; attend to nutrition
- Functional ability: assess ADLs, disease impact, quality of life
- Immunizations: influenza, pneumococcal
- Climacteric; peri/postmenopause
- Prostate cancer screening

Gynecological disorders:
- Osteoporosis
- Pelvic floor dysfunction; cystocele, rectocele, enterocele, urinary stress incontinence
- Endometrial cancer

Mental/emotional health:
- Personality changes
- Change in ability to perform ADLs
- Requires collaborative treatment
- Death & dying issues
- Decrease in social connectedness

Nursing Insight:
- Nurses can help women view menopause as a mid-life celebration

Complementary Care:
- Can use herbs for anxiety & depression: watch for S.E.
- Herbs/supplements used for menopause symptoms

Be Sure To:
- Provide accurate info on menopausal therapies

Optimizing Outcomes:
- Monthly BSE: clinical breast exam; mammograms all help to detect cancer early

Collaboration In Caring:
- Approach to senior care in community should be culturally sensitive

Now Can You:
- Discuss infant/child nutrition & safety issues
- List developmentally appropriate play for children
- Provide safety education for adolescents
- Discuss pelvic exam process & strategies for enhancing breast health

Across Care Settings:
- Many community resources available to keep seniors active
- Nursing-> encourage, give info

one
two
three
four
five
six
seven

The Process of Human Reproduction

Reproductive Anatomy and Physiology

 Since you are like no other being ever created since the beginning of time, you are incomparable.

— Brenda Ueland

LEARNING TARGETS *At the completion of this chapter the student will be able to:*

◆ Describe gender differentiation and differences in male and female embryos including timing of anatomical sexual differences.

◆ Identify anatomy of the female and male reproductive systems.

◆ Explain physiological functions of the reproductive organs.

◆ Analyze the actions and interactions of hormones from the hypothalamus, pituitary, gonads, and other hormones that affect the reproductive system.

◆ Describe the process of sexual maturation.

◆ Discuss various physiological events that accompany the menstrual cycle.

◆ Develop an understanding of physiological changes that occur during the menopause years.

◆ Identify several age-related issues for men.

---

 moving toward evidence-based practice Menstrual Cycle Variability

Fehring, R.J., Schneider, M., & Raviele, K. (2006). Variability in the phases of the menstrual cycle. *JOGNN, 35*(3), 376–384.

The purpose of this study was to determine the variability in the phases of the menstrual cycle among 165 healthy, regularly menstruating women. The sample consisted of 21- to 44-year-old women from four major U.S. cities. All participants reported having regular menstrual cycles that occurred every 21–42 days. None of the women had used depot medroxyprogesterone acetate (Depo-Provera) for the previous 12 months or oral or subdermal contraceptives for 3 months before the study. None of the women had known fertility problems. To be included in the study, breastfeeding mothers must have experienced at least three menstrual cycles after infant weaning.

The participants were taught how to monitor fertility by the use of the Clearblue Easy Fertility Monitor, a handheld electronic device designed to read wick-type urine test strips. The monitor notes "low," "high," or "peak" fertility status based on urine hormone levels. According to the manufacturer, the Clearblue Easy Fertility Monitor is accurate in detecting a hormone surge

98.8% of the time. The participants were also taught how to record monitor readings and the days of menstruation on a fertility chart. The fertility charts were reviewed with each participant at 1, 2, 6, and 12 months.

This prospective descriptive study utilized a data set with biological markers to estimate menstrual cycle parameters:

- Length of the follicular, fertile, luteal, and menstrual phases
- The estimated day of ovulation based on the "peak fertility" monitor reading (determined by the urinary luteinizing hormone surge)
- The cycle length, determined by counting the number of days beginning with the 1st day of menses to the beginning of the next menses
- The fertile phase, defined as a 6-day interval beginning with the 5 days preceding and including the second "peak fertility" day (the estimated day of ovulation)

(continued)

- The follicular phase, defined as the interval from the first day of menses up to and including the estimated day of ovulation
- The luteal phase, defined as the interval from the first day after the estimated day of ovulation up to and including the day before the next menstrual cycle
- The menses phase, defined as the interval beginning with the first day of bleeding through the last day of bleeding

Data analysis revealed the following:

- Mean age = 29.0 years; average number of children = 1.3
- Average number of menstrual cycles per 12 months = 5.2 (range 3–13)
- Mean frequency of menstrual cycles = 28.9 days; (range 22–36 days)
- Mean frequency of menstrual cycles in women over 35 years of age = 27.2 days
- On average, the fertile phase began on cycle day 13 and lasted for 6 days

- On average, the menstrual phase lasted for 5.8 days (range 3–8 days)
- On average, the follicular phase lasted 16.5 days (range 10–22 days)
- On average, the luteal phase lasted 12.4 days (range 9–16 days)

The study findings confirmed and expanded known information about the norms of menstrual cycle variability. There is considerable normal variability in the phases of the menstrual cycle among regularly menstruating women; the greatest amount of variability occurs in the follicular phase.

---

1. What might be considered as limitations to this study?
2. How is this information useful to clinical nursing practice?

See Suggested Responses for Moving Toward Evidence-Based Practice on the Electronic Study Guide or DavisPlus.

Introduction

This chapter provides an overview of the anatomy and physiology of the male and female reproductive systems. Growth and development over the life span is explored with a primary focus on females, and special issues related to male development. The menstrual cycle and events that occur in the absence of fertilization as well as those that take place soon after conception are explored. A discussion of key hormones that impact the menstrual cycle enhances understanding of the symphony of cyclic events during the reproductive years.

Sexual Differentiation in the Embryo

In humans, the course of gender maturation is quite lengthy, extending from embryonic development to full maturation in later adolescence. Although the gender of an individual is determined at the moment of conception, it takes about 8 weeks of development before the reproductive system becomes differentiated as male or female. Before 8 weeks' gestation, the embryo displays no distinguishing sexual characteristics. At 5 weeks after conception, the first reproductive tissue arises from the **mesoderm**, the embryo's middle layer. The first structure formed is a **gonad** (sex gland), which is composed of an internal portion called a medulla and an external portion known as the cortex. During the next few weeks, the gonad undergoes various developmental changes. Primitive reproductive ducts form during this undifferentiated period, and include a pair of mesonephric ducts and a pair of paramesonephric ducts. The mesonephric ducts are dominant in males and the paramesonephric ducts are dominant in females (Blackburn, 2003). Depending on the gender of the embryo, one ductal pair becomes dominant in genital development while the other genital pair regresses. Differing male/female developmental changes in the embryonic mesonephric/paramesonephric duct structure are the first gender changes that occur.

Male Gender

In a male embryo, the cortex of the gonad regresses and the medulla develops into a testis at around the 7th to 8th week of gestation. The mesonephric ducts evolve into the efferent ductule, vas deferens, epididymis, seminal vesicle, and ejaculatory duct. Collectively, these structures become the male genital tract. This process is stimulated by the production of testosterone in the testes. The testes also secrete Müllerian regression factor, which suppresses the paramesonephric ducts. The testes do not produce **spermatozoa** (sperm) until puberty. Beginning in the 12th developmental week, androgens begin to stimulate the growth of the external genitalia (Blackburn, 2003).

Female Gender

In a female embryo, the medulla of the first primitive gonad regresses while the cortex develops into an ovary at approximately 10 weeks. During fetal life, underdeveloped egg cells, **oogonia**, develop to become **oocytes**, (primitive eggs). At the time of birth, There are 2 to 4 million oocytes present in the ovary. The process of oocyte development that results in maturation of human ova is called **oogenesis**. External female genitalia develop in the absence of androgens. At approximately 12 weeks, the clitoris is formed and the labia majora and minora develop from the surrounding connective tissue. By 16 weeks, the paramesonephric ducts have evolved into the fallopian tubes, uterus, and vagina.

Female Reproductive System

EXTERNAL STRUCTURES (PUDENDUM MULIEBRE)

The external genital structures include the mons pubis, labia majora, labia minora, clitoris, vestibule of the vagina, urethral (urinary) meatus, Skene's glands, Bartholin's glands, vaginal introitus (opening), hymen, and the perineum (Fig. 5-1).

The **vulva** (pudendum femininum) is the portion of the female external genitalia that lies posterior to the mons pubis. It consists of the labia majora, labia minora, clitoris, vestibule of the vagina, vaginal opening, and Bartholin's glands (Venes, 2009).

Mons Pubis

The mons pubis, or mons veneris, is a layer of subcutaneous tissue anterior to the genitalia in front of the symphysis pubis. It is located in the lowest portion of the abdomen and typically is covered with pubic hair that grows in a transverse pattern. The texture and amount of pubic hair vary ethnically. In Asian women, the hair is fine and sparse. In women of African descent, the hair is thick and curly. The mons pubis is essentially a fatty pad that cushions and protects the pelvic bones, especially during intercourse.

Labia

The **labia majora** are the two folds of tissue that lie lateral to the genitalia and serve to protect the delicate tissues between them. The external labia are covered with pubic hair while the medial surfaces, which are moist and pink, are without pubic hair. During pregnancy, the labia majora are highly vascular due to hormonal influences. The labia majora share an extensive lymphatic network with other vulvar structures, leading to an enhanced capacity to spread diseases such as malignant carcinomas. The labia majora become less prominent after each pregnancy.

The **labia minora** are two folds of tissue that lie within the labia majora and converge near the anus to form the **fourchette** (a tense fold of mucous membrane at the posterior opening of the vagina). Similar to but smaller than the labia majora, these structures are moist and absent of hair follicles and resemble mucous membrane. The labia minora contain a number of sebaceous glands that provide lubrication and protective bacteriocidal secretions. During puberty the labia minora enlarge. After menopause they become smaller due to declining hormonal levels. The mons, labia majora, and labia minora all function to protect the clitoris and vestibule.

Clitoris

The clitoris is located at the upper junction of the labia minora. The **prepuce**, or clitoral hood, is a small fold of skin that partially covers the glans (head) of the clitoris. Composed of erectile tissue, the clitoris is primarily the organ of sexual pleasure and orgasm in women. The clitoris contains a rich blood and nerve supply, and is extremely sensitive. Sensory receptors located in the clitoris send information to the sexual response area in the brain. This message prompts the clitoris to secrete a cheese-like fatty substance with a distinctive odor called **smegma**. It is believed that smegma is a pheromone (chemical signal sent between individuals). Anatomically, the clitoral shape is similar to that of the urinary meatus, and the structural similarity of the two organs sometimes results in misguided and painful catheterization attempts. Some cultures remove the clitoris and other external genitalia in a ritualistic process called **female circumcision**.

Vestibule

The vestibule is essentially an oval-shaped space enclosed by the labia minora. It contains openings to the urethra and vagina, the Skene's glands, and the Bartholin's glands. This area of a woman's anatomy is extremely sensitive to chemical irritants. Nurses should be prepared to educate women about the potential discomforts associated with the use of dyes and perfumes found in soaps, detergents, and feminine hygiene products, and encourage their discontinuation if symptoms develop.

Urethral (Urinary) Meatus

The urethral or urinary **meatus** (opening) is located in the midline of the vestibule, approximately 0.4 to 1 inch (1 to 2.5 cm) below the clitoris. The small opening is often shaped like an inverted "V." The vaginal orifice or introitus lies in the lower portion of the vestibule posterior to the urethral meatus. It is essentially a boundary between the internal and external genitals. The **hymen**, a connective tissue membrane, encircles the vaginal introitus.

Skene's Glands and Bartholin's Glands

The Skene's glands (paraurethral glands), located on each side of the urethra, produce mucus that helps to lubricate the vagina. The Skene's glands are not readily visible. To facilitate examination, the margins of the urethra are drawn apart and the mucous membrane gently everted to reveal the small glandular opening on each side of the floor of the urethra (Venes, 2009).

The Bartholin's glands, also known as the greater vestibular or vulvovaginal glands, are located deep within the posterior portion of the vestibule near the posterior vaginal introitus. These glands secrete a clear mucus that moistens and lubricates the vagina during sexual arousal.

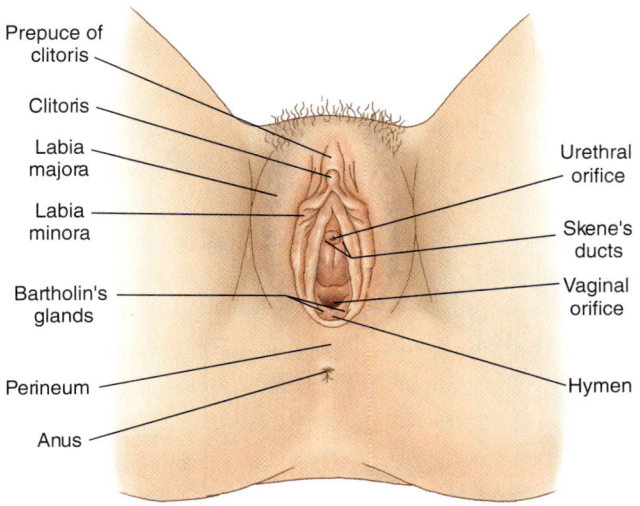

Prepuce of clitoris
Clitoris
Labia majora
Labia minora
Bartholin's glands
Perineum
Anus

Urethral orifice
Skene's ducts
Vaginal orifice
Hymen

Figure 5-1 Female external genitalia.

Hymen

Surrounding the opening of the vagina is a small portion of tissue called the hymen. The hymen typically forms a border around the entrance of the vagina in premenstrual girls. Hymenal tissue does not completely cover or occlude the vagina. Ultimately the hymen becomes widened, sometimes by tearing, which may be accompanied by bleeding. Widening of the hymen may also occur following a vulvar injury, tampon insertion, or at the time of the first sexual intercourse. It is a societal myth that the hymen must be intact for a female to be considered a virgin.

Perineum

The perineum, an anatomical landmark, is the skin-covered region between the vagina and the anus. The perineal body consists of fibromuscular tissue located between the lower part of the vagina and the anus. During the labor process, as the fetus descends through the vagina, the perineum stretches and becomes very thin, sometimes tearing as the baby is born. An **episiotomy** (incision made to enlarge the perineal opening to allow delivery of a fetus) may be performed to widen the external passage (see Chapter 12 for further discussion).

 Now Can You—Discuss aspects of development of the reproductive system and identify components of the female reproductive tract?

1. Identify the developmental week when differentiation of the embryo's reproductive system occurs?
2. Name three structures that arise from the mesonephric ducts?
3. Describe the anatomical locations and functions of the labia, Skene's glands, and Bartholin's glands?

PELVIC FLOOR

The bony pelvis contains a pelvic floor of soft tissues that provides support and stability for surrounding structures. Most of the perineal support comes from the pelvic diaphragm (musculofascial layer forming the lower boundary of the abdominopelvic cavity) and the urogenital diaphragm (musculofascial sheath lying between the ischiopubic rami surrounding the female vagina). The pelvic diaphragm includes fascia and the levator ani and coccygeus muscles (Cunningham et al., 2005).

Above the pelvic diaphragm lies the pelvic cavity; below and behind is the perineum. The urogenital diaphragm includes fascia, deep transverse perineal muscles, and the urethral constrictor (Cunningham et al, 2005). The muscles of the pelvic floor include the levator ani (consists of the iliococcygeal, pubococcygeal [pubovaginal], puborectal muscles) and the coccygeus. These structures create a "sling" that provides support for internal pelvic structures and the pelvic floor. The ischiocavernosus muscle extends from the clitoris to the ischial tuberosities on each side of the lower bony pelvis. Two transverse perineal muscles extend from fibrous tissue of the perineum to the ischial tuberosities to stabilize the perineum (Fig. 5-2).

INTERNAL STRUCTURES

The internal female reproductive structures consist of the ovaries, fallopian tubes (oviducts, or uterine tubes), uterus, adjacent structures (**adnexa**), and vagina (Figs. 5-3 and 5-4). The ureters, bladder, and urethra are structures of the internal urinary system.

Ovaries

The ovaries are sometimes referred to as the essential female organ because they produce **ova** (female gametes or eggs) that are required for reproduction. They are a pair of oval structures, each measuring approximately 1.5 inches (4 cm) long, located on each side of the uterus below and behind the fallopian tubes. The ovarian ligament extends from the medial side of each ovary to the uterine wall; the broad ligament is a fold of the peritoneum that provides a covering for the ovaries. These two ligaments help to keep the ovaries in place.

The ovaries are responsible for the production of ova and the secretion of female sex hormones. Both of these functions become activated at the time of puberty. **Oogenesis** (the process of meiosis for egg cell formation) results in the formation of mature eggs within the ovary. Oogenesis is a process that occurs at regular (usually monthly) intervals. The ovaries also secrete the female sex hormones estrogen

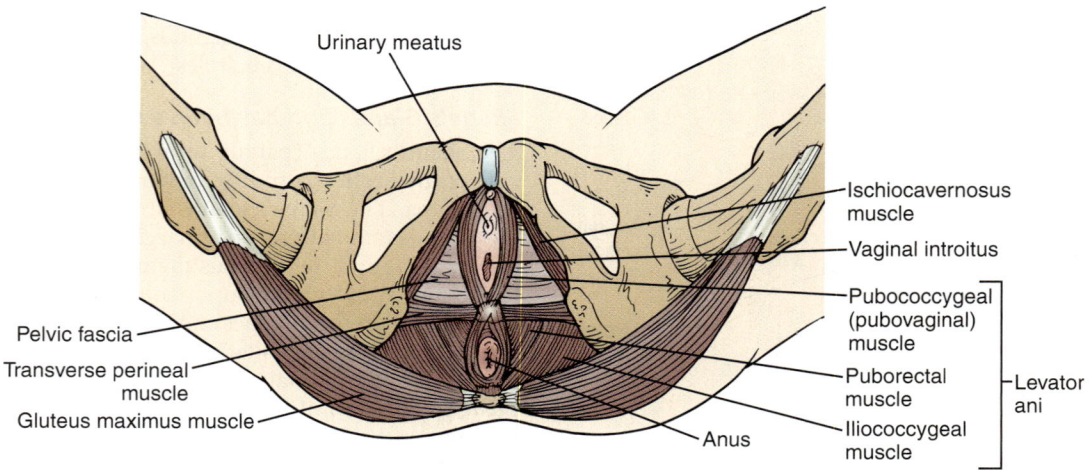

Figure 5-2 The muscles of the female pelvic floor.

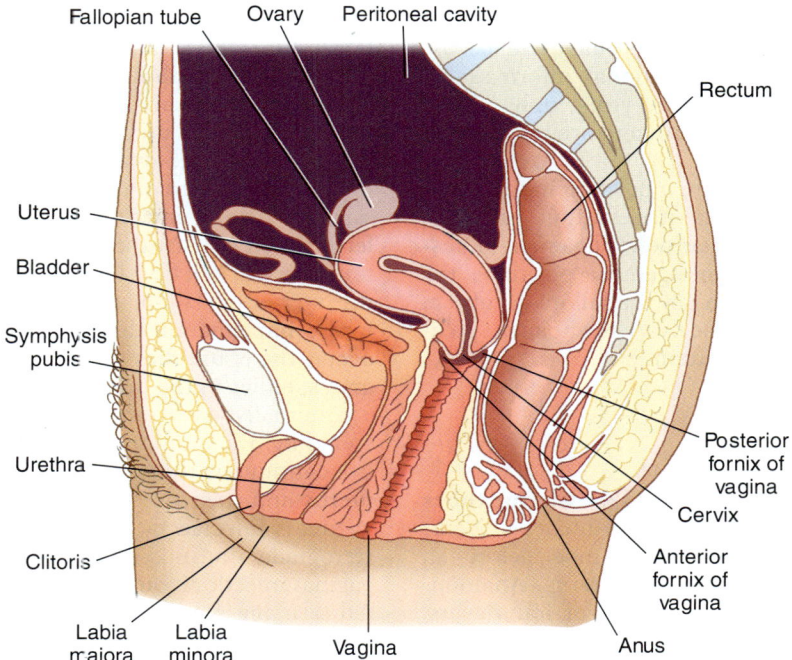

Figure 5-3 Internal female genitalia and cross section of the rectum.

and progesterone. This important endocrine function helps to regulate the menstrual cycle.

A & P review   Oogenesis

Oogenesis begins in the ovaries and is regulated by follicle stimulating hormone (FSH), which initiates the growth of ovarian follicles. Each follicle contains an **oogonium**, or egg-generating cell (Fig. 5-5). FSH also stimulates the follicle cells to secrete estrogen, which promotes maturation of the ovum. For each primary oocyte that undergoes the process of meiosis, only one functional egg cell is produced. The remaining three cells, termed polar bodies, have no function and deteriorate. A mature ovarian follicle, also called a **graafian follicle**, contains the secondary oocyte and if the egg is fertilized, the second meiotic division occurs and the ovum nucleus becomes the female pronucleus. ◆

Microscopically, the ovarian surface is termed the germinal epithelium. Each ovary has hundreds of thousands of follicles that contain immature female sex cells. All of the follicles in a woman's ovaries develop in utero and are present at birth. During a postpubertal woman's monthly

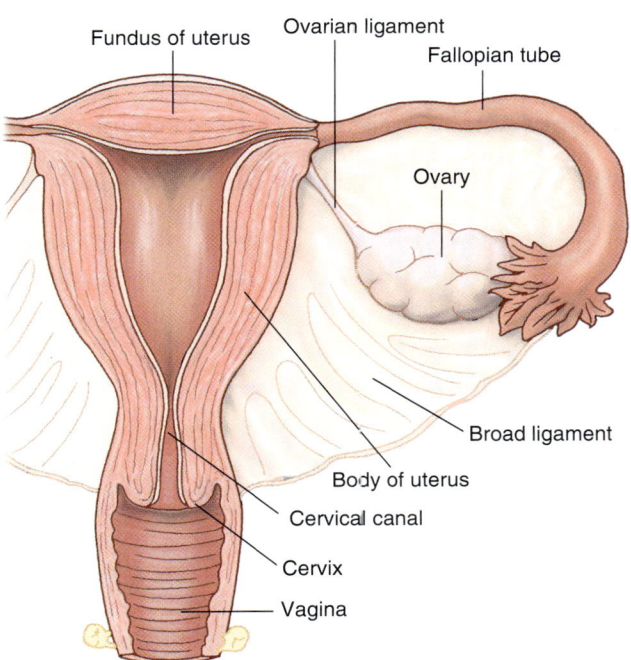

Figure 5-4 Internal structures of the adnexa.

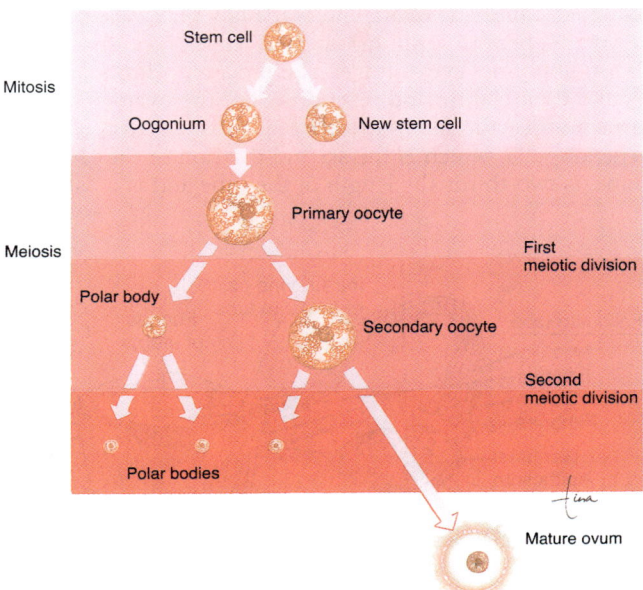

Figure 5-5 Oogenesis is the processes of mitosis and meiosis. For each primary oocyte that undergoes meiosis, only one functional ovum is formed.

menstrual cycle, one follicle develops and releases a mature ovum. (Please refer to the menstrual cycle discussion later in this chapter for additional information.) Throughout a woman's reproductive years, only 300 to 400 follicles develop into mature ova and are released for potential fertilization by a sperm.

The ovaries are supported in their position in the pelvis by three important ligaments: the mesovarium, the ovarian ligament, and the infundibular pelvic ligament or suspensory ligament. The ovarian ligament positions the fimbriae (finger-like projections) of the fallopian tube in contact with the lower pole of the ovary to enhance "pick-up" of the ovum following ovulation.

ACCESSORY ORGANS

Fallopian Tubes

The (two) fallopian tubes are also called the **uterine tubes** or **oviducts**. Measuring approximately 4 inches (10 cm) in length, the lateral end of each fallopian tube encloses an ovary; the medial end opens into the uterus. Anatomically, the fallopian tubes are composed of four layers. Beginning with the external layer and progressing inward to the internal layer, these include the peritoneal (serous), which is covered by the peritoneum, the subserous (adventitial), the muscular, and the mucous layers. The blood and nerve supplies are housed in the subserous layer. The muscular layer has an inner circular and an outer longitudinal layer of smooth muscle. It provides peristalsis that assists in transporting the ovum toward the uterus for potential implantation. The mucosal layer contains **cilia** (hairlike projections) that also assist in directing the ovum toward the uterus (Venes, 2009).

The fallopian tubes are attached at the upper outer angles of the uterus, and then extend upward and outward (Fig. 5-6). The diameter of each tube is approximately 6 mm. Anatomically, the tubes consist of three divisions: infundibulum, ampulla, and isthmus. The infundibulum is the funnel-shaped portion located at the distal end of the fallopian tube. The ovum enters the fallopian tube through a small opening (ostium) located at the bottom of the infundibulum. Several finger-like processes (fimbriae) surround each ostium and extend toward the ovary. The longest fimbria, the fimbria ovarica, is attached to the ovary. The ampulla, which is the second division of the fallopian tube, is two-thirds the length of the tube and is most often

the site of ovum fertilization. The third division of the fallopian tube, the isthmus, is nearest the uterus and is typically the site for **tubal ligation** (permanent sterilization).

A patent fallopian tube is able to convey the ovum from the ovary to the uterus and the spermatozoa from the uterus toward the ovary. Fertilization usually occurs in the outer one third of the fallopian tube, which provides a safe, nourishing environment for the ovum and sperm. If fertilization occurs, the fertilized ovum (termed a **zygote** until the first cell division) is slowly and gently swept into the uterus by fallopian peristalsis and cilia movement, where implantation takes place. If fertilization does not occur, the ovum dies within 24 to 48 hours and disintegrates, either in the tube or in the uterus.

Internally, each tube connects laterally with its corresponding ovary and medially with the uterus. Thus, there is a continuous route that passes from the vagina into the uterus and then on out to the tubes and ovaries. If the vagina is infected by a pathogen, the potential exists for retrograde transmission to the ovaries. Although most vaginal infections can be readily treated and cured, residual scarring from the inflammatory process can cause tubal narrowing leading to an increased risk for tubal pregnancies or infertility resulting from blockage.

Uterus

The uterus, centrally located in the pelvic cavity between the bladder (anteriorly) and rectum (posteriorly), is approximately 3 inches long by 2 inches wide (7.5 cm × 5 cm). It is a pear-shaped organ with the narrower end positioned closest to the vagina (Fig. 5-7). The uterine interior is hollow and forms a path from the vagina to the fallopian tubes. Because the uterine walls are very thick and collapsed upon each other, the interior cavity is, in actuality, a "potential space."

Two major functions of the uterus are to permit sperm to ascend toward the fallopian tubes and to provide a nourishing environment for the zygote until placental function begins. In addition, it provides a safe environment that protects and nurtures the growing embryo/fetus until the pregnancy has been completed. In the absence of conception, the uterus sheds the outermost layers of the inside of the endometrium (menstruation) in order to prepare for another menstrual cycle by regeneration of the endometrium.

The arteries of the uterus are the uterine, from the hypogastric arteries, and the ovarian, from the abdominal

Figure 5-6 Fallopian tube and ovary.

Figure 5-7 Uterus and surrounding structures of the female genitourinary system shown in a midsagittal section through the pelvic cavity.

aorta. This rich blood supply helps to ensure ample oxygenation and nutrition to facilitate the growing uterus and fetus during pregnancy. The uterine veins drain into the internal iliac veins. The vasculature of the uterus is twisted and tortuous and as the **gravid** (pregnant) uterus expands, these vessels straighten out, allowing a continued rich blood supply throughout pregnancy.

The uterus receives its nerve supply via the afferent (sensory) and efferent (motor) autonomic nervous systems. These two systems are important in regulating both vasoconstriction and muscle contractions. The uterus also has an innate intrinsic motility as well. Thus, a patient with a spinal cord injury above level T6 may still have adequate enough uterine contractions to deliver a fetus vaginally.

Uterine pain nerve fibers reach the spinal cord at levels T11 and T12. Because of this location and the presence of other pain receptors there, pain from the ovaries, ureters, and uterus may all be similar and may be reported by a woman who identifies pain in the flank, inguinal, or vulvar areas. Several sensory nerve fibers that contribute to **dysmenorrhea** (painful menstruation) are housed in the uterosacral ligaments.

Uterine Anatomy

The uterus is divided into three sections: the corpus, the isthmus, and the cervix.

The corpus of the uterus is the upper two-thirds of the uterine body and contains the cornua portion, where the fallopian tubes enter, and the fundus or uppermost section superior to the cornua (Fig. 5-8).

CORPUS

The layers of the corpus of the uterus include the perimetrium, the myometrium, and the endometrium. The perimetrium is the outer, incomplete layer of the parietal peritoneum (the serous membrane that lines the abdominal wall). The **myometrium**, or middle layer, is composed of layers of smooth muscle that extend in three directions—longitudinal, transverse, and oblique—and are continuous with the supportive ligaments of the uterus (Fig. 5-9). The tridirectional formation of the muscular layers is important in facilitating effective uterine contractions during labor and birth. The endometrium is the third and innermost uterine layer. It is composed of three layers, and of these, two are shed with each menses.

ISTHMUS

The isthmus is a slight constriction on the surface of the uterus midway between the uterine body (the corpus, or upper two-thirds), and the **cervix**, or "neck." During pregnancy, the isthmus becomes incorporated into the lower uterine segment and acts as a passive or noncontractile part of the uterus during the labor process. The isthmus is the site for the uterine incision when a low-transverse cesarean section is performed.

CERVIX

The cervix is the lower, narrow end of the uterus. It is similar to a neck or tube and extends from the inside of the uterus, opening into the vagina. The cervix secretes

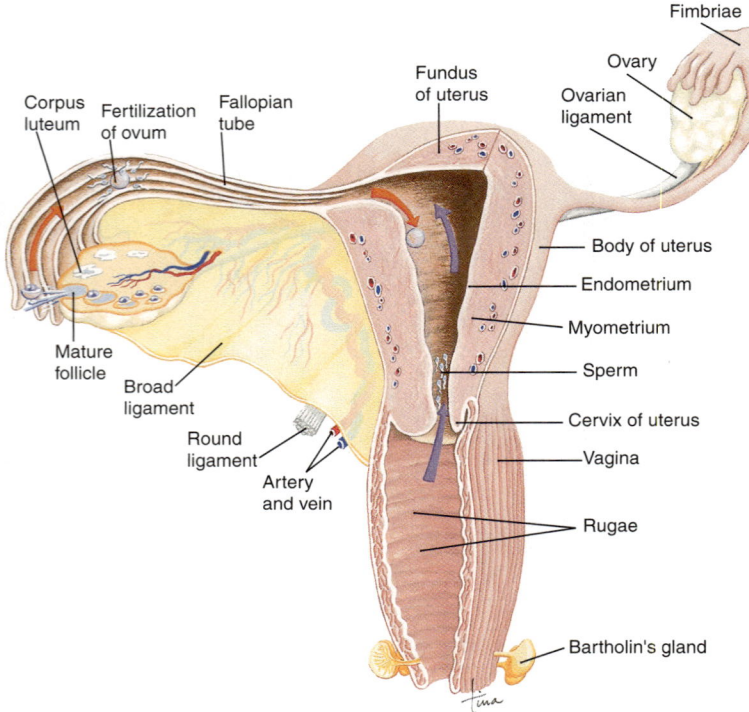

Figure 5-8 Female reproductive system shown in anterior view. The left ovary has been sectioned to show the developing follicles. The left fallopian tube has been sectioned to show fertilization. The uterus and vagina have been sectioned to show internal structures. Arrows indicate the movement of the ovum toward the uterus and the movement of sperm from the vagina toward the fallopian tube.

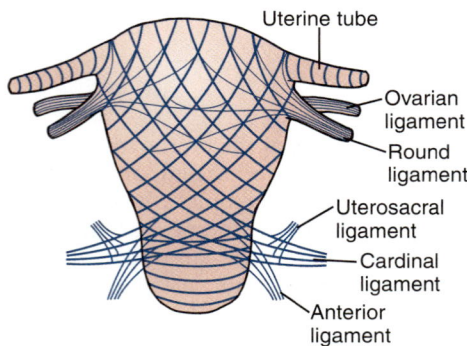

Figure 5-9 Arrangement of the directions of the smooth muscles of the myometrium. The uterine muscle fibers are continuous with the supportive ligaments of the uterus.

mucus, which serves several functions: (1) lubricates the vaginal canal, (2) forms a barrier to sperm penetration into the uterus during nonfertile periods, (3) provides an easy flowing pathway to facilitate sperm passage into the uterus during fertile periods, (4) provides an alkaline environment to facilitate the viability of sperm that have been deposited in the acidic vagina, (5) forms a solid plug called an **operculum** to protect a pregnancy from outside pathogens, and (6) functions as a bacteriostatic agent. The composition of cervical mucus changes during the menstrual cycle and these changes are important in the fertility assessment. During pregnancy, the cervical mucus forms a thick plug that creates a safe barrier between the developing embryo/fetus and the outside environment.

The vaginal portion of the cervix is composed of squamous (epithelial) cells. This portion of the cervix is fleshy pink in color. The canal portion of the cervix that leads into the uterine epithelium is composed of columnar cells. This tissue is bright red in color. The juncture of these two cell types is called the **squamocolumnar junction**. After puberty, this junction is active with cellular growth activity and cell turnover and it is the site where dysplasia (abnormal tissue development) may occur.

Uterine Support Structures

Uterine position in the body varies with age, pregnancy, and distention of related pelvic viscera. Typically, the uterus lies over the urinary bladder. The cervix points down and backward and enters the apex (the pointed extremity portion) of the vagina at a right angle. Several ligaments hold the uterus in place, but also allow for some movement.

The uterus is supported in the pelvis by several ligaments and muscles. These include the broad, round, cardinal, pubocervical, and uterosacral ligaments and the pelvic muscles (Fig. 5-10). The broad and round ligaments support the upper portion of the uterus, while the cardinal, pubocervical, and uterosacral ligaments provide support for the middle portion. The lower portion of the uterus is supported by the muscles of the pelvic floor.

The broad ligaments are supportive stretches of peritoneum that extend from the lateral pelvic sidewalls to the uterus. Within these structures are the fallopian tubes, arteries and veins, ligaments, ureters, and other tissues.

Figure 5-10 Uterine ligaments.

The round ligaments expand both in diameter and in length during pregnancy and this normal physiological change may be associated with maternal discomfort termed "round ligament pain." As the uterus expands, the round ligaments become stretched tight and sudden movements such as position changes, coughing or stretching may result in sharp pains that can be quite concerning until the woman understands the physiology for the discomfort. The round ligaments also play an important role during labor by pulling the uterus forward and downward, thereby holding it steady to facilitate the movement of the fetal presenting part toward the cervix. The cardinal ligaments prevent uterine prolapse and are the major support structures for the uterus and cervix.

Vagina

The vagina is a tubular organ approximately 4 inches (10 cm) in length that internally extends between the uterus and perineal opening. It is located between the rectum, urethra, and bladder. The collapsible vagina is composed of smooth muscle lined with mucous membrane arranged in **rugae** (small ridges), which allow distention during childbirth. The vagina has five functions: (1) to provide lubrication to facilitate intercourse, (2) to stimulate the penis during intercourse, (3) to act as a receptacle for semen, (4) to transport tissue and blood during menses to the outside, and (5) to function as the lower portion of the birth canal during childbirth.

The apex of the vagina, also termed the vaginal vault or fornix, is the upper, recessed area around the cervix. Following intercourse, sperm pool in the fornix, where they have close contact with the cervix and its alkaline pH. The vaginal pH is typically acidic (4.5 to 5.5) during the reproductive years. The acid environment, though harmful to sperm, helps to protect the genital tract from pathogens.

Ureters, Bladder, and Urethra

The ureters, bladder, and urethra and its external opening or meatus are part of the urinary system and are not reproductive organs. The urethra is a mucous membrane–lined tube that passes from the bladder to outside of the body to allow micturition. Its position is posterior to the symphysis pubis and anterior to the vagina. The urethra is approximately 1.2 inches (3 cm) in length.

 Now Can You— **Discuss various aspects of the female reproductive system?**

1. Identify the location of the perineum and describe its importance during childbirth?
2. Describe three functions of the uterus?
3. Name the five functions of the cervix?

Bony Pelvis

The pelvis forms a bony ring that transmits body weight to the lower extremities. In women, the bony pelvis is structured to adapt to the demands of childbearing. The pelvis functions to support and protect the pelvic contents and to form a relatively fixed axis for the birth passage (Cunningham et al., 2005).

The pelvis is composed of four bones: the sacrum, the coccyx, and two innominate (hip) bones. The bilateral innominate bones are formed by the fusion of the ilium, ischium, and pubis bones (Fig. 5-11).

True/False Pelves

The pelvis consists of two sections known as the "false pelvis" and the "true pelvis." These sections are divided by the **linea terminalis**, or pelvic brim. The false pelvis is superior to the linea terminalis. Its anterior boundary is the abdominal wall, its posterior boundary is the lumbar vertebra, and the lateral boundary is the iliac fossa. The false pelvis helps to support the gravid uterus and direct the fetal presenting part down toward the true pelvis.

The true pelvis, located below the linea terminalis, is important for childbearing. Its size and structure direct the fetus downward for delivery and its dimensions must be large enough to deliver the fetus for a vaginal birth. Its boundaries are partly bony and partly ligamentous. Superiorly, the true pelvis is bounded by the sacral promontory

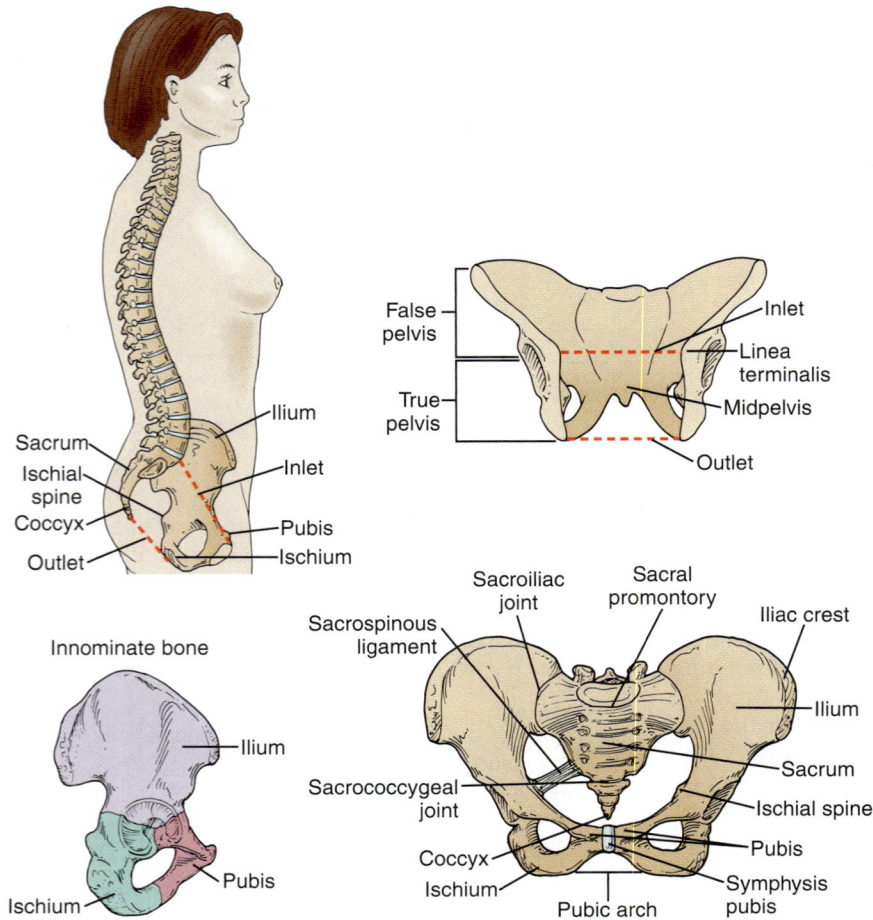

Figure 5-11 Female bony pelvis.

(anterior projecting portion of the base of the sacrum) and the sacral alae (broad bilateral projections from the base of the sacrum), the linea terminalis, and the upper margins of the pubic bones. Inferiorly, the lowest portion of the true pelvis is termed the **pelvic outlet**. The anterior landmarks of the true pelvis consist of the pubic bones, the ascending superior rami of the ischial bones, and the obturator foramen. The sacrum serves as the posterior landmark. Bilaterally, the true pelvis is bordered by the ischial bones and the sacrosciatic notches and ligaments. The true pelvis is divided into three sections: the inlet, the midpelvis, and the outlet, and each of these three components is important during the labor process.

Pelvic Diameters and Planes

In order to assess the adequacy of a woman's pelvis for delivery of a fetus of average size, health care providers may use **pelvimetry** (measurement of the pelvis to predict the feasibility of a vaginal birth). (See Chapter 9 for further discussion.) Measurements of the pelvis are approximate for two reasons: an inability to measure it directly and the presence of soft tissue covering the pelvis that can distort the actual size. Despite findings from clinical pelvimetry, in most situations, women in labor are allowed to experi-

ence a **trial of labor** (allowing uterine contractions in order to evaluate labor progress, i.e., cervical dilation and fetal descent) to assess the feasibility of vaginal birth.

Three portions of the true pelvis are measured during pelvimetry: the pelvic inlet, the midpelvis, and the pelvic outlet. The narrowest portion of the pelvic inlet is the line between the sacral promontory and the inner pelvic arch including the symphysis pubis. It is termed the **obstetrical conjugate** and should measure at least 4.5 inches (11.5 cm). Once the fetus passes this landmark, the presenting part is "engaged" in the pelvis. The midpelvis, which constitutes the area between the ischial spines, is the narrowest lateral portion of the female pelvis. This measurement needs to be at least 4.7 inches (12 cm) to allow for a vaginal birth. During labor, the ischial spines serve as a landmark for assessing the level of the fetal presenting part into the pelvis. At the pelvic outlet, two measurements are assessed: the angle of the ascending rami (pubic arch), which should be at least 90 to 100 degrees and the distance between the ischial tuberosities, which should be at least 3.9 inches (10 cm). These are the minimal measurements deemed necessary to allow the fetus to descend through the pelvis for birth. During pregnancy the joints of the pelvis soften and become more mobile due to effects of the hormone relaxin. This important physiological change creates additional space to accommodate childbirth (see Chapter 12 for further discussion).

Pelvic Types

There are four basic bony pelvic types that have a distinct shape that has distinct implications for childbirth (Caldwell & Moloy, 1933) (Fig. 5-12):

- Gynecoid: The gynecoid pelvic type is the typical, traditional female pelvis (present in 50% of women) that is best suited for childbirth. The anterior/posterior and lateral measurements in the inlet, midpelvis, and outlet of the true pelvis are largest in the gynecoid pelvis. The inlet is round to oval-shaped laterally, a characteristic that improves its adequacy for childbirth. In addition, the ischial spines are less prominent, the shortened sacrum has a deep, wide curve and the subpubic arch is wide and round. All of these characteristics enhance the feasibility for a vaginal birth. The other pelvic structures can pose problems for vaginal birth.

- Android: The android pelvis (found in 23% of women) resembles a typical male pelvis. The inlet is triangular or heart-shaped, and laterally narrow. The subpubic arch is narrow; there are more bony prominences, including the ischial spines, which are also prominent and narrow. These characteristics can cause difficulty during fetal descent.

- Anthropoid: The anthropoid pelvis (occurs in 24% of women) resembles the pelvis of the anthropoid ape. Similar to the gynecoid pelvis, the anthropoid pelvis is oval-shaped at the inlet, but in the anterior–posterior, rather than lateral, plane. The subpubic arch may be slightly narrowed. Fetal descent through an anthropoid pelvis is more likely to be in a posterior (facing the woman's front) rather than anterior (facing the woman's back) presentation (see Chapter 12 for further discussion).

- Platypelloid: The platypelloid pelvis (found in 3% of women) is broad and flat and bears no resemblance to a lower mammal form. The pelvic inlet is wide laterally with a flattened anterior–posterior plane and the sacrum and ischial spines are prominent. The subpubic arch is generally wide. Fetal descent through a platypelloid pelvis is usually in a transverse presentation and will not allow for a vaginal birth (see Chapter 12 for further discussion).

 Now Can You—Discuss aspects of the female bony pelvis?

1. Differentiate between the true and false pelves?
2. Name the three components of the true pelvis that are measured during pelvimetry?
3. Identify characteristics of the gynecoid pelvis and explain why this type is best suited for vaginal birth?

Breasts

The female breasts or mammary glands are considered to be accessory organs of the reproductive system (Fig. 5-13). The two breasts lie over the pectoral and anterior serratus muscles. Breast tissue consists primarily of glandular, fibrous, and adipose tissue suspended within the conical-shaped breasts by Cooper's ligaments that extend from the deep fascia.

The glandular tissue contains 15 to 24 lobes that are separated by fibrous and adipose tissue. Each lobe contains several lobules composed of numerous alveoli clustered around tiny ducts that are layered with secretory cuboidal epithelium called alveoli or acini. The epithelial lining of the ducts secretes various components of milk. The ducts from several lobules come together to form the lactiferous ducts, which are larger ducts that open on the surface of the nipple.

The wide variation in breast size among women is related to the differing amounts of adipose tissue that surrounds the mammary glands. At puberty, development of an adolescent's breasts is controlled by the hormones estrogen and

	Shape		Inlet	Midpelvis	Outlet
Gynecoid					
Android					
Anthropoid					
Platypelloid					

Figure 5-12 Comparison of the four Caldwell–Moloy pelvic types. The average woman has a gynecoid pelvis; others may have a variation or a mixture of types. Few women have pure android, anthropoid, or platypelloid types.

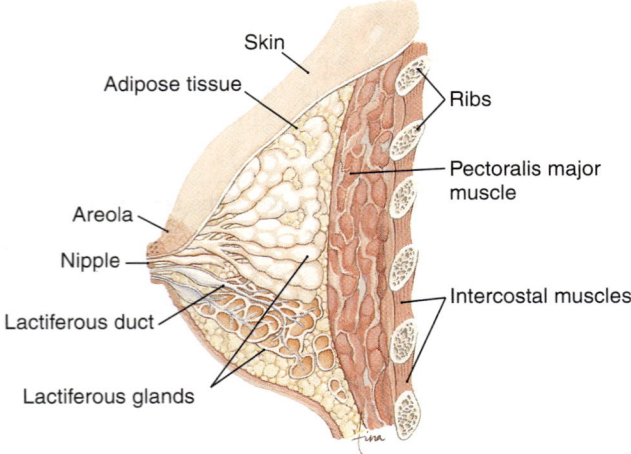

Figure 5-13 Mammary gland shown in a midsagittal section

progesterone. Interestingly, in most women, the left breast is often larger than the right.

The primary function of the breasts is to provide nutrition to offspring through the process known as lactation. Preparation for milk production takes place during pregnancy as the ovaries and placenta produce hormones (estrogen and progesterone) to prepare the breasts structurally for lactation by promoting growth of the ducts and secretory cells. After birth and delivery of the placenta, there is an abrupt decrease in estrogen. This event triggers an increased secretion of prolactin (the hormone that stimulates milk production) by the anterior pituitary gland. The posterior pituitary and hypothalamus play a role in the production and secretion of oxytocin, a hormone that causes release of milk from the alveoli.

PARTS OF THE BREAST

Nipples

Centrally located on the breast, the nipples contain several pores that secrete colostrum (breast fluid that precedes breast milk) and breast milk during lactation. The nipples consist primarily of erectile tissue to assist with infant latch-on during suckling (see Chapter 15 for further discussion).

Areola

The areola is a more deeply pigmented area that surrounds the nipple. Its diameter ranges from 1 to 3.9 inches (2.5 to 10 cm).

Montgomery Tubercles

The Montgomery tubercles are papillae located on the surface of the nipple and the areola. The Montgomery tubercles secrete a fatty substance that lubricates and protects the nipple and areola during breastfeeding.

 Now Can You— Discuss anatomy of the female breast?

1. Name three types of tissue that comprise the breast?
2. Identify the pituitary hormone responsible for initiation of lactation?
3. Explain the function of the Montgomery tubercles?

The Interplay of Hormones and Reproduction

Knowledge of the functions of key hormones associated with reproduction is essential to an understanding of the female menstrual cycle. The following discussion centers on hormones that play a major role in the process of human reproduction.

HORMONES RELEASED BY THE HYPOTHALAMUS

Since hormones released by the hypothalamus stimulate the release of other hormones, they are termed "releasing factors." Factor hormones act on the anterior pituitary and stimulate the release of hormones from the pituitary. Releasing factors from the hypothalamus include the following:

- *Gonadotropin-releasing hormone* (GnRH): Stimulates the release of the gonadotropins follicle-stimulating hormone (FSH) and luteinizing hormone (LH) from the anterior pituitary. These hormones are released when a decrease in ovarian hormones (estrogen and progesterone) is detected by the hypothalamus. In the premenopausal female, GnRH exerts an ovarian influence: it affects the cyclic process of follicular growth, ovulation, and maintenance of the corpus luteum. In the male, GnRH affects **spermatogenesis**, the process of meiosis in the testes to produce sperm cells.
- *Corticotropin-releasing hormone* (CRH): Regulates adrenocorticotropic-stimulating hormone (ACTH) secretion by the anterior pituitary to activate the sympathetic nervous system. CRH is also released by the pregnant woman and her embryo soon after implantation. CRH appears to provide a protective action by minimizing a maternal immunological rejection that could result in a miscarriage. Other effects of CRH relate to the woman's response to stress.
- *Growth hormone-releasing hormone* (GH-RH): Stimulates the production and release of growth hormone (GH) by the anterior pituitary.
- *Growth hormone-inhibiting hormone* (GH-IH), also known as somatostatin: Inhibits the release of GH.
- *Thyrotropin-releasing hormone* (TRH): Regulates thyroid hormones (T_3 and T_4) by stimulating the anterior pituitary to release thyroid-stimulating hormone (TSH). TRH also stimulates the release of prolactin.
- *Prolactin-inhibiting factor* (PIF), also known as prolactostatin: Inhibits the synthesis and release of prolactin by the pituitary gland. Dopamine, another hormone released by the hypothalamus, also inhibits prolactin.

HORMONES RELEASED BY THE PITUITARY GLAND

The anterior pituitary produces the following hormones:

- *Thyroid-stimulating hormone* (TSH), also known as thyrotropin: Regulates the endocrine function of the thyroid gland.
- *Adrenocorticotropic hormone* (ACTH), also known as corticotropin: Controls the development and functioning of

the adrenal cortex, including its secretion of glucocorticoids and androgens (Venes, 2009).

- *Prolactin* (PRL): Stimulates the maturation of the mammary glands during pregnancy; initiates milk production and provides some inhibition to the stimulation of FSH and LH.
- *Growth hormone* (GH), also known as somatotropin: Stimulates growth and cell reproduction (e.g., height growth during childhood) in humans. Growth hormone is also responsible for increased muscle mass, calcium retention and bone mineralization, the growth of various organ systems, protein synthesis, stimulation of the immune system, reduced uptake of glucose in the liver, and the promotion of lipolysis.
- **Gonadotropins** (gonad-stimulating hormones): Follicle-stimulating hormone (FSH) and luteinizing hormone (LH) stimulate and inhibit the ovaries. These two hormones help to regulate the menstrual cycle by producing a positive and negative feedback of estrogen and progesterone by the ovaries. The feedback systems stimulate the hypothalamic secretion of releasing hormones that act on the anterior pituitary gland.

The posterior pituitary releases oxytocin. Oxytocin stimulates uterine contractions and the release of milk from milk ducts in the breasts during lactation. A synthetic form of oxytocin can be administered during labor to enhance uterine contractions and after birth to promote expulsion of the placenta and minimize uterine bleeding.

Collectively, the pituitary hormones are essential in the regulation of gonadal, thyroid, and adrenal function, lactation, body growth, and somatic development (Moskosky, 1995; Venes, 2009).

A & P review **Hormonally Mediated Events and the Menstrual Cycle**

The menstrual cycle is hormonally mediated through events that take place in the hypothalamus, anterior pituitary gland, and the ovaries. The hypothalamus stimulates the anterior pituitary gland to produce gonadotropin. FSH, one of these hormones, stimulates the growth and development of the graafian follicle, which secretes estrogen. Estrogen stimulates proliferation of the endometrial lining of the uterus. After ovulation, the anterior pituitary gland secretes LH, which stimulates development of the corpus luteum. Progesterone secreted by the corpus luteum prompts further development of the lining of the uterus in preparation for the fertilized ovum. When pregnancy does not occur, the corpus luteum degenerates, and the levels of estrogen and progesterone decline. The decreased levels of estrogen and progesterone cause the uterus to shed its lining during menstruation. The decrease in estrogen and progesterone triggers a positive feedback to the hypothalamus, which stimulates the anterior pituitary gland to secrete FSH once again. A schema depicting the hormonal feedback mechanisms that regulate the menstrual cycle is presented in Figure 5-14. The interrelationships between the levels of hormone secretion, development of ovarian follicles, and changes in the uterine endometrium are presented in Figure 5-15. ◆

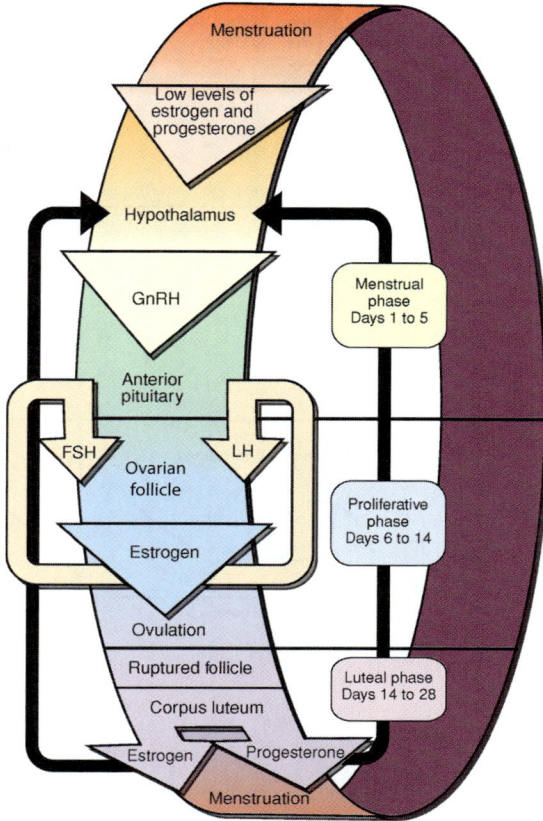

Figure 5-14 Hormonal feedback mechanisms that regulate the female menstrual cycle.

HORMONES RELEASED BY THE GONADS

The gonadal hormones are estrogen, progesterone, and testosterone. Estrogen and progesterone are primarily female hormones; testosterone is primarily a male hormone. These hormones are produced chiefly by the gonads (ovaries and testes) and have important influences on sexual characteristics and the menstrual cycle. Fluctuating levels of estrogen and progesterone stimulate or suppress the hypothalamus or pituitary gland to release or cease releasing their hormones in a complex orchestration of events that regulate the menstrual cycle.

Estrogen

Estrogen, the primary female sex hormone, is present in high levels in women of childbearing age, and is also present in much smaller levels in men. In females, estrogen is responsible for development of the secondary sex characteristics (i.e., breast development, widening of the hips, deposition of fat in the buttocks and mons pubis). It also helps to regulate the menstrual cycle by stimulating proliferation of the endometrial lining in preparation for a pregnancy.

Progesterone

Progesterone also plays a role in regulation of the menstrual cycle. It decreases uterine motility and contractility (caused by estrogen) and prepares the uterus for implantation after fertilization. During pregnancy, progesterone readies the breasts for lactation.

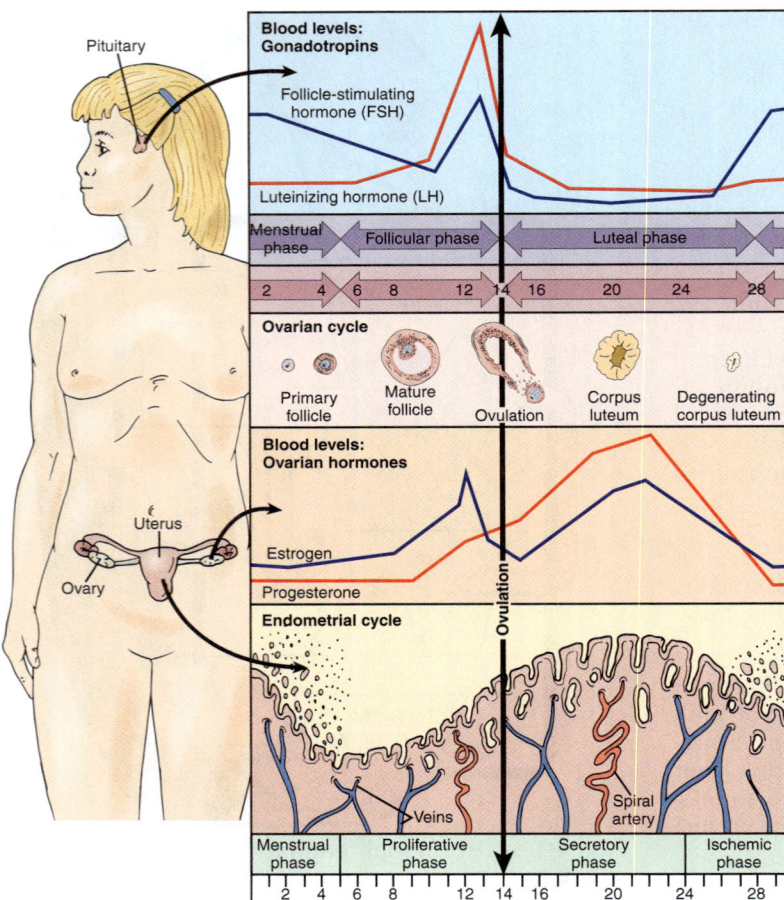

Figure 5-15 The female reproductive cycle. Levels of the hormones secreted from the anterior pituitary are shown relative to one another and throughout the cycle. Changes in the ovarian follicle are depicted. The relative thickness of the endometrium is also shown.

Testosterone

Testosterone, the primary male hormone, is produced by the testes (in men) and the ovaries (in women). Testosterone is responsible for the development of the male genital tract and the secondary sex characteristics (body hair distribution, growth and strength of the long bones, increase in muscle mass, deepening of the voice through enlargement of the vocal cords). In both genders, testosterone enhances the libido, increases energy, boosts immune function, and helps protect against osteoporosis.

HUMAN CHORIONIC GONADOTROPIN, PROSTAGLANDINS, AND RELAXIN

Human chorionic gonadotropin (hCG) is an important hormone during early pregnancy. It is produced by the **trophoblast** (outermost layer of the developing blastocyst) and maintains the ovarian **corpus luteum** (remainder of ovarian follicle after ovulation) by keeping levels of progesterone and estrogen elevated until the placenta has sufficiently developed to assume that function. Human chorionic gonadotropin may also play a role in limiting the maternal immune response to the pregnancy. Serum or urine hCG levels are measured to diagnose pregnancy.

Prostaglandins are unsaturated, oxygenated fatty acids classified as hormones. Prostaglandins are found in many body tissues, occurring in high concentrations in the female reproductive tract. Prostaglandins modulate hormonal activity and have an effect on ovulation, fertility, and cervical mucus viscosity. Premenstrually, the release of prostaglandins in the uterus causes vasoconstriction and muscle contractions that lead to the tissue ischemia and pain associated with premenstrual syndrome (PMS). During pregnancy, prostaglandins are believed to help maintain a reduced placental vascular resistance and most likely are involved in the biochemical process that initiates labor.

Relaxin is a hormone primarily produced by the corpus luteum, although the uterine decidua and the placenta are also believed to produce small amounts. Relaxin may be detected in maternal serum by the time of the first missed menstrual period. Although its role in pregnancy is not fully understood, relaxin aids in the softening and lengthening of the uterine cervix and works on the myometrial smooth muscle to promote uterine relaxation.

 Now Can You—— Discuss key hormones involved in reproduction?

1. Name two gonadotropins and describe their functions?
2. Explain the primary action of human chorionic gonadotropin (hCG)?
3. Identify one action of prostaglandins during pregnancy?

Sexual Maturation

PUBERTY

Puberty is the biological time frame between childhood and adulthood characterized by physical body changes that lead to sexual maturity. During this period, adolescents experience a growth spurt, develop secondary sexual characteristics, and achieve reproductive maturity. The timing of puberty onset and its progress are variable between individuals and are influenced primarily by genetics. However, other factors such as geographical location, exposure to light, nutritional status, and general health all influence the timing of puberty. It is known that the initiation of puberty is triggered by events that lead to the production of gonadotropin-releasing hormone (GnRH) in the hypothalamus. GnRH stimulates the manufacture of follicle-stimulating hormone (FSH) and luteinizing hormone (LH) in the anterior pituitary. The increasing levels of FSH and LH initiate a gonadal response, and this response varies between males and females.

In females, sexual maturation begins with **thelarche**, the appearance of breast buds. Thelarche, which occurs at approximately 9 to 11 years, is the first signal that ovarian function has begun. It is followed by the growth of pubic hair. During thelarche, the "growth spurt," or period of peak height velocity occurs. **Menarche**, the first menstrual period, begins approximately 1 year after the peak height velocity. It usually occurs between the ages of 9 and 15 years; the average age is 12.4 years (Chumlea et al., 2003).

Major hormonal events surrounding menarche involve the secretion of follicle stimulating hormone (FSH) from the pituitary gland. FSH stimulates the ovaries to begin follicular maturation and to produce estrogen. After maturation of an ovum, LH stimulates release of the ovum from the ovary (**ovulation**). Left behind is the **corpus luteum** ("yellow body" that remains in the ovary following ovulation), a structure that produces progesterone.

In males, LH stimulates the Leydig cells in the testicles to mature the testes and begin testosterone production. FSH and LH stimulate sperm production. Increasing levels of estrogen, progesterone, testosterone, and other circulating androgens stimulate the hypothalamus to continue to release GnRH, which perpetuates the cycle. As puberty progresses, the gonads become increasingly sensitive to hormone stimulation and begin to function. Testosterone secretion causes testicular enlargement, which is the first sign of pubertal changes in males.

Development of the secondary sexual characteristics begins around age 11 to 13 and puberty is completed when a young person reaches sexual maturity at approximately 18 to 20 years of age. The time frame from the first stages of puberty to full sexual maturation ranges from 1.5 to 9 years. In females, puberty is generally initiated about 2 years earlier in the life span than in males. Throughout the process of puberty, both genders experience a myriad of physical, psychological, and emotional changes. Alterations in body image and social interactions typically accompany these changes.

FEMALE SECONDARY SEXUAL CHARACTERISTICS

At birth, oocytes are present in the ovary as primary follicles in a state of suspended meiosis. With the onset of puberty, hormonal stimulation prompts the ovaries to secrete small amounts of estrogen. As the process of puberty progresses, estrogen levels rise and menarche occurs. However, estrogen levels at this time are usually insufficient to stimulate ovulation and the menstrual periods are generally unpredictable and irregular. As the gonadotropin cycles continue, the ovaries mature from sustained hormonal stimulation and eventually become capable of follicular maturation with increasing numbers of cycles. Over time, regular cyclic ovulation is established and each menstrual period becomes increasingly more predictable. Once a female reaches a weight of 105 pounds (47.8 kg) and 16% to 23.5% body fat, there is a high correlation with menarche (Garibaldi, 2004).

In addition to the cyclic hormonal changes associated with ovulation, sexual physical changes (secondary sexual characteristics) also occur during puberty. Hormones of the hypothalamic–pituitary–ovarian axis trigger most of the changes that take place in the young woman's body during this time. (Please see the menstrual cycle discussion). Examples of some of the pubertal changes that occur in the female are presented in Table 5-1.

Other female secondary sexual characteristic changes include growth and development of the vagina, uterus, and fallopian tubes, darkening and growth of the skin on the areola, and external genitals and widening of the hips. Appearance of the secondary sexual characteristics precedes menarche. Estrogen is primarily responsible for changes in the breasts although progesterone, thyroxine, cortisol, insulin, and prolactin also affect glandular development. Guidelines of secondary sexual characteristic

Table 5-1 Female Body Changes Associated with Puberty				
Type of Body Change	**Body Change**	**Definition**	**Average Age Initiated**	**Average Age Completed**
Growth spurt	Adolescent growth spurt	Height increase 2.4–4.3 inches (6–11 cm) in 1 year	10	11.8
Secondary	Thelarche	Breast budding	9.8	14.6
	Adrenarche	↑ Adrenal androgen secretion → axillary and pubic hair	10.5	
Primary	Menarche	First menstrual period	12.8	

Figure 5-16 Maturation states in females. *A*, Preadolescent. No pubic hair, just fine body hair similar to hair on abdomen. *B*, Sparse growth of long, downy hair, straight or slightly curled mainly along labia. *C*, Darker, coarser, curlier hair that spreads over pubic symphysis. *D*, Hair is coarse and curly and covers more area. *E*, Adult. Hair may spread over medial surfaces of thighs, but not over abdomen.

development, termed "Tanner stages" measure the predictable stages of pubertal body changes in both genders (Tanner, 1962). A sexual maturity rating concerning development of pubic hair in the female is presented in Figure 5-16.

 Now Can You— **Discuss concepts related to puberty?**

1. Trace the hormonal events associated with the onset of puberty in females?
2. Explain why the first few menstrual periods are often irregular?
3. Identify six female secondary sex characteristics that precede menarche?

The Menstrual Cycle and Reproduction

Menstruation is the periodic discharge of bloody fluid from the vagina that women experience during reproductive years. Menstrual flow begins at puberty and continues for approximately three to four decades. The **menstrual cycle** refers to the changes that occur in the uterus, cervix, and vagina associated with menstruation and during the interval between each menstruation, termed the "intermenstrual period." The average time for a menstrual cycle is 28 to 32 days, although there is considerable variation among women and monthly cycles. Factors such as stress, nutritional status, excessive exercise, fatigue, and illness can alter an individual's cycle intervals and length.

Menstruation and ovulation, key elements in the reproductive cycle, are controlled by positive and negative feedback systems associated with hormones released by the hypothalamus, pituitary, and ovaries. In synchrony, the hormones coordinate the complex biochemical events that result in the monthly menstrual cycle. Regulation of the menstrual cycle involves an overlapping of the uterine (endometrial), hypothalamic-pituitary and ovarian cycles (see Figs. 5-14 and 5-15).

Uterine (Endometrial) Cycle

The uterine, or endometrial, cycle has four phases: menstrual, proliferative, secretory, and ischemic.

MENSTRUAL PHASE

The menstrual phase is the time of vaginal bleeding (approximately days 1 to 6). The onset of menses signals the beginning of the follicular phase of the ovarian cycle. Menstruation is triggered by declining levels of estrogen and progesterone produced by the corpus luteum. The decrease in hormones results in poor endometrial support and constriction of the endometrial blood vessels. These changes lead to a decreased supply of oxygen and nutrients to the endometrium. Disintegration and sloughing of the endometrial tissue occurs. During menstruation, constriction of the endometrial blood vessels limits the likelihood of hemorrhage.

Prostaglandins also play a role in menstruation. The uterus releases prostaglandins that cause contractions of the smooth muscle and decrease the risk of hemorrhage. Prostaglandin-induced uterine contractions often produce **dysmenorrhea** (painful menstruation) in the days surrounding the onset of menstrual flow. Other systemic effects of prostaglandins include headache and nausea. Over-the-counter medications that inhibit prostaglandin synthesis such as nonsteroidal anti-inflammatory agents can be used to control the discomfort associated with dysmenorrhea and premenstrual syndrome.

Menstrual fluid is composed of endometrial tissue, blood, cervical and vaginal secretions, bacteria, mucus, leukocytes, prostaglandins, and other debris. The color of menstrual fluid is dark red, but variable throughout the days of menses. The amount of discharge is typically 30 to 40 mL and the duration of bleeding is 4 to 6 days ± 2 days.

PROLIFERATIVE PHASE

The proliferative phase is the end of menses through ovulation (approximately days 7 to 14). At the beginning of the proliferative phase, the endometrial lining is 1 to 2 mm thick. Circulating estrogen levels are low. Gradually increasing levels of estrogen, enlarging endometrial glands, and the growth of uterine smooth muscle characterize the proliferative phase. Endometrial receptor sites for progesterone are developed during this time. Systemic effects of the increasing amounts of estrogen include an increased secretion of thyroxine-binding globulin (TBG) by the liver, an increase in the breast mammary duct cells, thickening of the vaginal mucosa, and changes in cervical mucus (i.e., increased amount and elasticity) to facilitate sperm penetration at midcycle.

SECRETORY PHASE

The secretory phase is the time of ovulation to the period just prior to menses (approximately days 15 to 26). This phase of the endometrial cycle is characterized by changes induced by increasing amounts of progesterone. Progesterone functions to create a highly vascular secretory endometrium that is suitable for implantation of a fertilized ovum. Glycogen-producing glands secrete endometrial fluid in preparation for a fertilized ovum. At this time, endometrial growth ceases and the number of estrogen and progesterone receptors decrease. Other progesterone effects during the secretory phase include increased glandular growth of the breasts, thinning of the vaginal mucosa, and increased thickness and stickiness of the cervical mucus.

ISCHEMIC PHASE

The ischemic phase is from the end of the secretory phase to the onset of menstruation (approximately days 27 to 28). During the ischemic phase, estrogen and progesterone levels are low and the uterine spiral arteries constrict. The endometrium becomes pale in color due to a limited blood supply and the blood vessels ultimately rupture. Rupture of the endometrial blood vessels leads to the onset of menses (this event marks day 1 of the next cycle) and initiation of the menstrual phase of the cycle.

HYPOTHALAMIC–PITUITARY–OVARIAN CYCLE

The menstrual cycle is controlled by complex interactions between hormones secreted by the hypothalamus, anterior pituitary, and ovaries (see Fig. 5-14). Hormones from the hypothalamic–pituitary–gonadal (ovarian) axis interact with one another and influence the secretion of hormones from other sites. The hypothalamus and anterior pituitary communicate through the hypophyseal portal system (a system of venous capillary blood vessels that supplies blood and endocrine communication between the hypothalamus and pituitary). The major interacting hormones include GnRH (hypothalamus), LH, and FSH (pituitary), and estrogen and progesterone (ovaries).

HYPOTHALAMIC–PITUITARY COMPONENT

The pituitary receives GnRH input from the hypothalamus. GnRH stimulates the secretion of FSH and LH. FSH prompts the ovaries to secrete estrogen and progesterone and these hormones inhibit the continued secretion of hypothalamic GnRH. FSH also induces the proliferation of ovarian granulosa cells. LH stimulates the growth of the ovarian follicles and prompts ovulation and luteinization (formation of the corpus luteum) of the dominant follicle. The corpus luteum produces high levels of progesterone along with small amounts of estrogen.

OVARIAN COMPONENT

The ovarian portion of the hypothalamic–pituitary–ovarian axis occurs in two phases: the follicular phase and the luteal phase. The phases are distinguished by events in the ovarian cycle, especially those related to ovulation.

FOLLICULAR PHASE

Day 1 of the menstrual cycle begins with the onset of bleeding (menstruation). This event marks the beginning of the follicular phase, which lasts about 14 days, but can vary from 7 to 22 days. This variance often accounts for the irregularity in menstrual cycles in some women (Fehring, Schneider, & Raviele, 2006). The follicular phase is characterized by dominance in estrogen, follicle-stimulating hormone (FSH), and leutinizing hormone (LH). (Please refer to the earlier discussion concerning the role of estrogen and the endometrial cycle.)

FSH stimulates the ovary to prepare a mature ovum for release at ovulation. LH stimulates the theca cells of the ovary to produce androgens which convert to estrogen in the granulosa cells of the ovary. Immediately before ovulation, the hypothalamus secretes gonadotropin-releasing hormone (GnRH). This action prompts the anterior pituitary to release LH and FSH. The surge of LH stimulates the release of the ovum and ovulation generally occurs within 10 to 16 hours after the LH surge.

Ovulation signifies the end of the follicular phase of the ovarian follicular cycle. The ovum is capable of fertilization by a sperm cell for approximately 12 to 24 hours after ovulation. The follicle that contained the mature ovum remains in the ovary and becomes the corpus luteum, a structure that plays a major role during the second half, or luteal phase, of the ovarian cycle.

LUTEAL PHASE

The luteal phase of the ovarian cycle begins at ovulation and ends with the onset of menses. When pregnancy is not achieved following ovulation, the corpus luteum dominates over the second half of the menstrual cycle. In the absence of fertilization, the life span of the corpus luteum is 14 days. Thus, the luteal phase of the uterine cycle is predictable in length and lasts for 14 days. The corpus luteum secretes estrogen and progesterone, producing a negative feedback that signals the anterior pituitary gland to decrease production of FSH and LH. As the end of the luteal phase nears (approximately 8 to 10 days), low levels of FSH and LH cause regression of the corpus luteum. Degeneration of the corpus luteum is associated with declining levels of estrogen and progesterone. The resultant low progesterone levels stimulate the hypothalamus to secrete GnRH, while the decreased levels of estrogen and progesterone trigger endometrial sloughing. The corpus albicans ("white body") forms from the remnants of the corpus luteum and eventually disappears.

Body Changes Related to the Menstrual Cycle and Ovulation

Before ovulation, several events occur to indicate that the woman's body is preparing for fertilization of the released ovum. Increased estrogen secretion by the ovaries produces changes in the cervical mucus that assist the sperm in successfully locating the ovum. There is a dramatic increase in the amount and quality of the cervical mucus. It becomes watery and clear, creating a pathway for sperm to readily swim through the cervix. The elasticity (**spinnbarkheit**) of the cervical mucus increases and the woman can assess this change by stretching the mucus between her fingers (Fig. 5-17). Another method of assessment involves stretching the cervical mucus between two glass slides. At the time of ovulation, the cervical mucus can be stretched to 8 to 10 cm or longer. If the mucus is thin, watery, and stretchable the woman is ready to conceive.

There is also an increase in the **ferning** capacity (crystallization) of the cervical mucus (Fig. 5-18). Ferning, an indirect indicator of estrogen production, results from a decrease in the levels of salt and water that interact with glycoproteins in the mucus during midcycle. The clinician assesses for the presence of ferning by placing a sample of cervical mucus on a glass slide, allowing it to air dry and examining it under a microscope for a fernlike pattern.

Figure 5-17 Spinnbarkheit (elasticity).

Physiological changes also accompany ovulation. The basal body temperature (BBT) increases 0.3 to 0.6°C approximately 24 to 48 hours after ovulation and some women experience mittelschmerz (abdominal pain that occurs at the time of ovulation, typically described as a cramping sensation) and midcycle spotting. It is still possible to become pregnant at this point in the menstrual cycle, even when spotting is present.

Natural Cessation of Menses

CLIMACTERIC PHASE

The **climacteric** is a phase characterized by the decline in ovarian function and the associated loss of estrogen and progesterone production.

PERIMENOPAUSAL PHASE

Perimenopause, the time preceding menopause, is the period associated with declining fertility for two reasons: the number of ovarian follicles responsive to gonadotropins is decreased; and the responsive follicles do not develop as quickly as before. Because of these normal changes, many cycles during perimenopause are **anovulatory** (no ova are released from ovary). Anovulatory menstrual cycles are irregular and often variable in the amount of blood flow. Fewer functioning follicles are associated with lower estradiol (estrogen, E_2) levels. Decreased circulating estrogen levels prompt the anterior pituitary to secrete follicle-stimulating hormone (FSH). Elevated serum FSH levels combined with low estradiol levels are usually indicative of perimenopause/menopause.

The peri-/postmenopausal period is characterized by greatly decreased amounts of endogenous estrogen. During this time, estrone (E_1), created from the peripheral conversion of androstenedione, becomes the predominant form of estrogen. A number of physical changes may accompany the estrogen depletion. These include vasomotor instability (hot flashes/flushes/night sweats), atrophy of the urogenital sites (vaginal dryness, urinary disturbances), amenorrhea (cessation of menses), skin changes (hyper/hypopigmentation, decreased sweat and sebaceous gland activity, thinning of the epidermal and dermal skin layers, decrease in hair distribution), musculoskeletal changes (bone thinning and osteoporosis), and psychological changes (anxiety, depression, irritability, libido changes, insomnia).

The hot flashes associated with perimenopause usually occur at night and result from vasodilation associated with decreased estrogen levels. Vaginal atrophy, also related to estrogen deficiency, results in vaginal dryness and increased sensitivity and pain, particularly during sexual intercourse. Atrophy of the urinary tissues may cause urinary incontinence. Alterations in mood, such as depression, mood swings, and tiredness also result from decreased estrogen levels.

A number of long-term effects occur with the diminishing hormone levels during menopause. Decreased estrogen, associated with lower levels of high-density lipids and elevated levels of low-density lipids, increases the risk for cardiovascular disease. As estrogen diminishes, there is a loss in skeletal bone mass, which results in more brittle bones, and leads to the development of osteoporosis and a loss of spinal flexibility.

MENOPAUSE

Menopause simply refers to the last menstrual period.

POSTMENOPAUSAL PHASE

Postmenopause, the time after menopause, is characterized by estrogen production solely by the adrenal glands. Although controversial, menopausal hormone therapy (HT), prescribed on a highly individual basis, may be used to minimize the symptoms and improve quality of life. HRT

Figure 5-18 A fern-like pattern of cervical mucus occurs with high estrogen levels.

can be provided as estrogen only or estrogen and progestin. Estrogen-only HT reduces the symptoms of menopause. However, the continuous administration of estrogen with no progesterone to facilitate shedding of the endometrial lining should be used only after hysterectomy or after menopause is complete to reduce the risk of endometrial cancer. Estrogen-only HT also increases the risk of breast cancer. Estrogen-progestin therapy increases the risk of cardiovascular disease, stroke and deep vein thrombosis by decreasing protective factors.

Selective serotonin reuptake inhibitors may be prescribed for alleviation of symptoms. These medications decrease hot flashes in approximately half of the women who take them, and are also useful in managing the mood changes that occur during perimenopause. Gabapentin (Neurontin) and clonidine (Catapres) reportedly reduce hot flashes, but are associated with side effects including drowsiness, dizziness, and sexual dysfunction. Selective estrogen receptor modulators (SERMs) such as raloxifene (Evista) mimic the effects of estrogen without increasing the risk of breast cancer and endometrial cancer; however, hot flashes are a common side effect of SERMs.

Now Can You— Discuss characteristics of the uterine cycle?

1. Outline the four phases of the uterine cycle and describe the major physiological events that occur during each phase?
2. Trace the hormonal interplays that characterize the hypothalamic–pituitary–ovarian cycle?
3. Describe four physiological changes that occur in the female body around the time of ovulation?
4. Discuss the hormonal events that accompany perimenopause?

Male Reproductive System

EXTERNAL STRUCTURES

The external structures consist of the perineum, penis, and scrotum (Fig. 5-19).

Perineum

The male perineum is a roughly diamond-shaped area that extends from the symphysis pubis anteriorly to the coccyx posteriorly and laterally to the ischial tuberosity.

Penis

The penis is composed of three cylindrical masses of erectile tissue that surround the urethra. The function of the penis is to contain the urethra and serve as the terminal duct for the urinary and reproductive tracts by excreting urine and semen. During sexual arousal, the penis becomes erect to allow penetration for sexual intercourse.

The glans penis is the tip of the penis. It contains many nerve endings, is very sensitive and important in sexual arousal. The urethra is approximately 8 inches (20 cm) long and serves as a passageway for both urine and ejaculated semen. It extends from the urinary bladder to the urethral meatus at the tip of the penis. **Circumcision** is a surgical procedure in which the prepuce (epithelial layer covering the penis; foreskin) is separated from the glans penis and excised. (See Chapter 18 for further discussion.)

Scrotum

The scrotum is a two-compartment pouch covered by skin. It is suspended from the perineum and contains two testes, the epididymis, and the lower portion of the spermatic

Figure 5-19 The male reproductive system shown in a midsagittal section through the pelvic cavity.

cord. The scrotum functions to enclose and protect the two testes. A large component of the protection occurs through temperature regulation of the testes (maintained at about 5 degrees F below core body temperature), which is accomplished by the cartos and cremaster scrotal muscles. These muscles control elevation of the scrotal sac to help maintain the testes in a controlled temperature environment. When exposed to cold, the scrotal muscles contract, causing the testes to be elevated closer to the body to preserve warmth.

INTERNAL STRUCTURES

The internal male reproductive structures include the testes, epididymis, ducts (vas deferens, ejaculatory duct), urethra, spermatic cords, and accessory glands (seminal vesicles, prostate, bulbourethral glands and urethral glands) (Fig. 5-20).

Testicles/Testes

The male testes are considered "essential organs" because they manufacture sperm, which are necessary for reproduction. The two testicles are composed of several lobules, seminiferous tubules, and interstitial cells separated by septa. They are encased in the tunica albuginea capsule. The seminiferous tubules open into a plexus (rete testis) drained by efferent ductules located on the top of the testicle that enters the head of the epididymis. The seminiferous tubules contain spermatogonia, or sperm-generating cells that divide first by the process of mitosis to produce primary spermatocytes (Figs. 5-20 and 5-21).

One testicle is housed in each compartment of the scrotum. The function of the testicle is twofold and includes spermatogenesis and the production and secretion of the male hormone testosterone by the interstitial cells of Leydig.

A & P review   Spermatogenesis

Spermatogenesis, the formation of mature sperm within the seminiferous tubules, is a process that occurs in the following four stages:

1. Spermatogonia, the primary germinal epithelial cells, grow and develop into primary spermatocytes. Spermatogonia and primary spermatocytes both contain 46 chromosomes; these consist of 44 autosomes and the two sex chromosomes, X and Y.
2. The primary spermatocytes divide to form secondary spermatocytes. In this stage no new chromosomes are formed; instead, the pairs only divide. Each secondary spermatocyte contains half the number of autosomes—22—and one secondary spermatocyte contains an X chromosome and the other contains a Y chromosome.
3. Each secondary spermatocyte then undergoes another division to form spermatids.
4. In the final stage, the spermatids undergo a series of structural changes that transform them into mature spermatozoa (sperm), each containing a head, neck, body, and tail. The head houses the nucleus; the tail contains a large amount of adenosine triphosphate (ATP), which provides energy for sperm motility (Dillon, 2007). ◆

Epididymis

There are two epididymi, which are tightly coiled tubes positioned on the top of each testis. The epididymi store maturing sperm cells and convey sperm to the vas deferens. They also secrete seminal fluid and serve as the site where sperm become motile.

Ducts

There are two vas deferens/ductus deferens and two ejaculatory ducts. The vas deferens are two tubes that extend beyond the epididymis through the inguinal canal into the abdomen and over and behind the bladder. They serve as an excretory duct for seminal fluid. The vas deferens also connect the epididymis with the ejaculatory duct. The two ejaculatory ducts serve as the connection between the vas deferens and the seminal vesicle ducts. The ejaculatory ducts pass through the prostate gland and terminate in the urethra.

Urethra

The urethra is a mucus membrane–lined tube that passes from the bladder to the exterior of the body. It joins with the two ejaculatory ducts in the prostate gland. Its length is approximately 7.9 inches (20 cm). In males, the urethra functions in both the urinary and reproductive systems.

Spermatic Cords

The two spermatic cords are fibrous cylinders located in the inguinal canals. They enclose the seminal ducts, blood and lymphatic vessels, and nerves.

Accessory Glands

The accessory glands include the seminal vesicles, the prostate, the bulbourethral glands, and the urethral (Littre's) glands.

The two seminal vesicles are pouches located on the posterior surface of the bladder. They secrete the viscous nutrient-rich component of seminal fluid. This fluid, which accounts for 60% of semen volume, contains alkaline prostaglandin to help neutralize semen pH.

The prostate, located inferiorly to the bladder, is a donut-shaped structure that encircles the urethra. It secretes a thin, milky, alkaline fluid that is rich in zinc, citric acid, acid phosphatase, and calcium. Prostatic fluid helps protect sperm from the acidic environments of the vagina and male urethra and accounts for 30% of the semen volume.

Each of the two bulbourethral glands is a small pea-shaped organ that contains a 1-inch (2.5-cm) long duct leading into the urethra. These glands are located below the prostate gland and they function to secrete fluid to lubricate the end of the penis. This fluid makes up 5% of the semen volume.

The urethral or Littre's glands are multiple glands located along the urethra, especially in the penile section. They secrete mucus that is incorporated into the semen.

Characteristics of Semen and Sperm

Seminal fluid consists of secretions from the testes, the epididymi, the seminal vesicles, the prostate, the bulbourethral glands, and the urethral glands. Seminal fluid is

Figure 5-20 *A*, Midsagittal section of portion of a testis; the epididymis is on the posterior side of the testis. *B*, Cross section through a seminiferous tubule showing development of sperm.

Figure 5-21 Spermatogenesis. The processes of mitosis and meiosis are shown. For each primary spermatocyte that undergoes meiosis, four functional sperm cells are formed. The structure of a mature sperm cell is also shown.

secreted during ejaculation and is slightly alkaline with a pH of about 7.5. The typical amount present in one ejaculate is 2 to 5 mL. There are approximately 120 million sperm cells in each milliliter of ejaculate and, typically, around 40% of the sperm are motile. There are also about 5 million white blood cells in each milliliter of semen along with secretions from the testes, epididymi, seminal vesicles, prostate and bulbourethral glands. The following pathway traces the events from the formation of sperm to the ejaculation of semen:

1. The testes produce sperm that are transported to the epididymis.
2. Sperm and seminal fluid move to the vas deferens.
3. From there the seminal fluid moves to the ejaculatory duct before exiting the body through the urethra.

Sperm are capable of surviving in optimal favorable alkaline conditions for up to 72 hours postejaculation in a woman's body. The average length of time for sperm to locate from the cervix to the fallopian tubes is approximately 5 minutes under favorable conditions.

Male Hormonal Influences

TESTOSTERONE

The testes produce androgens, the male sex hormones. Testosterone is the dominant male hormone. At the time of puberty, testosterone stimulates enlargement of the testes and accessory organs and prompts development of the secondary sex characteristics. The male secondary sex characteristics include changes in body hair (coarse hair on face, chest, and pubic area and sometimes decreased hair on the head), a deepening of the voice, thickened skin, increased upper body musculature and narrow waist, and a thickening and straightening of bone (Shier, Butler, & Lewis, 2003). Testosterone also prompts a linear growth spurt.

Fertility

Male fertility is related to overall sperm number, size, shape, and motility. Decreased fertility is associated with insufficient sperm counts affected by active contact sports; smoking; and tight, constrictive clothing. Decreased fertility is also associated with an autoimmune disorder that results in the manufacture of antibodies to one's own sperm. The presence of varicose veins on the scrotum (varicocele) can cause testicular warming and adversely affect the life span of the sperm. Decreased sperm motility or "slow swimming" caused by an ineffective flagella also affects male fertility.

Age-related Development of the Male Reproductive System

Similar to embryological development in the female, the male genital organs develop in the abdomen of the fetus, but are immature. The testes develop near the kidneys and descend into the scrotum through the inguinal canal after 35 weeks' gestation. Scrotal examination is an important component of the male neonate's physical assessment to ensure that the testes have descended and do not remain in the inguinal canal. **Cryptorchidism** is the condition in which the testes fail to descend; sterility results unless the testes are surgically placed in the scrotum (Scanlon & Sanders, 2003) (See Chapter 18 for further discussion). It is important to locate both testes in a newborn as testicular failure to descend may indicate gonadal malgenesis, which can lead to testicular cancer and fertility issues in young adulthood.

The reproductive functions of the testes begin at the time of puberty. Once critical hormone levels have been reached, the final stages of reproductive system development take place. A gradual decline in hormone production normally occurs during late adulthood. Although the hormonal decline may be associated with a decrease in sexual desire and fertility, most men maintain the ability to reproduce into old age.

 Now Can You— **Discuss aspects of the male reproductive system?**

1. Identify the three external structures of the male reproductive system and describe one function for two of them?
2. Discuss the functions of the testicles, epididymis, vas deferens and prostate gland?
3. Trace the pathway from sperm production to semen ejaculation?
4. Name five male secondary sex characteristics that result from the influence of testosterone?

summary points

◆ Gender is determined at the moment of conception. Identifiable sexual characteristics are apparent in the embryo at 8 weeks of gestation.

◆ Gender maturation is a lengthy process that begins during embryonic development and reaches full maturity during late adolescence.

◆ External structures of the female reproductive system include the mons pubis, labia, clitoris, vestibule, urethral meatus, Skene's and Bartholin's glands, vaginal introitus, hymen and perineum.

◆ Internal structures of the female reproductive system include the ovaries, fallopian tubes, uterus, and vagina.

◆ The female bony pelvis supports and protects the contents of the pelvis and provides a fixed axis for the process of childbirth.

◆ The breasts or mammary glands are considered to be accessory organs of the female reproductive system.

◆ Hormones secreted by the pituitary gland are essential in the regulation of gonadal, thyroid and adrenal function, lactation, body growth, and somatic development.

◆ Menstruation and ovulation are controlled by a complex interplay of positive and negative feedback systems associated with hormones released by the hypothalamus, pituitary, and ovaries.

◆ The male reproductive system consists of the testes, where spermatogonia and male sex hormones are formed; a series of continuous ducts that allow spermatozoa to be transported outside the body; accessory glands that produce secretions to foster sperm nutrition, survival, and transport; and the penis, which functions as the reproductive organ of intercourse.

◆ Testosterone, the dominant male hormone, is responsible for the development of secondary sex characteristics in the male.

review questions

Multiple Choice

1. The perinatal nurse explains to the new nurse that a female fetus has a developed ovary by
A. 8 weeks
B. 10 weeks
C. 12 weeks
D. 16 weeks

2. The perinatal nurse describes to the prenatal class attendees that an incision for a cesarean birth is normally made in the uterine segment known as the:
A. Isthmus
B. Cervix
C. Apex
D. Corpus

3. The perinatal nurse knows that ova are produced and estrogen secreted at the time of:
A. Puberty
B. Birth
C. The climacteric
D. Pregnancy

4. The perinatal nurse teaches the new nurse that the assessment landmark for the fetal presenting part is the:
A. Ischial spines
B. Sacral promontory
C. Sacral alae
D. True pelvis

Fill-in-the-Blank

5. The clinic nurse teaches the new nurse that the fallopian tubes or _____ measure about _____ inches (_____cm) and are vulnerable to infection which can cause _____ and increase the risk of _____ pregnancy.

6. The perinatal nurse knows that uterine circulation is supplied by the _____ and _____ arteries, which are _____ until the uterus expands during pregnancy.

7. The clinic nurse is aware that when a woman is undergoing a Pap test and physical examination, it is not always possible to visualize the _____ glands located on either side of the _____. These glands are responsible for mucus production that _____ the vagina.

True/False

8. The perinatal nurse knows that beginning at the 12th gestational week, a male fetus produces androgens that stimulate growth of the external genitalia.

Select All that Apply

9. The perinatal nurse describes the multiple functions of the uterus as:
A. Providing a safe environment for a growing embryo
B. Providing a passageway for sperm
C. Providing nourishment for the zygote
D. Providing a blood supply for the accessory organs

10. The perinatal nurse knows that the internal urinary system is composed of:
A. Ureters
B. Urethra
C. Vagina
D. Bladder

See Answers to End of Chapter Review Questions on the Electronic Study Guide or DavisPlus.

REFERENCES
Blackburn, S.T. (2003). *Maternal, fetal, and neonatal physiology: A clinical perspective* (2nd ed.). St. Louis: W.B. Saunders.
Bulechek, G., Butcher, H.M., & Dochterman, J. (2008). *Nursing interventions classification (NIC)* (5th ed.). St. Louis, MO: C.V. Mosby.
Caldwell, W., & Moloy, H. (1933). Anatomical variations in the female pelvis and their effect in labor with a suggested classification. *American Journal of Obstetrics and Gynecology, 26*, 479–505.
Chumlea, W.C., Schubert, C.M., Roche, A.F., Kulin, H.E., Lee, P.A., Himes, J.H., & Sun, S.S. (2003). Age at menarche and racial comparisons in U.S. girls. *Pediatrics, 11*(1), 110–113.
Cunningham, F., Leveno, K., Bloom, S., Hauth, J., Gilstrap III, L. & Wenstrom, K. (2005). *Williams Obstetrics* (22nd ed.). New York: McGraw-Hill.
Dillon, P.M. (2007). *Nursing health assessment: A critical thinking, case studies approach* (2nd ed.). Philadelphia: F.A. Davis.
Fehring, R., Schneider, M., & Raviele, K. (2006). Variability in the phases of the menstrual cycle. *Journal of Obstetric, Gynecologic and Neonatal Nursing, 35*(3), 376–384.
Garibaldi, L. (2004). Physiology of puberty. In Nelson, W.E., Behrman, R.E., Kliegman, R.M., & Arvin, A.M. (Eds.). *Nelson textbook of pediatrics* (14th ed., p. 1862). Philadelphia: W.B. Saunders.
Johnson, M., Bulechek, G., Butcher, H., McCloskey Dochterman, J., Maas, M., Moorhead, S., & Swanson, E. (2006). *NANDA, NOC, and NIC Linkages: nursing diagnoses, outcomes, & interventions* (2nd ed.). St. Louis, MO: Mosby Elsevier.
Moorehead, S., Johnson, M., Mass, M., & Swanson, E. (2008) *Nursing outcomes classification (NOC)* (4th ed.). St. Louis, MO: C.V. Mosby.
Moskosky, S., Ed. (1995). *Women's health care nurse practitioner certification review guide.* Potomac, MD: Health Leadership Associates, Inc.
Scanlon, V.C., & Sanders, T. (2007). *Essentials of anatomy and physiology* (5th ed.). Philadelphia: F.A. Davis.
Shier, D., Butler, J., & Lewis, R. (2003). *Hole's essentials of human anatomy and physiology* (8th ed.). New York: McGraw-Hill.
Speroff, L., Glass, R., & Kase, N. (1999). *Clinical gynecology, endocrinology, and infertility* (6th ed.). Baltimore: Lippincott Williams & Wilkins.
Tanner, J.M. (1962). *Growth at adolescence* (2nd ed.). Oxford: Blackwell Scientific.
Venes, D. (2009). *Taber's cyclopedic medical dictionary* (21st ed.). Philadelphia: F.A. Davis.

CONCEPT MAP

Structures of the female reproductive system

At 5 weeks: Begin male/female differentiation in embryo

Structures of the male reproductive system

Internal:
• Ovaries=oogenesis
• Fallopian tubes
• Uterus
  - Corpus
  - Isthmus
  - Cervix
• Vagina
• Ligaments/muscles supporting uterus

External:
• Vulva
  - Labia majora/minora
  - Clitoris
  - Vaginal vestibule
  - Vaginal opening
  - Bartholin's glands
• Mons pubis
• Skene's glands
• Hymen
• Perineum

External:
• Perineum
• Pelvis
• Scrotum

Internal:
• Testes
• Epididymis
• Vas deferens
• Ductus deferens
• Ejaculatory ducts
• Urethra
• Spermatic cords
• Accessory glands

Other

Bony pelvis:
• Supports/protects pelvic contents
• Fixed axis for birth passage

Breasts:
• Nipples/areola
• Montgomery tubercles
• Alveoli/lactiferous ducts

Reproductive Anatomy & Physiology

Types:
• Gynecoid
• Android
• Anthropoid
• Platypelloid

Measurements/ Pelvimetry:
• Pelvic inlet
• Midpelvis
• Pelvic outlet

Hormonal influences on reproduction:
Hypothalamus: releasing factors → gonadotropin releasing hormone; corticotropin releasing hormone; growth hormone releasing factor/ inhibiting factor; thyrotropin releasing hormone; prolactin inhibiting factor
Pituitary: ACTH; prolactin; growth hormone; gonadotropins; oxytocin
Gonadal: estrogen; progesterone; testosterone
In addition: hCG, prostaglandins; relaxin

Puberty

Female   **Male**

Menstrual cycle:
• Begins in puberty
• Changes occur in uterus, cervix and vagina
• Controlled by hormones via positive and negative feedback

Uterine cycle:
• Proliferative phase
• Secretory phase
• Ischemic phase

Hypothalamic-pituitary-ovarian cycle:
• Interaction of GnRH, LH, FSH, estrogen and progesterone that promote:
  - Ovarian follicle growth, ovulation, luteinization
  - Onset of menstruation

• Thelarche
• Menarche
• Hypothalamus/pituitary/ ovarian axis → development of secondary sex characteristics

Physical, psychological & emotional changes

• Reproductive function of testes begins
• Enlargement of testes
• Development of secondary sex characteristics
• Growth spurt
• Sperm production

Now Can You:
• Discuss various aspects of the female and male reproductive systems
• Identify aspects of the bony pelvis and female breast
• Discuss key hormones involved in reproduction
• Discuss concepts related to puberty

Human Sexuality and Fertility

Cherish your human connections: Your relationships with friends and family.

—Barbara Bush

LEARNING TARGETS *At the completion of this chapter, the student will be able to:*

◆ Discuss the nurse's role in providing sexual and reproductive health care.

◆ Identify advantages and disadvantages of barrier and hormonal contraceptive methods, intrauterine devices, and permanent sterilization.

◆ Teach patients how to use various methods of contraception.

◆ Assess a patient for short-term complications after an induced abortion.

◆ Analyze the nurse's role in infertility care.

◆ Differentiate among the various advanced reproductive technologies.

◆ Identify potential alternatives to childbearing for the infertile couple.

---

moving toward evidence-based practice Therapy for Unexplained Infertility

Harrison, E.C., & Taylor, J.S. (2006). IVF therapy for unexplained infertility [Electronic version]. *American Family Physician, 73*(1), 63–66.

The purpose of this review was to determine whether in vitro fertilization (IVF) improves the probability of live births in the context of unexplained infertility, compared to alternative management approaches. Unexplained infertility was defined as failure to conceive after 1 year in couples in whom no abnormalities were found during an infertility work-up. IVF is a process that involves stimulation of the ovaries with gonadotropins, egg retrieval, and fertilization in the laboratory. Pregnancy rates achieved with IVF therapy have been reported to reach 30%.

Alternative management approaches to achieve live births included: (1) expectant management, (2) the administration of clomiphene citrate (Clomid), (3) intrauterine insemination (IUI) with or without controlled ovarian stimulation, and (4) gamete intrafallopian transfer (GIFT).

Of the ten randomized controlled trials (RCT) reviewed, six met the study criteria and were included in the meta-analysis. Significant variations among study outcomes and therapies were found; the live-birth rate per patient was considered to be the outcome of interest.

Data analysis revealed the following: (1) IVF was found to be significantly better than expectant management in two studies; (2) there were no significant differences in live-birth rates among patients who received IVF and those who received intrauterine insemination; and (3) one study reported a greater live-birth rate associated with IVF as compared with GIFT. The use of clomiphene citrate (Clomid) was not compared with other infertility therapies in any of the studies.

The researchers concluded that there were insufficient data to allow for the comparison of IVF with other methods of infertility treatment and recommended larger randomized trials.

It was noted that the cost of a single cycle of IVF reportedly exceeds $10,000.00. Insurance coverage for IVF varies from zero to 100% reimbursement.

Risks associated with infertility therapies include psychological stress (e.g., anxiety and depression), multiple gestations, operative risks, and ovarian hyperstimulation syndrome. Approximately 25% of IVF pregnancies involve multiple gestations, which are frequently associated with maternal–fetal complications.

(continued)

Introduction

Sexuality is a multidimensional concept that encompasses one's sexual nature, activity, and interest. Influenced by ethical, spiritual, cultural, and moral factors, sexuality constitutes an important component of women's health. A central role for nurses involves helping women to understand their sexual health and assist them with reproductive life planning. This chapter explores the nurse's roles in various aspects of reproductive health care and concludes with a brief overview of some of the legal and ethical issues that surround methods of advanced reproductive technology.

Sexuality and Reproductive Health Care

Women's health care is a broad term that encompasses the provision of holistic care to women within the context of their day-to-day lives. This approach to health recognizes that a woman's physical, mental, and spiritual states are interdependent and all affect the present level of wellness. In any therapeutic setting, eliciting the woman's view of her situation, and assessing her needs, values, beliefs, and supports constitute essential components in formulating an appropriate plan of care.

Nurses have an opportunity to work with women in a variety of settings. Teaching about health promotion can take place at community centers, schools, clinics, private offices, and senior centers. The majority of women's health care is delivered outside of the acute care setting. Approaching women's health from a community-based perspective enables nurses to recognize each person's autonomy and provide holistic care that is sensitive to physical, emotional, sociocultural, and situational needs.

Sexuality and its reproductive implications are woven into the fabric of human behavior. Because it is such an emotion-laden aspect of life, people have many concerns, problems, and questions about sex roles, behaviors, inhibitions, education, morality, and related components such as contraception. The reproductive implications of sexual behavior must also be considered. Some people desire pregnancy; others wish to avoid it. Health concerns constitute yet another issue that must be addressed. The rising incidence of sexually transmitted infections, especially HIV/AIDS and herpes virus, has prompted many individuals to modify their sexual practices. Women often ask questions and voice concerns about these issues to the

nurse in the ambulatory care setting. Hence, the nurse may need to assume the role of educator, counselor, or care provider when dealing with sexual and reproductive health matters.

It is essential that nurses who practice in reproductive care settings develop an awareness and understanding of personal feelings, values, and attitudes about sexuality. These insights allow the nurse to provide sensitive, individualized care to women who have their own set of values and beliefs. Nurses must have current, evidence-based information about anatomy and physiology and about topics related to sexuality and reproductive health. Nurses must also be sensitive to the relationship dynamics they may observe when women arrive for care accompanied by their partners.

THE HUMAN SEXUAL RESPONSE

In the 1960s, the research work of Masters and Johnson (1966) helped to define sexuality as a natural component of a healthy human personality. Before that time, human sexuality was often viewed as a negative or nonexistent, sometimes shameful, aspect that needed to be shrouded in secrecy. The work of the two sexuality researchers gave new insights into the physical components of human pleasure during sexual response and orgasm.

Masters and Johnson described four human sexual response phases: excitement, plateau, orgasmic, and resolution. The *excitement phase* is characterized by physiological responses to internal and/or external cues. Women experience vaginal lubrication, breast and pelvic engorgement, and increased heart rate, respiratory rate, and blood pressure. Clitoral and labial tissues become swollen, the nipples become erect, and the vagina becomes distended and elongated. Men experience penile engorgement with an increase in circumference and length (erection) along with scrotal thickening and elevation.

During the *plateau phase*, women experience the most heightened sense of sexual tension. The labia become more congested, the vagina becomes more fully expanded and the uterus rises out of the pelvis in preparation for intercourse. Most women also experience sexual flushing, tachycardia, and hyperventilation. In men, the testicles enlarge and become elevated and the coronal circumference of the penis increases. Both genders experience a generalized muscular tension.

The *orgasmic phase* is characterized by an intense desire for sexual release due to congestion of the blood vessels. Tachycardia, blood pressure, and hyperventilation are intensified. These sensations build until orgasm is reached.

Muscular contractions occur in the man's accessory reproductive organs (vas deferens, seminal vesicles, and ejaculatory duct). There is a relaxation of the bladder sphincter muscles along with contractions of the urethra and perirectal muscles followed by ejaculation as orgasm occurs.

An overall release of muscular tension takes place during the *resolution phase*. Both genders experience a feeling of warmth and relaxation and women may experience a brief refractory period or "rest time" before they are interested in sexual intercourse again. Women are capable of experiencing multiple orgasms.

Masters and Johnson were instrumental in opening the topic of human sexual response for discussion and study in the United States. The media often send the message that sexuality involves only a physical expression such as the act of sexual intercourse. In actuality, human sexuality is a multidimensional phenomenon that touches and permeates many aspects of human behavior.

EXPLORING DIMENSIONS OF SEXUALITY

Sexual Orientations

Even though it constitutes an integral and normal dimension of every human being, sexuality evokes controversy when it involves alternative sexual orientation or sexual expression at either end of the age spectrum. **Heterosexual** sexual orientation is the sexual attraction to or sexual activity with a person of the opposite sex or gender. Heterosexuality is often considered the norm in America, and any other form of sexual expression is viewed as being outside the realm of "normal."

Homosexuality is the sexual attraction to or sexual activity of a person with another individual belonging to the same sex or gender. The term "gay" is often used for homosexual males; "lesbian" is used for females. An estimated 2.3 million women in the United States presently identify themselves as lesbians (Marrazzo, 2004). Although a genetic factor has been linked with male homosexuality, no such etiology has been identified for lesbians (Ridley, 2000). Thus, the origin of this sexual orientation in women remains basically unknown.

Masters and Johnson (1966) refuted the idea that homosexuality is a mental health disorder. Yet lesbians and bisexuals (individuals who are sexually active with others of both sexes) are more likely to report that they experience poor physical and mental health (Mays, Yancey, Cochran, Weber, & Fielding, 2002). Although the exact etiology of diminished health status among this population is not clear, one factor may relate to homosexual/bisexual women's hesitancy in seeking health care. The mental and physical discomforts associated with seeking medical attention may translate into a failure to obtain timely professional help for health concerns or illnesses. Some lesbians may be reluctant to disclose their sexual orientation to their health care provider owing to fears related to hostility, inadequate health care, or breach of confidentiality. Also, in many health care settings, patient heterosexuality is assumed and interview questions are structured toward a heterosexual orientation.

Lesbians who decide to bear a child often must undergo a number of medical procedures in order to conceive. In general, lesbian women who choose to have children are firmly committed to their decision, for they must work

harder at achieving conception than other women. Significant health issues also exist for this population. Women who are lesbians are more at risk for breast cancer due to their lower rates of breastfeeding. They are also at risk for sexually transmitted infections (including HIV) and cervical cancer. However, woman-to-woman transmission of sexually transmitted infections is much lower than in heterosexual relationships. Since not all gynecological cancers are related to sexual activity, lesbian women who have never had children may be at an increased risk for endometrial and ovarian cancer. Further, their risk for other cancers (e.g., lung and colon) and heart disease is not different from that of heterosexual women. It is essential that health care providers give correct advice and conduct appropriate cancer and other disease screening for these women. The nurse should develop an approach that does not assume that all patients are heterosexual (Martinez, 2007; Stevens & Hall, 2001). As is true with any group, homosexual women deserve to have their health care concerns addressed by compassionate, nonjudgmental health care providers who are knowledgeable about the health care needs of women with alternative sexual preferences.

A Nursing Framework for Promoting Women's Sexual and Reproductive Health

Nurses who work with women in reproductive care settings must understand what is meant by healthy sexual function before they can begin to recognize and understand how a behavior becomes dysfunctional. A newer vision of sexuality in women (Basson, 2002; Katz, 2007) takes into account relationships for women by including emotional intimacy, sexual stimuli, and relationship satisfaction as a model of sexual response. Thus, women's sexual response is far more complex and complicated than the achievement of an orgasm with intercourse. Sexuality for women encompasses much more than the physical dimension of the sex act.

Sexual dysfunction for women is defined as any sexual situation that causes distress for the woman herself. If the woman is comfortable with a situation, there is no dysfunction. If she is distressed by any physical, emotional, or relationship aspect of her sexuality, she may be experiencing a dysfunction (Hicks, 2004). Dysfunction can be manifested in the form of pain, arousal disorder, orgasmic disorder, or desire disorder (American Psychiatric Association [APA], 2000).

ASSESSMENT

A first step in the sexual and reproductive health assessment involves the establishment of a trusting relationship where the patient feels safe asking questions and sharing concerns. Discussion of sexual issues can be embarrassing for women. Nurses need to be aware of their own sexual biases and beliefs and educate themselves about the many aspects of sexuality. When assessing women for sexual concerns, it is important not to make assumptions about partner preferences or sexual activity. Misguided assumptions can bring an abrupt ending to any therapeutic communications. For example, speaking with a woman about contraceptive choices may halt further dialogue with the patient who is lesbian and has sexual concerns unrelated to a heterosexual relationship (Martinez, 2007).

When working with very young patients, the nurse must avoid communicating personal views that adolescent sexual behavior is wrong or shameful. Regardless of involvement in sexual activity, teenagers need a reliable source of education and information. They must first feel accepted before they can ask questions and share concerns about sexuality and sexual behavior.

Assessing women for current or past problems that may interfere with or contraindicate pregnancy or the use of certain types of **contraception** (products that prevent pregnancy) is an important nursing role in reproductive health care. For example, women with chronic health problems such as diabetes, stroke, multiple sclerosis, cancer, or pain may be taking medications that are contraindicated with certain contraceptives or are associated with fetal anomalies (Table 6-1). Individualized counseling, guidance, and reliable information helps empower them to make informed, realistic choices about reproductive planning. Other chronic conditions, including endometriosis and polycystic ovarian disease, may interfere with fertility and create a sense of powerlessness in those who desire pregnancy. Nurses are in a unique position to listen generously to these women, make appropriate referrals, and assist them in resolving their grief and feelings of loss (Katz, 2007; Martinez, 2007).

Women also need to be counseled about the ideal age for childbearing and the implications of delaying pregnancy too long. Those who have not conceived by the mid- to late 30s may remain childless and burdened with guilt. Outside pressures exerted by cultural influences and family expectations often compound the feelings of remorse. Providing all women with current, factual information about the natural aging process and its influence on fertility empowers women of all ages to make informed decisions that best suit their needs.

Obtaining the Sexual History

The sexual history elicits information concerning prior treatment for sexually transmitted infections (STIs), pain with intercourse (**dyspareunia**), postcoital spotting or bleeding, and frequency of intercourse. Women who have intercourse more frequently and on a regular basis are more likely to become pregnant. The probability for pregnancy with each unprotected intercourse is about 20% (Nelson & Marshall, 2004). An important component of holistic reproductive care centers on helping women to understand their body's natural functioning in relation to the menstrual cycle, so that they can problem-solve about the timing of intercourse to achieve pregnancy, if desired.

The nurse also inquires about the number of past sexual partners. This information is useful in developing an estimate of the patient's risk for STIs and guides the nurse in providing appropriate education about safe sex practices. It is estimated that 4 out of 10 Americans between 18 and 59 years of age have had five or more partners (Haffner & Stayton, 2004). Since the risk of contracting a sexually transmitted infection increases with

each sexual partner, this information is very important for women whose reproductive life plan includes future pregnancy. Sexual health promotion includes providing correct information about the implications of multiple sexual partners; this information empowers women to make knowledgeable, informed choices. Depending on the situation and purpose of the visit, other appropriate components of the patient assessment may include a physical examination and diagnostic testing.

 Now Can You— Discuss the nurse's role in reproductive health care?

1. Explain why nurses who work in a reproductive health care setting must be comfortable with their own sexuality?
2. Develop six questions that will assist with taking a patient's sexual history?
3. Analyze the nurse's role in the reproductive health assessment?

NURSING DIAGNOSES FOR PATIENTS SEEKING CONTRACEPTIVE CARE

Depending on the purpose of the visit and analysis of the assessment findings, a number of nursing diagnoses may be appropriate. For women seeking contraception, diagnoses may include decisional conflict regarding choice of birth control because of a health concern, contraceptive alternatives, or the partner's willingness to agree on the contraceptive method. Other possible nursing diagnoses are listed in Box 6-1.

PLANNING AND IMPLEMENTATION OF CARE

Regardless of the patient's age and contraceptive method selected, the nurse must first seek the woman's confirmation that she truly wants contraception. Birth control is always an individual choice. Feelings of helplessness and manipulation may result when the woman believes that someone else has decided what is "best" for her or coerces her into contraceptive use.

One of the primary goals during the contraceptive care visit is to determine and provide the contraceptive method of "best fit" for the woman or couple. Obtaining the medical, social, and cultural history helps to safeguard the

---

Box 6-1 Possible Nursing Diagnoses for Reproductive Care

Ineffective Sexuality patterns related to fear of pregnancy

Knowledge Deficit related to new use of the contraceptive method of choice

Effective Therapeutic Management related to birth control method of choice

Risk for Spiritual Distress related to discrepancy between religious or cultural beliefs and choice of contraception

Risk for Infection related to use of contraceptive method or unprotected sexual intercourse

Broken skin or mucous membrane after surgery or intrauterine device (IUD) insertion

Fear related to contraceptive method side effects

Table 6-1 Drugs that Adversely Affect the Female Reproductive System

Drug Class	Drug	Possible Adverse Reactions
Androgens	Danazol	Vaginitis, with itching, dryness, burning, or bleeding; amenorrhea
	Fluoxymesterone, methyltestosterone, testosterone	Amenorrhea and other menstrual irregularities; virilization, including clitoral enlargement
Antidepressants	Tricyclic antidepressants	Changed libido, menstrual irregularity
	Selective serotonin reuptake inhibitors	Decreased libido, anorgasmia
Antihypertensives	Clonidine, reserpine	Decreased libido
	Methyldopa	Decreased libido, amenorrhea
Antipsychotics	Chlorpromazine, perphenazine, prochlorperazine, thioridazine, trifluoperazine, haloperidol	Inhibition of ovulation (chlorpromazine only), menstrual irregularities, amenorrhea, change in libido
Beta blockers	Atenolol, labetalol hydrochloride, nadolol, propanolol hydrochloride, metoprolol	Decreased libido
Cardiac glycosides	Digoxin	Changes in cellular layer of vaginal walls in postmenopausal women
Corticosteroids	Dexamethasone, hydrocortisone, prednisone	Amenorrhea and menstrual irregularities
Cytotoxics	Busulfan	Amenorrhea with menopausal symptoms in premenopausal women, ovarian suppression, ovarian fibrosis and atrophy
	Chlorambucil	Amenorrhea
	Cyclophosphamide	Gonadal suppression (possibly irreversible), amenorrhea, ovarian fibrosis
	Methotrexate	Menstrual dysfunction, infertility
	Tamoxifen	Vaginal discharge or bleeding, menstrual irregularities, pruritus vulvae (intense itching of the female external genitalia)
	Thiotepa	Amenorrhea
Estrogens	Conjugated estrogens, esterified estrogens, estradiol, estrone, ethinyl estradiol	Altered menstrual flow, dysmenorrhea, amenorrhea, cervical erosion or abnormal secretions, enlargement of uterine fibromas, vaginal candidiasis
	Dienestrol	Vaginal discharge, uterine bleeding with excessive use
Progestins	Medroxyprogesterone acetate, norethindrone, norgestrel, progesterone	Breakthrough bleeding, dysmenorrhea, amenorrhea, cervical erosion, and abnormal secretions
Thyroid hormones	Levothyroxine, sodium, thyroid USP, and others	Menstrual irregularities with excessive doses
Miscellaneous	Lithium carbonate	Decreased libido
	L-tryptophan	Decreased libido
	Spironolactone	Menstrual irregularities, amenorrhea, possible polycystic ovarian syndrome

Source: Dillon, P.M. (2007). *Nursing health assessment. Clinical pocket guide* (pp. 234–235). Philadelphia: F.A. Davis. Reprinted with permission.

patient's health and guide discussion of the contraceptive choices available to her. Patients often come for care with a specific birth control method in mind. However, it is essential that the nurse explore the woman's knowledge and understanding of contraceptive choices, her motiva-

tions for using a method, and her level of commitment to use the method consistently. On occasion, the desired contraceptive method is contraindicated or associated with side effects that outweigh the personal benefits. Open, honest discussion where appropriate information can be provided in a nonthreatening environment empowers the patient to make an informed choice of a birth control method that is best suited to her lifestyle (Fig. 6-1).

 Across Care Settings: **Enhancing contraceptive decision making**

The choice of a contraceptive method usually rests with the individual, although certain types of birth control may not be the best fit for special populations. Methods that require planning ahead, visiting a restroom for insertion, or are considered "messy" may not be the best choice for adolescents. Combination hormonal methods may be contraindicated in women with a history of breast cancer or diabetes, and these patients need assistance in finding another method that safely suits their lifestyle and health needs. An essential nursing role centers on obtaining a comprehensive history and educating patients about options, special considerations, and side effects. Often the nurse enlists the assistance of other health professionals such as health educators, social workers, translators, and home health workers in teaching about contraception and in managing appropriate follow-up care.

EVALUATION

When obtaining contraception is the purpose of the reproductive health visit, an immediate evaluation may take place at the conclusion of the patient encounter. This evaluation centers on mutually agreed upon outcomes that reflect the patient's understanding of, and comfort level with, the chosen method. Examples of possible outcomes are listed below.

The patient:

- Voices understanding about the selected contraceptive method.
- Voices an understanding of all information necessary to provide informed consent.
- Voices a comfort level with use of the contraceptive method selected.

Intermediate and long-term evaluation of outcomes is especially important in the area of contraceptive care because patients who discontinue use of a birth control

method are at risk for pregnancy. Ideally, patients should be reassessed within a few weeks after initiating a new method. At this time, appropriate outcomes may include the following.

The patient:

- Has used the contraceptive method correctly and consistently.
- Has experienced no adverse side effects from use of the contraceptive method.
- Voices continued satisfaction with the selected contraceptive method.
- Consistently uses the contraceptive method without pregnancy for the following year.

Toward Achieving the National Goals for Reproductive Life Planning

The *Healthy People 2010* national initiative includes a number of goals that directly address reproductive health (Box 6-2). Individuals and couples who seek assistance with this aspect of their lives may need counseling about fertility and methods of contraception. Seeking guidance and making decisions about contraception are prompted by a number of influences but generally center on a desire to take control over one's reproductive life.

Nurses can be instrumental in helping the nation to achieve the objectives by assisting women who want to practice safe sex and providing effective contraception when they do not desire to be pregnant. Women of all ages are capable of responsible sexual behavior when given enough education, motivation, and opportunity. One of the challenges for nurses in the community concerns poor women who are unable to afford contraception as well as those with fertility problems who cannot afford special treatments to achieve pregnancy. Nurses must advocate for all women to ensure that reproductive care is available to all persons, regardless of socioeconomic status.

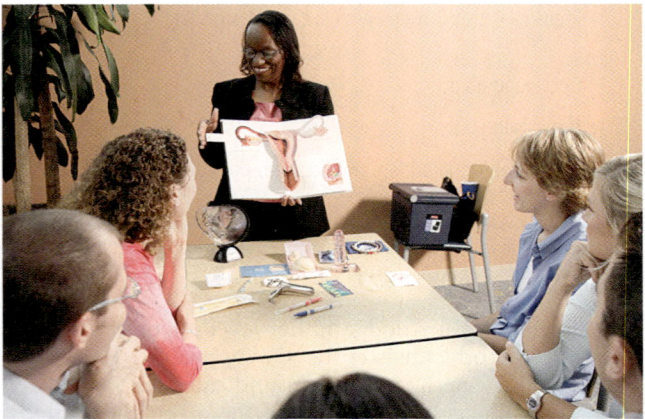

Figure 6-1 Teaching about contraception is an essential component of reproductive health care.

Box 6-2 *Healthy People 2010* **National Goals Related to Reproductive Life Planning**

Several of the National Health Goals are related to reproductive life planning. These include the following:

- Reduce the proportion of women experiencing pregnancy despite use of a reversible contraceptive method from a baseline of 13% to a target of 7%.
- Increase the proportion of pregnancies that are intended from a baseline of 51% to a target of 70%.
- Decrease the proportion of births occurring within 24 months of a previous birth from a baseline of 11% to a target of 6%.
- Increase the proportion of females at risk for unintended pregnancy (and their partners) who use contraception from a baseline of 93% to a target of 100%.
- Increase the number of health care providers who provide emergency contraception.
- Increase male involvement in pregnancy prevention and family planning efforts (new goal; baseline to be determined).

Source: Department of Health and Human Services (DHHS). (2000). *Healthy People 2010.* Washington, DC: DHHS.

Although the rate of unintended pregnancies in the United States has declined, the rate of unintentional pregnancy remains highest among young, less educated women with low income (American Medical Women's Association, 2005). These individuals, who may be less likely to afford birth control or reach a health care clinic, must be a major focus for education and support from nurses in the community. All women deserve holistic health care along with culturally, educationally, and developmentally appropriate information to empower them to make realistic decisions about reproductive life planning.

Providing Contraceptive Care: Methods of Contraception

MEDICATION-FREE CONTRACEPTION

- *Natural Family Planning* (NFP) is a contraceptive method that involves identifying the fertile time period and avoiding intercourse during that time every cycle. It is the only method of contraception acceptable to the Roman Catholic Church.
- *Fertility Awareness Methods* (FAMs) identify the fertile time during the cycle and use abstinence or other contraceptive methods during the fertile periods. These methods require motivation and considerable counseling to be used effectively. They may interfere with sexual spontaneity and require several months of symptom/cycle charting before they may be used effectively.

Effectiveness

The effectiveness in preventing pregnancy depends on the exact method used, but it is generally around 75% effective.

Optimizing Outcomes— When teaching about NFP and FAMs of contraception

The patient and her partner need to be fully committed to use these methods successfully. There are several variations: (1) the calendar, or rhythm method in which the fertile days are calculated; (2) the standard days method in which color-coded strung beads are used to track infertile days; (3) the cervical mucus method (also called the "ovulation detection method" or the "Billings method") where the changes in cervical mucus are used to track fertile periods; (4) the basal body temperature (BBT) method in which body temperature changes are used to detect the fertile period (Fig. 6-2; Box 6-3); and the symptothermal method that combines the BBT and cervical mucus methods and involves recording various symptoms such as changes in cervical mucus, mittelschmerz (abdominal pain at midcycle), abdominal bloating, and the BBT to recognize signs of ovulation (Hatcher et al., 2005). The woman needs to realize that stress or illness can affect her cycle and cause a variation in the fertile days. These methods are not best suited for adolescents or couples who would be devastated by an unplanned pregnancy. Since the "natural" methods identify fertile periods, couples who are attempting to conceive may also wish to use them.

Ovulation predictor kits detect the surge in luteinizing hormone (LH) that occurs 24–36 hours before ovulation.

The kits vary in price and procedure but most are similar to home pregnancy tests and are performed on the woman's urine. Intercourse can then be timed to avoid or achieve pregnancy.

COITUS INTERRUPTUS

Coitus interruptus or the "withdrawal method" involves the man withdrawing his penis from the vagina before ejaculation. However, ejaculation may occur before withdrawal is complete and spermatozoa may be present in the preejaculation fluid. Men with unpredictable or premature ejaculation have difficulty using this method successfully.

Effectiveness

The typical effectiveness rate for this method is about 71%.

LACTATIONAL AMENORRHEA METHOD (BREASTFEEDING)

Breastfeeding can be a form of contraception, although it is used more effectively in underdeveloped countries where mothers breastfeed their infants exclusively. Some lactating mothers may ovulate but not menstruate. It is difficult to determine when fertility is restored. This

Figure 6-2 A basal body temperature chart.

Box 6-3 Basal Body Temperature as an Indicator of Ovulation

During the preovulatory phase, the basal temperature is usually below 98°F (36.7°C). As ovulation approaches, estrogen production increases. At its peak, estrogen may cause a slight drop, then a rise, in the basal temperature. Before ovulation, a surge in luteinizing hormone (LH) stimulates the production of progesterone. The LH surge causes a 0.5°F–1°F (0.3°C–0.6°C) rise in the basal temperature. These changes in the basal temperature create the biphasic pattern consistent with ovulation. Progesterone, a thermogenic, or heat-producing hormone, maintains the temperature increase during the second half of the menstrual cycle. Although the temperature elevation does not predict the exact day of ovulation, it does provide evidence of ovulation about one day after it has occurred. Release of the ovum probably occurs 24–36 hours before the first temperature elevation.

method works best when the mother exclusively breast-feeds, has had no menstrual period since giving birth, and whose infant is younger than 6 months of age.

Effectiveness

When the above conditions are met, the effectiveness rate for this method is about 98% (Hatcher et al., 2005).

ABSTINENCE

Abstinence is the only contraceptive method with a 100% effectiveness rate. If a couple chooses to be **abstinent** (refrain from vaginal intercourse), intimacy and sexuality may be expressed in many other ways. Abstinence requires commitment and self-control, but success with this method can lead to increased self-esteem and enhanced communication about emotions and feelings. Abstinence can help adolescents learn negotiation skills (Hatcher et al., 2005).

BARRIER METHODS

Barrier methods are relatively inexpensive and some types can be used more than once. Although less effective than certain other forms of contraception, barrier methods have gained in popularity as a protective measure against the spread of STIs. If the woman is under 30 years of age, uses alcohol or recreational drugs, or has intercourse three or more times weekly, barrier methods are usually not as effective because of a decreased likelihood to use them consistently (Cates & Stewart, 2004).

Many women dislike barrier methods because they must be inserted or applied before intercourse. Most require a water-based lubricant and these should never be used with an oil-based lubricant (i.e., baby oil, petroleum jelly, vegetable oil) or vaginal yeast cream as these products cause latex deterioration. Barrier methods have few side effects, although latex allergy may lead to life-threatening anaphylaxis. There is evidence that consistent use of latex condoms reduces the rate of HIV transmission, and both condoms and diaphragms can reduce the risk of cervical STIs (Hatcher et al., 2005). Each of the barrier methods must be applied or inserted with clean hands. The key to success with these contraceptives is consistent and correct use, and the nurse must ensure that women know how to use their barrier method correctly and that they are satisfied with their choice.

Diaphragm

The **diaphragm** is a latex dome-shaped barrier device with a spring rim that resembles half a tennis ball. It is filled with spermicide and inserted up into the vagina to cover the cervix. Diaphragms are available in several sizes and types and must be fitted by a trained health care professional.

Use of the diaphragm requires some planning ahead, so this method may not be the best choice for adolescents. The diaphragm is inserted by the woman using her fingers or an inserter up to 6 hours before intercourse, and it must be filled with a spermicide applied inside and along the rim before insertion (Fig. 6-3). The diaphragm must remain in place for 6 hours after intercourse. If intercourse occurs again before 6 hours have elapsed, the diaphragm should be left undisturbed and another applicator-full of spermicide should be inserted into the vagina. The diaphragm should remain in place for 6 hours after the last act of intercourse. To ensure continued protection, the

Figure 6-3 Diaphragm insertion.

diaphragm should be replaced every 2 years, and it may need to be refitted after weight loss or weight gain, term birth or second trimester abortion (Hatcher et al., 2005).

SIDE EFFECTS. Other than occasional allergic reactions to the diaphragm or spermicide, there are no side effects from a well-fitted device. There is an increased risk of urinary tract infections due to pressure of the diaphragm against the urethra, which may interfere with complete emptying of the bladder. Thus, women with a history of frequent urinary tract infections (UTIs) should avoid this method. The diaphragm should not be used during menses due to the risk of **toxic shock syndrome** (TSS), a rare, sometimes fatal disease caused by toxins produced by certain strains of the bacterium *Staphylococcus aureus*. Women with pelvic relaxation syndrome or a large cystocele are not suitable candidates for the diaphragm.

EFFECTIVENESS. The effectiveness in preventing pregnancy for typical use is 84% (Bachmann, 2007). For this reason, the diaphragm may not be the best choice for a woman who would consider pregnancy a disaster in her life or for a woman who feels uncomfortable touching her genital area. Since it is made of latex, the diaphragm is contraindicated in women with latex allergies.

Optimizing Outcomes— **When teaching patients about use of the diaphragm**

The diaphragm must be in the correct position for it to be comfortable and work effectively as a contraceptive. The patient should practice insertion and removal of the diaphragm before leaving the clinic, and be instructed to return with it in place for a recheck of proper fit 1 week later. Before each use, the diaphragm is carefully inspected for tears, holes, or damage. After removal, the device is cleaned with mild soap and water, dried thoroughly, and stored in its case in a cool place. Oil-based vaginal medications or lubricants should never be used with the diaphragm (Hatcher et al., 2005).

Cervical Cap

The **cervical cap** is a thimble-shaped latex device that fits firmly around the base of the cervix close to the junction of the cervix and vaginal fornices (Hatcher et al., 2005, Fig. 6-4). The device has a pliable rim and is available in

Figure 6-4 Cervical cap insertion.

four sizes. It is somewhat more difficult to use than the diaphragm because it must be placed exactly over the cervix where it is held in place by suction. The seal provides a physical barrier to sperm and the spermicide placed inside the cap provides a chemical barrier. Women who choose the cervical cap should practice insertion and removal after the fitting and return in 1 week with the cap inserted to check for proper placement.

Nursing Insight— *When counseling patients about the cervical cap*

Certain women are not suitable candidates for the cervical cap. Patients who have a history of toxic shock syndrome, pelvic inflammatory disease (PID), cervicitis, papillomavirus infection, a previous abnormal Pap smear or cervical cancer, and undiagnosed vaginal bleeding should choose another contraceptive method. Also, women who have an abnormally short or long cervix may not be able to use a cervical cap satisfactorily.

SIDE EFFECTS. There is evidence that the cervical cap can cause cervical irritation and erosion and it is not recommended for women who are at high risk for HIV (Hatcher et al., 2005). Because the device is made of latex, it is contraindicated in women with latex allergies. Since the cervical cap is associated with a high failure rate, women who choose this method should also be given emergency contraception pills.

EFFECTIVENESS. With typical use, the FemCap cervical cap is about 74% effective in preventing pregnancy (Trussell, 2004), so it may not be the best choice for the woman who would consider a pregnancy to be a disaster in her life. It is not as effective for contraception in women who have had a pregnancy (Bachmann, 2007). Since proper use of the cervical cap requires planning ahead and strong motivation, it may not be the best contraceptive method for adolescents.

Optimizing Outcomes— **When teaching patients about use of the cervical cap**

Before insertion, approximately one-third of the cap is filled with spermicide. Taking care not to spill the spermicide, the woman inserts the cap into the vagina and places it

directly over the cervix. The woman is taught to use her finger to trace around the rim of the cap to make certain the entire cervix is covered. The cervical cap can be inserted up to 6 hours before intercourse and should remain in place for 6 hours after the last intercourse. No additional spermicide is necessary with repeated intercourse. The cap should never remain in place longer than 48 hours and it should never be used during menses or when a vaginal infection is present. To remove the cap, the woman pushes against the rim with her finger to dislodge it from the cervix, gently hooks her finger over the rim and removes it. The cap is then washed with mild soap and water. The cap should be dried thoroughly and stored in a cool, dry place. Oil-based vaginal medications or lubricants should never be used with the cervical cap (Hatcher et al., 2005).

Be sure to— **Inquire about latex allergy**

Before dispensing diaphragms, cervical caps, or male condoms, ask all patients about a personal or partner history of allergy to latex. Use of latex contraceptive devices is contraindicated in patients with latex sensitivity.

Condoms

Condoms are generally considered to be a male contraceptive device although the female condom (vaginal sheath) is also available. Male condoms may be made of latex rubber, polyurethane, or natural membranes. Latex male condoms are widely recognized for their role in preventing HIV infection and sexually transmitted infections (STIs). Natural skin condoms do not offer protection against HIV and STIs because they contain small pores that may permit the passage of viruses including HIV, hepatitis B, and herpes simplex. Although previous recommendations included combining condom use with the spermicide nonoxynol-9, recent data suggest that the spermicidal coating does not provide additional protection from pregnancy or STIs (Nelson & Le, 2007). Also, frequent use of condoms coated with nonoxynol-9 may increase the transmission of HIV and can cause genital lesions (Centers for Disease Control and Prevention [CDC], 2007; Warner, Hatcher, & Steiner, 2004). Condoms are non-reusable and act as a mechanical barrier between the female and male genitalia.

MALE CONDOMS. Male condoms are one of the oldest known methods of contraception. When used correctly, male condoms are placed over the erect penis before any genital, oral, or anal contact. Condoms are inexpensive, require no prescription, and are available in a variety sizes, shapes, and colors. To prevent pregnancy and the spread of STIs, they must be used correctly at every act of intercourse.

SIDE EFFECTS. Condoms may cause an anaphylactic reaction in patients who are allergic to latex. Individuals with latex allergies must choose condoms made of other materials.

EFFECTIVENESS. With typical use, male condoms are about 85% effective in preventing pregnancy.

Optimizing Outcomes— When teaching patients about use of the male condom

It is important to choose and use the correct size of condom. The condom is rolled onto the erect penis and should fit snugly. The reservoir tip should be left unobstructed or extra space at the end (of a condom with no reservoir tip) should be provided for collection of the semen. Care must be taken not to tear the condom or spill its contents during removal. When possible, patients should practice placing a condom on a penile model to enhance understanding of the proper technique. Immediately after intercourse, the man should hold the condom at the base of the penis and withdraw the penis while still erect, then check the condom for the presence of tears after removal. Expiration dates should be checked often and out-of-date condoms discarded. Condoms should always be stored in a cool, dry place and latex condoms only used with water-based lubricants (Nelson & Le, 2007).

FEMALE CONDOMS. Made of polyurethane in a "one size fits all," the female condom or vaginal sheath (Fig. 6-5) is less widely used than the male condom. The female condom resembles a sheath with a ring on each end: the closed end is inserted into the vagina and anchored around the cervix; the open end is placed at the vaginal introitus. Although no prescription is needed, female condoms are often difficult to find, and they are more expensive than male condoms. Because they contain no latex, female condoms are safe for use in individuals with latex allergies.

Optimizing Outcomes— When teaching patients about use of the female condom

Female condoms cannot be used at the same time as male condoms. The man must carefully direct his penis into the condom to keep from inserting it between the condom and the vaginal wall. The female condom can be used during oral sex. Some individuals complain that female condoms generate "noise" during intercourse, but lubricant seems to help alleviate this problem.

Figure 6-5 Insertion of a female condom.

Spermicides

Spermicides are available in the form of gels, creams, films, and suppositories. All are inserted into the vagina or used with diaphragms or cervical caps. Spermicidal condoms are no longer recommended for use. Spermicides act as chemical barriers that cause death of the spermatozoa before they can enter the cervix. Although spermicides can be messy, the lubrication afforded by the spermicide-based methods may improve sexual satisfaction for both partners.

Women who are at risk for HIV should not use spermicides as their only method of birth control (Hatcher et al., 2005). Since spermicidal suppositories and films require 15 minutes to become effective, women who feel they cannot comply with this time constraint may wish to use a spermicidal foam, cream, or gel instead. Because of the low effectiveness rates associated with spermicides, the woman who believes that pregnancy would be personally disastrous may wish to choose another contraceptive method.

SIDE EFFECTS. Spermicides should not be used in women with acute cervicitis because of the potential for further cervical irritation. Rarely, topical irritation may develop from contact with spermicides. When this occurs, the product should be discontinued and another contraceptive method selected.

EFFECTIVENESS. The typical use effectiveness of spermicides in preventing pregnancy is 71%.

Optimizing Outcomes— When teaching patients about the use of spermicides

The woman should wash her hands before inserting any spermicide. Spermicides are most effective when used with a diaphragm or cervical cap. Most contraceptive films and suppositories require a period of 15 minutes to elapse after insertion to become effective and they should be inserted no longer than one hour before intercourse. The spermicide should be inserted deep into the vagina so that it makes contact with the cervix. Although douching is never recommended, it should be avoided for 6 hours after intercourse to avoid washing the spermicide away (Hatcher et al., 2004). Douching in and of itself is not a reliable form of birth control.

Contraceptive Sponge

The contraceptive sponge was recently returned to the U.S. market. It is a soft, round disposable polyurethane device that fits over the cervix (one size fits all). The sponge is permeated with the spermicide nonoxynol-9. One side is concave to enhance fit over the cervix; the other side contains a woven polyester loop to facilitate removal.

SIDE EFFECTS. The contraceptive sponge is contraindicated in women who are allergic to the spermicide nonoxynol-9. The sponge should not be left in place for more than 30 hours (which includes the 6-hour waiting period after the last act of intercourse) due to the risk of toxic shock syndrome. It should not be used during menstruation or immediately after abortion or childbirth or if a woman has a history of toxic shock syndrome.

EFFECTIVENESS. The typical use effectiveness of the contraceptive sponge in preventing pregnancy is 84% to 87%.

Optimizing Outcomes— When teaching patients about use of the contraceptive sponge

The patient should wash her hands before inserting the sponge. The sponge is moistened thoroughly with tap water and inserted into the vagina prior to intercourse. It provides up to 24 hours of protection for repeated sexual intercourse. The sponge must remain in the vagina for at least 6 hours after the last act of intercourse. The contraceptive sponge offers no protection against STIs or HIV.

Be sure to— Teach about toxic shock syndrome

Women who use the diaphragm, cervical cap, or contraceptive sponge should be aware of the possible association between these devices and toxic shock syndrome (TSS). Common signs of TSS include fever of sudden onset greater than 101.1°F (38.4°C), rash, and hypotension with a systolic blood pressure less than 90 mm Hg.

HORMONAL METHODS

Hormonal contraceptive methods include oral medications, the transdermal patch, the vaginal ring, long-acting injectables, the subdermal implant, and the progestin-releasing intrauterine device. Estrogen and progestins decrease the pituitary's release of follicle-stimulating hormone and luteinizing hormone to prevent ovulation. Progestins also thicken cervical mucus to prevent sperm penetration.

Oral Contraceptives

This method, known as "the pill," or oral contraceptive pill (OCP), has been available for more than 40 years. Throughout that time, the dose of estrogen has significantly decreased and newer generation progestins have become safer with fewer side effects. It was once recommended that patients occasionally "take a break" from the pill because of the high hormonal dosages they contained. With today's formulations however, patients can continue to take oral contraceptives into the perimenopausal years. Oral contraceptives are the most extensively studied medications in history (Hatcher, 2004).

Hormonal contraceptives contain estrogen in the form of ethinyl estradiol or mestranol; ethinyl estradiol is the most common estrogen used. Estrogens work by preventing the release of follicle-stimulating hormone (FSH) from the anterior pituitary. When FSH levels are kept low, the ovarian follicle is unable to form and ovulation is prevented (Rice & Thompson, 2006).

Progestins provide effective contraception when used alone or in combination with estrogen. When combined with an estrogen, progestins inhibit the luteinizing hormone (LH) surge, which is required for ovulation. When used alone, progestins are believed to inhibit ovulation inconsistently. Progestin-only contraceptives are thought to function primarily by creating a thickened cervical mucus (which produces a hostile environment for sperm penetration) and by causing endometrial atrophy. These alterations inhibit egg implantation and decrease the penetration of sperm and ovum transport (Rice & Thompson, 2006).

In the United States, oral contraceptives are available in monophasic, biphasic, and triphasic preparations. Monophasic formulas provide fixed doses of estrogen and progestin throughout a 21-day cycle. Biphasic preparations provide a constant amount of estrogen throughout the cycle but there is an increased amount of progestin during the last 11 days. Triphasic formulas, designed to more closely mimic a natural cycle, provide varied levels of estrogen and progestin throughout the cycle. Triphasic preparations reduce the incidence of breakthrough bleeding (bleeding that occurs outside of menstruation) in many women.

Women who wish to use oral contraceptives are examined before the medication is prescribed and then yearly thereafter. The mandatory examination includes a history, weight, blood pressure, general physical and pelvic examination, and Pap smear. Most providers schedule women for a return visit approximately 3 months after initiating the medication to confirm patient acceptance and correct use of the method and to detect any complications.

Optimizing Outcomes— Counseling about medications that decrease the effectiveness of oral contraceptives

It is essential for the nurse to take a thorough history on any patient who wishes to use oral contraceptives for birth control. Certain medications such as rifampin (Rifadin, Rimactane), isoniazid, barbiturates, and griseofulvin (Fulvicin-U/F, Gris-PEG, Grifulvin V) can decrease the effectiveness of oral contraceptives, and higher doses of estrogen must be used. Vomiting and diarrhea affect the absorption of oral contraceptives, thus patients who experience these symptoms should use a back-up method such as condoms. Recent research indicates that antibiotics do not affect the effectiveness of oral contraceptives (Hatcher et al., 2005). Interactions with certain drugs such as acetaminophen, anticoagulants, and some anticonvulsants (e.g., phenytoin sodium, carbamazepine, primidone, topiramate), may reduce efficacy of the OCP.

Many noncontraceptive benefits are associated with OCPs (Box 6-4). Perimenopausal women who do not smoke, who maintain a normal blood pressure and who have a normal well-woman annual exam can safely use oral contraceptives. Oral contraceptives can moderate the irregular bleeding that often occurs during the perimenopausal period and provide contraception as well. When used on an extended cycle basis, hot flashes and vaginal dryness may also be alleviated (Clark & Burkman, 2006). The onset of menopause in women who use hormonal contraception may be difficult to detect.

CONTRAINDICATIONS. There are several absolute and relative contraindications to the use of combined oral contraceptive pills and the nurse must be fully aware of

> ### Box 6-4 Noncontraceptive Benefits of Oral Contraceptive Pills
>
> Oral contraceptive pills are associated with a decreased incidence of:
> - Fibrocystic breast disease
> - Iron-deficiency anemia, due to a reduced amount of menstrual flow
> - Colorectal, endometrial, and ovarian cancer and the formation of ovarian cysts
> - Mittelschmerz and dysmenorrhea, due to the lack of ovulation
> - Premenstrual dysphoric syndrome, due to increased progesterone levels
> - Acute pelvic inflammatory disease (PID) and scarring of the fallopian tubes
> - Ectopic pregnancy
> - Osteopenia and osteoporosis

them. Relative contraindications include hypertension, migraine headaches, epilepsy, obstructive jaundice in pregnancy, gallbladder disease, surgery with prolonged immobilization, and sickle cell disease (Rice & Thompson, 2006).

SIDE EFFECTS. A number of unpleasant and often troublesome side effects may accompany OCP use, especially during the first 3 months after initiation of the method. Nurses should teach patients that they might experience scanty periods, bleeding between periods (breakthrough bleeding), nausea, breast tenderness, headaches, and cyclic weight gain from fluid retention. If patients understand that these side effects may occur, they are more likely to seek health care provider advice before arbitrarily discontinuing use of the OCP. The symptoms often subside after a few months of use or they may be diminished with a change in routine or in the brand of contraceptive.

EFFECTIVENESS. The typical user effectiveness of combined oral contraceptives is 95% (Family Health International, 2006).

 Optimizing Outcomes— When teaching patients about use of oral contraceptive pills

The woman should identify a convenient and obvious place to keep her pills so that she will remember to take one every day. Ovulation suppressants work only when they are taken consistently and conscientiously. OCPs are not effective for the first 7 days, so a second form of contraception should be used during the first 7 days that the initial package of pills is taken. OCPs should be taken at approximately the same time each day. Many OCPs are available. Most are taken daily for 21 days, beginning on the Sunday after the first day of the menstrual cycle. Withdrawal bleeding usually occurs within 1–4 days after the last pill is taken. This schedule was developed on the assumption that women would desire to have monthly periods (Dominguez, Moore, & Wysocki, 2005). Seven days after taking the last pill, the woman begins a new package (she always begins a new pack on the same day). Some OCP packages contain seven inert or iron pills during the fourth week so that the woman never stops taking a pill. In addition to the nurse's verbal

instructions, it is imperative that all women receive written information to take home with them and encouraged to call if they have questions or experience any problems. Oral contraceptive pills offer no protection against STIs or HIV.

 critical nursing action Recognizing Contraindications to Oral Contraceptive Use

> When counseling patients about oral contraceptive pills, the nurse must be aware of the following *absolute* contraindications to use:
> - Smoking and age greater than 35 years
> - Moderate to severe hypertension (BP 160/100)
> - Undiagnosed uterine bleeding
> - Diabetes of more than 20 years' duration or with vascular complications
> - History of pulmonary embolism or deep venous thrombosis
> - Ischemic heart disease or stroke
> - Severe migraine headaches
> - Known or suspected breast cancer
> - Marked liver function impairment
> - Pregnancy
> - Major immobilizing surgery within the past month
> - Cholecystitis

A major emphasis in patient teaching concerns warning signs that must be immediately reported to the health care provider. The acronym "ACHES" can prompt the health care provider and patient to remember the warning signs. "ACHES" uses the first letter of each sign of cardiovascular, liver, gallbladder, or thromboembolic complications that are side effects of estrogen use and can be life-threatening. If patients experience any of these signs, they must stop taking the pill and promptly contact the health care provider. In addition to the "ACHES" signs, patients who become depressed or jaundiced, or who develop a breast lump should notify their health care provider.

 Be sure to— Teach the patient taking oral contraceptives to report ACHES

Abdominal pain (problem with liver or gall bladder)
Chest pain or shortness of breath (blood clot in lungs or heart)
Headaches: Sudden or persistent (hypertension, cardiovascular accident)
Eye problems (hypertension, vascular accident)
Severe leg pain (thromboembolism)

Nursing Insight— *Postponing initiation of OCPs in adolescents*

Adolescent girls should have well-established menstrual cycles before beginning OCPs. Waiting until 2 years of monthly cycles have occurred reduces the chance that the oral contraceptive will cause permanent suppression of the pituitary-regulating center. In addition, estrogen prompts closure of the long bone epiphyses; postponing initiation of OCPs ensures that the preadolescent growth spurt will not be prematurely halted.

Low-Dose Progestin-Only Contraceptive Pills

Low-dose progestin-only contraceptive pills are often referred to as the "mini pill" because they contain no estrogen. Although ovulation may occur, the progestins cause thickening of the cervical mucus and endometrial atrophy. These changes inhibit implantation and decrease the penetration of sperm and ovum transport (Rice & Thompson, 2006). The minipill is used primarily by women who have a contraindication to the estrogen component of the combination OCP. It must be taken at the same time every day. The minipill may be used during breastfeeding because it does not interfere with milk production.

SIDE EFFECTS. Irregular menses frequently occur with the progestin-only pills. Also, this type of oral contraceptive may be associated with an increased number of persistent ovarian follicles (Hatcher et al., 2005). Women with a history of functional ovarian cysts, a history of ectopic pregnancy or those with unexplained vaginal bleeding should not take the progestin-only oral contraceptive pills.

EFFECTIVENESS. The progestin-only contraceptive pills are 92% effective in preventing pregnancy (Hatcher et al., 2005).

 case study   Young Woman Who Believes She Is Infertile

Jana, who is 16 years old, arrives at the family planning clinic with her 17-year-old girlfriend who has brought her in for a "check up." During the health history, she tells the nurse that she believes she cannot have children. She confides that she has been having occasional unprotected sex with different boyfriends for the past year, and has never gotten pregnant. But she believes she should use "something," just in case.

1. What are the major teaching needs for Jana?

2. The nurse determines that this will be Jana's first gynecological examination. What are some teaching needs and strategies?

3. In addition to specific instruction about the prescribed oral contraceptive, what other information should be emphasized?

◆ See Suggested Answers to Case Studies in text on the Electronic Study Guide or DavisPlus.

Transdermal Contraceptive Patch

The transdermal contraceptive patch is applied to the abdomen, buttock, upper outer arm, or upper torso once weekly for 3 weeks, followed by one patch-free week. It should not be placed on the breasts. During the patch-free week, withdrawal bleeding occurs. The patch delivers low levels of estrogen and a progestin (norelgestromin) that are readily absorbed into the skin on a daily basis. The contraceptive patch costs slightly more than combined oral contraceptive pills.

SIDE EFFECTS. The side effects and contraindications and warning signs for the patch are the same as for the oral contraceptive pills. However, the patch exposes patients to higher steady-state concentrations and lower peak concentrations of ethinyl estradiol (the estrogen component). There is a potential for increased adverse events in women using the patch (Rice & Thompson, 2006).

EFFECTIVENESS. The patch is about 99% effective in preventing pregnancy. Due to concerns that excessive adipose tissue may be associated with inconsistent levels of hormonal absorption, it is not recommended for women who weigh more than 198 pounds. In general, patient compliance is enhanced because of the once-weekly administration (Potts & Lobo, 2005).

 Optimizing Outcomes— **When teaching patients about use of the transdermal contraceptive patch**

The patch can cause skin irritation, particularly if it is placed on damp skin or in the same location every time. Thus, rotating the application site is recommended. Hypopigmentation at the site of the patch placement has been reported (Hatcher et al., 2005). Some women have complained that the patch adhesive catches fibers from their clothing; placing the patch on the buttock under the underpants may be desirable. Bathing and swimming should not interfere with the patch. If the patch becomes detached for more than 24 hours, a new one should be applied and another form of contraception used for the following 7 days (Burki, 2005). The transdermal contraceptive patch offers no protection against STIs or HIV.

Vaginal Contraceptive Ring

The vaginal contraceptive ring contains estrogen and etonogestrel, a progestin. It is a flexible ring that is inserted deep into the vagina by the fifth day of the menstrual cycle, and left in place for 3 weeks. It is removed during the fourth week to allow withdrawal bleeding and a new ring is inserted at approximately the same time of day that the old ring was removed.

SIDE EFFECTS. The vaginal contraceptive ring is associated with a higher incidence of vaginitis, vaginal discomfort, and vaginal infections when compared to other forms of hormonal contraception. It is not recommended for patients with cystocele, rectocele, or uterine prolapse (Rice & Thompson, 2006).

EFFECTIVENESS. The ring slowly releases estrogen and progestin. Its effectiveness in preventing pregnancy is about 98% (Rice & Thompson, 2006).

 Optimizing Outcomes— **When teaching patients about use of the vaginal contraceptive ring**

The contraceptive ring should not be removed before, during, or after intercourse. The patient should not douche. If the contraceptive ring comes out of the vagina, it should be washed with plain hand soap and warm water before reinsertion. If the woman has a supply of more than four rings, they should be stored in the refrigerator (Hatcher et al., 2005). Before discarding a used contraceptive ring, the patient should take care to protect the environment by sealing the used ring in a closed plastic bag. If the ring is removed for more than 3 hours, it should be reinserted and another method of contraception should be used for the following 7 days (Burki, 2005). Unopened vaginal rings must be protected from sunlight and high temperatures. The vaginal contraceptive ring offers no protection against STIs or HIV.

Emergency Postcoital Contraception

Emergency contraception (EC) is available to women whose birth control methods fail or who have been the victims of sexual assault. Two forms of emergency postcoital contraception are available: hormonal methods, which include estrogen and progestin or progestin-only oral contraceptive pills; and the insertion of a copper releasing intrauterine device (IUD). Emergency contraception is available by prescription, office visit or, in some states, over the counter.

HORMONAL METHOD. Often referred-to as "the morning after pill," or the "emergency contraceptive pill" (ECP), there are two FDA-approved OC products specifically packaged for emergency contraception. Preven is a kit that contains four combination estrogen/progestin tablets and a pregnancy test. Plan B contains two progestin-only tablets. The hormonal preparations are most effective when taken as soon as possible after unprotected intercourse. The first dose should be taken within 72 hours (after intercourse); the second dose 12 hours later. Nausea and vomiting is a common side effect with both products and may be minimized by taking an antiemetic 1 hour before the first EC dose (Burki, 2005; Lever, 2005). Although regular OCPs can be taken for emergency contraception, the dose varies with the brand and may require taking a large number of tablets. The risk of pregnancy is reduced by 75% after completion of the EC dose.

IUD METHOD. The copper IUD can be inserted within 5 days of unprotected intercourse. Because of the product's cost and the need for insertion by a trained professional, the IUD is used less frequently than the ECPs. The IUD is not recommended for women who have been raped or are at risk for STIs and pelvic infections (Burki, 2005).

SIDE EFFECTS. Fewer side effects are associated with oral emergency contraceptive pills than with continuous oral contraceptives. Side effects include nausea and vomiting and bleeding within a few days after administration. The side effects for the IUD are the same whether it is being used as an emergency contraception method or as a long-term contraceptive. (See later discussion in this chapter.)

EFFECTIVENESS. Emergency contraceptive pills are 98.9% effective in preventing pregnancy if used correctly and the IUD is 99% to 100% effective (Hatcher et al., 2005).

💿 **Optimizing Outcomes**— **When teaching patients about postcoital emergency contraception**

Emergency contraception in either form (pills or IUD) does not cause abortion although it is often confused with the medical abortion procedure. The high hormone levels in the oral contraceptive pills prevent or delay ovulation,

thicken cervical mucus, alter sperm transport to prevent fertilization, and interfere with normal endometrial development. Emergency contraception is ineffective if implantation has already occurred and it does not harm a developing embryo (Smith, 2007).

The IUD is suitable for women who wish to have the benefit of long-term contraception. Insertion of the IUD within 5 days after intercourse causes an alteration in the endometrium to prevent implantation. Patients should contact their health care providers if no period occurs within 3 weeks after insertion (Lever, 2005). Emergency contraception offers no protection against STIs or HIV.

INJECTABLE HORMONAL CONTRACEPTIVE METHODS

Depo-Provera (DMPA), Depo-SubQ Provera 104 (Depot Medroxyprogesterone)

Depo-Provera (medroxyprogesterone acetate) is a progestin-only long-term contraceptive. Its effects last about 3 months, and it is injected either intramuscularly (150 mg) or subcutaneously (104 mg). The first injection should be given within the first 5 days of menstruation to ensure the patient is not pregnant. Medroxyprogesterone 150 mg is injected into the deltoid or gluteal muscle and functions by suppressing ovulation and altering the cervical environment (Rice & Thompson, 2006). The administration site should not be massaged after injection, as it may reduce the effectiveness of DMPA.

Depo-SubQProvera 104 was the first subcutaneous hormonal contraceptive product available. It is administered into the anterior thigh or the abdomen and functions by preventing ovulation and producing thinning of the endometrium. On average, ovulation is restored within 10 months after discontinuation of the medication (both dosages).

SIDE EFFECTS. Irregular bleeding is the most common side effect of Depo-Provera. Most women who use this method experience spotting during the first few months, usually until the second injection. Amenorrhea often occurs after about 6 months of use. Other side effects include weight gain, depression, headache, and breast tenderness. Although Depo-Provera may reduce bone mineral density, the subcutaneous injectable form may not be associated with a loss in bone density (Hatcher et al., 2005).

EFFECTIVENESS. The typical effectiveness for the 150-mg intramuscular dose of Depo-Provera is 98% to 99%. The typical effectiveness rate of the subcutaneous 104-mg Depo-Provera injection appears to be greater than 99% (Hatcher et al., 2005).

💿 **Optimizing Outcomes**— **When teaching patients about injectable hormonal contraception**

Women who desire pregnancy within the next year may wish to choose another contraceptive method that is more easily reversible. Depo-Provera is associated with weight gain and a reduction in bone mineral density. Patients who use DMPA should include adequate calcium in their diet

(1200 mg/day) and perform daily weight-bearing exercise to enhance bone density maintenance and to offset weight gain. Clinic visits must be scheduled every 3 months for the contraceptive injection. Providing a reminder card that includes the date of the next injection is helpful, and some women set their PDA calendars or cell phones to alarm on the date. Since DMPA is injected, it cannot be reversed or stopped abruptly. Women who wish to hide their use of contraception from a partner or others may find this method to be particularly appealing. Because it contains no estrogen, DMPA can be safely given to breastfeeding mothers. Injectable hormonal contraception offers no protection against STIs or HIV.

where research and practice meet:
Detrimental Effects of Depo-Provera on Bone Mineral Density in Adolescents

Findings from a 2005 prospective cohort trial established that adolescents are at increased risk for detrimental effects of Depo-Provera on bone mineral density (BMD). Study participants included 14- to 18-year-old women, in whom bone density is expected to increase due to continued bone growth and development. Those who used Depo-Provera experienced significant losses in bone mineral density at both the hip and spine in comparison to participants not using Depo-Provera, whose bone mineral density increased. After discontinuation of Depo-Provera, BMD significantly improved (Scholes et al., 2005). These findings suggest that the adverse effect is reversible in adolescents if therapy is withdrawn. Recommendations from professional organizations including the American College of Obstetricians and Gynecologists (ACOG), the Society for Adolescent Medicine (SAM), and the World Health Organization (WHO) state that for the majority of adolescents, the benefits of DMPA use outweigh the potential risks (Arias, Kaunitz, & McClung, 2007). During contraceptive counseling, nurses must empower young patients with information about decreased bone mineral density and Depo-Provera and assist them in making appropriate contraceptive choices (Rice & Thompson, 2006).

SUBDERMAL HORMONAL IMPLANT

Implanon

Implanon is a subdermal contraceptive that is effective for 3 years. The single-rod implant, which is inserted on the inner side of the woman's upper arm, contains etonogestrel (ENG), a progestin. It is simpler to insert and remove than the previously available six-capsule levonorgestrel implant (Norplant) (Schulman, 2007). Implanon functions to prevent pregnancy by suppressing ovulation and by creating a thickened cervical mucus that hinders sperm penetration. Etonogestrel is metabolized by the liver. Hepatic-enzyme inducers, including certain antiepileptic agents, may interfere with absorption and contraceptive effectiveness (*Clinician Reviews*, 2006; Darney & Mishell, 2006).

SIDE EFFECTS. Bleeding irregularities frequently occur during the first several months after insertion; amenorrhea becomes more common with increasing duration of use. Other symptoms include emotional lability,

weight increase, headache, depression, dysmenorrhea, and acne.

EFFECTIVENESS. Effectiveness rates approach 100%.

 Optimizing Outcomes—— When teaching patients about the contraceptive implant

The Implanon contraceptive is appropriate for women who desire long-term reversible contraception and who have no objections to the insertion/removal procedures or to palpating the implant when it is in place. It must be removed and replaced every 3 years if continued contraception is desired. After removal, ovulation occurs within 3 to 6 weeks. Contraceptive efficacy in obese women (>130% of ideal body weight) has not been studied (Darney & Mishell, 2006). The contraceptive implant offers no protection against STIs or HIV.

INTRAUTERINE DEVICES

The intrauterine device (IUD) is a small plastic device that is inserted into the uterus and left in place for an extended period of time, providing continuous contraception. The exact mechanism of action is not fully understood although it is believed that the IUD causes a sterile inflammatory response that results in a spermicidal intrauterine environment. Few sperm are able to reach the fallopian tubes and if fertilization does occur, the intrauterine environment is unfavorable for implantation (Epsey, 2005).

Two types of intrauterine devices (IUDs) are currently available in the United States: the levonorgestrel-releasing intrauterine system (LNG-IUS) (Mirena), which releases a progestin, and the copper T380A (ParaGard) (Fig. 6-6). The Dalkon Shield IUD was removed from the market in the 1970s due to pelvic infections associated with it. Today's IUD manufacturers have corrected the design problem that accompanied the Dalkon Shield, and IUDs are once again safe to use.

LNG-IUS (Mirena) slowly releases a small amount of levonorgestrel, a progestin, on a constant basis. It must be replaced every 5 years. The ParaGard IUD has copper wire

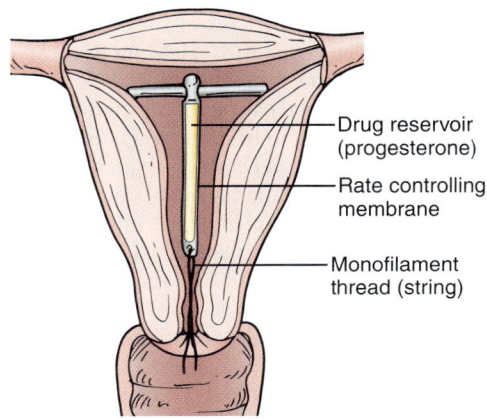

Figure 6-6 Intrauterine device (IUD) properly positioned in the uterus.

wrapped around it and this device may remain in place for 10 years. Both types of IUDs are shaped like the letter "T." They are inserted in a collapsed position and then expand into shape in the uterus once the inserter is withdrawn. The IUD is contained wholly within the uterus and the attached plastic string, or "tail," extends through the cervix and into the vagina. Both are impregnated with barium sulfate for radiopacity. The IUD is inserted during menses to ensure that pregnancy has not occurred; it may also be inserted immediately after childbirth or first trimester abortion (Clark & Arias, 2007; Hatcher et al., 2005).

Once in place, the IUD has several advantages over other methods of contraception. There is no continued expense, no daily attention is required and the device does not interfere with sexual enjoyment. The IUD may decrease the incidence of endometrial cancer. The IUD is appropriate for women who are at risk for developing complications related to OCPs or who desire to avoid the systemic effects of hormonal preparations. When pregnancy is desired, the IUD is removed by the health care provider.

SIDE EFFECTS. Irregular bleeding and/or spotting may occur about 3 months following insertion. The Mirena IUD may produce amenorrhea (Rice & Thompson, 2006). Pelvic infections may occur and the likelihood of occurrence is greatest during the first month after insertion (Epsey, 2005). Contraindications to IUDs include pregnancy, current sexually transmitted diseases, abnormal vaginal bleeding, cancer of the genital tract, known uterine anomalies or fibroid tumors (which may make insertion difficult), or allergy to any of the IUD components.

EFFECTIVENESS. Both types of IUDs have a failure rate of 1% to 2% (Hatcher et al., 2005).

 Optimizing Outcomes— **When teaching patients about the IUD**

The IUD should be considered a long-term form of contraception—it is relatively expensive if used for only a short period of time. Sharp cramping may occur at the time of insertion. The IUD offers no protection against STIs or HIV. Women who use the IUD may experience irregular bleeding, **menorrhagia** (heavy menstrual flow), or dysmenorrhea (painful menstruation) for several months following insertion. The progestin releasing IUD can decrease menstrual bleeding and dysmenorrhea; the copper-bearing IUD can increase menstrual flow and cramping (Clark & Arias, 2007). Women who become pregnant using the IUD are more likely to have an ectopic pregnancy or spontaneous abortion. All IUD patients must understand warning signs ("PAINS") that may indicate infection or ectopic pregnancy. A vaginal "string check" should be performed each month to ensure that the IUD remains in place. If the strings are not felt or if they seem to be longer or shorter than they were previously, the woman should return to her health care provider for evaluation. If pregnancy occurs with the IUD in place, the device is usually removed vaginally to decrease the possibility of infection or spontaneous abortion. IUD users should obtain a yearly pelvic examination and Pap smear.

 critial nursing action Teach "PAINS" Warning Signs to IUD Users

Period late (pregnancy)
Abdominal pain, pain with intercourse (infection)
Infection exposure or vaginal discharge
Not feeling well, fever, or chills (infection)
String missing, shorter or longer (IUD expelled)

Optimizing Outcomes— **With the IUD as a contraceptive choice**

Appropriate candidates for intrauterine contraception include nulliparas; women with previous ectopic pregnancies; women receiving treatment for pelvic inflammatory disease; lactating women; women testing positive for human immunodeficiency virus; and women immediately postpartum or postabortion (World Health Organization, 2004). Before insertion, patients should have a negative pregnancy test, treatment for dysplasia if present, cervical cultures to rule out STIs and a consent form that has been signed.

STERILIZATION

Sterilization should be considered a permanent and irreversible form of birth control. Although both the male and female procedures are theoretically reversible, the permanency of the method should be emphasized. An essential nursing role centers on counseling to empower the couple to make an informed decision. The nurse must also ensure that informed consent documentation has been obtained and is attached to the patient's chart.

Female Sterilization

Bilateral tubal ligation (BTL) or "tying the tubes" causes interruption in the patency of the fallopian tubes. This permanent birth control method is most easily performed during cesarean birth or in the first 48 hours following a vaginal birth because at this time, the uterine fundus is located near the umbilicus and the fallopian tubes are immediately below the abdominal wall. At other times, the procedure is performed in an outpatient surgery clinic, usually under general anesthesia.

Tubal ligation may be accomplished in various ways. In the postpartum period, a minilaparotomy incision is made near the umbilicus or just above the symphysis pubis at other times. The fallopian tubes are brought through the incision and a small segment is removed. The remaining ends are cauterized or tied, or both. Another method of tubal ligation is accomplished with a laparoscope. The surgeon locates the fallopian tubes and obstructs them with clips or rings or destroys a portion of them with electrocoagulation.

A nonincisional method, called a hysteroscopic tubal ligation, is also available. This procedure is performed in the physician's office or as an outpatient procedure with a local anesthetic to the cervix. Microinserts are placed into the openings of the fallopian tubes. During the following months, scar tissue grows into the inserts, causing tubal blockage. A **hysterosalpingogram** (dye test to evaluate tubal patency) is performed at 3 months to ensure that both tubes have been blocked. Patients are instructed to use an alternate form of contraception until bilateral tubal blockage has been confirmed (Holloway, Moredich, & Aduddell, 2006).

SIDE EFFECTS. As with any surgery, complications include infection, hemorrhage and blood vessel injury, damage to adjacent organs, and complications from anesthesia (Hatcher et al., 2005; Holloway et al., 2006).

EFFECTIVENESS. The effectiveness depends on the type of procedure used and ranges from 96.3% with the clip procedure to better than 99% with the postpartum procedure (Hatcher et al., 2005).

Male Sterilization

Vasectomy is a surgical procedure that involves a small incision in the scrotum. The vas deferens is cauterized, clipped, or cut to interrupt the passage of sperm into the seminal fluid. Following vasectomy, the semen no longer contains sperm. Vasectomy should be considered a permanent method.

SIDE EFFECTS. Complications following vasectomy include infection, hematoma, and excessive pain and swelling.

EFFECTIVENESS. Vasectomy is greater than 99% effective in preventing pregnancy.

Optimizing Outcomes— When teaching patients about permanent sterilization

There is a high rate of ectopic pregnancies in tubal ligation procedures that fail. BTL has been found to decrease the risk of ovarian cancer and ovarian cancer mortality (Schulman & Westhoff, 2006). Menstruation and menopause are unaffected. After vasectomy, the man should rest, apply ice to the scrotum, and wear snug underwear for scrotal support. Complete sterilization has not occurred until all sperm have left the system. This process may take several weeks. The man will need to submit semen specimens for analysis until two specimens show no sperm present; he should also plan to have periodic sperm counts every few years (Hatcher et al., 2005). Permanent sterilization methods offer no protection against STIs or HIV.

Now Can You— Teach about contraception?

1. Explain what is meant by "natural family planning"?
2. Compare and contrast barrier and hormonal methods of contraception?
3. Identify five danger signs associated with OCPs and intrauterine devices?

Clinical Termination of Pregnancy

A clinical termination of pregnancy, or abortion, is a procedure performed to deliberately end a pregnancy before the fetus reaches a viable age. The legal definition of viability (usually 20 to 24 weeks) varies from state to state. Abortion has been legal in the United States since the 1973 Supreme Court decision in *Roe v. Wade*.

An abortion performed at the patient's request is termed an **elective abortion**; when performed for reasons of maternal or fetal health or disease, the term **therapeutic abortion** applies. Abortions performed during the first trimester are technically easier and safer than abortions performed during the second trimester. Methods for performing early elective abortion include vacuum aspiration and medical methods. Second-trimester abortion is associated with increased complications and costs and involves cervical dilation and removal of the fetus and placenta.

NURSING CARE RELATED TO ELECTIVE PREGNANCY TERMINATION

Holistic nursing care for women who are considering abortion includes guidance for pregnancy testing, ultrasonography to accurately determine the weeks of gestation, and individualized counseling about the available options. Any woman who is unsure of her decision deserves emotional support and time to allow her to make the choice that she feels is the appropriate one for her. The decision for nearly every woman is difficult and complicated. Once a decision has been made for an abortion, a medical history and physical examination with appropriate screening tests (e.g., complete blood count [CBC], blood typing and Rh, gonococcal smear, serological test for syphilis (STS), urinalysis, and Pap smear) are obtained. Informed consent documents are signed and placed on the patient's chart. The nurse counsels the patient about potential complications such as excessive bleeding and infection, reinforces information about follow-up visits, and offers strategies for self-care. The nurse must ensure that the patient understands how to contact a health care provider if needed. Women who are Rh$_0$D-negative should receive Rh$_0$(D) immune globulin (RhoGAM) if they do not have a preexisting sensitivity to Rh-positive blood. Since fertility returns quickly after a pregnancy termination, the nurse should also provide information about contraception.

SURGICAL TERMINATION OF PREGNANCY

Vacuum Aspiration

Vacuum aspiration is the most common method for surgical abortion for pregnancies up to 12 weeks' gestation. Very early (5 to 7 weeks after the LMP) procedures, called menstrual extraction and endometrial aspiration, can be done with a small flexible plastic cannula with no cervical dilation or anesthesia. **Laminaria**, dried seaweed that swells as it absorbs moisture and mechanically dilates the cervix, may be inserted 4 to 24 hours before the pregnancy termination. Upon removal, the cervix has usually dilated two to three times its original diameter and further instrumental dilation is unnecessary.

Abortions performed between 8 and 12 weeks' gestation require mechanical cervical dilation after injection of a local anesthetic. A plastic cannula is then inserted into the uterine cavity. The contents are aspirated with negative pressure and the uterine cavity is often scraped with a curet to ensure that the uterus is empty. Patients may experience cramping for 20 to 30 minutes following the procedure. Complications include uterine perforation, cervical lacerations, hemorrhage, infection, and adverse reactions to the anesthetic agent.

Abortion during the second trimester involves cervical dilation with removal of the fetus and placenta. This procedure is termed "dilation and evacuation" (D & E). Similar to vacuum curettage, greater cervical dilation and use of a larger cannula are required because of the increased volume in the products of conception. Laminaria are inserted 24 hours before the procedure to dilate the cervix. D & E may be associated with long-term adverse effects from cervical trauma.

Nursing care during surgical abortion includes continued patient assessment and emotional support. The woman should be informed about what to expect: abdominal cramping and sounds emitted by the suction machine. After the procedure, the patient rests in a recovery area for 1 to 3 hours to ensure that no excessive cramping or bleeding occurs. The aspirated uterine contents are inspected to ascertain that all fetal parts and adequate placental tissue have been aspirated.

Although check-up visits are usually scheduled between 2 weeks and 6 weeks postabortion, serum levels of human chorionic gonadotrophin (hCG) may remain elevated even if the abortion successfully ended the pregnancy. Women whose hCG levels are still present in the urine (at the follow-up appointment) should be encouraged to return for urine hCG levels every 2 weeks until the test is negative. Persistently elevated hCG levels are associated with a delay in the return of menses.

 ### clinical alert

Signs of short-term complications after clinical termination of pregnancy

- Fever of 40°C (104°F)
- Abdominal pain or tenderness in the abdomen
- Prolonged or heavy bleeding or passing large clots
- Foul smelling vaginal discharge
- No menstrual period within 6 weeks

Source: Hatcher et al. (2004).

MEDICAL TERMINATION OF PREGNANCY

"Medical abortion" is an alternative for the surgical form of abortion, and for some women this method is more "natural" and more closely resembles a miscarriage (Stewart et al., 2004). A medical abortion can be performed for up to 63 days of gestation. The woman who considers medical abortion should be carefully educated about what to expect. Specific medications are used to induce uterine contractions to end the pregnancy. These include mifepristone (Mifeprex, originally called RU-486), an abortifacient, and methotrexate (amethopterin, Folex, Rheumatrex, Trexall), an antimetabolite used to treat certain types of cancer. Both medications may be followed by a vaginal administration of misoprostol (Cytotec), a prostaglandin

analogue that promotes expulsion of the pregnancy. Misoprostol is commonly associated with nausea, vomiting, and cramping.

Uterine bleeding begins several days after medication administration, and most patients experience a period of painless heavy bleeding along with the expulsion of tissue (the products of conception). This experience may trigger strong emotions. The nurse should advise the patient that she would most likely benefit from the presence of a caring, trusted close friend, or relative who can help her through the experience and lend emotional and physical support (Stewart et al., 2004). Follow-up visits include ultrasonography (to confirm that the uterus is empty) and assessment of hCG levels. A surgical abortion procedure may be necessary if medical attempts are unsuccessful.

Medical termination of pregnancy is probably not the ideal choice for adolescents, and for this reason, some clinics offer this method of abortion only to women 18 years of age or older. Interestingly, this method has been proven useful in evacuating pregnancies that occur in the fallopian tubes. Medical termination of a tubal pregnancy has enabled many women to avoid surgery and preserve the fallopian tubes for future pregnancy conceptions.

Medical termination during the second trimester most often includes an administration of prostaglandins via vaginal suppository, gel, or by intrauterine injection. Repeated doses are often needed and side effects including nausea, vomiting, diarrhea, and cramping usually occur. Rarely used methods include the intrauterine instillation of hypertonic solutions such as saline or urea and uterotonic agents (e.g., misoprostol and dinoprostone).

Complications

Legal abortion is actually safer than pregnancy, especially when performed early in pregnancy. All patients should be told to expect cramping and some bleeding after an abortion. Some of the rare complications associated with abortion include infection, incomplete abortion, hemorrhage, **Asherman syndrome** (condition characterized by the presence of endometrial adhesions or scar tissue), and postabortal syndrome (severe abdominal cramping and pain from intrauterine blood clots) (Hatcher et al., 2005). Patients should be cautioned to call the office should any signs of short-term complications (i.e., excessive bleeding, pain, fever) occur. Most complications develop within the first few days after the abortion. All patients should return in 2 weeks for a follow-up examination.

The Nurse's Role in Infertility Care

THE INITIAL ASSESSMENT

Fertility requires that the sperm and the ovum can meet, that the sperm is viable, normal, and able to penetrate a viable, normal egg, and that the lining of the uterus can support the implanted embryo. **Sterility** is the term applied when there is an absolute factor that prevents reproduction. **Infertility** is diagnosed if a woman has not conceived within 12 months of actively attempting pregnancy. At present, 10% to 15% of heterosexual couples in the United States are infertile (Nelson & Marshall, 2004). Approximately 40% of cases of infertility can be attributed to female problems, 40% can be attributed to male causes, and the remaining cases of infertility are attributable to a combination of male and female factors, or are undeterminable (Mooney, 2005). Delays in childbearing and increased consumer awareness of reproductive technology have prompted more heterosexual couples, single women, and same-sex couples to seek fertility assistance than ever before. The nurse's role in infertility care begins with education and counseling during the initial assessment.

 Nursing Insight— *Toward meeting the Healthy People 2010 national goals*

The *Healthy People 2010* goal that directly addresses infertility states: "Reduce the proportion of married couples whose ability to conceive or maintain a pregnancy is impaired from a baseline of 13% to a target of 10%" (DHHS, 2000). To help achieve this goal, nurses must be proactive in health promotion strategies for all childbearing aged individuals. Empowering young adults with knowledge about nutrition, exercise, stress reduction, and safe sex practices helps them to make lifestyle choices that foster optimal health and preservation of fertility.

Before extensive testing for infertility, it is important to establish that the timing of intercourse and length of coital exposure are adequate. The nurse assesses the couple's understanding about the most fertile times to have intercourse during the menstrual cycle. Teaching about the signs and timing of ovulation, the most effective times for intercourse (every 48 hours around ovulation) and positions to enhance sperm retention is an important nursing intervention during the initial evaluation.

 Ethnocultural Considerations— Obtaining a sexual history for infertility care

Culturally influenced practices and taboos may create feelings of discomfort for couples when asked specific details of their intimate lives during the infertility care interview. Nurses must be sensitive to these issues and aware of cultural variations. For example, Orthodox Jewish law forbids a couple from engaging in sexual intercourse for 7 days after the menstrual period. This tenet can create an infertility problem if ovulation occurs during the early days after menstruation.

Providing an overview of what to expect during the initial and subsequent visits empowers the couple to make an informed decision about their level of commitment to the evaluation and possible treatment and affords them some sense of control over their situation. The nurse explains what is involved in the basic infertility work-up in a sensitive, unhurried manner that conveys caring and promotes a trusting, therapeutic relationship. Depending on findings from the history and physical examination, the evaluation will most likely include an assessment of

ovarian function, cervical mucus (amount and receptivity to sperm), sperm adequacy, tubal patency, and the general condition of the pelvic organs.

Instructions about recording the basal body temperature are usually provided at the initial visit. An in-depth interview, preferably with both partners, may reveal medical problems (e.g., chronic illness), lifestyle patterns (e.g., substance abuse, sexual orientation) or other factors such as advanced age that can adversely affect fertility. The physical examination includes evaluation of the pelvis (bimanual and rectovaginal assessment) and laboratory testing.

LATER METHODS OF ASSESSMENT

A thyroid function test, glucose tolerance test, serum prolactin levels, and specific hormonal assays (i.e., estradiol, LH, progesterone, dehydroepiandrosterone [DHEA], androstenedione, testosterone, 17 alpha-hydroxy progesterone [17-OHP]) may also be ordered along with ultrasonography (abdominal or transvaginal) to visualize the pelvic structures. Other diagnostic tests may include an endometrial biopsy to assess the endometrial response to progesterone, a hysterosalpingography (transcervical instillation of a radiopaque dye to provide visualization of the interior dimensions of the uterine cavity and fallopian tubes), and a laparoscopy to allow direct visualization of the internal pelvic structures. Selected methods of fertility evaluation in the female along with nursing implications are presented in Table 6-2.

Evaluation of the man begins with a semen analysis to assess the quality and quantity of sperm. The nurse explains the purpose of the test and advises the man to collect the semen specimen by masturbation following a 2- to 3-day abstinence. He is instructed to note the time the specimen was obtained. This information allows the laboratory to evaluate liquefaction of the semen. The specimen should be transported near the body (to preserve warmth) and should arrive at the laboratory within 1 hour after collection. Additional testing may include serum samples for evaluation of endocrine function (testosterone, estradiol, LH, FSH), ultrasonography, testicular biopsy, and sperm penetration assay. Referral to a urologist may be indicated. A postcoital test (PCT) may be ordered to assess the cervical mucus, sperm, and degree of sperm penetration through the cervical mucus. The test is performed on a sample of cervical mucus obtained several hours after intercourse.

Labs: Basic Infertility Evaluation and Workup

Woman:	Man:
CBC	Semen analysis: sperm count should be:
Urinalysis	Volume of 2–6 mL of semen
Pap smear and wet mount	
Serology	>20 million sperm per 1 mL of semen
Luteinizing-hormone-surge ovulation predictor kit	>50% forward moving sperm
	>30% normal sperm
FSH cycle day 3 if >35 years old	
Rh factor, blood grouping	< 1 million WBCs per mL of semen
Hysterosalpingogram (to reveal uterine or tubal obstruction or abnormalities)	

Table 6-2 Common Diagnostic Methods Used in the Evaluation of Female Infertility

Type/Name of Test	Role of the Nurse
Prediction of Ovulation To identify the LH surge – precedes ovulation by 24–36 hours. Also identifies the absence of ovulation. Tests include basal body temperature, commercial ovulation predictor kits, and assessment of cervical mucus.	Teach the couple how the information helps to determine timing of intercourse to coincide with ovulation. Instruct the woman about recording the BBT and assessing cervical mucus; reinforce directions for using commercial ovulation predictor kits.
Postcoital Test (PCT); Huhner Test Assessment of the quality and quantity of cervical mucus and sperm function at the time of ovulation.	Instruct the patient to arrange to come in 6–12 hours after intercourse for evaluation of the cervical mucus.
Ultrasound Examination To evaluate structure of the pelvic organs; identify maturing ovarian follicles and the timing of ovulation.	Reassure the patient that sonography uses sound waves, not radiation, to evaluate the pelvic structures. The examination may be conducted transabdominally or transvaginally and specific instructions are given, depending on method.
Hysterosalpingogram (see Diagnostic Tools)	
Tests of Endocrine Function To evaluate the hypothalamus, pituitary gland and ovaries. Various assays determine levels of FSH, LH, estrogen, and progesterone. Depending on the history and physical findings, additional testing may be indicated.	Inform the patient that testing is performed on serum samples and timing is an important consideration in interpretation of the results. Explain that FSH and LH stimulate ovulation; and estrogen and progesterone make the endometrium receptive for implantation of the fertilized ovum.
Endometrial Biopsy Involves the removal of a sample of the endometrium with a small pipette attached to suction. Provides information about the effects of progesterone (produced by the corpus luteum after ovulation) on the endometrium.	Teach the patient about the purpose and appropriate timing of the test: it should be performed not earlier than 10–12 days after ovulation (2–3 days before menstruation is expected). Cramping, pelvic discomfort, and vaginal spotting may occur; a mild analgesic (e.g., ibuprofen) may be used to alleviate the discomfort.
Hysteroscopy and Laparoscopy Procedures that involve the use of an endoscope to examine the interior of the uterus and the pelvic organs under general anesthesia. Hysteroscopy may be performed without general anesthesia in the office. Abnormalities such as polyps, myomata (fibroid tumors) and endometrial adhesions are identified.	Explain the purpose of the test and other procedures that may be done at the same time. When general anesthesia is to be used, the patient should take nothing by mouth for several hours before the planned procedure. Advise her that since carbon dioxide gas will be instilled in the abdomen to enhance organ visibility, she may experience post-operative cramping and referred shoulder pain, which can be relieved with a mild analgesic.

diagnostic tools: Hysterosalpingography (HSG)

During hysterosalpingography, radiopaque dye is injected through the cervix. The dye enters the uterus and fallopian tubes and through x-ray examination, any abnormalities in the uterine structure or tubal patency can be identified.

- It is performed during the follicular phase of the menstrual cycle to avoid interrupting an early pregnancy. It may exert a therapeutic effect as well: instillation of the water-based dye may flush out debris or adhesions in the uterine cavity.
- Moderate to severe cramping and shoulder pain "referred" from the subdiaphragmatic collection of gas may occur. All patients should be warned about the possibility of pain during the test.
- The patient should be given a nonsteroidal anti-inflammatory drug (NSAID) (e.g., ibuprofen) 30 minutes to 1 hour before the procedure.
- Recurrence of pelvic inflammatory disease may result from the test; prophylactic antibiotics are recommended to prevent infection.
- The patient is instructed to report severe cramping, bleeding, fever or malodorous discharge that develops within a week following the procedure, although spotting and slight cramping for a few days may occur. She should be advised to take an NSAID after the procedure for these symptoms.

Treatment Options for Infertility

MEDICATIONS

Depending on the cause of infertility, a number of pharmacological methods are used to induce ovulation, supplement the woman's levels of follicle-stimulating hormone (FSH) and luteinizing hormone (LH), prepare the uterine endometrium for implantation, and support the pregnancy following conception and implantation (Table 6-3).

Induction of Ovulation

Medications are commonly used to stimulate follicle development in women who are anovulatory or who ovulate infrequently. Clomiphene citrate (Clomid) is frequently prescribed. It is an antiestrogenic agent that binds to hypothalamic estrogen receptors to trigger the release of FSH and LH. Patients who will be undergoing assisted

Table 6-3 Selected Medications Used in the Treatment of Infertility

Medication	Actions	Nursing Considerations and Side Effects
Clomiphene citrate (Clomid)	Antiestrogen that binds with estrogen receptors to trigger FSH and LH release.	Contraindicated with hepatic impairment. Patients may experience ovarian enlargement, vasomotor flushes, abdominal distention, nausea and vomiting, breast tenderness, blurred vision, headache, pelvic pain, abnormal uterine bleeding. May cause multiple ovulation.
Bromocriptine mesylate (Parlodel)	Reduces elevated prolactin secretion by the anterior pituitary, which improves gonadotropin-releasing hormone secretion and normalizes follicle-stimulating hormone and luteinizing hormone release. Ovulation is restored and increased progesterone by the corpus luteum supports early pregnancy.	Patients may experience nausea and vomiting, headache, dizziness, orthostatic hypotension, blurred vision, diarrhea, metallic taste, dry mouth, urticaria, rash.
GnRH agonists (gonadorelin); goserelin [Zoladex], leuprolide [Lupron], nafarelin [Synarel]	Stimulates release of pituitary FSH and LH in patients with deficient hypothalamic GnRH secretion. FSH and LH stimulate ovulation (female) and testosterone and spermatogenesis (male).	Advise patients of potential side effects: headache, depression, nasal irritation (Synarel), vaginal dryness, breast swelling and tenderness, hot flashes, vaginal spotting, decreased libido, and impotence.
GnRH antagonists; cetrorelix [Cetrotide], ganirelix [Antagon], abarelix [Plenaxis], histrelin [Supprelin]	Reduces extent of endometriosis; used with medications that stimulate ovulation by suppressing LH and FSH.	Patients are closely monitored for ovarian hyperstimulation (ascites with or without pain, pleural effusion, ruptured ovarian cysts, multiple births), headache, nausea.
Human chorionic gonadotropin (hCG) (Profasi HP, Pregnyl, Chorex)	Used after failure to respond to therapy with clomiphene citrate, induces ovulation; used in conjunction with gonadotropins (FSH and LH [Pergonal], [Repronex], [Humegon]); ovulation usually occurs within 18 hours. Also stimulates production of progesterone by the corpus luteum.	When used with menotropins, risk for ovarian hyperstimulation, and arterial thromboembolism; other side effects include headache, irritability, restlessness, and depression.
Progesterone (IM, intravaginal)	Provides luteal phase support—prepares the endometrial lining to promote implantation of the embryo.	Common side effects include nausea, weight gain, and fluid retention.

reproductive techniques including in vitro fertilization, gamete intrafallopian transfer, and tubal embryo transfer may also receive agents to induce superovulation, or the release of several ova. After adequate follicular stimulation, human chorionic gonadotropin (hCG) is administered to prompt ovulation.

Induction of ovulation increases the risk of multiple births because many ova may be released and fertilized. Depending on the medications used, daily ultrasound examinations and serum estrogen levels may be obtained to monitor ovarian response. **Ovarian hyperstimulation** is a serious complication that may result from ovulation induction. It is characterized by marked ovarian enlargement, ascites with or without pain, and pleural effusion. When detected, hCG is not given, and ovulation will not occur. The patient undergoes a "rest" period and postponement of the infertility treatment until the following cycle. Careful monitoring and medication titration are usually successful in preventing this complication as well as high-order (triplets or more) multifetal pregnancy. Throughout therapy, which often requires repeated office visits and testing, nursing interventions center on continued education and patient support. Emotional instability, anxiety, and depression are common reactions to the dramatic hormonal alterations and need for frequent surveillance.

SURGICAL OPTIONS

Surgical interventions using endoscopic techniques may be useful in correcting obstructions. Laparoscopic ablation (destruction) of endometrial implants may help patients with endometriosis achieve pregnancy, especially during the first few months immediately following the procedure. Newer laser surgical techniques are minimally invasive and useful in reducing adhesions that have resulted from infection, prior surgical procedures, and endometriosis. Microsurgical techniques may be successful in correcting obstructions in the fallopian tubes or in the male tubal structures. Transcervical tuboplasty (surgery for correction of fallopian tube abnormalities) is a minimally invasive technique that involves insertion of a catheter through the cervix, into the uterus and the fallopian tube. A balloon is inflated to clear any blockage.

THERAPEUTIC INSEMINATION

Therapeutic insemination (previously termed "artificial insemination") involves the placement of semen at the cervical os or directly in the uterus (intrauterine insemination [IUI]) by mechanical means. Partner sperm (termed "therapeutic husband insemination" [THI]) or donor sperm (termed "therapeutic donor insemination" [TDI]) is used. Clomiphene citrate and ultrasound monitoring for follicle development are frequently used to ensure timing of the insemination with ovulation. Fertilization most often occurs in the fallopian tube. The technique involves the insertion of a small catheter into the vagina and through the cervix to facilitate the deposition of sperm directly into the uterus. Since seminal fluid is rich in prostaglandins, IUI prevents the nausea, cramping, abdominal pain, and diarrhea that can result from the absorption of prostaglandins by the cervical lining.

Before the IUI, the sperm are "washed": they are removed from the seminal fluid and placed in a special solution that enhances motility and improves the chances for fertilization. An added advantage of washing sperm concerns sperm antibodies. After infection or surgery, a woman's immune system may produce antibodies that cause sperm clumping and adversely affect motility and ovum penetration. Sperm washing may correct the clumping, increase sperm motility and improve the likelihood of fertilization (Mooney, 2005).

ADVANCED REPRODUCTIVE TECHNOLOGIES

Gamete Intrafallopian Transfer

Advanced reproductive technologies (ARTs) are procedures intended to achieve pregnancy by placing gametes together to promote fertilization. Although assisted reproductive methods are more common today than in the past, they are very expensive, and are often unavailable to women of lower socioeconomic status. **Gamete intrafallopian transfer (GIFT)** is a technique that involves laparoscopy and ovulation induction. The patient must have at least one patent fallopian tube. Three to five oocytes are harvested from the ovary and immediately placed into a catheter along with washed, motile donor or partner sperm. The sperm and oocytes are injected into the fimbriated ends of the fallopian tube(s) through a laparoscope. Since fertilization normally takes place in the fallopian tube, this technique increases the likelihood of conception in situations where the sperm and ovum may be prevented from uniting. Supplemental progesterone is given to promote implantation and provide support for the early pregnancy.

Zygote Intrafallopian Transfer

Zygote intrafallopian transfer (ZIFT) is a procedure that evolved from the GIFT procedure. Following ovulation induction, retrieved oocytes are fertilized outside the woman's body and the subsequent zygotes are placed in the distal fallopian tube(s).

Tubal Embryo Transfer

Tubal embryo transfer (TET) involves placement at the embryo stage. The patient must have at least one patent fallopian tube. Exogenous progesterone is used to enhance endometrial preparation.

In Vitro Fertilization

In vitro fertilization (IVF) involves retrieval of the oocytes from the ovaries, usually via an intra-abdominal approach or a transvaginal approach under ultrasound guidance. The oocytes are then combined with partner or donor sperm in the laboratory. After fertilization, the normally developing embryos are placed in the uterus (Fig. 6-7). Success with IVF is dependent upon many factors, such as the woman's age and the indication for the procedure. On average, women who undergo three IVF cycles have a good chance of achieving pregnancy.

Embryo Cryopreservation

Cryopreservation, or freezing, is used in some instances to store sperm or ovarian tissue for future use or to freeze excess embryos that have resulted from an in vitro fertilization procedure. If no pregnancy results, the frozen embryos can be processed and replaced in the uterus. This option allows the couple to attempt another pregnancy without the need for ovarian stimulation and egg retrieval.

An initial fee is charged for the freezing process; additional fees are incurred for the continued preservation of the frozen reproductive tissues. One of the ethical and sociocultural issues involved with cryopreservation arises when excess embryos are no longer needed or desired by the woman or couple. In most situations, the embryos are destroyed although a social debate presently concerns an alternate use of the embryos for research.

Micromanipulation

Micromanipulation is a process that involves the use of micromanipulators—fine, specialized instruments—to handle individual sperm and ova. Intracytoplasmic sperm injection (ICSI) allows a sperm cell to be directly injected into an ovum. Assisted embryo hatching is used as an IVF adjunct for women in whom the normal "hatching process" is impeded because of a thickening of the zona pellucida. A small opening created in the zona pellucida facilitates the hatching process by allowing the embryo to escape from the zona pellucida to interact with the endometrium for implantation. Blastomere analysis allows for chromosomal analysis using a single cell from the six-to eight-cell embryo before implantation.

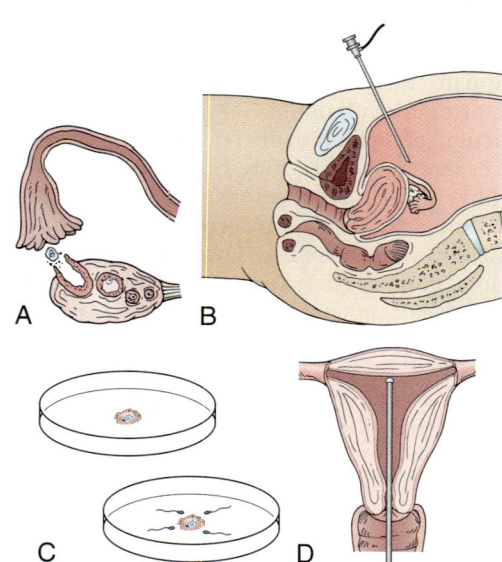

Figure 6-7 The process of in vitro fertilization.
A, Ovulation. B, Intra-abdominal retrieval of the ova.
C, Ova fertilization and growth in culture medium.
D, Fertilized ova is placed in the uterus.

ART and Legal Considerations

Before any ART procedure, patients must be given current, factual information about the advantages and limitations of techniques that involve the use of donor sperm or eggs for the purpose of conception. Informed consent must be obtained and documented in the patient record. Advanced reproductive technology is expensive (approximately $10,000.00 a cycle) and available only in specialized centers. Unfortunately, there is never a guarantee of a viable pregnancy that will result in a healthy child. Nursing responsibilities include ensuring that patients and their partners have ample opportunity to ask questions, thoughtfully explore available options, and freely express concerns. They must be able to verbalize an understanding of the chosen procedure(s), including the risks and potential complications. Ongoing support includes education, counseling, and strategies for continued follow-up.

When donor ova or sperm are to used, patients and their partners require additional information. They need to be reassured that all gamete donors have undergone psychological and physical examinations and screening for medical and genetic disease. Clinical findings from potential donors are made available to the woman or couple to allow them to make an informed decision. The donor's and the recipient's confidentiality are closely guarded, and in most instances, their identities are not revealed without their specific permission.

Infertility, ART, and Potential Effects on the Couple's Relationship

Infertility produces a great amount of emotional stress for most couples. Societal and cultural influences may intensify the feelings of disappointment and failure. It is not unusual for the woman and her partner to experience a sense of loss: loss of perceived good health, loss of self-esteem, loss of a "normal" relationship with the spouse, loss of security and self-confidence, and loss of the potential child. Affected individuals often move through the stages of grieving identified by Kubler-Ross: surprise, denial, anger, isolation, guilt, grief and resolution.

For heterosexual couples, intercourse can transition from a shared loving, intimate moment into a clinical, goal-oriented procedure. Unfortunately, some relationships do not survive the stress of infertility. Even under the best of circumstances, infertile couples are subjected to a loss of privacy and often a lack of spontaneity. During treatment for infertility, menstrual periods become a regular and repeated reminder of failure. Patients are asked to share with others their most personal and emotionally laden information concerning sexual preferences and sexual practices. It is imperative that the nurse and other members of the health care team maintain confidentiality and privacy for these patients as much as possible. The nurse's caring demeanor and expressions of genuine concern are essential qualities when dealing with the sensitive and emotional circumstances that surround infertility testing and treatment. Depending on the patient's unique situation, a number of nursing diagnoses may be appropriate (Box 6-5).

Box 6-5 Potential Nursing Diagnoses for the Patient Experiencing Infertility

- Risk for ineffective coping related to infertility
- Risk for posttrauma response related to infertility
- Risk for spiritual distress related to infertility
- Risk for situational low self-esteem related to infertility

Family Teaching Guidelines...
Fostering Relationships During Evaluation and Treatment for Infertility

Couples should be encouraged to spend quality time with one another and enjoy sexual intimacy outside of the "fertile times." Professional counseling may be appropriate if one member of a couple becomes depressed or obsessed with conceiving while the other remains less involved. The nurse may suggest involvement with infertility community support groups and contact with RESOLVE, a national education/support organization that is readily available at http://www.resolve.org/.

LIFESTYLE CHOICES AND INFERTILITY

Regular physical activity, adequate rest, stress reduction and balanced nutrition, essential strategies for health promotion, are especially important during the infertility work-up and treatment. Many seek holistic and complementary alternatives to enhance therapeutic regimens or promote a sense of personal control and well-being. Yoga is an example of a lifestyle choice that combines meditation, spirituality, exercise, and relaxation to promote balance and harmony. In addition, a number of herbal alternatives to fertility medications are available and this information may be shared with infertile couples.

 Complementary Care: *Herbal supplements and infertility*

Chaste berry tree is believed to promote ovulation; false unicorn root powder has been used to enhance fertility and prevent miscarriage. However, little research has been conducted to confirm the safety or effectiveness of these herbs and patients should be warned about the lack of scientific data about herbal preparations. Certain herbs, including blue or black cohosh, goldenseal, poke root, pennyroyal, and maloe can be detrimental to a pregnancy and should be avoided by couples who are attempting to conceive (see Table 6-4).

ADDITIONAL OPTIONS FOR THE INFERTILE COUPLE

For patients for whom advanced reproductive technologies are unsuccessful or undesirable, surrogacy, use of a gestational carrier or adoption may be the best option. Surrogate mothers contract to carry pregnancies for women who are unable to carry a pregnancy due to an

Table 6-4	Herbs to Avoid When Attempting to Achieve Pregnancy

Category	Herb
Anthraquinone Laxatives	Aloe
	Buckthorn
	Cascara sagrada
	Docks
	Meadow saffron
	Senna
Uterine Stimulants	American mandrake
	Black cohosh
	Blue cohosh
	Bloodroot
	Calamus
	Cayenne
	Fennel
	Feverfew
	Flax seed
	Goldenseal
	Lady's mantle
	Licorice
	Make fern
	Sage
	Tansy
	Thuja
	Thyme
	Wild cherry
	Wormwood
	Mayapple
	Mistletoe
	Passion flower
	Pennyroyal
	Periwinkle
	Poke root
	Rhubarb
Alkaloids/Bitter Principles	Barberry
	Bloodroot
	Celandine
	Cinchona
	Ephedra
	Goldenseal

Adapted from Herbs to avoid during pregnancy. *Pregnancy Today*. Retrieved from http://pregnancytoday.com/articles/medications-and-herbs-to-avoid-during-pregnancy-2293/

absent or anomalous uterus or medical condition that would be life threatening during pregnancy. A gestational carrier contracts to carry a pregnancy that is not genetically her own offspring. Adoption may be considered after repeated attempts for pregnancy. Today, there are fewer infants and children available for adoption. Consequently, the adoptive process is often prolonged and difficult unless the couple considers a foreign-born or physically or cognitively challenged child.

Surrogacy and the use of gestational carriers involve legal as well as ethical considerations. Financial resources, personal values, and religious beliefs are all factors that may prohibit these options from being viable alternatives to a traditional pregnancy. Individuals and couples who consider these options should be advised to see an attorney to ensure that their rights, the surrogate's/carrier's rights, and the rights of the child are protected. This very important visit for legal counsel may avoid later heartbreak and legal entanglements for the patient and her family. If the surrogate/carrier changes her mind or the parents change their minds, safeguards must be in place for all parties, including the child.

Remaining childless is another option for fertile and infertile couples. Many advantages, such as opportunity for career fulfillment, travel, and continued education make a child-free lifestyle the right choice for many couples. When working with couples who are exploring these alternative options, the nurse's role centers on education, advocacy, and empowerment. Using a framework that encompasses the cultural, spiritual, and environmental domains, the nurse provides information and guidance to community and national resources to assist the couple in dealing with these important issues.

Now Can You— **Provide sensitive, appropriate care for the infertile couple?**

1. Discuss emotions and stressors frequently experienced during infertility treatment?
2. Analyze the nurse's role in infertility care?
3. Create a teaching plan that describes the various reproductive technologies available?

summary points

◆ Sexuality is a multidimensional concept that is influenced by ethical, spiritual, cultural, and moral factors.

◆ A variety of contraceptives are available; contraceptive care should empower the patient to choose the method best suited for her.

◆ Tubal ligation and vasectomy are permanent sterilization procedures that have become increasingly popular.

◆ Infertility is the inability to conceive and carry a child when the couple wishes to do so.

◆ Abortion performed during the first trimester is safer than abortion performed during the second trimester.

◆ Reproductive alternatives include IVF, GIFT, ZIFT, oocyte/embryo donation, TDI, surrogate motherhood, and adoption.

review questions

Multiple Choice

1. The clinic nurse understands that according to Masters and Johnson's research about the four human sexual response phases, women experience the highest sense of sexual tension in the:
A. Excitement phase
B. Plateau phase
C. Orgasmic phase
D. Resolution phase

2. The Family Planning clinic nurse describes the contraceptive options for Janeen, an 18-year-old who has had a sexual partner who tested positive for HIV. Janeen has also been treated for gonorrhea. Janeen's best option for contraception would be:
A. Spermicide
B. Cervical cap
C. Latex male condom
D. Progestin-only pill

3. The clinic nurse schedules Tina for her initial dose of Depo-Provera (medroxyprogesterone acetate) within:
A. 24 hours of menstruation
B. 48 hours of menstruation
C. 3–4 days of menstruation
D. 5 days of menstruation

True/False

4. The contemporary perinatal nurse must become aware of personal feelings, values, and attitudes about sexuality in order to sensitively practice woman-centered care.

5. The clinic nurse explains to the new nurse that an intrauterine device (IUD) is believed to cause a sterile inflammatory response that results in a spermicidal intrauterine environment.

Fill-in-the-Blank

6. The first step that the clinic nurse takes when initiating the interview and sexual history from a woman is to form a _____ _____ with her.

7. During discussion about pregnancy options, the clinic nurse explains to a young couple that _____ is the term used after 12 months of unprotected intercourse with no pregnancy.

8. A young woman who is concerned about the possibility of an unwanted pregnancy inquires about emergency contraception. The nurse explains that with Plan B, ____ progestin-only pills are taken immediately with an ____-____ medication to minimize side effects.

Select All that Apply

9. When assisting a woman who is choosing a method of contraception, it is important for the clinic nurse to:
A. Assess the woman's knowledge of options.
B. Assess her motivation for different options.
C. Determine her level of commitment.
D. Ask about methods she has used in the past.

10. As a part of health promotion, the clinic nurse reviews the diet and activity levels of every woman who is using Depo-Provera (medroxyprogesterone acetate) as a contraceptive method. The clinic nurse recommends:
A. Daily weight-bearing exercise
B. 500 mg calcium daily
C. 1200 mg calcium daily
D. 1200 mg calcium daily with vitamin D

See Answers to End of Chapter Review Questions on the Electronic Study Guide or DavisPlus.

REFERENCES

American Medical Women's Association (2005). *AMWA's Statement on emergency contraception.* Retrieved from http://www.amwa-doc.org (Accessed August 9, 2005).

American Psychiatric Association (APA). (2000). *DSM IV: Diagnostic and statistical manual of mental disorders* (4th ed.). New York: American Psychiatric Press.

Arias, R.D., Kaunitz, A.M., & McClung, M.R. (2007). Depot medroxy-progesterone acetate and bone density. *Dialogues in Contraception* 11(1), 3–4.

Bachmann, G. (2007). Preventing pregnancy without hormones. *The Clinical Advisor,* 76–79.

Basson, R. (2002). A model of women's sexual arousal. *Journal of Sex and Marital Therapy,* 28(1), 1–10.

Bulechek, G., Butcher, H.M., & Dochterman, J. (2008). *Nursing interventions classification (NIC)* (5th ed.). St. Louis, MO: C.V. Mosby.

Burki, R.E. (May, 2005). Reversible hormonal contraceptives: Update. *Clinical Advisor,* 34–38.

Cates, W., & Stewart, F. (2004) Vaginal barriers. In Hatcher, R.A., Trussell, J., Stewart, F., Nelson, A., Cates, W., Guest, F. & Kowal, D. *Contraceptive technology* (18th ed.). New York: Ardent Media.

Centers for Disease Control and Prevention (CDC). (2007). *HIV and AIDS: Are you at risk?* Retrieved from http://www.cdc.gov/hiv/resources/brochures/at-risk.htm. (Accessed March 4, 2008).

Chen, P. (2004). Atrophic vaginitis. *MedlinePlus Medical Encyclopedia.* Retrieved from http://www.nlm.nih.gov/medlineplus/ency/article/000892.htm (Accessed March 2, 2006).

Clark, B., & Arias, R.D. (2007). Underuse of intrauterine contraception in the United States. *The Female Patient,* 32, 57–58.

Clark, B., & Burkman, R.T. (2006). Noncontraceptive health benefits of hormonal contraception. *The Female Patient,* 31, 42–45.

Clinician Reviews. (2006). "New Product – Implanon." 16(11), 55.

Darney, P.D., & Mishell, D.R., Jr. (2006). Etonogestrel-containing single-rod implant: A new contraceptive option. *Dialogues in Contraception,* 10(4), 6-7.

Department of Health and Human Services (DHHS). (2000). *Healthy People 2010.* Washington, DC: DHHS.

Dominguez, L., Moore, A., & Wysocki, S. (2005). The extended–cycle oral contraceptive: Six seasons and counting. *The American Journal for Nurse Practitioners,* 9(3), 55–66.

Epsey, E. (2005). Intrauterine device. *ACOG Practice Bulletin,* 59, 6.

Haffner, D.W., & Stayton, W.R. (2004). Sexuality and reproductive health. In Hatcher, R.A., Trussell, J., Stewart, F., Nelson, A., Cates, W., Guest, F., & Kowal, D. *Contraceptive technology* (18th ed.). New York: Ardent Media.

Hatcher, R.A. (2004). Depo-provera injections, implants, and progestin-only pills (minipills). In Hatcher, R.A., Trussell, J., Stewart, F., Nelson, A., Cates, W., Guest, F., & Kowal, D. *Contraceptive Technology* (18th ed.). New York: Ardent Media.

Hatcher, R., Zieman, M., Creinin, M., Stosur, H., Cwiak, C., & Darney, P. (2004a). Retrieved from http://www.managingcontraception.com/cmanager/publish/choices.shtml (Accessed April 6, 2007).

Hatcher, R.A., Zieman M., Cwiak, C., Darney, P.D., Creinin, M.D., & Stosur, H.R. (2004b). *A pocket guide to managing contraception.* New York: Ardent Media.

Herbs to avoid during pregnancy. *Pregnancy Today.* Retrieved from http://www.pregnancytoday.com/articles/medications-and-herbs-to-avoid-during-pregnancy-2293/ (Accessed September 16, 2008).

Hicks, K.M. (2004). *Women's sexual problems—A guide to integrating the "new view" approach* (Clinical Update). Retrieved from http://www.medscape.com/viewprogram/3437 (Accessed August 29, 2007).

Holloway, B., Moredich, C., & Aduddell, K. (2006). *OB peds women's health notes*. Philadelphia: F.A. Davis.

Interventions labels and definitions. *Nursing Interventions Classification (NIC)*. (4th ed.). Retrieved from http://www.nursing.uiowa.edu/centers/cncce/nic/labeldefinitions.pdf (Accessed March 2, 2006).

Johnson, M., Bulechek, G., Butcher, H., McCloskey Dochterman, J., Maas, M., Moorhead, S., & Swanson, E. (2006). *NANDA, NOC, and NIC Linkages: nursing diagnoses, outcomes, & interventions* (2nd ed.). St. Louis, MO: Mosby Elsevier.

Katz, A. (2007). Sexuality and women: The experts speak. *Nursing for Women's Health, 11*(1), 38–42.

Lever, K.A. (2005). Emergency contraception. *Lifelines, 9*(3), 218–227.

Marrazzo, J.M. (2004). Barriers to infectious disease care among lesbians. *Emerging Infectious Disease* [serial on the Internet]. Retrieved from http://www.cdc.gov/ncidod/EID/vol10no11/04-0467.htm (Accessed May 1, 2007).

Martinez, L. (2007). Effective communication: Overcoming the embarrassment. *The Female Patient, 32,* 33–35.

Masters, W., & Johnson, V.E. (1966). *Human sexual response*. Boston: Little Brown.

Mays, V.M., Yancey, A.K., Cochran, S.D., Weber, M., & Fielding, J.E. (2002). Heterogeneity of health disparities among African American, Hispanic, and Asian American women: Unrecognized influences of sexual orientation. *American Journal of Public Health, 92,* 632–639.

Mooney, B. (2005). Catalyzing conception. *Advance for Nurses, Southeastern States,* August, 25–27.

Moorehead, S., Johnson, M., Mass, M., & Swanson, E. (2008). *Nursing outcomes classification (NOC)* (4th ed.). St. Louis, MO: C.V. Mosby.

NANDA International (2007). *NANDA-I Nursing Diagnoses: Definitions and Classifications 2007-2008*. Philadelphia: NANDA-I.

Nelson, A.L., & Le, M.H.H. (2007). Modern male condoms: not your father's 'rubbers'. *The Female Patient 32,* 59–66.

Nelson, A.L., & Marshall, J.R. (2004). Impaired fertility. In Hatcher, R.A., Trussell, J., Stewart, F., Nelson, A., Cates, W., Guest, F., & Kowal, D. *Contraceptive technology* (18th ed.). New York: Ardent Media.

Potts, R.O., & Lobo, R.A. (2005). Transdermal drug delivery: clinical considerations for the obstetrician-gynecologist. *Obstetrics and Gynecology, 105*(5 pt 1), pp. 953–961.

Rice, C., & Thompson, J. (2006). Selecting a hormonal contraceptive that suits your patient's needs. *Women's Health Ob-GYN Edition*. (November–December), 26–34.

Ridley, M. (2000). *Genome*. New York: Harper Collins.

Scholes, D., LaCroix, A.Z., Ichikawa, L.E., et al. (2005). Change in bone mineral density among adolescent women using and discontinuing depot medroxyprogesterone acetate contraception. *Archives of Pediatric Adolescent Medicine, 159*(2), 139–144.

Schulman, L.P. (2007). New paradigms in hormonal contraception. *The Forum, 5*(1), 19–22.

Schulman, L.P., & Westhoff, C.L. (2006). Contraception and cancer. *Dialogues in Contraception, 10*(3), 5–8.

Smith, D.M. (2007). Emergency contraception: An update. *Dialogues in Contraception, 11*(1), 8–9.

St.Hill, P.F., Lipson, J.G., & Meleis, A.I. (2003). *Caring for women cross-culturally*. Philadelphia: F.A. Davis.

Stevens, P., & Hall, J. (2001). Sexuality and safer sex: The issue of lesbians and bisexual women. *Journal of Obstetric, Gynecologic and Neonatal Nursing, 30*(4), 439–447.

Stewart, F. H., Elbertson, C., & Cates, W. Abortion. In Hatcher, R.A., Trussell, J., Stewart, F., Nelson, A., Cates, W., Guest, F., & Kowal, D. *Contraceptive Technology* (18th ed.). New York: Ardent Media.

Trussell, J. (2004). Contraceptive efficacy. In Hatcher, R.A., Trussell, J., Stewart, F., Nelson, A., Cates, W., Guest, F., & Kowal, D. *Contraceptive technology* (18th ed.). New York: Ardent Media.

Warner, L., Hatcher, R.A., & Steiner, M.J. (2004). In Hatcher, R.A., Trussell, J., Stewart, F., Nelson, A., Cates, W., Guest, F., & Kowal, D. *Contraceptive technology* (18th ed.). New York: Ardent Media.

World Health Organization. (2004). *Medical eligibility criteria for contraceptive use* (3rd ed.). Geneva, Switzerland: World Health Organization; 2004. Retrieved from http://www.who.int/reproductive-health/publications/mec/index.htm (Accessed June 4, 2007).

 For more information, go to http://davisplus.fadavis.com/

CONCEPT MAP

Human Sexuality and Fertility

Sexual Response:
Phases:
- Excitement
- Plateau
- Orgasmic
- Resolution

Sexual Dysfunction:
Sexual stimulation that produces distress:
- Pain
- Arousal disorder
- Orgasmic disorder
- Desire disorder

Sexual Orientation:
- Heterosexual
- Homosexual
  - Gay, Lesbian

Nursing Assessment:
- Establish trusting relationship
- Be aware of own biases
- Don't make assumptions about sexual partners/ activity
- Avoid judgment → shame
- Elicit sexual history

Nursing Insight:
- Not every woman is a candidate for cervical cap
- Be proactive with health promotion strategies
- When to begin OCP in adolescents

Across Care Settings:
- Fit birth control method to the needs of special populations

Healthy People 2010 : Reproductive Life Planning
- **Decrease unwanted pregnancies**
- **Improve contraception access/use**

Infertility

Nursing Role: Infertility Care
- Assess: timing of intercourse & length of coital exposure; knowledge of fertile periods
- Assess for influencing factors: acute/chronic disease; lifestyle patterns; STIs; age
- Teach: signs of ovulation, positioning; recording basal temp
- Later assessment methods:
  - Labs: thyroid, glucose prolactin/other hormones
  - Endometrial biopsy
  - Hysterosalpingography
  - Laparoscopy
  - Semen analysis
  - Postcoital test

Managing Infertility

Fertility treatments:
Inducing ovulation:
- Medications
- Surgery
- Therapeutic insemination
- ARTs:
  - GIFT
  - ZIFT
  - TET
  - In vitro fertilization
- Embryo cryopreservation
- Micromanipulation

- Surrogacy
- Adoption
- Childless

Preventing Conception

Methods:
- NFP: Natural family planning
- Fertility awareness
  - Coitus interruptus
  - Breastfeeding
  - Abstinence
- Barriers
  - Diaphragm, cervial cap, condoms, sponge, spermaticides
- Hormones
  - OCP, patch, vaginal ring, emergency contraceptives; sub-dermal implant; injected: DMPA
- IUD
- Sterilization

Nursing: Assess Pt's
- Knowledge of method
- Comfort level
- Correct/consistent use of contraceptive
- Satisfaction with chosen method

Clinical Termination of Pregnancy

Elective and therapeutic methods:
- Surgical: D&E, vacuum suction
- Medical:
  - Mifepristone
  - Methotrexate

Nursing:
- Emotional support
- Labs; history; exam; determine gestation
- Assess for postprocedure complications
- Teach:
  - Birth control plan

Optimizing Outcomes:
- Accurate and thorough teaching about all contraceptive methods
- Specific teaching:
  - Drug/drug interactions with OCP
  - Permanent sterilization

Complementary Care:
- Use caution when trying herbs for infertility

Clinical Alert:
- Watch for short-term complications of abortion

Critical Nursing Actions:
- Teach absolute contraindications for OCP
- Teach "PAINS" to IUD users

Where Research And Practice Meet:
- Depo-Provera can decrease bone density in adolescents

Be Sure To:
- Ask about latex allergies
- Teach about toxic shock syndrome
- Teach "ACHES" for OCP users

Now Can You:
- Develop questions that will assist with taking a sexual history
- Analyze the role of the nurse in dealing with patients seeking a contraceptive method
- Discuss the nurse's overall role in reproductive health
- Provide teaching for patients regarding various reproductive technologies

chapter 7

Conception and Development of the Embryo and Fetus

 You are a child of the universe no less than the trees and the stars; you have a right to be here.
And whether or not it is clear to you, no doubt the universe is unfolding as it should.

—From the poem "Desiderata"

LEARNING TARGETS *At the completion of this chapter, the student will be able to:*

◆ Explain the basic concepts of inheritance.

◆ Outline the process of germ cell formation.

◆ Outline the process of fertilization, implantation, and placental development.

◆ Discuss the structure and function of the placenta and umbilical cord.

◆ Trace a drop of blood through the fetal circulatory system.

◆ Explain the origin and purpose of the fetal membranes and amniotic fluid.

◆ Identify the time intervals and major events of the pre-embryonic, embryonic, and fetal stages of development.

◆ Discuss threats to embryo/fetal well-being and development.

◆ Explain the nurse's role in minimizing threats to the developing fetus.

---

 moving toward evidence-based practice Vitamin E and Fetal Growth

Scholl, T.O., Chen, X., Sims, M., & Stein, T.P. (2006). Vitamin E: Maternal concentrations are associated with fetal growth. *American Journal of Clinical Nutrition, 84*(6), 1442–1448.

The purpose of this study was to examine the relationship between vitamin E and fetal growth. The researchers theorized that antioxidants such as vitamin E may decrease adverse maternal–fetal outcomes, such as preeclampsia, preterm birth, and low birth weight (LBW) by reducing oxidative damage to the mother and the fetus. Antioxidants are naturally produced by the body or are consumed in the diet. Naturally occurring vitamin E (α-tocopherol) and dietary-consumed vitamin E (γ-tocopherol) levels were examined.

The sample consisted of 1231 pregnant women from Camden, NJ who entered the study at approximately 16 weeks of gestation. Vitamin E plasma concentrations were measured at the time of entry into the study, at 20 weeks' gestation, and again at 28 weeks' gestation. The participants included women ≤18 years to 45 years of age who received prenatal care through local area clinics. Forty-nine percent of the participants were Hispanic and 39.7% were African American. Women with serious nonobstetric problems were excluded from the study.

Data collection methods included interviews and 24-hour dietary recalls along with serum concentration levels of vitamin E.

Multiple linear regression was used to examine the relationships among the plasma concentrations of vitamin E, the maternal diet, and the use of prenatal multivitamins.

Findings:

1. Women with the highest concentrations of naturally occurring and dietary vitamin E were generally older, multiparous, and tended to have a higher body mass index (BMI).

2. Obese women had lower concentrations of α-tocopherol and higher concentrations of γ-tocopherol.

(continued)

---

moving toward evidence-based practice (continued)

3. African American women had the lowest concentration of α-tocopherol compared to Hispanic, Asian, and Caucasian women.

4. Hispanic women had lower concentrations of γ-tocopherol compared to the other ethnic groups.

5. The concentration of α-tocopherol was lower in women who smoked; the serum levels rose with increasing age, intake of dietary vitamin E, and use of prenatal multivitamins.

The researchers found that: (1) plasma concentrations for the vitamin E isomers at the time of entry into the study and again at 28 weeks' gestation were positively associated with increased fetal growth, a decreased risk of small for gestational age infants, and an increased risk for large for gestational age infants. (2) Concentration of α-tocopherol was

positively associated with the maternal intake of prenatal multivitamins and a dietary intake of vitamin E. (3) The concentration of γ-tocopherol was positively associated with dietary fat intake and negatively associated with the use of multivitamins. (4) An early and late circulating concentration of α-tocopherol is positively associated with fetal growth.

---

1. This investigation was conducted in one of the poorest cities in the United States, and approximately 90% of the study participants were from minority populations. Do you believe that the study findings could be generalized to other populations?

2. How is this information useful to clinical nursing practice?

See Suggested Responses for Moving Toward Evidence-Based Practice on the Electronic Study Guide or DavisPlus.

Introduction

The beginnings of human life occur when a female gamete (ovum) unites with a male gamete (spermatozoa). The birth of a newborn signals the completion of a successful process that begins with conception (the union of a single egg and sperm) and continues throughout a remarkable period of fetal growth and development. During this time, many complex events take place. Fertilization of an ovum by a sperm creates a zygote, which must successfully implant into the hormonally prepared uterus for continued survival. The placenta plays an essential role in the ongoing transfer of oxygen and nutrients to the developing embryo and fetus. The umbilical cord that connects the developing fetus to the placenta is another key structure that facilitates the transfer of maternal oxygen and nutrients, and the removal of fetal waste products. The fetal circulatory system follows a unique pathway that allows the delivery of oxygen-rich blood from the placenta to all major organ systems while bypassing the lungs. The membranes and amniotic fluid are other important elements that are essential for successful fetal growth and development. During the gestational period, drugs, infections, and environmental hazards can have a negative impact on the developing embryo and fetus. This chapter examines the key events that take place during conception and fetal development. Threats to the embryo/fetus, influences of heredity and genetics, and the basics of multifetal pregnancy are also explored.

Basic Concepts of Inheritance

THE HUMAN GENOME PROJECT

The Human Genome Project began in 1990 with an overarching goal to identify the exact **DNA** (deoxyribonucleic acid) sequences and **genes** (segments of DNA that contain information needed to make protein) that occur in humans. The information obtained from the Human Genome Project has enabled scientists to read

the complete genetic blueprint of a human being. It is anticipated that the project findings will lead to new methods of diagnosing, treating, and perhaps even preventing a host of diverse human diseases and disorders. Additional information about the Human Genome Project can be found at http://www.genome.gov/10001772 and in Chapter 2.

 Nursing Insight— Differentiating between "genetics" and "genomics"

Genetics is the study of single genes and their effects. Genomics is the study of the functions and interactions of all genes in the **genome** (a complete copy of the genetic material in an organism) (Guttmacher & Collins, 2005). The shift from genetics to genomics may be viewed as a continuum that ranges from the concept of disease in genetics to the concept of genetic information in genomics (Khoury, 2003).

CHROMOSOMES, DNA, AND GENES

Before our present understanding of DNA, scientists noticed that traits were passed down from preceding generations. In the 19th century, Gregor Mendel proposed that the "strength" of some characteristics explains the variations in patterns of inheritance. Later in the 19th century, scientists identified **chromosomes** (threadlike packages of genes and other DNA) in the nucleus of the cell and found that one half of each pair was derived from the maternal **gamete** (mature germ cell) and one half from the paternal gamete. A number of influences help to determine who we are. These include heredity, the process of cellular division, and environmental factors.

The fundamental unit of heredity in humans is a linear sequence of working subunits of DNA called genes. DNA carries the instructions that allow cells to make proteins and transmit hereditary information from one cell to another. Most genes are located on chromosomes found in the nucleus of cells. Genes occupy a specific location along each chromosome, known as a locus. Genes come in pairs, with one copy inherited from each parent. Many genes come in a number of variant forms, known as alleles. Different alleles produce different characteristics such as hair color or blood type. One form of the allele (the dominant one) may be more greatly expressed than another form (the recessive one).

All normal somatic (body) cells contain 46 chromosomes that are arranged as 23 pairs of **homologous** or matched chromosomes. One chromosome of each pair is inherited from each parent. Twenty-two of the pairs are **autosomes** (nonsex chromosomes that are common to both males and females) and there is one pair of the sex chromosomes that determines gender (Fig. 7-1). The autosomes are involved in the transmission of all genetic traits and conditions other than those associated with the sex-linked chromosomes. The large **X chromosome** is the female chromosome; the small male chromosome is the **Y chromosome**. The presence of a Y chromosome causes the embryo to develop as a male; in the absence of a Y chromosome, the embryo develops as a female. Thus, a normal female has a 46 XX chromosome constitution; a normal male has a 46 XY chromosome constitution. The two distinct sex chromosomes carry the genes that transmit sex-linked traits and conditions. Because the chromosomes are paired, there are two copies of each gene. If the gene pairs are identical, they are **homozygous**; if they are different, they are **heterozygous**. In the heterozygous state, if one allele is expressed over the other, this allele is considered dominant. Recessive traits can be expressed when the allele responsible for the trait is found on both chromosomes.

 Nursing Insight— *Differentiating genotype from phenotype*

Although "**genotype**" refers to the genetic makeup of an individual when referring to a specific gene pair, it is sometimes used to refer to an individual's entire genetic makeup or all of the genes that a person can pass on to future generations. An individual's **genome** is the complete set of genes present (about 50,000 to 100,000). The term "**phenotype**" refers to the *observable* expression of a person's genotype: physical features, a biochemical or molecular trait, or a psychological trait. A trait or disorder is *dominant* if it is phenotypically apparent when only one copy of an allele associated with the trait is present. It is *recessive* if it is phenotypically apparent only when two copies of the alleles associated with the trait are present. Consider, for example, the inheritance of eye color. Although eye color is determined by many pairs of genes, with many possible phenotypes, one pair is considered the principal pair, with brown eyes dominant over blue eyes. A Punnett square (diagram drawn to determine the possible combinations of alleles in the offspring of a particular set of parents) may be used to illustrate inheritance of eye color (Fig. 7-2). Both parents are heterozygous for eye color; their genotype consists of a gene for brown eyes and a gene for blue eyes but their phenotype is brown eyes (Scanlon & Sanders, 2007).

The sex of the embryo is determined at fertilization and is dependent on the sperm (X or Y) that fertilizes the ovum (Fig. 7-3). The union of these highly specialized cells marks the beginning of the development of each unique human being. Clinical practice is based on a calculation of pregnancy weeks, beginning with the first day of the last normal menstrual period (LNMP). However, fertilization usually occurs approximately 2 weeks after

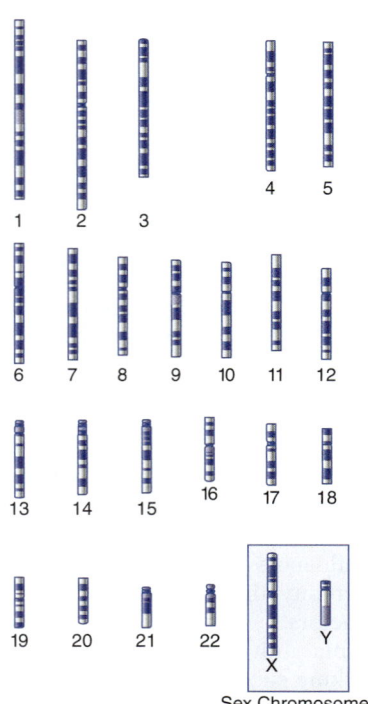

Figure 7-1 The sex chromosomes. (Courtesy of National Human Genome Research Institute.)

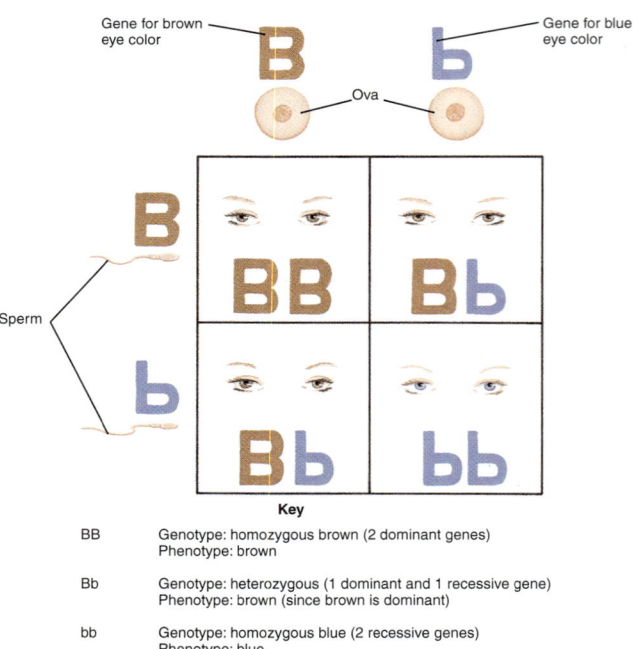

Figure 7-2 Use of a Punnett square to demonstrate inheritance of eye color.

the beginning of the woman's LNMP. **Gestation** is defined as the length of time from conception to birth. The gestational period in humans ranges from 259 to 287 days. In this chapter, the weeks of gestation are calculated from the time of fertilization.

 Nursing Insight— *Understanding abnormalities in sex chromosomes*

Turner syndrome, the most common sex chromosome deviation in females, is characterized by a chromosomal constitution of 45X: one X chromosome is missing (**monosomy X**). Affected females usually exhibit juvenile external genitalia, undeveloped ovaries, short stature, and webbing of the neck. Intelligence may be impaired. In males, *Klinefelter's syndrome*, or trisomy XXY, is the most common sex chromosome deviation. The presence of the extra X chromosome results in poorly developed male secondary sexual characteristics, small testes, and infertility. Intelligence may be impaired as well.

Inheritance of Disease

Heritable characteristics describe those that can be passed on to offspring. The manner in which genetic material is transmitted to the next generation is dependent on the number of genes involved in the expression of the trait. A number of phenotypic characteristics can result when two or more genes on different chromosomes act together (known as multifactorial inheritance). A trait or disorder may also be controlled by a single gene (referred to as unifactorial inheritance). A family pedigree, or map of family relationships, is useful for assessing the incidence of inherited disorders.

MULTIFACTORIAL INHERITANCE

The majority of congenital malformations result from multifactorial inheritance, a combination of genetic and environmental factors. Examples include malformations such as cleft lip, cleft palate, neural tube defects, pyloric stenosis,

and congenital heart disease that may range from mild to severe, depending on the number of genes for the particular defect and the amount of the environmental influence.

UNIFACTORIAL INHERITANCE

Unifactorial mendelian or single-gene inheritance describes a pattern of inheritance that results when a specific trait or disorder is controlled by a single gene. There are many more single-gene disorders than chromosomal abnormalities. Patterns of inheritance for single-gene disorders include autosomal dominant, autosomal recessive, and X-linked dominant and recessive modes of inheritance.

Autosomal Dominant Inheritance

Autosomal dominant inheritance disorders are caused by a single altered gene along one of the autosomes. In most situations, the affected individual comes from a family of multiple generations that have the disorder. The variant allele may also arise from a **mutation** (a spontaneous, permanent change in the normal gene structure). In this situation, the disorder occurs for the first time in the family. An affected parent who is heterozygous for the trait (i.e., has a corresponding healthy recessive gene for the trait) has a 50% chance of passing the variant allele to each offspring. Examples of autosomal dominant disorders include neurofibromatosis (a progressive disorder of the nervous system that causes the formation of nerve tumors throughout the body), Marfan's syndrome (a connective tissue disorder in which the child is taller and thinner than normal and has associated heart defects), Factor V Leiden mutation (a disorder that significantly increases the individual's risk for deep venous thrombosis and pulmonary emboli) (Foster, 2007; Moll, 2006), achondroplasia (dwarfism), Huntington's disease (a progressive disease of the central nervous system characterized by involuntary writhing, ballistic or dance-like movements), and facioscapulohumeral muscular dystrophy (a form of osteogenesis imperfecta, a disorder in which the bones are extremely brittle). A typical pedigree of a family with neurofibromatosis, a dominantly inherited autosomal disorder, is shown in Figure 7-4. Several human genetic diseases, with their patterns of inheritance, are described in Table 7-1.

Figure 7-3 Inheritance of gender.

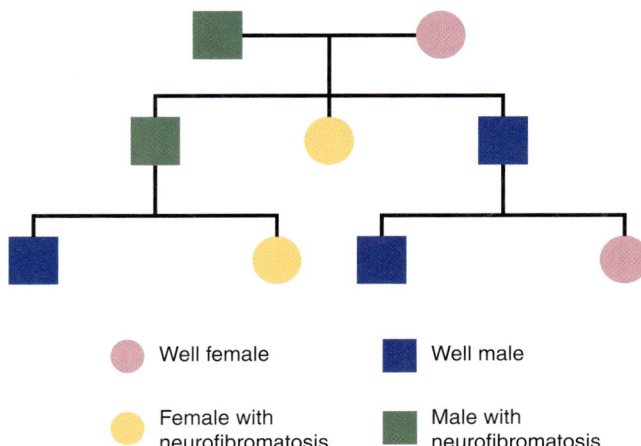

Figure 7-4 Family pedigree for neurofibromatosis, an autosomal dominant disorder.

Table 7-1 Human Genetic Diseases

Disease (Pattern of Inheritance)	Description
Sickle cell anemia (R)	The most common genetic disease among people of African ancestry. Sickle cell hemoglobin forms rigid crystals that distort and disrupt red blood cells; oxygen-carrying capacity of the blood is diminished.
Cystic fibrosis (R)	The most common genetic disease among people of European ancestry. Production of thick mucus clogs the bronchial tree and pancreatic ducts. Most severe effects are chronic respiratory infections and pulmonary failure.
Tay–Sachs disease (R)	The most common genetic disease among people of Jewish ancestry. Degeneration of neurons and the nervous system results in death by the age of 2 years.
Phenylketonuria of PKU (R)	Lack of an enzyme to metabolize the amino acid phenylalanine leads to severe mental and physical retardation. These effects may be prevented by the use of a diet (beginning at birth) that limits phenylalanine.
Huntington's disease (D)	Uncontrollable muscle contractions begin between the ages of 30 and 50 years, followed by loss of memory and personality. There is no treatment that can delay mental deterioration.
Hemophilia (X-linked)	Lack of Factor 8 impairs chemical clotting; may be controlled with Factor 8 from donated blood.
Duchenne's muscular dystrophy (X-linked)	Replacement of muscle by adipose or scar tissue, with progressive loss of muscle function; often fatal before age 20 years due to involvement of cardiac muscle.

R = recessive; D = dominant.
Source: Scanlon, V.C. and Sanders, T. (2007). *Essentials of anatomy and physiology* (5th ed., p. 490). Philadelphia: F.A. Davis.

Autosomal Recessive Inheritance

Autosomal recessive inheritance disorders are expressed in an individual when both members of an autosomal gene pair are altered. Although each parent carries the recessive altered gene, neither is affected by the disorder because each is heterozygous for the trait and the altered gene is not expressed. When two individuals carrying the same recessive altered gene reproduce, both may pass the altered gene to their offspring. Each parent, or **carrier,** of the autosomal recessive disorder, has a 25% risk of passing the disorder to each offspring, who will then have no normal gene to carry out the necessary function. Because parents must pass the same altered gene for expression of the disorder to occur in their children, an increased incidence of the disorder occurs in consanguineous matings (closely related parents). In addition, specific populations may have a greater frequency of recessive disorders than other populations. For example, sickle cell anemia occurs more frequently in African American populations than in Caucasian populations. A Punnett square illustrating the inheritance pattern of sickle cell anemia is presented in Figure 7-5. Other examples of autosomal recessive inheritance disorders include galactosemia, phenylketonuria (PKU), maple syrup urine disease, Tay–Sachs disease, and cystic fibrosis (CF).

X-Linked Dominant Inheritance

X-linked dominant inheritance disorders are the result of an alteration in a gene located along an X chromosome (Fig. 7-6). Since females have two X chromosomes, these disorders occur twice as frequently in females as in males. When the gene is dominant, it need be present on only one of the X chromosomes for symptoms of the disorder to be expressed. X-linked dominant disorders are passed from an affected male to all of his daughters, because the daughters receive the father's altered X chromosome. Conversely, none of the sons are affected because they receive only the father's Y chromosome.

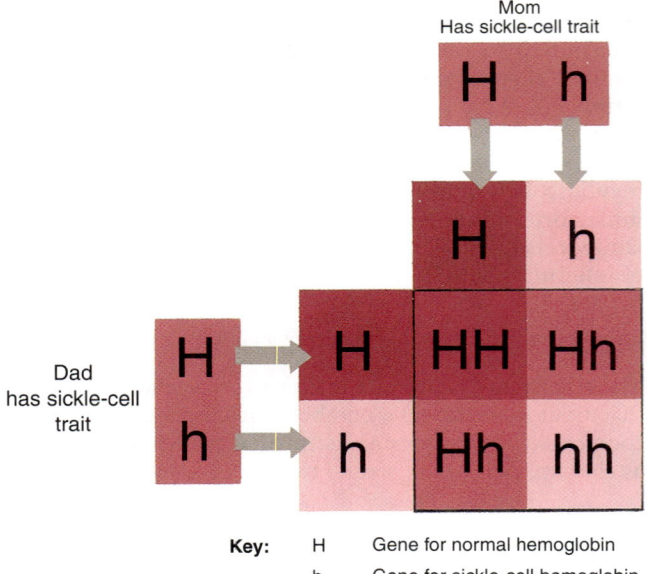

Figure 7-5 Inheritance of sickle cell anemia, an autosomal recessive disorder.

A female with an X-linked dominant disorder has a 50% chance of passing the altered genes to her offspring. Each child of a female with the X-linked dominant disorder has a 1 in 2 chance of expressing the disorder. Examples of X-linked dominant disorders include hypophosphatemia (vitamin D-resistant rickets) and cervico-oculo-acoustic syndrome.

X-Linked Recessive Inheritance

X-linked recessive inheritance disorders are more common than X-linked dominant disorders and occur more frequently in males because males have a single X chromosome and the single X chromosome carries the altered

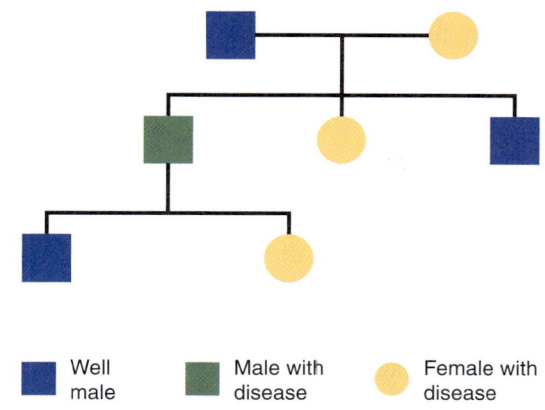

Figure 7-6 Family pedigree for X-linked dominant inheritance.

Key:
- Well male
- Male with disease
- Female with disease

Mom
Carrier of color blindness

Dad
Normal color vision

Key:

XX	X chromosome with gene for normal color vision
Y	Y chromosome (has no gene for color vision)
Xc	X chromosome with gene for red-green color blindness

Figure 7-7 Inheritance of red-green color blindness.

gene. Thus, when the male receives a "single dose" of the altered gene, the disorder is expressed. For the disorder to be expressed in the female, the altered gene must be present on both X chromosomes.

A female who is a carrier of a gene that causes an X-linked recessive disorder has a 50% risk of passing the abnormal gene to her male offspring. Each son has a 1 in 2 chance of expressing the disorder. The female carrier also has a 50% chance of passing the altered gene to her female offspring, who will have a 1 in 2 chance of becoming carriers of the altered gene. A son who is affected by an X-linked disorder has a 100% chance of passing the variant X to his daughters since the affected father has only one X to pass on. Fathers cannot transmit the altered gene to their male offspring because they transmit the Y instead of the X chromosome to their sons. The Punnet square in Figure 7-7 illustrates the inheritance pattern for red-green color blindness, an X-linked recessive inheritance disorder. Other X-linked recessive inheritance disorders include hemophilia A, Duchenne's (pseudohypertrophic) muscular dystrophy and Christmas disease, a blood-factor deficiency (Lashley, 2005).

 Now Can You— Discuss aspects of patterns of inheritance?

1. Differentiate between unifactorial and multifactorial patterns of inheritance?
2. Compare and contrast autosoma dominant, autosomal recessive, and X-linked inheritance disorders?
3. Construct a Punnett square to illustrate inheritance patterns for a dominant trait?

Cellular Division

Human cells can be categorized into either gametes (sperm and egg cells) or somatic cells (any body cell that contains 46 chromosomes in its nucleus). Gametes are haploid cells. They have only one member of each chromosome pair and contain 23 chromosomes. Somatic cells are diploid, which means that they contain chromosome pairs (a total of 46 chromosomes). One member of each pair comes from the mother, and one member comes from the father. Cells reproduce through either meiosis or mitosis. **Meiosis** is a process of cell division that leads to the development of sperm and ova, each containing half the number (haploid) of chromosomes as normal cells. **Mitosis** is the process of the formation of two identical cells that are exactly the same as the original cell and have the normal (diploid) amount of chromosomes.

Meiosis occurs during gametogenesis, the process in which germ cells, or gametes, are produced. During cell division, the genetic complement of the cells is reduced by one half. During meiosis, a sex cell containing 46 chromosomes (the diploid number of chromosomes) divides into two, and then four cells, each containing 23 chromosomes (a haploid number of chromosomes). The resulting "daughter cells" are exactly alike, but they are all different from the original cell. The process of meiosis includes two completely different cell divisions. During the first cell division, the chromosomes replicate each of the 46 chromosomes (diploid number of chromosomes). The chromosomes then become closely intertwined and the sharing of genetic material occurs. New combinations are produced, and this process accounts for the variations of traits in individuals. Next, the chromosomes separate and the cell divides and forms two daughter cells, each containing 23 double structured chromosomes (the same amount of DNA as a normal somatic cell).

In the second division, each chromosome divides and each half (or chromatid) moves to opposite sides of the cell. The cells divide and form four cells containing 23 single chromosomes each, a haploid number of chromosomes, or half the number of chromosomes present in the somatic cell. Gametes must contain the haploid number of chromosomes. When the female and male gametes unite to form a fertilized ovum (zygote), the normal (diploid) number of 46 chromosomes is reestablished. The entire process results in the creation of four haploid gamete cells from one diploid sex cell.

Mitosis is the phase in the cell cycle that permits duplication of two genetically identical daughter cells each containing the diploid number of chromosomes. The process of mitosis allows each daughter cell to inherit the exact human genome.

The Process of Fertilization

Fertilization is a complex series of events. Transportation of gametes must occur to allow the oocyte and the sperm to meet. Most often, this meeting takes place in the ampulla of the uterine (fallopian) tube (Fig. 7-8).

After completion of the first meiotic division, the secondary oocyte is expelled from the ovary during ovulation. The oocyte then makes its way to the infundibulum (funnel-shaped passage) at the end of the fallopian tube and passes into the ampulla of the tube. At the time of ejaculation, about 200 to 600 million sperm are deposited around the external cervical os and in the fornix of the vagina. During ovulation, the amount of cervical mucus increases and it becomes less viscous and more favorable for sperm penetration. Propelled by the flagellar movement of their tails, sperm travel into the uterus and upward through the fallopian tubes. Muscular contractions of the tubal walls, believed to be enhanced by prostaglandins in the semen, facilitate the sperm movement. The fallopian tubes are lined with **cilia**, hairlike projections from the epithelial cells that serve a dual action: movement of the ovum toward the uterus and movement of the sperm from the uterus toward the ovary. Of the 200 to 600 million sperm deposited, approximately 200 actually reach the fertilization site.

Sperm must undergo a process called capacitation, whereby a glycoprotein coat and seminal proteins are removed from the surface of the sperm's acrosome (the caplike structure surrounding the head of the sperm). The sperm become more active during this process of capacitation, which takes about 7 hours and usually occurs in the fallopian tube but may begin in the uterus. An acrosome reaction occurs when the capacitated sperm comes into contact with the zona pellucida surrounding the secondary oocyte. During the acrosome reaction, enzymes from the sperm's head are released. This helps to create a pathway through the zona pellucida, allowing the sperm to reach the egg and fertilization to occur.

Once a sperm penetrates through the zona pellucida, a reaction takes place to prevent fertilization by other sperm. The oocyte then undergoes its second meiotic division and forms a mature oocyte and secondary polar body. The nucleus of the mature oocyte becomes the female pronucleus. The sperm loses its tail within the cytoplasm of the oocyte, and then enlarges to become the male pronucleus. Fusion of pronuclei of both the oocyte and sperm create a single zygote containing the diploid number of chromosomes. The zygote is genetically unique in that it contains half of its chromosomes from the mother and half from the father.

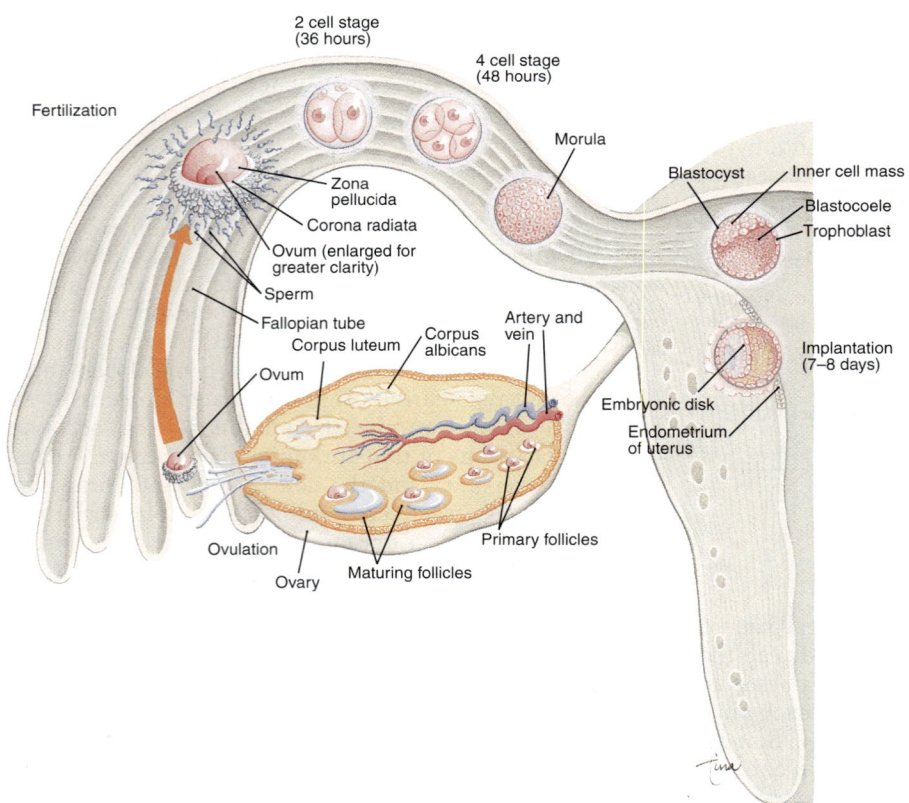

Figure 7-8 Ovulation, fertilization, and early embryonic development.

Collaboration in Caring— Impaired fecundity

According to the National Center for Health Statistics (NCHS), in 2002, 7.3 million women between the ages of 15 and 44 had "impaired fecundity," meaning it was difficult or impossible to get pregnant or carry a fetus to term (NCHS, 2006). Infertility is a widespread problem and treatment may include referrals to internal medicine, endocrinology, obstetrics, urology, and psychiatry. Infertility is usually first identified by the gynecologist/obstetrician. A referral to internal medicine may be recommended to optimize the health status of both partners. A reproductive endocrinologist specializes in infertility. Treatments offered by an endocrinologist include fertility drugs, infertility surgery, and assisted reproductive therapy. Routine screening (including laboratory tests) is conducted on both partners to identify the possible cause of infertility. Abnormalities identified in the male partner may involve the care of the urologist.

The Process of Implantation and Placental Development

After conception, the fertilized ovum, or zygote, remains in the ampulla for 24 hours and then, propelled by ciliary action, travels toward the uterus. During this time, cleavage (mitotic cell division of the zygote) occurs. By 3 to 4 days after fertilization, there are approximately 16 cells. The zygote is now called a **morula**, and enters the uterus. Once the morula enters the uterus, fluid passes through the zona pellucida, into the intercellular spaces of the inner cell mass and forms a large fluid-filled cavity. The morula is now called a **blastocyst** and contains an inner mass of cells called the embryoblast. The embryo develops from the embryoblast, and contains an outer cell layer called the trophoblast. The chorion and placenta develop from the trophoblast.

 Nursing Insight— Understanding the origin of embryonic stem cells

The cells of the inner cell mass are termed embryonic stem cells. In these cells, all of the DNA has the potential to develop into any of the 200 kinds of human cells that will be present at birth. As the cells continue to divide and increase in number, some DNA will be "switched off" in each cell, the genes will become inactive and the possibilities for specialization of each cell will decrease (Scanlon & Sanders, 2007).

The uterus secretes a mixture of lipids, mucopolysaccharides, and glycogen that nourishes the blastocyst. The zona pellucida degenerates approximately 5 to 6 days after fertilization. This process allows the blastocyst to adhere to the endometrial surface of the uterus (usually in the upper posterior portion) to obtain nutrients. Implantation begins as the trophoblast cells invade the endometrium. By the tenth day after fertilization, **nidation** (implantation of the fertilized ovum into the endometrium) has occurred and the blastocyst is buried beneath the endometrial surface.

The placenta develops from the trophoblast cells at the site of implantation. This important organ is essential for the transfer of nutrients and oxygen to the fetus and the removal of waste products from the fetus, and any alteration in its function can adversely affect growth and development. As the trophoblast cells invade the endometrium, spaces termed lacunae develop. The lacunae fill with fluid from ruptured maternal capillaries and endometrial glands. This fluid nourishes the embryoblast by the process of diffusion. The lacunae later become the intervillous spaces of the placenta. At about the same time, the trophoblast cells form primary **chorionic villi**, small nonvascular processes that absorb nutritive materials for growth. Blood vessels begin to develop in the chorionic villi around the third week and a primitive fetoplacental circulation is established.

The trophoblast cells continue to invade the endometrium until 25 to 35 days after fertilization, when they reach the maternal spiral arterioles. Spurts of maternal blood form hollows around the villi, creating **intervillous spaces** containing reservoirs of blood that supply the developing embryo and fetus with oxygen and nutrients. The placenta has become well established by 8 to 10 weeks after conception. By 4 months, the placenta has reached maximal thickness although circumferential growth progresses as the fetus continues to grow. The placenta is responsible for providing oxygenation, nutrition, waste elimination, and hormones necessary to maintain the pregnancy (Fig. 7-9).

The placenta is a metabolic organ with its own substrate needs. Metabolic activities of the placenta include glycolysis, gluconeogenesis, glycogenesis, oxidation, protein synthesis, amino acid interconversion, triglyceride synthesis, and lengthening or shortening of fatty acid chains. The placenta uptakes glucose, synthesizes estrogens and progesterone from cholesterol, and uses fatty acids for oxidation and membrane formation. Placental transport of gases, nutrients, wastes, and other substances occurs in a bidirectional movement from maternal to fetal circulation, and from fetal to maternal circulation. Transport across the placenta increases with gestation due to the decreased distance between the fetal and maternal blood, increased blood flow, and increased needs of the developing fetus.

There are several mechanisms by which substances are transported across the placenta. These include simple (passive) diffusion, facilitated diffusion, active diffusion, pinocytosis and endocytosis, bulk flow, accidental capillary breaks, and independent movement. Pinocytosis is the process by which cells absorb or ingest nutrients and fluid; endocytosis is a method of ingestion of a foreign substance by a cell wall (Venes, 2009).

- Simple diffusion: Substances transported via this mechanism include water, electrolytes, oxygen, carbon dioxide, urea, simple amines, fatty acids, steroids, fat-soluble vitamins, narcotics, antibiotics, barbiturates, and anesthetics.
- Facilitated diffusion: Substances transported are glucose and oxygen.

Figure 7-9 Placenta and umbilical cord.

- Active transport: Substances transported via this mechanism include amino acids, water-soluble vitamins, calcium, iron, and iodine.
- Pinocytosis and endocytosis: Globulins, phospholipids, lipoproteins, antibodies, and viruses use these mechanisms of transport.
- Bulk flow and solvent drag: Water and electrolytes use these mechanisms of transport.
- Accidental capillary breaks: Facilitate the transport of intact blood cells.
- Independent movement: Maternal leukocytes and microorganisms such as *Treponema pallidum* use this mechanism of transport.

Placental endocrine activity plays a crucial role in maintaining the pregnancy. The four main hormones produced by the placenta are human chorionic gonadotrophin (hCG), human placental lactogen (hPL), progesterone, and estrogens. Human chorionic gonadotropin maintains the corpus luteum (a structure that secretes progesterone) during early pregnancy until the placenta has sufficiently developed to produce adequate amounts of progesterone. Human placental lactogen regulates glucose availability for the fetus and promotes fetal growth by altering maternal protein, carbohydrate, and fat metabolism. Progesterone helps to suppress maternal immunological responses to fetal antigens, thereby preventing maternal rejection of the fetus. Progesterone has a number of additional functions: decreases myometrial activity and irritability, constricts myometrial vessels, decreases maternal sensitivity to carbon dioxide, inhibits prolactin secretion, relaxes smooth muscle in the gastrointestinal and urinary systems, increases basal body temperature, and increases maternal sodium and chloride secretion.

Estrogen production increases significantly during pregnancy. This essential hormone enhances myometrial activity, promotes myometrial vasodilation, increases maternal respiratory center sensitivity to carbon dioxide, softens fibers in the cervical collagen tissue, increases the pituitary secretion of prolactin, increases serum binding proteins and fibrinogen, decreases plasma proteins, and increases sensitivity of the uterus to progesterone in late pregnancy.

The placenta also plays an important role in protecting the fetus from pathogens and in preventing maternal rejection of the pregnancy. Although many bacteria are too large to pass through the placenta, most viruses and some bacteria are able to cross the placenta. Maternal antibodies (i.e., all subclasses of IgG) transit the placenta primarily by pinocytosis; others cross by the process of diffusion. Although the fetus has a unique genetic makeup that is different from the mother's, maternal rejection of the fetus usually does not occur. The exact reason for this phenomenon is not known.

Development of the Embryo and Fetus

THE YOLK SAC

Early in the pregnancy, the embryo is a flattened disk that is situated between the **amnion** (thick membrane that forms the amniotic sac that surrounds the embryo and fetus) and the yolk sac. The yolk sac is a structure that develops in the embryo's inner cell mass around day 8 or 9 after conception. It is essential for the transfer of nutrients to the embryo during the second and third weeks of gestation when development of the uteroplacental circulation is underway. **Hematopoiesis** (formation and development of red blood cells) occurs in the wall of the yolk sac beginning in the third week. This function gradually declines after the eighth gestational week when the fetal liver begins to take over this process. As the pregnancy progresses, the yolk sac atrophies and is incorporated into the umbilical cord. Key events that take place during early development of the embryo are shown in Figure 7-10.

Approximately 12 days
— Embryonic disk

Approximately 14 days
— Embryonic disk

Approximately 20 days
Head of embryo
Chorionic villi

Approximately 4–5 weeks
Head of embryo
Umbilical cord
Limb buds

Endometrium
Trophoblast
Amnion
Yolk sac
Embryo
Placenta
Chorion

Figure 7-10 Key events during early development of the embryo.

ORIGIN AND FUNCTION OF THE UMBILICAL CORD

During the time of placental development, the umbilical cord is also being formed. The body stalk connects the embryo to the yolk sac that contains blood vessels connecting to the chorionic villi. The vessels contract to form two arteries and one vein as the body stalk elongates and develops into the umbilical cord. Maternal blood flows through the uterine arteries and into the intervillous spaces of the placenta. The blood returns through the uterine veins and into the maternal circulation. Fetal blood flows through the umbilical arteries and into the villous capillaries of the placenta. The blood returns through the umbilical vein and into the fetal circulation. **Wharton's jelly** is a specialized connective tissue that surrounds the two arteries and one vein in the umbilical cord. This tissue, in addition to the high volume and pressure in the blood vessels, is important because it helps to protect the umbilical cord from compression. Most umbilical cords have a central insertion site into the placenta and at term are approximately 21 inches (55 cm) long with a diameter that ranges from 0.38 to 0.77 inch (1 to 2 cm).

Now Can You— Discuss characteristics of growth in the embryo/fetus?

1. Identify where the developing embryo obtains nutrients prior to development of the feto–maternal circulatory placental unit?

2. Describe seven mechanisms used for the transport of nutrients across the placenta?
3. Discuss how human placental lactogen (hPL) promotes fetal growth?

THE FETAL CIRCULATORY SYSTEM

The embryo receives nutrition from maternal blood by diffusion through the extraembryonic coelom (fluid-filled cavity surrounding the amnion and yolk sac) and the yolk sac by the end of the second week. Blood vessels begin to develop in the yolk sac during the beginning of the third week and embryonic blood vessels begin to develop about two days later. A primordial heart tube joins with blood vessels in the embryo, connecting the body stalk, chorion, and yolk sac to form a primitive cardiovascular system. The heart begins to beat and blood begins to circulate by the end of the third week.

During the third week, capillaries develop in the chorionic villi and become connected to the embryonic heart through vessels in the chorion and the connecting stalk. By the end of the third week, embryonic blood begins to flow through capillaries in the chorionic villi. Oxygen and nutrients from maternal blood diffuse through the walls in the villi and enter the embryo's blood. Carbon dioxide and waste products diffuse from blood in the embryo's capillaries through the wall of the chorionic villi and into the maternal blood. The umbilical cord is formed from the connecting stalk during the fourth week.

Blood travels through the fetus in a unique way. The umbilical cord contains three vessels: two arteries and one vein. Blood flows through the vein from the placenta to the fetus. A small amount of blood flows through the liver and then empties into the inferior vena cava. Most of the blood bypasses the liver and then enters the inferior vena cava by way of the **ductus venosus**, a vascular channel that connects the umbilical vein to the inferior vena cava. The blood then empties into the right atrium, passes through the **foramen ovale** (an opening in the septum between the right and left atrium) into the left atrium, then moves into the left ventricle and on into the aorta. From the aorta, blood travels to the head, upper extremities, and lower extremities. Blood returning from the head enters the superior vena cava, then the right atrium and the right ventricle before entering the pulmonary artery. Most of the blood that enters the pulmonary artery bypasses the lungs and enters the aorta through the **ductus arteriosus**, a vascular channel between the pulmonary artery and descending aorta. The remaining blood flows to the pulmonary circulation to support lung development. The blood then returns through the pulmonary vein to the left atrium, the left ventricle, to the aorta, and returns to the placenta through the two arteries. Most of the blood in the lower extremities enters the internal iliac artery and the umbilical arteries to the placenta to be re-oxygenated and re-circulated. Some of the blood in the lower extremities passes back to the ascending vena cava and is mixed with oxygenated blood from the placenta without being oxygenated.

The placenta is the site of oxygenation and waste elimination. Blood travels through the umbilical vein from the placenta to the fetus (Fig. 7-11). There are three shunts unique to fetal circulation:

1. Some blood circulates through the liver, but most bypasses the liver through the *ductus venosus* and enters the inferior vena cava.
2. Blood from the superior vena cava enters the right atrium, passes through the *foramen ovale*, through the right ventricle and into the aorta, supplying blood to the head and upper and lower extremities.
3. Blood returning from the head enters the right atrium, and then flows through the right ventricle and into the pulmonary artery. Most of this blood bypasses the lungs through the *ductus arteriosus*. A small amount of blood flows through the pulmonary circulation, back into the right atrium, right ventricle, and then into the aorta.

The arterial Po_2 of the fetus is about one-fourth of the maternal Po_2 because of the structure and function of the placenta (i.e., oxygenation of fetal blood takes place at a low Po_2), and because arterial blood in the fetal circulation is formed by the mixing of maternal oxygenated blood with fetal deoxygenated blood. Fetal hemoglobin has a lower oxygen content than that of the adult. The highest oxygen concentration (Po_2 = 30 to 35 mm Hg) is found in the blood returning from the placenta via the umbilical vein; the lowest oxygen concentration occurs in blood shunted to the placenta where re-oxygenation takes place. The blood with the highest oxygen content is delivered to the fetal heart, head, neck, and upper limbs, while the blood with the lowest oxygen content is shunted

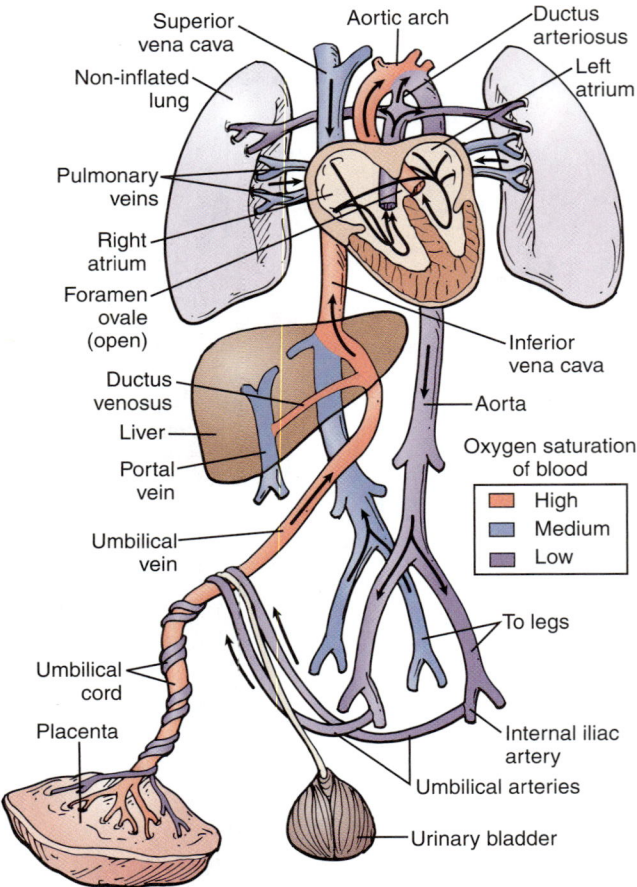

Superior vena cava — Aortic arch — Ductus arteriosus — Left atrium — Non-inflated lung — Pulmonary veins — Right atrium — Foramen ovale (open) — Ductus venosus — Liver — Portal vein — Umbilical vein — Umbilical cord — Placenta — Inferior vena cava — Aorta — To legs — Internal iliac artery — Umbilical arteries — Urinary bladder

Oxygen saturation of blood
- High
- Medium
- Low

Figure 7-11 Fetal circulation.

toward the placenta. The low Po_2 level is important in maintaining fetal circulation, as it keeps the ductus arteriosus open and the pulmonary vascular bed constricted. Fetal hemoglobin enables the fetus to adapt to the lowered Po_2. This unique type of hemoglobin has a high affinity for oxygen at low tensions, which improves saturation and facilitates oxygen transport to the fetal tissues. The increased perfusion rate (as compared to the adult) also helps to compensate for the lower oxygen saturations and increased oxygen–hemoglobin affinity.

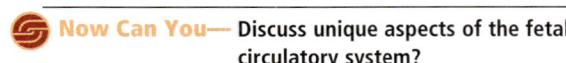 **Now Can You—** **Discuss unique aspects of the fetal circulatory system?**

1. Name the three shunts found in the fetal circulatory system?
2. Identify where the highest and lowest fetal oxygen concentrations are found?
3. Explain how fetal hemoglobin is unique?

FETAL MEMBRANES AND AMNIOTIC FLUID

The embryonic membranes (chorion and amnion) are early protective structures that begin to form at the time of implantation. The thick **chorion**, or outer membrane, forms first. It develops from the trophoblast and encloses the amnion, embryo, and yolk sac. The chorion contains fingerlike projections (chorionic villi) that may be used for genetic testing (chorionic villus sampling) during the first trimester. The villi beneath the embryo grow and branch out into depressions in the wall of the uterus, and from this structure, the fetal portion of the placenta is formed.

The amnion arises from the ectoderm during early embryonic development. This membrane is a thin, protective structure that contains the amniotic fluid. The amniotic cavity, or space between the amnion and the embryo, houses the embryo and yolk sac, except in the area where the developing embryo attaches to the trophoblast via the umbilical cord. With embryonic growth, the amnion expands and comes into contact with the chorion. The two fetal membranes are slightly adherent and form the amniotic fluid-filled sac (the **amniotic sac**), also called the bag of waters. The fetal membranes provide a barrier of protection from ascending infection.

Amniotic fluid is vital for fetal growth and development. It cushions the fetus and protects against mechanical injury, helps the fetus to maintain a normal body temperature, allows for symmetrical fetal growth, prevents adherence of the amnion to the fetus, and aids in fetal musculoskeletal development by providing freedom of movement. It is essential for normal fetal lung development. The amniotic fluid volume is dynamic, constantly changing as the fluid moves back and forth across the placental membrane.

Amniotic fluid first appears at about 3 weeks. Approximately 30 mL of amniotic fluid are present at 10 weeks' gestation, and this amount increases to approximately 800 mL at 24 weeks' gestation. After that time, the total fluid volume remains fairly stable until it begins to decrease slightly as the pregnancy reaches term.

During late gestation, fetal urine and fetal lung secretions are the primary contributors to the total amniotic fluid volume. Fetal swallowing and absorption through the placenta are the primary pathways for amniotic fluid clearance. The fetus swallows approximately 600 mL every 4 hours and up to 400 mL of amniotic fluid flows from the fetal lungs every 24 hours. Amniotic fluid is slightly alkaline and contains antibacterial and other protective substances similar to those found in maternal breast milk (e.g., transferrin, beta-lysin, peroxidase, fatty acids, immunoglobulins [IgG and IgA], and lysozyme). It also contains albumin, uric acid, creatinine, lecithin, sphingomyelin, bilirubin, vernix, leukocytes, epithelial cells, and **lanugo** (fine, downy hair).

 Now Can You— Discuss aspects of the amniotic sac and amniotic fluid?

1. Identify the origins of the embryonic membranes?
2. Name five functions of the amniotic fluid?
3. Discuss where amniotic fluid originates?

Human Growth and Development

Major organs are formed (organogenesis) during the first 8 weeks after fertilization. During this time, the developing organism is called an **embryo.** By the end of eight weeks, the embryo has sufficiently developed to be called a **fetus**. Human development proceeds in a cephalocaudal pattern of maturation: motor development, control, and coordination progress from the head to the feet.

The loss of a fetus before 20 to 22 weeks' gestation (less than 500 grams) is referred to as an abortion because the fetus is considered too immature to survive the **extrauterine** (outside of the uterus) environment. A fetus born before the completion of 37 weeks is considered to be preterm or premature.

PRE-EMBRYONIC PERIOD

The pre-embryonic period refers to the first 2 weeks of human development after conception. Rapid cellular multiplication, cell differentiation, and establishment of the embryonic membranes and primary germ layers occur during this time. Development takes place in a pattern that is cephalocaudal, proximal to distal and general to specific.

EMBRYONIC PERIOD

Critical development that occurs during the embryonic period involves cleavage of the zygote, blastogenesis (early development characterized by cleavage and formation of three germ layers that later develop into tissues and organs), and the early development of the nervous system, cardiovascular system, and all major internal and external structures. The pre-embryonic period refers to the first 2 weeks beginning at fertilization, which for most is approximately 2 weeks after the last normal menstrual period. The embryonic period is the time period beginning with the third week after fertilization and continuing until the end of the eighth week. This period is known as the organogenetic period that denotes the formation and differentiation of organs and organ systems.

Week 1

Fertilization usually occurs in the outer third portion of the uterine tube. The zygote then travels toward the uterus, while undergoing cleavage (series of mitotic cell division) and forming blastomeres (cells formed from the first mitotic division). Approximately 3 days after fertilization, a morula (a ball of 12 or more blastomeres) enters the uterus. A cavity forms within the morula, creating a blastocyst that consists of a trophoblast that encloses both the embryoblast (gives rise to the embryo and some extraembryonic tissues) and the blastocystic cavity (fluid-filled space). The trophoblast begins to invade the uterus and the blastocyst is superficially implanted by the end of the first week.

Week 2

The trophoblast undergoes rapid proliferation and differentiation as the blastocyst continues the process of uterine implantation. The yolk sac develops, the amniotic cavity appears, and the embryoblast differentiates into the bilaminar embryonic disk. Implantation of the blastocyst is completed by the end of the second week.

Week 3

The third week is characterized by the appearance of a primitive streak (proliferation and migration of cells to the central posterior region of the embryonic disk), the development of the notochord (cellular rod along the dorsal surface that will later be surrounded by vertebrae), and differentiation of the three germ layers: embryonic **ectoderm** (outer layer, gives rise to skin, teeth, and glands of the mouth and nervous system), **endoderm** (inner layer, gives rise to epithelium of the respiratory, digestive and genitourinary tracts), and **mesoderm** (lies between the ectoderm and endoderm; gives rise to the connective tissue) (Table 7-2).

A & P review Formation of the Primary Germ Layers

Implantation of the blastocyst occurs at approximately 7 to 8 days after conception. At this time, the cells of the embryonic disk are separated from the amnion by a fluid-filled space. The syncytiotrophoblast continue to erode the endometrium and implantation is completed by the ninth day. The extraembryonic mesoderm forms a discrete layer beneath the cytotrophoblast. By the 16th day, all three germ layers are present, along with a yolk sac and the allantois, an outpouching of the yolk sac that forms the structural basis of the body stalk, or umbilical cord. The chorion arises from the cytotrophoblast and associated mesoderm and contains many fingerlike projections (chorionic villi) on its surface. ◆

Week 4

At the beginning of the fourth week, the flat trilaminar embryonic disk folds into a C-shaped, cylindrical embryo. Development continues as the three germ layers differentiate into various organs and tissues. By 28 postovulatory days, four limb buds and a closed otic vesicle (later develops into labyrinth of inner ear) are present (Fig. 7-12).

During the third and fourth weeks, development of the nervous system is well underway. A thickened portion of the ectoderm develops into the neural plate. The top portion will differentiate into the **neural tube**, which forms the central nervous system (brain and spinal cord) and the neural crest, which will develop into the peripheral nervous system. Later, the eye and inner ear develop as projections of the original neural tube. During the early period of development, the embryo's nervous system is particularly vulnerable to environmental insults.

Figure 7-12 Embryo at 4 weeks' gestation (28 postovulatory days). All four limb buds are present. (Smith, B.R. (2008). The multidimensional human embryo, Carnegie Stages. Retrieved from http://embryo.soad.umich.edu/carnstages/)

⟳ Optimizing Outcomes— Preventing neural tube defects

Defective closure of the neural tube during the fourth week of development results in a condition known as a **neural tube defect** (NTD). This is a malformation that involves defects in the skull and spinal column and is primarily caused by failure of the neural tube to close. Tissues overlying the spinal cord including the meninges, vertebral arches, muscles, and skin may be affected as well. Neural tube defects include rachischisis (spina bifida), myelocele, myelomeningocele, and meningocele. Immediate surgical repair is often necessary after birth. NTDs are the second most frequent structural fetal malformation and occur in 1 to 2 per 1000 live births (Cunningham et al., 2005). Folic acid supplementation has been found to decrease the incidence of NTDs (Evans, Llurba, Landsberger, O'Brien, & Harrison, 2004). Currently, the United States Public Health Service recommends that all women of childbearing age who are capable of becoming pregnant consume 0.4 mg of folic acid daily to reduce the incidence of neural tube defects.

Week 8

By the end of the eighth week, there is a clear distinction between the upper and lower limbs, the external genitals are well developed, although not always well enough to distinguish the gender, and the embryo has a human appearance (Fig. 7-13). The main organ systems have also begun to develop by the end of 8 weeks. Except for the cardiovascular system, however, there is minimal function of most of the organ systems.

⟳ Now Can You— Discuss the pre-embryonic and embryonic periods of development?

1. Define the pre-embryonic period and identify the pattern of human development that occurs?
2. Identify what time frame is encompassed in the embryonic period?
3. Describe the major developmental events that have occurred by the end of the eighth week?

THE FETAL PERIOD

The beginning of the ninth week marks the beginning of the fetal period when the embryo has now developed into a recognizable human being. The fetal period is character-

Table 7-2 Derivatives of the Three Germ Layers		
Ectoderm	**Mesoderm**	**Endoderm**
Epidermis, epithelium of mouth, oral glands, teeth, and organs of special sense	Smooth muscle coats, connective tissues, and vessels associated with tissues and organs	Epithelium of the pharynx, thyroid, thymus, parathyroid, respiratory passages, gastrointestinal tract, liver and pancreas
Central nervous system	Blood	
Peripheral nervous system	Bone marrow	
Hypophysis	Muscular tissues	
Suprarenal medulla	Skeletal tissues	
	Suprarenal cortex	

Figure 7-13 The embryo at 8 weeks (56 to 57 postovulatory days) has a human appearance. (Smith, B.R. [2008]. The multidimensional human embryo, Carnegie Stages. Retrieved from http://embryo.soad.umich.edu/carnstages/)

ized by rapid body growth and differentiation of tissues, organs, and systems. The rate of head growth during this period of time slows down as compared to the rate of body growth. During the last 12 weeks of pregnancy there is a substantial increase in fetal size: the weight triples and the body length doubles.

Weeks 9 to 12

The fetal head is half the length of the crown–rump length at the beginning of the ninth week. The face is recognizably human at 10 weeks. Body growth increases, and as a result, the crown–rump length more than doubles by the twelfth week. Head growth does not keep pace with body growth and slows considerably by the twelfth week but remains proportionately large as compared to the rest of the body. Ossification centers appear in the skeleton. The intestines leave the umbilical cord and enter the abdomen. The external genitalia differentiate and are distinguishable by week 12. At 9 weeks, the liver serves as the major site for red blood cell production (erythropoiesis). However, by 12 weeks, the spleen begins to take over this process. Urine production commences between 9 and 12 weeks.

Weeks 13 to 16

There is very rapid growth during this period. Although coordinated movements of the limbs occur by the fourteenth week, they are too small to be felt by the mother. Ossification of the skeleton takes place and the bones become clearly visible on ultrasound examination. The external genitalia are recognizable by 12 to 14 weeks, the ovaries are differentiated, and the primordial (primitive) ovarian follicles are present by 16 weeks.

Weeks 17 to 20

Growth continues but slows during this period. Maternal awareness of fetal movements (**quickening**) is frequently reported during this time. The skin is now covered with a thick, cheese-like material called **vernix caseosa** that protects the fetal skin from exposure to the amniotic fluid. By 20 weeks, hair appears on the eyebrows and head. Fine downy hair (lanugo) is usually present by 20 weeks and covers all parts of the body except the palms, soles, or areas where other types of hair are usually found. Subcutaneous deposits of **brown fat,** used by the newborn for heat production, help to make the skin less transparent in appearance. The fetal

uterus is formed at 18 weeks in females, and in males, the testes have begun to descend but are still located in the abdominal wall. By 20 weeks, the fetus weighs about 300 grams and is approximately 7.3 inches (19 cm) long.

Weeks 21 to 25

The fetus gains much weight during this time. The skin appears pink or red as blood is now visible in the capillaries. Rapid eye movements begin at 21 weeks. By 24 weeks, the fetus has fingernails and the lungs have begun to secrete **surfactant**, a substance that decreases surface tension in the alveoli and is necessary for survival following birth.

Weeks 26 to 29

A fetus may survive if born during this time because the lungs can breathe air, and the central nervous system can regulate body temperature and direct rhythmic breathing. The eyelids are open, the toenails are evident, and subcutaneous fat is present under the skin. Erythropoiesis occurs in the spleen but ends at 28 weeks when the bone marrow takes over that function.

Weeks 30 to 34

At 30 weeks, the pupillary light reflex is present.

Weeks 35 to 40

At 35 weeks, the fetus has a strong hand grasp reflex and orientation to light. At 38 to 40 weeks, the average fetus weighs 3000 to 3800 grams, and is 17.3 to 19.2 inches (45 to 50 cm) long (Table 7-3).

 ### Across Care Settings: Empowering through education

The nurse who works in any perinatal setting can help to promote self-care and empowerment by increasing the pregnant woman's understanding of the prenatal journey and by encouraging her active involvement in safeguarding her pregnancy. Providing information regarding normal fetal growth and development constitutes an important component of the early and ongoing bonding process for many women. Displaying fetal growth charts in visible areas and discussing developmental landmarks throughout gestation facilitate discussion and enhance understanding for the patient and her family. Other professional resources including the nutritionist, social worker, and home health worker can be instrumental in helping to ensure healthy fetal growth and development.

 ### Nursing Insight— Preterm birth at less than 38 weeks' gestation

It is important to understand fetal growth and development so that the nurse can anticipate specific types of problems that may occur when infants are born prematurely. An infant born at 28 weeks will have significantly different needs from an infant born at 38 weeks' gestation.

Table 7-3 Embryonic and Fetal Growth and Development

Weeks	Weight	Length (crown to rump)	Characteristics
2 weeks	?	2 mm	Blastocyst implanted in uterus.
4 weeks	0.4 g	4 mm	Embryo is curved, tail prominent. Upper limb buds and otic pits present. Heart prominence evident.
8 weeks	2 g	3 cm	Head rounded with human characteristics. Unable to determine sex. Intestines still present in umbilical cord. Ovaries and testes distinguishable.
12 weeks	19 g	8 cm	Resembles human being, with disproportionately large head. Eyes fused. Skin pink and delicate. Upper limbs almost reached final length. Intestines in the stomach. Sex distinguishable externally.
16 weeks	100 g	13.5 cm	Scalp hair appears. External ears present. Lower limbs well developed. Arm to leg ratio proportionate. Fetus active.
20 weeks	300 g	18.5 cm	Head and body hair (lanugo) present. Vernix covers skin. Quickening felt by the woman.
24 weeks	600 g	23 cm	Skin reddish and wrinkled. Some subcutaneous fat present. Some respiratory-like movements. Fingernails present. Lean body.
28 weeks	1100 g	27 cm	Eyes open with eyelashes present. Much hair present. Skin slightly wrinkled, more fat now present.
32 weeks	1800 g	31 cm	Skin is smooth. Increase in weight gain more than length. Toenails present. Testes descending.
36 weeks	2200 g	34 cm	Skin pale, body plump. Body lanugo almost gone. Able to flex arm and form grasp. Umbilicus in center of body. Testes in inguinal canal, scrotum small with few rugae. Some sole creases present.
40 weeks	3200+ g	40 cm	Skin smooth and pink. Lanugo on upper back and shoulders. Ear lobes formed and firm. Chest prominent and breasts often protrude slightly. Testes with well defined rugae. Labia majora well developed. Creases cover soles of feet.

Now Can You— Discuss major events of the fetal period?

1. Identify the developmental week when the fetal face becomes human in appearance?
2. Name the cheese-like substance that covers and protects the skin?
3. List three developmental events that occur from 26 to 29 weeks?

Factors that May Adversely Affect Embryonic and Fetal Development

Damage to the developing embryo/fetus may result from genetic factors or from maternal exposure to various environmental hazards. In most circumstances, the uterus provides a safe and peaceful environment for the developing embryo and fetus. However, teratogens (drugs, radiation, and infectious agents that can cause developmental or structural abnormalities in an embryo) and a variety of internal and external developmental events may cause structural and functional defects.

CHROMOSOMES AND TERATOGENS

Genetic defects and congenital anomalies usually result from genetic factors, environmental hazards (e.g., drugs and viruses), or a combination of both (multifactorial inheritance). However, the exact cause of anomalies is unknown in approximately 50% to 60% of cases. Congenital anomalies may occur singularly or in combination with other defects (multiple anomalies) and they may be of little or of great clinical significance. Single, minor anomalies occur in approximately 14% of newborns. The greater the number of anomalies present, the greater the risk of a major anomaly. Statistically, 90% of infants with three or more minor anomalies will also have one or more major anomaly. Major developmental defects are more common in early embryos that are usually spontaneously aborted. It has been estimated that approximately one-third of all birth defects are caused by genetic factors.

Before fertilization, damage may have already occurred to the chromosomes of one or both parents, or they may carry defective genes inherited from their own parents. Alterations in the development of sperm or an ovum may also cause alterations in the development of the embryo. Teratogens or environmental factors may adversely affect the process of implantation and result in loss of the zygote. Teratogens may have specific effects associated with congenital anomalies (e.g., alcohol: fetal alcohol syndrome; rubella: cataracts; tetracycline: stained teeth) or they may produce dysmorphic (damage to the structure and form) features. The extent of the teratogenic effect depends on the developmental timing, duration, and dosage of exposure as well as the maternal genetic susceptibility. Greater exposure during early gestation is associated with more severe effects.

Teratogen Exposure During Organogenesis

The period of organogenesis lasts from approximately the second until the eighth week of gestation, during which time the embryo undergoes rapid growth and differentiation. During organogenesis the embryo is extremely vulnerable to teratogens such as medications, alcohol, tobacco, caffeine, illegal drugs, radiation, heavy metals, and maternal (TORCH) infections. Structural defects are most likely to occur during this period because exposure to teratogens either before or during a critical period of development of an organ can cause a malformation.

After 11 weeks, the fetus becomes more resistant to damage from teratogens because the organ systems have been established. However, organ function can still be adversely affected. Insults that occur later in fetal life or during early infancy may cause mental retardation, blindness, hearing loss, deafness, stillbirth, or malignancy.

The most critical time for brain development is between 3 and 16 weeks of gestation. However, the brain continues to differentiate and grow rapidly until at least the first 2 years of life. Diet and nutrition are important during this time because amino acids, glucose, and fatty acids are considered to be the primary dietary factors in brain growth.

Medications and Other Substances

It is estimated that approximately 82% of women between the ages of 18 and 44 regularly use at least one medication (prescription or over-the-counter) or vitamins, minerals, herbal supplements, topical medications, or eye drops. Forty-six percent take a prescription medication and the most commonly used drugs used include acetaminophen, ibuprofen, estrogen, pseudoephedrine, and aspirin (National Center for Health Statistics, 2006). Many women unintentionally take medications during early pregnancy when they do not yet know they are pregnant and approximately 59% of pregnant women receive a prescription for a medication other than a vitamin or mineral supplement. To identify drugs that are unsafe for maternal ingestion due to their teratogenic potential, the U.S. Food and Drug Administration (FDA) has established five categories of safety (Table 7-4).

A small number of medications and other substances are known or are strongly suspected to be human teratogens. These include fat-soluble vitamins, alcohol, tobacco, caffeine, cocaine, opiates, anticonvulsants, warfarin (Coumadin), cardiovascular agents (e.g., Lipitor, Mevacor, Pravachol), retinoids (e.g., Soriatane, Tegison, Accutane, Avage), certain hormones (e.g., Android, Androlone-D, Pitressin), antineoplastic agents (e.g., Targretin, Cascdex, Emcyt), certain anti-infective agents (e.g., Penetrex, Novo quinine, Virazole), thalidomide, and methyl mercury.

FAT-SOLUBLE VITAMINS. Both high and low doses of vitamin A (Retinol) can cause fetal malformations that include anomalies of the central nervous system, microtia (deformity of the outer ear), and clefts (a fissure or elongated opening that originates in the embryo, such as a branchial or facial cleft). Vitamin D deficiency may cause poor fetal growth, neonatal hypocalcemia, rickets, and poor tooth enamel. High doses of vitamin E (α-tocopherol) may increase the risk for bleeding problems, but neither deficiency nor excess has been associated with maternal or fetal complications during pregnancy (Tillett et al., 2003).

Table 7-4 FDA Pregnancy Categories	
Category	**Interpretation**
A	Adequate, well-controlled studies in pregnant women have not shown an increased risk of fetal abnormalities to the fetus in any trimester of pregnancy.
B	Animal studies have revealed no evidence of harm to the fetus; however, there are no adequate and well-controlled studies in pregnant women.
	OR
	Animal studies have shown as adverse effect, but adequate and well-controlled studies in pregnant women have failed to demonstrate a risk to the fetus in any trimester.
C	Animal studies have shown an adverse effect and there are no adequate and well-controlled studies in pregnant women.
	OR
	No animal studies have been conducted and there are no adequate and well-controlled studies in pregnant women.
D	Adequate well-controlled or observational studies in pregnant women have demonstrated a risk to the fetus.
	However, the benefits of therapy may outweigh the potential risk. For example, the drug may be acceptable if needed in a life-threatening situation or serious disease for which safer drugs cannot be used or are ineffective.
X	Adequate well-controlled or observational studies in animals or pregnant women have demonstrated positive evidence of fetal abnormalities or risks.
	The use of the product is contraindicated in women who are or may become pregnant.

ALCOHOL. Ethyl alcohol is one of the most potent teratogens known. The Surgeon General's advisory on alcohol use (February, 2005) found that in 2003, approximately 10% of pregnant women reported drinking, and of those, 4% reported having engaged in binge drinking (U.S. Department of Health and Human Services [USDHHS], 2005).

A safe threshold level for the use of alcohol during pregnancy has never been established. Current data suggest that children of mothers who chronically ingested large amounts of alcohol or who engaged in binge drinking (five or more drinks on one occasion) during pregnancy are at greatest risk for permanent damage. (See Chapter 10 for further discussion.)

TOBACCO. Approximately 25% of women smoke while pregnant. Cigarette smoking during pregnancy is associated with an overall reduction in fetal growth, cleft lip anomalies, impaired infant neurobehavior, and decreased babbling in infants (Chiriboga, 2003). Nicotine causes vasoconstriction of the uterine blood vessels, resulting in a decreased blood flow and supply of nutrients and oxygen to the fetus. Cigarette smoking doubles the risk of low birth weight and increases the likelihood of giving birth to a small for gestational age (SGA) infant (Reed, Aranda, & Hales, 2006). Cessation of smoking during pregnancy is beneficial to the developing fetus, and infants born to women who stop smoking during the first trimester have birth weights similar to those of infants born to nonsmoking women. (See Chapter 10 for further discussion.)

CAFFEINE. Caffeine, present in many beverages (sodas, coffee, tea, hot cocoa) and other substances including chocolate, cold remedies, and analgesics, is the most popular drug in the United States. Caffeine stimulates central nervous system and cardiac function and produces vasoconstriction and mild diuresis. The half-life of caffeine is tripled during pregnancy. Although caffeine readily crosses the placenta and stimulates the fetus, it is not known to be a teratogen. However, there is no assurance that maternal consumption of large quantities of caffeine is safe for the developing fetus. (See Chapter 10 for further discussion.)

COCAINE AND CRACK. Cocaine and crack (a form of freebase cocaine that can be smoked) use during pregnancy causes vasoconstriction of the uterine vessels and adversely affects blood flow to the fetus. Cocaine use in pregnancy is associated with spontaneous abortion, abruptio placentae, stillbirth, intrauterine growth restriction (IUGR), fetal distress, meconium staining, and preterm birth. Problems manifested in children born to women who use cocaine during pregnancy include altered neurological and behavior patterns, neonatal strokes and seizures, and congenital malformations (genitourinary anomalies, limb reduction deformities, intestinal atresia, and heart defects) (Chiriboga, 2003). (See Chapters 9 and 10 for further discussion.)

OPIATES. Morphine, heroin, and methadone are opiates sometimes used by pregnant women. Maternal effects from these substances include spontaneous abortion, premature rupture of the membranes, preterm labor, an increased incidence of sexually transmitted infections, hepatitis, an increased potential for HIV exposure, and malnutrition. Methadone is a habit-forming synthetic analgesic drug with a potency equal to that of morphine but with a weaker narcotic action. It is frequently given to pregnant women who enter drug addiction programs. Fetal death, intrauterine growth restriction, perinatal asphyxia, prematurity, intellectual impairment, and neonatal infection are associated with maternal opiate use. Neonatal withdrawal syndrome, characterized by hyperirritability, gastrointestinal dysfunction, respiratory distress, and autonomic disturbances, has been reported in 50 to 80% of infants born to opiate-dependent mothers (Chiriboga, 2003). (See Chapters 9 and 19 for further discussion.)

SEDATIVES. Barbiturates and tranquilizers produce maternal lethargy, drowsiness, and CNS depression. In the neonate, these substances are associated with withdrawal syndrome, seizures and delayed lung maturity.

AMPHETAMINES. Amphetamines are also known as "speed," "crystal," and "ice"; use of these substances during pregnancy is associated with maternal malnutrition, tachycardia, and withdrawal symptoms that include lethargy and depression. The fetus is at an increased risk for intrauterine growth restriction, prematurity, cardiac anomalies, cleft palate, and placental abruption. Following birth, affected neonates may exhibit hypoglycemia, sweating, poor visual tracking, lethargy, and difficulty feeding. (See Chapter 9 for further discussion.)

MARIJUANA. Δ-9-Tetrahydrocannabinol (THC), the active component in marijuana, passes through the placenta and may remain in the fetus for up to 30 days. The carbon monoxide levels produced with marijuana smoking are five times higher than amounts produced with cigarette smoking. Marijuana may cause intrauterine growth restriction, and research has indicated that maternal use of marijuana during pregnancy has adverse effects on neonatal neurobehavior (e.g., hyperirritability, tremors, photosensitivity) and can affect cognitive and language development in infants up to 48 months of age (Chiriboga, 2003). In addition, maternal marijuana use is often combined with other drugs such as cocaine and alcohol. Repeated marijuana use during pregnancy may increase the incidence of maternal anemia and low weight gain. (See Chapters 9 and 10 for further discussion.)

RADIATION. High levels of radiation during pregnancy may cause damage to chromosomes and embryonic cells. Radiation can adversely affect fetal physical growth and cause mental retardation. Unborn babies are particularly at risk to damage from radiation exposure during the first trimester. Consequences of radiation exposure during this time include stunted growth, deformities, abnormal brain function, or cancer that may develop sometime later in life (Centers for Disease Control and Prevention [CDC], 2005).

LEAD. Lead passes through the placenta and has been found to be associated with spontaneous abortion, fetal anomalies, and preterm birth. The nervous system is the most sensitive target of lead exposure. Fetuses and young children are especially vulnerable to the neurological effects of lead because their brains and nervous systems are still developing and the blood–brain barrier is incomplete (USDHHS, 1999). Fetal anomalies associated with lead exposure include hemangiomas, lymphangiomas, hydrocele, minor skin abnormalities (e.g., skin tags and papillae), and undescended testes (Gardella, 2001).

Optimizing Outcomes— Prenatal screening and questions regarding drug use

Due to the teratogenic effects of drugs and other substances on the developing embryo/fetus, prenatal screening for maternal drug use is an important component of the prenatal interview. The nurse should ask questions regarding maternal drug use in a nonjudgmental manner that conveys caring and concern. Questions should be specific, and begin with inquiries that concern innocuous drug use and then progress to the most harmful substances. Examples of questions to ask include the following:

Do you drink any caffeinated beverages? How many in a day?

Do you smoke cigarettes? How many in a day?

Do you drink alcohol? What kind, and how much in a day?

Do you use substances such as marijuana, cocaine, crack, or heroin? Which ones, and how often?

Are you currently, or have you ever been enrolled in a substance abuse program?

 Now Can You—Discuss substances that may adversely affect embryo/fetal growth and development?

1. Explain why the embryo is particularly vulnerable to teratogens during organogenesis?
2. Name two vitamins that are associated with fetal malformations?
3. List one fetal effect associated with maternal use of each of the following: tobacco, cocaine, heroin, and marijuana?

TORCH INFECTIONS

TORCH infections are a group of agents that can infect the fetus or newborn. These include **T**oxoplasmosis, **O**ther infections, **R**ubella virus, **C**ytomegalovirus, and the **H**erpes simplex virus. The fetal risks associated with the various TORCH infections are listed in Box 7-1. (See Chapters 4, 9, and 11 for further discussion about TORCH infections.)

Toxoplasmosis

Toxoplasma gondii, a single-celled parasite, is responsible for toxoplasmosis. This parasite is found throughout the world, and although more than 60 million people in the United States may be infected, most are unaware of the disease (CDC, 2004a). The majority of individuals who become infected with toxoplasmosis are asymptomatic, although when present, symptoms are described as "flu-like" and include glandular pain and enlargement (lymphadenopathy) and myalgia. Severe infection may cause damage to the brain, eyes, or organs. Toxoplasmosis is usually acquired by eating raw or poorly cooked meat contaminated with *Toxoplasma gondii*. This disease may also be acquired through close contact with feces from an infected animal (usually a cat) or from contact with soil that has been contaminated with *Toxoplasma gondii*.

Once maternal infection occurs, the *Toxoplasma gondii* organism crosses the placental membrane and infects the fetus, causing damage to the eyes and brain. If the infection is acquired early in the gestation, there is an increased risk of fetal death. To minimize the risk of infection, pregnant women should avoid raw or poorly cooled meats and contact with animals that may be infected with the toxoplasmosis parasite.

Other Infections

Other infections recognized as teratogens include varicella-zoster virus (chickenpox), human immunodeficiency virus (HIV), and syphilis. The varicella-zoster virus, a member of the herpes family, causes chickenpox and shingles. Infection with the varicella virus during the first 4 months of pregnancy is associated with a number of congenital anomalies including muscle atrophy, limb hypoplasia (underdevelopment), damage to the eyes and brain, and mental retardation. No proven teratogenic risks have

---

Box 7-1   TORCH Infections

TORCH infections can cause serious harm to the embryo-fetus, especially during the first 12 weeks when developmental anomalies may occur.

TOXOPLASMOSIS
Associated with consumption of infested undercooked meat and poor hand washing after handling cat litter. Fetal infection occurs if the mother acquires toxoplasmosis after conception and passes it to the fetus via the placenta. Most infants are asymptomatic at birth, but develop symptoms later.

Maternal Effects
Flu-like symptoms in the acute phase.

Fetal/Neonatal Effects
Miscarriage likely in early pregnancy. In neonates, CNS lesions can result in hydrocephaly, microcephaly, chronic retinitis, and seizures. Retinochoroiditis may appear in adolescence or adulthood.

OTHER INFECTIONS
Most commonly includes the hepatitis virus. Hepatitis A virus is spread by droplets or hands; transmission is rare but can occur. Hepatitis B virus can be transmitted via placenta, but transmission usually occurs when the infant is exposed to blood and genital secretions during labor and birth.

Maternal Effects
Fever, malaise, nausea, abdominal discomfort, may be associated with liver failure.

Fetal/Neonatal Effects
Preterm birth, hepatitis infection, intrauterine death.

RUBELLA (GERMAN MEASLES)
Spread by respiratory droplets.

Maternal Effects
Fever, rash, mild lymphedema.

Fetal/Neonatal Effects
Miscarriage, IUGR, cataracts, congenital anomalies, hepatosplenomegaly, hyperbilirubinemia, mental retardation, and death. Other symptoms may develop later. Infants born with congenital rubella are contagious and should be isolated. Patients are instructed not to become pregnant for 1 month after receiving the immunization; a signed consent form must be obtained before administration of the vaccine.

CYTOMEGALOVIRUS (CMV)
Respiratory droplets, semen, cervical and vaginal secretions, breast milk, placental tissue, urine, feces, and banked blood (nearly 50% of adults in United States have antibodies for this virus).

Maternal Effects
Asymptomatic illness, cervical discharge, and mononucleosis-like syndrome.

Fetal/Neonatal Effects
Fetal death or severe generalized disease with hemolytic anemia and jaundice, hydrocephaly or microcephaly, pneumonitis, hepatosplenomegaly, mental retardation, cerebral palsy, and deafness. The organs/tissues affected most often are blood, brain, and liver.

HERPES SIMPLEX VIRUS (HSV)
HSV II is sexually transmitted, infant usually infected during exposure to lesion in birth canal, most at risk during a primary infection in the mother (50% born vaginally will develop some form of herpes; 60% will die; half of survivors develop problems).

Maternal Effects
Blisters, rash, fever, malaise, nausea, and headache.

Fetal/Neonatal Effects
Miscarriage, preterm birth, stillbirth, transplacental infection is rare but can cause skin lesions, IUGR, mental retardation, microcephaly, seizures, coma.

been associated with varicella infection that occurs after 20 weeks' gestation (Moore & Persaud, 2003) although approximately 25% of infants born to mothers who become infected with varicella in the last 3 weeks of pregnancy will develop clinical varicella (Gershon, 2006).

The human immunodeficiency virus may be transplacentally transmitted to the fetus in utero. Infection may also occur intrapartally (during labor and birth) from exposure to maternal blood and body fluids, and postpartally (after birth), through breast milk. Without medical intervention, the risk of perinatal transmission of HIV is approximately 25%; with appropriate treatment, the rate of perinatal transmission can be reduced to 2% (Havens & Walters, 2004). (See Chapter 11 for further discussion.)

Treponema pallidum, the microorganism that causes syphilis, readily crosses the placenta. The fetus may become infected during any time of gestation. Serious fetal infection and congenital anomalies are almost always associated with primary maternal infections that occur during pregnancy. However, *Treponema pallidum* can be destroyed with adequate treatment that will prevent placental transmission and fetal infection. Secondary infections acquired before pregnancy rarely result in fetal disease and anomalies. Left untreated, only 20% of pregnant women with primary syphilis infections will give birth to a normal term infant. Neonatal manifestations of congenital syphilis infection include prematurity, skin rash, hydrops fetalis, failure to thrive, hepatosplenomegaly, lymphadenopathy, and bone lesions (osteochondritis, osteomyelitis, and periostitis). Late-onset manifestations of congenital syphilis infection include keratitis (inflammation of the cornea), deafness, and bowing of the shins (Woods, 2005).

Rubella

The virus that causes rubella (also known as German measles) can cause damage to the developing embryo/fetus. The earlier in the pregnancy that the disease is contracted, the greater the risk to the developing embryo. If the pregnant woman experiences a primary rubella infection during the first trimester, there is a 20% risk that the fetus will also become infected. When maternal rubella infection occurs during the first 4 to 5 weeks after fertilization, the majority of infants will demonstrate congenital anomalies. If rubella is contracted during the second and third trimesters, the risk of congenital anomalies is decreased to 10%, but mental retardation and hearing loss may result from infection that occurs late in the gestation. Birth defects associated with congenital rubella syndrome include hearing loss, eye defects causing vision loss or blindness, heart defects, and mental retardation.

Cytomegalovirus (CMV)

Approximately 50% to 80% of adults have antibodies to the cytomegalovirus (CMV) (Yudkin & Gonik, 2006). CMV produces no signs or symptoms of infection in the majority of affected individuals. However, CMV can cause disease in unborn babies or in persons with weakened immune systems. The cytomegalovirus is a member of the herpesvirus family, and is the most common viral infection in the fetus.

Spontaneous abortion (miscarriage) may result from maternal CMV infection during the first trimester. Infection that occurs later in the pregnancy may result in fetal intrauterine growth restriction, microphthalmia, chorioretinitis, blindness, microcephaly, cerebral calcification, mental retardation, deafness, cerebral palsy, and hepatosplenomegaly. In the neonate, asymptomatic CMV infections are often associated with audiological, neurological, and neurobehavioral disturbances.

Herpes Simplex Virus (HSV)

Spontaneous abortion is increased threefold if maternal infection from herpes simplex virus occurs in early pregnancy. Infection after the twentieth gestational week is associated with an increased rate of prematurity. The transmission of the herpes virus occurs at the time of delivery during passage through the birth canal, but may also occur transplacentally via ascending infection before labor or rupture of the membranes. Congenital anomalies associated with the herpes simplex virus include extensive dermatological scarring or bullae, microencephaly, hydrencephaly, encephalitis, microphthalmia, chorioretinitis, and hepatosplenomegaly (Pan, Cole, & Weintrub, 2005). (See Chapter 19 for further discussion.)

 Now Can You— **Discuss TORCH infections?**

1. Identify the components of the acronym "TORCH"?
2. Describe a teaching need for pregnant women who have indoor cats?
3. Explain why pregnant women should avoid individuals infected with chickenpox and rubella?

The Nurse's Role in Prenatal Evaluation

The clinical gestational period is divided into three trimesters that each last for 3 months. By the end of the first trimester, all major organs are developed. During the second trimester, the fetus continues to grow in size and most fetal anomalies can be detected using high-resolution real-time ultrasound. By the beginning of the third trimester the fetus has a chance for survival and most survive if born at or after 35 weeks' gestation.

At the initial prenatal visit, the nurse performs an assessment that includes careful consideration of cultural, emotional, physical, and physiological factors that may signal a need for genetics counseling and comprehensive fetal evaluation.

 Optimizing Outcomes— **Expanding nursing roles in genetics health care**

Roles for maternity, women's health, and pediatrics nurses in genetics health care have expanded significantly over the past few years as genetics education and counseling has become standard of care. Today, nurses may provide preconception counseling for women at risk for the transmission of a genetic disorder (Klipstein, 2005), prenatal care for women with genetically linked psychiatric disorders (Lamberg, 2005) or other conditions (e.g. congenital heart disease) that require specialized care (Khairy et al., 2006), or infant screening (Kenner & Moran, 2005). Nurses may also be involved in caring for families who have children with genetic conditions (Gallo, Angst, Knafl, Hadley, & Smith, 2005; Kenner, Gallo, & Bryant, 2005) or those who have lost a fetus or child affected by a genetic condition (Korenromp, 2005). In 2005, nursing leaders developed the document *Essential Nursing Competencies and Curricula Guidelines for Genetics and Genomics*. This publication, which presents minimal genetic and genomic competencies for all nurses, may be accessed at http://www.nursingworld.org/.

Prenatal care involves ongoing medical and psychosocial support. (See Chapter 9 for further discussion.) Common prenatal screening includes blood testing and ultrasound examination. Depending on maternal and familial risk factors, advanced screening tests may be indicated. Amniocentesis, chorionic villus sampling, and percutaneous umbilical blood sampling (PUBS) are examples of specialized prenatal diagnostic methods. (See Chapters 9 and 11 for further discussion.)

 Nursing Insight— *Specific methods for gene identification and testing*

Gene identification and testing involves the analysis of human DNA, RNA (ribonucleic acid), chromosomes, or certain proteins to identify abnormalities related to an inherited condition. Through direct or molecular testing, the DNA and RNA that make up a single gene are directly examined; with linkage analysis, markers that are co-inherited with a specific gene that causes a genetic condition are analyzed; through biochemical testing, scientists examine the protein products of genes; and with cytogenetic testing, individual chromosomes are examined. Commercially available genetic tests can be accessed online at GeneTests, http://www.genetests.org./

Genetic counseling should be offered to couples with a personal or family history of a heritable genetic disorder. The nurse must be aware of, and be able to provide education regarding the potential for an increased risk for various diseases found among certain racial and ethnic populations (Table 7-5). Testing for many common genetic diseases is now available. For diseases in which the responsible gene has not been identified, the risk can sometimes be estimated by comparing fetal DNA with that of affected and non-affected family members.

 Ethnocultural Considerations— Maintaining and communicating a caring and accepting attitude

It is important for the nurse to be knowledgeable of various cultural practices and beliefs that may impact on the development of the fetus. Culture and experience influence every aspect of individuals' lives and how they care for themselves and their families. For example, women from some ethnic groups choose to visit health healers and lay midwives throughout pregnancy.

The nurse should maintain an unbiased and accepting attitude when working with patients from populations with varying

Table 7-5 Racial and Ethnic Groups with Increased Risk for Diseases Caused by Recessive Genes	
Racial/Ethnic Group	**Disease**
African, Mediterranean, Caribbean, Latin American, or Middle Eastern descent	Hemoglobin gene mutations are more common in persons from these areas. African Americans have an increased incidence of sickle cell anemia. Southeast Asians have a greater likelihood of carrying hemoglobin E, an abnormal hemoglobin.
Mediterranean or Asian origin	These individuals have a higher risk of the hereditary anemia thalassemia.
Jewish ancestry	Individuals with Jewish ancestry have an increased risk for diseases associated with inborn errors of metabolism caused by different enzyme deficiencies (e.g., Tay–Sachs, Canavan, and Gaucher).
Caucasian or northern European descent	The most common disorder found among this population is cystic fibrosis.

beliefs and practices. Awareness and understanding of personal practices and beliefs constitutes the first step toward ensuring an unbiased disposition when providing patient care. Recognizing that cultural values and experiences shape an individual's likelihood to continue or discontinue familial beliefs and practices helps the nurse to develop a more accepting attitude and deliver appropriate care in a culturally sensitive manner.

Heredity and Genetics

According to the CDC, the leading cause of infant death in the United States in 2002 was related to problems associated with congenital malformations, deformations, and chromosomal abnormalities. These conditions accounted for 20% of all infant deaths (CDC, 2004b). Birth defects, or **congenital anomalies**, are structural abnormalities present at birth. Congenital anomalies may result from four different pathological processes: malformation, disruption, deformation, and dysplasia. **Malformation** is the alteration in embryonic development caused by genetic transmission, chromosomal anomalies, environmental factors, and multifactorial/unknown causes. This defect results from an intrinsic abnormal development that is present from the beginning of development, such as one that arises from a chromosomal abnormality. A disruption is caused by an external force that alters previously normal tissue and interferes with normal development. Maternal exposure to teratogens, such as drugs, viruses or environmental hazards, may also cause a disruption. Disruptions are not inherited although an individual may be predisposed to the development of a disruption. **Deformations** are physical alterations in form, shape, or position that are caused by extrinsic mechanical factors (e.g., clubfoot that results from intrauterine fetal restraint or fetal compression defects that result from decreased amniotic fluid [oligohydramnios]). **Dysplasia** (an abnormal development of tissue) is caused by an abnormal organization of cells that results in abnormal tissue formation. (See Chapter 11 for further discussion.)

Damage that may alter embryological development can occur to the chromosomes of one or both parents prior to conception. During the pre-embryonic period (up to 14 days after conception), while the zygote is protected by the zona pellucida, exposure to teratogens most likely causes either no harmful effects or produces severe damage that results in loss of the pregnancy.

"What to say" — *Prenatal identification of a fetal anomaly*

Prenatal testing may identify a fetus with a congenital anomaly. When this occurs, families are generally faced with a flood of emotions and difficult decisions. The nurse plays an important role in providing support and education regarding options available to these couples. A nonjudgmental and caring attitude is vital at this difficult and vulnerable time.

Therapeutic communication is enhanced when the nurse uses statements such as:

"It's normal to have fear, grief, or even be angry."

"It's normal to have concerns about your ability to have a normal baby."

"I am here to answer your questions and listen to your concerns. If I don't know the answers I will either find and share them or arrange for a colleague to meet with you."

The nurse should avoid using statements such as:

"You can always have other children."

"I know how you feel."

"At least you don't know the baby yet."

Optimizing Outcomes— **Including the father of the baby**

Health care providers frequently focus primarily on the pregnant woman. It is important that nurses remember to include fathers and care for the couple when providing patient education and support.

Maternal Age and Chromosomes

Advanced maternal age (age 35 and above at the time of birth) is associated with an increased risk of chromosomal abnormalities (1% risk beginning at age 35 and increasing each year, up to an 8% risk at age 46), with trisomy 21 **(Down syndrome)** consisting of half of these. The risk of giving birth to a child with Down syndrome increases with age: the incidence is approximately 1 in 1350 for a 25-year old woman; 1 in 400 for a 35-year-old woman; and 1 in 30 for a 45-year-old woman. However, children with Down syndrome may be born to mothers of any age: approximately 80% of children with Down syndrome are born to mothers younger than 35 years (National Down Syndrome Society, 2006).

A **trisomy** occurs when there are three particular chromosomes instead of the normal number of two. Figure 7-14 illustrates the extra chromosome that occurs with Down syndrome. The three most common trisomies found in live newborns are trisomy 18 (Edward syndrome), trisomy 21 (Down syndrome), and trisomy 13 (Patau syndrome).

Trisomy 13 and trisomy 18 are rare; each occurs only about once in every 5000 live births. Trisomy 21 is the most common trisomy and occurs in approximately every 650 live births (Scanlon & Sanders, 2007). The prognosis for both trisomy 13 and 18 is very poor; approximately 70% of infants with these chromosomal disorders die within the first 3 months of life from complications associated with respiratory and cardiac abnormalities. Neonatal effects from these three most common trisomies include central nervous system abnormalities, mental retardation, and hypotonia at birth. Although children with Down syndrome are mentally retarded, there is a wide range of mental ability among this group.

Deletion and translocation describe other chromosomal abnormalities. Women younger than 35 years of age who have previously given birth to a child with a chromosomal abnormality have a 1% increased risk of having another affected child. A **deletion** is a loss of a portion of DNA from a chromosome (Fig. 7-15). This alteration can be caused by an unknown event, mutation, or exposure to irradiation, or it may occur during cell division. When a gene necessary for cell function is absent, disease may result. A **translocation** occurs when all or a segment of one chromosome breaks off and attaches to the same or to a different chromosome (Fig. 7-16). Parents who have a chromosomal translocation or who have had a child with structural malformations are at increased risk for having another affected child.

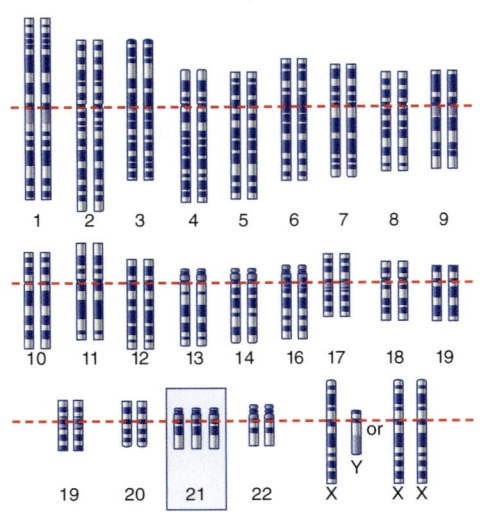

Figure 7-14 Trisomy 21. (Courtesy of National Human Genome Research Institute.)

Figure 7-15 Deletion. (Courtesy of National Human Genome Research Institute.)

Figure 7-16 Translocation. (Courtesy of National Human Genome Research Institute.)

Multifetal Pregnancy

Monozygotic (identical) twins develop from one fertilized oocyte (zygote) that divides into equal halves during an early cleavage phase (series of mitotic cell divisions) of development (Fig. 7-17). This type of twinning occurs in approximately 1 of 250 live births (Benirschke, 2004). Monozygotic twins are genetically identical, always the same gender, and very similar in physical appearance. The number of amnions and chorions depends on the timing of division (cleavage) of the zygote. If the division occurs during the two to eight cell stages, there will be two amnions, two chorions, and two placentas. For most monozygotic twins, the division occurs at the end of the first week after fertilization and results from the division of the singular embryoblast into two embryoblasts. When the division occurs during this time, each fetus has its own amnion, but resides within a single chorion and receives oxygen and nutrients from the same placenta. Depending on the timing of cleavage, the following multifetal combinations occur:

- Division that occurs during the first 72 hours after fertilization: two embryos, two amnions, and two chorions develop with two distinct placentas, or a single fused placenta.
- Division that occurs between the fourth and eight day: two embryos, each in a separate amnion sac covered by a single chorion.
- Division that occurs approximately 8 days after fertilization after the chorion and amnion have differentiated: two embryos in a common amniotic sac.
- Division that occurs after the embryonic disk has formed: cleavage is incomplete and conjoined twins result.

Conjoined twins occur when the embryonic disk does not divide completely, or when adjacent embryonic disks fuse. Conjoined twinning occurs in approximately 1 in 50,000 to 100,000 births. Twins may be connected to one another by the skin only or by cutaneous and other tissues. In many cases, surgical separation is possible but, depending on the anatomical region of attachment and the sharing of vital organs, may not be feasible.

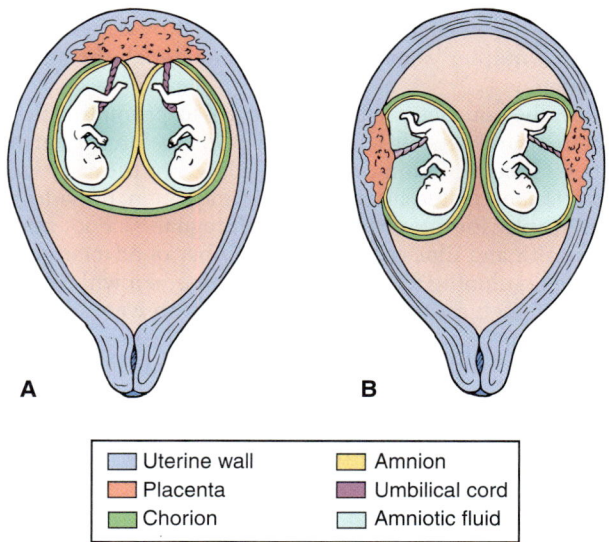

Uterine wall	Amnion
Placenta	Umbilical cord
Chorion	Amniotic fluid

Figure 7-17 Multiple gestations. *A,* Monozygotic twins with one placenta, one chorion and two amnions. *B,* Dizygotic twins with two placentas, two chorions and two amnions

Dizygotic (fraternal) twins develop from two zygotes and may be the same or different genders. Dizygotic twins are no more genetically similar than other siblings born to the same parents. There are separate amnions and chorions although the chorions and placentas may be fused. The incidence of dizygotic twinning is approximately 1 in 500 Asians, 1 in 125 Caucasians, and as high as 1 in 20 in some African populations. Triplets may result from the division of a single zygote into three zygotes (one original fertilized egg), or from the division of one zygote (identical twins are formed) plus another zygote (a total of two original fertilized eggs), or from three different zygotes (a total of three original fertilized eggs).

Now Can You— Discuss maternal age-related chromosomal problems and the origins of twinning?

1. Differentiate among the terms "malformation," "disruption," "deformation," and "dysplasia"?
2. Define "trisomy" and identify two of the most common trisomies?
3. Explain how twinning occurs?

The Nurse's Role in Minimizing Threats to the Developing Embryo and Fetus

Nurses provide holistic care to the family unit. The nurse must assess for environmental and lifestyle risks that may harm the fetus or mother. Ongoing evaluations should include assessment of the patient's knowledge, lifestyle patterns, environmental conditions, and physical and psychosocial well-being. Reduction of maternal–fetal risks and helping to ensure the birth of a healthy newborn to a healthy mother remains the essential goal throughout pregnancy.

Ideally, counseling about strategies to promote optimal maternal and fetal health should begin before pregnancy occurs. Preconception counseling allows for the early identification of maternal risk factors and often provides an opportunity for intervention before pregnancy. Poor maternal health and illness can have a number of adverse effects on the developing fetus. In years past, women with chronic illnesses such as diabetes and hypertension were unable to conceive or were advised not to become pregnant. The advent of insulin and antihypertensive medications has allowed these women to not only contemplate pregnancy but to successfully carry a pregnancy to maturity with healthy outcomes for both the mother and her baby.

 Nursing Insight— Karyotyping as a component of preconception counseling

Karyotyping of the parents as well as their child with a genetic disorder may be appropriate during the preconception period. A **karyotype** is a photomicrograph of the chromosomes of a single cell; the chromosomes are then arranged in numerical order (Venes, 2009) (Fig. 7-18). Cells, obtained from a sample of peripheral venous blood or a scraping of the buccal membrane tissue, are stained and photographed following a period of growth in the laboratory. *Fluorescence in situ hybridization* (FISH) is a rapid technique that allows for immediate karyotyping without a period of cell growth.

Through preventive strategies, preconception counseling can significantly decrease the incidence of birth defects and problems associated with preterm birth along with other disorders linked to maternal illness and nutritional deficiencies. Counseling should include discussion of possible fetal risks from exposure to teratogens. Factors that could potentially harm the developing fetus are identified and the woman is advised of her risks. When possible, strategies to reduce or prevent risk to the fetus are

Figure 7-18 Karyotype of human chromosomes of male and female.

discussed with the woman and her family. If exposure has occurred, every effort should be made to identify the timing of the contact and the amount of exposure. This information is essential, since the calculation of risk varies according to the particular teratogen, and the timing and dose of the exposure. (See Chapter 10 for further discussion.)

 Optimizing Outcomes— Formulating nursing diagnoses for women and couples seeking genetic screening and assessment

Nursing diagnoses that may be applicable for genetic screening and assessment include:

- Health-seeking behaviors related to potential for genetic transmission of disease
- Deficient knowledge related to inheritance pattern of the family's inherited disorder
- Fear related to outcome of genetic screening tests
- Decisional conflict related to testing for an untreatable genetic disorder

After the infant's birth, diseases that may increase the risk for infection, cause liver damage, mental retardation, or death can often be identified through newborn screening tests. Newborn screening, which was initiated in the 1960s, was the first population-based screening program to test for genetic conditions. Through screening, diagnosis and treatment for many diseases and disorders can take place before permanent damage occurs. One of the *Healthy People 2010* goals is to ensure that all newborns are screened at birth as mandated by their state-sponsored screening programs, that follow-up diagnostic testing for positive findings is performed in the appropriate time period, and that infants with diagnosed disorders are enrolled in appropriate service interventions in a timely manner. Additional information about the *Healthy People 2010* national initiative is available at http://www.healthypeople.gov/Publications.

summary points

◆ The Human Genome Project that ended in 2003 provided important insights into our understanding of the genetic complexity of humans.

◆ A genotype is an individual's gene composition; a phenotype refers to the observable expression of a person's genotype; a genome is a complete copy of the genes present.

◆ The developing embryo/fetus lives in a unique environment where all essential elements needed for normal growth and development is provided.

◆ The gestational period, which lasts an average of 40 weeks from the time of fertilization, occurs in three stages: the pre-embryonic stage; the embryonic stage; and the fetal stage.

◆ During the embryonic stage the heart begins to beat and the body's circulation is established.

◆ Structural refinement and perfection of function of all systems occur during the fetal stage.

◆ Teratogens, substances that cause harm to the developing fetus, may be in the form of chemicals, viruses, environmental agents, physical factors, and drugs.

◆ By educating pregnant women about fetal developmental events and avoidance of potential hazards, nurses can help to ensure a healthy outcome for the mother and her infant.

review questions

Multiple Choice

1. The nurse working in reproductive health is aware that the goal of the Human Genome Project was to:
A. Identify exact human DNA sequences and genes.
B. Identify human DNA and RNA sequences.
C. Measure exact human DNA sequences for chromosomal diseases.
D. Measure exact human DNA sequence maps for disease prevention.

2. At the obstetrician's office, a couple receives information about assisted reproductive technologies. The nurse explains that the in vitro fertilization procedure involves the following:
A. Approximately 35 to 60 hours after fertilization in the laboratory, an embryo is injected into the woman's cervix.
B. An embryo is injected into the fallopian tubes at 50 hours after fertilization in the laboratory.
C. Many sperm cells and ova are injected into the fallopian tubes to achieve fertilization inside the tubes, where it normally occurs.
D. Many sperm cells and ova are injected into the cervix to achieve fertilization inside the woman.

3. When describing fetal growth and development, the perinatal nurse correctly identifies the gestational week that the heart begins to beat as the:
A. Second
B. Third
C. Fourth
D. Sixth

4. The perinatal nurse provides information about fetal growth and development to parents in a prenatal class. The nurse explains that fetal urine production begins at:
A. 6 to 8 weeks
B. 9 to 12 weeks
C. 12 to 16 weeks
D. 15 to 18 weeks

5. During preconception counseling, the clinic nurse explains that the time period when the fetus is most vulnerable to the effects of teratogens is from:
A. 5 to 10 weeks
B. 2 to 8 weeks
C. 4 to 12 weeks
D. 6 to 15 weeks

True/False

6. The perinatal nurse describes the process of inception for identical twins as monozygotic or coming from one fertilized oocyte.

7. When describing fetal circulation to the student nurse, the clinic nurse explains that most of the fetus's blood bypasses the lungs by shunting through the ductus arteriosus.

Fill-in-the-Blank

8. The clinic nurse is aware that the primary sources of amniotic fluid in pregnancy are fetal _____ and _____ secretions.

9. The perinatal nurse explains to the student nurse that the growing embryo is called a _____ beginning at _____ weeks of gestational age.

10. The perinatal nurse defines a _____ as any substance that adversely affects the growth and development of the fetus.

See Answers to End of Chapter Review Questions on the Electronic Study Guide or DavisPlus.

REFERENCES

Benirschke, K. (2004). Multiple gestation. The biology of twinning. In R. Creasy, R. Resnik, & J. Iams (Eds.), *Maternal-fetal medicine: Principles and practice* (5th ed.). Philadelphia: W.B. Saunders.

Bulechek, G., Butcher, H.M., & Dochterman, J. (2008). *Nursing interventions classification (NIC)* (5th ed.). St. Louis, MO: C.V. Mosby.

Centers for Disease Control and Prevention (CDC), Division of Parasitic Diseases. (2004a). *Parasites and health: Toxoplasmosis.* Retrieved from www.dpd.cdc.gov/DPDx/HTML/Toxoplasmosis.htm (Accessed June 21, 2007).

Centers for Disease Control and Prevention (CDC). National Vital Statistics Reports (2004b), Vol. 53(10). *Infant mortality statistics from the 2002 period linked birth/infant death data set.* Retrieved from http://origin.cdc.gov/nchs/data/nvsr/nvsr53/nvsr53_10.pdf (Accessed June 21, 2007).

Centers for Disease Control and Prevention (CDC), Emergency Preparedness & Response. (2005). *Possible health effects of radiation exposure on unborn babies.* Retrieved from www.bt.cdc.gov/radiation/prenatal.asp (Accessed June 21, 2007).

Chiriboga, C.A. (2003, November). Fetal alcohol and drug effects. *The Neurologist, 9*(6), 267–279.

Cunningham, F.G., Leveno, K.J., Bloom, S.L., Hauth, J.C., Gilstrap III, L.C., & Wenstrom, K.D. (2005). Fetal growth and development. *Williams obstetrics* (22nd ed., pp. 129-166). New York: McGraw-Hill.

Evans, M.I., Llurba, E., Landsberger, E.J., O'Brien, J.E., & Harrison, H.H. (2004, March). Impact of folic acid fortification in the United States: Markedly diminished high maternal serum alpha-fetoprotein values. *Obstetrics & Gynecology, 103*(3), 474–479.

Foster, C. (2007). Factor V Leiden mutation: What is it? What are the implications for clinical practice? *The American Journal for Nurse Practitioners, 11*(6), 35–46.

Gallo, A., Angst, D., Knafl, K., Hadley, E., & Smith, C. (2005). Parents sharing information with their children about genetic conditions. *Journal of Pediatric Health Care, 19*(5), 267–275.

Gardella, C. (2001, April). Lead exposure in pregnancy: A review of the literature and argument for routine prenatal screening. *Obstetrical and Gynecologic Survey, 56*(4), 231–238.

Gershon, A. (2006). Chickenpox, measles and mumps. In J. Remington, J. Klein, C. Baker, & C. Wilson (Eds.), *Infectious diseases of the fetus and newborn infant* (6th ed., pp. 446-459). Philadelphia: W.B. Saunders.

Guttmacher, A., & Collins, F. (2005). Realizing the promise of genomics in biomedical research. *JAMA, 294*(11), 1399–1402.

Havens, P.L., & Walters, D. (2004). Management of the infant born to a mother with HIV infection. *Pediatric Clinics of North America, 51*, 909–937.

Johnson, M., Bulechek, G., Butcher, H., McCloskey Dochterman, J., Maas, M., Moorhead, S., & Swanson, E. (2006). *NANDA, NOC, and NIC Linkages: nursing diagnoses, outcomes, & interventions* (2nd ed.). St. Louis, MO: Mosby Elsevier.

Kenner, C., Gallo, A., & Bryant, K. (2005). Promoting children's health through understanding of genetics and genomics. *Journal of Nursing Scholarship, 37*(4), 308–314.

Kenner, C., & Moran, M. (2005). Newborn screening and genetic testing. *Journal of Midwifery & Women's Health, 50*(3), 219–226.

Khairy, P., Ouyang, D., Fernandes, S., Lee-Parritz, A., Economy, K., & Landzberg, M. (2006). Pregnancy outcomes in women with congenital heart disease. *Circulation, 113*(4), 517–524.

Khoury, M. (2003). Genetics and genomics in practice: The continuum from genetic disease to genetic information in health and disease. *Genetics in Medicine, 5*(4), 261–268.

Klipstein, S. (2005). Preimplantation genetic diagnosis: Technological promise and ethical perils. *Fertility and Sterility, 83*(5), 1347–1353.

Korenromp, M. (2005). Long-term psychological consequences of pregnancy termination for fetal abnormality: A cross-sectional study. *Prenatal Diagnosis, 25*(3), 253–260.

Lamberg, L. (2005). Risks and benefits key to psychotropic use during pregnancy and postpartum period. *JAMA, 294*(13), 1604–1608.

Lashley, F. (2005). *Clinical genetics in nursing practice* (3rd ed.). New York: Springer.

Moll, S. (2006). Thrombophilias – practical implications and testing caveats. *Journal of Thrombosis and Thrombolysis, 21*(1), 7–15.

Moore, K.L., & Persaud, T.V.N. (2003). *The developing human: Clinically oriented embryology* (7th ed.). Philadelphia: Elsevier.

Moorehead, S., Johnson, M., Mass, M., & Swanson, E. (2008). *Nursing outcomes classification (NOC)* (4th ed.). St. Louis, MO: C.V. Mosby.

National Center for Health Statistics (NCHS). (2006). Health data for allages. Retrieved from www.cdc.gov/nchs/health_data_for_all_ages. htm (Accessed June 21, 2007).

National Down Syndrome Society (2006). NDSS Statement on the CDC's new study on the prevalence of Down Syndrome. Retrieved from www.ndss.org/content.cfm?fuseaction_InfoResGeneralArticle&article_29 (Accessed June 13, 2007).

Pan, E.S., Cole, F.S., & Weintrub, P.S. (2005). Viral infections of the fetus and newborn. In H.W. Taeusch, R.A. Ballard, & C.A. Gleason. *Avery's diseases of the newborn* (8th ed., pp. 495–529). Philadelphia: Elsevier.

Reed, M., Aranda, J., & Hales, B. (2006). Developmental pharmacology. In R. Martin, A. Faranoff, & M. Walsh (Eds.), *Fanaroff and Martin's neonatal-perinatal medicine: Diseases of the fetus and infant* (8th ed., pp. 672–681). Philadelphia: C.V. Mosby.

Scanlon, V.C., & Sanders, T. (2007). *Essentials of anatomy and physiology* (5th ed.). Philadelphia: F.A. Davis.

Smith, B.R. (2008). The multidimensional human embryo, Carnegie Stages. Retrieved from http://embryo.soad.umich.edu/carnstages/ (Accessed June 8, 2007).

Tillett, J., Kostich, L., & VandeVusse, L. (2003, January/March). Use of over-the-counter medications during pregnancy. *The Journal of Perinatal & Neonatal Nursing, 17*(1), 3–18.

U.S. Department of Health and Human Services (USDHHS). (1999). Agency for Toxic Substances and Disease Registry (ATSDR). *Case studies in environmental medicine (CSEM) lead toxicity physiologic effects*. Retrieved from www.atsdr.cdc.gov/HEC/CSEM/lead/physiologic_effects.htm (Accessed June 21, 2007).

U.S. Department of Health and Human Services (USDHHS). (2005). Office of the Surgeon General, Advisory on Alcohol Use in Pregnancy. Retrieved from www.surgeongeneral.gov/pressreleases/sg02222005.htm (Accessed June 21, 2007).

Venes, D., Ed. (2009). *Taber's cyclopedic medical dictionary* (21st ed.). Philadelphia: F.A. Davis.

Woods, C. (2005). Syphilis in children: Congenital and acquired. *Seminars in Pediatric Infectious Diseases, 16*(4), 245–257.

Yudkin, M., & Gonik, B. (2006). Perinatal infections. In R. Martin, A. Fanaroff, & M. Walsh (Eds.). *Faranoff & Martin's neonatal-perinatal medicine: Diseases of the fetus and infant* (8th ed.). Philadelphia: C.V. Mosby.

 For more information, go to http://davisplus.fadavis.com/

CONCEPT MAP

Conception and Development of the Embryo/Fetus

Conception

Factors Affecting Fetal/Embryonic Development:
- Damage to parental chromosomes
  - Advanced maternal age
  - Inheriting defective genes
- Teratogens
  - Alcohol, nicotine
  - Caffeine
  - Medications
  - Environmental pollutants
  - "Street drugs"→ cocaine/crack, marijuana, opiates
- Infections
  - TORCH, rubella, CMV, HSV, toxoplasmosis

Potential for Inheriting a Disease:
- Multifactorial
  - Cleft lip, cleft palate, neural tube defects, pyloric stenosis, and congenital heart disease
- Unifactorial
  - Autosomal dominant
  - Autosomal recessive
  - X-linked dominant
  - X-linked recessive

Fertilization:
- Meeting of oocyte and sperm in fallopian tube
  - →Capacitation
  - →Acrosome reaction
  - →Zona pellucida penetration
- Zygote formation
- Potential for multifetal pregnancy

Implantation:
- Morula enters uterus→ blastocyst
  - Embryoblast = embryo
  - Trophoblast = placenta
- Nidation
- Formation of:
  - Chorionic villi; intervillous spaces
  - Embryonic membranes: amnion; chorion
  - Amniotic fluid

Placental Development:
- Oxygenation
- Nutrition
- Waste elimination
- Hormone production

Umbilical Cord Formation:
- Elongation of body stalk
- Development of 2 arteries; 1 vein from yolk sac vessels

Development of Fetal Circulation:
- Embryonic vessels→ after 3rd week
- Beating heart→ end of 3rd week
Unique features
- Bypasses liver via ductus venosus
- Flows from right atrium to left atrium via foramen ovale
- Bypasses lungs via ductus arteriosus

Pre-embryonic Period:
- First 2 wks after conception
Development:
- Cephalocaudal
- Proximal to distal
- General to specific

Embryonic Period:
- 3rd week after conception → end of 8th week
  - Blastogenesis
  - Development of neuro/CV systems
  - All major internal/external structures

The Fetal Period: 9th to 40th Week:
- 9–16 wks: recognizable face; increasing body growth; ossification centers appear; distinguishable genitalia; bones visible on ultrasound
- 17–20 wks: quickening; vernix caseosa present; lanugo; SQ brown fat; formation of uterus/testes
- 21–25 wks: weight gain; blood visible in capillaries; rapid eye movement; surfactant secreted
- 26–29 wks: eyelids open; CNS regulates temp/directs breathing; may survive after birth
- 30-40 wks: pupillary light reflex; hand grasp reflex; oriented to light

Leading Causes Of Infant Death:
- Congenital anomalies
- Malformation; disruption deformation; dysplasia
- Chromosomal abnormalities

Nurse's Role: Minimizing Threats:
- Preconception counseling
- Assessment → environmental risks, patient's knowledge, physical/psychosocial well-being
- Newborn screening→disease, genetic conditions

Ethnocultural Considerations:
- Caring/acceptance results from knowledge about cultural practices/beliefs

Nursing Insight:
- Stage of development guides care/needs in premature infants

Optimizing Outcomes:
- Prenatal screening for maternal drug use
- Use of folic acid to prevent neural tube defects

What To Say:
- Nonjudgmental and caring approach when congenital anomalies are identified

Across Care Settings:
- Any prenatal care setting; Education/active involvement → increases understanding and self-care

Now Can You:
?
- Discuss the characteristics of embryonic/fetal growth
- Identify the unique aspects of fetal circulation
- Identify the pattern of human development by periods
- Discuss substances that may adversely affect development

one
two
three
four
five
six
seven

The Prenatal Journey

Physiological and Psychosocial Changes During Pregnancy

chapter 8

Everything in nature bespeaks the mother. The sun is the mother of the earth and gives it its nourishment of heat; it never leaves the universe at night until it has put the earth to sleep to the song of the sea and the hymn of the birds and brooks. And this earth is the mother of trees and flowers. It produces them, nurses them, and weans them. The trees and flowers become kind mothers of their great fruits and seeds. And the mother, the prototype of all existence, is the eternal spirit, full of beauty and love.

—Kahlil Gibran

LEARNING TARGETS *At the completion of this chapter, the student will be able to:*

◆ Describe the physiological changes that occur during pregnancy and their etiologies.

◆ Identify nursing measures to relieve the discomforts caused by the physiological changes.

◆ Describe the psychosocial changes that occur during pregnancy and the factors that influence these changes.

◆ Identify nursing interventions to help families adapt to the psychosocial changes.

---

 moving toward evidence-based practice Parental Efficacy

de Montigny, F., & Lacharité, C. (2005). Perceived parental efficacy: Concept analysis. *Journal of Advanced Nursing, 49*(4), 387–396.

The purpose of this study was to (1) distinguish perceived parental efficacy from parental confidence and parental competence; (2) clarify perceived parental efficacy by identifying its attributes, antecedents, and consequences; (3) explore changes that have occurred in the concept over time; and (4) explore areas of agreement and disagreement across the nursing and psychology disciplines. A concept analysis of literature from psychology and nursing covering a 20-year period from 1980 to 2000 was completed to include the topics of parental self-efficacy, competence, and confidence. One hundred and thirteen articles were obtained. Of these, 30 were selected to represent each discipline based on the extent to which the concepts were represented in the discussion. Data analysis was carried out in a thematic manner similar to the content analysis suggested by Rodgers and Knafl (2000).

The researchers defined parental efficacy as "beliefs one holds in one's capabilities to organize and execute the courses of actions required to produce given attainments" as identified in Bandura's Social Cognitive Theory. The following theory concepts were selected to serve as the framework for the concept analysis: personal beliefs, capabilities and power, ability to organize and execute actions that produce results, and situation-specific tasks related to parenting a child.

Based on interpretation of Bandura's theory, concept definitions included:

- Parent's beliefs/judgment: Refers to judgments held by the parent and strength of that judgment
- Capabilities: Refers to what "one can do under a different set of conditions with whatever skills one possesses"
- Actions that are organized and executed to produce a set of tasks: Means "being able to integrate sub skills into appropriate courses of actions and to execute them well under difficult circumstances"
- Situation-specific tasks related to parenting a child: Refers to situation-specific tasks that are related to parenting, be they instrumental tasks such as feeding, or affective tasks, such as comforting" (de Montigny & Lacharité, 2005, p. 390).

The attribute "perceived parental efficacy" included positive enactive mastery experiences, vicarious experiences, verbal persuasion, and an appropriate physiological and affective state.

(continued)

"Enactive mastery experiences" provide information regarding an individual's capabilities and limitations and contribute to one's overall belief system. Mastery, which occurs as a result of successful parenting experiences, can include childcare experiences before becoming a parent. "Vicarious experiences" provide a reference point for comparison with others who have attained competencies. These experiences are transmitted through observation and role modeling. "Verbal persuasion" is important as a form of reinforcement of one's beliefs and the capacity of significant others in the relationship to believe in that parent's perception. "Physiological and affective states" refers to fluctuations, such as those caused by stress, which can lead to vulnerability and a decrease in feelings of being efficacious.

It was concluded that parental efficacy could be described as "beliefs or judgments a parent has about their capabilities to organize and execute a set of tasks related to parenting a child" (Rodgers & Knafl, 2000).

1. What research limitations can be identified from the above synopsis of this study?
   What additional research may be indicated?
2. How is this information useful to clinical nursing practice?

See Suggested Responses for Moving Toward Evidence-Based Practice on the Electronic Study Guide or DavisPlus.

Introduction

From the time just before conception, and then for the following 10 lunar months, the woman's body undergoes many complex alterations that prepare her to nurture a new life. The physical, psychological, and emotional changes that accompany pregnancy are all focused on the growth, development, and future envelopment of the baby into a new family. The beginning of a new life is a time of awe and amazement shaped by a myriad of events that bring about unique changes for the woman and her family.

This chapter explores the physiological and psychosocial changes that occur during pregnancy and their effects on the woman, the fetus, and her family.

Physiological Preparation for Pregnancy

HORMONAL INFLUENCES

Many hormones are responsible for the changes that take place during and beyond pregnancy. Each serves a specific function in the nurturing process for the embryo, fetus, and neonate. The pituitary gland secretes hormones that influence ovarian follicular development, prompt ovulation, and stimulate the uterine lining to prepare for pregnancy and maintain it until the placenta becomes fully functional. Other pituitary hormones alter metabolism, stimulate lactation, produce pigmentation changes in the skin, stimulate uterine muscle contractions, prompt milk ejection from the breasts, allow for vasoconstriction to maintain blood pressure, and regulate water balance.

After conception, ovulation ceases. The corpus luteum produces progesterone and, to a lesser degree, estrogen. Progesterone is the hormone primarily responsible for maintaining the pregnancy. Once implantation occurs, the trophoblast secretes human chorionic gonadotrophin (hCG) to prompt the corpus luteum to continue progesterone production until this function is taken over by the placenta. The ovarian hormones work in synchrony to maintain the endometrium, provide nutrition for the developing morula and blastocyst, aid in implantation,

decrease the contractility of the uterus to prevent spontaneous abortion, initiate development of the ductal system in the breasts, and prompt remodeling of maternal joint collagen.

The placenta provides hormones essential to the survival of the pregnancy and fetus. Placental hormones do the following:

- Prevent the normal involution of the ovarian corpus luteum
- Stimulate production of testosterone in the male fetus
- Protect the pregnancy from the maternal immune response
- Ensure that added glucose, protein, and minerals are available for the fetus
- Prompt proliferation of the uterus and breast glandular tissue
- Promote relaxation of the woman's smooth muscle
- Create a loosening of the pelvis and other major joints

Each of these hormones plays a vital role in the maintenance of the pregnancy, and all body systems are affected by the profound changes that prepare the woman to nurture the growing fetus and neonate.

A & P review   **The Major Pregnancy Hormones and Their Effects on the Reproductive System**

Estrogen and progesterone are the major hormones produced by the placenta during pregnancy. The effect of estrogen is one of "growth"; the effect of progesterone is one of "maintenance."

Estrogen prompts hyperplasia and hypertrophy (growth of cells in number and size) during pregnancy. Because of the effects of estrogen, breast tissue enlarges and becomes functional and the uterus expands, a process that allows for stretching of the muscles to accommodate the growing fetus. Estrogen also enhances uterine contractility to prepare the muscles for labor.

Progesterone enables the pregnancy to thrive by its relaxation effect on the smooth muscle. Progesterone causes vasodilation and an increased blood flow to all body tissues, it slows the gastrointestinal tract to ensure absorption of essential nutrients for fetal development, and it relaxes the uterine muscle to prevent the onset of labor until term. Progesterone has been called the "pro-pregnancy hormone." ◆

REPRODUCTIVE SYSTEM

The reproductive system undergoes the greatest changes in size and function and every organ within this system is affected by or focused on the needs of the growing fetus.

Uterus

The uterus provides a home for the growing fetus for its 10-lunar-month stay in the woman. Its pattern of growth is very predictable for the first 20 weeks of the pregnancy. Depending on fetal size, uterine growth over the next 20 weeks varies. The shape of the uterus changes dramatically. Very early in pregnancy the uterus is shaped like a "lightbulb" or inverted pear. By the end of the first trimester the uterus has developed into a soft, enlarged globular structure that has risen out of the pelvis and into the abdominal cavity (Fig. 8-1). Under the influence of estrogen and progesterone, the myometrial cells and muscle fibers undergo hyperplasia and hypertrophy, processes that allow the uterus to enlarge and stretch as the fetus grows. By term, the uterine wall thins to 0.6 inch (1.5 cm) or less and its weight will have increased from 1.8 oz. to 2.2 lb. (70 g to 1100 g).

Estrogen causes the uterine muscles to contract. Braxton-Hicks contractions are irregular and painless and may begin as early as the 16th week of gestation. As the pregnancy advances and the fetal size increases, the contractions become increasingly more frequent and intense and are easily felt by the woman. Until late in the second trimester the contractions serve to prepare the uterine muscles for the synchronized activity necessary for effective labor. As long as the contractions are irregular in frequency and last for less than 60 seconds, the patient may be reassured of their normalcy. However, if a pattern of contraction regularity is noted or if the contractions are associated with bleeding, nausea, vomiting, or intense pain, the patient should be instructed to promptly report to her health care provider for evaluation.

Blood flow is increased from the effects of progesterone on the smooth muscle of the vasculature to provide adequate circulation for endometrial growth and placental function. The enhanced uterine circulation is important for ensuring adequate fetal nutrition and the removal of waste products.

After implantation, the endometrium lining the uterus is termed the **decidua**. The decidua consists of three layers:

Decidua vera is the external layer and it has no contact with the fetus.
Decidua basalis is the uterine lining beneath the site of implantation.
Decidua capsularis is the endometrial tissue that covers the embryo (Fig. 8-2).

Cervix

One of the earliest signs of pregnancy is the discoloration, or bluish purple hue, that appears on the cervix, vagina, and vulva. This color change is known as **Chadwick's sign** (Fig. 8-3). High levels of circulating estrogen cause stimulation of the cervical glandular tissue, which increases in cell number and becomes hyperactive. Increased blood flow and engorgement produces the bluish discoloration.

Stimulation from the hormones estrogen and progesterone produces cervical softening (**Goodell's sign**). This physiological change is related to several events, including a decrease in the collagen fibers of the connective tissue, increased vascularity and edema, and slight tissue hypertrophy and hyperplasia. Before pregnancy, the cervix is firm and its texture resembles that of the tip of the nose. After conception, the cervix softens and its texture begins to resemble that of an ear lobe.

Estrogen and progesterone cause a proliferation of the mucus-producing cervical glands. Early in pregnancy, the endocervical tissue begins to take on a honeycomb appearance. Cervical mucus fills the endocervical canal and forms a mucus plug (**operculum**), which helps to keep harmful

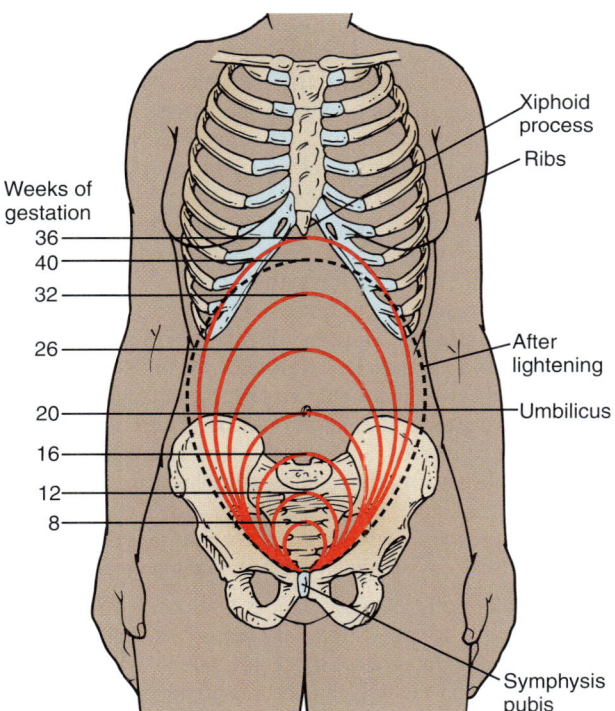

Figure 8-1 Pattern of uterine growth during pregnancy.

Figure 8-2 The layers of the decidua.

Figure 8-3 Chadwick's sign.

agents out of the uterus. **Leukorrhea**, an increased whitish vaginal discharge, results from hyperplasia of the vaginal mucosa and increased mucus production from the endocervical glands. The discharge is often profuse and may be worrisome. As the due date approaches, cervical effacement and dilation cause a breakdown of the mucus plug, resulting in an increased vaginal discharge. The nurse should reassure the patient about the normalcy of leukorrhea during pregnancy and instruct her to call her health care provider if the discharge appears thicker; becomes bloody or yellowish/green; is accompanied by a foul odor; or if it causes itching, irritation, or pain in the vulvar or vaginal area.

Vagina and Vulva

Changes that occur in the vagina and vulva are similar to those that take place in the cervix. An increased blood flow (hyperemia) produces a bluish-purple hue (Chadwick's sign). Thickening of the vaginal mucosa develops and the rugae (vaginal folds) become more prominent. The rugae deepen from hyperplasia and hypertrophy of the epithelial and elastic tissues and this change allows for adequate stretching of the vaginal vault during childbirth. As the pregnancy progresses, the area becomes edematous from poor venous return due to the weight of the gravid uterus. For some women, the increased pelvic congestion can lead to a heightened sexual interest and increased orgasmic experience (McKinney, James, Murray, & Ashwill, 2005). Leukorrhea results from increased cervical mucus along with elevated glycogen levels in the vaginal cells, which produces rapid sloughing of tissue. The increased glycogen levels also create a vaginal environment more susceptible to the growth of *Candida albicans*. Thus, during pregnancy the woman is more susceptible to the development of monilial vaginitis (yeast infections). The pH of the vaginal fluids becomes more acidic, and decreases from 6.0 to 3.5. This change results from the action of *Lactobacillus acidophilus* on the increased glycogen levels in the vaginal epithelium (Cunningham et al., 2005). The increased acidity helps to control the growth of most pathogens in the vaginal canal.

The nurse should discuss the importance of vulvar hygiene with the patient. Gentle external cleansing with plain soap and water is adequate. Douching, or internal cleansing of the vagina, should be avoided because this practice can alter the vaginal pH and allow pathogens to grow as well as disrupt the cervical mucus plug.

Ovaries

After ovulation, the pituitary hormone luteinizing hormone (LH) stimulates the corpus luteum (functional cyst that remains on the ovary) to produce progesterone for 6 to 7 weeks. Once the placenta is developed and functional, it begins to take over the task of progesterone production. At that time, the corpus luteum ceases to function and is gradually absorbed by the ovary. The corpus luteal cyst enlarges while functioning and may reach the size of a golf ball before it begins to recede. In some cases the cyst may rupture, causing the woman some pelvic discomfort associated with bleeding into the pelvic cavity. The pain should dissipate as the cyst and blood are absorbed. If the pain is persistent or if vaginal bleeding occurs, the nurse should advise the woman to seek medical care. Ovulation ceases during pregnancy due to the high circulating levels of estrogen and progesterone, which inhibit the pituitary release of follicle-stimulating hormone (FSH) and LH.

Breasts

Estrogen and progesterone produce a number of changes in the mammary glands. Breast enlargement, fullness, tingling, and increased sensitivity occur during the early weeks of gestation. The superficial veins become more prominent from the vascular relaxation effects of progesterone. Often the venous congestion is more noticeable in primigravidas. Melanotropin, a hormone secreted by the pituitary gland, causes the nipples to become tender and more pronounced with darkening of the areola. The **Montgomery tubercles** (sebaceous glands) on and around the areola enlarge and provide lubrication for the nipple tissue. **Striae gravidarum** (stretch marks) may develop as the breast tissue stretches (Fig. 8-4).

During the second trimester, pre-colostrum, a clear thin fluid, is found in the acini cells, the smallest parts of the milk glands. Pre-colostrum becomes **colostrum**, a creamy whitish-yellow liquid that may leak from the nipples as early as the 16th week of gestation. This pre-milk substance contains antibodies, essential proteins, and fat to nourish the baby and prepare his intestines for digestion and elimination. Colostrum is converted to mature milk during the first few days after birth.

During prenatal care, the nurse should discuss the need for changes in bra size, options for infant feeding, and, if the patient wishes to breast feed, strategies to help her prepare for successful breast feeding. The process of lactation should be reviewed and the woman should be given a list of lactation support resources. Soft cotton liners can be used to pad the bra if leaking of the nipples is troublesome.

 Now Can You— Describe major changes that occur in the reproductive system during pregnancy?

1. Identify four physiological changes that occur in the uterus and possible symptoms that may accompany these changes?
2. Explain the hormonal basis for changes in the vagina and vulva and identify patient teaching needs concerning the changes?
3. Describe three breast changes and identify the hormones responsible for the changes?

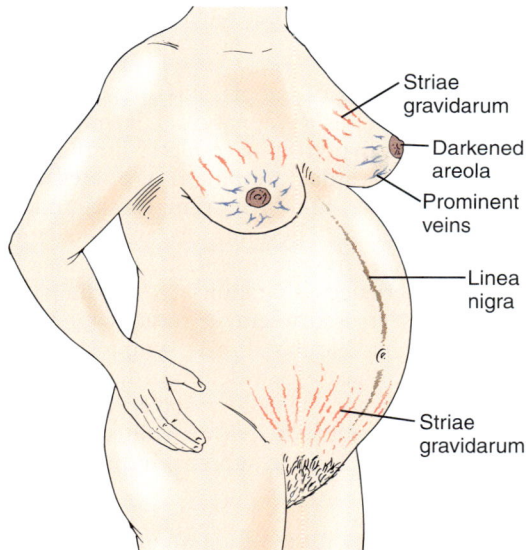

Figure 8-4 Integumentary system changes include darkening of the areolae, appearance of the linea nigra, and striae gravidarum.

Figure 8-5 Chloasma.

INTEGUMENTARY SYSTEM

Estrogen, progesterone, and alpha-melanocyte-stimulating hormones cause many changes in the appearance, structure, and function of the integumentary system. Though seldom serious, the outward changes in appearance may negatively affect the woman's self-concept and body image.

The skin undergoes a number of pigmentation changes related to the influence of estrogen. Moles (nevi), freckles, and recent scars may darken or appear to multiply in number. The nipples, areolae, axillae, vulvar area, and perineum also darken in color.

The linea alba, a light line that extends from the umbilicus to the mons pubis (and sometimes upward to the xiphoid process), darkens, becoming the **linea nigra** (see Fig. 8-4). The linea is more noticeable in the woman with a naturally darker complexion. Melasma gravidarum, also known as **chloasma**, forms the "mask of pregnancy" (Fig. 8-5). This dark, blotchy brownish pigmentation change occurs around the hairline, brow, nose and cheeks and often gives the appearance of "raccoon eyes." The heightened pigmentation fades after pregnancy but can recur after exposure to the sun. During pregnancy the skin becomes photosensitive and sunburn may occur in a shorter exposure time than usual for the individual. The nurse should teach the patient about the importance of regular sunscreen use and decreased sun exposure time.

Alterations in hair as well as nail growth and texture may occur. The nails may become stronger and grow faster. The number of hair follicles in the dormant phase may decrease, and this change stimulates new hair growth. Once the infant is born, this process is reversed and there is an increase in hair shedding for approximately 1 to 4 months. Although this change may be disconcerting, the nurse can reassure the patient that virtually all hair will be replaced within 6 to 12 months (Cuningham et al., 2005). During pregnancy, hair may react differently to dyes and chemicals.

Increased adrenal steroid levels cause the connective tissue to lose strength and become more fragile. This change can cause striae gravidarum, or "stretch marks" on the breasts, buttocks, thighs, and abdomen (see Fig. 8-4). Striae appear as reddish, wavy, depressed streaks that will fade to a silvery white color after birth but they do not usually disappear completely.

Increased levels of estrogen during pregnancy may cause **angiomas** and **palmar erythema**. Angiomas, also called "vascular spiders," are tiny, bluish, end-arterioles that occur on the neck, thorax, face, and arms. They may appear as star shaped or branched structures that are slightly raised and do not blanch with pressure. More common in Caucasian women, angiomas appear most often during the second to fifth month of pregnancy and usually disappear after birth. Palmar erythema is a condition characterized by color changes over the palmar surfaces of the hands (Fig. 8-6). Approximately 60% of Caucasian women and 35% of African American women experience palmar erythema during pregnancy, which presents as a diffuse, reddish-pink mottling of the palms. Increased blood flow, along with high levels of circulating hormones, can produce other skin changes such as inflammatory pruritus and acne vulgaris, a condition seen predominately in the first trimester. Hyperactivity of the sweat and sebaceous glands may cause some women to experience excessive perspiration, night sweats, and skin changes that can range from extreme dryness to extreme oiliness.

The nurse should offer reassurance and provide anticipatory guidance as these changes occur. Recommendations to the patient include daily bathing, the liberal use of lotions or oils for dry skin, the regular use of deodorant, and limited sun exposure with the diligent use of sunscreen.

NEUROLOGICAL SYSTEM

The central nervous system appears to be affected by the hormonal changes of pregnancy although the specific alterations other than those involving the hypothalamic–pituitary axis are less well known. Many women complain of a decreased attention span, poor concentration, and memory lapses during and shortly after pregnancy. Cunningham and colleagues (2005) identified a pregnancy sleep pattern phenomenon characterized by reduced sleep efficiency, fewer hours of night sleep, frequent awakenings, and difficulty

Figure 8-6 Palmar erythema.

going to sleep. Nurses can advise patients that afternoon napping may help alleviate the fatigue associated with the sleep alterations. Providing anticipatory guidance related to expected alterations is key in facilitating the woman's acceptance of these changes.

Edema from vascular permeability can lead to a collection of fluid in the wrist that puts pressure on the median nerve lying beneath the carpal ligament. This alteration leads to **carpal tunnel syndrome**, a condition that usually develops during the third trimester. It is manifested by pain and paresthesia (a burning, tingling, or numb sensation) in the hand that radiates to the elbow. The pain occurs in one (usually the dominant) or both hands and is intensified with attempts to grasp objects. Elevation of the hands at night may help to reduce the edema. Occasionally, a woman may need to wear a "cock splint" to prevent the wrist from flexing, an action that puts additional pressure on the median nerve. Carpal tunnel syndrome usually subsides after the pregnancy (and the accompanying edema) has ended although some women may require surgical treatment if symptoms persist.

Syncope (a transient loss of consciousness and postural tone with spontaneous recovery) during pregnancy is frequently attributed to orthostatic hypotension and/or inferior vena cava compression by the gravid uterus (Cunningham et al., 2005). It may also occur as increased intra abdominal pressure from the growing uterus places pressure on the vagus nerve. Coughing, straining during bowel movements, and upward pressure from the growing fetus can trigger a vasovagal response that produces faintness or loss of consciousness. Lightheadedness, sweating, nausea, yawning, and feelings of warmth are warning signs that often precede syncope. Educating the patient about signs and symptoms often helps to alleviate the fears that frequently accompany the fainting episodes. If lightheadedness or other warning signs are experienced, the woman is instructed to immediately assume a sitting or lying position. A left side-lying position is preferred to avoid compression of the vena cava (which can lead to supine hypotension) from the gravid uterus.

🌀 **Now Can You—** Discuss changes in the integumentary and neurological systems?

1. Identify four changes that occur in the integumentary system and discuss patient teaching needs for these changes?
2. Define carpal tunnel syndrome and identify two interventions to help alleviate the associated symptoms?
3. Discuss the physiological origins of syncope during pregnancy and patient education concerning syncope?

CARDIOVASCULAR SYSTEM

Heart

As growth of the fetus exerts pressure on the diaphragm, the maternal heart is pushed upward and laterally to the left (Fig. 8-7). Cardiac hypertrophy results from the increased blood volume and cardiac output. Exaggerated first and third heart sounds and systolic murmurs are common findings during pregnancy. The murmurs are usually asymptomatic and require no treatment. If symptomatic, the woman may experience palpitations, chest pain, shortness of breath, or a decreased tolerance to activity. The nurse should advise the patient that if these symptoms occur, she should see her health care provider immediately for evaluation. Systolic murmurs usually resolve within the first 2 weeks postpartum after the plasma volume levels return to normal. They may recur in subsequent pregnancies.

Blood Volume

An increase in maternal blood volume begins during the first trimester and peaks at term. The increase approaches 40% to 45% and is due primarily to an increase in plasma and erythrocyte volume. Additional erythrocytes, needed because of the extra oxygen requirements of the maternal and placental tissue, ensure an adequate supply of oxygen to the fetus. The elevation in erythrocyte volume remains constant during pregnancy.

Most of the increased blood flow is directed to the uterus, and of this amount, 80% is channeled to the placenta. Blood flow to the maternal kidneys is increased by 30% to 50%, and this alteration enhances the excretion of maternal and fetal wastes. Dilation of the capillaries and increased blood flow to the skin assist the woman in eliminating the extra heat generated by fetal metabolism. The extra blood volume decreases during the first 2 weeks postpartum and a substantial amount of fluid loss in the first 3 postpartal days occurs through maternal diuresis.

Iron

Iron is necessary for the formation of hemoglobin, the oxygen-carrying component of the erythrocyte. The increased need for oxygen requires the pregnant woman to increase her iron intake. The fetal need for iron is greatest during the last 4 weeks of pregnancy, when the fetal iron stores are amassed.

During pregnancy, the woman's hematocrit values may appear low due to the increase in total plasma volume

Figure 8-7 Growth of the uterus displaces the maternal heart upward and laterally to the left.

(on average, 50%). Since the plasma volume is greater than the increase in erythrocytes (30%), the hematocrit (a measurement of the red blood cell concentration in the plasma) decreases by about 7%. This alteration is termed "physiological anemia of pregnancy" or "pseudoanemia." The hemodilution effect is most apparent at 32 to 34 weeks. The mean acceptable hemoglobin level in pregnancy is 11 to 12 g/dL of blood. Some women experience symptoms of fatigue related to this phenomenon although altered sleep patterns may also contribute to the fatigue. The nurse should teach the patient to hydrate adequately by drinking 6 to 8 glasses of water each day, and also to ensure that her diet is high in protein and iron. Although gastrointestinal absorption of iron is enhanced during pregnancy, most women must add supplemental iron to meet the needs of the expanded erythrocytes and those of the growing fetus.

Leukocytes, Proteins, Platelets, Immunoglobulins

The number of leukocytes also increases and the average white blood cell count ranges from 5000 to 15,000 /mm^3. During labor and postpartum these levels may climb as high as 25,000/mm^3. Although the exact reason for this increase is unclear, it is known that leukocyte counts normally increase in response to stress and vigorous exercise (Cunningham et al., 2005). Normal laboratory values during pregnancy are presented in Table 8-1.

Plasma proteins also increase, although due to the hemodilution effect during pregnancy, there is a decrease

Table 8-1 Common Laboratory Values in Pregnancy		
Laboratory Values	**Usual Normal Female Value**	**Normal Value in Pregnancy**
Serum Values		
Hemoglobin	11.7–15.5 g/dL	Decreased by 1.5–2 g/dL
	(mean Hgb is 0.5–1.0 g lower in African Americans, Mexican and Asian Americans have a higher hemoglobin & hematocrit than Caucasians)	Lowest point occurs at 30–34 weeks
Hematocrit	38–44%	Decreased by 4–7%, lowest point at 30–34 weeks
Leukocytes	4.5–11.0 × 10^3/mm^3	Gradual increase of 3.5 × 10^3/mm^3
Platelets	150–400 × 10^3/mm^3	Slight decrease
Amylase	30–110 U/L	Increased by 50–100%
Chemistries		
Albumin	3.4–4.8 g/dL	Early decrease by 1 g/dL
Calcium (total)	8.2–10.2 mg/dL	Gradual decrease of 10%
Chloride	97–107 mEq/L	No significant change
Creatinine	0.5–1.1 mg/dL	Early decrease by 0.3 mg/dL
Fibrinogen	200–400 mg/dL	Progressive increase of 1–2 g/L
Glucose (fasting)	65–99 mg/dL	Gradual decrease of 10%
Potassium	3.5–5.0 mEq/L	Gradual decrease of 0.2–0.3 mEq/L
Protein (total)	6.0–8.0 g/dL	Early decrease of 1 g/dL then stable
Sodium	135–145 mEq/L	Early decrease of 2–4 mEq/L then stable
Urea nitrogen	8–20 mg/dL	Decrease in 1st trimester by 50%
Uric acid	2.3–6.6 mg/dL	First trimester decrease of 33%, rise at term
Urine Chemistries		
Creatinine	11–20 mg/kg per 24 hr	No significant change
Protein	10–140 mg per 24 hr	Up by 250–300 mg/day by the 20th week
Creatinine clearance	75–115 mL/min/1.73 m^2	Increased by 40–50% by the 16th week
Serum Hormones		
Cortisol	8–21 g/dL	Increased by 20 g/dL
Prolactin	3.3–26.7 ng/mL	Gradual increase, 5.3–215.3 ng/mL, peaks at term
Thyroxine (T$_4$) total	5.5–11.0 mcg/dL	5.5–16.0 mcg/dL
Triiodothyronine (T$_3$) total	70–204 ng/dL	Early sustained increase of up to 50%
		116–247 ng/dL (last 4 months of gestation)

in protein concentrations, especially in the level of albumins. Decreased plasma albumin leads to a drop in osmotic pressure, which causes body fluids to move into the second space. This change produces edema.

Although the platelet cell count does not change significantly, fibrinogen volume has been shown to increase by as much as 50%. This alteration leads to an increase in the sedimentation rate. Blood factors VII, VIII, IX, and X are also increased, and this change causes hypercoagulability. The hypercoagulable state, coupled with venous stasis (poor blood return from the lower extremities), places the pregnant woman at an increased risk for venous thrombosis, embolism, and when complications are present, disseminated intravascular coagulation (DIC). (See Chapter 11 for further discussion.)

The production of maternal immunoglobulins (IgA, IgG, IgM, IgD, IgE) is unchanged in pregnancy. Immunoglobulins protect the body from a variety of bacterial, viral, and parasitic infections. Three major types of immunoglobulins (IgG, IgA, and IgM) are primarily involved in immunity. Circulating levels of maternal IgG are decreased during pregnancy because of transfer across the placenta. As the only immunoglobulin transported across the placenta, IgG is active against bacterial toxins (Hacker, Moore, & Gambone, 2004). Although transport of IgG begins around the 16th week of gestation, the fetus does not acquire a significant amount of IgG until the last 4 weeks of pregnancy. At birth, the neonate's primary immunoglobulins (IgG) have been acquired from the mother via a process termed "passive acquired immunity" (Cunningham et al., 2005). Due to its large molecular size, IgM is unable to cross the placenta. IgA, IgD and IgE also remain in the maternal circulation. IgA, which is believed to provide protection to various secreting surfaces such as those in the respiratory tract, gastrointestinal tract, and eyes, is passed to the neonate in breast milk (Smeltzer & Bare, 2004). Immunoglobulins and their major actions are summarized in Table 8-2.

During pregnancy, resistance to infection is decreased as a result of depressed leukocyte function. Due to this normal physiological alteration, maternal autoimmune diseases such as lupus erythematosus may improve during pregnancy. (See Chapter 11 for further discussion.) Because of the increased susceptibility to infection, patients should be instructed to avoid crowds and individuals with active infections. Frequent, consistent hand washing and good respiratory hygiene should also be stressed.

Cardiac Output

Cardiac output increases, and peaks around the 20th to 24th week of gestation at about 30% to 50% above pre-pregnancy levels. It remains increased for the duration of the pregnancy. With the increased vascular volume and cardiac output, vasodilation (related to progesterone-induced relaxation of the vascular smooth muscle) prevents an elevation in blood pressure. The woman's pulse rate frequently increases up to 10 to 15 beats per minute to facilitate effective circulation of the increased blood volume.

During the first trimester, blood pressure normally remains the same as pre-pregnancy levels but then gradually decreases up to around 20 weeks of gestation. After 20 weeks, the vascular volume expands and the blood pressure increases to reach pre-pregnancy levels by term. Because of the relaxed vascular resistance and stasis of blood in the lower extremities, there is an increased risk of varicose veins and hemorrhoids. The nurse should instruct the woman to elevate her lower extremities by lying on her left side with the feet higher than her heart for 15 to 20 minutes daily to improve venous return from the lower extremities. Daily walks enhance circulation and also improve intestinal peristalsis, important in facilitating regular bowel function. Patients should be advised to drink at least 8 to 10 glasses of water each day and include adequate roughage in their diet. These strategies help prevent constipation and straining with bowel movements, both of which increase the likelihood of hemorrhoids.

Table 8-2 Immunoglobulins and Their Major Actions	
IgG (75% of Total Immunoglobulin)	Appears in serum and tissues (interstitial fluid)
	Assumes major role in blood borne and tissue infections
	Activates the complement system
	Enhances phagocytosis
	Crosses the placenta
IgA (15% of Total Immunoglobulin)	Appears in body fluids (blood, saliva, tears, **breast milk**, and pulmonary, gastrointestinal, prostatic and vaginal secretions)
	Protects against respiratory, gastrointestinal, and genitourinary infections
	Prevents absorption of antigens from food
	Is transferred to the neonate via breast milk
IgM (10% of Total Immunoglobulin)	Appears mostly in intravascular serum
	Appears as the first immunoglobulin produced in response to bacterial and viral infections
	Activates the complement system
	No placental transfer during pregnancy
IgD (0.2% of Total Immunoglobulin)	Appears in small amounts in serum
	Possibly influences B-lymphocyte differentiation, but its role is unclear
IgE (0.004% of Total Immunoglobulin)	Appears in serum
	Involved in allergic and some hypersensitivity reactions
	Combats parasitic infections

Adapted from Smeltzer, S.C., & Bare, B.G. (Eds.). (2004). *Textbook of medical-surgical nursing* (10th ed.). Philadelphia: Lippincott Williams & Wilkins.

Supine Hypotension Syndrome

The pregnant woman may experience **supine hypotension syndrome,** or **vena caval syndrome** (faintness related to bradycardia) if she lies on her back. The pressure from the enlarged uterus exerted on the vena cava decreases the amount of venous return from the lower extremities and causes a marked decrease in blood pressure, with accompanying dizziness, diaphoresis, and pallor (Fig. 8-8). Placing the woman on her left side can relieve the symptoms. Orthostatic hypotension is another condition that occurs frequently during pregnancy and results from stagnation of blood in the lower extremities. If the woman stands for too long or arises too quickly, gravity causes the blood to flow to the lower extremities, decreasing blood flow to the brain. **Mean arterial pressure** (MAP) indicates the average driving force for the movement of blood in the arterial system throughout the cardiac cycle (Darovic, 2004). The MAP is the same in all parts of the cardiovascular system when the patient is supine except during pregnancy, when the gravid uterus places pressure on the vena cava, and produces an alteration in the blood pressure. The change in the MAP leads to decreased blood flow throughout the body, particularly in the heart, brain, and uterus.

All of the changes in the circulatory system return to normal by the second to third week postpartum as the woman's body returns to a non-pregnant state. Reassurance can be given to the patient and she should be encouraged to arise slowly from a lying or sitting position. While standing, she should keep her feet moving to encourage adequate venous return from the lower extremities and avoid lying flat on her back.

Figure 8-8 Supine hypotension, or vena caval syndrome, may occur if the pregnant woman lies on her back. This causes compression of the vena cava.

 Now Can You—Discuss changes in the cardiovascular system?

1. Describe two changes in the heart and the physiological basis for these changes?
2. Discuss why there is a need for an increase in erythrocytes during pregnancy?
3. Explain what is meant by "passive acquired immunity"?
4. Differentiate between supine hypotension syndrome and orthostatic hypotension?

RESPIRATORY SYSTEM

During pregnancy, a number of changes occur to meet the woman's increased oxygen requirements. The tidal volume (amount of air breathed in each minute) increases 30% to 40%. This change is related to the elevated levels of estrogen and progesterone. Estrogen prompts hypertrophy and hyperplasia of the lung tissue. Progesterone decreases airway resistance by causing relaxation of the smooth muscle of the bronchi, bronchioles, and alveoli. These alterations produce an increase in oxygen consumption by approximately 15% to 20%, along with an increase in vital capacity (the maximum amount of air that can be moved in and out of the lungs with forced respiration).

The enlarging uterus creates an upward pressure that elevates the diaphragm and increases the subcostal angle. The chest circumference may increase by as much as 2.4 inches (6 cm). Although the "up and down" capacity of diaphragmatic movement is reduced (due to increasing pressure from the growing fetus), lateral movement of the chest and intercostal muscles accommodate for this loss of

movement and keep pulmonary functions stable. Many women verbalize an increased awareness of the need to breathe and may perceive this sensation as dyspnea (difficulty breathing). The nurse should offer reassurance and educate the woman about normal alterations and symptoms. Under normal circumstances, resting with the head elevated while taking slow, deep breaths causes an improvement in the symptoms. However, certain lung diseases including asthma and emphysema may be aggravated by the normal physiological changes as the oxygen demands of the pregnancy increase. If symptoms persist or worsen, the woman should contact her health care provider.

Eyes, Ears, Nose, and Throat

EYES Blurred vision, the most common visual complaint in pregnant women, is caused by corneal thickening associated with fluid retention and decreased intraocular pressure. These changes begin during the first trimester, persist throughout pregnancy, and regress by 6 to 8 weeks postpartum. As part of anticipatory guidance, the nurse teaches that since the changes are only temporary, a corrective lens prescription should not be changed until the pregnancy has been completed.

EARS No changes have been noted in auditory function during pregnancy.

NOSE An increase in mucus production results from the combined effects of progesterone (increased blood flow to the mucus membranes of the sinus and nasal passages) and estrogen (hypertrophy and hyperplasia of the mucosa). Nasal stuffiness and congestion (rhinitis of pregnancy) are common complaints. The nurse should educate the patient about these normal changes and offer reassurance. Increasing the oral fluid intake helps to keep the mucus thin and easier to mobilize.

Edema (an effect of estrogen) of the nasal mucosa, along with vascular congestion (an effect of progesterone) may cause epistaxis (nosebleeds). The woman should be advised to use caution when blowing her nose and to avoid probing the nasal cavities with a cotton swab. The use of nasal sprays designed to relieve congestion should be avoided due to their rebound effect that causes the congestion to worsen. Normal saline nasal sprays may be used sparingly to moisten the nasal passages.

THROAT Hyperemia (congestion) occurs from increased blood flow and relaxation of smooth muscle. Swallowing may be difficult if food is not chewed well.

GASTROINTESTINAL SYSTEM

The gastrointestinal system is probably the source of most of the woman's discomforts during pregnancy. Nausea and vomiting during the first trimester most likely are related to rising levels of human chorionic gonadotropin (hCG) and altered carbohydrate metabolism. Changes in taste and smell, due to alterations in the oral and nasal mucosa, can further aggravate the gastrointestinal discomfort. A nonspecific **gingivitis** (inflammation of the gums) occurs frequently due to the increased blood supply to the gums, along with estrogen-related tissue hypertrophy and edema. Although the gums may bleed from routine oral hygiene, the nurse should stress the importance of regular dental maintenance and its effect on good maternal nutrition.

On occasion, red, raised nodules (**epulis gravidarum**) appear at the gum line (Fig. 8-9). These growths bleed easily, and usually regress within 2 months after childbirth (Beckmann et al., 2006). If associated with excessive bleeding, local excision may be necessary. **Ptyalism**, excessive saliva production often with a bitter taste, may occur and can be unpleasant or embarrassing. Its cause is uncertain, although stimulation of the salivary glands from eating starch or decreased unconscious swallowing when nauseated may be contributing factors (Cunningham et al., 2005). Limited relief can be obtained with the use of chewing gum and lozenges. Patients can also be advised to eat small, frequent meals and avoid starchy foods such as potatoes, bread, and pasta.

The effect of progesterone on smooth muscle causes relaxation of the esophagus. The movement of food is slowed and the gastroesophageal, or cardiac sphincter (circular muscle located at the top of the stomach) weakens. This alteration prevents efficient closure when the stomach is emptying and allows the reflux of stomach contents into the esophagus, producing heartburn, or **pyrosis**. Pyrosis results from irritation to the esophageal lining by gastric secretions and acids. Eating small meals, avoiding lying down after meals for at least 1 hour, and limited use of antacids can alleviate some of these symptoms.

Nausea and vomiting of pregnancy, or "morning sickness," occurs because of high levels of hCG and relaxation of the stomach, esophagus, and gastroesophageal sphincters. Food remains in the stomach longer for enhanced digestion and moves more slowly through the small intestine to allow for complete absorption of nutrients. Since the large intestine is also sluggish from the effects of progesterone on the smooth muscle, more water is reabsorbed from the bowel and bloating and constipation can occur. Straining at defecation may cause or exacerbate hemorrhoids (vein varicosities in the lower rectum and anus).

Figure 8-9 Gingival hypertrophy; epulis.

Patients should be encouraged to drink at least 8 to 10 glasses of water each day, add fiber to their diets to produce bulk, and exercise to encourage peristalsis. They should be taught to avoid straining with bowel movements. Warm sitz baths may be helpful for hemorrhoid discomfort. (See Chapter 15 for further discussion.)

The liver, which breaks down maternal toxins, must deal with fetal waste products and toxins as well. The additional workload can lead to altered liver function tests, especially if accompanied by hepatic vessel vasoconstriction associated with preeclampsia. (See Chapter 11 for further discussion.)

The gall bladder, or storehouse for bile, is also composed of smooth muscle and becomes more relaxed, resulting in inefficient emptying. This alteration can lead to stasis of the bile (cholestasia) or inflammation and infection (cholecystitis). In addition, the progesterone-induced prolonged emptying time, combined with elevated blood cholesterol levels, may predispose the woman to gallstone formation (cholelithiasis). Pain in the epigastric region after ingestion of a high-fat meal constitutes the major symptom of these conditions. The pain is self-limiting and usually resolves within 2 hours. Cholelithiasis occurs more often in obese individuals with fair skin and in women older than 40 years of age.

Liver functions are only slightly altered during pregnancy. Stasis of bile in the liver (intrahepatic cholestasis) occasionally occurs late in pregnancy and can cause severe itching (**pruritus gravidarum**). This condition disappears soon after birth. Patients should be advised that avoiding high-fat meals can reduce the presence or frequency of these symptoms.

URINARY SYSTEM

Pregnancy leads to changes in the structure and function of the urinary system. These changes facilitate normal waste elimination for the woman and the increasing waste products of her fetus. During the first trimester, the bladder, a pelvic organ, is compressed by the weight of the growing uterus. The added pressure, along with progesterone-induced relaxation of the urethra and sphincter musculature, leads to urinary urgency, frequency, and nocturia. In the second trimester, when the uterus becomes an abdominal organ, bladder pressure is largely relieved, along with most of the frequency and urgency. By the third trimester, the fetal presenting part descends into the pelvis. At this time, increased pressure is again exerted upon the bladder and symptoms of frequency, urgency, and nocturia return (Fig. 8-10).

Ascension of bacteria into the bladder can cause asymptomatic bacteriuria (ASB) or urinary tract infections (UTIs). These infections occur more frequently in pregnancy due to relaxation of the smooth muscle of the bladder and urinary sphincter, changes that allow bacterial ascent into the bladder.

The ureters, composed of smooth muscle, are also affected by progesterone. Elongation and dilation, especially of the right ureter, occurs. Peristalsis that normally facilitates the movement of urine from the kidneys to the bladder is reduced. This change, coupled with pressure on the ureters from the enlarging uterus, causes an obstruction of urine flow. The stagnant urine becomes an excellent

Figure 8-10 Compression of the bladder results from the growing uterus.

medium for the growth of microorganisms. Patients should be encouraged to drink at least 8 to 10 glasses of water each day and empty their bladders at least every 2 to 3 hours and immediately after intercourse. These measures help to prevent stasis of urine and the bacterial contamination that leads to infection.

The glomerular filtration rate (GFR) and renal plasma flow are increased due to hormonal changes, blood volume increases, the woman's posture, physical activity level, and nutritional intake. During the second trimester, the GFR increases up to 50% in most women. This alteration prompts an increase in renal tubular reabsorption. During pregnancy, there is a greatly increased load of glucose presented to the renal tubules. As a result, glucose excretion increases in virtually all pregnant women (Beckmann et al., 2006). Although it may be a normal finding, glucosuria should always be investigated to rule out gestational diabetes, as the quantitative urine glucose does not accurately reflect blood glucose levels. (See Chapter 11 for further discussion.)

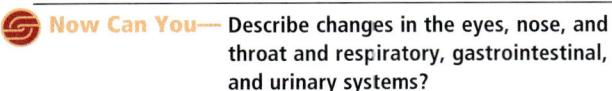 **Now Can You—** Describe changes in the eyes, nose, and throat and respiratory, gastrointestinal, and urinary systems?

1. Describe one alteration that occurs in each of the following: eyes, nose, throat and suggest interventions for relief from the accompanying symptoms?
2. Identify changes during pregnancy that compensate for the reduced diaphragmatic movement that results from the enlarging uterus?
3. Differentiate among epulis gravidarum, ptyalism, and pyrosis and delineate patient teaching needs concerning these symptoms?
4. Explain the physiological basis for glucosuria during pregnancy?

ENDOCRINE SYSTEM

Thyroid Gland

The thyroid gland changes in size and activity during pregnancy. On palpation, the increase in size is appreciated. Enlargement is caused by increased circulation from the progesterone-induced effects on the vessel walls, and by estrogen-induced hyperplasia of the glandular tissue. In early pregnancy, elevated levels of thyroxine-binding globulins cause an increase in the total thyroxine (T_4) and total 3,5,3-triiodothyronine (T_3) (Beckmann et al., 2006). The active hormones free T_4 and free T_3 remain unchanged from normal non-pregnant levels. Levels of total T_4 continue to be elevated until several weeks postpartum. Increased T_4-binding capacity is noted by an increase in the serum protein-bound iodine (PBI). These changes in thyroid regulation cause a progressive increase in the basal metabolic rate (BMR) of up to 25% by term. The BMR is the amount of oxygen consumed by the body over a unit of time (mL/min). Maternal effects of the increase in BMR include heat intolerance and an elevation in pulse rate and cardiac output. Within a few weeks following birth, thyroid function returns to normal levels (Hacker et al., 2004).

Parathyroid Glands

The parathyroid glands, which regulate calcium and phosphate metabolism, increase in size from estrogen-induced hyperplasia and hypertrophy. Maternal concentrations of parathyroid hormone increase as the fetus requires more calcium for skeletal growth during the second and third trimesters. Calcium intake is extremely important for the pregnant woman, whose daily intake should be at least 1200 to 1500 mg.

Pituitary Gland and Placenta

The anterior lobe of the pituitary gland, stimulated by the hypothalamus, increases in size and in weight. Pregnancy is possible because of the actions of FSH (stimulates growth of the graafian follicle) and LH, which prompts final maturation of the ovarian follicles and release of the mature ovum (Varney, 2004). If conception occurs, elevated levels of estrogen and progesterone (produced by the corpus luteum until about 14 weeks of gestation, when the placenta takes over this function) suppress production of FSH and LH. During pregnancy, ovarian follicle maturation may continue but ovulation does not occur.

Prolactin, also produced by the anterior pituitary gland, is responsible for initial lactation. Although this hormone increases 10-fold during pregnancy, the elevated levels of estrogen and progesterone inhibit lactation by interfering with prolactin-binding to the breast tissue. Prolactin may also play a role in fluid and electrolyte shifts across the fetal membranes (Hacker et al., 2004).

Oxytocin and vasopressin are produced in the posterior lobe of the pituitary. Oxytocin primarily causes uterine contractions but high levels of progesterone prevent contractions until close to term. Oxytocin also stimulates milk ejection from the breasts, or the **"let down" reflex**. Vasopressin causes vasoconstriction. Vasoconstriction leads to an increase in maternal blood pressure and exerts an antidiuretic effect that promotes maternal fluid retention to maintain circulating blood volume. The increased blood volume that occurs during pregnancy, along with changes in plasma osmolarity (the fluid-pulling capacity of the plasma to retain fluids) controls the release of vasopressin.

Maternal metabolism is altered to support the pregnancy by thyrotropin and adrenotropin. These hormones, produced by the anterior pituitary gland, exert their effects on the thyroid and adrenal glands. Thyrotropin causes an increased basal metabolism and adrenotropin alters adrenal gland function to increase fluid retention by the kidneys.

Human placental lactogen (hPL), also known as human chorionic somatomammotropin (hCS), is produced by the placental syncytiotrophoblasts. It is an insulin antagonist and acts as a fetal growth hormone. Human placental lactogen increases the number of circulating fatty acids to meet maternal metabolic needs and decreases maternal glucose utilization, which increases glucose availability to the fetus (Hacker et al., 2004).

Adrenal Glands

The adrenal glands, located above the kidneys, change little during pregnancy. The adrenal cortex produces cortisol, a hormone that allows the body to respond to stressors. Cortisol is increased during pregnancy due to decreased renal secretion (an alteration prompted by high estrogen levels). Cortisol regulates protein and carbohydrate metabolism and is believed to promote fetal lung maturation and stimulate labor at term. Following birth, it may take up to 6 weeks for maternal cortisol levels to return to normal.

By the second trimester, the adrenal cortex secretes increased levels of aldosterone, a mineral corticoid that causes the renal reabsorption of sodium. This physiological alteration promotes the reclaiming of water and helps to enhance circulatory volume. The increase in aldosterone may be a protective response to the increased renal and excretory gland sodium excretion that occurs due to the effects of progesterone.

Pancreas

The pancreas secretes insulin produced by the beta cells of the islets of Langerhans. Pregnancy prompts an increase in the number and size of the beta cells. These changes are responsible for the alterations that occur in carbohydrate metabolism during pregnancy.

Prostaglandins

Prostaglandins are lipid substances found in high concentrations in the female reproductive tract and in the uterine decidua during pregnancy. Their exact function in pregnancy is unknown although they may maintain a reduced placental vascular resistance. A decrease in prostaglandin levels may contribute to hypertension and preeclampsia. At term, an increased release of prostaglandins from the cervix as it softens and dilates may contribute to the onset of labor.

MUSCULOSKELETAL SYSTEM

As the pregnancy progresses, the abdominal wall weakens and the rectus abdominis muscles separate (**diastasis recti**) to accommodate the growing uterus. As the weight of the uterus shifts upward and outward, a lumbar lordosis (anterior convexity of the lumbar spine) develops (Fig. 8-11). This alteration compensates for the changing center of gravity and allows centering to remain over the woman's legs.

Figure 8-11 Lumbar lordosis.

Low back pain usually accompanies this physiological change. Separation of the rectus abdominis muscles along with an increase in intra-abdominal pressure from the growing uterus may exacerbate an abdominal wall hernia.

Relaxin, a hormone produced by the placenta, along with the action of progesterone, causes a relative laxity of the ligaments. The pubis symphysis separates at approximately 28 to 30 weeks gestation. These changes, coupled with the change in the maternal center of gravity, result in an unsteady gait and a greater tendency toward falls. The patient's gait takes on the appearance of a "pregnancy waddle" as the bones of the pelvis shift and move. The woman should be encouraged to maintain good posture and keep the abdominal muscles toned through exercise. Sitting in a firm chair and the use of a small pillow or blanket rolled and placed in the lumbar region (lumbar roll) for support can help decrease lower back pain.

Pregnant women frequently complain of sharp pain in the lower abdominal quadrants or in the groin area. Most often, the pain is related to stretching and hypertrophy of the round ligaments that support the uterus (round ligament pain). Because of dextrorotation of the gravid uterus as it rises out of the pelvis, the right maternal side is most commonly affected. Once a serious medical condition (e.g., appendicitis) has been ruled out, the nurse should offer reassurance and instruct the patient to sit in a chair or rest on her left side. The application of heat may also be helpful. A brief review of the anatomical changes that occur during pregnancy may alleviate the patient's fear of appendicitis. Since the appendix is pushed up and posterior by the gravid uterus, the typical location of pain (McBurney's Point) is not a reliable indicator for a ruptured appendix during pregnancy. The pain should gradually subside but if it persists or is accompanied by fever, a change in bowel habits, or decreased fetal movement, the patient should promptly contact her medical provider.

Mobilization of calcium stores occurs to provide for the fetal calcium needs necessary for skeletal grown. The total maternal serum calcium decreases, but the ionized calcium level remains unchanged from the prepregnant state. The increase in circulating maternal parathyroid hormone stimulates an increased absorption of calcium from the intestines and decreases the renal loss of calcium to maintain adequate calcium levels.

Calcitonin, a hormone important in the metabolism of calcium and phosphorus, suppresses bone resorption by inhibiting the activity of osteoclasts. Osteoclasts are a cell type that "digests" bone matrix, causing a release of calcium and phosphorus into the blood. Calcitonin is produced primarily in the thyroid gland, but it is also synthesized in a many other tissues, including the lungs and intestinal tract (Bowen, 2006). The activity of calcitonin, coupled with adequate nutrition, protect the maternal skeleton from a loss of bone density despite an increase in the turnover of bone mass. Calcium intake is of major importance during pregnancy, and women should be encouraged to increase their dietary calcium through the consumption of dairy products, calcium fortified orange juice, and dark green leafy vegetables.

Calcium supplementation may be advised for patients who are vegetarian or lactose intolerant. Pregnant women often complain of cramping in the lower extremities and calves, especially at night. The cramps, sometimes called "charleyhorses," can be extremely painful and are caused by poor circulation to the extremities. They have also been associated with imbalances in calcium and phosphorus. Increasing or decreasing calcium intake may be helpful. For immediate relief of the cramping, the woman should be instructed to stand and lean forward to stretch the calf muscle or have someone gently push her toes back toward her shin and hold this position for several seconds. Daily walks can also help because ambulation improves circulation to the muscles.

NURSING ASSESSMENT AND HEALTH EDUCATION

Nursing assessment must begin with a comprehensive history and examination at the first prenatal visit. The history should include information about the current pregnancy; the obstetric and gynecological history; a cultural assessment; and a medical, nutritional, social, and family (including the father's) medical history. A complete review of all of the physical systems should be conducted followed by a physical examination that includes appropriate nutritional assessments and diagnostic procedures. This information is essential to the formulation of appropriate nursing diagnoses (Box 8-1). Ongoing health education should focus on the current trimester and its physical changes. A trimester-by-trimester approach to teaching needs is presented in Table 8-3.

Now Can You— Discuss major changes in the endocrine and musculoskeletal systems during pregnancy?

1. Describe maternal symptoms associated with an increased basal metabolic rate (BMR)?
2. Identify where cortisol is produced and name two important actions of this hormone?
3. Discuss two physiological alterations that produce the "pregnancy waddle" and suggest two strategies for the relief of back pain?
4. Explain why adequate calcium intake is essential during pregnancy?

Box 8-1 Nursing Diagnoses Related to Physiological Adaptations to Pregnancy

- Deficient Knowledge related to normal physiological changes of pregnancy
- Constipation related to changes in gastrointestinal tract occurring in pregnancy
- Imbalanced Nutrition: More than Body Requirements related to excessive intake of calories
- Imbalanced Nutrition: Less than Body Requirements related to inadequate information about nutritional needs during pregnancy
- Activity Intolerance related to fatigue from the physiological changes of pregnancy

Psychosocial Adaptations During Pregnancy

For many women, pregnancy is a time of turmoil that affects the ability to deal with stress and cope with the changes that will take place over many months. These changes affect not only the woman but her partner and other family members as well. Pregnancy and childbearing constitute major developmental phases, and these events are often accompanied by ambivalence and conflicting emotions. The nurse must have a basic understanding of how the woman's progression through the developmental phases and the accompanying emotions affect her and her family's acceptance of the pregnancy and the unknown child. Nursing care for the woman and her family through each pregnancy milestone should be tailored with respect to personal and family values, cultural customs, and spiritual beliefs and health maintenance behaviors. Topics for health education related to the psychosocial adaptations to pregnancy are presented in Table 8-4.

DEVELOPMENTAL AND FAMILY CHANGES

According to Duvall's (1977) stages of family development, the expectant family sets about the task of preparing for its new role as childcare providers. The home must be reorganized to accommodate the infant; family member duties and responsibilities must often be realigned; and patterns of money management need to be altered. The couples' sexual relationship must adapt to the physical and emotional changes that accompany pregnancy. Family relationships with relatives are often reoriented as the couple gradually moves away from the former role of "child" and instead seek recognition as parents. Friendships and relationships with work associates also must adapt to the couple's changing lifestyle.

For both the expectant woman and her partner, emotional responses are often unpredictable and labile and require patience, understanding, and good communication. The couple needs to expand their knowledge about pregnancy, birth, and parenting to enhance their understanding of these life-altering events. Additional information also helps to empower them to better prepare for the major changes that will soon take place in their lives. With each subsequent pregnancy, the couple must adjust to the transitions in their relationship with one another and with each child. Each birth brings a new member who

Table 8-3 Health Education Topics Related to the Physiological Adaptations to Pregnancy

Topics to Include	First Trimester	Second Trimester	Third Trimester
Physiological Changes of Pregnancy and Related Discomforts	Pain and tingling in breasts	Enlargement of the abdomen	Dyspnea
	Nausea and vomiting (morning sickness)	Skin pigmentation	Leg and feet cramps
	Urinary frequency	Striae gravidarum	Constipation
	Fatigue	Vascular spiders	Indigestion, heartburn, gastric reflux
	Mood swings	Constipation	Pedal edema
		Heartburn or gastric reflux	Fatigue
		Leg cramps	Vaginal discharge
		Groin pain from round ligament stretching	Urinary frequency
		Leukorrhea	Braxton-Hicks contractions versus True labor
Danger Signs to Report to Health Care Provider	Vaginal bleeding	Vaginal bleeding	Visual disturbances
	Abdominal cramping or pain	Burning or painful urination	Headache
	Severe or prolonged vomiting	Fever, increased pulse rate	Hand and facial edema
		Decreased or absent fetal movements	Fever
		Unrelenting nausea and vomiting	Vaginal bleeding
		Abdominal pain or cramping	Abdominal pain; uterine contractions
		Swelling of face or fingers, headaches, visual disturbances or epigastric pain	Premature rupture of the membranes
			Decreased or absent fetal movement
General Health Teaching	Schedule of return visits for routine prenatal care	Reinforcement and reiteration of previous teaching	Signs and symptoms of labor/ preterm labor
	General hygiene	Comfort measures	When to call the health care provider, when to go to the birthing center or hospital
	Comfort measures	Anticipatory guidance	Comfort measures
	Anticipatory guidance	Choices of prenatal education classes	Anticipatory guidance
	Sexual activity and restrictions	Signs and symptoms of preterm labor	Reinforcement and reiteration of previous teaching
	Physical activities, exercise, and rest		Encouragement to attend a labor and birth class
	Nutritional guidance		
	Avoidance of alcohol, fetal alcohol effects		
	Effects of smoking, and smoking cessation strategies if indicated		

Adapted from Mattson, S., & Smith, J.E. (2004). *Core curriculum for maternal-newborn nursing.* St. Louis: W.B. Saunders.

Table 8-4   Health Education Topics Related to the Psychosocial Adaptations to Pregnancy

Topics to Include	First Trimester	Second Trimester	Third Trimester
Developmental Tasks of Pregnancy	Mother: Acceptance of pregnancy into her self-system	Mother: Binding-in to the pregnancy, ensuring safe passage, and differentiating the fetus from herself	Mother: Separating herself from the pregnancy and the fetus, trying various caregiving strategies
	Father: Announcement and realization of the pregnancy	Father: Anticipation of adapting to the role of fatherhood	Father: Role adaptation, preparation for labor and birth
	Couple: Realignment of relationships and roles	Couple: Realignment of roles and division of tasks	Couple: Preparation of the nursery
Psychosocial Changes During Pregnancy	Ambivalence about pregnancy	Active dream and fantasy life	Dislikes being pregnant but loves the child
	Introversion	Concerns with body image	Anxious about childbirth, but sees labor and birth as deliverance
	Passivity and difficulty with decision making	Nesting behaviors	The couple experiments with various mothering or fathering roles
	Sexual and emotional changes	Sexual behavior adjustment	Woman is introspective
	Changing self-image	Expanding to a variety of methods of expressing affection and intimacy	
	Ethical dilemmas of prenatal testing		

Adapted from Mattson, S., & Smith, J.E. (2004). *Core curriculum for maternal-newborn nursing.* St. Louis: W.B. Saunders.

must be introduced and incorporated into the existing family structure. Sibling rivalry, or competitiveness among the children, is common and can often be diminished by parental actions that actively involve each child with the pregnancy and anticipated birth.

MATERNAL TASKS AND ROLE TRANSITION

Rubin (1975) described specific tasks that a woman must accomplish to integrate the maternal role into her personality. The "tasks of pregnancy" generally occur concurrently during the pregnancy and help the woman develop her self-concept as a mother. To be successful in accomplishing these tasks, the pregnant woman must incorporate the pregnancy into her total identity. That is, she must "accept the reality of the pregnancy" and integrate it into her self concept, "accept the child," "reorder" her relationships, learn to "give of herself for the child," and "seek safe passage through the pregnancy, labor and birth" (Mattson & Smith, 2004). A summary of the maternal tasks of pregnancy is presented in Table 8-5.

Acceptance of the Pregnancy

The mother-to-be needs to accept the pregnancy and incorporate it into her own reality and self-concept. This process is known as "binding in." During the first trimester, the woman's focus centers on her physical discomforts (e.g., fatigue, nausea) and needs rather than on the developing child. By the second trimester, she feels fetal movement (quickening), has most likely seen the baby on ultrasound and heard his heartbeat, and begins to conceptualize the child as an individual within her. During the third trimester, as the due date approaches, the mother-to-be wants the child and just as strongly wants the pregnancy to be over. At this point, she is tired and needs a

considerable amount of emotional and physical support from her family and friends.

Acceptance of the Child

Acceptance of the child is critical to a successful adjustment to the pregnancy. Acceptance must come from the expectant woman as well as from others. During early pregnancy, announcements are made to one another and to family and friends. A positive response from those closest to the pregnant woman helps to foster her acceptance of the child. There is a great value attached to this unborn child and she wants and needs others in the family to accept the child as well. In the second trimester, the immediate family needs to exhibit behaviors consistent with relating to the child as a sibling, a son or a daughter. In the third trimester, the woman must develop an unconditional acceptance of the child or she and others may reject him for not meeting their expectations.

Reordering Relationships

To facilitate the necessary family transition, the pregnant woman must reorder her relationships to allow for the child to fit into the existing family structure and learn to give of herself to the unknown child. At this time, she becomes reflective and examines what things in her life may need to be given up or changed for the infant. If this is her first child, she may grieve the loss of her carefree life. As the pregnancy progresses, the woman begins to identify with the child and makes plans for their life together after the birth. During the last few weeks of the pregnancy, the woman must work through doubts of her ability to be a good mother. At this time, positive support from family and friends is essential in boosting her confidence and in assisting her in overcoming these feelings of self-doubt.

Table 8-5 Maternal Tasks of Pregnancy

General Principles	Pregnancy progressively becomes part of the woman's total identity.
	She feels unique because she can't share her sensory experience with others.
	Her focus turns inward and she is overly sensitive.
	She seeks the company of other women and pregnant women.
	Absence of a female support system during pregnancy is a singular index of a high-risk pregnancy.
Acceptance of Pregnancy	First trimester: She accepts the idea of pregnancy but not the child.
"Binding-in"	Second trimester: With sensation of fetal movement, or "quickening," she becomes aware of the child as a separate entity.
	Third trimester: She wants the child and is tired of being pregnant.
Acceptance of the Child	First trimester: Acceptance of the pregnancy by herself and others.
	Second trimester: The family needs to relate to the infant.
	Third trimester: The critical issue is the unconditional acceptance of the child; conditional acceptance may imply rejection by the mother or family members.
Reordering of Relationships, Giving of Self	First trimester: Examines what needs to be given up.
	Trade-offs for having the infant.
	May grieve the loss of a carefree life.
	Second trimester: Identifies with the child.
	Third trimester: Has decreased confidence in her ability to become a good mother to her child.
Safe Passage	First trimester: Focuses on herself, not on her infant.
	Second trimester: Develops a strong attachment and places great value on her infant.
	Third trimester: Has concern for herself and her infant as a unit, shares a symbiotic relationship. At the seventh month, she is in a state of high vulnerability.
	She views labor and birth as deliverance and as a hope, not as a threat.

Adapted from Mattson, S., & Smith, J.E. (2004). *Core curriculum for maternal-newborn nursing.* St. Louis: W.B. Saunders.

Seeking Safe Passage Through Pregnancy, Labor, and Birth

Seeking safe passage through the pregnancy, labor, and birth are maternal tasks that receive the most attention during the pregnancy. In the first trimester, the woman focuses on her own discomforts and places her needs before those of the fetus. Symptoms of fatigue, nausea, and breast tenderness can be overwhelming during this often difficult time. In the second and third trimesters, the woman develops an increasing sense of the value of her infant. She comes to conceptualize her fetus as a separate being (fetal distinction) and she accepts her changing body image. She becomes extremely vulnerable during her seventh month and increasingly worried about the impending labor and birth. As the due date approaches, the woman's fears about labor may diminish as she begins to view childbirth as an "end point." Participation in childbirth preparation classes can greatly assist the woman and her family in dealing with the anxiety and fears that often surround labor and birth.

Other developmental tasks take place during the passage of pregnancy as well. The woman needs to validate the pregnancy, and initial feelings of uncertainty or ambivalence are normal. When caring for expectant women, the nurse should never assume that the pregnancy was planned

or wanted. Instead, the nurse should facilitate discussion of uncertainties or concerns with the patient and her family to facilitate acceptance of the pregnancy. Many women fantasize and dream about their pregnancy and how it will change their lives. The woman must incorporate the fetus into her body image, a process termed "fetal embodiment." Accomplishing this task allows her to accept the changes in her body size and shape as the pregnancy progresses. The significant other plays an important role as the woman becomes increasingly dependent on that individual for helping to meet her daily needs.

As the pregnancy advances, the woman begins to conceptualize the fetus as a separate individual. She comes to view her changing body as a "vessel of new life" and often feels closer to her own mother at this time. This deeper relationship with her mother begins as one of dependency and progresses to one in which she identifies with her mother as a peer. If her mother is not available, she may reach out to another valued maternal figure for identification and support. As she reaches the end of the third trimester, the woman begins to give up her symbiotic relationship with the fetus. She harbors feelings of anxiety about the childbirth process and begins to gather supplies and prepare for the baby's entry into the home. This process is termed "nesting." At this point in pregnancy, the woman is often impatient with the awkwardness related to her increasing size and has a strong desire to see the pregnancy end so that she can begin her next phase as a mother.

 Now Can You— Discuss the "tasks of pregnancy"?

1. Describe why it is important for the pregnant woman to successfully accomplish the tasks of pregnancy?
2. Discuss the value of ongoing family support throughout pregnancy in fostering acceptance of the child?
3. Identify what is meant by "seeking safe passage"?
4. Explain why pregnant women often feel closer to their own mothers as the pregnancy progresses?

Developmental Tasks and the Pregnant Adolescent

For the pregnant adolescent, ongoing age-related developmental tasks can create conflict when coupled with the developmental tasks of pregnancy. Tasks associated with adolescence focus on growth and maturity. They include developing a personal value system, choosing a vocation or career, developing personal body image and sexuality, achieving a stable identity, and attaining independence from parents. Conflicts may arise when these tasks are overshadowed by the developmental tasks of pregnancy. While seeking safe passage, the adolescent may not seek prenatal care unless pressured by authority figures or peers to do so. By nature, adolescents are not future oriented. Hence, the pregnant adolescent may not be able to readily accept the reality of the unborn child. Because the adolescent's sense of identity is still incomplete, bodily changes often feel awkward. Because the family may not react positively to the pregnancy, acceptance of the pregnancy by self and others may be hindered. Many times, the adolescent's parents come to assume the role of parent. Although this may be helpful at times, this situation limits the young mother's involvement with the newborn and her ability to fully give of herself.

PATERNAL ADAPTATION TO PREGNANCY

Pregnancy is psychologically stressful for men. Expectant fathers often experience a variety of reactions to the pregnancy. Some enjoy the role of nurturer and marvel in the changes that occur in the woman. Others feel alienated and begin to stray from the relationship. Many men view pregnancy as positive proof of their masculinity and take steps to assume a dominant or more supportive role in the relationship. Others find no meaning or personal value in the pregnancy and consequently fail to develop any sense of responsibility toward the mother or the child. There are several styles of paternal involvement during pregnancy, including "observer," where the father is passive and detached; "expressive," where the expectant father attempts to experience the pregnancy as much as possible, and "instrumental," where the father is the caretaker (Callister, Matsumura, & Vehvilainnen-Julkunen, 2003).

Couvade, in the traditional sense, is the observance of certain rituals and taboos by the male to signify his transition to fatherhood. This action affirms the man's psychosocial and biophysical relationship to his partner and the child. In recent times, couvade has come to describe the unintentional development of pregnancy-related symptoms such as weight gain, nausea, back pain, difficulty sleeping,

and depression by the pregnant woman's partner. Men who experience the couvade syndrome often assume a more involved paternal role during the childbearing year.

The father of the baby also experiences specific tasks of pregnancy that correspond with the trimesters. During the first trimester, the father is in an "announcement phase." Similar to the woman's experience, the father may be ambivalent at this time. He must first accept the pregnancy as "real" in order to begin to incorporate the future child into his life and assume the expectant father role. In the second trimester, or "moratorium phase", the man's "binding in" usually takes longer to achieve than the woman's, and this is related to his "remoteness" to the fetus. At this time, involvement in prenatal visits, listening to the baby's heartbeat, and visualization of the fetus during ultrasound can make the fetus seem more real to the father. He begins to accept the woman's changing body and the reality of the fetus as a child when he can feel fetal movement.

 Optimizing Outcomes— Promoting prenatal paternal attachment

The nurse can be instrumental in promoting early paternal attachment. Encouraging the father to actively "engage" with the fetus through reflective journaling is one way to enhance prenatal bonding. One father later shared his recorded insights:

My earliest memories with Trina started the day she was born. No, they started before that. They started in the womb. I would come home and I would say, "Hello," and she would flick and flitter in the womb. She would start kicking. If I put my hand on my wife's tummy when she was carrying Trina, she would move over to where my hand was. If I put it on the other side, she would move to that side. I used to sing to her. It's always been that way and has just continued pretty much that way. I remember one night laying with my head on my wife's stomach and singing a lullaby or something, I can't remember exactly which song. She was very active but she settled down, and then I put my hand on her stomach and she moved my hand.

Excerpt from Callister, L.C., Matsumura, G., & Vehvilainnen-Julkunen, K. (2003). He's having a baby. The paternal childbirth experience. *Marriage & Families.* Retrieved from http://marriageandfamilies.byu.edu/issues/2003/January/baby.aspx

The couple's sexual relationship often changes as some men deal with fears of harming the fetus. The expectant father may also feel a rivalry with a male health care provider. Involvement of the father during examinations and tests with thorough explanations of the need for them can minimize the father's feelings of being left out. His partner's intense introspective nature may be confusing at times and he may feel pushed away. The man also fantasizes about being a father, although his fantasies are often centered on an older child rather than on an infant.

In the third trimester, the expectant father enters a "focusing phase." During this time he negotiates what his role in labor and birth will be; prepares for the reality of parenthood; alters his self-concept to reflect that of a more mature, or fatherly figure; becomes involved in setting up the nursery; and copes with his fears of the mutilation or death of his partner or child during birth. Fears and concerns are often lessened somewhat by participation in prenatal and parenting classes. The nurse should be aware of cues (e.g., lack of participation in prenatal care, behaviors that signal lack of interest in the woman, the fetus, or the pregnancy) that may indicate paternal detachment from the mother and the pregnancy. Referral for counseling, childbirth preparation classes, or other community resources may be appropriate. Pastoral care or local fathering support groups, if available, may also assist the father with his need for involvement. Problems such as a troubled relationship with his own father, a dysfunctional couple relationship, and sociocultural factors may be barriers that prevent the man from assuming a paternal role (Callister et al., 2003). Not uncommonly, the behavior associated with a "dead beat dad" stems from feelings of being pushed away or left out by the expectant woman and her other support systems.

ADAPTATION OF SIBLINGS AND GRANDPARENTS

The psychosocial reactions of other family members to the pregnancy and childbirth must also be explored, as these individuals often have a significant influence on the woman's passage through the developmental tasks of pregnancy. The reactions of siblings correlate closely to their age and level of involvement with the pregnancy. Children may express excitement, anticipation, anger, or despair. The toddler, characteristically involved in his own little world, may initially exhibit a reaction of indifference. However, the parents must be advised about the strong likelihood of a regression in age-appropriate behavior. For example, the child may want to nurse, drink from a bottle, or wear a diaper like the baby. The school-age child usually appears more interested but grasping the full reality of a baby in the family may not be realistic, since the process of concrete thinking is not fully developed until around age 10. Engaging the child in family discussions about the anticipated birth, encouraging the child to feel fetal movements, and listening to the fetal heart beat, sharing age-appropriate educational materials, and allowing him to attend sibling preparation classes are strategies that may help the child to feel that he is sharing in the pregnancy experience.

When a child reaches early adolescence, changing sexuality associated with this developmental phase may create a barrier between him and his mother. This sort of barrier makes it difficult for the adolescent to view his parent as a pregnant woman and may give rise to feelings of resentment toward the new child about to join the family. Parents need to be aware of ways to cope with potential negative behaviors and recognize that adolescents often appear to have knowledge and understanding about pregnancy and birth but their information may be incorrect and incomplete. The nurse can suggest that the child attend prenatal visits to listen to the baby's heartbeat and, if possible, view the fetus during ultrasound examinations. Parents should be assisted in developing other strategies to include the adolescent in the changes that are taking place during pregnancy and that will occur following the birth. Older children may benefit from attending prenatal classes or touring the birthing facility.

Grandparents are very often excited and eagerly await the birth of a grandchild, although this is not always the case. The grandparents' age at the time of the birth can exert a positive or a negative effect on their reactions. For example, if they will become first-time grandparents during their 30s or 40s, they may be ambivalent or feel they are not yet ready to assume the grandparent role. Conversely, those who are already grandparents may be excited with the prospect of another grandchild. Other factors (e.g., if the pregnancy was unplanned, if the mother is very young or unwed) may prompt feelings of anger and disappointment. Along with the woman's partner, the grandparents usually harbor concerns about the health and well-being of the expectant woman and her fetus. They also may be unsure about extent to which they should become involved in the childrearing process.

MATERNAL ADAPTATION DURING ABSENCE OF A SIGNIFICANT OTHER

If the woman has no involved significant other, she will need the presence of a strong support person to help her adapt to the pregnancy and the demands of parenting. The future she has planned for the child, such as the decision to place the child for adoption, can heavily influence her psychological needs. During prenatal visits, the nurse should ensure that the woman is given the opportunity to discuss her future plans for the child. After assessing the woman's needs, the nurse can make referrals to appropriate community resources that may include prenatal classes, psychological counseling, pastoral care or social services.

 Now Can You— Discuss pregnancy-related role transitions for the adolescent, father, siblings and grandparents?

1. Describe why the adolescent may have difficulty achieving the developmental tasks of pregnancy?
2. Explain what is meant by the couvade syndrome?
3. Discuss the "focusing phase" that occurs during the third trimester and identify two behaviors that may indicate a lack of paternal attachment?
4. Contrast behaviors of toddlers, school-age, and adolescent children in response to the pregnancy?
5. Identify two factors that may influence the grandparents' ability to make role transitions in response to the pregnancy?

CULTURAL INFLUENCES AND PSYCHOSOCIAL ADAPTATIONS

Universally, some type of ritual or ceremony is attached to important life events. In pregnancy and childbirth, this ritual may involve special care of the mother and baby, events planned to welcome the new member of the family, or rigid requirements that must be met by the family and health care providers. There are a multitude of cultural messages that may influence the woman's adaptation to pregnancy, birth, and the newborn. The nurse should explore these cultural influences with the patient and her family. By acknowledging and documenting specific beliefs and needs, the nurse can help guide the woman and her family through the prenatal and intrapartal care system more effectively. Through open discussion, erroneous or conflicting beliefs can be addressed and a plan can be developed to ensure a satisfactory, positive experience for the childbearing year.

HAZARDS OF HIGH-TECH MANAGEMENT ON MATERNAL ADAPTATION

The technology-focused society of today can lead to an increase in the level of anxiety and number of stressors experienced by the pregnant woman and her family. Moral and ethical dilemmas may arise from positive diagnostic tests. The pregnant woman's emotional and interpersonal needs may be overlooked by those caring for her as added importance is placed on the technology that surrounds the care. Full enjoyment of the pregnancy may not be possible, as the woman instead comes to focus on each test and its results. In this situation, the pregnancy becomes a "tentative pregnancy." A conflict of interest develops between the technology and the woman's trust of her own instincts and inner feelings. These conflicts can further undermine the woman's self-confidence. Collectively, these stressors interfere with the woman's ability to move through the tasks of maternal role development and delay her preparation for parenting.

SOCIETAL AND CULTURAL INFLUENCES ON FAMILY ADAPTATION

Cultural influences often affect how pregnancy is viewed and accepted by the woman and her family. Many cultures, such as the tribal Native Americans and most Latinos, consider pregnancy to be a normal and expected life event, not a state of illness. Some African nations impose rigid taboos concerning what a woman can eat, drink, wear, and do during her pregnancy. In some Middle Eastern cultures, pregnancy is viewed as "woman's work" and the father's involvement is minimal. In Korean and other southeastern Asian cultures, a harmonious balance such as yin/yang (masculine/feminine) or hot/cold must be closely observed. In the equilibrium model of health, achievement of balance allows for the normal growth of the baby and ensures the mother's recovery from the pregnancy. Some cultures place emphasis on certain behaviors designed to protect the pregnancy, such as avoidance of particular foods and harmful substances. Immigrants to America become acculturated to Western society. In so doing, they may give up their own health protective beliefs and behaviors and instead turn to the use of alcohol, drugs, and tobacco, or consume fast foods rather than a balanced diet. The nurse's role is to assess each patient's beliefs and develop a plan of care that is individualized and incorporates the woman's customs while providing comprehensive and safe care.

 Ethnocultural Considerations— **Myths, Taboos, and "Old Wives' Tales"**

In all cultures and subcultures there are myths, tales, and taboos associated with pregnancy. These have developed to explain the changes that occur during pregnancy or to link a cause to negative pregnancy outcomes. One myth concerns heartburn: if heartburn is experienced during pregnancy, the baby will be born with lots of hair. Another involves using the shape and height of the woman's belly or shape and fullness of her face as indicators to determine the baby's sex.

The Chinese and Malays believe that certain "cooling" foods—cucumber, cabbage, bananas, pineapples—and iced drinks—coconut water and tea—are taboo during pregnancy because they contribute to poor blood circulation. For the Chinese, other taboo foods are those considered to be "acidic," such as pineapple, mango, lime, sour orange, tapai (fermented tapioca rice), and concentrated coconut milk. These foods are believed to possibly induce bleeding or miscarriage.

Many "Old Wives' Tales" surround pregnancy. One suggests that raising the hands up over the head can cause the baby to become entangled in its cord. Another warns the pregnant woman not to take baths because germs may enter the vagina and pass to the baby. Another encourages abundant water intake so that the baby won't get dirty.

Adapted from Weiss, R.E. (2007). Old Wives' Tales. Retrieved from http://pregnancy.about.com/cs/myths/a/aa042299.htm

FACTORS THAT INTERFERE WITH PSYCHOSOCIAL ADAPTATIONS DURING PREGNANCY

Grief and loss during the perinatal period can be triggered by spontaneous abortion; elective termination; plans to relinquish the child for adoption or surrogacy; and loss of the perfect child through prematurity, illness, deformity, or less preferred gender. Parental reactions can produce a separation from the infant and delay attachment, prompt feelings of personal inadequacy concerning the inability to produce a healthy infant, and alter healthy methods of relating to the infant.

The importance of prenatal education, labor and birth preparation, and parenting classes cannot be stressed enough by the nurse. Many women bypass the courses offered by their health care providers or hospitals in lieu of watching birth stories on television. These programs are a good adjunct but must be placed into context by information obtained at the prenatal visits and during attendance at prenatal and childbirth education classes taught by nurses and certified personnel.

NURSING ASSESSMENT OF PSYCHOSOCIAL CHANGES AND PRENATAL HEALTH EDUCATION

Nursing assessment of the psychosocial changes that occur during pregnancy must include a thorough history including the family background, past obstetrical events, and the status of the current pregnancy. Each prenatal visit provides an opportunity to ask the patient about her pregnancy experience since the last visit, address current concerns, and offer anticipatory guidance of what to expect from the present visit to the next appointment. Based on this information, the nurse formulates appropriate nursing diagnoses related to the maternal psychosocial adaptation to pregnancy (Box 8-2). Health education should be focused according to the current trimester and evaluated by the patient's or couple's ability to verbalize the content presented, their efforts to seek assistance and support with psychological concerns, and indicators of satisfactory coping with the psychological transitions that are occurring. Suggested topics for health teaching during each trimester are presented in Table 8-5. Pregnancy represents a time of great physical and emotional change. The woman and her family require ongoing support and education to ensure that they safely and successfully move through the stages of pregnancy and, in the end, are prepared to welcome the new baby into their lives.

Box 8-2 Nursing Diagnoses Related to Psychosocial Adaptations to Pregnancy

- Risk for Disturbed Body Image related to anatomical and physiological changes of pregnancy
- Ineffective Role Performance related to taking on new roles; changes in roles
- Risk for Situational Low Self-esteem related to pregnancy complications, changes in body image, roles
- Ineffective Sexuality Patterns related to changes in libido during pregnancy
- Interrupted Family Processes related to developmental stressors of pregnancy or loss
- Anxiety related to fear of the unknown
- Readiness for Enhanced Family Coping related to opportunity for growth/mastery
- Risk for Impaired Parenting related to lack of knowledge, skills, support
- Health-seeking behaviors: developmental tasks needed to prepare for parenthood
- Dysfunctional grieving related to stillbirth, ill or preterm newborn, loss of the ideal of the perfect child, loss of pregnancy, or loss of desired labor or birth

Adapted from Mattson, S., & Smith, J.E. (2004). *Core curriculum for maternal-newborn nursing.* St. Louis: W.B. Saunders.

 Now Can You— **Discuss the effects of high technology and other influences on psychosocial adaptation during pregnancy?**

1. Explain how "high-tech" management can interfere with accomplishing the tasks associated with maternal role development?
2. Provide three examples of societal/cultural traditions that influence development of the maternal role?
3. Describe how assessment and education empower the pregnant woman and her family to successfully deal with the psychosocial changes that take place?

---

summary points

- Estrogen and progesterone are the major hormones produced by the placenta during pregnancy. Estrogen's effect is one of "growth"; progesterone's effect is one of "maintenance."

- The reproductive system undergoes the greatest changes in size and function and every organ within this system is affected by or focused on the needs of the growing fetus.

- Every system in the body experiences dramatic changes in structure and function as a result of the hormonal changes of pregnancy.

- Pregnancy is a time of turmoil in the woman's life that affects her ability to deal with stress and cope with the changes that will occur over many months. These changes affect not only the woman but also her partner and the other family members as well.

- Ethnocultural, familial, and spiritual beliefs exert a powerful influence on the woman's and her family's progress through the pregnancy and can enhance or interfere with routine prenatal care.

- The nurse's responsibility in prenatal care is to ensure that the patient and her family understand the physiological and psychosocial changes that occur due to pregnancy and equip them with strategies to cope with these changes.

review questions

Multiple Choice

1. The perinatal nurse knows that the hormone most responsible for maintaining pregnancy is:
   A. Estrogen
   B. Progesterone
   C. Relaxin
   D. Human chorionic gonadotrophin

2. The perinatal nurse explains to the woman in the assessment area who is experiencing painless, irregular contractions at 28 weeks' gestation that this is normal and is related to circulating levels of the hormone:
   A. Estrogen
   B. Progesterone
   C. Relaxin
   D. Prostaglandin

3. A speculum examination is performed during Kelly's first prenatal visit. The clinic nurse notes a bluish-purple coloration of the cervix. This finding is probably a sign of pregnancy termed:
   A. Goodell sign
   B. Chadwick's sign
   C. Striae gravidarum
   D. Linea nigra

4. During the prenatal class, the perinatal nurse explains to the expectant mothers and family members that one of the baby's protections during pregnancy is the cervical mucus or:
   A. Linea nigra
   B. Rugae
   C. Striae gravidarum
   D. Operculum

Fill-in-the-Blank

5. The perinatal nurse explains to the student nurse that during pregnancy, the hormones estrogen and _____ influence the myometrial cells and muscle _____ of the uterus by the processes of _____ and _____ .

Select All that Apply

6. The perinatal nurse talks with a pregnant woman at 20 weeks' gestation who has monilial vaginitis. The best information the perinatal nurse can provide is:
   A. Pregnancy is a time when women are at an increased risk for this type of infection.
   B. Your vaginal area has increased secretions and discharge that are normal to pregnancy but burning and itching are signs and symptoms that should always be reported.
   C. Gentle cleansing with plain soap and water is best during pregnancy.
   D. Douching may be required to ensure cleanliness.

7. The perinatal nurse sees Jenny for a prenatal clinic visit. Jenny is now at 36 weeks' gestation. The nurse teaches Jenny that she should go to the hospital if she is aware of vaginal discharge that includes:
   A. Blood
   B. A foul odor
   C. Yellow-green particulate
   D. Fleshy odor

8. During the prenatal class, the perinatal nurse describes breast changes that occur during pregnancy. Normal changes include:
   A. Leaking of colostrum
   B. Decreased nipple lubrication
   C. Darkening of the areola
   D. Presence of striae or stretch marks

9. The clinic nurse provides health teaching to Rachel, a 28-year-old woman in her tenth gestational week. This is Rachel's first pregnancy. Rachel is planning a trip and has many questions concerning sun exposure. The nurse explains to Rachel that:
   A. During pregnancy, the skin is photosensitive.
   B. She will need to use additional sunscreen.
   C. She will need to decrease her exposure time to the sun.
   D. The increased sun sensitivity will continue while she is breastfeeding.

True/False

10. The perinatal nurse is teaching the prenatal class attendees about the labor process. The ability of the vagina to accommodate the infant during childbirth is due to the hyperplasia of the vaginal rugae.

See Answers to End of Chapter Review Questions on the Electronic Study Guide or DavisPlus.

REFERENCES

Beckmann, C.R.B, Ling, F.W., Smith, R.P., Barzansky, B.M., Herbert, W.N.P., & Laube, D.W. (2006). *Obstetrics and gynecology* (5th ed.). Philadelphia: Lippincott, Williams & Wilkins.

Bowen, R. (2006). Pathophysiology of the endocrine system. Retrieved from http://www.vivo.colostate.edu/hbooks/pathphys/endocrine/thyroid/calcitonin.html (Accessed June 27, 2007).

Bulechek, G., Butcher, H.M., & Dochterman, J. (2008). *Nursing interventions classification (NIC)* (5th ed.). St. Louis, MO: C.V. Mosby.

Callister, L.C., Matsumura, G., & Vehvilainnen-Julkunen, K. (2003). He's having a baby. The paternal childbirth experience. *Marriage & Families.* Retrieved from http://marriageandfamilies.byu.edu/issues/2003/January/baby.aspx (Accessed June 27, 2007).

Cunningham, F.G., Leveno, K.J., Bloom, S.L., Hauth, J.C., Gilstrap III, L.C., & Wenstrom, K.D. (2005). Maternal adaptation to pregnancy. *Williams obstetrics* (22nd ed, pp. 167-200). New York: McGraw-Hill.

Darovic, G.O. (2004). *Handbook of hemodynamic monitoring* (2nd ed.). St. Louis: W.B. Saunders.

Duvall, E.M. (1977). *Marriage and family development* (5th ed.). Philadelphia: J.B. Lippincott.

Hacker, N.F., Moore, J.G., & Gambone, J.C. (2004). *Essentials of obstetrics and gynecology* (4th ed.). Philadelphia: W.B. Saunders.

Johnson, M., Bulechek, G., Butcher, H., McCloskey Dochterman, J., Maas, M., Moorhead, S., & Swanson, E. (2006). *NANDA, NOC, and NIC Linkages: nursing diagnoses, outcomes, & interventions* (2nd ed.). St. Louis, MO: Mosby Elsevier.

Mattson, S., & Smith, J.E. (2004). *Core curriculum for maternal-newborn nursing.* St. Louis: W.B. Saunders.

McKinney, E.S., James, S.R., Murray, S.S., & Ashwill, J.W. (2005). *Maternal-child nursing* (2nd ed.). Philadelphia: W.B. Saunders.

Moorehead, S., Johnson, M., Mass, M., & Swanson, E. (2008). *Nursing outcomes classification (NOC)* (4th ed.). St. Louis, MO: C.V. Mosby.

Rodgers, B.L., & Knafl, K. A. (2000). *Concept development in nursing* (2nd ed.). Montreal: W.B. Saunders.

Rubin, R. (1975). Maternal tasks in pregnancy. *MCN: The American Journal of Maternal-Child Nursing. 4*(3), 143–153.

Smeltzer, S.C., & Bare, B.G. (Eds.). (2004). *Textbook of medical-surgical nursing.* (10th ed.). Philadelphia: Lippincott Williams & Wilkins.

Van Leeuwen, A.M., Kranpitz, T.R., & Smith, L. (2006). *Davis's comprehensive handbook of laboratory and diagnostic tests with nursing implications* (2nd ed.). Philadelphia: F.A. Davis.

Varney, H. (2004). *Varney's midwifery* (4th ed.). Boston: Jones and Bartlett.

Weiss, R.E. (2007). Old Wives' Tales. Retrieved from http://pregnancy.about.com/cs/myths/a/aa042299.htm (Accessed June 27, 2007).

 For more information, go to http://davisplus.fadavis.com/

CONCEPT MAP

Reproductive System

Uterus/Cervix
- Change in size/shape
- Braxton Hicks contractions
- Chadwick's sign
- Formation of operculum
- Leukorrhea

Vagina
- Chadwick's sign
- Change in pH

Ovaries
- Initial progesterone from corpus luteum
- Cessation of ovulation

Breasts
- Enlarge; increased sensitivity
- Areola darkens; presence of pre-colostrum
- Striae

Endocrine
- Increased BMR
- Pituitary → FSH and LH make pregnancy possible; shut off after conception
- Lactation → oxytocin, prolactin
- Influences pubic symphysis separation and round ligament stretching

Neurological
- Decreased attention, concentration, memory
- Carpal tunnel syndrome
- Syncope

Integumentary
- Change in pigmentation
  - Linea nigra
  - Chloasma
- Striae gravidarum
- Angiomas; palmar erythema

Respiratory
- Increase in tidal volume; tidal capacity
- Change in diaphragmatic excursion

Gastrointestinal
- 1st trimester nausea/vomiting
- Epulis gravidarum and ptyalism
- +/– Glucosuria: (abnormal finding)
- Heartburn
- Hemorrhoids
- Predisposition to cholelithiasis

Cardiovascular
- Increased maternal volume/cardiac output; pseudoanemia
- Increased leukocytes/ fibrinogen volume
- Dilutional hypoalbuminemia
- Increased supine hypotension syndrome/orthostatic hypotension
- Increased need for iron

Musculoskeletal
- Separation of rectus abdominus
- Lumbar lordosis
- Potential changes in serum calcium levels

Urinary
- Frequency, urgency, nocturia
- Increased risk for UTI
- +/– Glucosuria: (abnormal finding)

Hormonal Influences: Major: estrogen and progesterone

Many mediated by

Physiological Changes

Physiological and Psychosocial Changes During Pregnancy

Psychosocial Changes

Factors Affecting Adaptation:
- Absence of significant others
- Pregnancy in adolescence
- Cultural and societal influences
- High-tech management

Family Adaptations:
- Reorganization of the home; realignment of duties
- Change in money management
- Interfamily role change: child to parent
- Incorporation of each new child into existing family structure

Maternal Adaptations:
- Incorporation of pregnancy into self-concept: fetal embodiment
- Unconditional acceptance of child
- Reorder relationships → accommodate child into family structure
- Nesting
- Participation in labor and birth
- Work through post-birth doubts

Paternal Adaptations:
- Varying degrees of involvement
  - Observer; expressive; instrumental
- Corresponding tasks: by trimesters
  - Announcement phase: acceptance
  - Moratorium phase: "binding in"
  - Focusing phase: increased involvement; role clarification
- Couvade syndrome

Factors that Interfere with Adaptation:
- Termination of pregnancy
  - Spontaneous abortion/elective termination
- Plan to relinquish child
- Loss of the "perfect" child

Optimizing Outcomes:
- Promote early paternal attachment through reflective journaling

 Now Can You:
- Identify the major physiological and psychosocial changes that occur during pregnancy

 Ethnocultural Considerations:
- Many cultural myths/tales exist that explain changes and negative outcomes that occur during pregnancy

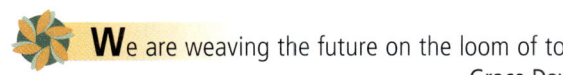

The Prenatal Assessment

chapter 9

 We are weaving the future on the loom of today.
—Grace Dawson

LEARNING TARGETS *At the completion of this chapter, the student will be able to:*

◆ Outline a schedule for and describe the benefits of prenatal care.

◆ Summarize the components of the first prenatal visit in relation to history taking, physical assessment, and risk assessment.

◆ Discuss factors that influence participation in prenatal care.

◆ Discuss how nurses can empower women to become shared decision makers and active participants in planning their prenatal care.

◆ Recognize lifestyle choices that may be detrimental to maternal and fetal well-being.

◆ Differentiate presumptive, probable, and positive signs of pregnancy.

◆ Determine the estimated date of delivery together with the woman's gravidity and parity.

◆ Describe components of the focused obstetric examination.

◆ Discuss aspects of prenatal care for the adolescent and for women over age 35.

---

moving toward evidence-based practice — Decline in Adolescent Pregnancy

Santelli, J.S., Lindberg, L.D., Finer, L.A., & Singh, S. (2007). Explaining recent declines in adolescent pregnancy in the United States: The contribution of abstinence and improved contraceptive use. *American Journal of Public Health, 97*(1), 150–156.

The purpose of this study was to explore the relationship among decreasing adolescent pregnancy rates, improved contraceptive use, and declining sexual activity. Data were analyzed from a national probability survey. The national survey is conducted every 7 years. For the purpose of this research, data from female respondents who were 15–19 years of age during the previous two survey years were used. Data were limited to include noninstitutionalized U.S. citizens 15–19 years of age, which included 1396 for the year of 1995 and 1150 for 2002. The analysis was based on two central measures: sexual activity and contraceptive use at the time of the most recent intercourse (within 3 months of the interview).

The researchers developed two indices: contraceptive risk index and overall pregnancy index. The "contraceptive risk index" was a summary of the overall effectiveness of contraceptive use among sexually active adolescents and included information concerning the nonuse of contraceptives. The "overall pregnancy index" was a calculation that included the contraceptive risk index and the percentage of those who reported sexual activity.

Declines in sexual activity among the 18–19 years-of-age group were considered to be nonsignificant. The contraceptive risk index declined 46% among teens 15–17 years of age. The pregnancy risk index among the same group also declined by 38% overall. Seventy-seven percent of the decline in pregnancy risk was attributed to improved contraceptive use and 23% (of the decline) to a decrease in sexual activity. The researchers concluded that the decline in pregnancy rates was related to an improved use of contraceptives.

1. What may be considered as limitations to this study?
2. How is this information useful to clinical nursing practice?

See Suggested Responses for Moving Toward Evidence-Based Practice on the Electronic Study Guide or DavisPlus.

Introduction

The objective of this chapter is to enhance understanding of the complexities and challenges involved in providing individualized, competent prenatal nursing care. The information presented serves as a knowledge base and introduction to clinical skills while promoting critical thinking and empathetic understanding. Framed in the nursing role, various components of the prenatal assessment throughout pregnancy are explored.

Each prenatal visit offers an opportunity for the nurse to provide a comforting, supportive environment for the expectant woman and her family members. During these visits, educational needs can be identified and addressed, concerns can be discussed, reassurance can be provided, and problems or potential problems can be discovered. Promoting maternal physical, psychological, and spiritual health and facilitating maternal empowerment are key to promoting and enhancing fetal well-being and a positive pregnancy outcome.

A Time of Wonder and Growth...and Ambivalence

For most women, pregnancy is a special time of wonder and personal growth. However, when faced with a positive pregnancy test result, many women experience ambivalence or begin to question their desire to be pregnant. This reaction is a normal response that occurs irrespective of how determined and committed the couple is to the goal of beginning or expanding a family. Part of the ambivalence relates to the sudden realization that life as it has been known is going to change dramatically and this change will be a life-long endeavor. The woman especially can anticipate role changes in relation to her career and relationships and a need to prepare for the role of being a mother to an infant who will be dependent upon her for survival. Recognizing ambivalence and its normalcy in relation to pregnancy during the first trimester and providing support and reassurance are essential in helping the woman positively embrace and celebrate her journey into motherhood.

Concerns over Self-Preservation

Pregnancy also raises issues of maternal self-preservation. Despite tremendous improvements in perinatal care, women still die in childbirth and it is not unrealistic for a woman to fear for her own safety. The World Health Report "Make Every Woman and Every Child Count" (World Health Organization [WHO], 2005b) focuses on making pregnancy safer and asserts that reaching this goal centers on providing excellent antenatal care and constructing societies that support pregnant women. Antenatal care must be consistently accessible and responsive while incorporating patient-centered interventions, thereby removing barriers that prevent access to care. Perhaps one of the most significant roles that nurses can play in helping to achieve this important goal lies in promoting optimal prenatal care for all women.

Women who receive prenatal care experience a fivefold decrease in pregnancy-related maternal deaths and have better pregnancy outcomes than those who do not receive prenatal care (Harper, Byington, & Espeland, 2003). Prenatal care should offer the patient evidence-based medical and nursing care together with an educational program specifically designed to meet that patient's needs. This approach to care enables informed and shared decision making (Kirkham, Harris, & Grzybowski, 2005).

Health care should begin during the preconception period and continue throughout the pregnancy and puerperium. Firmly grounded in an understanding of the physical, emotional, and psychological changes characteristic of the childbearing period, prenatal care should be focused on the early identification of deviations from the normal. Ideally, screening procedures are conducted where warranted, health maintenance and promotion are emphasized, and psychological support to facilitate optimal maternal and fetal outcomes is provided in a culturally sensitive setting. An integral aspect of all prenatal nursing care involves actively listening to the woman, providing individualized education, and respecting her choices. The woman has the right to expect continuity of care, clear explanations, consistent information, and the opportunity to discuss any aspect of her care at any time (Haire, 2000) (Fig. 9-1). A number of nursing diagnoses are applicable during the prenatal period. These are often related to maternal health-seeking behaviors (e.g., "health-seeking behaviors related to guidelines for activity and nutrition during pregnancy") and family support and coping (Box 9-1).

 Nursing Insight— *Goals that guide nursing care of the prenatal patient*

When providing care for the prenatal patient, essential nursing goals are:

- To recognize deviations from normal
- To provide individualized, evidence-based care
- To provide culturally appropriate prenatal education designed to meet the patient's learning style and needs
- To empower women to become actively involved in their pregnancy by being informed recipients and shared decision makers

Figure 9-1 Actively listening to the patient and providing individualized education is an essential component of prenatal care.

Prenatal care usually begins in the first trimester of pregnancy, when the patient is seen every 4 weeks until she reaches 28 to 32 weeks' gestation. At that time, the appointments are changed to visits every 2 weeks and then occur weekly from 36 weeks of gestation until birth. Although this schedule has to some extent become the "standard of care," it has not been possible to substantiate the necessity for such frequent visits. Interestingly, the number of total prenatal visits varies tremendously from as few as 3 to 4 visits for low-risk women in some European countries to 14 or more visits for women with uncomplicated pregnancies in the United States (Partridge & Holman, 2005).

A recent meta-analysis revealed that a reduction in the total number of prenatal visits did not negatively affect maternal or infant outcomes, but did negatively affect the women's level of satisfaction with the care received (Villar, Carroli, Khan-Neelofur, Piaggio, & Gulmezoglu, 2004). Based on these findings, a more patient-centered approach to care for low-risk women may entail fewer visits with a medical provider and more frequent visits with a nursing team who can provide continuity of care, psychological support, and individualized strategies to meet the patient's educational needs.

 Now Can You— **Discuss aspects of prenatal care?**

1. Discuss why ambivalence is frequently experienced during the first trimester?
2. Name three goals of prenatal care?
3. Describe the common prenatal visit schedule for a low-risk pregnancy?

Navigating the Health Care System

A woman's initial contact with the health care system may occur when she first seeks prenatal care. Attempts to navigate the system while becoming familiar with health

insurance or Medicaid coverage can result in an overwhelming, frightening experience. Many women have no financial resources for maternity care or for health care of any kind. Despite recent changes in legislation, approximately 45 million Americans remain without any source of health care insurance (Centers for Disease Control and Prevention [CDC], 2007). For uninsured women, pregnancy can create a major financial stress since health care for a single pregnancy may well exceed $20,000.00, depending on the type of birth and the development of complications.

CAREing for the Patient

Throughout the childbearing experience, the nurse's primary role is to "CARE" for the patient. The "CARE" principle centers on communicating, advocating, respecting and enabling/empowering the individual (Box 9-2). Some patients find both the health care system and the health care staff to be intimidating and nonreceptive when they attempt to voice concerns, doubts, or desires. There is a lack of effective communication between the patient and the nurse. When this occurs, many women adopt what is perceived as the "typical patient role"—one where the patient simply does as requested without question. Unfortunately, nurses sometimes have a tendency to facilitate and reinforce this behavior.

The nurse's role encompasses that of being an advocate for the patient. An advocate verbalizes the patient's wishes if the patient is unable to do so herself and ensures that the patient's questions are answered in an understandable and comprehensive way. It is also the advocate's responsibility to help the patient to become an informed recipient

---

Box 9-1 **Possible Nursing Diagnoses for the Prenatal Patient**

- Knowledge Deficit related to normal physiological changes of pregnancy
- Altered Nutrition Risk: less than body requirement
- Risk for Fatigue
- Risk for Disturbance in Body Image
- Risk for Altered Role Performance
- Altered sexual patterns
- Family coping
- Change in comfort level related to advancing pregnancy
- Change in sleep pattern disturbance
- Altered urinary elimination due to enlarging uterus or engagement of fetal part
- Anxiety
- Family coping
- Adolescent
- Family processes, altered

Adapted from Doenges (2005).

Box 9-2 **CARE Principles**

Communication
The exchange of information between individuals, for example, by means of speaking, writing, or using a common system of signs or behavior
A spoken or written message
The communicating of information
A sense of mutual understanding and sympathy

Advocate
One who argues for a cause; a supporter or defender
One who pleads in another's behalf; an intercessor: Advocates for abused children and spouses

Respect
To feel or show admiration and deference toward somebody or something
To pay due attention to and refrain from violating something
To show consideration or thoughtfulness in relation to somebody or something

Enable
To provide somebody with the resources, authority, or opportunity to do something
To make something possible or feasible

of care. Respecting the patient involves valuing her as an individual, listening attentively, and addressing all of her concerns.

Optimizing Outcomes— Being an advocate for the patient

The nurse is the ideal person to be an advocate for the pregnant patient. An advocate is a person who supports and represents the rights and interests of another individual in order to ensure the individual's full legal rights and access to services.

The nurse has the knowledge base to educate the patient and inform her of safe options or alternatives to meet her particular needs. The nurse also has the skills to communicate effectively with the patient, her family members, and her care provider. Thus, the nurse facilitates shared decision making and helps to promote patient satisfaction with the health care services received.

An informed recipient of care is an individual who has been made aware of available health care options and the possible consequences or outcomes of the choices made. Thus, the informed pregnant woman is able to discuss the advantages and disadvantages of various screening tools, diagnostic tests, and treatment options and she is empowered to make an informed choice that is right for her and her family. For the nurse, an important aspect of the advocate role involves remaining nonjudgmental and able to listen and respond accurately and objectively.

As health care professionals, nurses need to empower women by caring, actively listening, and recognizing their inner wisdom, strength, and abilities. In so doing, nurses gain insights to help them meet their patient's needs in relation to education; health promotion; and physical, psychological, emotional, and spiritual support. The pregnant woman has a journey ahead of her that should lead to greater self-understanding, enhanced feelings of self-worth, and the knowledge that she has the internal power to succeed.

Diminishing Stress and Improving Pregnancy Outcomes

Pregnancy is a developmental crisis that necessitates role adaptation and a restructuring of the tasks involved in daily living. It is a life-changing event that requires adjustments to the many physical and emotional changes that will take place. By nature, change is associated with stress. Eustress is defined as a normal, healthy level of stress. Most individuals are equipped with the resources needed to readily deal with eustress. However, when perceived stress exceeds the individual's resources, strategies, and abilities to effectively deal with it, the person moves into a state of distress.

Nursing Insight— *Diminishing maternal stress*

Women release oxytocin as a response to stress and when they engage in "tend and befriend" activities with friends. Oxytocin appears to buffer the stress response and produces a calming

effect. This physiological response to engagement in friendship behaviors helps women to dissipate stress (Taylor et al., 2002).

From a nursing perspective, there are a number of ways in which this information can be used. One strategy is to incorporate continuity of care, so that as the patient sees the same nursing staff throughout pregnancy, a professional relationship develops. This bond helps the patient to develop a sense of being cared for, appreciated and known as an individual by her care providers. Ultimately, this simple action can help to reduce maternal stress.

Maternal stress during pregnancy can be associated with difficulty accessing care. Transportation problems, appointment schedules that conflict with work commitments, and personal or family member illness may prevent the woman from keeping her prenatal appointments. Communication difficulties, perceptions of staff disinterest, and a lack of understanding about the importance of frequent prenatal visits are all potential sources of stress that may diminish the patient's ability to comply with the plan of care. By using an individualized approach with a focus on communication, personalized care, and education, nurses may help to reduce the patient's stress and increase her adherence to the care plan.

Pregnancy is a time of entering the unknown. The pregnant woman faces unpredictability and quite possibly the loss of control. Since the course of the pregnancy may differ from the anticipated experience, women need to be able to adapt to unexpected situations and meet unforeseen challenges as the pregnancy advances. The new stressors associated with pregnancy can become a deterrent to seeking or continuing prenatal care. Therefore, nurses must be cognizant of the fact that women, irrespective of culture, may face different stressors and often require a variety of resources and interventions to help them deal effectively with stress and improve their utilization of prenatal care.

Racial disparities exist in the provision and utilization of prenatal care. The effects of these discrepancies on pregnancy outcomes have been recognized for more than 90 years. One of the goals of the *Healthy People 2010* national initiative is to address these racial disparities and to increase the uptake of prenatal care in the first trimester of pregnancy for all women to 90% (Healy et al., 2006). By using the "CARE" principles, the nurse can provide individualized support to all patients irrespective of race or culture.

As an advocate, nurses can provide information about stress management for their patients. Social support is an important and positive factor in the reduction of stress (Fig. 9-2). If the pregnant woman has a good social support system, she is much more likely to have a venue to discuss issues of concern and gain morale support. It is important to note that a support system may be lacking for women who are trying to conceal a pregnancy or for women who are trying to keep the news of their pregnancy from relatives or friends until results from genetic tests are known. These individuals may need additional support from their nurses and other health care providers as they are placed in a powerless situation while awaiting results and face a pregnancy that may be in jeopardy.

Figure 9-2 Social support helps to reduce maternal stress.

Box 9-3 Definition of Certified Nurse Midwife and Sphere of Practice

DEFINITION OF CERTIFIED NURSE MIDWIFE AND SPHERE OF PRACTICE

A certified nurse midwife (CNM) is an individual educated in the two disciplines of nursing and midwifery who possesses evidence of certification according to the requirements of the American College of Nurse-Midwives (ACNM).

MIDWIFERY PRACTICE

Midwifery practice, as conducted by CNMs, is the independent management of women's health care, focusing particularly on common primary care issues; family planning and gynecological needs of women; pregnancy; childbirth; the post-period; and the care of the newborn. The CNM and certified midwife practice within a health care system that provides for consultation, collaborative management, or referral, as indicated by the health status of the client. CNMs practice in accord with the Standards for the Practice of Midwifery, as defined by the American College of Nurse-Midwives (ACNM), 2005.

Choosing a Pregnancy Care Provider

One of the first maternal tasks of pregnancy as described by Rubin (1984) is "Ensuring safe passage." This stage encompasses the active lifestyle choices that the woman makes, and the behaviors that she adopts to promote her own and her fetus's well-being. One of the early decisions the patient (and partner) makes concerns choosing a care provider. It is recommended that every patient arrange an appointment with a chosen care provider (obstetrician, family practice physician, certified nurse midwife) to discuss the management of pregnancy and childbirth as early as possible within the first trimester. The woman may seek childbearing care from an obstetrician, a family practice physician, or a certified nurse midwife (CNM) who is educated in the disciplines of nursing and midwifery and is certified by the American College of Nurse-Midwives (Box 9-3).

Approximately 90% of pregnant women choose an obstetrician as the primary care provider. Others use a CNM who can provide a more personalized, less routine approach to a normal, uncomplicated pregnancy and birth.

Healthy women who choose a CNM are as likely as those who choose an obstetrician to have an excellent outcome and they may also experience fewer medical interventions and a lower rate of cesarean births. Women who have complications related to the pregnancy or who are in a high-risk category should plan to meet with a perinatologist, an obstetrician with experience in managing high-risk pregnancies. The perinatologist works closely with the woman's obstetrician to determine the best plan for managing the pregnancy, labor, and birth.

A woman's journey through the pregnancy experience can have long-term effects on her self-perception and self-concept. Thus, it is especially important that the patient choose a care provider with whom she can openly relate and who shares the same philosophical views on the management of pregnancy. Continuity of prenatal care has been shown to be associated with increased maternal satisfaction and a need for fewer interventions during labor. The importance of developing a positive relationship with one's care provider and receiving personal, individualized care throughout the pregnancy is medically and psychologically advantageous (Hodnett, 2004).

During the initial interview with a care provider, it is helpful for the woman to discuss the provider's work schedule and how births that take place when the provider is not on call are managed. This is also an ideal time for the care provider to introduce the pregnant woman's Bill of Rights and to discuss the responsibilities the woman has to facilitate optimum health for herself and for her fetus (Appendix 9-1 in the Electronic Study Guide). Many pregnant women are not fully aware of their right of informed consent or of the obstetrician's legal obligation to obtain their patient's informed consent prior to treatment. The American College of Obstetricians and Gynecologists (ACOG) first publicly acknowledged the physician's legal obligation to obtain the pregnant patient's informed consent in its 1974 publication, Standards for Obstetric-Gynecological Services. The informed consent process is important in safeguarding the patient's autonomy (Box 9-4).

American patients are becoming increasingly aware that well-intentioned health professionals do not always have scientific data to support common American obstetric practices, and that many of these practices are carried out primarily because they are part of medical and hospital tradition. More than 20 years ago, the distinguished obstetrician Dr. Roberto Caldeyro-Barcia articulated clearly his concerns with the medical management of low-risk pregnancy and delivery:

In the last 40 years, many artificial practices have been introduced that have changed childbirth from a physiological event to a very complicated medical procedure in which all kinds of drugs are used and procedures carried out, sometimes unnecessarily, and many of them potentially damaging for the baby and even for the mother (Haire, 2000).

A growing body of research makes it alarmingly clear that every aspect of traditional American hospital care during labor and birth must now be questioned as to its possible effect on the future well-being of both the obstetric patient and her unborn child. Care needs to be individualized to meet each patient's particular needs, and

> ### Box 9-4   Informed Consent and Communication
>
> Informed consent is the willing and uncoerced acceptance of a medical intervention by a patient following the clinician's full disclosure of information that includes the nature of the intervention, the risks and benefits of the intervention, and the risks and benefits of any alternatives. The patient also has the right to informed refusal, that is, the right to refuse recommended medical treatment. Open, ongoing communication about relevant information empowers the patient to exercise personal choice, and is central to the patient-clinician relationship.
>
> *Source*: Amercian College of Obstetricians and Gynecologists (ACOG). (2007). Guidelines for Women's Health Care. A resource manual. (3rd ed.). Washington, DC, ACOG.

procedures performed only when the advantage to the patient outweighs any possible disadvantage.

The provision of prenatal care offers the nurse a unique opportunity to make a difference not only in the patient's life but also in the lives of her family. To truly take advantage of this opportunity, the nurse needs an expansive array of tools including the ability to communicate effectively with patients irrespective of cultural background, educational level, health care beliefs, or age, to understand family and group dynamics; and to accept diversity without prejudice or bias. Family care during the prenatal period centers on education and health promotion.

A number of issues affect a woman's willingness to use health care services. These include personal beliefs about pregnancy, cultural expectations, previous relationships with health care providers and perceived benefits of prenatal care, together with the more practical issues of access to care, medical insurance and/or financial support. By using therapeutic communication, the nurse can gain insights into the patient's belief system and manage care appropriately. Maintaining a nonjudgmental attitude is essential, for example, if the woman is a late recipient of prenatal care. Creating an atmosphere where the patient feels accepted and valued for seeking care is a therapeutic, positive approach and one that will hopefully foster patient adherence.

Through discussion, the nurse can gain an understanding of the availability and acceptability of traditional health care services and whether they meet the patient's individual health care needs. Each culture embraces different customs and health practices that need to be respected, and wherever possible, accommodated. These requirements may relate to the gender of the health care provider, the patient's clothing requirements, diet, and/or food preparation. The prenatal interview provides an opportunity to develop a positive relationship with the patient and emphasize the benefits of prenatal care for her and her unborn child.

In both the local and national arenas, nurses can empower women and their families by advocating for prenatal care that is readily available and affordable for all, especially for low-income and vulnerable populations. The "Health Care Safety Net" is one mechanism for providing health services for the needy. Despite the availability of these types of programs, there are still women who receive inadequate or no prenatal care. In 2005, close to four percent of women in the United States received inadequate prenatal care (National Center for Health Statistics [NCHS], 2007).

 Across Care Settings: **The health care safety net**

The health care safety net consists of a wide variety of providers who deliver care to low-income and other vulnerable populations, including the uninsured and those covered by Medicaid. Many of these providers have either a legal mandate or an explicit policy to provide services regardless of a patient's ability to pay.

Major safety net providers include public hospitals and community health centers as well as teaching and community hospitals, private physicians, and others who deliver a substantial amount of care to the targeted populations.

The health care safety net—the Nation's system of providing health care to low-income and other vulnerable populations—was recently described as "intact but endangered" (Agency for Healthcare Research and Quality 2003). Safety net monitoring initiative. Retrieved from http://www.ahrq.gov/data/safetynet/netfact.htm

 Now Can You— **Discuss health promotion strategies for pregnancy?**

1. Identify and describe each component of the "CARE" principle?
2. Discuss how stress adversely affects pregnancy and identify nursing interventions to help decrease patient stress?
3. Describe four important elements of a teaching plan for family health promotion during pregnancy?

The First Prenatal Visit

THE COMPREHENSIVE HEALTH HISTORY

Before initiating the interview, it is helpful for the nurse to review the paperwork to become familiar with the information to be gathered and to ensure an understanding of the relevance and appropriateness of the questions to be asked. The initial interview time with the patient should be used to build a positive, nonthreatening relationship and to gain her confidence. Strategies that are useful include active listening, validating responses when needed, maintaining eye-to-eye contact, and the use of humor as appropriate to relax the patient. Honesty is essential for effective communication. When uncertain of the answer to a question, the nurse should make a note to find the answer and report back to the patient at the end of the interview.

The first prenatal visit is an extremely important one that should take place as early in pregnancy as possible. Therapeutic communication skills are of paramount importance when obtaining the prenatal history. The information requested can often be of a very personal nature and it may be difficult for patients to disclose certain aspects of their past histories. Therefore, care must be taken to manage the environment to promote privacy and provide the patient with psychological and physical comfort.

It is important to avoid medical or technical jargon that may interfere with the patient's understanding, may intimidate her, or cause her to feel embarrassed due to a lack of

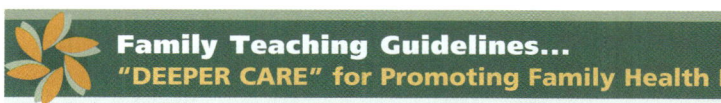

Family Teaching Guidelines...
"DEEPER CARE" for Promoting Family Health During Pregnancy

D	DIET	This is an ideal time to review the family diet and the way that foods are prepared. Encourage consumption of whole grains, dark green, yellow and orange vegetables, dry beans and peas; a variety of fresh or dried/canned fruit; increased low-fat and fat-free foods, milk and calcium-rich foods; poultry, low-fat meats, fish that are lowest in mercury (whitefish, haddock, pollock, sole, trout), nuts, and seeds.
E	EXERCISE	Aerobic exercise maintains physical fitness and promotes self-esteem and body image. It is a family activity that benefits all family members.
E	EDUCATION	Many childbirth education options are available to meet the needs of women and their families.
P	PLAY	Play is essential to health, happiness, and creativity. Fun family (couple) activities refresh, promote optimism, and provide an opportunity to "recharge and reconnect."
E	EXPECTATIONS	Pregnancy is a time of great expectations. Families need to know what changes are likely to occur and to be able to recognize normal from abnormal so they can recognize when to seek medical assistance.
R	RELAXATION	Relaxation benefits all family members by boosting immunity, lowering blood pressure, reducing stress, and increasing energy levels. Activities may include meditation, yoga, and visualization/positive thinking.
C	COMMUNICATION	Effective communication is essential to promote family cohesiveness. Communication includes both verbal and nonverbal language such as body posture, gestures, facial expressions, and tone of voice. Within the family, communication needs to be open and truthful and received in a nonjudgmental and accepting manner, ultimately affirming and supporting one other.
A	ATTITUDE	Positive thinking is under each individual's control but can be modeled. A positive attitude to life is associated with released stress, improved coping abilities, improved immunity, and a greater sense of well-being.
R	RESPECT	Healthy relationships require mutual respect, honesty, and trust. Compromise, negotiation, and shared responsibility are intrinsic to a positive relationship, as is equal distribution of power and control.
E	EMERGENCIES	Family members need to know the following danger signs of pregnancy and how to seek medical help: ◆ Reduction in fetal movements. ◆ Signs of preterm labor such as low, dull backache, pelvic pressure feelings, uterine contractions, or menstrual cramps. ◆ Vaginal fluid loss or vaginal bleeding. ◆ Maternal fever over 100.5°F (38.1°C). ◆ Persistent headache associated with blurred vision or flashing lights in front of the eyes. ◆ Continuous vomiting with weight loss, dehydration, weakness, dizziness, or fainting. ◆ Couple has an "inner feeling that something is just not right." It is always better to confirm normality rather than deal with an avoidable emergency.

comprehension. Questions should be phrased in a way to encourage the patient to discuss and share information rather than asking closed-ended questions that require only a "yes" or "no" response. The value the patient places on the care she receives and her interactions with personnel will determine whether she returns for subsequent prenatal care. Therefore, the prenatal team's objective is to provide a user-friendly service that is efficient, effective, caring, and patient centered. One major goal for this first visit is to explain the purpose of prenatal care and to establish specific goals. Care goals are determined through shared decision making with the patient and focus on promoting maternal and fetal health through assessment, education, screening, diagnosis, and treatment.

Biographical Data

Collection of the patient's biographical data, medical history, psychosocial history, and a medical examination are essential components of the first visit. To facilitate the collection of data, a number of prenatal forms such as the Prenatal Plus Program—Initial Assessment Form are available. This is a particularly in-depth and user-friendly tool produced by the Colorado Department of Public Health and Environment. This risk assessment form allows for the collection of information relating to the patient's pregnancy history, medical history, nutritional and exercise patterns, financial income, her vocational and educational goals, living arrangements, psychosocial history (includes depression and past suicidal tendencies), and lifestyle choices. It also provides an opportunity for the patient to request educational information on a variety of topics.

Completing the prenatal history form with the patient enables the nurse to provide personalized education that focuses on risk factors pertinent to that individual. For example, it may be appropriate to discuss the maternal and fetal effects of environmental substances to which the woman is exposed at home and in the work place. Common offenders include exposure to cigarette smoke (either directly or passively), alcohol consumption, recreational drugs, poor or inadequate diet, pollutants, viruses, and occupational hazards. It is estimated that approximately 10% of fetal malformations are related to exposure to environmental hazards (Silbergeld & Patrick, 2005).

The history should also include information concerning complementary and alternative therapies. An increasing number of individuals routinely use herbal or homeopathic remedies. Some of these substances, such as red raspberry tea, are safe and may be beneficial; others such as blue cohosh may be harmful if taken during pregnancy. Thus, it is essential to explore all nonprescription medications and supplements used.

 Complementary Care: *Red raspberry and blue cohosh*

For centuries, the leaves of the red raspberry plant (*Rubus idaeus*) have been used as a medicinal herb for menstrual problems, pregnancy, childbirth, and breastfeeding. Safe to use during pregnancy, raspberry leaf is believed to aid fertility, ease the symptoms of morning sickness, and assist with the birth of the baby and the placenta (Natural Standard, 2008).

Blue cohosh (*Caulophyllum thalictroides*) belongs to the Barberry family. It also has a long history of use as a medicinal herb. It was known as "papoose root" and used by the American Indians to induce labor or abortion. Blue cohosh should be avoided during pregnancy—it has been linked with cardiovascular emergencies in the woman and anoxia in the fetus (Dugoua, Perri, Seely, Mills, & Koren, 2008).

The biographical information usually includes contact information for the patient such as address and phone number(s), along with the patient's occupation and educational level, marital/relationship status, insurance data, and contact person information. Some forms also contain a section for recording special requests such as spiritual or cultural considerations. To ensure currency, it is important to reconfirm contact information at least every 2 months throughout the pregnancy. Maintaining a reliable and timely means for contacting the patient (e.g., to discuss screening or test results) is essential.

The woman's age and date of birth allow for easy recognition of potential risk factors (e.g., maternal age is one of the most commonly used indicators for initiating genetic testing). Teenage girls, who fall at the opposite end of the age spectrum, often need additional support and education throughout the prenatal period.

Social History

Together with the biographical details, additional information is obtained relating to the patient's educational level and occupation. These data help to establish the patient's socio-economic group and may provide some indication of family income, standard of housing and nutrition. Information regarding the patient's marital status is also obtained.

 Nursing Insight— *Homelessness and prenatal care*

Homelessness presents a significant barrier to receiving prenatal care. Homeless women may have fears related to acceptance, judgment, costs, and the philosophies and/or expectations of health care providers (Bloom et al., 2004). Nurses, especially those working in the community, need to advocate for homeless women and their children and explore avenues for bringing prenatal and child care in a nonthreatening environment to those in need.

History of Intimate Partner Violence

Intimate partner violence (IPV), formerly known as domestic violence, is the most common form of violence experienced by women worldwide; approximately one out of every six women has been a victim of domestic violence (World Health Organization [WHO], 2005a). In the United States, the reported incidence of physical abuse during pregnancy ranges from 4% to 30% (El Kady, Gilbert, Xing, & Smith, 2005). Up to 45% of victims of intimate partner abuse before pregnancy continue to be abused during the pregnancy (McFarlane, Campbell, Sharps, & Watson, 2002).

Shockingly, IPV may occur for the first time during pregnancy or the nurse may identify evidence during the

 where research and practice meet:
Marital Status and Perinatal Outcomes

A recent study of 720,586 births in Canada demonstrated that birth outcomes were improved when the mother was legally married as opposed to being in a common-law union. Women not involved in a close relationship with the father of the child experienced the worse perinatal outcomes in relation to preterm births, low birth weight, small for gestational age infants, and neonatal mortality rates (Luo, Wilkins, & Kramer, 2004). It is important to remember that this research is applicable to the group studied and may not be transferable to different social groups. Marital status alone cannot be used to place an individual into an "at risk" group but when combined with other factors, it may be a useful indicator of a pregnancy that warrants close surveillance.

physical examination that is suspicious of ongoing physical abuse. It is estimated that every day at least three women in the United States die as a result of intimate partner violence (Bureau of Justice Statistics, 2003). **Femicide** is presently the leading cause of pregnancy-associated death in the United States (Stevens, 2005). Femicide refers to the death of a woman resulting from an act of violence against that woman (Bull, 2003).

IPV is a difficult subject to discuss and the nurse may fear insulting or psychologically hurting the patient more. A nonthreatening approach is to ask patients directly whether they feel safe going home and whether they have been hurt physically, emotionally, or sexually by a past or present partner. If the partner has accompanied the woman to the prenatal visit, these questions are postponed until the nurse is alone with the patient, for obvious reasons.

An alternative method is to use a standardized form that has valid and reliable questions concerning IPV. The form could be incorporated into the intake assessment data obtained from all patients. Women who have been sexually abused as children are at greater risk of IPV in adult relationships. Sequelae of abuse include depression, anxiety, substance abuse and posttraumatic stress disorder (Coid et al., 2001). As a women's advocate, nurses have a duty to be observant, to actively listen and to use communication skills to gain clarification and understanding. The Centers for Disease Control and Prevention (CDC) have adopted the acronym "RADAR," a term originally developed by the Massachusetts Medical Society (Alpert, Freud, Park, Patel, & Sovak, 1992) to guide nurses as they interview patients about relationship violence:

- **R**outinely screen every patient
- **A**sk directly, kindly, and in a nonjudgmental manner
- **D**ocument your findings
- **A**ssess the patient's safety
- **R**eview options and provide referrals

 ### Nursing Insight— *Screening for intimate partner violence*

Domestic violence during pregnancy is more common than preeclampsia or gestational diabetes (Parson, 2000). Each year, approximately 324,000 pregnant women are abused by their intimate partner and that number increases by a factor of 2 to 4 if the pregnancy was unplanned (Gazmarian et al., 2000). Intimate partner violence can occur for a first time during pregnancy. Screening should be available to all pregnant women irrespective of social class or educational background.

Nurses need to promote screening for intimate partner violence so that it becomes a routine part of prenatal care.

Women may use a number of defenses to emotionally deal with abuse. One method may involve the use of recreational drugs. Irrespective of a history of intimate partner abuse, it is estimated that approximately 3% of pregnant women use nonprescription drugs such as cocaine, amphetamines, heroin, marijuana, or ecstasy (March of Dimes, 2006). Illegal or recreational drug use can have a number of detrimental effects (e.g., spontaneous abortion, low birth weight, placental abruption, and preterm labor) on maternal and fetal health during pregnancy. Selected recreational drugs and their effects on the pregnancy and the infant are presented in Table 9-1.

The nurse's role is to promote a healthy lifestyle for both the woman and her developing fetus. Recreational drug use puts both patients at increased risk, not only from the direct effects of the drugs but also from the behaviors needed to procure and maintain the supply of drugs. Women using drugs are more likely to have poor nutritional status and they are more prone to infection due to a lack of skin integrity and increased exposure to infective agents such as those responsible for sexually transmitted infections. Sex may be used as a bargaining tool or as a means of income to support a drug habit.

Developing a therapeutic nonjudgmental relationship with a drug-addicted woman is essential in order to provide education, support, and guidance. The majority of expectant women wish to do the best they can for their babies, so pregnancy is an ideal time to direct the woman to drug counseling, support groups, and medical care with the goal of reducing and eventually stopping the habit. For a woman to be successful in overcoming drug addiction, she must be internally motivated. The course to success with this problem is not an easy one and the nurse can be instrumental in helping her to achieve this goal.

Psychological Assessment

Pregnancy is a time of change, and usually change of any nature is linked with additional stress. How an individual deals with stress depends on learned behaviors, coping mechanisms, and support systems. Pregnancy is a major life change or developmental phase for all women. Each woman's approach to her pregnancy encompasses cultural values and family traditions and beliefs. One's status in relation to marriage or partnership, financial security, career, or educational achievements are influential factors that shape the overall childbearing experience. Past obstetric experiences including pregnancy outcomes, interactions with care providers, and level of physical health during and after pregnancy are instrumental in forming the woman's attitude toward this pregnancy. The loss of a previous pregnancy may adversely affect a woman's ability to bond with her present pregnancy. Understandably, she may be reluctant to invest in a pregnancy that she fears may not come to fruition. In other situations, acceptance of pregnancy may be delayed if it was unplanned or unwanted. Ambivalence is a normal initial reaction to pregnancy that usually diminishes as the woman accomplishes the developmental tasks of pregnancy.

Although the developmental tasks of pregnancy may be reviewed in a systematic way, it is important to remember that each woman is an individual who harbors a host of unique medical and psychological factors. For example, a woman with a history of a previous eating disorder may experience difficulty maintaining a healthy diet and achieving appropriate weight gain during pregnancy. Another woman may have struggled with anxiety and depression or alcohol or drug use or issues related to intimate partner violence prior to pregnancy. These are all factors that can have a significant impact on the prenatal course. Many tools such as "The Edinburgh Postnatal Depression Scale" are available to guide the nurse in conducting the prenatal and postpartal psychological assessment. (See Chapter 16 for further discussion.)

Table 9-1 Effects of Recreational Drug Use in Pregnancy

Name	Street Name	Route	Effect	Pregnancy	Newborn
Methamphetamines	Meth	Smoked	Stimulant	Spontaneous abortion	Withdrawal
	Crank	Snorted			Tremors
Dextroamphetamine	Speed	Swallowed		Prematurity	Poor muscle tone
	Ice	Injected			?↑SIDS
		Inhaled		Breastfeeding not recommended	http://otispregnancy.org/otis_fact_sheets.asp
Cocaine	Coke	Inhaled	Stimulant	Spontaneous abortion	Birth defects — abnormalities of brain, skull, face, eyes, heart, limbs, intestines, genitals and urinary tract.
		Smoked		Placental abruption	Neonatal withdrawal
				Preterm birth	Visual disturbances
				Breastfeeding not recommended	Delay in cognitive and/or learning ability
					http://otispregnancy.org/otis_fact_sheets.asp
Ecstasy	E, Adam, Roll, Bean, X and XTC· Clarity, Essence, Stacy, Lover's Speed, Eve	Pill form usually swallowed	Stimulant	Spontaneous abortion	Congenital abnormalities—cleft palate
(MDMA—compound may contain amphetamines and hallucinogens)		Crushed and Snorted	Mood enhancer	Placental abruption Preterm birth	Low birth weight (www.ravesafe.org.za/otherinfo/pregnancy.htm)
		Injected per rectum (known as "shafting") Smoked			Rats exposed to ecstasy showed memory and learning deficiencies (http://www.acde.org/common/ectasy.htm)
Marijuana Cannabis	Pot Weed Grass Mary Jane	Ingested Smoked Snorted Injected	Stimulant Psychedelic Depressant	Intrauterine growth restriction Preterm birth	Possible link to increased incidence of childhood cancers Withdrawal symptoms Decrease in verbal ability and memory, plus lower impulse control http://www.marchofdimes.com/professionals/14332_1169.asp
Heroin	Boy, brown, china white, dragon, gear, H, horse, junk, skag, smack	Swallowed	Sedative	Spontaneous abortion Intrauterine growth restriction Preterm labor/birth Stillbirth	Neonatal withdrawal syndrome http://www.patient.co.uk/showdoc/27000496/

THE OBSTETRIC HISTORY

Previous Pregnancies

One of the first steps in the prenatal interview process is to obtain an accurate and detailed obstetric history that provides the interviewer with essential information so that questions can be formulated and asked in a manner that respects and acknowledges the patient's past experiences with pregnancy. The history should cover the current pregnancy as well as all previous pregnancies and their outcomes, since complications experienced in a prior pregnancy often reoccur in subsequent pregnancies.

A history of preterm labor and delivery, defined as a birth that occurs before the 37th completed week of pregnancy, provides one example of the importance of the obstetric history in identifying potential problems during the current pregnancy. Preterm labor is the leading cause of perinatal mortality and morbidity in the United States, where the incidence is 11%, although this figure is much lower (5%) in some European countries including France and Finland. Once a woman has experienced a preterm birth, her risk of preterm labor in subsequent pregnancies is increased by 20% to 40%. Although the etiology for this condition remains largely unknown, there are a number of predisposing factors. Education, resources, and early interventions are important strategies since earlier diagnosis means earlier treatment and better outcomes. (See Chapter 11 for further discussion.)

A previous history of preeclampsia increases the woman's likelihood of a recurrence during subsequent pregnancies. (See Chapter 11 for further discussion.) Interestingly, if a woman did not experience preeclampsia with previous pregnancies but has a new partner for her current pregnancy, her risk of developing preeclampsia is similar to that of a woman who is pregnant for a first time. Although preeclampsia is a systemic disorder that occurs only during pregnancy, it is generally recognized via two classic symptoms: elevated blood pressure and proteinuria. The complication of preeclampsia places both the patient and her fetus at additional risk both during pregnancy and in the postpartum period.

A history of pregnancy-related diabetes or gestational diabetes mellitus (GDM) (carbohydrate intolerance that occurs during pregnancy) is also significant. GDM is estimated to affect up to 7% of pregnancies, and approximately one half of women who have had a previous pregnancy affected by GDM will develop this condition again in a subsequent pregnancy (American Diabetes Association, 2003). Since GDM is associated with a number of fetal and maternal complications, early screening is essential. (See Chapter 11 for further discussion.)

Patients who indicate a pattern of repeated spontaneous miscarriages most likely would benefit from genetic counseling, preferably during the preconception period. A family pedigree is often useful in determining the need for further screening and specific testing. Prenatal genetic screening questionnaires have been developed to guide counseling and intervention approaches. The Human Genome Project, completed in April 2003, provided information useful in facilitating the early diagnosis of genetic disorders and the timely initiation of medical care. For example, in April 2003, the gene for Hutchinson-Gilford Progeria Syndrome (HGPS) was identified. This finding prompted the development of a genetic test for the early diagnosis of the syndrome (National Human Genome Research Institute, 2003). Because of the rapid advances in the field of genetics, nurses must have a working knowledge of genetics terminology and recent findings so that they can initiate referrals when appropriate. The "Core Competencies in Genetics Essential for All Health Care Professionals" is a useful document with which all perinatal nurses should be familiar (Appendix 9-2 in the Electronic Study Guide).

 Nursing Insight— *Preconception genetics counseling*

Birth defects affect about one in every 33 babies born in the United States each year. They are the leading cause of infant deaths and account for more than 20% of all infant deaths.

Although it is never possible to guarantee a family a "perfect" baby, nurses can help recognize patients who may benefit from preconception or prenatal counseling and genetic testing. Keeping abreast of advances in prenatal genetic diagnosis or knowing where to seek pertinent information is a valuable asset in providing patient centered-care (CDC, 2007).

The loss of a previous pregnancy or the death of an infant brings a staggering cascade of emotions to a subsequent pregnancy. Fear of another fetal loss or infant death undoubtedly increases the couple's anxiety and stress. Although no couple is ever guaranteed a baby that is 100% perfect, the couple who has dealt with the death of a child or loss of a pregnancy faces the prospect of awaiting prenatal diagnostic test results with increased trepidation. Support and continuity of care are essential along with providing advice and listening to the woman's (couple's) concerns. As is true with any pregnant patient, emphasis on healthy lifestyles is of paramount importance. If the previous loss was a result of sudden infant death syndrome (SIDS), the nurse should provide the patient with information about strategies to reduce the incidence of SIDS, such as breast feeding if at all possible, avoiding cigarette smoke and positioning the baby on the back to sleep. Support groups may also help couples facing a new pregnancy after the loss of a previous one. (See Chapter 14 for further discussion.)

During the initial prenatal visit it is especially important to educate the woman about the developing embryo/fetus during the first few weeks of pregnancy. This is a time when the woman needs to be particularly conscious of potential **teratogens**. A teratogen is a substance that adversely affects fetal development. The vulnerability of the developing embryo/fetus during the early weeks of gestation underscores the importance of a healthy body and a healthy lifestyle.

 Now Can You— **Discuss various components of the prenatal assessment?**

1. Describe biographical information to be elicited from the prenatal patient?
2. Explain how to ask the patient about intimate partner violence?
3. Discuss why the psychological assessment is an important component of the prenatal assessment?
4. Explain the importance of past pregnancies in the obstetric history?

Current Pregnancy

When obtaining the medical history, the nurse should begin with the events of the current pregnancy. For the woman, the current pregnancy is the issue of most importance to her at this time and what has brought her to the office for prenatal care. Information is gathered to assist with confirmation of the pregnancy and to determine the expected date of birth (**EDB**). It is usually possible to determine from the patient's responses whether this was a planned or unexpected pregnancy. "Unexpected" does not necessarily mean "unwanted." Instead, this term refers to the fact that the pregnancy occurred when the couple was not actively trying to conceive. Often, pregnancy comes as a complete surprise when the menstrual period is missed or other signs of pregnancy appear. The diagnosis of pregnancy is based on the patient's reported symptoms and the presence of objective signs elicited by the health care provider. The signs and symptoms are traditionally divided into three classifications: presumptive (experienced by the patient), probable (observed by the examiner), and positive (attributable only to the presence of the fetus).

PRESUMPTIVE SIGNS OF PREGNANCY. The subjective signs of pregnancy are the symptoms that the patient experiences and reports. Because these symptoms may be caused by other conditions, they are the least indicative of pregnancy. In combination with other pregnancy symptoms, the following presumptive signs may serve as diagnostic clues:

- **Amenorrhea** (the absence of menses) is one of the earliest symptoms and is especially significant in a woman whose menstrual cycle is ordinarily regular. Amenorrhea may also be caused by chronic illness; infection; or endocrine, metabolic, or psychological factors.
- Nausea and vomiting ("morning sickness") may actually occur at any time and women who experience this symptom tend to have a decreased incidence of spontaneous abortion and perinatal mortality. Nausea and vomiting may also be caused by infection or gastrointestinal or emotional disorders.
- Frequent urination (urinary frequency) is caused by pressure exerted on the bladder by the enlarging uterus. Urinary frequency may also be caused by infection, cystocele, pelvic tumors, or urethral diverticuli.
- Breast tenderness results from hormonal changes during pregnancy. This symptom may also be associated with premenstrual syndrome, mastitis, and **pseudocyesis** (false pregnancy).
- Perception of fetal movement (quickening) occurs during the second trimester. The sensation of fetal movement may also result from flatus, peristalsis, and abdominal muscle contractions.
- Skin changes include stretch marks (striae gravidarum) and increased pigmentation. These changes may also result from weight gain and oral contraceptive pills.
- Fatigue may also be associated with illness, stress, or lifestyle changes.

PROBABLE SIGNS OF PREGNANCY. The probable signs of pregnancy are objective indicators that are observed by the examiner. These signs result from physical changes in the reproductive system. However, because they may be caused by other conditions, a positive diagnosis of pregnancy cannot be based on these findings alone.

- Abdominal enlargement may also be caused by uterine or abdominal tumors.
- **Piskacek sign** (uterine asymmetry with a soft prominence on the implantation side) may also be associated with uterine tumors.
- **Hegar's sign** (softening of the lower uterine segment) may also be caused by pelvic congestion.
- **Goodell's sign** (softening of the tip of the cervix) may also be caused by infection, hormonal imbalance or pelvic congestion.
- **Chadwick's sign** (violet-bluish color of the vaginal mucosa and cervix) may also be caused by pelvic congestion, infection, or a hormonal imbalance.
- **Braxton–Hicks sign** (intermittent uterine contractions) may also be associated with uterine leiomyomas (fibroids) or other tumors.
- Positive pregnancy test may occur from certain medications, premature menopause, choriocarcinoma (malignant tumors that produce human chorionic gonadotropin), or the presence of blood in the urine.
- **Ballottement** (passive movement of the unengaged fetus) may be due to uterine tumors or cervical polyps instead of the presence of a fetus.

POSITIVE SIGNS OF PREGNANCY. The positive indicators of pregnancy are attributable only to the presence of a fetus:

- Fetal heartbeat
- Visualization of the fetus
- Fetal movements palpated by the examiner

Establishing the Estimated Date of Birth

The antenatal period begins with the first day of the last normal menstrual period and ends when labor begins. This time frame is approximately 280 days in length or 40 weeks or 10 lunar months or 9 calendar months. Pregnancy is divided into three trimesters. Each trimester is approximately 14 weeks or 3 months in duration. A term pregnancy is defined as one that begins after the 37th completed week of pregnancy and ends before the 42nd week of pregnancy.

The **estimated date of birth** (EDB) or the **estimated date of delivery (EDD)** (formerly termed the "estimated date of confinement," or EDC) is based on the date of the last normal menstrual period with the assumption that the woman has a 28-day cycle. An important aspect of history taking involves collecting data that help to confirm the accuracy of the duration of the pregnancy. First, the date and a description of the last normal menstrual period are obtained to help determine if the LMP was a "normal" period rather than bleeding associated with implantation. The nurse should ask the patient if her last period was normal for her in relation to the amount and duration of blood loss. The length of the menstrual cycle and its predictability are also important factors. The EDB may be calculated using **Naegele's rule**. To use Naegele's rule, add 7 days, then subtract 3 months from the date of

Box 9-5 Naegele's Rule

Naegele's rule is used to calculate the Estimated Date of Birth (EDB) – Estimated Date of Delivery (EDD)

This calculation is based on the first day of the woman's last normal period.

7 days are added to the LMP and 3 months subtracted and where necessary a year added.

For example, if the woman's LMP was June 8, 2007
Add 7 days = June 15, 2007
Subtract 3 months = March 15, 2007
Add a year = March 15, 2008 EDB = March 15, 08

(An alternative way is to add 7 days and then add 9 months = year where needed)

Remember to ask the women about her last menstrual period (LMP).

Did her period start on the expected date?

Was blood loss normal (the same as her usual menstrual blood loss)?

Was her period different in any way?

What form of contraception had she been using and when was this method discontinued?

(Hormonal contraception may delay the return to a normal ovulation pattern.)

These questions will help you to determine an accurate date for the woman's last normal menstrual period.

Remember: Some women experience bleeding at the time of implantation, which normally occurs 7–9 days after fertilization. Care needs to be taken not to mistakenly use the date of implantation bleeding as the LMP.

Figure 9-3 A gestation wheel is a handy tool for determining the gestational age. The arrow labeled "first day of LMP" is placed on the date of the LMP. The date at the arrow labeled "expected delivery date" is then noted.

the patient's last normal menstrual period (LMP) and add a year where necessary (Box 9-5). Since Naegele's rule is based on a 28-day menstrual cycle, menstrual cycle irregularity and variations in cycle length most likely invalidate the use of Naegele's rule as the sole method for estimating gestational age. A gestation wheel is a useful tool for readily determining the gestational age during pregnancy (Fig. 9-3).

 Now Can You— Correctly calculate the EDB?

Calculate the estimated date of delivery/birth using Naegele's Rule?

Lynne is a 28-year-old woman who comes to the clinic with a history of amenorrhea and a positive home pregnancy test.

Her last menstrual period began on August 26, 2006. She bled for the usual amount of time and reports that the amount of blood loss was normal. Assuming that Lynne had a 28-day cycle, use Naegele's Rule to calculate her estimated date of birth.

Important to remember: The month of August has 31 days
August 26 + 7 days = September 2
(September) 9th month – 3 = 6th month (June)
EDD/EDC/EDB=June 2

Correct calculation of the EDB is dependent on a reliable date of the last menstrual period (LMP). Hormonal birth control methods such as combined oral contraceptive pills (OCP) and long-lasting progesterone injections can cause continued suppression of ovulation. Therefore, a discrepancy may exist between when the woman thought she ovulated and conceived and when these events actually occurred. Thus, the LMP may not be an accurate tool for estimating the due date.

Occasionally, pregnancy occurs in women who are taking oral contraceptives, usually as the result of a "pill failure" from forgotten pills or due to poor absorption that may result from various causes such as vomiting, diarrhea, or antibiotic use. Thus, contraceptive pill use may have unwittingly been continued during the early weeks of gestation. The nurse can assure the patient that prenatal hormone exposure associated with normal contraceptive use has not been shown to have any detrimental effects on the developing fetus (Kandinov, 2005).

THE PREGNANCY CLASSIFICATION SYSTEM

Another important task associated with the initial prenatal interview is to determine the patient's gravidity and parity. **Gravid** is the state of being pregnant; a **gravida** is a pregnant woman. **Gravidity** relates to the number of times that a woman has been pregnant, irrespective of the outcome.

 where research and practice meet:
Depo-Provera Use Before Pregnancy

Bone mass can be adversely affected by the use of depot medroxyprogesterone acetate (Depo-Provera). The extent to which bone mass is lowered appears to be linked to the length of use (Banks, Berrington, & Casabonne, 2001). Calcium has two main physiological functions: promoting skeletal growth and maintaining bone mass. Unfortunately, humans only absorb approximately 10% of the dietary calcium consumed. There are three periods in human life when calcium uptake is increased: during infancy, adolescence (growth spurt) and in the latter half of pregnancy (Heaney, 2006). To counsel prenatal patients appropriately, nurses should understand the benefits associated with meeting the recommended intake of daily calcium, and be knowledgeable about factors that increase absorption. Pregnancy is a time when maternal calcium absorption is increased. To take advantage of this physiological alteration, pregnant women should be encouraged to eat a well-balanced diet with adequate amounts of calcium, protein, and vitamin D and routinely participate in weight-bearing exercises (Heaney, 2006).

The term **nulligravida** is used to describe a woman who has never experienced a pregnancy. A **primigravida** is a woman pregnant for the first time and a **secundigravida** is a woman pregnant for a second time. Although officially correct, this term is seldom used and instead the term multigravida is used in its place. A **multigravida** describes a woman who is pregnant for the third (or more times). **Parity** refers to the number of pregnancies carried to a point of viability (generally accepted as 24 weeks of gestation), regardless of the outcome. For example, "para 1" indicates that one pregnancy reached the age of viability. A para 2 means that two pregnancies reached the age of viability. It is important to note that the term parity (or "para") denotes the number of pregnancies, not the number of fetuses/babies, and does not reflect whether the fetuses/babies were born alive or stillborn. Some facilities use a digital system (i.e., GTPAL) for recording the number of pregnancies and their outcomes.

G **G**ravida
T Number of **T**erm pregnancies
P Number of **P**reterm deliveries
A Number of **A**bortions, both spontaneous and induced
L Number of **L**iving children

PREGNANCY TESTING

A detectable level of human chorionic gonadotropin (hCG) must be present in the urine or blood for a pregnancy test to be positive. hCG is produced by the syncytiotrophoblastic cells found in the outer layer of the trophoblast and secreted into the maternal plasma and then excreted in the urine. Human chorionic gonadotropin levels peak between days 60 and 70 of pregnancy and then gradually decrease over approximately the next 40 days to reach a plateau that is maintained throughout the pregnancy. hCG can be detected in maternal blood as early as 1 day after implantation and in urine around day 26. The hCG molecule contains both an alpha-subunit and a beta-subunit. Because of the large number of commercial pregnancy tests available, women should be advised to use a home pregnancy test that is specific for the beta-subunit of hCG since this marker prevents cross reactions with other hormones. The alpha-subunit is very similar in molecular structure to luteinizing hormone (LH). Women with high LH levels (i.e., those experiencing perimenopause) who use a pregnancy test designed to detect the complete hCG molecule risk obtaining a false-positive result. If the over-the-counter pregnancy test used relies on urinary hCG, the patient should be advised to follow the manufacturer's recommendations carefully to avoid an unreliable result. If a home pregnancy test is negative and the signs and symptoms of pregnancy persist, the test should be repeated in a week or the woman should see her health care provider.

A "chemical pregnancy" is a term used to describe a situation that occurs when a home pregnancy test has confirmed the presence of hCG, but a late and often heavy menstrual period follows. In these instances, conception probably occurred but for some reason the pregnancy was unable to continue and develop into a viable embryo. The frequency of this occurrence is difficult to estimate accurately but it is thought to affect approximately 30% to 50% of all pregnancies. Before the development of sophisticated methods for detecting an early pregnancy, most of these early and unfruitful fertilizations would have gone undiagnosed.

where research and practice meet:
The Home Pregnancy Test

Despite advertising to the contrary, the majority of home pregnancy tests (HPTs) are not sensitive enough to detect pregnancy accurately at the time of the first missed period. In a study conducted in 2004, Cole and colleagues determined the levels of hCG from 25 women in New Mexico. The women were within a time period of 4 weeks and 4 weeks plus 3 days from the date of their last normal menstrual period. The investigators determined that to detect 95% of pregnancies at this gestation, a sensitivity of 12.5 mIU/mL hCG would be needed. Of the 18 types of HPTs tested, only one met this requirement (Cole, Khanlian, Sutton, Davies, & Rayburn, 2004).

Although this study had a small sample size, there are implications for nursing practice. Nurses should encourage women to recognize the limitations of early home pregnancy tests. Patients need to use the first urine sample of the day when hCG levels are most concentrated and they should also be encouraged to postpone testing until 1 week after the date of the expected (missed) period in order to obtain a more reliable result.

 Optimizing Outcomes— **Promoting a healthy beginning for the fetus**

The first few weeks of gestation are of paramount importance to the developing fetus. During this time, the fetus is most susceptible to teratogenic substances such as alcohol, drugs, and environmental toxins. If a woman suspects that she may be pregnant despite a negative home pregnancy test, the nurse should advise her to avoid substances that could be potentially harmful to the developing fetus.

The diagnosis of a multiple gestation places the pregnancy into a "high risk" classification. An early diagnosis of a multiple gestation allows for the development of a care plan that includes more frequent visits for maternal–fetal surveillance. As with any pregnancy, early and ongoing prenatal care offers an opportunity for the timely recognition of complications (more often associated with multiple gestations) and the initiation of interventions to maintain the pregnancy as long as possible. The woman expecting a multiple birth also needs additional psychological support, practical advice, and education. She may experience more intense discomforts of pregnancy and need to deal with upsetting and extreme body changes. In addition, she also faces the financial challenges associated with a potentially complicated pregnancy, possible preterm birth, and the economic burden of providing for multiple newborns.

 Now Can You— **Discuss essential aspects of the current pregnancy?**

1. Differentiate among the "presumptive," "probable," and "positive" signs of pregnancy?
2. Explain how to calculate the estimated date of birth using Naegele's rule?
3. Describe the GTPAL pregnancy classification system?
4. Explain what women should be taught about home pregnancy testing?

THE MEDICAL HISTORY

To provide the patient with appropriate care to meet medical needs during pregnancy, it is essential that a detailed medical history be obtained. This information gives insights into the patient's past and present health status and use of preventative services. The nurse should obtain contact information for the primary care provider in order to facilitate continuity of care. Lack of a family physician may be related to financial difficulties, lack of medical insurance, or cultural/value differences. The nurse can explore these issues through sensitive and respectful questioning and when appropriate, refer the patient and her family to local agencies that provide services such as the WIC (Women, Infants, and Children) program for nutritional support (Box 9-6).

Some European countries offer "shared" care for low-risk patients to serve as a link between the patient's primary care provider and her obstetrician. The pregnant woman visits her family physician for the majority of her prenatal care but also sees an obstetrician for two to three visits. If any complications arise, the patient is transferred for the remainder of the pregnancy to the care of the obstetrician. Since any complications that occur during pregnancy are associated with maternal and family stress, referral to a "known" obstetrician hopefully helps to diminish some of the anxiety.

Dental Health

Together with the overall evaluation of medical well-being, it is essential to explore dental health. The initial interview is an ideal time to provide education about the benefits of preventative dental care and to dispel common myths such as "for every pregnancy, a tooth is lost." It has been well established that the hormones of pregnancy predispose women to increased plaque and the development of gingivitis, or gum inflammation (Hey-Hadavi, 2002).

There is a link between periodontal disease in pregnancy, gingivitis, and preterm labor. It is believed that oral bacteria and their products travel via the bloodstream to the placental membranes, where an inflammatory response occurs. The inflammation may trigger the onset of preterm labor (López, Da Silva, Ipinza, & Gutiérrez, 2005). Oral caries may also pose a greater threat during pregnancy. This is especially true during early pregnancy, when vomiting from "morning sickness" causes the mouth to harbor an acid environment that favors cariogenic activity. Other investigators suggest that women's dental health practices suffer after pregnancy due to a lack of time and result in an increase in dental caries (Hey-Hadavi, 2002). To promote dental health among pregnant women, some European countries such as England offer free dental care during pregnancy and for the first year following childbirth. Part of the nurse's role during the prenatal period is to promote dental hygiene to reduce the incidence of periodontal disease such as gingivitis (which is reversible). Pregnant women need to receive regular dental examinations and appropriate treatment as determined by their dental practitioner.

 Optimizing Outcomes— **Promoting dental health during pregnancy**

- Encourage regular dental examinations.
- Promote twice daily brushing and flossing.
- Recommend the use of a fluoride toothpaste.
- Encourage a healthy diet.
- Encourage chewing gum containing xylitol after meals.

Eye Health

An ophthalmic evaluation is also recommended early in pregnancy, most often during the first trimester or at any time visual changes occur. This is especially important for women with medical conditions such as essential hypertension, Graves' disease, or diabetes mellitus, and for women who wear contact lenses. During pregnancy, a number of normal physiological ophthalmic changes occur, including corneal thickening, increased curvature of the cornea, and a decrease in corneal sensitivity and intraocular pressure. These changes usually resolve spontaneously during the postpartum period. Medical conditions peculiar to pregnancy such as pregnancy-induced hypertension, eclampsia, and gestational diabetes can also have detrimental effects on eye health and vision (Somani & Ahmed, 2004).

Box 9-6 WIC at a Glance

The WIC target population includes those who are low-income and nutritionally at risk:

- Pregnant women, and up to 6 weeks postpartum or after pregnancy ends
- Breastfeeding women (up to infant's first birthday)
- Non-breastfeeding postpartum women (up to 6 months after the birth of an infant or after pregnancy ends)
- Infants (up to first birthday). WIC serves 45% of all infants born in the United States
- Children up to their fifth birthday

BENEFITS

- Supplemental nutritious foods
- Nutrition education and counseling at WIC clinics
- Screening and referrals to other health, welfare, and social services

---

 where research and practice meet:
Eye Examinations During Pregnancy

During an eye examination, it is a relatively common practice to dilate the pupils to facilitate ocular assessment. Although occasional use of parasympatholytics (e.g., atropine) and sympathomimetics (i.e., epinephrine) is thought to be safe, repeated use is contraindicated because of possible teratogenic effects. Mydriatics (medications that dilate the pupils) are also contraindicated for breastfeeding mothers because they have a hypertensive and anticholinergic effect on the infant (Somani & Ahmed, 2005). This information is important to nurses who counsel prenatal and postpartal patients. All prenatal and breastfeeding patients should be advised that certain components of the eye examination may carry risks during pregnancy and they should make certain their eye care professional is aware that they are pregnant (or breastfeeding).

Immunizations

Another essential component of the medical history concerns patient immunizations. Nurses and their patients need to be aware that some infections contracted during pregnancy can be detrimental to the developing fetus. Rubella (German measles) is one of the most commonly recognized viral infections known to cause congenital problems. If a woman contracts rubella during the first 12 weeks of pregnancy, the fetus has a 90% chance of being adversely affected. Maternal exposure to rubella later in pregnancy is associated with a decreased fetal risk. If the pregnancy is between 12 and 16 weeks when rubella infection occurs, the fetal risk decreases to 20%. Typical symptoms of congenital rubella syndrome include intrauterine growth restriction, cardiac detects, sensorineural defects, cataracts, and microcephaly (Laartz, Gompf, Allaboun, Marinez, & Logan, 2006). According to the National Coalition for Adult Immunization, approximately 7 million childbearing-aged women in the United States are currently susceptible to the rubella virus (National Foundation for Infectious Diseases, 2007). A maternity patient who is not immune to rubella should be offered the rubella immunization after childbirth, ideally before hospital discharge. After the immunization, she needs to be advised against becoming pregnant for at least 4 weeks (Vaccine Information, 2005).

Other viruses known to cause complications during pregnancy include varicella (chickenpox) and rubeola (red measles). Information regarding the latest recommendations for immunizations can be found by visiting the Web site for the American Academy of Pediatrics: http://www.aap.org/family/parents/immunize.htm. (See Chapter 11 for further discussion.)

HEPATITIS B INFECTION. Although a vaccination is available to prevent hepatitis B, the rate of new cases of hepatitis B in the United States continues to rise and today approximately 1.25 million Americans are infected (Braun, Sanne, & Bartlett, 2006). During the prenatal period, it is important to screen for hepatitis B since a positive diagnosis will influence both the maternal and newborn medical management. When an acute infection occurs during pregnancy, the rate of vertical transmission from mother to fetus ranges from approximately 10% in the first trimester to 80% to 90% in the third trimester (ACOG, 1998).

From a nursing perspective, the patient will need support and education relating to both the present and long-term implications (Box 9-7). Clinical management focuses on the potential effects of hepatitis B on the pregnancy as well as the long-term maternal risks, including chronic liver disease. It is strongly recommended that household members and intimate partners of a positive hepatitis B carrier undergo screening, and, depending on the results, receive the vaccination.

Other populations at risk for hepatitis B infection include individuals from countries such as India, Africa, Asia, and the Pacific Isles. Due to needle sharing and a potentially high number of sexual partners (as payment for drugs), intravenous drug users are also at an increased risk for hepatitis B. Most adults in the United States contract hepatitis B through sexual contact, and it is estimated that about 25% of individuals who are sexually active with a hepatitis B infected individual will seroconvert (CDC, 2002). **Seroconversion** is the process whereby an individual develops antibodies in response to an infection and subsequently tests positive when screened, due to the presence of the antibodies.

Women who are considered to be at risk for hepatitis B also need to be screened for hepatitis C (HCV). The main route of transmission for this infection (previously known as "non-A, non-B hepatitis") is through intravenous drug use. Approximately 4 million Americans have HCV, which is now listed by the Institute of Medicine as an emerging infectious disease (Holloway & D'Acunto, 2006). Up to 80% of patients with acute HCV are asymptomatic, with seroconversion occurring in approximately 8 to 9 weeks. Preterm labor is the main pregnancy risk associated with HCV. However, there is a low (4% to 8%) risk of transmission to the neonate. If the mother is coinfected with HIV, the transmission rate to the newborn increases to around 13%. It is recommended that all infants born to mothers with HCV undergo testing at 12 to 18 months of age (CDC, 2006b).

Box 9-7 Educational Strategies for Patients Who Are Hepatitis Carriers

The nurse teaches prenatal patients who are hepatitis carriers to:

- Avoid drugs that are hepatotoxic such as acetaminophen (Tylenol).
- Avoid alcohol.
- Choose noninvasive prenatal diagnosis techniques, such as ultrasound and AFP screening rather than invasive procedures such as chorionic villus sampling (CVS) and amniocentesis (Boxall et al., 2004).
- Make certain that the pediatrician is aware of the maternal hepatitis B status.
- Practice "daily living" precautions to prevent transmission to household members. Strategies include covering cuts or skin lesions and not sharing toothbrushes or razors.
  Patients are also advised that:
- The neonate will need to receive hepatitis B immune globulin (HBIG) at birth. This action will provide antibodies to the hepatitis B virus and afford some initial protection to the newborn. The intramuscular injection must be administered within 12 hours of birth. The hepatitis B vaccine (Recombivax HB, Engerix-B), which induces protective anti-hepatitis B antibodies, may be administered at the same time as HBIG but at a different site. The hepatitis B vaccine is given again at 1, 2, and 12 months of age.
- There is at present no correlation between breastfeeding and the incidence of mother-to-infant transmission of hepatitis B (Reuters, 2005).
- The method of birth does not appear to influence the incidence of mother-to-child transmission (Reuters, 2005).

---

 where research and practice meet:
Gender and Neonatal Hepatitis C

There is no known method to prevent the vertical transmission of hepatitis C virus (HCV) from the mother to her infant. Presently, the transmission rate is approximately 4% to 8% and it is dependent on factors such as maternal viral load (Tajiri et al., 2001). A study conducted in 2005 with a population of 1787 HCV-infected pregnant women from 33 centers found that female infants were twice as likely as males to be infected with HCV. Variables such as mode of delivery, gestation, and infant feeding practices were examined. The Italian investigators speculated that the gender differences in the infection rate may be due to either genetic or hormonal factors (Reuters Health Information, 2005).

Screening for hepatitis should be available to individuals with a history of sexually transmitted infections or a history of incarceration. Since blood contact constitutes another high-risk factor, patients who receive blood products or are undergoing hemodialysis should also be screened and vaccinated. Due to their potential contact with bodily fluids, health care workers are also at risk and need to be screened and vaccinated.

Other Preexisting Medical Conditions

Preexisting maternal medical conditions such as diabetes, epilepsy, and phenylketonuria need to be managed appropriately to limit the risk of adverse fetal effects. For example, prenatal exposure to hydantoin (phenytoin) [Dilantin, DPH] has been associated with cleft lip and palate due to its folic acid antagonistic properties (Hernandez-Diaz, Werler, Walker, & Mitchell, 2000). Preconception care is important. The earlier that appropriate management/treatment is implemented, the better the pregnancy outcome.

Environmental Hazards

The developing fetus is at risk from maternal exposure to environmental toxins. Air pollution is one of the most common concerns for maternal and newborn health (Dyjack, Soret, Chen, Hwang, Nazari, & Gaede, 2005). Concentrations of air pollutants are approximately three to five times less outdoors than indoors, where the majority (up to 90%) of time is spent. Adverse birth outcomes including congenital anomalies, intrauterine growth restriction, and preterm birth have been linked to in utero exposure to various air pollutants (Bobak, 2000; Liu, Krewski, Shi, Chen, & Burnett, 2003; Maisonet, Bush, Correa, & Jaakkola, 2001).

Nurses can help to improve the fetal environment by educating women about the dangers of direct and passive smoking during pregnancy. Smoking cessation programs designed for pregnant women are readily available through the American College of Obstetricians and Gynecologists (ACOG, 2005). Effects of tobacco use during pregnancy are well documented and predispose to premature rupture of the membranes, preterm labor, placental abruption, placenta previa, and infants who are small for gestational age (SGA). The detrimental effects on the fetus/neonate continue well into childhood and are associated with problems such as upper respiratory infections, childhood asthma, and wheezing (Gilliland, Li, & Peters, 2001; Jaakkola & Gissler, 2004). Since chemicals, heavy metals, and other environmental hazards that pose a threat to the embryo–fetus may be present in the home or workplace, this information should be elicited and recorded in the prenatal assessment. (See Chapters 7 and 10 for further discussion.)

 Now Can You— Discuss how the prenatal patient's medical history guides care?

1. Explain why dental and eye care are important during pregnancy?
2. Identify three viruses known to adversely affect the developing fetus?
3. Name four essential guidelines that should be included in a teaching plan for pregnant women who test positive for hepatitis B?

THE GYNECOLOGICAL HISTORY

The nurse needs to obtain a concise gynecological (GYN) history primarily to determine if any event in the patient's past places the current pregnancy at risk or warrants further investigation. Women ages 35 and older and foreign-born women should be questioned about in utero exposure to **diethylstilbestrol** (DES). Diethylstilbestrol is a nonsteroidal, synthetic estrogen that is several times more potent than natural estrogens.

In the United States, diethylstilbestrol was widely prescribed during the late 1930s until the early 1970s as a preventative treatment to reduce the likelihood of spontaneous abortion (miscarriage) or preterm delivery (Smith, 1948). It is estimated that between 1 and 2 million pregnant women received this oral medication. Exposure to DES during intrauterine development produces both structural and functional gynecological abnormalities that are associated with numerous problems including infertility, increased incidence of ectopic pregnancies, preterm labor and birth, and vaginal adenocarcinoma (Smith, 1948; Cunningham et al., 2005). Unfortunately, DES is still being used during pregnancy in some countries (National Cancer Institute, 1999).

Screening and Diagnostic Tests During Pregnancy

Before prenatal testing it is essential to determine the gestational age accurately since a number of screening and diagnostic tests have different ranges of normality based upon the maturity of the pregnancy. Before a patient is asked to consent to any investigation, she should be counseled about the purpose of the test, its reliability, and the implications of a negative or positive result. The nurse also needs to explain the difference between a screening test and a diagnostic test.

 Nursing Insight— *Educating patients about screening and diagnostic tests*

To facilitate patient understanding of care options, nurses should explain the differences between screening and diagnostic tests.

A screening test: Identifies patients at increased risk for developing a disorder or disease

Identifies patients who need diagnostic testing

A diagnostic test: Confirms the presence of a disorder or disease

---

At the first prenatal visit, venous blood samples are taken so that abnormal findings can be identified and promptly treated. Blood is drawn for a number of tests: the patient's blood group and rhesus (Rh) factor; antibody screen (Kell, Duffy, rubella, varicella, toxoplasmosis, and anti-Rh), RPR (rapid plasma reagent)/VDRL (Venereal Disease Research Laboratory) screen for syphilis, and if the woman has not received the hepatitis B vaccine, she is tested for hepatitis B surface antigen (HbsAG) and hepatitis B surface antibody (HbsAB). A complete blood count (CBC) with hemoglobin, hematocrit, and differential cell count is obtained and assessed using laboratory values established for pregnancy. Testing for antibody to the human immunodeficiency virus (HIV) is recommended for all pregnant women (ACOG, 2004) and a sickle cell screen is recommended for women of African, Asian, or Middle Eastern descent. In the United States, sickle cell anemia is one of the most common genetic blood disorders and occurs most often in African American populations (NIH, 2006). (See Chapter 11 for further discussion.) During this visit, a Tine or purified protein derivative (PPD) tuberculin test may also be administered to assess for exposure to tuberculosis.

SEXUALLY TRANSMITTED INFECTIONS

Based on the patient's risk factors, screening for sexually transmitted diseases/infections (STDs/STIs) may need to be repeated during the pregnancy. The presence of an STI can predispose to a number of adverse pregnancy outcomes including ectopic pregnancy, spontaneous abortion, preterm labor, and increased neonatal morbidity. Taking a sexual history is an important component of the prenatal nursing assessment. Self-awareness and the use of effective communication techniques foster open, honest discussion of sensitive issues in a nonthreatening environment (Box 9-8).

The sexual history should include signs or symptoms (i.e., vaginal/rectal discharge, dyspareunia, ulcers, rashes, or anogenital itching) that may be indicative of infection. Information concerning recent sexual partners is also important so that when indicated, prior contacts can be notified and offered treatment. High-risk behaviors such as intravenous drug use, acquisition of tattoos, exposure to blood or blood products or sex with an individual from a high-risk category (e.g., a sex industry worker) should also be noted (Sexually Transmitted Diseases Services, 2005).

Human Immunodeficiency Virus

Infection with human immunodeficiency virus (HIV) leads to a progressive disease that results in acquired immunodeficiency syndrome (AIDS). (See Chapter 11 for further discussion.) Perinatal transmission may occur transplacentally, at birth from exposure to maternal blood and vaginal secretions and via breast milk. The incidence of perinatal transmission (HIV-positive mother to her fetus) ranges from 25% to 35%. Maternal treatment with zidovudine (AZT, Retrovir) reduces the risk of perinatal transmission and the risk of infant death. Elective cesarean birth has been shown to significantly reduce the risk of transmission from the mother to the infant (Brocklehurst & Volmink, 2002).

In 2004, the American College of Obstetricians and Gynecologists (ACOG) published a recommendation that all pregnant women be tested for HIV as part of the routine battery of prenatal tests, although patients may choose to opt out of this testing. Screening for HIV is done via an enzyme-linked immunosorbent assay (ELISA) on a blood sample. If the result from this test is positive, the finding is confirmed via a Western blot test.

Nurses need to be patient advocates and ensure that patients receive individualized and informed care. One aspect of the nurse's role in this situation is to make certain that each patient receives comprehensive pre- and post-counseling in relation to HIV testing. Clearly, it is medically advantageous for the pregnant patient to be diagnosed and treated (for HIV) during pregnancy to promote maternal well-being and to reduce the incidence of perinatal HIV transmission (Nielsen, 2006).

Syphilis

A syphilis infection during pregnancy can cause significant damage to the fetus after the 16th to 18th week of intrauterine life, when the cytotrophoblastic layer of the placental villi has atrophied and is no longer protective. Caused by the spirochete *Treponema pallidum*, syphilis is readily treated with penicillin or erythromycin. If the condition is treated before the 18th week, the fetus is rarely affected. Left untreated, transplacental transmission to the fetus is likely to occur (congenital syphilis) and may result in deafness, cognitive difficulties, osteochondritis, or fetal death.

Chlamydia trachomatis, Neisseria gonorrhoeae

Other routine screening tests including chlamydia and gonorrhea are obtained during the pelvic examination. Secretions from the cervix, vagina, and anus may be used to obtain samples for culture media. *Chlamydia trachomatis* is a bacterial infection that is prevalent in sexually active populations, especially those in the under 25-age group. Most patients with this infection are asymptomatic and consequently do not seek treatment. Complications of chlamydial infections include salpingitis, pelvic inflammatory disease, infertility, ectopic pregnancy, premature rupture of the membranes, and preterm birth. Transmission to the neonate may occur during birth and results in ophthalmia neonatorum and chlamydial neonatal pneumonia. During pregnancy, chlamydia is treated with oral anti-infectives or penicillin-based agents. (See Chapter 11 for further discussion). It is recommended that pregnant women be retested 3 weeks after treatment, although the validity of this practice has not yet been established (CDC et al., 2006a).

Gonorrhea is caused by the gram-negative intracellular diplococcal bacteria *Neisseria gonorrhoeae*. It is readily treated with antibiotics. When left untreated, ascending maternal infection may occur after rupture of the membranes. Transmission to the fetus can occur during vaginal delivery and may result in disseminated infection

---

Box 9-8 Tips for Taking A Sexual History

SELF-AWARENESS
Know your own comfort level and your ease at discussing sexual issues with patients.
Acknowledge areas of discomfort.

EFFECTIVE COMMUNICATION
If you are embarrassed, this will be apparent though body language, eye-to-eye contact, tone of voice, type of questioning chosen, for example, closed-ended questions as opposed to exploratory questions.
Use terminology: words/terms that the patient understands.
Environment: ensure privacy and confidentiality.
Never make assumptions or be judgmental in your response or attitude.

Source: Royal Adelaide Hospital Clinic, Sexually Transmitted Diseases Services. STD interview checklist (2005). Retrieved from http://www.stdservices.on.net/management/checklists/cl_interview.htm.

and ophthalmia neonatorum. (See Chapter 11 for further discussion.) Concomitant treatment for gonorrhea and *Chlamydia* is recommended because coinfection is common (CDC et al., 2006a).

Herpes Simplex Virus

Herpes simplex virus type 1 (HSV-1), transmitted nonsexually, is most commonly associated with fever blisters. Herpes simplex virus II (HSV-2) is usually transmitted sexually and is associated with genital lesions, although depending on sexual practices, both types are not exclusively associated with the respective sites. HSV-2 occurs more frequently in women (23%) than in men (11%), which most likely results from the greater likelihood of male-to-female transmission. Although HSV infection is not a reportable disease, it is estimated that 50 million Americans are infected with genital herpes (CDC, 2006a; Winer & Richwald, 2007).

The initial HSV genital infection generally produces flu-like symptoms including malaise, muscle aches, and headache accompanied by dysuria and the appearance of multiple painful blister-like lesions. The symptoms may persist for several weeks. A prodromal period characterized by marked skin sensitivity and nerve pain in the affected area may precede the outbreak of lesions (Gardner, 2006).

HSV-2 infection during pregnancy can have adverse effects on both the mother and her fetus. Primary infection during the first trimester is associated with congenital infection and an increased risk of pregnancy loss. In the neonate, herpes simplex virus infection is associated with a 60% mortality rate, and of those who survive, approximately 50% suffer serious neurological damage (Gardner, 2006). There is no cure for genital herpes. Care management centers on providing symptomatic relief. Although several antiviral agents are available, the safety of these medications during pregnancy and lactation has not been established (CDC, 2006a). (See Chapters 4, 11, and 19 for further discussion.)

CERVICAL CANCER

Cervical screening is usually a component of the first prenatal examination. Screening and treatment of cervical dysplasia (cancerous cellular changes) significantly reduces the chances that carcinoma will develop. This fact lends credence to the recommendation that screening via Papanicolaou testing be performed on all young adults. Furthermore, 50% of all women diagnosed with cervical cancer are diagnosed during the ages of young adulthood. (See Chapter 4 for further discussion.)

The Prenatal Physical Examination

PREPARING THE PATIENT

The patient should be given adequate private time to prepare for the examination and encouraged to void if needed (a urine specimen may also need to be collected). Before conducting the physical examination, it is essential to properly prepare the environment. The room should be warm, with a cover for the patient and a gown for her to wear. Ensure privacy for the patient, such as a "Do not disturb—exam in progress" sign affixed to the closed door.

Before the examination begins, the patient should receive an explanation of what the examination will involve and what she is expected to do. Obtain her consent to be examined. During a physical examination, the patient is usually scantily clothed and must remain on her back in a vulnerable position for the majority of the time. Gaining permission from the patient before proceeding gives her control, as she "allows" the examiner to continue. This action is especially important for women with a history of abuse, particularly, sexual abuse. Actively engaging the patient through dialogue during the examination process provides an excellent opportunity for teaching. Also, ongoing interaction while describing the findings and their relevance empowers the patient and dispels the oft-experienced feeling that something is being "done" to her. Before beginning the physical examination, the nurse should have collected all of the equipment that may be needed, along with any teaching literature that the patient should receive. It does not inspire confidence or relieve the patient's anxiety if the nurse is constantly leaving the room to retrieve forgotten items.

Optimizing Outcomes— Demonstrating professionalism during the physical examination

To convey respect and minimize the transmission of infection, the nurse should:
- Ensure that the fingernails are short and all jewelry items that may cause skin trauma have been removed.
- Wash hands thoroughly in the patient's presence. This simple act demonstrates respect and an understanding of and appreciation for the risk of cross-infection.
- Develop the habit of always washing the hands when entering and leaving a patient's room.

The physical examination should proceed in the same order each time (preferably head to toe) to reduce the likelihood of unintentionally omitting any component. The examination should be organized in a manner that reduces the movements the patient must make. Also, it is less threatening to the patient when less invasive procedures are performed first. Throughout the examination, it is essential for the nurse to use good communication skills and to advocate for and treat the patient with respect. These actions empower patients to participate actively in all health care decisions. The time before, during, and after the examination provides the nurse with an excellent opportunity to develop a good rapport while enhancing the patient's comfort level. Proper management of the clinical environment plays an important role in facilitating the patient's feelings of safety, privacy, and security.

PERFORMING THE GENERAL ASSESSMENT

The general assessment begins by simply observing the woman. Information that can be obtained includes her overall health/nutritional status; posture; ease of movement and gait; appearance (includes clothing and cleanliness); affect and speech pattern; eye contact; and general orientation to place, person, and time. As the pregnancy advances, changes in maternal gait become apparent due to increasing lordosis (curvature of the spine) in response to the increasing weight and size of the gravid uterus that changes the woman's center of gravity.

The nurse then obtains anthropometric measurements. When obtaining the weight it is valuable to ask the patient what her normal prepregnant weight was and to document this information (Fig. 9-4). The prepregnant weight gives an indication of how the patient is adapting to pregnancy. A dramatic, unintended weight loss can be indicative of severe nausea and vomiting (hyperemesis gravidarum). The height and weight are also recorded and used to calculate the patient's body mass index (BMI) and to determine nutritional needs. The BMI can be used to calculate whether the maternal weight is appropriate for height. (See BMI discussion in Chapter 10.) Woman who are underweight before pregnancy and have a low weight gain during the pregnancy are at a greater risk for preterm labor.

Obtaining Information and Promoting Good Nutrition

An important nursing goal is to promote appropriate weight gain during pregnancy through healthy nutrition. It may be helpful to use a 24-hour diet recall form to help provide pertinent information about the patient's nutritional intake and food preparation/cooking preferences. On average, during the second and third trimesters a woman's caloric need increases by 300 per day. A well-balanced diet that contains the necessary vitamins and nutrients is essential. It is important to educate women that prenatal vitamins are an option to ensure that their daily needs are being met, but megadoses of vitamins can be harmful. A woman's need for folic acid doubles during pregnancy and ideally supplementation with 400 mcg/day should be initiated prior to conception and continued at least through the first 3 months of pregnancy, to help reduce the incidence of open neural tube defects (NTDs) (CDC, 2005). (See Chapters 7 and 10 for further discussion.)

In the mid-1970s, nutritionist Agnes Higgins developed "The Higgins Method of Nutritional Rehabilitation During Pregnancy." This program focused on the individual woman's nutritional needs based on age, prepregnant weight, activity level, pregnancy weight gain, and risk factors. The Higgins Method, still relevant today, is grounded in the philosophy that each woman has specific dietary needs, and by meeting those needs, one can promote optimal growth and development of the fetus (Higgins, 1976). (See Chapter 10 for further information about dietary needs in pregnancy.)

 Optimizing Outcomes— **Vitamin C and premature rupture of the membranes**

Low levels of vitamin C may predispose women to premature rupture of membranes. As the cellular availability of vitamin C decreases, the rate of degradation of cervical collagen increases (Vadillo et al., 1995; Woods et al., 2001, cited in Modena, Kaihura, & Fieni, 2004). With decreased collagen, the cervix ripens more easily, prompting effacement and dilatation.

Recording Vital Signs

The vital signs are taken and documented. Blood pressure is a particularly important measurement and should be recorded under standardized conditions (making note of the arm used and the patient's position) and with the appropriate size blood pressure cuff. Since the initial prenatal visit may be the patient's first adult interaction with a health care professional, physiological indicators of anxiety (e.g., tachycardia, elevated blood pressure) may be present. In these situations, the nurse should record the first set of vital signs and then repeat the recordings later when the patient has had time to become familiar with her surroundings and is more relaxed.

 Ethnocultural Considerations— **Hypertension and pregnancy**

Nurses should be aware that hypertension is more prevalent in African American and Mexican American cultures, probably due to hereditary factors (Nabel, 2003). It is the most common medical condition affecting pregnancy and may worsen as the pregnancy progresses.

Obtaining the Urine Specimen

Before the physical examination, the nurse should ensure that the patient has had an opportunity to void and, if needed, a mid-stream urine sample is obtained (Procedure 9-1). A clean sample of urine should be cultured for asymptomatic bacteriuria during this first prenatal visit. As the name suggests, this type of urinary tract infection (UTI) does not cause symptoms but is present in more than 10% of pregnant women. Left untreated, a UTI may lead to a number of complications including preterm labor and pyelonephritis.

PERFORMING THE GENERAL PHYSICAL EXAMINATION

The general physical examination is then conducted with sensitivity to lifestyle choices, behaviors, and cultural beliefs. Together with physical data, the nurse should also gather

Figure 9-4 The weight is recorded and tracked throughout the pregnancy.

Procedure 9-1 Obtaining A Mid-Stream Urine Sample

Preparation

1. Complete the information requested on the container label. Include the patient's full name, and the date and time of collection of the specimen. If a requisition is needed, note the date and time on the requisition.

2. Explain the procedure to the woman to ensure she understands why a urine sample is requested, the purpose of any tests to be performed, and directions on how to obtain a mid-stream urine sample.

Equipment

- Approved empty sterile container for collection
- Towelette for cleaning in between the labia
- Tissue

Procedural Steps

Instruct the patient to do the following:

1. Wash and dry your hands thoroughly or use an alcohol-based hand-rub

   RATIONALE: To reduce the risk of specimen contamination. Alcohol-based hand-rubs are fast acting, reduce the number of microorganisms on the skin and may cause less skin irritation or dryness.

2. Remove the container cap and set it on a clean, even surface with the inner surface pointing up. Do not touch the inner surface of the lid or the container.

   RATIONALE: To reduce the risk of specimen contamination.

3. Sit on the toilet seat and separate the labia (vaginal lips) using your nondominant hand. Clean the urogenital area from the front to back with the towelette provided. Wipe for only one stroke and then discard the towelette.

   RATIONALE: To reduce the risk of specimen contamination and to reduce the number of microorganisms on the skin. Cleansing from front to back prevents bringing rectal contamination forward.

Patient cleansing labia.

4. Holding the labia apart, begin to pass urine. Allow the beginning urine to go directly into the toilet.

   RATIONALE: The initial stream of urine washes urethral microorganisms and other debris away from the urethral meatus. The midstream collection ensures that a sterile specimen is obtained.

5. Continue to urinate and hold the container under the urine stream Avoid touching the inside of the container. Remove the container when it is approximately half full.

Patient urinating into specimen cup.

6. Carefully replace the cap and secure tightly.

   RATIONALE: Placing the cap on the container prevents inadvertent spilling and possible contamination of the urine specimen.

7. Wash your hands again after the specimen collection.

Clinical Alert Pregnant women are at an increased risk for developing urinary tract infections, especially if they are diabetic or have gestational diabetes. Urinary tract infections may also predispose to the onset of preterm labor.

Teach Patient

Teach the patient to recognize common signs of a urinary tract infection:
Dysuria—pain (burning sensation) on urination
Urinary frequency associated with small amounts of urine
Hematuria—blood or red blood cells in the urine

Documentation

1/10/10 1100 Patient educated re midstream urine collection. Patient verbalized understanding. Sample obtained, labeled with name, date, time and type of specimen. Sent to lab at 1120 per Dr. Garner's order.

—M. D'Arcy-Evans, RN, CNM

information relating to the patient's usual state of health, her use of health promotion and maintenance strategies, and details of any present concerns or symptoms. The physical examination is a basic review of systems that includes ears, nose, mouth, and throat; cardio-respiratory; musculoskeletal; and neurological function with an in-depth evaluation of the maternal physical adaptation to the pregnancy.

 Now Can You— **Discuss aspects of the initial prenatal health assessment?**

1. Identify five screening tests routinely performed on the patient's serum during the initial prenatal examination?
2. Briefly discuss why screening for human immunodeficiency virus and *Chlamydia trachomatis* is recommended during pregnancy?
3. Identify four major components of the prenatal physical assessment?

THE FOCUSED OBSTETRIC EXAMINATION

Head, Neck, and Lungs

With the patient in a sitting position, the physical examination proceeds in a head to toe fashion beginning with a general evaluation of the skin and hair. Many women notice that their hair is healthier and more luxurious during pregnancy. Hair loss, common during the postpartum period, can be indicative of a vitamin or mineral deficiency. Increased levels of estrogen are responsible for a number of objective and subjective changes such as hypertrophy of the gingival tissue, nasal stuffiness, and an increased tendency for nosebleeds.

The thyroid gland is palpated while the patient remains in a sitting position. Enlargement is common during pregnancy due to increased vascularity and hyperplasia of the glandular tissue. The size and position of the thyroid are documented along with the presence of nodules or swelling (Koscica & Berstein, 2003). Anterior and posterior lung sounds are auscultated and the cardiac rhythm and rate are evaluated for adventitious sounds. During pregnancy, approximately 90% of women exhibit systolic heart murmurs due to an increase in blood volume. The systolic murmur may be clearer when the woman holds her breath. Heart sounds should be evaluated with the woman in both a sitting and lying position. Beginning late in the second trimester, the gravid uterus causes an upward and lateral displacement of the heart and the point of maximal impulse. Also, as pregnancy advances, the patient's breathing becomes thoracic in nature (rather than abdominal) due to the enlarged uterus.

The Skin

Assessment the skin may reveal pregnancy-associated changes such as chloasma (the mask of pregnancy) and hyperpigmentation of the areolae, vulva, abdomen, and linea (linea nigra). The skin is evaluated for color consistent with the woman's ethnic background, and for the presence of lesions or indicators of drug abuse (i.e., skin scratches, bruising or track marks, nasal discharge or irritated mucosa, constricted or dilated pupils).

The Breasts

The patient is assisted to a recumbent position for the breast examination. Depending on the gestational age, it may be advisable to place a wedge under one of her hips to prevent compression of the vena cava from the gravid uterus (supine hypotension syndrome). Inspection of the breasts usually reveals pregnancy-related changes including nodularity, striae, and enlargement and hyperpigmentation of the nipples and Montgomery tubercles. Areas of indentation or skin puckering are not normal findings. Colostrum, a precursor to breast milk, may be expressed from the nipples as early as the first trimester of pregnancy. The lymph nodes should not be palpable.

 Optimizing Outcomes— **Promoting breast comfort during pregnancy**

As a component of health teaching during pregnancy, the nurse should encourage patients to wear a firm, supporting bra. For some, professional fitting/measuring may be beneficial to promote both support and comfort. As the breasts increase in weight, bras with wider straps may be more comfortable. Some women choose to wear a "sleeping" bra during the night for added comfort.

The Abdomen

The obstetric abdominal examination focuses on recognizing signs and changes associated with pregnancy. It is not intended to replace a comprehensive abdominal examination. The patient should be appropriately draped to maintain her privacy, comfort, and body temperature. The abdominal shape is assessed and inspected for the presence of scars (previous surgery should be documented), linea nigra, striae gravidum, or signs of injury (e.g., bruising). As the pregnancy advances, visual inspection of the abdominal shape may reveal the fetal position, especially if transverse. Also, it may be possible to observe and palpate fetal movements. Patients generally become aware of fetal movements around the 16th to 20th week of pregnancy. A primigravida is usually able to identify fetal movements around 18 to 20 weeks; a multigravida may notice fetal movements as early as 16 weeks. This difference in awareness of fetal activity is most likely due to past experience in recognizing the movements along with a decrease in maternal abdominal muscle tone.

Uterine Size and Fetal Position

Abdominal palpation is used to evaluate the uterine size, to determine fetal position, and later in pregnancy, to determine whether the presenting part has engaged in the maternal pelvis. (See Chapter 12 for further discussion.) **Fundal height** is an indication of uterine size; periodic measurements of the fundal height should correlate strongly with fetal growth (Fig. 9-5). The relationship of the fundus (top part) of the uterus to specific maternal abdominal landmarks is used throughout pregnancy as a gauge to assess fetal growth. The fundal height measurement correlates to the weeks of gestation from approximately 22 to 34 weeks of gestation (Table 9-2). At 12 weeks of gestation, the fundus should be at the level of the

Table 9-2 Approximate Fundal Height in Relation to Weeks of Pregnancy	
Weeks of Gestation	**Approximate Expected Fundal Height**
12	Level of the symphysis pubis
16	Halfway between the symphysis pubis and the umbilicus
20	One to two finger-breadths below the umbilicus
24	One to two finger-breadths above the umbilicus
28–30	One-third of the way between the umbilicus and the xyphoid processs
32	Two-thirds of the way between the umbilicus and the xyphoid processs
36	At the xyphoid process
38	One to two finger-breadths below the xyphoid process
40	Three to four finger-breadths below the xyphoid process

Figure 9-5 Obtaining the fundal height measurement.

32 weeks · 24 weeks
36 weeks
28 weeks
20 weeks
16 weeks
40 weeks
12–13 weeks

Figure 9-6 Fundal measurement should approximately equal the number of weeks of gestation.

symphysis pubis; at 20 weeks, the fundus should be at the umbilicus. The fundal height can be measured by using a tape measure or finger-breadths in combination with known maternal landmarks. For example, two finger-breadths above the umbilicus would be equivalent to approximately 24 weeks of gestation. Although convenient, using finger-breadths as a measuring tool is subject to variations in finger size among different examiners. This method of fundal height measurement is appropriate only if the same examiner consistently assesses uterine size.

Most often, the fundal height is measured with a tape measure. This method is usually initiated at around 22 weeks of gestation. The end of the measuring tape with the zero mark is held on the superior border of the symphysis pubis. Using the abdominal midline as guide, the tape is stretched over the contour of the abdomen to the top of the fundus (McDonald's method; see Fig. 9-5). The measurement (in centimeters) is recorded and equals the weeks of gestation. For example, at 28 weeks of gestation, the fundal height should be approximately 11 inches (28 cm; Fig. 9-6).

LEOPOLD'S MANEUVERS The next step in abdominal palpation involves the use of **Leopold's maneuvers**, a four-part clinical assessment method. to determine the lie, presentation, and position of the fetus. The first maneuver determines which fetal body part (e.g., head or buttocks) occupies the uterine fundus. The examiner faces the patient's head and places the hands on the abdomen, using the palmar surface (not the fingertips) of the hands to gently palpate the fundal region of the uterus. The buttocks feel soft, broad, and poorly defined. It moves with the trunk. The head feels firm and round and moves independently of the trunk (Fig. 9-7).

The second maneuver determines the location of the fetal back or spine. Facing the maternal abdomen, the palmar surface of one hand is placed on one side of the patient's abdomen to provide support. The palmar surface of the opposite hand is used to palpate the fetal spine, which feels like a firm, continuous, smooth, convex structure. An irregular shape or fetal kicks indicate that the back is on the opposite side (Fig. 9-8).

The third maneuver ("Pawlik maneuver") compares the fetal part in the fundal region with the part in the lower uterine segment, primarily to confirm that the fetus is in a cephalic (head) presentation. The hands are placed just above the symphysis and the examiner notes whether the palpated part feels like the fetal head or the buttocks (breech; Fig. 9-9).

For the fourth maneuver, the examiner uses the fingertips of both hands. One hand is placed on each side of the women's lower abdomen with the palmar surfaces down. The hands are moved gently down the sides of the uterus toward the symphysis pubis as the fingertips palpate the presenting part to determine whether it is moveable (ballotable). If the presenting part is moveable, **engagement** (when the largest diameter of the presenting part reaches or passes through the maternal pelvic inlet) has *not* occurred. If the presenting part is fixed, engagement has occurred. With the first pregnancy, engagement occurs around 37 weeks gestation; with subsequent pregnancies, engagement may not occur until labor has begun (Figs. 9-10 and 9-11).

Figure 9-7 First Leopold's maneuver.

Figure 9-8 Second Leopold's maneuver.

Figure 9-9 Third Leopold's maneuver.

Figure 9-10 Fourth Leopold's maneuver.

Figure 9-11 Assessing fetal presentation/position.

Fetal Heart Auscultation

The information obtained during fetal palpation includes fetal presentation, lie, position, and engagement status (Table 9-3). (See Chapter 12 for further discussion.) Determining the fetal presentation facilitates fetal heart auscultation. The fetal heart rate (FHR) is heard most clearly directly over the fetal upper back (the maternal right or left lower abdominal quadrants) in a vertex presentation. The intensity of the fetal heart tones (FHT) varies according to the fetal position (Fig. 9-12). With a breech presentation, the fetal heart tones may be best heard in the patient's right or left upper abdominal quadrants. If fetal heart tones are auscultated most clearly in that location, the patient's care provider should be advised, as further assessment may be indicated to confirm the fetal presentation. This is especially important when the patient is in labor. However, before approximately 32 weeks of pregnancy, it is not uncommon for the fetus to be in a breech presentation. In most instances, by 36 to 37 weeks of gestation, the majority of fetuses will have spontaneously converted to a vertex (head down) presentation.

The normal heart rate for a fetus is approximately 120 to 160 beats per minute (bpm). If a slower heart rate is detected, the maternal pulse should first be evaluated to determine if the two heart rates are synchronous. If they are synchronous, the maternal pulse has inadvertently been auscultated through the abdomen and an attempt should be made to locate the fetal pulse. If the two pulses differ, the nurse should position the patient on her left side and seek assistance. Oxygen may be administered by mask and the patient should be instructed to take slow deep breaths. The nurse should continue to monitor the fetal heart rate and provide explanations and reassurance to the patient.

The fetal heart can be auscultated using a number of different devices. The least intrusive method involves the use of a Pinard stethoscope or a fetoscope (Fig. 9-13). Both of these devices are used without any additional equipment. However, they do require the examiner's ability to be able to palpate the woman's abdomen accurately to determine the fetal position and locate the fetal shoulder to ascertain the correct location for placement of the stethoscope. This method of fetal heart auscultation is ideal if the patient has expressed a desire to avoid an ultrasound (Doppler) stethoscope. Following the invention of the Doppler ultrasound stethoscope, use of the fetoscope and Pinard stethoscopes in clinical practice has decreased. The Doppler ultrasound stethoscope is a handheld device that uses ultrasound to

Table 9-3	Defining Terms in Relation to Maternal Abdominal Palpations
Lie of the Fetus	Where is the fetal spine in relation to the maternal spine? The maternal spine is always longitudinal. If the fetal spine is parallel to the maternal spine, the fetus is in a "longitudinal lie."
	If the fetal spine lies horizontally across the maternal spine, the fetus is in a "transverse lie."
	If the fetal spine lies obliquely across the maternal spine, the fetus is in an "oblique lie."
	"Lie" describes the relationship of the fetus to the long axis of the mother. Normal lie is longitudinal (the fetal long axis, or spine, is in line with the maternal long axis).
Presentation	Refers to the fetal part that would be delivered first in a vaginal birth.
	Normally, the fetal head is the part of the fetus that is presenting.
Position	The head is the most common presentation.
	When the fetus is in a well-flexed position (the fetal knees and chin against its body), the occiput area is determined to be the presenting part since this is the lowest part of the fetal head.
	To determine position, it is necessary to assess where the fetal occiput is, in relation to the maternal pelvis.
	If the fetal occiput faces toward the front near the symphysis pubis, the fetus is in an anterior position. If the occiput is on the maternal right side, the fetus is in a right occipito-anterior position (ROA). If on the maternal left side, the fetus is in a left occipito-anterior position (LOA).
	If the fetal occiput is toward the side of the maternal pelvis, the fetus is in a lateral (or transverse) position. If the occiput is on the maternal right, the fetus is in a right occipito-lateral position (ROL). If on the maternal left, it is a left occipito-lateral (LOL) position.
	If the fetal occiput is toward the maternal spine, the fetus is in a posterior position. If the occiput is on the maternal right, the fetus is in a right occipito-posterior position (ROP). If on the maternal left, it is a left occipito-posteror (LOP) position.
Engagement	When palpating the presenting part, is it moveable?
	If the presenting part is fixed (i.e., you are unable to move it) when palpating the maternal abdomen, the presenting part is said to be engaged.

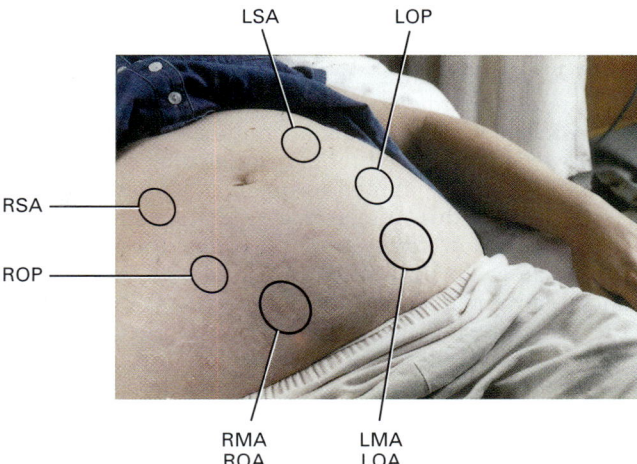

Figure 9-12 Fetal heart tone intensity varies according to the fetal position. RSA = right sacrum anterior; LSA = left sacrum anterior; ROP = right occipito-posterior; LOP = left occipito-posterior; RMA = right mentum anterior; LMA = left mentum anterior; ROA = right occipito-anterior; LOA = left occipito-anterior.

Figure 9-13 Auscultating the fetal heart tones with a fetoscope.

locate fetal heart sounds (Fig. 9-14). Use of the Doppler stethoscope to auscultate fetal heart tones is simple and requires no special skills since placement of the instrument in the general vicinity of the fetal heart will most likely produce audible heart tones. Although this approach may provide an easy, quick assessment, the nurse who uses this method may not be performing a detailed patient examination and may miss vital information. With the Doppler stethoscope, FHTs may be auscultated by 10 to 12 weeks or by 17 to 19 weeks with the fetal stethoscope.

Figure 9-14 Auscultating the fetal heart tones with a Doppler ultrasound stethoscope.

Some sophisticated Doppler models provide a printout similar to those of the more conventional fetal heart rate monitors. Beginning in the later weeks of the second trimester, standard electronic fetal monitors may be used to record the fetal heart rate in conjunction with uterine activity. Electronic fetal monitoring during the prenatal period is generally limited to pregnancies designated as being high risk due to maternal or fetal factors. In these situations, a **non-stress test** (NST) may be ordered to provide an evaluation of the fetal heart rate in response to fetal movement and/or uterine activity. A reactive test (the desirable result), is one in which the heart rate accelerates by at least 15 beats per minute for at least 15 seconds, with at least two "acceleration episodes" in a 20-minute period of monitoring. It is important to remember that a reactive non-stress test is only an indicator of the fetus's present condition rather than a test that can be used to predict future fetal well-being. (See Chapter 11 for further discussion.)

Nurses must be cautious not to place too much reliance on technology. Instead, nurses should use clinical skills coupled with evidence-based theory to transition from novice to expert practitioner. To attain this level of expertise, it is essential to maintain hands-on patient care. Experienced clinical nurses attain a sixth sense, or "specialty intuition," that enables them to quickly recognize deviations from normal and provide expert care in a timely manner. With regard to electronic fetal monitoring and other high-tech modalities, the nurse must be careful not to rely on imperfect tools and instead use sound clinical judgment and decision making.

 Now Can You— Discuss various methods of clinical fetal assessment?

1. Describe how to perform a fundal height measurement?
2. Identify how to perform each component of Leopold's maneuvers and explain what the findings indicate?
3. Compare and contrast the technique of fetal heart auscultation using a fetoscope and a Doppler ultrasound stethoscope?

The Vagina and Pelvis

A vaginal examination is usually performed at the initial prenatal visit following assessment of the maternal abdomen. Most women find this part of the examination to be intrusive and may fear being exposed, hurt, or embarrassed. An essential component of the nurse's role is to explain to the patient what to expect and to help her to verbalize any fears. The patient's permission to conduct a vaginal assessment must always be obtained before proceeding. Demonstrating awareness of the patient's feelings can be conveyed by simple strategies: remaining gentle and respectful; showing equipment that will be used with a demonstration of how it works; and ensuring privacy with appropriate drapes. Eye-to-eye contact maintains a connection between the nurse and the patient and allows the nurse to be aware of nonverbal communication. Some women feel less anxious if they are actively involved in the examination. For example, if desired, a mirror can be placed so that

the patient can view her cervix or be shown changes such as Chadwick's sign.

There are essentially four components to the examination, which begins with an assessment of the external genitalia (Fig. 9-15). Information can be obtained regarding secondary sexual characteristics by observing the pattern of hair growth. This is also an ideal time to check for the presence of **pediculosis**, or pubic lice. Signs of vaginal infection may be indicated by redness, edema, or an offensive vaginal discharge. The presence of lesions, condylomata (human papillomavirus), vesicles (herpes), ulceration (syphilitic chancre), or inflammation need to recognized and investigated. Bruising or tenderness may be present as a result of trauma or abuse. Observation of the perineal body may show evidence of a previous episiotomy or perineal tear. Women who have been subjected to female circumcision show varying degrees of genital mutilation. Women from cultures that support this practice may prefer to have a female care provider.

The second part of the examination includes visual inspection of the vaginal mucosa and cervix along with the collection of specimens such as the Papanicolaou test (Pap smear), cultures for gonorrhea or *Chlamydia* and, if indicated, wet smear slides to determine the cause of vaginal discharge. The examiner selects an appropriate size speculum. Specula may be constructed of metal or plastic and are generally available in two types: the Graves' speculum, useful for examining multiparous women, and the more narrow, flat Pedersen speculum, commonly used for children, women who have never been sexually active, nulliparous women and some postmenopausal women. The speculum is inserted into the vagina at an oblique angle, then rotated to a horizontal angle and gently advanced downward against the posterior vaginal wall. Once in position, the speculum blades are opened to allow visualization of the cervix (Fig. 9-16).

Figure 9-15 *A,* The vaginal examination begins with a visual inspection of the external genitalia. *B,* The thumb and index finger are used to separate the labia minora.

The cervix and vaginal mucosa are inspected for color and for the presence of inflammation, lesions, ulcerations, or erosion. The cervix is usually about 1 inch (2.5 cm) in length and the external cervical os is round in women who have never given birth (nulliparous) and appears "slit" shaped in the multigravida (Fig. 9-17).

The remaining part of the assessment includes clinical pelvimetry and the bimanual examination. Bimanual examination is an evaluation of uterine shape, position, and size (Fig. 9-18). The uterus is normally anteverted (tipped forward). As it enlarges during pregnancy, the uterus becomes more midline and globular in shape. The size of the pregnant uterus should be equal to the estimated weeks of gestation. If the uterus is larger than anticipated, this finding may be associated with a number of factors including miscalculation of the date of conception, multiple pregnancy, hydatidiform mole, uterine fibroid tumors or, later in pregnancy, a condition known as **hydramnios** (an increase in the volume of amniotic fluid). A uterus smaller than expected may indicate miscalculation of dates or a missed abortion. (See Chapter 11 for further discussion.) The manual examination provides an ideal time to evaluate vaginal and perineal muscle tone and to determine the presence of a cystocele (bladder prolapse), urethrocele (urethral prolapse), or rectocele (rectal prolapse). Women should be reminded to practice Kegel exercises to help maintain perineal muscle tone.

The rectovaginal examination is performed after completion of the bimanual examination. The examiner removes his or her hand from the vagina and dons a clean pair of gloves. A water-based lubricant is applied to the fingertips of the dominant hand. The index finger is reinserted into the vagina; the middle finger is inserted into the rectum. The rectal finger is advanced forward as the abdomen is depressed with the nondominant hand. Palpation of the tissue between the examining fingers allows for assessment of the strength and irregularity of the posterior vaginal wall. The fingers are withdrawn and any stool present on the glove may be tested for occult blood.

The final component of the physical examination involves the clinical evaluation of the pelvis, also known as clinical pelvimetry. The goal of this assessment is to recognize any abnormality in shape or size that may be associated with a difficult or traumatic vaginal birth. The four basic pelvic types include the gynecoid, found in more than 40% of women, the android (male), the anthropoid (most common in non-Caucasian races), and the platypelloid, which is the most rare type and is found in fewer than 3% of women. The internal pelvic measurements provide the diameters of the inlet and outlet through which the fetus must pass during birth. The measurements most commonly made include the diagonal conjugate, the true conjugate (conjugate vera), and the ischial tuberosity diameter. Clinical pelvimetry is performed by the physician, nurse midwife, or advanced practice nurse; it is generally not repeated in women who have previously given birth to an infant weighing 7 pounds or more (3.18 kg) unless there is a history of pelvic trauma in the intervening period between pregnancies.

The **diagonal conjugate** is the distance between the anterior surface of the sacral prominence and the anterior surface of the inferior margin of the symphysis pubis. This measurement, performed with the patient in a

Figure 9-16 *A,* Inserting the speculum. *B,* Opening the speculum. *C,* Proper position of speculum in the vagina. *D,* View through the speculum.

Figure 9-17 *A,* Circular cervical opening: nulliparous. *B,* Slit-shaped cervical opening: multiparous.

Figure 9-18 *A,* Palpating the uterus. *B,* Palpating the ovaries.

lithotomy position, indicates the anteroposterior diameter of the pelvic inlet—the most narrow diameter and the one most likely to create a problem with misfit of the fetal head. If the diagonal conjugate is greater than 12.5 cm, the pelvic inlet is considered to be adequate for childbirth (Fig. 9-19).

The **true conjugate** (conjugate vera) is the measurement between the anterior surface of the sacral prominence and the posterior surface of the inferior margin of the symphysis pubis. This measurement is estimated from the dimension made of the diagonal conjugate. It cannot be measured directly. The true conjugate is the actual diameter of the pelvic inlet through which the fetal head will pass. On average, the diameter of the true conjugate ranges from 4.1 to 4.3 inches (10.5 to 11 cm).

The **ischial tuberosity** diameter (also known as the intertuberous or biischial diameter) is a measurement of the distance between the ischial tuberosities (i.e., the transverse diameter of the outlet). Often assessed with a pelvimeter (a special device for measuring the pelvis), the diameter can also be measured with a ruler or with the examiner's clenched fist or handspan (the exact measurements of the fist and hand must be known). A diameter of 11 cm is considered adequate for passage of the widest diameter of the fetal head through the pelvic outlet. Using palpation, the examiner assesses the coccyx for mobility. A mobile nonprominent coccyx allows for some flexibility of the pelvic outlet during birth.

Subsequent Prenatal Examinations

The plan of care for the first prenatal visit should be amended to meet each individual woman's needs, based on medical, social, cultural, and individual factors. Subsequent prenatal visits are usually not as in depth, but should be designed to recognize any deviations from normal so that appropriate investigations can be ordered and care managed accordingly. Normally, patients are seen at a frequency of every 4 weeks until 28 to 32 weeks of pregnancy, then every 2 weeks until 36 weeks, and then weekly until childbirth. At each visit, standard of care includes an evaluation of the maternal weight gain, blood pressure, urine (for glucose and protein), uterine growth, fetal heart tones, fetal movements, and presentation (Box 9-9). The patient is also assessed for the presence of edema. Each prenatal appointment provides an ideal opportunity for education related to the patient's particular stage of pregnancy and what to expect before the next visit. A review of the warning signs of pregnancy is also essential and the nurse should confirm that the woman is able to verbalize when and how to seek professional assistance.

Evaluation of fetal well-being includes documentation of the patient's perception of fetal movements. Depending on the circumstances, fetal evaluation may also include electronic heart rate monitoring, ultrasonography to monitor growth patterns and/or placental aging and a biophysical profile. In addition, the patient may be offered various

A

B

Figure 9-19 *A,* The diagonal conjugate and the true conjugate (conjugate vera). *B,* Use of a pelvimeter to measure the ischial tuberosity diameter.

screening tests during pregnancy to detect fetal genetic or structural abnormalities. (See Chapters 10 and 11 for further discussion.)

 Now Can You— Discuss the vaginal examination, clinical pelvimetry, and assessments routinely made during each prenatal visit?

1. Compare and contrast the purpose of the vaginal speculum examination and the bimanual examination?
2. Explain the purpose of clinical pelvimetry and identify three measurements that are commonly included in this assessment?
3. Name seven maternal–fetal assessments routinely performed during each prenatal visit?

Assessing Special Populations

THE ADOLESCENT

Sexual Behavior and Pregnancy

Teenage pregnancy is not a new phenomenon. The transitional period of adolescence, which spans the years from 11 to 19, marks the biological and psychological passage from childhood into adulthood. Pregnancy during adolescence has far-reaching implications for society as well as for the young woman and her family.

In the American culture, the expectation is that women marry, ideally after having completed an acceptable level of education, before the couple plans the birth of their first child. Teenage pregnancy meets none of these expectations and as such is not condoned by American society in general. Despite this stigma, adolescent pregnancies continue to occur, are often fathered by teenage males or, in some cases, by men significantly older (Bunting & McAuley, 2004).

Not all teen pregnancies are accidents. For some adolescents, pregnancy provides a means of escape from an unpleasant situation, a method for achieving a goal, or someone to love. Relationships with the unequal power dynamics often present between an older male and a teenage female can predispose to coercion in sexual activity. Pregnancy may also result from sexual assault, incest, and dating violence that involves sexual intercourse (Silverman, Raj, & Clements, 2004).

Problems that develop in the wake of teen pregnancy are not limited to the duration of the pregnancy. Instead, they appear to be much longer lasting. For example, although many teenagers who become pregnant manage to complete high school, only a small percentage continue their education to earn a college degree. Without advanced education, their earning capacity and career opportunities are somewhat limited and this factor may become a life-long limitation.

In addition to the many developmental, social, educational, and life-long consequences for both the young mother and her child, the teenage patient is also at additional risk for a host of obstetric complications including anemia, preeclampsia, and preterm birth. Preterm birth and low-birth-weight infants are major causes of neonatal morbidity and mortality. Survival of a compromised infant may necessitate a lifetime of care and considerable economic resources.

The rate of adolescent pregnancy in the United States is almost double that of other developed countries. Clearly, teen pregnancy is a complex, multifaceted issue that must be addressed at the local, state, and national levels. One goal of the *Healthy People 2010* national health initiative directly addresses the number of pregnancies that occur in the adolescent population. It calls for a reduction in pregnancy rates among adolescent females to no more than 43/1000 adolescents from a baseline of 68/1000.

The Nurse's Role

Nurses can help the nation to achieve this goal by heightening public awareness of the complex personal and societal repercussions of adolescent pregnancy. Nurses can also empower women and their families with factual information and strategies to reduce unwanted pregnancies among this young population. In the community setting, nurses can advocate for responsible sexual behavior by providing educational programs for youth in schools, churches, clubs, and after school activities. In the clinical setting, nurses can listen to, counsel, and educate young patients to help prepare them for responsible sexual decision making. Nurses can also empower mothers and fathers of young adults with methods for facilitating open, honest family discussions about sexuality and sexual behavior.

Box 9-9 Essential Components of Subsequent Prenatal Visits

Review the Woman's Overall Health Status.
- Signs/symptoms of pregnancy
- Discomforts of pregnancy
- Changes in medications/over-the-counter/herbal/homeopathic
- Psychological assessment (emotional or psychological distress) including factors such as affect, sleep patterns, and diet

MATERNAL WELL-BEING
- Record vital signs.
  - Ensure blood pressure is recorded using an appropriately sized cuff and under the same conditions each visit (i.e., maternal position).
- Record maternal weight.
  - Weight gain is usually 1 pound per week during the second and third trimesters.
    - Excessive weight gain may be indicative of fluid retention and requires investigation.
    - Weight loss may be due to maternal disease or inadequate dietary intake: nursing assessment needed.
- Evaluate for edema: dependent edema especially in hot weather and at the end of the day is a normal finding.
- Where indicated, assess reflexes and check for clonus.
  - Assess for any signs of preterm labor such as uterine contractions or backache.
  - Ensure patient knows indicators of preterm labor and know how to seek medical advice.
- Assess for any signs of domestic/intimate partner abuse.

EVALUATE FETAL WELL-BEING
Listen to fetal heart tones, usually can be heard from approximately 12 to 14 weeks' gestation with a Doppler stethoscope: normal rate is 120 to 160 bpm
- Discuss pattern and frequency of fetal movements.
  - Encourage patient to monitor and record fetal movements daily.
  - Educate patient on the importance of fetal movements as an indicator of general fetal well-being.
  - Ensure the patient knows to immediately report a decrease in fetal movements.
- Evaluate uterine growth.
  - Measure fundal height.
  - Document findings and evaluate pattern of growth.
    - Weeks of gestation are equivalent to measurement in centimeters: McDonald Method (measure from the top of the symphysis pubis to fundus, from approximately 24 to 34 weeks' gestation)—for example, at 30 weeks' gestation the fundal height should be 11.8 inches (30 cm).
    - Measurement less than expected could indicate intrauterine growth restriction, oligohydramnios, or incorrect dates.
    - Measurement greater than expected could indicate multiple pregnancy, macrosomic infant, hydramnios, or incorrect dates.

PATIENT TEACHING
- Provide education related to stage of pregnancy (i.e., what physical changes to expect or danger signs that need to be reported, such as vaginal bleeding or fluid loss, abdominal pain, or visual disturbances).
- Encourage attendance in prenatal education classes.
- Encourage tour of facility where patient intends to give birth.
- Later in pregnancy, focus of education needs to include preparation for care of the newborn (e.g., car seats, male circumcision, immunizations) so that parents can make informed decisions.

Screening and laboratory testing may include:

Ultrasound	Some health care providers offer routine ultrasound examinations in the first trimester of pregnancy to confirm dates and ensure single pregnancy; may be repeated later in pregnancy.
Prenatal screening	MSAFP—screening for open neural tube defects and Down syndrome is done around 16 weeks—if indicated, follow-up may include amniocentesis.
Screening for gestational diabetes	Offered around 24–28 weeks' gestation.
	Patient drinks solution containing 50 g of glucose and then has blood drawn 1 hour later—results should be below 140 mg/dL.
Rh screening	Rh-negative woman: Check for Rh antibodies and if negative, 300 mcg of Rh_0 immune globulin (RhoGAM) is prescribed at 28 to 32 weeks' gestation.
Hemoglobin/hematocrit	Usually repeated mid-pregnancy and then as indicated.
Group B *Streptococcus* screening	Normally offered at 37 weeks' gestation to determine whether antibiotic coverage is needed during labor.

Confirm the patient's contact information (address/telephone numbers) and ensure she has a scheduled return appointment. Always provide time for the patient to ask questions, confirm her understanding and that she has no other concerns that need to be addressed.

Strategies that use a holistic family approach such as promoting open communication between parents/guardians and teenagers, together with teaching self-respect, setting boundaries, and providing appropriate supervision are essential components of any successful approach to reduce teenage pregnancy (Table 9-4).

"What to say" — *Dialoging with teens about sex*

When talking with teens about sex, it is important to use language with which they can relate. For example, the nurse may say:

"You would not give your $100 mobile phone to just anyone, so do not give your body to just anyone" (Harris, 2005, p. 15).

Some groups advocate mandatory sex education for all adolescents; others support programs that only teach sexual abstinence. There is little scientific evidence to determine which approach is most effective. Because individuals' responses and actions are shaped by personality, cultural norms, and observed social patterns and behaviors, any one doctrine is rarely applicable to every group.

Impact on Society

APPROACHES TO ADDRESSING THE PROBLEM OF ADOLESCENT PREGNANCY. Over the years, a variety of local and national efforts have attempted to dissuade adolescents from engaging in early sexual activity. Strategies have ranged from public awareness campaigns to public chastisement, conviction as a sex offender, and institutionalization for unacceptable moral behavior. The various approaches have met with some success, but usually on a short-term basis.

Table 9-4 A Holistic Family Approach to Preventing Teenage Pregnancies

Parental Influences	Strategies
• Parents have the strongest influence on teenage behavior.	• Promote open communication.
	• Foster safe and nonjudgmental environment to facilitate discussion of issues relating to vaginal and oral sex, relationships, self-esteem, self-worth and how to say "no" to unwanted sexual contact.
• Parents/adults need to model behaviors that are respectful, honest, nonaggressive, and healthy.	• Ways to interact and communicate are learned through observation. Observing a relationship between adults where each is given equal power and respect can help to initiate a sense of self-worth irrespective of gender.
• Promoting family values, caring behaviors and closeness.	• Shared family activities, eating meals together, taking time to be with one another to enjoy a shared interest.
• Build a trusting, loving relationship	• Take time to know teenagers' friends and their families.
	• Become involved, provide adequate supervision of activities.
	• Promote group activities rather than early dating.
• Providing accurate information to include both abstinence and contraception	• Parents may need help to increase their own comfort level and knowledge before being able to confidently help their child.
	• Need to develop active listening skills, and ensure it is a two-way conversation, not a mini lecture.
	• Dispel myths.
	• Don't promote double standards. Teenage sex is not to be encouraged irrespective of gender. Make expectations clearly known.
	• Use situations as they arise. For example, watching television together may provide an opportunity to discuss some relationship or sexual issue based on a program being viewed.
• Understanding developmental stages related to teenagers, such as egocentric thinking and their sense of invincibility	• Use scenarios within the family setting to demonstrate formal reasoning—the ability to recognize alternatives and the consequences of their choices, both short and long term.
	• Help the adolescent to see the "whole" picture and not just focus on their immediate needs (egocentric thinking).
	• Teenagers are generally unable to recognize and appreciate behavioral risk; they are more likely to ignore or fail to understand the logical laws of probability. "It won't happen to me" is the opinion much more likely to be believed.
• Future plans	• Discuss plans for the future—set goals.
	• Let it be known that education is essential to a bright future.

Source: The National Campaign to Prevent Teen and Unplanned Pregnancy (2004). Parent power: What parents need to know and do to help prevent teen pregnancy.

Current discussions center on the issue of whether providing sex education to children promotes early sexual activity. Rosengard and colleagues (2005) reported that although a majority of sexually active teenage boys did not intend to cause a pregnancy, they acknowledged that it was a possibility. Providing teenagers with sex education is an approach that endeavors to take the "secrecy" out of sex and instead provide basic, accurate information. It is believed that this strategy will empower adolescents with the knowledge needed to make informed decisions or, in the least, with the confidence necessary to seek guidance. When teenagers perceive sex to be a taboo subject, they are left to rely on friends, acquaintances, or peers who may not have a sound knowledge base to share. This paradigm supports the argument that knowledge reduces the need for experimentation and discovery. Experimentation without facts can lead to accidental pregnancy and sexually transmitted infections.

Teaching sexual abstinence before marriage can be effective in some cultures or populations, especially if the approach focuses on both genders. Discrepancy may exist between what is acceptable behavior or action for a teenage female and a teenage male. Interpretation of the phrase "sexual abstinence" may vary from no sexual contact of any description to simply maintaining virginity. In 1996, the U.S. Congress provided financial support of $87.5 million per year to states that provided abstinence-only education, irrespective of the lack of substantive data demonstrating the effectiveness of this approach.

Along with a tendency to behave impulsively, adolescents lack the ability to make informed, complex decisions or to accurately compare alternatives. Neurobiological factors may be responsible for this deficit. The brain's prefrontal cortex is responsible for all "executive functions." Maturity of this area is not fully attained until an individual has reached age 20 or older. Nurses need to incorporate this information into the design of health education classes that will enable teenagers to understand better the process of making an informed decision. Ensuring that the adolescent has a realistic perception of related risks and the potential short-term and long-term outcomes is an essential component of any educational effort.

Cultural Influences on Adolescent Pregnancy

Adolescent pregnancy exists within every culture although the prevalence varies and it is not always viewed negatively. Within the sub-Saharan African region, girls often as young as 12 or 14 years of age are still sold to prospective husbands in exchange for a negotiated amount of money or in exchange for animals. In this culture, arranging a good marriage for a young teenage girl can often be a solution to family poverty.

In the United States, African American and Hispanic adolescents represent the groups most likely to engage in early sexual activity, and not surprisingly, these groups have the highest rates of teenage pregnancy, although the discrepancy among different cultures is decreasing. In 2000, the rate of pregnancy among African American teenagers 15 to 19 years of age was 15.3%, compared to the national average of 8.3% (Box 9-10). **Pregnancy rate** is defined as the total number of pregnancies, including those that end in sponta-

---

Box 9-10 **Sexual Activity and Pregnancy Rates Among African American Teenagers in the United States**

- Have the highest pregnancy rate when compared with all major racial and ethnic groups
- Before the age of 20, approximately 57% will have experienced at least one pregnancy
- Have more sexual partners and are more sexually experienced
- As a group, African American teens demonstrated one of the highest reductions (31.5%) in teen pregnancy during the decade 1990-2000. The overall teen pregnancy rate during this time fell by 28.5%. In comparison, Hispanic teenage pregnancies decreased by 15%. (The Alan Guttmacher Institute, 2004).
- In 2002 almost 96% of African American women between the ages of 15 and 19 who gave birth were unmarried (Martin et al., 2003; National Campaign to Prevent Teenage Pregnancy, 2004).

---

neous abortion, elective abortion, or birth. In 2002, there were 425,000 births to girls 15 to 19 years of age, and of this group, approximately 25% were African American (National Campaign to Prevent Teenage Pregnancy, 2004).

Along with cultural influences, many other factors, such as education, spiritual beliefs and group support, family structure, and income also impact the occurrence of adolescent pregnancy. As educational level increases, the age at which first intercourse occurs also increases while the risk of pregnancy decreases. Teenagers from middle-class, two-parent families are more likely to delay their first sexual experience. This tendency is also documented among adolescents who report an affiliation with a church, synagogue, or other religious institution. These individuals benefit from the group support associated with their church-related activities.

In 2005, two national organizations, the National Campaign to Prevent Teen Pregnancy and the National Coalition of Pastors' Spouses, produced a document intended to heighten public awareness of the issues concerning pregnancy among African American teenagers. The collaborative effort underscored the value of family and the faith community on adolescent sexual behavior. The premise of the report holds that a teenager's religious and moral beliefs, personal experiences, and perception of family love and commitment are strongly reflected in sexual behaviors. Statistics concerning the long-term effects of teenage pregnancy were used to illustrate the magnitude of the problem:

- At age 27, 72% of African American girls who first gave birth at age 15 or younger were living in poverty, as were 59% of those who first gave birth at ages 16 or 17, compared to 45% of those who first gave birth at ages 20 to 21.
- Children of teen mothers are at great risk for a number of economic, social, and health problems. For example, compared to children with older mothers, children of adolescent parents are twice as likely to be abused and neglected; 22% more likely to become teen mothers themselves; and 50% are more likely to have children out-of-wedlock (The National Campaign to Prevent Teen Pregnancy, 2004, p. 2).

Identifying Adolescents at Greatest Risk for Unwanted Pregnancy

Adolescents who lack the support, security, and love of a family home are more likely to engage in high-risk behaviors including sex at an early age, multiple sexual partners, failure to use contraception, and unplanned pregnancy. Incarcerated juveniles constitute the most vulnerable group, especially when placed in an environment away from family support. These teenagers often have histories of physical neglect as well as severe physical, emotional, and sexual abuse. This group is more likely to experiment with high-risk behaviors, such as substance abuse, gang involvement, and violence. They may be more susceptible to peer pressure and are more likely to succumb to negative behaviors in an attempt to gain acceptance or peer status. Consequently, many begin sexual experimentation at a very early age and predictably experience unwanted teenage pregnancy (Carbone, 2001).

The Impact of Pregnancy on Meeting the Developmental Tasks of Adolescence

A pregnant teenager is required to be able to make informed decisions regarding continuing the pregnancy and, if the pregnancy comes to fruition, future plans for the child. This action hinges upon the premise that the adolescent has the necessary skills to appreciate the implications of these decisions as well as the potential life-long consequences associated with these decisions. Kaiser and Hays (2004) assert that pregnant adolescents face a dual task: meeting the developmental tasks of being a teenager, coupled with the developmental tasks associated with adapting to become a mother.

 Nursing Insight— *Pregnancy and the developmental tasks of adolescence*

According to Erikson (1963), there are four developmental tasks of adolescence:
- To establish a sense of self-worth and a value system
- To establish lasting relationships
- To emancipate from parents
- To choose a vocation

Pregnancy during adolescence creates an especially vulnerable situation because the developmental tasks of pregnancy are superimposed on those of adolescence.

For a teenager to successfully adapt and fulfill the role of being a mother, she must achieve four major developmental tasks:

- Gain acceptance of pregnancy: This involves disclosing the presence of the pregnancy to her family, the father of the child, and her friends; facing family reactions; and hopefully gaining support.
- Set goals: Make realistic and attainable plans for the future. These goals will be different from her original ones and will focus on her role as a mother of a dependent child.
- View self as mother: This task addresses self-image and redefining self as a woman with a child rather than as a teenager with the freedom to explore being an adolescent and the opportunity to mature gradually.
- Grow up: Being a competent mother demands maturity with the ability to place someone else's needs before one's own. Developmentally, teenagers are typically at an egocentric stage of development. Being a mother is demanding and requires the sacrifice of being a carefree teenager (Kaiser, 2002).

Delayed Entry into Care

Denial, a common reaction to an unplanned and unwanted pregnancy, is often the reason why adolescents do not seek early prenatal care. In some situations, even close family members do not suspect or recognize the signs of advancing pregnancy. Unfortunately, denial and postponement of care may place the teenager and her fetus at a greater risk for medical problems. Complications such as iron-deficiency anemia, preterm labor, and preeclampsia may progress without detection and treatment. Without ongoing emotional support and education throughout pregnancy, the teenager enters labor psychologically unprepared and lacking a knowledge base to understand the natural events that surround birth. (See Chapter 11 for further discussion.)

Dulit (2000) describes three clinical types of adolescent pregnancy denial. During the first of these clinical types, the teenager realizes that pregnancy is a possibility but continues to hope that it will not come to fruition, and if it does, that it will disappear on its own accord. As the pregnancy advances, the adolescent recognizes the need to acknowledge the pregnancy and will usually seek assistance.

The second type of denial is a continuation of the first except that the teenager actively conceals the pregnancy and deliberately uses whatever skills necessary to intentionally deceive and hide the changes taking place in her body. The third type is considered true denial. In this situation, the teenager is absolutely unaware of any of the physical or psychological signs or symptoms of pregnancy and experiences an unconscious denial of impeding motherhood. In this situation, the onset of labor is truly an unexpected event. A teenager who experiences this type of clinical denial is displaying psychopathology coupled with a significant ego pathology. The trauma of the birth may be sufficient to trigger a psychotic episode.

Infants born to this group of teenagers are at highest risk for being victims of neonaticide, as the mother fails to develop any form of attachment. Neonaticide is defined as the killing of a baby within the first 24 hours of birth. Active neonaticide is a deliberate action that occurs when the infant's death is the intended outcome of an act of violence. Passive (negligent) neonaticide results from an inability to provide the means for infant survival, for example, by maintaining an open airway, keeping the baby warm, or providing nutrition. Unfortunately, the victims are often the infants found abandoned in dumpsters or in public restrooms.

⚙ Be sure to— Advocate for newborns at risk

Nurses must actively advocate for newborns at risk. One way is by becoming knowledgeable about their practice state's Safe Haven laws and programs. This information may be accessed at: http://www.adopting.org/adoptions/legalized-abandonment-state-safe-haven-laws-and-programs.html

Nursing Care of the Pregnant Adolescent

For a teenager, pregnancy presents a number of issues: deciding whether to continue with the pregnancy; securing a means for gaining access to prenatal care; planning for infant/child care in a secure home environment; and arranging for economic resources to meet the needs of a dependent new family member. Social isolation may leave the expectant teen without peer support. When this occurs, the physical, emotional, and psychological transitions associated with pregnancy are more difficult for the teenager to accomplish successfully. Since the risk of pregnancy complications (e.g., iron-deficiency anemia, preeclampsia, intrauterine growth restriction, and cephalopelvic disproportion) are increased among this group, early and ongoing prenatal care is essential. A nursing approach that is designed to meet the special needs of the adolescent patient promotes adherence and an optimal pregnancy outcome.

ASSESSMENT. Assessment of the pregnant adolescent is similar to that of older women. The initial visit includes a personal health history and family history to determine whether medical problems such as diabetes or infectious diseases may threaten maternal or fetal health. Throughout the course of pregnancy, the young patient needs to be closely monitored for iron-deficiency anemia, STIs, and preeclampsia. She should also be assessed for high-risk behaviors such as tobacco, alcohol, and drug use and screened for sexual abuse. Therapeutic communication with the adolescent is enhanced when the interview is conducted in a warm, conversational style that conveys caring and acceptance.

It is important to assess the young patient's knowledge and level of understanding concerning personal care during pregnancy and care of the infant following birth. An educational plan individualized to meet the adolescent's specific needs can be developed during the initial visit and refined and altered as needed throughout the pregnancy. An approach that values the patient's support persons while recognizing the need to foster her personal sense of independence is essential. A plan of care that combines the collaborative efforts of various professionals including the physician, nurse, health educator, nutritionist, school counselor, and social worker is important in optimizing the outcomes for the young patient and her fetus. Reinforcing information, allowing ample time to discuss concerns, emphasizing the need to keep return appointments, and confirming that the patient can verbalize when and how to seek help are essential components of each visit.

Be sure to— Allow the pregnant adolescent to make health care decisions

Sometimes it is difficult for parents to allow an adolescent daughter to make health care decisions concerning her pregnancy. By law, a pregnant adolescent is an emancipated minor (a person capable of making health care decisions), so she may sign for her own care.

Framing the physical examination in a friendly, learning context helps to diminish the young patient's anxiety and fear and reinforces the information provided at each visit. Use of the Doppler stethoscope allows the patient to hear the fetal heart tones. This action reinforces the presence of the fetus and helps the teenager to acknowledge the reality of her pregnancy. Emphasizing the progression in the fundal height measurement at each visit confirms that her fetus is growing and reinforces that she is successfully nourishing her developing child.

DIAGNOSIS AND PLANNING. Because of unawareness or denial of the pregnancy, adolescents often do not enter the prenatal care system until the second or third trimester. They may be frightened, confused, and unsure where to go for care. They are usually unaware of maternal needs, such as nutritional requirements, during pregnancy. Prenatal care is often received sporadically in the adolescent population.

Optimizing Outcomes— Formulating a nursing diagnosis for the pregnant adolescent patient

Due to a lack of information about pregnancy, "Risk for Ineffective Health Maintenance related to lack of knowledge of measures to promote health during pregnancy and family stress" is an appropriate nursing diagnosis for most pregnant adolescent patients.

Expected outcomes are based on the situation. For example, the patient will: keep scheduled prenatal appointments; follow recommended strategies for health promotion; attend childbirth and child care classes; and the family will: voice emotions and concerns and provide consistent support throughout the childbearing experience.

INTERVENTIONS: STRATEGIES TO PROMOTE A HEALTHY PREGNANCY. Nursing interventions are structured to address the patient's identified needs. For example, the young patient may have difficulty accessing care due to her school schedule or transportation difficulties. The nurse helps to locate a prenatal clinic that schedules appointments in the late afternoon or evening and when needed, works with community resources to arrange for transportation to the clinic. Many facilities offer "teen clinics" that are geared to meet the special needs of young pregnant women. Some of these provide after-school transportation to the clinic, serve nutritious snacks, encourage patient participation in certain aspects of care (e.g., checking the urine with a dipstick; recording the weight), and provide education in small peer-oriented group settings that use repetition and reinforcement of information.

Optimizing Outcomes— with a CenteringPregnancy program

CenteringPregnancy is a group prenatal care program developed to improve pregnancy outcomes in the adolescent population. The CenteringPregnancy model incorporates a holistic approach that recognizes the adolescent's developmental need for socializing and peer support. Comprehensive prenatal care that includes risk assessment, education, and support is provided in a group-focused environment (Moeller, Vezeau, & Carr, 2007; Reid, 2007). Additional information may be found at: http://www.centeringpregnancy.com/

Referrals to other community resources such as WIC and home health nursing may be appropriate throughout pregnancy and during the puerperium.

 Nursing Insight— Adolescents and pregnancy outcomes with multiple gestations

Adolescents are at an increased risk for poor birth outcomes, particularly when multifetal pregnancies are involved. Adverse outcomes include low birth weight and very low birth weight, preterm and very preterm births, small-for-gestational age infants, and fetal and neonatal death (Shumpert, Salihu, & Kirby, 2004).

PROMOTING OPTIMAL NOURISHMENT FOR THE PATIENT AND HER FETUS. Pregnancy during adolescence is associated with a higher risk for maternal and fetal complications. Adolescents who are still growing and those who have recently experienced menarche are at greatest risk for pregnancy complications. Growing adolescents continue to add fat to their own bodies during the third trimester, and as a result, tend to have smaller infants.

Pregnant adolescents need more calcium, magnesium, and phosphorus to help meet their own growth needs. Teens often skip meals and have a tendency to choose convenience or "fast foods" that are high in calories, fat, and sodium and low in vitamins, minerals, and fiber. Educating the young maternity patient about the importance of nutrition during pregnancy, seeking her input in making simple dietary changes, and offering nutritious snacks during prenatal visits are examples of nursing interventions that have been successful in many settings.

The Adolescent Expectant Father

Although most partners of adolescent mothers are within 2 to 3 years of their age, approximately 7% are 6 or more years older. Many become "absent" parents who rarely see or assume any responsibility in childcare. The majority of adolescent fathers admit that they are not ready for fatherhood. Confusion, depression, and guilt may predominate as the young expectant father struggles with the conflicting tasks of adolescence and impending fatherhood.

The adolescent father may accompany the young woman to the clinic for pregnancy confirmation or for prenatal care. Some attend childbirth preparation classes and participate in the childbirth experience; others shy away and avoid contact with the young expectant girl. Often, support during the pregnancy and in the early months after birth diminishes as other interests and responsibilities become more important. However, nurses must guard against stereotyping young expectant fathers as being irresponsible and disinterested; many genuinely care and wish to be involved. When desired by the pregnant adolescent, the father's participation should be encouraged. It is a source of additional support for the young patient and allows the father an opportunity to work toward defining his role as a parent. Unfortunately, a large number of teenage expectant fathers come from low socioeconomic backgrounds and lack the resources, education, and job skills needed to be able to support their children.

 Be sure to— Recognize the adolescent father's lack of legal rights

If the adolescent father is not married to the pregnant teenager, he has no legal rights to participate in her decision making concerning the pregnancy, elective abortion, or plans for adoption.

Evaluation

Evaluation of the interventions is reflective of the expected outcomes. For example, did the patient keep her scheduled prenatal clinic appointments? Did she adhere to suggested health-promoting strategies? Did she attend the childbirth/child classes? Did her family remain supportive throughout the pregnancy?

 Now Can You— Discuss various aspects of adolescent pregnancy?

1. Explain how pregnancy affects the developmental tasks of adolescence?
2. Develop a plan of care that is appropriate for a pregnant adolescent?
3. Identify strategies for involving the adolescent father in the pregnancy?

THE PREGNANT WOMAN OLDER THAN AGE 35

Maternal age is an important factor in the management of pregnancy. Today, more and more first pregnancies are occurring in women over the age of 35, who are no longer referred to as the "elderly primigravida." As maternal age increases, there is a greater likelihood of pre-existing medical conditions such as diabetes and hypertension, which may be associated with maternal morbidity and poor fetal outcomes. Benign uterine leiomyomas (fibroids) occur with greater frequency in women over age 35 and may interfere with cervical dilation during labor and cause postpartum hemorrhage. Other obstetric complications including vaginal bleeding, preeclampsia, multiple gestation, gestational diabetes, preterm labor, dysfunctional labor, and cesarean birth are also increased in older primigravidas. The fetus is at greater risk for low birth weight, macrosomia, chromosomal abnormalities, and congenital malformations.

However, the risks are considerably reduced when the patient's preconception and prenatal care is managed by a team of nurses, medical specialists, perinatologists (obstetricians with a specialty in high-risk obstetrics), nutritionists, and other health professionals. Optimal maternal–fetal outcomes result from early and ongoing care along with healthy lifestyle factors that are appropriate for women of any age: being physically, psychologically, and emotionally well; remaining physically active, having an ability to access and utilize health care services; having received an adequate education, and belonging to a socioeconomic advantaged section of society.

Preconception and prenatal care for women in the over-35-age group is focused on recognizing chronic medical conditions (e.g., hypertension, diabetes) and identifying detrimental lifestyle habits such as alcohol, drug, and tobacco use. As is true with any population of women, a healthy lifestyle is an important first step toward achieving a good perinatal outcome. It is essential to listen actively to patients and their partners so that their concerns can be addressed, and, where appropriate, referrals can be made for counseling and screening or prenatal diagnostic procedures. Early prenatal care affords the opportunity for timely prenatal testing. Unfortunately, the older woman may mistake a scanty or missed period for signs of early menopause rather than pregnancy. When this occurs, entry for prenatal care is often delayed.

> ⚙ **Optimizing Outcomes**— **Early prenatal care facilitates prenatal diagnosis for the expectant couple older than age 35**
>
> After age 35, there is an increased risk of conceiving a child with Down syndrome. Genetic testing is routinely offered to older expectant couples to permit the early diagnosis of chromosomal abnormalities. .

Reactions to pregnancy in women 35 and older range from shock and disbelief to elation and joy. Many have reached the point in their lives where they have financial resources and economic stability, established careers, and the security of a stable interpersonal relationship. For women whose long-awaited pregnancy comes after months or years of attempts to conceive, pregnancy is a positive, exhilarating experience. Other women react with feelings of denial, uncertainty, and worry about how the pregnancy will affect their lives.

Nurses must be sensitive to each woman's situation and needs. Despite an abundance of other resources, peer support may be lacking. Often, the majority of the woman's contemporaries will have completed their childbearing many years earlier and are now the parents of almost-grown children. Effective nursing interventions include providing information and referral for genetics counseling and specialized diagnostic testing; structuring prenatal education to meet the unique needs of the older woman and her partner; and offering assistance in locating support groups, exercise, and childbirth preparation classes oriented toward the older woman. A timetable for screening for chromosomal abnormalities associated with advanced maternal age is presented in Table 9-5. Genetic abnormalities are also increased when the father is older than 40 years.

The physical examination should be conducted with a special focus on the identification of breast abnormalities and circulatory problems. After a careful breast examination, the patient should be encouraged to continue with monthly breast self-examination, as the incidence of breast cancer is increased in the older woman. Particular attention should be paid to inspection of the lower extremities because varicosities are also more common in older women. During the first trimester, the nurse should carefully assess for the presence of fetal heart sounds since the incidence of hydatidiform mole is increased in women over age 40. (See Chapter 11 for further discussion.)

Screening for Fetal Chromosomal Abnormalities

The American College of Obstetricians and Gynecologists (ACOG) now recommends that all pregnant women are offered a screening test for Down syndrome (ACOG, 2007).

Table 9-5 Timetable for Prenatal Diagnosis

Test	Significance
Maternal serum AFP screening	Sample of maternal blood obtained between 14 and 16 weeks of pregnancy.
	High levels may be indicative of an open neural tube defect, but may also result from incorrect dates, multiple pregnancy or fetal demise.
	Low levels of serum AFP are associated with Down syndrome. The incidence of Down syndrome increases with maternal age to approximately 1 in 100 at age 40 or older.
Triple test: alpha-fetoprotein (AFP), human chorionic gonadotropin (hCG), and unconjugated estriol	Levels of hCG are increased and levels of unconjugated estriol are decreased when a trisomy 21 (Down syndrome) is present.
	A low level of hCG can indicate trisomy 18. The sensitivity of the AFP test in detecting trisomy 21 is increased by 40% to 50% when hCG levels are added.

The incidence of having a child affected by Down syndrome (trisomy 21) increases dramatically with maternal age (Table 9-6). Although a variety of screening and diagnostic tests are available to detect a fetus with Down syndrome, it is essential that before implementing any of these, the patient and her significant other or family support person are provided with appropriate information concerning the tests. This information is valuable in helping them to understand the reliability of the screening or diagnostic test and the implications of the results. The early diagnosis of an affected pregnancy gives the patient and her family the opportunity to determine whether termination of pregnancy is an option for her. Alternatively, early discovery of

Table 9-6 Risk of Down Syndrome Related to Maternal Age

Maternal Age at Term	Risk of Down Syndrome
Younger than 25	1 : 1500
30	1 : 910
35	1 : 380
40	1 : 110
42	1 : 65
44	1 : 35
46	1 : 20
48	1 : 11
50	1 : 6

Source: Data from http://www.wolfson.qmul.ac.uk/epm/screening/calcrisk. shtml#markers a fetal problem provides time for the parents to become informed and make preparations for rearing a child with Down syndrome. If the patient chooses an elective termination of pregnancy, the earlier the gestation, the lower the maternal morbidity associated with the procedure.

Throughout the screening and diagnosis process, the patient deserves an unbiased counselor who can provide continuity of care and up-to-date, accurate, and in-depth information. The counselor also needs to be able to facilitate open discussion whereby the patient can voice concerns related to issues such as spiritual beliefs; financial constraints; family dynamics; emotional feelings; and cultural, philosophical, and ethical values. Whatever decision the patient makes regarding the pregnancy, she needs a sound support system that will help her and her family deal with the issues that arise during pregnancy and provide the appropriate aftercare.

Down syndrome screening may be initiated in the first or second trimester of pregnancy. In the first trimester, three "markers" (the Triple Screen or Triple Test) are evaluated: Pregnancy Associated Plasma Protein-A (PAPP-A), free β-human chorionic gonadotropin (free β-hCG), and nuchal translucency (NT). NT is an ultrasound-directed measurement of the swelling directly beneath the skin at the back of the fetal neck. A positive result for Down syndrome is associated with a decreased PAPP-A (approximately one half of the normal level), an elevated level of free β-hCG, (approximately twice the normal level), and a high measurement of the NT thickness (Reddy & Mennuti, 2006). In the second trimester, four "markers" (termed a Quad Screen) are used: α-fetoprotein (AFP), unconjugated estriol (uE3), free beta-human chorionic gonadotropin (free β-hCG), and inhibin A (inhibin). Inhibin is a hormone produced by the ovarian granulosa cells that suppresses the release of follicle-stimulating hormone (FSH). It is classified into subtypes inhibib-A and inhibib-B. Levels of inhibib-A are elevated in the presence of Down syndrome.

A diagnostic test such as an amniocentesis is usually offered if the calculated risk for Down syndrome is 1 in 150 or greater. If an open neural tube defect is suspected based on an elevated (2.5 times higher than the average for the number of gestational weeks) AFP, a diagnostic ultrasound examination can be obtained. All patients who have experienced prior pregnancies associated with fetal chromosomal abnormalities should be offered diagnostic testing such as chorionic villus sampling or amniocentesis (Barts and The London Queen Mary's School of Medicine and Dentistry, 2006). (See Chapter 11 for further discussion.) The most recent data now indicate that chorionic villus sampling carries no greater risk to pregnancy duration than amniocentesis (Caughey, Hopkins, & Norton, 2006).

 Nursing Insight— *Maternal age and Down syndrome screening results*

An older woman is more likely to have a screen-positive result than a younger woman because she starts with a higher age-specific risk of Down syndrome. Approximately 70% of pregnancies affected by Down syndrome is detected in women aged 25 or younger, while 99% of pregnancies affected by Down syndrome is detected in women older than the age of 45 (Wald & Rudnicka, 2004).

 where research and practice meet:
A Variety of Cultural, Medical, and Lifestyle Factors May Affect Prenatal Screening Tests

Prenatal screening tests results are affected by a number of factors.
- AFP levels tend to be about 20% higher and free ß-hCG levels about 10% higher in Afro-Caribbean women than in Caucasian women.
- Free ß-hCG levels tend to be about 10% higher and uE3 (estriol) levels about 10% lower in women who have become pregnant as a result of in vitro fertilization (IVF), as compared with non-IVF pregnancies.
- Free ß-hCG levels tend to be about 20% lower and inhibin levels are about 60% higher in women who smoke, as compared with women who do not smoke.
- Second-trimester serum marker levels are increased in twin pregnancies.
- Women with insulin-dependent diabetes mellitus usually have lower levels of AFP (decreased by 18%), inhibin (decreased by 12%), and uE3 (decreased by 6%) than women without insulin-dependent diabetes.
- Vaginal bleeding that occurs immediately before a second trimester blood sample is obtained can affect the screening result since bleeding may increase the maternal serum AFP level. When bleeding has occurred, it may be advisable to delay the screening test until a week after the bleeding has stopped.
- If an amniocentesis has been attempted in the pregnancy before obtaining a second-trimester blood sample, the result cannot be correctly interpreted due to the possibility of a feto–maternal transfusion, which can increase the maternal serum AFP level.
- Nurses should use this information to appropriately counsel patients who will be undergoing prenatal screening tests.

Data from http://www.wolfson.qmul.ac.uk/epm/screening

 Now Can You— **Discuss aspects of care for the pregnant woman older than age 35?**

1. Explain why women older than age 35 may experience more pregnancy complications than younger women?
2. Identify two components of the physical examination that merit special attention?
3. Identify three tests that are useful in the prenatal diagnosis of Down syndrome?

summary points

- Education and involvement in prenatal care empowers patients and their families to make informed decisions.

- The first prenatal visit includes a health history, physical examination, and laboratory testing. Establishing good rapport through effective communication is essential in creating an environment where the patient is more likely to return.

- Prenatal follow-up visits are shorter than the initial assessment, but they are important in monitoring maternal–fetal health and in providing anticipatory guidance for the patient and her family.

◆ Early and ongoing prenatal care is key to an optimal maternal–fetal outcome. Families should be involved in activities for health promotion and educated about strategies for self-care during the childbearing year.

◆ The diagnosis of pregnancy is based on three types of signs: presumptive, probable, and positive. Presumptive and probable signs may be caused by conditions other than pregnancy; positive signs can have no other cause.

◆ The teenage pregnant patient is at risk for a number of obstetric complications including anemia, preeclampsia, and preterm birth.

◆ Factors including education, culture, spiritual beliefs, and family support and income impact the occurrence of adolescent pregnancy.

◆ Preconception and prenatal care for the woman over 35 focuses on the recognition and management of chronic medical problems and strategies to promote a healthy lifestyle.

review questions

Multiple Choice

1. The clinic nurse informs the low-risk pregnant woman at 20 weeks' gestation that she should schedule her next routine prenatal appointment for:
A. 1 week
B. 2 weeks
C. 3 weeks
D. 4 weeks

2. Laura, a 38-year-old woman, calls the clinic to ask about a pregnancy test as she has missed her last period by 2 weeks. The clinic nurse recommends that Laura use a home pregnancy test:
A. That is specific to the beta subunit of hCG
B. That is specific to the alpha subunit of hCG
C. In 1 week
D. At the end of 2 weeks

3. The clinic nurse knows that a probable sign of pregnancy is:
A. Piskacek sign
B. Nausea and vomiting
C. Fetal heartbeat
D. Frequency of urination

4. The clinic nurse obtains information from Emma, a 22-year-old primigravida. Her last menstrual period was December 25th and it lasted 3 days (normal duration for Emma). The calculated Estimated Date of Birth (EDB) would be:
A. October 1
B. September 1
C. October 2
D. September 30

True/False

5. The perinatal nurse recognizes that the diagnosis of pregnancy may cause a woman to be afraid for her own safety.

6. The clinic nurse routinely includes information on genetic testing and diseases as a component of prenatal care to ensure informed choice for women and their families.

Fill-in-the-Blank

7. The clinic nurse encourages and schedules prenatal visits with patients because health care provided during pregnancy _____ mortality and _____ morbidity.

8. The clinic nurse uses the RADAR acronym as a tool for abuse screening. The "D" refers to _____ your _____.

9. The clinic nurse is aware that obtaining a woman's obstetric history is important to her care. A history of a _____ birth increases the woman's chances by 20% to 40% of a reoccurrence in a subsequent pregnancy.

10. The clinic nurse teaches pregnant women in their first trimester that frequency of urination is due to _____ on the bladder exerted by the _____.

See Answers to End of Chapter Review Questions on the Electronic Study Guide or DavisPlus.

REFERENCES

Agency for Healthcare Research and Quality (2003). Safety net monitoring initiative. Retrieved from http://www.ahrq.gov/data/safetynet/netfact.htm (Accessed April 1, 2008).

Alan Guttmacher Institute (2004). Facts on American Teens' sexual and reproductive health. Retrieved from http://www.guttmacher.org/sections/pregnancy.php (Accessed April 2, 2008).

Alliance for the Improvement of Maternity Services (AIMS). The Pregnant Patient's Bill of Rights. Retrieved from http://www.aimsusa.org/ppbr.htm (Accessed April 2, 2008).

Alpert, E.J., Freud, K.M., Park, C.C., Patel, J.C., & Sovak, M.A. (1992). Partner violence: how to recognize and treat victims of abuse. Massachusetts Medical Society, Waltham, MA.

American College of Nurse-Midwives (ACNM). (2005). Nurse-Midwifery in 2005: Evidence Based Practice. A Summary of Research on Nurse-Midwifery Practice in the United States. Author: Silver Spring, MD.

American College of Obstetricians and Gynecologists (ACOG). (1998). Viral hepatitis in pregnancy. Educational Bulletin No. 248. *International Journal of Gynaecology and Obstetrics, 63*, 195–202.

American College of Obstetricians and Gynecologists (ACOG). (2004). Prenatal and perinatal human immunodeficiency virus testing: Expanded recommendations. Committee Opinion No. 304. *Obstetrics and Gynecology, 104*(6), 1119–1124.

American College of Obstetricians and Gynecologists (ACOG). (2005). Smoking cessation during pregnancy. Committee Opinion No. 316. *Obstetrics and Gynecology 106*(2), 883–888.

American College of Obstetricians and Gynecologists (ACOG). (2007, January). Screening for fetal chromosomal abnormalities. *ACOG Practice Bulletin*, no. 77, 920–929.

Amercian College of Obstetricians and Gynecologists (ACOG). (2007). Guidelines for Women's Health Care. A resource manual. (3rd ed.). Washington, DC, ACOG.

American Diabetes Association (2003). Gestational diabetes mellitus. Retrieved from http://care.diabetesjournals.org/cgi/content/full/26/suppl_1/s103 (Accessed April 2, 2008).

Banks, E., Berrington, A., & Casabonne, D. (2001). Overview of the relationship between use of progestogen-only contraceptives and bone mineral density. *BJOG: An International Journal of Obstetrics & Gynaecology, 108*(12), 1214–1221.

Barts and The London Queen Mary's School of Medicine and Dentistry (2006). Antenatal screening services. Retrieved from http://www.wolfson.qmul.ac.uk/epm/screening/ (Accessed April 1, 2008).

Bloom, K.C., Bednarzyk, M.S., Devitt, D.L., Renaulty, R.A., Teaman, V., & Van Loock, D.M. (2004). Barriers to prenatal care for homeless pregnant women. *Journal of Obstetric, Gynecologic, and Neonatal Nursing, 33*(4), 428–435.

Bobak, M. (2000). Outdoor air pollution, low birth weight, and prematurity. *Environmental Health Perspectives 108*, 173–176.

Boxall, E.H., Sira, J., Standish, R.A., Davies, P., Sleight, E., Dhillon, A.P., Scheuer, P.J., & Kelly, D.A. (2004). Natural history of hepatitis B in perinatally infected carriers. *Archives of disease in Childhood (Fetal and Neonatal edition), 89*(5), F456–F460.

Braun, J.E.D., Sanne, I.M., & Bartlett, J. G., (2006). Treatment of chronic hepatitis B (HBV) and HIV-HBV coinfection. Medscape. Retrieved from http://www.medscape.com/viewprogram/5241 (Accessed January 12, 2007).

Brocklehurst, P., & Volmink, J. (2002). Antiretrovirals for reducing the risk of mother-to-child transmission of HIV infection (Cochrane Review). *The Cochrane Library*, Issue 3. Oxford: Update Software.

Bulechek, G., Butcher, H.M., & Dochterman, J. (2008). *Nursing interventions classification (NIC)* (5th ed.). St. Louis, MO: C.V. Mosby.

Bull, S.D. (2003, June). Violence against women: Media (mis)representation of femicide. Paper presented at the "Women Working to Make a Difference," IWPR's Seventh International Women's Policy Research Conference. Washington, DC.

Bunting, L., & McAuley, C. (2004). Research Review: Teenage pregnancy and parenthood: The role of fathers. *Child and Family Social Work, 9*, 295–303.

Bureau of Justice Statistics. (2003, February). Crime data brief. *Intimate Partner Violence, 1993–2001.*

Carbone, D.J. (2001). Under lock and key: Youth under the influence of HIV. *Body Positive Magazine.* Retrieved from http://www.thebody.com/bp/may01/feature_02.html (Accessed January 12, 2007).

Caughey, A.B., Hopkins, L.M., & Nortor., M.E. (2006). Chorionic villus sampling compared with amniocentesis and the difference in the rate of pregnancy loss. *Obstetrics & Gynecology, 108*, 612–616.

Centers for Disease Control and Prevention (CDC). (2002). Sexually transmitted diseases treatment guidelines. *MMWR* May 10, 2002/51(RR06); 1–80. Retrieved from http://www.cdc.gov/STD/treatment/4-2002TG.htm (Accessed May 21, 2006).

Centers for Disease Control and Prevention (CDC). (2005). Folic acid: PHS recommendations. Updated July 26, 2005. Retrieved from http://www.cdc.gov/ncbddd/folicacid/health_recomm.htm (Accessed April 2, 2008).

Centers for Disease Control and Prevention (CDC). (2006a). Sexually transmitted diseases treatment guidelines, 2006. *Morbidity and Mortality weekly Report, 55*(RR-11), 1–94.

Centers for Disease Control and Prevention (CDC). (2006b). Viral hepatitis C – Fact sheet. Retrieved from http://www.cdc.gov/ncidod/diseases/hepatitis/c/fact.htm (Accessed April 1, 2008).

Centers for Disease Control and Prevention (CDC). (2007). Birth defects. Retrieved from http://www.cdc.gov/ncbddd/bd/default.htm (Accessed April 1, 2008).

Coid, J., Petruckevitch, A., Feder, G., Chung, W.S., Richardson, J., & Moorey, S. (2001). Relation between child sexual and physical abuse and risk of re-victimisation in women: a cross-sectional study. *Lancet, 358*, 450–454.

Cole, L.A., Khanlian, S.A., Sutton, J.M., Davies, S., & Rayburn, W.F. (2004). Accuracy of home pregnancy tests at the time of missed menses. *American Journal of Obstetrics and Gynecology, 190*, 100–105.

Dugoua, J.J., Perri, D., Seely, D., Mills, E., & Koren, G. (2008). Safety and efficacy of blue cohosh (*Caulophyllum thalictroides*) during pregnancy and lactation. *The Canadian Journal of Clinical Pharmacology, 15*(1), e66–73.

Dulit, E. (2000). Girls who deny a pregnancy girls who kill the neonate. In: A.H. Esman, L.T. Flaherty, & H.A. Horowitz (Eds.), *Adolescent psychiatry: Developmental and clinical studies,* (vol. 25, p. 304). Hillsdale, NJ: The Analytical Press.

Dyjack, D., Soret, S., Chen, L., Hwaqng, R., Nazari, N., & Gaede, D. Residential environmental risks for reproductive age women in developing countries. *Journal of Midwifery & Women's Health, 50*, 309–314.

El Kady, D., Gilbert, W., Xing, G., & Smith, L. (2005). Maternal and neonatal outcomes of assaults during pregnancy. *Obstetrics and Gynecology, 105*(2), 356–363.

Erikson, E.H. (1963). *Childhood and society.* New York: W.W. Norton.

Gardner, J. (2006). What you need to know about genital herpes. *Nursing 2006, 36*(10), 26–29.

Gazmarrian, J.A., Lazorick, S., Spitz, A., Ballard, T.J., Saltzman, L.E., & Marks, J.S. (2000). Violence and reproductive health: Current knowledge and future research directives. *Maternal and Child Health Journal, 4*(2), 79-84.

Gilliland, F.D., Li, Y.F., & Peters, J.M. (2001). Effects of maternal smoking during pregnancy and environmental tobacco smoke on asthma and wheezing in children. *American Journal of Respiratory and Critical Care Medicine, 163*(2), 429–436.

Haire, D. (2000). Prepared for: American Foundation for Maternal and Child Health by Doris Haire. Alliance for the Improvement of Maternity Services (AIMS) The Pregnant Patient's Bill of Rights. Retrieved from http://www.aimsusa.org/ppbr.htm (Accessed May 25, 2006).

Harper, M.A., Byington, R.P., & Espeland, M.A. (2003). Pregnancy- related death and health care services. *Obstetrics and Gynecology, 102*, 273.

Harris, S. (2005). Under-12s have sex one night and play with Barbie dolls the next. *Nursing Standard, 19*(39), 14–16.

Healy, A.J., Malone, F.D., Sullivan, L.M., Porter, T.F., Luthy, D.A., Cornstock, C.H., Saade, G., Berkowitz, R., Klagman, S., Dugoff, L., Craigo, S.D., Timor-Tritsch, I., Carr, S.R., Wolfe, H.M., Bianchi, D.W., & D'Alton, M.E. (2006). Early access to prenatal care – Implications for racial disparity in perinatal mortailty. *Obstetrics and Gynecology, 107* (3), 625–631.

Heaney, R.P. (2006). Role and importance of calcium in preventing and managing osteoporosis. Medscape. Retrieved from http://www.medscape.com/viewprogram/5237?sssdmh=dm1.187248&src=nlcmealert (Accessed April 2, 2008).

Hernandez-Diaz, S., Werler, M.N., Walker, A.M., & Mitchell, A.A. (2000). Folic acid antagonists during pregnancy and the risk of birth defects. *New England Journal of Medicine, 343*(22), 1608–1614.

Hey-Hadavi. J.H. (2002). Women's oral health issues sex differences and clinical implications. *WOMEN'S HEALTH in Primary Care, 5*(3), 44–52.

Higgins, A.C. (1976). Nutritional status and the outcome of pregnancy. *Journal of the Canadian Diet Association, 37*, 17.

Hodnett, E.D. (2004). Continuity of caregivers for care during pregnancy and childbirth. *Cochrane Database System Review* (Issue 2), CD000062.

Holloway, M., & D'Acunto, K. (2006, June). An update on the ABCs of viral hepatitis. *The Clinical Advisor*, 29–39.

Jaakkola, J.J.K., & Gissler, M. (2004). Maternal smoking in pregnancy, fetal development, and childhood asthma. *American Journal of Public Health, 94*(1), 136–140.

Johnson, M., Bulechek, G., Butcher, H., McCloskey Dochterman, J., Maas, M., Moorhead, S., & Swanson, E. (2006). *NANDA, NOC, and NIC Linkages: nursing diagnoses, outcomes, & interventions* (2nd ed.). St. Louis, MO: Mosby Elsevier.

Kaiser, M.M. (2002). *Transition to motherhood in adolescence: The development of the Adolescent Prenatal Questionnaire.* Unpublished doctoral dissertation, University of Nebraska Medical Center.

Kaiser, M.M., & Hays, B.J. (2004). The adolescent prenatal questionnaire: Assessing psychosocial factors that influence transition to motherhood. *Health Care for Women International, 25*, 5–19.

Kandinov, L.D. (2005). Periconceptual exposure to oral contraceptives and risk for Down syndrome. Ask the experts about obstetrics and maternal-fetal medicine. *Medscape Ob/Gyn & Women's Health, 10*(1). Retrieved from http://www.medscape.com/viewarticle/498685 (Accessed April 2, 2008).

Kirkham, C., Harris, S., & Grzybowski, S. (2005). Evidence-based prenatal care: Part I. General prenatal care and counseling issues. *Amerian Family Physician, 71*(7), 32–41.

Koscica, K.L., & Berstein, P. (2003). Thyrotoxicosis in pregnancy: Ask the experts about obstetrics and maternal-fetal medicine. Retrieved from http://www.medscape.com/viewarticle/451718 (Accessed July 3, 2007).

Laartz, B., Gompf, S.G., Allaboum, K., Marinez, J., & Logan, J.L. (2006). Viral infections and pregnancy. Retrieved from http://www.emedicine.com/med/topic3270.htm (Accessed April 1, 2008).

Liu, S., Krewski, D., Shi, Y., Chen, Y., & Burnett, R.T. (2003). Association between gaseous ambient air pollutants and adverse pregnancy outcomes in Vancouver, Canada. *Environmental Health Perspectives, 111*, 1773–1778.

Lopez, N.J., DaSilva, I., Ipinza, J., & Gutierrez, J. (2005). Periodontal therapy reduces the rate of preterm low birth weight in women with pregnancy-associated gingivitis. *Journal of Periodontology, 76*(7 Suppl.), 2144–2153.

Luo, Z.C., Wilkins, R., & Kramer, M.S. (2004). Disparities in pregnancy outcomes according to marital and cohabitation status. *Obstetrics and Gynecology, 103*(6), 1300–1307.

Maisonet, M., Bush, T.J., Correa, A., & Jaakkola, J.J. (2001). Relation between ambient air pollution and low birth weight in the northeastern United States. *Environmental Health Perspectives 109*(Suppl 3), 351–358.

March of Dimes. (2006). Illicit drug use during pregnancy. Quick reference: Fact sheet. Retrieved from http://www.marchofdimes.com/professionals/14332_1169.asp (Accessed April 1, 2008).

Martin, J.A., Hamilton, B.E., Sutton, P.D., Ventura, S.J., Menacker, F., & Munson, M.L., (2003). Late or no prenatal care. Child Trends DataBank. Retrieved from http://www.childtrendsdatabank.org/indicators/25PrenatalCare.cfm (Accessed April 2, 2008).

McFarlane, J., Campbell, J., Sharps, P., & Watson, K. (2002). Abuse during pregnancy and femicide: Urgent implications for women's health. *Obstetrics and Gynecology, 100*(1), 27–36.

Modena, A.B., Kaihura, C., & Fieni, S. (2004). Prelabor rupture of the membranes: Recent evidence. *Acta Biologia Medica Ateneo Parmense, 75*(Suppl. 1), 5–10. Retrieved from http://www.actabiomedica.it/data/2004/supp_1_2004/bacchi.pdf (Accessed April 2, 2008).

Moeller, A.H., Vezeau, T.M., & Carr, K.C. (2007). CenteringPregnancy: A new program for adolescent prenatal care. *The American Journal for Nurse Practitioners, 11*(6), 48–58.

Moorehead, S., Johnson, M., Mass, M., & Swanson, E. (2008). *Nursing outcomes classification (NOC)* (4th ed.). St. Louis, MO: C.V. Mosby.

Nabel, E.G. (2003). Cardiovascular disease. *New England Journal of Medicine, 349*(1), 60–72.

NANDA International. (2007). *NANDA-I Nursing Diagnoses: Definitions and Classifications 2007-2008*. Philadelphia: NANDA-I.

The National Campaign to Prevent Teen Pregnancy. (2003). National campaign to prevent teen pregnancy 14 and younger. (2003). The sexual behavior of young adolescents. Author: Washington, DC. Retrieved from http://www.teenpregnancy.org/resources/reading/youngteens/default.asp (Accessed May 4, 2006).

The National Campaign to Prevent Teen Pregnancy. (2004, May). Fact Sheet: Teen sexual activity, pregnancy and childbearing among black teens in the US. Retrieved from http://www.teenpregnancy.org/resources/reading/fact_sheets/default.asp (Accessed May 4, 2006).

National Cancer Institute, National Institute of Environmental Health Sciences, Office of Research on Women's Health, US Public Health Service's Office on Women's Health, Centers for Disease Control and Prevention. (1999). DES research update: Current knowledge, future directions. Proceedings. Bethesda, MD: NIH.

National Center for Health Statistics. (2007). Prenatal care. Retrieved from http://www.cdc.gov/nchs/fastats/prenatal.htm (Accessed April 1, 2008).

National Human Genome Research Institute (2003). Researchers identify gene for premature aging disorder. Retrieved from http://www.genome.gov/11006962 (Accessed April 1, 2008).

National Foundation for Infectious Diseases. (2007). Facts about rubella for adults. Retrieved from http://www.nfid.org/pdf/factsheets/rubellaadult.pdf (Accessed April 1, 2008).

National Institutes of Health (NIH). (2006a). *Genetics home reference.* Bethesda, MD: Author.

National Institutes of Health. (2006b). NHLBL Scientists find blood test predicts common and severe complication of sickle cell disease, and identifies patients at highest risk of death. Retrieved from http://www.nih.gov/news/pr/jul2006/nhlbi-18.htm (Accessed August 25, 2006).

National Patient Advocate Foundation. (2006). CARE Principles. Retrieved from http://www.npaf.org (Accessed July 6, 2007).

Natural Standard (2008). Red raspberry. Retrieved from http://www.naturalstandard.com/ (Accessed April 1, 2008).

Nielsen, K.A. (2006). Prevention of mother-to-child HIV transmission: after 25 years, what have we learned? Retrieved from http://www.medscape.com/viewarticle/525167 (Accessed May 21, 2006).

Parson, L. (2000). Violence against women and reproductive health: Towards defining a role for reproductive health care services. *Maternal and Child Health Journal, 4*(2), 135.

Partridge, C. A., & Holman, J.R. (2005). Effects of a reduced-visit prenatal care clinical practice guideline. *The Journal of the American Board of Family Practice, 18*, 555–560.

Reddy, U.M., & Mennuti, M.T. (2006). Incorporating first-trimester Down syndrome studies into prenatal screening. *Obstetrics and Gynecology, 107*(1), 167–173.

Reid, J. (2007). CenteringPregnancy: A model for group prenatal care. *Nursing for Women's Health, 11*(4), 383–388.

Reuters Health Information. (2005) Vertical HCV transmission may occur more often among female infants. *Journal of Infectious Disease 192*, 1865–1866, 1872–1879. Retrieved from http://www.medscape.com/viewarticle/519850 (Accessed April 16, 2006).

Rosengard, C., Phipps, M.G., Adler, N.E., & Ellen, J.M. (2005). Psychosocial correlates of adolescent males' pregnancy intention. *Pediatrics, 116*(3), e114–e119.

Royal Adelaide Hospital Clinic, Sexually Transmitted Diseases Services. STD interview checklist (2005). Retrieved from http://www.stdservices.on.net/management/checklists/cl_interview.htm (Accessed April 2, 2008).

Rubin, R. (1984). *Maternal Identity and maternal experience.* New York: Springer.

Safety net monitoring initiative. Fact sheet. AHRQ Publication No. 03-P011, August 2003. Agency for Healthcare Research and Quality, Rockville, MD. http://www.ahrq.gov/data/safetynet/netfact.htm

Sexually Transmitted Diseases Services (Royal Adelaide Hospital). (2005). *STD interview checklist.* Retrieved from http://www.stdservices.on.net/links/default.htm (Accessed May 20, 2006).

Shumpert, M.N., Salihu, H.M., & Kirby, R.S. (2004). Impact of maternal anemia on birth outcomes of teen twin pregnancies: A comparative analysis with mature young mothers. *Journal of Obstetrics and Gynecology, 24*, 16–21.

Silbergeld, E., & Patrick, T. (2005). Environmental exposures, toxicologic mechanisms, and adverse pregnancy outcomes. *American Journal of Obstetrics and Gynecology, 192*(5), S11–121.

Silverman, J.G., Raj, A., & Clements, K. (2004). Dating violence and associated sexual risk and pregnancy among adolescent girls in the United States. *Pediatrics, 114*, 220–225.

Smith, O.W. (1948). Diethylstilbestrol in the prevention and treatment of complications of pregnancy. *American Journal of Obstetrics and Gynecology, 56*, 821–834.

Somani, S., & Ahmed, I.K. (2005). Pregnancy: Special considerations. Retrieved from http://www.emedicine.com/oph/topic747.htm (Accessed April 1, 2008).

Stevens, L. (2005). Improving screening of women for violence – basic guidelines for healthcare providers. Retrieved from http://www.medscape.com (Accessed April 2, 2008).

Tajiri, H., Miyoshi, Y., Funada, S., Etani, Y., Abe, J., Onodera, T., Goto, M., Funato, M., Ida, S., Noda, C., Nakayama, M., & Okada, S. (2001). Prospective study of mother-to-infant transmission of hepatitis C virus. *Pediatric Infectious Disease Journal, 20*(1), 10–14. Retrieved from http://www.pidj.com/pt/re/pidj/abstract.00006454 (Accessed April 16, 2006).

Taylor, S.E., Klein, L.C., Lewis, B.P., Gruenewald, T.L., Gurung, R.A., & Updegraff, J.A. (2002). Biobehavioral responses to stress in females: Tend-and-befriend, not fight-or-flight. *Psychology Review, 107*(5), 411–429.

U.S. Department of Health and Human Services (DHHS). National Center for Health Statistics (NCHS). (2007). Early release of selected estimates based on data from the 2006 National Health Interview Survey. Retrieved from http://www.cdc.gov/nchs/about/major/nhis/released200706.htm. (Accessed July 7, 2007).

Vaccine Information (2005). Rubella vaccine. Retrieved from http://www.vaccineinformation.org/rubella/qandavax.asp (Accessed August 25, 2006).

Vadillo, O.F., Pfeffer, B.F., Bermejo, M.M.L., Hernandez, M.M.A., Beltran, M.J., Tejero, B.E., Casanueva y Lopez, E. (1995). Dietetic factors and premature rupture of fetal membranes. Effects of vitamin C on collagen degradation in the chorioamnion. *Ginecologia Obstetrica Mexico, 63*, 15.

Villar, J., Carroli, G., Khan-Neelofur, D., Piaggio, G., & Gulmezoglu, M. (2004). Patterns of routine antenatal care for low-risk pregnancy. *Cochrane Database System Review* Issue 4, CD000934.

Wald, N., & Rudnicka, A. (2004). Antenatal screening for Downs syndrome. Retrieved from http://www.wolfson.qmul.ac.uk/epm/research/ (Accessed May 5, 2006).

Winer, S., & Richwald, G.A. (2007). Genital HSV update. *The Forum, 5*(2), 18-22.

Woodrow, N., Permezel, M., Butterfield, L., Rome, R., Tan, J., & Quinn, M. (1998). Cervical carcinoma associated with pregnancy. *Australia and New Zealand Journal of Obstetrics and Gynaecology, 38*, 161–165. Cited in Colposcopy and Programme Management – Guidelines for the NHS Cervical Screening Programme. NHSCSP Publication No. 20, April 2004.

World Health Organization (WHO). (2005a). WHO multicountry study on women's health and domestic violence against women. Summary report of initial results on prevalence, health outcomes, and women's responses. Geneva: Author.

World Health Organization (WHO). (2005b). Report: *Make every woman and every child count.* Retrieved from http://www.who.int/whr/2005/en/index.html (Accessed March 22, 2006).

CONCEPT MAP

The Prenatal Assessment

Pregnancy:
- Wonder/growth
- Ambivalence
- Self-preservation concerns

For best outcomes

Prenatal Care:
- Begins in first trimester
- Visits: once every 4 wks for 28–32 wks → q2wks
- Focus: early identification of deviations from the norm
- Facilitate health promotion/ health maintenance via screenings
- Psychosocial support

FIRST VISIT

Comprehensive Health History:
- Biographical data/social history
- History of intimate partner violence
- Psychological assessment
- OB history/past pregnancy
- Gynecological history

Current Pregnancy:
- Presumptive, probable and positive symptoms
- Establish estimated date of birth
- Determine gravidity and parity
- Complete pregnancy testing
- Identify multiple gestation

Medical History:
- Identifies present health status
- Dental and eye health
- Status of maternal immunizations
- Educate re: environmental hazards

Ethnocultural Considerations:
- HTN more prevalent in African American and Hispanic women

What To Say:
- Use language a teen can relate to during discussions about sex

Across Care Settings:
- Health care safety net for vulnerable populations

Family Teaching Guidelines:
- DEEPERCARE acronym

Nursing Insight:
- Continuity of care decreases maternal stress
- Homelessness is a barrier to prenatal care
- Domestic violence is more common than preeclampsia or gestational diabetes in pregnancy
- Identify couples who would benefit from genetic testing
- Educate re: difference between screening and diagnostic testing
- Adolescents have greater health risks with multiple gestation
- Developmental tasks of pregnancy superimposed on those of adolescence

Complementary Care:
- Do not use blue cohosh

Assist Patient With

Nursing Role: CARE ing:
Communicating
Advocating
Respecting
Enabling/empowering

Choosing a care provider
- Management of pregnancy/childbirth
- Individualized care

Eustress:
- Role adaptation
- Restructuring of tasks

Distress:
- Accessing care
- Unknown/loss of control
- Lack of social support

- Navigating the health care system
- Coping with financial concerns

Prenatal Physical Exam:
- Explain; obtain consent
- Ensure privacy
- Actively engage patient
- Same order each visit

Includes:
- General assessment → i.e., observation, weight, VS
- Focused OB exam → Skin; breasts, abdomen, uterine size, fetal position, fetal heart auscultation, vagina, pelvis

Pregnant Adolescents:
- Long term social and developmental consequences

Nursing:
- Heighten public awareness; ID those teens at greatest risk
- Advocate for responsible sexual behavior
- Empower families with information: provide age-appropriate health education classes
- Be aware of denial of pregnancy → neonaticide
- Assess in a caring/accepting manner; frame exam in a learning context
- Assist with access to prenatal care
- Promote optimal nutrition

Screening and Diagnostic Tests:
- Blood tests: blood type, Rh, antibody screens, RPR, VDRL, hepatitis, CBC, HIV, sickle cell anemia, PPD
- STI screening: HIV, syphilis chlamydia, gonorrhea
- Cervical cancer

Woman Older than 35:
- Increased risk of preexisting medical conditions/obstetric complications

Nursing:
- Be aware of varying responses to pregnancy
- Structure prenatal education to meet unique needs
- Special assessment for breast/circulatory abnormalities
- Education re: screening tests for chromosomal abnormalities

Where Research And Practice Meet:
- Legal marriage improves birth outcomes
- Increase calcium/weight bearing exercise when Depo-Provera used pre-pregnancy
- Limitations exist in home pregnancy tests
- Repeated use of eye exam meds can be teratogenic
- Female infants at increased risk for hepatitis C

Optimizing Outcomes:
- Be an advocate for patient rights/access
- Promote dental health/dental exams
- Demonstrate professionalism during exams
- Low vitamin C intake linked to PROM
- Encourage use of supportive bra
- Routine genetic testing for Down Syndrome in those >35 years

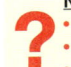

Be Sure To:
- Advocate for newborns at risk
- Allow adolescents to make health care decisions
- Recognize adolescent dad's rights

Now Can You:
- Discuss goals of prenatal care
- Discuss health promotion strategies for pregnancy
- Discuss components of prenatal assessment and various methods of clinical fetal assessment
- Discuss aspects of care for the pregnant adolescent and woman older than 35

Promoting a Healthy Pregnancy

 Little Seth, Precious One
What a miracle to be
A new life formed
Created from our deep love
And blessed by everyone above.

Our love combined as one
Creating a miracle of joy
Filling our hearts completely
Producing a baby boy.

Even though we have never seen your face
Or even heard your first cry
A special bond has been formed
Well deep from inside.

A bond that will never be broken
For as long as life shall be
Love will last forever
Far beyond than anyone can see.

As each day passes on
Your beginning edging nearer
We shield you from harm and
Pray for your well being
Until we may protect you in our arms.

You are our miracle soon to behold
For life is a beauty sometimes unseen
Ten tiny fingers, ten tiny toes
Perfection only to be seen.

You are so tiny, so small
So fragile, so sweet
A life not yet known
And yet loved so complete.

With all our love,
Mommy and Daddy
—Tamera and Daniel Ayriss

LEARNING TARGETS *At the completion of this chapter, the student will be able to:*

◆ Discuss holistic approaches for empowering women in planning for a healthy pregnancy.

◆ Describe factors that must be integrated to achieve optimal nutrition and weight gain during pregnancy.

◆ Assist a pregnant patient in formulating a daily food intake plan.

◆ Develop an exercise plan for women in the first, second, and third trimesters of pregnancy.

◆ Identify the signs of pregnancy and methods to manage the common associated discomforts.

◆ Recognize signs of impending complications of pregnancy and discuss interventions to decrease morbidity and mortality.

◆ Discuss the various methods of childbirth education.

◆ Assist a pregnant patient in developing a birth plan.

moving toward evidence-based practice Vitamin D Status During Pregnancy

Javaid, M.K., Crozier, S.R., Harvey, N.C., Dennison, E.M., Arden, N.K., Godfrey, K.M., & Cooper, C. (2006). Maternal vitamin D status during pregnancy and childhood bone mass at age 9 years: A longitudinal study. *The Lancet, 367*, 36–43.

The purpose of this longitudinal study was to investigate the effect of maternal vitamin D levels during pregnancy on childhood skeletal growth. The sample was composed of 198 Caucasian women who had participated in a previous study related to maternal nutrition and fetal growth. Other criteria for inclusion in the study were:

- Age greater than 16 years
- Initiated prenatal care before 17 weeks of gestation
- Delivered a singleton fetus at term

During the first and third trimesters the women completed a lifestyle questionnaire that included information concerning pre-pregnancy weight, smoking habits, and the use of dietary supplements during pregnancy. Assessments of maternal body build, nutritional status, and serum vitamin D levels were conducted. Beginning in the 7th month of gestation, personal exposure to ultraviolet B radiation was estimated from the number of hours of sunshine recorded by a local meteorological station.

After birth, each neonate's weight, crown–heel length, crown–rump length, and mid-upper-arm circumference were measured. Serum calcium levels were obtained from cord blood to provide a baseline indicator for vitamin D status, since vitamin D is essential for the metabolism of calcium.

Approximately 9 years later, the study participants and their children who continued to reside in the community were interviewed. At that time, nutritional status, physical activity patterns, and socioeconomic status were assessed for each mother and child. Each child's height, weight, whole body and lumbar-spine bone mineral content, bone area, and bone density were also obtained.

Findings from the study included the following:

Of the women participants:

- Average age was 27 years.
- 53% were primiparous.
- 31% smoked at the time of the last menstrual period; 20% continued to smoke during pregnancy.

- Vitamin D levels during late pregnancy were insufficient in 31% and deficient in 18%.
- All shared the same social class and general body build.

Of the offspring:

- Birth size and gestational length were similar.
- Birth weight, length, and abdominal and head circumference were unrelated to the maternal vitamin D level measured late in the pregnancy.
- Anthropometric characteristics at age 9 years were similar; the boys were slightly taller, heavier, and had a lower fat mass than the girls did.
- Those whose mothers had lower serum concentrations of vitamin D during late pregnancy had a reduced whole body bone mineral content and bone area at age 9 years.
- Neither height nor lean body mass were associated with the mother's vitamin D status during pregnancy.

Based on the findings, the researchers reached the following conclusions:

- Reduced maternal serum concentrations of vitamin D during late pregnancy were associated with decreased whole body and lumbar spine bone mineral content in the children at age 9 years.
- Bone mass in children and maternal vitamin D concentration were related to maternal use of vitamin D supplements and ultraviolet B radiation during late pregnancy.
- Insufficient vitamin D during pregnancy is associated with reduced bone-mineral accumulation during childhood.
- Vitamin D supplements taken during pregnancy may reduce the risk for osteoporosis-related fractures in the offspring.

1. What might be considered as limitations to this study?
2. How is this information useful to clinical nursing practice?

See Suggested Responses for Moving Toward Evidence-Based Practice on the Electronic Study Guide or DavisPlus.

Introduction

This chapter focuses on health promotion of childbearing women during preconception and throughout pregnancy. Counseling is an essential component of preconception care and provides information and education to women and families, which enables them to plan for their pregnancy and to develop a healthy body and a healthy mind surrounding the pregnancy.

Another important facet of health promotion during pregnancy is adequate nutrition and weight gain. Women need to have an understanding of essential elements required for a healthy pregnancy and of how to incorporate them into their daily diets. Along with diet and nutrition,

exercise, work, and rest must be balanced in order to achieve an optimal pregnancy outcome. Health care providers must provide guidelines for safe and beneficial exercise, which include teaching pregnant women about the effects of exercise and work.

This chapter also discusses the effects of medications during pregnancy and provides information concerning safe versus unsafe medications. Included in this section is information about over the counter medications, herbal therapies, and prescription medications. Certain medications are considered to be safe for use during pregnancy and these are incorporated into the discussion about the common discomforts of pregnancy.

Nurses and other health care providers can teach patients about common pregnancy discomforts to help alleviate anxiety and fear. Prenatal education also promotes empowerment that encourages women to manage pregnancy in a healthy manner. Pregnant women must also be knowledgeable about signs and symptoms of danger, including interventions that can be incorporated at home along with an understanding of when to seek professional care.

The course of a normal pregnancy, along with information concerning prenatal visits, is discussed in this chapter. Included in this section is a schedule for prenatal visits, information to be covered by the nurse at each visit, and laboratory tests that are completed with each visit. The nursing diagnosis: "*health seeking behaviors related to interest in maintaining optimal health during pregnancy*" is usually appropriate for women who regularly engage in prenatal care. Examples of other nursing diagnoses that address health promotion of the pregnant woman and her fetus are presented in Box 10-1.

Lastly, this chapter presents information about childbirth education, including a comparison of methods and strategies for finding information about various prenatal and childbirth education classes. As an integral part of promoting a healthy pregnancy and incorporating a holistic approach to care, women should be encouraged to develop a birth plan, which includes their preferences for care during the labor and birth of their child.

Planning for Pregnancy

Healthy People 2010 targets women of childbearing age with the goal of improving "the health and well-being of women, infants, children, and families" (U.S. Department of Health and Human Services [USDHHS], 2000, p. 16-3). To meet this goal, specific objectives are identified, focusing on the number of women receiving prenatal care, attendance at prepared childbirth education classes, delivery of low-birth-weight and very-low-birth-weight infants, preterm delivery, and maternal weight gain. One of the most important ways to facilitate meeting these objectives is for nurses and health care providers to promote healthy pregnancies in women through preconception counseling, individualized prenatal care, and identification and treatment of medical concerns and problems throughout the pregnancy.

Pregnancy care is a continuum that begins in adolescence. Once a female reaches menarche and is capable of reproduction, she should be cognizant of the fact that she could become pregnant and strive to achieve the best level of health that is possible. This time frame, which represents the earliest stage of the pregnancy continuum, is called **preconception**. The pregnancy continuum spans across the childbearing years and encompasses the prenatal period, birth, postpartum, and parenthood. **Periconception** is a term that generally refers to the time immediately before conception through the period of organogenesis, while **interconception** is the time period between the end of one pregnancy and the beginning of the next pregnancy. It is considered to be an optimal time to address problems that occurred with the previous pregnancy to minimize the likelihood of a repeated poor pregnancy outcome (Moos, 2006).

PRECONCEPTION COUNSELING: A TOOL TO HELP PROMOTE A POSITIVE PREGNANCY OUTCOME

It is during preconception that a woman builds the foundation for a healthy pregnancy long before she may ever even think of becoming pregnant. When a woman accesses her care provider during this time, it is known as preconception care. Ideally, health promotion for the pregnant woman should begin during the preconception period. Working with her health care provider during this time provides opportunities for empowering the woman for planning and carrying out a healthy pregnancy and birth.

The purpose of preconception care is to identify conditions, whether physical, psychological, or social, that could adversely affect a future pregnancy. By identifying these conditions early, interventions can be initiated to reduce or prevent potential complications that may be associated with them. Although certain conditions cannot be ameliorated, it may be possible to manage or treat them so that they have the smallest impact possible on future pregnancies. Each time a woman of childbearing age presents to her care provider for an annual gynecological exam, preconception counseling should be included, regardless of whether or not the woman is planning a pregnancy now or at any time in the foreseeable future.

Box 10-1 Possible Nursing Diagnoses Related to Health Promotion of the Pregnant Woman and Her Fetus

- Anxiety related to minor symptoms of pregnancy
- Disturbed Body Image related to change of appearance with pregnancy
- Fatigue related to metabolic changes of pregnancy
- Risk for Deficient Fluid Volume related to nausea and vomiting of pregnancy
- Constipation related to reduced peristalsis during pregnancy
- Deficient Knowledge related to inadequate information regarding nutritional needs during pregnancy
- Health-seeking Behaviors related to a lack of information about childbirth and newborn care
- Ineffective Coping related to lack of support people
- Risk for Fetal Injury related to maternal substance abuse

Optimizing Outcomes— Endorsing preconception care

The past decade has shown a growing trend among clinicians in women's health to expand the definition of prenatal care to include preconception counseling. National organizations such as the March of Dimes and the Centers for Disease Control and Prevention (CDC) endorse preconception counseling as an important component of care for women contemplating pregnancy or at risk of unintended pregnancy (Phillips, 2007). Nurses play a major role in endorsing preconception care for all women of childbearing age.

THE HEALTHY BODY

Preparing for pregnancy before becoming pregnant is the ideal, as it empowers women to become educated about the workings of their bodies and the benefits gained from pregnancy planning. During the preconception visit, the provider reinforces the importance of early and ongoing prenatal care and counsels the woman about establishing realistic expectations for pregnancy and its outcomes (American College of Obstetricians and Gynecologists [ACOG], 2005) (Fig. 10-1).

Menstrual and Medical History

When pregnancy is desired, the nurse can be instrumental in empowering the woman to take charge of her conception care by embracing a healthy lifestyle to ensure the best possible outcome. During the preconception visit, a review of the menstrual history guides the nurse in identifying specific needs so that an individualized conception plan can be developed. Determining the frequency and length of menstrual periods is essential information for teaching about the fertile period and how to enhance the likelihood of conception. The patient should be educated about the value of keeping an accurate menstrual calendar. She can be instructed to mark the first and every successive day of her menstrual periods on the calendar (Fig. 10-2). This information will help her to determine the length of each cycle and when to time sexual intercourse in succeeding months to increase the likelihood of conception. When pregnancy does occur, one of the first questions she will be asked is, "What was the first day of your last normal menstrual period (LNMP)?" If she has recorded this information, she can easily refer to her calendar for the accurate date.

There are times when charting a menstrual calendar also provides clues to menstrual and, perhaps, fertility problems. Some women have irregular cycles that are too close together or too far apart. This information, documented in a calendar, may signal the need for referral to a reproductive specialist.

A review of the family history is another important component of the preconception visit. Through the information gained, the woman's and her partner's extended families can be assessed for potential illnesses or diseases that tend to run in families. For this reason, it is desirable for the patient's partner to be present at the preconception visit so that he can accurately provide information about his family.

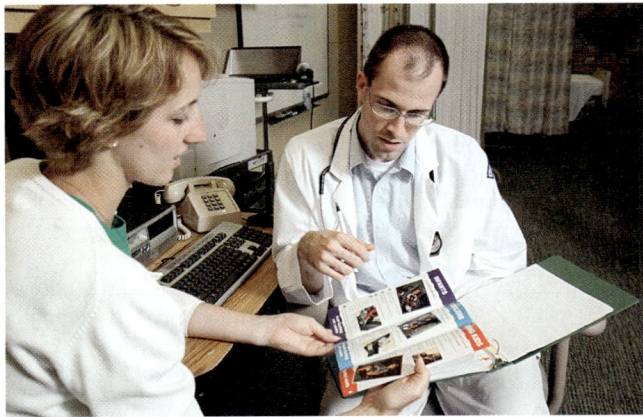

Figure 10-1 Health promotion for pregnancy begins during the preconception visit.

 Complementary Care: *Ayurveda to enhance the preconception period*

Ayurveda is a term derived from the words *ayur*, or life, and *veda*, or science. Developed hundreds of years ago in ancient India, Ayurveda is a system of natural and medical healing that includes diet, herbs, massage, exercise, music therapy, meditation, yoga, and aromatherapy. Practitioners of this modality believe that Ayurveda is beneficial during the preconception period in promoting optimal maternal and fetal health. According to Ayruveda, a healthy lifestyle is achieved by maintaining a mutually satisfying, harmonious emotional relationship while avoiding stress, tobacco, alcohol and drugs, meat, and dairy products (consume a vegetarian diet).

 Now Can You— Discuss preconception care?

1. Differentiate among preconception, periconception, and interconception?
2. Identify the purpose of preconception care?
3. Describe how to create a menstrual calendar?

INSTRUCTIONS: Shade in the appropriate box for every date of menstrual bleeding																														
January	1	2	3	4	5	6	7	8	9	10	11	12	13	14	15	16	17	18	19	20	21	22	23	24	25	26	27	28	29	30	31
February	1	2	3	4	5	6	7	8	9	10	11	12	13	14	15	16	17	18	19	20	21	22	23	24	25	26	27	28	{29}		
March	1	2	3	4	5	6	7	8	9	10	11	12	13	14	15	16	17	18	19	20	21	22	23	24	25	26	27	28	29	30	31
April	1	2	3	4	5	6	7	8	9	10	11	12	13	14	15	16	17	18	19	20	21	22	23	24	25	26	27	28	29	30	
May	1	2	3	4	5	6	7	8	9	10	11	12	13	14	15	16	17	18	19	20	21	22	23	24	25	26	27	28	29	30	31
June	1	2	3	4	5	6	7	8	9	10	11	12	13	14	15	16	17	18	19	20	21	22	23	24	25	26	27	28	29	30	
July	1	2	3	4	5	6	7	8	9	10	11	12	13	14	15	16	17	18	19	20	21	22	23	24	25	26	27	28	29	30	31
August	1	2	3	4	5	6	7	8	9	10	11	12	13	14	15	16	17	18	19	20	21	22	23	24	25	26	27	28	29	30	31
September	1	2	3	4	5	6	7	8	9	10	11	12	13	14	15	16	17	18	19	20	21	22	23	24	25	26	27	28	29	30	
October	1	2	3	4	5	6	7	8	9	10	11	12	13	14	15	16	17	18	19	20	21	22	23	24	25	26	27	28	29	30	31
November	1	2	3	4	5	6	7	8	9	10	11	12	13	14	15	16	17	18	19	20	21	22	23	24	25	26	27	28	29	30	
December	1	2	3	4	5	6	7	8	9	10	11	12	13	14	15	16	17	18	19	20	21	22	23	24	25	26	27	28	29	30	31

Figure 10-2 The menstrual calendar provides an accurate record for recording menstrual periods.

The Physical Examination

Using the patient history as a guide to help identify problems or special needs, the health care provider performs a complete physical examination. Along with the general physical assessment, a complete pelvic examination is also performed to evaluate the organs and bony structures of the pelvis. Abnormalities in this region can be crucial during pregnancy and childbirth. A Papanicolaou test (Pap smear), cultures for sexually transmitted infections (STIs), and cultures for other infections are often obtained during this exam as well. (See Chapter 9 for further discussion.)

Laboratory Evaluation

Every pregnant woman who presents for prenatal care is tested for various potential problems during the first visit and periodically throughout the antepartal period. The complete blood count (CBC) serves as the primary test for anemia via analysis of the hemoglobin and hematocrit. If the woman is anemic, the indices can aid in identifying the type of anemia (e.g., iron-deficiency, etc.). The patient can also be screened for infection by the white blood cell (WBC) count. If the WBCs are elevated, more information can be ascertained via the differential analysis. Platelets, essential components of the clotting mechanism, are also evaluated in a CBC.

Blood is also drawn for the identification of the woman's blood type, Rh status, and the presence of irregular antibodies. The blood type and Rh status are important in determining if the woman is at risk for developing isoimmunization during her pregnancy. This problem can occur if the woman's blood is Rh(D) negative and the fetus she is carrying is Rh(D) positive. Screening identifies the presence of antibodies that have been produced in response to exposure to fetal blood or other irregular antibodies that could potentially cause problems. (See Chapter 11 for further discussion.)

Exposure to Childhood Illnesses

Some of the routine maternal laboratory tests screen for childhood diseases that are known to cause congenital anomalies or other pregnancy complications if contracted during early pregnancy. Rubella, or German measles, was once a common childhood disease. Today, most women of childbearing age received rubella immunization during childhood. When contracted during the first trimester, rubella causes a number of fetal deformities. Therefore, all pregnant women are screened for rubella. A positive rubella screening test is indicative of immunity, and the woman cannot contract the disease. If the screening test is negative, the patient is advised to stay away from children who could possibly have the disease, and she is immunized for rubella after the infant is born.

Varicella (chickenpox) is another common childhood disease that may cause problems in the developing embryo and fetus. At present, an immunization for chickenpox is available and given to most children. If a woman presents for a preconception visit and her history reveals no prior chickenpox infection, she should be immunized before attempting pregnancy. Pregnant women should be questioned about childhood chickenpox, and a varicella titer may be obtained to confirm immunity. If nonimmune, the patient should be advised to avoid children who could potentially expose her to the chickenpox virus.

Finally, all adults should receive a tetanus booster immunization at least every 10 years. A booster can be given to the woman during the preconception period if she has not been immunized within the previous 10 years.

Exposure to Sexually Transmitted Infections

Sexually transmitted infections (STIs) may cause maternal and fetal complications during pregnancy. Routine screening for STIs aids in early detection and treatment. The Venereal Disease Research Laboratory (VDRL) test is a screening titer for syphilis that measures antibodies produced in mid-disease, but can produce a false positive result in women who are pregnant or who have rheumatoid arthritis or systemic lupus erythematosus. For these patients, a rapid plasma reagin (RPR) screening test may be used to confirm the presence of antibodies. In the event of a positive result, further testing is needed to confirm the findings and to determine whether the infection is in an active or latent phase.

In addition to screening for syphilis, all women should be screened for human immunodeficiency virus (HIV) during pregnancy (ACOG, 2004). If positive, therapy can be initiated to decrease the likelihood of transplacental viral transmission to the fetus. An important nursing role includes educating all women about HIV and the methods for decreasing the risk of infection.

Gonorrhea and chlamydia are cervical infections that can ascend through the cervix and increase the risk of premature rupture of the membranes and preterm labor. A cervical sample obtained during a speculum examination can be tested to determine if either of the pathogens is present.

Hepatitis B virus is a blood-borne infection that is acquired primarily by sexual contact or through exposure to infected blood. The Hepatitis B Surface Antigen (HBSaG) is used to screen for this infection. If the screening test is positive, further testing is indicated.

 Now Can You— Identify essential laboratory tests during preconception planning?

1. Discuss components of the CBC?
2. Explain the importance of identifying the woman's blood type and Rh status?
3. Identify routine screening tests performed for childhood diseases?
4. Describe the processes for sexually transmitted infection screening?

Genetic Testing

During the patient's first interview and visit, the nurse should ask questions that relate to the patient's and family's genetic history. Depending on the information gained, further blood work and testing may be indicated. For example, a positive family history of sickle cell disease or trait should be followed up with a maternal hemoglobin electrophoresis. If the patient tests positive, her partner should also be tested.

All women should be offered screening with maternal serum markers. Several different tests are available, such as the Triple Marker screen and the Quadruple Marker screen. Each tests for the presence of alpha-fetoprotein (AFP), estradiol, human chorionic gonadotropin (hCG), and other markers. These tests screen for potential neural tube defects, Down syndrome, and trisomy 18. If the screen is positive, the woman should be referred to a genetics specialist for counseling, and further testing, such as chorionic villus sampling (CVS) or amniocentesis, should be performed (ACOG, 2007).

While it is not possible to inquire about every inheritable disease or disorder, those most frequently encountered are addressed in Table 10-1.

ⓢ Optimizing Outcomes— Prenatal genetic testing

Prenatal nursing care is enhanced with the implementation of interventions for early diagnosis and treatment for the prevention of complications related to birth defects.

Best outcome: Provide prenatal interventions, including folic acid supplementation for all women of reproductive age, conduct rubella screening and immunization, teach women to avoid alcohol consumption during preconception and pregnancy, offer screening and detection of prenatal genetic disorders and early treatment of disorders when possible, and offer termination of pregnancy for severe defects.

Exposures Related to Lifestyle Choices

Several factors related to lifestyle choices can have detrimental effects on the developing fetus, including use of tobacco, alcohol, caffeine, artificial sweeteners, marijuana, and cocaine.

TOBACCO. Smoking during pregnancy causes a plethora of problems for the woman and the developing fetus. Carbon monoxide in the cigarette smoke binds more readily than oxygen to hemoglobin, thereby decreasing the oxygen-carrying capacity of the red blood cells. This alteration decreases the amount of oxygen traveling to the placenta, thereby decreasing the amount of oxygen available to the fetus for growth and development of tissues and organs.

The nicotine in the cigarette smoke also poses a significant risk to the developing fetus. Depending on the amount and the frequency of smoking, nicotine can act as either a stimulant or a relaxant. Nicotine causes the release of epinephrine, stimulating the "fight or flight" response that results in tachycardia, hypertension, and tachypnea. This response occurs in both the woman and her fetus. The stimulation of the sympathetic nervous system also prompts the release of cortisol from the adrenal glands, increasing blood glucose levels, and altering the body's immune response. Vasoconstriction results from stimulation of the sympathetic nervous system, causing decreased blood flow through the arteries and decreased oxygen transport to the placenta and the developing fetus.

Smoking is associated with spontaneous abortion, low birth weight, intrauterine growth restriction, preterm labor and birth, placenta previa, placental abruption, and premature rupture of the membranes. Infants born to mothers who smoke are more likely to be small for gestational age. Each of these complications predisposes the fetus to complications related to growth and physical and cognitive development. In fact, babies born to mothers who smoked during pregnancy are three times more likely to die from sudden infant death syndrome (SIDS) than babies born to women who do not smoke (U.S. Department of Health & Human Services [USDHHS], 2004).

Women who smoke should be encouraged to participate in a smoking cessation program. These programs are 50% to 70% effective in assisting and empowering women who smoke to be successful in quitting (March of Dimes, 2006). Smoking cessation during pregnancy reduces perinatal complications, even if the woman does not quit until the second or third trimester. (See Chapter 7 for further discussion.)

ALCOHOL. Alcohol consumption during pregnancy can cause physical and mental abnormalities in the developing fetus. Each year, more than 40,000 babies are born with complications resulting from alcohol use during pregnancy (March of Dimes, 2006). The current recommendation is that no alcohol consumption during pregnancy is safe, as no safe level has been determined.

Alcohol passes quickly through the placenta and reaches the fetal bloodstream much more rapidly than it does in adults. Fetal body system functions are immature and unable to metabolize alcohol, resulting in elevated alcohol levels and damage to developing organs and tissues. The resulting problems are manifested in the facial features associated with fetal alcohol syndrome (FAS): a low nasal bridge, short nose, flat midface, and short palpebral fissures. FAS is one of the most common causes of mental retardation. Body organs affected include the heart and the brain. Children born with lesser damage are diagnosed with fetal alcohol effects (FAEs), fetal alcohol spectrum disorder (FASD), or alcohol-related birth defects (ARBDs). (See Chapter 19 for further discussion.)

Heavy maternal drinking can result in spontaneous abortion or a low-birth-weight infant. In fact, heavy drinkers are two to four times more likely to have a spontaneous abortion than are nondrinkers (Centers for Disease Control & Prevention [CDC], 2002). While drinking alcohol should be discouraged for the duration of the pregnancy, many women do not know they are pregnant during the first few weeks. During this time, occasional alcohol consumption is not believed to harm the fetus. (See Chapter 7 for further discussion.)

ⓢ **Now Can You—** Discuss complications related to alcohol consumption during pregnancy?

1. Identify facial anomalies associated with FAS?
2. Identify fetal body organs affected by alcohol exposure?
3. Describe pregnancy complications related to alcohol consumption?

CAFFEINE. Caffeine acts as a central nervous system (CNS) stimulant, causing tachycardia and hypertension. Since caffeine readily passes through the placenta to the fetus, the effects of caffeine affect fetal heart rate and movement. High caffeine intake during pregnancy has been associated with preterm labor and birth as well as intrauterine growth restriction. However, no clear causation exists.

The primary sources of caffeine for most pregnant women include coffee, tea, and sodas. Other lesser known sources include chocolate, over-the-counter medications that contain

Table 10-1 Genetics Screening During Pregnancy

Disorder	Population Affected	Pathology	Pregnancy and Newborn Complications
Sickle cell disease	African Americans	• Autosomal recessive hemolytic disease	• Spontaneous abortion
	Persons of Mediterranean descent	• Involves an abnormal substitution of an amino acid in the structure of hemoglobin	• Preterm labor
		• Red blood cells assume abnormal, sickle shape in response to triggers, including hypoxia, infection, dehydration	• Intrauterine growth restriction
		• Results in inability to oxygenate tissues	• Stillbirth
		• Leads to occlusion and rupture of blood vessels	
Tay–Sachs disease	Ashkenazi Jews	• Lipid storage disease that results from a deficiency in hexosaminidase	• Infants appear normal at birth, until about 3–6 months of age
	Jewish people from eastern or central Europe	• Both parents must carry and pass on the trait to the child	• Neurological system begins to deteriorate
	French Canadians		• Death occurs between the ages of 2 and 4 years
	Cajuns		
Thalassemia	Greeks	• Disorder of hemoglobin synthesis	• Children appear normal at birth
	Italians	• Thalassemia minor: person is heterozygous for the trait; experiences fewer symptoms	• During first two years, become pale, lethargic, and develop jaundice
	Southeast Asians	• Thalassemia major: person is homozygous for the trait; experiences more severe symptoms	• Results in enlarged liver, spleen, and heart
	Filipinos		• Death results from heart failure and infection
Hemophilia	Males affected	• Mutation in the gene for coagulation factor VIII	• Males can have excessive bleeding when circumcised
	Females are carriers	• Causes a defect in blood clotting	• Increased incidence of intracranial hemorrhage
		• Leads to frequent bleeding episodes and hemorrhage	• Easy bruising and bleeding with injuries
Glucose-6-phosphate dehydrogenase (G6PD) deficiency	African Americans Seen mostly in males	• Causes drug-induced destruction of red blood cells when taking certain medications (e.g., sulfonamides)	• Increased incidence of pathological jaundice or hyperbilirubinemia due to destruction of red blood cells
Cystic fibrosis	Caucasians	• Autosomal recessive genetic disorder	• Results in chronic obstructive lung disease from thick mucous secretions in the lungs
		• Causes exocrine gland dysfunction	• Frequent lung infections occur
			• Causes a deficiency in pancreatic enzymes that prevents normal digestion

Data from: Cunningham et al., (2005); Kilpatrick & Laros (2004); & Lashley (2005).

caffeine as an ingredient, and dietary supplements. Women should be counseled that coffee and tea labeled "caffeine-free" still contain small amounts of caffeine.

Moderate intake of caffeine during pregnancy has not been found to cause perinatal problems. Women who are pregnant should limit their intake of caffeine to less than 300 mg/day, which is the equivalent of two (caffeinated) beverages per day (National Toxicology Program Center for the Evaluation of Risks to Human Reproduction, 2005). (See Chapter 7 for further discussion.)

ARTIFICIAL SWEETENERS. Aspartame (Nutrasweet®, Equal®), acesulfame potassium (Sunett®), and sucralose (Splenda®) have not been shown to have any negative effects associated with the developing fetus. However, because aspartame consists of two naturally occurring amino acids, women who have phenylketonuria (PKU) should not use this product. Saccharin, another artificial sweetener, is considered to be unsafe for use during pregnancy and should be avoided altogether.

MARIJUANA. No studies have documented fetal teratogenic effects associated with marijuana. Women who use marijuana, however, may engage in other high-risk behaviors (e.g., alcohol use) and the combination of effects may be associated with poor fetal outcomes. (See Chapters 7 and 9 for further discussion.)

COCAINE. It is difficult to determine the effects of cocaine use in pregnancy due to the high potential that the woman may be using other drugs and engaging in additional high-risk behaviors. Fetal exposure to cocaine is associated with an increased risk for congenital anomalies that most frequently occur in the cardiac and central nervous systems. The pregnant woman who uses cocaine is at risk for pregnancy complications that include stillbirth, abruptio placentae, preterm labor, preterm birth, and giving birth to an infant who is small for gestational age (SGA) (Stuart & Laraia, 2005). (See Chapters 7, 9, and 11 for further discussion.)

 Now Can You— Discuss substances to be avoided during pregnancy?

1. Name one harmful effect of caffeine during pregnancy?
2. Identify women who should be counseled to avoid the artificial sweetener aspartame?
3. Name three maternal/fetal complications that can result from cocaine use during pregnancy?

THE HEALTHY MIND

Maternal attachment to the fetus is an important area to assess and can be useful in identifying families at risk for maladaptive behaviors (Youngkin & Davis, 2004). The nurse should assess for indicators such as unintended pregnancy, intimate partner violence, difficulties in the partner relationship, sexually transmitted infections, limited financial resources, substance use, adolescence, poor social support systems, low educational level, and the presence of mental conditions that might interfere with the patient's ability to bond with and care for the infant (ACOG, 2006). It is important to remember that, depending on what is going on in her life at the time of the pregnancy, any woman has the potential for maladaptive behaviors.

Readiness for Motherhood

Motherhood is not necessarily instinctive for the pregnant woman. Each woman must work through the "process" of becoming a mother. Much of the woman's reservoir of beliefs about motherhood relate back to how she was parented as a child (Attrill, 2002). The pregnant woman must be able to see herself as a mother. To do so, she relies on her life experiences of how she was nurtured as a child and the types of relationships that she has developed over the years with other women (Lederman, 1996). The relationship with her own mother plays a significant role in how she views motherhood. If the woman's mother is available, accepting the pregnancy and respect for her daughter's autonomy play an integral role in assisting the woman to become a successful mother. Absence of some of these components may impede the pregnant woman's ability to develop into the motherhood role.

One way that a pregnant woman can demonstrate a positive attitude toward her pregnancy is by educating herself about maternal changes during pregnancy, fetal growth and development, and motherhood (Fig. 10-3). Many helpful books, brochures, online resources, and community programs on pregnancy and parenting are available for mothers-to-be.

Psychological Changes During Pregnancy

Hormone levels during pregnancy often play havoc with the pregnant woman's psyche. Progesterone exerts a depressant effect. Physical changes, changes in body image and fears related to becoming a mother, the impending labor and birth, and the increased responsibilities that accompany pregnancy and parenthood often produce anxiety or heighten depression during pregnancy (Youngkin & Davis, 2004). Providers must be aware of this potential and remain cognizant for signs and symptoms of mental illness in the pregnant woman. Referral to a mental health professional may be necessary.

The Healthy Relationship

The incidence of intimate partner violence (IPV) during pregnancy is high and, statistically, as many as 20% of pregnant women experience violence in the home (ACOG, 2006). Every woman should be screened for IPV during the initial visit and then as necessary (e.g., if bruises or other injuries are present) throughout the pregnancy. (See further discussion in Chapter 9.)

Maternal stress also has a negative effect on the developing fetus. Women who are anxious or stressed during their pregnancy are more likely to deliver preterm or to give birth to smaller babies. The nurse should assess all pregnant women for stressors and coping skills during pregnancy. (See Chapter 9 for further discussion.)

Figure 10-3 Learning about maternal changes, fetal growth and development and motherhood fosters a positive attitude toward the pregnancy.

Complementary Care: *Promoting stress management during pregnancy*

There are several complementary therapies that can safely be used during pregnancy, often recommended by nurse midwives and obstetricians:

- Massage therapy: Increases blood flow to maternal and fetal tissues; increases relaxation
- Chiropractic care: Treats lower back pain and headaches related to increased hormone levels
- Acupuncture and acupressure: Treat many physical ailments during pregnancy without the introduction of medications
- Relaxation exercises, meditation, and breathing techniques: Increase blood flow to maternal and fetal tissues; increase relaxation
- Light therapy: Enhances mood and treats depression
- Reflexology: Stimulates nerve pathways to increase blood flow and energy flow to corresponding areas of the body
- Aromatherapy: Increases relaxation

Readiness for Fatherhood

In preparation for parenthood, the male partner moves through a series of developmental tasks. During the first trimester, the father begins to deal with the reality of the pregnancy. At this time, he may worry about financial strain and his ability to be a good father. Feelings of confusion and guilt often surface with the recognition that he is not as excited about the pregnancy as is his partner. Couvade syndrome, the experience of maternal signs and symptoms, may develop. (See Chapter 8 for further discussion.)

In the second trimester, the pregnancy becomes more real for the father. The pregnancy begins to "show," and he is able to identify fetal movement through the maternal abdomen. Since there is an increased paternal willingness to learn about fetal growth and development during this time, the second trimester is the best time to provide prenatal education for the expectant couple.

During the third trimester, both parents are preparing for their new roles. Many of the father's early concerns regarding financial demands, personal parenting skills, and partner safety during birth return during this time. Conflicting feelings may emerge between excitement over the prospect of a new baby and the major lifestyle changes that will accompany the presence of a new family member. Most couples attend prenatal classes in preparation for the birth experience during the third trimester. The father may fear for the safety of his partner. How well the couple progresses through the developmental tasks of pregnancy has a major influence on their level of adaptation once the baby is born.

 Now Can You— **Discuss common paternal reactions and educational needs during pregnancy?**

1. Name two overriding concerns sometimes harbored by fathers during the first trimester?
2. Explain why pregnancy becomes more "real" for fathers during the second trimester?
3. Identify the trimester when education is likely to be most beneficial for the expectant couple?

Nutrition and Weight Gain

Nutrition and weight management play an essential role in the development of a healthy pregnancy. Not only does the patient need to have an understanding of the essential nutritional elements, but she must also be able to assess and modify her diet for the developing fetus and her own nutritional maintenance. To facilitate this process, it is the nurse's responsibility to provide education and counseling concerning dietary intake, weight management, and potentially harmful nutritional practices (Fig. 10-4).

 Optimizing Outcomes— **Resources for optimal nutritional counseling**

The document "Dietary Guidelines for Americans 2005" is an evidence-based resource guide for professionals and consumers that offers strategies for promoting health and reducing the risk for chronic diseases through diet and physical activity. Dietary guidelines, food composition, the food guide pyramid, dietary supplements, and resource lists are included in the guide (USDHHS & U.S. Department of Agriculture [USDA], 2005).

The nurse should obtain a nutritional history on all pregnant patients and patients of childbearing age. Information that is gained in a general nutritional assessment includes questions regarding eating patterns; changes in appetite, chewing, swallowing, and taste; presence of vomiting, diarrhea, or constipation; food allergies and intolerances; and self-care behaviors. In addition to these questions, the nurse needs to gain specific information related to the pregnancy, including:

- Foods that are preferred during pregnancy, which may provide information about cultural and environmental dietary factors
- Special diets, which will assist the nurse in planning for education or interventions for risk factors associated with dietary practices
- Cravings or aversions to specific foods

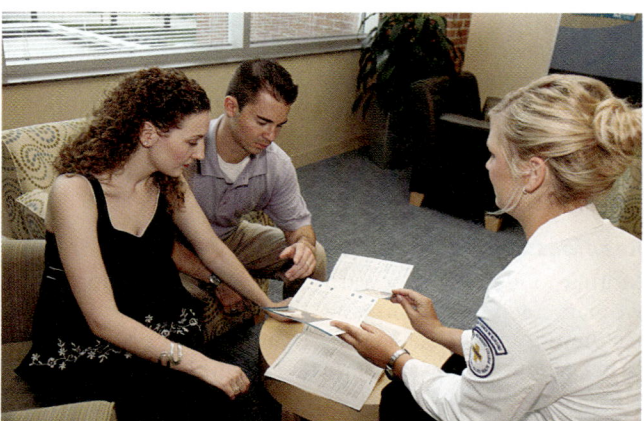

Figure 10-4 Nutritional counseling is an important component of prenatal care.

IMPORTANT NUTRITIONAL ELEMENTS

Many elements combine to facilitate a healthy pregnancy. Often pregnant women are told to eat as much as they want since "they are eating for two." However, this is not necessarily accurate advice. Practitioners must evaluate the amount as well as the nutritional value of the food consumed. Calories are an important consideration when planning the patient's daily food intake. Other essential nutritional elements are protein, water, iron, folic acid, and calcium. Maternal dietary practices that may exert a negative influence on the pregnancy must also be addressed.

Calories

A calorie, or unit of heat, signifies the energy expenditure of food. A kilocalorie (kcal) is equivalent to 1000 calories. It is the basic unit of measurement that more accurately defines the amount of energy needed to metabolize food and provide an energy source from this food (Venes, 2009). The body's energy needs are met by carbohydrate, fat, and protein in the diet.

The Recommended Daily Allowance (RDA) for caloric intake for nonpregnant women ranges from 1200 to 2400 kcal/day, depending on activity level. Women who are sedentary and who exercise less than 30 minutes per day should have a daily intake of 1200 kcal/day. Women who exercise vigorously for at least 30 minutes per day, 5 to 7 days per week, and engage in cardiovascular and strength training activities, should consume 2000 to 2400 kcal/day.

During pregnancy, the RDA for caloric intake increases only slightly, and requires only a 300 kcal/day increase from pre-pregnant needs. Growth during the first and second trimesters occurs primarily in the maternal tissues; during the third trimester, growth occurs mostly in the fetal tissues. An increase in maternal caloric intake is most important during the second and third trimesters. In the first trimester, the average maternal weight gain is 1 to 2.5 kg and thereafter the recommended weight gain for a woman of normal weight is approximately 0.4 kg per week. For overweight women, the recommended weekly weight gain during the second and third trimesters is 0.3 kg; for underweight women, it is 0.5 kg.

Pregnant women should be counseled about healthy ways to incorporate the additional 300 kcal needed in their daily diets. For example, adding an additional serving from each of the major food groups (skim milk, yogurt or cheese; fruits; vegetables; bread, cereal, rice or pasta) meets this need. It is essential for health care providers to stress to patients that the additional kilocalories should not be met through an increased intake of "empty calories" such as soda, candy, or simple carbohydrates.

Protein

Protein is necessary for tissue growth and repair. For pregnant women, protein is important for growth of maternal tissues, including the uterus and the breasts, and for development of fetal tissues and organs. Only a modest increase in protein is required; increasing intake of milk and dairy products by one or two servings per day meets the daily requirement for protein.

Protein is typically found in animal sources, specifically in meat, poultry, and fish. However, other protein sources are also available. Dairy products are a great source of protein, and include eggs, milk, cheese, and yogurt. For women who do not prefer dairy sources of protein, or who may be lactose intolerant, soy milk and soy cheese are available as protein-rich substitutes. In addition, beans and legumes provide a rich source of protein as well as fiber to the diet and can be substituted for protein servings in many meals. Peanut butter is another source rich in protein, but potentially high in fat. Beans and legumes are combined protein sources that provide carbohydrates with protein to supply the essential amino acids that may be missing when insufficient protein from animal sources is consumed.

A word of caution should be provided by health care providers to pregnant women with regard to microbial foodborne illness (USDHHS, 2005). Raw, or unpasteurized, milk, as well as partially cooked eggs and foods containing raw or partially cooked eggs should be avoided. Deli meats, luncheon meats, and frankfurters should be heated before consumption. In addition, raw shellfish and fish high in mercury, including shark, swordfish, tilefish, and king mackerel should be avoided. Fresh or frozen tuna, red snapper, and orange roughy contain moderate amounts of mercury and women who are pregnant or planning to become pregnant should limit their intake of these products to 12 ounces per week.

Water

Water is necessary for all body tissues and all body system functions. It is essential for the maintenance of life, and must be consumed in sufficient quantity to sustain homeostasis. All persons should consume six to eight (8-oz.) glasses of fluid daily; however, pregnant women should have an intake of eight to ten (8-oz.) glasses of fluid per day. The increased amount needed during pregnancy is necessary to meet the changing physiology of the maternal cardiovascular system and to maintain adequate blood flow to the fetus.

During pregnancy, blood volume increases about 1500 mL, which represents a 40% to 50% increase from the pre-pregnancy blood volume. The increase in maternal blood volume occurs for three primary reasons: to meet the needs of the hypertrophied vascular system of the enlarged uterus, to adequately hydrate maternal and fetal tissues, and to provide a fluid reserve for blood loss during childbirth. In addition, adequate blood flow to the fetus is necessary for oxygenation of body tissues and maintenance of a normal acid–base balance.

Water intake can be in the form of many different types of fluids, including fruit juice and vegetable juice. However, at least four to six glasses of the fluid consumed each day should be water. Patients should be cautioned to consume certain beverages, such as diet sodas (high in sodium and contain artificial sweeteners) and caffeinated drinks (promote diuresis) in moderation. Alcohol should be avoided entirely throughout the pregnancy, as no safe amount has been determined.

Minerals and Vitamins

Women who eat a balanced diet that includes recommended servings and serving sizes may meet the recommended nutritional needs during pregnancy without vitamin supplementation. However, the need for an increased intake of specific nutrients must be taken into consideration as the pregnant woman plans her diet. Specifically, the daily intake of calcium, iron, and folic acid must be adequate to meet the maternal–fetal needs for adequate growth and development.

CALCIUM AND VITAMIN D. The RDA for calcium is 1000 mg/day in pregnant and pre-pregnant women. Calcium requirements are increased in pregnant adolescents, who need an intake of 1300 mg/day. Without supplementation, most women fail to consume adequate amounts of dietary calcium. Calcium is essential for maintaining bone and tooth mineralization and calcification. During pregnancy, calcium must be available to the fetus for the growth and development of the skeleton and teeth.

Dairy products, especially milk and milk products, constitute the best nutritional sources of calcium. Three daily servings of dairy products are recommended for women; one to two additional daily servings of milk are recommended during pregnancy (USDHHS, 2005). Other rich sources of calcium include legumes, dark green leafy vegetables, dried fruits, and nuts.

 Optimizing Outcomes— **Teaching patients to avoid bone meal supplements**

Bone meal, sometimes used as a calcium source, should be avoided during pregnancy. This supplement is frequently contaminated with lead, a toxin that readily crosses the placenta and can result in high levels in the fetus.

Vitamin D is important in the absorption and metabolism of calcium. Milk and ready-to-eat cereals constitute the major food sources of vitamin D, which is also produced in the skin by the action of sunlight. Women who do not include milk in their diets should be taught about other vitamin D sources such as cereals, egg yolks, liver, and seafood. Also, since the use of sunscreens with a recommended SPF rating of 15 reduces the skin vitamin D production by up to 99% (Scanlon, 2001), all women should be taught about the need for vitamin D-fortified foods or supplements.

 Ethnocultural Considerations— **Vitamin D deficiency**

African Americans and other women with dark skin are at the greatest risk for vitamin D deficiency. Women who habitually cover most of their skin with clothing and those who live in northern latitudes with limited exposure to sunlight are also more likely to be deficient in vitamin D.

IRON AND VITAMIN C. As blood volume increases during pregnancy, the number of circulating red blood cells also increases. Maternal iron intake must be increased to maintain the oxygen-carrying capacity of the blood and to provide an adequate number of red blood cells. Fetal iron needs are increased during the last trimester. At this time, iron is stored in the immature liver for use during the first 4 months of life while the liver matures and liver enzymes are being produced. The newborn uses the stored iron to compensate for insufficient amounts of iron in the breast milk and in non-iron-fortified infant formula.

The iron RDA for pre-pregnant women is 18 mg/day, and for pregnant women, this amount increases to 30 mg/day, starting by 12 weeks of gestation (Institute of Medicine,

1992). Iron can be found in a variety of food sources. Many individuals may not be aware that adequate amounts of iron are found in fortified ready-to-eat cereals, white beans, lentils, spinach, kidney beans, lima beans, soybeans, shrimp, and prune juice. Red meats, including beef, duck, and lamb, contain moderate amounts of iron as well. Some of the best food sources for iron include oysters, organ meats (liver, giblets), and fortified instant cooked cereals. Interestingly, canned, drained clams provide the highest amount of iron per serving, with 23.8 mg of iron in each 3-ounce serving.

While most other necessary nutrients can be met through a balanced diet, it is almost impossible to meet the maternal daily requirements for iron without a dietary supplement. Consideration must be given, however, to the gastrointestinal side effects of supplemental iron, which include constipation, black tarry stools, nausea, and abdominal cramping. These side effects may exacerbate other pregnancy-related gastrointestinal discomforts. Daily iron supplementation is often initiated at around 12 weeks of gestation in order to avoid compounding the nausea commonly prevalent during the first trimester. Adequate water intake helps to decrease constipation, and patients may take the iron at bedtime if abdominal discomfort is experienced when taking iron between meals.

Nursing Insight— *When teaching about iron supplements*

Nurses can teach patients about substances known to decrease the absorption of iron. Women should be taught to avoid consuming bran, tea, coffee, milk, oxylates (found in Swiss chard and spinach), and egg yolk at the same time as they take the iron supplement. Also, iron is best absorbed when taken between meals with a beverage other than tea, coffee, or milk.

---

medication: Ferrous Sulfate

Ferrous sulfate (**fer**-us **sul**-fate)

Pregnancy Category B

Indications: Prevention/treatment of iron-deficiency anemia

Actions: An essential mineral found in hemoglobin, myoglobin, and many enzymes. Prevents iron deficiency.

Therapeutic Effects: Prevents/treats iron deficiency

Pharmacokinetics

ABSORPTION: Therapeutically administered PO iron may be 60% absorbed; absorption is an active and passive transport process.

CONTRAINDICATIONS AND PRECAUTIONS: Use cautiously in peptic ulcer, ulcerative colitis; indiscriminate chronic use may lead to iron overload.

Adverse Reactions and Side Effects: Constipation, dark stools, diarrhea, epigastric pain, gastrointestinal bleeding

Route and Dosage (mg elemental iron): 100–200 mg/day (2–3 mg/kg per day) in three divided doses

Nursing Implications:
1. Assess nutritional status and dietary history to determine possible cause of anemia and need for patient teaching.
2. Assess bowel function for constipation or diarrhea; notify care provider and use appropriate nursing measures if these symptoms occur.

Data from Deglin, J.H., & Vallerand, A.H. (2009). *Davis's drug guide for nurses* (11th ed.). Philadelphia. F.A. Davis.

Vitamin C (ascorbic acid), important in tissue formation, also enhances the absorption of iron. Women who take iron supplements should consume foods or beverages that contain vitamin C. Food sources rich in vitamin C include red and green sweet peppers, oranges, kiwi fruit, grapefruit, strawberries, Brussels sprouts, cantaloupe, broccoli, sweet potatoes, tomato juice, cauliflower, pineapple, and kale. Most pregnant women are able to meet the recommended daily allowance (80 to 85 mg) by including at least one daily serving of citrus fruit or juice or vitamin C-rich food source, although women who smoke need more.

Inadequate iron intake can lead to anemia, a decrease in the oxygen-carrying capacity of the blood. Physiological anemia, common during pregnancy, occurs when the plasma volume increases more than the red blood cell mass, producing a modest decrease in the hemoglobin concentration and hematocrit. True anemia, or iron-deficiency anemia, occurs when the hemoglobin level drops below 10 g/dL. The blood's decreased oxygen-carrying capacity causes a reduction in oxygen transport to the developing fetus. Decreased fetal oxygen transport has been associated with intrauterine growth restriction (IUGR) and preterm birth.

Ethnocultural Considerations— Anemia during pregnancy

In the United States, maternal anemia occurs most commonly among adolescents, African American women, and women of lower socioeconomic status (Siega-Riz & Savitz, 2001; Swensen, Harnack, & Ross, 2001).

In recent years, there has been some controversy surrounding the value of iron supplementation during pregnancy (Haram, Nilsen, & Schall, 2001; Mahomed, 2002; Scholl & Reilly, 2000). Although iron supplementation enhances maternal hematological values, its role in improving pregnancy outcomes is unclear. However, maternal iron supplementation is believed to improve fetal iron stores and reduce the risk of anemia in the infant during the first year of life (Haram et al., 2001). Furthermore, women who have iron-deficiency anemia during the early months of pregnancy are at an increased risk for preterm birth (Scholl, 2005).

FOLIC ACID   Vitamin B_9, or folic acid (folate), is a water-soluble vitamin that is closely related to iron. Working with vitamin B_{12}, folic acid helps to regulate red blood cell development and facilitates the oxygen-carrying capacity of the blood. Folic acid is essential in the production of DNA and RNA, and helps to maintain normal brain function and to stabilize mental and emotional health. Folic acid also works with vitamins B_6 and B_{12} to control blood levels of homocysteine, an amino acid that, in elevated amounts, has been linked to heart disease, depression, and Alzheimer's disease.

Increased estrogen production during pregnancy alters the absorption and metabolism of folic acid, producing an increased maternal susceptibility for folic acid deficiency. Folic acid deficiency is primarily responsible for the development of neural tube defects, including spina bifida, cleft lip and palate, and anencephaly. The neural tube is the embryonic structure that divides during embryo-fetal development to form the CNS, including the spinal cord

and the brain. (See Chapter 7 for further discussion.) The folic acid RDA for nonpregnant women is 400 mcg/day. During pregnancy, a minimum of 800 mcg/day of folic acid is recommended, and this amount is usually provided through supplementation. Childbearing aged women who have previously given birth to an infant with a neural tube defect or those who have a positive family history of neural tube defects are encouraged to consume 1 to 4 mg of folic acid each day (ACOG, 2003a; Veterans Health Administration, 2002).

The neural tube develops during the first 4 weeks after conception. During these early developmental weeks, the majority of women do not yet know that they have conceived. Because of the strong connection between folic acid deficiency and the subsequent development of neural tube defects, all women of childbearing age should take a folic acid supplement of at least 400 mcg/day. Research has indicated that an adequate intake of folic acid during the periconceptional period can reduce the incidence of neural tube defects by up to 50% (Krishnaswamy & Madhavan Nair, 2001; Lewis, Van Dyke, Stumbo, & Berg, 1998). Findings from studies also show an association between folic acid deficiency, elevated homocysteine, and the development of Down syndrome and childhood leukemia (Thompson, Gerald, Willoughby, & Armstrong, 2001).

Foods that are rich in folic acid include dark leafy greens, asparagus, Brussels sprouts, soybeans, liver, root vegetables, beans, and orange juice. Since 1998, all enriched grain products produced in the United States contain folic acid (Lewis et al., 1998), and this nutritional supplementation has decreased the incidence of neural tube defects by 19%. Current recommendations include consuming folic acid with vitamin C to enhance the absorption of iron and folic acid.

 Now Can You— **Discuss aspects of good nutrition during pregnancy?**

1. Identify two protein sources for women who wish to avoid dairy products?
2. Identify three calcium sources for women who wish to avoid dairy products?
3. Explain why adequate intake of vitamin C and folic acid are important during pregnancy?

WEIGHT GAIN DURING PREGNANCY

Weight gain is expected during pregnancy and results from a combination of maternal physiological changes and fetal growth. During early pregnancy, maternal weight gain is related to an increased blood volume, necessary to supply the enlarging uterus and support fetal growth and development. Dilation of the renal pelvis and ureters from increased blood flow adds volume to the bladder and results in an increased production of urine. Essential nutrients provided through the maternal blood supply enable fetal growth and development. As the pregnancy progresses, enlargement of the placenta and fetal body add to the woman's increase in weight. By term, maternal extracellular fluid, blood, uterine tissue, and breast tissue comprise 35% of the gestational weight gain; the maternal reserves comprise 27%; fetal tissue comprises 27%; and placental fluid comprises 11% of the total maternal weight gain (King, 2006).

Factors Affecting Weight Gain

In addition to maternal–fetal physiological factors, social influences are also important predictors of gestational weight gain (Stotland, 2006). Social factors related to an insufficient maternal weight gain may include an inability to purchase food, inadequate dairy intake, unplanned pregnancy, intimate partner violence, anorexia nervosa, shortened time period between pregnancies, and lack of prenatal care. Factors that may influence an excessive maternal weight gain during pregnancy include inadequate or inconsistent physical activity, a high carbohydrate or fat intake, excessive consumption of sweets, and lack of prenatal care.

An adverse outcome may result when the woman gains too much or too little weight during her pregnancy. Health care providers need to assess the patient's weight during the first prenatal visit and monitor the weight gain closely throughout the pregnancy. The amount of weight that is gained during the gestational period results from a combination of influences, including biological and social factors. Biological factors include genetic alleles that affect phenotypes responsible for regulating energy and fat metabolism. These, in turn, affect maternal weight and fat gain during pregnancy. High levels of insulin and leptin (a protein hormone that regulates energy metabolism and appetite) during the first trimester are also associated with higher maternal weight and fat gain during pregnancy (Stotland, 2006).

Women who gain too much weight during pregnancy are at an increased risk for gestational diabetes. This complication places the infant at risk for macrosomia (large body size), congenital anomalies, birth trauma, perinatal asphyxia, respiratory distress syndrome, hypoglycemia, hypocalcemia, cardiomyopathy, hyperbilirubinemia, and polycythemia. Gestational diabetes also increases the risk for maternal **preeclampsia**. Preeclampsia is a condition associated with a decreased blood supply to the maternal organs and to the developing fetus and may result in preterm birth, premature rupture of membranes, maternal organ damage, thrombocytopenia, intrauterine growth restriction, and an altered acid–base balance in the fetus (Mayo Foundation for Medical Education and Research, 2005). (See Chapter 11 for further discussion.)

Management of Weight During Pregnancy

Classification of weight is often based on **body mass index** (**BMI**), which is a method of evaluating the appropriateness of weight for height. The BMI is calculated using the formula:

$$BMI = \frac{Weight}{Height^2}$$

where the weight is recorded in kilograms and the height is in meters. For example, the calculated BMI for a woman who weighed 52 kg before pregnancy and is 1.58 m tall is:

$$BMI = \frac{52}{1.58^2} = 20.8$$

Persons with a BMI less than 18.5 are underweight; those with a BMI between 25 and 29.9 are overweight. Persons with a BMI between 30 and 34.9 are classified at Level 1 obesity; those with a BMI between 35 and 39.9 are classified at Level 2 obesity. Extreme obesity, or Level 3 obesity, includes persons with a BMI of 40 or above (Cogswell & Dietz, 2006). Given the increase in obesity in the United

States, one of the *Healthy People 2010* goals (USDHHS, 2000) is to increase the number of women who attain a recommended weight gain during their pregnancies, in consultation with their health care provider (Table 10-2).

There are also recommendations for specific populations of pregnant women. Pregnant adolescents and women of color should attempt to gain weight at the upper end of the appropriate range for their pre-pregnant BMI. Women of short stature (less than 62 inches [1.6 m] in height) should attempt to gain weight at the lower end of the appropriate range for the pre-pregnant BMI. Women pregnant with twins or triplets should gain a total of 35 to 45 lbs. (16 to 20.5 kg), primarily during the second and third trimesters.

Ideally, weight management begins before the pregnancy. At the preconception visit, women should be screened for height and weight, with the BMI calculated as a beginning point for determining an appropriate weight gain during pregnancy (Institute for Clinical Systems Improvement, 2005). The BMI and weight are then monitored at each prenatal visit. Throughout the pregnancy, counseling, educational interventions, and prophylaxis are provided (Table 10-3). Since excess weight gain during early pregnancy is associated with an increased incidence of gestational diabetes, new recommendations indicate that complications can be decreased if screening for gestational diabetes takes place during the first trimester (Riley, 2006).

PLANNING DAILY FOOD INTAKE

While planning daily food intake is based on individual preferences, consideration must be given to ensure that adequate nutrients are provided without an excessive increase in caloric intake. New guidelines indicate strategies for daily food consumption (USDHHS, 2005). The primary recommendations include the following:

- Including a variety of nutrient-dense foods and fluids while limiting saturated and trans fats, cholesterol, excessive sugar, salt, and alcohol
- Developing a balanced daily eating pattern, using the USDA Food Guide or the DASH Eating Plan (see below).

Specific recommendations for women of childbearing age and women who are pregnant incorporate the following strategies:

- Eating iron-rich foods or iron-fortified foods
- Including vitamin C to enhance the absorption of iron
- Including folic acid through consumption of fortified foods or supplemental folic acid

Table 10-2 Recommended Total Weight Gain During Pregnancy for a Single Birth	
Pre-Pregnancy BMI	**Recommended Total Weight Gain**
Underweight (<19.8)	28–40 lbs.
Normal weight (19.8–26)	25–35 lbs.
Overweight (>26–29)	15–20 lbs.
Obese (>29)	15+ lbs.

From the National Heart, Lung and Blood Institute (2006). Body mass index. Retrieved from www.nhlbi.nih.gov/guidelinesbmi_tbl.htm.

The *USDA Food Guide* visualized by the new Food Pyramid is based on individual factors, including age, gender, and activity level. No longer does "one size fit all." The new Food Pyramid is based on the guiding principles of overall health, up-to-date research, total diet, usefulness, realism, flexibility, practicality, and evolution. Using the name "MyPyramid" the Guide focuses the patient on developing an individual approach to daily dietary planning (see Fig. 4-1). The pyramid is color-coded to provide a visual view of the types and amounts of food that should be eaten. The bands are wide on the bottom and narrow on the top, indicating what nutrient-dense foods need to be consumed. The colors indicate the following:

- Orange: Grain group—make one half of the grain selections whole grains
- Green: Vegetable group—vary vegetables, and include green, red, and yellow vegetables
- Red: Fruit group—focus on fruits of various types
- Blue: Milk group—consume calcium-rich foods
- Purple: Meat and bean group—consume lean protein
- Yellow: Oils—not considered a food group, but essential as a source of essential fatty acids and vitamin E

The DASH (Dietary Approaches to Stop Hypertension) Eating Plan resulted from a study designed to investigate whether the typical American diet affected blood pressure (USDHHS, 2006). The diet plan includes the daily consumption of whole grain products, fish, poultry, and nuts. There is also a focus on reducing lean red meat, sweets, and added sugar found in foods and beverages. The DASH Eating Plan encourages an increased intake of potassium, magnesium, calcium, protein, and fiber. Table 10-4 compares the daily servings and serving sizes between the USDA Food Guide and the DASH Eating Plan.

 Now Can You— **Plan a Daily Menu for a Woman Who Is Pregnant?**

1. Identify proteins that meet pregnancy needs?
2. Suggest foods to increase daily intake of potassium, magnesium, calcium, protein, and fiber?
3. Describe foods that should be avoided by women who are pregnant?

 case study Excessive Weight Gain During Pregnancy

Tamara, a 24-year-old primigravida at 26 weeks' gestation, has presented for a routine second-trimester prenatal visit. During the interview with the nurse, Tamara voices no complaints. Her vital signs and laboratory data are assessed and all are within normal limits. However, her weight today is 155 lbs. (70.5 kg), which represents a 30-lb. (13.6 kg) weight gain from her pre-pregnancy weight. Tamara has no preexisting health conditions. She is married and lives in a mobile home. She works part time at a local fast food restaurant and readily admits that she enjoys eating the food served there.

Critical Thinking Questions

1. What are the major health concerns regarding Tamara at this time?
2. What patient education should the nurse provide for Tamara?
3. What additional care should be provided for Tamara?

◆ See Suggested Answers to Case Studies in the text on the Electronic Study Guide or DavisPlus.

Table 10-3 Recommendations for Weight Management During Pregnancy			
Time Frame	**Screening**	**Education**	**Prophylaxis**
Preconception Visit	Height Weight BMI calculation	Nutrition and weight	Folic acid supplementation
Initial Prenatal Visit: First Trimester	Height Weight BMI calculation	Lifestyle education on nutrition	Nutritional supplements
Subsequent Visits Up to 22 weeks	Weight	Follow-up on risk factors	Nutrition evaluation
Visit at approximately 22 weeks	Weight	Gestational diabetes	Nutrition evaluation
Visits from 28 to 36 weeks	Weight	Follow-up on risk factors	Nutrition evaluation
Visits from 38 to 41 weeks	Weight	Follow-up on risk factors	Discussion of postpartum nutrition

Adapted from: Institute for Clinical Systems Improvement (ICSI). (2005). Routine prenatal care. Bloomington, MN.

FACTORS AFFECTING NUTRITION DURING PREGNANCY

Several additional factors affect nutrition during pregnancy, and may lead to potentially adverse effects. These factors include eating disorders and certain cultural variations.

Eating Disorders

PICA. **Pica**, the consumption of non-nutritive substances or food, is a common eating disorder that can affect pregnancy. Substances that are most often ingested include clay, dirt, cornstarch, and ice (Fig. 10-5). Some individuals engage in poly-pica, the practice of consuming more than one of the non-nutritive substances. Pica occurs with greater frequency in developmentally disabled persons. There is also a cultural link that is considered nonpathological and is seen more commonly in African Americans and persons of mid-Eastern lineage (Mills, 2007).

Causes of pica are believed to include nutritional deficiencies, cultural and familial factors, stress, low socioeconomic status, and biochemical disorders. Specific nutritional deficiencies associated with pica include deficiencies in iron, calcium zinc, thiamine, niacin, vitamin C, and vitamin D. The consumption of clay and starch is most commonly seen in southern, rural, African American communities, and it is believed that this practice, especially the practice of eating starch, was first initiated to alleviate the discomfort of nausea in early pregnancy.

Treatment of pica focuses on the diagnosis and treatment of underlying nutritional deficiencies. The practice usually subsides after the birth of the baby.

 Ethnocultural Considerations— Consuming non-nutritive substances

Health care providers need to have an understanding of the cultural and religious factors associated with pica. In some cultures, non-nutritive food substances are thought to bring health or have positive spiritual effects for those who consume them. Some cultures believe that the consumption of specific non-nutritive substances plays a role in enhancing fertility or promoting luck within the family. The health care provider's knowledge and understanding about pica can provide opportunities for assessing complications in patients, providing education to reduce the behavior when harmful, or discussing alternatives for meeting the patient's needs.

ANOREXIA NERVOSA AND BULIMIA NERVOSA. Anorexia nervosa and bulimia nervosa are conditions characterized by a distorted body image. Both involve an intense fear of becoming obese and can have a major impact on the person's physical and psychological well-being. Patients with **anorexia nervosa** lose weight either by excessive dieting or by purging themselves of calories they have ingested. Patients with **bulimia nervosa** engage in recurrent episodes of binge eating, self-induced vomiting and diarrhea, excessive exercise, strict dieting, or fasting and display an exaggerated concern about body shape and weight (Venes, 2009).

Both of these eating disorders pose potentially harmful effects on the woman and the developing fetus, as nutrients are either not consumed or are quickly eliminated

Table 10-4 Comparison of USDA Food Guide and DASH Eating Plan

Food Groups and Subgroups	USDA Food Guide Amount	DASH Eating Plan Amount
Fruit Group	2 cups (4 servings)	2–2.5 cups (4–5 servings)
Vegetable Group	2.5 cups (5 servings)	2–2.5 cups (4–5 servings)
Dark green vegetables	3 cups/week	
Orange vegetables	2 cups/week	
Legumes	3 cups/week	
Starchy vegetables	3 cups/week	
Other vegetables	6.5 cups/week	
Grain Group	6 ounce-equivalents	7–8 ounce-equivalents (7–8 servings)
Whole grains	3 ounce-equivalents	
Other grains	3 ounce-equivalents	
Meat and Beans Group	5.5 ounce-equivalents	6 ounces or less of meat, poultry, fish
		4–5 servings/week of nuts, seeds, and dry beans
Milk Group	3 cups	2–3 cups
Oils	27 grams (6 tsp)	8–12 grams (2–3 tsp)

Source: U.S. Department of Agriculture. Dietary Guidelines for Americans 2005: Sample USDA Food Guide and the DASH Eating Plan at the 2,000-Calorie Level.

Box 10-2   Basic Prenatal Exercises

Basic prenatal exercises to help generate energy, diminish discomfort, and improve balance and stamina:

- **Arm and upper back stretch:** Raise your arms above your head, keeping the elbows straight, palms facing one another and hold for twenty second. Lower your arms to your sides. Bring the backs of your hands together behind your back and stretch.
- **Pelvic tilt:** Lie on your back with your knees slightly bent. Inhale through your nose while tightening your stomach muscles and buttocks. Flatten your back against the floor and tilt your pelvis slightly upward. Slowly exhale through your mouth while counting to five. Relax.
- **Sit-ups:** Lie on your back with your knees slightly bent. Inhale through your nose. While breathing out slowly through pursed lips, raise your head with your hands placed behind your head. Tuck your chin toward your chest and slightly lift your shoulders off the floor.
- **Kegels:** Before beginning this exercise for the first time, isolate the pubococcygeal (PC) muscle, which is the muscle used to start and stop the flow of urine. Practice stopping the flow of urine a few times; do not continue to do this as this may lead to a urinary tract infection. If you have difficulty isolating the muscle in this fashion, insert a clean finger into the vaginal opening and squeeze. This is the muscle that will tighten as the exercise is done properly. Kegel exercises will help to support the growing baby by strengthening the pelvic floor, assist during the birth process, decrease urinary problems during postpartum, and help to prevent hemorrhoids.
  - Squeeze the PC muscle for five seconds, then relax for five seconds. Repeat for a total of ten repetitions each day.
  - Squeeze and release the PC muscle as rapidly as possible for a total of ten times.
  - Increase this exercise up to 100 repetitions each day.
- **Squatting:** Move to a squatting position, with the knees located directly over the toes. Keeping your heels flat on the floor, stretch the back of the thighs. Hold for 20 to 30 seconds. Increase time to 60 to 90 seconds. Remember to keep your head and arms relaxed during this exercise.
- **Calf stretch:** Lean against a wall or flat surface with your hands against the surface. Move one leg behind you, keeping your heel flat on the floor. Lean into the wall to stretch the calf muscles. Hold for 20 to 30 seconds. Repeat with the other leg. This exercise will help to reduce leg cramps experienced during pregnancy.

with the health care provider, include general health and well-being, the overall progression of the pregnancy, present age, prior pregnancy complications, the type of work performed, the number of hours worked, and the environmental and safety risk factors associated with the work.

Evaluation of Work and Its Impact on the Pregnancy

The pregnant woman may be advised to reduce the number of hours worked if the job requires heavy lifting, prolonged standing, extensive walking, or physical exertion. When the nature of the work is physically demanding, safety concerns may require that she stop working altogether. The potential for maternal exposure to toxic substances such as chemotherapeutic agents, lead, and ionizing radiation (found in laboratories and health care facilities) or heavy machinery and other hazardous equipment should prompt reassignment to a different work

area. If reassignment is not possible, the woman may need to stop working until the pregnancy has been completed. Women who are currently experiencing pregnancy complications and those who have a history of pregnancy complications or other preexisting health disorders may be required to reduce their hours or stop working as well. Examples of problems and pregnancy complications that may necessitate a change in work hours include diabetes, kidney disease, heart disease, back problems, hypertension, and a history of spontaneous abortion or preterm labor.

Planning for Maternity Leave

Maternity leave provides the woman with time off from work during the pregnancy and after the birth of the child. While some companies may allow up to 6 weeks of paid time off, other companies may require that their pregnant employees use a combination of short-term disability, vacation time, sick time, and unpaid leave time. Health care providers can help women plan how much time they may need or wish to be away from work, and can provide them with options that may be available to them. All women who are employed outside of the home should be encouraged to meet with their employers to discuss the options that are provided by the workplace and to determine a satisfactory plan for their leave.

The Family and Medical Leave Act of 1993 (U.S. Department of Labor, 1995) guarantees most women, as well as men, 12 weeks of unpaid family leave following the birth or adoption of a child. By law, the employer is required to allow the family member to return to his or her job or a similar job with the same salary and benefits, without a reduction in seniority. Family members qualify for this benefit if they work for the federal, state, or local government or if the company has 50 or more employees working within 75 miles of the workplace. In addition, the family member must have worked for the employer at least 12 months or for at least 1250 hours in the previous year.

REST

Fatigue and tiredness are common symptoms associated with pregnancy. As the pregnancy progresses from one trimester to the next, the woman's level of fatigue changes along with the need for rest. An understanding of the expected alterations in maternal anatomy and physiology empowers the woman to anticipate and make changes in her daily routine to accommodate the necessary rest. Nurses should provide education about the anticipated need for additional rest and suggest strategies for managing fatigue and for promoting rest and relaxation.

Contributors to Fatigue During the First Trimester

During the first trimester, the woman's body begins to undergo changes that will support the developing fetus. One of the major changes is an increase in the production of progesterone, a hormone that causes increased fatigue and feelings of tiredness, especially during the day. The maternal blood volume also begins to increase and frequently results in physiological anemia. Women with decreased iron stores may develop "true" (iron-deficiency) anemia. As the fetus grows, oxygen requirements increase and cause an increased workload on the woman's body systems. These changes, along with the emotional stress often associated with adjustment to the news of the pregnancy, combine to produce fatigue. Strategies for coping with pregnancy-related fatigue should routinely be discussed with patients early in the pregnancy.

Contributors to Fatigue During the Second Trimester

During the second trimester the rapid physiological changes that occurred in the first trimester come into balance with the body's workload demands. Pregnant women experience increased energy and endurance during this time and are able to focus more on planning for the upcoming birth. Some women, however, may continue to experience fatigue that persists into the second trimester. Potential causes of the fatigue include depression, external stressors, and anemia. Other underlying medical causes may also be a factor and should be investigated by the woman's health care provider.

Contributors to Fatigue During the Third Trimester

The pregnant woman's level of fatigue increases as the fetus continues to grow and develop. The maternal weight-bearing load associated with the fetus is compounded by a corresponding increase in extracellular fluid and blood volume, maternal reserves, placental mass, and amniotic fluid. The enlarging fetus causes the maternal diaphragm to be upwardly displaced, decreasing lung expansion. Increased bladder pressure from the gravid uterus causes increased voiding, especially at night, when the woman is trying to sleep. Each of these factors plays a role in the overwhelming fatigue common during the third trimester.

Through education, the health care provider can empower the expectant mother throughout the pregnancy to better manage her rest demands and cope with fatigue. Planning and making healthy choices concerning rest enables the woman to feel more relaxed and energetic and better able to cope with and manage this common discomfort of pregnancy.

 Now Can You— Discuss work and fatigue during pregnancy?

1. Identify three situations in which women may need to stop working during pregnancy?
2. Name two reasons why fatigue is especially pronounced during the first and third trimesters?
3. Identify three strategies to help women cope with fatigue during pregnancy?

Medications

Medication use during pregnancy must be handled very carefully and the needs of the patient and her fetus should always be considered on an individual basis. Nurses need to be aware that their patients may be taking over-the-counter (OTC) medications and herbal preparations and often do not readily report this information during the prenatal interview. Thus, the nurse should ask specific questions regarding prescription and OTC medications and the use of any herbal therapies.

SAFE VERSUS TERATOGENIC MEDICATIONS

A **teratogen** is anything that adversely affects the normal cellular development in the embryo or fetus (Venes, 2009). Although some medications are safe, others are known teratogens or the safety of their use during pregnancy has not been demonstrated. The fetus is most vulnerable to the effects of teratogens from the third week of gestation through the third month. However, the risk for fetal developmental anomalies continues to exist throughout the pregnancy. The third trimester is the most vulnerable time for cognitive impairment from a teratogenic insult.

Over-the-Counter Medications

Nonprescription medications such as acetaminophen (Tylenol) and guaifenesin (Robitussin) are often taken for minor problems such as headaches, coughs, and colds. It is commonly assumed that a medication that requires no prescription must be safe to take. However, all medications, whether available by prescription or over the counter, have side effects, and many have adverse effects. The nurse needs to counsel women who are planning to become pregnant and those who are already pregnant not to take any medications (prescription or nonprescription) without first consulting with the primary health care provider. The provider will make a determination regarding the safety and necessity of the medication. Additional information (including a physical assessment) may need to be obtained and an alternate medication or therapy may be advised. When possible, all nonprescription drugs should be avoided during preconception and throughout pregnancy.

Herbal and Homeopathic Preparations

One of the most important facts about herbal and homeopathic preparations is that the U.S. Food and Drug Administration (FDA) has not approved these drugs and does not regulate or control them. Further, there are major drawbacks to the use of these substances. There is no regulation that controls product development, the dosages are not consistent between brands, and additives used in their composition may differ in type and amount. Also, since herbal and homeopathic products have not been subjected to rigorous research to determine their efficacy, effectiveness, side effects, therapeutic dosages, and adverse effects, there is no guarantee that the claims made about them are true. Although herbal and homeopathic treatments are considered to be "natural" because they have been developed from plants and other natural sources, many of these products are dangerous and toxic, and may cause effects that have not yet been discovered.

Several herbal products are recognized to be dangerous; others are known to have specific teratogenic effects. These substances need to be completely avoided during the periods of preconception and pregnancy. Nurses should warn patients about the use of these products,

Family Teaching Guidelines...
Common Herbs to Avoid During Preconception and Pregnancy

During preconception counseling and pregnancy, nurses should educate couples to avoid the following common herbs:

◆ Uterine stimulants that may cause preterm labor
  - Barberry
  - Black cohosh
  - Feverfew
  - Goldenseal
  - Mugwort
  - Pennyroyal leaf
  - Yarrow root

◆ Blood thinners and anticoagulants that may cause miscarriage
  - Dong quai

◆ Laxatives that may overstimulate digestion and metabolism and cause fluid and electrolyte imbalance
  - Blessed thistle
  - Cascara sagrada
  - Drug aloe
  - Senna

◆ Cardiovascular stimulants that may elevate blood pressure or cause abnormal heart rhythms
  - Ephedra
  - Licorice root

◆ Others that may damage the fetus during development
  - Gotu kola
  - Juniper berries

provide written information that can be taken home, and reinforce the teaching at each visit.

Prescription Medications

Certain prescription medications may be necessary during preconception and pregnancy. Women who suffer from life-threatening illnesses, such as seizure disorders, heart disease, respiratory disorders, or infections need to continue or initiate treatment in order to maintain their own health and safety. The health care practitioner must be aware of all prescription medications currently being taken in order to evaluate the safety of their continued use. In some instances, dosages can be adjusted or the medications can be replaced with safer medications.

Prenatal vitamins are usually given during preconception or at the beginning of a pregnancy. Prenatal vitamins provide the recommended daily allowance (RDA) for most vitamins and minerals as well as the additional calcium, iron, and folic acid needed during pregnancy.

Certain prescription medications must be avoided completely. Isotretinoin (Accutane), prescribed primarily for the treatment of acne, is associated with spontaneous abortions and congenital anomalies when taken early in pregnancy. Some antimicrobials cause altered fetal growth and development and should be avoided during the later months of gestation. Sulfonamides, for example, are associated with delayed fetal skeletal development while prenatal exposure to tetracycline causes staining of the child's teeth.

 Nursing Insight— Teaching childbearing aged women about Accutane

Isotretinoin (Accutane) is an extremely successful medication in the treatment of acne, and research demonstrates a successful remission (of acne) after only one treatment. However, there are significant adverse and teratogenic effects associated with the use of this medication. Isotretinoin is labeled as a pregnancy category X medication. Use during pregnancy may result in spontaneous abortion or stillbirth and there is a 50% chance of fetal anomalies that include physical deformities of the face, ears, heart, and brain and abnormal formation of internal organs (Goodheart, 2006). Women of childbearing age who are considering taking isotretinoin should use a reliable method of contraception for 1 month before treatment, during the entire course of treatment, and for 1 month after the cessation of treatment. Women who are considering pregnancy should not take isotretinoin (Encyclopedia of Genetic Disorders, 2008).

FDA CLASSIFICATION SYSTEM FOR MEDICATIONS USED DURING PREGNANCY

To determine the safety of medication use during pregnancy, the FDA devised a classification system according to known fetal risk, based on research findings. The following list summarizes the categories and associated fetal risk (see Chapter 7):

- Category A: No associated fetal risk; safe to take during pregnancy
- Category B: No associated fetal risk in animals; fetal risk in humans not identified
- Category C: Evidence of adverse effects in animal fetuses; fetal risk in humans not identified
- Category D: Evidence of adverse effects and fetal risk in humans; benefits and risks must be considered before prescribing
- Category X: Evidence of fetal risk and congenital anomalies in humans; risks outweigh the benefits; not prescribed during pregnancy

There are no absolutes when using any prescription or nonprescription drug during pregnancy. Each situation is different and requires individualized decision making that must be a mutual endeavor between the patient and her care provider. Cultural considerations, benefits, risks, and goals of all therapies must be assessed before any decisions are reached. Nurses play an essential role in gathering information for assessment and evaluation and in providing patient education and counseling.

Now Can You— Discuss the use of herbal preparations and prescription medications in pregnancy?

1. Identify two major concerns related to the use of herbal and homeopathic preparations?
2. Name four herbs that should be avoided during pregnancy?
3. Identify two types of prescription medications that should not be used during pregnancy?
4. Discuss what is meant by a Category B medication?

Common Discomforts During Pregnancy

Common discomforts experienced during pregnancy are caused by the major hormonal and anatomical changes that take place in the woman's body. (See Chapters 8 and 9 for further discussion.) As the pregnancy progresses, most patients report at least some of the common discomforts, which are presented in Table 10-5. Anticipatory guidance includes educating women about the normal physiological changes that occur during pregnancy, symptoms that frequently accompany the changes, and strategies for dealing with the discomfort.

NAUSEA

Nausea is often one of the first symptoms of pregnancy experienced. Although commonly known as "morning sickness," nausea can occur at any time of the day or night. While the exact cause of nausea is unknown, it most probably is related to the increased levels of the pregnancy hormones. Nausea is primarily noted during the first trimester of the pregnancy and usually resolves by 13 to 14 weeks, although it may persist throughout the pregnancy. Nausea during the early weeks of pregnancy is believed to be a reassuring indicator of embryo/fetal development with adequate hormonal support (Youngkin & Davis, 2004). Complaints of nausea should never be dismissed without further assessment to rule out pregnancy-related complications such as hyperemesis gravidarum, multiple gestation, gestational trophoblastic disease, or maternal gastrointestinal or eating disorders. (See Chapter 11 for further discussion.)

Nurses can suggest strategies to help offset the nausea, such as the avoidance of "trigger foods" (foods that cause nausea from sight or smell) and tight clothing that constricts the abdomen. The use of relaxation techniques (e.g., slow, deep breathing, mental imagery) can also help to decrease nausea. Other techniques that are often helpful include consuming plain, dry crackers or sucking on peppermint candy before arising; adhering to small, frequent meals; and remaining in an upright position after eating.

Medication is usually not necessary for the nausea of early pregnancy, although some women have found that taking vitamin B$_6$ or ginger tablets helps to lessen nausea. These oral supplements can be purchased over-the-counter and should be taken with meals. Acupressure bracelets, often used for the prevention of motion sickness, can also be purchased without a prescription and may be beneficial in reducing nausea during early pregnancy (Varney, Kriebs, & Gegor, 2004; Youngkin & Davis, 2004;).

Table 10-5	Common Discomforts During Each Trimester of Pregnancy
Trimester	**Common Discomforts**
First	Nausea
	Vomiting
	Fatigue
	Urinary frequency
	Nocturia
Second	Dyspepsia
	Gum hyperplasia and bleeding
	Dependent edema
	Leg varicosities
	Hyperventilation and shortness of breath
	Numbness and tingling of fingers
	Supine hypotensive syndrome
Third	Fatigue
	Urinary frequency
	Dyspepsia
	Flatulence
	Gum hyperplasia and bleeding
	Leg cramps
	Dependent edema
	Leg varicosities
	Dyspareunia
	Nocturia
	Round ligament pain
	Supine hypotensive syndrome
All Trimesters	Ptyalism
	Nasal congestion
	Back pain
	Leukorrhea
	Constipation
	Insomnia

VOMITING

Vomiting in early pregnancy often accompanies the nausea, although it is important to ascertain that the amount vomited is not excessive. During the assessment, nurses should question patients about vomiting frequency and amount, and their ability to consume and retain foods and liquids. It is important to assess for weight loss, dehydration, urine ketones, blood alkalosis, and hypokalemia, which are clinical findings that may be indicative of a more serious complication known as hyperemesis gravidarum (Youngkin & Davis, 2004). **Hyperemesis**

gravidarum is a pregnancy-related condition characterized by persistent, continuous, severe nausea and vomiting, often accompanied by dry retching (Venes, 2009). (See Chapter 11 for further discussion.)

PTYALISM

Ptyalism, or excessive salivation, can be quite distressing for the pregnant woman, who must frequently wipe her mouth or spit into a cup. Although the cause of ptyalism is unknown, it is most likely related to increased hormone levels. Ptyalism can also be a symptom of hyperemesis gravidarum and, when extreme, may be associated with maternal dehydration. While little can be done to reduce the amount of saliva, it is important to rule out dental abnormalities, upper gastrointestinal problems, and pica. Nurses can counsel patients to consume small, frequent meals; avoid starchy foods; drink plenty of water in small sips; suck on hard candies; and brush their teeth frequently (Youngkin & Davis, 2004).

FATIGUE

Fatigue occurs primarily during the first and third trimesters of pregnancy. In the first trimester, the fatigue is most likely related to physiological and hormonal changes. Psychological concerns may also lead to insomnia. During the third trimester, fatigue is usually related to physical discomforts and an increasing inability to sleep. Nurses can counsel patients to take naps during the day when possible, establish a bedtime "ritual" that includes going to bed at approximately the same time each night, increase daytime exercise, and practice relaxation techniques. If these strategies are not effective or the patient exhibits signs of psychosocial stress or depression, she should be referred for additional evaluation (Youngkin & Davis, 2004).

NASAL CONGESTION

Nasal congestion, a common maternal complaint, is known as rhinitis of pregnancy. Increased levels of estrogen and progesterone cause swelling of the nasal mucus membranes and produce symptoms of excess mucus and congestion. It is important to rule out colds and allergies. The nurse can suggest relief measures such as increasing fluids; taking a hot, steamy shower; using a vaporizer or humidifier; and the occasional administration of nasal saline drops. Decongestants should be avoided during the first trimester.

UPPER AND LOWER BACKACHE

Back pain during pregnancy results from the change in the center of gravity as the uterus enlarges. It is also related to high levels of progesterone, which cause a relaxation and softening of the connecting cartilage and joints. Low backache can be exacerbated by activities that require prolonged standing, walking, bending, or lifting. It is important to rule out other causes of backache, such as kidney stones, pyelonephritis, pancreatitis, ulcers, muscle sprain or strain, and preterm labor. For some women, a referral for physical therapy may be indicated (Varney et al., 2004).

 Optimizing Outcomes— Relief of backache during pregnancy

Best outcome: Nurses educate all patients about strategies that may prevent or relieve backache. Women can be taught to wear supportive, low-heeled shoes; use proper body mechanics; perform back strengthening and pelvic rock exercises; take frequent rest periods; sleep on a firm, supportive mattress; and wear a well-fitting, supportive bra. Body massage and warm tub baths may also be helpful.

LEUKORRHEA

High levels of estrogen stimulate vascularity and hypertrophy of the cervical glands, causing an increase in vaginal discharge. The discharge is usually yellow to white in color, thin, and more acidic than normal. It is important to rule out vaginal and sexually transmitted infections, and rupture of membranes. The nurse can counsel the patient to wear cotton underwear, avoid tight-fitting clothing, and follow strict hygiene to prevent infection. If a panty liner or sanitary pad is worn to absorb moisture, it should be changed frequently to prevent dampness and odor.

URINARY FREQUENCY

In early pregnancy, urinary frequency is caused by pressure exerted by the enlarging uterus on the bladder. During the second trimester, bladder pressure lessens once the uterus becomes an abdominal organ. In the third trimester, a number of physiological events cause urinary frequency. The fetal presenting part once again exerts pressure on the bladder. Progesterone relaxes the muscles of the urethra and may lead to incontinence, while an increase in the glomerular filtration rate causes increased urine production. It is important to rule out urinary tract infection, rupture of the membranes, kidney stones, gestational diabetes, and stress urinary incontinence. The nurse can suggest relief measures, including intake of adequate hydration, Kegel exercises, use of panty liners, frequent voiding, and decreasing fluid intake two to three hours before bedtime.

DYSPEPSIA

Dyspepsia, or heartburn, results from reflux of acidic gastric contents into the lower esophagus. Dyspepsia is caused by the progesterone-induced relaxation of the cardiac sphincter and delayed gastric emptying. Due to these changes, stomach contents remain in the stomach for a longer period of time and can reflux into the esophagus. As the pregnancy advances, the enlarging uterus pushes up on the stomach and compresses it, causing a reduced capacity. Making changes in the diet and eating patterns may be helpful in reducing heartburn although it is unlikely to disappear until after the baby is born.

Nursing Insight— *Relief measures for dyspepsia*

Nurses can suggest a number of relief measures for dyspepsia, a common complaint during pregnancy. Patients can be taught to consume small, frequent meals to avoid overloading the stomach, maintain good posture, remain upright after meals and avoid greasy and fatty foods, very cold foods and consuming beverages with meals. Drinking cultured or sweet milk and using over-the-counter antacids may also be helpful (Varney et al., 2004).

FLATULENCE

Flatulence (excessive gas in the stomach and intestines) is caused by decreased gastric motility that results from elevated levels of progesterone during pregnancy. Pressure of the enlarging uterus on the abdominal contents also contributes to the formation of gas. When excessive or particularly disturbing, other causes, such as irritable bowel syndrome or lactose intolerance should be ruled out. Patients can be counseled to avoid gas-forming foods, constipation, gum chewing, consuming large meals, and swallowing air.

CONSTIPATION

Elevated levels of progesterone relax the smooth muscles, causing decreased contractility of the lower gastrointestinal tract and slowed movement of the stool. As the uterus enlarges, the large intestines become compressed, further slowing movement of stool through the intestines. Supplemental iron may also be a contributor to the development of constipation. All patients should be taught about the importance of regular physical exercise and bowel habits, consuming a high-fiber diet with increased liquids, and to avoid straining at defecation and the use of mineral oil and bulk-forming laxatives.

DENTAL PROBLEMS

Elevations in pregnancy hormones cause the gums to become edematous and friable, which can lead to bleeding during brushing. Open lesions and other dental problems, such as caries, can open a direct pathway for pathogens to enter the bloodstream. Meticulous dental care during pregnancy is important to prevent infections and other dental complications. The dentist should be informed of the pregnancy so that an abdominal shield can be used if x-ray films are needed. If treatment is indicated, most local anesthetics can be used safely during pregnancy.

LEG CRAMPS

The actual cause of leg cramps is unknown, although decreased levels of calcium and phosphorus have been implicated. As the uterus enlarges, pressure is exerted on the major blood vessels, causing impaired circulation to the lower extremities. It is important to rule out thrombosed blood vessels, muscular strain, and other injuries to the lower extremities. The patient should be advised to engage in regular exercise and maintain good body mechanics; elevate the legs above the heart several times throughout the day; dorsiflex the foot; and consume a diet that includes adequate amounts of calcium and phosphorus (Varney et al., 2004; Youngkin & Davis, 2004).

DEPENDENT EDEMA

Edema in the lower extremities is caused by relaxation of the blood vessels (an effect of increased progesterone) and the increased pressure placed on the pelvic veins by the enlarging uterus. Tight, restrictive clothing that inhibits venous return from the lower extremities increases the edema. Once pathological conditions, such as gestational hypertension, renal disease, liver disease, cardiac disease, vascular disorders, trauma, and infection have been ruled out, the nurse can suggest relief measures. These include avoiding constrictive clothing, elevating the legs periodically throughout the day, and assuming a side-lying position when resting.

VARICOSITIES

A positive family history, coupled with the normal physiological changes of pregnancy, predisposes the patient to the development of varicose veins. Physiological changes of pregnancy include vascular relaxation from the effects of progesterone and impaired venous circulation from pressure exerted by the enlarged uterus. Constrictive clothing also increases the risk for varicose veins. Nursing care for patients with varicosities includes regular assessment of lower extremity peripheral pulses and education. Patients should be taught to avoid crossing their legs and the use of constrictive clothing such as knee-high stockings. They should also be encouraged to elevate their legs above the level of the heart at least twice a day. For some women, a maternity girdle may provide relief (Varney et al., 2004; Youngkin & Davis, 2004).

DYSPAREUNIA

Dyspareunia, or painful intercourse, may result from pelvic congestion and impaired circulation caused by the enlarging uterus. Also, as the pregnancy advances, finding a position of comfort for intercourse may become increasingly difficult due to the enlarging abdomen. Concerns that intercourse will harm the fetus may also interfere with sexual enjoyment and increase the likelihood of dyspareunia. Unless a medical condition contraindicates intercourse, the patient and her partner should be reassured that intercourse is safe during pregnancy. Education about sexual intimacy should include suggestions for comfortable positions for intercourse and alternative methods for mutual sexual satisfaction (Varney et al., 2004).

> **❝What to say❞** — *When asked about sexual activity during pregnancy*
>
> Couples have many questions regarding sexual activity during pregnancy. These questions relate to the safety of sexual intercourse, potential complications, when to stop having intercourse, and sexual positions that facilitate comfort. It is important for the health care provider to address sexual activity early in the pregnancy in an honest, open manner and to encourage the couple to communicate with each other. The nurse can address the couple's concerns with the following statements:
>
> "It is perfectly safe to continue sexual activity throughout your pregnancy unless your doctor or nurse midwife identifies risk factors that may preclude your activity (e.g., a risk for preterm labor). With no risk factors, sexual activity is safe for you and your baby as long as you continue to practice safe sex behaviors as you would if you were not pregnant. As you gain pregnancy weight, some sexual positions may be less comfortable; for comfort,

you can try woman on top and side-lying positions. A sexual activity to avoid during pregnancy includes oral sex during which water or air is placed in the vagina."

NOCTURIA

Nocturia, or excessive nighttime urination, is more common during the first and third trimesters. When the woman assumes a recumbent position, the gravid uterus no longer compresses the pelvic vessels, and blood flow to the kidneys is enhanced. This factor, combined with an increased glomerular filtration rate, increases the need to urinate. Although there is no remedy for nocturia, the nurse can teach the patient about the cause of nocturia and advise her that limiting fluids in the few hours before bedtime may be helpful.

INSOMNIA

Insomnia may have a variety of causes, including physical discomfort, nocturia, caffeine, or stress. The nurse can suggest strategies to enhance relaxation and comfort before bedtime. For example, the woman may incorporate sleep-inducing night time rituals such as taking a warm bath, enjoying a warm drink such as milk, engaging in a restful activity like reading, practicing meditation and other forms of relaxation, and arranging the bed covers and pillows in an inviting way that promotes rest.

ROUND LIGAMENT PAIN

The round ligaments support the uterus as it enlarges during pregnancy. These structures attach to the fundus on each side, pass through the inguinal canal, and insert into the upper portion of the labia majora. As the uterus enlarges, the round ligaments stretch and produce a painful sensation in the lower quadrants. Once pathological conditions such as preterm labor, rupture of an ovarian cyst, ectopic pregnancy, appendicitis, gallbladder disease, and peptic ulcer disease have been ruled out, the nurse can educate the patient about the cause of the pain and make suggestions for relief measures. Taking a warm bath, applying heat, supporting the uterus with a pillow when resting, and using a pregnancy girdle may help to diminish the discomfort (Varney et al., 2004; Youngkin & Davis, 2004).

HYPERVENTILATION AND SHORTNESS OF BREATH

Increased metabolic activity during pregnancy increases the amount of carbon dioxide in the maternal respiratory system. Hyperventilation decreases the amount of carbon dioxide and may trigger a feeling of "air hunger." Patients may also experience shortness of breath related to uterine enlargement and the upward pressure exerted on the diaphragm. Once pathological conditions such as upper respiratory infection, asthma, cardiac problems, and anemia have been ruled out, the nurse should explain the cause of hyperventilation to the patient and suggest that she consciously attempt to regulate her breathing. Other measures that may be helpful include breathing into a paper bag to decrease the symptoms of hyperventilation, maintaining good posture, and stretching the arms above the head (Varney et al., 2004; Youngkin & Davis, 2004).

NUMBNESS AND TINGLING IN THE FINGERS

Numbness and tingling in the fingers may be associated with hyperventilation or from nerve compression in the median and ulnar nerves in the arm. Maintaining good posture, elevating the hands on a pillow while sleeping, or wearing a wrist brace when sleeping may provide symptomatic relief.

SUPINE HYPOTENSIVE SYNDROME

Supine hypotension is caused by pressure of the enlarging uterus on the inferior vena cava while the woman is in a supine position. Vena caval compression impedes venous blood flow, reduces the amount of blood in the heart, and decreases cardiac output, causing dizziness and syncope. Pathological causes of supine hypotension include cardiac or respiratory disorders, anemia, hypoglycemia, dehydration, anxiety, and stress. Once these conditions have been ruled out, the nurse should educate the patient about the causes of supine hypotension and advise the woman to rest on her side and slowly move from a lying to a sitting to a standing position to minimize changes in blood pressure.

 Now Can You— Discuss Common Discomforts of Pregnancy?

1. Name four strategies to alleviate nausea during early pregnancy?
2. Identify four pathological causes of backache during pregnancy?
3. Explain how you would counsel couples regarding sexual intercourse during pregnancy?

Recognizing Signs and Symptoms of Danger

Complications can occur at any time during the pregnancy. Nurses need to educate the pregnant woman and her family about danger signs and symptoms, teach them about interventions that can be initiated at home, and provide specific instructions about when to notify the health care provider.

FIRST TRIMESTER

Nausea and Vomiting

During the first trimester, nausea and vomiting are common discomforts. However, when vomiting becomes severe, weight loss and dehydration can occur and place both the woman and her fetus at risk. Severe, persistent vomiting is indicative of hyperemesis gravidarum. Causes of hyperemesis gravidarum include multiple gestation; thyroid disorder; and **hydatidiform mole**, which is the growth of abnormal tissue that results from conception but does not give rise to a viable fetus. Nausea and vomiting are managed with oral fluids, small, frequent meals, and emotional support. Dehydration may require intravenous fluids and hospitalization. (See Chapter 11 for further discussion.)

Abdominal Pain and Vaginal Bleeding

Abdominal cramping and vaginal spotting or bleeding may indicate spontaneous abortion, or miscarriage.

Spontaneous abortion is the termination of pregnancy by natural causes before 20 weeks' gestation. The majority of spontaneous abortions are related to chromosomal defects. Approximately 10% to 20% of clinically recognized pregnancies end in spontaneous abortion (White & Bouvier, 2005). A woman may assume she is having a heavy period when she is actually experiencing a miscarriage. (See Chapter 11 for further discussion.) Treatment includes bedrest and emotional support. If bleeding and/or pain are excessive, the patient should contact her primary health care provider or report to the emergency department.

Infection

Generalized symptoms of infection include chills, fever, malaise, and anorexia. Burning on urination may indicate a urinary tract infection, which is treated with antibiotics. Patient education to prevent a urinary tract infection includes advising the woman to use white, unscented toilet paper; to avoid bubble baths or the addition of "additives" in the bath; to wear underwear with cotton crotches; to drink at least 8 to 12 glasses of liquid each day; and to urinate before going to bed and before and after sexual intercourse. Diarrhea may indicate a gastrointestinal infection, which may be treated with antibiotics if bacterial in origin.

SECOND TRIMESTER

Maternal Complications

Preeclampsia is one of the most common pregnancy complications during the second trimester. It is a pregnancy-specific systemic syndrome that is clinically defined as an increase in blood pressure (140/90) after 20 weeks' gestation accompanied by proteinuria (National High Blood Pressure Education Program Working Group, 2000; Peters & Flack, 2004). Early signs and symptoms of preeclampsia include headache, vision changes, elevated blood pressure, and edema. Patients who experience any of these symptoms should promptly notify their health care provider. Bedrest is the first intervention implemented in an effort to reduce blood pressure and alleviate the myriad of other problems that can be associated with this disorder. (See Chapter 11 for further discussion.)

Premature rupture of the membranes, which is rupture of the membranes before the onset of labor, can also occur during the second trimester. Patients are taught to promptly seek advice from their health care provider if vaginal discharge is present. Although increased vaginal discharge is normal during pregnancy, the provider will determine if the vaginal discharge is normal, is associated with a vaginal infection, or results from the leakage of amniotic fluid. Women who have experienced premature rupture of membranes must be closely monitored for signs of infection. (See Chapter 11 for further discussion.)

The presence of uterine contractions during the second trimester may indicate preterm labor (PTL). **Preterm labor** is defined as regular uterine contractions and cervical dilation before the end of the 36th week of gestation (ACOG, 2003b). All pregnant women are taught the signs and symptoms of preterm labor and instructed to contact their health care provider if the symptoms appear. True labor must be differentiated from Braxton-Hicks contractions (disorganized tightenings of the uterine muscles as they stretch to prepare for labor) so that appropriate interventions may be initiated. (See Chapters 11 and 12 for further discussion.)

Fetal Complications

During the second trimester the fetus is assessed for well-being. The fundal height measurement should correlate to the weeks of gestation from approximately 22 to 34 weeks of gestation. A decreased fundal height may indicate intrauterine growth restriction, while increased fundal height is suggestive of multiple gestation, fetal macrosomia, or hydramnios. The gestational age is also determined from a variety of sources that include the patient's menstrual history, contraceptive history, pregnancy test results, first documentation of fetal heart sounds, and ultrasonography. (See Chapters 9 and 11 for further discussion.)

A number of potential fetal problems may occur during the second trimester. These include hypoxia from maternal hypertension, irregular or absent heart rate, preterm birth, infection from premature rupture of membranes, and absence of fetal movements after quickening. If the woman experiences an absence of fetal movements, she is instructed to drink two full glasses of water, rest on her left side for 2 hours, and assess for fetal movements once again. If fewer than 10 fetal movements are noted after the liquid intake, the patient must be evaluated by her health care provider. (See Chapter 11 for further discussion.)

THIRD TRIMESTER

Maternal Complications

During the third trimester, the patient may develop the same problems that can occur during the second trimester, such as preeclampsia, premature rupture of the membranes, and preterm labor. Also, gestational diabetes may develop during this time. A Glucose Challenge Test (Glucola screening) is performed between 24 and 28 weeks of gestation and a positive test warrants further screening with a 3-hour oral glucose tolerance test (OGTT). A positive OGTT indicates the presence of gestational diabetes and patient care involves education and a team approach that usually includes the obstetrician, internist, endocrinologist, diabetes educator, neonatologist, dietitian, and nurse. (See Chapter 11 for further discussion.)

Hemorrhagic disorders may also develop during the third trimester. **Placenta previa** is an implantation of the placenta in the lower uterine segment, near or over the internal cervical os. The abnormal location of the placenta can cause painless, bright red vaginal bleeding as the lower uterine segment stretches and thins during the third trimester. Depending on the placental location, the patient may need to adhere to strict bedrest and a cesarean birth may be necessary. **Abruptio placentae**, or placental abruption, is the premature separation of a normally implanted placenta from the uterine wall. An abruption results in hemorrhage between the uterine wall and the placenta, causing abdominal pain and vaginal bleeding. Interventions may include hospitalization, bedrest, Trendelenburg position, intravenous fluids, and delivery. (See Chapter 11 for further discussion.)

Fetal Complications

Leopold maneuvers are used to determine the lie, presentation, and position of the fetus. (See Chapter 9 for further discussion.) To monitor fetal growth, the fundal height is measured and compared to the estimated date of delivery at each prenatal visit during the second and third trimesters. During the third trimester, non-stress tests may be performed to evaluate fetal well-being. (See Chapter 11 for further discussion.) Fetal complications during the third trimester are the same as for the second trimester although hypoxia related to poor placental perfusion may become more of a threat during this time.

 Optimizing Outcomes— **Fetal activity and well-being**

Maternal involvement in activities to monitor fetal well-being is an important component of prenatal care. Beginning in the second trimester, the patient should consistently assess fetal movements. Reassuring findings include a count of at least four movements within 1 hour, during rest after meals.

Best outcome: Fetal well-being is maintained during the third trimester, labor, and birth. The neonate is full term and appropriate for gestational age. Normal physiological transitions in the neonate occur without difficulty.

 Now Can You— **Identify danger signs during pregnancy?**

1. Discuss the significance of abdominal cramping and vaginal bleeding during the first trimester?
2. Identify two actions the pregnant woman should take if she experiences an absence of fetal movements?
3. Name two placental problems that can cause hemorrhage, especially during the third trimester?

Using a Pregnancy Map to Guide Prenatal Visits

A prenatal care map that includes a timetable for prenatal visits helps to ensure consistency of care, especially when many health care professionals are involved in the woman's care. The care map can be placed in the patient's chart during the initial visit and an abbreviated version that outlines the schedule for prenatal care visits may be given to the patient. Some facilities add a grid that provides additional space for entering scheduled appointment dates. An example of a prenatal care map is presented in Table 10-6. In other institutions, the care map consists of a comprehensive guide with check boxes and identifies counseling and education needs throughout pregnancy and during the postpartum period (Fig. 10-8).

Childbirth Education to Promote a Positive Childbearing Experience

Childbirth education provides a wealth of information to parents who are having a baby for the first time as well as to parents who have already experienced childbirth. The difficulty often lies in finding the right class to meet the specific needs of the expectant parents. Traditionally, childbirth education focused on managing labor and birth. Contemporary classes focus on a wide variety of topics, with the primary goal centered on facilitating a positive childbearing experience, including pregnancy, childbirth, postpartum, and newborn care. Topics typically discussed in childbirth classes include anatomy and physiology related to pregnancy; comfort measures during each trimester of pregnancy; the labor and birth process; relaxation and pain management, including pharmacological and nonpharmacological measures; complications related to pregnancy, labor, and birth; vaginal and cesarean births; postpartum care; newborn care; and newborn feeding, including bottle feeding and breastfeeding (Fig. 10-9).

METHODS OF CHILDBIRTH PREPARATION

Expectant parents can choose from a variety of available childbirth education classes. Ideally, they will select one that is in harmony with their beliefs and values about the childbearing experience and be able to engage in the educational process without reservation and with complete commitment. While different, all childbirth preparation classes incorporate a holistic approach to childbearing, which encompasses the biological, psychological, and social factors related to the experience. For many expectant parents, the experience of childbearing is more than just a physical and biological one; the experience can have emotional, mental, and spiritual meaning. This holistic approach to having a child allows the parents to assimilate all aspects of the experience in order to be prepared physically and mentally for becoming a parent.

Many childbirth education programs in the community combine aspects from the traditional stand-alone methods of childbirth preparation. Combining philosophies and activities into the classes allows the couple to identify more strongly with features that fit their individual and collective needs. The most common childbirth methods include the Lamaze and the Bradley methods of natural childbirth.

Lamaze Method

The Lamaze childbirth experience was started in 1960 by the American Society for Psychoprophylaxis in Obstetrics (ASPO) as a way to bring families together in the labor and delivery process while focusing on the normality of birth. The concepts were founded on principles and techniques used by Dr. Fernand Lamaze, giving rise to the familiar labeling of the association as ASPO/Lamaze. It was not until the 1970s that the organization officially changed its name to Lamaze International, becoming known as such throughout the United States.

The heart of the Lamaze method is empowerment, recognizing the woman's innate ability to give birth, while finding strength and support from her family and the members of the health care team during the labor and birth process. The Lamaze Philosophy of Birth (Box 10-3) identifies the core ideals of the organization and provides the template for the classes. Historically, Lamaze has focused on breathing techniques during labor and birth. As the philosophy indicates, this method incorporates the ideology of empowerment into the entire experience, providing more than just instruction on breathing.

Table 10-6 Example of a Prenatal Care Map

Trimester	Schedule for Return Visits	Components of the Nursing Interview	Lab Tests to Be Obtained
First	Every 4 weeks	• Reason for seeking care	• CBC with differential
		• Presumptive signs	• Blood type and Rh
		• Review of systems	• Rubella titer
		• Medical history	• VDRL or RPR
		• Family history	• HIV
		• Gynecologic and obstetric history	• Hemoglobin electrophoresis (sickle cell, thalassemia)
		• Nutritional history	• Urinalysis
		• Social history	• Pap test
		• Drug use	• Vaginal smear
		• Assessment of abuse risk	
		• Birth plan	
Second	Every 4 weeks	• Summary of relative events since last visit	• Hematocrit
		• General emotional state	• Urinalysis
		• Complaints/problems/questions	• Urine culture
		• Vital signs	• AFP or Triple Marker
		• Weight	
		• Presence of edema	
Third	Every 4 weeks through weeks 28–32	• Primary concerns	• Hematocrit
		• Attendance at childbirth education classes	• Urinalysis
		• Physical assessment	• Urine culture
		• Psychosocial responses	• Glucose tolerance test
	Every 2 weeks through week 36	• Vital signs	• Repeat, if needed: VDRL or RPR, HIV, CBC, sickle cell prep, vaginal smears
	Every week thereafter	• Weight	
		• Presence of edema	
		• Confirmation of gestational age	

As the Lamaze method has evolved over the years, many myths have continued to prevail regarding this method of childbirth preparation. The organization identified and addressed these myths (Lamaze International, 2005), and they include:

• *Lamaze is all about breathing*: In fact, Lamaze classes provide education on movement and position, massage, relaxation, and use of heat and cold in addition to the traditional focused-breathing techniques.

• *Lamaze promises painless childbirth*: Pain is a natural and normal part of childbirth. Instead of attempting to alleviate the pain, women are taught strategies for coping with the pain associated with labor and birth in positive ways. The strategies provide the woman with education to understand and respond to the pain signals and to facilitate the process of labor and birth.

• *Lamaze childbirth means you cannot have an epidural*: Education on epidural use is provided during Lamaze

INDIANA **PERINATAL** NETWORK
Lead/Convene/Collaborate
FOR MOTHERS & BABIES

INDIANA PRENATAL CARE GUIDE
Screening, Education & Counseling
2008

This Guide is intended as a resource for clinicians involved in the design and implementation of prenatal care services. This information should not be interpreted as excluding other acceptable course of care based upon medical judgement and patient preferences. The Guide reflects the current opinion of IPN for a standard approach to prenatal care. The use of pre-printed standardized antenatal record is recommended to reduce errors of omission.

Note: It is strongly recommended that prenatal care begin in the first trimester.

INITIAL VISIT	EACH VISIT	8-18 WEEKS	24-28 WEEKS	35-37 WEEKS	POSTPARTUM
HISTORY & PHYSICAL					
□ Assess for intent of pregnancy: "How are you/your partner feeling about being pregnant?" □ Medical and reproductive history □ Current pregnancy history □ Family history (including genetic history) □ Sexual History/practices □ Counsel and provide HIV information (required by IN law) □ Social history (including drugs, substance use, smoking, alcohol) □ Work history (including occupational hazards) □ Physical activity □ Domestic violence (physical, sexual, emotional abuse) □ Psychosocial stressors □ Dietary/nutritional assessment □ Physical examination (including dental, height, weight) □ Assign pregnancy risk status □ Other genetic counseling if needed □ Transportation availability □ Screen for health literacy	□ History since last visit; questions and problems □ Smoking status □ Weeks gestation □ Blood pressure □ Weight □ Cumulative weight gain/loss □ Fundal height (in cm) □ Fetal heart tones □ Edema □ Fetal presentation (when appropriate) □ Fetal movement □ Cervical exam (if indicated) □ Other physical exam as indicated Ask regarding: □ Uterine contractions/cramping □ Pain/pressure □ Change in vaginal discharge □ Vaginal bleeding □ Dysuria	□ Document beginning of fetal movement □ Document auscultation of fetal heart tones with fetoscope	□ Re-evaluate pregnancy risk status		□ Physical exam □ Nutritional assessment □ Lactation assessment if appropriate □ Psychosocial stressors □ Smoking status □ Perinatal Mood Disorders □ Family planning
ROUTINE BIOCHEMICAL EVALUATION					
□ Blood type □ Rh type □ Antibody screen □ CBC □ Rubella titre □ Syphilis screening (required by IN law) □ HbsAG* □ Offer/recommend HIV testing □ Cervical cytology □ Gonorrhea culture □ Chlamydia culture □ Urinalysis and culture □ Wet mount for bacterial vaginosis, if symptomatic or previous preterm delivery	Urine dipstick: □ Protein □ Sugar □ Leukocytes □ Nitrites □ Ketosis	□ Offer Maternal Multiple Marker at 15-18 weeks (labs may vary on timing of tests) □ Ultrasound as indicated	□ One hour GCT (if indicated) □ Hct/Hgb Syphilis screening > or = 28 weeks (as required by IN law)	□ Group B Beta Strep Culture (unless already plan to treat due to risk factors)	□ Cervical cytology
OTHER BIOCHEMICAL EVALUATION (when indicated)					
If indicated: □ Diabetes screen □ Hgb electrophoresis (sickle cell) □ Tay Sachs screen □ TB skin test □ TORCH titers □ Group B Beta Strep culture □ Toxoplasmosis titer □ Varicella titer □ Urine drug screen	*Other tests as indicated:* e.g. Antepartum Fetal Surveillance, wet prep for bacterial vaginosis, STD cultures and urine cultures as appropriate	□ Ultrasound as indicated	*If indicated:* □ Antibody screen (if Rh-) □ RhoGAM given (28 weeks if indicated) □ GTT	*If indicated:* □ GC/Chlamydia □ Herpes culture (if active lesion) □ Hepatitis B* □ HIV test	*If indicated:* □ Rubella immunization □ RhoGAM □ Varicella vaccine □ dt □ Hgb/Hct □ Gtt: 2 hour post 75 grams clucola if GDM during pregnancy

© 2008 Indiana Perinatal Network   www.indianaperinatal.org

* If positive, notify OB department at delivering hospital and physician caring for infant.

See reverse ▶

Figure 10-8 Prenatal Care Guide.

continued

chapter 10 Promoting a Healthy Pregnancy

INITIAL VISIT & EACH VISIT (AS NEEDED)	20-24 WEEKS	24-28 WEEKS	34-40 WEEKS	POSTPARTUM
COUNSELING & EDUCATION BY PROVIDER, PRENATAL CARE COORDINATOR OR OTHER EDUCATOR				
□ Emotional adaptation to pregnancy □ Screen for perinatal mood disorders (Edinburgh Postpartum Depression Scale) □ Physical changes during pregnancy □ Fetal growth and development □ Available options; Preference/plans for birth □ Benefits of and preparation for breastfeeding □ Violence-free environment □ Prenatal diagnosis □ "Smoke-free" pregnancy education □ Effects of drugs and alcohol □ Teratogen exposures □ Nutrition/prenatal vitamins/folate/calcium/iron □ Safety (seat belt, smoke detector) □ Communicable diseases/STDs/HIV □ Weight gain appropriate for body mass □ Minor discomforts □ Exercise and rest □ When to call, numbers to call, emergency plan □ Danger signs □ Adoption information if indicated	□ Preterm birth prevention education ———	——— Repeat as needed to 37 weeks ——— ► □ Signs and symptoms of pre-eclampsia ——— Repeat as needed ——— ► Repeat as needed ————————————— ► Repeat as needed ————————————— ► Repeat as needed ————————————— ►		□ Parenting and coping with a new baby □ Crying strategies □ Never shake a baby (Happiest Baby skills) □ Perinatal mood disorders (signs and symptoms) □ Domestic violence (physical, sexual, emotional abuse) □ Breastfeeding support □ If HIV positive, do not breastfeed □ Back to work/school □ Siblings □ Family planning/Tubal sterilization □ Safe sleep education □ "Smoke-free" home □ Car seat □ Safety/CPR □ Immunizations □ Feeding □ When to call health care provider □ ASK about tobacco exposure □ Developmental issues □ Child care arrangements
Referrals as indicated for: □ WIC □ Dietician/Nutritionist □ Medicaid/managed care □ Prenatal care coordination □ Childbirth education □ Smoking cessation □ HIV care coordination □ High risk management or pregnancy consultation □ Alcohol and drug cessation □ Home care □ Genetic counseling □ Food and housing assistance		□ Fetal movement/kick counts □ Preparation for labor and delivery-VBAC, counseling, labor signs and symptoms, pain management for labor, begin childbirth classes, induction of labor	**Consents signed:** □ VBAC, C-section, tubal (at least 30 days prior to EDD if on Medicaid)	Referral to early intervention as indicated
		Initiate Postpartum Education: □ Evaluate plans □ Preparation for breastfeeding/Lactation Consultant □ Home preparation □ Choosing/meeting a health care provider for baby □ Family planning □ Circumcision information	**Preparing to bring baby home:** □ Safe sleep education □ "Smokefree" home □ Car seat □ Breastfeeding/feeding □ Assistance after going home □ Safety/CPR □ Jandice □ Rashes □ Cord Care □ Circumcised/Uncircumcised Care □ Immunizations □ Crying strategies □ Never shake a baby □ Temperature taking □ When to call health provider □ Back to school/work □ Newborn hearing screening □ Newborn metabolic screening □ Family planning □ Touching/holding/cuddling	

This document reflects the consensus of the Indiana Perinatal Network (IPN) State Perinatal Advisory Board—a constituency of professional organizations (i.e. ACOG, AAP) and individuals (i.e. CNMs, MDs, consumers). It is intended to serve as recommendations—not as established standards or rigid rules. Health care providers must make the best decisions possible within the limitations of the particular situation.

© 2008 Indiana Perinatal Network   www.indianaperinatal.org

Figure 10-8 cont'd Prenatal Care Guide.

Figure 10-9 Childbirth education classes help to prepare the expectant couple for many aspects of the childbearing year.

Box 10-3 **Lamaze Philosophy of Birth**

- Birth is normal, natural, and healthy.
- The experience of birth profoundly affects women and their families.
- Women's inner wisdom guides them through birth.
- Women's confidence and ability to give birth is either enhanced or diminished by the care provider and place of birth.
- Women have a right to give birth free from routine medical interventions.
- Birth can safely take place in birth centers and at home.
- Childbirth education empowers women to make informed choices in health care, to assume responsibility for their health, and to trust their inner wisdom.

Source: Lamaze International (2005). *About Lamaze International, Inc.* Retrieved from www.lamazechildbirth.com/fact_sheet.html

education in addition to education on natural pain relief. Lamaze educators stress that women need to make the decision that is personally best for them, with the knowledge that elimination of the pain makes it difficult to respond appropriately to contractions. In addition, after an epidural is placed, hospitals usually require that women remain in bed, have continuous fetal monitoring, and use medication to augment their contractions. The addition of these added procedures takes away from the philosophy that childbirth is a natural process.

- *Lamaze does not work*: When the woman has a complete understanding of the process of birth, the strategies for coping with the pain of the birth process, and the support of her family and members of the health care team, she is able to experience the birth of her baby as a normal and natural experience.
- *Lamaze is not for everyone*: The strategies used by Lamaze educators stress the natural process of childbearing. The philosophy of birth according to Lamaze International provides education and strategies for coping with labor and delivery that can be used by anyone who chooses this method.

Controlled breathing is the primary coping strategy used by proponents of the Lamaze method. Different breathing techniques and continued childbirth partner coaching facilitate each stage of labor. During the first stage of labor, breathing is used to relax the abdominal muscles and enlarge the abdominal cavity to enhance fetal descent. The woman inhales slowly, expanding her chest and abdominal cavity, and focuses on energy entering her body. As she exhales slowly, she focuses on tension leaving her body.

As the woman enters the second phase of the first stage of labor, known as transition, contractions become stronger and more frequent. Often it becomes difficult to concentrate on breathing. During this time, the woman's partner watches for signs of hyperventilation and helps her to focus on slow-paced breathing. During the second stage of labor, the active or pushing stage, the woman uses her breathing patterns to increase abdominal pressure in order to expel the fetus. She takes a breath, holds it for several seconds,

and exerts downward pressure on her stomach muscles. As she releases her breath, she continues to focus on releasing tension from her body. Once the fetal head reaches the pelvic outlet, the partner coaches the woman to continue with bearing down and pushing efforts until the baby is born. (See Chapters 12 and 13 for further discussion.)

The Bradley Method of Natural Childbirth

While the Lamaze method uses techniques that focus the woman on recognizing the signals of labor and using controlled breathing and muscle relaxation to facilitate the birth, the Bradley method uses techniques that focus the woman on inward relaxation, by means of breathing control, abdominal breathing, and general relaxation. The partner facilitates the implementation of these techniques, through coaching, giving rise to the term "husband-coached childbirth." To assist the partner in coaching the laboring woman to relax, there is an emphasis on darkness, solitude, and quiet in order to reduce stimulation and enhance the calm and comfort needed to conserve energy that will be required for birth and to decrease anxiety and tension in the woman (Bradley, 1965).

Dr. Robert Bradley developed this method of childbirth in the 1960s after a decision that radically changed the traditional delivery room. Bradley became the first obstetrician to allow fathers into the delivery room and to seek out methods to involve them in the labor and birth of their child in order to provide the woman with another individual who could provide her with support. After noting the dramatic effects of having the father present during the labor and birth, educational programs were developed to teach the fathers to be labor coaches and have an active role in the experience. It is through this active participation by the fathers that the woman is able to remain relaxed, assume positions that are most comfortable, and experience the childbirth as a more natural and spiritual event.

One of the primary differences in the Bradley method when compared to the Lamaze method is the breathing technique. The Bradley method teaches that women should breathe normally throughout the labor and birth process in order to maintain a state of relaxation and to oxygenate the baby adequately. The concern with the breathing techniques taught in the Lamaze method is that they can lead to dizziness and hyperventilation, resulting in decreased oxygenation of the fetus.

Other Methods

While the Lamaze and Bradley methods remain the top childbirth education formats, with training to prepare educators to teach parents the strategies, other methods for childbirth exist. Prepared childbirth classes incorporate approaches from diverse methods to assist expectant couples in developing coping skills that will work best for them. Additional methods and techniques include the following:

- Dick-Read: The underlying philosophy in Dick-Read's approach to childbirth still focuses on the natural aspect of giving birth. After witnessing a birth in the 1920s, without the use of the traditional chloroform to render the laboring woman unconscious, he discovered that it was possible for women to experience pain-free birth. Through his study of physiology, he hypothesized that the pain associated with childbirth was caused by fear and tension, stimulating the sympathetic nervous system. This physiological event decreased blood flow to the uterus and created uterine muscle cell hypoxia. Through various relaxation techniques that consist of conscious and progressive relaxation of different muscle groups, the tension is reduced and blood flow to the uterus is restored. Although Dick-Read did not advocate the use of pharmacologic pain management during labor and delivery, he approved of its use when the woman was unable to relax or was experiencing complications (Dick-Read, 1987).
- HypnoBirthing: Classes using this method are based on Dick-Read's fear-tension-pain philosophy. Couples are taught, in four sessions, relaxation techniques to eliminate the pain associated with the fear and tension.
- LeBoyer method: Using this method, the baby is born in a dimly lit room that is conducive to relaxation and facilitates a tranquil entrance into the world. Immediately after birth, the newborn is placed in a warm water bath to enhance the transition from the intrauterine to the extrauterine environment. The infant is then moved to the mother's abdomen to initiate bonding. Through the gentle handling and the quiet, smooth transition, the newborn is able to open her eyes and breathe with minimal external stimulation.
- Odent method: This method arose from the LeBoyer method and includes moving the woman into a warm water bath for the birth. In addition to reducing labor pain, the warm water provides a comforting atmosphere to transition the newborn to extrauterine life. The underlying concept is that the infant can safely be born while submersed in water, without fear of drowning, since the fetus has lived in fluid for the duration of the pregnancy. Not all women are candidates for hydrotherapy. It is not an option for women who have rupture of the membranes or other complications that require continuous fetal monitoring.
- Birthing From Within: This method views childbirth as a rite of passage for parents and their infant. The underpinnings of this method focus on the psychological and spiritual aspects of birth, using art, writing, painting, and sculpting to encourage self-discovery. The focus is not on the birth process, but on the experience of birth.

FINDING INFORMATION ON CHILDBIRTH EDUCATION

There are many ways that expectant mothers and their partners can locate information on childbirth education. The best strategy is to begin with the health care provider, who can provide information about potential birth locations and childbirth education provided by the individual facilities. Internet sources can also assist couples in finding classes that are available to them locally. Expectant couples can engage in online childbirth education classes as well as home education through the purchase of comprehensive childbirth programs.

In determining the childbirth preparation class that will meet the individual needs of the parents, the following questions should be considered:

- Who sponsors the class?
- How many classes will we be expected to attend?
- How many couples are in the class?
- Can I bring more than one support person to the class?
- What types of teaching and learning strategies are used?
- What topics are covered in the course?
- Where will the classes be held?
- Is there a cost involved?
- Is the instructor certified? If so, with what organization is the instructor affiliated?

With the abundance of childbirth methods available and the different certifications that exist for childbirth educators, it is important for expectant parents to identify the approaches and methods that best meet their needs in order to make the childbirth experience as meaningful as possible to them. It is helpful not only to examine the questions listed above, but also to consider what the most important factors are with regard to personal values and beliefs. Using the list below, nurses can direct parents to the appropriate education program to meet their needs. The woman should identify which four of the following factors are most important in selecting a childbirth education class:

- Familiarize me with hospital routines
- Prepare me for a natural, nonmedicated birth
- Teach me breathing patterns and distraction techniques
- Give my partner the skills necessary to be an active and informed labor coach
- Teach us as parents to be childbirth consumers and to take responsibility for our child's birth
- Follow current medical policies
- Represent the most common type of childbirth education class in our area
- Teach relaxation and natural breathing
- Stress good nutrition and exercise
- Discuss medication options without making value judgments

CREATING A BIRTH PLAN

From the moment a woman discovers that she is pregnant, she begins to consider ideas for her birth experience. Although the birth is usually not imminent, previous knowledge and experience, along with information shared by friends and family, prompt her to seek out information on options that are available and choices that she can make to prepare for the birth. While the birth plan is not a concrete document from which to outline every step of the labor and birth, it provides written information that identifies preferences for labor and birth, empowering the expectant couple with the control that is needed to reduce the anxiety associated with labor. Birth plans can be tailored to meet the needs of expectant couples that anticipate a hospital delivery, a birthing center delivery, a home delivery, a cesarean delivery, or a multiple delivery. Developing a birth plan in conjunction with the health care provider assures that the woman's individual situation is considered, especially important for high-risk pregnancies.

Birth Plan Choices

There are many issues to consider when developing a personal birth plan. One concerns the presence of additional people in the birthing room. The woman may wish to include her partner, friends, relatives, a **doula** (a woman who is experienced in childbirth and provides physical and emotional support to the mother during the prenatal period, during labor, during birth, and during the postpartum period) or birthing coach, and children. She may desire to personalize the experience by wearing her own clothes, listening to music, and taking pictures or videotaping the birth. Fluids and food preferences can be noted, along with the woman's desire for a saline or heparin lock or an intravenous line. While most hospitals utilize continuous fetal monitoring, the woman can identify her wish for intermittent monitoring or no monitoring at all, unless an emergency develops. Preferences for laboring and birthing positions can also be noted. Choices regarding strategies for pharmacological and nonpharmacological pain management are identified, with the understanding that the woman has the right to change her mind and alter her plan at any time.

The woman who anticipates a vaginal birth should identify her preference regarding an episiotomy and the use of medication to augment labor contractions. The partner's desired level of involvement in the birth should also be identified. The woman can decide if she would like to hold her baby immediately after birth and, if she plans to breastfeed, whether she wishes to do so at that time.

Women who anticipate a cesarean birth or who discover that they need a cesarean birth can usually maintain some degree of control over this procedure as well. They may be allowed to have their partner present during the surgery. The partner may be permitted to hold the newborn during the first moments of life if there are no immediate health concerns. The mother may also choose to initiate breastfeeding in the recovery room. Other preferences regarding infant feeding, rooming-in and circumcision should be noted in the birth plan.

Choosing a Health Care Provider

Selecting a health care provider for the preconception, pregnancy, and birth experience is an essential first step that empowers the woman and her partner to become actively involved in care during the childbearing year. Approximately 90% of pregnant women choose an obstetrician as the primary care provider. Others use a certified nurse-midwife (CNM), who is trained in both nursing and midwifery and can provide a more personalized, less routine approach to a normal, uncomplicated pregnancy and birth. It is especially important that the patient choose a care provider with whom she can openly relate and who shares the same philosophical views on the management of pregnancy. (See Chapter 9 for further discussion.)

Choosing a Birth Location

A hospital is the most common birth location. In this setting, health care providers and patients have access to technology and individuals trained to manage any complications that may arise. Obstetricians and certified nurse midwives attend and facilitate childbirth in the hospital setting. When choosing the facility that best meets their needs, the expectant couple should identify the type of setting provided by the hospital. For example, some institutions have separate labor, delivery, recovery, and postpartum rooms. This arrangement requires the family to be moved from one location to another during their hospital stay. The newest facility models place emphasis on family-centered care and offer large, comfortable rooms where the woman remains for the duration of the childbirth experience.

Freestanding birthing centers were first opened in 1974 to provide women with a more homelike atmosphere in which to give birth. Although these facilities are located near the hospital in the event of an emergency, they are recommended for women with low-risk pregnancies. A major benefit of the birthing centers is that they have fewer restrictions and generally allow the parents more freedom to make personal decisions regarding labor and birth.

Home births are returning as an option for women with low-risk pregnancies and no known labor complications. Although obstetricians will not deliver babies at home, many CNMs are willing to do so. Many expectant couples believe that giving birth at home enriches the childbirth experience and allows them to better integrate the birth as a normal and natural event in their lives. However, the parents must be open to transfer to a hospital if complications arise.

 Now Can You— Discuss childbirth preparation, birth plans, and doulas?

1. Compare and contrast the Lamaze, Bradley, and LeBoyer methods of childbirth preparation?
2. Discuss the purpose of a birth plan?
3. Describe the role of a doula?

---

summary points

◆ Preconception counseling empowers families to plan for pregnancy and develop healthy bodies and minds to optimize birth outcomes.

◆ Nurses and other health care providers must collaboratively provide families with prenatal education and incorporate interventions for a holistic approach to pregnancy.

◆ A balance of diet and nutrition, exercise, work, and rest enhances the development of a healthy pregnancy.

◆ To determine safety of use during pregnancy, all medications, including prescription, over-the-counter, and herbal preparations, must be carefully evaluated. It is essential that the nurse obtain a comprehensive medication history during each prenatal visit.

◆ Ongoing prenatal education regarding pregnancy danger signs and symptoms, and appropriate home interventions is key in reducing complications.

◆ Nurses can help to empower families by providing information about childbirth education programs and other community resources.

◆ A holistic approach to a healthy pregnancy and birth includes all members of the family and the health care team. Encouraging the family to develop a birth plan is an important step in helping to create a positive, satisfying birth experience.

review questions

Multiple Choice

1. The perinatal nurse knows that the most ideal time to address issues related to a poor outcome in a past pregnancy is:
   A. Postpartum
   B. Prenatally
   C. Preconception
   D. Interconception

2. The prenatal nurse provides nutritional counseling during pregnancy to ensure adequate weight gain. The nurse teaches that the additional daily calories required are the equivalent of:
   A. One glass of skim milk
   B. Two servings of yogurt
   C. Two apples
   D. Three ounces of cheese

3. The perinatal nurse knows that the blood volume in pregnancy increases, on average, by:
   A. 20–30%
   B. 30–40%
   C. 40–50%
   D. 50–60%

Select All that Apply

4. The perinatal nurse knows that the *Healthy People 2010* national initiative suggests the use of specific outcomes to measure goals that are critical to the health of women and families. These outcomes include:
   A. The number of women receiving prenatal care
   B. The number of very low birth weight infants
   C. The level of maternal anxiety associated with prenatal care
   D. The preterm birth rate

5. The clinic nurse encourages all pregnant women to eat foods rich in folic acid such as:
   A. Cheese
   B. Chicken
   C. Brussels sprouts
   D. Orange juice

6. The clinic nurse offers smoking cessation programs to all prenatal women who smoke because cigarette smoking during pregnancy increases the risk for:
   A. Sudden infant death syndrome
   B. Spontaneous abortion
   C. Intrauterine growth restriction
   D. Postdate pregnancy

True/False

7. As part of preventive health care, the clinic nurse encourages all adults to have a tetanus booster every 10 years.

Fill-in-the-Blank

8. The clinic nurse includes tracking of a woman's _____ history as part of her preconception visit. Determining the _____ and length of _____ periods will enhance the likelihood of conception.

9. The clinic nurse is providing education to a pregnant woman who has come for her first prenatal visit at 8 weeks gestation. The nurse explains that _____ is common during the next few weeks but will usually resolve between thirteen and _____ weeks and is usually caused by adequate hormonal support for the pregnancy.

10. The clinic nurse knows that _____ is a hormone that acts as a depressant in pregnancy.

See Answers to End of Chapter Review Questions on the Electronic Study Guide or DavisPlus.

REFERENCES

American College of Obstetricians and Gynecologists (ACOG). (2001). Committee Opinion Number 264: *Air travel during pregnancy.* Washington, DC: Author

American College of Obstetricians and Gynecologists (ACOG). (2002). Committee Opinion Number 267: *Exercise during pregnancy and the postpartum period.* Washington, DC: Author.

American College of Obstetricians and Gynecologists (ACOG). (2003a). Neural Tube Defects (Practice Bulletin No. 44). Washington, DC: Author.

American College of Obstetricians and Gynecologists (ACOG). (2003b). Management of preterm labor (Practice Bulletin No. 43). Washington, DC: Author.

American College of Obstetricians and Gynecologists (ACOG). (2004). Committee Opinion Number 304: *Prenatal and perinatal Human Immunodeficiency Virus testing: expanded recommendations.* Washington, DC: Author.

American College of Obstetricians and Gynecologists (ACOG). (2005). Committee Opinion Number 313: *The importance of preconception care in the continuum of women's health care.* Washington, DC: Authors.

American College of Obstetricians and Gynecologists (ACOG). (2006). Committee Opinion Number 343: *Psychosocial risk factors: Perinatal screening and intervention.* Washington, DC: Author.

American College of Obstetricians and Gynecologists (ACOG). (2007). Screening for Fetal Chromosomal Abnormalities. (Practice Bulletin No. 77). Washington, DC: Authors.

Alexander, L.L., LaRosa, J.H., Bader, H., & Garfield, S. (2004). *New dimensions in women's health* (3rd ed., pp 191–240). Boston: Jones and Bartlett.

Attrill, B. (2002). The assumption of the maternal role: A developmental process. *Australian Journal of Midwifery, 15,* 21–25.

Bradley, R. (1965). *Husband-coached childbirth.* New York: HarperCollins.

Bulechek, G., Butcher, H.M., & Dochterman, J. (2008). *Nursing interventions classification (NIC)* (5th ed.). St. Louis, MO: C.V. Mosby.

Centers for Disease Control and Prevention (CDC). (2002). Alcohol use among women of childbearing age—United States, 1991–1999. *Morbidity and Mortality Weekly Reports, 51,* 273–276.

Cogswell, M.E., & Dietz, P.M. (2006). Maternal weight, before, during, and after pregnancy in the United States. *Workshop on the impact of pregnancy weight on maternal & child health, May 30–31, 2006.* The National Academies. Retrieved from www.bocyf.org/053006.html (Accessed June 12, 2006).

Cunningham, F., Leveno, K., Bloom, S., Hauth, J., Gilstrap, L., & Wenstrom, K. (Eds). *Williams obstetrics* (22nd ed.). New York: McGraw-Hill.

Deglin, J.H., & Vallerand, A.H. (2009). *Davis's drug guide for nurses* (11th ed.). Philadelphia. F.A. Davis.

Dick-Read, G. (1987). *Childbirth without fear* (5th ed.). New York: Harper & Collins.

Encyclopedia of genetic disorders. (2008). http://health.enotes.com/genetic-disorders-encyclopedia/accutane-embryopathy) (Accessed April 22, 2008).

Goodheart, H.P. (2006). Accutane for severe acne. *Women's Heath Ob-GYN Edition, 11*(12), 9–15.

Haram, K., Nilsen, S., & Schall, J. (2001). Iron supplementation in pregnancy: Evidence and controversies. *Acta Obstetrica et Gynecologica Scandinavica, 89,* 683–688.

Institute for Clinical Systems Improvement (ICSI). (2005). Routine prenatal care. Bloomington, MN: Author.

Institute of Medicine. (1992). *Nutrition during pregnancy and lactation: An implementation guide.* Washington, DC: National Academies Press.

Johnson, M., Bulechek, G., Butcher, H., McCloskey Dochterman, J., Maas, M., Moorhead, S., & Swanson, E. (2006). *NANDA, NOC, and NIC linkages: Nursing diagnoses, outcomes, & interventions* (2nd ed.). St. Louis, MO: Mosby Elsevier.

Kilpatrick, S., & Laros, R. (2004). Maternal hematologic disorders. In R. Creasy, R. Resnik, & J. Iams (Eds.), *Maternal-fetal medicine: Principles and practice* (5th ed.). Philadelphia: W.B. Saunders.

King, J.C. (2006). Biological determinants of gestational weight gain. *Workshop on the Impact of Pregnancy Weight on Maternal & Child Health, May 30–31, 2006.* The National Academies. Retrieved from www.bocyf.org/053006.html (Accessed June 12, 2006).

Krishnaswamy, K., & Madhavan Nair, K. (2001). Importance of folate in human nutrition. *British Journal of Nutrition, 85*(Supplement 2), S115–S124.

Lamaze International. (2005). *About Lamaze International, Inc.* Retrieved from www.lamazechildbirth.com/fact_sheet.html (Accessed April 22, 2008).

Lashley, F. (2005). *Clinical genetics in nursing practice* (3rd ed.). New York: Springer.

Lederman, R. (1996). *Psychosocial adaptation in pregnancy* (2nd ed.). Englewood Cliffs, NJ: Prentice-Hall.

Lewis, D.P., Van Dyke, D.C., Stumbo, P.J., & Berg, M.J. (1998). Drug and environmental factors associated with adverse pregnancy outcomes. Part II: Improvement with folic acid. *Annals of Pharmacotherapeutics (32),* 947–961.

Mahomed, K. (2002). Iron supplementation in pregnancy (Cochrane Review). *The Cochrane Library,* Issue 4. Oxford: Update Software.

March of Dimes Birth Defects Foundation (2006). *Smoking during pregnancy.* Retrieved from www.marchofdimes.com/printableArticles/14332_1171.asp (Accessed June 11, 2006).

Mayo Foundation for Medical Education & Research. (June 1, 2005). *Weight gain during pregnancy: What's healthy?* Retrieved from www.mayoclinic.com/print/pregnancy-weight-gain/PR00111/METHOD=print (Accessed June 11, 2006).

Mills, M.E. (2007). More than food: The implications of Pica in pregnancy. *Nursing for Women's Health, 11*(3), 266–273.

Moorehead, S., Johnson, M., Mass, M., & Swanson, E. (2008). *Nursing outcomes classification (NOC)* (4th ed.). St. Louis, MO: C.V. Mosby.

Moos, M.K. (2006). Preconception Care: Every Woman, Every Time. *AWHONN Lifelines, 10*(4), 332–334.

NANDA International. (2007). *NANDA-I Nursing Diagnoses: Definitions and Classifications 2007-2008.* Philadelphia: NANDA-I.

National High Blood Pressure Education Program Working Group. (2000). *Working group report on high blood pressure in pregnancy.* NHBPEP Publication No. 00-3029. Washington, DC: National Heart Lung and Blood Institute.

National Toxicology Program Center for the Evaluation of Risks to Human Reproduction (2005). Caffeine. Retrieved from http://cerhr.niehs.nih.gov/common/caffeine.html (Accessed July 16, 2007).

Peters, R.M., & Flack, J.M. (2004). Hypertensive disorders of pregnancy. *JOGNN: Journal of Obstetric, Gynecologic, and Neonatal Nursing, 33*(2), 209–220.

Phillips, O.P. (2007). Preconceptional care: Risk reduction starts before pregnancy. *The Forum, 5*(1), 12–18.

Riley, L.E. (2006). Recommended practices and policies for clinicians. *Workshop on the Impact of Pregnancy Weight on Maternal & Child Health, May 30–31, 2006.* The National Academies. Retrieved from www.bocyf.org/053006.html (Accessed June 12, 2006).

Scanlon, K. (Ed.) (2001). *Final report of the vitamin D expert panel.* Atlanta: Centers for Disease Control and Prevention.

Scholl, T. (2005). Iron status during pregnancy: Setting the stage for mother and infant. *American Journal of Clinical Nutrition, 81*(5), 1218S–1222S.

Scholl, T., & Reilly, T. (2000). Anemia, iron and pregnancy outcome. *Journal of Nutrition, 130*(25 Supplement), 443S–447S.

Siega-Riz, A., & Savitz, D. (2001). What are pregnant women eating? Nutrient and food group differences by race. *American Journal of Obstetrics and Gynecology, 186*(3), 480–486.

Stotland, N.E. (2006). Gestational weight gain: Social predictors or relationships. *Workshop on the Impact of Pregnancy Weight on Maternal & Child Health, May 30–31, 2006.* The National Academies. Retrieved from www.bocyf.org/053006.html (Accessed June 12, 2006).

Stuart, G., & Laraia, M. (2005). *Principles and practice of psychiatric nursing* (8th ed.). St. Louis: C.V. Mosby.

Swensen, A.R., Harnack, L.J., & Ross, J.A. (2001). Nutritional assessment of pregnant women enrolled in the special supplemental program for Women, Infants, and Children (WIC). *Journal of the American Dietetic Association, 101*(8), 903-908.

Thompson, J.R., Gerald, P.F., Willoughby, M.L., & Armstrong, B.K. (2001). Maternal folate supplementation in pregnancy and protection against acute lymphoblastic leukemia in childhood: A case-controlled study. *Lancet, 358,* 1935–1940.

U.S. Department of Health & Human Services (USDHHS). (2000). *Healthy People 2010: Understanding and improving health* (2nd ed.). Washington, DC: U.S. Government Printing Office.

U.S. Department of Health & Human Services (USDHHS). (2004). *The health consequences of smoking: A report of the Surgeon General—2004.* Atlanta, GA: CDC Office on Smoking and Health.

U.S. Department of Health & Human Services (USDHHS). (2005). *U.S. Department of Agriculture Dietary Guidelines for Americans, 2005.* Washington, DC: U.S. Government Printing Office.

U.S. Department of Health & Human Services (USDHHS). (2006). *Your guide to lowering your blood pressure with DASH* (NIH Publication No. 06-4082). Washington, DC: U.S. Government Printing Office.

United States Department of Health and Human Services (USDHHS), & United States Department of Agriculture (USDA). (2005). *Dietary Guidelines for Americans.* Retrieved from http://www.nal.usda.gov/fnic/.Hyattsville, MD: US Department of Agriculture.

United States Department of Labor. (1995). *Fact sheet #28: The Family and Medical Leave Act of 1993.* Retrieved from www.dol.gov/esa/regs/compliance/whd/printpage.asp?REF=whdfs28.htm (Accessed July 16, 2006).

Varney, H., Kriebs, J.M., & Gegor, C.L. (2004). *Varney's midwifery* (4th ed.). Boston: Jones and Bartlett.

Venes, D. (Ed.). (2009). *Tabers cyclopedic medical dictionary* (21st ed.). Philadelphia: F.A. Davis.

Veterans Health Administration. (2002). *Department of Defense/Veterans Administration clinical practice guideline for the management of uncomplicated pregnancy.* Washington, DC: U.S. Government Printing Office.

White, H., & Bouvier, D. (2005). Caring for a patient having a miscarriage. *Nursing 2005, 35*(7), 18–19.

Youngkin, E.Q., & Davis, M.S. (2004). *Women's health: A primary care clinical guide* (3rd ed.). Upper Saddle River, NJ: Pearson-Prentice Hall.

DavisPlus DavisPlus.fadavis.com **For more information, go to http://davisplus.fadavis.com/**

CONCEPT MAP

Promoting a Healthy Pregnancy

Preconception Counseling

Healthy Body: assess
- Medical/menstrual history
- Findings from physical/lab exams
- Exposure to STIs
- Lifestyle choices

Healthy Mind: assess
- Readiness for motherhood/fatherhood
- Healthy relationship
- Social support
- Educational level
- Mental illness

Nutrition

Factors Affecting:
- Eating disorders: pica, anorexia/bulimia
- Cultural influences
- Being vegan

Nursing:
- Obtain nutritional hx.
- Assess for nutritional elements: calories, proteins, water, minerals, vitamins, calcium, iron, vitamin C

Medications
- Encourage consultation with PCP to determine drug safety
- Know teratogens
- Assess for use of herbal/homeopathic preparations and OTCs

Activity

Work: assess impact
- What is the nature of the work?
- Is there exposure to toxins?
- What is the number of hours?
- Are there complications with pregnancy?
- Plan for maternity leave

Exercise:
- Focus on muscle strengthening
- Maintain adequate breathing rate; fluid intake during exercise
- Limit strenuous aerobics and increased body temperature
- Avoid exhaustion

Common Discomforts

Anticipatory guidance/care strategies for:
GI: nausea, vomiting, constipation, flatulence, dyspepsia, ptyalism
CV: dependent edema, varicosities, supine hypotensive syndrome
GU: frequency, nocturia
Pain: round ligament, paresthesias, backache, leg cramps
Other: leukorrhea, fatigue, shortness of breath, dyspareunia, dental issues, insomnia

Recognize signs of complications: Differentiate from discomforts

- Hyperemesis gravidarum
- Spontaneous abortion
- Infection
- Preeclampsia
- PROM
- Absence of fetal movement
- Placenta previa/abruptio placentae

Weight Gain

Factors Affecting:
Genetic/social hx.
Enlarging placenta
- Increased bladder volume
- Increased blood volume
- Fetal growth

Nursing:
- BMI screening
- Conscious planning of food intake: USDA food pyramid & DASH plan
- Patient education/counseling

Childbirth Education
- Class → harmonious with beliefs/values
- Goal → facilitate positive birth experience
- Topics: A&P, comfort measures, labor and birth process, childbirth methods, relaxation/pain management, types of births, postpartum care, newborn care/feeding
- Create a birth plan

Rest: tending to fatigue caused by:
- Increased progesterone production
- Physiological anemia
- Increased fetal oxygen needs
- Emotional stress
- Decreased maternal lung expansion
- Nocturia

 Complementary Care:
- Ayurveda during pre-conception period
- Manage stress with: massage, light and aromatherapy, reflexology, relaxation

Optimizing Outcomes:
- Prenatal interventions to prevent birth defects
- Educate re: strategies to relieve back pain
- Patient should participate in fetal movement assessment

Nursing Insight:
- Food/drug interactions with iron supplements
- Vegetarians at risk for B_{12} deficiency
- Significant teratogenic effects with Accutane
- Food choice and positioning can decrease dyspepsia

Now Can You:
? - Discuss preconception care
- Identify substances to be avoided
- Discuss aspects of good nutrition
- Discuss work, fatigue and medication use
- Identify common discomforts of pregnancy
- Identify danger signs in pregnancy

 Ethnocultural Considerations:
- Higher maternal anemia in adolescents, African American women/low socioeconomic status
- African Americans: higher vitamin D deficiency rate
- Pica associated with some cultural, religious beliefs

Caring for the Woman Experiencing Complications During Pregnancy

chapter
11

Apprehension, uncertainty, waiting, expectation, fear of surprise, do a patient more harm than exertion.

—Florence Nightingale, 1860

LEARNING TARGETS *At the completion of this chapter, the student will be able to:*

◆ Discuss the importance of ongoing assessment of the pregnant patient for potential complications throughout her pregnancy.

◆ Describe the roles of the perinatologist, neonatologist, obstetric nurse, visiting nurse, chaplain, nutritionist, and social worker in caring for the family experiencing complications during a pregnancy.

◆ Discuss the importance of understanding and respecting the cultural differences the nurse may encounter when caring for a diverse population experiencing a high-risk pregnancy.

◆ Plan nursing assessments and interventions for the woman experiencing complications of pregnancy.

◆ Discuss the importance of complete and accurate documentation in caring for the patient experiencing an obstetric emergency.

◆ Identify complications of pregnancy that require fetal surveillance.

◆ Describe fetal surveillance tests that may be warranted to evaluate fetal well-being.

◆ Relate the effects of antenatal bedrest to the physical, psychological, and social adjustment of a high-risk pregnancy.

---

 moving toward evidence-based practice Risk of Adverse Pregnancy Outcomes Related to Weight Changes

Villamor, E., & Cnattingius, S. (2006). Interpregnancy weight change and risk of adverse pregnancy outcomes: A population-based study. *The Lancet, 368*, 1164–1170.

The purpose of this study was to explore the relationship between overweight or obesity and adverse pregnancy outcomes. The association between the pre-pregnancy body-mass index (BMI) from the first to the second pregnancy and the risk of adverse outcomes during the second pregnancy were examined. The study sample consisted of data from 151,025 women who experienced first and second consecutive singleton births during the time interval from 1992 to 2001.

The participants' BMI was calculated during the first antenatal visit of each pregnancy. Interpregnancy changes in the BMI from the beginning of the first and second pregnancies were also calculated and the participants were placed in the following categories based on changes in BMI units:

- less than −1
- −1 to less than 1

- 1 to less than 2
- 2 to less than 3
- 3 or more units

The interpregnancy interval (months between birth of the first child and the estimated date of conception of the second child) included the following groups:

- 12–23 months
- 24–35 months
- 36 or more months

Based on the BMI at the beginning of the first pregnancy, participants were grouped using the following categories:

- Underweight (BMI <18.4)
- Healthy (BMI 18.5–24.9)

(continued)

moving toward evidence-based practice (continued)

- Overweight (BMI 25.0–29.9)
- Obese (BMI >30)

Demographic data included the number of years of formal education: 9 years or less; 10–11 years; 12 years; 13–14 years; and 15 years or more. Outcome measures included maternal complications (e.g., preeclampsia, gestational hypertension, gestational diabetes, and cesarean birth) and perinatal complications (e.g., stillbirth [fetal death at 28 weeks or later] and large for gestational age birth [more than 2 standard deviations above the mean for gestational age]) associated with the second pregnancy.

Data analysis revealed the following findings:

- On average, participants gained slightly more than one-half of a BMI unit during a mean pregnancy interval of 24 months.
- Weight gain declined between pregnancies with increasing maternal age and years of education.
- Weight gain (based on the BMI at the first pregnancy) and the incidence of complications increased with maternal tobacco use.
- There was an increased risk of adverse outcome associated with increased weight gain between pregnancies.

- The incidence of maternal/perinatal complications began to increase with a BMI of 1 to less than 2.
- The risk for preeclampsia and large for gestational age birth fell significantly in women who lost more than one BMI unit between pregnancies.
- After a gain of 3 or more BMI units between pregnancies, the risk for a stillbirth was 63%.
- An interpregnancy increase of 3 or more BMI units was associated with the following adverse pregnancy outcomes: preeclampsia, gestational hypertension, gestational diabetes, stillbirth, and large-for-gestational-age birth.
- Weight gain between pregnancies demonstrated a strong association between risk of a major maternal and/or perinatal complication and an increase in the interpregnancy BMI.

1. What might be considered as limitations to this study?
2. How is this information useful to clinical nursing practice?

See Suggested Responses for Moving Toward Evidence-Based Practice on the Electronic Study Guide or DavisPlus.

Introduction

Pregnancy is a normal physiological function of all living species. Couples (or, in more recent times, single individuals) who have chosen to become parents look forward to having a healthy, happy, and bright newborn enter their lives. They anticipate the arrival of a baby who they will be able to love and nurture over the years to grow into a happy, healthy and productive adult. However, pregnancies do not always progress smoothly and the pregnant woman and her family or significant other may experience a complication at some point during the childbearing year. Complications that arise during this time are often challenging and demand the perinatal nurse's skills, knowledge, and expertise combined with the nursing process to first identify the pregnant patient at risk and then formulate, implement, and evaluate an appropriate, holistic plan of care. Identification and activation of appropriate community resources is also an essential component of the care plan. Throughout the entire process, the nurse must remain cognizant of the unique individuality of the patient and her family and deliver care that is respectful of their diversity and culture.

Interviewing is a skill basic to nursing. A carefully conducted interview is a tool that enables nurses to collect data, recognize signs and symptoms of emerging problems, identify risks, and formulate nursing diagnoses and counseling strategies (Givens, Moore, & Freda, 2004). The signs and symptoms of the complications that may arise during pregnancy can be subtle. The nurse's need to elicit information from the patient through the interview and to process that information cannot be overemphasized. Anticipatory nursing care is invaluable in preventing a complication from becoming a major health crisis. Notifying the primary health care provider immediately of signs or symptoms of alterations from the expected clinical progression during pregnancy can facilitate early intervention and guide an appropriate management plan.

The complications described in this chapter can be extremely serious to both the patient and her fetus and result in severe morbidity or even death. It is essential that women feel comfortable and confident with the care they receive. Maternal health care often represents the first point of contact between immigrant women and the U.S. health care system. Since many do not speak and/or read English, the nurse must facilitate an interview in the woman's primary language. Use of the woman's native language greatly increases her level of comfort and acceptance and is paramount to establishing an accurate diagnosis and appropriate plan of care (Givens, Moore, & Freda, 2004). When indicated, every effort should be made to secure a female interpreter who is not a member of the family. In most cases, children are not suitable translators, as many assessment questions involve subjects that women may not wish to discuss with their children or with men. Friends and family members who serve as interpreters are not bound by a code of conduct and may breach confidentiality, editorialize, or omit information they find threatening or embarrassing. The woman's privacy may also be jeopardized (Givens, Moore, & Freda, 2004). By providing culturally competent nursing care to childbearing families, many potential complications can be identified in a timely manner to allow for effective treatment and improved outcomes.

Early Pregnancy Complications

PERINATAL LOSS

Perinatal loss can be divided into two major types: death of the fetus or newborn or birth of a less than a perfect child. The perinatal period encompasses the total embryonic, fetal, and neonatal life span. Because there is a greater danger to life during this period than at any other time during the life cycle, adverse outcomes can be expected. Loss of a child, whether it is an embryo, fetus, or neonate, can be totally devastating not only to the woman but to the entire family as well. Supporting the family through a perinatal loss can be very challenging to the obstetric nurse who must be in touch with personal feelings in order to help understand the family's response to their loss. (See Chapter 14 for further discussion.)

> ## 66 **What to say** 99 — *Communicating with the family who has experienced a perinatal loss*
>
> The nurse approaches the family with compassion and sincerity. Expressions of caring are conveyed in the following statements:
>
> "I understand this is a very difficult time for you and your family, but I want you to know that I am here and willing to listen if you want to talk. You let me know if and when you are ready."
>
> "It is normal for you to be sad and you will probably feel like this for some time. Losing a baby, no matter how far along in your pregnancy, is very difficult. I can recommend some support groups if you think you might be interested." If the patient says she does not want the information at this time, continue with "Please do not hesitate to call us if you change your mind. We can always give you the information."
>
> "Does your baby have a name?" The nurse would then refer to the fetus by name. Do not use the term "fetus" with the patient. To her the deceased fetus was her baby.

ECTOPIC PREGNANCY

An ectopic pregnancy is one that implants outside of the uterine cavity. Implantation may occur in the fallopian tube (99%), on the ovary, the cervix, on the outside of the fallopian tube, the abdominal wall, or on the bowel (Fig. 11-1). Patients who present with vaginal bleeding, a missed period, and abdominal tenderness or pain should always be evaluated for an ectopic pregnancy. Pain increases after rupture of the ectopic pregnancy and the woman may experience referred shoulder pain from diaphragmatic irritation caused by blood in the peritoneal cavity.

A number of factors place a woman at risk for experiencing an ectopic pregnancy. These include past and current medical and gynecological problems such as:

- History of sexually transmitted infections or pelvic inflammatory disease
- Prior ectopic pregnancy
- Previous tubal, pelvic, or abdominal surgery
- Endometriosis
- Current use of exogenous hormones (i.e., estrogen, progesterone)
- In vitro fertilization or other method of assisted reproduction
- In utero diethylstilbestrol (DES) exposure with abnormalities of the reproductive organs
- Use of an intrauterine device

Diagnosis

To prevent major morbidity or death, an ectopic pregnancy should be diagnosed before the onset of hypotension, bleeding, pain, and overt rupture. The patient's history (e.g., unilateral, bilateral or diffuse abdominal pain, missed period) and physical exam (a palpable mass is present on bimanual examination in approximately 50% of women) should alert the health care professional to the possible presence of an ectopic pregnancy. Active bleeding is associated with rupture; other symptoms of this complication may include hypotension, tachycardia, vertigo and shoulder pain. Diagnostic laboratory tests include a beta-human chorionic gonadotropin (β-hCG) that is low for gestational age (because an ectopic pregnancy has a poorly implanted placenta, the level of a β-hCG does not double every 48 hours as in normal implantation) and a white blood count (WBC) that can range from normal to $15,000/mm^3$. Transvaginal ultrasonography should be performed to confirm intrauterine or tubal pregnancy (Farquhar, 2005). Ultrasonographic identification of an intrauterine pregnancy rules out the presence of an ectopic pregnancy in most women (Murray, Baakdah, Bardell, & Tulandi, 2005).

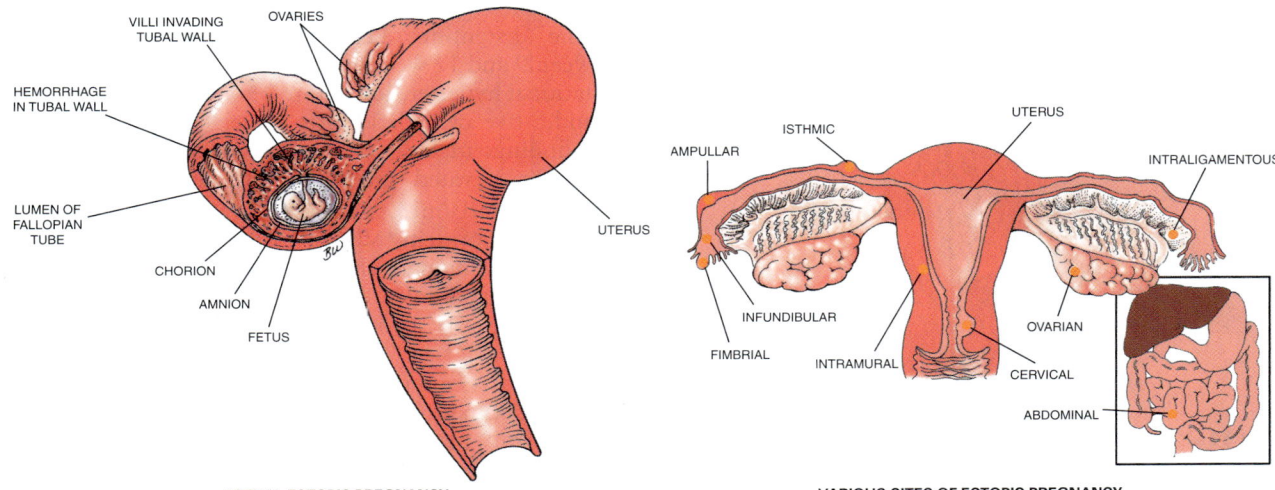

ACTUAL ECTOPIC PREGNANCY

VARIOUS SITES OF ECTOPIC PREGNANCY

Figure 11-1 Ectopic pregnancy.

Management

Salpingectomy (removal of the ruptured fallopian tube) by **laparotomy** (surgical procedure in which the abdomen is opened to visualize the abdominal organs) has long offered an almost 100% cure for the treatment of an ectopic pregnancy. However, current clinical emphasis is aimed not only on prevention of maternal death but also on the prompt restoration of health through a rapid recovery with preservation of fertility. To achieve this goal, **laparoscopic** (visualization of the reproductive organs using a laparoscope inserted into the pelvic cavity through a small incision in the abdomen), **salpingostomy** (incision into the fallopian tube to remove the pregnancy) and partial salpingectomy are replacing laparotomy as the treatment mode of choice. At present, laparotomy is performed only when a laparoscopic approach is too difficult, the surgeon is not trained in operative laparoscopy, or the patient is hemodynamically unstable.

Methotrexate, a chemotherapeutic drug and folic acid inhibitor that stops cell production and destroys remaining trophoblastic tissue, is used in the management of uncomplicated, non–life-threatening ectopic pregnancies. Patients are considered to be eligible for methotrexate therapy if the ectopic mass is unruptured and measures 1.6 inch (4 cm) or less on ultrasound examination. Patients with larger ectopic masses, embryonic cardiac activity, or clinical evidence of acute intra-abdominal bleeding (acute tender abdomen, hypotension, or falling hematocrit) are not eligible for this mode of treatment (Murray et al., 2005).

GESTATIONAL TROPHOBLASTIC DISEASE

Gestational trophoblastic disease (GTD) is a clinical diagnosis that includes the histologic diagnoses of hydatidiform mole ("molar pregnancy"), locally invasive mole, metastatic mole, and choriocarcinoma. It is a disease characterized by an abnormal placental development that results in the production of fluid-filled grapelike clusters (instead of normal placental tissue) and a vast proliferation of trophoblastic tissue (Fig. 11-2). It is associated with loss of the pregnancy and rarely, the development of cancer. GTD occurs in 1 in 1200 pregnancies (Berman, DiSaia, & Tewari, 2004).

Pathophysiology

The cause of molar pregnancy is unknown, but it is thought that complete moles result from the fertilization of an empty ovum (one whose nucleus is missing or nonfunctional) by a normal sperm. Since the ovum contains no maternal genetic material, all chromosomes in a molar pregnancy are paternally derived. The most common chromosomal pattern for complete moles is 46 XX. A complete mole is characterized by trophoblastic proliferation and the absence of fetal parts. Incomplete moles often appear with a coexistent fetus that has a triploid genotype (69 chromosomes) and multiple anomalies. Most fetuses associated with incomplete moles survive only several weeks in utero before being spontaneously aborted. Incomplete moles are almost always benign and have a much lower malignancy potential than complete moles. An invasive mole is similar to a complete mole but has invaded the myometrium layer of the uterus. Invasive moles rarely metastasize. Choriocarcinoma is invasive, malignant trophoblastic disease that is usually metastatic and can be fatal (Berman et al., 2004).

Risk Factors

The incidence of hydatidiform mole, whether complete or partial, increases with maternal age (especially in women 50 or older) and in those with a history of a previous molar pregnancy. The risk for a second molar pregnancy is 1% to 2% while the risk for a third molar pregnancy after two previous molar pregnancies is approximately 2.5 percent. Higher incidences have been found in geographical areas where the maternal diet is low in beta-carotene, animal fats, and folic acid and also in women with blood type A whose partners are of blood type O (Bess & Wood, 2006). There is also a higher incidence among women who have experienced prior miscarriages and in those who have undergone ovulation stimulation with clomiphene (Clomid).

Signs and Symptoms

More than 95% of patients experience vaginal bleeding which may be scant or profuse and ranges in color from dark brown to bright red. In early pregnancy, there is often a discrepancy between uterine size and dates. Uterine enlargement results from the rapidly proliferating trophoblastic tissue and the large accumulation of clotted blood. Anemia may result from the blood loss. Also, the patient may complain of excessive nausea and vomiting (hyperemesis gravidarum) and abdominal pain caused by uterine distention. Preeclampsia may occur, usually between 9 and 12 weeks of gestation but any symptoms of gestational hypertension before 24 weeks of gestation may be indicative of hydatidiform mole. Clinical and laboratory findings include an absence of fetal heart sounds, a markedly elevated quantitative serum hCG (may be >100,000 mIU/mL), and very low levels of maternal serum α-fetoprotein (MSAFP). Hyperthyroidism and trophoblastic pulmonary emboli are less common but serious complications of hydatidiform mole.

Diagnosis

The diagnosis of a molar pregnancy is made by an ultrasound examination. The placental tissue appears in a "snowstorm" pattern due to the profuse swelling of the chorionic villi. When a complete mole is present no fetus is identified in the uterus.

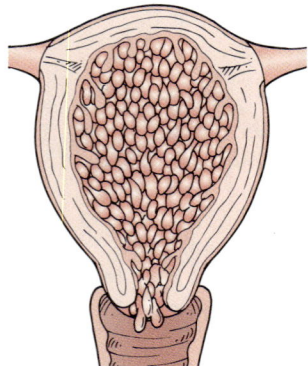

Figure 11-2 A hydatidiform mole pregnancy is one in which the chorionic villi degenerate into a mass of fluid-filled grapelike clusters.

Management

Clinical management involves removal of the uterine contents with meticulous follow-up that includes serial β-hCG levels. A sensitive marker, hCG is secreted by the molar cells and the amount of this hormone measured in maternal serum is directly related to the number of viable molar cells. The hCG levels should be assessed every 1 to 2 weeks until hCG is undetectable on two consecutive determinations. Thereafter, hCG should be measured every 1 to 2 months for at least a year (Cunningham et al., 2005). Effective contraception is needed during this time to prevent pregnancy and the resulting confusion about the cause of changes in the hCG levels. In addition, pregnancy could mask an hCG rise associated with malignant GTD. The perinatal nurse should carefully counsel the patient about different methods of contraception and stress the importance of avoiding pregnancy for a year.

 Collaboration in Caring— *Dealing with a molar pregnancy*

With any pregnancy loss, a challenging situation exists. However, the couple experiencing a molar pregnancy not only must realize that there will be no baby, but attempts at becoming pregnant must be delayed for at least a year. There is also the fear of malignant sequelae. The perinatal nurse's role is to support the couple, educate them regarding their contraceptive options, encourage them to voice their fears and concerns, and answer their questions appropriately. Involving community resources such as social services, support groups, and spiritual advisors can be of significant benefit.

Chemotherapy is initiated immediately if the hCG titer rises or plateaus during follow-up or if **metastases** (movement of cancer cells from the original site to another site) are detected at any time. Surgery may be indicated if chemotherapy is not successful or for patients who have completed their childbearing. Radiation therapy is usually reserved for treating brain and liver metastases (Cunningham et al., 2005).

Prognosis

Invasive moles are generally not metastatic and respond well to single-agent chemotherapy. Choriocarcinoma spreads to the lungs, vagina, pelvis, brain, liver, intestines, and kidneys. Since choriocarcinoma can occur weeks to years after any type of gestation, patients usually present with signs and symptoms of active metastases. The long-term prognosis depends on the degree of metastases and the patient's response to the chemotherapy.

SPONTANEOUS ABORTION

Not all conceptions result in a live-born infant. Of all clinically recognized pregnancies, 10% to 20% are lost, and approximately 22% of pregnancies detected on the basis of hCG assays are lost before the appearance of any clinical signs or symptoms (White & Bouvier, 2005). By definition, an early pregnancy loss occurs before 12 weeks of gestation; a late pregnancy loss is one that occurs between 12 and 20 weeks of gestation.

A **spontaneous abortion** (SAB) or miscarriage is a pregnancy that ends before 20 weeks gestation. The type of SAB that occurs is defined by whether any or all of the products of conception (POC) have been passed and whether or not the cervix is dilated.

Spontaneous abortions may be classified as the following:

- **Abortus**: Fetus lost before 20 weeks of gestation, less than 17.5 oz. (500 g), or less than 9.8 inches (25 cm) in size
- **Complete abortion**: Complete expulsion of all POC before 20 weeks of gestation
- **Incomplete abortion**: Partial expulsion of some but not all POC before 20 weeks of gestation
- **Inevitable abortion**: No expulsion of products, but bleeding and dilation of the cervix such that a pregnancy is unlikely
- **Threatened abortion**: Any intrauterine bleeding before 20 weeks of gestation, without dilation of the cervix or expulsion of any POC
- **Missed abortion**: Death of the embryo or fetus before 20 weeks of gestation with complete retention of the POC; these often proceed to a complete abortion within 1 to 3 weeks but occasionally they are retained much longer.

Etiology

It is estimated that 60% to 80% of all SABs in the first trimester are associated with chromosomal abnormalities (Griebel, Halvorsen, Goleman, & Day, 2005). Infections (e.g., bacteriuria and *Chlamydia trachomatis*), maternal anatomical defects, and immunological and endocrine factors have also been identified as causes of early pregnancy loss, although many have no obvious cause. Second-trimester spontaneous abortions (12 to 20 weeks) have been linked to chronic infection, recreational drug use, maternal uterine or cervical anatomical defects, maternal systemic disease, exposure to fetotoxic agents, and trauma (Cunningham et al., 2005).

Diagnosis

A woman who is experiencing a spontaneous abortion usually presents with bleeding and may also complain of cramping, abdominal pain, and decreased symptoms of pregnancy; cervical changes (dilation) may be present on vaginal examination. An ultrasound is performed for placental evaluation and to determine fetal viability. Laboratory tests include a quantitative level of β-hCG, which should show a lower value than when associated with a viable pregnancy (Fig. 11-3), hemoglobin and hematocrit, blood type and Rh status determination, and indirect Coombs' screen (Cunningham et al., 2005).

Management

Incomplete, inevitable, and missed abortions are usually managed via a dilatation and curettage (D & C: the cervix is dilated and a curette is inserted and used to scrape the uterine walls and remove the uterine contents). In the case of an incompetent cervix, an emergent **cerclage** (placement of ligature to close the cervix) may be performed. An unsensitized, Rh-negative woman should be given Rh₀(D) immune globulin (RhoGAM) to prevent

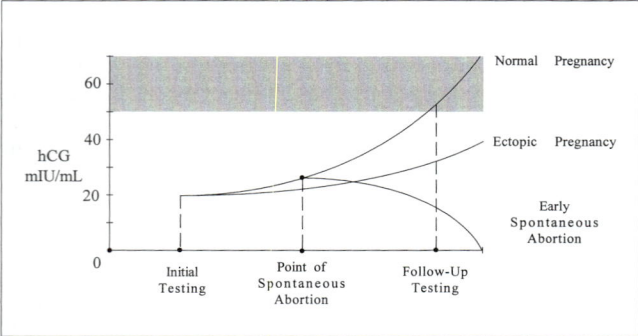

Figure 11-3 hCG levels.

antibody formation. (See discussion later in this chapter.)

Depending on the circumstances, the nurse can provide counseling or make an appropriate referral. Not all couples who suffer a pregnancy loss require formal assessment, but all couples should be offered a formal evaluation after several losses. The nurse should also allow the family to express as much grief as they are feeling at the moment and are willing to share, allow them to talk freely of what their hopes and expectations had been for this new life, and acknowledge that this is a very difficult time for them. The nurse may offer to enlist the assistance of social services, a chaplain, or rabbi or appropriate support groups if the couple so desires.

⊚ **Optimizing Outcomes—** **Follow-up for women who experience habitual abortions**

Patients who experience habitual (three or more) abortions may be offered these tests:

• A karyotype obtained from the products of conception and from both parents
• Examination of maternal anatomy, beginning with a hysterosalpingogram. If abnormal, hysteroscopy or laparoscopy
• Screening tests for maternal hypothyroidism, diabetes mellitus, antiphospholipid syndrome (APS; an acquired hypercoagulable state that involves venous and arteriole thrombosis) and systemic lupus erythematosus (SLE)
• Serum progesterone level during the luteal phase of the menstrual cycle
• Cultures of the cervix, vagina, and endometrium
• Endometrial biopsy during the luteal phase of the menstrual cycle (Cunningham et al., 2005)

INCOMPETENT CERVIX

Patients with cervical incompetence usually present with painless dilation and effacement of the cervix, often during the second trimester of pregnancy. They frequently give a history of repeated second trimester losses with no apparent etiology. Incompetent cervix is estimated to cause approximately 15% of all second trimester losses (Cunningham et al., 2005).

 Nursing Insight— *Identifying clues when taking the patient history*

The importance of knowing your patient's history cannot be overemphasized. Remember to read the prenatal records and also question your patient about all previous pregnancies and their outcomes. Since we live in such a mobile society, prenatal records may not always be available. A woman who is visiting on vacation or who has recently moved into the community often has no prenatal records with her. Many communities regularly see pregnant women seeking refuge from a war-torn country who arrive at the hospital with no records or who have had no prenatal care. You may also need to work with a medical interpreter to obtain an accurate history that can provide insights into present problems.

Etiology

Reduced cervical competence can be acquired (i.e., after trauma or surgery) or congenital (i.e., resulting from uterine anomalies or a history of DES exposure). Some women provide a typical history of painless cervical dilation in the first and every subsequent pregnancy, while others have experienced a progressively earlier delivery with each pregnancy until a typical "incompetent" history occurs.

The diagnosis of incompetent cervix is made when examination reveals cervical dilation in the absence of strong, regular contractions. The diagnosis may also be made before pregnancy or during the first trimester if a typical history of painless cervical dilation and effacement can be documented. Ultrasound examination may be useful in demonstrating funneling and shortening of the cervical length or effacement of the internal cervical os (ACOG, 2003b; Rust, Atlas, Kimmel, Roberts, & Hess, 2005).

Management

Management may include the vaginal placement of a **cerclage** or pursestring suture that is put beneath the cervical mucosa either at the cervical–vaginal junction (a McDonald cerclage) or at the internal cervical os (a Shirodkar cerclage). The intent of the cerclage is to close the cervix. The cerclage is usually removed in the office or clinic at 37 weeks of gestation to facilitate vaginal birth. A new cerclage will need to be placed with subsequent pregnancies. The cerclage may also be left in place, necessitating a cesarean delivery. Sometimes a cerclage is placed via an abdominal incision. It may be placed electively before pregnancy or at 12 to 14 weeks of gestation or as an emergency procedure (Rust & Roberts, 2005). Emergency cerclage may prolong pregnancy and increase the chance of a viable pregnancy outcome (Cockwell & Smith, 2005).

Patients who have an abdominal cerclage must give birth via cesarean section. Before and after cerclage placement, prophylactic **tocolytics** (medications used in an attempt to stop labor) may be given to prevent uterine contractions. Bedrest is an important part of the expectant management and patients may also be placed on home uterine activity monitoring. Depending upon the gestational age and imminence of delivery, patients may receive betamethasone, a glucocorticoid shown to decrease the chance of respiratory distress syndrome (RDS) in premature infants.

Now Can You— Discuss the care of the patient experiencing an early pregnancy loss?

1. Name three signs and symptoms associated with spontaneous abortion, ectopic pregnancy, and gestational trophoblastic disease?
2. Describe your plan of physical and emotional care for the patient who is suffering a pregnancy loss?
3. Identify other team members you would involve in your plan of care?

HYPEREMESIS GRAVIDARUM

Nausea and vomiting is a common condition of pregnancy that affects 70% to 85% of pregnant women and usually resolves by the 16th week of gestation. **Hyperemesis gravidarum** represents the extreme end of the nausea/vomiting spectrum in terms of severity. Criteria for the diagnosis of hyperemesis gravidarum include persistent vomiting unrelated to other causes, a measure of acute starvation (usually large ketonuria), and some discrete weight loss, most often 5% of the pre-pregnancy weight. Hyperemesis gravidarum is the most common indication for admission to the hospital during the first part of pregnancy and is second only to preterm labor as the most common reason for hospitalization during pregnancy (ACOG, 2004a; Hunter, Sullivan, Young, & Weber, 2007).

Etiology and Risk Factors

Although the exact etiology of nausea and vomiting of pregnancy is unknown, several theories have been proposed. Hyperemesis gravidarum may be related to the elevated levels of estrogen or hCG. Or, it may be associated with the transient elevation of thyroid hormone during pregnancy. Others have hypothesized a relationship between hyperemesis and the intrinsic hormones of the gastrointestinal tract (Cunningham et al., 2005). Psychological and metabolic causes have also been explored.

Risk factors include an increased placental mass associated with multiple gestation and molar pregnancy, a history of hyperemesis gravidarum in a previous pregnancy, and a history of motion sickness or migraine headaches. Daughters and sisters of women who experienced hyperemesis gravidarum and women who are pregnant with a female child are also considered to be at risk (ACOG, 2004a).

Maternal and Fetal Effects

In contrast to the early part of the 1900s, maternal mortality is rare today with very few cases reported. Serious complications of hyperemesis gravidarum for the woman and fetus arise in the group of women who cannot maintain their weight despite antiemetic therapy. In addition to increased hospital admissions, some women experience psychosocial morbidity of such significance that they feel compelled to terminate the pregnancy. Depression, **somatization** (the conversion of mental experiences into physical symptoms), and hypochondriasis can also be a problem for some women (ACOG, 2004a).

The effects on the embryo and fetus depend on the severity of the condition. Significant maternal weight loss may be associated with fetal intrauterine growth restriction (IUGR).

Management

Women with a history of nausea and vomiting in a previous pregnancy are advised to regularly take multivitamins before the next conception. Rest is encouraged. The nurse should counsel the woman to avoid foods and sensory stimuli that provoke symptoms (e.g., some women become nauseous when they smell certain foods being prepared) and also to eat small frequent meals of dry, bland foods and include high-protein snacks in their diet. Spicy foods should be avoided. Eating crackers before arising in the morning may be of benefit and ginger capsules have been shown to be effective. If the patient requires hospitalization, intravenous fluids containing dextrose and vitamins are given, and the patient is placed on an NPO status and treated with antiemetics (Box 11-1). Parenteral or enteral feedings may be ordered if the patient is unable to take oral nourishment and if normal weight gain parameters for the gestation of pregnancy are not being achieved (ACOG, 2004a).

 Complementary Care: *Nausea and vomiting of pregnancy*

Ginger, a perennial native to many Asian countries, has been found to be effective in treating nausea and vomiting during pregnancy. The antiemetic effect of this root (taken in a dosage of 1 g per day) is due to its ability to increase gastrointestinal motility. Ginger is available in tablet, capsule, and syrup form. Some concerns about taking ginger during pregnancy have been raised, but to date no significant side effects have been documented.

Elasticized wristbands (i.e., Sea-Bands®) that use a firm object to place pressure on the Neiguan point (acupressure P6 point) are a nonpharmacological, noninvasive method that may lessen the frequency and severity of nausea and vomiting during pregnancy (Hunter et al., 2007).

Hemorrhagic Disorders

Hemorrhagic disorders constitute an obstetric emergency and are a leading cause of maternal death in the United States. Third-trimester vaginal bleeding occurs in 3% to

---

Box 11-1 Medications for Nausea and Vomiting of Pregnancy

Pyridoxine (vitamin B_6), 25–75 mg (orally) per day, used alone or in combination with Doxylamine (Unisom), 25 mg (orally) per day

Promethazine (Phenergan) 12.5–25 mg (intravenously, intramuscularly, orally, or rectally) every 4 hours

Dimenhydrinate (Dramamine) 50–100 mg (orally or rectally) every 4–6 hours or 50 mg intravenously (in 50 mL of saline run over 20 minutes) every 4–6 hours

Metoclopramide (Reglan) 5–10 mg (intravenously, intramuscularly, or orally) every 8 hours

Sources: ACOG (2004a); Cunningham et al. (2005).

4% of all pregnancies and may be obstetric or nonobstetric in nature (Cunningham et al., 2005). Examples of nonobstetric causes include severe cervicitis, benign and malignant neoplasms, lacerations, and varices.

clinical alert

Early identification of maternal hemorrhage

During pregnancy, the woman's blood volume increases 50% and in the case of multiple gestation, as high as 100%. Due to this expanded blood volume, the patient may be asymptomatic and exhibit vital signs that remain within normal parameters despite a large amount of blood loss. Blood pressure is a very poor indicator of blood volume deficit. The maternal pulse (tachycardia) and/or fetal heart rate (bradycardia or tachycardia) may be the first indicators of maternal instability.

Obstetric Causes of Vaginal Bleeding

PLACENTA PREVIA

Placenta previa is an implantation of the placenta in the lower uterine segment, near or over the internal cervical os. This condition accounts for 20% of all antepartal hemorrhages. There are three recognized variations of placenta previa. With a **complete (total) placenta previa**, the placenta covers the entire cervical os. Since it is associated with the greatest amount of blood loss, a complete placenta previa presents the most serious risk. A **partial previa** describes a placenta that partially occludes the cervical os. A **marginal previa** is characterized by the encroachment of the placenta to the margin of the cervical os (Fig. 11-4). **Placenta accreta, percreta,** and **increta** are placentas with abnormally firm attachments to the uterine wall. Unusual placental adherence may accompany a placenta previa.

Placenta previa may be associated with conditions that cause scarring of the uterus such as a prior cesarean section, multiparity, or increased maternal age. A previa may also occur with a large placental mass as seen in multiple gestations and erythroblastosis. Other risk factors include smoking, cocaine use, a prior history of placenta previa, closely spaced pregnancies, African or Asian ethnicity, and maternal age greater than 35 years (Clark, 2004).

Signs and Symptoms

The most common symptom is painless vaginal bleeding. This is believed to occur from small disruptions in the placental attachment during normal development and the subsequent stretching and thinning of the lower uterine segment during the third trimester. Initially, the bleeding is usually a small amount that stops as the uterus contracts to close the open blood vessels. However, bleeding can reoccur at any time and may be associated with profuse hemorrhage and shock that leads to significant maternal and fetal morbidity and mortality. The blood is bright red (Cunningham et al., 2005).

Maternal and Fetal Morbidity and Mortality

Premature delivery is responsible for 60% of perinatal deaths associated with placenta previa. Other fetal risks

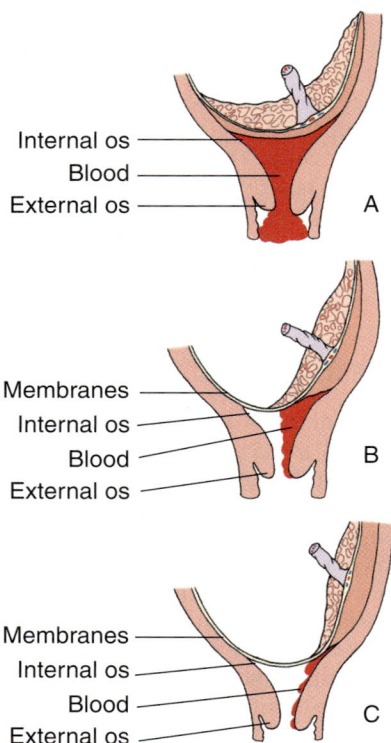

Figure 11-4 Placenta previa. *A*, Complete. *B*, Partial. *C*, Marginal.

include preterm premature rupture of the membranes (PPROM), intrauterine growth restriction (IUGR), malpresentation, congenital anomalies, and **vasa previa**. Vasa previa is a condition in which the umbilical cord is implanted into the membranes rather than the placenta. The vessels traverse within the membranes and cross the cervical os before reaching the placenta. The umbilical blood vessels are at risk for laceration. The appearance of bright red blood at the time of rupture of the membranes should alert the nurse to the possibility of a vasa previa. Maternal risks associated with placenta previa are shock, the potential for emergency hysterectomy, and death (Cunningham et al., 2005).

Diagnosis

The timing of the diagnosis of placenta previa has undergone significant change in the last decade. Although third-trimester bleeding was often the first indicator of placenta previa, today, most cases of placenta previa are detected antenatally before the onset of significant bleeding. The common practice of second-trimester abdominal ultrasound for the detection of fetal anomalies has led to this change. However, because most cases of placenta previa diagnosed in the second trimester tend to resolve as the uterus enlarges, management of placenta previa diagnosed in the second trimester differs from that for the same diagnosis made during the third trimester.

In patients diagnosed before 24 weeks' gestation, a repeat ultrasound should be scheduled between 24 and 28 weeks' gestation to confirm the diagnosis of placenta previa. However, if patients experience vaginal bleeding during this interval, they should be managed as presumed cases of placenta previa. Placenta previa should be suspected in all patients who present with bleeding after

24 completed weeks of gestation. Because of the risk of placental perforation, vaginal examinations are not performed. The nurse should advise any patient with a known or suspected previa to inform medical personnel that vaginal exams are prohibited. Abdominal examination generally shows a nontender, soft uterus with normal tone. Leopold maneuvers often reveal the fetus to be in a breech or oblique position or transverse lie because of the abnormal location of the placenta.

Management of the pregnant woman who is experiencing active bleeding associated with a placenta previa requires astute assessment skills so that there is no delay in treatment. Delay can mean the difference between an optimal or poor outcome for the patient and her fetus. Stabilization involves the administration of intravenous fluids and a laboratory workup that includes a complete blood count (CBC), prothrombin time (PT), partial thromboplastin time (PTT), fibrin split products, and fibrinogen. A blood type and crossmatch should be obtained in anticipation of the need for a transfusion. A maternal **Kleihauer–Betke** blood test may be ordered to determine if there has been a transfer of fetal blood cells into the maternal circulation. If the patient is Rh negative and unsensitized, $Rh_o(D)$ immune globulin (RhoGAM) should be administered even if the blood type of the baby cannot be determined (RhoGAM will cause no harm to the woman or her fetus if the fetus is Rh-negative). (See discussion later in this chapter.) The patient is placed on bedrest and the fetus is continuously assessed by electronic fetal monitoring. If time permits, betamethasone (a long-acting corticosteroid) may be administered (to the woman) to promote fetal lung maturity. Labor that cannot be halted, fetal compromise, and life-threatening maternal hemorrhage are indications for immediate delivery regardless of gestational age (Cunningham et al., 2005).

PLACENTAL ABRUPTION

Placenta abruption (**abruptio placentae**) is the premature separation of a normally implanted placenta from the uterine wall. An abruption results in hemorrhage between the uterine wall and the placenta. Fifty percent of abruptions occur before labor and after the 30th week, 15% occur during labor, and 30% are identified only on inspection of the placenta after delivery (Cunningham et al., 2005).

Etiology and Classifications

At the initial point of placental separation, nonclotted blood courses from the site of injury. The enlarging collection of blood may cause further separation of the placenta. Bleeding can be either concealed or revealed (apparent). A concealed hemorrhage occurs in 20% of cases and describes an abruption in which the bleeding is confined within the uterine cavity. The most common abruption is associated with a revealed or external hemorrhage, where the blood dissects downward toward the cervix (Fig. 11-5). Placental abruption may be broadly classified into three grades that correlate with clinical and laboratory findings (Box 11-2).

Perinatal and Maternal Morbidity and Mortality

Maternal mortality from abruptio placentae varies from 0.5% to 5%. The degree of hemorrhage that results from

| Partial separation (concealed hemorrhage) | Partial separation (apparent hemorrhage) | Complete separation (concealed hemorrhage) |

Figure 11-5 Abruptio placentae.

the torn placental vessels can vary from maternal anemia in mild cases to shock, acute renal failure, and maternal death in severe cases. Thirty-five percent of infants whose mothers require an antepartal transfusion will themselves be anemic and require a transfusion after birth. Fetal mortality occurs in about 35% of all placental abruptions and can be as high as 50% to 80% when associated with severe placental abruption. Death results from hypoxia that is related to the decreased placental surface area and maternal hemorrhage (Cunningham et al., 2005).

Signs and Symptoms

The classic presenting sign is third-trimester bleeding associated with severe abdominal pain. Other signs include uterine tenderness and abdominal or back pain, a boardlike abdomen and no vaginal bleeding, abnormal contractions and increased uterine tone, fetal compromise as evidenced by late fetal heart rate (FHR) decelerations, bradycardia and lack of variability on the electronic fetal monitor, and fetal demise.

Diagnosis

Vaginal bleeding in the third trimester of pregnancy is the hallmark of placental abruption or placenta previa and should always prompt an investigation to determine its etiology. Diagnosis is made by clinical findings and, when available, ultrasound examination. Recent advances in ultrasound imaging and interpretation have greatly

---

Box 11-2 Classifications of Abruptio Placentae

Grade 1: Slight vaginal bleeding and some uterine irritability are usually present. Maternal blood pressure is unaffected and the maternal fibrinogen level is normal. The fetal heart rate pattern is normal.

Grade 2: External uterine bleeding is absent to moderate. The uterus is irritable and tetanic or very frequent contractions may be present. Maternal blood pressure is maintained, but the pulse rate may be elevated and postural blood volume deficits may be present. The fibrinogen level may be decreased. The fetal heart rate pattern often shows signs of fetal compromise.

Grade 3: Bleeding is moderate to severe but may be concealed. The uterus is tetanic and painful. Maternal hypotension is frequently present and fetal death has occurred. Fibrinogen levels are often reduced or are less than 150 mg/dL; other coagulation abnormalities (thrombocytopenia, factor depletion) are present.

Source: Cunningham, F., Leveno, K., Bloom, S., Hauth, J., Gilstrap, L., & Wenstrom, K. (2005). *Williams obstetrics* (22nd ed.). New York: McGraw-Hill improved the diagnosis rate. On ultrasound examination, more than 50% of patients with a confirmed placental abruption will demonstrate evidence of hemorrhage. However, during the acute phase of placental abruption ultrasound findings may not be reliable, so a thorough clinical evaluation of any pregnant woman who presents with bleeding or acute abdominal pain is always indicated (Cunningham et al., 2005).

Management

The potential for rapid deterioration (hemorrhage, disseminated intravascular coagulation [DIC], fetal hypoxia) necessitates delivery in some cases of placental abruption. However, most abruptions are small and noncatastrophic, and therefore do not necessitate immediate delivery. Certain actions, including hospitalization, laboratory studies, continuous monitoring, and ongoing patient support should be initiated when placental abruption is suspected (Box 11-3).

 Optimizing Outcomes— **Religious beliefs and blood transfusions**

Members of Jehovah's Witness do not receive blood products or their derivatives. When bleeding occurs during pregnancy and blood is deemed necessary to save the woman's and/or fetus' life, a very challenging situation exists. Non-blood products may be given but are not always successful. Sometimes a court order is obtained so that blood can be administered to save the life of the woman and/or fetus. The perinatal nurse must be able to respect the family's beliefs and support them during this very difficult time when the health of both the woman and her fetus as well as their religious beliefs are being challenged.

Box 11-3 **Care for the Patient Experiencing an Abruptio Placentae**

- Hospitalization.
- Intravenous placement with a large-bore catheter (16-gauge).
- Labwork: Includes CBC, coagulation studies (fibrinogen, PT, PTT, platelet count, fibrin degradation products), type and screen for 4 units of blood, Kleihauer–Betke for Rh-negative patients. A "clot test" may be performed: a red top tube of blood is drawn, set aside, and checked for clotting. If a clot does not form within 6 minutes or if it forms and lyses within 30 minutes, a coagulation defect is probably present and the fibrinogen level is less than 150 mg/dL.
- Betamethasone may be given to the woman to promote fetal lung maturity when delivery is not imminent.
- Rh(D)-negative patients should receive RhoGAM to prevent isoimmunization.
- Continuous evaluation of intake and output.
- Continuous electronic fetal monitoring.
- Delivery (cesarean or vaginal birth) may be initiated depending on the status of the mother and the fetus.
- Nursing care is centered on continuous maternal–fetal assessment, with on-going information and emotional support for the patient and her family.

Source: Cunningham, F., Leveno, K., Bloom, S., Hauth, J., Gilstrap, L., & Wenstrom, K. (2005). *Williams obstetrics* (22nd ed.). New York: McGraw-Hill

---

 Now Can You— **Discuss the management of bleeding during pregnancy?**

1. Describe the differences between placenta previa and abruptio placentae?
2. Name three initial steps in the management of the bleeding pregnant patient?
3. Explain why it may be difficult to identify an early maternal hemorrhage?

Preterm Labor

Preterm labor (PTL) is defined as cervical changes and regular uterine contractions occurring between 20 and 37 weeks of pregnancy. Many patients present with preterm contractions, but only those who demonstrate changes in the cervix are diagnosed with preterm labor (ACOG, 2001).

INCIDENCE

Preterm birth, which is a birth that occurs before the completion of 37 weeks of pregnancy, is considered the most acute problem in maternal–child health (American College of Obstetricians and Gynecologists [ACOG]/American Academy of Pediatrics [AAP], 2002). The sequelae of preterm birth has a profound effect on the survival and health of about one in every eight infants born in the United States each year (Freda & Patterson, 2004). From 1981 to 2001, the rate of preterm births in the United States increased by 27%. In 2001, more than 476,000 infants were born at least 3 weeks before their due date (National Center for Health Statistics [NCHS], 2002). In spite of advances in obstetric care, the rate of prematurity has not decreased over the past 40 years and in most industrialized countries, it has slightly increased. The preterm delivery rate in the United States is approximately 11%; in Europe the rate varies between 5% and 7%. A very preterm birth is a birth that occurs before the completion of 32 weeks of pregnancy. In 2003, the very preterm birth rate in the United States was 1.97% (Martin et al., 2005).

ETIOLOGY AND RISK FACTORS

The defining physiological mechanism that triggers the onset of preterm labor is largely unknown but may include decidual hemorrhage (abruption), mechanical factors (uterine overdistention or cervical incompetence), hormonal changes (perhaps mediated by fetal or maternal stress) and bacterial infections (ACOG, 2001). However, a number of risk factors have been associated with preterm labor (Box 11-4).

 Collaboration in Caring— *Increasing public awareness of the problems of prematurity*

The Association of Women's Health, Obstetric and Neonatal Nurses (AWHONN), the American College of Obstetricians and Gynecologists (ACOG), and the American Academy of Pediatrics (AAP) have partnered with the March of Dimes in a multi-million-dollar research, education and awareness campaign to address the problem of prematurity. Educating all women of childbearing age about preterm labor is a crucial component of prevention (March of Dimes, 2005).

MORBIDITY AND MORTALITY

As a result of high-tech neonatal intensive care, advanced technology, and improved medications, the morbidity of babies born after 34 to 35 weeks has decreased and the definition of viability has changed dramatically throughout the past several decades (ACOG, 2002b). The limits of viability keep moving downward in gestation time, and this factor contributes to the increasing numbers of preterm births.

With appropriate medical care, neonatal survival dramatically improves as gestational age increases, with more than 50% of neonates surviving at 25 weeks' gestation, and more than 90% at 28 to 29 weeks' gestation. Short-term neonatal morbidities associated with preterm birth are numerous and include respiratory distress syndrome, intraventricular hemorrhage, periventricular leukomalacia, necrotizing enterocolitis, bronchopulmonary dysplasia, sepsis, and patent ductus arteriosus. Long-term morbidities include cerebral palsy, mental retardation, and retinopathy of prematurity. The risk of these morbidities is directly related to the infant's gestational age and birth weight.

DIAGNOSIS

The diagnosis of preterm labor can be very challenging since many of the symptoms are subtle and common during pregnancy. For example, women experiencing preterm labor may complain of backache, pelvic aching, menstrual-like cramps, increased vaginal discharge, pelvic pressure, urinary frequency, and intestinal cramping with or without diarrhea.

Box 11-4 Various Risk Factors Associated with Preterm Labor and Birth

- History of preterm birth
- Uterine or cervical anomalies
- Multiple gestation
- Hypertension
- Diabetes
- Obesity
- Clotting disorders
- Infection, especially urinary tract infections
- Fetal anomalies
- Premature rupture of membranes
- Vaginal bleeding, especially in the second trimester or in more than one trimester
- Late or no prenatal care
- Illicit drug use
- Smoking
- Alcohol
- Diethylstilbestrol (DES) exposure
- Domestic violence
- Non-Hispanic African American race
- Age <17 years or >35 years
- Low socioeconomic status
- Stress
- Long working hours with long periods of standing
- Periodontal disease

Sources: ACOG (2001); Freda & Patterson (2004).

A diagnosis of preterm labor is made when the following criteria are met (ACOG/AAP, 2007):

- A gestation of 20 to 37 weeks
- Documented persistent uterine contractions (4 every 20 minutes or 8 in 1 hour)
- Documented cervical effacement of 80% or greater
- Cervical dilation of more than 0.4 inch (1 cm) or a documented change in dilation

Infection has been implicated as a contributing factor in preterm labor. Prostaglandin production by the amnion, chorion, and decidua is stimulated by cytokines (extracellular factors) that are released by activated macrophages. Group B streptococci, chlamydia, and gonorrhea have been associated with preterm labor and preterm premature rupture of the membranes (Cunningham et al., 2005). It is always prudent for the nurse to obtain a clean-catch, midstream, or catheterized urine specimen to identify and treat infection if the patient presents with signs of preterm labor or preterm premature rupture of the membranes.

BIOCHEMICAL MARKERS

Early predictive factors for preterm labor and birth include fetal fibronectin (fFN) and salivary estriol. Fetal fibronectins are proteins produced by the fetal membranes. They are normally secreted in the cervicovaginal fluid until 20 weeks of gestation. Fetal fibronectins are best described as the "glue" that attaches the fetal membranes to the underlying uterine decidua. Their presence between 24 and 34 weeks in a patient with intact membranes suggests an increased risk for preterm labor in both symptomatic and asymptomatic women (Bernhardt & Dorman, 2004). The fFN is retrieved with a sterile cotton-tipped swab placed in the posterior vaginal fornix or in the ectocervical region of the external cervical os for a minimum of 10 seconds. The collection swab is then removed, placed into a manufacturer-supplied medium, and sent to a laboratory that performs the test. Results are reported in 24 to 48 hours. For women whose fetal fibronectin test is negative (i.e., no fFN is detected) the likelihood of giving birth in the following week is less than 1% (Iams & Creasy, 2004).

Observational studies have shown that maternal levels of serum estradiol and salivary estriol increase before the spontaneous onset of term and preterm labor (PTL). Salivary estriol (a biochemical marker under study for its predictive value in preterm labor) is an estrogen produced by fetal trophoblasts. The estriol is derived from adrenal and liver steroid precursors and then converted into estriol in the placenta. Levels of estriol present in maternal saliva have been shown to increase just before preterm labor begins. However, this test has not proven to be very effective since maternal estriol levels normally peak at night. The negative predictive value of both tests is high (95% for fFN; 98% for salivary estriol). Therefore, the tests are better indicators of who will not experience preterm labor rather than of who will experience PTL (ACOG, 2001; Bernhardt & Dorman, 2004).

MANAGEMENT

The two major goals in the management of preterm labor are to inhibit or reduce the strength and frequency of contractions, thus delaying the time of delivery, and to optimize the fetal status before preterm delivery (ACOG,

2003c; Cunningham et al., 2005). **Tocolysis** is the use of medications to inhibit uterine contractions. Drugs used for this purpose ("tocolytics") include the beta-adrenergic agonists (also called beta-mimetics), magnesium sulfate ($MGSO_4$), prostaglandin synthetase inhibitors (indomethacin [Indocin]) and calcium channel blockers (nifedipine [Procardia]). The most commonly used tocolytics are the beta-mimetics ritodrine (Yutopar) and terbutaline sulfate (Brethine) and magnesium sulfate, a CNS depressant. Although ritodrine is FDA approved for tocolysis, it is not used for this purpose as frequently as is terbutaline sulfate, which is not FDA approved for tocolysis. The use of these medications is contraindicated under certain conditions (Box 11-5). At present, it is believed that the best reason to use tocolytic drugs is to allow an opportunity to begin the administration of antenatal corticosteroids to accelerate fetal lung maturity. Also, delaying the birth provides time for maternal transport to a facility equipped with a neonatal intensive care unit (ACOG, 2003b). Caring for the patient receiving tocolytic therapy requires the nurse to be cognizant of not only the safety aspects of administering the medication to the pregnant woman but also to the emotional needs of the patient as attempts to halt the preterm labor are being made (Box 11-6).

 Now Can You— Care for the patient experiencing preterm labor?

1. Identify five symptoms of preterm labor?
2. Discuss the use of tocolytics in preterm labor?
3. Develop a teaching plan about preterm labor for pregnant women?

Box 11-5 **Contraindications to the Use of Tocolytics in Preterm Labor**

- Significant maternal hypertension (eclampsia, severe preeclampsia, chronic hypertension)
- Antepartum hemorrhage
- Cardiac disease
- Any medical or obstetric condition that contraindicates prolongation of pregnancy
- Hypersensitivity to a specific tocolytic agent
- Gestational age >37 weeks
- Advanced cervical dilation
- Fetal demise or lethal anomaly
- Chorioamnionitis
- In utero compromise
  - Acute: nonreassuring fetal heart rate pattern
  - Chronic: IUGR or substance abuse

Source: Cunningham, F., Leveno, K., Bloom, S., Hauth, J., Gilstrap, L., & Wenstrom, K. (2005). *Williams obstetrics* (22nd ed.). New York: McGraw-Hill

---

 Family Teaching Guidelines...
Preventing Prematurity

Freda and Patterson (2004) suggest that nurses be proactive by educating women about preterm labor and teaching them how to recognize the warning signs and symptoms.

- Encourage all pregnant women to obtain prenatal care.
- Educate all pregnant women as to the signs and symptoms of preterm labor.
- Eliminate the term "Braxton-Hicks" from teaching (women may delay seeking treatment if they believe they are only experiencing Braxton-Hicks contractions).
- Ask all pregnant women if they have had any symptoms of preterm labor.
- Screen for vaginal and urogenital infections and treat appropriately.
- Teach women about the dangers of douching.
- Assess all pregnant women for intimate partner violence and intervene.
- Discuss stress levels early in pregnancy, and intervene.
- Assess all pregnant women for nutritional status and weight gain in pregnancy and intervene as necessary.
- Assess for illicit drug use, and help the woman get into treatment.
- Encourage women who have preterm labor symptoms to drink fluids, lie down for 1 hour, and go to the hospital for a vaginal exam if symptoms continue.
- Remind the woman with symptoms that she should not hesitate to call her provider repeatedly if her symptoms recur.

Box 11-6 **Nursing Care of the Patient Receiving Tocolytic Therapy**

- Explore the woman's understanding of what is taking place.
- Include the woman's partner in all discussions about medications and their effects.
- Provide anticipatory guidance regarding what is likely to happen during medication administration.
- Position the woman on her side for better placental perfusion.
- Explain the side effects and contraindications of the drug.
- Assess blood pressure, pulse, and respirations regularly according to hospital policies (in many institutions every 15 minutes).
- Notify the health care provider if systolic blood pressure is >140 mm Hg or <90 mm Hg.
- Notify the health care provider if diastolic blood pressure is >90 mm Hg or <50 mm Hg.
- Assess for signs of pulmonary edema (chest pain, shortness of breath).
- Assess for the presence of deep tendon reflexes (DTRs).
- Assess output every 1 hour.
- Notify provider if output is <30 mL/hr.
- Limit intake to 2500 mL/day (90 mL/hr).
- Provide psychosocial support and opportunities for the patient to express anxiety.

Source: March of Dimes Nursing Module: Preterm Labor: Prevention and Nursing Management (2004).

Premature Rupture of the Membranes

To facilitate an understanding of premature rupture of the membranes (PROM), it is helpful to first define the various terms used:

- **Premature** rupture of the membranes (PROM) is defined as rupture of the membranes before the onset of labor at any gestational age.
- **Preterm** rupture of membranes is defined as rupture of the membranes before 37 completed weeks of gestation. It is a common cause of preterm labor, preterm delivery, and chorioamnionitis.
- **Preterm premature** rupture of the membranes (PPROM) is defined as a combination of both terms—rupture occurs before the 37th completed week of gestation and in the absence of labor. PPROM accounts for 25% of all cases of premature rupture of the amniotic membranes and is responsible for 30% to 40% of all preterm deliveries (Cunningham et al., 2005).

PATHOPHYSIOLOGY

Premature rupture of the membranes is multifactorial. Choriodecidual infection or inflammation appears to play an important role in the etiology of PPROM, especially at early gestational ages. Other factors include decreased amniotic membrane collagen, lower socioeconomic status, cigarette smoking, sexually transmitted infections, prior preterm delivery, prior preterm labor during the current pregnancy, uterine distention (e.g., multiple gestation, hydramnios), cervical cerclage, amniocentesis, and vaginal bleeding in pregnancy (Mercer, 2003). In many cases, the cause is not known.

DIAGNOSIS

Most often, the patient reports a gush or leakage of fluid from the vagina. However, any increased vaginal discharge should be evaluated. The diagnosis is based on the patient's history of leaking vaginal fluid and the finding of a pooling of fluid on sterile speculum examination. Nitrazine and fern tests confirm the diagnosis of PROM. Easily performed, these tests are used to discriminate between vaginal discharge and amniotic fluid. (See Procedure 12-2.) The tampon test may also be used to diagnose PROM. With this test, a blue dye (indigo carmine) is injected into the uterus via amniocentesis. A previously inserted vaginal tampon is then checked in 30 minutes for the presence of blue dye. The level of amniotic fluid in the uterus may also be checked via an abdominal ultrasound examination. Leakage of amniotic fluid is consistent with findings of **oligohydramnios** (decreased amniotic fluid).

MANAGEMENT

The risk of perinatal complications changes dramatically according to the gestational age when rupture of the membranes occurs. Clinical practice varies, and, at present, considerable controversy exists concerning the optimal management of PPROM. However, there is general consensus in regard to the following factors:

- Gestational age should be established based on clinical history and prior ultrasound assessment when available.
- Ultrasound should be performed to assess fetal growth, position, and residual amniotic fluid.
- The woman should be assessed for evidence of advanced labor, chorioamnionitis (intrauterine infection), abruptio placentae, and fetal distress.
- Patients with advanced labor, intrauterine infection, significant vaginal bleeding, or nonreassuring fetal testing are best delivered promptly, regardless of gestational age.

There is further debate over the use of tocolytics, corticosteroids, and antibiotics in patients with PPROM. Tocolysis appears to be of little benefit in PPROM and may be harmful when chorioamnionitis is present. However, in many hospitals, tocolytic therapy is instituted for 48 hours, especially with earlier gestational ages, in order to administer a course of corticosteroids to enhance fetal lung maturity (Cunningham et al., 2005).

Conservative management includes inpatient observation unless the membranes reseal and the leakage of fluid stops. This approach initially consists of prolonged continuous fetal and maternal monitoring combined with modified bedrest to promote amniotic fluid reaccumulation and spontaneous membrane sealing. Delivery of the fetus should be accomplished if signs of infection are present: maternal temperature of 100.4°F (38°C) or greater, foul-smelling vaginal discharge, elevated white blood count, uterine tenderness, and maternal and/or fetal tachycardia.

Without intervention, approximately 50% of patients who have ROM will go into labor within 24 hours, and up to 75% will do so within 48 hours. These rates are inversely correlated to the gestational age at the time of rupture of the membranes. Thus, patients with ROM before 26 weeks' gestational age are more likely to gain an additional week than those greater than 30 weeks' gestation. While maintaining the pregnancy to gain further fetal maturity can be beneficial, prolonged PPROM has been correlated with an increased risk of chorioamnionitis, placental abruption and cord prolapse (Cunningham et al., 2005).

The nurse's role in caring for the patient with PPROM includes explaining to the patient that she will be on full or modified bedrest and her vital signs will be checked at least every 4 hours to detect early signs of a developing infection. If the patient does not exhibit signs of labor, intermittent fetal monitoring is appropriate. Frequent ultrasound examinations are performed to assess amniotic fluid levels. An important component of the nursing care plan centers on providing emotional support to the patient who is understandably worried about the outcome for her baby. The nurse should encourage the woman and her family members to ask questions and express fears and concerns. When the nurse does not have enough information to respond adequately, another health team member who can appropriately answer the patient's questions and address her concerns should be contacted.

Now Can You— **Discuss the care of the patient with premature rupture of the membranes?**

1. Name three factors associated with premature rupture of membranes?
2. Discuss three major complications that accompany premature rupture of membranes?
3. Describe the Nitrazine, fern, and tampon tests?
4. Formulate a plan of care for the patient who has experienced premature rupture of membranes?

Hypertensive Disorders of Pregnancy

Hypertensive disorders are the most common medical complication of pregnancy. The incidence of hypertensive disorders is between 5% and 10%, and this complication is the second leading cause of maternal death in the United States (embolic events are the leading cause) (Martin et al., 2005). Hypertensive disorders contribute significantly to stillbirth and neonatal morbidity and mortality (National High Blood Pressure Education Program Working Group [NHBPEP], 2000; Sibai, Dekker, & Kupfermine, 2005) and can result in maternal cerebral hemorrhage, disseminated intravascular coagulation (DIC), hepatic failure, acute renal failure, pulmonary edema, adult respiratory distress syndrome, aspiration pneumonia, and abruptio placentae (ACOG, 2002a).

CLASSIFICATIONS AND DEFINITIONS

The terminology used to describe the hypertensive disorders of pregnancy is generally associated with imprecise usage. This misuse of terminology often creates confusion for health care professionals who care for women who experience hypertensive complications during pregnancy and childbirth (Sibai et al., 2005). Numerous attempts have been made to accurately describe pregnancy-related hypertensive disorders. The NHBPEP has recommended the following classifications (NHBPEP, 2000):

- Chronic hypertension
- Preeclampsia–eclampsia
- Chronic hypertension with superimposed preeclampsia
- Gestational (or transient) hypertension

Clinically, there are two basic types of hypertension during pregnancy. Distinction between chronic hypertension and pregnancy-induced hypertension (PIH) is based on the timing of the onset of the hypertension. However, NHBPEP advocates discarding the term pregnancy-induced hypertension because it does not differentiate between gestational hypertension, a relatively benign disorder, and the more serious condition of preeclampsia (Peters & Flack, 2004).

Chronic Hypertension

Chronic hypertension is defined as hypertension that is present and observable before pregnancy or hypertension that is diagnosed before the 20th week of gestation. Hypertension is defined as a blood pressure greater than 140/90 mm Hg. Hypertension for which a diagnosis is confirmed for the first time during pregnancy, and which persists beyond the 84th day postpartum, is also classified as chronic hypertension (Roberts, 2004).

Preeclampsia and Eclampsia

Preeclampsia is a pregnancy-specific systemic syndrome clinically defined as an increase in blood pressure (140/90) after 20 weeks' gestation accompanied by proteinuria (NHBPEP, 2000; Peters & Flack, 2004). This increase in blood pressure represents a change from the usual blood pressure findings during pregnancy. Under normal conditions, the blood pressure increases during the first trimester, decreases in the second trimester, and

then returns to nonpregnant values by the end of the third trimester.

At one time, the presence of edema was included in the definition of preeclampsia, but this criterion has been removed since edema is common during pregnancy. However, the sudden onset of severe edema always warrants close evaluation to rule out preeclampsia or other pathological processes such as renal disease. **Eclampsia** is the occurrence of a grand mal seizure in a woman with preeclampsia who has no other cause for seizure (ACOG, 2002a; Roberts, 2004).

 ***Nursing Insight*—** *Recognizing variations in the onset of eclampsia*

Approximately one third of cases of eclampsia develop during pregnancy; one third during labor and one third within 72 hours postpartum (Emery, 2005).

Chronic Hypertension with Superimposed Preeclampsia

There is ample evidence that preeclampsia can occur in women who are already hypertensive and that the prognosis for the woman and her fetus is worse for these patients than when either condition exists alone. Distinguishing superimposed preeclampsia from worsening chronic hypertension tests the skills of the clinician and the obstetric nurse. According to Roberts (2004), the following criteria are necessary to establish a diagnosis of superimposed preeclampsia:

1. Hypertension and no proteinuria early in pregnancy (prior to 20 weeks' gestation) and new-onset proteinuria, (defined as the urinary excretion of 0.3 g of protein in a 24-hour specimen) *or*
2. Hypertension and proteinuria before 20 weeks' gestation:
   - A sudden increase in protein—urinary excretion of 0.3 g protein or more in a 24-hour specimen, or two dipstick test results of 2+ (100 mg/dL), with the values recorded at least 4 hours apart, with no evidence of urinary tract infection
   - A sudden increase in blood pressure in a woman whose blood pressure has been well controlled
   - Thrombocytopenia (platelet count lower than 100,000/mm^3)
   - An increase in the liver enzymes alanine transaminase (ALT) or aspartate transaminase (AST) to abnormal levels

Gestational (or Transient) Hypertension

This is a nonspecific term used to describe the woman who has a blood pressure elevation detected for the first time during pregnancy, without proteinuria. This term is used only until a more specific diagnosis can be assigned postpartum. If preeclampsia does not develop (e.g., protein does not become present in the urine), and the woman's blood pressure falls into a normal range by 12 weeks postpartum, the diagnosis of transient hypertension of pregnancy can be made (Roberts, 2004).

Preeclampsia

PATHOPHYSIOLOGY

The normal physiological adaptations to pregnancy are altered in the woman who develops preeclampsia. Preeclampsia is a multisystem, vasopressive disease process that targets the cardiovascular, hematologic, hepatic, renal, and central nervous systems.

Preeclampsia is associated with a clinical spectrum of events that range from mild to severe with a potential endpoint of eclampsia. Patients do not suddenly "catch" severe preeclampsia or develop eclampsia but rather progress in a fairly predictable course through the clinical spectrum. In most cases, the progression is relatively slow, and the disorder may never proceed beyond mild preeclampsia. In other situations, the disease can progress more rapidly, and change from a mild to a severe form in a matter of days or weeks. In the most serious cases, the progression can be rapid: mild preeclampsia evolves to severe preeclampsia or eclampsia over hours or days (Roberts, 2004). Hence, the nurse must alert the patient to signs and symptoms that signal a worsening condition and continuously assess the patient for any change.

Although the pathophysiology is poorly understood, it is clear that the blueprint for its development is laid down early in pregnancy. Preeclampsia is a disease of the placenta because it has been documented in pregnancies that involve trophoblastic tissue but no fetus (i.e., a molar pregnancy). In a normal pregnancy, the endovascular trophoblast cells of the placenta transform uterine spiral arteries to accommodate an increased blood flow. In the presence of preeclampsia, the arterial transformation is incomplete. Women with preeclampsia have a distinctive lesion in the placenta termed "acute atherosis" (fat accumulation in the placental arteries). Their placentas also exhibit a greater degree of infarction (necrosis related to decreased blood supply) than are found in placentas of normotensive women. These pathological changes can lead to decreased placental perfusion and placental hypoxia (Cunningham et al., 2005; NHBPEP, 2000).

Vasospasm and endothelial cell damage are the major underlying pathophysiological events in preeclampsia. Vasospasm may be associated with an elevation in arterial blood pressure and resistance to blood flow. It is unclear whether vasospasm produces damage to the vessels or if damage to the vessels produces vasospasm. Regardless, the restriction of blood flow is associated with endothelial cell damage, and this tissue insult prompts the systemic utilization of platelets and fibrinogen. The widespread vascular changes alter blood flow and result in hypoxic damage to vulnerable organs. Over time, the alterations produce widespread maternal vasospasm that results in decreased perfusion to virtually all organs, including the placenta. Associated physiological events include decreased plasma volume, activation of the coagulation cascade, and alterations in the glomerular endothelium. The increased platelet activation and markers of endothelial activation can predate clinically evident preeclampsia by weeks or even months (Sibai et al., 2005) (Fig. 11-6).

In addition to endothelial damage and vasospasm, women with preeclampsia show an exaggerated response

Figure 11-6 Pathophysiological changes of preeclampsia.

to angiotensin II. Angiotensin II is produced by the renin-aldosterone pathway in the kidney when enzymes are released to convert angiotensin I to angiotensin II. Angiotensin II is a potent vasoconstrictor that can trigger arterial hypertension. During a normal pregnancy, the patient's physiological response to angiotensin II is blunted or decreased. In women with preeclampsia, the normal "blunting" does not occur (Sibai et al., 2005).

Pregnancy is normally associated with a low sensitivity to pressor agents, which increase blood pressure. Women with preeclampsia, however, demonstrate an exaggerated response to pressor agents. An imbalance between prostacyclin, a prostaglandin and potent vasodilator, and thromboxane (a compound synthesized in platelets from a prostaglandin), is also thought to occur. Prostacyclin exerts a direct effect on the tone of the arterial smooth muscles. It decreases blood pressure, prevents platelet aggregation (clumping) and promotes uterine blood flow. Thromboxane exerts the opposite effect. It is a potent vasoconstrictor that causes an increase in blood pressure and platelet aggregation (NHBPEP, 2000; Sibai et al., 2005).

 Nursing Insight— *SPASMS: A memory enhancer when caring for a patient with preeclampsia*

S **S**ignificant blood pressure changes may occur without warning.

P **P**roteinuria is a serious sign of renal involvement.

A **A**rterioles are affected by vasospasms that result in endothelial damage and leakage of intravascular fluid into the interstitial spaces. Edema results.

S **S**ignificant laboratory changes (most notably, liver function tests [LFTs] and the platelet count) signal worsening of the disease.

M **M**ultiple organ systems can be involved: cardiovascular, hematologic, hepatic, renal and central nervous system.

S **S**ymptoms appear after 20 weeks of gestation

RISK FACTORS FOR PREECLAMPSIA/ECLAMPSIA

Preeclampsia is a subtle and insidious disease process. Signs and symptoms become apparent relatively late in the course of the disease, usually during the third trimester of pregnancy. Preeclampsia occurs in about 5% to 8% of pregnancies and there is no truly "typical" patient (ACOG, 2002a; Martin et al., 2005).

Risk factors associated with preeclampsia are presented in Box 11-7. Throughout the world, an estimated 50,000 women die each year from preeclampsia. Preeclampsia is more likely to develop in women whose mothers had preeclampsia than in women whose mothers did not. Nulliparity has been confirmed as a risk factor in both large-scale epidemiological studies and in detailed clinical studies. Although some studies have shown an increased risk for preeclampsia in multiparous women with new partners for subsequent pregnancies (Longo et al., 2003) other investigators found that a change of partner did not increase the recurrence rate of preeclampsia (Hjartardottir et al., 2004). Approximately 40% to 50% of multiparous women with a diagnosis of preeclampsia have experienced preeclampsia during a previous pregnancy. Among nulliparous women,

---

> **Box 11-7** **Risk Factors for Preeclampsia**
>
> - Primigravida (6–8 times greater risk)
> - Age extremes (<17 years and >35 years)
> - Diabetes
> - Preexisting hypertension
> - Multiple gestation (5 times greater risk)
> - Fetal hydrops (10 times greater risk)
> - Hydatidiform mole (10 times greater risk)
> - Preeclampsia in a previous pregnancy
> - Family history
> - Obesity
> - Immunological factors
> - Chronic renal disease
> - Rh incompatibility
> - African American ethnicity
> - Pregnancies that result from donor insemination, oocyte donation, embryo donation
>
> *Sources*: ACOG Practice Bulletin No. 33 (2003); Duckitt & Harrington (2005); Sibai, Dekker, & Kupferminic (2005).

African American women have a risk of preeclampsia that is twice as high as that of Caucasian women; they are also more likely to have hypertension that is independent of pregnancy. Obese women (a body mass index of 29 or greater) are three times more likely to develop preeclampsia than are nonobese women (Sibai et al., 2005).

Immunological factors, genetic disposition and environmental factors may also contribute to the development of preeclampsia. The high incidence of preeclampsia in many poor countries suggests that an inadequate diet may constitute a risk factor. Dietary inadequacies that have been proposed as relevant to the development of preeclampsia include deficiencies of calcium, zinc, vitamins C and E, and n-3 essential fatty acids (Sibai et al., 2005).

MATERNAL AND FETAL MORBIDITY AND MORTALITY

A number of maternal and fetal complications are likely to develop if preeclampsia progresses from a mild to a severe form. These include placental abruption, acute renal failure, seizures, pulmonary edema, cerebral hemorrhage, hepatic failure, disseminated intravascular coagulation (DIC), IUGR, non-reassuring fetal heart rate pattern on antepartum testing and fetal death. The maternal complications associated with preeclampsia are related to the widespread arteriolar vasoconstriction that affects the brain (seizure and stroke), kidneys (oliguria and renal failure), liver (edema and subcapsular hematoma), and small blood vessels (small ruptures within the walls of the vessels use up large amounts of platelets in an effort to correct the bleeding. This results in thrombocytopenia and DIC) (Cunningham et al., 2005).

The perinatal outcome in preeclampsia is dependent on one or more of the following factors: the gestational age at the onset of the disease process, the presence of a multiple gestation, and the presence of underlying maternal hypertension or renal disease. In patients with mild preeclampsia at term, the perinatal mortality, incidence of fetal growth restriction, and neonatal morbidity are similar to those associated with normotensive pregnancies. In contrast, both perinatal and maternal morbidity are increased when the disease is severe, particularly when disease develops in the second trimester, and the fetus is quite immature. Maternal death and severe complication rates from preeclampsia are also lowest among women who receive regular prenatal care and are managed by experienced physicians in tertiary centers (August, 2004).

MANAGEMENT OF PREECLAMPSIA/ECLAMPSIA

Once the diagnosis of preeclampsia has been made, delivery of the fetus is the only cure. The primary considerations of therapy must always be the safety of the patient and the delivery of a live, mature newborn who will not require intensive and prolonged neonatal care. Mild preeclampsia, which presents as a maternal blood pressure of 140/90 and +1 to +2 proteinuria on urine dipstick, can often be managed at home after the patient has had a careful assessment of her signs and symptoms, a physical examination, laboratory tests, and evaluation of fetal well-being.

However, the National High Blood Pressure Education Program recommends that for patients with new-onset preeclampsia, the initial examination be performed in the hospital. If the woman's blood pressure and laboratory test results indicate that her care may be safely managed at home, the nurse must make certain that the patient fully understands the signs and symptoms associated with a worsening of the condition. The effects of illness, language, age, culture, beliefs, and support systems must be considered for each patient and appropriate community resources should be explored (Poole, 2004b).

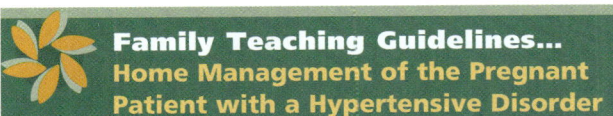

Family Teaching Guidelines...
Home Management of the Pregnant Patient with a Hypertensive Disorder

Before discharge, it is important to ascertain that the home environment is conducive to rest and the patient will be able to rest frequently throughout the day. It is essential that the patient can verbalize understanding of the importance of keeping all prenatal appointments and that she must immediately notify her physician or midwife at the first appearance of:

- Blood pressure values greater than those at the time of hospital discharge—M.D. or CNM should provide parameters
- Visual changes
- Epigastric pain
- Nausea and vomiting
- Bleeding gums
- Headaches
- Increasing edema, especially of the hands and face
- Decreasing urinary output
- Decreased fetal movement
- "Just not feeling right"

 Across Care Settings: **Promoting bedrest at home**

Obtaining an adequate amount of bedrest is not always easy, especially for women who have other children at home and no extended family to help. The nurse may offer suggestions such as lying down and resting while the other children nap or bringing young children into bed and reading them a story or asking a neighbor to watch the children. The woman's partner should also be involved in formulating a plan to help facilitate rest. Church groups may be able to help out with childcare, running errands, or preparing meals for the family. When friends ask what they can do to help, suggest that the woman have a prepared "wish list" of specific actions that would make it easier for her to maintain bedrest. The hospital's social services department should also be contacted and asked for assistance. They are a useful resource that can share information about organizations that can be called upon to help.

Since lying in the lateral side position decreases pressure on the vena cava, the woman is instructed to maintain this position as much as possible. This position also increases venous return, circulatory volume, and placental and renal perfusion. Improving renal blood flow helps decrease angiotensin II levels, promotes diuresis, and lowers blood pressure. Antihypertensive medications have not been shown to improve perinatal outcomes in mild to moderate preeclampsia (blood pressure 140 to 160/90 to 110) and should not be routinely prescribed (NHBPEP, 2000).

 critical nursing action Facilitating Effective CPR for the Pregnant Patient

Always instruct pregnant patients never to lie on their backs and explain that the weight of their baby exerts pressure on the large blood vessels and impedes blood flow back to the heart. If the pregnant patient experiences a cardiac arrest, this information is essential. CPR will not be effective if the fetus remains on the large blood vessels. One nurse must take responsibility to displace the uterus to the left while the cardiac compressions are being performed.

The clinical course of severe preeclampsia may be characterized by a progressive deterioration in both the maternal and fetal conditions. Pregnancies complicated by severe preeclampsia have been associated with increased rates of perinatal mortality and significant risks for maternal morbidity and mortality. Because of this fact, there is universal agreement that all patients should be promptly delivered if the disease develops after 34 weeks' gestation or before that time if there is evidence of maternal or fetal compromise. Management of severe preeclampsia includes the following clinical actions (Cunningham et al., 2005; Sibai et al., 2005):

1. Seizure prophylaxis with magnesium sulfate, which has been universally accepted as the drug of choice because of its CNS-depressant action.
2. Antihypertensive medications (Tables 11-1 and 11-2)
   - The use of antihypertensive agents in severe preeclampsia is generally indicated when diastolic blood pressures reach or exceed 110 mm Hg.

Table 11-1 Medications Used to Treat Chronic Severe Hypertension in Pregnancy

Agent (trade name)	Class	Dose	Contraindications and Adverse Effects	Breastfeeding
Alpha-methyldopa (Aldomet)	Central alpha-adrenergic inhibitor	Starting dose = 250 mg po, tid or qid. Maximum dosage of 2–4 g/24 hr	Methyldopa hypersensitivity, history of hepatitis, autonomic dysfunction, lethargy or syncope. Can cause liver damage, fever, Coombs-positive hemolytic anemia.	Safe
Labetalol (Trandate, Normodyne)	Alpha-/beta-adrenergic blocker	100–400 mg po, bid or tid maximum dose 2400 mg a day	Labetalol hypersensitivity, bradycardia, asthma, heart block, heart failure. Can cause maternal and fetal bradycardia, hypotension, bronchospasm.	Safe
Nifedipine (Adalat, Procardia)	Calcium channel blocker	10–30 mg po tid slow release once a day. Maximum of 90 mg/day	Hypersensitivity to calcium channel blockers, persistent dermatologic reactions, congestive heart failure. Can potentiate cardiac depressive effect of magnesium sulfate.	Safe
Furosemide (Lasix)	Loop diuretic	20–80 mg po, qd or bid	Hypersensitivity to furosemide, anuria, or depleted blood count. Can cause profound diuresis with water and electrolyte depletions, sun sensitivity to exposure to sunlight, hyperuricemia and gout, exacerbation of SLE, abdominal cramping, diarrhea, tinnitus, dizziness, pancreatitis, and cholestasis.	Safe
Hydrochlorothiazide (HydroDIURIL)	Loop diuretic	25–50 mg po, qd	Anuria, renal disease, liver disease, SLE, hypersensitivity to hydrochlorothiazide or other sulfonamide derived drugs. Can cause weakness, hypotension, pancreatitis, cholestasis, anemia, allergic reactions, electrolyte disturbance, hyperglycemia, hyperuricemia, dizziness, renal dysfunction.	Risk is remote, but there are concerns about potential thrombocytopenia in infants.

Source: Yankowitz, J. (2004). Pharmacologic treatment of hypertensive disorders during pregnancy. *The Journal of Perinatal & Neonatal Nursing, 18*(3), 230–240. Reproduced with permission.

Table 11-2 Medications Used to Acutely Treat Severe Hypertension in Pregnancy

Agent (Trade Name)	Class	Dosage
Labetalol hydrochloride (Normodyne, Trandate)	Alpha-/beta-adrenergic blocker	IV bolus 20 mg; if no response, double dose and repeat every 15 min, up to a cumulative maximum dose of 300 mg
Hydralazine (Apresoline, Nepresol)	Peripheral/arterial vasodilator	IV bolus 5–10 mg every 15–20 minutes to a maximum dose of 30 mg
Nifedipine (Adalat, Procardia)	Calcium channel blocker	Nifedipine can be given po in doses of 10 mg repeated every 15 minutes to a maximum of 30 mg
Sodium nitroprusside (Nipride, Nitropress)	Vasodilator	0.25 mcg/kg per minute (increase by 0.25 mcg/kg/min every 5 minutes) to a maximum of 5 mcg/kg per minute

Source: Yankowitz, J. (2004). Pharmacologic treatment of hypertensive disorders during pregnancy. *The Journal of Perinatal & Neonatal Nursing, 18*(3), 230–240. Reproduced with permission.

The goal of therapy is to reduce the risk of cerebral vascular accident, while maintaining uteroplacental perfusion. A decrease in the diastolic pressure to less than 90 mm Hg in the patient with severe hypertension will decrease placental blood flow, often with a decrease in the fetal heart rate (FHR). Management is directed at reducing the diastolic blood pressure to a value of less than 110 mm Hg, but greater than 95 to 100 mm Hg.

3. Invasive hemodynamic monitoring may be required if any of the following are present:
   - Oliguria unresponsive to a fluid challenge
   - Pulmonary edema
   - Hypertensive crisis refractory to conventional therapy
   - Cerebral edema
   - Disseminated intravascular coagulation (DIC)
   - Multisystem organ failure

medication: Magnesium Sulfate

Magnesium sulfate (mag-nee-zhum sul-fate)

Pregnancy Category: D
Indications:
Anticonvulsant in severe eclampsia or preeclampsia

Unlabeled Use: Preterm labor

Actions: Plays an important role in neurotransmission and muscular excitability

Therapeutic Effects: Resolution of eclampsia

Pharmacokinetics:
ABSORPTION: IV administration results in complete bioavailability; well absorbed from IM sites
DISTRIBUTION: Widely distributed; crosses the placenta and is present in breast milk.
METABOLISM AND EXCRETION: Excreted primarily by the kidneys
HALF-LIFE: Unknown

Contraindications and Precautions:
CONTRAINDICATED IN: Hypermagnesemia/hypocalcemia/anuria/heart block/active labor or within 2 hours of labor (unless used for preeclampsia or eclampsia)
USE CAUTIOUSLY IN: Any degree of renal insufficiency

Adverse Reactions and Side Effects:
Central nervous system: Drowsiness
Respiratory system: Decreased respirations
Cardiovascular system: Arrhythmias, hypotension, bradycardia
Gastrointestinal system: Diarrhea
Dermatology system: Flushing, sweating
Metabolic: Hypothermia

Interactions: Potentiates neuromuscular blocking agents

Route and Dosage (Eclampsia/Preeclampsia): Piggyback a solution of 40 g of magnesium sulfate in 1000 mL of lactated Ringer's solution—use an infusion control device (pump) at the ordered rates; loading dose: initial bolus of 4–6 g over 15–30 min; maintenance dose: 1–3 g/hr.
IM: 4–5 g given in each buttock, can be repeated at 4-hour intervals; use Z-track technique. (Note: IM route rarely used because the absorption rate cannot be controlled and injections are painful and may result in tissue necrosis.)

Time/Action Profile for Anticonvulsant Effect:
IM: Onset is 60 minutes with peak unknown and duration is 3–4 hours IV: onset is immediate with peak unknown and duration is 30 minutes.

Nursing Implications: Remember that this is a very potent, high alert drug!
Explain purpose and side effects of the medication to the patient and her companion.
Explain that she may feel very warm and become flushed and experience nausea and vomiting, visual blurring, and headaches.
Magnesium sulfate must never be abbreviated (i.e., MgSO₄ is not acceptable) and requires a written order by the physician for administration.
Always use an infusion pump for administration and run the medication piggyback, not as the main line.
Monitor pulse, blood pressure, respirations, and ECG frequently throughout parenteral administration. Respirations should be at least 16/min before each dose.
Monitor neurological status before and throughout therapy.
Institute seizure precautions.
Keep the room quiet and darkened to decrease the likelihood of triggering seizure activity.
Patellar reflexes should be tested before each parenteral dose of magnesium sulfate. If absent, no additional dose should be administered until a positive response returns.
Monitor intake and output. Urine output should be maintained at a level of at least 100 mL/4 hr.

Serum magnesium levels and renal function should be monitored periodically throughout administration of parenteral magnesium sulfate.
Have 10% calcium gluconate available should toxicity occur. Administer 10 mL intravenously over 1–3 minutes until signs and symptoms are reversed.
After delivery, monitor the newborn, for hypotension, hyporeflexia, and respiratory depression.

Data from Deglin, J.H., & Vallerand, A.H. (2009). *Davis's drug guide for nurses* (11th ed.). Philadelphia: F.A. Davis.

clinical alert

Accidental overdose of magnesium sulfate administration can pose a significant risk to both mother and newborn

Current recommendations to prevent magnesium sulfate accidents:

- A standardized unit protocol should be consistent and include: standing orders addressing the initial bolus and maintenance dose to be administered; how the pump should be programmed; the maintenance IV solutions that will be used and the frequency that the fetus and mother will be assessed.

- Administer IV magnesium sulfate (including the initial bolus) only through a controlled infusion device with free-flow protection.

- Use universal standardized dose prepackaged magnesium sulfate.

- Have a second nurse check the initial magnesium sulfate IV bag and pump settings (and every magnesium sulfate IV bag that is added and each subsequent rate change).

- Use a 100-mL (4 g) or 150-mL (6 g) IV piggyback (IVPB) for the initial bolus instead of bolusing from the main bag with a rate change on the pump.

- Use color-coded tags on the lines as they go into the pumps and into the IV ports.

- Provide 1:1 nursing care for women in labor who are receiving magnesium sulfate.

- When care is transferred to another nurse, have both nurses together at the bedside review the pump settings for both the magnesium sulfate and mainline IV fluids and review written physician orders for magnesium sulfate infusion orders.

- Implement periodic magnesium sulfate overdose drills with airway management and calcium administration with the physician and nurse team members participating together.

- Maintain the calcium antidote in the patient's room in a locked box (Simpson & Knox, 2004).

NURSING ASSESSMENTS

Nursing care centers on extremely accurate, astute observations and assessments. An in-depth understanding of the pharmacological regimens, management plans, and potential complications associated with this disease is also essential. The clinical manifestations of preeclampsia are directly related to the presence of vascular vasospasms. Vasospasms cause endothelial injury, red blood cell destruction, platelet aggregation, increased capillary permeability, increased systemic vascular resistance, and renal and hepatic dysfunction. Hypertension and proteinuria are the most significant indicators of preeclampsia (Poole, 2004b).

IDENTIFYING HYPERTENSION

Preventing hypertension-induced problems in pregnancy requires nurses to use their assessment, advocacy, and counseling skills. Assessment begins with accurate blood pressure measurements. Checking blood pressures should never be treated as a routine, mundane task.

In the past, hypertension indicative of preeclampsia had been defined as an elevation of more than 30 mm Hg systolic or more than 15 mm Hg diastolic above the patient's baseline blood pressure. However, this definition has not been a good prognostic indicator of outcome. The frequently cited "30–15" rule is not part of the criteria for preeclampsia according to the National High Blood Pressure Education Program Working Group. Instead, women who demonstrate a blood pressure elevation of more than 30 mm Hg systolic or more than 15 mm Hg diastolic above the pre-pregnancy baseline "warrant close observation" (ACOG, 2002a; Peters & Flack, 2004).

The nurse needs to remember that blood pressure presents differently in women with preeclampsia. Preeclamptic patients often demonstrate labile (unstable) pressures and a flattening or reversal of normal circadian blood pressure rhythms, with the highest values recorded at night (Cunningham et al., 2005). Because of this variation, hospitalized patients should routinely have a nocturnal blood pressure assessment unless otherwise ordered by the physician. A daily cardiovascular assessment is also an important monitoring component for the hospitalized patient.

 Be sure to— Perform a daily cardiovascular assessment on patients with preeclampsia

During the assessment, the nurse should include the following parameters:

- Auscultation of heart sounds, lungs, and breath sounds
- Presence and degree of edema
- Early signs or symptoms of pulmonary edema, such as tachycardia and tachypnea
- Daily weight taken at the same time of the day and on the same scale
- Skin color, temperature, and turgor
- Capillary refill, which may indicate decreased perfusion or vasoconstriction if >3 seconds

SIGNIFICANCE OF PROTEINURIA

Proteinuria is defined as the excretion of 300 mg or more of protein every 24 hours. If 24-hour urine samples are not available, proteinuria is defined as a protein concentration of 300 mg/L or more (>1+ on dipstick) in at least two random urine samples taken at least 4 to 6 hours apart and no more than 7 days apart. However, studies have shown that urinary dipstick determinations as well as random protein to creatinine ratios correlate poorly with the amount of protein found in a 24-hour sample of women with gestational hypertension. Therefore, the definitive test to diagnose proteinuria should be quantitative protein excretion over 24 hours (Sibai et al., 2005).

The purpose of the renal assessment is to identify renal compromise. Due to the vasospasm that accompanies preeclampsia, the expected increases in the glomerular filtration rate and renal blood flow may not occur, nor the expected decrease in serum creatinine, especially if the disease is severe. Preeclampsia may be associated with a profuse swelling in the kidney glomerular endothelial cell cytoplasm. This pathological change causes glomerular endotheliosis, a lesion that correlates with proteinuria (ACOG, 2002a).

As an important component of hospital care, the nurse assesses urine output every 1 to 4 hours to confirm adequate renal perfusion and oxygenation. A urinary output of 25 to 30 mL/hr or 100 mL/4 hr is normal; a downward trend in output should be reported immediately. A urimeter attached to the Foley catheter tubing is useful in the accurate assessment of the hourly urine output. A 24-hour urine test for total protein may be ordered to monitor for an increase in the excretion of protein, a finding indicative of increasing kidney impairment. The nurse should be aware that if the 24-hour urine specimen (for total protein) shows the presence of protein, a dipstick is not appropriate. Once protein is evident in a 24-hour urine collection, protein will always be present when the urine is tested by the dipstick. Therefore, no new information is obtained. The 24-hour urine sample yields more accurate information because it shows whether or not the urine protein is increasing, decreasing, or remaining the same. When indicated, a high-protein diet may be needed to replace the protein excreted in the urine.

ASSESSING EDEMA

At one time, edema was an important component of the triad considered along with hypertension and proteinuria to diagnose preeclampsia. However, edema is a common finding in pregnancy. Dependent edema in the absence of hypertension or proteinuria is generally related to changes in the interstitial and intravascular hydrostatic pressures that facilitate the movement of intravascular fluid into the tissues. When preeclampsia is present, continuous capillary leakage combined with a decreased colloidal pressure can lead to pulmonary edema. In this situation, intravascular fluid leaks out through holes (caused by vasospasms) in the endothelial lining of the blood vessels. Pulmonary edema can occur very suddenly, especially if the patient receives an overload of intravenous fluid. Because of the potential for rapid development of this life-threatening complication, the nurse must frequently perform a careful assessment of the patient's pulmonary status and meticulously monitor the total intake and output.

CENTRAL NERVOUS SYSTEM ALTERATIONS

Preeclampsia may quickly develop into eclampsia, the convulsive phase of preeclampsia. Before the onset of seizure activity, the patient may complain of headaches, visual disturbances, blurred vision, scotomata (specks or spots in the vision where the patient cannot see; "blind spots"), and, in rare cases, cortical blindness (August, 2004). These symptoms can be indicators of increased CNS irritability that precedes the onset of seizures. A retinal examination often reveals vascular constriction and narrowing of the small arteries. These changes are reflective of the widespread vasoconstriction that is occurring throughout the body. Deep tendon reflexes (DTRs) are also routinely assessed for evidence of irritability and clonus (rapidly alternating muscle contraction and relaxation), two additional signs of increased CNS irritability.

 Optimizing Outcomes— **Grading reflexes and checking for clonus**

During the assessment, grade maternal reflexes on a 0–4+ scale:

4+   Very brisk, hyperactive; often indicative of disease; often associated with clonus

3+   Brisker than average; possibly but not necessarily indicative of disease

2+   Average; normal

1+   Somewhat diminished

0   No response

If the reflexes are hyperactive, test for ankle clonus. Support the knee in a partly flexed position. With your other hand, dorsiflex and plantar flex the foot a few times while encouraging the patient to relax, and then sharply dorsiflex the foot and maintain it in dorsiflexion. Look and feel for rhythmic oscillations between dorsiflexion and plantar flexion. Normal is no reaction to this stimulus. Sustained clonus indicates upper motor neuron disease. The ankle plantar flexes and dorsiflexes repetitively and rhythmically (Fig. 11-7) (Dillon, 2007). Clonus is usually noted as "absent" or "present" but it may be rated as:

• Mild (2 movements)
• Moderate (3 to 5 movements)
• Severe (6 or more movements)

A neurological assessment of the patient with preeclampsia includes establishing her level of consciousness (LOC). Determining if the patient is alert and oriented can be accomplished by asking if she knows why she is in the hospital and if she can correctly identify the name of the hospital. It is also important for the nurse to assess for any change in the patient's behavior or personality. Preeclampsia is an insidious condition and symptoms associated with worsening of the disease can be very subtle. Maintaining a quiet, darkened environment reduces stimuli that may trigger seizure activity. Ensure that seizure precautions (e.g., suction equipment, oxygen administration equipment, emergency medication tray) are in place.

Eclampsia

Eclampsia is the occurrence of grand mal seizures in women who have either gestational hypertension or preeclampsia (Sibia et al., 2005). It is the most common CNS

complication of hypertension, and most maternal deaths attributable to hypertension occur in women with eclampsia. Although patients with severe preeclampsia are at the greatest risk for developing seizures, the onset of eclampsia-related seizures in women with mild preeclampsia have been reported. Women in whom eclampsia develops exhibit a wide spectrum of signs and symptoms, ranging from extremely high blood pressure, 4+ proteinuria, generalized edema, and 4+ patellar reflexes to minimal blood pressure elevation, no proteinuria or edema, and normal reflexes (Sibai, 2002).

Maternal complications of eclampsia include cerebral hemorrhage, aspiration pneumonia, hypoxic encephalopathy, coma, thromboembolic events, and maternal death (incidence 0.4% to 14%) (Poole, 2004b). The perinatal death rate in pregnancies complicated by eclampsia is 9% to 23%. Perinatal deaths are closely related to gestational age and most often result from premature delivery, abruptio placentae, and intrauterine asphyxia (Cunningham et al., 2005).

The exact cause of eclamptic seizures is unknown but many etiologies, including cerebral vasospasm with local ischemia, hypertensive encephalopathy with hyperperfusion, vasogenic edema, and endothelial damage, have been proposed (Cunningham et al., 2005). Eclamptic seizures are clonic–tonic in nature and are almost always self-limiting. They seldom last longer than 3 to 4 minutes.

 critical nursing action   Care of the Pregnant Patient Post-seizure

• Do not attempt to shorten or abolish the initial seizure. Attempts to administer anticonvulsants intravenously without secure venous access can lead to phlebitis and venous thrombosis.
• Prevent maternal injury.
• Maintain adequate oxygenation; administer oxygen via face mask at 10 L/min.
• Minimize the risk of aspiration. Position the patient on her side to facilitate drainage. Suction equipment should be ready and working.
• Give adequate magnesium sulfate to control seizures. As soon as possible following the seizure, venous access should be secured with a 4- to 6-g loading bolus of magnesium sulfate given over 15–20 minutes. If the patient seizes following the loading dose, another 2-g bolus may be given intravenously, over 3–5 minutes.
• Correct maternal acidemia. Blood gas analysis allows monitoring of oxygenation and pH status. Respiratory acidemia is possible after a seizure.
• Avoid polytherapy. Maternal respiratory depression, respiratory arrest, or cardiopulmonary arrest is more likely in women who receive polytherapy to arrest a seizure. Remember that anticonvulsants are respiratory depressants and may interact.
• **Be sure to check the fetus or fetuses** (all must be accounted for). After a seizure there may be loss of FHR variability and bradycardia on the fetal monitoring tracing.
• Check the patient for ruptured membranes, contractions, and cervical dilation.
• Prepare for delivery as indicated.
• Support the patient and her family. This is a very frightening event for them and they will need reassurance and to be kept aware of the plan of care and the well-being of their baby (Poole, 2004b).

Figure 11-7 Testing for clonus.

Be sure to— Document after a patient seizure

Time and length of seizure

Associated symptoms

Vital signs including fetal heart assessment

Presence or absence of uterine contractions

Any untoward results such as rupture of the membranes or signs of placental abruption

Medications that were given. Remember to have the physician write or co-sign any verbal orders that were given during the emergency (Poole, 2004b).

 case study Kimberly Stallings

Kimberly Stallings is a 25-year-old Caucasian married woman pregnant with her first child. Kimberly's family practice physician has been caring for her since her first prenatal visit at 11.4 weeks' gestation. During the initial prenatal visit, the following data was obtained:

Vital signs: temperature: 98.6°F (37.0°C); pulse: 78 beats/ min; respirations: 20 breaths/min; blood pressure: 110/70; weight: 146 lbs. (66.4 kg)

A complete physical exam was performed with normal findings and prenatal labs including a thyroid-stimulating hormone level (TSH, because of a positive family history for hypothyroidism) were drawn. During the interview, the nurse inquired about any other family medical problems. Kimberly reported that both her sister and her mother had experienced preeclampsia during pregnancy.

An ultrasound was ordered for pregnancy dating because Kimberly had experienced irregular menstrual periods since discontinuing oral contraceptives.

Kimberly was seen by her doctor every 4 weeks and the pregnancy progressed uneventfully until 4 months later, when she presented to the office with increased blood pressure and swollen legs. Kimberly had noticed an increased swelling that extended up to the knees of both legs. She denied hand or facial swelling, headaches, visual problems, or right upper quadrant (RUQ) pain. Her sister, a chiropractor, had been checking her blood pressure and noted it to be as high as 160–170/100 to 110. At this visit, the following data was obtained:

Blood pressure: 144/96 (sitting). Repeat on left side: 130/76. Weight: 172.5 lbs. (78.4 kg)

Physical exam: General: In no acute distress; abdomen: nontender; fundus at 28–11.8 inches (30 cm) above the symphysis pubis; FHR 150 bpm; cardiovascular: 1+ pedal edema; neurological: reflexes 3+ with no clonus.

Assessment: Mild preeclampsia.

The following lab tests were ordered: CBC with platelet count; liver enzyme determination (AST, ALT, LDH), alkaline phosphatase (ALP); prothrombin time (PT); a chemistry panel (electrolytes: Na^+, K^+, Cl^-, HCO_3^-, Ca^{2+}, Mg^{2+}), blood urea nitrogen (BUN), creatinine (Cr), uric acid and a 24-hour urine collection for protein and creatinine clearance. A sonogram (ultrasound) was also ordered to monitor the status of the fetus.

Kimberly was instructed to go home, observe modified bedrest, rest on her left side as much as possible, and call the nurse if she experienced increased edema, headaches, visual disturbances, or RUQ pain. She was told to continue with twice daily blood pressure monitoring and return to the office in 1 week.

On her next office visit 8 days later, Kimberly reported that she had been observing bedrest at home and had noticed that her leg edema was improved. She stated "I can see my ankle

bones again." Her sister had continued to monitor the blood pressure. According to the blood pressure log, Kimberly's systolic blood pressure measurements had been in the 160s and the diastolic measurements were in the 60–70 range. Kimberly denied headaches, visual disturbances, or abdominal pain and remarked that the fetus had been active. At this visit, the following data were obtained:

Blood pressure: 158/98 (sitting); 150/100 (left side); weight: 160 lbs. (72.7 kg); fundal height: 27 cm; FHR: 150–170 bpm; reflexes: 3–4+ with no clonus; urinary protein: 4+ (2000+ mg/dL) on dipstick

Assessment: Severe preeclampsia at 29 4/7 weeks' gestational age

At this point, Kimberly's physician consulted with a maternal fetal medicine specialist, who advised transferring Kimberly to a tertiary care center located 50 miles away. Kimberly was promptly transferred to the tertiary care center and admitted to the obstetrical service.

Critical Thinking Questions

1. What are Kimberly's risk factors for developing preeclampsia?

2. Why did the nurse ask Kimberly about headaches, blurred vision, and right upper quadrant (RUQ) pain?

3. What signs and symptoms prompted Kimberly's physician to consult with the maternal–fetal specialist and arrange for a transfer to a tertiary care center?

◆ See Suggested Answers to Case Studies in the text on the Electronic Study Guide or DavisPlus.

HELLP Syndrome

HELLP is an acronym for: **H**emolysis, **E**levated **L**iver enzymes and **L**ow **P**latelets

Due to the arteriolar vasospasms in the cardiovascular system that occur in preeclampsia, the circulating red blood cells (RBCs) are destroyed as they try to navigate through the constricted vessels (Hemolysis). Vasospasms decrease blood flow to the liver, resulting in tissue ischemia and hemorrhagic necrosis (Elevated Liver enzymes). In response to the endothelial damage caused by the vasospasms (small openings develop in the vessels), platelets aggregate at the site and a fibrin network is set up, leading to a decrease in the circulating platelets (Low Platelets).

HELLP syndrome is a serious complication of preeclampsia that can manifest itself at any time during pregnancy and the puerperium, but like preeclampsia, it is rare before 20 weeks' gestation. However, unlike preeclampsia, HELLP syndrome occurs more often in Caucasians, multiparas, and in women older than 35 years. One third of all cases of HELLP syndrome occur during postpartum, and only 80% of these patients are diagnosed with preeclampsia before delivery (Sibai et al., 2005).

HELLP syndrome is actually a laboratory diagnosis for a variant of severe preeclampsia. The primary presentation is consistent with hepatic dysfunction evidenced by findings from the patient's liver function tests (ACOG, 2002a; Poole, 2004b). HELLP syndrome is characterized by rapidly deteriorating liver function and thrombocytopenia. Liver capsule distention often produces epigastric pain. Though rare, liver rupture is one of the most ominous consequences of severe preeclampsia/HELLP syndrome, with a reported maternal death rate of more than 30%. The precise cause of liver rupture is unknown, but the prevailing theory postulates that the increased hepatic pressure leads to rupture. It is theorized that endothelial dysfunction with intravascular fibrin deposits and hepatic sinusoidal obstruction leads to intrahepatic vascular congestion, increased intrahepatic pressure, and distention of Glisson's capsule. This pathological process progresses to the development of a subcapsular hepatic hematoma and subsequent liver rupture (ACOG, 2002a; Cunningham et al., 2005).

Therapy for HELLP syndrome centers on improving the platelet count by transfusion of fresh-frozen plasma or platelets and delivery as soon as feasible by vaginal or cesarean birth. Intrapartum nursing care involves continuous maternal–fetal monitoring. Measurement of central venous pressure or pulmonary arterial wedge pressure (Swan–Ganz catheter) may be required to monitor fluid status accurately when pulmonary edema or acute renal failure are present (ACOG, 2002a).

 Now Can You— **Discuss HELLP syndrome?**

1. State what the acronym HELLP stands for?
2. Describe the basic pathology of HELLP syndrome?
3. Discuss the significance of epigastric pain in the patient with HELLP syndrome?

 Now Can You— **Discuss Hypertensive Complications of Pregnancy?**

1. Differentiate among the following conditions: chronic hypertension, preeclampsia, eclampsia, chronic hypertension with superimposed preeclampsia and gestational hypertension?
2. Describe the pathophysiology of preeclampsia?
3. Discuss the indications for use, action, dosage, and side effects of magnesium sulfate?
4. State the specific nursing actions required when caring for the patient receiving magnesium sulfate?

Disseminated Intravascular Coagulopathy

Disseminated intravascular coagulopathy (DIC) is a hematological disorder characterized by a pathological form of clotting that is diffuse and consumes large amounts of clotting factors. DIC causes widespread external or internal bleeding or both (Cunningham et al., 2005). The most common causes of DIC in pregnancy are excessive blood loss with inadequate blood component replacement, placental abruption, amniotic fluid embolism, and severe preeclampsia/HELLP syndrome. Because DIC is a consumptive coagulopathy that results in depletion of the platelets and clotting factors, early diagnosis and prompt and appropriate management are critical in reducing maternal and perinatal death and complication rates (Cunningham et al., 2005; Labelle & Kitchens, 2005).

NURSING CARE

Nursing care includes continued meticulous assessment for signs of bleeding (e.g., petechiae, oozing from injection sites, hematuria). Use of an indwelling catheter for monitoring urinary output is essential because renal failure is a potential consequence of DIC. Vital signs and fetal assessments are monitored frequently and the patient is maintained in a side-lying tilt to enhance blood flow to the uterus. Oxygen may be administered through a rebreathing mask at 8 to 10 L/min and blood and blood products are administered according to physician orders (Labelle & Kitchens, 2005). The patient and her family are emotionally supported and kept informed about the maternal–fetal status. (See Chapters 14, 16, and 33 for further discussion.)

Multiple Gestation

Multiple gestation occurs when a fertilized ovum divides into two separate ova or if ovulation produces two separate ova and each is fertilized. The terminology used to describe the different characteristics of multiple gestations includes the following:

- **Monozygotic**: "Identical twins," the product of one ovum that split around the end of the first week after fertilization. Accounts for one-third of all twins.
- **Dizygotic**: "Fraternal twins"—two separate ova have been fertilized by two sperm
- **Dichorionic/diamnionic**: Two chorions and two amnions
- **Monochorionic/diamnionic:** One chorion and two amnions
- **Monochorionic/monoamnionic**: One chorion and one amnion—the fetuses share the same living quarters. Associated with a very high (40% to 60%) mortality rate due to cord accidents from entanglement (Cunningham et al., 2005).

INCIDENCE

Multiple gestation (also known as multifetal pregnancy) has increased significantly during the past 10 years and is largely due to advanced maternal age at childbirth and the widespread availability of assisted reproductive technology. "Multiples" account for 3% of all births in the United States. During the past decade there has been a 25% increase in the number of twin births, a 116% increase in triplets, a 149% increase in quadruplets, and a 250% increase in the number of quintuplet or higher order births (Malone & D'Alton, 2004; Martin et al., 2005). Dizygotic twins tend to run in families and are more common in people of African descent. Around the world, the rate of dizygotic twins ranges from 1 in 1000 in Japan to 1 in 20 in several tribes in Nigeria (Cunningham et al., 2005).

ASSOCIATED COMPLICATIONS

Because multiple gestations are associated with a number of maternal and fetal complications, they are considered to be a high-risk pregnancy. Complications may occur during the antepartal, intrapartal, or postpartal period. Preterm labor often results from uterine overdistension and frequently necessitates an early operative delivery. Other complications include gestational diabetes, increased urinary tract infections, preeclampsia/eclampsia, placenta previa, fetal intrauterine growth restriction (IUGR), abnormal presentation, and umbilical cord prolapse (Cunningham et al., 2005).

MATERNAL AND FETAL MORBIDITY AND MORTALITY

Maternal morbidity is higher in women with multiple gestations and seems to be related to the number of fetuses present. Twin pregnancies are associated with significantly higher risks of hypertension, placental abruption, anemia, and urinary tract infections than are singleton pregnancies (Malone & D'Alton, 2004). Monochorionicity (one chorion instead of separate chorions surrounds the developing multiple gestation), growth restriction, and prematurity pose the main risks to fetuses and neonates in a multiple gestation. The mean duration of a twin gestation is 37 weeks; for triplets and quadruplets the mean duration of gestation is 33 and 31 weeks, respectively. The mean gestational age at delivery for multiple gestations can be misleading because the classification does not reveal the true incidence of extreme prematurity, which has great clinical significance. The incidence of preterm delivery prior to 28 weeks for singletons is 0.7% in the United States. For twins, the incidence increases to 5% and for triplet gestations the incidence is 14%. The perinatal mortality rate for twins is at least threefold higher than with singletons (Malone & D'Alton, 2004).

Perinatal morbidity is also more likely in a multiple gestation. The incidence of a severe handicap in neonatal survivors of multiple gestation is increased from 19.7 per 1000 for singleton survivors to 34.0 and 57.5 per 1000 twin and triplet survivors, respectively. Twins account for between 5% and 10% of all cases of cerebral palsy in the United States (Malone & D'Alton, 2004).

DIAGNOSIS

A positive diagnosis of a multiple gestation can be confirmed by ultrasound examination. Sonography reveals multiple gestational sacs with yolk sacs by 5 weeks of gestation and multiple embryos with cardiac activity by 6 weeks of gestation (Malone & D'Alton, 2004). Rapid uterine growth, excessive maternal weight gain, or palpation of three or more fetal large parts (cranium and breech) on Leopold maneuvers are clinical findings suggestive of multiple gestation. Laboratory tests show elevated levels of human chorionic gonadotropin (hCG), human placental lactogen (hPL), and maternal serum α-fetoprotein (MSAFP) (Cunningham et al., 2005).

MANAGEMENT

Since multiple gestation pregnancies are considered to be high risk, an appropriately trained specialist should ideally manage the obstetric care. Delivery should be planned to take place at a Level III facility that has trained personnel who are prepared to deal with maternal or neonatal complications. When a pregnancy is complicated by a multiple gestation, the normal maternal physiological adaptations to pregnancy are heightened. Complications that are associated with these changes help to guide the clinical management. Consideration of maternal–fetal physiological parameters along with ongoing surveillance is essential in developing an appropriate plan of care.

NURSING IMPLICATIONS

Caring for the patient with a multiple pregnancy can be challenging, especially when complications arise. Hospitalization may be needed due to the increased risk of complications, and the nurse needs to remain cognizant of this fact. As an example, the patient with a multiple gestation who requires tocolytic therapy to prevent preterm birth is at greater risk for complications related to the tocolytic therapy than the patient with a singleton gestation. There is an increased risk of pulmonary edema due to the expanded plasma volume and increased cardiac output. Also, nutritional requirements are increased. Maternal caloric needs are approximately 40% greater for a woman expecting twins and 80% greater for a woman pregnant with triplets or higher multiples (Luke, 2005). Early in the pregnancy, the patient may suffer from severe hyperemesis gravidarum due to higher levels of pregnancy hormones found in multiple pregnancies as compared to singleton pregnancies. This condition can lead to dehydration and poor nutrient intake and require hospitalization for rehydration. At this time, the nurse can refer the patient to a nutritionist and also review foods that might be more appealing to the patient (Bowers & Gromada, 2006).

The nurse must also remain aware that the patients being cared for are the woman (the primary patient) as well as each individual fetus. Serial ultrasounds, nonstress tests, and biophysical profiles will be part of the ongoing assessment for fetal well-being and growth. Fetal surveillance with electronic fetal monitoring may be difficult, especially when there are more than two fetuses. Triplet monitors are available that allow for the tracing of three separate FHRs on a single channel, or two heart rate tracings and a digital read-out for the third fetus. It is best to monitor all fetuses simultaneously and the nurse should label which line corresponds to which ultrasound transducer so that it is clear which fetus is being monitored. The presenting twin is always "A," with the remaining fetuses ("B," "C," etc.) identified by relative ascending positions. Although not common, late pregnancy changes in fetal positions (e.g., male fetus B now in the position of female fetus A) should be noted in the patient record. If no recent ultrasound has been obtained, the nurse should identify each FHR by the appropriate abdominal quadrant (Bowers & Gromada, 2006).

A multiple pregnancy can cause many concerns for the family. They often fear for the well-being of the babies, especially since preterm labor is a major complication with multiples. The thought of the everyday rigors of caring for several newborns at one time can constitute another major cause of stress. If there are other children in the household, the expectant couple may question how they are going to be able to give the older siblings the care and time they will also need. Family finances can be a great concern as well as the affordability of childcare when it is necessary for the mother to return to work. The nurse can be supportive in encouraging families to voice their concerns and address them as appropriately as possible. Helping the family to prepare for the birth of the babies can be of great benefit. The nurse may offer suggestions that include giving the older children household chores appropriate for their age, alerting the partner's employer of a potential need to adjust the work schedule in order to help out at home or finding someone to help with housekeeping, grocery shopping, laundry, cleaning, and/or childcare. Other team members such as social service can also provide valuable solutions to these concerns. Referring the couple to a "multiples" support group may also be appropriate and welcomed.

 Now Can You— Discuss care of the pregnant patient with a multiple gestation?

1. Name five complications associated with a multiple gestation?
2. Describe your plan of care, taking into consideration the maternal-fetal physiological parameters of the multiple gestation pregnancy?
3. Identify other team members you would include in your plan of care?

Infections

URINARY TRACT INFECTION

Urinary tract infection (UTI) is the most common bacterial infection in pregnancy. The three most common clinical syndromes associated with UTI are asymptomatic bacteriuria, acute cystitis and acute pyelonephritis (Savoia, 2004).

Pathophysiology

The physiological dilatation of the urinary collecting system that occurs normally during pregnancy is associated with an increase in ascending urinary infections. Mechanical and hormonal changes may lead to hydroureter, decreased peristalsis, bladder distention, and incomplete emptying. These events can result in urine stasis or reflux in the bladder and ureters (Cunningham et al., 2005; Savoia, 2004).

The most common infecting organism is *Escherichia coli* (*E. coli*), which is responsible for 75% to 90% of all bacteriuria during pregnancy. Other organisms frequently responsible for UTIs include *Klebsiella, Proteus, Pseudomonas,* Group B streptococcus, and coagulase-negative staphylococci (Davison & Lindheimer, 2004).

Morbidity

Bacteriuria in pregnancy predisposes the patient to the development of acute pyelonephritis, a condition that poses significant risk to the woman and her fetus (Savoia, 2004). Asymptomatic and untreated bacteriuria has been associated with a number of complications during pregnancy including low birth weight, intrauterine death, preeclampsia, and maternal anemia (Davison & Lindheimer, 2004).

Asymptomatic Bacteriuria

Asymptomatic bacteriuria is defined as the presence of at least 10^5 colony-forming units of bacteria per milliliter of clean, voided, midstream urine in specimens obtained on two separate occasions. As the name implies, the patient does not express any symptoms of a UTI. Asymptomatic bacteriuria occurs in 2% to 11% of pregnancies and if left untreated, approximately 40% of those infected will develop an acute symptomatic UTI. Treatment includes anti-infectives such as ampicillin (Marcillin) for a 7- to 10-day period. Screening women for asymptomatic bacteriuria on the first prenatal visit constitutes a standard of obstetric care (Davison & Lindheimer, 2004; Savoia, 2004).

Acute Cystitis

Symptomatic lower UTI occurs in 1.3% to 3.4% of pregnant women. Symptoms include urinary frequency, urgency, dysuria, and suprapubic pain. The treatment is the same as for asymptomatic bacteriuria (Savoia, 2004).

 Nursing Insight— *Anti-infective medications contraindicated during pregnancy*

Medications including amoxicillin (Amoxil), ampicillin (Marcillin), and cephalosporins (cephalexin [Keflex]) are safe antibiotics during pregnancy. Sulfonamides should not be used near term because they interfere with protein binding of bilirubin and tetracyclines should never be used because they cause retardation of fetal bone growth and staining of fetal teeth.

Acute Pyelonephritis

Pyelonephritis, an inflammation of the kidney substance and pelvis, occurs in 1% to 2% of pregnant women. This condition presents as flank tenderness on the affected side and is associated with nausea, vomiting, fever, and chills along with the symptoms of a lower UTI. Significant pyuria and bacteriuria are present. Pyelonephritis is treated aggressively with hospitalization and intravenous antibiotics. If left untreated or inadequately treated, septic shock, adult respiratory distress syndrome and/or preterm labor may result (Cunningham et al., 2005; Davison & Lindheimer, 2004).

 Optimizing Outcomes— When caring for the patient with a UTI

During pregnancy, a urine specimen is more likely to be contaminated by bacteria that originate in the urethra, vagina, or perineum. This occurs due to a change in pH during pregnancy: the urine becomes more alkaline due to the maternal excretion of bicarbonate; the vagina also becomes alkaline and the vaginal secretions have increased glycogen content, which aids bacterial growth). Before collecting a mid stream specimen, the nurse should instruct the patient about the importance of proper cleansing.

A urinalysis and urine culture and sensitivity (C & S) should be obtained on all patients who present with signs of preterm labor and the nurse must remember that signs of UTI often mimic normal pregnancy complaints (i.e., urgency, frequency). It is important to remind the patient to take **all** of the medication that has been prescribed, even if the symptoms subside and she feels better. A Test of Cure (repeat urine test to evaluate whether or not bacteria is still present) should be obtained once the treatment has been completed.

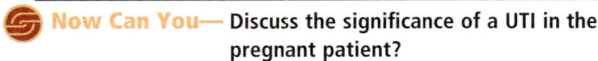

Now Can You— Discuss the significance of a UTI in the pregnant patient?

1. Describe anatomical and physiological renal system changes during pregnancy that place women at risk for UTIs? Identify the most common organism responsible for a UTI?
2. Explain why pyelonephritis must be treated aggressively?
3. Discuss nursing responsibilities when obtaining a urine specimen from a pregnant patient and identify instructions that should be given to the patient who is treated for a UTI?

Group B Streptococcal Infection

Group B streptococcus (GBS) is a frequent cause of urinary tract infections and chorioamnionitis during pregnancy and a significant cause of endometritis after the pregnancy has ended. It is a major pathogen in neonatal sepsis that can result in significant neonatal morbidity and mortality. Women harbor GBS as part of the normal fecal and vaginal flora. It is estimated that 10% to 30% of women are asymptomatic carriers of the organism. However, the rates vary according to the culture technique used, the number of samples cultured, and the nature of the populations studied. When maternal GBS colonization is present, transmission to the neonate is estimated to occur in approximately 60% of cases. The incidence is approximately 1.8 per 1000 live births (Cunningham et al., 2005; Savoia, 2004).

The onset of neonatal infection may be early (within the first 6 days of life) or late. Infants with early-onset infection generally develop signs (i.e., respiratory distress, septic shock) during the first 12 hours of life. Exposure to the organism occurs either in utero or during labor as the fetus travels down the colonized birth canal. Risk factors for contracting the infection include prematurity, low birth weight, premature rupture of the membranes, prolonged labor, maternal chorioamnionitis, multiple gestation, and GBS bacteremia during pregnancy. The overall rate of neonatal mortality from early onset GBS has declined from 50% in 1977 to approximately 6% currently, although infants of low birth weight continue to be at a substantial risk. Late-onset GBS is community acquired (the route of transmission is less clear and can be nosocomial [acquired while in the hospital], environmental, or maternal) and presents more than a week after birth. The majority of infants with community-acquired GBS are full term and 85% exhibit signs and symptoms of meningitis (Savoia, 2004).

In an effort to protect infants from Group B streptococcus infections, the Centers for Disease Control and Prevention (CDC) has issued guidelines that advocate obtaining vaginal and rectal cultures from all pregnant women between 35 and 37 weeks of pregnancy. Women with positive cultures and those with unknown GBS, ruptured membranes greater than 18 hours, previous preterm delivery (<37 weeks) or a history of a previous infant with GBS disease are treated with a penicillin-based anti-infective agent (Savoia, 2004).

TORCH INFECTIONS

TORCH refers to a group of maternal infectious diseases that cause harm to the embryo–fetus (Table 11-3). The TORCH acronym stands for **To**xoplasmosis, **R**ubella,

Cytomegalovirus (CMV), and **H**erpes simplex virus type 2 (HSV-2). (Some sources identify the "O" as "other" infections, such as hepatitis B, syphilis, and human immunodeficiency virus.) Maternal exposure to the TORCH infections during the first 12 weeks of gestation is associated with fetal developmental anomalies.

SEXUALLY TRANSMITTED INFECTIONS

Sexually transmitted infections (STIs) can cause serious morbidity and, in some cases, mortality in the mother, fetus, and infant. Following perinatal exposure, newborns are at risk for a number of minor and major complications that include congenital anomalies, mental impairment, and death. Women exposed to STIs are at risk for infertility, ectopic pregnancy, and pregnancy complications (Cunningham et al., 2005).

Chlamydia trachomatis

Chlamydia trachomatis is the most prevalent sexually transmitted infection in the United States. An estimated 3 million cases occur annually (CDC, Workowski, & Berman, 2006). *C. trachomatis* causes genital infections that can be asymptomatic and thus difficult to treat. However, infected women who do experience symptoms usually complain of vaginal discharge, dysuria, and, on occasion, abnormal vaginal bleeding. On speculum examination, the cervix exhibits a distinct mucopurulent discharge along with marked inflammation of the endocervix. Some women also experience an acute urethral syndrome manifested by dysuria, urinary frequency, and the presence of pyuria in a sterile urine specimen. Oral anti-infectives such as erythromycin or penicillin-based agents are used to treat *Chlamydia trachomatis* during pregnancy (Yudkin & Gonik, 2006).

Neonatal infection, most commonly manifested as conjunctivitis and pneumonia, results from exposure to the pathogen during birth. Typically, conjunctivitis occurs during the first 5 to 12 days of life whereas pneumonia does not develop until 1 to 3 months after birth (Rawlins, 2001). Topical antibiotic therapy, routinely administered during the immediate neonatal period, is inadequate for the treatment of a chlamydial infection. Since treatment with erythromycin is only about 80% effective, the newborn requires careful follow-up by the pediatrician (Yudkin & Gonik, 2006).

Neisseria gonorrhoeae

Neisseria gonorrhoeae (gonococci [GC], gonorrhea), a gram-negative diplococcus, is one of the oldest known sexually transmitted infections. It often coexists with chlamydia. The most common site of infection is the genitourinary tract. Infection sites unique to women include the Skene's and Bartholin's glands, endocervix, endometrium, and fallopian tubes. Symptoms of infection include vaginal discharge, dysuria, and abnormal vaginal bleeding. A speculum examination often reveals an inflamed, friable (easy to bleed) cervix. Treatment includes either oral or intramuscular cefixime (Suprax) or ceftriaxone (Rocephin) (CDC et al., 2006). Infants born to untreated, infected mothers are at risk for disseminated infection (bacteremia) and **ophthalmia neonatorum** (an eye inflammation) that can result in permanent blindness from perforation of the globe of the eye.

The amniotic infection syndrome is an additional manifestation of gonococcal infection in pregnancy. This entity manifests as placental, fetal membrane, and umbilical cord inflammation that occurs after premature rupture of the membranes (PROM) and is associated with infected oral and gastric aspirate, leukocytosis, neonatal infection, and maternal fever. The syndrome is characterized by PROM, premature delivery, and a high rate of infant morbidity (Gibbs, Sweet, & Duff, 2004).

Syphilis

Syphilis is an acute and chronic infection caused by the spirochete *Treponema pallidum*. It has a long clinical course that begins with an incubation period followed by primary, secondary and tertiary infection. Throughout this time, there is progressive damage to the CNS, cardiovascular system, and musculoskeletal system. Syphilis is transmitted primarily through sexual contact or fetal infection may occur transplacentally. During pregnancy, syphilis usually occurs in women who are young and unmarried and in those who receive little or no prenatal care (Savoia, 2004).

The onset of primary syphilis is usually heralded by the appearance of a chancre, a painless, round, ulcerated lesion with a raised border and indurated (hardened) base. In women, the chancre most commonly appears on the vulva, cervix, and vagina. Penicillin is the treatment of choice for all stages. If left untreated, the disease progresses, becomes chronic, and may lead to death.

Prompt maternal treatment eliminates most fetal syphilis infections, but delayed treatment or failure to obtain treatment may result in fetal effects that range from minor anomalies to preterm birth or fetal death. Damage to the fetus depends on when during gestation the infection occurred and the amount of time elapsed before treatment. Neonatal infection may be present at birth, but not expressed for up to 2 years ("silent infection") (Askin, 2004). Manifestations of congenital syphilis include rhinitis (snuffles), macular rash on the palms and soles of the feet, osteochondritis (inflammation of the bony epiphysis), perichondritis (inflammation of the membrane that covers the surface of cartilage), hepatosplenomegaly, jaundice, anemia, and thrombocytopenia (Savoia, 2004).

Human Papillomavirus Infection

Human papillomavirus (HPV) is a sexually transmitted virus that causes **condylomata acuminata** (genital warts) and is the primary cause of cervical neoplasia (American Cancer Society, 2006). Approximately 70% of cervical cancers result from infection with HPV (ACOG, 2006). Risk factors associated with HPV infection include early onset of sexual activity, multiple sex partners, cigarette smoking, and long-term use of oral contraceptives (Gibbs et al., 2004).

The prevalence of genital warts is highest among the 16- to 25–year-old age group, which is also the age group with the highest rate of pregnancy. The warts grow more rapidly during pregnancy and may involve the cervix, vagina, or vulva so extensively that vaginal delivery is precluded. The reason for the increase in size and number of the lesions is not known but has been postulated to be the decrease in cell-mediated immunity that occurs during pregnancy (Landry, 2004). Management of these lesions in pregnancy presents difficult problems and treatment includes trichloroacetic acid, dichloroacetic acid, cryotherapy, and surgical excision. None of these therapies has been shown to be superior to the others. The best approach to treatment during pregnancy may be the excision of the lesions by cautery or the use of cryosurgery. Care must be taken to prevent extensive scarring or sloughing of tissue (CDC et al., 2006; Gibbs et al., 2004).

The risk for transmission of the virus from maternal condylomata acuminata to the neonate has not been established. HPV is present in maternal blood and can be transmitted transplacentally to the fetus, but the incidence is very low according to reported studies (Gibbs et al., 2004).

 Nursing Insight— *Preventing HPV through vaccination with Gardasil*

Nurses can be instrumental in preventing infection caused by the human papillomavirus. The American College of Obstetricians and Gynecologists (ACOG) Committee on Adolescent Health Care and the ACOG Working Group on Immunization recommend that females 9–26 years of age receive vaccination against HPV. Although obstetricians-gynecologists are not likely to care for many girls in this initial vaccination group, ACOG has recommended that the first adolescent reproductive health care visit take place between 13 and 15 years of age. These visits are a strategic time to discuss HPV and the potential benefit of the HPV vaccine and to offer vaccination to those who have not already received it (ACOG, 2006).

HIV and AIDS

Human immunodeficiency virus (HIV) type 1 (HIV-1) infection, with rare exception, causes a slow but relentless destruction of the immune system that ultimately results in acquired immunodeficiency syndrome (AIDS). HIV type 2 (HIV-2) infection has a more variable and benign course. HIV-2 has remained largely confined to West Africa, whereas HIV-1 strains are causing increasing epidemics around the world (Landry, 2004).

HIV-1 infection is an increasing problem among women of childbearing age. AIDS is the fifth leading cause of death among women 25 to 44 years of age and has become a leading cause of death for young children in many parts of the world. Without identification of HIV-infected women and the aggressive use of preventive therapy, 20%-30% of these children will become infected with HIV (CDC, 2006a; Landry, 2004; Moran, 2004a).

TRANSMISSION. Heterosexual unprotected sexual contact now poses the greatest risk to women. Because vaginal mucus can harbor the retrovirus, women are more likely than men to contract HIV infection through heterosexual activity. Factors that increase the risk of transmission include (Moran, 2004a):

- Unprotected sexual intercourse (no condom is used)
- Sexual intercourse during menses
- Increased number of sexual contacts
- Presence of genital sores
- Advanced disease state

The risk of vertical transmission to the fetus or newborn is proportional to the concentration of virus in maternal plasma (viral load). Vertical transmission occurs antepartally when the virus crosses the placenta, intrapartally

Text continued on page 322

Table 11-3 TORCH Disease

Infection	Agent	Mode of Transmission	Detection	Maternal Effects
Toxoplasmosis	Single-celled protozoan parasite *Toxoplasma gondii*	Transplacental Eating raw meat, especially pork, lamb or venison Touching the hands or the mouth after handling undercooked meat containing *T. gondii* Secreted in feces of infected cats Cyst is destroyed with heat	Serologic antibody testing IgM specific antibody IgG seroconversion from negative to positive Most accurate confirmation of active infection is a rise in IgG titer in two appropriately spaced tests	Most infections in humans are asymptomatic However, may include fatigue, muscle pains, and sometimes lymphadenopathy In the immunocompetent person, toxoplasmosis can be a devastating infection
Other **Hepatitis B**	HBV Incubation usually 60–90 days	Direct contact with the blood or body fluids of an infected person Sexual Perinatal Percutaneous Transplacental Blood, stool, amniotic fluid, and saliva transmission Shared razors, toothbrushes, towels, and other personal items	HBsAg identified 7–14 days after exposure Hepatitis B surface antibody present with HBsAg indicates non infectious HBcAg, HBeAg, and AntiHBc evaluate stage and progression of the infection	Course of the disease is not altered during the pregnancy Symptoms are seen in only 30%–50% of patients; these include low-grade fever, nausea, anorexia, jaundice, hepatomegaly, malaise, preterm labor, and preterm birth No specific treatment, but may include bedrest and a high-protein, low-fat diet Mother to child transmission of HBV occurs in 10%-20% of women who are seropositive for HBsAg and in 90% of women who are seropositive for both HBsAg and HBcAg Transmission to the neonate appears to occur as a result of exposure to infected blood and genital secretions during delivery

Neonatal Effects	Treatment	Incidence and Prevention	High Risk Potential
Severity varies with gestational age Congenital infection can occur if a woman develops acute toxoplasmosis during pregnancy (most likely in the third trimester) May have miscarriage if acquired early Fetal infections more virulent the earlier the infection is acquired but less frequent Sequelae include low birth weight, hepatosplenomegaly, icterus, anemia, neurological disease, and chorioretinitis Clinically significant congenital toxoplasmosis occurs in approximately 1 in 8000 pregnancies	Pyrimethamine and sulfadiazine may reduce incidence of congenital toxoplasmosis Treatment of the mother has shown to reduce the risk of congential infection *Pyrimethamine is not recommended for use during the first trimester of pregnancy*	ACOG does not recommend routine screening except for pregnant women with HIV infection Incidence varies throughout the world (1–4 infants per 1000 live births) 30% of U.S. women have been exposed Approximately 40%–50% of U.S. adults have antibody to this organism Frequency of seroconversion during pregnancy is <5% and approximately 3 in 1000 infants show evidence of congenital infection Incidence of congenital toxoplasmosis infection in the U.S. is 1 in 1000–8000 More than 60 million people in the U.S. carry a parasite Cook meat to a safe temperature Peel or wash fruits and vegetables	People who consume raw or poorly cooked meat *High risk gestational age 10–24 weeks Toxoplasmosis is more common in Western Europe, particularly France*
Infants infected at birth have a 90% risk of becoming chronically infected with HBV (carrier) and 25% risk of developing significant liver disease—yet if they receive prophylaxis at birth, 95% can be prevented Increased risk of transmission to infant if mother is HBeAg-positive (indicating acute infection) Stillbirth Clinical illness is relatively infrequent Most (90%–95%) of those infected are symptomatic and become chronic hepatitis B carriers Infants born to women who have hepatitis B infection during pregnancy should be given HBIG within 12 hours of delivery	Mother: rest Infant: vaccine if mother is carrier, infant receives HBIG HBV vaccine recommended (three doses)	Screen all pregnant women; the incidence of hepatitis B in the U.S. declined by >60% from 1985 to 1995 Estimated that 1 to 1.25 million people in the U.S. are chronically infected with HBV Estimated that 300 million people worldwide are chronically infected with HBV Approximately 8000 acute HBV infections were reported to CDC HBV vaccine has been available since 1982 *Acute infection occurs in 1–2 per 10000 pregnancies* Minimize exposure of close physical contact Heptavax-B (pregnancy does not contraindicate vaccination)	High-risk categories: Pregnant women from China, Southeast Asia, Africa, Philippines, and Indonesia Eskimos Prostitutes Homosexuals IV drug users Hemophiliacs Transfusion recipients People with other sexually transmitted diseases or multiple sex partners CDC recommends universal screening of all prenatal patients

Continued

Table 11-3 TORCH Disease—cont'd

Infection	Agent	Mode of Transmission	Detection	Maternal Effects
Rubella (3-day German measles)	Rubella virus incubation is 2–3 weeks	Nasopharyngeal secretions Transplacental	Virus isolated from throat Rubella-specific IgM antibodies Hemagglutination-inhibition antibodies Complement-fixing antibodies Rubella antibody titer of 1:8 or more indicates immune status	Erythema Maculopapular rash on face, neck, arms, and legs lasting 3 days Lymph node enlargement Slight fever, malaise, headache, and arthralgia History of exposure 3 weeks earlier
Cytomegalovirus (CMV)	DNA virus of the herpesvirus group	Transmitted horizontally by droplet infection and contact with saliva and urine, vertically from mother to fetus-infant, and as a sexually transmitted disease Intimate contact with infected secretions (breast milk, cervical mucus, semen, saliva, tears and urine) Transplacental Organ transplacental	Isolation of virus from urine or endocervical secretions	Most infections are asymptomatic, but approximately 15% of adults have a mononucleosis-like syndrome characterized by fever, pharyngitis, lymphadenopathy, and polyarthritis

Neonatal Effects	Treatment	Incidence and Prevention	High Risk Potential
Overall risk of congenital rubella syndrome is approximately 20% for primary maternal infection in the first trimester	Women with rubella require no special therapy other than mild analgesics and rest	Last epidemic in 1965—since introduction of vaccine in late 1960s, rubella is rare	
High incidence of congenital abnormalities in newborns whose mother contracted rubella within the first 4 months of pregnancy	Infants born with congenital rubella may shed virus for many months and thus be a threat to other infants, as well as to susceptible adults	Absence of rubella antibody indicates susceptibility	
Approximately 50% of infants exposed to the virus within 4 weeks of conception will manifest signs of congenital infection		Estimated that 6%–25% of women are susceptible	
When infection occurs in second 4 week period after conception, approximately 25% of fetuses will be infected; when infection develops in third month, approximately 10% of fetuses will be infected		Occurs more commonly in the spring	
Spectrum anomalies:		Vaccinate immediately post partum and use contraception for a minimum of 1 month after vaccination	
Deafness (60%–75%)		Vaccination is contraindicated during pregnancy	
Eye defects (10%–30%)			
CNS anomalies (10%–25%)			
Cardiac malformation (10%–20%)			
Risks appear to be almost exclusively associated with women who previously have not been infected with CMV	Mother: treat symptoms	Maternal immunity to CMV does not prevent recurrence	Day-care centers are a common source of infection
Even in this case, 2/3 of infants will not become infected and only 10%–15% of the remaining will have symptoms	Infant: no satisfactory treatment is available	Found in 0.5%–2.0% of all neonates	Prevalence:
Infection is most likely to occur with primary maternal infection	Isolate infant	Incidence of primary CMV infection in pregnant women in the United States varies from 1%–3%	Depends on age, sex, SE class, sexual behavior, and occupational or institutional exposure
The timing of the infection during pregnancy is major determinant of outcome (first and second trimester being more severely affected)	Approximately 50% of females in the U.S. have antibodies	Rigorous personal hygiene throughout pregnancy	Serologic screening is not recommended by ACOG
CID includes low birth weight, IUGR, microcephaly	Estimates are that approximately 2% of susceptible pregnant women acquire primary CMV infection during pregnancy in the U.S.		Vaccine is experimental
CNS abnormalities, mental and motor retardation, intracranial calcifications, sensorineural deafness, blindness with chorioretinitis, mental retardation, hepatosplenomegaly and jaundice			

Continued

Table 11-3 TORCH Disease—cont'd

Infection	Agent	Mode of Transmission	Detection	Maternal Effects
Herpes simplex virus (HSV)	Herpes virus type 1 (more common with oral lesions) and type 2 (more common in genital lesions) Incubation is 2–10 days	Ascending infection Intimate mucocutaneous exposure Transmission is more likely to occur from men to women Passage through an infected birth canal Transplacental (although rare) if initial infection occurs during pregnancy	Tissue culture (swab specimen from vesicles) and immunofluorescent staining of the cell can differentiate HSV-1 from HSV-2 Swelling, redness, and painful lesions	Painful genital vesicle lesions Vesicles on the cervix, vagina, or external genitalia area Primary infection is commonly associated with fever, malaise, and myalgia; numbness, tingling, burning, itching, and pain with lesions; lymphadenopathy; and urinary retention

ACOG, American College of Obstetricians and Gynecologists; AntiHBc, antibody to hepatitis B core antigen; CDC, Centers for Disease Control; CID, cytomegalic inclusion disease; CNS, central nervous system; DNA, deoxyribonucleic acid; HBV, hepatitis B virus; HIV, human immunodeficiency virus; HbsAg, surface antigen to HBC; HbcAg, core antigen to HBV; HbeAg, hepatitis B early antigen; HBIg, hepatitis B immunoglobulin; IgG, immunoglobulin G; IgM, immunoglobulin M; IUGR, intrauterine growth restriction; IV, intravenous
Source: Moran, B. (2004). Maternal infections. In S. Mattson & J. Smith (Eds.), *Maternal-child nursing core curriculum* (3rd ed., pp 419-448). Philadelphia: W.B. Saunders. Reproduced with permission.

when it travels (via the bloodstream) from the vagina up into the uterus during labor or following rupture of the membranes or postpartally through transfer in the breast milk (Lawrence & Lawrence, 2005; Riordan, 2005). Transmission of HIV to the fetus or infant is believed to most often occur late in pregnancy or during labor and birth. Increased rates of transmission also occur with advanced maternal disease and ruptured membranes and after events during labor and delivery that increase fetal exposure to maternal blood (ACOG, 2000). In 2000, ACOG established guidelines to prevent HIV transmission; these guidelines were updated in 2004 (Box 11-8).

Optimizing Outcomes— Decreasing the incidence of STIs in women and children

Nurses should be aware of the signs and symptoms of STIs in order to recognize them and appropriately counsel patients about them.

- Alert the pediatrician to the patient's positive history of an STI.
- Counsel women in a nonjudgmental and compassionate manner about safe sex habits (i.e., the use of condoms).
- Encourage women to obtain routine checkups and promptly report any signs or symptoms of an STI to their provider.
- Instruct the woman undergoing treatment that she must take all of the medication prescribed and keep any follow-up appointments.
- Remind the patient that her partner must also be treated and if he refuses, she must abstain from sex with him until he is treated.
- Remember to always use Universal Precautions.

Box 11-8 Management to Prevent Transmission of HIV Infection

- Patients should be counseled that in the absence of antiretroviral therapy, the risk of vertical transmission is approximately 25%. With zidovudine (ZDV) therapy, the risk is reduced to 5–8%. When care includes both ZDV therapy and scheduled cesarean delivery, the risk is approximately 2%. A risk of 2% or less is seen in those women with viral loads of <1000 copies per milliliter even without delivery via cesarean section.
- Plasma viral loads should be determined at baseline and then every 3 months or following changes in therapy. The patient's most recently determined viral load should be used to direct counseling regarding the mode of delivery.
- Women infected with HIV whose viral loads are >1000 copies per milliliter should be counseled as to the benefits of a scheduled cesarean section in reducing the risk of vertical transmission to the infant.
- Patients should receive antiretroviral chemotherapy during pregnancy according to the accepted guidelines for adults. This therapy should not be interrupted around the time of cesarean delivery. For those patients receiving ZDV, adequate levels of the drug in the blood should be achieved if the infusion is begun 3 hours preoperatively.
- Best clinical estimates of gestational age should be used for planning cesarean delivery. Amniocentesis to determine fetal lung maturity should be avoided whenever possible.
- All women should be clearly informed of the risks associated with cesarean delivery as the preoperative maternal health status affects the degree of the risk of maternal morbidity associated with cesarean delivery.
- The patient's autonomy in making the decision regarding the route of delivery must be respected. A patient's informed decision to undergo vaginal delivery must be honored, with cesarean delivery performed only for other accepted indications and with patient consent.

Source: American College of Obstetricians and Gynecologists (ACOG) Committee Opinion (2000, 2004).

Neonatal Effects	Treatment	Incidence and Prevention	High Risk Potential
Rare transplacental transmission have resulted in miscarriage	Protect neonate from exposure at time of delivery	Estimated 1 million Americans are newly infected with genital HSV annually	Risk factors include female sex, African American, or Mexican American ethnic background, older age, low educational level, poverty, cocaine use, and a greater number of lifetime sexual partners
Mortality of 50%–60% if neonatal exposure is with active primary infection	Cultures are done when mother has active lesions	Seroprevalence of HSV is approximately 25%	
Neurologic morbidity such as chorioretinitis, microcephaly, mental retardation, seizures, and apnea	Avoid routine use of scalp electrodes	Approximately 1%–2% of pregnancies	
	If lesions are visible, delivery by cesarean section is the current standard of care	1 in 3000–20,000 live births for the development of neonatal herpes	Unprotected sex and having a sexual partner with genital herpes
	Acyclovir has been used near term to suppress outbreak	Up to 70% of women delivering infected infants have no history of genital herpes	
		Prophylactic treatment with oral acyclovir may be appropriate in women with frequent recurrent infections in pregnancy	
		If symptoms or lesions are present, cesarean delivery should be performed	
		Avoid genital contact when male partner has penile lesions	
		Use condoms	

TUBERCULOSIS

Tuberculosis (TB) is an infectious, communicable disease caused by the tubercle bacillus, *Mycobacterium tuberculosis*. The disease causes inflammatory infiltrations most commonly in the respiratory tract although TB may also affect the gastrointestinal and genitourinary tracts, bones, joints, nervous system, lymph nodes, and skin. Tuberculosis is the most common infectious disease in the world. Since 1992, the number of cases of TB has decreased. However, health care professionals caring for pregnant women and newborns are challenged to remain skilled in screening, identifying, and treating TB infection because the disease remains at epidemic levels in certain areas of the country and in certain populations. Women who are homeless, infected with HIV, IV drug users, or those who have emigrated from countries with a high rate of TB (i.e., Latin America, Asia, Africa) are at highest risk (Cunningham et al., 2005).

Although maternal tuberculosis does not appear to cause congenital malformations, it may lead to fetal infection. TB can spread to the fetus from the maternal blood if the bacilli cross the placenta and enter the umbilical vein. Fetal blood then passes through the liver, and this organ serves as the primary focus for the disease in the fetus and newborn. If the bacilli bypass the fetal liver, the lungs may become the primary infection site. Neonates may become infected at the time of birth by aspiration of infected amniotic fluid or by aspiration of infected blood and tissue if the mother has tuberculosis endometritis. They may also become infected through the traditional airborne route if individuals in the infant's environment have pulmonary tuberculosis (Cunningham et al., 2005; Savoia, 2004).

Initial treatment of active tuberculosis in pregnancy includes isoniazid (INH), ethambutol, and rifampin, medications that are considered to be safe during pregnancy.

Therapy should be continued for 9 months. Breastfeeding is not contraindicated and can begin or can continue during anti-TB therapy since the medications do not cross into the breast milk. However, if the infant is concurrently taking oral antituberculosis therapy, excessive drug levels may be reached in the neonate, and breastfeeding should be avoided (Savoia, 2004).

 Optimizing Outcomes— **Immunizations during pregnancy**

The ideal time to immunize women in order to prevent the spread of disease to the fetus is during the preconceptional period. However, the maternal and fetal benefits of immunization during pregnancy usually outweigh the theoretical risks of adverse effects. The risk for exposure to disease and its deleterious effects on the pregnant woman and the fetus must be balanced against the efficacy of the vaccine and any beneficial effects that may result from it. Nurses can educate their patients regarding the importance of immunizations and documentation of the patient's immunization status should be a part of the permanent medical record.

Inflammatory Disease and Pregnancy

SYSTEMIC LUPUS ERYTHEMATOSUS

Systemic lupus erythematosus (SLE) is a chronic multisystem inflammatory disorder. It is characterized by an autoimmune antibody production that results in an inflammation of the connective tissue in various organs or systems in the body (Yancy, 2004). The disease tends to affect young women in the second, third, and fourth decades of life but may occur in any age group. The prevalence of SLE is 100 per 100,000 in the general population (Laskin, 2004).

Pathophysiology

The immune system is composed of specialized cells that destroy invading organisms by phagocytosis and antibody and lymphocyte production. When a foreign organism or antigen enters the body, it is consumed by macrophages and then passed on to lymphokines, which present the antigens to the T and B lymphocytes. The B lymphocytes are activated, resulting in the production of an increased number of circulating antibodies that target their specific antigen. The antigen–antibody complex either promotes destruction of the antigen or activates the normal inactive proteins in the complement system. With SLE, the body fails to recognize its own proteins. The clinical manifestations result from inflammation of multiple organ systems, especially the joints, skin, kidneys, nervous system, and serous membranes (Laskin, 2004).

Effects During Pregnancy

Adverse pregnancy outcome is more common in SLE than in any other rheumatic disease. In the pre-steroid era, it was common practice to terminate pregnancy in patients with active SLE. However, with successful treatment of active disease with corticosteroids, this practice has become less frequent. Patients are more likely to have inactive SLE at the onset of pregnancy because of earlier disease diagnosis and more effective pre-pregnancy therapy, as well as appropriate pre-pregnancy counseling (Laskin, 2004). According to Yancy (2004), pregnancy outcome is improved in the following circumstances: SLE has been in remission for at least 6 months; there is no active renal involvement; superimposed preeclampsia does not develop; or there is no evidence of antiphospholipid antibody activity.

The patient with SLE should be seen frequently by both an internist-rheumatologist and a perinatologist specializing in high-risk cases. Assessment of the signs and symptoms of an impending SLE flareup should be elicited on the patient's history and physical examination, and blood samples obtained for serological evaluation. A rise in the anti-dsDNA antibody titer and a decrease in complement may be predictive of an exacerbation of SLE. The onset of edema and hypertension in pregnancy in these patients is characteristic of both preeclampsia and active SLE-associated nephritis. Since the treatment of these conditions is very different, the importance of an accurate diagnosis is essential (Laskin, 2004).

Perinatal Morbidity and Mortality

When SLE complicates the pregnancy, there is an increased risk of spontaneous abortion, premature rupture of the membranes, preterm labor, preterm birth, stillbirth, and neonatal death (Laskin, 2004; Yancy, 2004). Congenital heart block or congestive heart failure of the fetus or newborn is of particular concern. Maternal autoantibodies may cross the placenta and form immune complexes with fetal autoantigens, promoting fetal tissue destruction. Autoantibodies may initiate injury to fetal cardiac tissue, resulting in conduction disturbances that may be temporary or permanent (Laskin, 2004).

Management

Management of SLE is aggressive and includes immunosuppression of lupus flare with corticosteroid therapy, nonsteroidal anti-inflammatory drugs (NSAIDs), antimalarial agents, azathioprine (AZA), and careful fetal surveillance. If the disease flares during the pregnancy, treatment must be implemented as quickly as possible. The physician assesses the manifestations and extent of the disease exacerbation and selects the safest, most effective therapy. The patient's health must be deemed the first priority and the treatment is planned accordingly (Laskin, 2004). When caring for patients with SLE, nurses should offer support and remain alert for early indicators of SLE exacerbation and pregnancy complications. Patients and their families should be educated about the plan of care, the need for close surveillance, and the importance of effective family planning after the birth.

Hemoglobinopathies of Pregnancy

The major function of the red blood cell (RBC) is to carry hemoglobin, which transports oxygen from the lungs to the tissues. The ability of hemoglobin to bind to oxygen is determined by its structural composition. Normal hemoglobin consists of a heme molecule, which is an iron protoporphyrin, combined with two pairs of globin chains. Significant shortening of RBC survival occurs due to alterations in the structure (e.g., sickle hemoglobin) or quantity (e.g., thalassemia) of the hemoglobin chains. These alterations result from inherited disorders. In their most severe forms, these disorders are associated with hemolytic anemia and progressive multi-organ failure (Duffy, 2004).

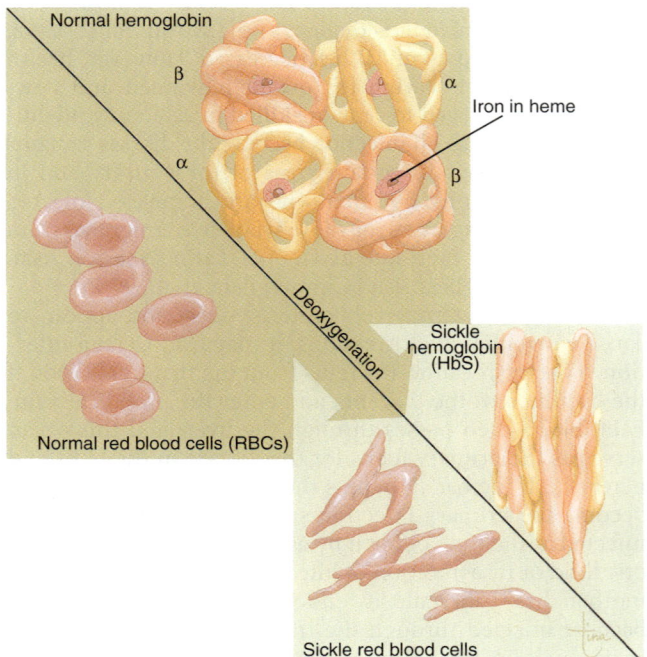

Figure 11-8 Comparison of normal hemoglobin and normal red blood cells to sickle hemoglobin (HbS) and sickle red blood cells.

SICKLE CELL DISEASE

Sickle cell disease is the most common hemoglobinopathy in the United States. It is of recessive inheritance and occurs when the gene for the production of hemoglobin S (HbS) is inherited from both parents (homozygous). It is seen most frequently in those of African and Mediterranean descent. Sickle cell anemia is the most prevalent and severe form of the sickle cell diseases (Yancy, 2004).

Pathophysiology

Patients with sickle cell anemia (SCA) suffer from lifelong complications, in part as a result of the markedly shortened life span of their RBCs (Kilpatrick & Laros, 2004). When HbS is exposed to low oxygen tension, it precipitates into long crystals, or polymers, within the red blood cell. With the lowered or absent amount of oxygen, the sickle cell hemoglobin molecule becomes rigid and dehydrated and assumes an abnormal crescent (sickled) shape (Fig. 11-8). The sickled erythrocytes cannot change their shape and are unable to squeeze through the microcirculation. Obstruction results, leading to hypoxia. Progressive tissue and organ damage occur along with painful vasoocclusive crises and an increased susceptibility to infection (Fig. 11-9). The signs and symptoms, which are related to vascular occlusion, hemolysis (lysis of the RBCs), and infection, are associated with a number of laboratory and clinical findings. Hemoglobin levels usually fall within the range of 6 to 8 g/dL, there is an increase in bilirubin levels due to hemolysis and folate, or iron deficiency results from bone marrow suppression. Clinical signs may include hepatomegaly, cardiomegaly, conjunctival vessel changes, systolic murmurs, and arthritis (Kilpatrick & Laros, 2004).

Effects During Pregnancy

Many pregnancies complicated by sickle cell anemia are associated with poor perinatal outcomes. Severe anemia and frequent vasoocclusive crises may occur during pregnancy and these problems are associated with an increased maternal and perinatal morbidity and mortality. Although maternal mortality is rare in patients with sickle cell anemia, maternal morbidity is great. Infections are common and occur in 50% to 67% of affected women. The respiratory and urinary tracts are the most common sites of infection, and all infections must be promptly treated since fever, dehydration, and acidosis results in further sickling and painful crises (Cunningham et al., 2005).

The rate of spontaneous abortion in pregnancies complicated by sickle cell anemia may be as high as 25% and stillbirth rates have been reported to reach 8% to 10%. Poor perinatal outcome is related to an increased frequency of preterm labor, premature birth, intrauterine infection, preeclampsia and poor placental perfusion (Cunningham et al., 2005).

Management

The care of the maternity patient with sickle cell anemia must be individualized. Ideally, care should be provided in a medical center experienced in treating the multitude of problems that can complicate these pregnancies. Management of care includes the following (Duffy, 2004; Kilpatrick & Laros, 2004):

- Promotion of good dietary habits with a folate supplement of at least 1 mg/d. Iron supplements are not

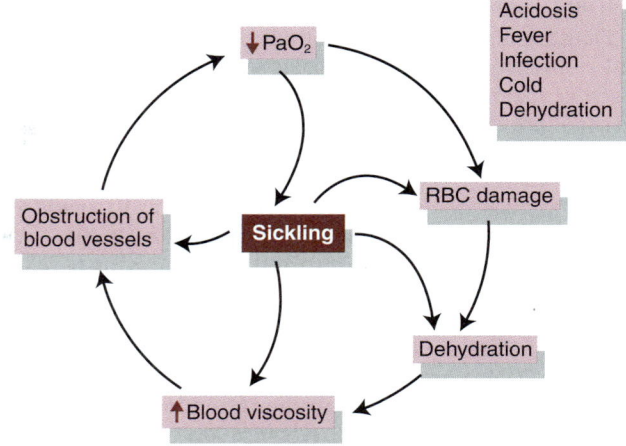

Figure 11-9 The sickling cycle.

routinely given, but serum iron and ferritin levels should be checked monthly and iron supplementation initiated only when the levels are diminished. Of note, the incidence of pica appears to be significantly increased in sickle cell patients. This non-nutritional practice may compromise the iron available for hemoglobin synthesis.
- Early detection of infection and treatment. Urine cultures are performed routinely to detect asymptomatic bacteriuria.
- Prevention of dehydration; intravenous fluids may be indicated.
- Prompt treatment of sickle cell crisis with oxygen, fluids, and pain management; intravenous morphine is usually the drug of choice.

Blood transfusions may be given to increase the hemoglobin to the 10 g/dL range and to reduce the percentage of sickle hemoglobin. This goal is best accomplished by an exchange transfusion: 2 units of blood are removed from the patient and 3 to 4 units of blood are transfused in. With this maneuver, the sickle hemoglobin percentage usually falls to approximately 40%.

- Fetal surveillance. Nonstress tests, biophysical profiles, and Doppler velocimetry begin as early as 26 weeks. Assessment of fundal height and ultrasound are used to monitor appropriate intrauterine growth (Cunningham et al., 2005).

THALASSEMIA

The thalassemia syndromes are named and classified by the type of globin chain that is inadequately produced. The defective chains damage the developing red blood cells by oxidative injury, resulting in chronic hemolysis and, ultimately, in iron overload (Duffy, 2004). The two most common types are α- or β-thalassemia, both of which affect the synthesis of hemoglobin A (Kilpatrick & Laros, 2004).

Thalassemia, also called "Mediterranean anemia," predominately affects African Americans and individuals of Italian, Greek, Middle Eastern, Indian, Asian, and West Indies descent. However, with the increased interethnic mixing and increasing immigration patterns of today, the at-risk populations are changing (Duffy, 2004; Kilpatrick & Laros, 2004).

β-Thalassemia

β-Thalassemia is the most common form of thalassemia. The homozygous state of β-thalassemia is known as "thalassemia major" or "Cooley's anemia." Patients with this disorder are transfusion dependent and have marked hepatosplenomegaly and bone changes secondary to increased hematopoiesis. Death generally is caused by infectious or cardiovascular complications before the third decade of life. Female infants who survive to puberty usually have amenorrhea and severely impaired fertility (Kilpatrick & Laros, 2004).

Heterozygous β-thalassemia minor results in various degrees of illness, depending on the rate of β-chain production. The characteristic findings of this disorder include a relatively high RBC count, moderate to marked microcytosis, and a peripheral smear that resembles iron deficiency (Kilpatrick & Laros, 2004). However, there may actually be a severe overload of iron due to the increased iron absorption that results from ineffective erythropoiesis (Poole, 2003).

β-THALASSEMIA AND PREGNANCY. The thalassemia syndromes constitute a group of inherited hemoglobinopathies that require close maternal and fetal surveillance during pregnancy. Ongoing consultations and appropriate treatment by maternal–fetal medicine and hematology specialists are essential throughout the pregnancy. The management is similar to care of patients with sickle cell disease. As with sickle cell disease, iron supplementation should be given only if necessary, because indiscriminate use of iron can lead to hemochromatosis (Cunningham et al., 2005; Poole, 2003).

Rh$_o$(D) Isoimmunization

Hemolytic disease of the fetus and newborn is a condition in which the life span of the fetal or neonatal RBCs is shortened by the action of maternal antibodies against antigens present on the fetal and neonatal RBCs. Antigens provoke an immune reaction if an incompatible blood cell enters the circulation. The RBCs are agglutinated and destroyed. The two most problematic types are those of the Rh (rhesus) system and the ABO system. Maternal antibodies form in the Rh-negative mother after exposure to Rh-positive fetal blood. Theoretically, no mixing of fetal and maternal blood occurs during pregnancy and childbirth. In reality, however, drops of fetal blood most likely enter the maternal circulation after small placental "accidents." The development of maternal antibodies, which destroy the fetus' Rh-positive blood, is termed **isoimmunization** or **sensitization**. In addition to the Rh (rhesus) system, there are more than 400 different antigens found on the surface of red blood cells. The incidence of hemolytic disease in the newborn has dramatically declined with the advent of Rh$_o$(D) immune globulin (RhoGAM) in the 1960s (Moise, 2004).

PATHOPHYSIOLOGY

For Rh(D) maternal isoimmunization to occur, at least three circumstances must exist:

- The fetus must have Rh(D)-positive erythrocytes, and the mother must have Rh(D)-negative erythrocytes.

- A sufficient number of fetal erythrocytes must gain access to the maternal circulation. This amount can be as little as 0.1 mL.
- The mother must have the immunogenic capacity to produce antibodies directed against the D antigen.

Fetal red blood cells gain access to the maternal circulation during pregnancy, childbirth, and in the immediate postpartum period. Clinical factors such as cesarean birth, multiple gestation, bleeding placenta previa or abruption, manual removal of the placenta, and intrauterine manipulation may increase the chance of substantial hemorrhage.

Rh$_o$(D) immune globulin (such as RhoGAM) works by coating and destroying fetal cells in the maternal circulation. Rh$_o$(D) immune globulin (RhoGAM) *must* be given within 72 hours and its effects last for 3 months. To ensure that the correct amount of Rh$_o$(D) immune globulin (RhoGAM) (sometimes more than one 300-mcg vial is required) is given to the patient, a fetal screen or Kleihauer–Betke blood test is performed on the woman's blood after it has been determined that the baby is Rh(D) positive. This test estimates the number of fetal RBCs in the mother's circulation. In most situations, exposure of maternal blood to fetal blood occurs during the third stage of labor at the time of placental separation. The woman's first child is usually unaffected because the maternal antibodies form after the infant's birth. However, subsequent Rh(D)-positive fetuses may be affected unless the woman receives Rh$_o$(D) immune globulin (RhoGAM) to prevent antibody formation. Rh$_o$(D) (RhoGAM) must be given after the birth of *every* Rh(D)-positive infant (Fig. 11-10). The information presented in Box 11-9 helps to simplify what can be a very confusing clinical situation.

When antibodies to the Rh factor are present in the pregnant patient's blood (i.e., the woman is sensitized), they freely cross the placenta and destroy the RBCs of the Rh(D)-positive fetus. Over time, the fetus develops an RBC deficiency, the fetal bilirubin levels rise ("icterus gravis") and severe neurological disease ("bilirubin encephalopathy") may result. In the fetus, this patho-

♂ Rh⁺ father   ♀ Rh⁻ mother   ▲ Anti-Rh(O) antibodies

Figure 11-10 The Rh isoimmunization sequence. Rh-positive father and Rh-negative mother; Rh-positive fetus. During pregnancy or childbirth, a small amount of fetal blood enters the mother's circulation. The mother's immune system produces anti-Rh$_o$(D) antibodies (triangles). In subsequent pregnancies with an Rh+ fetus, the antibodies cross the placenta, enter the fetal circulation and attack the fetal red blood cells, causing hemolysis.

medication: Rh₀(D) Immune Globulin

Rh₀(D) immune globulin (arr aych oh dee im-yoon glob-yoo-lin)

(RhoGAM, HypRho-D, BayRho-D, Gamulin Rh, Rhophylac)

Pregnancy Category: C

Indications: Administered to Rh-negative women who have been exposed to Rh-positive blood by:
Delivering an Rh₀(D)-positive infant
Aborting an Rh₀(D)-positive fetus
Having chorionic villus sampling, amniocentesis, or intraabdominal trauma while carrying an Rh₀(D)-positive fetus
Accidental transfusion of Rh₀(D)-positive blood

Action: Prevents production of anti Rh₀(D) antibodies in Rh₀(D)-negative patients who were exposed to Rh₀(D)-positive blood by suppressing the immune reaction of the Rh₀(D)-negative woman to the antigen in the Rh₀(D)-positive blood.

Therapeutic Effects: Prevents antibody response and subsequently prevents hemolytic disease of the newborn (erythroblastosis fetalis) in future pregnancies of women who have conceived an Rh₀(D)-positive fetus. Prevention of Rh₀(D) sensitization following transfusion accident.

Pharmacokinetics:

ABSORPTION: Well absorbed from IM sites.

Contraindications and Precautions:

CONTRAINDICATED IN: Rh₀(D)- or Du-positive patients; patients previously sensitized to Rh₀(D) or Du.

Adverse Reactions and Side Effects: Pain at IM site

Route and Dosage: One vial *standard* dose (300 mcg) administered intramuscularly:
- At 28 weeks of pregnancy and within 72 hours of delivery.
- Within 72 hours after the termination of a pregnancy of 13 weeks or more of gestation.
- After an accidental transfusion, dosage is calculated based on the volume of blood that was erroneously administered.

One vial *microdose* (50 mcg) within 72 hours after chorionic villus sampling (CVS) or the termination of a pregnancy of less than 13 weeks of gestation.

Note: (1) More than 300 mcg of RhoGAM may be indicated after a large transplacental hemorrhage or after a mismatched blood transfusion; (2) Rhophylac can be given IM or IV (prefilled syringes are available).

Nursing Implications:
1. Do not give to infant, to Rh₀(D)-positive individual or to Rh₀(D)-negative individual previously sensitized to the Rh₀(D) antigen. Note: There is no more risk than when given to a woman who is not sensitized—if in doubt, administer Rh₀(D) immune globulin.
2. Administer into the deltoid muscle. Should be given within 3 hours but may be given up to 72 hours after delivery, miscarriage, abortion, or transfusion.
3. Explain to the patient the purpose of this medication to protect future Rh₀(D)-positive infants; prior to administering, obtain a signed consent form if required by the agency.
4. Special considerations may be indicated for women who are members of Jehovah's Witnesses because this medication is made from human plasma.

Data from Deglin, J., & Vallerand, A. (2009). *Davis's drug guide for nurses* (11th ed.). Philadelphia: F.A. Davis.

Box 11-9 **Simplifying and Understanding the Rh Factor**

RH FACTOR

Rh D-positive: Persons who have the D genotype: the Rh antigen is present on their erythrocytes

RhD-negative: Persons who DO NOT possess the antigen on their red blood cells

Anti-Rh antibodies do not spontaneously occur and are only formed if there is sensitization by RhD-positive cells entering the circulation of the RhD-negative person. The RhD-negative person develops antibodies against the RhD-positive cells. This is why the first pregnancy is not affected, UNLESS the mother was previously sensitized during a miscarriage, amniocentesis, or antepartum hemorrhage.

EXAMPLE

RhD-negative mother gives birth to an RhD-positive baby and some of the baby's blood enters the mother's system at the time of delivery. (It takes only 0.1 mL.) Mother develops antibodies against any future RhD-positive babies.

During the prenatal period, all Rh(D)-negative women receive an antibody titer (indirect Coombs' test) to determine whether they are sensitized from a previous exposure to Rh(D)-positive blood. If the test is negative, another antibody titer is obtained at 28 weeks of gestation to rule out sensitization that may have occurred later in the pregnancy. If the woman remains unsensitized, Rh₀(D) immune globulin (RhoGAM) is given as a preventive measure to prevent formation of active antibodies during the remainder of pregnancy. After birth, if the infant is Rh(D) positive, another dose of Rh₀(D) immune globulin is administered. If the infant is Rh(D) negative, no Rh₀(D) immune globulin is necessary.

If the prenatal patient's indirect Coombs' test is positive, sensitization has occurred and antibodies against Rh(D)-positive erythrocytes are present in the maternal circulation. In this situation, the patient's antibody titer is repeated frequently throughout pregnancy to identify a rising level. A rise in the maternal antibody titer is indicative of ongoing antibody formation and an increased likelihood of fetal erythrocyte destruction.

When sensitization has occurred, an amniocentesis may be performed periodically throughout pregnancy to assess change in the optical density (ΔOD_{450}) of amniotic fluid. The ΔOD_{450} reflects the amount of bilirubin (bile pigment that remains after RBC destruction) in the amniotic fluid. When the fluid optical density remains low, it could indicate: (1) that the fetus is Rh(D) negative (and thus in no jeopardy) or (2) that the fetus is Rh(D) positive and is presently in no jeopardy. If the ΔOD_{450} is elevated, the fetus is experiencing RBC destruction and is in jeopardy.

Ultrasound evaluations may also be performed to assess for evidence of severe fetal anemia that has occurred due to hemolysis: edema, ascites, an enlarged heart, and hydramnios. An invasive procedure such as percutaneous umbilical blood sampling (discussed later in this chapter) may be performed to quantitatively determine the amount of fetal erythrocyte destruction. When necessary, an intrauterine transfusion of O-negative blood through the umbilical cord may be carried out or, as an alternative, erythrocytes may be transfused into the fetal abdominal cavity for absorption into the circulation.

logical process triggers a rapid production of erythroblasts (immature red blood cells) that are unable to carry oxygen. The syndrome associated with this hemolytic process is termed **erythroblastosis fetalis**. Fetal anemia and generalized edema ("hydrops fetalis") develop and lead to fetal congestive heart failure. (See Chapter 19 for further discussion.)

Be sure to— Administer and document RhoGAM when clinically indicated

Administering and properly documenting $Rh_o(D)$ immune globulin (RhoGAM) is an important nursing action.

If the mother is Rh negative and unsensitized and the baby is Rh positive, always check to be sure the patient has received $Rh_o(D)$ immune globulin (RhoGAM) if indicated before discharge. Make certain that she has received the appropriate dose.

Patients who have miscarried also must be treated. In cases where it is not possible to determine the fetus' or baby's blood type, $Rh_o(D)$ immune globulin (RhoGAM) is still given. Question if an order has not been written.

MANAGEMENT

Prevention of isoimmunization (a rising anti-Rh antibody titer in an Rh-negative woman) is the goal throughout pregnancy. All pregnant women should be tested for ABO and RhD type along with an antibody screen during their first prenatal visit. It is essential that these determinations be made during each subsequent pregnancy, as previous maternal antibody screening is not an adequate assessment. $Rh_o(D)$ immune globulin (RhoGAM) should also be given at any time during the pregnancy when a possibility exists that a patient may be exposed to fetal blood (i.e., CVS, amniocentesis, miscarriage, vaginal bleeding, abortion, ectopic pregnancy).

 Optimizing Outcomes— Safe administration of $Rh_o(D)$ immune globulin (RhoGAM)

In a RhD-negative woman who is **non**sensitized, RhoGAM should be given:

After delivery of an RhD-positive infant. In the United States the standard dose is 300 mcg and it is given within 72 hours of delivery.

Remember to educate your patient as to the reason why she is receiving RhoGAM.

Be sure to give your patient documentation that she has received RhoGAM.

Never give RhoGAM to:

- A Rh(D)-positive woman
- A sensitized Rh(D)-negative woman
- A Rh(D)-negative woman who has given birth to an Rh(D)-negative baby
- The baby or father of the baby!

SUMMARIZING CARE FOR THE SENSITIZED RhD-NEGATIVE PATIENT

Patients with an anti-D antibody titer of greater than 1:4 should be considered Rh sensitized and their pregnancies managed accordingly. The goal is to minimize fetal and neonatal morbidity and mortality. Management includes serial ultrasounds, serial amniocenteses to analyze bilirubin levels in the amniotic fluid, percutaneous umbilical blood sampling (PUBS) to obtain a fetal hematocrit, and intrauterine blood transfusions for a fetal hematocrit less than 30% (Moise, 2004). A delayed manifestation of Rh isoimmunization is

neonatal **kernicterus**, a condition characterized by CNS damage after exposure of the infant brain to hyperbilirubinemia. (See Chapter 19.) The nurse's identification of infants at risk anticipates this danger after birth and allows for early intervention with phototherapy or exchange transfusion before any damage may occur (Duffy, 2004).

ABO

In this condition the **mother is blood group O** and the **baby is either A or B.** This form of blood incompatibility is unrelated to the Rh factor. It is important for nurses to remember that blood group O carries no antigens; group A carries A antigen, and group B carries B antigen. Since the mother already has anti-A and anti-B antibodies present during the first pregnancy, the first child may be affected. IgG antibodies (immunoglobulins that respond to a specific antigen-in this case, A or B) can cross the placenta and cause hemolysis of the fetal RBCs.

The Coombs' test is performed on the baby's cord blood obtained at the time of birth. A **direct Coombs** identifies the presence of maternal antibodies in the neonate's blood and hemolysis or lysis of RBCs while the **indirect Coombs** detects antibodies against RBCs in the maternal serum. The results are reported as either positive or negative. A positive direct Coombs' test must be reported to the pediatrician.

 Now Can You— Discuss RhD and ABO isoimmunization?

1. Describe the pathophysiology of RhD isoimmunization?
2. Discuss the importance of preventing maternal isoimmunization?
3. Discuss the action of RhoGAM and the nursing responsibilities required in administering this medication?
4. Explain why ABO sensitization may occur during a first pregnancy?

Respiratory Complications

Pulmonary diseases have become more prevalent in the general population and, therefore, in pregnant women. The normal physiological changes of pregnancy can cause a woman with a history of compromised respirations to develop significant problems. The outcome for a pregnant woman with respiratory complications depends on the adequacy of ventilation and oxygenation as well as the early detection of respiratory compromise. Hypoxia poses a major threat to the fetus (Yancy, 2004).

PNEUMONIA

Although pneumonia is a rare complication of pregnancy, it is the most common nonobstetric infection that causes maternal mortality during the peripartum period. The overall frequency of pneumonia during pregnancy ranges from approximately 1 per 400 to 1 per 1200. The incidence may be increasing primarily as a reflection of the declining general health status of certain segments of the childbearing population (i.e., individuals with AIDS, cystic fibrosis, obesity, and those who smoke) (Mandel & Weinberger, 2004).

Etiology

Streptococcus pneumoniae, Mycoplasma pneumoniae, Chlamydia pneumoniae, and viruses (e.g., Influenza A and Varicella) are the major causative agents.

Effects on Pregnancy

Pneumonia can complicate pregnancy at any time during gestation. Maternal bacteremia, empyema, a need for mechanical intervention, and death have all been reported. Pneumonia may be associated with poor fetal growth (IUGR), preterm birth, and perinatal loss (Mandel & Weinberger, 2004).

Management

The normal physiological changes in the respiratory system that occur during pregnancy result in a loss of ventilatory reserve. These changes, coupled with pregnancy-related immunosuppression, place the woman and her fetus at an increased risk for respiratory infection. Any pregnant patient suspected of having pneumonia should be managed aggressively with appropriate laboratory testing, clinical surveillance, and medications.

ASTHMA

Asthma is the most common form of lung disease that affects pregnancy; from 0.5% to 8% of pregnant women have this condition (Gardner & Doyle, 2004). Asthma is characterized by a limitation of airflow that is generally more marked during expiration than during inspiration. The obstruction associated with asthma is a reversible process caused by airway inflammation and an increased responsiveness of the airways to a variety of stimuli (e.g., dust, pollen, grass, and cold temperature). The airway response to the stimuli involves contraction of the bronchial smooth muscle, hypersecretion of mucus, and edema of the mucosal surfaces. Collectively, these events contribute to the pathophysiological processes associated with the reversible airway obstruction characteristic of asthma (Mandel & Weinberger, 2004).

Effects on Pregnancy

Asthma is associated with significant risks for both the patient and her fetus. Maternal complications reported among asthmatics include hyperemesis, vaginal bleeding, hypertensive disorders, a predisposition to infections, gestational diabetes, preterm rupture of the membranes and preterm labor, and delivery of a low-birth-weight infant. There is little risk to the fetus with well-controlled maternal asthma and it is safer for pregnant asthmatics to be treated with appropriate medications than to have asthma symptoms and exacerbations. Exacerbations that cause hypoxia and decreased uterine blood flow increase the incidence of intrauterine growth restriction (IUGR), preterm birth, and neonatal mortality (Yancy, 2004).

Signs and Symptoms

A number of classic symptoms are associated with an exacerbation of asthma. These include dyspnea, coughing, wheezing, voice changes, chest tightening, and the presence of scant or copious clear sputum. Lung auscultation usually reveals bilateral expiratory wheezing.

Management

Careful monitoring along with appropriate adjustments in therapy may be required to maintain maternal lung function and ensure an adequate oxygen supply to the fetus. Failure to control asthma during pregnancy may result in hypoxia in both the patient and her fetus. A Po_2 of less than 60 mm Hg places the fetus in jeopardy (National Asthma Education and Prevention Expert Panel, 2005). Guidelines for asthma management have been developed to help ensure maternal–fetal safety and well-being during pregnancy. Goals of therapy include optimal control of asthma symptoms; attainment of normal pulmonary function; prevention and reversal of asthma attacks; and prevention of maternal and fetal complications (Guy, Kirumaki, & Hanania, 2004). Asthma therapy is based on a stepwise classification system designed to control symptoms, avoid acute attacks, and help patients achieve unhampered life styles (Kennedy, 2005).

Medications currently used for asthma are generally well tolerated during pregnancy and appear to be safe for the fetus. Therefore, the management of asthma in the pregnant woman differs little from management in the nonpregnant patient. It is also widely accepted that the fetal risk is higher with poorly controlled maternal asthma than with medications necessary to gain optimal symptom control. Nevertheless, nurses must be aware of available data concerning the use of these drugs during pregnancy (Gluck & Gluck, 2005; Mandel & Weinberger, 2004).

CYSTIC FIBROSIS

Cystic fibrosis (CF) is a chronic, progressive, genetic multisystem disease. It affects nearly 30,000 children and young adults, and occurs in approximately one out of every 3000 Caucasian live births (Brennan & Geddes, 2004). One thousand new cases are diagnosed each year, usually by the age of 3; however, nearly 10% of newly diagnosed cases involve individuals age 18 or older. Since CF is a recessive disorder, a child must inherit a defective gene from each parent. Each time two CF carriers conceive, there is a 25% chance that the child will have CF; a 50% chance that the child will be a carrier; and a 25% chance the child will be a noncarrier. One in 20 Americans (more than 20 million total) is an unknowing carrier of the defective gene for CF (Cystic Fibrosis Foundation, 2005).

The last several decades have witnessed a dramatic increase in the survival of patients with CF. This trend is attributable in large part to earlier diagnosis and intervention, the introduction of pulmonary therapies such as dornase-alpha and high-dose ibuprofen, new airway clearance techniques, effective antipseudomonal antibiotics such as tobramycin for inhalation, improved nutritional management, and dietary recommendations (Kulich et al., 2003). In the United States, the median survival age for persons with CF has increased to 31.1 years for men and 28.3 years for women (Cystic Fibrosis Foundation, 2005; Yankaskas, Marshall, Sufian, Simon, & Rodman, 2004). An increasing number of women with CF are now surviving into the reproductive years and, with meticulous management of their pulmonary function, usually maintain their fertility.

Pathophysiology

The major CF gene product is the protein cystic fibrosis transmembrane regulator (CFTR). When CFTR is not produced or is altered in structure or function as a result of mutations in the CF gene, viscid secretions are produced that primarily affect the respiratory and gastrointestinal systems. An absence or abnormality of the protein results in a blocked or altered chloride channel in the epithelial cell membranes. Chloride ions are trapped within the cell and cause sodium ions and water to diffuse back into the cell, leading to dehydration of the mucus secretions.

Effects on Pregnancy

Factors that may predict a poor outcome for a pregnant woman with CF include prepregnancy evidence of poor nutritional status, significant pulmonary disease with hypoxemia, and pulmonary hypertension. The risk of maternal mortality for those with cor pulmonale and deteriorating pulmonary function in the first trimester is exceptionally high and the couple may be advised to consider termination of the pregnancy. Risks to the fetus include preterm birth, growth restriction due to uteroplacental insufficiency, and CF. The couple must also consider the long-term psychosocial and physical assistance needs that may ensue because of the potential for maternal physical deterioration and/or premature death (Whitty & Dombrowski, 2004).

Optimizing Outcomes— Counseling women with cystic fibrosis

Preconception counseling is essential for women with CF. Because of extremely thick cervical mucus, fewer than one in five women with CF are able to conceive. Women who achieve pregnancy should be advised of the risks, according to their health status. If possible, women should be 90% of their ideal body weight before conception (Whitty & Dombrowski, 2004).

Management

When caring for a pregnant woman with cystic fibrosis, it is important for the nurse to recognize that the fetus is at risk for uteroplacental insufficiency and intrauterine growth restriction. The maternal nutritional status and weight gain during pregnancy greatly affect fetal growth. Ongoing collaboration with the nutritionist is essential, and close attention must be paid to the patient's nutritional status since maldigestion, malabsorption, and malnutrition are all complications of CF (Whitty & Dombrowski, 2004). An early nutritional consultation should be included in the nursing care plan developed for every CF patient. Throughout pregnancy, the nurse and other members of the care team must work closely with the nutritionist to ensure that the caloric requirements are being met. This component of care is especially important when the pregnant patient with CF experiences hyperemesis gravidarum.

Early recognition and prompt treatment of pulmonary infections are also important in the management of the pregnant woman with CF. Diagnostic tests that are helpful for assessing and guiding therapy with CF patients include sputum and culture sensitivity, chest films, spirometry, pulse oximetry, and complete blood counts with a chemistry panel (Whitty & Dombrowski, 2004).

Respiratory management during the preconception and the antenatal period includes baseline pulmonary function tests such as forced vital capacity (FVC), forced expiratory volume (FEV_1) lung volumes, pulse oximetry, and arterial blood gases as indicated. Laboratory values are closely monitored during pregnancy and any deterioration in pulmonary function is promptly addressed. Fetal growth should be monitored by fundal height measurements along with serial ultrasound evaluations of fetal growth and amniotic fluid volume. Doppler flow studies are also used to assess fetal growth and development and general health status. Maternal kick counts should begin at 28 weeks and non-stress tests initiated at 32 weeks to assess fetal well-being (Whitty & Dombrowski, 2004). Management of the pregnant woman with CF requires the involvement of an entire team of professionals: the perinatologist, pulmonologist, neonatologist, nutritionist, social worker, and nurse. When difficulties arise and the family is further challenged, spiritual guidance can be of great comfort and support to the family.

Maternal and consequently fetal oxygenation is of paramount importance during labor and birth. Continuous monitoring of maternal oxygen saturation using pulse oximetry is used to gauge the need for and response to supplemental oxygen therapy. Respiratory depressants, anticholinergic drugs, and inhalation anesthesia should be avoided. Lumbar epidural analgesia is the preferred mode of labor pain relief. The fetal heart rate (FHR) should be continuously monitored during labor and any signs of fetal intolerance (i.e., decelerations and/or a lack of FHR variability) must be promptly addressed (Whitty & Dombrowski, 2004). A critical intrapartal nursing issue centers on the recognition that high-risk couples may have depleted their coping skills due to perinatal complications. The nurse needs to be aware that the anxiety coupled with the stress of labor may be extremely difficult for the patient and her family. The nurse can provide assistance by encouraging the couple to express their emotional concerns, by keeping them informed of changes as the labor progresses, and by encouraging them to freely ask questions.

 Now Can You— Discuss respiratory complications during pregnancy?

1. Describe the normal anatomical and physiological changes in the respiratory system during pregnancy and how they affect the patient with asthma and cystic fibrosis?
2. Discuss the fetal effects of maternal oxygen deprivation?
3. Formulate a plan of care for the pregnant patient with a respiratory complication?

Cardiovascular Disease

Cardiovascular disease in women affects 1% to 4% of all pregnancies and remains the primary cause of nonobstetric maternal mortality in the United States (Foley, 2004; Setaro & Caulin-Glaser, 2004). Care of the patient with cardiovascular disease continues to be a great challenge to the obstetrical team despite advances in surgical techniques, medications, and technology, owing to three broad trends (Setaro & Caulin-Glaser, 2004):

- Successful treatment of congenital heart disease has created a new population of clinically complex patients who are able to reach childbearing age.

- There is an increasing trend toward pregnancies in older women who are susceptible to heart diseases acquired in adulthood.
- Immigration from underdeveloped nations has reacquainted Western medicine with a cohort of young childbearing patients who have rheumatic heart disease.

Signs and symptoms of cardiac disease can be similar to physiological changes that normally occur during pregnancy. For example, the pregnant patient may experience heart palpitations associated with the normal increase in blood volume. Women with heart disease may experience heart palpitations due to an arrhythmia. Fatigue, a common complaint during pregnancy, may result from poor cardiac output and myocardial ischemia in patients with heart disease. The incidence of maternal and fetal morbidity and mortality associated with cardiac disease during pregnancy depends on the specific cardiac lesion, the functional abnormality produced by the lesion, and the development of pregnancy-related complications, such as infection, hemorrhage, or preeclampsia (Yancy, 2004).

Categories of cardiac disease during pregnancy include congenital cardiac disease (e.g., atrial septal defect, ventricular septal defect, pulmonic stenosis, congenital aortic stenosis, coarctation of the aorta, tetralogy of Fallot, and Eisenmenger's syndrome) and acquired cardiac disease (i.e., lesions that are rheumatic in origin and valvular lesions such as mitral and aortic stenosis). Rheumatic mitral stenosis is the most common clinically significant valvular abnormality in pregnant women and may be associated with pulmonary congestion, edema, and atrial arrhythmias during pregnancy and soon after childbirth. Ischemic cardiac disease (coronary artery disease and myocardial infarction) is rare in pregnancy.

The New York Heart Association (NYHA) classification system is often used to assess the functional ability of the pregnant cardiac patient (Criteria Committee of the NYHA, 1979). Patient cardiac function is divided into four classes:

Class I	The patient is asymptomatic and there is no limitation on physical activity.
Class II	The patient is asymptomatic at rest, symptomatic with heavy physical activity, and requires slight limitation of activity.
Class III	The patient is asymptomatic at rest, symptomatic with minimal physical activity, and physical activity is considerably limited.
Class IV	The patient may be symptomatic at rest, is symptomatic with any activity, and has severe limitations on physical activity.

Patients classified as NYHA I and II generally do well during pregnancy, but those classified as III or IV have a significantly increased risk of morbidity and mortality with pregnancy. However, it must be remembered that any patient with a cardiac history, regardless of classification, must be thoroughly assessed for any signs of decompensation at each prenatal visit.

MANAGEMENT

Management of cardiac disease in pregnancy is frequently complicated by unique social and psychological concerns. Patients with congenital heart disease may have experienced multiple hospitalizations over the years and be fearful of the medical environment. Some of them never expected to bear children. Often, women with a history of rheumatic heart disease have lived outside the traditional medical care system due to conditions of poverty and cultural differences. Not uncommonly, they are recent immigrants. When caring for any patient with special needs, it is imperative for the nurse to collaborate with other health professionals and community support systems to facilitate the patient's access to care and to ensure her comfort with the health care environment (Easterling & Otto, 2002).

 Optimizing Outcomes— **Caring for the pregnant woman with cardiac disease**

Antepartally, continuity of care with a single provider, frequent prenatal visits, routine screening for bacteriuria, and prophylaxis against anemia are essential. Intrapartal care includes the induction of labor when cervical favorability is present, the avoidance of prolonged labor, second stage pushing and maternal blood loss, and prophylactic antibiotics when the woman is at risk for endocarditis. Postpartal care centers on strict management of blood volume and careful but aggressive diuresis (Easterling & Otto, 2002).

Labor, birth, and the immediate postpartum period provide a time of increased risk due to the rapid volume changes that occur. During labor and birth, epidural anesthesia may be used for most patients with cardiac disease, but care must be taken to avoid hypotension. Positioning the patient in a lateral recumbent position as well as careful administration of intravenous fluids will help to balance the patient's blood pressure. Continuous invasive hemodynamic monitoring is beneficial in evaluating rapid changes in heart rate, cardiac output, and pulmonary capillary wedge pressure (PCWP) (an estimation of left atrial pressure) so that fluid, diuretic, vasodilator, or pressor therapy may be guided (Setaro & Caulin-Glaser, 2004).

Medications that may be indicated for the pregnant cardiac patient include diuretics (e.g., Lasix) to prevent congestive heart failure, digitalis, nitrates (to reduce after-load, the resistance the ventricles must overcome to eject blood during systole), antiarrhythmic agents (e.g., lidocaine), beta blockers (e.g., labetalol), calcium channel blockers (e.g., nifedipine), antibiotics and anticoagulants (heparin–warfarin [Coumadin] is contraindicated because it crosses the placenta). As with any medication being considered for the pregnant patient, a thorough investigation of side effects and potential fetal harm must be evaluated before administration.

Nursing Insight— *Recognizing cardiac effects of various obstetric drugs*

Obstetric medications such as tocolytics and uterine stimulants can have a major impact on circulatory function. Terbutaline, administered to suppress premature uterine contractions, may stimulate the heart. Adverse effects include chest discomfort, dyspnea, irregular pulse, EKG changes, or pulmonary edema. The nurse should question the use of this medication with any patient with a cardiac history. Prostaglandin is a vasodilator and should not be used in patients with certain cardiac conditions. Oxytocin can cause hypertension and fluid retention and lead to congestive heart failure.

Vaginal birth is advisable for most patients with cardiac disease with care taken to avoid causing stress on the heart during the second stage of labor (pushing). Elective low or outlet forceps may be used to shorten this stage. Cesarean section may limit the stress of vaginal birth in patients with cardiac disease, but this method involves major surgery, blood loss, and the possibility of maternal stress from intubation. Cesarean birth is reserved for situations such as fetal compromise and failure of labor progression.

NURSING IMPLICATIONS FOR THE PREGNANT CARDIAC PATIENT

Due to the intense cardiovascular demands of pregnancy, care of the pregnant cardiac patient presents one of the greatest challenges to the obstetrical nurse. Nursing care should focus on assessment, early detection of problems, and treatment and prevention of complications to both mother and baby. Ideally, these women are cared for in a tertiary care center, but when this is not possible, there should be collaboration between critical care nurses and obstetric nurses. Nursing interventions include:

- Antenatal assessment of weight gain to ensure proper fetal growth while avoiding excessive weight gain which causes increased cardiac workload
- Nutritional counseling (a diet high in iron to prevent anemia and low in sodium to prevent fluid retention)
- Education to avoid/reduce stress and anxiety
- Encouragement of frequent rest periods
- Explanation of fetal surveillance testing
- Stressing the importance of keeping prenatal appointments
- Education regarding the signs and symptoms of complications; when to call the provider

 Nursing Insight— *Understanding hemodynamic changes in pregnancy*

A patient with a cardiac disorder is at greatest risk when hemodynamic changes reach their maximum, between the 28th and 32nd weeks of gestation. The nurse must have knowledge of the disease process and be able to assess the hemodynamic changes that occur during pregnancy.

Intrapartal interventions focus on assessing the patient and fetus for decreased cardiac output and oxygenation and intervening as needed.

 critical nursing action Assessing the Cardiac Patient During Labor and Birth

The nurse needs to assess the patient for signs and symptoms of decreased cardiac output:

- Decreased and/or irregular pulse
- Increased respiratory rate
- Dyspnea
- Chest pain
- Abnormal breath sounds: crackles at the base of the lungs
- Decreased blood pressure
- Decreased urinary output (less than 30 mL/hr)
- Edema of the hands, face and feet
- Abnormal heart sounds: diastolic murmur at the heart's apex
- Signs of air hunger: anxiety

- Decreased oxygen saturation: <95%
- Cool, clammy, cyanotic skin
- Increased capillary refill time: >3 seconds
- EKG changes
- Mental changes: disorientation; fatigue; syncope

Oxygen, if required, should be supplied via a re-breather mask at 10 L per minute, intravenous fluids are administered via a pump, and intake and output are meticulously monitored throughout labor. Antibiotic prophylaxis may be indicated for selected patients with cardiac disease because of their increased risk for developing endocarditis as a result of invasive procedures (e.g., invasive hemodynamic monitoring; intrauterine pressure catheter; fetal scalp electrode). Continuous fetal monitoring during labor is also a nursing responsibility. With decreased maternal cardiac output, the fetus will show signs of poor placental perfusion, as evidenced by late decelerations and/or the loss of baseline variability. (See Chapter 12 for further discussion.) Should these indicators develop, improved oxygenation must be delivered to the fetus by giving oxygen to the woman, who should be maintained in a lateral position. Intravenous fluids should be increased with caution to avoid maternal fluid overload.

After delivery of the baby and placenta, large quantities of fluid are rapidly mobilized. The patient with cardiac disease must be continually assessed for decompensation (inability of the heart to maintain a sufficient cardiac output) during the puerperium. Ambulation should be encouraged, as ordered, as soon as possible after birth to prevent deep vein thrombosis. If the mother who is receiving cardiovascular medications chooses to breastfeed, careful clinical observation of the newborn is warranted. Digoxin and beta–adrenergic blockers are generally regarded to be safe during lactation (Setaro & Caulin-Glaser, 2004).

MITRAL VALVE PROLAPSE

Mitral valve prolapse (MVP) is a common condition that affects 2% to 3% of reproductive-aged women; however, it generally does not affect pregnancy (Cunningham et al., 2005). The hemodynamic changes associated with pregnancy may alleviate the murmur of MVP as well as its symptoms. In rare cases, patients experience chest discomfort or rhythm disturbances and should be managed with reassurance. Therapy with beta-adrenergic blockers may be initiated in highly symptomatic patients. If a murmur is audible, antibiotic prophylaxis should be administered at the time of childbirth (Cunningham et al., 2005; Setaro & Caulin-Glaser, 2004).

PERIPARTUM CARDIOMYOPATHY

Peripartum cardiomyopathy (PPCM) is a rare syndrome of heart failure that occurs in late pregnancy or within the first 5 months postpartum. The patient typically has no history of cardiac disease and presents with dyspnea, fatigue, and peripheral or pulmonary edema. Radiological findings are consistent with cardiomegaly. Acute treatment is directed at improving cardiac function. Treatment includes diuretics to decrease preload and relieve pulmonary congestion; digoxin to improve contractility and facilitate rate control when atrial fibrillation is present; beta-adrenergic blockers; anticoagulation with heparin if the woman is antepartum and Coumadin if postpartum; and fluid and sodium restriction (Easterling & Otto, 2002; Klein & Galan, 2004).

The mortality rate associated with peripartum cardiomyopathy is reported to be 25% to 50%. Within 6 months after childbirth, half of the patients will demonstrate resolution of left ventricular dilation. Of those who do not, 8.5% will die within 4 to 5 years. Death is usually due to progressive heart failure, arrhythmia, or thromboembolism (Easterling & Otto, 2002).

Now Can You— Discuss cardiac complications during pregnancy?

1. Describe the normal anatomical and physiological changes that occur in the cardiovascular system during pregnancy and their impact on the pregnant woman with a cardiac disease?
2. State three important factors in the management of cardiac disease in pregnancy?
3. Identify team members you would include in your plan of care?

Diabetes in Pregnancy

Diabetes during pregnancy encompasses a range of disease entities that include gestational diabetes mellitus (GDM) and overt diabetes mellitus. Diabetes complicates more than 200,000 pregnancies each year in the United States (American Diabetes Association [ADA], 2006; Wallerstedt & Clokey, 2004). Diabetes is a complex health care problem that requires a comprehensive, multidisciplinary approach to ensure a healthy outcome for both the patient and her infant. When working with this population, perinatal nurses are challenged to provide care and education that incorporates diabetes management principles into obstetric care during all phases of childbearing, from preconception through the postpartum period.

DEFINITION AND CLASSIFICATION OF DIABETES MELLITUS

Pregestational diabetes mellitus is a chronic metabolic disease characterized by hyperglycemia that results from limited or absent insulin production, deficient insulin action, or a combination of the two (Expert Committee on the Diagnosis and Classification of Diabetes Mellitus [ECDCDM], 2003). Diabetes is divided into two broad categories—type 1 and type 2—that are differentiated according to the primary underlying etiology. Type 1 diabetes (formerly termed "insulin-dependent diabetes mellitus," or IDDM), is characterized by an autoimmunity directed at the pancreatic beta cells. With Type 1 diabetes, there is an absolute insulin deficiency and the following characteristics are typically present (ECDCDM, 2003):

- It is usually diagnosed in those younger than 30 years of age.
- Acute symptoms precede the diagnosis and include polyuria, polydipsia, and significant weight loss.
- It has an abrupt onset that requires emergency medical attention.
- It accounts for approximately 10% of those diagnosed with diabetes.

Type 2 diabetes, the most prevalent form of the disease, is characterized by a combination of insulin resistance and inadequate insulin production (ECDCDM, 2003). Characteristics of type 2 diabetes include:

- It is diagnosed primarily in adults older than age 30, but with the current obesity epidemic, it is now seen in children.
- The disease is typically symptom free for many years, with a slow onset and a gradual progression of symptoms.
- Individuals with type 2 are not ketosis prone.
- It does not always require insulin and can often be treated with diet, exercise, and/or oral hypoglycemic agents.

GDM is an impairment in carbohydrate metabolism that first manifests during pregnancy. This category may include a small number of previously undiagnosed type 1 and type 2 diabetic women. The following characteristics apply (ECDCDM, 2003):

- Estimated to occur in approximately 4% to 7% of pregnancies; however, the prevalence may range from 1% to 14%, depending on the population studied and the diagnostic test used (ADA, 2006).
- Develops in the latter half of pregnancy as a result of the altered hormonal milieu (Kenshole, 2004).
- Symptoms are usually mild and not life threatening.
- May be treated by either diet or insulin, depending on the blood glucose levels.
- Women diagnosed with GDM are at an increased risk for developing diabetes later in life.

RISK FACTORS FOR GESTATIONAL DIABETES

- Women older than 25 years of age
- Obesity
- Insulin resistance
- Polycystic ovary syndrome
- History of pregnancy-related diabetes mellitus
- History of a large-for-gestational age infant, hydramnios
- Stillbirth, miscarriage, or an infant with congenital anomalies during a previous pregnancy
- Family history of type 2 diabetes (first-degree relative)
- Ethnicity

 Ethnocultural Considerations— **Gestational Diabetes**

An increased incidence of gestational diabetes occurs in Native Americans, African Americans, Hispanic Americans, Asian Americans, and Pacific Islanders (ADA, 2006).

PATHOPHYSIOLOGY

The body requires a constant source of energy, provided mainly by glucose. Once glucose enters a cell, it may undergo oxidative (glycolysis) or nonoxidative metabolism (glycogen synthesis). In response to glucose ingestion, the pancreatic beta cells of the islets of Langerhans secrete insulin, a hormone that promotes the uptake of glucose into the cells. The regulation of plasma glucose levels and the entry of glucose into the cells are of critical importance.

Changes in carbohydrate, protein, and fat metabolism in normal pregnancy are profound, mediated in part by the developing fetus and the production of placental hormones. The first half of pregnancy is considered an "anabolic phase." It is associated with an increased storage of fat and protein, along with an increase in the secretion of estrogen and progesterone. These physiological events lead to maternal hyperplasia and hyperinsulinemia. The increased insulin production prompts an increased tissue response to insulin and the increased uptake and storage of glycogen and fat in the liver and tissues.

The second half of pregnancy is characterized by a "catabolic phase" associated with the breakdown of protein and fat. During this time there is also an increased insulin resistance due to the heightened production of placental hormones (insulinase and human placental lactogen), cortisol, and growth hormones. These hormones are diabetogenic and act as insulin antagonists. In women who cannot meet the increasing needs for insulin production, this change leads to an altered carbohydrate metabolism and progressive hyperglycemia.

During this time, the developing fetus continuously removes glucose and amino acids, substances that can easily cross the placenta, from the maternal circulation. Because insulin does not cross the placenta, the fetus must increase its own insulin production. Fetal hyperinsulinemia develops and acts as a growth hormone that contributes to an increase in fetal size (macrosomia), and a decrease in pulmonary surfactant production. Macrosomia occurs in 20% to 25% of diabetic pregnancies. When the pregnant woman's blood glucose levels remain abnormally elevated, there is a constant transport of maternal glucose across the placenta. This "glucose load" prompts the fetus to produce insulin at a greater rate in order to utilize the glucose.

 Nursing Insight— *Anticipating changes in insulin needs during pregnancy*

During the first trimester, maternal blood glucose levels are normally reduced and the insulin response to glucose is enhanced. The woman with well-controlled pregestational diabetes may need a decrease in her insulin dosage to avoid hypoglycemia. During the second and third trimesters, as the insulin requirements steadily increase, the insulin dosage must be adjusted to prevent hyperglycemia. Maternal insulin resistance begins around 14 weeks of gestation and continues to increase until it stabilizes during the final weeks of pregnancy.

MATERNAL AND PERINATAL MORBIDITY AND MORTALITY

The changes in the maternal milieu that characterize the diabetic state can have profound effects on the growth and development of the fetus, increase the risk of perinatal morbidity and mortality, and exert adverse effects throughout life. The physiological adaptations induced by pregnancy can unmask latent maternal diabetes or result in transient worsening of preexisting vascular compromise (Kenshole, 2004). Diabetic women are four times more likely to develop preeclampsia or eclampsia than are nondiabetic women and twice as likely to experience a spontaneous abortion. The rates of infection, hydramnios, postpartum hemorrhage, and

cesarean birth are increased. In the long term, GDM is also associated with impaired insulin tolerance and the manifestation of diabetes in later life (Cunningham et al., 2005).

Major fetal effects associated with diabetes include a fivefold increase in perinatal death and a two to threefold increase in the rate of congenital malformations. Early in pregnancy, the fetus is at risk for congenital malformations and poor fetal growth. The risk of major congenital defects is 4% to 8% greater with type 1 or 2 diabetes. Congenital defects result from the teratogenic effects of hyperglycemia during the time of organogenesis during the early gestational weeks. Late in pregnancy, the fetus is at risk for growth abnormalities and sudden intrauterine death (Cunningham et al., 2005).

Control of maternal glucose levels (<7.0% in overtly diabetic women) is an important factor in determining fetal outcome. The **glycosylated hemoglobin A$_{1c}$** (HbA$_{1c}$) level is commonly assessed to guide adjustments in the treatment plan throughout pregnancy. Since the maternal serum HbA$_{1c}$ reflects the degree of glycemic control during the preceding 5 to 6 weeks, the test is repeated every trimester. Good diabetic control is reflected by a HbA$_{1c}$ value of 2.5% to 5.9%; a HbA$_{1c}$ value greater than 8% is indicative of poor diabetic control. In the absence of pre-pregnancy and prenatal care, the rate of perinatal mortality for the diabetic patient and her fetus may be as high as 40%. However, with close, meticulous care, the perinatal mortality rate can be reduced to 3% to 5% (Cunningham et al., 2005).

Ketoacidosis

Diabetic ketoacidosis (DKA) is an accumulation of ketones in the blood that results from hyperglycemia. This condition, which can lead to metabolic acidosis, has become a less common occurrence since the implementation of meticulous antenatal care and protocols that stress the strict metabolic control of maternal blood glucose levels. Early recognition of the signs and symptoms of DKA helps to improve both maternal and fetal outcome. As occurs in the nonpregnant state, clinical signs of volume depletion follow the symptoms of hyperglycemia, which include polydipsia and polyuria. Malaise, headache, nausea, and vomiting are common patient complaints. A distinctive feature of diabetic ketoacidosis during pregnancy is that it can occur with remarkably low blood glucose levels (barely exceeding 200 mg/dL, compared with 300 to 350 mg/dL in the nonpregnant state) and requires emergency management to prevent maternal coma or death. Ketoacidosis that occurs at any time during pregnancy may result in fetal death and it is a common cause of preterm labor (Cunningham et al., 2005).

 clinical alert

Maternal diabetes and preterm labor

Magnesium sulfate is the drug of choice for diabetic women who experience preterm labor. The use of terbutaline sulfate (Brethine) or antenatal corticosteroids to accelerate fetal lung maturation can cause significant maternal hyperglycemia and precipitate DKA. Patients must be closely followed in an acute care setting for at least 48 to 72 hours after corticosteroids have been given. An intravenous insulin infusion will usually be required and is adjusted on the basis of frequent capillary glucose measurements (Landon, Catalano, & Gabbe, 2002).

SCREENING AND DIAGNOSIS

Since 1970, much has been learned about the important relationship between maternal glycemic control before and during pregnancy and fetal outcomes. The perinatal mortality rate has simultaneously improved as an intensive approach to the diabetic pregnancy has become standard. The American College of Obstetricians and Gynecologists (ACOG) recommends that all pregnant women should be screened for diabetes during the 24th and 28th weeks of gestation. Women with risk factors (age >40, family history of a first-degree relative with diabetes; prior macrosomic, malformed, and/or stillborn infant; obesity; hypertension; or glycosuria) should be screened earlier in pregnancy (ACOG, 2001a). The American Diabetes Association (ADA) recommends selective diabetes screening during pregnancy, eliminating the need to screen women who have no risk factors. Screening is recommended for pregnant women with risk factors that include age greater than 25 years, obesity, family history of type 2 diabetes, and a history of a poor obstetric outcome (ADA, 2006).

In the United States, most centers use the following diagnostic recommendations and criteria established by the National Diabetes Data Group:

- The Glucose Challenge Test (Glucola screening): A 50-g oral glucose solution is administered to the woman and a blood sample is taken 1 hour after it is consumed. Patients with a 1-hour plasma glucose value of 140 mg/dL or higher should be further evaluated with the formal 3-hour oral glucose tolerance test (OGTT).
- The 3-hour OGTT requires the fasting patient to ingest 100 g of glucose with blood drawn at 1-hour intervals. Before the test, the woman should avoid caffeine (it may increase glucose levels) and refrain from smoking at least 12 hours before and during the test. The diagnosis of GDM is made when two values or more of the threshold are above the norm. According to the American Diabetes Association (2006), the normal plasma values are:

Fasting blood sugar	<95 mg/dL
1 hour	<180 mg/dL
2 hour	<155 mg/dL
3 hour	<140 mg/dL

MANAGEMENT

The goal of modern glycemic management during the diabetic pregnancy is to maintain blood glucose levels as close to normal (euglycemia) as possible. Euglycemia is a normal blood glucose level in the range of 65 to 105 mg/dL preprandially. Two-hour postprandial blood glucose levels should be less than 130 mg/dL (ADA, 2006). Metabolic monitoring during pregnancy is directed at detecting hyperglycemia and making all necessary pharmacological, dietary, or activity adjustments in order to minimize any adverse effects to the fetus. Home blood glucose monitoring with a glucose reflectance meter or biosensor monitor is a widely accepted method for monitoring blood glucose levels and an essential tool for helping the woman to assess her degree of blood glucose control. Patients monitor their blood glucose levels daily, record the findings, and bring their blood glucose logs with them to each prenatal appointment.

Ongoing fetal surveillance is of utmost importance. Maternal care requires the cooperative efforts of a clinical team that includes the obstetrician, internist, endocrinologist, diabetes educator, neonatologist, dietitian, and nurse. Patient education is essential to ensure that the woman understands her diabetic state and the need to adhere to treatment so that an optimal outcome is achieved (Fig. 11-11). Social services, home nursing visitation, and spiritual support are often involved as well.

 Optimizing Outcomes— Diet and exercise for the patient with GDM

Diet and exercise are important components of care for the woman with GDM. Typically, the patient is placed on a standard diabetic diet that is calculated to include 30 kcal/kg per day, based on a normal preconceptional weight. For the obese woman, the diet may be calculated to include up to 25 kcal/kg per day (Chan & Winkle, 2006). Ongoing nutritional counseling is essential. Physical activity such as walking and swimming is also important for the woman with GDM. Exercise helps to lower blood glucose levels and may decrease the need for insulin (ADA, 2006).

 Nursing Insight— *Planning care for the woman with GDM*

Although diet and exercise are the mainstays of care for the woman with gestational diabetes mellitus, up to 20% will require insulin during pregnancy to maintain euglycemia. If fasting blood glucose levels exceed 105 mg/dL, insulin therapy is initiated (ADA, 2006). (Oral hypoglycemic agents are contraindicated during pregnancy.)

 Now Can You— Discuss diabetes management during pregnancy?

1. State three risk factors for gestational diabetes?
2. Discuss the effects of maternal diabetes on fetal growth and development?
3. Describe how you would educate the pregnant patient about the importance of diabetes screening?

The Thyroid Gland and Pregnancy

Thyroid disorders are relatively common among pregnant women. The hormonal changes and increasing metabolic demands of pregnancy bring about complex compensatory alterations in maternal thyroid function. Human chorionic gonadotropin (hCG), which is at its highest levels in early pregnancy, possesses intrinsic, weak thyroid-stimulating activity. Thyroid-stimulating hormone (TSH) levels fall during the first trimester, and this decrease parallels the rise in the production of hCG.

HYPERTHYROIDISM

Signs and Symptoms

The signs and symptoms of mild to moderate hyperthyroidism are common during pregnancy (heat intolerance, diaphoresis, fatigue, anxiety, emotional lability, tachycardia,

Nursing Care Plan Gestational Diabetes Mellitus

Nursing Diagnosis: Nutrition, Imbalanced: Less than Body Requirements related to impaired carbohydrate metabolism during pregnancy

Measurable Short-term Goal: The patient will plan a balanced diet and exercise program to follow during pregnancy.

Measurable Long-term Goal: The patient will obtain and metabolize sufficient nutrients for maternal and fetal needs and to maintain appropriate blood glucose levels during pregnancy.

NOC Outcomes:
Diabetes Self-Management (1619) Personal actions to manage diabetes mellitus and prevent disease progression.
Nutritional Status: Nutrient Intake (1009) Adequacy of usual pattern of nutrient intake

NIC Interventions:
Nutrition Therapy (1120)
Nutrition Counseling (5246)

Nursing Interventions:

1. Assess the patient's understanding of gestational diabetes and provide additional information as needed about changes in carbohydrate metabolism during pregnancy and how these may affect the patient and her fetus.

   RATIONALE: Teaching is based on the patient's need for information to help promote active participation in self-care.

2. Refer patient to a registered dietician and reinforce the recommended diet parameters with patient at each visit: an additional 300 calories per day are needed in the second and third trimesters; 40%–50% from complex carbohydrates, 10%–20% from protein, and 30% from fats; avoid concentrated sweets; nutrients should be divided each day between three meals and three snacks.

   RATIONALE: The diet is planned to maintain a normoglycemic state during pregnancy based on the patient's lifestyle and individual food preferences.

3. Encourage the patient to engage in 30 minutes of daily exercise appropriate for her pregnancy such as walking or swimming.

   RATIONALE: Regular exercise helps maintain lower blood glucose levels.

4. Ask patient to keep a daily log of her diet and exercise. Review at each prenatal visit and offer support and encouragement to continue regimen.

   RATIONALE: A written log allows the patient to monitor her own progress as well as providing a record of interventions to compare with blood glucose levels.

5. Inform patient that she will need to have her blood glucose checked weekly in the office and if it is still high after about 2 weeks of diet and exercise, she may need to begin insulin therapy.

   RATIONALE: Dietary changes and exercise may not be enough to maintain carbohydrate balance. Anticipatory guidance helps motivate the patient and prepare her for possible change.

6. Monitor fetal growth and well-being. Instruct patient in a method for fetal kick counts beginning at 28 weeks and prepare her for weekly NSTs from 34 weeks until birth.

   RATIONALE: Maternal hyperglycemia may result in fetal macrosomia. The fetus of a diabetic mother is at higher risk for complications.

---

and a wide pulse pressure). However, weight loss, tachycardia greater than 100 beats per minute, and diffuse goiter are clinical features suggestive of hyperthyroidism. Gastrointestinal symptoms (i.e., severe nausea, excessive vomiting, and diarrhea), cardiomyopathy, lymphadenopathy, and congestive heart failure can also accompany thyrotoxicosis (excessive thyroid activity) in pregnancy (Cunningham et al., 2005; Nader, 2004). Establishing a diagnosis of maternal hyperthyroidism can be challenging due to the myriad of metabolic and hormonal changes that normally take place during pregnancy. However, a depressed maternal serum TSH concentration and an elevated free thyroxine (T_4) level are useful in confirming the diagnosis. Although difficult,

prompt diagnosis of hyperthyroidism is imperative because of the potential for serious maternal and fetal complications. Research suggests that uncontrolled hyperthyroidism during pregnancy may be associated with increased preeclampsia, preterm labor, low birth weight, and neonatal mortality (Cunningham et al., 2005; Nader, 2004).

Treatment

Treatment for hyperthyroidism includes the use of antithyroid medications such as the thioamides, propylthiouracil (PTU—the drug of choice), or methimazole (Tapazole). Symptomatic improvement usually occurs within 2 weeks after the initiation of therapy although the

| Name _____ | Date of birth _____ Age _____ |
| Diabetes type _____ Age @ diagnosis _____ Expected date of confinement _____ Educator _____ |
| Blood pressure _____ Height _____ Weight _____ Urine: Protein _____ Glucose _____ Ketone _____ |
| Glucose tolerance test: Fasting blood sugar _____ 1h _____ 2h _____ 3h _____ |

The pregnant woman with diabetes will demonstrate the following:

Expected Outcome	Date
Understands diabetes, role of glucose and insulin transport	
Understands significance to pregnancy of 3-hour glucose tolerance test results (GDM)	
Understands effect pregnancy has on diabetes control, including role of placental hormones	
Understands potential outcomes of uncontrolled blood glucose—macrosomia, polyhydramnios, respiratory distress syndrome, preterm delivery, intrauterine fetal death, neonatal hypoglycemia, ketoacidosis, birth trauma, cesarean delivery	
Understands significance of hemoglobin A1C for spontaneous abortion and congenital defects	
Uses glucose meter, including quality controls	
Uses autolancet to obtain blood sample with appropriate disposal	
Understands diabetes/diet/diary and role of exercise, with safety guidelines	
Records technique of blood glucose values and abnormal reactions	
Understands glycemic goals for treatment	
Knows onset and peak times of prescribed insulin	
Inspects and stores insulin correctly	
Draws up insulin correctly (single and mixed)	
Identifies timing of injection, injection sites, rotation and technique, and appropriate syringe disposal	
Identifies signs and symptoms of hypoglycemia	
Treats hypoglycemia with documented low (written guidelines)	
Has support person with knowledge of glucagon use and appropriate administration—provided Rx with two refills	
Identifies signs and symptoms of ketoacidosis; reports persistent nausea/vomiting, illness, infection, persistent hyperglycemia, or recurrent insulin reactions	
Checks ketones daily with first void (pregestational) and with blood glucose values >180 mg/dL	
Understands sick day management (written guidelines)	
Schedules antepartum testing	
Understands significance of GDM for future pregnancy, development of overt diabetes mellitus later in life, appropriate follow-up, need for follow-up testing, preconception control, and risk-minimizing interventions	
Understands significance of diabetes and development of long-term complications related to poor control	

Level of comprehension _____ Learning impediments _____

Family support _____ Previous education _____ Meter _____

Figure 11-11 Diabetic education checklist.

medication does not become fully effective for 6 to 8 weeks. During treatment, the patient's free T_4 levels are obtained on a monthly basis and the findings are used to taper the dosage to achieve the smallest effective level to prevent unnecessary fetal hypothyroidism. When unresponsive to drug therapy, surgery (subtotal thyroidectomy) may be necessary. Since the surgery is associated with an increased risk of pregnancy loss and preterm labor, it is performed only for cases of severe hyperthyroidism. The use of radioactive iodine for diagnosis or treatment of hyperthyroidism is contraindicated during pregnancy because it may adversely affect the fetal thyroid (Golden & Burrow, 2004). When caring for patients with hyperthyroidism, the nurse must carefully monitor maternal weight gain and fetal growth.

HYPOTHYROIDISM

Symptoms

The symptoms of hypothyroidism are insidious and can be masked by the hypermetabolic state associated with pregnancy. Maternal symptoms can include modest weight gain, a decrease in exercise capacity, lethargy, cold intolerance, constipation, hoarseness, hair loss, brittle nails and dry skin. Laboratory confirmation is made from an elevated TSH level and low to normal T_3 and T_4 values (Cunningham et al., 2005; Nader, 2004).

Treatment

Hypothyroidism must be treated promptly as there is an increased risk for maternal preeclampsia, placental abruption, and stillbirth. Fetal neurological development can be severely affected by decreased levels of thyroid hormone. Treatment involves the use of a thyroid hormone supplement (i.e., levothyroxine [Synthroid]) with the dose adjusted every 4 weeks until the TSH level reaches the lower end of the normal range for pregnancy (Nader, 2004).

Venous Thrombosis and Pulmonary Embolism

Venous thromboembolic diseases include superficial and deep vein thrombophlebitis (DVT), pulmonary embolus (PE), septic pelvic thrombophlebitis, and thrombosis. These conditions account for one half of all obstetric morbidity. Pulmonary embolism, the leading cause of maternal mortality, accounts for 17% of all maternal deaths (Whitty & Dombrowski, 2004). The most common form of thrombosis that occurs during pregnancy involves veins of the calf, thigh, and pelvis. The most important aspect of lower extremity and pelvic venous thrombosis is that it can lead to pulmonary embolism, which poses a major threat to the pregnant woman (Cunningham et al., 2005).

PATHOPHYSIOLOGY

Thrombosis is thought to be the consequence of alterations in the vessel wall, slowing of blood flow (or stasis), and changes in blood components. Pregnancy presents the ideal state in which all three of these components may exist. Trauma to the vessel wall may occur during childbirth with alterations in the clot-inhibiting endothelial surface. Blood flow from the legs and pelvic veins are slowed during pregnancy because of pressure exerted on the iliac veins by the gravid uterus and by the relaxation of the smooth muscles in response to increased progesterone.

Finally, changes in blood components occur during pregnancy whereby some clotting factors are increased while other anticoagulant and fibrinolytic system factors are decreased.

INCIDENCE AND RISK FACTORS

When compared with nonpregnant women of similar age, the likelihood of venous thromboembolism during normal pregnancy and the puerperium is increased by a factor of five. Venous thromboembolism (VTE) occurs in 0.5 to 3 per 1000 pregnancies. An untreated DVT is associated with a 15% to 25% incidence of pulmonary embolus, which is associated with a 12% to 15% maternal mortality rate (McPhedran, 2004). A number of factors such as preeclampsia, advanced age, increased parity, multiple gestation, obesity, and dehydration place women at high risk for thromboembolic disease during pregnancy. When assessing the pregnant patient, the nurse must be aware of the characteristic signs and symptoms associated with thromboembolic disease.

 Critical Nursing Action Recognizing Thromboembolism

During the examination, the nurse assesses for the presence of the following signs and symptoms that may be indicative of thromboembolism (Cunningham et al., 2005; McPhedran, 2004):

- Pain, tenderness, warmth.
- Swelling of the lower extremity which is asymmetric with a difference of greater than 0.8 inch (2 cm) between the normal and affected leg. Swelling of the thigh is especially relevant because the risk of pulmonary embolism is associated with femoral or iliac phlebitis.
- Color change, especially in the left leg.
- A palpable cord underlying the region of pain and tenderness.
- Positive Homans' sign.

Symptoms of a pulmonary embolism:

- Tachypnea
- Dyspnea
- Pleuritic chest pain
- Atelectatic rales
- Cough
- Fever
- Diaphoresis
- Tachycardia
- Hemoptysis
- Cyanosis
- Heart gallop or murmur
- Anxiety
- Apprehension

The diagnosis can be very challenging as some of the signs and symptoms are normal during pregnancy (e.g., lower extremity edema). Doppler ultrasound technique has become the diagnostic study of choice in cases of proximal vein occlusion. Venography has not been used often in pregnancy because of possible hazards to the fetus, but it is a useful tool when results of other studies are equivocal (Laros, 2004). If there is a suspicion of PE, the ventilation–perfusion (VQ) scan results in minimal radiation exposure to the fetus. An entirely normal perfusion scan rules out PE (Refuerzo, Hechtman, Redman, & Whitty, 2004). Management involves a combination of strategies including medications (i.e., anticoagulant therapy with heparin), bedrest with elevation of the involved extremity, and the application of warm, moist heat.

 Now Can You— Discuss thromboembolism during pregnancy?

1. Describe why pregnancy is an ideal state for the development of thromboembolism?
2. Name five signs and symptoms to consider when assessing your pregnant patient for thromboembolism?
3. Formulate a plan of care for the patient with a diagnosis of thromboembolism?

Psychiatric Complications During Pregnancy

The recognition and management of depression and psychoses during pregnancy and the puerperium are of critical importance. Particularly in the United States, these disorders often are underrecognized and undertreated, and this factor potentially contributes to the likelihood of devastating effects on the child, the mother, the family, and society (Parry, 2004).

CONSULTING WITH THE PREGNANT PSYCHIATRIC PATIENT

Psychiatric complications during pregnancy can represent an exacerbation of an ongoing psychiatric disorder, a resurgence of previously remitted symptoms, or the onset of a new illness. Millions of women suffer from mental illness during their childbearing years, and more than 50% of pregnancies are unplanned in this population. These facts highlight the importance of prenatal counseling with regard to the natural history of various psychiatric disorders during pregnancy as well as the potential associated with fetal exposure to psychotropic agents and /or maternal mental illness (Epperson & Czarkowski, 2004).

Consultations with pregnant women who suffer from a psychiatric disorder, regardless of the diagnosis, should include discussion of the following facts (Epperson & Czarkowski, 2004):

- Psychoactive medications readily cross the placenta.
- There are potential risks associated with untreated maternal psychiatric illness as well as exposure to psychotropic medications. (Risks may include poor attention to prenatal care, substance abuse, and deliberate self-harm).

- Many women experience relapse or worsening of symptoms if pharmacologic treatment is not continued or instituted when necessary. (Maternal anxiety and stress have been shown to have adverse effects on pregnancy outcome, infant/child neurodevelopment, and maternal postnatal mental health.)

DEPRESSION

The incidence of depression during pregnancy is estimated to be 10% to 13%. Women at risk for antepartum and/or postpartum depression are those with a personal or family history of affective disorders (unipolar and bipolar), few social supports, marital conflict, or significant life events (Epperson & Czarkowski, 2004; Records & Rice, 2007).

Bipolar Disorder

The course of bipolar disorder is particularly unpredictable during pregnancy. There have been reports of heightened risk of depressive or manic relapse in women who rapidly discontinued their lithium treatment, in comparison with those who underwent a slow, controlled tapering off over 4 weeks. Regardless of how rapidly lithium doses were tapered, the risk of relapse illness in these women was 52% during pregnancy and 70% during the puerperium (Pigarelli, Kraus, & Potter, 2005).

Anxiety Disorders

Anxiety disorders including panic disorder, generalized anxiety disorder, obsessive–compulsive disorder (OCD), and posttraumatic stress disorder (PTSD) are common during the childbearing years. Childbearing has been associated with the onset or worsening of panic disorder or OCD (Epperson & Czarkowski, 2004).

Eating Disorders

Eating disorders in pregnant women have both physiologic and psychologic effects on the outcome of the pregnancy and on subsequent infant development. Anorexia nervosa has been associated with higher rates of perinatal mortality, obstetric complications, and congenital anomalies. Bulimia nervosa has been associated with extreme maternal weight gain, and preeclampsia and eclampsia (Epperson & Czarkowski, 2004).

MANAGEMENT

The importance of the detection of psychiatric problems in the pregnant population cannot be overemphasized. The health and welfare of not only the mother is at stake but also that of the entire family. Nurses are often the first care providers to recognize indicators of psychiatric difficulties in their patients. Strategies to help identify mental health problems during pregnancy may include (Epperson & Czarkowski, 2004; Parry, 2004):

- Placing psychoeducational materials throughout all patient areas
- Routinely inquiring about the patient's and her family's psychiatric history during the initial interview
- Administering the Edinburgh Postnatal Depression Scale (or a similar tool)
- Assessing the woman's access to social and family supports

- Referring the woman to community resources such as home health visitation and the local mental health agency

"What to say" — *When screening for depression during pregnancy*

The U.S. and Canadian Task Forces on Preventive Health Care recommend using the following two "probe questions" to screen women for depression during pregnancy:

- "Over the past two weeks have you felt down, depressed or helpless?"
- "Over the past two weeks have you felt little interest or pleasure in doing things?" (Records & Rice, 2007).

Substance Abuse in Pregnancy

Drug and alcohol use during pregnancy is a common phenomenon and a significant public health issue. Studies of substance abuse during pregnancy have documented a high incidence of adverse and, sometimes, catastrophic perinatal outcomes associated with intrauterine drug and alcohol exposure. Nurses are responsible for having up-to-date knowledge of the effects of alcohol, tobacco, and other drugs in pregnancy and for performing skilled and compassionate assessments of pregnant and postpartum women without criticizing their behavior or alienating them from their sources of health care.

According to the National Pregnancy and Health Survey, approximately 19% of women used alcohol during pregnancy; 5% used an illicit drug at least once during pregnancy, including marijuana (3%) and cocaine (1%). The Pregnancy Risk Assessment Monitoring System (PRAMS) estimated that women's alcohol use during pregnancy ranged from 3% to 10%. Findings from the Maternal Life Study, which oversampled very low-birth-weight infants, revealed that 35% of pregnant females reported alcohol use and 8% reported marijuana use during pregnancy. Meconium toxicology screens tested positive for cocaine or opioids in 11% of infants screened (Brady & Ashley, 2005).

SUBSTANCE ADDICTION

Pregnancy does not occur in a vacuum but rather it is an event that is superimposed on the context and circumstances of women's lives. Substance abusing women have a high incidence of social (intimate partner violence, risk-taking sexual behaviors) and psychologic (low self-esteem) conditions that affect their health status, their ability to engage in prenatal care, and their ability to succeed in drug abuse treatment. These social and psychologic conditions become more important considerations when the biologic and psychologic stress of pregnancy is added to an already fragile system (Mason & Lee, 2004).

Nurses face difficult ethical dilemmas when caring for pregnant and parenting women who use harmful substances. The conflict may be viewed as one that exists between the women's right to autonomy over her body and behavior and the nurse's obligation to prevent harm to the fetus or child (Kearney, Wellman, & Freda, 1999). Nurses in prenatal care and acute care settings are responsible for thoroughly assessing psychosocial risks and conducting mutual goal setting with pregnant patients to minimize the harm associated with these risks. Support and respect should be offered regardless of the woman's decisions about her health care or self-care. A nonjudgmental, concerned, and empathetic environment should be provided so that the patient feels encouraged to express her feelings and concerns about herself, her drug use, and her unborn child (Kearney et al., 1999; Moran, 2004b).

 Now Can You— Discuss issues associated with substance abuse during pregnancy?

1. Name five behaviors that may signal a substance abuse problem?
2. Discuss how substance abuse can affect the course and outcome of pregnancy?
3. Discuss the ethical dilemmas faced by the perinatal nurse who is caring for the pregnant woman with a substance abuse problem?

Antepartum Fetal Assessment

Fetal assessment is an integral component of prenatal care. Careful assessment of fetal well-being enhances perinatal outcome through early identification and intervention for fetal compromise. The goal of antepartum fetal surveillance is to prevent fetal death and to help ensure the best possible fetal outcome. A number of tests can be performed during pregnancy to monitor fetal growth, development, and well-being. Antenatal assessment during the first and second trimester is directed primarily at the diagnosis of fetal congenital anomalies while the goal of third trimester assessment is to determine the quality of the intrauterine environment for the maturing fetus.

CHORIONIC VILLUS SAMPLING

Chorionic villus sampling (CVS) is an invasive procedure that can be used to obtain a fetal karyotype. Because the villi arise from trophoblast cells, their chromosome structure is identical to that of the fetus. CVS is performed between 10 and 12 weeks' gestation and results are available quickly due to the rapid proliferation of the chorionic villi cells. Using ultrasound guidance to locate the chorion cells, a thin catheter is inserted vaginally into the intrauterine cavity. An alternative technique involves the abdominal or intravaginal insertion of a biopsy needle. A small quantity of chorionic villi is then aspirated from the placenta. The risk of complications associated with CVS is 1 in 200. Risks include infection (in 0.5% of cases), fetal loss (in 0.3% of cases), rupture of membranes (in 0.1% of cases), Rh isoimmunization, and possible fetal limb reduction (Gilbert & Harmon, 2003).

PERCUTANEOUS UMBILICAL BLOOD SAMPLING

Percutaneous umbilical blood sampling (PUBS) is an invasive procedure that is performed to obtain a sample of fetal blood for karyotyping and to test for anemia, isoimmunization, metabolic disorders, and infection. Under ultrasound guidance, a needle is inserted through the maternal abdomen and into the fetal umbilical cord. Use of a fetal blood sample for karyotyping allows for more rapid test results than when fetal skin cells are used, as with amniocentesis. Complications include cord laceration, thromboembolism, preterm labor, premature rupture of the membranes, and infection (Jenkins & Wapner, 2004).

AMNIOCENTESIS

Amniocentesis is an invasive procedure that involves the removal of amniotic fluid. Under ultrasound guidance, a needle is inserted through the maternal abdomen and into the amniotic sac (Fig. 11-12). Amniocentesis may be performed beginning at 12 weeks' gestation. Components of the amniotic fluid, including fetal cells, may be analyzed for chromosomal abnormalities, fetal lung maturity, infection, and the presence of bilirubin in Rh-sensitized pregnancies. Later in the pregnancy, amniotic fluid reduction (via amniocentesis) may be performed for temporary alleviation of maternal symptoms associated with hydramnios (excessive amniotic fluid). Complications associated with amniocentesis include rupture of the membranes, preterm labor, infection, fetal injury, and fetal death. If the woman has $Rh_o(D)$-negative blood, $Rh_o(D)$ immune globulin should be administered following the amniocentesis to prevent isoimmunization.

Amniocentesis is frequently performed late in pregnancy to provide information concerning fetal lung maturity. **Lecithin** and **sphingomyelin** are the protein components of surfactant, the lung enzyme that is formed by the alveoli beginning around the 22nd week of gestation. After amniocentesis, the **lecithin/sphingomyelin ratio** (L/S ratio) may be quickly determined by a "shake test" or sent to the laboratory for a quantified analysis. An L/S ratio of 2:1, which typically occurs by 35 weeks' gestation, is traditionally accepted as lung maturity (a ratio of 3:1 in the infant of a diabetic mother).

Phosphatidylglycerol and **desaturated phosphatidylcholine** are two other compounds that are found in surfactant after approximately 35 to 36 weeks of gestation. Since these two substances are present only with

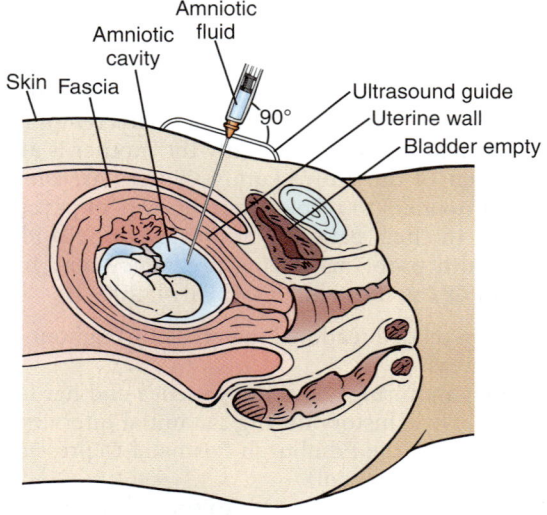

Figure 11-12. Amniocentesis.

lung maturity, their presence in the amniotic fluid sample is another indicator that respiratory distress syndrome will not occur in the neonate.

ADDITIONAL INVASIVE TESTS

Amnioscopy

Amnioscopy involves the use of an amnioscope (a small fetoscope) to visually inspect the amniotic fluid through the cervix and membranes. Most often this procedure is performed to detect meconium staining. It carries a risk of membrane rupture.

Fetoscopy

Fetoscopy is a method of visualizing the fetus with a fetoscope, an extremely narrow, hollow tube inserted through an amniocentesis technique. It is sometimes used to assess fetal well-being, obtain fetal tissue and blood samples, and perform fetal surgery, but not before 17 weeks of gestation. The procedure carries a risk of premature labor and infection.

ULTRASONOGRAPHY

Ultrasonography is the use of high-frequency (>20,000 Hz) sound waves to detect differences in tissue density and visualize outlines of structures in the body. Widely used in modern obstetrics, ultrasonography is an important component of antepartum fetal assessment and surveillance. The examination can be done abdominally (after application of a transmission gel, a transducer is moved over the skin) or transvaginally (a lubricated transducer probe is placed in the vagina) during pregnancy. The abdominal technique is more useful after the first trimester when the gravid uterus becomes an abdominal organ. The sound frequencies that bounce back from the uterus are displayed on an oscilloscope screen as a three-dimensional visual image. During the painless examination, the patient should be positioned so that she (and her support person, if present) can observe the images, if they wish to do so.

 Nursing Insight— *Levels of ultrasonography*

There are three levels of ultrasonography examinations: standard, limited, and specialized.

Ultrasonographers or other health care professionals who have received special training may perform the *standard* examination, which is used to detect fetal viability, assess the gestational age, determine the presentation of the fetus, locate the placenta, assess amniotic fluid volume (AFV), and examine the fetus for certain anatomic abnormalities. The *limited* examination is performed for a specific indication, such as determining the fetal presentation during labor or evaluating fetal heart activity when it cannot be detected by other methods. The *specialized* examination is performed to evaluate a fetus suspected to have an anatomical or physiological abnormality. This level of examination is generally performed by specialists in high-risk perinatal centers (ACOG, 2004).

During the first trimester, ultrasound may be used to confirm the viability and age of the pregnancy, determine the number, size, and location of the gestational sacs, identify uterine abnormalities (and rule out an ectopic pregnancy), and locate the presence of an intrauterine contraceptive device. Fetal heart rate activity can be observed as early as 6 to 7 weeks via real-time echo sonography. In the second and third trimesters, ultrasound is frequently used to confirm fetal viability and gestational age, monitor fetal growth, AFV, placental location and maturity, and assess uterine fibroid tumors and cervical length. Serial measurements are useful in providing an accurate determination of fetal age. Ultrasound is an essential component of the biophysical profile and fetal Doppler studies (discussed later).

 Optimizing Outcomes— **Accurately determining fetal age with ultrasonography**

Ultrasonography examinations provide an accurate estimate of fetal age during the first 20 weeks of gestation because most normal fetuses grow at approximately the same rate. Throughout the gestational period, fetal age determination may be made by the following sonographic measurements: (1) gestational sac dimensions (around 8 weeks); (2) crown–rump length (CRL) (around 7–12 weeks); (3) biparietal diameter (BPD) (after 12 weeks); and (4) femur length (after 12 weeks). The accuracy of gestational age assessment increases as the fetus ages because more than one structure is measured.

KICK COUNTS

Counting fetal movements or "kick counts" has been proposed as a primary method of fetal surveillance for all pregnancies. This method of fetal assessment has many benefits. It is easy to perform, readily available to the woman, and has no associated costs. The patient is instructed to lie on her side and count the number of times that she feels the fetus move. Many variations have been developed but there are two major methods for performing kick counts:

- The first method is done while the woman lies on her side. She counts and records 10 distinct movements in a period of up to 2 hours. Once 10 movements have been perceived, the count may be discontinued.
- With the second method, the patient counts and records fetal movements for 1 hour three times per week. The count is to be considered reassuring if it equals or exceeds the woman's previously established baseline.

DOPPLER ULTRASOUND BLOOD FLOW STUDIES (UMBILICAL VELOCIMETRY)

Doppler ultrasound is used to study blood flow in the umbilical vessels of the fetus, placental circulation, fetal cardiac motion, and maternal uterine circulation. This technology is useful in managing pregnancies at risk because of hypertension, diabetes mellitus, IUGR, multiple fetuses or preterm labor. A noninvasive Doppler wave measures the velocity of red blood cell movement through the uterine and fetal vessels. Assessment of the blood flow through the uterine vessels is useful in determining vascular resistance in women at risk for developing placental insufficiency. Decreased velocity is associated with poor neonatal outcome (Jasper, 2004).

FETAL BIOPHYSICAL PROFILE

The fetal **biophysical profile** (BPP) is a noninvasive "fetal physical examination" that is more accurate in predicting fetal well-being than any single assessment. It combines electronic fetal heart rate monitoring with ultrasonography to evaluate fetal well-being. The fetus responds to central hypoxia by alterations in movement, muscle tone, breathing, and heart rate patterns. A finding of normal fetal biophysical parameters indicates that that the central nervous system is functional and therefore the fetus is not hypoxemic. The BPP comprises the following five components and is based on a 30 minute time period (Harmon, 2004):

- Nonstress test
- Fetal breathing movements (one or more episodes of rhythmic fetal breathing movements for 30 seconds)
- Fetal movement (three or more discrete body or limb movements)
- Fetal tone (one or more episodes of extension of a fetal extremity with return to flexion, or opening or closing of a hand)
- Determination of the amniotic fluid volume (a single vertical pocket of amniotic fluid exceeding 0.8 inch (2 cm) is considered evidence of adequate amniotic fluid)

Each of the five components is assigned a score of 2 (normal or present) or 0 (abnormal). A score of 8 to 10 is reassuring while a score of 6 is considered "equivocal" and the test should be repeated within 24 hours in the case of a preterm infant; the term infant should be promptly delivered. When the score is 0 to 4/10, especially in the fetus with IUGR that has reduced amniotic fluid and in whom serial observations have previously been normal, delivery should commence without any delay (Harmon, 2004).

NONSTRESS TEST

The nonstress test (NST) is one of the most common methods of antenatal screening. It involves the use of electronic fetal monitoring (EFM) for approximately 20 minutes. The NST is based on the premise that a normal fetus moves at various intervals and that the CNS and myocardium responds to movement. The response is demonstrated by an acceleration of the FHR (the FHR "reacts"). Loss of heart rate reactivity is associated most commonly with a fetal sleep cycle but may result from any cause of central nervous system depression, including fetal hypoxia, acidosis, and some congenital anomalies (Harmon, 2004; Tucker, 2004).

Reactivity is also based on gestational age; 32 to 34 weeks is considered to be the appropriate age for reactivity to occur. Before this gestational age, a very large percentage of fetuses will not meet the acceptable criteria: a FHR acceleration of 15 beats per minute (bpm) that lasts for 15 seconds (ACOG, 1999). Fetuses less than 32 weeks are more likely not to meet the criteria for a reactive nonstress test. When the preterm fetus is monitored, consideration should be given to the effect of the gestational age on the size of the accelerations: a FHR acceleration of 10 bpm that lasts for 10 seconds is acceptable at 32 weeks. Once a fetus has a reactive tracing, however, it should remain reactive. Women with risk factors (e.g., diabetes,

uteroplacental insufficiency) undergo frequent non stress testing, often twice weekly (Cunningham et al., 2005).

With the patient in the lateral tilt position, the nurse applies the external electronic fetal monitor and observes the tracing for evidence of fetal heart rate accelerations of at least 15 bpm above the baseline heart rate. At least two FHR accelerations sustained for at least 15 seconds should occur over a 20-minute time period. If these criteria are met, the test is satisfactory and termed a "reactive test." The test may be extended for another 20 minutes if needed. If the reactive criteria are not met (e.g., the FHR accelerations do not reach 15 bpm or do not last for 15 seconds) over a 40-minute period, the test is considered to be "nonreactive." Depending on the fetal age, a nonreactive NST result should be followed by a contraction stress test or a biophysical profile (ACOG, 1999). An "unsatisfactory" NST result occurs if there is inadequate fetal activity or if the data cannot be interpreted.

ACOUSTIC STIMULATION/VIBROACOUSTIC STIMULATION

Acoustic (sound) **stimulation** and **vibroacoustic** (vibration and sound) **stimulation** may be used as an adjunct to the NST to elicit an acceleration of the fetal heart rate. A hand-held instrument such as an artificial larynx (especially designed for this purpose) is positioned on the maternal abdomen and a low-frequency vibration and a buzzing sound are emitted. The stimulus is applied for 1 to 3 seconds in an attempt to awaken the fetus and may be repeated up to three times with a 1-minute rest period between attempts. A fetus that shows no response to the applied stimulus may be neurologically compromised or acidotic and requires further evaluation (ACOG, 1999).

CONTRACTION STRESS TEST

The **contraction stress test (CST)** evaluates the FHR response to uterine contractions. The CST is based on the premise that fetal oxygenation that is only marginally adequate with the uterus at rest is transiently worsened by uterine contractions (Jasper, 2004). The nurse uses the electronic fetal monitor to obtain a baseline FHR tracing for 20 minutes. If spontaneous uterine contractions do not occur during this time, uterine stimulation is produced through IV oxytocin infusion (beginning with 0.5 milliunits/min and increasing the dose by 0.5 milliunits/min at 15- to 30-minute intervals) or patient nipple self-stimulation, until three contractions of at least 40 seconds duration occur within a 10-minute time frame. CSTs are evaluated according to the presence or absence of late FHR decelerations. A late deceleration, associated with fetal hypoxia, is one that begins at the peak of the contraction and persists after the conclusion of the contraction. The test is considered negative (normal) if there is no evidence of late or significant variable decelerations; a positive CST (abnormal) is one in which there are late decelerations after 50% of contractions, even if the frequency is less than three in 10 minutes. An equivocal or suspicious result indicates the presence of nonpersistent late decelerations or decelerations associated with hyperstimulation (contractions occur less than 2 minutes apart or last longer than 90 seconds) (ACOG, 1999; Harmon, 2004). Additional information is needed when this finding occurs.

Since the CST is based on the presence of uterine contractions, there are several contraindications to the test. Patients who have experienced third trimester bleeding from placenta previa or marginal abruptio placentae, women who have had a previous cesarean birth with a classical incision (vertical incision that extends into the uterine fundus), and those with premature rupture of the membranes, cervical incompetence or multiple gestation are not candidates for a CST.

ELECTRONIC FETAL HEART RATE MONITORING

Electronic fetal heart rate monitoring (EFM) uses electronic techniques to give an ongoing assessment of fetal well-being. EFM provides information related to the response of the fetal heart rate in the presence or absence of uterine contractions. Electronic monitoring of the fetal heart rate can be accomplished by either external or internal means. EFM is discussed in greater detail in Chapter 12.

 Now Can You— Discuss methods of antepartum fetal surveillance?

1. Differentiate among chorionic villus sampling, percutaneous umbilical sampling and amniocentesis?
2. Identify two methods for conducting kick counts?
3. List the fetal parameters assessed in a biophysical profile?
4. Discuss how the NST is performed and describe what is meant by a "reactive" and a "nonreactive" test result?

Special Conditions and Circumstances that May Complicate Pregnancy

THE PREGNANT WOMAN WHO REQUIRES ANTENATAL BEDREST

The patient whose antenatal course is compromised by obstetrical complications that require bedrest faces even more challenges. Maloni (2002) has written extensively about the deleterious effects of bedrest on body systems and addresses problems such as muscle wasting, failure to gain weight, and cardiovascular and psychological difficulties. Lack of weight bearing and inactivity make muscles weak. Dizziness, difficulty regulating blood pressure, and fainting are common symptoms in the patient confined to bedrest.

In most situations, regular home visitation by a community health nurse is an important component of care (Fig. 11-13). The nurse caring for the patient with a high-risk pregnancy needs to remain cognizant of the fact that depending on the circumstances, the woman's libido is often unaffected and she and her partner will need guidance regarding "safe" practices that promote intimacy without threatening the pregnancy. Also, as the pregnancy progresses, the woman on bedrest is presented with the same maternal tasks (Rubin, 1976), as is any other woman who is approaching motherhood. The woman's physical condition may cause difficulty in mastering the tasks. For example, Rubin observed that a pregnant woman is drawn to the company of other pregnant women, not only for acceptance but also to promote a greater understanding of interpersonal behavior during this special stage of her life.

Figure 11-13 Visiting patients confined to bedrest at home is an important nursing intervention.

These normal feelings and activities can be jeopardized by hospitalization and the woman's subsequent removal from the comforting patterns and rhythm of day-to-day life. Hospitalization, especially when prolonged, can create many additional problems, since hospitalized patients often suffer from loneliness, boredom, powerlessness, anxiety, anger, and depression.

Maloni, Brezinski-Tomasi, and Johnson (2001) reported that women confined to bedrest felt like prisoners and often experienced guilt over the extra responsibilities foisted upon their partners. In addition, childcare, with the necessary involvement of multiple providers and the disruption of usual routines, was viewed as a major concern. Financial strain and its impact on family well-being was also an issue. Referral to social services and other community resources may be helpful in assisting the couple with financial matters and other aspects of home care.

Nursing interventions that can be instituted to help the family adjust to the stress of a complicated pregnancy include the involvement of high-risk pregnancy or other specialty support groups, professional counseling when appropriate, and religious support when desired. The educational needs of the pregnant woman who is experiencing a high risk pregnancy are essentially the same as those of any childbearing woman. Whenever possible, nurses should encourage their patients to participate in prenatal classes, seek lactation counseling, learn about infant care, and attend self-care classes. The nurse may arrange for the couple to attend childbirth education classes in either a group or private setting. For most, participating in a group promotes a feeling of normalcy. Family members, particularly the woman's partner, should be included, as they can share infant care responsibilities and provide emotional support.

"Sidelines," a national support group, provides resources such as a helpful bedside checklist that describes a variety of activities for women confined to bedrest. This organization may be contacted at www.sidelines.org.

The recognition that high-risk couples may have depleted their coping skills due to perinatal complications constitutes an important nursing issue, especially during the intrapartal period. The nurse needs to be aware that the anxiety and stress of labor may be extremely difficult for the couple. The nurse can assist and empower the patient and her partner by encouraging them to express their emotional concerns, by keeping them informed of changes in the woman's condition and by encouraging them to ask questions.

Depending on the circumstances, the postpartum period may be very difficult as well, due to physical and emotional exhaustion, especially if antenatal hospitalization was required. Adverse symptoms associated with weeks of bedrest are often not resolved by 6 weeks postpartum (Maloni & Park, 2005). The woman may not be able to care for her infant as she would like, and this situation can quickly lead to feelings of helplessness, frustration, and disappointment. The nurse needs to remain supportive, conduct an ongoing assessment of the family's coping skills, monitor the extent of maternal–infant attachment, and engage the appropriate hospital and community resources.

 Now Can You— **Discuss care for the patient on antenatal bedrest?**

1. State six complications of antenatal bedrest?
2. Formulate a plan of care to meet the physiological, psychological and social needs of the pregnant patient on bedrest?
3. Identify team members to be included in your plan of care when caring for the pregnant patient on bedrest?
4. Describe how antenatal bedrest can affect the patient after childbirth (postpartum)?

ADOLESCENT PREGNANT PATIENT

Although teen pregnancies have been decreasing steadily during the past decade, the United States still has the highest teen pregnancy rate among all developed countries (Hoyert, Mathews, Menacker, Strobino, & Guyer, 2006). With early and thorough prenatal care, adolescents older than the age of 15 years experience no greater risks than those of the general pregnant population. Although the incidence of certain complications may be higher because of age extremes, the nursing diagnoses, interventions, and evaluations remain relatively unchanged from those for the general pregnant population with the same complications (Smith, 2004). Examples of nursing diagnoses for several complications of pregnancy are presented in Box 11-10.

Box 11-10 **Examples of Nursing Diagnoses for Selected Complications of Pregnancy**

- Risk for injury, maternal or fetal, related to inadequate prenatal care and screening
- Fear related to uncertain outcome of the pregnancy
- Risk for deficient fluid volume related to bleeding during pregnancy
- Risk for infection related to preterm rupture of the membranes
- Risk for injury to fetus related to uteroplacental insufficiency
- Ineffective tissue perfusion related to hypertension
- Risk for injury to self and fetus related to chronic substance abuse
- Interrupted family processes related to adolescent pregnancy
- Deficient diversional activity related to imposed bedrest

Prenatal medical and behavioral risk factors can severely complicate adolescent pregnancy and result in poor birth outcomes, particularly when late or inadequate prenatal care occurs. Prenatal medical and behavioral risks for the adolescent population include (Gilliam, Tapia, & Goldstein, 2003):

- Preterm labor and birth—especially when combined with low socioeconomic status, single parent, smoker, illicit drug use, pre-pregnant weight less than 100 lbs. (45.5 kg), poor weight gain during pregnancy, and inadequate prenatal care.
- Anemia
- Preeclampsia/eclampsia
- Repeated exposure to sexually transmitted infections
- Chronic or asymptomatic urinary tract infections
- Acute pyelonephritis
- Intrauterine growth restriction

The nurse's need for good communication skills when working with adolescents cannot be overstated since these young women often lack trust in medical personnel and fear that their behaviors might be judged. Without good communication, the nurse is unable to make an accurate assessment of the adolescent's knowledge about the importance of quality, consistent prenatal care. Without good communication, the professional nurse–patient relationship is neither established nor developed and the prenatal plan of care is jeopardized.

ADVANCED AGE PREGNANT PATIENT

Many women are now choosing to delay childbirth until later years. The implementation of infertility technology has broadened the boundaries of the reproductive age. Both socioeconomic circumstances and the nature of the older mother have changed with time. The older maternity patient today is at significantly lower risk than her contemporary of two decades ago, who tended to be the mother of many children, having commenced childbearing many years earlier. However, the nurse must be aware of special considerations such as an increased likelihood of chronic diseases (e.g., diabetes, hypertension) when planning care for the woman who has become pregnant after the age of 35 years. (See Chapter 9 for further discussion.)

 Nursing Insight— Recognizing potential problems associated with mature mothers

Pregnant women older than age 35 are more likely to experience obstetric complications such as placenta previa, abruptio placentae, prolonged labor, cesarean birth, and mortality. The fetus is at a greater risk for low birth weight, macrosomia, chromosomal abnormalities, congenital malformations, and neonatal mortality.

THE PREGNANT PATIENT WHO HAS SUFFERED TRAUMA

Trauma is the fourth leading cause of death worldwide and the leading nonobstetric cause of maternal death during pregnancy (Weinberg et al., 2005). Motor vehicle accidents account for more than one half of maternal trauma incidents. About 50% of fetal deaths result from maternal trauma, and most of these are due to motor vehicle accidents (Mattox & Goetzl, 2005). Blunt trauma is caused by the following conditions (Haney, 2004):

- Motor-vehicle collisions in which force is applied to the abdomen from direct impact or as a result of secondary injury from abdominal organs. Abruption of the placenta and/or preterm labor may result from the trauma.
- Accidental falls are usually more common in the third trimester as the woman's center of gravity becomes increasingly displaced.
- Assaults involving intimate partner violence (the incidence increases during pregnancy), gunshot and stabbing wounds.

Optimizing Outcomes— Considerations when caring for the obstetric trauma patient

Maternal stabilization is the initial goal in resuscitation. Resuscitation during pregnancy proceeds as with any other trauma. Trauma in pregnancy involves at least two patients (more in the case of multiple gestation). The fetal heart rate is often the first vital sign to change. All pregnant trauma patients need continuous fetal monitoring. Risk factors predictive of fetal death include ejection during an automobile crash, motorcycle and pedestrian collisions, abnormal heart fetal heart rate patterns, maternal tachycardia, and maternal death (Haney, 2004).

Be sure to— Take care with documentation

Document your nursing care by writing accurate and factual notes. Make certain you have described your assessment, plan of care, interventions, and evaluation for your plan of care. Frequently, trauma cases involve litigation. Well-documented records protect both the patient and the health care system.

SURGERY DURING PREGNANCY

Surgery for nonobstetric reasons occurs in about 1% to 2% of pregnant women. This figure is most likely an underestimated number since many women may not know that they are pregnant at the time of surgery (Callahan, 2004).

Maternal and Fetal Risks During Surgery

Anesthetic considerations are of prime importance when surgery becomes necessary during pregnancy. General anesthesia is a more complex issue during pregnancy because of the increase in maternal blood volume and cardiac output. Surgery risks are related to the possibility of increased maternal morbidity associated with pregnancy-induced changes in the cardiovascular, respiratory, hematologic, and gastrointestinal systems. Normal physiological changes that occur during pregnancy can adversely affect the use of anesthesia and the safety of the surgical procedure. Surgery carries a possibility of increased fetal risks due to an intraoperative decrease in uteroplacental blood flow (leading to fetal hypoxia), along with possible

teratogenic effects from the anesthetic agents. The risk of spontaneous abortion associated with maternal surgery is approximately 8% during the first trimester and 6.9% in the second trimester. Extra-abdominal surgery is less likely to be complicated by spontaneous abortion (Burtness, 2004; Callahan, 2004).

CANCER DURING PREGNANCY

The incidence of cancer is low during the childbearing years. During pregnancy, the incidence of cancer is similar to that of nonpregnant women of childbearing age. Cancer complicates 1 out of 1000 pregnancies and accounts for 5% of deaths that occur during pregnancy. Because more women today choose to delay childbearing, the co-occurrence of pregnancy and cancer may increase (Burtness, 2004). The prognosis best correlates with the anatomic extent of the disease at the time of diagnosis. Cancer in the pregnant woman does not appear to metastasize to the fetus because of the placenta's effectiveness as a barrier against spread and also because the fetus may be capable of resisting the invasion of malignant cells.

During pregnancy the diagnosis of cancer can be difficult for the following reasons: many of the presenting symptoms of cancer are often attributed to the pregnancy; many of the physiologic and anatomic alterations of pregnancy can compromise the physical examination; many serum tumor markers (β-hCG, α fetoprotein, CA 125) are normally increased during pregnancy; and the ability to perform either imaging studies or invasive diagnostic procedures is often altered (Gabbe, Niebyl, & Simpson, 2007).

Care of the pregnant patient with cancer is related to a number of factors:

- Gestational age of the pregnancy
- Stage of the cancer and the associated prognosis
- Potential for the cancer treatment to have adverse effects on the fetus, including the potential for long-term occult problems
- Risk to the patient of delaying therapy to permit fetal viability
- Risk to the fetus of early delivery to allow more timely cancer therapy; and the possible need to terminate an early pregnancy to allow an optimal opportunity to treat the patient and cure the malignancy.

OBESITY

Obesity has reached epidemic proportions in the United States, and nearly one third of reproductive-aged women are considered to be obese. In pregnancy, obesity is associated with a higher incidence of antepartum complications such as diabetes and hypertension, and with peripartum complications including macrosomia, prolonged labor, shoulder dystocia, and higher cesarean rates. Cesarean delivery is often complicated by excessive operative blood loss (greater than 1000 mL), difficult anesthesia intubations and operative times greater than 2 hours duration. Postoperative wound complications, including infection, delayed healing, operative injury, the need for blood transfusions, thromboembolism, and hysterectomy are also increased in obese women and result in prolonged hospitalization and increased costs.

Nursing Insight— *Differentiating between "overweight" and "obese"*

A pregnant woman is considered *overweight* if she is 20% above ideal weight or has a BMI over 25; she is considered *obese* if her weight exceeds 200 lbs. (91 kg), if she is 50% over ideal body weight for height or if her BMI is above 29.

Dieting for weight loss during pregnancy is not recommended because if carbohydrates are restricted too much, the body will burn fat and protein for energy. This can result in inadequate protein available for the fetus and lead to ketoacidosis. Dietary counseling should focus on reduced carbohydrates (daily caloric intake should not go below 1500 to 1800 calories per day), education to recognize nutritious food choices and the value of daily exercise. During the postpartum period, the woman should receive continued nutritional counseling and support with realistic goals for weight loss.

Be sure to— Voice concerns about difficulties with FHR monitoring

As a nurse using electronic fetal monitoring, you must be able to obtain a FHR strip that can be interpreted. Monitoring the obese patient can be very challenging. If you are having difficulty monitoring the fetal heart and/or uterine contractions, bring your concerns to the physician or midwife. In the event of a malpractice claim, the fetal monitoring strips can be used as evidence as to whether the standard of care was or was not met.

Obese patients often suffer from low self-esteem and are embarrassed by their size. Health care providers must always strive to preserve the patient's dignity and treat her with respect. Remarks should never be made as to the need for a "bigger bed" or blood pressure cuff. Requesting that extra personnel be available in the labor room to aid with a fetal shoulder dystocia or to help the patient to get out of bed postpartum should be made discreetly.

THE PATIENT WITH A DISABILITY

The pregnant woman with a disability often faces two major concerns: her ability to maintain her own health and her fetus' health throughout pregnancy, childbirth, and during the postpartum period; and the fear of not being able to physically care for her baby. The first concern, universally shared by all mothers, has added significance for the woman with a disability due to the possible interactions between the pregnancy and her disability. The disabled woman's experience of pregnancy, birth, and postpartum is shaped by what she brings to this period of transition as well as her prior experiences with the health care system. The woman's specific disability, her resources, and unique approach to pregnancy and birth are all factors that help shape her overall childbearing experience (Carty, 1998).

While pregnancy and childbirth can be very challenging for the woman with a disability, it provides the nurse with a wonderful opportunity to help make this event a special, memorable time in her life. Care must be well planned and individualized because many women with disabilities face unpredictability in their symptoms and in their day-to-day abilities. The nurse can develop a well organized plan of care by ensuring that there is documentation of the patient's specific needs, concerns, and desires for her labor and birth and that this information is readily available to all appropriate personnel.

Early in the pregnancy, a referral to the clinical nurse specialist or nurse manager on the birth unit allows the care plan and specific needs to be noted and prepared. Special equipment (e.g., mattress, commode) may need to be ordered and if there are mobility issues, a notation made that this patient will need assignment to a handicap accessible room. Staff nurses may also need to be educated about how to appropriately care for the patient. Advance notice may facilitate development of a nursing schedule that allows the same team to provide continuity of care throughout the woman's hospital stay. Other members of the health team (e.g., physical therapist, occupational therapist, lactation consultant, visiting nurse) should also be involved in the plan of care and kept aware of the patient's needs. If the patient has a service dog, all staff should be aware that it is permissible for the dog to be in the hospital. Furthermore, the staff should understand that the dog provides an important service for the patient, is "working" and should not be played with. While the woman and her dog are in the hospital, a family member should assume responsibility for the dog's needs. Many special devices are available to assist new mothers who have hearing or mobility impairments.

INTIMATE PARTNER VIOLENCE DURING PREGNANCY

Intimate partner violence (IPV), family violence, battering, and spousal abuse are all terms used to describe a pattern of assaultive and coercive behaviors. The true incidence of IPV perpetuated against women in the United States is unknown because much of it remains undetected and unreported. However, it is estimated that battered women account for up to 35% of all women seeking care in an emergency room (Mattson, 2004). Pregnancy is often the trigger for the beginning or escalation of violence in a relationship, and many chronically abused women report an increase in violence directed at them during pregnancy. There are many theories to account for this behavior. For example, the stress of pregnancy may strain a troubled relationship beyond normal coping abilities. The abuser may harbor jealousy against the fetus. Physical violence may be an attempt to end the pregnancy; and frequently, the battered pregnant woman is unlikely to have a strong social support network upon which she can rely (Mattson, 2004).

Characteristically, the abuser targets different maternal body parts during pregnancy. Pregnant women are likely to have more multiple injury sites than nonpregnant women and the abuse is often directed to the breasts, genitalia, and abdomen. The risk of injury to the fetus is very high due to the chance of placental injury that can result in an abruption.

Pregnant teenagers are particularly vulnerable because of their need to rely on others for the basics of life. Often those they rely on are their abusers. Incest, rape, child abuse, gang (group) fighting, stalking, and IPV from both male and female partners have been described. Nurses can help teenagers with violence only if they know that the teenagers are experiencing it. Thus, nurses need to be able to gain their young patients' trust and confidence so that they feel comfortable sharing their problems. Assessment, safety planning, documentation, and follow–up are all essential components of providing care for women who are experiencing violence, no matter what their age. The medical record is often the source of information that can raise suspicions of abuse, and a number of assessment forms specifically designed to elicit information regarding patterns of abuse have been developed. (See Chapter 9 for further discussion.)

 Now Can You— Discuss abuse during pregnancy?

1. Explain why pregnancy is often the trigger for the beginning or escalation of intimate partner violence?
2. Describe the body areas that are usually targeted during pregnancy?
3. Discuss your nursing plan of care when you suspect that your patient has been abused?

---

summary points

◆ Complications that arise during pregnancy are often challenging and demand the perinatal nurse's skills, knowledge, and expertise, combined with the nursing process, to first identify the pregnant patient at risk and then formulate, implement, and evaluate an appropriate, holistic plan of care.

◆ Anticipatory nursing care is invaluable in preventing a complication from becoming a major health crisis.

◆ Alterations of signs and symptoms from the expected clinical progression during pregnancy must be immediately conveyed to the primary health care provider so that an appropriate management plan may be activated.

◆ The nurse must always remain cognizant of the important role the patient's family, culture, language, and religious beliefs play in her adjustment to motherhood and overall well-being.

◆ By providing culturally competent care to childbearing families, many potential complications can be identified in a timely manner to allow for effective treatment and improved outcomes.

◆ Meticulous documentation of the patient's plan of care and response to the plan of care cannot be overemphasized.

review questions

Multiple Choice

1. The perinatal nurse describes for the woman/family who have experienced an 11-week miscarriage and desire information that the majority of miscarriages are caused by:
A. Nausea and vomiting in early pregnancy
B. Prenatal stress
C. Chromosomal abnormalities
D. Umbilical cord accidents

2. The perinatal nurse uses the acronym "SPASMS" to teach a new nurse about preeclampsia. The "P" refers to:
A. Pregnancy
B. Proteinuria
C. Pelvic circulation
D. Pressure

True/False

3. The perinatal nurse knows that the most common medical complications of pregnancy are those related to hypertension.

4. The perinatal nurse is aware that the most accurate determination of gestational age is based on the date of the last menstrual period and an early ultrasound examination.

Select All that Apply

5. The clinic nurse recognizes that a woman's risk factors for an ectopic pregnancy include:
A. The use of oral contraceptive pills
B. A previous history of a dilatation and curettage
C. A history of *Chlamydia trachomatis* infection
D. A history of rubella

6. The perinatal nurse provides additional time for the clinic appointment for Janet and her partner. Janet has just experienced a spontaneous abortion. The perinatal nurse knows that it is critical to provide:
A. Time to listen to their grief
B. Information about support groups
C. A referral to an obstetrician if requested
D. Appropriate contraceptive information

7. The perinatal nurse knows that risk factors for preeclampsia include:
A. Maternal history of preeclampsia
B. Body mass index (BMI) greater than 30
C. Nulliparity
D. History of a previous cesarean birth

Fill-in-the-Blank

8. As part of the surgical follow-up for removal of a molar pregnancy, the nurse schedules _____ hCG levels beginning at biweekly, then monthly for at least _____ months.

9. The perinatal nurse completes a _____ test on fluid obtained from a speculum examination on a woman at 35 weeks' gestation who describes a spontaneous rupture of the membranes.

10. The perinatal nurse knows that _____ bleeding related to disruption in _____ attachment is the most common presentation for _____ _____.

See Answers to End of Chapter Review Questions on the Electronic Study Guide or DavisPlus.

REFERENCES
American Cancer Society (ACS). (2006). *Cancer facts and figures 2006.* New York: Author.
American College of Obstetricians and Gynecologists (ACOG). (1999). *Antepartum fetal surveillance* (Practice Bulletin No. 9). Washington, DC: Author.

American College of Obstetricians and Gynecologists (ACOG). (2000). *Scheduled cesarean delivery and the prevention of vertical transmission of HIV infection* (Committee Opinion No. 234, pp 592-602). Washington, DC: Author.

American College of Obstetricians and Gynecologists (ACOG). (2001a). *Gestational diabetes.* (Practice Bulletin No. 30, pp. 525–538). Washington, DC: Author.

American College of Obstetricians and Gynecologists (ACOG). (2001b). *Assessment of risk factors for preterm birth* (Practice Bulletin No. 31, pp. 709–716). Washington, DC: Author.

American College of Obstetricians and Gynecologists (ACOG). (2002a). *Diagnosis and management of preeclampsia and eclampsia* (Practice Bulletin No. 33, pp. 717–725). Washington, DC: Author.

American College of Obstetricians and Gynecologists (ACOG). (2002b). *Prenatal care at the threshold of viability* (Practice Bulletin No. 38, pp. 751–758). Washington, DC: Author.

American College of Obstetricians and Gynecologists (ACOG). Committee on Clinical Practice. (2003a). *Immunization during pregnancy* (Committee Opinion No. 282, pp 434-439). Washington, DC: Author.

American College of Obstetricians and Gynecologists (ACOG). (2003b). *Cervical Insufficiency* (Practice Bulletin No. 48, pp. 793–801). Washington, DC: Author.

American College of Obstetricians and Gynecologists (ACOG). (2003c). *Management of Preterm Labor* (Practice Bulletin No. 43, pp. 765–773). Washington, DC: Author.

American College of Obstetricians and Gynecologists (ACOG). (2004a). *Nausea and vomiting of pregnancy.[miscellaneous]* (Practice Bulletin No. 52, pp. 812–823). Washington, DC: Author.

American College of Obstetricians and Gynecologists (ACOG). (2004b). Ultrasonography in pregnancy. (Practice Bulletin No. 58). *Obstetrics and Gynecology, 104*(6), 1149–1158.

American College of Obstetricians and Gynecologists (ACOG). Committee Opinion (2004c). *Prenatal and perinatal human immunodeficiency virus testing: Expanded recommendations* (Committee Opinion No. 304). Washington, DC: Author.

American College of Obstetricians and Gynecologists (ACOG). Committee Opinion (2006). *Human papillomavirus vaccination* (Committee opinion number 344). Washington, DC: Author.

American College of Obstetricians and Gynecologists & American Academy of Pediatrics (ACOG/AAP). (2007). *Guidelines for perinatal care* (6th ed.). Washington, DC: Author.

American Diabetes Association (ADA). (2006). Diagnosis and Classification of diabetes mellitus. *Diabetes Care, 29*(Supplement), S543–S548.

Askin, D. (2004). Intrauterine infections. *Neonatal Network,* 23(5), 23–29.

August, P. (2004). Hypertensive disorders in pregnancy. In G. Burrow, T. Duffy, & J. Copel (Eds.), *Medical complications during pregnancy* (6th ed., pp. 43–67). Philadelphia: W.B. Saunders.

Berman, M., DiSaia, P., & Tewari, K. (2004). Pelvic malignancies, gestational trophoblastic neoplasia, and nonpelvic malignancies. In R. Creasy, & R. Resnick (Eds.), *Maternal-fetal medicine: Principles and practice* (5th ed., pp. 1213–1242). Philadelphia: W.B. Saunders.

Bernhardt, J., & Dorman, K. (2004). Pre-term birth risk assessment tools. Exploring feal fibronectin and cervical length for validating risk. *AWHONN Lifelines, 8*(1), 38–44.

Bess, K., & Wood, T. (2006). Understanding gestational trophoblastic disease: How nurses can help those dealing with a diagnosis. *AWHONN Lifelines, 10*(4), 320–326.

Bowers, N., & Gromada, K. (2006). Care of the multiple birth family: Pregnancy and birth. March of Dimes Nursing Module. New York: March of Dimes.

Brady, T., & Ashley, O. (2005). *Women in substance abuse treatment: Results from alcohol and drug services study* (ADSS). DHHS Publication SMA 04-3968 analytic series A 26. Rockville, MD: Substance and Mental Health Services Administration, Office of Applied Studies.

Brennan, A., & Geddes, D. (2004). Bringing new treatments to the bedside in cystic fibrosis. *Pediatric Pulmonology, 37*(1), 87–98.

Bulechek, G., Butcher, H.M., & Dochterman, J. (2008). *Nursing interventions classification (NIC)* (5th ed.). St. Louis, MO: C.V. Mosby.

Burrow, G., Duffy, T., & Copel, J., Eds. (2004). *Medical complications of pregnancy.* Philadelphia: W.B. Saunders.

Burtness, B. (2004). Neoplastc diseases. In G. Burrow, T. Duffy, & J. Copel (Eds.), *Medical complications during pregnancy* (6th ed., pp. 479–504). Philadelphia: W.B. Saunders

Callahan, L. (2004). Surgery in pregnancy. In S. Mattson, & J. Smith (Eds.), *Core curriculum for maternal-child nursing* (3rd ed., pp. 727–749). Philadelphia: W.B. Saunders.

Carty, E. (1998). Disability and childbirth: meeting the challenges. *Canadian Medical Association Journal,* 159(4), 363–369.

Centers for Disease Control and Prevention (CDC). (2006a). HIV/AIDS Update: A glance at the epidemic. Retrieved from www.cdc.gov/hiv/pubs/facts/at-a-glance.htm (Accessed August 7, 2007).

Centers for Disease Control and Prevention, Workowski, K., & Berman, S. (2006b). Sexually transmitted diseases treatment guidelines 2006. *MMWR Morbidity and Mortality Weekly Report,* 51(RR11), 1–23.

Clark, S. (2004). Placenta previa and abruptio placentae. In R. Creasy, R. Resnik, & J. Iams (Eds.), *Maternal-fetal medicine: Principles and practice* (5th ed.). Philadelphia: W.B. Saunders.

Cockwell, H., & Smith, G. (2005). Cervical incompetence and the role of emergency cerclage. *Journal of Obstetrics and Gynecology Canada,* 27(2), 123–129.

Criteria Committee of the New York Heart Association. (1979). Nomenclature and criteria for diagnosis of diseases of the heart and great vessels (8th ed.). New York: New York Heart Association.

Cunningham, F., Leveno, K., Bloom, S., Hauth, J., Gilstrap, L., & Wenstrom, K. (2005). *Williams obstetrics* (22nd ed.). New York: McGraw-Hill.

Cystic Fibrosis Foundation. (2005). What is CF? Retrieved from http://www.cff.org (Accessed April 6, 2008).

Davison, J., & Lindheimer, M. (2004). Renal disorders. In R. Creasy, R. Resnick, & J. Iams (Eds.), *Maternal-fetal medicine: Principles and practice* (5th ed., pp. 901–923). Philadelphia: W.B. Saunders.

Deglin, J., & Vallerand, A. (2009). *Davis's drug guide for nurses* (11th ed.). Philadelphia: F.A. Davis.

Dillon, P.M. (2007). *Nursing health assessment.* Philadelphia: F.A. Davis.

Duffy, T. (2004). Hematologic aspects of pregnancy. In G. Burrow, T. Duffy, & J. Copel (Eds.), *Medical complications of pregnancy* (6th ed., pp. 69–86). Philadelphia: W.B. Saunders.

Easterling, T., & Otto, C. (2002). Heart disease. In S. Gabbe, J. Niebyl, & J. Simpson (Eds.), *Obstetrics normal and problem pregnancies* (4th ed., pp. 1005–1032). Philadelphia: Churchill Livingstone.

Emery, S. (2005). Hypertensive disorders of pregnancy: Over-diagnosis is appropriate. *Cleveland Clinic Journal of Medicine,* 72(4), 345–352.

Epperson, C., & Czarkowski, K. (2004). Psychiatric complications. In G. Burrow, T. Duffy, & J. Copel (Eds.), *Medical complications of pregnancy* (6th ed., pp. 505–513). Philadelphia: W.B. Saunders.

Expert Committee on the Diagnosis and Classification of Diabetes Mellitus. (2003). Report of the expert committee on the diagnosis and classification of diabetes mellitus. *Diabetes Care,* 26(Supplement 1), S5–S20.

Farquhar, C. (2005). Ectopic pregnancy. *Lancet,* 366(9485), 583–591.

Foley, M. (2004). Cardiac disease. In G. Dildy, M. Belfort, G. Saade, J. Phelan, G. Hankins, & S. Clark (Eds.), *Critical care obstetrics* (4th ed.). Malden, MA: Blackwell Science.

Freda, M., & Patterson, E. (2004). In R. Wieczorek (Ed.), *Preterm labor: Prevention and nursing management* (3rd ed.). White Plains, NY: March of Dimes.

Gabbe, S.G., Niebyl, J.R., & Simpson, J.L. (Eds). (2007). *Obstetric normal and problem pregnancies* (5th ed.). New York: Churchill Livingstone.

Gardner, M., & Doyle, N. (2004). Asthma in pregnancy. *Obstetrics and Gynecology Clinics of North America,* 31(2), 385–413.

Gibbs, R., Sweet, R., & Duff, P. (2004). Maternal and fetal infections. In R. Creasy, & R. Resnick (Eds.), *Maternal-fetal medicine; Principles and practice* (5th ed., pp. 741–801). Philadelphia: W.B. Saunders.

Gilbert, E., & Harmon, J. (2003). *Manual of high risk pregnancy and delivery* (3rd ed.). St. Louis: C.V. Mosby.

Gilliam, M., Tapia, B., & Goldstein, C. (2003). Adolescent girls' attitudes toward pregnancy. *Hispanic Journal of Behavioral Sciences,* 29(1), 50-67.

Givens, S., Moore, M., & Freda, M. (2004). *Interviewing by the perinatal nurse* (1st ed.). White Plains, NY: March of Dimes.

Gluck, J., & Gluck, P. (2005). Asthma in pregnancy. *Obstetrics and Gynecology,* 192(2), 369–380.

Golden, L. & Burrow, G. (2004). Thyroid disease in pregnancy. In G. Burrow, T. Duffy, & J. Copel (Eds.), *Medical complications of pregnancy* (6th ed., pp. 131–161). Philadelphia: W.B. Saunders.

Griebel, C., Halvorsen, J., Golemon, T., & Day, A. (2005). Management of spontaneous abortion. *American Family Physician,* 72(7), 1243–1250.

Guy, E., Kirumaki, A., & Hanania, N. (2004). Acute asthma in pregnancy. *Critical Care Clinics,* 20(4), 731–745.

Haney, S. (2004). Trauma in pregnancy. In S. Mattson, & J. Smith (Eds.), *Core curriculum for maternal-child nursing* (3rd ed., pp. 703–726). Philadelphia: W.B. Saunders.

Harmon, C. (2004). Assessment of fetal health. In R. Creasy, R. Resnik, & J. Iams (Eds.), *Maternal-fetal medicine: Principles and practice* (5th ed., pp. 357–401). Philadelphia: W.B. Saunders.

Hjartardottir, S., Leifsson, B., Geirsson, R., & Steinthorsdottir, V. (2004). Paternity change and the recurrence risk in familial hypertensive disorders in pregnancy. *Hypertension in Pregnancy, 23*(2), 219–225.

Hoyert, D., Mathews, T., Menacker, F., Strobino, D., & Guyer, B. (2006). Annual summary of vital statistics: 2004. *Pediatrics, 117*(1), 168–183.

Hunter, L.P., Sullivan, C.A., Young, R.E., & Weber, C.E. (2007). Nausea and vomiting of pregnancy: Clinical management. *The American Journal for Nurse Practitioners, 11*(8), 57–67.

Iams, J., & Creasy, R. (2004). Preterm labor and delivery. In R. Creasy, R. Resnik, & J. Iams (Eds.). *Maternal-fetal medicine: Principles and practice* (5th ed.). Philadelphia: W.B. Saunders.

Jasper, M. (2004). Antepartum fetal assessment. In S. Mattson, & J. Smith (Eds.), *Core curriculum for maternal-child nursing* (3rd ed., pp. 161–200). Philadelphia: W.B. Saunders.

Jenkins, T., & Wapner, R. (2004). Prenatal diagnosis of congenital disorders. In R. Creasy, R. Resnik, & J. Iams (Eds.), *Maternal-fetal medicine: Principles and practice* (5th ed.). Philadelphia: W.B. Saunders.

Johnson, M., Bulechek, G., Butcher, H., McCloskey Dochterman, J., Maas, M., Moorhead, S., & Swanson, E. (2006). *NANDA, NOC, and NIC linkages: Nursing diagnoses, outcomes, & interventions* (2nd ed.). St. Louis, MO: Mosby Elsevier.

Kearney, M., Wellman, L., & Freda, M. (1999). *Perinatal impact of alcohol, tobacco and other drugs* (1st ed.). White Plains, NY: March of Dimes.

Kennedy, M.S. (2005). Stepwise approach to managing asthma in pregnancy.[miscellaneous]. *AJN, American Journal of Nursing, 105*(4), 20.

Kenshole, A. (2004). Diabetes and pregnancy. In G. Burrow, T. Duffy, & J. Copel (Eds.), *Medical complications during pregnancy* (6th ed., pp. 15–42). Philadelphia: W.B. Saunders.

Kilpatrick, S., & Laros, R. (2004). Maternal hematologic disorders. In R. Creasy, R. Resnik, & J. Iams (Eds.), *Maternal-fetal medicine: Principles and practice* (5th ed., pp. 975–1021). Philadelphia: W.B. Saunders.

Klein, L., & Galan, H. (2004). Cardiac disease in pregnancy. *Obstetrics and Gynecology Clinics of North America, 31*(2), 429–459.

Kulich, M., Rosenfeld, M., Goss, C., & Wilmott, R. (2003). Improved survival among young patients with cystic fibrosis. *The Journal of Pediatrics, 142*(6), 631–636.

Labelle, C., & Kitchens, C. (2005). Disseminated intravascular coagulation: Treat the cause, not the lab values. *Cleveland Clinic Journal of Medicine, 72*(5), 377–397.

Landon, M., Catalano, P., & Gabbe, S. (2002). Diabetes mellitus. In S. Gabbe, J. Niebyl, & J. Simpson (Eds.), *Obstetrics: Normal and problem pregnancies* (4th ed., pp. 1081–1116). Philadelphia: Churchill Livingstone.

Landry, M. (2004). Viral infections. In G. Burrow, T. Duffy, & J. Copel (Eds.), *Medical complications of pregnancy* (6th ed., pp. 347–374). Philadelphia: W.B. Saunders.

Laros, R. (2004). Thromboembolic disease. In R. Creasy, R. Resnik, & J. Iams (Eds.), *Maternal-fetal medicine: Principles and practice* (5th ed., pp. 845–857). Philadelphia: W.B. Saunders.

Laskin, C. (2004). Pregnancy and the rheumatic diseases. In G. Burrow, T. Duffy, & J. Copel (Eds.), *Medical complications of pregnancy* (6th ed., pp. 429–449). Philadelphia: W.B. Saunders.

Lawrence, R., & Lawrence, R. (2005). *Breastfeeding: A guide for the medical profession* (6th ed.). Philadelphia: C.V. Mosby.

Longo, S., Dola, C., & Pridjian, G. (2003). Preeclampsia and eclampsia revisited. *Southern Medical Journal, 96*(9), 891–898.

Luke, B. (2005). Nutrition in multiple gestations. *Clinics in Perinatology, 32*(2), 403–429, vii.

Malone, F., & D'Alton, M. (2004). Multiple gestation: Clinical characteristics and management. In R. Creasy, R. Resnik, & J. Iams (Eds.), *Maternal-fetal medicine: Principles and practice* (5th ed., pp. 513–536). Philadelphia: W.B. Saunders.

Maloni, J.A. (2002). Astronauts & pregnancy bed rest: What NASA is teaching us about inactivity. *AWHONN Lifelines, 6*(4), [318–319], 320–323.

Maloni, J.A., Brezinski-Tomasi, J.E., & Johnson, L.A. (2001). Antepartum bed rest: Effect upon the family. *JOGNN: Journal of Obstetric, Gynecologic, and Neonatal Nursing, 30*(2), 165–173.

Maloni, J., & Park, S. (2005). Postpartum symptoms after antepartum bedrest. *Journal of Obstetric, Gynecologic and Neonatal Nursing, 34*(2), 163–171.

Mandel, J., & Weinberger, S. (2004). Pulmonary diseases. In G. Burrow, T. Duffy, & J. Copel (Eds.), *Medical complications of pregnancy* (6th ed., pp. 375–414). Philadelphia: W.B. Saunders.

March of Dimes. (2005). *March of Dimes prematurity campaign.* Retrieved from www.marchofdimes.com (Accessed August 6, 2007).

Martin, J., Hamilton, B., Sutton, P., Ventura, S., Menacker, F., & Munson, M. (2005). Births: Final data for 2003. *National Vital Statistics Report, 54*(2), 1–115.

Mason, E., & Lee, R. (2004). Substance abuse. In G. Burrow, T. Duffy, & J. Copel (Eds.), *Medical complications of pregnancy* (6th ed., pp. 515–537). Philadelphia: W.B. Saunders.

Mattox, K., & Goetzl, L. (2005). Trauma in pregnancy. *Critical Care Medicine, 33*(10S), S385–S389.

Mattson, S. (2004). Intimate partner violence. In S. Mattson, & J. Smith (Eds.), *Core curriculum for maternal-child nursing* (3rd ed., pp. 537–553). Philadelphia: W.B. Saunders.

McPhedran, P. (2004). Venous thromboembolism during pregnancy. In G. Burrow, T. Duffy, & J. Copel (Eds.), *Medical complications of pregnancy* (6th ed., pp. 87–101). Philadelphia: W.B. Saunders.

Mercer, B. (2003). Preterm premature rupture of the membranes. *Obstetrics and Gynecology, 101*(1), 178–193.

Moise, K. (2004). Hemolytic disease of the fetus and newborn. In R. Creasy, R. Resnik, & J. Iams (Eds.), *Maternal-fetal medicine: Principles and practice* (5th ed., pp. 537–561). Philadelphia: W.B. Saunders.

Moorehead, S., Johnson, M., Mass, M., & Swanson, E. (2008) *Nursing outcomes classification (NOC)* (4th ed.). St. Louis, MO: C.V. Mosby.

Moran, B. (2004a). Maternal infections. In S. Mattson, & J. Smith (Eds.), *Core curriculum for maternal-newborn nursing* (3rd ed., pp. 592–629). St. Louis: W.B. Saunders.

Moran, B. (2004b). Substance abuse in pregnancy. In S. Mattson, & J. Smith (Eds.), *Core curriculum for maternal-child nursing* (3rd ed., pp. 750–770). Philadelphia: W.B. Saunders.

Murray, H., Baakdah, H., Bardell, T., & Tulandi, T. (2005). Diagnosis and treatment of ectopic pregnancy. *Canadian Medical Association Journal, 173*(8), 905–912.

Nader, S. (2004). Thyroid disease in pregnancy. In R. Creasy, R. Resnik, & J. Iams (Eds.), *Maternal-fetal medicine: Principles and practice* (5th ed., pp. 1063–1081). Philadelphia: W.B. Saunders.

NANDA International. (2007). *NANDA-I Nursing Diagnoses: Definitions and Classifications 2007-2008.* Philadelphia: NANDA-I.

National Asthma Education and Prevention Expert Panel. (2005). Managing asthma during pregnancy: Recommendations for pharmacologic treatment—2004. *The Journal of Allergy and Clinical Immunology, 115*(1), 34–46.

National Center for Health Statistics (NCHS). (2002). *Report of final mortality statistics, 2000.*

National High Blood Pressure Education Program Working Group. (2000). Working group report on high blood pressure in pregnancy No. NHBPEP Publication No. 00-3029. Washington, D.C.: National Heart Lung and Blood Institute.

Norwitz, E., Hsu, C., & Repke, J. (2002). Acute complications of preeclampsia. *Clinical Obstetrics and Gynecology, 45*, 308–329.

Parry, B. (2004). Management of depression and psychoses during pregnancy and the puerperium. In R. Creasy, R. Resnick, & J. Iams (Eds.), *Maternal-fetal medicine: Principles and practice* (5th ed., pp. 1193–1200). Philadelphia: W.B. Saunders.

Peters, R.M., & Flack, J.M. (2004). Hypertensive disorders of pregnancy. *JOGNN: Journal of Obstetric, Gynecologic, and Neonatal Nursing, 33*(2), 209–220.

Pigarelli, D., Kraus, C., & Potter, B. (2005). Pregnancy and lactation: Therapeutic considerations. In J. DiPiro, R. Talbert, G. Yee, G. Matzke, B. Wells, & M. Posey (Eds.), *Pharmacotherapy: A pathophysiologic approach* (6th ed., pp 72–76). New York: McGraw-Hill.

Poole, J. (2003). Thalassemia and pregnancy. *The Journal of Perinatal & Neonatal Nursing, 17*(3), 196–208.

Poole, J. (2004a). Hemorrhagic disorders. In S. Mattson & J. Smith (Eds.), *Core curriculum for maternal-child nursing* (3rd ed., pp. 630–659). St. Louis: W.B. Saunders.

Poole, J. (2004b). Hypertensive disorders in pregnancy. In S. Mattson, & J. Smith (Eds.), *Core curriculum for maternal-newborn nursing* (3rd ed., pp. 554–591). St. Louis: W.B. Saunders.

Rawlins, S. (2001). Nonviral sexually transmitted infections. *Journal of Obstetrical, Gynecological and Neonatal Nursing, 30*(3), 324–331.

Records, K., & Rice, M. (2007). Psychosocial correlates of depression symptoms during the third trimester of pregnancy. *Journal of Obstetric, Gynecologic and Neonatal Nursing, 36*(3), 231–242.

Refuerzo, J.S., Hechtman, J.L., Redman, M.E., & Whitty, J.E. (2004). Venous thromboembolism during pregnancy: Clinical suspicion warrants evaluation. *Obstetrical & Gynecological Survey, 59*(4), 239-240.

Riordan, J. (2005). *Breastfeeding and human lactation* (3rd ed.). Boston: Jones & Bartlett.

Roberts, J.M. (2004). Pregnancy-related hypertension. In R. Creasy, & R. Resnik (Eds.), *Maternal-fetal medicine: Principles and practice* (5th ed., pp. 859–899). Philadelphia: W.B. Saunders.

Rubin, R. (1976). Maternal tasks of pregnancy. *Journal of Advanced Nursing, 1*, 367–376.

Rust, O., Atlas, R., Kimmel, S., Roberts, W., & Hess, I. (2005). Does the presence of a funnel increase the risk of adverse perinatal outcome in a patient with a short cervix? *American Journal of Obstetrics and Gynecology, 192*(4), 1060–1066.

Rust, O., & Roberts, W. (2005). Does cerclage prevent preterm birth? *Obstetrics and Gynecology Clinics of North America, 32*(3), 441–456.

Savoia, M. (2004). Bacterial, fungal, and parasitic disease. In G. Burrow, T. Duffy, & J. Copel (Eds.), *Medical complications of pregnancy* (6th ed., pp. 305–345). Philadelphia: W.B. Saunders.

Setaro, J., & Caulin-Glaser, T. (2004). Pregnancy and cardiovascular disease. In G. Burrow, T. Duffy, & J. Copel (Eds.), *Medical complications in pregnancy* (6th ed., pp. 103–129). Philadelphia: W.B. Saunders.

Sibai, B.M., Dekker, G., & Kupfermine, M. (2005). Preeclampsia. *The Lancet. 365*(9461), 785–799.

Simpson, K., & Knox, E. (2004). Obstetrical accidents involving intravenous magnesium sulfate: Recommendations to promote patient safety. *The American Journal of Maternal/Child Nursing, 29*(3), 161–171.

Smith, J. (2004). Age-related concerns. *Core curriculum for maternal-child nursing* (3rd ed., pp. 147–160). Philadelphia: W.B. Saunders.

Tucker, S.M. (2004). *Pocket Guide to fetal monitoring and assessment* (5th ed.). St Louis: Elsevier Health Sciences.

Wallerstedt, C., & Clokey, D. (2004). Endocrine and metabolic disorders. In S. Mattson, & J. Smith (Eds.), *Core curriculum for maternal-newborn nursing* (3rd ed., pp. 660–702). St. Louis: W.B. Saunders.

Weinberg, L., Steele, R., Pugh, R., Higgins, S., Herbert, M., & Story, D. (2005). The pregnant trauma patient. *Anaesthesia and Intensive Care, 33*(2), 167–180.

White, H., & Bouvier, D. (2005). Caring for a patient having a miscarriage. *Nursing 2005, 35*(7), 18–19.

Whitty, J., & Dombrowski, M. (2004). Respiratory diseases in pregnancy. In R. Creasy, R. Resnik, & J. Iams (Eds.), *Maternal-fetal medicine: Principles and practice* (5th ed.). Philadelphia: W.B. Saunders.

Yancy, M. (2004). Other medical complications. In S. Mattson, & J. Smith (Eds.), *Core curriculum for maternal-newborn nursing* (3rd ed., pp. 771–817). St. Louis: W.B. Saunders.

Yankaskas, J., Marshall, B., Sufian, B., Simon, R., & Rodman, D. (2004). Cystic fibrosis adult care: Consensus conference report. *Chest, 125*(1), 1–39.

Yudkin, M., & Gonik, B. (2006). Perinatal infections. In R. Martin, A., Fanaroff, & M. Walsh (Eds.). *Fanaroff & Martin's neonatal-perinatal medicine: Diseases of the fetus and infant* (8th ed., pp. 118–131). Philadelphia: C.V. Mosby.

 For more information, go to http://davisplus.fadavis.com/

CONCEPT MAP

Caring for the Woman Experiencing Complications During Pregnancy

Complications of Early Pregnancy
- Hyperemesis gravidarum
- Spontaneous abortion/ miscarriage
- Gestational trophoblastic disease
- Ectopic pregnancy
- Perinatal loss
  - Fetal death
  - Less than perfect child

Miscellaneous Complications
- Multiple gestation
- Premature rupture of membranes
- Preterm labor
- Incompetent cervix

Endocrine
- Diabetes
  - Type I & II
  - DKA
- Hyper/hypothyroid

Unique Conditions That Complicate Pregnancy
- Antenatal bedrest
- Adolescence
- Blunt abdominal trauma
- Surgery
- Cancer
- Obesity
- Physical disability
- Intimate partner violence
- Rh sensitization
- Systemic lupus

Cardiovascular/ Hematological
C/V
- Mitral valve prolapse
- Peripartum cardiomyopathy

Hematological
- Sickle cell anemia
- Thalassemia

Hypertensive disorders
- Chronic hypertension
- Preeclampsia/eclampsia
  - Proteinuria, edema, CNS alterations, HELLP
- Chronic hypertension with preeclampsia
- Gestational hypertension

Bleeding Disorders
- Placenta previa
- Placental abruption
- DIC

Psychiatric
Exacerbation: Resurgence: New onset:
- Depression
- Anxiety
- Eating disorder
- Substance abuse or addiction

Infections
- UTIs
  - Bacturia, cystitis pyelonephritis
- Group B strep
- TORCH
- STIs
  - Gonorrhea, syphilis, HPV, HIV/AIDS
- TB

Respiratory
- Pneumonia
- Asthma
- Cystic fibrosis

Family Teaching Guidelines:
- Preventing preterm birth
- Home care for patient with hypertensive disorder

Critical Nursing Actions:
- Maternal positioning in CPR
- Correct maternal/fetal care post maternal seizure
- Assess for decreased cardiac output during labor in maternal cardiovascular disease hx

Nursing Insight:
- Pneumonic for preeclampsia: SPASMS
- Vaccine for HPV
- OB meds that can affect maternal C/V diseases
- Risk for hemodynamic changes greater in wks 28–32

Ethnocultural Considerations:
- Beliefs related to pregnancy itself
- Preferences for provider's gender
- Culturally significant foods
- Need for interpreter
- Gestational diabetes → more prevalent in certain ethnic groups

Optimizing Outcomes:
- Offer tests with history of habitual spontaneous abortions
- Support religious beliefs related to transfusions
- Administer RhoGAM correctly

Complementary Care:
- Ginger for nausea and vomiting

Clinical Alert:
- Expanded volume in pregnancy can mask sx of hemorrhage
- Serious consequences occur with overdose of magnesium sulfate
- Have calcium gluconate (antidote) at bedside

Now Can You:
- Discuss the management of bleeding during pregnancy
- Identify 3 symptoms of preterm labor/PROM
- Discuss Rh$_o$(D) and ABO isoimmunization
- Discuss major disease processes that affect maternal health during pregnancy
- Identify how unique conditions complicate pregnancy

one
two
three
four
five
six
seven

The Birth Experience

The Process of Labor and Birth

To my labor and delivery nurse:
On February 24th you helped us welcome our darling daughter into the world. In fact you practically delivered her yourself. My labor and delivery moved along quite quickly. Through it all you somehow managed to always say and do the right thing. I have taken great pleasure in telling people what a really good labor and birth experience I had. You played a key role in that. While we know it's your job and all that, we thought you still deserved to know that your contribution to our daughter's birth was important and will always be a part of our memory. Years from now when we are telling her about her birth, your name is sure to come up. Thanks again!

—Anonymous

LEARNING TARGETS *At the completion of this chapter, the student will be able to:*

◆ Discuss various theories concerning the onset of labor.

◆ Describe signs and symptoms of impending labor.

◆ Distinguish between true and false labor.

◆ Contrast advantages and disadvantages of various childbirth settings.

◆ Describe the "5 Ps" and how each influences labor and birth.

◆ Differentiate among the four stages of labor according to the duration and work accomplished, contraction patterns, and maternal behaviors.

◆ Identify nursing interventions for each stage of labor.

◆ List five nursing diagnoses applicable to childbearing women.

---

 moving toward evidence-based practice Choice of Elective Cesarean Birth

Wax, J. R., Cartin, A., Pinette, M. G., & Blackstone, J. (2005). Patient choice cesarean—Maine experience. *Birth, 32*(3), 203–206.

The literature, as reported by the researchers, states that there has been a 42% increase in the number of elective cesarean procedures performed from 1999 to 2002, which accounted for 1.5–2.21% of all live births during that period.

The purpose of this study was to examine obstetricians' attitudes and practices with respect to patient choice of elective cesarean section. Questionnaires were sent to all (110) American College of Obstetricians and Gynecologists (ACOG) practicing Fellows and Junior Fellows in one northeastern state.

Physicians were asked whether they had ever performed a patient-requested cesarean section and, if so, how many were performed during the previous year. They were also asked what they considered as acceptable reasons for performing the procedure.

In addition, the physicians were also asked whether they would prefer this method of childbirth for themselves (if female) or for their partner (if male) and reasons for their choice.

If the respondent physicians had not performed any patient-requested cesarean deliveries, they were asked if they would be

(continued)

moving toward evidence-based practice (continued)

willing to perform the procedure if requested, if they had ever refused a request to perform the procedure, and, if so, the number of refusals during the previous year.

The questionnaires were completed and returned by 78 of the 110 physicians. Sixty respondents reported that they had previously performed or would be willing to perform an elective cesarean section.

Acceptable indications for performing elective cesarean deliveries included (in descending order of choice):

- Avoidance of damage to the woman's urinary tract system
- A woman who had experienced a previous adverse birth experience
- Avoidance of damage to anal continence
- Concern regarding fetal injury or death
- Maternal fear of childbirth
- Preservation of sexual function (26.7%); pelvic organ prolapse
- Pain
- Convenience
- Certainty of the delivering practitioner

The data also revealed that:

- Thirty-one physicians reported that they had performed elective cesarean deliveries and had averaged fewer than five procedures during the previous year.

- Of the 40 physicians who reported that they had not performed an elective cesarean delivery, 29 stated that they would be willing to do so if asked.
- The remaining 11 stated that they would be unwilling to perform any elective cesarean delivery.
- Of those who were willing to perform elective cesarean deliveries, only 15 stated that they would choose this surgery for themselves or for their partner.
- Female physician respondents younger than 35 years of age were more likely to select an elective cesarean birth for themselves than female physician respondents older than 35 years of age.
- The majority of the respondents stated that medical evidence supporting elective cesarean delivery was available.

The researchers concluded that even though the majority of physicians were willing to perform elective cesarean procedures for their patients, few preferred this method for themselves or for their partners.

1. What might be considered as limitations to this study?
2. How is this information useful to clinical nursing practice?

See Suggested Responses for Moving Toward Evidence-Based Practice on the Electronic Study Guide or DavisPlus.

Introduction

The journey from conception to birth is one of ongoing development and adaptation for the woman, the fetus, and the family. Physiological, psychological, and emotional changes that take place during pregnancy help to prepare the woman for labor and birth. Near the end of the pregnancy, the fetus continues to develop physiological abilities that facilitate successful adaptation for the transition from in utero life to the outside environment.

Each woman's labor and birth experience is uniquely shaped by a myriad of factors. Throughout this journey, the actions of nurses play a vital role in supporting the patient, the fetus, and the family. This chapter presents the processes of labor and birth, and the important roles of nurses during each stage.

Theories Concerning Labor Onset

For the majority of women, the onset of labor usually occurs between the 38th and 42nd weeks of pregnancy. For most of the pregnancy, the uterus stays in a relaxed state and the cervix remains closed and firm to maintain the pregnancy. Toward the end of pregnancy, there is a complete reversal where the uterus becomes more excitable and cervical softening (ripening) occurs. The cervical changes result from the breakdown of collagen fibers, which produce a decrease in the binding capacity. This

change, coupled with an increase in cervical water content, causes weakening and softening. Although many theories regarding the origin of labor have been proposed, no one theory can account for the onset of labor in all women. Instead, a combination of maternal and fetal factors most likely interacts to bring about the initiation of labor (Box 12-1).

The Process of Labor and Birth

A number of forces affect the progress of labor and help to bring about childbirth. These critical factors are often referred to as the "Ps" of labor:

- Powers (physiological forces)
- Passageway (maternal pelvis)
- Passenger (fetus and placenta)
- Passageway + Passenger and their relationship (engagement, attitude, position)
- Psychosocial influences (previous experiences, emotional status)

Position of the laboring patient is sometimes designated as a separate critical "P." In this chapter, maternal positions to facilitate labor and enhance comfort are included in the discussion under promoting comfort during labor. The coordination of the various factors that affect labor is essential for the labor and birth to progress in a successful manner.

POWERS

The powers are the physiological forces of labor and birth that include the uterine contractions and the maternal pushing efforts. The uterine muscular contractions, primarily responsible for causing cervical effacement and dilation, also move the fetus down toward the birth canal during the first stage of labor. Uterine contractions are considered the primary force of labor. Once the cervix is fully dilated, the maternal pushing efforts serve as an additional force. During the second stage of labor, use of the maternal abdominal muscles for pushing (the *secondary force* of labor) adds to the primary force to facilitate childbirth.

Characteristics of Uterine Contractions

Contractions are a rhythmic tightening of the uterus that occurs intermittently. Over time, this action shortens the individual uterine muscle fibers and aids in the process of cervical effacement and dilation, birth, and postpartal **involution** (the reduction in uterine size after birth). Each contraction consists of three distinct components: the **increment** (building of the contraction), the **acme** (peak of the contraction) and the **decrement** (decrease in the contraction).

Between contractions, the uterus normally returns to a state of complete relaxation. This rest period allows the uterine muscles to relax and provides the woman with a short recovery period that helps her to avoid exhaustion. In addition, uterine relaxation between contractions is important for fetal oxygenation as it allows for blood flow from the uterus to the placenta to be restored.

Contractions bring about changes in the uterine musculature. The upper portion of the uterus becomes thicker and more active. The lower uterine segment becomes thin-walled and passive. The boundary between the upper and lower uterine segments becomes marked by a ridge on the inner uterine surface, known as the "physiological retraction ring."

With each contraction, the uterus elongates. Elongation causes a straightening of the fetal body so that the upper body is pressed against the fundus and the lower, presenting part is pushed toward the lower uterine segment and the cervix. The pressure exerted by the fetus is called the fetal axis pressure. As the uterus elongates, the longitudinal muscle fibers are stretched upward over the presenting part. This force, along with the hydrostatic pressure of the fetal membranes, causes the cervix to dilate (open).

Assessment of Uterine Contractions

Contractions are often described in terms of their frequency, duration, and intensity. The **frequency** of a contraction is measured from the beginning of one contraction to the beginning of the next contraction. The **duration** of a contraction is measured from the start of one contraction to the end of the same contraction. The **intensity** of a contraction is most frequently measured by uterine palpation and is described in terms of mild, moderate, and strong (Fig. 12-1).

Palpation is a noninvasive procedure, and requires the nurse to place the fingertips of one hand on the fundus of the uterus where most contractions can be felt. The nurse applies gentle pressure and keeps the hand in the same place (moving the hand over the uterus may stimulate additional contractions, therefore interfering with the ability to accurately assess labor progress). Gentle palpation of the uterine fundus can determine the firmness of the uterus and whether there is an ability to indent the uterus at the acme (peak) of the contraction. Palpating the intensity of contractions is often compared to palpating one's nose (mild intensity), chin (moderate intensity), or forehead (strong intensity). When the uterine fundus remains soft at the acme of a contraction, the contraction intensity is described as "mild." Conversely, when there is an inability to indent the uterus at the acme of a contraction, the contraction intensity is described as "strong." "Moderate" contraction intensity falls somewhere in between and is characterized by a firm fundus that is difficult to indent with the fingertips. Several contractions must be evaluated to accurately determine the frequency, duration, and intensity.

Contractions may also be measured via electronic monitoring. Monitoring may be external or internal, and this modality can provide a continuous assessment of uterine activity. External contraction monitoring uses a **tocodynamometer**, which is a pressure-sensitive device that is applied against the uterine fundus. When the uterus contracts, the pressure that is exerted against the "toco" is measured and recorded on graph paper. External monitoring may be continuous or intermittent. It provides information about the frequency and duration of contractions, but may not give accurate data regarding the intensity of contractions because there are many variables (i.e., maternal position, obesity, and the placement of the monitor on the uterus) that can affect the tracing. Contraction intensity is best assessed with palpation.

Figure 12-1 Counting contractions. Contraction frequency is the time from the beginning of one contraction to the beginning of the next contraction. Contraction duration is the time from the beginning to the end of the same contraction.

Another method to measure the intensity of uterine contractions is an invasive procedure that involves the use of an internal monitor. If the amniotic membranes have ruptured, an internal pressure catheter is inserted through the cervix and into the uterus to measure the internal pressure generated during the contraction. Normally, the resting pressure in the uterus (between contractions) is 10 to 12 mm Hg. During the acme, contraction intensity ranges from 25 to 40 mm Hg during early labor, 50 to 70 mm Hg during active labor, 70 to 90 mm Hg during transition, and 70 to 100 mm Hg during maternal pushing in the second stage. Internal uterine pressure monitoring is most often used with high-risk pregnancies when accurate measurement of uterine activity is required. Since internal monitoring is an invasive procedure, it is associated with a slight risk of infection. (See Chapter 14 for further discussion.)

During early labor, uterine contractions are characteristically weak and irregular. They usually last for about 30 seconds and occur every 5 to 7 minutes. As the labor pattern becomes established, the uterine contractions typically become regular in frequency, longer in duration, and increased in intensity. The duration of contractions increases to about 60 seconds, and they occur every 2 to 3 minutes. The contractions are involuntary and are most efficient when there is a regular, rhythmic, coordinated labor pattern. The woman in labor is unable to control contraction frequency, duration, or intensity.

Uterine contractions also bring about changes in the pelvic floor musculature. The forces of labor cause the levator ani muscles and fascia of the pelvic floor to draw the rectum and vagina upward and forward. During descent, the fetal head exerts increasing pressure and causes thinning of the perineal body from 5 cm to less than 1 cm in thickness. Continued pressure causes the maternal anus to evert and the interior rectal wall is exposed as the fetal head descends forward (Cunningham et al., 2005).

Now Can You— Evaluate uterine contractions?

1. Discuss what is meant by the "powers" of labor?
2. Describe the terms used to evaluate contractions?
3. Identify two methods used to assess the intensity of contractions?

The coordinated efforts of the contractions help to bring about effacement and dilatation of the cervix. **Effacement** is the process of shortening and thinning of the cervix. As contractions occur, the cervix becomes progressively shorter until the cervical canal eventually disappears. The amount of cervical effacement is usually expressed as a percentage related to the length of the cervical canal, as compared to a noneffaced cervix. For example, if a cervix has thinned to half the normal length of a cervix it is considered to be 50% effaced. **Dilation** is the opening and enlargement of the cervix that progressively occurs throughout the first stage of labor. Cervical dilation is expressed in centimeters and full dilation is approximately 10 cm. With continued uterine contractions, the cervix eventually opens large enough to allow the fetal head to come through. At this point, the cervix is considered fully dilated or completely dilated and measures 10 cm (Fig. 12-2).

The first stage of labor, which begins with the onset of true labor, concludes when cervical effacement and dilation are complete. Effacement and dilation occur concurrently but at different rates. In a nulliparous patient, most cervical effacement is completed early during the process of cervical dilation whereas the multiparous cervix is often patulous (distended) before effacement begins.

Effacement and dilation are evaluated by a vaginal examination performed by a qualified practitioner such as a maternity nurse who has received specialized training in this procedure (Procedure 12-1). The vaginal examination provides important information regarding the diameter of the opening of the cervix, which ranges from 1 cm (not dilated) to 10 cm (fully dilated), the status of the amniotic membranes (ruptured or intact), and the fetal presentation and the station, or

Figure 12-2 Cervical effacement and dilation. The membranes are intact. *A.* Before labor. *B.* Early effacement. *C.* Complete (100%) effacement. The fetal head is well applied to the cervix. *D.* Complete dilation (10 cm). Note the overlapping of the cranial bones.

the extent of the fetal descent through the maternal pelvis. Once the cervix is fully dilated and retracted up into the lower uterine segment, it can no longer be palpated.

Maternal Pushing Efforts

After the cervix has become fully dilated, the laboring woman usually experiences an involuntary "bearing down" sensation that assists with the expulsion of the fetus. At this time, the woman can use her abdominal muscles to aid in the expulsion. It is important to remember that the cervix must be fully dilated before the patient is encouraged to push. Bearing down on a partially dilated cervix can cause cervical edema and damage and adversely affect the progress of the labor. For most women, the urge to bear down generally occurs when the fetal head reaches the pelvic floor. Women who have a strong urge to push often do so more effectively than women who force themselves to push without experiencing any sensations of pressure.

PASSAGEWAY

The passageway consists of the maternal pelvis and the soft tissues. The bony pelvis through which the fetus must pass is divided into three sections: the inlet, midpelvis (pelvic cavity), and outlet. Each of these pelvic components has a unique shape and dimension through which the fetus must maneuver to be born vaginally. In human females, the four classic types of pelvis are the gynecoid, android, platypelloid, and anthropoid. (See Chapter 5 for further discussion.)

PASSENGER

The passenger is referred to as the fetus and the fetal membranes. In the majority (96%) of pregnancies, the fetus presents in a head-first position. The fetal skull, usually the largest body structure, is also the least flexible part of the fetus. However, because of the sutures and fontanels, there is some flexibility in the fetal skull. These structures allow the cranial bones the capability of movement and they overlap in response to the powers of labor. The overlapping or overriding of the cranial bones is called **molding**.

A & P review   **The Fetal Skull**

The fetal skull, or cranium, consists of three major components: the face, the base of the skull, and the vault of the cranium (roof). The facial bones and the cranial base are fused and fixed. The cranial base is made up of two temporal bones and each has a sphenoid and ethmoid bone.

The cranial vault is composed of five bones: two frontal bones, two parietal bones, and the occipital bone. These bones, which are not fused, meet at the **sutures**. The sutures of the fetal skull are composed of strong but flexible connective tissue that fills the spaces that lie between the cranial bones.

The sagittal suture lies between the parietal bones and runs in an anteroposterior direction between the fontanels, dividing the head into a right and a left side. The lambdoidal suture extends from the posterior fontanel and separates the occipital bones from the parietal bones. The coronal sutures are located between the frontal and parietal bones. They extend from the anterior fontanel laterally and separate the parietal from the frontal bones. The frontal (mitotic) suture lies between the frontal bones and extends from the anterior fontanel to the prominence between the eyebrows.

Two membrane-filled spaces are present where the suture lines meet. These spaces are referred to as the anterior and posterior **fontanels**. The anterior fontanel is the larger of the two and measures approximately 0.8 × 1.2 inch (2 × 3 cm). It is diamond shaped and is positioned where the sagittal, frontal, and coronal sutures intersect. The anterior fontanel remains open until approximately 18 months of age to allow normal brain growth to occur. The posterior fontanel is triangular in shape and is much smaller than the anterior fontanel. It measures approximately 0.8 inch (2 cm) at its widest point. The posterior fontanel is positioned where the lambdoidal and sagittal sutures meet. Shaped like a small triangle, it closes at approximately 6 to 8 weeks after birth. The location of the fontanels assists the examiner in determining the position of the fetal skull during a

Procedure 12-1 Performing the Intrapartal Vaginal Examination

Purpose

Vaginal examination may be performed during the intrapartal period for many reasons including: assessment of cervical dilation, effacement and station, position and presentation of fetus, rupture of the membranes, and prolapse of the umbilical cord.

Equipment

- Sterile examination gloves (clean gloves may be used if the membranes are intact)
- Sterile lubricant
- Antiseptic solution and light source (if required)
- Disposable wipes

Steps

1. Wash and dry your hands. Explain the procedure and purpose of the examination to the patient.

   RATIONALE: *Hand washing helps to prevent the spread of microorganisms. Explanations help to decrease anxiety and promote patient understanding and cooperation.*

2. Assess for latex allergies.

   RATIONALE: *To prevent injury from latex exposure; if patient has a latex allergy, use nonlatex gloves.*

3. Ensure privacy.

   RATIONALE: *Privacy promotes comfort and self-esteem.*

4. Assemble necessary equipment including clean gloves (if the membranes are intact) or sterile examination gloves (if the membranes are ruptured), sterile lubricant, antiseptic solution (if required).

5. Position the patient in a supine position with a small pillow or towel under her hip to prevent supine hypotension. Instruct the patient to relax and position herself with her thighs flexed and abducted.

   RATIONALE: *Relaxation decreases muscle tension and enhances patient comfort. Proper positioning facilitates the examination by providing access to the perineum.*

6. Don sterile gloves (clean gloves may be used if the membranes are intact).

7. Inspect the perineum for any redness, irritation, or vesicles.

8. Using the nondominant hand, spread the labia majora and continue assessment of the genitalia. Note the presence of any discharge including blood or amniotic fluid.

   RATIONALE: *Positioning the hand in this manner facilitates good visualization of the perineum. The presence of lesions may be indicative of an infection and possibly preclude a vaginal birth. The presence of amniotic fluid implies that the membranes have ruptured. Bleeding may be a sign of placenta previa. Do not perform a vaginal examination if a placenta previa is suspected.*

9. Gently insert the lubricated gloved index and third fingers into the vagina in the direction of the posterior wall until they touch the cervix. The uterus may be stabilized by placing the nondominant hand on the woman's abdomen.

RATIONALE: *This position facilitates the examination by allowing the fingertips to point toward the umbilicus and find the cervix.*

10. Assess the cervix for effacement and the amount of dilation.

11. Assess for intact membranes; if fluid is expressed, test for amniotic fluid.

12. Palpate the presenting part.

    RATIONALE: *It is necessary to determine the presenting part in order to assess fetal position and evaluate fetal descent.*

13. Assess fetal descent and station by identifying the position of the posterior fontanel.

14. Withdraw the fingers. Assist the patient in wiping her perineum from front to back to remove lubricant or secretions. Help her to resume a comfortable position.

    RATIONALE: *Wiping from front to back prevents the transfer of rectal contamination toward the vagina.*

15. Inform the patient of the findings from the examination.

16. Wash hands.

17. Document the procedure on the patient's chart and on the fetal monitor strip (if a fetal monitor is being used). Include the assessment findings and the patient's tolerance of the procedure.

    RATIONALE: *Documentation provides a record for communication and evaluation of patient care.*

Documentation

6/8/09. 1235: Vaginal examination performed for assessment of labor. Cervix 4 cm dilated, 100% effaced, station 0. No membranes felt, patient leaking clear fluid from the vagina, position OA. Procedure tolerated well by patient, fetal heart rate 152 bpm post examination.

—L. Lopez, RN

vaginal examination. Important landmarks of the fetal skull are presented in Figure 12-3. ◆

The fetal skull contains several important landmarks (Box 12-2). There is much variation among the skull diameters. As molding occurs during labor, some skull diameters shorten while others lengthen. The head diameters are measured between the various skull landmarks. Most fetuses enter the maternal pelvis in the cephalic presentation but a number of variations are possible. The biparietal diameter is the major transverse diameter of the fetal head. It is measured between the two parietal bones and averages 3.7 inches (9.5 cm) in a term fetus. The anteroposterior diameter of the fetal head varies according to the degree of flexion. During labor, the most favorable situation occurs when the head becomes fully flexed and the anteroposterior diameter is the suboccipitobregmatic, which averages 3.7 inches (9.5 cm).

 Now Can You— **Discuss various factors associated with the process of labor?**

1. Define effacement and dilation?
2. Explain what is meant by the "passageway"?
3. Describe anatomical landmarks of the fetal skull?

Fetal Lie

The **fetal lie** refers to the relationship of the long axis of the woman to the long axis of the fetus (Fig. 12-4). If the head to tailbone axis of the fetus is the same as the woman's, the

> **Box 12-2** **Landmarks of the Fetal Skull**
>
> **Mentum:** fetal chin
> **Sinciput:** anterior area known as the "brow"
> **Bregma:** large, diamond-shaped anterior fontanel
> **Vertex:** the area between the anterior and the posterior fontanels
> **Posterior fontanel:** the intersection between the posterior cranial sutures
> **Occiput:** the area of the fetal skull that is occupied by the occipital bone, beneath the posterior fontanel (Fig. 12-3).

Figure 12-4 The fetal lie refers to the relationship of the long axis of the woman to the long axis of the fetus. *A.* Longitudinal lie. *B.* Transverse lie. *C.* Oblique lie.

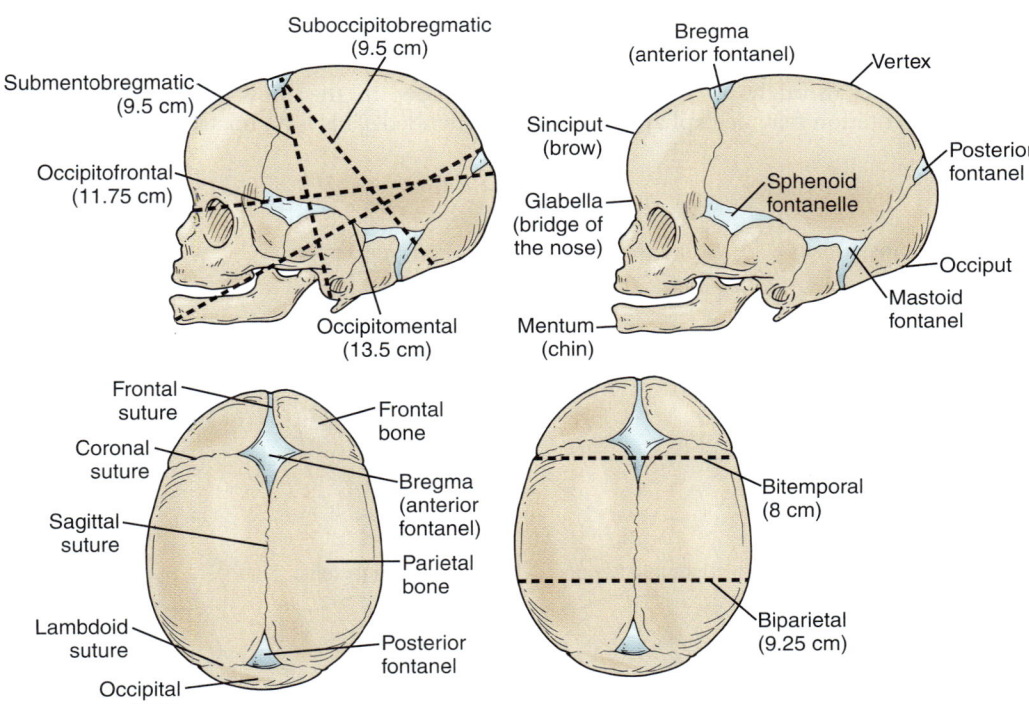

Figure 12-3 Bones, fontanels, and sutures of the fetal head. An understanding of the placement and relationships of these structures is essential in making an accurate assessment during the labor process.

fetus is in a **longitudinal lie**. In more than 99% of pregnancies, the lie is longitudinal. In the longitudinal lie, either the fetal head or the fetal buttocks enter the pelvis first. If the head to tailbone axis of the fetus is at a 90-degree angle to the woman, the fetus is in a **transverse** (horizontal) **lie**. A transverse lie occurs in fewer than 1% of pregnancies. An **oblique lie** is one that is at some angle between the longitudinal and the transverse lie.

Fetal Attitude

The fetal **attitude** describes the relationship of the fetus' body parts to one another. The fetus normally assumes an attitude of flexion. In this attitude, the fetal head is flexed so that the chin touches the chest, the arms are flexed and folded across the chest, the thighs are flexed on the abdomen, and the calves are flexed against the posterior aspects of the thighs. This is commonly referred to as the "fetal position."

In moderate flexion, the fetal chin is not touching the chest but is in an alert of "military position." This position causes the occipital frontal diameter to present to the birth canal. An attitude of moderate flexion usually does not interfere with labor because during descent and flexion the fetal head flexes fully. The fetus in partial extension presents the brow or face of the head to the birth canal.

Flexion of the fetal head (where the chin touches the chest) is the preferred position for birth because it allows the smallest anteroposterior diameter of the fetal skull to enter into the maternal pelvis. Any other position of the fetal head (other than that of complete flexion) will present with a larger anteroposterior diameter, which can ultimately contribute to a longer, more difficult labor (Fig. 12-5).

Fetal Presentation

The fetal **presentation** refers to the fetal part that enters the pelvic inlet first and leads through the birth canal during labor. The fetal presentation may be cephalic, breech,

Figure 12-5 The fetal attitude describes the relationship of the fetal body parts to one another. *A.* Flexion (vertex). *B.* Moderate flexion (military). *C.* Extension.

or shoulder. The part of the fetal body first felt by the examining finger during a vaginal examination is the "**presenting part.**" The presenting part is determined by the fetal lie and attitude.

CEPHALIC PRESENTATION. A **cephalic presentation** identifies that the fetal head will be first to come into contact with the maternal cervix. Cephalic presentations constitute the most desirable position for birth and occur in approximately 95% of pregnancies. There are four types of cephalic presentations (Fig. 12-6):

Vertex. The fetal head presents fully flexed. This is the most frequent and optimal presentation as it allows the smallest suboccipitalbregmatic diameter to present. It is called a "vertex presentation."

Military. In the military position, the fetal head presents in a neutral position, which is neither flexed nor extended. The occipitofrontal diameter presents to the maternal pelvis and the top of the head is the presenting part.

Brow. In the brow position, the fetal head is partly extended. This is an unstable presentation that converts to

Vertex presentation	Military presentation	Brow presentation	Face presentation
Complete flexion	Moderate flexion	Poor flexion (extension)	Full extension

Figure 12-6 There are four types of cephalic presentation; the vertex presentation with complete flexion is optimal. Fetal presentation refers to the fetal body part that first enters the maternal pelvis.

a vertex if the head flexes, or to a face presentation if the head extends. The occipitomental diameter (the largest anteroposterior diameter) presents to the maternal pelvis and the sinciput (fore and upper part of the cranium) is the presenting part.

Face. In the face presentation, the fetal head is fully extended and the occiput is near the fetal spine. The submentobregmatic diameter presents to the maternal pelvis and the face is the presenting part.

The following advantages are associated with a cephalic presentation:

- The fetal head is usually the largest part of the infant. Once the fetal head is born, the rest of the body usually delivers without complications.
- The fetal head is capable of molding. There is sufficient time during labor and descent for molding of the fetal head to occur. Molding helps the fetus to maneuver through the maternal birth passage.
- The fetal head is smooth and round, which is the optimal shape to apply pressure to the cervix and aid in dilation.

Other presentations (e.g., breech, shoulder) are associated with difficult, prolonged labor and often require cesarean births. They are called malpresentations.

 Now Can You— **Discuss passenger characteristics important during labor?**

1. Define "fetal lie" and identify three types of fetal lie?
2. Explain what is meant by "fetal attitude"?
3. Describe three advantages associated with a cephalic presentation?

BREECH PRESENTATION. A **breech** presentation occurs when the fetal buttocks enter the maternal pelvis first. Breech presentations occur in approximately 3% of births and are classified according to the attitude of the fetal hips and knees. Breech presentations are more likely to occur in preterm births or in the presence of a fetal abnormality such as hydrocephaly (head enlargement due to fluid) that prevents the head from entering the pelvis. They are also associated with abnormalities of the maternal uterus or pelvis. Since many factors can compromise the normal labor and birth process associated with breech presentations, delivery is usually accomplished via cesarean section. There are three types of breech presentations (Fig. 12-7):

Frank. The frank breech is the most common of all breech presentations. In the frank breech position, the fetal legs are completely extended up toward the fetal shoulders. The hips are flexed, the knees are extended, and the fetal buttocks present first in the maternal pelvis.

Complete (Full). The complete, or full, breech position is the same as the flexed position with the fetal buttocks presenting first. The legs are typically flexed. Essentially, this position is a reversal of the common cephalic presentation.

Footling. In the footling breech position, one or both of the fetal leg(s) are extended with one foot ("single footling") or both feet ("double footling") presenting first into the maternal pelvis.

Figure 12-7 There are three types of a breech presentation. *A.* Frank. *B.* Complete or full. *C.* Footling breech (single or double).

Several disadvantages are associated with a breech presentation:

- An increased risk for umbilical cord prolapse because the presenting part may not be covering the cervix (i.e., footling breech)
- The presenting part (buttocks, feet) is not as smooth and hard as the fetal head and is less effective in dilating the cervix
- Once the fetal body (abdomen) is delivered, the umbilical cord can become compressed. The fetus must then be delivered expeditiously to prevent hypoxia. Rapid delivery may be difficult since the fetal head is usually the largest body part and in this situation, there is no time to allow for molding.

In response to adverse outcomes that have been associated with vaginal breech births, the American College of Obstetricians and Gynecologists (ACOG, 2006) has published a Committee Opinion concerning planned breech deliveries.

SHOULDER PRESENTATION. The shoulder presentation is a transverse lie (Fig. 12-8). This presentation is rare and occurs in fewer than 1% of births. When a transverse lie is present, the maternal abdomen appears large from side to side, rather than up and down. In addition, the woman may demonstrate a lower than expected (for the gestational age) fundal height measurement. Although the shoulder is usually the presenting part, the fetal arm back, abdomen, or side may present in a transverse lie. This presentation occurs most often with preterm birth, high parity, prematurely ruptured membranes, hydramnios, and placenta previa. It is important for the nurse to promptly identify a transverse lie or shoulder presentation since the infant will almost always require a cesarean birth.

Figure 12-8 Shoulder presentation.

where research and practice meet:
The Planned Vaginal Breech Delivery

The American College of Obstetricians and Gynecologists (ACOG) published a Committee Opinion in July 2006, advising that in light of recent published studies that further clarify the long-term risks of vaginal breech delivery, "the mode of delivery should depend on the experience of the health care provider…Cesarean delivery will be the preferred mode for most physicians because of the diminishing expertise in vaginal breech delivery". A Randomized Controlled Trial (RCT) that included 2088 women found that perinatal mortality, neonatal mortality, or serious neonatal morbidity was significantly lower for the planned cesarean section group than for the planned vaginal birth group (Hannah et al., 2000). Currently, the standard of care in most practices is to deliver all breeches by cesarean section to avoid the potential complications of vaginal breech deliveries such as cord prolapse, head entrapment, birth asphyxia and birth trauma (Hacker, Moore, & Gambone, 2004).

 Now Can You— Discuss the breech and shoulder presentations?

1. Identify three types of breech presentations?
2. Explain three disadvantages of a breech presentation?
3. Describe how the nurse could identify a shoulder presentation?

PASSAGEWAY + PASSENGER

The passageway and the passenger have been identified as two of the factors that affect labor. The next "P" is the relationship between the passageway (maternal pelvis) and the passenger (fetus and membranes). The nurse assesses the relationship between the two when determining the engagement, station, and fetal position.

Engagement

Engagement is said to have occurred when the widest diameter of the fetal presenting part has passed through the pelvic inlet. In a cephalic presentation, the largest diameter is the biparietal; in breech presentations, it is the intertrochanteric diameter. Engagement can be determined by external palpation or by vaginal examination. In primigravidas, engagement usually occurs approximately 2 weeks before the due date. In multiparas, engagement may occur many weeks before the onset of labor or it may take place during labor. Although engagement confirms the adequacy of the pelvic inlet, it is not an indicator of the adequacy of the midpelvis and outlet.

Station

Station refers to the level of the presenting part in relation to the maternal ischial spines. In the normal female pelvis, the ischial spines represent the narrowest diameter through which the fetus must pass. The ischial spines, blunted prominences located in the midpelvis, have been designated as a landmark to identify station zero. To visualize the location of station zero, an imaginary line may be drawn between the ischial spines. Engagement has occurred when the presenting part is at station zero. When the presenting part lies above the maternal ischial spines, it is at a minus station. Therefore, a station of minus 5 (–5) cm indicates that the presenting part is at the pelvic inlet. Positive numbers indicate that the presenting part has descended past the ischial spines. A presenting part below the level of the ischial spines is considered to be a positive station. A station of +4 cm indicates that the presenting part is at the pelvic outlet (Fig. 12-9). During labor, the presenting part should continue to descend into the pelvis, indicating labor progress. As labor advances and the presenting part descends, the station should also progress to a numerically higher positive station. If the station does not change in the presence of strong, regular contractions, this finding may indicate a problem with the relationship between the maternal pelvis and the fetus ("cephalopelvic disproportion").

Position

Position refers to the location of a fixed reference point on the fetal presenting part in relation to a specific quadrant of the maternal pelvis (Fig. 12-10). The presenting part can be right anterior, left anterior, right posterior, and left posterior. These four quadrants designate whether the presenting part is directed toward the front, back, right, or left of the passageway.

Figure 12-9 Station.

Right occiput anterior (ROA)   Right occiput transverse (ROT)   Right occiput posterior (ROP)

Left occiput anterior (LOA)   Left occiput transverse (LOT)   Left occiput posterior (LOP)   Right mentum anterior (RMA)

Right mentum posterior (RMP)   Left mentum anterior (LMA)   Left sacrum anterior (LSA)   Left sacrum posterior (LSP)

Figure 12-10 Fetal presentations and positions. The position refers to how the presenting fetal part is positioned in relation to a specific quadrant of the maternal pelvis: front, back, or side.

Four landmarks of the fetus are used to describe the relationship of the presenting part to the maternal pelvis. In a vertex presentation, the occiput (O) is used. For a face presentation, the chin (M for mentum) is used. In a breech presentation, the sacrum (S) is used, and for a shoulder presentation, (A) for acromion process of the shoulder is used. Fetal position may be described as:

• Right (R) or left (L) side of the maternal pelvis
• The landmark of the presenting part: occiput (O), mentum (M), sacrum (S), acromion process (A)
• Anterior (A), posterior (P), transverse (T): This designation depends on whether the landmark is in the front, back, or side of the maternal pelvis

It is important for the nurse to assess the position of the fetus to identify whether the fetus is in an optimal position for a vaginal birth. To do so, the nurse uses inspection and palpation of the maternal abdomen and vaginal examination. Use of the abbreviated notations (listed above) helps to convey essential information to other members of the health care team. For example, when the fetal occiput is directed toward the maternal back (a posterior lie) and to the right of the birth passageway, the nurse would chart "ROP," to indicate right occiput–posterior. The fetal position most common, and most favorable for birth, is the right occiput–anterior (ROA). Identification of a malpresentation such as a footling breech or transverse lie is important, as the presence

of a malpresentation may signal the need for a cesarean delivery. Identification of a posterior lie may identify the potential for a longer labor as the fetus may attempt to rotate to an OA position. In addition, the nurse must be aware that the fetal position will vary as the fetus changes position to move through the different diameters of the maternal pelvis.

In some situations, the physician may have the option to attempt a fetal rotation. Prenatally, an external cephalic version may be performed in an attempt to rotate an identified breech presentation. A forceps rotation from a transverse or posterior position to an anterior position may also be indicated during a prolonged second stage of labor. However, as with any procedure, these maneuvers are associated with risks and benefits that must be presented to the patient for informed consent. (See Chapter 14 for further discussion.)

 critical nursing action Determining and Documenting Fetal Position

During the assessment, the nurse determines that the fetal occiput is in the right anterior quadrant of the maternal pelvis. The position is correctly documented as ROA. If the fetus were presenting in the frank breech position with the buttocks positioned to the left maternal posterior quadrant, the position would be correctly documented as LSP (left sacrum posterior).

Now Can You— Discuss the passageway and passenger?

1. Define engagement and identify when engagement has occurred?
2. List the four fetal landmarks used to describe the relationship of the presenting part?
3. Discuss why it is important for the nurse to assess fetal position during labor?

 Now Can You— Discuss the psychosocial influences of labor?

1. Describe why maternal psyche and cultural influences are important factors during labor?
2. Identify three culturally oriented nursing assessments for the laboring woman?
3. Discuss how maternal emotions can adversely affect the process of labor?

PSYCHOSOCIAL INFLUENCES

The first four Ps discussed address the physical forces of labor. The last "P" (psychosocial influences) acknowledges the many other critical factors that have an effect on parents such as their readiness for labor and birth, level of educational preparedness, previous experience with labor and birth, emotional readiness, cultural influences, and ethnicity. Transition into the maternal role, and most likely, into the paternal role as well, is facilitated by a positive childbirth experience. A number of internal and external influences can affect the woman's psychological well-being during labor and birth.

Culturally oriented views of childbirth help to shape the woman's expectations and ongoing perceptions of the birth experience. The nurse's understanding of the cultural values and expectations attached to childbirth provide a meaningful framework upon which to plan and deliver sensitive, appropriate care. Cultural considerations for the laboring woman encompass many elements of the birth experience including choice of a birth support person, strategies for coping with contractions, pain expression and relief and food preferences.

 Nursing Insight— Assessing cultural influences of the laboring patient

To provide culturally sensitive care to the laboring patient, the nurse should consider:

- The patient's and family's level of comfort with the nurse's "language" and whether an interpreter is needed
- Who is the designated birth support person and what will be the extent of this person's role
- The patient's level of comfort with touch
- If any special rituals or practices will be used during the childbirth experience

Studies have revealed that marked anxiety, fear, and fatigue can adversely affect the woman's ability to cope with the demands of labor. A negative childbirth experience can have far-reaching implications, interfering with bonding and maternal role attainment.

Emotional factors can have physiological implications as well. Maternal catecholamines (chemicals that affect the nervous and cardiovascular systems, metabolic rate, temperature, and smooth muscle) are often stimulated as a response to anxiety and fear and can inhibit uterine contractions and impede placental blood flow. During labor, the nurse's ongoing assessment of the maternal psyche along with appropriate interventions can help facilitate therapeutic communication to decrease or eliminate anxiety and fear through discussion and support.

Signs and Symptoms of Impending Labor

Before the onset of labor, a number of physiological changes occur that signal the readiness for labor and birth. These changes are usually noted by the primigravid woman at about 38 weeks of gestation. In multigravidas, they may not take place until labor begins. It is important for nurses to empower pregnant women and their families by teaching them about the signs and symptoms of impending labor. Providing guidelines about when to contact the health care provider or come to the birth facility helps to demystify the sometimes confusing events that surround birth and lessen the anxieties that can accompany the onset of labor.

LIGHTENING

At about 38 weeks in the primigravid pregnancy, the presenting part (usually the fetal head) settles downward into the pelvic cavity, causing the uterus to move downward as well. This process, called **lightening**, marks the beginning of engagement. As the uterus moves downward, the woman may state that her baby has "dropped." She may also report changes in the appearance of her abdomen such as a flattening of the upper area and an enhanced protrusion of the lower area. This downward settling of the uterus may decrease the upward pressure on the diaphragm and result in easier breathing. The downward settling may also lead to the following maternal symptoms:

- Leg cramps or pains
- Increased pelvic pressure
- Increased urinary frequency
- Increased venous stasis, causing edema in the lower extremities
- Increased vaginal secretions, due to congestion in the vaginal mucosa

BRAXTON-HICKS CONTRACTIONS

As the pregnancy approaches term, most women become more aware of irregular contractions called Braxton-Hicks contractions. As the contractions increase in frequency (they may occur as often as every 10 to 20 minutes), they may be associated with increased discomfort. Braxton-Hicks contractions are usually felt in the abdomen or groin region and patients may mistake them for true labor. It is believed that these contractions contribute to the preparation of the cervix and uterus for the advent of true labor. Braxton-Hicks contractions do not lead to dilation or effacement of the cervix, and thus are often termed "**false labor.**"

CERVICAL CHANGES

In the nonpregnant woman, the cervix is normally rigid. In preparation for passage of the fetus, the cervix undergoes many physiological changes. The cervix softens ("cervical ripening"), stretches, and thins, and eventually is taken up into the lower segment of the uterus. This softening and thinning is called cervical effacement.

BLOODY SHOW

During pregnancy the cervix is plugged with mucus. The mucus plug acts as a protective barrier for the uterus and its contents throughout the pregnancy. As the cervix begins to soften, stretch, and thin through effacement, there may be rupture of the small cervical capillaries. The added pressure created by engagement of the presenting part may lead to the expulsion of a blood-tinged mucus plug, called **bloody show**. Its presence often indicates that labor will begin within 24 to 48 hours. Late in pregnancy, vaginal examination that involves cervical manipulation may also produce a bloody discharge that can be confused with bloody show.

RUPTURE OF THE MEMBRANES

About 12% of pregnant women experience spontaneous rupture of the amniotic sac ("ruptured membranes" or "ruptured bag of waters") prior to the onset of labor. In the majority of pregnancies, the amniotic membranes rupture once labor is well established, either spontaneously or by **amniotomy**, the artificial rupture of the membranes by the primary care provider. Rupture of the membranes is a critical event in pregnancy. Assessment by the woman if rupture occurs at home, or by the nurse if it occurs in the birthing unit, is essential. If the membranes do rupture at home, the woman should be taught to immediately contact the nurse at the provider's office or at the birthing center who will advise her to report for an examination. It is important for the woman to note the color, amount, and odor of the amniotic fluid. The fluid should be clear and odorless. Often it contains white specks (vernix caseosa) and fetal hair (lanugo). A yellow-green tinged amniotic fluid may indicate infection or fetal passage of meconium and this finding always signals the need for further assessment and fetal heart rate monitoring. Urinary incontinence (frequently associated with urgency, coughing, and sneezing) is sometimes confused with ruptured membranes. The presence of amniotic fluid can be confirmed by a Nitrazine tape test or by a fern test (Procedure 12-2).

ENERGY SPURT

Toward the end of the pregnancy, some women experience a sudden increase in energy coupled with a desire to complete household preparations for the new baby. Some refer to this energy spurt as "nesting." The energy spurt may be related to an increase in the hormone adrenaline, which is needed to support the woman during the work of labor. Women should be cautioned not to overexert themselves doing household chores and instead to "store up" their energy for the childbirth process.

WEIGHT LOSS

Before the onset of labor, changes in the levels of estrogen and progesterone can lead to electrolyte shifts and may result in a reduction in fluid retention. The increased fluid loss can lead to a weight loss of up to 3 pounds (0.5 to 1.5 kg).

GASTROINTESTINAL DISTURBANCES

Some women experience gastrointestinal disturbances (diarrhea, nausea, vomiting or indigestion) as a sign of impending labor. The etiology of the gastrointestinal disturbances is generally unknown.

Distinguishing True Labor from False Labor

Recognizing the difference between true and false labor is important for the pregnant woman and her nurse (Table 12-1). True labor contractions lead to progressive dilation and effacement of the cervix. True labor contractions occur with regularity, and increase in frequency, duration, and intensity. The pain of true labor usually begins in the woman's lower back region, and radiates to the abdomen. The pain often intensifies with activity such as walking. In contrast, false labor contractions are irregular and usually do not change in intensity and duration. False labor does not lead to dilation and effacement of the cervix. The pain of false labor is usually felt in the abdominal region, and often stops with activities such as walking, position changes, and hot showers or other comfort measures.

Determining whether labor is true or false is an important assessment. Depending upon the findings, the nurse can help validate the next steps the woman should take. Any pregnant woman who arrives at the birth unit complaining of contractions must be carefully evaluated. After the assessment, if the maternity nurse confirms normal findings and intact membranes, the woman is sent home. For many, this can be a disappointing and frustrating experience. It is important for the nurse to provide reassurance that distinguishing true from false labor is difficult. Signs and symptoms of true labor should be reviewed in a sensitive, supportive manner, and the patient should be instructed about when to return to the birth unit.

Table 12-1 Distinguishing True from False Labor

True Labor	False Labor
• Contractions are at regular intervals.	• Contractions are irregular.
• Contractions increase in frequency, duration, and intensity.	• Usually there is no increase in frequency, duration, or intensity of contractions.
• Pains usually begin in lower back, radiating to the abdomen.	• Pains usually occur in the abdominal region.
• Dilation and effacement of the cervix are progressive.	• There is no change in the cervix.
• Activity such as walking usually increases labor pains.	• Walking may lessen the pain.

Procedure 12-2 Assessing for Amniotic Fluid

Purpose

Assessing for the presence of amniotic fluid helps determine whether the membranes have ruptured. There are two tests commonly used to detect amniotic fluid: the Nitrazine tape test and the fern test.

Equipment

- Nitrazine test tape
- Sterile gloves
- Sterile speculum
- Sterile cotton swab and glass slide
- Microscope

Steps

1. Wash and dry hands and explain the procedure and purpose of the examination to the patient, noting what she will experience, and what the results will indicate.

    RATIONALE: *Hand washing helps to prevent the spread of microorganisms. Explanations help to decrease anxiety and promote patient understanding and cooperation.*

2. Assess for latex allergies.

    RATIONALE: *To prevent injury from latex exposure; if the patient has a latex allergy, use nonlatex gloves.*

3. Ask the patient if she has noticed any leakage of fluid from her vagina.

4. Assess for the presence of amniotic fluid before other tests that require the use of lubricant (such as vaginal examination).

    RATIONALE: *Lubricant may alter the pH of amniotic fluid and contaminate the test result.*

5. Don sterile gloves. With one hand, spread the labia to expose the vaginal opening. With the other hand, place a 2-inch (5 cm) piece of Nitrazine tape against the vaginal opening, ensuring contact with enough fluid to wet the tape. Alternately, a sterile cotton-tipped applicator may be used to obtain fluid from the vagina. The applicator is then touched to the Nitrazine tape.

6. Remove the tape. Compare the color of the tape with the color guide on the Nitrazine tape container. If the tape turns blue-green, gray or deep blue, amniotic fluid is present. If the tape remains beige, no amniotic fluid has been detected.

    RATIONALE: *Amniotic fluid is alkaline, with a pH of 6.5 to 7.5. Urine and vaginal secretions are usually acidic.*

    Caution: Blood, Trichomonas vaginalis, and other substances may also turn the nitrazine test strip alkaline or blue.

7. When the Nitrazine test has not confirmed the presence of amniotic fluid, the nurse may insert a speculum and sterile cotton swab to collect a sample of fluid from the posterior vagina. The swab is smeared on a glass slide and allowed to dry. The glass slide is then placed on the microscope. The presence of a ferning pattern confirms the presence of amniotic fluid. The fern test is often indicated if premature rupture of the membranes (PROM) is suspected.

    RATIONALE: *Dried amniotic fluid shows a fern pattern due to its high estrogen content.*

8. Document the findings on the admission or labor record.

9. Inform the patient of the findings.

Documentation

8/30/09. 0430 Sterile speculum exam performed, large amount of clear, nonmalodorous fluid noted in vagina. Specimen obtained, fern test positive. Procedure tolerated well by patient, fetal heart rate 148 bpm by auscultation.

                                –L. Lopez, R.N.

"What to say" — *Questions to ask the patient who calls the birth unit*

A pregnant woman calls the birth unit to determine if she should come in for an evaluation or remain at home. The nurse conducts the telephone assessment by asking the following questions:

- "What is your due date?"
- "Are your membranes ruptured?" or "Did your water break?" and "Are you having any bleeding or vaginal discharge?"
- "Describe your contractions: When did they start? How frequent? How long? How strong?"
- "Is the fetus active?"
- "What helps with the discomfort?"
- "Who is with you?"

Now Can You— Identify true labor?

1. List four signs that may signify impending labor?
2. Compare and contrast signs of true labor versus false labor? Discuss how they can be differentiated?
3. Explain when a woman experiencing contractions at term should be instructed to go to the hospital?

Childbirth Settings and Labor Support

The decision about where to give birth is influenced by several factors: geographical location, socioeconomic status, the patient's preference, and the absence or presence of pregnancy complications. The size of the community often dictates the type and number of maternity health care facilities and the available primary care providers who may include family physicians, obstetricians, and certified nurse midwives (CNMs).

Large urban centers have hospitals with birthing units or birthing centers. Some of the units may offer labor options such as whirlpool baths. Other settings may provide a home-like environment for the expectant couple. Taking a tour of the available birth settings as part of prenatal education classes can help the pregnant woman and her partner develop an understanding of what to expect during the childbirth experience.

The woman's socioeconomic status and whether or not she has health insurance also affect the choices available for labor and birth. Some pregnant women who have no pregnancy complications may choose to have their prenatal care and birth managed by a CNM, and they may also plan for a home birth.

The patient usually determines whether or not a support person accompanies her to the birthing unit and remains throughout the labor and birth. This decision is based on personal preferences, and may reflect cultural or religious practices. The woman's partner or the baby's father is the most common labor support person, although the woman's mother or friend may also serve as a support person especially if the patient is single. The nurse can identify the patient's preference for a support person by asking a question such as, "Who is the main person that you want to stay with you during labor?"

In some centers, women may use a **doula** as a labor support person. The doula is a woman who has received professional training and is experienced in childbirth. The doula's role is to provide continuous information and physical and emotional support to the woman and her partner before, during, and immediately after the birth. She does not function in a clinical role but instead specializes in providing comfort measures to decrease the woman's anxiety. Breathing techniques, application of hot and cold, and massage are strategies often used to enhance comfort and the progress of labor.

The doula assists the family in gathering information concerning the labor process and available options before childbirth. If a cesarean birth is required, the doula may accompany the laboring woman into the surgical suite. Doulas also provide some postpartum services. In some situations, the family hires the doula. Doulas can be paid hospital employees or volunteer doulas may be available in certain settings. When needed, the bilingual doula can be an essential team member in helping to promote a positive childbirth experience for the woman and her family.

 Now Can You— **Discuss childbirth settings and support persons?**

1. Discuss various childbirth settings and factors that may influence the woman's choice?
2. Describe the role of a doula?

Routine Hospital and Birth Center Admission Procedures

In the third trimester it is important for the prenatal care nurse to explain the differences between true and false labor, and to teach the patient about when to go to the birthing center. Table 12-2 summarizes the circumstances that warrant going to the birthing center. The nurse should reinforce this information during each prenatal visit.

 Be sure to— **Understand federal regulations that relate to obstetric care**

The federal regulation known as *The Emergency Medical Treatment and Active Labor Act (EMTALA)* was created to ensure that all women receive emergency treatment or active labor care whenever such treatment is sought. Under the EMTALA regulation, true labor is considered to be an emergency medical condition. Thus the nurse working in a birthing unit must be familiar with the full range of responsibilities included in the EMTALA regulations: (1) provide services to pregnant women when an urgent pregnancy problem such as labor, rupture of the membranes, decreased fetal movement, or recent trauma is experienced and (2) fully document all relevant information to include assessment findings, interventions implemented and the patient's response to the care provided. Any pregnant woman who presents to an obstetric triage is considered to be experiencing "true labor" until a qualified health care provider determines that she is not (Angelini & Mahlmeister, 2005; Caliendo, Millbauer, Moore, & Kitchen, 2004).

where research and practice meet:
Home-like Birth Settings

In this Cochrane review of home-like versus conventional institutional settings for birth, Hodnett, Downe, Edwards, and Walsh (2005) reviewed six trials of 8677 women. The findings revealed a number of benefits associated with home-like settings for childbirth: increased maternal satisfaction with the intrapartum care; increased initiation and continuation of breastfeeding; an increased incidence of spontaneous vaginal births; and a reduced likelihood of medical interventions including analgesia/anesthesia and episiotomies. Despite these positive findings, the review also demonstrated an association between home-like birth settings and increased perinatal mortality. The authors concluded that although a home-like birth setting with its focus on normality is associated with modest benefits, care providers need to monitor patients closely for complications, regardless of the setting for labor and birth.

Table 12-2 Providing Patient Guidelines for Reporting to the Birthing Center

Questions to Ask the Patient	Guidelines for Admission
Describe your contractions: frequency, duration, and intensity?	Primigravida: Contractions are regular, occur about every 5 minutes for at least 1 hour.
	Multipara: Contractions are regular, occur about every 10 minutes for at least 1 hour.
Have your membranes ruptured?	*Any* gush of fluid needs to be evaluated, even if there are no contractions.
Is there any vaginal bleeding?	The mucus plug or "bloody show" is usually pink or dark red. Any bright red bleeding requires immediate evaluation.
Has there been a decrease in the movement of the baby?	Any decrease in fetal movement signals the need to report to the birthing center.
Has there been any change in your health?	Any cause for worry or anxiety in the pregnant woman needs to be explored by the nurse and may lead to admission.

Once the woman arrives at the birthing center, the role of the nurse is twofold: to establish a positive relationship with the patient and her family and support person and to assess the status of the patient and her fetus.

ESTABLISHING A POSITIVE RELATIONSHIP

The onset of labor is a time of many emotions for the woman and her family. There can be excitement, fear, and anxiety. The role of the nurse in recognizing these emotions and creating a caring, trusting relationship is paramount to a positive birth experience. The nurse needs to respect individual differences in the woman's knowledge and understanding of childbirth, as well as recognize the cultural or religious practices that may influence the experience. The nurse needs to remain nonjudgmental, particularly with patients who have not had adequate prenatal care or who have made unhealthy lifestyle choices during the pregnancy.

To foster a positive and therapeutic relationship, the nurse creates an atmosphere that encourages questions and the sharing of information. Some women have prepared written childbirth plans that describe their expectations of the experience. Getting to know each patient's expectations for her childbirth experience constitutes an important element in the relationship. The nurse must also recognize when an interpreter is needed to assist in the understanding and exchange of information.

Touch is an integral aspect of the nurse–patient relationship during labor and birth. Touch can convey caring and provide comfort. The nurse continuously assesses the patient's response to touch and provides intimate care that is culturally sensitive.

COLLECTING ADMISSION DATA

The nurse uses multiple sources and data collection methods to compile a comprehensive database to plan and deliver individualized care to the woman in labor. The prenatal record provides data regarding the current pregnancy and previous pregnancies and birth outcomes for the multiparous woman. Measurements such as maternal weight gain, fundal height, blood pressure, fetal heart rate patterns, laboratory values such as blood type and Rh factor, results from diagnostic tests such as amniocentesis, non-stress tests, and ultrasound examinations provide the basis for determining intrapartal risk.

The admission interview provides the nurse with information about the woman's reason for coming to the birthing center, her understanding and expectations of the labor and birth process, her subjective experience of the labor, as well as psychosocial and cultural factors that can impact her birth experience. The fetal assessment, including presentation, fetal heart rate (FHR), and movement provides essential data regarding fetal well-being. Maternal vital signs, particularly blood pressure and temperature, as well as the assessment of current labor status (uterine contraction patterns, cervical dilatation, and effacement, fetal station, rupture of membranes) provide important baseline labor data. A systematic physical assessment provides the nurse and other care providers with overall health data, and various laboratory tests, such as hematocrit, blood glucose, and HIV status, give further direction for the individual plan of care.

Initial Admission Assessments

For women who have received prenatal care, the prenatal care record is sent to the birthing center prior to the expected due date. The information is stored and readily available when the laboring patient reports there for care. Women without a prenatal care record require a more extensive assessment upon admission to the birth setting.

THE FOCUSED ASSESSMENT

On admission to the birthing unit, the nurse initiates a focused assessment to determine the condition of the mother and fetus and the progression of the labor. The data collected answers these critical questions and helps the nurse to establish priorities for care:

- Is this true labor, and if so, is birth imminent?
- Are there any factors that increase risk to the mother or fetus?

The nurse assesses the fetus' well-being by recording the FHR and noting the FHR in response to uterine contractions. The nurse also assesses fetal movement. If the woman reports that her membranes have ruptured, the nurse validates the presence of amniotic fluid using Nitrazine tape (see Procedure 12-2), and examines the amniotic fluid for color and odor.

The nurse assesses the patient's vital signs to establish a baseline for comparison during the labor and birth. An elevation in blood pressure may be a sign of pregnancy-induced hypertension (PIH). An elevated temperature may signal infection. The nurse also assesses the progression of the labor by monitoring the pattern of uterine contractions for frequency, duration, and intensity. The nurse further assesses the labor status by evaluating cervical dilatation and effacement, and fetal station, presentation, and position.

A patient who states "I feel like pushing" may be indicating that the birth is imminent. Important questions to ask this patient upon admission include the following:

- What is your name? Your support person's name?
- Have you received prenatal care? Who is your care provider?
- How many pregnancies and births have you had? Were the deliveries vaginal or cesarean? Were there any difficulties with previous deliveries?
- What is your due date? When was your last normal menstrual period?
- Have your membranes ruptured? What time? Describe the fluid.
- Have you had any complications with this pregnancy?
- Do you have any allergies?
- Describe your contractions—mild, moderate, or intense. When did your contractions begin? How are you coping?
- Are you taking any medications—prescribed and/or over-the-counter? Do you use illegal/street drugs? Do you smoke? Do you drink alcoholic beverages?
- When did you last eat or drink anything and what was it?
- Have you prepared a birth plan? Do you have any cultural preferences related to your labor and birth?

If the nurse determines that the fetal or maternal assessments are not normal, or that the birth is imminent, the physician or primary care provider is notified immediately. If the assessments are normal, and birth does not appear to be imminent, the nurse can then complete a more thorough admission assessment, which would include a systematic physical assessment.

THE PSYCHOSOCIAL ASSESSMENT

An important, yet sometimes challenging part of the data collection is the psychosocial assessment. Understanding the woman's behavioral responses to the pregnancy and childbirth experience allows the nurse to support and strengthen the identified coping mechanisms. Obtaining information that addresses questions such as "What was the previous birth experience like?" "How is the patient handling the labor pain?" and "Who is providing labor support for her?" helps the nurse to better meet the patient's and her support person's needs.

The nurse completes a social assessment, collecting information about the woman's family and support systems and living conditions. Questions about family violence can be particularly difficult. If the nurse suspects partner abuse, the patient should be interviewed alone in a private place where she feels safe.

Assessing the woman's social and lifestyle habits can also be difficult. Questions about drug and alcohol use and sexually transmitted infections are often embarrassing. The nurse can facilitate the sharing of this information through the establishment of a caring and nonjudgmental relationship with the patient.

❝What to say❞ — *Asking the difficult questions*

Asking closed-ended questions such as "Do you drink alcohol?" may elicit a quick "No" response. Asking more directed and open questions such as "How many drinks do you have each day?" may encourage a more detailed response. The nurse should remember that a caring and nonjudgmental attitude, in a private, nonthreatening environment, helps to foster a trusting nurse–patient relationship.

THE CULTURAL ASSESSMENT

To provide care that is culturally relevant, the nurse must assess the patient's cultural preferences, practices, and values related to labor and childbirth. Issues such as care provider gender preference, comfort level with intimate touch, and the presence or absence of a labor support person may be culturally determined. The woman's responses to the labor pain, her acceptance or rejection of labor support interventions, and her emotional responses to the newborn can be culturally based.

LABORATORY TESTS

Laboratory testing is a routine component of the admission process. Tests for blood type and Rh factor, complete blood count, hemoglobin and hematocrit, and blood glucose are generally obtained. Blood tests for syphilis, hepatitis B, and HIV are also collected. The urine specimen is tested for the presence of protein, glucose, and ketones.

Documentation of Admission

Each birth setting has documentation forms and set protocols to be completed with patient admissions. Collecting a complete health and childbirth history and performing a physical examination of the patient and her fetus provide an essential foundation for the care and support to be given during labor and birth. Once the admission assessments have been completed, the nurse documents the information using the birth setting's recording procedures, notifies the patient's primary care provider of the admission status, and receives orders. Critical information to relay to the physician or nurse-midwife includes:

- Patient's name and age
- Gravidity and parity
- Gestational age and estimated date of delivery
- Labor status: pattern of contractions, cervical dilatation and effacement, fetal presentation and station
- Status of membranes
- Fetal heart rate and response to contractions
- Patient's vital signs, especially blood pressure and temperature
- Any identified risk to maternal or fetal well-being
- Patient's coping ability in response to labor

After admission, the patient and her fetus are assessed frequently to monitor both the progression of labor and the responses of both to the labor. Throughout each stage of labor, ongoing maternal assessments include vital signs, intake and output, pattern of contractions, cervical dilatation and effacement, and response to labor. Fetal assessments, which primarily center on the response to labor, involve intermittent or continuous FHR monitoring.

First Stage of Labor

The first stage of labor is often referred to as the stage of dilation. This stage begins with the onset of regular uterine contractions and ends with complete dilation of the cervix. The onset of labor is often made retrospectively since the woman may not always recognize when true labor actually begins. The contractions often start slowly and are fairly tolerable. Over time, contractions tend to increase in frequency, duration, and intensity as the first stage of labor progresses. The first stage of labor is most often the longest stage and its duration can vary considerably among women. The first stage of labor is divided into three distinct phases: latent, active, and transition. Multiparous women tend to progress through the childbirth process much more rapidly than do nulliparous women. Factors such as analgesia, maternal and fetal position, the woman's body size and her level of physical fitness can also affect the length of labor.

LATENT PHASE

The **latent phase** of labor begins with the establishment of regular contractions (labor pains). Labor pains are often initially felt as sensations similar to painful menstrual cramping and are usually accompanied by low back pain. Contractions during this phase are typically about 5 minutes apart, last 30 to 45 seconds, and are considered to be mild. During this phase, the woman is usually excited about labor commencing and she remains chatty and sociable. Often this phase of labor is completed at home. During the latent phase cervical effacement and early dilation (0 to 3 cm) occurs. The latent phase of labor can last as long as 10 to 14 hours as the contractions are mild and cervical changes occur slowly.

ACTIVE PHASE

The **active phase** of labor is characterized by more active contractions. The contractions become more frequent (every 3 to 5 minutes), last longer (60 seconds), and are of a moderate to strong intensity. During the active labor phase, the woman becomes more focused on each contraction and tends to draw inward in an attempt to cope with the increasing demands of the labor. Cervical dilation during this phase advances more quickly as the contractions are often more efficient. While the length of the active phase is variable, nulliparous women generally progress at an average speed of 1 cm of dilation per hour and multiparas at 1.5 cm of cervical dilation per hour.

TRANSITION PHASE

The **transition phase** is the most intense phase of labor. Transition is characterized by frequent, strong contractions that occur every 2 to 3 minutes and last 60 to 90 seconds on average. Fortunately, this phase often does not take long because dilation usually progresses at a pace equal to or faster than active labor (1 cm/hr for a nullipara and 1.5 cm/hr for a multipara). During the transition phase, the laboring woman may feel that she can no longer continue or she may question her ability to cope with much more. Other sensations that a woman may feel during transition include rectal pressure, an increased urge to bear down, an increase in bloody show, and spontaneous rupture of the membranes (if they have not already ruptured). Table 12-3 presents a summary of the characteristics of the first and second stages of labor.

A labor curve assessment tool, often referred to as a "Friedman curve," is a graph used to help identify whether a patient's labor is progressing in a normal pattern (Fig. 12-11). Composite normal labor patterns are graphically presented for the multiparous and nulliparous patient. The labor curve assessment tool contains categories that include the time of day, amount of cervical dilation, and effacement and hours of labor that have elapsed. The patient's own labor progress is plotted on the graph to allow a comparison between her progress and the norm.

 Now Can You— **Identify characteristics of the first and second stages of labor?**

1. Define the characteristics of the first and second stages of labor including contractions, dilation, and maternal response?
2. Describe the three phases of the first stage of labor and the changes that occur during each phase?
3. Explain the value of using a labor curve assessment tool?

NURSING CARE DURING THE FIRST STAGE OF LABOR

Cunningham and associates (2005) noted that there are two opposing priorities in the ideal management of labor:

- Birthing should be recognized as a normal physiological process and should be treated as such.
- Intrapartum complications can arise quickly and unexpectedly and therefore should be anticipated.

There are several key roles for the nurse who is providing care for the woman in labor. It is essential that the nurse continually assess the patient and her fetus to ensure a safe delivery, help to facilitate a positive birth experience, assist in the satisfactory management of pain, and advocate for the patient's needs.

It is important to remember that nursing interventions must first be safe and consistent with the current standard of care. Interventions are also tailored to meet the individual needs and preferences of the woman in labor. The patient's needs may quickly change throughout the process of labor. For example, during early labor the woman may be very independent and in little need of assistance. During active labor or transition, the needs often become very different. Research has shown that during labor, support by nurses has a positive effect on maternal and fetal outcomes.

Table 12-3   Characteristics of the First and Second Stages of Labor

	First Stage	Second Stage
Definition	Commences with the onset of regular contractions and ends with full dilation (10 cm) of the cervix.	Begins with full dilation of the cervix (10 cm) and ends with the expulsion (birth) of the fetus.
Contractions	Latent: 5–10 minutes, may be irregular in frequency, duration 30–40 seconds, mild to moderate strength. Active: Regular pattern established (2–5 minutes apart), 40–60 seconds duration and moderate to strong by palpation. Transition: 2–3 minutes apart lasting 60–90 seconds, strong by palpation.	Contractions continue at a similar rate as during the transition phase; 2–3 minutes apart lasting 60 seconds and strong by palpation.
Dilation	Latent: 0–3 cm Active: 4–7 cm Transition: 8–10 cm	Fully dilated
Physical discomforts	Latent: Contractions often begin as painful menstrual-like cramps or low backache. Active: Increasing discomfort as contractions become stronger and more regular. May have backache. Transition: Increasing discomfort as contractions are very strong with little time for relaxation in between. As the fetal head descends there may be an increase in rectal pressure and the urge to push.	May have an urge to push that increases as the fetal head descends. Many women prefer to push so that they can use the contractions and work with them. When head is crowning may feel intense pain, burning.
Maternal behaviors	Latent: Pain often well controlled; various behaviors may be present: excited, talkative, confident, anxious, withdrawn Stage may be completed at home. Active: Needs to focus more on staying in control and managing the pain; often requires coaching at this stage; quieter and more inwardly focused. Transition: Most intense phase. Often difficult to cope; may experience various emotions: irritable, agitated, hopeless ("can't do it"); tired (sleeps between contractions).	Often during this stage many women get a "second wind" as they see that they are making progress and are embarking on a new (labor) phase. Intense concentration with pushing efforts.

Figure 12-11 A labor curve assessment tool, often referred to as a "Friedman curve," helps to identify whether a patient's labor is progressing in a normal pattern.

A recent systematic review that included 15 trials involving 12,791 women in 11 countries was conducted to assess the effects of continuous one-to-one labor support on mothers and their infants (Hodnett, Gates, Hofmeyr, & Sakala, 2006). The researchers found that women who were provided with one-to-one continuous support in labor were more likely to give birth without using analgesia or anesthesia, more likely to experience a spontaneous vaginal birth, and less likely to report dissatisfaction with their childbirth experience. Additional findings were that the positive effects of continuous one-to-one support increased when the support occurred from women who did not have any other responsibilities other than providing support to the laboring woman. Further, support begun early in the labor process appeared to be more effective than support initiated later in labor. Early and continuous support for women in labor should be encouraged whenever possible as an essential component of standard care.

Labor Support

Whenever possible, continuous labor support should be given to women in labor. Providing this level of care has been associated with positive outcomes for mothers and infants and there have been no documented harmful or adverse effects. Continuous labor support can be provided by professional nurses or by lay people.

PRESENCE

Presence is one method of providing continuous support. Offering one's presence in labor can be defined simply as "physically being with the woman." Women find that having a nurse present can be reassuring because they recognize that assistance is available when needed. Studies have demonstrated that "women want the nurse to be available, to be emotionally involved, to help create a special moment, to hear and respond to their concerns, to share the responsibilities for keeping them safe, and to act as a go-between for their family and the medical institution" (MacKinnon, McIntyre, & Quance, 2005, p. 32). Unfortunately, other studies have demonstrated that nurses may not be actually providing this type of care for several different reasons such as inadequate staffing, lack of time, lack of training, hospital practices that emphasize technological care, and resistance from physicians (Simkin, 2002). Nurses are especially adept in providing therapeutic labor support because their educational background emphasizes a caring, holistic approach that centers not only on knowledge of the labor process and supportive techniques but also on empowerment of the woman experiencing childbirth.

PROMOTION OF COMFORT

Position Changes

In labor, frequent position changes are beneficial in helping to promote the descent of the fetus. The nurse may assist the laboring woman to various positions and activities such as walking, standing, sitting, squatting, leaning over a piece of furniture, or assuming a hands and knees position (Fig. 12-12). Maternal preferences can guide the nurse in assessing which positions or activities the woman finds most comfortable. Each position is associated with advantages and disadvantages (Box 12-3). During early labor, women are often encouraged to remain ambulatory since activity has been shown to enhance the normal progression of labor.

As labor advances the woman may feel tired and in need of some relaxation between contractions. Sitting in a chair and reclining on the side are two positions that often bring comfort. Changes in the patient's status such as continuous fetal monitoring, premature rupture of the membranes, or epidural analgesia may necessitate a need for bedrest. In these situations, the nurse should encourage the laboring woman to rest on her left side

Figure 12-12 Various positions for labor and birth.

Box 12-3 Advantages and Disadvantages of Various Positions for Labor

WALKING/STANDING
Utilizes gravity, facilitates descent, places fetus in alignment with pelvis, may decrease the length of labor by enhancing the effect of contractions.
　May be tiring, requires telemetry for continuous electronic fetal monitoring, may not be possible with regional anesthesia.

SITTING
Utilizes gravity, increases pelvic diameter and shortens second-stage labor, avoids supine hypotension syndrome, decreases back pain, enhances communication with partner and allows for ready access to back and sacrum for massage and counterpressure.
　Labor may be slowed if not alternated with other positions, may intensify suprapubic pain and cause edema of the vulva or cervix.

HANDS AND KNEES POSITION
Stimulates rotation of fetus from a posterior to an anterior position, relieves backache and rectal pressure, facilitates pelvic rocking and pelvic mobility.
　May be tiring or embarrassing, difficult to keep external fetal monitor in place, may not be possible with regional anesthesia.

SQUATTING
Utilizes gravity, increases pelvic diameter, relieves backache, promotes fetal descent and rotation, facilitates second-stage pushing.
　May impede descent before engagement has occurred, may be tiring, uncomfortable, or embarrassing, may increase perineal and cervical edema.

---

to facilitate optimal uteroplacental blood flow. In addition, position changes should be encouraged even if the woman must remain in bed. If bedrest is necessary, the nurse may be able to assist the woman into a variety of positions in bed. Sitting, getting on hands and knees, or resting on alternate sides may be desirable, depending on the patient's condition and preferences. It is important to avoid the supine position since the pressure of the uterus on the maternal spine can cause compression of the inferior vena cava and lead to decreased blood pressure and diminished uteroplacental blood flow.

Personal Comfort Measures

Nurses can provide personal comfort measures for the laboring woman based on her preferences and needs. For example, assistance with basic hygiene, back rubs, ice chips, or application of a cold cloth may be quite comforting. Family members and support persons should be encouraged to remain with the woman and help to meet her personal comfort needs.

ENVIRONMENT. The woman or her family may prefer to have the lights dimmed to create a relaxing atmosphere. Conversely, other women and families may prefer to have the sun streaming into the room. During active labor the woman may verbalize heat intolerance (being too hot) due to the physical work and energy expenditure required in labor. An electric fan may be beneficial in providing a cooling breeze. Nurses must remember to turn off the fan or assess the room temperature during childbirth to ensure that the infant does not get unnecessarily chilled.

PERSONAL HYGIENE. As needed, the nurse can help promote the patient's sense of cleanliness and well-being by changing pads, linens, or gown especially if the woman is leaking amniotic fluid or bloody show. Many women who remain ambulatory are able to perform their own personal care. However, if the laboring woman is confined to bed or exhausted from the exertion of labor, full assistance should be provided.

Frequent mouth care should be encouraged since dry mouth is common during labor. Providing fluids to drink, ice chips, popsicles, or hard candy may help to alleviate the symptoms. In addition, the use of mouthwash or brushing the teeth may be especially beneficial following vomiting. Nurses should be aware that different institutional policies exist regarding oral intake in labor and remain knowledgeable of the policies and procedures that affect their practice.

ELIMINATION. A full bladder can inhibit the descent of the fetus and contribute to increased pain with contractions. Encouraging and assisting the woman to the toilet (or bedpan) to void at least every 2 hours is recommended. If the woman is unable to void and has a distended bladder a urinary catheter may be required.

SUPPORTIVE RELAXATION TECHNIQUES. During labor, the nurse may encourage, assist, or teach the woman about different interventions to help decrease pain and relieve anxiety. Relaxation techniques may include visualization, focal points, imagery, hydrotherapy, and breathing techniques. In addition, patients may bring items from home to enhance relaxation such as music, a picture, or a stuffed animal. (See Chapter 13 for further discussion.)

---

where research and practice meet:
Taiwanese Women's Perceptions of Helpful and Nonhelpful Nursing Behaviors During Labor

A major role of the labor and delivery nurse is to create a positive and satisfying birth experience. In order to determine what nursing interventions laboring women found most helpful, a study of Taiwanese women's perspectives about their encounters with obstetric nurses during labor was conducted. The results indicated that the majority (68%) of the women reported having received only helpful nursing behaviors, as compared with other study participants who reported both helpful and nonhelpful nursing interventions. Nursing interventions that were identified as helpful include: performing roles of emotional support provider, comforter, information/advice provider, professional technical skills provider, and advocate. The women who reported having received both helpful and nonhelpful nursing interventions (38%) stated that their nurses failed to provide emotional support or comfort measures, give adequate or correct information/advice, or perform technical duties. The results of this research are similar to findings from other studies conducted with North American women. The findings suggest that nursing interventions can have either a positive or negative effect on women's overall birthing experiences. This research identifies desirable personal qualities of labor nurses and many professional tasks that they should perform. During the birth experience, ideal nursing interventions should include the provision of ongoing emotional support and comfort, information and advice, professional and technical skills, and, in every activity, the nurse should serve as a patient advocate (Chen, Wang, & Chang, 2001).

Now Can You— **Provide comforting nursing care during labor?**

1. List four examples of nursing interventions that patients have identified as helpful in promoting comfort and relaxation?
2. Identify three beneficial positions for the laboring woman who is confined to bedrest?
3. Describe what is meant by "presence"?

ANTICIPATORY GUIDANCE

Providing anticipatory guidance for the woman and her family constitutes an essential role of the obstetric nurse. Regardless of whether or not they have attended prenatal classes, most women and their families have many questions. Anticipatory guidance should be provided throughout the childbirth experience. Women and families usually want to know what to expect. While the nurse cannot predict exactly what will happen, helpful information can be provided in general terms. For example, a woman in early active labor may comment: "These contractions are getting stronger, how strong will they get?" The nurse can empower the woman by identifying the progress she has made to that point. Explaining how the contractions have gradually become stronger and emphasizing how successful the patient has been in adjusting to the changes provides factual feedback and positive reinforcement of the progress made. In addition, the nurse may suggest comfort measures such as relaxing in a whirlpool bath or shower for later on when the contractions become stronger.

 ❝What to say❞ — *Positive, encouraging words during labor*

During labor the patient needs encouragement with positive words regarding what she is doing well even when she may not be coping at her optimal ability. Nurses must be careful not to use language that may be discouraging for the woman such as "This is just the beginning. It is going to get much worse." Instead, nurses should offer comments such as "Try focusing on one contraction at a time" or "See if you can concentrate on relaxing more between the contractions" followed by "That is really great, keep going, excellent, now let's try that again with the next one."

Keeping the woman and her family informed about the process of labor and birth is a constant and ever changing task. For example, during the transition phase the nurse may be teaching the woman breathing techniques to avoid pushing with a partially dilated cervix. In a matter of minutes, the patient can reach full cervical dilation. The nurse then teaches her how to push and may need to assist the woman into an effective pushing position.

CARING FOR THE BIRTH PARTNER

Obviously, most of the nurse's attention focuses on the woman in labor. Efforts also should be made to help the support person feel welcome and included whenever possible according to the woman's wishes. Orientation to the birth unit is helpful in identifying where to locate items such as towels and washcloths, kitchen supplies (ice chips), and the restroom.

Assessment of the degree of involvement the support person would like to assume is also important. It is helpful to determine whether or not the patient and labor partner have attended childbirth preparation classes and give respect to the support person for their identified wishes and or limitations. In some cultures, assistance at the birth might be considered "woman's work" and the laboring woman instead seeks support from a sister, mother, and aunt while the husband stays at home or assumes more of an observational role.

ENSURING CULTURE-CENTERED CARE

Providing care that is culturally appropriate is as important in caring for laboring women and their families as with any other patients. It is unrealistic to expect nurses to be knowledgeable about the cultural traditions and customs of all patients. However, it is important for nurses to remain open minded and aware that there are a myriad of values, attitudes, beliefs, and practices regarding childbearing that vary among cultures just as there may be wide variations within cultures. Body language and communication approaches provide examples of how differences in cultural practices can be applied when caring for a woman and her family during the childbirth experience.

 Ethnocultural Considerations— Cultural differences in communication

Eye contact: North American nurses have been taught that eye contact is an integral part of the communication process when communicating with patients. Some cultures do not maintain eye contact as they consider eye contact to be impolite or aggressive.

Silence: Some individuals find silence to be uncomfortable and may make efforts to communicate when there are gaps in a conversation. However, labor may be a time where it is inappropriate to be carrying on a conversation. Silence can be seen as a sign of respect for the laboring woman and the effort that she may be using to stay focused.

Touch: Often during the care of laboring women, nurses will use touch as a sign of caring and empathy. Wide variations in meaning can be attributed to touch among cultures. It is recommended to always ask the patient prior to touching her and assess her response to being touched.

Space: The concept of personal space varies among individuals and cultures. An awareness of personal space boundaries is essential; the individual patient will help the nurse to identify what she finds acceptable.

Care provider and labor support gender: Variations exist within cultures regarding norms relating to gender. Some cultures require a female care provider for the woman in labor. Other cultures require that a female labor companion accompany the woman in labor while the husband assumes a passive role.

Sick role behavior: Sick role behavior can vary among individuals and cultures. In some cultures it may be unacceptable to shout out during labor and the woman may be very stoic even though she is in extreme pain. Other cultures consider the childbearing year to be a time that requires intense assistance. In these situations, it is appropriate for the mother or sister to come live with the family to help care for the mother and infant.

Nursing Care Plan Young Primigravida in Labor

Allison is a 16-year-old gravida 1 para 0 who presents to the birth unit in early active labor accompanied by her mother. Allison appears quite fearful as she frequently asks, "what is that for?," "what are you going to do with that?," and "will it hurt?" On further questioning the nurse determines that Allison did not attend prenatal classes and has never been hospitalized.

Nursing Diagnosis: Deficient Knowledge related to hospitalization for labor and birth as manifested by frequent questions, no attendance at prenatal classes, and no previous hospitalizations.

Measurable Short-term Goal: The patient will have increased knowledge about labor and birth/hospital procedures.

Measurable Long-term Goal: The patient will have decreased anxiety related to hospitalization.

NOC Outcome:

Knowledge: Labor and Delivery (1817) Extent of understanding conveyed about labor and vaginal delivery

NIC Interventions:

Childbirth Preparation (6760)
Teaching: Individual (5606)

Nursing Interventions:

1. Establish rapport with the patient and her mother.

   RATIONALE: The support and understanding of the nurse will help decrease the patient's anxiety to facilitate learning. Including the mother in teaching provides an additional source of information and comfort for the patient.

2. Describe aspects of the admission process and standard care for labor patients with rationales.

   RATIONALE: Explaining to the patient what will occur and the reasons why they are important will increase the patient's knowledge and may alleviate some of her anxiety.

3. Orient the patient to the unit/room/birthing area.

   RATIONALE: Orientation to the hospital environment may assist in making the patient feel more comfortable with her surroundings.

4. Describe any procedures before performing them, including rationales, risks, and benefits.

   RATIONALE: This allows the patient to participate in her own care and make decisions based on knowledge.

5. Explain the nature of uterine contractions, cervical dilation, and labor progress.

   RATIONALE: This knowledge will reduce the patient's anxiety, which may also reduce perceived pain.

6. Teach the patient and her mother breathing and relaxation techniques that may be used as labor advances.

   RATIONALE: Anticipatory guidance provides the patient with tools to use during labor.

7. Teach support person(s) measures to comfort the patient during labor (specify, e.g., back rub, cool cloth, position changes, massage, imagery, use of birthing ball).

   RATIONALE: Providing presence conveys support and respect for the patient. Continuous support should be ongoing to prevent the patient from being left alone during labor.

8. Offer words of encouragement and suggestions for coping strategies as labor advances.

   RATIONALE: Empowers the patient to gain better control over her situation and helps to diminish fear and anxiety.

Assessment of the Fetus During Labor and Birth

Assessment of the fetus during labor and birth is a fundamental component of caring for a woman in labor. Intrapartal assessment of the fetus should be included in the maternal assessments at admission and remain ongoing throughout the intrapartal period. Fetal assessments include the identification of fetal position and presentation, and the evaluation of the fetal status.

Nurses use a variety of assessment techniques including observation, palpation, and auscultation. When assessing a woman in labor, the nurse is able to use observation and interview skills from the moment the woman comes through the door. Astute observation assists the nurse in assessing the patient's level of pain, her coping abilities, her contraction frequency, and the effectiveness of her support person. However, the nurse is unable to use direct observation skills to assess the status of the fetus. Therefore, it is critical that fetal assessment be a priority when the patient enters the intrapartal unit.

FETAL POSITION

There are four central ways to identify fetal position and some methods are more accurate than others. The nurse may attempt to identify the fetal presentation in the following ways:

• Abdominal palpation (Leopold's maneuvers)
• Location of the point of auscultation of the FHR
• Vaginal examination
• Ultrasound

Leopold's Maneuvers and Point of FHR Auscultation

Leopold's maneuvers are a systematic way of palpating the maternal abdomen to assess the fetal position. In addition, through the identification of fetal position, Leopold's maneuvers can also assist the nurse to identify the location in which to auscultate the fetal heart tones. Performing Leopold's maneuvers is a skill that requires practice and is not always accurate in identifying fetal position. Factors such as maternal obesity, hydramnios, and multiple gestation can increase the difficulty of identifying fetal position by Leopold's maneuvers. (See Chapter 9 for further discussion.)

 Critical Nursing Action Prevent Supine Hypotension

Much of the fetal assessment involves the maternal abdomen. Avoid positioning the patient flat on her back. Instead, slightly elevate the head of the bed or place a wedge under the patient's hip to prevent compression of the maternal vena cava caused by the gravid uterus.

Vaginal Examination

Another method of assessing the fetal position is by vaginal examination (see Procedure 12-1). The examiner may be able to palpate the fontanels or cranial suture to identify that the fetus is in a cephalic presentation. The landmarks may also be used to further identify the degree of flexion and the specific presentation such as vertex. If the membranes are intact or if the cervix is minimally dilated the examiner may not be able to identify the position of the fetus.

Ultrasound Examination

Ultrasound may be used when the practitioner is unable to identify the position by abdominal palpation or when it is necessary to determine the fetal position with the most accuracy. If a breech presentation is suspected during labor, an ultrasound examination may be performed to confirm the fetal presentation prior to performing a cesarean section.

 Now Can You— Discuss determination of fetal position during labor?

1. Identify and describe three methods used to determine fetal position?
2. Outline the major steps involved in performing an intrapartal vaginal examination?

ASSESSMENT OF THE FETAL HEART RATE

Much debate exists regarding the optimal method for evaluating the FHR in labor with the use of continuous or intermittent electronic fetal monitoring and intermittent auscultation. In addition, there is considerable variation among the methods of fetal monitoring used routinely in practice and the scientific evidence to support clinical practice. There is no consensus in the literature that electronic fetal monitoring provides superior assessment over intermittent auscultation (IA) in low-risk women. However, in practice, many low-risk women continue to be electronically monitored during labor. In addition, there is evidence to support the assertion that continuous electronic fetal monitoring can be associated with negative outcomes (Thacker, Stroup, & Chang, 2005).

 Across Care Settings: **Variations in practice environments for perinatal nurses**

Since diverse policies are found in different practice environments, nurses are encouraged to seek relevant policies and procedures within their individual health care organizations to guide their practice. It is important that the nurse practice within the standards set by the employer institution. The nurse is professionally accountable and has a legal responsibility to be knowledgeable of the current standards that affect practice. Perinatal nurses should be fully cognizant of the institutional policies concerning fetal heart surveillance during labor. Pertinent information generally includes the method of assessment, qualifications for those performing the technique, nurse to patient ratio, frequency and duration of assessment for specific stages of labor and defined risk categories, indications for specific methods, when to notify the primary care provider, and documentation (Goodwin, 2000).

Table 12-4 identifies recommendations for fetal monitoring generated by various professional organizations. This information further underscores the diversity of professional standards related to the issue of FHR monitoring.

Auscultation of Fetal Heart Sounds

Fetal heart sounds are best heard over the fetal back when the fetus is in the flexed position, as this is the part in closest contact with the uterine wall. Where to auscultate the

Table 12-4 Professional Organizations and Fetal Monitoring Recommendations	
Professional Organization	**Recommendations**
AWHONN (Association of Women's Health, Obstetric and Neonatal Nurses, 2000, 2003b)	Supports both the use of IA and uterine palpation as an appropriate method of fetal assessment for both antepartum and intrapartum patients and the judicious, appropriate application of EFM intrapartally.
	Risk assessment of the mother and fetus should guide the use of technology.
ACOG (American College of Obstetrics and Gynecology, 2005)	Recommends that either EFM or electronic IA be used during the labors of low-risk pregnant women.
SOGC (Society of Obstetricians and Gynaecologists of Canada, 2005)	Recommends IA as the preferred method of fetal surveillance of low-risk pregnancies and that there is insufficient evidence to justify the use of continuous EFM in routine practice.

IA = intermittent auscultation; EFM = electronic fetal monitoring.

fetal heart sounds depends on the fetal position (back to maternal left or right side; breech versus cephalic) (Fig. 12-13). Finding the best location to auscultate fetal heart sounds facilitates another method to identify or confirm fetal position. Typically, with a cephalic presentation, the fetal heart sounds are heard below the level of the maternal umbilicus. In a ROA position, the heart sounds are heard loudest in the right lower quadrant. Conversely, with a breech presentation, the fetal heart sounds are often auscultated above the level of the umbilicus. In a LSA position, the fetal heart sounds should be heard loudest in the upper left quadrant.

Regardless of the method used to assess fetal well-being in labor, nurses need to be extremely attentive to the fetal heart sounds. In addition, nurses must be knowledgeable regarding the identification of reassuring versus non-reassuring FHR sounds and the appropriate interventions that may be required.

INTERMITTENT AUSCULTATION. Intermittent auscultation (IA) of the fetal heart rate is frequently the recommended method for evaluating fetal status in women who have been identified as low risk. The fetal heart rate can be auscultated with a fetoscope or Doppler instrument and should be assessed for the baseline FHR, regular or irregular rhythm pattern, and the presence of accelerations (discussed later). In addition, the nurse should be able to identify reassuring and non-reassuring FHR patterns and recognize the implications and interventions that may be required. Intermittent auscultation is conducted using a fetoscope or Doppler instrument (Procedure 12-3).

Figure 12-13 Identifying where to auscultate fetal heart sounds depends on the fetal position.

Optimizing Outcomes— Recognizing reassuring and non-reassuring FHR patterns

The use of intermittent auscultation to monitor FHR during labor requires the nurse to recognize characteristics of reassuring and non-reassuring patterns.

Reassuring FHR characteristics:

- Normal FHR baseline (110–160 bpm)
- Presence of accelerations

Non-reassuring FHR characteristics:

- Abnormal FHR baseline (<110 or >160 bpm)
- Presence of decelerations (ACOG, 2005)

Now Can You— Assess FHR by auscultation?

1. Describe situations in which intermittent auscultation of the FHR is indicated?
2. List the characteristics of a reassuring FHR monitored by intermittent auscultation?

Electronic Fetal Monitoring

Electronic fetal monitoring (EFM) may be conducted on an intermittent or continuous basis. In a large number of American and Canadian hospitals, women are routinely monitored on admission for a short period of time to assess fetal well-being and then the monitoring is conducted periodically throughout labor. This practice is referred to as "intermittent" fetal monitoring. However, the evidence base supporting this practice has not demonstrated improved outcomes (Thacker, Stroup, & Chang, 2005). Thacker and colleagues (2005) reported that EFM, as compared to IA, has not been associated with a decrease in neonatal mortality or morbidity although EFM has been associated with increased rates of cesarean section, operative vaginal birth and the use of obstetrical anesthesia. At present, more than 85% of laboring women in the United Sates are monitored electronically for at least part of their labor (Martin et al., 2005). The continued use of EFM over intermittent FHR auscultation is believed to be related to concerns about liability and the increased nurse-to-patient ratio required with IA (Wood, 2003). In view of the fact that all fetal surveillance methods have limitations, some professionals assert that the current evidence supports a return to the use of IA for low-risk laboring women (Dildy, 2005).

Situations where EFM is recommended continuously for assessing fetal well-being include the presence of a high-risk pregnancy, induction of labor with oxytocin, when IA identifies a non-reassuring FHR or if the institution is unable to provide IA. EFM can be performed externally or internally. The external EFM involves a process that is very similar to the non-stress test (NST) (see Chapter 11). The external monitor is composed of a Doppler ultrasound transducer and tocodynanometer that is applied to the maternal abdomen to monitor and display the FHR and contractions (Fig. 12-14). Although the use of an external transducer requires that the woman remain confined to a bed or chair, portable telemetry units allow patients to ambulate during electronic monitoring. The nurse is able to observe the FHR and uterine contraction patterns at a centrally located electronic display station. Some facilities are equipped with monitoring units that can be used when the woman is submerged in water.

The internal fetal monitor is composed of a spiral electrode that must be inserted into the fetal scalp or presenting part during a vaginal examination (Fig. 12-15). The cardiac signal is transmitted through the spiral electrode and a fetal electrocardiogram tracing is produced. Uterine activity is assessed by a solid or fluid-filled intrauterine pressure catheter (IUPC) that is introduced into the uterine cavity. The IUPC can measure contraction frequency, duration, and

Procedure 12-3 Auscultating the Fetal Heart Tones During Labor

Purpose

Auscultation, an auditory method of monitoring the fetal heart tones, is performed intermittently during labor to assess the fetus. Auscultation allows the laboring woman greater freedom because she is not attached to a machine and does not have to wear belts to secure the ultrasound transducer and the tocotransducer. Intermittent auscultation does not provide a printed record of the fetal heart rate for other members of the health care team to review. Auscultation also does not provide an assessment of fetal heart rate variability or of other subtle changes in the fetal heart rate.

Equipment

- Fetoscope or hand-held Doppler ultrasound with gel ("Doppler")
- Disposable wipes

Steps

1. Wash and dry hands and explain procedure and purpose of the examination to the patient.

   RATIONALE: *Hand washing helps to prevent the spread of microorganisms. Explanations help to decrease anxiety, and promote patient understanding and cooperation.*

2. Help the patient assume a comfortable position that provides access to the abdomen.

3. Palpate the maternal abdomen using Leopold's maneuvers to identify the fetal position to aid in obtaining the location of the fetal heart tones. Note that the fetal heart tones are heard most loudly over the fetal back.

4. Palpate the fundus of the uterus for the presence of uterine contractions. At the end of a uterine contraction, place the fetoscope or Doppler over the location of the fetal back. Adjust the fetoscope or Doppler if necessary to obtain a clearly audible FHR. Depending on fetal position, the fetal heart sounds may be soft and muffled or loud and clear.

5. Listen for audible fetal heart sounds. Note that two distinctly different sounds can be heard: fetal heart tones that result from blood moving through the placenta and umbilical cord (funic soufflé) and the uterine soufflé, which is the same rate as the maternal pulse.

6. Palpate the maternal radial pulse to ensure that the auscultated fetal heart sounds are at a different rate than the maternal pulse.

7. Auscultate the fetal heart sounds for the rate and rhythm. The greatest accuracy for assessment of the fetal heart rate occurs when listening for 1 minute.

Note: During active labor, 30-second intervals may be more feasible.

8. Count the FHR for 30–60 seconds between contractions to determine the baseline rate.

   RATIONALE: *The baseline rate can be assessed only during the absence of uterine activity.*

9. Interpret the fetal heart rate: Is the baseline normal between 110 and 160 bpm? Is there tachycardia (baseline >160 bpm) or bradycardia (baseline <110/bpm)? Is the rhythm regular or irregular? Can you note the presence of accelerations or decelerations?

10. Repeat the procedure as indicated according to agency policy.

11. Inform the patient of the findings.

12. Document the fetal heart rate according to agency policy.

Documentation

5/5/09 1030: Fetal heart rate obtained by fetoscope at 144 bpm and regular. Acceleration of the fetal heart rate noted. Patient coping well in active labor. Contractions 3 min apart, 60-second duration with moderate intensity.

—L. Lopez, RN

---

intensity. The internal method is a more accurate form of fetal monitoring. However, owing to the invasive nature of the procedure, internal EFM is often reserved for high-risk pregnancies (situations in which external fetal monitoring is insufficient in obtaining the FHR or in situations where there is evidence of a non-reassuring fetal heart rate). The application of an internal electrode requires that the membranes be ruptured and that the cervix has sufficiently dilated.

The interpretation of the fetal heart rate pattern requires a holistic assessment of the maternal risk factors, uterine activity, and FHR patterns including baseline, variability and the presence of accelerations, and the identification of any decelerations. Members of the obstetrical team must maintain close communication and reach mutual consensus regarding interpretation of fetal heart patterns. Often, nurses who practice in labor and delivery units obtain advanced training and education regarding fetal monitoring to aid in accurate interpretation.

 Optimizing Outcomes— **Standards for the interpretation of FHR patterns**

In 1997, the National Institute of Child Health and Human Development (NICHD) published a proposed nomenclature system for EFM interpretation. Standardized definitions for FHR monitoring were presented (NICHD, 1997). Concerns regarding enhancing communication among various caregivers and patient safety (Simpson, 2004) as well as concerns about research validity have led to the

Toco transducer (uterine contractions) — Ultrasound transducer (FHR)

Figure 12-14 External fetal monitor.

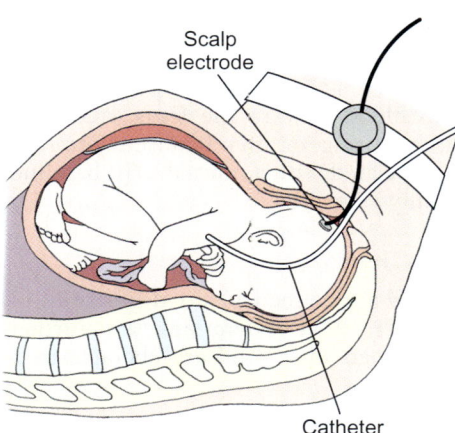

Scalp electrode — Catheter

Figure 12-15 Internal fetal monitor.

adoption of the NICHD terminology by the American College of Obstetricians and Gynecologists (ACOG, 2005) and Association of Women's Health, Obstetric and Neonatal Nurses (AWHONN, 2003a).

Baseline Fetal Heart Rate

The **baseline fetal heart rate** (FHR) is referred to as the average fetal heart rate observed between contractions over a 10-minute period (Fig. 12-16). The recorded baseline excludes periodic FHR changes that are evidenced by increased variability or accelerations. The normal baseline fetal heart rate at term is 110 to 160 beats per minute (bpm). There are two abnormal variations of the baseline: tachycardia (baseline above 160 bpm); and bradycardia (baseline below 110 bpm) (ACOG, 2005).

TACHYCARDIA. **Tachycardia** is generally defined as a sustained baseline fetal heart rate greater than 160 beats per minute for a duration of 10 minutes or longer. A number of conditions are associated with fetal tachycardia:

- Fetal hypoxia: The fetus attempts to compensate for reduced blood flow by increasing sympathetic stimulation of the central nervous system (CNS).

Figure 12-16 The normal baseline fetal heart rate at term is 110 to 160 bpm. *Top.* Fetal heart rate. *Bottom.* Uterine contractions.

- Maternal fever: An increase in maternal temperature accelerates fetal metabolism, thus increasing the FHR. This situation may be seen in a laboring woman who becomes dehydrated or has an increased temperature following prolonged exposure in a warm bath or whirlpool.
- Maternal medications: Both parasympathetic drugs (i.e., atropine, scopolamine) and beta-sympathetic drugs (tocolytic drugs used to halt contractions) can have a stimulant effect and increase the fetal heart rate.
- Infection: Tachycardia may be an initial sign of uterine infection (amnionitis) and may precede an increased maternal temperature by 1 to 2 hours.
- Fetal anemia: In response to a decrease in hemoglobin, the FHR increases to compensate and improve tissue metabolism.
- Maternal hyperthyroidism: Thyroid-stimulating hormone (TSH) may cross the placenta and stimulate the fetal heart rate (Tucker, 2004).

BRADYCARDIA. **Bradycardia** is defined as a sustained (greater than 10 minutes) baseline FHR of less than 110 to 120 bpm. Fetal bradycardia may be associated with:

- Late hypoxia: Myocardial activity becomes depressed and lowers the fetal heart rate.
- Medications: Beta-adrenergic blocking drugs (e.g., propanolol [Inderal]).
- Maternal hypotension: Results in decreased blood flow to the fetus and can lower the FHR. Maternal hypotension can result from positioning (i.e., supine hypotension) and is a common side effect associated with an epidural or spinal anesthetic.
- Prolonged umbilical cord compression: Stimulates fetal baroreceptors that cause vagal stimulation and a decreased FHR.
- Bradyarrhythmias: With complete heart block, the FHR baseline is often as low as 70 to 90 bpm (Tucker, 2004).

VARIABILITY

Variability of the FHR is manifested by fluctuations in the baseline fetal heart rate observed on the fetal monitor. The pattern denotes an irregular, changing FHR rather than a straight line that indicates few changes in the rate. The variability of the FHR is a result of the interplay between the fetal sympathetic nervous system, which assists to increase the heart rate and the parasympathetic nervous system, which acts to decrease the heart rate.

Variability can further be classified as short-term or long-term variability. Short-term variability is the beat to beat changes in the FHR and is most accurately assessed with an internal electrode. Long-term variability refers to the changes in fetal heart rate over a longer period of time such as 1 minute. The absence of or undetected variability is considered non-reassuring. Health care providers are able to assess the overall amount of (long-term) variability and describe it as absent, minimal, moderate, or marked (Table 12-5).

The presence of adequate (moderate) variability is an important indicator of fetal well-being. FHR variability is indicative of an adequately oxygenated neurological pathway in which impulses are transmitted from the fetal brain to the cardiac conduction system (Fox, Kilpatrick, King, & Parer, 2000). An electronic fetal monitor tracing that records the FHR as a changing, jagged line is reflective of an adequately oxygenated, responsive fetal brain and fetal heart.

Conversely, the absence of variability may indicate normal variations such as fetal sleep (the sleep state should not last longer than 30 minutes), a response to certain drugs that depress the CNS, such as analgesics (meperidine [Demerol], tranquilizers (diazepam [Valium]), barbiturates (secobarbital [Seconal] and pentobarbital [Nembutal]), ataractics (promethazine [Phenergan]), and general anesthetics or a pathological condition such as hypoxia, a CNS abnormality, or acidemia.

ACCELERATIONS

An **acceleration** is defined as an increase in the FHR of 15 bpm above the fetal heart baseline that lasts for at least 15 to 30 seconds. Accelerations are considered a sign of fetal well-being when they accompany fetal movement. Thus, when a fetus is active in utero, accelerations are

Figure 12-17 *Top.* Fetal heart rate accelerations. *Bottom.* Uterine contractions.

normally present. Consequently, when the fetus is sleeping or not moving, limited FHR accelerations may be noted.

When contractions are present, accelerations are often noted as a response to the contraction. This type of periodic FHR acceleration with contractions is thought to be a compensatory accelerative response to a transient decrease in blood flow to the fetus. Accelerations may occur before, during, or after a contraction. Accelerations are often associated with a normal FHR baseline and normal variability (Fig. 12-17).

DECELERATIONS

Decelerations are defined as any decrease in FHR below the baseline FHR. Decelerations are further defined according to their onset and are characterized as early, variable, and late.

Early Decelerations

Early decelerations are characterized by a deceleration in the FHR that resembles a mirror image to the contraction. Therefore, the onset of the deceleration begins near the onset of the contraction, the lowest part of the deceleration occurs at the peak of contraction, and the FHR returns to baseline by the end of the contraction. Early decelerations are usually repetitive and are commonly observed during active labor and descent of the fetus (Fig. 12-18).

Table 12-5	Classifications of FHR Variability and Possible Causes	
Variability	**Amplitude of FHR Changes**	**Causes**
Absent	Undetectable	May represent fetal cerebral asphyxia. Warrants immediate evaluation.
Minimal	>2–<5 beats per minute (bpm)	May be related to narcotics, tranquilizers, magnesium sulfate, barbiturates, anesthetic agents, prematurity or fetal sleep.
Moderate	6–25 bpm	Reassuring; indicates fetal well-being.
Marked	>25 bpm	Marked variability is believed to be a less common response to fetal hypoxia.

Source: Simpson, K.R., and Creehan, P.A. (2001). *AWHONN Perinatal Nursing* (2nd ed.). Philadelphia: Lippincott.

Figure 12-18 *Top.* Early decelerations. *Bottom.* Uterine contractions.

Early decelerations are considered benign and are usually well tolerated by the fetus. They are believed to be related to fetal head compression and the resulting vagal stimulation that slows the FHR. They may occur during vaginal examinations, uterine contractions, and during placement of the internal mode of fetal monitoring. Early decelerations are viewed as a reassuring FHR pattern when accompanied by normal baseline FHR and normal variability.

Variable Decelerations

Variable decelerations, as the name implies, are decelerations that are variable in terms of their onset, frequency, duration, and intensity. The decrease in FHR below the baseline is 15 bpm or more, lasts at least 15 seconds, and returns to the baseline in less than 2 minutes from the time of onset (NICHD, 1997) (Fig. 12-19). The deceleration is unrelated to the presence of uterine contractions. Variable decelerations are thought to be a result of umbilical cord compression. Thus, the degree by which the cord is compressed (partially versus completely) can affect the severity of the deceleration. For example, a cord that is briefly compressed by the fetus may be manifest as a very abrupt decrease in the FHR with a rapid return to baseline. Conversely, a cord that is tightly wrapped around the fetal neck (**nuchal cord**) progressively becomes more compressed as the fetus descends into the maternal pelvis. This situation is most likely to result in longer, more severe decelerations. In general, brief, occasional decelerations are often considered benign whereas repetitive, worsening variable decelerations are cause for concern and always warrant further investigation.

The American College of Obstetricians and Gynecologists (ACOG, 2005) classifies variable decelerations as significant when the FHR falls below 70 bpm and lasts longer than 60 seconds. In addition, the Society of Obstetricians and Gynaecologists of Canada (SOGC, 2005) concurs and further identifies "non-reassuring" or "atypical" variable decelerations as:

- Deceleration to less than 70 bpm lasting greater than 60 seconds
- Loss of variability in the baseline FHR and in the trough of the deceleration
- Biphasic deceleration
- Slow return to baseline

- Continuation of a baseline at a lower level that before the deceleration
- The presence of fetal tachycardia

 Optimizing Outcomes— Amnioinfusion to relieve cord compression

Amnioinfusion is the infusion of warmed normal saline into the uterus via sterile catheter (IUPC). Amnioinfusion may be used in an attempt to reduce the severity of variable decelerations caused by cord compression. The nurse assists with the procedure by assembling the equipment; monitoring the FHR, contraction status, and maternal temperature; and by verifying that the infused fluid is exiting the uterus.

Late Decelerations

The patterns of late decelerations typically mirror the contraction, and this characteristic is similar in appearance to early decelerations. With late decelerations, the deceleration has a late onset and begins around the peak of the contraction (Fig. 12-20). This type of deceleration does not resolve until after the contraction has ended. Late decelerations indicate the presence of **uteroplacental insufficiency**, a decline in placental function. Normally, the fetus can withstand repeated contractions with sufficient oxygenation. However, in this circumstance a decrease in blood flow from the uterus to the placenta results in fetal hypoxia and late decelerations.

Late decelerations require prompt attention and reporting. The longer the late decelerations persist, the more serious they become. Immediate attempts should be made to correct the cause of the late decelerations if possible. For example, late decelerations in the presence of an oxytocin infusion may signal a need to immediately discontinue the oxytocin infusion, especially if uterine hyperstimulation is suspected. Nursing interventions that should be implemented immediately include reporting the late decelerations, changing the maternal position, discontinuing the oxytocin infusion, increasing the intravenous fluids, and administering oxygen by mask.

Figure 12-19 *Top.* Variable decelerations. *Bottom.* Uterine contractions.

Figure 12-20 *Top.* Late decelerations. *Bottom.* Uterine contractions.

It is important to note that late decelerations can present very obviously or very subtly. In addition, late decelerations are often accompanied by other non-reassuring fetal heart patterns such as a loss of or decrease in variability.

 Nursing Insight— Potential causes of uteroplacental insufficiency

Late decelerations that are caused by uteroplacental insufficiency may be related to uterine hyperstimulation with oxytocin, postdate or preterm pregnancy, amnionitis, preeclampsia, small for gestational age (SGA) fetus, placenta previa, abruptio placentae, maternal diabetes, conduction anesthesia that causes maternal hypotension, maternal cardiac disease and maternal anemia.

INTERPRETATION OF FHR TRACINGS

A systematic approach to the interpretation of FHR tracings ensures that all possibilities are considered. Most institutions have established protocols to guide electronic fetal heart monitoring methods and to maintain consistency in the interpretation of FHR patterns. When assessing FHR tracings, nurses should consider factors such as contraction frequency and intensity, stage of labor, and the earlier FHR pattern.

 critical nursing action Interpreting Fetal Monitor Tracings

To aid in the interpretation of EFM tracings, the nurse should consider the following parameters:

* **Uterine activity:** What is the frequency, duration, and intensity of contractions?
* **Labor progress:** What is the stage of labor? What is the dilation, effacement, station, presentation, and position?
* **Baseline FHR:** What is the baseline FHR? Is tachycardia or bradycardia present?
* **Baseline variability:** What is the variability of the FHR (absent, minimal, moderate, marked, or other)?
* **Periodic changes in FHR:** Are there any FHR changes from the baseline? Are accelerations present? Are any decelerations present? If decelerations are present are they early, variable, late, or prolonged?
* **Maternal history and condition:** Are there any pre-existing conditions that increase risk for this pregnancy? Are there any intrapartum high-risk factors (e.g., meconium) that should be noted?

Based on a systematic interpretation, FHR tracings are generally classified as reassuring or non-reassuring (Box 12-4). This classification helps to determine the need for interventions. In general, a reassuring (normal) FHR tracing is generally associated with fetal well-being. Routine assessment of the fetal heart rate is conducted according to the birth center protocol. A non-reassuring tracing indicates an urgent need to notify the physician (or nurse midwife) and implement appropriate interventions.

It is important to note that when non-reassuring FHR patterns are identified, there is often a combination of more than one non-reassuring feature such as late decelerations and decreased variability or tachycardia and absent variability. When a non-reassuring FHR pattern is present, it is imperative to intervene immediately in an effort to correct the problem and prevent the worsening of symptoms.

 Optimizing Outcomes— Communicating about FHR patterns

In clinical practice, various guidelines exist concerning the management of FHR tracings. Accurate, consistent, and timely communication among health care providers is always required to optimize outcomes for the patient and her fetus.

 Be sure to— Use appropriate terminology during documentation of FHR auscultation

When documenting the findings from FHR auscultation, descriptive terms associated with EFM such as "marked variability" or "variable deceleration" should be avoided because these terms reflect visual descriptions of the patterns produced on the monitor tracing. Terms that are *numerically* defined (i.e., "bradycardia," "tachycardia") may be used. When auscultated, FHR must be described as a baseline number or range and as having a regular or irregular rhythm. The presence or absence of accelerations or decelerations that occur during and after contractions should be noted (AWHONN, 2000; 2003b).

NURSING INTERVENTIONS AND DIAGNOSES

Early decelerations are considered to be benign and no action is necessary. However, it is important to identify them so that they can be differentiated from late or variable decelerations. Depending on the cause, interventions for variable and late decelerations include lateral position changes (to displace the weight of the gravid uterus off the inferior vena cava), oxygen administration at 8 to 10 L per minute by face mask, palpation of the uterus for hyperstimulation, discontinuation of oxytocin if infusing, increasing the rate of the maintenance intravenous solution, and assisting with fetal oxygen saturation monitoring if ordered. Possible nursing diagnoses include impaired fetal gas exchange related to umbilical cord compression or placental insufficiency; decreased maternal cardiac output related to supine hypotension secondary to position; and anxiety related to lack of knowledge concerning fetal monitoring/fetal well-being during labor.

 Now Can You— Assess FHR patterns detected by EFM?

1. Describe situations when electronic fetal monitoring instead of intermittent auscultation is indicated?
2. Define the following frequently used terminology: baseline fetal heart rate, variability, acceleration, deceleration?
3. Describe the assessment of a reassuring and a non-reassuring fetal heart rate?
4. List four nursing interventions for variable and late decelerations?

Second Stage of Labor

The second stage of labor commences with full dilation of the cervix and ends with the birth of the infant. Often the woman or nurse may suspect that the woman has entered the second stage of labor because of the patient's urge to push or the presence of involuntary bearing down efforts. The contractions often remain very similar to those experienced during the transition stage. They continue to occur frequently and are very intense. The woman may exhibit varying emotions during the second stage. Some patients may get a spurt of energy or a "second wind" to help them get through the second stage. Others may be nervous or fearful of the new sensations that they are feeling. Encouragement and support from the labor nurse and support person are crucial at this stage. The woman is not to be left alone during this time, and continuous support should be provided. It is important to encourage the patient to rest between pushing in order to maintain her energy throughout the second stage.

The duration of the second stage is variable and may be influenced by several factors such as parity; the type and amount of analgesia or anesthesia administered; the frequency, intensity, and duration of contractions; maternal efforts in pushing, and the support the patient receives. For nulliparous women, the second stage often involves 1 to 2 hours of pushing. Multiparous women typically experience a much shorter second stage and childbirth may occur within minutes following full cervical dilation.

PROMOTING EFFECTIVE PUSHING

Women push most effectively when they experience the urge to bear down and push. The urge to push is believed to be stimulated by the Ferguson reflex as the presenting part stretches the pelvic floor muscles. Thus, the maternal urge to push may be more related to the station of the presenting part rather than to the dilation of the cervix.

Differing practices exist regarding the promotion of pushing during the second stage. Many practitioners believe that pushing should be encouraged only when the woman has the urge to push, instead of when full cervical dilation has been reached. Some women (i.e., those with an epidural analgesia or other types of anesthesia) may have no urge to bear down. When this situation occurs, a process called "laboring down" may be used. "Laboring down" allows the woman to rest as the fetus descends. Pushing is postponed until the urge to push is experienced. Research suggests that there is a decrease in maternal fatigue and an increase in fetal oxygenation when women delay pushing until they feel the urge (Minato, 2000; Roberts, 2003). It has been proposed that the decision concerning when to initiate pushing should be based on the individual maternal response rather than on standardized routine practices. Furthermore, the duration of active maternal pushing has been found to be more closely related to the neonate's condition at birth than the duration of the second stage of labor (Cesario, 2004; Minato, 2000; Roberts, 2002).

There are generally two methods of pushing during the second stage of labor: closed-glottis and open-glottis pushing. Closed-glottis pushing, also referred to as "directed pushing," is the traditional method, in which women are encouraged to begin pushing at full cervical dilation regardless of the urge to bear down. The woman is encouraged to take a deep breath and hold it for at least 10 seconds while pushing as hard and as long as she is able throughout the contraction. Simpson and Creehan (2001) identify this practice as outdated and physiologically inappropriate. They assert that there is a lack of scientific evidence to support closed-glottis pushing and point out that this practice has been associated with adverse outcomes including fetal hypoxia, acidemia, and lower neonatal Apgar scores. The poor outcomes are believed to result from prolonged maternal breath holding that ultimately affect uteroplacental blood flow.

Open-glottis pushing, also referred to as "involuntary pushing", is another method of pushing. With this technique, the laboring woman is encouraged to hold her

 where research and practice meet: Use of EFM

Researchers evaluated nine randomized controlled trials that included 18,561 low- and high-risk pregnant women from diverse countries to compare the efficacy and safety of routine continuous EFM during labor with intermittent auscultation. Overall, there was a statistically significant decrease in the incidence of neonatal seizures in infants subjected to EFM. They found no significant differences between patients who received electronic fetal monitoring or intermittent auscultation during labor on: Apgar scores of infants at 1 minute of less than 7 or less than 4, rate of admission to neonatal intensive care units, perinatal deaths, or the development of cerebral palsy. However, there was an increased rate of cesarean delivery and operative vaginal delivery with the use of EFM. Implications for clinical practice include the following: (1) EFM may exert a preventative effect on neonatal seizures and (2) the use of EFM appears to increase the rate of maternal operative deliveries, a factor that may balance or outweigh the potential benefits of its use (Thacker, Stroup, & Chang, 2005).

breath for only 5 to 6 seconds during pushing and to take several breaths between each bearing down effort. In addition, women are allowed to exhale throughout the bearing down attempts. This process is believed to produce no compromise to the uteroplacental blood flow and therefore is thought to invoke less stress on the fetus.

Variations in pushing techniques are found in clinical practice. Regardless of the process used for second-stage pushing, laboring women require continuous support and encouragement from their health care provider(s). It is important to calmly provide easy-to-understand, consistent information to avoid confusion. It is also important to remember that the patient and her partner can become anxious and confused if several people attempt to give directions at the same time.

ACHIEVING A POSITION OF COMFORT

During the second stage, comfort measures remain equally important and many of the interventions and positioning identified for the first stage of labor can be implemented during the second stage as well. Many factors (e.g., the woman's personal preferences, the use of analgesia or anesthesia, the preferences of the health care practitioner, and the imminence of birth) have an influence on the optimal maternal position during this stage. When pushing, women are encouraged whenever possible to maintain an upright or semi-upright position, such as squatting, sitting, standing, kneeling, on all fours, or sitting on the toilet.

Pushing when in an upright position allows the use of gravity to promote fetal descent and has been associated with a shortened labor. Positions such as squatting and kneeling may also help to increase the dimensions of the maternal pelvis. Assuming a hands and knees position or leaning over a table or chair helps to take pressure off the maternal spine and often reduces backache commonly associated with a fetal occipital–posterior position (see Fig. 12-12).

 Now Can You— Discuss comfort measures and pushing techniques for the second stage of labor?

1. List three comfort measures used during the first stage of labor that would also be effective during the second stage of labor?
2. Discuss how the nurse can advocate for a patient who does not have the urge to push in the second stage?
3. List two positions for pushing and provide one advantage of each?

PREPARATION FOR THE BIRTH

As the fetus descends, the woman experiences an increasing urge to bear down due to pressure of the fetal head on the sacral and obturator nerves. As the patient pushes, contraction of the abdominal muscles exerts intra-abdominal pressure. With the maternal bearing down efforts and further descent of the fetus, the nurse may notice bulging of the perineum and rectum. As the fetal head progresses downward, the perineum begins to stretch, thin out, and move anteriorly. The amount of bloody show may increase at this time and the labia begin to part with each contraction. The fetal head, which may be observable at the vaginal

introitus, often appears to recede between contractions. As the contractions and maternal pushing efforts continue, the presenting part descends farther.

Crowning, which means that birth is imminent, occurs when the fetal head is encircled by the vaginal introitus (Fig. 12-21). Some women may complain of a burning sensation as the perineum is stretched. This experience can be frightening for the woman and it is important for the nurse to identify it as a normal sensation. The woman may also feel intense pressure in the rectum and a need to evacuate her bowels. Again, the nurse should confirm the normalcy of these sensations and continue to offer encouragement and support. If the woman does pass stool, she should be cleaned in a timely manner. Some women may feel as though they are losing control and a variety of emotions (e.g., irritability, fear, embarrassment, and helplessness) may be displayed. These behaviors can be frightening to the support person as well. The nurse needs to continue to encourage and reinforce to the woman and her support person that these reactions are normal and that progress is being made.

EPISIOTOMY

Episiotomy is a surgical incision of the perineum that is performed to enlarge the vaginal orifice during the second stage of labor (Carroli & Belizan, 2006). The frequency of routine episiotomy has decreased over the last 20 years as the benefits of performing routine episiotomy began to be questioned. In the 1980s, the episiotomy rate was reported to be approximately 64 out of 100 births. At that time, many physicians routinely performed episiotomies based on the belief that surgical enlargement of the vaginal opening would prevent intrapartal complications such as protracted second stage of labor, fetal trauma, and severe lacerations, and later maternal problems such as cystocele, rectocele, dyspareunia, and uterine prolapse.

Many women questioned the use of routine episiotomy and current practices have changed to reflect existing evidence that routine episiotomy has not been associated with better outcomes over selective episiotomy. In studies where episiotomy had been performed for medical indications, the results demonstrated positive benefits. When medically indicated, episiotomy was associated with decreased posterior perineal trauma and suturing and

Figure 12-21 Crowning.

fewer complications. No differences were found in maternal pain experience or the incidence of severe vaginal or perineal trauma when routine and selective episiotomies were compared. There was an increased risk of anterior perineal trauma associated with selective episiotomy (Carroli & Belizan, 2006). Many practitioners currently reserve the use of episiotomy for medical indications, which include instrumentation during birth (forceps or vacuum), a need to expedite the birth (evidence of fetal compromise), or in the event of maternal exhaustion.

Two different methods are used for the episiotomy. The most common method is the midline or median episiotomy. An incision is made from the vaginal opening downward toward the rectum. A midline episiotomy is easily repaired, heals quickly, and is associated with less postoperative pain than a mediolateral episiotomy. However, the primary disadvantage of a midline episiotomy is the risk of third- and fourth-degree lacerations with extension through the rectal sphincter. The mediolateral episiotomy is less common. An incision is made from the vagina to the 5 o'clock or 7 o'clock position (the maternal left mediolateral or right mediolateral position). Compared to a midline incision, the mediolateral episiotomy is associated with a smaller risk of fourth-degree lacerations although third-degree lacerations may occur. The amount of blood loss is usually greater, the surgical repair is more difficult, and there is increased pain postpartum (Fig. 12-22).

✺ Complementary Care: *Methods to decrease perineal trauma*

Various strategies to decrease the risk of perineal trauma during the second stage of labor have been implemented and evaluated. These include perineal massage (antenatal and intrapartal), application of warm compresses, use of lubricating oils, and manual support. However, research has demonstrated variable results and further investigation is indicated. Maternal positioning for birth has also shown variable results regarding its effect on perineal trauma. Soong and Barnes (2005) found that women who gave birth in a semirecumbent position had an increased need for sutures for perineal lacerations than women who gave

birth in an "all fours" position. In addition, women who received regional anesthesia also demonstrated an increased need for suturing than women who gave birth in a lateral position.

Nurses should be aware of the potential benefits and risks associated with various techniques intended to help minimize perineal trauma. It is important for nurses to remain open-minded, encouraging, and supportive of patients who wish to utilize alternate methods to help facilitate perineal stretching.

 Now Can You— Discuss factors associated with impending childbirth?

1. Explain the significance of crowning?
2. Discuss the controversies surrounding routine episiotomy?
3. Identify three strategies that may be effective in reducing perineal trauma during childbirth?

Birth

As the fetal head is crowning, the perineum is stretched very thin and the anus stretches and protrudes. With continued maternal pushing efforts, the fetal head extends under the symphysis pubis and is born. The practitioner assisting at the birth may prefer to coach the patient regarding pushing and breathing, as the birth of the head should occur in a controlled manner in an attempt to limit injury to the perineum. Once the anterior shoulder reaches the pelvic outlet, it rotates to the midline and is delivered from under the pubic arch. The posterior shoulder is guided over the perineum, and the body follows.

THE CARDINAL MOVEMENTS

The **cardinal movements**, or mechanisms of labor, have been used to describe how the fetus (in a vertex presentation) passes through the birth canal and the positional changes required to facilitate birth (Fig. 12-23). The cardinal movements are presented in the order in which they occur.

Descent

Four forces facilitate **descent**, which is the progression of the fetal head into the maternal pelvis: (1) pressure of the amniotic fluid; (2) direct pressure of the uterine fundus on the fetal breech; (3) contraction of the maternal abdominal muscles; and (4) extension and straightening of the fetal body. The fetal head enters the maternal inlet in the occiput transverse or the oblique position because the pelvic inlet is widest from side to side. The sagittal suture is equidistant from the maternal symphysis pubis and sacral promontory. The degree of fetal descent is measured by stations.

Flexion

Flexion occurs as the fetal head descends and comes into contact with the soft tissues of the pelvis, the muscles of the maternal pelvic floor, and the cervix. The resistance encountered with these structures causes the fetal chin to flex downward onto the chest. This position allows the smallest fetal diameters to enter the maternal pelvis.

Fetal head
Perineal body
Mediolateral
Midline

Figure 12-22 An episiotomy is a surgical incision of the perineum that is performed to facilitate birth. The most common method is the midline or median episiotomy. An incision is made from the vaginal opening downward toward the rectum.

Engagement, descent, flexion

Internal rotation

Extension beginning (rotation complete)

Extension complete

External rotation (restitution)

External rotation (shoulder rotation)

Expulsion

Figure 12-23 The cardinal movements, or mechanisms of labor.

Internal Rotation

To fit into the maternal pelvic cavity, which is widest in the anteroposterior diameter, the fetal head must rotate. As the occiput of the fetal head comes into contact with the levator ani muscles and surrounding fascia, it meets with resistance. This causes the occiput to rotate, usually from left to right, and the sagittal suture aligns with the long axis of the maternal pelvis (the anteroposterior pelvic diameter).

Extension

As the fetal head passes under the maternal symphysis pubis, it meets with resistance from the pelvic floor. The head pivots and extends with each maternal pushing effort. The head is born in extension as the occiput slides under the symphysis and the face is directed toward the rectum. The fetal brow, nose, and chin then emerge.

Restitution

Internal rotation causes the fetal shoulders to enter the maternal pelvis in an oblique position. After the head is delivered in the extended position, it rotates briefly to the position it occupied when it was engaged in the inlet. This movement is termed restitution. The 45-degree turn of the fetal head facilitates realignment with the long axis of the body.

External Rotation

As restitution continues, the shoulders align in the anteroposterior diameter, causing the head to continue to turn farther to one side (external rotation). The fetal trunk moves through the pelvis with the anterior shoulders descending first.

Expulsion

After external rotation, maternal pushing efforts bring the anterior shoulder under the symphysis pubis. Lateral flexion of the shoulder and head occurs and the anterior, then posterior, shoulder is born. Once the shoulders are delivered, the rest of the body quickly follows.

CLAMPING THE UMBILICAL CORD

Much controversy exists concerning the issue of when and how to clamp the umbilical cord. When the newborn is held above the level of the placenta, a transfer of blood occurs from the newborn back to the placenta. Conversely, delaying the umbilical cord clamping and holding the newborn below the level of the placenta can result in a transfer of 50 to 100 mL of blood from the placenta to the newborn. The additional blood may be beneficial in reducing infant iron deficiency, although this practice may also contribute to polycythemia and potential hyperbilirubinemia.

The primary care provider places two Kelly clamps on the umbilical cord, and may invite the father or birth support person to cut the cord between the two clamps. Either the primary care provider or the nurse then places a plastic clamp on the umbilical cord approximately 0.5 to 1 inch (1.2 to 2.5 cm) from the newborn's abdomen, being careful to not catch the abdominal skin in the clamp. The nurse observes the cut cord for the presence of three blood vessels: two arteries and one vein. Samples of cord blood are collected for laboratory analysis. Some parents request to have their newborn's cord blood "banked" in the event that the stem cells in the cord blood may be required in the future for the treatment of a family illness. A vaginal birth sequence is presented in Figure 12-24.

Possible Nursing Diagnoses for the Intrapartal Patient

Examples of common nursing diagnoses during labor and birth are listed below. It is important to be cognizant of individual differences among patients. While these are common nursing diagnoses, they will vary among individuals and stages of labor.

• Pain related to increasing frequency, duration, and intensity of contractions
• Knowledge deficit related to pain management techniques for active labor
• Anxiety related to the previous birth experience
• Fatigue related to a prolonged latent phase labor
• Risk for infection related to prolonged rupture of membranes

• Impaired fetal gas exchange related to umbilical cord compression
• Deceased maternal cardiac output related to supine hypotension secondary to maternal position

---

Now Can You— **Discuss cardinal movements and umbilical cord clamping?**

1. Describe what is meant by the cardinal movements?
2. Compare and contrast early versus late clamping of the umbilical cord?

Third and Fourth Stages of Labor

Nursing care during the third and fourth stages of labor is focused on providing immediate care for the newborn in the adjustment to extrauterine life, assisting with the delivery of the placenta, monitoring and assisting the mother with the physiological adjustments of labor and birth, and facilitating the attachment between the mother and baby. Characteristics of the third and fourth stages of labor are presented in Table 12-6.

Third Stage of Labor

The third stage of labor is the period of time from the birth of the baby to the complete delivery of the placenta. This stage usually lasts 5 to 10 minutes, and may last up to 30 minutes. Once the baby is born, the uterine cavity immediately becomes smaller. The change in the interior dimension of the uterus results in a reduction in the size of the placental attachment site. This event leads to the

---

Table 12-6 Characteristics of the Third and Fourth Stages of Labor

	Third Stage	Fourth Stage
Description	Begins with the birth of the infant and ends with the delivery of the placenta. Usually takes 5–10 minutes, and may take up to 30 minutes.	A time of physiological adaptation that begins following delivery of the placenta and lasts 1–2 hours.
Contractions	The uterus should be firmly contracted.	The uterus should be firmly contracted.
Assessment	Uterus becomes globelike.	Uterus remains firmly contracted.
	Uterus rises upward.	Lochia rubra, bright red blood flow with occasional small clots.
	Umbilical cord descends further.	Vital signs return to prelabor values.
	Gush of blood as placenta detaches.	
Physical discomforts	Some discomfort or cramping as the placenta is expelled.	Some experience perineal discomfort usually related to trauma from the episiotomy or tearing, or hemorrhoids.
Maternal behaviors	Focus on infant well-being.	Excited, tired.
	Crying common. Expressions of relief.	Bonding and attachment with infant.
	Culturally influenced.	Initiation of breastfeeding.
		Culturally influenced.

Figure 12-24 Vaginal birth sequence. *A.* Pushing in an upright position allows the use of gravity to promote fetal descent. *B.* Crowning. *C.* Birth of the head. *D.* Birth of the shoulders. *E.* The infant is shown to the new parents. *F.* The baby's father cuts the umbilical cord.

separation of the placenta from the uterus. The following clinical indicators signal that separation of the placenta from the uterus has occurred:

- The uterus becomes spherical in shape.
- The uterus rises upward in the abdomen due to the descent of the placenta into the vagina.
- The umbilical cord descends further through the vagina.
- A gush of blood occurs once the placenta detaches from the uterus.

The placenta is expelled in either the Schultze or Duncan manner (Fig. 12-25). The **Schultze mechanism** ("shiny Schultze") occurs when the placenta separates from the inside to the outer margins with the shiny, fetal side of the placenta presenting first. It is the most common method of placental expulsion. The **Duncan mechanism** occurs when the placenta separates from the outer margins inward, rolls up, and presents sideways. Since the placental surface is rough, the Duncan mechanism is commonly called "dirty Duncan."

As the placenta separates from the uterine wall, it is important that the uterus continues to contract. The contractions minimize the bleeding that results from the open blood vessels left at the placental attachment site. Failure of the uterus to contract adequately with separation of the placenta can result in excessive blood loss or hemorrhage. To enhance the uterine contractions after expulsion of the placenta, oxytocic medications are often given. Oxytocin is administered either by the intravenous (IV) route or by intramuscular (IM) injection.

NURSING CARE OF THE MOTHER DURING THE THIRD STAGE OF LABOR

After the birth of the infant, the nurse observes for signs that the placenta has separated from the wall of the uterus. The uterus is palpated to determine the rise upward as well as the characteristic change in shape from one resembling a disk to that of a globe. The nurse may ask the woman to push again, to facilitate in the delivery of the placenta. If 30 minutes have elapsed from completion of

medication: Oxytocin

Oxytocin (ox-i-**toe**-sin)

Pitocin, Syntocinon

Pregnancy Category: X (intranasal), UK (IV, IM)

Indications:
Induction of labor at term
Facilitation of uterine contractions at term
Facilitation of threatened abortion
Control of postpartum bleeding after expulsion of placenta

Actions: Stimulates uterine smooth muscle producing uterine contractions similar to those in spontaneous labor (administered intravenously). Stimulates mammary gland smooth muscle facilitating lactation (administered intranasally). Has vasopressor and diuretic effects.

Therapeutic Effects: Induces labor. Reduces postpartum bleeding. Induces breast milk letdown.

Pharmacokinetics:
ABSORPTION: Well-absorbed from the nasal mucosa when administered intranasally.
DISTRIBUTION: Through extracellular fluid. Small amounts reach fetal circulation.
METABOLISM: Metabolized rapidly in kidneys and liver.
EXCRETION: Small amounts excreted in urine, half-life 3–9 minutes.

Contraindications and Precautions:
Contraindicated in CPD or deliveries that require conversion (i.e., transverse lie). Use with caution in first and second stages of labor.

Adverse Reactions and Side Effects: Maternal adverse reactions are associated with IV use only. Painful contractions and increased uterine motility most common. May contribute to maternal coma, seizures, hypotension. May contribute to fetal asphyxia or arrhythmias.

Route and Dosage: May be added to IV for labor induction or given IV or IM to control postpartum bleeding (do not administer IM and IV routes simultaneously). Intranasal spray is administered 2–3 minutes before planned breastfeeding.

Nursing Implications:
Fetal maturity, presentation, and maternal pelvic adequacy should be assessed before administration to induce labor.
Monitor contractions, resting uterine tone, and FHR frequently.
Monitor uterus for firmness and early detection of bogginess.
Monitor lochia for signs of excessive bleeding.

Adapted from Deglin, J.H., and Vallerand, A.H. (2009). *Davis's drug guide for nurses* (11th ed.). Philadelphia: F.A. Davis.

Figure 12-25 Third stage of labor: separation and expulsion of the placenta. *A.* Schultze mechanism. *B.* Duncan mechanism.

the second stage of labor and the placenta has not yet been expelled, it is considered to be "retained". (See Chapter 14 for further discussion.)

Oxytocic medications such as Pitocin and Syntocinon are often administered at the time of the delivery of the placenta. These drugs are used to stimulate uterine contractions, thereby minimizing the bleeding from the placental attachment site and reducing the risk of postpartum hemorrhage. The nurse administers oxytocic medications according to institutional protocol. If a peripheral intravenous infusion has been established, oxytocin 10 to 20 units may be added to the intravenous infusion. If no intravenous infusion is present, 10 units of oxytocin may be administered intramuscularly. In situations where there is excessive blood loss, the physician may order up to 40 units of oxytocin per liter of intravenous infusion fluid. Other medications such as methylergonovine maleate (Methergine) or carboprost tromethamine (Hemabate) may be given intramuscularly to control blood loss. During this time the nurse continues to assess the volume of blood loss and monitor the patient's vital signs, paying close attention to the blood pressure and heart rate.

Once the placenta has been delivered, the nurse carefully examines it to ensure that all cotyledons are intact (Fig. 12-26). If any part of the placenta is missing, the nurse immediately reports this finding to the attending physician. Because retained placental fragments can contribute to postpartum hemorrhage or infection, the physician may perform a manual exploration of the uterus to remove any remaining placental tissue.

Emotional Support

The birth of the newborn is an emotional experience for the patient and her support person. Hearing the infant's first cry can evoke tears, laughter, and feelings of relief, accomplishment, and amazement. The nurse can support the mother and birth partner by promoting contact with the infant. The stable newborn can be placed on the maternal abdomen, and as soon as possible, the nurse can help the mother into a comfortable position to hold the infant.

Initiating Infant Attachment

Once the birth has taken place, the time that immediately follows is ideal for fostering attachment between the mother, her birth partner, and the newborn. The infant is in a stage of alertness during the first hour after birth and is responsive to voice, touch, and gaze. The nurse can facilitate eye-to-eye contact between the patient and her neonate by dimming the room lights. This occasion also provides an excellent time to initiate breastfeeding if the mother wishes to do so.

Immediate Nursing Care of the Newborn

Once the newborn has been born, the primary care provider (physician or certified nurse midwife) places the infant on the mother's abdomen (if the infant is stable), in a modified Trendelenburg position. This immediate contact between mother and newborn provides reassurance to the mother regarding the overall well-being of the baby, and begins the attachment process.

Birth signals the transition from fetus to newborn. Several physiological adaptations must occur to facilitate the adjustment of the newborn to the extrauterine environment. Of primary importance is the initiation of the newborn's respirations, a process that results in the replacement of fetal lung fluid with air. In most situations, the actions of drying the newborn and performing nasopharyngeal suctioning, if needed, provide adequate stimulation to initiate the newborn's respiratory effort. While respirations are being established, the newborn's cardiovascular system is also undergoing major adaptations to allow the flow of deoxygenated blood into the lungs for gas exchange. Fetal circulation transitions to neonatal circulation after closure of the ductus arteriosus, the foramen ovale, and the ductus venosus. (See Chapter 17 for further discussion of the physiological transitions in the newborn.)

The modified Trendelenburg position facilitates the drainage of mucus from the newborn's nasopharynx and trachea. The nurse suctions the newborn's nose and mouth with a bulb syringe as needed. Preventing heat loss in the neonate constitutes an important nursing role. Before the infant is placed on the mother's abdomen, the nurse dries the infant, discards the wet linens, and applies warm blankets. Skin-to-skin contact between the mother and baby also helps to maintain the newborn's temperature.

THE APGAR SCORING SYSTEM

The nurse assesses this transition stage after one minute and again after 5 minutes, using the **Apgar Scoring System** (Apgar, 1966). The Apgar scoring system evaluates

Figure 12-26 Examination of the placenta.

five signs of newborn cardiopulmonary adaptation and neuromuscular function: heart rate, respiratory effort, muscle tone, reflex irritability, and color (Table 12-7).

HEART RATE. The priority assessment of the newborn is the heart rate. On auscultation or palpation, the nurse recognizes an absent heart rate or heart rate less than 100 bpm as a signal for resuscitation.

RESPIRATORY EFFORT. The newborn's vigorous cry best indicates adequate respiratory effort, the next most important assessment after birth. A weak or absent cry is a signal for intervention.

MUSCLE TONE. The nurse determines the newborn's muscle tone by assessing the response to the extension of the extremities. Good muscle tone is noted when the extremities return to a position of flexion.

REFLEX IRRITABILITY. The nurse assesses reflex irritability by observing the newborn's response to stimuli such as a gentle stroking motion along the spine or flicking the soles of the feet. When this stimulation elicits a cry, the score is 2. A grimace in response to stimulation scores 1, and no response is a score of 0.

COLOR. The nurse assesses skin color for pallor and cyanosis. Most newborns exhibit cyanosis of the extremities at the 1-minute Apgar check, and this normal finding is termed **acrocyanosis**. A score of 2 indicates that the infant's skin is completely pink. Newborns with darker pigmented skin are assessed for pallor and acrocyanosis.

IDENTIFICATION OF THE NEWBORN

Another important nursing action involves placing matching identification bands on the infant and the mother. Some hospitals also provide identification bands for the father or other designated birth support person. The infant's identification bands are placed snugly enough so that when the initial weight loss occurs, the ID band does not fall off. Agency protocols may also direct the nurse to footprint the newborn. (See Chapter 18 for further discussion.)

While the newborn rests upon the mother's abdomen, the nurse performs a head-to-toe assessment to detect any abnormalities. The nurse observes the infant's overall size relative to the gestational age, noting the shape and size of the head and chest. The color of the skin, presence of vernix and lanugo, and any evidence of trauma are also noted. (See Chapter 18 for further discussion.)

> **Now Can You—** Discuss essential nursing actions during the third stage of labor?
>
> 1. Name three clinical indicators that signal placental separation during the third stage of labor?
> 2. Explain what is meant by "shiny Schultze" and "dirty Duncan"?
> 3. Describe essential nursing actions concerning the oxytocin infusion, placenta inspection, and immediate newborn care?

Fourth Stage of Labor

The fourth stage of labor is the period of maternal physiological adjustment that occurs from the time of delivery of the placenta through the first 1 to 2 hours after birth. Monitoring of the mother and infant takes place frequently during this time.

NURSING CARE DURING THE FOURTH STAGE OF LABOR

While the physician examines the mother's perineum, cervix, and vagina for evidence of tears, the nurse assesses the uterus for firmness, height, and position. To perform fundal palpation, the left hand is placed directly above the symphysis pubis and gentle downward pressure is exerted. The right hand is cupped around the uterine fundus (Fig. 12-27). On palpation, the uterus is expected to feel firm and be positioned in the midline, at or just below the umbilicus. It can be described as closely

Figure 12-27 Fundal palpation during the fourth stage of labor. The left hand is placed directly above the symphysis pubis and exerts gentle downward pressure; the right hand is cupped around the uterine fundus.

Table 12-7 The Apgar Scoring System			
Physiological Parameter	**Score**		
	0	**1**	**2**
Heart Rate	Absent	Slow: below 100	Above 100
Respiratory Effort	Absent	Slow: irregular, weak cry	Good; strong cry
Muscle Tone	Flaccid	Some flexion of extremities	Well flexed
Reflex Irritability	No response	Grimace	Vigorous cry
Color	Blue, pale	Pink body, blue extremities	Completely pink

Range of Apgar Score: from 0 to 10
A score of 8–10 reflects a newborn in good condition that usually requires only nasopharyngeal suctioning. A score less than 8 may warrant further resuscitation measures.

approximating the size of a grapefruit. A full bladder or excessive blood in the uterus may cause it to be displaced from the midline.

If the uterus feels soft or "boggy" on palpation, this finding may indicate that excessive blood and/or clots have pooled in the uterus. The nurse immediately begins to massage the uterus until it becomes firm. To perform uterine fundal massage correctly, the nurse uses two hands. One hand applies firm pressure to the fundus to express the blood clots; the other hand supports the lower aspect of the uterus to protect the ligaments from damage.

While monitoring the firmness and position of the uterus, the nurse also assesses the bloody vaginal discharge or **lochia**, noting the color, amount, and presence of clots. The first lochia that appears is bright red, and is called **lochia rubra**. The amount of lochia is determined by examining the soaking of the perineal pads and the frequency of pad changes required. One soaked pad within the first postpartal hour is considered the normal maximum flow. Small blood clots are common; large clots are not normal. A steady trickle of blood or blood pooling under the mother's buttocks can be a sign of trauma to the perineum or birth canal.

The nurse also assesses the mother's vital signs frequently, generally every 5 to 15 minutes. The blood pressure should return to the prelabor level and the pulse rate should be slower than that recorded during the labor experience. A rising pulse rate or a decreasing blood pressure are indicators of excessive blood loss. The temperature is also assessed at the beginning of the fourth stage of labor, and on transfer from the birthing room to the postpartum area. A rise in temperature and an increase in the pulse may be early indicators of postpartum infection.

The nurse monitors maternal urine output. A full, distended bladder can displace the uterus and impede its ability to contract adequately, potentially leading to hemorrhage. Trauma to the urethra or bladder during childbirth may impair the mother's perception of the urge to void.

 critical nursing action Fourth-Stage Risk Signs

The nurse must be alert to the following risk signs that may occur during the fourth stage of labor: hypotension, tachycardia, excessive bleeding, or a boggy noncontracting uterus. These signs are associated with hemorrhage and must be reported immediately. If the uterus is boggy, the nurse must immediately initiate fundal massage and continue until the uterus becomes firm.

Comfort

It is not unusual for the mother to experience extreme shivering during the fourth stage of labor. The nurse can offer a heated blanket or warm beverage as comfort measures. The work of labor has expended considerable maternal energy, and providing a light meal and fluids can help replace lost calories. The process of labor is also extremely fatiguing, and the nurse can encourage both the mother and her birth partner to rest.

Figure 12-28 Family members share a special time with the newborn.

Promoting Attachment and Breastfeeding

The first hour after the birth is an ideal time to promote parent–infant attachment. During this time the stable newborn is in a state of alertness and is responsive to voice and touch. The nurse can support this attachment by completing many maternal and newborn assessments while the infant is held by the parents. Providing a private, quiet environment enhances the opportunity for parent–infant eye contact. Some parents may wish to include siblings or other family members in this experience (Fig. 12-28).

The mother may wish to initiate breastfeeding at this time. The nipple stimulation associated with maternal breastfeeding is beneficial in two ways: it initiates the process of lactation and assists in the process of uterine involution by triggering the release of endogenous oxytocin. As with any interactions with childbearing families, it is important for the nurse to be aware of and respect the family's cultural practices.

 Now Can You— Discuss the fourth stage of labor?

1. Explain what is meant by the fourth stage of labor?
2. Describe essential nursing assessments and appropriate interventions during the fourth stage of labor?
3. Name two nursing actions to promote infant attachment during the fourth stage of labor?

 case study The Birth Experience of a Multigravida

Tina Sanchez is a 26-year-old Mexican-American gravida 2 para 1 who comes to the birthing unit with her husband Thomas. On arrival, Tina describes her contractions as starting approximately 2 hours earlier, regular and of moderate strength. You note that while she is walking to her room she has two contractions that are approximately 4 minutes apart and 60 seconds long. Tina is coping well with the contractions. She tells you in between contractions that with her first baby 3 years ago she was induced and confined to bed with an electronic monitor and does not want that this time if possible.

critical thinking questions

1. What type of information do you need to obtain from Tina and her husband?

2. What are your priority nursing assessments?

3. How would you respond to Tina's request not to be confined to bed?

   The nurse completes the assessment of Tina and the admission history between contractions. Tina has experienced a healthy pregnancy and is considered low risk. The institution policy promotes intermittent auscultation for low-risk patients in active labor. Tina's contractions are growing longer in duration and becoming stronger in intensity. Tina states: "I don't know how long I am going to be able to do this, it is getting harder."

4. What evaluation of the FHR would you make during intermittent auscultation?

5. How would you respond to Tina, considering that at this time she appears to be coping well?

6. What type of comfort measures could you suggest?

   While ambulating in the room, Tina experiences a large gush of greenish-brown fluid from her vagina.

7. What are your priority nursing assessments?

   The amniotic fluid is noted to be meconium stained, a finding that is an indication for continuous fetal monitoring. The nurse explains the findings to Tina and Thomas and places Tina on the electronic FHR monitor. The fetal heart tracing shows a baseline rate of 140 bpm with accelerations to 160 bpm. The variability is normal and no decelerations are noted.

8. Are these findings normal or pathological? What further interventions are required?

   Thirty minutes later Tina is fully dilated and begins to push with each contraction. The FHR is now decreasing with each contraction and resembles the mirror image of the contraction.

9. What stage of labor has Tina now entered?

10. What is your interpretation of the FHR at this time?

11. What type of nursing interventions would you anticipate for Tina?

    Tina gives birth to a healthy baby girl 20 minutes later. The infant is suctioned well at the perineum and examined by the pediatrician due to the presence of meconium in the amniotic fluid. The infant is pink with acrocyanosis and does not demonstrate any signs of respiratory difficulties and is quickly returned to the proud parents.

12. Considering that the newborn infant has acrocyanosis, what is the highest possible Apgar score this infant could receive?

13. What are your priority nursing interventions for the newborn, Tina, and the family?

◆ See Suggested Answers to Case Studies in the text on the Electronic Study Guide or DavisPlus.

summary points

◆ Each patient's labor and birth experience is unique, and nurses play a vital role in facilitating a positive outcome for the patient, infant, and family.

◆ Nurses recognize that the labor and birth experience is influenced by a myriad of factors such as maternal age and well-being, social support, and cultural and religious beliefs and practices.

◆ Nurses need a strong knowledge base about the physiological processes of labor and birth in order to provide safe and effective care.

◆ In each of the four stages of labor, the nurse uses well-developed assessment skills to recognize the normal progression of labor, to identify potential risks to the patient and fetus, and to identify how and when to intervene and consult with other health care providers.

◆ The overall goal of intrapartal nursing care is to promote comfort and safety of the patient, the fetus, and the newborn infant.

◆ A positive nurse–patient relationship in which the woman feels cared for and informed will empower her in coping with her labor.

◆ Nurses include the patient and her support person(s) in the planning and delivery of care.

◆ The nursing care given throughout labor and birth is an important determinant of the woman's overall perception of her childbirth experience.

review questions

Multiple Choice

1. When describing the "powers" of labor to a new nurse, the perinatal nurse discusses the uterine contractions and the:
   A. Woman's pushing efforts
   B. Unique musculature of the uterus
   C. Position of the fetus
   D. Hormonal influences regulating labor

2. The perinatal nurse assesses Diane, a 22-year-old primigravida who has just arrived at the birth facility for labor assessment. Diane describes contractions that are 7 to 10 minutes apart, and felt in the abdomen. She states that the contractions "feel better" when she is walking. This is most likely:
   A. True labor
   B. Transition
   C. Early labor
   D. False labor

3. The perinatal nurse describes for the student nurse the lettering used to designate fetal position. The correct use includes:
   A. "P" indicating fetal pelvis location
   B. "P" indicating posterior maternal pelvis
   C. "M" indicating fetal mandible
   D. "A" indicating maternal anus

Fill-in-the-Blank

4. The perinatal nurse describes labor contractions as composed of three distinct parts: an increment or _____, an _____ or peak and the decrement or _____ in the contraction.

5. The perinatal nurse teaches the new nurse about fetal lie. The perinatal nurse describes fetal lie as the relationship of the _____ axis of the woman to the _____ axis of the fetus.

6. The perinatal nurse knows that offering relaxation techniques such as massage and assistance with breathing can decrease the production of _____, which can _____ uterine blood flow during labor.

True/False

7. The perinatal nurse knows that the fetus is normally in a flexed position prior to birth.

Select All that Apply

8. The perinatal nurse knows to assess for the uterine relaxation that occurs between contractions. This period of uterine relaxation is important for:
A. Fetal oxygenation
B. Maternal rest
C. Lactic acid production
D. Oxytocin production

9. The perinatal nurse describes the latent phase of labor to the new nurse. Characteristics of this phase include:
A. Cervical dilation from 0 to 3 cm
B. Excitement and nervousness
C. Moderate to strong contractions
D. Admission to the hospital

10. The perinatal nurse describes for the student nurse the risks associated with a breech birth which include:
A. Cord prolapse
B. Birth trauma
C. Shoulder dystocia
D. Vaginal bleeding

See Answers to End of Chapter Review Questions on the Electronic Study Guide or DavisPlus.

REFERENCES

American College of Obstetricians and Gyneologists (ACOG). (2005). Intrapartum fetal heart rate monitoring. Practice Bulletin Number 70. Washington, DC: ACOG.

American College of Obstetricians and Gynecologists (ACOG). (2006). Mode of term singleton breech delivery. Committee Opinion Number 340. Washington, DC: ACOG.

Andrews, M., & Boyle, J. (2003). *Transcultural concepts in nursing care* (4th ed.). Philadelphia: Lippincott.

Angelini, D., & Mahlmeister, L. (2005). Liability in triage: Management of EMTALA regulations and common obstetric risks. *Journal of Midwifery & Women's Health, 50*(6), 472–478.

Apgar, V. (1966). The newborn scoring system: Reflections and advice. *Pediatric Clinics of North America, 13,* 645–650.

Association of Women's Health, Obstetric and Neonatal Nurses (AWHONN). (2000). *Fetal assessment* (position statement). Washington, DC: Author.

Association of Women's Health, Obstetric and Neonatal Nurses (AWHONN). (2003a). *Fetal heart monitoring principles and practice* (3rd ed). Dubuque, IA: Kendall/Hunt.

Association of Women's Health, Obstetric, & Neonatal Nurses (AWHONN). (2003b). *Standards for professional nursing practice in the care of women and newborns* (6th ed.). Washington, DC: Author.

Bulechek, G., Butcher, H.M., & Dochterman, J. (2008). *Nursing interventions classification (NIC)* (5th ed.). St. Louis, MO: C.V. Mosby.

Caliendo, C., Millbauer, L., Moore, B., & Kitchen, E. (2004). Obstetric triage and EMTALA: Practice strategies for labor and delivery nursing units. *AWHONN Lifelines, 8*(5), 442–448.

Carroli, G., & Belizan, J. (2006). Episiotomy for vaginal birth. *The Cochrane Database of Systematic Reviews,* No. 2. Chichester, UK: John Wiley & Sons, pp 178–180.

Cesario, S. (2004). Reevaluation of the Friedman labor cure: A pilot study. *Journal of Obstetric, Gynecologic and Neonatal Nursing, 33*(6), 713–722.

Chen, C-H., Wang, S-Y., & Chang, M-Y. (2001). Women's perceptions of helpful and unhelpful nursing behaviors during labor: A study in Taiwan. *BIRTH, 28*(3), 180–185.

Cunningham, G., Leveno, K., Bloom, S., Hauth, J., Gilstrap, L., & Wenstrom, K. (2005). *Williams obstetrics* (22nd ed.). New York: McGraw-Hill.

Deglin, J.H., & Vallerand, A.H. (2009). *Davis's drug guide for nurses* (11th ed.). Philadelphia: F.A. Davis.

Dildy, G. (2005). Intrapartum assessment of the fetus: Historical and evidence-based practice. *Obstetrics and Gynecology Clinics of North America, 32*(2), 255–271.

Fox, M., Kilpatrick, S., King, T., & Parer, J. (2000). Fetal heart rate monitoring: Interpretation and collaborative management. *Journal of Midwifery & Womens Health, 45*(6), 498–507.

Goodwin, L. (2000). Intermittent auscultation of the fetal heart rate: A review of general principles. *Journal of Perinatal and Neonatal Nursing, 14*(3), 53–61.

Hacker, N., Moore, J., & Gambone, J. (2004). *Essentials of Obstetrics and Gynecology.* (4th ed.). Philadelphia: W.B. Saunders.

Hannah, M., Hannah, W., Hewson, S. Hodnett, E., Saigal, S., & Willan, A.R. (2000). Planned cesarean section vs vaginal birth for breech presentation at term: A randomized multicenter trial. *Lancet, 356,* 1375–1383.

Hodnett, E.D., Downe, S., Edwards, N., & Walsh, D. (2005). Home-like versus conventional institutional settings for birth. *The Cochrane Library,* No. 1. Chichester, UK: John Wiley & Sons, pp 367–372.

Hodnett, E.D., Gates, S., Hofmeyr, G.J., & Sakala, C. (2006). Continuous support for women during childbirth. *Cochrane Database of Systematic Reviews,* No. 3. Chichester, UK: John Wiley & Sons, pp 103–105.

Johnson, M., Bulechek, G., Butcher, H., McCloskey Dochterman, J., Maas, M., Moorehead, S., & Swanson, E. (2006). *NANDA, NOC, and NIC linkages: Nursing diagnoses, outcomes, & interventions* (2nd ed.). St. Louis, MO: Mosby Elsevier.

MacKinnon, K., McIntyre, M., & Quance, M. (2005). The meaning of the nurse's presence during childbirth. *Journal of Obstetrics, Gynecology and Neonatal Nursing, 34*(1), 28–36.

Martin, J., Hamilton, B., Sutton, P., Ventura, S., Menacker, F., & Munson, M. (2005). Births: Final data for 2003. *National Vital Statistics Report, 54*(2), 1–116.

Minato, J. (2000). Is it time to push? *AWHONN Lifelines, 46*(6), 20–23.

Moorehead, S., Johnson, M., Maas, M., & Swanson, E. (2008). *Nursing outcomes classification (NOC)* (4th ed.). St. Louis, MO: C.V. Mosby.

NANDA International (2007). *NANDA-I nursing diagnoses: Definitions and classifications 2007–2008.* Philadelphia: NANDA-I.

National Institute of Child Health and Human Development (NICHD) Research Planning Workshop. (1997). Electronic fetal heart rate monitoring: Research guidelines for interpretation. *American Journal of Obstetrics and Gynecology, 177*(6), 1385–1390.

Roberts, J. (2002). The "push" for evidence: Management of the second stage. *Journal of Midwifery and Women's Health, 47*(1), 2–15.

Roberts, J. (2003). A new understanding of the second stage of labor: Implications for care. *Journal of Obstetric, Gynecologic and Neonatal Nursing, 32*(6), 794–801.

Simkin, P. (2002). Supportive care during labor: A guide for busy nurses. *JOGGN, 31,* 721–732.

Simpson, K. (2004). Standardized language for electronic fetal heart rate monitoring. *MCN American Journal of Maternal/Child Nursing, 29*(5), 336.

Simpson, K.R., & Creehan, P.A. (2001). *AWHONN Perinatal Nursing* (2nd ed.). Philadelphia: Lippincott.

Society of Obstetricians and Gynaecologists of Canada (SOGC). (2005). Clinical Practice Guidelines: Fetal health surveillance in labor. *Journal of Gynecology Canada, 24*(3), 250–262.

Soong, B., & Barnes, M. (2005). Maternal position at midwife-attended birth and perineal trauma: Is there an association? *Birth, 32*(3), 164–169.

Thacker, S., Stroup, D., & Chang, M. (2005). Continuous electronic heart rate monitoring for fetal assessment during labor. *Cochrane Database of Systematic Reviews*, No. 4. Chichester, UK: John Wiley & Sons, (5th ed.).

Tucker, S.M. (2004). *Pocket Guide to Fetal Monitoring and Assessment* (5th ed., pp 73–86). St Louis: C.V. Mosby.

Wood, S. (2003). Should women be given a choice about fetal assessment in labor? *MCN American Journal of Maternal/Child Nursing, 28*(5), 292–298.

 For more information, go to http://davisplus.fadavis.com/

CONCEPT MAP

The 5 Ps of Labor

Powers
Uterine contractions
- Increment; acme; decrement
- Responsible for cervical:
  - Effacement
  - Dilation

Maternal pushing
- Facilitates expulsion of fetus

Passageway
- Maternal bony pelvis
  - Inlet
  - Midpelvis
  - Outlet
- Pelvic soft tissue

Passenger/Passageway: Relationship Between
- Determined by assessing
  - Engagement
  - Station
  - Position

Passenger: Fetus and Fetal Membranes
Fetal considerations:
- Fetal lie
- Fetal attitude
- Fetal presentation
  - Cephalic
  - Breech
  - Shoulder

Psychosocial Influences
- Readiness for labor/birth
- Level of educational preparedness
  - Prior experience
  - Emotional readiness
  - Culture

The Process of Labor and Birth

Complementary Care:
- Perineal massage, warm compresses, lubricating oils, semi-recumbent position ⟶ potentially decrease perineal trauma

Where Research And Practice Meet:
- Planned vaginal delivery of singleton term breech may no longer be appropriate
- Despite benefits of home birth, patient also at risk for complications
- More positive outcomes found with continuous labor support
- EFM: may prevent neonatal seizures

Critical Nursing Actions:
- Determine/document fetal position
- Assess for 4th stage signs of hemorrhage
- Prevent maternal supine hypotension
- Interpret fetal monitor tracings correctly

Fetal Assessment: Labor/Birth
- Fetal position
  - Leopold's maneuvers
  - Point of FHR
  - Vaginal exam/Ultrasound
- Fetal heart rate
  - Variability
  - Accelerations/decelerations
  - Interpret FHR pattern ⟶ requires holistic assessment
  - Interpret FHR tracings: use protocol
- Fetal heart sounds
- Electronic fetal monitoring

Stages of Labor:
1st Stage: regular contractions to complete cervical dilation
  - Latent phase
  - Active phase
  - Transition
2nd Stage: full dilation to birth
  - Urge to push/"bearing down"
  - Duration variable
Birth: fetal cardinal movements
  - Descent; flexion; internal rotation; extension; restitution; external rotation; expulsion
3rd Stage: birth to delivery of placenta
  - Decrease in uterine size
  - Placenta separates from uterus
4th Stage: delivery of placenta through first four hours post birth

Impending Labor: Signs/Symptoms
- Lightening
- Braxton-Hicks contractions
- Cervical ripening
- Bloody show/ruptured membranes
- Energy spurt
- Weight loss/GI disturbances

Nursing Considerations: Labor
- Stage 1: continual monitoring mother/fetus; facilitate positive experience; manage pain
- Stage 2: promote effective pushing; position for comfort
- Stage 3: facilitate delivery of placenta; promote infant bonding; immediate infant care; ID infant
- Stage 4: promote comfort, attachment and breastfeeding

General Labor Support:
- Offering presence
- Promote comfort/position changes/relaxation
- Provide relaxed environment
- Attend to hygiene/elimination needs
- Provide anticipatory guidance
- Support birth partner

True labor vs. false labor: ⟶ **differences in**
- Regularity, intensity, duration; whether effacement/dilation occurs
- Back pain that radiates and worsens with activity vs. abdominal pain that eases with activity

What To Say:
- Questions for telephone assessment of a laboring woman
- Use direct, open questions for difficult topics ⟶ drug, alcohol use

Now Can You:
- Evaluate uterine contractions
- Identify and discuss the 5 Ps of labor
- Identify the characteristics of nursing care for each stage of labor
- Identify the critical elements of fetal assessment during and after labor

Promoting Patient Comfort During Labor and Birth

Natural childbirth means that no drugs will be put into the mother's body during delivery—the father can have all he wants.

—Bill Cosby

LEARNING TARGETS *At the completion of this chapter, the student will be able to:*

- ◆ Describe the unique characteristics of pain associated with childbirth.
- ◆ Discuss sociocultural factors that shape the woman's pain experience during labor and childbirth.
- ◆ Identify nonpharmacological methods to promote comfort during labor and birth.
- ◆ Compare pharmacological interventions used for discomfort and pain during different stages of labor.
- ◆ Summarize the possible complications associated with regional and general anesthesia.
- ◆ Discuss the nurse's role in ensuring maternal-fetal safety while promoting comfort during labor and birth.

---

 moving toward evidence-based practice Use of a Doula to Support Women in Labor

Campbell, D.A., Lake, M.F., Falk, M., & Backstand, J.R. (2006). A randomized control trial of continuous support in labor by a lay doula. *JOGNN, 35*(4), 456–463.

Previous meta-analysis of randomized clinical trials have found that there is a reduction in the number of cesarean deliveries, length of labor, and use of analgesia along with increased infant Apgar scores in women who receive continuous support during labor. One form of support can be provided by a doula, who is a female support for women in labor. She is not a physician, nurse, or midwife and does not provide medical treatment. In addition, her presence is not intended to take the place of the male partner or other family members who may be present during labor.

The purpose of the study was to compare labor outcomes of nulliparous women accompanied by a doula with the labor outcomes of nulliparous women who received standard care and did not have the support of a doula, regardless of support from the male partner or other family members. The outcomes under investigation included:

- Length of labor, which was defined as the time from the onset of regular contractions to the birth of the neonate.

The onset of regular contractions was determined by the nurse or reported by the patient. The actual time of birth was obtained from the woman's medical record.

- Type of birth
- Type and timing of administration of analgesia or anesthesia
- Apgar scores at 1 and 5 minutes.

The study took place in a tertiary perinatal care hospital that provides care for underinsured low-income women. A convenience sample of 600 nulliparous women met the criteria for the study: low-risk, singleton pregnancy. Male partners and/or additional family members were allowed to provide support during labor.

Three hundred women who were randomly assigned to the experimental group identified a female friend or family member who was willing to serve as a lay doula.

(continued)

---

moving toward evidence-based practice (continued)

A research assistant who was certified as a doula met with the pregnant women and their female support for two-2-hour sessions to teach traditional doula supportive techniques.

Data analysis of the 586 women who completed the study revealed the following:

Of the 586 of the original 600 women who completed the study,

- Fifty-six percent of the women in each group were Caucasian.
- Thirty-six percent of women in the experimental (doula) group and 29% in the control (non-doula) group were African American.
- Fewer than 1% in both groups described themselves as Indian, Chinese, or Filipino; 6.4% in the experimental (doula) group and 12% in the control (non-doula) group described their ethnicity as "other."
- The participants' ages ranged from 14 to 40 years at the time of birth. The mean age was 22.2 years for the

experimental (doula) group and 22.6 years for the control (non-doula) group.

- The experimental (doula) group experienced shorter labors, greater cervical dilation at the time of administration of epidural anesthesia (if used), and higher infant Apgar scores at 1 and 5 minutes.
- No difference was found between the two groups in the number of cesarean births, duration of the second stage of labor or type of analgesia/anesthesia administered.

The researchers concluded that providing low-income pregnant women with an option to choose a female friend to train and serve as a doula shortens the labor process and improves maternal and neonatal outcomes.

---

1. What might be considered as limitations to this study?
2. How is this information useful to clinical nursing practice?

See Suggested Responses for Moving Toward Evidence-Based Practice on the Electronic Study Guide or DavisPlus.

Introduction

When a laboring woman experiences discomfort and pain, there are many interventions that nurses can implement to help reduce anxiety and promote comfort. There is an increasingly accepted perspective that certain physiological processes are normally associated with a certain level of pain, and that the pain serves a useful purpose. The pain of childbirth, for example, may serve to warn the woman to seek a safe haven and obtain help. Ideally, these actions help to ensure that the birth takes place in safe surroundings and facilitate a positive outcome, whether childbirth takes place at home, in a free-standing birth center, or at a hospital. However, this perspective should not be confused with the belief that childbirth should not be painful. To deny that discomfort or pain exists during childbirth is patently unrealistic. The nurse, the laboring woman, and her support person(s) all benefit from an understanding of the physiological and psychological processes that underlie the experience of pain. Becoming familiar with strategies for managing or diminishing the pain of childbirth empowers the laboring woman to make informed decisions about the various pain management measures she will use. This chapter discusses the physiology of childbirth pain, theories related to pain perception, cultural and psychological factors that affect childbirth pain, non-pharmacological and pharmacological pain management interventions, and implications for nursing care.

⟲ **Optimizing Outcomes—** Helping to achieve *Healthy People 2010* national goals

Because the use of anesthesia and analgesia during childbirth can increase maternal mortality, several of the *Healthy*

People 2010 national goals relate to pain relief during labor. One such goal is:

- Reduce the maternal mortality rate to no more than 3.3 per 100,000 live births from a baseline of 7.1 maternal deaths in 1998.

Nurses can help the nation achieve this goal by educating women about the benefits of prepared childbirth. During labor, nurses can educate, reassure, and continuously monitor patients and assist them in the use of nonpharmacological pain relief methods to enhance comfort and reduce the total amount of analgesics needed.

The Physiology of Pain During Labor and Birth

DEFINING PAIN

Pain is a complex, multidimensional experience. According to Padfield and colleagues (2003), pain is defined as whatever the person who is experiencing it says it is. The International Association for the Study of Pain defines pain as an unpleasant sensory and emotional experience arising from actual or potential tissue damage or described in terms of such damage. Pain includes not only the perception of an uncomfortable stimulus but also the response to that perception (Venes, 2009). The expression of pain is influenced by a number of psychosocial and cultural factors. For example, in some cultures it is permissible for the woman in labor to freely verbalize her pain. In others, the laboring woman must be stoic and keep her emotions to herself.

The pain experienced during childbirth is an unpleasant sensation that is usually localized to the back and the abdomen. For most, the pain associated with childbirth intensifies an already highly emotional experience for both the laboring woman and her support person. How well the laboring woman is able to cope with her pain significantly affects the overall birth experience.

During the assessment, the nurse may identify physiological and psychological changes that are indicative of maternal pain. These include an increased pulse rate and blood pressure, changes in mood, increased anxiety and stress, marked agitation, confusion, decreased urine output, decreased intestinal motility, and guarding of the target area of discomfort. Pain affects the patient's physiologic, behavioral, sensory, and cognitive responses. It is frequently intensified by fear, anxiety, and fatigue.

The experience of pain is shaped by many factors such as the patient's age, educational background, state of wellness, prior experiences, sociocultural background, degree of family and social support, and mastery of coping mechanisms. Nurses must simply accept what the patient says about her pain experience. The pain is real for each woman and occurs wherever she reports it to hurt. Despite the presence or absence of physiological indicators of pain, only the patient can validate with certainty her present level of discomfort.

Nursing Insight— *Recognizing the unique characteristics of childbirth pain*

When caring for laboring women, nurses must recognize that unlike other sources of pain, childbirth pain:

- Is part of a normal process (not associated with illness or injury)
- Can be anticipated, and thus prepared for (through childbirth education and the practice of distraction techniques and comfort measures)
- Has an end point (the baby's birth brings relief on a physical and emotional level)

PHYSICAL CAUSES OF PAIN RELATED TO LABOR AND BIRTH

Pain Neurology

The pain associated with labor and birth has both visceral and somatic origins (Lowe, 2002). Uterine contractions during the first stage of labor bring about cervical dilation and effacement. During each contraction, arteries that supply the myometrium are compressed, causing uterine ischemia (oxygen deficit that results from decreased blood flow). During the first stage of labor, pain impulses are transmitted via the T11 and T12 spinal nerve segments and accessory lower thoracic and upper lumbar sympathetic nerves. These nerves originate in the uterus.

Visceral pain describes the predominant discomfort experienced during the first stage of labor. It is related to changes in the cervix (i.e., dilation and effacement), distention of the lower uterine segment and uterine ischemia. Visceral pain is a slow, deep, poorly localized pain that occurs over the lower abdomen. It is commonly described as a dull aching pain. Laboring women may also experience **referred pain**. Referred pain describes pain that originates in the uterus and then radiates to the

abdominal wall, the lumbosacral area of the back, the iliac crests, the gluteus maximus, and down the thighs. Usually, the discomfort is felt only during contractions. A period of pain relief occurs between contractions although some women report continued nonremitting pain even during the interval between contractions (Lowe, 2002).

Somatic pain, a faster, well localized intense, sharp, burning, prickling pain, occurs during the second stage of labor. Somatic pain is associated with stretching and distention of the perineal body to allow for birth. It is also related to distention and traction placed on the peritoneum and uterocervical supportive tissue during contractions and can result from soft tissue lacerations that frequently occur in the cervix, vagina, or perineum. Somatic pain may also occur from the maternal expulsive forces during the second, or "pushing" stage of labor or by fetal pressure on the bladder, bowel, or other pelvic structures. During the second stage of labor, pain impulses are transmitted via the pudendal nerve through S2 to S4 spinal nerve segments and the parasympathetic system (Lowe, 2002).

During the third stage of labor, and in the early post-partum period, discomfort is associated with uterine contractions. The pain experienced during this time is similar to that associated with the first stage of labor.

PAIN PERCEPTION AND EXPRESSION

Although pain is a universal experience, how a woman reacts to and expresses pain is highly personal and subjective. One's perception of and response to pain is colored by many factors including gender, culture, ethnicity, and past experiences. Research from the disciplines of psychology, anthropology, and sociology has offered insights into the influence of one's primary social group on the meaning of pain and verbal and nonverbal expressions of pain.

Optimizing Outcomes— Recognizing cultural influences on the experience of pain

When providing care, nurses must recognize that culture strongly influences how one perceives and copes with pain. Women from certain cultures seek pain relief through prayer; others rely on herbal remedies, the application of cold or warmth, acupuncture, the "laying on of hands," and therapeutic massage. Assessment of cultural beliefs and practices, questions to identify specific needs and encouragement and support to use safe interventions is key in providing culturally sensitive care that empowers the patient to maintain her sense of control over her labor and childbirth experience.

For example, a primigravid Haitian woman may respond to painful uterine contractions with crying, loud screams, and hysteria (Colin & Paperwalla, 2003). Laboring Cambodian women, usually attended by a female relative rather than the male partner, tend to be quiet and sedate during labor and birth (Kulig, 2003). The Mexican American woman in labor is likely to be very vocal. Family members other than the baby's father frequently assist with emotional and verbal support (Lagana & Gonzalez-Ramirez, 2003). In any clinical setting, it is helpful for the nurse to identify the ethnic groups most often cared for and develop an awareness of culturally specific childbirth practices and pain behaviors. However, the nurse should be cautious not to stereotype patients and must remain sensitive to individual variations in women's choices for dealing with pain during the childbirth process. Approaching each woman's response to her labor and pain with acceptance and support is key to a therapeutic nursing relationship.

✾ *Ethnocultural Considerations*— Realities of the cultural model

When caring for women, nurses must be aware that a potential limitation of relying solely on a cultural perspective comes from neglecting to recognize women's individuality in how they conform to traditional values and norms. Cultural models of health care frequently stereotype women who share the same cultural heritage. In so doing, they may immobilize health providers who seek to change unfavorable health care situations in the name of protection of the cultural heritage (Meleis, 2003).

Pain is expressed in a number of physiological and affective ways. During labor and childbirth, the sympathetic nervous system responds to pain with increased levels of catecholamines (e.g., epinephrine and norepinephrine— biologically active substances that produce a marked effect on the nervous and cardiovascular systems, metabolic rate, temperature, and smooth muscle). There is a rise in blood pressure and heart rate. Increased maternal oxygen consumption results in an altered respiratory pattern that may produce hyperventilation and respiratory alkalosis. The woman may become diaphoretic, and nausea and vomiting are common during the active phase of labor. Throughout this process, decreased placental perfusion and uterine activity can potentially prolong labor and adversely affect fetal well-being.

Visceral and somatic pain has been described as burning, prickling, stabbing, heavy, pulling, pointing, sharp, stinging, and throbbing. On an emotional, or affective level, maternal pain during childbirth has been characterized as exhausting, nauseating, annoying and sickening (Lowe, 2002). Outward signs of suffering tend to be universal and are exhibited in varying degrees. Patients in pain cry, scream, clench and wring their hands, moan, groan, clench their jaws, and in other ways demonstrate increasing anxiety with a reduced perceptual field.

FACTORS THAT AFFECT MATERNAL PAIN RESPONSE

Physical, physiologic, and psychological influences affect the laboring woman's perception and tolerance of pain. Physical factors include labor intensity, cervical readiness, fetal position, pelvic dimensions, fatigue, and medical interventions.

Physical Factors

A brief, intense labor is often associated with a greater level of discomfort and pain because the contractions are highly efficient in accomplishing cervical changes (effacement and dilation) and fetal progress (descent). Also, a shortened labor may diminish the woman's options for pharmacological methods of pain relief. When cervical changes (softening, some dilation and effacement) have occurred before the onset of labor, the cervix opens more readily. Theoretically, fewer contractions are needed to achieve dilation and effacement.

When the fetus is in an unfavorable position, the labor is likely to be longer and associated with a greater amount of discomfort. For example, when the fetus is in an occiput posterior position, the woman experiences intense pain during contractions as the fetal occiput is pressed against the maternal sacrum. The pain associated with "back labor" persists between contractions and is unremitting until the fetus rotates to a more favorable position (e.g., occiput anterior). The size and shape of the maternal pelvis influences the progress, and thus the level of discomfort and pain associated with the labor. Structural abnormalities may cause the labor to be prolonged and may contribute to fetal malpresentation.

Maternal fatigue adversely affects the ability to tolerate pain and the effective use of coping techniques and strategies to remain in control. Fatigue can hamper the woman's ability to concentrate and prevent her from using imagery, focal points, breathing techniques, and other methods of distraction. Lack of refreshing sleep is not unusual during the last weeks of pregnancy; a well-rested woman who experiences a prolonged labor can quickly become exhausted long before the birth takes place.

Certain care provider interventions, such as intravenous and fetal monitoring equipment, can intensify the discomfort naturally associated with labor. At times, these methods may also interfere with maternal mobility and the ability to assume a position of comfort. Labor induction and augmentation, amniotomy and vaginal examinations may also be associated with intensifying labor discomfort.

Physiological Factors

Physiological forces influence the laboring woman's pain response. If there is a history of dysmenorrhea, increased childbirth pain may be related to higher levels of circulating prostaglandins. Laboring in an upright, instead of supine, position may help alleviate discomfort. Freedom to ambulate and assume a position of comfort during labor has been shown to be beneficial in reducing pain and muscle tension. Furthermore, the opportunity to choose positions for labor empowers the woman with a greater sense of control over her situation. In addition, the fetal size in relation to the maternal pelvic dimensions may also affect the level of pain intensity (Lowe, 2002; Simkin & O'Hara, 2002).

Although the physiological role is not well understood, the level of circulating endorphins is believed to have an important effect on the laboring woman's sense of well-being. **Endorphins** are endogenous opioids secreted by the pituitary gland. Endorphins act as opiates and produce analgesia by binding at opiate receptor sites involved in pain perception. In this manner, endorphins increase the threshold for pain. Beta-endorphin is the most active compound. When present in higher levels, endorphins are believed to increase the laboring woman's ability to tolerate pain; increased endorphin levels have been demonstrated with spontaneous, natural childbirth (Righard, 2001).

Psychological Factors

A number of psychological forces such as anxiety, fear, previous experiences, support systems, and childbirth preparation influence perception of and response to pain. Maternal anxiety during labor triggers the release of catecholamines, which increase the amount of pelvic pain stimuli sent to the brain, resulting in an intensified perception of pain (Lowe, 2002). As muscle tension increases, the effectiveness of the uterine contractions decreases and maternal discomfort and pain are intensified. Over time, the cycle of anxiety → tension → pain diminishes the progress of labor. At the same time, the woman's self-confidence in her ability to cope with the pain erodes and therapeutic interventions to help reduce pain and discomfort become less effective.

The woman's previous experience with pain and childbirth also influences her pain perception and ability to cope during labor. For most young, healthy women, childbirth often represents the first exposure to prolonged, intense pain. During early labor, sensory pain tends to be more pronounced in the nulliparous patient because the reproductive tract structures are less pliant and flexible. Multiparous patients may experience greater sensory pain during the transition phase of the first stage of labor because their pliable reproductive tract structures allow for a more rapid fetal descent accompanied by a heightened intensity in pain. During the first stage of labor, affective pain is usually greater for nulliparous women but is decreased for both nulliparous and multiparous women during the second stage (Lowe, 2002).

The patient's personal experience with a previous childbirth also influences her pain perception. A prior negative experience marked by misery and pain may produce an expectation of a repeated negative experience that is filled with fear and dread. A woman whose prior childbirth experience was satisfying is more likely to approach the present birth with a positive attitude and confidence in her ability to cope with the pain and discomfort.

The physical environment that envelops the birth experience should be considered as well. "Environment" encompasses those present as well as the physical space where the labor takes place. When indicated, labor support persons should be encouraged to serve as the patient's advocate in communicating desires, expectations and concerns and in providing physical comfort measures. Women prefer to be cared for in a home-style setting by trusted, familiar caregivers (Hodnett, 2002).

 Nursing Insight— *Environmental strategies to enhance comfort during labor*

The labor environment should provide privacy, comfort, and a sense of security. Allowing patients to determine the amount of noise, light, and temperature in their room fosters relaxation and a sense of control over their situation. Ideally, the room has an abundance of space that freely allows for patient and staff mobility, equipment (preferably hidden from view unless needed) and comfort measures such as birth balls, reclining chairs, tubs, and showers.

 Now Can You— Discuss characteristics of pain during labor and birth?

1. Identify three distinct characteristics of childbirth pain?
2. Differentiate among visceral, somatic, and referred pain and discuss when these pain types are most likely to occur during labor?
3. Discuss the physical, physiological, and psychological factors that influence the laboring woman's experience of pain?

THE EFFECTS OF PREPARED CHILDBIRTH ON PAIN PATHWAYS

Prepared childbirth provides the patient and her partner with an understanding of what to expect during childbirth and empowers them to become knowledgeable consumers of health care who can make informed choices concerning their childbearing experience. Accessible through many avenues, childbirth education is offered by most care providers, and may also be obtained in written or online materials, or through participation in formal childbirth education classes. In most areas, a variety of classes are available to provide general or specialized information. Prenatal classes focus on fetal growth and maternal changes and often place emphasis on health promotion through nutrition, exercise, stress reduction, and adequate rest. Other classes are intended to prepare the expectant couple for the labor process, and much time is spent exploring nonpharmacological and pharmacological measures for pain relief. These classes generally focus on educating the woman and her support person(s) about strategies such as position changes, breathing techniques, massage, and other methods to achieve relaxation and enhance comfort during labor. Classes for women with a planned cesarean birth are also available, and for those who wish to breastfeed, hospital maternity programs and local lactation support groups frequently provide focused breastfeeding classes.

To enhance understanding of how methods learned through prepared childbirth work to promote comfort during labor, it is helpful to review pain pathways and the gate control theory of pain. Pain may be viewed as a multidimensional phenomenon that encompasses the following five dimensions: affective, physiologic, behavioral, sensory, and cognitive. The neural pathway for pain involves four processes: transduction, transmission, perception, and modulation. Transduction is the conversion of a mechanical, thermal, or chemical stimulus into a neuronal action potential. Transduction occurs at the nociceptors, nerves that receive and transmit painful stimuli. Stated another way, incoming noxious stimuli are converted to electrical activity at the sensory endings of the peripheral nerves. Transmission is the movement of the pain impulse from the site of transduction (e.g., uterine contractions) to the brain. Perception is the development of the sensory, subjective and emotional experience identified by the individual as pain. Perception occurs when the patient feels the pain and responds to it, and modulation involves the activation of descending pathways that exert either inhibitory or facilitatory effects on the transmission of pain (Lowe, 2002).

Sometimes it is possible for painful stimuli to be ignored. Groups of certain nerve cells located in the spinal cord, brainstem, and cerebral cortex have the ability to modulate, or alter, pain impulses through a blocking mechanism. According to the **gate-control theory** of pain control (Melzack & Wall, 1965), pain sensations travel along sensory nerve pathways to the brain—but only a certain number of sensations, or "messages" can pass through the nerve pathways at one time. Methods of distraction learned and practiced in prepared childbirth classes such as breathing patterns, massage, music, and the use of focal points and imagery reduce or completely block the capacity of the nerve pathways to transmit pain. It is believed that these physical and psychological distractions work by "shutting the gate" in the spinal cord so that pain signals are unable to reach the brain.

When the laboring woman is actively involved in neuromuscular and motor activity, there is an increase in spinal cord activity that further modifies the transmission of pain. For example, the cognitive effort channeled into concentration on breathing patterns, focal points, and imagery requires selective and directed cortical activity that activates and closes the gating mechanism. The gate-control theory helps to explain how methods such as hypnosis and the various pain relief techniques taught in childbirth education classes help to diminish the laboring woman's perception of pain.

BENEFITS OF COMFORT AND SUPPORT ON PAIN PERCEPTION

In the traditional medical model, pain and discomfort during labor have largely been viewed as a negative component that should be eliminated. An alternative approach views labor as a natural process that challenges women to seek activities of comfort that will allow them to transcend the pain to achieve the satisfaction and contentment of birth. Feeling safe, secure, comforted, and in control empowers the laboring woman to find strength in dealing with her discomfort and pain. Nurses can facilitate comfort by providing a caring, supportive, therapeutic presence.

Support during labor and birth has a major impact on the woman's birth experience. Support includes both nonpharmacological and pharmacological measures. The nurse's attitude, expressions of caring, and supportive actions play a significant role in the woman's perception of pain and in her overall childbearing experience. Patients who feel they have control over their situation (self-efficacy) and who are actively engaged in the decision-making process concerning interventions and pain relief measures during labor and birth report a greater sense of satisfaction with their birth experience (Hodnett, 2002). When support is perceived to be ongoing and individualized throughout labor, women require fewer pain medications and interventions and experience improved outcomes (Simkin & O'Hara, 2002).

 Optimizing Outcomes— Assessment of pain during labor

Throughout the process of labor and birth, the nurse continuously assesses the patient and addresses her needs for comfort measures. Conducting an initial and ongoing pain assessment lays the foundation for intrapartal nursing care. Once the beginning assessment has been completed, the nurse uses the information to develop an individualized plan of care that includes pain relief interventions acceptable to the patient. A number of tools have been developed to facilitate pain assessment during labor; these may be modified or adapted as needed (Fig. 13-1).

Providing Comfort and Pain Relief

Methods to provide comfort and relieve pain are of paramount importance for the childbearing couple. The woman's perception of her overall birth experience is greatly influenced by her ability to cope with pain in whatever manner is acceptable to her. Nonpharmacological pain relief measures are for the most part inexpensive, easy to use, safe, and readily available. They also allow the patient to gain an enhanced sense of control over her childbirth experience. Despite their effectiveness, however, none of the various techniques are more effective than methods of epidural analgesia. Nurses play a key role in educating women and their support persons about the various nonpharmacological and pharmacological pain relief methods available. During labor, women should be encouraged to try a variety of pain relief measures, including pharmacological methods, if needed. Factual information and ongoing support empowers the patient to make informed choices and to participate fully in the decision-making process.

Another important component of childbirth preparation concerns the choice of the birth setting. Many communities offer several options for where the childbirth

---

Pain Assessment During Labor

Patient's Name _____ Date _____ Age _____ Room _____

Diagnosis _____ Physician/Midwife _____

Gravida _____ Para _____

Location of pain _____ Intensity of pain (scale of 0–10) _____

Present pain _____ The worst pain has been _____

Quality _____ Onset and duration _____

What has the patient done at home to cope with the pain? _____

What comfort measures would the patient like to use now? _____

How is the pain affecting the patient? _____

Other _____

Nurse's Plan for Pain Management _____

Signature of Nurse completing form _____

Figure 13-1 Assessment tool to gauge pain during labor.

will take place. Often during the first prepared childbirth class, expectant couples are encouraged to explore community options for the childbirth setting that best "fits" with their desired childbirth experience.

 Across Care Settings: **Childbirth options in the local community**

Encouraging expectant couples to explore options for the childbirth setting is an important component of prenatal education. As consumers of health care, patients should seek a primary care provider and facility that will safely meet their childbirth needs. Depending on the locale, the community may have a large city hospital, a small community hospital, a birth center, or a practicing group of certified nurse midwives (CNMs) that provides care during home births. When considering a birth facility, the woman may wish to ask the following questions:

1. Where does my primary care provider have childbirth privileges?
2. Does the facility offer personal Jacuzzis? Traditional bathtubs? Showers?
3. Does the facility have birth balls? Could I bring my own birth ball?
4. Would the facility allow me to play my own music during labor and birth?
5. How many labor support persons may be with me when I give birth?
6. Does the facility permit the use of aromatherapy?
7. Does the facility have transcutaneous electrical nerve stimulation (TENS) units available?
8. At what point would I be allowed to receive an epidural?
9. What medications would be available during my labor?

 Now Can You— Discuss a pain control theory, pain perception, and considerations for the childbirth setting?

1. Discuss the basic premise of the gate control theory of pain control?
2. Explain how comfort and support during labor decrease the woman's perception of discomfort and pain?
3. Identify four questions the expectant couple may wish to ask to help determine their choice of childbirth setting?

NONPHARMACOLOGICAL PAIN RELIEF MEASURES

Maternal Position and Movement

One way the nurse can facilitate relaxation is by helping the patient to find a position of comfort. Movement and changes in maternal position are important strategies for facilitating labor and childbirth. As the patient changes positions, gravity assists the fetus' descent down the birth canal. Slow dancing during labor is an activity that the expectant couple may enjoy. Most find slow dancing to special music from their own collection to be comforting and relaxing. When the couple assumes the slow dance position, the woman can lean on her coach (this helps to support her), and they can sway and dance together through the contractions.

Laboring women may also wish to use a "squatting bar" or assume a squatting position at the edge of the bed. The

squatting position helps to open the pelvic outlet, which facilitates the fetus' downward movement. Assuming a hands and knees position is comforting for women who have back labor or whose fetus is in a posterior position. The hands and knees position decreases the patient's back pressure and helps the fetus to rotate into an anterior position. Many hospital birthing suites offer wireless telemetry units that provide continuous monitoring while the patient ambulates at her leisure (Fig. 13-2).

The "birth ball" may be also used to promote comfort during labor. Essentially, the birth ball is a large, firm yet pliable physical therapy ball or gymnastic ball that provides support for the laboring woman. The patient carefully sits on the birth ball and rhythmically rocks back and forth or moves the ball around in a circular motion. Assuming a sitting position on the birth ball facilitates a supported squatting position that opens the pelvis to allow fetal descent in preparation for birth. Warm compresses applied to the back and perineum while balancing on the ball enhance relaxation and promote comfort (Fig. 13-3). The birth ball should be large enough to allow the woman to sit comfortably on it with her knees bent at a 90-degree angle with her feet flat on the floor and approximately 2 feet apart (Perez, 2000). The woman may also place the birth ball against the wall behind the small of her back and gently lunge from side to side to open the pelvis. When needed, assuming a kneeling position while leaning forward on the birth ball may encourage the rotation of the fetus from a posterior to an anterior position.

Breathing Techniques

During childbirth education classes, the pregnant woman and her labor coach learn about conscious breathing patterns that involve slowed respirations to enhance relaxation. Specific breathing methods are also taught as attention

Figure 13-2 Use of a wireless telemetry unit allows the woman to ambulate during labor.

Figure 13-3 The coach applies counterpressure and warm compresses to the woman's lower back as she balances on the birth ball.

focusing and distraction techniques to help relieve discomfort and pain during labor. Distraction helps to reduce the woman's perception of pain. The labor "coach," or support person, assists the woman by learning to palpate her body to identify muscle tenseness, by signaling the onset of contractions, and by monitoring her effective use of the breathing techniques. Techniques learned in class are practiced at home so that when labor begins, the couple is prepared to use relaxation and breathing patterns as a strategy to help diminish discomfort and pain (Fig. 13-4).

Figure 13-4 Practice of relaxation techniques and breathing exercises help to prepare the couple for labor and birth.

The woman is instructed to take a slow, deep cleansing breath in through the nose and out through the mouth at the beginning of every contraction. During early labor, when the woman is no longer able to walk or talk through contractions, she may wish to begin using *slow-paced* breathing. With this pattern, following a cleansing breath, the woman begins to slowly breathe in and out through her mouth while her coach slowly counts out loud. The breathing rate is approximately half the woman's normal breathing rate—6 to 8 breaths per minute. With this pattern, she is prompted to slowly breathe in while the coach counts "one, two, three, four," and then slowly breathe out to the same rhythm as the coach counts "one, two, three, four."

As the labor progresses, and the contractions increase in frequency and intensity, the patient may need to change to a *modified-paced* breathing pattern. This breathing technique is shallower and approximately twice the woman's normal rate of breathing—32 to 40 breaths per minute. After a deep cleansing breath, the woman inhales slowly, but exhales at faster pace. For example, the coach may instruct her to take a cleansing breath, then breathe in to a count of one, two, three, four and breathe out to a count of one, two, three. All contractions should end with another deep cleansing breath. The modified paced breathing pattern requires more concentration and is believed to block more painful stimuli than the slow-paced breathing pattern (Perinatal Education Associates, 2006). The woman may wish to combine the slow and modified paced breathing: use the slow-paced breathing at the beginning and end of the contractions; and the modified-paced breathing during the contraction intensity. Combining the patterns helps to conserve maternal energy and lessens fatigue and the likelihood of hyperventilation.

During the transition phase of labor, when contractions are most intense, patients usually find it difficult to concentrate on breathing techniques. At this time, the *pattern-paced* breathing technique, which requires increased concentration, is helpful. With this breathing pattern, following a cleansing breath, the woman begins with a 3:1 pattern: breathe in, breathe out; breathe in, breathe out; breathe in, then blow (as if blowing out a candle). This sequence is repeated throughout the contraction. As needed, the ratio may be increased to 4:1. As with the other breathing patterns, a cleansing breath is taken at the end of the contraction. The patient can use and modify any of the breathing techniques that work best for her at any stage of her labor.

❝What to say❞ — *When the patient needs assistance refocusing during labor*

While in the transition phase of labor, the laboring patient screams out "I quit, I cannot do this anymore, I have no more energy, I can't do this." At this point, comfort measures are ineffective. Instead, the nurse can help the patient stay focused on dealing with each contraction by offering words of support and encouragement with statements such as:

"You are doing a great job!"
"You are almost there!"
"I can see your baby's head—reach down and feel it!"
"You can do it!"

ⓢ Optimizing Outcomes— Recognizing hyperventilation

The pattern-paced breathing technique may result in maternal hyperventilation. The nurse should alert the patient and her support person to symptoms of respiratory alkalosis: light-headedness, dizziness, tingling of the fingers, or circumoral numbness. Strategies to eliminate respiratory alkalosis focus on replacement of the bicarbonate ion by rebreathing carbon dioxide. This can be accomplished by instructing the woman to breathe into a paper bag held tightly around the mouth and nose or, if no bag is available, instructing her to breathe into her cupped hands.

During the second-stage pushing phase of labor, patients should be encouraged to use whatever breathing pattern is comfortable and relaxing. To ensure optimal blood flow to the fetus, prolonged breath holding during pushing should be avoided. When needed, the urge to push may be controlled by a breathing pattern that consists of panting breaths or by slow exhalation through pursed lips (Perinatal Education Associates, 2006).

It is important for the pregnant woman and her coach to practice all breathing techniques before the onset of labor. The practice helps to increase their comfort level with the techniques and increases the likelihood that they will be able to use them effectively during labor. The breathing and relaxation techniques can be practiced together at home and at any time to reduce stress. When necessary, couples that are unfamiliar with breathing strategies can be taught during labor. Breathing techniques offer a form of distraction since the woman who is concentrating on slow paced breathing cannot focus on her pain. The breathing patterns are also beneficial in increasing blood flow to the fetus.

Music

Music can help to create a relaxing environment and boost spirits. During labor, music provides comfort and decreases maternal anxiety by stimulating the release of endorphins. For most couples, quiet, soothing music works best. Compact disc players are often available in hospital birthing suites and freestanding birth centers and patients are encouraged to supply music of their choice. A headset or earphones used with the compact disc player or patient's personal iPod may be even more effective because environmental sounds are tuned out. Comforting music during labor promotes maternal relaxation, thereby increasing oxygen intake. Some women find that music enhances their ability to remain focused during contractions. Music alone may also provide pain relief during labor, although further research is needed (Smith, Collins, Cyna, & Crowther, 2005). In some birth settings, patients are allowed to bring personal videos or DVDs from home to enjoy as another strategy for distraction during labor.

Relaxation

Various relaxation techniques are used to help decrease anxiety during labor. When the nurse, patient, and her labor support person(s) are successful in diminishing the patient's level of anxiety, stress and tension are also reduced. When tension is reduced, the woman breathes more deeply, resulting in improved maternal and fetal oxygenation. When the laboring woman experiences increased anxiety, stress levels and tension build and trigger a cascade of events that heighten the sensation of pain. Pain also impedes the patient's ability to relax. The nurse's ongoing assessment of maternal pain should be conducted throughout labor and birth. The use of a standardized pain assessment tool facilitates the evaluation and allows for an easy reassessment of pain following therapeutic interventions. Use of a patient self-assessment tool is preferable because it ensures that the management of pain is based on the subjective nature of the woman's pain rather than on the nurse's judgment alone.

 Nursing Insight— Use of a visual analog scale for the assessment of pain

A visual analog scale for pain assessment is helpful because the patient is able to indicate on a line how intense she perceives her pain to be: the choices range from "no pain" to "pain as bad as it could possibly be." Other scales that present drawings that range from happy, smiling faces to sad, crying faces are also available. The nurse should ask the woman to rate her pain on the scale before and after pain-relief measures to evaluate their effectiveness.

Other Attention-Focusing Strategies

Guided imagery is a state of intense, focused concentration that one uses to create persuasive mental images. Guided imagery distracts the laboring woman and transports her to a place that is special to her. The nurse or labor support person assists with guided imagery by asking the laboring woman to focus on a place where she likes to be. Many patients choose the beach or the mountains as their special locale. Next, the nurse or the labor support person verbalizes sights and sounds of that unique place in an attempt to relax and distract the patient. Often, the labor support person can describe the special place in a meaningful, calming way. For example, the coach may say:

> Close your eyes, get comfortable in your chair (or bed), take yourself to the beach. You are standing on the edge of the water. You hear the sounds of the waves rolling in. The water gently laps at your feet. The waves roll in, and the waves roll out. You smell the salty air. Feel the warm sun on your face, the sun is getting warmer and warmer. The waves roll in and out, and the sun is getting warmer. Listen, the sea gulls are flying overhead, you hear them crying out, and you hear the peaceful sound of the waves rolling in and out. You glow with the warm sun on your face, and you feel the gentle breezes against your skin. The waves roll in and out.

Focal points also distract the patient. A focal point may be a picture, photograph, stuffed animal, piece of needlework, or clock on the wall. The laboring woman concentrates or "focuses" on the object while breathing during the contractions. Patients are encouraged to bring the object that will serve as a focal point with them to the hospital or birth center. Focal points enhance concentration and help distract from the discomfort associated with contractions.

Massage and Touch

Massage and touch are techniques that have long been used to facilitate comfort and relaxation during labor. The patient's labor support person or nurse can perform simple hand massage to help decrease tension. Back massage is especially beneficial for the discomfort of back labor.

Effleurage, taken from the French word *effleurer* (to touch lightly) is a gentle stroking technique performed in rhythm with contractions. The patient or her labor support person massages the abdomen using light circular motions. Effleurage is helpful in distracting the patient from her contractions. Massage of the hands, feet, and back may be effective in diminishing tension and in enhancing comfort. Throughout the labor experience, patients and their partners should be encouraged to experiment with various techniques to determine what methods work best for them.

Counterpressure is often effective in enhancing the woman's ability to cope with discomfort from internal pressure and lower back pain. This technique involves use of the labor support person's fist or heel of the hand to apply steady pressure to the sacral area. Counterpressure is especially helpful when maternal back pain results from pressure of the occiput against spinal nerves when the fetal head is in a posterior position. This technique brings pain relief as the counterpressure lifts the occiput off of the spinal nerves.

Therapeutic touch is based on the use of "prana," the body's energy fields. Prana is believed to be deficient in some individuals who experience pain. Specially trained persons use laying-on of hands to provide therapeutic touch to redirect the energy fields thought to be associated with the pain (Scheiber & Selby, 2000). Although the benefits of therapeutic touch in enhancing relaxation and in reducing anxiety and pain have been documented (Marks, 2000), the effectiveness of this modality for pain relief during labor is not known.

Healing touch is also based on use of the body's energy fields. This modality employs a combination of techniques from multiple disciplines. Persons trained in healing touch are taught energetic diagnosis and treatment forms and how to document the patient's response and progress. It is believed that the various techniques align and balance the human energy field, enhancing the body's ability to heal itself. Although healing touch has been used during labor, no studies have been published to document its effectiveness (Hover-Kramer, Mentgen, & Scandrett-Hibdon, 2001).

Hydrotherapy

Hydrotherapy (water therapy) is the use of warm water to promote comfort and relaxation. Hydrotherapy may involve showering or soaking in a regular tub or whirlpool bath. When showering is the selected method of hydrotherapy, the patient stands in a warm shower and allows the water to gently glide over her abdomen. Alternatively, she may wish to sit in a shower chair. The nurse or labor coach may use a handheld sprayer to direct a steady stream of water over the abdomen or back. Throughout this time, the support person provides reassurance and encouragement, assists with breathing techniques during contractions, and offers touch and massage. The flow of warm water enhances feelings of relaxation and helps to decrease muscle tension. Reduced discomfort and increased relaxation often empowers the woman to have more control over her labor.

Immersion in a tub of warm water filled up to shoulder level is also beneficial in promoting comfort and relaxation. For most, the buoyancy provided by the water provides welcomed relief from labor discomfort and pain. The production of maternal catecholamines is decreased, prompting an increase in the release of oxytocin (stimulates uterine contractions) and endorphins (reduces the perception of pain). If the woman is experiencing "back labor" from a fetal occiput posterior or transverse position, she may be assisted into a side-lying or hands-and-knees position in the tub. These positions enhance comfort and help to facilitate fetal rotation into an occiput anterior position.

Whirlpool tubs ("jet hydrotherapy") are available in many birth settings, although some institutions require prior approval for use from the patient's primary care provider. The pulsating flow of warm water from the whirlpool jets is soothing and delivers continuous massage to the patient's legs, abdomen, and back. The rhythm of the water flowing in the shower or whirlpool tub provides a soothing sound that aids in relaxation.

During hydrotherapy, fetal heart rate (FHR) monitoring may be intermittent or continuous. It may be conducted via Doppler technique, fetoscope, or use of a wireless external monitor device. Internal electrode placement may not be used with whirlpool baths. In some settings, women with ruptured membranes are allowed to use jet hydrotherapy, provided that the amniotic fluid is clear.

Patients may stay in the tub as long as desired; most remain for 40 to 60 minutes. During that time, if the maternal temperature or FHR increase, if the labor slows or becomes too intense, or if the comforting effects of the water are diminished, patients may come out of the tub and return at a later time. For many, repeated immersions are more effective in relieving pain than a long, continuous exposure to the water. During tub hydrotherapy, the nurse or labor partner can offer comforting, cool washcloths for the face and fluids to promote hydration (Mackey, 2001; Simkin & O'Hara, 2002). To avoid overheating, the water temperature should be maintained at 96.8° to 100.4°F (36° to 38°C) (Florence & Palmer, 2003).

Hypnotherapy

Hypnotherapy is a structured technique that enables the patient to achieve a state of heightened awareness and focused concentration that can be used to alter the perception of pain. With this modality, emphasis is placed on promoting maternal relaxation while decreasing fear, anxiety, and the perception of pain. To accomplish this, the woman may be given direct suggestions about pain relief or indirect suggestions that she is experiencing decreased discomfort (Ketterhagen, VandeVusse, & Berner, 2002). Education about the method and continued practice during the prenatal period are essential in the successful use of hypnotherapy during labor and birth (Gentz, 2001). Hypnotherapy involves the induction of a state of great mental and physical relaxation that can be therapeutic in the management of pain control (Potter, 2006).

Aromatherapy

Aromatherapy is the use of essential oils, derived from plants, flowers, herbs, and trees, whose aroma is thought to have a therapeutic effect in treating illnesses and promoting health and well-being. The fragrances of rose, lavender, frankincense, and bergamot oils are believed to promote comfort and relaxation and decrease pain. Patients may use the scented oils by adding a few drops to a warm tub bath, or to body compresses and massage lotions or to an aromatherapy lamp used to add fragrance to the room. Drops of lavender and other essential oils may also be massaged into the woman's temples or forehead or placed on a pillow to induce relaxation (Simkin & Bolding, 2004).

 clinical alert

When using aromatherapy

Nurses must be aware that the essential oils used in aromatherapy should never be applied to the skin in a full-strength form. Instead, the oils must be diluted, usually in a vegetable oil base, before application. Patients should be cautioned that not all aromatherapy oils are safe to use during pregnancy; some oils, when inhaled, cause side effects such as nausea and headache (Gentz, 2001).

Figure 13-5 A cool washcloth placed on the forehead provides comfort during labor.

 Complementary Care: *Yoga to reduce discomfort during labor*

Prenatal yoga classes, which focus on breathing techniques and enhanced relaxation, are becoming increasingly popular. Physiologically, yoga increases the efficiency of the heart, slows the respiratory rate, and lowers blood pressure. For many, yoga helps decrease stress and anxiety during the prenatal period and provides coping strategies that can be used during labor. The practice of yoga during pregnancy helps women learn to decrease the urge to tighten muscles in response to pain. This response promotes the release of oxytocin to enhance the progress of labor. Poses used in prenatal yoga also facilitate the descent of the fetus and often decrease back pain. Women should always check with their primary care provider before beginning prenatal yoga. For many, attending a prenatal yoga class in the community is a healthy way to meet other women who are beginning a new chapter in their life.

Application of Heat and Cold

The application of heat and cold can promote comfort and help decrease pain during labor and birth. The two modalities may be used alternately to enhance their effects. Heat exerts a therapeutic effect by relieving muscle ischemia and increasing blood flow to the area of discomfort. Warm washcloths applied to the perineum help to relieve the discomfort associated with stretching. Socks or bags that are sewn from cloth can be filled with uncooked rice and heated in a microwave oven. Once warmed, the bags radiate soothing heat that helps to diminish pain. The rice bags may be placed on the patient's neck, back, or wherever the discomfort is felt. When desired, lavender oil, a comforting aroma to many, may be added to the homemade rice bag before heating.

Cold washcloths or ice packs placed on the forehead, chest, or face may be comforting to laboring women who feel warm (Fig. 13-5). Cold packs may also be applied to areas of pain where they exert a therapeutic effect by reducing muscle temperature and relieving muscle spasms. The nurse should be aware that some patients' cultural beliefs may not permit the use of cold therapy during labor (Simkin & Bolding, 2004).

 Optimizing Outcomes— **When using heat and cold for pain relief during labor**

Nurses should avoid the application of heat or cold over body areas that have been anesthetized because of the risk for tissue damage. Hot and cold packs should be used only after one to two layers of cloth have been placed between the pack and the patient's skin (Simkin & Bolding, 2004).

Biofeedback

Biofeedback has been used for many years to enhance relaxation and help patients to gain control over their pain. It is based on the concept that the mind controls the body: if one can recognize physical signals, certain internal physiological events can be changed. During the prenatal period, the woman is taught body awareness, how to recognize responses to stimuli, and various relaxation techniques. She practices using strategies such as concentration, focal points, and breathing to control her response to uncomfortable stimuli. The labor partner learns to recognize cues (e.g., grimacing, tensing, frowning, moaning, and breath holding) indicative of pain and uses verbal feedback and touch to help the woman to achieve relaxation. Formal biofeedback, which involves the use of a recording device to measure physiological responses, requires special training by a skilled biofeedback therapist. Body signals (e.g., skin temperature, blood flow, and muscle tension) that indicate pain and stress are sent via attached electrodes back to the biofeedback unit. The unit then alerts the patient who uses various techniques to decrease the tension and discomfort.

Transcutaneous Electrical Nerve Stimulation

Transcutaneous electrical nerve stimulation (TENS) involves the delivery of an electric current through electrodes that are applied to the skin over the painful region of a peripheral nerve (Simkin & Bolding, 2004). The TENS unit relieves pain by producing counterirritation on the nociceptors. Normally, two pairs of flat electrodes are placed on either side of the patient's thoracic and sacral spine. Continuous low-intensity electrical impulses are delivered through a battery-operated device. During a contraction, patients are instructed to turn the knobs on the unit to increase the degree of stimulation from a low intensity to a high intensity. High-intensity levels maintained for at least 1 minute facilitate the release of endorphins. Most women report a pleasant buzzing or tingling sensation that offsets the pain. The TENS unit is especially beneficial for relief of low back pain. The doctor or certified nurse midwife prescribes the use of a TENS unit, which may initially be applied by a physical therapist. The nurse explains the use of the device, assists with its application, and evaluates its effectiveness.

Intradermal Water Block

Intradermal water block is a technique that involves the use of a small (e.g., 25-gauge) needle to inject small amounts (e.g., 0.05 to 0.1 mL) of sterile water into four locations on the patient's lower back to relieve back pain. This method may be used during early labor to delay the initiation of pharmacological pain relief methods. Patients experience a brief stinging sensation immediately after the injections, but the back pain is generally relieved for 45 minutes to 2 hours. Although the mechanism of action is not fully understood, the technique is believed to work by producing counterirritation (pain in one specific area is reduced while skin in close proximity is irritated), gate control, or by increasing circulating endorphins. Once the beneficial effects have diminished, the treatment may be repeated or another pain relief method may be instituted (Gentz, 2001; Simkin & O'Hara, 2002).

Acupressure and Acupuncture

Acupressure, sometimes called "Chinese massage," involves the application of pressure, or heat or cold to identified acupuncture points to decrease the sensation of pain. The points contain an increased density of neuroreceptors and increased electrical conductivity. It is believed that the technique's effectiveness is related to the gate-control theory of pain and an increased release of endorphins. Pressure may be applied by the support person's hands, tennis balls, or by the application of pressure bands–cloth-covered elastic bands that contain rigid plastic inserts–to provide the pressure. During labor, pressure is applied to various acupressure points, which are located on the neck, shoulders, wrists, lower back, hips, area below the kneecaps, ankles, toenails, and soles of the feet. A commonly identified point used for women in labor is Co4 (Hoku or Hegu point), which is located between the first and second metacarpal bones on the back of the hand. Another acupressure point is located between the inner anklebone and the Achilles' tendon. Applying pressure for 1 minute on each ankle is believed to be beneficial in relieving labor pain.

Acupuncture is a therapy used in traditional Chinese medicine for healing and comfort. It is based on the theory that illness results from an imbalance of energy. This method involves the insertion of fine, sterile, stainless steel needles into specific points in the body (i.e., those associated with labor pain) to control the flow of "chi," or life energy. Activation of the insertion points is believed to trigger the release of endorphins. Acupuncture should be performed only by a trained, certified acupuncturist. Although acupuncture is considered to be safe, it is an invasive therapy that carries a risk of infection (Smith et al., 2005).

 Collaboration in Caring— *Acupressure and acupuncture as modalities for labor pain relief*

Not as widely accepted in the United States as in some countries, interest in acupressure and acupuncture as a method of inducing labor and relieving labor pain is increasing as more individuals seek holistic practices and alternative medicine (Allaire, 2001). Today, there are more than 40 schools and colleges of acupuncture that offer training in the technique. While the practice of acupuncture requires a considerable amount of education and training, the certified nurse midwife may work with an acupressurist/acupuncturist to become skilled in the manual massage of acupuncture and acupressure points, as well as shiatsu (the application of pressure to acupuncture sites) and other touch therapies.

 Now Can You— Discuss nonpharmacological methods of pain relief during labor?

1. Demonstrate three breathing patterns for labor and explain when each is likely to be of most benefit?
2. Identify four signs of hyperventilation and describe nursing interventions to facilitate restoration of the patient's oxygen–carbon dioxide balance?
3. Briefly discuss the use of guided imagery, touch, hydrotherapy, application of heat and cold, and transcutaneous electrical nerve stimulation as nonpharmacological methods to reduce discomfort and pain during labor?

Pharmacological Pain Relief Measures

Pharmacological methods of pain control should be initiated before the pain intensifies to the point that catecholamines are released and labor is prolonged. A combination of nonpharmacological and pharmacological measures provides pain relief, enhances the patient's comfort and sense of control over her situation, and promotes a positive childbearing experience for the woman and her family. During early labor, nonpharmacological methods alone are often satisfactory for relaxation and pain relief. As labor progresses, contractions and discomfort intensify, often necessitating the addition of pharmacological agents for pain control. Because nonpharmacological measures promote relaxation and potentiate the effects of analgesic agents, less pharmacological intervention is usually required (Faucher & Brucker, 2000).

 Be sure to— Ensure the patient is informed about available pharmacological methods of pain relief

The nursing role of patient advocate includes ensuring that the woman understands the alternative methods of pain relief that are available in the birth facility and, when indicated, by asking the primary care provider for further details or clarification. Obtaining an informed consent for interventions means that the procedure and its advantages and disadvantages are fully explained; the patient must agree with the plan of care as it is described

Nursing Care Plan Patient Who Plans to Use Nonpharmacological Methods of Pain Relief During Labor

Ann is a 28 year old gravida 2, para 1, who was admitted 45 minutes ago. Ann's cervix is 4 cm dilated and 100% effaced, the station is –2 and her membranes are intact. Uterine contractions occur every 3 minutes, last 45–50 seconds and are of moderate intensity. The fetal heart rate averages 140–145 beats per minute and has no non-reassuring patterns. Ann complains of low back pressure and pain. She and her husband Raul have prepared a birth plan; they attended childbirth preparation classes and state they feel comfortable with using the methods learned.

Nursing Diagnosis: Coping, Readiness for Enhanced related to intention and preparation to meet the demands of childbirth

Measurable Short-term Goal: Ann will demonstrate a relaxed facial and body posture during contractions.

Measurable Long-term Goal: Ann will successfully use relaxation and breathing techniques learned in childbirth class throughout her labor.

NOC Outcomes:
Personal Well-Being (2002) Extent of positive perception of one's health status and life circumstances
Coping (1302) Personal actions to manage stressors that tax an individual's resources

NIC Interventions:
Coping Enhancement (5230)
Support System Enhancement (5440)

Nursing Interventions:

1. Review the birth plan with Ann and Raul, answering any questions and providing additional information as needed. Inform other caregivers of the couple's plans for their labor and birth.

   RATIONALE: Appraisal of the couple's expectations allows the opportunity to provide factual information and offer support in an accepting environment.

2. Ensure a comforting environment: offer warmed blankets, an electric or handheld fan; adjust the room thermostat as needed.

   RATIONALE: A comfortable environment enhances relaxation and increases the patient's ability to focus on her coping skills.

3. Provide Ann's preferred music as desired; use soft lighting; ensure the focal point is within easy view; avoid conducting assessments and procedures during contractions; ensure that bed linens are soft, clean, and dry.

   RATIONALE: Listening to favorite music may distract the patient from discomfort and external noises. Environmental distractions and unnecessary stimulants interfere with the successful use of learned techniques to manage labor discomfort.

4. Assist Raul in helping Ann to find a position of comfort; encourage position changes every 30–60 minutes and unless contraindicated, encourage ambulation, sitting in a chair or use of a birth ball.

   RATIONALE: Assistance empowers Raul to participate actively in the labor and birth experience. Position changes enhance maternal comfort by reducing muscle tension and facilitate fetal descent.

5. Encourage Raul to perform back rubs or provide counterpressure as learned in childbirth classes, according to Ann's desires.

   RATIONALE: Back rubs and counterpressure provide comfort from pain associated with back labor by stimulating the large-diameter fibers and interfering with the transmission of pain impulses to the brain.

6. Keep Ann and Raul informed of the progress of labor.

   RATIONALE: Ongoing information helps to decrease anxiety and fear, which increase the perception of pain and decrease pain tolerance; news of labor progress provides an incentive to continue with efforts to cope with labor.

---

to her; and the patient's consent must be given freely without coercion or manipulation from her health care provider (Lowe, 2004).

SEDATIVES AND ANTIEMETICS

Sedatives are agents that relieve anxiety and induce sleep. They are primarily used during the early latent phase of labor, when the cervix is long, closed, and thick and rest has been prescribed for the patient. Sedatives may also be used to augment analgesics and reduce nausea after the administration of opioids. Sedatives induce sleep for a few hours. Once the woman awakens, either the contractions have ceased (i.e., the patient had experienced false labor) or regular, effective contractions that produce cervical change occur. Sedatives should not be used during active labor because they can cause respiratory depression in the neonate (Faucher & Brucker, 2000).

Be sure to— Assess and reassess during the intrapartal period

During the intrapartal period, it is important to assess the laboring patient and her fetus following each intervention to promote comfort. Specifically, nurses should:

• Assess for risk factors: bleeding, infection, ruptured membranes, fetal presentation, prolapsed cord, precipitous labor, meconium-stained amniotic fluid, postmaturity, prematurity, or fetal heart rate irregularities.
• Assess maternal vital signs per facility protocol.
• Assess the patient's anxiety level, coping mechanisms, and labor support.
• Assess the progress of labor.
• Assess the fetal heart rate, lie, and presentation.
• Assess the maternal and fetal response to each comfort measure.
• Carefully document all findings.

Barbiturates

Secobarbital is the most commonly used barbiturate in labor. It a fast-acting oral agent that produces mild sedation within 15 minutes after administration; its effects last for 3 to 4 hours. Undesirable effects include maternal and neonatal respiratory and vasomotor depression. These effects are intensified if a barbiturate is administered with another central nervous system (CNS) depressant. However, when given without an analgesic to a woman experiencing pain, the pain is increased. For these reasons, barbiturates are rarely used in labor (Faucher & Brucker, 2000; Hawkins, Chestnut, & Gibbs, 2002).

Benzodiazepines

Benzodiazepines are agents primarily used to treat anxiety (e.g., diazepam [Valium]; lorazepam [Ativan]). Their mechanism of action is similar to that of barbiturates. When given with an opioid analgesic, benzodiazepines enhance pain relief and decrease nausea and vomiting, although some have an amnesic effect that may be unacceptable for women in labor (Bricker & Lavender, 2002; Lehne, 2006).

 clinical alert

Flumazenil to reverse the effects of benzodiazepine sedatives

Flumazenil (Romazicon) is an agent that reverses the effects of benzodiazepine sedatives. This intravenously administered medication should be readily available in any childbirth setting where benzodiazepines are used.

H₁-Receptor Antagonists

H₁ receptor antagonists are medications that block the action of histamines at the receptor sites. These medications produce sedative, anti-Parkinson, and antiemetic effects. They cause drowsiness and are often used during early labor to promote sleep and decrease anxiety. During labor, the H₁ receptor antagonists commonly used include promethazine (Phenergan), hydroxyzine (Vistaril), and diphenhydramine (Benadryl) (Hawkins et al., 2002).

Promethazine (Phenergan), a phenothiazine, produces marked sedation and has strong antiemetic effects. It is frequently combined with opiates because it potentiates their effects. Phenothiazines readily cross the placenta, and may produce decreased FHR beat-to-beat variability. They also bind to bilirubin binding sites in the neonate and may cause increased hyperbilirubinemia and jaundice in term infants who were exposed to the drug during the intrapartal period (Hawkins et al., 2002).

Hydroxyzine (Vistaril), a piperazine subtype, is used during early or prodromal labor to decrease nausea and anxiety. It also exerts a sedative effect. Often, women who receive this intramuscular medication awaken to increased contraction intensity that produces cervical changes (i.e., active labor).

Diphenhydramine (Benadryl) is a nonprescription medication with sedative and antiemetic properties that is given during early labor. Because the drug is readily available, nurses can advise women to use it at home although it may cause agitation in some patients. The half-life of diphenhydramine is 1 to 4 hours and its effects may last up to 8 hours.

 Nursing Insight— *Recognizing the anxiety–tissue anoxia–pain connection*

Pain can trigger the body's general stress response, called the "fight or flight" reaction. The release of epinephrine causes peripheral and uterine vasoconstriction, which results in tissue anoxia and increased pain. Decreasing the patient's anxiety through assistance with relaxation techniques or administration of antianxiety medications reduces vasoconstriction and helps to decrease pain.

 Now Can You— Discuss informed consent and the use of sedatives and antiemetics during labor?

1. State the three components of an informed consent that must be assured before instituting pharmacological interventions for pain relief during labor?
2. Describe the indications for the use of sedatives and antiemetics during labor and identify two commonly prescribed H₁-receptor antagonists?
3. Explain how diminishing maternal anxiety helps to relieve pain?

DIFFERENTIATING ANALGESIA FROM ANESTHESIA

To enhance understanding of the pharmacological methods of pain relief, it is important to distinguish between the concepts of analgesia and anesthesia. **Analgesia** is relief, to some degree, from pain. Pain may be entirely eliminated or only lessened. Analgesia may be accomplished via many methods, including medications, the application of heat or cold, massage, or electrical stimulation. **Anesthesia** is the partial or complete loss of sensation with or without the loss of consciousness. There are many types of analgesia and anesthesia and a number of methods for administering it. The analgesic or anesthetic selected is determined, to some degree, by the patient's stage of labor and by the method of birth anticipated (Boxes 13-1 and 13-2). When given too early, analgesia may prolong the labor and cause fetal depression. When administered too late, analgesia provides no benefit to the woman and may cause depression in the neonate.

The nurse's role involves continuous patient assessment to monitor the progress of labor and to identify cues that indicate that the patient would benefit from the administration of analgesic medications prescribed by the physician, certified nurse-midwife (CNM), or certified registered nurse-anesthetist (CRNA). Depending on institutional policy, the CNM or physician may evaluate the woman in the birthing facility or rely on the nurse's assessment and instruct the nurse to administer the ordered medications. In most facilities, the CRNA monitors analgesia-related complications and conducts continuous monitoring for patients who receive epidural anesthesia. In some institutions, an anesthesiologist (physician who specializes in the administration of anesthesia) is available to provide these services.

Box 13-1 **Pharmacological Interventions for Intrapartal Pain Control According to Stage of Labor**

FIRST STAGE OF LABOR
Systemic Analgesia
Opioid agonists (e.g., hydromorphone hydrochloride [Dilaudid]; meperidine hydrochloride [Demerol]; fentanyl citrate [Sublimaze]; sufentanil citrate [Sufenta])

Opioid agonist–antagonists (e.g., butorphanol [Stadol]; nalbuphine [Nubain])

Nerve Block Analgesia
Epidural

Combined spinal–epidural

SECOND STAGE OF LABOR
Nerve Block Analgesia and Anesthesia
Local infiltration

Pudendal block

Spinal block

Epidural block

Combined spinal–epidural

Box 13-2 **Pharmacological Interventions for Intrapartal Pain Control According to Birth Method**

VAGINAL BIRTH
- Local infiltration anesthesia
- Pudendal block
- Epidural block analgesia/anesthesia
- Spinal block anesthesia
- Combined spinal–epidural analgesia/anesthesia

CESAREAN BIRTH
- Spinal block anesthesia
- Epidural block anesthesia
- General anesthesia

SYSTEMIC ANALGESIA

Systemic analgesic agents provide central analgesia to the patient and fetus, since they readily cross the placenta. Although this method of pain control during labor has declined, it is still used in facilities where specialists trained in administering regional analgesia (e.g., epidural analgesia) are not available (Bricker & Lavender, 2002; Bucklin, Hawkins, Anderson, & Ulrich, 2005). Fetal–neonatal effects include respiratory depression, decreased alertness, and delayed sucking, depending on the agent used, the dosage given, and the route and timing of administration. Intravenous administration is preferred over intramuscular injection because the onset of action is more rapid and predictable, pain relief is obtained with smaller doses of the drug, and the duration of the effect is more predictable. The medication is administered into the intravenous tubing port nearest the patient while the IV solution is stopped.

 Optimizing Outcomes— **When administering intravenous medications during labor**

Intravenous analgesics are given slowly, in small doses during a contraction. When necessary, the medication may be given over a period of four to five consecutive contractions in order to complete the dose. Administering the medication during a contraction decreases fetal exposure to the drug because uterine blood vessels are constricted during contractions and the medication remains in the maternal vascular system for several seconds before the uterine blood vessels reopen.

In many institutions, patient-controlled analgesia (PCA) is available. The laboring woman self-administers small amounts of an opioid analgesic using a pump previously programmed for dose and frequency. As a result, a smaller amount of medication is required and women are generally pleased with the level of pain control achieved (Bricker & Lavender, 2002). Analgesic agents available for the intrapartum period include opioid (narcotic) agonists and opioid (narcotic) agonist–antagonists.

✦ *Nursing Insight*— *Differentiating between agonist agents and antagonist agents*

Analgesic medications used intrapartally include opioid agonists and opioid antagonists.

Agonist agents stimulate receptors to act. Antagonist agents block receptors or medications designed to activate receptors.

Opioid Agonist Analgesics

Opioid agonist analgesics include hydromorphone hydrochloride (Dilaudid), meperidine hydrochloride (Demerol), fentanyl citrate (Sublimaze), and sufentanil citrate (Sufenta) (Table 13-1). These agents work by stimulating the major opioid receptors mu and kappa. They promote feelings of euphoria and exert no amnesic effects. Because they delay gastric emptying time, nausea and vomiting are common side effects; bladder and bowel elimination may also be diminished. Results from a national survey of women's childbearing experiences revealed that women were not satisfied with the level of pain relief achieved with opioid analgesics given intrapartally. Nearly 40% of women who received parenteral opioids during labor rated them as being not very helpful or not helpful at all. However, intrapartum opioid administration is associated with shorter labors, less use of oxytocin, and fewer instrumented vaginal births (e.g., forceps-assisted, vacuum-assisted) than intrapartal epidural administration (Bricker & Lavender, 2002; Caton et al., 2002; Leighton & Halpern, 2002; Maternity Center Association, 2002). Ideally, opioid agonist analgesics should be given either less than 1 hour or greater than 4 hours before birth to minimize neonatal depression. Fentanyl citrate and sufentanil citrate require more frequent administration because of their relatively short duration of action (30 to 60 minutes, compared with 2 to 4 hours for hydromorphone hydrochloride and meperidine hydrochloride). Consequently, these agents are often administered intrathecally or epidurally, alone or in combination with a local anesthetic medication (Faucher & Brucker, 2000; Florence & Palmer, 2003; Lehne, 2006).

 Optimizing Outcomes— Safety measures for women who receive opioid analgesics

Opioid analgesics may cause bradycardia/tachycardia, hypotension, and respiratory depression and should be administered cautiously in women with respiratory or cardiovascular disorders (Lehne, 2006). Because patients may experience sedation and dizziness following administration, nurses should assist with ambulation and observe for adverse effects.

Opioid Agonist–Antagonist Analgesics

Opioid agonist–antagonist agents include butorphanol (Stadol) and nalbuphine (Nubain), which are agonists at kappa opioid receptors and either antagonists or weak agonists at mu opioid receptors. During labor, these medications provide satisfactory pain control without inducing respiratory depression in the woman or neonate. They are also associated with less nausea and vomiting and are used more often during labor than the opioid agonist analgesics. They may be administered intravenously or intramuscularly; the parenteral route is preferred. Opioid agonist–antagonists should not be given to women with an opioid dependence because the antagonist activity may precipitate maternal/neonatal withdrawal symptoms (Deglin & Vallerand, 2009; Florence & Palmer, 2003; Lehne, 2006).

medication: Fentanyl

Fentanyl (**fen**-ta-nil)
Sublimaze

Schedule II Pregnancy Category: C

Indications: Supplement to regional/local anesthesia; often administered epidurally or intrathecally to relieve moderate to severe labor pain and postoperative pain after cesarean birth.

Actions: Binds to opiate receptors in the CNS, alters the response to and perception of pain; produces CNS depression

Therapeutic Effects: Supplement to anesthesia; decreased pain

Contraindications and Precautions:
CONTRAINDICATED IN: Hypersensitivity; known intolerance

Adverse Reactions and Side Effects: Confusion, drowsiness, dizziness, rash, maternal and fetal/neonatal respiratory depression, nausea and vomiting, urinary retention

Adjunct for Regional Anesthesia: IM 50–100 micrograms (using the symbol for micrograms); IV 2–20 micrograms/kg over 1–2 min up to 50 micrograms/kg.

For Postoperative Pain: IM 50–100 micrograms q 1–2h prn.

Nursing Implications:
Assess for respiratory depression; naloxone should be readily available as antidote.

Adapted from Deglin, J.H., and Vallerand, A.H. (2009). *Davis's drug guide for nurses* (11th ed.). Philadelphia: F.A. Davis.

Table 13-1 Opioid Agonist Analgesics

Opioid–Agonist Analgesic	Route and Dosage	Nursing Considerations
Hydromorphone hydrochloride (Dilaudid)	IV: 1 mg q3h prn IM: 1–2 mg q3–6h prn	Monitor vital signs, FHR pattern and uterine activity prior to and during administration; observe for maternal respiratory depression; encourage voiding q2h, palpate for bladder distention; if birth occurs within 1–4 hours after administration, observe neonate for respiratory depression
Meperidine hydrochloride (Demerol)	IV: 25 mg q1–3h prn IM: 50–100 mg q1–3h prn	
Fentanyl citrate (Sublimaze)	IV: 25–50 mcg; 1–2 mg with 0.125% bupivacaine at rate of 8–10 mL/hr epidurally	
Sufentanil citrate (Sufenta)	IV: 1 mg with 0.125% bupivacaine at rate of 10 mL/hr	

medication: Butorphanol

Butorphanol (byoo-**tor**-fa-nole)
Stadol

Schedule IV Pregnancy Category: C

Indications: Moderate to severe labor pain; postoperative pain after cesarean birth

Actions: Stimulates kappa opioid receptors and blocks or weakly stimulates mu opioid receptors; alters pain perception, produces generalized CNS depression

Therapeutic Effects: Decreased severity of pain

Contraindications and Precautions:
CONTRAINDICATED IN: Hypersensitivity; patients dependent on opioids (may precipitate withdrawal)

Adverse Reactions and Side Effects: Confusion, drowsiness, sedation, blurred vision, headache, dysphoria, hallucinations, sweating, maternal palpitations/tachycardia or bradycardia, respiratory depression, transient nonpathologic sinusoidal-like FHR rhythm, urinary retention and urgency

Route and Dosage: 1 mg (range 0.5–2 mg) IV every 3–4 hours as needed; 2 mg (range 1–4 mg) IM every 3–4 hours as needed

Nursing Indications: May precipitate withdrawal symptoms in woman/neonate

Adapted from Deglin, J.H., and Vallerand, A.H. (2009). *Davis's drug guide for nurses* (11th ed.). Philadelphia: F.A. Davis.

critical nursing action When Combining Butorphanol with Other CNS Depressants

Butorphanol is associated with respiratory depression in both the mother and fetus. When administering butorphanol with other CNS depressants (e.g., hypnotic agents, phenothiazides, sedatives, other tranquilizers, and general anesthetics), the nurse should closely monitor the patient's respiratory and cardiac status for signs of respiratory depression. Ongoing observation of the maternal level of consciousness, vital signs, and pulse oximetry as well as continuous electronic FHR monitoring is recommended. Naloxone (Narcan), the specific antagonist for this medication, should be readily available to reverse the drug effects if needed.

Opioid Antagonists

Opioid antagonists, such as naloxone (Narcan), reverse the CNS depressant effects of opioids. Administered intravenously or intramuscularly, they are of benefit when labor progresses more rapidly than anticipated and birth is expected to occur when the opioid is at its peak effect. Placental transfer of naloxone is variable; the neonate may not require treatment with an opioid antagonist (Lehne, 2006).

 Now Can You— Discuss characteristics of systemic analgesia used during labor?

1. Explain how systemic analgesia should be administered during labor?
2. Identify three advantages and one major disadvantage associated with the use of opioid agonist agents during labor?
3. Explain specific precautions that should be taken when administering opioid agonist–antagonists to a woman in labor?

NERVE BLOCK ANALGESIA AND ANESTHESIA

Local anesthetics used in obstetrics may produce regional analgesia, which provides some degree of pain relief and motor block; and anesthesia, which provides complete pain relief and motor block. Regional analgesia may be obtained by the injection of a narcotic agent such as fentanyl along with a small amount of a local anesthetic agent. **Regional anesthesia,** a temporary and reversible loss of sensation, is produced by the injection of an anesthetic agent (a local anesthetic) into an area that brings the medication into direct contact with nervous tissue. Regional anesthetic agents block sodium and potassium transport in the nerve membrane, causing stabilization of the nerve(s) in a polarized resting state, which prevents the initiation and transmission of nerve impulses. Rarely, serious reactions (e.g., respiratory depression, hypotension) to local anesthesia may occur from one or more anesthetic agents. The nurse should ensure that emergency measures, including epinephrine, antihistamines, and oxygen are readily available in all patient areas where these medications are used. When caring for patients receiving analgesia/anesthesia by catheter, nurses must be aware of institutional policy and national standards. The Association of Women's Health, Obstetric and Neonatal Nurses (AWHONN) has developed a clinical position statement (AWHONN, 2002; available at http://www.awhonn.org/awhonn/content.do?name= 05HealthPolicyLegislation/5HPositionStatements.htm) to guide safe practice.

 Nursing Insight— Recognizing local anesthetic agents

Because most local anesthetic agents are chemically related to cocaine, their names end with the suffix "-caine." Examples of such medications include lidocaine, mepivacaine, bupivacaine, ropivacaine, and chloroprocaine.

The regional anesthetic blocks commonly used in obstetrics include epidural, spinal, or combined epidural–spinal. Epidural blocks may be administered for analgesia during labor and vaginal birth and for anesthesia during cesarean birth. Alternately, a combined epidural–spinal block may be used—the epidural provides analgesia for labor; the spinal provides anesthesia for birth or analgesia after the birth. During the first stage of labor, an epidural relieves pain by blocking the sensory nerves that supply the uterus. Pain experienced during the second stage of labor and with birth can be alleviated with epidural, combined epidural–spinal, and pudendal blocks. A summary of commonly used regional blocks is presented in Table 13-2.

Local Perineal Infiltration Anesthesia

Local perineal infiltration anesthesia is used to provide pain control when an episiotomy is to be performed or when suturing of lacerations is necessary in a patient who does not have regional anesthesia. Epinephrine, which causes vasoconstriction, may be added to the anesthetic agent to intensify the anesthesia effect and to minimize bleeding and prevent systemic absorption (Lehne, 2006).

Table 13-2 Commonly Used Regional Blocks for Labor and Birth

Type of Block; Areas Affected	When Used During Labor and Birth	Nursing Implications
Local Perineal Infiltration *Affected area:* **Perineum**	Immediately before birth for episiotomy; after birth for repair of lacerations.	Assess patient's knowledge and understanding; provide information as needed. Observe perineum for bruising or discoloration during the recovery period.
Pudendal Nerve Block *Affected areas:* **Perineum and lower vagina**	Late in the second stage for episiotomy, forceps, or vacuum extraction; during third stage for repair of episiotomy or lacerations.	Assess patient's level of knowledge and understanding; provide additional information as needed.
Spinal Anesthesia Block *Affected areas:* **Uterus, cervix, vagina, and perineum**	First stage for both elective and emergent cesarean births; low spinal anesthesia block may be used for vaginal birth—not suitable for labor.	Assess patient's level of knowledge and understanding; provide additional information as needed. Monitor maternal vital signs and FHR status.
Lumbar Epidural Block *Affected areas:* **Uterus, cervix, vagina, and perineum**	First and second stages.	Assess patient's level of knowledge and understanding; provide additional information as needed. Monitor maternal blood pressure—major side effect is hypotension. Provide ongoing support.
Combined Spinal–Epidural *Affected areas:* **Uterus, cervix, vagina, and perineum**	Spinal analgesia may be administered during the latent phase for pain relief. Epidural is given when active labor begins.	Assess patient's level of knowledge and understanding; provide additional information as needed. Monitor maternal vital signs and FHR status. Provide ongoing support.

 Nursing Insight— *Recognizing the value of natural pressure anesthesia*

Pressure anesthesia is the natural numbing effect caused by pressure of the fetal head against the woman's stretched perineum. For some, pressure anesthesia is adequate enough to allow an episiotomy to be performed without feeling the sensation of the actual surgical cut. Others require additional medication to help reduce the pain associated with childbirth.

Pudendal Nerve Block

A pudendal nerve block provides pain relief in the lower vagina, vulva, and perineum (Fig. 13-6). It should be administered 10 to 20 minutes before perineal anesthesia is needed and may be used late in the second stage of labor if an episiotomy is to be performed or if forceps or vacuum extraction will be used to facilitate birth. The anesthetic effect diminishes or completely removes the maternal bearing-down reflex. It may also be used during the third stage of labor for laceration repair.

Spinal Anesthesia Block

Spinal anesthesia block involves the injection of a solution containing a single local anesthetic or an anesthetic combined with fentanyl through the third, fourth, or fifth lumbar interspace into the subarachnoid space, where it mixes with cerebrospinal fluid. The subarachnoid space is a fluid filled area located between the dura mater and the spinal cord. At present, the spinal anesthesia block is used more often for elective and emergent cesarean births than epidural

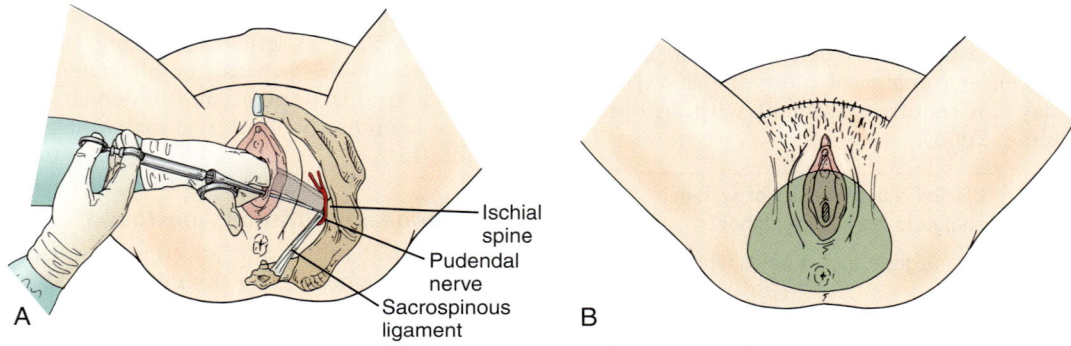

Ischial spine
Pudendal nerve
Sacrospinous ligament

A   B

Figure 13-6 *A.* Administration of a pudendal block. *B.* The areas of the perineum affected by a pudendal block.

Figure 13-7 *A.* The spinal column: levels of the sacral, lumbar, and thoracic nerves. *B.* Levels of anesthesia necessary for vaginal and cesarean births.

anesthesia (Bucklin et al., 2005). The differences in the levels of spinal anesthesia for vaginal and cesarean birth are created by the dosage of the anesthetic agent administered, and the position of the patient after placement of the medication in the dural sac. For vaginal birth, a low spinal anesthesia block provides anesthesia from level T10 (hips) to the feet; patients remain in a sitting position for a brief period of 1 to 2 minutes after administration to facilitate downward migration of the anesthetic solution toward the sacral area. For cesarean birth, the level of anesthesia coverage extends from the nipples (T6) to the feet; after administration of the anesthetic solution, patients are immediately assisted to a supine position with a left lateral tilt to enhance a cephalad spread of the anesthesia (and a higher level of sensory blockade). The anesthetic agent may be "weighted" with glucose to make it heavier than CSF. This prevents the medication from rising too high in the spinal canal and interfering with motor control of the uterus or with the maternal respiratory muscles (Fig. 13-7).

Spinal anesthesia block has several advantages: it is easy to administer; has an immediate onset of anesthesia; requires a smaller volume of medication; produces excellent muscular relaxation; allows for maintenance of maternal consciousness; and is associated with minimal blood loss. However, because uterine contraction sensation is lost, the patient must be instructed when to bear down during a vaginal birth. Since voluntary maternal expulsive efforts are compromised, there is an increased likelihood of an operative (e.g., episiotomy, forceps-assisted; vacuum-assisted) birth. After childbirth, there is an increased incidence of bladder and uterine atony and postdural puncture headache.

Nursing care during administration of a spinal anesthesia block includes proper positioning of the patient in a lateral or sitting position with the back curved outward to widen the intervertebral space (Fig. 13-8). After injection of the anesthetic solution, the patient is positioned upright to allow downward flow of the solution to provide a lower level of anesthesia suitable for a vaginal birth. For a cesarean birth, the patient is placed in a supine position with the head and shoulders slightly elevated with a wedge placed under one of the hips to displace the uterus (to obtain a higher level of anesthesia coverage). Effects from the anesthesia occur within 1 to 2 minutes after injection and last 1-3 hours, depending on the anesthetic agent used (Hawkins et al., 2002) (Procedure 13-1).

Figure 13-8 *A.* Lateral position for spinal and epidural block. *B.* Sitting position for spinal and epidural block.

Procedure 13-1 Assisting with the Administration of Spinal Anesthesia

Purpose

To facilitate administration of a spinal anesthesia block for the relief of pain during labor and birth.

Equipment

- Blood pressure cuff
- Stethoscope
- Fetal monitor

Steps

1. Wash and dry your hands. Explain the procedure and purpose of the examination to the patient.

   RATIONALE: *Hand washing helps to prevent the spread of microorganisms. Explanations help to decrease anxiety and promote patient's understanding and cooperation.*

2. Assist the patient to a sitting position on the edge of the bed or operating table (as directed by the nurse anesthetist or anesthesiologist).

3. Provide support, promote comfort, and limit motion during the procedure.

   RATIONALE: *Proper positioning (e.g., head bowed so that the back arches outward to widen the intervertebral space) and restricted movement are essential to successful anesthesia administration. Support prevents the patient from falling forward (she is "top heavy" from the gravid uterus).*

4. Check the intravenous infusion for patency.

   RATIONALE: *Hypotension from sympathetic blockage in the lower extremities may occur immediately after anesthesia administration. For this reason, IV fluids such as lactated Ringer's solution (500–1000 mL) are usually given before the injection to ensure maternal hydration; confirming the patency of IV tubing ensures that the fluid is infusing well before the anesthesia is administered and facilitates the rapid infusion of fluids if needed for postadministration hypotension.*

5. Assist the patient to lie down on her back after anesthesia administration (as directed by the nurse anesthetist or anesthesiologist).

6. Place a pillow under her head and a wedge under her right hip.

   RATIONALE: *Remaining in an upright position for too long prevents the anesthetic from rising high enough up the spinal canal to achieve pain relief. Conversely, lying down too soon allows the anesthetic to rise too high in the spinal canal. Lying with a pillow under the head helps to ensure that the anesthesia will be confined to the lower spinal canal. A wedge placed under the right hip displaces the uterus and helps to prevent compression of the vena cava.*

7. Monitor the pulse, blood pressure, and respirations every 1 to 2 minutes for the first 10 minutes, then every 5 to 10 minutes. Use electronic monitoring to continuously monitor the FHR.

   RATIONALE: *Frequent assessment of maternal vital signs is essential for recognizing hypotension (from sympathetic blockage in the lower extremities) or an adverse reaction. Ongoing assessment of the fetal heart rate and pattern provides evidence of fetal well-being.*

8. Document the procedure on the patient's chart.

   RATIONALE: *Documentation provides a record for communication and evaluation of patient care.*

Nursing Consideration

The nurse informs the nurse anesthetist or anesthesiologist when a contraction is beginning so that the anesthetic will not be administered during a contraction.

Documentation

8/30/09. 0425: Spinal anesthesia administered by J. Chen, CRNA. 1000 mL lactated Ringer's solution infused IV prior to administration per protocol. Procedure tolerated well by patient. Vital signs: Preanesthesia administration, BP: 116/78 mm Hg, Pulse: 84 bpm, Respirations: 14 breaths/min, FHR: 146 bpm and regular; Postanesthesia administration, BP: 110/72 mm Hg, Pulse: 80 bpm, Respirations: 12 breaths/min, FHR: 148 bpm and regular.

—S. Rinaldi, RNC

Complications that may occur with spinal anesthesia block include maternal hypotension, decreased placental perfusion, and an ineffective breathing pattern. Before administration, the patient's fluid balance is assessed and intravenous fluids are administered to reduce the potential for sympathetic blockade (decreased cardiac output that results from vasodilation with pooling of blood in the lower extremities). After administration of the anesthetic, the patient's blood pressure, pulse, and respirations and FHR must be taken and documented every 5 to 10 minutes. If indicators of severe maternal hypotension (e.g., a drop in the baseline blood pressure of more than 20%) or fetal compromise (e.g., bradycardia; decreased variability; late decelerations) develop, emergency measures must be instituted.

critical nursing action Severe Maternal Hypotension and Decreased Placental Perfusion

In the event of severe maternal hypotension, the nurse takes the following actions:

- Place the patient in a lateral position or use a wedge under the hip to displace the uterus; elevate the legs.
- Maintain or increase the IV infusion rate, according to institution protocol.
- Administer oxygen by face mask at 10–12 L/min, or according to institution protocol.
- Alert the primary care provider, anesthesiologist, or nurse anesthetist.

- Administer an IV vasopressor (e.g., ephedrine 5–10 mg) according to institutional protocol, if the above measures are ineffective.
- Remain calm, offer reassurance, and continue to assess maternal blood pressure and FHR every 5 minutes until stable or per order from the primary care provider.

Postdural puncture headache, a complication that may develop within 48 hours after the puncture, is believed to occur from leakage of cerebrospinal fluid (CSF) from the puncture site in the dura mater. Typically, the headache is intensified when the patient assumes an upright position and relieved when she assumes a supine position. Accompanying symptoms include auditory (tinnitus) and visual (blurred vision, photophobia) problems. Interventions usually center on oral analgesics, bedrest in a darkened room, caffeine, and hydration. If these measures are not effective, an autologous epidural blood patch may be administered. Approximately 10–20 mL of the patient's blood is slowly injected into the lumbar epidural space. A clot forms in the tear or hole in the dura mater around the spinal cord, effectively sealing the area from further CSF leakage.

 Optimizing Outcomes— Discharge instructions after autologous epidural blood patch

Discharge planning after administration of an autologous epidural blood patch includes providing the following instructions:

- Maintain bedrest for 24–48 hours.
- Apply cold packs to the area as needed for pain relief.
- Increase oral fluids.
- Avoid the use of analgesics that affect platelet aggregation (e.g., nonsteroidal anti-inflammatory drugs) for 2 days.
- Observe for signs of infection at the site.
- Observe for signs of neurological complications (pain, numbness, tingling in the legs; difficulty with ambulation).

 Now Can You— Discuss local infiltration, pudendal nerve block, and spinal block anesthesia?

1. Discuss the indications for and timing of administration for local infiltration anesthesia and a pudendal nerve block?
2. Name four advantages and two disadvantages associated with spinal block anesthesia?
3. Describe the immediate nursing actions to be taken for severe maternal hypotension with decreased placental perfusion?

Epidural Anesthesia or Analgesia Block

Injection of a local anesthetic such as bupivacaine, an opioid analgesic such as fentanyl or sufentanil, or both into the epidural space (between L4 and L5) provides pain relief from uterine contractions and vaginal or cesarean birth. The degree of analgesic or anesthetic effect obtained is related to the specific medication used. Combining an opioid with a local anesthetic agent reduces the total amount of anesthetic required and helps to preserve a greater amount of maternal motor function (McCool, Packman, & Zwerling, 2004).

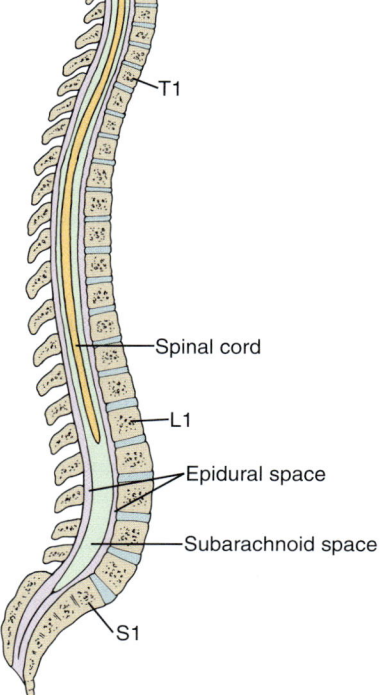

Figure 13-9 The epidural space is located between the dura mater and the ligamentum flavum and extends from the base of the skull to the end of the sacral canal.

Figure 13-10 The spinal canal: injection sites for regional anesthesia.

A & P review **The Epidural Space**

The nerves located in the spinal cord are covered and protected by several tissue layers. The pia mater is the membrane that adheres to the nerve fibers. It is surrounded by CSF. The next layer is the arachnoid membrane; the dura mater is the protective covering that lies outside of this membrane. An anesthetic agent administered into the CSF in the subarachnoid space is called *spinal anesthesia*. The epidural space is a vacant space located outside the dura mater; beyond the epidural space, the ligamentum flavum, which extends from the base of the skull to the end of the sacral canal, provides another protective layer. With *epidural anesthesia*, an anesthetic agent is placed just inside the ligamentum flavum in the epidural space (Figs. 13-9 and 13-10). ◆

 Nursing Insight— *Methods for administering an epidural block*

Epidural blocks, administered by a nurse anesthetist or anesthesiologist, may be given in different ways. For analgesia and anesthesia during labor, the block may be administered as a single dose with an epidural needle. It may also be administered as a single dose through an epidural catheter, with additional doses ("top-offs") given as needed, or given as a continuous epidural. Patients may be required to remain in bed; other blocks allow ambulation ("walking epidural") (Mayberry, Clemmens, & De, 2002).

LUMBAR EPIDURAL ANESTHESIA AND ANALGESIA BLOCK. The lumbar epidural anesthesia and analgesia block is the most commonly used method of pain control during labor; nearly two thirds of women in the United States incorporate this intervention for discomfort and pain into their birth plan (Bucklin et al., 2005). Advantages of this method include maternal relaxation, enhanced comfort and pain relief, and an ability to remain alert and participate in the birth. Also, there is little blood loss, the respiratory reflexes remain intact, there is no delay in gastric emptying, and only a partial degree of motor paralysis occurs. Fetal complications are rare and are related to maternal hypotension or effects from the rapid absorption of the medication. Postdural puncture headaches, caused by leakage of CSF, rarely occur because with epidural anesthesia, the CSF space is not entered.

Epidural blocks are advantageous for patients with diabetes, heart disease, pulmonary disease, and, in some cases, pregnancy-induced hypertension because they essentially eliminate the pain associated with labor and thus reduce the maternal stress associated with labor discomfort. The patient's energy level is preserved because she does not feel the contractions. Epidural blocks may be used with preterm pregnancies because there is minimal effect on the fetus. A gentle, controlled birth is associated with minimal trauma to the immature fetal skull and there are no systemic narcotic analgesics to cause depression in the premature neonate.

Maternal hypotension is the most common complication of epidural anesthesia. Preloading the patient with a rapid infusion of intravenous fluids, which increases the blood volume and cardiac output, can usually prevent this complication. Intravenous fluids are then infused continuously. Most institutions use dextrose-free solutions because dextrose can cause fetal hyperglycemia with rebound hypoglycemia during the first several hours after birth. The nurse should be in continuous attendance after administration of an epidural anesthetic. To detect hypotension, blood pressure should be continuously monitored for at least the first 20 minutes and after each new injection of the anesthetic. Blood pressure should be monitored during the entire time the anesthetic is in effect to ensure that the

systolic pressure does not fall below 100 mm Hg or decrease 20 mm Hg in a hypertensive patient. A drop greater than this may be life-threatening to the fetus unless effective interventions (e.g., maternal position change; administration of antihypotensive agents) are instituted.

Other disadvantages include limited mobility due to medical interventions such as the intravenous infusion and electronic monitoring equipment. Patients may experience orthostatic hypotension, dizziness, sedation, and lower extremity weakness. The accidental injection of a local anesthetic into a blood vessel can cause CNS effects including bizarre behavior, disorientation, excitation, and convulsions. Severe maternal hypotension resulting from sympathetic blockade can cause a significant decrease in uteroplacental perfusion and the delivery of oxygen to the fetus (Anim-Somuah, Smyth, & Howell, 2005).

 Nursing Insight— *Shiver response after epidural block administration*

The patient may exhibit a shiver response after administration of epidural block anesthesia. This physiological reaction can result from heat loss related to increased peripheral blood flow. It may also be related to an alteration of thermal input to the CNS when warm but not cold sensations have been suppressed. Essentially, the body believes that the temperature is lower than the true temperature and raises the "thermostat" to generate heat by shivering. The nurse should apply warm blankets for comfort and offer reassurance.

The nurse must perform frequent assessments of the maternal bladder to avoid bladder distention. Although the patient may be unable to void and require catheterization, the bedpan should always be offered initially to minimize the potential for a urinary tract infection. Urinary retention and stress incontinence may also occur immediately postpartum. Intense pruritus is a common side effect of opioid use; this symptom is usually treated with diphenhydramine (Benadryl), 25 mg administered intravenously or 50 mg administered intramuscularly. A temporary elevation in temperature may occur after administration of epidural anesthesia (Hawkins et al., 2002).

Optimizing Outcomes— **During the second stage of labor after administration of an epidural block**

The patient who has received an epidural block may require assistance with pushing because of an inability to feel the contractions or experience the urge to push. She may also need someone to hold or control her legs in order to push. After birth, the nurse must ensure that full sensation has returned and the patient is able to control her legs before ambulation is permitted. Depending on the agent used and the dose administered, this may take several hours.

For relief of labor pain and a vaginal birth, a block from T10 to S5 is performed, usually when the cervix has dilated to 5 to 6 cm. For a cesarean birth, a block from T8 to S1 is required. The patient is positioned on her side with her legs slightly flexed or she is asked to sit on the edge of the bed. She is instructed to drop her shoulders, round out the small of her back ("arch the back like a cat"), and put her chin into her chest. The medication is injected between contractions to minimize the risk of tachycardia that can occur if the drug is unintentionally injected directly into a vessel. The diffusion of the epidural anesthesia is dependent on the placement of the catheter tip, the dose and volume of medication used, and the patient's position (e.g., horizontal or upright). Once the epidural has been administered, a side-lying position (alternating sides each hour) is maintained to prevent compression of the vena cava. Depending on the degree of motor impairment, ambulation may be encouraged.

 ### Nursing Insight— *Methods for epidural anesthesia block*

Most often, a continuous epidural anesthesia block, a method achieved by the use of a pump to infuse solution into an indwelling catheter, is used. In many areas, patients are allowed to control the dosing with a programmed pump (patient-controlled epidural analgesia [PCEA]). This method empowers the patient to achieve some degree of control over her labor comfort and has been shown to decrease the total amount of medication needed. A lock-out period after each self-administration prevents overdosage. Less commonly, an intermittent block that relies on repeated injections of anesthetic solution is performed.

COMBINED SPINAL–EPIDURAL ANALGESIA. A combination of spinal–epidural analgesia may be used to block pain transmission without interfering with motor ability. Pain relief is immediate, unlike the 20- to 30-minute delay associated with an epidural alone. With the combined approach, an opioid such as fentanyl or sufentanil is injected into the subarachnoid space to rapidly activate the opioid receptors. A catheter inserted in the epidural space extends the duration of the analgesia by using a lower dose of a local anesthetic agent alone or in combination with an opioid agonist analgesic (Hawkins et al., 2002). Although patients may ambulate, they often choose not to do so because of fatigue, sensations of weakness in the legs, and a fear of falling. They should be encouraged to change positions frequently and assisted to an upright position to enhance bearing-down efforts. Because this method is associated with puncture of the dura and placement of a catheter in the epidural space, there is a greater risk for infection and postdural puncture headache (Lieberman & O'Donoghue, 2002; McCool et al., 2004). A combined spinal–epidural block may be used for both labor analgesia and for cesarean birth; the anesthetic and analgesic agents used vary according to the purpose of the procedure. Additional medication may be added to increase its effectiveness or if an instrument-assisted or cesarean birth is needed.

EPIDURAL AND INTRATHECAL OPIOIDS. Another approach for nerve block analgesia/anesthesia involves the use of opioids alone. This method eliminates the effects of a local anesthetic. Advantages of epidural or intrathecal (injected into the subarachnoid space) opioids without local anesthetics include the following: there is no maternal hypotension or alteration in vital signs; the patient is aware of

contractions but does not feel pain—thus she is able to bear down during the second stage of labor; and her motor power remains intact.

Opioids such as fentanyl, sufentanil (short-acting agents—effects last 1.5 to 4 hours) and preservative-free morphine (long-acting—effects last up to 7 hours) may be used. A drawback of this method concerns the potential need for a pudendal nerve block or local perineal infiltration anesthesia since intrathecal opioids do not provide adequate anesthesia for second-stage labor pain, episiotomy, or birth for most women (Cunningham et al., 2005). More often, epidural and intrathecal opioids are used for postoperative pain control. After cesarean birth, women are comfortable enough to freely ambulate and care for their newborns. Early ambulation is associated with enhanced bladder emptying, more rapid return of peristalsis, and a decreased risk of respiratory complications and thrombophlebitis. Side effects are more common when preservative-free morphine is used. These include nausea and vomiting, pruritus, urinary retention, and delayed respiratory depression.

 ### Optimizing Outcomes— **When epidural and intrathecal opioids are administered**

The nurse should monitor and record the patient's respiratory rate every hour for 24 hours (or per institutional protocol) after administration of epidural or intrathecal opioids. Naloxone (Narcan) should be administered if the maternal respiratory rate decreases to less than 10 breaths per minute or if the maternal oxygen saturation rate decreases to less than 89%. Oxygen may be administered by face mask and the anesthesiologist should be notified.

 ### Now Can You— **Discuss epidural and intrathecal anesthesia?**

1. Name six advantages of epidural anesthesia and identify the most common complication associated with this method?
2. Describe the benefits of combined spinal–epidural anesthesia?
3. Identify an essential component of nursing assessment after the administration of epidural or intrathecal opioids?

GENERAL ANESTHESIA

General anesthesia (induced unconsciousness) may be used for unplanned, rapid (emergency) cesarean birth, when there are contraindications to an epidural or spinal block, or when surgical intervention is required for certain obstetric complications (Box 13-3). The major risks

---

> **Box 13-3 Contraindications to Spinal/Epidural Block Anesthesia**
>
> - Maternal refusal
> - Local or systemic infection
> - Coagulation disorders
> - Actual or anticipated maternal hemorrhage
> - Allergy to specific anesthetic agents
> - Lack of trained staff available (Cunningham et al., 2005)

associated with general anesthesia administered for childbirth are hypoxia and the possible inhalation of vomitus during administration. Pregnant women are particularly prone to gastric reflux due to increased stomach pressure from the gravid uterus beneath it. In addition, the gastroesophageal valve may be displaced, allowing the upward passage of stomach contents. The aspiration of stomach contents that have an acid pH may cause chemical pneumonitis and secondary infection of the respiratory tract.

Fetal depression is directly related to the depth and duration of the anesthesia. Most general anesthetic agents reach the fetus in approximately 2 minutes. General anesthesia is not recommended when the fetus is considered to be high risk, especially in preterm birth. Measures to reduce respiratory depression in the neonate include reducing the time from induction of the anesthesia until the umbilical cord is clamped and using a minimum of sedating drugs and anesthetics until after the cord has been clamped.

To prepare the patient for general anesthesia, the nurse ensures that an IV infusion is in place, and if time permits, premedicates her with an oral antacid (e.g., sodium citrate, Bicitra, Alka-Seltzer) to neutralize the acidic contents of the stomach. Some anesthesiologists order ranitidine hydrochloride (Zantac) IV or cimetidine (Tagamet) to decrease the production of stomach acid; metoclopramide (Reglan) may also be prescribed to increase gastric emptying (Hawkins et al., 2002). Before administration of the anesthesia, a wedge is placed under the right hip to displace the uterus (to prevent aortocaval compression and decreased placental perfusion). When possible, the patient is preoxygenated with 3 to 5 minutes of 100% oxygen.

Thiopental sodium (Pentothal), an ultra-short-acting barbiturate, is usually given. This agent causes rapid induction of anesthesia and minimal postpartal bleeding. Succinyl choline (Anectine) is a muscle relaxant used to facilitate passage of the endotracheal tube. To prevent gastric reflux and aspiration before the woman fully loses consciousness, the nurse may be asked to assist with applying cricoid pressure. This maneuver seals off the esophagus by compressing it between the cricoid cartilage and the cervical vertebrae. The cricoid ring, which is the only tracheal cartilage that forms a complete ring, is located immediately below the thyroid bone. The cricoid cartilage is depressed 2 to 3 cm posteriorly and pressure is maintained until the cuffed endotracheal tube is securely in place (Fig. 13-11). While applying pressure, the nurse should use the other hand to support the patient's neck.

After intubation, a 50:50 mixture of oxygen and nitrous oxide is usually administered. Small amounts of a halogenated agent such as isoflurane or methoxyflurane may also be given to enhance pain relief and to reduce maternal awareness and recall (Hawkins et al., 2002). The halogenated agents produce rapid uterine relaxation to facilitate intrauterine manipulation and extraction. However, at high concentrations they readily cross the placenta and can produce fetal narcosis and an increased risk for postpartal maternal hemorrhage due to uterine relaxation.

Recovery room care is focused on maintenance of an open airway, continuous monitoring of cardiopulmonary function, and the prevention of postpartum hemorrhage. Postpartal care should be arranged to facilitate parent–infant bonding as soon as possible. The nurse offers

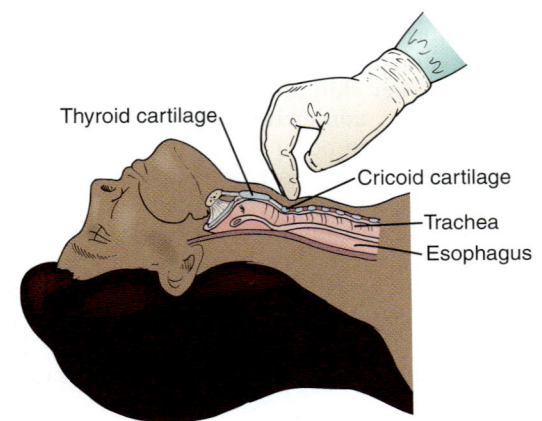

Figure 13-11 Correct position for applying cricoid pressure until endotracheal tube placement has been completed.

emotional support, answers questions concerning the birth, provides updates regarding maternal/neonatal status, and assesses the patient's readiness to interact with her newborn.

 Now Can You— Discuss implications of general anesthesia used during childbirth?

1. Identify two major risks associated with the use of general anesthesia for childbirth?
2. Demonstrate how to apply cricoid pressure and explain the importance of this intervention?
3. Describe two major nursing responsibilities for recovery room patient care following the use of general anesthesia?

Nursing Care for the Patient Receiving Interventions to Promote Comfort During Labor and Birth

The patient's methods of pain relief are influenced by several factors: her wishes and desires; the phase and stage of labor; the availability of the chosen modalities in the birth center; and the knowledge and expertise of the health care team with the various pharmacological and nonpharmacological methods.

NURSING ASSESSMENT AND DIAGNOSES

Assessment during labor is an ongoing process that requires a collaborative approach from the primary care provider, the nurse, the patient, and her labor support person(s). Factors such as maternal/fetal status, the progress of labor, and the patient's level of comfort must be taken into consideration before a decision is made concerning whether nonpharmacological methods, pharmacological methods, or a combined approach will be used. The nurse never assumes that all pain experienced during labor is uterine in origin. Instead, a physical assessment that includes an evaluation of the characteristics of the patient's pain (location, intensity, quality, frequency, duration, and effectiveness of all relief measures) must be performed. The patient's prenatal record is reviewed to identify pertinent obstetrical information; drug allergies; a history of tobacco, alcohol, or other substance abuse; as well as spinal or neurological disorders.

The patient interview focuses on information concerning the onset of labor; the most recent oral intake (time, amount), present illnesses, allergies, and events that have occurred since her last visit with her primary care provider. She is asked about attendance in childbirth education classes and preferences for intrapartum comfort measures. When available, the birth plan is reviewed and updated or modified as needed.

The physical examination includes assessment of maternal vital signs, fetal heart rate and pattern, uterine contractions, amniotic membranes and fluid, cervical effacement and dilation, and fetal descent. The nurse also evaluates the patient's hydration status and palpates for bladder distention. After the administration of pharmacological agents, the nurse provides ongoing assessment of the patient, fetus, and labor progress according to institutional policy and professional standards (Association of Women's Health, Obstetric and Neonatal Nurses [AWHONN], 2001; Mahlmeister, 2003). Maternal assessment for evidence of allergic reaction to medications includes monitoring vital signs, respiratory status, platelet, and white blood cell count and observing for integumentary changes. Laboratory data are analyzed to identify anemia, coagulopathy or bleeding disorders, or infection. Fetal status is also assessed and non-reassuring changes in heart rate or pattern are promptly reported to the patient's primary health care provider.

A number of nursing diagnoses are relevant to anxiety, discomfort, and pain relief during labor and birth:

• Anxiety related to lack of knowledge about the labor experience
• Ineffective coping related to the combination of uterine contractions and anxiety
• Acute pain related to the processes of labor and birth

Expected outcomes of nursing interventions include:

• The patient verbalizes understanding of what is happening with her labor; she is able to identify the beginning and ending of contractions and demonstrates confidence instead of confusion with the labor process.
• The patient verbalizes confidence in her ability to participate actively in her labor experience, she demonstrates effective breathing techniques, guides her labor support person in providing effective comfort measures, readily engages in position changes and other strategies to enhance comfort and remain in control, and expresses confidence in her labor nurse and other care providers.
• The patient verbalizes that with the methods used, her pain has been relieved to a tolerable level; she is responsive to questions and suggestions and demonstrates an ability to deal with her contractions

A plan of care individualized to each patient is developed and modified as needed. A collaborative approach that includes the patient, her primary care provider, and labor support person is important in ensuring that safe, effective care is provided that promotes a positive childbirth experience for the woman and her family.

summary points

◆ Pain during labor is unique in that it is normal, can be anticipated and prepared for, and ends with a birth.

◆ Although a universal phenomenon, every individual perceives pain differently.

◆ The better prepared a woman is for childbirth, the less likely is the need for analgesia and anesthesia.

◆ Relaxation, massage, breathing techniques, and other nonpharmacological strategies should be encouraged in conjunction with prescribed analgesics.

◆ The type of analgesic or anesthetic to be used depends, in part, on the stage of labor and the method of birth.

◆ Sedatives are used during a prolonged early labor when there is a need to decrease anxiety or promote rest.

◆ Regional anesthesia can be extremely effective for pain; the nurse must ensure adequate maternal hydration and normal blood pressure before administration.

◆ General anesthesia is rarely used for vaginal birth because of risks for both the woman and her neonate.

review questions

Multiple Choice

1. In the first stage of labor, the perinatal nurse is aware that pain impulses are transmitted via:
   A. T11, T12 spinal nerve segments
   B. T9, T10 spinal nerve segments
   C. L4, L5 spinal nerve segments
   D. Sacral spinal nerve segments

2. The perinatal nurse is aware that a woman's history of past painful experiences with labor and birth are part of which neural pathway process for pain?
   A. Transduction
   B. Transmission
   C. Perception
   D. Modulation

3. Marianne, a 29 year old multigravid woman, was given promethazine (Phenergan) and meperidine hydrochloride (Demerol) during labor as part of her pain management. The perinatal nurse is aware that during the first 24 hours after birth, Marianne's infant will have an increased risk for:
   A. Hyperbilirubinemia
   B. Tachypnea
   C. Irritability
   D. Tremors

Fill-in-the-Blank

4. The perinatal nurse teaches the laboring woman and her partner about the cycle of _____, _____, and _____ that can escalate to decrease labor progress.

5. The perinatal nurse knows that evidence-based care in labor includes providing _____ and a _____ presence.

6. In providing care to the laboring woman, the perinatal nurse must balance the knowledge that the analgesia/

anesthesia chosen is determined by the _____ of _____ and the woman's available _____ at the birth facility.

True/False

7. Childbirth education is encouraged by the perinatal nurse as it increases the information that women and families have about labor, birth, and options for pain relief.

Case Study

8. The perinatal nurse assists Teresa, a laboring woman, and her partner between contractions to increase their knowledge and ability to use breathing methods during the contractions. Teresa's use of breathing techniques during a contraction may decrease pain by:
A. Reducing the capacity of nerve pathways to transmit pain
B. Increasing the capacity of nerve pathways to transmit endorphins
C. Decreasing her anxiety about labor
D. Decreasing her distraction during her contractions

Select All that Apply

9. The perinatal nurse is aware that one of the *Healthy People 2010* goals is to:
A. Educate women in the use of nonpharmacological pain management in labor.
B. Decrease mortality related to pharmacological methods of pain relief in labor.
C. Increase informed use of pharmacological methods of pain relief in labor.
D. Increase availability of pharmacological pain relief in labor.

10. The perinatal nurse understands that the advantages to a spinal anesthetic for a woman in labor include:
A. Easy administration
B. Immediate pain relief
C. Minimal blood loss
D. Good voluntary maternal expulsive efforts

See Answers to End of Chapter Review Questions on the Electronic Study Guide or DavisPlus.

REFERENCES

Allaire, A.D. (2001). Complementary and alternative medicine in the labor and delivery suite. *Clinical Obstetrics and Gynecology, 44*(4), 681–691.

Anim-Somuah, M., Smyth, R., & Howell, C. (2005). Epidural versus non-epidural or no analgesia in labor. *The Cochrane Database of Systematic Reviews, 2006*, No. 3. Chichester, UK: John Wiley & Sons.

Association of Women's Health, Obstetric, and Neonatal Nurses (AWHONN). (2001). *Evidence-based clinical practice guidelines: Nursing care of the woman receiving regional analgesia/anesthesia in labor.* Washington, DC: Author.

Association of Women's Health, Obstetric, and Neonatal Nurses (AWHONN). (2002). *The role of the registered nurse (RN) in the care of pregnant women receiving analgesia/anesthesia by catheter techniques (epidural, intrathecal, spinal, PCEA catheters).* Clinical Position Statement. Retrieved from http://www.awhonn.org (Accessed April 12, 2008).

Bricker, L., & Lavender, T. (2002). Parenteral opioids for labor pain relief: A systematic review. *American Journal of Obstetrics and Gynecology, 186*(5), S94–S109.

Bucklin, B., Hawkins, J., Anderson, J., & Ulrich, F. (2005). Obstetric workforce survey. *Anesthesiology, 103*(3), 645–653.

Bulechek, G., Butcher, H.M., & Dochterman, J. (2008). *Nursing interventions classification (NIC)* (5th ed.). St. Louis, MO: C.V. Mosby.

Caton, D., Corry, M., Frigoletto, F., Hopkins, D., Lieberman, E., Mayberry, L., et al. (2002). The nature and management of labor pain: Executive summary. *American Journal of Obstetrics and Gynecology, 186*(5), S1–S15.

Colin, J.M., & Paperwalla, G. (2003). Haitians. In St. Hill P., Lipson, J.G., & Meleis, A.I. (Eds.), *Caring for women cross-culturally* (pp. 172–187). Philadelphia: F.A. Davis.

Cunningham, F., Leveno, K., Bloom, S., Hauth, J., Gilstrap, L., & Wenstrom, K. (2005). *Williams' obstetrics* (22nd ed.). New York: McGraw-Hill.

Deglin, J.H., & Vallerand, A.H. (2009). *Davis's drug guide for nurses* (11th ed.). Philadelphia: F.A. Davis.

Faucher, M., & Brucker, M. (2000). Intrapartum pain: Pharmacologic management. *Journal of Obstetric, Gynecologic and Neonatal Nursing, 29*(2), 169–180.

Florence, D., & Palmer, D. (2003). Therapeutic choices for the discomforts of labor. *Journal of Perinatal and Neonatal Nursing, 37*, 238.

Gentz, B. (2001). Alternative therapies for the management of pain in labor and delivery. *Clinical Obstetrics and Gynecology, 44*(4), 704–732.

Hawkins, J., Chestnut, D., & Gibbs, C. (2002). Obstetric anesthesia. In Gabbe S., Niebyl, J., & Simpson, J. (Eds.), *Obstetrics: Normal and problem pregnancies* (4th ed.). Philadelphia: Churchill Livingstone.

Hodnett, E. (2002). Pain and women's satisfaction with the experience of childbirth: A systematic review. *American Journal of Obstetrics and Gynecology 186*(5), S160–172.

Hover-Kramer, D., Mentgen, J., & Scandrett-Hibdon, S. (2001). *Healing touch; A resource for health care professionals.* Albany, NY: Delmar.

Johnson, M., Bulechek, G., Butcher, H., McCloskey Dochterman, J., Maas, M., Moorehead, S., & Swanson, E. (2006). *NANDA, NOC, and NIC linkages: Nursing diagnoses, outcomes, & interventions* (2nd ed.). St. Louis, MO: Mosby Elsevier.

Ketterhagen, D., VandeVusse, L., & Berner, M. (2002). Self-hypnosis: Alternative anesthesia for childbirth. *MCN American Journal of Maternal/Child Nursing, 27*(6), 335–340.

Kulig, J.C. (2003). Cambodians. In St. Hill, P., Lipson, J.G., & Meleis, A.I. (Eds.), *Caring for women cross-culturally* (pp. 78–91). Philadelphia: F.A. Davis.

Lagana, K., & Gonzalez-Ramirez, L. (2003). Mexican Americans. In St. Hill, P., Lipson, J.G., & Meleis, A.I. (Eds.), *Caring for women cross-culturally* (pp. 218–235). Philadelphia: F.A. Davis.

Lehne, R. (2006). *Pharmacology for nursing care* (6th ed.). Philadelphia: Saunders.

Leighton, B., & Halpern, S. (2002). The effects of epidural analgesia on labor, maternal, and neonatal outcomes: A systematic review. *American Journal of Obstetrics and Gynecology, 186*(5), S69–S77.

Lieberman, E., & O'Donoghue, C. (2002). Unintended effects of epidural anesthesia during labor: A systematic review. *American Journal of Obstetrics & Gynecology, 186*(5), S31–S68.

Lowe, N. (2002). The nature of labor pain. *American Journal of Obstetrics and Gynecology, 186*(5), S16–S24.

Lowe, N. (2004). Context and process of informed consent for pharmacologic strategies in labor pain care. *Journal of Midwifery & Women's Health, 49*(3), 250–259.

Mackey, M. (2001). Use of water in labor and birth. *Clinical Obstetrics and Gynecology, 44*(4), 733–749.

Mahlmeister, L. (2003). Nursing responsibilities in preventing, preparing for, and managing epidural emergencies. *Journal of Perinatal and Neonatal Nursing, 17*(1), 19–32.

Marks, G. (2000). Alternative therapies. In Nichols, F., & Humernick, S. (Eds.), *Childbirth education: Practice, research and theory* (2nd ed.). Philadelphia: W.B. Saunders.

Maternity Center Association. (2002). *Listening to mothers: Report of the first national U.S. survey of women's childbearing experiences executive summary and recommendations issued by the Maternity Center Association.* New York: Maternity Association. Retrieved from http://www.maternitywise.org (Accessed April 11, 2008).

Mayberry, L., Clemmens, D., & De, A. (2002). Epidural anesthesia side effects, co-interventions, and care of women during childbirth: A systematic review. *American Journal of Obstetrics and Gynecology 186*(5) Supplement S, S81–93.

McCool, W., Packman, J., & Zwerling, A. (2004). Obstetric anesthesia: changes and choices. *Journal of Midwifery & Women's Health, 49*(6), 505–513.

Meleis, A. (2003). Theoretical considerations of health care for immigrant and minority women. In St. Hill, P., Lipson, J.G., & Meleis, A.I. (Eds.), *Caring for women cross-culturally* (pp. 1–10). Philadelphia: F.A. Davis.

Metzack, R., & Wall, P. (1965). Pain mechanisms: A new theory. *Science, 150*(2), 971–982.

Moorehead, S., Johnson, M., Maas, M., & Swanson, E. (2008). *Nursing outcomes classification (NOC)* (4th ed.). St. Louis, MO: C.V. Mosby.

NANDA International (2007). *NANDA-I nursing diagnoses: Definitions and classifications 2007–2008.* Philadelphia: NANDA-I.

Padfield, D., Hurwitz, B., & Pither, C. (2003). *Perceptions of pain.* Stockport, England: Dewi Lewis Publishing.

Perinatal Education Associates. (2006). *Breathing.* Retrieved from http://www.birthsource.com (Accessed April 6, 2007).

Perez, P. (2000). *Birthballs: The use of physical therapy balls in maternity care.* Johnson, VT: Cutting Edge Press.

Potter, G. (2006). RN teaches expectant parents the power of hypnosis. *Nursing Spectrum* (Greater Philadelphia/Tri-State Edition), *5*(3), 14-15.

Righard, L. (2001). Making childbirth a normal process. *Birth, 28*(1), 1–4.

Scheiber, B., & Selby, C. (Eds.). (2000). *Therapeutic touch.* New York: Prometheus Books.

Simkin, P., & Bolding, A. (2004). Update on nonpharmacologic approaches to relieve labor pain and prevent suffering. *Journal of Midwifery & Women's Health, 49*(6), 489–504.

Simkin, P., & O'Hara, M. (2002). Nonpharmacologic relief of pain during labor: Systematic reviews of five methods. *American Journal of Obstetrics and Gynecology, 186*(5), 5131–5159.

Smith, C., Collins, C., Cyna, A., & Crowther, C. (2005). Complementary and alternative therapies for pain management in labour. *The Cochrane Database of Systematic Reviews,* 2006, Issue 3. Chichester, UK: John Wiley & Sons.

Venes, D. (Ed.). (2009). *Taber's cyclopedic medical dictionary* (21st ed.). Philadelphia: F.A. Davis.

 For more information, go to http://davisplus.fadavis.com/

CONCEPT MAP

What To Say:
- Offer encouraging words to help patient refocus in transition

Complementary Care:
- Can use Yoga for discomfort in labor

Collaboration In Caring:
- Use of acupressure/acupuncture more widely accepted to relieve labor pain

Types of Pain

Visceral: 1st stage of labor
- r/t change in cervix, lower uterine segment, uterine ischemia
- Radiates to abdominal wall/lumbosacral area/gluteus maximus/thighs

Somatic: 2nd stage of labor
- r/t stretching/distention of perineal body; traction on peritoneum; soft tissue lacerations; expulsive forces; fetal pressure

- Multidimensional experience
- Unique to each individual
- Includes perception of and response to

Perception/Expression:
- Influenced by
  - Primary social group; culture; ethnicity; past experience
- Psychological/emotional response:
  - crying; screaming; quiet; exhaustion; clenching teeth; groaning; wringing hands
- Physiological response:
  - elevated BP, heart rate, respirations; diaphoresis nausea/vomiting+

Influencing factors

Physical:
- Duration/intensity of labor
- Position of fetus
- Pelvic size/shape
- Maternal fatigue
- Presence of equipment
- Induction of labor

Psychological:
- Anxiety/fear
- Previous experience/childbirth preparation
- Support systems

PAIN

Across Care Settings:
- Encourage investigation of available childbirth settings

Promoting Comfort In Labor and Birth

Critical Nursing Actions:
- Combining butorphanol (Stadol) with other CNS depressants increases respiratory suppression
- Respond quickly/correctly to maternal hypotension/decreased placental perfusion

Nursing Insight:
- Childbirth pain is unique
- Allow patient to dictate labor environment as much as possible
- Use visual analogue pain scale
- Decreasing anxiety can reduce vasoconstriction/pain
- Know the difference between opioid agonist/antagonists; recognize local anesthetic agents
- Recognize value of natural pressure anesthesia
- Be aware of different methods to administer epidural blocks
- Recognize shiver response

Optimizing Outcomes:
- Non-pharmacological comfort measures can decrease maternal mortality
- Recognize cultural influences on pain
- Continually assess pain throughout labor
- Recognize hyperventilation
- Do not apply "heat/cold" on anesthetized areas
- Give IV analgesics in small dose, during contraction
- Use opioids with caution/monitor for safety; have Narcan and oxygen ready
- Give complete D/C instructions after autologous epidural blood patch
- Epidural block ⟶ assist to push; assess return of sensation

Nonpharmacological
- Positioning ⟶ squatting, "slow-dance"
- Breathing techniques
- Relaxation ⟶ music, guided imagery, massage/touch
- Hydro; hypno; aroma therapies
- Use of heat and cold
- Biofeedback
- TENS
- Acupressure/-puncture
- Intradermal water block

Pharmacological
- Sedatives: barbiturates; benzodiazepines
- Antiemetics: H₁ antagonist
- Analgesics: opioids, regional, epidural block
- Anesthesia: local perineal infiltration, pudendal block, spinal/epidural, general

Be Sure To:
- ☑ Inform patient about pharmacological pain relief and obtain consent
- Assess/reassess during intrapartal period

Now Can You:
- Discuss characteristics of pain during labor/birth
- Discuss a pain control theory
- Discuss non-pharmacologic/pharmacologic pain relief methods and all of the nursing implications
- Discuss different types of blocks/anesthetics and associated nursing considerations

Caring for the Woman Experiencing Complications During Labor and Birth

 And when our baby stirs and struggles to be born it compels humility, what we began is now its own.

—Anne Ridler

LEARNING TARGETS *At the completion of this chapter, the student will be able to:*

◆ Differentiate critical factors associated with nursing care of women experiencing dysfunctional labor patterns.

◆ Discuss pharmacological and nonpharmacological interventions used for the induction and augmentation of labor.

◆ Discuss collaborative care of the woman experiencing an induction of labor.

◆ Compare and contrast methods of instrumentation assistance of birth.

◆ Describe the management of selected maternal complications during the intrapartal period.

◆ Discuss how fetal malpresentation and malposition affect labor and birth.

◆ Compare and contrast the intrapartal management for placenta previa and abruptio placentae.

◆ Describe emergency nursing care for various uterine, placental, umbilical, and amniotic complications during labor and birth.

◆ Plan appropriate nursing care for a family experiencing a fetal loss.

◆ Discuss maternal and fetal factors associated with cesarean birth.

◆ Describe the controversies associated with vaginal birth after cesarean birth.

---

moving toward evidence-based practice Maternal placental syndrome as it relates to cardiovascular health

Ray, J.G., Vermeulen. M.J., Schull, M.J., & Redelmeier, D.A. (2005). Cardiovascular health after maternal placental syndromes (CHAMPS): Population-based retrospective cohort study. *The Lancet, 366,* 1797–1803.

Research indicates that the presence of maternal placental syndromes, which include hypertensive disorders of pregnancy and abruption or infarction of the placenta, probably originate from diseased placental vessels. These conditions occur more often in women with metabolic risk factors for cardiovascular disease such as obesity, hypertension, diabetes, and hyperlipidemia. The purpose of this study was to assess for the risk of premature vascular disease in women who experienced maternal placental syndrome during pregnancy.

The population-based retrospective cohort study included 1.03 million women who had no evidence of cardiovascular disease before their first documented delivery. The sample, obtained through multiple databases, consisted of women admitted to the hospital for the first obstetrical delivery of a live or stillborn infant after 20 weeks of gestation. Women younger than age 14, older than age 50, and those with a preexisting diagnosis of cardiovascular disease in the 24 months preceding the birth were excluded.

Maternal placental syndrome included preeclampsia, gestational hypertension, placental abruption, and placental infarction. A history of hospitalization for cardiovascular, coronary artery, or peripheral artery disease a minimum of 90 days after the delivery discharge date was identified as the point for determining the composite for the development of cardiovascular disease.

(continued)

moving toward evidence-based practice (continued)

Data analysis revealed the following findings:

- The mean age of the participants was 28.2 years at the time of the infant's birth.
- Maternal placental syndrome was diagnosed in 75,380 (7%) of the women.
- The incidence of cardiovascular disease was 500 per one million person-years in women with a placental syndrome, as compared to 200 per one million-person years in those who did not have a placental syndrome.
- The risk of cardiovascular disease was higher with the combined presence of maternal placental syndrome and either poor fetal growth or intrauterine fetal death.
- Of those diagnosed with the maternal placental syndrome, risk factors were more commonly present before delivery than in those participants who were not diagnosed with the maternal placental syndrome.

- The median period for follow-up was 8.7 years. The mean age of the participants at the time of the first cardiovascular event was 38.3 years; the maximum age of the participants was 60.2 years.
- The risk of cardiovascular disease increased with the number of risk factors present.
- The risk of premature cardiovascular disease is higher in women who have experienced maternal placental syndrome, especially in the presence of fetal complications.

1. What might be considered as limitations to this study?
2. How is this information useful to clinical nursing practice?

See Suggested Responses for Moving Toward Evidence-Based Practice on the Electronic Study Guide or DavisPlus.

Introduction

The nurse who cares for women and their families experiencing complications during labor and birth is responsible for creating a supportive environment that provides complex nursing care. Under normal circumstances labor and birth places stress on the family unit and when problems are superimposed during this time frame, another layer of complexity is added. The woman often needs to respond rapidly to changing health conditions for which she might not be prepared. The nurse has to be proactive and reassuring in support of the woman and her family unit. It is critical to empower the woman and encourage her to take control as much as possible. The nurse acts as her advocate in collaborative care when the woman is unable to have her voice.

Complications arise from a variety of factors. Women experience problems with uterine dysfunction often referred to as the powers of labor. The presentation and position of the fetus is integral to a positive labor outcome. When the fetus is not in a favorable lie, the labor process may lengthened, require instrumentation assistance, or necessitate an operative birth. Multiple fetuses are more prone to these issues because of their locations within the uterus. Placenta obstruction or an inadequate bony pelvis may hinder fetal progress through the birth canal and require more extensive medical intervention. Medical emergencies and complications from maternal disease also place the patient at increased risk for a complicated and intervention-driven labor and birth.

Cesarean or operative birth is one of the outcomes associated with a complicated labor. In the United States, the cesarean birth rate has steadily increased. Controversy surrounds this statistic while at the same time more women are requesting an elective cesarean birth. The nurse working in perinatal care has to be concerned with ethical issues and be prepared to foster evidence-based research studies to examine the multiple factors involved with cesarean deliveries.

Perinatal loss necessitates a collaborative response from all professionals involved in the care of the patient. Nurses can lead others in providing support. Spiritual, emotional, psychological, and physical needs are important considerations that need to be met during this time. Although this situation cannot be normalized, the nurse can encourage the woman to hold her infant, give her a baby picture, and provide a memory book to acknowledge the existence of the child.

The nurse serves in many capacities when managing the care of patients experiencing a complicated labor and birth. Use of the nursing process combined with a strong theoretical background provides a foundation for the critical decision making that exists in the clinical unit. Nursing diagnoses specific to the woman experiencing a complication during the intrapartal period refer to specific problems and often relate to the broad concepts of fear, anxiety, coping, and fatigue. Examples of possible nursing diagnoses are presented in Box 14-1. The nurse has the unique opportunity to empower the woman and assist her in taking control as much as possible in these difficult situations. Since patients are unique in their responses, it is incumbent upon the nurse to be sensitive to all individuals and be culturally competent. Finally, the nurse must constantly examine practice and promote research initiatives that give evidence to optimal outcomes in complex perinatal care.

Optimizing Outcomes— Helping to meet *Healthy People 2010* national goals

Nurses who work with birthing mothers can be instrumental in helping the nation to meet *Healthy People 2010* goals that address intrapartal complications:

- Reduce the maternal mortality rate to no more than 3.3 per 100,000 live births from a baseline of 7.1 per 100,000.
- Reduce cesarean births among low-risk women to no more than 15 per 100 deliveries from a baseline of 18 per 100 by carefully monitoring laboring women to

---

Box 14-1 Possible Nursing Diagnoses for the Woman Experiencing Complications During Labor and Birth

- Fear related to unknown high-risk condition of labor
- Anxiety related to loss of control during labor
- Coping, Ineffective, related to inadequate opportunity to prepare for high-risk labor
- Fatigue related to increased physical exertion during a long labor
- Powerlessness related to lack of control over decisions in a complicated birth
- Deficient Knowledge related to unknown high-risk condition
- Communication, Verbal Impaired, related to cultural differences
- Risk for Spiritual Distress related to emotional response to high-risk labor and birth
- Risk for Ineffective Tissue Perfusion related to excessive loss of blood
- Risk for Injury related to damage of tissue during a complicated birth
- Pain, Acute, related to tissue damage
- Fluid Volume, Deficit, related to decreased urinary output
- Fluid Volume, Excess, related to compromise of the cardiovascular system
- Risk for Trauma related to instrumentation-assisted birth
- Anticipatory Grieving related to fetal demise

---

identify early signs of potentially life-threatening events (i.e., placental abruption, uterine rupture) and by assisting women with fetal malpresentations amenable to rotation with positional changes to help reduce the number of cesarean births.

Dystocia

Dystocia, defined as a long, difficult or abnormal labor, is a term used to identify poor labor progression. Dystocia may arise from any of the three major components of the labor process—the powers (uterine contractions), the passenger (fetus), or the passageway (maternal pelvis). In addition, various medical interventions used during labor and birth may create problems that complicate the birth process.

Dystocia may be related to maternal positioning during labor, as well as fetal malpresentation, anomalies, macrosomia and multiple gestation. Also, maternal psychological responses to the labor, based on past experiences, cultural influences, and the woman's present level of support may play a role in the normal progress of labor.

 Nursing Insight— *Recognizing indicators of dystocia*

Nurses should suspect dystocia when there is a lack of progress in the rate of cervical dilation; fetal descent and expulsion; or an alteration in the pattern of normal uterine contractions.

DYSFUNCTIONAL LABOR PATTERNS

Dysfunctional labor patterns are deviations from the normal pattern of labor as illustrated by a labor curve assessment tool. (See Chapter 12.) Labor alterations occur more frequently during the first stage of labor (cervical dilation and effacement) than during the second stage (maternal expulsive efforts). Nulliparous women have a higher incidence of abnormalities than do multiparous women. Dysfunctional labor is the fourth most common complication of labor and birth, and several factors may increase a woman's risk for dystocia (Box 14-2). There are two general types of labor dysfunction: hypertonic and hypotonic (Fig. 14-1). These contraction patterns are classified according to when they occur in labor and the nature of the uterine contractions.

HYPERTONIC LABOR

Hypertonic labor contractions are strong and often painful but are ineffective in producing cervical effacement and dilation. An increase in maternal catecholamine release (i.e., epinephrine, norepinephrine) can result in poor uterine contractility (Cunningham et al., 2005). Uterine pacemakers (the energy source of contractions located in the uterine wall) do not initiate a good myometrial response needed for progressive cervical change. Instead, irregular spasmodic episodes occur that do not result in effective contractions or assist in bringing the fetus into a more favorable downward position (Gilbert, 2006).

Maternal anxiety plays a major role in hypertonic labor. Anxiety is known to produce high levels of catecholamines. Many factors contribute to a woman's fear related to labor and birth:

- Primiparous labor
- Loss of control
- Sexual abuse
- Lack of support
- Cultural differences
- Fear of pain

An occiput–posterior malposition of the fetus, which occurs in approximately 15% of labors, also leads to hypertonic labor contractions. In approximately one half of all cases of hypertonic labor patterns, however, there is no apparent cause (Gilbert, 2006).

Although the management of hypertonic labor contractions varies, in general, the emphasis is on establishing a more effective labor pattern. Rest, hydration, and sedation reduce the irritability of the uterus and help to diminish the ineffective contractions. Medications that may be prescribed to induce therapeutic rest include meperidine (Demerol),

---

Box 14-2 Factors Associated with an Increased Risk for Uterine Dystocia

- Uterine abnormalities, such as congenital malformations and overdistention (e.g., hydramnios, multiple gestation)
- Fetal malpresentation or malposition
- Cephalopelvic disproportion (CPD)
- Maternal body build (>30 lbs. [13.6 kg] overweight, short stature)
- Uterine overstimulation with oxytocin
- Inappropriate timing of administration of analgesic/anesthetic agents
- Maternal fear, fatigue, dehydration, electrolyte imbalance

Source: Gilbert, E.S. (2006). *Manual of high risk pregnancy and delivery.* St. Louis, MO: C.V. Mosby.

Figure 14-1 Uterine contraction patterns. *A.* Normal uterine contraction pattern. *B.* Hypertonic uterine contraction pattern. *C.* Hypotonic uterine contraction pattern.

hydromorphone (Dilaudid), and morphine (Cunningham et al., 2005). Natural labor with effective contractions often resumes after this simple intervention. Nonpharmacological techniques to reduce anxiety such as relaxation techniques, massage, a warm shower or tub bath, and increased emotional support are also helpful for some women.

For a woman whose fetus is in an occiput–posterior position, the major goal of care is to facilitate rotation of the fetal head into a more favorable position. The nurse can encourage the laboring woman to walk and change positions frequently throughout the course of labor. The descent of the fetus into an anterior lie creates a better environment for normal labor progression.

Nursing care begins with a thorough assessment. It is critical to identify factors that contribute to increased maternal anxiety. Careful monitoring of contractions may provide early information regarding poor labor progression and lead to timely interventions. While frequent checks for cervical dilation are not advisable, this assessment, when performed at proper intervals, provides a strong indicator of labor progression. Along with continued assessment of the contraction pattern, the nurse can use this information to validate the finding of hypertonic labor. Once any intervention has occurred, the nurse evaluates the plan of care and, depending on the results, initiates appropriate measures.

 Ethnocultural Considerations—
Communication difficulties during labor

Nurses need to be sensitive to cultural differences among women experiencing hypertonic labor—those who are unable to speak or understand the English language may have difficulty communicating their feelings.

HYPOTONIC LABOR

Hypotonic labor is a more common type of uterine dysfunctional pattern that contributes to poor labor progression. With hypotonic dystocia, the uterine contractions decrease in frequency and intensity. A hypotonic labor pattern usually occurs during the active phase of labor. It is defined as fewer than two to three contractions during a 10-minute period. The uterus can be easily indented, even at the peak of the contraction, and the intrauterine pressure (IUP) is insufficient for the progression of cervical effacement and dilation (Gilbert, 2006).

Hypotonic labor may be associated with a number of maternal and fetal factors that produce excessive uterine stretching and overdistention. For example, fetal macrosomia, multiple gestation, and hydramnios are all risk factors for hypotonic labor. Grand multiparity may also be a contributing cause.

Fetal **macrosomia** occurs in one fourth of all pregnancies and is the leading cause of uterine hypotonia. Macrosomia, defined as a fetus whose birth weight is above the 90th percentile on an intrauterine growth chart for that gestational age, often results from a fetal imbalance between glucose and insulin in women diagnosed with any type of diabetes. Over time, as increased amounts of glucose are absorbed from the mother, the fetus produces pancreatic insulin which results in an increase in fat deposits.

Maternal obesity unaccompanied by diabetes also contributes to a larger fetus. Hall and Neubert (2005) define obesity as a woman who has a body mass index (BMI) of greater than 30 kg/m². In their review of studies that examined obesity and pregnancy, direct links were found between maternal obesity and fetal macrosomia. The study findings are consistent with data from Young's and Woodmansee's (2002) research, which demonstrated a positive relationship between an increased maternal BMI and fetal macrosomia.

Pharmacological agents used to alleviate pain during labor may also contribute to the risk of uterine hypotonia. If a labor pattern is not well established, these medications often halt or significantly slow down the progress of labor. Various studies have produced conflicting data concerning a clear link between the use of analgesia, anesthesia, and the progress of labor. After administration of epidural anesthesia, some women may experience a longer second stage of labor. The effects of the epidural may make it difficult for the patient to identify when to push and how long to push because the contractions are not always detected. However, nulliparous women who experience long and painful labors are more likely to choose epidural anesthesia for pain relief. Often it is difficult to document which factors contribute most significantly to a protracted labor.

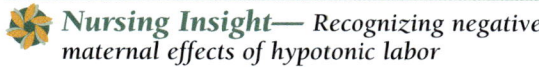

> ### *Nursing Insight*— *Recognizing negative maternal effects of hypotonic labor*
>
> As an ineffective labor pattern continues, the woman is likely to become fatigued and may be at an increased risk for infection.

Depending on the cause, labor hypotonia is managed in different ways. Careful, ongoing assessments are key. If a diagnostic modality such as ultrasound examination has demonstrated that the woman's pelvis is adequate for vaginal birth, measures to produce effective contractions are implemented. Walking and position changes in labor assist in fetal descent through the maternal pelvis and therefore need to be encouraged. The use of relaxation techniques, massage, and water treatments can decrease the need for pharmacological agents for pain.

Augmentation of labor contractions is considered when either the natural measures are unsuccessful or when it is deemed the best approach. At certain points in the labor, an amniotomy, or artificial rupture of the membranes, may be successful in increasing uterine contractility. Other measures to enhance the progress of labor include membrane stripping, nipple stimulation, and oxytocin infusion. Maternal and fetal assessments including vital signs, contraction patterns, and cervical changes need to be documented on a regular basis.

PRECIPITATE LABOR AND BIRTH

Contrary to both hypertonic and hypotonic labor, **precipitate labor** contractions produce very rapid, intense contractions. By definition, a precipitate labor lasts less than 3 hours from the beginning of contractions to birth. Church and Hodgson (2003) report that multiparous women with little soft tissue resistance are at the greatest risk for this labor pattern. Patients often progress through the first stage of labor with little or no pain and may present to the birth setting already advanced into the second stage. In a nulliparous patient, cervical dilation that occurs faster than 5 cm per hour is defined as precipitous labor. In a multiparous woman, cervical dilation may occur as rapidly as 10 cm in 1 hour. Precipitous labor may result from hypertonic uterine contractions that are tetanic in their intensity (Church & Hodgson, 2003).

Complications from a precipitate labor pattern result from trauma to maternal tissue and to the fetus because of the rapid descent. Hemorrhage may occur from uterine rupture and vaginal lacerations. Most women are ill prepared for the rapid advancement of their labor and become alarmed, highly anxious, and fearful. The fetus may suffer from hypoxia related to the decreased periods of uterine relaxation between the contractions and intracranial hemorrhage related to the rapid birth (Cunningham et al., 2005).

Nursing Considerations

Initial assessments are paramount to establishing the pattern of precipitous labor. A multiparous patient with a previous history of rapid labors needs to alert her physician or certified nurse midwife (CNM) as soon as she recognizes any signs of labor. Her prenatal record should include this information and be readily accessible to nursing personnel managing her care. In a nulliparous patient, careful examination for cervical dilation and effacement is required. Since a previous labor pattern is an unknown variable in the nulliparous patient, the nurse must be alert in recognizing signs of abnormally rapid cervical dilation (Church & Hodgson, 2003).

The woman and her support person need reassurance throughout the rapidly advancing labor. Breathing and relaxation techniques are helpful tools that the nurse can use to assist the woman to cope with labor. If the patient and her family do not speak or understand the English language, it is incumbent on the nurse to request a translator. Precipitate labor is an anxiety-producing situation that is compounded by the woman's inability to understand what is happening to her body. Although some precipitate labors occur with little or no pain, the patient is nevertheless aware of contractions that are occurring more quickly than normal. This experience can be frightening. The woman may also have concerns regarding a loss of control over her labor. Continuous surveillance, frequent updates on her status, and reassurance about her condition can help to allay the patient's anxiety. Medical management includes readiness on the part of the entire health team for the birth, particularly when the patient has a history of rapid labor. In most circumstances, a planned induction is part of the plan. Small dosages of intravenous analgesics may be used to help decrease pain.

The nurse can assist the woman in breathing through her contractions to avoid pushing and to help prevent tearing. If the nurse is alone with the patient during a precipitous delivery, the nurse follows delivery protocols when assisting in the birth of the infant. At the same time, the nurse uses the call bell to alert others for assistance. The nurse supports the perineum, assists the fetal head as it emerges, and checks for the umbilical cord as the head rotates. The newborn's nose and mouth are suctioned; the shoulders and then the rest of the newborn's body are supported during the birthing process. The nurse assesses the neonate's respiratory and cardiac rates.

After birth, whether assisted by the nurse or physician, the maternal soft tissue and placenta need to be carefully examined. The patient may require suturing of the cervix or vagina for lacerations. During the immediate postpartum period, the woman must be continuously monitored for hemorrhage. Providing ongoing information and support assists the patient and helps her support person cope with this unexpected event (Church & Hodgson, 2003).

critical nursing action Assisting with a Precipitous Birth

The nurse who assists with a precipitous birth should take the following actions:

- Request a translator to interpret for patients unable to speak or understand English.
- Assist the laboring woman to breathe through each contraction to prevent pushing.
- Provide continuous emotional support.
- Provide perineal support with warm cloths.
- Frequently monitor the maternal and fetal vital signs and immediately report any abnormal findings to the physician or certified nurse midwife.
- After birth, carefully monitor the patient for signs of hemorrhage; assess for trauma to the perineum.
- Assess the neonate for evidence of trauma and report and document all findings.

PELVIC STRUCTURE ALTERATIONS

Pelvic Dystocia

Pelvic dystocia occurs when contractures of the pelvic diameters reduce the capacity of the bony pelvis, the midpelvis, the outlet, or any combination of these planes. Contractures of the maternal pelvis may result from malnutrition, neoplasms, congenital abnormalities, traumatic spinal injury, or spinal disorders. In addition, immaturity of the pelvis may predispose some adolescent mothers to pelvic dystocia. During labor, contractures of the inlet, midplane, or outlet can cause interference in engagement and fetal descent, necessitating cesarean birth (Cunningham et al., 2005).

Soft Tissue Dystocia

Soft tissue dystocia occurs when the birth passage is obstructed by an anatomical abnormality other than that involving the bony pelvis. The obstruction, which prevents the fetus from entering the bony pelvis, may be caused by placenta previa, uterine fibroid tumors (leiomyomas), ovarian tumors, or a full bladder or rectum. **Bandl ring** is a pathological retraction ring that develops between the upper and lower uterine segments. It is associated with protracted labor, prolonged rupture of the membranes, and an increased risk of uterine rupture (Cunningham et al., 2005).

TRIAL OF LABOR

A **trial of labor** (TOL) is the surveillance of a woman and her fetus for a set amount of time (usually 4 to 6 hours) during spontaneous active labor to assess the safety of a vaginal birth. Indications for a trial of labor include situations when the maternal pelvis is of questionable size or shape, when the fetus is in an abnormal presentation, and when the woman desires to have a vaginal birth after a previous (low-segment transverse) cesarean birth. Before the TOL, an assessment of the adequacy of the maternal pelvis for vaginal birth (to rule out cephalopelvic disproportion [CPD]) is conducted with sonography or maternal pelvimetry. The cervix must be favorable (soft, dilatable), and throughout the TOL, the woman is assessed for the presence of adequate contractions, engagement and descent of the fetal presenting part and cervical dilation and effacement.

 Optimizing Outcomes— Providing support during a trial of labor

Nursing responsibilities during a TOL include assessment of maternal vital signs and FHR and pattern. If complications arise, the nurse notifies the primary health care provider, and evaluates and documents the maternal–fetal responses to the interventions. Offering support and encouragement to the woman and her labor partner and ongoing information about labor progress are essential components of care.

 Now Can You— Discuss factors that impede the progress of labor?

1. Describe why maternal anxiety contributes to a lack of labor progression?
2. List three ways the nurse can reduce maternal anxiety?
3. Identify which synthesizing enzymes are significant to the lack of myometrial contractility?

Obstetric Interventions

AMNIOINFUSION

Pregnancy outcome in patients experiencing variable fetal heart rate (FHR) decelerations caused by cord compression is improved through the use of amnioinfusion, which is the instillation of normal saline or lactated Ringer's solution into the uterine cavity. Amnioinfusion is used to supplement the amniotic fluid volume in patients with oligohydramnios due to uteroplacental insufficiency, premature rupture of the membranes, and postmaturity; it may also be done to dilute meconium-stained amniotic fluid (Fraser et al., 2005). Risks of the procedure include infection, overdistention of the uterus, and increased uterine tone.

 Nursing Insight— *Understanding amnioinfusion as an intervention for meconium-stained amniotic fluid*

When there is evidence of moderate to thick meconium in the amniotic fluid, amnioinfusion is used to dilute and help wash out the meconium to avoid neonatal meconium aspiration syndrome (Parer & Nageotte, 2004).

In most circumstances, the fluid is instilled through an intrauterine pressure catheter (IUPC); the amniotic membranes must be ruptured for catheter placement. The fluid may be warmed with a blood warmer before administration and the infusion may be given by bolus or continuous flow. When possible, a double-lumen IUPC is used because the intrauterine pressure can be monitored without stopping the amnioinfusion.

Nursing considerations include careful monitoring of the infusion, the intensity and frequency of uterine contractions, and the maternal vital signs. In some institutions, patients are required to sign an informed consent prior to the intervention. It is important for the nurse to educate the woman and her support person regarding the need for the infusion and its purpose. Nurses must document the amount of the solution infused and the presence of any vaginal discharge (Gilbert, 2006).

critical nursing action When Caring for a Patient Undergoing Amnioinfusion

When caring for a patient undergoing amnioinfusion, the nurse must:

1. Assess the patient's response to the fluid infusion.
2. Continually monitor the frequency and intensity of uterine contractions.
3. Stop the infusion if the following signs and symptoms are noted: maternal shortness of breath, an over distended uterus, hypotension, or tachycardia.

AMNIOTOMY

Amniotomy, or the artificial rupture of membranes (AROM), is a nonpharmacological intervention that may be done to augment or induce labor or to facilitate the placement of internal monitors during labor. The procedure involves the insertion of an Amnihook or other sharp instrument into the lower segment of the fetal membranes; following rupture, the fluid is allowed to drain slowly (Fig. 14-2). The rupture of the membranes causes a release of arachidonic acid, which converts to prostaglandins, known inducers of labor through the stimulation of oxytocin in the uterus (Gilbert, 2006). Labor usually commences within 12 hours after artificial rupture. However, if labor does not ensue, there is an increased risk of infection; other risks include fetal injury and umbilical cord prolapse. Because of the risk for infection, amniotomy is frequently used in combination with oxytocin induction to facilitate delivery.

The nurse carefully monitors the patient who will undergo an amniotomy. Vital signs, cervical effacement and dilation, station of the presenting part, FHR, and contractions are documented. The presenting part must be engaged and well applied to the cervix to prevent **umbilical cord prolapse** (protrusion of the umbilical cord in advance of the presenting part). There should be no evidence of active infection of the genital tract (e.g., herpes) or human immunodeficiency virus (HIV) infection (Norwitz, Robinson & Repke, 2002).

⬣ Optimizing Outcomes— Preparing the Patient for an Amniotomy

The nurse provides information, assesses the woman's understanding of the procedure, and assures her that the membrane rupture will be painless to her and her fetus although she may experience some discomfort when the instrument is inserted through the vagina and cervix. The nurse ensures that the necessary equipment has been assembled: sterile gloves, lubricant, and the Amnihook or Allis clamp. After placing hip pads under the buttocks to absorb the fluid, the nurse positions the woman on a padded bedpan or with rolled up linens to elevate the hips. The nurse assists the health care provider performing the procedure by unwrapping and passing the equipment.

Immediately after the artificial rupture, the nurse notes and records the FHR and pattern. The color, odor, consistency, and clarity (and amount, if unusual) of the amniotic fluid are also documented, along with the time of rupture

Amniotic membrane

Figure 14-2 An Amnihook is used to rupture the membranes.

and the indication for the amniotomy. The patient may request analgesia or epidural anesthesia before the procedure. If she has not requested any medication, the nurse assists her with relaxation and breathing techniques during the contractions following the amniotomy because they are likely to be stronger.

⬣ Be sure to— Monitor and document FHR during AROM

The nurse needs to assess the FHR immediately before and after the artificial rupture of membranes. Changes such as transient fetal tachycardia may occur and are common. However, other FHR patterns such as bradycardia and variable decelerations may be indicative of cord compression or prolapse.

Maternal temperature is assessed frequently (at least every 2 hours) after amniotomy to rule out infection. A temperature of 100.4°F (38°C) may be indicative of an infection and the health care provider should be notified. Other signs and symptoms of infection include the presence of chills, uterine tenderness on palpation, foul-smelling vaginal discharge, and fetal tachycardia (Simpson, 2005b).

Pharmacological Induction of Labor

INDICATIONS FOR INDUCTION

Induction of labor describes the use of chemical or mechanical modalities to initiate uterine contractions (before their spontaneous onset) to bring about childbirth. Induction of labor is considered when either a maternal or fetal condition exists that dictates the need for medical intervention in the labor process. According to Simpson and Atterbury (2003), labor induction often leads to an increase in interventionist care including the use of intravenous therapy, amniotomy, internal monitoring, epidural anesthesia, and a longer stay in the labor unit. Martin et al. (2005) reported that since the year 1989, when data were first collected, there has been a 125% increase in labor induction and a 75% increase in labor augmentation. Interestingly, non-Hispanic Caucasian women experience the highest rate of inductions. In 2003, the rate was 24.7%, while Asian or Pacific Islanders (14%) and Hispanic women (13.8%) experienced the lowest induction rates.

According to the American College of Obstetricians and Gynecologists (ACOG) the following maternal/fetal conditions serve as some of the indications for induction (ACOG, 1999):

- Postterm pregnancy
- Maternal medical conditions (e.g., diabetes mellitus, renal disease, chronic pulmonary disease, chronic hypertension)
- Pregnancy-induced hypertension (PIH)
- Fetal demise
- Chorioamnionitis
- Premature rupture of membranes
- Fetal compromise (e.g., severe fetal growth restriction, isoimmunization)
- Preeclampsia, eclampsia

Since induction carries certain risks, it is not performed without careful consideration and evaluation of the maternal–fetal status. However, due to the rise in the U.S. cesarean rate over the last two decades, medical management of labor is commonly practiced in many hospitals to prevent the need for surgical delivery. This practice often involves admission of the patient with complete cervical effacement, rupture of the membranes, or expulsion of the mucus plug who is begun on a series of protocols that frequently include amniotomy combined with oxytocin infusion.

Induction of labor is more successful when the cervix is "favorable," or inducible. The **Bishop score** is a rating system that may be used to determine the level of cervical inducibility. A series of points is awarded to cervical dilation, effacement, station, consistency, and position (Table 14-1). In general, labor induction is more likely to be successful with a higher score (9 or more for nulliparous women; 5 or more for multiparous women) (Cunningham et al., 2005; Gülmezoglu, Crowther, & Middleton, 2006).

Cervical Ripening Agents

If it is determined that the cervix is not favorable for oxytocin induction, a chemical cervical ripening agent using prostaglandin E$_1$ PGE$_1$ (Misoprostol) or prostaglandin E$_2$ (PGE$_2$) (Dinoprostone [Prepidil, Cervidil]) may be prescribed (Table 14-2). These agents are most beneficial when the patient's Bishop score is greater than 6, although they are commonly used when the Bishop score is 4 or less. Before administration, informed consent may be required, according to agency protocol.

Misoprostol (Cytotec) is an analogue of prostaglandin E$_1$. Available in tablet form, the medication is inserted into the posterior vaginal fornix. Misoprostol ripens the cervix, causing it to begin to dilate and efface. The U.S. Food and Drug Administration (FDA) has not approved the use of misoprostol for cervical ripening. Wing (2002) found misoprostol to be an effective agent for cervical ripening and induction of labor that also decreases the amount of oxytocin required. Culver et al. (2004) concurred that misoprostol is an effective cervical ripening agent but cited higher failure rates in nulliparous women with a low Bishop score and reported an increased incidence of uterine hyperstimulation with the medication. At least 4 hours after the last dose, oxytocin may be initiated for the induction of labor if cervical ripening has occurred and labor has not begun.

Dinoprostone, marketed as Cervidil Insert and Prepidil Gel, is an analogue of (PGE$_2$). This cervical ripening agent makes the cervix softer, causing it to begin to dilate and efface and stimulate uterine contractions. PGE$_2$ is used for preinduction cervical ripening when the Bishop score is 4 or less. Cervidil is applied into the posterior vaginal fornix; Prepidil is inserted through a syringe into the cervical canal just below the internal cervical os or into the posterior fornix. Cervidil acts more quickly. Uterine contractions usually begin in 5 to 7 hours after administration. When necessary, induction with oxytocin can be initiated 30 to 60 minutes after removal of the Cervidil insert. When using Prepidil gel, oxytocin induction must be delayed until 6 to 12 hours after the last instillation of the medication. Cervidil has an added advantage—the insert can be removed if uterine hyperstimulation occurs. Dinoprostone is FDA approved for cervical ripening.

Contraindications to the PGE$_1$ and PGE$_2$ cervical ripening agents include the presence of a non-reassuring FHR pattern, maternal fever, infection, vaginal bleeding, hypersensitivity, regular, progressive uterine contractions, and a history of cesarean birth or uterine scar. The medications should be cautiously used in women with a history of asthma, glaucoma or renal, hepatic, or cardiovascular disorders. After insertion, the nurse should clearly document all assessment findings and administration procedures.

Mechanical Methods

Mechanical methods provide another approach to cervical ripening. Dilators placed in the cervix cause cervical ripening by stimulating the release of endogenous prostaglandins. Rai and Schreiber (2005) cite the use of a balloon catheter (e.g., Foley catheter) placed into the intracervical canal to increase pressure exerted on the lower uterine segment. Hydroscopic dilators (those that enlarge as they absorb moisture from the surrounding tissue) such as laminaria tents (made from desiccated seaweed) and synthetic dilators containing magnesium sulfate (Lamicel) may be inserted into the endocervix without rupturing the membranes. The dilators remain in place for 6 to 12 hours before removal for assessment of cervical dilation. Fresh dilators may then be inserted if necessary. Amniotomy and membrane stripping (the physician or midwife inserts a gloved finger into the cervical os to gently "strip" the membranes) can be also be used to ripen the cervix.

Oxytocin

Oxytocin, a hormone produced by the pituitary gland, stimulates uterine contractions. (See Chapter 12.) It can be used to induce labor or augment a labor that is progressing slowly due to ineffective uterine contractions. Administration of the medication is closely monitored according to institutional protocols. An intravenous infusion of 0.5 to 2 milliunits per minute of oxytocin is used for labor induction or augmentation. The dose is increased 1 to 2 milliunits per minute at intervals no less than 30 to 60 minutes until adequate labor progress is achieved. The patient should be reevaluated if the dose reaches 20 milliunits per minute (Deglin & Vallerand, 2009).

Table 14-1 The Bishop Score

	Score			
	0	1	2	3
Dilation (cm)	0	1–2	3–4	>5
Effacement (%)	0–30	40–50	60–70	>80
Station (cm)	−3	−2	−1	+1, +2
Cervical consistency	Firm	Medium	Soft	
Cervix position	Posterior	Midposition	Anterior	

Adapted from Rai, J., & Schreiber, J.R. (2005). Cervical ripenning. *EMedicine.* Retrieved from http://www.emedicine.com.

Table 14-2 Cervical Ripening Agents

Medication	Action	Adverse Effects	Dosage
Prostaglandin E$_1$ Misoprostol (Cytotec)	Induces labor contractions	Diarrhea, abdominal pain, headaches, fever, tachysystole, uterine hyperstimulation.	Intravaginally: 25 mcg—repeat every 4–6 hours until Bishop score equals 8 or greater.
Prostaglandin E$_2$ Dinoprostone (Cervidil Insert, Prepidil Gel)	Promotes initiation of cervical ripening	Uterine hyperstimulation, fever, back pain, headache, nausea and vomiting, diarrhea, hypotension, tachysystole.	Cervidil Insert: (10 mg dinoprostone gradually released over 12 hours). Remove after 12 hours or at labor onset. Keep insert frozen until ready to use.
	May stimulate labor contractions	*Adverse effects are more common with intracervical administration.*	Prepidil Gel: (2.5-mL syringe containing 0.5 mg of dinoprostone). Repeat gel insertion in 6 hours as needed (maximum = 1.5 mg or 3 doses/24 hr). Allow gel to reach room temperature before administration; do not heat. Continue administration until maximum dose is reached, or uterine contractions are established (3/10 min) or Bishop score equals 8 or greater or adverse reactions occur.

Teaching: Patient Education

- Assess knowledge of the medication.
- Explain purpose of medication and side effects.
- Discuss comfort options to offset side effects.
- Instruct the patient to void before insertion.
- Instruct the patient to maintain a supine position with a lateral tilt or side-lying position for 30–40 minutes after insertion.

Sources: Deglin & Vallerand (2009) and Turkoski et al. (2004).

Optimizing Outcomes— Through the safe administration of oxytocin

First, the patient's primary health care provider writes an order for oxytocin for labor induction or augmentation. After an explanation and assessment of the patient's level of understanding, the nurse assists the woman to a side-lying or upright position. Assessment of the patient and fetus is conducted and documented. The solution is prepared and administered with a pump delivery system according to the prescribed orders. The piggyback solution is connected to the intravenous infusion at the port nearest the point of venous insertion. The medication is administered as ordered; ongoing assessments are conducted according to institutional protocol. The nurse documents the medication (kind, amount, times of beginning infusion, increasing the dose, maintaining the dose, discontinuing the infusion), maternal–fetal reactions (FHR and pattern, maternal vital signs, pattern and progress of labor, nursing interventions, and maternal response) and when notification of the primary health care provider takes place.

Oxytocin acts on receptors in the myometrium to create an increase in the strength, duration, and frequency of the contractions. These same receptors are susceptible to uterine hyperstimulation, which constitutes a major risk associated with the medication. Signs of uterine hyperstimulation include the following:

- Uterine contractions that last greater than 90 seconds and occur more frequently than every 2 minutes
- Uterine resting tone greater than 20 mm Hg
- Non-reassuring fetal heart and pattern (baseline less than 100 or greater than 160 beats per minute; Absent variability; Repeated late decelerations or prolonged decelerations)

Higher doses are associated with an increased incidence of hyperstimulation; however, low dosages result in an increased rate of cesarean births due to failure of labor progression (Dudley, 2003). Uterine hyperstimulation causes reduced blood flow through the placenta and results in FHR decelerations, fetal asphyxia, and neonatal hypoxia. Because of the potential for life-threatening adverse complications associated with the use of oxytocin during the intrapartal period, the FDA has issued a number of restrictions to its use.

clinical alert

Contraindications to the use of oxytocin to stimulate labor

Nurses should be aware of contraindications to the use of oxytocin to stimulate labor, which include, but are not limited to (ACOG, 1999):

- Vasa previa or complete placenta previa
- Transverse fetal lie
- Umbilical cord prolapse
- Previous transfundal uterine surgery

Conditions that necessitate special precaution during oxytocin administration include:

- Breech presentation
- Multifetal pregnancy
- Presenting part above the pelvic inlet
- Severe hypertension
- Maternal heart disease
- Polyhydramnios
- One or more previous low-transverse cesarean deliveries
- Abnormal fetal heart rate patterns not necessitating emergent delivery

Augmentation of labor is used to stimulate uterine contractions after labor has begun spontaneously but is not progressing satisfactorily. It is most commonly indicated for the management of hypotonic uterine dysfunction. Labor augmentation may be accomplished with amniotomy, oxytocin infusion, and nipple stimulation. Noninvasive approaches include ambulation, hydration, relaxation, and hydrotherapy and these methods should be attempted before the initiation of invasive measures.

Nipple stimulation has been used for labor augmentation and induction. The action of nipple rolling produces an increase in the release of oxytocin from the anterior pituitary gland. The nurse instructs the woman to roll her nipple through her clothing for ten minutes on one side and then proceed to the other side, resting during a contraction. A breast pump may also be used. Nipple stimulation rarely causes hyperstimulation of the uterus. However, the results of nipple stimulation are less predictable than the administration of specified dosages of oxytocin. Sexual intercourse has also been helpful as a method of induction because semen contains prostaglandins (Gilbert, 2006). Both of these methods require additional evidence-based research before their endorsement as viable alternatives for labor induction.

Complementary Care: *Measures for induction of labor*

Several nonpharmacological methods or alternative methods have been used to induce labor. Herbal remedies such as black haw, primrose oil, black and blue cohosh, chamomile, and red raspberry leaves are prescribed as labor inducers in some cultures. Technically these substances are medicinal agents with some properties similar to those of oxytocin. Use of these agents creates problems because of the lack of scientific research and validation of their effectiveness. Much of the information about how they work is anecdotal, which also makes it difficult to evaluate the risks and the benefits, critical information for patients and their health care providers (Tenore, 2003). Nonherbal methods include acupuncture, the ingestion of a laxative (e.g., castor oil), and the stripping of membranes.

NURSING CONSIDERATIONS

The nurse's responsibilities during labor induction or augmentation begins with obtaining informed consent for the procedure after physician explanation. Patient education regarding the procedure and its consequences is critical. Monitoring of the labor is essential since hyperstimulation of the uterus may lead to uterine rupture. Oxytocin protocols in many institutions require that the nurse remain at the patient's bedside at all times for careful surveillance. The following data should be placed on a flow sheet in the patient record:

- Patient's vital signs (blood pressure, pulse and respirations every 30 to 60 minutes and with every increment in medication dose)
- FHR (via electronic monitoring)
- Frequency, duration, and strength of contractions (note contraction pattern and uterine resting tone every 15 minutes and with every increment in medication dose during first stage; then monitor every 5 minutes during second stage)
- Cervical effacement and dilatation
- Fetal station and lie
- Rate of oxytocin infusion
- Intake and urine output (limit intravenous fluid intake to 1000 mL/8 hr; output should be 120 mL or more every 4 hours)
- Any untoward effect of the medication administration (nausea, vomiting, headache, hypotension)
- Psychological response of the patient (ACOG, 1999; Gilbert, 2006; Simpson, 2005b).

critical nursing action Recognizing and Responding to Problems During Labor Induction with Oxytocin

During induction of labor with oxytocin, the nurse remains alert to signs indicative of complications such as uterine hyperstimulation, non-reassuring FHR pattern, and suspected uterine rupture. Immediate emergency measures include: discontinuing the oxytocin per institutional protocol; positioning the patient on her side; increasing the primary IV rate up to 200 mL/hr (unless there is evidence of water intoxication—in this situation, the rate is decreased to one that keeps the vein open); administering oxygen by face mask at 8–10 L/min or per physician order or institutional protocol.

The nurse needs to discuss pain relief options with the patient before oxytocin administration. The information presented should include prescribed medications as well as natural options. If the woman declines pharmacological analgesia or anesthesia, the nurse must work closely with her and her support person in the effective use of relaxation and breathing techniques. The woman placed on bedrest as a result of the induction needs frequent position changes. Massage may enhance her comfort during the procedure. The nurse should keep the patient and her support person informed of her progress as this information reassures the patient and gives her confidence.

 Now Can You— Discuss labor induction?

1. Identify eight indicators for labor induction?
2. Explain the relationship between the Bishop score and induction of labor?
3. Identify and discuss the implications of pertinent data recorded on the maternal flow sheet during labor induction with oxytocin?

INSTRUMENTATION ASSISTANCE OF BIRTH

Forceps and vacuum extraction are used to decrease the length of the second stage of labor when indicated because of maternal exhaustion or epidural anesthesia, suspected fetal distress, and the need to rotate the fetal head. In the United States there has been a decrease in the overall use of instrumentation as a birth assist while there has been an increase in operative deliveries. Speculation as to the reason for this trend has been attributed to a fear of malpractice related to complications associated with the methods as well as a lack of physicians' training in the use of delivery instrumentation (Patel & Murphy, 2004).

Forceps-Assisted Birth

A forceps-assisted birth is one in which a steel instrument with two curved blades is used to facilitate the birth of the infant's head. **Forceps** is an instrument consisting of cephalic-curved blades similar to the shape of the fetal head (Fig. 14-3). The two blades slide together at the shaft to form a handle. The first blade is inserted into the maternal vagina next to the fetal head. The second blade is then inserted and applied to the opposite side of the fetal head. The shafts of the forceps are brought together in the midline and secured to form a handle. Forceps prevent pressure from being exerted on the fetal head and facilitate birth.

Maternal indications for a forceps-assisted birth include a need to shorten the second stage of labor for the following reasons: dystocia; an inability to push with contractions (e.g., due to exhaustion, spinal or epidural anesthesia, spinal cord injury); to prevent worsening of serious

medical complications such as cardiac compensation. Fetal indications include an abnormal presentation, arrest of rotation, immaturity, and distress from a complication such as prolapsed cord.

There are various applications and several different types of forceps for forceps-assisted birth. Outlet forceps are used when the fetal scalp is visible on the maternal perineum without manual separation of the labia. Low forceps are used when the fetal head is at a +2 station or more. Midforceps are used when the fetal head is engaged but at less than a +2 station. Because birth trauma has been associated with the use of midforceps, this procedure has been largely replaced by cesarean birth, which poses less risk to the fetus. Forceps are never applied to an unengaged presenting part. Piper forceps are used to facilitate delivery of the head in a breech birth. Some form of anesthesia is administered before forceps application to achieve pelvic relaxation and decrease pain. An episiotomy is usually performed to prevent perineal tearing. Before forceps application, the following criteria must be met:

- The cervix must be fully dilated; bladder empty; presenting part engaged
- The membranes must be ruptured
- Cephalopelvic disproportion must not be present

 critical nursing action When Attending a Forceps-Assisted Birth

The FHR and pattern are assessed and recorded before the forceps application. When the forceps are applied, there is a danger of compression of the cord between the fetal head and the forceps blade. Cord compression causes a decrease in FHR. Therefore, assess and record the FHR and pattern again *immediately* after the forceps application.

Perineal trauma is one of the major complications associated with the use of forceps. Since hemorrhage may result from cervical lacerations and vaginal tearing, the woman requires close observation during the postpartum period. To rule out maternal bladder injury, the nurse documents the time and amount of the first postbirth voiding. Some women have reported fecal incontinence following forceps injury. Women who experience forceps-related problems may suffer fear and anxiety regarding the birth experience in subsequent pregnancies (Patel & Murphy, 2004).

Fetal morbidity occurs in direct response to occipital trauma. Superficial scalp and facial markings are the most common complications and are rarely significant. However, it is important for the nurse to clearly discuss this possibility with the family. Once the parents understand that the trauma marks gradually disappear, they are usually more accepting of the baby's (usually) superficial injuries. Other forceps-related complications that rarely occur include facial nerve injury, cephalhematoma, retinal hemorrhage, and ocular trauma. Neonatal intracranial bleeding constitutes a major concern but it is often difficult to ascertain whether the hemorrhage resulted from the forceps or it was related to the difficult birth (Belfort, 2003).

Figure 14-3 caption block:

Fenestrated blades · Shank · Handle
Simpson forceps (outlet)

Solid blades · Shank · Handle · Lock
Tucker-McLean forceps (outlet)

Fenestrated blades · Shank · Handle
Piper forceps (aftercoming head in breech)

Direction of gentle traction for outlet forceps delivery

Figure 14-3 Forceps are instruments with curved blades that are used to facilitate the birth of the fetal head.

 Now Can You— Discuss issues surrounding the use of forceps?

1. Identify three maternal indications and three fetal indications for a forceps-assisted birth?
2. Describe maternal–fetal complications associated with the use of forceps instrumentation?
3. Discuss key information the nurse provides the parents regarding a forceps-assisted birth?

Vacuum-Assisted Birth

Vacuum-assisted birth, also termed vacuum extraction, is an alternative method used in an assisted vaginal delivery (Fig. 14-4). The vacuum extractor consists of a soft plastic cup that is attached to the fetal head over the posterior fontanel and a suction apparatus that uses negative pressure to facilitate the birth of the head. This modality is used for a patient who is unable to voluntarily push during the second stage of labor (most often due to exhaustion or pharmacological agents), fetal distress or failure to progress. The same conditions apply to the use of the vacuum as for forceps: vertex presentation, ruptured membranes, and absence of CPD. Vacuum-assisted birth has certain advantages over forceps-assisted birth: little anesthesia is required (the fetus is less depressed at birth) and it is associated with fewer lacerations of the maternal birth canal. Vacuum extraction should not be used

following fetal scalp blood sampling. The suction pressure can cause excessive bleeding at the sampling site. It is also not recommended for preterm fetuses whose skulls are extremely soft.

To prepare the patient for a vacuum-assisted birth, the nurse provides education and support and encourages the woman's continued participation in childbirth by pushing during contractions. The FHR is assessed before and throughout the procedure. The nurse assists the woman to a lithotomy position to allow sufficient traction. The primary care provider applies the cup to the fetal head and a caput (swelling of the soft tissue) develops inside the cup as the pressure is initiated. Gentle traction is applied to facilitate descent of the fetal head. An episiotomy may be performed as the head crowns.

 Be sure to— Assume nursing responsibilities associated with a vacuum-assisted birth

The nurse is responsible for management of care during a vacuum-assisted procedure. Although the physician applies the vacuum to the infant head, the nurse controls the vacuum gun and the pressure and is responsible for all of the required documentation. The perinatal team must communicate frequently during the procedure as they each assess progress or the lack of progress. The nurse, following protocols, can advocate for cesarean birth if maternal exhaustion and/or failure of descent indicates that the

A

B

Figure 14-4 Vacuum extraction also facilitates the delivery of the fetal head and is associated with fewer lacerations of the maternal birth canal. A. Vacuum extractor is applied with a downward and outward traction. B. A caput succedaneum, or chignon, is formed from the suction cup.

vacuum assistance is not effective. If the nurse fails to communicate concerns and there is an untoward event, the nurse can be held liable. Liability is also incurred if the nurse fails to document the sequence of events during the vacuum assistance along with the maternal–fetal response. After an assisted birth, the nurse who assesses the neonate is also liable with regard to the documentation of vital signs and the neonatal assessment (Mahlmeister, 2005).

The caput that has formed on the neonate's scalp begins to disappear in several hours but may persist for up to 7 days after birth. Appropriate education of the parents before the vacuum application helps them to understand that the caput swelling is not harmful to the infant and the markings will decrease rapidly. Neonatal complications include cephalhematoma, scalp lacerations, and subdural hematoma. The infant should be carefully observed for signs of trauma and infection at the application site.

Maternal Conditions that Complicate Childbirth

HYPERTENSIVE DISORDERS

Management of hypertensive disorders during parturition is based on two goals: preventing further deterioration of affected organs and fostering a positive maternal-infant outcome. Women who have been diagnosed with severe

preeclampsia or HELLP syndrome (**H**emolysis, **E**levated **L**iver enzymes, and **L**ow **P**latelets; see Chapter 11) may be placed in an obstetric critical care unit or a medical intensive care unit for hemodynamic monitoring. Maternal vital signs, FHR, urine output, deep tendon reflexes, level of edema, and mental orientation and neurological status are assessed. Fetal–maternal factors that may necessitate immediate interventions to facilitate birth are presented in Box 14-3.

When severe preeclampsia is diagnosed at less than 34 weeks' gestation, the approach to care may include an observational period and conservative management. If the gestational age is 32 to 35 weeks, induction of labor is usually initiated. Vaginal birth is considered safer than cesarean birth and is attempted if cervical favorability is present. Antenatal glucocorticoids such as betamethasone may be given (12 mg IM 24 hours apart) to promote lung maturity if the gestational age is less than 34 weeks and delivery can be delayed for 48 hours (ACOG, 2002a; Cunningham et al., 2005; Sibai, Dekker, & Kuperminic, 2005). (See Chapter 11.)

Nursing Considerations

The nurse is the manager of care for the woman with preeclampsia during the intrapartal period. Careful assessments are critical. The nurse plans and evaluates all interventions on a continuous basis. The patient with severe preeclampsia is in an extremely fragile condition. Since any change in condition may require an emergency intervention, the nurse must be prepared to provide the necessary care immediately. The nurse is responsible for the continuous monitoring of several key parameters (Box 14-4). Laboratory tests include a complete blood count (CBC) with platelets, coagulation profile to assess for disseminated intravascular coagulation (DIC), metabolic studies for determination of liver enzymes (aspartate aminotransferase [AST], alanine aminotransferase [ALT], lactate dehydrogenase [LDH]) and electrolyte studies to establish renal functioning (ACOG, 2002). (See Chapter 11 for further discussion.)

Box 14-3 **Factors that May Necessitate Immediate Intervention to Facilitate Birth in Patients with Hypertensive Disorders**

- Uncontrolled severe hypertension
- Eclampsia
- Persistent oliguria (< 500 mL/24 hr)
- Abruptio placentae
- Platelet count less than 100,000/mm³
- Elevated liver enzyme levels with epigastric pain or right upper quadrant tenderness
- Pulmonary edema
- Persistent severe headache or visual changes
- Spontaneous labor
- Fetal death
- Rupture of the membranes
- Gestational age less than 34 weeks (an observational period may be initially attempted as a conservative management approach)
- Evidence of fetal compromise

Box 14-4 Intrapartal Nursing Care for Patients with Preeclampsia

BLOOD PRESSURE

The blood pressure is taken every 4 hours or more frequently according to physician orders or institutional protocol. Blood pressure should be taken in the same arm at each assessment. Encourage the patient to assume a side-lying position to enhance uterine perfusion. Record the data. Notify the physician of an increase in blood pressure.

MEDICATION ADMINISTRATION

Administer medication as ordered and evaluate its effect. Adhere to hospital protocol for magnesium sulfate infusion. Monitor maternal vital signs, FHR, urine output, DTRs, IV flow rate and serum magnesium levels to assess for magnesium sulfate toxicity (e.g., depressed respirations, hyporeflexia, sudden onset of hypotension, oliguria, indicators of fetal compromise). Administer calcium gluconate (the antidote for magnesium sulfate toxicity) for respirations below 12 breaths/min and discontinue the magnesium sulfate infusion.

RENAL BALANCE

Edema is rated on scale of 1 to 4. A score of 4 is generalized massive edema that includes the face, abdomen and sacrum. Assess and record urinary output. An indwelling urinary catheter may be inserted to more accurately measure urinary output. A urine output less than 30 mL/hr is indicative of oliguria and the physician must be notified. A dipstick measurement is performed every 4 hours or more frequently to assess urinary protein on a scale of 1–4. A dipstick reading over 2+ is indicative of a worsening condition.

NEUROLOGICAL STATUS

Deep tendon reflexes (DTRs) are assessed every 4 hours (or more frequently) and rated on a scale of 1 to 4. Reflexes greater than 2+ are a sign of worsening status. If dorsiflexion of the foot produces clonus (convulsive spasm), this finding provides an additional indication of a deteriorating maternal condition.

PULMONARY STATUS

Auscultation of the lungs is performed every 4 hours (or more frequently) to assess for dyspnea, crackles and diminished breath sounds, which may be indicative of pulmonary edema. The respiratory rate is assessed every 4 hours (or more frequently). Patients who are receiving magnesium sulfate require more frequent respiratory assessments since a respiratory rate below 12 is an indicator of magnesium toxicity. Hemoglobin oxygen saturation can be assessed with a pulse oximeter.

PSYCHOLOGICAL STATUS

Assess the woman for indicators of anxiety and fear. Provide information to the patient and family about the treatment protocols and status of the maternal condition. Assess their level of understanding and provide updates when indicated.

ADVANCING SYMPTOMS

Headaches, blurred vision, severe right upper quadrant epigastric pain, and restlessness are all indicators of impending eclampsia. Prepare for immediate delivery.

SEIZURES

Protect the patient. Keep the airway patent: turn head to one side and place pillow or folded linen under one shoulder or back. Call for assistance. Ensure that the siderails have been raised. Observe and document all seizure activity. Notify the physician and prepare for delivery. Administer oxygen.

FETAL STATUS

Monitor the fetal heart rate every 4 hours or more frequently as indicated. Assess fetal movements. Notify the physician if indicators of fetal compromise are noted.

The nurse must also monitor the laboratory values for impending HELLP syndrome during labor. The nurse follows the plan of care for the patient with severe preeclampsia.

Special precautions need to be considered to prevent adverse outcomes in a patient with the HELLP syndrome who requires a cesarean birth. The nurse is responsible for administering 5 to 10 units of platelets on the physician's order before the birth to prevent thrombocytopenia. Providing ongoing information to the patient and her family is an essential nursing intervention to help decrease anxiety and fear (Sibai et al., 2005).

DIABETES

Women with the metabolic disorder of diabetes that is under control may safely give birth spontaneously at term provided there are no indications of severe cephalopelvic disproportion (CPD). When a possibility of CPD exists, the diabetic woman may be given a trial of labor. If successful, a cesarean birth, which always presents a higher risk than a vaginal birth for the fetus, has been avoided.

 Nursing Insight— *Recognizing medical indications for elective preterm birth in women with diabetes*

As long as she remains in good metabolic control and all parameters of fetal surveillance are within normal limits, the woman whose pregnancy is complicated by diabetes may safely carry the pregnancy to 38.5–40 weeks of gestation. However, the presence of poor metabolic control, a worsening hypertensive disorder, fetal macrosomia (often defined as weight >4500 g) or fetal growth restriction are all indications for elective preterm birth (ACOG, 2001; Cunningham et al., 2005).

The physician may plan an elective induction of labor between 38 and 40 weeks of gestation. An amniocentesis performed between 37 and 38.5 weeks of gestation is performed to confirm fetal lung maturity. Fetal lung maturation is better predicted by an amniotic fluid phosphatidylglycerol level of greater than 3% than by an amniotic fluid lecithin/sphingomyelin ratio (3:1) in the pregnancy complicated by diabetes. If the fetal lungs are immature, birth may be delayed as long as all parameters of the maternal and fetal assessment remain reassuring (Moore, 2004). (See Chapter 11.)

Intrapartum management for the woman with pregestational diabetes centers on the close surveillance of maternal hydration and blood glucose levels to prevent complications associated with dehydration, hypoglycemia, and hyperglycemia. An intravenous infusion of a maintenance fluid such as lactated Ringer's solution or 5% dextrose in lactated Ringer's solution may be ordered. Insulin is usually administered by continuous infusion; only regular insulin may be administered intravenously. Blood glucose levels are assessed every hour and fluid/insulin adjustments are made as needed to maintain maternal blood glucose levels between 80 and 120 mg/dL (Bernasko, 2004). It is essential that maternal hyperglycemia during the intrapartal period be avoided to prevent neonatal metabolic problems such as hypoglycemia.

The laboring patient is maintained in an upright or side-lying position with continuous FHR monitoring. Nursing care involves close surveillance for indicators of normal labor progression along with a stable maternal–fetal unit. Failure to progress may be related to fetal macrosomia or CPD and necessitate a cesarean birth. Diabetes-related complications such as hyperglycemia, ketosis, and ketoacidosis may develop and must be promptly managed. Shoulder dystocia associated with fetal macrosomia may complicate the second stage of labor. A team that consists of the obstetrician and neonatologist, pediatrician, or neonatal nurse practitioner should attend the birth to provide immediate neonatal assessment and care.

When a cesarean birth has been planned, the surgery is scheduled for the early morning to achieve optimal glycemic control. Depending on physician orders, the nurse may be instructed to withhold the morning insulin. Other protocols allow administration of an intermediate-acting insulin in the morning and every 8 hours until surgery (Chan & Winkle, 2006). The patient is allowed nothing by mouth. Epidural anesthesia is preferred because hypoglycemia can be detected earlier if the woman remains awake. After the surgery, maternal blood glucose levels are assessed at least every 2 hours; target plasma levels are between 80 and 160 mg/dL (Moore, 2004).

The first 24 hours postpartum are remarkable for the dramatic decrease in insulin requirements that occurs after removal of the placenta. Depending on the amount of food consumed, women with type I diabetes may require only one fourth to one third of the prenatal insulin dose (Bernasko, 2004). Some women may not require insulin for 24 to 72 hours postpartum (Chan & Winkle, 2006). Throughout the postpartal period, blood glucose levels continue to be monitored and insulin dosage adjustments are made as needed, often using a sliding scale.

 Nursing Insight— *Increased risk of postpartal complications in diabetic women*

Women whose pregnancies have been complicated by diabetes have an increased risk for complications such as preeclampsia/eclampsia, hemorrhage, and infection (i.e., endometritis) during the postpartal period. Hemorrhage is more likely if the uterus was overdistended due to fetal macrosomia or hydramnios. (See Chapter 16.)

The nurse should encourage mothers with pregestational and gestational diabetes to breastfeed. However, because glucose levels are lower, especially during early postpartum, breastfeeding women are at an increased risk for hypoglycemia. Also, the mother with poor metabolic control may have a delay in lactogenesis that results in decreased milk production (Moore, 2004).

Discharge planning for women with diabetes should include discussion about contraceptive information as appropriate. Because women with gestational diabetes are at increased risk for developing diabetes later in life, the nurse should counsel them about the importance of maintaining a healthy weight and undergoing glucose testing during routine health maintenance visits.

PRETERM LABOR AND BIRTH

Preterm labor that is not arrested leads to preterm birth. In the United States, preterm birth has increased over the last decade despite the use of preventive pharmacological therapies. Martin et al. (2005) reports that in 2002, 12.3% of infants born were preterm. This figure is the highest number recorded since preterm birth data have been collected. Accompanying this dramatic increase in preterm births is a 50% increase in premature infants born with neurological deficits (ACOG, 2003a).

 Ethnocultural Considerations— **Preterm labor and birth**

Race and ethnicity cannot be disregarded in any discussion of preterm labor. African American women are at a higher risk for preterm birth than are Caucasian women. When preterm birth rates of married, educated African American women are compared with those of matched Caucasian women, a disparity continues to be noted in the African American women. The increase in cases of preterm labor results in a greater percentage of infant mortality in the African American population (Moore, 2003).

The causes for preterm birth are often a series of overlapping conditions such as premature rupture of membranes combined with cervical incompetence. Canavan, Simhan, and Cartis (2004) reported that premature rupture of the membranes accounts for approximately 3% of all preterm births. In many cases, patients experience "silent" (asymptomatic) uterine contractions throughout pregnancy that contribute to progressive cervical effacement and dilation. (See Chapter 11.)

Although interventions including bedrest, hydration, and tocolytic therapy are used to inhibit contractions, in many situations the labor cannot be halted. If the woman's membranes have ruptured or if the cervix is greater than 50% effaced and 3 to 4 cm dilated, it is unlikely that the labor can be stopped. If the fetus is very immature and birth is deemed to be inevitable, a cesarean birth may be planned to reduce pressure on the fetal head and decrease the possibility of subdural or intraventricular hemorrhage.

Nursing Considerations

In addition to careful maternal monitoring, FHR monitoring is one of the most important nursing responsibilities when caring for a patient in preterm labor. A number of perinatal complications such as preeclampsia, intra-amniotic infection, oligohydramnios, umbilical cord compression, placental abruption, intrauterine growth restriction, uteroplacental insufficiency, and multiple gestation occur more often with preterm labor. This combination of complications may result in FHR patterns that differ from the norm. Because of the increased incidence of neurological deficits in premature infants, it is essential that the nurse be able to identify and report data suggestive of hypoxia as early as possible (Simpson, 2004).

Best clinical practice for fetal monitoring begins with correct application of the tocodynamometer and the fetal heart monitor. Leopold's maneuvers are used to identify the fetal back and presenting part. Since multiple gestations are often associated with preterm labor, it is important to identify and monitor each fetus. The tocodynamometer needs to be placed at the height of fundus to ensure the best interpretation of the labor contractions (Simpson, 2004).

Optimizing Outcomes— Providing pain relief during preterm labor and birth

The length of the first stage of labor for a woman who is preterm is essentially the same as for a woman with a full term gestation although the second stage may be shorter—the smaller fetal size can be pushed through the dilated cervix more easily. Maternal analgesia is used cautiously due to the immaturity of the fetus, who may have considerable difficulty breathing without the additional burden of sedative effects from maternal analgesic agents. If the patient desires analgesia, the nurse can explain why epidural pain relief is most likely preferable. An episiotomy is often performed at the time of birth to lessen trauma on the fragile fetal head; forceps may also be used.

Because of the patient's medical complications and related fetal issues, she and her support person often experience increased anxiety and fear during the labor and birth. The nurse is there to offer clinical expertise; provide a calming presence; and inform, support, and assist the patient and her partner throughout the birth experience. A careful assessment of the patient's psychological status can help direct the care. Expressions of caring coupled with dialog that includes specific questions help to identify the patient's main concerns.

Optimizing Outcomes— Exploring concerns of the woman experiencing preterm labor

The nurse should use active listening and remain nearby. The patient should be encouraged to participate in decision making as much as possible throughout the labor process. Women who have anticipated an uncomplicated labor and birth experience often feel out of control when events occur that differ from their expectations. The nurse can play a vital role in keeping the patient informed and helping her to remain an active participant throughout the birth process. One approach involves teaching the patient and her partner what to expect during each phase and how they can help one another throughout the process. If the patient so wishes, the nurse involves the support person in the care as much as possible.

🌼 *Ethnocultural Considerations*— Minority women and level of care received

The Institute of Medicine (2003) reported that minorities do not receive the same level of quality care as do Caucasian Americans. A nurse working in the birth unit needs to be attentive to this problem. It is incumbent on all nurses to advocate for patients any time there appears to be an ethnic bias in treatment. The nurse also must be aware of any of personal prejudices that could affect care. In institutions that serve minority populations, it is essential that all hospital staff members undergo frequent in-service educational offerings that focus on heightening cultural sensitivity.

 Now Can You— **Discuss aspects of various maternal conditions that complicate childbirth?**

1. Discuss critical aspects of intrapartal care for the woman with diabetes?
2. Describe one critical nursing responsibility in the patient experiencing a nonarrested preterm labor?
3. Identify three teaching needs for the patient experiencing preterm labor and birth?

Complications of Labor and Birth Associated with the Fetus

FETAL MALPRESENTATION

Fetal malpresentation is the second most commonly reported complication of labor and birth. In 2003, it occurred at a rate of 38.5 per 1000 live births (Martin et al., 2005). The fetal occiput is the most favorable presenting part for a vaginal birth. Face, brow, shoulder, compound, and breech constitute malpresentations. A breech presentation, in which the buttocks or legs present first, occurs in approximately 3% of all births and is considered the most common malpresentation. (See Chapter 12.) It is important that these conditions be identified during the antepartum period since a malpresentation may place the woman and fetus at risk for complications during labor and birth. Diagnosis is made by abdominal palpation (i.e., Leopold's maneuvers) and vaginal examination and is usually confirmed by ultrasonography.

During labor, descent of the fetus in a breech presentation may be slow. This is because the breech is not as effective as a dilating wedge as the fetal head. There is an increased risk of prolapsed cord if the membranes rupture during early labor (Fig. 14-5).

Nursing Insight— *Breech presentation and meconium in the amniotic fluid*

When the fetus is in a breech presentation, the presence of meconium in the amniotic fluid may not be indicative of fetal distress. Pressure exerted on the fetal abdomen during the birth process may cause the passage of meconium. It is important to assess the FHR and pattern to ensure there are changes indicative of fetal hypoxia. When the fetus is in a breech position, the FHR is best auscultated at or above the maternal umbilicus.

During the vaginal birth of a fetus in a breech presentation, the physician uses labor mechanisms that manipulate the buttocks and lower extremities. Piper forceps are sometimes applied to facilitate delivery of the head. Before the birth, the physician may attempt an external cephalic version to rotate the fetus to a vertex presentation. (See later discussion.) Cesarean birth is commonly performed when the following circumstances exist: the fetus is estimated to be larger than 3800 g or smaller than 1500 g; the labor is ineffective; this is the woman's first pregnancy; or there are additional maternal–fetal complications.

Face and brow presentations are examples of **asynclitism** (the fetal head is presenting at a different angle than

Figure 14-5 The mechanisms of labor in a breech presentation. The aftercoming fetal head delivers last.

expected). Face and brow presentations hyperextend the neck and increase the overall circumference of the presenting part. These presentations are uncommon and are usually associated with fetal anomalies (i.e., anencephaly), macrosomia, CPD, and contractures of the maternal pelvis. Vaginal birth may be accomplished if the fetus flexes to a vertex presentation. Forceps are often used. Cesarean birth is indicated if the presentation persists, if there is evidence of fetal compromise, or if there is an arrest in the progression of labor. Shoulder and compound presentations (e.g., a hand combined with the head) contribute to fetal and vaginal trauma and usually require cesarean birth (Cunningham et al., 2005).

VERSION

Version (turning of a fetus from one presentation to another) may be done either externally or internally by the physician.

External Version

An external cephalic version (ECV) is used as an attempt to turn the fetus from a breech presentation to a vertex presentation to allow a vaginal birth (Fig. 14-6). Since cesarean birth is a major surgical procedure associated with numerous maternal and fetal risks, ECV may offer an alternative to surgery. The procedure, performed in a birth unit, may be attempted after 37 weeks' gestation. Contraindications to ECV include previous cesarean birth,

uterine anomalies, CPD, placenta previa, multifetal gestation, and oligohydramnios (Cunningham et al., 2005).

Before the version, ultrasonography is obtained to confirm the fetal position, locate the umbilical cord; rule out placenta previa; assess the maternal pelvic dimensions and the amniotic fluid volume, fetal size and gestational age, and the presence of anomalies. Before the version, a non-stress test (NST) is performed to confirm fetal well-being, or the FHR may be electronically monitored for a brief period (e.g., 10 to 20 minutes).

Ultrasound guidance is used as the physician slowly applies gentle, steady pressure over the fetal head and buttocks to rotate the position. Complications associated with version include umbilical cord compression, placental abruption, maternal hemorrhage, and fetal bradycardia (Vadhera & Locksmith, 2004).

The procedure of rotating the fetus (version) requires uterine relaxation. Tocolytic agents such as magnesium sulfate or terbutaline are used to facilitate this process. Acoustic stimulation of the fetus has also resulted in successful versions (Vadhera & Locksmith, 2004).

Optimizing Outcomes— Assisting with ECV

The nurse is responsible for obtaining written informed consent from the patient after physician explanation, providing teaching regarding the procedure, administering medications as ordered, and conducting constant surveillance of the maternal–infant dyad. The patient

Intravenous tocolytic drug

Figure 14-6 External cephalic version is a maneuver performed through the maternal abdominal wall in an attempt to change the fetal position from a breech to a cephalic presentation.

needs to know not only that the version attempt might not be successful; she must also be aware of the associated complications that may occur such as rupture of the membranes, fetal bradycardia, and discomfort. During the version, if there is any indication of significant fetal or maternal compromise, the nurse prepares the woman for a cesarean birth. Women who are Rh-negative are given Rh immune globulin because the manipulation may cause fetomaternal bleeding (Bowes & Thorp, 2004; Vadhera & Locksmith, 2004).

Internal Version

With internal version, the physician rotates the fetus by inserting a hand into the uterus and changes the fetal presentation to cephalic (head) or podalic (foot). Internal version is used with multifetal gestations to deliver the second fetus. However, the safety of this procedure has not been documented. Cesarean birth is usually performed for malpresentation in multiple gestations. Nursing responsibilities center on maternal–fetal monitoring and providing support to the woman.

SHOULDER DYSTOCIA

Shoulder dystocia is an uncommon obstetric emergency that occurs in 0.5% to 1.5% of all births (Jevitt, 2005). In this type of dystocia, the head is born but the anterior shoulder cannot pass under the maternal pubic arch. The problem is often not identified until the head is born. Risk factors for shoulder dystocia include maternal pelvic abnormalities, a history of shoulder dystocia in a previous pregnancy, obesity, diabetes, prolonged labor, postdate pregnancy, and fetal macrosomia (greater than 4000 g) (Gherman, 2005).

Although there are no methods to predict or prevent shoulder dystocia, the nurse should be alert to clinical

indicators: slowed labor progression and formation of a caput succedaneum that increases in size. When the fetal head emerges on the perineum (crowning), it retracts instead of protruding with subsequent contractions (termed the "turtle sign"), and external rotation does not occur (ACOG, 2002b; Bowes & Thorp, 2004; Jevitt, 2005). Fetal/neonatal injuries are related to birth asphyxia; damage to the brachial plexus; and fractures, usually of the humerus or clavicle. Maternal injury is most commonly associated with excessive blood loss that results from uterine atony or rupture; other risks include lacerations, extension of the episiotomy, and postpartum endometritis.

A number of maneuvers have been attempted to free up the anterior shoulder and facilitate delivery. The McRoberts maneuver is one approach. The woman is placed in a dorsal lithotomy position, and her thighs are sharply flexed on her abdomen. This position increases the angle between the symphysis pubis and the sacral promontory, allowing for greater room in fetal descent. Suprapubic pressure applied immediately above the symphysis pubis may be needed along with the McRoberts maneuver to loosen the trapped shoulders (Baxley & Gobbo, 2004; Camune & Brucker, 2007) (Fig. 14-7).

Other methods of delivery assistance for shoulder dystocia center on maternal positional changes: a hands-and-knees position, a squatting position, or a lateral recumbent position (Bowes & Thorp, 2004; Camune & Brucker, 2007; Jevitt, 2005).

 Optimizing Outcomes— When birth is complicated by shoulder dystocia

When childbirth is complicated by shoulder dystocia, the nurse's role is to assist the woman in assuming the positions, assist the physician with the maneuvers, and to document all procedures. The nurse also provides careful

Figure 14-7 Methods to relieve shoulder dystocia. *A.* Pressure is applied immediately above the maternal symphysis pubis to push the fetal anterior shoulder downward. *B.* McRoberts maneuver. The woman's thighs are sharply flexed on her abdomen to straighten the pelvic curve. *C.* Angle of pelvis before maneuver. *D.* Angle of pelvis after maneuver.

instruction to the patient to facilitate cooperation and understanding (Jevitt, 2005). After birth, the woman is closely observed for signs of hemorrhage and soft tissue trauma of the birth canal; the neonate is assessed for fracture of the clavicle or humerus, brachial plexus injuries, and asphyxia (Bowes & Thorp, 2004).

CEPHALOPELVIC DISPROPORTION

Although there are true problems that create issues between the head of the fetus and the pelvis of the mother, in the United States, **cephalopelvic disproportion** (CPD) is often used to describe unsuccessful attempts at vaginal birth. When CPD is present, the fetus cannot fit through the maternal pelvis to allow a vaginal birth. Often related to excessive fetal size (macrosomia), CPD occurred at a rate of 14.6 per 1000 live births in 2003 (Martin et al., 2005). A macrosomic infant (birth weight greater than 4000 grams) is likely to have a large head that can prevent descent into the maternal pelvis.

Despite ultrasound evaluation, it is difficult to predict the safest mode of birth for the macrosomic infant. A trial of

labor is suggested if the woman is nulliparous. Women with a previous history of cesarean birth for CPD may also be offered a trial of labor although a prompt cesarean birth is recommended at the earliest sign of maternal or fetal compromise.

The maternal pelvis is assessed before the onset of labor to determine type and size. A gynecoid pelvis is considered to be the most common female pelvic type and most amenable to vaginal birth although markedly small dimensions may preclude a vaginal birth. Other pelvic types are the android, anthropoid, and platypelloid. (See Chapter 5 for further discussion.) Although the other types of pelvises may not contraindicate a trial of labor, vaginal birth may not be possible for the woman with a platypelloid pelvis because its markedly shortened anterior–posterior diameter prevents fetal descent (Cunningham et al., 2005).

Nursing Care

A thorough nursing assessment including a review of present and past pregnancies is important in guiding care. Women with a history of cephalopelvic disproportion are at increased risk during the present labor. Slow progression of effacement and dilation, lack of fetal descent, and excessive pain are all possible indicators of CPD. Nursing interventions such as maternal position changes, particularly to an upright posture (e.g., sitting or squatting) to widen the pelvic girdle, relaxation, and water therapy are strategies to facilitate labor progression. The use of analgesic agents may alleviate pain-creating tension that is interfering with fetal descent. Supportive care includes information related to labor status and encouragement when progress has been made.

MULTIPLE GESTATION

Managing the births of more than one fetus is complex and requires the expert collaboration of medical and nursing personnel. The gestational age, number, health and presentation of the fetuses determine the mode of birth, whether vaginal or cesarean.

 Nursing Insight— *Fetal presentations with multiple gestations*

Both fetuses present in the vertex position (most favorable for vaginal birth) in only one half of all twin pregnancies. In one third of multifetal pregnancies, one twin may present in the vertex position and one in the breech position (Cunningham et al., 2005).

Multiple births are associated with more complications than singleton births. The woman's health status may be compromised by problems such as hypertension of pregnancy, anemia, or gestational diabetes. She is also at increased risk for hemorrhage related to atony from uterine overdistention, abruptio placentae, and multiple or adherent placentas. Because of the multiple fetuses, abnormal fetal presentation may occur. Increased fetal/newborn complications are related primarily to problems associated with low-birth-weight infants due to preterm birth and intrauterine growth restriction. Intrapartal fetal distress may result from cord prolapse and the onset of placental separation after the birth of the first fetus. Because of these problems, the risk for long-term disabilities such as cerebral palsy is greater among multiple births.

Women who present at 38 weeks with a twin pregnancy are less likely to experience fetal morbidity and mortality and may be appropriate candidates for a vaginal birth. It is recommended, although it is not always possible, that women with a multiple gestation, particularly triplets or higher-order multiples, deliver at a tertiary care center where facilities are available in the event of an emergency. Birthing centers must have transport ready for infant transfer to neonatal intensive care units. Patients who will undergo labor or a trial of labor require careful monitoring. Ultrasound is used to determine position and presentation of the fetal parts. Electronic fetal monitoring (EFM) is applied. It is important to identify each of the individual FHRs and the use of a separate monitor for each fetus is preferable. Interventions, such as analgesia, anesthesia, and intravenous infusions are determined on a case-by-case basis. The stimulation of labor with oxytocin, and epidural anesthesia, forceps, and vacuum assistance and fetal version may all be used to facilitate the vaginal birth of twins. Women in good health and with no evidence of fetal distress should be given the opportunity to participate in medical decision management.

When the woman is fully dilated and ready to push, she is moved to the birthing suite, where personnel, equipment, and supplies are readily available in the event there is a need for a cesarean birth. The woman may safely give birth in a labor, delivery, recovery, postpartum (LDRP) suite provided there is quick access to the surgical area. The nurse prepares the woman and her support for the possibility that she may experience both a vaginal and a cesarean birth depending on the fetal presentation. The nurse also explains the external version procedure in case this intervention is necessary. Patient education is carried out in a timely manner when the patient is capable of participation.

The majority (approximately 80%) of vertex, vertex twins are delivered with success vaginally. The first infant born is identified as "A" and neonatal care is initiated. Oxytocin, usually given to halt contractions and minimize bleeding, is withheld to avoid compromising circulation to the unborn fetus. In the vertex, breech presentation, an external version of the second twin is attempted provided that the conditions are favorable. If the second fetus is a footling breech, has a hyperextended head, or exhibits signs of compromise, a cesarean birth is considered the better option. The birth of the second twin normally occurs within 15 minutes of the birth of the first twin. Although there has been concern over complications associated with a longer time period between births, studies have shown that with proper fetal monitoring and maternal surveillance, a safe vaginal birth can take place in an indefinite amount of time (Cunningham et al., 2005; Vadhera & Locksmith, 2004). The nurse documents the time of birth for the first infant and all subsequent infants who are born.

Across Care Settings: Planning the multiple gestation birth

Together, the obstetrician, anesthesiologist, and patient discuss the anesthetic options available for childbirth. This collaborative meeting is best done in an office visit before the onset of labor. Epidural anesthesia is considered a safe method for providing relief of pain and it allows prompt intervention in case the second twin requires an external version or a cesarean birth (Vadhera & Locksmith, 2004). The woman may experience an unmedicated birth provided she understands that if it is necessary to proceed to a cesarean birth she will receive a general anesthetic to facilitate uterine relaxation.

There is controversy over the medical management in twin births where the second twin is not in a vertex position. Data from a retrospective cohort study with 15,185 participants that studied twin births of vertex, nonvertex pairs showed that there is a higher risk of neonatal mortality and morbidity with vaginal birth of the nonvertex twin (Yang et al., 2005). The acknowledged limitations of large cohort studies lies in the fact that they are chart reviews and therefore do not examine complications associated with the birth of the second twin (Wen et al., 2004).

Triplets and higher order multiples generally require a cesarean birth. This mode of birth decreases the risk that the second fetus will experience anoxia as well as other complications such as cord entanglement and premature placental separation. While there are reports of triplet vaginal births, these successes are tempered with the strong possibility that both the second and the third neonates may be in breech presentations and require operative interventions. If it is deemed possible for the woman to give birth to triplets vaginally, the medical team must be on ready standby for an immediate cesarean surgery (Cunningham et al., 2005).

 Now Can You— Discuss birth options for a woman with a multiple gestation?

1. Identify what factors determine whether a woman with multiple gestation may be allowed to attempt a vaginal birth?
2. Describe the primary recommendations concerning the childbirth options available for a woman with a multiple gestation?
3. Discuss controversies that surround the medical management of twin births?

NON-REASSURING FHR PATTERNS

Fetal heart monitoring is one type of assessment that provides the nurse, the patient, and her support(s) feedback concerning the well-being of the fetus. Families often request to increase the volume of the fetal monitor so that they hear the reassurance of a strong heartbeat. It is essential that the nurse understand actions that should be taken when decelerations or other ominous FHR patterns are detected. (See Chapter 12.)

 Optimizing Outcomes— Responding to a non-reassuring FHR pattern

- Provide information to the woman; assist her to a lateral position.
- Encourage relaxation and mental imagery to reduce anxiety.

- Assess for and correct maternal hypotension by elevating the legs.
- Increase the rate of the maintenance IV fluids.
- Assess for hyperstimulation by palpating the uterus.
- Discontinue oxytocin if infusing.
- Administer oxygen at 8-10 L/min by mask.
- Consider internal monitoring to obtain more accurate fetal/uterine assessments.
- Apply fetal scalp or acoustic stimulation.
- Assist with fetal oxygen saturation monitoring if ordered.
- Assist with birth (cesarean or vaginal-assisted) if a non-reassuring FHR pattern cannot be corrected.

It is important that the nurse immediately notifies the physician or certified nurse midwife and initiate appropriate interventions for non-reassuring FHR patterns. (See Chapter 12.) A **prolonged deceleration** is the presence of a decrease in the FHR below the baseline 15 beats per minute or more that lasts more than 2 minutes, but less than 10 minutes. A deceleration that lasts more than 10 minutes is considered a baseline change (National Institute of Child Health and Human Development [NICHD], 1997). Benign causes of prolonged FHR decelerations include pelvic examination, application of a fetal spiral electrode, rapid fetal descent, and prolonged maternal Valsalva maneuver. Less benign causes include progressive severe variable decelerations, umbilical cord prolapse, hypotension associated with spinal or epidural analgesia/anesthesia, paracervical anesthesia, tetanic uterine contractions, placental hemorrhage, uterine rupture, and maternal hypoxia. A prolonged FHR deceleration that occurs late in the course of severe variable decelerations or a series of prolonged decelerations may occur immediately before fetal death.

 critical nursing action Assisting with Intrauterine Resuscitation

Intrauterine resuscitation, a term used to describe interventions initiated when a non-reassuring FHR pattern is detected, centers on improving uterine and intervillous space blood flow and cardiac output (Simpson & James, 2005). When intrauterine resuscitation is underway, nursing priorities are: (1) to open the maternal and fetal vascular systems; (2) to increase the blood volume; and (3) to optimize oxygenation of the circulating blood volume. These interventions are accomplished by maternal positional changes, increasing the rate of the primary IV, and providing oxygen by face mask.

When non-reassuring FHR patterns are detected by EFM, other methods of assessment may be initiated:

- Fetal scalp and vibroacoustic stimulation
- Fetal oxygen saturation monitoring
- Fetal scalp blood sampling

Fetal Scalp and Vibroacoustic Stimulation

Fetal stimulation is done to elicit an acceleration of the FHR (15 beats per minute for at least 15 seconds) that occurs in response to a tactile stimulus (Tucker, 2004). Acceleration of the FHR will not occur in the presence of fetal distress and acidosis; thus, fetal stimulation is an assessment of the fetal acid–base balance. Scalp stimulation is conducted by applying pressure with the fingers to the fetal scalp during a vaginal examination. Vibroacoustic stimulation is accomplished by placing an artificial larynx or fetal acoustic stimulation device on the maternal abdomen directly over the fetal head for 1 to 2 seconds. Acceleration of the FHR in response to the stimulation is usually indicative of fetal well-being; lack of a FHR acceleration does not necessarily indicate fetal compromise but warrants further evaluation.

Fetal Oxygen Saturation Monitoring

Fetal pulse oximetry (FPO), or continuous monitoring of fetal oxygen saturation, is similar to pulse oximetry used in children and adults. A small sensor designed to assess oxygen saturation is inserted next to the fetal cheek or temple area. The sensor is connected to a monitor; incoming data are continuously displayed on the uterine activity panel of the fetal monitor tracing. The normal range for oxygen saturation in the healthy fetus is 30% to 70%. Before this modality can be used, certain criteria (e.g., 36 weeks' gestation or greater; singleton fetus; vertex presentation; non-reassuring FHR pattern; ruptured membranes; fetal station less than or equal to –2) must be met. The American College of Obstetricians and Gynecologists (ACOG) has not endorsed FPO in clinical practice and recommends further clinical research for this assessment modality (ACOG, 2005).

Fetal Scalp Blood Sampling

Fetal scalp blood sampling is conducted to assess the fetal pH, P_{O_2} and P_{CO_2}. A small sample of capillary blood is taken from the fetal scalp as it presents at the dilated cervix. If the fetus is hypoxic, there is a drop in the pH (acidosis). A scalp blood pH greater than 7.25 is considered normal for a fetus during labor; a scalp blood pH below 7.20 is acidotic and is recognized as an indicator of fetal distress. However, because of the frequent variations in fetal blood gas values associated with transient circulatory changes, fetal blood sampling is rarely performed except in tertiary centers that have a capability for repetitive sampling and the rapid report of results.

Depending on the situation, watchful waiting with continuous monitoring conducted by the nurse may provide the best option for assessment of fetal well-being. Since non-reassuring FHR patterns constitute a risk indicator for cesarean birth, the nurse and all members of the health care team must be ready for this outcome at all times. It is important to provide ongoing support for the laboring woman and keep her informed of her labor progress and fetal status.

" What to say " — *When a non-reassuring FHR pattern is detected via electronic monitoring*

When electronic monitoring reveals a non-reassuring FHR pattern, the nurse needs to maintain a calming presence and offer factual, simple explanations for all actions. For example, the nurse may say:

"We are concerned about your baby's heart rate pattern."

"I am going to change your position to your side to increase oxygen flow to your baby."

"I am also going to place this oxygen mask on your face to increase the oxygen flow to you and to your baby, and increase your IV rate."

"Do you have any questions?"

"I am here to help in any way and I will stay here with you. Please let me know what concerns you have."

Amniotic Fluid Complications

Oligohydramnios (less than 300 mL of amniotic fluid), **hydramnios** (polyhydramnios) (greater than 2 L of amniotic fluid), and the presence of **meconium** (the first stools of the infant) in the amniotic fluid complicate labor and birth.

OLIGOHYDRAMNIOS

Oligohydramnios may result from fetal renal abnormalities, poor placental perfusion, or premature rupture of the membranes. During labor, the absence of the amniotic fluid buffer may lead to cord compression during contractions and decreased fetal blood flow as evidenced by variable heart rate decelerations. Women with pregnancies complicated by oligohydramnios require careful nursing and medical surveillance; amnioinfusion may be indicated to replace the cushion of fluid for the cord and relieve the frequency and intensity of variable decelerations. (See Chapter 12.)

HYDRAMNIOS

Hydramnios occurs in multiple gestations, fetal anomalies, and as a complication of maternal disease such as diabetes. During labor, the nurse needs to be aware that the excessive volume of fluid may obscure the fetal heart tracings. Hydramnios can cause fetal malpresentation because of the extra uterine space for the fetus to turn that it provides. The mother is also at risk for prolapse of the umbilical cord because the increased amount of fluid pushes the fetus high into the uterine cavity. Preterm rupture of the membranes, another complication associated with hydramnios, increases the risks of both infection and prolapsed cord.

MECONIUM

Meconium-stained amniotic fluid during intrapartum is an indication for careful fetal surveillance by EFM and possibly fetal scalp blood sampling. Although not always a sign of fetal distress, its presence, which occurs during fetal loss of sphincter control, is highly correlated with its occurrence. Reasons for the passage of meconium during labor include:

- Hypoxia-related peristalsis and sphincter relaxation
- Breech presentation or normal physiological function that occurs with fetal maturity
- Following umbilical cord compression-induced vagal stimulation in the mature fetus

Meconium staining, which occurs in approximately 20% of births, is observed more frequently in prolonged pregnancies. A decrease in amniotic fluid (oligohydramnios) increases the viscosity of the meconium and the risk of neonatal aspiration during delivery. The nurse must carefully document the presence of meconium stained fluid at the time of rupture of the membranes. In addition, the nurse should note the occurrence of variable decelerations and immediately notify the physician or certified nurse midwife regardless of whether or not meconium is present. Amnioinfusion has been shown to be effective in decreasing the fetal mortality associated with variable FHR decelerations.

 Optimizing Outcomes— Intrapartal neonatal suctioning and meconium-stained amniotic fluid

The nasopharynx and oropharynx of the neonate born in the presence of meconium-stained amniotic fluid are often suctioned before the first breath to reduce the incidence and severity of meconium aspiration syndrome (MAS). However, because research does not support the efficacy of routine intrapartum suctioning to prevent MAS, this practice is no longer recommended (Vain et al., 2004).

NUCHAL CORD

Nuchal cord (a cord that is wrapped around the infant's neck) and cords with true knots are observed in approximately 1% of all births. Nuchal cord, which rarely causes hypoxia, occurs most often in fetuses with long umbilical cords. When a tight knot is present in the cord, variable heart rate decelerations associated with fetal asphyxia may be noted on EFM. Nursing interventions follow protocols used for other abnormal variations of the fetal heart tracing.

Once the head is born, gentle palpation is used to feel for the cord. If the cord is present, it is loosened and carefully slipped over the head. If it is too tightly coiled to allow this intervention, the cord is clamped twice, cut between the clamps, and unwound from around the neck before the shoulders are delivered. Otherwise, the cord could tear and interfere with the fetal oxygen supply.

Complications Associated with the Placenta

Critical nursing actions are required when the woman's intrapartum course is complicated by bleeding related to placenta previa (a low implantation of the placenta) or abruptio placentae (a premature separation of the placenta). (See Chapter 11.) Either condition places the woman at risk for hemorrhage and shock. A deteriorating physiological status of the mother impacts the fetus and often results in hypoxia. The nurse faces the challenge of helping to manage this intrapartum emergency. Guidelines for nursing care of the patient experiencing an intrapartal hemorrhage are presented in Table 14-3.

PLACENTA PREVIA

With placenta previa, bleeding occurs when the lower uterine segment begins to differentiate from the upper segment late in pregnancy and the cervix begins to dilate. If the bleeding has stopped, the maternal vital signs are stable, the fetal heart sounds are of good quality, and the fetus has not yet reached 36 weeks, the woman is usually managed by expectant watching. If the woman is at term (greater than 37 weeks of gestation) and in labor or bleeding persistently, immediate birth by cesarean is almost always indicated. Women diagnosed with partial or marginal placenta previa who have no bleeding or minimal bleeding may be allowed to attempt a vaginal birth.

When cesarean birth is planned, nursing responsibilities include continuous maternal–fetal assessment while preparing the woman for surgery. Maternal vital signs are

Table 14-3 Care of the Patient Experiencing an Intrapartal Hemorrhage

Assessment	Plan	Intervention	Evaluation
Vital Signs	Establish maternal stability.	Take every 5 minutes if unstable, or every 15 minutes if stable.	Vital signs are within normal range.
		Use pulse oximetry.	Pulse is between 60 and 120 beats/min.
		Auscultate respirations.	Respirations are between 14 and 26 breaths/min.
			Temperature is less than 100.4°F (38.0°C).
			Blood pressure is greater than 90/60.
Bleeding	Resolve hemorrhage.	Start two large-bore IV sites.	Bleeding is minimized.
	Prevent shock.	Infuse normal saline and lactated Ringer's solution.	Homeostasis is established.
		Estimate blood loss	
		(1 g = 1 mL) for replacement.	
		Infuse blood products as necessary.	
		Monitor circulatory volume using CVP/Swan-Ganz catheter as needed for extreme bleeding.	
		Send blood sample to lab for analysis of gases.	
		Document blood loss.	
Intake/Output	Prevent volume depletion.	Insert indwelling urinary catheter.	Urine output will be greater than 30 mL/hr.
		Measure and record output every hour.	
		Measure and record input every hour.	
Fetal Status	Prevent fetal injury.	Continuous electronic fetal monitoring.	Fetal heart rate tracings remain between 120 and 160 beats/min. No evidence of abnormal tracings.
Emotional Response	Assist patient to cope with condition.	Educate the patient regarding all procedures.	Patient verbalizes an understanding of her condition.
		Inform the patient of her status throughout the bleeding crisis.	Face displays no grimace.
		Provide relaxation and breathing techniques.	Muscles remain relaxed.
		Provide spiritual support as necessary.	
Pain	Reduce pain.	Provide relaxation and breathing techniques.	Patient reports pain on a scale of 1–10 as between 3 and 5.
		Use guided imagery.	
		Offer massage.	
		Monitor contractions.	
		Offer limited pain medication as ordered.	

Adapted from MacMullen et al. (2005); Curran (2003); and Mandeville & Troiano (1999).

assessed for indicators of hemorrhage (decreasing blood pressure, tachycardia, changes in the level of consciousness (LOC), and oliguria). Continuous EFM is used to assess the fetus for signs of hypoxia.

There is an increased risk for postpartal hemorrhage because the placental site is in the lower uterine segment, which does not contract as efficiently as the upper segment. Also, because the uterine blood supply is less in the lower uterine segment, the placenta tends to grow larger than when implanted in the upper segment. Thus, a larger denuded surface area is exposed after removal of the placenta. Nursing care throughout the intrapartal course centers on providing emotional support for the woman and her family and collaborating with and supporting medical management.

PLACENTAL ABRUPTION

Placental abruption (abruptio placentae), which tends to occur in late pregnancy, may occur as late as the first or second stage of labor. Although the primary cause of premature placental separation is unknown, predisposing factors include maternal hypertension, cocaine use (associated with vasoconstriction), direct trauma, and a history of previous placental abruption (Ananth, Oyelese, Yeo, Pradhan, & Vintzileos, 2005).

Treatment for abruptio placentae depends on the severity of maternal blood loss and the fetal maturity and status. If the abruption is mild and the fetus is less than 36 weeks and not in distress, expectant management may be implemented. (See Chapter 11.) When the fetus is at term gestation or if the bleeding is moderate to severe and the woman of fetus is in jeopardy, delivery is facilitated. Nursing care includes continuous maternal-fetal monitoring and emotional support. The patient is maintained in a lateral position to prevent pressure on the vena cava and to facilitate placental blood flow. To avoid further damage to the injured placenta, no vaginal or pelvic examinations are performed and no enemas are administered.

Blood and fluid volume replacement are implemented to maintain the urine output (assessed by indwelling Foley catheter) at 30 mL/hr or more and the hematocrit at 30% or more. Hemodynamic monitoring may be necessary. If the premature placental separation occurs during active labor, the physician may elect to rupture the membranes or augment the labor with intravenous oxytocin to hasten birth. Rupturing the membranes prevents large amounts of blood from collecting in the myometrium, which can interfere with uterine contractions. Artificial rupture of the membranes allows a slow, steady escape of amniotic fluid, preventing a sudden change in intrauterine pressure that may encourage further placental separation. Vaginal birth is desirable, especially in cases of fetal death. If birth does not appear to be imminent, a cesarean birth is the delivery method of choice. However, cesarean birth should be reserved for cases of fetal distress or other obstetric indications and should not be attempted if the woman has severe and uncorrected coagulopathy (i.e., disseminated intravascular coagulation [DIC]).

The patient with unresolved bleeding from a placental abruption is most vulnerable to severe complications. Maternal problems resulting from abruptio placentae include a **Couvelaire** uterus (the accumulation of blood between the separated placenta and the uterine wall) and DIC. Although a Couvelaire uterus is rare, its implications are severe. The uterus takes on a bluish tinge as blood extravasates from the clot into the myometrium. Contractility is lost. The condition is so severe that a hysterectomy may be necessary to control the bleeding (Cunningham et al., 2006).

If DIC has developed, surgery poses a major maternal risk due to the possibility of hemorrhage during surgery and later from the incisional site. The administration of intravenous fibrinogen or cryoprecipitate (which contains fibrinogen) may be given to increase the maternal fibrinogen level.

The maternal prognosis depends on how quickly interventions are initiated and how effective they are in halting the hemorrhage. Death can occur from massive hemorrhage that leads to shock or renal failure from circulatory collapse. The fetal prognosis depends on the extent of the abruption and the severity of the accompanying hypoxia.

 case study A Pregnant Adolescent in the Emergency Department

Maria Selles is a 14-year-old girl who arrives in the emergency department (ED) complaining of severe abdominal pain. She is pale and diaphoretic. A small amount of bright red blood is slowly trickling from her vagina. On assessment, her blood pressure is 120/70; pulse, 100; respirations 22 breaths/minute; temperature 99°F (37.2°C). Her physical examination reveals an enlarged abdomen, which is rigid and board-like with extreme tenderness. Maria is known to the ED because of a history of repeated drug abuse including cocaine. She has been living on the street since she was kicked out of her house several months ago.

critical thinking questions

1. Based on this initial information, what is the nurse's assessment of the possible problem?

2. Since Maria is in such extreme distress, the nurse is aware of a need to limit the number of questions asked. What critical questions should be asked at this point?

3. What laboratory tests would be important to check?

◆ See Suggested Answers to Case Studies in the text on the Electronic Study Guide or DavisPlus.

The nurse's further assessment reveals dark red vaginal bleeding and clinical signs consistent with pregnancy (the presence of abdominal enlargement, deeply pigmented areolae, linea nigra, and striae gravidarum). The young patient has said very little in response to the questions but Maria does admit to sexual intercourse and no recent periods.

Given this information, the nurse formulates the care priorities for Maria. Although her physical condition and that of the fetus warrant immediate priority, the nurse needs to support this young girl psychologically in order to proceed with any plan. Any support people who have come with her to the ED should be identified. If there is no one with her, the nurse explains the plan of care and describes what she should expect. The nurse places Maria on the electronic fetal monitor and immediately notifies the physician of her condition. Because cocaine is associated with placental abruption, the nurse must identify any recent drug use. The care plan should be developmentally oriented. The nurse implements strategies to keep Maria warm, provides emotional support and a calming presence, and continues to monitor her vital signs and her vaginal flow until the physician arrives.

DISSEMINATED INTRAVASCULAR COAGULATION

Disseminated intravascular coagulation (DIC) is an acquired disorder of blood clotting. Affected individuals can experience widespread internal and external bleeding and clotting. Clinical symptoms may include easy bruising, the appearance of multiple petechiae, and bleeding from intravenous sites. DIC is most often triggered by the release of large amounts of tissue thromboplastin, which occurs in abruptio placentae, and in retained dead fetus (the fetus has died and is retained in the uterus for 6 or more weeks) and amniotic fluid syndromes (Cunningham et al., 2005).

 Optimizing Outcomes— **Prompt identification of clinical signs that may indicate DIC**

When conducting a physical assessment of the pregnant woman at risk for DIC, the nurse must be alert to the following clinical signs:

- Bleeding from multiple sites: intravenous access site, venipuncture site, site of urinary catheter insertion
- Spontaneous bleeding from the gums and nose
- Widespread petechiae and bruising
- Gastrointestinal bleeding
- Tachycardia
- Diaphoresis

With DIC, the anticoagulation and procoagulation factors are activated simultaneously. Thromboplastin (a clotting factor) is released into the maternal circulation as a result of placental bleeding and the consequent clot formation. Circulating levels of thromboplastin activate widespread clotting throughout the microcirculation. This process consumes or "uses up" other clotting factors such as fibrinogen and platelets. The condition is complicated further by the activation of the fibrinolytic system to lyse (destroy) the clots. As a result, there is a simultaneous decrease in clotting factors and an increase in circulating anticoagulants, leaving the circulating blood unable to clot. Laboratory results reveal low hemoglobin, hematocrit, platelets, and fibrinogen and elevated fibrin split/degradation products.

The priority in treatment of DIC is to correct the underlying cause and replace fluids and essential clotting factors. When premature placental separation has triggered the coagulopathy, delivery of the fetus and placenta must be accomplished so that the production of thromboplastin, which is driving the process, is halted. This is accomplished with intravenous administration of heparin to stop the clotting cascade. Heparin is cautiously given close to the time of birth to decrease the likelihood of postpartum hemorrhage after the delivery of the placenta. The administration of blood and platelets is usually delayed until after completion of the heparin therapy so that the newly infused blood factors are not consumed by the widespread coagulation process. Depending on the clinical setting, antithrombin III factor, fibrinogen, or cryoprecipitate may also be used to restore blood clotting (Labelle & Kitchens, 2005).

Nursing care includes continuous maternal–fetal assessment, administering the prescribed fluids, blood, and blood products; and assessing for signs of complications from the replacement products. The woman is positioned in a side-lying tilt to maximize placental perfusion, and oxygen may be administered via rebreathing mask at 8 to 10 L/min or according to physician or institutional protocol. Because renal failure may result from DIC, urinary output is closely monitored; it should be maintained at more than 30 mL/hr. The patient and her family should be provided with ongoing information and emotional support (Labelle & Kitchens, 2005). (See Chapters 11, 16, and 33 for further discussion on DIC.)

RUPTURE OF THE UTERUS

Rupture of the uterus during labor is a rare but life-threatening obstetric complication that occurs in 1 to 1500 to 2000 births (Fig. 14-8). It is most often associated with the tearing of a uterine scar (usually from a previous classic cesarean birth), uterine trauma (e.g., accidents, surgery), and a congenital uterine anomaly. Rupture of the uterus occurs more often in multigravidas than in primigravidas. Intrapartal uterine rupture may result from overdistention (e.g., multiple gestation), hyperstimulation (e.g., oxytocin, prostaglandin), external or internal version, malpresentation, or a difficult forceps-assisted birth (Cunningham et al., 2005).

 Nursing Insight— *Understanding types of uterine rupture*

Uterine rupture may be classified as complete or incomplete. A complete rupture extends through the endometrium, myometrium, and peritoneum. When this occurs, uterine contractions stop. The woman complains of sudden, severe abdominal pain during a strong contraction followed by cessation of the pain. There is bleeding into the abdominal cavity and possibly into the vagina. An incomplete rupture extends into the peritoneum but not into the peritoneal cavity or broad ligament. Bleeding is usually internal and the woman may be asymptomatic (a "silent" rupture) or complain of localized tenderness and aching pain over the lower uterine segment.

Changes in fetal heart tracings such as late decelerations, decreased variability, and increased or decreased heart rate may or may not be present. Maternal signs and symptoms may include faintness, vomiting, abdominal tenderness, hypotonic uterine contractions, and lack of labor progress. As blood loss continues, the woman may exhibit signs of hypovolemic shock (hypotension; tachypnea; pallor; and cool, clammy skin). Fetal parts may be readily palpable through the abdomen.

Rupture of the uterus constitutes an obstetric emergency; the type of medical management depends on the severity. A small rupture may be safely managed with a laparotomy and birth of the infant, repair of the tear, and volume replacement with fluids and blood transfusions if needed. A complete uterine rupture requires hysterectomy and blood replacement.

Nursing Care Plan The Patient with Abruptio Placentae

Nursing Diagnosis: Deficient Fluid Volume related to active losses from premature separation of the placenta.

Measurable Short-term Goal: The patient and her fetus will maintain fluid balance during the intrapartum period.

Measurable Long-term Goal: The patient and newborn will have stable homeostatic conditions upon discharge.

NOC Outcomes:
Fluid Balance (0601) Water balance in the intracellular and extracellular compartments of the body
Blood Loss Severity (0413) Severity of internal or external bleeding/hemorrhage
Fetal Status Antepartum (0111) Extent to which fetal signs are within normal limits from conception to the onset of labor

NIC Interventions:
Fluid Management (4120)
Bleeding Reduction: Antepartum Uterus (4021)
Electronic Fetal Monitoring: Intrapartum (6772)

Nursing Interventions:

1. Monitor vital signs every 5–15 minutes with active bleeding or if the vital signs are not stable.

   RATIONALE: The vital signs provide important information about the response of the cardiac system to active bleeding and possible development of shock.

2. Provide continuous monitoring of the FHR and pattern.

   RATIONALE: The fetus reacts directly to an assault on the mother's system. Bleeding from the placenta places the fetus in distress, which is manifested by changes in the FHR.

3. Observe the perineum and behind the patient's back at least every hour for signs of active bleeding. Weigh pads as needed to estimate losses.

   RATIONALE: Observation of active bleeding may indicate the need for an emergency cesarean delivery. One gram of weight can be estimated to equal 1 mL of blood lost.

4. Assess for abdominal pain, palpate fundal tone, and measure abdominal girth at the umbilicus at least each hour.

   RATIONALE: Concealed bleeding into the myometrium may result in a painful, rigid, board-like uterus that becomes enlarged over time.

5. Review baseline and ongoing laboratory data including: complete blood count (CBC), clotting studies, serum electrolytes, and renal function tests.

   RATIONALE: Baseline information is used to alert the care providers to changes in the patient's condition as additional lab tests are obtained.

6. Maintain intravenous access with a large-bore catheter and administer intravenous fluids as directed.

   RATIONALE: Intravenous access is required to maintain and replace fluid volume. Large catheters facilitate the infusion of large volumes of fluid quickly.

7. Administer blood replacement products in a timely manner as directed.

   RATIONALE: The hematocrit level should be 30% or greater to prevent severe shock.

8. Assess hourly intake and output with an indwelling urinary catheter.

   RATIONALE: A decrease in urine output below 30 mL/hr indicates that the patient may be developing shock.

9. Monitor for development of abnormal clotting studies, bleeding from gums, oozing from injection sites, bruising, or petechiae and notify caregiver.

   RATIONALE: The patient is at risk for developing DIC because of excessive bleeding. Fibrinogen levels should be greater than 150 mg/dL.

10. Facilitate delivery as necessary to prevent maternal–fetal injury.

    RATIONALE: If the patient is actively bleeding, or there is any indication that she has concealed bleeding, she must be delivered to prevent hemorrhage, shock, and death.

Adapted from Gilbert, E., & Harmon, J. (2003). *High-risk pregnancy and delivery* (3rd ed.). St. Louis, MO: C.V. Mosby.

Figure 14-8 Rupture of the uterus in the lower uterine segment.

Nursing responsibilities include administering intravenous fluids, blood products, and oxygen and helping to prepare the woman for immediate surgery. Since the patient is anxious and fearful, it is important for the nurse to attempt to provide emotional support for the woman and her support person throughout the process. The nurse must maintain a calm demeanor while organizing critical care for the patient. As much as possible, the patient and her support person should be involved in decision making and informed of all procedures. Depending on the circumstances, it may be appropriate to provide information about chaplain support services. The associated fetal mortality rate ranges from 50% to 75% and the maternal mortality rate may be high if treatment is not initiated immediately (Cunningham et al., 2005).

UTERINE INVERSION

Uterine inversion (uterus is turned inside out) is a rare but potentially life-threatening complication that most often results from excessive pulling on the umbilical cord in an attempt to hasten the third stage of delivery. Other contributing factors include fundal implantation of the placenta, vigorous fundal pressure, uterine atony,

and abnormally adherent placental tissue (Bowes & Thorp, 2004). When complete inversion occurs, a large, red, globular mass (that may contain the still-attached placenta) protrudes 20 to 30 cm outside the vaginal introitus. A partial or incomplete inversion is not visible; instead, a smooth mass is palpated through the dilated cervix. Maternal symptoms include pain, hemorrhage, and shock. Management involves manual replacement of the fundus (under general anesthesia) by the physician, followed by oxytocin to facilitate uterine contractions and antibiotic therapy to prevent infection. Prevention (by not pulling strongly on the cord until the placenta has fully separated) is the safest and most effective therapy (Cunningham et al., 2005).

UMBILICAL CORD PROLAPSE

Umbilical cord prolapse occurs when a loop of the umbilical cord slips down below the presenting part of the fetus (Fig. 14-9). Prolapse of the umbilical cord may be *occult* (hidden; not visible) at any time during labor whether or not the membranes have ruptured—the cord lies beside the presenting part in the pelvic inlet. With a *complete* cord prolapse, the cord descends into the vagina, where it is felt as a pulsating mass on vaginal examination. It may or may not be seen. Frank (visible) prolapse most commonly occurs immediately after rupture of membranes as gravity washes the cord in front of the presenting part. Risk factors associated with cord prolapse include a long (greater than 100 cm) cord, malpresentation (e.g., breech), transverse lie, hydramnios, preterm or low-birth-weight infant, multiple gestation, and unengaged presenting part (Cunningham et al., 2005). If the presenting part does not fit snugly into the lower uterine segment, the sudden gush of amniotic fluid that accompanies rupture of the membranes may cause the cord to be displaced downward.

🌀 **Optimizing Outcomes—** **Actions to reduce the risk of umbilical cord prolapse**

If spontaneous rupture of the membranes (SROM) has occurred, the woman should be kept on bedrest until the fetal presenting part is engaged. Artificial rupture of the membranes (AROM) should not be attempted until engagement has occurred. To rule out umbilical cord prolapse, the nurse should assess the fetal heart sounds immediately after spontaneous or artificial rupture of the membranes.

Figure 14-9 Umbilical cord prolapse. *A.* Occult. The cord cannot be seen or felt during a vaginal examination. *B.* Complete. During a vaginal examination, the cord is felt as a pulsating mass. *C.* Frank. The cord precedes the fetal head or feet and can be seen protruding from the vagina.

It is imperative that the nurse recognizes indicators of umbilical cord prolapse: fetal bradycardia with variable decelerations during contractions; observing or palpating the cord in the vagina; woman's statement that she "feels the cord" after membrane rupture. Prolonged cord compression causes fetal hypoxia; occlusion of blood flow to and from the fetus for greater than 5 minutes is likely to result in central nervous system damage or fetal death.

To relieve pressure on the cord, the examiner places a sterile gloved hand into the vagina and manually lifts the presenting part off of the umbilical cord. The patient is assisted into a position such as a modified Sims, extreme Trendelenburg, or knee–chest position, which uses gravity to cause the presenting part to fall back from the cord (Fig. 14-10). The nurse administers oxygen at 10 L/min by face mask to improve oxygenation to the fetus; the physician may order administration of a tocolytic agent to reduce uterine activity and relieve pressure on the fetus. If the cord is protruding from the vagina, the exposure to room air will cause drying, which leads to atrophy of the umbilical vessels. No attempts should be made to place the cord back into the vagina. Instead, the nurse should cover the exposed segment of umbilical cord with warm, sterile saline compresses to prevent drying. Prompt delivery, often with forceps assistance, is facilitated if the cervix is fully dilated. Otherwise, the

nurse or other care provider continues to manually maintain upward pressure on the presenting part (using a hand in the vagina) until a cesarean birth can be accomplished.

 critical nursing action After Prolapse of the Umbilical Cord

After prolapse of the umbilical cord, immediate nursing interventions are essential:

- Call for assistance; notify the primary health care provider.
- Using the gloved examining hand, insert two fingers into the vagina to the cervix. Place one finger on either side of the cord or both fingers to one side and quickly exert upward pressure against the presenting part to relieve compression of the cord.
- Assist the woman into an extreme Trendelenburg, modified Sims, or knee–chest position.
- If the cord is protruding from the vagina, wrap it loosely in a sterile towel saturated with a warmed, sterile normal saline solution.
- Administer oxygen at 10 L/min by face mask.
- Increase the IV fluids; administer a tocolytic agent as ordered.
- Continuously monitor the FHR by internal fetal scalp electrode if possible.
- Provide information and support to the woman and her birth partner.
- Prepare for an immediate vaginal birth if the cervix is fully dilated or for cesarean birth if it is not.

Figure 14-10 Interventions to relieve pressure on a prolapsed umbilical cord until birth can be effected. *A.* A gloved hand is placed in the vagina to lift the presenting part off the cord. *B.* The maternal hips are elevated with two pillows; this intervention is often combined with a Trendelenburg position. *C.* The knee–chest position uses gravity to shift the fetus out of the maternal pelvis.

VARIATIONS RELATED TO UMBILICAL CORD INSERTION AND THE PLACENTA

Velamentous Cord Insertion/Vasa Previa

A *velamentous* insertion of the umbilical cord occurs when the fetal vessels separate at the distal end of the cord and insert into the placenta at a distance away from the margin (Fig. 14-11). The vessels are not protected by Wharton's jelly and are subject to compression, rupture, and thrombosis, major complications that may lead to severe fetal distress and death. This form of cord insertion most frequently occurs with placenta previa and multiple pregnancies; it may also be associated with fetal anomalies. Rupture of the membranes or traction on the umbilical cord may tear the fetal vessels. This event produces rapid, usually fatal, fetal hemorrhage. **Vasa previa** occurs when the unprotected fetal vessels cover the cervical os and precede the fetus. It is usually seen with a velamentous insertion of the umbilical cord. Because the vessels are not covered with Wharton's jelly, the examiner may be able to feel pulsations of the umbilical cord. Lacerations of the vessels, which can occur at any time, cause sudden fetal blood loss. The onset of sudden, painless bleeding at the beginning of cervical dilation or during rupture of membranes (ROM) may signal the presence of vasa previa; diagnosis may be confirmed by sonogram (Clark, 2004; Cunningham, 2005).

Without ultrasound assessment, velamentous cord insertion is not easily detectable. The nurse may note a drop in FHR during a vaginal exam. A ready FHR return to the baseline after the exam may be indicative of a velamentous cord insertion. With any episode of vaginal bleeding, the alum-precipitated toxoid (APT) test may be used to determine the presence of fetal blood cells. After the rupture of blood vessels, fetal blood leaks into the vagina and can be readily sampled for examination. Despite the rarity of this condition, velamentous cord insertion should always be suspected and ruled out via a careful vaginal exam with cervical palpation for detection of exposed vessels. Immediate action by the medical team, prompted by the nurse's critical assessments, can result in an emergency cesarean birth; best outcomes occur with early prenatal diagnosis and cesarean birth at 35 weeks or earlier (Oyelese et al., 2004).

Circumvallate, Succenturiate, and Battledore Placenta

Other placental variations and problems related to the umbilical cord insertion site include **circumvallate** placenta (placenta circumvallata), **succenturiate** placenta (placenta succenturiata), and **battledore** placenta. These conditions are associated with variations that occurred during placentation (formation and attachment of the placenta). The circumvallate placenta is one in which a ring composed of a double fold of amnion and chorion has formed near the fetal surface. This placental aberration has been reported to be associated with antepartum hemorrhage, preterm delivery, and fetal malformations. The succenturiate placenta contains one or two separate lobes, each with its own circulation. After childbirth, one of the separate lobes may be retained in the uterus and impede contractions, resulting in severe maternal hemorrhage. The remaining lobes must be manually removed from the uterus to prevent hemorrhage. Battledore insertion of the cord describes a condition in which the umbilical cord is implanted near the margin of the placenta. Battledore placenta may be associated with fetal hemorrhage, especially after marginal separation of the placenta (Cunningham et al., 2005).

Placenta Accreta, Placenta Increta, Placenta Percreta

Abnormal adherence of the placenta is rare and its causes are unknown. After birth, the usual maneuvers to remove the placenta are unsuccessful and laceration or perforation of the uterine wall may result. When this occurs, the woman is at high risk for hemorrhage and infection. The placental adherence may be partial or complete. **Placenta accreta** describes a slight penetration of the myometrium by the trophoblast. **Placenta increta** describes a deep placental penetration of the myometrium and **placenta percreta** describes placental perforation of the uterus. Depending on the degree of placental adherence (and the severity of the hemorrhage), the patient will require blood replacement and a vaginal hysterectomy may be indicated (Clark, 2004; Cunningham et al., 2005).

A   B   C   D

Figure 14-11 Variations related to umbilical cord insertion in the placenta. *A.* Velamentous insertion of the umbilical cord. *B.* Circumvallate placenta. *C.* Succenturiate placenta. *D.* Battledore placenta.

AMNIOTIC FLUID EMBOLISM

Amniotic fluid embolism (AFE) (obstruction of a blood vessel by amniotic fluid) is a rare complication of the intra- and postpartum periods that is associated with a high incidence of maternal and fetal death. For mothers, the mortality rate is as high as 80%; approximately 50% of neonates who survive this event have neurological impairment (Schoening, 2006). The origins of the problem are not clear, but it is hypothesized that amniotic fluid containing particles of fetal debris (meconium, hair, vernix, skin cells) escapes into the maternal circulation and causes the release of endogenous mediators such as histamine, prostaglandins, and thromboxane. Obstruction of the pulmonary vessels leads to respiratory distress and circulatory collapse. Hemorrhage, disseminated intravascular coagulation, and pulmonary edema are present to some extent in women who experience an amniotic fluid embolism. AFE is not preventable because it cannot be predicted although maternal factors (including multiparity, abruptio placentae, tumultuous labor) and fetal problems (including macrosomia, meconium passage, death) have been associated with an increased risk for development (Cunningham, 2005).

The nurse must recognize the rapidly deteriorating maternal condition and seek immediate help. Frequently, the first symptom is acute dyspnea, followed by severe hypotension. Other symptoms include restlessness, cyanosis, tachycardia, respiratory arrest, shock, and cardiac arrest (Schoening, 2006).

 critical nursing action   When Amniotic Fluid Embolism Develops

The immediate management includes the administration of oxygen by face mask or cannula at a rate of 8–10 L/min; or resuscitation bag to deliver 100% oxygen. Nursing interventions center on support of resuscitation efforts:

- Prepare for intubation and mechanical ventilation.
- Initiate or assist with cardiopulmonary resuscitation (CPR). Position the pregnant woman in a 30-degree lateral tilt to displace the uterus.
- Administer intravenous fluids and blood (e.g., packed cells; fresh frozen plasma).
- Insert indwelling urinary catheter; measure hourly urine output.
- Continuously monitor maternal–fetal status.
- Prepare for emergency birth once the woman is stable.
- Provide ongoing information and emotional support to the woman and her family.

The maternal prognosis depends on the size of the embolism and speed and skill of the responding perinatal team. If the woman survives, she will most likely be transferred to a critical care unit for hemodynamic monitoring, blood replacement, and coagulopathy treatment. Although rapid delivery is paramount to save the fetus, a delay in delivery usually occurs to stabilize the mother. In the event of maternal cardiopulmonary arrest, for optimal fetal survival, a perimortem cesarean delivery should occur within 5 minutes (Curran, 2003).

This type of a situation is very difficult for all health professionals involved in the care of the patient. An ethical conflict may arise when the health of the mother is given consideration over the fetus. While there are no easy answers to these dilemmas, the nurse can serve as a leader by organizing regular meetings during which issues of this nature can be discussed in a calm, open manner. The nurse is in a key position to help create an environment where health professionals can resolve or work through difficult dilemmas.

Collaboration in Perinatal Emergencies

Approximately 1% to 2% of pregnancies are complicated by an obstetrical emergency and require a multidisciplinary approach to provide an effective, rapid response. Communication is an essential component in all patient environments but it is critical in emergency obstetrical nursing. Team members need to collaborate to provide timely interventions that promote patient safety. Learning how to present information in a way that is non-threatening but effective is key to promoting positive communication patterns (Clements, Flohr-Rincon, Bombard, & Catanzarite, 2007).

Miller (2005) identifies the hierarchical communication that often exists between physicians and nurses as detrimental to good perinatal outcomes. The need to employ healthy communication patterns to effect safe and healthy outcomes for the patient is tantamount. Effective communication does not mean that there are no followers of orders or directives. Instead, it is important for both the leaders and the followers to employ critical thinking skills. Use of the word "we" promotes collaboration and underscores the nurse's role as a patient advocate in this effective communication style.

"What to say" — *Communicating concerns with members of the health care team*

Simpson (2005a) emphasizes the critical need for effective communication among the health care team. Problems in care are encountered when people fail to collaborate or communicate. Teamwork is enhanced when everyone knows the expectations of their role in the obstetric emergency (Box 14-5). Standardization of protocols allows everyone to function more effectively and prevent poor outcomes.

Box 14-5 **Collaborative Care Principles in Perinatal Nursing**

To facilitate the team process when providing care in emergency situations, the perinatal nurse should:

- Employ effective communication techniques.
- Advocate for the patient through assertive statements.
- Conduct interdisciplinary reviews of all cases to identify risks.
- Promote team collaboration by rotating leadership roles in the case reviews.
- Assist in the evaluation process of all emergency cases.
- Use outcome measurements to evaluate safe and effective care.

Perinatal Fetal Loss

The World Health Organization definition of **perinatal death** is death of the offspring "occurring during late pregnancy (at 22 completed weeks gestation and greater), during childbirth and up to seven completed days of life" (Smith, 2005, p. 17). Perinatal deaths can occur during the antepartum, intrapartum, or postpartum periods. A variety of causes may lead to the death of the fetus or the newborn and these are often related to obstetric complications such as placental abruption or neonatal prematurity related to genetic disorders or congenital malformations (Smith, 2005). Perinatal death is rare because the majority of the childbearing population consists of young healthy women who expect to give birth to healthy babies. This prevailing expectation among the general population constitutes a major reason why it is so difficult for all involved when a perinatal death occurs.

Nursing practice has changed over the years in regard to caring for families who are dealing with a perinatal loss. During the 1960s through the 1980s, women who experienced a perinatal loss were often placed on a medical–surgical unit to prevent them from hearing the sounds of infants crying. One problem with this approach lies in the fact that the most experienced professionals in perinatal nursing are not located in the medical–surgical areas. The patient who has suffered a loss still requires all assessments and interventions involved in normal postpartum care. A nurse in the perinatal practice area can better focus on therapeutic interventions to assist the woman and her family in the grieving process.

The nurse organizes and coordinates a team approach to bereavement. Different members may participate but there should be key individuals such as spiritual or religious representatives, social workers, and physicians, in addition to the nurse. It is important to identify which hospital routines associated with perinatal death might interfere with allowing the family to have options concerning decisions made regarding their infant. As an example, in some cases, the infant's body might be moved to the funeral home before the family has had the opportunity to hold him or her. Many parents wish to hold their child prior to an autopsy, and they should be encouraged to do so. Before presenting the parents with their infant, the nurse should make certain the infant has been cleaned and is wrapped in a soft blanket. Depending on the cause of death, it may also be prudent to give the parents an idea of their infant's appearance. Usually, parents' preconceived perceptions concerning how their infant will look is much worse than the reality. Individuals from the hospital morgue or a funeral home who are involved with regular bereavement team meetings can be instrumental in developing a perinatal bereavement plan that is grounded in compassion and sensitivity.

When healthy infants are discharged, it is common practice to take their picture. Photographs should also be taken when an infant has died. Parents should always be encouraged to view, touch, and hold the deceased infant. However, if they do not wish to see the infant while in the hospital, the picture provides a way for them to see their infant at a future time when they are ready. Photographs can be stored in a file and given to the parents upon their request. Use of an experienced photographer is preferred, since the infant may not always be in the most favorable condition. The maternity unit should always have a supply of clothing and new blankets available for these infants.

To provide the family as much privacy as possible from hospital workers who might not know that the family has experienced a loss it is best to have some sort of indicator outside of the room. One hospital unit places a single red rose across the door. Another places a special "remembrance card" outside the doorframe. Both provide an immediate identification to any hospital worker entering the room that the patient and her family have experienced a loss.

All of these practices stem from the development of hospital protocols regarding bereavement. The team develops a list of critical actions and specific plans to respond to each point. There is flexibility to allow the parents to be active participants in the decision making but it is also organized so that as nursing and hospital personnel change, there is consistency in the approach.

Communication is another critical factor in providing care for the family who has experienced a fetal or neonatal loss. Parents report that comforting words, touch, and directed speech are helpful to them. Nurses need to avoid using phrases such as:

- "It's God's will."
- "You can always have another."
- "There was a problem with this baby."
- "There's always next time."

Parents respond better to acknowledgment of the infant's death than to avoidance. A simple "I'm sorry" and a touch of the hand can convey the nurse's care and concern when the right words are hard to find. It is also important for the nurse to sit and listen. Parents often have multiple feelings, which they need to share. The nurse, as the objective individual, can help interpret feelings and recommend resources to assist the family as they deal with their grief. It is essential that the perinatal care team remain sensitive to the cultural and spiritual beliefs and practices of the bereaved parents and families. (See Chapter 11 for further discussion.)

" What to say " — *To the mother whose newborn has died*

When caring for the mother whose infant has died, the nurse conveys compassion by simply being available. Often, the mother finds comfort in talking about the birth experience, her infant, and how she will cope with her loss. The nurse can gain insights into the mother's support systems by asking the following questions:

"What are you most worried or fearful about?"

"How supportive is the baby's father and your family or friends?"

"What coping techniques have been helpful for you in the past?"

(Gilbert, 2006)

A perinatal loss might be the first experience a family has with death. It is a confusing, anxiety-provoking time that often creates a fear that it will happen again. Death of a child of any age is also viewed as unnatural. Parents expect their children to die after them—not before them. Dreams and expectations for the lost child will now never be realized. A resource guide given to the family on discharge is an important tool to help them cope with their loss. Since much of the grieving work is done after the hospitalization, family members need to know where to call for help.

A support group that includes someone from the bereavement team can offer the parents a connection to the hospital. Some parents find this helpful in acknowledging the existence of their child while others feel more comfortable with the support of a close family network. The key is that the family is supported through their loss and is able to move through the grief process toward resolution. It is important to understand that many families will never totally come to terms with the untimely death of a child, regardless of the age of the infant or fetus.

CULTURAL ASPECTS OF LOSS

In a cultural context, death has many views. There are different ways of grieving. Tears and emotional outbursts are common to some cultures while others are quiet and introspective. The nurse needs to have an awareness and understanding of how different cultural groups interpret the meaning of death and the factors that govern their response to death. The Hispanic culture that includes Mexicans, Puerto Ricans, and Cubans views children as their future. The loss of a child denies that future. They welcome touch from others and expect health care professionals to respect their need for extended family during this time frame. All cultures should be treated with sensitivity, respect and caring (Gilbert, 2006).

 Now Can You— Discuss Issues Concerning Perinatal Death?

1. Identify significant members of the bereavement team?
2. Discuss interventions for families experiencing a perinatal loss?
3. Voice some comments that would be helpful for a grieving family?

Cesarean Birth

DEFINITION AND INCIDENCE

Cesarean birth is the birth of a fetus through an abdominal incision into the uterus; it is performed to preserve the life of the mother and her fetus. In 1965, the rate of cesarean births in the United States was less than 5% (Hamilton et al., 2005). Preliminary data for 2005 indicate that 30.2% of all live births in this country were cesarean births, marking the highest U.S. total cesarean rate ever reported. Since 1996, the number of cesarean births has increased by 46%, driven by both an increase in the percentage of all women having a first cesarean and a decline in the percentage of women who gave birth vaginally after a previous cesarean birth (CDC, 2007). Modern surgical advances and the use of antibiotics have resulted in a decrease in maternal and fetal morbidity and mortality. However, despite these advances, cesarean birth is a major surgical procedure that poses threats to the health of the mother and her infant.

INDICATIONS

Cesarean birth is performed when the health of the mother or her fetus is jeopardized. Maternal medical risk factors most closely associated with cesarean birth include hypertensive disorders, active genital herpes, positive HIV status, and diabetes. Fetal complications most closely associated with cesarean birth include CPD, malpresentations (i.e., breech, shoulder), placental abnormalities (e.g., abruptio, previa), dysfunctional labor patterns, fetal distress, multiple gestation, and umbilical cord prolapse. In actuality, few absolute indications exist for cesarean birth and most are primarily performed for the benefit of the fetus (Martin et al., 2005).

Elective cesarean births have been on the rise since 1985. In contemporary society, women are requesting cesarean births for reasons other than medical, obstetric, or fetal complications. One reason is related to a fear of vaginal birth, or tocophobia. Others are concerned about the potential for future problems with pelvic support or sexual dysfunction related to perineal or rectal injury. Some women view cesarean birth to be an empowering experience and wish to choose the birth method and date rather than have it selected for them (Tillett, 2005; Williams, 2005). At issue is the question of whether or not an elective cesarean birth is more beneficial or harmful to a woman and her baby than a vaginal birth (Hannah, 2004). The Association of Women's Health, Obstetric and Gynecologic and Neonatal Nurses (AWHONN) supports the need to learn more about the nature of elective cesarean birth. AWHONN calls for continued research into strategies to decrease traumas associated with vaginal birth and subsequently decrease the need for elective cesarean birth due to maternal fear (Simpson & Thorman, 2005; Wax, Cartin, Pinette, & Blackstone, 2004; Williams, 2005).

Cesarean birth is a major surgical procedure that carries risks and complications. It is associated with a host of potential postoperative problems such as hemorrhage, thromboembolism, and infection during the postpartum period. The surgery can result in adhesions, dehiscence of the wound, and problems with the placenta in subsequent pregnancies (Porter & Scott, 2003). Zelop and Heffner (2004) report that women face a higher incidence of death during a surgical procedure with the use of general anesthesia. Women are also at greater risk for intraoperative surgical complications such as lacerations of the uterus and bladder. In addition, there is a greater likelihood for hysterectomy associated with cesarean birth than with vaginal birth.

ETHICAL CONSIDERATIONS OF ELECTIVE CESAREAN BIRTH

If it is more dangerous to have an elective cesarean birth than a vaginal birth, is it ethical to allow the woman to select this as her birth method of choice? Wax (2004) discusses the contrast between beneficence (the principle of doing good) and the physician's responsibility to do no harm and the patient's right to autonomy. The American College of Obstetricians and Gynecologists (ACOG) Committee on Ethics maintains that if a patient requests a cesarean birth, and the physician believes that the overall health of the mother and fetus will benefit, then the elective cesarean delivery has merit (ACOG, 2003b). If the physician does not think a cesarean method of birth is in the best interest of the patient, the patient should be informed and given the right to select another physician. However, the issue is far more complex than this simple example.

Williams and Shah (2003) plead for a return to common sense. Birth is a normal and natural event. These authors raise the following questions: "Have we become a nation so obsessed with expediency and control that we are willing to relinquish our humanity to technology? Are we truly willing to sacrifice our health and future childbearing for the lure of 'birth by appointment'? Are our demands for perfection or compensation unnecessary interventions (p. 284)?" All women are entitled to unbiased information and a safe, supportive environment. Continued studies that examine the myriad issues concerning aspects of benefit versus harm including the economic ramifications of elective cesarean birth are in order.

SURGICAL PROCEDURES

There are two main types of cesarean operations: the classic (vertical) incision and the lower-segment transverse (LST) incision (Fig. 14-12). The surgeon chooses the incision type based on the patient's condition and the fetal status. Rarely used today, the classic cesarean incision is reserved for some cases of shoulder presentation, placenta previa, and when birth must take place immediately. Since this type of uterine incision is associated with complications including considerable blood loss, infection, and uterine rupture with subsequent pregnancies, women who undergo classic cesarean births may not attempt future vaginal births.

The lower segment cesarean (preferred by women for cosmetic reasons) may involve either a vertical or a transverse uterine incision. The transverse incision, more commonly performed, is associated with less blood loss, fewer postoperative infections, and a decreased likelihood of uterine rupture during subsequent pregnancies (Bowes & Thorp, 2004; Cunningham et al., 2005). The skin incision made into the abdomen is either transverse (sometimes called a "Pfannenstiel" or "bikini" incision) or vertical (sometimes called a "midline" incision). The skin incision may or may not be the same type of incision that is made into the abdomen. After the skin incision, the surgeon carefully moves through the tissue layers to the uterus. An incision is made into the uterus and the fetal head is gently elevated through the opening. A patent airway is established and the rest of the fetus is delivered. The cord is clamped and the newborn is placed, depending on the circumstances, either in the arms of the parent or in the neonatal warmer. After removal of the placenta, the incision is sutured at each layer and a sterile bandage is placed over it (Cunningham et al., 2005; Porter & Scott, 2003).

The nurse documents all components of patient care including the time of birth and offers ongoing encouragement and support to the mother. Once the birth has taken place, the nurse facilitates attachment with the new family. When complications are present, the nurse provides information including a description of the newborn to the family. If the newborn requires resuscitation or a transfer to the neonatal intensive care unit, the family is allowed to view the neonate in the isolette before transport. When the newborn's condition is satisfactory, the newborn is presented to the parent or support person to hold. Although the mother is restrained by surgical equipment, the parent or support person can hold the baby close to the mother's face so that she can see her child. This initial bonding experience can usually take place while the surgeon completes the suturing process. The family is then moved to the recovery room for post-surgical care.

NURSING CARE

In most instances, the patient scheduled for a planned cesarean birth is admitted on the day of surgery. When the need for an emergency or unplanned cesarean arises, the patient undergoes the same procedures but in a more timely manner. Blood work, including type and cross match and a complete blood count, is obtained before admission and the results are entered in the chart. The woman has been instructed to remain NPO since midnight before admission. The nurse orients the patient to the unit, reviews the prenatal history, and responds to any questions or concerns. An informed consent is signed. A fetal monitor is placed on the patient's abdomen for a 20- to 30-minute baseline assessment. Vital signs are taken and charted. In preparation for the surgery, the abdomen is cleaned and shaved, an intravenous line is placed, and an indwelling urinary catheter is inserted to keep the bladder empty during the operation. Medications are administered according to the physician's orders. If an epidural anesthetic is to be used, the nurse properly positions the patient and supports her during its administration. If a general anesthetic is to be used, an oral antacid may be prescribed to neutralize gastric secretions in the event of aspiration. The woman is then transported to the operative suite (Simpson & Creehan, 2001).

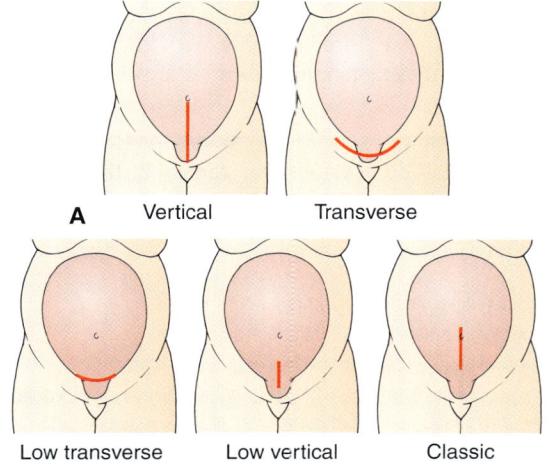

A Vertical Transverse

B Low transverse Low vertical Classic

Figure 14-12 Abdominal wall and uterine incisions for cesarean births. *A.*Skin (abdominal wall) incisions. Vertical and transverse (Pfannenstiel). *B.*Uterine wall incisions. Low transverse, low vertical, classic.

🌀 **Optimizing Outcomes—** **Enhancing maternal anesthesia knowledge and choice**

Spinal, epidural, and general anesthesia are used for cesarean births. Although epidural anesthesia is a popular choice because the woman may remain awake during the birth experience, the type of anesthesia used depends on factors such as the maternal medical history and current status, and how quickly the birth needs to take place. In addition, the woman is a factor—she may harbor fears about having an anesthetic injected into her back. Patients should be given information including the risks and benefits associated with the different types of anesthesia to empower them to make an informed decision whenever there is a choice.

SURGICAL CARE

The nurse's role varies during the surgical procedure. Depending on the hospital setting and protocols, one nurse assists the physician during the procedure while another nurse circulates. A team consisting of a neonatal nurse and a neonatologist or nurse skilled in neonatal resuscitation is in attendance to provide care for the infant. The patient is placed on the surgical table with a hip wedge to slightly elevate the hips. The fetal heart rate is continuously monitored until the patient's abdomen is ready for surgical preparation according to hospital protocol. The support person, dressed in appropriate surgical attire, may be present at any point in the process but is usually asked to wait until the surgical drapes are in place before being seated by the patient's head. The anesthesiologist monitors the maternal vital signs and the intravenous solutions.

When the woman remains awake during the procedure, the nurse and other members of the care team provide information about the events taking place and sensations that the woman may be experiencing. Continued support and explanations help to decrease anxiety, enhance feelings of comfort, and help the woman to maintain a sense of control in the unfamiliar and perhaps frightening, environment.

POSTOPERATIVE CARE

After the completion of the surgery, the woman is transferred to a recovery room or to her labor room. According to agency protocol, the nurse assesses various aspects of the recovery progress, including effects from the anesthesia, the status of the postoperative/postbirth uterus, and the degree of pain. If a general anesthetic was used, special attention is given to maintenance of a patent airway. The patient is positioned to prevent aspiration and vital signs are assessed every 15 minutes for the first 2 hours, or until stable. The nurse frequently inspects the incisional dressing and assesses the fundus, the amount of lochia, the intravenous infusion, and the urinary output. The woman is assisted to turn, cough, deep breathe, and perform leg exercises. Pain medications are administered as needed.

If the neonate is with the mother and her labor support, time is provided to facilitate family bonding and attachment. If the woman wishes to breastfeed, she is encouraged to do so. Patients generally remain in the recovery area for 1 to 2 hours before transfer to the postpartum unit for continued care. (See Chapter 15.)

VAGINAL BIRTH AFTER CESAREAN

There is an old adage, "once a cesarean, always a cesarean." During the 1970s and 1980s, women challenged this rule and fought for the opportunity to attempt a **vaginal birth after a cesarean birth** (VBAC). Dauphinee (2004)

reported that research conducted during that time provided evidence that a VBAC was safe and a more cost-effective birth alternative. This movement also coincided with the growing concern in the United States over the dramatic increase in cesarean birth rates, especially among women requiring a repeat cesarean birth.

In 1988, the American College of Obstetricians and Gynecologists (ACOG), having concluded that women with a low transverse incision could safely be allowed a trial of labor and possible vaginal birth, released a statement in support of VBAC. ACOG endorsed the practice of oxytocin administration, epidural anesthesia, and early ambulation for women with previous cesarean births who met certain criteria. A standby team prepared to perform a cesarean birth in the event of an emergency was to be available at all times (Dauphinee, 2004). Numerous studies supported the success of VBAC. During the 1990s, approximately 60% to 80% of women who underwent a trial of labor following a previous cesarean were able to give birth vaginally with minimal complications (Porter & Scott, 2003). Safety concerns arose although data showed that uterine rupture, the most serious of complications, was a rare event. In response to these concerns, physicians began to more closely restrict the types of patients allowed to attempt a trial of labor. Criteria for the selection of candidates for a trial of labor have been developed (Box 14-6). A critical point confirmed by the studies was that VBACs needed to be performed in large hospitals or tertiary level centers since these institutions offer continued 24-hour anesthesia coverage necessary to prevent perinatal mortality and morbidity if uterine rupture occurs (Porter & Scott, 2003).

NURSING IMPLICATIONS

To provide safe, effective care, it is essential that nurses who care for patients in the labor and birth suite have received extensive training in fetal monitoring interpretation. At the first sign of any abnormality in the fetal heart rate tracing, the nurse must alert the physician or certified nurse midwife. Meticulous documentation is critical, as it provides essential information to other members of the health care team. For the elective cesarean birth, informed consent is obtained in the physician's office before admission and the nurse confirms this with the patient. Once patients actually experience labor, it is possible for them

---

Box 14-6 Selection Criteria for Vaginal Birth After Cesarean Birth (VBAC)

- One previous low-transverse cesarean birth (If two prior cesarean births, only those who have also had a vaginal birth as well should be considered candidates for a spontaneous labor)
- Clinically adequate pelvis in relation to fetal size
- No other uterine scars, anomalies, or previous rupture
- Physician immediately available throughout active labor capable of monitoring labor and performing an emergency cesarean birth
- Availability of anesthesia and personnel for emergency cesarean birth

Source: American College of Obstetricians and Gynecologists (ACOG). (2004a). *Vaginal birth after previous cesarean delivery* (Practice Bulletin No. 54). Washington, DC: Author.

to change their minds and, depending upon the circumstances, they may choose not to have a vaginal birth. As in other situations, the nurse responds to questions and concerns and ascertains the patient's understanding of the associated benefits and risks (Dauphinee, 2004).

During the entire labor process the nurse is alert for any changes in the maternal–fetal condition. The FHR pattern and uterine activity are usually monitored electronically during the active phase of labor. Non-reassuring FHR patterns such as prolonged decelerations, late decelerations, and variable decelerations, may precede uterine rupture or herald its occurrence. The nurse continuously evaluates the woman's level of pain. Uterine rupture may be accompanied by abdominal, shoulder, or back pain even when epidural anesthesia has been administered. However, the nurse should frequently palpate the uterus for signs of rigidity since the patient may report no pain. Since there is always the possibility of an emergency at any time, the nurse must be prepared to react in a calm manner. As the labor progresses, the patient and her support(s) should receive reassurance and information regarding any change in the plan of care (Dauphinee, 2004).

 Now Can You— **Discuss VBAC?**

1. Name five criteria for a patient to be allowed to attempt a vaginal birth after a previous cesarean birth?
2. Discuss possible patient concerns regarding VBAC and how the nurse should appropriately respond to them?
3. List three specific nursing implications associated with the care of the woman who is experiencing a VBAC?

RESEARCH FINDINGS AND IMPLICATIONS

The rising rate of cesarean births and the decrease in the number of vaginal births after cesarean births (VBAC) are related. The higher the number of first-time mothers who experience a cesarean delivery, the higher the number of women who may not have a choice for a vaginal delivery the next time if their physician is reluctant to attempt a VBAC. Medical studies currently question the rising cesarean birth rate. Kabir and colleagues (2004) evaluated a large database of U.S. patients and concluded that a high proportion of unnecessary cesarean births occur. For study purposes, an "unnecessary cesarean birth" was defined as one that occurred when there were no identified medical risks or adverse circumstances. The adverse consequences of higher cesarean birth rates contribute to an increase in maternal morbidity and mortality. In addition, there are significant economic costs related to the prolonged hospital stays and the increased need for expensive surgery-related technologies. Although the greatest concern centers on the health and safety of the mother and her fetus, burgeoning health care costs cannot be discounted as a problem (Kabir et al., 2004).

Nurse researchers should continue to examine evidence to provide a better understanding of the factors that impact the cesarean birth rate. A few of the modifiable variables include maternal obesity, fear of labor and delivery, physiological pushing techniques, fear of injury, and convenience in planning a birth. Nurses need to engage in clinical research designed to offer evidence identifying the myriad of factors that contribute to the rise in cesarean births. The results of such studies may lead to a decrease in the overall cesarean birth rate, which has risen steadily throughout the last decade. Nurse educators in the community can provide supportive interventions for all of these issues. Counseling during the prenatal period to allay anxieties and fears is critical. Families also need realistic plans for the childbirth along with thorough explanations of procedures and what they should expect (Tillett, 2005).

Prepared childbirth classes have increased in numbers and variety in the United States. Although many health educators serve an important role, the nurse with a clinical practice in obstetrics and women's health is in an ideal position to offer constructive guidance to families. Families need to learn to advocate for themselves through increased knowledge and understanding of the issues surrounding operative deliveries. If women's fears concerning childbirth are lessened, they become more open to teaching and can begin to function as collaborators in their own care. For example, perinatal education and selective tension-reducing labor techniques may reduce the woman's fear of labor and birth. Perhaps women who are able to overcome their fear of labor will choose to attempt vaginal birth instead of an elective cesarean birth. Nurses who serve as childbirth educators have a unique opportunity to empower women and their families through education and this new knowledge and self confidence may translate into a reduction in the rate of cesarean births.

Postterm Pregnancy/Prolonged Pregnancy

A **postterm pregnancy** is defined as one that extends beyond 294 days or 42 weeks past the first day of the last normal menstrual period. Stated another way, a postterm pregnancy has gone at least 1 day past 42 completed weeks (gestational age 42+1). A similar term, **postdate**, identifies a pregnancy that has gone past the estimated date of birth. It is estimated that postterm pregnancies occur in approximately 3% to 12% of all pregnancies.

Prolonged pregnancies are at risk for a number of problems including fetal macrosomia associated with shoulder dystocia and fetal injury, oligohydramnios, meconium aspiration, intrapartum fetal distress, and stillbirth. Neonatal problems may include asphyxia, meconium aspiration syndrome, hypoglycemia, polycythemia, respiratory distress, and dysmaturity syndrome (Gilbert, 2006).

Maternal risks such as trauma, hemorrhage, infection, and labor abnormalities are also associated with postterm pregnancy. Labor interventions including induction with prostaglandins or oxytocin, forceps- or vacuum-assisted birth and cesarean birth are more likely to be needed. In addition, the woman may experience fatigue and psychological responses such as depression, frustration, loss of control, and feelings of inadequacy as the pregnancy extends beyond the estimated date of birth (ACOG, 2004b; Moore & Martin, 2003).

The exact cause of postterm pregnancy is unknown. However, a possible cause may be related to a deficiency of placental estrogen and the continued secretion of progesterone. Low levels of estrogen may result in a decrease in prostaglandin precursors and the reduced formation of myometrial oxytocin receptors (Gilbert, 2006). A woman with a history of one postterm pregnancy is more likely to experience another with subsequent pregnancies (Divon, 2002).

Because the placenta ages rapidly past the fortieth week of gestation, it becomes inefficient and cannot adequately support the fetus. A decrease in oxygen and nutrients results in fetal hypoxic episodes. Hypoxic events that occur on a regular basis stress the fetus. When labor commences, the postterm compromised fetus is at a greater risk for severe distress than the nonstressed term infant (Gilbert, 2006).

Antenatal testing combined with careful expectant management is used to monitor fetal status beyond the fortieth week of gestation. Antenatal testing is not viewed as a predictor of an untoward event but as a way to identify the fetus that demonstrates signs of compromise. The antenatal assessments most often obtained include non-stress tests (NST), biophysical profiles (BPP), amniotic fluid volume (AFV) measurements and maternal daily fetal movement counts. Other tests include the contraction stress test (CST), which relies on oxytocin-stimulated contractions to identify FHR decelerations associated with fetal hypoxia and Doppler flow measurements. The tests are usually performed on a weekly or twice-weekly basis (Cunningham et al., 2005; Divon, 2002). (See Chapter 11 for further discussion.)

MEDICAL MANAGEMENT

If a woman does not experience spontaneous labor by the 42nd week (sometimes earlier), induction is considered the primary medical management choice. Expectant management, including daily kick counts, weekly monitoring of the amniotic fluid index, and non-stress testing provide information regarding fetal well-being but are not always conclusive. If the gestational age is documented by ultrasound to be beyond 42 weeks and the cervix is favorable, most physicians proceed with labor induction. A cervix that is favorable (i.e., one that has begun to efface and dilate) is more conducive to the induction. If the cervix is not favorable, a cervical ripening agent (e.g., prostaglandin insert or gel) may be administered, followed by oxytocin induction (ACOG, 2004b; Resnik & Resnik, 2004). Some women with an unfavorable cervix may choose to continue with careful daily monitoring instead of the induction. As long as the physician considers the surveillance to be a safe option, the patient may be allowed to continue with the process of expectant management. However, if spontaneous labor does not begin by the 42nd or 43rd week, most physicians proceed with induction (Beckman et al., 2002).

NURSING IMPLICATIONS

The nurse conducts the non-stress and nipple stimulation contraction stress tests in the antepartum clinical setting, interprets information for the patient and provides reassurance. The nurse must be cautious in providing only the factual information. Since there is a possibility of false readings, the nurse must avoid offering unfound reassurances and immediately notify the physician if test results are not normal. Understandably, patients often experience increased anxiety when their due date has passed and they are still pregnant. The nurse is in a position to provide a consistent presence and respond to any questions or concerns. If induction is decided as the treatment option, the nurse explains the procedure to the patient and again responds to questions and concerns.

Intrapartal nursing care centers on close maternal–fetal surveillance and continued emotional support. During labor, the fetus should be monitored electronically to obtain an accurate assessment of the FHR and pattern. Umbilical cord compression, which is more likely to occur in the presence of decreased amniotic fluid, results in fetal hypoxia. Variable or prolonged deceleration patterns and the passage of meconium are reflective of fetal hypoxia. If oligohydramnios is present, amnioinfusion may be performed to restore the amniotic fluid volume to provide a fluid cushion for the umbilical cord (Cunningham et al., 2005).

summary points

- The nurse serves in many capacities when managing the care of women experiencing a complicated labor and birth; a strong theoretical background provides a foundation for the necessary critical decision making.

- Dystocia, a long, difficult or abnormal labor, may arise from any of the three major components of the labor process: the powers, passenger or passageway.

- During a trial of labor, nursing responsibilities center on assessment of maternal vital signs and fetal heart rate and pattern.

- Oxytocin used during labor induction and augmentation should always be administered as a "piggyback" solution, and a uterine and FHR monitor should be used continuously during the infusion.

- Forceps and vacuum extraction are methods to assist birth; the mother and the infant require special observation during and after these procedures.

- The management of hypertensive disorders during intrapartum is focused on preventing further deterioration of affected organs and fostering a positive maternal–fetal outcome.

- Cesarean birth, which may be a scheduled or emergency procedure, is associated with increased risk for the mother and her infant and should be undertaken only when medically necessary.

- Perinatal loss necessitates a collaborative response from all professionals involved in the care of the patient.

review questions

Multiple Choice

1. When reviewing hypotonic labor, the perinatal nurse explains to a student nurse that the leading cause of this dysfunctional labor pattern is:
   A. Fetal macrosomia
   B. Maternal android pelvis
   C. Inadequate uterine pacemakers
   D. Fetal occiput posterior position

2. The perinatal nurse is aware that the minimal amount of fluid that would be infused for an amnioinfusion is:
A. 500 mL
B. 300 mL
C. 250 mL
D. 800 mL

3. The perinatal nurse understands that one of the risks of oxytocin infusion includes fetal heart rate changes related to:
A. Decreased placental perfusion
B. Oligohydramnios
C. Maternal hypotonic contractions
D. Maternal hypotension

True/False

4. The perinatal nurse understands the definition of hypotonic labor to be one that has fewer than five contractions in a 10-minute period.

5. The perinatal nurse is aware that clinical signs that require discontinuation of an amnioinfusion include maternal shortness of breath or tachycardia.

6. The perinatal nurse recognizes that the presence of hydramnios, which occurs when there is an excessive amount of amniotic fluid, may increase the risk of prolapsed umbilical cord following rupture of membranes.

Fill-in-the-Blank

7. The perinatal nurse knows that fetal macrosomia is significantly related to maternal _____ measurement and _____ _____.

8. After a precipitous birth, the perinatal nurse carefully assesses the mother and her neonate for signs or symptoms of _____.

9. In providing information to a woman in labor who is to have an amniotomy, the perinatal nurse identifies _____ to be one of the procedure's risks, which means that there will be a commitment to have this birth occur in a timely manner.

Case Study

10. The perinatal nurse is caring for Christy, a 22-year-old G3 TPAL 1011, who is 9 cm. dilated and contracting every 2 to 3 minutes. Her labor has been rapid and she has been admitted in the last 30 minutes. Christy's membranes rupture spontaneously and the perinatal nurse is not able to auscultate the fetal heart. The most immediate nursing action is to:
A. Check the perineum for the possibility of a prolapsed umbilical cord.
B. Reposition the Doppler to attempt to auscultate the fetal heart rate.
C. Reposition Christy to a left lateral position.
D. Reassure Christy that her labor is progressing well.

See Answers to End of Chapter Review Questions on the Electronic Study Guide or DavisPlus.

REFERENCES

American College of Obstetricians and Gynecologists (ACOG). (1999). *Induction of labor* (Practice Bulletin No. 10, pp 603–612). Washington DC: Author.

American College of Obstetricians and Gynecologists (ACOG). (2001). *Gestational diabetes* (Practice Bulletin No. 30, pp 695–708). Washington, DC: Author.

American College of Obstetricians and Gynecologists (ACOG). (2002a). *Diagnosis and management of preeclampsia and eclampsia* (Practice Bulletin No. 33). Washington, DC: Author.

American College of Obstetricians and Gynecologists (ACOG). (2002b). *Shoulder dystocia* (Practice Bulletin No. 40). Washington, DC: Author.

American College of Obstetricians and Gynecologists (ACOG). (2003a). *Management of preterm labor* (Practice Bulletin No. 43). Washington, DC: Author.

American College of Obstetricians and Gynecologists (ACOG). (2003b). *New ACOG opinion addresses elective cesarean controversy,* ACOG news release, October 31, 2003. Washington, DC: Author.

American College of Obstetricians and Gynecologists (ACOG). (2004a). *Vaginal birth after previous cesarean delivery* (Practice Bulletin No. 54). Washington, DC: Author.

American College of Obstetricians and Gynecologists (ACOG). (2004b). *Management of postterm pregnancy* (Practice Bulletin No. 55). Washington, DC: Author.

American College of Obstetricians and Gynecologists (ACOG). (2005). *Intrapartum fetal heart rate monitoring* (Practice Bulletin No. 70). Washington, DC: Author.

Ananth, C., Oyelese, Y., Yeo, L., Pradhan, A., & Vintzileos, A. (2005). Placental abruption in the United States, 1979 through 2001: Temporal trends and potential determinants. *American Journal of Obstetrics and Gynecology, 192*(1), 191–198.

Baxley, E., & Gobbo, R. (2004). Shoulder dystocia. *American Family Physician, 69*(7), 57–68.

Beckman, C., Ling, F., Laube, D., Smith, R., Barzansky, B., & Herbert, W. (2002). *Obstetrics and Gynecology* (4th ed.). Philadelphia: Lippincott Williams & Wilkins.

Belfort, M. (2003). Operative vaginal delivery. In J.R. Scott, R.S. Gibbs, B.Y. Karlan, & A.F. Haney (Eds.), *Danforth's obstetrics and gynecology* (9th ed., pp. 419–447). Philadelphia: Lippincott Williams & Wilkins.

Bernasko, J. (2004). Contemporary management of type I diabetes mellitus in pregnancy. *Obstetrical and Gynecological Survey, 59*(8), 628–636.

Bowes, W., & Thorp, J. (2004). Clinical aspects of normal and abnormal labor. In R. Creasy, R. Resnik, & J. Iams (Eds.), *Maternal-fetal medicine: Principles and practice* (5th ed.). Philadelphia: W.B. Saunders.

Bulechek, G., Butcher, H.M., & Dochterman, J. (2008). *Nursing interventions classification (NIC)* (5th ed.). St. Louis, MO: C.V. Mosby.

Camune, B., & Brucker, M.C. (2007). An overview of shoulder dystocia. *Nursing for Women's Health, 11*(5), 490–498.

Canavan, T., Simhan, H., & Cartis, S. (2004). An evidenced-based approach to the evaluation and treatment of premature rupture of membranes. Part II. *Obsterical & Gynecological Survey, 59*(9), 678–689.

Centers for Disease Control and Prevention (CDC). (2007). Quick Stats: Percentage of all live births by cesarean delivery—National vital statistics system, United States, 2005. *MMWR Morbidity and Mortality Weekly Report, 56*(15), 1–2.

Chan, P., & Winkle, C. (2006). *Gynecology and obstetrics: Current clinical strategies.* Laguna Hills, CA: CCS Publishing.

Church, S., & Hodgson, T. (2003). Disordered uterine action In J.R. Scott, R.S. Gibbs, B.Y. Karlan, & A.F. Haney (Eds.), *Danforth's obstetrics and gynecology* (9th ed., pp. 876–883). Philadelphia: Lippincott Williams & Wilkins.

Clark, S. (2004). Placenta previa and abruptio placentae. In R. Creasy, R. Resnik, & J. Iams (Eds.), *Maternal-fetal medicine: Principles and practice* (5th ed.). Philadelphia: W.B. Saunders.

Clements, C.J., Flohr-Rincon, S., Bombard, A.T., & Catanzarite, V. (2007). OB team stat: Rapid response to obstetrical emergencies. *Nursing for Women's Health, 11*(2), 194–198.

Culver, J., Strauss, R., Brody, S., Dorman, K., Timlin, S., & McMahon, M. (2004). A randomized trial of intracervical Foley catheter with concurrent oxytocin compared to vaginal misoprostol for labor induction in nulliparous women [Supplement]. *American Journal of Obstetrics & Gynecology, 185*(6), S203.

Cunningham, F., Leveno, K., Bloom, S., Hauth, J., Gilstrap, L., & Wenstrom, K. (2005). *Williams' obstetrics* (22nd ed.). New York: McGraw-Hill.

Curran, C. (2003). Intrapartum emergencies. *Journal of Obstetric, Gynecologic, and Neonatal Nursing, 32*(6), 802–813.

Dauphinee, J. (2004). VBAC: Safety for the patient and the nurse. *Journal of Obstetric Gynecologic and Neonatal Nursing, 33*(1), 105–115.

Deglin, J.H., & Vallerand, A.H. (2009). *Davis's drug guide for nurses* (11th ed.). Philadelphia: F.A. Davis.

Divon, M. (2002). Prolonged pregnancy. In S. Gabbe, J. Niebyl, & J. Simpson (Eds.), *Obstetrics: Normal and problem pregnancies* (4th ed.). New York: Churchill Livingstone.

Dudley, D. (2003). Complications of labor. In J.R. Scott, R.S. Gibbs, B.Y. Karlan, & A.F. Haney (Eds.), *Danforth's obstetrics and gynecology* (9th ed., pp. 397–417). Philadelphia: Lippincott Williams & Wilkins.

Fraser, W.D., Hofmeyr, J., Lede, R., Faron, G., Alexander, S., Goffinet, F., Ohisson, A., et al. (2005). Amnioinfusion for the prevention of meconium aspiration syndrome. *New England Journal of Medicine, 353*(9), 909–917.

Gherman, R.B. (2005). Shoulder dystocia prevention and management. *Obstetrics and Gynecology Clinics of North America, 32,* 297–305.

Gilbert, E.S. (2006). *Manual of high risk pregnancy and delivery.* St. Louis, MO: C.V. Mosby.

Gilbert, E., & Harmon, J. (2003). *High-risk pregnancy and delivery* (3rd ed.). St. Louis, MO: C.V. Mosby.

Gülmezoglu, A.M., Crowther, C.A., & Middleton, P. (2006). Induction of labor for improving birth outcomes for women at or beyond term. *Cochrane Database of Systematic Reviews* 2006, Issue 4. Art. No.: CD004945. DOI: 10.1002/14651858.CD004945.pub2

Hall, L., & Neubert, A. (2005). Obesity and pregnancy. *Obstetrical and Gynecological Survey, 60*(4), 253–260.

Hamilton, B., Martin, J., Ventura, S., Sutton, P., Menaker, F., & Division of Vital Statistics. (2005). Births: Preliminary data from 2004. *National Vital Statistics Report, 54*(8), 1–18.

Hannah, M. (2004). Planned elective cesarean section: A reasonable choice for some women? *Canadian Medical Association Journal, 170*(5), 1–7.

Institute of Medicine. (2003). *The future of the public's health in the 21st century.* Washington, DC: National Academy Press.

Jevitt, C. (2005). Shoulder dystocia: Etiology, common risk factors and management. *Journal of Midwifery & Women's Health, 50*(6), 485–497.

Johnson, M., Bulechek, G., Butcher, H., McCloskey Dochterman, J., Maas, M., Moorhead, S., & Swanson, E. (2006). *NANDA, NOC, and NIC linkages: Nursing diagnoses, outcomes, & interventions* (2nd ed.). St. Louis, MO: Mosby Elsevier.

Kabir, A., Steinmann, W., Myers, L., Khan, M.M., Herrera, E.A., Yu, S., & Jooma, N. (2004). Unnecessary cesarean delivery in Louisiana: An analysis of birth certificate data. *American Journal of Obstetrics and Gynecology, 190*(1), 10–19.

Labelle, C., & Kitchens, C. (2005). Disseminated intravascular coagulation: Treat the cause, not the lab values. *Cleveland Clinic Journal of Medicine, 72*(5), 377–397.

MacMullen, N., Dulski, L., & Meagher, B. (2005). RED ALERT: Perinatal hemorrhage. *The American Journal of Maternal Child Health, 30*(1), 46–51.

Mahlmeister, L. (2005). Nursing responsibilities in preventing, preparing for and managing epidural emergencies. *Journal of Perinatal and Neonatal Nursing, 17*(1), 19–34.

Mandeville, L., & Troiano, N. (1999). *High-risk and critical care: Intrapartum nursing* (2nd ed.). Philadelphia: Lippincott.

Martin, J.A., Hamilton, B.E., Sutton, P.D., Ventura, S.J., Menacker, F., & Munson, M.L. (2005). Births: Final data for 2003. (Electronic version). *National Vital Statistics Report, 52*(10), 1–114.

Miller, L. (2005). Patient safety and teamwork in perinatal care: Resources for clinicians. *The Journal of Perinatal & Neonatal Nursing, 19*(1), 46–51.

Moore, L., & Martin, J. (2003). Prolonged pregnancy. In J.R. Scott, R.S. Gibbs, B.Y. Karlan, & A.F. Haney (Eds.), *Danforth's obstetrics and gynecology* (pp. 219–223). Philadelphia: Lippincott Williams & Wilkins.

Moore, M. (2003). Preterm labor and birth: What have we learned in the past two decades? *Journal of Obstetric Gynecological and Neonatal Nursing, 32,* 638–649.

Moore, T. (2004). Diabetes in pregnancy. In R. Creasy, R. Resnik, & J. Iams (Eds.), *Maternal-fetal medicine: Principles and practice* (5th ed.). Philadelphia: W.B. Saunders.

Moorehead, S., Johnson, M., Mass, M., & Swanson, E. (2008). *Nursing outcomes classification (NOC)* (4th ed.). St. Louis, MO: C.V. Mosby.

NANDA International. (2007). *NANDA-I nursing diagnosis: Definitions and classifications 2007–2008.* Philadelphia: NANDA-I.

National Institute of Child Health and Human Development (NICHD) Research Planning Workshop. (1997). Electronic fetal heart rate monitoring: Research guidelines for interpretation. *American Journal of Obstetrics and Gynecology, 177*(6), 1385–1390.

Norwitz, E., Robinson, J., & Repke, J. (2002). Labor and delivery. In S. Gabbe, J. Niebyl, & J. Simpson (Eds.), *Obstetrics: Normal and problem pregnancies* (4th ed.). New York: Churchill Livingstone.

Oyelese, Y., Catanzarite, V., Prefumo, F., Lashley, S., Schachter, M., Tovbin, Y., et al. (2004). Vasa previa: The impact of prenatal diagnosis on outcomes. *Obstetrics and Gynecology, 103*(5), 937–942.

Parer, J., & Nageotte, M. (2004). Intrapartum fetal surveillance. In R. Creasy, R. Resnik, & J. Iams (Eds.), *Maternal-fetal medicine: Principles and Practice* (5th ed.). Philadelphia: W.B. Saunders.

Patel, R., & Murphy, D. (2004). Forceps delivery in modern obstetric practice. *British Medical Journal, 328*(7451), 1302–1305.

Porter, F., & Scott, J. (2003). Cesarean delivery. In J.R. Scott, R.S. Gibbs, B.Y. Karlan, & A.F. Haney (Eds.), *Danforth's obstetrics and gynecology* (9th ed., pp. 449–460). Philadelphia: Lippincott Williams & Wilkins.

Rai, J., & Schreiber, J.R. (2005). Cervical ripening. *EMedicine.* Retrieved from http://www.emedicine.com (Accessed September 19, 2005).

Resnik, J., & Resnik, R. (2004). Post-term pregnancy. In R. Creasy, R. Resnik, & J. Iams (Eds.), *Maternal-fetal medicine: Principles and practice* (5th ed.). Philadelphia: W.B. Saunders.

Schoening, A.M. (2006). Amniotic fluid embolism: Historical perspectives and new possibilities. *MCN: The American Journal of Maternal Child Nursing, 31*(2), 78-83.

Sibai, B., Dekker, G., & Kuperminic, M. (2005). Pre-eclampsia. *Lancet, 365*(9461), 785–799.

Simpson, K. (2004). Monitoring the preterm fetus during labor. *American Journal of Maternal Child Health, 29*(6), 380–390.

Simpson, K. (2005a). Failure to rescue: Implications for evaluating quality of care during labor and birth. *Journal of Perinatology & Neonatal Nursing, 19*(1), 24–36.

Simpson, K. (2005b). The context and clinical evidence for common nursing practices during labor. *MCN American Journal of Maternal/Child Nursing, 30*(6), 356–363.

Simpson, K., & Atterbury, J. (2003). Trends and issues in labor induction in the United States: Implications for practice. *Journal of Obstetric Gynecologic and Neonatal Nursing, 32*(6), 767–779.

Simpson, K., & Creehan, P. (2001). *Perinatal nursing.* Philadelphia: Lippincott.

Simpson, K., & James, D. (2005). Efficacy of intrauterine resuscitation techniques in improving fetal oxygen status during labor. *Obstetrics and Gynecology, 105*(6), 1362–1368.

Simpson, K., & Thorman, K. (2005). Obstetric "conveniences": Elective induction of labor, cesarean birth on demand, and other potentially unnecessary interventions. *The Journal of Perinatal & Neonatal Nursing, 19*(2), 134–144.

Smith, G. (2005). Estimating risks of perinatal death. *American Journal of Obstetrics and Gynecology, 192*(1), 17–22.

Tenore, J. (2003). Methods for cervical ripening and induction of labor. *American Academy of Family Physicians, 67*(10), 2123–2128.

Tillett, J. (2005). The labor progress handbook: Early interventions to prevent and treat dystocia. *Journal of Perinatal & Neonatal Nursing, 14*(3), 97.

Tucker, S.M. (2004). *Pocket guide to fetal monitoring and assessment* (4th ed.). St. Louis, MO: C.V. Mosby.

Turkoski, B.B., Lance, B.R., & Bonfiglio, M.F. (2004). *Lexi comp's drug information for nursing: Including assessment, administration, monitoring guidelines, and patient education* (6th ed.). Hudson, OH: Lexi-Comp.

U.S. Department of Health and Human Services (USDHHS). (2000). *Healthy People 2010.* Washington, DC: Author.

Vadhera, R., & Locksmith, G. (2004). Breech presentation, malpresentation, and multiple gestation. In S. Datta (Ed.), *Anesthetic and obstetrics management of high-risk pregnancy* (3rd ed., pp. 67–85). Boston: Springer.

Vain, N., Szyld, E., Prudent, L., Wiswell, T., Aguilar, A., & Vivas, N. (2004). Oropharyngeal and nasopharyngeal suctioning of meconium-stained neonates before delivery of their shoulders: Multicentre, randomized, controlled trial. *Lancet, 364*(9434), 597–602.

Wax, J. (2004). Gravid uterus exteriorization at cesarean delivery for prenatally diagnosed placenta previa-accreta. *American Journal of Perinatology, 21*(6), 311–313.

Wax, J., Cartin, A., Pinette, M., & Blackstone, J. (2004). Patient choice cesarean: An evidence-based review. *Obstetrical & Gynecological Survey, 59*(8), 566–567.

Wen, S., Rusen, I., Walker, M., Liston, R., Kramer, M., Baskett, T., et al. (2004). Comparison of maternal mortality and morbidity between trial of labor and elective cesarean section among women with previous cesarean delivery. *American Journal of Obstetrics and Gynecology, 191*(4), 1263–1269.

Williams, D. (2005). The top 10 reasons elective cesarean section should be on the decline. *AWHONN Lifelines, 9*(1), 23–24.

Williams, D., & Shah, M. (2003). Soaring cesarean section rates: A cause for alarm. *Journal of Obstetric Gynecological and Neonatal Nursing, 32,* 283–284.

Wing, D.A. (2002). A benefit-risk assessment of Misoprostol for cervical ripening and labour induction. *Drug Safety, 25*(9), 665-676.

Yang, Q., Wen, S., Chen, Y., Krewski, D., Fung, K., & Walker, M. (2005). Occurrence and clinical predictors of operative delivery of the vertex second twin after normal vaginal delivery of the first twin. *American Journal of Obstetrics and Gynecology, 192*(1), 178–184.

Young, T., & Woodmansee, B. (2002). Factors that are associated with cesarean delivery in a large private practice: The importance of pre-pregnancy body mass index and weight gain. *American Journal of Obstetrics & Gynecology, 187*(2), 312–320.

Zelop, C., & Heffner, L. (2004). The downside of cesarean delivery: Short- and long-term complications. *Clinical Obstetrics and Gynecology, 47*(2), 386–393.

 DavisPlus
DavisPlus.fadavis.com **For more information, go to http://davisplus.fadavis.com/**

CONCEPT MAP

Caring for the Woman Experiencing Complications During Labor and Birth

Complications of Labor

Dysfunctional labor
- Hypertonic labor
- Hypotonic labor
- Precipitate labor

Nursing
- ID labor pattern
- Frequent monitoring:
  – Vital signs
  – Reflexes
  – Cervical dilation, effacement
  – Contractions
- Teach breathing, relaxation
- Provide information, reassurance

Nursing
- Obtain consent
- Monitor labor: vitals, fetal heart tones, contractions, cervical changes, fetal station/lie
- Monitor oxytocin rate, side effects, urine output
- Pain management
- Positioning

Placental Complications

Placenta Previa
- Collaborate with medical treatment plan

Placental Abruption
- Continuous fetal monitor
- Frequent vital signs
- Assess perineum, urine output, labs

May necessitate

Obstetric Interventions
- Amnioinfusion
- Amniotomy
- Pharmacological induction
- Complementary measures
- Instrumentation assistance

Maternal Complications

Preeclampsia
- Manage HTN
- Fetal monitoring
- Vitals/neurological
- Urine output/edema
- Watch labs for HELLP
- MgSO$_4$ monitoring

Diabetes
- FSBG q 2 hours
- Possible insulin drip
- Prepare for C-birth

Preterm labor
- Maternal and fetal monitoring
- Correct application of monitoring equipment and interpretation of tracings

Perinatal Fetal Loss
- Often due to obstetric complications
- Team approach to bereavement: organized, culturally sensitive, flexible plan
- Allow parental decisions
- Communication
- Support groups

Fetal Complications

Fetal Malpresentation
- Consent for version
- Prep for C-birth

Cephalopelvic Disproportion
- Position changes
- Relaxation, water therapy
- Pain management

Multiple Gestation
- Careful monitoring
- Assess individual fetal heart rates

Fetal compromise
- Immediate MD notification
- Assess acid/base
- Position change

Oligohydramnios

Hydramnios

Meconium Staining

Nuchal cord

Cesarean Birth
- When health of mother/fetus in jeopardy
- Major surgical procedure
- Ethical concerns
- Involves care of the postoperative patient
- Concerns re:VBAC

Other Complications

- Uterine rupture
- Uterine inversion
- Prolapse of the umbilical cord
- Vasa previa/velamentous insertion
- Amniotic fluid embolism

Across Care Settings:
- Collaborative care for multiple gestation birth

Critical Nursing Actions:
- Assisting with precipitous birth
- Caring for the patient undergoing amnioinfusion
- Responding to umbilical cord prolapse

Ethnocultural Considerations:
- Level of quality of care differs between Caucasian and non-Caucasian populations

What To Say:
- For preterm labor: active listening, explore concerns
- Calm, factual explanation during fetal distress
- Effective team communication during obstetric emergencies
- Conveying compassion in fetal loss

? Now Can You:
- Identify factors that impede labor progression
- Explain the difference between labor induction and augmentation
- Explain correct procedure for application of the fetal monitor
- Discuss care and medical management of twin births
- Discuss issues and appropriate communication concerning perinatal death

Care of the
New Family

Caring for the Postpartal Woman and Her Family

Within a period of one day, most of what has been carefully accumulated over nine months is eliminated as no longer necessary by the body.

—Rubin, 1984, p. 753

LEARNING TARGETS *At the completion of this chapter the student will be able to:*

◆ Discuss the physiological and psychological changes that occur in the postpartal woman.

◆ Assess the physiological and psychosocial status of the postpartal woman.

◆ Plan holistic nursing care for the postpartal woman and her family that includes strategies for home follow-up.

◆ Implement nursing interventions to promote positive breast and formula feeding outcomes for the mother and her infant.

◆ Describe effective maternal self-care measures to be implemented during the puerperium.

◆ Discuss methods for assessing and treating pain in the postpartal period.

◆ Conduct appropriate nursing assessments and plan interventions for the patient who has experienced a cesarean birth.

◆ Discuss dimensions of postpartal care for the multicultural family.

◆ Plan postpartal nursing care with interventions to assess and foster maternal/infant/family bonding.

---

 moving toward evidence-based practice The Influence of Norms on Breastfeeding Decisions

Swanson, V., & Power, K.G. (2005). Initiation and continuation of breastfeeding: theory of planned behavior. *Journal of Advanced Nursing, (50)*3, 272–282.
Rimal, R.N., & Real, K. (2003). Understanding the influence of perceived norms on behaviors. *Communication Theory 13*(2), 184–203.

The purpose of this study was to investigate the subjective norms of new mothers in relation to the decision to breast or bottle feed. Norms were defined as "group identity-based codes of conduct that are understood and disseminated through group interaction" (Rimal & Real, 2003). The Theory of Planned Behavior (TPB), a social cognition model, was used as a framework for the study, which explored how attitudes, norms, and perceived behavior control (PBC) predicted mothers' feeding behaviors at birth.

Specifically, the research was designed to measure changes in norms and attitudes on the selected infant feeding method from birth to 6 weeks postpartum. Follow-up for both breast- and bottle-fed infants and a decision to discontinue breastfeed-

ing during this period was examined. The researchers also explored the views held by significant persons in the women's environment (partner, own mother, and nurses) in relation to the mother's decision about a method of feeding.

An initial interview and self-administered questionnaire were completed by 203 new mothers after childbirth. At 6 weeks postpartum, 118 of the participants completed a follow-up questionnaire. The sample included primiparous and multiparous women who experienced a vaginal or cesarean birth. At the time of delivery, 103 participants planned to breastfeed; 100 planned to bottle feed.

(continued)

Data analysis revealed the following findings:

- One half of the sample were multiparas; the majority of these mothers chose to use the same feeding method used with their previous children.
- Eight mothers who had breast fed their first child chose to bottle feed the newborn; 11 mothers who had bottle fed their first child chose to breastfeed the newborn.
- Mothers who bottle fed their children tended to be younger, single, less educated, of lower socioeconomic status, and more likely to live in a rental unit.
- At the 6-week follow-up, 48% who initially planned to breastfeed continued to do so; 47% continued to bottle feed; and 12% combined breast and bottle feeding methods.
- Mothers who were breastfeeding reported positive beliefs toward breastfeeding. In addition, mothers who were bottle-feeding also reported positive beliefs.
- No significant differences were found in the mothers' perceived level of control over their choice of infant feeding methods.

- Both breast-feeding and bottle-feeding mothers were in agreement with social norms as expressed by their partner, mother, close female friends, and nurses or midwives.
- At 6 weeks postpartum, the breastfeeding mothers indicated that significant persons were more in favor of bottle feeding than breastfeeding. Ratings of the bottle-feeding mothers did not change.
- The partners, nurses, and nurse midwives were considered to have the most influence in relation to the mother's decision about a method of feeding.
- Mothers who discontinued breastfeeding by 6 weeks perceived more overall social pressure to bottle feed.

The researchers concluded that nurses and midwives have a crucial role in communicating positive views on breastfeeding to new mothers.

1. What might be considered as limitations to this study?
2. How is this information useful to clinical nursing practice?

See Suggested Responses for Moving Toward Evidence-Based Practice on the Electronic Study Guide or DavisPlus.

Introduction

Postpartum care begins immediately after childbirth. During this time, the nurse assists the new mother in learning how to care for herself and her baby. This 6-week period of time, also known as the **puerperium**, is filled with a myriad of changes that require careful nursing assessments for the mother, the newborn, and the family. The nurse's knowledge and care provided during this **"fourth trimester"** of pregnancy can have a life-long impact in shaping the future plans and choices for the new family.

The *Healthy People 2010* national initiative includes several goals that encompass the time period of the early puerperium:

- Reduce the maternal mortality rate to no more than 3.3/100,000 live births from a baseline of 7.1/100,000.
- Reduce the proportion of births occurring within 24 months of a previous birth to 6% from a baseline of 11%.
- Increase to at least 75% the proportion of mothers who breastfeed their babies in the early postpartum period from a baseline of 64% (DHHS, 2000).

Nursing actions to help the nation achieve these goals center on close observation to identify hemorrhage and related complications during the critical first hour after childbirth and ongoing education and support for women and families. Teaching about normal physiological changes during the puerperium, signs of danger, contraceptive methods, and benefits of breastfeeding empowers them to make informed decisions and choices.

Current trends reflect a shortened hospital stay for the new mother and her infant. However, there are several drawbacks to this approach. A longer (greater than 24 hours) hospital stay provides more rest and recuperation

time for the mother; a greater opportunity for postpartal education about self and infant care; and time for infant observation and assessment for anomalies, defects, or other problems, and improved maternal outcomes. Early hospital discharge has advantages as well. These include a decreased risk of nosocomial infections for the mother and infant, reduced medical expenses, and an opportunity for enhanced infant—family bonding.

Providing care during this period requires knowledge of the physiological and psychosocial aspects of the puerperium. The transitions that occur as the changes of pregnancy are reversed are considered to be a normal, but distinct, process. Protecting this process requires the nurse who cares for the postpartum patient to be equipped with special knowledge and skills. This chapter will discuss the physiological and psychosocial adaptations that occur during the postpartum period and the nursing assessments and interventions required to promote positive, healthy outcomes.

Ensuring Safety for the Mother and Infant

Early newborn discharge began as a consumer-initiated movement and as an alternative to home births in the 1980s. In the 1990s, third-party payers began to refuse reimbursement for hospital stays that extended beyond 24 hours, particularly after an uncomplicated vaginal birth. Congress responded to the growing concern over the safety of this practice by signing into law the Newborns' and Mothers' Health Protection Act of 1996. This legislation prohibits third-party payers from restricting benefits for hospital stays of less than 48 hours after a vaginal birth or less than 96 hours after a cesarean birth. Forty-eight hours is an incredibly short amount of time to assess, assist, and educate new mothers about matters concerning personal, newborn, and family health. Information provided by the postpartum nurse can protect the newborn and his family from unnecessary morbidity and mortality.

Fears surrounding infant abductions have long been a common concern among hospital staff and families. These concerns have created the need for the electronic tracking of infants. The growing need for fail-proof mechanisms to ensure infant safety has prompted the development of a variety of systems designed to foil infant abduction attempts. In response to increased litigation and pressure from The Joint Commission, it has become mandatory for hospitals to offer state-of-the-art security protection for their patients, mother/baby units, and visitors.

To meet The Joint Commission mandatory infant safety requirements, hospitals have instituted policies and procedures that nurses and mothers must follow to ensure their newborn's safety. Infant security experts agree that an informed mother is the baby's first line of defense while in the hospital as well as after returning home. It is essential that nurses educate new mothers about measures designed to protect their newborns from potential abductors.

⬤ Be sure to— Check identification bracelets

The safety and security of the infant must be maintained at all times during hospitalization. This process involves the placement of identification bands on both the mother and infant shortly after birth. On bringing the infant to the mother, it is essential for the nurse to verify that the bracelets match. At discharge, it may be necessary for the nurse to retain both the infant's and parent's identification bracelets as part of the permanent record. This safety measure serves a twofold purpose: to prevent the unauthorized removal of the infant from the hospital unit and to prevent the inadvertent mix-up or switching of newborns.

⬤ Be sure to— Protect the infant from abduction

Protecting the infant from abduction is an extremely important consideration during hospitalization. Personnel, parents, and significant others must be educated regarding the various measures implemented to protect the safety of the infant. Any time the infant is transported from the nursery to the mother's room, it is essential for staff to follow the hospital's protocol. In most facilities, infants may be transported only in a bassinet and parents are prohibited from carrying the infant in the halls. When identification bracelets are used, they are matched before giving the infant to the mother. Mothers should be instructed to release the infant only to properly identified hospital personnel. After birth, admission photographs and footprints are most likely taken and affixed to the permanent record. When two or more infants have a similar or same last name, it is common practice for the infants' cribs and charts to indicate the mother's first name, and bear a label that designates a "NAME ALERT." When there are multiple births, the infants' cribs may be labeled with the infant's name followed by a letter of the alphabet (i.e., A, B, C, or D).

Hospital personnel are typically required to wear visible photo identification when working in the maternal child unit. All employee photo badges should be similar in appearance to facilitate the ready identification of individuals posing as hospital employees. Visitors may be required to wear identification badges while on the unit. Hospital staff should be empowered to question any suspicious activity or individuals who are present on the maternal child unit.

 Now Can You— **Discuss strategies to ensure maternal–infant safety?**

1. Identify three measures the hospital nurse can implement to ensure the safety of both the infant and the mother?
2. Suggest a strategy to decrease the potential for confusing infants whose last names are similar or identical?
3. Describe two actions that hospital personnel can take to help prevent infant abduction?

Early Maternal Assessment

VITAL SIGNS

During the postpartum period, vital signs are a reflection of the body's attempts to return to a pre-pregnant state. Vital signs can alert the nurse to the presence of hemorrhage or infection and should be monitored according to hospital policy. After a vaginal birth, vital signs are typically monitored every 15 minutes during the first hour after childbirth, then every 30 minutes during the second hour, once during the third hour, and then every 8 hours until discharge or until they are stable. A different protocol is followed for vital sign assessment after a cesarean birth (e.g., q30min × 4 hours; then q1h × 3; then q4–8h).

Temperature

During the first 24 hours postpartum, some women experience an increase in body temperature up to 100.4°F (38°C). The exertion and dehydration that accompany labor are the primary causes for the temperature elevation, and increased fluids usually return the temperature to a normal range. Increased breast vascularity may also cause a transient increase in temperature. After the first 24 postpartal hours have passed, however, the patient should be afebrile. A temperature above 100.4°F (38°C) at this time may be indicative of infection. (See Chapter 16 for further discussion).

Pulse

Heart rates of 50 to 70 beats per minute (bradycardia) commonly occur during the first 6 to 10 days of the postpartum period. During pregnancy, the weight of the gravid uterus causes a decreased flow of venous blood to the heart. After childbirth, there is an increase in intravascular volume. The elevated stroke volume leads to a decreased heart rate. Postpartal tachycardia may result from a complication, prolonged labor, blood loss, temperature elevation, or infection.

Blood Pressure

Postpartal blood pressure values should be compared with blood pressure values obtained during the first trimester. Decreased blood pressure may result from the physiological changes associated with the decrease in intrapelvic pressure, or it may be indicative of uterine hemorrhage. An increase in the systolic blood pressure of 30 mm Hg or 15 mm Hg in the diastolic blood pressure, especially when associated with headaches or visual changes, may be a sign of gestational hypertension. Further assessment is indicated.

In the puerperium, plasma renin and angiotensin II levels return to normal, nonpregnant levels. These physiological changes produce a decrease in vascular resistance. Orthostatic hypotension may occur when the patient moves from a supine to a sitting position. Otherwise, maternal blood pressure should remain stable (Cunningham et al., 2005).

Respirations

The respiratory rate should remain within the normal range of 12 to 20 respirations per minute. However, slightly elevated respirations may occur due to pain, fear, excitement, exertion, or excessive blood loss. Careful nursing assessment for causes of an elevated respiratory rate is indicated, along with appropriate interventions. Tachypnea, abnormal lung sounds, shortness of breath, chest pain, anxiety, or restlessness are abnormal findings that must be reported immediately. These signs and symptoms may be indicative of pulmonary edema or emboli. (See Chapter 16 for further discussion.)

 Nursing Insight— *Promoting comfort during the immediate postpartum period*

It is not unusual for women to experience shaking chills during the time immediately after childbirth. This physiological response results from: (1) pressure changes in the abdomen after the reduction in the bulk of the uterus and (2) temperature readjustments after the diaphoresis of labor. Feelings of excitement and exhaustion may also play a role. Nurses should reassure patients of the normalcy of this temporary reaction and offer warm blankets and beverages as comfort measures.

FUNDUS, LOCHIA, PERINEUM

Within a few minutes after birth, the firmly contracted uterine fundus should be palpable through the abdominal wall halfway between the umbilicus and the symphysis pubis. Approximately 1 hour later, the fundus should have risen to the level of the umbilicus, where it remains for the following 24 hours.

 Optimizing Outcomes— Uterine assessment crucial during the first hour postpartum

Because the first postpartal hour represents the most dangerous time for the patient, it is essential that the nurse conduct frequent uterine assessments during this time. Relaxation of the uterus (atony) results in rapid, life-threatening blood loss because no permanent thrombi have yet formed at the placental site.

The fundus then descends one fingerbreadth (1 cm) per day in size. The fundus, **lochia** (puerperal discharge of blood, mucus, and tissue), and perineum need to be assessed every 15 minutes during the immediate postpartum period. To facilitate the perineal assessment, the nurse assists the patient into a Sims' (side-lying) position with her back facing the nurse.

 Nursing Insight— *Perineal assessment*

Protecting the patient's privacy and ensuring adequate lighting are essential components of the perineal assessment. Although some edema of the vulva and perineum is a common finding during the first few postpartum days, excessive swelling, discoloration, incisional separation, or discharge other than lochia should be reported, along with the patient's complaints of pain or discomfort.

With adequate lighting in place, the nurse gently lifts the buttock cheeks to visualize the perineum. Use of the acronym REEDA guides the nurse to assess for **R**edness, **E**dema, **E**cchymosis, **D**rainage or discharge, and **A**pproximation of the episiotomy if present (Table 15-1). The episiotomy and/or laceration repairs should appear intact with the tissue edges closely approximated. Hemorrhoids

Table 15-1 The REEDA Acronym to Guide the Perineal Assessment

Points	Redness	Edema	Ecchymosis	Discharge	Approximation
0	None	None	None	None	Closed
1	Within 0.25 cm of incision bilaterally	Less than 1 cm from incision	1–2 cm from incision	Serum	Skin separation 3 mm or less
2	Within 0.5 cm of incision bilaterally	1–2 cm from incision	0.25–1 cm bilaterally or 0.5–2 cm unilaterally	Serosanguineous	Skin and subcutaneous fat separated
3	Beyond 0.5 cm of incision bilaterally	Greater than 2 cm from incision	Greater that 1 cm bilaterally or 2 cm unilaterally	Bloody, purulent	Skin, subcutaneous fat and fascial separation

may also be present. The nurse should note and document the number, appearance, and size (in centimeters) of the hemorrhoids.

HEMORRHOIDS

Hemorrhoids that may be present before pregnancy or develop during pregnancy can become enlarged due to pressure on the lower bowel during the second stage of labor. The application of ice packs and/or pharmaceutical preparations such as topical anesthetic ointments or witch hazel pads helps to relieve discomfort. Frozen tea peripads may also be used as a comfort measure for hemorrhoids and labial swelling. The tannic acid decreases edema and is soothing. Other actions to minimize hemorrhoidal discomfort include assisting the patient to a side-lying position in bed and teaching her to sit on flat, hard surfaces and to tighten her buttocks before sitting. Soft surfaces and pillows such as donut rings should be avoided because they separate the buttocks and decrease venous flow, intensifying the pain. If the hemorrhoids are severe, the patient can be taught how to manually reposition the hemorrhoids back into the rectum. Hemorrhoids that developed during pregnancy generally disappear within a few weeks after childbirth.

 Now Can You— **Discuss postpartum vital signs and perineal assessment?**

1. Describe the expected vital sign findings during the postpartum period?
2. Identify potential causes for increased blood pressure, pulse, and respirations during the postpartum period?
3. Explain what is meant by the REEDA acronym to facilitate the perineal assessment?

A Concise Postpartum Assessment Guide to Facilitate Nursing Care

THE *BUBBLE-HE* MNEMONIC

Use of a systematic assessment process helps the nurse ensure that the special needs of postpartum patients are met. As with all nursing care, a complete head-to-toe assessment must be completed for the postpartum patient who has unique needs not found in any other nursing environment. To assist with the postpartum assessment, the mnemonic BUBBLE-HE is commonly used to guide nursing practice. BUBBLE-HE reminds the nurse to assess the breasts, uterus, bladder, bowel, lochia, and episiotomy. Assessment of maternal pain, Homans' sign, the patient's emotional status and initiation of infant bonding are other important components to be included in the postpartum evaluation (Table 15-2). Medications commonly prescribed during the puerperium are presented in Table 15-3.

Breasts

A number of physiological changes occur during pregnancy to prepare the breasts for the process of lactation. The mammary glands, or milk producing system, are unlike any other organ system. Throughout the woman's growth and development, no other human organ undergoes the dramatic changes in size, shape, and function that take place in the breasts (Riordan, 2005). Essentially, the breasts serve no function other than to nourish the child. Breast size has no bearing on the woman's ability or capacity to nourish her infant. Instead, the infant's appetite and frequent emptying of the breasts dictate the quantity of milk produced.

A & P review **Hormonal Changes to Prepare the Breasts for Lactation**

Up until the onset of puberty, the breasts are much the same in males and females and their internal structure is similar: they consist of a collection of ducts that empty into the nipple. In the female, breast tissue responds to the release of the female sex hormones estrogen and progesterone during puberty. Estrogen stimulates the formation of additional ducts, the elongation of existing ducts and the formation of a system of milk secreting glands. These changes are associated with an increase in volume and elasticity of connective tissue, deposition of adipose tissue and increased vascularity. Progesterone stimulates the formation of lobules, the glands in the breast which produce milk.

Table 15-2	BUBBLE-HE: Components of a Postpartum Assessment	
Letter	**Assess**	**Assessment Includes**
B	Breasts	Inspection of nipples: everted, flat, inverted? Breast tissue: soft, filling, firm? Temperature and color: warm, pink, cool, red streaked?
U	Uterus	Location (midline or deviated to right or left side) and tone (firm, firm with massage, boggy)
B	Bladder	Last time the patient emptied her bladder (spontaneously or via catheter)? Palpable or nonpalpable? Color, odor, and amount of urine?
B	Bowels	Date/time of last BM; presence of flatus and hunger (unless the colon was manipulated, do not need to auscultate for bowel sounds)
L	Lochia	Color, amount, presence of clots, any free flow?
(I) E	(Incision) Episiotomy	Type as well as other tissue trauma (lacerations, etc.); assess using REEDA
L/H	Legs (Homans' sign)	Pain, varicosities, warmth or discoloration in calves; presence of pedal pulses; sensation and movement (after cesarean birth)
E	Emotions	Affect, patient-family interaction, effects of exhaustion
(B)	Bonding	Interaction with infant—"taking in" phase—presence of finger tipping, gazing, enfolding, calling infant by name, identifying unique characteristics

Table 15-3 Commonly Used Medications in the Postpartum Period

Classification	Medication	Dose / Safety of Use in Breastfeeding	Indication for Use in Postpartum Phase
Stool softener	Docusate sodium (Colace)	50 mg to 500 mg by mouth daily until bowel movements are normal. Not contraindicated in breastfeeding mother.	Used in the treatment of constipation
Stool softener	Bisacodyl (Dulcolax)	10 mg to 30 mg by mouth until bowel movements are normal. Not contraindicated in breastfeeding mother.	Used in the treatment of constipation
Topical anesthetic	Lidocaine spray	Spray to perineal area after sitz bath or perineum care. Not contraindicated in breastfeeding mother.	Used on the skin to relieve pain and itching
Hemorrhoid care	Witch hazel (Tucks)	Apply to perineal area after sitz bath or perineum care. Not contraindicated in breastfeeding mother.	Used on the skin to relieve the itching, burning, and irritation associated with hemorrhoids
Nonsteroidal anti-inflammatory drugs	Ibuprofen (Motrin)	400 mg by mouth every 4–6 hours as needed for pain. Not contraindicated in breastfeeding mother.	Used for the treatment of mild to moderate pain
Opioid analgesics	Darvocet (propoxyphene and acetaminophen)	Take one tablet by mouth every four hours as needed for pain. Not contraindicated in breastfeeding mother.	Used for the treatment of moderate to severe pain
Opioid analgesics	Percocet (oxycodone and acetaminophen)	Take one to two tablets every 4–6 hours as needed for pain. Not contraindicated in breastfeeding mother.	Used for the treatment of moderate to severe pain

Source: Deglin, J.H., & Vallerand, A.H. (2009). *Davis's Drug Guide for Nurses* (11th ed.). Philadelphia: F.A. Davis.

By the time the breasts are fully formed, typically by the age of 15, breast tissue extends medially from the second or third rib to the sixth or seventh rib, and laterally from the breastbone to the edge of the axillae. Although genetic factors, body size and ethnicity account for some variations, on average, the breasts weigh approximately 200 grams. During pregnancy, each breast increases in size and weight to reach approximately 600 grams and 600 to 800 grams during lactation (Lawrence & Lawrence, 2005).

Until menopause, when menstrual periods cease, the woman's breast tissue continues to respond to the changing hormonal environment that accompanies each menstrual cycle. Throughout the majority of the woman's life, the breasts remain in a resting state except for the time during pregnancy and lactation. ◆

Regardless of whether the woman plans to breast or bottle feed, the breasts require careful assessment. After ensuring privacy, the nurse asks the patient to remove her bra. The chest area is covered with a sheet or towel and the woman is instructed to raise her arms and rest her hands on her head. The nurse inspects and palpates each breast for size, shape, tenderness, and color. During the first 2 postpartal days, the breast tissue should feel soft to the touch. By the third day, the breasts should begin to feel firm and warm. This change is described as "filling." On the fourth and fifth days postpartum, breastfeeding mothers' breasts should feel firm before infant feeding, then become soft once the baby is satiated. The noticeable changes in breast firmness are indicative of milk transfer.

The process of lactation is established in all postpartum women, regardless of their intention to breast or formula

feed. Tense, painful breasts in a breastfeeding mother are indicative of poor transfer of milk to the infant. This finding should prompt a breastfeeding assessment and, when appropriate, referral to an international board-certified lactation consultant. (See discussion later in this chapter.)

Occasionally, small, firm nodules can be palpated in the filling breasts. The nodules result from incomplete emptying of the breasts during the previous feeding. Usually, a nodule arises from a blocked milk duct or from milk contained in a gland that is not flowing forward to the nipple. Although the nodules typically disappear after a satisfactory feeding, their location should be noted and monitored. Persistence of any breast mass may be indicative of fibrocystic disease or malignant growths unrelated to the pregnancy. The nurse also documents the appearance of the nipples, noting the presence of fissures, cracks, blood, or dried milk, and whether they are erect or inverted.

Uterus

Involution is a term that describes the process whereby the uterus returns to the nonpregnant state. The uterus undergoes a dramatic reduction in size although it will remain slightly larger than its size before the first pregnancy. Immediately after expulsion of the placenta, the uterus rapidly contracts to prevent hemorrhage. The uterus weighs approximately 1000 g in the immediate postpartal period and by the end of the first week, its weight has diminished to 500 g. Uterine size and weight continue to decrease and on average, the uterus weighs 300 g by the end of the second week and thereafter the weight is 100 g or less (Cunningham et al., 2005).

After the birth of the infant, placental expulsion spontaneously occurs within 15 minutes in approximately 90% of women. To prevent hemorrhage, rapid uterine contractions seal off the placental site, effectively pinching off the massive network of maternal blood vessels that were attached to the placenta (Cunningham et al., 2005).

The original site of placental implantation covers a surface area that is approximately 8 to 10 cm in size. By the end of the second postpartal week, the site has shrunk to about 3 to 4 cm; complete healing takes approximately 6 to 7 weeks. The uterus is predominantly composed of a muscle layer, the myometrium. The myometrium is covered by serosa and lined by the decidua basalis. The process of uterine involution results from a decrease in the *size* of the myometrial cells rather than from a decrease in the *number* of myometrial cells. The decrease in cell size results in myometrial thickening and ischemia from reduced blood flow to the contracted uterus.

Phagocytosis (the engulfment and destruction of cells) contributes to the process of uterine involution by removing elastic and fibrous tissue from the uterus. The process is further hastened by autolysis (self-digestion) that results from migration of macrophages to the uterus.

Subinvolution is the failure of the uterus to return to the nonpregnant state. Uterine involution may be inhibited by multiple births, hydramnios, prolonged labor or difficult birth, infection, grand multiparity, or excessive maternal analgesia. In addition, a full bladder or retained placental tissue may prevent the uterus from sustaining the contractions needed to prevent hemorrhage or to facilitate involution. (See Chapter 16 for further discussion.)

The placental site heals by a process called exfoliation. Exfoliation is the scaling off of dead tissue. New endometrial tissue is generated at the site from the glands and tissue that remain in the lower layer of the decidua after separation of the placenta. This physiological process results in a uterine lining that contains no scar tissue, which could impede implantation in future pregnancies. Regeneration of the endometrium is complete by the 16th postpartum day, except at the placental site, where regeneration is usually not complete until approximately 6 weeks after childbirth.

To perform the uterine assessment, the nurse assists the patient to a supine position so that the height of the uterus is not influenced by an elevated position. The patient's abdomen is observed for contour to detect distention and the presence of striae or a diastasis (separation), which appears as a slightly indented groove in the midline. When present, the width and length of a diastasis are recorded in fingerbreadths. The uterine fundus is palpated by placing one hand immediately above the symphysis pubis to stabilize the uterus and the other hand at the level of the umbilicus (Fig. 15-1). The nurse presses inward and downward with the hand positioned on the umbilicus until the fundus is located. It should feel like a firm, globular mass located at or slightly above the umbilicus during the first hour after birth.

clinical alert

Proper technique for uterine palpation

The uterus should never be palpated without supporting the lower uterine segment. Failure to do so may result in uterine inversion and hemorrhage.

FUNDUS. Immediately after childbirth, the uterus rapidly contracts to facilitate compression of the intra myometrial blood vessels. The uterine fundus can be palpated midline, midway between the umbilicus and symphysis pubis. Within an hour, the uterus settles in the midline at the level of the umbilicus. Over the course of days, the uterus descends into the pelvis at a rate of about 1 cm/day (one fingerbreadth) (Fig. 15-2). After 10 days, the uterus has descended into the pelvis and is no longer palpable.

The fundus is assessed for consistency (firm, soft, or boggy), location (should be midline), and height (measured in finger breadths). During the fundal assessment, the nurse notes whether it is located midline or deviated to one side. On occasion, the fundus can be palpated slightly to the right because of displacement from the sigmoid colon during pregnancy. Assessment of the fundus should be made shortly after the patient has emptied her bladder. A full bladder prevents the uterus from contract-

Figure 15-1 To palpate the uterus, the upper hand is cupped over the fundus; the lower hand stabilizes the uterus at the symphysis pubis.

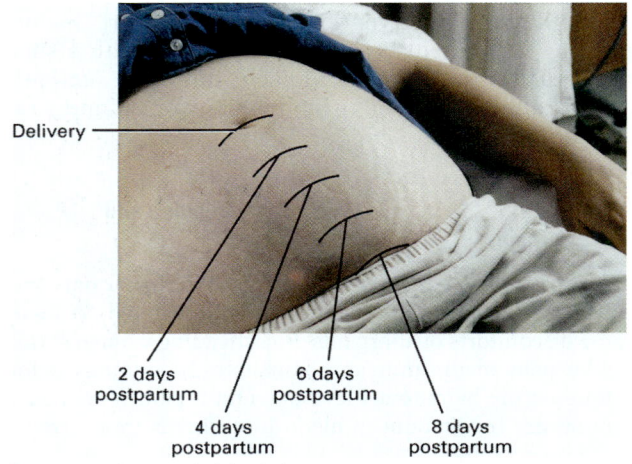

Delivery

2 days postpartum

4 days postpartum

6 days postpartum

8 days postpartum

Figure 15-2 Fundal heights postpartum.

Table 15-4	Assessment and Documentation of Uterine Involution	
Time	**Location of Fundus**	**Documentation**
Immediately after birth	Midline, midway between umbilicus and symphysis pubis	
1–2 hours	At the level of the umbilicus	at U (umbilicus)
12 hours	1 cm above umbilicus (1 fingerbreadth)	U + 1
24 hours	1 cm below umbilicus	U − 1
2 days	2 cm below umbilicus (2 fingerbreadths)	U − 2
3 days	3 cm below umbilicus (3 fingerbreadths)	U − 3
7 days	Palpable at the symphysis pubis	
10 days	Not palpable	

ing and instead pushes the uterus upward and may deviate it from the midline, due to laxness of the uterine ligaments. A flabby, noncontracted, boggy uterus is associated with increased bleeding. A well-contracted fundus is firm, round, and midline. The nurse documents the location of the fundus according to fingerbreadths above or below the umbilicus (Table 15-4).

Afterpains (afterbirth pains) are intermittent uterine contractions that occur during the process of involution. Patients often describe the sensation as a discomfort similar to menstrual cramps. The primiparous woman typically has mild afterpains, if she notices them at all, because her uterus is able to maintain a contracted state. Multiparas and patients with uterine overdistention (e.g., large baby, multifetal gestation, hydramnios) are more likely to experience afterpains, due to the continuous pattern of uterine relaxation and vigorous contractions. When the uterus maintains a constant contraction, the afterpains cease. Breastfeeding and the administration of exogenous oxytocin usually produce pronounced afterpains because both cause powerful uterine contractions. Afterbirth pain is often severe for 2 to 3 days after childbirth. Nursing interventions for discomfort include assisting the patient into a prone position with a small pillow placed under her abdomen, initiating sitz baths (for warmth), encouraging ambulation, and administrating mild analgesics.

 Optimizing Outcomes— **Breastfeeding and afterpains**

Analgesics such as ibuprofen (Advil, Motrin) or naproxen (Aleve, Anaprox) are frequently administered to lessen the discomforts of afterpains. Breastfeeding women should take pain medication approximately 30 minutes before nursing the baby to achieve maximum pain relief and to minimize the amount of medication that is transferred in the breast milk.

 Now Can You— Discuss changes in the breasts and uterus during the postpartum period?

1. Name each component of the BUBBLE-HE mnemonic for the postpartum assessment?
2. Explain normal breast changes that occur during the first few postpartal days?
3. Explain what is meant by "involution"?

Bladder

After childbirth, spontaneous voiding should occur within 6 to 8 hours and the first few voiding amounts should be monitored. Urinary output of at least 150 mL/hr is necessary to avoid urinary retention or stasis. Generalized edema is often present in the early puerperium. It is related to the fluid accumulation that normally occurs during pregnancy combined with intravenous fluids frequently administered during labor and birth. Maternal diuresis occurs almost immediately after birth and urinary output reaches up to 3000 mL each day by the second to fifth postpartum days.

Decreased bladder tone is normal during pregnancy, and results from the effects of progesterone on the smooth muscle, edema from pressure of the presenting part, and mucosal hyperemia from the increase in blood vessel size. Prolonged labor, the use of forceps, analgesia, and anesthesia may intensify the changes in the immediate postpartum period. Pressure caused by the fetal head pressing on the bladder during labor can result in trauma and a transient loss of bladder sensation during the first few postpartal days or weeks. These changes can result in incomplete bladder emptying and overdistention.

Bladder and urethral trauma is not uncommon during the intrapartal period and may be associated with a decreased flow of urine immediately after a vaginal birth. An increase in the voided volume, the total flow time (how long it takes to empty the bladder) and the time to peak urine flow (the maximum urinary flow rate) begins to occur during the first postpartum day. Urine volume and flow time should return to pre-pregnant levels by 2 to 3 days after childbirth. Epidural anesthesia, catheterization before birth, and an instrument-facilitated birth are associated with an increased risk of postpartum urinary retention. Urethral and bladder trauma and lacerations may accompany vaginal or cesarean birth.

Urinary retention can also result from bladder hypotonia after childbirth since the weight of the gravid uterus no longer limits bladder capacity. Assessment of the maternal bladder is an extremely important component of the nursing evaluation (Table 15-5). An overdistended bladder, which displaces the uterus above and to the right of the umbilicus, can cause uterine atony and lead to hemorrhage. Other assessment findings may include presence of the bladder palpated as a hard or firm area just above the symphysis pubis and a urinary output that is disproportionate to the fluid intake. Bladder percussion enhances the assessment. To percuss the bladder, the nurse places one finger flat on the patient's abdomen over the bladder and taps it with the finger of the other hand. A full bladder produces a resonant sound. An empty bladder has a dull, thudding sound. Patients may express an urge to void but be unable to void. Fortunately, spontaneous voiding typi-

Table 15-5 Nursing Assessment and Interventions for the Urinary System	
Patient's Signs and Symptoms	**Nursing Interventions**
• Location of fundus above baseline level • Fundus displaced from midline • Excessive lochia • Bladder discomfort • Bulge of bladder above symphysis pubis • Frequent voiding of less than 150 mL of urine; urinary output disproportionate to fluid intake	• Promote hydration • Promote ambulation • Administer an analgesic before voiding, as prescribed • Place ice on perineum to reduce swelling and pain • Encourage the use of a sitz bath • Provide privacy • Turn on the bathroom faucet

Box 15-1 Nursing Interventions to Facilitate Normal Bowel Function During the Puerperium

To facilitate the return of normal bowel function in the puerperium, the nurse should:

• Encourage the patient to drink at least six to eight 8-oz. glasses of water every day to help keep the stool soft.
• Encourage the patient to eat a high-fiber diet that includes an abundance of fruits and vegetables, oat and bran cereal, whole-grain bread, and brown rice.
• Encourage the patient to avoid ignoring the urge to defecate.
• Encourage the patient to avoid straining to have a bowel movement.
• Encourage the patient to initiate early ambulation.
• Administer stool softeners and/or laxatives as ordered.
• Explain that after hospital discharge, over-the-counter medications may be helpful for hemorrhoidal symptoms of pain, itching, or swelling but encourage the patient to consult with her caregiver before using such medications.

cally returns within 6 to 8 hours after childbirth. Until this time, the nurse should support and enhance the woman's attempts to void. Nursing interventions may include assisting the patient to the toilet, providing privacy and a unhurried environment, turning on the lavatory faucet, and assisting the patient into a sitz bath.

Bowel

The gastrointestinal system becomes more active soon after childbirth. The patient often feels hungry and thirsty after the food and fluid restrictions that usually accompany the intrapartal experience. The peptide hormone relaxin, which reaches high circulating levels during pregnancy, depresses bowel motility (Cunningham et al., 2005). The relaxed condition of the intestinal and abdominal muscles, combined with the continued effects of progesterone on the smooth muscles, diminishes bowel motility. These factors commonly result in constipation during the early puerperium. After childbirth, bowel movements are typically delayed until the second or third puerperal day and hemorrhoids (distended rectal veins), perineal trauma, and the presence of an episiotomy may be associated with painful defecation. Early ambulation, abundant fluids, and a high-fiber diet are a few strategies to help prevent constipation (Box 15-1).

Lochia

Separation of the placenta and membranes occurs in the spongy or outer layer of the decidua basalis. The uterine decidua basalis reorganizes into the basal and superficial layers. The inner basal layer becomes the foundation from which new layers of endometrium will form. The superficial layer becomes necrotic and sloughs off in the uterine discharge, called lochia. Lochia is composed of erythrocytes; epithelial cells; blood; and fragments of decidua, mucus, and bacteria (Cunningham et al., 2005). The characteristics of the lochia are indicative of the woman's status in the process of involution.

During the first few days postpartum, the lochia consists mostly of blood, which gives it a characteristic red color known as **lochia rubra**. Lochia rubra also contains elements of amnion, chorion, decidua, vernix, lanugo,

and meconium if the fetus had passed any stool in utero. These components cause the fleshy odor associated with lochia rubra.

After 3 to 4 days, the lochia becomes the pinkish-brownish **lochia serosa**. Lochia serosa contains blood, wound exudates, erythrocytes, leukocytes, and cervical mucosa. After approximately 10 to 14 days, the uterine discharge has a reduced fluid content and is largely composed of leukocytes. This combination produces a white or yellow-white thick discharge known as **lochia alba.** Lochia alba also contains decidual cells, mucus, bacteria, and epithelial cells. It is present until about the third week after childbirth but may persist for 6 weeks.

The pattern of lochia flow, from lochia rubra to serosa to alba, should not reverse. A return of lochia rubra after it has turned pink or white may indicate retained placental fragments or decreased uterine contractions and new bleeding. Lochia should contain no large clots, which may indicate the presence of retained placental fragments that are preventing closure of maternal uterine blood sinuses. The odor of lochia is similar to that of menstrual blood. An offensive odor is indicative of infection.

After assessment of the lochia, the nurse may find it difficult to document the findings correctly. Lochia is typically documented in amounts described as *scant, small, moderate,* or *heavy.* The amount of vaginal discharge is not a true indicator of the lochia flow unless the time factor is also considered. For example, a perineal pad (peripad) that accumulates less than 1 cm of lochia in 1 hour is associated with scant flow (Fig. 15-3). Nurses must also be certain to take into account the specific type of peripad used, since some are more absorbent than others. At times, visually assessing the amount of lochia flow can be difficult and inaccurate.

 Optimizing Outcomes— Abnormal findings in a postpartal patient

During a routine postpartal assessment conducted 2 hours after childbirth, the nurse records the following vital signs: pulse = 102 beats/minute; blood pressure = 130/86 mm Hg;

Scant: Blood only on tissue when wiped or 1- to 2-inch stain

Light: 4-inch or less stain

Moderate: Less than 6-inch stain

Heavy: Saturated pad

Figure 15-3 Assessment of lochia flow in one hour.

respirations = 21 breaths/minute; temperature = 98.9°F (37.1°C). The nurse's first action is to assess the fundus. With the cupped palm placed directly over the uterine fundus, the nurse uses palpation to assess for the state of contraction (e.g., soft, boggy, or firmly contracted), along with the location and height of the fundus. If soft, the fundus is massaged in a circular motion with the cupped palm until the uterus is well contracted. The nurse inspects the peripad for the lochia amount and color, and the presence of odor. The physician or nurse midwife is notified of the findings. If excessive blood loss has occurred or if the uterus is not well contracted, the nurse administers appropriate prn medication(s) (e.g., Methylergonovine [Methergine]) as ordered.

Episiotomy

An episiotomy is a 1- to 2-inch surgical incision made in the muscular area between the vagina and the anus (the perineum) to enlarge the vaginal opening before birth. The midline episiotomy is a straight incision extending toward the anus. A mediolateral episiotomy extends downward and to the side. (See Chapter 12.) Typically, the episiotomy edges have become fused (the edges have sealed) by the first 24 hours after birth. Although the patient's perineal folds may interfere with full visualization of a midline episiotomy, it is important for the nurse to carefully assess the episiotomy for redness, edema, ecchymosis, discharge, and approximation (REEDA) and then document all findings.

 clinical alert

Hematoma After an Episiotomy

Severe hemorrhage after an episiotomy is possible. Maternal complaints of excessive perineal pain should alert the nurse to the possibility of a perineal, vulvar, vaginal, or ischiorectal **hematoma** (a blood-filled swelling that occurs from damage to a blood vessel).

 medication: Methylergonovine

Methylergonovine (meth-ill-er-goe-**noe**-veen)

Methergine

Pregnancy Category: C

Indications: Prevention and treatment of postpartum and postabortion hemorrhage caused by uterine atony or subinvolution

Actions: Directly stimulates uterine and vascular smooth muscle.

Therapeutic Effects: Uterine contraction

Pharmacokinetics:
ABSORPTION: Well absorbed after oral or IM administration
ONSET OF ACTION: Oral: 5–10 minutes; IM: 2–5 minutes; IV: Immediately
DISTRIBUTION: Oral: 3 hours; IM: 3 hours; IV: 45 minutes. Enters breast milk in small quantities.
METABOLISM AND EXCRETION: Probably metabolized by the liver
HALF-LIFE: 30–120 minutes

Contraindications and Precautions
CONTRAINDICATED IN: Hypersensitivity. Should not be used to induce labor.
USE CAUTIOUSLY IN: Hypertensive or eclamptic patients (more susceptible to hypertensive and arrhythmogenic side effects); severe hepatic or renal disease; sepsis
EXERCISE EXTREME CAUTION IN: Third stage of labor

Adverse Reactions and Side Effects:
CENTRAL NERVOUS SYSTEM: Dizziness, headache
EYES, EARS, NOSE, THROAT: Tinnitus
RESPIRATORY: Dyspnea
CARDIOVASCULAR: Hypotension, arrhythmias, chest pain, hypertension, palpitations
GASTROINTESTINAL: Nausea, vomiting
GENITOURINARY: Cramps
DERMATOLOGICAL: Diaphoresis

Route and Dosage:
PO: 200–400 mcg (0.4–0.6 mg) q6–12h for 2–7 days
IM, IV: 200 mcg (0.2 mg) after delivery of fetal anterior shoulder, after delivery of the placenta, or during the puerperium; may be repeated as required at intervals of 2–4 hours up to five doses.

Nursing Implications:
1. Physical assessment: Monitor blood pressure, heart rate and uterine response frequently during medication administration. Notify the primary health care provider if uterine relaxation becomes prolonged or if character of vaginal bleeding changes.
2. Assess for signs of ergotism (cold, numb fingers and toes, chest pain, nausea, vomiting, headache, muscle pain, weakness)

Data from Deglin, J.H., and Vallerand, A.H. (2009). *Davis's drug guide for nurses* (11th ed.). Philadelphia: F.A. Davis.

To assess for perineal hematoma, the nurse should:
1. Look for discoloration of the perineum.
2. Listen for the patient's complaints or expression of severe perineal pain.
3. Observe for edema of the area.
4. Listen for the patient's expression of a need to defecate (the hematoma may cause rectal pressure).
5. Don sterile gloves, gently palpate the area, and observe for the patient's degree of sensitivity to the area by touch.
6. Call the physician or nurse-midwife to report the findings immediately. The bleeding that has produced the hematoma must be promptly identified and halted.

Optimizing Outcomes— **Early episiotomy care**

The nurse should apply an ice bag or commercial cold pack to the perineum during the first 24 hours after childbirth. The ice bag should be wrapped in a towel or disposable paper cover to prevent a thermal injury. Application of cold provides local anesthesia and promotes vasoconstriction while reducing edema and the incidence of peripheral bleeding. Later (after 24 hours), the nurse encourages the use of moist heat (sitz bath) between 100° and 105°F (37.8–40.5°C) for 20 minutes three to four times per day. The sitz bath increases circulation to the perineum, enhances blood flow to the tissues, reduces edema, and promotes healing. Dry heat, in the form of a commercial perineal "hot pack," may also be used. The packs are "cracked" to generate heat. Women should be cautioned to apply a washcloth or gauze square between the hot pack and their skin to prevent a potential burn.

ASSESSMENT OF PAIN. Pain, sometimes considered the fifth "vital sign," must be recognized as an important assessment focus throughout the postpartum period. Nurses play an important role in assessing, planning, and implementing interventions to manage maternal pain effectively. Pain should be recognized and treated in a timely manner. The failure to manage pain effectively has been associated with numerous complications, including prolonged recovery, increased length of hospital stay, depression, anxiety, poor coping, and altered sleep patterns.

Discomfort and pain may occur from several sources. Afterpains, which most commonly occur in the multiparous patient, can be quite intense, especially after breastfeeding. Analgesics such as acetaminophen (e.g., Tylenol) or nonsteroidal anti-inflammatory agents (NSAIDs) such as ibuprofen (e.g., Motrin, Advil) are effective and safe for use. Heat is not applied to the abdomen because of the potential for uterine relaxation and bleeding.

Muscular aches and cramps related to the physical exertion expended during labor and birth may be relieved with back rubs and massage. When necessary, acetaminophen (e.g., Tylenol) may be used to alleviate the discomfort. Pain occurring in the calf of the leg must be carefully evaluated for thromboembolic disease. Episiotomy pain and discomfort may be associated with sitting, walking, bending, urinating, and defecating. It may interfere with the woman's ability to comfortably hold and feed her infant. Interventions to decrease discomfort from the episiotomy include the application of cold (first 24 hours) and heat, and the use of topical anesthetic creams, sprays, and sitz baths. The **sitz bath** is a portable unit with a reservoir that fits on the toilet. When filled with warm water, the swirling action of the fluid soothes the tissue, reduces inflammation by promoting vasodilation to the area, and provides comfort and healing. The nurse prepares and assists the patient to the sitz bath, which should be used for 20 minutes three to four times a day (Procedure 15-1).

 Optimizing Outcomes— **Enhancing comfort and healing with a sitz bath**

A sitz bath is a warm-water bath taken in the sitting position that covers only the perineum and buttocks. It can be placed in the toilet, with the seat raised. Other mechanisms for taking a sitz bath include sitting in a tub filled with 4–6 inches of warm water or the use of a nonportable sitz bath unit (similar to a toilet that fills up with warm water). A sitz bath may be used for either healing or hygiene purposes. The water may contain medication. Sitz baths are used to relieve pain, itching, or muscle spasms.

The patient likely has expectations regarding pain management during the postpartum phase. She should be encouraged to express her requests or concerns regarding pain control. Education regarding the available modalities is essential and will likely enhance the patient's perception of control, as well as her level of satisfaction with the nursing care received. The nurse should regularly assess for pain and medication side effects and actively involve the patient in her pain management regimen. Use of a standardized pain rating scale enhances the assessment by allowing the patient to select the pain intensity level being experienced.

The nurse assesses and documents the patient's pain behavior regarding the:

- Location of the pain
- Type of pain: stabbing, burning, throbbing, aching
- Duration of pain: intermittent or continuous

Nursing interventions include the administration of analgesics and patient education about other measures to promote comfort.

- Suggest nonpharmacological methods for pain relief such as imagery, therapeutic touch, relaxation, distraction, and interaction with the infant.
- Provide pain relief by administering prescribed agents such as ibuprofen, propoxyphene napsylate/acetaminophen (Darvocet-N), or oxycodone/acetaminophen (Percocet).
- Suggest over-the-counter medications and alternative therapies such as tea tree oil for self-care after hospital discharge. Teach the patient that medications such as acetaminophen or ibuprofen may be equally as effective as narcotic analgesics.
- Reassure the patient that the pain and discomfort should not persist beyond 5 to 7 days and that since the episiotomy sutures are made of an absorbable material, they will not need to be removed.

 Complementary Care: *Tea tree oil to facilitate episiotomy healing*

Tea tree (*Melaleuca alternifolia*) oil applied to the perineum is believed to be beneficial in facilitating healing of the episiotomy site. *Melaleuca alternifolia* oil has been in use as a botanical medicine in various forms for centuries. For hundreds of years, the Australian aboriginal people have used tea tree oil as an antiseptic, antimicrobial, and anti-inflammatory agent. The anti-inflammatory properties are believed to be particularly helpful in promoting incisional healing (Halon & Milkus, 2004) although allergic contact dermatitis may occasionally occur (Stonehouse & Studdiford, 2007).

Postpartum women with episiotomies may be taught to fill an applicator with tea tree oil and then apply the oil directly to the wound. A few drops of the oil provide cooling to the wound, relieve pain, enhance comfort, and promote healing.

Procedure 15-1 Preparing a Sitz Bath

Purpose

To facilitate healing through the application of moist heat.

Equipment

- Sitz bath tub/toilet insert with water receptacle
- Medications to be added to water or saline, as ordered
- Towels for drying the perineal area after the treatment
- Clean perineal pad to be applied after the treatment

Steps

1. Wash your hands, identify the patient, and explain the procedure.

   RATIONALE: *Hand washing helps to prevent infection. Patient identification ensures that the procedure is performed on the correct patient. Providing an explanation educates the patient and helps to alleviate anxiety.*

2. Assess the patient to confirm that she is able to ambulate to the bathroom.

   RATIONALE: *A sitz bath can cause dizziness and increase the potential for injury. It is important to ascertain that the patient can safely ambulate to the bathroom before initiating the procedure.*

3. Assemble equipment and ensure that all equipment is clean.

   RATIONALE: *Gathering all equipment before the procedure enhances efficiency.*

4. Raise the toilet seat in the patient's bathroom.

5. Insert the sitz bath apparatus into the toilet. The overflow opening should be directed toward the back of the toilet.

6. Fill the collecting bag with water or saline, as directed, at the appropriate temperature (105°F [41°C]).

7. Test the water temperature. It should feel comfortably warm on the wrist.

   RATIONALE: *Ensuring a correct water temperature reduces the chance of thermal injury. The flow of warm water to the perineum promotes healing by increasing circulation and reducing inflammation.*

8. If prescribed, add medications to the solution.

9. Hang the bag overhead to allow a steady stream of water to flow from the bag, through the tubing, and into the reservoir.

10. Assist the ambulating patient to the bathroom. Help with removal of the perineal pad from front to back. Assist the patient to sit in the basin.

    RATIONALE: *Assistance with ambulation reduces the chance for patient injury. Removal of the pad from front to back decreases the risk for infection transmission. Proper placement on the seat ensures comfort and effectiveness of the treatment.*

11. Instruct the patient to use the tubing clamp to regulate the flow of water. Ensure that the patient is adequately covered with a robe or blankets to prevent chilling.

    RATIONALE: *The swirling warm water helps to reduce edema and promote comfort. Clothing and extra blankets for warmth prevent chilling and enhance patient comfort.*

12. Verify that the call bell is within reach and provide for privacy.

    RATIONALE: *Easy access to the call bell reassures the patient that prompt assistance is readily available when needed.*

13. Encourage the patient to remain in the sitz bath for approximately 20 minutes.

    RATIONALE: *After 20 minutes, vasoconstriction occurs and heat is no longer therapeutic.*

14. Provide assistance with drying the perineal area and applying a clean perineal pad by grasping the pad by the ends or bottom side.

    RATIONALE: *Holding the pad correctly decreases the risk for contamination and subsequent infection.*

15. Assist the patient back to the room.

    RATIONALE: *After the procedure, the patient may be fatigued or light headed from the warm water; assistance minimizes the risk of injury.*

16. Assess the patient's response to the procedure. Reinforce teaching about continued perineal care at home.

    RATIONALE: *Assessment helps to determine the effectiveness of the procedure; teaching enhances understanding and promotes continuity of care after discharge.*

17. Record completion of the procedure, the condition of the perineum, and the patient's tolerance.

    RATIONALE: *Documentation provides evidence of the intervention and an additional opportunity for evaluation of care and the patient's tolerance of the procedure.*

Clinical Alert The warm environment associated with a sitz bath may cause the patient to feel light-headed or dizzy. It is important to monitor the patient frequently throughout the intervention to ensure safety and tolerance.

(continued)

Procedure 15-1 Preparing a Sitz Bath (continued)

Teach the Patient

1. The benefits of using the sitz bath, which include enhanced hygiene, comfort, and improved circulation.

2. To use the sitz bath as often as recommended—usually three to four times per day or as needed for discomfort.

3. To contact the nursing staff immediately if she becomes light-headed or dizzy.

4. To check the temperature of the solution before use. Applying water or solution that is too warm may result in local trauma or burns to the area.

Note

If the patient prefers to prepare a sitz bath in the tub at home, she should be instructed not to use the same water for bathing. Instead, fresh water should be drawn for washing to diminish the potential for infection.

Caution: The nurse must check the temperature of the water before administration of the sitz bath to ensure that it is not too warm.

Documentation

6/29/09 1500 Patient reported perineal discomfort. Mild perineal edema noted. Patient assisted into bathroom for sitz bath. Tolerated sitz bath with warm water for 20 minutes. She denied any discomfort or syncope throughout treatment. Perineal care was provided and a new peripad was applied. The patient was assisted back into bed. She denies perineal pain at present.

—Olga Sanchez, RN

Homans' Sign

Homans' sign is often used in the assessment for deep venous thrombosis (DVT) in the leg. To assess for Homans' sign, the patient's legs should be extended and relaxed with the knees flexed. The examiner grasps the foot and sharply dorsiflexes it (Fig. 15-4). No pain or discomfort should be present. The other leg is assessed in the same manner. If calf pain is elicited, a positive Homans' sign is present. The pain occurs from inflammation of the blood vessel and is believed to be associated with the presence of a thrombosis. Pain on dorsiflexion is indicative of DVT in approximately 50% of patients. Thus, a negative Homans' sign does not rule out DVT. A diagnosis based solely on the evaluation of clinical signs that include pain in the calf, erythema, warmth greater in one calf than the other, and unequal calf circumference has proven to be unreliable. Instead, specific diagnostic procedures (e.g., venography, real-time and color Doppler ultrasound) should be performed when DVT is suspected. (See Chapter 16 for further discussion.)

Figure 15-4 Assessing for Homans' sign.

Emotional Status

The birth of a child is associated with a range of emotional experiences in the new mother. During the early puerperium, it is not unusual for patients to have periods of happiness that are intermingled with sadness, insecurity, and depression. Continued assessment of the woman's emotional status is an important nursing action that begins immediately after childbirth and continues throughout the hospital stay. The nurse should offer support to the new mother, which may include listening to her share her labor experience or reassuring her about her ability to effectively care for the newborn. The nurse should also provide information regarding the "baby blues," and emphasize that these feelings are common and temporary (Horowitz & Goodman, 2005).

 Now Can You— Discuss essential components of postpartum nursing care?

1. Identify three types of lochia and explain the characteristics and duration of each?
2. Describe nursing interventions to promote healing, enhance comfort, and prevent infection in the patient with an episiotomy?
3. Discuss the nurse's role in pain assessment of the postpartal patient?

Maternal Physiological Adaptations and Continued Assessment of the Patient

HEMATOLOGICAL AND METABOLIC SYSTEMS

During the immediate postpartum period, a decrease in blood volume correlates with the blood loss experienced during delivery. During the next few days after childbirth, the maternal plasma volume decreases even further as a

Nursing Care Plan Acute Pain/Discomfort in the Postpartal Patient

Nursing Diagnosis: Acute Pain related to tissue damage secondary to childbirth

Measurable Short-term Goal: The patient will report decreased pain to a level that is acceptable to her.

Measurable Long-term Goal: The patient will report minimal or no pain upon discharge from the hospital.

NOC Outcomes:
Pain Level (2102) Severity of observed or reported pain
Pain Control (1605) Personal actions to control pain

NIC Interventions:
Pain Management (1400)
Analgesic Administration (2210)
Heat/Cold Application (1380)

Nursing Interventions:

1. Perform routine, comprehensive pain assessments to include: onset, location, intensity, quality, characteristics, and aggravating and alleviating factors of the discomfort. Note verbal and nonverbal indications of discomfort.

   RATIONALE: Routine, comprehensive pain assessments enable the nurse to provide interventions in a timely manner to enhance effectiveness of medications and ensures early identification of complications resulting in painful stimuli.

2. Ask the patient to rate her pain on a standard 0 to 10 pain scale before and after interventions and to identify her own acceptable comfort level on the scale.

   RATIONALE: Use of a consistent pain scale provides objective measurement of the patient's perception of pain, the effectiveness of interventions, and the acceptable comfort level for the individual.

3. Identify cultural or personal beliefs about the experience of pain and the use of pain interventions, including prescribed medications.

   RATIONALE: Expression of pain and use of pain relief interventions may vary according to culture and personal beliefs. Patients may prefer a stoic response to pain or fear becoming addicted to narcotics.

4. Provide factual, nonjudgmental information regarding pain interventions that are available to the patient. Encourage use of culturally based comfort measures when appropriate.

   RATIONALE: Accurate information and respect for the individual's experience and preferences empowers the patient and reduces psychic discomfort.

5. Offer an ice pack to the perineum if the patient experienced perineal trauma or episiotomy. Apply for 20 minutes followed by removal for 10 minutes.

   RATIONALE: Cold therapy causes vasoconstriction and reduces edema resulting in decreased pain. Periodic removal avoids thermal injury.

6. Assist the patient with a sitz bath as ordered if the patient experiences perineal discomfort.

   RATIONALE: Cool water in the sitz bath decreases pain associated with edema while warm water promotes vasodilation and increased circulation to promote healing and provide comfort.

7. Teach the patient to apply topical medications for perineal or hemorrhoid pain as ordered.

   RATIONALE: Topical anesthetics, such as Dermoplast spray, produce localized pain relief by inhibiting conduction of sensory nerve impulses. Tucks pads contain witch hazel, which has astringent properties to shrink hemorrhoids and reduce perineal edema.

8. Teach the patient about the sources of pain and the effects of prescribed medications and interventions. Encourage her participation in developing a pain management plan.

   RATIONALE: Information and involvement increases the patient's perception of control and increases her personal satisfaction with postpartum pain management.

result of diuresis. The 500-mL blood loss that typically accompanies a vaginal birth (1000 mL for a cesarean birth) usually results in a 1 gram (2 grams for a cesarean birth) drop in hemoglobin. It is important for the nurse to remember that as the body's excess fluid is excreted, the hematocrit may rise due to hemoconcentration. However, the hematocrit should have returned to pre-pregnancy levels by 4 to 6 weeks postpartum.

The white blood cell (WBC) count, which increases during labor and in the immediate postpartum period,

returns to normal values within 6 days. Levels of plasma fibrinogen tend to remain elevated during the first few postpartal weeks. Although this alteration exerts a protective effect against hemorrhage, it increases the patient's risk of thrombus formation. Overall, the hematologic system has usually returned to a nonpregnant status by the third to fourth postpartal week.

Circulating levels of estrogen and progesterone decrease dramatically after delivery of the placenta. The decline in these two hormones signals the anterior pituitary gland to produce prolactin in readiness for lactation. In nonlactating (formula feeding) women, prolactin levels return to normal by the third to fourth postpartal week.

After childbirth and expulsion of the placenta, circulating levels of other hormones, including placental lactogen, cortisol, growth hormone, and insulinase, also fall. During the early postpartum period, the decline in the serum levels of these substances reduces the anti-insulin effects that occur during pregnancy. Hence, insulin requirements are reduced for insulin dependent women during this time, sometimes termed a "honeymoon phase." For many insulin-dependent diabetics, glucose levels remain in a normal range (without intervention) during the first few days after childbirth (Chan & Winkle, 2006).

NEUROLOGICAL SYSTEM

Fatigue and discomfort are common complaints after childbirth. The demands of the newborn frequently create altered sleep patterns that contribute to increased maternal fatigue. Anesthesia and analgesia received during labor and birth may cause transient maternal neurological changes such as numbness in the legs or dizziness. When these changes are present, the nursing priority is to safeguard the patient and her infant and prevent injury from falls.

Complaints of headaches require further nursing assessment. Patients who received epidural or spinal anesthesia may experience headaches, especially when they assume an upright position. After spinal or epidural anesthesia, headaches may result from the leakage of cerebrospinal fluid into the extradural space. Labor-induced stress or gestational hypertension may also cause headaches. It is essential that the nurse assess the quality and location of the headache and carefully monitor maternal vital signs. Headaches that are accompanied by double or blurred vision, photophobia, epigastric or abdominal pain, and proteinuria may be signs of a developing or worsening preeclampsia. Report these findings immediately to the primary health care provider. Implement environmental interventions such as reducing the room lighting and noise levels and limiting visitors. The physiological edema of pregnancy is dramatically reversed during postpartum diuresis. Patients who experienced medial nerve compression and carpel tunnel syndrome during pregnancy often obtain relief of symptoms.

RENAL SYSTEM, FLUID, AND ELECTROLYTES

The renal plasma flow, glomerular filtration rate (GFR), plasma creatinine and blood urea nitrogen (BUN) return to pre-pregnant levels by the second to third month after childbirth. Urinary glucose excretion increases in pregnancy by 100-fold over nonpregnant values. These values return to nonpregnant levels after the first postpartal week. Pregnancy-associated proteinuria (up to 1+ on a urine dipstick or less than 300 mg in 24 hours) is common during pregnancy and generally returns to pre-pregnancy values by 6 weeks postpartum (Cunningham et al., 2005).

During the postpartum period, there is a rapid, sustained natriuresis (excessively large amount of sodium in the urine) and diuresis as the sodium and water retention of pregnancy is reversed. The physiological reversal is particularly pronounced during the second to fifth puerperal days. In most women, the body's fluid and electro-

lyte balance has been restored to a nonpregnant homeostatic state by the third postpartal week.

After childbirth, a decrease in levels of oxytocin and estrogen naturally occurs and contributes to diuresis. As the serum levels decline, the diuresis becomes more pronounced. Nurses often note a maternal urinary output that reaches 3000 mL excreted in a 24-hour period. For the postpartum patient, a single voiding may contain 500 to 1000 mL of urine.

 Now Can You— **Describe early postpartal physiological adaptations in the metabolic, neurological, and renal systems?**

1. Explain what is meant by the "honeymoon phase" and why this may occur?
2. Identify possible causes and describe appropriate nursing assessments for patients who complain of headache?
3. Discuss physiological adaptations in the renal system and identify one patient teaching need related to these adaptations?

RESPIRATORY SYSTEM

Respiratory alkalosis and compensated metabolic acidosis occur during labor and may persist into the postpartum period. In most situations, however, after delivery of the placenta and the decline in levels of progesterone, the respiratory system quickly returns to a pre-pregnant state. In addition, the immediate decrease in intra-abdominal pressure associated with the birth of the baby allows for increased expansion of the diaphragm and relief from the dyspnea usually associated with pregnancy. By the third postpartal week, the respiratory system has returned to a pre-pregnant state.

INTEGUMENTARY SYSTEM

Changes in the skin during pregnancy and in the postpartum period are related to the major alterations in hormones. Women may experience alterations in pigmentation, connective and cutaneous tissue, hair, nails, secretory glands, and pruritus. Most pregnancy-related skin changes disappear completely during the postpartum period although some, such as striae gravidarum (stretch marks) fade but may remain permanently.

 Ethnocultural Considerations— **Pregnancy-related skin changes in the puerperium**

Although abdominal stretch marks (striae gravidarum) appear more pronounced immediately after childbirth, they tend to fade over the following 6 months. In Caucasian women, striae become pale and white in color; in African American women, they will appear as a slightly darker pigment.

CARDIOVASCULAR SYSTEM

During pregnancy, the heart is displaced slightly upward and to the left. As involution of the uterus occurs, the heart returns to its normal position. Dramatic changes in the maternal hemodynamic system result from birth of the baby, expulsion of the placenta, and loss of the amniotic fluid. These abrupt alterations can create cardiovascular instability during the immediate postpartum period. Despite the usual blood loss (500 mL with a vaginal birth; 1000 mL with a cesarean birth), the maternal cardiac output is significantly elevated above prelabor levels for 1 to 2 hours postpartum and remains high for 48 hours postpartum. The cardiac output returns to pre-pregnant levels within 2 to 4 weeks after childbirth.

On average, a 3-kg weight loss occurs during the first postpartal week. Diuresis takes place between the second and fifth day. A major fluid shift involves the movement of extracellular fluid back into the venous system for excretion through urine and perspiration. If the physiologic diuresis does not occur, there is an increased risk of pulmonary edema. The cardiac output and stroke volume remain elevated for at least 48 hours after childbirth. Within 2 weeks, the cardiac output has decreased by 30% and then reaches pre-pregnant values by 6 to 12 weeks postpartum in most women (Cunningham et al., 2005).

IMMUNE SYSTEM

The WBC count is increased during labor and birth and remains elevated during the early postpartum period, gradually returning to normal values within 4 to 7 days after childbirth. Depending on the patient's blood type and immune status, administration of RhoGAM (see below) may be indicated. Women who are rubella susceptible during pregnancy should receive the MMR (measles–mumps–rubella) vaccine at the time of hospital discharge; varicella vaccine should also be encouraged (American College of Obstetricians and Gynecologists [ACOG], 2003).

Rh₀(D) Immune Globulin

Nonsensitized women who are $Rh_o(D)$-negative and have given birth to an Rh(D)-positive infant should receive 300 mcg of $Rh_o(D)$ immune globulin (RhoGAM) within 72 hours after giving birth. RhoGAM should be given whether or not the mother received RhoGAM during the antepartum period. In some situations, depending on the extent of hemorrhage and exchange of maternal–fetal blood, a larger dose of RhoGAM may be indicated. (See Chapter 11 for further discussion.)

Rubella Vaccine

Before discharge, the patient needs to be assessed for rubella immunity. If nonimmune (rubella titer less than 1:8, or antibody negative on the enzyme-linked immunosorbent assay [ELISA]), the MMR vaccine should be administered. The nurse should counsel the patient about the need to avoid pregnancy for 1 month after receiving the vaccine (due to the teratogenic effects associated with congenital rubella syndrome) and advise her that she may briefly experience rubella-type symptoms such as lymphadenopathy, arthralgia, and a low-grade fever. The vaccine may be safely given to breastfeeding mothers. A signed consent form must be obtained before administration of the vaccine (ACOG, 2003).

REPRODUCTIVE SYSTEM

The uterus undergoes a rapid reduction in size (involution) and returns to its pre-pregnant state in about 3 weeks. The former site of the placenta heals by the process of exfoliation, which ensures that the placental site heals without leaving a fibrous scar. Formation of scar tissue would limit areas for future implantation and adversely affect the potential for future pregnancies. After a vaginal birth, the vagina often appears edematous or bruised and superficial lacerations may be present. Although swelling is resolved during the healing process, the vagina does not return to its nulliparous size and the labia majora and labia minora remain more flaccid in the multiparous woman (Cunningham et al., 2005).

During the postpartum phase, the return of ovulation and menstruation varies according to the individual. Menstruation usually resumes within 6 to 8 weeks after childbirth in women who are not breastfeeding. Seventy-five percent menstruate by the twelfth postpartal week. The first cycle is often anovulatory. The return of ovulation and menstruation is typically prolonged in lactating women. Those who exclusively breastfeed may not ovulate or menstruate for 3 or more months. It is important to educate patients that since ovulation can precede menstruation, breastfeeding is not a reliable method of contraception.

GASTROINTESTINAL SYSTEM

Owing to hormonal effects, gastric motility is decreased during pregnancy. It is further decreased during labor and in the first few postpartal days due to decreased abdominal wall tone. Abdominal discomfort results from gaseous distention related to decreased motility and abdominal muscle relaxation. Constipation, a common nursing diagnosis for the postpartal patient, is associated with abdominal discomfort and decreased hunger. Straining to pass hard stool can cause hemorrhoids and tear episiotomy sutures. Although spontaneous bowel movements usually resume by the second or third day after childbirth, it is important to educate the patient about strategies to prevent constipation. Stool softeners may be necessary. Additional nursing diagnoses for the postpartal patient focus on a variety of other problems such as pain, fatigue, and sleep disturbances, infant feeding difficulties and knowledge deficit (Box 15-2).

Box 15-2 Common Nursing Diagnoses During the Puerperium

- Breastfeeding, ineffective/effective
- Risk for constipation
- Sleep-pattern disturbed
- Fatigue
- Pain, acute
- Activity intolerance
- Skin integrity, risk for impaired
- Knowledge, deficient regarding self-care or care of infant
- Risk for infection
- Family processes parenting impaired
- Risk for situational low self-esteem related to body image changes
- Risk for urinary retention

MUSCULOSKELETAL SYSTEM

During pregnancy, the pelvic joints and ligaments have increased laxity. The hormones relaxin and progesterone are believed to contribute to the relaxation of the soft tissues (muscles, ligaments, and connective tissue) in the maternal pelvis to create room for the birthing process. In some women, the loosening of the pelvic joints causes pain and functional limitations.

During the first few days after childbirth, the woman may experience muscle fatigue and general body aches from the exertion of labor and delivery of the baby. Muscle fatigue can be exacerbated by the extended lack of nutrition and fluids throughout the course of labor. The maternal expenditure of glucose during **parturition** (the act of giving birth) can also add to muscle fatigue and may interfere with the patient's ability to ambulate and initiate postpartum exercises. The nurse needs to assure the patient that the muscular discomforts are temporary and not indicative of a serious medical problem.

During pregnancy, the abdominal walls are stretched to accommodate the growing fetus. The progressive stretching causes a decrease in the muscle tone of the rectus muscles of the abdomen and results in the soft, flabby, and weak muscles experienced after birth. Rectus abdominis diastasis is a conventional term used to define the split between the two rectus abdominis muscles that can occur from pregnancy. Women should be aware that during the early postpartal period, the abdominal wall may not be sufficiently protected to withstand additional stress from increased activities. Nurses should teach them to maintain correct posture when performing activities such as lifting, carrying, and bathing the baby for at least 12 weeks after birth. Performing modified sit-ups during this time is beneficial in helping to strengthen the abdominal muscles.

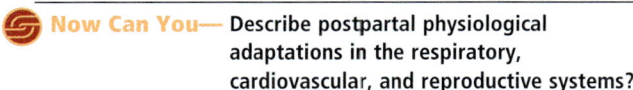 **Now Can You—** Describe postpartal physiological adaptations in the respiratory, cardiovascular, and reproductive systems?

1. Explain why pregnancy-related dyspnea is relieved in the early postpartal period?
2. Describe three intra-postpartal events that cause dramatic changes in the maternal hemodynamic system?
3. Identify when ovulation and menstruation usually occur in the postpartal woman and explain specific information that should be given to lactating mothers?

Care for the Multicultural Family

ENHANCING CULTURAL SENSITIVITY

According to the United States Census Bureau (2001), ethnic and racial diversity in the U.S. population has reached new levels. At present, the population includes 77.1% Caucasians, 12.9% African Americans, 12% Hispanics, 4.2% Asians, 1.5% Native Americans/Alaska Natives, 0.3% Native Hawaiian/other Pacific Islanders, and 2.4% as persons who describe themselves as members of other races. Diversity in the population reaches into the health care sector and has prompted emphasis on cultural awareness in nursing education curricula and mandatory in-service offerings for hospital staff.

Culturally competent care involves knowledge of the various dimensions of care, including moving beyond the biomedical needs of the patient. Rather, a holistic approach is one that expands knowledge, changes attitudes, and enhances clinical skills. To provide optimal care in a variety of clinical settings, it is important for health care professionals to conduct cultural assessments and expand their knowledge and understanding of culturally influenced beliefs, common health care practices, customs, and rituals (Taylor, 2005). In preparation for the cultural assessment, health care providers should:

* Assess their own cultural beliefs, identifying personal biases, stereotypes, and prejudices.
* Make a conscious commitment to respect and value the beliefs of others.
* Learn the customs and rituals of the common cultural groups within the community.
* Seek input from patients regarding health-related traditions and practices.
* Evaluate if what is about to be taught is really better than what the patient is already doing for herself.
* Adapt care to meet the special needs of the patient and her family, as long as standards of health and safety are not compromised.
* Include cultural assessment as a routine part of perinatal health care.

CULTURAL INFLUENCES ON THE PUERPERIUM

In certain multicultural populations such as India, Thailand, and China, the woman's postpartum confinement lasts for 40 days. During this time, prolonged rest with restricted activity is believed to be essential. The postpartum period is an important time for ensuring future good health; thus great emphasis is placed on allowing the mother's body to regain balance after the birth of a child.

During the 40-day confinement, support for the mother is provided by the female family members, usually the woman's mother, sister(s), and mother-in law, who perform household chores such as cooking and caring for the siblings and new baby. The woman's mother or older female relative often prescribes cultural remedies to aid in recovery and promote good health in the future. The female family members also provide the new mother with information on caring for herself and activities to avoid. Lack of adequate rest and poor diet are believed to result in poor eyesight, varicose veins, digestive disorders, headache, and backache (Davis, 2001).

Certain beliefs regarding hot and cold exist among several multicultural groups. Blood is considered "hot," and because the postpartum woman loses blood, she is considered to be in a "cold" state. To avoid illness, the mother must restore her health status by moving from a cold to hot state. The mother accomplishes this by:

* Adopting a diet that includes drinking/eating hot foods (foods such as black pepper, ginger, and garlic are believed to improve blood circulation). Sour foods such as lemons, grapefruits, and oranges are discouraged because they are thought to cause urinary incontinence later in life if eaten too early during the puerperium.

- Avoiding the consumption of ice water or cold water. These cold beverages are believed to cause weakness and delay healing.
- Avoiding cold temperatures, which are thought to be detrimental to the mother's recovery. To maintain warmth, the mother dresses warmly and stays in bed for several days. Bathing, showering, and washing the hair is delayed for 40 days because water cools the body.
- Avoiding drafts by keeping doors and windows closed and avoiding fans and air-conditioning.

CLINICAL IMPLICATIONS OF CULTURALLY APPROPRIATE CARE

To provide sensitive, appropriate care, nurses need to adopt a flexible approach when caring for women who embrace non-Western health beliefs and practices. Inquiring about cultural beliefs, and, when possible, incorporating the beliefs into the plan of care are important strategies to help achieve this goal. For example, to demonstrate sensitivity to beliefs regarding hot and cold, the nurse may offer a warm sponge bath instead of a shower, adjust the thermostat in the room and provide extra blankets for warmth; offer warm drinks instead of cold beverages; and allow female family members as much access to the mother as possible.

 Now Can You— **Provide culturally sensitive postpartal care?**

1. Identify at least five ways that health care providers can enhance cultural sensitivity before conducting a cultural assessment?
2. Describe several cultural beliefs concerning "hot" and "cold" and identify specific nursing interventions that allow women to adhere to these beliefs?

Promoting Recovery and Self-Care in the Puerperium

ACTIVITY AND REST

In the postpartum period, it is important for the new mother to begin ambulating as soon as her condition permits. Despite recent advances in diagnosis and treatment, deep vein thrombosis after birth continues to constitute a leading cause of maternal morbidity and mortality. Venous stasis and hypercoagulation, conditions that exist in pregnancy, are continued into the postpartum period. Early postpartum ambulation is key in preventing maternal thromboembolic events.

The type of birth and overall health status determines how soon the patient is allowed to resume exercise. The woman should be taught to begin with mild exercises, such as Kegel exercises, to strengthen the pelvic floor muscles. Nonambulating patients may begin with leg exercises. All exercise methods should be increased gradually.

Many women enter labor fatigued from the discomforts of pregnancy and lack of satisfying sleep associated with the third trimester. The length of labor and demands of the new mothering role further increase the feelings of exhaustion. During the hospital stay and later at home, all patients should be encouraged to obtain adequate sleep and frequent rest periods to help facilitate an optimal recovery.

NOURISHMENT

A weight loss of approximately 10 to 12 lbs. (4.5 to 5.5 kg) occurs immediately after childbirth, and this amount is directly related to the collective weights of the baby, placenta, and amniotic fluid. An additional 5 lbs. (2.3 kg) is lost over the following week as a result of puerperal diuresis and uterine involution. How quickly the woman returns to her pre-pregnancy weight depends on her physical activity level, eating habits, and lifestyle. Olson, Strawderman, Hinton, and Pearson (2003) noted that women whose weight increase was within the recommended limit of 25 to 30 lbs. (11.4 to 13.6 kg) during pregnancy could anticipate a return to the pre-pregnancy weight by 6 to 8 weeks postpartum. Factors associated with weight changes during the postpartum period include gestational weight gain, frequency of exercise, dietary intake, and breastfeeding for longer than 1 year.

Because of the restriction of food during labor, most patients demonstrate a hearty appetite after childbirth. All parturient women should be encouraged to eat a balanced, nutritious diet with multivitamin supplements. Iron is recommended only if the patient's hemoglobin is low.

ELIMINATION

Voiding should occur within 4 hours of childbirth. Patients should be encouraged to empty the bladder every 4 to 6 hours and to expect to excrete large volumes of urine. In addition to the extra- to intravascular fluid shift that follows childbirth, there is a decrease in the production of the adrenal hormone aldosterone. Declining levels of aldosterone are associated with a decrease in sodium retention and an increase in urinary output.

An intake and output record should be maintained to monitor the volume of urine passed during the first 24 hours. The woman who has recently given birth is prone to urinary stasis and retention. Incomplete bladder emptying or urinary retention may result from trauma to urethral tissue sustained during the "pushing phase" of a vaginal birth. Also, patients who were catheterized or who received regional anesthesia during childbirth sometimes experience an absence of the sensation to void. Bladder hypotonia during labor may also lead to postpartal urinary retention or stasis, factors that increase the risk of infection.

Incomplete emptying of the bladder is suspected when the patient experiences urinary frequency and passes 100 to 150 mL of urine with each voiding. The nurse's assessment includes careful palpation of the lower abdomen to identify a distended or displaced uterus. The uterine fundus is felt above the symphysis pubis with a lateral displacement of the uterus. The nurse also notes an increase in the amount of lochia since the uterus is unable to contract effectively. The bladder is displaced, bulges above the symphysis pubis, and feels "boggy" on palpation. Patients experiencing urinary retention due to absence of the urge to void can be helped by assisted early ambulation to the toilet and other measures such as running the water from the lavatory faucet. If ambulation is not possible, the nurse can pour warm water over the vulva and perineal area to help relax the urethral sphincter. Owing to the risk of urinary infection associated with urinary stasis, catheterization may be necessary if the patient is unable to void.

Constipation commonly occurs because of slowed peristalsis associated with pregnancy hormones and childbirth anesthesia. In addition, perineal discomfort, fear of suture separation at the episiotomy site, and incisional pain (after a cesarean birth) may contribute to decreased frequency in bowel movements. To prevent constipation, nurses should encourage patients to consume foods high in fiber and roughage. Adequate fluid intake that includes drinking at least six to eight glasses of water or juice daily is another important strategy to prevent constipation. Early ambulation is also encouraged to improve peristalsis and relieve abdominal gas pain. If these measures are not effective, the primary care provider may prescribe a stool softener, suppository, or enema to alleviate the symptoms.

PERINEAL CARE

The perineum is susceptible to infection because of impaired tissue integrity resulting from bruising, laceration, or an episiotomy. The proximity of the perineum to the anus increases the risk of the incision becoming contaminated with fecal material; continuous drainage of blood creates a favorable medium for the proliferation of bacteria. To minimize infection, patients should be taught about perineal hygiene. A teaching approach that incorporates a return demonstration, encouragement, and positive reinforcement is most likely to be successful. Instructions should be given about properly cleansing the perineal area and the value of sitz baths, which not only cleanse but also provide relief from discomfort during the first 24 to 48 hours postpartum.

Patients should be educated about the importance of cleansing the perineum after each voiding and bowel movement. Hand washing before and after perineal care ("pericare") is essential for the prevention of infection. The nurse instructs the patient to gently rinse her perineum with fresh warm water after use of the toilet and before a new perineal pad is applied. The patient is taught to fill the peri-bottle (handheld squirt bottle) with warm tap water and gently squirt the water toward the front of the perineum and allow the water to flow from front to back. Consistent use of the peri-bottle is soothing, cleansing, and helps to relieve discomfort. Peri-pads should be changed often and secured in the underwear to allow for free drainage of the lochia. Tampons are contraindicated due to the risk of infection.

The nurse provides pericare for patients recovering from cesarean births until they are ambulatory and able to perform personal self-care. To provide pericare for the bedbound patient, a plastic-covered pad is placed under the patient's buttocks to protect the bed during the procedure. With the woman in a supine position, the nurse carefully removes the perineal pad in a front-to-back direction. This prevents the portion of the pad that touched the rectal area from sliding forward and contaminating the vagina. Next, a bedpan is positioned under the buttocks. The movement associated with lifting the buttocks helps to expel clots and/or pooled blood in the vaginal canal. This also serves as a good time to assess the fundus for tone. Uterine palpation may be beneficial in helping the patient expel additional blood or clots. The nurse uses a peri-bottle filled with warm water (or other solution used according to hospital policy) and gently squirts the perineum from front to back while allowing the water to collect in the bedpan. The labia are not separated because they prevent the solution from entering the vagina. The perineal area is then gently dried and a clean peripad is applied from front to back.

⬡ Optimizing Outcomes— Teaching about perineal care

To enhance the patient's understanding about proper perineal care, the nurse provides the following instructions:

1. Fill the squeeze/peri bottle with tap water. The water should feel comfortably warm on your wrist.
2. Sit on the toilet with the bottle positioned between your legs so that water can be squirted directly on the perineum. Aim the bottle opening at your perineum and spray so that the water moves from front to back. Do not separate the labia and do not spray the water into your vagina. Empty the entire bottle over the perineum— this should take approximately 2 minutes.
3. Gently pat the area dry with toilet paper or cotton wipes. Move from front to back, use each wipe once, then drop it in the toilet.
4. Grasping the bottom side or ends of a clean perineal pad, apply it from front to back.
5. Stand before flushing the toilet to prevent the water from the toilet from spraying onto your perineum.

Ice Packs

To reduce perineal swelling and pain that result from bruising, ice packs may be applied every 2 to 4 hours. Application of cold is beneficial because of its vasoconstriction and numbing effects. The ice pack should always be covered and applied from front to back. It should be left in place for no longer than 20 minutes to minimize the complications associated with prolonged vasoconstriction. Patients obtain the most relief when ice packs are applied within the first 24 hours after childbirth.

DISCOMFORT RELATED TO AFTERPAINS

Afterbirth pains describe intermittent uterine contractions that occur during the process of involution. In general, the pains are more pronounced in patients with decreased uterine tone due to overdistention. Uterine overdistention is associated with multiple gestation, multiparity, macrosomia, and hydramnios. Afterpains also tend to be more intense in breastfeeding women because infant suckling and/or pumping the breasts triggers an endogenous release of oxytocin, the hormone that initiates the milk-ejection reflex. Oxytocin causes powerful uterine contractions. Afterbirth pain maybe severe for 2 to 3 days after childbirth. Mild analgesics should provide relief.

SPECIAL CONSIDERATIONS FOR WOMEN WITH HIV/AIDS

Women who have the human immunodeficiency virus (HIV) or acquired immunodeficiency syndrome (AIDS) require special precautionary care during the puerperium.

All personnel who come in close contact with the patient should wear latex gloves (unless the patient has a latex allergy). In that situation, nonlatex gloves are used, as well as safety glasses to prevent the transmission of blood and body fluids. Patients need to be taught to avoid contact of personal body fluids with the infant's mucous membranes and open skin lesions. Breastfeeding is not advised due to the risk of transmission of HIV to the infant. (See Chapter 11 for further information.)

 Now Can You— **Promote recovery and self-care in the puerperium?**

1. Identify factors that determine how quickly patients should return to the pre-pregnant weight?
2. Describe the essential components of patient teaching about perineal care?
3. Describe special precautions that should be taken for postpartal HIV-positive women?

Care of the Postpartal Surgical Patient

PERMANENT STERILIZATION (TUBAL LIGATION)

A postpartum tubal ligation is a procedure that blocks the fallopian tubes to prevent the woman from becoming pregnant. When requested, the procedure, called a minilaparotomy, is performed after childbirth while the mother is still hospitalized. The size and position of the uterus during the early puerperium facilitates the surgical procedure. When a cesarean birth has been performed, the tubal ligation may be done at the same time. Patients need to be informed that while it is typically considered to be a permanent form of fertility control, there is a small chance that a future pregnancy may occur. (See Chapter 6 for further discussion.)

Patients scheduled for a tubal ligation are NPO before the surgical procedure. If epidural anesthesia was used for childbirth, the catheter is often left in place so that the patient can be re-anesthetized easily. When no epidural was previously placed, general anesthesia will most likely be used during surgery.

CARE OF THE PATIENT AFTER A CESAREAN BIRTH

Nursing care of the postoperative postpartum patient is similar to the care provided to all postoperative patients. The nurse must complete the BUBBLE-HE assessment previously discussed. Because the woman is confined to bed until full sensation has returned to the lower extremities, interventions for the prevention of deep vein thrombosis (DVTs) must be implemented. Preventive strategies include leg exercises (flexion and extension of the knee) and application of compression boots as ordered by the physician.

How the patient reacts to her surgery is often tied to the circumstances surrounding the birth—that is, whether the cesarean section ("c-section") was a planned procedure or an emergency event. Women who experience an emergency or unplanned cesarean birth may suffer from extreme disappointment, feelings of inadequacy, guilt, and personal failure. They may also harbor hostilities directed toward the medical and nursing staff. (See Chapter 16 for further discussion.)

After a cesarean birth, especially when unplanned, nurses must be aware of the myriad of potential psychological issues that may arise. Research suggests that women may perceive cesarean birth to be a less positive experience than a vaginal birth. Vaginal birth has been shown to be associated with enhanced maternal satisfaction and perceptions of greater personal control over the birth. Women who experience vaginal birth describe feelings of empowerment, elation, and achievement (Lavender, Hofmeyr, Nielson, Kingdon, & Gyte, 2007). Particularly for unplanned or emergent cesarean deliveries, the experience of cesarean birth may be associated with more negative perceptions of the birthing experience. However, research regarding the psychological outcomes associated with cesarean birth remains mixed (Patel, Murphy, & Peters, 2005).

The benefits of maternal–child interaction during the early postpartal hours are well documented. The first few hours after childbirth constitute a critical time for the initiation of a healthy maternal–infant interaction. For most mothers, a successful vaginal birth is psychologically better tolerated and avoids the need for additional recovery time that is necessary after a cesarean birth. In addition, early breast feeding (for those who wish to breast feed) is more easily implemented after a vaginal birth.

Additional challenges faced by patients during recovery from a cesarean birth include recovery from the anesthesia, a need to cope with incisional and gas pain, and slow ambulation. Mother–infant bonding may be delayed and patients are at an increased risk for hemorrhage, surgical wound infection, urinary tract infections, and DVT. (See Chapter 16 for additional information.)

CARE OF THE INCISIONAL WOUND

The surgical incision requires ongoing nursing assessment after a cesarean birth. The nurse should assess for approximation of the wound edges, and make note of any redness, discoloration, warmth, edema, unusual tenderness, or drainage. If a dry sterile dressing has been applied, the surrounding tissue should be carefully evaluated for evidence of a reaction to the tape used to secure the dressing. Assessing for and effectively treating incisional pain is also of paramount importance.

RECOVERY FROM ANESTHESIA

Ambulation is encouraged as soon as the patient's vital signs are stable. If a spinal or epidural anesthesia was used, ambulation is delayed until full sensation has returned to the lower extremities. Common side effects of anesthesia include paresthesias (sensation of pins and needles in the legs) and headache. Assistance is required when the patient gets out of bed for the first time. Nurses should administer pain medication 30 minutes before the patient attempts ambulation. To minimize dizziness from orthostatic hypotension, the nurse should instruct the patient to sit on the side of her bed for several minutes before moving into a standing position.

Respiratory Care

Incisional pain and abdominal distension often cause patients to adopt shallow breathing patterns that can lead to decreased gas exchange and a reduced tidal volume. To facilitate adequate lung functions, patients should be taught how to perform pulmonary exercises. After being placed in a high Fowler's position, the patient is shown to use a pillow to support her incision and instructed to take a deep breath and cough. Respiratory therapists are often included in the team approach to care for postoperative patients. Expectoration of secretions and deep breathing help prevent common complications including atelectasis and pneumonia. The nurse should administer pain medication 15 to 30 minutes before the patient begins her respiratory exercises.

Abdominal distension and gas pains are common after abdominal surgery and result from delayed peristalsis. Breakdown of digested food in the colon produces a buildup of gas that results in distension and discomfort. Anesthesia also causes a delay in the return of peristalsis and it usually takes several days for the intestinal function to return.

Until bowel sounds are present, the nurse should offer the patient ice chips and small sips of water only. The diet is slowly advanced as tolerated. To minimize gas pains and stimulate the return of peristalsis, frequent ambulation is encouraged.

An indwelling Foley catheter connected to a closed drainage system remains in place for approximately 24 hours after a cesarean birth. While the catheter is in place, the nurse must assess for urine output of at least 150 mL/hr and maintain appropriate perineal care to reduce the risk of urinary tract infection. Once the catheter has been removed, the patient is at risk for urinary retention and her output must be closely monitored. The nurse can help facilitate the return of normal voiding patterns by encouraging early ambulation to the toilet, ensuring privacy, allowing water to run in the lavatory, and pouring warm water on the perineum. If the patient is unable to void within 6 hours, a diagnosis of urinary retention should be considered and catheterization may be necessary.

Now Can You— **Provide nursing care for the surgical postpartal patient?**

1. Identify nursing assessments appropriate for the postoperative postpartum patient?
2. Describe maternal psychological issues that may accompany a cesarean birth?
3. Discuss nursing interventions to facilitate ambulation and lung expansion?

Facilitating Infant Nourishment: Educating Parents to Make Informed Choices

Holistic care during the puerperium includes educating women and their partners about infant nutrition and providing support to facilitate success with the feeding method chosen. By the time they enter the postpartum phase of childbearing, most women have already made a decision about infant feeding. Providing current, evidence-based information, offering clinical guidance, and identifying appropriate resources when needed empowers patients to achieve success in nourishing and nurturing their newborn.

Breastfeeding has long been established as the optimal method of infant feeding and current trends are reflective of the public's awareness of its value. Today, more women in the United States are breastfeeding their babies than at any time in modern history. While the rate of breastfeeding has increased in all demographic groups, certain populations of women are less likely to breastfeed. These include women younger than 25 years of age; those with a lower income; primiparas; African Americans; those who participate in the special Supplemental Nutrition Program for Women, Infants, and Children (WIC); those with a high school education or less; and those who are employed full time outside of the home (Johnston & Esposito, 2007).

Human breast milk is the ideal infant food choice. It is bacteriologically safe, fresh, readily available and balanced to meet the infant's needs. According to the American Academy of Pediatrics, "human milk is species-specific, and all substitute feeding preparations differ markedly from it, making human milk uniquely superior for infant feeding" (Gartner et al., 2005). When discussing infant feeding options with parents, nurses can share factual information about the physiological and psychological benefits of breastfeeding (Box 15-3). There are economic benefits as well: breastfeeding reduces the cost of feeding and preparation time. Providing such information may reinforce the mother's decision to breastfeed or help women and their partners in the decision-making process. The partner's level of support with the infant feeding method is an important factor in the woman's decision and success. There are only a few situations in which breast feeding is contraindicated:

- Infants with galactosemia (due to an inability to digest the lactose in the milk)

Box 15-3 **Selected Breastfeeding Benefits**

FOR MOTHERS
- Decreased risk of breast cancer
- Lactational amenorrhea (LAM) (although breastfeeding is not considered an effective form of contraception)
- Enhanced involution (due to uterine contractions triggered by the release of oxytocin) and decreased risk of postpartum hemorrhage
- Enhanced postpartum weight loss
- Increased bone density
- Enhanced bonding with infant

FOR INFANTS
- Enhanced immunity through the transfer of maternal antibodies; decreased incidence of infections including otitis media, pneumonia, urinary tract infections, bacteremia and bacterial meningitis
- Enhanced maturation of the gastrointestinal tract
- Decreased likelihood of developing insulin-dependent (type 1) diabetes
- Decreased risk of childhood obesity
- Enhanced jaw development
- Protective effects against certain childhood cancers

- Mothers with active tuberculosis or HIV infection
- Mothers with active herpes lesions on the nipples
- Mothers who are receiving certain medications, such as lithium or methotrexate
- Mothers who are exposed to radioactive isotopes (e.g., during diagnostic testing)

Despite knowledge of the benefits of breastfeeding some women choose to formula feed. Concerns about convenience, opportunity to involve the father in the baby's care, and modesty and embarrassment may be factors that influence the mother's decision. An unsuccessful breastfeeding experience during a previous pregnancy may also play a role. Some women anticipate that breastfeeding will interfere with plans to return to work. Whatever the reasons, the nurse must provide information and support in a caring, nonjudgmental manner. Postpartal women who planned to bottle feed may still benefit from education about the benefits of breast milk over formula (Miller, Cook, Brooks, Heine, & Curtis, 2007). The nurse's offer of breastfeeding support and assistance may encourage some women to change their chosen feeding method. The importance of the nurse's role in the promotion of breastfeeding has been underscored in an AWHONN clinical position statement (1999; available at http://www.awhonn.org/awhonn/content.do?name=05HealthPolicyLegislation/5HPositionStatements.htm).

Optimizing Outcomes— **Supporting women in their infant feeding choice**

Although breast milk provides the best nutrition choice for infants, the decision to breastfeed is always one that must be made by the woman. She should make the choice based on what pleases her and makes her feel most comfortable. If the woman is pleased and comfortable with her choice, the infant will also be pleased and comfortable and both will benefit from the experience.

ENHANCING UNDERSTANDING OF THE PROCESS OF LACTATION

Normal Structure of the Breast

The breast is composed of glandular, connective, and fatty tissue. The lactating breast contains lobes that house the milk production cells called aveoli (alveolus), fatty tissue, and a series of small and main ducts. The ducts converge into 9 to 10 duct openings in the nipple (Fig. 15-5). According to most published literature, each breast contains 15 to 20 lobes although recent ultrasound studies have demonstrated variations that range from 4 to 18 lobes per breast (Ramsay, Kent, Hartmann, & Hartmann, 2005). Each lobe has a small duct that unites with others to form a main duct. The lobes are connected by areolar tissue and blood vessels. The ducts function to collect milk from the alveolus and transport it toward the nipple. The Cooper's ligaments, along with the fatty adipose tissue, give shape to the breasts and provide support to the ductal system (Fig. 15-6).

The areola, a 15- to 16-mm circular pigmented structure, darkens and enlarges with pregnancy. The Montgomery tubercles are small sebaceous glands in the areola that enlarge during pregnancy. They secrete a waxy substance

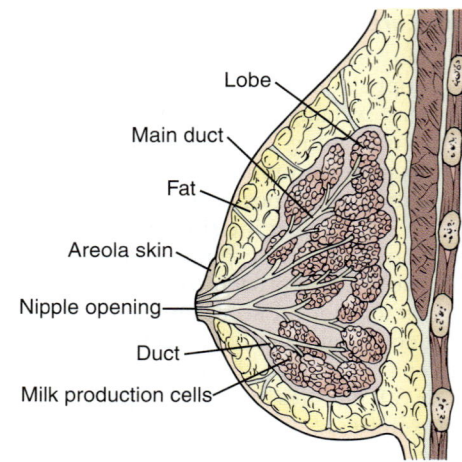

Figure 15-5 Cross section of a lactating breast.

that acts as a lubricant and contains anti-infective properties that protect the nipples. The nipple, a mass of conical erectile tissue, is located in the center of the areola and projects a few millimeters from the center of the breast. Circular smooth muscles surround the areola and cause the nipple to become erect with stimulation. The main ducts converge and open into the nipple (Riordan, 2005).

Blood and Nerve Supply and Lymphatic Drainage

There is an abundant vascular supply to the breasts. Approximately 60% of the blood supply to the breasts comes from the internal mammary artery. The remainder is supplied by branches of the intercostal, subclavian, and axillary arteries (Lawrence & Lawrence, 2005). Branches from the mammary arteries anastomose around the nipples and areolae and provide blood to those structures.

The fourth, fifth, and sixth intercostal nerves provide innervation to the breasts. The fourth nerve enters into the posterior aspect of the breast (anatomically, in the position of 4 o'clock on the left breast; 8 o'clock on the right breast) and provides maximum sensation to the nipple and the areola. The areola is the most sensitive area of the breast; the nipple itself is the least sensitive area. Damage to the intercostal nerves can result in some loss of sensation to the breast (Riordan, 2005). Loss of sensation may prevent the nipple from protruding and becoming erect in preparation for a baby's latching-on to breastfeed.

The breasts contain an extensive lymphatic network. The skin covering the breasts houses superficial lymph

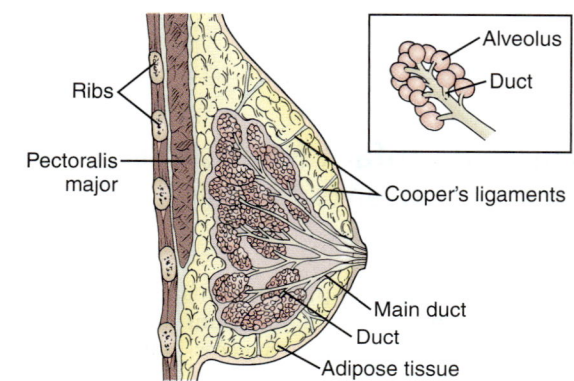

Figure 15-6 The ductal system of the breast.

channels that serve the chest wall and are continuous with the superficial lymphatics of the neck and abdomen. A rich network of lymphatics is also present deep in the breasts. The primary deep lymphatics drain laterally toward the axillae.

The Physiology of Lactation

MILK PRODUCTION AND LET-DOWN. **Lactogenesis,** the process by which the breasts secrete milk, is dependent on the release of the hormones prolactin and oxytocin. The process of milk synthesis begins after the delivery of the placenta. This event results in a dramatic decrease in plasma progesterone and estrogen and an increase in the secretion of prolactin from the anterior lobe of the pituitary gland. Prolactin stimulates the alveoli, or milk-producing cells, to secrete milk. Stimulation from infant suckling or pumping the breasts triggers the release of oxytocin from the posterior lobe of the pituitary gland. Oxytocin prompts contraction of the smooth muscle myo-epithelial cells surrounding the alveoli to eject milk from the alveoli into the lactiferous (main) ducts (Fig. 15-7). Movement of milk into the large lactiferous ducts for removal is called the **"milk ejection reflex"** or the **"let-down" reflex.** Lactating mothers describe "let-down" as a tingling or pins and needles sensation that occurs immediately before or during breastfeeding. Frequent stimulation and release of milk from the breasts are necessary for the continued release of prolactin.

The initiation of milk production is divided into three stages. Stage 1 occurs in late pregnancy and is characterized by the maturation of the alveoli, the proliferation of the secretory alveoli ductal system, and the increase in size and weight of the breast. Stage 2 begins during the postpartum period. Reduced plasma progesterone levels lead to an increase in prolactin levels that cause a copious milk production by the fourth to fifth postpartal day. Stage 3, the establishment and maintenance of the milk supply, is governed by a principle of "supply and demand"

and continues until breastfeeding ceases. The "weaning" stage, sometimes referred to as "Stage 4," begins when breast stimulation ceases. This stage is characterized by a significant reduction in milk volume.

A lack of breastfeeding (in breastfeeding or non breast-feeding mothers), or a failure to empty the breasts by pumping, results in an accumulation of inhibiting peptides, or hormones released from the hypothalamus. Inhibiting peptides act on the breast secretory cells, causing a gradual decrease in milk volume and the eventual death of the epithelial cells.

ASSISTING THE MOTHER WHO CHOOSES TO BREASTFEED: STRATEGIES FOR BREASTFEEDING SUCCESS

The most important information that the nurse can give to a mother is that breastfeeding should not be painful. When the baby is feeding at the breast, the woman should experience a strong tugging sensation and occasional mild discomfort. However, pain associated with breastfeeding is not a normal finding. The nurse should refer women who experience breastfeeding pain or other difficulties to a board-certified lactation consultant (IBCLC) for help and assistance. Although the pediatrician is responsible for the health care of the infant, the IBCLC is a lactation expert who offers the most current, up-to-date, accurate information on breastfeeding using a "hands-on" approach. Mothers should be encouraged to consult with an IBCLC when they have any questions, are having difficulty with the latch-on process, or express concerns about their milk production. Ideally, all breastfeeding mothers should be discharged with an appointment to an IBCLC.

 Collaboration in Caring— *Partnering with an IBCLC and other community resources*

An IBCLC is a health care professional who specializes in the clinical management of breastfeeding. IBCLCs are certified by the International Board of Lactation Consultant Examiners Inc. under the direction of the US National Commission for Certifying Agencies. IBCLCs work in a variety of health care settings including hospitals, pediatric offices, public health clinics, and private practice. The IBCLC credential is primarily an add-on qualification that brings together health professionals from different disciplines who share a common knowledge base in human lactation. Among those who become IBCLCs are midwives, nurses, family practitioners, pediatricians, obstetricians, educators, dietitians, and occupational, speech, and physical therapists. Most of these health care professionals have spent at least 4 years acquiring the experience and education required for certification.

Costs for services provided by IBCLCs depend upon the environments in which they work. Charges for inpatients are typically incorporated into the hospital stay. Follow-up visits in a hospital-based lactation department may or may not be included as a benefit for giving birth at that facility. Other consultations are fee-for-service. Most insurance companies do not pay for lactation services unless the service is provided within a physician's office under the supervision of the physician. Under these circumstances, the office visit charges may apply.

Figure 15-7 Mechanism for milk production.

Many government sponsored health programs such as the Special Supplemental Nutrition Program for Women, Infants, and Children (WIC) provide breastfeeding support services that are staffed by breastfeeding peer counselors. A mother who indicates that she is breastfeeding and is part of the WIC program will be provided with a special food package for herself and for her newborn. The La Leche League, an international support organization for breastfeeding mothers, is another resource that may be available in the community.

Optimizing Outcomes— Care of the breasts during lactation

The nurse should teach breastfeeding mothers to wash the nipples with warm water. Soap, which can have a drying effect and cause cracked nipples, should be avoided. Breast creams are also to be avoided. They may block the natural oil secreted by the Montgomery tubercles on the areolae; others contain alcohol, a drying agent. Creams or oils that contain vitamin E should also be avoided because the infant may absorb toxic amounts of the fat-soluble vitamin.

Initiating the Feeding

The optimal time to breastfeed is when the baby is in a quiet alert state. Crying is usually a late sign of hunger and achieving satisfactory latch-on at this time is difficult. **Latch-on** is proper attachment of the infant to the breast for feeding. The neonate is most alert during the first 1 to 2 hours after an unmedicated birth, and this is the ideal time to put the infant to the breast. Bathing the neonate before the first breastfeeding should be avoided. The smell of the amniotic fluid on the infant matches the smells of the mother and serves as a "homing device" for the baby. Cesarean deliveries and medicated births, including those with epidural anesthesia, may require more mother–infant skin to skin contact before a successful latch-on occurs.

To assist the breastfeeding mother, the nurse must understand that a baby latched on to the breast is not necessarily transferring milk. A baby that breastfeeds effectively cues (shows readiness) for feedings, is in a good feeding position, latches-on (attaches) deeply at the breast, and moves milk forward from the breast and into the mouth. When the infant is properly latched-on to the breast, the tip of his nose, cheeks and chin should all be touching the breast (Fig. 15-8).

To feed effectively, the infant must awaken and let his mother know that he wants to eat. When possible, mother-baby rooming-in creates an optimal situation for breastfeeding. When the infant is in the mother's room at all times, she is able to observe "feeding-readiness cues" that signal the infant's readiness to feed (Box 15-4).

❝ What to say ❞ — *To assist the mother whose infant won't awaken to breastfeed*

During hospitalization, nurses provide much information and coaching regarding breastfeeding. One new mother expresses her concern that her infant is too sleepy to breastfeed.

Figure 15-8 When properly latched-on, the tip of the infant's nose, cheeks and chin should all be touching the breast.

The nurse may ask:

- Have you tried to unwrap the baby's swaddling? Doing this will increase skin-to-skin contact and help to awaken the infant and promote feeding.
- Have you tried to rest with the baby by your breast? Doing this may allow the infant to feel and/or smell the breast, which may promote feeding.
- Are you familiar with feeding cues? Watching for feeding cues may help you to recognize when your baby is ready to breastfeed. Examples of infant feeding cues are vocalizations, movements of the mouth, and moving the hand toward the mouth. Hunger-related crying is a late sign of hunger and should not be used as the cue for feeding.

An optimal breastfeeding experience begins with the mother's prompt response to her infant's feeding readiness cues (Cadwell et al., 2006). The mother should hold the baby so that his nose is aligned with the nipple and watch

---

Box 15-4 **Infant Feeding-Readiness Cues**

The infant demonstrates readiness for feeding when she:
- Begins to stir.
- Bobs the head against the mattress or mother's neck/shoulder.
- Makes hand-to-mouth or hand-to-hand movements.
- Exhibits sucking or licking.
- Exhibits rooting.
- Demonstrates increased activity; arms and legs flexed; hands in a fist.

for an open mouth gape. At the height of the gape, when the mouth is open widest, the mother should aim the bottom lip as far away as possible from the base of the nipple. With this action, the infant's chin and the lower jaw meet the breast first and the nipple is pointed to the roof of the mouth. To facilitate a proper latch-on, it is desirable that the nipple be aligned with the baby's nose. This position allows the baby to tilt his head upward slightly so that the chin and lower jaw drops, creating the wide open gape desired. Next, the infant's mouth should be placed 1 to 2 inches beyond the base of the nipple. Depending on the areola size, most of the areola should be visible from the infant's top lip but not from the bottom lip. The top and bottom lips should be flanged outward. When properly positioned, there should be no slurping or clicking sounds or dimpling of the cheeks. Also, the mother should report a tugging sensation but no pain or pinching. If any of these are present, the infant should be removed from the breast by instructing the mother to insert her finger into the corner of the baby's mouth to break the seal. As an alternative, the mother can gently lift up and push back on the baby's upper lip (Fig. 15-9).

Optimizing Outcomes— Assessing for milk let-down

The nurse assesses for cues that indicate that the milk let-down reflex has occurred:

- The mother reports a tingling sensation in the nipples (not always present).
- The infant's quick, shallow sucking pattern transitions to a slower, more drawing pattern.
- The infant exhibits audible swallowing.
- The mother reports uterine cramping; increased lochia may be present.
- The mother states she feels extremely relaxed during the feeding.
- The opposite breast may leak milk.

Once the baby is latched on correctly, he must suckle and transfer milk. There should be a 2:1 or 1:1 suck/swallow ratio with audible swallowing to indicate that milk transfer is occurring. A 5:1 or higher suck/swallow ratio is indicative of non-nutritive suckling. Non-nutritive suckling can result in poor milk supply and lead to poor infant weight gain.

Figure 15-9 Infant latch-on. *A.* Nipple is aligned with the baby's nose. *B, C.* As the baby latches to the nipple, the baby's mouth is placed one to two inches beyond the base of the nipple. *D.* To remove the baby from the breast, the mother inserts her finger into the corner of the baby's mouth to break the seal.

Feedings that last less than 10 minutes or continue for longer than 40 minutes are not satisfactory and require consultation and assessment by a lactation consultant.

Optimal feeding results in the infant coming off the breast without assistance. Once the feeding has ended, the infant should be in a relaxed state with hands open; he may or may not be asleep. After a successful breastfeeding experience, mothers often describe their baby as having a "drunken stupor" look. The nipple should be everted and round, never flat or pinched on any side. The mother should report no pain and the infant should appear satiated.

EVALUATION OF NOURISHMENT: INFANT WEIGHT GAIN

All newborns are expected to lose weight during the early days of life. A newborn who is feeding frequently and effectively, in general, may lose an average of 5% of his birth weight (American Academy of Pediatrics [AAP], 2004). Any infant who loses more than 7% of his birth weight should be carefully evaluated to make sure that the he is being fed frequently enough and that the feeding technique is effective in transferring milk from the mother's breast.

An infant weight loss of greater than 7% is not an "automatic" reason to supplement breast feedings with formula. The administration of formula may interfere with the baby's interest in feeding at the breast and his ability to learn appropriate breastfeeding techniques.

 Nursing Insight— *Preventing nipple confusion*

Nipple confusion may result when breast fed infants receive supplemental feedings. Essentially, the infant exhibits difficulty in knowing how to latch-on to the breast. Nipple confusion occurs because breastfeeding and bottle feeding require different skills. Sucking and swallowing patterns as well as the way the tongue, cheeks, and lips are used vary considerably between breast and bottle feeding. The infant's tongue is pulled backward when sucking from the breast; it is thrust forward when sucking from a rubber nipple. Parents should be taught to avoid bottles until breast feeding is well established (usually 3 to 4 weeks).

Once the mother's milk production increases and the volume of milk consumed increases, most infants begin to gain 15 to 30 g or 1/2 to 1 oz. per day (AAP, 2004). This rate of gain continues for the first several months of life. Loss of excessive weight or failure to begin a steady pattern of weight gain indicates that the mother is not producing adequate milk, or the infant is not ingesting adequate milk, or, much less commonly, the infant has other organic problems. In most instances, correcting latch-on difficulties and proper positioning improves milk transfer from the breast to the baby. As long as the baby continues to feed well and is gaining weight the mother can be reassured not to worry.

POSITIONS FOR BREASTFEEDING

Common positions for nursing a baby include cradle hold, cross-cradle hold, football, and side-lying (Fig. 15-10). In the cradle hold position, the infant is cradled

in the arm, close to the maternal breast. The infant's abdomen is placed against the mother's abdomen with the mother's other hand supporting the breast. The cross cradle hold is similar to the cradle hold, although in this hold, the infant is laying in the opposite direction. In the

Figure 15-10 Common positions for breastfeeding. *A.* Cradle hold position. *B.* Football hold position. *C.* Side-lying position.

football hold, the infant's back and shoulders are held in the palm of the mother's hand. The infant is tucked up under the mother's arm, keeping the infant's hip, shoulder, and ear in alignment. The mother supports the breast to touch the infant's lips. Once the infant's mouth is open, the mother pulls the infant toward the breast. In the side-lying position, both the mother and the infant lay on their sides. Facing one another, the mother should place a pillow behind the infant's back for support. The nipple should be placed within easy reach for the infant with the mother guiding the nipple into the infant's mouth (Lawrence & Lawrence, 2005).

Now Can You— Discuss the physiology of lactation and assist the breastfeeding mother?

1. Describe the four stages involved in the process of lactation?
2. Discuss techniques the breastfeeding mother can use to promote proper "latch-on"?
3. Explain what the mother should be taught regarding the infant's weight?
4. Demonstrate four common breastfeeding positions?

PROBLEMS THAT RESULT IN INEFFECTIVE BREASTFEEDING

Sore nipples are related to an incorrect latch-on and positioning of the infant at the breast. If a mother complains of pain when the infant is nursing, it is important to observe the baby for correct latch-on during feeding. The nurse can assess for proper latching by making the following observations when the infant is at the breast: maternal–infant positioning is optimal for feeding; the infant exhibits a flanged lower lip, there is a good seal between the mouth and nipple, and an audible swallow. Successful latch-on is essential to prevent trauma to the nipple. The shape of the nipple at the conclusion of the feeding also provides a good indicator for correct latching. If the nipple shape has changed at the end of the feeding, the nurse should troubleshoot for specific problems and teach the mother about correct latch and positioning techniques.

Optimizing Outcomes— Breast shells for flat, inverted, or sore nipples

Breast shells, which are plastic "nipple cups," or inserts that fit into the bra, are useful for women with flat or inverted nipples because they help the nipples to become more protuberant. They may also be used to prevent sore nipples from making contact with the woman's clothing or bra.

Breast **engorgement** is described as excessive swelling and overfilling of the breast and areola and is a physiological response to an increase in blood flow and an increase in milk production. Engorgement, which may occur from infrequent feeding or ineffective emptying of the breasts, results in congestion and overdistension of the collecting ductal system and obstruction of lymphatic drainage. It typically lasts about 24 hours. Symptoms of engorgement usually occur between the third and fifth day after childbirth (when the milk "comes in")

and vary from minimally engorged (patients complain of breast fullness and discomfort) to severe engorgement, characterized by symptoms of pain, tenderness, hardness and warmth to the touch. With severe engorgement, swelling of the breasts is profuse and extends from the clavicle to the tail of Spence and the lower rib cage. The breasts may have a shiny, taut appearance. The areolae become very firm and the nipples may flatten, making it difficult for the infant to latch-on. Back pressure exerted on full milk glands inhibits milk production. Thus, if milk is not removed from the breasts, the milk supply may decrease. Treatment involves relieving the patient's discomfort by removal of the milk (via breast feeding or pumping) to decrease stasis, which reduces the swelling and discomfort.

Because the infant is very efficient in the removal of milk, frequent feeding (at least every 2 to 3 hours) is advised to minimize the stasis of milk. The infant should feed at each breast at least 15 to 20 minutes until at least one breast softens after the feeding. To help reduce the swelling and enhance milk flow, the nurse should instruct the mother to use warm compresses and perform hand expression before nursing. This action softens the areola, initiates the let-down reflex, and allows the infant to more easily grasp the areola. Massaging the breasts during feedings is also beneficial. Other methods to enhance milk flow and help facilitate infant latch-on include taking a warm shower or leaning over a bowl of warm water and hand-expressing some milk before nursing. Since breast swelling is related to increased blood flow, cold ice packs may be used after breastfeeding or pumping to constrict blood flow and reduce the edema.

✿ Complementary Care— *Cabbage leaves to diminish breast swelling*

Patients can be taught to place raw cabbage leaves over their breasts between feedings to help reduce swelling. First, several large cabbage leaves are washed, then stored in the refrigerator until they become cool. The leaves are then crushed and placed directly on the breasts for 15 to 20 minutes. This process may be repeated two to three times only; frequent application of the cabbage leaves may decrease the milk supply. Women who are allergic to cabbage, sulfa drugs, or who develop a skin rash should not use cabbage leaves (Lactation Education Resources, 2004).

A nonprescription anti-inflammatory medication such as ibuprofen (e.g., Motrin, Advil) may be taken for the pain and swelling related to engorgement. It may be particularly helpful for the mother to take the medication before breastfeeding in anticipation of postfeeding discomfort. Because of the significant increase in breast size during lactation, patients should be advised to wear well-fitting supportive bras with no underwire for comfort. Bras that are too small may compress the ducts and obstruct milk flow. If the infant is unable to breastfeed, warm soaks, breast massage and the use of a manual or electric pump for the expression of milk help to reduce milk stasis and swelling.

Ethnocultural Considerations— Cultural influences and interventions for breastfeeding discomfort

When educating mothers regarding management of breast-feeding-related discomfort, the nurse must consider the cultural background of the patient. Many non-Western cultures such as Asian, Latin, and African cultures embrace a hot and cold "humoral theory." Breastfeeding mothers from these cultures may choose not to utilize a cold modality for the relief of breast engorgement or discomfort. Although the nurse may explain the clinical rationale for applying ice packs to the breasts, the patient is culturally bound to adhere to her beliefs. Nurses must remain sensitive to culturally influenced customs and allow patients to use relief measures that do not conflict with their personal beliefs.

COLLECTING AND STORING BREAST MILK

Collecting and storing breast milk is a necessity for mothers who are separated from their infants due to problems such as prematurity or illness. In other situations, women may elect to return to school or work and wish to have breast milk available for feeding by another individual. Freshly pumped breast milk can be safely stored at room temperature for four hours or refrigerated at 34 to 39°F (0°C) for 5 to 7 days after collection. Milk kept in a deep freezer at 0°F (−19°C) can be stored for 6 to 12 months (Lawrence & Lawrence, 2005).

The oldest milk should be used first, unless the pediatrician recommends the use of recently expressed milk. Women should be taught to thaw breast milk by placing the collection container in the refrigerator. The thawing process may be accelerated by holding the collection container under warm running water or by placing it in a cup, pot, bowl, or basin of warm water. Breast milk should not be allowed to thaw at room temperature, in very hot water, or in the microwave oven. Microwaving the breast milk container can create "hot spots" and use of the microwave oven or heating the container in very hot water may decrease the milk's anti-infective properties. Breast milk separates during storage. The cream rises to the top, because breast milk is not homogenized. To mix the milk after storage, the collection container should be gently swirled, or rotated; vigorous shaking should be avoided. After the feeding, any milk that remains in the feeding container should be discarded and not saved for a later feeding. Thawed milk should never be refrozen.

Optimizing Outcomes— With manual (hand) and electric expression of breast milk

Performing manual or electric expression of breast milk is sometimes necessary because of medical complications or for occupational reasons. During the early postpartum period, the woman should be encouraged to frequently express her breast milk. This action helps to establish and increase the milk supply for later breastfeeding needs. Once lactation has been established, the mother should be encouraged to express milk, either manually or with an electric breast pump, whichever method is most convenient or effective for her (Miller et al., 2007).

Electric Expression of Breast Milk

Women should be encouraged to avoid pumping the breasts until the infant is breastfeeding comfortably. Although the mother can help her baby learn to take a bottle once breastfeeding has been well established, it is best to wait for 3 to 4 weeks before introducing bottle feeding. The American Academy of Pediatrics (2004) recommends exclusive breastfeeding with no supplements, for the first 6 months of life.

The nurse teaches the woman to use hot, soapy water to wash her hands, all components of the breast pump that will touch her breasts and all collecting bottles before proceeding. Most equipment may also be safely cleaned in an automatic dishwasher. If soap and water are not available, many "quick clean" products may be safely used instead. Collecting bottles should be allowed to air dry on a clean towel.

The woman is encouraged to carefully read the instruction manual and practice pumping when she is rested, relaxed, and when her breasts feel full. The nurse can teach employed mothers to begin to pump and store breast milk 2 to 3 weeks before returning to work. The breasts should be pumped once a day, every day, 7 days a week. The first morning pumping usually produces the largest quantity of milk. If possible, the woman should nurse the baby on one breast while pumping the other breast. The breast milk may be stored in the refrigerator or freezer. The 7-day-a-week pumping schedule should continue even after the woman has returned to work (Tully, 2005).

Many employed mothers use the fresh breast milk they pump while at work for infant feedings the following day. For example, the breast milk pumped at work on Monday should be refrigerated and used on Tuesday. Mothers should be counseled to breastfeed the infant before leaving for work and then adhere to a set schedule of pumping and feeding each day. Breast milk collected (by pumping) on Friday and Saturday can be frozen for future use. Ideally, mothers should pump the breasts for each missed feeding, but two pumpings per work day during an 8-hour work shift is realistic for most women. The breasts should be pumped for 15 to 20 minutes or until the milk flow stops. Breastfeeding should be resumed during the evening and throughout weekends (Johnston & Esposito, 2007).

Types of Breast Pumps

A variety of manual and electric breast pumps are available, and, for most women, the choice is made according to needs, preferences, and financial resources. Hospital-grade electric breast pumps are designed for complete mother–baby separation. In these situations, the infant will not be able to breastfeed for an indeterminate period of time due to problems such as prematurity, surgery, or illness. Hospital-grade electric pumps are typically considered to be multiple-user rental equipment. Retail or "personal use" electric breast pumps are excellent alternatives to the rented hospital-grade pump (Fig. 15-11). These single-user electric breast pumps usually work well for the

Figure 15-11 Personal use electric breast pump.

working mother or in situations in which consistent pumping is needed. Occasional use battery powered or manual breast pumps are designed for the mother who needs to have extra milk only once in a while.

INFANT WEANING

When a mother decides to wean the baby from the breast, it is recommended that she begin by eliminating one feeding at a time. Usually the least favorite nursing time is the first one that is discontinued (Cadwell et al., 2006). After waiting for a few days, an alternate feeding time (not the one immediately before or after the one already discontinued) may be eliminated. Mothers should be advised to carefully observe the baby for signs of emotional or physical reactions (i.e., cow's milk allergy if formula is introduced). Babies sometimes choose to stop nursing although this does not usually occur with infants younger than 1 year of age. The American Academy of Pediatrics (2004) currently recommends breastfeeding for the first 12 months of life.

ASSISTING THE MOTHER WHO CHOOSES TO FORMULA-FEED HER INFANT

Information regarding formula choices should be offered to mothers who choose not to breastfeed. Formula preparations come in ready-to-feed cans that can be poured directly into a bottle, liquid concentrates that require dilution before feeding and powder formulas that are mixed with water.

A variety of bottles and nipples are also available, and selection is usually based on the parent's preference. For example, the mother may choose from glass bottles or plastic bottles with angled or straight nipples or convenience bottles with disposable liners. The nurse should remind the parents to periodically check the nipple integrity to ensure that the formula flows freely one drop at a time. If the formula flows too quickly, the nipple should be discarded because it poses a risk for infant choking and aspiration.

Parents should also be advised to read and follow the manufacturer's instructions explicitly when preparing the formula. For example, no water should be added to the ready-to-feed preparations and care should be taken to correctly dilute the concentrate and powder preparations. Poorly prepared formula that is too concentrated (from adding an incorrect amount of water) may result in infant hypernatremia and dehydration. Formula that is too dilute may cause the infant to demonstrate symptoms of undernourishment and water intoxication.

Bottles and nipples must be thoroughly washed in hot soapy water with dishwashing detergent and then rinsed in hot clean water. They may also be cleaned in an automatic dishwasher. Some parents prefer to sterilize their equipment and a variety of commercial sterilizers that can be placed in a microwave oven are available for purchase at most baby stores. If boiling is the preferred cleaning method, parents should be instructed to wash the bottles, nipples, rings, discs and all other equipment used to prepare the formula in hot soapy water. The items are then well rinsed in hot, clean water, placed in a pot filled with enough water to cover the equipment and boiled for 5 to 10 minutes.

Although formula can be fed to the baby at room temperature, if warmed formula is preferred, the parents are instructed to place the prepared bottle of formula in a bowl of hot (not boiling) water for a few minutes. Alternatively, the prepared bottle of formula can be warmed in an electric bottle warmer available at most baby stores. It is important to emphasize to parents the need for testing the temperature of warmed formula before feeding. Parents are instructed to shake a few drops of formula on the inside of the wrist. The liquid should feel warm, but not hot.

When feeding the baby, parents should choose a comfortable chair, and hold the baby in their arms close to them with the baby's head higher than the rest of the body to prevent aspiration and minimize ear infection. Holding the baby skin-to-skin and maintaining full eye contact throughout the feeding helps to facilitate the bonding process. To prevent the baby from swallowing too much air, the bottle should be kept in an angled position with the nipple continuously filled with formula. Burping is usually performed midway and at the end of the feeding to remove excess air from the infant's stomach. To burp the baby properly, parents are taught to either hold the baby over their shoulder or on their lap with the baby's head supported. The baby's back is gently rubbed until air is expelled (Fig. 15-12).

Parents should be advised that babies usually spit up during burping and that this is normal. However, the pediatrician must be consulted if the baby vomits large amount of formula with burping or after feeding. Since babies eat more efficiently and take in the desired amount of formula when they are hungry, a "baby-driven" demand feeding schedule rather than a regimented feeding schedule is desirable. The pediatrician can provide guidelines regarding the volume of formula the baby needs.

Safe Practices for Bottle Feeding

When informing parents about the safety of formula, it is important for health care professionals to be aware that

Figure 15-12 One infant burping technique.

liquid formulas have been subjected to high temperatures to make the product sterile. Powdered formulas are not sterile because high temperatures destroy vital nutrients. The microorganism *Enterobacter sakazakii*, known to cause meningitis, has been identified in powdered formula. To minimize the risk of infection, health care professionals must provide accurate instructions to parents regarding the correct procedure for formula preparation, storage and reconstitution. Instructions given should emphasize the importance of good handwashing techniques before handling the equipment that is to be used to reconstitute the powder. The formula should never be mixed in a blender or stored in large amounts for longer than 24 hours. Cold water should be used to mix the powder, only the amount to be used for each feeding should be prepared, and any unused formula should be discarded. Parents should be cautioned not to use a microwave oven to prepare or warm the formula due to the potential for "hot spots" that can burn the infant's mouth. They should also be taught to never prop the bottle to allow the infant to feed alone or put the infant to bed with a bottle. These practices may result in choking, ear infections, and tooth decay.

Optimizing Outcomes— Safely preparing infant formula

Nurses can provide the following safety instructions to parents who plan to formula feed their infant:

- Wash hands before beginning to prepare formula and after any interruptions.
- Always shake and wash tops of liquid formula cans before opening.
- Reconstitute the formula according to the manufacturer's recommendations.
- Store the ready-to-feed formula according to the manufacturer's recommendations.

- Shake the bottle well before feeding.
- Discard any formula that the infant does not drink.
- Wash thoroughly/sterilize all equipment used to prepare the infant formula and use a bottle and nipple brush to remove milk residue.
- Replace the nipples regularly.

 Now Can You— Discuss breast milk storage and assist the mother who is bottle feeding her infant?

1. Explain what the breastfeeding mother should be taught about pumping and storing breast milk?
2. Discuss appropriate cleaning techniques for bottles and nipples?
3. Describe special precautions to be used with powdered formulas?

Promoting Family and Infant Bonding

FACILITATING THE TRANSITION TO PARENTHOOD

The transition to parenthood can be an especially difficult and challenging time for primiparous mothers with limited experience in infant care and for new parents who are experiencing social isolation from family or friends. Feelings of anxiety and inadequacy regarding parenting skills, lack of knowledge and confidence about providing baby care, emotional concerns, depression, and detachment toward the infant are all symptoms not infrequently expressed by first-time mothers. This information underscores the importance patients place on nurses and other health care professionals to provide emotional support and accurate information about self care and baby care.

An essential goal of nursing care at this time is to create a supportive teaching environment that increases the parents' knowledge and confidence in caring for themselves and their infants. Using the principles of Family-Centered Care as a guideline, nurses can help parents cope with the emotional and physical changes that accompany the childbearing year. To create a supportive teaching environment, the nurse can:

- Perform a needs assessment to identify the parents' knowledge/skill deficits.
- Utilize good communication and listening skills to provide support.
- Empower the parents by assisting them in recognizing their own strengths.
- Facilitate parents' actions to participate in the decision making process.
- Provide learning opportunities that move the parents from dependence to independence and self-reliance.

ASSUMING THE MOTHERING ROLE

Rubin (1975) described three distinct phases that are associated with the woman's assuming the mothering role. She labeled these phases "Taking-in," "Taking-hold," and "Letting-go" (Table 15-6). At the time of Rubin's work, women were traditionally hospitalized for 5-7 days after childbirth and nurses could readily observe their patients'

Table 15-6 Phases Associated with the Mothering Role		
Phase 1: Taking-In	**Phase 2: Taking-Hold**	**Phase 3: Letting-Go**
First 1–2 days	**Second and/or third day**	**First 2–6 weeks postpartum**
The mother is recovering from the immediate exhaustion of labor.	The mother starts to initiate action and to begin some of the tasks of motherhood. She may:	This is the time during which the mother redefines her new role.
She is relatively dependent on others to meet her physical needs.	a) Ask for help with self-care.	She:
Characteristics of her behavior include:	b) Begin caring for the baby.	a) Moves beyond the mother–infant symbiosis of pregnancy and early postpartum and begins to see her infant as an emerging individual.
a) Physical exhaustion.	c) Be anxious about her mothering abilities.	b) Starts to focus on issues larger than those associated directly with herself and her newborn. (She begins to focus on her partner, other children, and family issues.)
b) Elation, excitement, and/or anxiety and confusion.		
c) Reliving, verbally and mentally, the events of her labor and birth.		

Adapted from Rubin R. (1975). Maternal tasks in pregnancy. *MCN: The Amercian Journal of Maternal-Child Nursing, 4*(3), 143–153.

transitions through each phase. Today, however, with shortened hospital stays, women seem to move through the transitions much more rapidly and often there is overlapping of the phases.

In the first day or two after birth, the mother is exhausted and should be encouraged to rest. During this time she is reflecting and clarifying, or "*taking-in*" her birth experience. Many mothers want to talk about their labor, discuss with family members the detailed events of the labor, seek clarification if unexpected events occurred, and share joys or disappointments associated with the birth. Mothers who hold specific expectations for their birth experience and are unable to follow a birth plan or who are required to transfer from a birth center to a hospital setting may experience feelings of loss and mourn for the hoped for birth experience.

As the mother's physical condition improves, she begins to take charge, and enters the *taking-hold* phase where she assumes care for herself and her infant. At this time, the mother eagerly wants information about infant care and shows signs of bonding with her infant. During this phase, the nurse should closely observe mother–infant interactions for signs of poor bonding and if present, implement actions to facilitate attachment.

 critical nursing action Assessing for Maternal–Infant Attachment

When observing the mother with her newborn, the nurse should look for clues that indicate successful bonding. The nurse should assess for the following indicators:

Does the mother show eagerness to care for her infant?

What is her response when the baby cries?

Does she make eye contact when holding and feeding her baby?

In the *letting-go phase*, seen later in the mother's recovery, the woman begins to see the infant as an individual separate from herself. At this point, she can leave the baby with a sitter, set aside more time for herself, become more involved with her partner, and begin adapting to the reali-

ties of parenthood. Maladjustment during this phase may occur with an overprotective mother who has difficulty accepting help with infant care from others and who excludes the partner from her affections.

 Across Care Settings: **Successful maternal transition into the letting-go phase**

During the letting-go phase, the mother may have difficulty with the tasks associated with viewing the infant as a separate individual. This phase occurs after the mother has been discharged from the hospital or birthing center. Postpartum and community health nurses who suspect that patients may have difficulty making a successful transition into this phase must communicate their concerns with the infant's pediatric care team so that appropriate assessments and interventions can be carried out.

Bonding and Attachment

Bonding is described by Klaus (1982) as the promotion of a unique and powerful relationship between the parent and the infant. **Attachment** refers to the tie that exists between the parent and infant and is recognized as a feeling that binds one person to another.

MATERNAL

Bonding begins at the moment the pregnancy is confirmed and continues through the birth experience, during the postpartal period and throughout the early years of the child's life. Bonding is critical for the infant's survival and development. Providing parents with a model of caring during labor, birth, and in the early postpartum period enhances the bonding process and helps to lay the foundation for the nurturing care that the child will later receive.

Touch is recognized as an important communication tool between humans. Touch is an essential element in the creation of a loving relationship and lasting attachment between the parents and their child. Nurses can be

Figure 15-13 Bonding is enhanced with mother–infant eye-to-eye contact.

instrumental in enhancing the bonding process by minimizing the time that the infant is separated from the mother. Fostering a positive mother–child relationship begins in the delivery/birthing room when the infant is placed directly on the mother's chest and is held skin-to-skin. The nurse should encourage the mother to initiate early eye contact during the first 30 minutes after childbirth when both the mother and her baby are alert (Fig. 15-13). This special quiet time provides an opportunity for connecting and communicating with one another. Early initiation of breastfeeding for mothers who wish to breastfeed and utilizing a rooming-in protocol are important nursing interventions that contribute to a positive maternal–child relationship (Dabrowski, 2007).

> **Optimizing Outcomes—** Providing couplet care as an alternative to rooming-in
>
> Rooming-in is a common strategy to enhance bonding. With this arrangement, the mother and her infant share a room and the mother and her nurse share the care of the infant. Some facilities offer a variation termed **couplet care**. In these settings, the nurse has been educated in both mother and infant care and serves as the primary nurse for the mother and the infant, even when the infant is kept in the nursery.

PATERNAL

Historically, mothers have been considered to be the major nurturer of children. By tradition, the mother took care of the child's needs while the father, in the "breadwinner" role, worked and formed little attachment during the infant's early years. Changes in women's roles, couples' participation in childbirth preparation classes, allowing fathers in the delivery room and encouraging early contact with the infant have all been instrumental in promoting and fostering early paternal–infant bonding. Other researchers (St. John, Cameron, & McVeigh, 2005) have documented the benefits of early and ongoing contact between fathers and infants (Fig. 15-14). When the primary caregiver is able to touch, hold, and attach with the newborn infant, this special interaction helps to build the

Figure 15-14 The father gets acquainted with his newborn.

foundation for a nurturing and protective relationship. Fathers should be encouraged to assume an active role in infant bonding by participating in the care giving activities. For example, fathers can change diapers, engage in skin-to-skin holding and infant massage, and feed the bottle-fed infant.

FACTORS THAT MAY INTERRUPT THE BONDING PROCESS

Stress associated with insufficient finances to purchase infant supplies, a chaotic home life, concerns about child care if the mother must return to work, lack of family support, and substance abuse may negatively interfere with the bonding process. An essential nursing role involves identifying obstacles to optimal bonding and coordinating with appropriate community resources such as social services to explore the mother's eligibility for Medicaid, the Women's Infants and Children's (WIC) program, and Healthy Start. Other resources may include counseling and support services, financial aid, and pastoral care.

Adolescent mothers may not demonstrate attachment behaviors because they have unrealistic expectations of the infant's level of functioning and may not be aware of the infant's vulnerability. It is important for nurses to create a supportive environment that allows the young mother close and frequent interaction with her infant. The nurse must also provide anticipatory guidance and education about infant care that includes how to recognize and respond appropriately to infant cues. With today's shortened hospital stays, it becomes imperative that appropriate home follow-up and social work referrals are established before discharge for this vulnerable population.

case study Adolescent Primipara with a Possible Bonding Difficulty

Sarah, a 17-year-old primipara, gave birth to a healthy 7 lb., 8 oz. (3.4 kg) baby boy yesterday. Although Sarah has been pleasant during her hospitalization, she has expressed little interest in her infant. When the nurses offer to bring the infant to the room, Sarah typically asks them to keep the infant in the nursery so that she can "relax and sleep." She plans to bottle feed her son but has repeatedly found excuses not to feed the baby. The nursery personnel have been feeding the infant instead. The nurses are becoming very concerned because Sarah is to be discharged home with the infant tomorrow.

1. How would you initially respond to the situation? Based on your understanding of the developmental tasks of adolescence, how will you initiate dialog with Sarah?

2. How can the nurse help Sarah begin to feel comfortable holding her baby and also promote maternal–infant bonding?

3. What other nursing actions are indicated?

◆ See Suggested Answers to Case Studies in text on the Electronic Study Guide or DavisPlus.

Women from diverse cultural groups who reside in extended families may be comfortable enlisting the help of their mother, mother-in-law, or a female relative in caring for the infant while they recuperate from childbirth. It is important for the nurse to explore the mother's cultural values and mores before reporting a lack of bonding and attachment between the mother and her infant.

An interruption in the bonding process may occur when infants must be separated from their parents for medical or surgical interventions. To promote optimal bonding in these special circumstances, it is important to allow the parents early and frequent access to the infant. The staff in the neonatal intensive care unit (NICU) can enhance parental attachment and bonding by encouraging the parents to touch, speak to and hold their neonate skin-to-skin as soon as is medically safe. If the mother is unable to visit, photographs of the infant should be sent to her as soon as possible and frequent telephone calls made to keep her advised of the infant's status. The mother must be reassured that the bonding process is ongoing and that lack of early contact will not interfere with the development of a positive relationship with her infant.

ADJUSTMENT OF SIBLINGS TO THE NEWBORN

The arrival of a new baby into the family results in many emotional changes for the siblings. Feelings of hurt and jealously, sibling rivalry, and behavioral regression are all common among younger siblings. For example, a toilet trained toddler may once again require diapers or a 2-year-old who has been weaned may now wish to breastfeed.

Parents should be prepared for these common emotional upheavals and formulate strategies that will help the sibling(s) adjust and accept the baby. Many hospitals offer sibling classes for young (ages 2 to 8) children that introduces the concept of having a new addition to the family and provides parents with specific information about how to make the transition easier.

Family Teaching Guidelines...
Helping Older Siblings Adjust to the New Baby

Nurses can be instrumental in arming parents with strategies to help their children accept and adjust to a new infant. The following tips may be useful:

◆ Talk with the child(ren) about their feelings regarding the new baby. Listen and validate their feelings.

◆ Teach the older sibling how to play with the new baby; encourage gentleness.

◆ Help develop the child's self-esteem by giving him/her special jobs, for example, bringing the diaper when you are changing the baby. Praise each contribution.

◆ Praise age-appropriate behaviors and do not criticize regressive behaviors.

◆ Set aside a special time each day for you to be alone with the older child; remind the child that he/she is loved very much.

TOPIC: **Warning signs indicative of poor sibling adjustment**

Professional help may be needed when the child:

◆ Continually avoids or ignores the baby

◆ Shows the baby no affection

◆ Is consistently angry, taunting or demonstrating aggressive behavior toward the baby or other family members

◆ Experiences nightmares and sleeping difficulties

Adapted from International Childbirth Education Association (2003).

ADJUSTMENT OF GRANDPARENTS TO THE NEWBORN

Grandparents can provide much support to the new family and the degree of their involvement is often linked to cultural expectations. Many cultures (i.e., Hispanics, Asians, and Caribbeans) strongly value the extended family. In these settings, the grandparents are intimately involved in the fabric of family dynamics and frequently exert a strong influence on child-rearing practices. Grandparents' classes, offered by most hospitals, usually focus on defining grandparenting roles such as helping with sibling care during the mother's hospitalization and providing assistance with household activities and cooking and shopping during the first few postpartal weeks. Other class themes include current recommendations concerning infant positioning, feeding and clothing, responding to behavior cues, and positive strategies for assuming a supportive, rather than a parenting role.

 Now Can You— Facilitate family bonding with the newborn?

1. Identify and describe Rubin's three phases associated with assuming the mothering role?

2. Describe strategies to facilitate maternal and paternal bonding?
3. Discuss five specific activities that parents can use to help older siblings adjust to the newborn?

Emotional and Physiological Adjustments During the Puerperium

EMOTIONAL EVENTS

Many mothers experience a roller coaster of emotions after childbirth. These feelings stem from a number of influences and are often linked to perceptions concerning the fulfillment of expectations surrounding the childbirth experience. A complicated birth, a premature birth or a sick infant, as well as the woman's parity, age, marital status and stability of family finances are some of the many factors known to shape emotions experienced during the postpartum period.

The first 3 months after birth are recognized as the most vulnerable emotional period for mothers. Insecurity about infant care, the constant demands associated with caring for the baby, sleep deprivation, and minimal social support create the potential for frequent and dramatic mood changes. Rapid hormonal changes during the first few postpartal days and weeks may give rise to mood disorders. The most common of these is often termed "the blues." Other less common puerperal mood disorders include post partum depression and post partum psychosis. (See Chapter 16 for further discussion.)

Maternity Blues/Baby Blues/Postpartum Blues

The "maternity blues" are considered to be a normal reaction to the dramatic changes that occur after childbirth including abrupt withdrawal of the hormones estrogen, progesterone and cortisol. Women experience a range of symptoms that include tearfulness, mood swings, insomnia, fatigue, anxiety, difficulty concentrating, irritability and poor appetite. The symptoms usually begin during the first few postpartal days, peak on the fifth day, and then subside over the next several days. Blues do not affect the woman's ability to care for herself or her newborn and family.

The "blues" are treated with support and reassurance (Beck, Records, & Rice, 2006). Proactive education to prepare the woman and her family for the possibility of postpartum blues is important. The nurse needs to explore what resources the new mother will have available when she goes home. The discussion should focus on whether the patient has adequate food, clothing, shelter, and transportation, and whether there are relational concerns that need to be addressed before discharge. Incorporating community resources such as the woman's church, a Mother's Day Out group, a hobby club, or La Leche League can help the new mother realize she is not alone in the experience of nurturing a newborn, while also caring for herself and her family. Referral to a health care provider is appropriate for women whose symptoms persist for more than ten days, as this pattern is suggestive of postpartum depression.

Postpartum Depression

Postpartum depression, which affects 10% to 13% of women, usually appears around two weeks after child-

birth. The symptoms associated with this condition are often insidious and include sleep disturbances, guilt, fatigue, and feelings of hopelessness and worthlessness. In severe instances, suicidal ideation may occur. Patients who demonstrate symptoms of post partum depression must be promptly referred for evaluation and intervention. (See Chapter 16 for further discussion.)

Postpartum Psychosis

Postpartum psychosis develops in approximately one or two women for every 1000 births and is unlikely to manifest itself during the early postpartum period. Symptoms include delusions; hallucinations; agitation; inability to sleep; and bizarre, irrational behavior. Before hospital discharge, patients with a history of mood disorders or depression should be referred to appropriate resources for community support and follow-up. (See Chapter 16 for further discussion.)

PHYSIOLOGICAL RESPONSES TO EMOTIONAL EVENTS

Tiredness and Fatigue

Postpartum tiredness and fatigue have long been considered a natural physiological and psychological response to the stresses of labor and childbirth coupled with the additional responsibilities of motherhood. Although new mothers are often confident that tiredness will improve upon returning home, this phenomenon is not supported by the nursing literature. Rather, the multiplicity of demands associated with motherhood augments the experience of physical and mental exhaustion. While changes in societal trends in the care of children suggest that fathers are taking a more active role, mothers continue to hold the main responsibility for care. Thus, it is essential for the nurse to encourage new mothers to enlist the support and assistance of family and friends in an effort to promote time for rest and recovery (Runquist, 2007).

 Nursing Insight— *Persistent fatigue during the puerperium*

Feelings of fatigue that extend beyond the 6-week postpartal period may be indicative of a more serious condition. Persistent, pervasive fatigue may be indicative of postpartum depression (Troy, 2003). The woman and her family should be provided with guidelines about normal feelings and reactions during the puerperium and encouraged to report excessive tiredness or fatigue to the health care provider.

Contributors to fatigue and tiredness in the postpartum period include physical, psychological, and situational variables. Physical contributors include the length of labor, maternal hormone shifts, maternal anemia, episiotomy or surgical incision healing, breast feeding, and pain. Psychological contributors include difficulty sleeping, depression, and a non supportive partner. The challenge of managing multiple roles, cultural influences and expectations, a lack of assistance with housework or childcare, having more than one child under the age of 5 in the home, and returning to outside employment are situational variables that can readily lead to fatigue. Insights into the multiple contexts that shape the patient's environment allow nurses to provide anticipatory guidance regarding fatigue and its relationship with diminished quality of life in the postpartum period (Runquist, 2007).

Postpartal Discharge Planning and Teaching

PROMOTING MATERNAL SELF CARE

Because of early postnatal discharge, all postpartal women must be taught strategies for self-care. A self-assessment sheet completed before discharge helps to identify areas of deficits. When possible, parents are encouraged to attend a discharge teaching class. Topics reviewed usually include infant bathing, breastfeeding, perineal hygiene, physical activity, rest and expected emotional changes. This information is useful because it empowers the family to identify normal events and to promptly recognize complications that should be reported to the health care provider. Many institutions also distribute home care booklets that provide written information about maternal and newborn care and available community resources. Often, home visitation by a community health nurse is arranged before the patient's discharge. The community health nurse visit typically includes an examination of the mother and infant, an opportunity for discussion about problems or concerns and breastfeeding or formula feeding support. Additional areas of focus during the postpartal visit include education regarding basic maternal and infant care, plans for follow up visits and contraception counseling (Fig. 15-15).

Optimizing Outcomes— When early postpartum discharge is planned

Women and their families may have the option of early discharge with postpartum home care. Maternal criteria for early discharge includes an uncomplicated perinatal course, no evidence of PROM, no difficulties with voiding or ambulation, normal vital signs, hemoglobin > 10 g and no sig-

Figure 15-15 The postpartum home visit usually involves an examination of the mother and baby. It provides an opportunity for teaching and promotes continuity of care.

nificant vaginal bleeding. The infant must also meet certain criteria (i.e., full term, normal vs and physical examination, feeding, urinating, stooling, laboratory/screening tests completed). Early follow-up visits are an essential component of safe care for mothers and their infants (AAP Committee on Fetus and Newborn, 2004; Meara, Kotagal, Atherton, & Lieu, 2004).

COMPONENTS OF MATERNAL SELF-ASSESSMENT

Fundus

The woman is taught how to locate and palpate the fundus and how to determine the progression of the fundal height as it involutes into the pelvis. After months of abdominal enlargement, many women are delighted to be able to rest in a prone position. Nurses can explain that lying on the abdomen is beneficial because this position supports the abdominal muscles and aids involution because the uterus is tipped into its natural forward position.

clinical alert

Avoiding the knee–chest position

The nurse teaches the patient to avoid a knee–chest position until at least the third postpartal week. This position causes the vagina to open. Since the cervical os is still open to some extent, there is a danger that air can enter the vagina, pass into the cervix and enter the open blood sinuses inside the uterus. Entry of air into the circulatory system can cause an air embolus.

Lochia

The nurse reinforces to the patient that the lochia (vaginal discharge) may continue for 3 to 6 weeks after birth. During this time, it is important for her to examine the peripads for color, amount and odor each time she visits the toilet. The woman should be provided with guidelines concerning the anticipated color and amount of the lochia and reminded to promptly report abnormal findings such as heavy bleeding, the passing of large clots and foul smelling odor.

Hygiene

The patient is advised to continue to use her perineal squeeze bottle until the bleeding stops and to use the prescribed medications and/or sitz bath for episiotomy discomfort. After each visit to the toilet she is reminded to carefully wipe from front to back and thoroughly wash her hands before and after changing the peri pads.

Abdominal Incision

Nurses should instruct the postoperative patient to shower as normal and to carefully pat the incision dry. If staples were applied at the incision site, the obstetrician will inform her when to come into the office for removal. Steri-strips used for incision closure should remain undisturbed until they eventually fall off. The woman is advised to avoid the application of cream or powder to the incision site and to notify her obstetrician if she experiences fever or develops signs of incisional infection such as redness, offensive odor or discharge.

Body Temperature

Some women experience a transient increase in body temperature along with breast heaviness on the third to fourth postpartum day when the milk supply is established. They should be reminded that temperatures above 100.4°F (38.0°C) and flu-like symptoms (e.g., chills, body aches, severe pain) may indicate infection and should be promptly reported to the health care provider.

Urination

Before discharge, all patients should be able to pass urine without difficulty. Women should be taught the signs and symptoms of a urinary tract infection (UTI). Specifically, burning on urination (dysuria), frequent voiding with only a small amount of urine passed, the presence of a "fishy" odor to the urine and lower abdominal or flank pain are symptoms that must be reported to the health care provider. To reduce the likelihood of a urinary tract infection, patients are advised to drink at least eight 8-oz. glasses of water each day, avoid delays in emptying the bladder, wipe the perineum from front-to-back after each use of the toilet, change peripads after toileting, and to wash their hands frequently.

Bowel Function

The nurse teaches about the importance of maintaining good hydration and consuming a healthy diet abundant in fiber and roughage. An exploration of the woman's dietary preferences facilitates discussion about specific types of foods (e.g., fruits, vegetables, whole-grain cereals) that promote bowel regularity. The patient should consult with her obstetrician or certified nurse midwife if laxatives or other medications become necessary. Stool softeners are usually prescribed for women with third or fourth degree episiotomies or vaginal lacerations.

Nutrition

Most women are concerned about weight increase during the pregnancy and how quickly they can expect to return to their pre-pregnancy weight. A well-balanced diet that includes high-energy foods is essential to recovery in the puerperium. Patients should be counseled about the need for adequate protein to promote tissue repair and healing and encouraged to select a healthy, low-fat diet that contains protein along with carbohydrates, fruits, and vegetables.

Fatigue

Patients should be reminded that since the first six postpartal weeks are devoted to infant care and recovery from childbirth, energy depletion, usually manifested as extreme tiredness and fatigue, often occurs. They should be encouraged to limit visitors and whenever possible to rest when the baby sleeps. Patients may wish to cook easily prepared meals in advance and freeze foods for later use. When possible, the new mother should solicit help from her partner, family members and friends to assist with the household chores, shopping and child care.

Weight Loss

Weight loss at the time of childbirth is precipitous. Within minutes after birth, the parturient woman loses half of the weight gained during the previous nine months. On average, the weight loss amounts to 10 to 12 lbs. (4.5 to 5.5 kg). This loss comes from the infant, the placenta, amniotic fluid, and blood. Rapid diuresis and diaphoresis occur during the second to fifth postpartum days and result in an additional weight loss of about 5 lbs. (2.3 kg). By the sixth to eighth postpartal week, many women will have returned to their pre-pregnant weight. The amount of weight lost during the puerperium is primarily related to the amount of weight gained during pregnancy and the woman's level of physical activity.

Exercise

The patient is advised to resume activities gradually, beginning with Kegel exercises to strengthen the pelvic-floor muscles. After a vaginal birth, patients may begin modified sit-ups to strengthen the abdominal muscles and perform knee and leg roll exercises to firm the waist. Modified sit-ups are especially beneficial for women with diastasis recti.

 Optimizing Outcomes— Postnatal exercises to promote physical fitness

Teaching patients about exercises to help return the body to its pre-pregnant state is an important component of postpartal care. Exercises to strengthen the back, abdominal muscles, thighs, and shoulders are particularly beneficial at this time.

Supple Spine

Begin on all fours. Inhale. Lift your head, keeping your back straight or arching slightly (avoid strain). Then exhale, round your back, tighten abdominals, tuck in tail and head. Repeat the sequence eight times. This exercise strengthens the back and abdominals.

Tighter Abdominals

Lie on your back in a straight line. Then exhale, lowering the back, vertebra by vertebra. Repeat sequence five times. This exercise helps develop a strong back and abdominals.

Stronger Back

Sit upright, knees bent, feet flat on the floor, back straight, arms forward at shoulder level. Inhale, then exhale and lean back halfway. Inhale again and sit up slowly. Repeat five times. This exercise strengthens the back and abdominals.

Flexible Body

Stand upright with arms raised, elbows slightly relaxed. Inhale, then exhale and bend forward, keeping back straight and swinging arms down and back. Then relax your head and stretch your arms up behind you. Inhale as you swing arms and body up again, returning to your original position. Repeat eight times. Go carefully and do not strain. This exercise is good for thighs, hips, back, arms, shoulders, and neck.

Pain Management

Medications for pain relief (nonsteroidal antiinflammatory medications or analgesics) may be prescribed, especially for postoperative patients. The nurse should ensure that medications prescribed for breastfeeding patients are not contraindicated. Information regarding therapeutic modalities such ice packs, sitz baths, or topical anesthetics may be helpful for the relief of perineal discomfort from hemorrhoids or the episiotomy incision. Patients are instructed to notify their health care provider if pain persists or increases in intensity, and the nurse also reviews other danger signs and symptoms that must be promptly reported (Box 15-5).

Mood

The nurse should provide support and empower the family by discussing the often overwhelming responsibilities associated with newborn care. Information shared with the mother and her partner includes the emotional changes such as feelings of sadness and weepiness that often appear on the second or third postpartal day. Patients can

---

> **Box 15-5** Postpartum Discharge Teaching: Danger Signs to Be Reported
>
> An important component of discharge teaching focuses on alerting patients to signs and symptoms that must be reported to the health care provider. The nurse should ensure that the patient is given written information and knows how to reach her care provider. The patient should immediately report:
>
> - Temperature greater than 100.4°F (38.0°C), chills, or flu-like symptoms.
> - Abdominal incision that is red, tender to touch, or painful, or if edges of the incision have separated.
> - Difficulty initiating urination, urinary frequency or painful urination.
> - Increased vaginal bleeding with or without clots, or foul-smelling vaginal discharge.
> - Persistent pain or marked swelling at the site of a perineal laceration or episiotomy.
> - Swelling or masses in the breasts, red streaks, shooting pain in the breasts, or cracked, bleeding nipples.
> - Swelling, warmth, tenderness or painful areas in the legs.
> - Blurred vision or persistent headache that is not relieved by pain medication.
> - Overwhelming feelings of sadness or an inability to care for self or the baby.

be assured that "mood swings" and periods of unexpected crying, moodiness or anxiety are common and occur in 70% to 80% of women. If the following symptoms persist for more than 2 weeks after childbirth, the woman, her partner, a family member or a support person should contact the health care provider for assistance:

- Crying excessively
- Significant changes in appetite
- Feeling helpless
- Experiencing extreme worry, concern
- Unable to sleep/wanting to sleep all the time
- Unable to care for herself or the baby
- Panic attack
- Fear of harming self or the baby

Sexual Activity and Contraception

To maximize healing and prevent infection, patients are discouraged from resuming sexual activity until after the six week postpartum check-up with the obstetrician or midwife. It is important for the nurse to inform the woman and her partner that since ovulation may resume as early as two weeks after childbirth, pregnancy can occur if no contraceptive is used.

Although advised to abstain from sexual intercourse until the postpartum examination, many couples wish to resume intimate relations before this time. Coitus is safe once the woman's lochia has transitioned to alba and the episiotomy (if present) has healed. This usually occurs after the first week after childbirth. The patient should be warned that she may experience vaginal discomfort because the cells lining the vagina may not be as thick as before, due to a hormonal imbalance. A contraceptive foam or lubricating jelly may be used to enhance comfort.

Exploring previously used methods of contraception may be helpful in identifying a starting place for the discussion. The couple's religion and cultural background often dictates their contraceptive choice. Discussing contraception options with the patient and her partner (if present) before discharge allows the couple time to make informed decisions before resuming sexual intercourse. The breastfeeding mother should be warned that she can become pregnant during lactation and that breastfeeding is not a substitute for birth control. If the breastfeeding patient wishes to use an oral contraceptive the nurse must inform the health care provider so that a progesterone-only pill can be prescribed. (See Chapter 6 for further information.)

PLANNING FOR THE FOLLOW-UP EXAMINATION

Most health care providers schedule a 6-week follow-up appointment ("postpartal check"). Women who have had cesarean births are often scheduled for a return visit to the physician's office 2 weeks after hospital discharge. It is helpful to indicate the date and time of the return appointment in the patient's discharge instructions.

The nurse can explain that during the 6-week follow-up visit, fundal palpation and a vaginal examination will be performed to evaluate the size of the uterus. The episiotomy or abdominal incision site will be evaluated for healing and a breast examination will be performed. If desired, a contraceptive method or prescription will also be given. The nurse should encourage the patient to discuss any concerns during this visit.

The parents should also schedule a newborn follow-up appointment before hospital discharge. Most physicians and clinics wish to see the infant within the first week or by age 2 weeks.

Now Can You— Promote self-care for the puerperium?

1. Outline postpartal teaching guidelines that include information about self-assessment of the fundus, lochia, hygiene, incisional site, body temperature, and elimination?
2. Demonstrate appropriate exercises for the postpartal patient?
3. Identify at least six symptoms indicative of poor emotional adjustment that, if present for more than 2 weeks, should be reported to the health care provider?

Patients with Special Needs During the Puerperium

CARE OF THE ADOLESCENT

The period of adolescence is a time to form important relationships with peers – these close connections help to facilitate self-growth and development. Adolescents who are thrust into an untimely motherhood role must also deal with their own personal and social development. Adjusting to pregnancy and impending motherhood can be emotionally and physically challenging for a mature woman; the adolescent requires special assistance from the nurse.

Many adolescents enter motherhood with unrealistic expectations. They lack mothering and child care skills.

Fatigue and sleep deprivation, common in all new mothers, coupled with the responsibility of caring for an infant who requires constant attention often results in limited time for social activities and subsequent social isolation from their peers.

Nurses who care for the adolescent mother must be cognizant of personal prejudices or feelings of disapproval and avoid expressing negative feelings toward the teen mother. It is important for the nurse to provide emotional support for the postpartum adolescent that will help her adjust to role changes, foster feelings of positive self-esteem and assist her in developing a new identity and sense of self (Logsdon & Koniak-Griffin, 2005). The nurse must create a supportive environment by recognizing the adolescent as the infant's primary caregiver, irrespective of her age. The nurse models and facilitates infant caring behaviors that will promote bonding and teaches about infant care and child safety. Before discharge, arrangements should be made for a community health nurse follow-up visit within a week.

" What to say " — *When planning the adolescent mother's hospital discharge*

The adolescent mother has unique needs for discharge planning. The nurse can best explore the young patient's immediate plans for herself and the baby by initiating dialog in a supportive, nonthreatening environment. Examples of appropriate questions that the nurse may ask include the following:

"Do you have someone available to offer you help and/or support?"

"Do you feel a sense of closeness or attachment to your baby?"

"After you leave the hospital, will anyone be helping you to care for your baby?"

"Will anyone be taking care of the baby so that you can go back to school?"

"Where will you take the baby for follow-up care?"

To facilitate a supportive home and family environment, the community health nurse will conduct a social support assessment to identify the significant family member or other person who will be assisting with parenting responsibilities and financial support. If the adolescent's mother is identified as the primary support person, the nurse explores the mother's and grandmother's expectations in caring for the newborn in order to provide anticipatory guidance regarding each person's new role before discharge.

A supportive family environment is the single most important element in facilitating the adolescent mother's successful transition to motherhood. When appropriate, referrals should be made for social services and other community resources such as home health nursing care, pastoral care, teen parent support groups, and economic assistance. Guidance and support provided by these professionals help to reinforce infant care skills and identify additional resources to enable the young mother to complete her education. Professional and family support has proven to be effective in helping adolescents delay a subsequent pregnancy, stay enrolled in school, find work and complete the developmental tasks of adolescence (Logsdon & Koniak-Griffin, 2005; Secco et al., 2007).

THE WOMAN WHO IS PLACING HER INFANT FOR ADOPTION

The relinquishment of an infant triggers a host of emotions for the woman and her family. Nurses must be sensitive to the myriad of psychological stressors and social stigmas associated with placing a child for adoption. Depending on hospital policy, the patient may be admitted to the postpartum unit where she can be attended to by nurses who are experienced in perinatal care. The nurse should offer support, a "listening ear," and a compassionate environment where the patient feels safe in expressing her feelings. The woman will likely experience a range of emotions such as grief, loneliness, and guilt. After birth, the patient should have access to her newborn if she so desires. The opportunity to see, hold, and feed the infant may help her to accept the reality that she has given birth to a healthy child. This affirmation may foster feelings of self-esteem and provide a foundation for emotional healing. Postpartum care may continue well beyond hospital discharge for women who choose to give up the infant. Referrals to various community resources may be appropriate (Cunningham et al., 2005). In some cases, the adoptive couple may come into the hospital to meet the new infant. The new parents will need the same instruction in infant care and safety as the biological parents.

THE OLDER WOMAN

Today, it is not uncommon for women over age 35 to experience their first pregnancy, and when pregnancy occurs among this population, it is deemed "advanced maternal age".

The older patient may have preexisting medical conditions (e.g., hypertension, diabetes) and experience greater health risks and pregnancy complications such as gestational diabetes and preeclampsia. In these situations, pregnancy and puerperal care involve a collaborative approach that includes a physician with special training in high-risk obstetrics (perinatologist) and medical specialists (e.g., endocrinologist, rheumatologist, cardiologist).

Women experience pregnancy after the age of 35 for a number of reasons. Some postpone pregnancy in order to make advancements in careers; others have struggled with infertility and become pregnant following advanced reproductive techniques while others report contraceptive failure. There is a wide range of attitudes and emotions that accompany parenthood during midlife. Some women believe that delaying motherhood enhances the adaptation to the parental role. They cite qualities such as maturity, patience, and understanding and greater life experiences as positive influences for assuming the parental role. For others, parenthood at an older age can be disruptive to intimate relationships, interfere with career goals, and create a perception of loss of control. Reassurance, support, and referral, when appropriate, help to facilitate transitions during the puerperium for the older couple.

Community Resources for the New Family

SUPPORT GROUPS

The birth of a newborn constitutes a major life transition. For the new parent, attending a support group can provide a venue for sharing experiences and challenges with other new parents. Information about "essential" parenting topics, such infant feeding and nutrition, behavior, sleeping patterns, and strategies for fostering family relationships is readily available during the meetings. Specific support groups may also be available for unique populations, such as single parents, working mothers and parents of infants with special needs. Parents who participated in childbirth education classes together often reunite to form a support group after childbirth.

HOME VISITS

Some facilities routinely schedule home visits for maternal and baby assessment. This visit provides the nurse with an opportunity to assess bonding, conduct patient teaching, answer questions, correct learning deficits, reinforce hospital discharge instructions and make appropriate community referrals.

TELEPHONE FOLLOW-UP

Facilities that offer home follow-up services usually call parents approximately two to three days after discharge. Making personal contact with the family provides early support and reassurance, allows for questions to be answered and discharge instructions to be reviewed and clarified.

OUTPATIENT CLINICS

Outpatient clinics provide another option for facilities that do not offer home visitation. The clinics are often nurse-managed and allow the mother and her baby to receive further information about maternal-infant care. The patient's additional questions or concerns can also be dealt with at this time.

A list of community resources and phone numbers is often provided to the couple before discharge. These services may include professional lactation services, nursing mother's support groups, "Mommy and Me" classes, postnatal exercise classes, parenting education and support groups, medical care, crisis lines/counseling, emergency and financial assistance, and bereavement support.

 Now Can You— Care for postpartal patients with special needs and identify community resources for the postpartal family?

1. Identify nursing interventions that foster the postpartal adolescent's self-esteem and empower her to bond with and care for her infant?

2. Describe nursing interventions to provide appropriate emotional support for the woman who chooses to place her infant for adoption?

3. Identify at least three sources of community support for the postpartal family and discuss the benefits of each?

summary points

- During the postpartum period, the nurse assumes the responsibility of facilitating the integration of the newborn into the family unit.

- The postpartum patient has unique assessment needs that include physical and psychosocial considerations.

- The new mother should be given the opportunity to discuss her birth experience.

- The postpartum woman who has experienced a cesarean birth is also considered to be a surgical patient who has special needs for additional nursing care.

- Effective pain management should be an integral component of the postpartal nursing assessment.

- The breastfeeding mother should be provided with sufficient support to facilitate success.

- The nurse should provide anticipatory guidance that includes family members whenever possible.

review questions

Multiple Choice

1. In the preadmission clinic, the perinatal nurse describes the advantages to a short hospital stay as including:
   A. Decreased risk of nosocomial infection
   B. Increased rest and recuperation
   C. Increased opportunity to initiate successful breastfeeding
   D. Increased teaching about infant care

2. In the immediate postpartum period, the perinatal nurse knows that the postpartum woman most often has a:
   A. Bradycardia
   B. Tachycardia
   C. Pulse within the normal adult range
   D. Tachycardia then a pulse rate that returns to normal in 4 hours

3. The postpartum nurse expects a postpartum woman's bladder function to return to normal within which length of time:
   A. 4–6 hours
   B. 6–8 hours
   C. 2–4 hours
   D. 8–12 hours

Fill-in-the-Blank

4. The perinatal nurse knows that the first 6 weeks after birth is described as the _____.

5. The perinatal nurse works with the health care facility's unit council to develop policies to promote patient safety. The policy on infant safety particularly focuses on the challenge of two infants/families with the same _____ to ensure that there are specific strategies to protect each family.

6. The perinatal nurse recognizes that it is common for women using insulin to have _____ insulin requirements postpartum. This finding is due to a _____ in levels of placental lactogen and insulinase.

True/False

7. The perinatal nurse teaches the student nurse about the use of the acronym REEDA for wound assessment. The "R" stands for Redness and the "A" stands for Approximation of the wound edges.

Select All that Apply

8. The perinatal nurse teaches a new nurse about the *Healthy People 2010* initiative, which includes postpartum teaching that focuses on:
   A. Warning signs during the postpartum period
   B. Benefits of breastfeeding
   C. Use of infant soothers
   D. Contraceptive methods

9. The postpartum nurse recognizes that after birth, the patient is at risk for decreased bladder tone and function if her labor/birth included:
   A. Forceps
   B. Vacuum extraction
   C. Prodromal labor
   D. Prolonged second stage

Case Study

10. The perinatal nurse is assessing Ruth, who has given birth 2 hours ago. The nurse notes a discoloration of the perineum and Ruth complains of pain and rectal pressure. The most appropriate action for the nurse is to:
    A. Call the health care provider to assess immediately.
    B. Increase IV fluids and request an order for ergonovine (Ergotrate).
    C. Reassure Ruth and her family that postpartum pain is normal and medication is available.
    D. Apply ice packs to the perineum as quickly as possible.

See Answers to End of Chapter Review Questions on the Electronic Study Guide or DavisPlus.

REFERENCES

American Academy of Pediatrics (AAP) Committee on Fetus and Newborn. (2004). Hospital stay for healthy term infants. *Pediatrics, 113*(5), 1434–1436.

American College of Obstetricians and Gynecologists (ACOG). (2003). ACOG Committee Opinion No. 282. Immunization during pregnancy. *Obstetrics and Gynecology, 101*(4), 207–212.

Association of Women's Health, Obstetric and Neonatal Nurses (AWHONN). (1999). *Clinical position statement: The role of the nurse in the promotion of breastfeeding.* Washington, DC: Author.

Beck, C., Records, K., & Rice, M. (2006). Further development of the postpartum depression predictors inventory-revised. *Journal of Obstetric, Gynecologic, & Neonatal Nursing, 35*(6), 735–745.

Bulechek, G., Butcher, H.M., & Dochterman, J. (2008). *Nursing interventions classification (NIC)* (5th ed.). St. Louis, MO: C.V. Mosby.

Cadwell, K., Turner-Maffei, C., O'Conner, B., Cadwell-Blair, A., Arnold, L., and Blair, E. (2006). *Maternal and infant assessment for breastfeeding and human lactation: A guide for the practitioner* (2nd ed.). Sudbury, MA: Jones and Bartlett.

Chan, P., & Winkle, C. (2006). *Gynecology and obstetrics: Current clinical strategies.* Laguna Hills, CA: CCS Publishing.

Cunningham, F., Leveno, K., Bloom, S., Hauth, J., Gilstrap, L., & Wenstrom, K. (2005). *Williams' obstetrics* (22nd ed). New York: McGraw-Hill.

Dabrowski, G.A. (2007). Skin to skin contact: Giving birth back to mothers and babies. *Nursing for Women's Health, 11*(1), 64–71.

Davis, R. (2001). The postpartum experience for Southeast Asian women in the United States. *The American Journal of Maternal Child Nursing, 26*(4), 208–213.

Deglin, J.H., & Vallerand, A.H. (2009). *Davis's drug guide for nurses* (11th ed.). Philadelphia: F.A. Davis.

Gartner, L., Morton, J., Lawrence, R., Naylor, A., O'Hare, D., Schanler, R., et al. (2005). Breastfeeding and the use of human milk. *Pediatrics, 115*(2), 496–506.

Halon, L., & Milkus, K. (2004). *Staphylococcus aureus* and wounds: A review of tea tree oil (Melaeuca alternifolia) as a promising antimicrobial. *American Journal of Infection Control, 32*(7), 402–408.

Horowitz, J.A., & Goodman, J.H. (2005). Identifying and treating postpartum depression. *Journal of Obstetric, Gynecologic & Neonatal Nursing, 34*(5), 264–273.

International Childbirth Education Association (ICEA). (2003). *Siblings and the new baby.* (Brochure). Minneapolis, MN: Author.

Johnson, M., Bulechek, G., Butcher, H., McCloskey Dochterman, J., Maas, M., Moorehead, S., & Swanson, E. (2006). *NANDA, NOC, and NIC linkages: Nursing diagnoses, outcomes, & interventions* (2nd ed.). St. Louis, MO: Mosby Elsevier.

Johnston, M.L., & Esposito, N. (2007). Barriers and facilitators for breastfeeding among working women in the United States. *Journal of Obstetric, Gynecologic & Neonatal Nursing, 36*(1), 9–20.

Klaus, M. (1982). *Parent-infant bonding* (2nd ed.). St. Louis, MO: C.V. Mosby.

Lactation Education Resources. (2004). *Breast engorgement.* Retrieved from www.leron-line.com/handouts/Breast_Engorgement.htm (Accessed December 2, 2006).

Lavender, T., Hofmeyr, G.J., Nielson, J.P., Kingdon, C., & Gyte, G.M. (2007). Depressive symptoms in mothers of prematurely born infants. *Journal of Developmental and Behavioral Pediatrics, 28*(1), 36–44.

Lawrence, R., & Lawrence, R. (2005). *Breastfeeding: A guide for the medical profession* (6th ed.). Philadelphia: Elsevier Mosby.

Logsdon, M.C., & Koniak-Griffin, K. (2005). Social support in postpartum adolescents: Guidelines for nursing assessments and interventions. *Journal of Obstetric, Gynecologic, & Neonatal Nursing, 34*(6), 761–768.

Meara, E., Kotagal, U., Atherton, H., & Lieu, T. (2004). Impact of early newborn discharge legislation and early follow-up visits on infant outcomes in a state Medicaid population. *Pediatrics, 113*(6), 1619–1627.

Miller, L.C., Cook, J.T., Brooks, C.W., Heine, A.G., & Curtis, T.K. (2007). Breastfeeding education: Empowering future health care providers. *Nursing for Women's Health, 11*(4), 375–380.

Moorehead, S., Johnson, M., Maas, M., & Swanson, E. (2008). *Nursing outcomes classification (NOC)* (4th ed.). St. Louis, MO: C.V. Mosby.

NANDA International (2007). *NANDA-I nursing diagnoses: Definitions and classifications 2007–2008.* Philadelphia: NANDA-I.

Olson, C., Strawderman, M., Hinton, P., & Pearson, T. (2003). Gestational weight gain and postpartum behaviors associated with weight change from early pregnancy to 1 year postpartum. *International Journal of Obesity, 27*(1), 117–127.

Patel, R.R., Murphy, D.J., & Peters, T.J. (2005). Operative delivery and postnatal depression: A cohort study. *British Medical Journal, 330*(4), 879–886.

Ramsay, D., Kent, J., Harmann, R., & Harmtann, P. (2005). Anatomy of the lactating human breast redefined with ultrasound imaging. *Journal of Anatomy, 206*(6), 525–534.

Riordan, J. (2005). *Breastfeeding and human lactation* (3rd ed.). Sudbury, MA: Jones and Bartlett.

Rubin, R. (1984). *Maternal identity and the maternal experience.* New York: Springer.

Rubin, R. (1975). Maternal tasks in pregnancy. *MCN: The American Journal of Maternal-Child Nursing, 4*(3), 143–153.

Runquist, J. (2007). Persevering through postpartum fatigue. *Journal of Obstetric, Gynecologic & Neonatal Nursing, 36*(1), 28–37.

Secco, M.L., Profit, S., Kennedy, E., Walsh, A., Letourneau, N., & Stewart, M. (2007). Factors affecting postpartum depressive symptoms of adolescent mothers. *Journal of Obstetric, Gynecologic & Neonatal Nursing, 36*(7), 47–54.

St. John, W., Cameron, C., & McVeigh, C. (2005). Meeting the challenge of new fatherhood during the early weeks. *Journal of Obstetric, Gynecologic & Neonatal Nursing, 34*(2), 180–189.

Stonehouse, A., & Studdiford, J. (2007). Allergic contact dermatitis from tea tree oil. *Consultant, 42*(4), 781.

Taylor, R. (2005). Addressing barriers to cultural competence. *Journal for Nurses in Staff Development, 21*(4), 135–142.

Troy, N. (2003). Is the significance of postpartum fatigue being overlooked in the lives of women? *MCN American Journal of Maternal/Child Nursing, 28*(4), 252–257.

Tully, M.R. (2005). Working & Breastfeeding. *AWHONN Lifelines 9*(3), 198–203.

U.S. Census Bureau. (2001). Mapping Census 2000: The Geography of U.S. Diversity. Retrieved from http://www.census.gov/ (Accessed August 21, 2007).

U.S. Department of Health and Human Services. (2000). *Healthy People 2010.* Washington, DC: Author.

 For more information, go to http://davisplus.fadavis.com/

CONCEPT MAP

Caring for the Postpartal Woman and Her Family

Discharge: Planning/Teaching:
- Maternal self-care
- Infant bathing, breastfeeding, activity/rest, perineal hygiene, emotional changes
- Teach self-assessment
- Teach: nutrition, weight loss, exercise, pain management, sexual activity, follow-up exams
- Identify community resources

Promoting Recovery/Self-Care
- Early ambulation; adequate sleep/frequent rest; balanced and nutritious diet
- Promote bowel and bladder function: monitor for urinary retention, possible catheterization prn, stool softeners/enemas prn
- Peri-care: ice packs, sitz bath
- Analgesics for afterpains
- Routine post-op care for patient having sterilization/cesarean birth: wound care, anesthesia recovery, pain control, Foley catheter; psychological issues with cesarean

Physiological Adaptations/Con't Assessments
- Decreased blood volume/elevated cardiac output
- WBC: increased with labor, decreased after 6 days
- Estrogen/progesterone decrease; prolactin released
- Fatigue/discomfort: further assess headaches
- GFR/creatinine/BUN decreased by 2–3 months
- Decreased urine protein and glucose
- Natriuresis/diuresis/possible urinary retention
- Stretch marks
- Involution/uterine contractions; in 6–8 wks resumption of menstruation and ovulation
- Muscle/body aches; rectus abdominis diastasis

Emotional Adjustments
- Linked to childbirth preconceptions, parity, age, maturity, finances, complications
- Insecurity
- Potential mood changes
- Postpartum blues
- Refer for indicators of postpartum depression or psychosis

Complementary Care:
- Tea tree oil for episiotomy healing
- Cabbage leaves to decrease breast swelling

Critical Nursing Action:
- Assessing for maternal–infant attachment

Formula Feeding
- Correct, safe preparation
- Cleaning bottles/nipples
- No microwaving or propping
- Skin-to-skin/full eye contact
- Watch for large emesis of formula

Across Care Settings:
- Community health nurse should refer patient if "letting-go" becomes an issue

Clinical Alert:
- Proper uterine palpation
- Avoid knee-chest position × 3 weeks

Be Sure To:
- Check ID bands
- Prevent abduction

Promoting Breastfeeding:
- Teach: lactation/lactogenesis
- Success strategies: IBCLC
- ID feeding readiness cues
- Facilitate latching-on/suckling
- Proper positioning
- Care: sore nipples/breast engorgement
- Teach about collection/storage of breast milk and weaning

Collaboration
In Caring:
- IBCLCs/LaLeche League
- WIC program

Now Can You:
- Discuss important physiological changes in the postpartum period and essential components of postpartum nursing care
- Discuss physiological adaptations during the postpartum period
- Provide care to the surgical postpartal patient
- Promote recovery and self-care
- Support and care for the breastfeeding mother
- Care for postpartal mothers with special needs

Nursing Insight:
- Perineal assessment: lighting/privacy
- Prevent nipple confusion
- Persistent fatigue may indicate depression

Maternal Assessments
- Vital signs
- Fundus; lochia; perineum: REEDA
- Hemorrhoids
- BUBBLE-HE: breasts, uterus, bladder, bowel, lochia, episiotomy, Homans' sign, emotions
- Pain assessment

Multicultural Family Care
- Holistic and flexible approach
- Know and understand rites/customs/beliefs
- Cultural assessment
- Affects: longevity of confinement/activity during/degree of family involvement
- Hot/cold beliefs: affect diet and environmental temperature

Family–Infant Bonding
- Create positive environment
- Provide emotional support/accurate information
- Maternal: taking-in/ taking-hold/letting-go; promote bonding/ attachment
- Paternal: encourage participation
- Siblings: formulate strategies to increase acceptance
- Grandparents: involvement linked to culture

Ethnocultural Considerations:
- Striae color varies among races
- Use culturally appropriate methods for breast feeding discomfort

Optimizing Outcomes:
- Uterine assessment critical in 1st hr
- Deal quickly with abnormal findings
- Early episiotomy care: ice pack
- Teaching peri-care
- Support feeding choice
- Breast care during lactation
- Preparing formula safely
- Couplet care

Maternal Care — **Infant** — **Nutrition**

Caring for the Woman Experiencing Complications During the Postpartal Period

Do all the good you can. By all the means you can.
In all the ways you can. In all the places you can.
At all the times you can. To all the people you can.
For long as ever you can.

—John Wesley

LEARNING TARGETS *At the completion of this chapter, the student will be able to:*

◆ Describe the causes and collaborative management of postpartum hemorrhage.

◆ Discuss the signs and symptoms of postpartum hematoma; describe nursing care for a patient experiencing a postpartum hematoma.

◆ Describe the collaborative management for infections during the puerperium.

◆ Discuss the collaborative management of thrombophlebitis and thrombosis in postpartum women.

◆ Describe the signs, symptoms, and management of a pulmonary embolism.

◆ Summarize important interventions in meeting psychosocial needs of postpartum women and their families.

◆ Describe current community and governmental services that are available to vulnerable postpartum women and their families.

---

 moving toward evidence-based practice Postpartum Depression

Dennis, C.L., & Ross, L. (2005). Relationship among infant sleep patterns, maternal fatigue, and development of depressive symptomatology. *Birth, 32*(3), 187–193.

Through the replication of a previous study, the purpose of this longitudinal study was to examine the relationship among infant sleep patterns, maternal fatigue, and the development of postpartum depression in women with no major depressive symptomatology.

Depression was defined in the previous study as either meeting the criteria for the diagnosis of a major depression or scoring above 15 on the Edinburgh Postnatal Depression Scale. Variables in the original study and considered to be predictive of depression included maternal age, depression during pregnancy, thoughts of death and dying at 1 month postpartum, and difficulty falling asleep at 1 month postpartum. Prenatal participants in the study were recruited through family physician, obstetrician, and nurse midwife offices. Postnatal participants were obtained through the input of public health nurses during the standard 48-hour discharge telephone call to new mothers. Participation was voluntary and included mothers who were at least 18 years of age and at more than 32 weeks of gestation. Data was obtained through an initial questionnaire and follow-up questionnaires at 4 and 8 weeks postpartum. From a potential population of 857 candidates, 667 agreed to participate. Of that total, 585 returned the questionnaire at 1 week, with 505 (86.3%) scoring less than 13 on the Edinburgh Postnatal Depression Scale (EPDS), qualifying them to participate in this study.

The EPDS assessed symptoms of depression through ratings of 10 items on a four-point scale; a high score indicated a more depressed mood. Depressive symptomatology was defined as a score >12.

(continued)

Sleep outcomes were assessed based on the infant's sleep patterns and their impact on the mother. Examples of those questions included: how well the baby slept; how many times the baby usually awoke during the night; and how many hours of sleep the mother usually had in a 24-hour period. High ratings indicated an increased likelihood of depressive symptoms.

Data analysis revealed the following findings about the mothers and their scores on the EPDS:

- Ages of the mothers ranged from 18 to 43; the mean age was 29 years.
- Ninety-three percent of the mothers were Caucasian; 92% were married; 42% were primiparous; 77% experienced a vaginal birth.
- Twenty-two percent of the mothers had a university degree or higher; 39% graduated from a technical school or college; 34% graduated from high school; and 4% did not have a high school diploma.
- Thirty-six percent of the mothers reported an annual household income greater than $60,000; 26% between $40,000 and 60,000; 37% less than $40,000.
- Scores on the EPDS were as follows: 21 (4.6%) scored >12 at 4 weeks postpartum, 20 (4.7%) scored >12 at 8 weeks. These findings were consistent with the previous study's meta-analysis.

Results at 4 weeks: Mothers who reported that their baby cried often and woke up three times or more during the night, and who slept less than 6 hours in a 24-hour period were more likely to exhibit EPDS scores of >12.

Results at 8 weeks: Mothers who reported that their baby cried often, woke up three times or more during the night, and slept less than six hours in a 24-hour period were more likely to exhibit EPDS scores of >12. These mothers were also three times more likely to report that their baby did not sleep well and six times more likely to report that their baby's sleep pattern did not allow them to obtain a reasonable amount of sleep in a 24-hour period.

Mothers with scores of >12 were more likely to report feeling tired at 4 weeks and at 8 weeks.

The researchers concluded that mothers who demonstrated depression symptoms on the EPDS at 4 and 8 weeks were more likely to report that their baby cried often and woke up three times or more during the night. Mothers who demonstrated depression symptoms were also more likely to sleep less than 6 hours in a 24-hour period and indicated that their baby did not sleep well, a factor that prevented them from getting more sleep. Mothers who scored >12 on the EPDS were also more likely to report feeling tired.

The researchers stated that their findings suggest that infant sleep patterns and maternal fatigue are strongly associated with the onset of depressive symptoms during the postpartum period.

1. What might be considered as limitations to this study?
2. How is this information useful to clinical nursing practice?

See Suggested Responses for Moving Toward Evidence-Based Practice on the Electronic Study Guide or DavisPlus.

Introduction

Most childbearing women have healthy babies and recover from the physiological and psychological adaptations to pregnancy without difficulty. Physiological complications and psychosocial complications are rare, especially in industrialized nations such as the United States, Japan, Australia, and in European countries. Because perinatal care focuses on wellness, health promotion-maintenance, and education for healthy women in multiple settings across the childbearing cycle, the danger of minimizing or misinterpreting pathological signs and symptoms is ever present. Delayed or absent communication between care provider call groups combined with this wellness focus can lead to suboptimal outcomes for women and their families.

When prenatal care begins, whether in a private practice or clinic setting, nurses can serve as liaisons between patients, families, care providers, and community agencies. In this role, the nurse is often the first health care provider to identify physiological signs and symptoms or recognize psychosocial concerns that need to be addressed by the health care team. Synthesizing knowledge with clinical data and thinking critically about the meaning of these data are vitally important.

This chapter describes postpartum physiological and psychosocial complications and concerns from a nursing process perspective. The nurse's role in the collaborative treatment of patients and their families who experience these complications is multifaceted and cannot be overly emphasized. More than any other health care team member, the nurse uses vigilance to apply nursing knowledge and implement informed nursing actions. Vigilance involves combining careful observation, knowledge, and expectations with cues from the patient and her family (Meyer & Lavin, 2005) and is a critical component of nursing care, particularly in the perinatal area where patients are assumed to be healthy. Whether functioning as an independent practitioner or as a member of the health care team, the nurse's judgments and actions affect both present and future generations for years to come.

Postpartum Hemorrhage

INCIDENCE AND DEFINITION

Postpartum hemorrhage (PPH) is a leading cause of maternal morbidity and mortality in the United States and around the world. Approximately 5% of all women who give birth vaginally experience a postpartum hemorrhage. Internationally, postpartum hemorrhage accounts for one of the three major causes of maternal mortality. According to The World Health Organization, 25% of all pregnancy related deaths result from postpartum hemorrhage (Cunningham et al., 2005; Magann, Hutchinson, Collins, Howard, & Morrison, 2005). Historically, practitioners have defined postpartum hemorrhage as a blood loss greater than 500 mL after a vaginal birth and 1000 mL or more after a cesarean birth (Mac-Mullen, Dulski, & Meagher, 2005). Hematocrit levels that decrease 10% from pre- to postbirth measurements are also included in the definition (Cunningham et al., 2005), along with a need for a red blood cell transfusion due to anemia or hemodynamic instability (Magann et al., 2005). Cunningham and colleagues (2005) emphasize that postpartum hemorrhage is a description "of an event, not a diagnosis" (p. 635).

As is often the case with other clinical events, most definitions of postpartum hemorrhage contain a subjective component. Caregivers rarely measure actual blood loss after childbirth. Instead, the physician, nurse midwife, or nurse attendant estimates the amount of blood soaked on the bedding and pads or collected in the placenta basin and suction canister. This nonscientific method is frequently inaccurate and may lead to an underestimation of actual blood loss by as much as 40% to 50% (Cunningham et al., 2005). Accuracy in determining true blood loss is possible if a member of the health care team carefully weighs the placenta basin and all bloody items such as pads, linens, and clothing with a gram scale (1 mL = 1 gram). If in doubt, the nurse should err on the side of safety until objective data can be obtained and confirmed.

critical nursing action Accurately Determining Blood Loss

After childbirth, the nurse carefully weighs all pads, linens, clothing, and clots in the placenta basin on a gram scale to accurately determine the patient's blood loss.

EARLY VERSUS LATE HEMORRHAGE

Although the criteria for a diagnosis of postpartum hemorrhage may vary from practitioner to practitioner, the definition of an early and a late postpartum hemorrhage is straightforward. An early hemorrhage occurs within the first 24 hours after birth. A late hemorrhage occurs more than 24 hours but less than 6 weeks postpartum. The greatest likelihood for occurrence of an early hemorrhage is within the first 4 postpartum hours. During this time, the blood flow to the uterus is between 500 and 800 mL/minute, and the placental site contains multiple exposed venous areas and low resistance (Smith & Brennan, 2006). One researcher suggests the use of the acronym "LARRY" to serve as a memory prompt for the common causes of early PPH (Flamm, 2003): **L**acerations, **A**tony, **R**etained placental tissue, **R**uptured uterus, and "**Y**ou pulled too hard on the cord (thereby creating an inversion of the uterus)." More commonly, the 4 "T's" serve as a reminder of factors associated with PPH: **t**one, **t**rauma, **t**issue, and **t**hrombin (Cunningham et al., 2005; Smith & Brennan, 2006). A lack of uterine tone (**atony**) and genital tract trauma are the most common conditions that cause postpartum hemorrhage.

 Nursing Insight— *Using a standardized assessment for blood loss after childbirth*

According to Luegenbiehl, Brophy, Artigue, Phillips, and Flack (1990), nurses may use the following definitions to accurately describe the amount of blood saturation on a perineal pad:

Scant: Peripad blood stain <2 inches (<10 mL) within 1 hour

Small: Peripad blood stain >2 inches, <4 inches (10–25 mL) within 1 hour

Moderate: Peripad blood stain >4 inches but <6 inches (25–50 mL) within 1 hour

Large: Peripad blood stain >6 inches to saturated peripad (50–80 mL) within 1 hour

UTERINE ATONY

Uterine atony is a failure of the uterine myometrium to contract and retract following birth. Normally, the uterine muscle fibers contract firmly around the blood vessels during placental separation. A lack of contraction and retraction results in noncompression of the uterine arteries and veins at the placental implantation site, thereby preventing hemostasis. The hallmark of uterine atony is a soft uterus filled with clots and blood. Multiple factors place the childbearing woman at risk for hemorrhage from uterine atony. An understanding of the factors that increase the risk of uterine atony allows the nurse to anticipate hemorrhage and intervene to prevent excessive blood loss (Box 16-1).

TRAUMA

During the second stage of labor, soft tissue trauma from a number of causes (e.g., rapid labor, operative delivery, episiotomy) can result in genital tract lacerations (Box 16-2). While PPH from uterine atony is evident from a soft,

---

Box 16-1 Risk Factors for Uterine Atony

- Uterine overdistention
- Large baby
- Multiple gestation
- Hydramnios
- Bladder distention
- Prolonged first and/or second stage labor
- Precipitous labor
- Labor induction/augmentation with Pitocin
- Tocolytic therapy (especially with magnesium sulfate)
- High parity*
- Retained placental fragments
- Halogenated anesthetic agents
- Prolonged/mismanaged third stage of labor**

———————
*Magann et al. (2005) found no correlation between PPH from uterine atony and maternal parity in their large study (18,735 women).
**In his review of PPH risk factors, Hobbins (2005) determined that a third stage >18 minutes increased the risk of PPH and that there is a six time greater risk of PPH if the third stage is >30 minutes.

Box 16-2 **Risk Factors for Postpartum Hemorrhage from Tissue Trauma**

- Rapid second stage labor
- Rapid/precipitous labor (< 3 hours from onset to delivery)
- Operative vaginal deliveries (forceps, vacuum extraction)
- Fetal manipulation (extrauterine or intrauterine version, corkscrew maneuver for shoulder dystocia [corkscrew maneuver: a progressive 180 degree manual rotation of the baby's posterior shoulder to release the impacted anterior shoulder]) (Cunningham et al., 2005, p. 512)
- Large episiotomies, including extensions
- Large baby
- Cesarean birth
- Uterine rupture (increased incidence with previous uterine surgery, tetanic contractions, labor stimulation, versions, placental attachment abnormalities)

blood-filled uterus, if the source of hemorrhage is genital tract lacerations, the uterus remains firm. One large or several small lacerations can adversely affect hemodynamic stability.

clinical alert

Postpartal blood loss

The nurse and other practitioners must remember that in the presence of a firm uterus, continual vaginal bleeding in a slow but steady trickle, with or without clots, can result in significant blood loss (MacMullen et al., 2005; Smith & Brennan, 2006).

Lacerations are usually internal and are not visible when the nurse examines the perineum. Identifying either a vaginal wall or cervical laceration usually requires that the physician or midwife examine the patient while she is in the lithotomy position. Not infrequently, the doctor locates and repairs a laceration before the patient's transfer to the postpartum unit.

TISSUE

Careful examination of the placenta after delivery is a component of standard care. Hence, retained placental tissue is an uncommon cause of early PPH. If the pregnancy included problems with placental implantation (e.g., previa, accreta), the primary care provider is aware of these risks before the birth takes place. Should the practitioner note that lobes of the placenta are missing during the placental examination, the physician or certified nurse midwife explores the patient's uterus to remove them. More often, a soft uterus with bright red bleeding later in the postpartum course identifies the source of a late postpartum hemorrhage (Cunningham et al., 2005; MacMullen et al., 2005).

THROMBIN

Thrombin refers to problems with maternal coagulation. Disorders of the coagulation system and platelets do not usually result in excessive bleeding during the immediate postpartum period. Preexistent maternal factors such as low fibrinogen levels and idiopathic thrombocytopenia

(ITP) and acquired pathology such as HELLP syndrome (condition characterized by **H**emolysis, **E**levated **L**iver enzymes, and **L**ow **P**latelet count) disseminated intravascular coagulation (DIC), sepsis, and abruptio placentae require vigilant care and anticipation of possible hemorrhage after birth (Smith & Brennan, 2006).

LATE POSTPARTUM HEMORRHAGE

Late postpartum hemorrhage occurs in only 1% to 2% of all childbearing women, usually within the first 2 weeks after birth (Franzblau & Witt, 2006). Retained placental fragments are the most common cause of late PPH. Other causes include subinvolution (failure of the uterus to return to its pre-pregnant size) and uterine infection. Regardless of the cause, treatment usually includes ergonovine medication (Ergotrate or Methergine 0.2 mg orally every 4 hours for 48 hours), antibiotics, and, if necessary, dilation and curettage to remove placental fragments. Since *Chlamydia trachomatis* is a common organism for postpartum uterine infection that causes subinvolution (Cunningham et al., 2005), tetracycline anti-infective agents such as Tetracap, Tetracyn and Sumycin are often prescribed. After birth and before discharge, the nurse is responsible for educating the patient and her family about the signs and symptoms of subinvolution. Signs and symptoms of subinvolution include lower abdominal (uterine) tenderness with or without fever, continuation of red vaginal drainage beyond 1 week, and foul smelling vaginal drainage, regardless of color.

 Nursing Insight— *Recognizing characteristics that point to the source of postpartal bleeding*

The color and character of the blood and the consistency of the uterus can often identify the source of postpartal bleeding. When bleeding is associated with uterine atony or retained placental fragments, the blood is dark red with clots and the uterus is soft and boggy. When bleeding is associated with lacerations from the perineum, cervix, or vagina, the blood is bright red and the uterus remains firmly contracted.

HYPOVOLEMIC SHOCK

Hypovolemic (hemorrhagic) shock can result if PPH is not managed aggressively. Most women can tolerate a 1000 mL blood loss because they are healthy, have a 35% to 45% increase in the plasma and red blood cell (RBC) volume (2 pints of blood), and give birth in positions that "pool blood" in the pelvis (Cunningham et al., 2005).

clinical alert

Blood loss and vital signs

Normal physiological adaptations in pregnancy mean that a large loss of blood can occur before changes in vital signs (decreased blood pressure and increased pulse) are evident. The lack of objective signs and symptoms may lead to a delay in treatment.

The nurse, physician, or midwife may not see the usual signs of shock—restlessness, anxiety, pallor, cool, clammy skin, increased pulse, tachypnea, shaking, decreased blood pressure—until 30% to 40% of the patient's total circulating blood volume has been lost.

COLLABORATIVE MANAGEMENT OF PPH

After birth, standard care requires frequent measurement of vital signs and fundal massage to check the location and condition of the uterine fundus. Most hospitals and birthing centers require that the registered nurse perform these checks at least every 15 minutes for the first postpartal hour. Thereafter, the frequency of assessment varies from one institution to another. As the primary caregiver and the one completing these assessments, the registered nurse may be the first person to identify excessive blood loss. When identified, immediate actions are necessary. While another member of the team calls the physician or nurse midwife, the nurse can obtain some important assessment data. The nurse must be cognizant of risk factors in the patient's history. After locating the uterine fundus and initiating fundal massage, the nurse can also begin frequent vital sign measurements with an automatic device. The nurse should also palpate the bladder for distention. The length of time it takes for blood loss to saturate a perineal pad is an important parameter to record, as is a measurement of total intake and output up to that point. Keeping in mind that the pulse and blood pressure may remain unchanged until a large volume of blood has been lost, the nurse must pay particular attention to the mean arterial pressure (MAP). A decrease in this measurement may be the first indicator of hypovolemia (Cunningham et al., 2005). Of importance, also, is to note the patient's behavior, in particular her level of consciousness, the presence of restlessness, vague complaints, and her pain level. Possible nursing diagnoses and goals for postpartum hemorrhage are listed in Boxes 16-3 and 16-4.

 Optimizing Outcomes— **Using time intervals and weight to improve accuracy of the estimate of perineal pad saturation**

It is difficult to estimate the amount of blood required to saturate a perineal pad. When fully saturated, a perineal pad can hold between 50 and 80 mL. The nurse can use distinct time intervals for measurement, such as every 15 or 30 minutes, to increase the accuracy of the estimated blood loss. For example, six pads saturated in 30 minutes is much more alarming than six pads saturated in 6 hours. It is also essential to differentiate between the terms "saturated" and "used" when performing a pad count. An accurate way to measure vaginal blood loss is to weigh the perineal pad before and after use and subtract the difference. One gram (1 g) in weight equals one milliliter (1 mL) in volume of blood because grams and milliliters are comparable measures. The woman should be positioned on her side when observing for blood loss. Otherwise, large amounts of pooled blood under her buttocks may go undetected.

Once the physician or nurse identifies a postpartum hemorrhage, interventions quickly follow. If the cause of the hemorrhage is uterine atony, continual fundal massage *with lower uterine segment support* is mandatory (Procedure 16-1). While one member of the team massages the fundus, another nurse establishes intravenous access with a large-bore needle (usually an 18-gauge or larger) and administers oxytocic drugs. The usual order of oxytocic drug administration is oxytocin (Pitocin), followed by methylergonovine (Methergine) or ergonovine (Ergotrate), carboprost (Hemabate), and recently, misoprostol (Cytotec). See Table 16-1 for further information and nursing implications concerning these medications.

Box 16-3 Possible Nursing Diagnoses for Postpartum Hemorrhage

Fluid volume deficit related to decreased circulating blood volume secondary to uterine atony (genital tract trauma, uterine rupture, retained placental fragments, inversion of the uterus)

- Altered tissue perfusion related to hypovolemia
- Fear related to threat to health and powerlessness
- Pain related to uterine massage and invasive procedures
- Risk for infection related to invasive procedures

Box 16-4 Possible Goals for the Patient Experiencing a Postpartum Hemorrhage

- The patient's circulating blood volume will be maintained and/or the blood volume will be restored to a physiologically adequate level.
- Peripheral pulses and oxygenation will be maintained.
- The patient/family will express their fears.
- The patient's pain will be managed at a level acceptable to her.
- The patient will maintain normal vital signs and laboratory values.

Adapted from Wilkinson, J.M. (2005). *Nursing diagnosis handbook*. Upper Saddle River, NJ: Pearson Education.

---

 clinical alert

Off-label use of misoprostol for postpartum hemorrhage

Misoprostol (Cytotec), a prostaglandin E$_1$ analogue, is neither marketed by its maker (Pfizer) for obstetrical use nor approved by the FDA for obstetrical use. However, its effectiveness in abating postpartum hemorrhage (and ripening of the cervix for the induction of labor) is now generally accepted. Since first introduced in 1985, it has been approved for use in the prevention and treatment of PPH in more than 85 countries. Misoprostol may be administered orally, sublingually, and intravenously. Maternal pyrexia and shivering are the most common side effects; nausea, vomiting, and diarrhea may also occur (Walters & Wing, 2007).

---

 critical nursing action Immediate Intervention for Uterine Atony

As soon as excessive blood loss is noted, the nurse's most important intervention is to begin fundal massage. Support the lower uterine segment by placing a hand in a slight "C" position just above the symphysis pubis. *Do not* express clots if the uterus does not become firm with massage. The clots may protect the patient from an even greater blood loss.

Procedure 16-1 Performing Fundal Massage

Purpose

Fundal massage is used as an emergency measure to contract the uterus that is soft and boggy due to atony. It is performed to promote uterine tone and consistency and minimize the risk of hemorrhage. Uterine atony may result from prolonged labor, rapid or precipitous labor and birth, high parity, medications during labor (e.g., oxytocin, magnesium sulfate, inhalation anesthesia), intra-amniotic infection, operative delivery and uterine overdistention from multiple gestation, hydramnios, or macrosomia.

Equipment

- Clean examination gloves
- Disposable cleansing wipes
- Two clean peripads

Preexamination Preparation

1. Wash and dry hands, explain the procedure and its purpose to the patient; ensure privacy.

   RATIONALE: *Hand washing helps to prevent the spread of microorganisms. Explanations help to decrease anxiety; providing privacy helps to promote the patient's comfort and self-esteem.*

2. Assemble necessary equipment, including clean examination gloves, disposable cleansing wipes, clean peripads.

3. Ask the patient to void, unless fundal massage must be performed immediately due to excessive bleeding.

   RATIONALE: *An empty bladder prevents uterine displacement and facilitates an accurate assessment of uterine tone.*

4. Assist the woman to a supine position with the knees flexed and the feet placed together.

   RATIONALE: *Proper positioning facilitates easy visualization and enhances the effectiveness of the procedure.*

Steps

1. Don gloves, remove the peripad, and inspect the perineum. Observe the character and amount of drainage on the pad and the presence of clots. Apply a clean peripad.

   RATIONALE: *Gloves serve as a barrier against possible infection from the vaginal drainage. Obtaining a baseline assessment provides information for future assessments; it also provides a means for evaluating the effectiveness of the procedure.*

2. Place one hand on the abdomen, just above the symphysis pubis.

   RATIONALE: *This location provides support for the lower uterine segment.*

3. Place the other hand around the top of the fundus.

   RATIONALE: *This location helps to locate and assess the fundus and the fundal height.*

4. With the lower hand maintained in a stable position, rotate the upper hand and massage the uterus until it is firm. Avoid overmassaging the uterus.

RATIONALE: *The uterus should be massaged only when it is not firm. Massaging a firm uterus may result in muscle fatigue and uterine relaxation. Overly aggressive fundal massage may result in uterine prolapse.*

5. Once the uterus has become firm, *gently* press the fundus between the hands. Apply a slight downward pressure against the lower hand.

   RATIONALE: *Gentle squeezing with downward pressure assists in the expulsion of blood or clots that have collected in the uterine cavity.*

6. Observe the perineum for the passage of clots and the amount of bleeding.

   RATIONALE: *This action helps to assess the presence of clots and the degree of bleeding.*

7. Once the uterus remains firm, cleanse the perineum and apply a clean peripad. Dispose of the soiled gloves and pads according to institutional policy.

   RATIONALE: *This action promotes maternal comfort and hygiene and reduces the risk for infection.*

8. Document the findings. Continue to assess the fundus and vaginal drainage according to institutional protocol. Alert the physician or nurse midwife if the fundus does not remain contracted or if bleeding persists.

   RATIONALE: *Documentation serves as a means for evaluation. Continued assessment allows for the early identification of problems and facilitates timely intervention with additional measures such as medications (i.e., oxytocin) to prevent hemorrhage.*

Documentation

7/27/10 0550: Fundal massage performed with a moderate amount of bright red lochia and small clots expressed. Uterus remained firm and contracted below the umbilicus. Procedure tolerated well by the patient.

—Sejal Patel, RNC

Table 16-1 Medications and Nursing Considerations for Postpartum Hemorrhage				
Name	**Action**	**Dosage/Route**	**Contraindications**	**Nursing Considerations**
Oxytocin (Pitocin)	Stimulates uterine smooth muscle and produces contractions similar to those that occur during spontaneous labor	10 units IM if no IV access; 10–40 units in 1000 cc crystalloid IV fluid (lactated Ringer's or normal saline)	Hypersensitivity	Monitor uterine response. DO NOT administer a bolus of undiluted oxytocin, as it can cause hypotension and cardiac arrhythmias. Consider administration of pain medication for uterine cramping.
Methylergonovine (Methergine)	Causes uterine contractions by stimulating uterine and vascular smooth muscles.	0.1–0.2 mg IM followed by 0.2 mg PO q4–6h × 24 hours	Hypersensitivity History of, or current elevation of blood pressure	Keep refrigerated. DO NOT add it to IV solutions or mix in a syringe with other medications.
Carboprost* (Hemabate)	Stimulates contractions of the myometrium	250 mcg IM or directly into the uterus (by MD or CNM) may repeat dosage	Asthma or glaucoma	Do not administer if patient demonstrates shock, as it will not be well absorbed. Keep refrigerated. This medication is VERY expensive.
Misoprostol (Cytotec)	Acts as a prostaglandin analogue; stimulates powerful contractions of the myometrium	400–1000 mcg rectally	Hypersensitivity to prostaglandins	Stable at room temperature. Rectal absorption is likely slower than IV medication. Monitor uterine response.

*Eighty to ninety percent effective in stopping postpartum hemorrhage when patient is unresponsive to Pitocin or Methergine (Smith & Brennen, 2006).
Data from Adams et al. (2005); Cunningham et al. (2005); Smith & Brennan (2006); and Tucker (2004).

If the patient has a distended bladder, an indwelling urinary catheter needs to be inserted and all intake and output carefully recorded. The nurse also needs to weigh pads, linens, and other bloody items on a gram scale to obtain an accurate picture of blood loss. It may be necessary to administer oxygen at 10 to 12 L/min to treat compromised tissue perfusion. Additional baseline information that should be obtained includes a complete blood count (CBC) and coagulation studies (PT [prothrombin time] partial thromboplastin time [PTT], fibrinogen, and fibrin degradation products). The physician or nurse midwife orders the blood tests, along with a type and cross match for replacement blood as an anticipatory measure in the event a transfusion is necessary. The patient is carefully assessed for indicators of disseminated intravascular coagulation (DIC).

DIC is a diffuse clotting pathology that involves the consumption of large amounts of clotting factors including platelets, fibrinogen, prothrombin, and factors V and VII. The pathological process may cause both internal and external bleeding. Vascular occlusion of small vessels occurs as small clots form in the microcirculation. Although DIC may occur during the postpartum period, it is most likely to be associated with abruptio placentae, severe preeclampsia, amniotic fluid embolism, septicemia, cardiopulmonary arrest, hemorrhage, and dead fetus syndrome (a complication that may occur when the fetus has died and is retained in the uterus for 6 or more weeks). Diagnosis is made according to clinical findings and laboratory results. (See Chapters 11, 14, and 33 for further discussion.)

Labs: Findings with DIC

Low hemoglobin	Low fibrinogen
Low hematocrit	Elevated fibrin split/degradation products
Low platelets	

The physician or midwife may also perform bimanual compression in an effort to empty the uterus of clots and restore its tone. To perform this procedure, the physician inserts one hand in the vagina while pushing against the fundus through the abdominal wall with the other hand (Fig. 16-1). If these interventions fail to stabilize the patient by restoring tone to the uterus and decreasing the blood loss, an invasive procedure performed in the operating room will be necessary. Invasive procedures include the placement of uterine packing, embolization occlusion of a vessel with a clot, usually in a radiological procedure), or uterine artery ligation (a simple, highly effective treatment to control bleeding that involves stitching the artery/vein to narrow its lumen and significantly decrease blood flow to the involved organ).

Optimizing Outcomes— **Holistic care during management of a PPH**

Best outcome: The nurse provides physiologic care in a timely manner and also serves as an advocate for the patient's pain control and reassures the patient and her family by explaining interventions as they occur. These actions help control not only the blood loss but also the patient's pain and the patient's/family's anxiety.

Figure 16-1 Bimanual compression.

Collaborative interventions for hemorrhage from genital tract lacerations are essentially the same. Patients who are experiencing hemorrhage from genital tract lacerations need a large-bore intravenous site, frequent recording of vital signs, accurate measurements of intake and output from all sources (including blood), lab work, an indwelling urinary catheter, oxygen, and pain medication. In addition, the physician or nurse midwife examines the perineum, vagina, and cervix in an attempt to locate the source of bleeding. The postpartum nurse needs to help the patient assume a lithotomy position, obtain bright lighting and examination instruments, and prepare suction equipment. The nurse continually provides support and reassurance to the patient and her family. Most physicians or midwives choose to repair lacerations in the operating room with an anesthesiologist present and the patient anesthetized.

Once the crisis has passed and immediate interventions have been completed, a debriefing of the health care team's response to the situation can be helpful as a learning opportunity. The patient's outcomes will be evident as she recovers from the postpartum hemorrhage event. Of significance is to note the family's response to the unforeseen events and include them, as appropriate, in the discussion. Because most families expect childbirth to be uneventful, a postpartum hemorrhage can provoke widely differing emotional responses. The prudent and compassionate clinician takes the time to let both the patient and the family express their feelings and affirm their concerns. The nurse must be sure to include care of and bonding with the newborn in the recovery process.

⟳ Now Can You— Discuss postpartum hemorrhage?

1. State the four "T's" that lead to postpartum hemorrhage?
2. Describe five standard nursing interventions for managing postpartum hemorrhage?
3. Discuss holistic care in the management of a woman/family experiencing a postpartum hemorrhage?

Hematomas

DEFINITION, INCIDENCE, AND RISK FACTORS

A **hematoma** is a localized collection of blood in connective or soft tissue under the skin that follows injury of or laceration to a blood vessel without injury to the overlying tissue. At the time of injury, pressure necrosis and inadequate hemostasis occurs. This complication can result in a large amount of blood loss and patient discomfort if not recognized rapidly. Risk factors for hematoma formation include genital tract lacerations, episiotomies, operative vaginal deliveries, a difficult or prolonged second stage of labor, and nulliparity. Hematomas occur most frequently in the vulva, but they can also occur in the vagina and in the retroperitoneal area (Figs. 16-2 and 16-3).

SIGNS AND SYMPTOMS

The most common sign or symptom of a hematoma is unremitting pain and pressure. The pain and pressure worsen if active bleeding continues. On examination of the perineal or vulvar areas, the nurse may notice discoloration and bulging of the tissue at the hematoma site. If touched, the patient complains of severe tenderness, and the clinician generally describes the tissue as "full." If the hematoma is large, signs of shock may be evident and the patient may exhibit an absence of lochia, and an inability to void. Possible nursing diagnoses and goals for a patient experiencing a hematoma are presented in Box 16-5.

COLLABORATIVE MANAGEMENT

Assessment for the presence of a hematoma involves listening to the patient's subjective complaints, measuring vital signs, and examining the perineal and vulvar areas to identify a bulging mass. To examine the perineal and vulvar areas, the nurse assists the patient to a side lying position, gently lifts the upper buttock, and asks her to bear down. The nurse also needs to watch for behavioral signs and symptoms of shock (previously described) and assess the patient's and family's understanding of what is occurring.

Figure 16-2 Vulvar hematoma.

Figure 16-3 Vaginal wall hematoma.

Box 16-5 **Possible Nursing Diagnoses and Goals for Patients with a Postpartum Hematoma**

Pain related to tissue trauma and pressure.
   Patient's pain will be managed to an acceptable level.
Anxiety and/or fear related to knowledge deficit of procedures and plan of care.
   Patient will express her fears.
Altered family processes related to physiological crisis.
   Patient and her family will support one another verbally and behaviorally.
Powerlessness related to loss of control of physiological functions.
   Patient will make choices over which she has control.
At risk for infection related to invasive procedures.
   Patient will remain afebrile and her WBC will be within normal limits.
   Patient's perineum will heal without evidence of drainage or separation.
At risk for fluid volume deficit.
   Patient's blood loss will be minimized.
At risk for altered attachment related to separation from infant.
   Patient will demonstrate concern for and care of infant before discharge.

If findings from the assessment are strongly suggestive of a hematoma, the nurse needs to immediately notify the physician or nurse midwife and implement pain relief measures. If the hematoma is less than 3 to 5 cm in diameter, the physician usually orders palliative treatments such as ice to the area for the first 12 hours along with pain medication, and close observation of the area for extension of the hematoma. After 12 hours, sitz baths are prescribed to replace the application of ice. Sitz baths are therapeutic in providing comfort and in facilitating reabsorption of the clot. A hematoma larger than 5 cm may require incision and drainage with the possible placement of a drain. This invasive procedure is performed in the operating room while the patient is sedated with an anesthetic.

The health care team must be particularly sensitive to the fact that large hematomas can lead to shock. In this case, the physician orders aggressive treatment that includes intravenous fluids, oxygen, frequent measurement of vital signs, urinary catheter placement, and strict intake and output measurements to stabilize the patient before taking her to the operating room.

In the midst of the important interventions implemented to deal with the hematoma, the nurse needs to remember that the family is watching and responding to events as they unfold. Neither the patient nor the family may understand what they are seeing or experiencing. As the various treatments and medications are administered, the nurse should explain each action, along with the rationale for it. If the patient and her family can be involved, it is important to allow them to make choices, so that they do not feel as powerless. The nurse can assist the family by encouraging them to care for and bond with the infant as much as possible.

case study Patient Experiencing a Vulvar Hematoma

Molly is a 20-year-old gravida 1, para 1 who gave birth to a term, healthy baby boy, weighing 9 lbs 1 oz (4.1 kg) at 23:32 hours. She received an epidural for labor pain control, pushed for 3 hours, and required a vacuum-assisted delivery. Her perineum required repair of a third-degree laceration. After birth, the nurse discontinued the continuous epidural pump, placed ice on the perineum, completed the required 15-minute checks (× 5), helped Molly breastfeed, and assisted Molly's boyfriend in holding the baby and taking pictures. On arrival to the mother–baby unit, Molly requests pain medication and states that the ice is helping some but that she wants to "stay on top of it." She rates the pain as a 5 on a 10-point scale. The admission vital signs and fundal location are within normal limits. An examination of Molly's perineum reveals mild swelling and a normal amount of vaginal bleeding. Molly is tired and asks that she be allowed to sleep. Her boyfriend goes home to sleep, and the baby is taken to the nursery.

Two hours later, Molly calls for her nurse and complains of intense burning, pain, and pressure "where I had my stitches." You examine her perineum and note an 8 cm bulging mass on her left vulva. When you touch it with a gloved hand, Molly says, "Oh, that is so tender! That hurts!"

critical thinking questions

1. What factors during birth placed Molly at risk for development of a hematoma?

2. Name two appropriate nursing diagnoses for Molly.

3. What are the expected outcomes for Molly?

4. List four nursing interventions along with rationales.

◆ See Suggested Answers to Case Studies in the text on the Electronic Study Guide or DavisPlus.

 Now Can You— **Discuss implications of a postpartum hematoma?**

1. Describe the classic signs and symptoms of a puerperal hematoma?

2. Identify the most common anatomical locations for a postpartum hematoma?

3. Differentiate between the collaborative management for a small and a large hematoma?

Puerperal (Postpartum) Infections

DEFINITION AND INCIDENCE

Puerperal infection is a bacterial infection of the genital tract, usually of the endometrium (**endometritis**) that occurs within 28 days after miscarriage, induced abortion, or childbirth. The presence of fever often indicates puerperal infection. In the United States, the definition continues to be a temperature of 100.4°F (38°C) or greater on 2 successive days of the first 10 postpartum days (omitting the first 24 hours) measured orally at least four hours apart. A fever of 102.2°F (39°C) or greater within the first 24 hours is often associated with severe pelvic sepsis, usually resulting from Group A or B *Streptococcus* (Cunningham et al., 2005; Table 16-2).

Throughout the world, puerperal infection probably constitutes the major cause of maternal morbidity and mortality; in the United States, the postpartum infection rate is 1% to 8%, with a mortality of 4% to 8% from complications (Kennedy, 2007). Cesarean birth mothers have a greater incidence (5% to 15%) of postpartum infection than do mothers who give birth vaginally (1% to 3% incidence) (Franzblau & Witt, 2006). If a cesarean birth mother experiences a prolonged labor prior to delivery, the incidence of postpartum infection increases to 30% to 35%.

🔵 Optimizing Outcomes— Educating patients about risk factors for puerperal infection

Shorter hospital stays after birth make the nurse's role in educating the new mother and her family about signs and symptoms of postpartum infection vitally important. The nurse should alert the patient about antepartum or intrapartum events that are risk factors for the development of a postpartum infection and make certain the family understands the importance of promptly notifying their care provider if any symptoms occur.

TYPES OF PUERPERAL INFECTIONS

Infections during the puerperium most commonly involve the endometrium (endometritis), operative wound (cesarean incision; episiotomy), urinary tract, and breasts (**mastitis**). Septic pelvic thrombophlebitis may also occur.

Endometritis

During the immediate postpartum period, the most common site of infection is the uterine endometrium (Fig. 16-4). This infection presents with a temperature elevation over 101°F (38.4°C), often within the first 24 to 48 hours after childbirth, followed by uterine tenderness and foul-smelling lochia. Since urinary tract infections can occur during any part of the pregnancy and puerperium, differentiating the various signs and symptoms is important. As noted in Tables 16-2 through 16-6, other infections are more likely to occur following discharge from the hospital. Therefore, follow-up in the home or clinic by a nurse or primary care provider may offer the first opportunity to identify infectious processes.

Mastitis

Mastitis is usually unilateral and develops after the flow of milk has been established. The most common causative organism is *Staphylococcus aureus*, introduced from the infant's mouth through a fissure in the nipple. The infection involves the ductal system, causing inflammatory edema, enlarged axillary lymph nodes, and breast engorgement with obstruction of milk flow (Fig. 16-5). Without treatment, mastitis may progress to a breast abscess. Symptoms include fever, malaise and localized breast tenderness. Management centers on antibiotic therapy (e.g., cephalosporins and vancomycin), application of heat or cold to the breasts, hydration, and analgesics. To maintain lactation, the woman may empty the breasts every 2 to 4 hours by breast feeding, manual expression, or breast pump. Since mastitis usually occurs after hospital discharge, an important component of nursing care includes teaching the breastfeeding mother about signs of mastitis and strategies to prevent cracked nipples.

NURSING ASSESSMENT

Assessment is central to the delivery of safe, effective postpartal nursing care. Ongoing, careful attention must be paid to the patient's mental status and to her vital signs, breasts, fundus, lochia, incisions, and urinary status. Temperature elevation may be the first indication of an infection. If an elevated temperature is combined with any of the following signs and symptoms, the nurse must notify the primary care provider immediately: tachycardia, uterine or fundal tenderness or pain, foul-smelling lochia, an absence or decrease in lochia, chills, decreased appetite, malaise, elevated white blood cell count (WBC), back pain (costovertebral angle tenderness [CVAT]), generalized aching, headache, dysuria, urinary frequency or retention, wound drainage, erythema, edema. Early, ongoing collaborative treatment can then be initiated.

🔵 Optimizing Outcomes— Tests to help identify a postpartum infection

To detect sources of puerperal infection, the nurse can anticipate that the following samples are likely to be obtained:

- Complete blood count (CBC) with differential
- Blood cultures if sepsis is suspected
- Urinalysis with culture and sensitivity
- Cervical, uterine, or wound culture as needed

COLLABORATIVE MANAGEMENT

All bacterial puerperal infections require treatment with antibiotics. The nurse can encourage rest and increased fluid intake and instruct the patient about the importance of increasing protein and vitamin C in her diet. In many hospitals, a nurse can refer a patient to a dietitian for instruction without a physician's order.

Comfort measures are as important in facilitating the patient's full recovery as the administration of antibiotics. Cool showers, sitz baths, warm compresses applied to the breasts, therapeutic touch and massage, soothing music, relaxation techniques, pain medications, and antipyretics are all strategies to promote patient well-being. Because of their anti-inflammatory effect, many physicians order a nonsteroidal anti-inflammatory medication (NSAID) to serve as an antipyretic and analgesic. Throughout the course of treatment, health care team members also need to provide education to the patient and her family regarding her diagnosis and prognosis, treatment plan, measures to promote good hygiene, and follow-up care.

Table 16-2 Postpartum Infection: Endometritis

Type of Infection	Risk Factors	Onset	Signs and Symptoms	Causative Organisms	Diagnosis Based on	Collaborative Treatment	Prognosis and Complications

Endometritis (inflammation and infection of the inner lining of the uterus)
 	
Incidence:
 	
vaginal birth 1–3% and cesarean birth 10–20% (Kennedy, 2005)
	Cesarean birth Prolonged rupture of the membranes, multiple vaginal examinations, internal electronic FHR monitoring, low socio-economic status, poor nutrition, young age, diabetes, prior genital infection, lapse in aseptic technique, anemia, smoking, nulliparity, operative vaginal delivery, poor postpartum perineal care	2–4 days following childbirth	Prolonged fever > 100.4°F (38°C), foul smelling lochia, uterine or abdominal tenderness, chills, poor appetite, malaise, increased pulse rate, cramping pain, increased white blood cell count (WBC) (above 20–30,000 mm³)	Normal vaginal flora and enteric bacteria	Clinical signs and symptoms
					
					Vaginal and bimanual examination
					
					Laboratory test results: culture of lochia; elevated white blood cell count (WBC)
					
					(Must also rule out urinary tract infection)
						1. MD/CNM: order antibiotics.
						2. Treat symptoms:
						  a. Rest
						  b. Antipyretics
						  c. Increase fluid intake
						  d. Encourage high protein, high vitamin C foods
						  e. Promote uterine drainage via ambulation and Fowler's position
						  f. Instruct in perineal care
						3. Explain treatments to patient/family.
						4. Home antibiotic therapy may need to be arranged with follow-up by a home care nurse.
						5. Promote infant attachment.
							90–95% improvement within 48–72 hours after treatment.
							
							May be discharged on oral antibiotics.
							
							Complication:
							
							Extension of infections via lymphatic system to connective tissues (pelvic infection)
							
							Dehiscence of cesarean section incision or episiotomy
							
							Peritonitis

Data from American Academy of Pediatrics & American College of Obstetricians and Gynecologists (2002); Cunningham et al. (2005); and Gibbs et al. (2004).

Figure 16-4 Postpartum endometritis.

Family Teaching Guidelines...
Prevention of Infection

- Wash your hands before and after going to the bathroom, when changing pads, changing the baby's diaper, etc. Hand washing with friction removes infection-causing microorganisms.

- Use a squeeze bottle with warm water to cleanse the perineum, pat the perineum dry, and remove and replace pads from front to back. Front to back patting and pad removal/application prevents bringing rectal organisms forward to the perineum and vagina.

- Drink extra fluids (eight 8-ounce glasses of water) to increase urine production. The increased blood flow and urine production will decrease the stagnation of microorganisms in the urinary tract.

- Wash incisions with soap and water. Be sure to dry the incision completely. If necessary, use a hair dryer set on low heat to be sure the incision is dry. A dry incision is less likely than a wet one to promote bacterial growth.

- If breastfeeding, feed the infant every 2–3 hours and alternate feeding positions. Be sure the baby gets as much of the nipple and areola in his mouth as possible. These actions reduce the likelihood of injury to the nipple.

- For a breast infection to occur, a cracked or blistered nipple is necessary. Use lanolin, vitamin E, cod liver oil, or express breast milk and rub any of these into the nipple to help reduce soreness and to protect the nipple from trauma.

- Echinacea is an herb that can boost the immune system. It has anti-inflammatory effects and stimulates the production of interleukin and interferon (both of which help the body fight infection, bacterial and viral) (Lincoln & Kleiner, 2004).

ESSENTIAL INFORMATION

- Notify your health care provider if you develop pain, redness, or swelling at the site of any incision.

- Notify your health care provider if you develop a fever of 100.4°F (38°C). (If you are breastfeeding, a temperature elevation to 100.4°F [38°C] may occur when your milk production begins) (Lincoln & Kleiner, 2004).

herbal medication: Echinacea Purpurea

Echinacea (Ek-i-neigh-sha)

Pregnancy Category: Injectable form not recommended during pregnancy

Indications: Treatment of wounds, injuries, enlarged lymph nodes; prevent and reduce symptoms and duration of common cold and bacterial infections of the upper respiratory tract; used by Native Americans to treat burns and insect and rattlesnake bites.

Actions: Boosts the immune system by increasing phagocytosis of the WBCs and by inhibiting the bacterial enzyme hyaluronidase; also stimulates the production of interleukin and interferon; exerts an anti-inflammatory action.

Therapeutic Effects: Used by proponents to both prevent and treat infections; juice from leaves used as a supportive treatment for vaginal yeast infections; approved in Germany for treatment of the common cold and influenza.

Contraindications and Precautions: Herb–drug interactions with amiodarone, anabolic steroids, ketoconazole, methotrexate (possible increased hepatic toxicity) Possible exacerbation of autoimmune diseases (rheumatoid arthritis, lupus, multiple sclerosis, etc.) because of its immune system stimulation properties (no clinical evidence to support).

Is a member of the Daisy family: possible crossover allergic reaction

Adverse Reactions and Effects: No toxicity noted with even extremely high doses of oral Echinacea; most common side effects from oral form—gastrointestinal symptoms and increased urination.
INJECTIONS SIDE EFFECTS: short-term nausea, vomiting, shivering, headache, fever

Route and Dosage: Tincture, oral, injection (dosage individualized)

Nursing Implications:
1. Be sure to ask every patient if she uses herbal remedies.
2. Instruct the patient that daily dosages of Echinacea in an attempt to prevent infections may decrease the immunostimulating effects of this herb.
3. Since the U.S. Food and Drug Administration (FDA) has not approved herbal treatments/remedies, encourage the patient to be sure that she uses a reputable form of the herb to ensure its quality.

Data from Adams et al. (2005); Deglin & Vallerand (2009); and Lincoln & Kleiner (2004).

Although the infection may be easily treated and short lived, any postpartum complication can psychosocially affect a patient and her family. Prolonged treatment or hospitalization may create financial hardships, negatively impact family relationships and attachment with the infant, or result in psycho-emotional or spiritual crises. Referrals to the social worker, hospital chaplain or pastor, financial counselor, lactation consultant, community health nurse, or counselor need to be considered as an essential component of holistic care. As the health care team member who is most consistently present, the nurse has a responsibility to help the patient and her family identify when such referrals would be beneficial and to serve as an advocate to ensure that the patient receives these services.

Text continued on page 527

Table 16-3 Postpartum Infection: Wound Infections

Type of Infection	Risk Factors	Onset	Signs and Symptoms for ALL	Causative Organisms	Diagnosis Based on	Collaborative Treatment	Prognosis and Complications
Wound infections Perineal Incidence: 0.35%–10% Cesarean incision Incidence: 3%–5%	Endometritis (infected lochia), poor hygiene, fecal contamination, hematoma ALL wound infections: obesity, diabetes, hypertension, immunosuppression, malnutrition, anemia, hemorrhage, prolonged labor, chorioamnionitis prolonged rupture of membranes, hematoma	Early: 48 hours Late: 6–8 days	Pain, foul smelling discharge, edema, low grade fever Sudden chills, high fever, abdominal tenderness, erythema, edema, warmth of incision, drainage from the incision	Polymicrobial, normal vaginal flora *Staphylococcus aureus,* aerobic streptococci, aerobic and anaerobic bacilli	Clinical signs and symptoms, subjective complaints Clinical signs and symptoms, along with a poor response to antibiotics given for endometritis Laboratory test results: elevated white blood cell count (WBC)	1. Antibiotics per order. 2. May require incision and drainage with placement of drain to facilitate healing by secondary intention.* If packing has been placed in the wound to keep it open and maintain drainage, alert the patient to exercise caution when changing her perineal pads to avoid dislodging the packing. 3. Perineal: sitz baths; instruct in perineal care. 4. Cesarean: wet to dry dressing changes 3+ times/day. 5. Pain medication per order (usually nonsteroidal anti-inflammatory drugs [NSAIDs]). 6. Instructions to patient and family about wound care. 7. Possible referral for home health or community health nurse visits.	Improvement usually within 24–48 hours; may require long term antibiotic therapy Complication: necrotizing fasciitis, abscess, wound dehiscence

*Secondary intention: healing from the inside of the wound out to the skin.
Data from Cunningham et al. (2005); Franzblau & Witt (2006); Gibbs et al. (2004); and Kennedy (2007).

Table 16-4 Postpartum Infection: Urinary Tract Infections (UTI)

Type of Infection	Risk Factors	Onset	Signs and Symptoms	Causative Organisms	Diagnosis Based on	Collaborative Treatment	Prognosis and Complications

Urinary tract infections
 	
Incidence: 2%–4%
	Catheterization, multiple vaginal exams, poor postpartum hygiene, genital tract trauma, epidural anesthesia, cesarean birth, premature rupture of the membranes, poor nutritional status, history of UTIs during pregnancy, diabetes, decreased bladder sensation following birth	Any time during pregnancy or after birth	May have none
			
			Dysuria (painful urination), frequency, burning on urination, difficulty voiding and/or retention, costovertebral angle tenderness (CVAT), back or suprapubic pain, hematuria (blood in the urine); fever, fatigue, nausea, vomiting
				Most common:
				
				Escherichia coli (60–90% of all UTIs); *Proteus mirabilis, Klebsiella pneumoniae,* group B hemolytic streptococcus, *Staphylococcus saprophyticus*
					Clinical signs and symptoms
					
					Laboratory test results: urine C&S, presence of leukocytes and blood on urine dipstick
						1. Antibiotics per order (usually sulfonamides, aminopenicillins, anti-infectives, nitrofurantoin, or cephalosporins × 3–10 days depending on symptoms). Teach importance of taking all medication.
						2. Encourage increased fluid intake, including cranberry juice.
						3. Encourage rest.
						4. Instruct in perineal care.
						5. Instruct in monitoring temperature, bladder function, normal appearance of urine.
						6. Instruct in/administer antipyretics, antispasmodics, analgesics, and antiemetics.
						7. Educate patient to avoid recurrence:
						  a. When intercourse resumes, void following.
						  b. Clean from front to back.
							Improvement within 48–72 hours following initiation of antibiotic therapy
							
							Can reoccur with bacteremia and scarring of the kidney followed by hypertension and kidney damage

Data from Cunningham et al. (2005); Franzblau & Witt (2006); and Kennedy (2007).

Table 16-5 Postpartum Infection: Mastitis

Type of Infection	Risk Factors	Onset	Signs and Symptoms	Causative Organisms	Diagnosis Based on	Collaborative Treatment	Prognosis and Complications
Mastitis	Milk stasis, plugged milk duct, infrequent breastfeeding, fatigue, nipple trauma, primiparity	3–4 weeks postpartum	Warm, tender, hardened area on breast (usually only one), enlarged axillary lymph nodes, fever (up to 102°F [38.9°C]), chills, generalized aching, headache, malaise	Most common: *Staphylococcus aureus;* also: *Haemophilus parainfluenzae* (from infant's mouth and nose), *Candida albicans, Streptococcus viridans*	Clinical signs and symptoms Laboratory test results: culture of breast milk	1. Notify MD/CNM. 2. Initiate antibiotics. 3. Continue breastfeeding or manual/electrical expression of milk to maintain lactation. May be instructed to discard the milk. 4. Promote rest. 5. Increase fluid intake. 6. Pump breast after infant feeding to ensure breast is empty. 7. Warm compress or ice to breast for comfort. 8. Antipyretics. 9. Instruct in high protein, high vitamin C diet. 10. Educate regarding hygiene and prevention of future recurrence. 11. Assess the infant's mouth for signs of thrush (oral *Candida*), an overgrowth of fungal organisms related to the mother's antibiotic therapy.	Improvement within 24–48 hours following initiation of antibiotics Complication: breast abscess If breast abscess occurs: must discontinue breastfeeding on the affected side—may lead to decreased maternal-infant attachment, low self-esteem and feelings of disappointment and guilt

Data from Lawrence, R., & Lawrence, R. (2005). *Breastfeeding: A guide for the medical profession* (6th ed.). Philadelphia: C.V. Mosby.

Table 16-6 Postpartum Infection: Septic Pelvic Thrombophlebitis

Type of Infection	Risk Factors	Onset	Signs and Symptoms	Causative Organisms	Diagnosis Based on	Collaborative Treatment	Prognosis and Complications
Septic pelvic thrombophlebitis	Cesarean birth, genital tract lacerations, history of varicosities, immobility, operative vaginal delivery, prolonged labor, multiple vaginal exams	48 hours to 4–6 weeks postpartum	Fever > 102.2°F (39°C) with spikes after initiation of antibiotic therapy, abdominal and/or back pain, chills, increased pulse (resting tachycardia), few or absent bowel sounds	Normal vaginal flora and enteric bacteria—is usually an extension of endometritis	Clinical signs and symptoms Pelvic CT or MRI to confirm the clinical picture; Laboratory test results: CBC; coagulation profile; blood chemistries	1. MD/CNM: prescribe antibiotics. 2. Add heparin therapy to increase APTT (activated partial thromboplastin time) to 1.5–2 times the normal value. 3. Rest in Fowler's position. 4. High-protein, high-vitamin C diet. 5. Increased fluids. 6. Comfort measures: pain medications, antipyretics. 7. Complementary therapies: heat, cold, relaxation, music, touch, etc. 8. Explain treatments. 9. Promote infant attachment.	Improvement usually within 48–72 hours of heparin initiation; may need to continue anticoagulant therapy for 6 months (7–10 days of heparin followed by warfarin [Coumadin]) Complication: Pulmonary embolism Possible decreased infant attachment; prolonged hospitalization

Data from Cunningham et al. (2005) and Gibbs et al. (2004).

Figure 16-5 Mastitis usually occurs several weeks after childbirth. The axillary lymph nodes are enlarged and there is a warm, tender, hardened area on the affected breast.

 Across Care Settings: Care collaboration to prevent postpartum infection after discharge

If the postpartum patient is at risk for the development of a postpartum infection, the nurse needs to communicate this information to health care providers and family members who may be involved in helping her after she goes home. Some hospitals routinely follow new mothers into the home with a postpartum and newborn visit by a registered nurse. The lactation consultant or breastfeeding support group, newborn's physician, or public health nurse should also be notified of events during labor, birth, or postpartum that they should address the first time they see the new mother following discharge.

 Now Can You— Discuss infections that occur during the puerperium?

1. List six risk factors for the development of a postpartum infection?
2. Describe nursing assessment findings that should be reported to the physician or nurse midwife that indicate the patient has an infection?
3. Discuss ways the nurse can promote healthy family dynamics for the woman hospitalized with a postpartum infection?

Thrombophlebitis and Thrombosis

DEFINITION, INCIDENCE, AND RISK FACTORS

Thrombophlebitis and **thrombosis** are terms that describe an inflammation of the venous circulation and blood clot formation that typically occur in the lower extremities. The depth of the inflammation and the location of the involved veins determine the severity of this complication. Veins located above the fascia, such as the saphenous vein system, are superficial, and distend easily, while veins below the fascia, such as the popliteal system, are deep and less elastic.

The incidence of postpartal thrombophlebitis and deep vein thrombosis (DVT) is low and varies from approximately 0.5 to 3 per 1000 women. The decline in incidence over the past two decades is largely attributable to early postpartum ambulation, which has become the standard of care. Venous stasis and hypercoagulation, normal changes during pregnancy, are the major causes of thromboembolic disease. After the third month of pregnancy, fibrinogen levels increase, and in the second half of pregnancy, clotting factors VII, VIII, IX, and X increase in preparation for minimizing normal blood loss during birth. A decreased breakdown of fibrin, which forms the protein mesh of a clot, also occurs (Cunningham et al., 2005).

Lower extremity venous stasis results from the weight of the gravid uterus on the maternal inferior vena cava and pelvic veins. If the woman smokes, is obese, older (greater than 35 years), immobile, or a grand multigravida, the risk of DVT also increases. Chronic health problems such as inflammatory bowel disease, lupus erythematosus, antiphospholipid syndrome, varicose veins, and pregnancy-related conditions such as preeclampsia, an operative vaginal delivery, cesarean birth, hemorrhage, and sepsis are all possible precursors to the development of DVT . A woman with a positive history of DVT is also at greater risk than one with no DVT history (Colman-Brochu, 2005; Cunningham et al., 2005).

 Ethnocultural Considerations— Ethnicity and factor V Leiden mutation

Ethnicity influences coagulation patterns. Approximately 5% to 7% of North American Caucasians, 2% of Hispanics, and 1% of African Americans have a deficiency of coagulation inhibitors, termed the factor V Leiden mutation. Individuals need factor V to convert prothrombin to thrombin. Protein C inhibits the conversion of prothrombin to thrombin. Normally, protein C levels remain constant during pregnancy. When a factor V Leiden mutation occurs, protein C is lower than normal, and the body converts prothrombin to thrombin more readily. Women with factor V Leiden mutation have an increased risk for the development of a DVT during the puerperium (Cunningham et al., 2005; Foster, 2007).

PATHOPHYSIOLOGY

DVT develops from several key factors: a hypercoagulable state, venous stasis, and vein injury. A hypercoagulable state and venous stasis routinely exist in a normal pregnancy. Vessel injury can occur from trauma to an extremity, from birth events such as operative vaginal deliveries or cesarean births, and from simple invasive procedures such as an intravenous catheter insertion or venous blood sampling. Once vessel injury occurs, platelets begin to clump, then stick to one another. Thrombus formation follows.

SIGNS AND SYMPTOMS

Superficial venous thrombosis involves the superficial saphenous venous system. The most common form of postpartum thrombophlebitis, superficial venous thrombosis is characterized by pain and tenderness in the lower extremity. Deep vein thrombosis is more common during pregnancy and may extend from the foot to the iliofemoral region. It is associated with unilateral leg pain, calf tenderness, and swelling. However, up to 50% of all individuals with a DVT are asymptomatic. Signs and symptoms depend on the size, location, degree of vessel occlusion, and development of collateral circulation around the clot. The classic presentation of DVT involves pain, tenderness, edema, redness, and localized heat. The presence of a palpable cord, changes in skin color ("milk" or "blue leg"), a decreased peripheral pulse, and a circumference that is 2 cm larger (or more) in the affected extremity assists in the DVT diagnosis. Dorsiflexing the woman's foot while her knee is extended may elicit a positive Homans' sign (pain in the foot or leg) in the presence of thrombophlebitis and thrombosis (Colman-Brochu, 2005; Cunningham et al., 2005) (Fig. 16-6).

 Nursing Insight— Recognizing signs and symptoms indicative of DVT

Additional signs and symptoms that may be associated with DVT include elevated temperature, cough, tachycardia, hemoptysis, pleuritic chest pain, and increasing apprehension. The presence of dyspnea and tachypnea may signal pulmonary embolism. Pulmonary embolism is a complication of DVT that occurs when part of a blood clot breaks away and travels to the pulmonary artery, where it occludes the vessel and obstructs blood flow to the lungs.

DIAGNOSTIC TESTS

Because pregnancy is frequently accompanied by various aches and lower extremity edema, the clinical presentation of thrombophlebitis and DVT may be difficult to identify. The venogram, an invasive test used to confirm deep vein thrombosis, is contraindicated in pregnancy. No specific laboratory tests can confirm or exclude deep or superficial venous thrombosis. Venous duplex ultrasonography (real-time imaging and Doppler flow studies) is the appropriate test to confirm the diagnosis of DVT.

Figure 16-6 Deep vein thrombophlebitis.

If the result of this test is equivocal, **magnetic resonance imaging** (MRI) (a diagnostic test that uses electromagnetic energy to provide images of the heart, large blood vessels, brain, and soft tissues) may be ordered to determine the extent of any pelvic vein involvement (Colman-Brochu, 2005; Cunningham et al., 2005).

COLLABORATIVE MANAGEMENT

Routine interventions for either superficial or DVT include the administration of analgesics; rest with elevation of the affected extremity; elastic support to the affected leg; increased fluid intake; and the local application of moist, warm packs. The nurse should ensure that the weight of the warmed pack does not rest on the leg, causing obstruction of blood flow. Analgesics are prescribed for pain.

 clinical alert

Avoiding extremity massage when DVT is suspected

If DVT is present or suspected, it is essential to refrain from massaging the affected area. This action could loosen the clot and result in a pulmonary or cerebral embolism.

Possible nursing diagnoses for the patient with DVT are presented in Box 16-6. The patient usually is given bathroom privileges for elimination needs. If the thrombosis is located in a deep vein, hospitalization for either intravenous or subcutaneous heparin therapy is generally required. The patient is usually placed on complete bedrest until the anticoagulation therapy is effective. The goal in heparin dosing is to increase the prothrombin time (PT) to 1.5 to two times higher than the control. The pregnant patient has a greater plasma volume and an increased renal clearance (due to increased blood flow to the kidneys). The combination of normally occurring heparin-binding proteins along with the breakdown of heparin often results in the need for higher doses of heparin during pregnancy. The primary purpose of heparin therapy is to prevent extension of the current clot and to prevent new clot formation (Colman-Brochu, 2005).

During hospitalization, the nurse needs to monitor the patient for any signs of unusual bleeding and make certain that the antidote for heparin (protamine sulfate) is readily available. Vital signs should be measured at least every 4 to 6 hours, analgesics administered as needed, and circulation to the affected extremity checked during every nursing shift. The circumference of the affected extremity

---

Box 16-6 Possible Nursing Diagnoses for Thrombophlebitis and Thrombosis

- Pain
- At risk for injury
- Altered peripheral tissue perfusion
- Altered family processes
- Self-care deficit
- Fear
- Altered individual/family coping

should be measured and recorded daily. As the therapy continues, the nurse should assist the patient in increasing her level of activity and in assuming self-care activities. Equally as important, the nurse must assess the patient and her family for signs and symptoms of depression, anger, or decreased attachment to the newborn. Many insurance companies require that the infant be discharged, even if her mother needs to stay in the hospital. Some families may choose to care for the infant at home during the first few postpartum days while the mother is acutely ill. This decision may negatively impact the new mother's ability to feed, care for, and bond with her infant and may also create family conflicts that require the assistance of a spiritual advisor, financial counselor, social worker, home health nurse, lactation consultant, or family therapist. All members of the health care team need to encourage family involvement in the patient's care. If a family member can bring the infant to the hospital daily, the patient can be assisted in holding and caring for her infant and maternal attachment can be promoted.

Warfarin (Coumadin), an oral anticoagulant, is introduced before the patient's discharge, and during this time, the heparin therapy is tapered. Since warfarin is excreted in breast milk, the breastfeeding mother is maintained on subcutaneous heparin, and the warfarin is omitted. Either medication (heparin or warfarin) is continued for a minimum of 3 months after birth. Use of this long-term therapy regimen mandates specific patient–family education and support from a variety of health care providers. An important component of the discharge teaching conducted by the nurse, dietician, or pharmacist includes a discussion about medications, side effects, and potential interactions.

Optimizing Outcomes— Teaching patients about aspirin and anticoagulants

During discharge teaching, the nurse cautions the patient on anticoagulant therapy to avoid medications that contain aspirin (salicylic acid). Aspirin, which acts as an antiplatelet agent and prevents blood clotting, can lead to prolonged clotting time and an increased risk of bleeding.

Collaboration in Caring— *Education about food–drug interactions*

The nurse, pharmacist, or dietitian can initiate patient and family education about food and drug interactions. Nurses do not always feel comfortable providing education on dietary topics, and the dietitian has the knowledge to discuss this information with the patient and her family. Likewise, the pharmacist has greater knowledge than the nurse about drug effects and side effects. A team approach works well with topics such as this one. Be sure to obtain an interpreter if needed, and have written information available that the patient and her family can take home.

The nurse should emphasize the importance of follow-up care for laboratory tests and medication dosage adjustments. Avoiding trauma that may result in extensive bruising, using safe care practices to avoid bleeding, and instructing the patient and her family to be alert for signs that indicate the

---

medication: Warfarin

Warfarin (**war**-fa-rin)

Coumadin

Pregnancy Category: X

Indications: Prevention of thrombosis (clot) formation

Actions: Inhibits the hepatic synthesis of coagulation factors II, VII, IX, and X; inhibits the action of vitamin K

Therapeutic Effects: Used in patients who are at high risk for development of or who have a history of deep vein thrombosis or other thrombophilia (love of clot formation) conditions

Pharmacokinetics: 99% binds to plasma proteins, thereby delaying the effects of warfarin.

Route and Dosage: Orally; dosage adjusted on the basis of international normalized ratio (INR) results (range is 2.5 to 10 mg daily)

Contraindications and Precautions: Drug–drug interactions occur with NSAIDs, diuretics, antidepressants, steroids, some antibiotics, vaccines, and vitamin K. Concurrent use with NSAIDs may increase the risk of bleeding.

Herbal supplements such as garlic, ginger, and feverfew may increase the risk of bleeding. Arnica may increase the anticoagulant effect of warfarin.

Even after the drug is discontinued, its effects may continue for up to 10 days. Warfarin dosage must be individualized on the basis of prothrombin time results. The INR is now used for dosage adjustments. A normal INR is 2.0–3.5.

Adverse Reactions and Effects: Overdosage leads to excessive blood loss that may appear via gastrointestinal bleeding, bleeding from the gums, nosebleeds, petechiae, excessive bruising, etc. The patient begins with heparin therapy for anticoagulation and transitions to warfarin. Because normal clotting factors circulate in the patient's blood stream routinely, several days of both heparin and warfarin therapy may be required for the anticoagulant effect

Nursing Implications:
1. This drug is dangerous. The patient and family must receive detailed information regarding follow-up care and drug–drug, drug–herb, and food–drug interactions.
2. Instruct the patient to notify the doctor of excessive bruising, take warfarin at the same time each day, and to avoid activities that could result in a bleeding injury.
3. Be sure the patient receives instructions on foods to minimize/avoid. (Involve the dietitian).

Data from Deglin, J.H., & Vallerand, A.H. (2009). *Davis's drug guide for nurses* (11th ed.). Philadelphia: F.A. Davis.

---

anticoagulation therapy is excessive are also important topics for instruction. Short-term referral to a home health nurse should be considered; the hospital nurse may need to mention the need for this referral to the physician.

Be sure to— Document family education

The importance of clear, concise, complete chronological documentation of all patient/family education cannot be overly emphasized. The current litigious society in the United States lends itself to lawsuits against all health care providers. The nurse has primary responsibility for both routine/standard patient/family education as well as specialized education. If another health care provider, such as a dietitian, social worker, or pharmacist is involved in any aspect of patient/family education, the nurse should note this collaboration in the medical record as soon as possible.

PULMONARY EMBOLUS

The abrupt onset of chest pain, dyspnea, shock, diaphoresis, syncope, and anxiety in a patient with DVT signals a major complication, pulmonary embolus (PE). PE is a life-threatening emergency that results from the breakup of the clot with migration of pieces through the heart to the lungs. Emergency treatment for this potentially fatal complication involves the "ABC" response used for any cardiorespiratory event. The nurse should immediately call for assistance, administer oxygen, obtain the crash cart, and begin CPR if necessary. Both the physician and respiratory therapist are important responders. Assuming that chest compressions are not needed, the nurse should elevate the head of the bed and apply an automatic blood pressure machine, cardiorespiratory monitor, and pulse oximeter. If not already in place, a large-bore intravenous line must be started immediately, so that fluids, heparin, and pain medication (usually morphine) can be readily administered. Once stabilized, patients with a PE are routinely transferred to a critical care unit for further care.

If the PE occurs while the patient is still recovering from childbirth, ensuring care for the newborn and support for the patient's family are paramount. Until the patient's condition improves, limitations are placed on visitors. This arrangement usually means that the family can remain with the infant. In this situation, the postpartum nurse can debrief and provide explanations to the family about events and possible future care requirements. If the patient survives, both she and her family will need detailed instructions concerning the prevention of thrombus reoccurrence. They also need to understand that the patient is at a much greater risk for the subsequent development of a DVT, even in the absence of another pregnancy.

 Now Can You— Discuss deep vein thrombosis?

1. Describe why the postpartum patient is at risk for development of a deep vein thrombosis (DVT)?
2. Discuss routine nursing care for the postpartum patient hospitalized with a DVT? (Remember to include the baby and family in this answer.)
3. Develop a postpartum teaching plan for the postpartum patient who is discharged on warfarin (Coumadin)?

Postpartum Psychosocial Complications

The focus on physiological recovery and health in the childbearing woman and her infant can easily result in an inaccurate assumption that all is well with the new family. Beyond the physical needs of the new mother lies a gamut of emotional, spiritual, relational, and socioeconomic concerns to which the nurse must be sensitive. Because most people consider childbearing a joyful time in life, the new mother who experiences negative emotions or who cannot cope with new demands on her time, energy, or priorities may struggle to recognize her need for help. Moreover, even if she recognizes her limitations and knows she needs help, the new mother may be reluctant to ask for help. Whether working in the hospital, in home care, in a clinic, or in a physician's office, the nurse can be a lifeline for the woman who experiences postpartum psychosocial complications.

These complications include postpartum blues, depression, psychosis, panic disorder, and the long-term sequelae from abusive relationships, homelessness, and access to care.

POSTPARTUM BLUES

Postpartum blues are common. Fifty to eighty percent of all postpartum women experience some degree of postpartum blues within the first 2 weeks after childbirth. Blues are usually self-limiting, last several days, and often peak by the end of the first week. Signs and symptoms include tearfulness, mood swings, anxiety, fatigue, sadness, insomnia, forgetfulness, and confusion (American Academy of Pediatrics [AAP] & American College of Obstetricians and Gynecologists [ACOG], 2007; Franzblau & Witt, 2006). Often, extra rest, reassurance, and therapeutic listening encourage the new mother to see beyond the immediate crisis and realize that better days lie ahead. (See Chapter 15 for further discussion.)

POSTPARTUM DEPRESSION

Incidence, Definition, and Risk Factors

Fortunately, most postpartum women recover from the blues and are able to enjoy their newborns and families. However, 8% to 15% of postpartal women progress to postpartum depression (PPD). According to the American Psychiatric Association (APA, 2000), a diagnosis of depression requires that one of two symptoms exist most or all of the day: a depressed mood or decreased interest/pleasure in previously enjoyable activities. Recognized risk factors for PPD include an undesired/unplanned pregnancy, a history of depression, recent major life changes such as the death of a family member or moving to a new community, lack of family or social support, financial stress, marital discord, adolescent age, and homelessness (APA, 2000; Cunningham et al., 2005; Nonacs, 2005).

 Collaboration in Caring— *Resources for the postpartal patient*

A woman who presents to the hospital with no prenatal care, gives birth, and prepares to go home should be closely screened for and warned about PPD. Often these women do not have the financial resources for perinatal care. They could also be homeless or lack social support. The nurse should ensure that the social worker is involved in the screening process. To facilitate ongoing care and follow-up for the new mother and her infant, appropriate community resources should be contacted and arrangements made before discharge.

Signs and Symptoms and Diagnosis

Symptoms of PPD resemble those of other depressions (Box 16-7). The difference between PPD and other types is that the depression affects not only the woman and her adult family members, but also her newborn. The woman may have a decreased interest in the baby or may be overly concerned that "something bad" is going to happen to the baby. These fears may be expressed in a panic attack with hyperactivity and an inability to make decisions or prioritize. Male partners of women suffering from PPD

Box 16-7 **Signs and Symptoms of Postpartum Depression**

Decreased appetite	Excessive fears about the infant's health/safety
Insomnia or fragmented sleep	Hopelessness
Fatigue	Negativity
Inability to concentrate Confusion	Complaints about "loss of self" and a "sense of loneliness" (Clemmens et al., 2004)
Withdrawal	Guilt
Decreased self-esteem	Decreased interest and functioning in both self and infant care
Suicidal thoughts	
Infant neglect or abuse	

---

report feelings of being overwhelmed, isolated, stigmatized, and extremely frustrated. The combined negative effects of maternal and paternal depression on infant development places the child at risk (Beck, Records, & Rice, 2006; Davey, Dziurawiec, & O'Brien-Malone, 2006).

The greatest barrier in diagnosing PPD lies in differentiating it from other types of major depression. Since the presenting symptoms are similar to those of other types of depression, and the onset of the symptoms varies within the first year after childbirth, PPD is often under-diagnosed. The reasons for this are varied. Many women believe that labile feelings are a normal part of adjusting to parenthood. They fear the stigma associated with a diagnosis of depression, as well as the possible negative consequences, such as the involvement of local Child Protective Services. In addition, the emphasis on physiological recovery frequently results in an unwillingness on the part of health care providers and the woman's support systems to explore psychosocial concerns (Clemmens, Driscoll, & Beck, 2004; Logsdon, Birkimer, Simpson, & Looney, 2005; Stoops & Mann, 2004).

Etiology

PPD is a multifactorial problem. While there may be a genetic propensity toward depression, environmental factors such as financial stress and poor living conditions or psychological factors such as difficult adaptation to parenthood may push the woman toward previously unexperienced depression. Physiological factors involving changes in endorphins and the production and processing of neurotransmitters are also implicated in the onset of depression.

Assessment

Screening for the presence of PPD risk factors should begin with the first prenatal visit. The office or clinic nurse may be the first health care provider to obtain basic information, such as educational level, living conditions, financial stressors, whether the pregnancy was planned or unplanned, support systems available for the pregnant woman, and family involvement and attitudes of its members toward the pregnancy. If the nurse, physician, social worker, or other health care team member identifies risk factors, these should be noted in detail on the prenatal record. If prenatal support groups are available, the woman should be referred to one of them in an attempt to minimize the risk for PPD.

The postpartum nurse needs to be aware of previously identified risk factors. A personal history of a mood disorder or a family history of a mood disorder, mood or anxiety symptoms during the prenatal period, and postpartum blues are factors that increase the risk for PPD. Moreover, as the nurse carefully assesses the new mother and her interaction with the baby, other risk factors may be noted. Some of these may include unmet pregnancy or labor and birth expectations resulting in feelings of failure, a delay in a prolonged sleep and rest period, and a demanding newborn without the presence of family members to help. A new mother's continued dependency on caregivers despite adequate sleep and apparent control of postpartum discomforts may constitute another signal that requires close observation. If the new mother does not respond to her infant's needs or demonstrate bonding or attachment behaviors, these actions require follow-up. The hospital nurse's primary responsibility is to detect comments or behaviors that need to be referred to the social worker, home health nurse, physician, chaplain, lactation consultant, and community agencies (Goodman, 2004, Jesse & Graham, 2005; Linter & Gray, 2006).

If a home health nurse does not visit the newborn and mother within the first week, the well baby checkup that follows 1 to 2 weeks after the hospital discharge may offer the first opportunity to assess the mother-baby dyad. In this setting, the nurse needs to be alert for subtle cues from the new mother, such as making negative comments about the baby or herself, ignoring the baby's or other children's needs, as well as the mother's physical appearance. Does she look unkempt or exhausted? Is the baby clean and dry? Does the new mother say something about needing more help at home? Did she come to the office or clinic with the baby (and other children) or by herself?

❝What to say❞ — *Exploring the new mother's feelings*

In a private area, the nurse should take time to explore the new mother's feelings. A non-threatening way to open the dialogue might be to say: "Tell me how the first few days at home have gone." This statement provides the new mother with an opportunity to share both positive and negative impressions. Do not "fill the silence" if the new mother does not respond immediately. She may need to process her thoughts before speaking. Be aware, too, of nonverbal cues and body language, such as affect, eye contact, and open or closed posture.

If the nurse believes that the new mother is demonstrating signs and symptoms of PPD, several depression screening tools are available. These include the Edinburgh Postnatal Depression Scale, Postpartum Depression Predictors Inventory, Center for Epidemiological Studies—Depression, and Beck Depression Inventory II. Because they are highly predictive, these scales are valuable tools that can be combined with the informal interview during a routine postbirth checkup (Beck et al., 2006; Franzblau & Witt, 2006; Goodman, 2004; Nonacs, 2004). Nursing diagnoses for PPD may incorporate psychological, circumstantial, and physiological factors (Box 16-8).

Box 16-8 Possible Nursing Diagnoses for Postpartum Depression

Ineffective coping	Situational low self-esteem
Compromised family coping	Compromised family coping
Anxiety	Injury to the newborn
Impaired parent/infant attachment	
Impaired parenting	
Hopelessness	
Impaired sleep pattern	

---

where research and practice meet:
Screening Tools for PPD

Jesse and Graham (2005) tested a two-item depression screen to determine if it would correlate well with the 21-item Beck Depression Inventory (BDI). The two questions they asked were: "Are you often sad and depressed?" and "Have you had a loss of interest in pleasurable activities?" (These are the two symptoms required for a diagnosis of depression, according to the American Psychological Association.) Their findings indicated that this short questionnaire predicted those at low risk for PPD 94% of the time and at high risk for PPD 42% of the time. These statistics are similar to the predictive value of the longer BDI.

Collaborative Management

An important first step in the collaborative management of PPD involves ruling out a physical cause such as hypothyroidism. Once a physical cause has been eliminated, both traditional and complementary therapies can begin. Most often both the woman and her family will begin psychotherapy (interpersonal and group) as soon as possible. If the depressive symptoms are moderate to severe and do not respond to nonpharmacological treatment, the physician often prescribes a selective serotonin reuptake inhibitor (SSRI) or serotonin-norepinephrine reuptake inhibitor (SNRI) antidepressant. If the woman is experiencing sleep disturbances, tricyclic antidepressants may be useful (Cunningham et al., 2005; Franzblau & Witt, 2006; Nonacs, 2005) (Box 16-9).

Each of the medication groups is associated with side effects, and all antidepressants pass into the breast milk. If the woman is breastfeeding, the physician and nurse must monitor both the desired effects on the mother and any possible undesired effects on the baby. Medication dosage adjustments may be necessary, and the pharmacological treatment needs to continue for at least 6 months, even if rapid improvement occurs. If the woman does not respond to medications or psychotherapy, electroconvulsive therapy (ECT) may be used for the most severe cases of PPD (Cunningham et al., 2005; Nonacs, 2005).

Not to be discounted are complementary therapies for PPD. These therapies enhance the effects of traditional treatments, but Synder and Lindquist (2001) assert that "merely adding additional therapies to a system of care without implementing a holistic, caring approach to the care of patients will do little to improve

---

Box 16-9 Medications Used to Treat Postpartum Depression

SSRIs	**SNRIs**	**TRICYCLICs**
Fluoxetine (Prozac)	Venlafaxine (Effexor)	Pamelor (Nortriptyline)
Paroxetine (Paxil)	Duloxetine (Cymbalta)	Imipramine (Tofranil)
Sertraline (Zoloft)		Doxepin (Sinequan)

---

health" (p. 1). Since many complementary therapies can be used without a physician's prescription, they can also empower the woman and her family in self-care and help them to feel that they are actively involved in the treatment plan.

 Complementary Care: *Therapies for postpartum depression*

The nurse may be asked about various complementary therapies that may help new mothers and their families deal with PPD. Hypnosis enhances relaxation and an ability to focus on daily tasks. Exercise has been shown to increase levels of neurotransmitters that communicate with brain cells to increase feelings of euphoria. St. John's wort (*Hypericum perforatum*) is an herb that has been approved in Germany for the treatment of anxiety and depression, skin inflammation, blunt injuries, wounds, and burns. It is believed to bind with neuroreceptors in the brain to prevent a response to the "depression" neurotransmitters (Lincoln & Kleiner, 2004). *St. John's wort cannot be used in combination with SSRI antidepressants.* Biofeedback promotes relaxation and decreases anxiety, meditation helps the woman to focus on "being rather than doing," thereby relieving stress and tension and humor has been shown to decrease anxiety, fear, tension, anger, and frustration and stimulate the immune system. Acupuncture, aromatherapy, and massage are other complementary therapies that may be beneficial.

Prognosis

The earlier that PPD is recognized and treatment begun, the better the prognosis for a full recovery. However, the woman must be prepared for a relapse should she choose to have another baby. A previous history of any type of depression places a woman at a 25% risk of PPD; those who experienced PPD with a previous birth have a 50% to 90% recurrence rate (Nonacs, 2005; Stoops & Mann, 2004). Preconception counseling with a physician, nurse, social worker, or spiritual advisor and the initiation of antidepressants early in the pregnancy (after the first trimester) are preventative strategies.

POSTPARTUM PSYCHOSIS

Definition, Incidence, and Onset

Postpartum psychosis is a rare but severe form of mental illness that seriously affects not only the new mother but also the entire family. The incidence is low, occurring in one to four women per 1000 births. Though rare, postpartum women have a 10 to 15 times greater risk of psychosis

Nursing Care Plan The Woman Experiencing Postpartum Depression

Nursing Diagnosis: Ineffective Individual Coping related to multiple factors, including hormonal changes, addition of a newborn to the family, and time management constraints

Measurable Short-term Goal: The patient will acknowledge that she is depressed and agree to participate in individual and family therapy.

Measurable Long-term Goal: The patient will participate in activities she previously enjoyed and her affect will demonstrate positive feelings.

NOC Outcome:
Coping (1302) Personal actions to manage stressors that tax an individual's resources

NIC Interventions:
Coping Enhancement (5230)
Counseling (5240)
Medication Management (2380)

Nursing Interventions:

1. Approach the patient in a calm, nonthreatening, and concerned manner.

   RATIONALE: This approach may encourage the patient to be open about her thoughts and feelings.

2. Ask open-ended questions and wait for a response.

   RATIONALE: Open-ended questions require more than a one-word answer, which may encourage verbalization. Waiting for an answer indicates that what she says is worth the silence.

3. Affirm the woman's feelings and allow her to cry should she desire.

   RATIONALE: These responses demonstrate genuine concern.

4. Notify the patient's primary caregiver about the patient's depressed affect.

   RATIONALE: PPD may require medication or therapy.

5. Provide information about PPD and gently correct any misinformation or misconceptions the patient has about depression.

   RATIONALE: Correct information may instill hope and encourage the woman to continue therapy.

6. Provide instructions about medications (antidepressants) that may be ordered.

   RATIONALE: The patient needs to know the effects and side effects of medications so that she can report unusual symptoms.

7. Ask the patient what activities she no longer enjoys that were previously enjoyable.

   RATIONALE: This baseline information allows you and the patient to establish some goals for therapy.

8. Involve the family in helping the patient cope with her feelings and assisting with infant care.

   RATIONALE: Involvement of the patient's support system is vitally important. She needs to know that she is not alone in her struggle with depression.

9. Help the patient/family establish an activity goal that she can achieve within the next week.

   RATIONALE: This intervention involves the patient in her care, allows her some control, and encourages her to focus on a positive action/behavior.

---

than they do at any other time in their lives. Its onset may be dramatic, often occurring within the first 24 to 48 hours following birth, but it always appears within the first 8 postpartum weeks. Women with preexisting psychosis, especially bipolar disorder, are at the greatest risk for postpartum psychosis (Sadock & Sadock, 2004; Nonacs, 2005).

Postpartum psychosis may present with symptoms of PPD. However, the distinguishing signs of psychosis are hallucinations, delusions, agitation, confusion, disorientation, sleep disturbances, suicidal and homicidal thoughts, and a loss of touch with reality. This condition may also resemble a sudden manic attack. Mothers who are in a manic state require constant supervision when caring for their infant; they are frequently too preoccupied to tend to their infant's needs (Franzblau & Witt, 2006; Nonacs, 2005).

 Nursing Insight— Recognizing behavioral cues that signal postpartum psychosis

When providing hospital and community care for postpartum women, the nurse should be alert to behavioral cues that may signal psychosis:

- Hyperactivity
- Agitation
- Confusion
- Suspiciousness
- Excessive complaints

Collaborative Management

Infanticide (the killing of an infant) is as high as 4% in women with postpartum psychosis. Because of this danger and the loss of touch with reality, postpartum psychosis is a true emergency. The woman must be hospitalized, and mental health experts must become involved in her care as quickly as possible. Immediate treatment usually includes a mood stabilizer (lithium [Lithobid] or valproic acid [Depakene]), antipsychotic medications (Thorazine, Mellaril, Serentil), and anti-anxiety medications (benzodiazepines—Xanax, Libruim, Tranxene, Lorazepam). If required, electroconvulsive therapy (ECT) often leads to rapid improvement. Long-term psychotherapy and pharmacological treatment follows the immediate care (Adams et al., 2005; Franzblau & Witt, 2006; Nonacs, 2005).

Women who are taking mood stabilizers need extensive counseling about the side effects associated with these medications. Patients on lithium must have serum lithium levels drawn every 6 months. Most antipsychotic medications can cause orthostatic hypotension and sedation, side effects that pose a major risk for mothers providing child care. Because the woman's thought processes may be altered, the nurse should share specific information about medication side effects with a close family member. If the mother wishes to breast feed, some sources recommend that no pharmacological agents be prescribed (Sadock & Sadock, 2004), while others advise caution when prescribing some medications (Schatzberg & Nemeroff, 2004). Current recommendations are that although most medications pass into breast milk, there are very few instances in which breastfeeding must be discontinued (Pigarelli, Kraus, & Potter, 2008). The infant's daily dose of medications is less than the maternal daily dose. With lithium, however, serum concentrations in the infant may reach 50% of maternal levels. Thus, breastfeeding is usually discouraged in mothers who are taking lithium; the American Psychiatric Association considers lithium incompatible with breastfeeding (Fankhauser & Freeman, 2005). Long-term neurobehavioral effects on the infant related to exposure to psychotropic medications in breast milk are unknown.

Prognosis

Women with postpartum psychosis have a 25% to 50% chance of reoccurrence in future pregnancies (APA, 2000; Nonacs, 2005). These women are also at greater risk for a future psychotic event unrelated to pregnancy. Counseling and educational roles of the health care team for these patients and their families is paramount to health promotion and maintenance.

 Now Can You— Discuss postpartum blues, depression and psychosis?

1. State the difference between postpartum blues and postpartum depression?
2. Discuss what you would tell a woman with a history of postpartum depression about future pregnancies and the probable plan of care?
3. Describe the signs and symptoms of postpartum psychosis?

SUMMARIZING POSTPARTUM PSYCHOSOCIAL NURSING CARE

Perinatal nursing offers an opportunity to develop a therapeutic relationship with a woman and her family during one of the most vulnerable times in their lives. Most pregnancies are both planned and desired, but physiological and psychosocial adaptations to the pregnancy, birth, and expanded family present challenges that require maturity and flexibility. The nurse can become involved with the childbearing family during the first prenatal visit. As the pregnancy progresses, the nurse becomes increasingly familiar with the woman and her family's lifestyle, stressors, successes, disappointments, and challenges. The postpartum nurse is at a distinct disadvantage because of the limited time a woman remains hospitalized after birth. However, any nurse, regardless of care setting or time constraints, can develop an attentive ear and sensitivity. By doing so, the nurse is then able to promote health and well-being for the new mother, her newborn, and the family.

During the postpartum period, the nurse can provide information that stresses the importance of asking for help if the patient feels overwhelmed. Promoting care and activities that allow the new mother and her family to attach to the infant is vitally important. Examples of bonding-oriented nursing care include rooming-in, decreasing sensory stimuli so that the family can focus on one another, and limiting visitors (if the patient desires). The postpartum nurse should note negative comments the patient makes about herself, her family, or the newborn and encourage the patient to talk about her expectations for both herself and the family. If the pregnancy and birth were difficult, the patient may be disappointed in herself and "blame" the baby for the difficulties.

Moreover, if the patient is exhausted and requires extra rest, the nurse can help her inform her friends and family about this need. The nurse should give the patient permission to send her newborn to the nursery without feeling guilty, so that when she awakens, she can enjoy the newborn rather than becoming frustrated by his demands. It is paramount for the nurse to remain sensitive to patients who are not coping well in the hospital, and advocate for follow-up by a home health nurse or social worker.

After discharge, the nurse in the office or clinic can utilize waiting time for conversation and make note of any physical characteristics that may indicate the need for some respite time from the demands and responsibilities of parenthood. The nurse should become familiar with available community support services such as a Mother's Day Out to which the mother can be referred. It is also important to involve the collaborative team—the physician, lactation consultant, social worker, and spiritual advisor—in the patient's care.

Postpartum Nursing for Vulnerable Populations

While caring for women and their families after birth, the postpartum nurse may be informed about or discover that special needs exist. If the woman received prenatal care, the prenatal history and physical examination may contain information that indicates the patient is in an abusive relationship, is living in a homeless shelter, has no transportation, is a migrant worker, or did not initiate care until the second or third trimester. These social risk factors are of concern and always require follow-up. In addition, a woman who gives birth with no prenatal care requires support from health care professionals to ensure that both she and her newborn will have their basic needs of food, clothing, and shelter met. Though many in the world view the United States as an international social welfare agency and wish to live here, some American citizens, visitors, and undocumented immigrants live in fear, poverty, poor health, or oppression. The nurse caring for childbearing women and their families has a mandate to address these needs whether these patients are in a hospital, clinic, or private physician's office.

VICTIMS OF ABUSE

Abuse can take several forms: physical, emotional, verbal, or sexual. Unfortunately, most often someone the woman loves is the perpetrator, and the abuse may take more than one form. Physical violence during pregnancy has far-reaching effects for the infant as well as the mother. Battery during pregnancy is associated with a greater incidence of low-birth-weight neonates, preterm birth, and neonatal death (Yost, Bloom, McIntire, & Leveno, 2005). (See Chapters 9 and 11 for further discussion.) No stereotypes exist for women who are abused because the problem crosses all socioeconomic, ethnocultural, and educational lines. The National Center for Injury Prevention and Control and other researchers list multiple factors that place an individual at risk for committing intimate partner abuse and for being a victim of intimate partner abuse (Tables 16-7 and 16-8).

"What to say" — *Inquiring about intimate partner violence during pregnancy*

Physicians routinely screen pregnant women for gestational diabetes and pregnancy induced hypertension. However, more pregnant women are battered by their intimate partners than the combined total of pregnant women who develop these physiological complications (Family Violence Prevention Fund, 2008). Regardless of the setting, the nurse caring for perinatal patients at any time before or after birth can initiate a conversation about intimate partner violence. Many victims want to tell someone about the violence they are experiencing, but they must be asked directly. After establishing privacy, the nurse should be direct and say, "In this office, a part of our routine care is to ask about domestic violence. Do you currently feel safe with your partner? Have you been kicked, hit, slapped, or otherwise physically hurt within the last year? Do you have concerns about how your partner treats you emotionally or treats you sexually?" *Be sure to wait for the answer to each question. Do not rush the answers.*

Table 16-8 Risk Factors for Being a Victim of Intimate Partner Abuse

Individual Factors	Relationship Factors
History of child abuse	Marital conflict
History of physical abuse	Marital instability
History of sexual abuse	Male dominance in the family
Prior injury from the same partner	Poor family functioning
Having a verbally abusive partner	Partner history of alcohol or drug abuse
Economic stress, low income	
Tobacco, alcohol and illicit drug use	
Depression or suicide attempts	
History of sexually transmitted infections	
Young age (less than 24 years, especially adolescents)	
Lack of high school diploma	
Unplanned pregnancies (often as a result of birth control sabotage)	

 ***Ethnocultural Considerations*— Women and battering**

- In New York City, a 1999 study found that 51% of intimate partner homicide victims were foreign born.
- Sixty percent (60%) of Korean women surveyed reported battering by their husbands.
- Forty-eight percent of Latina women stated that since immigrating to the United States partner violence had increased.
- Many cultures accept battering and violence as a way of life. Women from these cultures may feel that U.S. laws and protection do not apply to them.
- If battered immigrant women attempt to flee the violence, they may not have access to bilingual shelters, financial assistance, or food.
- McCosker, Barnard, and Gerber (2003) reported from a review of literature that one in five Australian women experienced domestic violence during their lifetimes and that one in ten experienced violence during pregnancy.
- Reuters Health (2005) reported that two thirds of Native Americans overall experience some type of trauma during their lives. Native American women reported high rates of physical abuse, often by a spouse, more rape, and more sexual assault.
- Bohn, Tebben, and Campbell (2004) found that for "lifetime abuse by a current partner" (p. 565) African American and Puerto Rican women had the highest odds ratio and that African American, Puerto Rican, and Mexican/Mexican American women had a higher incidence of abuse during pregnancy.

Table 16-7 Risk Factors for Committing Intimate Partner Violence

Individual Factors	Relationship Factors
Young age	Marital conflict
Low self-esteem	Marital instability
Low income	Male dominance in the family
Low academic achievement	Poor family functioning
Aggressive or delinquent behavior as a child	Emotional dependence and insecurity
Alcohol or drug use	Belief in strict gender roles
Witnessing or experiencing childhood violence	Desire for power and control in relationships
Social isolation	Angry or hostile behavior toward a partner
Unemployment	

When a postpartum nurse determines that a postpartum patient and her infant are possibly returning to an abusive environment, several interventions can occur. The nurse must first confirm the suspicions by asking direct questions. If the patient confirms that she is a victim of intimate partner violence (regardless of the form), the nurse needs to immediately enlist the help of a social worker and a chaplain. These professionals are more knowledgeable about community resources such as safe houses, churches, and child protective services to which the patient can be referred. The health care team can help empower the patient to have an action plan to escape the abuse at a later time, should she choose to delay this decision.

It is important to remember that if the patient chooses to return to the abusive environment, the nurse's role does not end. Follow-up after discharge may include a home visit or a well-baby checkup, during which time further interventions can occur. When a patient has only herself to think about, she may be less likely to take protective action. However, maternal instincts may empower the woman to protect her baby and other children from abuse or violence. Even if the nurse is only able to be a therapeutic listener, this role may allow the patient to rehearse her action plan, ask questions, share information, and affirm her decisions regarding the future.

Lack of personal contact does not mean that interventions cannot occur. McFarland et al. (2004) used telephone interviews to conduct a longitudinal study on abused women. After an initial personal contact with abused women to ask about inclusion in the study and to obtain informed consent, researchers contacted the women with either six intervention and four follow-up calls (experimental group) or four follow-up calls only (control group). During the phone calls, the interviewers asked women in the experimental group to answer yes or no to a series of safety promoting behaviors. These behaviors included such actions as hiding money, hiding house and car keys, removing weapons from the house, asking neighbors to call police if violence begins, establishing a code with family and friends, and obtaining items such as birth certificates, important phone numbers, identification cards, and rent and utility receipts. The research findings indicated that women in the intervention group (those who received six additional phone calls) practiced more safety-promoting behaviors than did those in the control group and that the required nursing time was minimal. Such research findings are significant in supporting the important role that nurses and other members of the health care team can have in helping victims of intimate partner violence take control of their environments and practice positive behaviors that can break the cycle of abuse.

UNDOCUMENTED IMMIGRANTS AND MINORITY HEALTH CARE

As a nurse provides care for postpartum women and their families, ethical and legal concerns inevitably arise. One of these issues often concerns undocumented immigrants and minority health. The United States continues to attract a cosmopolitan population and to be viewed as a haven for those in search of a better life. Not all who come to the United States seek American citizenship or a legal visa for employment purposes. In particular, citizens in states that border Mexico (Texas, New Mexico, Arizona, and California) routinely fund and provide care for undocumented immigrants. Wrongly, many Americans believe that the primary reason Latinos come to the United States is to receive free medical care, which can include delivering a baby in this country in order to have a United States citizen in the family. Berk, Schur, Chavéz, and Frankel (2000) studied undocumented Latinos in Houston and El Paso, Texas and in Fresno and Los Angeles, California. They studied Latinos because this group represents an estimated 70% of all undocumented immigrants. The sample size began with 7352 households and eventually resulted in 973 participants. From surveying and interviewing one member of each household, the investigators found that the primary reason undocumented Latinos come to the United States is to find jobs. Only in El Paso was this not the primary reason. In El Paso, 49% of respondents cited "uniting with family members and friends" as their main reason for immigrating, and this primary reason was followed by "finding work" (p. 49).

Recently, the Centers for Medicare and Medicaid Services (CMS) proposed a plan whereby those states bearing the highest cost of health care services for undocumented immigrants under EMTALA (Emergency Medical Treatment and Active Labor Act) requirements would receive reimbursement over 4 years for these services. Though this plan would help defray state costs for these services, health care providers would be expected to document the immigration status of their patients. Immediately after this proposal, the American Nurses Association leadership shared its concerns with CMS officials. Requiring this documentation would likely lead to illegal immigrants avoiding health care settings, even when seriously ill or injured (Trossman, 2004). While intended to help state budgets with the high cost of emergency health care for undocumented immigrants, many providers have also expressed concern. They assert that the need to establish immigration status may create not only a public health crisis, but also a greater financial burden, since preventative care (including prenatal care) would not be included in the reimbursement plan. Statistically, immigrant and minority women have higher rates of disability and mortality, and their overall health status is lower than that of Caucasian women (AHRQ, 2006).

The nurse needs to provide unbiased, excellent care to all patients, regardless of immigration or minority status. A new mother and her family's immigration status or nationality does not change her needs or her family's need for compassionate, holistic, and quality care. If the patient has received minimal or no prenatal care, physical and psychosocial needs may be greater and may result in complications that require greater skill on the part of every involved individual. Direct care nurses are not primarily policy experts, nor do many desire this role. A vital factor in being able to provide ongoing perinatal care is to ensure women and their families they can trust those with whom they share information and concerns. While the United States and individual state politicians debate the financial implications and resources required to provide health care for those in this country who need it, the mandate for nurses is that they be one of the most valuable resources available to meet the needs of all new mothers and families for whom they care. Nursing is as much a "calling" as it is a profession.

Now Can You— Discuss issues related to the care of minority and undocumented immigrant women?

1. State the most common reason undocumented immigrants come into the United States?
2. Describe a major nursing role when caring for immigrant and minority women?
3. State some potential outcomes for women and their babies who obtain minimal or no prenatal care?

HOMELESSNESS AND LIMITED ACCESS TO CARE

Women and newborns who are homeless and without an established health care provider for follow-up constitute a particularly vulnerable population after childbirth. Better health care outcomes are positively correlated with having a usual or principal source of care. African American and Hispanic American women are much less likely than others to have a primary source of care, and this population is also more likely to be uninsured (Partnership for the Homeless, 2008).

Often these same women are those who are homeless. Whether migrant workers who follow the crops they help to harvest or individuals with socioeconomic and interpersonal challenges, homeless women and their children represent a population that requires sensitive, skilled discussions, so that they can receive appropriate follow-up care. The fact that the pregnancy rate among homeless women is almost twice that of the general population (Gelberg et al., 2001) is a statistic that requires action. The *Healthy People 2010* indicators include access to prenatal care for all women as a major initiative.

Studies designed to address barriers to perinatal care have noted similar findings. The research of both Mikhail (1999) and Bloom et al. (2004) examined barriers among homeless, pregnant women (in California and Florida, respectively). There are several barriers pregnant, homeless women face when considering whether to begin or continue prenatal care (e.g., waiting time to see a practitioner, especially when compared to the time the practitioner actually spent with the patient; lack of transportation, care for older children, or encouragement to get prenatal care from family members; concern about having their children removed from their care; and finances). Maupin, Fatsis, and Prystowiski (2004) described women who give birth with no prenatal care as those who are more likely to be multiparous, living with at least one child, less educated, uninsured, and tobacco or recreational drug users. Most pregnant, homeless women surveyed did not intend to become pregnant. Ethnically, more African American and Hispanic women are likely to bypass prenatal care than are their Caucasian counterparts (Bloom et al., 2004; Frisbie, Echevarria, & Hummer, 2001).

If a woman presents to a hospital in labor and has not received prenatal care, EMTALA requires that a physician and hospital staff members deliver her baby and provide her and her newborn with care until they can be safely discharged. If it is determined that the mother is homeless, once again the nurse must solicit the help of the interdisciplinary team, including the social worker and chaplain. The physician caring for the mother and baby needs to satisfy legal requirements before discharging the patient and newborn. Often, the nurse needs to collect newborn urine and/or meconium samples for drug screening. If the hospital or birthing center employs a nurse who conducts a follow-up visit to check on the new mother and baby and immediate housing is available, the physician may elect to discharge them with an early visit arranged.

If the woman has absolutely nowhere to go after discharge, the nurse and others have an ethical and legal responsibility to ensure that the newborn is adequately fed and clothed. Child Protective Services, the United Way Agency, or church-affiliated social programs may be sources of help for this family. Immediate solutions are required. Longer-term arrangements will take additional resources and time. Ultimately, because the newborn is completely dependent on others for his needs to be met, the best situation for the baby often drives the final decisions.

POSTPARTUM CARE OF VULNERABLE POPULATIONS

Most commonly, postpartum nurses care for women and families who are functional and healthy (physically, psychosocially, spiritually). If the nurse knows a couple or family who is unable to have children and who is exploring the option of adoption, handling dilemmas such as abuse or homelessness may be especially difficult. When a childbearing woman faces difficult challenges and requires additional support, her only source of this support may be the health care community. Regardless of personal impressions, the nurse needs to be receptive to lessons that can be learned from this patient's situation. Most new mothers want the best life possible for their newborns. Armed with this fact, nurses can grow in their ability to understand and respond with sensitivity to all families for whom they care.

 Now Can You— Discuss strategies in caring for vulnerable populations?

1. List important members of the health care team to involve in the continuum of care for vulnerable pregnant women or new mothers and their babies?
2. State a *Healthy People 2010* goal for pregnant women?
3. List characteristics of pregnant women who are most unlikely to get prenatal care?

summary points

◆ Postpartum hemorrhage may occur early (within the first 24 hours after birth) or late (after the first 24 hours but within 6 weeks after childbirth).

◆ Puerperal infections may involve the uterus, urinary system, incisions, and breasts. Each type of infection has common and unique risk factors, onset, signs and symptoms, causative organisms, and complications.

◆ Thrombophlebitis is an inflammation of the venous circulation and blood clot formation that typically occurs in the lower extremities. Treatment involves bedrest with elevation of the affected extremity, application of moist heat, and anticoagulant therapy. If thromboembolic disease is suspected, the affected area should never be massaged because this action may cause dislodgement of the clot and the potential for a pulmonary embolism.

◆ Postpartum "blues" are common and usually self-limiting. Postpartum depression is a multifactorial problem that requires prompt assessment and intervention.

◆ Vulnerable populations include homeless, minority, and undocumented immigrant women, as well as those who are victims of abuse. Providing holistic, quality postpartal nursing care for vulnerable populations requires self-examination, sensitivity, and compassion.

review questions

Multiple Choice

1. The perinatal nurse, when using the acronym "LARRY" to remember the common causes of postpartum hemorrhage, is aware that the "L" refers to:
A. Lacerations
B. Loss of blood > 500 mL
C. Low platelet count
D. Low hemoglobin

2. As part of a postpartum woman's assessment, the perinatal nurse observes for signs and symptoms of hematoma formation. The most common anatomical location is in the:
A. Rectum
B. Vulva
C. Cervix
D. Episiotomy site

3. The perinatal nurse promotes postpartum health and prevents infection with the inclusion of critical information about:
A. Good hand washing
B. Early ambulation
C. Minimal fluid intake
D. Restricted protein intake

4. The perinatal nurse is providing information to a postpartum woman who is being discharged from the hospital on warfarin (Coumadin) therapy. Instructions would include restrictions of which drug due to concern about interactions:
A. Acetaminophen
B. Ibuprofen
C. Prenatal vitamins
D. Docusate sodium

True/False

5. The perinatal nurse is aware that there is an increased risk of minimizing pathological symptoms during the childbearing process because of a focus on health promotion and wellness.

6. The perinatal nurse routinely screens for intimate partner violence as part of the hospital admission history, as studies have shown that women wish to be asked directly.

Fill-in-the-Blank

7. The amount of blood loss postpartum is frequently _____ estimated by perinatal nurses and other health care providers.

8. The perinatal nurse explains to a student nurse that the development of an endometrial infection following childbirth is called a _____ infection.

Case Study

9. Julia, a G4, TPAL 4004, experienced a normal vaginal birth approximately 60 minutes ago. No episiotomy was made at the time of birth. Her daughters, 5, 3, and 2 years of age have now come to visit. Julia states that her pad feels "very wet." As the perinatal nurse, you assess the tone of Julia's uterus and it is firm. Your next action would be to:
A. Massage her uterus to ensure that it remains firm
B. Change and weigh her pads to accurately determine her blood loss
C. Request that the physician come and check for internal lacerations
D. Request that her family members leave immediately

10. The perinatal nurse is caring for Maria, a 23-year-old G2 TPAL 1011 woman, who experienced 14 hours of labor prior to a cesarean birth for failure to progress. She is now 48 hours postbirth and is complaining of abdominal pain that is not relieved with medication given two hours ago. Her temperature is 100.8°F (38.2°C). The perinatal nurse is expected to obtain:
A. An accurate blood pressure
B. Incisional swab for culture and sensitivity
C. An accurate pain assessment
D. Additional orders for pain management

See Answers to End of Chapter Review Questions on the Electronic Study Guide or DavisPlus.

REFERENCES

Adams, M.P., Josephson, D.L., & Holland, L.N. (2005). *Pharmacology for nurses: A pathophysiologic approach.* Upper Saddle River, NJ: Pearson Education.

Agency for Healthcare Research and Quality (June, 2006). *Health care for minority women.* Program Brief. AHRQ Publication No. 06-P017. Rockville, MD: Author. Retrieved from http://www.ahrq.gov/research/minority.htm (Accessed October 2, 2007).

American Academy of Pedatrics (AAP) & The American College of Obstetricians and Gynecologists (ACOG). (2007). *Guidelines for perinatal care.* (6th ed.) Washington, DC: Author.

American Psychiatric Association (APA). (2000). *Diagnostic and statistical manual (DSM-IV).* Washington, DC: Auhor.

Beck, C.T., Records, K., & Rice, M. (2006). Further development of the Postpartum Depression Predictors Inventory-Revised. *Journal of Obstetric, Gynecologic, & Neonatal Nursing, 35*(6), 735–745.

Berk, M.L., Schur, C.L., Chavez, L.R., & Frankel, M. (2000). Health care use among undocumented Latino immigrants. *Health Affairs, 19*(4), 44057.

Bloom, K.C., Bednarzyk, M.S., Devitt, D.L., Renault, R.A., Teaman, V., & Van Loock, D.M. (2004). Barriers to prenatal care for homeless pregnant women. *Journal of Obstetric, Gynecologic, and Neonatal Nursing, 33*(4), 428–435.

Bohn, D.K., Tebben, J.G., & Campbell, J.C. (2004). Influences of income, education, age, and ethnicity on physical abuse before and during pregnancy. *Journal of Obstetric, Gynecologic, and Neonatal Nursing, 33*(5), 561–571.

Bulechek, G., Butcher, H.M., & Dochterman, J. (2008). *Nursing interventions classification (NIC)* (5th ed.). St. Louis, MO: C.V. Mosby.

Clemmens, D., Driscoll, J.W., & Beck, C.T. (2004). Postpartum depression as profiled through the postpartum depression screening scale. *The American Journal of Maternal/Child Nursing, 29*(3), 180–185.

Colman-Brochu, S. (2005). Deep vein thrombosis in pregnancy. *The American Journal of Maternal/Child Nursing, 29*(3), 186–192.

Cunningham, F., Leveno, K., Bloom, S., Hauth, J., Gilstrap, L., & Wenstrom, K.D. (2005). *Williams' obstetrics* (22nd ed.). New York: McGraw-Hill.

Davey, S.J., Dziurawiec, S., & O'Brien-Malone, A. (2006). Men's voices: Postnatal depression from the perspective of male partners. *Qualitative Health Research, 16*, 206–220.

Deglin, J.H., & Vallerand, A.H. (2009). *Davis's drug guide for nurses* (11th ed.). Philadelphia: F.A. Davis.

Family Violence Prevention Fund. (2008). Domestic violence and health care. Retrieved from www.endabuse.org (Accessed April 17, 2008).

Fankhauser, M., & Freeman, M. (2005). Bipolar disorder. In J. DiPiro, R. Talbert, G. Yee, G. Matzke, B. Wells, & M. Posey (Eds.), *Pharmacotherapy: A pathophysiologic approach* (6th ed., 216–233). New York: McGraw-Hill.

Flamm, B.L. (Nov. 15, 2003). Postpartum hemorrhage (Clinical Pearls). *ObGyn News. 38*(22), 39. Retrieved from http://80-galenet.galegroup.com (Accessed May 12, 2005).

Foster, C. (2007). Factor V Leiden Mutation: What is it? What are the implications for clinical practice? *The American Journal for Nurse Practitioners, 11*(6), 35–46.

Franzblau, N., & Witt, K. (June 26, 2006). Normal and abnormal puerperium. Retrieved from http://www.emedicine.com/med/topic3240.htm (Accessed October 1, 2007).

Frisbie, W.P., Echevarria, S., & Hummer, R.A. (March, 2001). Prenatal care utilization among non-Hispanic whites, African-Americans, and Mexican Americans. *Maternal and Child Health Journal, 5*(1), 21–33.

Gelberg, L., Leake, B.D., Lu, M.C., Anderson, R.M., Wenzel, S.L., & Morgenstern, H. (2001). Use of contraceptive methods among homeless women for protection against unwanted pregnancies and sexually transmitted diseases: Prior use and willingness to use in the future. *Contraception, 63*, 277–281.

Gibbs, R., Sweet, R., & Duff, P. (2004). Maternal and fetal infectious disorders. In R. Creasy, R. Reznik, & J. Iams (Eds), *Maternal-fetal medicine: Principles and practice* (5th ed., 955–986). Philadelphia: W.B. Saunders.

Goodman, J.H. (2004). Postpartum depression beyond the early postpartum period. *Journal of Obstetric, Gynecologic, and Neonatal Nursing, 33*(4), 410–420.

Healthy People 2010: Understanding and improving health. (2000). Retrieved from http://www.health.gov/healthypeople/Publications (Accessed September 23, 2005).

Hobbins, J.C. (April 1, 2005). The length of the third stage of labor and risk of postpartum hemorrhage. *OB/GYN Clinical Alert (Comment).* Retrieved from http://80-galenet.galegroup.com (Accessed May 12, 2005).

Jesse, D.E., & Graham, M. (2005). Are you often sad and depressed: Brief measures to identify women at risk for depression in pregnancy. *The American Journal of Maternal/Child Nursing, 1*(1), 40–45.

Johnson, M., Bulechek, G., Butcher, H., McCloskey Dochterman, J., Maas, M., Moorhead, S., & Swanson, E. (2006). *NANDA, NOC, and NIC linkages: Nursing diagnoses, outcomes, & interventions* (2nd ed.). St. Louis, MO: Mosby Elsevier.

Kennedy, E. (August 8, 2007). Pregnancy, postpartum infections. Retrieved from http://www.emedicine.com/emerg/topic482.htm (Accessed October 1, 2007).

Lawrence, R., & Lawrence, R. (2005). *Breastfeeding: A guide for the medical profession* (6th ed.). Philadelphia: C.V. Mosby.

Lincoln, V., & Kleiner, K. (2004). Holistic health: Complementary therapeutic disciplines and remedies. In M.Condon (Ed), *Women's health: An integrated approach to wellness and illness* (pp. 195–225). Upper Saddle River, NJ: Pearson Education, Inc.

Linter, N., & Gray, B. (2006). Childbearing and depression: What nurses need to know. *AWHONN Lifelines, 10*(1), 50–57.

Logsdon, M.C., Birkimer, J.C., Simpson, T., & Looney, S. (2005). Postpartum depression and social support in adolescents. *Journal of Obstetric, Gynecologic & Neonatal Nursing, 34*(1), 46–54.

Luegenbiehl, D.L., Brophy, G., Artigue, G., Phillips, K., & Flack, R. (1990). Standardized assessment of blood loss. *MCN: American Journal of Maternal-Child Nursing, 15*(4), 241–244.

MacMullen, N.J., Dulski, L., & Meagher, B. (2005). Red alert: Perinatal hemorrhage. *The American Journal of Maternal/Child Nursing, 30*(1), 46–51.

Magann, S.E., Hutchinson, M., Collins, R., Howard, B.C., & Morrison, J.C. (April, 2005). Postpartum hemorrhage after vaginal birth: An analysis of risk factors. *Southern Medical Journal 98*(4), 419–424. Retrieved from http://80-galenet.gale-group.com (Accessed May 12, 2005).

Mass, S. (2004). Breast pain: Engorgement, nipple pain, and mastitis. *Clinical Obstetrics and Gynecology, 47*(3), 676–682.

Maupin, R., Fatsis, J., & Prystowiski, E. (2004). Characteristics of women who deliver with no prenatal care. *Journal of Maternal-Fetal and Neonatal Medicine 16*(1), 45–50.

McCosker, H., Barnard, A., & Gerber, R. (Nov. 21, 2003). A phenomenographic study of women's experiences of domestic violence during the childbearing years. *Online Journal of Issues in Nursing.* Retrieved from http://www.ana.org/ojin/topic17/tpc17_6.htm (Accessed May 4, 2005).

McFarland, J., Malecha, A., Gist, J., Watson, K., Batten, E., Hall, I., & Smith, S. (2004). Original research: Increasing the safety promoting behaviors of abused women. *American Journal of Nursing, 104*(3), 40–51.

Meyer, G., & Lavin, M.A. (2005). Vigilance: The essence of nursing. *Online Journal of Issues in Nursing.* Retrieved from http://nursing-world.org/ojin/topic22/tpc22_6.htmon (Accessed October 5, 2006).

Mikhail, B.I. (1999). Perceived impediments to prenatal care among low-income women. *Western Journal of Nursing Research, 21*(3), 335–348.

Moorehead, S., Johnson, M., Mass, M., & Swanson, E. (2008). *Nursing outcomes classification (NOC)* (4th ed.). St. Louis, MO: C.V. Mosby.

NANDA International. (2007). *NANDA-I nursing diagnoses: Definitions and classifications 2007-2008.* Philadelphia: NANDA-I.

National Center for Injury Prevention and Control. (2008). Intimate partner violence: Fact sheet. Retrieved from http://www.cdc.gov/ncipic/factsheets/ipvfacts.htm (Accessed April 17, 2008).

Nonacs, R.M. (August 8, 2005). Postpartum depression. Retrieved from http://www.emedicine.com/med/topic3408.htm (Accessed October 1, 2007).

Partnership for the Homeless. (2008). The Partnership's programs work to break the cycle of homelessness. Retrieved from http://www.partnershipforthehomeless.org/ (Accessed April 17, 2008).

Pigarelli, D., Kraus, C., & Potter, B. (2008). Pregnancy and lactation: Therapeutic considerations. In J. DiPiro, R. Talbert, G. Yee, G. Matzke, B. Wells, & M. Posey (Eds.), *Pharmacotherapy: A pathophysiologic approach* (7th ed., pp 1297–1312). New York: McGraw-Hill.

Reuters Health (2005). Trauma common feature of American Indian life. From *American Journal of Public Health, May, 2005.* Retrieved from http://www.nlm.gov/medlineplus/news/fullstory_24951.html (Accessed June 9, 2005).

Sadock, B.J., & Sadock, V.A. (2004). *Kaplan & Sadock's comprehensive textbook of psychiatry.* Philadelphia: Lippincott Williams & Wilkins.

Schatzberg, A., & Nemeroff, C. (Eds.). (2004). *The American Psychiatric Publishing textbook of psychopharmacology.* (3rd ed.). Washington, DC: American Psychiatric Publishing.

Smith, J.R., & Brennan, B. (June 13, 2006). Postpartum hemorrhage. Retrieved from http://emedicine.com (Accessed June 13, 2006).

Stoops, J., & Mann, N. (2004). Psychological/emotional wellness and illness. In M. Condon (Ed.), *Women's health: An integrated approach to wellness and illness* (pp. 538–556). Upper Saddle River, NJ: Pearson Education.

Trossman, S. (November–December, 2004). No easy answers: Addressing the needs of undocumented immigrants. *The American Nurse, November–December, 2004.* Retrieved from http://www.NursingWorld.org (Accessed May 4, 2005).

Walters, K.C., & Wing, D.A. (2007). Misoprostol and postpartum hemorrhage. *The Female Patient, 32*(7), 53–60.

Wilkinson, J.M. (2005). *Nursing diagnosis handbook.* Upper Saddle River, NJ: Pearson Education.

Yost, N., Bloom, S., McIntire, G., & Leveno, K. (2005). A prospective observational study of domestic violence during pregnancy. *Obstetrics and Gynecology, 106*(1), 61–65.

CONCEPT MAP

• Assess safety
• Therapeutic listening
• Trusting relationship/ non-judgmental
• Address barriers to care

Vulnerable Populations
• Victims of abuse
• Undocumented immigrants
• Homeless women

Physical

Caring for the Woman Experiencing Complications During the Postpartal Period

Psychosocial

Thrombophlebitis; Thrombosis

Collaborative Management
• Analgesics; rest; elevate extremity
• Elastic support hose
• Encourage fluids; apply heat
• Possible SQ heparin
• Monitor for bleeding
• Assess vital signs
• Measure calf circumference
• Monitor for pulmonary embolus
• Do not massage affected extremity!

Hematoma

Collaborative Management
• Assess for c/o unremitting pain and pressure; vital signs; examine perineum/vulva; assess for shock; notify MD or CNM; ice for 12 hours then sitz bath; analgesics; greater than 12 cm → I&D

Postpartum hemorrhage

Early: within first 24 hours; higher in first 4 hours

Late: within first 6 weeks

Collaborative Management
• Locate source of bleeding; establish IV access
• Assess for: hypovolemic shock; vital signs; MAP; LOC
• Fundal massage; bladder palpation
• Observe rate of pad saturation; calculate I&O
• Monitor for bleeding
• Possible surgical intervention

Postpartum Blues
• Common, self-limiting
• Teary, moody, sadness
• Related to abrupt hormone changes

Nursing
• Education; Assess resources
• Rest, reassurance, therapeutic listening

Puerperal infections

Collaborative Management
• Assess for: fever, tachycardia, uterine/fundal pain or tenderness, foul smelling lochia, chills, malaise, dysuria, inflammatory breast edema
• Antibiotic therapy; analgesics
• Encourage rest
• Increase fluids, protein, vitamin C

Postpartum Depression
• Decreased interest in infant or overconcern
• Panic attacks
• Inability to make decisions

Nursing
• Prenatal screening
• Assess mother–infant interaction, bonding, prior risk factors
• Continue assessment during well-baby checkup; negativity, neglect, social needs

Across Care Settings:
• Communicate risk for infection to family and community health providers

Best Outcome
• Weigh pads for accurate blood loss
• Explain interventions; control pain

Clinical Alert:
• Firm uterus plus slow steady blood trickle = significant loss
• Large blood loss can occur without change in vital signs

Postpartum Psychosis
• Rare, severe mental illness
• Involves hallucinations, delusions, agitation, confusion, suicidal/homicidal thoughts

Management
• Mental health emergency: hospitalize
• Immediate and long-term pharmacotherapy

Where Research And Practice Meet:
• Education regarding puerperal infections r/t early discharges
• Jesse/Graham 2 item depression screen

Critical Nursing Action:
• Fundal massage for uterine atony

Now Can You:
• Discuss holistic care of the woman experiencing postpartum hemorrhage
• Discuss routine care of the postpartum patient hospitalized with a DVT
• Describe the signs and symptoms of postpartum psychosis

Physiological Transition of the Newborn

 Our journey begins and ends with the development of a family. Becoming a mother is the beginning of a wondrous journey… The transition of that little living being within you to that amazing, beautiful newborn you will love and loves you back unconditionally…

—D. Teeple

LEARNING TARGETS *At the completion of this chapter, the student will be able to:*

◆ Explain the importance of the development of surfactant and its role in the successful transition of the neonate.

◆ Identify the four factors that influence the initiation of respirations.

◆ Discuss how the four anatomical structures that enable in utero survival must undergo significant transition following birth.

◆ Explain the importance of administering vitamin K to the neonate after birth and describe its effect on the hematopoietic system.

◆ Describe the process of nonshivering thermogenesis and the importance of brown adipose tissue in the neonate.

◆ List neonatal liver functions that allow for successful physiological transition.

◆ Name the enzymes present in the neonate's gastrointestinal system and describe their role in digestion.

◆ Identify the factors that influence kidney adaptation to allow for the management of bodily fluids and urine excretion.

◆ Identify the three primary immunoglobulins that are important in strengthening the neonate's immunological system.

◆ Discuss normal neonatal patterns of behavior during the first several hours after birth.

---

 moving toward evidence-based practice Maternal Engagement

Sanders, L.W., & Buckner, E.B. (2006). The newborn behavioral observations system as a nursing intervention to enhance engagement in first-time mothers: Feasibility and desirability. *Pediatric Nursing, 32*(5), 455–459.

The purpose of this study was to explore with first-time mothers the feasibility and desirability of the Newborn Behavioral Observation (NBO) system as a nursing intervention in assisting mothers to establish engagement with their newborn. Engagement was defined as "the social process of maternal transition that enables growth and transformation and is linked to attachment and bonding." The NBO was developed by Nugent, Keefer, O'Brien, Johnson, and Blanchford (Brazelton Institute, n.d.; Nugent et al., in press) as a tool to promote positive parent–infant relationships that could be included as part of routine maternal–child care. The tool assists the nurse in orienting parents to the characteristics and competencies of the newborn through neurobehavioral assessment items.

(continued)

The convenience sample consisted of 10 first-time mothers recruited from a mother–baby unit in a large university hospital. Characteristics of the participants were as follows:

- Six mothers were African American, two mothers were Caucasian, one mother was Asian, and one mother was Indian.
- All gave birth to healthy babies and participated in rooming-in.
- Their ages ranged from 19 to 27 years.
- Their incomes ranged from under $15,000 to $30,000.
- Six mothers reported a greater than a high school education; four mothers attended prenatal classes.

Methods: An NBO session was followed by an interview to determine the mother's perception of the intervention. The interview consisted of both open-ended and closed-ended questions regarding the mother's opinions of the effectiveness of the NBO in enhancing activities to increase engagement. After the interview the mothers completed an NBO Parent Questionnaire designed to assess "the usefulness of the NBO in teaching parents and enhancing engagement."

Using a 4-point scale (1 = nothing; 4 = a lot), the mothers gave the NBO a high rating in regard to increasing their

knowledge of what their infants can do and how they can interact with their infants. The mothers' participation in the intervention was also rated to determine if a relationship existed between the observed and the reported level of effectiveness in increasing engagement activities. Eight maternal behaviors, which were indicative of interest, were rated on a 3-point scale. The mothers were also asked what they liked about the intervention, what they learned about their infants, and what they knew about how to provide care. Themes that emerged from the mothers' qualitative responses included two of the activities of engagement: experiencing the infant and active participation in care.

The researchers concluded that the NBO is an effective nursing intervention for enhancing maternal engagement during the early postpartum period.

1. What might be considered as limitations to this study?
2. How is this information useful to clinical nursing practice?

See Suggested Responses for Moving Toward Evidence-Based Practice on the Electronic Study Guide or DavisPlus.

Introduction

Once the umbilical cord is clamped and the infant takes the first breath, the transition from intrauterine to extrauterine life begins. Transition is one of the most intense and dynamic periods in the human life cycle. The transition from total dependence on another for every life-sustaining need from oxygenation and nutrition to total independence requires dramatic changes. For the neonate, the transitional phase may take minutes, hours, or days.

This chapter explores the physiological changes that take place in the newborn during the process of transition. Alterations that occur in each major body system are discussed, with emphasis on nursing assessment and interventions to facilitate a normal transition.

A & P review   **Normal Respiratory Function**

The primary function of the respiratory system is twofold: the exchange of oxygen and carbon dioxide through respiration and maintenance of the acid–base balance.

The mechanical process of respiration is accomplished via the exchange of air between the lungs and the atmosphere (pulmonary ventilation). The two phases of pulmonary ventilation are inspiration and exhalation.

The physiological processes involved in pulmonary ventilation take place on three levels: external, internal, and cellular. External respiration is the exchange of gases (oxygen, carbon dioxide) between the alveoli and the blood through the alveolar–capillary membrane. Internal respiration is the exchange of gases between the systemic capillaries and the tissue at the cellular level. The cellular physiological process is the exchange of gases within the cell (Dillon, 2007). ◆

Adaptations of the Respiratory System

INTRAPULMONARY FLUID, FETAL BREATHING MOVEMENTS, AND SURFACTANT

After birth, the initiation of respirations constitutes the first important step in neonatal transition. Many forces that occur during pregnancy and childbirth facilitate this essential process. The amniotic fluid plays an important role in fetal lung development. Inhalation of the amniotic fluid into the lungs helps to promote growth and differentiation of the lung tissue. Normal pulmonary functioning is dependent on two factors: the alternating in and out fetal breathing movements and the formation of intrapulmonary fluid.

 Nursing Insight— *Fetal breathing movements*

Breathing efforts are first initiated in utero as the fetus spends months practicing coordinated inhalation and exhalation movements. Fetal breathing movements (FBMs) can be observed by ultrasonography as early as 11 weeks of gestation. The breathing movements serve as an important mechanism that helps to develop the muscles of the chest wall and the diaphragm.

As the fetus approaches term, there is a decrease in the secretion of intrapulmonary fluid. The absorption of fetal lung fluid is accelerated during labor and delivery and for up to a few hours after birth. This fluid shift constitutes an important physiologic event: it assists in reducing the pulmonary resistance to blood flow (necessary while in utero) and facilitates the initiation of air breathing (Hernandez, Zabloudil, & Hernandez, 2004). During a vaginal birth, approximately one third of the fetal lung fluid is expelled due to the "thoracic squeeze" that occurs during passage through the birth canal. Infants of cesarean births are at a higher risk for pulmonary transitional difficulties because they do not receive the lung compression benefits associated with a vaginal birth.

Lung expansion after birth stimulates the release of **surfactant**, a slippery, detergent-like lipoprotein. Surfactant causes a decreased surface tension within the alveoli, which allows for alveolar re-expansion after each exhalation. Under normal circumstances, by the 34th to 36th weeks of gestation, surfactant is produced in sufficient amounts to maintain alveolar stability (Bloom, 2006).

Many factors such as acidemia, hypoxia, shock, mechanical ventilation, and hypercapnia (an increased level of serum carbon dioxide) may interfere with surfactant metabolism. Surfactant production is decreased in infants of diabetic mothers (classes A, B, and C), infants with hemolytic disorders (e.g., erythroblastosis fetalis), and in multiple gestations. Conversely, surfactant production may be accelerated in other infants such as those of mothers with class D, F, and R diabetes, hypertension, and heroin addiction. Fetal exposure to maternal infections and placental insufficiency may also accelerate the production of surfactant.

THE FIRST BREATH

Four factors influence the initiation of the newborn's first breath. These include internal stimuli: the chemical changes; and external stimuli: the sensory, thermal, and mechanical changes (Fig. 17-1). Each factor stimulates the respiratory center located within the medulla of the brain.

Chemical Factors

Chemical factors that initiate respirations are hypercarbia, acidosis, and hypoxia. These conditions, brought about by the stress of labor and birth, stimulate the respiratory center in the brain to initiate breathing. Hypoxia causes blood oxygen levels (PO_2) and pH to drop. Subsequently, blood carbon dioxide levels (PCO_2) begin to rise and prompt the respiratory center within the medulla to initiate breathing. This brief period of asphyxia occurs in all newborns during the birth process. However, prolonged asphyxia that accompanies a traumatic birth is abnormal and may cause a central nervous system (CNS)-mediated respiratory depression.

Sensory Factors

The newborn experiences a vast amount of stimuli when leaving a familiar, comfortable, warm environment to enter into an extremely sensory overloaded one—filled with a multitude of tactile, visual, and auditory stimuli. These sensory experiences aid in the initiation of respirations.

Thermal Factors

After months of development in a warm (98.6°F [37°C]) fluid-filled environment, the newborn abruptly enters into a thermal environment that ranges from 70 to 75°F (21 to 23.9°C). The drastic change in temperature helps to stimulate the initiation of respirations. Sensors in the skin respond to the temperature changes and send signals to the respiratory system in the brain. Physiological changes in the neonate's temperature may occur and as long as the temperature remains within the normal range of 97.7 to 98.6°F (36.5 to 37.0°C), no problems related to the thermal environment should develop. However, to prevent cold stress and respiratory depression, it is imperative for the nurse to immediately dry and either place the infant (skin to skin) with the mother or in a radiant warmer.

Mechanical Factors

Removal of fluid from the lungs with the subsequent replacement of air constitutes the primary mechanical factors involved in the initiation of respirations. The fetal chest compression that occurs during a vaginal birth increases the intrathoracic pressure and helps to push fluid out of the lungs. Recoil of the chest wall after delivery of the neonate's trunk creates a negative intrathoracic pressure. This facilitates a small, passive inspiration of air, which replaces the fluid that has been squeezed out.

Figure 17-1 Chemical, sensory, thermal, and mechanical factors involved in the initiation of respirations.

Nursing Insight— *Recognizing normal neonatal lung sounds during early auscultation*

Continuation of respirations occurs when the pressure within the neonate's lungs increases and pushes the remaining fetal lung fluid into the lymphatic and circulatory systems. Most of the fluid is reabsorbed within the first few hours, but in some infants this process may take up to 24 hours (Fig. 17-2). The neonate's lung sounds may sound moist during early auscultation, but should become clear as the fluid is absorbed.

 Now Can You— **Discuss elements of pulmonary function in the neonate?**

1. Discuss why intrapulmonary fluid and fetal breathing movements are important for normal pulmonary functioning?
2. Explain why surfactant is important for respirations and identify two prenatal conditions that may be associated with a decrease in surfactant production?
3. Describe the four factors that are essential for the initiation of respirations?

FACTORS THAT MAY INTERFERE WITH INITIATION AND MAINTENANCE OF RESPIRATIONS

A number of factors may interfere with the neonate's ability to initiate respirations. Conditions such as prematurity or birth asphyxia can adversely affect lung compliance (elasticity) and surfactant production. Childbirth events including trauma, maternal medications, and the mode of delivery can interfere with normal pulmonary transition.

Because of the low levels of surfactant normally present in infants less than 36 weeks' gestation, preterm infants are more likely to develop **respiratory distress syndrome** (RDS). RDS is a developmental disorder of the respiratory system that begins at birth or very soon afterward. It occurs most frequently in infants born with immature lungs. Lack of adequate surfactant leads to the sequelae associated with RDS: progressive atelectasis, loss of functional residual

Figure 17-2 The process of absorption of fetal lung fluid once breathing has been initiated after birth. *A.* Before labor, alveolar fluid fills the lungs and circulates with amniotic fluid. During labor, air sacs and airways remain filled with fluid. *B.* During vaginal birth, the fetal thorax is compressed (thoracic squeeze) and approximately one third of the lung fluid is expelled. *C.* After vaginal birth, the neonate's first breath expands the lungs and fluid is displaced. Spontaneous respirations happen over the next 24 hours. Air displaces the remaining fluid, which is removed by the capillaries and lymphatics.

capacity, alterations in the ventilation perfusion ratio, and poor lung compliance (MacDonald, Mullett, & Seshia, 2005). (See Chapters 18 and 19 for further discussion.)

When there is a strong likelihood that a preterm delivery will occur, the pregnant patient may receive tocolytic medications (inhibit uterine contractions) to postpone birth. The delay allows for the administration of glucocorticoids (e.g., betamethasone) to boost fetal lung maturation in an effort to improve the neonate's outcome. Betamethasone is given to the woman at least 24 hours before birth, if possible, to prompt the production of fetal surfactant and hopefully improve respiratory functioning in the neonate.

 medication: Betamethasone, Dexamethasone

Betamethasone (bay-ta-**meth**-a-sone)

Dexamethasone (dex-a-**meth**-a-sone)

Pregnancy/Category: C

Indications: To prevent or reduce the severity of respiratory distress syndrome in preterm infants between 24 and 34 weeks of gestation (unlabeled use).

Action: Stimulates fetal lung maturation by promoting the release of enzymes that induce the production or release of lung surfactant.

Classification(s):
Therapeutic: Stimulates fetal lung maturation
Pharmacological: Glucocorticoids (corticosteroids)

Pharmacokinetics:
ABSORPTION: Preferred method of absorption is via injection.
DISTRIBUTION: Crosses the placenta; enters the breast milk.
METABOLISM AND EXCRETION: Metabolized in the liver and excreted by the kidneys
HALF-LIFE: 6.5 hours

Contraindications and Precautions: Contraindicated in women in whom there is a medical indication for delivery (i.e., severe pregnancy-induced hypertension [PIH], cord prolapse, chorioamnionitis, abruptio placentae), and in women with systemic fungal infection.

Adverse Reactions and Side Effects: Seizures, headache, vertigo, hypertension, increased perspiration, petechiae, ecchymoses, facial erythema, maternal infection, pulmonary edema (if administered with beta-adrenergic medications). May worsen certain maternal conditions such as diabetes and hypertension.

Route and Dosage: 12 mg IM q24h × 2 doses

Nursing Implications:
1. Inform the woman of the benefit of medication and the need to administer to prevent RDS in her preterm infant.
2. Teach the woman the signs and symptoms of pulmonary edema; assess lung sounds.
3. Shake the suspension well; prolonged exposure to heat and light must be avoided.
4. Administer the medication into a large muscle; avoid the deltoid to prevent local atrophy.
5. Vital signs must be monitored frequently and fetal monitoring should be performed according to institution policy.
6. Accurate intake and output must be monitored and recorded.
7. Monitor blood sugars if the woman is diabetic or at risk for diabetes.
8. Do not administer if the woman has an infection
NOTE: The FDA has not approved the medication for this use.

Data from Deglin, J.H., & Vallerand, A.P. (2009). *Davis's drug guide for nurses* (11th ed., pp. 350–360). Philadelphia: F.A. Davis; and Hayes, E., Kee, J., & McCuistion, L. (2006). *Pharmacology: A nursing process approach* (5th ed., pp. 674–678). St. Louis, MO: W.B. Saunders/Elsevier.

CARDIOPULMONARY TRANSITIONS

Cardiopulmonary adaptations must also occur during the transition from fetal to neonatal pulmonary functioning. As air enters the lungs, the P_{O_2} rises in the alveoli. This normal physiologic response causes pulmonary artery relaxation and results in a decrease in pulmonary vascular resistance. As the pulmonary vascular resistance decreases, pulmonary blood flow increases, reaching 100% by the first 24 hours of life. The increased pulmonary blood volume contributes to the conversion from fetal to newborn circulation (Fig. 17-3). Once the pulmonary circulation has been functionally established, blood is distributed throughout the lungs.

Although a variety of hemoglobins are present in the fetus and newborn, the most significant types are fetal hemoglobin (HbF) and adult hemoglobin (HbA). Since HbF has a greater affinity for oxygen than does HbA, the newborn's blood oxygen saturation is greater than that found in adults. However, there is less oxygen available to the tissues. Before birth, this situation is beneficial— the fetus must maintain an adequate oxygen uptake despite low oxygen tension levels since the umbilical venous P_{O_2} cannot exceed the uterine venous P_{O_2}.

Assessment of the neonate's cardiopulmonary system must occur immediately after birth. Overall skin color provides one of the most important indicators of how well the neonate is making the transition to extrauterine life. Caucasian infants typically exhibit a central pink hue with **acrocyanosis**, a bluish coloration of the hands and feet that may persist for up to 24 hours until peripheral circulation improves. In dark skinned infants, the mucus membranes provide a better indication of cyanosis than skin color.

The normal respiratory rate for a healthy term newborn is 40 to 60 breaths per minute. The breathing pattern is often shallow, diaphragmatic, and irregular. Abdominal movements should be synchronous with the chest movements. The breathing pattern may include brief pauses that last 5 to 15 seconds. Termed **periodic breathing**, this pattern is usually not associated with any change in skin color or heart rate and it has no prognostic significance. **Apnea** is cessation of breathing that lasts more than 20 seconds. It is abnormal in the term neonate and may or may not be accompanied by changes in skin color or a decrease in the heart rate below 100 beats per minute. Apnea should be reported immediately. Other indicators of respiratory difficulties include expiratory grunting and retractions when the neonate is at rest or a breathing rate that is outside of the normal range.

> **? case study** Baby Girl Emily
>
> Baby girl Emily is a 2-hour-old infant born at 40 weeks' gestation via a normal spontaneous vaginal birth. Her mother is a 20-year-old Caucasian primipara who experienced an uneventful pregnancy and has a strong support system. Baby Emily has remained with her parents in the birthing suite since her birth. Her mother expresses concern about Emily's hands and feet and asks the nurse why they are "bluish" in appearance, when the rest of Emily's body is nice and pink. She also states that at times, Emily seems to "stop breathing."
>
> **critical thinking questions**
>
> 1. What would you tell Emily's parents about the bluish appearance of Emily's hands and feet?
>
> 2. What would you tell Emily's parents about Emily's breathing pattern?
>
> ◆ See Suggested Answers to Case Studies in the text on the Electronic Study Guide or DavisPlus.

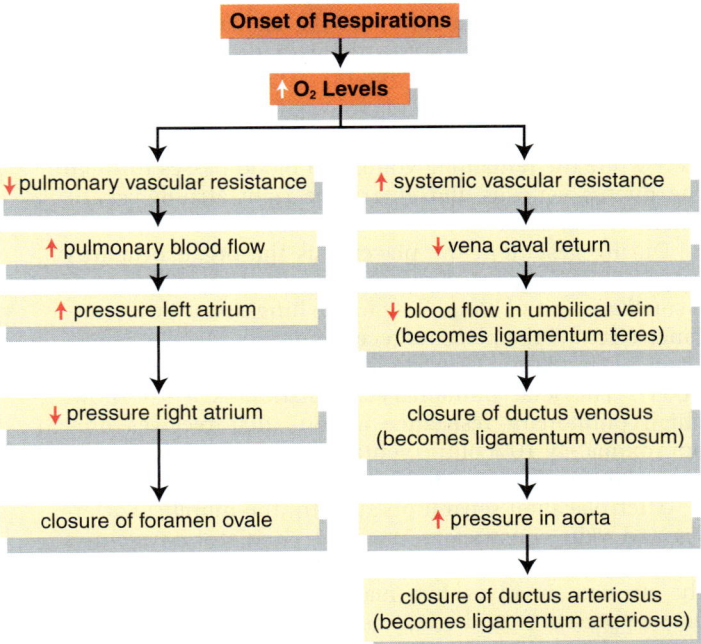

Figure 17-3 Major events that occur during the transition from fetal to neonatal circulation include closure of the foramen ovale, the ductus arteriosus, and the ductus venosus.

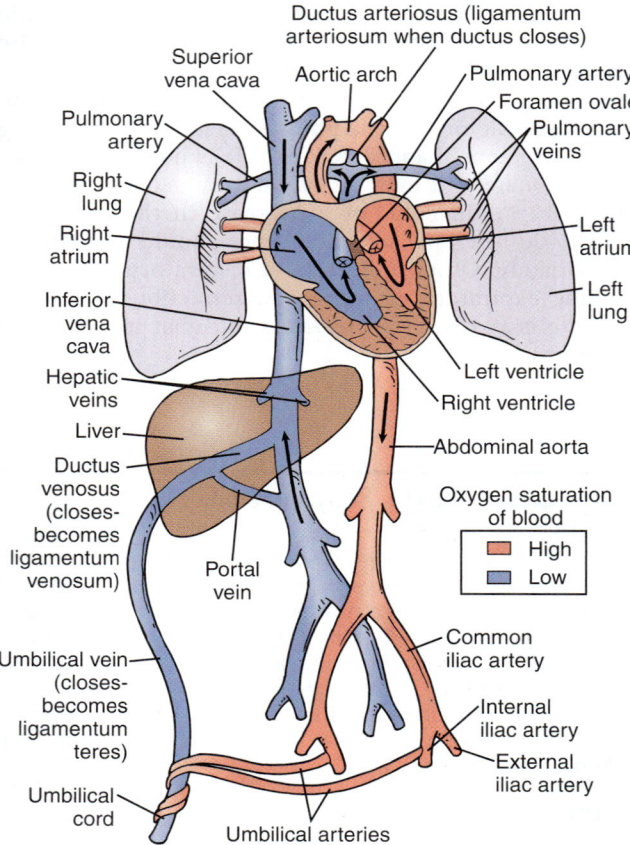

Superior
vena cava

Ductus arteriosus (ligamentum
arteriosum when ductus closes)

Aortic arch

Pulmonary artery

Foramen ovale

Pulmonary
artery

Pulmonary
veins

Right
lung

Left
atrium

Right
atrium

Left
lung

Inferior
vena
cava

Left ventricle

Hepatic
veins

Right ventricle

Liver

Abdominal aorta

Ductus
venosus
(closes-
becomes
ligamentum
venosum)

Portal
vein

Oxygen saturation
of blood

High
Low

Umbilical vein
(closes-
becomes
ligamentum
teres)

Common
iliac artery

Internal
iliac artery

External
iliac artery

Umbilical
cord

Umbilical arteries

Figure 17-4 Neonatal circulation.

Cardiovascular Adaptation

CHANGES AFTER PLACENTAL EXPULSION

Expulsion of the placenta following childbirth triggers important physiological events in the transition process. In utero, the placenta serves as the exchange organ for oxygen and nutrients and for the excretion of fetal waste products such as carbon dioxide. Maternal oxygenated blood enters the fetal circulation via the umbilical vein. Approximately 40% to 60% of the blood perfuses the fetal liver while the remaining volume of blood passes through the ductus venosus and enters the right atrium via the inferior vena cava.

During gestation, the placenta is the organ primarily responsible for gas exchange in the fetus although there is a small amount of blood flow to the lungs. As a "low resistance circuit," the placenta receives approximately 50% of the fetal circulation (Hernandez, Zabloudil, & Hernandez, 2004). The fetal pulmonary circulation is a low flow, "high pulmonary resistance circuit" that receives only approximately 10% of the ventricular output (MacDonald et al., 2005). (See Chapter 7 for further discussion.)

After placental separation at birth, the umbilical arteries and vein constrict as the fetal circulatory system is interrupted. Successful cardiopulmonary adaptation in the neonate involves five major changes: an increased aortic pressure and decreased venous pressure; an increased systemic pressure and decreased pulmonary

pressure; and closure of the foramen ovale, the ductus arteriosus, and the ductus venosus (Hernandez & Hernandez, 2004) (Fig. 17-4). A summary of the structural changes in circulation that take place in the neonate is presented in Table 17-1.

Closure of the Foramen Ovale

The foramen ovale is a flap in the septum of the fetal heart that allows blood flow between the left and right atria. Oxygen-rich blood returning to the heart from the inferior vena cava crosses from the right atria to the left atria across the foramen ovale. This pathway allows most of the oxygenated blood to bypass the nonfunctioning lungs and supply the aorta and vessels of the heart and head with oxygen. Blood flowing through the foramen ovale accounts for approximately one third of the fetal cardiac output; less than 10% is used for lung perfusion (Barzansky et al., 2006).

The right-to-left shunting ceases once the umbilical cord has been clamped. The ventricular and aortic pressures in the left side of the heart rise. The systemic vascular resistance increases while pressure in the right side decreases. The pulmonary blood vessels respond to the increase in PO_2 during lung expansion and aeration with vasodilation and a decrease in pulmonary vascular resistance. These changes cause an increase in blood flow through the pulmonary veins to the left atrium and lead to an increased left atrial pressure that results in closure of the foramen ovale (MacDonald et al., 2005). Since the foramen ovale is capable only of shunting from right to left, this physiological event closes the shunt. Because of unequal pressures within the heart, the foramen ovale is functionally closed within 1 to 2 hours after birth. Deposits of fibrin and cells seal the shunt and it is physiologically closed by 1 month of age. Permanent closure occurs by the sixth month of life. If the infant experiences difficulties such as asphyxia, acidosis, or cold stress during the physiological transition period, the shunt may reopen and allow for continued right to left shunting due to the increased pressure in the right atria.

Closure of the Ductus Arteriosus

In utero, most of the fetal blood flow occurs across the ductus arteriosus. This structure functions as the pathway between the pulmonary artery and the descending aorta. Blood flow through the ductus arteriosus occurs in a right-to-left direction due to a high pulmonary vascular resistance and low placental resistance. Once the umbilical cord is clamped, placental blood flow ceases and there

Table 17-1 Structural Changes in Circulation After Birth	
Fetus	**Neonate**
Umbilical vein	Ligamentum teres
Ductus venosus	Ligamentum venosum
Foramen ovale	Closed atrial septum
Ductus arteriosus	Ligamentum arteriosum
Umbilical artery	Superior vesical (bladder) artery
	Lateral vesicoumbilical ligaments

is an increase in the systemic blood pressure and vascular resistance. At this point, the lungs oxygenate the blood and the increased PaO_2 stimulates the closure of the ductus arteriosus.

During pregnancy, the placenta produces prostaglandin E_2 (PGE_2), a hormone-like substance that causes vasodilation of the ductus. After birth, declining PGE_2 levels contribute to the closure of the ductus arteriosus. In the neonate, a small amount of blood flowing through the ductus may produce a soft murmur. When present, it can be auscultated at the left sternal border in the area of the second intercostal space. Considered innocent, the functional murmur occurs in the absence of any cardiac anomalies and is generally asymptomatic (Miller & Newman, 2005).

Functional closure of the ductus arteriosus in a term infant typically occurs within the first 72 hours of life. Once permanent closure occurs at 3 to 4 weeks, the structure is termed the **ligamentum arteriosum.** Permanent closure results from endothelial destruction, connective tissue formation and subintimal proliferation (MacDonald et al., 2005).

The infant whose birth transition has been complicated by factors such as asphyxia or prematurity has an increased risk of a return to fetal circulation. This event results from continued blood flow through the partially opened ductus arteriosus. Low levels of oxygenated blood flowing through the shunt cause it to dilate, creating a serious transitional complication (MacDonald et al., 2005).

Closure of the Ductus Venosus

The ductus venosus links the inferior vena cava with the umbilical vein. The umbilical vein delivers approximately 50% of the placental blood flow through the ductus venosus into the inferior vena cava and then mixes with the systemic venous drainage from the lower body. Blood flow through the left hepatic vein mixes with blood in the inferior vena cava and flows toward the foramen ovale. Oxygenated blood traveling through the umbilical vein enters the left ventricles and supplies the carotid arteries with oxygen (Barzansky et al., 2006). Once the umbilical cord is clamped, cessation of umbilical venous blood return, along with mechanical pressure changes, lead to closure of the ductus venosus. Closure of the bypass route forces enhanced blood flow to the liver. Fibrosis occurs in the nonfunctional ductus venosus and the structure, which is termed the **ligamentum venosum**, usually closes by the end of the first week.

 Now Can You— Discuss cardiopulmonary transitions in the neonate?

1. Explain characteristics of periodic breathing in the neonate?
2. Identify when the ductus venosus functionally closes?
3. Describe the physiological event that causes closure of the foramen ovale?

ASSESSING THE CARDIOVASCULAR TRANSITION

It is important to continually monitor the newborn's cardiovascular status during transition. Immediately after birth, the newborn's pulse rate may reach 160 to 180 beats per minute but during the first 30 minutes of life, the rate should decline to 120 to 160 beats per minute. This normal fluctuation occurs in response to the cardiovascular transition and the newborn's behavioral states.

On assessment, the systemic circulation is deemed adequate if the newborn exhibits a brisk capillary refill and stable blood pressure. Capillary refill in less than 3 seconds is considered adequate. A refill time greater than 4 seconds may be indicative of an underlying condition such as sepsis, hypoxia, or cardiovascular or central nervous system compromise.

 Across Care Settings: **Facilitating newborn transition in a birth center**

It is essential that the nurse who assists with an unexpected birth in a nonhospital setting such as a minor care clinic or physician office be able to recognize behaviors associated with normal and abnormal physiological transition in the newborn. Since resources outside of the hospital are usually limited, the nurse must be alert to signs of transitional difficulties. As much as is possible, the environment should be manipulated to provide immediate care for the newborn during transition from the intra- to the extrauterine environment. After ensuring effective respirations, facilitating a neutral thermal environment is an essential nursing action. Ideally, a supply of warm, dry linens should be available to prevent neonatal cold stress. In the optimal situation, the nurse has time to evaluate the mother prior to delivery and can be alert to any potential maternal complications during childbirth. A reliable mechanism for the safe transport of the mother and her newborn to the hospital should be established as soon as possible. The nurse must manage care of the neonate and the mother until the transport team arrives.

Thermogenic Adaptation

Neonatal thermoregulation is essential for life sustaining physiologic adaptation. The newborn's ability to maintain a normal body temperature after birth is dependent on factors in the external environment as well as internal physiologic processes. Newborns are characteristically **homeothermic**—that is, they attempt to regulate and maintain their internal core temperature regardless of varying external environmental temperatures.

THE NEUTRAL THERMAL ENVIRONMENT

Thermogenic adaptation is closely related to the infant's rate of oxygen consumption and metabolism. The **neutral thermal environment** (NTE) is the range of temperature in which the newborn's body temperature can be maintained with minimal metabolic demands and oxygen consumption. To maintain a neutral thermal environment, the neonate may need to make certain vasomotor adjustments, such as vasoconstriction to conserve heat or vasodilation to release heat.

Factors such as the infant's body size and gestational age can affect the ability to maintain a neutral thermal environment. Although the term newborn's protective subcutaneous fat helps to maintain a barrier for prevention of heat loss, neonates have less than half of the amount of subcutaneous fat normally present in adults. Preterm infants are born with very little adipose tissue and lack the muscle development needed to maintain a flexed position for heat conservation. Although full-term newborns have a large body area in relation to the total body mass, their normal position of flexion facilitates maintenance of body heat.

As the newborn transitions to extrauterine life, the core body temperature decreases in response to the environmental temperature. A term infant's core temperature can fall by approximately 0.5°F (0.3°C) per minute up to a total of 5.4°F (3°C) before ever leaving the birthing area. However, most term newborns are able to restore the initial decline in body temperature and stabilize at a normal temperature of 97.7°F (36.5°C) to 98.6°F (37°C) within 2 to 3 hours after birth (Hernandez & Hernandez, 2004).

FACTORS RELATED TO COLD STRESS

Exposure to low environmental temperatures, especially for a prolonged period of time, causes an increase in oxygen consumption and an increased rate of metabolism. These metabolic events lead to cold stress. All newborns are at high risk for cold stress and ineffective thermal regulation due to the following factors:

• Large body area in relation to body mass
• Limited subcutaneous fat
• Limited ability to shiver
• The skin is thin and their blood vessels are close to body surface

PHYSIOLOGICAL ADAPTATIONS FOR HEAT PRODUCTION

When the infant is exposed to a cold environment, several physiological adaptations help him to increase heat production. These include increasing the basal metabolic rate and muscle activity to generate heat, peripheral vasoconstriction to conserve heat, and **nonshivering** (or chemical) **thermogenesis** (NST) (heat production). Unlike children and adults, newborns are unable to shiver to generate heat. Instead, they must produce heat via NST and this process becomes the key mechanism for maintaining a neutral thermal environment.

The sympathetic nervous system responds to skin receptors programmed to recognize a drop in the environmental temperature. Once low temperatures are detected, the receptors alert the sympathetic nervous system. Nonshivering thermogenesis utilizes the newborn's stores of **brown adipose tissue** (BAT) to provide heat in the cold-stressed newborn. Formation of brown adipose tissue in the fetus begins at around 26 to 30 weeks of gestation. The deposits of BAT steadily increase until 2 to 5 weeks after birth unless they have been depleted by cold stress. Stores of brown adipose tissue are located in the midscapular area, around the neck, and in the axillae. Deeper deposits are found around the trachea, esophagus, abdominal aorta, kidneys, and adrenal glands (Fig. 17-5).

Brown adipose tissue, also known as "brown fat," is a unique highly vascular fat found only in newborns. BAT derives its name from the rich abundance of blood

Figure 17-5 Sites of brown adipose tissue stores in the newborn.

vessels, cells, and nerve endings that cause it to appear dark in color. The masses of brown fat cells accelerate triglyceride metabolism, triggering a process that produces heat. Rapid metabolism, along with the generation of heat, quickly sends heat to the peripheral circulation. However, fatty acids are released from metabolized BAT and can cause a life-threatening metabolic acidosis. When the elevated fatty acids are released into the blood stream, the infant is at risk for jaundice due to interference with the transport of bilirubin to the liver (Sedin, 2006).

Optimizing Outcomes— **Preventing cold stress in the newborn**

An important factor in neonatal resuscitation is the prevention of cold stress. Several body systems are affected when the infant has difficulty maintaining a normal temperature and becomes hypothermic. During nonshivering thermogenesis, the newborn metabolizes brown fat, a process that increases the metabolic rate and oxygen consumption. Over time, the newborn uses all available glucose and glycogen stores while attempting to maintain a neutral thermal environment. Utilization of the brown fat stores places the infant at risk for metabolic acidosis. Decreased oxygen causes peripheral vasoconstriction and increases the likelihood of respiratory distress. Peripheral vasoconstriction can lead to increased pulmonary vascular resistance and a return to fetal circulation as a compensatory mechanism. Elevated fatty acids can interfere with the transport of bilirubin to the liver and increase the risk of jaundice (Sedin, 2006) (Fig. 17-6).

MECHANISMS FOR NEONATAL HEAT LOSS

The nurse's role in preventing neonatal cold stress is critical. Supporting thermoregulation after birth allows the newborn to have a successful transition from intrauterine to extrauterine life. Thorough assessments of all of the newborn's systems should be aimed at maintaining a neutral thermal environment. The newborn has four mechanisms by which heat is lost after birth: evaporation, conduction, convection, and radiation (Fig. 17-7).

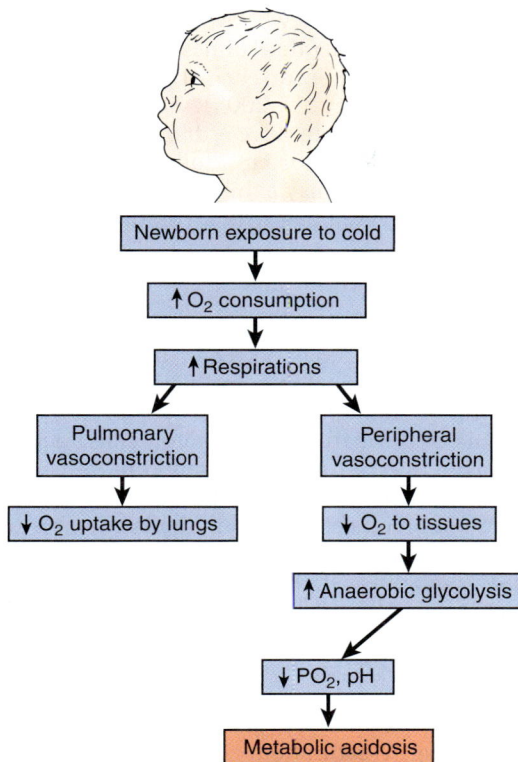

Figure 17-6 Metabolic events associated with cold stress in the neonate.

Evaporation

Evaporation is the loss of heat that occurs when water is converted into a vapor. If not adequately dried after birth, the neonate loses heat through the evaporation of amniotic fluid on the skin. This invisible process is termed **insensible water loss** (IWL). Nursing interventions geared toward preventing evaporative heat loss include thoroughly drying the neonate after birth, promptly removing wet linens, and immediately placing a hat on the head to prevent evaporation through the scalp.

Conduction

Conduction is the loss of heat to a cooler surface via direct skin contact. Conductive heat loss occurs when the infant is placed on a cold surface, such as a cold scale, mattress, or examining table. Nursing interventions to minimize conductive heat loss include placing the infant on a prewarmed radiant warmer, using warmed blankets, covering scales with blankets prior to weighing, and avoiding the use of cold instruments (e.g., stethoscope). The newborn can also be placed skin to skin with the mother to facilitate body warming and bonding.

Convection

Convection is the loss of heat from the warm body surface to the cooler air currents. Convective heat loss occurs when the neonate is exposed to drafts and cool circulating air. The nurse can help minimize neonatal heat loss through convection by preventing drafts in the birth area (e.g., no ceiling fans) and by placing the newborn away from doors or windows. Also, depending on the environment, the neonate should be warmly clothed and possibly swaddled to prevent cooling from air currents.

Radiation

Radiation heat loss occurs when there is a transfer of heat between objects that are not in direct contact with each other. The walls of the nursery or the incubator may serve as potential sources of heat loss through radiation. Nursing interventions to prevent heat loss through radiation include having a prewarmed radiant warmer present at the birth, avoiding placement of the crib or incubator by a cold window, and keeping cold objects well away from the neonate.

PREVENTING HYPERTHERMIA

It is also important to prevent neonatal **hyperthermia** (elevated core body temperature). Although sweating is the full-term infant's initial response to elevated body temperature, the sweat glands are not fully functional until after the first month of life. Before that time, the body loses heat through peripheral vasodilation and the evaporation of insensible water loss. An increase in oxygen consumption and the metabolic rate are associated with hyperthermia and when severe, brain damage, or death may result.

During the first few minutes of life, neonatal hyperthermia is most often associated with maternal fever (Hertz, 2005). An elevated core body temperature can

Figure 17-7 The four mechanisms of heat loss in the newborn. *A.* Evaporation. *B.* Conduction. *C.* Convection. *D.* Radiation.

also result from an ambient environment that is too hot for the newborn to successfully maintain a neutral temperature. Other causes of hyperthermia include infection, CNS impairment, dehydration, and medications.

Radiant warmers, essential equipment in the birth area, must be monitored closely to ensure they are in proper working order with reliable heating mechanisms. Caution must be exercised with the use of servo-controlled radiant warmers since they may cause an undesirable elevation in the neonate's temperature if not monitored correctly. In addition, if programmed to maintain a set temperature, these units may the mask the signs and symptoms of an infection if the neonate is not appropriately assessed. On discharge, the nurse needs to teach parents to closely monitor body temperature when placing the newborn in a sunny location to decrease elevated bilirubin levels. (See Chapters 18 and 19 for further discussion.)

 Now Can You— Discuss thermoregulation in the newborn?

1. Define nonshivering thermogenesis and discuss its effect on thermoregulation in the newborn?
2. Identify three nursing interventions to prevent heat loss by evaporation and convection after birth?
3. Explain how depletion of the brown adipose tissue stores places the term newborn at risk for respiratory distress?

Hematopoietic Adaptation

As with most of the neonate's other body systems, the hematopoietic system is not fully mature at birth. Instead, in the days following birth, the neonate's hematopoietic system transitions from an in utero oxygenation pathway to an extrauterine perfusion pathway.

BLOOD VOLUME

The full-term infant's average blood volume ranges from 80 to 90 mL/kg of body weight, as compared with a blood volume of 90 to 105 mL/kg of body weight in the preterm infant. The neonate's blood volume is determined in large part by the timing of umbilical cord clamping. At birth there is a transfer of blood from the placenta to the neonate: approximately one fourth of the fetal blood volume is transferred within the first 15 seconds; approximately one half of the fetal blood volume is transferred by the end of the first minute of life. The umbilical vessels carry approximately 75 to 125 mL of blood at birth and the neonate's total blood volume may be increased by as much as 61%, depending on a delay in cord clamping (MacDonald et al., 2005).

Currently, much debate surrounds the issue of how long the umbilical cord should be allowed to pulsate before it is clamped. Holding the neonate below the level of the placenta and delaying the clamping of the cord may allow up to a 100 mL/kg increase in the neonate's total blood volume. The increase in blood volume may facilitate an improved transition due to enhanced pulmonary perfusion and the gain of additional iron stores. A disadvantage of this practice concerns the increased risk of jaundice due to the higher volume of erythrocytes and possible resultant polycythemia.

Blood volume in the newborn varies according to gestational age, a factor that determines the amount of circulating volume, and the occurrence of prenatal or postnatal hemorrhage (Bloom et al., 2005). Maternal prenatal or perinatal hemorrhage can have a dramatic impact on the infant's hematopoietic system; following a significant hemorrhage the infant may exhibit decreased hemoglobin and hematocrit levels along with a risk of hypovolemia.

BLOOD COMPONENTS

Erythrocytes and Hemoglobin

At birth, the neonate has a greater number of erythrocytes and higher hemoglobin and hematocrit levels than those found in an adult. During early fetal development, erythropoiesis (formation of red blood cells) occurs primarily in the liver. At approximately 6 months of gestation, the bone marrow becomes the site for hematopoiesis (formation of blood cells). During the later stages of fetal development, fetal hemoglobin (HbF) is slowly replaced by adult hemoglobin (HbA) (MacDonald et al., 2005). Fetal hemoglobin carries 20% to 50% more oxygen than adult hemoglobin.

The process of erythropoiesis is stimulated by the renal hormone erythropoietin. Red blood cell (RBC) production increases in response to a rise in erythropoietin after low fetal oxygen saturation. This physiological event facilitates adequate tissue perfusion and oxygenation. After the initiation of normal respirations at birth, the neonate's oxygen saturation rises, causing an inhibition in the secretion of erythropoietin. This event inhibits the production of red blood cells. The neonate's erythrocytes (fetal RBCs) have a shorter life span (90 days) than do adult erythrocytes (120 days). As the neonate's red blood cell count decreases from deterioration of the fetal erythrocytes, physiological anemia of infancy may develop and persist for 2 to 3 months. The life span of erythrocytes in the full term neonate is 60 to 70 days; for the preterm neonate, the RBC life span is only 35 to 50 days. In the event of hemolysis, the hemoglobin is broken down and bilirubin is released into the systemic circulation. If large numbers of RBCs are involved, blood levels of bilirubin rise and the newborn becomes jaundiced (Pagana & Pagana, 2006). (See Chapter 19 for further discussion.)

Hematocrit

Hematocrit is defined as a percentage of red blood cells within a certain unit volume of blood. Normal neonatal blood values vary according to gestational age and the volume of placental blood that was transfused at the time of birth (i.e., delayed cord clamping) (Table 17-2). Hematocrit levels are generally higher in peripheral blood samples due to peripheral vasoconstriction and the stasis of blood cells. A peripherally drawn hematocrit for a normal infant ranges from 48% to 64%. If the hematocrit drawn from a central site is greater than 65%, the infant is considered to be polycythemic. **Polycythemia**, an abnormally high erythrocyte count, is a condition that can place the infant at high risk for jaundice and organ damage due to increased viscosity of the blood cells. Polycythemic infants are also at an increased risk for hypoglycemia and respiratory distress. Under routine circumstances, unless the infant exhibits signs and symptoms associated with

Table 17-2	Laboratory Values for the Normal Term Neonate: Blood
Blood Component	**Normal Range**
Albumin	3.6–5.4 g/dL
Amylase	0–1000 IU/hr
Bicarbonate	20–26 mmol/L
Bilirubin, direct	Less than 0.5 mg/dL
Bilirubin, total	Less than 2.8 mg/dL (cord blood)
0–1 days	2.6 mg/dL (peripheral blood)
1–2 days	6–7 mg/dL (peripheral blood)
3–5 days	4–6 mg/dL (peripheral blood)
Bleeding time	2 Minutes
Arterial blood gases	
pH	7.35–7.45
$Paco_2$	35–45 mm Hg
Pao_2	50–90 mm Hg
Venous blood gases	
pH	7.35–7.45
$Paco_2$	41–51 mm Hg
Pao_2	20–49 mm Hg
Calcium, ionized	2.5–5 mg/dL
Calcium, total	7–12 mg/dL
Glucose	30–125 mg/dL
Hematocrit	48%–64%
	53% (cord blood)
Hemoglobin	17–18.4 g/dL
	16.8 g/dL (cord blood)
Platelets	150,000–300,000/mm³
Immunoglobulins, total	660–1439 mg/dL
Iron	100–250 mcg/dL
Red blood cell count	4,800,000–7,100,000/mm³
White blood cell count	9000–30,000/mm³

Adapted from Nettina (2007) and Pagana & Pagana (2006).

transitional difficulties, hematocrit and hemoglobin levels are not routinely assessed (Pagana & Pagana, 2006).

Leukocytes

Leukocytes (white blood cells [WBCs]) serve as the major defense against infection in the neonate. The WBCs are classified into five categories: neutrophils, eosinophils, basophils, lymphocytes, and monocytes. Neutrophils act as phagocytes that ingest and destroy small particles of bacteria and cellular debris. Eosinophils perform similar duties but are less effective. However, eosinophils survive for longer periods of time and are important mediators in an allergic and anaphylactic response. Basophils play an important role as responders to allergic and inflammatory reactions. Lymphocytes respond to graft versus host allergic diseases and allergic reactions. Monocytes clean up old blood cells and cellular debris and remove activated clotting factors from the circulation.

An elevated leukocyte count in a normal newborn does not always indicate infection. During the first 12 hours after birth, the leukocyte count typically remains elevated before it begins to decline. The average white blood cell count in the term newborn is 18,000/mm³, but ranges from 9000 to 30,000/mm³ are considered to be within normal limits. Infection is usually associated with a decrease in the leukocyte count. Neonatal sepsis is accompanied by an increased number of immature leukocytes along with a decrease in the total platelet count (Roberts, 2005). (See Chapter 19 for further discussion.)

Platelets

Due to the absence of vitamin K at birth, the neonate is at risk for developing a blood clotting deficiency during the first few days of life. To facilitate clotting, the following blood factors must be present: factor II (prothrombin) and factors VII, IX, and X. Vitamin K, synthesized in the infant's intestinal tract, is not produced in the intestines until food and normal intestinal flora are present.

The infant is given an intramuscular injection of vitamin K_1 phytonadione (AquaMEPHYTON) during the initial care and assessment to prevent hemorrhagic disease of the newborn. (See Chapter 19 for further discussion.) The normal newborn's platelet (thrombocyte) levels range from 150,000 to 300,000/mm³ and are essentially the same as in adults. Small for gestational age (SGA) infants may have platelet counts up to 25% lower than those found in appropriate for gestational age neonates. Circulating platelets are hypoactive during the first few days of life. Although this physiological phenomenon prevents the newborn from developing thrombosis, there may be an increased risk for bleeding and coagulopathy (Pagana & Pagana, 2006).

Hepatic Adaptation

The newborn's liver is a large organ that accounts for about 40% of the total abdominal area. It is palpable approximately 2 to 3 cm below the right costal region. An essential organ, the liver is responsible for the regulation of blood glucose, iron storage, bilirubin conjugation, and coagulation of the blood.

GLYCOGEN AND BLOOD GLUCOSE MAINTENANCE

Throughout pregnancy, the fetus receives glucose by way of the placenta. During the last 4 to 8 weeks of gestation, the glucose is stored as glycogen in the fetal liver and skeletal system for use after birth. Glucose is utilized more rapidly in the newborn than in the fetus because of the metabolic events that occur during the normal transitional phase. The newborn requires added energy to accomplish several essential tasks to offset the stress of birth, to initiate breathing, to activate muscular activity, and to produce heat.

The stressful events associated with the birth process prompt the conversion of fats and glycogen to glucose. After delivery, an increase in circulating catecholamines triggers the release of glycogen from the neonate's liver. Glycogen provides a ready source of glucose to the brain and other vital organs. During the first three hours of life, a healthy term newborn may utilize up to 90% of his liver's glycogen stores (Hernandez & Hernandez, 2004). Although the brain's primary source of fuel is glucose, ketones, lactic acids, fatty acids, and glycerol can also be utilized if necessary to maintain an adequate supply of energy. The liver's ability to adequately convert glycogen to glucose for fuel is essential for a successful physiologic transition.

The blood glucose of a term infant should be 70% to 80% of the maternal blood glucose level. The maternal glucose level is influenced by a number of factors including the timing and contents of the last meal consumed, the duration and mode of delivery and the components of any intravenous fluids or medications administered during labor and birth.

During the first 4 to 6 hours of life, the newborn's main source of energy is glucose. The serum blood glucose level drops during the first 3 hours of life and then gradually rises over the next 3 to 4 hours to reach a steady state of 40 to 80 mg/dL. **Glycogenolysis,** the breakdown of glycogen into the more usable form of glucose within the body tissues, can occur if the newborn does not receive any exogenous glucose before the initial hepatic and skeletal glycogen stores have been depleted. This process prompts the release of glucose into the bloodstream as needed to maintain normal blood levels.

Hypoglycemia

Hypoglycemia can occur after any stressful events (e.g., hypothermia, hypoxia) that increase metabolic demands. Nurses must be aware of risk factors associated with neonatal hypoglycemia (Box 17-1). For example, preterm and SGA infants may not have accumulated the glycogen stores necessary to maintain serum glucose levels required for energy needs. Large for gestational age (LGA) and infants of diabetic mothers (IDM) may produce too much insulin postnatally and rapidly metabolize their glucose stores (Kalhan & Parimi, 2006). Postterm or intrauterine growth restricted (IUGR) fetuses can develop hypoglycemia related to poor intrauterine nourishment from a deteriorating placenta. Consequently, they have depleted glucose stores before birth. Neonates exposed to postbirth stressors such as asphyxia, infection, or cold stress rapidly utilize their glucose stores to assist with the transition process (Hertz, 2005). (See Chapter 19 for further discussion.)

 critical nursing action Recognizing Hypoglycemia in the Neonate

When assessing the neonate during the transitional period, the nurse should be alert to signs and symptoms of hypoglycemia. These include jitteriness, diaphoresis, poor muscle tone, poor sucking reflex, temperature instability (low temperature), respiratory distress, tachycardia, dyspnea, apnea, high-pitched cry, irritability, lethargy, seizures, or coma. However, the infant may be asymptomatic. Therefore, awareness of prenatal and perinatal risk factors that may predispose to postnatal hypoglycemia is essential.

Labs: Neonatal Blood Glucose Assessment

Capillary blood obtained from the neonate's heel is commonly used to assess blood glucose. When available, a heel warmer is used to increase blood flow to the sample site. The area is cleansed with a sterile alcohol pad and the heel is gently punctured, taking care to avoid the middle area where there is a risk for nerve damage or puncture of the plantar artery. A large drop of blood is placed on the test strip and a sterile bandage is used to apply pressure on the sample site.

IRON STORAGE

During the last few weeks of pregnancy, iron is stored in the fetal liver. As RBCs are destroyed after birth, the neonatal liver stores additional iron until needed for the production of new RBCs. At term, the newborn has approximately 270 mg of iron, and of this amount, 140 to 170 mg of iron is contained in the hemoglobin. Adequate maternal iron intake during pregnancy ensures that a sufficient amount of iron is available in the infant to last up to 6 months of age. Term infants who are exclusively breastfed do not need additional iron until at least 6 months of age. However, formula-fed infants should be given an iron-fortified formula, and beginning at 6 months, all infants should receive iron supplements or iron-rich foods to prevent anemia (Luchtman-Jones, Schwartz, & Wilson, 2006).

CONJUGATION OF BILIRUBIN

Conjugation of bilirubin constitutes a major function of the newborn's liver. Conjugation is a process that converts the yellow lipid-soluble (nonexcretable) bilirubin pigment (present in bile) into a water-soluble (excretable) pigment. **Jaundice** is a condition characterized by a yellow (icteric) coloration of the skin, sclera, and oral mucous membranes. Jaundice results from the accumulation of bile pigments associated with an excessive amount of bilirubin in the blood (**hyperbilirubinemia**). This condition occurs in approximately 60% of full-term infants and in up to 80% of preterm infants. The presence of jaundice is directly related to the liver's maturity and its ability to conjugate bilirubin (MacDonald et al., 2005).

Bilirubin is produced from the hemolysis (breakdown) of erythrocytes. Removal of bilirubin begins in the reticuloendothelial system, where mononuclear phagocytes remove aging RBCs from the circulation. Heme, the oxygen-carrying component of hemoglobin, is broken down into

---

Box 17-1 Risk Factors for Hypoglycemia in the Neonate

- Prematurity
- Postmaturity
- Intrauterine growth restriction (IUGR)
- Large or small for gestational age (LGA or SGA)
- Asphyxia
- Difficult transition at birth
- Cold stress
- Maternal diabetes
- Maternal intake of ritodrine (Yutopar) or terbutaline (Brethine)
- Infections

three elements: iron, carbon monoxide, and biliverdin. Iron, stored in the hemoglobin, is used for a number of essential bodily functions. Carbon monoxide is exhaled through the lungs as a waste product, and biliverdin is further broken down into lipid-soluble bilirubin.

During the process of normal conjugation, bilirubin attaches to the blood albumin and is transported to the liver. In the liver, the unbound bilirubin detaches from the albumin, and is conjugated with glucuronide in the presence of the enzyme glucuronyl transferase. This process produces water-soluble **direct bilirubin**, which is excreted into the common duct and duodenum. Normal intestinal flora reduce the direct bilirubin into urobilinogen and stercobilinogen. This product is then excreted as a yellow-brown pigment in the stools, and a small amount is excreted through the kidneys. The physiological pathway for the excretion of bilirubin is presented in Figure 17-8.

The breakdown of 1 gram of hemoglobin yields approximately 34 mg of bilirubin. The normal term newborn produces 6 to 10 mg of bilirubin per kilogram per day. In comparison, adults produce 3 to 4 mg of bilirubin per kilogram per day. The increased bilirubin production in the newborn is related to the high concentration of RBCs at birth and the shortened life span of fetal erythrocytes (Hernandez & Hernandez, 2004).

Conjugated or "direct" bilirubin has been converted from a lipid-soluble, nonexcretable pigment into a water-soluble, excretable pigment. Unconjugated, or "indirect" bilirubin is fat-soluble and nonexcretable. The newborn's liver must be able to convert the fat-soluble (nonexcretable) bilirubin into a water-soluble (excretable) form by way of conjugation. Elevated blood levels of unconjugated bilirubin can be toxic and result in **kernicterus**, a life-threatening condition caused by the deposition of unconjugated bilirubin in the brain and spinal cord. (See Chapter 19 for further discussion.)

The total serum bilirubin level (TSB) is a measurement of both the conjugated and unconjugated bilirubin. At birth, the normal total serum bilirubin level is 3 mg/dL or less. Before birth, the fetus does not need to conjugate bilirubin; instead, unconjugated bilirubin is transferred across the placenta for maternal excretion. After birth, the neonate's liver must be able to satisfactorily conjugate bilirubin (MacDonald et al., 2005).

 Nursing Insight— Maternal medications may decrease neonatal albumin-binding sites

Maternal ingestion of medications such as aspirin and sulfa drugs may reduce the number of albumin-binding sites in the infant and result in neonatal hyperbilirubinemia.

Risk Factors for Hyperbilirubinemia

Neonatal jaundice that occurs during the first week of life most often results from excessive levels of unconjugated bilirubin. Unlike pathologic jaundice (present at birth or occurring during the first 24 hours), the signs of physiologic jaundice do not occur until *after* the first 24 hours of life. Jaundice is usually first noted on the face and sclera when the serum bilirubin levels reach approximately 4 to 6 mg/dL. The yellow coloration then progresses caudally as the total serum bilirubin level rises to 6 to 7 mg/dL (Bhutani, Johnson, & Keren, 2005). Many maternal and neonatal factors such as ethnicity, diabetes, prematurity, and delay in feeding place the infant at risk for hyperbilirubinemia (Box 17-2). (See Chapter 18 for further discussion.)

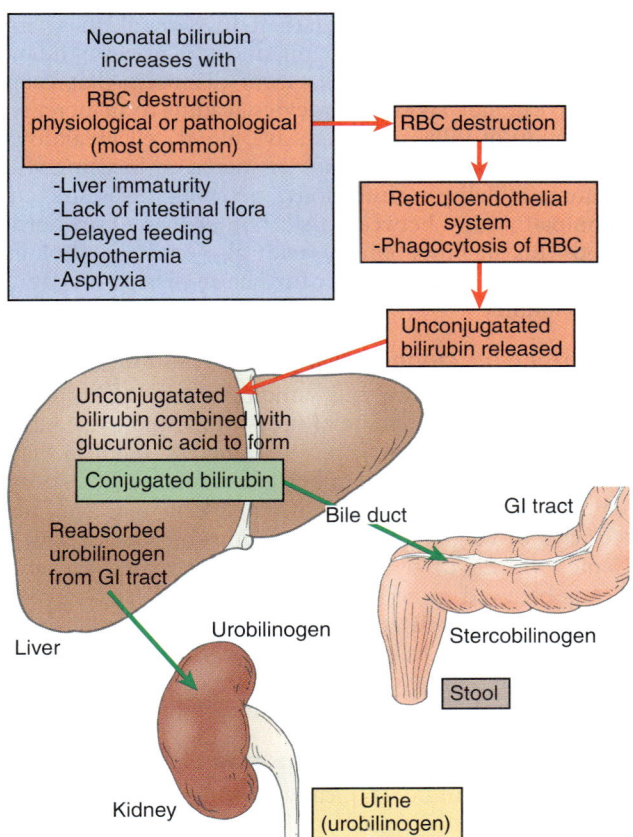

Figure 17-8 Physiological pathway for the excretion of bilirubin.

Box 17-2 **Factors that May Influence Bilirubin Levels in the Neonate**

- Cultural background: Chinese, Japanese, Korean, and Native American neonates exhibit higher bilirubin levels than do European and American Caucasian neonates. The elevated levels of bilirubin persist for a longer period of time and cause no apparent adverse effects.
- Perinatal events (i.e., delayed cord cutting, breech presentation, the use of Pitocin).
- Prematurity.
- Maternal diabetes.
- Excess bilirubin production (e.g., hemolytic diseases such as Rh isoimmunization and ABO incompatibility; sepsis; metabolic disorders).
- Delayed feedings.
- Liver immaturity (i.e., prematurity; glucose-6-phosphate dehydrogenase deficiency).
- Birth trauma.
- Family history of jaundice or previous child with jaundice.
- Neonatal complications (i.e., asphyxia neonatorum, cold stress, hypoglycemia).

Ethnocultural Considerations— Neonatal jaundice and RBC enzyme defects

Jaundice occurs with greater frequency in infants of Chinese, Japanese, Korean, Native American, and Greek descent. In these populations, there is an increased incidence of red blood cell enzyme defects, including glucose-6-phosphate dehydrogenase (G6PD) deficiency and pyruvate kinase deficiency. G6PD deficiency, an X-linked recessive disorder, represents one of the most common autosomal recessive traits. It occurs most frequently in Mediterranean, Middle-Eastern, Southeast Asian, and African infants. An estimated 11% to 13% of African American infants who are born in the United States are affected as well (Hernandez & Hernandez, 2004). Pyruvate kinase deficiency, also an autosomal recessive trait, is the next most common enzyme deficiency. Affected infants typically display symptoms of jaundice, anemia, and reticulocytosis (MacDonald et al., 2005).

Perinatal events, such as delayed clamping of the umbilical cord, increase the volume of circulating erythrocytes and predispose the neonate to an increased breakdown of RBCs and the subsequent development of jaundice. Traumatic births that involve the use of forceps or vacuum extraction, and fetal presentations that increase the likelihood of bruising, all lead to erythrocyte destruction. Although the mechanism is unclear, there is evidence to suggest that the use of oxytocin and epidural medications may lead to hemolysis of RBCs and serve as an increased source of jaundice (Verklan & Walden, 2004).

Infants who begin feeding early and are feeding well soon establish normal intestinal flora and the regular passage of meconium, which contains large amounts of bilirubin. Infants with delayed or poor feedings have a prolonged exposure to the enzyme beta-glucuronidase, which converts conjugated bilirubin back into deconjugated bilirubin, which is then reabsorbed into the blood. Premature infants, whose livers and blood–brain barriers are immature, do not yet produce the enzymes necessary for bilirubin conjugation and thus are at an increased risk for jaundice (Hertz, 2005).

Development of Physiological Jaundice

Physiological jaundice occurs in more than 60% of term newborns and in up to 80% of preterm newborns. Physiological jaundice is the transient form of jaundice that typically occurs after the first 24 to 48 hours of life and becomes visible when the total serum bilirubin level is greater than 5 mg to 7 mg/dL. The rate at which the bilirubin level climbs and peaks in relation to the weight and gestational age of the infant is an important parameter of assessment in terms of treatment (MacDonald et al., 2005). In the presence of physiological jaundice, bilirubin levels typically peak between days 5 to 7 and then gradually decline after 10 to 14 days of life. Peak bilirubin levels are reached between the 3rd and 5th days in the term infant and between the 5th and 7th days in the preterm infant. The interaction of the following four factors can lead to the development of physiological jaundice:

• There is an increased amount of bilirubin presented to the liver. This is related to an increase in blood volume (following a delay in cord clamping) and

accelerated RBC destruction due to their shortened life span. Newborns produce and break down two to three times more bilirubin than do adults.

• There is a decreased reabsorption of bilirubin from the intestines. This is related to the decreased caloric intake common in most infants during the first few days of life. When the caloric intake is inadequate, the production of hepatic binding proteins is decreased and the levels of bilirubin rise.

• Defective bilirubin conjugation related to a decrease in glucuronyl transferase activity (as occurs in hypothyroidism, for example) coupled with inadequate caloric intake may cause saturation of the intracellular binding proteins and result in increased blood levels of unconjugated bilirubin. Also, fatty acids present in breast milk are believed to compete with bilirubin for albumin binding sites and interfere with bilirubin metabolism.

• A defect in bilirubin excretion may result from a congenital infection. A delay in the introduction of normal bacterial flora coupled with decreased intestinal motility may cause delayed excretion and increase the bilirubin deconjugation process via the enterohepatic circulation (MacDonald et al., 2005).

Development of Nonphysiological or Pathological Jaundice

Pathological jaundice occurs within the first 24 hours of life. The infant may exhibit a total serum bilirubin concentration (TSB) that increases by 0.5 mg/dL per hour or 5 mg/dL per day. The diagnosis is usually made when TSB concentrations climb greater than 12.9 mg/dL in a term infant and greater than 15 mg/dL in a preterm infant. Pathological jaundice results from disorders that cause excessive hemolysis of erythrocytes, leading to an increased production of bilirubin. Excessive blood cell breakdown may result from polycythemia or increased bruising after a traumatic delivery. Infections, metabolic disorders, and incompatibilities between the mother's and newborn's blood (Rh incompatibility) may also cause pathologic jaundice. (See Chapter 19 for further discussion on pathologic jaundice.)

Breastfeeding Jaundice (Early-Onset Jaundice)

Breastfeeding jaundice is a condition that occurs when there is a decreased intake of breast milk and a decreased passage of meconium. Breastfed infants tend to have higher bilirubin levels than bottle-fed infants. Breastfeeding jaundice generally occurs between the 2nd and 4th days of life. The total serum bilirubin levels peak at 15 mg to 19 mg/dL by 72 hours of life. Breastfeeding jaundice is believed to be associated with poor feeding practices and is not related to the composition of the breast milk. Early and frequent feedings with avoidance of formula and glucose supplementation constitutes the primary therapy for breastfeeding jaundice (Hertz, 2005).

Breast Milk Jaundice (Late-Onset Jaundice)

Breast milk jaundice typically occurs in the full-term infant, with an incidence of approximately 2% to 4%. This condition has a later onset than breastfeeding jaundice and usually appears after the first week of life and peaks around day 10. Unlike physiological jaundice, a condition characterized by declining bilirubin levels within the first week, bilirubin levels associated with breast milk jaundice continue to rise and peak at 2 to 3 weeks of life. Meanwhile, infants typically are thriving, stooling appropriately, and gaining weight without any evidence of hemolysis (Hertz, 2005).

At one time, it was thought that breast milk jaundice was related to an enzyme in the breast milk that inhibited the action of glucuronyl transferase. Today the appearance of breast milk jaundice is believed to be related to a factor in human milk that increases the intestinal absorption of bilirubin. In most circumstances, no intervention is necessary. If the infant continues to breastfeed, the TSB gradually declines over the course of a few weeks. Some experts recommend temporarily halting breast feeding for 48 hours to allow the serum bilirubin levels to decline. It is important to carefully monitor infants and provide phototherapy or supplemental nutrition when needed (Verklan & Walden, 2004). (See Chapter 18 for further discussion.)

COAGULATION OF BLOOD

Another important function of the liver involves the production of coagulation factors to enable the newborn to effectively clot blood after birth. The coagulation factors are activated by vitamin K (AquaMEPHYTON), given to the newborn within one hour following birth. An intramuscular injection of Vitamin K (AquaMEPHYTON) given prophylactically within this first hour of life prevents hemorrhagic diseases of the newborn. Coagulation factors synthesized in the liver include prothrombin and factors II, VII, IX, and X. Circulating levels of the coagulation factors vary according to the gestational age of the infant (MacDonald et al., 2005).

 Now Can You— Discuss neonatal jaundice?

1. Identify two factors that may place an infant at risk for physiological jaundice?
2. Explain why infants of Mediterranean descent are at a higher risk for jaundice?
3. Discuss why delayed cord clamping at birth can affect the development of jaundice?

Gastrointestinal Adaptation

STOMACH AND DIGESTIVE ENZYMES

The neonate's stomach capacity is approximately 6 mL/kg at birth and by the end of the first week of life, the capacity has increased to hold approximately 90 mL. In utero, the fetal gastrointestinal system reaches maturity around 36 to 38 weeks of gestation when there is sufficient enzymatic activity for digestion and the transport of nutrients throughout the body. To nutritionally thrive, newborns must be able to digest essential carbohydrate disaccharides that include lactose, maltose and sucrose. Lactose, the primary carbohydrate in breast milk, is easily digested and readily absorbed (Hertz, 2005). A deficiency of pancreatic amylase, the only enzyme lacking at birth and during the first few months of life, makes it difficult for infants to digest fats efficiently. Newborns also have a decreased production of pancreatic lipase and bile acids, which further limits their ability to absorb fats.

Production of pancreatic lipase gradually increases during the first few weeks of life.

INTESTINAL PERISTALSIS

Fetal peristalsis can be influenced by anoxia, which triggers the expulsion of meconium into the amniotic fluid. Immediately after birth, air enters the stomach and reaches the small intestine within 2 to 12 hours. Bowel sounds are present within the first 15 to 30 minutes of life due to the air that has entered the stomach and small intestines. The gastrocolic reflex is stimulated when the stomach fills, and this process helps to enhance intestinal peristalsis. The stomach empties intermittently, usually at the beginning of a feeding and up until 2 to 4 hours after a feeding. The salivary glands are immature at birth; little saliva is produced for the first 3 months of life. The cardiac sphincter (located between the esophagus and the stomach) is immature, and it is not unusual for newborns to regurgitate small amounts following feedings (Hertz, 2005).

Compared to the overall body size, the newborn's intestines are long, a feature that provides an increased surface area for the absorption of nutrients. However, if diarrhea occurs, the additional surface area places the infant at an increased risk for dehydration and water loss. Infants born at term generally pass their first meconium stool within 8 to 24 hours of life. An important nursing function includes documentation of the first meconium stool. Absence of passage of a bowel movement by 72 hours of age may be indicative of an obstructive bowel problem (Miller & Newman, 2005).

Meconium consists of particles found in the amniotic fluid such as vernix, skin cells, hair, and cells that have been shed by the intestinal tract. Meconium stools, which are characteristically greenish-black and viscous, gradually change to transitional stools that are thinner and greenish-brown to yellowish-brown. The newborn may pass stools from one to ten times a day over a 24-hour period. Following the transitional stools, stool appearance and frequency varies, depending on whether the infants is breast- or bottle-fed.

 Now Can You— Discuss gastrointestinal functioning in the newborn?

1. Describe the fetal to newborn transition process that takes place in the gastrointestinal tract?
2. Identify the enzymes that aid in digestion and those that are deficient at birth?
3. Identify when bowel sounds become present in the newborn?

Genitourinary Adaptation

KIDNEY FUNCTION

In the term newborn, the following three major physiological factors enable the kidneys to manage bodily fluids and excrete urine:

- The nephrons are fully functional by 34 to 36 weeks of gestation.
- The glomerular filtration rate is lower than that of the adult.
- There is a limited capacity for the reabsorption of HCO_3^- and H^+.

Although the fetal kidneys contain working nephrons by 34 to 36 weeks of gestation, the kidneys are not mature and fully functional until after birth when the newborn becomes responsible for the elimination of waste products. The neonate's elevated hematocrit (related to the high concentration of RBCs) and low blood pressure may lead to a decreased glomerular filtration rate (GFR) (the volume of glomerular filtrate that is formed over a specific period of time). With a low GFR, the newborn's kidneys are unable to dispose of fluid rapidly and tend to reabsorb excess sodium. As the kidneys mature and enlarge, the GFR rapidly increases during the first 4 months of life. Adult GFR values are reached at around 2 years of age (MacDonald et al., 2005).

In the neonate, urine specific gravity normally ranges from 1.002 to 1.010. Term newborns are unable to adequately concentrate urine (reabsorb water back into the blood) because the kidney tubules are short and narrow. This alteration may lead to an inappropriate loss of substances such as amino acids and glucose. By 3 months of age, infants are able to fully concentrate their urine (Modi, 2005). Normal laboratory values for components in the neonate's urine are presented in Table 17-3.

Along with the lungs and circulatory system, the kidneys perform an important function in helping the body maintain a normal acid–base balance. Several factors can interfere with the newborn's ability to maintain homeostasis in this system. The limited capacity for tubular reabsorption of HCO_3^- and H^+ can lead to a loss of essential substances (e.g., amino acids, bicarbonate, glucose, sodium) in the filtrate. Due to immaturity of the newborn's kidneys, there is a greater capacity for glomerular filtration than for tubular reabsorption and secretion (Cloherty, Eichenwald, & Stark, 2004).

It is important for the nurse to carefully monitor the newborn's intake and output to prevent overhydration and/or dehydration. Most newborns void immediately after birth or within the first few hours, although some may not void for up to 24 hours. On average, approximately 68% of normal newborns void within the first 12 hours, 93% by 24 hours, and 100% will have voided by 48 hours. Recording the neonate's first voiding is an important nursing action. If voiding has not occurred by 24 hours of life, the nurse must alert the pediatrician or neonatal nurse practitioner. The infant may be experiencing hypovolemia related to an insufficient fluid intake. Failure to void during the first 24 hours of life may also indicate the presence of an obstruction in the urinary outflow system and the infant should be carefully assessed for bladder distention, restlessness, and symptoms of pain (Hernandez & Hernandez, 2004).

Initially, the newborn's bladder capacity ranges from 6 to 44 mL of urine. During the first 2 days of life, infants normally void two to six times in a 24-hour period, with a total output of 15 mL/day. Urine output is significantly higher in infants with edema. By the fourth day, the frequency of voiding should have increased to more than six voids in a 24 hour period. Since the kidneys have difficulty concentrating urine and removing waste products from the blood immediately after birth, small amounts of protein and glucose are frequently present in the urine. Urate crystals, which are pink-red in color, are excreted in the urine and can be mistaken for blood. The crystals (sometimes referred to as "brick dust spots") disappear after the first few days of life as kidney function matures.

During the first 24 to 48 hours, full-term newborns require 60 to 80 mL/kg of fluids to maintain an adequate fluid balance. This requirement increases to 100 to 150 mL/kg per day after the first few days, and a urine output of 1 to 3 mL/kg per hour is indicative of adequate fluid maintenance (Hertz, 2005). Because the neonate's kidneys are unable to tolerate large changes in volume, careful monitoring of fluid balance is essential. Large changes in fluid balance can create a problem if the infant becomes ill and needs to receive intravenous fluids during that time. Nursing diagnoses for the neonate experiencing difficulty during the transitional period may be related to the specific organ system(s) involved, environmental factors, or medical interventions (Box 17-3).

Assessing the appearance of the newborn's urine is important when evaluating genitourinary system function. When necessary, the nurse may need to apply a urine collection bag to obtain a urine sample from the infant.

Table 17-3 Laboratory Values for Urine in the Normal Term Neonate

Urine Component	Normal Range
Casts, WBC	Normal to be present for the first 2–4 days
Osmolality (maximum concentration ability)	800 mOsmol/L*
(Maximum diluting ability)	25–30 mOsmol/L
pH	4.5–8.0
Phenylketonuria	No color changes
Specific gravity	1.002–1.010
Protein	May be present during first 2–4 days
Glucose	Negative
Blood	Negative
Leukocytes	Negative

Adapted from Cloherty, Eichenwald, & Stark (2004) and Nettina (2007).

Box 17-3 Possible Nursing Diagnoses Related to Newborn Physiological Transitions

- Altered Health Maintenance related to separation from the maternal support system.
- Risk for Infection related to the newborn's immature immunological system.
- Risk for Ineffective Airway Clearance related to excessive fluid present in lungs during neonatal transition.
- Risk for Pain related to increased environmental stimuli.
- Risk for Ineffective Thermoregulation related to the newborn's immature temperature regulation systems.
- Altered Nutrition: Less than Body Requirements related to limited nutritional and fluid intake and increased caloric expenditure.

After the first voiding the urine may be cloudy (from mucus) and contain (innocuous) urate crystals. The urine should be odorless and straw colored to clear in appearance as the newborn's fluid intake increases.

Immunological Adaptation

The newborn's immunological system remains immature after birth and may not adequately react to an infectious process. Signs of infection in the newborn can be very subtle and often are not as obvious as they would be in an older child. The newborn receives immunity through two types of methods: active acquired immunity and passive acquired immunity. The pregnant woman's exposure to illness and immunizations prompts the development of antibodies in a process termed **active acquired immunity.** The infant receives **passive acquired immunity** through antibodies that have been passed through the placenta by way of the IgG immunoglobulins.

There are three primary immunoglobulins: IgG, IgA, and IgM. These immunoglobulins, also referred to as humoral antibodies, are proteins that are synthesized in response to a specific antigen. Humoral immunity is important in protecting the newborn against bacterial and viral infections. Low levels of immunoglobulins and immature leukocyte function in destroying pathogens render the newborn especially vulnerable to infections.

IgG is the only immunoglobulin able to pass through the placenta before birth. Placental transfer of this immunoglobulin occurs primarily during the third trimester. At birth, full-term infants have already acquired immunity to tetanus, diphtheria, smallpox, measles, mumps, poliomyelitis, and a host of other bacterial and viral diseases. Preterm infants born before 34 weeks of gestation are at a greater risk for infection. Passive acquired immunity typically disappears by 6 months of age. The infant continues to develop antibodies by active acquired immunity either by direct exposure to an infection with the subsequent development of antibodies or through the immunization schedule recommended by the American Academy of Pediatrics (AAP) and the Centers for Disease Control and Prevention (CDC) (Cant & Gennery, 2005; Kapur, Yoder, & Poplin, 2006).

IgA is important in protecting the infant against gastrointestinal and respiratory infections. Colostrum and breast milk are important sources of IgA, and this factor constitutes yet another benefit of breastfeeding. IgA is not detectable in the newborn's system until at least 2 to 3 weeks of life, unless elevated levels are present from a viral infection (Cant & Gennery, 2005).

IgM immunoglobulins are produced in response to blood group antigens, gram-negative enteric pathogens, and certain maternal viruses. This immunoglobulin is synthesized early in utero, beginning at approximately 10 to 15 weeks of gestation. Detectable levels are reached by 30 weeks of gestation and IgM serum concentrations increase rapidly after birth. Elevated levels at birth may result from placental leaks or, more likely, from antigenic stimulation that occurred in utero. Thus, an increased IgM titer is suggestive of exposure to an intrauterine infection such as syphilis or one of the TORCH infections (toxoplasmosis, rubella, cytomegalovirus, herpes virus) (Kapur et al., 2006). (See Chapter 11 for further discussion.)

 Nursing Insight— *Preventing newborn infections*

Newborns are especially susceptible to infections due to their immature immune system and their poor ability to fight infections. During the birth process, the neonate is exposed to a vast number of potential infectious agents, such as *Staphylococcus* and group B *Streptococcus*. Newborns do not exhibit signs and symptoms of infection in the same manner as do older infants and children. Instead, they may demonstrate subtle behavior changes and poor feeding patterns, develop respiratory distress, or become hypothermic. Maintenance of skin integrity is crucial, especially in the preterm infant, because the skin is thin and fragile. The nurse's awareness of potential risk factors (e.g., maternal group B *Streptococcus* exposure) and thorough assessment skills are essential in the prevention and early detection of newborn infections. Circumcision sites, healing heel sticks, and umbilical stumps are all potential areas for infection that can challenge the newborn's immature immune system. Providing parents with thorough discharge instructions regarding infant hygiene, proper skin care, and awareness of signs and symptoms of infection is an important component of the nursing care plan.

 Now Can You— **Discuss aspects of the genitourinary and immunological systems?**

1. Identify three physiological factors that enable the newborn's kidneys to produce and excrete urine?
2. Explain the origin and significance of "brick dust spots" in the neonate's urine?
3. Describe what is meant by "humoral immunity"?

Psychosocial Adaptation

EARLY STAGES OF ACTIVITY

Full-term infants experience several "activity" stages during the early hours after birth. It is important to educate parents about normal neonatal behavior during this period and encourage them to enjoy this opportunity to become acquainted with their newest family member. An understanding of normal neonatal activities during the first hours of life provides reassurance and empowers them to promptly recognize and seek assistance for any signs of difficulty. The infant's psychosocial adaptation begins with two stages of activity followed by a period of sleep.

The First Period of Reactivity

This stage is the first period of active, alert wakefulness that the infant displays immediately after birth (Fig. 17-9). It may last from 30 minutes to 2 hours and is a wonderful time for parents to get to know their baby, and to perform their first full "inspection" of their infant. The newborn is very alert during this stage and moves around energetically while taking in the new surroundings. The heart rate and respirations are rapid and the infant may exhibit occasional nasal flaring and grunting that can last for up to 15 minutes. Muscle tone and motor activity are increased. Body temperature is decreased. Bowel sounds tend to be absent during this period and there is minimal saliva

Figure 17-9 The mother and her newborn become acquainted during the first period of reactivity.

production (Hernandez & Hernandez, 2004). This first period of reactivity is an opportune time for the mother to initiate breastfeeding if she wishes to do so.

Optimizing Outcomes— Promoting initial bonding in the breastfeeding mother

Best outcome: The nurse places the infant on the mother's chest for skin-to-skin contact and eye-to-eye contact for early bonding. The infant nuzzles the mother's breast, smells colostrum, and attempts to latch-on to the breast during the first period of reactivity.

The Period of Inactivity and Sleep

After being awake and alert for the first 30 minutes to 2 hours after birth, the neonate settles in to the sleep phase. At this time the infant displays decreased muscle activity and is difficult to awaken, instead resting quietly and recovering from the stress of birth. The heart rate and respirations return to a normal range. Central perfusion and general coloring should be excellent at this time, although acrocyanosis is not unusual (Hernandez & Hernandez, 2004). The sleep period may last from a few minutes to 2 to 4 hours.

The Second Period of Reactivity

At this time, the newborn awakens and becomes alert once again. Most infants show signs for feeding readiness (e.g., sucking, rooting) and are eager to begin feeding if not previously fed. During the second period of reactivity the newborn becomes increasingly more responsive to exogenous and endogenous stimulation, which can cause the heart rate to become labile. The infant may exhibit brief periods of tachycardia, tachypnea, and rapid changes in color and muscle tone. The nurse needs to be aware of normal newborn behaviors during this period that may last for minutes up to several hours. Careful and ongoing assessment allows for differentiation between normal reactions and symptoms that signal difficulty with transition (Hernandez & Hernandez, 2005).

Bowel sounds are usually present and the infant may have increased oral mucus, causing transient episodes of gagging and vomiting. The nurse should monitor the infant closely, assess for a clear airway and have suctioning equipment readily available. Parents should be taught how to use a bulb syringe correctly in the event of gagging or vomiting episodes (Hernandez & Hernandez, 2004). (See Chapter 18 for further discussion.) The gastrointestinal system becomes more active during the second period of reactivity and it is not unusual for newborns to pass their first meconium stool or void if they have not already done so.

Newborn Behavioral States

SLEEP STATES

According to Brazelton (1999), newborn behavior can be divided into the sleep state and the alert state. Two sleep states are exhibited: the deep or quiet sleep and the period of active rapid eye movement (REM). The length of time spent in each sleep cycle is dependent on the newborn's age. At term, REM active and quiet sleep occurs in intervals of approximately 50 minutes. Approximately one half of the infant's total sleep is "active" sleep. Forty-five percent is "quiet" sleep and 10% is transitional sleep occurring between the two periods. It has been suggested that REM sleep is instrumental in promoting growth of the neural system. As the infant matures, the sleep–wake cycle adjusts to a diurnal pattern of sleeping during the night and remaining awake during the day.

Nursing Insight— *Recognizing sleep states in the neonate*

Nurses who care for newborns should be aware of behaviors typically exhibited during deep, quiet sleep and active rapid eye movement (REM) sleep. During deep sleep, the infant's eyes are closed, no eye movements occur, and breathing is regular and even. Jerky motions are common although behavioral responses to external stimuli are delayed. The heart rate ranges from 100 to 120 beats per minute.

During REM sleep, the infant's respirations are irregular, the eyes are closed with REMs visible through the lids, and irregular sucking motions are common. There is minimal activity. Environmental and internal stimuli may prompt a startle reaction and a change of state.

ALERT STATES

The quiet alert state, which generally occurs during the first 30 minutes to 1 hour after birth, characterizes the first period of reactivity. This period is an excellent time for parents to enjoy bonding with their infant. The periods of alertness are fairly brief during the first 2 days of life as the infant recovers from the events associated with birth. After that time, the infant's alert states result from choice or necessity. Stimuli that may prompt wakefulness include hunger, cold, and heat. Once the triggering stimuli are removed, the infant tends to fall back asleep. The alert state has been subcategorized into four distinct

Nursing Care Plan Normal Newborn Transition

Nursing Diagnosis: Readiness for Enhanced Organized Infant Behavior related to effective modulation of the physiological and behavioral systems of functioning

Measurable Short-term Goal: The newborn will transition to necessary extrauterine cardiorespiratory, feeding, and elimination functions without complications.

Measurable Long-term Goal: The newborn and mother (family) will experience successful interactions and psychosocial adaptation to each other.

NOC Outcomes:

Newborn Adaptation (0118): Adaptive response to the extrauterine environment by a physiologically mature newborn during the first 28 days.

Parent–Infant Attachment (1500): Parent and infant behaviors that demonstrate an enduring affectionate bond.

NIC Interventions:

Newborn Monitoring (6890)
Environmental Management (6480)
Breastfeeding Assistance (1054) or
    Bottle Feeding (1052)
Attachment Promotion (6710)

Nursing Interventions:

1. Before birth, review maternal record for antenatal or intrapartal complications, events, or medications that may affect the neonate. Prepare room and equipment for the birth.

   RATIONALE: Review allows anticipation and preparation for complications that may occur at birth.

2. Dry newborn with prewarmed blankets while on mother's abdomen. Assess respiratory effort, clear airway and stimulate as needed. Discard wet blankets, cover mother and infant with a warm, dry blanket, and place a cap on the infant's head.

   RATIONALE: Prevents heat loss by evaporation and convection and helps open the airway and initiate respirations.

3. Assess newborn's heart rate and color. Complete Apgar scoring at 1 and 5 minutes of age. If the score is 7 or greater, continue to monitor infant.

   RATIONALE: Heart rate and color provide information about cardiovascular transition to extrauterine function. Infants with Apgar scores of 7 or higher are considered stable.

4. Once the umbilical cord has been cut, assess the number of cord vessels and encourage mother to put the baby in kangaroo care (skin-to-skin) at the breast.

   RATIONALE: It is easiest to note the cord vessels in a freshly cut cord. Kangaroo care helps the newborn maintain temperature and facilitates breastfeeding.

5. Offer instruction about breast feeding if needed and give praise and encouragement. Provide time and space for first feeding.

   RATIONALE: During the first period of reactivity, the unmedicated infant is alert and ready to breastfeed. The mother should not be overwhelmed with teaching and nursing activity but encouraged to get to know her baby.

6. Continue to monitor infant's vital signs per protocol. Encourage stable infant to remain with mother in kangaroo care for first period of reactivity.

   RATIONALE: The stable infant benefits most from maternal contact. Vital signs can be monitored in the mother's arms.

7. At a convenient time during the first 2 hours, place the infant under a radiant warmer with a servo-controlled skin probe in place. Perform a brief physical exam and administer vitamin K and eye prophylaxis as ordered. Place identification bands on the infant and mother.

   RATIONALE: The radiant warmer and probe provide a safe source for external heat as the infant is examined. Vitamin K prevents neonatal hemorrhage and eye prophylaxis is required to prevent eye infection. Two forms of identification applied before separation help ensure that the right mother and infant are together.

8. Monitor for passage of urine and first meconium and document. Teach parents about elimination and diapering as needed.

   RATIONALE: The passage of urine and meconium provides information about the normal newborn's anatomy and physiology. Every opportunity for teaching should be appreciated during the short hospital stay.

9. Observe the parents' interactions with the newborn: eye contact, stroking, talking to baby. Point out attractive features and infant's responses to parents. Offer encouragement to fathers to touch and hold their newborn.

   RATIONALE: Observation helps the nurse identify appropriate behaviors related to attachment and bonding with the newborn. Encouragement provides the novice father with "permission" to parent.

phases: drowsy or semidozing, wide awake, active awake, and crying (Brazelton, 1999).

Drowsy or Semidozing

Physical manifestations include open or closed eyes; fluttering eyelids; semidozing appearance; and slow, regular movement of the extremities. There is a delayed response to external stimuli.

Wide Awake

The infant is alert and follows and fixates on attractive objects, faces, or auditory stimuli. There is minimal motor activity and a delayed response to external stimuli.

Active Awake

The eyes are open, motor activity is intense and the infant displays thrusting movements of the extremities. Environmental stimuli increases the motor activity.

Crying

Jerky movements accompany intense crying. Crying often serves as a distraction from unpleasant stimuli such as hunger and pain. It allows the infant to discharge energy and elicits a helpful response from the parents.

 Now Can You— Discuss psychosocial adaptation in the newborn?

1. Compare and contrast the first period of reactivity and the period of inactivity/sleep?
2. Identify two behavioral characteristics associated with deep, quiet sleep and REM sleep?
3. Name four phases of the quiet alert state and identify two behavioral characteristics of each phase?

---

summary points

◆ Surfactant, a lipoprotein that reduces surface tension, is essential in keeping the lungs expanded during expiration.

◆ Initiation of the neonate's first breath is influenced by chemical, sensory, thermal, and mechanical factors.

◆ Successful cardiopulmonary adaptation in the neonate is dependent on five major changes related to aortic, venous, and pulmonary pressures and closure of the foramen ovale and ductus arteriosus and ductus venosus.

◆ A number of factors, including body size and gestational age, affect the neonate's ability to maintain a neutral thermal environment.

◆ Heat loss may occur through the processes of evaporation, conduction, convection, and radiation.

◆ The neonate's liver has essential roles in iron storage, carbohydrate metabolism, bilirubin conjugation, and blood coagulation.

◆ The neonate receives immunity through active acquired immunity and passive acquired immunity.

◆ The newborn exhibits two periods of reactivity and two behavioral states that may be divided into sleep states and alert states.

review questions

Multiple Choice (Select all that apply.)

1. The perinatal nurse explains to the new nurse that some infants have increased surfactant production prior to birth that facilitates their transition including:
   A. Infants of mothers with gestational hypertension
   B. Infants of mothers with placental insufficiency
   C. Infants of mothers with abruptio placentae
   D. Infants of mothers with a multiple gestation

2. The perinatal nurse describes a typical newborn breathing pattern to the new parents as:
   A. Shallow
   B. Irregular
   C. About 40 to 60 breaths per minute
   D. About 60 to 80 breaths per minute

3. The perinatal nurse understands that many factors stimulate the newborn to begin breathing including:
   A. Hypercarbia, acidosis, and hypoxia
   B. Sensory stimuli
   C. Decreased temperature in the environment
   D. Cutting the umbilical cord

4. The perinatal nurse recognizes that the infant that develops respiratory distress syndrome is at risk for further complications such as:
   A. Loss of functional residual capacity
   B. Atelectasis
   C. Poor lung compliance
   D. Hypoglycemia

5. The perinatal nurse is caring for Sarah, a primigravid antenatal patient at 32 weeks' gestation. Betamethasone 12 mg IM q24h × 2 is ordered. Appropriate nursing care includes:
   A. Assessing Sarah's temperature and white blood count
   B. Conducting continuous fetal monitoring for 30 minutes pre and post injection
   C. Providing information to Sarah and her family about the benefits of this medication as well as information about the signs and symptoms of pulmonary edema
   D. Monitoring Sarah's intake and output

Fill-in-the-Blank

6. The perinatal nurse understands that pulmonary ventilation in the newborn takes place on three levels: _____ respiration, _____ respiration and at the _____ level.

7. The perinatal nurse explains to the student nurse that _____ _____ is a brief pause between breaths of 5 to 15 seconds while _____ is cessation of breathing for _____ seconds or more.

True/False

8. The perinatal nurse explains to the woman who has given birth to a preterm infant that part of the infant's care is to provide a dose of surfactant, a phospholipid that increases lung compliance.

9. The perinatal nurse prepares for newborn care at a cesarean birth. The nurse knows that this infant is at a higher risk for pulmonary transition difficulties due to the absence of a "thoracic squeeze" during birth.

10. The perinatal nurse assesses the newborn at 2 hours of age. The findings include: respiratory rate of 48 breaths per minute, irregular, no abdominal or chest retractions or grunting. These findings would be normal.

See Answers to End of Chapter Review Questions on the Electronic Study Guide or DavisPlus.

REFERENCES

Barzansky, B., Beckmann, C., Herbert, W., Laube, D., Ling, F., and Smith, R. (2006). *Obstetrics and gynecology* (5th ed.). Philadelphia: Lippincott.

Bhutani, V., Johnson, L., & Keren, R. (2005). Treating acute bilirubin encephalopathy – before it's too late. *Contemporary Pediatrics, 22*(5), 57–70.

Bloom, R. (2006). Delivery room resuscitation of the newborn: Part 1: Overview and initial management. In R. Martin, A. Fanaroff, & M. Walsh (Eds.), *Fanaroff and Martin's neonatal-perinatal medicine: Diseases of the fetus and infant* (8th ed., pp. 483–489). Philadelphia: C.V. Mosby.

Bloom, S., Cunningham, F., Gilstrap, L., Hauth, J., Leveno, K., & Wenstrom, K. (2005). *Williams' obstetrics* (22nd ed.). New York: McGraw-Hill.

Brazelton, T.B. (1999). Behavioral competence. In G.B. Avery, M.A. Fletcher, & M.G. MacDonald (Eds), *Neonatology: Pathophysiology and management of the newborn* (5th ed, pp. 321–332). Philadelphia: Lippincott.

Brazelton Institute. (n.d.). The Newborn Behavioral Observations (NBO) system: What is it? Retrieved from http://www.brazelton-institute.com/cinbas.html (Accessed September 28, 2008).

Bulechek, G., Butcher, H.M., & Dochterman, J. (2008). *Nursing interventions classification (NIC)* (5th ed.). St. Louis, MO: C.V. Mosby.

Cant, A., & Gennery, A. (2005). Neonatal infection. In J. Rennie (Ed.), *Robertson's textbook of neonatology* (4th ed., pp. 509–522). Philadelphia: Churchill Livingstone.

Cloherty, J., Eichenwald, E., & Stark, A. (2004). *Manual of neonatal care* (5th ed.). Philadelphia: Lippincott.

Deglin, J.H., & Vallerand, A.P. (2009). *Davis's drug guide for nurses* (11th ed.). Philadelphia: F.A. Davis.

Dillon, P.M. (2007). *Nursing health assessment: A critical thinking, case studies approach.* Philadelphia: F.A. Davis.

Hayes, E., Kee, J., & McCuistion, L. (2006). *Pharmacology: A nursing process approach* (5th ed.). St. Louis, MO: W.B. Saunders/Elsevier.

Hernandez, J., Zabloudil, C., & Hernandez, P. (2004). Adaptation to extrauterine life and management during transition. In P. Thureen, D. Hall, J. Deacon, & J. Hernandez. *Assessment and care of the well newborn* (2nd ed., pp. 83–100). St. Louis, MO: W.B. Saunders.

Hernandez, P., & Hernandez, J. (2004). Physical assessment of the newborn. In P. Thureen, D. Hall, J. Deacon, & J. Hernandez. *Assessment and care of the well newborn* (2nd ed., pp. 114–125). St. Louis, MO: W.B. Saunders.

Hertz, D. (2005). *Care of the newborn, A handbook for primary care.* Philadelphia: Lippincott.

Johnson, M., Bulechek, G., Butcher, H., McCloskey Dochterman, J., Maas, M., Moorhead, S., & Swanson, E. (2006). *NANDA, NOC, and NIC linkages: Nursing diagnoses, outcomes, & interventions* (2nd ed.). St. Louis, MO: Mosby Elsevier.

Kalhan, S., & Parimi, P. (2006). Metabolic and endocrine disorders. In R. Martin, A. Fanaroff, & M. Walsh (Eds.), *Fanaroff and Martin's neonatal-perinatal medicine: Diseases of the fetus and infant* (8th ed., pp. 1254–1272). Philadelphia: C.V. Mosby.

Kapur, R., Yoder, M., & Poplin, R. (2006). Developmental immunology. In R. Martin, A. Fanaroff, & M. Walsh (Eds.), *Fanaroff and Martin's neonatal-perinatal medicine: Diseases of the fetus and infant* (8th ed., pp. 806–824). Philadelphia: C.V. Mosby.

Luchtman-Jones, L., Schwartz, A., & Wilson, D. (2006). Hematologic problems in the fetus and neonate. In R. Martin, A. Fanaroff, & M. Walsh (Eds.), *Fanaroff and Martin's neonatal-perinatal medicine: Diseases of the fetus and infant* (8th ed., pp. 756–789). Philadelphia: C.V. Mosby.

MacDonald, M., Mullett, M., & Seshia, M. (2005). *Avery's neonatology, pathophysiology & management of the newborn* (6th ed.). Philadelphia: Lippincott.

Miller, C., & Newman, T. (2005). Routine newborn care. In H. Taeusch, R. Ballard, & C. Gleason (Eds.), *Avery's diseases of the newborn* (8th ed., pp. 239–246). Philadelphia: W.B. Saunders.

Modi, N. (2005). Fluid and electrolyte balance. In J. Jennie (Ed.), *Robertson's textbook of neonatology* (4th ed.). Philadelphia: Churchill Livingstone.

Moorehead, S., Johnson, M., Mass, M., & Swanson, E. (2008). *Nursing outcomes classification (NOC)* (4th ed., pp 264–275). St. Louis, MO: C.V. Mosby.

NANDA International. (2007). *NANDA-I nursing diagnoses: Definitions and classifications 2007-2008.* Philadelphia: NANDA-I.

Nettina, S. (2007). *Lippincott manual of nursing practice.* Philadelphia: Lippincott Williams & Wilkins.

Nugent, J.K., Keefer, C.H., O'Brien, S., Johnson, L., & Blanchard, Y. (in press). *Handbook for the newborn behavioral observations (NBO) system.* Baltimore: Paul H. Brookes.

Pagana, K., & Pagana, T. (2006). *Mosby's manual of diagnostic and laboratory tests* (3rd ed.). St. Louis, MO: C.V. Mosby.

Roberts, I. (2005). Haematological values in the newborn. In J. Rennie (Ed.), *Robertson's textbook of neonatology* (4th ed., pp. 204–222). Philadelphia: Churchill Livingstone.

Sedin, G. (2006). Physical environment: Part 1. The thermal environment of the newborn infant. In R. Martin, A. Fanaroff, & M. Walsh (Eds.), *Fanaroff and Martin's neonatal-perinatal medicine: Diseases of the fetus and infant* (8th ed., pp. 146–158). Philadelphia: C.V. Mosby.

Verklan, M., & Walden, M. (2004). *Core curriculum for neonatal intensive nursing* (3rd ed.). St. Louis, MO: Elsevier/W.B. Saunders.

Wong, R., DeSandre, G., Sibley, E., & Stevenson, D. (2006). Neonatal jaundice and liver disease. In R. Martin, A. Fanaroff, & M. Walsh (Eds.), *Fanaroff and Martin's neonatal-perinatal medicine: Diseases of the fetus and infant* (8th ed., pp. 578–586). Philadelphia: C.V. Mosby.

 For more information, go to http://davisplus.fadavis.com/

CONCEPT MAP

First Breath→
Initiating Factors:
- Chemical:
  - Hypercarbia
  - Acidosis
  - Hypoxia
- Sensory changes
- Dramatic temp changes
- Mechanical: lung fluid replaced by air → thoracic squeeze

After 1st Inspiration
- + intrathoracic pressure → establish FRC
- Fetal lung fluid enters circulation
- Progressive decrease in pulmonary vascular resistance

Blood volume: influenced by placental transfer/timing of cord clamp
- HbF replaced by HbA
- Hematocrit: varies by gestational age/placental transfer
- Leukocytes: elevation can be normal
- Platelets: hypoactive at birth: administer vitamin K

Associated CV
- Increased PO_2
- Decreased PVR
- Increased pulmonary blood flow/volume
- Fetal circulation → newborn circulation

Five Major Changes - Facilitated by Cord Clamping
- Increased aortic pressure; decreased venous pressure
- Increased systemic pressure; decreased pulmonary pressure
- Closure of foramen ovale
- Closure of ductus arteriosus
- Closure of ductus venosus

- Stores glucose → blood glucose maintenance
- Birth stress = glycogenolysis, risk for hypoglycemia
- Storage of iron
- Conjugation of bilirubin
- Production of coagulation factors

Essential Transitions

Respiratory System | **Cardiovascular System** | **Hematopoietic** | **Hepatic**

Intrauterine — **BIRTH** → **Physiological Transition of the Newborn**

Optimizing Outcomes:
- Proper infant position to enhance bonding with breastfeeding

Immune | **Thermogenic** | **Gastrointestinal/Genitourinary**

- Loss of passive acquired immunity at 6 months
- Begin active acquired immunity via exposure or immunization
- IgA → from breast milk
- Immature immune system = risk for infection

Thermogenic
- Factors affecting maintenance of NTE:
  - Body size, gestational age, subcutaneous fat
- Factors related to cold stress:
  - Large body area r/t mass, limited subcutaneous fat, limited ability to shiver, thin skin, superficial vessels
- Mechanisms for heat loss:
  - Evaporation; conduction; convection; radiation
- Mechanisms to increase heat production:
  - Increased BMR/muscle activity; peripheral vasoconstriction; non-shivering thermogenesis; utilization of brown adipose tissue

Gastrointestinal
- Increasing production of digestive enzymes
- Passage of meconium stool
- Increasing peristalsis

Genitourinary
- Increasing GFR
- Inability to concentrate urine until 3 months of age
- At risk for acid/base imbalances
- Should void within 12-48 hrs
- Maintain fluid intake → 100–150 mL/kg/24 hrs

Across Care Settings:
- Recognize signs of abnormal physiological transition in infant following home birth

Nursing Insight:
- Be aware of behaviors exhibited in various neonatal sleep states

Now Can You:
- Discuss elements of pulmonary function after birth
- Assess cardiovascular functioning after birth
- Discuss aspects of GU, GI, immune system
- Discuss thermoregulation in the newborn

Critical Nursing Action:
- Be aware of signs and symptoms and risk factors for neonatal hypoglycemia

Caring for the Normal Newborn

 A new baby is like the beginning of all things—wonder, hope, a dream of possibilities.

—Eda J. Le Shan

LEARNING TARGETS *At the completion of this chapter, the student will be able to:*

◆ Identify the components of the immediate newborn assessment.

◆ Describe methods for determining the gestational age of the neonate.

◆ Discuss how to perform a newborn behavioral assessment.

◆ List at least four actions to assess the neonate's transition to extrauterine life.

◆ Identify three sources of heat loss in the neonate and suggest strategies to prevent the heat loss for each.

◆ Describe strategies to prevent neonatal infection.

◆ Describe four activities to promote early infant bonding.

◆ Develop a discharge teaching plan for the mother and her newborn infant.

---

 moving toward evidence-based practice Informing Parents About Newborn Screening

Kemper, A.R., Fant, K.E., & Clark, S.J. (2005). Informing parents about newborn screening. *Public Heath Nursing, 22*(4), 332–338.

The purpose of this cross-sectional study was to evaluate current rules and regulations for educating parents about newborn screening. The sample included 51 newborn screening program coordinators from all 50 states and the District of Columbia. A 20-item telephone survey was used to obtain data about policies, rules, and regulations along with specific topics, such as types of information given to families, and strategies for informing the general public and primary care providers about newborn screening.

Data analysis revealed the following information about newborn screening programs:

• Fifty state programs use standard information to inform parents about newborn screening.
• Thirty-two state programs offer the information in languages other than English.
• Twenty-five state programs have specific requirements for informing parents about the screening; of these, 12 state programs specified who should inform the family and 9 state programs were unclear about how parents should be informed.

• No state program had specific rules or regulations about how to inform parents about newborn screening before birth although 36 state programs indicated the parents should be informed by the obstetrician.
• Thirty state programs indicated that parents should be offered information prenatally and again after delivery.
• Five state programs require parental consent before infant screening.
• Thirty-three state programs do not routinely screen for all conditions recommended by the March of Dimes and the National Newborn screening and Genetic Resource Center. These conditions include but are not limited to phenylketonuria (PKU), congenital hypothyroidism (CH), galactosemia (GALT), maple sugar disease, sickle cell disease, and cystic fibrosis.
• No state program has requirements that parents should be informed about the availability of additional screening.

(continued)

---

moving toward evidence-based practice (continued)

- Thirty-eight state programs have a formal process for parents who wish to refuse screening. Of these, 15 state programs do not require that parents be informed of their right to refuse; 29 state programs have a standardized refusal form; and 6 state programs offer the (refusal) form in languages other than English. Among state programs with no standardized refusal form, documentation of the refusal is left to the individual agency.
- Thirty-nine state programs use outreach education (i.e., press releases, agency Web site) to inform the general public about newborn screening. All but one state program direct educational efforts toward physicians through mailings, medical education activities, and information posted on the agency website.

The researchers concluded that although standardized information is available for parents, few agencies specify how this information is provided and there is much variation in policy language among the screening programs. Although the majority of programs have educational outreach efforts, little information is available regarding the effectiveness of those efforts and how the information can be disseminated to increase the parents' understanding of newborn screening. The investigators suggest that parent education about newborn screening should be initiated during the prenatal period. Providing information at this critical time offers a unique opportunity and challenge for nurses in both obstetric and public health settings.

---

1. What might be considered as limitations to this study?
2. How is this information useful to clinical nursing practice?

See Suggested Responses for Moving Toward Evidence-Based Practice on the Electronic Study Guide or DavisPlus.

Introduction

Most nurses who care for newborns and their families view their specialty to be the most exhilarating and rewarding of any area in nursing. Childbirth marks the beginning of profound changes in the lives of the mother, her infant, and the family. From the moment of the parents' first interaction with their newborn, a journey of growth and exploration begins for each of them. After ensuring that the neonate is physiologically stable, the infant's nurse plays a pivotal role in preserving and protecting this most special time by not intruding or allowing any interruptions as the new family becomes acquainted.

During the transitional period after birth, nursing care focuses primarily on two goals: to safeguard and support the neonate's physical well-being and to promote the establishment of a healthy family unit. The first goal is met by close observation coupled with skilled assessment throughout the time the infant remains in the health care facility. The nurse meets the second goal by educating the family about care of their newborn. Ongoing interaction with the parents provides insights concerning the family's ethnic influences and cultural values, and this information helps to direct and guide the teaching plan. By providing culturally appropriate education along with expressions of support of parenting efforts, the nurse empowers the parents with information and knowledge about their infant's needs. Furthermore, the nurse's teaching efforts can be instrumental in heightening parents' awareness of family adjustments that may need to occur during this time of family transition and role changes (Hisley, 2006). This chapter focuses on the healthy neonate. A system-by-system guide to physical assessment of the infant is provided along with a discussion of nursing measures intended to meet the newborn's needs. Methods to determine the neonate's gestational age are presented. The chapter concludes with infant discharge planning; a list of possible nursing diagnoses for the healthy neonate is presented in Box 18-1.

Box 18-1 **Possible Nursing Diagnoses for the Normal Neonate**

- Risk for Altered Nutrition, Less than Body Requirements, related to inadequate formula intake
- Risk for Altered Body Temperature related to evaporative, conductive, radiant, and convective heat losses
- Risk for Ineffective Airway Clearance related to excessive secretions in the airway
- Risk for Ineffective Thermoregulation related to an immature thermoregulatory system
- Risk for Infection related to parents' lack of knowledge concerning umbilical cord care
- Acute Pain related to circumcision
- Risk for Injury related to lack of parental knowledge about normal newborn needs

---

The Immediate Neonatal Assessment

The newborn infant's physical condition is assessed immediately at the time of birth. If necessary, suctioning of the oral, pharyngeal, or endotracheal area is conducted according to the health facility's policy, procedure, and protocol (Procedure 18-1). The infant is carefully handed to the nurse, who receives the neonate into a sterile baby blanket and, in the ideal situation, places him upon the mother's abdomen. For most, this simple action is a deeply satisfying source of comfort for the mother and her infant and the warmth of the mother's body helps to maintain the neonate's body temperature. In addition, heated blankets placed over the neonate minimize heat loss by evaporation. In other situations, the nurse places the infant in an incubator or directly beneath a radiant heater unit to prevent evaporative heat loss. After being carefully dried off, a cap is placed on the head for extra warmth.

Procedure 18-1 Suctioning the Infant's Oral and Nasal Passages

Purpose

To clear secretions from oral and nasal passages

Equipment

- One bulb syringe
- Tissue

Steps for Oral Suctioning

1. Assess the infant for oral secretions.
2. Position the infant's head to the side or downward if he is vomiting or gagging.
3. Compress the bulb syringe.

   RATIONALE: *Removing the air prevents forcing secretions deeper into the respiratory tract.*

4. Insert the bulb syringe approximately 1 inch into one side of the infant's cheek. Avoid contact with the roof of the mouth and the back of the throat.

   RATIONALE: *To prevent stimulation of the gag reflex.*

5. Gently release compression of the bulb syringe and allow it to fill with oral secretions.
6. Gently remove the bulb syringe; expel drainage into a tissue.
7. Repeat the process on the other side of the infant's cheek.
8. Repeat as needed.

   Clinical Alert Always suction the mouth before suctioning the nares because fluids and secretions that could obstruct the respiratory tract may be present in the mouth or the nares or both. Placing the syringe in the nares first may trigger an inspiratory gasp, causing the infant to pull mucus further into the respiratory tract.

Steps for Nasal Suctioning

1. Assess the infant for nasal congestion.
2. Position the infant's head to the side or downward if he is vomiting or gagging.
3. Compress the bulb syringe.

   RATIONALE: *Removing the air prevents forcing secretions deeper into the respiratory tract.*

4. Insert the bulb syringe into the tip of the infant's nostril. Avoid obstructing the nasal passageway.

   RATIONALE: *To prevent respiratory distress.*

5. Gently release the compression of the bulb syringe to allow it to fill with mucus or nasal drainage.
6. Gently remove the bulb syringe; expel drainage into a tissue.
7. Repeat as needed.

   Clinical Alert An increasing respiratory rate is often the first sign of respiratory comprise or obstruction. If this occurs, measures must be initiated to maintain effective ventilation.

Teach Parents

- Proper technique for use of the bulb syringe; ask for return demonstration.
- Proper care of the bulb syringe: wash in warm, soapy water each day and after each use.
- Store the bulb syringe at the infant's bedside.

Note

Instruct the parents to position the infant's head to the side or downward if he is vomiting or gagging.

Caution: The nurse must emphasize to the parents that the bulb syringe must be compressed first and then inserted into the infant's nostril or mouth. If they insert the bulb syringe and then compress the bulb syringe, they may actually force secretions further back into the nose or throat and possibly cause an obstruction.

Documentation

6/29/10 0300 Baby boy Smith had a small amount of clear thick mucus draining from both nares, respirations 40 per minute, breathing without difficulty, and no retractions noted. Both nares suctioned with bulb syringe with a return of a small amount of clear thick mucus, procedure tolerated without difficulty.

—S. Chang, RN

Optimizing Outcomes— Placing the infant under the radiant heater

Best outcome: The nurse dries the infant before placing him unclothed on a clean, dry blanket under the radiant-heater unit. Since the generated heat from the unit warms only the outer surface of objects, it is counterproductive to cover or clothe the infant, as he will get no benefit from the radiant heat.

While performing these actions, the nurse observes the infant's respiratory effort, color, and muscle tone, and makes sure that the activities underway are stimulating the neonate to breathe deeply and cry. If needed, lightly flicking the infant's soles prompts a crying response.

 Nursing Insight— Observing standard precautions when handling the neonate

Because there is a possibility of transmission of viruses such as hepatitis B (HBV) and human immunodeficiency virus (HIV) from maternal blood and blood-stained amniotic fluid, the neonate is considered a potential contamination source. Nurses must observe Standard Precautions by wearing gloves when handling the neonate until blood and amniotic fluid are removed by bathing.

During the initial assessment, the nurse remains alert for any signs of respiratory difficulty, such as rib or sternal retractions, "grunting" sounds, or nasal flaring. To check the heart rate, the nurse places the thumb and two fingers at the base of the umbilical cord and counts the pulsations. The infant's body temperature may be assessed by recording the axillary temperature or by attaching a thermoprobe and recording monitor to the skin. At this time, the infant is usually crying and turning pink, although the hands and feet remain slightly blue due to acrocyanosis, a condition related to vasomotor insufficiency and poor peripheral perfusion. If necessary, respiratory support is initiated according to hospital protocol. Oxygen may be administered via bag or mask. Obvious abnormalities are noted and the nurse also checks and records the number of vessels in the umbilical cord, which should have two arteries and one vein. If the cord contains only two vessels (one artery, one vein), the physician should be notified immediately since this finding may be associated with renal and cardiac anomalies. Further testing is indicated. A two-vessel cord may be indicative of renal agenesis, a condition in which one kidney fails to develop normally during the gestational period. The infant's weight and length are determined and recorded. Normal newborn parameters are presented in Table 18-1.

A numerical expression of the neonate's well-being, the Apgar score is assigned at 1 and 5 minutes after birth. This score provides an objective means for assessing the neonate's immediate adaptation to extrauterine life. Five categories, including respiratory effort, heart rate, muscle tone, reflex irritability, and skin color are assessed, and each component is given a score ranging from 0 to 2. If neonatal resuscitation is required, it should be initiated before the 1-minute Apgar score (American Academy of

Table 18-1	Normal Neonatal Parameters at Birth
Parameter	**Normal Finding**
Respirations	Rate 30–60 breaths per minute, irregular
	No retractions or grunting
Apical pulse	Rate 120–160 beats per minute
Temperature	97.8°F (36.5°C)
Skin color	Pink body, blue extremities
Umbilical cord	Contains two arteries and one vein
Gestational age	Full term: >37 completed weeks (should be 38–42 weeks to remain with parents for an extended time period)
Weight	2500–4300 grams
Length	45–54 cm

Pediatrics [AAP] & American College of Obstetricians and Gynecologists [ACOG], 2007). (See Chapter 12 for further discussion.)

Various newborn laboratory tests may be routinely ordered according to hospital protocol. One test may be a sample of the cord blood if the mother is Rh negative or has type O blood group. The cord blood for the infant's blood type and Rh factor is obtained by the birth attendant while awaiting placental separation. If the infant's Apgar score is low, cord blood gas analysis may be ordered as well.

When the Apgar score is less than 9 at 5 minutes of life, it is important to stabilize the infant rather than allowing him to remain with his mother in the birthing unit. Other conditions that would necessitate immediate infant stabilization include observations of nasal flaring, grunting respirations, rib retractions, heart rate below 120 beats per minute or above 160 beats per minute, pallor, serious congenital anomalies (such as a neural tube defect), preterm infant (less than 38 weeks' gestational age), infant of a diabetic mother, or an infant who appears to be small for gestational age.

 critical nursing action Recognizing Immediate Neonatal Respiratory Distress

During the neonatal assessment, the nurse is alert to the following signs and symptoms that are indicative of respiratory distress. If any of these symptoms are present, the nurse must immediately notify the physician:

- Generalized cyanosis
- Tachycardia (heart rate >160 beats per minute)
- Tachypnea (respiratory rate >70 breaths per minute)
- Rib retractions
- Expiratory grunting
- Flaring nostrils

IDENTIFICATION

After the Apgar evaluation, the nurse completes the mother–infant identification process according to hospital policy. This procedure usually includes obtaining infant footprints and a fingerprint and thumbprint of the mother along with

Nursing Care Plan Maintaining Newborn Thermoregulation

Nursing Diagnosis: Risk for Imbalanced Body Temperature

Measurable Short-term Goal: The newborn will maintain a body temperature between 97.7° and 99.4°F (36.5°–37.5°C) in the first 24 hours postbirth.

Measurable Long-term Goal: The newborn will maintain a body temperature between 97.7° and 99.4°F (36.5°–37.5°C) (wrapped in blankets in an open crib) after the first 24 hours postbirth.

NOC Outcome:

Thermoregulation: Newborn (0801) Balance among heat production, heat gain, and heat loss during the first 28 days of life

NIC Interventions:

Newborn Care (6880)
Temperature Regulation (3900)
Vital Sign Monitoring (6680)

Nursing Interventions:

1. Place newborn under radiant warmer or skin-to-skin with mother after birth and dry well, discarding wet linens.

   RATIONALE: The radiant warmer or maternal skin provides a heat-gaining environment. Drying the infant reduces heat loss from evaporation.

2. Monitor newborn's axillary temperature per protocol until stabilized.

   RATIONALE: Monitoring the temperature will assess the effectiveness of the therapy.

3. Apply stockinet cap and instruct parents to keep infant's head covered.

   RATIONALE: A cap helps prevent heat loss by convection from the large surface area of the head to the cooler room air.

4. Place the newborn under the radiant warmer with temperature probe attached and alarms turned on as needed to maintain temperature >97.6°F (36.5°C).

   RATIONALE: The radiant warmer provides a heat-gaining environment and prevents heat loss from contact with a cool surface (conduction). Active alarms and use of the temperature probe assure the infant will not be under- or overheated.

5. When the temperature stabilizes, wrap the infant in two blankets and place him in an open crib. Instruct the parents to keep the crib away from windows and drafts.

   RATIONALE: Keeping the crib away from windows and drafts helps to prevent heat loss by radiation and convection.

---

appropriate labeling. Most institutions employ a system of waterproof matching identification bracelets that show the mother's name, the baby's gender, the name of the physician or nurse midwife of record, and the date and time of birth. Two bracelets are worn by the neonate while the mother and her partner wear the others. Careful and continuous monitoring of infants is essential to prevent misidentification, baby switching, or abduction. Alerting staff about mothers who share identical last names helps to decrease the likelihood of mistakes, and special security measures such as sensing devices, video cameras, and door alarms on all mother-baby units helps allay parents' concerns about their infants' safety. (See Chapter 15 for further discussion.)

INFECTION AND INJURY PREVENTION

The prevention of infection and injury constitute important aspects of newborn care. Hand washing is essential in preventing cross contamination by all individuals caring for the newborn. In many facilities, nursery personnel are required to wear scrub clothes, remove nail polish, and keep fingernails trimmed. Other measures to prevent infection include infant bathing, umbilical cord care, care of the circumcision, and eye care. Soon after birth, the newborn receives a prophylactic ophthalmic agent to prevent ophthalmia neonatorum, eye inflammation from

gonorrheal or chlamydial infection contracted during passage through the mother's birth canal. Medications most often used are erythromycin, tetracycline, or silver nitrate.

 Optimizing Outcomes— Eye prophylaxis to prevent ophthalmia neonatorum

In some birth facilities, neonatal eye prophylaxis is delayed up to an hour to allow eye contact to facilitate parent-infant bonding. However, the Centers for Disease Control and Prevention (CDC) recommends that the medication be administered as soon as possible after birth. If instillation is delayed, the facility should have a monitoring system in place to ensure that all infants receive the prophylaxis (CDC, Workowski, & Berman, 2006).

During the first few days of life, the newborn has low levels of vitamin K due to sterile intestinal contents. Vitamin K acts as a catalyst to synthesize prothrombin, needed for blood clotting, in the liver. To prevent the neonatal injury caused by hemorrhage, a single dose (0.5 to 1.0 mg) of vitamin K_1 phytonadione (AquaMEPHYTON) is administered via an intramuscular injection in the vastus lateralis or the ventrogluteal muscle.

medication: Erythromycin

Erythromycin (eh-rith-roe-**mye**-sin)

Ilotycin

Pregnancy Category: B

Indications:

INFANTS: Prophylaxis of ophthalmia neonatorum

Actions: Suppresses protein synthesis at the level of the 50S ribosome

Therapeutic Effects: Bacteriostatic action against susceptible bacteria spectrum: Streptococci, staphylococci, gram-positive bacilli

Pharmacokinetics:

ABSORPTION: Minimal absorption may follow topical or ophthalmic use.

Contraindications and Precautions:

CONTRAINDICATED IN: Hypersensitivity

Adverse Reactions and Side Effects: Irritation

Route and Dosage: Apply a thin strip to each eye as a single dose.

Nursing Implications:

- Inform parents of medication administration.
- Prepare to administer the eye ointment to the infant 1 hour after birth.
- Apply a thin strip to each eye as a single dose.
- Start at the inner canthus and move to the outer canthus.
- Dab excess medication off gently; do not wash away the medicine.

Adapted from Deglin, J.H., & Vallerand, A.H. (2009). *Davis's drug guide for nurses* (11th ed). Philadelphia: F.A. Davis.

 Optimizing Outcomes— Newborn immunization to prevent hepatitis B

Vaccination for hepatitis B, given in a series of three doses beginning at birth, is recommended for all infants. Before administration, the nurse obtains written parental consent. After injection of hepatitis B vaccine (Recombivax HB, Enerix-B) into the vastus lateralis muscle, the nurse massages the site with a gauze square to enhance absorption. Additional doses are administered at 1 and 6 months of age.

Assessment of blood glucose helps to prevent newborn injury related to hypoglycemia. In healthy term infants after an uneventful pregnancy and delivery, blood glucose monitoring often takes place within the first hour after birth. During the early newborn period of a term infant, hypoglycemia is defined as a blood glucose concentration of less than 35 mg/dL or a plasma concentration of less than 40 mg/dL. Infants with a low blood glucose level or those who exhibit signs and symptoms of hypoglycemia (jitteriness, apnea, seizures or lethargy) require immediate attention to prevent brain cell damage. Hypoglycemia is usually resolved with feeding. If the newborn continues to display signs and symptoms of hypoglycemia along with low blood glucose laboratory results, transfer to the neonatal intensive care unit for intravenous administration of glucose may be necessary.

A heel stick blood sample for hematocrit and hemoglobin may be performed to detect anemia or polycythemia (an excess number of red blood cells). Anemia can result from hypovolemia associated with complications such as placenta previa, abruptio placentae, or cesarean birth.

 medication: AquaMEPHYTON

Phytonadione (fye-**toe**-na-dye-one)

AquaMEPHYTON, Mephyton, vitamin K

Classification(s):

THERAPEUTIC: Antidotes, vitamins

PHARMACOLOGICAL: Fat-soluble vitamins

Pregnancy Category: UK

Indications: Prevention and treatment of hypoprothrombinemia, which may be associated with excessive doses of oral anticoagulants, salicylates, certain anti-infective agents, nutritional deficiencies, and prolonged total parenteral nutrition. Prevention of hemorrhagic disease of the newborn.

Action: Required for hepatic synthesis of blood coagulation factors II (prothrombin), VII, IX, and X. Therapeutic effects: Prevention of bleeding due to hypoprothrombinemia

Pharmacokinetics:

ABSORPTION: Well absorbed after oral, IM, or subcutaneous administration

DISTRIBUTION: Crosses the placenta; does not enter breast milk.

Metabolism and excretion: Rapidity metabolized in the liver

HALF-LIFE: Unknown

Contraindications and Precautions:

CONTRAINDICATED IN: Hypersensitivity, hypersensitivity or intolerance to benzyl alcohol (injection only)

USE CAUTIOUSLY IN: Impaired liver function

EXERCISE EXTREME CAUTION IN: Severe life-threatening reactions have occurred after IV administration; use other routes unless IV is justified.

Adverse Reactions and Side Effects:

GASTROINTESTINAL: Gastric upset, unusual taste

DERMATOLOGICAL: Flushing, rash, urticaria

HEMATOLOGICAL: Hemolytic anemia

LOCAL: Erythema, pain at injection site, swelling

MISCELLANEOUS: Allergic reactions, hyperbilirubinemia (large doses in very premature infants), kernicterus

Route and Dosage: IV use of phytonadione should be reserved for emergencies.

Prevention of hemorrhagic disease of the newborn:

IM (NEONATES): 0.5–1 mg, given within 1 hour of birth. May be repeated in 2–3 weeks if the mother received previous anticonvulsant/anticoagulant/anti-infective/antitubercular therapy. 1–5 mg may be given IM to the mother 12–24 hours before delivery.

Nursing Implications:

- Inform parents of medication administration.
- Prepare to administer the injection to the infant 1 hour after birth.
- Administer IM injection into the anterolateral muscle of the newborn's thigh.
- Report any symptoms of unusual bleeding or bruising (bleeding gums; nosebleed; black, tarry stools; hematuria; bleeding from the base of the umbilical cord or other open wounds).
- A decrease in hemoglobin and hematocrit levels or any bleeding may indicate that the effects of the medicine have not been achieved and that more vitamin K may be necessary. Call the physician for further instruction.

Adapted from Deglin, J.H., & Vallerand, A.H. (2009). *Davis's drug guide for nurses* (11th ed). Philadelphia: F.A. Davis.

Polycythemia may be related to excessive blood flow from the umbilical cord into the infant at birth. A normal hematocrit at 1 hour of life is 50% to 55%. A normal hemoglobin is 14.5 to 22.5 g/dL. Early detection of abnormal laboratory results can ensure immediate treatment.

Be sure to— Document appropriate birth information

After the baby's birth, many pieces of important information are collected during the nursery admission process. The nurse records the actual time of birth, the status of infant's respirations—whether spontaneous or assisted, the 1- and 5-minute Apgar scores, the birth weight in pounds and kilograms, the axillary temperature, and the number of vessels in the umbilical cord. Also documented is the type and amount of medication instilled for eye prophylaxis, the injection sites for vitamin K and hepatitis B vaccine administration, the findings from the general physical assessment, observations of voiding or stooling, and all laboratory testing obtained, such as blood glucose or cultures. It is the responsibility of the physician, midwife, or the birth facility to legally register the neonate. All infants are registered at the State Bureau of Vital Statistics in the state in which they were born. Essential information including the mother's name; the father's name (if the mother gives permission); and the date, time, and place of birth is required. Birth registration information is important because as the child grows older, this information is required to enter school, obtain a Social Security card, register to vote, and obtain a passport and a driver's license.

Infants who are stable may remain with their parents in the birthing area to facilitate family bonding and attachment. Newborns experiencing complications are taken to the nursery for further evaluation. After the immediate neonatal assessment, a later examination is conducted within the first 4 hours after birth. At this time, the nurse performs a brief physical assessment to estimate the infant's gestational age and evaluate the neonate's transition to extrauterine life (AAP & ACOG, 2007). Problems that place the neonate at risk are identified and evaluated. At some point before the infant's discharge, a complete physical examination and behavioral assessment are conducted to detect any emerging or potential problems. Depending on birthing facility protocol, this evaluation may be performed by the nurse, with certain components completed by a physician, certified nurse-midwife, or nurse practitioner.

 Now Can You— Discuss components of the neonate's initial adaptation?

1. Recognize what constitutes normal vital signs in the infant?
2. Use the following information to calculate Baby O'Leary's Apgar score. At 1 minute of life, Baby O'Leary is crying quietly in a radiant warmer. Her hands and feet are blue and her extremities are floppy. Her heart rate is 122 beats per minute and her respiratory rate is 28 breaths per minute and irregular. The Apgar score at 1 minute is _____?
3. Identify six indicators of neonatal respiratory distress?

The Later Neonatal Assessment

The neonate is usually greeted with a whirlwind of activities immediately after birth. However, many other activities and assessments will take place later in the newborn nursery. In the initial setting, the nurse conducts a brief physical assessment, carefully making note of body position, skin color, overall body size and symmetry, and level of interaction with the environment.

BODY POSITIONING

Not surprisingly, many infants seek comfort and security by resuming their dominant in utero position following birth. The normal newborn baby assumes a position of flexion of the upper and lower extremities. Flexed arms enable infants to use their hands to touch their faces, suck their fingers, and explore their world (Fig. 18-1).

The legs may be extended, arranged in the position assumed at the time of birth, or flexed. Most often, the infants' body positioning is symmetrical. Nurses should recognize that asymmetrical positioning at the time of the assessment may indicate injury from birth trauma. An infant's failure to move one or more extremities also signals that further investigation is warranted. When positioning the infant, nurses must be sure to follow the guidelines established by the American Academy of Pediatrics (2005a) to prevent sudden infant death syndrome (SIDS). (See Chapter 19.)

 critical nursing action Safe Positions to Prevent SIDS

• All newborns should be put to sleep on their backs; avoid placing the infant in a prone position.
• When using a side-lying position, place the infant's dependent arm forward to lessen the likelihood that the infant will roll into a prone position.

✿ *Nursing Insight— Helping to meet the Healthy People 2010 national goals*

One National Goal directly addresses the reduction in SIDS-related infant deaths: "increase the percentage of healthy full-term infants who are put to sleep on their backs from a baseline of 35% to 70%." Nurses can help to meet this goal by teaching parents and all infant care providers the advantage of placing the newborn on their back to sleep.

Figure 18-1 The full-term infant assumes a flexed position.

SKIN COLOR

Assessment of the infant's skin color constitutes an essential component of the general physical examination. Jaundice (hyperbilirubinemia), a yellow coloration of the skin, may be apparent in the neonate. Normally, jaundice develops gradually over several days in a head-to-toe, or cephalocaudal pattern. Any term infant less than 24 hours old who demonstrates visual jaundice is considered to have "pathological jaundice" or "hemolytic jaundice," a condition that most often results from a serious blood incompatibility between the mother and her newborn. (See Chapter 19 for further discussion of physiological and pathological jaundice.)

When conducting the skin assessment, the nurse must remember that certain characteristics of the nursery or mother's postpartum room can affect the accuracy of the exam. For example, pink walls and artificial lighting may mask the early detection of jaundice, and interfere with an accurate assessment of the degree of severity of the condition. It is best to examine the neonate's skin in natural daylight, if possible. When jaundice is suspected, the nurse can readily assess the skin coloring by pressing on the infant's forehead or nose with a finger. When blanching occurs, the nurse can observe for the yellow coloration associated with jaundice.

"Physiological jaundice" or "nonhemolytic" jaundice describes the more commonly occurring yellowing of the skin in neonates that becomes apparent after the first 24 hours of life and usually peaks by the third to fifth day. Physiological jaundice often has a nonhemolytic cause and frequently results from a failure to adequately process bilirubin due to inadequate intake or elimination, birth trauma, or from minor blood incompatibilities.

Breastfed infants may develop early-onset or "breastfeeding jaundice," which is associated with insufficient feeding and infrequent stooling. Since colostrum has a natural laxative effect that stimulates the passage of meconium, frequent breastfeeding during the early days of life is beneficial in reducing the neonate's serum bilirubin levels. Late-onset or "breast milk jaundice" sometimes affects breastfed infants during the second week of life. This type of jaundice usually develops around the fourth day when the mother's mature breast milk comes in and peaks around day 10. Breast milk jaundice is believed to be related to a factor in human milk that causes an increased intestinal absorption of bilirubin. Although usually no treatment is necessary, some physicians advise mothers to discontinue breastfeeding for 12 to 24 hours to allow the infant's bilirubin levels to decrease (Verklan & Walden, 2004).

Nurses can implement several actions to decrease the likelihood of high bilirubin levels in the neonate. Maintaining the infant's skin temperature at or above 98.7°F (36.5°C) is beneficial since cold stress can cause acidosis, a condition linked with an elevated serum bilirubin. Also, careful monitoring of the infant's intake and output, with special attention to stool characteristics and frequency is important. Since bilirubin is excreted in the feces, inadequate elimination can result in the reabsorption and recycling of bilirubin. Finally, the nurse should encourage early (within the first hour of life) feedings when possible to promote rapid and continuous intestinal evacuation and provide the calories necessary for the production of hepatic binding proteins.

Understandably, the presence of physiological jaundice in the infant can be distressing for parents. Nurses can address these concerns by providing ongoing emotional support along with accurate explanations of the condition. Parents should be taught about the importance of adequate hydration and how to assess the infant for signs of jaundice. If the baby undergoes phototherapy (exposure to high-intensity lights) for treatment, additional days of hospitalization may be required, and the mother may have to leave the birth center without her baby. Parents should be encouraged to help meet their infant's emotional needs by holding, feeding, touching, and interacting with the baby. When the mother must leave the hospital without her infant, the nurse can support the bonding process by providing the nursery telephone number and name(s) of the baby's primary caregiver(s). Mothers should also be encouraged to call for updates and return for feedings as often as possible. Breastfeeding mothers may wish to remain in the hospital until the infant is released. In other situations, initiation of home phototherapy for the jaundiced infant may be an option. When the infant is treated in the home, nurses monitor the phototherapy regimen and obtain serum bilirubin levels as dictated by hospital or agency policy. (See Chapter 19.)

Infants with congenital heart defects often exhibit skin pallor that does not improve with time. All infants should exhibit pink skin, which is an important indicator of satisfactory perfusion to the extremities. Acrocyanosis, a common finding, is confined to the hands and feet. Neonates with central cyanosis may demonstrate a blue tint to the lips, gums, tongue, fingertips, and toes, as well as pallor under the eyes and on the cheeks. These findings are indicative of a circulatory problem and warrant immediate investigation into the suspected cause of the cyanosis. The diagnostic work-up for infants with central cyanosis may include echocardiography and cardiac catheterization. Depending on the findings, treatment may involve medical or surgical intervention. (See Chapters 19 and 26.)

When stimulated by physical contact, infants should demonstrate a rapid pinking of the skin that progresses to a red color. These changes are reflective of an increased respiratory and heart rate. Observing how long it takes for the infant to return to the previous skin color after stimulation is an important component of the nurse's visual assessment of the neonate's cardiovascular system. Making an accurate assessment of the infant's "true" skin color is of paramount importance when observing for color changes related to pathological conditions. For the nurse to accurately assess the color of the neonate's skin, it is necessary to know what constitutes the "normal" skin color for that individual. It is important to remember that skin color is influenced by ethnicity. For example, the natural skin colors of African American and Hispanic infants may be infused with yellow tones that make it difficult for the nurse to determine normal skin color.

Optimizing Outcomes— Obtaining an accurate assessment of the infant's true skin color

- Use a variety of light sources (helps to ascertain the "true" color).
- Examine the infant's entire skin surface.
- Carefully inspect the palms, soles of the feet, lips, and areas behind the ears.
- Gently palpate bony prominences (nose, sternum, sacrum, wrists, ankles).
- Apply slight pressure for 1 second ("blanching").
- Observe for true skin color, reflective of the infant's ethnic heritage.
- Record true skin color: yellow is indicative of jaundice; white is indicative of pallor.

BODY SIZE

At the time of birth, the neonate's weight and length are measured and recorded. The nurse also visually inspects the infant for symmetry of head-to-toe length along with abdominal girth. Later, the neonate's actual body measurements are correlated with a development graph to ascertain appropriateness of the physical size. As a component of the visual inspection, the nurse confirms that the infant's head appears to be the largest body part.

 Now Can You— Discuss essential nursing actions associated with newborn safety and skin color assessment?

1. Describe and demonstrate how the infant should be positioned to prevent SIDS?
2. Name three nursing actions that can help minimize physiological jaundice?
3. Discuss four techniques that should be used to assess the infant's true skin color?

LEVEL OF REACTIVITY

The infant's reaction to the environment is an important indicator of the level of neuromuscular development. The nurse routinely assesses the infant's state of responsiveness and reactivity. During the exam, it is helpful to consider these questions, designed to ensure a thorough assessment:

"Is the neonate awake and quiet, or restless and crying?"
"Does the infant respond by looking and moving all extremities?"
"Is the infant's sleep pattern best characterized by quiet slumber or agitated restlessness?"

According to Brazelton (1973), neonates exhibit several discrete behavioral levels or "states" of awareness and normally progress or regress smoothly from one to the other. The distinct states include deep sleep, light sleep, drowsy, quiet alert, considerable motor activity, and crying. The neonatal behavioral assessment is an important component of the overall evaluation, since it validates a mature neurological–organizational system that allows the term infant to readily transition from one behavioral state to another. Certain conditions such as in utero exposure to cocaine disrupt this normal development; affected neonates exhibit erratic, disorganized behavior, an excessive response to stimuli and lengthy or absent transition periods between behaviors. (See Chapter 19 for further discussion.)

The nurse may assess the infant's response to voices and physical presence to confirm the level of responsiveness and behavioral organization. An infant who displays irritability and an overreaction to voices, touch, or movement needs to be comforted and special care must be taken to provide calming measures such as swaddling the neonate in blankets, cuddling, rocking, and gentle holding. It is best to postpone the physical examination because the manipulation and handling will most likely cause further disruption and behavioral disorganization.

OBTAINING MEASUREMENTS AND DETERMINING THE GESTATIONAL AGE

Routine assessment of the neonate's vital signs is important before the physical examination and throughout the infant's hospital stay. It is essential that the nurse recognizes the normal parameters for temperature, pulse, respirations, and blood pressure so that any change in the neonate's status can be readily identified.

 critical nursing action Recognizing Normal Newborn Vital Signs

When assessing newborn vital signs, the nurse must be aware of the following normal parameters:

Temperature:
Normal range: 97.7°–99.4°F (36.5°–37.0°C)
Axillary: 97.5°–99°F (36.5°–37.2°C)

Pulse:
120–160 beats per minute (count pulse rate for one full minute)
During sleep, the pulse rate can be as low as 80 beats per minute.
During crying the pulse rate can be as high as 180 beats per minute.

Respirations:
30–60 respirations per minute (count respiratory rate for one full minute)
Abdominal breathing is normal. Periodic breathing is considered normal and classified as short pauses in the breathing of the newborn that last only approximately 3 seconds. Apneic episodes are significant if they last more than 15 to 20 seconds; they may be accompanied by abrupt pallor, hypotonia, cyanosis, and bradycardia. Apnea must be differentiated from periodic breathing, which is normal in the newborn.

Caution: Withhold oral feeding if the respiratory rate is >60 respirations per minute.

Blood pressure:
Systolic: 60–80 mm Hg; diastolic: 40–50 mm Hg at birth
Systolic: 95–100 mm Hg; diastolic: slight increase at 10 days of age

Procedure 18-2 Measuring the Newborn's Body Length

Purpose

To establish and document the newborn's body length

Equipment

- Standard paper tape measure

Steps

1. Place the infant on a paper-covered flat surface.
2. Fully extend the infant's body by holding the head midline.

   RATIONALE: *The newborn normally assumes a flexed position and must be fully extended to obtain an accurate measurement.*

3. Gently grasp the knees and place them together.
4. Push down gently on the knees until they are fully extended and flat against the table surface.
5. Measure the crown-to-heel recumbent length by placing the paper tape measure beside the infant with the 0 end of the tape at the top of the head.

Keep the infant's body in alignment and carefully extend one leg. Ensure that the tape measure remains straight. Note the length and record it in the infant's chart. As an alternate measurement method, make a slash mark with a pen at the end points by the top of the infant's head and the heels of the foot. While providing continuous support, gently roll the infant to the side and measure between the two points with a paper tape measure that has increments designated in tenths.

RATIONALE: *Careful body positioning and use of a tape measure gradated in tenths ensures an accurate measurement. Measurements are taken and recorded to note abnormalities and to provide a baseline value.*

Documentation

3/4/10 0800 – Infant length: 50 cm.

                  –J. Yamoto, RN

The neonate's weight, recorded in grams, and the length, recorded in centimeters, are measured in the birthing room and again during the transitional period (Figs. 18-2 and 18-3). On average, a term newborn infant weighs 3400 grams, with a normal range of 2500 to 4300 grams. Recumbent length is a crown-to-heel measurement taken with the infant in a supine position (Procedure 18-2). The recumbent length is recorded on a regular basis until the infant reaches 24 months of age. Normal length parameters for newborns are approximately 18 to 22 inches (45 to 55 cm).

The nurse also obtains and records the frontal–occipital circumference (FOC), or head measurement (Fig. 18-4). A paper tape measure with increments marked in tenths of a centimeter is used to ensure an accurate measurement.

To obtain the head circumference, the tape measure is placed on the area immediately above the eyebrows and pinna of the ears and then wrapped around to the occipital prominence at the back of the head. This location represents the area of the greatest head circumference. After obtaining the head measurement three times, the nurse records the largest finding. The normal head circumference for a full-term neonate ranges from 13 to 15 inches (33 to 38 cm). Measurement of the head circumference is repeated at subsequent physical exams until the infant reaches 36 months of age.

To obtain the chest measurement, the paper tape measure is placed on the nipple line and then wrapped around the entire thoracic area (Fig. 18-5). The head and chest measurement may be equal during the first

Figure 18-2 Weighing the infant.

Figure 18-3 Measuring the infant's body length.

Figure 18-4 Measuring the head circumference.

Figure 18-5 Measuring the chest circumference.

few days of life. A normal chest measurement is 12 to 13 inches (30.5 to 33 cm). The abdominal circumference may be obtained by encircling the infant's body with the paper tape measure placed directly above the umbilicus (Fig. 18-6). The abdomen should be approximately the same size as the chest (Dillon, 2007). Once all measurements have been obtained, the nurse plots the weight, length, and head circumference against the infant's gestational age to determine the appropriate size category (Fig. 18-7). Size categories are small for gestational age (SGA), appropriate for gestational age (AGA), and large for gestational age (LGA). If at any time the physical measurements fall outside of the normal growth parameters, the physician should be notified. Information concerning normal growth parameters for infants, children and adults is available at the CDC National Center for Health Statistics Web site: http://www.cdc.gov/nchs/about/major/nhanes/growthcharts/charts.htm.

 Nursing Insight— *Understanding classifications for newborn weight*

Large for gestational age (LGA): Weight is above the 90th percentile at any week.

Appropriate for gestational age (AGA): Weight falls between the 10th and 90th percentiles for the infant's age.

Small for gestational age: (SGA): Weight falls below the 10th percentile for the infant's age.

Figure 18-6 Measuring the abdominal circumference.

In 1967, the American Academy of Pediatrics recommended that all newborns be classified by birth weight and gestational age. Since that time, a scoring system developed by Ballard and colleagues (1991), which represents a modification of the Dubowitz system, has been the most commonly used method for determining the neonate's gestational age. With this assessment system, the infant examination yields a score of neuromuscular and physical maturity that can be extrapolated onto a corresponding age scale to reveal the infant's gestational age in weeks. Additional methods used to determine gestational age are fundal height measurement before delivery, ultrasonography, and eye lens vascularity. A rough approximation of the gestational age at birth can be calculated according to the date of the mother's last normal menstrual period. Since these other sources of age determination are not as accurate as the neonatal physical examination, gestational age assessments are frequently performed by the nurse and recorded on the infant's chart.

 Optimizing Outcomes— **Use of the Ballard Gestational Age by Maturity Rating tool**

The Ballard Gestational Age by Maturity Rating tool includes a neuromuscular maturity and a physical maturity component (Fig. 18-8) that contains six characteristics to be assessed. At the conclusion of the examination, the scores from each component are added together, then mathematically extrapolated onto the maturity rating scale to determine the infant's gestational age by examination. The scoring system is designed to identify the decreased levels of muscle and joint flexibility characteristic of the premature infant, as well as the mature term infant's ability to return to the original position after movement. The nurse usually performs this assessment within the first 12 hours of the infant's life. The Ballard scoring system is more accurate when conducted on term infants who are between 10 and 36 hours of life. The order in which the assessment is conducted is unimportant.

Interestingly, gestational age maturity may occur at different rates among the various categories. For example, a score of 4 (full maturity) in one category does not indicate

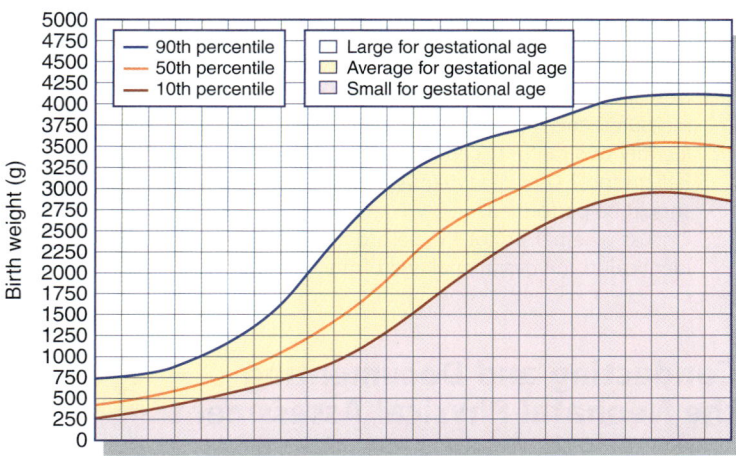

Figure 18-7 Gestational age assessment.

Neuromuscular Maturity

	-1	0	1	2	3	4	5
Posture							
Square Window (Wrist)	-90°	90°	60°	45°	30°	0°	
Arm Recoil		180°	140°-180°	110°-140°	90°-110°	<90°	
Popliteal Angle	180°	160°	140°	120°	100°	90°	<90°
Scarf Sign							
Heel To Ear							

Physical Maturity

Skin	sticky friable transparent	gelantinous red translucent	smooth pink visible veins	superficial peeling or rash, few veins	cracking pale areas rare veins	parchment deep cracking no vessels	leathery cracked wrinkled	
Lanugo	none	sparse	abundant	thinning	bald areas	mostly bald		
Plantar Surface	heel-toe 40–50 mm:-1 <40 mm:-2	>50 mm no crease	faint red marks	anterior transverse crease only	creases ant. 2/3	creases over entire sole		
Breast	imperceptible	barely perceptible	flat areola no bud	stippled areola 1–2 mm bud	raised areola 3–4 mm bud	full areola 5–10 mm bud		
Eye/ear	lids fused loosely:-1 tightly:-2	lids open pinna flat stays folded	sl. curved pinna; soft; slow recoil	well-curved pinna; soft but ready recoil	formed and firm instant recoil	thick cartilage ear stiff		
Genitals (Male)	scrotum flat, smooth	scrotum empty faint rugae	testes in upper canal rare rugae	testes descending few rugae	testes down good rugae	testes pendulous deep rugae		
Genitals (Female)	clitoris prominent labia flat	prominent clitoris small labia minora	prominent clitoris enlarging minora	majora and minora equally prominent	majora large minora small	majora cover clitoris and minora		

Maturity Rating

Score	Weeks
-10	20
-5	22
0	24
5	26
10	28
15	30
20	32
25	34
30	36
35	38
40	40
45	42
50	44

Figure 18-8 The New Ballard score.

that all subsequent categories must also reflect a score of 4. "Half-scores" are often recorded if the examiner believes that the infant exhibits a characteristic that falls between two scoring options during the assessment. It is important to remember that the infant's maturity scoring does not directly translate to the gestational age in weeks.

 Now Can You— Obtain neonatal measurements and determine gestational age?

1. Describe and demonstrate how to obtain neonatal body measurements?
2. Identify two maturity components that are assessed in the Ballard tool? Describe when and why the Ballard assessment should be performed?
3. Discuss whether or not the Ballard maturity score should be identical to the gestational age of the neonate?

Conducting and Documenting the Neonatal Physical Assessment

The nurse conducts the neonatal physical examination with the review of systems following the general nursing assessment of the newborn. This examination should not be initiated if the infant is crying or appears to be upset. Instead, it is best to postpone the assessment until the infant is calm. Infant registration and documentation of findings from the physical examination, along with other pertinent information (i.e., site and dosage of the vitamin K and hepatitis B vaccine injections, instillation of medication for eye prophylaxis) must be completed for each infant before hospital discharge.

ASSESSMENT OF THE NEONATE: A SYSTEMS APPROACH

Once the assessment of the infant's general physical growth parameters and gestational age has been completed, the nurse systematically examines each body system, beginning with the skin and proceeding in a head-to-toe direction. This assessment may take place in the nursery with the infant resting comfortably in a crib, under a radiant warmer (to maintain temperature stability), or if stable, in the mother's room. Carrying out the assessment by the mother's bedside has several advantages. For most, the bedside is a nonthreatening environment where the mother and the nurse can "explore" the baby's special and unique characteristics. Also, conducting the evaluation in this relaxed setting gives the nurse an opportunity to observe the mother's ease in interacting with and touching and holding her infant. Appropriate positive reinforcement by the nurse affirms and validates the mother's actions, enhances her sense of maternal worthiness, and strengthens the bonding relationship. For the infant, the evolving sense of trust and perception of a secure environment are two essential developmental milestones first established during these early contacts with caregivers. These experiences lay the foundation for the child's life-long development of self-esteem and self-love. A spiritual health promotion strategy for the family with a newborn centers on encouraging the parents and caregivers to shower their infants and toddlers with love and comfort (Tucker, 2002).

With the infant in a supine position, the nurse follows the steps of inspection, light palpation, deep palpation, and auscultation to facilitate the examination. When assessing the abdomen, the proper sequence is inspection, auscultation, and light palpation followed by deep palpation.

Assessment of the Integumentary System

Wearing gloves, the nurse examines the neonate's skin, scalp and body hair, and nails for color, texture, distribution, disruptions, eruptions, and birthmarks. It is important that the assessment take place in a well-lit room and additional light sources may be needed to confirm accuracy of findings. The infant's skin should be pink, a finding that indicates adequate peripheral cardiac perfusion. Blanching the skin over bony prominences should yield a pink-white color before returning to natural pigmentation.

As previously described, acrocyanosis, a bluish coloration to the hands and feet, is a normal condition related to vasomotor instability and poor peripheral circulation. To differentiate between acrocyanosis and true cyanosis, the nurse can vigorously rub the sole of the neonate's foot. If the sole turns pink, the diagnosis is acrocyanosis. If the sole remains blue, it is true cyanosis. Also, acrocyanosis disappears when the infant cries. Visual inspection of the infant's mouth, tongue, and gums confirms the skin color assessment, as these areas should be pink-red in color and darken to bright red with crying. True cyanosis produces a bluish coloration and pallor (paleness) of the lips and on the area around the mouth.

Careful, daily assessment of the newborn's skin constitutes an important nursing action that may lead to early detection of potential problems. If pallor, **plethora** (a deep purplish color related to an increased number of circulating red blood cells), **petechiae** (pinpoint hemorrhagic areas), central cyanosis, or jaundice is detected, further evaluation is warranted. The nurse describes and records in the infant's medical chart the location of any birth injuries such as forceps marks or fetal monitoring lesions. Infants born with a nuchal cord (umbilical cord around the neck) or those who assumed a face presentation commonly exhibit bruises or petechiae on the head, neck, and face. If extensive bruising is present, the infant's bilirubin level may be elevated. Although focal petechiae may be related to injury from increased pressure, the presence of petechiae scattered throughout the infant's body can be indicative of an underlying problem such as a low platelet count or infection. Periauricular papillomas, or skin tags, are a benign common finding that often run in families and usually are insignificant and require no intervention.

The term infant's skin should feel smooth and soft. In the postterm infant, the skin is often tough and leathery, with cracking and peeling. Disruptions or breaks in the skin may be related to electrode marks or lacerations. Infants delivered by forceps or vacuum extraction may have skin disruptions or bruising on the scalp and face. Often, infants are born with pustular melanosis, a condition in which small pustules are formed prior to birth. As the pustule disintegrates, a small residue or "scale" in the shape of the pustule is formed. This lesion later develops into a small (1 to 2 millimeter) macule, or flat spot. Macules, which are brown in color, appear similar to freckles and are frequently located on the chest and extremities. Pustular melanosis occurs more commonly on African American infants than on Caucasian infants (Miller & Newman, 2005).

Another common skin condition is **milia**, small white papules or sebaceous cysts on the infant's face that resemble pimples (Fig. 18-9). Inclusion cysts may be seen singularly or in pairs on the penis or scrotum of male infants or on the areola of female infants. Acne, a skin condition common in adolescents, may also be present in newborns and is related to excessive amounts of maternal hormones. Over time, neonatal acne disappears spontaneously from the infant's cheeks and chest. **Erythema toxicum**, a transient rash that covers the face and chest with spread to the entire body, is the most common normal skin eruption in term neonates. It is also called "erythema neonatorum," "newborn rash," or "flea bite" dermatitis. Typically, the rash consists of small, irregular, flat red patches on the checks that develop into singular, small yellow pimples appearing on the chest, abdomen, and extremities. The cause of this skin condition is unknown, and it may persist for up to 1 month of life. There is no treatment available to hasten the resolution of the rash, which, because of its frequently unsightly appearance, can be quite disturbing to parents.

Blisters related to repetitive sucking may form on the fingers, wrists, and upper lips of infants who often perpetuate a habit begun in utero. Although these lesions may appear to be serious, parents can be assured that they will resolve over time without intervention.

Many neonatal skin variations are characterized by color changes that are different from normal pigmentation. For example, **Mongolian spots** are areas that appear gray, dark blue, or purple and are most commonly located on the back and buttocks, although they may also be found on the shoulders, wrists, forearms, and ankles (Fig. 18-10).

Figure 18-9 Milia.

Figure 18-10 Mongolian spots.

Mongolian spots are seen most often in infants whose ethnic backgrounds include the Mediterranean area, Latin America, Asia, or Africa. Parents can be assured that these skin changes will fade and disappear as the infant grows older. Since they may be mistaken for bruises, it is important that the nurse document Mongolian spots on the infant's chart. Another condition, "cutis marmorata," or mottling, is common in neonates and is most often caused by the infant's vasomotor response to the lower environmental temperature outside of the uterus. Mottling may also be related to prolonged apnea. Usually, the mottling disappears once the newborn adjusts to the extrauterine environment. A deepened coloration of the genital skin in males and females may occur due to the influence of maternal hormones. This color change also diminishes over time.

Birthmarks are distinct areas of color that may be tan, brown, white, or red. Their appearance varies but generally these lesions are small and flat. It is important to distinguish birthmarks from skin lesions that result from birth trauma. The nurse documents the location, size, and color of the birthmark, and if the lesion contains hair or is located along the anterior or posterior midline, further investigation is warranted to rule out underlying tissue involvement. Hypopigmentation refers to a white or pale area of skin. When it occurs as a single lesion, hypopigmentation is not a cause for worry. However, if multiple hypopigmented areas, including lesions in a leaf pattern are present, the infant should be referred for further evaluation. These lesions, which sometimes appear on the chest, back, extremities and axilla, may be associated with tuberous sclerosis, a neurological condition. Café-au-lait marks are flat, tan spots that are quite common and insignificant unless the infant exhibits six or more marks that are greater than 1 cm in diameter. In this circumstance, the neonate should be carefully evaluated during infancy for tumors that develop beneath the skin, as he may be at risk for developing type 1 neurofibromatosis. The nurse should be aware that because café-au-lait spots and other skin pigment variations can be very difficult to identify in African American infants, extra care must be taken when performing the integumentary system assessment (Miller & Newman, 2005).

Brown **nevi** are brown skin marks, or birth marks whose color can vary from brown to deep black. Since a nevus may represent a very early form of a precancerous lesion, the nurse should teach parents to routinely check the lesion for changes in color, shape, size, shape, or elevation from the skin surface. The careful observation of this skin lesion should be ongoing and continuous throughout the child's lifetime.

A **nevus flammeus**, often referred to as a "port wine stain," is a capillary angioma located directly below the epidermis. Usually apparent at birth, the nevus flammeus is a non-elevated, red to purple network of dense capillaries that varies in size, shape and location, although it commonly appears on the face. It does not blanch on pressure, disappear or grow in size. Sturge-Weber syndrome, a clinical condition involving the fifth cranial nerve, may be present when a nevus flammeus is accompanied by convulsions or other indicators of neurological problems (Miller & Newman, 2005).

A **telangiectatic nevus** is a red birthmark often seen at the nape of the neck and commonly referred to as a "stork bite" or "angel kiss" (Fig. 18-11). This lesion may also occur on the face between the eyebrows, on the eyelids, nose, or upper lip. It is usually irregular in shape and pale red, often turning bright red when the infant cries. The telangiectatic nevus tends to fade as the infant grows older and usually disappears by the second birthday. A **nevus vasculosus**, or "strawberry mark," is a red, raised capillary hemangioma that can occur anywhere on the neonate's body. This birthmark usually has sharp borders and a rough surface that resembles a strawberry. Although often alarming due to its appearance, the nurse can reassure parents that over time this lesion will eventually undergo a process of involution and disappear during the first year of life. Unless they interfere with a vital organ system or are located on the face, surgical removal of capillary hemangiomas is not recommended. The blue nevus appears as a distinct blue or blue-black birthmark often found on the buttocks, hands, and feet. Although sometimes mistaken for a Mongolian spot when it appears on the buttocks, nurses can differentiate the blue nevus by noting its distinct borders and brighter color, as compared to the Mongolian spot, which covers a larger area. The blue nevus is usually 1 cm or less in size.

CONDITIONS THAT MAY WARRANT FURTHER ASSESSMENT. Blemishes and other marks on an infant's skin that are related to birth trauma most often mirror the traumatizing

 where research and practice meet:
The Neonatal Skin Condition Score

Providing timely, evidence-based skin care to neonates is of major importance to nurses. Nurses can implement various interventions to reduce injury to skin integrity, prevent absorption of potentially toxic agents, and promote the development of healthy skin (Lund & Osborne, 2004). The Neonatal Skin Condition Score (NSCS) is an assessment tool developed by investigators involved in the Neonatal Skin Care Project, a clinical study designed to develop guidelines for the examination and evaluation of neonatal skin care (Lund, Kuller, et al., 2001; Lund, Osborne, et al., 2001). The NSCS consists of a 9-point scale that evaluates three broad categories: dryness, erythema, and breakdown/excoriation. A score ranging from 1 (normal) to 3 (extensive) is assigned to each category; a perfect score = 3 and the worst possible score = 9. The NSCS is designed to provide a concise, objective method of accurately reporting skin conditions in the hospitalized neonate and a timely means for identifying infants with need for interventions such as monitoring for systemic candidiasis and application of emollients.

Figure 18-11 Stork bite.

instrument such as forceps or scalp electrodes. Characteristically, the color of these lesions progresses through the various skin color changes commonly associated with bruising. When assessing for birth injuries, the nurse pays close attention to the scalp, face, shoulders, arms, legs, and feet. Large infants frequently exhibit marks from trauma sustained during a difficult vaginal birth. Infants born with a nuchal cord (umbilical cord around the neck) may demonstrate considerable bruising of the neck and face. Also, neonates whose presenting part was the legs, feet, or buttocks may have extensive edema or bruising of the lower extremities. Sometimes the full extent of tissue damage cannot be appreciated by routine inspection and palpation. Instead, the nurse may note that the infant responds to positional changes and other gentle manual manipulation with excessive crying or irritability. In these circumstances, further assessment should be conducted with the infant placed in the supine and prone positions. Since excessive bruising may be associated with elevated bilirubin levels, the infant should be closely observed for signs of jaundice. Widespread petechiae or petechiae unrelated to birth trauma should be reported to the pediatrician because these findings may be associated with infection, low platelets, or congenital problems such as rubella.

Abnormally pigmented skin lesions and variations in hair patterns are other findings that may signal underlying problems. Infants who exhibit hairy pigmented skin lesions containing two distinct areas of color should be evaluated by a dermatologist. Since these findings may be related to an underlying structural defect, diagnostic ultrasound is often performed to evaluate the tissue beneath the skin surface. Hairy nevi describe skin nevi that contain individual hairs or a full tuft of hair. The presence of hairy nevi located in the posterior midline area near the spinal column may indicate a vertebral defect. When present, ultrasound examination of the spinal column is necessary in order to confirm any defects related to spina bifida or spina bifida occulta.

The nurse may identify an infant whose skin color remains deep pink or red during quiet rest or sleep. This finding may indicate plethora, a condition most often caused by polycythemia vera or hyperthermia. Polycythemia vera, a condition characterized by an excessive number of red blood cells, occurs from the transfer of maternal blood into the neonate's circulation during the time when the umbilical cord was cut. Polycythemia vera can be confirmed by a capillary hematocrit value of 65 or greater or a venous hematocrit of 60 or more. Treatment for this condition usually involves a partial exchange transfusion. (See Chapter 19 for further discussion of neonatal exchange transfusions.) Hyperthermia can be detected by checking the infant's body temperature.

Careful examination of the infant's hair pattern constitutes another essential component of the nursing assessment. Special attention should be paid to the hair texture, color, and distribution, noting any disruptions to the hair distribution or areas of asymmetry on the scalp. Hair that covers the forehead and creates a shortened distance between the hairline and the eyebrows may be indicative of a congenital syndrome. The nurse notes any variations such as hair that is lighter in color than the surrounding hair, or hair that appears to grow in a circular pattern or whorl. Sections of white hair embedded in darker scalp hair may indicate an underlying structural defect or the presence of a congenital syndrome.

Ongoing observation and assessment of the neonate's skin allows the nurse an opportunity to confirm normalcy, identify potential problems, and prepare for possible interventions. It also provides an opportunity to educate and reassure parents about normal neonatal skin characteristics and findings that might indicate problems. Parents are often fearful about "body marks" and the nurse can allay anxieties and stress the importance of conducting routine skin observations throughout childhood.

Now Can You— Discuss neonatal skin conditions?

1. Explain what parents should be taught about treatment for their infant's erythema toxicum?
2. Identify when the presence of café-au-lait spots in the neonate warrants further investigation?
3. Discuss the significance of hairy, pigmented skin lesions in the newborn?
4. Describe why the nurse should carefully assess the neonate's hair pattern?

Assessment of the Infant's Head

Following the skin assessment, the infant's head, eyes, ears, nose, and throat are evaluated next. The nurse methodically assesses the face for symmetry, noting the placement of the eyes, nose, lips, mouth, and ears (Fig. 18-12). Eye shape and size are noted along with assessment for coordinated movement of the lids. Eye color and placement on the forehead are recorded. The lips are also assessed for movement. Birth-related damage to the 7th cranial (facial) nerve can result in a number of findings such as unilateral drooping of the tongue or mouth, unequal movement of the cheek muscles, or inappropriate eyelid movement. Special attention is paid to the shape, size, and placement of the ears. Low-set ears may signal the need for further assessment and evaluation for chromosomal abnormalities (Fig. 18-13). Placement of

Figure 18-12 The face is examined for symmetry, noting placement of the eyes, nose, lips, mouth, and ears.

Figure 18-14 Palpating the fontanel borders.

one ear slightly lower than the other is a common finding that generally has no clinical significance. Nostrils should be open bilaterally and the nasal bridge should be centered with no lateral deviations. Lip color should be consistent with the tongue and buccal mucosa of the mouth. The upper and lower lips should be approximately uniform in size. The infant's chin should be readily apparent when viewed in a profile position. Micrognathia, or small jaw, may interfere with tooth development, sucking, swallowing and tongue movement inside the mouth during speech (Dillon, 2007).

The nurse carefully palpates the infant's head to assess the fontanels, the cranial suture lines, and the presence of any birth-related edema. The anterior fontanel is readily identifiable as a diamond-shaped open space formed by the anterior–posterior sagittal and frontal sutures and the lateral coronal suture (Fig. 18-14). Assessment of the fontanel includes an estimation of the overall fontanel

size. The nurse can readily determine this dimension by palpation of the fontanel borders with use of the finger for measurements (the distance from the tip of the finger to the first finger joint is roughly 1 inch, or 2.5 cm). Variations in anterior fontanel size are common and range from 0.4 to 2.8 inches (1 to 7 cm). The posterior fontanel, located toward the back of the cranium, is a small, triangular-shaped space formed by the sagittal suture and the posterior lateral suture. At its widest point, the posterior fontanel is usually only 0.4 inch (1 cm) and may be closed at initial examination. The anterior fontanel must remain open during the first year of life to accommodate skull bone expansion that accompanies normal brain growth. Open spaces between the suture lines result from cranial molding during the birth process. Assessment of the fontanels for intracranial pressure is an important component of the examination. Normal intracranial pressure is characterized by a finding of fontanel fullness without bulging, either on visual inspection or palpation. Bulging, tense fontanels in an infant with a large head circumference are indicative of increased intracranial pressure, often associated with hydrocephalus.

The nurse may note the presence of swelling or soft tissue edema of the head that has resulted from trauma during the birth process. **Caput succedaneum** is diffuse edema that crosses the cranial suture lines and disappears without treatment during the first few days of life. **Cephalhematoma**, a more serious condition, results from a subperiosteal hemorrhage that does not cross the suture lines (Fig. 18-15). It appears as a localized swelling on one side of the infant's head and persists for weeks while the tissue fluid is slowly broken down and absorbed. During this time, the infant may exhibit signs of jaundice related to the metabolism of damaged red blood cells from the subperiosteal hemorrhage.

The nurse next palpates the neonate's eyes, ears, and nose to confirm shape and size. The eyelids are manually opened and the iris, sclera, and conjunctiva are examined. It is not unusual to detect tiny pinpoint scleral hemorrhages (related to birth trauma) in the outer canthus of the eyes. Swollen eyelids and a yellow discharge that adheres to the eyelashes may provide evidence of eye prophylaxis medication. The nurse uses an ophthalmoscope to check for bilateral red reflexes and records the findings on the infant's chart. Absence of bilateral red reflexes constitutes a medical emergency; this finding warrants immediate attention.

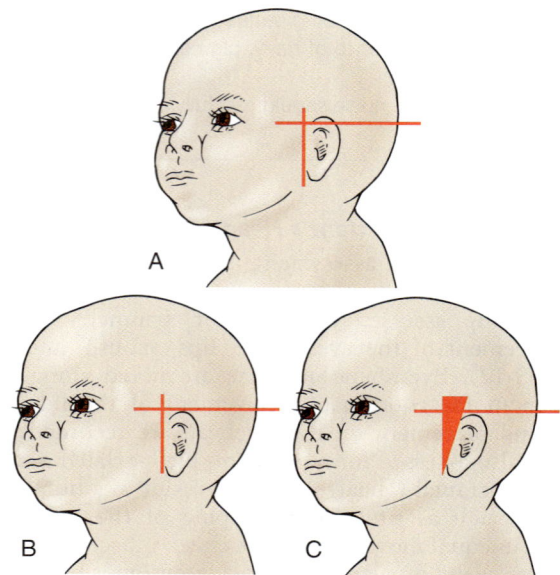

Figure 18-13 To determine ear placement, an imaginary line is drawn from the inner to the outer canthus of the eye and then to the ear. *A.* Normal ear position. *B.* Low-set ear. *C.* Slanted low-set ear.

critical nursing action Recognizing an Ophthalmic Emergency in the Infant

When using an ophthalmoscope to examine an infant's eyes, the nurse notes the following finding: Right eye: red reflex present. Left eye: red reflex absent.

What is the significance of these findings? What action should the nurse take next?

Absence of the red reflex indicates an interference with the transmission of light to the retina. This finding constitutes an ophthalmic emergency that requires immediate medical attention, since optic nerve suppression from obstructed light pathways may result in permanent blindness. The nurse must immediately notify the physician.

The nurse may assess the infant's gross vision by determining the infant's ability to direct his or her gaze at the examiner when positioned approximately 10 inches from the infant's face. The examiner then moves and notes whether or not the infant is able to appropriately readjust the gaze. The infant's nose is assessed by careful palpation of the nasal bridge to determine symmetry and the presence of fracture that may have occurred during birth. The nurse gently opens the infant's mouth and visually inspects, then palpates the gums for the presence of onatal teeth above or beneath the gum surface (Fig. 18-16). Teeth that have emerged through the gums should be checked for looseness and may need to be extracted because of the risk of aspiration. Since the presence of natal teeth may be associated with a congenital defect, further evaluation may be indicated (Dillon, 2007).

Epstein's pearls, whitish hardened nodules on the gums or roof of the mouth, may be visualized or palpated (Fig. 18-17). These pearl-like inclusion cysts are not an unusual finding and disappear within a few weeks. The presence of the uvula in the midline is noted; a bivalve or double lobed uvula may indicate a cleft in the palate. The infant's ability to suck can also be assessed during the oral examination. The nurse inserts a gloved finger into the infant's mouth and notes and records the strength of the sucking motion. Also, at this time the hard and soft palates can be examined for size, shape, and cleft formations. When present, a cleft defect is felt as an open space or as a notched ridge. A high, arched palate may be associated with difficulty swallowing or with later speech development. Next, the gag reflex is elicited and the back of the throat, tongue, and uvula are visualized. The infant's throat is also externally palpated to check for enlargement of the thyroid gland and to ensure that the trachea is located in the midline. The nurse checks for neck rotation by observing the infant's head movement and by gently turning the head from side to side. Torticollis is a deviation of the neck to one side caused by a spasmodic contraction of neck muscles. In the neonate, a torticollis is

Figure 18-15 *A.* Normal head. *B.* Caput succedaneum. Localized soft tissue edema present at birth. It does not increase in size. Swelling crosses the suture lines. *C.* Cephalhematoma. A collection of blood from a subperiosteal hemorrhage appears after birth. It increases in size. Swelling does not cross the suture lines.

Figure 18-16 Natal teeth.

Figure 18-17 Epstein's pearls usually disappear within a few weeks.

apparent when the head is positioned on one side while the chin points to the opposite side. Torticollis or the presence of a congenital cervical spine defect are two serious conditions that may produce limitations in neck movement and should be reported immediately.

The nurse palpates and inspects the neonate's ears to determine the thickness of the ear lobe and pinna. Ear pits and ear tags are common preauricular ear malformations. Ear pits, tiny pinholes found near the upper curved border of the pinna, arise from the imperfect fusion of the tubercles of the first and second brachial arches during early fetal development. Since they may signal a small sinus tract between the skin and underlying structures, they should be carefully evaluated to determine whether a layer of skin covers the opening or if the pit is open at the bottom. When signs of infection (i.e., redness, edema, draining fluid) are present, the ear pits should be surgically repaired. Ear tags, fleshy bulb-shaped growths that project from the surface of the skin, should be removed for cosmetic purposes by a plastic surgeon since they frequently contain microcapillaries that bleed when cut. The ear canals are assessed for patency and gross hearing may be evaluated by softly ringing a bell near each ear.

Most states in the United States require routine hearing screening before a newborn's discharge from the hospital. The goal of newborn screening is to identify congenital hearing loss and to refer those affected for early intervention. Screening is done using automated auditory brainstem response (AABR) in which electrodes are placed on the forehead and neck and soft earphones on the ears of a sleepy, calm infant. A series of clicks are introduced, usually at the 30- to 40-decibel level. If an infant has normal hearing, the response is detected by the electrodes (Kaye, 2007). Infants whose test results are unsatisfactory should be referred for repeated testing to take place no later than 8 weeks of age. Early hearing screening allows for timely identification of problems and reduces the age at which affected infants may be treated (Johnson et al., 2005; Joint Committee on Infant Hearing, 2000; U.S. Preventive Services Task Force, 2001).

Assessment of the nose begins with an observation of the placement of the nose, normally located in the middle of the face. The nurse can draw an imaginary line from the center of the bridge of the nose downward to the notch of the upper lip. The nose should lie exactly vertical to this line. Each side of the nose should be symmetrical. It is important to note any deviation to one side, as well as asymmetry in relation to the size and dimensions of the nostrils. Remember that the bridge of the nose in African American or Asian children is normally flat.

CONDITIONS THAT MAY WARRANT FURTHER ASSESSMENT. When conducting an assessment of the head, ears, eyes, nose, and throat, the nurse is alert to findings of asymmetry, unusual shape or evidence of defects in underlying structures or congenital syndromes. Generally, findings that are immediately apparent to the nurse examiner pose the greatest problems for the neonate. For example, Down syndrome is frequently identified during the assessment of the head when the nurse notes a flattened (instead of round) occiput, a broad nasal bridge, upward slanted eyes with epicanthal folds, low-set ears, an enlarged tongue, high arched palate, and a small chin. Open separations of the lip, mouth, nose, and hard or soft palate are indicative of cleft lip or cleft palate. Since facial disfigurement accompanies these defects, nurses should be extremely sensitive to the feelings of parents and other family members who interact with the infant.

The eye examination may provide an early indicator of several conditions that can affect the infant's well-being. For example, sclera, normally white, may appear to be blue or yellow in color. Bluish colored sclera may signal a congenital condition known as osteogenesis imperfecta, which is characterized by a loss of bone structure and integrity. Infants with this condition must be handled with extreme gentleness, and may have already suffered fractures during the birth process. Yellowing of the sclera, related to elevated bilirubin levels, is a late manifestation of jaundice in the neonate. The nurse should seek immediate medical assistance for the infant and plan for rapid intervention such as intravenous fluids and phototherapy. A disruption in the iris, called a coloboma, appears as a keyhole in the circle of the iris and pupil and will affect vision in that eye. Congenital cataracts are noted when white or pale yellow tissue covers the pupil and iris and occludes the red reflex. This finding warrants prompt referral. Occasionally, the red reflex (normally red or reddish orange in color) appears to be white, a finding that requires immediate attention since it may signal the presence of a neuroblastoma. Congenital glaucoma is an ophthalmic emergency that requires the timely instillation of eye drops to prevent blindness caused by increased intraocular pressure. This condition is characterized by protuberant eyes that appear to extend beyond the orbits and feel firm on gentle palpation.

Careful examination of the infant's facial features may provide evidence of birth defects associated with maternal alcohol use. Characteristic findings include short palpebral fissures; a flattened nasal bridge with a small, upturned nose; flat midface, thin upper lip and smooth philtrum. Alcohol-related birth defects (ARBD) also include poor growth, mental retardation (often associated with **microcephaly**, or small head), and small chin (micrognathia). This condition, also called fetal alcohol syndrome (FAS) or fetal alcohol effects (FAE), describes the range of physical and mental effects that are related to the mother's alcohol use during fetal growth and development. After birth, affected infants are often jittery, irritable, and poor feeders. Nursing interventions focus on providing a calming, quiet, nurturing environment with minimal stimulation. (See Chapter 19 for further discussion.)

The nurse's careful assessment of the infant's head, face, eyes, ears, nose, and throat constitutes an essential component of the neonatal physical examination. Since infants are frequently bundled in blankets when presented to parents and loved ones, initial impressions are often formed based on the appearance of the neonate's face and head. Because many congenital malformations affect these body parts, the nurse must be sensitive to parents' feelings and approach the initial "viewing" prepared to provide immediate emotional support and subsequent referral to appropriate resources as indicated. It is important to remember that a wide range of normal variations (i.e., birth marks, hair patterns, large eyes, nose, or ears) commonly occur and result from familial characteristics and inheritance patterns rather than from congenital syndromes.

Now Can You— Describe the assessment related to the infant's head?

1. Describe the location of the fontanels? Explain why it is important to assess them?
2. Differentiate between caput succedaneum and cephalhematoma and discuss how each is treated?
3. Describe how to conduct an assessment of the neonate's mouth and explain why this assessment is important?
4. Identify neonatal features that are characteristic of Down syndrome and maternal alcohol use?

 case study Baby Boy Goldman

Baby Boy Goldman was born via a normal spontaneous vaginal birth 4 hours ago. His parents are of eastern Mediterranean descent. His mother's prenatal care was initiated during the third month of gestation and the pregnancy was uncomplicated. He is awake and resting quietly in the nursery bassinet. During a review of the infant's medical record, the nurse notes the following information, recorded approximately 1 hour earlier: axillary temperature: 98.0°F (36.7°C) pulse: 136 beats per minute; respirations: 40 breaths per minute; weight: 8 lbs. 2 oz. (17.7 kg); length: 20.5 inches (8.1 cm). At birth, Baby Goldman's heart rate was 92 beats per minute and he was crying and moving all extremities. The nurse now observes that the infant's hands and feet are bluish in color and his face contains several white "bumps" that are scattered over his nose and forehead. Dark gray areas are seen on his lower back and buttocks. On palpation of Baby Goldman's head, the nurse notes a small degree of swelling that is symmetrical and crosses the suture lines.

critical thinking questions

1. Are these findings normal or pathological?
2. What actions should the nurse take?

◆ See Suggested Answers to Case Studies in the text on the Electronic Study Guide or DavisPlus.

Assessment of the Respiratory System

When assessing the neonate's respiratory efforts, the nurse first observes for symmetry in chest movement, and at the same time notes the placement and size of breast tissue. Enlargement of the breasts in male infants is common and only a temporary condition since it is related to maternal hormones. The breast tissue and nipples should be located in the midclavicular line. This anatomical landmark is actually an imaginary line that is one-half of the distance from the midline (the lower border of the sternum) to the lateral border of the chest wall formed by the rib cage. If the breast tissue is located between the midclavicular line and the lateral chest wall, the nurse documents this finding as "wide-spaced nipples." The presence of wide-spaced nipples may signal a congenital syndrome, such as Down syndrome. Extra or "accessory" nipples may be located above or below the primary nipples. This finding is not associated with a congenital syndrome and parents can be assured that the accessory nipples will not enlarge during puberty and if desired, they may be safely removed at a later date (Dillon, 2007).

To assess for nasal patency, the nurse carefully occludes one naris while the infant's mouth is closed. A rise in the infant's chest confirms that the nasal passageway is open and air has been inhaled. The assessment may be repeated with the other naris. If the infant demonstrates difficulty with this maneuver, he may have a developmental anomaly known as **choanal atresia** (a malformation of the bucco-nasal membrane). When present bilaterally, cyanosis is noted when the infant's mouth is closed but disappears when the mouth is open. An inability to pass a small catheter into the nares confirms the diagnosis. Since choanal atresia may be associated with other developmental anomalies, a positive finding should be reported immediately.

With the infant in a supine position, the nurse can readily assess his ease with overall breathing efforts. Respirations are counted and the pattern and any use of accessory muscles are noted. Slight sternal retractions may occur; this is a normal finding. Prominence of the xiphoid process is not unusual and with normal growth and development, the prominence will diminish. The lungs are auscultated anteriorly and posteriorly (Fig. 18-18). Infants may exhibit irregular breathing patterns accompanied by periods of apnea that can persist for up to 15 to 20 seconds. While not worrisome, it is important to alert parents that a brief cessation in respirations is common in neonates. The nurse also teaches the infant's caregivers how to recognize signs of respiratory distress: flaring of the nares, **retractions** (in-drawing of tissues between the ribs, below the rib cage or above the sternum and clavicles), or grunting with expirations. For healthy full-term neonates, a respiratory rate below 60 breaths per minute is considered normal. To obtain an accurate respiratory rate, it may be necessary to count the infant's respirations at several different times during the physical assessment. If the respiratory rate remains above 60 to 70 breaths per minute during rest, further evaluation is warranted.

Figure 18-18 *A.* The lungs are auscultated anteriorly. *B.* The lungs are auscultated posteriorly

Family Teaching Guidelines...
How to Recognize Breathing Difficulties

As a component of newborn care, the nurse provides the following information to parents:

Your baby may be experiencing breathing difficulty if she:

◆ Has above normal respirations.

◆ Has prolonged (greater than 15 seconds) periods of breath holding.

◆ Shows sucking-in and seesaw movements around her rib cage.

◆ Flares her nostrils.

◆ Makes grunting sounds.

CONDITIONS THAT MAY WARRANT FURTHER ASSESSMENT. If the infant appears to be expending considerable energy to breathe or shows other signs of breathing difficulty, prompt evaluation of the respiratory status must be immediately sought. Signs of respiratory distress may be manifested by marked sternal or intercostal retractions. During the assessment, the nurse should gently palpate the anterior lung field to identify birth injuries, such as fractures of the clavicle or ribs. These injuries can cause an increased respiratory rate due to pain. Asymmetry of the chest wall during respirations may also signal the presence of a rib fracture. The nurse next inspects the chest wall to confirm symmetry and shape. Anatomical deformities such as pectus carinatum (pigeon chest) and pectus excavatum (funnel chest) arise from abnormal development of the ribs and sternum and may interfere with normal lung expansion. All lung fields should be auscultated anteriorly and posteriorly and the respiratory rate is counted from the auscultation, rather than from observation of abdominal movements (Dillon, 2007). Auscultation of the infant's nose can help differentiate upper airway congestion (from mucus, amniotic fluid) from lower airway congestion. When the nasal passages, throat, or upper bronchus is congested, noisy breath sounds are often detected. Using a bulb syringe, the nurse gently removes fluid and mucus from the infant's nasal and throat passages to facilitate easy respirations. After this intervention, any retractions should disappear.

If the infant continues to exhibit retractions and other signs of breathing difficulty, prompt investigation is warranted, as this finding may constitute a life-threatening event. Respiratory distress is associated with a number of conditions that may be related to the lungs or heart. Narrowing of the airways is associated with many congenital respiratory conditions while congenital heart defects often interfere with the lungs' capacity to oxygenate the blood. Congenital or acquired infection in the neonate may also cause respiratory distress. If the infant's respiratory rate remains elevated (60 to 70 breaths per minute) during periods of rest, the nurse must provide continuous observation. While the increased respiratory rate may represent a transitional period of adjustment to extrauterine life, the development of other symptoms such as nasal flaring, grunting, or intercostal retractions is indicative of respiratory distress. (See Chapter 19 for further discussion.) To complete the assessment, the nurse should also note the infant's skin color and assess the capillary refill of his extremities, actions that provide additional information concerning the status of respiratory system functioning.

 Now Can You— Discuss components of the neonatal respiratory system assessment?

1. Discuss what parents should be told about breast enlargement in their male infant?

2. Describe the significance of wide spaced or accessory nipples in a neonate?

3. Discuss why palpation is an important component of the neonatal respiratory assessment?

4. Identify the indicators of neonatal respiratory distress?

Assessment of the Cardiovascular System

The nurse assesses the neonate's circulatory system by visual inspection and auscultation. Careful inspection of the skin, lips, gums, and buccal mucosa provides reliable evidence of cardiac perfusion. At rest, the infant's skin should be pink in color and progress to red during crying or physical activity. The nurse palpates the chest to detect any thrills or heaves and the point of maximum impulse (PMI), which is auscultated at the apex of the heart near the third or fourth left intercostal space (Dillon, 2007) (Fig. 18-19). For infants, the normal heart rate should be between 120 and 160 beats per minute. A heart rate above 160 beats per minute is termed tachycardia.

To assess capillary refill in the extremities, the nurse gently pinches the end of the infant's finger or toe and then counts the number of seconds required for the skin to return to its normal color. The average refill time is 3 seconds. If more than 3 seconds lapse, there may be shunting of blood from the periphery toward the infant's trunk.

The nurse palpates all peripheral pulses for bilateral symmetry, strength, and rate. The femoral pulses on each side are carefully checked and compared to the brachial pulses (Fig. 18-20). If a decrease in the strength of the pulse between the brachial pulses and femoral pulses is noted, this finding may be indicative of coarctation of the aorta, a cardiac condition associated with a narrowing of the aortic arch. Since the aorta is the main vessel for transporting oxygenated blood to the upper and lower body, a narrowing of the aortic arch produces a compromise in blood flow and should be suspected when decreased femoral pulses are detected. (See Chapter 19 for further discussion of coarctation of the aorta.)

Figure 18-19 Auscultating the heart.

Figure 18-20 Palpating the femoral pulse.

COMMON FINDINGS. The nurse carefully auscultates all areas of the heart, including the aortic, pulmonic, tricuspid, and mitral valves, along with the base and apex. Since the normal infant heart rate is between 110 and 160 beats per minute, rates higher than 160 beats per minute are consistent with tachycardia; rates lower than 100 beats per minute are termed bradycardia. Either condition, if persistent, warrants further investigation. Heart rate auscultation in the neonate is often difficult due to the thinness of the chest wall combined with the noisiness of heart sounds that are often obscured by respirations. The nurse should listen carefully and take time in counting the heart rate. It is not uncommon to hear murmurs in infants less than 24 hours old. The murmurs are characterized by a sound (best heard near the sternal border at the second or third intercostal space on the left side) that grows louder during systole. Although a heart sound arising from a patent ductus arteriosus may be heard initially, the sound disappears within 2 to 3 days when the ductus closes. If a murmur remains audible after the second day of life and intensifies to a "whoosh" sound, further investigation is warranted, as this finding is not characteristic of a patent ductus and may indicate the presence of another type of heart lesion.

CONDITIONS THAT MAY WARRANT FURTHER ASSESSMENT. Ventricular septal defect (VSD), a condition in which a small hole exists in the ventricle wall between the right and left chambers of the heart, is the most common heart murmur in infants. The VSD produces a sound created by the leaking of blood through the small defect. Interestingly, smaller defects are associated with louder murmurs due to the buildup of pressure in the heart chambers as the blood leaks through with each contraction. Large defects are associated with softer murmurs because the ease with which blood flows through the opening produces little pressure buildup. Most ventral septal defects close with normal cardiac growth during the first year of life and require no surgical intervention. (See Chapter 19 for further discussion.)

Cardiac insufficiency describes a condition that occurs when an infant cannot adequately oxygenate and circulate blood. This condition is characterized by pallor, rapid breathing, and cyanosis around the lips. Pulse oximetry readings should be obtained immediately. Readings of less than 94% oxygen saturation are of major concern and if an infant's oxygen saturation drops below 90%, rapid transfer to an intensive care unit for continuous respiratory and cardiac monitoring should be accomplished. Cardiac evaluation is carried out and, depending on the findings, treatment may be medical, surgical, or both.

Infants who demonstrate cardiac instability within the first 2 days of life are usually those with a genetic karyotype of trisomy 13, 18, or 21 or **tetralogy of Fallot**. Tetralogy of Fallot is a congenital heart defect that involves four distinct cardiac anomalies: transposition of the aorta and pulmonary artery, right ventricular hypertrophy, pulmonary stenosis, and ventricular septal defect. Infants born with tetralogy of Fallot demonstrate no difficulties until the ductus begins to close after the first 24 hours of life. At that point, the infant experiences severe cardiac instability and develops central cyanosis. Transfer to an intensive care unit allows for intravenous fluids, medications, and continuous cardiac monitoring to be carried out until surgical and medical evaluation can take place. (See Chapter 19 for further discussion.) When any infant is diagnosed with a cardiac problem, the nurse should be sensitive to the parents' frequently overwhelming feelings of fear and inadequacy and be prepared to offer reassurance, support, and accurate information.

Now Can You— Identify cardiac problems in the neonate?

1. Demonstrate how to assess capillary refill and discuss why this assessment is important?
2. Identify when auscultation of a heart murmur in a neonate is considered to be a normal finding?
3. Describe a ventricular septal defect and discuss the treatment for this condition?

Assessment of the Gastrointestinal System

The nurse begins the assessment by placing the infant in a supine position to facilitate the abdominal inspection. The abdomen should be round and bilaterally symmetrical. The clamped umbilical cord should show no evidence of active bleeding or oozing. It is inspected to confirm the presence of three vessels: two arteries and one vein. If fewer than three vessels are seen, the nurse documents the findings and notifies the physician since this finding may be associated with congenital anomalies. Wharton's jelly, the gelatinous substance that prevents compression of the blood vessels, may appear as areas of varying amounts of thickness. The abdomen may appear distended due to stool that has not yet been emptied from the bowel. The nurse carefully auscultates all four quadrants of the abdomen for bowel sounds (Fig. 18-21). To facilitate thorough auscultation, each quadrant is divided into small sections to lessen the likelihood that any one area is overlooked. Bowel obstruction in the neonate is often first identified by an absence of bowel sounds in a small, distinct section of the intestines. The nurse completes the assessment with auscultation of the upper abdomen for the gastric bubble and the heart sounds of the abdominal aorta.

COMMON FINDINGS. The nurse uses light, then deep palpation of the abdomen to assess the structure and contents of the abdomen. Light palpation is initiated at the lower sternal border and proceeds along the midline down to the umbilicus. Diastasis rectus, a thinning of the abdominal wall, may be detected. Diastasis rectus can also be identified by the presence of a long, raised "lump" along the midline that becomes prominent when the infant is crying. The nurse assesses the area surrounding the umbilicus for the presence of an umbilical hernia. Using the fingertips to

Figure 18-21 Auscultating bowel sounds.

determine the hernia size, the nurse notes whether it appears to be large or small, and documents this information in the medical record. Small umbilical hernias are common in newborns and often close without surgical intervention as the infant grows. The nurse continues palpation along the midline toward the symphysis pubis to detect any inferior extension of the hernia. Light palpation from the midline is then extended laterally toward the rib cage to assess for masses or enlarged organs.

Deep palpation facilitates examination of the organs. The border of the liver should be smooth and firm and located just below the right costal margin. The spleen, which lies beneath the left costal margin, should be palpable only at the tip. If a larger segment of spleen is palpated, this finding is reason for concern, since it is indicative of organ enlargement. Due to their small size, the kidneys may be difficult to detect. They are located approximately 1 to 2 cm above the umbilicus and are at a right angle to the umbilicus at the midline. The bladder should be present as a smooth organ in the midline below the umbilicus.

CONDITIONS THAT MAY WARRANT FURTHER ASSESSMENT. Findings indicative of a serious abdominal problem in the neonate include the following: abdominal distention, absence of bowel sounds, discharge from the umbilical cord or cord site, and palpation of an abdominal mass. Abdominal distention may involve the entire abdomen or it may be confined to small areas. Abdominal blood vessels may be readily visible in the distended abdomen. The presence of stool in the intestines is frequently detected, and this finding is not a cause for concern. Abdominal bulging that shifts when the infant's position is changed may be indicative of fluid in the abdomen. Absence of bowel sounds indicates an area of bowel that is not functioning; this finding must be immediately reported.

Necrotizing enterocolitis is a life-threatening condition that occurs when a lack of blood flow to the bowel results in destruction of the intestinal mucosa. Loss of bowel function results and toxins are released from the damaged, necrotic tissue. Immediate surgical intervention is required. (See Chapter 19 for further discussion.)

Discharge from the umbilical cord or cord site indicates the presence of infection. Unless a bacteriostatic dye has been used to paint the area, the cord should be pale yellow in appearance. An extra clamp may be applied if blood is actively leaking from the umbilical cord. If meconium was passed in utero, the cord may be stained a gray-green color. The area around the base of the cord should be kept clean and dry. During diapering, care must be taken not to allow stool or urine to come in contact with the cord or the cord base. If this occurs, the nurse should carefully clean and dry the site. The tissue surrounding the base of the cord should be inspected for redness, a finding that may indicate **omphalitis** (an infection that is readily treated with antibiotics).

Palpation to detect an abdominal mass or enlarged organ is usually facilitated by the infant's small abdominal girth. Positive findings require immediate referral for evaluation. Often, an ultrasound examination is conducted to determine the source of the clinical findings and to guide the management. In infancy, abdominal masses are frequently a form of neuroblastoma, a type of tumor that is confirmed by biopsy. The kidneys, liver, and spleen are the organs most commonly enlarged, and these findings can be confirmed with ultrasound. Enlargement may result from obstruction or it may be associated with a congenital malformation.

critical nursing action Recognizing Acute Abdomen in the Neonate

During the neonatal assessment, the nurse is alert to the following symptoms that may indicate acute abdomen:

- Rigid, board-like abdomen
- Inability to palpate abdominal organs
- Indicators of pain (continuous crying, facial changes, gross motor movements)

 Now Can You— **Identify gastrointestinal problems in the neonate?**

1. Demonstrate how to perform the abdominal assessment on the neonate?
2. Identify findings that are associated with serious abdominal problems?
3. Describe two nursing interventions to minimize the risk of infection at the umbilical cord site?

Assessment of the Genitourinary System

The nurse begins the assessment by placing the infant in a supine position with the hips abducted. With the male neonate, the scrotum is examined to confirm that both testicles have descended. If flat or depressed areas are identified, this finding may indicate that a testis has not descended. Palpation of the scrotum is accomplished by placement of the examiner's second finger at the posterior scrotal midline with the thumb on the anterior midline (Fig. 18-22). Using the index finger and the thumb, the nurse palpates the left side of the scrotum for the presence of a testis and then uses the third finger and thumb to palpate for a testis on the right side of the

Figure 18-22 Palpating the scrotum.

scrotum. Proceeding in this pattern helps to ensure that one testis is not mistakenly being "counted" twice. If a testis is not detected, the nurse can softly stroke the inguinal canal in an attempt to locate an undescended testis. Warm soapy water applied to the inguinal area may enhance testicular prominence and help it to be more easily identified. Any infant older than 35 weeks' gestation who has undescended testicles should be referred for a urological consultation (Dillon, 2007).

Inspection of the female genitalia begins with the labia majora. The extent to which the labia cover the surrounding tissues corresponds with the developmental maturity of the female neonate. For most term infants, the borders of the labia majora touch and the clitoris is covered completely. Occasionally, a full-term infant has delayed genital development, and on examination, the nurse can easily view the labia minora and exposed clitoris.

The anus and anal opening are also assessed at this time. While stooling confirms anal patency, it is beneficial to actually witness the passage of meconium, as it provides an opportunity for the nurse to confirm that the stool passes through only one opening. Stool in the vagina indicates the presence of a rectovaginal fistula, an opening between the rectum and vagina. To palpate the anus, the nurse gently touches the tissue around the anal opening and assesses the musculature surrounding the opening. Tiny rectal tears from the passage of stool in the anal ring are noted and the anal wink reflex is assessed. The infant is placed in a prone position and, using the index finger, the nurse gently strokes the buttocks from side to side. In response, the buttocks draw together and "wink" at the point of the anal opening. This response validates the correct anatomical position of the anal opening. In females, the anal wink reflex is useful in assessing anal openings that are positioned less than 1 cm from the vaginal opening. When the anal opening is located too close to the vaginal opening, proper muscle strength needed to evacuate the rectum as the child grows older does not develop. The wink reflex is also useful in facilitating proper placement of the anal opening during future surgical correction (Dillon, 2007).

COMMON FINDINGS. Careful assessment of genitalia is essential in both males and females. First, the nurse visually inspects, then palpates the male genitalia. Infants of various ethnic backgrounds, especially those of African American heritage, have dark-colored scrotal skin. Scrotal swelling may interfere with an accurate palpation. If swelling is present, it is important to auscultate the scrotum to ensure that it does not hold entrapped bowel.

If no bowel sounds are heard, transillumination can be used to verify the presence of fluid in the scrotal sac. The nurse secures a penlight or ophthalmoscope, which will be used as a light source; darkens the room; and gently presses the light source against the scrotum. Fluid appears as a reddish yellow reflection. Masses do not transilluminate, and if detected, must be reported immediately. Scrotal fluid is slowly reabsorbed during the first weeks of life and no treatment is necessary. The nurse can reassure the parents that any swelling will resolve over time and the scrotum will gradually take on a more normal appearance.

 clinical alert

Bowel sounds in the scrotum

To confirm that no bowel is entrapped in the scrotum, the nurse carefully auscultates the scrotum for bowel sounds. If bowel sounds are present, immediate assistance must be obtained. This is a medical emergency.

The penis is palpated to estimate the approximate length. Penile length in the full-term newborn male is approximately 2 cm. The nurse gently retracts the prepuce, or foreskin, to inspect the urethral opening and to determine the location of the opening on the glans. Smegma, a waxy substance, may be present on the glans beneath the foreskin. Instead of the normal round urethral opening, or meatus, a vertical opening may be seen. When present on the ventral (instead of central) surface, this finding is indicative of **hypospadias**. Hypospadias requires surgical repair by a physician. Since the excess foreskin is used to create a properly positioned meatus, males with suspected hypospadias should not be circumcised. **Epispadias** is a similar condition. When present, the vertical urinary opening is located on the dorsal surface of the penis instead of on the glans. Epispadias is also repaired surgically with the use of excess foreskin.

During the inspection of the female genitalia, the nurse may identify vernix caseosa, a whitish, cheesy substance, covering the tissue between the labia. This is a normal finding. The hymenal tag, a small piece of triangle-shaped tissue, may also be present between the labia. The nurse gently palpates the labia majora and labia minora, an action that facilitates examination of the hymenal area. Small amounts of blood and whitish mucoid discharge ("pseudomenstruation"), related to the maternal hormones, may be noted in the vaginal area. Parents can be assured that this discharge is normal and will disappear in about a week. Smegma may also be present between the labia.

CONDITIONS THAT MAY WARRANT FURTHER ASSESSMENT. When examining the male genitalia, the nurse may note the presence of bruising or swelling, especially if the infant was delivered in a breech presentation. Careful palpation facilitates the scrotal assessment, conducted to confirm that both testes have descended. Inspection and palpation of the penis includes assessment of the penile length. Micropenis, a penis that is less than 2 cm in length, may be associated with a pituitary tumor. Ambiguous genitalia describes a condition where the male has genital structures that mimic labia or the female has a structure similar to a penis. If the definite genitalia cannot be determined, the infant is referred for genetic studies and evaluated for adrenal gland insufficiency. In situations of ambiguous genitalia, the nurse must be careful not to prematurely label an infant as a "boy" or "girl," to avoid compounding the parents' confusion. It is important that the nurse approach the parents with sensitivity and compassion.

66 What to say 99 — *Infant with ambiguous genitalia*

Despite the initial birthing room determination of the neonate's gender, careful later examination of the genitalia may prompt concerns regarding the true sex assignment. It is important to promptly alert parents of the need for further testing for gender determination. The nurse can address the parents' concerns with reassuring statements such as:

"Since there is some question regarding your baby's sex organs, the doctor has asked a specialist to examine your baby. Additional testing may be indicated. You may want to wait to name your baby until we know for sure. For now, it is important to spend as much time as possible with the baby as you get to know one another."

In the assessment of the female genitalia, most concerns center around the presence of an enlarged clitoral hood and the finding of an imperforate hymen. Although maternal hormones may produce slight clitoral enlargement, a hood-shaped, grossly enlarged clitoris may be related to excessive androgen production. Since this condition may signal congenital adrenal hyperplasia, further evaluation and testing should be performed. The infant's genitalia may also be edematous from birth trauma, making the examination difficult. The nurse should gently separate the labia and inspect the area for the location of the urethral and vaginal openings. Imperforate hymen is present when tissue obstructs the vaginal opening, necessitating later surgical correction to allow for the discharge of menstrual blood.

Male and female infants may have anal ring skin tags or an anal ring that has no opening. The skin tags are hemorrhoid-like tissues that can cause discomfort or bleeding when the infant stools. The absence of an opening in the anal ring is a condition known as **imperforate anus**.

The finding of imperforate anus constitutes a medical emergency since the infant is unable to pass stool through the anus. In approximately half of the infants with this condition, the imperforate anus occurs as an isolated event unrelated to any congenital syndrome. In the other half of occurrences, the imperforate anus is a part of a congenital syndrome associated with anal malformations, called the VATER association. At least three of the major abnormalities must be present for diagnosis. The overall prognosis is improved following the surgical correction of each anomaly. Characteristics of VATER association in the newborn include:

V = vertebral abnormalities
A = anal abnormalities (imperforate anus)
T = tracheal abnormalities
E = esophageal abnormalities (tracheal-esophageal fistulas)
R = renal and radial abnormalities

 critical nursing action Recognizing the Infant with Imperforate Anus

The nurse observes that Infant Gracie has not passed a meconium stool since her birth 26 hours ago. Infant Gracie has been breastfed several times and her mother reports that her baby is a "ready feeder" who is "always hungry." The mother states that she has not changed her baby's diaper. The infant's abdomen appears distended and feels firm on palpation. The nurse recognizes that these clinical findings may be indicative of imperforate anus and immediately notifies the physician.

The nurse's careful assessment of the neonate's genitalia has far-reaching implications. The findings from this examination form the foundation for future parental interaction with their newborn. While gender determination is briefly addressed at the time of birth, the nurse who later conducts the thorough assessment is responsible for identifying any problems and seeking appropriate consultation. The nurse must remain sensitive to the parents' concerns and be ready to correct any misinformation that might affect the parents' ability to relate to their infant in a positive manner.

Now Can You— Identify genitourinary conditions in the neonate?

1. Describe how to assess for undescended testes in the male infant and discuss the significance of this finding?
2. Describe the procedure for performing a transillumination of the scrotum and identify when this examination is used?
3. Name the two most common problems that affect the female genitalia?
4. Discuss how the infant is assessed for imperforate anus and describe the treatment for this condition?

Assessment of the Musculoskeletal System

The nurse can readily assess the functioning of the musculoskeletal system by observing the newborn in the crib where the infant has the freedom to continue and expand movements first initiated in utero. By flexing and extending the arms and legs, sucking on the fingers, and moving the head from side to side, the neonate provides a visual display of his musculoskeletal status. Any compromise in movement alerts the nurse to the location of possible birth trauma or other injury. Inspection of the extremities for differences in length or size is an important component of the assessment. Positive findings may be indicative of achondroplasia, a congenital condition characterized by a small thoracic area, an inability to extend the elbows and a marked shortening of the femurs and humerus. Often referred to as "dwarfs," individuals with achondroplasia frequently have neurological and respiratory problems in addition to their skeletal deformities.

To assess muscle tone and strength, the nurse first places the infant in a supine position and then in a prone position. If the infant is unable to move the lower extremities, damage to the spinal cord is suspected. Asymmetry in movement suggests nerve damage or fracture related to birth trauma. If the infant does not move or appears floppy when repositioned, the nurse suspects hypotonia, or diminished muscle tone. Hypotonia may be related to an episode of anoxia, either during birth or while in utero. Increased muscle tone, or hypertonia, is characterized by muscle tremors, twitches or jerkiness, and this finding is often associated with neonatal abstinence syndrome. Symptoms of drug withdrawal are manifest through the increased muscular movements.

COMMON FINDINGS. After the visual inspection, the nurse begins palpation of the musculoskeletal system. Starting with the shoulders, the examination progresses downward toward the lower extremities. The muscles and joints are assessed for symmetry and gentle passive range of motion is used to evaluate joint rotation. Rotation of the neck is the first and most important rotation assessed. Passive range of motion should confirm the infant's ability to accomplish full rotation of the neck. Failure to achieve full rotation may be related to torticollis or to the congenital absence of portions of the cervical vertebra. Normal growth and development in infants is enhanced by their ability to turn the head toward the location of sound and then follow the auditory cue with their eyes. Thus, normal neck rotation plays an important role in the refinement of hearing and in the development of sight. To assess head lag, the nurse carefully pulls the infant up while watching the head gently fall back (Fig. 18-23). This maneuver also provides an opportunity to inspect the neck for bulging of the thyroid gland and for assessing the muscle tone of the upper body along with shoulder and arm strength.

The nurse's attention is next directed toward assessment of the hip joint, the second most important joint evaluation in the neonate. **Developmental dysplasia of the hip** (DDH) is a congenital condition that, left untreated, can affect the infant's future ability to walk and maintain balance. It occurs when the acetabulum is flat, rather than round and cup-like in shape. DDH most often results when the developing fetus assumed a dominant breech position with upwardly extended legs during the period of bone growth. The assessment begins with inspection of the skin folds on the infant's thighs in both the prone and supine positions (Fig. 18-24).

Asymmetry of the skin folds may signal the presence of hip dysplasia. The nurse also assesses the leg length and knee height for unevenness. Next, the nurse slowly moves the infant's lower extremities in a kicking motion while observing for signs of pain or distress. The nurse's hands are placed on the infant's thigh with the fingertips around the femur head while the thumb and index finger stabilize the knee joint. While maintaining this position, the nurse performs the Barlow's maneuver by exerting a downward pressure on the head of the femur in an attempt to dislodge the femur head from the acetabulum (Procedure 18-3). The Ortolani's maneuver involves a circular rotation of the femoral head or an inward–outward action that attempts to

Figure 18-24 Inspecting gluteal skin folds.

reposition the femur head that was displaced by the Barlow's maneuver. In the normal neonate, the hip joints move easily and it is not uncommon to detect crepitus, or a slight grinding (known as a "hip click") when the femur head is manipulated in the socket (Dillon, 2007).

It is not unusual to detect hip dysplasia in infants who maintained a breech position in utero or who were delivered vaginally in a breech position. Hip dysplasia can be confirmed by a noticeable difficulty when moving the leg in the hip joint and also by feeling the head of the femur pop out of the hip socket, sometimes referred to as a "hip clunk." Often, infants who were in a breech position in utero have hyperextended knee joints that can give the appearance of hip dysplasia. However, subsequent examination confirms that the head of the femur remains firmly secured in the acetabulum. Parents can be assured that over time, the infant's legs will return to the normal flexed position. The nurse may also detect a "looseness" in the infant's hip joint despite a normal evaluation that shows no evidence of hip dysplasia. This finding is related to the maternal hormones that create a joint flexibility not only in mothers but in their infants as well.

Dysplasia is not confirmed by x-ray but by ultrasound or CT Developmental dysplasia of the hip, once confirmed by x-ray exam, is managed by the placement of a special splint to keep the infant's legs in a position of abduction. The Pavlik harness, the most widely used device, does not rigidly immobilize the hip but acts to prevent hip extension or abduction. The harness is worn continuously for approximately 3 to 6 months, until new bone growth has formed around the head of the femur and a normal cup-shaped hip joint has been created.

To assess the remaining joints, the nurse performs passive range of motion and also continues to observe the infant's spontaneous movements in his crib. It is not uncommon to identify unusual positions of the foot, and these findings are most often related the infant's position in utero. Pronation, or inward turning, of both feet is common and the nurse can demonstrate to the parents how gentle stroking of the infant's insoles prompts a ready return to a normal position. When the foot is severely pronated, spontaneous normal alignment may be unattainable. In this instance, an evaluation of the posterior alignment of the infant's heel and knee is conducted. Club foot, suspected when there is a medial displacement of the heel from the posterior knee alignment, can be confirmed by x-ray exam. Soon after a diagnosis of clubfoot, a cast is placed on the affected extremity to restore proper alignment. The nurse should demonstrate how to safely stabilize the cast when holding the infant and teach the parents how to care for the cast.

Figure 18-23 To assess head lag, the infant is gently pulled up as the nurse observes his head fall back.

Procedure 18-3 Performing the Barlow–Ortolani Maneuver

Purpose

To assess for developmental dysplasia of the hips

Equipment

None

Steps

1. Place the infant supine on a flat surface.

2. Place your thumbs on the infant's inner thighs and your fingers on the outside of the greater trochanters of the hips.

3. Flex the infant's knees and move the legs inward until your fingers touch.

4. Using gentle but firm pressure, rotate the hips outward so that the knees touch the flat surface. No clicking or crepitus should be detected.

RATIONALE: *The presence of clicking or crepitus indicates joint instability.*

Documentation

3/4/10 1500 – Barlow-Ortolani maneuver negative

— J. Yamoto, RN

CONDITIONS THAT MAY WARRANT FURTHER ASSESSMENT. Before performing the musculoskeletal assessment, the nurse first must determine that there are no broken bones. It is important that the infant not be moved or repositioned until this has been accomplished. In the neonate, the clavicle is the bone most commonly fractured. The injury occurs during birth when the infant's shoulders do not readily rotate. The nurse should palpate the clavicles to check for a separation between the bone ends or for the presence of crepitus. Signs and symptoms of fractures include swelling at the fracture site, bruising, or discoloration of the affected area and the infant's expression of discomfort when moved. Other common sites for neonatal fractures are the ribs, humerus, and skull. An x-ray exam is used to confirm the diagnosis. Clavicular fractures heal over time without intervention and the nurse can teach the parents to position the infant on the side opposite the injury and how to hold and support the infant's head and shoulders until healing is complete. Casts are usually applied to humeral fractures while rib fractures are generally wrapped. Infants with skull fractures are most often cared for in the intensive care unit where they can be continuously monitored.

Sometimes, infants are born with extra digits (fingers) and toes (**polydactyly**) or with what appears to be webbing of the skin between the digits and toes (**syndactyly**). On the hand, the extra digits often are located below the fourth finger and are attached to the palm by a thin line of skin. They may resemble the fourth finger and may even contain a fingernail. The nurse should palpate all extra digits for the presence of bone, which must be surgically removed. If no bone is present, the digit may be tied off with suture silk to occlude the capillary to cause necrosis and loss of the digit. Polydactyly is often a family characteristic and parents may recall other family members who were born with extra digits or toes. Webbing of the toes does not interfere with balance or walking, and parents may not wish to have their infant's toes surgically released from one another. Webbing of the fingers is often surgically corrected to facilitate dexterity and for cosmetic reasons.

The nurse inspects the palms of the hands for the presence of palmar creases. The hands of a normal neonate usually contain three or four curved palmar creases. A **simian crease** is a single, straight crease that appears in the middle of the palm on one or both hands (Fig. 18-25). When unaccompanied by other findings, the simian crease is insignificant. However, when detected along with other symptoms, a simian crease may be associated with other syndromes, such as Down syndrome.

Figure 18-25 *A.* Normal palmar crease. *B.* Simian crease.

 Now Can You— **Complete a neonatal musculoskeletal assessment?**

1. Identify the most important joints to assess in the neonate and describe how the assessments are performed?
2. Discuss the management options for an infant with developmental dysplasia of the hip?
3. Describe the significance of polydactyly and syndactyly?
4. Recognize why the discovery of a simian crease prompts further investigation?

Assessment of the Neurological System

The physical assessment of the neonate concludes with the nervous system and reflexes. During this assessment, the nurse focuses on the reflexes and other movements that provide an indication of the infant's level of neurological function. It is helpful to divide the reflexes into two broad categories: major reflexes (reflective of normal neurological function) and minor reflexes (finger grasp, toe grasp, rooting, sucking, head righting, stepping and tonic neck). The major reflexes include the gag, Babinski, Moro, and Galant reflexes. Methods for assessing the various reflexes are displayed in Table 18-2.

The finger or palmar grasp reflex is assessed by observing the infant curl the fingers around an object (often the nurse's finger) that has been placed in the palm. The toe or plantar grasp is assessed in the same manner, by placing an object across the sole of the foot. The nurse observes the rooting and sucking reflexes by stroking the infant's cheek and watching him turn toward the finger, open the mouth, and suck on an object placed in the mouth. The head righting reflex is elicited by lifting the neonate in the prone position and then gently stroking the back in the midline, along the spinal cord. With this action, the normal infant attempts to raise the head and arch the back at the same time. To assess the stepping reflex, the nurse holds the infant in an upright position with the legs flexed. The soles of the feet are lightly brushed against a flat surface. In response to the stimulation, the infant lifts his feet and then places them back down in a stepwise pattern that imitates walking. The tonic neck or "fencing" reflex is observed with the infant in a supine position. The nurse observes the infant extend the arm and leg on the side to which the head and jaw are turned while flexing the arm and leg on the opposite side.

To assess the major reflexes, the nurse progresses methodically, taking care to document and record each finding. For the infant to successfully eat and move fluid away from the back of the throat without choking, the gag reflex must be intact. The Babinski reflex is demonstrated by lightly stroking the plantar surface of the foot from the heel toward the toes. The infant responds to this stimulation by first incurving the toes, then uncurling and stretching them out. The nurse can assess the **Moro reflex** at the same time as the head righting reflex is elicited. As the infant's head is lifted, the nurse mimics a release and watches for extension of both arms along with flexion of the legs, movements that confirm the Moro reflex. In the past, the examiner often assessed the Moro reflex by creating a loud clapping sound near the infant in an attempt to startle him. This method of assessment is not reliable. The infant's response to the clapping stimulus may not be consistent with the Moro movements because the infant could be reacting to the movement of air across his body as the examiner makes the clapping sound, or to the sound of the clap itself. The Galant reflex, also called the trunk incurvation reflex, is elicited as the infant is held or supported in a prone position. One side of the vertebral column is then stroked. The infant responds to this stimulus by moving the buttocks in a curving motion toward the side that is being stroked.

CONDITIONS THAT MAY WARRANT FURTHER ASSESSMENT. The most frequently seen neurological injuries in the neonate involve the brachial plexus and are related to difficulties with shoulder rotation and delivery at the time of birth. The nurse must differentiate these injuries from shoulder dystocia, which is identified by a temporary decrease in the movement and muscle tone of a shoulder and upper arm. Injury related to shoulder dystocia rapidly improves after delivery.

Erb's palsy is one form of brachial plexus injury that is readily identified from the positioning of the infant's arm while in the supine position. When Erb's palsy is present, one or both arms and hands are extended and do not move into a flexed position. On palpation, the nurse notes a decrease in muscle tone, a decreased grasp reflex and an absence of arm recoil on the affected side. Sometimes called the "waiter's position," the position is reminiscent of a waiter who keeps one arm by the side while the other is held out for a tip.

Most injuries involving the brachial plexus resolve in approximately 2 weeks without treatment. The infant should be positioned with the arm in a gently flexed position and when held, care should be taken to support the arm on the affected side. The nurse should teach parents how to use gentle exercise to facilitate the healing process. Simple arm strengthening exercises that passively flex and extend the infant's arm can be practiced during each parent–infant interaction.

Infants with major neurological problems that have occurred during embryonic or fetal development, or result from events during the birthing process are assessed in the neonatal intensive care unit. Severe damage that affects the brain or muscle movement may be associated with periods of anoxia (lack of oxygen) that occurred during fetal growth or during the birth process. Cerebral palsy is one condition that results from oxygen deprivation. Infants with cerebral palsy often demonstrate a number of motor difficulties, such as difficulty swallowing, breathing, or moving. The length of the anoxic period corresponds with the severity of brain damage. When caring for infants with cerebral palsy, the nurse may deal with a spectrum of difficulties that ranges from minimal limitation to a total loss of reflexes and controlled body movements.

Table 18-2 Newborn Reflexes

Palmar Grasp

The infant curls his fingers around an object.

Toe or Plantar Grasp

The infant curls his toes around an object that has been placed at the sole of the foot.

Rooting and Sucking Reflexes

Stroke the infant's cheek and watch him turn toward the finger, open his mouth and suck on an object placed in his mouth.

Extrusion Reflex

Touch the tip of the infant's tongue and the tongue will protrude outward.

Table 18-2 Newborn Reflexes—cont'd

Stepping Reflex

Hold the infant in an upright position with the legs flexed. The soles of the feet are lightly brushed against a flat surface. In response to the stimulation, the infant lifts his feet and then places them back down in a stepwise pattern that imitates walking.

Tonic Neck or Fencing Reflex

Observe the infant, in a supine position, extend his arm and leg on the side to which his head and jaw is turned while flexing his arm and leg on the opposite side.

Glabellar Reflex

Tap on infant's forehead and observe him blink for the first few taps.

Babinski Reflex

Lightly stroke the plantar surface of the foot from the heel toward the toes. The infant responds to this stimulation by first incurving the toes, then uncurling and stretching them out.

Moro Reflex

Observe the infant's head as it is lifted while the nurse mimics a release and watches for extension of both arms along with flexion of the legs.

Continued

Table 18-2 Newborn Reflexes—cont'd

Magnet Reflex

With the infant in a supine position, flex the leg and apply pressure to the soles of the feet. Observe the infant extend his legs against the pressure.

Galant Reflex or Trunk Incurvation Reflex

Observe the infant while supported in a prone position. Stroke one side of the vertebral column. The infant responds to this stimulus by moving his buttocks in a curving motion toward the side that is being stroked.

Crawling Reflex

Place infant on his abdomen; observe him attempt to crawl.

Crossed Extension

With the infant in a supine position, stimulate one foot; observe flexion, adduction, and then extension of the opposite leg.

In utero development of the brain and spinal cord is a process initiated during the embryonic period. During the first 30 days of gestation, the primitive neural tube closes. A failure of the tube to close at the posterior end results in an open area that may be filled with fluid or with a section of the spinal cord. This condition, called spina bifida, is usually detected during routine maternal–fetal antenatal testing. When the infant is born, the lesion of spina bifida resembles a skin-covered sac located between the fifth lumbar and first sacral vertebrae. The sac, which may contain the dura mater and spinal fluid, is called a **meningocele**. This condition usually does not cause any loss of motor function, or paralysis, below the waist. A more serious lesion is the **myelomeningocele**. When present, a myelomeningocele is a sac that contains dura mater, spinal fluid and a portion of the spinal cord. Individuals with a myelomeningocele have no bladder or bowel control and there is a loss of motor function below the waist.

Treatment of spina bifida is related to the location and extent of the lesion. Most often, the sac is surgically closed to prevent infection. Spina bifida occulta is a mild variation of spina bifida. In this condition, there is a small defect in the spinal vertebrae. However, since there is no protrusion of the dura mater, spinal fluid, or spinal cord, all motor activity remains intact.

An incomplete closure of the anterior portion of the neural tube causes a condition known as **anencephaly**. Lack of closure in this location causes portions of the brain, forehead, skull, and occiput to be missing. Infants born with anencephaly are usually placed on respirators and monitored to assess viability. When caring for the mother and her family, the nurse must be extremely sensitive to the emotional impact associated with this condition and offer the parents privacy and support.

Now Can You— Complete a neonatal neurological assessment?

1. Identify the major and minor reflexes in a neonate?
2. Demonstrate how the Moro reflex is elicited and describe why this assessment is performed?
3. Recognize the signs of a brachial plexus injury?
4. Describe two types of neural tube defects?

Enhancing the Neonate's Transition to Extrauterine Life

The newborn's adaptation to extrauterine life is an amazing and complex process. In the early days of adjustment as well as through infancy, newborns need significant physical, emotional, and spiritual care. Mothers and other caregivers must learn the essential aspects of newborn care in order to promote optimal infant growth and development. Critical aspects of physical care include bathing, clothing, diapering, and feeding the infant. It is also important that parents' discharge instructions provide easy to understand information about the proper care of the infant's nails, umbilical cord, and, when appropriate, the circumcision. Bonding with the newborn is essential for emotional care and the beginnings for spiritual development are established by building trust through relationships with the primary caregiver. Parents must be educated about the importance of timely metabolic screening for the newborn, since many life-threatening problems can be detected early enough for effective intervention.

TEMPERATURE ASSESSMENT

To prevent dangerous heat loss in the infant, nurses, mothers, and other caregivers need to understand how to protect the infant from extreme temperature fluctuations during bath time. In the hospital before the bath is given, it is important to take the newborn's temperature to ensure stability.

Temperature may be assessed by several methods. The axillary skin method, which is reflective of the infant's core temperature and the body's compensatory response to the environment, is the preferred noninvasive method that provides a close estimation of the rectal temperature. Although rectal temperature represents the closest approximation of core temperature, this route is not recommended because of the possibility of irritation and perforation of the rectal mucosa. The infant's temperature may also be assessed with a continuous skin probe (especially useful with small newborns or infants placed in incubators or under radiant warmers) or via tympanic thermometer, a portable sensor probe that is placed in the ear canal. This method employs infrared technology to measure the temperature of the internal carotid artery blood flow. As long as the temperature is maintained between 97.5° and 99°F (36.4°–37.2°C), the bath can be given. At home, it is not necessary to take the temperature before bath time.

BATHING THE NEWBORN

When bathing the newborn, the bath should take place in a warm area free from drafts. The newborn can be given a sponge bath using only warm water for the first few days of life. After the cord stump has dried completely and fallen off in approximately 2 weeks, the infant can be immersed in a small tub filled with about 4 to 5 inches of water.

Optimizing Outcomes— Ensuring safety for the newborn

It is paramount to remember that wet newborns are slippery! The nurse and parents must keep a firm hold on the baby, and continuously support the head up out of the water. When instructing new parents about the bath it is important that they understand that it is never acceptable to leave any child unattended near water, even a small amount of water. Submersion injury is the second leading cause of accidental death in children.

Newborns do not require a daily bath; bathing them once a week is adequate. However, the face and hands can be wiped off daily. The infant's bottom and genital area should be cleansed several times during the day. Because the newborn's skin may be sensitive, a mild, unscented soap is recommended for the bath. The initial bath after birth takes place after temperature stabilization. The procedure for the bath after birth and at home is fairly simple. The bath should proceed from head to toe. Parents must understand that good hygiene, including clean clothes, hair, nails, and teeth is important in promoting proper growth and development for their infant. At home, newborns can be placed in 4 to

5 inches of water in a small nonskid surface infant bathtub. Infants who are immersed in water for bathing have a tendency to be calmer and quieter and experience less heat loss than infants who are sponge bathed. Immersing the infant's body with water facilitates thorough distribution of the water to ensure even temperature and decreased evaporative heat loss. Benefits of immersion include a soothing feeling, hydration to the skin, and tactile stimulation.

If dry skin is a problem, baths may be given less frequently and a moisturizing lotion can be applied after the infant is dried. Since the newborn's skin can be sensitive to scented lotion, it is best to use an unscented product. Bath time is an ideal time for the nurse to assess the newborn's physical condition, muscular activity, behavior, state of arousal and alertness, and the act of showing parents how to properly bathe their infant provides a perfect opportunity to observe and encourage maternal and family bonding.

NAIL CARE AND UMBILICAL CORD CARE

Newborn nails are rarely trimmed in the hospital or birthing center in the initial days of life due to the increased potential for injury to surrounding tissue that may result in infection. After about a week, the nails more readily separate from the skin and often break off naturally. In the early days, to prevent the infant's nails from scratching the face, filing the nails with a fine emery-textured board or covering the infant's hands with a cuffed T-shirt or mittens are safer options. However, covering the hands should be avoided if possible because this action prevents the infant from sucking on the fingers for self-consolation. In the home, parents may continue to file their newborn's nails or they may be taught how to carefully trim them, often while the infant sleeps.

The umbilical cord appears as a gelatinous white stump with two arteries and one vein. Immediately after birth, the cord is cut with a sterile scissors and clamped. Goals of cord care center on the prevention and early detection of hemorrhage or infection. Because it provides an excellent medium for bacterial growth, the cord stump is a potential source of infection (Miller & Newman, 2005). The Association of Women's Health, Obstetric and Neonatal Nurses (AWHONN) recommends that the cord initially be cleaned with sterile water or a neutral pH cleanser and thereafter with water (AWHONN, 2001). The cord begins to dry out in approximately 1 to 2 hours. The cord clamp must remain in place for 24 hours when it can be removed with a special cord clamp remover. By the third day, the cord appears to be discolored and shrunken. By 10 to 14 days, the cord has usually detached completely and parents often find the remnants in the infant's diaper or on the bedding.

⊙ Optimizing Outcomes— Teaching parents about umbilical cord care

Information regarding umbilical cord care should be included as a component of discharge teaching. Parents are taught about the cord's normal appearance and shown how to fold and position the diaper below the cord stump. Remind parents to keep the area free from urine and wetness during bathing and when to expect complete cord detachment. It is also helpful to alert them to potential danger signs such as bleeding or a foul odor.

CLOTHING

Understanding the concepts of thermoregulation is also important when clothing the newborn. In the hospital or birthing center, the infant often wears a T-shirt, diaper, and booties. Frequently, two or three blankets and a hat are required to help the newborn maintain body temperature within a normal range.

 Nursing Insight— *Importance of temperature assessment*

If the newborn's temperature drops to 97.5°F (36.4°C) or below, it is essential that the nurse immediately initiate temperature stabilization measures such as skin-to-skin contact by placing the infant directly on the mother's unclothed arms, chest, or abdomen or move him to a radiant warmer. When the newborn's temperature reaches 98.6°F (37.0°C) or above, he can safely be dressed in a T-shirt and hat and covered with two or three blankets.

At home, the type and amount of clothing for the newborn is dependent on the local climate and temperature. The infant can be dressed like other family members are dressed; that is, appropriate for the temperature and season. Special attention should be given when the newborn is outdoors. A cap or bonnet decreases body heat loss and protects the newborn from dangerous sun rays and wind drafts to the ears. During warm weather, babies should be covered in lightweight clothing and placed in shady spots when outdoors.

 clinical alert

Protecting the infant from the sun

While specially formulated sunscreens especially made for infants are available, it is important to advise parents to check with their health care provider about use of these products Many health care providers do not recommend use of sunscreens until the infant is at least 6 months of age.

DIAPERING

Many families prefer the convenience of disposable diapers, which vary in style, size, functionality, and cost. It is important to remember that the infant's sensitive skin may react adversely to the perfume in the diaper. If diaper rash or dermatitis occurs, parents can be advised to try another brand of diaper, but should contact their health care professional if the problem persists. Other parents prefer cloth diapers, which may be provided by a commercial diapering service or personally purchased and laundered. Parents need to be taught that cloth diapers must be laundered separately from other clothing articles, using ¼ cup detergent. Presoaking is often necessary to remove stains. When teaching parents about the advantages of breastfeeding, remember to include information that a breastfed baby's stools do not have an odor or cause diaper stains.

Ethnocultural Considerations— Diapering Practices

While diapering practices vary widely according to personal preference, custom, or culture, the nurse can teach the caregiver from any culture how to prevent diaper rash:

- Keep the baby's diaper area clean and dry.
- Change the baby's diaper often.
- Carefully clean the baby's bottom between diaper changes, using a mild soap and plain warm water.
- During a wet or soiled diaper change, allow the baby's skin to dry completely before putting on another diaper.
- Allow the baby to go without a diaper whenever possible to let the air dry the skin.
- If diaper rash persists, contact the health care provider.

FOSTERING ATTACHMENT

Attachment describes a mutually reciprocal relationship that takes place between the parents and their infant during the moments after birth. Attachment is critical to the child's ongoing optimal growth and development. One of the nurse's most important roles is observing for healthy attachment behaviors and helping the family to establish a good relationship with their infant. By observing parental behaviors and engaging in meaningful dialogue with the mother and father, the nurse may uncover important cues that could have an impact on the infant's growth and development. Remember that after 9 months of pregnancy and perhaps a difficult labor and birth, parents often feel tired and overwhelmed with the realization that their newborn is totally dependent on them. They may be too embarrassed to ask questions or clarify information previously given to them. The nurse must create a non-threatening and nonjudgmental environment in which parents can openly express ideas and ask questions. An important concept for the nurse, mother, and other caregivers to understand is that healthy bonding is essential for adequate physical, emotional and spiritual growth. Early infancy is an ideal time to establish a trusting relationship between the newborn and the primary caregiver.

❝ **What to say** ❞ — *Questions the nurse can ask the mother to assess attachment*

On the first day after giving birth, a the mother states that she doesn't want to hold her baby. The nurse responds by asking…

- Can you tell me more? Are you in pain? Are you feeling sleepy? Are you afraid?
- Does your baby have a name yet?
- Do you have any concerns about basic care for your baby such as holding, feeding, diapering, or bathing?
- How will you respond when your baby fusses or cries?

Minutes after the infant's birth, most parents are given an opportunity to spend quality bonding time with their newborn. To accurately assess this first expression of

Family Teaching Guidelines... Promoting Family Attachment

Nurses can promote family attachment in many ways:

- Provide time in the first few hours after birth for privacy and time for the new family to get to know one another.
- Delay any unnecessary procedures immediately after birth, such as measurements and other admission procedures. Instead, allow the family adequate time alone after birth to spend time getting to know one another.
- Encourage early breastfeeding by providing proper education and support.
- Teach parents about infant behavioral cues for feeding (rooting, sucking on fingers or fist, increasing motor activity, or crying) and how to respond to their infant.
- Help parents understand that crying is the infant's way of communicating, and all newborns have distinguishable cries for hunger, pain, tiredness, fussiness, or getting attention.
- Teach parents that newborns have a built-in capacity to console themselves and do so by sucking, motion, and distraction.
- Help parents to recognize the joys and frustrations that go along with ongoing parenting. Assure them it takes time to feel comfortable in meeting their newborn's unique needs.
- Introduce the concept of anticipatory guidance to help prepare parents for important developmental milestones that will occur.
- Encourage the parents to invite siblings and other family members to visit for short periods of time to share the joy and to provide support.
- Provide consistent nurses during the hospital or birthing center stay.

parent–infant attachment, it is important for the nurse to watch for and understand the behaviors commonly observed. Mothers and fathers usually begin with an exploration of their infant's physical characteristics. First, they examine each tiny fingertip. Next, they carefully explore their baby's extremities. Finally, they view and softly stroke the full length of the infant's trunk. During this entire process, the parents assume the **en face** position where they establish and maintain direct visual contact with their infant (Fig. 18-26). This initial exploration of gentle touch, coupled with reciprocal eye contact, helps to lay the foundation for a loving bond between the parents and their infant.

Nurses can be instrumental in facilitating a healthy parent–infant attachment. Taking time to teach, provide assistance when needed and listen to concerns help encourage and foster healthy parenting skills and enhance the newborn's potential for optimal growth and development.

Figure 18-26 The en face position allows parents and their newborn eye-to-eye contact.

 Ethnocultural Considerations— Accepting customs and traditions

It is important for nurses who work with childbearing families from various ethnic backgrounds to be aware of differences in cultural beliefs and practices related to pregnancy and newborn care. While many facets of the Western lifestyle may be readily adopted, families from other countries often wish to preserve certain customs and traditions brought from their native countries. Not surprisingly, valued health beliefs frequently extend to the area of infant care. For example, persons of the Latin American or Filipino cultures may apply an abdominal binder or protective "belly band" to the infant's umbilical stump to protect against dirt, injury, or hernia. Cradle boards may be used by Native American mothers, notably the Navajos, to carry the infant and maintain close contact. Persons of Iranian heritage may breastfeed female infants longer than male infants. Some Asians, Hispanics, Eastern Europeans, and Native Americans delay the initiation of breastfeeding because of the belief that colostrum is "bad" (D'Avanzo & Geissler, 2003; Dillon, 2007).

CIRCUMCISION

Circumcision is a surgical procedure that involves removal of the foreskin on the glans penis. Although commonly done to promote hygiene and easier cleaning, circumcision may primarily be requested because of family tradition or social and cultural factors. Historically based on a religious rite of passage from the Jewish and Muslim traditions, circumcision has gained widespread acceptance in the United States.

The 1999 American Academy of Pediatrics circumcision policy statement indicated that it is important that parents be knowledgeable about this surgical procedure. The policy advises that physicians give parents correct and impartial information about the benefits and risks and that they understand that circumcision is an elective procedure. Parents need to have the opportunity to examine all of the facts surrounding circumcision, ask questions,

and then without pressure from health care professionals, decide whether or not to have their baby circumcised (Ressler-Maerlender & Sorensen, 2005). The American Academy of Pediatrics Task Force on Circumcision: Circumcision Policy Statement (1999) also recommends that if parents choose to circumcise their infant, appropriate analgesia be provided. Bleeding, infection, dehiscence (separation of the approximated edges of skin), and trauma are complications that can be associated with the procedure.

 Nursing Insight— *Factors that may influence the parental decision for infant circumcision*

The American Academy of Pediatrics Task Force on Circumcision (1999) concludes that although there are associated risks (i.e., hemorrhage, infection, penile injury), circumcision does provide some benefits for the infant (e.g., reduced incidence of urinary tract infections and decreased risk for sexually transmitted infections, penile cancer, and human papilloma virus [HPV] infection). Additional reasons for choosing infant circumcision may include the parents' desire to ensure that their son's body likeness is consistent with that of peers from the same area, region, or country, and to avoid complications that are associated with circumcision performed on a child who is older than 1 month of age.

While the surgical removal of the foreskin is a fairly simple procedure that can take place in either in the hospital or community setting, it must be performed using sterile technique. The infant is restrained on a board or chair. Hospitalization is necessary if the infant is older than 1 month. The newborn must be stable and a physical examination by a physician or other health care provider should have been completed before the circumcision. The procedure involves removing the prepuce, which is the epithelial layer of skin on the penis. This small piece of skin is separated and removed from the glans penis. Newborn circumcision is frequently performed with the use of a surgical device such as the Gomco or Yellen clamp or the Mogen clamp. Once the procedure is completed, a

 where research and practice meet:
Providing Pain Management During Circumcision

Three types of pain management can be used for circumcision. A ring block is considered the most effective method (buffered lidocaine is subcutaneously injected on each side of the penile shaft). Alternatively, a dorsal penile nerve block (DPNB) (buffered lidocaine is subcutaneously injected at the 2 o'clock and 10 o'clock positions at the base of the penis) may be used. In other settings, a topical anesthetic such as prilocaine-lidocaine cream (i.e., eutectic mixture of local anesthetic [EMLA]) is applied to the base of the penis 1 hour before the procedure (Weise & Nahata, 2005). Nonpharmacologic interventions such as non-nutritive sucking, swaddling, and containment, along with oral acetaminophen and a concentrated oral glucose solution may also be used. Research has shown that a combination of swaddling, ring block or DPNB, topical anesthetic, non-nutritive sucking, oral acetaminophen, and a concentrated solution of oral sucrose given during the procedure by syringe or applied to a pacifier or nipple provides the most effective pain relief (Anand et al., 2005).

petrolatum gauze dressing is applied for 1 to 2 days to prevent the diaper from adhering to the surgical site. Another method involves use of the PlastiBell device, which is fitted over the glans and remains there until it falls off in approximately 5 to 7 days (Fig. 18-27). No petrolatum gauze dressing is used after circumcision with a PlastiBell device (Glass, 2005). Nursing care for the circumcised newborn focuses on alleviation of pain and the prevention of infection. Parent/caregiver education is also an important component of care. Therapeutic touch is a beneficial comfort measure for all infants and is especially useful following painful procedures.

❋ Complementary Care: *Therapeutic touch enhances comfort*

The use of touch to promote healing and comfort dates back to more than 5000 years ago, when Asian therapists used a variety of touching methods as an important strategy in the healing ritual. Over the ages, other ancient cultures, such as the East Indians and Native Americans, also found value in the power of "hands on" healing. Many spiritual traditions, including the Judeo–Christian doctrine, view healing by the "laying on of hands" as a key element in the promotion and restoration of physical and mental health.

Touch plays an important role in fostering healthy human development. It has been shown to boost the functioning of the immune system and enhance overall feelings of well-being. Touch is a basic human expression that conveys caring and nurturing. The mother intuitively places a comforting hand to her child's feverish head, pinched finger, or scraped knee. Friends instinctively reach out to touch one another in an expression of caring and compassion. Nurses have long recognized and embraced the value of touch as an important therapeutic tool useful with patients of all ages.

For the neonate, life's initial impressions, wrapped in a halo of warmth, love, and pleasure, are all conveyed through touch. The infant's growing knowledge and awareness of those around him is directly shaped by the way in which he is handled. His sense of comfort, security, and well-being are powerfully influenced by the nature of his mother's or caregiver's touch. Touch experiences occurring during the hours and days after birth, and the infant's feelings that are shaped by these experiences, serve to set the foundation for feelings about people throughout life. Premature and sick infants in the intensive care unit can also benefit from a light, calming touch that promotes a sense of security and warmth.

Reasons for not circumcising a newborn may be related to the surgical risks and/or pain associated with the procedure. If the parents choose not to have their son circumcised, they need to receive information about how to keep their son's penis clean.

❝ What to say ❞ — *Teaching parents who choose not to have their son circumcised*

When parents who have decided against infant circumcision inquire about personal hygiene for their son, the nurse may make the following suggestions:

"When your son is 4–5 years old, he can learn how to keep his penis clean just as he will learn to keep other parts of his body clean. The foreskin usually does not fully retract for several years and should not be forced. For an infant, the uncircumcised penis is easy to keep clean by gently washing the genital area while bathing. You do not need to do any special cleansing, such as with cotton swabs or antiseptics.

Around the age of 4–5 years, when the foreskin fully retracts, boys should be taught how to wash underneath the foreskin every day. Teach your son to clean his foreskin by gently pulling it back away from the head of the penis and then rinsing the head of the penis and inside fold of the foreskin with soap and warm water. After washing, the foreskin should be pulled back over the head of the penis."

Figure 18-27 Removal of the prepuce during circumcision. *A.* Yellen clamp procedure. *B.* PlastiBell procedure.

⟳ **Now Can You**— **Discuss aspects of circumcision?**

1. Discuss the benefits and risks of circumcision?
2. Explain how to promote parents' increased knowledge and understanding about circumcision?

ENSURING OPTIMAL NUTRITION

Most parents begin to consider feeding options for their baby during the prenatal period. How to feed a newborn after birth is an important decision with implications for the entire family. Two feeding choices are available for newborns: breastfeeding with the mother's natural milk or bottle-feeding with a commercially prepared cow's milk formula. It is paramount that the infant's diet be sufficient to optimally meet his rapidly changing physical and psychosocial needs and adhere to the current recommended dietary allowances. The diet must include essential nutrients such as protein to support rapid cellular growth, carbohydrates to provide energy, and fat to supply the needed calories, regulate fluid and electrolyte balance, and sustain development of the brain and neurological system. Water intake, essential for tissue hydration, should amount to 140 to 160 mL/kg per day. Because the bioavailability of iron in breast milk is much greater than in formula preparations, full-term infants who are breastfed do not need supplemental iron until they reach 6 months of age. At that time, breastfed babies require iron-fortified formula in combination with the breast milk. Infants who are bottle-fed should be given a commercial formula fortified with iron from the beginning. Adequate calories are also necessary and daily requirements of 105 to 108 kcal/kg per day have been established. (See Chapter 15 for further discussion about infant feeding.)

Discharge Planning for the Infant and Family

The new family is discharged from the hospital or birthing center as early as 24 hours after birth, so early initiation of the discharge planning process is crucial. If this is the couple's first child, discharge planning becomes even more important. The nurse must use every opportunity, beginning during the prenatal period, to teach the family about newborn care. The astute nurse gathers cues about family adaptation to the new baby by observing how the members interact with one another and their level of comfort when holding, feeding, diapering, and dressing the newborn. Questions such as "Tell me how you will care for your new baby?" or "Who is available to help you care for your new baby?" may give the nurse insight as to the type of information the family may need.

 Across Care Settings: **Providing parenting information**

Offering essential information in any setting through individual instruction, educational videos, or parenting classes about such topics as health promotion, growth and development, handling, nasal and oral suctioning, hygiene, diapering, dressing, comforting, nutrition and elimination, rest and sleep, safety and anticipatory guidance may help the mother and family gain confidence about caring for their baby. It is also helpful to educate parents about routine laboratory screening tests that may be performed in the hospital, home, doctor's office, or community clinic.

Discharge from the hospital or birthing center is an ideal time to discuss and implement car seat safety measures as automobile accidents are a safety concern for new parents. In moving vehicles, infants and older children must always be transported in a safe seating device.

Infants up to 20 pounds must be placed in a rear-facing position in the back seat of the car. Infants must not be placed in the front seas as inflating front seat air bags may cause suffocation (AAP Committee on Safety, 2002).

 Across Care Settings: **Car seat safety**

The nurse can assist the new family by providing information and guidance to resources on car seat safety:

- When purchasing a car seat, parents need to be aware that the seat must meet certain federal guidelines. A label on the seat tag or packaging box states whether the product has met these guidelines. The American Academy of Pediatrics Web site (www.AAP.org) also lists the guidelines. It is important to emphasize that the car seat instructions must be followed when installing the car seat.
- Several community resources are available to the family that will rent or loan a car seat for the initial dismissal. The hospital or birthing center may have a car seat program. Other resources include the American Red Cross, the Local Health and Safety Council, and the State Department of Health.
- The infant must be dressed so that the clothing facilitates ease of positioning and strap placement. To ensure correct fit, the infant can wear a single layer of clothing, preferably pants, so that the strap can fit between the legs. Sack sleepers are not recommended and bundling is discouraged because the strap may not fit snugly. Head support is recommended. Parents can use a commercially made product or place a rolled-up receiving blanket around the head and neck area. To protect the infant from burns and overheating in warm weather, parents should check the temperature of the car seat by touching the surface.
- Trained professionals may be available to perform safety checks to help parents with proper car seat installation and use. New cars are required to be equipped with tethers and lower anchors to ensure child safety.

CHILD CARE

When the new family arrives home, they have many decisions to make about the new baby. One important decision is who will care for the child when the parent(s) return to work.

Over the past 35 years, caring for children has shifted from home care to care away from the home. It is essential that the child care facility offer an environment of trust along with safe and competent care. In addition, the child care provider must offer ways to stimulate growth and development as well as meet the physical and psychosocial needs of the developing child. The nurse's responsibility is to help guide the family when choosing a child care facility. There are several options available for families today. In-home care refers to a child care provider such as a nanny, baby sitter, family member, or friend who comes into the family home. Work-based group care occurs when the child is placed in a facility that is directly associated with the parent(s)' employment. Another child care option involves placement of the child in another family's home. This type of care can be licensed or unlicensed and may be considered more informal. Established business day care centers offer more formal licensed care settings that comply with set standards and follow state regulations. These day care centers have specific policies that include minimum child to worker ratios. Sick-child care may also be available to the family in times of illness. These care facilities are often offered in community or hospital settings.

 Collaboration in Caring— *Child care for* *new families*

The nurse can encourage the family to:

- Communicate their needs and express their concerns about child care.
- Interview the facility director along with other individuals who may be involved in the child's care.
- Evaluate the educational programs related to qualification of teachers and structure of the learning environment (structured or unstructured).
- Investigate the provision of meals, nutrition, and related sanitation.
- Visit the child care facility on a few occasions, announced and unannounced.
- Identify practical aspects of child care such as location, hours of operation, fee requirements and payment schedule, child to worker ratio, environmental safety, indoor and outdoor space, sick day policies, and availability of care during a holiday or inclement weather.
- Evaluate the infection control and injury prevention measures.
- Gain broader information about the facility related to breast feeding, discipline, nurturing, diapering/toileting, stimulating growth and development, play, nap/rest time, and field trips.
- Discover state regulations and read the care facility's policies and related public records.
- Become familiar with early childhood program that offer voluntary accreditation such as the National Academy of Early Childhood Programs.

Newborn Metabolic Screening Tests

Newborn screening, designed to identify newborns with genetic, metabolic, and/or infectious conditions, is an essential part of preventative care. Through screening, many life-threatening problems can be detected early enough for effective intervention. Conditions commonly discovered through early screening include biotinidase deficiency, hemoglobinopathies, medium-chain acyl Co-A dehydrogenase deficiency, phenylketonuria (PKU), galactosemia, cystic fibrosis, congenital adrenal hyperplasia, congenital hypothyroidism, sickle cell anemia, and phenylketonuria (PKU). PKU, which occurs in approximately 1 in 10,000 to 25,000 births, is a genetic metabolic disorder. It is characterized by a deficiency of the enzyme phenylalanine hydroxylase, which the body needs to convert phenylalanine to tyrosine. A lack of proper conversion results in a build-up of toxic blood levels of phenylalanine, a condition that causes central nervous system (CNS) damage (Edwards, Howell, & Lloyd-Puryear, 2006). (See Chapter 19 for further discussion.)

Under state law requirements, screening of neonates has been routinely performed in the United States since the 1960s. However, no universal screening policy has been in place to assure uniformity. Instead, policies concerning routine neonatal screening vary from state to state and are frequently based on local demographics, cost, reimbursement, politics, and ready availability of resources. To address the lack of uniformity in screening practices, the American Academy of Pediatrics (AAP) convened a national Task Force on Newborn Screening. An important outcome of this work was the directive that each newborn have a medical home. A medical home means that every newborn should receive the benefit of a pediatrician or other primary care health professional who works in partnership with the newborn's family to ensure that appropriate screening is completed, test results are reported, and appropriate follow-up is conducted (AAP, 2000; AAP, 2005b).

On the federal level, members of congress recently directed the U.S. General Accounting Office to compile information related to newborn screening programs and state variations. The report revealed that most states screen newborns for only eight or fewer disorders. Furthermore, most states selected the disorders for screening according to whether or not they were treatable. Based on these findings, the Department of Health and Human Services (DHHS) suggested that a common set of disorders be established for all states, along with selection criteria for which disorders would be tested (U.S. General Accounting Office, 2003).

It is essential that nurses recognize that early detection of various disorders allows for timely intervention that can prevent or minimize complications. Before mothers and their infants are discharged from the hospital or birthing center, the nurse should educate the family about the importance of newborn screening. Emphasis should be placed on the long-term benefits of neonatal screening since early detection can allow for the initiation of timely treatment and the development of a plan for ongoing follow-up care. From a community perspective, universal screening and timely intervention can lead to a national reduction in infant disabilities, morbidity, and mortality.

While a positive screening test may indeed indicate that the newborn has a disorder, a diagnosis is generally not made from a single laboratory result. Instead, subsequent testing is conducted since "false positives" (a positive finding although the infant does not have the disorder) can occur. A false-negative result can occur if the specimen was collected at too young of an age, or if the quality of the specimen was in some way jeopardized.

 Optimizing Outcomes— Newborn metabolic screening

Best Outcome: Understand the effects of various disorders detected by metabolic screening and advocate for universal routine screening of all newborns. At present, the minimum mandatory newborn screening tests in most states in the United States are for inborn errors of metabolism such as PKU, galactosemia, hemoglobinopathy (sickle cell disease and thalassemias), and hypothyroidism. In Canada, newborn screening testing varies by province (CDC, 2005).

diagnostic tools Newborn Metabolic Screening

Approximately 24 hours following birth, a small sample of blood is taken from the infant's heel. The specimen should be obtained as close to the time of the infant's hospital discharge as possible and not later than 7 days. A blood sample taken before 24 hours of age may be unreliable in detecting several conditions. However, if the newborn is discharged from the hospital or birthing center before completing the first 24 hours of life, a sample must be obtained and the infant's parents must be instructed to contact the physician within 2 weeks to arrange to have another specimen drawn.

Neonates born at home must also be screened for disease. The parents or the person registering the birth must make the proper arrangements with a doctor or health care provider to have the tests completed prior to completion of the first week of life. If the 1-week time period is missed, the infant should be tested anyway, as he may still benefit from early intervention for certain disorders.

Now Can You— Discharge the new family?

1. Identify cues that may indicate how the family is adapting to the newborn?
2. Develop a discharge teaching plan for the family of a normal neonate?
3. Counsel parents about metabolic screening for their new baby?

---

summary points

◆ Key components of the immediate nursing assessment of the neonate center on ensuring adequate respiratory function and the prevention of heat loss.

◆ The later assessment of the newborn is conducted in a systematic manner that includes careful evaluation of each body system.

◆ Important aspects of newborn care focus on the prevention of infection and injury.

◆ The nurse provides newborn care in an environment that is safe and protective, enhances the transition to extrauterine life and one that fosters parent–infant bonding.

◆ Parents must be given correct and impartial information that includes the risks and benefits of circumcision, an elective surgical procedure.

◆ Neonatal pain must be readily identified, assessed, and appropriately managed.

◆ An essential role for nurses involves teaching and discharge planning for the new family.

review questions

Multiple Choice

1. The nurse's use of prewarmed blankets to wrap the newborn at birth is intended to decrease heat loss by which mechanism:
   A. Evaporation
   B. Convection
   C. Conduction
   D. Radiation

2. During the reflex assessment, the nurse places the infant in the prone position and strokes one side of the vertebral column. The nurse is assessing which reflex?
   A. Moro
   B. Galant
   C. Babinski
   D. Stepping

3. The perinatal nurse understands that soft tissue diffuse edema of the infant's head is a condition best described as:
   A. Caput succedaneum
   B. Cephalhematoma
   C. Subperiosteal hemorrhage
   D. Periorbital edema

Select All that Apply

4. During Baby G.'s initial examination, the nurse observes a two-vessel cord. The nurse's immediate response is to notify the health care provider as this finding can be a sign of abnormality in which system?
   A. Renal
   B. Cardiac
   C. Neurological
   D. Musculoskeletal

5. Infant admission documentation completed by the perinatal nurse includes information concerning the following:
   A. Passage of meconium
   B. Vitamin K injection site
   C. Ballard score
   D. Rectal temperature recording

6. The perinatal nurse observes for behaviors reflective of the early expression of parent–infant attachment, which include:
   A. Assuming an en face position with the infant
   B. Examining the infant's fingertips
   C. Stroking the infant's trunk
   D. Exploring the infant's extremities

True/False

7. The nurse recognizes that the noisy breath sounds heard during an infant's examination are caused by mucous or amniotic fluid in the upper airway.

Fill-in-the-Blank

8. The nurse recognizes that behavioral assessment in the neonate is measured by the infant's response to _____.

9. _____ is a normal finding in the assessment of the infant's head, eyes, ears, and nose.

10. The perinatal nurse explains to the new parents that the normal healthy term infant's usual position of comfort is _____ of the upper and lower extremities.

See Answers to End of Chapter Review Questions on the Electronic Study Guide or DavisPlus.

REFERENCES

American Academy of Pediatrics (AAP). (2000). Serving the family from birth to the medical home: Newborn screening: A blueprint for the future: Executive summary: newborn screening task force report. *Pediatrics, 106*(2) (Supplement), 389–427.

American Academy of Pediatrics (AAP). (2002). Policy Statement: Selecting and using the most appropriate car safety seats for growing children – guidelines for counseling parents. *Pediatrics, 109*(3), 550–553.

American Academy of Pediatrics (AAP). (2003). Controversies concerning vitamin K and the newborn: committee on fetus and newborn: Policy statement. *Pediatrics 112*(1), 191–192.

American Academy of Pediatrics (AAP). (2005a). The changing concept of sudden infant death syndrome: Diagnostic coding shifts, controversies regarding the sleeping environment and new variables to consider in reducing risk. *Pediatrics, 116*(5), 1245–1255.

American Academy of Pediatrics (AAP). (2005b). The national center of medical home initiatives: Metabolic/genetic screening activities. Retrieved from http://www.medicalhomeinfo.org/screening/newborn.html (Accessed September 6, 2007).

American Academy of Pediatrics (AAP) Task Force on Circumcision. (1999). Circumcision policy statement. *Pediatrics, 103*(3), 686-693.

American Academy of Pediatrics (AAP) Committee on Fetus and Newborn & American College of Obstetricians and Gynecologists (ACOG) Committee on Obstetrics (2002). *Guidelines for perinatal care* (5th ed.). Evanston, IL: Author.

American Academy of Pediatrics (AAP) and American College of Obstetricians and Gynecologists (ACOG). (2007). *Guidelines for perinatal care* (6th ed.). Elk Grove Village, IL: AAP.

Anand, K., Johnston, C., Oberlander, R., Taddio, A., Lehr, V., & Walco, G. (2005). Prevention and management of pain and stress in the neonate. *Pediatrics, 27*(6), 884–876.

Association for Women's Health, Obstetric and Neonatal Nurses (AWHONN). (2001). *Evidence-based clinical practice guideline: Neonatal skin care.* Washington, DC: Author.

Askin, D.F. (2007). Physical assessment of the newborn. Parts 1 and 2. *Nursing for Women's Health, 11*(3), 294–315.

Ballard, J.L., Khoury, J.C., Wedig, K., Wang, L., Eilers-Waisman, B.L., & Lipp, R. (1991). New Ballard score, expanded to include extremely premature infants. *Journal of Pediatrics, 119*, 417–423.

Brazelton, T.B. (1973). *Neonatal behavioral assessment scale.* Philadelphia: Lippincott.

Bulechek, G., Butcher, H.M., & Dochterman, J. (2008). *Nursing interventions classification (NIC)* (5th ed.). St. Louis, MO: C.V. Mosby.

Centers for Disease Control and Prevention (CDC). National Center for Health Statistics. (2007). *National health and nutrition examination survey.* Retrieved from http://www.cdc.gov/nchs/about/major/nhanes/growthcharts/charts.htm (Accessed April 20, 2008).

Centers for Disease Control and Prevention (2005). Retrieved from http://www.phppo.cdc.gov (Accessed August 9, 2007).

Centers for Disease Control and Prevention, Workowski, K., & Bergman, S. (2006). Sexually transmitted disease treatment guidelines, 2006. *MMWR Morbidity and Mortality Weekly Report, 55*(RR-11), 1–94.

D'Avanzo, C., & Geissler, E. (2003). *Pocket guide to cultural assessment* (3rd ed.). St. Louis, MO: C.V. Mosby.

Deglin, J.H., & Vallerand, A.H. (2009). *Davis's drug guide for nurses* (11th ed.). Philadelphia: F.A. Davis.

Dillon, P.M. (2007). *Nursing Health Assessment: A critical thinking, case studies approach* (2nd ed.). Philadelphia: F.A. Davis.

Edwards, S.E., Howell, R.R., & Lloyd-Puryear, M.A. (2006). A look at newborn screening: Today and tomorrow. *Pediatrics* (Supplement), 117(5), i

Glass, S. (2005). Circumcision. In P. Thureen, J. Deacon, J. Hernandez, & D. Hall (Eds.), *Assessment and care of the well newborn* (2nd ed., pp. 456–464). St. Louis, MO: W.B. Saunders.

Hisley, S.M. (2006). Care of the mother and neonate during the postpartum period. In *Lippincott manual of nursing practice* (8th ed., pp. 1233–1258). Philadelphia: Lippincott Williams & Wilkins.

Johnson, J., White, K., Widen, J., Gravel, J., James, M., Kennalley, T., et al. (2005). A multicenter evaluation of how many infants with permanent hearing loss pass a two-state otoacoustic emissions/automated auditory brainstem response newborn hearing screening protocol. *Pediatrics, 116*(3), 663–672.

Johnson, M., Bulechek, G., Butcher, H., McCloskey Dochterman, J., Maas, M., Moorehead, S., & Swanson, E. (2006). *NANDA, NOC, and NIC linkages: Nursing diagnoses, outcomes, & interventions* (2nd ed.). St. Louis, MO: Mosby Elsevier.

Joint Committee on Infant Hearing, American Academy of Audiology, American Academy of Pediatrics, American Speech-Language-Hearing Association, and Directors of Speech and Hearing Programs in State Health and Welfare Agencies. (2000). Year 2000 position statement: Principles and guidelines for early hearing detection and intervention programs. *Pediatrics, 106*(4), 798–817.

Kaye, C.I. (2007). Introduction to the newborn screening fact sheets. *Pediatrics, 118*(3), 1304–1312.

Lund, C., Kuller, J., Lane, A., Lott, J., Raines, D., & Thomas, K. (2001). Neonatal skin care: evaluation of the AWHONN/NANN research-based practice project on knowledge and skin care practices. *JOGNN, 30*, 30–40.

Lund, C., & Osborne, J. (2004). Validity and reliability of the neonatal skin condition score. *JOGNN, 23*(3), 320–327.

Lund, C., Osborne, J., Kuller, J., Lane, A.T., Lott, J.W., & Raines, D.A. (2001). Neonatal skin care: Clinical outcomes of the AWHONN/NANN evidence-based clinical practice guideline. *JOGNN, 30*, 41–51.

Miller, C., & Newman, T. (2005). Routine newborn care. In H. Taeusch, R. Ballard, & C. Gleason (Eds.), *Avery's diseases of the newborn* (8th ed., pp. 239–246). Philadelphia: W.B. Saunders.

Moorehead, S., Johnson, M., Maas, M., & Swanson, E. (2008). *Nursing outcomes classification (NOC)* (4th ed.). St. Louis, MO: C.V. Mosby.

NANDA International (2007). *NANDA-I nursing diagnoses: Definitions and classifications 2007–2008.* Philadelphia: NANDA-I.

National Newborn Screening and Genetic and Resource Center; *National newborn screening status report.* Retrieved from http://genes-r-us.uthscsa.edu/nbsdisorders.pdf (Accessed April 18, 2008).

Recommended Childhood and Adolescent Immunizations Schedule—United States (2007). Approved by the Advisory Committee on Immunization Practices (www.cdc.gov/nip/acip), the American Academy of Pediatrics (www.aap.org), and the American Academy of Family Physicians (www.aafp.org). http://www.cdc.gov/vaccines/recs/acip/default.htm (Accessed September 9, 2007).

Ressler-Maerlender, J., & Sorensen, R. (2005). Circumcision: An informed choice. *AWHONN Lifelines, 9*(2), 146–150.

Scanlon, V.C. (2007). *Essentials of anatomy and physiology* (5th ed.). Philadelphia: F.A. Davis.

Tucker, B.A. (2002). Promoting health of the infant and child. In J.A. Maville, & C.G. Huerta (Eds.), *Health promotion in nursing.* Albany, NY: Delmar.

U.S. General Accounting Office (2003). Report to congressional requestors: Newborn screening characteristics of state programs. Retrieved from www.gao.gov/new.items/do3449.pdf (Accessed August 9, 2005).

U.S. Preventive Services Task Force (USPSTF) (2001). *Screening for newborn hearing. Recommendation statement.* Retrieved from www.ahrq.gov/clinic/uspstf/uspsnbhr.htm (Accessed April 19, 2008).

Verklan, M., & Walden, M. (2004). *Core curriculum for neonatal intensive nursing* (3rd ed.). St. Louis, MO: Elsevier/Saunders.

Weise, K., & Nahata, M. (2005). EMLA for painful procedures in infants. *Journal of Pediatric Health Care, 19*(1), 42–47.

CONCEPT MAP

Immediate
• Airway/respirations
• Body temperature maintenance
• Heart rate
• Weight/length
• Apgar score
• Cord assessment
• Mother/infant identification
• Labs
• Pharmacotherapy
• Bonding

Integumentary: skin, scalp, body hair, nails
Head: eyes, ears, nose, throat, fontanels
Respiratory: respiratory effort, rate, pattern, breast tissue, nipple spacing
Cardiovascular: chest palpation, heart rate, heart sounds, perfusion/skin inspection
Gastrointestinal: abdominal inspection, cord, bowel sounds
Genitourinary: genitalia, anus
Musculoskeletal: muscles, limb length/size, joints
Neurological: nervous system, reflexes

Later
• Body positioning
 - Symmetry
 - Movement
• Color
 - Jaundice
 - Cultural norms
 - Acrocyanosis/ central cyanosis
• Body size
• Reactivity
• Determining gestational age

Optimizing Outcomes:
• Use of radiant warmer
• Newborn metabolic screening

Nursing Assessment

Critical Nursing Actions:
• Recognizing:
 - Respiratory distress
 - Ophthalmic emergency
 - Acute abdomen
 - Imperforate anus
• Prevent heat loss

Assessment tools/research
• Neonatal skin condition
• Ballard tool

Caring for the Normal Newborn

Be Sure To:
• Complete birth documentation/registration

Ethnocultural Considerations:
• Color
• Diapering
• Customs/traditions related to health beliefs

Family Education

Physical Care

Across Care Settings:
• Parenting information
• Car seat safety
• Child care

Emotional Care

• Temperature assessment
• Bathing: warm water; every week; mild soap; unscented lotion
• Nail/cord care: file/trim nails; cuffed shirt; normal cord appearance; diaper position; cord care; signs to report
• Clothing: maintaining body temperature; dress for climate
• Diapering: disposable versus cloth
• Nutrition: breast versus bottle
• Oral/nasal suctioning

Miscellaneous:
• Growth and development
• Rest and sleep
• Metabolic screening

Attachment:
• Arranging time
• Breast feeding
• Responding to cues
• Dealing with crying
• Handling

Now Can You:
• Recognize normal neonatal vital signs
• Complete a neonatal head-to-toe assessment
• Identify characteristics of Down syndrome and fetal alcohol syndrome
• Identify neonatal respiratory distress
• Develop a discharge teaching plan for the family of a normal neonate

Complementary Care:
• Use of therapeutic touch

Caring for the Newborn at Risk

 Be gentle with the young.

—Juvenal, *Roman poet & satirist (55 AD–127 AD)*

LEARNING TARGETS *At the completion of this chapter, the student will be able to:*

◆ Identify the criteria for classification of high-risk newborns such as gestational age factors, birth weight, and intrauterine growth restricted parameters.

◆ Describe the conditions for a small for gestational age newborn.

◆ Describe the conditions for a large for gestational age newborn.

◆ Discuss the physical assessment of the premature infant.

◆ Explain the conditions affecting the premature newborn.

◆ Explain the conditions affecting the postmature newborn.

◆ Describe other conditions affecting the high-risk newborn.

◆ Prioritize nursing care interventions for the high-risk newborn.

◆ Develop a discharge-teaching plan for the parents of the high-risk newborn.

---

moving toward evidence-based practice End-of-Life Care for the Neonate

Moro, T., Kavanaugh, K., Okuno-Jones, S., and VanKleef, J. A. (2006). Neonatal end-of-life care: A review of the research literature. *Journal of Neonatal Nursing, 20*(3), 262–273.

The purpose of this integrative review of the literature was to synthesize existing empirical research about neonatal end-of-life care. The neonatal period was defined as the time from birth to 27 days of life. Articles published before 1997 and those that dealt with ethics or considered to be clinical in nature were not included in the review.

Two readers reviewed all of the research studies and mutually agreed on a total of 10 articles that met the study criteria, based on the definitions of palliative and end-of-life care in neonates. Prematurity was the most common infant diagnosis for end-of-life care. The following four categories were included in the synthesis:

• Practices for withdrawing or withholding life-sustaining treatment
• Pain management during ventilator withdrawal
• Parents and the decision-making process
• The dying process

The sample consisted of more than 800 participants. The following were practices for *withdrawing* or *withholding* life-sustaining treatment:

"*Withholding* of treatment" was defined as refusing to administer cardiopulmonary resuscitation. The decision to withhold treatment has increased in the recent past and occurred in up to 69% of the cases reviewed. Decisions to *withhold* treatment were made in situations where treatment attempts were believed to have been futile (74%), and these cases primarily involved a diagnosis of extreme prematurity and/or extreme neurological damage.

"*Withdrawal* of treatment" was defined as the removal of mechanical ventilation. Decisions to *withdraw* treatment primarily included situations where continued support was considered to be futile (74%). Most deaths occurred after the decision to *withdraw* treatment had been made.

(continued)

---

moving toward evidence-based practice (continued)

Pain management during ventilator withdrawal consisted of the following: Opioid analgesia was used in up to 84% of the cases after life support was withdrawn or withheld. Sixty-five percent of the infants receiving opioid analgesia were diagnosed for major congenital anomalies/chromosomal abnormalities and necrotizing enterocolitis. (A previous study on these conditions found that although analgesia was used when mechanical ventilation was removed, only 22% of the infants continued to receive analgesia after ventilation withdrawal.)

In most cases, the parents were involved in the decision-making process although the level of involvement varied. One study found that parental participation in the decision-making process was not documented in 17% of the cases.

- In the cases where the physician made the decision alone, most infants (67%) were treated with a maximum effort.
- In the cases where parents were involved, the more likely decision was to limit, withhold, or withdraw treatment.
- Several studies found that parents' perceptions and experiences with providers had a major impact on the decision-making process. Parents were more likely to accept the decision if they believed that they were well informed and had a good level of interaction with the care provider.
- Parents also believed that it was important for the provider to be perceived as honest and a clear communicator. Overall, the parents who felt involved with the decision-making process were more inclined to trust the provider when considering treatment limitations.

With regard to the dying process, the studies reported:

- Most parents were present by choice at the time of their infant's death.
- A few parents (4%) did not wish to watch their baby die.
- 17% of the time there was no documentation about whether the parents were present or the reason for their absence.
- Parents were often unprepared for the neonatal dying process; 22% found the experience to be very distressing.
- The parents' specific concerns related to not knowing what to expect, e.g., how long the dying process would take, changes in breathing patterns and skin color following removal of the ventilator.
- Parents of infants whose death was prolonged after removal of the ventilator more often questioned whether or not the correct decision had been made.

The researchers concluded that an increased availability of palliative care services may help parents resolve some of the issues surrounding the understanding of neonatal pain control, continuity of care, and acceptance of the infant's end-of-life experience.

1. What might be considered as limitations to this study?
2. How is this information useful to clinical nursing practice?

See Suggested Responses for Moving Toward Evidence-Based Practice on the Electronic Study Guide or DavisPlus.

Introduction

Newborns can be put at risk any time during their intrauterine (in utero), intrapartum (from the beginning of the first stage of labor to the end of the third stage of labor), or extrauterine development (once the newborn is born). They can be placed at risk in their prenatal or intrauterine environment by genetic disorders (associated with inheritance), congenital anomalies (an abnormality a newborn acquires in utero), or maternal factors such as disease states, trauma, and drug use. Newborns are at risk based on a stressful intrapartum environment resulting in conditions of asphyxia (lack of oxygen) and birth injuries (trauma associated with delivery) or they can be placed at risk in the immediate neonatal or extrauterine environment as a result of conditions such as hypothermia (low body temperature), poor oxygenation, prematurity, or congenital anomalies (Table 19-1 and Box 19-1).

A & P review

It is important that the high-risk newborn have lung, circulatory, and neurological maturity.

Lung Maturity: Fetal lung maturity develops in utero progressively until term. Fetal lung maturity is determined by the L/S ratio (lecithin and sphingomyelin) and PG (phosphatidylglycerol) values, which are essential in

Table 19-1 Risk Factors that Compromise the Newborn

Intrauterine	Intrapartum	Extrauterine
Genetic disorders	Asphyxia	Hypothermia
Congenital anomalies	Birth injuries	Poor oxygenation
Maternal disease	Complications of labor	Prematurity
Trauma	Multiple gestation	Congenital anomalies
Drug use	Poor presentation	Metabolic disorders
	Maternal infection	

promoting oxygenation of the lung alveoli. They act on the pulmonary surface and are needed for lung stabilization. L/S ration and PG values are often mature at 35 weeks' gestation, before this time newborns are at risk for respiratory distress syndrome (RDS).

Circulatory Maturity: Fetal circulation functions in utero to oxygenate the organs needed for intrauterine growth. Blood is shunted away from the lungs and liver because the placenta performs those functions and more blood is circulated to the brain and heart to accommodate

Box 19-1 Risk Factors for Premature Delivery

Mother smokes

Mother older then 35 years at delivery and younger than 20 years

Maternal drug abuse

Female partner abuse

Multiple gestations

Maternal uterine abnormalities

Fetal anomalies

Maternal infection (especially: chlamydia, gonorrhea, and bacterial vaginosis)

Maternal cervical anomalies

History of previous preterm birth (carries twice the risk)

African American descent

Genetic susceptibility

rapid growth. The circulatory system of the fetus also develops strength and resiliency with increasing gestational age. At birth the fetal shunts (ductus arteriosus, foramen ovale, and ductus venosus) close and circulation converts to adult circulation to accommodate oxygen intake by the lungs and filtering of blood by the liver. If the shunts fail to respond to extrauterine oxygen and pressure levels, there is a structural deformity in the circulatory system and the newborn is at risk. The preterm newborn is at increased risk because of a fragile circulatory system that is overexerted by the stress of the extrauterine environment.

Neurological Maturity: The neurological system, including the central and peripheral nervous systems and the parasympathetic and sympathetic nervous systems, are underdeveloped at birth. Neurologically, newborns are immature due to limited synaptic and dendritic interconnections in the brain and immature myelination of the nerve cells. The preterm newborn has an increased risk resulting in the inability to cope with the extrauterine stimuli at birth. Neurological deficits are experienced both short and long term in newborns at risk due to interrupted neuronal development (Klaus & Fanaroff, 2005). ◆

The High-Risk Newborn

Nursing care of the high-risk newborn has become an extremely technologically enhanced specialty over the past 50 years and has rapidly evolved into a dynamic field of nursing care. Advances in neonatal intensive care units (NICUs) are steadily increasing the survival rate of newborns at risk but they still have a significantly higher mortality and morbidity rate when compared to uncomplicated, full-term newborns. The majority of newborns who are cared for in NICUs are preterm newborns (newborns born at 37 weeks of gestation or earlier). The preterm rate in the United States is 12.1% as of 2002, which shows an increase over previous years, and this has been associated with increased multiple gestations. In 2001, 41% of newborns born before 28 weeks of gestation did not survive 1 year. The mortality rate decreases to 5% for preterm newborns born between 28 and 31 weeks of gestation. Currently, the age of viability or the gestational age at which a newborn can survive is approximately 23 to 24 weeks' gestation. Newborns less than 22 weeks do not survive and those between 22 and 23 weeks rarely survive (Klaus & Fanaroff, 2005).

CLASSIFICATION OF HIGH-RISK NEWBORNS

High-risk newborns are classified according to two main criteria: gestational age (GA; length of time in utero) and birth weight (recorded in grams in the NICU). Another classification is intrauterine growth restriction (IUGR). It is important to consider all criteria when assessing a newborn.

Gestational Age

Term newborns are neonates delivered at or after 38 through 42 weeks of gestation because this is the optimal developmental time for adjustment to the extrauterine environment. A neonate born at or before 37 weeks of gestation is preterm and behaves differently and has different nursing care needs than does a full-term newborn. A newborn delivered on or after 42 weeks of gestation is postterm and also has different nursing care needs than a full-term newborn. Some clinicians use the terms postconceptual age (PCA) or postmenstrual age (PMA) to designate the gestational age of a newborn (Sahni et al., 2005).

 Nursing Insight— Understanding newborn classification

Preterm newborn: A newborn born before 37 completed weeks of gestation

Term newborn: A newborn born between weeks 38 and 42 of completed gestation

Postterm newborn: A newborn born after week 42 of completed gestation.

VIABILITY. Only 10% of newborns at 23 weeks of gestation survive, whereas 33% of 24-week gestational age newborns survive. At 25 weeks, 58% of newborns survive (Box 19-2). These criteria do not address the developmental and neurological delays of the extremely premature or preterm newborn (Taeusch, Ballard, & Gleason, 2005).

Box 19-2 Viability Related to Newborns Classified According to Gestational Age (GA)

Viable: Newborns whom all neonatal clinicians agree should be treated (GA greater than or equal to 25 weeks)

Nonviable: Newborns that nearly all neonatal clinicians agree should not be treated (GA less than or equal to 22 weeks)

Viability uncertain: Newborns in which clinicians debate, discuss, and often disagree whether they should undergo resuscitation or treatment (GA 23–24 weeks)

Source: Taeusch, H., Ballard, R., & Gleason C. (2005). *Avery's diseases of the newborn.* (8th ed.). Philadelphia: Elsevier Saunders.

Table 19-2 Newborn Classification by Birth Weight and Gestational Age	
SGA: Small for gestational age	Weight below the 10th percentile for gestational age
AGA: Average for gestational age	Weight between the 10th and 90th percentile for gestational age
LGA: Large for gestational age	Weight above the 90th percentile for gestational age

Birth Weight

Previously, newborns were classified as high-risk solely on the basis of birth weight. Now birth weight is compared to gestational age for a more accurate assessment of risk factors and specific growth patterns. Newborns born with a weight between the 10th and 90th percentile on the developmental growth chart have less mortality and morbidity than those above the 90th percentile or below the 10th percentile. Birth weight must be compared to gestational age to make an accurate assessment of risk for each newborn. Newborn classification by birth weight and gestational age is shown in Table 19-2.

 Ethnocultural Considerations— Converting weights

Record the newborn's weight into pounds if the parents are from North America and kilograms if they are European or Asian.

There are other classification systems that use newborn weight as a criterion for classifying premature newborns but do not consider the gestational age in relation to weight (Fig. 19-1). This clinical terminology uses low birth weight (LBW) or very low birth weight (VLBW) or extremely low birth weight (ELBW). Low birth weight (LBW) refers to a newborn weighing less than 2500 grams (7.8% of all births), and very low birth weight (VLBW) refers to a

Figure 19-1 A high-risk newborn in the neonatal intensive care unit.

 where research and practice meet:
Measurement of Growth and Gestational Age

The measurement of growth and gestational age of the newborn is dependent on graphs developed during research trials. Some current research indicates that birth weight may be increasing in the general population and that growth charts may not consider specific populations and obstetrical conditions (Fok, Wong, Chang, Lau, & Lee, 2003).

newborn weighing less than 1500 grams (1.46% of all births). Extremely low birth weight refers to newborns who weigh less than 1000 grams. The numbers of LBW and VLBW newborns have been steadily increasing owing to the increased incidence of multiple births. LBW newborns die at a rate five times higher than an AGA newborn, and VLBW babies have a 100 times higher risk of dying than a normal birth weight newborn (NCHS, 2004).

Intrauterine Growth Restriction

Intrauterine growth restriction (IUGR) is a term used to denote a lack of intrauterine fetal growth which usually results in an SGA newborn. An older term previously used in clinical practice was "intrauterine growth retardation," but it is no longer used because the lay person may equate the word "retardation" with cognitive (intellectual) development, whereas in fact it was a reference to somatic (body) development of the newborn.

Small-for-Gestational-Age Infants

Small-for-gestational-age (SGA) infants are those born at any gestational age who have a birth weight that falls below the 10th percentile on the growth charts. The SGA condition is a result of intrauterine growth restriction (IUGR) and can be classified into two categories: asymmetrical and symmetrical. Asymmetrically small newborns have an appropriate size head circumference that measures between the 10th and 90th percentile for their gestational age when plotted on the head circumference chart but their weight falls below the 10th percentile. Asymmetrical SGA is sometimes called "brain sparing" SGA. Symmetrically small newborns are not only below the 10th percentile for weight but also have a small head circumference that measures below the 10th percentile for their gestational age. Symmetrical SGA is sometimes called "non-brain-sparing" SGA.

SGA newborns are small because they have suffered a nutritional or oxygenation deficit in utero due to maternal causes, fetal causes, or a placental or cord malfunction. If the fetus experienced the deficit in the first trimester, the newborn is usually symmetrically SGA but if the deficit started after the 20th week of gestation he is more likely to be asymmetrically SGA. Interestingly, in developed countries, such as the United States, one of the most common factors related to intrauterine fetal growth restriction is maternal smoking. In developing countries, the leading causes are maternal nutritional deficits and infections such as malaria. Some conditions that can produce an intrauterine environment leading to a SGA newborn are listed in Box 19-3.

SGA newborns are not only smaller but often have a characteristic appearance. In asymmetrical SGA newborns the head appears large in relation to the body. The body of both types (symmetrical and asymmetrical) of SGA newborns looks wasted because of lack of brown fat. The chest is often scaphoid and the eyes appear large with a "wise old man" look. The fingernails are often long and a meconium-stained thin cord is often present (Klaus & Fanaroff, 2005).

CONDITIONS AFFECTING THE SGA NEWBORN

Morbidity and mortality are significantly higher for SGA newborns. Delivery problems include asphyxia and low Apgar scores (see Chapter 18). Four immediate conditions in SGA newborns that are frequent nursing concerns are hypothermia, pain, hypoglycemia, and polycythemia (Doctor, O'Riordan, & Kirchner, 2001).

Hypothermia

SGA newborns have decreased brown fat and subcutaneous tissue to protect them from the cold. They also have higher caloric needs and rest needs are increased to conserve energy needed for growth. They have high metabolic rates and low glycogen stores which predispose them to hypothermia.

SIGNS AND SYMPTOMS. Hypothermia occurs when the baby becomes cold and loses heat at faster rate than the body can create heat. Hypothermia in the newborn is a body temperature below 36.2°C (97°F). Other signs and symptoms include shivering and cold, pale or bluish skin.

DIAGNOSIS. Diagnosis is based on the infant's temperature, nursing assessment, and signs and symptoms.

 Nursing Insight— **Cold stress**

Cold stress is more likely in SGA and preterm newborns because they not only have less brown fat but are also less flexed and have thinner skin. In VLBW newborns, water loss can be 8 to 10 times greater than in an adult and heat loss 5 to 6 times greater. Cold stress increases metabolic needs and places the SGA and preterm newborn at further risk for respiratory distress and metabolic acidosis. The nurse understands the need to assess for the signs of cold stress: poor feeding, lethargy, central cyanosis or pallor, respiratory distress, and bradycardia (Klaus & Fanaroff, 2005). Nursing care can prevent cold stress by maintaining a thermoneutral environment using artificial heat source and reducing heat loss related to convection, radiation, conduction, and evaporation

NURSING CARE. Nursing care includes providing a thermoneutral environment via an artificial heat source if the newborn cannot maintain an adequate temperature. After rewarming, the infant is then bundled (wrapped in blankets) in an open crib. The most commonly used artificial heat sources include radiant warmers and incubators.

A radiant warmer that is used in the newborn nursery is an overhead heater that accommodates an open crib underneath. The nurse can assess and bathe a newborn under the warmer and then remove the crib from the warmer once the newborn's body temperature is stable. The radiant warmers used primarily in the NICU have a flat table-like mattress with low sides that can be taken down for easy accessibility to the newborn. During warming, the infant's temperature is monitored continuously with a skin probe.

 Nursing Insight— **Temperature**

Normal skin temperature: 97–98°F (36.2–36.8°C)
Normal axillary temperature: 97.7–99.5°F (36.5–37.5°C)
Normal rectal temperature: 97.9–100.4°F (36.6–38°C)

Incubators are used to provide longer periods of artificial heat. They are double-walled containers with port holes that are covered in plastic to allow caregiver access. They can also be set on two different modes: skin (servo) or air (ambient). The skin mode works via the same mechanism as the radiant warmer servo mode. The servo mode uses a skin probe on the newborn (which should not be placed over the liver or a bony prominence). The probe is attached to the newborn with a reflective adhesive to help the heat source record the temperature of the skin. The probe should be positioned on the newborn's body so the adhesive piece is exposed to the heat source above. The air mode maintains a set temperature within the incubator and the newborn regulates his own body temperature in the warmer environment. The newest models of incubators open from the top, thereby maintaining some of the heat, as does a radiant warmer. Incubators are often covered with a baby blanket to protect the newborn from excessive light (Fig. 19-2).

Figure 19-2 Incubator used in the NICU.

critical nursing action Weaning the Newborn from the Incubator

When the newborn is being "weaned" from the servo (skin) mode of the incubator the temperature is decreased gradually every few hours while the body temperature is checked. Once the newborn can maintain his temperature above 97.7°F (36.5°C) axillary; he is switched to air mode and dressed. The newborn's temperature, weight gain, and behavioral status are observed closely during the weaning process.

Another way to provide a temporary heat source is to wrap the newborn in blankets that were warmed in a blanket warmer. This is a temporary method since the blankets cool fairly rapidly. To prevent cold stress in a newborn, a head covering, such as a stockinet hat, is also effective in preventing heat loss.

The nurse can also have a parent provide kangaroo care (skin-to-skin holding of the baby who is dressed only in a diaper). The baby is held next to the mother's or father's chest, preferably with an ear over the parent's heart to allow the baby to hear the familiar heartbeat (Johnson, 2005). Kangaroo care is an effective way of maintaining newborn temperature and is recommended for a growing newborn who is stable and can tolerate periods of time out of the incubator. Kangaroo holding has been found to produce benefits for both the mother and the baby by enhancing mother–baby interaction as well as promoting bonding and newborn growth and development (Johnson, 2005; McCall, Alderdice, Halliday, Jenkins, & Vohra, 2005).

 Across Care Settings: **The Linus Project**

Growing newborns in the NICU use a large amount of clothing, blankets, and linens. Volunteer groups such as the Linus Project (http://www.projectlinus.org/index.shtml), senior groups, and local high school home economics classes are often happy to crochet or knit warm blankets and hats for NICU newborns that can often be sent home with the family when the newborn is discharged.

Pain

High-risk newborns undergo much life-saving interventions, many of which produce pain. Pain should be assessed during both procedural and routine care.

SIGNS AND SYMPTOMS. Pain has detrimental physiological effects on the newborn's cardiovascular, respiratory, endocrine, metabolic, immunological, and coagulation systems that lead to an increase in heart rate, blood pressure, and respiratory rate. Pain in the newborn also produces shallow respirations, pallor, flushing, diaphoresis, palmar sweating, and decreased oxygen saturation. The newborn also displays pain in facial expressions, including lowering the brows and drawing them together, crunching the forehead and revealing vertical furrows between the brows, closing the eyes tightly and squaring off the mouth while holding the lips tight. The newborn's cry can also be an indicator of pain because it becomes higher pitched with long pauses in breathing before it eventually becomes a rhythmic rising and falling pattern of crying. The newborn's body movements also display pain reactions by limb withdrawal from touch, rigidity or flaccidity, and clenched fists. Pain alters the wake–sleep cycles of newborns.

DIAGNOSIS. A pain diagnosis can be based on the Premature Infant Pain Profile (PIPP) or other neonatal pain scale.

NURSING CARE. Pain management is an important nursing consideration in the NICU. Pain is considered the fifth vital sign in the NICU and is assessed every 3 hours or with nursing care. Pain can be accurately assessed using a verified pain scale. More than 35 different pain scales are available for assessing newborn pain (Duhn & Medves, 2004). Some pain assessment scales are for the term newborn while others are specific to the preterm newborn. A commonly used pain assessment in the NICU is the Premature Infant Pain Profile (PIPP) (Stevens, Johnston, Petryshen, & Taddio, 1996). The PIPP rates six

 where research and practice meet: **The Pain Assessment Tool (PAT)**

The Pain Assessment Tool (PAT) was recently developed for all newborns cared for in the NICU regardless of gestational age. It is user-friendly and has been tested on 144 newborns. The PAT score was shown in this study to be a valid, reliable, and clinician-friendly pain assessment measurement tool for all newborns in the NICU that may increase the consistency of nursing assessment (Spence, Gillies, Harrison, Johnston, & Nagy, 2005)

Premature Infant Pain Profile (PIPP)

	0	1	2	3
GA	>/= 36 Wks	32–36 6/7 Wks	28–31 6/7 Wks	</= 28 Wks
Behavioral state	Active/awake	Quiet/awake	Active/sleep	Quiet/sleep
HR	0–4 beats/ minute Inc	5–14 beats/ minute Inc	15–24 beats/ minute Inc	25 beats or > Inc
O2 Sats	0–2.4% Decrease	2.5–4.9% Decrease	5–7.4% Decrease	7.5% or Decrease
Brow bulge	None	Minimum	Moderate	Maximum
Eye squeeze	None	Minimum	Moderate	Maximum
Nasolabial furrow	None	Minimum	Moderate	Maximum

Figure 19-3 A commonly used pain assessment in the NICU is the Premature Infant Pain Profile (PIPP).

parameters within four different age groups (Fig. 19-3). Many NICUs have protocols that treat a newborn for a PIPP score higher than 6 or 7. A score of 12 indicates severe pain and requiring immediate attention (Pasero, 2002) (Fig. 19-4).

 Nursing Insight— Newborn pain

Many people have myths about newborn pain [e.g., newborns do not feel or react to pain, newborns do have memory of pain]. The response to pain is subjective and determined very early in life and is in part a socially learned reaction. Not adequately medicating newborns and children for pain can have life-long effects (Young, 2005).

Hypoglycemia

Hypoglycemia occurs more rapidly in newborns. SGA and preterm newborns have higher glucose needs than do term newborns. In utero, glucose is provided by continuous placental transfer from maternal circulating glucose. After the umbilical cord is cut and the glucose supply is halted, the newborn has to use liver glycogen and adipose tissue stores for glucose control. Gluconeogenesis and ketogenesis are underdeveloped and glucose levels can fall rapidly after birth.

SIGNS AND SYMPTOMS. Hypoglycemic symptoms in the newborn may range from no symptoms at all to lethargy, jitteriness, poor feeding, cyanosis, high pitched or weak cry, eye rolling, and seizures.

DIAGNOSIS. When glucose levels fall below 60 mg/dL a diagnosis of hypoglycemia can be made. The newborn may also start building up ketones.

NURSING CARE. The nurse must provide proper nursing care to the newborn experiencing hypoglycemia to ensure the best outcome and long-term good health.

Figure 19-4 Many NICUs have protocols which treat a newborn for a PIPP score higher than 6 or 7. A score of 12 indicates severe pain and needs immediate attention.

 critical nursing action Hypoglycemia in the Newborn

The nurse must understand the dynamics of hypoglycemia and remember not all newborns are symptomatic:

- Glucose levels should be monitored carefully in SGA newborns. Many times glucose testing is done by heelstick (capillary blood sampling). A heelstick is done by pricking the heel and scooping the dripping heel blood into the appropriate neonatal laboratory tubes that require approximately 1 mL of blood for testing (Fig. 19-5).
- Optimal glucose levels are 70–100 mg/dL, as they are in adults. The lowest clinically acceptable level is 60 mg/dL. At a level of 40 mg/dL the newborn may become symptomatic.
- Many NICUs have protocols requiring blood glucose levels at specific intervals for SGA newborns. Many nurseries have protocols that continue to check newborn glucose levels at birth and 1, 2, 4, and 8 hours of age (Klaus & Faranoff, 2005). Some NICUs even repeat glucose levels at 12 and 24 hours of age.
- For newborns on IV therapy, since a basic component of the parenteral fluid is glucose, nurseries maintain routine blood glucose checks. IV therapy consists of providing glucose at a rate of 4 to 8 mg/kg per minute.
- If a stable newborn is found to be hypoglycemic on routine blood glucose check, enteral feedings should be started immediately. After the feeding the glucose level should be rechecked at 30 minutes.

Polycythemia

Polycythemia is a condition of too many circulating red blood cells (RBCs) in the newborn and can have several causes. Newborns who experience oxygen deprivation in utero produce additional RBCs to increase the circulation of oxygen. Some of the common conditions in utero that produce polycythemia in the newborn are listed in Box 19-4. Polycythemia may also occur when a newborn (either SGA or LGA) is exposed to an intrapartum environment that allows the blood in the cord and placenta to enter his circulation by gravity or "milking the cord" at delivery. Polycythemia greatly increases the viscosity of the circulating volume, which can produce multiple organ damage.

SIGNS AND SYMPTOMS. Polycythemia includes plethoric (ruddy) skin and delayed capillary refilling, hematuria, proteinuria, necrotizing enterocolitis (NEC), pulmonary hypertension, thrombocytopenia, jaundice, and neurological sequelae including central nervous system irritability, seizures, and cerebral infarction (Klaus & Fanaroff, 2005).

DIAGNOSIS. Diagnosis is made when the venous hematocrit is 65% or greater.

NURSING CARE. The nurse initiates care by performing a urine analysis. Macroscopic urine analysis can be done by dipsticking urine for a rapid assessment. Hemoglobin, hematocrit, and bilirubin levels can be done by peripheral blood drawing or heelstick. Nursing care consists of assessment, feeding the infant (breast for formula) or giving an intravenous glucose infusion for infants who are unable to tolerate oral feedings or are unable to maintain adequate glucose levels.

 critical nursing action Hemoglobin and Hematocrit Levels

Hemoglobin and hematocrit levels need to be monitored closely, as do bilirubin levels. To prevent neurological deficits in newborns, exchange transfusions may be ordered for hematocrits greater than 65% in the

Figure 19-5 A heel stick is done by pricking the heel and scooping the dripping heel blood into the appropriate neonatal laboratory tubes that require approximately a mL of blood for testing.

first 24 hours of life. Exact hematocrit values at which complications will occur are difficult to determine since different newborns become symptomatic at different levels. Nursing care should include monitoring questionable hematocrit levels via venous blood because capillary hematocrits are less exact. Assess the newborn for neurological symptoms such as high-pitched cry, feeding problems, irritability, and apnea. Testing urine for blood and macroscopic analysis is also recommended (Klaus & Fanaroff, 2005).

Optimizing Outcomes— **Preventing hemolysis**

Best outcome: To prevent hemolysis, transport the blood specimen to the lab as soon as possible.

 nursing diagnoses The SGA Newborn

- Risk for activity intolerance related to increased metabolic needs
- Possible ineffective feeding pattern related to increased metabolic needs
- Nutritional imbalance related to hypoglycemia
- Risk for impaired parenting related to increased care needs
- Caregiver role strain related to increased care needs
- Risk for growth and developmental delays related to intrauterine nutritional and oxygenation status
- Risk for imbalanced body temperature related to decreased subcutaneous tissue and brown fat (Doenges, Moorhouse, & Geissler-Murr, 2005)

Box 19-4 **Conditions that May Produce Polycythemia in the Newborn**

- Placental insufficiency
- Maternal hypertension
- Pregnancy at high altitudes
- Maternal diabetes
- Trisomies

Large-for-Gestational–Age Infants

Newborns who are large for gestational age (LGA) are over the 90th percentile on the growth chart (this is a newborn who weighs approximately 3750 grams or 8 pounds and 4 ounces at 40 weeks gestation). A macrosomic newborn weighs more than 4050 grams and is always LGA. Excessive fetal size is found in 9% to 13% of all deliveries. LGA newborns have a higher morbidity rate than AGA newborns.

There are two reasons why newborns may grow to a larger than average size in utero. They can be genetically large or, more commonly, they are exposed to an imbalance of nutrients in utero. The most common energy and growth source in utero is glucose. It is easily transported by diffusion across the placental barrier. If the maternal circulation contains excessive glucose levels the fetus' circulation will have a higher than normal glucose level also. The intrauterine conditions that place a newborn at risk for LGA are listed in Box 19-5. Delivery of a LGA newborn places the newborn at a greater risk for complications (Box 19-6).

Infants of diabetic mothers are often LGA. LGA newborns are also at risk for transient tachypnea, hypoglycemia, hypocalcemia, hypomagnesemia, birth injuries, brachial plexus injuries, and fractures (Klaus & Fanaroff, 2005).

Box 19-5 **Risk Factors Contributing to LGA Newborns**

- Increasing parity
- Increased maternal age
- Increased maternal height
- History of other LGA newborns
- Prolonged pregnancy
- Maternal obesity
- Maternal glucose intolerance
- Large pregnancy weight gain

Box 19-6 **Complications Associated with LGA or Macrosomic Newborns**

- Shoulder dystocia at delivery
- Brachial nerve plexus
- Asphyxia
- Hyperinsulinemia and hypoglycemia
- Hypocalcemia

CONDITIONS AFFECTING THE LGA NEWBORN

Infant with a Diabetic Mother

Infants of diabetic mothers may experience a chronic hyperglycemic state (greater than 125 mg/dL in the full-term infant and 150 mg/dL in the preterm infant) in utero due to elevated maternal glucose levels. The effects of the maternal glucose levels on the newborn depend on several factors such as the maternal glucose control, the onset of the diabetic state, and the length of gestation. Glucose readily passes through the placenta but insulin, due to its molecular size, does not. Therefore, the fetus produces larger than normal amounts of insulin to keep up with the extra glucose. This makes the glucose accessible to the cells, producing a large newborn. When the cord is cut at delivery the glucose supply is abruptly stopped but the newborn's pancreas is still hyperstimulated and producing insulin resulting in a severe hypoglycemic state.

SIGNS AND SYMPTOMS. The nurse must determine if the infant is in a hypoglycemic or hyperglycemic state. Hyperglycemia is usually asymptomatic but can be detected by routine screening (heel sticks) soon after birth, many times within 15 to 30 minutes, and be completed at regular intervals.

 Nursing Insight— *Hyperglycemia in the high-risk newborn*

Hyperglycemia is rarer than hypoglycemia but is still significant. A blood glucose level above 150 mg/dL is considered hyperglycemia and can cause dehydration and weight loss. Severe hyperglycemia may also cause cerebral hemorrhage (Taeusch et al., 2005).

NURSING CARE. If the infant is in a hyperglycemic state, insulin infusion is sometimes started and urinary output is carefully monitored to detect glycosuria and possible osmotic diuresis. It is important to communicate the baby's condition to the parents.

 nursing diagnoses The Infant with a Diabetic Mother

- Impaired physical mobility related to possible fractures
- Nutrition: Imbalanced, less than body requirements related to somatic size and glucose needs
- Pain (chronic) related to possible birth injuries
- Impaired gas exchange related to transient tachypnea of the newborn

- Infection, at risk or related to increased hospital procedures
- Parenting, impaired related to newborn with special needs
- Disturbance in sensory perception related to eye covers for phototherapy (Doenges & Moorhouse, 2005)

Hypoglycemia

One of the most important nursing actions for an LGA newborn is the close monitoring of glucose levels. A glucose level below 60 mg/dL is cause for immediate action. Feeding of 5% glucose, formula or encouraging breastfeeding is often the best way to raise the glucose level. Many nurseries have protocols that check LGA newborn glucose levels at birth and 1, 2, 4, and 8 hours of age similar to the protocol used for the SGA newborn.

Transient Tachypnea of the Newborn

Respiratory distress syndrome type II or transient tachypnea of the newborn (TTN) is common in infants of diabetic mothers. TTN is a delayed clearance of fetal lung fluid as a result of hyperaeration of the fetal lungs and transient pulmonary edema from the fetal lung fluid (which is different from amniotic fluid) in the alveoli. The air is trapped in the alveoli and hypoxia results due to poor lung ventilation. The onset of labor appears to be the mechanism by which the lungs reabsorb fluid which puts newborns who have not experienced labor at even a greater risk for TTN. Many LGA and IDM newborns are delivered by scheduled cesarean section and do not experience labor.

SIGNS AND SYMPTOMS. Clinical signs of TTN include a high respiratory rate of 60 to 120 breaths/minute, grunting, retractions, and nasal flaring (Fig. 19-6).

DIAGNOSIS. Blood gas usually shows respiratory acidosis (Table 19-3).

 Nursing Insight— *Metabolic acidosis*

Metabolic acidosis increases pulmonary resistance. Bicarbonate therapy is used less now that oxygenation of newborns is better through ventilation methods. Bicarbonate is given IV push 1–2 mEq/kg in a maximum concentration of 0.5 mL (Taeusch et al., 2005) (see Table 19-3).

NURSING CARE. The treatment is often continuous positive airway pressure (CPAP) at 40% oxygen for 24 to 48 hours. Complete resolution takes 2 to 3 days. TTN is self-limiting with no reported long-term complications (Taeusch et al., 2005).

 Nursing Insight— *Continuous positive airway pressure (CPAP)*

CPAP is oxygen most often delivered through nasal prongs to avoid intubation with an ET tube. CPAP maintains the patency of the upper airway and is usually set at pressures of 2–6 cm H_2O. The nasal prongs fit snuggly into the newborn's nose and are usually held in place by pinning the tubing to a stockinette cap.

Observation of Retractions

	Upper chest	Lower chest	Xiphoid retractions	Nares dilation	Expiratory grunt
Grade 0	Synchronized	No retractions	None	None	None
Grade 1	Lag on inspiration	Just visible	Just visible	Minimal	Stethoscope only
Grade 2	See-Saw	Marked	Marked	Marked	Naked ear

Figure 19-6 The Silverman and Andersen Index Evaluation of Respiratory Status.

critical nursing action Transient Tachypnea of the Newborn

The nurse must perform an accurate assessment of the respiratory system because immediately after birth or into the transitional period (within 1–2 hours) the neonate's respiratory rate should be below 60 with *no* retractions, nasal flaring, grunting and a peripheral pulse oximeter reading of greater than 92%. If any of these clinical signs appear immediately after birth or persist into the transitional period, immediate attention and supplemental oxygen are warranted.

Hypocalcemia

Calcium levels should be above 7.5 mg/dL in preterm newborns and 8 mg/dL in term newborns. Low calcium level can produce seizures in the newborn and may be present along with hypoglycemia. Other reasons for hypocalcemia in the newborn are trauma, hemolytic disease, asphyxia, and maternal hypocalcemia (Taeusch et al., 2005).

SIGNS AND SYMPTOMS. Symptoms of hypocalcaemia can range from asymptomatic to seizures and are similar to the symptoms of hypoglycemia and often difficult to

Table 19-3 The Relationship Between pH and Concentration of Arterial Blood Gases

	pH	P_{CO_2}	Pa_{O_2}	$P_{HCO_3}^-$
	Measures blood acidity.	Partial pressure of carbon dioxide in blood.	Partial pressure of oxygen in blood.	Partial presure of bicarbonate (alkaline or base) in blood.
Normal Neonatal Values	pH = 7.25–7.45	P_{CO_2} = 35–40 mm Hg	Pa_{O_2} = 50–80 mm Hg	$P_{HCO_3}^-$ = 20–22 mEq/L
Respiratory Acidosis (due to poor ventilation)	↓ pH	↑ P_{CO_2}	WNL	WNL
Metabolic Acidosis (anaerobic metabolism from hypoxia, diarrhea or kidney disease)	↓ pH	WNL	WNL	↑ $P_{HCO_3}^-$
Respiratory Alkalosis (hyperventilation)	↑ pH	↓ P_{CO_2}	↑ Pa_{O_2}	WNL
Metabolic Alkalosis (vomiting, diarrhea, hypocalcemia)	↑ pH	WNL	WNL	↑ $P_{HCO_3}^-$

WNL= within normal limits.
Adapted from Noerr, B. (2000). Neonatal respiratory disease and management strategies, May 18. Hershey, PA. A continuing education service of Penn State's College of Medicine at the Milton S. Hershey Medical Center.

differentiate. Often a hypoglycemic newborn may also be hypocalcemic. Other symptoms may include jitteriness, hyperalertness, increased tone, poor feeding, and a high-pitched cry.

DIAGNOSIS. The diagnosis is made by laboratory study, where the calcium level is below 7.5 mg/dL in preterm newborns and 8 mg/dL in term newborns (Klaus & Fanaroff, 2005).

NURSING CARE. The nurse understands that return to a normal calcium level is facilitated by feeding the infant soon after birth. Other treatment can include physiological correction of hypoparathroidism, administration of calcium supplements, and in severe cases the administration of 10% calcium gluconate.

Hypomagnesemia

Magnesium is necessary for proper parathyroid function. Hypomagnesemia frequently coexists with hypocalcaemia.

SIGNS AND SYMPTOMS. The decreased magnesium in the blood is usually accompanied by increased neuromuscular irritability.

DIAGNOSIS. Hypomagnesemia is present when the magnesium levels are below 1.5 mg/dL (normal newborn range is 1.5 to 2.8 mg/dL). It can be caused by low maternal magnesium levels, SGA or LGA growth patterns, and hypoparathyroidism.

NURSING CARE. Nursing care consists of magnesium replacement by giving magnesium sulfate. Magnesium may be given orally (PO) in the form of citrate, gluconate, and chloride. Levels should be checked every 24 hours to prevent hypomagnesemia that can produce hypotonia, poor feeding, and respiratory distress (Klaus & Fanaroff, 2005).

Birth Injuries

A thorough physical assessment is warranted for the LGA newborn to assess for birth injuries related to difficult deliveries. Birth injuries or traumas are usually one of two types: neurological injuries or bone fractures.

SIGNS AND SYMPTOMS. Signs and symptoms are directly related to the specific birth injury or trauma.

DIAGNOSIS. Diagnosis can be made by a thorough nursing assessment, x-ray exam, or appropriate laboratory studies.

NURSING CARE. Nursing care includes neurological assessment for intracranial bleeding and includes assessing posture, cry, seizure activity, and coordination of sucking and swallowing. Any abnormalities in these signs must be reported immediately. Head circumference should be measured in centimeters every hour if neurological symptoms are present. The nurse also assesses for bone fractures and can suggest an x-ray exam to the pediatrician if suspicious.

Brachial Plexus Injuries

Brachial plexus injuries (BPI) affect 5400 newborns in the United States each year. The brachial plexus is a complex nerve supply that is responsible for the movement of the shoulders, chest, and arms. Shoulder dystocia in labor is the leading cause of BPI.

SIGNS AND SYMPTOMS. BPI is classified by type and degree. A first-degree injury consists of stretching of the nerve fibers called neurapraxia, and recovery is usually complete within a few days. Second-degree BPI is called axonotmesis and the nerve is compressed and becomes edematous. Recovery of second-degree BPI takes longer but is often complete. In third-degree injuries, axonotmesis, the sheath is damaged and full recovery is never achieved. Fourth-degree injury is caused by formation of a neuroma that prevents full nerve regeneration, and fifth-degree injury is a disruption of the nerve at the spinal cord and results in complete loss of nerve function.

DIAGNOSIS. Diagnosis is made through a complete neurological assessment to determine the exact damage including the type and degree as well as the extent of nerve impairment.

NURSING CARE. Nursing care focuses on assessment, resolution of the trauma, and addressing any complications. The nurse can assess the Moro, biceps, and radial reflexes. The grasp reflex is usually intact. It is important to prevent contractures that usually involve limb immobilization. The limb is gently placed across the abdomen, where the hand cuff of the T-shirt is pinned so that the arm is in a flexed position to produce a loose splint. Passive range-of-motion (ROM) exercises usually begin soon. This condition usually improves rapidly without long-term consequences.

 Nursing Insight— *Erb's or Erb-Duchenne palsy*

Upper root injuries produce Erb's or Erb-Duchenne palsy, and the newborn usually holds the affected arm limp and turned inward (often called the "waiter's tip" position). Lower root injury is called Klumpke's palsy and produces a weak turned out arm and limp hand. Complete nerve injury is called Erb-Klumpke's or total paralysis. An assessment will reveal lack of flexion and movement in the affected arm. The position in which the newborn holds his arm may indicate the sight of the BPI (Benjamin, 2005).

Fractures

Fractures are also common birth injuries and usually involve the clavicle, humerus, or femur.

CLAVICLES. Broken clavicles are the most common fractures from birth (2 to 35:1000 births). Fractured clavicles can occur alone, with brachial plexus injury, or with a fractured humerus. Risk factors for a broken clavicle include LGA newborns, forceps use, and shoulder dystocia.

Signs and Symptoms. Symptoms of a broken clavicle include asymmetrical arm movement, asymmetrical Moro reflex, swelling, and "crepitus" detected on palpation of the bone. Crepitus describes the assessment of bone rubbing against bone which can be felt and sometimes even heard on examination. Clavicles heal spontaneously with very little intervention.

Diagnosis. If a course crackling is heard or felt during the physical examination. An x-ray exam will confirm the diagnosis. In addition, a palpable soft mass (hematoma or edema) may also be a sign of a fractured clavicle.

clinical alert

Fractured clavicles

The T-shirt is sometimes pinned so that the arm is in a flexed position to produce a loose splint. The affected arm is pinned to the opposite shoulder by the hand cuff of the newborn T-shirt. Pain management may be needed if the newborn appears uncomfortable. Keep the newborn off the injured side to decrease pain and promote alignment.

LONG BONE FRACTURES. The incidence of a fractured humerus is less than that of clavicle fractures. When they occur they are often treated with soft splinting to immobilize the arm for approximately 2 weeks. Healing is rapid and complete in most cases. Femoral fractures happen at a rate of 0.13/1000 and most often occur in twin gestations. Other risk factors for long bone fractures are breech presentation, prematurity, and osteoporosis. Femoral fractures can be treated with a Pavlik harness which immobilizes the hip and leg and allows the femur to heal. All long bones should be examined by inspection and palpation.

Signs and Symptoms. Some of the symptoms to observe for any birth fractures are crepitus on palpation, pain on palpation, asymmetrical movement or Moro reflexes, swelling and discoloration, or malalignment of the extremity.

Diagnosis. Definitive diagnosis is made by x-ray exam (Taeusch et al., 2005).

Nursing Care. The nurse understands that the fractured humerus must be immobilized immediately. The nurse must conduct neurovascular checks frequently. Elevation of the extremity above the level of the heart can facilitate circulation. Cold therapy can help reduce swelling, and pain medication administration is essential. The nurse must remember to communicate the infant's condition to parents and what care measures will be implemented.

 Now Can You— Discuss SGA and LGA?

1. Can you discuss conditions affecting SGA infants?
2. Can you discuss conditions affecting LGA infants?

The Premature Newborn

Premature delivery before 37 weeks is still a major health problem in the United States because each year 12.3% of newborns are premature. Prematurity is classified by the weeks of gestation. Severe prematurity is classified as birth at 23 to 26 weeks; moderate prematurity is birth at 26 to 30 weeks. The risk factors increase as the size and gestational age of the newborn decrease. A newborn can be SGA as well as preterm. Premature newborns are at risk for a number of complications and are responsible for more than half of the 36.7 billion dollars spent each year on newborn care in the United States (March of Dimes, 2006). Premature deliveries have increased over the past 20 years.

 Ethnocultural Considerations— **Racial disparities**

Healthy People 2010 calls for a reduction in preterm deliveries to a national average of 7.6%. The United States is well off that mark and obvious racial disparities exist. Caucasian and Asian women have preterm newborns at a 10.7% rate while African American women have premature births at a 17.6% rate. Hispanic women deliver preterm newborns at a rate of 11.4% (Cuevas et al., 2005).

PHYSICAL ASSESSMENT OF THE PREMATURE NEWBORN

The preterm newborn is not only smaller than a term newborn but also has specific characteristics due to his abbreviated development in utero (Table 19-4).

 case study Premature Newborn

Ms. Jones, an 18-year-old G-1, comes into the labor and delivery suite at 6 cm cervical dilatation. She is 33 weeks' gestation by last menstrual period (LMP). Baby girl Jones is delivered within the hour and weighs 2000 grams. She breaths spontaneously and her heart rate is 166 beats per minute. She is thoroughly dried, suctioned with a small size bulb syringe for excessive nasal pharyngeal fluid, placed under the radiant warmer, and an initial assessment is done. Her rectal temperature is 98.2°F (36.8°C). Her PIPP pain score is 2 (1 for gestational age and 1 for increased HR). The results of a skin assessment are no skin lesions, birthmarks, or reddened areas. Respirations are 70 per minute with slight nasal flaring, intercostal retractions, and an expiratory grunt. Her extremities have full ROM but poor flexion.

critical thinking questions

1. What classification by gestational age is baby girl Jones?

2. What condition is associated with her respiratory assessment?

3. What are important nursing interventions for baby girl Jones?

◆ See Suggested Answers to Case Studies in text on the Electronic Study Guide or DavisPlus.

CONDITIONS AFFECTING THE PREMATURE NEWBORN

Premature newborns are at risk for respiratory distress syndrome, apnea of prematurity, jaundice, retinopathy of prematurity, anemia of prematurity, and sudden infant death syndrome.

Respiratory Distress Syndrome

Respiratory distress syndrome (RDS) is a developmental respiratory disorder affecting preterm newborns due to lack of lung surfactant. In RDS there is diffuse atelectasis with congestion and edema in the lung spaces. On deflation the alveoli collapse and there is decreased lung compliance. Lecithin-sphingomyelin (L/S) ratio and phosphatidylglycerol (PG) levels are low and inadequate to keep the immature alveoli of the lungs open. Preterm newborns may also have underdeveloped alveoli.

Nursing Insight— *Respiratory Distress Syndrome*

Respiratory distress syndrome (RDS) affects 40,000 newborns a year in the United States. Respiratory distress may also be referred to as hyaline membrane disease (HMD), surfactant deficiency, or idiopathic respiratory distress. As gestational age decreases the incidence of RDS increases (at 29 weeks of gestation, 60% of newborns experience RDS while at 39 weeks of gestation almost no newborn will experience RDS). RDS has an increased incidence in males, Caucasians, and newborns delivered by cesarean birth (Taeusch et al., 2005).

SIGNS AND SYMPTOMS. The clinical signs of RDS begin shortly after birth. Premature newborns are often cyanotic in room air. Breathing is rapid (tachypnea) with labored retractions, and is often accompanied by an expiratory grunt. If untreated the arterial blood gas values show oxygenation deficits with hypercarbia and metabolic acidosis.

DIAGNOSIS. A pulse oximetry can assist with diagnosis to determine hypoxia. Laboratory studies such as blood glucose (hypoglycemia) serum calcium (hypocalcemia), and Pao_2 (hypoxia) blood gas measurements for serum pH (acidosis) also help in the diagnosis of RDS.

Collaboration in Caring— *Radiology*

The x-ray findings of RDS reveal a reticulogranular pattern that looks like "ground glass," possible atelectasis which looks like "white out," and obscure heart boarders (Noerr, 2000).

NURSING CARE. Oxygenation is the priority intervention for the newborn with RDS. The first action to promote oxygenation is mechanical ventilation via endotracheal intubation. Mechanical ventilation is used for preterm newborns with respiratory distress who have very little capacity to oxygenate their alveoli on their own.

An endotracheal tube is placed by a clinician certified in intubations and neonatal resuscitation for delivery of mechanical ventilation. Endotracheal intubation (ET) is done by inserting an endotracheal tube orally or nasally to create an open secure airway in which to ventilate the newborn. Mechanical ventilation with positive end-expiratory pressure (PEEP) is usually needed when newborns weigh less than 1000 g at birth.

After an airway has been established, the administration of synthetic surfactant within 15 to 30 minutes of birth is required. The synthetic surfactant is administered through a catheter in the endotracheal tube. For newborns less than 1000 g it is given to coat the alveoli to keep them open so that they can perfuse with oxygen. Newborns larger than 1000 g benefit from surfactant therapy at any time during the first 2 to 6 hours of life. Continued mechanical ventilation after administration helps the medication to be spread throughout the lung tissue.

medication: Beractant (Survanta)

Classification(s): Sterile nonpyrogenic pulmonary surfactant.

Indications: Lowers minimum surface tension and increases pulmonary compliance and oxygenation in preterm newborns. Prevent and treat RDS in premature newborns.

Action: Lowers surface tension at alveoli level.

Storage: Refrigerate and protect from light.
PHARMACOKINETICS: Absorption: Absorbed only in lungs.
DISTRIBUTION: Does not get absorbed systemically.

Contraindications and Precautions: Monitor heart rate and respiration.

Adverse Reactions and Side Effects: Transient bradycardia, oxygen desaturation, possible increased nosocomial infections.

Route and Dosage: Intratracheal 4 mL/kg q 6 h × 4 (maximum of four doses in first 48 hours)

Nursing Implications:
1. Give within 15 minutes of birth to premature newborns.
2. Naso-oral suction before administration.
3. Warm vial 20 minutes to room temperature.
4. Do not suction for 1 hour after administration.
5. Discard vial after use—do not re-refrigerate once it is warmed.

Data from Deglin, J.H., & Vallerand, A.H. (2009). *Davis's drug guide for nurses* (11th ed.). Philadelphia: F.A. Davis.

Newborns are generally "weaned" from mechanical ventilation as soon as possible to avoid complications of oxygen such as bronchopulmonary dysplasia (BPD) and retinopathy of prematurity (ROP). Often they are placed on an alternative oxygen source such as continuous positive airway pressure (CPAP).

Another mode of delivering oxygen is via nasal cannula, which is continuous flow of low-level oxygen to supplement the newborn's own intake. Oxygen by mask is an unreliable method for a newborn.

On occasion an oxygen hood is used to keep a baby in an oxygen-rich environment for a short period of time. Hoods are easy to use and provide easy access to the newborn for procedures and assessment. The newborn with RDS will require blood gas monitoring as well as blood analysis for electrolytes, calcium, and glucose levels.

Optimizing Outcomes— Oximeter

Best Outcome: To ensure adequate oxygenation (above 92%) keep the newborn on a pulse oximeter whenever oxygen is being used.

Apnea of Prematurity

Apnea, a spontaneous pause in breathing, is a common occurrence in preterm newborns. The inspiratory center in the medulla oblongata of the brainstem, the central and peripheral chemoreceptors, and the neuroregulators are immature and do not provide the normal negative feedback loop to hypoxia and hypercapnia.

Table 19-4 Assessment of the Preterm Infant

Skin	Head	Chest	Cardiac
Skin tags	Irregular shaped head, molding after delivery, caput succedaneum cephalhematoma	Funnel or pigeon chest	Apical heart rate is assessed for a full minute
Translucent	Large anterior and posterior fontanels present Fused sutures Bulging or depressed fontanels	Supernumerary nipples or nipples are flat on the chest wall	The heart rate may normally be above 160 bpm but it should not be above 180 bpm
Lanugo covering the shoulders, back, thighs, forehead, and ears	Ear pinnas are flat and readily fold upon themselves	Ribs are visible	Heart auscultation is done in the second and fourth right and left intercostal spaces as well as the apex and axillae area
Little subcutaneous fat	Eyes are fused before 24 weeks' gestation	Grunting, nasal flaring, or retractions (subcostal, sternal or suprasternal) are signs of respiratory distress	Auscultation of heart sounds should be done routinely to detect murmurs, which may or may not be innocent
Fragile and easily injured	Nose flattened or bruised Nasal patency Low placement of ears	Auscultate anterior, posterior, and at the sides of the chest	Blood pressures on all four extremities are done to determine any wide variations that may be indicative of a ductal defect
Mottled related to poor peripheral perfusion	Facial anomalies	Auscultate respiratory rate for a full minute	Persistent central cyanosis
Prominent veins		Respiratory rate is between 60 and 80 respirations per minute	Displacement of apex
Covered in vernix		Respiratory rate above 80 respirations per minute are not within normal limits	Cardiomegaly
Pale (pallor) related to anemia from blood loss		Asymmetrical chest movement may suggest respiratory conditions such as pneumothorax or diaphragmatic hernia	
Congenital strawberry hemangiomas		Excessive secretions will affect the oxygen intake	
Diaper rash is common related to the increase in irritation of the stool when the newborn is on antibiotics and due to the fragility of the skin			
Soles of the feet are smooth			

 Nursing Insight— Apnea verses periodic breathing

Apnea must be differentiated from periodic breathing which is normal in the newborn. Periodic breathing is classified as short pauses in the breathing of the newborn that only last approximately 3 seconds. The incidence of apnea increases as the gestational age of the newborn decreases. The apneic spells many times is accompanied by a bradycardiac episode which has led to the clinical term "A&B spell."

SIGNS AND SYMPTOMS. Apnea spells are significant if they last more than 15 to 20 seconds and many times are accompanied by abrupt pallor, hypotonia, cyanosis, and bradycardia. Apnea, and many times the resulting bradycardia and desaturation, is due to several factors, such as neurological immaturity, increased resistance to rising P_{CO_2} blood levels, and immaturity of the respiratory receptors, which respond normally to increasing CO_2 levels.

DIAGNOSIS. Apnea is diagnosed if the spell lasts more than 20 seconds and is accompanied by the other signs and symptoms.

Abdomen	Musculoskeletal	Genitalia	Neurological/Sensory
Cord does not have two arteries and 1 vein	No flexion of extremities, resulting in increased susceptibility to heat loss and skin breakdown	Male scrotum has no rugae and the testes are often undescended	Marked head lag in all positions
Palpate for masses	Assess for fractures or developmental hip dysplasia or fractured clavicle	Female clitoris is often prominent and not covered by the labia minora; the labia majora is also small	Consistent caregivers read the cues and notice subtle changes
Auscultate bowel sounds		Inguinal hernias are common	Sucking and gagging reflexes are often absent until 32 to 34 weeks' gestation
Abdominal circumference is done to assess for distention that may indicate necrotizing enterocolitis (NEC)		Female absence of vaginal or male urethral opening covered by prepuce	Moro reflex may be absent to weak
		Meconium found in the vaginal opening	Any signs or symptoms of increased intracranial pressure may be related to cerebral insults
Enlarged liver or spleen		Ambiguous genitalia	Hypotonia or hypertonia
		Bladder exstrophy	Twitches, jittery, myclonic jerks
			Eye lids edematous, drainage present, minimal reactivity to light, congenital cataracts, absence of red reflex, inability to follow object or bright light
			Eyes have nystagmus strabismus ruptured capillaries

NURSING CARE. Most preterm newborns are on a cardio-respiratory (C-R) monitor (Fig. 19-7). The C-R monitor is attached to the newborn by three electrodes. Two electrodes are placed on either side of the chest and the third on the abdomen. The electrodes are changed often based on NICU protocol. Every time the electrodes are changed they are applied to a new area of skin to prevent breakdown from the adhesive. The C-R monitor is set to alarm if the newborn fails to breathe spontaneously for 20 seconds, the respiratory rate falls below a certain rate (usually 20 respirations/min) or the heart rate drops below a certain rate (usually 80 to 100 beats per minute). An alarm notifies the nurse of an impending apnea or bradycardic spell or combined A&B episode.

Preterm apnea usually resolves at 37 to 38 weeks postconceptual age (PCA) but may last longer. Many preterm newborns are sent home on home monitoring systems that alarm if respirations stop longer than 20 seconds or the heart rate drops (Stokowski, 2005). If newborns are discharged without monitors they usually need to be A&B spell free in the hospital for at least 5 to 7 days (Hummel & Cronin, 2004).

The pulse oximeter is a small plastic light-emitting probe that is noninvasive and can be secured to the newborn's extremity. The newborn is maintained on

Figure 19-7 Most preterm newborns are on a cardio-respiratory monitor.

Figure 19-8 Some newborns need aggressive stimulation to regain cardiorespiratory control which includes increasing existing oxygen flow or using positive pressure through bag and mask ventilation.

continuous pulse oximeters to guard against desaturation episodes. Oxygen saturation is calculated from the hemoglobin flowing under the light and then the percent is displayed on the monitor. It is easy to use and the saturation measurements are fairly reliable when compared to arterial samples of blood. The saturation should be maintained above 92% (Klaus & Faranoff, 2005).

The pulse oximeter is also set to alarm during a low peripheral O_2 saturation (usually below 88%). If the newborn desaturates without a corresponding A&B spell, it is called a desaturation episode. An apneic, bradycardic, or desaturation episode requires immediate attention. There are different severities of A&B spells. Some newborns take a deep breath and regulate themselves back into a normal cardiorespiratory pattern without intervention, which is often called a self-limiting episode. Some newborns continue the apnea, bradycardia, and desaturation spell and need mild stimulation to induce them to take a deep breath and regain a normal cardiorespiratory pattern. Stimulation is done by rubbing their backs or flicking their feet. Periodically, newborns need aggressive stimulation to regain cardiorespiratory control which includes increasing existing oxygen flow or using positive pressure through bag and mask ventilation (Fig. 19-8).

 Nursing Insight— *Bronchopulmonary Dysplasia*

Bronchopulmonary dysplasia (BPD) or Chronic lung disease (CLD) is a condition in which the newborn becomes oxygen dependent past 36 weeks gestation (Sahne et al., 2005). BPD is a complication produced by long-term oxygen use. Although oxygen is needed by the preterm to maintain proper tissue perfusion until the maturing lungs can resume that function, supplemental oxygen can also damage lung tissue by suppressing compliancy. Because oxygen is administered, the lungs fail to develop the normal compliancy needed to force adequate levels of air in and out. Sometimes the preterm newborn ends up with noncompliant lungs that need oxygen via cannula for an

extended period of time, sometimes up to a few years, in order to properly oxygenate their growing bodies. Newborns with BPD are often sent home on O_2 after the parents have been educated in oxygen administration. The amounts of oxygen needed through the cannula vary with the severity of the BPD but often it is a small flow at anywhere from ¼ to 1 liter flow rate with anywhere from 21% to 30% of oxygen.

Jaundice

Newborn physiological jaundice (hyperbilirubinemia) is common and occurs because of the newborn's immature liver (especially the preterm newborn). The liver cannot conjugate the bilirubin as quickly as needed. The excess bilirubin in the circulatory system moves into the skin, sclerae, nails, body fluids, as well as other body tissues resulting in jaundice. Jaundice that appears on the second or third day of life usually peaks on day four and declines on day five.

Nursing Insight— *Jaundice*

Bilirubin is a byproduct of the breakdown of hemoglobin. Newborns have higher levels of fetal hemoglobin at birth which breaks down faster because it has a shorter life span than adult hemoglobin.

The fetal hemoglobin is broken down by the reticuloendothelial system and bilirubin is released into the circulation. The circulating bilirubin or total serum bilirubin (TSB) binds to plasma albumin. This circulating bilirubin is unconjugated (UCB) and not water soluble. The bilirubin is then converted in the liver to conjugated (water-soluble) bilirubin. The conjugated bilirubin is excreted in the bile by the gastrointestinal tract and then excreted in the stool.

The two categories of jaundice are physiological and pathological.

Premature infants develop physiological jaundice at a rate of 90% compared to 60% of full-term newborns due to the extreme immature liver functions and polycythemia. Physiological jaundice occurs in the first 24 hours of life and lasts about 5 days. The infant does not display any other signs of illness.

Pathological jaundice usually happens at less than 24 hours of age and lasts for longer than the first week of life.

More serious conditions, such as obstructive (biliary atresia) or metabolic disorders, hemolysis, infections, or toxic disorders, are the reasons for this type of jaundice.

If jaundice is suspected, a total serum bilirubin level (the sum of conjugated and unconjugated bilirubin) blood specimen is collected stat and then care is given as determined by the medical doctor's order.

Transcutaneous bilirubinometry (TcB) is a noninvasive way of monitoring bilirubin in the skin. Over time, multiple readings at a consistent site (forehead or sternum) provide the most accurate measurement of the bilirubin. However, once phototherapy has begun the TcB monitor is no longer a useful screening tool and serum blood specimens must be drawn every 6 to 12 hours.

In addition, other laboratory samples, such as liver enzymes (GGT), alkaline phosphatase, prothrombin time (PT), and partial thromboplastin time (PTT), are drawn. If a more serious abnormality is suspected a radiological evaluation is done.

 Nursing Insight— Jaundice in breastfeeding infants

Early jaundice in breastfed infants begins at 2–4 days and most likely results from decreased fluid intake and caloric intake. After the milk supply is well established this type of jaundice resolves.

Late jaundice in breastfed infants begins at 4–7 days and can peak during the second week of life. Factors in the breast milk are thought to inhibit the conjugation or decrease the excretion of excess bilirubin. This type of jaundice may resolve on its own or the infant may need further care.

SIGNS AND SYMPTOMS. Normally unconjugated bilirubin values are between 0.2 and 1.4 mg/dL. Visible jaundice (a yellowish discoloration) is usually seen at a level of 5 mg/dL within the first 24 hours of birth.

DIAGNOSIS. Jaundice is diagnosed in term infants with a serum bilirubin level greater than 12.9 mg/dL and in preterm infants with a serum bilirubin greater than 15 mg/dL. In addition to serum blood levels other factors that help determine the extent of the jaundice is evidence of hemolysis, gestational age at birth, family history (including maternal Rh factor), timing of the appearance, and method of feeding. If jaundice appears, a bilirubin level to determine the bilirubin risk factor is plotted on the bilirubin graph in relation to hours of age (American Academy of Pediatrics [AAP], 2004) (Fig. 19-9).

NURSING CARE. Treatment of jaundice is based on the underlying cause. Infants who are plotted on the graph in the high-risk zone on the bilirubin risk chart undergo phototherapy (bilirubin lights). Phototherapy uses daylight, cool white, blue, or "special blue" fluorescent light tubes. Fluorescent lights are the most effective form of phototherapy and are placed around and above the newborn (Fig. 19-10). The level of bilirubin in the blood determines if the newborn is placed under single, double, or triple phototherapy. Fiberoptic systems (Bili-blanket) can also deliver phototherapy in a blanket form placed under or around the newborn.

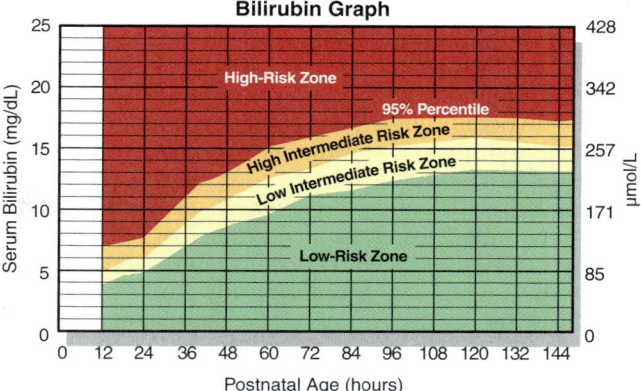

Figure 19-9 Laboratory evaluation of the jaundiced infant of 35 or more weeks' gestation.

Figure 19-10 The eyes and genitalia of the newborn are always covered to prevent tissue and retinal damage.

 critical nursing action Care of the Jaundiced Infant

The nurse must remember that when a newborn is under phototherapy the eyes must be shielded by an opaque mask. The nurse assesses the newborn's eyes every 4 hours to assess for discharge or corneal irritation. It is important to remove the mask during feedings so the infant can receive visual stimulation. The infant's genitalia area must also be covered. Also, during phototherapy or use of the Bili-blanket, the newborn should be kept warm. The infant is susceptible to hypothermia due to skin exposure and the temperature needs to be monitored closely. In addition, it is important that the infant receive proper nutrition to ensure the clearance of the bilirubin. The breast or formula feeding mother can be encouraged to feed the child as often as every 2 hours. These treatment measures must be explained to parents to help decrease their anxiety. Parents need to report any changes in the infant's condition such as an increase in jaundice, poor feeding, lethargy, or vomiting.

Other treatments for hyperbilirubinemia include hydration with an electrolyte solution if the newborn shows signs of dehydration such as dry skin and mucus membranes, poor intake, concentrated urine, or limited urine output and irritability (AAP, 2004).

Without appropriate screening and treatment of hyperbilirubinemia in the newborn, complications can occur.

Bilirubin encephalopathy describes the clinical findings when the serum bilirubin level is so elevated that the central nervous system is affected. The newborn becomes lethargic, hypotonic, and has feeding difficulty. This is a severe hyperbilirubinemic condition that warrants exchange transfusions to prevent a condition called kernicterus (AAP, 2004).

An infant with untreated jaundice is at risk for kernicterus. If bilirubin crosses the blood–brain barrier it can permanently damage a newborn's brain (Shapiro, 2005). Not all newborns with bilirubin encephalopathy progress to kernicterus, and the exact level of serum bilirubin required to cause damage is not yet known. The damage caused by kernicterus can be cerebral palsy, auditory dysfunction, dental-enamel dysplasia, upward gaze, as well as intellectual and other handicaps (AAP, 2004).

Retinopathy of Prematurity

The retinal vessels of the preterm newborn are frail and immature. Retinopathy of prematurity (ROP) is a result of immature retinal vasculature followed by hypoxia. The concentration and duration of supplemental oxygen are thought to play a role in the development of ROP.

ROP is inversely related to gestational age. Therefore, the younger the infant the greater the likelihood he has of developing this condition. Risk factors include gestational age of less than 32 weeks, birth weight of less than 1500 g, hypothermia, sepsis, and high-intensity lighting. The extent of retinal damage in the preterm newborn is dependent on three criteria: (1) the gestational age of the newborn, (2) the length of exposure to oxygen, and (3) arterial pressure.

SIGNS AND SYMPTOMS. In the first stage of ROP, the retinal vessels react to oxygen administration with vasoconstriction. If the vasoconstriction of the vessels is prolonged, abnormal vessel growth ensues. In the second stage vessel hemorrhages and edema into the vitreous occur. In the third stage the vessels fibrose. The fourth stage is severe and is classified by retinal detachment.

DIAGNOSIS. Retinopathy of prematurity is diagnosed based on five stages, ranging from mild to severe.

Stage   I — abnormal blood vessel growth is mild.
Stage   II — abnormal blood vessel growth is moderate.
Stage III — abnormal blood vessel growth is severe.
Stage IV — the retina is partially detached.
Stage   V — completely detached retina. This is the end stage of the disease.

NURSING CARE. During oxygen administration, fluctuations in arterial concentrations of oxygen must be prevented. The nurse understands that the PaO_2 should not be set greater than 80 mm Hg and that the preterm newborn should be weaned off oxygen as soon as possible. In addition, the nurse can decrease the constant bright lights in the infant's environment. A blanket can be placed over the incubator during the day. Nap time can be designated where the lights are lowered and other environmental stimuli are decreased.

The preterm newborn should be checked routinely for signs of ROP by a specialist. Examinations should be started at 4 to 6 weeks of age and continue until vascularization of the retina to reduce the risk of visual impairment (usually myopia) and blindness. Most babies who develop retinopathy of prematurity have stages I or II. If ROP is untreated it will destroy the infant's vision (National Eye Institute, 2008). Cryotherapy is used to treat ROP (Kraus & Fanaroff, 2005).

critical nursing action Retinopathy of Prematurity

Because retinopathy of prematurity (ROP) may be a complication of oxygen therapy, the nurse must maintain the lowest level of oxygen as possible to maintain the pulse oximeter reading above 92%.

Anemia of Prematurity

Premature newborns are often anemic for several reasons. One reason is that the newborn undergoes many lab evaluations. Even though small amounts of blood are taken for each study, multiple studies are done and it reduces circulatory volume. A second reason for anemia is the rapid growth a preterm newborn undergoes in a short period of time. A third reason has to do with erythropoietin release. Erythropoietin is not released until 34 to 36 weeks of gestation and then responds when hematocrit levels are low. There is an approximate 1-week delay between erythropoietin release and the production of reticulocytes.

SIGNS AND SYMPTOMS. Typical signs and symptoms include fatigue, shortness of breath, headache, dizziness, and pale skin.

DIAGNOSIS. A drop in hemoglobin below the average hematocrit value (between 35% and 45%) is the definitive signs of anemia.

NURSING CARE. Nursing care consists of transfusions of blood, although many times necessary, actually delay the erythropoietin mechanism. Anemia of prematurity is treated with recombinant human erythropoietin (r-HuEPO) subcutaneous to stimulate erythropoiesis. It is given until 34 to 35 weeks of gestation (Fike, 2004; Klaus & Fanaroff, 2005). The nurse assesses hematocrit levels per hospital policy.

Sudden Infant Death Syndrome

"Back to sleep" is the American Academy of Pediatric (AAP) campaign to educate parents and families who are involved in newborn care to prevent sudden infant death syndrome (SIDS). Since US public education started in the early 1990s there has been a 50% reduction rate in SIDS deaths. The current incidence of SIDS is 1:2000 newborns.

NURSING CARE. Priority nursing care includes education about sudden infant death.

The following recommendations are incorporated into the care of the preterm newborn in the NICU. Newborns who have been in the NICU and are preparing for discharge in the near future must be taught to sleep on their backs even though the prone position may have been used as a care intervention to increase gastric motility. Home monitors are not recommended for SIDS prevention although preterm newborns may be sent home on monitoring for other reasons. Most preterm newborns are well acquainted with a pacifier long before their discharge date to assist with their sucking and swallowing coordination, so this practice should be continued.

Family Teaching Guidelines...
Preventing Sudden Infant Death Syndrome

◆ Put all newborns on their backs to sleep.

◆ Use a firm mattress.

◆ Ensure there are no toys, soft bedding, or extra linen in the newborn's sleeping area.

◆ Encourage the use of pacifiers as they decrease the incidence of SIDS (although the exact reason why is not known).

◆ Do not allow smoking in the home.

◆ Be aware that commercial home monitoring devices do not decrease the incidence of SIDS.

◆ Never allow newborns to sleep in parental beds.

◆ Newborns should sleep in close proximity of their parents/guardian (usually interpreted as in the same room).

◆ Avoid overheating the newborn.

Essential information: The current guidelines of the American Academy of Pediatrics (AAP) apply to all newborns, but it is important to remember that the preterm newborn is at a higher risk for SIDS. These recommendations have been made by the AAP as of October 10, 2005.

The Postterm Newborn

Postterm newborns are also considered high-risk. Although fewer pregnancies are carried to post-term today due to elective inductions there are still incidences where a newborn is born after 42 weeks of gestation. Postterm newborns may or may not be LGA. The newborn may have actually lost weight in utero because of declining placental ability to transport nutrients and oxygen.

Because these newborns are in utero after the optimal growth time they undergo developmental changes including skin desquamation or peeling. The skin of a post-term infant is often parchment-like and is often cracked on the abdomen and extremities. The fingers appear long and are often peeling and sometimes general muscle wasting is evident.

Postterm newborns are at risk for passing meconium stool in utero, which increases their chances of meconium aspiration pneumonia and persistent pulmonary hypertension (PPHN). Often the cord is meconium stained on assessment indicating that meconium was passed in utero at some time well before delivery (Klaus & Fanaroff, 2005).

CONDITIONS AFFECTING THE POSTTERM NEWBORN

Meconium Aspiration Pneumonia

Meconium aspiration pneumonia occurs in 10% to 26% of all deliveries and the incidence increases directly with gestational age (before 37 weeks of gestation there is a 2% incidence and at 42 weeks of gestation a 44% incidence). The passage of meconium in utero is believed to be either a response to intrauterine hypoxia or a maturational occurrence for the newborn. Meconium can be aspirated at birth if it is not removed from the trachea at delivery.

Meconium in the lungs causes obstruction in the small airways and hyperinflation with areas of atelectasis (collapse of a portion or the entire lung due to blockage of air passage) leading to hypoxia. Some newborns with meconium aspiration pneumonia have elevated pulmonary arterial pressures and develop persistent pulmonary hypertension (PPHN).

SIGNS AND SYMPTOMS. Signs of meconium aspiration are meconium-stained skin, nails, and umbilical cord. The newborn usually has initial respiratory distress tachypenia and often has a barrel shaped chest from overinflated lungs. Rales and rhonchi are heard on auscultation.

The respiratory symptoms get progressively worse over the first 12 to 24 hours. Meconium aspiration pneumonia is often complicated by pneumothorax (collection of gas in the space surrounding the lungs) and pneumomediastinum (condition in which air is present in the space in the chest between the two lungs). Pneumothorax is an emergency situation and requires chest tubes.

DIAGNOSIS. Meconium aspiration pneumonia can be visualized in the infant's vocal cords and respiratory passages using a laryngoscope. Diagnosis is confirmed through a chest x-ray exam.

 diagnostic tools X-Ray Films

The chest x-ray film usually shows: patchy infiltrates, overexpansion, atelectasis, flattened diaphragm, and bulging intercostal spaces (Noerr, 2000).

NURSING CARE. Nursing care of meconium aspiration pneumonia consists of chest physiotherapy (PT) and oxygen administration. Chest physiotherapy can be done by percussion with a small cup, base of a feeding nipple, or specifically made neonatal chest PT device or vibration by a battery-operated vibrator. Chest PT should be done every 3 to 4 hours to help maintain a clear airway. Postural drainage with percussion or vibration is followed by suction.

CPAP is frequently used to provide oxygen. Oxygen by noninvasive means such as hood or cannula is often not sufficient. If the newborn cannot maintain a PaO_2 of 50 mm Hg or higher in 100% oxygen then mechanical ventilation is used.

Because the newborn is postterm and neurologically more mature than ventilated preterm newborn, neuromuscular medications such as Pavulon (Pancuronium) or vecuronium (Norcuron) may be used to increase the effectiveness of ventilation efforts. Analgesic and sedative medications may also be used such as fentanyl (Sublimaze), lorazepam (Ativan), morphine sulfate (Astramorph), or demerol (Meperidine) so the newborn does not "fight "the ventilator (Taeusch et al., 2005).

Persistent Pulmonary Hypertension of the Newborn

Persistent pulmonary hypertension of the newborn (PPHN) was once termed persistent fetal circulation because there is right-to-left shunting of blood across the foramen ovale and through the ductus arteriosus. The meconium in the newborn's lung induces platelet aggregation in the microcirculation of the pulmonary system, keeping the arterial pressure elevated. The PPHN is vascular resistance in the pulmonary system which can be caused by sepsis or pneumonia but the most common cause of newborn PPHN is meconium aspiration pneumonia. This occurs when pulmonary vascular resistance does not decrease after birth so the transition to normal adult-type circulation to the pulmonary system is resisted, forcing fetal circulation to persist. PPHN produces a right ventricular overload and poor left ventricular filling. The critical cycle of PPHN is shown in Figure 19-11.

SIGNS AND SYMPTOMS. PPHN usually affects term or postterm newborns because they frequently are born through meconium stained amniotic fluid. The newborn has brief respiratory distress at birth and then responds normally. By 12 hours after birth the signs of PPHN are displayed. The newborn is centrally cyanotic and tachypneic. Grunting and retracting is usually not evident. They may have an audible murmur due to tricuspid insufficiency but their blood pressure remains normal.

DIAGNOSIS. Diagnosis is confirmed from the clinical signs and symptoms and chest x-ray exam. There is often hypoglycemia and hypocalcemia. Arterial blood gases show oxygen desaturation. Ultrasonography of the heart is done to rule out cardiac anomalies and to visualize any right-to-left shunting (Taeusch et al., 2005).

NURSING CARE (SEE NURSING CARE PLAN, P. 619). Nursing care of the newborn with (PPHN) is critical with the optimal outcome of good oxygen saturation as well as overall stabilization.

 critical nursing action Extracorporeal Membrane Oxygenation

Extracorporeal membrane oxygenation (ECMO) is used for newborns who are not responding to conventional or high-frequency ventilation (Fig. 19-12). ECMO has only an 80% success rate and it is used as a last resort for respiratory support. Delivering ECMO is a complicated procedure and is a heart and lung bypass procedure used mainly for newborns with meconium aspiration pneumonia, neonatal pneumonia, and congenital diaphragmatic hernias. Newborns less than 34 weeks' gestation or 2000 g are not candidates due the need for heparinization of the blood which can cause a cerebral hemorrhage in small or preterm newborns. ECMO is accomplished by inserting a catheter into the right internal jugular vein that extends into the right atrium and another catheter inserted into the right carotid artery into the aorta arch. The system drains venous blood and replaces arterial blood with oxygenated packed red blood cells, platelets, and fresh frozen plasma. The procedure is expensive, work intensive, and carries a multitude of complications. It is available only at select Level III neonatal centers (Taeusch et al., 2005).

Additional Conditions Affecting the High-Risk Newborn

Many conditions are now diagnosed prenatally with ultrasound. High-risk newborns may have several conditions that impact their health. Any condition can be devastating for the family and may require emergency treatment. Some significant conditions include metabolic, neurological, and gastrointestinal anomalies as well as abdominal

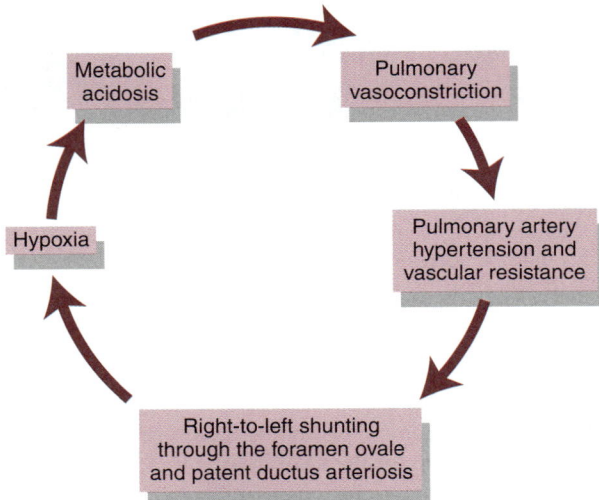

Figure 19-11 Persistent pulmonary hypertension of the newborn.

Figure 19-12 Extracorporeal membrane oxygenation (ECMO) is used for newborns that are not responding to conventional or high frequency ventilation.

wall defects, infections, and a condition that causes developmental delay. The nursing care for the infant is holistic and individualized.

METABOLIC CONDITIONS

Metabolic disorders are diagnosed after birth, and 4 million newborns undergo metabolic and genetic screening each year. Four thousand identified newborns are then diagnosed

Nursing Care Plan   Persistent Pulmonary Hypertension of the High-Risk Newborn

Nursing Diagnosis: Ineffective Tissue Perfusion: Cardiopulmonary, related to persistent pulmonary hypertension of the newborn (PPHN).

Measurable Short-term Goal: The newborn will maintain peripheral oxygen saturation levels of 92–95%.

Measurable Long-term Goal: The newborn will maintain adequate tissue perfusion on room air.

NOC Outcomes:

Tissue perfusion: Pulmonary (0408) Adequacy of blood flow through pulmonary vasculature to perfuse alveoli/capillary unit

Respiratory status: Gas Exchange (0402) Alveolar exchange of carbon dioxide and oxygen to maintain arterial blood gas concentrations

NIC Interventions:

Respiratory Monitoring (3350)
Oxygen Therapy (3320)

Nursing Interventions:

1. Monitor respiratory rate, lung sounds, effort of respirations, color, and oxygen saturation frequently (specify how often) for 24–48 hours after meconium-stained delivery.

   RATIONALE: PPHN sometimes develops after the first 12–24 hours of life.

2. Notify the caregiver of signs of respiratory distress: tachypnea, grunting, nasal flaring, retracting, cyanosis, or decreased oxygen saturation.

   RATIONALE: Respiratory distress related to PPHN can occur rapidly.

3. Record a preductal (right radial) pulse oximeter reading and postductal (left radial or either foot) pulse oximeter reading simultaneously.

   RATIONALE: A difference of 5% may be helpful in diagnosing the right-to-left shunt produced by PPHN.

4. Take four extremity blood pressures.

   RATIONALE: A difference of >10–15 mm Hg preductal and postductal may suggest a right-to-left shunt.

5. Provide and monitor oxygen and respiratory support as ordered (specify) to maintain a pulse oximetry reading of >92%.

   RATIONALE: Oxygen therapy may be needed to maintain adequate saturation levels.

6. Maintain infant in a neutral thermal environment without excessive noise or stimulation.

   RATIONALE: A thermoneutral environment decreases metabolic needs and decreased environmental stimuli may avoid excess neurological stimulation.

7. Administer sedation as ordered (specify drug, dose, route, and time).

   RATIONALE: (Specify action of the drug) Sedation may reduce metabolic needs.

8. Closely monitor intake and output. Restrict fluids as ordered (specify).

   RATIONALE: Excessive fluids can increase pulmonary workload and increase respiratory distress.

9. Provide information and support to the family.

   RATIONALE: These newborns can become critically ill and are often transferred out to the most technologically advanced Level III NICU for extracorporeal membrane oxygenation (ECMO) support.

---

with metabolic disorders. All 50 states (and Puerto Rico) screen for phenylketonuria and hypothyroidism, 46 states screen for galactosemia and 43 for hemoglobinopathy. Maple syrup urine is included in the screening for 25 states. Other disorders are screened for in various states such as homocystinuria, biotinidase deficiency, congenital adrenal hyperplasia (CAH), cystic fibrosis (CF), and toxoplasmosis. The screening that is done for these conditions can promote early intervention, thereby decreasing devastating complications (AAP, 2005). States vary greatly among the different tests screened for and new tests that can be included in regular screening are being discovered on a regular basis (Kenner & Moran, 2005) (Box 19-7).

Box 19-7   Metabolic Diseases of the Newborn

- Tyrosinemia
- Adenosine deaminase deficiency (ADA)
- Arginase deficiency (AD)
- Urea cycle defects
- Duchenne muscular dystrophy (DMD)
- Glucose-6-phosphate dehydrogenase (G-6PD) deficiency
- Pyroglutamic aciduria
- Medium-chain acyl-CoA dehydrogenase deficiency (MCAD)

Phenylketonuria

As early as 1961, Dr. Robert Guthrie developed a blood test to diagnose newborns with phenylketonuria (PKU). It was the first metabolic disease that prompted universal screening for metabolic diseases and it is currently screened for in all U.S. states/territories. It is a disease transmitted by an autosomal recessive gene. The incidence varies greatly by race from 1:6000 in Caucasian to 1:60,000 in newborns of Japanese descent. There is a deficiency of phenylalanine hydroxylation and phenylalanine cannot be broken down.

SIGNS AND SYMPTOMS. There are no signs or symptoms at birth. Accumulations of phenylalanine eventually cause developmental delays, mental retardation, and seizures.

DIAGNOSIS. Phenylketonuria is diagnosed through a blood test.

NURSING CARE. The nurse communicates to the parents that phenylketonuria is controlled by a phenylalanine-free diet with the elimination of proteins (including breast milk and formula). The diet is continued for the child's entire life. Parents can find information about this condition and diet at Centers for Disease Control and Prevention (PKU) (http://www.cdc.gov/; AAP, 2008).

Galactosemia

Galactosemia is screened in 46 U.S. states/territories. The incidence is 1:60,000-80,000. It is an inherited metabolic deficiency. Children with galactosemia cannot metabolize galactose, and it results in failure to thrive, vomiting, liver disease, cataracts, mental retardation, and even death.

SIGNS AND SYMPTOMS. The signs and symptoms of galactosemia cause the inability to use galactose to produce energy.

DIAGNOSIS. Galactosemia is diagnosed through a blood test.

NURSING CARE. Children diagnosed with galactosemia are placed on a galactose-free diet that needs to be maintained for life (AAP, 2008).

Maple Syrup Urine Disease (Branched-Chain Ketoaciduria)

Maple syrup urine disease is screened for in 25 U.S. states/territories. It is an autosomal recessive disorder that results in high body fluid levels of ketoacids and can lead to lethargy, irritability, and then progress to coma and death. This specific metabolic deficiency has a high incidence in the Mennonite population (1 in 760) but should be considered for any newborn with severe acidosis in the first 10 days of life.

SIGNS AND SYMPTOMS. There are no symptoms at birth. Urine has a characteristic odor. If left untreated the newborn will show neurological signs, poor feeding, vomiting, increased reflexes, and seizures.

DIAGNOSIS. Maple syrup urine disease is diagnosed through a blood test.

NURSING CARE. A low-protein diet is initiated and thiamine supplements may be given. The parents are told that the dietary treatment must begin as soon as possible and continued throughout life (AAP, 2008).

Homocystinuria

Homocystinuria is screened for in 22 U.S. states/territories. The incidence is 1:50,000. It is an autosomal recessive genetic transmission. There is a deficiency in cystathionine beta-synthase which causes high levels of serum methionine. Children with homocystinuria have ocular abnormalities and thromboembolisms that affect both legs.

SIGNS AND SYMPTOMS. Signs of homocystinuria can include skeletal abnormalities, displacement of the eye lens, an increase risk for blood clots, and as the child grows problems with learning and development.

DIAGNOSIS. Homocystinuria is diagnosed through a blood test.

NURSING CARE. Diet therapy includes high doses of vitamin B_6 and methionine and cystine restriction (AAP, 2008).

Biotinidase Deficiency

Biotinidase deficiency is screened for in 21 U.S. states/territories. It is an autosomal recessive metabolic disorder that leads to carboxylase deficiency due to faulty biotin recycling.

SIGNS AND SYMPTOMS. Without treatment, symptoms show at 7 weeks to 3 years and include developmental delay, hypotonia, uncoordinated movement, alopecia, rash, hearing loss, optic nerve atrophy, seizures, and mental retardation. Untreated cases progress to metabolic acidosis that can lead to death.

DIAGNOSIS. Biotinidase deficiency is diagnosed through a blood test.

NURSING CARE. The nurse communicates to the family the infant must receive Pantothenic acid or biotin (types of B vitamins). These vitamins must be replaced every day because they are essential to growth and help the body break down and use food. Pantothenic acid and biotin are also found in foods such as eggs, fish, milk and milk products, whole grain cereals, lean beef, legumes, and broccoli (AAP, 2008).

NEUROLOGICAL CONDITIONS

Intraventricular and Periventricular Hemorrhage

Acute intracranial hemorrhage (ICH) of the newborn is bleeding into the epidural, subdural, or subarachnoid areas of the brain. An ICH can be minimal or extensive and present clinically from asymptomatic to seizures activity.

SIGNS AND SYMPTOMS. The ICH is often categorized by extent and involvement. Grade I hemorrhages bleed into the subependymal only; grade II hemorrhages bleed into the subependymal and the ventricles but do not produce distention of the ventricles. Grade III hemorrhages bleed into the ventricles and produce dilatation of the ventricles which can lead to hydrocephalus. Grade IV hemorrhages produce the same bleeding as in grade III but the bleeding extends to the parenchymal.

DIAGNOSIS. ICH are diagnosed by cerebral ultrasound and followed up with magnetic imaging or CT scan (Taeusch et al., 2005). Diagnosis can also be made by observing altered states of consciousness in the preterm newborn as well as behavioral changes. In addition, an enlarging head circumference needs immediate attention and is indicative of a worsening IVH or periventricular hemorrhage (PVH).

NURSING CARE. Priority nursing care centers on recognition of infant seizures so treatment can begin immediately. Phenobarbital (Luminal Sodium) is the drug of choice as well as phenytoin (Dilantin), lorazepam (Ativan), and diazepam (Valium). It is also essential to prevent cerebral damage as well as maintain adequate oxygenation. Parents will need information about their infant's status and subsequent care.

Neurological sequelae related to IVH and PHV are associated with the severity of the bleed. Severe bleeds can lead to seizures, mental deficiencies, and cerebral palsy. Head ultrasounds are done routinely in the nursery, usually every week in order to evaluate the presence of IVH and PVH in the preterm population. If the bleed causes obstruction of cerebral spinal fluid (CSF), a shunt is needed to prevent hydrocephalous.

 critical nursing action Intraventricular and Periventricular Hemorrhage

When caring for a neonate with intraventricular or periventricular hemorrhage, the nurse must observe for neurological symptoms, including poor oxygenation readings on pulse oximeter, poor feeding (if the newborn is being fed), and lethargic behavior. Increased apnea, bradycardic spells, and seizures may also occur. Critical nursing actions include keeping accurate and frequent measurements of head circumference in centimeters, reporting any sudden increase in head circumference, and monitoring fontanels to ensure they are soft, flat, and open on palpation.

Anencephaly

Anencephaly is a condition in which the skull and cerebrum is malformed but the anterior lobe of the pituitary is intact. These newborns can be born alive but the condition is lethal so they die in a short period of time. Anencephaly has a higher incidence in girls than boys. The defect is visually disturbing because most of the skull is not present (Taeusch et al., 2005). Nurses provide palliative and spiritual care with no effort at resuscitation. The family requires emotional support to cope with the infant's devastating condition.

Encephalocele

Encephalocele is a neural tube defect that is noticeable at birth because there is protrusion of the brain through a skull defect. Sixty to 80% of the time it occurs in the occipital area but it can also occur in the parietal, frontal or nasal regions. This defect often accompanies other congenital anomalies and surgical repair is attempted to close the defect and prevent infection. The mortality rate is higher than 30% and many of the survivors have neurological deficits. Encephalocele requires care that is directed at the defect, including the neurological and developmental effects (Taeusch et al., 2005).

Microcephaly

Microcephaly may be caused by an autosomal recessive disorder, toxic stimulus during prenatal development, or a chromosomal abnormality. Microcephaly means the infant

has a smaller than normal head circumference. It is defined as a head circumference 2 standard deviations below the mean for gestational age and is identified by progressive head circumference measurements. Microcephalic newborns may have other congenital malformations but in many cases do not show a recognizable syndrome (Vargas, Allred, Leviton, & Holmes, 2001). There is no treatment for microcephaly and nursing care is supportive. The nurse teaches parents how to rear the child according to the most realistic developmental level.

 clinical alert

Microcephaly

It is critical to maintain accurate and consistent head circumference measurements by plotting on the growth chart and monitoring the newborn for neurological symptoms.

Holoprosencephaly

Holoprosencephaly is a condition in which the cerebral matter fails to form as two distinct hemispheres. There is no fissure between the brain's hemispheres and often the ventricular system of the brain is malformed. These newborns often have facial deformities from the midline. These defects can be as severe as having one eye or nostril. These newborns are often stillborn or die shortly after birth (Taeusch et al., 2005). Nursing care includes the perinatal bereavement nurse that is sensitive to the grieving needs of the family.

GASTROINTESTINAL CONDITIONS

Cleft Lip and Cleft Palate

Cleft lip (CL), cleft palate (CP), or both is a multifactorial congenital defect that has genetic and environmental predispositions. It is the fourth most common congenital birth defect. During intrauterine fetal life the primary palate does not fully fuse and any one of several variations of clefts can occur depending on the timing of the insult. Cleft lip is sometimes detected prenatally on ultrasound.

SIGNS AND SYMPTOMS. A cleft lip can occur unilaterally or bilaterally. Either type can occur with or without a cleft of the hard and/or soft palate. Also, both or either of the palates can be cleft without the lip. The uvula can also contain a cleft.

DIAGNOSIS. Cleft lip is obvious but cleft palates call for a thorough examination of the newborn's mouth with a good light source.

NURSING CARE. The focus of nursing care is on maintaining adequate nutrition because cleft lip and palate present feeding difficulties. The nurse understands that newborns with cleft lip and palate can be successfully breastfed. Breastfeeding may be interrupted for a period of time based on the need for surgical repair. Bottle feeding is usually initiated with a special nipple that is longer than a regular newborn nipple to help prevent aspiration. One type of nipple is the Haberman nipple, which is longer and has a reservoir to regulate the flow of formula.

Newborns with clefts are fed in an upright position to decrease the incidence of regurgitation. Surgical repair of cleft lip is typically done at 3 months of age and cleft palates are usually repaired before 18 months. Some clefts require more than one surgical procedure to reconstruct. Parents must be supported by having all the treatments, feeding methods, and course of care explained. Emotional support is needed to assist in the grieving process of dealing with the reality of the nonperfect child with surgical needs (Merritt, 2005).

"What to say" — *Communicating to parents about cleft lip and palate repair*

The nurse can provide parents emotional support related to their newborn's cleft lip and palate repair. The nurse can also refer parents to Web sites that contain valuable information. Some Web sites provide the parents with suggestions on wording for the birth announcement so that family and friends are informed about this issue prior to seeing the baby.

March of Dimes: http://www.marchofdimes.com/ pnhec/4439.asp

Wide Smiles: http://www.widesmiles.org/

CLAPA (Cleft Lip and Palate Association): http:// www.clapa.com/

American Society of Plastic Surgeons: http://www. plasticsurgery.org/public_education/procedures/ CleftLipPalate.cfm

---

Necrotizing Enterocolitis

Necrotizing enterocolitis (NEC) is another complication that affects mostly preterm newborns. It is due to an ischemic episode of the bowel. When a lack of oxygen occurs in any human, blood is shunted from the nonessential organs (bowel) to the essential organs: lungs and brain. If the ischemic attack is severe it can decrease the circulation to the bowel to the point of ischemia. The extent that any portion of the bowel is affected depends on the severity of the ischemic attack. Once the bowel is necrotic or the tissue dies from lack of O_2 there is no peristalsis to move food or gas and it builds up in that section of the bowel. NEC is dangerous because it can easily produce septicemia in the preterm newborn (full-term newborns who experience a severe asphyxia can also experience NEC).

SIGNS AND SYMPTOMS. NEC is suspected if there is lack of bowel movements, abdominal distention, or an increase of 1 to 2 cm in abdominal circumference from the last feed, or newborn irritability or lethargy.

DIAGNOSIS. NEC is diagnosed via x-ray exam where a sausage-shaped dilation of the intestine is present. Laboratory findings show leukopenia, metabolic acidosis, anemia, electrolyte imbalance, and leukocytosis. A dangerous sign is free air in the abdomen that may indicate perforation.

NURSING CARE. When providing care to an infant suspected with NEC oral feedings are immediately stopped and the primary care provider is notified.

The nurse understands that if only a small portion of the bowel is affected, a rest period may reinstate enough

circulation for future functioning. If a large section of the bowel is affected, a surgical bowel resection may be warranted and sometimes it can lead to a colostomy that may or may not be permanent.

> **critical nursing action** Necrotizing Enterocolitis (NEC)
>
> When caring for a child with necrotizing enterocolitis the nurse must measure and record frequent abdominal circumferences, auscultate bowel sounds before every feeding, and observe abdomen for distention (observable loops or shiny skin indicating distention).
>
> Before a feeding, the nurse must check for aspirates at each feed for undigested formula or breast milk. If excessive (20%) undigested breast milk or formula is found, the nurse must follow the hospital's protocol, which may suggest that the next feeding be held and the primary care practitioner notified. All bowel movements must be recorded: amount, consistency, and frequency. Hematesting stools may be needed to detect occult (nonvisible) fecal blood.

ABDOMINAL WALL DEFECTS

Gastroschisis and Omphalocele

Gastroschisis is a congenital anomaly that is usually diagnosed during a prenatal ultrasound. In gastroschisis, the stomach and intestine herniate through the abdominal wall (Fig. 19-13).

Omphalocele (exomphalos) is a congenital condition in which the intestines protrude into the umbilical cord region of the abdominal wall. It is often associated with trisomy 13 and 18, and urinary tract anomalies.

SIGNS AND SYMPTOMS. In gastroschisis the abdominal wall fails to close, usually on the right side of the umbilicus, and the intestines are exposed (DiTanna, Rosano, & Mastroiacovo, 2002).

In omphalocele, if the abdominal wall defect is less then 4 cm it is usually considered an umbilical hernia and does not usually require repair.

DIAGNOSIS. Diagnosis can be made by visualization and assessment of the defect.

Figure 19-13 The newborn with gastroschisis.

NURSING CARE. Surgery is performed immediately on the infant with gastroschisis to prevent intestinal atresia resulting in obstruction. Surgical repair should be done within 2 to 4 hours of birth if the repair can be accomplished in one stage. The amount of displaced intestines determines the course of treatment of an omphalocele (Taeusch et al., 2005).

In gastroschisis, the nurse keeps the abdominal contents sterile by covering them with moist gauze and wrapped in plastic. Extreme care should be taken to position the newborn supine and prevent the mesenteric vessels from kinking so adequate blood supply continues to flow to the bowel.

Both conditions may require either a nasogastric or orogastric tube to eliminate air in the bowel. The nurse replaces fluids intravenously at 1.5 times the normal maintenance volume due to insensible water loss from the exposed bowel. Antibiotics are started preoperatively to prevent against infection.

 Nursing Insight— Gastroschisis

For larger bowel exposure a silo device is used to cover the abdominal contents and they are pushed back into the abdominal cavity gradually over 7–10 days, then repair is accomplished (Taeusch et al., 2005).

Postoperative care for either condition should be focused on fluid and electrolyte balance, nutritional support with total parental nutrition (TPN) through a central line, infection protection, and pain management. Supportive care is given to all other related problems as well as the infant who requires mechanical ventilation. Parents must be kept informed about the infant's condition and treatment regimes.

INFECTIONS IN THE NEWBORN

Herpes Simplex

Genital herpes simplex virus (HSV-2) is one of the fastest growing sexually transmitted infections in the United States. Mothers who contract a primary infection in the third trimester are more likely to transmit the infection to the newborn. A small percentage of newborns can acquire an HSV-2 infection transplacentally in utero or through a reoccurring genital infection. Newborns can acquire HSV type 1 infections from people in the environment with herpes lesions of the mouth.

SIGNS AND SYMPTOMS. Genital HSV-2 may be asymptomatic but can be activated anytime because the virus persists in the dorsal root ganglia for the lifetime of an infected individual. This neonatal infection can be disseminated or involve multiple organs, or localized involving the brain or skin, eyes and mouth. Disseminated infections carry a high mortality rate and chance for neurological sequelae.

DIAGNOSIS. HSV is cultured from the stool, urine, cerebrospinal fluid (CSF) conjunctivae, nasopharynx, and skin.

NURSING CARE. Nursing care involves the administration of acyclovir (Avirax) for a minimum of 14 days (Klaus & Fanaroff, 2005). In addition, the nurse pays attention to other associated needs of the infant and family. The nurse can ensure that the infant receives proper developmental stimulation.

Neonatal Sepsis

The incidence of sepsis is 1 to 10:1000 for newborns but is increased in the high-risk newborn population to 13 to 27:1000. Mortality rates can be anywhere from 13% to 50%.

Newborn sepsis is a systemic infection and can be due to any number of causes. The most common causes include preterm delivery, prolonged labor, rupture of membranes greater than 18 hours, maternal fever, amnionitis, or maternal group B streptococcal infection. Sepsis is classified according to the time of onset. Early onset occurs within the first 5 to 7 days of life and can progress rapidly. Late-onset sepsis is most common after a week of life and it often results in meningitis. Nosocomial sepsis occurs in high-risk newborns who have extended periods of stay in the NICU. The most common causes of neonatal sepsis according to onset of symptoms are listed in Table 19-5.

SIGNS AND SYMPTOMS. Sepsis in the newborn may be asymptomatic, so risk factors and maternal history need to be evaluated carefully. When symptoms do appear the first indications of sepsis may be behavioral changes which is a good reason to have consistent nursing care in the nursery and NICU because a nurse who "knows the newborn" may pick up subtle changes earlier than someone who has not previously cared for the newborn.

Newborns respond differently to systemic infections than adults. Some newborns may get hypothermia while others become hyperthermic. Lethargy, hypoglycemia, and poor feeding are other signs of sepsis.

DIAGNOSIS. If a newborn displays signs of sepsis or is from an environmental condition that is predisposing him to sepsis, the appropriate laboratory tests should be done and interpreted for a definitive diagnosis.

NURSING CARE. The diagnostic workup includes a complete blood count with differential, C-reactive protein level (CRP), platelet count, and blood culture. Some septic workups may include a spinal tap and urinalysis. No one test is sensitive so an evaluation of all the data is important. Neutropenia (low neutrophils in the blood) may be a significant sign because neutrophils battle bacterial infections and may be depleted if the newborn has an infection. Many nurseries use a formula that analyzes the ratio of immature to total neutrophils (I/T ratio) in the white blood cell (WBC) count.

Table 19-5	Most Common Causes of Neonatal Sepsis Broken Down into Onset of Symptoms	
Early Onset and Late Onset	**Nosocomial Onset**
Group B streptococci (GBS)	Staphylococci epidermidis
Listeria monocytogenes	*Pseudomonas*
Staphylococcus	*Klebsiella*
Streptococci	Serratia
Haemophilus influenzae	Proteus

Labs: Differential White Blood Cell Count

The formula for an I/T ratio is bands divided by segs + bands or

$$\frac{bands}{segs + bands}$$

$$\frac{7\ bands}{54 + 7} = 0.11\ shift$$

Example:
This is < 0.3 shift and is not indicative of an infection.

Most neutrophils should be segmented (SEGS) or mature cells. When 20% to 25% of the neutrophils are immature or bands (sometimes called juveniles or stabs) or unsegmented neutrophils it is suspicious of an infection. If a shift of 0.3 or greater is detected, the newborn is treated for sepsis.

Antibiotic treatment is started for a minimum of 48 hours at which time the reports on the cultured specimens should be known. A broad spectrum antibiotic or a combination of antibiotics is started as soon as possible. The usually antibiotics of choice are ampicillin (Marcillin) and gentamicin (Garamycin) (Klaus & Fanaroff, 2005).

 Nursing Insight— *Group B Streptococcus (GBS) infection in the newborn*

Group B Streptococcus (GBS) is the leading cause of neonatal sepsis in the United States. One in three women has colonized GBS in her vagina and it can be spread to the newborn during the labor process, which is vertical transmission. Before the recognition of GBS as a cause of newborn sepsis in the 1970s the mortality rate was 55%. Today mortality rate is less than 5% of those newborns contracting GBS because of protocols in place to treat women in labor or to treat the newborn if the woman was not adequately treated in labor. All women should be screened for GBS at 35 to 37 weeks of gestation. For newborns delivered in which the maternal GBS status is unknown due to premature delivery or inadequate prenatal care the newborn should be carefully observed for signs of sepsis including poor feeding, inability to maintain body temperature, inability to maintain blood glucose level over 60 mg/dL, lethargy, and seizure activity (Dremer, Lee, & Few, 2004).

DEVELOPMENTAL DELAY

Neonatal Abstinence Syndrome

There are 250,000 to 300,000 female IV drug abusers in the United States. More than 50% of them are in the childbearing age group (Coyle, Ferguson, LaGasse, Liu, & Lester, 2005). An infant of a drug-abusing mother (IDAM) is a newborn who has been exposed to drugs in the intrauterine environment which can cause withdrawal symptoms in the extrauterine environment (Gomella, 1999) (Table 19-6). Drugs that are abused have low molecular weight and transfer easily across the placenta. These drugs have a long half-life in the fetus and bind to CNS receptors, causing fetal cell damage. Some drugs such as cocaine are vasoconstrictors and affect blood flow to the fetus.

SIGNS AND SYMPTOMS. The signs and symptoms of withdrawal or neonatal abstinence syndrome (NAS) to deter-

Table 19-6 Drugs that Can Cause Withdrawal Symptoms

Opiates	Barbiturates	Others
Codeine	Butalbital	Alcohol
Heroin	Phenobarbital	Amphetamine
Meperidine	Secobarbital	Chlordiazepoxide
Methadone		Clomipramine
Morphine		Cocaine
Pentazocine		Desmethylimipramine
Propoxyphene		Diazepam
		Diphenhydramine
		Ethchlorvynol
		Fluphenazine
		Glutethimide
		Hydroxyzine
		Imipramine
		Meprobamate
		Phencyclidine

Box 19-8 Signs of Neonatal Abstinence Syndrome

Irritability	Hypertonia
Tremors	Seizures
Wakefulness	Exaggerated rooting reflex
Uncoordinated feeding pattern	Regurgitation and vomiting
Loose stools	Tachypnea or apnea
Yawning or hiccups	Sneezing and stuffy nose
Poor weight gain	Lacrimation

mine if a newborn is an IDAM are listed in Box 19-8 (Gomella, 1999).

DIAGNOSIS. Laboratory tests are often done to reveal if the drugs are in the newborn's system. Urine tests are most frequently done but reflect only the last few days of intrauterine environmental exposure. Meconium is being used more and more to test for drugs in the newborn's system. It can be obtained up to 3 days and reflects a longer period of time of intrauterine exposure than urine testing.

NURSING CARE. These newborns are a nursing challenge because they sleep very little and are irritable. Newborns that have tested positive for drugs or display neonatal abstinence syndrome should be assessed using a neonatal abstinence scoring tool for signs and signs and symptoms approximately every 3 hours.

Newborns with neonatal abstinence scores greater than 7 for 3 consecutive scorings are uncomfortable and need to be treated with medication to decrease the severity of the withdrawal effects (Box 19-9).

> **Box 19-9** Medications Used to Treat IDAM
>
> Paregoric (camphorated tincture of opium)   Chlorpromazine (Thorazine)
> Phenobarbital (Luminal)   Diazepam (Valium)
> Clonidine (Catapres)

 Nursing Insight— *Using naloxone (Narcan) in a newborn with neonatal abstinence syndrome*

Naloxone (Narcan) use may increase the severity of drug withdrawal in IDAMs. If the mother is a suspected drug abuser it should not be used.

Care of the High-Risk Newborn

Care of the high-risk newborn is multifaceted and complex. The nurse provides general care measures, interventions tailored to specific conditions, holistic and developmental care, as well as ensuring a safe nurturing environment. A thorough physical assessment is completed and vital signs are monitored frequently. Vital signs include temperature, pulse, respiration, and blood pressure. Pain is considered the fifth vital sign.

BLOOD PRESSURE

Blood pressure measuring in newborns is an indicator of cardiovascular function. In high-risk newborns hypotension is encountered more often than hypertension. Hypertension although rare is usually related to neonatal renal dysfunction.

Systolic, diastolic, and mean arterial pressure (MAP) should be assessed on the high-risk newborn. MAP is the average pressure during the entire cardiac cycle and it is reported on cardiac monitors and may differ by birth weight. Arterial pressure can be calculated by internal blood pressure monitoring done through an umbilical vessel. Pulse pressure is the difference between the systolic and diastolic pressures and is another, less significant, cardiac indicator. A wide pulse pressure is sometimes indicative of a patent ductus (the average values are 25 to 30 mm Hg in term newborns and 15 to 25 mm Hg in preterm newborns).

Most NICUs use oscillometry methods to take noninvasive blood pressure readings in the neonate. Studies have shown that non invasive blood pressure readings by oscillation are consistent with invasive blood pressure readings.

To take a blood pressure reading accurately on a neonate several things need to be considered. The equipment needs to be reliably and calculated correctly for neonates. The appropriate cuff size needs to be chosen. Blood pressures can be greatly affected by the newborn's temperature, activity, or posture (newborns that are awake and sucking average 10 to 20 mm Hg higher). Single and four extremity blood pressures can be done (Stebor, 2005).

Single blood pressure reading should be done for all high-risk newborns on a regular basis. Four extremity blood pressures are done if a cardiac murmur is heard to determine if the MAP of the upper and lower extremities are similar. Blood pressure is normally slightly greater in the lower extremities. A difference (20 mm Hg or higher in the upper arms) may indicate aortic coarctation (Procedure 19-1).

NUTRITIONAL CARE

Adequate nutritional intake is a major concern for the preterm newborn. Feeding readiness in preterm newborns is determined by each individual newborn's behavioral states. Alert states around feeding time are assessed to determine newborn feeding readiness. Preterm newborns spend less time in wake states than full-term newborns (White-Traut, Berlbaum, Lessen, McFarlin, & Cardenaas, 2005).

The nutritional needs of the preterm newborn are complicated for three reasons:

1. They have not had the time in utero to build up nutritional stores.
2. They have extrauterine complications such as RDS which increases their metabolic expenditure.
3. They should be gaining weight daily at rates double those of a full-term newborn. In addition the preterm newborn may not be able to feed due to regurgitating the feeding, losing weight, or cold stress. If an infant is not ready to feed by mouth, the nurse uses alternative ways to ensure proper nutrition such as intravenous or enteral feeding.

Intravenous Feedings

Initially fluids are given parenterally. Peripheral lines are used for shorter periods of time and most preterm newborns are placed on parenteral fluids for the first few days of life The goal for the infant in the first few days of life is to provide sufficient fluid to result in an urine output of 1 to 3 mL/kg per hour, and a urine specific gravity of no greater than 1.012.

A central line placed in the umbilical artery (UA) or vein (UV) is used for longer periods of time and provide the high-risk newborn with fluids, nutrients, blood components and medications. Another type of line called a peripherally inserted central catheter (PICC) line is also used for long term parenteral therapy.

Total Parenteral Nutrition

Total parenteral nutrition (TPN) is the initial essential nutritional support for high-risk newborns and is used to establish positive nitrogen and energy balance to promote growth (Premji, 2005). TPN also increases protein synthesis and reversal of any negative nitrogen effects that may take place in the first days of life.

The TPN solution is a calculated combination of glucose, amino acids, and electrolytes. TPN is usually started by the third or fourth day. After the first days of TPN intravenous lipid emulsions are added to the parenteral therapy as a piggybacked or secondary solution in concentrations of 10% to 20% over a slow continuous infusion. This is done to reverse fatty acid deficiency and provide energy for tissue healing and growth.

Procedure 19-1 Taking a Newborn's Blood Pressure

Purpose

Taking the blood pressure is an indicator of a newborn's state of health. Blood pressure means the pressure of blood as it is forced against the arterial walls during a cardiac contraction.

Equipment

Appropriate size cuff
Blood pressure (B/P) machine
Method to record results

Steps

1. Choose the appropriate size cuff by measuring the midpoint of the limb.

   RATIONALE: *Cuffs that are either too narrow or too small affect the accuracy of the blood pressure measurement. Choose a cuff that has a width that is approximately 40% of the arm's circumference. A properly fitting cuff will cover about 2/3 or entire upper arm (or other extremity).*

2. Do not use an extremity that has an IV.

   RATIONALE: *This prevents trauma or damage to the IV site.*

3. Do not apply to broken skin areas.

   RATIONALE: *This prevents further damage to the skin.*

4. Do not extend cuff over a joint.

   RATIONALE: *This prevents an inaccurate measurement.*

5. Inspect the cuff for intactness and decompress it to ensure it is not leaking.

   RATIONALE: *Proper function equipment is essential for accurate blood pressure measurement.*

6. If the cuff has an arterial mark, palpate the artery and line up the mark.

7. Wrap cuff snugly.

   RATIONALE: *A properly fitting cuff is essential for accurate blood pressure measurement.*

8. Connect the cuff to the air hose.

9. Start the blood pressure device.

10. Remove the cuff and inspect the skin (Stebor, 2005).

Clinical Alert Attempt to take blood pressure while the newborn is sleeping or use a pacifier to quiet the newborn for the procedure.

Note

The B/P is usually slightly higher in the legs.

Caution

A wide pulse pressure may indicate A-V malformation, truncus arteriosus, or PDA. A narrowed pulse pressure may indicate: peripheral vasoconstriction and cardiac failure. A systolic pressure in the arms that is 20 mm Hg or higher may indicate aortic coarctation.

Teach Parents:

The nurse can teach the parents that the blood pressure is an indicator of a newborn's state of health.

Documentation
2/17/10 1300 Murmur auscultated, HR 160 BPM, pulse O₂ = 97%, 4 extremity B/Ps done.   —R. Wittmann-Price, RN

Enteral Feedings

Enteral feedings of prescribed formula or breast milk given through either a nasogastric or orogastric tube are started as soon as the preterm newborn is stable. A continuous infusion pump method ensures safe administration of the feeding. As the infant grows and becomes more stable, bolus feedings every 3 hours are eventually started because the newborn can now tolerate this kind of feeding. As the feedings are increasingly tolerated by the preterm newborn the parenteral therapy can be decreased.

Bottle- and Breastfeeding

Once the newborn reaches 32 weeks of gestational age and is stable, bottle and or breastfeeding is attempted usually once a day and increased as tolerated. The feedings should start slowly and advance over several days.

clinical alert

Aspiration

Newborns with greater than 60 respirations/minute should *never* be PO fed because they have an increased risk of aspiration pneumonia.

There are many different types of formulas used for newborns. Each type of formula has a different nutritional goal. When preparing a formula feeding for high-risk newborns the procedure should be done on a clean surface with only one formula preparation being done at a time with proper labeling.

Breastfeeding should be encouraged for families who choose it as soon as the newborn is able to spend limited amounts of time out of the incubator and is more than 32 to 34 weeks postconceptual age. Preterm newborns can be successfully taught to breastfeed if there is a planned approach that supports the family's decision (Callen & Pinelli, 2005).

Breast milk has benefits for the preterm newborn. Breast milk can supply IgA and other proteins that decrease the incidence of infection in the preterm newborn. Neurological benefits have also been suggested with the use of breast milk (AAP, 2005).

Non-nutritive Sucking

Non-nutritive sucking (NNS) is promoted for the preterm and high-risk newborn for physiological and psychological reasons. Using a pacifier promotes comfort (Klaus & Fanaroff, 2005) and NNS may promote breastfeeding in

where research and practice meet:
Breastfeeding

The number one issue related to unsuccessful breastfeeding after discharge from the NICU was low milk supply. Mothers who decide to breast feed must be encouraged to pump regularly and often in order to maintain their milk supply until their premature newborn can be regularly breastfed (Callen, Pinelli, Atkinson, & Saigal, 2005).

the high-risk newborn (Spatz, 2005). Pacifiers are made in different sizes to accommodate the size of the newborn.

Other Nutrients Needed for High-Risk Newborn Growth

Calcium phosphate and magnesium is needed to prevent undermineralization of bones, fractures, and rickets. Calcium is given at 185 to 200 mg/kg per day, phosphorus at 100 to 113 mg/kg per day and magnesium 5.3 to 6.1 mg/kg per day as the recommended doses and is usually started after the first day or so of TPN. Vitamin D is also required for metabolism of calcium, phosphate, and magnesium for the preterm newborn. Trace elements of copper, zinc, selenium, manganese, and chromium are also added to parenteral nutrition to prevent deficiencies.

Vitamin intake for the preterm newborn is calculated on weight and can be delivered in the TPN or lipid solution. Vitamin A is also placed in the TPN.

Intake and Output

High-risk newborns are maintained on strict intake and output (I & O) until they are growing adequately. Adequate growth means a sustained pattern of weight gain. The actual intake of a newborn is calculated on total daily amount of calories (kcal/kg per day) and fluid requirements (mL/kg per day). To maintain adequate growth newborns need a caloric intake of 100 to 120 kcal/kg per day and a fluid intake of 150 to 180 mL/kg per day.

! clinical alert

Calculating standard newborn formulas

$$kcal/kg/day = \frac{kcal/mL \times \text{Total mL of formula}}{\text{Weight}}$$

The normal output for a preterm newborn is 1 to 3 mL/kg per hour. Oliguria is defined as <0.5 to 1 mL/kg per hour (Fig. 19-14).

 where research and practice meet:
Non-nutritive Sucking

A recent study by Pinelli and Symington (2005) showed a significant decrease in length of stay (LOS) for newborns who were provided with non-nutritive sucking (NNS). There was no significant difference in weight gain between newborns who had NNS and those without NNS.

Figure 19-14 Newborn output is calculated by weighing the diaper on a gram scale.

DEVELOPMENTAL CARE

Although more preterm newborns are surviving, many still have negative consequences, including developmental disabilities and delays, as well as vision and hearing deficits (Cuevas, Silver, Brooten, Younglut, & Bobo, 2005). Appropriate developmental care in the NICU may be a key to decreasing long-term developmental disabilities for the preterm newborn. There is increasing evidence in the literature that environmental issues, such as excessive noise and uncontrolled lighting, is detrimental to the developing preterm newborn (Graven, 2000). The NICU environment should replicate a smooth transition from the intrauterine environment as much as possible and limit excessive stimuli to ensure maximum developmental growth.

Preterm newborns do not have the neurological and social development needed to deal with the sudden stimuli of extrauterine life. Cortical organization in the preterm newborn is immature and preterm newborns are poorly equipped to self-modulate their behavior. Overstimulation from environmental factors can have long-term detrimental developmental effects.

Providing an environment for optimal growth is the primary philosophy of developmental care. Developmental care assists to modulate the preterm newborn's behavioral states. Some of the environmental issues that can be controlled by the nurse in order to promote developmental growth include noise, lighting, handling, and positioning.

Noise

Sensory systems of the fetus develop in sequences. The sensory modalities develop in the third trimester. Premature birth exposes the newborn to excessive stimuli before this sensory sequencing is established. The preterm newborn is suddenly in an unnatural environment that demands use of the different systems out of sequence and ultimately becomes a source for developmental problems.

The most vulnerable period of development occurs during neuronal differentiation. It has been argued that the harsh and noisy NICU environment may affect normal development and that the auditory system is the most vulnerable. Noise can cause damage to the cochlea, and cause outer hair cell loss with significantly lower intensity levels than would be expected.

The noise level in the traditional NICU may be very disruptive to a premature newborn compared to the intra-uterine environment. Noise in NICUs can easily exceed acceptable limits for optimal growth and development. The Report of the Fifth Consensus Report of the Newborn ICU Design Committee states that noise should not exceed an overall background limit of 50 to 55 decibels (dB) and maximum intermittent sound should not exceed 70 dB (Understanding Decibels, 2005).

Prevalent neurological and behavior deficits such as disruptive sleep, poor motor function, attention deficit, and sensorineural hearing loss could be the results from the traditional noisy NICU environment. Environmental changes can be made to decrease in the noise level and off-set adverse effects (Thear & Wittmann-Price, 2006). The nurse can provide a quiet environment to prevent hearing loss, neurological and behavior deficits, and stress in the high-risk newborn.

Lighting

Most NICUs keep the lights subdued to mimic the intra-uterine environment. Studies are now showing that newborns with light–dark cycles imposed in the external environment have better weight gain and better sleep patterns then those newborns cared for in non cyclic lighting (Rivkees & Hao, 2000). The nurse can provide an environment that promotes a natural sleep wake cycle for the infant. Creating a designated nap time during which incubators are covered with a small blanket may help regulate the infant's circadian rhythm.

Handling

Minimal stimulation is advised to reduce oxygen consumption and prevent rapid increases in blood pressure that may cause cerebral hemorrhage (Taeusch et al., 2005). This has prompted most NICUs to organize nursing care into "cluster care." Cluster care is a concept in which all the nursing care for a high-risk newborn is done at one time, usually at 3-hour intervals. With cluster care there are 1 to 3 hours of undisturbed time in between vital signs, feedings, and treatments. Organization and collaboration of multidisciplinary care to enhance minimal disturbance of the high-risk newborn is a goal in NICU. Current philosophy, such as that being taught by the Newborn Individualized Developmental Care and Assessment Program (NIDCAP), view the newborn as an active participant in care. Care is regulated not by task and time but by the behavioral assessment of the newborn (NIDCAP, 2006).

Parents should be included as a partner in discharge planning for the preterm newborn and this is initiated as soon as the newborn is admitted. Many aspects of care must be taught to the family before discharge. The nurse can ensure that cluster care is used, along with including the parents in the care of the child.

 ## Complementary Care: *Preemie massage*

Preemie massage as an adjunct therapy to developmental care has shown great benefits including increased weight gain, improved nervous system development, lower levels of cortisol, increased muscle tone, better sleep–wake patterns, shortened length of stay (LOS) and improved cognitive and motor development at 8 months of age. Massage is done to simulate the tactile stimulation the newborn would have felt in utero (Molloy, 2006).

Positioning

Positioning is done with the goal of providing comfort and modulation. Premature newborns have normally extended extremities compared to flexed full-term newborns. "Nesting" is a concept in which the linen is used to safely contain the newborn in a flexed position. Specially made bean bag rolls and "frogs" are use to provide security to body parts and keep them in position. The nurse can use nesting as an intervention to promote comfort to the high-risk newborn.

The Neonatal Intensive Care Unit

The NICU is a frightening place for parents. The first visit to the NICU is extremely difficult and the parents must be prepared for what they are about to experience. The rules of the unit must be outlined and the expectations gently discussed. The newborns are extremely small and fragile and there are several pieces of highly technical equipment, all with alarms. The nurse can explain that the NICU keeps the lighting dimmed and voices low to increase rest for the newborn to promote developmental care. Care is done in clustering and the nurse tries to schedule all the procedures needed on the newborn during the assessment period, which is usually every 1 to 3 hours depending on the acuity of care for the threatened newborn. The nurse can also explain that NICU tries to simulate an intrauterine environment as much as possible. This means decreasing the stimulus to the newborn as much as possible to allow normal growth and development.

Some of the NICU care concepts create a difficult adjustment for parents. Most parents are back to work long before their newborn is discharged. Many parents have an overwhelming desire to interact with their newborn but are not available during the care times. Creating partnership in care between the NICU staff and family benefits the newborn and every effort needs to be made in order to communicate and collaborate with parents. The family of the NICU newborn is encouraged to bond with their newborn just as if it was in the newborn nursery. NICU nurses must encourage them to visit and assist with care whenever possible.

Parents of NICU newborns actually go through some developmental phases until they can become partners with the staff in their newborn's care. First, the environment of the NICU is overwhelming but most parents are able, after a short time, to focus on the baby and keep the environmental distractions in the background. Second, the parents begin to develop a relationship with the newborn and take ownership of their infant. This is sometimes difficult because the nurses are providing the care. Third, the parents eventually take an active role in the newborn's care and become the voice of the newborn. This stage lends itself to parents as partners in providing the best individual developmental care for the newborn (Heermann, Wilson, & Wilhelm, 2005).

Most NICUs practice primary care nursing in order for the parents to have a consistent contact person to ask questions and to call when they are home. Some NICU staffs make routine phone calls to the family to give updates.

From the very first visit onward, the parents are encouraged to touch the newborn. Touch is a very important act for bonding with the newborn. Kangaroo care is also encouraged as soon as the newborn is stable enough to be taken out of the incubator. Many parents have the need to stay at the bedside for extended periods of time. The NICU nurse must assist the parents in finding a realistic routine that enhances the newborn's health care needs. Fathers should be included in the educational and care process of the newborn. Studies show that parents of NICU newborns report stress and anxiety about the future of the newborn years after discharge. Education about developmental care and continuity of care that includes home care are most important to the high-risk newborn (Bakewell-Sachs & Gennara, 2004). Parents also have anxiety about the newborn's discharge, so the nurse must prepare them to care for their child at home.

 critical nursing action   The Neonatal Intensive
                                          Care Unit

- Orient the parents to the NICU environment and policies and procedures and HIPAA regulations.
- Assign one primary care nurse as the main contact for the parents.
- Explain the rationale for policies and procedures.
- Listen to the parent's expectation of their role in the NICU.
- Explain the integration of caretaking roles between parents and staff.
- Use a white board at the newborn's bed to relay messages back and forth.
- Encourage parents to call the NICU and inquire about their newborn 24/7.
- Encourage parents to bring in the newborn's personal clothes when the newborn can be dressed.
- Encourage parents to verbalize dissatisfaction with newborn's care.
- Try to incorporate parent's suggestions into care when possible.

 Be sure to— Explain HIPAA

Explain to parents that HIPAA [Health Insurance Portability and Accountability Act of 1996 from the U.S. Department of Health and Human Services (HHS)] is taken seriously within the unit and should be addressed during parent orientation to the unit including:

- Parents may be asked to step out of the unit during medical rounds, nursing report times, and possibly in emergencies to protect the privacy of all newborns.

- Phone inquiries can only be done by the parents after they identify themselves by the infant's medical record or bracelet number and they have signed a consent permitting nursing and medical personnel to discuss information on the phone with them.
- Nurses and physicians will not answer questions regarding the condition of other newborns in the unit.
- Pictures of their own newborn are allowed but they cannot photograph other newborns in the unit.

For more information on Protecting the Privacy of Health Information go to: http://www.hhs.gov/news/facts/privacy.html

CLASSIFICATION OF THE NEONATAL INTENSIVE CARE UNIT

NICUs are classified according to level of care. Regionalization is a concept in care that arose in the 1980s to conserve health care dollars, consolidate services, and improve outcomes. Today hospitals often compete within the same geographic area to have the largest and most recognized services in specialty care areas. Level I nursery care is for well newborns and can stabilize high-risk newborns for transport. Level II nurseries can provide the same care as Level I nurseries plus provide premature care, give oxygen by hood and start intravenous therapy. Level III NICUs are the most sophisticated of the nurseries because they ventilate newborns (Klaus & Fanaroff, 2005).

TRANSPORTING THE PRETERM NEWBORN

Newborn transport is done if more technologically advanced care is needed than can be safely provided at the institution (Fig. 19-15). Most Level III NICUs have a specially trained transport team who go to the referring institution, stabilize the newborn, and bring the high-risk newborn back to the regional Level III center by ambulance or helicopter. The terrain, location, and weather of each referring NICU determine the safest transport mode.

Figure 19-15 Neonatal transporter.

Transport of newborns is traumatic for the newborn and family and should be avoided when at all possible (Klaus & Fanaroff, 2005).

The Transport Team

Neonatal transport teams are comprised of a physician or nurse practitioner from the Level III nursery along with nursing and respiratory staff that are educated in stabilizing the newborn. Specific protocols are followed and the team should be able to contact the referring neonatologist during transport for any unanswered questions.

The S.T.A.B.L.E. Program is a program designed to assist health care professionals in the post resuscitation/pre transport phase of neonatal care. It is an acronym for aspects critical to stabilization of the high-risk newborn (Box 19-10). It is a program promoted by the March of Dimes and American Academy of Pediatrics as an adjunct to neonatal resuscitation to improve neonatal outcomes (STABLE program, 2006).

"What to say" — *Communicating to parents about transporting the newborn*

Parents often ask if it is necessary for the newborn to be transported. The nurse can explain the advantages of treatment offered at the referring hospital and make sure the parents have a direct number to the unit and the name and number of the admitting neonatologist.

Discharge Planning

Discharge planning must be started as soon as the newborn is admitted. Most NICUs use standards for discharge such as respiratory stability, consistent weight gain, and successful oral feedings as discharge criteria (McGrath & Braescu, 2004). Studies show that nursing follow-up and phone calls decrease parental anxiety and hospital readmission (Monsen, 2005). Parent information on discharge topics can be obtained at www.advanceinneonatalcare.org.

The newborn at risk may have immediate and long-term disabilities. Newborns are extremely resilient but the lack of neurological development associated with interrupted intrauterine growth affects them not only physically but socially and developmentally. NICU "graduates" often need intensive follow-up care. They are sometimes referred to specialists for sight and hearing

follow-up (Wittmann-Price & Pope, 2002). They often need intervention from developmental and educational specialists, physical therapists, and occupational therapists. Case management is an invaluable resource in the NICU when coordinating follow-up efforts with insurance reimbursements plans. Many NICU units host social events that increase parent-to-parent support after discharge.

summary points

- Newborns can be put at risk any time during their intrauterine or extrauterine development, by genetic disorders, congenital anomalies, maternal factors, asphyxia or birth injuries resulting from conditions such as hypothermia, poor oxygenation, prematurity or congenital anomalies.

- Small-for-gestational-age (SGA) infants are newborns born at any gestational age and have a birth weight that falls below the 10th percentile on the growth chart and have suffered a nutritional or oxygenation deficit in utero due to maternal causes, fetal causes or a placenta or cord malfunction.

- Newborns who are large for gestational age (LGA) are over the 90th percentile on the growth chart because of genetics or, more commonly, have been exposed to an imbalance of nutrients in utero.

- Infants of diabetic mothers are often LGA. LGA newborns are also at risk for transient tachypnea, hypoglycemia, hypocalcemia, hypomagnesemia, birth injuries, brachial plexus injuries, and fractures.

- Premature newborns are at risk for respiratory distress syndrome, apnea of prematurity, jaundice, retinopathy of prematurity, anemia of prematurity, and sudden infant death syndrome.

- Postterm newborns are at high-risk for complications such as meconium aspiration pneumonia and persistent pulmonary hypertension.

- Appropriate developmental care in the NICU may be a key to decreasing long-term developmental disabilities for the preterm newborn.

- Discharge planning includes respiratory stability, consistent weight gain, and successful oral feedings as discharge criteria. Discharge planning must be started as soon as the newborn is admitted to the NICU.

Box 19-10 **Steps Emphasized in the Stable Program**

S Sugar
T Temperature
A Airway
B Blood pressure
L Lab work
E Emotional support

Source: STABLE Program. (2006). http://www.stableprogram.org/addinfo.html.

---

review questions

Multiple Choice

1. Immediate conditions that pose nursing concerns for the small for gestational age (SGA) newborn include which of the following?
   A. Long-term chronic or end of life care
   B. Bronchopulmonary dysplasia and ischemia
   C. Muscle contractures and hyperthermia
   D. Hypothermia and pain management

2. Upon assessing the newborn, the nurse notes shallow rapid respirations, palmar sweating, decreased oxygen saturation, and a high-pitched cry. These clinical assessments are indicative of which of the following?
   A. A neurological problem
   B. Hypoglycemia
   C. Pain
   D. Transient tachypnea of the newborn (TTN)

3. A 24-hour-old newborn is being treated for hyperbilirubinemia with phototherapy bilirubin lights. The patient is in an incubator fully undressed. All EXCEPT which of the following measures should be included in the nursing plan of care?
   A. Apply eye patches to prevent retinal damage and a covering over the genital area.
   B. Receive proper nutrition to ensure the clearance of bilirubin.
   C. Apply a head covering (stockinet hat) to prevent heat loss.
   D. Maintain adequate hydration to promote excretion.

4. A 42-week gestational aged newborn is assessed 20 hours after delivery by the nurse. On assessment the nurse auscultates rales and rhonchi, notes the newborn is tachypneic and has meconium stained nails. The nurse suspects that the newborn has:
   A. Sepsis
   B. Meconium aspiration pneumonia
   C. Transient tachypnea of the newborn (TTN)
   D. Respiratory distress syndrome (RDS)

5. A 30-week gestational aged neonate has anemia of prematurity. The neonatologist has ordered recombinant human erythropoietin 250 U/kg subcutaneous 3 times a week. The nursing implication related to this medication include:
   A. Administering the medication prior to feedings
   B. Applying pressure to the injection site for 5 min
   C. Assessing hematocrit levels as per hospital policy
   D. Assessing electrolyte levels weekly

True/False

6. When discussing survival rates with nursing students the NICU nurse teaches that newborns who are 25 weeks of gestational age have a 58% chance of survival.

7. The nursery nurse is aware that the infant with a diabetic mother may experience a chronic hyperglycemic state.

8. The NICU nurse recognizes that the infant born at 29 weeks of gestational age has a greater chance of developing respiratory distress syndrome (RDS) than the infant born at 36 weeks gestational age.

9. The NICU nurse understands that the administration of synthetic surfactant is the first line of defense to treat and prevent bronchopulmonary dysplasia (BPD).

10. Nonnutritive sucking is promoted for the preterm and high-risk newborn for physiological and psychological reasons.

Fill-in-the-Blank

11. A nurse should perform an accurate respiratory assessment of the infant with a diabetic mother to assess for transient tachypnea of the newborn (TTN) 1 to 2 hours post delivery. The neonate's respiratory rate must be below _____, without any _____, nasal flaring, _____ and a peripheral pulse oximeter of greater than _____% in room air. Otherwise immediate attention and supplemental _____ should be administered.

12. Abdominal circumference of the preterm newborn should be measured frequently by the nurse in order to assess for distention which may indicate the development of _____.

13. The NICU nurse must perform a neurological assessment of the preterm newborn, which includes measuring the ____ _____ and assessing for a bulging _____ _____.

14. The nursery nurse alerts a group of nursing students that newborns with a respiratory rate of greater than 60 should never be fed orally because of the risk of _____ _____.

15. One of the main nursing priorities for a preterm infant is assessing adequate intake and output. Adequate urine output for a preterm infant is _____. Oliguria is defined as _____.

See Answers to End of Chapter Review Questions on the Electronic Study Guide or DavisPlus.

REFERENCES

American Academy of Pediatrics (AAP). (2004). Clinical Practice Guidelines. Management of Hyperbilirubinemia in the Newborn Infant 35 or More Weeks of Gestation, Subcommittee on Hyperbilirubinemia. *Pediatrics, 114* (1), 297–316.

American Academy of Pediatrics (AAP). (2005). Breastfeeding made easier at home and work. Retrieved from http://www.aap.org/pubed/ZZZRYZIYKRD.htm?&sub_cat=1 (Accessed October 24, 2008).

American Academy of Pediatrics. (AAP). (2008). Retrieved from http://medicalhomeinfo.org/screening/newborn%20condion%20specific.html (Accessed March 9, 2008).

Bakewell-Sachs, S., & Gennara, S. (2004). Parenting the post-NICU premature infant. *MCN, 29*(6), 398–403.

Benjamin, K. (2005). Part 1. Injuries to the brachial plexus: Mechanisms of injury and identification of risk factor. *Advances in Neonatal Care, 5*(4), 181–189.

Bulechek, G., Butcher, H.M., & Dochterman, J. (2008). *Nursing interventions classification (NIC)* (5th ed.). St. Louis, MO: C.V. Mosby.

Callen, J., & Pinelli, J. (2005). A review of the literature examining the benefits and challenges, incidence and duration, and barriers to breastfeeding in preterm infants. *Advances in Neonatal Care, 5*(2), 72–92.

Callen, J., Pinelli, J., Atkinson, S., & Saigal, S. (2005). Qualitative analysis of barriers to breastfeeding in very-low-birth weight infants in the hospital and post discharge. *Advances in Neonatal Care, 5*(2), 93–103.

Coyle, M., Ferguson, A., LaGasse, L., Liu, J., & Lester, B. (2005). Neurobehavioral effect of treatment for opiate withdrawal. *Archives of Diseases in Childhood, 90,* F73–F74.

Cuevas, K., Silver, D., Brooten, D., Younglut, J., & Bobo, C. (2005). The cost of prematurity: hospital charges at birth and frequency of rehospitalizations and acute care visits over he first year of life. *AJN 105*(7), 56–64.

Deglin, J.H., & Vallerand, A.H. (2009). *Davis's drug guide for nurses* (11th ed.). Philadelphia: F.A. Davis.

DiTanna, G., Rosano, A., & Mastroiacovo, P. (2002). Prevalence of gastroschisis at birth: Retrospective study. *BMJ, 325,* 1389–1390.

Doctor, B., O'Riordan, M., & Kirchner, H. (2001). Perinatal correlates and neonatal outcomes for small for gestational age infants born at term gestation. *American Journal of Obstetrics and Gynecology, 185,* 652–659.

Doenges, M., Moorhouse, M., & Geissler-Murr, A. (2005). *Nursing Diagnosis manual: Planning Individualizing and Documenting Client Care.* Philadelphia: F.A. Davis.

Dremer, P., Lee, E., & Few, B. (2004). A history of neonatal group B streptococcus with its related morbidity and mortality rates in the United States. *Journal of Pediatric Nursing, 19*(5), 357–363.

Duhn, L., & Medves, J.(2004). A systematic integrative review of infant pain assessment tools. *Advances in Neonatal Care,* 4(3), 126–140.

Fike, D. (2004). Recombinant erythropoietin for the treatment of anemia of prematurity: Is it beneficial? *Newborn and Infant Nursing Reviews,* (3), 156–161.

Fok, T., Wong, H., Chang, A., Lau, C., & Lee, W. (2003). Updated gestational age specific birth weight, crown-heel length, and head circumference of Chinese newborns. *Archives of Diseases in Childhood, 88,* F229–F236.

Gomella, T. (1999). *Neonatology.* Stamford, CT: Appleton & Lange.

Graven, S. (2000). The full-term and premature newborn. *Journal of Perinatology, 20,* S88–S93.

Heermann, J.A., Wilson, M.E., & Wilhelm, P.A. (2005). Mothers in the NICU: Outsider to partner. *Pediatric Nursing, 31*(3), 176–181.

Hummel, P., & Conin, J. (2004). Home care of the high-risk infant. *Advances in Neonatal Care, 4*(6), 354–364.

Johnson, A. (2005). Kangaroo holding beyond the NICU. *Pediatric Nursing* 31(1), 53–56.

Johnson, M., Bulechek, G., Butcher, H., McCloskey Dochterman, J., Maas, M., Moorehead, S., & Swanson, E. (2006). *NANDA, NOC, and NIC linkages: Nursing diagnoses, outcomes, & interventions* (2nd ed.). St. Louis, MO: Mosby Elsevier.

Kenner, C., & Moran, M. (2005). Newborn screening and genetic testing. *Journal of Midwifery and Women's Health, 50*(3), 219-226.

Klaus, M., & Fanaroff, A. (2005). *Care of the high-risk neonate* (5th ed.). Philadelphia: W.B. Saunders.

March of Dimes. (2006). Perinatal Overview. Retrieved from http://www.marchofdimes.com/peristats/tlanding.aspx?reg=99&top=1&lev=0&slev=1 (Accessed October 24, 2008).

Merritt, L. (2005). Part 2: Physical assessment of the infant with cleft lip an/or palate. *Advances in Neonatal Care, 5*(3), 125–134.

McCall, E., Alderdice, F., Halliday, H., Jenkins, J., & Vohra S. (2005). Interventions to prevent hypothermia at birth in preterm and/or low birth weight babies. *The Cochrane Library,* No. 2. Chichester, UK: John Wiley & Sons.

McGrath, J., & Braesu, A. (2004). State of the science: Feeding readiness in preterm infants. *Journal of Perinatal and Neonatal Nursing, 18*(4), 353–370.

Molloy, C. (2006). Preemie massage. *Premature Magazine,* (winter), 64–68.

Moorehead, S., Johnson, M., Maas, M., & Swanson, E. (2008). *Nursing outcomes classification (NOC)* (4th ed.). St. Louis, MO: C.V. Mosby.

NANDA International (2007). *NANDA-I nursing diagnoses: Definitions and classifications 2007–2008.* Philadelphia: NANDA-I.

National Center for Health Statistics (NCHS). (2004). NCHS FASTATS. Retrieved from http://www.cdc.gov/hchs/fastats/birthwt.htm (Accessed October 24, 2008).

National Eye Institute. (2008). Retinopathy of Prematurity (ROP). Retrieved from http://www.nei.nih.gov/health/rop/ (Accessed March 10, 2008).

NIDCAP Federation International. (2006). Retrieved from http://www.nidcap.com/ (Accessed October 24, 2008).

Noerr, B. (2000). Neonatal respiratory disease and management strategies, May 18. Hershey, PA. A continuing education service of Penn State's College of Medicine at the Milton S. Hershey Medical Center.

Pasero, C. (2002). Pain control. Pain assessment in infants and young children: Premature Infant Pain Profile. *American Journal of Nursing,* 102(9), 105–106.

Pinelli, J., & Symington, A. (2005). Non-nutritive sucking for promoting physiologic stability and nutrition in preterm infants. The Cochrane Library. (Oxford) (ID no. CD001071.

Premji, S. (2005). Enteral feeding for high-risk neonates. *Journal of Perinatal and Neonatal Nurses, 19*(1), 59–71.

Rivkees, S., & Hao, H. (2000). Developing circadian rhythmicity. *Seminars in Perinatology, 24*(4), 232–242.

Sahni, R., Ammari, A., Suri, M., Milisavljevic, V., Ohira-Kist, K., Wung, J., et al. (2005). Is the new definition of bronchopulmonary dysplasia more useful? *Journal of Perinatology, 25,* 41–46.

Shapiro, S. (2005). Definition of the clinical spectrum of kernicterus and bilirubin-induced neurological dysfunction (BIND). *Journal of Perinatology, 25,* 54–59.

Sharts-Hopko, N, (2005). Why every nurse should be concerned about prematurity. *AJN, 105*(7), 60–61.

Spatz, D. (2005). Report of a staff program to promote and support breastfeeding in the care of vulnerable infants at a children's hospital *Journal of Perinatal Education,* 14(1), 30–38.

Spence, K., Gillies, D., Harrison, D., Johnston, L., & Nagy, S. (2005). A reliable pain assessment tool for clinical assessment in the neonatal intensive care unit *JOGNN: Journal of Obstetric, Gynecologic, and Neonatal Nursing, 34*(1), 80–86.

STABLE Program. (2006). http://www.stableprogram.org/addinfo.html (Accessed August 15, 2006).

Stebor, A.D. (2005). Basic principles of noninvasive blood pressure measurement in infants. *Advances in Neonatal Care, 5*(5), 252-261.

Stevens, B., Johnston, C., Petryshen, P., & Taddio, A. (1996). Premature Infant Pain Profile: development and initial validation. *Clinical Journal of Pain, 12*(1):13–22.

Stokowski, L. (2005). A primer on apnea of prematurity. *Advances in Neonatal Care, 5*(3), 155–170.

Taeusch, H., Ballard, R., & Gleason, C. (2005). *Avery's diseases of the newborn.* (8th ed.). Philadelphia: Elsevier Saunders.

Thear, G., & Wittmann-Price, R.A. (2006). Project Noise Buster in the NICU. *AJN, 106*(5), 64AA-EE.

Understanding Decibels. Retrieved from http://www.jimprice.com/prosound/db.htm (Accessed October 24, 2008).

Vargas, J., Allred, E., Leviton, A., & Holmes, L. (2001). Congenital microcephaly: phenotypic features in a consecutive sample of newborn infants. *Journal of Pediatrics,* 139(2), 210–214.

White-Traut, R., Berbaum, M., Lessen, B., McFarlin, B., & Cardenaas, L. (2005). Feeding readiness in preterm infants. *MCN 30* (1), 52–59.

Wittmann-Price, R.A., & Pope, K.A. (2002), Universal newborn hearing screening. *AJN, 102*(11), 71–77.

Young, K.D. (2005). Pediatric procedural pain. *Annals of Emergency Medicine, 45*(2), 160–71.

 For more information, go to http://davisplus.fadavis.com/

CONCEPT MAP

Nursing Considerations
- Thermoneutral environment
- Pain management
- Heelstick (capillary) blood glucose monitoring
- Monitor lab results
- Accurate physical assessment

Across Care Settings:
- Linus Project

What To Say:
- Explain:
  - Color r/t polycythemia
  - Health risks r/t LGA
- Support with birth injuries

Nursing Considerations
- Blood glucose monitoring
- Calcium gluconate
- Positioning for fractures
- Monitoring lab results
- Assessing extremities/behavior

- Hypothermia
- Hypoglycemia
- Polycythemia

Critical Nursing Action:
- Gestational age and weight accuracy
- Incubator weaning
- Closely monitor H&H
- Assess head circumference
- Glucose monitoring protocols

Nursing Insight:
- Use of stockinette caps
- Risks r/t hyperglycemia
- Newborn phlebotomy
- Fontanel assessment r/t HCP
- Glucose meter maintenance

- Hypoglycemia
- Hypocalcemia
- Birth injuries
  - Intracranial hemorrhage
  - Brachial plexus injuries
  - Fractures

SGA: Small for gestational age

LGA: Small for gestational age

Caring for The Newborn at Risk

Where Research And Practice Meet:
- Number one issue related to unsuccessful breast feeding after discharge from NICU is low milk supply

Infection   **Congenital Anomalies**

Clinical Alert:
- Fractured clavicles–T-shirt is pinned so arm is in flexed position
- Microcephaly–Accurate head circumference measurement
- Aspiration–Newborns with respirations over 60 breaths/minute should never be fed PO

Genetic Disorders
- Trisomies: 21,18 13, metabolic

Infants of Diabetic Mom/ Insulin-Dependent Mom

- Hypoglycemia
- Hypocalcemia
- Hypomagnesemia
- Polycythemia
- Hyperbilirubinemia; possible jaundice, encephalopathy, kernicterus
- Transient tachypnea

Nursing Considerations
- Phototherapy
- Glucose/bilirubin monitoring
- Magnesium sulfate, calcium gluconate
- Monitor for seizures/dehydration
- CPAP; ABGs

Critical Nursing Action:
- R/T phototherapy:
  - Temperature check
  - Cover eyes/genitalia
  - Adequate hydration
  - Bilirubin monitoring

Preterm Infant

- Cold stress
- Respiratory distress syndrome
- Apnea of prematurity
- Bronchopulmonary dysplasia
- Patent ductus arteriosus
- Anemia of prematurity
- GERD
- Necrotizing enterocolitis
- Intra/periventricular hemorrhage
- Retinopathy of prematurity
- SIDS

Nursing Considerations
- Thorough, ongoing physical assessment
- Oxygenation issues: mechanical ventilation; cannulas; CPAP
- C-R monitor; BP monitoring
- Nutritional support; parenteral; naso/orogastric, fortified breast or bottle
- Hydration status; I&O
- "Back to sleep"
- Transportation issues to and from the NICU

Postterm Infant

- Meconium aspiration pneumonia
  - Pneumothorax
  - Pneumomediastinum
- Persistent pulmonary hypertension

Nursing Considerations
- Chest physiotherapy
- CPAP
- Mechanical ventilation
- Extracorporeal membrane oxygenation

Critical Nursing Action:
- Assess for signs of cold stress
- Correct positioning; suction equipment; ongoing respiratory assessment
- Breastfeeding teaching
- Monitor growth rate; weight gain; head circumference
- Abdominal circumference; bowel sounds; stools
- Lowest oxygen level

Collaboration In Caring:
- Radiology: RDS, ET tube placement
- Teach home monitor/CPR
- "Eye rounds"

Now Can You:
- Identify a clavicle fracture by palpating for crepitus
- Correctly interpret ABG results: to identify acid–base imbalances

one
two
three
four
five

six

seven

Caring for the Child and Family

Caring for the Developing Child

You rose into my life like a promised sunrise, brightening my days with the light in your eyes.
—Maya Angelou

LEARNING TARGETS *At the completion of this chapter, the student will be able to:*

◆ Describe the principles inherent in the developmental process.

◆ Identify and explain physical, emotional, cognitive, moral, and spiritual theories of growth and development.

◆ Discuss the important Touchpoints in the development of infants, toddlers, and preschoolers.

◆ Address the discipline needs for each developmental stage.

◆ Develop a care plan for the child and family across care settings.

---

moving toward evidence-based practice Grandparents

Butler, F.R., & Zakari, N. (2005). Grandparents parenting grandchildren: Assessing health status, parental stress and social supports. *Journal of Gerontological Nursing, 31*(3), 43–54.

The purpose of this study was to describe the physical and emotional health of grandparents who were raising grandchildren and the extent to which their health was impacted by this role. The study consisted of both qualitative and quantitative data obtained from a sample of 17 grandparents 46 to 83 years of age. All of the actual participants were women, although grandfathers were present in five of the homes. The sample included 15 African American grandmothers and 2 Caucasian grandmothers. The participants resided in a three-state metropolitan area of the United States.

The following were criteria for inclusion in the study: (1) the children lived with the grandparent on a daily basis; (2) the grandparent had responsibility for raising the children; (3) the children were younger than 18 years of age; and (4) the birth parent who also may have resided in the home was considered a minor.

Strategies for data collection included: (1) a self-report questionnaire to obtain demographic characteristics; (2) an in-depth interview that was audiotaped; and (3) an observation about the home environment. In addition, the grandparents completed a Parenting Stress Index (PSI) Likert scale tool (Abidin, 1995) as well as a personal home assessment. Home visits, which lasted 1–2 hours, were made over a 10-month period by the primary investigator.

Frequency distribution and Pearson's Product-Moment Correlation were used to determine the relationship among the variables including age, income, physical and mental health, socioeconomic resources, and stress level. Qualitative analysis was used to identify codes and categories, which were further collapsed into themes.

Demographic data indicated that 47% of the participants reported being married. Their incomes ranged from $3,600 to $94,900 per year, with an average of $31,605. The mean for educational achievement was completion of 12th grade; 35% of participants were employed; 65% were retired or unemployed. In 66% of the families, incarceration of the birth parent as a result of drug addiction led to the grandparent's role change. For the remainder (24%) of the participant families, the birth mother died as a result of addiction or terminal illness.

The researchers reported that although there was wide variation in the participants' physical and mental health status, most scored high in the area designated as "parental stress." Analysis of the PSI scores revealed that 47% of the participants had exceptionally high stress scores. Areas of significant concern included to the participants were financial problems, disrupted

(continued)

moving toward evidence-based practice (continued)

social activities, and alterations in family processes. All but three participants indicated a need for child support, medical benefits, and transportation resources. The participants rated social support, provided by other family members or friends, as very good to excellent. However, finding time for personal social activities was reported to be difficult.

Sixty-four percent of the participant grandparents reported high blood pressure as the most common health concern, followed by arthritis (52.9%), circulatory problems (41.1%), and

diabetes (29.4%). Eight grandparents rated their mental health to be good to excellent; eight considered their mental health to be impaired.

1. Based on this study, do you believe that the results can be generalized to other populations?
2. How is this information useful to clinical nursing practice?

See Suggested Responses for Moving Toward Evidence-Based Practice on the Electronic Study Guide or DavisPlus.

Introduction

It is important for the pediatric nurse to have a good knowledge base of growth and development in order to tailor care to the specific needs of the child and help the family understand normal limits. It is impossible to divide the stages of development into discrete age groups. The following groupings are acceptable standards. *Newborn* refers to the stage immediately after birth until 1 month. *Infancy* is the period from 1 month until 12 months. The *toddler* stage is from 12 months until approximately 3 years. The next developmental stage is interchangeably referred to as *Early childhood* or *Preschool*. Children in this group range from 3- to 6-year-olds. *School-age* children are 6 to 12 years old. *Adolescence* begins around 12 or 13 and lasts until the beginning of adulthood.

Influences on Growth and Development

The debate over nature versus nurture is longstanding. Which is the more powerful influence in the formation of a person's essence? Nature describes the traits inherent in the infant: biologically imposed idiosyncratic factors that create what and how each person "is." Nurture, on the other hand, refers to the influence of external events such as parenting received, culture, or the "times" in which a child lives. It appears that both are intrinsically influential. "Generally speaking, genes are responsible for the basic wiring plan – for forming all of the cells (neurons) and general connections between different brain regions – while experience is responsible for fine-tuning those connections, helping each child adapt to the particular environment (geographical, cultural, family, school, peergroup) to which he belongs. Genetic potential is necessary, but DNA alone cannot teach a child to talk" (Zero to three. Brain Wonders, n.d).

Principles of Childhood Growth and Development

It is inherently pleasurable to watch a baby grow and develop. Each child moves at her own pace and in her own way. One child may move quickly through physical tasks, only to be slower with words. Another child may be emotionally tuned into the needs of others while peers are still very self-focused. Despite these differences, a nurse needs to be aware of certain universal factors in addressing the developmental needs of children. Growth refers to the continuous adjustment in the size of the child, internally and externally. Development, on the other hand, refers to the ongoing process of adapting throughout the life span. Growth and development is a continuous process from conception to death. Although development advances in an orderly sequence, each child progresses through the predictable stages within a certain timeframe. The established guidelines are just that, guidelines that have been developed through observation over time. In addition, within each individual, body systems develop at differing rates. For the child, growth "spurts" tend to be followed by periods of relative "rest" as it takes plenty of energy to continue the growth process. The periods of rest allow the child to incorporate the new growth or the newly developed skill into their personal repertoire more completely before attempting the next level.

Regardless of the rate of growth and development, children progress developmentally in a prescribed fashion. There are three primary considerations related to growth and development. First, development proceeds in a cephalocaudal direction. Cephalocaudal is a progression from head to tail; top to bottom. For example, the baby's brain develops quickly; therefore, the head grows first in comparison to the rest of the body. The child gains control of his head and neck before learning to grasp or to sit up. The baby's sensory and motor skills also begin developing from the head down. Second, development proceeds proximodistally, meaning from near to far and midline to periphery. For example, the torso develops before the arms and legs. Development proceeds to the hands and feet, and then fingers and toes. The third consideration is that development proceeds from gross motor skills (e.g., walking, jumping, riding a bike) to fine motor skills. Gross motor skills provide the foundation for fine motor developments such as eating, coloring, or buttoning a shirt.

T. Barry Brazelton, a renowned pediatrician, developed the Touchpoints model of child development (Box 20-1). Brazelton described Touchpoints as "periods during the

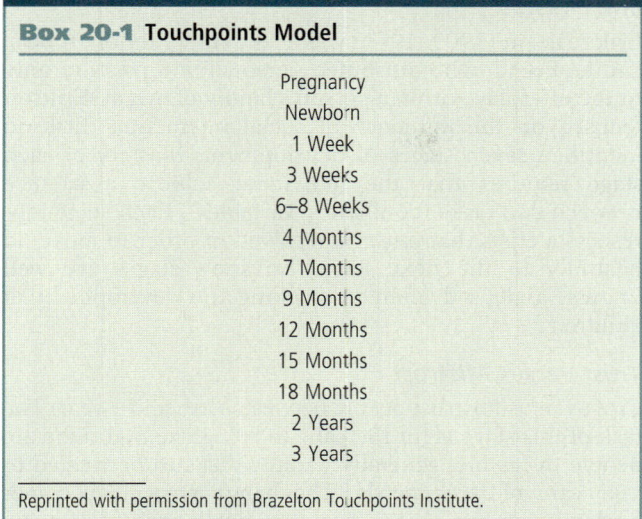

Box 20-1 Touchpoints Model

Pregnancy
Newborn
1 Week
3 Weeks
6–8 Weeks
4 Months
7 Months
9 Months
12 Months
15 Months
18 Months
2 Years
3 Years

Reprinted with permission from Brazelton Touchpoints Institute.

first three years of life during which children's spurts in development resulted in pronounced disruption in the family system" (Brazelton, 1992, p. xvii). Brazelton mapped the psychological development of children, focusing on the periods of regression that occur just prior to periods of growth. "The cost of each new achievement can temporarily disrupt the child's and even the whole family's progress" (Brazelton, 1992, p. xvii). Brazelton tracked the variations in these Touchpoints and offered anticipatory guidance for parents and professionals in moving through the stages with the child.

Brazelton and Sparrow went on to develop specific aspects about the Touchpoints that related to temperament, learning, moral development, relationships, independence, and separation issues for each of the years from ages 3 to 6. Responding to these Touchpoints gives parents the tools to help the child develop healthily.

It is important to know that Touchpoints represents a positive and well-integrated way of conceptualizing developmental progress. Its perspective assumes, among other things, that parents know their child better than they know anyone else (Brazelton & Sparrow, 2002). With that in mind, the nurse works with the family at the various Touchpoints to help them anticipate and move through the periods of disequilibrium (Box 20-2).

Box 20-2 A Paradigm Shift

FROM	TO
• Deficit model	• Positive model
• Linear development	• Multidimensional development
• Prescriptive	• Collaborative
• Objective involvement	• Empathic involvement
• Strict discipline boundaries	• Flexible discipline boundaries

Reprinted with permission from Brazelton Touchpoints Institute.

 Optimizing Outcomes— Understanding growth and development

Best outcome: The nurse can use the multidimensional developmental framework of Drs. Brazelton and Sparrow (2002) to anticipate developmental transition points to help both families and caregivers deal with the difficulties that may arise during these times.

Growth and Development Theories

Growth and development can be discussed in terms of theoretical approaches or developmental domains. A theoretical approach explains, describes, and predicts the various aspects of growth and development. A developmental domain refers to a way of understanding the total child in relation to the mind, body, and spirit. Understanding both the theoretical and developmental aspects is important because each contributes to a broader understanding about the child. A variety of theories will be discussed as well as the following developmental domains: Physical, Psychosocial (emotional, psychological, and social), Cognitive (including language and intelligence), Moral/Spiritual, and Family Development. Some of the theories are stage-related, meaning that the theorist identified specific stages and ages through which a child progresses.

Each child develops at her own pace and the stages are not rigid. It is also important to note that there is variability within each child. For example, a child may be ahead or behind physically and within normal cognitive and emotional limits, or any combination of these patterns. Growth and development takes energy. How each child expends that energy is a result of individual, family, and social variables. In contrast to the stage theories that are described, the non-stage theories are less concerned with specific ages or timeframes, but focused on the process or trajectory of developing maturity.

PSYCHOSOCIAL DEVELOPMENT THEORIES

The psychosocial domain refers to the psychological and emotional progression of the child as well as the relationships with others who are involved in the child's life. While there are many psychosocial theorists, this chapter describes the well-known theories of Sigmund Freud and Erik Erikson.

Sigmund Freud, Psychosexual

Sigmund Freud (1856–1939) believed that development was most influenced by biological instincts. Freud observed that these instincts were psychosexual in nature, meaning that a child progresses through developmental stages based on resolution of conflicts surrounding urges and rules (Box 20-3). Through observation, Freud developed a framework that is widely known today and that set the stage for modern psychoanalysis.

Freud also described the development of three essential aspects of the human personality. The initial aspect, the id, is the emotional part of the personality. The id is present at birth and is predominantly unregulated. For instance,

Box 20-3 Freud's Stages of Psychosexual Development

ORAL STAGE (BIRTH–1 YEAR)
The infant is fixated on oral curiosity (whatever he can put in the mouth). The infant derives pleasure from and relieves anxiety through oral sensations; for example, the infant sucks on his mother's breast or his bottle and is fed and pleasured. The infant puts his fist in his mouth, or uses a teething ring. Children at this stage often use pacifiers or thumbs to decrease anxiety and increase comfort.

ANAL STAGE (1–3 YEARS)
By the time the child reaches this stage; the child is ready to control elimination. Some children readily use the "big kid" potty; others resist. This is a time of increasing control in other areas of the life of the child. The child recognizes that this newfound control can run a collision course with the world, hence the term "the terrible twos." For example, the child explores, asserts, and learns boundaries about where to play safely. The child may struggle against these boundaries by escaping the backyard and running down the block.

PHALLIC STAGE (3–6 YEARS)
By early childhood, sexual difference is discovered. The child begins to compare both the male and female bodies simply out of curiosity. For example, the child notices that girls are physically different from boys. During this time, a girl child wants to push mommy aside and marry daddy or vice versa.

LATENCY STAGE (6–12 YEARS)
Freud believed that the child "takes a break" psychosexually during this period of development. This allows the child to focus more intently on other aspects of growth and learning. For example, the child spends time with his same-gender friends, excelling in sports or video games. At this age, the child presumably has little interest in issues of sexuality.

GENITAL STAGE (12–18 YEARS)
By the time the child reaches puberty, sexuality and relationships are the focus. For example, this is a time for exploring relationships and of developing a sense of romanticism.

---

the infant responds to all stimuli emotionally. The infant cries, laughs, or coos automatically and without thought. The id is the part of the personality that relies solely on instinct. During the baby's first year, the ego begins to develop to provide balance between the competing id and reality. The ego provides a sense of identity separate from others and promotes the ability of the child to function individually. During infancy, the ego helps the baby begin to learn that the mother is not simply an extension of his body. They are separate. Between the ages of 3 and 6 a superego, which serves to help regulate behavior, is developed. In this stage, the child develops cognitively and learns about rules and the needs of others. The superego functions as not only a center for conscience, but as a sense of what and how the child perceives self. An example of the superego is the young child obeying the parents' rules by picking up toys even though the child would rather continue playing. The child is learning that there is a difference between right and wrong and that they are not the "center of the universe" as previously believed. The child knows that a "good" boy obeys his parents.

During adolescence, the ego again provides a balance, this time between the id and the superego. When the adolescent refuses to drink alcohol with friends because it is against the child's conscience and the law, it shows that the ego has prevailed.

Erik Erikson

Erik Erikson (1902–1994) was a contemporary of Freud's. Unlike Freud, who attributed personality formation only to the interplay within a person's family of origin, Erikson focused on the influence of social interaction. Erikson identified seven stages of development. Mastery of each stage requires that the individual achieve a balance between two tasks (conflicting variables). Each stage represents a crisis that must be resolved in order to move on healthily to the next stage. Erikson's stages are well known, and used often in tracking the development of children.

Trust versus Mistrust

Trust versus mistrust occurs between birth and 1 year. The task of this stage is for the baby to recognize that there are people in his life, generally parents that can be trusted to take care of basic needs. The baby's struggle becomes evidenced in the recognition that not everyone or every situation is "safe." Through trust the baby learns to have confidence in personal worth and well-being along with connectedness to others. Failure to master this stage leaves a sense of hopelessness and disconnectedness. Examples of this disconnect can be seen in infants with failure to thrive or with attachment disorders. Difficulty in trusting can be seen even in adults who have problems maintaining significant relationships.

Autonomy versus Shame and Doubt

Autonomy versus Shame and Doubt occurs between 1 and 3 years. The task of this stage is for the child to balance independence and self-sufficiency against the predictable sense of uncertainty and misgiving when placed in life's situations. It is the time for the child to establish will-power, determination, and a can-do attitude about self. An example of this stage happens when the toddler wants to choose clothing and dress independently. The struggle happens when the parents allow the child to make personal choices yet expect the choices to be socially acceptable. At this age, the child is able to do many new things and wants to explore everything. This newfound independence is accompanied by new rules that may cause internal conflict. The child must develop personal abilities while struggling with both fears and wishes.

Initiative versus Guilt

Initiative versus guilt occurs between 3 and 6 years. The child's task during this stage is to develop the resourcefulness to achieve and learn new things without receiving self-reproach. It is difficult for a young child to resolve the conflict between wanting to be independent and needing to stay attached to parents. The child's writing plays or new songs, games, or jokes are good examples of initiative. The child feels confident to try new ideas. It is important that parents and teachers encourage this initiative to help the child develop a sense of purpose. If initiative is discouraged or ignored, the child may feel guilt and lack of resourcefulness.

Industry versus Inferiority

Industry versus inferiority occurs between the ages of 6 and 12. In this stage, the child develops a sense of confidence through mastery of tasks. This sense of accomplishment can be counterbalanced by a sense of inadequacy or inferiority that comes from not succeeding. The realization that the child is competent is one of the important building blocks in the development of self-esteem. Industry is evident when the child is able to do homework independently and regulate social behavior. Performing the prescribed tasks at school or home also show industry. If the child cannot accomplish realistic expected tasks, the feeling of inferiority may result.

Identity versus Role Confusion

Identity versus role confusion occurs between the ages of 12 and 18. This is a time of forging ahead and acquiring a clear sense of self as an individual in the face of new and at times conflicting demands or desires. During this stage the adolescent wants to define "what to be when I grow up." She begins to concentrate on goals and life plans separate from those of peers and family. At this point, the child has the ability to think about self as well as others and proceeds accordingly.

> **"What to say"** — *When a parent inquires about the development of their child*
>
> When parents ask the nurse about a delay in their child's development the nurse can respond by saying "It is important to note that your child may not have reached the 'appropriate' developmental stage based on chronological age alone. There may be events or variables that stunt your child's attempts to move forward such as an illness."

ATTACHMENT THEORIES

Attachment refers to the bond or emotional and physical connection that develops between an infant and caregiver that tends to endure (Ainsworth, 1978). Early theorists associated attachment with the mother who met the infant's innate drive to be fed and nurtured. Other examples of attachment behaviors are dressing, bathing, diapering, cuddling, loving, playing, and comforting. In contrast, Bowlby in 1978 and Ainsworth in 1978 refocused on the attainment of and subsequent quality of the bonding relationship between the infant and caregiver. Both the infant and the caregiver rely on the quality of the interaction between them. In other words, a healthy infant–mother relationship is contingent on the characteristic value of the communication between them. While researchers generally concentrated on the birthmother as the primary attachment figure in the infant's world, Bowlby (1978) also referred to attachment with a "mother-substitute" (p. xxvii).

John Bowlby

In the early 1900s, John Bowlby, a British psychologist (1907–1990), was fascinated with children and the influence that separation had on their ability to bond with their caregivers. Bowlby became particularly interested in the impact of separation of young children from their mothers, identifying three phases of response to that separation: *protest* (in response to the anxiety produced by separation), *despair* (related to the grief and mourning caused by prolonged separation), and *detachment* (a defense against the feelings associated with despair). Bowlby viewed attach-

ment as biological and evolutionary adaptation. The infant develops an attachment to his mother as a means of surviving the vulnerability of infancy, rather than as a simple response to having his biological needs met. As the infant begins to explore the world and the other people in it the mother is perceived as "home base." When the infant becomes frightened or threatened, home base is found. If the infant feels secure in the knowledge that the home base is reliable, the infant can move on to develop additional relationships and attachments.

Mary Ainsworth

Mary Ainsworth (1913–1999) was a colleague of Bowlby's and added to the work with studies about infants in unfamiliar situations. Through the use of the "strange situation" room, the researcher introduced infants (10 to 24 months old) to a series of situations that tested the strength of their attachment to their mothers. The situations demonstrated three patterns:

- Secure attachment: Baby cries when the mother leaves and is happy when the mother returns.
- Avoidant attachment: Baby rarely cries when the mother leaves and avoids the mother upon return.
- Ambivalent attachment: Baby becomes anxious prior to the mother leaving, is very upset when the mother leaves, and seeks contact with her while pushing her away on return.

Ainsworth's research in Uganda, and later in Baltimore was important because it was the first truly empirical studies related to Bowlby's original attachment theory.

 Ethnocultural Considerations — **Attachment**

Infants from various cultures bond with parents and caregivers in the manner appropriate to each culture. Some cultures are more comfortable with physical touch; others with verbal exchange. Infants respond based on the cultural norms.

LEARNING THEORIES

Beginning with the Ivan Pavlov work in 1890 about "classical conditioning," learning theorists began to understand development as a cognitive/learning process. There were two main types of learning theorists, behavioral and

 where research and practice meet:
Attachment

Relationships are important in the development of humans. Bowlby (1978) and Ainsworth (1978) pioneered the study of the initial relationship between the birthmother and the baby. Understanding attachment theory provides a base from which researchers can study the development of relationships throughout the life span. Research has substantiated that bonding and attachment is important for normal development to occur where the infant is born into a loving home. Each theoretical perspective adds to this important body of knowledge and it is important to note that the ability to connect with others is vitally important throughout the life of a child (Table 20-1).

Table 20-1 Phases of Attachment

Phase	Bowlby (1978)	Ainsworth (1978)	Manifestation
Phase I (birth–2 months)	Orientation and signals without discrimination of figure	The initial preattachment phase	The infant responds to everyone in his environment without discrimination.
Phase II (8–12 weeks)	Orientation and signals directed toward one or more discriminated figures	Attachment-in-the-making phase	The infant responds most to those significant caretakers in his life.
Phase III (6–7 months)	Maintenance of proximity to a discriminated figure by locomotion and signals	Clear-cut attachment	The baby attaches to his caretaker crawling toward the caregiver, reaching for or cooing at the caregiver.
Phase IV (around age 3)	Implications of the partnership for the organization of attachment behavior during the preschool years	Goal-corrected partnership	The preschool child begins to develop an understanding of the caregiver's goals. The child knows that a tantrum might get the mother to fulfill demands.

Source: Ainsworth, M. (1978). Patterns of attachment: *A psychological study of the strange situation.* Hillsdale, NJ: Lawrence Erlbaum Associates.

social learning scientists. Behavioral scientists saw the learner as passive, while social learning scientists emphasize the interplay of the individual within his environment. J.B. Watson, a behavioral scientist, sought to understand observable behavior. B.F. Skinner, also a behavioral scientist, described growth and development as a process of responding to stimuli within the environment (positive and negative reinforcement) that created new learning along with adaptive behaviors. While both types of scientific investigation are important, this chapter discusses the theories of the social learning theorists, Albert Bandura, Lev Vygotsky, and Urie Bronfenbrenner.

Social Theories

Albert Bandura

Albert Bandura's (1925–present) theory of development does not rely on predetermined stages. Bandura proposed that learning occurs within a social context through observation and modeling. The child pays attention to a new concept/task, retains that image, and then reproduces the action physically. Each successful approximation (reproduction) of the action increases the child's perception of personal effectiveness, which then contributes to the development of new social skills. For example, a newborn has no sense of self as separate from others. As the infant develops new skills, inadvertently at first, he becomes motivated to continue learning. Bandura also describes self-efficacy (sense of self) and refers to several foundations for developing self-efficacy. They are mastery (being successful), modeling by others (imitation), "social persuasion" (pairing situations in which success is likely to occur after positive feedback), and being able to decrease the perception of stress and threat (a conscience willingness to continue using the senses for learning rather than simply for surviving).

As the infant acquires this sense of self and begins to differentiate himself from others, the infant develops new skills, and, hopefully, resilience in the face of life's difficulties along with adaptations to surviving developmental transitions. Conversely, children who have not had adequate positive modeling, or who have not had access to success-inducing experiences, may suffer negative consequences and lack good self-efficacy.

Lev Vygotsky

Vygotsky (1896–1934) was a Russian psychologist who studied the influence of culture on development. Vygotsky was a contemporary of Albert Bandura. He emphasized that culture and certain factors within the child's environment have a dramatic impact on language development. He believed that development occurs on two levels: personal (intrapsychological) and social (interpsychological). Vygotsky coined the term "zone of proximal development," which means that one learns much more successfully when assisted by another person. In other words, a child left alone to their own devices would accomplish fewer developmental tasks, not nearly to the degree if the child had assistance of another person.

Urie Bronfenbrenner

Urie Bronfenbrenner (1917–2005) studied the effects that social environment has on a child's development (1979). Within this ecological approach, Bronfenbrenner defined three systems in each child's life. The microsystem refers to the systems where the child is actively involved. Typically, in a child's life, the microsystem would be family, school, and peer group. Mesosystem refers to the interaction between two microsystems, such as the interplay between a child's home and school. The exosystem refers to those systems that may have an impact on the child, but with which the child is not intimately involved, for instance, the parent's work. The parent's work affects the child's life, yet he is not directly involved in it.

COGNITIVE THEORIES

Cognitive theory focus on how an individual thinks and how thinking influences worldview. The capacity to think develops over time and with experience. Jean Piaget discussed cognition (thought) and how it influences development.

Jean Piaget

Jean Piaget (1896–1980), a Swiss psychologist, studied the development of cognition in children. In Piaget & Inhelder's book, *The Psychology of the Child* (1969), information was presented about how children think and learn. Thinking and learning for children takes place through four distinct stages. The initial period, the sensorimotor stage, takes place from birth to age 2. During this time, the infant's primary means of cognition is through the senses. The child takes in and processes information strictly on a physiological or emotional level.

At the age of 2, the child begins to use cognitive processes to respond to the world physically. The preoperational stage (ages 2 to 7 years) takes into account the development of motor skills and is divided into two substages: *preconceptual* and *intuitive*. The child is still not capable of logical thinking, but due to increased ability to use words and actions together, the child is increasingly able to connect cognitively with the world.

The third stage is the concrete operational stage. At this stage, the 7- to 11-year-old child is much more able to organize thought in logical order. The child is able to categorize and label objects. It is also possible at this stage for the child to solve concrete problems.

Piaget's final stage of cognitive development is the formal operational stage during which time the 11- to 15-year-old child uses abstract reasoning to handle difficult concepts and can analyze both sides of an issue.

INTELLIGENCE THEORIES

Intelligence is defined in the Merriam-Webster's Online Dictionary (n.d.) as "the ability to learn or understand or to deal with new or trying situations by using reason, which is the ability to apply knowledge to manipulate one's environment or to think abstractly as measured by objective criteria (as tests)." Intelligence has been studied mostly in terms of how it is measured. As in all other developmental dimensions, intelligence does not exist in a vacuum. The ability to bring in and retain new information and skills relies on the interconnectedness of cognitive, emotional, and environmental factors. Traditional standardized measures of intelligence have relied on assessing cognitive abilities, most specifically math and verbal. Many of these measures are criticized as not taking into account varying cultural and socioeconomic factors. In other words, a child may test as less intelligent than the norm, when in fact his test responses are based on his experience culturally. Standardized IQ tests have also been criticized for not measuring varying learning styles.

✿ Ethnocultural Considerations— Perception of intelligence

When providing nursing care it is important to understand that culture or ethnicity can influence perception of intelligence. For example, a Hispanic immigrant child in grade school may not understand his food choices in the school cafeteria based on his cultural knowledge about food. The child may be misinterpreted as unintelligent rather than growing up with different food choices than his peers.

Howard Gardner studied intelligence from a different vantage point. In his book, *Frames of Mind* (1993), he describes eight forms of intelligence: bodily-kinesthetic, interpersonal, intrapersonal, linguistic, logical-mathematical, musical, naturalistic, and spatial (Davidson, 2005; Gardner, 1993). The particular type of intelligence people have varies and Gardner believes these types of intelligence are equally important (Table 20-2).

MORAL DEVELOPMENT THEORIES

Study of moral development deals with a child's perception about right and wrong. Piaget, Lawrence Kohlberg, and Carol Gilligan are the three of the most well known theorists in this area. Of these, Kohlberg is the most often cited for understanding moral development in children.

Piaget (1896–1980) studied the progression of moral thinking in children based on the ability to reason and understand the environment. Piaget identified two stages of moral judgment. The first stage describes the way in which children younger than 11 years old experience right and wrong as concrete, black-and-white concepts. Simply put the child understands that an act is good or bad, right or wrong. The second stage coincides with Piaget's Formal Operational Stage of cognitive development during which the child is better able to think abstractly. Rules are important, but not always absolute or "carved in stone" (Table 20-3).

Table 20-2 Multiple Intelligences	
Bodily–Kinesthetic	A child who learns through movement or touch. The child excels in physical tasks and may love to dance and move, or touch.
Interpersonal	A child who learns through relating to others. The child has good use of verbal and nonverbal communication skills.
Intrapersonal	A child who learns through self-reflection. This child pays attention to the moods of others as well as to his own.
Linguistic	A child who learns by auditory means. The child will hear and say things in order to understand and remember them.
Logical–Mathematical	A child who learns through making connections. The child will work to figure things out by applying logic and systems.
Musical	A child who learns through making a song. The child may excel by singing songs or playing a musical instrument.
Naturalistic	A child who learns best in the natural or animal world. This child loves spending time with animals or plants or nature.
Spatial	A child who learns visually using charts, maps, movies, pictures. This child enjoys picture books and videos.

Source: Gardner, H. (2004). Audiences for the theory of multiple intelligences. *Teachers College Record, 106*, 212–220.

Table 20-3 Summary of Theorists

Domain	Theorist(s)	Key Points
Psychosocial	Sigmund Freud	<u>Psychosexual stages</u> • Oral (birth–1 year) • Anal (1–3 years) • Phallic (3–6 years) • Latency (6–12 years) • Genital (12–18 years)
	Erik Erikson	<u>Psychosocial stages</u> • Trust vs. Mistrust (birth–1 year) • Autonomy vs. Shame and Doubt (1–3 years) • Initiative vs. Guilt (3–6 years) • Industry vs. Inferiority (6–12 years) • Identity vs. Role Confusion (12–18 years)
Attachment	John Bowlby	<u>Three phases of responses to separation</u> • Protest • Despair • Detachment
	Mary Ainsworth	<u>Patterns of attachment</u> • Secure attachment • Avoidant attachment • Ambivalent attachment
Learning	Ivan Pavlov (mentioned)	<u>Classical conditioning</u>
	J.B. Watson (mentioned)	<u>Observable behavior</u>
	B.F. Skinner (mentioned)	<u>Stimulus-response</u>
	Albert Bandura	<u>Social context of learning</u> • Approximation • Self-efficacy • Mastery • Modeling • Social persuasion • Decreased perception of stress and threat
	Lev Vygotsky	<u>Levels of development</u> • Personal (intrapsychological) • Social (interpsychological) • Zone of proximal development
	Urie Bronfenbrenner	<u>Ecological definition of development</u> • Microsystem • Mesosystem • Exosystem

Cognitive	Jean Piaget	<u>Stages of cognitive development</u>
		• Sensorimotor (birth–2 years)
		  • Use of reflexes
		  • Primary circular reactions
		  • Secondary circular reactions
		  • Coordination of secondary schemes
		  • Tertiary circular reactions

Table 20-3 Summary of Theorists—cont'd

Domain	Theorist(s)	Key Points
		• Mental combinations
		• Preoperational (2–7 years)
		• Preconceptual (2–4 years)
		• Intuitive (4–7 years)
		• Concrete Operational (7–11 years)
		• Formal Operational (11–15 years)
Intelligence	Howard Gardner	<u>Multiple Intelligences</u>
		• Bodily–kinesthetic
		• Interpersonal
		• Intrapersonal
		• Linguistic
		• Logical–mathematical
		• Musical
		• Naturalistic
		• Spatial
Moral	Lawrence Kohlberg	<u>Moral Development</u>
		• Preconventional Morality
		• Obedience & Punishment
		• Individualism & Exchange
		• Conventional Morality
		• Good interpersonal relationships
		• Maintaining the social order
		• Postconventional morality
		• Social contract & individual rights
		• Universal principles
	Carol Gilligan	<u>Moral development</u>
		• Orientation of individual survival
		• Goodness as self-sacrifice
		• Shift from goodness to truth
Spiritual	James Fowler	<u>Spirituality stages</u>
		• Undifferentiated (infancy)
		• Intuitive–projective (2–6 or 7 years)
		• Mythical–literal (6–12 years)
		• Symbolic–convention (12+ years)
		• Individuation–reflexive (late adolescence +)
Family	E.R. Duvall	<u>Family development</u>
		• Marriage
		• Family with infants
		• Family with preschool children
		• Family with school children
		• Family with adolescent
		• Family launching young adult
		• Middle-age family
		• Aging family

Lawrence Kohlberg

Lawrence Kohlberg (1927–1987) based the theory of moral development (1984) on the thinking processes involved when making moral decisions. Kohlberg identified three levels of moral development: preconventional, conventional, and postconventional. Each level of moral development represents a major modification in the child's thinking and is further separated into stages (Table 20-4). Within Level I, Preconventional Level, the child's thinking is concrete and egocentric. Obedience and punishment are unquestioned and understood as either good or bad. The child behavior is based on which actions are rewarded or punished. Individualism and exchange occurs when the child begins to define right and wrong and develops an individual sense of fairness and personal justification. As the child matures and is confronted with opposing views, he begins to recognize that not everything is black and white. The child's sense of morality is still concrete but the child begins to take into account personal reasoning. If the child can justify an action, then, in his mind, it is acceptable to bend or break rules.

Transition to the Level II, Conventional Level for the child, is marked by the child's incorporation of social and interpersonal relationships. The good interpersonal and relationships stage is where the child's actions are justified by personal motivation to "do good" for family members or other individuals. The child understands that maintaining the social order means that society as a whole may benefit by her actions.

Level III, Postconventional Morality, is divided into social contract and individual rights and universal principles both of which require significant degrees of personal deliberation and maturity. These stages are sequential and require a level of cognitive development, they are not necessarily age-related. In fact, an adult may have reached only the preconventional level of moral development and has not reached the postconventional level of moral development because progression through the levels is influenced by a variety of factors such as experience, health, socioeconomic status, family structure, and culture.

Carol Gilligan

Carol Gilligan (1936–present) initially worked with Kohlberg as a research assistant. Gilligan became concerned that Kohlberg's studies of moral development were based only on norms for males. When girls were compared to boys using Kohlberg's framework, girls appeared morally weaker or slower to develop than their male counterparts. In Gilligan's book, *In a Different Voice* (1982), previously held beliefs about female moral development were questioned by interviewing both women and men about their life experiences. Gilligan identified two tracts of moral development. One was based on autonomy and justice (Gilligan, 1982), as seen in Kohlberg's interviews with men. The other was based on caring and relationship (Gilligan, 1982), which Gilligan attributed to women. Gilligan's work helped to define moral development for women in a different way than men. Even though Gilligan later withdrew the charge of gender bias, Gilligan continued to champion the study of female moral development (Box 20-4).

Table 20-4	Lawrence Kohlberg's Stages of Moral Development
Level I. Preconventional Morality Morality is determined by external sources—rules, laws, possibility of punishment.	Stage 1: Obedience and Punishment—The child will obey in order to avoid being punished. Stage 2: Individualism and Exchange—The child thinks that it may be okay to do something wrong if a good comes from it (in other words, the end justifies the means).
Level II. Conventional Morality Morality is determined by being a "good person." The intent is to please others and to do the "right thing."	Stage 3: Good Interpersonal Relationships—The child's moral decisions are based on the "goodness" of motivation and on what others expect. Stage 4: Maintaining the Social Order—The child's good moral decisions are those that preserve the needs of society.
Level III. Postconventional Morality	Stage 5: Social Contract and Individual Rights—The individual's thinking is characterized by a deeper questioning of social order versus an individual's personal rights. A person in this stage would work tirelessly to change unjust laws. Stage 6: Universal Principles—An individual incorporates a deep awareness of justice. An example would be breaking an unjust law to save lives of innocent people.

SPIRITUAL DEVELOPMENT THEORIES

James Fowler (1981) identified seven stages related to faith and spiritual development. Fowler defined faith outside the usual "religious" definition. Fowler believed that faith is commonly experienced and that it is the individual striving for something "more than the self." The development of faith depends on a certain level of cognitive achievement. Deepening levels of belief rely on the ability to think abstractly. Understanding Fowler's stages are important in providing complementary care to children and their families (see Complemenatry Care: Understanding Spirituality).

Box 20-4 **Gilligan's Three Levels of Moral Development**

Level 1: *Orientation of individual survival.* As the girl *transitions* through this level, they move from *selfishness to responsibility* where they consider other people.

Level 2: *Goodness as self-sacrifice.* This level involves looking at the world through the needs of others. The girl sacrifices her own needs and considers herself responsible for others.

Level 3 (*the transition level*) requires movement from *goodness to truth.* In other words, the woman recognizes that choice is important when doing for herself or others, rather than focusing on being good for the sake of being good.

Complementary Care: *Understanding spirituality*

Stage 0: Undifferentiated (infancy): Prestage during which the infant is learning "fundamentals of basic trust and the relational experience of mutuality with the one(s) providing primary love and care" (Fowler, 1981, p. 121). This foundation of trust sets the stage for developing a spiritual faith.

Stage 1: Intuitive-projective (ages 2–6 or 7): Corresponds with the child's imaginative period. Beliefs and faith are unquestioning. It is a time of fantasy and magical thinking.

Stage 2: Mythical-literal (ages 6–12): The child retells the spiritual stories and takes them literally and concretely.

Stage 3: Synthetic-convention (typically begins around 12 or 13 years): The young person begins to personalize beliefs. The youth looks beyond his family to include values encountered in relationships, in school, and in society in general. Sometimes adults remain in this stage.

Stage 4: Individuating–reflexive (may begin late adolescence or early adulthood, or not at all): The individual takes responsibility for personal beliefs and commitments. The individual invests personal energy in what spiritually makes sense, regardless of what others believe.

Fowler goes on to describe two additional stages of faith that may occur in adulthood, *Conjunctive Faith* and *Universalizing Faith.*

FAMILY DEVELOPMENT THEORIES

There are many theories describing family interaction. Duvall's (1977) theory is based on Erikson's individual stages of psychosocial development and is the most well known. The family development stages are as follows:

Marriage. The task of couples in this stage is to establish themselves as a pair and to prepare for parenting. This is also a time for realigning with both families of origin from the position of a new family.

Family with Infants. During this stage, the family adjusts to its new structure while the couple begins to adjust to their new role as parents. Grandparents adjust to their new role too.

Family with Preschool Children. As the oldest child enters the stage of early childhood, the family functions to socialize the children, helping them to cope with separation involved in starting school.

Family with School Children. As the children develop friendships and launch socially outside the family, the system must adjust.

Family with Adolescent. The oldest child turns toward launching and independence. At this point, the parents begin to refocus on their marriage.

Family Launching Young Adult. This stage begins when the oldest child leaves home. If there are other children, it ends when the youngest leaves home. Family tasks during this stage center on the development of individual and independent identities, both children and parents. The marriage continues to be a major area of energy.

Middle-age Family. The family continues to focus on reinvesting in the couple relationship. Relationships with extended family are realigned.

Aging Family. During this stage, the family copes with the process of and losses involved in retirement and aging.

 Nursing Insight— *Applying Duvall's theory*

Duvall's theory provides a framework for observing the development of families. It is important to understand that this framework applies to specific family types and styles such as those families with children who remain married and whose children leave home in the appointed timeframe. Remember, when caring for children from other family types the nurse must consider family make-ups such as divorced families, single parent families, child-free families, children who return home after launching, and culturally diverse families. The nurse needs to consider a multitude of factors and approach families using a non-judgmental demeanor and help the family understand and explore solutions based on their unique family.

 Collaboration in Caring— *The health care team*

Various members of the health care team oversee growth and development across care settings throughout the life of a child. Both nurses and physicians assess a newborn while in the hospital and a lactation consultant may be involved if the newborn is breastfed. Well-child visits to the family physician or health care provider at the child's medical home at regular intervals help track a child's growth and development and intervene if problems arise. Public health nurses may also assess the child, particularly at times of immunizations. Complementary and alternative health practitioners such as chiropractors, massage therapists, and naturopaths may also play a role in caring for a child.

 Now Can You— **Apply theories to nursing practice?**

1. Describe the importance of using theoretical based knowledge in the care of children and families?
2. Discuss the different types of theories used in the care of children and families?
3. Educate families about what to expect during growth and development?

Temperament

Children come in all shapes and sizes and represent all temperamental profiles and personality styles. Children are not simply "miniature adults." They require professional assessment and attention across care settings based on their level of development.

Temperament refers to those characteristics present at birth that govern the way in which an infant responds to their surroundings. There is a strong biological and environmental basis for temperament. Likewise, the baby's temperament generally has a profound influence on their interactions with caretakers and the environment itself.

Thomas & Chess (1977) studied temperament. Nine temperamental traits present at birth that persist throughout life were identified. These traits exist on a continuum depending on the infant's reaction to the environment. To help ensure effective parenting the nurse can teach parents about their infant's temperament traits.

 Across Care Settings: **Infant temperament**

During a normal daily routine the child may be exposed to a variety of settings and exposed to several people; a day care center, visiting extended family, physician's office or in public places in the community. Understanding an infant's temperament is essential in the care of the child to help both the parent and child adapt to these experiences. Based on the work by Thomas, Chess, and Brich (1968) the following descriptors are used to help recognize the infant's unique personality.

Regularity: The child needs regularity in sleeping, eating, and bowel habits. A child who is "easy" is one who can adapt to relatively flexible schedules. A child who is "difficult" has difficulty when the schedule has been disrupted.

Reaction to new people and situations: The "easy" child responds easily to new people in their environment. Another child may stand back or withdraw when something or someone new is present.

Adaptability to change: This trait refers to a child's willingness to change routine. An "easy" child makes transitions with little or no discomfort. A slow-to-adapt child will become distressed with even the smallest changes, for instance, taking a different route home from school.

Sensory sensitivity: An "easy" child with lower sensitivity will appear much less meticulous or disturbed by her senses. A "difficult" child with high sensitivity may react strongly when exposed to sensory stimuli. The child may chafe against certain textures, tastes, smells, or sounds.

Emotional intensity: An "easy" child shows little or no response to a situation. An intense child reacts dramatically and profoundly, whether that reaction is loud or withdrawn.

Level of persistence: This trait refers to the child's willingness to stay engaged regardless of setbacks. A persistent child has difficulty giving up until the goal is reached. A less persistent child is more flexible and may give up easier.

Activity level: An "easy" child will generally be less frenetic with activity. A "difficult" child has difficulty with inactivity, preferring to always be on the move.

Distractibility: The distractible child has difficulty concentrating on tasks in which they are not immersed; not the same as Attention Deficit Disorder (ADD). A less distractible child stays with a task longer.

Mood: An "easy" child tends to see the world in a more positive way. A "difficult" child will react more negatively.

The ability to recognize these traits is helpful for determining the goodness of fit between the caregiver(s), family members, and the child along with helping families strategize to improve the fit. This way of understanding the child takes into account that each person in the child's life has also a unique temperamental style, which complements, becomes enmeshed with, or antagonizes that of the child.

Newborn and Infant

The entire infant period of development encompasses the development from 1 to 12 months of life. This period of development continues to be a time of rapid change in all aspects of development. The baby develops on all levels, at a varying pace. It is important for the nurse to remember that each infant moves at his pace and with his own style.

The neonate's movements are random and erratic. The neonate can move the head from side to side, but has little control of her neck and back muscles.

REFLEXES AND NEUROLOGICAL DEVELOPMENT

Primitive reflexes are those adaptive and innate mechanisms that protect the developing infant while the brain is maturing (see Chapter 18 for more information). The reflexes are controlled by the lower brain centers. There are several reflexes present at birth or shortly after. They naturally disappear by 9 months.

 clinical alert

Reflexes

As the nurse performs an assessment it is imperative to note important infant reflexes:

- Rooting baby's head turns and begins to suck when her cheek or lower lip is stroked.
- Sucking motion of lips, mouth, and tongue allowing infant to take in sustenance.
- Moro: Startle response with sudden jarring causes extension of the head. The arms abduct and move upward. The hands form a "C."
- Grasping: When palm of hands or soles of feet are stroked.
- Babinski: Turning in of foot and out of toes when sole of foot is stroked.

At birth, the lower portions of the nervous system (spinal cord and the brainstem) are already developed. They are necessary for the infant to sustain life (basic body functions and primitive reflexes). As the infant matures, the higher sections of the nervous system become more developed. For instance, the limbic system and the cerebral cortex are responsible for ongoing learning that occurs during the life span.

SENSORY DEVELOPMENT

Touch is an extremely important sense and is the first sense to develop. The ability to feel objects, textures, and other people opens up the newborn's world of learning. It is important for the infant to experience soft comforting textures. The ability to experience pain is also an extremely important element, particularly as a protective device. If the infant has a pain experience, he reacts to pain with the whole body by quickly extending and then retracting the extremities. Along with this reaction, the infant cries.

Smell and taste begin developing in utero and intrinsically connected. Infants respond to smells within the first

Figure 20-1 At 3 months of age an infant can lift her head and chest while on her belly *(top)* and roll on her side *(bottom)*.

A newborn's head is proportionally larger than the rest of the body, which is in keeping with the cephalocaudal course of development. The newborn's head grows rapidly during the first month as the brain grows. By the time the baby reaches 1 year of age, the head and chest circumferences are about the same.

In order for the infant to move or to perform actions (motor skills), he must have adequate muscle development. At birth, the newborn's movement is involuntary. It takes the infant time to mature physically in order to be able to demonstrate motor skills. Gross motor skills (the ability to use large muscles for movement) are the first to develop in the newborn and infant. Generally, by the end of the first 3 months of life, she can raise her head and chest while lying on her belly and stretch the legs out and kick from a prone position, and roll from side to side (Fig. 20-1). She can turn over completely at about 6 or 7 months of age. By 8 to 9 months of age, the infant begins to crawl and then by using high objects the infant can begin pulling up. Once the infant has mastered an upright position, he may begin to then cruise (walking while holding on to furniture) or even attempt to walk. Again, development is variable on each individual child. One child may be walking before his first birthday, while another does not walk until later.

Fine motor skills (the use of muscles to accomplish minute tasks like pinching or picking up food) build on the gross motor skills (Fig. 20-2). Other fine motor skills that develop between 6 and 12 months include the ability to stack large objects, scribble, bang on pots and pans, and transfer objects from one hand to another and back again.

COGNITIVE DEVELOPMENT

Infancy corresponds to Piaget's sensorimotor stage of development. The infant uses the five senses to explore and to learn about the world. For instance, the infant learns that lip smacking when hungry leads to a full

few days and have an innate preference for sweet tastes. The nurse is aware that infants can recognize their mother's smell long before they achieve visual recognition.

Hearing is well developed at birth. A newborn can immediately recognize the difference between male and female voices and will generally turn toward the female voice. By the second week, the newborn can recognize the sound of the mother's voice. A newborn's ability to discriminate sounds develops quickly, contributing to language development. By the time the infant is 3 months, the infant jabbers and begins to imitate sounds. During the next few months, the infant becomes more adept at responding to and imitating familiar sounds by smiling and cooing.

Vision is the least developed of the senses at birth. Newborns are fascinated with faces and with designs or objects that resemble faces. While a newborn is able to remember an object, he remembers it only in the exact form originally seen (e.g., if the child sees his sister in pigtails, the child does not recognize the sister with her hair down). Infants are most attracted to bright colors and to black and white because of the limited nature of their vision. The newborn generally has poor peripheral vision until 10 weeks of age. Within the first 3 months, the infant can watch faces intently, follow moving objects, and recognize familiar objects and people at a distance. There can also be the beginnings of eye–hand coordination. Binocular vision (ability to use both eyes to see) develops about 4 or 5 months of age. The capacity to distinguish colors and to see things in the distance develops throughout the first 7 to 12 months.

PHYSICAL DEVELOPMENT

Growth is rapid. Infants gain 1.5 pounds (680 g)/month, double their weight by 6 months and triple it by 1 year. Height increases by 1 inch (2.5 cm) for the first 6 months.

Figure 20-2 One of the first fine motor skills to develop is the ability to pinch to pick up small objects like food.

Family Teaching Guidelines...
Introducing Solid Foods to Infants

TOPIC: Introducing Solid Foods:

The baby is ready for the introduction of solid foods at approximately 6 months of age. To help determine if the baby is ready for solid foods, look for developmental cues such as the ability to sit well with support. The baby may watch very intently as you eat, and may seem hungry between bottles or breastfeeding.

◆ Iron-fortified rice cereal is recommended as the baby's first solid food for a couple of reasons. It is the least allergenic of the grains, and the iron will help the baby replenish the iron stores received in utero. The term "solid food" is something of a misnomer. When introducing the rice cereal to the baby, you can mix it with formula, breast milk, or boiled and cooled water until it is very soupy. As the baby adapts to solids, you can increase the consistency of the cereal.

◆ When the baby is eating about 4 tablespoons of cereal twice per day, begin to introduce vegetables and fruits. Starting with vegetables may help to increase acceptance by the infant not yet exposed to the sweet taste of fruits.

◆ Introduce one food at a time, waiting 3–5 days between new foods so you will be able to identify any reactions to particular foods.

◆ Introduce food before formula or breastfeeding when the infant is hungry, and follow each solid food meal with a bottle or breast.

Seeking Additional Help: If the infant is not growing or gaining weight, cannot suck or swallow or shows any sign of allergic reaction, it is important to seek help from the primary health care provider, nearby clinic, or emergency room if the problem is emergent.

ESSENTIAL INFORMATION

◆ Avoid salt, sugar, and additives.

◆ Never put food in bottles or mix with formula (to avoid aspiration).

◆ Pay close attention while feeding and keep bites small to avoid choking.

Source: American Academy of Pediatrics (2008).

stomach. When the infant's belly is full, physical needs are met and the infant can then begin to explore the environment. Ultimately, the infant learns that he can have an impact within that environment. The infant must achieve three major tasks during this phase of development:

Separation. Recognizing that there is no merging with or attachment to familiar people (family members)

Object Permanence. The infant knows that an object or person still exists even if covered up or removed from sight; this is why babies respond so strongly to peek-a-boo.

Mental Representation. The ability to use symbols to communicate.

Piaget also identified six substages within the sensorimotor stage that describes mental representation. It is important to note that four of these substages occur during the first year of life. The first substage, Use of reflexes is present at birth. The majorities of the reflexes are necessary for survival and disappear during the first 9 months. The second substage, Primary circular reactions (1 to 4 months), takes place when the infant responds to things that give pleasure. The infant's response encourages caregivers to continue providing pleasurable experiences. The third substage, Secondary circular reactions, begins when the infant recognizes cause and effect. For example, the actions that the infant can perform independently begin to capture their attention (e.g., shaking a rattle). The fourth substage begins around 8 to 12 months when the infant becomes deliberate with their actions. During substage 4, Coordination of secondary schemes, the infant intentionally seeks out objects. The infant now knows that punching the button starts the music on a toy. During this substage, the infant also develops object permanence. The remaining substages, Tertiary circular reactions, and Mental combinations happen during the toddler stage of development.

LANGUAGE

Babies initially communicate through cries (a universal language) that indicate physical discomfort or loneliness. As a mother or father responds to the cries, the infant learns to communicate more deliberately. The nurse must recognize that an infant's early speech is evidenced by crying, babbling, and imitation. Influences on language development include maturation of the brain and the degree and quality of social interaction. If families respond favorably to baby's sounds, like "ba" for bottle or "da" for daddy, the baby is more likely to repeat these sounds bringing the infant closer to the native language.

PSYCHOSOCIAL DEVELOPMENT

In infants, the first displays of emotions, crying and smiling, are related to physiological needs rather than psychological stimuli. For example, the newborn wails loudly when uncomfortable physically and smiles involuntarily during sleep. However, by the time the baby is two weeks of age, the smiles begin to signify contentment and elicit positive family response. The infant's smile then becomes social and interaction with the environment occurs.

Corresponding with Erikson's psychosocial stage of trust versus mistrust, the nurse knows that it is a critical time for the newborn to absorb the whole environment and the related experiences. The caretaker's task is to respond to the infant in such ways as to engender a sense of security and well-being. Essentially, the baby's mission is to develop a sense that caretakers are reliable and present.

Ainsworth described four stages of attachment. During the first stage (birth to two months), the newborn and infant randomly responds to anyone. By the second stage (8 to 12 weeks), the infant begins to respond more to the mother than to anyone else, but the infant continues to respond indiscriminately to others. It is not until the third stage (6 or 7 months) that the infant demonstrates a strong connection to the mother and possibly develop a fear of strangers. Not all babies develop stranger anxiety as was historically thought. Throughout the first year, the infant is developing attachments to all of the important people in the family. Achieving the necessary milestones is essential for the infant to move on to the next stage of psychosocial development. An example of psychosocial development is the infant becoming more aware of others and responding to people (or animals) that are physically on the same level (Fig. 20-3).

DISCIPLINE

Discipline plays an important role in the psychosocial development of the infant. Merriam-Webster's Online Dictionary (n.d.) defines discipline as "training that corrects, molds, or perfects mental capacities or moral character." The definition additionally identifies teach as a synonym. In the best of all worlds, discipline and teaching would be the same. In reality, much of what is designated as discipline is in fact punishment. Punishment, as defined in Merriam-Webster's online dictionary, is "suffering, pain, or loss that serves as retribution." It is important for the nurse to be aware of these definitions when helping parents and caretakers determine how they plan to provide for the correction, molding, and refining of their children's mental capacities and moral characters.

It is important for the nurse to include information about discipline when teaching the parents about the infant. Teaching parents about discipline helps the infant learn about maintaining safety measures, develop satisfying relationships, and become a good global citizen. The American Academy of Pediatrics (1998, 2004) indicates that early forms of discipline take place when the caregiver molds and structures the infant's daily routines and by responding to the infant's needs. Limit-setting functions to acclimate the infant to the world and to keep the infant out of harm's way. It is important to note that parents often learn how to discipline from their own

Figure 20-3 An example of psychosocial development is when an infant becomes more aware of others by responding to people or animals that are physically on the same level.

experiences as children. It is essential that parents be taught what to expect at each of the developmental stages and how to recognize appropriate strategies for teaching and limit-setting.

> **critical nursing actions** Anticipatory Guidance
>
> Anticipatory guidance is a way of providing caregivers with information and examples about what to expect in the future regarding their child's next developmental phase. A few examples of important topics may include discipline, nutrition, safety, schooling, elimination, immunizations, or play.
>
> It is important that the nurse teach parents that infants do not misbehave on purpose. Exploration and crying are normal behaviors for infants. The purpose of discipline at this age is to keep the child safe. Using a firm tone of voice or facial expression while telling the child "no" or "stop" as he or she reaches for the stove helps the infant know that there are limits to his actions. The infant can then be redirected to a similar experience such as reaching instead for a toy off a countertop.

Toddler (1 to 3 years)

PHYSICAL DEVELOPMENT

By the time, the infant reaches 1 year of age, physical growth has slowed. Between ages 1 and 3, each year the typical toddler gains 4 to 6 pounds (1.8 to 2.7 kg) and grows 3 inches (7.5 cm) taller. Much of the toddler's energies during this period are directed to other realms of development. As the physical growth rate slows, the toddler develops skills (physical, cognitive, and emotional) that help him to become more independent. As the toddler develops mobility, he explores how things work and his senses become more refined. The toddler uses newly acquired gross motor skills to run, jump, and move up and down stairs with increasing ease. Around age 3, he may learn to ride a tricycle or slide down the slide in the park without help. All this newfound freedom and movement create many opportunities for danger as the toddler moves quickly from one new experience to another.

Fine motor skills continue to develop rapidly also. The toddler can hold a spoon or a large crayon appropriately and continues to make artwork that is more representative of the object she is trying to depict. He is increasingly able to manipulate smaller toys.

COGNITIVE DEVELOPMENT

Early toddlerhood corresponds with Piaget's fifth substage of cognitive development, Tertiary circular reactions, during which the toddler experiments and learns new behaviors. The toddler then moves into Piaget's sixth substage, Mental combinations, during which she begins to understand cause and effect and is able to imitate others.

The toddler loves to imitate (Fig. 20-4). Much of the toddler's behavior is through replicating what she sees and hears. The toddler also learns through repetition. This is why a toddler may want the same book to be read over and over, staying engrossed in the story every time.

Figure 20-4 Toddlers love to imitate.

A toddler also likes order and often responds with difficulty to any disruption in routine. The level of response is related to the temperament of the child. Some toddlers may revolt with pure temper tantrum while others can calmly transition. Regardless of temperament, most children at this stage respond favorably to predictable routines.

LANGUAGE DEVELOPMENT

Because toddlers are increasing in cognitive development, they are able to listen to and understand short explanations. This is a time when the child develops a more understandable language system. Language is about fulfilling needs; "I do" or "want drink." The toddler moves from using single words to short phrases. Some parents worry when their child does not fall exactly within what are considered normal language parameters. The nurse can reassure parents that it is important to assess what the child understands and what the child is able to communicate, with or without words, rather than exact correctness in pronunciation.

PSYCHOSOCIAL DEVELOPMENT

Toddlers typically exemplify characteristics of Freud's *anal stage*. The child begins to develop a sense of self as separate from his mother. The toddler's task is to move away from the primary caregiver while in some way maintaining enough connection to feel secure. This process, called rapprochement, is healthy and expected.

Toddlerhood also corresponds with Erikson's stage of autonomy versus shame and doubt. It is a time when the child makes every effort to "do it myself." Mastery is an extremely important task of this stage of development. Since the toddler's abilities begin to surpass cognitive judgment, it is also a time of potential hazard for the developing child. Caregivers must walk the fine line between allowing exploratory independence and "mastery" on one hand and vigilance on the other. It is often a time of bumps and "boo boos."

Often dubbed as the "terrible twos," this entire stage can be a tumultuous time for both caregivers and toddlers. The child must begin to internalize behavioral standards at a time when establishing independence is important. The nurse can help parents understand that the toddler does not set out to make life miserable. The toddler simply has few internal mechanisms in place to accomplish what needs to be done safely. It is frustrating to the toddler when confronted with blocks to budding mastery. The word "no" begins to signify the toddler's simple response to frustrated emotions encountered.

MORAL DEVELOPMENT

Cognitively, the toddler is still a very concrete thinker and knows that something is "good" or "bad," but does not know why. At this stage, the toddler identifies good and bad, right and wrong by virtue of whether or not it is rewarded or punished. This corresponds to Kohlberg's preconventional level of moral development.

DISCIPLINE

The purpose of discipline is to teach the child socialization and safety. It is the responsibility of the parent to provide a firm structure so the toddler can explore the world while offering safe limits. Most children will repeatedly test rules, while also unconsciously learning to rely on the security those limits provide. Having a structured environment for the child does not necessarily mean rigid or inflexible. Parents must learn to structure the toddler's surroundings that allow enough flexibility to test limits.

A child at this stage needs much guidance in determining how to act appropriately. The toddler thinks concretely and must rely on others to help give realistic parameters. Some parameters may create a great deal of conflict when what the toddler *can* do does not match what the toddler *wants* to do, which may result in a temper tantrum. Praise becomes an excellent component of discipline as most children want to please the parent.

TEMPER TANTRUMS

Because this is a time of intense exploration and discovery and a time when the toddler is establishing a sense of herself as a competent doer, there will be "bumps in the road." A tantrum is a normal way for a toddler of working things out internally. Parents and caregivers need to know that tantrums are normal for the toddler. It may be possible for parents to anticipate when tantrums are most apt to occur (e.g., when the toddler is tired, hungry, or overwhelmed by new situations, reserves are low and therefore, he may be more likely to explode or "meltdown"). Tantrums may be avoided or minimized if anticipated. Get a tired child to rest or feed a hungry child to decrease his frustration level. If a tantrum does develop, there are coping strategies that a nurse can teach a parent. When the child is wailing and thrashing, but not doing any harm, ignore her. Often this is not possible, and it may be necessary for the parent to intervene quickly and decisively to remove the child to a quieter or safer place. Touching and distractions may help soothe a tantrum; while another child may need to continue the tantrum under the watchful eye of the parent. The latter requires that the parent be present, but not engaged in direct communication with the child. The goal is for the child to feel (and be) safe without being reinforced (positively or negatively) for having a tantrum.

When faced with the sometimes daunting task of caring for a "willful" toddler (one who is regularly asserting her power), parents are often confused. It is indeed difficult to know how and when to avoid the power struggles inherent in a clash of wills. It is essential to be able to create boundaries that limit the toddler's scope of power. Inevitably, there are times when the toddler must be disciplined, so seeking help from a professional child counselor is essential (Box 20-5).

66 **What to say** 99 — *Tips for effective discipline*

During effective discipline, allow for negotiation and flexibility, which can help build the child's social skills. Also, allow the child to experience the consequences of behavior.

- Speak to the child as you would want to be spoken to if someone were reprimanding you.
- Never resort to name-calling, yelling, or disrespect.
- Be clear about what you mean.
- Be firm and specific.

Note: Whenever possible, the consequences must be delivered immediately, relate to the rule broken, be short enough in duration and emphasize the positives. In addition, the consequences must be fair and appropriate to the situation and the child's age.

Box 20-5 Discipline Strategies

Distraction: Provide a toy to divert the child's attention.
Time-out: Move the child to a "cooling-off" place where the child can calm down.
Removal of privileges: Withhold a favorite toy until the child's behavior is appropriate.
Verbal reprimands: Give spoken warnings or disapprovals without berating the child or judging the child as "bad."
Corporal punishment (e.g., spanking, swatting, grabbing): Not recommended.

Early Childhood (Preschooler) (3 to 6 years)

PHYSICAL DEVELOPMENT

Children at this age come in various sizes, shapes, and body types. As a rule, preschoolers begin to grow taller and thinner. Their bellies flatten as they grow and their abdominal muscles strengthen, and their pelves straighten. The physical growth rate for this stage of development is slow but steady. The preschooler average weight gain is about 4.5 to 6.5 pounds (2 to 3 kg) and growth is 2.5 to 3.5 inches (6.2 to 8.7 cm) per year. The 4-year-old's posture straightens and the young child is able to move around in a more balanced fashion. Preschoolers become stronger as their muscles become more developed. Their faces become more like they will be when they grow up with narrowing of the face, enlargement of the nose, and a more adult-like appearance to the skin.

The preschooler is much more agile. The preschooler can climb stairs using alternating feet and is able to ride his tricycle. At 4, the preschooler can climb up and down the stairs comfortably using alternating feet. The preschooler can skip and hop and is much more coordinated on the balance beam.

Fine motor skills rely on the use of the forefinger and the thumb. As the brain becomes more developed, she is better able to pick things up with the fingers. Hand dominance (whether or not the child is right- or left-handed) begins to develop around the age of 3. At this time, the preschooler may show a preference in using one hand over the other. By the age of 4, that preference is established.

COGNITIVE DEVELOPMENT

This period of development corresponds with Piaget's pre-operational stage (2 to 4 years). During this time, the preschooler increases the ability to verbalize. The preschooler can symbolically use language to represent concepts that need to be conveyed. The young child is still egocentric (focused only on his own sense of things) and therefore is limited socially. This is in large part due to concrete thinking processes and the inability to abstractly shift focus from self to others. The preschooler is also not able to transfer attention from one aspect of an object to another (e.g., a child at this stage can identify a dog's collar, but is not able to describe its texture).

LANGUAGE

The preschooler has increased ability to verbalize; vocabulary increases from 1500 to 2000 words between the ages 3 and 5. The preschooler uses sentences and is much more able to convey an intended message. When the young child is more able to use words, tantrums generally begin to subside. The preschooler loves silly words, rhymes, and asks many questions, generally those that begin with "why?" To meet the needs of the preschooler, keep answers simple and avoid giving too much information. Bombarding the preschooler with overwhelming answers can be quite disconcerting for the child. The nurse can tell the parent that a preschooler may stutter as he tries to get out all of the words faster than he is able to speak them. Stuttering generally resolves fairly quickly.

case study Early Childhood Development

Mrs. James brings Steven, her three-year-old son, into the clinic for a well-child visit. She states she is concerned because Steven does not talk as well as his peers. She describes how at play group, the other 3-year olds talk more than Steven, and states that Steven barely says a word. When asked how Steven communicates what he wants, Mrs. James states that he points to things and sometimes says one word such as "more" or "juice." Mrs. James added that Steven often gets frustrated when his parents do not understand what he wants. A review of his medical history reveals that Steven was born 39 weeks, weighed 8 lbs, 1 oz (3.7 kg) and had an unremarkable delivery. He has had no difficulties with feeding or sleep. He began babbling at 6 months but did not speak his first word until 14 months. By 19 months he could say "mama," "dada, and "juice." Presently, Mrs. James states he uses approximately 10 words but does not combine them.

critical thinking questions

1. What further assessments would you complete for Steven?

2. What would you say to Mrs. James about Steven?

3. What nursing interventions would be appropriate at this time?

◆ See Suggested Answers to Case Studies in text on the Electronic Study Guide or DavisPlus.

PSYCHOSOCIAL DEVELOPMENT

Early childhood is a wonderful time of exploration of new skills and about finally being able to figure out how to get and do things for oneself. As the preschooler develops, he is presented with many situations where he can truly excel. The preschooler has learned many new skills and is becoming a "big kid." The preschooler enjoys positive feedback for accomplishments. The fact that the preschooler is able to do many new things creates a dilemma and the preschooler must decide which things are most important. Parents may not approve of the decisions made by the preschooler and he may become conflicted when limits are set. Often times the preschooler ponders doing "the right thing" or doing "the wrong thing" and risking the mother's dismay. Conscience develops and begins to guide the child through the maze of wants versus cans.

The preschool child has a good deal of magical thinking. In a preschooler's desire to do what she wants to do, she may angrily wish something bad would happen to another person, often a parent. If something bad actually does happen, the preschooler will believe that her thinking caused the outcome.

Freud described this period as the phallic or oedipal period. The child is becoming more aware of gender differences. The preschooler may want to marry mom or the girl in preschool, rather than relate to his best male friend.

Family is very important to the preschooler. However, the preschooler is now discovering the joys of having friendships. The young child looks to his peers for new ideas and information and begins to develop an understanding of what it means to be kind. The preschooler is more social and is often more willing to share toys with others than when he was a toddler.

MORAL DEVELOPMENT

Early childhood typically corresponds with Kohlberg's preconventional morality stage (4 to 10) when the major impetus for moral judgment is to avoid punishment. It is not uncommon for the child in this age group to tell lies to avoid consequences. A child at this age may judge an action to be wrong only if caught. The young child is only guilty if the parent has seen the actions.

DISCIPLINE

Since the preschooler is beginning to understand that actions have consequences, caregivers can take advantage of this understanding. The preschooler is able to understand that there are rules and that not obeying those rules leads to consequences. It is best if rules are explained before infractions occur. At the very least, the rules should be addressed before disciplining the child. This helps the preschool child to learn more clearly how to behave. Consequences can, as much as possible, follow naturally and fit the behavior being punished (e.g., having the child clean up his own messes, or miss a favorite show if he dawdles).

A typical discipline strategy instituted at this stage of development is having the child take a time-out. Whether that time-out is in a specified chair, or section of the room, it is important to help the child know that the purpose of the time-out is to calm himself and to shift gears and act appropriately.

Many parents begin using behavioral charts (charts constructed to praise positive behavior) at this age to help their toddler visually see what is expected and to be rewarded when "good" behavior is shown. For many preschoolers, simply getting a star or sticker on the chart is reward enough to encourage behavior. For others, a more sophisticated measure of rewards is needed. Again, the goal of discipline and limit-setting at this stage of development is to begin teaching preschoolers to begin regulating their own behavior.

School-Age Child (6 to 12 years)

PHYSICAL DEVELOPMENT

Early in this stage (ages 6 to 9), boys and girls follow similar growth trajectories. Both begin to grow taller, reducing their "baby fat" even more. Children at this age gain about 4 to 6 pounds (1.8 to 2.7 kg) and grow 2 inches (5 cm) per year. As their abdominal muscles strengthen, their posture straightens. Facial features become more refined. Still, there are many variations in size and shape of children in this period. These variations are influenced not only by familial and cultural genetics, but also by environmental factors (e.g., diet and exercise).

Most school-age children (boys and girls) begin to develop axillary sweating. In girls, hips begin to broaden and the pelvis widens in preparation for childbearing. Breasts begin to enlarge and become tender. The vaginal ph changes from alkaline to acidic and the vagina develops a thick mucoid lining. Usually, pubic hair begins to develop between the ages of 8 and 14. While menarche can begin as early as 8 to 10 years of age, the average age in the United States is 12 years of age.

Ethnocultural Considerations— **Puberty**

African American girls tend to develop secondary sexual characteristics and begin menses somewhat earlier than Caucasian girls.

---

 clinical alert

Privacy

At this age, it is important to guard the child's privacy. As a nurse be aware of self-conscious behavior related to physical changes occurring in the body. Along with privacy the nurse must be aware of other issues affecting the child and family related to menstruation, secondary sexual characteristics, hormone imbalances, mood swings, social needs well as other specific areas identified by the child and family.

Boys also begin sexual development at these ages. Their bodies become more muscular. About 10 to 12 years of age, a boy's testes begin to change. During this stage, the testes are more sensitive to pressure, the skin of the scrotum darkens, and pubic hair begins to develop. Boys often experience gynecomastia, a temporary enlargement of breasts. This can be embarrassing and should be explained to the child and family as a temporary condition.

COGNITIVE DEVELOPMENT

The school-age child is better able than the younger child to use logical thinking. This logic in thinking corresponds with Piaget's concrete operations stage of cognitive development. While the child's thinking is still quite concrete, she can begin to solve problems. During this childhood stage, she begins to replace this ever-present "why" with "how?" Mastery is in the arena of figuring out how things work. The school-age child builds on experience and begins to recognize consequences of actions. In school, she works on tasks requiring awareness of space (where things are in relation to other things), causality (logical consequences), categories (how things fit together), conservation (physical quantity can remain constant even when state is altered), and numbers. She is also capable of metacognition, the ability to think about thinking. At this age the child is aware of her own thinking and is able to assess how she came to conclusions, eventually leading to critical thinking.

Memory deepens as the child grows. She becomes more adept at processing and working through information. Memory improves because the brain developmentally retains more information. A child in this age group is also more able to determine what is important to remember and what is not. This helps her filter out irrelevant data, leaving memory space available.

LANGUAGE DEVELOPMENT

Language improves considerably. The child uses words more accurately, particularly verbs, metaphors, and similes. The child is able to elaborate on concepts that she wants to get across.

PSYCHOSOCIAL DEVELOPMENT

There is vast emotional growth during the middle child years. Erikson described this stage as one of industry versus inferiority. Unlike the younger child who believes he can do almost anything, the 6- to 10-year-old child begins to assess what they can and cannot accomplish. A school-age child has a more definite sense of self-esteem or competence based on the ability or lack of ability to perform.

Early in the middle childhood period (ages 6 to 9), the child is still self-focused. School-age children continue to exhibit magical thinking, in that they still may feel responsible for bad things happening. Later (ages 9 to 12) children at this stage are increasingly independent, although they want approval and validation. Competing and winning become important in the growing sense of self-competence. Friendships are exceptionally important at this stage. The school-age child looks more to friends than family, but family is still important. Best friends tend to be of the same gender, although mixed gender groups of school-age children become common as they reach the preteen and early teen years (Fig. 20-5).

MORAL DEVELOPMENT

For the first several years, the school-age child is still operating within preconventional morality. The younger child sees things as black and white and as self-referenced, rather than connected with more generalized rules and concepts. By the age of 10, the child enters Kohlberg's conventional morality stage. During this time, the child has internalized rules and is intently gaining approval. The older child operates within a morality of cooperation that implies recognition of the interaction between the self and a "bigger" worldview. Most children at this age are motivated by adhering to laws as a way to keep order.

Figure 20-5 Establishing strong friendships is very important to school-age children.

DISCIPLINE

Since the child in this stage of development is beginning to internalize rules, it is important to allow the child more independence, and thus more awareness of the natural consequences of behavior. An effective parent technique is to refrain from "rescuing" their child from the consequences of their behavior (e.g., do not rush home to retrieve a forgotten piece of homework whenever the child calls rather than allowing her to learn a valuable lesson).

While many school-age children respond appropriately to natural consequences, some do not yet understand responsibility. In addition, most children opt at some time to ignore the natural consequences. Parents may need to impose the previously discussed time-out strategy (e.g., grounded for a period of time or pleasures restricted).

Adolescence (12 to 19 years)

PHYSICAL DEVELOPMENT

Adolescence technically begins with the onset of puberty when the pituitary gland relays messages to sex glands to manufacture hormones necessary for reproduction. It is a period of great growth, second only to infancy. While the growth rate is not as dramatic as that of the earlier stage, it is still significant. It is not unusual for girls to gain 15 to 55 pounds (6.8 to 25 kg) and grow 2 to 8 inches (5 to 20 cm) and boys to gain 15 to 66 pounds (6.8 to 30 kg) and grow 4 to 12 inches (10 to 30 cm) before they reach maturity. While girls develop earlier than boys, they tend to have a smaller overall physical structure. Both boys and girls develop primary and secondary sex characteristics at this stage. The timing of development is variable.

COGNITIVE DEVELOPMENT

Adolescence corresponds with Piaget's formal operations stage. The teenager is able to think abstractly and uses logic to solve problems and to test out hypotheses. In addition, the teen uses deductive reasoning and can think about thinking. Teenagers are often beginning to be concerned with such things as philosophy, morality, and social issues. They are able to project their thoughts over the long term, thus making plans and setting life goals. They often compare their beliefs with those of peers.

LANGUAGE

By adolescence, children have highly developed language skills. They have the ability to speak and write correctly as well as communicate alternative points of view. They have sophisticated communication skills.

PSYCHOSOCIAL DEVELOPMENT

According to Erikson, the adolescent crisis is concerned with identity versus role confusion. The adolescent must begin to identify who they are and who they will be in life. The three major issues that must be confronted: an occupation, establishing and subscribing to a set of values, and developing a satisfactory sexual identity.

 Be sure to— Include the adolescent in the informed consent process

An informed consent is a way to elicit permission that is given freely that protects a person's right to autonomy and self-determination. Informed consent is given when the person understands the usual procedures, their rationales, and associated risks. A legal parent or guardian customarily gives informed consent on behalf of the child. As children gain critical thinking skills they can become more active in the consent process. Depending on state law, children 18–21 years of age can give legal informed consent under these circumstances: when they are minor parents of the child patient, when they are between 16 and 18 years old seeking birth control, counseling or help for substance abuse or when the are self-supporting (emancipated). In many states, a pregnant teen is considered emancipated and can provide informed consent. The physician is ultimately responsible for explaining the procedure and related risks while the nurse's role is to serve as a witness to the parent's signature for the child or an emancipated adolescent's signature. The nurse is responsible to notify the physician if the parent (or legal guardian) does not understand the procedure or related risks.

MORAL DEVELOPMENT

At this stage, conflicts emerge between what the adolescent has believed to be right or wrong, and what others may believe. This is a time of great questioning and consternation as the adolescent learns that it is possible for several views of morality to exist. Kohlberg defines this stage as postconventional morality.

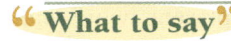 **❝What to say❞** — *Helping the teen make good decisions*

The nurse can be influential in helping the teenager make healthy decisions. This can be accomplished by the employing the following techniques:

- Listen: Pay close attention not only to what the adolescent is saying, but also to his nonverbal cues. Try to understand his view of the world and stay open minded.
- Discuss without judging: The nurse can share her understanding of the issues and her perspectives while respecting those of the teenager.
- Encourage critical thought: Allow the teenager to explore and further develop his options.

DISCIPLINE

The adolescent is at the stage where she begins to internalize responsibility for behavior. The adolescent still needs parental input and guidance in terms of rules (curfew, homework, chores, etc.) and possible consequences for infractions, but the adolescent is much more able than in any previous stage to monitor and regulate her own actions based on her own critical thinking. It is important in this stage, as in all others, that the parent focus on the positives of the teen's behavior. Natural consequences are powerful motivators, but by this time, the adolescent may have learned that he can avoid consequences by being crafty. Removing privileges may be an effective consequence for the teen's poor decisionmaking.

summary points

◆ Information about growth and development, newborn through adolescence, is important information for the nurse and family.

◆ Principles of growth and development can assist the nurse when teaching the family about their child.

◆ While all children grow and develop in their own manner, each child typically follows a designated pattern or trajectory.

◆ Characteristics of children can help the nurse and family understand about the uniqueness of the child.

◆ Prominent theories of development allow the nurse and family to have a deeper understanding of the "why'" behind developmental tasks and stages.

◆ Understanding growth and development provides the nurse with tools to develop a plan care for the family across care settings.

review questions

Multiple Choice

1. The pediatric nurse assesses the toddler's fine motor skills by observing which one of the following?
   A. Buttoning a shirt
   B. Writing with a pencil
   C. Holding a spoon to eat
   D. Using the pincer grasp

2. According to Piaget, an infant uses his senses to learn and explore the environment. The pediatric nurse understands the concept of object permanence by:
   A. Playing the game of peek-a-boo
   B. Encouraging the infant to shake a rattle
   C. Pushing a button on an overhead mobile
   D. Placing the child in a stroller and going for a walk

3. The pediatric nurse is promoting anticipatory guidance about safety to the mother of a 10-month-old infant. Included in the teaching, the pediatric nurse includes all of the following except:
   A. "Do not leave small objects on the floor as your baby will be crawling soon."
   B. "Keep the side rails up to prevent your baby from falling out of the crib."
   C. "Put safety locks on all cabinets to prevent accidents."
   D. "Allow your baby to stay alone for short periods of time to promote independence."

4. The mother of a 26-month-old toddler tells the pediatric nurse that she is having trouble disciplining her daughter. The mother states; "She really knows how to push me to my limit. I don't know what to do

with her!" What is the best therapeutic response the nurse can make?
   A. "The terrible two's are a difficult time. You have to show her that you are the boss!"
   B. "When she does something wrong, tell her she is a bad girl and has to be punished for her actions."
   C. "Grab her by the arm and give her a time out on a chair in the corner."
   D. "Take away her favorite doll and tell her that she cannot have it back until she changes her behavior."

5. The parents of a toddler ask the nurse how to best prepare the toddler for a planned medical procedure. The pediatric nurse recognizes that:
   A. The toddler is too young to understand what will happen and does not need an explanation.
   B. The use of short explanations can best help the toddler understand the planned procedure.
   C. Allowing the toddler to explore the procedure room may be helpful.
   D. It is beneficial for the nurse to demonstrate the upcoming procedure to the toddler.

6. The father of a 4-year-old is concerned about his son's reaction to an injury of his friend. He told the nurse that the child stayed in his room over the weekend and cried himself to sleep. When the pediatric nurse questioned the child, he described an argument that he and his friend had about a week prior to his friend's injury. The nurse recognizes that the preschooler is suffering from:
   A. Magical thinking
   B. Inferiority
   C. Guilt complex
   D. A morality issue

7. Key aspects in a teen's environment that help him make good decisions include all of the following except:
   A. Ability to think abstractly
   B. Ability to use deductive reasoning
   C. Ability to make long-term plans
   D. Ability to use logical thinking

True/False

8. The pediatric nurse is aware that although developmental advances occur in an orderly fashion, each child progresses through the predicted stages within her own time frame.

9. The nurse is teaching parents of a school-age child about discipline. The nurse stresses to the parents that if the child does not follow family rules they should use corporal punishment.

10. The use of a pacifier or thumb/sucking is a concern during toddler years.

Fill-in-the-Blank

11. According to Erikson's psychosocial stage of _____ vs. _____, the infant will learn to trust his environment if his needs are consistently met.

12. When caring for the developing child, _____ refers to the continuous adjustment in the size of the child and _____ refers to the ongoing process of adaptation.

See Answers to End of Chapter Review Questions on the Electronic Study Guide or DavisPlus.

REFERENCES

Abidin, R. (1995). *Parenting stress index manual* (3rd ed.). Odessa, FL: Psychological Assessment Resources.

Ainsworth, M. (1978). *Patterns of attachment: A psychological study of the strange situation*. Hillsdale, NJ: Lawrence Erlbaum Associates.

American Academy of Pediatrics (AAP). (2008). Children's health topics. Retrieved from http://www.aap.org (Accessed October 1, 2008).

American Academy of Pediatrics (AAP). (2005). Policy statement: The changing concept of sudden infant death syndrome: Diagnostic coding shifts, controversies regarding the sleeping environment, and new variables to consider in reducing risk. *116* (5):1245–1255. Retrieved from http://www.aap.org/ (Accessed September 9, 2007).

American Academy of Pediatrics (AAP) Policy Statement. (1998, 2004). Guidance for effective discipline. *Pediatrics, 101* (4), 723–728. Retrieved from http://www.aap.org/ (Accessed May 16, 2008).

Bowlby, J. (1978). *Attachment and loss*. Harmondsworth: Penguin Education.

Brazelton, T.B. (1992). *Touchpoints: Emotional and behavioral development*. Reading, MA: Addison–Wesley.

Brazelton, T.B., & Sparrow, J. (2002). *Touchpoints: 3–6: Your child's emotional and behavioral development*. Cambridge, MA: Perseus.

Bronfenbrenner, U. (1979). *The ecology of human development*. Cambridge, MA: Harvard University Press.

Bulechek, G., Butcher, H.M., & Dochterman, J. (2008). *Nursing interventions classification (NIC)* (5th ed.). St. Louis, MO: C.V. Mosby.

Davidson, J. (2009). Multiple intelligences. Retrieved from http://childdevelopmentinfo.com/learning/multiple_intelligences.htm (Accessed September 29, 2009).

Duvall, E.R. (1977). *Marriage and family development*. Philadelphia: Lippincott.

Fowler, J.W. (1981). *Stages of faith: The psychology of human development and the quest for meaning*. San Francisco: Harper & Row.

Gardner, H. (2004). Audiences for the theory of multiple intelligences. *Teachers College Record, 106*, 212–220.

Gilligan, C. (1982). *In a different voice: Psychological theory and women's development*. Cambridge, MA: Harvard University Press.

Johnson, M., Bulechek, G., Butcher, H., McCloskey Dochterman, J., Maas, M., Moorhead, S., & Swanson, E. (2006). *NANDA, NOC, and NIC linkages: Nursing diagnoses, outcomes, & interventions* (2nd ed.). St. Louis, MO: Mosby Elsevier.

Kohlberg, L. (1984). *Essays on moral development*. San Francisco: Harper & Row.

Merriam-Webster Online Dictionary (n.d.) Retrieved from http://www.m–w.com (Accessed Ocotber 1, 2005).

Moorehead, S., Johnson, M., Mass, M., & Swanson, E. (2008) *Nursing outcomes classification (NOC)* (4th ed.). St. Louis, MO: C.V. Mosby.

NANDA-International (2007). *NANDA-I nursing diagnoses: Definitions and classifications 2007–2008*. Philadelphia: NANDA-I.

Pfeiffer, E., Johnson, T., & Chiofolo, R. (1981). Functional assessment of elderly subjects in four service settings. *Journal of American Geriatrics Society, 29*, 433–347.

Piaget, J. (1969). *The moral judgment of the child*. New York: Free Press.

Piaget, J., & Inhelder, B. (1969). *The psychology of the child*. New York: Basic Books.

Thomas, A., & Chess, S. (1977). *Temperament and development*. New York: Brunner/Mazel.

Thomas, A., Chess, S., & Birch, H. G. (1968). *Temperament and behavior disorders in children*. New York: New York University Press.

Zero To Three Brainwonders (n.d.). *Brain development: Frequently asked questions* Retrieved from http://www.zerotothree.org/brainwonders/FAQ–body.html (Accessed May 16, 2008).

DavisPlus DavisPlus.fadavis.com **For more information, go to http://davisplus.fadavis.com/**

CONCEPT MAP

Nature
• inherent traits
Nurture
• influence of external events

Collaboration In Caring:
• Growth and development is assessed by a variety of health care team members

• Cephalocaudal
• Proximodistally
• Gross to fine motor

Theories:
• Psychosexual: Sigmund Freud
• Psychosocial: Erik Erikson
• Attachment: John Bowlby, Mary Ainsworth
• Social learning: Albert Bandura, Lev Vygotsky; Uri Bronfenbrenner
• Cognitive: Jean Piaget
• Moral development: Lawrence Kohlberg, Carol Gilligan
• Spiritual development: James Fowler
• Family development: Duvall & Hill

Influence   *Directions*

Ethnocultural Considerations:
• Some cultures are more comfortable with touch
• Important to understand cultures
• Secondary sex characteristics in African American girls begin earlier than Caucasian girls

Growth   Development

Critical Nursing Action:
• Use anticipatory guidance

Newborn/Infant
Physical:
• Reflexes: moro, sucking, rooting
• Sensory: touch first; vision last
• Motor: involuntary to gross motor
Cognitive:
• Sensorimotor; use senses
Psychosocial:
• Trust vs. mistrust
Play:
• reflexive to manipulative
Safety:
• Falls, suffocating, poisoning; SIDS
Nutrition:
• Up to 6 months; breast milk or formula
Sleep:
• 15–20 hours per day; no co-sleeping; back to sleep

Toddler
Physical:
• Growth slows; increased mobility
Cognitive:
• Tertiary circular reactions; mental combinations
Psychosocial:
• Autonomy vs. shame and doubt
Moral:
• Preconventional
Play:
• Parallel play; imitative
Safety:
• Accidents related to exploration
Nutrition:
• Small portions; nutritious foods and snacks
Sleep:
• 14 hours with naps; bedtime routine important

Early Childhood
Physical:
• Vertical growth; increasing muscle strength, agility, fine motor skills
Cognitive:
• Preoperational stage; increased verbal skills
Psychosocial:
• Initiative vs. guilt
Moral:
• Preconventional
Play:
• Associative; imaginary; physical activity, reading
Safety:
• Motor vehicle and bike accidents, drowning; fire
Nutrition:
• Small portions of nutritious foods and snacks
Sleep:
• 11 hours with naps; regular bed time

School-Age
Physical:
• Reduced baby-fat; defined facial features; begin sexual development
Cognitive:
• Concrete operations; metacognition; improved memory/language
Psychosocial:
• Industry vs. inferiority
Moral:
• Conventional
Play:
• Cooperative play; teams; creative activities; independent enjoys reading
Safety:
• Fractures, fights; motor vehicles
Nutrition:
• Education related to healthy foods
Sleep:
• 10–12 hours

Adolescence
Physical:
• Significant growth; secondary sex characteristics
Cognitive:
• Formal operations; think abstractly
Psychosocial:
• Identity vs. role confusion; occupation focus
Moral:
• Postconventional
Play:
• Social interaction; peer identification; sports; sexual exploration
Safety:
• Motor vehicle accidents; self-mutilation; suicide and alcohol abuse
Nutrition:
• Issues related to fast food, eating disorders, body image concerns
Sleep:
• Sleep deprivation common

What To Say:
• Delays in development can be attributed to many factors
• Tips for effective discipline
• Listen, discuss and encourage

Where Research And Practice Meet:
• Attachment; Relationships are important in development

Across Care Settings:
• Infant temperament

Be Sure To:
• include the adolescent in the informed concert process

Nursing Insight:
• Duvall's theory: only speaks to traditional family group

Optimizing Outcomes:
• Anticipate developmental transition points

Clinical Alert:
• Reflexes
• Remember privacy for school age child due to physical changes

Complementary Care:
• Care delivery enhanced by understanding of Fowler's 7 stages of faith and spiritual development

Family Teaching Guidelines:
• Introducing solid foods

Now Can You:
• Identify the importance of using growth and development theories as the basis for care of children and families

Caring for the Child in the Hospital and in the Community

 It is when we include caring and love in our science, we discover our caring-healing professions and disciplines are much more than a detached scientific endeavor, but a life-giving and life-receiving endeavor for humanity.

—Jean Watson (from *Caring Science as Sacred Science,* p. 3)

LEARNING TARGETS *At the completion of this chapter, the student will be able to:*

- ◆ Discuss how to gather the history of the child and family.
- ◆ Discuss the physical assessment of an infant, toddler, pre-schooler, school-aged child and adolescent, as well as resources available for families.
- ◆ Identify general care measures for the child in the hospital or clinic setting.
- ◆ Examine ways to prevent injuries in children.
- ◆ Identify common procedures for the child in the hospital or clinic setting.
- ◆ Explore the common practices when medicating the child.
- ◆ Discuss the child in pain.
- ◆ Identify the needs of the child in the family who is living with disabilities.

---

 moving toward evidence-based practice Parent Satisfaction with Care of Developmentally Disabled Children

Liptak, G.S., Orlando, M., Yingling, J.T., Theurer-Kaufman, K.L., Malay, D.P., Tompkins, L.A., & Flynn, J.R. (2006). Satisfaction with primary health care received by families of children with developmental disabilities. *Journal of Pediatric Health Care, 20*(4), 245–252.

The purpose of this study was to examine the perceptions of families who had children with developmental disabilities in relation to care and differences based on a specific condition. The sample included patients and their families who received services through a developmental center at a children's hospital in New York. This center provided care to children with both physical and developmental disabilities, such as spina bifida, cerebral palsy, autism, and mental retardation.

Three hundred potential participants with the aforementioned four conditions were identified through the hospital database and received mailed surveys; responses were returned from 121 families. The survey consisted of three parts: demographic information, the Multidimensional Assessment of Parental Satisfaction for Children with Special Needs (MAPS) developed by Ireys and Perry (1999), and general questions regarding health care.

The MAPS was described as a valid tool for measuring satisfaction with provider care in five areas: coordination of care, family-centered care, developmentally appropriate care, and interpersonal and technical competence of the provider. The MAPS has been shown to have a standardized alpha coefficient (a measure of internal consistency) of 0.87. The Pearson correlation coefficient ranged from 0.85 to 0.91 in terms of validity between the satisfaction scale and the mean score of the three items used in the study. Seven general questions regarding health care, including baseline attitudes toward providers in general, were added. The questions measured the attitudes toward physicians in primary care as described by Hulka, Zyzanski, Cassel, and Thompson (1970). Data from the MAPS were scored using the method established by Ireys and Perry (1999), i.e., those answering fair or poor were combined into one group

(continued)

---

moving toward evidence-based practice (continued)

and those answering very good to excellent were placed in another group.

Thirty-three percent of the sample rated the primary care physician's ability to put them in touch with other parents as fair or poor, a finding that was lower than data from previous studies. Twenty percent of the sample rated physicians as "fair" or "poor" in: understanding the impact of the condition on the family; their ability to answer questions regarding the condition; and their ability to provide preventive guidance. Physicians' knowledge about complementary and alternative medicine and their ability to manage the care of the disabled child were also ranked below satisfactory. The parents of

children with autism ranked overall care including community support and the use of alternative or complementary medicine lower than did the parents of children with other disabilities. Providers received the highest ratings for their sensitivity to the needs of the children and in their ability to keep up with new aspects of care.

1. What implications for the care of the developmentally disabled child and families can be drawn from this study?
2. How is this information useful to clinical nursing practice?

See Suggested Responses for Moving Toward Evidence-Based Practice on the Electronic Study Guide or DavisPlus.

Introduction

The standards of nursing practice describe a competent level of care for the nursing profession (American Nurses Association [ANA], 2004). Several themes that are fundamental to many of the standards include providing age-appropriate and culturally sensitive care, maintaining a safe environment, educating patients about healthy practices, and assuring continuity of care (ANA, 2004). For a pediatric nurse, these themes are fundamental to a holistic and caring practice.

Registered nurses are held accountable for thinking critically through conclusions derived in the course of their practice. The judgments made and actions taken are based on a core body of knowledge. This chapter provides the basis of that core in several areas.

First, the chapter presents a complete assessment of the child and family. Age-appropriate and culturally sensitive topics are interspersed throughout the chapter in relation to history-taking and the physical assessment of the child.

Second, the chapter presents an assessment of developmental milestones and the patterns of daily life for the developing child. The nurse becomes acquainted with the norms of pediatric nursing practice and must also understand that the nurse's practice must be individualized for the unique needs of the patient. Since each patient has a personal story to share, nurses are in a privileged position to guide and educate that patient.

Last, the chapter presents the fundamentals of general care measures the nurse provides in the clinic and hospital setting. Maintaining a safe environment is an essential component for some general care practices, such as the use of restraints and infection-control measures. Explaining procedures gives nurses the opportunity to educate the patient about healthy practices, to relieve anxiety and to promote well-being.

Caring for the developing child is an ongoing task and the day-to-day responsibilities of childrearing can be formidable. Families must adapt emotionally as well as financially to the new responsibilities. Processes of adaptation continually evolve as the child grows and develops and parents learn to nurture the child. Along the way, parents must also adapt parenting skills to meet daily challenges. Often, the parents are unprepared for the parenting role,

with no frame of reference other than the role-modeling of their own parents. Raising a family can be a time of both intense joy and intense angst, especially when confronted with unfamiliar developmental challenges such as temper tantrums, or a more serious illness or injury.

Parents caring for the developing child born with or who develops an emotional or physical condition are faced with even greater challenges. They must learn to cope with multiple "out of the norm" aspects of child care, especially when the child's condition necessitates frequent clinic or hospital visits, or when clinical assessments define future challenges faced by the child. For instance, if a child is born with a physically disfiguring or mental condition such as Down syndrome, the parents and child must overcome both social attitudes and possible ongoing medical challenges. No matter what the configuration or situation of the family, the nurse can assist the family to meet the physical, emotional, and spiritual needs of the developing child.

Gathering the Child's Health History

ESTABLISHING A RELATIONSHIP WITH THE PATIENT AND THE FAMILY

Assessing a child's health history can be a daunting task. Children vary in language skills, clarity of speech, cognitive abilities, and social skills. Some children can verbalize where they hurt while others may only react by crying. Each child must be approached with these differences in mind, while note must be taken of any differences that fall out of the realm of what is considered normal growth and development. In addition, the nurse must remember to use the Health Insurance Portability and Accountability Act of 1996 ("HIPAA"). This privacy act ensures that the child's health information is protected while allowing the flow of health information needed to ensure high-quality health care (U.S. Department of Health and Human Services, 2007).

For an infant or a nonverbal child, the nurse begins the health history with an interview of the parent. Grandparents, foster parents, step-parents, nannies, older siblings, and adult guardians also may accompany the child to the office or hospital. After introductions are made, it is important to clarify the identity of the person who has brought the child in for care.

Young children need to feel secure before engaging in conversation with the nurse. In this instance, the nurse should establish a rapport with the parent first. Once the child feels comfortable with the nurse present, the child may be more apt to contribute to the interview process. The child may be able to add an important piece of information needed for optimum care.

The older child may elect to be interviewed without the parent in the room. In this case, the nurse should speak with the parent separately to determine if the child has specific concerns or issues that may need to be addressed during the visit.

With the preadolescent and adolescent, the nurse may ask the parent to leave the room during the discussion of issues related to social and sexual content. The older child needs to know that a discussion can take place without the parent's knowledge. In this way, appropriate medical and nursing care can be given to ensure the safety of the child. Exceptions to maintaining confidentiality involve situations concerning abuse or a life-threatening situation.

 Ethnocultural Considerations— **Avoiding stereotyping**

Stereotyping an individual or family based on a specific racial or cultural background, or assuming that all members of a particular culture subscribe to the traditions, beliefs, and customs associated with that culture, must be avoided. Length of time in the country, level of education, level of acculturation, and economic status all affect the degree to which the culture shapes the parent's approach to health care (Salimbene, 2005).

ASKING QUESTIONS

The interview is conducted in a comfortable room with available seating for the parent, and with eye-level interaction with both the parent and the child. An unhurried environment encourages the parent to ask questions appropriate to the health of the child. The nurse projects a genuine interest in and a desire to help the child and family. This lays the foundation for a positive therapeutic relationship.

Beginning with open-ended questions allows for concerns to be explored, as the nurse invites the child or parent to tell his story by asking, "How can I help you today?" or, for a problem-oriented visit, "What made you come in today?" (Bickley & Szilagyi, 2007). This type of question allows the parent to recount the history of the present condition, also known as the chief complaint. A focused or problem-oriented health history is then obtained.

When clarifying the child's history, the nurse may use the mnemonic **OLD CAT** (Bickley & Szilagyi, 2007, p. 31) to ask the appropriate questions:

Onset: "When did the child become ill?"
Location: "Where is the pain?"
Duration: "How long does the pain last?"
Character: "Can you tell me on a scale of 1 to 10 how bad it is?" Or, for a younger child, "How much pain do you think the child is experiencing?"
Aggravating/Alleviating: "What has made the pain better or worse?"
Timing: "When does the pain start/stop?"

After the chief complaint is determined, the child's past medical history is reviewed. This includes past acute illnesses and history of chronic illnesses, immunization history, hospitalizations, emergency room visits, serious injuries, operations, and current medication usage. Inquiries are made as to the use of any over-the-counter medications, herbal preparations, or folk remedies, as well as any history of allergic reactions to food, medications, and environmental allergens. Information regarding reactions experienced by the child to a reported allergen is noted on the patient's chart.

The impact of the current illness is evaluated by inquiring about the child's daily activities, using the mnemonic **SODA** to ask the appropriate questions:

Sleep: "How has your child been sleeping?"
Output: "How many times per day do you _____?" (Use the expression the family has adopted to convey urine/stool output). Or, for the younger child ask, "How many wet diapers has he had today?"
Diet: "How much fluid has your child taken in today?" "Has the illness affected the child's appetite or diet?"
Activity: "Has the child's activity level changed since he has been ill?"

Interviews are commonly concluded by asking if the parents have any other concerns or problems they would like to discuss.

COMPREHENSIVE HEALTH HISTORY

When a child is seen for a well-child visit, a comprehensive health history is necessary. Components of a child's health history include family medical and social history, immunizations, past medical history, developmental milestones achieved, patterns of daily activities, and a review of systems.

Family Medical and Social History

The family medical and social history includes documenting the current household make-up as well as the age and health of each family member. Document the following:

- Ages and cause of death of any deceased parents, grandparents, and siblings
- Chronic illnesses experienced by family members
- Inherited diseases
- Parents' professions, religious affiliations or spiritual beliefs, and family activities
- For the older child, interviewed without the presence of the parent, the social history must also include information regarding grade level, friendships, drug or alcohol use, smoking, sexual activity, and safe sex practices

Past Medical History

A thorough birth history can provide valuable information about the health status of a younger child. The history of the pregnancy, labor and delivery, and the health of the baby at birth are documented, including the birth weight and APGAR scores, if available. In addition, any difficulties with feeding, breathing, jaundice, or other medical problems in the early neonatal period must be documented.

The past medical history in children includes documentation of all acute illnesses. Chronic illnesses and the medications that have been prescribed are listed, as well as the use of any herbal products and home remedies. If the child's chart is available, all encounter forms are reviewed to determine the reason for the visits, resultant medical diagnoses, and outcomes of previous treatments.

✿ Complementary Care: *Commonly used herbal preparations*

Herb	Use	Concerns
Aloe vera	Minor skin wounds and irritations.	No known side effects for topical applications.
Bilberry	The tea form is used for the treatment of diarrhea.	Can affect clotting time by decreasing platelet aggregation.
Cayenne pepper	Relief of pain associated with tonsillitis (capsule form) and sore muscles (ointment).	Ointment may cause burning sensation when used topically.
Chamomile	Pain associated with colic, teething, and stomach aches.	Hypersensitivity reaction. Contraindicated in those allergic to daisies, marigolds or ragweed.
Echinacea	Symptoms of the common cold and mild infections.	Do not use for autoimmune disorders, diabetes, AIDS, HIV. Use for short-term illnesses only.
Fennel	Colic, stomach spasms, and cough associated with respiratory infections.	May have a laxative effect.
Feverfew	Migraines.	Not safe for children younger than 2 years of age. Administration of NSAIDs inhibits effect of feverfew.
Licorice	The oral form treats cough; the topical form is used in the treatment of eczema.	Safe for children if taken for short-term illness. Contraindicated in diabetes, hypertension, liver and kidney disease.
Nettle	Asthma and allergy symptoms.	May increase blood sugar.
St. John's Wort	Mild depression.	May cause photosensitivity; many herb–drug interactions.
Tea Tree Oil	The topical form is used as an antibacterial.	Use restricted to topical application.
Valerian	Mild to moderate insomnia.	May potentiate sedative effects of barbiturates, anesthetics, and CNS depressants. May cause GI upset.

Adapted from Bascom, A. (2002). *Incorporating herbal medicine into clinical practice.* Philadelphia: F.A. Davis.

where research and practice meet:
Use of Herbal Products

The use of herbal products and home remedies is common (Lanski, Greenwald, Perkins, & Simon 2003). Often, however, parents do not divulge herbal product use for their children in encounters with health care providers. Likewise, Woolf, Gardiner, Whelan, Alpert, and Dvorkin (2005) found that only 42% of pediatric nurses and physicians surveyed felt confident initiating the topic of herbal product use with parents. In addition, only 7% felt that the use of herbs was appropriate as adjunct therapy for the hospitalized child, even if some herbs form the basis of approved pharmaceuticals: Digoxin (Lanoxin), for example, comes from the foxglove plant. It is important, however, to ask about the use of herbal products to avoid inadvertent drug interactions.

Immunizations

Common childhood diseases the child may have had, as well as any immunizations received, are documented, and the chart is reviewed before the interview to determine if the immunizations are current. Maintaining current immunization status protects the child and family against preventable communicable diseases. The Centers for Disease Control and Prevention (CDC) reviews and updates the immunization schedule regularly, so it is important for the nurse to be aware of and follow the most current guidelines (CDC, 2007). The following Web site provides the most current child immunization schedules: http://www.cdc.gov/vaccines.

Developmental Milestones

A good foundation in growth and development is a necessity for the nurse working in a pediatric setting. Developmental assessment is important to determine if a child's development is within the normal range. It is also useful in identifying children at risk. Developmental milestones can be assessed using the Denver II Screening Test in children from birth to 6 years of age (Denver Developmental Materials, 1990). The Denver II assesses personal–social, fine motor–adaptive, gross motor, and language skills (Frankenburg, Dobbs, Archer, Shapiro, & Bresnick, 1992). The nurse also documents the child's behaviors during administration of the test, including compliance during testing, interest in surroundings, fearfulness, and a subjective measure of the child's attention span. After the test has been administered, the parents may be asked if the child's performance was characteristic of his normal behaviors. Referral is needed when the child has "failed" the test with two or more delays, if there is no improvement in areas of concern 3 months after the initial screen, or if the child is determined to be "untestable" at two consecutive screenings.

Administering the 125-item test requires training. Information on training sessions and testing materials can be obtained through the following link: http://www.denverii.com/DenverII.html.

Due to the training process involved and the time required to administer the Denver II, a more focused and concise assessment can be employed instead. Table 21-1 provides a synopsis of the various age groups' gross and fine motor skills and sensory development. Language and play are also listed.

Table 21-1 Developmental Milestones

Age	Gross Motor	Fine Motor	Sensory/Language/Play
Newborn: Birth–1 Month	*Birth–1 month* Reflexes present Absence of head control, but can momentarily hold the head in midline Head lag when the newborn is pulled from a lying to a sitting position Assumes flexed position When supine assumes tonic neck flex position Kicks legs and waves arms Rounded back when sitting Rolls over accidently	*Birth–1 month* Hands predominately closed Strong grasp reflex	*Birth–1 month* Touch: First sense to develop Smell: Recognizes mother and has a taste preference for sweets Hearing well developed: Becomes quiet when hears a familiar voice Limited visual acuity 20/100, fascinated with faces, follows moving objects, contrasting colors (black and white) Language: Cries and smiles during sleep Play: Interaction with parents and caregivers
Infant: 1–2 Months	*1–2 months* Less head lag when pulled to sitting position When prone can slightly lift head off of floor Improved head control, turns and lifts head from side to side when prone	*1–2 months* Holds hands open Grasp reflex absent Can pull at clothes and blanket, bats at objects	*1–2 months* When supine follows dangling toys Visually searches for sounds Turns head to sound Language: Coos, has social smile Play: Interaction with parents and caregivers, through gross and fine motor skills and senses
Infant: 3–6 Months	*3–6 months* Can hold head more erect when sitting, still some bobbing, by 6 months sturdy head control Only slight head lag, by 6 months no head lag Raises head to 45°–90° off of floor In sitting position (tripod) back is straight and balances head well, sits alone by 8 months When held in a standing position can bear some weight, by 8 months readily bears weight Rolls from back to side and then abdomen to back When supine puts feet to mouth Begins to creep on hands and knees	*3–6 months* Plays with toes Clutches own hands, inspects and plays with hands Pulls blanket over face Rakes objects Grasps objects with both hands (palmer grasp) Shakes rattle and holds bottle Eventually able to put objects in container and bang them together Carries objects to mouth Transfers objects from hand to hand Reaches and bangs toys on table Likes mirror images	*3–6 months* Follows object 180° Good vision Locates sound by turning head Beginning eye–hand coordination Pursues dropped object visually Sees small objects Responds to name Language: Coos and babbles Play: Interaction with parents and caregivers, through gross and fine motor skills and senses
Infant: 9–12 Months	*9–12 months* Creeps on hands and knees Pulls self to standing position Stands while holding onto furniture and begins to cruise Stands alone Changes from prone to sitting position Can reach backwards while sitting Can sit down from standing position alone Begins to walk holding hand and then independently, takes first step	*9–12 months* Uses pincer grasp Hand dominance now evident Releases and rescues an object When sitting, purposely reaches around back to retrieve object Can randomly turn pages in a book Can make a simple mark on paper Waves bye-bye and plays pat-a-cake Begins to feed self finger foods	*9–12 months* Increasing depth perception Moves toward sound Thoroughly explores and experiences objects Points to simple objects Language: Says "mama" and "dada" Play: solitary play (play alone), and continued interaction with parents and caregivers, through gross and fine motor skills and senses

Table 21-1	Developmental Milestones—cont'd		
Age	**Gross Motor**	**Fine Motor**	**Sensory/Language/Play**
Toddler: 1–3 Years	Stands without support Walks independently Creeps upstairs Pulls toys while walking Runs with wide stance Jumps in place with both feet Climbs Begins to stand on one foot momentarily Can walk up and down stairs with alternate feet	Holds a pencil or a large crayon Makes artwork that is more representative of the object Copies a circle Knows colors Feeds self with a spoon and drinks from a cup Constantly throws objects on floor Builds tower of 3–4 cubes eventually building tower of 7–8 cubes Screws/unscrews Turns pages in a book one page at a time Turn knobs Removes shoes and socks, learns to undress self	Well developed vision Can identify geometric objects Intense interest in book's pictures Distinguishes food preferences based on senses Language: Single words and simple phrases, "I do" or "Want drink." By 15 months knows 15 words. Play: Parallel play (play along side another child)
Early childhood (preschooler): 3–6 Years	Dresses self Throws and catches ball Pedals tricycle Kicks ball forward Stands on one foot for 5–10 seconds Skips and hops on one foot Walks down steps with alternate feet Jumps from bottom step Balances on alternate feet with eyes closed	Moves around in a more balanced fashion Builds tower of 9–10 cubes Draws stick figure with 6 parts Uses scissors to cut outline of picture Copies and traces geometric patterns Ties shoe laces Uses fork, spoon and knife with supervision Colors, prints letters Mostly independent toileting	Well developed senses Preferences based on the use of senses Language: Vocabulary has increased, from 1500 to 2000 words, eventually speaks in complete sentences Play: Cooperative play (play with peers), make believe, dramatic play
School-age: 6–12 Years	Gradual increase in dexterity and becomes limber Improves coordination and balance, rhythm Climbs, bikes, skips, jumps rope and swings Learns to swim, dance, do somersaults and skate	Good eye–hand coordination Balance improves Can sew, draw, make arts and crafts, build models, play video games Prints and writes Likes activities that promote dexterity such as playing a musical instrument	20/20 Visual acuity Color discrimination fully developed Mature sense of smell Hearing deficits may be discovered as language develops Language: Accelerated, vocabulary expands to 8000–15,000 words Play: Cooperative play (play with peers), solitary activities and active play (e.g., dance or karate)

Continued

Table 21-1 Developmental Milestones—cont'd			
Age	**Gross Motor**	**Fine Motor**	**Sensory/Language/Play**
Adolescence: 12–19 Years	Begin to develop endurance Speed and coordination Focuses skills on interest area	Manipulates complicated objects High skill level playing video games and computer Good finger dexterity for writing and other intricate tasks Precise eye–hand coordination	Increased concentration so can follow complicated instructions Senses tied into body image Develops adult preferences based on senses Language: Continues to develop and refine with increased vocabulary up to 50,000 words. Improved communication skills "Play": Peer groups, team sports, solitary time, school or community activities, dating

Patterns of Daily Activities

SLEEP. The nurse must determine both the number of hours and the quality of sleep the child receives each night. Sleep requirements change as the child grows and each child's sleep requirements are different. Newborns sleep about 16 or 17 hours a day, typically in stretches of 2 to 3 hours at a time. Babies are typically able to sleep through the night by age 6 months (http://www.mayo-clinic.com/). Children also differ in their ability to sleep. Some can sleep anywhere under any conditions while others suffer sleepless nights if there is even the slightest change in their normal routine. Naps may be a part of a child's life up to the preschool years. Children may experience nightmares or night terrors that can disrupt sleep. Nightmares may reflect the struggles children experience during the day, or the fears a child has regarding separation, impulses, or conflicts. Night terrors occur during the first few hours of sleep. Nightmares and night terrors can be frightening experiences for a child; a child can recount her nightmares. However, with night terrors the child has no recollection.

Nutrition

The questions a nurse asks regarding nutrition are based on the child's age. If the infant is breastfed, information is gathered as to how often and for how long the child is fed at each feeding, and how many wet diapers are changed in the course of one day. With sufficient breast milk intake, the infant will have six or more wet diapers and gain weight. Newborns often lose 10% of their birth weight. This weight loss is usually by the 12th day of life (Wright & Parkinson, 2004).

For the infant who is receiving formula, information is gathered as to the type of formula, the amount taken at each feeding, and the number of feedings per day. It is also important to note if and when juices or solid foods have been started, and whether supplements or vitamins have been prescribed.

When assessing children and adolescents, a 24-hour recall elicits the food items eaten in a typical day and reflects sociocultural trends. The nurse can document the amount and type of milk, juices, and all other liquids. In addition, the nurse must document food allergies for all children. Analysis of the food intake is compared to the foods suggested in the Food Guide Pyramid for Young Children. (Go to http://www.mypyramid.gov/kids/index.html.)

PLAY, ACTIVITIES, AND SCHOOLWORK. Patterns of play and children's activities reflect the interests of the child, the family financial circumstances, and work schedules of the parents, environmental safety, and the availability of after-school activities. Throughout infancy, learning takes place in the context of sensory stimulation. The parent can provide insight into whether there is sufficient stimulation in the immediate environment to help the child learn. For example, talking and singing adds auditory stimulation. Holding, cuddling, and consoling the infant provides the tactile sensory stimulation for developing a sense of trust and facilitates the bonding process.

As the child matures, continued supervision of the child's activities is needed to encourage social competence and healthy habits. Information is gathered about the daily routine of the child, the contact the child has with playmates, older siblings, and adults, and whether the child has an opportunity to develop gross and fine motor skills or has attended community programs such as Head Start. For school age children, additional information is gathered regarding achievement with schoolwork, special education needs, extracurricular activities, and interaction with peers.

A good understanding of the patterns of daily activities allows the nurse to make suggestions for a healthy lifestyle to the parent or child, alert the primary care provider of potential problems, and provide anticipatory guidance as appropriate to the situation.

Review of Systems

Much like the physical examination, the review of systems is best conducted with a "head-to-toe" approach, starting with a general question regarding each body system. It can also be conducted by asking questions during the physical

Nursing Care Plan Imbalanced Nutrition

Nursing Diagnosis: Imbalanced Nutrition: Less Than Body Requirements related to inadequate intake

Measurable Short-term Goal: Child will ingest adequate nutrients.

Measurable Long-term Goal: Child will demonstrate appropriate growth for age on normal curve.

NOC Outcomes:
Appetite (1014) Desire to eat when ill or receiving treatment
Nutritional Status (1004) Extent to which nutrients are available to meet metabolic needs

NIC Interventions:
Nutrition Therapy (1120)
Nutritional Monitoring (1160)
Nutrition Management (1100)

Nursing Interventions:

1. Monitor weight daily on same scale and at same time during hospitalization and at every encounter in community-based care.

   RATIONALE: Monitoring assists in early identification and correction of nutritional deficiencies to prevent complications from malnutrition.

2. Provide favorite high-protein, high-calorie, nutritious foods and drinks in small frequent meals (specify for child).

   RATIONALE: Child is more likely to eat familiar foods and small frequent meals may be better tolerated during illness.

3. Ensure that mealtime is pleasant and uninterrupted. Be sure to schedule treatment and procedures at times other than feeding time. Do not mix medications in food offered during mealtimes.

   RATIONALE: Child may refuse to eat essential foods if they have been associated with unpleasant activities, smells, or tastes.

4. Encourage additional nutritious, high-calorie snacks as tolerated by child (e.g., milkshakes, string cheese).

   RATIONALE: Supplemental nutrition may provide the additional calories and nutrients via the preferred oral route.

5. Initiate oro- or nasogastric supplementation as appropriate.

   RATIONALE: The ill child may be unable to ingest adequate calories and nutrients orally.

---

examination. The review of systems includes the following areas:

- General: usual weight, change in weight, weakness, fatigue, fever or allergies
- Skin: rashes, pruritus, turgor, changes in color, indications of injury, acne, changes in nails or hair
- Head, Eyes, Ears, Nose, Throat (HEENT): injury to head, headaches, dizziness; eye infections, itching or watering eyes, behaviors indicating change in visual acuity, use of glasses, date of last eye exam; ear infections, behaviors indicating change in hearing; nose bleeds, colds, hay fever, sinus infections; sore throats, tonsils, dentition, caries
- Neck: neck pain, enlarged lymph glands, neck range of motion
- Chest: respiratory infections, asthma, chronic cough, wheezing, shortness of breath, breast changes
- Cardiovascular: heart murmur, palpitations, date of last blood work
- Gastrointestinal: regurgitation, vomiting, changes in bowel habits, constipation, diarrhea, food intolerance, abdominal pain, changes in appetite or eating pattern
- Genitourinary: *General*—dysuria, urgency, odor to urine, date of last urinalysis, signs of puberty, urethral or vaginal discharge, presence of lesions, sexual habits, contraceptive use, and symptoms or history of sexually transmitted infections; *males*—changes in groin/scrotum/glans, presence of circumcision; *females*—

menarche, date of last menstrual period, dysmenorrhea, and date of last Pap smear (if appropriate)
- Musculoskeletal: injuries, fractures, weakness, clumsiness, gait, muscle pains
- Neurological: seizures, tics, psychiatric diseases, anxiety, depression
- Endocrine: history or symptoms of thyroid disease or diabetes or diseases that affect normal growth.

 Nursing Insight— *Family dynamics*

Family dynamics are assessed by observing the behaviors between the child and his parent.

Questions to consider:

- During a health care visit, does the parent or caregiver seem sufficiently concerned about the problem? Or, does the parent or caregiver seem overly concerned about the problem?
- Does the parent or caregiver have the information that a responsible parent would know regarding the child's illness, past medical history and immunizations? Is the parent or caregiver a reliable historian?
- Is the parent or caregiver providing comfort to the child if the child is frightened?
- Does the parent or caregiver appear angry about being in the office?
- Is the parent or caregiver aware of the needs of the child?
- Does the child look well cared for?

Now Can You— Discuss the health history for the child?

1. State the major components of a thorough health history for the child?
2. Ask salient questions about the child's health?

Health Assessment

When examining children, the approach to the physical assessment is based on the child's age, cognitive level, and degree of illness. Infants can be examined from head to toe without difficulty. Some children are fearful of any examiner and are uncooperative. Others seem to enjoy the experience as something new. As a guideline, an exam starts with the least invasive actions and concludes with the most distressful actions. For example, it is easier to examine the posterior lung fields with the caregiver holding the child on her lap early in the exam while leaving the examination of the ears and mouth for the end of the exam (see Chapter 18 for assessment of the newborn).

ANTHROPOMETRIC MEASUREMENTS

Before the physical assessment, vital signs and growth measurements of length, weight, head circumference, and skinfold thickness are taken and recorded. Growth charts from the National Center for Health Statistics (NCHS) were revised in 2000 to include body mass index-for-age (BMI-for-age) (see Chapter 18). These growth charts can be found at http://www.cdc.gov/nchs/about/major/nhanes/growthcharts/charts.htm.

Length

Length is measured in the infant while he is lying supine on a measuring tray or board. If a measuring board is not available, the nurse holds the head in midline while an assistant holds the hips and knees extended flat on a paper-covered table. Points are marked at the top of the head and the heels of the feet, the child is moved, and the distance between markings is measured. For the older child a stadiometer is used to obtain a standing height. The child removes his shoes and stands with his back to the stadiometer, with the back of the heels and shoulders touching the wall.

Weight

The weight of an infant is measured using an infant scale lined with a thin paper cover. After the scale setting is balanced, the infant's clothing is removed and the child is weighed in either a supine or sitting position. The nurse protects the child from an accidental fall by placing a hand over the infant without direct contact. Older children are weighed on a standing scale. The same scales should be used to measure height and weight at each visit.

Body Mass Index

Once weight and height are assessed, body mass index (BMI) can be calculated. The BMI is used to assess total body fat and nutritional status. In children, the BMI is represented as a percentile, allowing a comparison to other children of the same age and gender.

 diagnostic tools Body Mass Index (BMI)

A BMI-for-age plotted below the 5th percentile indicates a child who is underweight; a BMI-for-age between the 5th and 85th percentile is considered a healthy weight; children with a BMI-for-age between the 85th and 95th percentile are considered at risk for obesity; and those with a BMI-for-age >95% are considered obese.

 assessment tools Body Mass Index (BMI)

The BMI-for-age is calculated by dividing the weight in kilograms by the meter height squared. However, since most health care providers obtain height in centimeters, an alternative calculation is to divide the weight in kilograms by the centimeter height squared multiplied by 10,000. For example, the BMI for an 8-year-old boy who weighs 26 kg with a height of 135 cm is calculated as follows: 26 divided by 135^2 (18,225) $\times$ 10,000 = 14.26. A BMI of 14.26 plots on the growth chart between the 10th and 25th percentile, which is a healthy weight. The nurse can help the family calculate their child's BMI by accessing the CDC Web site. This Web site has a BMI Percentile Calculator for the Child and the Teen: http://apps.nccd.cdc.gov/dnpabmi/Calculator.aspx.

Head Circumference

For children 2 years of age and younger, head circumference measurements are done at routine well-child visits. The head's largest circumference is measured by placing the tape over the lower forehead, above the pinna of the ears, and over the occipital prominence (Fig. 21-1). This measurement is recorded in centimeters and displayed as a percentile. As with weight and height, evidence of growth within the percentiles remains consistent over time, with normal values according to age and gender reflecting normal development. When there is a deviation, either below or above the percentile from the previous visit, it may signify a potential problem. The nurse informs the primary care provider of these findings

Skinfold Thickness Measurements

Skinfold thickness measurements indicate the degree of adipose tissue or body fat. In addition to calculating and plotting the BMI once yearly, as recommended by the American Academy of Pediatrics (AAP, 2003), skinfold thickness measurements can add to the objective assessment of obesity in children and adolescents who are at risk. The nurse might measure the degree of skinfold thickness in the tricep or abdominal areas. The average of two consecutive readings is used as the skinfold thickness measurement. The reliability of the skin fold measurement is entirely dependent on correct measurement technique.

Figure 21-1 Measuring head circumference.

VITAL SIGNS

Temperature

Vital signs consist of temperature, pulse, respirations, and blood pressure (Table 21-2). Due to the toxic nature of the chemical, mercury thermometers should not be used in assessing temperature. A variety of digital and tympanic thermometers are available. The route used for assessing temperature depends on the age and developmental level of the child. Newborn temperature is assessed via the axillary route. The tip of a digital thermometer is placed in the axilla with the arm held against the side of the body until the temperature registers. Rectal temperatures are not routinely measured. If a rectal temperature is desired, caution is taken not to insert the thermometer more than ½ inch. In older children, tympanic membrane temperatures are obtained (Fig. 21-2). Since temperatures register within seconds, this route is a convenient one in pediatrics. The route used is charted when recording the temperature (see Appendices A and B).

Pulse

Assessing the pulse in newborns and children requires concentration. The heart rate is variable and changes with illness. The pulse is counted for a full minute while the infant or child is quiet. The most accurate pulse in children of all ages is the apical pulse, and it is also the one assessed prior to giving many medications. With an uncooperative infant, the femoral arteries are palpated in the inguinal area, or the brachial arteries in the antecubital fossa.

Respirations

Respirations are to be counted for one full minute and can be assessed accurately only when the infant or child is not crying. A good time to count them is when a child is sleeping or resting quietly in a parent's arms. If possible, it is wise to start the vital sign assessment with respirations. There is a great deal of variability in the respiratory rate in children. Infants and young children are diaphragmatic breathers. The nurse can visually count the number of respirations by observing the abdomen as the child breathes.

Blood Pressure

Blood pressures are measured during well-child visits or routine physicals beginning when the child reaches 3 years of age. Readings are especially important for children with cardiac, pulmonary or kidney disease, dehydration, or complaints of dizziness, regardless of age. Selection of the cuff size is an important consideration. A good rule of thumb is to use a cuff with a bladder width that is approximately 40% of the arm circumference. With this approximation, an accurate radial blood pressure can be assessed (Clark et al., 2002). Electronic blood pressure devices with varying cuff sizes are also available.

PHYSICAL ASSESSMENT

General Impression

As the nurse meets the child and the parents and engages in conversation with them, an impression begins to take form. This subjective feeling about the child encompasses many areas of assessment. As the nurse conducts the health history and performs the physical assessment, additional notions regarding the child and family develop. Not only is the uniqueness of the child portrayed, but a reflection of the family life that the child is a part of also becomes evident.

Take note of the behaviors of the child as he interacts with his parents. How does the child react to questions? What is the child's speech like? Is the child quiet, pleasant, talkative, uninterested or angry? For the younger child, does the child listen to parents, interact in a meaningful way, or engage in age-appropriate behavior?

Hygiene and nutritional status are also examined. Is the child clean and appropriately dressed for the season? Body size, skin color, eyes, and the condition of the hair are observed for evidence of a good overall nutritional state.

Skin Assessment

The skin is assessed for color, turgor, and lesions. Skin color reflects ethnicity, diet, disease, and injury. Variations in tone are due to genetic composition. Carotenemia, a benign yellowing of the skin due to excessive carotene in the blood, may be present in the child with a diet high in yellow and orange vegetables. Pallor may indicate anemia, cyanosis may indicate a compromised cardiorespiratory state, and yellowing of the skin and sclerae may indicate a dysfunction of the liver. Petechial lesions may be indicative of an infectious process or a blood disorder. Ecchymotic lesions may also indicate a blood disorder or be a tell-tale sign of past accidental or non-accidental injuries.

The nurse can assess the child's skin for evidence of dehydration by grasping a small area of skin and pulling

Table 21-2	Average Range for Pediatric Vital Signs			
Age Group	**HR**	**RR**	**BP Systolic**	**BP Diastolic**
Infant	80–150	25–55	65–100	45–65
Toddler	70–110	20–30	90–105	55–70
Preschooler	65–110	20–25	95–110	60–75
School-age	60–95	14–22	100–120	60–75
Adolescent	55–85	12–18	110–125	65–85

Figure 21-2 Taking tympanic temperature.

up. Once released, the skin should quickly return to its normal position. Skin that remains in the "tenting" position for several seconds indicates absence or presence of skin turgor and inadequate hydration.

If a rash is present or if jaundice is suspected, the nurse determines if the skin blanches or turns pale. The nurse applies pressure to the skin with the thumbs about 1 to 2 inches apart. This presses the normal pink and darker colors out. In the presence of jaundice, there is a yellowish underlying color. Petechial lesions do not blanch, which may indicate a serious bacterial infection in an ill child. The primary health care provider should be notified immediately.

The skin examination concludes with the inspection and documentation of the texture of the hair and the condition of the scalp, palms, and nails. Cradle cap is most common in newborns and is identified by thick, crusty scales over the scalp. The older child is monitored for lice or ticks.

Normal nails are pink and convex, with white edges extending over the end of the fingers. In children with cardiac disease, nails are examined for evidence of clubbing. Nail biting is a nervous habit that is evidenced by very short nails without the normal white edges.

The palms are examined for the normal flexion creases. Normally there are three creases. In a small section of the population, the two horizontal creases fuse to form a single horizontal palmar crease. This is a common finding in many genetic disorders, particularly Down syndrome. If this palmar crease is evident on only one hand, the child may have no genetic disorders.

✺ *Ethnocultural Considerations*— Skin assessment

In light-skinned individuals, the sclera is white. In darker-skinned individuals, the sclera can be slightly yellow with small black marks. This is a normal finding.

Head Assessment

The head is observed for symmetry and shape. Beyond the newborn period, head shape abnormalities in the infant may be due to craniosynostosis, a premature fusing of one or more of the cranial sutures, or from gravitational influences caused by the infant's head being kept in the same position for an extended period of time. An odd head shape can

develop due to the malleability of the skull bones. The supine sleep position has greatly reduced the incidence of sudden infant death syndrome (SIDS). However, infants who are placed in the recommended supine position for sleep are at increased risk for deformational posterior plagiocephaly, or flattening, of the occiput (Nield & Kamat, 2006). Head repositioning techniques, especially during play times, may be useful when the first signs of plagiocephaly occur (Persing, James, Swanson, & Kattwinkel, 2003).

The skull is palpated to evaluate fontanels, sutures, contusions, or other swellings. Fontanels are fibrous-membrane-covered areas where two or more skull bones converge. Although there are six fontanels, the two most commonly evaluated are the posterior and anterior fontanels. The posterior fontanel closes within 1 to 3 months after birth, while the diamond-shaped anterior fontanel remains open until 12 to 18 months of age.

The anterior fontanel is the most significant fontanel for evaluation (Fig. 21-3). The average width is 2.1 cm (Kreisler & Ricter, 2003). A larger fontanel or one with a delayed closure may signify an infant with hypothyroidism, Down syndrome, achondroplasia (congenital dwarfism) or increased intracranial pressure. Assess the fontanels when the infant is held in a sitting position. Depression of the fontanel may be indicative of dehydration; fullness of the fontanel is a potential sign of increased intracranial pressure.

The face is examined for general appearance and the comparison of features to those of the parents. Unusual features are noted, such as a micrognathia (shortened chin), low-set ears, flattened nasal bridge, enlarged or protruding tongue, allergic shiners (dark, under-eye rings) or a wide and flattened philtrum (the vertical groove from the bottom of the nose to the upper lip).

Neck Assessment

Lymph nodes of the head and neck are palpated systematically, starting at the preauricular area, proceeding to the postauricular area, and then to the occipital nodes (Fig. 21-4). Next, the tonsillar nodes at the angle of the mandible are examined, followed by the submandibular and submental nodes under the chin, the cervical chain of lymph nodes, and finally the supraclavicular area. Size, shape, mobility and tenderness are documented. It is

Figure 21-3 Anterior and posterior fontanels.

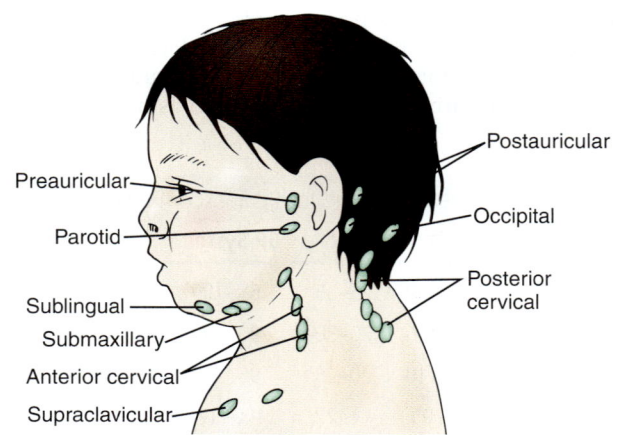

Figure 21-4 Lymph nodes of the head and neck.

common for young children to have palpable, painless, movable nodes up to 1 cm in diameter. Pain upon palpation may be indicative of an upper airway infection. The trachea is palpated for midline placement and masses. A lateral deviation of the trachea may be due to a mass or a collapsed lung. The thyroid gland is examined for enlargement, nodules, and goiters.

Eye Assessment

Observation of the eyes includes assessment of symmetry, shape, and placement in relation to the nose. In addition, the nurse can assess for symmetry and size of the pupils and their response to light. The conjunctiva and lids are observed for conjunctivitis, styes, or chalazions (small discrete swellings of the upper lid that develop when a meibomian oil gland becomes blocked). The sclerae are inspected for color. The nurse notes erythema, swelling, or discharge from the eye. Documentation of the presence of discharge includes type (watery, purulent), color, amount, and associated symptoms. Treatment depends on the cause, which may be bacterial, viral, or an allergen.

 assessment tools Visual Acuity

Visual screening for children can begin at the age of 2 ½ years. There are a variety of charts that will assist in the assessment of visual acuity. Visual acuity for each eye is assessed by occluding the contralateral eye with a plastic paddle. With all charts the objects, letters and numbers decrease in size. The Allen chart requires the child to identify common objects; the "tumbling E" requires the child to identify in which direction each E is facing; and the Snellen charts require the child to identify letters or numbers.

To ensure optimal eye health in children, testing for ocular alignment and visual acuity is essential (Bickley & Szilagyi, 2007). Assessment of visual acuity depends on the age of the child. Infants begin to use a steady gaze to regard faces or objects with interesting patterns. The nurse observes for and documents this finding during the physical exam. Any difference in visual acuity between one eye and the other is abnormal and should be referred. In addition, children are referred for further evaluation if they have a visual acuity reading of less than 20/50 or after failing a second screening.

TESTING FOR OCULAR ALIGNMENT. A common method for assessing ocular alignment is the Hirschberg corneal light reflex test, in which a light is shone directly into the child's eyes and note is taken of the position of the corneal light reflection in both eyes. The reflection should fall in the same location on the cornea of each eye. Displacement of the corneal light reflection in one eye is indicative of strabismus.

The second screening test is the cover–uncover test, in which the child is asked to focus on a distant object across the room. The nurse covers the first eye while watching the second eye for any movement. The cover is then removed from the first eye, which is observed for any movement. If no movement is detected, ocular alignment is intact. The examination is repeated on the opposite eye.

The red reflex is tested by viewing the pupil through an ophthalmoscope from a distance of ten inches. If the pupil appears red, the finding is normal. A white retinal reflex may indicate cataracts, retinoblastoma, or chorioretinitis.

TESTING FOR COLOR BLINDNESS. Children should be screened at least once during the school-age years for the ability to discriminate between red, yellow, and green. A common method for detecting color blindness is the use of the Ishihara pseudochromatic charts. Each chart consists of a field of colored dots, each with a number in the center of the colored field: the inability to identify these numbers indicates color blindness (see chapter 29).

Ear Assessment

The external ears are examined for size, shape, placement, pain, and presence of drainage from the ear canal. The pinna of the ear should be above the imaginary horizontal line drawn from the medial and lateral canthi toward the occiput. Low-set ears may indicate a congenital anomaly such as Down syndrome. To assess for pain, the nurse moves the pinna of the ear up and down. If the child complains of pain when pressure is applied to the tragus, the canal is examined for evidence of otitis externa. Cerumen (ear wax) may be seen on the external ear or in the external canal with an otoscope. Purulent drainage may indicate a foreign body in the external ear canal or a ruptured tympanic membrane. Any clear drainage noted from the ear, particularly after head trauma or with cranial infections, should be reported to the health care provider immediately as this fluid may indicate a cerebrospinal fluid leak.

❝What to say❞ — *Use of a small cotton swab to clean the ear*

The nurse can instruct parents on the use of a small cotton swab to clean the ear. A small cotton swab should be used to clean only the external ear, and not the ear canal. When a small cotton swab is used in the ear canal, the cerumen is pushed back into the canal where it cannot be moved out by the mechanical action of the tiny ear hairs. Cerumen tends to dry, harden, and become difficult to remove over time. Impacted cerumen in the ear canal may lead to hearing deficits.

When an otoscope is used, the canal should be positioned for the optimal viewing of the tympanic membrane and canal. As a general rule, the pinna is pulled down and back for children younger than 3 years, and up and back for older children. The child is positioned to prevent injury or discomfort. With the parent's help to gently restrain the child from moving, the otoscopic examination can take place either with the child either sitting on the parent's lap or in the supine position.

The nurse understands that holding the otoscope upside down allows the nurse the use of one hand to help hold the child's head and the other to position the stem of the otoscope against the child's head for more stability. The tympanic membrane is examined for the presence of normal anatomical landmarks (Fig. 21-5).

Visual loss of these landmarks may be due to erythema, fullness behind the tympanic membrane, inflammation, purulent exudate, or fluid. Due to the anatomic structure of their ears, infants and young children are prone to developing otitis media. The eustachian tubes are shorter and more horizontally positioned, enabling viruses and bacteria to travel to the middle ear. Infants who are breastfed, do not attend daycare, and are fed in an upright position have decreased rates of otitis media.

HEARING SCREENING.
In the older cooperative child, a tuning fork is utilized to assess bone and air conduction of sound. The Weber test involves striking the tines of the tuning fork and immediately placing the handle of the tuning fork midline on top of the child's head. The nurse asks the child in which ear he hears the sound best. If hearing is normal, sound is heard equally in both ears. Sound heard in one ear better than the other indicates a conductive hearing loss.

The Rinne test assesses both air and bone conduction of sound. Bone conduction is tested by placing the handle of the vibrating tuning fork on the mastoid process behind the ear. The child informs the nurse when he no longer can hear the sound of the vibrating tuning fork and the nurse immediately moves the tines forward to within 1 to 2 inches of the auditory meatus. The child should hear the air-conducted sound of the vibrating tines twice as long as he heard the bone-conducted sound.

Tympanometry assesses the status of the middle ear. The nurse places a probe into the ear canal. The amount of sound that is reflected by the tympanic membrane is measured along with the pressure in the canal. The tympanogram delineates the movement of the eardrum as stiffness, floppiness, or normal eardrum movement.

Early detection of hearing loss is important to prevent delayed hearing, speech, and language development (Box 21-1). Hearing loss may affect both the academic success and psychosocial development of the child. Since hearing loss in childhood is associated with middle ear disease, it is recommended that children with positive results from office screening exams be referred to an audiologist for further evaluation and treatment.

 Nursing Insight— *Screening techniques for children*

Screening tests require cooperation of the child. Hearing screening should be performed before any injections, vaccines, or laboratory work. With testing, the nurse assesses for frequency (pitch) and the decibel level (loudness). Frequency is defined as the number of vibrations a sound creates per second. As the frequency increases, the pitch of the sound also increases. The frequency range is 250–6000. For a normal finding, the child should hear at all frequencies at the 20-dB range.

Conditioned play audiometry (CPA) is a common test for children older than 3 years. In this test, the child is asked to engage in a play-oriented activity, like placing a colorful block in a box each time a sound is heard. The child is subjected to sounds of different frequencies that a child with normal hearing could hear.

A conventional audiogram assesses hearing acuity by asking the child to raise her hand or press a button each time a sound is heard. The child must be able to understand the language spoken, be able to follow directions, pay attention, and wait to listen to the sounds.

 Optimizing Outcomes— **Hearing screening**

Children should be screened for hearing loss as needed. A hearing impairment may interfere with normal psychosocial development, communication among friends, and educational pursuits. The best outcome to detect hearing loss includes periodic screenings because of the increased potential for hearing loss due to overexposure to high levels of noise associated with yard work, listening to music at concerts and via earphones, and through chronic ear infections, ototoxic drugs, head injuries, including abuse, or diseases.

Figure 21-5 Tympanic membrane landmarks.

- Malleus
- Tympanic membrane
- Umbo
- Cone of light

Box 21-1 **Risk Factors for Hearing Loss in Preschoolers**

- Family history of childhood hearing loss
- Parental concerns regarding hearing, speech, or language development
- Prior infections with meningitis, mumps, or otitis media
- Head trauma

Nose/Sinus Assessment

The nasal mucosa is inspected for color and inflammation. Pale, boggy mucosa is a typical finding in a child with allergic rhinitis. The nasal mucosa appears erythematous with upper respiratory infections. Any bleeding of the mucosal lining is noted. Purulent discharge from the nose may indicate a viral or bacterial condition. Purulent discharge occurring in one nostril is suggestive of a foreign object in the other nostril. The septum is inspected for the midline position. Maxillary sinuses are detected via x-ray exam by age 4, with other sinuses radiologically evident by age six (Bickley & Szilagyi, 2007). These areas are palpated for tenderness, using the thumbs of both hands and holding the child's head.

Throat/Mouth Assessment

The examination of the throat and mouth is saved for last in younger, less cooperative children. The nurse may ask the child to see "all of the tongue." Eliciting the sound "eeehh" flattens the tongue better than "aaahh" and visualization of the posterior pharynx is possible without the use of the tongue blade. The palate, uvula, tonsils, and mucous membranes are observed and assessed for color, exudate, and odor. The lips are observed for shape, symmetry, color, dryness, fissures at the corners of the mouth indicative of B_2 (riboflavin) deficiency, and clefts.

The teeth are inspected for number present, condition, color, alignment, and caries. Tooth eruptions occur at varying rates. Generally, when counting teeth on visual examination, the nurse can expect one tooth per month after 6 months of age until all 20 deciduous teeth are in place. The gingival tissue is inspected for color and condition. The gingival tissue is the same color as the surrounding mucous membranes and should not be hypertrophied or show evidence of bleeding.

Chest Assessment

The nurse inspects the chest for size, shape, symmetry, respiratory effort, and breast development. In infants, the anteroposterior diameter is fairly equal to the lateral diameter. By 2 years of age, the lateral diameter is greater than the anteroposterior diameter. Equal anteroposterior and lateral diameter after the age of 2 years may indicate chronic lung disease. A chest that is larger on the left than on the right may indicate an enlarged heart or a collapsed right lung. Pectus carinatum (pigeon chest) and pectus excavatum (funnel chest) are abnormal chest shapes caused by sternal deviations. Pectus carinatum is a protrusion of the sternum. Pectus excavatum is a depression of the lower portion of the sternum.

 Nursing Insight— *Retractions*

With any increased work of breathing, retractions are observed. When the trachea or the smaller airways of the lungs experience air flow restriction, the pressure within the chest is reduced. As a result, the intercostal muscles are drawn inward in an attempt to assist in breathing. This drawing inward is visible as intercostal retractions. Retractions may also be seen in the substernal, subcostal, and suprasternal notch regions.

Normal breast development begins in girls between 10 and 14 years of age. Boys also undergo breast changes and many show evidence of breast development. For the female, the breast development is documented using the Tanner Staging Guidelines.

Breast enlargement in the neonate is normal, and is a result of maternal hormones. This enlargement subsides over the first 30 days of life. Breast assessment is important at every well-child visit for early detection of precocious puberty. Girls must be taught breast self-exam when breast tissue begins to develop.

Lung Assessment

Lung sounds are best auscultated with the child in a sitting position. The nurse instructs the child to take slow deep breaths through an open mouth. Using a stethoscope with an appropriately sized pediatric diaphragm, the nurse systematically auscultates the five lobes of the lungs, anteriorly and posteriorly, beginning with the apices and then moving side to side to compare bilateral lung sounds. In an infant, auscultation of lung sounds is best done early in the exam, while the child is quiet.

Direct observation of breathing can also indicate inadequate oxygenation. For instance, a child with tachypnea (rapid respiratory rate, 80 to 120 breaths/minute), shallow breathing, and use of accessory muscles means respiratory distress. On the other hand, the child with slow breathing means the child does not have the energy for adequate oxygenation. Quiet breath sounds with an increased work of breathing means that air is not entering into the lung fields. An alteration in depth hyperpnea (too deep) is associated with fever and hypopnea (to shallow) is associated with central nervous system depression.

The child's posture can also indicate adequate or inadequate oxygenation. The child in respiratory distress sits in a tripod position sitting upright, leaning forward on outstretched arms with the jaw thrust forward. This particular position helps maximize opening up the airway and use of accessory muscles of respiration. Because a child with respiratory difficulties is often anxious, it is important to allow him to assume the position of comfort, which is usually the position that is easiest for the child to breathe.

 Nursing Insight— *Lung Assessment*

The nurse will more accurately assess the lungs by creating a quiet environment, placing the child in the best position for auscultation, warming the diaphragm of the stethoscope before auscultation, placing the stethoscope on the child's bare skin, and comparing bilateral breath sounds.

BREATH SOUNDS. Normal breath sounds can be classified as bronchial, bronchovesicular, or vesicular. Adventitious sounds of these three classifications are described as crackles, wheezes, and rhonchi, respectively. Bronchial breath sounds are loud, high-pitched, and heard only over the trachea. The inspiratory and expiratory sounds are equal in length. Bronchovesicular breath sounds are of intermediate intensity and pitch, with equal inspiratory and expiratory phases. These sounds are best heard between the scapulae and over the mainstem bronchi. If bronchial or bronchovesicular sounds are heard elsewhere, it is indicative of an area of consolidation. Vesicular breath sounds are heard throughout the lung fields. These soft and low-pitched sounds have a longer inspiratory phase than an expiratory one. Decreased or absent breath sounds indicate a serious condition such as asthma, atelectasis, emphysema, pneumothorax, or acute respiratory distress syndrome (ARDS).

clinical alert

Important respiratory signals

The nurse must recognize that normal breath sounds are equal bilaterally in intensity, rhythm, and pitch. The following respiratory signals may indicate that a respiratory condition is present in a child:

- Noisy breathing or snoring (air passing through a narrowed upper airway) may indicate nasal polyps, foreign body obstruction, choanal obstruction, hypertrophied adenoid tissue or obesity.

- Grunting is caused by the glottis closing at the end of expiration and may suggest respiratory distress or pneumonia.

- Nasal flaring (intermittent outward movement of the nostrils) happens on inspiration and is a form of accessory muscle use found in a variety of conditions such as respiratory distress syndrome (Venes, 2009).

- Coughing (a forceful expiratory effort) is a normal process that clears the throat, but can indicate an infection, asthma, lung disease, or sinusitis.

- Stridor (a high-pitched, harsh sound occurring during inspiration) results from air moving through a narrowed trachea and larynx and can indicate croup (Venes, 2009).

- Wheezing (a musical noise) results from air moving through mucus or fluids in a narrowed lower airway that is associated with asthma.

- Hoarseness is a rough quality in the child's voice and can mean that the airway is inflamed.

- Crackles is a fine, high-pitched sound heard on inspiration or expiration produced by air passing over retained airway secretions or the sudden opening of collapsed airways found in several respiratory conditions (Venes, 2009).

- Rhonchi is a low-pitched wheezing, snoring, or squeaking sound indicating a partial airway obstruction. Mucus or other secretions in the airway, bronchial hyperreactivity, or tumors that occlude respiratory passages can cause the airway obstruction (Venes, 2009).

- Color changes in the skin (pallor, mottling, and cyanosis) are significant respiratory signals and usually indicate cardiac involvement.

- Chest pain is caused by alteration in chest structures, nonpulmonary involvement, or a variety of respiratory conditions.

- Clubbing (excessive growth of the soft tissues at the ends of the fingers or toes) is usually associated with chronic hypoxia and pulmonary disease.

critical nursing action Adventitious Lung Sounds

A 3-year-old child is brought into the clinic with a chief complaint of recent coughing. The mother states that the child has no fever or cold symptoms, but began to cough that day. The nurse auscultates all lung fields and hears wheezing and localized rhonchi on the left side, but normal vesicular sounds on the right side. The nurse must notify the health care provider immediately for further evaluation and treatment.

Cardiac Assessment

The chest is inspected for symmetry and pulsations and all peripheral pulses are palpated (Table 21-3). In slim children, pulsations from the heart may be visible. The nurse begins palpation with the carotid pulse, making note of any distended neck veins, and continues with the brachial and radial pulses. Capillary refill is assessed as well as changes in the fingernails, e.g., clubbing of the fingers is noted. Peripheral edema and cyanosis are assessed during palpation of the femoral, popliteal, posterior tibial, and dorsalis pedis pulses.

Continued palpation of the chest can identify the presence of thrills, which are a consequence of blood flowing rapidly from high pressure to low pressure. The rough vibrating sensations are felt by placing the palm of the hand over the chest. Some ventricular septal defects result in thrills at the lower left sternal border. Pulmonary stenosis may cause a thrill at the upper left sternal border, whereas aortic stenosis is frequently palpable in the suprasternal notch.

Nursing Insight— Point of Maximum Impulse (PMI)

The point of maximal impulse (PMI), or area of most intense pulsation, and the point of apical impulse, or the impulse corresponding to the apex of the heart, are usually located in the same area of the chest. Generally, the apical impulse is found just lateral of the left midclavicular line (MCL) and fourth intercostal space (ICS) in children younger than 7 years. For children older than 7 years, it is found in the fifth ICS. The stethoscope is placed over this area for auscultation of the apical pulse.

Auscultation begins with the diaphragm of the stethoscope and further evaluation of the heart sounds is done with the bell of the stethoscope (Fig. 21-6). To assess for the first heart sound (S_1—the "lub" sound), the nurse begins at the fourth or fifth *left* ICS at the MCL. The first heart sound reflects the closure of the mitral and tricuspid valves and signifies the beginning of ventricular contraction or systole. The second heart sound (S_2—the "dub" sound) reflects the closure of the pulmonary and aortic valves and signifies the beginning of atrial contraction or diastole. The nurse hears "lub dub."

During inspiration, the S_2 sound may be audible as a split sound as the pulmonary valve closes slightly later than the aortic valve. This physiological splitting is heard as a "lub-dub" and is within the context of normal. If splitting is also heard during expiration, this is suggestive of pulmonary valve pathology.

Two other heart sounds may be heard during the cardiac cycle. The S_3 and S_4 heart sounds are both heard in diastole. A physiological S_3 is heard frequently in children and young adults. It is heard best at the apex in a left lateral lying position by listening for the sound in early diastole

Table 21-3 Cardiac Assessment Techniques

Assessment Technique	What to Look for	Normal Findings	Abnormal Findings	Rationale
Inspection	Skin color, shape and symmetry of chest, clubbing	Pink, symmetrical chest	Pallor, cyanosis, asymmetry of chest shape and movement, hyperdynamic precordium	Poor cardiac output; deoxygenated circulating blood, ventricular failure or hypertrophy, tachycardia
Palpation	Skin and body temperature, moisture, chest movement, point of maximal impulse (PMI)	Warm, dry, symmetrical movement, PMI at 4th or 5th ICS at midclavicular line	Cold extremities, dry flaky skin, diaphoresis; thrills or heaves	Poor circulation, heart failure, ventricular hypertrophy
Percussion	Heart shape and size	Normal size and shape for age and weight	Enlarged heart, axis deviation	Heart failure and hypertrophy
Auscultation	Murmurs, other sounds	No murmurs, innocent murmurs; quiet precordium	Murmurs, clicks, rubs, snaps	Structural defects, increased workload of heart and volume overload

© Judith M. Marshall (2006).

right after the S_2. It is called a ventricular gallop and, due to the cadence of the rhythm, sounds like the word "Kentucky." Although an S_3 is most likely a finding not associated with heart disease, the finding should be documented and reported. S_4, heard in late diastole, is heard only in children who have congenital heart disease such as pulmonary hypertension and pulmonic stenosis. It is never a normal finding and must be reported to the primary health care provider. The sound is sometimes compared to the word "Tennessee."

Murmurs are attributed to turbulent blood flow within the vessels. The nurse assesses for intensity, location, radiation, timing, and quality. Innocent murmurs are systolic, musical, or vibratory and of low intensity. The Still's murmur is the most common murmur and is located over the mid or lower left sternal border. This murmur may be heard in well children, those with fever, after exercise, or in children with anemia when cardiac output is increased. A venous hum is a continuous soft, hollow sound that disappears when the child is supine. Diastolic murmurs usually indicate pathology.

Abdominal Assessment

The child should lie quietly in the supine position. The assessment begins with an inspection of the abdomen and its contour, which may be flat, round, protuberant, or scaphoid (shaped like a boat). Visible peristalsis may be noted in a thin child, and should be documented and reported. The umbilicus and inguinal areas are inspected for bulging, and note is made of any scars, rashes, and lesions or piercings.

The abdomen is divided into four quadrants: right upper quadrant (RUQ), left upper quadrant (LUQ), right lower quadrant (RLQ), and left lower quadrant (LLQ) (Fig. 21-7). The terms epigastric, umbilical, periumbilical, and suprapubic can also be used to describe symptoms and physical findings that are specific to these areas. The nurse must listen for up to 1 minute before determining the absence of bowel sounds in any one quadrant.

After inspection, the abdomen is auscultated in all four quadrants to assess for bowel motility. These high-pitched sounds occur every 5 to 10 seconds, so it is important for the nurse to allow enough time to adequately assess frequency and character of the bowel sounds. The absence of bowel sounds or high-pitched tinkles in the presence of abdominal distention and/or peritoneal signs suggest an acute abdominal condition. A child who is experiencing signs of a bowel obstruction has absent bowel sounds below the obstruction.

Figure 21-6 Four points of cardiac auscultation.

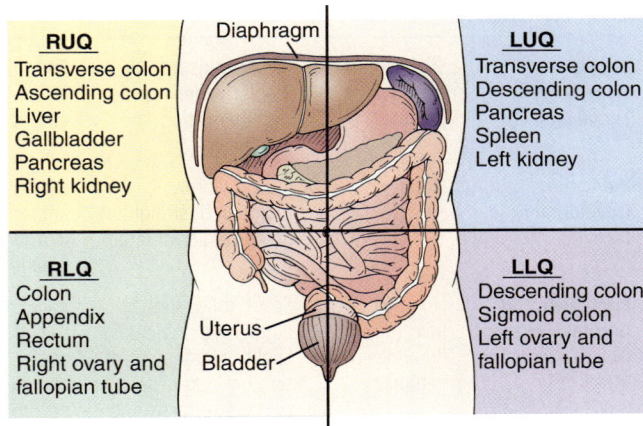

Figure 21-7 Abdomen divided into quadrants and organs in each quadrant.

Palpation of the abdomen occurs last so as not to disrupt bowel sounds. Palpation is divided into light palpation and deep palpation. Light palpation assists in identifying abdominal tenderness. Deep palpation is useful when assessing for the liver, kidneys, spleen, inguinal lymph nodes, and abnormal masses. If a mass is encountered, it is reported, noting its location, size, shape, consistency, and tenderness. Throughout the abdominal assessment, the nurse observes for changes in facial expression, guarding, and tensing of the abdominal muscles.

 Nursing Insight— *Palpation of the abdomen*

To minimize the sensation of tickling during palpation of the abdomen the nurse may palpate through a layer of light clothing or place the child's hand on top of the nurse's hand while palpating. To relax the abdominal muscles, bend the child's knees until feet are flat on the exam table. Palpate any tender or painful areas last. The suprapubic area may feel tender if the child's bladder is full. Consider having the child empty their bladder before the abdominal assessment.

Genitourinary and Perineal Assessment

Both males and females are assessed for Tanner staging of hair growth, evidence of normal development for the age of the child, signs of sexual abuse, and precocious puberty (Table 21-4).

FEMALE GENITALIA. The femoral nodes should be palpated. Enlarged nodes may indicate the presence of a sexually transmitted infection or something as simple as an inflamed hair follicle after shaving. The external genitalia of the female (the labia minora, labia majora, clitoris, vaginal opening, and urinary meatus) are examined for the presence of lesions, discharge, and irritation. The nurse must be able to visualize the vaginal and urethral openings. Occasionally the labia minora are fused due to adhesions, making this assessment difficult to impossible; this finding must be reported to the primary health care provider for further evaluation and separation of the labia minora. A malodorous vaginal discharge may indicate the presence of a foreign body, especially in young children, or an infection. In the neonate, the labia majora is often under developed and does not cover the labia minora. This is even more pronounced in the premature. Vaginal exams in young children need to be completed by trained examiners. The American Academy of Pediatrics recommends the first annual pelvic exam between the ages of 18 and 21 or when the girl becomes sexually active, regardless of age (AAP, 2007).

MALE GENITALIA. The penis is inspected for size, presence of foreskin, placement of the urinary meatus, and signs of inflammation and infections. The penis should be straight, the glans clean and smooth, and the slit-shaped urinary meatus near the end of the glans.

 Nursing Insight— *Uncircumcised Males*

The foreskin of uncircumcised males should not be forcibly retracted until after 1 year of age. After 1 year of age, genital retraction and subsequently replacing the foreskin to its neutral position is possible.

Palpate the penis for masses and nodules. Inspect the scrotum for size, shape, symmetry, and presence of testicles. An enlarged scrotum should be transilluminated to assess for hydrocele versus a possible hernia. The nurse places a penlight under the scrotum; the scrotum will exhibit a red glow with a hydrocele, but not with a hernia. The testicles are palpated for size and shape. Testicles are roughly the same size and smooth in contour. A testicle that is hard or in which a nodule is palpated must be reported to the primary health care provider to further rule out a tumor. The nurse must also report if one or both testicles have not descended. Males are instructed in testicular self-examination by the age of 14 years. Testicular cancer, while rare, is the most common cancer in men age 15 to 35 years (Nemours Foundation, 2007).

Table 21-4 Tanner Staging of Development of Secondary Sex Characteristics					
Sex Characteristics	**Scoring**				
	1	**2**	**3**	**4**	**5**
Breast Development in Females	Slight to no elevation of papilla	Breast buds appear; areolar widening with slight elevation	Entire breast enlarged with no protrusion of the papilla or nipple	Enlargement of the entire breast with formation of secondary mound of areola and papilla	Mature breast with protrusion of nipple only. No protrusion of the papilla
Pubic Hair Development in Females	None	Sparse, lightly pigmented, straight along border of labia	Darker and increasing amount on labia and pubis. Distribution in typical female inverted triangle	Coarse, thicker, curly. Increasing amount, less than adult.	Adult female triangle with extension of hair onto medial thighs
Pubic Hair and Genital Development in Males	No pubic hair. Preadolescent genitalia	Scant, long, slightly pigmented pubic hair. Slight enlargement of scrotum and testes; scrotum reddens and becomes more textured	Pubic hair darker, starting to curl and extends across pubis. Scrotum and testes continue to enlarge. Penis becomes longer and slightly wider	Pubic hair is coarse, curly, less quantity than adult. Scrotum is darker; penis increases in length and breadth. Glans is broader.	Adult distribution of pubic hair with extension to medial thighs; genitalia adult in size and shape

Adapted from Tanner, J.M. (1962). *Growth at adolescence* (2nd ed.). Oxford: Blackwell Scientific.

ANAL EXAMINATION. The anus is not routinely examined in children unless indicated by abdominal, bowel, rectal, or stool abnormalities. If an anal examination is indicated, the child is placed in a side-lying position with the knees flexed. The area is examined for anal placement, lesions, trauma, irritation, fissures, bleeding, leakage of stool, and hemorrhoids, as well as general cleanliness. Tone can be assessed by lightly touching the anus and observing for the anal reflex. If a digital exam is necessary, educate the child about the procedure in an age-appropriate manner, provide distraction during the procedure, and ask the child to "push down like he is trying to poop" to help relax the anal sphincter.

Musculoskeletal Assessment

Much of the musculoskeletal exam can be done while observing the child enter and move about the exam room. The child is observed for range of motion, symmetry of movement, general alignment, and any deformities. Each joint is palpated for range of motion and the presence of any erythema or swelling.

The child's muscles are assessed for strength of movement. For upper extremity strength, the child is asked to hold both arms out to the sides and then out to the front. The child is asked to hold these positions as the nurse applies downward pressure to both arms. The symmetry of strength in both hands can be assessed by having the child squeeze the nurse's index fingers. The strength of the legs can be tested by asking the child who is lying supine to raise his legs while the nurse applies downward pressure on the legs. Screening for scoliosis is usually done at age 14. A scoliometer can be used to assess for the condition as well as noting if the back appears straight and the hips are even.

Neurological Assessment

Mental status can be assessed by observing the infant interact with the parent, or by asking the older child to answer questions and listening for clear speech in the responses. This can be assessed in the course of a normal interview. Most of the assessment of motor functioning is done during the skeletal examination. In addition, the child can be asked to hop, skip, or jump to assess symmetry of movement. The nurse might suggest a game such as 'hop on one foot.' Sensory testing is done if there is a question regarding sensory functioning.

Cerebellar function is checked by observing the child's posture and gait or by using the finger-to-nose test. Young children perceive this test as a game and readily cooperate. The Romberg test assesses cerebellar functioning; the child stands with eyes closed and arms outstretched and is assessed for the ability to stand without swaying.

The child is also assessed for persistence of primitive reflexes, which normally disappear during infancy. Babinski, Moro, palmar, plantar, and tonic neck reflexes are a few that are seen in the neonate but that disappear over time. Persistence of these reflexes may indicate cerebral dysfunction. Deep-tendon reflexes (DTRs) are elicited using the reflex hammer. DTRs are difficult to elicit in some children and a distraction may be needed while testing reflexes.

Cranial nerve assessment is an integral part of the physical examination and may be completed throughout the exam or as a separate part of the exam (Table 21-5). For instance, the nurse can assess the muscles for facial expression during the interview. The nurse also examines

Table 21-5	Cranial Nerve Testing
Cranial Nerve	**How to Test**
I. Olfactory	Ask the child to close both eyes and have the child identify smells. Rarely done during a routine examination.
II. Optic	Perform vision screen for test of visual acuity and color vision, test for peripheral vision, and examine the optic disc with the ophthalmoscope.
III. Oculomotor	Ask the child to follow an object through the six cardinal positions of gaze. Assess for pupillary response and drooping of upper lids.
IV. Trochlear	CN III, IV, and VI are tested together.
V. Trigeminal	Observe child chewing on a cracker. With eyes closed, gently stroke different areas of the face with a cotton ball to assess sensory function.
VI. Abducens	CN III, IV, and VI are tested together.
VII. Facial	Observe child's facial expressions during the interview and exam. May need to ask child to frown and then smile.
VIII. Acoustic	Cause a loud sound and assess if child turns to the sound.
IX. Glossopharyngeal	Stimulate gag reflex.
X. Vagus	Assess uvula in midline. Assess ability to swallow by asking child to do so.
XI. Accessory	As the nurse provides resistance, ask child to shrug shoulders and turn head side to side.
XII. Hypoglossal	Observe infant sucking on a bottle. Ask child to stick out the tongue. Listen for clarity of speech.

the pharynx, tongue, and muscles of mastication during the examination of the mouth. The nurse understands that abnormal results of the cranial nerve exam may indicate a brain injury, infection, or compression of a particular nerve.

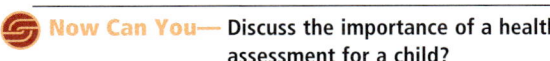 **Now Can You**— Discuss the importance of a health assessment for a child?

1. State the major components of a health assessment for the child?
2. Describe alterations in a health assessment for the child?

ROUTINE HEALTH SCREENING

Children are screened for lead poisoning and iron-deficient anemia during well-child care visits. Children with a positive family history for acquired cardiac disease or hypercholesterolemia may be screened for elevated cholesterol levels. High-risk children are screened for tuberculosis.

Lead Poisoning Screening

Routine screening for lead poisoning occurs during the latter part of infancy. The incidence of lead poisoning has decreased with the removal of sources of lead in gasoline, lead paint, and water supplies. However, lead can be found in tap water and in some folk medicines. Visit http://www.cdc.gov/nceh/lead/publications/books/plpyc/chapter3.htm#top for more information on the prevention of lead poisoning in children.

Ethnocultural Considerations— Lead exposure in folk medicines

Folk medicines used by Indian, Middle Eastern, West Asian, and Hispanic cultures may contain high levels of lead. During a health assessment interview, inquire as to the use of Greta, Azarcon (coral, luiga, maria luisa, or rueda), Ghasard, or Ba-baw-san.

Across Care Settings: Decreasing exposure to lead

Nurses can promote decreased lead exposure in tap water by encouraging parents to contact the water authority to determine the lead content in the water. The EPA states that 15 parts per billion is acceptable. If mixing formula from powder or concentrate, advise parents to flush water from the system by running the tap for 1–2 minutes before using the water. Most of the lead comes from the corrosion of older pipes that leach into the water supply after sitting in the pipes for several hours.

Iron-Deficiency Anemia Screening

Iron-deficiency anemia is screened in children by hemoglobin and hematocrit measurements. Since children are at risk for anemia in infancy, screening is done in the latter stage of infancy. However, the incidence of iron-deficiency anemia is declining with an overall prevalence of 7% in children 1 to 2 years of age. The U.S. Preventive Services Task Force (USPSTF) has determined that there is insufficient evidence to recommend for or against routine screening for iron deficiency anemia in asymptomatic children 6 to 12 months of age. Continued screening of high-risk children is recommended (USPSTF, 2006).

Cholesterol Screening

Children from families with hypercholesterolemia are candidates for cholesterol screening. For children with cholesterol levels greater than or equal to 200, weight loss is recommended (Newman & Garber, 2003). Further, the discontinuance of saturated fat from the diet of a child may decrease the cholesterol. A child should not be placed on a weight reduction diet without proper guidance from a health care professional.

Tuberculosis Screening

Tuberculosis (TB) screening is recommended for children at high risk; those who are foreign-born; those who travel to or have household visitors from a country with a high prevalence of TB; and those in contact with people who are homeless, incarcerated, infected with HIV, or are intravenous drug users. Other risk factors include living with a household member who has an active case of TB, a chronic condition such as diabetes or renal failure, or who is immunocompromised. Tuberculin skin testing (TST) for latent TB infection is administered to children who have one or more risk factors (Reznik & Ozuah, 2006).

General Care Measures for the Child in the Hospital or Clinic Setting

The child who requires general care in the hospital or clinic setting may be admitted for testing or treatment of an illness or disease. Parents may wish to provide much of the care their child needs in regard to bathing and feeding. These measures are comforting to the child and parent and reduce anxiety in both. The nurse is responsible for these activities in addition to the child's safety. General care measures include: bathing, feeding, rest and safety, infection control, and fever reducing measures. The nurse also provides emotional and spiritual support as needed.

BATHING

Family home practices and preferences for bathing are assessed on admission of the child. Bathing of infants can be accomplished at the bedside using a portable tub. For infants younger than 6 months or for those who have head lag, the nurse supports the head and neck with one hand while using the other hand to wash. If a tub bath is contraindicated, a bed bath can be given. Precautions are taken to control the water temperature so that it does not exceed 100°F (37.8°C), and to quickly cover areas of the body after washing. The parent may welcome the respite from caring for the child or may wish to continue bathing the child in the hospital. Toddlers and preschoolers may enjoy a bath in a larger tub. Although they can wash some body areas without supervision, most children need reminders or prompting to wash. A child is never left alone while tub bathing. Older children may be able to shower and groom themselves with little assistance. Privacy is valued by the older child. A child who is feeling ill or who has tubes, drains, or dressings may be unable to ambulate to the bathroom for washing or to immerse herself in water. A sponge bath is appropriate in this case.

Shampooing hair during the bath may be part of daily care for children. Again, the nurse can assess family preferences and practices. Shampoo basins can be used at the bedside to wash hair. African American children or those with braiding or dreadlocks require special care. Braids are left in place for several weeks and care of the hair and scalp is individualized for each child. Parents may be asked for instructions in hair care.

The nurse can use bath time to observe parent–child interaction and to assess the child. Language skills and social skills can also be assessed during the bath. The skin is assessed for lesions, rashes, turgor, color, and circulatory integrity. Muscle tone is easily assessed along with adequate respiratory status. This can also be a time for the child to become acquainted with the nurse as a caring, supportive person.

critical nursing action Key Actions in Caring for the Child Confined to Bed

The child confined to bed is at risk for skin breakdown. The nurse should do the following:

- Keep the skin clean and dry.
- Assess nutritional status for adequate protein.
- Use the draw sheet for position changes.
- Assess skin for irritated areas.
- Assess for pressure ulcers by looking for the "red flush" (the first sign of tissue compromise and ischemia).

FEEDING

Basic knowledge of nutritional requirements is essential when working with children. Formula-fed infants require no more than 24 to 32 ounces of iron-fortified formula daily. For infants who have a gastrointestinal disturbance, pulmonary failure, or are in congestive heart failure, it may be difficult to ingest the required amount of calories without tiring and gavage feedings may be necessary.

For the older child, assess preferences by taking a diet history and asking about routines at mealtimes. Children are often prescribed an "as tolerated" diet and they are able to select foods that appeal to them. It is best to gently encourage the intake of wholesome and nutritious foods and snacks. Foods ingested are also important for their fluid content (e.g., gelatin and ice pops). Parents can be encouraged to bring in favorite foods from home. Cultural preferences may make a difference in whether or not a child eats while hospitalized. Foods and caloric intake should be appropriate for age and developmental level (Table 21-6).

 Nursing Insight— Encouraging adequate food and fluid intake

- Offer small portions at frequent intervals.
- Host a "tea party" using medicine cups filled with the child's favorite drink.
- Make food into fun shapes (trace a smile face with a spread on a sandwich; use a cookie cutter to make different shapes for sandwiches).
- Offer incentives of more time doing a favored activity.
- Offer two choices ("Would you like to use a straw or a colored cup for your drink?"). This allows autonomy.

Table 21-6 Average Daily Caloric Requirements for Children

Age	Daily Caloric Requirements
0–1 month	100–110 kcal/kg per day
2–4 months	90–100 kcal/kg per day
5–60 months	70–90 kcal/kg per day
>5 years	1500 kcal for first 20 kg + 25 kcal for each additional kg

Source: Hay W.W. Jr. (2005). *Current pediatric diagnosis & treatment* (17th ed.). New York: Lange Medical Books/McGraw-Hill.

REST

Hospitalization disrupts a child's normal daily routine as well as their sleep pattern. The pediatric nurse can assess normal sleep patterns, including information on both nighttime hours of sleep and daytime naps. Most pediatric units allow parents to "sleep-in." This provides both the parent and child with comfort and creates an environment with decreased levels of unfamiliarity and anxiety. The nurse understands that children up to the age of 5 may take an afternoon nap. If the child's condition allows, uninterrupted naptimes should be included in the plan of care.

SAFETY MEASURES

Safety measures instituted on a pediatric unit are based on the developmental level of each child to protect him from harm. Safety measures include keeping toxic materials out of reach, identifying children with name bands, and knowing the whereabouts of children on the unit. The nurse must also provide a safe environment in the hospital room and in the transport of children from their room to other departments in the hospital.

clinical alert

Keeping children safe in the home or hospital

In the home, parents must think like a child thinks. Suggest that parents get down on the floor in their home to see what their child sees (e.g., electrical plugs and outlets, tablecloths ready to be pulled, hot coffee mugs on the edge of the table).

In the hospital, toxic and nontoxic materials should be stored in a locked utility room, on the top shelf of a cabinet, or in another location where children do not have ready access. Utility rooms, kitchens, medication carts, treatment rooms, and supply rooms are locked, denying access to children. Play areas should be locked unless the child is accompanied by an adult.

The nurse verifies the child's identity by checking the name band before any treatment or medication is administered. Name bands can be removed by the child easily or they may inadvertently fall off leaving the nurse with no means to verify a child's identity. If a child is found without a name band, the child's name must be verified and a new name band applied to an extremity. The nurse cannot depend on all children to correctly identify themselves. Younger children may answer to any name or may not answer at all. When a name band is not on a child's extremity, medications or treatments are administered only after a parent or nurse has identified the child and the name band has been replaced.

The nurse is responsible for keeping children safe on the pediatric unit. Many pediatric units have alarms and restricted access at stairways, elevators, and the entrance to the unit. The nurse can review with the older child the places she is allowed to go and the activities she can engage in while a patient on the unit. Limits must be set and enforced. To prevent child abduction, pediatric personnel need to be vigilant about visitors.

In the child's room, safety features are used on high chairs and strollers, and beds are kept in the locked position with the height of the bed in the lowest position. Crib side rails are elevated when the child is in the bed. Bubble tops may be needed to prevent a child from climbing over the rails. Check the room for any small articles that may be left behind in a bed, such as syringe covers and alcohol wipes. All items must be removed from the bed.

Safety concerns regarding the transport of children are based on their developmental level. Infants can be carried short distances in the room or on the unit. For longer transports to other areas of the hospital, bassinets, cribs, strollers, wheelchairs, or special vehicles are used (e.g., wagon with raised sides). The wagon can be painted in bright colors, and some have plastic bubble tops in the shape of small automobiles. Children enjoy this type of transport. It is important to check that restraint devices like a seat belt in a stroller are securely fastened and that the child is not left unattended during transport.

INFECTION CONTROL MEASURES

Transmission of infection requires three essential elements: an offending microorganism, a susceptible host, and a method of transmission to infect the host. The offending microorganism can be brought into the hospital setting with the ill child or can be part of the new environment. Main routes of transmission include contact, droplet, airborne, common vehicle, and vector borne. Fundamental isolation precautions include handwashing and gloving, the appropriate placement of a patient, and the use of barrier gear to protect the caregiver and prevent further transmission of infection.

The Healthcare Infection Control Practices Advisory Committee (HICPAC, 2008) lists two tiers of isolation precautions. The first tier is "standard precautions" that integrate the features of universal precautions designed to reduce the risk of transmission of blood borne pathogens. The second tier is "transmission-based precautions" that are intended to prevent the transmission of pathogens from those with infectious diseases. Transmission-based precautions include airborne, droplet, and contact precautions (Schulster et al., 2004). When caring for children in a hospitalized setting, the specific guidelines from the CDC should be followed for procedures related to precautions (Schulster et al., 2004).

clinical alert

Hand washing

The nurse knows that hand washing is essential prior to patient care. Hand washing removes microorganisms and can minimize infection to the patient. Meticulous hand washing also allows antimicrobial products to be effective against the transmission of infection.

The experience of isolation for a child can be perceived in negative ways. In the preschool years, when magical thinking is the predominant manner of processing information, the child may perceive the situation as a punishment for some previous thought or action. Koller, David, Goldie, Gearing, and Selkirk (2006) found that children placed in isolation because of the SARS (severe acute respiratory syndrome) outbreak in Canada experienced emotional upheaval. The authors recommended that nurses be aware of the difficult situation that existed and continue to provide family-centered care.

Once the precautions are in place, and the child and family are coping with the restrictions, children may need diversional activities. Child life specialists can assist in the selection of age-appropriate games and toys. Once a toy is brought into a precaution room, it must be cleaned before other children can play with the toy. Visitors need not be restricted from the room but they do need specific instructions on how to protect themselves and the patient. Guidelines are placed on the door with step-by-step instructions on what is required prior to entering the room. Hand washing before and after leaving the room is essential.

FEVER-REDUCING MEASURES

Fever (a temperature greater than 100.4°F [38.0°C]) accompanies many childhood illnesses. A fever is a natural and beneficial response to the invasion of an offending organism and can help "kill" the virus or bacteria. If a child with a fever is very uncomfortable and irritable his fever may be treated with antipyretics or by using environmental measures. Antipyretics work to lower the set point at the thermoregulatory center in the hypothalamus. Antipyretic drugs commonly administered to children include acetaminophen and nonsteroidal anti-inflammatory drugs (NSAIDs).

clinical alert

Aspirin (Salicylates)

Aspirin (Salicylates) is not given due to the correlation between the use of aspirin and the development of Reye's syndrome in children with viral infections.

Acetaminophen (Children's Tylenol) is available in suppository, liquid, and capsule form. It can be given every 4 hours with no more than five doses in a 24-hour period; there is little risk of hepatic toxicity. Ibuprofen (Children's Advil), a common NSAID, is given to children as a fever-reducing measure. This drug is given every 6 hours and may be an advantage when rest is crucial or when administering medications to the child is a challenging task. Dyspepsia and nausea are common side effects of ibuprofen. The medication, taken as a chewable tablet, caplet, or liquid, can be given with food or after meals if gastrointestinal (GI) upset occurs. The child should be monitored for GI bleeding. Dosing for ibuprofen is dependent on the

medication: Dosage Recommendations for Acetaminophen (Children's Tylenol)

Acetaminophen (a-seet-a-**min**-oh-fen)

Age:	Dosage (mg):
0–3 months	40
4–11 months	80
12–23 months	120
2–3 years	160
4–5 years	240
6–8 years	320
9–10 years	400
11 years	480

Data from Karch, A. (2006). *Lippincott's Nursing Drug Guide*. Philadelphia: Lippincott Williams & Wilkins.

temperature of the child. A fever below 102.6°F (39.2°C) warrants a dose of 5 mg/kg of body weight. If a child's temperature is over 102.6°F (39.2°C), the dose is increased to 10 mg/kg of body weight. The efficacy of antipyretic medication is assessed by retaking the child's temperature one hour after administration.

Environmental measures can be effective in reducing fevers in children. Measures that do not cause shivering are essential. Shivering produces heat, which is counterproductive in reducing fever. Cooling measures, such as reducing room temperature, applying cool compresses to the skin, and wearing a light layer of clothing, are effective alone or when administered 1 hour after an antipyretic is given.

A cooling blanket, which has coils through which a refrigerated solution circulates, may be necessary to control hyperthermia. The cooling blanket is placed on the bed, covered with a sheet, connected, and set to a temperature of 98.6°F (37°C). The temperature is decreased according to the child's response to cooling. Rectal temperature must be monitored every 15 minutes while the child is on the machine, and the child must be assessed for shivering. Cooling blankets are only used in circumstances warranting an immediate drop of a very high fever.

EMOTIONAL AND SPIRITUAL SUPPORT

Parents may be in need of emotional and spiritual support when a child is hospitalized. It is important for the nurse to be "in the moment" with parents and other family members. Conveying a caring attitude and listening closely to what the parent is really saying is important in making a connection with them. The relationship that the nurse creates with parents and family members is basic to healing and is an expression of spirituality (Dossey, Keegan, Guzzetta, & Kolkmeier, 2005).

The nurse helps family members by listening to their concerns, clarifying any misconceptions, and helping the family develop coping strategies to decrease stress and optimize functioning. Coping resources include using both the strength from within and the support from resources in the community.

Collaboration in Caring— *Spiritual care*

The parents and child may find comfort in talking with a priest, monk, chaplain, deacon, rabbi, imam, or other trusted person with religious ties. Spiritual care may come from a particular faith community that has shared beliefs and values. At times when parents ask "why is this happening to my child?" it may be beneficial for the nurse to arrange a meeting with people from their faith community to discuss the parents concerns and issues.

Common Procedures for the Child in the Hospital or Clinic Setting

EXPLAINING PROCEDURES

As a child develops cognitively, his understanding of the world changes. To an adolescent, a venipuncture may be an annoyance, but to a toddler, it may be a frightening

experience that is stressful not only to the child but to the parent as well. Developmental characteristics dictate how to approach the child and what to say to the child. What the nurse conveys to the patient and the parents can diminish the anxiety and fearfulness associated with common procedures.

 critical nursing action Preparing an Infant for a Procedure

- Describe the procedure to the parents, explaining what will happen and how long it will take. Encourage the parent to stop you at any point if there is a question.
- Remind parents that infants often cry for reasons other than discomfort, but be honest about any discomfort the infant may experience with the procedure.
- Identify what restraints may be used and give an explanation as to why they are needed.
- Allow parents to decide whether they would like to be present for the procedure. Parents may prefer to leave the room and return immediately following the procedure to comfort their child.

 critical nursing action Preparing a Toddler for a Procedure

- Describe the procedure to the parents, explaining what will happen and how long it will take.
- Use play to demonstrate the procedure to the toddler; encourage him to demonstrate/practice with a doll or teddy bear.
- Use simple, concrete language to describe the procedure and how it might feel to the toddler. Limit preparation to 5–10 minutes due to the short attention span of the toddler.
- Identify what restraints may be used and give an explanation as to why they are needed.
- Allow parents to decide whether they would like to be present for the procedure. Parents may prefer to leave the room and return immediately after the procedure to comfort their child. Allow the parents to stroke their child or speak soothingly to their child if they remain in the room.

 critical nursing action Preparing a Preschooler for a Procedure

Explain the procedure in terminology the child can understand. *Begin* preparation immediately prior to the procedure so the child will not worry for hours or days. *Use* play to demonstrate the procedure to the child; encourage her to demonstrate/practice with a doll or teddy bear.

Set limits for the child so she is aware of expectations. For example, tell her she can yell and scream as much as she wants, but must hold very still. *Give* legitimate choices to the child whenever possible. *Allow* parents to decide whether they would like to be present for the procedure. Parents may prefer to leave the room and return immediately after the procedure to comfort their child. Allow the parents to stroke their child or speak soothingly to their child if they remain in the room. *Use* distraction techniques such as deep breathing, singing, or squeezing a parent or nurse's hand.

Nursing Insight— Distraction

A distraction kit is a set of materials that help divert the child's attention to a more pleasant experience than the painful experience.

- Appropriate for any age
- Use before, during and after procedure
- Can also suggest holding someone's hand really tight, say 'ouch' really loud, count to 10 or count backwards, sing a song, pretend to be somewhere else.

Environment:

- Use designated treatment rooms when possible.
- Child's inpatient room should be kept as a 'safe area' whenever possible.
- Optimal lighting for a procedure should be sufficiently bright and focused on safety, but otherwise without glare.

Preparations:

- Parent: Relieve parental anxiety so they can help prepare and reassure the child/youth. Provide an explanation of what they will see and hear.
- Patient: Relieve patient anxiety. Use simple explanations that are developmentally appropriate to explain how, why, where and when.

Source: Stollery Children's Hospital, Edmonton, Alberta, Canada.

 critical nursing action Preparing a School-Age Child for a Procedure

Explain the procedure in terminology that the child can understand. Children in this stage of development have a good concept of time, so preparation can begin in advance of the procedure.

For the younger school-age child, *use play to demonstrate* the procedure and if possible have the child demonstrate on and practice positioning with a doll or teddy bear. *Allow* the child to touch and explore equipment to be used in the procedure, and involve the child in simple tasks during the procedure when possible. *Set limits* for the child so she is aware of expectations. For example, tell her she can yell and scream as much as she wants, but must hold very still. Give legitimate choices to the child whenever possible. *Allow* parents and the child to decide together whether parents will be present for the procedure. Some school-age children may be modest about exposing body parts in front of family members. Allow the parents to stroke their child or speak soothingly to their child if they remain in the room. *Teach* the child techniques such as deep breathing, counting, reciting a silly rhyme, or anything else that might help distract and relax the child during the procedure.

 critical nursing action Preparing an Adolescent for a Procedure

Describe the procedure, explaining exactly what will happen and how long it will take.

Encourage the adolescent to stop you at any point if she has a question. *Be honest. Describe* potential risks and pain associated with the procedure, but don't dwell on it. *Allow* the adolescent to take as active a role as possible in the procedure. Practicing positioning or demonstrating the equipment prior to the procedure will help give the adolescent

sense of control. Provide a peer video of the procedure if possible. *Allow* the adolescent to make decisions such as when the procedure should take place, if possible. Allow the adolescent the option of having a parent present. *Offer* tips for distraction such as deep breathing, relaxation, counting, or squeezing an object or parent's hand.

 critical nursing action Before, During, and After a Procedure

Before:

1. Think through the procedure in advance and anticipate problems.
2. Gather all equipment and check to make sure it functions properly.
3. Establish trust. Get to know the child first.
4. Through the use of play, allow the child to "perform" the procedure on her doll, teddy bear, or other appropriate surrogate.
5. Offer a coping strategy such as guided imagery or relaxation breathing.
6. Give the child realistic choices.
7. Be sure informed consent is signed.
8. Wash hands.
9. Let the child know that it is "OK" to cry.

During:

1. Whenever possible, all treatments need to be scheduled away from the child's bed or "safe area."
2. Expect the child to do well.
3. Talk to the child and ask how he is doing.
4. Keep the child informed as to the progress of the procedure.
5. Use distraction techniques such as pop-up picture books, bubbles, "shutting off the pain switch," or other techniques that have been practiced before the procedure.
6. When appropriate, give the child some control by allowing him to make some of the decisions.
7. Involve the parent to provide comfort to the child, if the parent is able. Sometimes a parent's presence at the procedure may not be beneficial for the child.

After:

1. Praise the child for completing the procedure.
2. Provide an opportunity for the child to verbalize feelings.
3. If the parents were not involved in the procedure, comment on a positive aspect involving the child during the procedure. "Jill was able to help out and keep still when she was asked to do so! She did a great job!"
4. Give a reward (stickers, small toy, previously agreed-upon reward negotiated with parents).
5. Document the child's response to procedure and outcomes.

❝ What to say ❞ — *Using developmentally appropriate words*

For children with beginning language skills, use simple terms that are familiar to the child, such as "go potty," "owie," and "boo boo." For the concrete thinker who takes what is said literally, do not use words that may frighten the child (e.g., "*dye* in your vein," "*shot* in the arm," "*cut* out the tonsils," and "*take* your temperature"). Instead, use "*special medicine* in your vein," "*special medicine* in your arm," "*make* your tonsils *better*," "*check* to see if your temperature *is working*." For all children, be honest and they will learn to trust you.

INFORMED CONSENT

Informed consent involves providing the patient with the necessary knowledge to make a decision regarding health care. Informed consent implies that the person understands the benefits and risks of treatment or the refusal of treatment. The person must also be legally able to give consent by virtue of his age. In most of the United States and Canadian provinces, the age of majority is 18. An exception is made for the adolescent younger than 18 who is married, a parent, self-supporting, or a member of the military (Feldman-Winter & McAbee, 2002). Informed consent can be obtained from these emancipated minors. In some jurisdictions, the age of consent varies for girls aged 14 years and older for contraception advice and gynecological procedures. For most children, the parent or legal guardian is the person who gives consent for their care.

Written informed consent is required before diagnostic procedures, medical treatments, or surgical procedures. It is also required prior to immunizations or any treatment with inherent risks.

 Be sure to— Obtain written consent before a procedure

Informed consent must be obtained before a procedure is performed. It is the physician's responsibility to explain the procedure and the risks and benefits of treatment. In addition, alternatives to the prescribed treatment should be discussed. When signed by the emancipated minor or parent, an informed consent is a legal document denoting that the emancipated minor or parent understands the nature of the procedure, risks, and benefits. The nurse serves as a witness to the signature.

 nursing diagnoses The Child Undergoing Procedures or Surgery

- Anxiety related to the procedure
- Pain related to break in skin integrity
- Knowledge Deficit related to unfamiliarity of procedure
- Interrupted Family Process related to demand of surgery
- Risk for Fluid Volume Deficit related to NPO status, nausea, vomiting, or bleeding

INTRAVENOUS LINES

Children may require intravenous therapy for treatment of dehydration. In the hospital, children may require intravenous therapy for fluid maintenance or replacement, before diagnostic testing, blood product replacement, or medication administration or preoperatively. Intravenous fluids may be administered through a peripheral line, a central venous access, or a peripherally inserted central catheter.

A peripheral line with a normal saline lock is used to keep the vein open (KVO) for the possibility of future intravenous therapy, or for the child who requires intermittent medication administration. The tubing is capped at the end with an injection cap that allows for multiple punctures. Once the medication is disconnected from this tubing, and the line flushed, the child can ambulate unencumbered by the IV pole and tubing. The hospital's protocol for flushing the peripheral intermittent infusion device is followed. The normal saline lock is secured to prevent accidental dislodgement. For the younger child who has a normal saline lock inserted in the dorsum of the hand, a cover with cling wrap may be necessary to prevent the child from manipulating or pulling out the normal saline lock (Fig. 21-8).

Children with a condition necessitating long-term intravenous access are candidates for central venous access devices. The intravenous catheter is inserted into a large vein such as the vena cava, subclavian, jugular, or femoral vein. Broviac, Hickman, and Groshong catheters are used for access. These catheters are multilumen and accommodate more than one intravenous therapy. After insertion, a chest x-ray exam is done to confirm proper positioning of the catheter. With a central venous access device, the child is not subjected to multiple intravenous "sticks." It is easily accessed for medication and fluid administration as well as blood draws, without the pain associated with further needle punctures.

The peripherally inserted central catheter line (PICC line) can be left in place for up to 4 months. It is inserted above the antecubital fossa into the median, cephalic or basilic vein and threaded into the superior vena cava. PICC lines are most often used for long-term antibiotic and analgesic therapy (Fig. 21-9). These lines may also be threaded just to the head of the clavicle. This is considered a midline placement and is often used for antibiotic therapy. The hospital's protocol for PICC line flushing and dressing changes over the insertion site is followed.

A vascular access port is another central venous access device that is implanted under the skin and is used for

 where research and practice meet: **Informed consent**

For children who are part of a research study, consent needs to be obtained (Lee, Haven, Sato, Hoffman, & Leuthner, 2006). Assent seeks to obtain the child's agreement to participate in the study and assurance that he understands all the material presented to him regarding the study. Depending on the age of the child, the material is presented in terms that the child can comprehend. Assent implies that sufficient education about the project, the process, and the consequences have been explained fully and that the child is sharing in the decision-making process.

Figure 21-8 Normal saline lock.

Figure 21-9 PICC line.

Figure 21-10 Infus-a-port.

long-term fluid or medication administration. The Infus-A-Port or Port-A-Cath is not visible and no dressing is required (Fig. 21-10). Although the child may be restricted from contact sports, he can swim or shower without restrictions. To access this device, the nurse palpates for placement, cleanses the area, and uses the Huber needle to puncture the port's central diaphragm.

 clinical alert

Risk of infection

With any procedure where the skin barrier is compromised, adhere to sterile techniques for dressing changes over IV sites and to monitor for signs and symptoms of infection: change in temperature, erythema, edema, pain at IV site, and tenderness on palpation.

Table 21-7	Calculation of Daily Maintenance Fluid Requirements	
Child's Weight	**Daily Maintenance Fluid Requirement**
0–10 kg	100 mL/kilogram of body weight
11–20 kg	1000 mL + 50 ml/kilogram for each kg >10
>20 kg	1500 mL + 20 ml/kilogram for each kg >20
Example:	
A child weighs 48 kg. For the first 20 kg the child needs 1500 mL. For the next 28 kg, the child needs 20 mL/kg. So,	
1500 mL + (28 kg × 20 mL) = 1500 mL + 560 mL = 2060 mL/day	

MEASURING INTAKE AND OUTPUT

The pediatric nurse carefully assesses the intake and output in children, especially those with vomiting, diarrhea, fever, nasogastric suctioning, draining wounds, and burns; presurgical patients; and children with cardiac, renal, or respiratory illnesses. Calculation of daily maintenance fluid requirements is described in Table 21-7. The nurse measures intake for the breastfed infant by recording "breastfed" (or by weighing the infant before and after the feeding and recording the increase in weight as ounces or milliliters consumed) on the intake sheet. For infants with congestive failure or a respiratory illness like bronchiolitis, the nurse also asks about the length of time the feeding took to complete. Expending too much energy in feeding may be deleterious to the child's health. Gavage feedings may be necessary for the child in congestive failure. Intravenous fluids may be required for the child struggling to breathe with a dyspneic respiratory condition.

For the child who wears diapers, the diaper can be weighed before and after use to determine urinary output. Diapers are weighed on a gram scale and output is determined by subtracting the weight of a dry diaper from the weight of a wet one. Each gram is equal to about one milliliter; therefore the difference is the amount of urine output in milliliters. The method used to measure normal urinary output is 1 to 2 mL/kg per hour.

X-RAY EXAMS

Children require x-ray exams for diagnostic purposes. They are also essential when checking for the placement of a chest tube, central line, or a feeding tube. For the younger child needing an x-ray exam the nurse may be asked to help position the child for an optimal view. A lead apron is worn to protect against unnecessary exposure to radiation. Pregnant women should not assist since fetal tissue is especially sensitive to damage by x-rays.

SPECIMEN COLLECTION

Urine Sample Collection

To collect a urine sample, children may require either catheterization or a clean-catch specimen. A catheterized specimen is obtained using sterile technique. Bladder catheterization can be a traumatic experience for both the child and the parents. Distraction techniques can be helpful in decreasing anxiety and fear. A lubricant with 2% lidocaine is used to eliminate the discomfort of catheterization. If a clean-catch specimen is requested, the nurse places a urine collection bag around the perineal area after cleaning the perineum and surrounding skin (Fig. 21-11). The infant is diapered and the bag monitored for urinary output. The urine must be removed from the bag and sent to the lab within 30 minutes of voiding.

Figure 21-11 Urine collection bag.

Stool Sample Collection

Stool samples are frequently obtained for ova and parasites (O & P), to determine the causative agent for a diarrheal condition, or to check for the presence of occult blood. If the child is toilet-trained, he can use the potty chair or the toilet with a collection hat under the seat. In a non-potty trained child, stool from the diaper is collected. Samples are transferred into a collection cup using tongue blades. O&P samples are sent to the lab as soon as possible. When lab services are not provided 24 hours a day, the sample should be refrigerated as soon as possible.

Blood Sample Collection

Having blood drawn can be a traumatic event. Preparation and support during the procedure will alleviate some of the fear and pain associated with venipuncture. Trauma can be alleviated by using distraction techniques with the child prior to the venipuncture. Application of EMLA cream, a topical analgesic containing lidocaine and prilocaine, anesthetizes the skin before any painful procedure. The cream is applied to the site, covered with a transparent dressing for one hour, and removed prior to the venipuncture.

Throat Culture Collection

A rapid strep test or a throat culture can be used to diagnose group A streptococci as the cause of sore throat. If the rapid strep test is positive, an antibiotic is prescribed. If the rapid strep test is negative, a culture to grow the bacteria is done to confirm the results. A throat culture is more accurate than the rapid strep test, but it may take several days to obtain results. Most children do not tolerate throat cultures very well. For younger children it may be helpful to place the child on the parent's lap facing forward, and have the parent place one arm across the child's chest and over his arms, and one hand on the child's forehead. The child is now sufficiently restrained to obtain a specimen safely. The nurse uses a tongue blade to push the tongue downward and swabs the posterior pharynx with two sterile cotton-tipped applicators.

 clinical alert

Epiglottitis

One caveat exists regarding throat cultures. Throat examinations and cultures should not be performed on a child who has suddenly developed a high fever; is drooling; has severe sore throat, hoarseness, stridor; and sits in a tripod position. This history indicates the possibility of epiglottitis. Eliciting the gag reflex, as happens with a throat culture, in this child may cause the inflamed epiglottis to completely obstruct the airway.

Cerebrospinal Fluid Collection

A lumbar puncture (LP) is a necessary procedure to rule out sepsis or meningitis. It can also be scheduled as a procedure for children undergoing treatment for cancer. The nurse prepares the child for a LP by telling the family and the child the reason for the procedure, showing them how to help out with positioning, and teaching some distraction methods. Practicing the position required for the procedure can be helpful. An hour before the lumbar puncture, EMLA cream can be applied to the skin at the designated site. This makes the procedure less painful. With the lumbar puncture, a needle is inserted into the subarachnoid space at the level of L4 or L5 to withdraw cerebrospinal fluid (CSF) for analysis. An infant is seated upright with the head bent forward. An older child must lie on his side with the head flexed, hips and knees flexed, and the back arched while being firmly held to make sure he does not move. CSF samples are sent for culture, glucose, red blood cells, and protein.

After CSF test, vital signs are taken. The child is encouraged to lie flat for 1 hour and drink fluids. The child may complain of a headache or pain at the site of the lumbar puncture. Neurological signs are observed for any changes. Complications such as nerve trauma, infection, bleeding, or pressure effects are rare.

Enteral Tube Feedings

When a child is unable to take adequate nutrition by mouth, an alternate feeding method is used to maintain and promote growth in the child. The type of feeding method selected depends on the child's medical condition. Children can be nourished through an oro- or nasogastric feeding tube or a gastrostomy tube. Feedings may be administered as a bolus or a continuous infusion. Bolus feedings are given at relatively the same rate as an oral feeding would normally be taken and are the preferred method to deliver formula in children who cannot tolerate oral feedings. Formula given as a continuous infusion is placed on a feeding pump and regulated to be administered over a predetermined number of hours. Continuous infusions are often preferred in children with serious cardiac defects to decrease the workload of the heart while providing enteral nutrition. To allow underweight infants

Labs: Analysis of Cerebrospinal Fluid

	Pressure (mm Hg)	Protein (mg/dL)	RBCs	Glucose (mg/dL)	WBCs
Infant	<200	20–170	None	34–119	0–30
Child	<200	5–40	None	60–80	0–20

RBCs = Red blood cells, WBCs = White blood cells.
Data from Van Leeuwen, A.M., Kranpitz, T.R., & Smith, L.S. (2006). *Davis's comprehensive handbook of laboratory and diagnostic tests with nursing implications.* Philadelphia: F.A. Davis.

Procedure 21-1 Inserting an Oro- or Nasogastric Tube

Purpose

To maintain the child's nutrition using a feeding tube that is passed through the mouth or nares and into the stomach

Equipment

- Oro- or nasogastric tube
- Tap water or a water soluble lubricant
- Syringe
- pH indicator paper

Steps

1. Wash hands and don gloves

2. Determine tube length required by measuring from the nose to the earlobe and to the midway point between the end of the xiphoid process and the umbilicus.

   RATIONALE: *Proper measurement determines the distance that the catheter is inserted.*

3. Note the measurement by finding the manufacturer's black mark on the appropriately sized feeding tube.

4. Lubricate the tube with tap water or a water-soluble lubricant. Follow manufacturer guidelines.

   RATIONALE: *Lubrication eases catheter insertion.*

5. Using the dominant hand, gently direct the tube toward the back of the throat or, if using the nose, toward the occiput.

6. Aspirate stomach contents.

   RATIONALE: *Indicates proper placement.*

7. Check for proper placement using the method following the institution's policy:
   a. Use pH indicator paper for assessment of gastric aspirate.
   d. Inject a small amount of air into the tube while auscultating over the stomach; the nurse should hear a "swoosh" as the air enters the stomach.
   c. Obtain an x-ray film to verify placement. This method is not practical for every feeding, but is often used after initial placement of the oro- or nasogastric feeding tube when used for continuous feeding.

   RATIONALE: *Indicates proper placement.*

   Clinical Alert There are some risks with an oro- or nasogastric tube. The liquid from the feeding or medication may enter the lungs and possibility cause pneumonia. In addition, the feeding tubes may cause the child discomfort. The tube can also become plugged, causing pain, nausea, or vomiting.

Teach Parents

It is important to teach parents about artificial nutrition and hydration as well as the function of the oro- or nasogastric tube. Parents can be encouraged to report displacement of the tube, noted distress in the child and tube placement if necessary.

> **Documentation**
>
> 6/18/10 1300 Nasogastric tube inserted in left nostril without difficulty. Placement of the tube confirmed. Nasogastric tube secured.
>
> —D. Naccarini, RN

---

or children to gain weight, a continuous feeding may be given during hours of sleep to boost calorie intake without interfering with a normal daily feeding/eating schedule.

OROGASTRIC AND NASOGASTRIC FEEDING TUBES. For newborn infants requiring gavage feedings (a feeding done using a tube that is passed through the nares and into the stomach; the food is in liquid form, usually at room temperature), the orogastric route is preferred because newborns are obligate nose breathers. The tube is inserted and then removed at the end of the bolus feed. If the tube is to be left in place, the nasogastric route should be considered. Nasogastric tube feedings are preferred over total parenteral nutrition since they preserve the stomach's mucosa, allow the digestive process to continue, and are cost-effective (Procedure 21-1).

Nursing Insight— *Psychosocial needs of the infant receiving gavage feedings*

The time taken to administer a gavage feeding can be used in the same way as in a regular feeding. Place the infant comfortably in the mother's arms with the head elevated. Provide the infant with a pacifier to help simulate an actual feeding.

Non-nutritive sucking has been shown to increase weight gain and decrease crying, and to allow for the normal muscular development of the mouth and tongue.

Once placement of the tube is confirmed and the child is in position, the nurse administers a bolus feeding of room-temperature formula via gravity through an appropriately sized syringe attached to the feeding tube. The formula-filled syringe is held less than 12 inches above the infant. When the feeding is complete, the tubing is flushed with tap water to prevent clogging of the lumen, the syringe is removed, and the feeding port capped. To decrease the chance of regurgitation, the infant is burped after the bolus is infused. Follow hospital guidelines for nasogastric gavage feedings. The nurse must remember that the amount of water should be only the amount required to successfully flush the length of tubing; excess water may result in overfeeding.

GASTROSTOMY FEEDING TUBES. When a child requires enteral tube feedings over a longer period of time, such as those with oral feeding aversions or neurological dysfunction, a gastrostomy tube (GT) is an alternative to the nasogastric tube. A GT is inserted through the abdominal

Figure 21-13 Child with an ostomy.

Figure 21-12 Gastrostomy tubes. *A.* PEG. *B.* Mic-Key.

wall into the stomach. The GT is secured internally and externally with a variety of bumpers depending on the manufacturer of the GT. Some physicians also secure the GT in place with external sutures for the first 7 to 10 days postoperatively.

After the initial insertion, the GT is left open to gravity drainage for 12 to 24 hours and the wound site observed for signs of infection. Stoma care and assessment are important nursing interventions due to the potential for leakage of gastric secretions onto the periostomal skin. Guidelines for feeding the child through a gastrostomy tube are similar to nasogastric tube feedings. Two of the many types of gastrostomy tubes available are shown in Figure 21-12.

 clinical alert

Gastrostomy tubes

A gastrostomy tube may move into the duodenum and cause an obstruction as it occludes the pyloric sphincter. Mark the tube with indelible ink to make it is easy to observe for migration. The nurse must report any vomiting, abdominal distention, or evidence of bile drainage as aspirate.

Ostomies

An ostomy is a surgical opening from either the small or large bowel to the surface of the abdomen to allow for fecal elimination (Fig. 21-13). An ostomy may be needed for a variety of reasons, including trauma, obstruction, disease, and infection. It may be needed on a temporary basis to allow the bowel sufficient time to heal, or permanently when the child's condition does not allow for ostomy reversal.

For infants and toddlers, the parent assumes all responsibility for the care of the ostomy. The nurse assists the parents by clarifying misconceptions, addressing concerns about caring for the child with an ostomy, and providing teaching guidelines regarding ostomy care. It is necessary

for the nurse to feel comfortable discussing difficult issues with the child. If the child is unable or unwilling to verbalize his feelings, the nurse may attempt to engage the child through the use of play or art by bringing crayons and paper to the child's room and giving the child time to process the current events in his life. The child may be able to express himself through art or play more readily than through words. A Child Life Specialist may provide additional ways for the child to communicate his "stories" about how the ostomy is affecting his everyday life. Nurses must be aware of community resources and refer the parents and child to appropriate support groups. Through participation in support groups, the parents and child will be able to talk with others who face the same issues and have struggled with similar concerns.

Older children must be encouraged to become independent in the care of their ostomy. A school-aged child needs to learn all aspects of ostomy care, including removal and reapplication of the ostomy appliance and periostomal skin care. The child must be aware of the signs and symptoms of potential complications to report to the school nurse or parents. Nurses and parents must be aware of the special needs of all adolescents (peer group and self-acceptance, sexuality, and depression) and how those needs may be further affected in the presence of an ostomy. When the child is in the school setting, there should be an arrangement made with the school nurse to allow for adequate time and privacy for maintenance of the ostomy and for storage of ostomy supplies.

RESTRAINING THE CHILD

Physical Restraint

Restraining a child may be a necessary intervention to ensure a child's safety during a procedure or to prevent injury to an operative site. Parents as well as the child need to be informed as to why a restraint is necessary. Once the restraint is applied, the child must be checked and documentation made as to the condition of the skin and circulation of the affected extremity. The extremity is checked every 15 minutes for 1 hour after initial application and then every 1 to 2 hours to ensure the child's safety.

Be sure to— Use of restraints

The Joint Commission has specific information about restraint and seclusion http://www.jointcommission.org/

 critical nursing action Care of the Child in Restraints

1. Remove restraints every 2 hours to assess skin and provide range of motion to the affected extremity.
2. Provide supervised time with restraints off, if appropriate, to allow the child to engage in activities of daily living (toileting, feeding, reading a book, watching TV, etc.).
3. Encourage games and activities that promote growth and development.
4. Reapply restraints.
5. Document condition of skin, nursing care given with restraints off, removal and reapplication of restraints.
6. Teach parents how to remove and reapply restraints.

Common types of restraints used for children are the elbow restraint and the mummy restraint. The elbow restraint prevents the child from flexing the elbow, therefore preventing the child's hands from reaching the head. They prevent the child from pulling out an intravenous (IV) line in a scalp vein or other peripheral line. If the child is recovering from cleft lip repair, the elbow restraint prevents the child from touching the incision area. Most children tolerate this type of restraint without problems related to skin integrity or circulatory compromise.

The mummy restraint temporarily immobilizes an infant or small child for an examination or procedure that involves the head, neck, or throat. This is ideal to keep the child safe during venipuncture, throat examination, insertion of a nasogastric tube, or administration of ophthalmic, otic, or oral medications. The mummy restraint is much like swaddling an infant. It is a total body restraint.

Pharmacological Restraint

In addition to physical restraints, pharmacological restraints can be administered to children during diagnostic and therapeutic procedures. Sedation of children is administered to allow the safe completion of a procedure. Chlo-

 medication: Chloral Hydrate (Aquachloral)— Points to Remember

Chloral Hydrate (**klor**-al **hye**-drate)

- As a sedative, administer 25 mg/kg per day PO up to 500 mg per single dose.
- As a hypnotic, administer 50 mg/kg per day PO up to 1 g per single dose.
- Administer 1 hour before the procedure.
- Peak time is 1–3 hours.
- Duration of action is 4–8 hours.
- Provide juice, ginger ale, or water for administration of liquid chloral hydrate
- Monitor for dizziness, confusion, and delirium.

Data from Karch, A. (2006). *Lippincott's Nursing Drug Guide*. Philadelphia: Lippincott Williams & Wilkins.

ral hydrate (Aquachloral) is a nonbarbiturate sedative–hypnotic drug commonly used in children to produce sedation. The drug decreases anxiety and induces sleep without respiratory depression or suppression of the cough reflex.

The Child in Pain

Whether hospitalized, in a clinic, or in the home, a child may experience pain related to an acute injury, medical or surgical condition, or disability. A child's pain may be either acute or chronic. All pain is not the same for all people. The skill of the nurse lies in helping the child to convey the kind and intensity of the pain he is experiencing and then determining the best way to manage pain (pharmacological and nonpharmacological).

 Nursing Insight— *The definition of pain*

A key point to remember is: *pain is whatever the child says it is*. What one person experiences as mild pain, another may experience as severe pain. With the use of pediatric pain scales, most children are able to communicate their level of pain very clearly. The important thing is for the nurse to listen to the child rather than prejudge what the child should feel.

PAIN ASSESSMENT AND MANAGEMENT

Ongoing assessment is essential for the child experiencing pain. Proper pain assessment requires identification of the type of pain the child is experiencing, the origins of either physiological or psychological pain, and the behavioral patterns associated with the pain. Pain assessment tools are invaluable for obtaining a child's perception and for the younger or disabled child as well as the parent's view of pain levels. There are several statistically reliable pain scales available for use with children of different ages and stages of cognitive development. The most commonly used pain scales are the numeric scale, the Wong Faces Scale, and the FLACC pain scale (Fig. 21-14 and Table 21-8).

The nurse should familiarize the child and family with an appropriate pain scale during hospitalization or a clinic visit, when the child is injured or ill, or for a medical procedure or surgery. The nurse understands that it is important to use the same pain scale according to age, developmental stage, and cognitive function level. In addition to the pain scales, the nurse asks about intensity, duration, and location of the pain; the effects of movement on

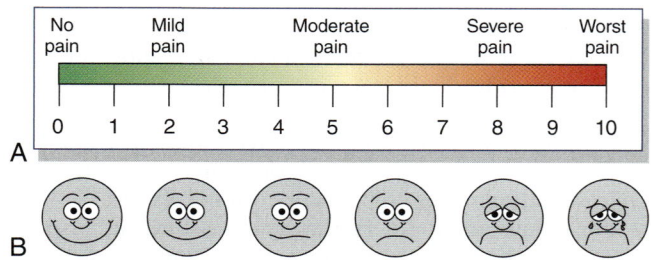

Figure 21-14 Pain scales. *A.* Numeric pain scale (about 12 years or older). *B.* Wong-Baker Faces pain scale (preschool through schoolage).

Table 21-8   FLACC Pain Scale

	Scoring		
Categories	0	1	2
Face	No particular expression or smile; disinterested	Occasional grimace or frown; withdrawn	Frequent to constant frown, clenched jaw, quivering chin
Legs	Normal position or relaxed	Uneasy, restless, tense	Kicking, or legs drawn up
Activity	Lying quietly, normal position, moves easily	Squirming, shifting back and forth, tense	Arched, rigid, or jerking
Cry	No cry (awake or asleep)	Moans or whimpers, occasional complaint	Crying steadily, screams or sobs, frequent complaints
Consolability	Content, relaxed	Reassured by occasional touching, hugging, or talking to; distractible	Difficult to console or comfort

Each of the 5 categories—(F) Face; (L) Legs; (A) Activity; (C) Cry; (C) Consolability—is scored from 0 to 2, which results in a total score between 0 and 10.

the severity of pain; any aggravating and alleviating factors; and, if appropriate, previous interventions that alleviated the pain. It is useful to know what experiences the child has had with pain, including previous surgeries, illnesses, or congenital conditions. A child's ability to manage pain is sometimes related to the child's position in the family or his experience of illnesses in other close family members. Pain has many descriptors: mild, moderate, severe, chronic, stabbing, burning, pricking, aching, throbbing, or dull. Pain is also expressed nonverbally with facial expressions, guarding, and muscle tension.

Mild pain is a slight discomfort. Its management may include minor analgesics along with comfort measures or distraction. However, engaging in a distraction does not mean that the child has no pain. It is simply a coping mechanism that diverts a child's attention from the pain for a finite period of time. Pharmacological intervention for mild pain starts with analgesics such as children's acetaminophen (Tylenol) or ibuprofen (Advil, Motrin), and is administered on a scheduled or as-needed basis.

Although moderate pain may also be relieved by using distraction, the child experiences much stronger unpleasant sensations. Using a child's vivid imagination is very effective in pain management, as long as it is used in conjunction with regularly timed analgesic administration, including milder opioids such as codeine in varying combinations of acetaminophen (Children's Tylenol).

Severe pain causes pallor, sweating, piloerection (elevation of the hair above the skin), dilated pupils, increased respiration and blood pressure, and muscle tension. However, if pain has been prolonged then the child's body may have become accustomed to it, in which case marked increases in vital signs may not be noted. Again, that does not mean that the child is not experiencing pain. When brief, intense pain subsides, the child's body may respond with a lower BP or pulse rate.

Management of severe pain, often associated with surgical interventions, usually calls for strong analgesics like morphine (Astramorph). The maximum allowable dosage may be started in the recovery room and followed by regular dosing, within the allowable limit for the specific child, to ensure adequate pain coverage.

Acute pain occurs 24 to 48 hours after trauma or surgery. It is initially experienced as severe pain, and gradually subsides over time. With orthopedic trauma, a short period of auto-anesthesia can occur that belies the extent of the injury. As narcotics do not relieve all of the pain following surgery, they can be accompanied with some success by comfort measures, such as holding a hand or encouraging the child "to send his pain to you by squeezing your hand tightly."

Chronic pain in children is any pain lasting more than 3 months. It can result in fear of re-injury, anorexia, weight loss, changes in sleep patterns, guarded movements, a rigid facial expression, and an overall diminishment of the child's joy of living. Management of chronic pain involves careful observation of which pain relief measures work best for a particular child. Decreasing pain to acceptable levels allows the child to carry on with as many age-appropriate activities as possible given the circumstances of his illness or condition. Table 21-9 shows a comparison of acute and chronic pain.

Clinical Alert

Naloxone (Narcan)

When giving morphine sulfate (Astramorph), be sure to have the opioid antagonist Naloxone (Narcan) available. Narcan completely blocks the effects of opioids including CNS effects and respiratory depression. The dose for children is 5–10 mcg/kg (0.01 mg/kg).

Data from Deglin, J.H., & Vallerand, A.H. (2009). *Davis's drug guide for nurses* (11th ed., pp. 862–864). Philadelphia: F.A. Davis.

medication: Morphine Sulfate (Astramorph)

Morphine (**mor**-feen)

Morphine sulfate (Astramorph) is an opioid analgesic. It is frequently used for children with chronic pain. It can be given PO, IV, IM, epidurally, or via a patient-controlled analgesia pump (PCA). For children less than 50 lbs. (22.7 kg) the dose is:

   0.3 mg/kg PO every 3–4 hours, or
   0.1 mg/kg IV or IM every 3–4 hours.

Data from Deglin, J.H., & Vallerand, A.H. (2009). *Davis's drug guide for nurses* (11th ed., pp. 843–847). Philadelphia: F.A. Davis.

Table 21-9 Characteristics of Acute and Chronic Pain

Acute Pain	Chronic Pain	Chronic Cancer Pain
Identifiable cause	Cause hard to find	Usually identifiable cause
Short duration	Lasts longer than three months	Duration varies
Sudden onset	Begins gradually and persists	Onset varies
Well defined	May or may not be well defined	May or may not be well defined
Limited	Unlimited	Unlimited
Decreases with healing	Persists beyond healing time	May persist beyond healing
Reversible	Exhausting and useless	Exhausting and useless
Objective signs and symptoms	Objective signs absent	Objective signs absent
Anxiety	Depression and fatigue	Depression, fatigue, and anxiety

Nursing Insight— *Myths about pain management*

- Children do not feel pain with the same intensity as adults.
- Neonates do not feel pain because their nervous systems are not mature.
- Children cannot tell where they hurt.
- Children will tell you if they are really having pain.
- Children become accustomed to pain.
- Narcotic analgesics are dangerous for children because they become addicted or go into respiratory distress.
- If children can be distracted, they are not in pain.
- If children say they are in pain, but do not look in pain, they do not need to be medicated.
- Being in pain for only a little while is not that bad.
- After children have undergone surgery they should not be given analgesia until they can vocalize pain, because they received enough anesthetic to "cover" their pain.
- The best way to give analgesics is intramuscularly.
- Children with neurological impairments do not feel pain as much as other children.
- Children, especially boys, should learn to tolerate pain; they will make better, stronger adults.

Children react to pain and its management in individual ways that also correspond to their developmental level (Table 21-10). Responses to analgesia, time, route, and dose are documented to enable nurses across all shifts to provide a continuum of care for the child.

Now Can You— Discuss important aspects for the care of the child in the hospital or clinic setting?

1. Discuss general care measures for the child in the hospital or clinic setting.
2. Discuss the important aspects of preparing the infant and child for a procedure.
3. Describe developmentally appropriate assessments of pain in children?

The Child with Disabilities

Disabilities may be congenital or develop from illness, injury, or disease progression. Regardless of the cause, families of children with disabilities are beset with emotional upset and confusion about the reality of not having the child they expected (i.e., one without a disability). In addition, the family is often distressed about the child's pain and her experiences with surgery, treatments, procedures, and repeated clinic appointments. The child is apt to have ongoing physical, occupational, or speech therapy, and parents often need to perform physically painful procedures at home in order to promote their child's development. Other ongoing treatments and procedures include respiratory therapy, gavage feedings, medication administration, using assistive devices, planning special diets, taking care of elimination needs, and implementing special techniques to maintain the musculoskeletal system.

EMOTIONAL CONCERNS

Raising a child with a disability is distressing due to the disruption of the normal routine, the conveyance of continuous "bad news" or prognostics, the reconfirmation of future emotional and physical concerns, and the awareness of financial implications the diagnosis and treatment provoke. These financial concerns include medical care that is not covered by insurance or government-sponsored health care programs, as well as expenses incurred for child care or respite care. Often, a parent is required to stop working and become a full-time caregiver resulting in further economic distress.

Across Care Settings: Insurance for children

The nurse can teach the family about how to obtain health insurance for their child. Health insurance provided to children through state and national programs is free or low-cost. The costs are different depending on the state and the family's income. When there are charges for health care the charges are minimal. Children who have health insurance generally have better health throughout their childhood. Benefits of insurance for children include: (1) receiving

Table 21-10 Pain Management Strategies

Age (Guidline Only)	Concerns/Reactions	Distraction	Environment	Parental Involvement	Preparation	Positions	Post Procedure Comforting
Infant /Toddler (0–3 Years)	Separation anxiety Protest Despair Denial	Pacifier Swaddling Rocking Eye contact Music Picture books	Controlled lighting and noise Use treatment room	Encourage parental presence, provide guidance and if possible, comfort/cuddle baby during procedure	Prepare parent: offer explanations of what they will see and hear Develop a plan "who will do what"	Swaddle Cuddle	Soothe Swaddle Hold and rock Soft music Soothing voice
Preschool (3–6 Years)	Separation anxiety Concerns with body image Develops fantasies with illness and treatment Battle for control	Distraction kit Deep breathing Bubble blowing Counting Singing	Use treatment room Music Controlled lighting and noise	Encourage parental presence and provide guidance in encouraging participation during strategies	Medical play with relevant medical equipment and participation Pre-procedural teaching Reassurance of what child is to expect—focus on senses	Lap Parent or staff may support patient or have other close physical contact Present patient with choices	Praise and reward (stickers) Medical play Play Stories
School Age (6–11 Years)	Has questions regarding body and illness Concerns of helplessness, passivity, and dependency Tend to be phobic and develop fears Anger	Deep breathing Hand squeezing Riddles/trivia Pretend games Talking Distraction kit	Use treatment room Music Controlled lighting and noise	Encourage parental presence and provide guidance Encourage parents to be part of the team	Simple medical terms to describe what will happen Allow appropriate play with medical equipment Explain reasons for various components of tests and allow appropriate participation by patient	Lap Parent may support patient or have other close physical contact Present patient with choices	Praise, reward (stickers) Play, medical play Stories Evaluate procedures and discuss suggestions for next time
Teens (12 and older)	Illness interferes with struggle for independence Illness is a major threat to developing self-image Very threatened by helplessness and loss of privacy Denial, withdrawal, anger, hostility, disappointment	Imagery Walkman Deep breathing Hand squeezing Talking Jokes Distraction kit	Use treatment room Music Controlled lighting and noise	Ask permission of patient for parental involvement Encourage parents to be part of the team	Clarify misconceptions and initiate discussions about the past experiences with procedures Allow appropriate participation by patient Pre-procedural teaching utilizing medical play	Present patient with choices Plan positioning with teen	Praise, reward (stickers) Play, medical play Stories, evaluate procedures and discuss suggestions for next time

needed immunizations that prevent disease, (2) receiving treatment for acute as well as recurring illnesses and (3) receiving preventative care to keep the child healthy.

The nurse can encourage the family to call 1-877 KIDS NOW (1-877-543-7669) or go to your state's program: http://www.insurekidsnow.gov/states.asp

It is important to note that children who are eligible for Medicaid cannot enroll in the state program because Medicaid provides comprehensive health benefits.

DEVELOPMENTAL CONCERNS

Many congenital problems are repaired surgically either shortly after birth or once the child is physically developed and strong enough to withstand the rigors of surgery. Parents and the child need constant support from health care personnel to sustain a loving environment for the child with a disability who may be undergoing the same growth and development changes as any other child of the same age. However, due to constant medical and surgical interventions, the child may demonstrate either signs of regression to more immature behaviors, or surprising evidence of what some call a "maturity beyond their years." The latter has been observed in children with cancer who are faced with pain and/or body image disturbances, such as alopecia or extreme weight loss, and with their own mortality as they might understand it at their age.

PHYSICAL CONCERNS

The child with a disability undergoing surgery, especially at a younger age, may experience rapid fluid and electrolyte changes (see Chapter 32). These conditions may require intensive care procedures that are worrisome to parents and often painful for the children. Children with severe congenital heart problems (see Chapter 27) face a lifetime of corrective procedures to augment initial surgeries or pharmacological therapy that consume time, energy, and finances. In addition, both parents and child need to learn physical self-care techniques, such as diabetes or anticoagulation monitoring. Often, abnormalities affect several body systems so that visits must be made to several different medical specialists who may require multiple pharmacotherapeutic regimens. Throughout all this, families must learn to care for the physical needs of the child.

CAREGIVER FATIGUE

Caring for a child with a significant disability takes its toll on the entire family. Respite care agencies were developed in response to the needs of parents of extremely disabled children to give short-term relief from the 24-hour surveillance and care often required in cases of severe disability. As medical advancements have increased the life expectancy of disabled children, so too have the number of disabled children or premature births resulted in larger numbers of children and families requiring long-term medical care and social systems to support their needs.

Most disabilities in childhood result in multiple visits to clinics, hospitals, or rehabilitation centers, thus disrupting normal activity and sleep patterns. It requires much more energy for a disabled child to perform even the simplest task than it does for a healthy child. It has been estimated that a severely disabled child needs to perform a simple task, such as getting into "puppy position" or standing independently for 15 seconds, 10,000 more times than a physically healthy child in order to accomplish it. These children have extra requirements for stamina, calories, vitamins, minerals, and protein in order to accomplish normal daily activities, let alone learning developmentally appropriate mental skills. These children also need additional sleep, but may have more trouble getting enough sleep if the demands of their care interfere with a normal sleep pattern. All of these factors contribute to caregiver fatigue.

RESILIENCY

Coping mechanisms give rise to resiliency in children and their families. Resiliency theory defines the protective factors in families, schools, and communities that exist in the lives of children. Four common attributes of resilient children include social competence, problem-solving skills, autonomy, and a sense of purpose and future. Nurses can help parents and children develop resiliency and positive self-esteem by fostering a mix of love and nurturing in the face of overwhelming stressors (DuHoux, 2004). Emotional security and maturity provide the foundation for resiliency (Box 21-2).

 nursing diagnoses The Developing Child

Family Processes, altered—related to health condition (specify), injury, violence
Growth and Development, altered—related to trauma, hospitalization, congenital defects, prolonged pain, separation from family
Injury, high risk for—related to lack of awareness of environmental hazards
Pain, Chronic—related to effects of condition (specify)
Poisoning, high risk for—related to age-specific environmental hazards
Self-esteem, chronic low—related to disfigurement, separation, ineffective relationship with parents or peers
Sleep Pattern Disturbance—related to pain, fear, desire to sleep with parents at night
Social Isolation—related to physical handicap, hospitalization, terminal illness
Violence, high risk for—related to verbal threats of physical assault, perceived threat to self-esteem

 Family Teaching Guidelines...
Caring for the Child with a Disability

How to: Care for the child with a disability
Topic: The nurse will improve the care of the family and a child with a disability
Essential information:

- Maintain a respectful attitude toward the parent and the child

- Listen carefully to the parent's concerns, realizing that parents often "know their child best"

- Evaluate how social and health care agencies can assist parents and the child to manage the disability—financial, medical, community services

- Assess the child's skills for coping with pain or fatigue

- Evaluate the need for respite care and reliable community resource providers

---

Box 21-2 Ways to Promote Resiliency

- Express love and gratitude
- Foster competency and positive attitudes
- Nurture positive emotions
- Encourage helping others
- Teach peace-building skills
- Reinforce positive behaviors
- Reduce stress

summary points

◆ When examining infants, children, and adolescents, the approach to the physical assessment will be based on the child's age, developmental and cognitive level, and, when ill, the extent of the illness.

◆ Vision and hearing screening are important ongoing assessments in children to promote normal psychosocial development, communication among friends, and academic success.

◆ Screening for lead poisoning, iron deficiency anemia, cholesterolemia, and tuberculosis are important assessments in the at-risk developing child.

◆ Explanations of procedures must be given at a developmentally appropriate level, avoiding words that may be unintentionally frightening.

◆ Regardless of a child's age, the nurse works to gain the trust of both the child and the family to help establish a therapeutic relationship.

◆ Children react to pain and its management in ways that correspond to their developmental level. Accurate pain assessment depends on the consistent use of an assessment tool both familiar to the child and parent.

◆ Disabled children expend a great deal of energy to perform the simple activities of daily life; therefore, children need age-appropriate care.

◆ Caring for the child with a physical or mental disability exacts its toll on the entire family. The pediatric nurse must be aware of all available resources within the community to assist the family in the care of the disabled child.

review questions

Multiple Choice

1. When preparing a 4-year-old child for a procedure, the pediatric nurse must be aware of the child's developmental status. The nurse would best demonstrate this awareness by:
   A. Demonstrating the procedure on the child's teddy bear
   B. Providing a peer video of the procedure for the child to view
   C. Explaining the procedure to the child the day before the actual procedure occurs
   D. Discussing the procedure at length with the child

2. The 10-year-old child is receiving preoperative teaching prior to a tonsillectomy. The pediatric nurse should teach the child about the operation and use developmentally appropriate explanations such as:
   A. "Don't worry; the doctor will cut your tonsils out while you are asleep."
   B. "The shot that you will receive in your arm will only help the pain a little bit."
   C. "Don't worry about the operation; it is really not a big deal."
   D. "The doctor will give you special sleeping medicine before she operates."

3. There are many myths regarding children and pain levels. The pediatric nurse is aware that the following is true of pain management in pediatrics.
   A. Children cannot tell where they hurt.
   B. The child who is neurologically impaired does not feel pain.
   C. Children should not receive narcotics because they will become addicts.
   D. The use of special pain scales allows children to better express their level of pain.

4. The pediatric nurse utilizes the "head to toe" approach when conducting a physical assessment on an infant. The correct technique is demonstrated in which of the following sequences? Assessing the....
   A. Heart rate, urine output, respiratory rate, and presence of bowel sounds.
   B. Head circumference, lung sounds, presence of bowel sounds, urine output
   C. Presence of eye drainage, abdominal pain, lung sounds, and urine output
   D. Urine output, skin color, skin turgor, heart rate and bowel sounds.

Select All that Apply

5. A 24-month-old child comes to the clinic for a well-visit assessment. The pediatric nurse is orienting a new graduate nurse and begins the assessment. The assessment will include which of the following components?
   A. Visual screening by having the child identify certain objects
   B. Viewing the tympanic membrane by pulling the pinna down and back
   C. Auscultation of bowel sounds in all 4 quadrants
   D. Taking the child's vital signs.

Fill-in-the-Blank

6. The pediatric nurse is preparing to administer ibuprofen (Children's Motrin) to a 12-kg (26.4 lbs.) child with a fever of 103.6°F (39.8°C). The nurse understands that a child with this degree of temperature elevation can receive the medication at a dose calculated to 10 mg/kg of body weight. The nurse understands the importance of safe medication administration by giving _____ mg.

7. The 2-month-old child who requires intermittent gavage feedings will have an _____ tube inserted because infants are obligatory _____ _____. The infant should be positioned in the parent's arms with the _____ elevated.

8. The pediatric nurse is aware that the posterior fontanel closes at approximately ___ to ___ months of age and that the anterior fontanel remains open until approximately ___ to ___ months of age.

True/False

9. It is not necessary for the pediatric nurse to ask the parent questions related to the use of herbal products because this is not a common finding in pediatrics.

10. An accurate and effective way to assess the pediatric patient's respiratory rate is by counting the respirations while the child is sleeping and by observing the abdominal area.

11. According to the Centers for Disease Control and Prevention, handwashing is not necessary if the pediatric nurse is wearing gloves when providing care.

12. It is important for the pediatric nurse to incorporate developmental theory when working with children. The preschool-age child who is on isolation precautions will perceive isolation as a punishment for a previous thought or action because of the developmental stage of magical thinking.

See Answers to End of Chapter Review Questions on the Electronic Study Guide or DavisPlus.

REFERENCES

American Academy of Pediatrics (AAP). (2005). Recommendations for Preventive Pediatric Health Care (RE9353). Retrieved from http://www.aappolicy.aappublications.org/sub-journals/pediatrics/html (Accessed May 28, 2007).

American Academy of Pediatrics (AAP). (2003). Health supervision recommendations: Prevention of pediatric overweight and obesity, *Pediatrics, 112*, 424–430.

American Nurses Association (ANA). (2004). *Nursing: Scope and standards of practice.* Washington, DC: Nursesbooks.org

Bascom, A. (2002). *Incorporating herbal medicine into clinical practice.* Philadelphia: F.A. Davis.

Berger, K.S. (2005). *The developing person through the life span* (6th ed). New York: Worth.

Bickley, L.S., & Szilagyi, P.G. (2007). *Bates' guide to physical examination and history taking* (9th ed). Philadelphia: Lippincott Williams & Wilkins.

Bulechek, G., Butcher, H.M., & Dochterman, J. (2008). *Nursing interventions classification (NIC)* (5th ed.). St. Louis, MO: C.V. Mosby.

Centers for Disease Control and Prevention (CDC). (2007). Recommended immunization schedule for persons aged 0–6 years. Retrieved from http://www.cdc.gov/nip/recs/child-schedule-color-print.pdf (Accessed April 15, 2007).

Clark, J., Lieh-Lai, M., Sarnaik, A., Mattoo, T. (2002). Discrepancies between direct and indirect blood pressure measurements using various recommendations for arm cuff selection. *Pediatrics, 110* (5), 920–923.

Deglin, J.H., & Vallerand, A.H. (2009). *Davis's drug guide for nurses* (11th ed.). Philadelphia: F.A. Davis.

Denver Developmental Materials. (1990). *Denver II developmental test.* Denver, CO: Denver Developmental Materials.

Dossey, B.M., Keegan, L., Guzzetta, C.E., & Kolkmeier, L.G. (2005). *Holistic nursing: A handbook for practice* (4th ed.). Sudbury, MA: Jones & Bartlett.

DuHoux, M. (2004). Building resiliency: Helping children to weather tough times. Retrieved from http://www.nasponline.org/communications/topicalresources.aspx

Feldman-Winter, L., & McAbee, G.N. (2002). Legal issues in caring for adolescent patients: Physicians can optimize healthcare. *Postgraduate Medicine, 111*(3), 15–21.

Frankenburg, W.K., Dobbs, J.B., Archer, P., Shapiro, H., & Bresnick, B. (1992).The Denver II: A major revision and restandardization of the Denver developmental screening test. *Pediatrics, 89*(1), 91–97.

Hay, W.W. Jr. (2005). *Current pediatric diagnosis & treatment* (17th ed.). New York: Lange Medical Books/McGraw-Hill.

Healthcare Infection Control Practices Advisory Committee (HICPAC). (2008). Department of Human Service, Center for Disease Control and Prevention. Retrieved from http://www.cdc.gov/ncidod/dhqp/hicpac.html (Accessed May 22, 2008).

Hulka, B.S., Zyzanski, S.J., Cassei, J.C., & Thompson, S.J. (1970). Scale for the measurement of attitudes toward physicians and primary medical care. *Medical Care, 8,* 429–436.

Ireys, H.T., & Perry, J.J. (1999). Development and evaluation of a satisfaction scale for parents of children with special health care needs. *Pediatrics, 104,* 118–1191.

Johnson, M., Bulechek, G., Butcher, H., McCloskey Dochterman, J., Maas, M., Moorehead, S., & Swanson, E. (2006). *NANDA, NOC, and NIC linkages: Nursing diagnoses, outcomes, & interventions* (2nd ed.). St. Louis, MO: Mosby Elsevier.

Karch, A. (2006). *Lippincott's Nursing Drug Guide.* Philadelphia: Lippincott Williams & Wilkins.

Koller, D., David, N., Goldie, R.S., Gearing, R., & Selkirk, E.K. (2006). When family-centered care is challenged by infectious disease: Pediatric health care delivery during the SARS outbreak. *Qualitative Health Research, 16*(1), 47–60.

Kreisler, J., & Ricter, R. (2003). The abnormal fontanel. *American Academy of Family Physicians, 67*(12), 2547–2552.

Lanski, S.L., Greenwald, M., Perkins, A., & Simon, H.K. (2003). Herbal therapy use in a pediatric emergency department population: Expect the unexpected. *Pediatrics, 111*(5), 981–986.

Lee, K.J., Haven, P.L., Sato, T.T., Hoffman, G.M., & Leuthner, S.R. (2006). Assent for treatment: Clinical knowledge, attitudes, and practice, *Pediatrics, 118*(2), 723–731.

Mayo Clinic Tools for healthier lives. Retrieved from http://www.mayoclinic.com (Accessed May 22, 2008).

Moorehead, S., Johnson, M., Maas, M., & Swanson, E. (2008). *Nursing outcomes classification (NOC)* (4th ed.). St. Louis, MO: C.V. Mosby.

NANDA International (2007). *NANDA-I nursing diagnoses: Definitions and classifications 2007–2008.* Philadelphia: NANDA-I.

Nemours Foundation. (2007). How to perform a testicular self-examination. Retrieved from http://kidshealth.org (Accessed May 21, 2007).

Newman, T.B., & Garber, A.M. (2003). Cholesterol screening in children and adolescents, *Pediatrics, 105*(3), 637–639.

Nield, L.S., & Kamat, D.M. (2006). Odd skull shapes: Heads up on diagnosis and therapy, *Consultant for Pediatricians, 5*(11), 701–709.

Persing, J., James, H., Swanson, J., & Kattwinkel, J. (2003). Prevention and management of positional skull deformities in infants. American Academy of Pediatrics Committee on Practice and Ambulatory Medicine. *Pediatrics, 111*, 199–202.

Reznik, M., & Ozuah, P.O. (2006). Tuberculin skin testing in children. *Emergency Infectious Disease.* Retrieved from http://www.cdc.gov/ncidod/EIF/vol12no05/05-0980.htm (Accessed February 24, 2007).

Salimbene, S. (2005). *What language does your patient hurt in?* St. Paul, MN: EMCParadigm.

Schulster, L.M., Chinn, R.Y.W., Arduino, M.J., Carpenter, J., Donland, R., Ashford, D., Besser, R., Fields, B., McNeil, M.M., Witney, C., Wong, S., Juranek, D., & Cleveland, J. (2004). *Guidelines for environmental infection control in health-care facilities: Recommendations from CDC and the healthcare infection control practices advisory committee (HICPAC).* Chicago: American Society for Healthcare Engineering/American Hospital Association.

Stollery Children's Hospital, 8440-112 Street, Edmonton, Alberta, Canada.

Tanner, J.M. (1962). *Growth at adolescence* (2nd ed.). Oxford: Blackwell Scientific.

U.S. Department of Agriculture. (2007). Steps to a healthier you. Retrieved from http://www.mypyradmid.gov/kids/index.html (Accessed May 1, 2007).

U.S. Department of Health and Human Services. (2002). Bright futures: Guidelines for health supervision of infants, children, and adolescents. Retrieved from http://www.brightfutures.org (Accessed December 13, 2006).

U.S. Department of Health and Human Services. (2007). CDC growth charts: United States. Retrieved from http://www.cdc.gov/nchs/about/major/nhanes/growthcharts/charts.htm (Accessed April 3, 2007).

U.S. Department of Health and Human Services. (2007). Insure kids now! Retrieved from http://www.insurekidsnow.gov/questions.asp#why1 (Accessed June 7, 2007).

U.S. Preventive Services Task Force (2006). Screening for iron deficiency anemia—including iron supplementation for children and pregnant women. *The American Journal for Nurse Practitioners, 10*(10), 79–84.

Van Leeuwen, A.M., Kranpitz, T R., & Smith, L.S. (2006). *Davis's comprehensive handbook of laboratory and diagnostic tests with nursing implications*. Philadelphia: F.A. Davis.

Venes, D. (Ed.). (2009). *Taber's cyclopedic medical dictionary* (21st ed.). Philadelphia: F.A. Davis.

Watson, J. (2005). *Caring science as sacred science*. Philadelphia: F.A. Davis.

Wong, D.L., Hockenberry-Eaton, M., Wilson, D., Winkelstein, M.L., & Schwartz, P., (2001). *Wong's essentials of pediatric nursing* (6th ed.). St. Louis: C.V. Mosby.

Woolf, A.D., Gardiner, P., Whelan, J., Alpert, H.R., & Dvorkin, L. (2005). Views of pediatric health care providers in the use of herbs and dietary supplements in children. *Clinical Pediatrics, 44*(7), 579–584.

Wright, C.M., & Parkinson, K.N. (2004). Postnatal weight loss in term infants: What is normal and do growth charts allow for it? *Archives of Disease in Childhood. Fetal and Neonatal Edition, 89*(3), 254–257.

 For more information, go to http://davisplus.fadavis.com/

CONCEPT MAP

General Care Measures
- Bathing: shampooing
- Feeding: nutritional needs; diet hx/routines; home food
- Rest: parents sleeping-in; naps
- Safety: store toxics; name bands; alarm exits; transportation issues
- Infection control: isolated child
- Fever reduction: antipyretics; manage environment

Caring for the Child in the Hospital and in the Community

Routine Screenings:
- Lead poisoning
- Iron-deficiency anemia
- Cholesterol
- Tuberculosis

Comprehensive Health History
- "OLDCAT" ; "SODA"
- Family/social/past medical history
- Immunizations
- Developmental milestones
  – Fine/gross motor; language
- Patterns of daily activity
  – Sleep; nutrition
  – Play/activity/schoolwork
- Review of body systems

Where Research And Practice Meet:
- Issues r/t providers asking about/using herbs in treatment

Across Care Settings:
- Teach family how to obtain insurance for child

Health Assessment:
- Anthropometric measurements: length; weight/BMI; head circumference; skin fold
- Physical assessment: Vital signs.
  – Skin → color; turgor; lesions; includes hair/nails
  – Head & neck → symmetry; shape; fontanels; facial features; thyroid, lymph
  – Chest → shape; symmetry; respiratory effort; breast development
  – Lungs → adventitious breath sounds; stridor
  – Cardiac → pulses; PMI; heart sounds; edema; murmurs
  – Abdomen → contour; umbilicus; inguinal area; bowel sounds; organ palpation
  – GU/perineal → male/female genitalia; anus; Tanner staging/hair; sexual abuse
  – Musculoskeletal → symmetry of movement; ROM; alignment; strength
  – Neurological → mental status; motor functioning; sensory functioning

Restraining a Child
- Instruct parents
- Follow assessment and documentation policies
- Types: elbow; mummy; pharmacological

Ethnocultural Considerations:
- To establish therapeutic relationship: avoid stereotyping
- Color of sclera can vary
- Lead found in some folk medicine

Common Procedures
- IV access: peripheral; central venous access; PICC; ports
- I&O: includes breastfeeding/gavage feeding; weighing diapers
- X-ray exam help with positioning
- Consents: give parent information to decide

Specimen Collection:
- Stool/urine: depends on potty training
- Blood: address fears and discomfort
- Throat cultures: NOT in epiglottitis
- Lumbar puncture: positioning for and assessments after procedure

Enteral Feedings
- Tube routes: oro/nasogastric; G-tube
- Types: bolus; intermittent

Pain Management:
- Peds specific scales: numeric; FLACC; Wong Faces
- Descriptors: mild; moderate; severe; acute; chronic
- Pharmacologic; distraction; verbal comforting

Managing Sleep/Fatigue
- Fatigue has physical/emotional causes
- Assess infant for physical cues of fatigue
- Older child: can signal underlying disorder

What To Say:
- Correct use of Q-tips
- Age appropriate approach to prepare child for procedure
- Use developmentally appropriate words in speaking

Nursing Insight:
- Parent/child interaction gives cues to family dynamics
- Lung assessment: position, quiet, warm diaphragm
- Palpate abd through clothes to decrease tickling sensation
- To increase fluid intake: "Tea party," fun shapes, colored straws
- Non-nutritive sucking is important beneficial during gavage
- Know myths about children's pain

Clinical Alert:
- Understanding key respiratory signals
- Strategies to keep children safe at home and hospital: Think like the child
- Gloves don't replace hand washing
- G-tube can migrate: cause obstruction
- Pain is whatever the child says it is
- Naloxone (Narcan) reverses opioid toxicity

Collaboration In Caring:
- Call religious leader for spiritual care

Critical Nursing Action:
- Notify provider of adventitious breath sounds ASAP
- Child confined to bed at risk for skin breakdown
- Know nursing responsibility before and after a procedure done on child
- Be aware of infection risk with all procedures
- Follow skin assessment/removal and documentation policies when using restraints

Now Can You:
- Identify the major components of the health history
- Discuss all components of hosp/clinical care for the developing child

Caring for the Family Across Care Settings

A Link in the Chain

Nurses assist in making the lives of children better.
Nurses work in hospitals, in intensive care units with alarms everywhere, in clinics with toys all around, in community settings or behind desks in offices.
Nurses assist in making the lives of children better.
Nurses help repair children's bodies when they are broken or not made just right.
Nurses help children smile when they are receiving medication that might make them sicker before they become better.
Nurses deliver treatments to open up their airways, change dressings and deliver IV fluids.
Nurses assist in making the lives of children better.
Nurses must be creative and make medical situations fun rather than frightening.
Nurses cradle the children in their hearts and hands to help them feel secure and safe in a strange environment.
Nurses assist in making the lives of children better.
Nurses give of themselves by opening up their hearts to the families - letting them know that they genuinely care.
Nurses truly make a difference.
Nurses together are a long and strong chain that embraces many children.
Each nurse is an individual link in that chain.

— Megan Connelly, MSN, APRN, CCRN, CPNP-AC, Children's Hospital in Omaha, Nebraska

LEARNING TARGETS *At the completion of this chapter, the student will be able to:*

- Identify the effects of hospitalization on the child and his or her family.
- Discuss ways in which nurses can decrease the stress of hospitalization for the child and family.
- Discuss the concept of across care settings.
- Identify various community settings.
- Determine the nurse's role in assisting children and families in the various care settings.

---

 moving toward evidence-based practice Dental Care

Kenny, G.M., McFeeters, J.R., & Yee, J.Y. (2005). Preventive dental care and unmet dental needs among low-income children. *American Journal of Public Health, 95*(8), 1360–1366.

The purpose of this study was to examine variations in the level of dental care and unmet dental needs among low-income children. Data for the study were drawn from the 2002 National Survey of America's Families (NSAF). The NSAF is a national household survey that provides information on more than 100,000 children and adults younger than the age of 65 in the United States. Each survey respondent is allowed to provide data on up to two children regardless of the number of children residing in the household. The data must be from two categories: children 5 years of age or younger and/or children ages 6 through 17 years.

(continued)

Introduction

Nursing care for mothers, families, and children has "matured from providing simple basic care to providing highly scientific and technological care both in the hospital and community settings. Currently, there is a body of knowledge that supports early diagnosis, disease prevention along with health promotion, shorter hospital stay, increased outpatient services, community health care, and a holistic approach. Advances in knowledge have supported a healthier lifestyle and longer life expectancy but have also contributed to the complexity of issues that nurses face in providing safe and competent nursing care to mothers, children, and families across care settings. Regardless of the positive or negative consequences of the complexity of issues, families are demanding better health care in more a humanized and compassionate environment.

Pediatric nurses today must find a balance between advanced scientific and technological care and humanized compassionate care. Now, pediatric nurses have an opportunity to guide child health care of the future by integrating attitudes of human caring, supporting a holistic perspective, and shifting nursing care from the popular curative view of health care to an attitude of health promotion, illness prevention and a more family centered care environment" (Ward, 2006, pp. 15–16).

Pediatric nursing occurs in multiple settings, including hospitals, clinics, home health settings, rehabilitation centers, schools, and other supportive services. Because children and families have a variety of unique needs throughout the life cycle, the pediatric nurse must be knowledgeable and highly skilled in meeting them, which requires a broad base of knowledge about growth and development, family functioning, and environmental influences (Fig. 22-1). The concepts outlined in this chapter present innovative nursing care across care settings.

Across Care Settings

Currently there are myriad options for the delivery of nursing care ranging from the traditional hospital inpatient environment to the broader community setting. Pediatric nursing care for families is holistic, based on normal growth and development, emphasizing the optimization of preventative health and safety measures yielding positive health outcomes. Family-centered care across all settings, from community to acute care, is the underpinning for contemporary nursing and parallels today's trend for the child and family to obtain health care in diverse familiar settings in which they live, grow, play, work, or go to school.

Based on the many options available for children and families today there is need for an ongoing source of health care. A medical home provides comprehensive primary care services on an ongoing basis, in a manner encouraging

Figure 22-1 Pediatric nurse holding a child.

a positive relationship with the child, family, and the health care team. The concept of a medical home has gained attention, particularly in the care of children who have special needs, which comprise approximately 1 in 5 households (American Academy of Pediatrics, 2008). The care is provided in a manner that is family-centered, coordinated, culturally sensitive, and accessible (Alberg & Kerr, 2004). Quality of life can be improved for all children, especially those with special needs, with the collaboration of families, insurers, employers, government, medical educators, and other components of the health care system, through the care provided in a medical home.

 critical nursing action Outcomes of a Medical Home and Coordinated Care

Children with special needs receive coordinated ongoing comprehensive care within a medical home based on these outcomes

- Families of children with special health care needs will have adequate private and/or public insurance to pay for the services needed.
- Children will be screened early and continuously for special health care needs and will have increased wellness.
- Services for children with special health care needs will be organized in a manner that fosters trust, considers the family's cultural and religious beliefs, and builds support for the child and family.
- Families of children with special needs will partner in decision making at all levels, and will be satisfied with the services they receive.
- All youth with special needs will receive the services necessary to make appropriate transitions to adult heath care, work, and independence.
  Families will have increased satisfaction with their health care.
  (The National Center for medical home initiatives for children with special needs, 2008)

 Nursing Insight— *Benefits of a medical home*

- A child regularly sees the same primary care physician and staff.
- There is coordination of care for the child.
- There is an open exchange of information in an honest and respectful manner.
- There is support for finding resources and information related to all stages of growth and development and medical conditions.
- The family is connected to information and family support organizations.
- The medical home partnership promotes health and quality of life as the child grows and develops.

PRIMARY HEALTH CARE PROVIDER OR CLINIC SETTING

When a child becomes ill, pediatric nursing care traditionally takes place in a primary health care provider's office or clinic setting. The primary health care provider's office is a private medical office or clinic facility where diagnosis and treatment are offered, related to a variety of acute and chronic conditions (Wheeler, 2005). Health information is also provided and discussions are held with the family about how to take care of the child at home, providing well childhood check-ups and administering scheduled immunizations. It is important that caregivers understand the importance of accessing a primary health care provider to receive comprehensive care and education about their child's condition. The pediatric nurse in this setting can recommend additional community resources for the family (Fig. 22-2). Advantages for this type of care include a reasonable cost of care, continuity of care by remaining in a medical home, and the fact that the child remains in the care of the family. Because it is generally episodic and short-term care, it can decrease the risk of exposure that the child may have to other infectious or communicable conditions.

Figure 22-2 The nurse provides community resources to parents.

Family Teaching Guidelines...
Teaching Tips for Families

How To: The nurse can tell the family to bring a list of questions or concerns to discuss when visiting the primary care physician's office (WebMD, 2008).

ESSENTIAL INFORMATION

◆ Bring a list of any allergies that the child has along with medications the child is currently taking.

◆ Be ready to share information as to how the child is growing and changing. Keep track of the child's developmental progress.

◆ Inquire about resources including community organizations that may provide assistance.

◆ Ask about how to receive care after normal business hours or emergency care.

◆ Request to meet the health team members who will be working with the child (a nurse, a referral coordinator, or a medical assistant).

THE HOSPITALIZED CHILD

Hospitalization is required when the child becomes ill and the level of care requires more in-depth treatment than can be provided by a primary health care provider in the office or clinic. When a child enters the hospital, it may be an entirely new experience where both the child and family are exposed to an unfamiliar medical environment. The hospital may be a specialty hospital located in a separate building especially designed for children or may be part of a general care hospital.

 Collaboration in Caring— *Types of hospitals*

Hospitals: Acute care settings that provide many health care services, such as emergency care, specialized in-patient care, surgery, critical care, diagnostic tests and treatments, therapies, patient education, and other specialized services.

Children's Hospital: A specialty pediatric hospital that is specially designed and managed specifically for children that provides various health care services, such as emergency care, specialized in-patient care, surgery, critical care, diagnostic tests and treatments, patient education, and other specialized services where physicians, nurses, child life specialists, other health care providers, and employees are specially trained to work with children.

Day Hospital: A specialized hospital that serves children who require medical treatments such as blood transfusions, chemotherapy, steroid pulse therapy, intravenous hydration, intravenous antibiotic therapy, immunoglobulin therapy, or Remicade infusions.

Ambulatory Surgery Centers: A surgical center is where children receive minimal surgical treatment, recover from the procedure, and are discharged soon after the surgery.

Children are more vulnerable to the stress of hospitalization because they do not have a full range of coping mechanisms such as highly developed problem-solving

skills. The child and family are also introduced to an entirely new group of people, and are exposed to uncomfortable or painful treatments and procedures, to other cultures and languages, and to many new and difficult stressors (Leininger, 1988). The pediatric nurse must provide skilled, safe, and competent care and be supportive in their adaptation to this unfamiliar and potentially frightening environment (Gurwitch, Kees, Becker, Schreiber, Pfefferbaum, & Diamond, 2004).

In a family-centered care environment, it is essential that the pediatric nurse understands that the family is the primary caregiver and decision maker in the care of their child. It is paramount that pediatric nurses have access to and provide education about the child's condition, diagnostic testing, and procedures and, lastly, provide important discharge and teaching instructions. The nurse must also provide emotional support and take extra time to communicate effectively and therapeutically with the child and family. An important role of the pediatric nurse is to support and care for the child and family so that the child may function at the highest level possible. The nurse is committed to nurturing the child's development; supporting the child's need for family; recognizing that the child has a unique perception of the world; and respecting the child's and family's individual rights, thoughts, and feelings. The child reacts to hospitalization in a manner that reflects the wide range of development and differences of the age group. To provide effective pediatric nursing care to the child, the nurse must be keenly aware of all of these issues and seek to understand and incorporate these and the developmental level into the plan for provision of care.

When caring for children and their families in hospitals, nurses must use evidence-based theory and provide care that takes into account the effects of hospitalization and separation on the child and family (Hopia, Tomlinson, Paavilainen, & Astedt-Kurki, 2005). Typically, healthy children have a single and brief encounter when hospitalized. The stressors are real, but not as pronounced as for children who have chronic illnesses. Some of the issues experienced during hospitalization include separation from the child's parents and family, fear of the unfamiliar, and sometimes events that are painful or disturbing. Children who have chronic illness and have repeated experiences with hospitalization often experience stress over loss over the routine or regimen related to the child's condition, trying to maintain activities of daily living that are often more complex (e.g., feeding and mobility), multiple personnel with whom to communicate, and attempting to maintain a routine family life during repeated hospital stays.

Based on age and developmental milestones, the effects of separation can be more or less profound. Specifically, infants 6 months of age and younger have not developed a clear and selective attachment to their parents. For this reason, hospitalization may not cause severe direct psychological trauma to the infant. As long as the infant has contact with a nurturing caretaker, such as a nurse, he or she may not experience adverse effects. Long-term absence can also affect the parents. They may withdraw and become less attached to their infant.

A toddler's reactions to separation may become more intense and emotional (e.g., biting, kicking, crying, and hitting). In addition, any disruptions in routines may cause stress for the toddler that then may contribute to the continuation of naughty behavior. Another reaction to this stress may be that regression occurs in their bowel and bladder control and the toddler who was once potty trained may revert to diapers for a short period. Older children also may exhibit negative responses to hospitalization through the display of negative behavior and verbal expressions of anger or sadness. They begin to associate certain health care providers with specific treatments or procedures that cause stress, such as a laboratory technician drawing their blood or a nurse giving an intramuscular injection.

Regardless of age or separation from family, a child who is hospitalized will exhibit three stages: protest, despair, and detachment. The *protest phase* begins when the child realizes his or her parent is leaving or that he or she is separated from them, even if for a brief period. Depending on the child's age, the child could cry, cling, and act aggressively. This is then followed by the *despair phase* in which the child seems to withdraw from the environment and becomes very apathetic. If the parent does not return, the child begins to show renewed interest in his or her surroundings and begins to form new relationships with others. During this formation of new relationships, the child begins detaching his or her feeling from their parents. Sometimes, in this *detachment phase*, health care providers see this as a good sign of the child's adjustment; however, it is really an important clue for intervention. These children have simply repressed their pain at the sense of loss of their about their parents' absence. This may help explain why children sometimes show disinterest on the return of their parents, as a way of acting out their anger. It is encouraging to note that this process is reversible but potentially may leave permanent emotional scars if the parents are away for an extended length of time. Detachment is the final phase, when the child has begun to internalize the stressor and seems outwardly happy, although the stressors are still present.

 Now Can You— Describe the effects of hospitalization on a child?

1. Describe how family-centered care impacts hospitalization?
2. Discuss developmental differences related to reactions to hospitalization?
3. Describe protest, despair, and detachment in relation to hospitalization?

Ways to Decrease the Stress of Hospitalization

Family visitation and the family-centered care have dramatically helped children and families cope with the stress of a hospitalized child. Despite the availability of parental rooming in, the parent may also be coping with other children at home or the need to work, which could lead to separation from the child, even though family visitation is encouraged. It is important to remember that the ill child depends on his parents as the primary source of coping and comfort. To help a child of any age adapt to the stress of hospitalization, the pediatric nurse can suggest rooming-in to the parents, where they stay in the room both during the day and through the night (Table 22-1).

The nurse can also use creativity in helping the child to gain control over the environment by encouraging the child to bring something from home to familiarize the room and make it personal. They might also encourage the child to draw a picture or design that can be hung up in the hospital room or give him or her a choice to watch a movie or select a game that he or she would like to play.

THERAPEUTIC PLAY. Therapeutic play otherwise known as play therapy or medical play has been shown to help to ease the stress of hospitalization and provide children with a means for dealing with their concerns and feelings.

 Nursing Insight— *Therapeutic play*

Therapeutic play is the use of play as therapy to help children who have had or will have a stressful experience. Therapeutic play may decrease the child's fear and anxiety. It also may help to correct misconceptions the child may have about being in the hospital. There are two types of play techniques: directed and nondirected. Directed therapeutic play is guided by an adult who facilitates the play, including determination of the goals. In nondirected therapeutic play, the child is in control of the activity, although an adult may select the materials. Both types of play allow the child to demonstrate his or her emotions regarding the hospitalized experience.

Often, a child life therapist may be available to assist with therapeutic play and offer age appropriate toys or distraction such as music or games. Therapeutic play also may help the child to cope with, and master, stressful experiences (Fig. 22-3). Pediatric nurses are encouraged to incorporate the use of therapeutic play in their everyday care of the child. By using play techniques and activities in all settings, including the emergency and outpatient departments, children benefit even if it means only that they are able to watch other children at play.

Therapeutic play happens when a child is preparing to receive an injection. The nurse or child life therapist encourages the child to play with equipment such as a needle-less syringe filled with water, a doll, and an alcohol prep pad. After the injection, the nurse can then provide a bandage and a sticker for a reward. Another example is an older child simulating the medical procedure (administering IV antibiotics), a therapeutic play technique that the nurse uses

Figure 22-3 Child life specialist playing with child.

Table 22-1 Erikson's Developmental Tasks and What May Happen During Hospitalization

Age	Developmental Task	What May Happen During Hospitalization	The Nurse Can
Infant	Trust vs. mistrust	Separation anxiety Stranger anxiety Disruption in normal routine	Encourage consistency among caregivers. Encourage the parents to stay with the infant. Encourage bonding. Allow the infant's home routine whenever possible. Comfort the infant; rock, hold cuddle, swaddle. Encourage parents to bring familiar toys/blanket from home. Communicate with parents.
Toddler	Autonomy vs. shame and doubt	Regression Separation anxiety Negative behavior Increase in tantrums Fearfulness	Encourage consistency among caregivers. Encourage the parents to stay with the toddler. Allow the child's home routine whenever possible. Encourage parents to bring familiar toys/blanket from home. Communicate with parents. Allow the child to participate in care whenever possible. Use therapeutic play. Offer praise. Ensure a safe environment.
Preschool	Initiative vs. guilt	Play restrictions Fearfulness Thinks that hospitalization is a punishment	Encourage consistency among caregivers. Encourage the parents to stay with the preschool child. Allow the child's home routine whenever possible. Encourage parents to bring familiar toys from home. Communicate with parents. Allow the child to participate in care whenever possible. Use therapeutic play. Offer praise. Ensure a safe environment. Encourage use of the playroom and interaction with other children. Explain a procedure, treatment and/or surgery in simple terms. Allow the child to ask questions. Encourage realistic choices whenever possible.
School Age	Industry vs. inferiority	Play restrictions Questions identity Increased need for attention Regression Fear of bodily mutilation	Encourage the parents to stay with the school age child. Allow the child's home routine whenever possible. Encourage parents to bring familiar toys from home. Communicate with parents. Allow the child to participate in care whenever possible. Use therapeutic play. Offer praise. Ensure a safe environment. Encourage use of the playroom and interaction with other children. Explain a procedure, treatment and/or surgery in simple terms. Allow the child to ask questions. Encourage realistic choices whenever possible. Encourage the child to verbalize feelings. Alleviate fears about changes in body image. Respect the child's privacy.

Table 22-1 Erikson's Developmental Tasks and What May Happen During Hospitalization—cont'd

Age	Developmental Task	What May Happen During Hospitalization	The Nurse Can
Adolescent	Identity vs. role confusion	Concerns about body image	Encourage visits or contact from peers.
		Separation from peers	Explain a procedure, treatment and/or surgery in understandable terms.
		Loss of independence	Be honest.
		Decrease in socialization	Allow the teen to ask questions.
			Encourage realistic choices whenever possible.
			Encourage the teen to verbalize feelings.
			Alleviate fears about changes in body image.
			Respect the teen's privacy.
			Encourage parent's involvement in care.
			Recognize the teen's tendency to reject authority.

to discuss the process with the child, clarifying what is going to happen and allowing him or her to release anxiety and decrease fears of the imminent situation.

GUIDED IMAGERY. Another way to help a child cope with the stress of hospitalization is the use of guided imagery.

 Complementary Care: *Guided imagery*

- Guided imagery is a relaxation technique that aims to ease stress and to promote a sense of peace and harmony during a difficult time.
- Guided imagery can be used by persons of all ages.
- Guided imagery encompasses the power of the mind, to help heal the body, while maintaining a relaxed state including all of the body's senses (touch, smell, sound, sight and visual). (Tusek, 2008)

ROLE MODELING. Role modeling is another way to decrease the stress of hospitalization and refers to a process by which the child learns certain behaviors by observing the behavior of others. Role modeling can help to decrease fears and anxieties as well as teach coping skills. Role models can be the people who are involved in the child's life, such as parents, grandparents, siblings, or teachers. Role models can also come from videotapes, movies, or even their peers. Role models who are similar in age, sex, race, and attitudes are more likely to be imitated as well as models who have a caring demeanor (Watson, 1996). For example, a child might view a video about another child and his or her experience preparing for hospitalization and surgery. Viewing how the child in the video prepares for surgery may help the child who is facing surgery to find ways to cope with the anxiety and stress of the procedure.

 critical nursing action   The Nurse Role Models for the Child

The pediatric nurse says "I am going to give you medicine that will help you get better." The nurse may need to role model by pretending to drink the medicine, encouraging the child to take the medicine.

The child may be still somewhat hesitant after the role modeling but may eventually drink the medicine. The nurse then offers praise and allows the child to select a colorful sticker.

Effects of a Hospitalized Child on Parents

Parenting an ill child can be stressful and demanding on both the child and the parent. During the period of illness, the child can begin to recover, become gradually sicker, or suddenly begin to exhibit behaviors that give the parents cause for great concern. Symptoms such as withdrawal, lack of activity, or irritability in performing basic functions may be a signal that the child's condition is worsening. During these times, continued parenting of a hospitalized child has many dimensions, such as interpreting the child's behaviors, teaching the child new skills or how to perform basic functions again, helping a child understand the words and language of health care providers, and offering support during frightening experiences. Hospitalization has been demonstrated to be equally stressful for the parent as for the child. Parents may describe themselves as feeling incapable due to their loss of control over the situation and their inability to be able to protect their child. Some observed behaviors of parents include anxiety, denial and withdrawal, guilt and fear (including concerns by the parents that they may have had a causal effect on their child's illness). There are ways that the nurse can help parents cope with the stressful situation during a child's hospitalization.

The pediatric nurse has a critical role in assisting parents in adapting to the child's hospitalization. The plan of care for the hospitalized child begins with the admission process when the pediatric nurse includes the parents in a conversation about important information about the child while at the same time offering support. The planning stage, with parental involvement, includes setting goals and objectives that are used to evaluate overall care. The plan of care also includes home routines, preferences, developmental needs, and identification of special needs.

Parents with a hospitalized child often need to debrief and tell their story about the events that led to their child's hospitalization. Nursing assessment of parental needs,

Nursing Care Plan The Hospitalized Child

Nursing Diagnosis: Anxiety related to unfamiliar environment and procedures

Measurable Short-term Goal: The child will experience decreased feelings of apprehension and anxiety.

Measurable Long-term Goal: The child will not experience unavoidable anxiety during hospitalization.

NOC Outcomes:

Anxiety Level (1211) Severity of manifested apprehension, tension, or uneasiness arising from an unidentifiable source

Anxiety Self-Control (1402) Personal actions to eliminate or reduce feelings of apprehension, tension, or uneasiness arising from an unidentifiable source

NIC Interventions:

Anxiety Reduction (5820)
Security Enhancement (5380)
Calming Technique (5880)

Nursing Interventions:

1. Approach the child and parent(s) in a calm and reassuring manner, providing teaching and anticipatory guidance as appropriate.

   RATIONALE: Feelings of anxiety or apprehension in the caregiver are easily transmitted to the patient and family. Knowledge reduces fear of the unknown.

2. Encourage the family to stay overnight, bring the child's favorite toys or security objects, and maintain routines as appropriate.

   RATIONALE: Familiarity enhances the child's feeling of safety in a strange environment.

3. Provide a pacifier for an infant or rock, hold, or comfort an older child as needed.

   RATIONALE: Comfort measures will vary by age, culture, and individual preference.

4. Perform any invasive or painful procedures in a place other than the patient's room.

   RATIONALE: The patient's room should become and remain a safe place where the child is able to relax.

5. Encourage the family, and the child, if age-appropriate, to participate in care activities such as bathing, feeding, medication administration, or help with dressing changes.

   RATIONALE: Reduces unnecessary anxiety from having a stranger perform tasks. An older child will feel less anxiety if allowed some control over how things are done.

---

knowledge, concerns, expectations, and coping abilities is imperative to direct nursing actions that ease parental role stress. Parental stressors include sights and sounds of the hospital, changes in the child's behavior or appearance, changes in the parental role, unknown outcome, financial concerns, guilt or anger over the situation, and frustration about the function of the entire family (Fig. 22-4). Seeking parental advice about the best way to approach their child, acknowledging parental need for involvement, and anticipating stressful events are integral to appropriately caring for the child in a family-centered manner. The communication between the pediatric nurse and family members must be genuine and the plan of care must include resources available in the hospital as well as the community.

Nursing Insight— *Nursing interventions to help parents cope with the child's hospitalization*

Parents suggest that nurses may perform common interventions to help them cope with their child's hospitalization.
- Before admission, if possible, visit the hospital to see where the child will be staying.
- Encourage constant and open communication with the health care team.
- Encourage visitation of parents, friends, and family members. The number of visitors may be limited depending on the child's condition.

- Perform ongoing assessment to ensure that the nurse fully understands any changes in the plan of care for the child.
- Observe for the need for crisis intervention, should the child's condition deteriorate or change.
- Encourage the parents to participate in the child's care, while being supportive of the child and family.

Figure 22-4 Parents at the bedside of a child in the hospital.

"What to say" — *Developing a plan of care*

Admission to the hospital is a critical period for both the child and parents. The nurse can ease the experience by including the parents in the plan of care. The nurse can request information from the parents about the child's personal routine as well as the child's perception of hospitalization.

- What are your child's daily routines related to eating, elimination, sleeping, bathing, and play?
- Who are the important people in your child's life?
- Does your child have a favorite toy or attachment object?
- Has your child had previous hospitalizations?
- What has your child been told about hospitalization?
- Does your child have any fears that the staff should know about?
- Have there been any recent changes or problems in your child's life?
- How does your child usually react to pain or when frightened?

The nurse must recognize the parent's concerns, including possible guilt, fear, or other anxieties about the child's hospitalization. The pediatric nurse plans care ensuring the promotion of trust by the child and parents through prompt attention to the child's needs. The nurse provides opportunities for the child and family to participate in care and by including parental preferences and home schedules so that care is provided in a familiar and consistent manner. The nurse can also provide positive reinforcement for the parents that may help alleviate some stress. Finally, the nurse ensures an ongoing evaluation of the plan of care is necessary in order to make needed adaptations and modifications.

TWENTY-FOUR-HOUR OBSERVATION UNIT

A short-stay hospitalization experience is also known as 24-hour observation. A 24-hour observation occurs when a child becomes suddenly ill and will most likely recover quickly. The child may need a shortened hospital stay for observation and specifically for treatments such as rehydration, aerosol treatment for acute asthma, or medication for an allergic reaction. At the conclusion of the 24-hour period the child is reassessed and it is then determined whether continued hospitalization is needed or whether the child can be discharged home. The pediatric nurse provides acute nursing care and then quickly begins to prepare the child and family for discharge. As a part of discharge process, the nurse explains specific medical orders as well as when to notify the primary health care provider with any questions, concerns, or change in condition.

AMBULATORY SURGERY CENTER

An ambulatory surgery center is a place where children receive minimal surgical treatment, recover from the procedure, and then are discharged home soon after the

surgery. This type of experience minimizes the separation between child and family and can be emotionally less stressful. Although the surgery is usually minor, it is essential to teach the family about what the surgery entails and ways to care for the child at home. Some of the recovery takes place in the surgery center, but the longer recovery process continues at home. At home, parents need to be informed about the exact recovery process along with how to care for the child and when the child can resume normal daily activity. The nurse assesses the family's knowledge in order to determine their ability to care for the child independently at home or if additional support is needed.

 critical nursing action Caring for the Child at Home After Minor Surgery

Nurses can teach parents how to care for their child at home after minor surgery:

- Taking the child's axillary temperature
- Assessing the child's level of consciousness
- When to offer liquids based on type of surgery, prescribed diet, and age
- When to offer solid food based on type of surgery, prescribed diet, and age
- What type of activity is expected or should be encouraged
- What are the actions and side effects of medications
- What are the signs and symptoms of infection
- What are signs of poor airway exchange
- How to use assistive devices and medical equipment and perform home treatments
- How to contact a nurse, pharmacist, health care professional, or community agency
- When to call the doctor

CRITICAL CARE UNIT

When critical care of the child is required, the child is admitted to the critical care unit, usually through the emergency department or the operating room. A child who becomes very ill on a medical–surgical floor is transferred into a pediatric critical care unit (Hohenhaus, 2005). After delivery, a newborn who requires intensive care is transferred to a neonatal intensive care unit. Other types of critical care units where children might receive care include cardiac, surgical, or psychiatric critical care units. In any of these units, the child is extremely ill and receives specialized care, medication, intravenous fluid, respiratory, or ventilator support (Fig. 22-5).

 clinical alert

Common problems of critical illness

Common problems of critical illness are shock, acute respiratory failure, chronic respiratory failure, infection, sepsis, renal failure, neurological conditions, bleeding and clotting disorders, or multiorgan dysfunction.

Figure 22-5 Child in critical care unit.

Nursing interventions for the illness is complex and ongoing. In this type of setting, the pediatric nurse usually cares for just one or two patients at a time in order to meet the multifaceted health care and emotional support needs of the child and family.

EMERGENCY DEPARTMENT

Emergency care is provided in a hospital or health care facility that provides quick treatment for children who have become suddenly ill or experienced a severe injury. Emergency departments are open 24 hours per day and 7 days per week. Children who arrive in the emergency department first receive a rapid screening or triage assessment to establish the nature and severity of their presenting illness. If the illness or injury is severe, the child is treated in an urgent manner and all necessary procedures, treatments, and tests are preformed immediately. The emergency department may have several areas of treatment, including a general and minor care area; a resuscitation room; or specialty areas for specific populations such as children, women, or persons requiring mental health care.

Usually, children who have a minor illness such as an ear infection are sent to a less acute area, sometimes termed non-urgent. In some hospitals there is a "fast track" system were less urgent children are quickly assessed, treated by a physician, and then discharged home. Sometimes after the child receives an initial assessment and treatment, he or she is admitted to a hospital depending on the diagnosis and subsequent treatment.

Community Settings

Children have special health care needs where families, nurses, and other health care providers collaborate to create a family-centered plan of care. Today children are apt to receive the majority of their health care in a community setting. Community settings are on the front line of prevention and early detection and these settings may be located in neighborhood clinics, schools, shopping malls, or health care centers.

 Collaboration in Caring— *Caring for children in the community: Where they live, play, and go to school*

There are many places in the community where children and their families can access health care:

Community Centers: A community-based center where the pediatric nurse provides health screening and education; emphasizing health promotion and disease prevention

Preventative Medicine Center: A community-based center that provides a comprehensive menu of pediatric testing, diagnosis, and treatment related to acute and chronic conditions

Home Health Care: Health care services provided by nurses and other health care professionals in the child's home

Medical Home: An ongoing source of health care providing primary care services that is both ongoing and comprehensive

Mobile Health Care Units: A portable van that visits neighborhoods, schools, and other community locations where children can obtain screening, diagnosis, and treatment related to a variety of medical conditions, receive immunizations, and receive well childhood check-ups or basic care

Primary Physician's Office: A medical facility that provides diagnosis and treatment related to a variety of acute and chronic conditions as well as education, dissemination of information, well childhood check-ups, and administration of immunizations.

Rehabilitation Services: Services that can be provided in a community-based center or hospital where children can receive occupational, physical, audiology, and/or speech therapy.

School Setting: Schools offer basic nursing care for minor acute conditions, disease management, and teaching about health promotion and disease prevention, as well as play a role in advocacy, screening, and counseling services.

State Health Program: Each state works with its federal and local partners to help children remain healthy and safe. The programs and services help prevent illness and injury, promote healthy places to live and work, provide education to help people make good health decisions, and ensure that states are prepared for emergencies or natural disasters (National Center for Injury Prevention and Control, 2008).

The Department of Health and Human Services: The United States government's principal agency for protecting the health of all Americans and providing essential human services, especially for those who are least able to help themselves (U.S. Department of Health and Human Services Health Resources and Services Administration, Maternal and Child Health Bureau, 2008).

In the care of children and families, the focus for health care is early identification, assessment, and referral. Community settings often provide primary care along with health screening and surveillance. Health screening means to test or examine children for the presence a disease, illness, chronic condition, developmental delays, or mental health issue. Health screening plays an important role in the early diagnosis and management of selected illnesses or conditions and the initiation treatment which can then prolong and improve lives (The National Academy Press, 2008). **Health surveillance** is the continuous observation related to tracking health conditions and risk behaviors. Nurses, physicians, and other health care professionals gather ongoing information about disease incidence, demographics of an illness, and implementation of policies that may prevent further spread of diseases.

 Collaboration in Caring— *The nurse's role in health screening and surveillance*

The nurse has a key role in health screening and surveillance:

- Pay attention to voiced parental concerns.
- Ask questions about the child's growth and development.
- Observe the child's mental, physical, and spiritual state (not just a diagnosed condition).
- Note any risk factors that may be present.
- Document specific observations and findings.
- Provide community resources and make appropriate referrals.
- Track disease incidence and demographics of illnesses.
- Implement policies that may prevent further spread of diseases.
- Initiate follow-up care for any concerns and conditions.

CLINICS

When a child comes to a community setting such as a clinic to receive health care services, her symptoms are noted and she may undergo a physical assessment by a primary health care provider or nurse practitioner to diagnose the condition. In the community setting, children can receive treatment for the condition and may experience diagnostic testing such as x-ray exam or blood sampling. In a small town or rural area only one community clinic might be available. In a large urban area there can be many specialty sites. Clinics can also be housed in an acute care setting such as a hospital.

 Across Care Settings: Clinics

In a community, there can be one general care clinic or many types of specialty clinics:

Allergy & Asthma Clinic: A clinic for children that provides comprehensive services for diagnosis and treatment of allergy and asthmatic conditions

Audiological Clinic: A clinic for children where they are assessed for auditory conditions, may receive newborn hearing screenings, obtain treatment for otitis media, or receive hearing aids

Cardiology Clinic: A clinic for children that provides comprehensive services for diagnosis and treatment of congenital and acquired heart conditions

Dermatology Clinic: A comprehensive clinic for the evaluation of children with conditions related to acute, chronic, or genetic integumentary conditions

Diabetes Clinic: A consultation and management clinic for children who are diagnosed and are living with diabetes

Eating Disorders Clinic: A consultation clinic employed by physicians, psychologists, dietitians, and social workers

that is specifically designed for children with eating disorders, such as anorexia nervosa or bulimia

Endocrinology Clinic: A clinic for children that provides comprehensive services for diagnosis and treatment of endocrine and metabolic conditions

Gastroenterology—Nutrition Clinic: A clinic for children that provides comprehensive services for diagnosis and treatment of gastrointestinal, nutritional, and liver conditions

Genetic Clinic: A clinic for children that provides comprehensive services for diagnosis and treatment of inborn errors of metabolism and biochemical genetic conditions along with genetic counseling of patients and prenatal testing

Immunology Clinic: A clinic for children that provides comprehensive services for diagnosis and treatment of children with unusual infections, primary immune deficiencies, or complement deficiencies

Infectious Disease Clinic: A clinic for children that provides comprehensive services for diagnosis and treatment of acute infections or chronic infections

Neurology Clinic: A clinic for children with neurological conditions such as spina bifida, cerebral palsy, or autism who require comprehensive care and treatment

Oncology Clinic: A clinic for children that provides comprehensive services for diagnosis and treatment of cancer

Ophthalmology Clinic: A clinic for children that provides comprehensive services for diagnosis and treatment of ophthalmologic conditions

Orthopedics: A clinic for children that provides comprehensive services for diagnosis and treatment of acute and chronic musculoskeletal and bone conditions

Pulmonary/Cystic Fibrosis Clinic: A clinic for children that provides comprehensive services for diagnosis and treatment for acute and chronic respiratory conditions

Rheumatology Clinic: A clinic for children that provides comprehensive services for diagnosis and treatment of arthritis, lupus, and inflammatory conditions

Urology Clinic: A clinic for children that provides comprehensive services for diagnosis and treatment of acute, chronic, and congenital genitourinary conditions

SPECIALTY CAMPS

Specialty camps are a recreational, educational, and supportive resource where children can play, learn how to care for and cope with their condition, and meet other children who share the same medical condition (e.g., Asthma Camp, Arthritis Camp, Diabetes Camp, Ventilator Assistive Camp). In specialty camps, activities are planned that help children alleviate stress, interact with their peers, achieve mastery over planned activities, and provide a diversion from the challenges of coping with their illness or condition.

CHURCHES, SYNAGOGUES, MOSQUES

Faith communities can offer a wide variety of health-related services including teaching about health promotion and disease prevention, administration of immunizations and flu shots, provision of sick-day care, as well as daycare, preschool, and after-school care programs. In addition, prenatal classes including newborn care and information about normal growth and development may be taught in the faith community setting (Walker-Brown, 2005).

Nursing Insight— *Maternal and Child Health Bureau*

This U.S. Department of Health and Human Services Web site offers information about equal access for all to quality health care in a supportive, culturally competent, family and community setting (U.S. Department of Health and Human Services Health Resources and Services Administration, Maternal and Child Health Bureau, 2008).

After a child has received the needed health care, parents may wonder how to continue to care for their child and his or her special needs. Families must be given information about follow-up care especially related to rehabilitation. Follow-up care can help ensure that the child returns to normal functioning, learns to adapt to his or her condition, or reaches the highest most realistic level of health.

"What to say" — *When a family asks about follow-up care*

When a family asks about follow-up care related to rehabilitation services for the child, the pediatric nurse responds by saying:

Rehabilitation services generally happen in a hospital or community center where the child can begin to recuperate and receive physical, occupational, audiology, or speech assessment and therapy. Other health care professionals will assist the child in working toward the achievement of optimal function and the relief of pain. The ultimate goal is to assist the child's physical recovery and reentry into the community, home, and school. A social worker may also be involved in the child's care to assess the capacities of the family's ability to cope with the impact of the condition and situation. A social worker can also offer a broad range of community services and may serve as emotional support to referrals for community resources.

CARE IN SCHOOL SETTINGS

Care in school settings is provided by nurses who specialize in the prevention of illness, help children with special health care needs, and assist in the early identification of health concerns for children. The National Association of School Nurses (NASN)'s purpose is to advance the delivery of professional school health services to promote optimal health and learning in students. School nursing is a speciality practice that helps children maintain good health practices, along with academic success. The school nurse's role is to facilitate normal development, promote health and safety, and intervene with actual and potential health problems. The school nurse also provides case management services and collaborates with other professionals to maintain the family unit, instill self management skills, as well as promote self advocacy (National Association of School Nurses, 2008).

School nurses also focus on supporting the families of these children by working with children who do not have access to primary care, are uninsured, or are homeless (Meadows-Oliver, 2003). Nurses in the school settings can be an advocate for children and encourage parents to immunize the child as well as keep track of immunizations.

The school health nurse also plays a leadership role in the support of a coordinated school health initiative. There are eight potential areas in which the school health nurse may be involved:

- Provide the experience and resources in health education including developing health information and health programs
- Provide activities and health information including increasing the awareness and education of staff and faculty of the school and keep accurate health records
- Assess the health of students and providing access to health care
- Counsel and advise staff in the early identification of psychological or social issues
- Providing health education about nutrition, encourage healthy eating and snacking behaviors, and review and improve offerings of school menus
- Work with students and physical education teachers to encourage physical activity including students who may have special health care needs
- Report and intervene when there are hazardous situations within the school, including crisis intervention
- Provide leadership and collaborative partnerships with community agencies to meet the health care needs of children and their families.

Nursing Insight— *School nurses are the link between health and education*

- Provide education on health related topics such as nutrition.
- Assist special needs children with their unique needs.
- Help families access health care.
- Complete important screenings such as vision, hearing, and scoliosis.
- Offer counseling, primary health care services, and emergency care.
- Ensure communicable disease control by tracking immunizations and tuberculin skin test.
- Work with teachers in the identification of children at high health risk.
- Supply information for community referral and follow-up.
- Serve as advocates for children through medical case management, child abuse recognition, and crisis intervention/triage.
- Assist in the creation of community-wide disaster plans.
- Use individualized care plans and individualized family service plans.

summary points

- Family-centered care across all settings, from community to acute care settings, is the underpinning for contemporary nursing and parallels today's trend for the child and family to obtain health care in diverse familiar settings in which they live, grow, play, work, or go to school.

- Pediatric nursing occurs in multiple settings, including hospitals, clinic settings, home health settings, rehabilitation centers, schools, and other supportive services.

◆ Hospitalization can occur when the child becomes ill and his or her care requires more in-depth treatment than can be provided by a primary health care provider in the office or clinic.

◆ The pediatric nurse must possess a broad base of knowledge about growth and development, family functioning, and environmental influences in order to care for children and their families across care settings.

review questions

Multiple Choice

1. During a well baby visit, the pediatric nurse initiates teaching related to health promotion and prevention of illness. Which of the following suggestions should the nurse include in the teaching session?
A. "Call the pediatrician if the baby has a temperature of 99°F (37.2°C)."
B. "If you smoke be sure to blow the smoke away from the baby's face."
C. "Call the pediatrician if you notice a change in the baby's activity level or feedings."
D. "We want to watch the baby's weight gain, so feed the baby when she cries."

2. The pediatric nurse utilizes Erikson's developmental model to help the 2-year-old master the stage of autonomy. Which of the following will help the toddler to accomplish this task?
A. Allow the child to dress herself as much as possible.
B. Tell the parents to keep the child in view at all times.
C. Suggest colored mobiles be placed above the bed.
D. Instruct the parents to rock the child once a day.

Select All that Apply

3. What is the nurse's responsibility in educating families about how to care for their child at home after minor surgery.
A. Taking the child's axillary temperature.
B. Assessing their child's level of consciousness.
C. Teaching about the signs and symptoms of infection.
D. Teaching about the signs of poor air exchange.

Fill-in-the-Blank

4. In order to provide effective pediatric nursing care to a child, the nurse must incorporate the child's _____ _____ into the plan of care.

5. Pediatric nurses utilize _____ _____ to help decrease the stress and fear of hospitalization.

True/False

6. Providing culturally competent care means that a pediatric nurse can integrate the family's cultural elements to enhance communication and work effectively with one another.

7. Effective parenting children can help meet children's physical, emotional, and spiritual needs.

See Answers to End of Chapter Review Questions on the Electronic Study Guide or DavisPlus.

REFERENCES

Alberg, J., & Kerr, I. (2004). Meeting challenges of the 21st century: Multicultural populations. *Volta Voices: Early Intervention Issue*, November, 16–17.

American Academy of Pediatrics (2008). The National Center of Medical Home Initiatives for Children with Special Needs. Retrieved from http://www.medicalhomeinfo.org/ (Accessed June 10, 2008).

Bulechek, G., Butcher, H.M., & Dochterman, J. (2008). *Nursing interventions classification (NIC)* (5th ed.). St. Louis, MO: C.V. Mosby.

Gurwitch, R.H., Kees, M., Becker, S.M., Schreiber, M., Pfefferbaum, B., & Diamond, D. (2004). When disaster strikes: Responding to the needs of children. *Prehospital and Disaster Medicine*, 19(1), 21–28.

Healthy People 2010. Retrieved from http://www.healthypeople.gov/ (Accessed March 1, 2008).

Hohenhaus, S.M. (2005). Practical considerations for providing pediatric care in a mass casualty incident. *Nursing Clinics of North America, 40*, 523–533.

Hopia, H., Tomlinson, P.S., Paavilainen, E., & Astedt-Kurki, P. (2005). Child in hospital: Family experiences and expectations of how nurses can promote family health. *Journal of Clinical Nursing, 14*, 212–222.

Johnson, M., Bulechek, G., Butcher, H., McCloskey Dochterman, J., Maas, M., Moorehead, S., & Swanson, E. (2006). *NANDA, NOC, and NIC linkages: Nursing diagnoses, outcomes, & interventions* (2nd ed.). St. Louis, MO: Mosby Elsevier.

Leininger, M. (1988). Leininger's theory of nursing: Cultural care diversity and universality. *Nursing Science Quarterly, 1*(4), 152–160.

Meadows-Oliver, M. (2003). Mothering in public: A meta-synthesis of homeless women with children living in shelters. *Journal of the Society of Pediatric Nursing, 8*(4), 130–136.

Moorehead, S., Johnson, M., Maas, M., & Swanson, E. (2008). *Nursing outcomes classification (NOC)* (4th ed.). St. Louis, MO: C.V. Mosby.

NANDA International (2007). *NANDA-I nursing diagnoses: Definitions and classifications 2007–2008*. Philadelphia: NANDA-I.

National Academy Press: Children's health, the nation's wealth (2008). Retrieved from http://www.nap.edu/openbook/0309091187/html/1.html (Accessed November 12, 2008).

National Association of School Nurses. Retrieved from http://www.nasn.org/ (Accessed March 1, 2008).

National Center for Injury Prevention and Control. Retrieved from http://www.cdc.gov/ncipc/cmprfact.htm (Accessed March 1, 2008).

National Center for Medical Home Initiatives for Children with Special Needs. Retrieved from http://www.medicalhomeinfo.org/ (Accessed November 12, 2008)

Tusek, D. (2008). What is guided imagery? Retrieved from http://www.guidedimageryinc.com/guided.html (Accessed June 10, 2008).

U.S. Department of Health and Human Services. Retrieved from http://www.hhs.gov/about/whatwedo.html/ (Accessed March 1, 2008).

U.S. Department of Health and Human Services Health Resources and Services Administration, Maternal and Child Health Bureau (2008). Retrieved from http://www.mchb.hrsa.gov/programs/ (Accessed June 10, 2008).

Walker-Brown, T. (2005). Parish nursing/health ministry: An emerging health delivery system. *Alabama Nurse, 32*(2), 7.

Ward, S. (2006). What healing means to nursing students: A phenomenological study. *Health Ministry Journal, 2*(1), 15–27.

Watson, J. (1996). Watson's theory of transpersonal caring. In P. H. Walker & B. Neuman (Eds.). *Blueprint for use of nursing models: Education, research, practice, and administration* (pp. 141-184). New York: National League for Nursing Press.

WebMD. Retrieved from http://www.webmd.com. (Accessed June 10, 2008).

Wheeler, H.J. (2005). The importance of parental support when caring for the acutely ill child. *Nursing in Critical Care, 10*(2), 56–62.

CONCEPT MAP

What To Say:
- When a family asks about follow-up care related to rehabilitation services
- Admission to the hospital is a critical time for both the child and parents

Clinical Alert:
- Common problems of the child with a critical illness
  - Shock
  - Respiratory failure
  - Infection
  - Sepsis
  - Renal failure
  - Neurological conditions
  - Bleeding/clotting
  - Multiorgan dysfunction

Caring for the Family Across Care Settings

When

Issues Affecting Children/Families
- Hospitalization
  - Effects of hospitalization on child and parents
- Ways to decrease effects of hospitalization
  - Family-centered care
  - Therapeutic play
  - Help child gain control
  - Compensatory care
  - Role modeling
  - Assist parent to adapt

Who

Concerns of Care Across Settings
- Pair advanced technology with humanized care
  - Provide ➝ family-centered care
  - Ensure continuity of care
  - Facilitate optimal health
  - Provide anticipatory guidance

Nursing Goals

Children:
- Have distinct health care needs

Health Promotion

What

Illness Prevention
- Teaching tips for families

Health Restoration
- Early disease detection Nurse: collaborative approach
- Evaluate financial concerns and baseline knowledge
- Family education
- Support medical/rehab services

Where

- Primary care provider
- Hospital/ICU/ER
- Ambulatory surgery/ 24-hour observation
- Community/ school-based care/ specialty camps

How

Collaboration In Caring:
- Create a family-centered plan of care
- Places in community where care is delivered
- Nurse's role in screening/surveillance

Why

Optimizing Outcomes:
- Emphasize optimization of preventative health and safety measures

Nursing Insight:
- Benefits of a medical home
- Use of therapeutic play
- Maternal/Child Health Bureau
- School nurses are the link between health and education

Critical Nursing Action:
- Use key principles to collaborate with families, patients and providers
- Comprehensive coordinated care
- Care for special needs children
- Teach parents to care for post-surgical child at home
- Nursing care for spiritual distress
- The nurse role models for the child

Be Sure To:
- Ensure a safe environment

Now Can You:
- Describe the effects of hospitalization on a child

one
two
three
four
five
six
seven

Ongoing Care of the Child in the Hospital and in the Community

Caring for the Child with a Psychosocial or Cognitive Condition

The thing most people want is genuine understanding. If you can understand the feelings and moods of another person you have something to offer.

—Paul Brock

LEARNING TARGETS *At the completion of this chapter, the student will be able to:*

◆ Explain the importance of integrating aspects of developmental psychopathology, and intergenerational transmission of vulnerability and resilience to form a framework to understand how to promote children's cognitive and psychosocial health.

◆ Explore intervention options for children with cognitive and psychosocial problems/disorders.

◆ Describe the influence of ethnicity and culture on the promotion of children's cognitive and psychosocial health.

◆ Examine the incidence of the various cognitive and psychosocial problems/disorders.

◆ Relate how developmentally sensitive approaches are used in identification of disorders and strengths used to devise a care plan.

◆ Describe criteria for referring children for mental health evaluation or psychological testing.

---

 moving toward evidence-based practice Childhood Depression and Alcohol Use

Wu, P., Bird, H.R., Liu, X., Fan, B., Fuller, C., Shen, S., Durate, C.S., & Canino, G.J. (2006). Childhood depressive symptoms and early onset of alcohol use. *Pediatrics, 118*(5), 1907–1915.

The purpose of this study was to examine the relationship between depressive symptoms and the early onset of alcohol use in children and adolescents.

The investigation was based on data from a longitudinal study of psychopathology in 2491 children and early adolescents, ages 5–13 years. A subsample of 1119 children ages 10–13 years who reported never having used alcohol at the initiation of the study also completed the baseline and follow-up interviews. All of the children in the study had a Puerto Rican background.

Data collection included several types of measurements:

A structured interview was conducted with both parents and children. The interview included assessing the children for affective disorders, anxiety disorders, disruptive behavior disorders, and substance abuse and dependence disorders using the Diagnostic Interview Schedule for Children (DISC-IV) and based on the criteria identified in the *Diagnostic and Statistical Manual of Mental Disorders*, 4th ed. (DSM-IV).

For study purposes, alcohol use was defined as "drinking a full can or bottle of beer, a glass of wine or wine cooler, a shot of liquor, or a mixed drink with liquor in it."

Depressive symptoms were considered positive if reported by either the parent or child. The numbers of depressive symptoms were measured in categories: <2 (low level depressive symptoms); 2–9 (medium-level depressive symptoms); and >10 (high-level depressive symptoms). Parents were asked about the presence of emotional, alcohol, or drug problems in either parent.

Parents completed a "parental monitoring" Likert-type scale that consisted of nine questions. The purpose of the tool was to determine how often the parent monitored the child's television watching, video game playing, and other activities in or outside of the home. A high score indicated a high level of parental monitoring.

The parents' use of discipline was measured through an interview that consisted of six items regarding the use of physical

(continued)

---

moving toward evidence-based practice (continued)

and verbal abuse, various forms of punishments and the with-holding of affection.

Maternal warmth and support was evaluated using a 13-item Likert-type scale. A high score indicated a close maternal–child relationship.

A four-item tool that related to parental behaviors including hitting, beating, or badly hurting the child was used to assess physical abuse. A positive response to any of the four questions was considered to be consistent with physical abuse.

Measured socioeconomic factors included the age of the child, gender, highest level of parental education, and family structure/composition (i.e., the number of parent figures).

Data analysis revealed the following findings:

- One hundred and ten (9.8%) of children who had not used alcohol at the time of the initial interview reported the use of alcohol at the first follow-up.
- The rates of alcohol use varied according to the level of depression: at the baseline interview, those with <1 depressive symptoms reported an alcohol use rate of 4.1%; those with 2–9 depressive symptoms reported an alcohol use rate of 10.2%; and those with >10 symptoms reported an alcohol use rate of 14.1%.
- Sociodemographic factors revealed that the age of the child was positively associated with the timing of the onset of alcohol use and that parental education made little difference in the child's use of alcohol.
- No association was found between alcohol use and the child's gender or whether the child lived in a single-parent home.

- Parent psychopathology and child physical abuse were positively associated with alcohol use in the child.
- No association was found between alcohol use and a close maternal relationship or the level of parental discipline.
- Sensation seeking, exposure to violence, and antisocial behaviors were identified as risk factors for child alcohol use.
- No relationship was found between the child's alcohol use and church attendance or the presence of stressful live events.

Children with high-level depressive symptoms and medium-level depressive symptoms were more likely to use alcohol than those with low-level symptoms. Children with fewer than two depressive symptoms were less likely to begin drinking than those with two or more depressive symptoms.

An early onset of alcohol use may be impacted by early life depressive symptoms. In addition, the presence of parent psychopathology, exposure to violence, and antisocial behaviors were also found to be significant risk factors for the early onset of alcohol use in children.

---

1. What might be considered as limitations to this study?
2. How is this information useful to clinical nursing practice?

See Suggested Responses for Moving Toward Evidence-Based Practice on the Electronic Study Guide or DavisPlus.

Introduction

Understanding the normal neurological, cognitive, and emotional development of children is important in determining if they are functioning within their appropriate developmental level. For example, developmentally expected anxiety in infants and young children may suddenly arise as a fear of strangers or in response to separation from caregivers. This typically occurs between 7 to 12 months and peaks between 9 to 18 months, but decreases for most children by age 2 1/2 (Zero to Three, 2005a). Also, a child may have an inherent anxious temperament and may be inhibited when encountering new situations, people, or objects and may respond to these with fear and withdrawal. Likewise, nurses should note that normal behaviors for young children (imaginary friends, concrete thinking, etc.) are interpreted differently when displayed in adults (as signs of schizophrenia). Awareness of language development is important in determining learning disabilities, developmental disabilities, or autism.

Most children do not develop cognitive or psychosocial disorders. However, it is important for the nurse to have a good history of developmental milestones, including language development, sensory perception, emotion regulation, motor skills, attention, and memory (Denham, 2006; Heffelfinger & Mrakotsky, 2006).

Developmental Psychopathology

This chapter uses a framework based on developmental psychopathology, which draws on multiple theoretical models and literature across scientific disciplines, to help explain the interaction between normality and pathology at various stages of child and adolescent development. **Developmental psychopathology** is an actual discipline that evolved from the contribution of multiple fields of study with the goal to provide understanding between psychopathology and normal adaptation (Cicchetti & Posner, 2005). It combines developmental, biological, and social theories to track deviations from developmental norms as they relate to psychological pathologies. This reflects an understanding that adaptive and maladaptive (mental illness) patterns can occur in infancy, childhood, or adolescence. In addition, and most importantly, it is thought that individuals with psychopathologies have the ability to function in an adaptive way. It is expected through the use of this framework that the nurse will gain understanding into individual patterns of cognitive and psychosocial child/adolescent health. Understanding of developmental psychopathology may aid in the prevention and early intervention of mental illness (maladaptive patterns).

Vulnerability and Resilience

Vulnerability and resilience are important topics in the care of children. The intergenerational transmission model is based on the premise that vulnerability toward maladjustment or resilience in the face of adversity may be passed on from one generation to the next. It is important that the nurse working with children and their families have a good understanding of the key concepts of intergenerational transmission of vulnerability and resilience. Vulnerability is defined as "a predispositional factor, or set of factors, that makes a disorder state possible" (Ingram & Luxton, 2005, p. 34). Children with resilience show positive adaptation despite significant life adversity (Cicchetti, 2003).

Optimizing Outcomes— Understanding resilience in the face of vulnerability

It is important to keep in mind that not all offspring of parents with mental health issues go on to develop mental health-related problems themselves. In fact, the children of parents or caregivers with mental health issues who do not exhibit any maladjustment or symptoms of mental health problems during childhood are known to be resilient children (Hammen, 2003). Researchers in this area of study found that much can be learned about mental health wellbeing from these children. The best outcome gained from this knowledge can be used to prevent and promote good mental health for all children.

Culture, Diversity, and Health Disparities

The anthropological model of culture, ethnicity, and race disputes beliefs that culture and race are innate (Smedley & Smedley, 2005). Within an anthropological framework, culture and race are learned behaviors. This dynamic view can be used to illustrate the value of how culture and diversity influence children's and families' cognitive and psychosocial health. Culture is considered to be an external and acquired phenomenon. It is the complex set of beliefs and attributes passed on within a group. Ethnicity refers to groups of people who share similar cultural characteristics (i.e., common language, religion, food, and

beliefs about health). Race is used to describe categories of people, mostly based on physical characteristics (e.g., skin color, shape of nose).

Another issue that deserves a great deal of attention from the nursing community involves health disparities. There is vast information research indicating that health care disparities in racial and ethnic minorities are widespread compared to those in non-minorities, and barriers such as mistrust, fear, and discrimination stand in the way of optimal mental health outcomes in ethnically diverse families (Heffernan, 2004). For instance, the nurse must recognize that new immigrants may be concerned with learning the language and getting and keeping a job, and may focus only on their children's basic health care needs (e.g., vaccines, treatment for ear infection) and may not at all attend to children's cognitive and psychosocial health needs. It is important that the nurse do a thorough assessment of health care needs, including cognitive and psychosocial wellbeing.

Given the magnitude of mental health disparities in children and adolescents, nurses at all levels of practice along with other health care providers must become better prepared to implement strategies designed to reduce health care disparities. In particular, nurses are well positioned to take a leadership role in the movement toward abating and eliminating health care disparities (Heffernan, 2004).

Nursing Insight— *Understanding mental health disparities in children*

In contrast to younger children, adolescents have the necessary cognitive and social structures to be able to perceive discrimination. In a study with Latino children and adolescents, researchers found that adolescents who perceived severe discrimination had poorer mental health outcomes compared with their peers (Szalacha et al., 2003). This indicates that children's perceptions about how they are treated make an important difference in their own mental health outcomes. It is therefore important for the nurse to assess children's perceptions of how they are viewed by others, including health care professionals.

Ethnocultural Considerations— Promoting understanding of culture in diverse families

It is important that nurses gain an in-depth understanding regarding the culture of various people; acquire sensitivity and empathy in working with diverse families (e.g., give up preconceived notions or generalizations about particular ethnic or racial groups); and attain skills in relationship building with children, adolescents, and parents/caregivers of various ethnic and racial backgrounds. It is recommended that nurses working with children and families of diverse socioeconomic backgrounds take an approach of listening, providing as much positive feedback as possible for what families are doing well and keep resilience-promoting strategies in mind. Using anticipatory guidance, nurses working with children and their families may be most effective suggesting alternative ways of handling a specific cognitive or psychosocial-related concern.

where research and practice meet: Is Mental Illness Passed Along to Children?

In a study of 166 low-income and racially diverse adolescent children of mentally ill mothers, Mowbray et al. (2004) discovered that the majority of children (30.1%) were actually socially and academically proficient, whereas, 15.1% of the children showed anxiety and depression with poor social and academic competence. In addition, 27.1% of the children were delinquent and peer-oriented, and 4.8% were classified as isolated noncomformists. Of the total children, 22.3% were in the middle of these groups (Mowbray et al., 2004). The intergenerational transmission of vulnerability and resilience model is important to consider while the nurse conducts assessment, formulates a nursing diagnosis, devises preventive interventions or plan of care for the child or family, and finally executes evaluation.

In this way, nurses can provide health and psychoeducation in a nonthreatening way to help families decide what works best for them.

There is also a flawed belief that poverty predisposes children and families to mental illness. Although it needs to be studied more thoroughly, there is evidence suggesting that poverty by itself does not cause mental health problems in children and families (Rutter, 2003). Strategies outlined above for nurses to decrease health care disparities also apply in working with families who may be poor, disenfranchised, affected by substance abuse, family violence, and child maltreatment.

Barriers to Child and Adolescent Mental Health

There are a number of barriers to the diagnosis and treatment of children's cognitive and psychosocial health. A brief overview is provided here to help the nurse gain an understanding of the issues in order to intervene to minimize these barriers. Though there are increasing efforts to educate the public, the *stigma* of mental illness continues to be a major barrier to accessing mental health services for children and their families (Hinshaw, 2006). The health care community and the lay public have long been skeptical about whether young children, in particular, experience clinically significant mental health disorders, such as depression. There is a prominent belief that childhood is a "sacred" happy time free of problems. Health care providers have also had a role in perpetuating barriers by minimizing or dismissing parents' or caregivers' concerns. Parents may be told that the child is simply going through a stage that will pass, when there are indeed grounds for concern (e.g., early signs of autism spectrum disorder). It is important for the nurse to understand that this type of thinking may lead to several issues for children, adolescents, and their families such as: (1) not getting screened on a timely basis for disordered behaviors and emotional difficulties that often can be attenuated or resolved if early intervention is sought in a timely fashion; (2) having a sense of shame for the family if a child or adolescent is eventually diagnosed with a mental health problem that might have been prevented or attenuated earlier; and (3) inability to receive adequate mental health or psychosocial treatment when indicated because of lack of resources (Hinshaw, 2005).

⊖ where research and practice meet:
Injury Control Research Centers (ICRC)

The Department of Health and Human Services Center for Disease Control and Prevention; Injury Control Research Centers (ICRC) serves to conduct research about injury control in the areas of prevention, acute care, and rehabilitation. In addition, the ICRC serve as training and public information centers. This valuable research can help nurses to understand violent behaviors in youth today (U.S. Department of Health and Human Services, Centers for Disease Control and Prevention, 2008).

Psychopathology in Children

Children and adolescents are not immune to mental and emotional illnesses. Mental illness in children and adolescents may be confusing and frightening for children and families. The disorders can be quite devastating, particularly if they are not detected and treated.

ANXIETY

Anxiety disorders are among the most common psychiatric complaints in children. While children commonly experience transient anxieties at various developmental points, clinically significant anxiety must be recognized as a problem. It is important to distinguish between developmentally expected anxiety, anxious temperament, and symptoms of a disorder. The following diagnostic categories related to anxiety disorders have been identified in the *Diagnostic and Statistical Manual* (DSM-IV-TR): separation anxiety disorder (SAD), generalized anxiety disorder (GAD), specific phobia, panic disorder, social phobia, selective mutism, posttraumatic stress disorder, and obsessive–compulsive disorder (OCD) (American Psychiatric Association [APA], 2000). In separation anxiety disorder, children experience overwhelming fear of becoming separated from or losing a caregiver (Fig. 23-1). The nurse understands that some degree of separation anxiety is normal at various stages of development and during transitions, but if the anxiety is severe and excessively disruptive, and if it persists for longer than 4 weeks, the child should be evaluated by a mental health professional. In GAD, children experience excessive worry about everything, including peer relationships, social acceptance, and pleasing others. Specific phobia refers to unrelenting fear of certain objects or situations (i.e., spiders, storms, snakes, water). These may be difficult to evaluate because

Figure 23-1 This child is displaying signs of separation anxiety.

at each developmental stage children and adolescents have various expected fears. Panic disorder usually begins in adolescence but may start earlier. Symptoms of a panic attack might include palpitations, sweating, shaking, nausea, dizziness, fear of dying, tingling sensations, chills, or hot flushes. Selective mutism refers to a child's enduring refusal to speak in certain situations. This refusal interferes with the child's functioning and development and is not due to physiological or deficit of knowledge. Posttraumatic stress disorder occurs in response to a perceived or actual threat to one's life or safety. There is a clear precipitant and a reaction is generally understandable. The response may persist for weeks, months, or years and is accompanied by panic symptoms. In obsessive–compulsive disorder (OCD), the child experiences sometimes debilitating recurrent worries or thoughts (obsessions) and repetitive actions or thoughts that bind the anxious thoughts (compulsions).

It is estimated that 13% of children between the ages of 9 and 17 suffer with some type of anxiety disorder (Substance Abuse and Mental Health Services Administration [SAMHSA], n.d.). Nearly 50% of children with anxiety disorders have at least one other psychiatric disorder (SAMSHA, n.d.).

Signs and Symptoms

It is important for the nurse to understand normal developmental anxiety. This understanding provides a baseline from which to judge the occurrence of clinically significant distress. Anxiety is an important factor in motivation and alertness. Worries and fears are a part of every developmental stage, even throughout adulthood. An occasional bout of feeling nervous accompanied by sweating, nausea, diarrhea, worry, and/or tearfulness is well within normal limits. But when the anxiety does not abate or it gets worse with time, it may be indicative of an anxiety disorder. The nurse should question a child's or adolescent's level of anxiety if it does not respond to reassurance or closeness with a safe person or if it interferes with functioning.

Anxiety often presents in the form of somatic complaints like stomachaches and restlessness (Ginzburg, Riddle, & Davies, 2006). The school nurse can recognize anxiety problems when a child persistently presents with symptoms that do not have a recognizable physical cause.

Children or adolescents with clinically diagnosable anxiety disorders may suffer from persistent worry, unfounded fears, separation difficulties, sleep problems, or obsessions or compulsions (Cleveland Clinic, 2007). Anxious children may also resist going to school or staying there after arriving. They may avoid play time, even with good friends, and not be able to explain why.

Diagnosis

As with any emotional or psychiatric difficulty, a complete physical, psychosocial and family history helps reveal genetic, biological, and familial contributors to anxiety.

Nursing Care

There are specific interventions that a nurse may do to help prevent anxiety disorders from occurring or to lessen their impact on children. Simply paying attention to any signs of anxiety (SAMSHA, n.d.) is the first step in recognizing clinically significant symptoms. The nurse should refer a child to a mental health professional if the child's anxiety interferes with normal functioning or if it persists regardless of attempts to reassure the child. The nurse can provide health teaching related to what makes the child anxious or worried and how to cope with such worries. Teaching may involve teaching relaxation and deep breathing as well as problem-solving techniques (Tomb & Hunter, 2004). Young people are more likely to respond to someone who takes the time to listen and care.

Current Western culture is filled with scary images, whether in the form of games, movies, television, or actual events in the news. It is important for the nurse to understand and to help parents think about how and when to protect children from the influx of information that might be overwhelming.

There are several evidence-based therapies provided by qualified advanced practice clinicians. The pediatric nurse can be aware of some of these therapies in order to assist parents in finding a referral. The Coping Cat program is designed for children ages 7 to 13 with anxiety disorders and the CAT program is for adolescents (Kendall, Aschenbrand, & Hudson, 2003). Both of these cognitive–behavioral programs are designed to help the child develop skills to cope with anxiety, as well as techniques to decrease fears through systematic exposure to the feared object. These programs are intended to be used with children and adolescents who have SAD, GAD, and social phobia.

The FRIENDS program was designed for the parents as well as their children with anxiety disorders (Barrett & Shortt, 2003). It is similar to the Coping Cat in that it uses cognitive–behavioral techniques to help children and their families cope with anxiety. FRIENDS is an acronym for **F**eeling worried? **R**elax and feel good. **I**nner thoughts. **E**xplore plans. **N**ice work so reward yourself. **D**on't forget to practice. **S**tay calm, you know how to cope. This program has proved to be useful in reducing the risk of development of anxiety disorders in children (Barrett, Farrell, Ollendick, & Dadds, 2006), but has proven less useful when used to prevent depression (Spence & Shortt, 2007).

✿ Complementary Care: *Mindful breathing*

Mindfulness means paying attention in the present moment. Paying attention to one's breathing may be a way of coping with anxiety. The teaching works best before an anxiety episode.

The nurse teaches slow breathing by telling the child to (Fig. 23-2):

- Consciously direct your attention to your breathing.
- Breathe in slowly, paying attention as the air enters nose and mouth and filling your lungs.
- Breathe out slowly, paying attention as the air leaves your body.
- Allow your mind to follow the breath in and out.
- Imagine yourself in a rubber raft riding the gentle waves of your breath.

Figure 23-2 The nurse teaches the child how to reduce anxiety with slow breathing.

POSTTRAUMATIC STRESS DISORDER

Posttraumatic stress disorder (PTSD) is an anxiety disorder that occurs in response to a real or perceived trauma or threat to one's life or safety. PTSD in young children has been the subject of great debate at professional meetings because not all children who have endured trauma present with a neat and simple set of symptoms (Scheeringa, 2006).

It is known that the types of events that are experienced by young children as traumatic are similar to those of older children, adolescents, adults, and elderly (e.g., automobile crashes, natural disasters, war, witnessing brutal deaths) (Scheeringa, 2006). Other types of trauma, like physical or sexual abuse, or witnessing of domestic violence can be devastating for the child and can cause PTSD that persists even into adulthood if not treated.

Children who endure trauma often exhibit additional symptomatology to that of PTSD and frequently may suffer from comorbid disorders such as depression, conduct disorders, and other anxiety disorders as well as physical disorders. While the current DSM-IV-TR (APA, 2000) criteria are not developmentally sensitive for young children, they are used by most clinicians to help develop a diagnosis. Many children do not experience all of the criteria required to meet the DSM diagnosis, but children can still suffer greatly with the anxiety resulting from the original trauma.

 Nursing Insight— *Posttraumatic stress disorder in adolescence*

Adolescence is a time of experimentation and of a sense of invincibility. For those reasons, adolescents may be more likely to be in a position to experience traumatic events, thus being exposed to the possibility of PTSD. In a survey of American adolescents, researchers found that 23% had been both a victim and witness to a traumatic event (i.e., assault) and more than 20% had symptoms that met criteria for PTSD (Commission on Adolescent Anxiety Disorders, 2005).

Signs and Symptoms

After a trauma, a child with PTSD exhibits symptoms within each of the following sets of reactions:

- Re-experiencing the trauma, perhaps in the form of a flashback (intense "remembering" of the event while feeling as if it were happening at the present moment), nightmares, or sensations.
- Avoidance of anything that could trigger the memories, through dissociation (a sense of being detached emotionally, mentally, and perhaps even physically) or avoiding places or events reminiscent of the trauma.
- Physiological symptoms of anxious arousal (insomnia, startle response, sense of panic) (Commission on Adolescent Anxiety Disorders, 2005).

The hallmark symptoms of PTSD in children are nightmares, flashbacks, dissociative experiences, psychological and/or physiological distress at reminders of the traumatic event, irritability, anger, hypervigilance, new fears and anxieties and many other symptoms that may interfere with adjustment and daily functioning (Scheeringa, 2006).

Diagnosis

A complete history reveals a traumatic event(s) that may help diagnosis PTSD. Diagnosis is based on the symptoms and reaction(s) to the event.

Nursing Care

Many children who endure posttraumatic distress may not be brought into a health care facility for clinical intervention. A significant number of seriously traumatized children enter treatment through the court system after having experienced abuse or serious loss within the family of origin (Osofsky, 2004). The nurse may come in contact with these children in primary care or in school or other settings.

In the community, the nurse can be instrumental in educating parents about the symptoms and helping the family and child by making referrals for appropriate services. The nurse can reinforce that it is important to provide a secure base for the child, one that includes family or caregiver's willingness to be available to and comfort the child without judgment.

Be aware of resources available that might provide play therapy for young children and their parents (Van Horn & Lieberman, 2006) or cognitive behavioral therapies (CBTs) for older children. The nurse can also teach the family that pharmacotherapy with selective serotonin reuptake inhibitors (SSRIs) has also been known to be effective in adolescents (Commission on Adolescent Anxiety Disorders, 2005).

Implementing nursing care similar to that given with any anxious child may help to allay fears. During an acute panic episode when the child is re-experiencing the triggering event or feels completely out of control, the nurse must remain with him, talk soothingly, and reassure the child that the nurse is providing personal safety.

Mood Disorders

Similar to adult psychiatric disorders, pediatric mood disorders may take the form of major depression (serious, time-limited depression), dysthymic disorder (longer-term, less intense depression), or bipolar disorder (consisting of mood swings between depression and mania). These disorders are sometimes more difficult to diagnose in children and adolescents than in adults because of developmental phases and the lack of language and cognitive skills to describe symptoms and experiences. Health care providers may also not have adequate knowledge about prior symptoms.

DEPRESSION

Infants born of mothers who have been significantly depressed or stressed during pregnancy can exhibit depressive symptoms (listlessness, failure to attach, irritability) (Commission on Adolescent Depression & Bipolar Disorder, 2005). Likewise, infants who are unable to attach securely or who are listless or irritable may be difficult for the mother to care for and show attachment. This behavior can perpetuate disengaged attachment and depression in the infant. Some studies have indicated that children as young as 3 years old are capable of experiencing depressive disorders (Luby et al., 2003, 2006). These depressions may be related to environmental factors combined with genetic and biological factors.

Depressive symptoms are estimated to occur in 10% to 15% of children and adolescents. Untreated depression in a young person often increases the likelihood of recurrent depression or bipolar illness later in life. For this reason it is important to recognize and treat depression early on (SAMHSA, n.d.).

Signs and Symptoms

Five key features must be present and persistent for most days during a period of 2 weeks for the diagnosis of a major depressive disorder in children and adolescents. The nurse must remember that children can have just a few of these depressive symptoms that will interfere with optimal functioning. This list of symptoms was compiled based on several diagnostic classification publications to reflect a developmentally sensitive criterion (APA, 2000; Greenspan, 2005; Zero to Three, 2005b):

* Persistent sad or irritable mood—by subjective report (e.g., sad or empty) or observed by others (e.g., appears tearful). This mood is different from the child's baseline emotional and behavioral state, and is unrelated to events that may cause temporary distress or sadness (e.g., getting a time-out).
* Loss of interest in activities once enjoyed (anhedonia)—reported by child or observed by others.
* Significant change in appetite or body weight—weight loss or gain reflected by more than a 5% change in body weight.
* Difficulty sleeping or oversleeping—insomnia or hypersomnia (excessive sleep).
* Physical agitation or slowing—observed by others and the child's subjective report of being restless or "slowed down."
* Fatigue or loss of energy.
* Feelings of worthlessness or excessive/inappropriate guilt.
* Decreased ability to think or concentrate or to make decisions as self-reported or observed by others, and in younger children this sign may appear as difficulty

in solving problems, responding to caregivers or sustaining attention. An example is a drop in grades and/or school performance.
* Recurrent thoughts of death or suicide with or without a suicide plan, and in younger children consistent engagement in activities or play that involve themes of death and suicide.

Depression in infants may include:

* Listlessness without physical cause
* Failure to respond to caregiver

The nurse understands that symptoms in the infant and very young child mirror the symptoms of attachment disorders and failure to thrive.

Diagnosis

Diagnosis is based on the exhibited depressive symptoms.

Nursing Care

The most important aspect of helping a depressed child is to ensure safety. It is recommended that any nurse working with a child who is depressed understand how to deal with the potential suicide ideation or intent.

Since depression often goes unrecognized in children or adolescents, the nurse can be instrumental in determining its presence. Pediatric and school nurses are in a position to observe changes in a child's behavior and demeanor as well as grades. Developing a trusting relationship with a child and asking about feelings or thoughts may provide evidence of underlying depression and provide the child with a first step in feeling better. Nurses should talk with the parent(s) or caregiver(s) of a child about suspected depression and suggest referral to a counselor for evaluation and treatment.

BIPOLAR DISORDER

Bipolar disorder (BPD), also known as manic–depression, is a mood disorder that is evidenced by significant mood swings (from depression to mania). It is thought that childhood or adolescent onset bipolar disorder may have an extended early course and may respond less

---

medication: Somatic Therapies for Depression

Serotonin Selective Reuptake Inhibitors (SSRIs):
Open-label studies suggest that fluoxetine (Prozac) is an effective medication in the treatment of pediatric major depression and dysthymia in patients with and without co-occurring mental health disorders (Findling, Feeny, Stansbrey, Delorto-Bedoya, & Demeter, 2001). This type of medication has been used in children as young as 8 years old (National Institute of Mental Health [NIMH], 2001). Other SSRIs are used off-label (meaning use other than specifically approved for by the Food & Drug Administration [FDA]) such as sertraline (Zoloft), paroxetine (Paxil), citalopram (Celexa), escitalopram (Lexipro), or fluvoxamine (Luvox) have also been prescribed by some clinicians (NIMH, 2001).
NOTE: Recent evidence that SSRIs can contribute to suicide ideation in adolescents and children have left many parents and physicians leery of using this medication to treat depression in young people.

Nursing Care Plan Depressed Child

Nursing Diagnosis: Self-Esteem: Situational Low related to cognitive and perceptual distortions

Measurable Short-term Goal: Child will use positive talk to interrupt negative thinking about self.

Measurable Long-term Goal: Child will demonstrate increased self-esteem by accepting positive feedback from others.

NOC Outcome:
Self-Esteem (1205) Personal judgment of self-worth

NIC Interventions:
Self-Esteem Enhancement (5400)
Active Listening (4920)

Nursing Interventions:

1. Listen actively to child, displaying interest without judgment or responding too quickly.

   RATIONALE: Active listening shows attention to the message and respect for the child's thinking and perceptions.

2. Monitor and help the child to identify statements reflecting perceived self-worth.

   RATIONALE: Provides information about distorted or negative perceptions.

3. Assist the child to examine perceptions of self reflected in negative "self-talk" and turn these into positive statements of self-worth.

   RATIONALE: Allows replacement of negative self-evaluations with positive statements that enhance self-esteem.

4. Encourage the child to identify personal strengths and accept valid positive responses from others.

   RATIONALE: Helps the child develop positive self-esteem.

5. Assist child to set realistic goals to enhance self-esteem, providing appropriate praise or rewards for progress.

   RATIONALE: Positive reinforcement supports progress in meeting realistic personal goals.

---

favorably to treatment. Children and adolescents with bipolar disorder may have coexisting mental health disorders as well (e.g., attention-deficit/hyperactivity disorder, oppositional defiant disorder, conduct disorder, anxiety disorder, and substance abuse) (Kowatch et al., 2005).

There are three recognized types of bipolar disorder. Bipolar disorder I (BD-I) is defined by the presence of depressive and manic episodes. Bipolar disorder II (BD-II) is characterized by episodes of hypomania (a lesser degree of mania) and depression. Bipolar disorder not otherwise specified (BD-NOS) is commonly the diagnosis given to children when the DSM-IV-TR (APA, 2000) criteria for BD-I and II are not specifically met but who show symptoms of bipolar illness.

There are little definitive data related to incidence of BD-I since many of the studies done to date have not used standardized criteria to explain the onset of symptoms. The overall lifetime pervasiveness of BD beginning between 15 and 17 is 1.3%. Typically the disorder is diagnosed in early adulthood. While BD was originally thought to be relatively rare in children, more research efforts are aimed at identifying and understanding this disorder.

Signs and Symptoms

Since BPD is a combination of major depression and mania, the nurse must be aware of symptoms associated with BPD. Both manic and depressive symptoms, as described by the National Institute of Mental Health (2000) are listed.

Nursing Insight— *Bipolar disorder*

Mania	**Depression**
Severe changes in mood—either extremely irritable or overly silly and elated	Persistent sad or irritable mood
Overly inflated self-esteem; grandiosity	Loss of interest in activities once enjoyed
Increased energy	Significant change in appetite or body weight
Decreased need for sleep—able to go with very little or no sleep for days without tiring	Difficulty sleeping or oversleeping
Increased talking—talks too much, too fast; changes topics too quickly; cannot be interrupted	Physical agitation or slowing
Distractibility—attention moves constantly from one thing to the next	Loss of energy
	Feelings of worthlessness or inappropriate guilt
Hypersexuality—increased sexual thoughts, feelings, or behaviors; use of explicit sexual language	Difficulty concentrating
Increased goal-directed activity or physical agitation	Recurrent thoughts of death or suicide
Disregard of risk—excessive involvement in risky behaviors or activities	

Source: NIMH (2000). *Child & adolescent bipolar disorder: An update from the National Institute of Mental Health. (NIH Publication Number: 00–4778). Retrieved from http://www.nimh.nih.gov/publicat/index.clm*

Although young children do not have distinct episodes of mania, children may have severe mood dysregulation with multiple, intense, prolonged mood swings each day (Kowatch et al., 2005). Also, children are more likely to display irritability or destructiveness than adults who display euphoria.

Diagnosis

Diagnosis is based on a thorough history and physical as well as the identification of the significant mood swings (from depression to mania). Often family members or significant others can describe the behavior that may help lead to a diagnosis.

Nursing Care

It is important for the nurse to recognize that if a child is in an acutely manic state, the child is struggling against an internal force and is not being a "bad child." The nurse can teach the family and the child, as well as model the following therapeutic parenting techniques presented by the Child and Adolescent Bipolar Foundation (CABF, 2008):

- Practice and teach relaxation techniques
- Use firm restraint holds to control rages
- Prioritize battles and let go of less important matters
- Reduce stress in the home
- Use good listening and communication skills
- Use music and sound, lighting, water, and massage to assist the child with waking, falling asleep, and relaxation
- Become an advocate for stress reduction and other accommodations at school
- Help the child anticipate and avoid, or prepare for stressful situations by developing coping strategies beforehand
- Engage the child's creativity through activities that express and channel gifts and strengths
- Provide routines, structure and freedom within limits
- Remove objects from the home (or lock them in a safe place) that could be used to harm self or others during a rage, especially guns
- Keep medications in a locked cabinet or box

It is also important to note that a person should be present to care for a child experiencing a depressed phase of bipolar disorder. Just in case the diagnosis of bipolar disorder is missed, and an antidepressant is prescribed, the nurse understands that an antidepressant could trigger mania. It is important to fully assess history of symptoms and to teach the family what to watch for in terms of the child's reaction to the medication(s). The nurse can have the family visit the following Web site for more information about bipolar disorder: http://www.bpkids.org, a parent-led organization that provides supportive information for children, caregivers, and families.

 Now Can You— Differentiate between depression and bipolar disorder?

1. Describe the signs and symptoms of depression and bipolar disorder?
2. Describe nursing care for the child with depression or bipolar disorder?

SUICIDE

Suicide represents a devastating consequence resulting from any number of psychiatric difficulties. What was relatively rare before the mid-1950s has now become an alarmingly frequent occurrence. Barrio (2007) summarized potential factors that might influence a child or adolescent to consider or attempt suicide: (1) certain psychiatric disorders that may be related to a sense of helplessness (depression, substance abuse, anxiety disorders, or aggressive disorders); (2) a history of family or friend having attempted or actually committed suicide; (3) personal or familial biological factors (related to depression and/or impulsivity); (4) environmental factors, such as accessibility of a means (guns, poison, etc.), or lack of connection or supervision; previous suicide attempts; and/or (5) disenfranchised status (sexual orientation, minority status).

According to the National Center for Health Statistics, suicide is the third leading cause of death in young people 10 to 24 years of age, which in 2004 translated in into the following statistics: 1.3 children (ages 10 to 14) per 100,000, 8.2 adolescents (ages 15 to 19) per 100,000, and 12.5 young adults (ages 20 to 24) per 100,000. Younger children more often resorted to suffocation as a method to kill themselves while older children tended to use firearms or poison. There were gender differences that identified males as four times more likely in their adolescents and six times more likely in early adulthood to succeed at suicide than females (Centers for Disease Control and Prevention [CDC], n.d.). This difference may be due to the choice of method (males tend to choose more lethal means).

Signs and Symptoms

The nurse should suspect suicide potential when faced with any of the following in the child or adolescent:

- Symptoms of depression or other mental illness
- Alienation or withdrawal from friendships or relationships
- Personality changes
- Decline in schoolwork
- Giving away personal possessions that were once prized
- Preoccupation with death in writing or drawings
- References to dying or no longer being around
- Access to a method of suicide (e.g., medications, weapons)

---

medication: Valproate (Depakote)

The nurse needs to be aware that most medications used for the treatment of bipolar disorder have not been studied specifically with children. Lithium carbonate (Eskalith, Lithobid) has been the most common treatment. It is a mood stabilizer that calms the manic symptoms.

Diagnosis

Nursing Insight— *Assessing the child for suicide risk*

If the nurse is concerned that a child or adolescent might be suicidal, the nurse must ask the child about suicidal thoughts or behaviors. This information may help to save the child's life.

- "Have you thought about doing something to hurt yourself or take your life?"
- "Do you ever wish you were not alive?"
- "What would you do if you were to hurt yourself?"

When a child or adolescent gives information that indicates risk for suicidal behavior, the nurse must take steps to keep the child or adolescent safe and make a referral for immediate mental health evaluation.

Nursing Care

The school nurse is in a position to recognize children or adolescents who might be suicidal. This care involves awareness of the signs of suicide ideation and the risk factors that may precede suicide ideation. The nurse must ask about suicide ideation. The nurse can discern: Does the child have a plan? Is that plan possible (i.e., is the means to self-harm accessible)? Has the child attempted suicide before? Foremost, if any of these factors are present, the nurse must refer the child (and family) to a mental health professional that can assess the level of risk. The child or adolescent may need immediate hospitalization to remain safe.

If danger is not imminent, the nurse can assist the child or adolescent and the family in identifying and further developing the protective factors available to them. The nurse can identify family strengths and resources available in the community (crisis or suicide hot lines, counseling, inpatient treatment facilities) to help protect the child. The nurse can also talk with the family about other measures that can be implemented to keep their child safe (e.g., remove all guns or other weapons from the home, ridding cupboards of poisons, locking medicines away, monitor the child closely).

Specific psychotherapeutic approaches like cognitive behavior therapy (CBT) or dialectical behavior therapy (DBT) focuses on helping the child and adolescent develop skills for coping with emotional intensity and impulsivity (Katz, Cox, Gunasekara, & Miller, 2004). Both types of therapy are performed by specifically educated clinicians, but the nurse, particularly in the hospital, can be supportive. Pharmacological treatments include medications to treat the underlying psychiatric difficulty (Table 23-1).

In the community, the nurse can raise awareness about the programs that seek to prevent suicidal behavior in adolescents. There are some school-based programs that target students who are at-risk for dropping out of school and assist the child or adolescent to remain involved in school. Once a child or adolescent has dropped out of school, economic and social changes also might play a role in suicidal thoughts. In addition, the child or adolescent may be more susceptible to feelings of hopelessness and isolation.

clinical alert

Suicidal behavior related to antidepressant therapy

In 2006, the Food and Drug Administration (FDA) requested that pharmaceutical companies manufacturing SSRIs add a "black box" warning to the packaging. This warning is related to an apparent rise in suicide in children and adolescents recently prescribed an SSRI for depression. Subsequent studies discussed by Goodman, Murphy, & Storch (2007) related that the increased incidence of suicide ideation and attempt was not universal, nor was it related only to those diagnosed with depression, but also in children taking SSRIs for other disorders. The evidence is controversial because other studies have shown antidepressants to be very effective in decreasing the suicide risk by effectively dealing with the underlying causes. Several factors have been proposed to explain the occurrence of suicidal ideation in children treated with these medications. (1) The prescription may be an inadequate dose and therefore the depression is not treated. (2) An energizing phenomenon, which describes a situation in which the depressive symptoms related to energy decrease before the mood symptoms, may occur, thus making it more possible for the depressed individual to have the energy to attempt suicide. (3) The emergence of an activation syndrome may be related to a toxic reaction to the medication. (4) Motor restlessness related to akathisia (motor restlessness that may appear as a side effect of antipsychotic medication) may occur. (5) A shift from depression to mania in a not-yet-diagnosed bipolar child may occur. (6) Idiosyncratic reactions (perhaps related to gene-drug reactions) may occur (Goodman et al., 2007).

SCHIZOPHRENIA

Schizophrenia is a serious chronic mental health disorder that is thought to be the result of abnormalities in neuro-developmental processes that occur early (prenatal, infancy, early childhood) as well as later (late childhood and adolescence) in life (Bearden, Meyer, Loewy, Niendam, & Cannon, 2006). The disorder typically begins in late adolescence or early adulthood, but it is possible for children as young as 5 or 6 to exhibit signs. Researchers have found that the age at onset of schizophrenia plays an important role in the course and outcome of illness. The earlier the onset of symptoms occur, the greater the impairment (Bearden et al., 2006). Although schizophrenia is a chronic mental illness, early recognition and treatment can vastly improve the outcome for the child. Untreated, schizophrenia can be devastating for the individual and the family.

Schizophrenia is rarer in children younger than pre-adolescence. About 1% of the world's population (adult, adolescent, and child) is identified with a diagnosis of schizophrenia (Nicholson & Rapoport, 1999, cited in NIMH, 2001). Further complicating the diagnosis is that early symptoms are similar to those of pervasive developmental disorders such as autism. In some cases, it is thought that a pervasive developmental disorder is a precursor of schizophrenia.

Signs and Symptoms

The nurse knows that discerning the signs and symptoms of schizophrenia begins with a mental health interview that includes a comprehensive developmental and family history. Schizophrenia typically has a gradual onset, is difficult to identify in young children, and may

Table 23-1 Pharmacological Treatments for Psychological Difficulties

Category	Medications	Uses
Antianxiety	Beta blockers	Anxiety
	Propanolol (Inderal)	
	Alpha blockers	
	Clonidine (Catapres)	
Antidepressants	**Selective serotonin uptake inhibitors (SSRIs)**	Depression
		Anxiety
	Fluoxetine (Prozac)	OCD
	Sertraline (Zoloft)	Elective mutism
	Paroxetine (Paxil)	
	Citalopram (Celexa)	
	Escitalopram (Lexapro)	
	Fluvoxamine (Luvox)	
	Tricyclics	Enuresis
	Imipramine (Tofranil)	Autism
	Clomipramine (Anafranil)	
	Other	
	Bupropion (Wellbutrin)	
	Venlafaxine	
Mood Stabilizer	Lithium carbonate	Bipolar disorder
	(Lithobid, Lithane, or Eskalith)	Mania
		ODD
		ADHD
Anticonvulsants	Valproate (Depakote)	Bipolar disorder
		Mania
Antipsychotics	**Traditional**	Autism
	Haloperidol (Haldol)	Psychosis
	Atypical	Tourette's syndrome
	Risperidone (Risperdal)	Behavioral problems related to other psychiatric disorders (conduct disorder, ADHD, MR)
	Olanzapine (Zyprexa)	
	Quetiapine (Seroquel)	
	Ziprasidone (Geodon)	
	Aripiprazole (Abilify)	
Stimulants	Methylphenidate (Ritalin and Concerta)	ADHD
	Dextroamphetamine	
	(Dexedrine and Adderall)	
Nonstimulants	Atomoxetine (Strattera)	ADHD

be indistinguishable from other disorders. The nurse understands that it is important to recognize early signs and symptoms and begin treatment as early as possible (Commission on Adolescent Schizophrenia, 2005).

There are two types of symptoms in the presentation of schizophrenia. Positive symptoms are those that are generally seen after observing and listening to the parent or the child. These symptoms include hallucinations (hearing voices, seeing things, experiencing strange sensations), delusions (false beliefs, i.e., beliefs that the radio is sending special messages), and disorganized speech and behavior (APA, 2000). Negative symptoms are less obvious. These symptoms include a decrease or "flattening" of affect (visible expression of mood), speech, and motivation (APA, 2000).

Diagnosis

A diagnosis of schizophrenia is based on a mental health interview that includes a comprehensive developmental and family history. If the child has had has a gradual onset of the signs and symptoms this condition may be suspected. Before the actual evidence of diagnostic symptoms there is often a prodromal (period marked by a shifting in personality) and the emergence of "odd" behaviors (i.e., withdrawal, obsessions, aloofness), thoughts (distractibility), or emotions (lability, anxiety).

Diagnosis may be confirmed by the presence of initial and subsequent psychoses such as hallucinations, delusions, disorganized thinking and speech, lack of motivation and interest in life, and aberrant emotional expressions (Bearden et al., 2006).

Nursing Care

Early treatment for schizophrenia usually involves pharmacological agents (e.g., atypical antipsychotics), adolescent and family psychoeducation, and brief psychotherapy aimed at increasing level of functioning. Treatment is usually divided into the acute and maintenance phase. To obtain the best outcome, the adolescent and family should always stay in treatment (Commission on Adolescent Schizophrenia, 2005). Acute treatment for active psychosis (hallucinations, delusions, fearfulness, acting out) consists of maintaining the safety of the child and others. It is frightening to lose sight of reality. The child may act out against misperceived threats and injure self or others. The majority of treatment at this point is pharmacological adjustment. The nurse uses therapeutic communication to convey a sense of security to the child and family. It is also important to approach the child in a calm and reassuring manner. If the symptoms are severe the child may be hospitalized.

The schizophrenic child will always need to take medications to control symptoms. Pharmacological treatment involves the use of antipsychotic medications such as risperidone (Risperdal), olanzapine (Zyprexa), or quetiapine fumarate (Seroquel). Other forms of care for the child include group training in social skill acquisition (as most schizophrenic children have inadequate social skills) and cognitive behavioral therapy (CBT). Nursing care also includes educating the child and family about the importance of taking the medications and related side effects. Families of children with schizophrenia, like those with any chronic difficult illness, may need ongoing support. There are organizations that offer support and advocacy for families of the mentally ill. One such organization is the National Alliance for the Mentally Ill (NAMI; www.nami.org) that provides parents and families with important information. The nurse is in an ideal position to help identify children and adolescents with early prodromal signs and refer for further evaluation, family psychoeducation, and other interventions such as understanding the importance of medication.

AUTISM SPECTRUM DISORDERS

Autism spectrum disorder (ASD) can be first diagnosed in infancy or childhood. The DSM-IV-TR defines autism spectrum disorder as a continuum of disorders that involve limitations in social relatedness, verbal and nonverbal communication, and the range of interests and behaviors (APA, 2000). There are five specific autism spectrum diagnoses. Pervasive developmental disorder (PDD) is the term used by DSM-IV-TR and is synonymous with autism spectrum disorders. The five pervasive developmental disorders include autistic disorder (serious deficits in the development of social and communication skills accompanied by significant repetitive behaviors), Asperger's disorder (a milder form of autistic disorder), Rett's disorder (a rare disorder that predominantly affects girls; development is normal until around 6 to 18 months when autistic symptoms appear), childhood disintegrative disorder (a rare disorder in which the child usually develops normally until age 2 before developing symptoms of autism; predominantly affects boys), and pervasive developmental disorder not otherwise specified (a disorder in which either autism or Asperger's is suspected but the diagnostic criteria are not fully met) (APA, 2000; Ozonoff, Rogers, & Hendren, 2003).

Signs and Symptoms

Three clusters of symptoms characterize autism spectrum disorder (ASD). The first symptom cluster involves qualitative impairment in social reciprocity which means the child is unable to engage in socially appropriate communication. This impairment is marked by poor eye contact, lack of interest in other people, and failure to interact appropriately with others.

The second symptom cluster is characterized by communication impairment. The child either uses no language at all, or exhibits deviant speech with errors in tone, prosody, pitch, grammar, or pragmatics. Errors in pragmatics, such as difficulty taking turns in conversation, are particularly common in higher functioning individuals.

Restrictive and repetitive behaviors, interests, or activities characterize the third symptom cluster. Specifically, restrictive interests are narrow in focus, overly intense, and/or unusual. An example might include experiencing sensory qualities of objects in unusual ways (e.g., sniffing objects or playing with toys in unusual ways). Another example of unusual interests would be a preoccupation with the parts of a toy rather than enjoying the toy. Restrictive behavior is characterized by unreasonable insistence on sameness or following familiar routines in a very rigid or extreme way.

Repetitive behavior is a common symptom that is displayed by children with autism spectrum disorder through repetitive motor mannerisms such as hand flapping or spinning or rocking; these movements are called *stereotypies* or tics (sudden uncontrollable movement or vocalization).

Nursing Insight— *Autism spectrum disorders*

The reported number of children with autism spectrum disorders has increased since the early 1990s. Whether there is a true increase in prevalence or whether past rates were underreported is a matter of debate. The factors involved in understanding the potential increase in prevalence include that the true prevalence rates 10 or 20 years ago are difficult to ascertain retrospectively; changes in diagnostic criteria, e.g., the concept of autism is now viewed as a spectrum of disorders; a heightened public awareness of autism; and increased media coverage of affected children and families. Also relevant is that in 1991, the US Department of Education added autism as a category for special education services. It is speculated that this change led to increases in the number of children classified as autistic, because a diagnosis would allow children to take part in available educational services (Yeargin-Allsopp et al., 2003). The CDC estimates that 1 in 166 children are diagnosed with an autism spectrum disorder (CDC, 2004).

 critical nursing action Understanding Autism Spectrum Disorder

The "First Signs" program uses the acronym Autism A.L.A.R.M. to highlight important clinical guidelines:

Autism is prevalent (Wiseman, 2006):

- 1 out of 6 children are diagnosed with a developmental disorder and/or behavioral problem.
- 1 in 166 children are diagnosed with an autism spectrum disorder.
- Developmental disorders have subtle signs and may be easily missed.

Listen to patients:

- Early signs of autism are often present before 18 months.
- Parents usually do have concerns that something is wrong.
- Parents generally do give accurate and quality information.
- When parents do not spontaneously raise concern, ask if they have any concerns.

Act early:

- Make screening and surveillance an important part of your practice (as endorsed by the AAP).
- Know the subtle differences between typical and atypical development.
- Learn to recognize red flags.
- Improve the quality of life for children and their families through early and appropriate intervention.

Refer:

- To Early Intervention or a local school program (do not wait for a diagnosis).
- To an autism specialist, or team of specialists, immediately for a definitive diagnosis.
- To audiology and rule out a hearing impairment.
- To local community resources for help and family support.

Monitor:

- Schedule a follow-up appointment to discuss concerns more thoroughly.
- Look for other features known to be associated with autism.
- Educate parents and provide them with up-to-date information.
- Advocate for families with local early intervention programs, schools, respite care agencies, and insurance companies.
- Continue surveillance and watch for additional or late signs of autism and/or other developmental disorders.

Diagnosis

In 2003, a partnership between the American Pediatric Association and the Center for Disease Control created a program called First Signs (see critical nursing action Understanding Autism Spectrum Disorder). This widely disseminated public awareness campaign was designed to increase pediatric primary care provider and parental awareness about the signs and symptoms of autism. Based on this awareness, a thorough developmental history can be conducted that can lead to an early diagnosis.

Nursing Care

Nurses who work in primary care settings can provide care for children with autism. Awareness of the need for early intervention is important because of the substantial cortical plasticity (the ability of tissues to grow during early brain development). There are many successful nonmedical treatments for children with autism. One of the most important interventions involves early language development. Ozonoff et al. noted that "language functioning is the strongest predictor of outcome in autism and very limited language at age five is a powerful indicator of severe handicap in adulthood" (2003, p. 134). Poor functional communication skills also contribute significantly to the problematic behaviors that some autistic children display (e.g., poor frustration tolerance and aggression toward self or others). Equally important are interventions that address social competence. The nurse can teach parents that social skills training and acquisition groups provide the child with an opportunity to learn and practice appropriate social relatedness.

Using the actions suggested in the mnemonic A.L.A.R.M., the nurse can assist the child and family in coping with this disorder. Children with autistic spectrum disorders respond best to structure and predictability. Learning and social interactions should be approached systematically and gradually, allowing the child to develop comfort with the concepts (Wiseman, 2006). As with the schizophrenic child, it is important to stay aware of the child's physical boundaries and reluctance to be touched by others.

Psychosocial and Cognitive Disorders

REACTIVE ATTACHMENT DISORDER

Reactive attachment disorder (RAD) mirrors the information on attachment theory. It is important to note that developmental research in attachment is vast and growing but that clinical research regarding attachment disorders is just beginning to emerge and there is much yet to be learned about assessment, prevention, and treatment (Stafford & Zeanah, 2006). There are few if any statistics citing the incidence of RAD. It is reportedly a rare disorder (APA, 2000). Adoptive and foster parents are most frequently faced with attachment difficulties in children placed after the first 11 months of life.

There are two types of RAD: emotionally withdrawn/ inhibited and indiscriminately social/disinhibited. The inhibited RAD children usually lack the ability to seek and accept comfort, and to respond to or show affection. These children may have problems with emotion regulation evidenced by withdrawal, avoidance, and "frozen watchfulness" (APA, 2000).

The disinhibited RAD children usually show more ability to interact with caregivers but seek comfort and affection from strangers indiscriminately (APA, 2000). This describes the child who arbitrarily wanders off with any stranger, not even thinking to turn back to ensure that the caregiver is near.

 Nursing Insight— *Understanding reactive attachment disorder*

The nurse must first understand how the attachment system works. Basically, the goal of the attachment system is designed "to ensure survival of offspring by promoting mutual proximity of infants and caregivers, thereby providing protection from danger" (Stafford & Zeanah, 2006, p. 231). Another role of the attachment system is to help with regulation of developing emotion in the infant and child (Stafford & Zeanah, 2006). The attachment system works in conjunction with other systems that include affiliate, exploratory, and wariness (temperament) systems.

Signs and Symptoms

Infants and children diagnosed with attachment disorders have usually endured neglect or maltreatment or have experienced severe trauma. Many of these children have been institutionalized during the first year of life when the ability to connect with another is forming. The main sign/symptom is children who experience difficulties attaching or bonding (even to a parent).

Diagnosis

There are currently no established tools to use to make a diagnosis of RAD, but a thorough clinical interview and observation is essential in identifying behaviors that suggest a diagnosis of attachment disorder (Stafford & Zeanah, 2006). Infants typically exhibit attachment patterns around 9 to 12 months of age. The pediatric nurse can aid in the diagnostic process by observing how the child interacts around parents and strangers.

The medical diagnosis of RAD as per DSM-IV-TR (APA, 2000) requires that marked disturbances and developmentally inappropriate social relatedness symptoms start before the age of 5 and must be evident in most situations.

Nursing Care

Since attachment disorders in infants and children result from the lack of opportunity to experience a caring relationship, this opportunity should be offered as a first step

 where research and practice meet:
Patterns of Attachment

Through the Strange Situation procedure (Ainsworth, Blehar, Waters, & Wall, 1978) researchers are able to assess the infant's or child's organizational patterns of attachment during low- and high-stress episodes involving a caregiver. The patterns are divided into three categories of strategies: secure organized, insecure organized (avoidant, resistant, dependent), and insecure not organized (disorganized, controlling, defended/coercive, unclassified) (Stafford & Zeanah, 2006).

in treatment. Developing trust through meeting the child's basic needs or responding to cries or tantrums or listlessness with patience and consistency is exceptionally important. A child with RAD has no true concept about which basic needs will be met.

When a caring person is available to the infant or child that person should receive support and education from professionals. Nurses can work with all types of families such as foster care families, families with children adopted from institutions, and children in other situations to help the family with RAD. It is important to let the families know that while the children need loving and nurturing, they may rebuff the care that is offered. Nurses can also identify barriers to intervention that might include parental mental health needs, substance abuse, family violence, and trauma. They can then mobilize the appropriate resources to involve children and families into recovery. Child–parent psychotherapy is a respected intervention that should be considered and nurses can connect families with these services (Van Horn & Lieberman, 2006).

 clinical alert

Dangerous "attachment therapies"

Nurses should know that there is a group of therapies to avoid for children with attachment disorders because of coercive techniques employed, and in fact these therapies have been dangerous as there have been child deaths related to treatment. These therapies are usually known as "attachment therapy," "holding therapy," "rage reduction," and "rebirth" (Barth, Crea, John, Thoburn, & Quinton, 2005; Stafford & Zeanah, 2006).

FAILURE TO THRIVE

Failure to thrive (FTT) is not a diagnosis but a description of a condition that usually happens early in life when the infant does not meet age-appropriate weight gain (Locklin, 2005). It is known that FTT infants do not obtain or are unable to take in enough nutrition to adequately meet standard growth and weight expectations.

Certain situations from a mental health perspective are related to the development of FTT. Families in vulnerable situations (e.g., poverty, young and/or single parent, mentally ill or substance-abusing parents), or those in which child abuse or neglect exist, are at risk for FTT.

Bassali and Benjamin (2007) reported that in the 1980s, 1% to 5% of the admissions to tertiary care for children younger than 1 year were related to FTT and 10% of outpatient visits were related to FTT. This condition is more common in underdeveloped countries where poverty and hunger are more rampant. Poverty is by far the greatest determinant in FTT (Block & Krebs, 2006).

Signs and Symptoms

Assessment of the signs and symptoms of failure to thrive is accomplished by tracking the growth rate of the infant or child to determine if an actual lack of adequate progression exists. Physical examination and evaluation of the child's developmental status is also important, since lack of sufficient nutrition on an ongoing basis will affect the child's cognitive and emotional development. Beyond that, it is important to develop an understanding of the underlying cause(s).

Historically, health care providers distinguished FTT according to organic (medical conditions or illnesses that would affect the child's ability to take in or use nutrition) versus nonorganic (related to abuse, neglect, or attachment difficulties) classifications. In recent years, however, these distinctions have been less useful as many children with FTT exhibit symptoms of both causes (Block & Krebs, 2006). As a result, there is much less emphasis on attributing FTT to a problematic infant–caregiver relationship or maternal deprivation (Locklin, 2005). Still, psychosocial factors cannot be ruled out without assessing the family situation as well as potential physiological causes.

Diagnosis

Infants that have weights below the 3rd percentile or are two standard deviations below the mean for their gestational age on standardized growth charts are commonly diagnosed with FTT (Locklin, 2005) (Fig. 23-3).

 Nursing Insight— *Failure to thrive*

During a nursing assessment the nurse can discern:

- How does the caretaker interact with the child?
- Are there signs of abuse or neglect?
- Does the caretaker understand appropriate feeding amounts and routines?
- Does the caretaker mistakenly believe that a healthy adult diet (i.e., lower fat) is also healthy for an infant?

Nursing Care

A comprehensive history and physical examination are vital in identifying the source of the problem and developing a plan of care. There are sometimes challenging cases of FTT that require specialized intervention by developmental pediatric or mental health care providers. Nurses can help identify these cases and provide education regarding feeding practices and the importance of support for caregivers and families. The nurse can also provide support and reassurance to new mothers and caregivers who are struggling with FTT infants and young children. While nursing care must address the physiological needs

Figure 23-3 Failure to thrive.

of the child, it must also encompass the emotional needs. If the nurse suspects neglect or abuse, steps must be taken to the appropriate child protection agency.

 nursing diagnoses Failure to Thrive

- Imbalanced Nutrition: less than body requirements related to inability to ingest or digest food or absorb nutrients because of biological or psychological factors
- Delayed Growth and Development related to inadequate caretaking, environmental and stimulation deficiencies, or physical/psychosocial conditions
- Risk for Impaired Parenting related to unmet social and emotional needs of parental caregivers, ineffective role modeling, insufficient knowledge or crisis

ATTENTION-DEFICIT/HYPERACTIVITY DISORDER

Attention-deficit/hyperactivity disorder (ADHD) is familiar to parents, school teachers, and others who know the child. Images of the overactive, talkative child "bouncing off the walls," and always in trouble are likely portrayed. ADHD is one of the most publicized and perhaps overdiagnosed psychiatric conditions of childhood. A child can have attention-deficit disorder with or without hyperactivity. The category of ADHD without hyperactivity typically has symptoms of distractibility. While ADHD without hyperactivity garners much less attention than ADHD with hyperactivity, it can cause just as much difficulty in the life of the child and the family.

The CDC indicated that a total of 4 million children between the ages of 3 and 17 have been diagnosed with ADHD. This comprises 6.5% of the children of the number of U.S. children born since the diagnosis of ADHD has been used.

Signs and Symptoms

Symptoms of ADHD may include hyperactivity, impulsivity, distractibility, and inattention. Although ADHD is most often diagnosed in early school-age children, symptoms can be seen in much younger children. Children with these symptoms often have difficulty with school performance as well as social and peer interaction. While poor school performance is usually the driving factor in seeking help for children with these symptoms, difficulty with peer groups and family relationships are just as evident. Many children with ADHD also have comorbid conditions such as depression, anxiety, oppositional defiant disorder, and learning disabilities.

Diagnosis

Evaluations for ADHD are conducted by advanced practice nurses, physicians, and other heath care providers. For appropriate assessment of ADHD, the child must first meet the diagnostic criteria outlined in the DSM-IV-TR (APA, 2000) (Table 23-2).

When the criterion is met, the final diagnosis requires evidence of the child's behavior in a variety of settings, such as classroom, during homework, or playtime. Evidence is obtained by asking parents, teachers, and other caregivers to complete rating scales about behavior. Additional information needed includes the age at onset of symptoms, duration of symptoms, and degree of impaired functioning.

Table 23-2 Characteristics of Attention Deficit/Hyperactivity Disorder	
Developmentally inappropriate or maladaptive symptoms consisting of either inattentive symptoms (1st column), hyperactive or impulsive symptoms (2nd column), or a combination (both columns).	
Inattention	**Hyperactivity or Impulsivity**
Distractibility	Excessive energy and activity
Inability to complete projects	Restlessness
Easily bored	Overactivity
Disorganized	Inability to sit still or stay in one place for long
Inattentiveness	Excessive talking
Avoidance of detailed tasks	Poor boundaries—interrupts or intrudes
Forgetfulness	Difficulty delaying

Nursing Care

The nurse understands that ADHD is evaluated by using a variety of rating scales. Specific rating scales are the DuPaul ADHD Rating Scale, the Connors Parent/Teacher Rating Scale and the Child Behavior Checklist (teacher, parent versions) (Achenbach, 2001; Achenbach & Rescorla, 2000) that have been validated as useful in diagnosing ADHD. Each of these rating scales asks the caregiver or teacher to rate the child's behavior (e.g., behavior occurs extremely often, often, sometimes, rarely or never). A school nurse may be trained to perform observations of the child while in class to assist in the information gathering. These scales in combination with a clinical family interview provide the examiner with valuable information to determine a diagnosis. A thorough clinical interview with the child is also important in determining the appropriate diagnosis and treatment.

The most effective treatment for ADHD is a combination of pharmacological and psychosocial interventions. Using both modalities allows for the control or abatement of symptomatic behavior by the medication while at the same time working on changing maladaptive behavior patterns through therapy with the child and family. When recommending psychosocial intervention, clinicians must keep in mind the developmental level of the child and family. Also, from a developmental psychopathology perspective it is important to inform the family that early intervention works best and that the child and family may have periods of adaptive and maladaptive behavior.

PHARMACOLOGICAL INTERVENTION. Stimulants are the most commonly used medication for this condition. Ritalin and other forms of methylphenidate, Adderall (amphetamine salts), and atomoxetine (Strattera), a nonstimulant medication, are commonly used in this condition. The FDA recently approved a transdermal methylphenidate patch for children 6 years and older. This patch was designed for children who were unable to swallow any tablets or capsules.

PSYCHOSOCIAL INTERVENTION. The nurse recognizes that children often respond to therapeutic approaches that include behavioral therapy, rewards (sticker charts), as well as positive versus negative reinforcement (used as often as possible when child demonstrates acceptable behavior). School nurses are in a position of supporting teachers and other staff in the use of behavioral charts. Pediatric nurses in the community can offer support to parents and families in ongoing use of behavior modification.

Some families may resist medications. Other families may put all of their faith into medications, thus not following through with the entire treatment plan. It is important for the nurse to help the family make use of all of the treatment options available to them and to participate actively with their health provider(s) in developing a plan for their child.

OPPOSITIONAL DEFIANT DISORDER AND CONDUCT DISORDER

Antisocial behavior is at the core of disordered behavior that can often explode into clinical disorders most often known as oppositional defiant disorder (ODD) and conduct disorder (CD).

ODD and CD have multifactorial and complex etiologies. Studies have identified a number of biological and psychosocial factors that may be associated with the development of CD and ODD in children and adolescents. Among the biological factors is temperament, hormonal changes (especially in adolescence), neurotransmitter dysfunction, and prenatal toxin exposures (e.g., fetal alcohol exposure). Psychosocial factors include less competence in problem-solving skills, less ability to take on another's viewpoint, family or parental history of depression, antisocial personality, criminal behavior, disruptions in family functioning (e.g., parental conflict, parenting practices), peer group rejection, and lower-socioeconomic background. Specifically, there is evidence showing that parental hostile attributions and parental harsh discipline styles may lead to child behavioral problems (Dishion & Patterson, 2006).

Signs and Symptoms

There is evidence indicating that early childhood problem behaviors may include noncompliance, oppositional behavior, and temper tantrums. Sometimes it can be difficult to distinguish between normative and problematic behavior in young children. It is important that the nurse become familiar with normal development stages and not to overpathologize negative behavior during childhood (Wakschlag & Danis, 2004).

In middle childhood, children may show overt (e.g., hitting) and covert (e.g., saying mean things about a friend) antisocial behavior (experienced by others as aversive, disruptive and unpleasant), and relational aggression (aggression toward people who have a relationship with the child). It may be less clear about what behavior problems demonstrated in middle childhood may be grouped into either ODD or CD.

Later in adolescence, behavior may include delinquency, substance abuse, and high-risk sexual behavior. The set of behavior problems typically exhibited in early childhood are often identified as oppositional defiant disorder (ODD). Finally, behaviors observed later in adolescence are often identified as CD (Dishion & Patterson, 2006).

where research and practice meet:
Oppositional Defiant and Conduct Disorder

Disruptive, aggressive, and antisocial behaviors in children are often the type of behaviors that lead families to seek help for psychosocial-related problems. These behaviors are often difficult to tolerate by parents, family members, peers, teachers, and others. The nurse will encounter families with children exhibiting these behaviors. There are a number of preventive intervention studies that show promise for clinical application.

One such study is the Family Check-UP (FCU), a randomized trial of parental management strategies used in the context of increasing young children's autonomy. The FCU also addresses other familial issues including parental depression, housing and daycare needs, and feedback sessions using motivational interviewing approach. These management strategies were administered to the families of young children (enrolled when children were 17–27 months old) and showed promising results. The findings included decreased Child Behavior Check List [CBCL] Destructive Scale scores for 3-year-old boys and improved maternal engagement when children were 2 years of age (Shaw, Dishion, Supplee, Gardner, & Arnds, 2006).

Diagnosis

Improvement in self-report measures (Achenbach & Rescorla, 2000), and better criteria in the DSM-IV-TR as well as the help of other tools (Greenspan, 2005), has made it easier for clinicians to diagnose behavior disorders.

What is less well known is the difference between ODD and CD. It is important to note that many children who meet the criteria for ODD or CD often have comorbid mental health problems and may also function poorly in interpersonal relationships with peers and caregivers (Dishion & Patterson, 2006).

Nursing Care

Early assessment of these conditions is important, using multimethod and multi-informant approaches that include: self-report scales (e.g., CBCL), child interview, parent interview, physical assessment, observation of child–parent interaction, and thorough family assessment (e.g., history of exposure to violence in the family and community).

When working with children and adolescents who exhibit ODD or CD, it is important for the nurse to be aware and manage personal feelings that may be aroused by the patient and family. The nurse can educate the family about the family-based prevention and intervention programs.

 Nursing Insight— Prevention and intervention programs using a family-based approach for oppositional defiant disorder and conduct disorder

The Nurse–Family Partnership (Olds, 2002): Incorporates nurse home visits by specially trained nurses to low-income first-time families and their support systems. The nurse helps the family learn about preventive prenatal and postnatal health and offers support in maintaining optimum health. (Another resource is www.nursefamilypartnership.org.)

The Incredible Years program (Baydar, Reid, & Webster-Stratton, 2003): This program was developed by Carolyn Webster-Stratton, a pediatric nurse practitioner as well as a clinical psychologist. The program is an evidence-based intervention program designed to help parents and young children (ages 3–10) who have or are at-risk to develop aggressive, disobedient, hyperactive and inattentive behaviors.

The Family Check-UP (FCU) (Dishion & Kavanagh, 2003; Shaw, Dishion, Supplee, Gardner, & Arnds, 2006): This intervention program assesses families to identify those with children at risk for substance abuse or antisocial behavior. These families are then offered support and therapeutic and case management services to decrease the risk factors.

Evidence-based programs have been found to be effective across various socio-demographic and ethnic samples in the United States and northern European countries (Webster-Stratton, Reid, & Hammond, 2004). Some of the programs have also been implemented from a preventive perspective with at risk preschool and school-age families (Baydar et al., 2003). Although it takes special training, the programs are comprehensive and intensive. The programs are valuable for nurses to learn about in order to help families find proper resources.

The nurse can also help parents learn some basic behavioral techniques. For example, the nurse can teach the parent about the value of ignoring annoying behaviors exhibited by the child. If the behaviors do not present safety issues, ignoring the behavior can be one of the best ways of extinguishing it because the child does not garner the desired attention. The nurse can tell the parent that it is also important to offer positive verbal feedback when behaviors are within acceptable limits.

 Nursing Insight— Youth violence: Fact sheet

The Youth Violence: Fact Sheet at http://www.cdc.gov/ncipc/factsheets/yvfacts.htm offers a comprehensive resource about the problem of violence (compiled and referenced from research and refereed articles). The nurse can access this information to be used as an educational tool when talking to youth and families about violence. Examples of fact sheet topics are the following:

- Occurrence
- Consequences
- Groups at Risk
- Risk Factors
- Individual Risk Factors
- Family Risk Factors
- Peer/School Risk Factors
- Community Risk Factors
- Protective Factors
- Individual Protective Factors
- Family Protective Factors
- Peer/School Protective Factors

Nursing care for this condition also includes educating the family about medications. It is important that the child and family understand the action, potential side effects, and additional information about prescribed medications. Children with ODD or CD may be prescribed medications from a number of categories such as stimulants for ADHD symptoms; antipsychotics for behavior regulation; mood stabilizers for regulation of high and low mood presentations; as well as antianxiety agents.

Nurses who work with families that have children with ODD or CD must be mindful of the stress that these disorders have on the whole family. It may be exhausting for parents to cope with the defiant behaviors. Siblings may be put at risk simply spending time with the misbehaved child. Respite care (short-term care) can give the family a "rest" from the child who has the disorder. Encouraging family members to take care of personal needs as well as the child's may be useful in helping them to find balance in daily living.

 nursing diagnoses Oppositional Defiant Disorder and Conduct Disorder

- Ineffective coping related to personal vulnerability
- Impaired social interaction related to hostile, negative, and defiant behavior
- Chronic low self-esteem related to difficulties with positive social interactions
- Compromised family functioning related to inadequate information and family disorganization

Tic Disorders

A tic is a sudden seemingly uncontrollable movement or vocalization. Many children in the elementary school age group experience motor tics (facial or bodily twitches or shrugs) that are mild and eventually spontaneously resolve. Generally, tics are manageable when the child concentrates on controlling them, but they become worse when the child is under stress. Vocal (phonic) tics are characterized by bursts of yelling out words, grunts, and throat-clearing (APA, 2000). Tics are more common in boys than in girls.

TOURETTE'S SYNDROME

There are a number of tic disorders, including Tourette's syndrome, which is a motor and vocal tic disorder that may have a chronic motor or sometimes transient tic (APA, 2000). Specifically, Tourette's syndrome most often includes chronic motor and phonic tics that vary in frequency, intensity, and complexity (Spessot & Peterson, 2006). Children may not initially know they exhibit tics but over time become aware of the behavior. By adolescence most children have become aware of the

premonitory urge (warning signal) (Spessot & Peterson, 2006). Tics occur more frequently in children than in adults. The incidence is estimated to be 5 to 30 per 10,000. The tic can begin as early as 2 years of age and can last throughout the lifetime with asymptomatic periods (APA, 2000).

Signs and Symptoms

Children with Tourette's syndrome often exhibit symptoms of other disorders, similar to obsessive–compulsive disorder (APA, 2000; Leckman et al., 2006; Snider & Swedo, 2003), autism spectrum disorders (Canitano & Vivanti, 2007), and ADHD (Leckman et al., 2006). Many of the symptoms are similar. Children with co-existing disorders are more likely to suffer depression, low self-esteem, negative peer acceptance, and poor school performance than those with tics alone (Leckman et al., 2006).

Diagnosis

 diagnostic tools Tourette's Syndrome

The nurse can help the family recognize certain features of Tourette's syndrome to assist in the diagnosis of the condition:

- The child may have both multiple motor and one or more vocal tics present at some time but not necessarily concurrently.
- The tics occur several times a day
- The tics occur almost every day or intermittently throughout a period of more than 1 year.
- The onset of tics is before age 18 years.
- The disturbance is not due to the direct physiological effects of a substance or a general medical condition.

(Canitano & Vivanti, 2007).

Nursing Care

The nurse working with a child with Tourette's syndrome must recognize the impact the disorder has on the child's functioning and social relationships. The child becomes self-conscious and worried that he will blurt out words or utterances at inopportune times. The child may also be shunned or laughed at by peers who do not understand the behavior. The nurse can help the parents watch for signs that the child is being bullied by peers or siblings. In addition, the nurse can help teachers understand that the child cannot control the tics. Robertson et al. (1999, cited in Leckman et al., 2006) referenced two interesting features of Tourette's: (1) suggestible, meaning talking about tics can trigger the tic, (2) suppressible, meaning that if the child is told to stop the tic or can focus on the tic, the tic might be stopped momentarily.

Tic disorders do not often cause impairment of daily living. In fact, many of the manifestations are actually mild. Nursing interventions are predominantly geared toward helping the child and family cope with the disorder. Tourette's and other tics can create stress for the child as the child may experience low self-esteem. The nurse can also help the family watch for signs of coexisting disorders such as ADHD or OCD. Behavioral skills training and stress management can be helpful in teaching the child to recognize the warning signs and to better decrease stressful situations that might lead to tic episodes. Pharmacological interventions include the use of haloperidol (Haldol) or clonidine (Catapres).

 where research and practice meet:
Parenting Patterns

In a study, Dishion and Patterson (2006) differentiated the parenting patterns in families with children who exhibit antisocial and disruptive behavior from those of families whose children do not show these behavior problems. It was found that proactive parenting (engaging children in positive and joint activities, use of verbal cues that promote positive behavior in children) distracted children from misbehavior.

Maltreatment of Children

Child maltreatment is considered to be any action or failure to act by a person that endangers a child's physical or emotional health and development. A person is abusive if he or she fails to nurture the child, physically injures the child, or relates sexually to the child (U.S. Department of Health and Human Services [USDHHS], 2007). Child abuse may include physical, sexual, emotional abuse, and neglect.

Child physical abuse may result in injury inflicted by beating, pushing, kicking, pinching, burning, or choking. Physical abuse includes shaken baby syndrome, which manifests as symptoms related to head trauma as a result of forceful shaking of the infant or young child.

Child sexual abuse involves any sexually related act, usually between a child and an adult (related or not) that can include fondling, forced, or assented oral sex or intercourse, sodomy, exposing children to adult sexual behavior (showing pornography to children), and exploiting through child pornography or prostitution.

Child emotional abuse includes any behavior, attitude, or failure to act that disrupts children's socio-emotional development and mental health. Some examples include shaming or humiliating (ascribing derogatory labels to the child, "you are worthless"), intimidating (threatening and frightening).

Child neglect involves failure to provide emotional and physical care as well as opportunity for education. Neglect is most common but also the most difficult to identify.

Other types of abuse include Munchausen-by-proxy syndrome (a person, usually the mother, deliberately makes the child sick) as well as the electronic sexual luring (enticing via computer) of children.

 Nursing Insight*— *Incidence of child maltreatment

Statistics gathered routinely by the U.S. Department of Health and Human Services (DHHS) track the incidence of child maltreatment and give a breakdown of the incidence of the various types of maltreatment. In 2005, it was estimated that of the 899,000 U.S. (including Puerto Rico and the District of Columbia) children abused, 62.8% were neglected, 16.6% were physically abused, 9.3% had been sexually abused, and 7.1% were emotionally abused (DHHS, 2007). Of these children, 1460 children died related to their abuse or neglect (1.96 children per 100,000). These statistics reflect only the cases that were reported and does not address those children subjected to other forms of domestic violence (parents abusing parents or elders). It also does not address the numbers of children and adolescents who are lured into online abuse experiences. Unfortunately, those responsible for maltreatment of children in the U.S. (perpetrators) are most often parents (79.4%). Other offenders include relatives (6.8%) or unrelated caregivers (10.1%) (DHHS, 2007).

Signs and Symptoms

Children from any family can exhibit any signs and symptoms of abuse, but there are certain children who are in a more vulnerable position. Child rearing can be difficult in normal circumstances, but additional stressors can contribute to child maltreatment. Children with disabilities or with difficult temperamental characteristics may be abused by frustrated or unprepared parents. Children of very young parents or young single mothers who live in poverty or in situations that are stressful may be more apt to abuse a child. Parents who suffer from mental or chronic physical illness may not have adequate resources available to deal with parenting. Other parents who have extremely stringent ideas of discipline may use harsh punishment. The signs and symptoms of abuse are multifaceted (Table 23-3).

Diagnosis

Abuse may be difficult to diagnosis. However, the health care provider can pay close attention to circumstances where the child is exposed to situations where there is excessive stress, marital conflict, parental substance abuse and psychopathology, intergenerational history of abuse, beliefs that children need to be "toughened up," and in families who experience hardships. Diagnosis of physical, sexual, or emotional abuse or neglect may take time, and a thorough family history, physical examination, and developmental assessment are necessary for diagnosis.

Nursing Care

The nurse can be instrumental in the care of children who have experienced any type of abuse including family education, support, referral, and initiatives to help abate and ultimately stop child abuse (Lieberman & Van Horn, 2005).

Educating parents about what to expect from parenthood and from child rearing may help the parents understand how to cope with some of the difficult times related to raising a child. Helping the parents develop resources for support such as babysitters, family members, community sites, and health care resources may help them find ways to cope with parenting. In addition, the nurse can provide parents with information regarding "normal" stages of growth and development which may help the parents to avoid pressuring the child to develop faster than physiologically able. It may also be helpful to discuss with parents ways to discipline the child that does not involve physical or verbal aggression.

The nurse can educate children and adolescents about the body and personal boundaries. The community nurse is sometimes the first person who recognizes abuse or the person with whom a child is comfortable sharing information. The nurse understands that it is important to develop a safe and trusting relationship with children.

It is also important that the nurse understands what steps to take in reporting maltreatment in children as well as implementing steps toward prevention and intervention. Efforts to stop abuse against children should include the following measures: decrease unintended pregnancies, stop the use of alcohol or drugs during pregnancy, decrease the use of drugs or alcohol by new parents, improve availability of and access to health care across the spectrum of the family's life, and help parents and caregivers learn about nonviolent parenting and discipline. The nurse can also be involved politically and educationally to promote these efforts.

Health care professionals cite several reasons for underreporting suspected child abuse. For instance, despite the availability of education and training regarding how to

Table 23-3 Physical, Sexual, Emotional Abuse and Neglect		
Type of Abuse	**Tactics of Abuse**	**Possible Signs and Symptoms in the Child**
Physical: Bodily injury caused by intentional or unintentional physical aggression.	Beating, hitting, slapping, poisoning, kicking, pinching, biting, shoving, choking, pulling hair, burning	Suspicious bruises, welts, or burns
		Unexplained fractures or dislocations
	Excessive corporal punishment	New and healing or healed lacerations or abrasions
		Wariness of adults or caregivers
		Fearful of going home
		Acting out with aggression
	Shaken baby syndrome	Retinal hemorrhages
		CNS injury
	Munchausen by proxy	Prolonged or recurrent illnesses or injuries that cannot be explained
Sexual: Sexual acts involving an adult and a child.	Penetration, incest, rape, oral sex, sodomy, fondling	Inappropriate or precocious interest in or knowledge of sexuality
	Violations of bodily privacy	Poor peer relationships
	Exposing children to adult sexuality	Sudden changes in behavior (regressive, acting out, sexual)
	Commercial exploitation	Running away from home or substance abuse
	Sexual exploitation (prostitution or pornography)	Rapidly declining school performance
		Suicide attempts
Emotional: Attitude, behavior, or failure to act that interferes with a child's mental health or social development.	Intimidation, belittling, shaming, lack of affection and warmth, habitual blaming, ignoring or rejection, extreme punishment, exposure to violence, child exploitation, child abduction	Apathy, depression
		Hostility
		Difficulty concentrating
Neglect: Pattern of failing to meet basic needs.	Physical, educational, emotional	Clothing unsuited to the weather
		Poor hygiene
		Hunger
		Lack of supervision

report cases of child abuse and neglect, many professionals feel ill equipped to handle the situation once a case is identified. Contrary to current belief, professionals who report child abuse are not revealed to the family in question unless the caller chooses to disclose this information. Also, while all reports are taken seriously, not all reports result in the removal of the child from the home. Every reports is investigated but any action may or not be taken depending on the assessment (Childhelp National Child Abuse Hotline, n.d.). It is also important to note that the nurse is required to report any suspicion of child abuse or neglect.

 Be sure to— Report cases of child abuse

To report suspected child abuse, the nurse can call the local enforcement agency and/or follow the clinical setting's guidelines for reporting abuse. All U.S. states have mandatory reporting guidelines for professionally licensed health care workers/providers. It can be a difficult experience to report child abuse because of possible consequences to the child, family, and professional. It is important to remember that all allegations of child abuse must

first be investigated before confirmed. After documented confirmation the child will be placed in a safe environment free of abuse.

National Hotline in USA: 1-800-4-A-Child

For more information consult the link:

http://www.helpguide.org/mental/child_abuse_physical_emotional_sexual_neglect.htm#online

See also Vieth, Bottoms, & Perona (2006).

Substance Use and Abuse

Substance abuse refers to the repeated use of illicit substances (drugs or alcohol or inhalants) despite the negative consequences (APA, 2000). Substance dependence/addiction refers to the physiological and/or emotional reliance on that substance (APA, 2000). The incidence of substance abuse by young people has waxed and waned over the decades, but its significance cannot be ignored. It is known that 80% of deaths in adolescents involve accidents, homicides and suicides and in many of these cases drugs and alcohol are involved (Mayes & Suchman, 2006).

Clearly, the problem of alcohol and drug use and abuse in children and adolescents is a grave concern. Youth in the United States are exposed to drug or alcohol abuse at significant rates. It is estimated that 8.2% of U.S. children, age 12 and older used an illicit substance (SAMHSA, 2003).

 ### Nursing Insight— *Substance use and abuse*

The literature and research is vast regarding drug and alcohol abuse and risk factors. An interesting body of literature involves studies examining biological and genetic factors, especially related to alcohol abuse (Mayes & Suchman, 2006). In studies of twins and family behaviors, researchers found evidence suggesting that both genetic predisposition and behavior were important in adolescents' initial use of marijuana (Mayes & Suchman, 2006). These data seem to suggest that there may be an important link between genetic and environmental circumstances (Mayes & Suchman, 2006).

Young people may abuse any of the substances abused by adults. The major factors determining which substances are used are availability and cost. Some of the more common substances of abuse for children and adolescents include alcohol, tobacco, marijuana, cocaine, ecstasy (MDMA), methamphetamine, other forms of stimulants, prescription medications (the child's own prescription, or medications stolen from a family member), and inhalants (e.g., glue, gasoline, white-out). It is essential that nurses not be naive about the possibility of substance abuse.

Signs and Symptoms

Signs and symptoms of a child who is using and abusing may be surprisingly similar to those of depression and/or suicide. In fact, psychiatric disorders and the possibility of suicide ideation go hand in hand with the abuse of or addiction to illicit substances. The American Academy of Child & Adolescent Psychiatry (AACAP, n.d.) published a list online of some of the warning signs that a young person might be abusing alcohol or drugs:

- Physical: fatigue, repeated health complaints, red and glazed eyes, and a lasting cough
- Emotional: personality change, sudden mood changes, irritability, irresponsible behavior, low self-esteem, poor judgment, depression, and a general lack of interest
- Family: starting arguments, breaking rules, or withdrawing from the family
- School: decreased interest, negative attitude, drop in grades, many absences, truancy, and discipline problems
- Social problems: new friends who are less interested in standard home and school activities, problems with the law, and changes to less conventional styles of dress and music

Diagnosis

Diagnosis of substance use and abuse is based on the physical, emotional and social factors exhibited by the child. A thorough family history is essential along with information about the child's physical and emotional health.

Nursing Care

Initial nursing care involves the use of screening tools to assess drug and alcohol use in children. The nurse is in an ideal position to identify adolescents at-risk for substance abuse, especially if there is a strong family and genetic history of abuse. Two tools that can be used in the identification of substance abuse are the CRAFFT (Knight, Sherritt, Shrier, Harris, & Chang, 2002) and the CAGE (Ewing, 1984). Both of these tools use simple acronyms to assist in the evaluation of drinking or drug use.

After a thorough assessment is done the nurse can help the child and family find community resources that may help conquer the substance abuse problem. Research indicates that nearly 80% of adolescents with substance abuse receive treatment (Commission on Adolescent Substance and Alcohol Abuse, 2005). There are many different types of treatment, but the most promising appears to be a family-based approach, as it shows the best outcomes for reduction in substance abuse in adolescents (Commission on Adolescent Substance and Alcohol Abuse, 2005). Family treatment means that the entire family receives psychoeducation regarding substance abuse.

Eating Disorders

Eating disorders that are mostly apparent in adolescence are classified into four categories that include anorexia nervosa (purging or withholding), bulimia nervosa (binging and purging), binge eating disorder (binging without purging), and eating disorder not otherwise specified (EDNOC) (APA, 2000; Commission on Adolescent Eating Disorders, 2005). Eating disorders most often affect females but adolescent males are also known to suffer from these illnesses. Eating disorders are mostly a phenomenon of Westernized society and thus it is thought that Western media plays a role in these problems (Commission on Adolescent Eating Disorders, 2005).

From a developmental psychopathology perspective, there are a number of risk factors that may cause the adolescent to develop an eating disorder. The physiological factors include hormonal and physical changes associated with puberty in conjunction with temperamental factors. In addition, possible genetic factors might contribute to the development of eating disorders (Steiner et al., 2003). Certain experiences can protect the adolescent from eating disorders, including participation in high school sports that focus on the sport rather than on pursuit of thinness (Steiner et al., 2003) as well as supportive families and peer groups.

The prevalence of data found in community samples report rates of 0.3% to 0.58% in female and 2% in male children and adolescents 11 to 20 years old (Commission on Adolescent Eating Disorders, 2005). These data provide limited information for several reasons. The research has ignored populations that have well documented incidences of eating disorders (e.g., children of ethnic minorities in Westernized countries and generally in children of non-Westernized society). Also, studies have not used uniform tools to measure the disorders.

Signs and Symptoms

In general, adolescents with eating disorders (anorexia or bulimia nervosa) have an inordinate concern with body image and body weight. Adolescents with eating disorders often hide behaviors related to food and caloric intake from others. It is also not unusual for these adolescents to have other co-occurring or resultant mental health and family psychosocial problems (e.g., depression, anxiety, and family discord) as well.

Adolescents with anorexia nervosa usually lose up to 85% of ideal body weight by either restricting food or caloric intake or by consuming caloric intake but then purging by vomiting or vigorous physical activity (Commission on Adolescent Eating Disorders, 2005). These behaviors can result in physical symptoms including amenorrhea, weakness, or fatigue that interfere with general health and well-being. In some cases, symptoms may result in a life-threatening situation and even death.

 clinical alert

Anorexia nervosa

Anorexia nervosa can become a life-threatening problem or cause death because of severe weight loss that can result in electrolyte imbalance and hemodynamic instability.

Diagnosis

The diagnosis of anorexia nervosa or bulimia can be challenging and based on both physical and emotional signs and symptoms. Adolescents with this disorder are below their ideal body weight and are often preoccupied with food. During an interview, the adolescent may express that he or she refuses to eat or consumes very large amounts of calories and then purges by self-induced vomiting or using laxatives or other means (Commission on Adolescent Eating Disorders, 2005).

Nursing Care

The nurse can communicate to the family that treatment of anorexia nervosa and bulimia involves contacting a physician to address the physical symptoms based on the dangerously low body weight. In some instances, adolescents may require hospitalization to correct electrolyte imbalance and homodynamic stability. Because this condition has both physical and psychological implications, nurses caring for children with anorexia nervosa must have the appropriate education and training. Often, once the child's physical health has been stabilized the child is admitted to a psychological unit or directed to outpatient psychological care.

Antidepressant and antipsychotic medications have yielded some promising results. Research shows that antidepressant medication in combination with cognitive behavior therapy has been effective in the treatment of adolescents with bulimia nervosa (Commission on Adolescent Eating Disorders, 2005). The nurse can provide support to the adolescent and family.

Along with physical and mental care, adolescents with bulimia nervosa may need dental care for repair of dental erosion and cavities that result from vomiting.

The nurse may be in the best position to identify early cases of eating disorders and refer for preventive individual and family treatment. The nurse has to keep in mind that the assessment needs to be conducted within a growth and developmental perspective and that intervention should be considered within a family-based approach. When making referrals for treatment, it is important to consider the skill level of the treatment clinician and often a team approach with expertise in this area of health and mental health

works best. For guidelines and further information, the nurse should consult the American Academy of Pediatrics: Committee on Adolescence Identifying and Treating Eating Disorders http://aappolicy.aappublications.org/cgi/reprint/pediatrics;111/1/204.pdf.

Obesity

The definition of obesity in children and adolescents has been debated a great deal by professionals in the field. Recently researchers and care providers have agreed upon certain criteria. Youth are considered overweight if they reach a body mass index (BMI) above the 85th percentile and obese when the BMI is above the 95th percentile. These definitions take into account the child's or adolescent's age and gender (Anderson & Butcher, 2006).

While obesity is not technically classified as an eating disorder, the psychological factors involved are significant. Being overweight or obese deserves the collaborative attention of pediatric primary care providers, nurses, nutritionists, educators, mental health specialists, public health researchers and clinicians, policy makers, parents and children, and others (Anderson & Butcher, 2006; Caprio, 2006).

Daniels (2006) describes many of the physiological problems that go along with obesity including hypertension, diabetes, sleep disorders related to breathing difficulties, and increased risk for cardiovascular disease. In addition to the physiological problems encountered, children who are overweight or obese may be teased or bullied by peers, leading to difficulties with self-esteem and social development.

Obesity in children and adolescents is widespread and is considered to be an important US and International public health problem. In the United States, 17% of children between the ages of 2 and 19 are obese. The breakdown of these statistics shows that 13.9% of 2- to 5-year-olds, 19% of 6- to 11-year-olds, and 17% of teens between 12 and 19 years old fall above the 95th percentile for weight related to their height. These statistics show a dramatic increase since the late 1980s and early 1990s (Ogden et al., 2006). Childhood obesity is of epidemic proportions.

Signs and Symptoms

The nurse understands that it is important to identify obesity as early as possible in the child. The nurse can begin with a comprehensive individual and family history (diabetes, dyslipidemia, cardiovascular disease) and physical assessment as well examining a set of laboratory tests (e.g., metabolic profile). The height, weight, and body mass index (BMI) should be assessed and plotted on the charts identified by the CDC (Caprio, 2006).

Currently there is research assessing the possible link between the environment (physical space available for children to be physically active) and obesity (Epstein, 2003). The link between environment and obesity is not yet conclusive (Sallis & Glanz, 2006).

Golan and Crow (2004) present information about the obesogenic factors present in Western society. **Obesogenic** refers to the role that environment plays in the development of obesity (Pearce, Blakely, Witten, & Bartie, 2007; Swindburn & Egger, 2004). Certain factors found in modern Western lifestyles contribute to eating disorders in general, including the availability of high-density, high-caloric energy foods, decreased physical activity, inactivity, media (constant barrage of food commercials targeting children), and the glorification of thinness and diets (Golan & Crow, 2004).

It is also important to assess individual and family attitudes and practices related to food and weight. Parents who are fearful that their child will become fat may inadvertently overrestrict food to the point that the child hoards food or uses it for comfort. On the other hand, parents who do not understand or cannot afford a healthy diet may reinforce poor dietary habits.

 ### *Ethnocultural Considerations—* **Disparities in childhood obesity**

Despite the fact that African American and Latino children and adolescents have higher prevalence rates of obesity compared to Caucasian children and adolescents, researchers have found that African American and Latino children receive much less attention related to obesity. It is also known that African American and Latino children are also more likely to develop obesity-related problems, such as type 2 diabetes (Caprio, 2006).

Children in low-income families also experience higher levels of obesity. Access to high-quality, low-fat foods is limited, as is often the education of the parents in providing such foods. Lower-income families often have less access to programs than more privileged families have (Kumanyika & Grier, 2006).

Nurses and especially nurses of African American and Latino backgrounds are well positioned to close the gap and help eliminate these disparities by becoming involved or taking leadership roles in programs that identify and involve these youngsters and their families in interventions.

Diagnosis

Diagnosis of obesity is based on an excess of fat in proportion to lean body mass. Basically, the child is considered obese when his or her weight is greater than what is considered healthy for his or her height (BMI above the 95th percentile).

Nursing Care

An important role of the nurse is assessing the risk factors and early onset of obesity (family history, sedentary lifestyle, availability of healthy nutritional resources) in order to begin preventive teaching efforts. The nurse can communicate to families that the Women Infants and Children (WIC) program educates families and provides food packages to underprivileged families. In addition, clinic nurses have the opportunity to help new parents learn healthful attitudes about food and feeding. The nurse can use the information from *Healthy People 2010* obesity prevention to guide family teaching.

Improving the activity level of children and adolescents should be included in teaching. The nurse can be instrumental when working with school programs to offer adequate physical education along with academics. Nurses can also encourage parents to monitor their child's nutrition and activity levels, particularly passive entertainment (computer, television, or video games).

The nurse should also be aware that dieting is not suggested for young people. In fact, in the long run restrictive eating often contributes to boomerang overweight or to other eating problems. Nevertheless, focusing on healthy eating habits that can last throughout the lifetime is essential. It is important to empathize with the child who expresses dissatisfaction with his or her weight and provide education and guidance related to healthful eating and exercise.

 ### *Across Care Settings:* **Prevention of childhood obesity in schools**

The school environment is a good community site to begin implementing prevention of obesity programs because it is the place where most children spend most of their waking hours. The nurse can help ensure that the school provides healthy meals; replaces soda machines with water; promotes and improves physical activity; and provides education about nutrition, physical activity, and acceptable weight (Story, Kaphingst, & French, 2006). The nurse can become involved in school-based programs by providing health education that is known to promote healthy eating, physical activity, and well-being. The nurse can also become involved at other levels, including as a parent, researcher, and advocate for change in school policy.

Sleep Disorders

Sleep and lack of sleep is a complex issue. Reports of sleep problems in children are often identified by the parents or caregivers because children do not usually complain of sleep issues (Kryger, 2005). The child's sleep problem is an issue that can affect the entire family. Often, the nurse encounters sleep-deprived parents based on the child's sleeping difficulties.

During the nursing assessment, the nurse discovers that a variety of daytime difficulties can contribute to sleeplessness at night. These difficulties include the child taking long naps during the day, excessive caffeine consumption, worry and stress, or childhood illness. In addition, parents may communicate that teachers complain about the child's irritability or hyperactivity or about the child falling asleep during class. There are few studies about childhood sleeping patterns that include infants, children, and adolescents but the existing evidence provides some understanding into this important area of study (Owens & Mindell, 2005).

It is estimated that about 25% of all children experience sleeping issues during childhood and the degree of problems varies from mild to severe difficulties with falling asleep or staying asleep. Studies of childhood sleep disturbances, using mostly caregiver-reported data, suggest that 6% to 50% of preschool- and school-age children have sleeping problems (Owens & Mindell, 2005).

Signs and Symptoms

It is thought that the problem of sleep disorders stems from an interaction between neurodevelopment and behavior (Sheldon, 2005). Temperamental tendency for being awake at night, developmental issues, the quality of the child's health, and the way parents or caregivers manage the child's sleep routines are all thought to play important roles in the outcome of sleep related difficulties. Signs and symptoms of a child having a sleep disorder might include sleepwalking, difficulties getting to sleep or staying asleep, nightmares, excessive daytime sleepiness, or irregularity of sleep routine (Owens & Mindell, 2005).

Family Teaching Guidelines...
Sleep Hygiene

Shelton (2005), a pediatric sleep medicine specialist, recommends the following sleep hygiene guidelines for children:

◆ Provide a quiet, dark, and comfortable environment or bedroom.

◆ Set a strict bedtime and awake routine that remains consistent on a daily basis.

◆ Avoid long daytime naps.

◆ Allow a long space of time between daytime nap and bedtime.

◆ Provide a healthy snack before bedtime so the child is not hungry.

◆ Avoid substances such as caffeine, chocolate, and medications that contain alcohol or other foods/beverages that are stimulating to children.

◆ Cut down on fluids before bedtime so that a full bladder or wetness does not interrupt sleep.

◆ Avoid a high level of activity and television viewing before bedtime and replace it with quiet activities (e.g., reading books).

◆ Encourage children to fall asleep without the parent/ caregiver in the room.

Diagnosis

Sleep disorders can be diagnosed based on a positive answer by the caregiver to one or more of these questions:

• Is it hard for your child to fall asleep?
• Is it hard for your child to stay asleep through the night?
• Does your child wake up feeling tired?
• Is your child sleepy during the day?

Nursing Care

The nurse must listen carefully to the parents' concerns about the child's sleeping issues. The nurse knows that it is important to discover this problem early, understand the causes of sleep disturbances, as well as to implement prevention and intervention strategies. Sheldon (2005) found that children who slept longer had higher intelligence test scores and performed better in school.

The nurse can perform a thorough physical assessment of the child. Certain health conditions can interfere with sleeping, including cow's milk allergies, otitis media, neurological disorders, attention-deficit/hyperactivity disorder (ADHD), and some chronic illnesses.

It is also important that the nurse conduct a thorough assessment of the child's sleeping patterns and how these patterns influence the child's well-being and family functioning. A comprehensive assessment also includes development and behavior history. Sometimes diagnostic data conducted in a sleep laboratory can help confer a sleep-related diagnosis. The electroencephalogram (EEG) is a diagnostic test that provides important data about stages of sleep as well as the integrity and development of the central nervous system (Sheldon, 2005).

The nurse can help the family by providing support while listening without passing judgment and then provide information on sleep hygiene.

 What to say — *Bathing before bedtime is not recommended*

Did you know that a bath before bedtime is no longer considered to have a calming effect? The literature says that a bath before bedtime can have the opposite effect as it stimulates the child and therefore it is not recommended (Sheldon, 2005). The most important principles that nurses can suggest to parents are that there be a consistent bedtime and standard routines (Sheldon, 2005). The nurse can ask parents to describe the bedtime routines and help parents create good sleep hygiene habits for the child. Medications such as hypnotics may be prescribed for children, but it is thought that over time medications do not improve sleeping patterns in otherwise healthy children (Sheldon, 2005).

 case study Sleeping Issues

Paul is 4 years old, and according to his mother he has had sleeping difficulties since he was born. He voices many fears, makes demands, and sometimes has tantrums at bedtime. He says he is afraid of the dark even though he has a night light in his room. Paul complains of being hungry as soon as he lies down in bed. Unless his mother stays in the room with Paul until he falls asleep, he does not stop crying and often becomes upset for no apparent reason. Paul takes an afternoon nap until 5:00 P.M. Now that the family is expecting a new baby they wish to have Paul's sleeping difficulties under control. He has a bedtime of 8:00 P.M. but he does not get to sleep until 11:00 P.M. or midnight unless he has not napped during the day.

critical thinking questions

1. Name the priority nursing diagnosis related to this situation.

2. Discuss the importance of parental education and specific sleep hygiene techniques that the nurse can teach.

◆ See Suggested Answers to Case Studies in text on the Electronic Study Guide or DavisPlus.

Now Can You— **Discuss sleep disorders?**

1. Explain how a nurse would assess a child who complains of sleep disorders.
2. How can sleep disorders be diagnosed?
3. Explain sleep hygiene.

Developmental Conditions

DEVELOPMENTAL DISABILITIES

Children and adolescents who are diagnosed with developmental disabilities are affected by the disparities in health care (Fisher, 2004). Goals related to developmental disabilities have been included in the *Healthy People 2010* initiative as a step toward reducing those disparities. Developmental disabilities is a term that encompasses a number of disorders, including Down syndrome (DS), fragile X syndrome, and fetal alcohol spectrum disorders (FASD). Developmental disabilities may also co-occur with a variety of physical symptoms (seizures, sensory impairments, speech and language problems, and cerebral palsy).

A number of factors that cause genetic conditions, such as Down syndrome or fragile X syndrome, result when abnormal genes are inherited from parents or when there are errors in genetic combinations. Metabolic conditions such as phenylketonuria (PKU) can lead to developmental disabilities if not recognized and treated early. Pregnancy-related problems include alcohol ingestion or viral infection such as rubella. In addition, trauma or asphyxia during the birth process can lead to inadequate oxygen availability and may cause developmental disabilities. Certain illnesses or events that may occur during childhood or adolescence (e.g., whooping cough, measles or meningitis, extreme malnutrition, lack of medical care or exposure to toxins like lead or mercury, as well as head trauma) can contribute to the development of developmental disabilities (National Information Center for Children and Youth with Disabilities [NICHCY], 2004).

As many as 3 out of every 100 people in the United States have developmental disabilities (The Arc, 2001, revised 2004). More than one half million children ages 6 to 21 have developmental disabilities and require special educational services in school.

 ### Nursing Insight— *Fragile X syndrome*

Fragile X syndrome (FXS) is the most common cause of developmental disabilities. It is caused by "an expansion mutation in the fragile X gene (*FMR1*) located on the X chromosome" (Wattendorf & Muenke, 2005, p. 111). FXS is known to affect 1 in 4000 male and 1 in 6000–8000 female children. This genetic disorder is typically not tested for unless there is a family history of developmental disabilities or dysmorphic physical features (e.g., elongated face, large ears, and macroorchidism in boys) associated with the disorder. It is estimated that about 25% of children with FXS also meet the criteria for autism spectrum disorder (ASD) as these children show difficulties with relatedness, play, and communication and demonstrate repetitive behaviors. It can be difficult to distinguish between infants who have FXS and infants with other disorders as the physical features are not known to be the best marker of diagnosis. There is new research attempting to look at how best to differentiate these infants from others early on. A group of researchers have sought to examine early sensory-motor patterns through videotape analysis of infants with FXS vs. ASD in retrospective types of research (Baranek et al., 2005). It is imperative that early identification of the disorder be made and that early intervention with the child and family begin so there is the best opportunity to maximize positive outcomes for the child and family. The nurse has an important role to help identify the disorder and then provide family education, support, and connecting families with appropriate special education and health services.

Signs and Symptoms

Three criteria must be present for the diagnosis of developmental disabilities to be made: (1) an intelligence quotient (IQ) score significantly below average (i.e., below 70—average score is 100); (2) limitations in functions of daily life, such as communication, social situations, and school activities (APA, 2000; CDC, 2005b); and (3) onset before the age of 18.

There are four levels of developmental disabilities:

- Mild: IQ between 55 and 69; person generally able to live independently; by far the largest group of developmentally disabled children
- Moderate: IQ between 40 and 54; person able to function semi-independently with help
- Severe: IQ between 25 and 39; person generally requires institutionalization or very close monitoring
- Profound: IQ below 25; person requires total care

The incidence of each type of developmental disability decreases with the severity of the difficulty.

Diagnosis

Diagnosis of developmental disabilities is based on IQ and on the signs and symptoms seen during infancy based on the baby's physical characteristics (facial features, head circumference) or significant delays in reaching developmental milestones.

Official diagnosis of developmental disabilities is performed by a qualified clinician or a collaborative team of clinicians. These clinicians assess developmental progress at various stages of development as well as perform intelligence and achievement testing. With a confirmed diagnosis of developmental disabilities, the nurse can assess the level of functioning of the child and the family and determine their current level of need. The nurse can communicate to parents that using standardized tests can further suggest a diagnosis.

Nursing Care

Nursing assessment for developmental disabilities should entail prenatal history, birth history, and developmental progress. Each of these assessment categories provides the nurse and family with valuable information.

The nurse understands that there is not one portrait of a developmentally disabled child. Some mildly disabled children may not appear "different." The nurse must remember that each type of disability has unique needs.

An important aspect of nursing care is communication. The nurse can communicate to families that the most preventable forms of developmental disabilities are related to prenatal nutrition and abstinence from alcohol (CDC, n.d.). Genetic counseling may also be helpful, particularly in families where the parents are older or where there is history of fragile X. Promoting good prenatal care as well as encouraging parents to have their children immunized (CDC, n.d.), and enforcing safe practices when bike-riding or playing may help prevent developmental disabilities.

Another focus of nursing care is educational and directed toward building life skills for the child based on the degree of disability. The goal is for the child or adolescent to develop the greatest level of functioning and skills possible to maintain daily living. The nurse can encourage the family to use physical therapy, speech and language therapy, and special educational opportunities. The nurse can teach the family about community resources such as the Special Olympics or schools for therapeutic horseback riding instruction. Group activities can build both motor and learning skills as well as provide socialization.

For eligible school-aged children (including preschoolers), special education and related services are available most often through the public school system. The school teacher, nurse, and parents work together to develop an Individualized Education Plan (IEP). This plan addresses the child's unique needs and provides the services to meet the needs of each child.

DOWN SYNDROME

Down syndrome (DS) is the most common and readily identifiable chromosomal abnormality associated with developmental disabilities. During cell development, the fetus receives 47 chromosomes instead of the normal 46. The extra chromosome changes the development of the body and the brain.

Down syndrome affects approximately 1 in every 800 live births in the United States each year. Although a woman of any age can have a child with Down syndrome, the chances increase for women older than 35 years of age.

Signs and Symptoms

The most common physical characteristics of DS are poor muscle tone, slanting eyes with folds of skin at inner corners (epicanthal folds), hyperflexibility, short, broad hands with a single crease across the palm of one or both hands, broad feet with increased space between the first and second toes, flat bridge of the nose, short, low-set ears, short neck with extra folds of skin, small head, small oral cavity and airway, and short, high-pitched cries in infancy.

In addition to distinct physical appearance, children with DS frequently have health-related issues. Approximately one third of babies with DS have heart defects, which can be surgically corrected, while some have gastrointestinal anomalies that require surgery. Visual and hearing problems are also common, along with speech difficulty, as are sleep-related issues often due to sleep apnea. Assessment of sleep issues should be conducted usually beginning with asking the caregiver if the child snores and has pauses in breathing during sleep. If that is the case, then further evaluation is needed and it begins with sleep studies that include electroencephalography (EEG). Children with DS are also prone to hypothyroidism and should be evaluated yearly. While this condition is potentially serious, proper diagnosis through an x-ray exam by age 3 can prevent serious injury.

Diagnosis

The diagnosis of DS is usually made from a chromosomal blood test shortly after birth. In addition, just as intelligence varies in the normal population, there is a wide variation in the DS population as well regarding cognitive abilities, behavior, and developmental progress.

Nursing Care

Nursing care of a child with DS is similar to that of any developmental disorder. The nurse must be sensitive to the needs of parents who have learned the newborn has the disorder. Helping parents cope and providing them with resources is an important nursing intervention.

Early intervention with children who have DS has become much more sophisticated. Early intervention

serves to provide the best possible individualized care to children with DS so these individuals can make the most of personal capabilities. Nursing care should be geared to the special physical, developmental, and emotional needs of each child. The nurse can coordinate programs designed to help children with DS. These programs offer speech therapy, cognitive and social skills, self-help skills, as well as occupational and physical therapies that may improve gross and fine motor development. The nurse is also in a good position to help families cope emotionally with living with a child with this disability.

 Collaboration in Caring— *Raising public awareness*

The nurse has a responsibility to raise public awareness and acceptance about children with Down syndrome. Children with DS can be included in mainstream educational curriculum and society. The parent, nurse, school personnel, and other individuals in the community can develop an Individualized Education Plan (IEP). The nurse can also communicate to the family and public sector that the National Information Center for Children and Youth with Disabilities at www.nichcy.org is a good resource. The nurse can help the child with DS throughout the life span as the child grows into adulthood. Through improved public acceptance and increased community resources more opportunities for persons with disabilities to live and work independently in the community is possible.

FETAL ALCOHOL SPECTRUM DISORDER

The teratogenic effects (causing abnormal development of the embryo) of alcohol have long been recognized. Warnings against drinking while pregnant are carried on all alcoholic beverages. Still, fetal alcohol spectrum disorder (FASD) is a common disorder with a range of physical and neurodevelopmental problems that are known to be completely preventable. The term FASD is more commonly used now than fetal alcohol syndrome (FAS) to describe the effects on infants and children caused by maternal alcohol intake during pregnancy (Caley, Kramer, & Robinson, 2005). FASD describes a spectrum of alcohol-related disorders that includes FAS, alcohol-related neurodevelopmental disorder (ARND), alcohol-related birth defects (ARBD), and fetal alcohol effects (FAE).

Epidemiological studies report that the prevalence of FASD is 1 to 1.5 per 1000 live births, but alcohol-related neurodevelopmental disorders (ARND) (i.e., associated problems that do not fully meet the criteria for FASD) are six to eight times more common than FASD (Klug & Burd, 2003). FASD results from maternal consumption of alcohol during pregnancy. Data show that alcohol intake at any time of pregnancy can be harmful.

Signs and Symptoms

Nurses working in the nursery or in the neonatal intensive care may be able to identify traits of FASD. Characteristics of FASD include facial dysmorhic features (e.g., epicanthal folds, flat mid-face, short nose, short eye openings, thin upper lip, underdeveloped jaw, groove in upper lip), low birth weight, failure to thrive and microcephaly. Later on developmental delays, hyperactive behavior, learning and attention difficulties, poor motor skills, and developmental disabilities are noted (Caley, Kramer, & Robinson, 2005).

Diagnosis

Early diagnosis is important, but often very difficult without definitive evidence of maternal alcohol ingestion. A diagnosis of FASD requires a good history, including information on maternal consumption of alcohol during pregnancy.

Nursing Care

The nurse can communicate to families that FASD and ARND are 100% preventable, and as such, it is important to develop prevention programs to reduce the rates of these disorders. It is known that prevention programs designed to prevent these disorders would save money that is currently being used to treat children with FASD (Klug & Burd, 2003). Nurses can provide information to families about the effects of alcohol on the fetus. School nurses especially can facilitate early education regarding alcohol consumption during pregnancy (Caley, Kramer, & Robinson, 2005). Since there are no guidelines about safe consumption rates for pregnant women, the public should know that the safe amount is no alcohol intake during pregnancy. Material can be obtained from National Institute on Alcohol Abuse and Alcoholism (NIAAA) Web site (www.science.education. nih.gov). In addition, nurses can help to identify cases of FASD and help families seek appropriate services.

Learning Disorders and Cognitive Impairment

The Interdisciplinary Council on Developmental and Learning Disorders–Diagnostic Manual for Infancy and Early Childhood (ICDL-DMIC) (Greenspan, 2005) prefers to label learning disorders as learning challenges. The nurse understands that a child may manifest challenges in more than one specific learning area, including math, reading, and organizing skills (Greenspan, 2005). It is known that early learning challenges are influenced by emotional and social competencies, auditory processing and language skills (memory, ability to retrieve), perceptual motor skills, motor planning (sequencing, visual memory), visual/spatial processing skills, and ability to modulate sensory information (Greenspan, 2005). The ability to learn involves many of these skills working together. Increased information about learning issues may help identify this condition early and initiate preventive interventions.

There are several disorders in this area including

- Reading Disorder (Dyslexia—significantly impaired ability to read; words or letters may be "mixed up" or distorted, making it impossible to recognize what others see)
- Arithmetic Disorder (Dyscalculia—significant inability to understand or recognize numbers or functions of numbers, or copy them correctly, or follow sequences)
- Writing Disorder (dysgraphia)
- Graphomotor Disorder (related to poor fine motor skills)
- Disorder of Written Expression (related to significantly poor spelling, grammar, handwriting)
- Language Disorder (delays in or lack of ability to understand or express verbal communication)

It is estimated that nearly 5% of the children currently in the U.S. school system have a learning disorder. Overall population statistics point to prevalence between 2% and 10% (APA, 2000).

Signs and Symptoms

The nurse understands that a multi-dimensional approach is used to assess early learning patterns. The recommended areas for assessment include functional emotional developmental capacities, auditory processing and language, visuospatial capacities, and regulatory-sensory processing patterns (Greenspan, 2005). The Diagnostic Manual for Infancy and Early Childhood has a comprehensive section with details regarding each area of assessment and the interested reader is encouraged to consult this original source (Greenspan, 2005).

Diagnosis

Diagnosis is made through comprehensive assessments involving interviews and observation. Definitive testing is recommended before a learning disorder or challenge is diagnosed. The DSM-IV-TR identifies reading disorder, mathematics disorder, disorder of written expression, and learning disorder not otherwise specified. It also specifies that each disorder must be diagnosed as a result of a standardized test administered on an individual basis (APA, 2000).

Nursing Care

Early identification of learning challenges should be conducted before a child is fully immersed in an academic environment so that early intervention can begin. Early identification and treatment gives the child the greatest potential for a good outcome (Greenspan, 2005). The nurse can communicate to the family that the child's strengths should be incorporated as part of assessment, early prevention, and intervention. The nurse can fully inform the parents about their child's rights and entitlements in the public school sector. Often, children who enter public education with a learning challenge or disability will have an IEP (Individualized Education Plan) that is revised every few months. School nurses can provide education and support to children and their families.

Elimination Disorders

ENURESIS

Most children have experienced toileting "accidents" based on waiting too long to use the bathroom or drinking too much liquid before going to bed. For the most part, these experiences, while embarrassing, are not overly concerning. Parental worries about toilet learning can often be allayed when the nurse instructs parents on the normal growth and development that makes toilet learning possible.

Enuresis refers to the occurrence of wetting clothing or the bed at least two times per week for at least 3 months, or that causes significant embarrassment or restriction of activities for the child, like not attending sleepovers or camp (APA, 2000). Children and adolescents can exhibit either diurnal (daytime), nocturnal (nighttime), or *both* types of enuresis. Primary enuresis is diagnosed in children who are at least 5 years of age and have not yet achieved toileting control. Secondary enuresis occurs in children who have been successful in using the toilet for a significant period of time (6 to 12 months) and then become regularly incontinent.

Causes of enuresis range from physiological problems (urinary tract infections or diabetes) to anatomical problems (genitourinary malformations) to psychological problems (stress or trauma) or disturbances in the sleep cycle (American Academy of Child and Adolescent Psychiatry [AACAP], 2004).

Enuresis tends to run in families. Seventy-five percent of all children with enuresis have a first-degree relative who has also suffered from the disorder (APA, 2000).

Signs and Symptoms

The nurse performs a complete history when assessing the child with enuresis. This history will be helpful in the development of a differential diagnosis. First the diagnosing clinician (nurse practitioner or physician) rules out medical conditions, like urinary tract infections, structural problems, diabetes, or kidney disease. Since there is a familial pattern, understanding its presence in biological relatives is an important clue.

Diagnosis

In considering the child's toilet learning history, age of learning, and difficulties experienced, the nurse can help the family document the onset of the disorder and situations when "accidents" happen. The nurse can also assess recent and chronic stressors that may be affecting the child such as the birth of a sibling, divorce, or other family disruption that might contribute to regression and lead to a diagnosis.

Nursing Care

Initially, the nurse can recognize that it is important to understand parental attitudes about toilet training. Parents who expect their child to be potty trained before the child is physically or emotionally able may stymie their efforts by their insistence.

"What to say" — *Toilet training*

The nurse can communicate to parents that toilet training can begin when both the parents and child are ready. Parents are ready when they can devote about 3 months of time offering lessons and encouragement. The child is ready to be toilet trained when he or she can indicate that his or her diaper is soiled or wet or can communicate that he or she would like to use the toilet. The child can communicate this information at about 18–24 months of age. Other indicators that the child is ready include the child showing interest in other people using the bathroom or in underwear, noticing a small toilet in the bathroom, or even playing with the toilet paper. The nurse can remind parents that sometimes the child is not ready to be toilet trained until 2 ½ or 3 years of age (American Academy of Family Physicians [AAFP], 2006).

The nurse can also communicate to parents that treatment falls into two categories: behavioral and pharmacological. Behavioral treatments are common and effective. An example of a behavioral treatment is using the bell and pad method, in which a pad that is attached to an alarm is placed under the child at bedtime. If the child urinates, the alarm

rings. Other behavioral methods parents can easily employ are to make sure the child stops drinking liquids early in the evening and the child urinates before going to bed. The parent may also choose to awaken the child during the night to use the bathroom. In time, the problem generally resolves.

Early pharmacological treatments include the use of the tricyclic antidepressant, Imipramine (Tofranil). It is important to note that other tricyclics do not stop bedwetting. More recently, DDAVP (desmopressin), a vasopressin analog, has been shown to work to decrease nighttime enuresis. This medication is administered either nasally or orally.

ENCOPRESIS

The DSM-IV-TR describes **encopresis** as the "repeated passage of feces into inappropriate places (e.g., clothing or floor)" (APA, 2000, p. 116). Encopresis can be primary (in children who have not become consistently continent by age 5) or secondary (children who have been continent and then become incontinent for a period of time). The child may present with either constipation with fecal incontinence due to overflow of feces, or without constipation.

Signs and Symptoms

Signs and symptoms of encopresis in the child can be observed or noted as the child may withhold the feces involuntarily due to constipation which may set into motion a cycle of fearfulness of the pain of defecation. The child may also suffer from encopresis related to psychological stressors. If the potty training period is difficult, or if the child uses a toilet that is too tall to get good enough leverage to force the feces out properly, defecation may become associated with pain.

Diagnosis

As with enuresis, children may be diagnosed when they exhibit regression in bowel habits when confronted with stressful situations.

Nursing Care

It is important for the nurse talk to the parents about the child's defecation patterns during a medical appointment. The nurse also understands that it is important to take a thorough history of bowel habits and toilet training. Monitoring the occurrence of constipation will give an indicator of the cause(s). It is also important to evaluate the child's dietary habits, focusing on the amount of fiber and liquids the child consumes. The nurse can also talk to the parents to determine any transitions that may be happening in the child's life such as moving, a new baby in the household, or loss of a caregiver.

---

where research and practice meet:
Encopresis

There are few statistics available for encopresis. A study of 13,111 parents and children of various cultures in Amsterdam found that encopresis occurred in 4.1% of 5- to 6-year-olds, and 1.6% of 11- to 12-year-olds. Twenty-five percent of the children seen by pediatric gastroenterologists present with symptoms of encopresis or constipation. It is estimated that encopresis occurs six times more prominently in boys than in girls (kidshealth.org).

As with enuresis, it is important for the nurse to help the family understand healthy toilet training. Making defecation nonstressful and rewarding may help the child change the behavior. A child's potty is recommended to help the child position him- or herself to push stool out adequately. Nurses can also encourage families to provide a high-fiber diet for their child both for prevention and for intervention with constipation. Since family stress and change can contribute to encopresis, referral of the family for counseling may be in order.

summary points

◆ Developmental psychopathology is a discipline that evolved from the contribution from multiple fields of study with the goal of providing an understanding of psychopathology and normal adaptation.

◆ Vulnerability is defined as a predispositional factor, or set of factors, that makes a disordered state possible. Resilience is a dynamic developmental process reflecting evidence of positive adaptation despite significant life adversity.

◆ There is vast research indicating that health care disparities in racial and ethnic minorities are widespread compared to those in non-minorities, and barriers such as mistrust, fear, and discrimination stand in the way of optimal mental health outcomes in ethnically diverse families.

◆ Though there are increasing efforts to educate the public, the stigma of mental illness continues to be a major barrier to accessing mental health services for children and their families.

◆ Psychopathology in children includes conditions such as anxiety, depression, posttraumatic stress disorder, suicide, bipolar disorder, schizophrenia, and autism spectrum disorder.

◆ The most effective treatment for attention-deficit/ hyperactivity disorder (ADHD) is a combination of pharmacological and nonpharmacological interventions. Using both modalities allows for the control or abatement of symptomatic behavior.

◆ Child maltreatment is considered to be any action or failure to act by a person that endangers a child's physical or emotional health and development. A person is abusive if the person fails to nurture the child, physically injures the child, or relates sexually to the child.

◆ The nurse is in an ideal position to identify adolescents at risk for substance abuse, especially if there is a strong family and genetic history of abuse; referring for treatment as early as possible. Treatment might involve family psychoeducation regarding substance abuse.

◆ Anorexia nervosa can become a life-threatening problem or cause death because of severe weight loss that can result in electrolyte imbalance and hemodynamic instability.

◆ A number of factors can cause developmental disabilities: genetic conditions, such as Down syndrome or fragile X syndrome; metabolic conditions such as phenylketonuria (PKU); or pregnancy-related problems, including alcohol ingestion or viral infections such as rubella.

◆ The nurse recognizes that it is important to take a complete nursing history when assessing the child with elimination disorders.

review questions

Multiple Choice

1. In the emergency room, a 10-year-child complains of dizziness, palpitations, sweating, and tingling sensations. The child's mother tells the nurse that recently her child has been talking about death. The pediatric nurse analyzes these behaviors as signs and/or symptoms related to what condition?
A. Selective mutism
B. Panic disorder
C. Posttraumatic stress disorder
D. Suicidal tendencies

Select All that Apply

2. A nurse working in the newborn nursery admits a newborn with facial dysmorphic features. What other clinical manifestations leads the nurse to believe that this neonate was born to a mother who consumed a large amount of alcohol during her pregnancy?
A. Low birth weight
B. Hypoactive behavior
C. A high pitched cry
D. Microcephaly

3. When developing a nursing care plan for a 26-month-old toddler with inorganic failure to thrive, the pediatric nurse determines which diagnosis as the priority?
A. Imbalanced Nutrition Less than Body Requirements related to the inability to absorb nutrients
B. Delayed Growth and Development related to inadequate ingestion of nutrients
C. Risk for Impaired parenting related to insufficient knowledge or crisis
D. Imbalanced Nutrition Less than Body Requirements related to vomiting and diarrhea.

4. An infant comes to the genetic clinic to be evaluated for Down syndrome. While performing a nursing assessment, the pediatric nurse documents several clinical manifestations that are suspicious of Down syndrome. Which of the following clinical manifestations are indicative of this genetic disorder?
A. Epicanthal folds
B. Flattened nose
C. Short, low set ears
D. Short neck with extra skin folds

Fill-in-the-Blank

5. An infant born to a mother who consumes alcohol during her pregnancy is at risk for developing _____ _____ _____ _____.

6. Researchers have found that the age at onset of schizophrenia plays an important role in the outcome of this condition. It is believed that the _____ the onset, the _____ the impairment.

True/False

7. The pediatric nurse is aware that while performing an adolescent assessment, he or she should not be fearful of asking the adolescent questions related to suicidal thoughts.

8. The pediatric nurse must keep in mind when working with children whose parents have mental health problems that these children will likely go on to develop mental health problems.

9. Attention-deficit/hyperactivity disorder is one of the most commonly recognized psychiatric childhood conditions.

10. The pediatric nurse working in a clinic must be able to identify appropriate developmental milestones in order to facilitate expected outcomes for the child.

See Answers to End of Chapter Review Questions on the Electronic Study Guide or DavisPlus.

REFERENCES

Achenbach, T. (2001). Child behavior checklist for ages 6–18: ASEBA, University of Vermont.

Achenbach, T., & Rescorla, L. (2000). Child behavior checklist for ages 1 1/2–5. ASEBA, University of Vermont.

Ainsworth, M., Blehar, M., Waters, E., & Wall, S. (1978). *Patterns of attachment: A psychological study of the strange situation.* Oxford: Lawrence Erlbaum.

American Academy of Child & Adolescent Psychiatry (AACAP). (2004). Summary of the practice parameter for the assessment and treatment of children and adolescents with enuresis. *Journal of the Academy of Child and Adolescent Psychiatry, 43*(1), 123-125.

American Academy of Family Physicians (AAFP). (updated 2006). Toilet training your child. Retrieved from http://familydoctor. org/online/famdocen/home/children/parents/toilet/179 (Accessed July 7, 2007).

American Psychiatric Association (APA). (2000). *Diagnostic and statistical manual of mental disorders (DSM-IV-TR)* (4th, text revision ed.). Washington, DC: Author.

Anderson, P.M., & Butcher, K.F. (2006). Childhood obesity: Trends and potential causes.*The Future of Children. Special Issue: Childhood Obesity, 16*(1), 19–45.

The Arc (2001, revised 2004). Retrieved from http://www.thearc.org/ NetCommunity/Page.aspx?&pid=403&srcid=270 (Accessed August 11, 2007).

Baranek, G.T., Danko, C.D., Skinner, M.L., Bailey, D.B., Hatton, D.D., Roberts, J.E., & Mirrett, P.L. (2005). Video analysis of sensory-motor features in infants with fragile X syndrome at 9–12 months of age. *Journal of Autism and Developmental Disorders, 35*(5), 645–656.

Barrett, P. M., Farrell, L. J., Ollendick, T. H., & Dadds, M. (2006). Long-Term Outcomes of an Australian Universal Prevention Trial of Anxiety and Depression Symptoms in Children and Youth: An Evaluation of the Friends Program. *Journal of Clinical Child and Adolescent Psychology, 35*(3), 403-411.

Barrett, P.M., & Shortt, A.L. (2003). Parental involvement in the treatment of anxious children. In A.E. Kazdin & J.R. Weisz (Eds.), *Evidence-based psychotherapies for children and adolescents* (pp. 101–119). New York: Guilford Press.

Barrio, C.A. (2007). Assessing suicide risk in children: Guidelines for developmentally appropriate interviewing. *Journal of Mental Health Counseling, 29*(1), 50–66.

Barth, R. P., Crea, T. M., John, K., Thoburn, J., & Quinton, D. (2005). Beyond attachment theory and therapy: Towards sensitive and evidence-based interventions with foster and adoptive families in distress. *Child and Family Social Work, 10*(4), 257-268.

Bassali, R.D., & Benjamin, J. (2007). Failure to thrive. *E-medicine from WebMD.* Retrieved from http://www.emedicine.com/ped/topic738. htm (Accessed August 2, 2007).

Baydar, N., Reid, M., & Webster-Stratton, C. (2003). The role of mental health factors and programs engagement in the effectiveness of a preventive parenting program for Head Start mothers. *Child Development, 74*(5), 1433–1453.

Bearden, C.E., Meyer, S.E., Loewy, R.L., Niendam, T.A., & Cannon, T.D. (2006). The neurodevelopmental model of schizophrenia: Updated. In D. Cicchetti & D.J. Cohen (Eds.), *Developmental psychopathology: Risk, disorder, and adaptation* (Vol. 3, pp. 542–569). Hoboken, NJ: John Wiley & Sons.

Block, R., & Krebs, N. (2006). Failure to thrive as a manifestation of child neglect. *Journal of the American Academy of Child & Adolescent Psychiatry, 45*(5), 595.

Bulechek, G., Butcher, H.M., & Dochterman, J. (2008). *Nursing interventions classification (NIC)* (5th ed.). St. Louis, MO: C.V. Mosby.

Caley, L.M., Kramer, C., & Robinson, L.K. (2005). Fetal alcohol spectrum disorder. *The Journal of School Nursing, 21*(3), 139–146.

Canitano, R., & Vivanti, G. (2007). Tics and Tourette syndrome in autism spectrum disorders. *Autism, 11*(1), 19–28.

Caprio, S. (2006). Treating child obesity and associated medical conditions. *The Future of Children, 16*(1), 209–224. Retrieved from www. futureofchildren.org (Accessed August 2, 2007).

Centers for Disease Control and Prevention (CDC) Center for Health Statistics (n.d.). Retrieved from http://www.cdc.gov/nchs/Default. htm (Accessed July 15, 2007).

Centers for Disease Control and Prevention (CDC). (2004). Autism A.L.A.R.M. Brochure from the American Academy of Pediatrics and the National Center on Birth Defects and Developmental Disabilities at the Centers for Disease Control and Prevention (CDC). Retrieved from http://www.medicalhomeinfo.org (Accessed June 12, 2008).

Centers for Disease Control and Prevention (CDC). (2005a). Summary Health Statistics for U.S. Children: National Health Interview Survey, 2005, Appendix III, Table VI. Retrieved from http://www.cdc.gov/ nchs/Default.htm (Accessed July 15, 2007).

Centers for Disease Control and Prevention (CDC). (2005b). Developmental disabilities: mental retardation. Retrieved from http://www. cc.gov/ncbddd/dd/mr3/htm (Accessed June 22, 2007).

Child and Adolescent Bipolar Foundation. Retrieved from http://www. bpkids.org/site/PageServer (Accessed June 12, 2008).

Childhelp National Child Abuse Hotline. (n.d.). Misconceptions of reporting child abuse. Retrieved from http://www.childhelp.org/get_ help (Accessed August 1, 2007).

Child Welfare Information Gateway. (2007). Surviving toilet training. Retrieved from http://www.childwelfare.gov/preventing/supporting/ resources/toilettrining.cfm (Accessed July 8, 2007).

Cicchetti, D. (2003). Foreword. In S.S. Luthar (Ed.), *Resilience and vulnerability: Adaptation in the context of childhood adversities* (pp. xix–xxvii). Cambridge, UK: Cambridge Press.

Cicchetti, D., & Posner, M.I. (2005). Cognitive and affective neuroscience and developmental psychopathology. *Development & Psychopathology, 17*(3), 569–575.

Cleveland Clinic. (2007). Treating anxiety disorders in children and adolescents. Retrieved from http://www.clevelandclinic.org/health/ health-info/docs/0700/0772.asp (Accessed July 7, 2007).

Commission on Adolescent Anxiety Disorders. (2005). Anxiety disorders. In D.L. Evans, E.B. Foa, R.E. Gur, H. Hendin, C.P. O'Brien, M.E.P. Seligman, & B.T. Walsh (Eds.), *Treating and preventing adolescent mental health disorders: What we know and don't know: A research agenda for improving the mental health of our youth* (pp. 162–253). New York: Oxford University Press.

Commission on Adolescent Depression & Bipolar Disorder. (2005). Depression and Bipolar Disorder. In D.L. Evans, E.B. Foa, R.E. Gur, H. Hendin, C.P. O'Brien, M.E.P. Seligman, & B.T. Walsh, *Treating and preventing adolescent mental health disorders: What we know and don't know: A research agenda for improving the mental health of our youth* (pp. 4–74). New York: Oxford University Press.

Commission on Adolescent Eating Disorders. (2005). Eating disorders. In D.L. Evans, E.B. Foa, R.E. Gur, H. Hendin, C.P. O'Brien, M.E.P. Seligman, & B.T. Walsh. *Treating and preventing adolescent mental health disorders: What we know and don't know: A research agenda for improving the mental health of our youth* (pp. 257–332). New York: Oxford University Press.

Commission on Adolescent Schizophrenia. (2005). Schizophrenia. In D.L. Evans, E.B. Foa, R.E. Gur, H. Hendin, C.P. O'Brien, M.E.P. Seligman, & B.T. Walsh (Eds.), *Treating and preventing adolescent mental health disorders: What we know and don't know: A research agenda for improving the mental health of our youth* (pp. 75–156). New York: Oxford University Press.

Commission on Adolescent Substance and Alcohol Abuse. (2005). Substance use disorders. In D.L. Evans, E.B. Foa, R.E. Gur, H. Hendin, C.P. O'Brien, M.E.P. Seligman, & B.T. Walsh (Eds.), *Treating and preventing adolescent mental health disorders: What we know and don't know: A research agenda for improving the mental health of our youth* (pp. 333–429). New York: Oxford University Press.

Daniels, S.R. (2006). The consequences of childhood overweight and obesity. The Future of Children/Center for the Future of Children, the David and Lucile Packard Foundation. *16*(1), 47–67.

Denham, B. (2006). Emotional competence: Implications for social functioning. In: J. Luby (Ed.), *Handbook of preschool mental heath: Department, disorders and treatment* (pp. 23-44). New York: Guilford Press.

Dishion, T., & Kavanagh, K. (2003). *Intervening in adolescent problems behavior: A family-centered approach.* New York: Guilford Press.

Dishion, T., & Patterson, G. (2006). *The development and ecology of antisocial behavior in children and adolescents.* Hoboken, NJ: John Wiley & Sons.

Epstein, L.H. (2003). Development of evidence-based treatments for pediatric obesity. In A. Kazdin & J. Weisz (Eds.), *Evidence-based psychotherapies for children and adolescents* (pp. 374–387). New York: Guilford Press.

Ewing, J.A. (1984). Detecting alcoholism: The CAGE questionnaire. *Journal of the American Medical Association, 252*(14), 1905–1907.

Findling, R.L., Feeny, N.C., Stansbrey, R.J., Delporto-Bedoya, D., & Demeter, C. (2004). Special articles: Treatment of mood disorders in children and adolescents: Somatic treatment for depressive illnesses in children and adolescents. *Psychiatric Clinics of North America, 27*(1), 113–137.

Fisher, K. (2004). Health disparities and mental retardation [Electronic version]. *Journal of Nursing Scholarship, 36*(1), 48–53.

Ginzburg, G.S., Riddle, M.A., & Davies, M. (2006). Somatic symptoms in children and adolescents with anxiety disorders. *Journal of the American Academy of Child and Adolescent Psychiatry, 45*(10), 1179–1187.

Golan, M., & Crow, S. (2004). Parents are key players in the prevention and treatment of weight-related problems. *Nutrition Reviews, 62*(1), 39–50.

Goodman, W.K., Murphy, T.K., & Storch, E.A. (2007). Risk of adverse behavioral effects with pediatric use of antidepressants [Electronic version]. *Psychopharmacology, 191*(87), 87–96.

Greenspan, S. (2005). *Diagnostic manual for infancy and early childhood.* Bethesda, MD: Interdisciplinary Council on Developmental and Learning Disorders.

Hammen, C. (2003). Risk and protective factors for children of depressed parents. In S.S. Luthar (Ed.), *Resilience and vulnerability: Adaptation in the context of childhood adversities* (pp. 50–75). New York: Cambridge University Press.

Heffelfinger, A.K., & Mrakotsky, C. (2006). Cognitive Development. In J.L. Luby (Ed.), *Handbook of preschool mental health: Development, disorders, and treatment* (pp. 45–50). New York: Guilford Press.

Heffernan, J. (2004). The right to equal treatment: Ending racial and ethnic disparities in health care. *Journal of Ambulatory Care Management, 27*(1), 84–86.

Hinshaw, S. (2005). The stigmatization of mental illness in children and parents: Developmental issues, family concerns, and research needs. *Journal of Child Psychology and Psychiatry, 46*(7), 714–734.

Hinshaw, S. (2006). *Stigma and mental illness: Developmental issues and future prospects* [e-book]. Hoboken, NJ: John Wiley & Sons. Available from: PsycINFO, Ipswich, MA (Accessed August 11, 2007).

Ingram, R., & Luxton, D. (2005). Vulnerability-stress models. In B. Hankin & J. Abela (Eds.), *Development of psychopathology: A vulnerability-stress perspective* (pp. 32–46). Thousand Oaks, CA: Sage Publications.

Johnson, M., Bulechek, G., Butcher, H., McCloskey Dochterman, J., Maas, M., Moorehead, S., & Swanson, E. (2006). *NANDA, NOC, and NIC linkages: Nursing diagnoses, outcomes, & interventions* (2nd ed.). St. Louis, MO: Mosby Elsevier.

Katz, L.Y., Cox, B.J., Gunasekara, S., & Miller, A.L. (2004). Feasibility of dialectical behavior therapy for suicidal adolescent inpatients. *Journal of the American Academy of Child and Adolescent Psychiatry, 43*(3), 276–282.

Keep Kids Healthy (n.d.). Encopresis. Retrieved from http://www.keepkidshealthy.com/welcome/conditions/encopresis.html (Accessed August 11, 2007).

Kendall, P.C., Aschenbrand, S.G., & Hudson, J.L. (2003). Child-focused treatment of anxiety. In A.E. Kazdin & J.R. Weisz (Eds.), *Evidence-based psychotherapies for children and adolescents* (pp. 81–100). New York: Guilford Press.

Kidshealth.org Retrieved from http://kidshealth.org/PageManager.jsp?dn=KidsHealth&lic=1&ps-107&cat_id-128&article (Accessed July 8, 2007).

Klug, M.G., & Burd, L. (2003). Fetal alcohol syndrome prevention: annual and cumulative cost savings. *Neurotoxicology & Teratology 25*(6), 763–765.

Knight, J.R., Sherritt, L., Shrier, L.A., Harris, S.K., & Chang, G. (2002). Validity of the CRAFFT Substance Abuse Screening Test Among Adolescent Clinic Patients. *Archives of Pediatrics and Adolescent Medicine, 156*, 607–614.

Kowatch, R.A., Fristad, M., Birmaher, B., Wagner, K.D., Findling, R.L., Hellander, M., et al. (2005). Treatment guidelines for children and adolescents with bipolar disorder.[see comment]. *Journal of the American Academy of Child & Adolescent Psychiatry, 44*(3), 213–235.

Kryger, M.H. (2005). Differential diagnosis of pediatric sleep disorders. In S.H. Sheldon, R. Ferber, & M.H. Kryger (Eds.). *Principles and practice of pediatric sleep medicine* (pp. 17–26). Philadelphia: Elsevier Saunders.

Kumanyika, S., & Grier, S. (2006). Targeting interventions for ethnic minority and low-income populations. *The Future of Children, 16*(1), 187–207.

Leckman, J.F., Bloch, M.H., Scahill, L., & King, R.A. (2006). Tourette syndrome: The self under siege. *Journal of Child Neurology, 21*(8), 642–649.

Lieberman, A.F., & Van Horn, P. (2005). *Don't hit my mommy: A manual for child-parent psychotherapy with young witnesses of family violence.* Washington, DC: Zero to Three.

Locklin, M. (2005). The redefinition of failure to thrive from a case study perspective. *Pediatric Nursing, 31*(6), 474–495.

Luby, J.L., Heffelfinger, A.K., Mrakotsky, C., Brown, K.M., Hessler, M.J., Wallis, J.M., et al. (2003). The clinical picture of depression in preschool children.[see comment]. *Journal of the American Academy of Child & Adolescent Psychiatry, 42*(3), 340–348.

Luby, J.L., Sullivan, J., Belden, A., Stalets, M., Blankenship, S., & Spitznagel, E. (2006). An observational analysis of behavior in depressed preschoolers: Further validation of early-onset depression. *Journal of the American Academy of Child & Adolescent Psychiatry, 45*(2), 203–212.

Mayes, L.C., & Suchman, N.E. (2006). Developmental pathways to substance abuse. In D. Cicchetti & D.J. Cohen (Eds.), *Developmental psychopathology: Risk, disorder, and adaptation* (Vol. 3, pp. 599–619). Hoboken, NJ: John Wiley & Sons.

Moorehead, S., Johnson, M., Maas, M., & Swanson, E. (2008). *Nursing outcomes classification (NOC)* (4th ed.). St. Louis, MO: C.V. Mosby.

NANDA International (2007). *NANDA-I nursing diagnoses: Definitions and classifications 2007–2008.* Philadelphia: NANDA-I.

National Advisory Mental Health Council Workgroup on Child and Adolescent Mental Health Intervention Development and Deployment. (2001). *Blueprint for change: Research on child and adolescent mental health.* Washington, DC: NIMH.

National Institute on Alcohol Abuse and Alcoholism (NIAAA). (n.d.). CAGE Questionnaire. Retrieved from http://pubs.niaaa.nih.gov/publications/Assesing%20Alcohol/InstrumentPDFs/16_CAGE.pd (Accessed August 1, 2007).

National Information Center for Children and Youth with Disabilities. Retrieved from www.nichcy.org (Accessed June 12, 2008).

National Institute of Mental Health (NIMH). (2000). *Child & adolescent bipolar disorder: An update from the National Institute of Mental Health.* (NIH Publication Number: 00-4778). Retrieved from http://www.nimh.nih.gov/publicat/index.cfm.

National Institute of Mental Health (NIMH). (2001). *Blueprint for change: Research on child and adolescent mental health: Report of the National Advisory Mental Health Council's Workgroup on Child and Adolescent Mental Health Development and Deployment* (pp. 23-29). Washington, DC: Office of Communications and Public Liaison (ERIC Document Reproduction Service No. ED462650).

Ogden, C.L., Carroll, M.D., Curtin, L.R., McDowell, M.A., Tabak, C.J., & Flegal, K.M. (2006). Prevalence of overweight and obesity in the United States, 1999–2004. *Journal of the American Medical Association, 295*, 1549–1555.

Olds, D. (2002). Prenatal and infancy home visiting by nurses: From randomized trials to community replication. *Prevention Science, 3*, 153–172.

Osofsky, J.D. (2004). *Young children and trauma: Intervention and treatment.* New York: The Guilford Press.

Owens, J. (2005). Epidemiology of sleep disorders during childhood. In S.H. Sheldon, R. Ferber, & M.H. Kryger (Eds.), *Principles and practice of pediatric sleep medicine* (pp. 27–34). Philadelphia: Elsevier Saunders.

Owens, J., & Mindell, J. (2005). *Take charge of your child's sleep: The all-in-one resource for solving sleep problems in kids and teens.* New York: Marlowe & Company.

Ozonoff, S., Rogers, S., & Hendren, R. (2003). *Autism spectrum disorders: A research review for practitioners.* Washington, DC: American Psychiatric Publishing.

Pearce, J., Blakely, T., Witten, K., & Bartie, P. (2007). Neighborhood deprivation and access to fast-food retailing. *American Journal of Preventive Medicine, 32*(5), 375–382.

Pinto-Martin, J.A., Souders, M.C., Giarelli, E., & Levy, S.E. (2005). The role of nurses in screening for autistic spectrum disorder in pediatric primary care. *Journal of Pediatric Nursing, 20*(3), 163–169.

Reynolds, C.R., & Kamphaus, R.W. (2002). *The clinician's guide to the Behavior Assessment System for Children (BASC).* New York: Guilford Press.

Rutter, M. (2003). Poverty and child mental health. *Journal of the American Medical Association, 290*(15), 2063–2064.

Sallis, J.F., & Glanz, K. (2006). The role of built environments in physical activity, eating, and obesity in childhood. *The Future of Children* (Special issue), *16*(1), 89–108.

Scheeringa, M.S. (2006). Posttraumatic stress disorder: Clinical guidelines and research findings. In J.L. Luby (Ed.), *Handbook of preschool mental health: Development, disorders, and treatment* (pp. 165–185). New York: Guilford Press.

Shaw, D.S., Dishion, T.J., Supplee, L., Gardner, F., & Arnds, K. (2006). Randomized trial of a family-centered approach to the prevention of early conduct problems: 2-year effects of the family check-up in early childhood. *Journal of Consulting and Clinical Psychology, 74*(1), 1–9.

Shaw, D.S., Gilliom, M., Ingoldsby, E., & Nagin, D. (2003). Trajectories leading to school-age conduct problems. *Developmental Psychology, 39,* 189–200.

Sheldon, S.H. (2005). Introduction to pediatric sleep medicine. In S.H. Sheldon, R. Ferber, & M.H. Kryger (Eds.), *Principles and practice of pediatric sleep medicine* (pp. 1–16). Philadelphia: Elsevier Saunders.

Shelton, D., & Pearson, G. (2005). ADHD in juvenile offenders: Treatment issues nurses need to know. *Journal of Psychosocial Nursing and Mental Health Services, 43*(9), 38–46.

Shortt, A.L., & Spence, S.H. (2006). Risk and protective factors for depression in youth. *Behaviour Change, 23*(1), 1–30.

Smedley, A., & Smedley, B.D. (2005). Race as biology is fiction, racism as a social problem is real: Anthropological and historical perspectives on the social construction of race. *American Psychologist, 60*(1), 16–26.

Snider, L.A., & Swedo, S.E. (2003). Childhood-onset obsessive-compulsive disorder and tic disorders: Case report and literature review. *Journal of Child and Adolescent Psychopharmacology, 13*(S1), S18–S88.

Spence, S.H., & Shortt, A.L. (2007). Can we justify the widespread dissemination of universal, school-based interventions for the prevention of depression among children and adolescents? *Journal of Psychology and Psychiatry, 48*(6), 526–542.

Spessot, A.L., & Peterson, B.S. (2006). Tourette's syndrome; developmental psychopathology. In D. Cicchetti, & D.J. Cohen (Eds.), *Developmental psychopathology, Vol 3: Risk, disorder and adaptation* (2nd ed., pp. 436–469). Hoboken, NJ: John Wiley & Sons.

Stafford, B.S., & Zeanah, C.H. (2006). Attachment disorders. In J.L. Luby (Ed.), *Handbook of preschool mental health: Development, disorders, and treatment,* (pp. 231–251). New York: Guilford Press.

Steiner, H., Kwan, W., Shaffer, T.G., Walker, S., Miller, S., Sagar, A., & Lock, J. (2003). Risk and protective factors for juvenile eating disorders. *European Child & Adolescent Psychiatry* (Supplement 1), *12,* 38–46.

Story, M., Kaphingst, K., & French, S. (2006). The role of child care settings in obesity prevention. *The Future of Children, 16*(1), 143–168.

Substance Abuse and Mental Health Services Administration [SAMHSA], (n.d.). How families can help children cope with fear and anxiety. Retrieved from http://mentalhealth.samhsa.gov/ (Accessed June 12, 2008).

Substance Abuse and Mental Health Services Administration [SAMHSA], (n.d.). Major depression in children and adolescents. Retrieved from http://mentalhelath.samhsa.gov/publicaions/allpubs/Ca-0011/default.asp (Accessed July 7, 2007).

Swindburn, B., & Egger, G. (2004). The runaway weight gain train: Too many accelerators, not enough brakes. *British Journal of Medicine, 329,* 736–739.

Szalacha, L.A., Erkut, S., Garcia Coll, C., Alarcon, O., Fields, J.P., & Ceder, I. (2003). Discrimination and Puerto Rican children's and adolescents' mental health. *Cultural Diversity & Ethnic Minority Psychology, 9*(2), 141–155.

Tomb, M., & Hunter, L. (2004). Prevention of anxiety in children and adolescents in a school setting: The role of school-based practitioners. *National Association of Social Workers, Inc.* (CCC Code: 1532-8759/04).

U.S. Department of Health and Human Services (USDHHS) (2000). *Healthy People 2010* (conference edition) Washington, DC: US Government Printing Office.

U.S. Department of Health and Human Services (USDHHS). (2007). Administration on Children, Youth, and Families. (2005). *Child Maltreatment, 2003.* Washington, DC: U.S. Government Printing Office. Online summary: http://www.acf.hhs.gov/programs/cb/publications/

U.S. Department of Health and Human Services, Centers for Disease Control and Prevention, 2008. Retrieved from http://www.cdc.gov/ (Accessed June 12, 2008).

Van Horn, P., & Lieberman, A. (2006). Using play in child-parent psychotherapy to treat trauma. In J.L. Luby (Ed.), *Handbook of preschool mental health: Development, disorders, and treatment* (pp. 372–387). New York: Guilford Press.

Vieth, V.I., Bottoms, B.L., & Perona, A.R. (2006). *Ending child abuse: new effort in prevention, investigation, and training.* Binghamton, NY: The Haworth Maltreatment & Trauma Press.

Wakschlag, L., & Danis, B. (2004). Assessment of disruptive behavior in young children: a clinical-developmental framework. In R. DelCarmen-Wiggins & A.S. Carter (Eds.), *Handbook of infant, toddler, and preschool mental health assessment* (pp. 421–440). New York: Oxford University Press.

Wattendorf, D.J., & Muenke, M. (2005). Diagnosis and management of fragile X syndrome. *American Family Physician, 72*(1), 111–113.

Webster-Stratton, C., Reid, M.J., & Hammond, M. (2004). Treating children with early-onset conduct problems: Intervention outcomes for parent, child, and teacher training. [References]. *Journal of Clinical Child and Adolescent Psychology, 33*(1), 105–124.

Wiseman, N.D. (2006). *Could it be autism? A parent's guide to the first signs and next steps.* New York: Broadway Books.

Yeargin-Allsopp, M., Rice, C., Karapurkar, T., Doernberg, N., Boyle, C., & Murphy, C. (2003). Prevalence of Autism in a US Metropolitan Area. *Journal of the American Medical Association,, 289,* 49–55.

Zero to Three. (2005a). Research diagnostic criteria – preschool age. (RDC-PA). Document retrieved from Tulane Institute of Infant and Early Childhood Mental Health, http://www.infantinstitute.com/RDC-PA.htm

Zero to Three (2005b). Diagnostic classification of mental health and developmental disorders of infancy and early childhood, Revised (DC:0-3R), Washington, DC: Zero to Three: National Center for Infants, Toddlers, and Families.

CONCEPT MAP

Developmental Psychopathology

Factors affecting

- Vulnerability
- Resilience
  - Intergenerational transmission
- Culture/race/ethnicity
- Health care disparities
  - mistrust/fear/discrimination

Caring for the Child with a Psychosocial or Cognitive Condition

Barriers

- Stigma of mental illness
- Beliefs about childhood
- Dismissal/minimizing parental concerns
- Lack of resources

Miscellaneous Disorders

- Tic disorders
  - Tourette's syndrome
- Maltreatment of children
  - Child abuse: physical/emotional
  - Child neglect
  - Shaken baby syndrome
- Substance use/abuse
- Eating disorders
  - anorexia; bulimia; obesity
- Sleep disorder
- Elimination disorders
  - enuresis; encopresis

Developmental Conditions

- Developmental disabilities
  - Mild; severe; profound
- Fragile X syndrome
- Down syndrome
- Fetal alcohol spectrum disorder
- Learning disorders and cognitive impairment, e.g., dyslexia; dyscalculia

Psychosocial/Cognitive

- Reactive attachment disorder
- Failure to thrive
  - organic/nonorganic
- ADHD
- ODD/conduct disorder

Psychopathology

- Anxiety → e.g., SAD, GAD, phobias, OCD, PTSD
- Mood disorders → e.g., depression, bipolar disorder
- Suicide
- Schizophrenia
- Autism spectrum disorders → autistic disorder; Asperger's; Rett's; childhood disintegrative disorder

General Potential Nursing Care

Assess: Observe for behavioral abnormalities; use active listening; develop trust; be aware of/manage personal feelings

Implement: ID positive characteristics; encourage coping behaviors; use age specific therapies → e.g., "FRIENDS"; cognitive behavioral therapy; behavior modification; pharmacotherapy; refer to mental health care providers; report neglect/abuse

Teach Parents/Child: Prevention e.g., normal stages of growth and development; therapeutic parenting; support organizations/community resources; disease versus "bad" child; medication compliance/side effects; how to provide a secure base

Optimizing Outcomes:

- Understand resilience in the face of vulnerability

Across Care Settings:

- Obesity prevention can be promoted in schools

Where Research And Practice Meet:

- Encopresis is six times more prominent in boys than girls
- Is mental illness passed along to children?
- Research can help nurses understand violent behaviors in youth
- Researchers are able to assess children's patterns of attachment
- "Family Check-Up" – Strategy to promote autonomy in ODD/CD
- Proactive parenting and use of verbal cues can distract children from misbehavior

Ethnocultural Considerations:

- Understand cultural diversity r/t treatment
- Disparity in treating obesity

Clinical Alert:

- Suicide may occur in children on SSRIs
- Avoid dangerous attachment therapies
- Anorexia can be fatal

Collaboration In Caring:

- Raising awareness/acceptance of Down Syndrome

Critical Nursing Action:

- "A.L.A.R.M." as Guideline for ASD

What To Say:

- Bathing at bedtime not recommended
- Toilet train when ready

Nursing Insight:

- Understanding mental health disparities
- Posttraumatic disorder in adolescents
- Bipolar disorder
- Assessing suicide risk
- Autism spectrum disorders
- Reactive attachment disorder
- Failure to thrive
- Family-based prevention/intervention in ODD/CD
- Youth violence: fact sheet
- Incidence of maltreatment
- Fragile X most common cause of inherited MR

Complementary Care:

- Mindful breathing for Anxiety

Be Sure To:

- Report cases of child abuse

Now Can You:

- Discuss nursing care of the child with depression
- Assess a child with a sleeping disorder
- Plan care for a child with a mental health disorder

chapter
24

Caring for the Child with a Respiratory Condition

 When the breath wanders the mind also is unsteady. But when the breath is calmed the mind too will be still…

— Svatmarama

LEARNING TARGETS *At the completion of this chapter, the student will be able to:*

◆ Describe the anatomy and physiology of the respiratory system.

◆ Identify congenital respiratory conditions and structural anomalies in children that affect respiratory function.

◆ Explore upper and lower airway disorders in children.

◆ Examine infectious and noninfectious agents and allergens that affect children's respiratory health.

◆ Plan nursing care for children with respiratory conditions across care settings.

---

 moving toward evidence-based practice Use of Antibiotics for Acute Otitis Media

Rovers, M. Glasziou, P., Appelman, C., Burke, P., McCormick, D., Damoiseaux, R., et al. (2006). Antibiotics for acute otitis media: A meta-analysis with individual patient data. *The Lancet.* 368 (9545), 1429–1435.

The study examined data from six randomized controlled trials that compared antibiotics with placebo or no treatment in 1643 children ages 0–12 years (mean age 3.4 years) with acute otitis media. All participants were assessed for pain and fever control. Forty-two percent had evidence of bulging tympanic membranes. Two of the trials used a low dose of antibiotics for the treatment regimen; one trial excluded children younger than 2 years of age, one trial included only nonsevere cases, and two trials excluded children determined to need immediate antibiotics.

Among children younger than 2 years of age diagnosed with bilateral, acute otitis media, 55% of the control group and 30% of the group taking antibiotics continued to have pain,

fever, or both at 3–7 days. The researchers concluded that treatment with antibiotics reduced both pain and fever at 3–7 days and is most beneficial in children younger than 2 years of age diagnosed with bilateral acute otitis media and otorrhea. Observation was recommended for older children with mild disease.

1. Based on the above synopsis do you believe it is justified to use observation with children younger than 2 years old who do not present with bilateral otitis media or otorrhea?
2. How is this information useful to clinical nursing practice?

See Suggested Responses for Moving Toward Evidence-Based Practice on the Electronic Study Guide or DavisPlus.

Introduction

Pediatric respiratory conditions can be very frightening for children and parents. Nurses equipped with the necessary knowledge and skills can be instrumental in providing the competent care needed for these conditions. Nurses are in a position to comfort a frightened child, reassure parental anxieties, and ensure timely nursing interventions.

Gas exchange is the main function of the respiratory system. Body cells need to consume oxygen and discharge carbon dioxide. Respiration is needed both internally at the cellular level and externally through breathing. To accomplish this, the respiratory system undergoes periods of development from the newborn period through late childhood. Major changes in the respiratory system occur immediately after birth and within the first 4 weeks of life. Other changes occur over the course of 12 years of life resulting in lengthening of the airways and expansion of the alveoli. This chapter describes the important differences in the anatomy and physiology of the respiratory system between the adult and the child, provides respiratory assessment in formation, discusses treatments and procedures, and explains a variety of respiratory conditions experienced in childhood.

A & P review The Respiratory System

The anatomy and physiology of the respiratory system in children differs from that of the adults in many ways. There are anatomical and physiological differences; the most obvious difference is size. Anatomically, the respiratory system consists of the upper respiratory tract, which comprises the nose, nasal cavity, sinuses, pharynx, larynx, and trachea, and the lower respiratory tract, which includes the lungs, bronchi, bronchioles, and alveoli.

Ventilation (breathing) involves taking in oxygen through the nose and mouth and then delivering it to the lungs. The nose has cilia (small hair-like projections) and mucus-producing cells that line the nostrils to prevent small particles from entering the nasal cavity. Foreign matter entering the nasopharyngeal cavities are trapped in the mucus.

The oxygen passes from the pharynx to the larynx. To prevent any food or liquid from entering the larynx, the epiglottis closes over the opening of the larynx during swallowing. A cough reflex expels foreign bodies. From the larynx, air passes through the trachea which branches into the left and right bronchi. The bronchi divide into smaller branches called bronchioles. The bronchioles end in a cluster of air sacs called the acinus.

Individual air sacs called alveoli exchange oxygen and carbon dioxide. Oxygen exchange with the bloodstream occurs in the capillaries. Oxygen attaches to the red blood cells and is transported to the rest of the body. Carbon dioxide diffuses from the bloodstream into the alveolus where it is transported out of the body during exhalation. ◆

The Child's Respiratory System

The differences between adult and children's respiratory systems affect function and subsequent respiratory conditions. In infants, the nares are much smaller and more easily occluded than in adults. Until about 4 weeks of age, infants are obligate nose breathers and do not open their mouths to breathe. Nasal patency is essential for inhalation and exhalation to occur in the infant.

The epiglottis in a younger (usually age 8 and under) child is longer and flaccid (floppy), making it more susceptible to swelling which may lead to airway occlusion. The epiglottis is small and does not close properly, and the larynx and the glottis are higher in the younger child's neck, which makes the child more prone to aspiration. The thyroid, cricoid, and tracheal cartilages are immature and are easily collapsible with flexion of the neck. There are fewer functional muscles in the neck and the increased amount of soft tissue makes the younger child more susceptible to infection and edema.

The trachea in children is much shorter and narrower in diameter than in adults. To compare, the child's trachea is about 4 mm in diameter, about the diameter of a drinking straw (or as a general rule, the size of the infant's or child's little finger) while the adult's trachea is about 20 mm in diameter. The child's trachea bifurcates (separates into two branches) at the third thoracic vertebra, while the adult's trachea bifurcates at the sixth thoracic vertebra. In addition to the higher level of bifurcation, the angle of the right bronchus (one of the two large branches of the trachea) is much sharper.

Because of the differences in the child's airway, the force needed for ventilation is greater. There is increased friction and resistance, making it more difficult to generate ventilation in the presence of airway edema that may result from hypersensitivity reactions or infectious process.

Lung tissue is also immature at birth and continues to grow and develop until about the age of 12. The alveoli also increase in number from 25 to 300 million during this time, along with increasing size and functionality. The maturity of the alveoli enhances ventilation and respiration, thereby promoting more effective gas exchange.

Children younger than the age of 6 are abdominal breathers instead of thoracic breathers. The intercostal muscles are too weak to facilitate respiration, causing the child to rely on the use of the diaphragm for inspiration. As the diaphragm moves downward, negative pressure is created, expanding the alveoli and filling the lungs with air. The downward movement of the diaphragm places pressure on the abdominal contents. With increased airway resistance, the weak musculature of the thorax is pulled inward, causing retractions, as if sucking on a collapsed straw.

 clinical alert

Retractions

Retractions are a drawing back of the chest wall with inspiration and occur when the accessory muscles are used for breathing. In the chest, common sites for retractions include suprasternal, supraclavicular, intercostal, subcostal, and substernal.

Since the system is undergoing a process of development during childhood, the child is more prone to develop respiratory problems. In addition, the child does not have the immunity that adults have to many infectious agents. Respiratory infections are especially frequent during the years of growth. Because children are prone to respiratory illness, it is important for the nurse to know the normal

Table 24-1	Normal Values for Arterial Blood Gases		
Component	**Definition**	**Normal Values**	**Interpretation**
pH	Acid–base status of the body	Preterm: 7.3–7.4	Acidosis <7.35
		Full term: 7.3–7.4	Alkalosis >7.45
		Children: 7.35–7.45	
Paco$_2$	Pressure exerted by CO$_2$ in blood	Newborn: 30–40 mm Hg	Acidosis >45 mm Hg
		Infant: 30–41 mm Hg	Alkalosis <35 mm Hg
		Children: 35–45 mm Hg	
HCO$_3^-$	Buffers effect of acid in blood	Children >7 yr	Acidosis: 22 mEq/L
		20-22 mEq/L	Alkalosis: 26 mEq/L
Base excess	Status of bases in blood	Newborn: (−10) (−2) mEq/L	Acidosis more +
		Infant: (−7) (−1) mEq/L	Alkalosis more −
		Children: (−4) (+2) mEq/L	
		Thereafter: (−3) (+3) mEq/L	
Pao$_2$	Pressure exerted by dissolved O$_2$ in blood	Newborn: 60–90 mm Hg	Acidosis: <80 mm Hg
		Infant: 80–100 mm Hg	
		Children: 80–100 mm Hg	Alkalosis: >100 mm Hg

values for arterial blood gases in order to deliver effective care (Table 24-1). Pediatric nurses must consider these factors when caring for pediatric patients.

Congenital Respiratory Conditions and Structural Anomalies

There are a variety of congenital respiratory conditions and structural anomalies in children. It is essential that the nurse have a good understanding of the diagnosed condition along with an understanding of signs and symptoms and prescribed care.

CHOANAL ATRESIA

Choanal atresia is a congenital malformation of the nose in which there is blockage of the posterior side of the nose. It often is associated with bony abnormalities and may affect one side or both sides of the nose. A child with bilateral choanal atresia usually displays respiratory problems during development. Choanal atresia occurs in approximately one in 7000 live births (Haddad, 2004).

Signs and Symptoms

After 4 weeks of age, neonates have the ability to breathe through their mouths so that symptoms may not be apparent at birth. In unilateral cases, the neonate may be asymptomatic until signs of respiratory infection, nasal discharge, or persistent nasal obstruction occur. Children with bilateral choanal atresia may have difficulty with nasal breathing and make vigorous attempts to inspire, suck with their lips, and develop cyanosis. A newborn who is pink in color when crying, yet turns bluish when quiet, should be suspected of having bilateral choanal atresia or another defect impeding the nasal airway.

The deformity of the nose may lead to involvement of other systems as the child grows, so the child may exhibit multiple problems. The child has a history of difficulty in breathing, and because of this may not eat properly. During feeding, the child may choke or regurgitate the formula or breast milk. The infant may have difficulty coordinating chewing, breathing and swallowing which may also cause regurgitation or aspiration. Weight gain may also be slow or poor. A child with this condition must be evaluated for cardiopulmonary and gastrointestinal involvement.

Diagnosis

Diagnosis of choanal atresia is established by the inability to pass a firm catheter through each nostril 3–4 cm into the nasopharynx. The diagnosis is confirmed by computerized tomography (CT) scan with intranasal contrast that shows narrowing of the posterior side of the nose.

Nursing Care

Immediate care of a child with choanal atresia includes inserting an oral airway and starting gavage feeding to prevent aspiration and malnutrition in later life. The child will have definitive repair which involves transnasal puncture and stenting, or through endoscopy, resection may be done. After any type of surgery, the child may have recurrent stenosis necessitating dilatation, reoperation, or both.

Nurses caring for children with choanal atresia need to teach the parents to keep the child's nostrils clean by gently cleansing the rim of the nostrils with a warm soft cloth. A clean nasal area prevents dry mucus from accumulating in the child's nostrils to facilitating breathing. Since the child may have difficulty with feeding, aspiration precautions must be observed. The baby is fed in a semi-upright position with periods of rest to facilitate breathing. The nurse also instructs the mother to protect the child against respiratory infection by using good hand washing and keeping the child warm and dry. The nurse must also communicate to parents to keep the child away from densely populated public places such as day cares, grocery stores, and malls. The nurse can encourage the parents to opt for early treatment, especially if the condition is bilateral.

ESOPHAGEAL ATRESIA AND TRACHEOESOPHAGEAL FISTULA

Esophageal atresia (EA) is failure of the esophagus to develop as a continuous passage, at times leading to a blind pouch. Tracheoesophageal fistula (TEF) is an abnormal communication between the trachea and the esophagus. This condition may lead to serious effects in ventilation. EA is the most frequent congenital anomaly of the esophagus, affecting about 1 in 4000 neonates. Of these, more than 90% have an associated tracheoesophageal fistula (Orenstein et al., 2004). In the neonate, EA is an emergency medical condition necessitating immediate action to protect the airway and respiratory system.

clinical alert

Checking the Mother's Obstetric History

When the nurse is caring for a newborn and observes the baby to be drooling excessively and/or having persistent choking spells and color change with feedings, it is important for the nurse to check the mother's obstetric history. If there is history of polyhydramnios, the nurse must report the observed symptoms to the baby's pediatrician at once. These symptoms are highly suspicious of esophageal atresia and tracheoesophageal fistula.

Nursing Insight— *Variations of esophageal atresia with or without tracheoesophageal fistula*

The nurse understands that there are different anatomical variations of EA with or without tracheoesophageal fistula:

- Esophageal atresia with distal tracheoesophageal fistula (87% of the cases)
- Isolated esophageal atresia
- Isolated tracheoesophageal fistula
- Esophageal atresia with proximal tracheoesophageal fistula
- Esophageal atresia with double tracheoesophageal fistula

This anomaly develops during fetal development when failure of separation takes place in the long tube in the neck when the tracheoesophageal groove fails to close. The esophagus and trachea are made up from the foregut in the 4- to 6-week-old embryo. The caudal part of the foregut forms a ventral diverticulum that develops into the trachea. The horizontal part of the trachea and esophagus fold then join together to form the septum that divides the foregut into ventral larynx and trachea. and dorsal part of the long tube called the esophagus. During this process of formation of the respiratory tract and passage for the food, the posterior deviation of the tracheoesophageal septum leads to failure of closure between the trachea and esophagus.

The exact cause of TEF is not known but approximately 17% to 70% children exhibit associated developmental anomalies, like chromosomal abnormalities, duodenal

atresia, and cardiovascular defects with TEFs (Sharma, 2006). The severity of the anomaly is analyzed on the basis of involvement of other organs. TEF can affect the trachea alone or it may affect the esophagus and other systems.

Signs and Symptoms

On assessment the nurse may observe frothing and bubbling at the mouth and nose, excessive drooling and salivation, episodes of coughing, cyanosis, and respiratory distress. With feeding, the symptoms may intensify and may lead to regurgitation, choking, and aspiration, so the infant should be NPO. In cases of isolated TEF, symptoms may occur later in life with the child having chronic respiratory problems and abdominal distension due to air building up in the stomach. Since EA and TEF have been associated with other congenital anomalies that occur in the musculoskeletal, gastrointestinal, cardiac, and genitourinary systems a thorough assessment by the nurse is necessary.

Diagnosis

If not diagnosed with prenatal sonogram, most neonates are diagnosed soon after birth or during infancy because TEF is life-threatening condition. A neonate is diagnosed on the basis of prenatal history of maternal polyhydramnios (excessive amniotic fluid). TEF may be confirmed by observing for an early onset of respiratory distress accompanied by signs and symptoms described earlier and possibly the inability to pass a nasogastric or orogastric tube. Confirmatory diagnosis is made through radiography. A radio-opaque dye is administered to assess the extent of the anomaly. Chest films are taken to determine the patency of the esophagus or the presence and level of the blind pouch.

nursing diagnoses Esophageal Atresia with or without Tracheoesophageal Fistula

- Ineffective Airway Clearance related to excessive secretions
- Altered Nutrition: Less than Body Requirement related to inadequate ingestion of nutrients
- High Risk for Infection related to accumulation of secretion in the lungs
- Altered Family Processes related to frequent hospitalization/prolonged sickness
- Impaired Family Social Interaction related to situational crisis
- High Risk of Aspiration related to excessive drooling and poor swallowing and inability to clear secretions

Nursing Care

Immediately after birth treatment is aimed at maintaining a patent airway and preventing aspiration of secretions. Although EA and TEF are surgical emergencies, discretion should be used about performing immediate surgical corrections. Highly compromised neonates such as those who are premature, those with concurrent congenital anomalies, and those who are in poor physical condition should not be operated on immediately. After life-sustaining measures are given, surgical corrections may come in stages that may be palliative in nature (i.e., gastrostomy and drainage of esophageal pouch). A child may be assisted with artificial ventilation in the beginning and could be weaned off the artificial ventilation as the condition improves. However, endotracheal intubation may be avoided because it may worsen abdominal distention due to the connection between the trachea and esophagus.

critical nursing action Nursing Assessment

The nurse must use a complete nursing assessment to assess the child's condition. A complete nursing assessment includes watching for subtle changes in the child's color, respiration, behavior, heart rate, and general health. The nurse understands that subtle changes can occur before technology is able to recognize the changes. The nurse also understands the importance of using innate instincts when caring for the child; if the nurse senses impending crisis it is important to pay attention to this instinct and act accordingly (getting emergency equipment ready). It is also important to remember that the child has an uncanny ability to compensate. When the child is no longer able to compensate the child "crashes" and then may then have a poor probability of recovery.

Before surgical correction, the nurse understands that the neonate is not given oral feedings but instead intravenous fluids are given. The nurse positions the neonate at a 30-degree elevation to protect the trachea from secretions and the head is turned to the side to prevent aspiration and drain secretions. Suctioning is done regularly and at frequent intervals. A nasogastric or orogastric tube with continuous suctioning is likely to be placed into the blind pouch, usually by the surgical team. Often antibiotic therapy is started because aspiration pneumonia is inevitable.

Immediately after the surgical correction, nurses must monitor vital signs at regular intervals. The site requiring correction is usually in the thoracic cavity, so the nurse should expect the baby to return with a chest tube, and possibly still be intubated with an ET tube. Infants with chest tubes are carefully handled to avoid dislodging of the tube. Suctioning of the oropharyngeal area is kept to a minimum to avoid disruption of the surgical repair.

Initially, nutrition is given parenterally. Oral feeding can be started when the child is both surgically and medically ready. It is also important to prevent infection; therefore vigilant nursing care should be observed at all times.

After corrective surgery, the majority of the infants lead normal lives. If complications do occur, they are challenging, especially during infancy. Prognosis depends on the presence or absence of other associated anomalies.

CONGENITAL DIAPHRAGMATIC HERNIA

Congenital diaphragmatic hernia (CDH) is a life-threatening congenital abnormality characterized by a variable degree of pulmonary hypoplasia associated with a decrease in cross-sectional area of the pulmonary vasculature and dysfunction of the surfactant system. In the United States, CDH occurs in 1 of every 2000 to 4000 live births and accounts for 8% of all major congenital anomalies (Hekmatnia, 2003). Population-based studies report survival rates ranging from 25% to 60%. Infants with multiple anomalies have much lower survival rates than those with isolated defects (Steinhorn, 2004).

While CDH is frequently found among newborns, the child may exhibit signs and symptoms after the newborn period or even during adulthood. Prognosis is better with late presentations, with low or no mortality.

Closure of the posterolateral pleuroperitoneal canals during the 8th week of gestation causes separation of the developing thoracic and abdominal cavities. The failure of these canals to close causes the classical posterolateral

Family Teaching Guidelines...
Esophageal Atresia with or without Tracheoesophageal Fistula

In many hospitals, the nurse takes responsibility in preparing parents for discharge and home management. There are several topics that the nurse must teach parents in order to care for the child who has a diagnosis of EA or TEF:

◆ In the case of tracheotomy, nurses must teach parents proper sterile technique of suctioning and how to handle the equipment appropriately.

◆ Ensure all emergency calling numbers are written down so emergency care could be provided in a serious situation.

◆ Ensure parents know how to identify respiratory distress.

◆ Ensure parents know feeding techniques for gastrostomy tube and how to handle tube plugging and dislodging.

◆ Instruct parents in performing CPR before the child goes home.

◆ Encourage parents to use different toys and games to promote stimulation during regular care (e.g., encourage mobilization or action play to help the child reach developmental milestones and divert the child's mind, which may help the child cope during the prolonged sickness). Mobilization can be as simple as holding or rocking while action play can be games, toy figures, or crafts.

◆ Involve other siblings in adapting the young child with EA or TEF. It is essential that the family help the child with EA or TEF learn socialization and interaction with others.

◆ Ensure the family knows how to operate equipment and knows proper maintenance of the equipment used at home.

diaphragmatic hernia where the herniation is through the foramen of Bochdalek. The effect on the diaphragm may be small, slit-like, or include the entire hemidiaphragm. Both lungs are small, with the lung on the side of the defect more severely affected. There is a decrease in the number of alveoli and bronchial generations. The pulmonary vasculature is abnormal, with a decrease in volume and a marked increase in muscular mass in the arterioles. The pulmonary abnormalities may be due to the compression of the intrathoracic abdominal viscera although this is not the primary cause. Because of lung hypoplasia, poor gas exchange, and surfactant dysfunction, the whole pulmonary function is disrupted.

The three basic types of CDH are the posterolateral Bochdalek hernia (left sided) which occurs in utero at approximately 6 weeks of gestation. Left-sided Bochdalek hernia occurs in approximately 90% of the cases. It affects both the small and the large bowel, causing herniation of these organs that extends into the thoracic cavity. The anterior Morgagni hernia occurs in the anterior midline through the sternocostal hiatus of the diaphragm, with 90% of cases occurring on the right side; and the hiatus hernia, a less common form in which the stomach hernia occurs through the esophageal hiatus.

Signs and Symptoms

Newborns with CDH usually have severe respiratory distress, typically developing within the first several minutes of life.

Diagnosis

The condition may be diagnosed during the prenatal period through ultrasonography. Features found in utero pointing to CDH include polyhydramnios, absent or intrathoracic stomach bubble, and mediastinal and cardiac shift away from the side of the herniation. It is suggested that parents whose baby has been diagnosed with CDH prenatally be counseled to deliver their infant at an institution able to appropriately care for the mother and newborn, and have a realistic understanding about the severity of this diagnosis. Postnatally, children suspected with CDH or those with symptoms of respiratory distress require a chest x-ray exam after emergency stabilization measures are taken.

Nursing Care

While CDH was once considered a surgical emergency, today, a delayed surgical approach enables preoperative stabilization and decreases morbidity and mortality. The presence of pulmonary hypoplasia, pulmonary hypertension, and surfactant deficiency has negative effects on the neonate if early surgery is performed, especially if the neonate is premature.

The ideal time to repair a CDH is unknown. Some authors suggest that repair 24 hours after stabilization is ideal, but delays of up to 7 to 10 days are often well tolerated. Many surgeons now prefer to operate on these neonates when echocardiographic evidence for normal pulmonary artery pressures is maintained for at least 24 to 48 hours (Steinhorn, 2004).

Immediate medical management is aimed at stabilizing the patient, optimizing oxygenation, and preventing further trauma. First, an endotracheal intubation rather than mask ventilation is inserted to optimize oxygenation (Fig. 24-1). The nurse sees to it that the endotracheal tube is patent.

Then an orogastric or nasogastric tube connected to a continuous suction is inserted to prevent bowel distention

Figure 24-1 Child with an endotracheal tube.

Figure 24-2 Continuous pulse oxymetry is an important nursing intervention.

and avoid further lung compression. The administration of exogenous surfactant a few hours after delivery alleviates the existing surfactant deficiency. The use of extracorporeal membrane oxygenation (ECMO) may be recommended for full-term infants if ventilator and medical therapy do not maintain acceptable oxygenation and ventilation.

Nursing care requires skillful and cautious monitoring of oxygenation, blood pressure, and perfusion while maintaining the principle of minimal handling. Patients with CDH require a specially trained group of medical and nursing personnel both before and after surgery.

Before surgery, the child is cared for in an intensive care unit with close monitoring of the pulmonary and cardiac functions. Continuous pulse oxymetry is essential (Fig. 24-2). The nurse must perform orogastric or nasogastric suctioning (to prevent abdominal distention) at regular intervals if the child is not already on continuous suction. As much as possible, the child is turned on the affected side so that the unaffected lung may expand to the fullest.

 clinical alert

Preoperative and postoperative suctioning

Preoperatively, any nasogastric or orogastric tube placement for suctioning must be done extremely carefully and gently, and progression stopped immediately if any resistance is met, as it is very easy to perforate the esophageal tissue of an infant with an anomaly.

Postoperative oral or nasal suctioning of the infant with EA, TEF, or CDH must also be done extremely carefully to avoid disruption of the repairs. Carefully measure the catheter and do not insert any further than the distance from the nares to the ear lobe.

Postoperatively, nursing care plays a vital role in the child's recovery. The nurse must perform vigilant assessments on all body systems to detect any complications or new problems. Because the child may have low blood counts and decrease in fluid volume the nurse must regulate plasma or blood transfusion and the intravenous infusions adequately. To maintain adequate nutrition, gavage feeding may be initiated by the second or third postoperative day. The nurse understands that gavage feedings must be administered slowly while watching the child closely for any untoward manifestations such as aspiration. The child requires prolonged hospitalization, so the family must be informed about the lengthy hospital stay and the myriad ongoing treatments. After the child has recovered, he may be discharged to the care of the parents. The nurse must emphasize to the family the need for frequent follow-up visits to ensure that no complications or problems are present.

RESPIRATORY DISTRESS SYNDROME

Respiratory distress syndrome (RDS) or hyaline membrane disease (HMD) are the terms used to refer to respiratory dysfunctions mostly among the preterm neonates related to the developmental delay in lung maturation. It occurs in 60% to 80% of infants less than 28 weeks of gestational age, in 15% to 30% of those between 32 and 36 weeks, in about 5% beyond 37 weeks, and rarely at term (Stoll & Kliegman, 2004). RDS is associated with infants of diabetic mothers, delivery before 37 weeks of gestation, deliveries by caesarean section, multifetal pregnancies, precipitous deliveries, asphyxia, cold stress, and a history of previously affected infants.

Decreased production and secretion of lung surfactant is the main cause of RDS. Surfactant is a surface-active phospholipid secreted by the alveolar epithelium. This substance reduces the surface tension of fluids that line the alveoli and respiratory passages, resulting in uniform expansion and maintenance of lung expansion at low intraalveolar pressure. Immature development of these functions produces consequences that seriously compromise respiratory efficiency. Adequate levels of surfactant are present after 35 weeks of gestation.

Deficiency in surfactant leads to unequal inflation of alveoli on inspiration and the collapse of the alveoli on end expiration. The neonate is unable to keep the lungs inflated and exerts extensive effort to re-expand the alveoli on each breath due to surfactant deficiency. This leads to atelectasis, increased pulmonary vascular resistance, hypoperfusion to the lung tissue, and consequently, hypoxemia and hypercapnia. These series of events cause hypoventilation with increased $PaCO_2$, decreased PaO_2, and decreased pH. The combination of hypercapnia, hypoxia, and acidosis produces pulmonary arterial vasoconstriction, resulting in further alveolar hypoperfusion, impaired cellular metabolism, and consequently diminished production of surfactant. This vicious cycle continues unless prompt treatment is initiated.

Signs and Symptoms

The symptoms are apparent within a few minutes after birth although in larger premature neonates, the onset of symptoms may occur several hours later. Rapid, shallow, respiration with a rate of 60 breaths/min or greater should alert the nurse. Tachypnea (80 to 120 breaths/min), audible grunting, intercostal and subcostal **retractions**, nasal flaring, and cyanosis are accompanying symptoms. As the condition worsens, flaccidity and apnea occur. Respiratory failure may occur with the rapid progression of the disease.

Diagnosis

Diagnosis of RDS is based on the signs and symptoms of this condition, x-ray exam of the chest, and blood gas and acid-base values. Radiographic findings include granular appearance of the lungs, bronchograms (dark streaks), and an air-filled esophagus. Laboratory findings are characterized by hypoxemia and variable metabolic acidosis.

Nursing Care

Most cases of RDS are self-limiting. Immediate establishment of oxygenation, ventilation, and supportive care are needed to prevent complications. Treatments of these neonates are best carried out in a specially staffed and equipped neonatal intensive care unit (NICU). Principles of supportive care in any preterm neonate should be adhered to, such as gentle handling and minimum disturbance, avoidance of hypothermia, and minimizing oxygen consumption. The nurse is advised to plan care appropriately so that these principles are followed.

The nurse understands that rescue therapy with surfactant is initiated as soon as possible in the first 24 hours of life. Administration of exogenous surfactant to neonates requiring 30% oxygen and mechanical ventilation dramatically improves survival and reduces the incidence of bronchopulmonary dysplasia. A physician who is qualified for neonatal resuscitation and respiratory management administers exogenous surfactant. The physician is supported by well-trained nurses and a respiratory therapist experienced in ventilatory management. Nursing responsibilities include assistance in the delivery of surfactant, collection and monitoring of arterial blood gases, conscientious monitoring of oxygenation with pulse oximetry, and reporting any adverse reactions to therapy.

Immediately after delivery, the neonate is placed in an incubator or a radiant warmer. The nurse ensures that the child's core body temperature is maintained at 97.9 to 98.6°F (36.6 to 37°C) through frequent monitoring. Nursing care also includes administering warm humidified oxygen at a concentration sufficient to keep arterial oxygen levels between 55 and 70 mm Hg (>90% saturation) to maintain normal tissue oxygenation while minimizing the risk of oxygen toxicity. Humidity of the air in the incubator is maintained at 30% to 60%.

When completing a respiratory assessment, if the child's PaO_2 cannot be maintained above 50 mm Hg at inspired oxygen concentration of 60% or greater, apply continuous positive airway pressure (CPAP) at a pressure of 6 to 10 cm H_2O via nasal prongs (Fig. 24-3). CPAP prevents collapse of surfactant-deficient alveoli and improves ventilation perfusion. Caring for children on CPAP requires advanced training and technical skills, so it is appropriate that nurses who are highly trained in neonatal intensive care handle children on CPAP.

Certain laboratory values such as oxygen and carbon dioxide tension and the ph of the arterial and capillary blood are monitored from time to time. Nurses must schedule laboratory testing at intervals that allow for maximum periods of rest for the child.

Nursing management for children with RDS also requires a vigilant nursing assessment and monitoring of vital signs. The nurse must accurately record and report significant changes in vital signs to the physician. Calories and fluids are provided intravenously; therefore, the nurse must monitor exact intake and output.

Figure 24-3 Child on continuous positive airway pressure.

clinical alert

Assisted mechanical ventilation

Neonates with severe RDS and those with complications require assisted mechanical ventilation.

case study Respiratory Distress Syndrome

Lara Smith, a 42-year-old primigravida with type 2 diabetes and in her 28th week of gestation, was admitted into the delivery room. She was complaining of lumbosacral pain 2 hours before admission. The labor and delivery nurse begins to monitor the progress of labor as well as provide emotional support since Lara appears to be quite anxious. The neonatal intensive care unit has been notified about a possible admission of a neonate at risk for respiratory distress syndrome.

critical thinking questions

1. What maternal conditions place the newborn at risk for respiratory distress syndrome?

2. What possible treatment can be given to Lara to prevent respiratory distress syndrome?

◆ See Suggested Answers to Case Studies in text on the Electronic Study Guide or DavisPlus.

BRONCHOPULMONARY DYSPLASIA

Bronchopulmonary dysplasia (BPD), also known as chronic lung disease (CLD), is a chronic obstructive disease of the lungs that occurs as a complication of prolonged oxygen therapy, especially in preterm infants who are on assisted ventilation. It was first described by Northway and associates in 1967 in a review of chest radiographs of preterm infants who were treated with positive pressure ventilation and oxygen for respiratory distress syndrome (Driscoll, 2003).

Immature lungs are one of the most important factors in the development of BPD; however, the mechanism by which this occurs is not yet completely understood. What is known about BPD is that its multiple factors are responsible. Available views on BPD suggest that it is a complex disorder resulting from more than solely lung injury related to oxygen toxicity and trauma from mechanical ventilation. Consistent pathological findings are decreased alveolarization, decreased septation, and minimal airway disease, all of which suggest arrest in lung development. Atelectasis, together with mechanical ventilation, induces increased lung volume and overdistention of the lungs, resulting in injury. The mechanically ventilated oxygen produces injury by producing free radicals that cannot be metabolized by the immature antioxidant system of the neonates. Several clinical factors, including immaturity, infection, symptomatic patent ductus arteriosus (PDA), and malnutrition, contribute to the development of BPD.

Signs and Symptoms

Signs and symptoms of BPD include tachypnea, wheezing, rales, retractions, and episodes of cyanosis. Respiratory rates are increased by as much as 20 to 30 breaths/min from the regular rates based on age. There is prolonged exhalation and increased use of abdominal and accessory muscles. Due to the increase in abdominal pressure from high airway resistance and use of accessory muscles, umbilical and inguinal hernia may occur. Feeding, handling, and activity intolerance make the infant prone to develop undernutrition leading to stunted growth and development.

Diagnosis

Neonates are diagnosed based on signs, symptoms, and radiographic findings. Radiographic examination shows thickened and fibrotic changes in the airways and alveoli.

Nursing Care

critical nursing action Assessing Respiratory Status

The nurse needs to assess the infant's respiratory status including increasing respiratory rate and decreasing oxygenation. The child who has a severe case of BPD may need recurrent hospitalization; therefore, the nurse must be able to provide emotional support to parents during these crucial moments.

The aim of management is to provide supportive care and minimize additional injury to the respiratory system by decreasing the workload of breathing and normalizing gas exchange, thus permitting improvements in growth and development. Infants with BPD who remain ventilator dependent for several weeks should be weaned gradually. An adjustment could be made to the small tidal volumes to prevent mechanical injury. In addition, a positive end-expiratory pressure (PEEP) of 6 to 7 cm H_2O may reduce the effects of atelectasis. A slightly prolonged inspiration duration of 0.5 to 0.6 seconds may improve lung function. Infants who can maintain their own breathing while weaning from the ventilator should be supplemented with oxygen therapy. Oxygen therapy should maintain arterial

PaO_2 above 50 to 55 mm Hg, since this level helps in adequate function of the tissues oxygenation and prevents pulmonary vascular resistance related to hypoxemia.

The nurse understands that wheezing is managed with bronchodilators. If the child responds to bronchodilators, the medication should be continued. Inhaled, Albuterol (Ventolin) increases air movement and improves the comfort of breathing. Corticosteroids may be administered to reduce inflammation and improve lung function. Different routes of medication administration such as intravenous or inhalation therapy are used according to the severity of the disease.

When caring for a child with BPD, the nurse uses pulse oximetry to monitor fluctuation in oxygen saturation. In addition, an arterial blood sample can be drawn to monitor hypoxemia in the tissue. As changes in the neonate's condition occur, the nurse anticipates that x-ray studies will help determine the respiratory status of the infant.

If an infant is placed on diuretics, careful replacement of calcium, chloride, and potassium must be ensured through regular electrolyte tests. Essential nursing care includes monitoring and maintaining fluid intake because infants with BPD are at high risk for developing pulmonary edema.

The nurse can ensure a proper nutritional plan to promote recovery, growth, and development. Caloric requirements increase to 150 kcal/kg per day in infants with BPD. If the infant can tolerate sucking, breast feeding is encouraged. If formula feeding is used, supplemental fortified formula should be given via nasogastric, orogastric, or gastrostomy tubes. The nurse can also observe the mother or both parents during feeding time to promote support and increase the mother's confidence in caring for the child.

critical nursing action Prevention of Respiratory Illnesses in Patients with BPD

The nurse should instruct all visitors to wash their hands before touching the neonate. The nurse should politely ask visitors with current respiratory infections to leave the room, explaining that the infant is at an increased risk for infection.

nursing diagnoses Bronchopulmonary Dysplasia

- Impaired Gas Exchange related to alveolar damage
- Ineffective Airway Clearance related to fatigue associated with poor oxygen to the tissues
- High Risk for Infection related to deformity in the lungs
- Altered Nutrition: Less than Body Requirements related to feeding difficulties and fatigue
- Fluid Volume Excess related to intestinal fluid edema
- Ineffective Family Coping related to chronic disease

CYSTIC FIBROSIS

Cystic fibrosis (CF) is an inherited autosomal-recessive disorder that causes the production of thick mucus that blocks exocrine glands and affects several body systems, including respiratory, gastrointestinal, and reproductive. CF is the most common cause of chronic respiratory disease in children, and is accompanied by multiple, severe respiratory infections. The increased mucus production in the airways causes obstruction and stasis of fluid, providing a rich habitat for bacterial growth. In addition, the pancreatic ducts are often blocked by mucus, prohibiting the secretions of pancreatic enzymes necessary for the metabolism of food nutrients. In later childhood, the reproductive system is affected, as ovarian ducts and the vas deferens may be occluded, leading to infertility. There is also an increased loss of sodium, causing salt depletion in children with CF.

CF is most common in Caucasian individuals with fair skin, affecting approximately 30,000 children and adults in the United States. More than 10 million persons are carriers of the defective gene (Porth, 2005).

CF is transmitted as an autosomal-recessive trait, which means that the child can receive a defective gene from either parent. When both parents carry the defective gene, there is a 25% chance that the child will inherit one CF gene from each parent and manifest the disease. There is a 50% chance that the child will inherit one defective gene from each parent and just be a carrier of the disease. There is a 25% chance that the child will inherit only normal genes and be completely free of CF.

The CF genes have been found on chromosome 7, which encodes cystic fibrosis transmembrane conductor regulator (CFTR) protein. CFTR normally regulates the chloride channel and facilitates the activity of other chloride and sodium channels at the cell surface. Abnormal functions of CFTR cause a disruption of sodium ion transport across the exocrine and epithelial gland cells and make the cell walls impermeable to chloride ions (Porth, 2005). This causes an excess of sodium and chloride found in the sweat of children affected by CF. In addition, the loss of sodium and water from the airways increases the viscosity of the mucus and disrupts the ciliary mechanism (hair-like process) that is intended to clear the airways, predisposing the child to recurrent respiratory infections.

A similar transport defect occurs in the pancreatic and bile ducts. With inadequate excretion of pancreatic enzymes for food breakdown, children experience varying levels of protein and fat absorption. With reduced protein and fat absorption, there is weight loss and failure to thrive, requiring children's diets to be high in protein and calories. Fat is excreted in the stool, resulting in abnormal bowel patterns, including steatorrhea, diarrhea, and abdominal pain.

The mucus gland produces thin, free-flowing secretions, but in CF it produces thick mucus that accumulates and obstructs the different organs. In newborns, thick secretions may plug the small intestine and lead to failure in passing meconium (the first feces of a newborn infant, which is greenish black, odorless, and tarry) (Venes, 2009). In the gastrointestinal system thick secretions impair the digestive system and lead to malnutrition in childhood.

Signs and Symptoms

CF affects the different vital organs of the body, and children with the condition show a wide range of signs and symptoms. The severity of the symptoms varies from child to child. Since CF is a multisystem disease (failure of two or more organ systems), the symptoms are presented according to the body system affected.

The initial presentation of CF in the neonate appears in the gastrointestinal system. The newborn may have a meconium ileus, with meconium so thick that it causes obstruction and requires surgical removal. The infant may initially have bulky stools that are frothy and foul smelling. Prolapse of the rectum may also occur in infancy and childhood. Malnutrition, anemia, and growth failure persists despite normal caloric intake. Children with CF are usually thin and underweight. Of children diagnosed as having CF, 50% are classified in the less than the 10th percentile for height and weight. Protuberant abdomen, barrel chest, wasted buttocks, and thin extremities are common features in children with CF.

In the respiratory system, the child exhibits crackles, wheezes, and diminished breath sounds with a dry, nonproductive cough. There may be repeated bouts of pneumonia and bronchitis because thick secretions provide favorable flora for the bacteria to grow. In addition, the child has a history or recurrent attacks of infection and persistent cough. With increasing severity, difficulty in breathing, tachypnea, hypoxia, and cyanosis may occur. In advanced cases, the child may show emphysema and atelectasis as the airways become increasingly obstructed with secretions. Prolonged hypoxia in the child may lead to digital clubbing.

In the integumentary system, there is a persistent high concentration of sodium and chloride in sweat. The mother may report that the skin of her baby is always wet or salty when kissed. The child may show wrinkled skin because of dehydration or dry skin. Prolonged or untreated electrolyte imbalance may lead to a listless or inactive child. Mothers may report long sleep and nap times. The nurse may assess dehydration by looking at the mouth of a child (dry mouth, ulceration, or rash in the mouth).

Later, children with CF are potentially at greater risk of delayed development of secondary sex characteristics. The male's vas deferens may be occluded and the female's ovarian ducts may also be occluded, leading to infertility. In addition, due to pancreatic damage, there is also an increased risk of diabetes.

Diagnosis

The diagnosis of CF is based on the child's signs and symptoms, including a positive history of the disease in the family, absence of pancreatic enzymes, increase in the electrolyte concentration of sweat, and chronic pulmonary involvement. Chest x-ray films show patchy atelectasis and obstructive emphysema. A quantitative sweat chloride test is performed on sweat obtained by iontophoresis of pilocarpine. A chloride concentration of greater than 60 mEq/L is diagnostic of CF. The normal values of sweat chloride test are usually less than 40 mEq/L. In infants, a value greater than 40 mEq/L is highly suggestive of CF (Winkelstein, 2005). Pancreatic dysfunction is also clinically apparent. Tests for direct documentation of enzyme secretion are invasive and are not routinely done for children. Pulmonary function tests are done in older children. These tests help to evaluate the progression of the disorder and provide direction for suitable treatment.

Nursing Care

The goal of treatment is to ensure respiratory function, enhance nutrition, promote growth and development, and encourage independence in an individual child and family.

Across Care Settings: **Promoting respiratory function**

To ensure respiratory function, a multidisciplinary approach should be taken. A physician, nurse, respiratory therapist, social worker, dietitian, and psychologist are the important professionals in the management of a child with CF.

The nurse understands that ensuring respiratory function in children entails controlling infection and improving aeration. These care measures are achieved via medicated aerosol therapy, chest physiotherapy (percussion and postural drainage), and antibiotic therapy (Fig. 24-4). Some children with CF may have a central venous access device for frequent antibiotic administration.

Most children with CF have a complete loss of pancreatic function and inadequate digestion of fats and protein; therefore, an important aspect of management is to replace the pancreatic enzymes. The nurse should remember that enzyme replacement is administered with meals and snacks so the digestive enzymes are mixed with food in the duodenum. Enzyme replacement should not exceed 2500 lipase units/kg per meal. The nurse must explore the best way of administering oral capsules with the family and the child.

Optimizing Outcomes— Nutrition

The best outcome for a child with CF is a well-balanced, high-protein, high-caloric diet. Pancreatic insufficiency results in malabsorption of fat-soluble vitamins (vitamins A, D, E, K). Daily vitamin supplementation is recommended. The nurse can also work closely with family to prevent infection as well as optimize nutrition and growth of a child.

Figure 24-4 Chest physiotherapy is performed to loosen and remove lung secretions. Percussion and vibration are used over the affected areas of the lungs.

Nursing Care Plan The Child with Cystic Fibrosis

Nursing Diagnosis: Risk for infection related to impaired body defense system

Measurable Short-term Goal: The child will remain free from symptoms of infection during hospitalization.

Measurable Long-term Goal: The parents will implement measures to prevent infection.

NOC Outcomes:

Risk Control (1902) Personal actions to prevent, eliminate, or reduce modifiable health threats

Immune Status (0702) Natural and acquired appropriately targeted resistance to internal and external antigens

NIC Interventions:

Health Education (5510)

Infection Protection (6550)

Medication Management (2380)

Nursing Interventions:

1. Wash hands or use approved alcohol-based hand rubs, before and after providing care.

   RATIONALE: Appropriate hand hygiene helps prevent infection outbreaks, reduces transmission of antimicrobial resistant organisms and reduces overall infection rates.

2. Monitor temperature every 4 hours. Report a single temperature greater than 101.3°F (38.5°C) or three temperatures greater than 100°F (38°C) in 24 hours to the care provider.

   RATIONALE: Fever is often the first indication of infection.

3. Observe for and report additional signs of infection such as increased mucus production, persistent cough, tachypnea, difficulty breathing, or cyanosis.

   RATIONALE: Increased mucus production in the airways causes obstruction and stasis of fluid, providing a rich habitat for bacterial growth. Early detection of infection allows for prompt and appropriate intervention.

4. Monitor and report laboratory values as ordered, such as complete blood count (CBC) with differential, serum protein, serum albumin, and cultures.

   RATIONALE: Laboratory values are correlated with the child's history and physical examination to provide a global view of the patient's immune function and nutritional status.

5. Encourage fluid intake and a high-calorie balanced diet, emphasizing proteins, fatty acids, and vitamins.

   RATIONALE: Nutrients benefiting the immune system include essential amino acids, linoleic acid, vitamin A, folic acid, vitamin B_6, vitamin B_{12}, vitamin C, vitamin E, Zn, Cu, Fe, and Se. Efficient immune function may be affected by deficiencies in one or more of these nutrients.

6. Instruct the child and parents on principles of medication management: prophylactic antibiotics, medicated aerosol therapy, chest physiotherapy (CPT), and deep breathing and cardiovascular exercise.

   RATIONALE: Instruction empowers the child and family to manage care. Medicated aerosol therapy, CPT, and deep breathing exercises help reduce atelectasis and risk for infection and promote healing.

7. Encourage use of community resources such as the Cystic Fibrosis Foundation.

   RATIONALE: The use of community resources may help support the family to find ways to prevent infection and increase the possibility of a positive adjustment to the condition.

The nurse must help the parents understand that caring for a child with CF can be challenging. There are sufficient resources and help lines that can assist parents. The nurse should use these existing resources and facilities to provide adequate health education to parents and older children.

 nursing diagnoses Cystic Fibrosis

- Ineffective Airway Clearance related to thickened secretions.
- Ineffective Breathing Patterns related to tracheobronchial obstructions.
- Altered Nutrition: Less than Body Requirement related to inability to digest and/or loss of appetite.
- Altered Growth and Development related to inadequate thickening of nutrients.
- High Risk for Infection related to impaired body defense system.
- Altered Family Processes related to frequent hospitalization/prolonged sickness.

 Across Care Settings: **Caring for the child with cystic fibrosis at home**

It is essential that the nurse teach parents how to care for their child at home. After the diagnosed and acute phase of illness, the family is prepared for home management and assists in promoting child growth and development with limitations.

- Teach the family about the nature of disease and prepare them to manage day-to-day minor complaints.
- Assist the family in arranging for the portable suction machine and about the proper technique suctioning at home.
- Instruct the family to do the respiratory therapy before a meal because chest physiotherapy may induce vomiting "of the thick tenacious mucus."

- Teach the family different techniques used for chest physiotherapy and postural drainage and coughing exercises based on their child's age. The child needs to be suctioned followed by chest physiotherapy and inhalation to liquefy the thick secretions.
- Teach the family about preferred meal plans, high-caloric diet, and mixing pancreatic enzyme with meal.
- Instruct the family to monitor the child's weight to ensure proper growth patterns.
- Teach the family how to administer medications properly.
- Inform the family how to access community resources and how to contact their home health nurse.

 Be sure to— Use ethical considerations when conducting research involving children

In conditions such as CF, it is important for the pediatric nurse to conduct research for the advancement of knowledge. It is also important for the nurse to protect the children when doing research. Children are under the legal age limit and research requires the consent of the parent or legal guardian. Children are especially vulnerable due to their immaturity and inability to decide for themselves.

When conducting research in the pediatric setting, be sure to:

- Obtain written consent from the parents or legal guardians.
- Obtain written assent from mature children (generally age 12–13 and older).
- Use the ethical principles of beneficence, nonmalfeasance, autonomy, veracity, justice, fidelity, and professional integrity.
- Review the institutional protocols carefully, ensuring that the highest standards of research are addressed.
- Secure clearance from the Institutional Review Board at the institution

Be sure to design the research so that:

- Children's rights are respected.
- Children are protected from harm and discomfort.
- Children's parents or legal guardians are provided the information necessary for them to give their informed consent.
- Children's rights to anonymity and confidentiality are ensured.

(Code of Federal Regulations Subpart A Sec. 46.102 (2005). *Basic HHS Policy for Protection of Human Research Subjects.* Office of Human Subjects Research. National Institute of Health: Bethesda, MD).

Now Can You— Describe congenital respiratory conditions and structural anomalies?

1. Identify the symptoms of the various congenital respiratory conditions and structural anomalies.
2. Prepare home care and management plans for children with congenital respiratory conditions and structural anomalies.

Upper Airway Disorders

SINUSITIS

Sinuses are hollow air spaces in the human body. In relation to the respiratory system, each sinus cavity has an opening into the nose for free exchange of air and mucus and is joined with the nasal passages by a continuous mucous membrane lining. The maxillary (behind the cheek) and ethmoid (between the eyes) sinuses are small but present at birth. The child's sinus cavities are not fully developed until 20 years of age, which makes the child vulnerable to sinus infection. Sinusitis is an infection of the sinus cavities.

Anything that causes a swelling in the nose such as an infection or an allergic reaction can affect the sinus causing problems. Normally, mucus collects in the sinuses and drains into the nasal passages. When children have a cold or an allergy attack, the sinuses become inflamed and drainage is difficult. In addition, air is trapped within the already blocked sinus along with pus or other secretions. This inflammation and accumulation of secretions can lead to congestion and infection. There is usually accompanying facial pain, headache and fever. If sinusitis persists for more than 3 months is it called chronic sinusitis.

Signs and Symptoms

The nurse can observe the following signs and symptoms in a child that is indicative of sinusitis:

- A cold lasting more than 10 to 14 days, sometimes with low-grade fever
- Thick yellow-green nasal discharge
- Postnasal drip leading to sore throat, cough, bad breath, nausea, and vomiting
- Headaches (usually not before age 6)
- Irritability and fatigue
- Swelling around the eyes

Diagnosis

When the child comes to the health care facility, diagnosis of acute sinusitis is determined by a physical examination with emphasis on the above listed symptoms. Sinus aspirate culture is the only accurate method of diagnosis but is not practical for routine use.

 Nursing Insight— *Diagnosing sinusitis*

Sinusitis is difficult to diagnose in children because respiratory infections are more frequent during childhood.

Nursing Care

Medical management for bacterial sinusitis includes a prescription of antibiotics. An oral or nasal spray or drop decongestant also may be used to relieve congestion. The nurse can communicate to the parents that steam inhalation and use of saline nasal sprays can help relieve sinus discomfort. If the child shows symptoms of chronic sinusitis, the primary care provider initiates an intensive regimen of antibiotic therapy. Surgery is sometimes necessary to remove a physical obstruction. The nurse can teach the child and parents the importance of how to avoid sinusitis during a cold or allergy attack.

Complementary Care: *Chiropractic care and chronic sinusitis*

Complementary and alternative care has been increasingly used for children. A good knowledge and understanding of these approaches helps the pediatric nurse provide information about these therapies.

Chiropractors are one of the professional complementary care providers most often used for children. Chiropractors are licensed in all states and their professional fees are covered by third-party payers including Medicare and most leading insurance carriers. Chiropractors do not prescribe pharmaceuticals or perform surgery. Spinal manipulation is the principal therapeutic option. Spinal manipulation is a form of manual therapy that involves the movement of a joint beyond its usual end range of motion but not past its anatomic range of motion. Chiropractors engage in health promotion and treatments of pediatric conditions such as otitis media, asthma, allergic rhinitis, sinusitis, infantile colic, and enuresis. An initial visit to the chiropractic clinic lasts for about 45 minutes; follow-up visits are generally 15 to 20 minutes. Adverse effects from chiropractic adjustments are rare. Families who use this complementary therapy rarely abandon their mainstream pediatricians; as they are used as an adjunct therapy.

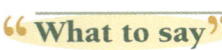 ## " What to say " — *How to talk to parents about chiropractic therapy*

Pediatric nurses are in a position to be asked by parents about chiropractic therapy. When asked, the nurse can provide parents with the basic knowledge in nontechnical terms. The nurse can speak in an open minded, nonjudgmental fashion, avoiding terms such as "unproven" or "unconventional." The nurse can also elicit values, beliefs, and influences that led the parents to opt for the complementary therapy. When possible, the nurse can support the parents' decisions and offer to obtain more information.

NASOPHARYNGITIS

Nasopharyngitis (the common cold) is a viral infection of the respiratory tract that involves the nose and throat. It occurs throughout the year but the highest incidence occurs during the early fall until the late spring and lasts for about 7 days. Young children have an average of six to seven colds per year but 10% to 15% of them have at least 12 infections per year. The incidence of illness decreases with age, with two to three illnesses per year by adulthood (Turner & Hayden, 2004).

Causative agents include rhinovirus in the early fall and late spring season, the respiratory syncytial virus (RSV) primarily in the winter and spring, and the parainfluenza virus in autumn. Adenovirus and coronavirus produce epidemics during the winter and spring. The common cold spreads easily from one person to another. Viruses causing the ailment are spread by small and large particle aerosols.

Signs and Symptoms

The common cold begins with dryness and stuffiness affecting the nasopharynx and is accompanied with increased

 ## Family Teaching Guidelines...
How to Avoid Sinusitis

HOW TO KEEP THE CHILD'S SINUSES CLEAR

- Use an oral decongestant or a nasal spray decongestant when initial signs and symptoms appear. Gently have the child blow the nose, blocking one nostril while blowing through the other one. It is also important to remember that a nasal spray decongestant can cause rebound swelling after 3 days of usage.

- Ensure that the child drinks plenty of fluids to keep nasal discharges thin.

- Apply heat via warm compresses or heating pad (on low heat) over the inflamed area.

- Use a cool mist humidifier in the same room or area occupied by the child.

ESSENTIAL INFORMATION

- Avoiding air travel during the symptomatic period is recommended. In the event that there is a need for the child to fly, a nasal spray decongestant may be used before airplane take-off to help prevent blockage of the sinuses and allowing mucus secretions to drain.

- Avoiding contact with known allergens is important.

- Using air conditioners to help ensure even room temperature is helpful.

- Using electrostatic filters attached to heating and air conditioning equipment to help remove allergens from the air is necessary.

(Academy of Otolaryngology, Head and Neck Surgery, 2008).

 ### medication: Erythromycin

Erythromycin (eh-rith-roe-**mye**-sin)

Indications:
IV, PO: Infections caused by susceptible organisms including upper and lower respiratory tract infections and otitis media

Action: Suppresses protein synthesis at the level of the 50S ribosome.

Therapeutic Effects: Bacteriostatic action against susceptible bacteria spectrum: streptococci, staphylococci, gram-positive bacilli

Pharmacokinetics:
ABSORPTION: Variable absorption from the duodenum after oral administration.

Contraindications and Precautions:
CONTRAINDICATED IN: Hypersensitivity

Adverse Reactions and Side Effects: Irritation

Route and Dosage:
CHILDREN PO: 30–50 mg/kg in divided doses q 6–8 hr.
NEONATES PO: 20–50 mg/kg per day divided q 6–12 hr.

Nursing Implications:
Inform parents of medication administration.
Prepare to administer around the clock.
Use calibrated measuring device for liquid preparations.
Do not crush or chew delayed-release capsules or tablets; swallow whole.

Data from Deglin, J.H., & Vallerand, A.H. (2009). *Davis's drug guide for nurses* (11th ed., pp. 498–501). Philadelphia: F.A. Davis.

clear and watery nasal secretions and lacrimation (discharge of tears). At times the pharynx and larynx are also affected, which brings on sore throat and hoarseness. The child complains of headache and general malaise.

Diagnosis

Diagnosis is based on the presenting symptoms. It is important to rule out other conditions that are possibly more harmful than the common cold. Routine laboratory examinations are not generally necessary in diagnosing a common cold. Pathogens associated with colds may be detected by culture, antigen detection, or serological methods. A specific etiological diagnosis is useful only when treatment with antiviral agents is being considered.

Nursing Care

The management of the common cold consists mainly of symptomatic treatment and good hand washing and cleaning of toys, tables, and other items used by the child to prevent the spread. Symptomatic treatment includes antipyretics and rest. Antihistamines help in drying up nasal secretions. They should be administered with caution as they dry up the bronchial secretions, which in turn may make the cough worse. Antihistamines can also cause dizziness and drowsiness. Decongestants are given to infants older than 6 months. They cause vasoconstriction and are usually given in the form of nasal drops. Antibiotics are not recommended for the dry hacking cough. Most cough mixtures contain alcohol so the medication needs to be administered with caution.

Nasopharyngitis causes discomfort especially for the infant. The nurse can elevate the head or crib, which helps with the child's drainage of secretions. Maintaining adequate fluid intake in the child is important because it prevents dehydration and keeps secretions thinned for easier expulsion. Fruit juices and gelatins may be offered to the child to increase their fluid intake. The nurse can communicate to the parents to avoid milk and milk products in excess, as this makes secretions thick and sticky. It may be helpful if nurses offer these fluids in tiny colorful cups or glasses with straw so they are more attractive for the child. The nurse can also stress the importance of rest. Children may be given play activities such as puzzle games, story books, crayons, and art materials to decrease boredom.

Because the hands are the primary vehicle for transmission of the cold virus the nurse should tell the family that hand washing must be strictly adhered to in order to prevent the spread of infection. The nurse must advise the parents that disposable wipes and tissue papers used for secretions should be disposed in sealed plastic bags.

The nurse, during health teachings, must reiterate the importance of good health as the major preventive measure for children not to catch cold. Prevention means that children are given adequate nutrition, rest, and sleep.

PHARYNGITIS

Pharyngitis is an inflammation of the pharynx that frequently results in sore throat. It occurs most commonly in winter and is spread by close contact. The incidence is high among children and declines in late adolescence and adulthood.

Pharyngitis can either be a short illness with no symptoms or could result is severe toxicity. In the case of the latter the causative agent is group A Beta-Hemolytic streptococci, which is also known as GABHS infection of the upper airway and may lead to acute rheumatic fever (ARF), scarlet fever, or acute glomerulonephritis (AGN). Colonization of the pharynx by GABHS may produce either asymptomatic or acute infection. The M protein is the major virulence factor of GABHS and facilitates resistance to phagocytosis by polymorphonuclear neutrophils. Type-specific immunity develops during infection and provides protective immunity to subsequent infection with that particular M serotype.

Signs and Symptoms

This illness in a child is abrupt and is accompanied by headache, fever, and abdominal pain. The tonsils and pharynx are inflamed, large, red, and often covered with yellow exudate (fluid released from the body). The anterior cervical lymph nodes are enlarged and tender and the child experiences pain on swallowing. Symptoms usually subside in 3 to 5 days unless superimposed by sinusitis, parapharyngeal, or peritonsillar abscess.

Diagnosis

Throat culture remains a good way to diagnose streptococcal pharyngitis (Fig. 24-5). A false-positive culture can occur if other organisms are misidentified as GABHS and children who are streptococcal carriers may have positive cultures. False-negative cultures are attributed to a variety of causes, including an inadequate throat swab specimen and a patient's covert use of antibiotics (Turner & Hayden, 2005). Diagnostic test kits with rapid identification of GABHS are available for use at the office or clinic settings. These rapid tests have high specificity. Therefore, a positive result generally does not need a throat culture confirmation. The throat culture does give information about susceptibility of the organism to specific antibiotics.

Nursing Care

Most untreated cases of streptococcal pharyngitis resolve in a few days. The objective of antibiotic therapy is to hasten clinical recovery and prevent acute rheumatic

Figure 24-5 Use a long, sterile cotton swab to swab a culture from the back of the child's throat.

fever. Antibiotics may be started immediately without culture. Oral penicillin is the prescribed treatment of choice. Oral penicillin is inexpensive and is given two or three times a day for 10 days. Oral amoxicillin (Amoxil) is suitable for children since it is available as chewy tablets. A once daily 750-mg dose of amoxicillin (Amoxil) given orally for 10 days is as effective as 250 mg of penicillin given three times per day for 10 days (Turner & Hayden, 2004). Oral erythromycin (Erythrocin) is indicated in children allergic to penicillin.

The nurse instructs parents about administering oral penicillin and analgesics as prescribed. Emphasize bedrest especially during the acute phase of the illness. A cold or warm compress to the neck is helpful to relieve pain. If the child is old enough, warm saline gargles are offered to the child to soothe the painful throat. Food and fluids are given as tolerated because swallowing is painful. Cool and bland liquids are less painful to swallow than hot and solid foods. The child should not be forced to eat if there is intense pain on swallowing. Rather, foods that are high in nutrients and energy can be offered when the child can tolerate eating. Hand washing by the caregivers, both nurses and parents, should be done to prevent the spread of the infection.

For children who are cared for at home, it is important that the nurse instruct the parents to give the full dose of the antibiotic prescribed even though the child shows signs of improvement. This is a very important aspect in the management of pharyngitis to prevent valvular damage of the heart.

TONSILLITIS

Tonsillitis is an inflammation of the tonsils, which are two masses of lymphoid tissue located within the pharynx. Tonsils protect the respiratory and alimentary tracts from infection by inducing secretory immunity and regulating the production of secretory immunoglobulin. Tonsils normally enlarge progressively between 2 and 10 years of age and reduce progressively during preadolescence, which makes the tonsils of children larger than those of adults. Nearly all children in the United States experience at least one episode of tonsillitis.

Viruses and group A Beta-Hemolytic *Streptococcus* are the most common cause of infection in tonsillitis. Children who have been treated continually with antibiotics can become immunocompromised.

Signs and Symptoms

There are several types of tonsillitis: acute, recurrent, chronic, and peritonsillar abscess. The signs and symptoms differentiate the types of tonsillitis. The presenting symptoms in acute tonsillitis are fever and chills, foul breath, dry throat, dysphagia (difficulty in swallowing), referred otalgia (pain in the ears), headache, malaise (fatigue), muscular pains, and enlarged cervical nodes. Airway obstruction due to swelling causes the patient to breathe through the mouth. Symptoms usually resolve in 3 to 4 days; however, some patients may remain symptomatic for up to 2 weeks, even during therapy. Recurrent tonsillitis presents with multiple episodes of the illness in a year. Patients with chronic tonsillitis frequently present with halitosis, chronic sore throats, foreign body sensation, or a history of expelling foul tasting and smelly cheesy lumps. Severe throat pain, fever, drooling

foul breath, difficulty opening the mouth, and changes in voice quality are the symptoms of peritonsillar abscess. The inflammatory process brought about by the infectious process within these areas interferes with breathing, swallowing, and may cause partial deafness.

Diagnosis

Diagnosis is based on the presenting symptoms and inspection of the throat.

Nursing Care

Two treatment modalities are used for the management of tonsillitis: medical management and tonsillectomy. Medical management consists of antibiotics, antipyretics, and analgesics. Penicillin, erythromycin (Erythrocin), and amoxicillin (Amoxil) are the commonly prescribed antibiotics. Cephalosporins or clindamycin (Cleocin) are more effective for patients with chronic conditions.

Tonsillectomy (surgical removal of the tonsils) is used for recurrent or chronic tonsillitis. There are no criteria for the number of infections before tonsillectomy is carried out (Wetmore, 2004). The American Academy of Otolaryngology and Head and Neck Surgery (2008) suggests the occurrence of three or more treated infections per year as sufficient to necessitate a surgical intervention. Surgery is performed 6 weeks after an acute infection has been resolved.

Nursing care after surgery involves provision of comfort and reducing activities that may bring on bleeding. Vaporizers keep the mucous membrane moist during periods of mouth breathing. Warm saline gargles, throat lozenges, and antipyretics are given. A soft or liquid diet is preferred.

After the surgery, children are kept on their side to facilitate drainage of secretions. Coughing, clearing the throat, and blowing the nose are to be avoided. Secretions and vomitus are checked for fresh blood. Since the throat is very sore after surgery, the nurse can apply ice packs and an ice collar to provide relief. Food and fluids are offered when the child is alert: cool water, crushed ice, and flavored ice-pops are the initial foods to be given. However, red or brown colored fluids should not be given to be able to distinguish fresh or old blood. As the child begins to tolerate food, gelatin, cooked fruit, sherbet, soup, and mashed potatoes are offered. Foods to avoid include milk, ice cream, and pudding as they coat the mouth and throat and cause the child to clear the throat, which may cause bleeding.

Family Teaching Guidelines...
Home Discharge Instructions Following a Tonsillectomy

The nurse can teach the parents to:

♦ Keep the child away from highly seasoned food and "sharp" foods (e.g., nacho chips) for a period of 2 weeks. The scab is most likely to be dislodged at 8–12 days.

♦ Have the child avoid gargling and vigorous tooth brushing.

♦ Instruct the child that he or she should not cough or clear the throat.

♦ Limit the child's activities that may result in bleeding.

CROUP OR LARYNGOTRACHEOBRONCHITIS

Croup is a generic term encompassing a heterogeneous group of illnesses affecting the larynx, trachea, and bronchi. Croup is described according to the main anatomical area affected. Epiglottitis, supraglottitis, laryngitis, laryngotracheobroncholitis and bacterial tracheitis encompass the croup syndrome.

Croup commonly affects children between 3 months and 5 years of age, most often at around 2 years of age. The incidence is higher in boys and it is most frequent during the winter months. The incidence of epiglottitis has dramatically decreased since the introduction of the Hib vaccine in the late 1980s.

where research and practice meet:
Nurse–Child–Parent Interaction

In the pediatric setting, the nurses' interactions and communications with both the child and the parents are important components of nursing outcomes. It has been observed that the nurse tends to communicate with parents rather than with the child. This leaves the child an inactive or passive participant in his or her own care. Positive interactions and communication with patients and families who are experiencing crisis during illness and hospitalization are essential for the nurses to provide the highest quality of care.

Shin and White-Traut (2005) conducted a study to evaluate patterns of nurse–child–parent interaction and identify the characteristics of nurse–child and nurse–parent interaction in an inpatient pediatric unit. Eight triads of nurses, patients, and their mothers were videotaped for 4 hours each day over a 2-day period for 3 months as they interacted with each other. Data gathered were coded and analyzed via the Bales Interaction Process Analysis. The average time per interaction was 2 to 24 minutes. Interaction episodes consisted of nursing activities such as rounds, patient monitoring, and patient care. Nurses initiated the majority of the interactions between patients and mothers. Both positive and negative behaviors were more frequent between nurses and children whereas neutral behaviors were more common between nurses and mothers. Children remained passive participants in the interaction. Interaction strategies are needed to help children to learn how they can actively interact with their nurses. These strategies may contribute to the children feeling more in control in these interactions and in their care.

Now Can You— Enhance communication?

1. What activities can the nurse perform to increase the child's communication and interaction with the nurses during illness and hospitalization?

2. How can the nurse enhance the children's feelings of control over their care?

Viral agents, particularly the parainfluenza viruses 1, 2, and 3, which account for 75% of the cases, are the most common cause of croup (Knutson & Aring, 2004). *Streptococcus pyogenes, S. pneumoniae,* and *Staphylococcus aureus* are the common causes of epiglottitis while *Haemophilus influenzae, Staphylococcus aureus,* and *Corynebacterium diphtheriae* are involved in bacterial tracheitis.

Signs and Symptoms

The symptoms of croup can be explained in terms of the anatomic structure of the children. The subglottic region of the larynx is held within the rigid ring of the cricoid cartilage. In children with croup, viral infections cause this area to become inflamed and edematous. This condition leads to obstruction because children have a narrow larynx such that a decrease in airway diameter causes a decrease in airflow, leading to the symptoms of croup.

Hoarseness, a resonant cough described as barking or brassy accompanied by varying degrees of respiratory distress resulting from swelling or obstruction in the region of the larynx and inspiratory stridor, are the major symptoms of croup. Most children have mild symptoms of an upper respiratory tract infection such as rhinorrhea, cough, and low-grade fever for 1 to 3 days before the symptoms of croup become evident.

Nursing Insight— Acute epiglottitis or supraglottitis; a medical emergency

Acute epiglottitis or supraglottitis is a sudden, potentially lethal condition characterized by high fever, sore throat, dyspnea, and rapidly progressing respiratory obstruction. The nurse understands acute epiglottitis is considered a serious obstructive inflammatory condition, which requires immediate attention as this condition is a medical emergency. A common scenario is that the child goes to bed asymptomatic and awakens with complaints of sore throat and pain on swelling accompanied by a febrile state. The child typically assumes the tripod position: leaning forward and sitting upright with chin thrust, mouth open while bracing on the arms, and tongue protruding with drooling of saliva. The child is irritable and restless with a thick and muffled voice and there is a froglike croaking sound on inspiration. Suprasternal and substernal retractions may be visible. The nurse notes that the child breathes slowly, the throat is red and inflamed, and there is a distinctive large, cherry red edematous epiglottis.

Laryngitis is more common in older children. Viruses are also the usual causative agents. The principal complaint is hoarseness, which may be associated with other upper respiratory symptoms including coryza, sore throat, and nasal congestion and generalized symptoms such as malaise, fever, headache, myalgia, and malaise.

Laryngotracheobronchitis (LTB) is a viral infection of the glottic and supraglottic regions. Some clinicians use the term laryngotracheitis for the most common and most typical form of croup and reserve the term laryngotracheobronchitis for the more severe form. LTB is preceded by an upper respiratory tract infection and is characterized by onset of low-grade fever, inspiratory stridor (a high-pitched, harsh sound), barking cough, and hoarseness.

Bacterial tracheitis is an infection of the lining of the trachea but does not involve the epiglottis. Like epiglottitis, it is capable of causing life-threatening airway obstruction severe enough to cause respiratory arrest. It is considered a bacterial complication of a viral disease. It begins with an upper respiratory tract infection with croupy cough, stridor unaffected by position, toxicity, and high fever. The child does not have the dysphagia associated with epiglottitis. A major symptom of bacterial tracheitis is the production of thick purulent tracheal secretions, which brings about respiratory difficulties.

Diagnosis

Diagnosis of the croup syndrome is based on the signs and symptoms along with the history. Owing to the severity of the respiratory distress, immediate treatment takes priority over testing.

Nursing Care

The most important goals in the treatment of children with croup is maintaining the airway and providing adequate respiratory exchange.

Commonly, mild cases of croup are treated with cool mist. A high-humidity cool air vaporizer may be used at home in the child's room. In the hospital setting, oxygen hoods for infants and oxygen tents for toddlers are used. Cool mist is thought to moisten airway secretions to facilitate clearance, soothe inflamed mucosa, and provide comfort and reassurance to the child thereby lessening anxiety. Nebulized racemic epinephrine (MicroNefrin or Vaponefrin) (0.25 to 0.75 mL in 3 mL of a normal saline solution) or l-epinephrine (5 mL of 1:1000 solution) are equally effective to cause mucosal vasoconstriction and consequently decrease subglottic edema, thus relieving the symptoms. This treatment is indicated for those with moderate to severe stridor at rest or when stridor does not respond to cool mist. The nurse must observe the child after nebulization to assess the airway and side effects of the delivered medication.

Corticosteroids are also given to children to decrease the edema in the laryngeal mucosa through their anti-inflammatory action. Intramuscular dexamethasone (Decadron) and nebulized budesonide (Pulmicort) are widely used.

Antibiotics are not used in the management of croup since it is primarily viral in nature. Symptoms which warrant hospitalization are: progressive stridor, severe stridor at rest, respiratory distress, hypoxia, cyanosis, and depressed mental status.

Epiglottitis and bacterial tracheitis are considered pediatric emergencies and may require artificial airways. **The nurse must never assess the child's throat with a tongue blade, unless a respiratory therapist or medical doctor is present, because of the possibility of laryngeal spasm and emergent need of artificial airway; emergent intubation and tracheostomy may be necessary.** Artificial airways usually improve the child's status. Antibiotic therapy is indicated for these two conditions. Combinations of ampicillin and sulbactam (Unasyn) are the drugs most often prescribed.

Monitoring the child's respiratory and cardiac system is a priority nursing care measure. Changes in condition are based on observations and assessment of the child's response to therapy, including careful observation of the child's response to his or her surroundings (changes in level of consciousness).

✿✿ nursing diagnoses Upper Respiratory Disorders

- Risk for Ineffective Airway clearance related to excessive secretions, inflammation or obstruction in the airway
- Risk for Ineffective Breathing Pattern related to tracheobronchial inflammation or obstruction
- Risk for Imbalanced Nutrition: Less than Body Requirements related to discomfort with swallowing
- Anxiety related to perceived threat of hospitalization, or to invasive procedures or changes in health status of the child
- Risk for Deficient Fluid Volume related to inadequate fluid intake or excessive losses through abdominal route
- Pain related to procedures or increased pressure in the middle ear (specific to otitis media)
- Disturbed Sensory Perception: Auditory related to inflammation and edema in the middle ear (specific to otitis media)
- Fatigue related to increased respiratory effort

OTITIS MEDIA/EXTERNA

External otitis, also known as otitis externa, is an inflammation, irritation, or inflammation of the outer ear and ear canal. Although it is popularly called swimmer's ear, it can occur in situations that do not involve swimming. It usually affects older children and teens whose ears are exposed to persistent excessive moisture. It occurs more often in warm climates and during summer.

External otitis is commonly caused by *Pseudomonas aeruginosa*. Fungal infections with *Candida* and *Aspergillus* may also be the causative agents. Excessive wetness as in swimming or bathing, dryness of the air canal, lack of cerumen, presence of other skin pathology, digital trauma, and a foreign body make the skin of the ear canal vulnerable to infection.

Signs and Symptoms

The main symptom is ear pain, which is often severe. It is accentuated when the pinna of the ear is pulled or pressed. There can be itching and drainage of yellow to yellow-green secretions. On inspection, there is erythema and edema of the ear canal. Cerumen (wax) may become whitish instead of its usual yellow color. Severe cases may lead to hearing loss.

Diagnosis

Examination of the ear and the occurrence of the presenting symptoms including a positive history confirm the diagnosis. On otoscopy (the use of the otoscope in examining the ear), the eardrum appears red or there may be difficulty in visualizing the eardrum.

Nursing Care

Antibiotic ear drops are prescribed for a course of 7 to 10 days. Corticosteroids are also effective in treating most forms of external otitis. If the ear canal is swollen, a cotton wick is inserted into the ear canal so that the ear drops travels into the end of the canal. Analgesics are given to relieve pain.

During the course of treatment, the nurse can advise the child avoid wetting the ears. During bathing, shower caps or ear plugs with petroleum jelly may be used.

 Nursing Insight— Preventing external otitis

Nurses can teach parents and older children ways to prevent infections. Children are advised to limit their stay in the water to less than an hour and ears should be completely dry before entering the water again. Shaking the head and judicious use of the corner of a towel can remove most excess water. The ear canal can also be dried with a small tuft of cotton. To keep the ear dry the parent can pull the auricle up and out to straighten the canal, then use a conventional hair dryer set on low or no heat held at a distance of 18 to 24 inches for 30 seconds, three times a day. Earplugs may be recommended by the physician. Children can also be advised to avoid swimming in dirty water and in public swimming pools that do not maintain good control of their chlorine and pH pool testing and treatment.

OTITIS MEDIA

Otitis media (OM) is basically an infection of the middle ear. It is one of the most prevalent conditions of early childhood. The incidence is highest among children between 6 months to 2 years. By 6 years of age, 75% of children have had one or more episodes of otitis media. In addition to the physical discomfort and economic costs related to otitis media, there is evidence that children with recurrent otitis media are at risk for both hearing loss and speech delay.

Otitis media presents in many forms: otitis media, acute otitis media (AOM), otitis media with effusion (OME), and chronic otitis media with effusion. Otitis media is an inflammation of the middle ear without reference to etiology or pathogenesis. Acute otitis media is inflammation of the middle ear space with the rapid onset of the signs and symptoms of acute infection such as fever and ear pain. Otitis media with effusion occurs when there is fluid in the middle ear space without symptoms of acute infection. Chronic otitis media with effusion is a persistent middle ear infection with discharge through a tympanic membrane perforation. An unresolved AOM that persists for more than 3 months leads to chronic otitis media.

The pathology of otitis media is better understood by reviewing the structure and functions of the Eustachian tube in children. The Eustachian tubes in children are shorter, wider, and more horizontal in infants than in adults. The Eustachian tube carries out three functions:

- Protection of the middle ear from nasopharyngeal secretions
- Drainage of secretions produced in the middle ear
- Ventilation of the middle ear to equalize air pressure within the middle ear with atmospheric pressure in the external ear canal and replenishment of oxygen that has been absorbed.

Because of this structure in children, drainage as a function is often impaired, which results in retention of secretions and air in the middle ear. The horizontal position also facilitates the movement of pathogens up the Eustachian tube from the pharynx into the middle ear.

Edema resulting from upper respiratory infection, allergic rhinitis, or hypertrophic adenoids interferes with the functions of the Eustachian tube.

Streptococcus pneumoniae, Haemophilus influenzae, and *Moraxella catarrhalis* are the three most common causes of infection in otitis media (Winklestein, 2005). Tobacco smoke as well as passive or second hand smoke aggravates the otitis media by impairing mucociliary function with subsequent congestion of soft nasopharyngeal tissues.

A direct link has been established between OM and infant feeding methods. Infants who have been breastfed have a lower incidence of OM than those who have been bottle fed. The number of episodes of OM decreases significantly with increased duration and exclusive breast feeding. Breast milk contains immunoglobulin A (IgA), which offers protection against allergies and viruses. Due to the position of the infant during breastfeeding there is less likelihood of reflux of milk in the ear, whereas during bottle feeding the chances of milk getting into the ear is increased.

The following factors lead to otitis media in children:

- The Eustachian tubes are short, wide, and straight and lie in a horizontal plane.
- The cartilage lining is undeveloped, making the tubes more distensible. The normally abundant pharyngeal lymphoid tissue readily obstructs the Eustachian tube openings in the nasopharynx.
- Immature humoral defense mechanisms increase the risk of infections.
- The lying down position of infants favors the pooling of fluid, such as formula, in the pharyngeal cavity.

Signs and Symptoms

The accumulation of fluids in the small space of the middle ear chamber results in pressure on surrounding structures, bringing about pain. Infants become irritable and express discomfort and pain by either holding and pulling on the affected ear or rolling their head from side to side. The child is febrile with a temperature as high as 104°F (40°C). Lymph gland enlargement may arise particularly in the post auricular and cervical lymph glands. Rhinorrhea, vomiting, and diarrhea may also be present. Loss of appetite is often present and chewing and sucking are known to aggravate the condition. In children with OME, exudate may accumulate and pressure increases, leading to tympanic membrane rupture. Often the child may not appear ill and only exhibits a feeling of fullness in the ear and a popping sensation during swallowing.

Diagnosis

Diagnosis is based on signs and symptoms as well as an otoscopic examination. An otoscopic examination reveals that in AOM the intact membrane appears bright red and bulging with no visible landmarks or light reflex. The usual landmarks of the bony prominences from the long and short processes of the malleus are obscured by the outwardly bulging membrane. In OME, otoscopic examination reveals a slightly injected, dull gray membrane, obscured landmarks, and a visible fluid level or meniscus behind the eardrum if air is present above the fluid.

Nursing Care

Antibiotics are used judiciously in the management of otitis because of the increasing resistance of the pathogens. Health education from the nurse is important if a decision is made to treat the condition with an antimicrobial agent. The full course of the antimicrobial therapy should be followed strictly. The nurse can tell the parents that if the child fails to respond to this initial antimicrobial management within 48 to 72 hours, another assessment must be done to confirm AOM and exclude other causes of illness or ineffective antibiotic response.

The American Academy of Pediatrics published guidelines in the management of AOM in 2004 recommending that pain should be treated with either acetaminophen (Children's Tylenol) or ibuprofen (Children's Advil). The cause of AOM has changed from primarily bacterial to primarily viral in recent years due to increasing administration of vaccines that decrease the incidence of bacterial infections, so withholding the use of antimicrobials is advised unless a bacterial cause is clearly evident. The nurse understands that the first line of drug choice is amoxicillin (Amoxil) given at 80 to 90 mg/kg per day.

Care may also include high doses of cefdinir (Omnicef) in combination with tympanocentesis (drainage of fluid from the middle ear by using a small-gauge needle to puncture the tympanic membrane) (Venes, 2009). The fluid is then cultured to determine the identity of any microbes that may be present. The use of complementary therapies is not recommended since there is insufficient evidence of its effectiveness. Finally, prevention through the reduction of risk factors is highly encouraged. To minimize the recurrence of otitis media, the nurse can teach parents to eliminate identified environmental allergens, feed infants in upright position, and encourage medical follow-up to check for complications such as chronic hearing loss.

 clinical alert

Rupture of the tympanic membrane

The rupture of the tympanic membrane brings immediate relief of pain, a gradual decrease in temperature, and the presence of a purulent discharge in the external auditory canal. Rupture of the tympanic membrane may lead to scarring and hearing loss.

Lower Airway Disorders

BRONCHITIS

Bronchitis is a nonspecific bronchial condition in which there is inflammation of the bronchial tubes. Tracheobronchitis is the term used when the trachea is prominently involved. Bronchitis may be acute or chronic. Acute bronchitis is commonly preceded by a viral upper respiratory tract infection and may last for 1 to 3 weeks. The incidence of acute bronchitis is highest during the winter months. Children are usually affected in their first 4 years of life. Chronic bronchitis lasts for months or years and is more common among adults, particularly smokers.

Viruses are usually the causative organism. The tracheobronchial epithelium is invaded by the infectious agent, and this leads to activation of inflammatory cells and release of cytokines, giving way to the occurrence of symptoms. If the tracheobronchial epithelium becomes significantly damaged or hypersensitized, then a protracted cough may last for 1 to 3 weeks.

Signs and Symptoms

Cough is the first prominent symptom for bronchitis, with rhinorrhea occurring 3 to 4 days later. The child also has a dry, hacking cough that is worse at night. In a few days, the cough becomes productive and purulent. This does not necessarily imply a bacterial infection but rather it indicates leukocyte migration.

Diagnosis

Based on the fact that a virus is usually the causative organism, bronchitis is diagnosed based on the child's symptoms. In children older than 6 years of age, *M. pneumoniae* can be a common cause and bronchitis can then be determined by the identification of this bacterium.

Nursing Care

Bronchitis requires symptomatic treatment, including antipyretics, analgesics, and humidity. Cough suppressants are administered with caution as they interfere with clearance of secretions. The condition is self limiting, and antibiotics, although frequently prescribed, do not hasten improvement in uncomplicated cases.

The nurse must remember that adequate oxygenation is a very important aspect of care in patients with bronchitis. To be able to provide oxygenation, the nurse must see to it that the airway is open and free of obstruction. The airway can be open by administering prescribed bronchodilators. The nurse can encourage the child to clear the airway from secretions by coughing. The nurse may also provide a cool-mist vaporizer by the bedside, especially at night, to help liquefy secretions, which can then be coughed out easily. The nurse understands that secretions must be disposed in sealed plastic bags. Parents should be told that the young child may swallow secretions instead of coughing them out, and may vomit these accumulated secretions during the night.

The nurse encourages the child to take in fluids such as clear liquids and fruit juices. The nurse recommends bedrest to the parents. Tell parents to avoid exposing the child to second-hand smoke and to provide a clean environment with adequate nutrition.

RESPIRATORY SYNCYTIAL VIRUS

Respiratory syncytial virus (RSV) is an acute viral infection involving the bronchioles and alveoli. The infection is common among children who are 2 years or younger. By the age of 2 years, nearly every child has been exposed to the virus (Polark, 2004). The ailment is seasonal, with peaks during winter and early spring. It spreads from hand to eye, nose, and mucous membranes.

RSV most often begins as an infection in the nasal epithelial cells. The RSV virus then replicates in the host cell. The peak period for RSV is December through March. The host cell is destroyed and virus particles are released to propagate the infection. The infection results in the destruction of the epithelial cells of the respiratory tract. Exposure to RSV triggers a humoral immune response.

Primary RSV infection results in only a weak antibody response with IgM, IgG, and IgA produced. This response is not enough to destroy the virus completely or to prevent upper respiratory tract replication of the virus. Consequently, an upper respiratory tract illness develops. High levels of neutralizing antibodies are required to prevent the progression of infection from the upper respiratory tract to lower respiratory tract (Polark, 2004).

Signs and Symptoms

As the virus replicates in the nasopharynx, symptoms such as mild cough, nasal congestion, clear rhinorrhea, and increase in the oral secretion (drooling) occur. Low-grade fever may also be present. The thick mucus, exudate, and mucosal edema obstruct the smaller airways (bronchioles). This obstruction leads to a reduction in expiration, air trapping, and hyperinflation of the alveoli. The obstruction interferes with the gas exchange, which may lead to hypoxemia (decreased oxygen) and hypercapnia (increased carbon dioxide in the blood), which in turn leads to respiratory acidosis. Often RSV is accompanied by otitis media and conjunctivitis. RSV can result in hospitalization with infected infants and children.

Diagnosis

Positive identification of RSV is accomplished by either of two methods: enzyme linked immunosorbent assay (ELISA) or rapid immunofluorescent antibody (IFA) from direct or aspiration of nasal secretions or nasopharyngeal washings. The nurse understands that chest x-ray films reveal hyper-aeration, hyperinflation, atelectasis, areas of collapse, and flattened diaphragm indicating air trapping.

Arterial blood gases (ABG) reveal decreased pH and a $PaCO_2$ greater than 45 mm Hg, indicating respiratory compromise and potential failure. Complete blood count shows increased WBC, which is indicative of infectious processes.

Nursing Care

The monoclonal antibody palivizumab (Synagis) has been shown to be effective in reducing the complications of RSV. Palivizumab (Synagis) is given intramuscularly to high-risk infants. The clinical goal is to return the child to a normal respiratory status. Medical therapy is aimed at relief of respiratory distress, improvement in oxygenation, and alleviation of airway obstruction.

Nurses must keep in mind that RSV is treated symptomatically with maintenance of hydration, oxygenation, and keeping the mucous membranes clear of mucus. Children may be managed at home. The nurse can tell the parents that hospitalization is recommended for children who have some other underlying illness or are in a debilitated state. In the hospital, nursing care includes mist therapy combined with oxygen administered by hood or tent in concentrations sufficient to alleviate dyspnea and hypoxia. The nurse administers intravenous fluids until the child shows signs of improvements.

Strict isolation is required for patients infected with RSV virus because it is easily spread from hand to eyes or nose and other mucous membrane. The nurse emphasizes hand washing and that contact precautions such as the use of gown, gloves, and masks are required (Fig. 24-6). Parents need to know that the first 24 to 72 hours is the critical time and in most cases there is complete recovery.

Figure 24-6 When a child has respiratory syncytial virus, contact precautions, such as the use of a gown, gloves, and masks, are required.

An antiviral agent such as RSV-IGIV or RespiGam has been used as a prophylactic to prevent RSV in high-risk children. This antiviral agent may be administered via endotracheal tube, hood, or tent. When an antiviral agent is administered, the nurse understands that crystallization of the medication can occur in the nares, endotracheal tube, or eyes. The nurse also understands that an antiviral agent can be teratogenic (an environmental agent capable of producing a birth defect) to the fetus of a pregnant woman.

 Nursing Insight— *Preventing RSV*

For preventive purposes, RSV immunoglobulin (RSV-IGIV), an intravenous preparation of immunoglobulin G that provides neutralizing antibodies against RSV, may be given as an intravenous infusion just before the start of the RSV season. It is a monthly injection given to infants at high risk of severe disease such as those born prematurely or those with chronic lung disease and those fitting the AAP criteria throughout the RSV season.

PNEUMONIA

Pneumonia is a lower respiratory tract infection of the pulmonary parenchyma. It is more common in infancy and early childhood. It may occur as a primary infection or secondary to another illness or infection. Pneumonias are classified as lobar, bronchopneumonia, and interstitial.

Lobar pneumonia involves lobes of the lungs. Bronchopneumonia begins with involvement of the terminal bronchioles that become clogged with mucopurulent exudate and forms consolidated patches in the lungs, while interstitial pneumonia is more or less confined to the alveolar walls.

Viral pneumonia, a more common form, involves RSV infection in infants and parainfluenza and adenoviruses in older children, whereas *Streptococcus pneumoniae* is the common pathogen causing bacterial pneumonia. The nurse must remember that a viral infection can have a secondary bacterial infection 6 to 8 days after initial onset due to viral insult of protective mechanisms.

Most often, pneumonia is a complication of a pre-existing infection or a condition produced when a patient's defense mechanisms have been weakened. Interference in normal clearing mechanisms from the nasopharynx, epiglottis, epithelial cells, and mucociliary flow by allergy, viral infections, or irritants may allow colonization and subsequent infection with the organisms causing pneumonia. This depresses the function of alveolar macrophages and neutrophils. Phagocytosis is impeded by respiratory secretions and alveolar exudates. In the tissues, the causative agent multiplies and is spread through the lymphatics, bloodstream, and sinuses. The severity is related to the virulence of the invading microorganism.

Signs and Symptoms

The symptoms of pneumonia are variable depending on the site affected; however, the general symptoms are high fever, cough, rapid respirations, chest pain, retractions, and nasal flaring and body malaise. Rhonchi or fine crackles are heard on auscultation.

Diagnosis

Clinical features and chest x-ray exams aid in the diagnosis of pneumonia. It is not always possible to identify the causative agents based on x-ray exams alone. Clinical history, the child's age, and laboratory examinations help in identifying the causative agent. Radiographic examination shows diffuse or patchy infiltration with peribronchial distribution.

 diagnostic tools Chest Radiograph

The nurse must recognize the importance of chest radiograph in the diagnosis of pneumonia. Opacities, seen as white areas on the x-ray plate, represent consolidation and are typical in cases of pneumonias.

Nursing Care

Most cases of pneumonia can be treated at home with rest and fluids and symptomatic management with analgesics and antipyretics. Antibiotics are given for bacterial pneumonia and not for viral pneumonia. If antibiotics are given, the drugs may range from amoxicillin (Amoxil) to the third-generation cephalosporins, depending on the severity of the condition.

Oxygen administration via nasal canula with cool mist, chest physiotherapy, and postural drainage are initiated for patients requiring hospitalization (Fig. 24-7). Bronchodilators also might be used. Treatment of a child with pneumonia is supportive depending on the severity of the symptoms.

Labs: Sputum Culture and Sensitivity

To be able to establish the causative organism and the appropriate antibiotic that works best, culture and sensitivity test of the sputum are performed. Coughed out sputum is difficult to obtain from children, especially those who are very young. A specimen may be obtained via a direct throat swab immediately after coughing. In some cases, a sterile catheter may be inserted directly into the trachea through the endotracheal tube or during direct laryngoscopy. During sleep, children usually swallow their sputum; therefore, an early morning fasting specimen obtained via gastric aspiration may also be obtained. The gastric content can be collected before breakfast by inserting the naso-oral tube into the stomach.

The nurse must place the specimen in the appropriate container and properly label it with the patient's name, the nature of the specimen, date and time collected, and the examination desired. Ideally, the specimen must be sent immediately to the laboratory. If this is not feasible, the specimen is kept in a refrigerator until it is taken to the laboratory. Results of the test may be reported in 2 or more days.

Nursing care revolves around administration of oxygen and antibiotics. Fluids are given to prevent dehydration. The nurse can administer an antitussive medication at bedtime for cough. Nursing care measures such as changing the child's clothes and linen should take place frequently to prevent chills. The nurse must remember that positioning the child on the affected side naturally splints the chest and reduces pleural rubbing that causes discomfort. It is also helpful to elevate the child's head to expand the ribcage.

The nurse can assess the child's sputum for color, amount, and consistency. The sputum assessment must be adequately recorded in the child's record.

To detect any change in condition, the nurse assesses vital signs and breath sounds. The nurse must also assist the child and the parents in alleviating anxieties through continuous emotional support and reassurance. It is important for the nurse to inform the parents that complete recovery from pneumonia may occur in about 2 weeks. Even if the child is feeling better after treatment, gradual return to normal activities like school and play are encouraged. The nurse can reinforce to parents that adequate food, fluids, and rest are important during convalescence.

Figure 24-7 Oxygen administration via nasal canula.

SEVERE ACUTE RESPIRATORY DISTRESS SYNDROME

Acute respiratory distress syndrome (SARS) was first reported in Asia in 2003. The coronavirus SARS Co-V is its main causative agent.

Signs and Symptoms

Fever of greater than 100.4°F (38°C) is the most common symptom and the main criterion in the current WHO case definition for suspected or probable SARS. Fever is accompanied by other symptoms including chills, cough, rigor (stiffness of some body parts), headache, dizziness, malaise, and myalgia. Initial symptoms may resemble those of an atypical pneumonia. Often the symptoms increase in severity, which necessitates intubation and mechanical ventilation. The SARS coronavirus is spread by droplets shed from respiratory secretions of an infected person.

Diagnosis

The diagnosis of SARS continues to be based on clinical and epidemiological findings until standardized reagents for virus and antibody detection become available and methods have been adequately field tested. At present, there are no defined criteria for SARS CoV test results to confirm or reject the diagnosis of SARS (Kamps & Hoffman, 2003).

In patients reported with SARS, laboratory investigation shows the presence of lymphopenia, leukopenia, thrombocytopenia, elevated lactate dehydrogenase, aspartate aminotransferase, and creatinine kinase levels.

Nursing Care

The treatment for SARS is still developing because the condition is relatively new and research is still underway. SARS has been treated with antibiotics because the signs and symptoms are nonspecific and because confirmatory laboratory testing has not yet been established. Antibiotics are then necessary to cover respiratory pathogens for community-acquired or nosocomial pneumonia. Antiviral drugs and steroids together with noninvasive mechanical ventilation have also been used as treatment modalities.

Vigilant nursing care is vital in caring for children with SARS. Since the treatment for SARS is still being studied, it is important to prevent its transmission. Three important points are to be considered by the nurse to prevent SARS: case detection, patient isolation, and contact tracing. If a child with a suspected case of SARS is admitted in the hospital, he or she must be isolated because SARS is transmitted through droplet infection. All health care providers, especially nurses caring for the child, should observe strict infection control measures, which include wearing masks, gloves, caps, and gown. Hand washing is essential before and after entering the child's room. Similarly, the nurse should instruct the child's visitors to observe proper infection control measures. If the admitted child is placed on assisted ventilation, the nurse must assist and monitor the child accordingly.

The nurse can be active in SARS case detection, and suspected cases must be reported immediately for proper management. Contact tracing can be achieved by identifying exactly who had close contact with the child. The most likely contacts are members of the same household, friends, and other relatives. People who had contact with the child must be monitored even at home during home health visits. The nurse encourages these people to seek medical consultation.

 nursing diagnoses Lower Respiratory Disorders

- Risk for Ineffective Airway clearance related to excessive secretions in the airway, tracheobronchial inflammation, or obstruction
- Risk for Ineffective Breathing Pattern related to tracheobronchial inflammation or obstruction
- Risk for Impaired Gas Exchange related to ventilation perfusion imbalance
- Anxiety related to perceived threat of hospitalization, or to invasive procedures or changes in health status of the child
- Risk for Deficient Fluid Volume related to inadequate fluid intake or excessive losses through abdominal route
- Fatigue related to increased respiratory effort

Infectious Conditions

PERTUSSIS

Pertussis or whooping cough is a highly contagious bacterial infection of the respiratory tract that causes paroxysmal cough. A "whooping" sound is produced as the child tries to take a breath. The disease is still a major cause of morbidity and mortality in children younger than 2 years. Sixty million cases a year occur worldwide (Long, 2004). In the United States, 11,647 cases were reported between 1976 and 2003 (Bocka, 2005).

The causative organism is *Bordetella pertussis*, a gram-negative coccobacillus. The disease is spread via droplet infection and direct contact with discharges from respiratory mucous membranes of an infected child. Pertussis is highly contagious; approximately 80% to 90% of susceptible individuals exposed to the infection develop the disease.

In this condition, *B. pertussis* attaches to and multiplies on the respiratory epithelium, starting in the nasopharynx and ending primarily in the bronchi and bronchioles (Bocka, 2005). A tracheal cytotoxin is produced that is responsible for the local epithelial damage that produces the respiratory symptom.

Signs and Symptoms

Pertussis lasts for 6 weeks and is divided into three stages: catarrhal, paroxysmal, and convalescent stages. Each of the stages lasts for 1 to 2 weeks. The incubation period ranges from 3 to 12 days.

 where research and practice meet:
Severe Acute Respiratory Distress Syndrome (SARS)

Two studies have reported SARS among children. In the first study, Hon et al. (2003) reported persistent fever, cough, progressive chest radiograph changes, and lymphopenia. In 10 teen-age patients, symptoms of malaise, chill, and rigor were similar to those of adults. Younger children presented chiefly with cough, runny nose, rigor, or myalgia.

Fever was the presenting symptom in the second study; with 19 out of the 21 patients having the symptom. Prodromal symptoms included malaise, loss of appetite, chills, dizziness, and rhinorrhea. During the respiratory phase of the illness, half of the children had cough, of which one third was productive (Chiu et al., 2003).

The catarrhal stage presents like the common upper respiratory infection with the presence of nasal congestion, rhinorrhea, sneezing, lacrimation, and conjunctival suffusion. This is the most communicable stage, but pertussis remains communicable up to 3 weeks after the onset of cough.

The paroxysmal stage presents with intense coughing lasting for several minutes. In older infants and toddlers, the characteristic "whoop" follows coughing as the child attempts to breathe. Infants younger than 6 months may not exhibit the "whoop." Instead, they may have episodes of apnea. Apnea occurs because the airway is still partially closed. The child turns red while coughing and vomiting usual follows the coughing episodes.

The convalescent stage presents with chronic cough lasting for weeks. Older children and adolescents may not show signs of the three stages; instead, the symptoms are an uninterrupted cough, feelings of suffocation or strangulation, and headache.

The child with pertussis typically does not have a fever. The presence of conjunctival hemorrhage and facial petechiae is visible and is due to the forceful, intense coughing.

Diagnosis

It is not easy to diagnose pertussis because the initial symptoms are similar to those of other upper respiratory tract infections. The diagnosis of pertussis is based on a history of severe coughing with or without a whoop, reddening of the face during coughing and incomplete or absent pertussis vaccination.

When blood testing is performed there is profound lymphocytosis, usually more than 70% of the total WBC count, which often increases to 20,000 to 40,000 or even 100,000 cells/mm^2. Chest radiography may show focal atelectasis and/or peribronchial cuffing.

The criterion standard for diagnosis of pertussis is isolation of *B. pertussis* in a culture from a swab taken from nasopharyngeal secretions. Polymerase chain reaction (PCR) testing to detect DNA is also commonly done. The Centers for Disease Control and Prevention (CDC) recommends both culture and PRC tests if a child has a cough lasting longer than 3 weeks. Many health care professionals now consider serological testing with ELISA to be the criterion testing standard (Bocka, 2005).

Nursing Care

The goals of therapy include limiting the number of paroxysms; observing the severity of cough; and maximizing nutrition, rest, and recovery (Guinto-Ocampo, Bennett, & Attia, 2008).

Antibiotic therapy is given to eradicate the infection, reduce morbidity, and prevent complications. Erythromycin (Erythrocin) is the drug of choice for pertussis. It is given at 40 mg/kg per day (not to exceed 2 g) qid for 14 days. Children allergic to erythromycin (Erythrocin) are given trimethoprim sulfamethoxazole (Bactrim).

The nurse can communicate to parents that the most important preventive measure is vaccination against the disease with DTaP. The vaccine is a combination of diphtheria and tetanus toxoids. The child must be immunized before the age 7. Children who are younger than 5 years of age must complete three doses of DTaP. The vaccine may not prevent the illness entirely, but it has been shown to lessen disease severity and duration.

Hospitalization is required when the child younger than 1 year of age who has developed pneumonia, has apnea, cyanosis, or hypoxia, and with moderate to severe dehydration. While in the hospital, the nurse can implement droplet precaution. Droplet precaution is an isolation technique that decreases transmission of organisms when an infected child coughs, sneezes, or spits (Venes, 2009). Droplet precautions are recommended for 5 days after the commencement of therapy or 3 weeks after the onset of paroxysmal cough if no antimicrobial therapy has been given.

During hospitalization, the nurse must vigilantly monitor the child's vital signs and oxygen saturation. Nursing care also centers on the child's hydration and nutritional status. If the child is unable to drink, an intravenous infusion is given. The nurse should accurately record coughing, feeding, vomiting, and weight changes. The nurse also instructs the parents that no special diet is required for the child, as the child is fed according to what is tolerated. The same is true for the child's activities. For as long as the child can tolerate, he or she can participate in regular activities and play. The prognosis for recovery is good for children who are well managed. It is important for the nurse to emphasize the importance of follow-up check-ups.

 Nursing Insight— *Pertussis vaccination*

In December 2005, the American Academy of Pediatrics approved recommendations from the Committee on Infectious Disease (COID) for universal vaccination of DTaP for adolescents at the 11 or 12 year visit to boost protection against pertussis.

TUBERCULOSIS

Tuberculosis (TB) is a chronic bacterial infection, usually of the lungs that is spread through the air. *Mycobacterium tuberculosis*, its most common causative agent, may also attack other organs and body parts. The CDC reported 14,093 cases of active TB in 2005 in the United States. In addition, an estimated 10 to 15 million people have latent TB. There was a declining rate of TB until the mid-1980s, when outbreaks drew new attention to TB. This outbreak was brought about by the increase in immunosuppressed individuals, particularly those with HIV and increased drug-resistant strains.

M. tuberculosis remains a public health concern. The World Health Organization (WHO) estimates that approximately one third of the world's population is infected with *M. tuberculosis*. The global burden of tuberculosis continues to grow due to factors like HIV epidemics, population migration patterns, increasing poverty, social upheavals, crowded living conditions in developing countries and inner city populations in developed countries, inadequate health coverage, poor access to health services, and inefficient tuberculosis control programs (Munoz & Stark, 2004).

Aside from *M. tuberculosis*, *Mycobacterium bovis* may also affect children as the microorganism may be present in unpasteurized milk or milk products. Latent tuberculosis infection (LTBI) occurs after the inhalation of infective droplet nuclei of *M. tuberculosis*. Conditions such as lowered body resistance, HIV infection, malnutrition, untreated upper respiratory tract infection (URTI), and other debilitating conditions increase the chance acquiring an active infection.

Transmission of tuberculosis is person-to-person through airborne droplet nuclei. It rarely occurs by direct contact with infected discharge or a contaminated fomite (any substance that adheres to and transmits infectious material) (Venes, 2009). Young children with tuberculosis rarely infect other children or adults because the tubercle bacilli are sparse in the endobronchial secretions of children and cough is often absent or lack the force necessary to suspend the infectious particles (Munoz & Stark, 2004).

When the organism enters the lungs, there is proliferation of epithelial cells that surrounds and encapsulates the multiplying bacilli as a way of warding it off. This process forms the typical tubercle. The extension of the primary lesion causes progressive tissue destruction as it spreads within the lungs. The tubercle bacilli are carried to most tissues of the body through the blood and lymphatic vessels. Multiplication of the bacilli is likely to occur in organs with conditions that favor their growth such as the brain, kidneys, and bones.

Signs and Symptoms

Many children with TB do not develop symptoms early in the infection. Low-grade fever, mild cough, and flu-like symptoms that resolve within a week may be observed. Anorexia and weight loss may follow as the disease progresses.

Diagnosis

The diagnosis of TB in children is challenging because children exhibit a variety of symptoms. Exact diagnosis of TB is based on the child's physical signs and symptoms, the history of exposure to TB, x-ray films that may show evidence of *M. tuberculosis* infection, and laboratory culture that may confirm the diagnosis. Early morning gastric contents from the stomach may be helpful in diagnosing TB. However, it takes about 4 weeks for the culture test to confirm the diagnosis because the bacillus grows slowly on a culture medium.

 ***Ethnocultural Considerations*—** Bacille Calmette-Guérin vaccine

Bacille Calmette-Guérin (BCG) vaccine is a preparation of a dried, living but attenuated culture of *Mycobacterium bovis*. It is used worldwide in areas with a high incidence of tuberculosis (TB) to provide passive TB immunity to infants and to protect adults who have an unavoidable risk of TB infection. In many foreign countries where BCG vaccination is widely used, the TST skin test is not useful because patients vaccinated with BCG will have a positive skin test (Venes, 2009).

The BCG vaccine is not routinely given in the United States because researchers have shown that BCG vaccine has worked well in some situations but poorly in others. The best use of BCG vaccination appears to be the prevention of life threatening forms of tuberculosis in infants and young children.

Nursing Care

The basic principles of management of tuberculosis are the same for children and adults. They consist of proper nutrition, anti-TB drugs, supportive care, and prevention of reinfection.

The American Academy of Pediatrics recommends a combination of isoniazid (INH), rifampicin, and pyrazin-

Labs: Tuberculin Skin Test

The tuberculin skin test (TST) is an exact indicator whether a child has been infected with the tubercle bacillus. The skin test consists of injecting a measured amount of the intermediate strength of 5 tuberculin units of tuberculin purified protein derivative (PPD) intradermally to form a small wheal in the forearm. In 48–72 hours, a positive reaction is marked by an area of red induration (an area of hardened tissue). Reactions greater than 10 mm in size are considered positive in non-immunocompromised patients (NIAID, 2006). The American Academy of Pediatrics recommends that administration and interpretation of skin test be performed and read by trained health care professionals (Fig. 24-8).

amide (PZA) given daily for the first 2 months followed by INH and rifampicin (Rifadin) given two to three times a week by direct observation of therapy for the next 4 months. Direct observation therapy (DOT) means that a health care worker or other responsible, mutually agreed-on individual is present when medications are administered to the child. DOT has been recommended for treatment for children and adolescents with TB in the United States because it decreases the rate of relapse, treatment failures, and drug resistance.

Children with TB are usually treated in outpatient clinics. However, in case of serious infection and involvement of other organs, children may need hospitalization. Children started with drug therapy are not contagious and require only standard precautions. Children with no cough and negative sputum smears may be cared for without isolation. Children with contagious infections must be placed in isolation.

During the child's hospitalization, the nurse must work closely with the family and the child to ensure that optimal care is provided. The nurse can explain the nature of disease and how children are at high risk of getting the infection. The nurse must emphasize good hand washing to reduce the chance of transmission from one person to another person. Nurses can also teach children to cover their nose and mouth with tissue paper when sneezing

Figure 24-8 Nurse is performing a tuberculin skin test.

and coughing. Proper disposal of the tissue paper in waste baskets must also be emphasized.

During hospitalization, the nurse must assist the child in collecting different specimens for the diagnosis, which includes sputum for culture. Children are unable to cough properly, so sputum may be difficult to collect from the young child.

The family of the child can be informed about the benefits of DOT. Nurses can discuss with the family about the ways of giving the medicines (e.g., tablets may need to be crushed well to facilitate its oral intake). The availability of liquid preparation in syrup form may be explored. The nurse can tell the family that they need to follow precautionary measures to prevent latent infection. The nurse should emphasize regular follow-up visits and regular intake of medications.

INFLUENZA

Influenza or flu is a common infection of the respiratory system caused by viruses. Infants and children are most vulnerable to the influenza virus. It is estimated that children are three times more likely to become ill with influenza than adults are. Each year, more than 36,000 persons, especially older individuals and those with chronic medical conditions, die from influenza in the United States (American Lung Association's Influenza Prevention, Program, 2008). The disease rapidly spreads worldwide in seasonal epidemics. Influenza is most common during the winter months.

Three types of virus cause influenza. Influenza types A and B are the major influenzal pathogens and cause epidemics. These viruses mutate and create different strains. Influenza type C causes mild symptoms and does not cause epidemics.

Influenza is spread through droplets when an infected person coughs, sneezes, or speaks. Indirectly, articles contaminated by nasopharyngeal secretions may spread the infection. Influenza causes a lytic (cellular destruction) infection of the respiratory epithelium with loss of ciliary function, decreased mucus production, and desquamation of the epithelial layer. These changes may permit secondary bacterial invasion directly from the epithelium or through the middle ear space. The rapid multiplication of the virus in the mucosa causes problems in the immune response mechanism (Torpy, 2005).

Signs and Symptoms

With the influenza virus there is the sudden onset of fever and chills accompanied by a flushed face, photophobia (intolerance to light), myalgia (pain in the muscles), hyperesthesia (sensitivity to sensory stimuli), and prostration (exhaustion). Complications include severe viral pneumonia, encephalitis, and secondary bacterial infections such as otitis media, sinusitis, or pneumonia. Flu symptoms in children are similar to that of adults except that children have higher degrees of fever of up to 105.1°F (40.6°C).

Diagnosis

The diagnosis of flu is based on the child's signs and symptoms and epidemiologic considerations. In the presence of a known epidemic, a child who has symptoms of fever, malaise, and respiratory illness may easily be diagnosed. Laboratory tests may also isolate the virus from the nasopharynx if done early in the course of illness.

Nursing Care

In uncomplicated cases, influenza is treated symptomatically since symptoms usually recede in 48 to 72 hours. Adequate rest and fluid intake are important components of the regimen. For fever and pain, acetaminophen (Children's Tylenol) or ibuprofen (Children's Advil) is given. Antiviral drugs such as oseltamivir (Tamiflu), amantadine (Symmetrel), and rimantadine (Flumadine) are currently used to manage influenza. Theses medications are usually given in the first 48 hours to decrease the severity and duration of the illness. Antibiotics are given when there is evidence of a superimposed bacterial infection like prolonged fever and deterioration of the condition.

Influenza vaccines are now widely used for prevention. There are two routes for the vaccines: intramuscular and nasal spray. Vaccination is recommended annually to populations at risk since the flu virus is continuously changing. Katz and Hall (2005), in a cost–benefit analysis for the recommended universal influenza immunization in children age 6 to 23 months found that influenza vaccine is less costly than hospitalization for the child.

Since influenza is a self-limiting condition, nursing care is supportive. Depending on the severity of influenza, the child recovers within 1 to 2 weeks. The nurse must emphasize to the parents the importance of adequate rest and sleep. When the child has the flu, more fluids should be offered. An electrolyte solution is recommended. The nurse can reiterate the importance of having an annual vaccination.

❝ What to say ❞ — *Salicylates (aspirin)*

The nurse can instruct the parents to avoid giving salicylates (aspirin) because of the possibility of Reye syndrome. Reye syndrome is an encephalitis-like illness following a viral infection. Reye syndrome is highly associated with the intake of salicylates (aspirin) during the course of the viral disease. The symptoms include nausea, vomiting, lethargy, and indifference; in severe cases, there may be irrational behavior, delirium, and rapid breathing. Warn parents to watch out for these symptoms, especially if aspirin has been given to the patient prior to consultation.

Pulmonary Noninfectious Irritation

FOREIGN BODY ASPIRATION

Anything that is caught in the respiratory tract and blocks the air passage is called foreign body (FB) aspiration. Young children are at greater risk of aspirating foreign bodies based on curiosity and the habit of putting things in the mouth. Foreign body aspiration may occur at any age but it is most common among toddlers. Almost 2.5 million children are affected each year in the United States, and FB aspiration leads to 300 deaths annually. The most frequently aspirated objects are organic food items such as peanuts, popcorn, hot dogs, or vegetable matter and fruit gel snacks. Nonfood objects include balloons, coins, pen tops, and pins (Qureshi & Mink, 2003).

medication: Oseltamivir (Tamiflu)

Oseltamivir (o-sel-**tam**-i-vir)

Pregnancy Category: C

Indications: Uncomplicated acute illness due to influenza infection in adults and children >1 year who have had symptoms for < 2 days
   Prevention of influenza in patients > 13 years

Actions: Inhibits the enzyme neuraminidase, which may alter virus particle aggregation and release.

Therapeutic Effects: Reduced duration of flu related symptoms

Pharmacokinetics:
ABSORPTION: Rapidly absorbed from the GI tract and converted by the liver to the active form, oseltamivir carboxylate, 75% reaches systemic circulation as the active drug.

Contraindications and Precautions:
CONTRAINDICATED IN: Hypersensitivity and children <1 year old

Adverse Reactions and Side Effects:
CNS: Insomnia, vertigo. Respiratory bronchitis. GI: nausea, vomiting

Route and Dosage:
PO:
Children >88 lb (40 kg): 75 mg twice daily for 5 days
Children 50.6–88 lb (23–40 kg): 60 mg twice daily
Children 33–50.6 lb (15–23 kg): 45 mg twice daily
Children < 33 lb (15 kg) and >1 year: 30 mg twice daily

Nursing Implications:
- Monitor influenza symptoms. Additional supportive treatment may be indicated to treat symptoms. Treatment should be started as soon as possible from the first sign of flu symptoms. Administer with food or milk to minimize GI irritation.
- Drug should be used within 10 days of constitution.
- Caution patients/parents that Tamiflu should not be shared with anyone even if they have the same symptoms.
- Tamiflu is not a substitute for flu shots according to immunization guidelines.
- Advise patient to consult health care professional before taking any medications concurrently with Tamiflu.

Data from Deglin, J.H., & Vallerand, A.P. (2009). *Davis's drug guide for nurses* (11th ed., pp. 916–917). Philadelphia: F.A. Davis.

In the child, the aspirated object may stay in the same place of obstruction or move with air. There is a possibility that if the child forcefully coughs the object may be spit out. During the presence of FB the bronchioles and bronchi may become larger during inspiration and smaller during expiration. Small objects may cause little damage and large objects may occlude the whole airway passage, causing more severe symptoms. A sharp object not only blocks the airway but also may lead to severe trauma and the child may have complications such as inflammation and abscess, atelectasis, and emphysema.

Signs and Symptoms

After aspiration, the child patient exhibits symptoms of choking, gagging, wheezing, or coughing. Dyspnea, cough, stridor, and hoarseness are present when the obstruction is in the laryngotracheal area. If the obstruction is in the larynx, the child may be unable to speak and breathe. If the object is in the bronchioles, the child may show difficulty in breathing and unequal breath sounds. The child's condition may worsen with the total obstruction and the

child may become cyanotic or unconscious. The nurse understands that any delay in removal of the foreign body may be fatal.

Diagnosis

The child's history and physical signs help in the diagnosis of foreign body aspiration. In children, a foreign body should be suspected in the presence of acute or chronic pulmonary lesions. The nurse can communicate to the family that an x-ray exam with fluoroscopic examination can be helpful in locating the site of the aspirated object. Definitive diagnosis of FB aspiration is through bronchoscopic examination.

The nurse who is knowledgeable in assessing respiratory emergencies can make a difference in saving the child's life. The CUPS (critical, unstable, potentially unstable and stable) assessment method may be a useful tool for the nurse as it includes actions that the nurse can take for each level of emergency.

assessment tools Pediatric Respiratory Emergencies

Assessment	Critical	Unstable	Potentially Unstable	Stable
Airway	Completely or severely obstructed	Partially obstructed, excessive secretions or blood	Open with secretions	Open
Breathing rate	May be slow, absent, or very fast with periods of slowing	Increased	Occasionally increased	Normal
Breathing effort	Absent or greatly increased with periods of weakness	Increased	Normal	Normal
Breath sounds	Grunting, faint, or absent	Wheezing or stridor, decreased breath sounds	Normal or slight wheezing	Normal
Skin color	Pale, mottled, or blue	Pink or pale	Pink	Pink
Inspection	Normal, decreased, or absent chest movement	Normal or decreased chest movement	Runny nose, red eyes, fever	Runny nose
Actions	Immediately open airway, suction, give high concentration oxygen with assisted ventilation, and transport	Move at moderate pace; give high concentration oxygen; prepare for transport; reassess frequently	Move at moderate pace; help into position of comfort; give high concentration oxygen; prepare for transport	Begin focused history and physical exam

Data from Rahm, N.S., Hansen, J.D., & Sanddal, N.D. (1997). *Critical trauma care by the basic EMT.* Bozeman, MT: Critical Illness and Trauma Foundation, Inc.

Nursing Care

If a large object has been swallowed then it may be difficult for the child to remove the foreign body spontaneously by coughing. In this case, the child will need instrumental assistance to remove the obstruction. The nurse understands that delays in the treatment may lead to swelling in the obstructed site and inflammation may set in, hampering the removal of the object. The foreign body may also adhere to the lumen of the air passage.

Medical management involves the removal of foreign bodies from the respiratory tract by direct laryngoscopy or bronchoscopy. The child is hospitalized during and after the procedure for observation of laryngeal edema and respiratory distress.

In the hospital, the nurse must closely monitor the child's vital signs and assess the level of consciousness. The nurse can explain any procedures to the parents to help allay anxieties. Initially, the child may be placed on NPO and the family should be encouraged to follow the medical regimen. The nurse can provide a cool mist vaporizer and administer antibiotic therapy if deemed appropriate.

The nurse, especially in the community, plays very important roles in foreign body aspiration since the community nurse is involved in health care in the home setting where the accidents commonly occur. In the community setting, the nurse must be skillful in Heimlich maneuver and can provide health education to parents regarding the procedure. Parents can be taught about safety precautions to avoid foreign body aspiration. For instance, the nurse can communicate to the parents that toys should not have small detachable parts and food size should be appropriate for age.

✿ Collaboration in Caring— *The Heimlich maneuver*

The Heimlich maneuver is a life saving way of removing the foreign body. In a choking child older than 1 year of age, abdominal thrusts are necessary. In a choking infant back blows and chest thrusts are performed. The community health nurse can encourage the parents to complete a cardiopulmonary resuscitation course (CPR) at the American Red Cross (ARC), the American Heart Association (AHA), or other community agencies that teach CPR.

Heimlich maneuver on a conscious child older than 1 year of age:

1. Give five blows to the child's back with heel of your hand with the child sitting, kneeling, or lying.
2. If the obstruction persists, go behind the child and pass your arms around the child's body; form a fist with one hand immediately below the child's sternum. Place the other hand over the fist and pull upwards into the abdomen. Repeat five times.

3. Check the child's mouth for any obvious obstruction that can be removed.

4. If necessary, repeat the sequence and ask for help to call 911 or rush to the nearest hospital

Heimlich maneuver on an infant:

1. Lay the infant on your arm or thigh with the infant's head down.
2. Give five blows to the infant's back using the heel of your hand.

3. If the airway obstruction continues, turn the infant over with head down and give five chest thrusts using two fingers at a distance of 1 fingerbreadth below the nipple level in midline.

4. Check the infant's mouth for any obvious obstructions that can be removed.
5. If necessary, repeat the sequence and ask for help to call 911 or rush to the nearest hospital (The AHA Subcommittee on Pediatric Resuscitation, 2006. http://pediatrics.aappublications.org/cgi/content/full/117/5/e989)

SMOKE INHALATION

Fires continue to be one of the most hazardous forms of manmade disasters and are responsible for approximately 5000 deaths per year in the United States. The majority of these deaths are due to smoke inhalation rather than to surface burns (Mandel & Hales, 2005). Smoke is a mixture of gases and aerosolized particulate matter generated by combustion. Incomplete combustion produces noxious substances that when inhaled are toxic to humans.

Smoke inhalation may cause three types of injury: heat, chemical, and systemic. Smoke tends to be dry but with high temperature. Heat produces immediate injury to the mucosa resulting in erythema, ulceration, and edema, thus compromising the upper airway. If significant edema ensues, symptoms related to obstruction such as dyspnea, stridor, and cyanosis occur. Chemical injury is related to the inhalation of substances generated during combustions. Irritant gasses such as carbon dioxide combine with water in the lungs to form corrosive acids; aldehyde cause denaturation of proteins, cellular damage, and edema of pulmonary tissues (Winklestein, 2005).

Systemic injury occurs from gases formed during combustion that are nontoxic to the airways but may cause injury or death by interfering with oxygen utilization. Carbon monoxide and hydrogen cyanide are substances that can be formed when materials such as silk, nylon, polyurethane, and organic matters are burned. These substances are considered as asphyxiant and lead to neurological symptoms (Clardy & Manaker, 2006).

Signs and Symptoms

Symptoms from heat injury are proportionate to the damage to the upper airway. Burns in the face and neck may accentuate the symptoms. Edema of the upper airway usually manifests within 24 hours of injury. Dyspnea and stridor are the initial symptoms. Chemical injury may result in erythema, edema, and ulceration of the airways. Cough, bronchorrhea, dyspnea, and wheezing may not appear until 12 to 36 hours after the exposure. Moderate carbon monoxide (CO) poisoning presents with constitutional symptoms like headache, malaise, nausea, dizziness, and alterations in mental status. Severe CO poisoning can produce seizures, syncope, cherry red mucous membranes, falsely high Po_2 readings, or coma.

Diagnosis

Diagnosis of smoke inhalation is based on the signs and symptoms of the injury, especially in survivors of the fire. However, the nurse understands that diagnosis of CO poisoning requires careful neurological examination and should be based on compatible history and clinical findings.

Nursing Care

Treatment is aimed at managing upper airway obstruction and possible CO poisoning. Urgent attention to the adequacy of airway, breathing, and circulation is obligatory. The immediate administration of 100% oxygen via a high flow system is important to reverse tissue hypoxia. If the child is comatose, intubation is recommended to deliver the highest possible Fio_2 and to prevent CO_2 retention. After the initial stabilization, treatment of concomitant burns injury is initiated.

It is important for the nurse to remember that nursing care of children with smoke inhalation involves prioritizing life-sustaining systems of respiration and circulation. Nurses assist in emergency intubation and monitor the patients accordingly. Signs of carbon monoxide poisoning should be recorded and reported without delay.

Recovery for children with minor burns and smoke inhalation is good provided adequate nutrition is provided when the patient is medically cleared to have oral intake. The nurse should offer foods that are attractively served so that the child is encouraged to eat. Favorite toys may be placed at the bedside so that the child is not bored and will maintain normal development. For infants, a child life specialist can offer stimulation and calming music. Nurses can encourage parents to participate in the care of the child.

PASSIVE SMOKING

Passive smoking is defined as a nonsmoker's inhalation of the smoke coming from the smoker. The smoke inhaled by nonsmokers is called environmental tobacco smoke (ETS). The term was first used by the German physician Fritz Lickint in 1939. Since then, numerous studies were conducted about the effects of cigarette smoking on nonsmokers. There is conclusive evidence about the ill effects of smoking and ETS on health. The findings on passive smoking and disease have been the foundation of the drive for smoke-free environments and for educating parents concerning the effects of their smoking on their children's health (Samet & Sokrinder, 2006).

The nonsmoker breathes "sidestream smoke" from the burning tip of the cigarette and "mainstream smoke" that has been inhaled then exhaled by the smoker. ETS contains more than 4000 chemicals, some of which have irritant properties and some 60 known or suspected carcinogens. Inhalation of ETS may bring both short-term and long-term effects. The short-term effects are manifested as irritation to the upper airways, while the long-term effects are related to the consequences of inhaling the chemicals in ETS such as nicotine and carbon monoxide for prolonged periods of time.

Signs and Symptoms

Short-term effects are manifested in symptoms such as stuffy, runny nose, watery eyes, sneezing, coughing, and wheezing. Headache and nausea may also be felt. The long-term effects are the negative results of frequent and long-term exposure. Numerous studies found strong relationships between passive smoking and lung cancer, heart disease, miscarriage, birth defects, lung infection, ear infection, and worsening asthma and other allergic conditions.

Diagnosis

The diagnosis of conditions related to passive smoking is based on history and evidence of exposure to ETS. At present, 1.1 billion adults worldwide are smokers, implying that some ETS exposure is almost unavoidable for children and for the two thirds of adults who do not smoke (Samet & Sockrider, 2006). Measurements of several components of ETS have been made in homes, workplaces, and public places to characterize the contribution of smoking to indoor air pollution. Dangerous levels of ETS components usually come within those measures.

Nursing Care

Treatment for children is focused on the specific ailments that exposure to ETS has produced. One most important component to be addressed in passive smoking is its control. Strategies to control ETS are currently being undertaken by both the government and private sectors through education, regulation, legislation, and litigation.

The nurse plays an active role through health education, especially to parents. The nurse, through health education, must emphasize the negative effects of smoking, both for the smokers and the recipients of environment tobacco smoke. To support "stop smoking campaigns" means the nurse must be a good role model and give up any personal smoking habits.

Nurses must also support the call of the World Health Organization (WHO) for the right of every child to grow up in an environment free of tobacco smoke. Efforts should be made by the nurses to persuade parents, especially pregnant women, to give up smoking. This is one way of advocating for the rights of children.

Respiratory Conditions Related to Allergens

ALLERGIC RHINITIS

Allergic rhinitis is an inflammation of the nasal membranes predominantly in the child's nose and eyes. Airborne particles of dust, dander, or plant pollens in children who are allergic to these substances cause allergic rhinitis. It appears alone or in combination with a cold.

 Nursing Insight— *How does inflammation of the nasal membranes occur?*

Inflammation of the mucous membranes is characterized by a complex interaction of inflammatory mediators and is triggered by an immunoglobulin E (IgE)-mediated response to an extrinsic protein.

The mediators that are released immediately include histamine, tryptase, chymase, kinins, and heparin. The mast cells quickly synthesize other mediators including leukotrienes and prostaglandin D_2. These mediators then lead to the symptoms of rhinorrhea.

Next mucous glands are stimulated, leading to increase for secretions produced. Vasodilatation then leads to congestion and pressure. Sensory nerves are also stimulated, leading to sneezing and itching. This sequel happens in a matter of minutes and is called the early phase response.

In the next 4–8 hours there is a complex interplay of neutrophils, eosinophils, lymphocytes, and macrophages. This interplay brings about continued inflammation, termed as late phase response. The phase may persist for days and systemic effects range from fatigue to sleepiness to malaise to generalized weakness.

Signs and Symptoms

Symptoms associated with allergic rhinitis range include sneezing, itching (of nose, eyes, ears, palate), rhinorrhea, postnasal drip, congestion, headache, earache, tearing, red eyes, eye swelling, fatigue, drowsiness, and malaise. There is nasal itching and so to relieve the itching the child performs what is called allergic salute by rubbing the nose upwards.

Diagnosis

A thorough history and physical examination of the child confirm allergic rhinitis. A nasal smear is done to determine the number of eosinophils in the nasal secretions. A radioallergosorbent test (RAST) is done to determine specific IgE antibodies. Skin testing is often done to identify the specific allergen.

Nursing Care

Treatment for allergic rhinitis in the child involves pharmacological management. Pharmacological management includes short-acting antihistamines, longer acting histamines, nasal corticosteroid sprays, decongestants, and leukotriene inhibitors. There is evidence to prove that high-dose allergy shots are recommended if the allergen cannot be removed and if the child's symptoms are hard to control. This includes regular injections of the allergen

given in increasing doses, which in turn help the body to adjust to the allergen.

Nursing care for the child with allergic rhinitis falls under three broad categories:

- Identify triggers in the environment both outdoors and indoors that bring about allergic rhinitis. Pollen tends to be very high from late spring until summer, so reduce the child's outdoor exposure. Keep windows and doors shut during this season. Bathing after being outdoors helps to reduce the pollen present on hair and skin.
- Indoor measures include covering mattresses and pillows with dust covers. Bed linen should be washed more frequently every 2 weeks in hot water. Carpets and stuffed toys that harbor dust mites should be removed. If the allergen identified is a pet, it should be removed.
- Carry out prescribed drug therapies when necessary.
- Encourage parents about the benefits of allergy shots.

 Across Care Settings: **Education**

Education about environmental control measures involves both the avoidance of known allergens (substances to which the patient has IgE-mediated sensitivity) and the avoidance of nonspecific irritants and triggers. In the clinic setting, the nurse can explore possible allergens of the child with the parents to obtain important information that might determine the cause of the allergic rhinitis. Parents must understand the possible complications that allergic rhinitis may cause. These complications range from otitis media, eustachian tube dysfunction, and acute sinusitis to chronic sinusitis.

ASTHMA

Asthma is a chronic disorder of the airway characterized by the triad symptoms of bronchial smooth muscle spasm, inflammation and edema of the bronchial mucosa, and production and retention of thick, tenacious, pulmonary secretions leading to airway obstruction. The term **status asthmaticus** is used to refer to persistent and intractable asthma in which the child does not respond to therapy and a medical emergency ensues.

 Ethnocultural Considerations— **Asthma**

In the United States, the poor, especially of African American or Hispanic background, experience disproportional high rates of both asthma prevalence and morbidity (Castro, Schechtman, Halstead, & Bloomberg, 2001; Mannino et al., 2002). There is great worldwide variability in prevalence, with industrialized areas having consistently high rates.

Genetic, environmental/extrinsic factors and intrinsic factors predispose the child to develop asthma. Although allergens play an important role in asthma, 20% to 40% of children with asthma have no evidence of allergic disease. Among the extrinsic factors are allergens such as dust; pollen; animal hairs; chemical sprays; perfumes; baby powder; molds; and foods such as nuts, chocolates, oranges, and chicken. Conditions such as changes in weather, pollution, and smoke may also trigger an attack. Intrinsic factors include exercise, anxiety, strong emotions such as fear and laughter, and infections.

When any of the factors trigger an asthma attack, the response comes in 10 to 20 minutes. The allergen/antigen binds to the allergen-specific immunoglobulin E (IgE) surface, causing activation of resident airway mast cells and macrophages. Proinflammatory mediators, such as histamine and leukotrienes, are released. They provoke contraction of the airway's smooth muscles, increased mucus secretion, and vasodilatation. Consequently, microvascular leakage and exudation of plasma into the airway walls cause them to become thickened and edematous with subsequent lumen constriction (Kieckhefer & Ratcliffe, 2004).

Signs and Symptoms

Signs and symptoms in the child during the early phase are wheeze; paroxysmal, irritative, and nonproductive cough; prolonged expiratory phase; tachypnea; retractions; and nasal flaring. As the disease becomes chronic, cough persists especially at night. There may be enlarged AP diameter of the chest wall or barrel chest and elevated shoulders.

Diagnosis

The asthma diagnosis for the child is based on clinical symptoms, history, physical examination, and to a lesser extent, laboratory tests. The nurse can explain to the parents that radiographic examinations are done to rule out the presence of coexisting disease or infection and to evaluate the condition of the lungs. Generally, chronic cough in the absence of infection, wheezing, and prolonged expiratory phase is sufficient to establish a diagnosis (Winkelstein, 2005).

Nursing Care

Treatment consists of early relief of symptoms through drug therapy and prevention of further attacks through allergen control, environmental manipulation, and health education. The goal is to enable the child to have as regular a life as possible by keeping the lung function within normal limits. The nurse provides adequate health education about the use of a Peak Flow Meter to help the parents increase their capacity to care for the child (Procedure 24-1).

Drug therapy depends upon the level of severity of the disease. There are two approaches to this therapy; one is the quick-relief or rescue medications and the second is the long-term control medications.

The U.S. Department of Health and Human Services 2007, the National Asthma Education and Prevention Program, expert panel report 3: Guidelines for the diagnosis and management of asthma has provided a revised classification scheme for asthma severity (Table 24-2).

The guidelines recommend daily anti-inflammatory agents to control the levels of persistent asthma, with increasing doses of medication as necessary. The use of low-dose control medications such as inhaled steroids, cromolyn sodium (Intal), nedocromil (Tilade), or an anti-leukotriene agent such as a montelukast sodium (Singulair) tablet usually taken at night is recommended for children with mild persistent asthma (Fig. 24-9). A higher dose of steroids with the addition of long-acting beta agonist may be needed for moderate and severe persistent asthma. For quick relief of bronchospasm and for children with asthma, short-acting inhaled beta antagonists are recommended. For more detailed information of the guidelines visit http://www.nhlbi.nih.gov/guidelines/asthma/index.htm.

The Asthma Action Plan (http://www.lungusa.org/atf/cf/%7B7A8D42C2-FCCA-4604-8ADE-7F5D5E762256%7D/AAP.PDF) is an educational communication tool used between the health care provider and the patient, with their family and caregivers, to properly manage asthma, and respond to asthma episodes. The Asthma Action Plan is completed by the child's primary care provider. It includes the symptoms and management for each color zone including peak flow measurements appropriate for each color zone. Nurses can provide adequate instructions on how to use, interpret, and complete the form.

A peak flow meter, which can be purchased over the counter, is an essential companion for the Asthma Action Plan for children older than 6 years old. The peak flow meter is a portable handheld device that is used to measure the ability to push air out of the lungs. To determine the child's zone for children younger than 6 years old, the symptoms alone are used. The "personal best" peak flow is determined when the child is symptom free. A peak flow meter package usually contains a form where peak flow readings are recorded regularly. A personal best normal may be obtained from measuring the patient's own peak flow rate. Therefore, it is important for the patient, parents, and the doctor to discuss what is considered "normal."

Nursing care for children with asthma involves assisting with relief of symptoms and providing health education to patients and family. Asthma attacks are frightening and stressful both for the child and family; therefore, the nurse should have a calm approach in its initial management. Administering quick relief medications without delay is important. Essential nursing interventions include giving medications on time, liquefying secretions through

Figure 24-9 The respiratory therapist helps the child use a metered dose inhaler to control asthma.

Procedure 24-1 Using a Peak Flow Meter

The peak flow meter is a portable handheld device that is used to measure the child's ability to push air out of the lungs. The American Lung Association recommends the following steps in using the peal flow meter (http://www.lungusa.org).

Purpose

The purpose of a Peak Flow Meter is to keep track of the results and help the parents and child to learn about asthma. Keeping a daily record may also help determine if the child's asthma is getting worse.

Equipment

Peak Flow Meter
Peak Flow Record

Steps

1. Before each use, make sure the sliding marker or arrow on the Peak Flow Meter is at the bottom of the numbered scale (zero or the lowest number on the scale).

   RATIONALE: *Initial calibration ensures an accurate reading.*

2. Instruct the child to stand up straight and to remove gum or any food from the mouth.

   RATIONALE: *Proper body alignment is essential for an accurate reading.*

3. Instruct the child to take a deep breath and to put the mouthpiece of the Peak Flow Meter into the mouth. Close the lips tightly around the mouthpiece. Be sure to keep the tongue away from the mouthpiece.

   RATIONALE: *A tight seal is necessary for measuring an accurate reading.*

4. Instruct the child to take in one breath and to then blow out as hard and as quickly as possible. Blow a "fast hard blast" rather than "slowly blowing" until all of the air is emptied from the lungs.

   RATIONALE: *A fast hard blast empties all the air from the lungs. This helps ensure an accurate measurement.*

5. Teach the parents that the force of the air coming out of the lungs causes the marker to move along the numbered scale. Record the number where the marker landed on a *Peak Flow Record*.

   RATIONALE: *Teaching the parents about how to use and record the measurement of the Peak Flow Meter increases their capacity to care for the child.*

6. Repeat the entire routine three times (if the routine is done correctly the numbers from all three tries are very close together).

   RATIONALE: *Repeating the entire routine three times helps ensure accurate data collection.*

7. Record the highest reading. Do not calculate an average.

   RATIONALE: *The highest reading provides the most accurate data.*

8. Measure the peak flow rate at the same time each day. A good time to measure the peak flow rate is between 7 and 9 A.M. and between 6 and 8 P.M. Note, It may be a good idea to measure the peak flow rate before or after using asthma medicine.

   RATIONALE: *A consistent time of day provides the best information about the child's ongoing lung function.*

7. Keep a chart of the peak flow rates on a *Peak Flow Record*.

   RATIONALE: *Having written documentation records information about the lung function from day to day and may help with early identification of problems.*

Clinical Alert A Peak Flow Meter package usually contains a *Peak Flow Record* where the peak flow readings are recorded regularly.

Teach Parents

Teach parents about the child's personal best. The "personal best" peak flow is determined when the child is symptom free. It is important for the child, parents, and the doctor to discuss what is considered "normal." Remind parents of the need to discuss the readings with the physician.

Documentation

10/12/10 0900 Peak flow meter used. Green zone, good control; 80% of personal best, no symptoms noted. Continues to take usual medication.
—I. Bustamante-Gavino, RN

---

adequate hydration and positioning the child properly (head of bed elevated 30 degrees) to provide comfort, and lung expansion. The side lying and semi-prone positions are also recommended. It is vital that the nurse reports and records the child's respiratory assessment as well as responses to medications so that appropriate management may be initiated immediately. The nurse can also ensure that respiratory treatments happen in timely manner and

that ordering a p.r.n. (as needed) treatment may be necessary.

The community nurse can offer health education to families that emphasizes adherence to the treatment regimen correctly, preventing infection, and avoiding asthma triggers. Nurses are in the best position to provide health education because they are in contact with the patients and the parents most of the time.

Table 24–2 Criteria for Classification of Asthma Severity in Children 0–4 Years of Age				
Severity	**Day Symptoms**	**Night Awakenings**	**SABA Use***	**Limit to Activity**
Intermittent	≤2 days/week	None	None	≤2 times/week
Mild Persistent	3–6 days/week	1–2 times/month	>2 days/week	Minor
Mod. Persistent	Daily	3–4 times/month	Daily	Some
Severe Persistent	Several times/day	>1 time/week	Several times/day	Extremely

*Short-acting beta 2 agonists (SABA) such as albuterol use does not include prevention of exercise-induced bronchospasm (EIB).
Source: The U.S. Department of Health and Human Services (2007). National asthma education and prevention program. Expert panel report 3: Guidelines for the diagnosis and management of asthma.

 ### Nursing Insight— *Spacers*

The nurse understands that for children less than 5 years of age, a spacer or a valved holding chamber (VHC) is recommended which is attached to the MDI. A spacer may deliver the medication to the child's lungs better than an inhaler alone and may be easier for the child to use than an MDI alone. In addition, for ease of delivery, child sized masks are available that fit the VHC. With this device there is more medication deposited in the lungs and less systemic side effects. After VHC use, the nurse can have the child follow with mouth washing and spitting to decrease swallowing medication and side effect including, in the case of inhaled corticosteroids (ICS), prevention of oral *candidiasis* (U.S. Department of Health and Human Services, 2007).

 ### Across Care Settings: What to do in cases of an acute asthma attack

An asthma attack may occur anytime and anywhere. It may happen in the home, at a school, in a mall, or in a park. To guide parents, teachers, and people who work in places where children go, the nurse can provide the following tips:

Teachers and school administrators should be familiar with the health history of the child. It is important to coordinate care and share information with the school health nurse. The nurse should also know the school district's rules and regulations regarding carrying asthma medications to school, including where the medications are to be kept and how to use the medications. In coordination with the child's physician and parents the nurse can fill out an emergency asthma action plan, including the child's triggers. The nurse needs to post emergency phone numbers in case of an attack. In addition, the nurse must know the child's peak flow readings, the child's personal best, and when the child runs into trouble. The nurse can also educate the teachers and other personnel who come in contact with the child.

Parents: Be sure that you carry the child's quick relief medications. It is helpful if the school-age child carries it too, along with the instructions about how the medication is used.

Nurses can give information on environmental control and creating an allergen-free environment. In addition, through community health education, the nurse can emphasize that when a child exhibits difficulty breathing, wheezing, and coughing, it is important to be calm and reassure the child. It is important to find out if the child's medicine is available; if not, call 911.

Personnel in parks, mall, and play areas should be briefed about possible pediatric emergencies including management in an emergency situation.

summary points

- The differences between the adult and child respiratory system affect function and subsequent respiratory conditions.

- It is essential that the nurse have a good understanding of congenital respiratory conditions and structural anomalies in children along with an understanding of signs and symptoms and prescribed treatment.

- Nurses must provide adequate emotional support to parents whose children have life-threatening respiratory conditions.

- The diagnosis, signs and symptoms, and nursing care measures are important in caring for children with respiratory conditions.

- Nursing care for children with infectious respiratory conditions includes close monitoring and correct treatment to prevent spread of infection.

- Nursing care for noninfectious respiratory conditions is aimed at managing the upper airway to prevent obstruction and further damage.

- During health teachings, nurses should emphasize to parents an awareness of the ill effects of the different forms of air pollutants, including environmental tobacco.

- The goal for children with asthma is to enable the child to have as normal a life as possible by keeping the lung functioning within normal limits.

- The nurse can educate the family about the child wearing a medical alert bracelet.

review questions

Multiple Choice

1. The pediatric nurse is aware that the child with cystic fibrosis (CF) has discharge planning needs. Which of the following is important to include in the discharge-teaching plan?
   A. Communicating to the family about a well balanced, low-protein, high-calorie diet

B. Communicating to the family about when to administer pancreatic enzymes

C. Communicating to the family that vitamin supplements are not necessary

D. Communicating to the family that cystic fibrosis (CF) a self limiting illness

2. A 2-year-old child is discharged from the out-patient surgical unit after having had a tonsillectomy. The pediatric nurse knows that the discharge teaching is effective after the parents verbalize which of the following statements as the most important aspect of the teaching?

A. "I will administer cherry flavored acetaminophen (Children's Tylenol) for pain."

B. "It's important to have my child gargle to prevent an infection."

C. "I will bring my child to the emergency room if I see excessive swallowing."

D. "I will offer my child ice cream to help soothe the pain in the throat."

Select All that Apply

3. A 5-month-old infant is admitted to the hospital's pediatric unit with a history of Bronchopulmonary Dysplasia (BPD). What are the nurse's priority nursing actions?

A. Administer Albuterol (Ventolin) nebulizer as ordered.

B. Monitor the infant's oxygen saturation levels.

C. Calculate the infant's intake and output.

D. Administer antibiotic therapy as ordered.

4. When caring for the pediatric patient, the nurse is aware that there are differences in the anatomy and physiology between the child's and the adult's airway that predispose the child to contracting a respiratory condition.

A. Infants are obligatory nose breathers until about 4 weeks of age so it is essential to maintain nasal patency.

B. The trachea of the adult is shorter and narrower in diameter than the trachea of the child.

C. The epiglottis of the child is longer and flaccid, making it more susceptible to swelling which may lead to airway occlusion.

D. The increased amount of soft tissue in the child's neck makes the child more susceptible to infection and edema.

5. Which assessment must the pediatric nurse include when evaluating the respiratory status of a child?

A. Skin turgor

B. Oxygen saturation levels

C. Skin color and moisture

D. Respiratory rate and depth

True/False

6. The best time for the pediatric nurse to assess the child's respiratory status is when the child is awake and active.

7. Excessive drooling in the newborn with a history of polyhydramnios in the mother's obstetrical history may be indicative of a diaphragmatic hernia.

8. The pediatric nurse understands that two primary goals in caring for a child with cystic fibrosis are to control infection and improve aeration.

Fill-in-the-Blank

9. In the newborn diagnosed with a congenital diaphragmatic hernia (CDH), the nurse understands that there is an opening between the _____ and _____ cavities through which the abdominal organs can herniate into the thoracic cavity and present with symptoms of _____.

Matching

Match the appropriate signs and/or symptoms the nurse would observe in each of the following respiratory conditions. Write the letters on the blank provided before the item number.

_____ **10.** Croup

_____ **11.** Pharyngitis

_____ **12.** Sinusitis

_____ **13.** Bronchitis

_____ **14.** Asthma

_____ **15.** Severe acute respiratory distress syndrome (SARS)

a. Dry, hacking cough

b. Facial pain, headache, and fever

c. Rigor, chills, and myalgia

d. Hoarse, barky cough

e. Pain on swallowing

f. An irritating, nonproductive cough, nasal flaring, retractions

See Answers to End of Chapter Review Questions on the Electronic Study Guide or DavisPlus.

REFERENCES

American Academy of Family Physicians. (2005). Asthma Action Plan. Retrieved from http://familydoctor.org/online/famdocen/home.html (Accessed June 20, 2008).

American Lung Association's Influenza Prevention Program. (2008). Faces of influenza. Retrieved from http://www.facesofinfluenza.org/home.php?utm_source=yahoo&utm_medium=cpc&utm_campaign=Influenza (Accessed June 20, 2008).

American Academy of Otolaryngology, Head and Neck Surgery. (2008). Retrieved from http://entmd.org/healthinfo/sinus/sinusitis.cfm (Accessed June 20, 2008).

The AHA Subcommittee on Pediatric Resuscitation. (2006). *Pediatrics 117*(5) pp. e989-e1004 (doi:10.1542/peds.2006-0219). (Accessed February 27, 2007).

American Lung Association. (2008). Asthma management. Retrieved from http://www.lungusa.org/ (Accessed November 2, 2008).

Asthma Action Plan. (2008). Asthma management Retrieved from http://www.lungusa.org/ (Accessed November 2, 2008).

Bocka, J. E-medicine. (2006). Pediatric pertussis, *Web MD*. Retrieved from http://www.ama-assn.org/ (Accessed July 9, 2008).

Bulechek, G., Butcher, H.M., & Dochterman, J. (2008). *Nursing interventions classification (NIC)* (5th ed.). St. Louis, MO: C.V. Mosby.

Castro, M., Schechtman, K., Halstead, J., & Bloomberg, G. (2001). Risk factors for asthma morbidity and mortality in a large metropolitan city. *Journal of Asthma, 38*(8), 625–635.

Chiu, W.K., Cheung, P.C., Ng, K.L., Ip, P.L., Sugunan, V.K., Luk, D.C., et al. (2003). Severe acute respiratory syndrome in children: experience in a regional hospital in Hong Kong. *Pediatric Critical Care Medicine: A Journal of the Society of Critical Care Medicine and the World Federation of Pediatric Intensive and Critical Care Societies, 4*(3), 279–283.

Clardy, P.F., &. Manaker, S. (2006). Carbon monoxide poisoning. Retrieved from http://www.uptodate.com (Accessed November 2, 2008).

Code of Federal Regulations Subpart A Sec. 46.102 (2005). *Basic HHS Policy for Protection of Human Research Subjects*. Office of Human Subjects Research. National Institute of Health: Bethesda, MD: http://www.nihtraining.com/ohrsite/guidelines/graybook.html

Deglin, J.H., & Vallerand, A.H. (2009). *Davis's drug guide for nurses* (11th ed.). Philadelphia: F.A. Davis.

Driscoll, W. (2003). Bronchopulmonary dysplasia, *Web MD*. Retrieved from http://www.ama-assn.org/ (Accessed July 7, 2006).

Guinto-Ocampo, H., Bennett, J., & Attia, M. (2008). Predicting pertussis in infants. *Pediatric Emergency Care, 24*(1), 16–20.

Haddad, J. (2004). Congenital disorders of the nose. In Behrman, R.E., Kliegman, R.M., & Jenson, H.B. (Eds.), *Nelson textbook of pediatrics,* 17th ed. Philadelphia: Elsevier, pp. 1386–1387.

Hekmatnia, A. (2003). Congenital diaphragmatic hernia. *Web MD.* Retrieved from http://www.ama-assn.org/ (Accessed November 5, 2008).

Hon, K.L., Leung, C.W., Cheng, W.T., Chan, P.K., Chu, W.C., Kwan, Y.W., et al. (2003). Clinical presentations and outcome of severe acute respiratory syndrome in children. *Lancet, 361*(9370), 1701–1703.

Hoffman, C., & Kamps, B. S. (2003). *SARSReference.* [S.l.]: Amedeo. Retrieved from http://www.sarsreference.com (Accessed November 5, 2008).

Johnson, M., Bulechek, G., Butcher, H., McCloskey Dochterman, J., Maas, M., Moorehead, S., & Swanson, E. (2006). *NANDA, NOC, and NIC linkages: Nursing diagnoses, outcomes, & interventions* (2nd ed.). St. Louis, MO: Mosby Elsevier.

Katz, J.I., & Hall, B.Z. (2005). Cost of influenza hospitalization at a tertiary care children's hospital and its impact on the cost–benefit analysis of the recommendation for universal influenza immunization in children age 6 to 23 months. *Journal of Pediatrics, 147*(6), 801–811.

Kieckhefer, G., & Ratcliffe, M. (2004). Asthma. In P.J. Allen, & J. Vessey, *Primary care of a child with chronic condition* (4th ed., pp. 174–197). St. Louis: C.V. Mosby.

Knutson, A., & Aring, D. (2004). Viral croup. *American Family Physician, 69*(3), 535–540. Retrieved from www.aafp.org/afp (Accessed November 5, 2008).

Long, S. (2004). Pertussis (*Bordetella pertussis* and *B. parapertussis*). In R.E. Behrman, R.N. Kliegman, & H.B. Jenson (Eds) *Nelson textbook of pediatrics* (17th ed., pp. 908–912). Philadelphia: Elsevier.

Mandel, A., & Hales, C. (2005). Smoke inhalation. Retrieved from http://www.uptodate.com (Accessed November 5, 2008).

Mannino, D.M., Homa, D.M., Akinbami, L.J., Moorman, J.E., Gwynn, C., & Redd, S.C. (2002). Surveillance for asthma—United States, 1980-1999. *MMWR. Surveillance Summaries: Asthma action plan: Morbidity and Mortality Weekly Report. Surveillance Summaries / CDC. 51*(1), 1–13.

Maryland Department of Health and Mental Hygiene. (2007). Asthma action plan. Retrieved from http://www.fha.state.md.us/mch/asthma/pdf/Asthma_Action_Plan.pdf (Accessed November 5, 2008).

Moorehead, S., Johnson, M., Maas, M., & Swanson, E. (2008) *Nursing outcomes classification (NOC)* (4th ed.). St. Louis, MO: C.V. Mosby.

Munoz, F.M., & Starke, J.F. (2004). Tuberculosis. In R.E. Behrman, R.M. Kliegman, & H.B. Jenson (Eds.), *Nelson textbook of pediatrics* (17th ed, pp. 958–972). Philadelphia: Elsevier.

NANDA International (2007). *NANDA-I nursing diagnoses: Definitions and classifications 2007–2008.* Philadelphia: NANDA-I.

National Heart, Lung, and Blood Institute: National Asthma Education and Prevention Program. (2007). Expert Panel Report 3 : Guidelines for the diagnosis and management of asthma. Retrieved from http://www.nhlbi.nih.gov/guidelines/asthma/asthgdln.pdf (Accessed November 5. 2008).

Orenstein, S., Peters, J., Khan, S., Yousef, N., & Hussain, S.Z. (2004).The esophagus. In R.E. Behrman, R.M. Kliegman, & H.B. Jenson (Eds.), *Nelson textbook of pediatrics* (17th ed, pp. 1217–1218). Philadelphia: Elsevier.

Panel on Definition and Description. (1995). *Defining and describing complementary and alternative medicine.* CAM Research Methodology Conference April 1995. Retrieved from www.ncbi.nlm.nih.gov/entrez/query.fcgi? cmd=Retrieve&db=PubMed&list_uids=9061989&adopt=Abstract (Accessed November 5, 2008).

Pfeiffer, W. (2005). A multicultural approach to a patient who has a common cold. *Pediatrics in Review, 26*(5), 171–175.

Polark, M.J. (March 2004). Syncytial virus (RSV): Overview, treatment and prevention strategies. *Newborn and Infant Nursing Reviews, 4*(1). Retrieved from http:www.nursingconsult.com/das/article/body (Accessed November 5, 2008).

Porth, C.M. (2005). *Pathophysiology: Concepts of altered health states* (5th ed., pp. 545–546). Philadelphia: Lippincott.

Qureshi, S., & Mink, R. (2003). Aspiration of fruit gel snacks. *Pediatrics 111*, 687–688.

Rahm, N.S., Hansen, J.D., & Sanddal, N.D. (1997). Critical trauma care by the basic EMT. Bozeman, MT: Critical Illness and Trauma Foundation, Inc.

Rovers, M., Glasziou, P., Appelman, C., Burke, P., McCormick, D., Damoiseaux, R., et al. (2006). Antibiotics for acute otitis media: A meta-analysis with individual patient data. *The Lancet, 368*(9545), 1429–1435.

Samet, J.M., & Sockrider, M. (2006). Environmental tobacco smoke exposure in children. Retrieved from http://www.uptodate.com (Accessed November 5, 2008).

Sharma, S. (2006). Tracheoesophageal fistula. *Web MD.* Retrieved from http://www.ama-assn.org/ (Accessed November 5, 2008).

Shin, H., & White-Traut, R. (2005). Nurse-child interaction on an inpatient paediatric unit. *Journal of Advanced Nursing, 52* (1), 56–62.

Steinhorn, R. (2004). Congenital diaphragmatic hernia. *Web MD.* Retrieved from http://www.ama-assn.org/ (Accessed November 5, 2008).

Turner, R.B., & Hayden, G.F. (2004). The common cold. In R.E. Behrman, R.M. Kliegman, & H.B. Jenson (Eds.), *Nelson textbook of pediatrics* (17th ed., pp. 1389–1391). Philadelphia: Elsevier.

Torpy, J.M. (2005). Influenza. *Journal of the American Medical Association, 293*(8), 1024.

U.S. Department of Health and Human Services. (2007). National asthma education and prevention program. Expert panel report 3: Guidelines for the diagnosis and management of asthma. Full report 2007. NIH Publication No. 07–4051. Bethesda, MD: NHLBI Health Information Center. Retrieved from http://www.nhlbi.nih.gov/guidelines/asthma/asthgdln.htm (Accessed July 8, 2008).

Venes, D. (Ed.). (2009). *Taber's cyclopedic medical dictionary* (21st ed.). Philadelphia: F.A. Davis.

Wetmore, R.F. (2004). Tonsils and adenoids. In R.E. Behrman, R.M. Kliegman, & H.B. Jenson (Eds.), *Nelson textbook of pediatrics* (17th ed., pp. 1396–1397). Philadelphia: Elsevier.

WHO, *WER 20/2003.* SARS outbreak in the Philippines. 78, 198–192.

Winklestein, M. (2005). The child with respiratory dysfunction: Smoke inhalation injury. In M.J. Hockenberry, *Wong's Essential of Pediatric Nursing* (7th ed., pp. 787–833). St. Louis, MO: C.V. Mosby.

CONCEPT MAP

Caring for the Child With a Respiratory Condition

Diagnostics / **Anatomical differences**

Could Precipitate a Condition:
- Smaller nares
- Epiglottis: longer, higher, flaccid
- Trachea: shorter, narrower, higher bifurcation
- Increased friction and resistance → difficult ventilation
- Lung tissue immature at birth
- < 6 yrs: abdominal breather
- Less mature immune system

Oxygenation
- Pulse oximetry
- Arterial blood gases

Function
- Pulmonary Function Test
- Slow vital capacity
- Lung volume and capacity

Infectious Conditions
- Pertussis/Whooping Cough
- Tuberculosis
- Influenza

Noninfectious Irritation
- Foreign body aspiration
- Smoke inhalation/passive smoking

Radiological
- X-rays
- CT scan
- Fluoroscopy

Visualization
- Laryngoscopy
- Bronchoscopy
- Thoracoscopy
- Endoscopy
- Otoscopy

Lab studies
- Lung tissue biopsy
- Blood cultures

Upper Airway Disorders
- Sinusitis/nasopharyngitis/pharyngitis
- Tonsillitis
- Croup/croup syndrome
- Otitis media/externa

Lower Airway Disorders
- Bronchitis/Bronchiolitis
- Pneumonias
- SARS

Congenital Conditions
- Choanal atresia
- Esophageal atresia and TEF
- Diaphragmatic hernia
- RDS
- Bronchopulmonary dysplasia
- Cystic fibrosis

Disorders Related to Allergens
- Allergic rhinitis
- Asthma

General Potential Nursing Care
- Assessment: airway patency; color; LOC; cardiac assessment; posture; respiratory rate; chest symmetry percussion/palpation; auscultation; sputum
- Promote adequate oxygenation: clean nasal area; suction; chest PT; vaporizer; oximetry/ABG results; CPAP/mechanical ventilation; stat rx for asthma
- Aspiration precautions; watch feeding position
- Monitor vital signs
- Maintain adequate nutrition and fluid balance
- Protect against infection; hand washing
- Infection processes: possible strict isolation; antibiotic therapy; prevent transmission
- Care of the post-op child
- Promote normal development

Critical Nursing Action:
- Keep child calm during assessments
- Nursing instinct can ID subtle changes before technology
- Prevent resp. infection in BPD

Clinical Alert:
- Retractions indicate use of accessory muscles/trouble
- Respiratory rate >60 endangers air exchange
- Signals such as stridor, grunting, hoarseness can indicate certain conditions
- Maternal polyhydramnios is associated with esophageal atresia
- Use great care/accurate technique with p.o. suctioning
- RDS necessitates assisted mechanical ventilation
- Continuous swallowing might indicate p.o. tonsillectomy bleed
- Rupture tympanic membrane → decrease in pain, temperature, + purulent ear discharge

Nursing Insight:
- Know normal HR/RR
- Chest landmarks help ID conditions
- There are different variations of esophageal atresia
- How to prevent P.O. bleed after tonsillectomy
- Preventing otitis media
- RSV-IGIV: can prevent RSV
- 11-12 y/o needs pertussis booster

Complementary Care:
- Use of chiropractic care for asthma/rhinitis/sinusitis
- Encourage parents to learn Heimlich maneuver

Ethnocultural Considerations:
- Bacille Calmette-Guérin (BCG) vaccine is used worldwide
- Higher asthma rate in African Americans/Hispanics

Across Care Settings:
- Cystic fibrosis → multidisciplinary collaboration/extensive family teaching
- Teach how to avoid/control allergens
- Asthma → requires awareness by multiple community partners/collaborative treatment

Where Research And Practice Meet:
- Nurse needs to interact with child → increases their control/improves outcomes
- 2 studies have found SARS in children

Now Can You:
- Discuss anatomical differences and respiratory assessment in the child
- ID signs, symptoms, care for the child with a congenital respiratory disorder
- Prepare home care and management plans

Caring for the Child with a Gastrointestinal Condition

chapter 25

It's all right to have butterflies in your stomach. Just get them to fly in formation.
—*Laura Moncur's Motivational Quotations:* Dr. Rob Gilbert

LEARNING TARGETS *At the completion of this chapter, the student will be able to:*

◆ Identify the organs in the gastrointestinal system.

◆ Describe the functions (ingestion, digestion, absorption, metabolism, and elimination) of the gastrointestinal system.

◆ Describe the nursing diagnoses, goals, and priority interventions related to children with various gastrointestinal conditions.

◆ Plan nursing care for children with gastrointestinal tract conditions.

◆ Develop and implement specific teaching plans for parents whose children have various gastrointestinal conditions.

◆ Explore treatment and pharmacological options for various gastrointestinal tract conditions.

---

 moving toward evidence-based practice Probiotic Use in Antibiotic-Associated Diarrhea Prevention

Johnston, B.C., Supina, A.L., & Vohra, S. (2006). Probiotics for pediatric antibiotic-associated diarrhea: A meta-analysis of randomized placebo-controlled trials. *CMAJ, 175*(4), 377–383.

The purpose of this study was to assess the efficacy of probiotics in the prevention of antibiotic-associated diarrhea in children. Adverse events associated with coadministration of probiotics and antibiotics were also explored. The incidence of antibiotic-associated diarrhea in children who received broad-spectrum antibiotics was reported as 11% to 62%. A systematic review of probiotic trials was completed. The analysis included six pediatric trials with a total of 707 patients. A significant reduction in the incidence of antibiotic-associated diarrhea in children was reported in all studies. Four of the six studies reported use of *Lactobacillus GG, L. sporogenes,* or *Saccharomyces boulardii* and showed evidence of preventive effects with no reported adverse

events. None of the studies provided a definition for adverse events although four reported minor events to include rash, gas, vomiting, increased phlegm, and chest pain. "The potential protective effects of probiotics to prevent diarrhea in children do not withstand intention-to-treat analysis" (p. 377). Further studies are needed.

1. Based on the findings from this study, are probiotics effective in the treatment and prevention of antibiotic associated diarrhea?
2. How is this information useful to clinical nursing practice?

Suggested Responses for Moving Toward Evidence-Based Practice on the Electronic Study Guide or DavisPlus.

Introduction

Children who experience a gastrointestinal (GI) tract condition can have an isolated condition or may encounter several disorders because the GI tract involves numer-ous organs. In addition, any alteration in the GI tract can affect the child's overall growth and development. Normal growth and development relies on the healthy functioning of the GI tract. The function of the GI tract is to ingest and absorb nutrients and to eliminate waste products. An understanding of the basic anatomy and physiology of the GI tract and common disorders will help the nurse care for the child experiencing alterations in GI tract functioning.

A & P review The Gastrointestinal System

The GI system is responsible for ingestion, digestion, absorption, metabolism, and elimination of solid and liquid nutrients. Each organ in the system performs a specific function in this process. The system is divided into the upper and lower portions. The upper portion includes the mouth (teeth, gums), the esophagus, and the stomach. The lower portion consists of the small intestine, large intestine (colon), rectum, and anus. In addition, other organs are a significant part of the GI system: the liver, pancreas, and gallbladder.

The upper portion of the GI system is responsible for nutrient intake or ingestion: the mouth and esophagus. The tongue senses the taste and texture of food, which initiates salivation. Digestion begins in the mouth with the release of the enzymes amylase and ptyalin, which begin the breakdown of complex starches into disaccharides. The esophagus transports food to the stomach by the process of peristalsis. In the stomach food mixes with gastric fluids and is then propelled into the small intestine.

The lower portion of the GI system handles the remainder of the digestion, absorption, and metabolism processes with the assistance of the liver and pancreas. The small intestine does most of the work of absorption through a system of villi and folds, which increases the absorptive surface. The small intestines further convert disaccharides into monosaccharides. Hindrance of this process can lead to diarrhea. The small intestine is primarily responsible for absorption of carbohydrates, fats, proteins, minerals, and vitamins into the systemic circulation. The duodenum forms the first portion of the small intestines. Pancreatic and bile ducts empty in the upper portion of the duodenum. The duodenum is followed by the jejunum, where the majority of water, protein, carbohydrates, and vitamins are absorbed. Fat breakdown occurs mainly in the jejunum through the secretion of lipases by the pancreas. The lymphatic system then absorbs fats. Proteins are converted to amino acids by the pancreatic enzyme trypsin and are absorbed via the capillary walls of the villi and into the systematic circulation. The last and longest segment of the small intestines is the ileum, which absorbs bile salts, vitamins C and B_{12}, and chloride.

The large intestine takes care of elimination. The content of the intestines enters the cecum through the ileocecal valve, which is located in the right lower quadrant of the abdomen and forms the beginning of the large intestines. The appendix, which is described as a blind tube containing lymphoid tissue, is attached to the cecum. The ascending colon rises along the right anterior portion of the abdomen, followed by the transverse colon, which lies horizontally across the abdomen and then forms the descending colon along the left lateral abdomen. The sigmoid colon follows the descending colon into the pelvic cavity. The sigmoid colon then connects to the rectum, where stool is stored until it is expelled through the anal canal and through the anus. Elimination culminates in the removal of solid waste products through defecation.

Accessory Structures

The liver is located below the right diaphragm and is the largest and heaviest organ in the body. The liver is a vascular organ composed of right and left hepatic lobes. The liver is responsible for metabolizing carbohydrates, fats, and proteins and also breaks down toxic substances such as drugs. In addition, the liver stores vitamins and iron and produces antibodies, bile, prothrombin, and fibrinogen for coagulation.

The gallbladder, which lies within the inferior surface of the liver, excretes and stores bile. The bile is then secreted into the duodenum through the cystic duct and common bile duct, where it assists in the digestion of fats.

The pancreas can be found between the spleen and stomach in the left upper quadrant of the abdominal cavity. The pancreas produces pancreatic enzymes, which are excreted into the duodenum by way of the pancreatic duct. The pancreatic enzymes assist in the metabolism of proteins, fats, and carbohydrates. Insulin and glucagon are also produced by the pancreas and secreted directly into the blood stream. ◆

Developmental Aspects of the Gastrointestinal System

The GI system plays an essential role in a child's growth and development. Because the GI system is complex, the nurse must understand the ways in which each developmental stage contributes to the promotion of the health of the child.

The infant has several physiological mechanisms in place to ensure the adequate intake of nutrients. The infant has a built-in safeguard to prevent choking while swallowing and sucking. The posterior portion of the tongue that separates the mouth and throat is raised against the soft palate while the infant sucks. This allows the infant to suck and breathe at same time. The infant also has a longer posterior soft palate, which assists him or her in swallowing milk. In addition, the passage from mouth to pharynx is smaller, which helps to control the amount of liquid that is taken in. The nurse can teach the parents that the infant's stomach usually empties in 2.5 to 3 hours and this is the reason that the infant has frequent feedings. Digestion takes place in the intestines so it is important that the intestines function properly. In addition, the liver and pancreas do not mature until 6 months of age. The nurse can therefore tell the parents that infants younger than 6 months of age do not require solid foods. Pancreatic lipase is essential for fat and protein metabolism but is not adequately secreted until age 1 year, which limits the body's ability to absorb fats, such as those present in cow's milk and reinforces the need to carefully introduce foods into the infant diet, limiting foods to those that are specially prepared for infant digestion.

Nursing Insight— Infant stools

Infant stools are watery and frequently related to food passing quickly with not enough time to absorb water. Infants do not absorb water as rapidly as older children do. When defecating (evacuation of the bowels, feces), the infant may appear to be straining because of immature muscle coordination (Venes, 2009).

By 2 years, the child's salivary glands reach adult size (Murphy, 2004). The average toddler gains 5 to 6 lb. (2.3 to 2.7 kg) per year. The stomach capacity increases to about 500 mL and the liver matures to become more efficient in vitamin storage, glycogenesis (the formation of glycogen from glucose [Venes, 2009]), and amino acid changes (Murphy, 2004). The growth of the child's digestive system slows during the toddler years, which leads to a reduction in caloric needs from those of the infant period. The average toddler needs approximately 102 kcal/kg (46 kcal/lb) as opposed to 108 kcal/kg (50 kcal/lb) during infancy. Since the toddler characteristically has a decreased appetite and reduced metabolic rate, his or her appetite may be sporadic or appear finicky. Because of this sporadic behavior, the toddler may also go on food fads or "jags," preferring only one item and refusing others that he or she has preferred in the past.

By age 4 to 5, the GI system is mature enough for the child to eat a full range of food, with stools becoming more like those of adults (Murphy, 2004). The preschool-age child continues to have appetite fluctuations, with periods of overeating or refusal to eat. The preschool-age child gains about 4 to 5 lb (1.8 to 2.3 kg) per year.

By the time the child reaches the middle school age years, the GI tract has become relatively stable. The digestive system is adult size and functioning. Stools are usually passed once per day and are well formed.

Nursing Insight— Infant bowel sounds

In the newborn, bowel sounds are audible within the first few hours of life. A newborn with a scaphoid abdomen or signs of respiratory distress should be evaluated carefully for bowel sounds and/or decreased breath sounds in the chest, which may be evidence of congenital diaphragmatic hernia. A congenital diaphragmatic hernia is an opening between the chest and abdominal cavities through which abdominal organs may herniate into the chest cavity, compromising respiratory and cardiac structures.

clinical alert

Abdominal pain in children

In children, abdominal pain can be referred from an extra-abdominal source such as pneumonia, a urinary tract infection, or testicular torsion or can be associated with a systemic disease. Abdominal pain is a common complaint in ill children and can be found in conditions such as streptococcal pharyngitis, lower lobe pneumonia, sickle cell disease, cystic fibrosis, as well as in other conditions.

A child's abdominal pain experience is usually limited and the child may be unable to accurately describe or pinpoint the location or sensation.

Structural Gastrointestinal Disorders

INGUINAL HERNIA

Inguinal hernia is the most common type of hernia in children, accounting for 80% of all childhood hernias, or approximately 10 to 20 in 1000 live births (Mao, 2005). An inguinal hernia arises from the failure of the processus vaginalis to atrophy and close during the eighth month of gestation. This provides a canal that allows for abdominal fluid or structure (bowel, ovary, or Fallopian tube) to extend up to or through the inguinal ring into the scrotum or labia.

This type of hernia is five times more common in males with a 30% incidence among premature children (Mao, 2005). An inguinal hernia is defined as the protrusion of bowel through the inguinal canal and is usually evident by a protrusion in the inguinal area and a bulging of the scrotal sac (Mao, 2005). In females, the hernia may involve a protrusion through the round ligament into the labia. Inguinal hernias in the pediatric population are generally considered indirect, meaning that the hernia "passes through the internal abdominal ring, traverses the spermatic cord through the inguinal canal and emerges at the external inguinal ring".

Signs and Symptoms

Most inguinal hernias are painless and may be more apparent with coughing, crying, or straining and disappear during quiet periods.

Diagnosis

An inguinal hernia is identified by a painless swelling in the inguinal area that extends toward or into the scrotum. Most inguinal hernias are observed by 6 months of age with more than 50% diagnosed before 1 year of age.

Nursing Care

Elective surgical correction is the treatment of choice for the healthy child.

Nursing Insight— Incarcerated Hernia

An incarcerated hernia is a portion of the intestine that cannot be returned to the abdominal cavity. The condition causes obstruction or pain and if left untreated can lead to strangulation (Venes, 2009) and requires prompt referral and correction to prevent the bowel from becoming strangulated and necrotic.

The majority of inguinal hernias are managed on an outpatient basis. The initial nursing care of the child hospitalized for the hernia repair involves parental education and preoperative preparation of the child.

"What to say" — *Inguinal hernia*

If the child has an inguinal hernia, the nurse can tell the parents that the surgery will repair the defect caused by the hernia. Recovery for an inguinal hernia is usually rapid and the child will return home the same day as the surgery. After surgery, the nurse can inform the parents that the child's vital signs are monitored frequently and that the child's position will be changed often to avoid undue stress on the surgical area. Postoperative care includes keeping the wound clean and dry and managing the child's pain. For a child who is not toilet trained, changing diapers as soon as possible is important to prevent wound irritation and infection.

Discharge instructions include informing the parents on wound care and the importance of keeping the surgical site clean and dry. The nurse can also tell the parents that the child can resume normal activity within 4–6 weeks and that they may be given a prescription for stool softeners for the child to prevent straining during defecation (Venes, 2009).

UMBILICAL HERNIA

The nurse understands that umbilical hernia is the most common type of hernia in infants. An umbilical hernia is the protrusion of the intestine through the abdominal fascia, which is often identifiable during crying, defecation, or coughing (Fig. 25-1). An umbilical hernia occurs as a result of failure of the umbilical ring to close, which normally begins at the end of the first trimester. The incidence of umbilical hernias is estimated at one out of every six live births. Umbilical hernias are more common in premature and low-birth-weight infants and ten times more common in African American children. Umbilical hernias are also more common in children with Down syndrome and in children with hypothyroidism.

Signs and Symptoms

The majority of umbilical hernias are asymptomatic. Umbilical hernias may also appear be more prominent when the infant is crying.

Figure 25-1 An umbilical hernia is the protrusion of the intestine through the abdominal fascia.

Diagnosis

Umbilical hernias can be identified as a soft midline swelling in the umbilical area, which can be reduced with pressure.

Nursing Care

Most umbilical hernias resolve spontaneously by 3 to 5 years of age, though there is a decreased likelihood of spontaneous closure for hernias, larger than 1.5 cm in diameter or for those with a large, proboscis-like defect (elongated or extensible tubular process). Surgery is considered for persistent hernias beyond the age of 5, incarcerated hernias, and hernias that enlarge dramatically. Postoperative complications of umbilical hernia repair are rare.

The nurse should instruct the parents about umbilical hernia and prognosis for the spontaneous resolution of the umbilical hernia. The initial nursing care of the child hospitalized for the repair of an umbilical hernia involves parental education and preoperative preparation of the child. The majority of umbilical hernias are managed on an outpatient basis. Postoperative care includes keeping the wound clean and dry and managing the child's pain. A pressure dressing is generally maintained for 48 hours postoperatively. The child may resume a normal diet and activity postoperatively, although parents should be instructed to have the child avoid strenuous activities for 2 to 3 weeks after the surgery.

ANORECTAL MALFORMATIONS

Anorectal malformations range from simple, such as an imperforate anus to include other associated anomalies of not only the GI systems but also the GU system and pelvic organs. The incidence of anorectal malformation is approximately one in 4000 to 5000 births and is more common in males. As one of the most common groups of congenital defects, these abnormalities are caused by abnormal or arrested development. The location of the abnormality and actual organ systems involved is related to the week of gestation at which the development was disrupted (Potts, 2002). The etiology of anorectal malformations is unknown.

Signs and Symptoms

Anorectal abnormalities are generally apparent at birth. Rectal atresia (closure) and stenosis (constriction or narrowing of a passage) may initially present as a normal appearing anal opening but is later detected as an abnormal situation. Additional signs of rectal stenosis include vomiting, abdominal distention, and difficult stooling. Rectal atresia is defined as a complete obstruction that precludes the passage of stool. Immediate surgical intervention is mandatory for rectal atresia. On the other hand, rectal stenosis may present with a ribbon-like or narrow stool, which is not always readily apparent at birth. More extensive defects may present with evidence of a rectal connection to the vagina or urethra as the opening through which the stool passes.

Absence of a rectal opening is referred to as an imperforate anus. This defect can be manifested in several forms, which include a fistula or connection from the distal rectum to the perineum or GU system. Passage of meconium through the vagina, urethra, or an opening under the scrotum is early evidence of an imperforate anus though the presence of a fistula may not be evident at birth. In this condition, as peristalsis increases the meconium is forced through the abnormal passage.

Diagnosis

Diagnosis is made by physical examination and radiological imaging, which indicates the level of the defect and location of fistula formation (Potts, 2002). The visualization of gas in the bladder or urethra during imaging also indicates the presence of a fistula connection between the bowel and associated structure (Potts, 2002). Magnetic resonance imaging (MRI) of the lumbosacral spinal cord is required for all children presenting with an imperforate anus to rule out the presence of a tethered spinal cord, which is common in children with this malformation (Bishop, 2006). An ultrasound (outlines the shape of tissues and organs) of the abdomen and pelvis, an intravenous pyelogram (provides information about the structure and function of the kidney, ureter, and bladder), and voiding cystogram (radiography of the bladder) are performed to evaluated associated defects of the urinary tract.

Nursing Care

Management of anorectal malformations may require extensive treatment, depending on the extent of the defect and associated organ involvement, including GI, urinary, and reproductive systems. Repeated manual dilation can be used to treat anal stenosis. The creation of a new anal opening may be used to correct anatomically lower anorectal defects.

A two-stage repair is generally necessary for anatomically higher anorectal defects. The first stage of anorectal repair involves resection and the creation of a temporary colostomy. The second stage involves "the closure of the colostomy and a pull through procedure in which the blind pouch of the rectum is anastomosed to the anus" (Potts, 2002, p. 668).

Nursing care for anorectal malformation may involve the initial diagnosis of an anorectal defect by observation of the passage of meconium and assessment of the patency of the rectum through the insertion of a rectal thermometer (Potts, 2002). Overall nursing care depends on the type of defect and the extent of surgical correction. Care of the infant before surgery includes caregiver education and maintenance of intravenous fluids while the child is kept NPO.

In addition to basic needs of the child undergoing surgery of the GI tract, pain control and the importance of infection control must be stressed related to the location of the surgical incision and the potential for fecal or urinary contamination. For high anorectal malformations colostomy care is also required. With the presence of a colostomy the nurse should stress the importance of good skin care in the postoperative period. Nasogastric decompression is often required early in the postoperative period. Oral feedings are generally initiated with the reestablishment of peristalsis and once stooling has begun.

Discharge instructions include colostomy care, wound care, prevention of infection, and the procedure for anal dilation if appropriate for the defect. The importance of adequate fluids is also stressed. The caregiver should be instructed on the potential need for dietary fiber and the possible use of stool softeners or bulking agents in the future. In addition, the caregiver should be advised of the potential for delayed toilet training.

Obstructive Gastrointestinal Disorders

HYPERTROPHIC PYLORIC STENOSIS

The etiology of hypertrophic pyloric stenosis is unknown. Suggested causal theories include a deficiency in inhibitory neuronal signals or molecular causes, such as a mechanism similar to that of Hirschsprung's disease discussed later in this chapter (Bishop, 2006). Ganglionic cell immaturity has also been suggested as a causative factor.

 Ethnocultural Considerations— *Occurrence of hypertrophic pyloric stenosis*

Hypertrophic pyloric stenosis occurs in approximately 6–8 of 1000 live births in the United States (Bishop, 2006). The incidence of pyloric stenosis is more common in the Caucasian population compared to 1.8 per 1000 live births in the Hispanic population and 0.7 in the African American population. Males, especially firstborns, are affected two to four times more often than females are and there may be a positive family history.

Signs and Symptoms

Hypertrophic pyloric stenosis typically occurs in a healthy male infant with a pattern of normal feedings and new onset of nonbilious vomiting. The vomiting usually begins with episodes of regurgitation during the first few weeks of life (Parks & Yetman, 2004). Vomiting usually occurs immediately after a feeding and may become projectile in nature. The infant generally appears hungry immediately after vomiting and eagerly wants to feed again. Weight loss, dehydration, and constipation may also be seen. During palpation, in an infant between 3 and 12 weeks with projectile, nonbilious vomiting and an olive-shaped mass, pyloric stenosis may be suspected.

Visible reverse, or left to right, peristalsis may be observable in the left upper quadrant upon abdominal assessment and the stomach may become enlarged with retained food and secretions (Parks & Yetman, 2004). Jaundice and hiatal hernia are associated secondary features, which may occur in a small percentage of affected infants (Reichard & Lake, 2005).

clinical alert

Vomiting

Projectile vomiting is the classic and most common symptom of hypertrophic pyloric stenosis.

Diagnosis

Diagnosis of hypertrophic pyloric stenosis can be made by palpating the pyloric mass. The mass is olive-shaped, movable, firm, and best palpated from the left side and located above and to the right of the umbilicus in the mid-epigastrium (the superior central portion of the abdomen) beneath the liver edge (Bishop, 2006). An abdominal x-ray film may show an enlarged stomach with diminished or absent gas in the intestine (Bishop, 2006). Examination of the pylorus on ultrasound shows elongation and thickening of the pylorus, which may be confirmed by a barium upper GI series. Confirmation by an upper GI series demonstrates a "string sign," which is caused by the barium passing through narrowed pylorus (Bishop, 2006).

 diagnostic tools Ultrasound

A diagnosis is often made after the history and physical examination. The diagnosis can be established 60% to 80% of the time by an experienced examiner. If the diagnosis of hypertrophic pyloric stenosis is inconclusive an ultrasound can be used to demonstrate an elongated muscular mass surrounding a long pyloric canal. Ultrasound confirms the diagnosis of hypertrophic pyloric stenosis.

Nursing Care

Treatment for hypertrophic pyloric stenosis is surgery. The surgical procedure of choice is the Ramstedt pyloromyotomy (incision and suture of the pyloric sphincter) and is performed by laparoscopy (abdominal exploration) with an endoscope. The pyloric mass is split without cutting the mucosa and the incision is closed (Bishop, 2006). The operative mortality rate is very low, 0 to 0.5%. Endoscopic balloon dilation has also been successful in infants with persistent vomiting.

Initial care of the child with the diagnosis of pyloric stenosis should include a careful history and assessment of the child. The nurse needs to be alert to signs of dehydration, such as changes in skin turgor, appearance of the mucous membranes, depressed fontanel, presence or absence of tears, urine output, and changes in vital signs as well as weight loss and evidence of discomfort.

Before surgery, the child is given nothing by mouth (NPO) and a nasal gastric tube is inserted to provide gastric decompression (the removal of pressure). Surgery may be performed without delay in infants without dehydration and electrolyte imbalances. If dehydration is present, the dehydration imbalance is corrected with intravenous fluids and administration of appropriate electrolyte therapy.

Postoperative care includes maintaining fluid and electrolyte balance. The nurse should communicate to the family that it is common for the infant to experience some vomiting in the first 24 to 36 hours after surgery (Parks & Yetman, 2004). Fluid balance is maintained through administration of intravenous fluids and oral liquids as tolerated. Small, frequent, clear liquid feedings, such as electrolyte solutions, are begun about 4 to 6 hours postoperatively. Formula or breast feedings may be resumed in 24 hours if clear liquids are tolerated. It is important for the nurse to continue to monitor for signs of dehydration and for the infant's response to oral fluids. After surgery, the family members can be instructed on the importance of saving wet diapers that are weighed in order to measure output. Postoperative care also includes monitoring the surgical site for signs of infection, keeping the wound clean and dry, and providing pain relief.

Discharge instructions include care of the incision and observation for signs of infection. The nurse must instruct caregivers to observe the infant's response to feedings, as some vomiting may still occur within the first 48 hours postoperatively. Vomiting beyond 48 hours must be reported to the child's health care provider.

 nursing diagnoses Hypertrophic Pyloric Stenosis

- Fluid Volume Deficit related to the effects of frequent vomiting
- Nutritional Imbalance: Less than Body Requirements related to vomiting and gradual reintroduction of feedings.
- Pain related to surgical trauma
- Risk for Infection related to surgical incision.
- Caregiver Knowledge deficit related to postoperative care of the infant

INTUSSUSCEPTION

Intussusception is a condition that occurs when a proximal section of the intestine and the mesentery (the peritoneal fold that encircles the small intestine and connects it to the posterior abdominal wall) "telescopes" into a distal section of the intestine (Mow, 2005; Venes, 2009). Most intussusception conditions occur between the ages of 5 and 9 months but children can be susceptible until early school age. The incidence of intussusception is 1 to 4 per 1000 live births and is four times more common in males (Mow, 2005). Suggested predisposing factors to the development of intussusception include the presence of polyps, Meckel's diverticulum, Henoch–Schönlein purpura, constipation, lymphomas, lipomas, parasites, rotavirus, adenovirus, and the presence of foreign bodies. Intussusception may also occur as a complication of cystic fibrosis (Petersen-Smith, 2004).

Signs and Symptoms

The most characteristic symptom of intussusception is acute abdominal pain caused by the spasm of the telescoping bowel. This pain frequently mimics the pain experienced by "colicky" infants because it is acute, causing the infants to cry and pull their legs up toward the abdomen. The pain is relieved once the abdomen relaxes. The other classic symptom is the presence of currant jelly stools. Vomiting may or may not be present and it may or may not be projectile. Other symptoms of intussusception include fever, dehydration, abdominal distention, lethargy, and grunting due to pain.

Diagnosis

Diagnosis of intussusception is based on a history of the characteristic symptoms and the physical findings during examination. The presence of a "sausage-shaped" mass in the upper right quadrant (Danca's sign) during palpation of the abdomen is indicative of intussusception (Petersen-Smith, 2004). Although the upper right quadrant is the most common site, the mass may be felt in other abdominal areas too. The abdomen is distended and tender on palpation and bowel sounds may be either increased or decreased.

 assessment tools Classic Symptomatic Triad for Intussusception

The classic symptomatic triad for intussusception includes:

- "Paroxysmal, episodic abdominal pain with vomiting every 5–30 minutes.
- Screaming and drawing up legs with periods of calm, sleeping, or lethargy between episodes (Fig. 25-2).
- Stool, possible diarrheal in nature, with blood (currant jelly)" (Petersen-Smith, 2004, p. 862).

 diagnostic tools Intussusception

A flat-plate x-ray film of the child can appear normal early in the course of the disorder. However, an abdominal "ultrasound establishes the diagnosis in 90% of the cases" (Petersen-Smith, 2004, p. 862).

Nursing Care

A barium or air enema is used to both diagnose and treat intussusception. In radiological reduction, the barium (contrast media) or air allows visualization of the telescoped bowel. The pressure applied by the enema may cause the telescoped bowel to return to its normal position, thus relieving the obstruction. Reduction rates are reported as high as 65% to 90% through the instillation of barium or air. If radiological reduction is ineffective or if peritonitis, perforation, or shock is evident, prompt surgical correction is required (Petersen-Smith, 2004). The surgical procedure either repairs the bowel or removes any portion that has been permanently damaged.

When the child has been diagnosed with intussusception, the nurse can provide information about the condition and reassurance to the parents. If the treatment is managed through radiological reduction, the child should be observed for passage of stool and barium or contrast material as indicated.

Figure 25-2 Infant with paroxysmal, episodic abdominal pain displays screaming and drawing up the legs.

If the child is having surgery, preparation before surgery includes placing the child NPO, inserting a nasogastric tube, and initiating intravenous fluid therapy. The nurse is responsible for monitoring the infant for signs of perforation (a hole), peritonitis (inflammation of the abdominal cavity), or shock in addition to evidence of increased pain. The nurse also monitors and records the child's stools. The nurse understands that the spontaneous passing of a stool may indicate a resolution of the obstruction. Postoperative care and discharge instructions will be similar to that of the child surgery for pyloric stenosis.

 clinical alert

Signs of perforation and peritonitis

The child with perforation has acute pain, beginning over the perforated area and spreading over the abdomen. The abdomen may become rigid and the child may experience nausea and vomiting, tachycardia, fevers, chills, sweats, confusion, and decreased urinary output (Venes, 2009).

The child with peritonitis has moderate or mild abdominal pain that worsens with movement. Fever, change in bowel habits, and malaise are also common. In addition, the child has nausea, loss of appetite, and fever or hypothermia. During the nursing assessment, the nurse notes that the abdomen is distended with decreased bowel sounds (Venes, 2009).

MALROTATION AND VOLVULUS

Abnormal rotation of the intestine around the superior mesenteric artery during fetal development may lead to malrotation of the intestine. Malrotation may present in utero or remain asymptomatic throughout life. Malrotation is the most serious type of intestinal obstruction because it may lead to intestinal necrosis, peritonitis, perforation, and death related to a complete twisting of the intestine around itself or volvulus. The incidence of malrotation is approximately one in 500 live births.

Signs and Symptoms

Symptoms of malrotation or volvulus may occur at any age but are most common in the first month of life. Fifty percent to 75% of children who become symptomatic do so in the first month of life, with approximately 90% becoming symptomatic within the first year.

A major symptom is intermittent bilious or green vomit. Additional symptoms include abdominal distention, recurrent abdominal pain, lower GI bleeding, a palpable epigastric mass, dehydration, lethargy, and shock.

 clinical alert

Shock

Signs of shock include tachycardia; tachypnea; hypotension; and cool, clammy, or cyanotic skin (Venes, 2009).

The child's stools may be bloody, which suggests ischemia and possibly gangrene of the bowel. Without surgical correction, ischemia can lead to infarction of the bowel, which is demonstrated by painful abdominal

Nursing Care Plan A Child Who Has Undergone Abdominal Surgery

Nursing Diagnosis: Imbalanced Nutrition: Less than body requirements related to inability to ingest nutrients by mouth

Measurable Short-term Goal: The child will receive adequate fluid intake.

Measurable Long-term Goal: The child will receive adequate nutrients to meet metabolic needs and for healing.

NOC Outcomes:
Nutritional Status (1004) Extent to which nutrients are available to meet metabolic needs

NIC Interventions:
Nutrition Therapy (1120)
Diet Staging (1020)

Nursing Interventions:

1. Maintain NPO status as ordered by caregiver.

   RATIONALE: To promote bowel rest and healing related to the surgical procedure.

2. Assist mother with pumping and storing breast milk if appropriate.

   RATIONALE: Pumping helps to maintain milk production. Breast milk contains maternal antibodies, which may aid healing.

3. Maintain intravenous access and administer fluids and medications as prescribed. Monitor intake and output.

   RATIONALE: To provide short-term fluid, electrolyte, and caloric support (specify actions of medications) and maintain fluid balance.

4. Auscultate for presence of bowel sounds each shift.

   RATIONALE: Adequate bowel motility is required before the reintroduction of oral fluids and foods.

5. Collaborate with the care provider to introduce oral clear liquids and progress to small, frequent feedings as tolerated. (For infants, progress from glucose water or oral rehydration solution to half-strength formula, to full-strength formula.)

   RATIONALE: To determine tolerance of oral fluids and foods by introducing in small amounts.

---

distension and shock. Older children show recurrent abdominal pain, intermittent vomiting, chronic diarrhea, and symptoms related to failure to thrive or malabsorption (inadequate absorption of nutrients from the intestinal tract) (Venes, 2009).

Thirty percent to 60% of children with malrotation have associated anomalies, such as diaphragmatic hernia, omphalocele, gastroschisis, intestinal atresia, imperforate anus, Meckel diverticulum, Hirschsprung disease, and congenital heart disease.

Diagnosis

Diagnosis is based on history, physical examination, and radiographic studies such as barium enema and upper GI series, which is the definitive procedure to diagnose the condition. "The abnormality has a characteristic 'corkscrew,' 'coiled,' or 'bird's beak appearance.'"

Nursing Care

Surgical treatment for malrotation and volvulus includes resection of nonviable intestinal segments with anastomosis (surgical connection). Short bowel syndrome is a potential postoperative complication because extensive portions of the bowel are either reconstructed or removed. For the asymptomatic child younger than 2 years of age, timely repair is indicated to prevent potential complications.

Preoperatively nursing care includes intravenous hydration to restore fluid and electrolyte balance, nasogastric suction, and administration of intravenous antibiotics. Postoperative care is comparable to that of an infant or child undergoing abdominal surgery.

 Now Can You— **Identify obstructive gastrointestinal disorders?**

1. Identify obstructive GI disorders?
2. Identify signs and symptoms of obstructive GI disorders?
3. Identify nursing care for obstructive GI disorders?

Inflammatory Disorders

INFLAMMATORY BOWEL DISEASE

Inflammatory bowel disease (IBD) is a general term often used to refer to two major forms of chronic intestinal inflammatory conditions, Crohn's disease and ulcerative colitis, which have common epidemiology and clinical features. Both Crohn's disease and ulcerative colitis are characterized by extraintestinal and systemic features, yet they are distinct disorders as described in the following sections.

Crohn's Disease

Crohn's disease is a chronic inflammatory disease characterized by periods of exacerbations and remissions. Crohn's disease can affect any portion of the GI tract. The bowel may present with a combination of nonsequential areas of pathology and disease-free sections of bowel. Crohn's disease rarely affects the oropharynx, esophagus, and stomach;

the small bowel is affected 25% to 30% of the time; the colon and anus are affected 25% of the time; the ileocolonic region is affected up to 40% of the time; and diffuse disease occurs 5% of the time (Petersen-Smith, 2004). The majority of Crohn's disease occurs in the terminal ileum, with resultant potential nutritional deficiencies.

The incidence of Crohn's disease in the Western population is 16 out of 100,000 and has increased during the past few decades. It is more common in Caucasians, and affects males and females equally. The age at onset is between 10 and 20 years, and the condition occurs throughout the life span with peaks in the second, fourth, and sixth decades of life. Although the cause of Crohn's disease is unknown, it is thought that the susceptibility to Crohn's is most likely inherited and "is most likely a genetically determined response that is immunologically mediated" (Petersen-Smith, 2004, p. 869). The incidence in siblings is as high as 35% (Petersen-Smith, 2004).

SIGNS AND SYMPTOMS. Children with Crohn's disease may have an acute or insidious onset. Common signs and symptoms include abdominal pain, diarrhea, anorexia, and weight loss. Clinical presentation of Crohn's disease varies extensively depending on the area of the intestine that is involved and the severity of the inflammation (Campbell & Balistreri, 2005). If the disease is limited to the colon, symptoms are similar to those of ulcerative colitis. Upper GI tract involvement is manifested by vomiting and epigastric pain. Small bowel involvement is manifest by cramplike pain commonly located in the right lower quadrant and is associated with tenderness and a feeling of fullness.

Extraintestinal symptoms may include, but are not limited to, fever, growth delay, delayed sexual development, arthralgias (joint pain) or arthritis in the large joints, stomatitis (inflammation of the mouth lips, tongue, and mucous membranes), apthous ulcers, uveitis (inflammation of the eye), conjunctivitis, renal stones, and erythema nodosum (a tender, red, nodular rash on the shins) (Petersen-Smith, 2004; Venes, 2009).

DIAGNOSIS. Diagnosis is based on client history, physical findings, and laboratory results. Laboratory findings may include leukocytosis, microcytic anemia, low serum iron and total iron-binding capacity, low serum albumin, thrombocytosis, and elevated sedimentation rates and C-reactive protein.

NURSING CARE. In children, the treatment for Crohn's is pharmacological, nutritional, and surgical. The goals of treatment include "controlling the disease, including remission and preventing relapses," while maintaining adequate nutrition (Potts, 2002, p. 678). Corticosteroids are effective for reduction of inflammation in moderate to severe disease and may be given orally, rectally, or intravenously for acute exacerbations. Metronidazole (Flagyl) and ciprofloxacin (Cipro) have demonstrated effectiveness in the treatment of perianal complications. Antibiotics such as ampicillin (Marcillin), gentamicin (Garamycin), clindamycin (Cleocin), and metronidazole (Flagyl) are effective during acute exacerbations (Petersen-Smith, 2004). Immunosuppressive medications are useful with corticosteroid-resistant disease (Potts, 2002).

where research and practice meet: Crohn's disease

Research exploring the use of an enteric-coated fish oil preparation in adult Crohn's disease patients found that those who received the fish-oil preparation were less likely to have relapses than patients who received placebos. Fish oil has been found to not only have anti-inflammatory actions but also to increase the absorption of nutrients resulting in improved nutrition.

Nursing care includes the administration of medication and nutritional management, emotional support, and community referral (Potts, 2002). The focus of care during periods of remission involves monitoring compliance. As symptoms resolve, the child may resist taking medications. The adolescent with Crohn's disease presents unique challenges in the treatment of his or her disease. Adolescents have a natural desire to be "normal" and to be like their peers. This may lead the adolescent to resist taking prescribed medications that cause obvious side effects, such as those experienced with prolonged use of steroids.

Surgery for a child with Crohn's disease may be indicated if the child does not respond to medical treatment, or in the case of bowel strictures, obstruction, perforation or intractable bleeding or diarrhea. Surgical correction involves removal or resection of the diseased segment with resection or anastomosis (connection). The nurse should communicate to the family that surgical repair does not cure Crohn's disease (Potts, 2002).

Across Care Settings: Promoting growth

The nurse understands that no special diet is indicated for children with Crohn's disease. Nutritional therapy may be helpful in correcting malnutrition and promoting growth. A well-balanced, high-protein diet is recommended for children whose symptoms do not prohibit oral intake. Fiber-containing foods, such as seeds, popcorn, and corn, may produce symptoms and obstructions in children with intestinal stricture though there is no evidence that avoiding specific foods influences severity of the disease in most children. A dietitian teaches the family how to provide for adequate nutrition to promote growth. High-calorie liquid supplements may be recommended as well as supplemental vitamins, especially the fat-soluble vitamins, and minerals.

medication: Steroid Side Effects

CARDIOVASCULAR: Edema hypertension, congestive heart failure
CENTRAL NERVOUS SYSTEM: Vertigo, seizures, psychoses, headache
DERMATOLOGICAL: Acne, skin atrophy, impaired wound healing, petechiae, bruising
ENDOCRINE AND METABOLIC: Cushing's syndrome, growth suppression, glucose intolerance, and sodium and water retention
GASTROINTESTINAL: Peptic ulcer, nausea, vomiting
GENITOURINARY: Menstrual irregularities
NEUROMUSCULAR AND SKELETAL: Muscle weakness, osteoporosis, fractures
OCULAR: Cataracts, elevated intraocular pressure, glaucoma

Data from Deglin, J.H., & Vallerand, A.H. (2009). *Davis's drug guide for nurses* (11th ed.). Philadelphia: F.A. Davis.

Emotional support is another important nursing intervention for both the child and family in the management of this chronic condition. The nurse can communicate to the family that the child with Crohn's disease may experience depression, anxiety, and low self-esteem. Early detection of psychological problems requires referral, which often involves both the child and family (Potts, 2002).

 nursing diagnoses The Child with Crohn's Disease

- Imbalanced Nutrition: Less than Body Requirements related to inability to ingest, and absorb food and nutrients
- Risk for Fluid Volume Deficit related to excessive losses through diarrhea
- Pain related to inflammation and irritation of the bowel
- Potential for Delayed Growth and Development related to effects of physical illness and inability to maintain nutritional needs
- Anxiety related to threat to self–concept from change in health status

Ulcerative Colitis

Ulcerative colitis is an acute or chronic inflammation of the colon, which is characterized by recurring bloody diarrhea (Petersen-Smith, 2004). Unlike Crohn's disease, ulcerative colitis involves a continuous segment of the colon. The pathology of ulcerative colitis is described as a superficial, acute inflammation of mucosa with microscopic crypt abscess (Petersen-Smith, 2004).

The cause of ulcerative colitis is unknown. The probability of a genetically determined and an altered immunologically mediated response to the intestinal mucosa is likely (Petersen-Smith, 2004). Infectious agents, autoimmune responses, and environmental factors play a role though no specific responsible agents have been identified (Bishop, 2006).

The incidence of ulcerative colitis is increasing, especially in industrialized countries, though it is relatively uncommon in tropical and underdeveloped countries (Bishop, 2006). Ulcerative colitis is more common in the Jewish population. In addition, there is a higher risk in families who have a close relative with ulcerative colitis (Bishop, 2006). The overall incidence of ulcerative colitis is 0.05 of every 1000 persons. The peak onset occurs between ages 16 and 20, with approximately 20% of the cases occurring in children and adolescents younger than 20 years (Bishop, 2006).

SIGNS AND SYMPTOMS. Ulcerative colitis is characterized by abdominal pain, bloody diarrhea, urgency, and tenesmus (a painful spasmodic contraction of the anal sphincter leading to the sensation of constantly needing to empty the bowel). Children experience left lower quadrant pain with cramping, which increases before defecation and passing flatus (Petersen-Smith, 2004). Weight loss and delays in growth and sexual maturation may also occur. Other manifestations, though not present in all cases, may include arthritis/arthralgias of the large joints, oral ulcera, primary sclerosing cholangitis (chronic liver inflammation leading to scarring of hepatic ducts), uveitis, and skin lesions such as those found in pyoderma gangrenosum (a rare, ulcerating skin disease) and erythema nodosum (a tender, red, nodular rash) (Bishop, 2006; Petersen-Smith, 2004).

DIAGNOSIS. Diagnosis of ulcerative colitis in a child is based on history and physical findings. Radiological and

Labs: Laboratory Findings for Ulcerative Colitis

Laboratory findings for ulcerative colitis may include elevated sedimentation rate, microcytic anemia, and elevated white blood cell count with left shift, antineutrophil cytoplasmic antibodies (ANA) present in 80% (Petersen-Smith, 2004).

endoscopic examinations are used to evaluate the characteristics and location of the lesions.

NURSING CARE. Goals of the treatment of ulcerative colitis include disease control, inducing remission, preventing relapse, and achieving normal growth and lifestyle (Petersen-Smith, 2004). Pharmacological, nutritional, surgical, and psychosocial management may be included in the plan of care. Intravenous or oral steroids are used for moderate to severe ulcerative colitis, with dosages tapered when the child is in remission. Immunomodulatory agents (alternative medications such as vitamins, minerals, and natural foods) are given as well as medications such as azathioprine (Imuran) or 6-mercaptopurine (Purinethol), are used to wean the patient off of steroids. Aminosalicylates relieve symptoms and inflammation in the intestines and help IBD go into remission. Iron supplementation is given to correct anemia and antispasmodics may be given before meals (Petersen-Smith, 2004).

The nurse can communicate to the family that nutritional recommendations include use of a diet high in protein and carbohydrates with normal fat and decreased roughage. Vitamin and iron supplements are recommended. Nutritional supplements may also be used.

Ulcerative colitis is curable surgically with a total mucosal proctocolectomy with the ileal pouch–anal anastomosis as the most common restorative surgery. Failed medical therapy and persistent hemorrhage are the most common indications for surgical correction.

As with Crohn's disease, nursing care includes medication and nutritional management, emotional support, and community referral (Potts, 2002). A referral should be made to an ophthalmologist to rule out ophthalmologic manifestations of the disease. Psychosocial therapy may be indicated, as depressive disorders are common (Petersen-Smith, 2004). Refer to care of the child with Crohn's disease for general nursing management.

 Now Can You— Distinguish between Crohn's disease and ulcerative colitis?

1. Discuss the differences between Crohn's disease and ulcerative colitis.
2. Discuss nursing care for Crohn's disease and ulcerative colitis.

APPENDICITIS

Appendicitis is an inflammation of the appendix, which is a small sac-like structure at the end of the cecum. Appendicitis is considered the most common condition requiring abdominal surgery in childhood (Potts, 2002). In appendicitis the lumen of the appendix becomes obstructed with fecal matter, lymphoid tissue, tumor, parasite, foreign body, or inspissated (thickened) cystic fibrosis secretions, which cause the appendix to become distended and subject to ischemia and necrosis (Petersen-Smith, 2004).

The characteristic symptoms are caused by the inflammation around the infected appendix with approximately "a 36-hour period from the onset of pain to the rupture of the appendix, with 80% of children perforating within 48 hours" (Petersen-Smith, 2004, p. 856).

The incidence of appendicitis increases with age, with the average age of occurrence at 10 years. The incidence is slightly higher in boys than in girls and more common in Caucasians (Potts, 2002). The risk of perforation is twice as likely for children younger than 8 years of age. Perforation occurs in approximately one third of children before treatment is initiated (Petersen-Smith, 2004). Appendicitis occurs in approximately 7% to 9% of the population and accounts for 1% to 8% of children presenting to emergency departments with a complaint of abdominal pain (Fig. 25-3).

SIGNS AND SYMPTOMS. The most reliable diagnosis of appendicitis is gained through an evaluation of the sequencing of the symptoms (Petersen-Smith, 2004). One of the earliest symptoms is periumbilical pain (pain around the umbilicus). This pain often awakens the child peaking at 4-hour intervals. The periumbilical pain subsides and then is followed by the classic sign of right lower quadrant pain. In appendicitis, vomiting generally follows periumbilical pain, unlike the vomiting associated with gastroenteritis, which precedes the pain. Anorexia is common and stools may be described as low in volume and mucus-like.

Figure 25-3 Appendicitis physical examination reveals rebound tenderness.

 clinical alert

Appendicitis

Children with suspected appendicitis who respond yes to being hungry most likely do not have appendicitis since in most cases the child does not feel like eating (Potts, 2002).

Heel-drop jarring test	Stands on toes for 15 seconds, then drops on heels—inability to stand straight or climb stairs; winces when getting off examination table.
Psoas sign	Abdominal pain with right hip flexion against resistance
Obturator sign	Pain on passive internal rotation of the flexed right thigh
Rovsing sign	Deep pressure in lower left quadrant elicits pain with a sudden release (Petersen-Smith, 2004).

DIAGNOSIS. The child diagnosed with appendicitis experiences a progression of symptoms with no single test providing overall confirmation of the diagnosis. Laboratory findings may demonstrate an elevated white blood cell count. An elevated white blood cell count does not distinguish simple appendicitis from perforated appendicitis. Children with appendicitis may also have a normal white blood cell count. An abdominal radiograph may reveal fecal matter, or some other obstruction, although this rarely confirms the diagnosis. If there is uncertainty in young children, ultrasound and computed tomography (CT) scan may help differentiate abdominal pain from other causes though the usefulness is variable (Mow, 2005).

NURSING CARE. Treatment for children who have appendicitis is surgical and an appendectomy is curative if performed before perforation. If perforation occurs, a course of postoperative antibiotics is needed (Bishop, 2006).

 Ethnocultural Considerations— Empacho

Empacho is a Spanish word for indigestion, stomach pains, and cramps. A common belief in the Hispanic culture is that the symptoms are caused by a "ball of undigested food clinging to some part of the GI tract and are due to being forced to eat against one's will or lying about the amount of food eaten" (Potts, 2002, p. 673). Treatment includes massaging and pinching the spine (Potts, 2002).

Nursing care of the child with appendicitis who has undergone an appendectomy includes monitoring intake and output, wound care, and pain control. The child will be NPO for 24 hours or until peristalsis returns. Most children are discharged to home in 2 to 3 days. If the procedure is performed by laparoscope (abdominal exploration with an endoscope) (Venes, 2009), the child may remain in the hospital overnight or be discharged the day of surgery. If perforation occurred, drains may protrude from the incision or the wound and remain open to prevent

 Nursing Insight— Appendicitis physical examination

Rebound tenderness	Presence of involuntary guarding, rebound tenderness with pain over McBurney's point, which is located 1.5–2 inches in from the right anterior superior iliac crest on a line toward the umbilicus—best elicited on palpation.

infection and allow healing (Potts, 2002). In the case of a perforated appendix, intravenous antibiotics are given for 7 to 10 days. The child generally remains NPO with a nasogastric tube in place until bowel function returns.

OMPHALITIS

Omphalitis is an infection of the umbilical stump. This occurs once the umbilicus is colonized with streptococci, staphylococci, or gram-negative organisms, which may cause a local infection (Thilo & Rosenberg, 2007).

SIGNS AND SYMPTOMS. Omphalitis is manifested by redness and edema of the soft tissue around the umbilical stump.

DIAGNOSIS. Local and systemic cultures should be obtained to confirm diagnosis (Thilo & Rosenberg, 2007).

NURSING CARE. Prevention through good perinatal care and caregiver education is paramount to the occurrence of omphalitis. Intravenous broad-spectrum antibiotics, such as nafcillin (Unipen), vancomycin (Vancocin), or third-generation cephalosporins (Cefotaxime), are used to treat omphalitis (Thilo & Rosenberg, 2007).

Nursing care of omphalitis is aimed at prevention and education of the parent or caregiver. The potential for infection can be minimized by keeping the cord clean and dry. Several methods may be used to provide cord care, which include use of an antimicrobial such as bacitracin (Baciguent) or use of triple dye. Other experts suggest the use of alcohol, cleansing with soap and water, cleansing with sterile water or a neutral pH cleanser, povidone-iodine, or natural healing with no treatment. Before discharge, the parent or caregiver needs to be instructed on the recommended method of cord care and the importance of placing the diaper below the level of the cord to avoid irritation. Parents should also be instructed regarding the expected process for stump deterioration and symptoms of infection that should be reported to their heath care provider. Cord separation generally takes place in 10 to 14 days.

MECKEL DIVERTICULUM

Meckel diverticulum arises from a remnant of the fetal development in the midgut, which normally is obliterated by the seventh to eighth week of gestation. Failure of this destructive process results in an omphalomesenteric problem (referring to the umbilicus and mesentery fistula or fibrous band [Venes, 2009]). The fibrous band, known as Meckel diverticulum, connects the small intestine to the umbilicus. A Meckel diverticulum averages 1 to 10 cm in length and is the most common congenital malformation of the GI tract, present in 1% to 4% of the population. Meckel diverticulum is twice as common in males, who are also more likely to experience complications than females.

SIGNS AND SYMPTOMS. Symptoms of Meckel diverticulum are recognized in childhood, with 65% in children younger than 5 years of age and the peak at 2 years of age. Meckel diverticulum is manifested by abdominal pain. Pain may be described as periumbilical or lower abdominal. The pain is similar to appendicitis or volvulus and may be vague and recurrent. A major manifestation in the older child includes painless rectal bleeding with stools described as bright or dark red with mucus or of a "currant jelly" appearance. Rectal bleeding in infants may be accompanied by pain. If Meckel diverticulum goes undetected, severe anemia and shock can occur.

DIAGNOSIS. Diagnosis in the child is based on history, physical examination, and radiography, specifically a nuclear medicine scan. A radionuclide scintigraphy or Meckel scan detects the presence of gastric mucosa and has an overall diagnostic accuracy of 90%. A radionuclide or Meckel scan is an imaging study that uses injection and detection of radioactive isotopes to create images of body parts (Venes, 2009). A Meckel scan is more effective in the identification of diverticulum, which may be difficult to visualize with plain films, CT, or barium studies. Abdominal radiographs and barium enema are not useful for diagnosis. The child should also be screened for anemia.

NURSING CARE. Treatment for symptomatic Meckel's diverticulum involves surgical removal of the diverticulum or pouch to prevent hypovolemic shock from hemorrhage (Potts, 2002). Surgical repair is more common in children younger than 2 years of age, which accounts for 50% of those requiring surgery. Preoperative antibiotics may be ordered if diverticulitis (inflammation of the diverticulum [Venes, 2009]) has occurred. If obstruction has occurred, fluid and electrolyte imbalances are corrected before surgery.

Nursing care is similar to that of any child undergoing surgery as well as monitoring for shock and blood loss and providing rest. Postoperative care includes fluid replacement and gastric decompression and evacuation via nasogastric tube.

Functional Gastrointestinal Conditions

IRRITABLE BOWEL SYNDROME

Irritable bowel syndrome (IBS) is a common cause of recurrent abdominal pain in children. IBS affects boys and girls equally, with diagnosis usually during school-age and adolescence. The cause of IBS is thought to involve a combination of factors, including motor, autonomic, and psychological functions. A diagnosis of IBS is generally made by ruling out organic causes for the symptoms, such as other inflammatory diseases, lactose intolerance, and parasitic infections.

Signs and Symptoms

IBS is a GI disorder that causes a variety of symptoms, including abdominal pain, flatus, bloating, constipation, or diarrhea or a combination of both constipation and diarrhea. IBS is sometimes referred to as "nervous stomach" or spastic colon. IBS is classified as a functional GI disorder because the symptoms occur when the intestines or bowels function improperly. When the intestines are exposed to certain "triggers," the bowels respond with muscle spasms instead of normal peristalsis. These muscle spasms result in one of more of the symptoms of IBS. Triggers that can cause the symptoms of IBS to "flare" include eating large amounts of food at one time; eating spicy, high-fat or gas-causing foods; or stress. Most children with IBS have various symptoms including variable stool patterns, alternating between constipation and diarrhea.

Children with IBS have pain beginning with a change in stool frequency or consistency (Bishop, 2006). IBS does not cause constant symptoms. Exacerbations can occur at any time and cause one or more symptoms. Perhaps the most common symptom seen in IBS is abdominal pain. There are a variety of reasons and causes for abdominal pain in children. Most children have abdominal pain at some point.

Diagnosis

Since there is no specific test or procedure to diagnose IBS, the diagnosis is based on clinical signs and symptoms. A diagnosis of IBS is made when other GI disorders are ruled out.

 assessment tools Irritable Bowel Syndrome

Abdominal pain *and* any two of the following:

- Pain is relieved with bowel movement.
- Onset of pain coincides with a change in stool frequency.
- Onset of pain coincides with a change in stool consistency.
- The symptoms of IBS must be present for at least 3 months in the preceding 12 months.

Additional symptoms may appear if the classic symptoms are severe or the child has frequent exacerbations. Children with frequent bouts of IBS or those who suffer several symptoms simultaneously may experience headache, nausea, mucus in the stools, anorexia, and weight loss.

Nursing Care

Treatment for IBS is almost always purely dietary. Discovering what foods trigger symptoms is most important. Food diaries are very useful in helping determine what foods should be avoided. In addition, eating more fiber and less fatty foods seems to help prevent intestinal muscle spasms. Drinking plenty of liquids, including water, can promote regular stool elimination patterns. Healthy toilet training and toileting patterns can control some symptoms. Promoting a healthy routine for regular bowel elimination can decrease the symptoms as well as the stress related to worry about bowel movements at school or at other inconvenient times. Encouraging positive strategies for managing stress can prevent exacerbations. Children need a balance of school, physical activity, socialization, and other age-appropriate activities. Children need to be taught to share feelings, concerns, and other typical growth and development issues with a parent or other interested caring adult. Medications are rarely used in the treatment of IBS in children. If constipation becomes a chronic problem, stool softeners may be indicated for short-term use. Antispasmodics such as hyoscyamine (Levsin), atropine (Atriopine-Care), scopolamine (Isopto), and phenobarbital (Donnatol), and propantheline bromide (Pro-Banthine) may be used in severe cases.

 clinical alert

Irritable Bowel Syndrome

Symptoms of IBS accompanied by fever, severe abdominal pain, and/or vomiting blood require immediate attention. Surgical evaluation and/or intervention may be necessary.

Family support and education are the primary goals in nursing care. The nurse can assist the caregiver and child in developing strategies that will decrease symptoms. Nutritional strategies include eating more slowly, avoiding carbonated drinks, and including fiber in the diet. The child also needs support and assistance in developing strategies to reduce environmental stressors.

"What to say" — *Irritable bowel syndrome*

The nurse should communicate to the family and school that stress can trigger the symptoms of IBS in many children.

Often, family circumstances present stressful situations. Parents may need help in dealing with certain situations that are stressful to their child and exacerbate the symptoms of IBS. Family counseling may be an option. At home, parents and children can be taught to keep a food diary so they can determine the triggers that cause "flares" of IBS.

Teachers must also be aware of the condition and may need to be involved in helping the child reduce or cope with the stress related to school. The school counselor can be a good resource for the child.

INFANTILE COLIC

The cause of infantile colic is unknown. Several factors have been implicated in the development of colic, including both physical and psychological factors such as allergy, cow's milk intolerance, over or underfeeding, inadequate burping, cigarette smoke, maternal anxiety, and familial stress (Petersen-Smith, 2004). A stressful pregnancy and birth experience have also been suggested as potential underlying factors in the development of colic.

Signs and Symptoms

Colic is described as persistent, unexplained crying or fussing in infants younger than 3 months of age (Petersen-Smith, 2004). Episodes generally occur at the same time each day, usually during the late afternoon or evening. The infant is fussing and appears to be pulling both legs and arms into a flexed position.

Diagnosis

Diagnosis is based on a report of the symptoms occurring for more than 3 weeks, during which the crying episodes occurred for more than 3 days of the week with crying for 2 to 3 hours a day. The incidence of colic is estimated to be about one third of all infants (Petersen-Smith, 2004).

> **Box 25-1** **Management Strategies for Infantile Colic**
>
> - Support parents.
> - Assure parents that the child is in good health.
> - Reinforce parents' efforts to comfort the child.
> - Instruct parents on strategies to calm infant, such as swaddling, decreasing environmental stimulation, and rocking.
> - Assess feeding techniques and instruct as needed.
> - Provide an opportunity for parents to express frustrations.
>
> ---
>
> *Source:* Petersen-Smith, A.M. (2004). Gastrointestinal disorders. In C.E. Burns, A.M. Dunn, M.A. Brady, N.B. Starr, & C.G. Blosser (3rd ed.). *Pediatric primary care: A handbook for nurse practitioners* (3rd ed.). St Louis: Elserier, pp. 839–884.

Nursing Care

Management of colic begins with ruling out acute conditions that cause abdominal pain. The goal of treatment for infantile colic is to manage the situation until the symptoms resolve as no cure exists (Box 25-1). Though anticholinergics, barbiturates, motility enhancing agents, and antiflatulents have been prescribed, practitioners generally avoid using these drugs because of their limited success and the lack of scientific data to support their effectiveness (Petersen-Smith, 2004).

 ### Ethnocultural Considerations— *Israel*

Chamomile, vervain, licorice, fennel, and balm mint, which have antispasmodic properties, are found in herbal teas and are used as a remedy for colic in Israel.

ACUTE DIARRHEA

Acute diarrhea also refers to acute enteritis or acute gastroenteritis (Jensen & Baltimore, 2006). Acute diarrhea is defined as excessive loss of fluid and electrolytes in the stool. Stool loss is considered excessive when it is more than 10 g/kg per day in infants and more than 200 g/day in children (Petersen-Smith, 2004, p. 875). Acute diarrhea with or without vomiting has multiple causes, which may include infections in or outside the intestinal tract, diet, medications, or toxic substances. Four kinds of diarrhea have been defined in the literature.

- "Osmotic diarrhea results when osmotically active particles in the intestine draw excess fluid into the stool; this condition occurs with dumping syndrome, lactose deficiency, overfeeding, malabsorption syndromes, and excess ingestion of hypertonic juices" (Petersen-Smith, 2004, p. 875).
- Secretory diarrhea happens when there is an increase in the active secretion, or there is an inhibition of absorption. The most common cause of this type of diarrhea is bacterial endotoxins that stimulate the secretion of chloride ions. There is little to no structural damage.
- "Motility disorders cause diarrhea but not malabsorption. Bile salt and pancreatic enzyme deficiency can cause diarrhea by deletion or inhibition of the normal absorption process" (Petersen-Smith, 2004, p. 875).

- "Inflammatory processes such as bacterial invasion, celiac sprue, and irritable bowel syndrome or surgical procedures can change the anatomy and functional ability of the intestine. Abnormal peristalsis for any reason can result in acute diarrhea" (Petersen-Smith, 2004, p. 875).

Infectious agents associated with diarrhea include bacteria: *Campylobacter jejuni*, *Clostridium difficile*, *Yersinia enterocolitica*, *Salmonella*, *Shigella*, enterohemorrhagic *Escherichia coli*, and viruses: human rotavirus and adenovirus (Petersen-Smith, 2004) (Table 25-1).

Approximately 20% of office visits of children younger than 2 years of age and eight of 1000 hospitalizations of children younger than 1 year of age are for acute diarrhea. Acute diarrhea causes 10% of preventable deaths in the United States, including 500 deaths in children between the ages of 1 and 4 (Petersen-Smith, 2004). The literature suggests that the cause of morbidity and mortality from this illness is related to poverty and poor access to care.

Signs and Symptoms

The clinical manifestations of diarrhea include increased frequency and fluid content of the stools with or without associated symptoms. Signs of systemic illness may also be evident. The caregiver should be asked about the presence of other signs and symptoms, such as vomiting, fever, and pain with special attention to the number of wet diapers within the previous 24-hour period.

Diagnosis

Diagnosis of diarrhea should include a history of recent travel, day care or school illness contacts, family members with similar illnesses, ingestion of medications and toxic substances, and a dietary history. In addition, information regarding the number of stools, frequency, and quality should be elicited and include when the symptoms began.

The physical examination focuses attention to the abdomen and perineum in addition to state of alertness, changes in the growth pattern, and the hydration status of the child. Laboratory tests are selected based on the suspected etiology and the overall health and appearance of the child. No blood tests may be indicated for an essentially well appearing child. For a child demonstrating symptoms of toxicity, stool for culture and sensitivity (C & S), serum electrolytes, and a complete blood count (CBC) with differential are suggested. Diarrhea with weight loss suggests the need for serum electrolytes and CBC with differential. Evidence of blood in the stool with or without a history of antibiotic use suggests a need to assess stool for C & S, CBC with differential, and serum electrolytes.

Nursing Care

Most incidences of acute diarrhea are self limiting. Management of viral and most bacterial causes is primarily supportive (Jensen & Baltimore, 2006). Treatment of acute diarrhea is determined by extent of the illness and the cause, with attention to hydration and dietary needs as appropriate and with prevention as a priority. Initially the priority is to restore and maintain hydration. Oral rehy-

Table 25-1 Rotavirus

Rotavirus	Incidence	Protecting Children	Dehydration Secondary to Gastroenteritis
Viral gastroenteritis causes approximately 80% of all cases of diarrhea in children younger than 1 year with rotavirus, accounting for 50% of the cases of acute diarrhea in children. Rotavirus is the most common cause of diarrhea illness among children worldwide and accounts for approximately one third of hospitalizations of children in industrialized countries. It is estimated that by 5 years of age, nearly every child will have had at least one episode of rotavirus-induced illness. Epidemiological studies conservatively estimate that rotavirus caused gastroenteritis is responsible for 352,000–592,000 deaths annually in children younger than 5 years, with 82% of these deaths occurring in the poorest of countries. The primary transmission of this virus is via the fecal–oral route; however, the virus is very hearty and stable on surfaces for long periods of time, increasing the risk for transmission through contaminated surfaces or food. In addition, the virus has been found in the respiratory tract of infected individuals, raising concern for transmission via infectious secretions.	The incidence for rotavirus does not vary between industrialized and developing countries, nor has incidence been shown to decrease with increased sanitation in developing nations. The incubation period for rotavirus is approximately 1–3 days. This is followed by a 3- to 8-day period of fever, vomiting, diarrhea, and abdominal pain. The disease is self-limiting. However, the vomiting and diarrhea in rotavirus may be severe enough to require intervention to prevent dehydration. A primary factor in survival of rotaviral induced gastroenteritis is access to adequate medical care. Worldwide children have limited access to rehydration therapy. Most often, therapy primarily consists of oral rehydration. In the case of rotavirus, vomiting may limit the usefulness of oral rehydration and in the absence of access to intravenous hydration, death occurs secondary to fluid and electrolyte imbalances.	Surviving an episode of rotaviral gastroenteritis confers partial immunity. Subsequent cases are possible but tend to be milder and less life-threatening. In 1998 a rotavirus vaccine was introduced, RotaShield. The vaccine was shown to be 100% effective in prevention of rotavirus infection but was quickly withdrawn after it was demonstrated that the vaccine was associated with a slightly higher risk of intussusception in infants. The recommended 2007 immunization schedule for 0–6 years of age now currently includes a recommendation for a three-dose series of rotavirus vaccine (Rota). The first dose is recommended to be administered between 6 and 12 weeks of age, with the initial dose not to be started later than age 12 weeks (American Academy of Pediatrics Committee on Infectious Disease. [November, 2006]).	Rotaviral gastroenteritis is a self-limiting disease. Deaths from rotavirus are due to dehydration. As most children with a diarrhea type illness are cared for in the home it is critical that the nurse educate the families on early signs of dehydration requiring medical treatment. Specific indicators of dehydration in infants include: • Decreased number wet diapers • Sunken fontanel and eyes • Listlessness • Cool, pale skin Families should be given specific instructions regarding oral intake goals during treatment for rotavirus and instructed to return for follow-up if a child is unable to meet the goals or the appearance of any of the above symptoms of dehydration.

dration is generally attempted before intravenous hydration is initiated and is again related to the acuity of the illness and its affect on the child. Recent trends in rehydration of the child who is not experiencing vomiting is to allow the child to drink what he or she desires, which may include formula or milk, although other authors may consider this controversial. Traditional treatment of children with mild to moderate dehydration (less than 10%) includes oral rehydration for 24 hours (Jensen & Baltimore, 2006). The rehydrating solutions generally recommended include glucose and electrolytes, such as Pedialyte and Infalyte. Fruit juices, soda, sports drinks, and powered drinks are generally not recommended by those employing traditional treatments. Returning to full-strength formula is recommended as quickly as possible. If the infant does not tolerate full-strength formula, a diluted formula (one-fourth to half strength) may be used for a short time, often 4 to 6 hours. Breast-fed infants may be fed more frequently for shorter periods of time.

Solid food is generally started within the first 24 to 48 hours and starts with bland, soft foods. Care needs to be taken to avoid foods with a high fat content and simple sugars. Foods generally well tolerated include vegetables, fruits, yogurt, complex carbohydrates, and lean meat.

Depending on the cause of the diarrhea, pharmacological treatment in general is not ordered for young children. Although antidiarrheals are generally not recommended they may be used with caution in older children if the diarrhea persists beyond the initial infection. The use of *Lactobacillus* (gram-positive, anaerobic, non–spore-forming bacilli) has been found to shorten the duration of the illness if used early in the process (Petersen-Smith, 2004).

Intravenous fluids are essential with "impaired circulation and possible shock; weight less than 8.8 to 11 lb (4 to 5 kg) or a child younger than 3 months; intractable diarrhea, lethargy, anatomic anomalies; failure to gain weight or continued weight loss despite oral fluids" (Petersen-Smith, 2004, p. 876).

Complementary Care: *Diarrhea*

Products containing *Lactobacillus acidophilus*, such as yogurt, can be used to decrease the incidence of rotavirus diarrhea in infants 5–24 months of age (Blosser, 2004). *Lactobacillus* is a nonpathogenic bacteria that produces lactic acid from carbohydrates and is normally found in milk, feces of infants fed by bottle, and adults. The addition of *Lactobacillus acidophilus* to the diet changes the bacterial flora of the GI tract, hence treating the overgrowth of pathogenic or diarrhea-causing organisms in the GI tract.

Care of the child hospitalized for acute diarrhea includes monitoring fluid intake and output, observing for signs of dehydration, offering fluids as indicated, and monitoring intravenous infusions if ordered. The skin integrity of the perineal and buttock areas must be monitored for irritation related to frequent stooling and good perineal skin care must be provided. Nursing care also includes education on preventive measures. The child and caregivers need to be instructed on good hand washing in addition to appropriate care of soiled clothing and diapers. The nurse must reinforce proper hand washing to include not only that which follows toileting or diaper changes but also before and after eating and in the preparation of foods.

 Across Care Settings: Schools, day care, and community

The most effective treatment for gastroenteritis is prevention through good hand washing.

CHRONIC DIARRHEA

Chronic diarrhea is defined as "one or more liquid to semiliquid stools passed per day for 14 days or longer" (Petersen-Smith, 2004, p. 878). Chronic diarrhea is usually associated with a chronic condition, such as inflammatory bowel disease, malabsorption syndromes, overfeeding, formula protein intolerance, lactose intolerance, food allergies, viral, bacterial or parasitic agents, radiation therapy, or immunodeficiencies (Jensen & Baltimore, 2006). Inadequate management of acute diarrhea can also lead to chronic diarrhea. Chronic nonspecific diarrhea (CNSD) or toddler's diarrhea is the most common cause of chronic loose stools in childhood. The child with toddler's diarrhea generally has a normal growth and weight gain. The cause of toddler's diarrhea may be from "excessive intake of fruit juices which contain non-digestible carbohydrates" (Jensen & Baltimore, 2006, p. 587).

Signs and Symptoms

Clinical manifestations reflect the underlying pathology. The nurse should obtain information regarding the history of the diarrhea, including frequency and appearance. Information regarding weight loss, medications, and presence of associated symptoms should be determined. Special consideration needs to be taken to determine the dietary history with special attention to the amount of fruit juice ingested per day. The caregiver also should be asked whether the child has had stool incontinence and what treatments have been attempted at home in addition to recent travel and school exposure.

During the physical health assessment, the nurse should observe for evidence of abdominal distention or tenderness and the presence of hyperactive bowel sounds. Signs of weight loss and dehydration should also be included in addition to the condition of the perineal area. The child with toddler's diarrhea has no evidence of mal-nutrition or growth failure. Stools are described as loose and are often found to have undigested food particles present. There should be no evidence of blood in the stool of the child with toddler's diarrhea.

Diagnosis

Diagnostic assessment may include stool for culture and sensitivity, ova and parasites, pH occult blood, fat stain, and Clinitest for reducing substances. Sweat chloride and lactose tolerance tests may be ordered to rule out cystic fibrosis or lactose intolerance. In addition, a CBC with differential, erythrocyte sedimentation rate (ESR), serum electrolytes, albumin level, and a urinalysis with culture as used as nonspecific indicators of illness (Procedure 25-1).

Nursing Care

Management of chronic diarrhea involves treating the underlying cause. Enteral (by way of the intestine) or total parenteral nutrition (TPN) is provided for the child who is unable to maintain adequate oral nutritional intake (Petersen-Smith, 2004) (Fig. 25-4). The treatment for toddler's diarrhea is a change or reduction in the child's intake of fruit juices.

The general nursing care of the child with chronic diarrhea is similar to that of acute diarrhea with special focus related to the underlying cause. As with acute diarrhea the child and caregiver need to be educated on primary prevention.

VOMITING

Vomiting is the forceful expulsion of stomach contents. The type of emesis assists in identifying the cause. "Nonbilious vomit is generally caused by infection, metabolic, neurologic, or psychological problems" (Petersen-Smith, 2004, p. 842). Bilious (vomit containing bile) vomiting is more likely caused by an obstructive process. Bloody emesis is usually evidence of active bleeding in the GI tract. The nurse communicates to the family that nausea and retching often accompany vomiting. Regurgitation in contrast is a more passive and effortless phenomenon. Table 25-2 lists the most common causes of vomiting related to origin.

Signs and Symptoms

Specific manifestations and diagnosis vary as greatly as the causes and origin of the illness. A thorough history and assessment must include a description of the onset, duration, quality and quantity, appearance, presence of undigested food, odor, and evidence of a precipitating event. The child's recent exposure to illness, injury, or stress, in addition to family history of a similar illness, needs to be determined. The caregiver or child should be asked about the relation of the vomiting to the time of day, meals, or other activities. Associated symptoms, such as fever, diarrhea, ear pain, headache, and signs of increased intracranial pressure or urinary tract infection, should also be evaluated. Vomiting upon arising in the morning is often associated with neurological involvement. The nurse should also ask the caregiver or child about medications currently being taken to include over the counter, herbal, cultural, and homeopathic remedies (Petersen-Smith, 2004).

Procedure 25-1 Collecting Stool for Culture and Sensitivity and Ova and Parasites

Purpose

Collecting stool for culture and sensitivity and ova and parasites is used to detect the presence of bacterial overgrowth; to confirm bacterial gastroenteritis; and to assess sensitivity of specific antimicrobials.

Equipment
- Gloves
- Patient identification label
- Sterile culture tube and cotton swab to collect specimen
- Biohazard container

Steps

1. Don gloves.

   RATIONALE: *Prevents the spread of bacteria.*

2. Using the sterile cotton swab collect (scrape) a fresh, warm specimen of stool from the diaper or stool receptacle and place it into the sterile culture tube.

3. Label both the sterile culture tube and the biohazard bag with the patient's identification information.

   RATIONALE: *Accurate labeling is essential for correct patient identification.*

4. Place the sterile culture tube into the biohazard bag.

   RATIONALE: *To ensure that the properly identified specimen is safely transported to the laboratory.*

5. Deliver the fresh specimen of stool to the laboratory promptly after collection.

   RATIONALE: *Delays in transfer of the specimen may affect viability of the organism.*

Clinical Alert
- Avoid external contamination of stool and deliver to laboratory promptly.
- Provide samples from several areas of the stool to ensure that organisms are isolated. Failure to do so may yield a false-negative result.
- Inform the lab of antimicrobial or antiamebic therapy within 10 days as it may yield false-negative results.
- Medications such as antacids, antibiotics, antidiarrheals, iron, and castor oil may interfere with analysis.

Teach Parents

Teach the parents that a stool for culture and sensitivity is used to detect the presence of bacterial overgrowth; confirm bacterial gastroenteritis; and to assess sensitivity of specific antimicrobials.

Teach parents that a stool for ova and parasites (O & P) is used to aid in diagnosis of parasites or their eggs.

Documentation

10/12/10 0900 Stool for culture and sensitivity and ova and parasites collected from the diaper, labeled, placed in biohazard bag and sent to laboratory via laboratory collection personnel.

N. Kramer, RN

Source: Schnell, Van Leeuwen, & Kranpitz (2003).

Figure 25-4 Total parenteral nutrition (TPN) is provided for the child who is unable to maintain adequate oral nutritional intake.

The nurse should assess the abdomen for the presence of distention, visible peristalsis, and presence of bowel sounds. Depending on the cause of the vomiting, bowel sounds may be hyperactive or hypoactive. With a history of persistent vomiting, it is essential for the nurse to assess the child's hydration status in addition to evidence of malnutrition.

Diagnosis

In addition to a thorough history and physical examination diagnostic studies may include urinalysis and culture, CBC, serum electrolytes, blood culture, liver function tests, and select abdominal imaging depending on suspected cause of the vomiting. Plain radiograph or ultrasonography of the abdomen may detect anatomic abnormalities. Endoscopy of the upper GI tract can be used if esophagitis is suspected. Further studies may include a toxicology screen, rapid strep test/throat culture, pregnancy test, or electroencephalogram depending on the suspected origin of the vomiting.

Table 25-2 Common Causes of Vomiting

Origin	Cause
Upper GI	• Gastritis • Esophagitis • Pyloric stenosis
Small intestine	• Intestinal malrotation with volvulus
Colon	• Hirschsprung's disease • Intussusception • Fecal impaction
Liver or pancreas	• Hepatobiliary dysfunction
Infections	• Bacterial enteritis • Otitis media • Urinary track infection • Viral gastroenteritis • Hepatitis • Sepsis
Neurologic	• Hydrocephalus • Brain tumor • Migraine headache • Head trauma • Congenital malformation
Other	• Cow's milk protein allergy • Maternal drug exposure and withdrawal • Toxic ingestion • Appendicitis • Inborn error of metabolism • Pneumonia • Drug or alcohol ingestion • Eating disorders • Pregnancy

Nursing Care

Management is directed toward the treatment of the cause and prevention of complications. The degree of dehydration is determined and treated. For self limiting causes of vomiting in childhood the bowel is allowed to rest. Rehydration is generally initiated after 1 to 2 hours with nothing by mouth. Plain water, apple juice, soda, milk, and sports drinks are avoided. Breastfed infants may be nursed more frequently for shorter periods. Solids are avoided for 4 to 6 hours after which reintroduction is begun with bland solids, which may include complex carbohydrates, such as rice, wheat, cereals, yogurt, cooked vegetables, and lean meats. Fatty foods and those high in simple sugars are avoided. Though the recommendation is a change from the BRAT diet, which consisted of bananas, rice, applesauce, and toast, it is still well tolerated though low in density, fat, and protein sources.

When vomiting is of a limited duration and the cause is known, antiemetic drugs may be indicated. Adverse affects are rare with antiemetic use in children. Antiemetic drugs that block chemoreceptor triggers include ondanse-tron (Zofran) or trimethobenzamide (Tigan). The nurse understands that metoclopramide (Reglan) enhances peristalsis and, therefore, gastric emptying. Phenothiazine (Phenergan) is used cautiously per rectum every 6 hours if vomiting is excessive, dehydration is imminent, and GI disease has been excluded.

Nursing care is determined by cause and generally focuses on careful observation and support. Care is taken to carefully position the child who is vomiting to prevent aspiration. The nurse assesses for signs of dehydration and carefully monitors fluid intake and output. Oral hygiene may include rinsing the mouth or brushing the teeth after vomiting to dilute the hydrochloric acid that comes in contact with the teeth. If vomiting has been determined to be related to improper feeding technique, the caregiver needs instruction on food or formula preparation and a demonstration of correct positioning during and after feeding in the care of an infant.

CYCLIC VOMITING SYNDROME

Cyclic vomiting syndrome (CVS) is a recurrent stereotypical spell of vomiting followed by periods of wellness. One third of recurrent vomiting in children is caused by CVS, with a female to male ratio of 5:4. The average age at onset is 5.3 years of age. Petersen-Smith (2004) suggests that it often takes more than 2 years to diagnosis and lasts on average 3.4 years. CVS is generally outgrown before or during the preteen years.

The typical child presents as well 90% of the time. However, during exacerbations significant costs are incurred and children miss an average of 20 days of school per year. Medical costs are related to intravenous rehydration, diagnostic studies, procedures, emergency room costs, and time taken off of from work by the caregiver.

Signs and Symptoms

The following diagnostic criteria were defined by the International Scientific Symposium on Cyclic Vomiting Syndrome as cited by Petersen-Smith (2004):

- Essential criteria include recurrent, severe, discrete episodes of vomiting; varying intervals of normal health between episodes; duration of vomiting lasts hours to days; and there is no apparent cause of vomiting (negative laboratory, radiographic, and endoscopic testing).
- Supportive criteria include a pattern that is stereotypical (each episode is similar as to onset, intensity, duration, frequency, associated symptoms, and signs within individuals) and self-limited (episodes resolve spontaneously if left untreated).
- Associated symptoms include nausea, abdominal pain, headache, motion sickness, photophobia, and lethargy.
- Associated signs include fever, pallor, diarrhea, dehydration, excess salivation, and social withdrawal (p. 846).

The primary clinical manifestation is recurrent episodic vomiting, usually lasting 24 to 48 hours. The vomiting occurs at regular intervals, usually every 2 to 4 weeks. The condition may include a prodromal (initial or indicative of an approaching illness [Venes, 2009]) period during which the child may demonstrate signs of pallor, anorexia, nausea, abdominal pain, and lethargy. Once the episode resolves a brief recovery period occurs during which the child returns to normal activities. Episodes generally occur in the middle of the night or early morning. Vomiting occurs as often as every 5 to 10 minutes. Seventy-six percent of the time the emesis is described as bilious with hematemesis (vomiting of blood) occurring approximately 32% of the time. Associated GI symptoms may include abdominal pain, retching, anorexia, nausea, or diarrhea. Systemic symptoms include headache, photophobia (light intolerance), phonophobia (intolerance or fear of sound), or vertigo (sensation of moving in space or having objects move). Infection, psychological stress, diet changes, or menstruation may be precipitating factors. A positive family history of migraine headaches may be present. On examination, the child may appear pale and listless, often lying in a position to decrease the pain, such as in a fetal position. Dehydration may be evident.

Petersen-Smith (2004) describes three questions that are essential to make the diagnosis.

- Has the child had at least three episodes?
- Is the child completely asymptomatic between episodes?
- Are the episodes stereotypical? (p. 846)

Additional diagnostic red flags may include "severe headache, GI bleeding, unilateral abdominal pain, weight loss, failure to respond to any treatment, progressive worsening, prolonged episodes requiring repeat hospitalizations, and a change in pattern or symptoms" (Petersen-Smith, 2004, p. 846).

Diagnosis

Diagnostic studies are used to rule out other conditions. Laboratory studies may include CBC with differential, electrolytes, glucose, liver function tests, metabolic screening (lactate, ammonia, amino acids, and porphobilinogen), urinalysis, urine culture, and urine organic acids. Imaging studies may include small bowel radiography, abdominal ultrasound, MRI or CT of the head or sinuses and endoscopy.

Nursing Care

Management is generally supportive care and includes fluid replacement, rest, and pharmacotherapy as needed. Careful monitoring and documentation of fluid intake and output during vomiting episodes are essential. Accurate assessment includes the type and appearance of the vomiting in addition to associated behavior. A calm stress-free environment should be provided. Although up to 28% of children with cyclic vomiting suffer with migraines as adolescents and adults, most children outgrow cyclic vomiting before or during the preadolescent years. A psychiatric evaluation may be indicated for cyclic vomiting as the symptoms can be associated with psychological stress.

CONSTIPATION

Constipation is the difficult or infrequent passage of hard stool, which is often associated with straining, abdominal pain, or withholding behaviors. Frequency alone is not a good diagnostic criterion as children vary greatly in their stooling frequency.

Constipation accounts for 3% of office visits and 25% of pediatric gastroenterologist visits (Potts, 2002). Constipation peaks between the ages of 2 and 4 and is more common in males than in females until adolescence, after which it is seen more frequently in females.

Constipation can occur secondary to an organic cause or in association with a systemic condition. Strictures and Hirschsprung disease are included among organic causes. Systemic conditions that may be a factor in the development of constipation include hypothyroidism, hypercalcemia caused by hyperparathyroidism or vitamin D excess, and chronic lead poisoning. Drugs such as antacids, diuretics, iron supplements, opioids, antihistamines, and antiepileptics are also associated with constipation as a side effect. Children with spinal cord pathology may experience a loss of rectal tone and sensation.

Most constipation is considered idiopathic or functional with no clear underlying cause. Environmental and/or psychosocial factors, such as travel, illness, dietary changes, and emotional factors, may cause chronic constipation. Children may also experience constipation during toilet training, which is related to not wanting to take time from play or from overenthusiastic toilet training. Dilation and stretching of the rectum may come from repeated withholding. This leads to a decreased sensation or urge to pass stool.

Onset of constipation during infancy is generally associated with dietary causes. Constipation is less common in breastfed infants. Environmental changes and attention to controlling the passage of stool are more common causes of constipation in early childhood. Any feeling of discomfort during stooling may lead the child to deliberately withhold stool in the future.

In the school-age child, organic and environmental factors are considered. Fear of using school restrooms or embarrassment in asking the teacher is a common cause of constipation in early school age children. Separation, change in routine, and change in eating and sleeping patterns may all contribute to the change seen in bowel habits. These children may try to "hold" their stool until a later time. When they do finally try to eliminate the stool, it may be very hard and painful. The longer the child holds the stool and delays elimination, the harder and larger the stool becomes and the more painful the process.

> **medication:** Medications Used for Vomiting
>
> A combination of medications is used for sedation and the relief of pain and nausea and vomiting, which may include a combination of diphenhydramine (Benadryl), lorazepam (Ativan), promethazine (Phenergan), and meperidine (Demerol). Metoclopramide (Reglan) is a prokinetic agent that accelerates gastric emptying. Migraine relief includes sumatriptan (Imitrex) for acute episodes; amitriptyline (Elavil), cyproheptadine (Periactin), phenobarbital (Luminal), propranolol (Inderal) for prophylaxis; and ethinyl estradiol (Loestrin) for menstrual pain relief. Erythromycin (E-Mycin, E.E.S., EryPed) as a prokinetic is not used much in children secondary to the gastric effects and questionable efficacy.

Nursing Insight— *Constipation*

The majority of children have idiopathic or functional constipation. This classification is used when there is no identifiable reason or underlying cause for their constipation.

Signs and Symptoms

The major symptoms associated with constipation are poor appetite and straining with stools. Soiling is more common with the diagnosis of encopresis. Stools are hard and blood may occasionally be seen in the outer surface of the stool. Additional signs include a potential for tenderness in the area of the colon and small intestines and rectal fissures.

Diagnosis

Diagnosis is based on the symptoms. An abdominal radiography and barium enema may be ordered for children who do not respond to treatment.

 clinical alert

Abdominal Pain

Most children who are constipated usually have some abdominal pain due to cramping. However, if the onset of constipation and severe abdominal pain is acute and/or accompanied by fever, vomiting or other symptoms, the child must be evaluated for a bowel obstruction.

Nursing Care

The management of simple constipation can generally be accomplished by focusing on dietary intake and keeping the bowel relatively empty. Occasional constipation caused by dietary intake can be treated with adequate intake of water and other fluids, which assist in regulating elimination. A regular diet, rich in all nutrients coupled with an adequate amount of water and other fluids, is the best way to ensure normal bowel elimination patterns. Fresh fruit adds fiber and can relieve constipation. Limiting dairy products such as cheese can also provide relief. However, many children can be "picky eaters" at times, preferring fast food or the same food for every meal. This type of eating can lead to disruptive bowel patterns including constipation. Occasionally, stool softeners may be needed to "train" the child and the bowels into a regular pattern of elimination. Giving the stool softener at bedtime allows it to work gently overnight to foster a morning elimination pattern. No medication should be used on a long-term basis without a physician's prescription or health care provider's guidance.

 Nursing Insight— *Constipation*

Not all fruits contribute to soft stools. Applesauce and bananas are two fruits that can be used when children have diarrhea because they make stools firmer.

Chronic constipation may require strategies to restore a regular stooling pattern, hence shrinking the distended rectum to a normal size and promoting regular toileting practices. Therapy for chronic constipation may include bowel cleansing and maintenance therapy to prevent further stool retention. Initial treatment of chronic constipation includes removing hard, impacted stool, which may be accomplished through use of "suppositories, enemas, and occasionally the use of polyethylene glycol electrolyte solution (GoLYTELY) administered orally or by NG tube". A combination of mineral oil and enemas may be used for severe impaction for which suppositories are not effective. Rarely surgical removal is needed.

Once the impaction is removed, maintenance therapy includes use of mineral oil, stool softeners, and laxatives. Stool softeners may not be effective for severe constipation. The safest laxatives are milk of magnesia and polyethylene glycol (MiraLax).

Bowel retraining includes developing good toileting habits and reinforcement of sitting on the toilet for defecation. A regular toileting time should be established once or twice per day. The child should be allowed to sit on the toilet 5 to 10 minutes with positive behaviors reinforced.

 Optimizing Outcomes— **Constipation**

A 2½-year-old child has not passed a stool in 5 days. The parents report that the child has been eating and growing well and has no other symptoms of illness. They report that the last stool passed was firm and appeared to cause the child some discomfort. The parents also report no evidence of blood has been noted in the stool. In addition, the parents began toilet training the child approximately 3 weeks ago.

The best outcome for the family is to understand that the child is normal. The nurse can discuss toilet training readiness to include not only physical readiness but also mental and psychological readiness. In addition, the nurse can include instructions regarding the importance of water and high fiber in the diet and the avoidance of excessive refined carbohydrates.

Care of the child with constipation begins with a careful assessment of bowel patterns, diet history, drug history, and environmental factors. The nurse should ask the

 Family Teaching Guidelines—
Dealing with Food Jags with Young Children

- Reassure the parents that food jags are normal at this age and that the tendencies will pass. Stress that a little patience will keep both parents and child from further gastrointestinal upsets.

- Suggest that the parents not force the child to eat foods he is not interested in but to provide a variety of nutritious foods during meals and for between meals snacks in the amount appropriate for the child's age.

- Inform the family about treatments and when they need to seek additional help (www.nal.usda.gov/fnic/; www.mypyramid.gov; www.aap.org).

caregiver to describe the color, consistency, frequency, and characteristics of the stool. Caregiver education is an important part of nursing care and should include instruction on dietary needs, toileting practices, and bowel cleansing as needed.

Now Can You— **Discuss functional gastrointestinal conditions?**

1. Discuss functional gastrointestinal conditions?
2. Discuss signs and symptoms of functional gastrointestinal conditions?
3. Discuss nursing care for functional gastrointestinal conditions?

ENCOPRESIS

Encopresis is stool incontinence beyond the age when children should normally be able to control their bowels, which is usually beyond the age of 4. Encopresis is considered primary in children who have never obtained stool continence and secondary in the child who has been previously trained and then becomes incontinent of stool (Dunn, 2004). Encopresis is divided into two types: "encopresis with constipation, associated with stool retention, constipation, and incontinence and encopresis without constipation" (Dunn, 2004, p. 291). In encopresis with constipation, the pathophysiology is similar to that of regular constipation (i.e., stool retention leads to distention of the colon and stretching of the rectum). This distention is followed by ineffective peristalsis and decreased sensation to defecate, which can lead to impaction. Eventually the rectal and sphincter muscles become weakened. Once the rectum becomes impacted with hard stool, semiformed or liquid stool from higher in the intestines may leak around the impacted stool and pass through the rectum causing soiling. Encopresis with constipation is involuntary and the child may be unaware of the passage of stool. Children with encopresis without constipation have voluntary stools in inappropriate places (Dunn, 2004).

Encopresis is more common in boys than in girls. The etiology is unclear and includes both physiological and psychosocial factors. Physiological factors may include inadequate fluid intake; dehydration (caused by illness, fever, or an active exercise during hot weather); dietary changes; inappropriate use of laxatives, suppositories or enema; and retention and constipation secondary to anal fissures, neurogenic conditions, medications, and painful stools. Psychosocial factors may include major family or life changes or loss; inappropriate toilet training techniques; irregular toileting patterns; and physical and sexual abuse (Dunn, 2004).

Signs and Symptoms

Manifestations include a history of stained underwear, difficult or painful defecation, large and/or hard stools, reports of bloating or pain, streaks of bright blood, anorexia, evidence of attempts to retain stool (i.e., grimacing, shifting position or crossing legs, and urinary tract infection). Physical symptoms may include abdominal distention and tenderness, overflow soiling, impaction, a midline palpated mass, and anal fissures.

Diagnosis

Radiography and laboratory tests may be performed to rule out structural or organic causes, they are not routinely needed (Dunn, 2004).

Nursing Care

The nurse understands that the main goal of treatment is to establish regular bowel habits, is often multidisciplinary, and requires child and caregiver education. Basic treatment of encopresis without constipation includes dietary monitoring to ensure adequate fiber and water intake. Milk is decreased to 16 oz./day with limited cheese, rice, applesauce, and bananas. Stool softeners and laxatives are avoided. The child and caregiver are instructed on the need to establish a routine for toileting in addition to encouraging the child to take responsibility for his or her own toileting habits. Incentives or rewards may be used to reinforce positive behaviors.

Management of children with constipation is more complicated and begins with a catharsis phase, during which thorough bowel cleansing is accomplished through the use of enemas, suppositories, and laxatives. The catharsis phase takes approximately 2 weeks, after which a follow-up abdominal radiograph is done to confirm catharsis.

The catharsis phase is followed by a maintenance phase. The goals of maintenance include no soiling, regular, soft stools at least every other day to three-times/week, and increased awareness of the need to defecate. Laxatives may be substituted or alternated with stool softeners in order to maintain soft bowel movements. Toileting time should be planned around the times when the child is most likely to have a stool.

During the maintenance phase, behavioral changes are addressed, which include toilet sitting 3 to 4 times per day for 10 minutes (Dunn, 2004). An increase in physical activity is encouraged. Dietary changes include an increase in fluids other than milk, increase in fiber, and a decrease in constipating foods. Bowel movements are documented for time, quality, amount, and location. The maintenance phase may take up to 6 months before the bowel regains full function.

The follow-up phase involves regular visits from approximately every 4 to 10 weeks depending on the severity of the condition and the family need for support. Counseling or referral may be ordered for psychosocial and developmental needs as appropriate. The goals of follow-up visits are to monitor compliance, provide encouragement and support, and to detect and treat relapse.

Nursing care involves anticipatory guidance, child and caregiver support, and education. Instruction needs to be provided regarding appropriate dietary needs and toileting. The caregiver may need a demonstration on the use of enemas and suppositories if this is part of the treatment plan.

❁ Collaboration in Caring— *Encopresis*

The school nurse needs to collaborate with the child, family, and teachers in setting up an effective plan of care for the child while he is attending school. School personnel should be instructed about the child's need for emotional support, privacy, and timing of stool elimination. In addition, there should be sensitivity to the child's concerns about soiling and odors, allowing the child to attend to toileting needs as requested. Successful reconciliation of this disorder involves collaboration from the adults in the child's immediate environment.

GASTROESOPHAGEAL REFLUX AND GASTROESOPHAGEAL REFLUX DISEASE

Gastroesophageal reflux (GER) is the return of gastric contents from the stomach through the lower esophageal sphincter into the esophagus. Research suggests that up to "50% of infants younger than 2 months are reported to have symptoms of reflux, defined clinically as more than two episodes per day of regurgitation or emesis".

Classifications of reflux include physiological, functional and pathological.

Physiological reflux or GRE is described as infrequent and episodic vomiting and is a common occurrence in many healthy infants. A decrease is seen as the esophagus elongates and matures. Suwandhi and colleagues (2006) suggest that the occurrence of physiological GER is present in 60% to 70% of infants ages 3 to 4 months and usually resolves by 1 year.

 Nursing Insight— Functional GER

Functional GER involves painless, effortless vomiting with no physical sequelae (Petersen-Smith, 2004).

Pathological reflux or GERD is frequent with associated physical dysfunction. Though the diagnosis of GERD is generally considered when reflux persists beyond 18 months of age and involves an increased frequency and duration of episodes, GERD occurs in approximately 5% to 8% of all newborns and has been associated with apnea and other life-threatening events. GERD is often associated with esophagitis, failure to thrive, and aspiration pneumonia and is noted after there is a pathological and/or histological change due to reflux (Potts, 2002). Children with GERD beyond 18 months are more likely to experience symptoms similar to an adult's.

The incidence of GER in healthy infants is approximately 40% to 50% as demonstrated by regurgitation followed by crying. The incidence of GER peaks at approximately 4 months of age, then steadily declines.

GERD is more common in premature infants and those born with neurological impairments (Potts, 2002). GERD can be identified in as many as 70% of low-birth-weight infants ($\leq$1700 g) with up to 85% of those infants becoming symptom free by 1 year of age (Petersen-Smith, 2004). Up to 10% of very-low-birth-weight infants have reflux associated apnea, bradycardia, or bronchopulmonary dysplasia exacerbations. Reflux disease remains significant in 1% to 3% of older children.

The cause of GER is unknown and considered multifactorial. Neuromuscular immaturity of the lower esophagus, age, hormones, and intraabdominal pressure are suggested as factors in the development of GERD. The following information will focus mainly on GER with some integration of information about GERD.

Signs and Symptoms

The most common symptoms of GER are vomiting and regurgitation that is nonbilious and includes undigested formula or food (Potts, 2002). The infant may also appear fussy related to irritation from the acidic gastric contents. The child may also refuse to feed because of the discomfort (Potts, 2002). Other manifestations include choking, coughing, wheezing, apnea, weight loss, frequent respiratory infections, and bloody vomit.

Diagnosis

Diagnosis of GER is through history and physical exam. An upper GI series may be used to rule out anatomical abnormalities but it does not provide information about the physiological function of the esophagus and is considered an unreliable diagnostic test for pathological GERD. Post-swallowing reflux can be observed through a barium swallow. A 24-hour intraesophageal pH monitoring study is essential in the diagnosis of GERD. If esophagitis, strictures, or Barrett esophagus are suspected, an endoscopy with biopsy may be completed to confirm the diagnosis.

case study Gastroesophageal Reflux

Two-month-old Ella was born via a normal spontaneous vaginal delivery. Her birth weight was 10 lb, 2 oz. (4.6 kg) and she was 22 inches (55.8 cm) long. Her parents are of Caucasian descent. Her mother's prenatal care was initiated during the third month of gestation and the pregnancy was uncomplicated. Her mother states that Ella spits up four or five times per day. She reports that Ella has four or five soft yellowish-brown stools daily. Ella is breast-fed and her mother reports that Ella nurses every 3–5 hours. No solids have been initiated.

Ella is awake and resting quietly in her mother's arms. During the initial assessment the nurse notes the following information: axillary temperature: 98.6°F (37°C); pulse, 106 beats per minute; respirations, 28 breaths per minute; weight is 13 lb. 10 oz. (6.2 kg); and length is 23.5 inches (59.7 cm). Ella appears pink, well nourished, and well hydrated. After the assessment, Ella began to fuss, at which time her mother offered her a bottle of Enfamil, which she takes eagerly. After completion of the bottle, Ella regurgitates a small amount of partially digested nonbilious liquid. Ella then closes her eyes and quietly falls asleep. The mother proceeds to tell the nurse that this is what normally occurs when Ella vomits.

1. Are these findings normal or pathological?

2. What actions should the nurse take?

3. What should be included in parent teaching?

◆ See Suggested Answers to Case Studies in text on the Electronic Study Guide or DavisPlus.

Nursing Care

Healthy, well-nourished infants need no treatment for physiological reflux. Common interventions include providing caregiver support and anticipatory guidance. The caregiver needs to be reassured that there is no underlying disease.

Steps in managing reflux with no underlying structural problems may begin with evaluating and changing the volume of the feeding such as offering small amounts more often and burping frequently. Thickening of feedings with cereal can provide sufficient calories while reducing the volume. One teaspoon per ounce of dry infant cereal may be added to 1 to 2 ounces of formula. Care must be taken when adding cereal to formula as it increases the caloric density of the formula and decreases the amount of fluid intake. Intra-abdominal pressure increase can be avoided by positioning the infant in an upright position (generally no higher than a 45 degree angle) after feeding. Several studies have reported that a prone position decreases episodes of reflux. Since prone positioning has been associated with sudden infant death syndrome (SIDS) this should only be considered with extreme caution and when complications from GER exceed the risk of SIDS. In addition, right side-lying positioning facilitates gastric emptying.

If the infant experiences complications, pharmacological therapy may be offered (Bishop, 2006). Proton-pump inhibitors, such as omeprazole (Losec) and lansoprazole (Prevacid), provide effective medical therapy for heartburn and esophagitis. H₂ inhibitors such as cimetidine (Tagamet) and ranitidine (Zantac) may also reduce heartburn though are considered less effective (Bishop, 2006). Prokinetic drugs, such as metoclopramide (Reglan), offer enhanced stomach emptying and increase lower esophageal sphincter control though the benefit is considered minimal (Bishop, 2006). Surgical treatment may be recommended for severe symptoms, such as those that are life threatening or unresponsive to nonsurgical interventions.

The surgical intervention of choice for the treatment of GERD is a **Nissen fundoplication** (wrapping the gastric cardia with adjacent portions of the gastric fundus) (Venes, 2009). A feeding jejunostomy (a surgical creation of an opening into the jejunum) may be used for infants with severe neurological defects who cannot tolerate oral or gastric tube feedings (Bishop, 2006).

Nursing care for either GER or GERD includes a thorough assessment of the infant's growth measurements and developmental patterns. Feeding patterns should be evaluated, and the amount, type, and frequency of feedings should be established with the pattern of regurgitation or emesis related to the feedings. In addition, information about positioning and burping after feedings should be determined. A baseline respiratory status is important because of the risk of aspiration associated with GERD (Potts, 2002). Much of the initial nursing management focuses on educating the caregiver regarding dietary modifications, positioning, and pharmacological therapy if prescribed. The importance of frequent burping and suggested positions for burping should also be discussed with the caregiver. Depending on the age of the child and the nature of the diet, education may also include information about dietary irritants (e.g., chocolate, caffeine products, citrus fruits, fruit drinks, tomatoes). If treatment includes use of thickened feedings, the nurse should demonstrate how to enlarge the hole in the nipple to better facilitate this type of feeding (Potts, 2002). Caregivers may also need to be reminded to avoid vigorous playing after feeding.

Nursing Insight— *Gastroesophageal reflux*

Frequent use of an infant seat for positioning should be avoided as it reduces truncal tone in infants and increases intraabdominal pressure, which can promote reflux (Potts, 2002).

nursing diagnoses The Child with Gastroesophageal Reflux (GER and GERD)

- Imbalanced Nutrition: Less than Body Requirements related to chronic vomiting or regurgitation
- Risk for Fluid Volume Deficit related to excessive losses through normal route
- Risk for Aspiration related to increased intragastric pressure with an incompetent cardiac sphincter
- Potential for Parental Knowledge Deficit related to lack of information concerning the child's care

HIRSCHSPRUNG DISEASE

Hirschsprung disease, also known as congenital aganglionic megacolon, is caused by a congenital absence of Meissner's and Auerbach's autonomic plexus in the bowel wall. This absence of ganglion cells results in lack of motility in the affected portion of the bowel (Parks & Yetman, 2004). Hirschsprung disease is usually limited to the distal colon. The absence of ganglion cells in the affected portion of the bowel results in lack of nervous system stimulation to that portion of the colon. This leads to abnormal or absence of peristalsis in the involved segment and an inability of the internal sphincter to relax. A complete or partial bowel obstruction may occur as a result of this inability of the smooth muscles to relax. This in turn leads to an accumulation of bowel contents and an innervated bowel. The obstruction may extend proximally to involve varying portions of the colon.

The incidence of Hirschsprung disease is 1 in 5000 births. It is the most common cause of neonatal obstruction of the colon and accounts for up to 33% of all neonatal obstructions (Parks & Yetman, 2004). The condition is familial, four times more common in males, and more common in children with trisomy 21 (Down syndrome) (Parks & Yetman, 2004).

Signs and Symptoms

The history of the child with Hirschsprung disease may include a failure to pass meconium within the first 48 hours of life, failure to thrive, poor feeding, chronic constipation, and Down syndrome (Parks & Yetman, 2004). Physical findings include vomiting, abdominal obstruction, failure to pass stools, diarrhea, flatus, or explosive bowel movements. In older children, the initial symptom is chronic constipation (Potts, 2002). The child's stools may be described as ribbon or pellet shaped and foul smelling.

Enterocolitis (inflammation of the small intestine and colon) is the most ominous presentation of Hirschsprung disease. Enterocolitis may present in an otherwise well infant with a history of constipation. The child with enterocolitis may present with an abrupt onset of foul-smelling diarrhea, abdominal distention, and fever. Rapid progression may indicate perforation of the bowel and sepsis. The major cause of death in Hirschsprung disease is related to enterocolitis and sepsis, accounting for up to 30% of cases (Potts, 2002).

Diagnosis

Diagnosis in the newborn is suspected based on clinical presentation or intestinal obstruction and failure to pass meconium. Radiographic studies show evidence of a dilated loop of bowel. A barium enema often demonstrates the transition between the dilated proximal colon and the aganglionic distal segment, though this may not be evident until age 2 months or later. Absence of ganglion cells is determined by a biopsy. Rectal manometry and rectal suction biopsy are the easiest and most reliable indicators of Hirschsprung disease. In anorectal manometry a balloon is distended in the rectum and measures the pressure of the internal anal sphincter. In normal patients, rectal distention initiates a reflex decline in internal sphincter pressure. In patients with Hirschsprung disease, the pressure fails to drop or there is a rise in pressure with rectal distension.

Nursing Care

Correction of Hirschsprung disease involves surgical resection of the affected bowel with or without a colostomy (Parks & Yetman, 2004). Surgical interventions generally include a temporary colostomy to be performed with an ostomy takedown and reanastomosis at age 6 to 12 months. Other surgical options include excising the aganglionic segment and anastomosing the normal proximal bowel to the rectum 1 to 2 cm above the dentate line.

Another procedure includes creating a neorectum. A neorectum involves bringing down normally innervated bowel behind the aganglionic rectum. The endorectal pull-through procedure involves stripping the mucosa from the aganglionic rectum and bringing normally innervated colon through the residual muscular cuff. This bypasses the abnormal bowel from within. Advances in techniques have led to successful laparoscopic pull-through (Potts, 2002).

Initial care of the child with Hirschsprung disease involves preoperative assessment of the child's fluid and electrolyte status. The child is placed NPO and a nasogastric tube is inserted. Intravenous fluids and electrolytes are administered to prevent and/or correct imbalances (Potts, 2002).

Postoperative care includes routine post-abdominal surgical intervention. Patency of the nasogastric tube is maintained along with monitoring for abdominal distention and assessing for return of bowel sounds. Proper placement of the NG tube can be checked by instillation of air and listening for a "pop" or aspiration of gastric contents. Accurate intake and output is maintained to include colostomy and nasogastric tube drainage.

The nurse must instruct the caregiver how to care for the temporary colostomy. The instructions should include care of the skin, appliance application, and referral to community resources. The caregiver also needs to be instructed on the symptoms of complications, such as enterocolitis, leaks, and strictures at the site of anastomosis. Signs of leaks include abdominal distention and irritability. Constipation, vomiting, and diarrhea may indicate strictures (Potts, 2002). Signs of enterocolitis may include abdominal distention and pain in addition to fever, diarrhea, or shock-like symptoms (Lee & Kocoshis, 2005).

Malabsorption Disorders

LACTOSE INTOLERANCE

Lactose intolerance is an inability to digest milk and some dairy products, which leads to symptoms of bloating, cramping, and diarrhea (Venes, 2009). This condition results from a deficiency in the enzyme lactase, which is necessary for the digestion of lactose in the small intestine where lactose is hydrolyzed into glucose and galactose. Hydrolysis is a chemical decomposition in which a substance is split into simpler compounds by taking up the elements of water (Venes, 2009). Lactose intolerance can be categorized into at least three different entities. Congenital lactase deficiency is an inborn error of metabolism, which becomes evident once the newborn consumes a lactose-containing product, such as human milk or formula products. This deficiency results from reduced or absence of lactase. Congenital lactose deficiency is rare and requires lifelong dietary restrictions.

Primary lactase deficiency, also referred to as late-onset lactase deficiency, is the most common type of lactose intolerance. Primary lactase deficiency usually becomes evident around three to seven years of age.

 Ethnocultural Considerations— Occurrence of Lactose Intolerance

Asians, southern Europeans, Arabs, Israelis, and African Americans experience a high incidence of primary lactase deficiency.

Secondary lactase deficiency, or lactose intolerance, can also occur secondary to intestinal lumen injury. Damage to the intestine can decrease or destroy the enzyme lactase. Temporary or permanent lactose intolerance can be caused by disorders such as cystic fibrosis, celiac disease, and kwashiorkor (severe protein-deficiency form of malnutrition of children), as can various infectious processes such as giardiasis (infection with a flagellate protozoan), rotavirus (a RNA virus), or HIV (human immunodeficiency virus).

Signs and Symptoms

The major symptoms of lactose intolerance are bloating, cramping, abdominal pain, and flatulence. Pain and diarrhea occur often within 30 minutes of the ingestion of lactose-containing products. Children with lactose intolerance may have a recent history of viral gastroenteritis. Signs in infants include vomiting, distention, abdominal pain after ingesting lactose-containing formula or the ingestion of cow's milk by the breast-feeding mother. Severe watery diarrhea with stools positive for reducing substance may be evident in infants with congenital lactase deficiency.

Diagnosis

Lactose intolerance is diagnosed on the basis of the history and a decrease in symptoms with elimination of lactose products from the diet. Diagnosis is further confirmed with the reintroduction of lactose-containing foods and a flare of symptoms. The nurse can communicate to the family that "the breath-hydrogen test is used to positively diagnose the condition". The breath-hydrogen test measures hydrogen in the breath after a challenge with the ingestion of 50 grams of lactose (Venes, 2009).

 Nursing Insight— *Diagnosing lactose intolerance in infants and toddlers*

An endoscopic visualization of the gastric mucosa and a digestive fluid sample may be needed with infants and toddlers due to the difficulty of performing the breath hydrogen test.

Nursing Care

Eliminating dairy products or the use of enzyme replacement may be used for the treatment of lactose intolerance. Reducing the amounts of dairy products instead of eliminating them is recommended by others. Soy-based formula can be substituted for formula or breast milk in infants. Most individuals can tolerate small amounts of lactose and should be encouraged to include it in their diets. Milk products are better tolerated when taken at meal times. Enzyme tablets, such as Lactaid, Lactrase, and Dairy Ease, can be used to predigest the lactose in milk or supplement the child's own lactose. The enzyme tablets can be added to milk or sprinkled on dairy products.

 critical nursing action Lactose Intolerance

The nurse understands that dairy products are a major source of calcium and that vitamin D supplements are needed to prevent deficiency. Hard cheese, cottage cheese, or yogurt may be taken in place of milk.

 clinical alert

Probiotics

Concern regarding the potential for decreased bone mineral density and osteoporosis in children and adolescents with lactose intolerance reinforces the recommendations for the ingestion of small amounts of dairy products with meals. **Probiotics** (food preparations containing microorganism) such as *Lactobacillus* can improve lactose intolerance when live cultures are fermented in dairy products. Lactobacillus is a nonpathogenic bacteria that produces lactic acid from carbohydrates and is normally found in milk, feces of infants fed by bottle, and adults. The active culture in yogurt provides a source of calcium for persons with lactose intolerance in addition to producing some of the lactose enzyme required for proper digestions.

Care of the child and family dealing with lactose intolerance is primarily directed at diagnosis, support, and education. Dietary education should include identification of the restrictions and alternative sources of dairy products, which can be included in the diet. Caregivers also need to be made aware of hidden sources of lactose such as its use as a bulk agent in certain medications. Caregivers need to consult with pharmacists regarding the avoidance of lactose-containing medications. The caregiver should be directed to alternative sources of calcium, such as yogurt, that are appropriate for the child's diet.

CELIAC DISEASE

Celiac disease, also known as celiac sprue, gluten-induced enteropathy, and gluten-sensitive enteropathy, is a disorder in which the proximal small bowel mucosa is damaged as a result of dietary exposure to gluten and is the second only to cystic fibroses as a cause of malabsorption disease in children (Bishop, 2006). The disorder does not present until gluten products have been introduced into the diet, usually between 6 months and 2 years of age as table foods are introduced into the diet. Celiac disease is a permanent intolerance to gluten. Gluten consists of two protein components, glutenin and gliadin. The toxic protein component is thought to be that of gliadin (Potts, 2002). Gluten is found in wheat, rye, barley, and related grains. Rice does not contain toxic gluten and can be eaten freely, as can a special preparation of oats (Bishop, 2006).

The pathology shown with celiac disease reveals a diffuse lesion of the upper small intestinal mucosa. Short, flat villi, deepened crypts, and irregular vacuolated surface epithelial layer and crypt hyperplasia are seen via light microscopy (Potts, 2002). As the villi flatten out and atrophy there is a decrease in the absorptive surface of the intestine. Malabsorption with a decreased fat absorption eventually impacts the absorption of proteins; carbohydrates; and the fat-soluble vitamins A, D, E, and K (Potts, 2002).

It is estimated that approximately 1 in 250 and up to 1% of the population in the United States has celiac disease, of which only a few are diagnosed (Gelfond & Fasano, 2006). The disease is also more common in persons with type 1 diabetes, autoimmune thyroiditis, trisomy 21, Turner syndrome, and IgA deficiency (Bishop, 2006).

 Ethnocultural Considerations— *Occurrence of Celiac Disease*

Celiac disease primarily affects people of northern European descent. The average incidence of celiac disease in Europe is 1:1000 live births with a range of 1:250 in Sweden to 1:4000 in Denmark (Potts, 2002).

Signs and Symptoms

Early manifestations of celiac disease are nonspecific and include anorexia, irritability, weight loss, and listlessness. Classic presentation in the pediatric population begins around age 6 months to 2 years and is characterized by gastrointestinal manifestations as gluten products are introduced into the diet. As the disease begins to progress, symptoms include diarrhea and abdominal distention. The diarrhea becomes chronic and is bulky, greasy, foul-smelling, and putty colored due to the large amount of undigested fat content (Potts, 2002). The presence of high fat content in the stool is called steatorrhea and may also cause the stool to float. Due to protein losses the child develops a protuberant abdomen, loss of subcutaneous fat, hypotonia, anorexia, lethargy, and muscle wasting. Inadequate vitamin K absorption leads to the development of anemia and bruising. Growth retardation and osteoporosis, in addition to delayed puberty development, are considered late signs. A less typical presentation occurs in children between ages 5 and 7 years and may include unusual intestinal complaints, such as recurrent abdominal pain, nausea, vomiting, bloating, constipation, and extraintestinal manifestations. In addition to delay in puberty and short stature the child may experience iron deficiency, abnormal liver function, and dental enamel defects. An atypical presentation of celiac disease may delay diagnosis until adult years as the extraintestinal manifestations overshadow the GI symptoms, which may be mild or entirely absent.

Diagnosis

The combination of clinical symptoms and serologic markers may suggest the diagnosis of celiac disease though a small bowel biopsy is essential to confirm the diagnosis and should be performed before gluten is eliminated from the diet (Bishop, 2006; Potts, 2002). A positive biopsy reveals atrophy of the villi and deep crypts on the intestinal mucosa is the definitive test (Potts, 2002). Laboratory tests can detect antigliadin and antiendomysial antibodies in addition to evidence of malabsorption and nutritional deficiencies. The nurse understands that the presence of antigliadin and antiendomysial antibodies and their disappearance when gluten is removed from the diet are important findings in the diagnosis.

Nursing Care

The treatment of celiac disease is a gluten-free diet. Since gluten is found mainly in wheat and rye and to a smaller extent in barley and oat products it is recommended that they be eliminated from the diet. Corn, rice, and millet are grains that are allowed in the diet. Dietary consultation is helpful as well as referral to a celiac support group (Bishop, 2006). The child and caregivers need to be instructed on the hidden sources of gluten, which may be found in many processed foods, such as thickening agents, soups, and luncheon meats. Gluten is added to many foods as hydrolyzed vegetable protein. Supplemental calories, vitamins, and minerals are recommended during the acute phase. The nurse should communicate to the caregiver that normal amounts of fat are suggested. Improvement is generally demonstrated within a week though complete recovery and histologic normality may require from 3 to 12 months (Sondheimer, 2007). Assessment of symptoms, growth, and adherence to the gluten-free diet (GFD) should be assessed and monitored with periodic visits. The Celiac Disease Guideline Committee recommends measurement of transglutaminase (TTG) after 6 months of treatment with a GFD to demonstrate a decrease in antibody titer as an indirect indicator of dietary adherence

and recovery. Measurement of TTG levels is also recommended in individuals with recurrent or persistent symptoms at any time after initiation of the GFD. Intervals of a year or longer in the asymptomatic patient serve as a monitor of adherence to the GFD.

 Optimizing Outcomes— Celiac disease

Best Outcome: Celiac disease requires a life-long commitment to diet control. Providing optimal outcomes for the child with celiac disease involves dietary guidance. Instruct the child and parents on the importance of carefully reading labels for hidden sources of gluten-based products. These can often be found in common foods, such as ice cream, hot dogs, luncheon meats, soups, and cookies.

Children with more severe mucosal damage have impaired digestion of disaccharides, especially in relation to lactose. This may also necessitate the need for temporary lactose restriction in the diet. General dietary needs include high calories and proteins with simple carbohydrates, such as fruits and vegetables. High-fiber foods, such as raw vegetables and fruits with skins, nuts, and raisins are avoided until bowel inflammation has been reduced. It is important to stress the life-long need for diet control. Once the gluten-free diet has been introduced and symptoms are resolved the child, and possibly the caregivers, may believe that the condition has been corrected.

 Be sure to— Obtain consent for genetic testing

In the case of genetic testing of children, the risks and benefits of testing should be discussed with the child as appropriate for their level of development. Most testing requires only a blood sample with little physical risk, although there can be psychological risks to the child that include decreased self-worth, anxiety, and disruption of family bonds (Chasson, Gutt, & Ihlenfeld, 2002). The best interest of the child should be the primary consideration when genetic testing is ordered with counseling provided before the testing. Where possible both parents and the child should provide informed consent.

SHORT BOWEL SYNDROME

Short bowel syndrome (SBS) is a malabsorptive disorder that results from decreased mucosal surface area, which is usually caused by surgical resection of the small bowel. Factors such as dysmobility and overgrowth of bacteria can exacerbate the malabsorption. Volvulus, gastroschisis, necrotizing enterocolitis, and atresias are the most common causes of SBS in children. Crohn's disease is also a cause in older children. Trauma to the GI tract is a less common cause of SBS. The small intestine may be congenitally short in conditions in which bowel is lost in utero. Loss of a large portion of the bowel produces malabsorption and malnutrition. Short bowel syndrome results in compromised bowel function.

Signs and Symptoms

Malnutrition and diarrhea are the most common manifestations of SBS. Steatorrhea and carbohydrate malabsorption result in diarrhea and failure to thrive. The potential for dehydration, acidosis, hyponatremia, and hypokalemia results from an inadequacy of the short bowel to reabsorb fluid and electrolytes.

 Nursing Insight— Short bowel syndrome

The major symptoms are diarrhea, malabsorption, malnutrition, and dehydration. Electrolytes are abnormal secondary to diarrhea and malabsorption.

Diagnosis

Diagnosis is confirmed by abdominal x-ray exam, abdominal ultrasound, endoscopy, colonoscopy, and complete blood count (CBC) that reveals anemia.

A stool sample may reveal presence of infection; blood; or nonabsorbed sugar, fats, and protein.

Nursing Care

Nursing care focuses on maintaining adequate nutrition and preventing complications (Potts, 2002). The use of total parenteral nutrition (TPN) via a central line is part of the initial treatment of SBS. Enteral feedings are begun via nasogastric or gastrostomy tube (Potts, 2002). The nurse should communicate to the caregiver that the "main purpose of enteral nutrition is to stimulate the adaptive growth of the small intestine" (Potts, 2002, p. 692). Oral feedings may be started as tolerated in order for the infant to learn to suck and swallow. Pacifiers are also encouraged for this purpose. TPN may be gradually decreased as enteral and oral feedings are increased.

One main focus of nursing care includes administration and monitoring of the nutritional therapy. Care must be taken to avoid the complications of a central venous line (a venous access device inserted into the vena cava to infuse fluids and medicines) and TPN therapy (Venes, 2009).

 clinical alert

Complications of a Central Venous Line

When the child has a central line placement, the nurse observes the infusion site at least every 4 hours for complications such as infiltration, thrombophlebitis, fluid or electrolyte overload, or air embolism. The site dressing and administration set are also changed according to the institution's policies (Venes, 2009).

The care of enteral feeding tubes is also an important part of nursing care. Care must be taken to observe for signs of dislodgement, infection, or occlusion.

Feeding tolerance must also be included as part of nursing care. Input, output, specific gravity, and weights are assessed daily by the nurse. Stools are tested for occult blood, pH, and reducing substances in addition to monitoring for vomiting, changes in the appearance of the stools, and abdominal distention.

With prolonged hospitalization, the nurse needs to consider the child's emotional and developmental needs. Caregivers also need to be provided with psychosocial support and education to assist them in coping with the long-term effects of SBS. The plan of care should include attention to interventions to promote family adaptation.

Home-care services provide the opportunity for children with SBS to receive carefully monitored care at home. The nurse may serve as a resource for connecting the family to the appropriate home-care agencies, nutritional support services, and supply sources.

Hepatic Disorders

BILIARY ATRESIA

Biliary atresia, or extrahepatic biliary atresia (EHBA), is an idiopathic, progressive, inflammatory process that causes both intrahepatic and extrahepatic bile duct fibrosis and obstruction. Biliary atresia is the second most common liver disease diagnosed in infants with an incidence that ranges from 1 in 8000 to 21,000 live births and is fatal within the first 2 years of life if not corrected. The disease is more common in girls and premature infants. In the United States, the incidence is twice as high in African American infants as in Caucasian infants. The exact cause of biliary atresia is unknown. EHBA has two distinct presentations, postnatal and fetal, with differing mechanisms of development suggested. Infections and immune-related mechanisms are implicated in postnatal EHBS, which represents 65% to 90% of cases. In the fetal form there is a congenital absence of patent biliary ducts.

Signs and Symptoms

The earliest clinical manifestations of EHBS and most outstanding features include jaundice, which can be first observed in the sclera. Jaundice may also be evident at birth but usually is not apparent until age 2 to 3 weeks of age. Urine is dark and stains the infant's diaper. Stools are lighter than normal and often tan to white in color. The infant demonstrates poor weight gain and symptoms of failure to thrive resulting from poor fat metabolism. Pruritus (itching, burning, or tingling of the skin) and irritability are present, which are often evident by an infant who is difficult to comfort. Hepatomegaly (enlarged liver) is an early symptom and the liver is firm upon palpitation. Splenomegaly (enlargement of the spleen) occurs later.

Diagnosis

Early diagnosis is the key to survival of the child with EHBA. Infants who have surgery within the first 60 days of life have an 80% chance of establishing bile flow, with the potential for successful correction. CBC, electrolytes, bilirubin, and liver enzymes are included in the diagnostic workup as well as a TORCH titer (lab test for presence of antibodies for Toxoplasmosis, Other infections, Rubella, Cytomegalovirus, Herpes simplex, and urine cytomegalovirus) and sweat test (measures electrolytes excreted in a sweat test to rule out cystic fibrosis) to rule out other conditions with symptoms of jaundice and cholestasis. Biliary patency may be demonstrated by hepatobiliary scintigraphy (HIDA scan) but is not diagnostic. Endoscopic retrograde cholangiopancreatography (ERCP) can be performed in a very young infant and has an 80% accuracy. A percutaneous liver biopsy is also highly reliable.

Nursing Care

Medical care is primarily supportive and focuses on providing nutritional support. Formula with medium-chain triglycerides and essential fatty acids is recommended as well as supplemental minerals including iron, zinc, and selenium and the fat-soluble vitamins A, D, E, and K. For the infant with moderate to severe failure to thrive, aggressive nutritional support in the form of continuous tube feedings or TPN may be required. For advanced liver dysfunction, management is similar to that of the child with cirrhosis.

Management also involves surgical resection to correct the obstruction and provide for the drainage of bile from the liver into the intestines. The Kasai procedure, which is a hepatic portoenterostomy, may be performed to slow pathological changes that take place in the biliary duct (Potts, 2002). In surgery done before 8 weeks of age bile flow drainage is achieved approximately 90% of the time. A hepatic portoenterostomy involves resecting a section of the jejunum to the liver at the normal exit site of the hepatic duct to allow bile drainage into the small intestine. The jejunum may be looped to form a cutaneous double-barreled ostomy (Venes, 2009). Approximately one-third of infants regain normal liver function and become jaundice free after the Kasai procedure. A middle third demonstrate liver damage and must be supported by medical and nutritional interventions and the last third eventually require a liver transplant.

Preoperative care involves educating the family regarding the plan of care and the long-term nature of the condition. Nursing care immediately after a hepatic portoenterostomy is similar to that of the child following other major abdominal surgery. To help the child regain optimal health, providing nutritional support postoperatively involves special formulas, vitamins, and mineral supplements parenterally and through tube feedings. For the infant with a double-barreled ostomy bile is obtained from one site and refed into the other site after feeding. The child's family needs to be instructed on and demonstrate skin and stoma care to be continued after discharge. The family also needs instruction on how to monitor and administer nutritional therapy. Side effects such as pruritus can be addressed through drug therapy and comfort measures. Postoperative risks and long-term complications should be explained so as to include symptoms to observe for such as indications of GI bleeding, ascites (accumulation of fluid in the peritoneal cavity), and cholangitis. Psychosocial support should be provided to the child and family to assist them in coping with the long-term nature of the condition, financial burden, uncertain prognosis, and potential waiting for transplant.

CIRRHOSIS

Cirrhosis is a pathological condition that occurs as an end stage to many liver and inflammatory conditions such as biliary atresia and chronic hepatitis (Potts, 2002). Autoimmune factors, infection, and chronic diseases such as hemophilia and cystic fibrosis can cause severe liver disease, which can lead to cirrhosis or irreversible damage. Cirrhosis is rare in the pediatric population but may develop as a result of chronic inflammation or disease, which causes scar tissue formation. Scar tissue leads to impaired intrahepatic blood flow and ongoing necrosis, which results in further cirrhotic changes.

Signs and Symptoms

Manifestations vary depending on the cause. General manifestations include jaundice, growth failure, muscle weakness, anorexia, and lethargy. Impaired intrahepatic blood flow leads to anemia, abdominal pain, edema, ascites, and GI bleeding. If the cirrhosis is secondary to a disorder of fat metabolism, steatorrhea may be observed (Potts, 2002). Portal hypertension and ascites are common symptoms of cirrhosis in the child with biliary anomalies. Splenomegaly is the most important sign of portal hypertension (Potts, 2002). Splenomegaly may be demonstrated by the presence of anemia, leukopenia, thrombocytopenia, and esophageal varices. These conditions lead to easy bruising, epistaxis, and GI hemorrhage (Potts, 2002). Jaundice, dark urine, and pruritis are symptoms of biliary obstruction.

Diagnosis

Diagnosis of cirrhosis is based on history, physical examination, laboratory values, and liver biopsy. Ascites, blood flow through the liver and spleen, and patency of the portal vein can be confirmed by Doppler ultrasonography of the liver and spleen. Laboratory evaluation includes liver function tests, such as bilirubin, aminotransferase, ammonia, albumin, cholesterol, and prothrombin time.

Nursing Care

Goals of care are directed at preventing and treating complications as there is no successful treatment of cirrhosis. Malabsorption problems are treated with nutritional support, such as a low-fat, low-protein diet and supplemental fat-soluble vitamins. Fluid restrictions, diuretics, and low-sodium diet are used to treat ascites. Blood and blood products are administered for the treatment of bleeding complications and hepatic encephalopathy is treated with reduced protein diet (Potts, 2002).

The only definitive treatment for end-stage liver disease and cirrhosis is a liver transplant, which improves the prognosis for many children (Potts, 2002). A 90% 1-year survival rate has occurred as a result of a combination of new surgical techniques and the use of immunosuppressive therapy.

Nursing care of the child with cirrhosis is similar to that of any child with a severe life-threatening disease. Interventions include monitoring for complications of malnutrition, hemorrhage, and hepatic failure in addition to providing comfort measures and emotional support.

HEPATITIS

Hepatitis may be acute or chronic and involves an inflammation of the liver. Hepatitis may be caused by virus or bacterial infections, fungal or parasitic infections, or chemical or drug toxicity (Potts, 2002). Six distinct viruses have been identified as causing hepatitis: hepatitis A virus (HAV), hepatitis B virus (HBV), and hepatitis C virus (HCV) in addition to hepatitis D virus (HDV), hepatitis E virus (HEV), and hepatitis G (HGV), which are not common (Potts, 2002). HAV, HEV, and HGV cause only acute infection. HBV and HCV cause chronic infections, whereas HDV has both acute and chronic forms. HAV and HEV are transmitted via the fecal–oral route, which is referred to as an enteral form of hepatitis (Potts, 2002). HBV, HCV, HDV, and HGV are transmitted via blood transfer or through intimate sexual contact, which is referred to as a parenteral form (Potts, 2002). Vaccines are available for the prevention of HAV and HBV. While each type of hepatitis has unique characteristics, assessment findings and treatments have many similarities (Table 25-3).

Most cases of hepatitis in children are caused by HAV and are most common in ages 5 to 14 years (Potts, 2002). HAV is found in the stool of infected individuals and transferred by oral ingestion, which is easily spread in areas with poor sanitation. Poor hygiene is also an important factor in the spread of HAV. High-risk areas also include settings where there are a number of children and infants in a common area, such as a day care center. Contact may occur directly through infected feces or indirectly through food and water contamination (Potts, 2002). Outbreaks have occurred in areas that have experienced sewage-contaminated water, infected food handlers with poor hygiene, and shellfish caught in water contaminated by sewage (Potts, 2002). The incubation period is 15 to 40 days (Sokol & Narkewicz, 2007).

HDV occurs only in patients with acute or chronic HBV infection, which causes it to be severe. The risk of HDV is reduced with hepatitis B vaccination. HDV is also more common in Mediterranean countries and among hemophiliacs and IV drug users. HEV is more common in adults and uncommon in developed countries and is rare in the United States (Sokol & Narkewicz, 2007). High-epidemic areas include Southeast Asia; China; the Middle East; and parts of Africa, Mexico, and Central America (Sokol & Narkewicz, 2007). HEV produces a high incidence of mortality in pregnant women. The high-risk group for HGV includes transfusion recipients, IV drug users, and persons infected with HCV. Individuals infected with HGV are usually asymptomatic for liver involvement.

Signs and Symptoms

Characteristics for HAV, HBV, and HCV overlap considerably. Headache, anorexia, malaise, abdominal pain, nausea, and vomiting are characteristic of the preicteric phase, which lasts approximately 1 week and usually precedes the onset of clinically detectable disease (Jensen & Baltimore, 2006). Dark urine precedes the jaundice phase (Sokol & Narkewicz, 2007). The most common symptoms of the icteric phase are jaundice and hepatomegaly, which may last several weeks. Stools may appear clay-colored during this phase (Sokol & Narkewicz, 2007). Prodromal symptoms (initial stages of the disease) often decline in children during the icteric phase (Jensen & Baltimore, 2006). Young children are often asymptomatic or have a mild, nonspecific illness without icterus hepatitis A virus (HAV), hepatitis B virus (HBV), and hepatitis C virus (HCV) (Table 25-4).

Diagnosis

Diagnosis is based on history of exposure, symptoms, and serologic testing for markers of hepatitis A, B, and C, and liver function tests, specifically an elevation of ALT (alanine aminotransferase—an intracellular enzyme involved in amino acid and carbohydrate metabolism [Venes, 2009]), AST (aspartate aminotransferase—an intracellular enzyme involved in amino acid and carbohydrate metabolism [Venes, 2009]) and serum total bilirubin. Liver biopsy may be required to establish the diagnosis and degree of disease, although it is rarely indicated in the

Table 25-3 Hepatitis Viruses					
	HAV	**HBV**	**HCV**	**HDV**	**HEV**
Type of Virus	Enterovirus	Hepadnavirus	Flavivirus	Incomplete	Calicivirus
Transmission	Fecal–oral	Parenteral, sexual, vertical	Parenteral, sexual, vertical	Parenteral, sexual	Fecal–oral
Incubation period	15–40 days	50–150 days	30–150 days	20–90 days	14–65 days
Diagnostic tests	Anti-HAV IgM	HBsAg, anti-HBc IgM	Anti-HCV, PCR-RNA test	Anti-HDV	Anti-HEV
Mortality rate	0.1–0.2%	0.5–2%	1–2%	2–20%	1–2% (20% in pregnant women)
Carrier state	No	Yes	Yes	Yes	No
Vaccine available	Yes	Yes	No	Yes (HBV)	No
Treatment	None	Interferon-α, nucleoside analogues (lamivudine, tenofovir, adefovir, entecavir)	Interferon-α (pegylated interferon in adults) plus ribavirin	Treatment for HBV	None

Source: Sokol, R.J., & Narkewicz, M.R. (2007). Liver and pancreas. In W.W. Hay, M.J. Levin, J.M. Sondheimer, & R.R. Deterding (Eds.). *Current diagnosis & treatment in pediatrics* (18th ed.). New York: Lange Medical Books/McGraw-Hill, pp. 638–683.

Table 25-4 Comparison of Hepatitis A (HAV), Hepatitis B (HBV), and Hepatitis C (HCV)			
Clinical Features	**HAV**	**HBV**	**HCV**
• Onset	Usually rapid, acute	More insidious	Usually insidious
• Fever	Common and early	Less frequent	Less frequent
• Anorexia	Common	Mild to moderate	Mild to moderate
• Nausea & vomiting	Common	Sometimes present	Mild to moderate
• Rash	Rare	Common	Sometimes present
• Arthralgia	Rare	Common	Rare
• Pruritus	Rare	Sometimes present	Sometimes present
• Jaundice	Present	Present	Present

Source: Sokol, R.J., & Narkewicz, M.R. (2007). Liver and pancreas. In W.W. Hay, M.J. Levin, J.M. Sondheimer, & R.R. Deterding (Eds.). *Current diagnosis & treatment in pediatrics* (18th ed.). New York: Lange Medical Books/McGraw-Hill, pp. 638–683.

diagnosis of HAV (Sokol & Narkewicz, 2007). The nurse understands that the presence of antigens or antibodies confirms and differentiates the diagnosis HAV, HBV, and HCV. Serum immunological tests are not available to detect HAV, but there are two HAV antibody tests, anti-HAV IgG and immunoglobulin M (IgM). Anti-HAV is present at the onset and persists throughout life. A positive anti-HAV test indicates the presence of a current infection, immunity from a past infection or immunization.

Nursing Care

The goal for management of viral hepatitis includes early detection, support, and monitoring of the disease, recognition of chronic liver disease, and prevention of spread of the disease. Management of hepatitis is primarily supportive as there is no specific treatment (Potts, 2002). Management includes measures to provide rest to the liver, hydration, adequate nutrition, and the prevention of complications. Severe dehydration, vomiting, a prolonged prothrombin time, or signs of encephalopathy are indications for hospitalization (Jensen & Baltimore, 2006).

Immune globulin should be given to children who have been exposed to a person with HAV within 2 weeks of exposure. Immune globulin is up to 90% effective when given during this time period (Potts, 2002). The prognosis for children with hepatitis A virus (HAV) is usually good as most cases are mild and in most cases carrier states do not occur. Prevention of HBV infection after a one-time exposure such as a needle stick can be effectively prevented by the use of hepatitis B immune globulin (HBIG).

Nursing care is directed at maintaining comfort, providing adequate nutrition, and educating the family regarding prevention measures. Children with mild symptoms can be cared for at home, which necessitates the need to instruct the family regarding infection control, providing a well balanced diet, and providing rest. Children with hepatitis A virus (HAV) are not considered infectious within a week after the onset of jaundice and school attendance may be resumed. The family also needs to be instructed to avoid administering any medication to the child since normal doses of drugs may become dangerous because of the liver's inability to process them. Preventive measures include instructing the family on good hand washing (the single most effective preventive measure), food handling, and careful disposal of excreta and stool-contaminated objects. Hepatitis A vaccine is recommended for children ages 2 through 18 years who may be living in high-risk communities (Potts, 2002).

 critical nursing action Prevention of Hepatitis A and Hepatitis B

- Wash hands after changing diapers and using the toilet.
- Wash hands before food preparation and eating.
- Carefully dispose of soiled diapers.
- Wash linen or clothing contaminated with stool separately in hot water.
- Clean contaminated household surfaces with bleach and water (1/4 cup of bleach to 1 gallon of water).
- HAV and HBV vaccination.

Source: Potts, N. (2002). Gastrointestinal alterations. In N.L. Potts & B.L. Mandleco (Eds.). *Pediatric nursing: Caring for children and their families.* Clifton Park, NY: Delmar-Thomson Learning, pp. 653–696.

Abdominal Trauma: Injuries

The leading cause of death in children and adolescents after the first year of life is caused by injuries. Injuries are responsible for more than 50% of all deaths in the 15- to 24-year age group (Brayden, Daley, & Brown, 2007). Motor vehicle injuries are the primary cause of accidental death in the United States with nearly 60% occurring with unrestrained children (Brayden et al., 2007). Ten percent of serious trauma to children occurs as a result of abdominal and genitourinary injury, which include contusion or laceration to liver, spleen, and kidneys (Ruddy, 2005) (Table 25-5). Injuries to hollow organs are increasing partly related to the increasing number of improperly restrained children involved in motor vehicle accidents (Ruddy, 2005).

Table 25-5 Injuries Caused by Abdominal Trauma

Organ	Incidence and Description	Management
Abdomen	• Approximately 8% of pediatric trauma • Risk of blunt trauma injuries increased because of relative size and close proximity of organs • Penetrating trauma accounts for <10% of pediatric abdominal trauma • Gunshot wounds involve multiple organs in 80% of the cases	• Serial examination is primary in decisions regarding surgical interventions • Surgical intervention may be required if persistent unstable vital signs along with aggressive fluid replacement • Laparoscopy may be indicated with peritoneal irritation and abdominal wall discoloration • CT is valuable for assessing intra-abdominal trauma
Spleen	• Most frequently injured abdominal organ in children • Positive Kehr sign (pressure on the left upper quadrant eliciting left shoulder pain) related to diaphragmatic irritation from ruptured spleen • Spleen injury suspected with left upper quadrant abrasions or tenderness • Splenic injury may include capsular tear to a complete rupture	• CT scan can be used to grade splenic injury • Treatment of choice is nonoperative management • Surgery indicated for blood loss greater than 40 mL/kg or transfused blood in 24–36 hours or evidence of hemodynamic instability • With splenectomy penicillin prophylaxis is recommended
Liver	• Accounts for 40% of all deaths associated with blunt abdominal trauma in children • Right lobe injuries are more common • Diagnosis based on Kehr sign (pressure on the right upper quadrant eliciting right shoulder pain) • Severe hemorrhage is more common with liver injury than with other abdominal organs	• Conservative management is recommended with ongoing monitoring of blood loss, hepatic function, and liver structure with serial CR scans or ultrasound • Operative management is reserved for life-threatening situation
Pancreas and duodenum	• Less common in children than adults • Seen in bicycle handlebar injuries, motor vehicle crashes and nonaccidental trauma • Diagnosis difficult unless obvious injury to overlying structures • Diffuse abdominal tenderness, pain and vomiting accompanied by elevation of amylase and lipase may be indicative of injury though often does not occur for several days after injury • Duodenal injuries include hematomas and perforation • Perforations are difficult to diagnose	• Management includes nasogastric suction and parenteral nutrition • Nonoperative management is appropriate for contusions • Surgical interventions may be required with distal transection • Perforation is not always obvious with a CT
Intestinal	• Injury occurs less often than with solid intra-abdominal organs • Risk varies with the amount of intestinal contents, i.e., a full bowel is likely to shear more easily than an empty bowel • Lap belt or seatbelt in a motor vehicle crash results in a sudden deceleration and increase in intraluminal pressure and can lead to perforation	• Presence of a contusion over the seatbelt area and abdomen or back pain indicates a need to pursue the diagnosis of intestinal injury • Pneumoperitoneum in association with intestinal perforation occurs in about 20% of patients

Source: Marcdante, K.J. (2006). The acutely ill or injured child. In R.M. Kliegman, K.J. Marcdante, H.B. Jenson, & R.E. Behrman (Eds.). *Nelson: Essentials of Pediatrics* (5th ed.). Philadelphia: Elsevier, pp. 179–216.

summary points

◆ The gastrointestinal (GI) system of the child is immature compared to that of an adult, leading to variations in response to illnesses.

◆ Pyloric stenosis is characterized by projectile vomiting and a palpable olive-shaped mass in the epigastrium.

◆ One of the most common causes of intestinal obstruction in infancy is from intussusception.

◆ Anorectal malformations are usually evident at birth.

◆ The most common type of hernia in children is an umbilical hernia.

◆ Signs and symptoms of appendicitis include abdominal pain that begins in the periumbilical area and moves to the right lower quadrant, accompanied by a low-grade fever, nausea, and occasionally vomiting.

◆ Treatment focus for inflammatory bowel disease includes medication, nutrition, and often surgery.

- Nursing care of the child with celiac disease includes education about the gluten free diet.

- The complications of peritonitis and perforation from appendicitis can be prevented by prompt recognition and diagnosis.

- Care of the child with gastroesophageal reflux (GER and GERD) can be managed by teaching the caregiver feeding and positioning methods to prevent or reduce reflux.

- Correction of Hirschsprung disease involves surgical resection of the affected bowel with or without a colostomy.

- Malabsorption disorders include lactose intolerance, celiac disease, and short bowel syndrome.

- Progressive cirrhosis and death occur from untreated biliary atresia in most children by age two.

- Cirrhosis is a pathological condition that occurs as an end stage to many liver and inflammatory conditions such as biliary atresia and chronic hepatitis.

- Hepatitis may be acute or chronic and involves an inflammation of the liver. Hepatitis may be caused by virus or bacterial infections, fungal or parasitic infections, or chemical and drug toxicity.

- Ten percent of serious trauma to children occurs as a result of abdominal and genitourinary injuries, which include contusion or laceration to liver, spleen, and kidneys

review questions

Multiple Choice

1. A 6-week-old infant is admitted to the hospital with the possible diagnosis of hypertropic pyloric stenosis. The nurse asks the parents about the infant's feeding history. Which of the following symptoms is most descriptive of pyloric stenosis in the infant?
   A. Abdominal peristaltic waves passing from right to left
   B. Frequently appearing hungry with projectile vomiting
   C. Periodic bilious forceful vomiting after feedings
   D. Decrease interest in feedings with weight loss

2. The pediatric nurse is monitoring a child for signs of bowel perforation. On assessment, the nurse notes which of the following as an important sign of bowel perforation?
   A. Acute pain over the affected area
   B. Frequent bradycardia
   C. Increased urinary output
   D. An episode of bloody diarrhea

Select All that Apply

3. It is important for the pediatric nurse to have keen assessment skills in order to monitor a child who may display signs of shock. Which signs should be immediately brought to the attention of the pediatrician?
   A. Hypotension
   B. Hypertension
   C. Cyanosis
   D. Tachycardia

Case study (Questions 4 and 5 refer to the same scenario.)

4. A 10-year-old boy is admitted to the pediatric unit where the nurse is suspicious of appendicitis. During the interview process, the child tells the nurse that the pain woke him up in the morning and that although he has not eaten in the past 24 hours, he does not feel hungry at all.
   Which of the following signs are indicative of appendicitis?
   A. Constant pain in the left lower quadrant
   B. History of vomiting before the onset of the pain
   C. History of pain around the umbilicus
   D. History of diarrhea in the past 48 hours

5. Shortly after admission to the pediatric unit, the child complains of severe acute pain that spreads over the entire abdomen. On assessment, the pediatric nurse finds that the child has a rigid and tense abdomen. The child is also tachycardic and has a fever. Perforation of the appendix is suspected. The child is taken to the operating room immediately. Immediate postoperative care for appendectomy includes which of the following? (Select all that apply.)
   A. A nasogastric tube is inserted to decompress the stomach.
   B. Bowel sounds are not assessed as to prevent further damage.
   C. Fluids are given to the child when awake.
   D. Intravenous antibiotics are given for 7 to 10 days.

True/False

6. The nurse teaches the mother of a newborn that her baby has been born with an absent vaginal opening and that this condition is called an imperforate anus.

7. A 14-year-old child has just been admitted to the emergency room. The pediatric nurse is teaching the family about peritonitis. The nurse explains that peritonitis in children includes moderate pain that worsens with movement.

8. A 12-year-old child has just been diagnosed with Crohn's disease. The nurse explains to the family that surgical treatment can cure the child.

Fill-in-the-Blank

9. During the abdominal assessment, the nurse is aware that a classic sign of hypertrophic pyloric stenosis is the _____ to _____ movement of peristalsis.

10. The nurse teaches the parents of a 3-month-old infant with gastroesophageal reflux to place the infant _____ following feedings ensuring that the infant is awake and well supervised.

11. The nurse needs to be alert to signs of dehydration, such as changes in _____ _____, appearance of the _____ _____, depressed fontanel, presence or absence of _____, urine output, and changes in _____ _____.

12. When comparing the adolescent with Crohn's disease to the adolescent with ulcerative colitis, the patient with _____ _____ will have continuous patchy areas in the intestine, as opposed to the

patient with _____ _____ who will have diffuse, segmented areas of involvement.

See Answers to End of Chapter Review Questions on the Electronic Study Guide or DavisPlus.

REFERENCES

Bishop, W.P. (2006). The digestive system. In R.M. Kliegman., K.J. Marcdante, H.B. Jensen, & R.E. Behrman (Eds.). *Nelson essential of pediatrics* (5th ed.). St. Louis, MO: Elsevier, pp. 579–624.

Blosser, C.G. (2004). Complementary medicine. In C.E. Burns, A.M. Dunn, M.A., Brady, N.B. Starr, & C.G. Blosser (Eds.). *Pediatric primary care: A handbook for nurse practitioners* (3rd ed.). St. Louis, MO: Elsevier, pp. 1211–1248.

Brayden, R.M., Daley, M.F., & Brown, J.M. (2007). Ambulatory & commuity pediatrics. In W.W. Hay, M.J. Levin, J.M. Sondheimer, & R.R. Deterding (Eds.). *Current diagnosis & treatment in pediatrics* (18th ed.). New York: Lange Medical Books/McGraw-Hill, pp. 225–245.

Bulechek, G., Butcher, H.M., & Dochterman, J. (2008). *Nursing interventions classification (NIC)* (5th ed.). St. Louis, MO: C.V. Mosby.

Campbell, K.M., & Balistreri, W.F. (2005). Inflammatory bowel disease. In L.M. Osborn, T.G. DeWitt, L.R. First, & J.A. Zenel (Eds.). *Pediatrics*. St. Louis, MO: Elsevier, pp. 947–953.

Chasson, C., Gutt, C., & Ihlenfeld, J.T. (2002). Legal and ethical issues. In N.L. Potts, & B.L. Mandleco (Eds.). *Pediatric nursing: Caring for children and their families*. Clifton Park, NY: Delmar-Thomson Learning, pp. 33–54.

Deglin, J.H., & Vallerand, A.H. (2009). *Davis's drug guide for nurses* (11th ed.). Philadelphia: F.A. Davis.

Dunn, A.M. (2004). Elimination patterns. In C.E. Burns, A.M. Dunn, M.A. Brady, N.B. Starr, & C.G. Blosser (Eds.). *Pediatric primary care: A handbook for nurse practitioners* (3rd ed.). St. Louis, MO: Elsevier, pp. 285–300.

Jensen, H.B., & Baltimore, R.S. (2006). Infectious diseases. In R.M. Kliegman., K.J. Marcdante, H.B. Jenson, & R.E. Behrman (Eds.). *Nelson essential of pediatrics* (5th ed.). St. Louis, MO: Elsevier, pp. 445–578.

Johnson, M., Bulechek, G., Butcher, H., McCloskey Dochterman, J., Maas, M., Moorehead, S., & Swanson, E. (2006). *NANDA, NOC, and NIC linkage: Nursing diagnoses, outcomes, & interventions* (2nd ed.). St. Louis, MO: Mosby Elsevier.

Lee, P., & Kocoshis, S.A. (2005). Congenital anatomic disorders of the gastrointestinal tract. In L.M. Osborn, T.G. DeWitt, L.R. First, & J.A. Zenel (Eds.). *Pediatrics*. St. Louis, MO: Elsevier, pp. 938–940.

Mao, C.S. (2005). Genital disorders in preadolescent boys. In L.M. Osborn, T.G. DeWitt, L.R. First, & J.A. Zenel (Eds.). *Pediatrics*. St. Louis, MO: Elsevier, pp. 742–746.

Marcdante, K.J. (2006). The acutely ill or injured child. In R.M. Kliegman, K.J. Marcdante, H.B. Jenson, & R.E. Behrman (Eds.). *Nelson: Essentials of pediatrics* (5th ed.). Philadelphia: Elsevier, pp. 179–216.

Moorehead, S., Johnson, M., Maas, M., & Swanson, E. (2008). *Nursing outcomes classification (NOC)* (4th ed.). St. Louis, MO: C.V. Mosby.

Murphy, M.A. (2004). Developmental management of toddlers and preschoolers. In C.E. Burns, A.M. Dunn, M.A. Brady, N.B. Starr, & C.G. Blosser (Eds.). *Pediatric primary care: A handbook for nurse practitioners* (3rd ed.). St. Louis, MO: Elsevier, pp. 107–126.

Mow, W. (2005). Disorders of the intestine. In L.M. Osborn, T.G. DeWitt, L.R. First, & J.A. Zenel (Eds.). *Pediatrics*. St. Louis, MO: Elsevier, pp. 670–677.

NANDA International (2007). *NANDA-I nursing diagnoses: Definitions and classifications 2007–2008*. Philadelphia: NANDA-I.

Parks, D.K., & Yetman, R.J. (2004). Perinatal conditions. In C.E. Burns, A.M. Dunn, M.A. Brady, N.B. Starr, & C.G. Blosser (Eds.). *Pediatric primary care: A handbook for nurse practitioners* (3rd ed.). St. Louis, MO: Elsevier, pp. 1083–1128.

Petersen-Smith, A.M. (2004). Gastrointestinal disorders. In C.E. Burns, A.M. Dunn, M.A. Brady, N.B. Starr, & C.G. Blosser (Eds.). *Pediatric primary care: A handbook for nurse practitioners* (3rd ed.). St. Louis, MO: Elsevier, pp. 839–884.

Potts, N. (2002). Gastrointestinal alterations. In N.L. Potts, & B.L. Mandleco (Eds.). *Pediatric nursing: Caring for children and their families*. Clifton Park, NY: Delmar-Thomson Learning, pp. 653–696.

Reichard, K., & Lake, A.M. (2005). Disorders of the gastrointestinal tract and liver. In L.M. Osborn, T.G. DeWitt, L.R. First, & J.A. Zenel (Eds.). *Pediatrics*. St. Louis, MO: Elsevier, pp. 938–970.

Ruddy, R.M. (2005) Injuries and trauma. In L.M. Osborn, T.G. DeWitt, L.R. First, & J.A. Zenel (Eds.). *Pediatrics*. St. Louis, MO: Elsevier, pp. 279–285.

Sokol, R.J., & Narkewicz, M.R. (2007). Liver and pancreas. In W.W. Hay, M.J. Levin, J.M. Sondheimer, & R.R. Deterding (Eds.). *Current diagnosis & treatment in pediatrics* (18th ed.). New York: Lange Medical Books/McGraw-Hill, pp. 638–683.

Sondheimer, J.M. (2007). Gastrointestinal tract. In W.W. Hay, M.J. Levin, J.M. Sondheimer, & R.R. Deterding (Eds.). *Current diagnosis & treatment in pediatrics* (18th ed.). New York: Lange Medical Books/McGraw-Hill, pp. 605–637.

Thilo, E.H., & Rosenberg, A.A. (2007). The newborn infant. In W.W. Hay, M.J. Levin, J.M. Sondheimer, & R.R. Deterding (Eds.). *Current diagnosis & treatment in pediatrics* (18th ed.). New York: Lange Medical Books/McGraw-Hill, pp. 1–64.

Venes, D. Ed. (2009). *Taber's cyclopedic medical dictionary* (21st ed.) Philadelphia: F.A. Davis.

DavisPlus For more information, go to **http://davisplus.fadavis.com/**

CONCEPT MAP

Malabsorption disorders:
- Lactose intolerance
- Celiac disease
- Short bowel syndrome

Care Of The Child With A GI Disorder

Hepatic disorders:
- Biliary atresia
- Cirrhosis
- Hepatitis

Structural disorders:
- Inguinal hernia
- Umbilical hernia
- Anorectal malformation
  - Rectal atresia/stenosis
  - Imperforate anus

Potential Nursing Care:
Depends on → type and severity of disease
May include:
- Assessments
  - Stool pattern; growth and development; diet/eating pattern; medications
- Care
  - Correct prep for diagnostics
  - Preoperative care → prepare child/family
  - Postoperative → wound care, I&O/fluid status, pain management
  - Nutritional support → TPN; dietary restrictions
  - Prevent infection
  - Treat underlying cause of condition
  - Correct administration of medication(s)
  - Ostomy care
- Teaching
  - Compliance
  - Life-long dietary changes
  - Toileting/enemas
  - Spontaneous resolution
  - Umbilical cord care
  - Prevention/vaccination

Inflammatory disorders:
- IBD → Crohn's; ulcerative colitis
- Appendicitis
- Omphalitis
- Meckel diverticulum

Functional disorders:
- Irritable bowel syndrome
- Infantile colic
- Acute/chronic diarrhea
- Vomiting
- Constipation
- Encopresis
- GER & GERD
- Hirschsprung disease

Obstructive disorders:
- Hypertrophic pyloric stenosis
- Intussusception
- Malrotation/volvulus

Critical Nursing Action:
- Know alternate sources of calcium and vitamin D
- Hepatitis A and B prevention
- Lie child down to palpate abdomen
- Skin turgor is a critical assessment

What To Say:
- Surgery repairs for hernia defect: give post op care instructions
- School stress can trigger IBS

Collaboration In Caring:
- Plan of care for child with encopresis requires collaboration with school nurse

Clinical Alert:
- Abdominal pain can be referred
- Hypertrophic pyloric stenosis → classic sign projectile vomiting
- Know symptoms of IBS, perforation; peritonitis and shock
  - Most constipation is idiopathic
  - Major signs of short bowel syndrome are diarrhea and malabsorption

Across Care Settings:
- A balanced diet promotes growth
- Hand-washing in the community decreases gastroenteritis
- A food diary can identify triggers for IBS

Where Research Meets Practice:
- Using enteric-coated fish oil decreases relapses of Crohn's

Complementary Care:
- *Lactobacillus* decreases diarrhea associated with rotavirus in infants

Nursing Insight:
- Watery stools are normal in infants
- Congenital diaphragmatic hernia = bowel sounds heard in chest
- Appendicitis signs: periumbilical pain; vomiting
- Not all fruits decrease constipation
- IBS can include ulcerative colitis and Crohn's

Ethnocultural Considerations:
- Hypertrophic pyloric stenosis more common in Caucasian males
- "Empacho" = indigestion
- Occurrence of primary lactose deficiency and celiac disease culturally linked

Now Can You:
- Identify the general signs of GI obstruction
- Discuss various treatments for IBD
- Discuss the management of constipation
- Differentiate between regurgitation and GERD
- Differentiate between hepatitis A, B and C

Caring for the Child with an Immunological or Infectious Condition

Integrating the Science and Art of Nursing

Nursing is a learned profession built upon a core body of knowledge reflective of its dual components of science and art. Nursing requires judgment and skill based upon principles of the biological, physical, behavioral, and social sciences. Registered nurses use critical thinking to apply the best available evidence and research data to the processes of diagnosis and treatment. Nurses continually evaluate quality and effectiveness of nursing practice to seek to optimize outcomes.

—American Nurses Association (2004). *The Scope and Standards of Nursing*, p. 10.

LEARNING TARGETS *At the completion of this chapter, the student will be able to:*

◆ Discuss why infectious and immune diseases represent a significant pediatric health concern for the child, family, and public.

◆ Describe the body's first and second lines of defense.

◆ Explain the congenital immunodeficiency disorders.

◆ Examine the goals of treatment for HIV-positive children.

◆ Discuss why post-cell-transplant children are placed in a medically induced state of immunosuppression.

◆ Explore autoimmune disorders together with related nursing care.

◆ Discuss the three types of infections together with related nursing care.

◆ Describe the importance of immunizations and the role of the nurse.

◆ Explain why animals serve as a reservoir for certain infectious diseases.

◆ Describe possible solutions for the increase in the incidence of infections with antibiotic-resistant organisms.

---

 moving toward evidence-based practice Maintaining Peripheral Intravenous Locks

Mok, E., Kwong, T.K., & Chan, M.F. (2007). A randomized controlled trial for maintaining peripheral intravenous lock in children. *International Journal of Nursing Practice, 13*, 33–45.

The purposes of this study were to compare the effectiveness and safety of three intravenous flush solutions in maintaining peripheral locks and to evaluate differences in the incidence of complications among them. The methods compared were a normal saline flush, a 1 unit/mL heparin–saline flush, and a 10 units/mL heparin–saline flush.

The study, conducted in a hospital pediatric unit, included a sample of 123 children whose ages ranged from 1 year to 10 years. The participants were randomly assigned to one of the three treatment groups; each group consisted of 43 children. Each child was selected to receive one of the three flush solutions.

Study inclusion criteria included:

- Presence of a 22-gauge or a 24-gauge peripheral intravenous (IV) catheter that was anticipated to remain beyond the day of insertion
- IV flush or medication ordered every 6 or 8 hours
- Written consent obtained from a parent or guardian
- Verbal consent obtained from the patient as appropriate

(continued)

---

moving toward evidence-based practice (continued)

Study exclusion criteria included:

- Presence of a known bleeding disorder
- Abnormal platelet count or clotting factors
- Received medication that affected coagulation
- Received a transfusion of blood products or IV cytotoxic drugs.

The researchers developed an IV site assessment form that was used every 8 hours or with each administration of medication or IV flush through the peripheral lock. The form assessed the following signs of complications: redness, swelling, pain, coolness to the touch, and/or leakage at the insertion site.

Before the initiation of the study, the pediatric unit nurses who would be performing the peripheral flush and completing the IV site assessment form received education and hands-on practice on a standard method for flushing a peripheral lock.

All IV peripheral flushes were documented in the treatment records as Heparin Flush A or B or C. Since the study was a double-blind design, the nurse providing the flush only knew that the participant belonged to group A, group B, or group C and did not know the type of flush administered. All doses were prepared by two nurses who were not involved in the IV site assessments.

The study found no statistically significant differences among the three groups in:

- Length of catheter use
- Estimated catheter survival
- Incidence of intravenous complications
- Types of flushing solution in terms of the catheter longevity
- Incidence of intravenous complications

However, the researchers determined that children older than 2 years of age had a greater incidence of backflows (abnormal backward flow of fluid) that required additional flushes. This increase in incidence of backflows may be related to the child's mobility and play, which has been supported in the literature.

The researchers concluded that the type of flush used was not a significant predictor of catheter longevity and incidence of intravenous complications.

---

1. What might be considered as limitations to this study?
2. How is this information useful to clinical nursing practice?

See Suggested Responses for Moving Toward Evidence-Based Practice on the Electronic Study Guide or DavisPlus.

Introduction

Infectious and immune diseases represent a significant pediatric health concern for the child, family, and public. Prevention and control of infections and communicable diseases is a primary goal of national, state, and local health agencies, addressed largely through surveillance, public education, and immunization programs. Pediatric nurses are at the forefront of these efforts and are responsible for nursing care of children and families and in assisting families to become informed and educated so that they can take an active role in caring and advocating for their children.

Pediatric immune disorders are complex and require the pediatric nurse to work closely with the family to develop a plan of care that will promote healthy growth and development while addressing health needs related to the illness. An intact immune system has a profound effect on the vulnerability of the child to infectious disease. Disorders of the immune system in children, either absence of a component of immunity or a failure to differentiate self from nonself, may be either congenital or acquired.

The nurse's role in health promotion and prevention of immune and infectious diseases is explored, with an emphasis on the role of the nurse as caregiver and educator. Information on nurse–family partnership addresses immune system dysfunction in children.

The Immune System

The immune system protects the child from an attack of foreign intruders. Although the purpose of the immune system is identical for children and adults, in the child much of the immune response is as yet untested, or naïve, making the response somewhat less efficient (Hoffjan et al., 2005).

A & P review   **An Important Line of Defense**

The immune system is made up of cells, tissues, and organs that work in an organized manner to protect the body against invaders and infectious organisms.

The white blood cells (leukocytes) are part of the defense system. There are two basic types: phagocytes (neutrophils are the most common and fight bacteria) and lymphocytes (B lymphocytes and T lymphocytes), which seek out and destroy organisms that might cause disease.

Leukocytes are produced or stored in the lymphoid organs: lymph nodes, bone marrow, thymus, spleen, and tonsils. The leukocytes circulate throughout the body via the blood.

Antigens are foreign substances that invade the body. When an antigen is detected several types of cells work together to recognize and respond to the invader. Mature B lymphocytes independently identify foreign antigens and differentiate into antibody-producing plasma cells (memory cells). Once the B lymphocytes have produced antibodies, these antibodies remember so if the same antigen is presented to the immune system again, the antibodies can respond. Although antibodies can recognize an antigen they are not capable of destroying it without the help mature T cells that are antigen specific.

Antibodies can also neutralize toxins and activate a group of proteins that assist in killing bacteria, viruses, or infected cells.

The protection offered by the immune system is called immunity. There are three types of immunity: innate, adaptive, and passive. Innate immunity (or natural) is a general protection and includes the physcial barriers of the body, like the skin and mucous membranes. The skin is the first line of defense in preventing diseases from entering the body. Adaptive (or active) immunity develops as children are exposed to diseases or immunized against diseases through vaccination. Passive immunity is acquired by the introduction of preformed antibodies into an unprotected individual and it lasts for a short period of time. For example, passive immunity can occur from antibodies that pass from the mother to the fetus through the placenta or newborns that acquire immunity through breastfeeding. ◆

The Body's Defense

The skin is the most important physical barrier and the body's first line of defense. It is the largest organ of the body and has several major functions:

1. Protects the deeper tissues from injury
2. Protects the body from foreign matter invasion
3. Regulates temperature
4. Aids in water retention
5. Aids in synthesis of vitamin D
6. Initiates the sensations of touch, pain, heat, and cold
   - The mucous membranes provide a protective barrier against the entry of pathogens.

Mechanical and chemical barriers also help protect the child. For instance, tears, urine, vaginal secretions, and semen have a role in primary defense against infection. The nurse understands that the mechanical action of these fluids flowing out from the body carries with it unwanted intruders that may cause disease. An example of a chemical barrier is the acidic secretions of the stomach and digestive enzymes that serve to neutralize organisms taken into the body through the mouth. Chemical barriers in the gastrointestinal system can be maintained with good nutrition.

 Clinical Alert

Increased risk for infection

The nurse understands that something as simple and common as diaper rash is more than a simple irritation; it is also a potential portal entry for microorganisms.

The body's second line of defense is the **immune response**. The overall purpose of the immune response is to defend the body against microorganisms, parasites, and foreign cells such as cancer cells and transplanted cells. Key to a normal immune response is the body's ability to recognize foreign substances as nonself and then to mobilize defenses and attack the invaders. A deficiency in the immune response may lead to serious illness in the pediatric patient.

 Nursing Insight— Immunoglobulins

Immunoglobulins, also known as antibodies, are substances made by the body's immune system in response to diseases and other insults. The major types of immunoglobulins are:

IgM is the first type of antibody made by the body in response to an infection. This antibody also helps other immune system cells destroy foreign substances. An adult level is attained by 9–12 months of age.

IgG antibodies are important in fighting bacterial and viral infections. An adult level is attained by 1 year of age.

IgA antibodies protect the body's surface from foreign substances. An adult level is attained by 5 years of age.

IgE causes the body to react against foreign substances such as fungus spores, animal dander, and pollen. An adult level is attained by early childhood

 Nursing Insight— Children are more vulnerable to infection

There are important aspects about children that make them more vulnerable to infection:

1. The skin has a thinner texture that is more susceptible to external irritants and a greater risk for the absorption of microorganisms because of the greater body surface area.
2. Immunoglobulin A (IgA) secreted by the epithelial cells of the mucous membranes does not reach adult levels until the child is 5 years of age, making children less resistant to organisms.
3. The endocrine glands that secrete sweat are not capable of mature function until 3 years of age, making children less able to regulate body temperature.

A way to help ensure a healthy immune system is to educate the family about the role of the immune system and the natural processes that help the body maintain resistance to disease. Nurses can support the child's immune system through nursing interventions, such as meticulous skin care and measures that target the maintenance of important barriers (Fig. 26-1).

Congenital Immunodeficiency Disorders

Congenital immunodeficiency disorders are rare but include more than 70 specific types of disorders that result in life-long impairment of immune system function. The impairment causes an increase in incidence, severity, and recurrence of infections.

Symptoms of congenital immunodeficiency disorders begin in infancy, and the actual onset of symptoms

Figure 26-1 Assessing and maintaining skin care is an important role of the nurse.

depends on the exact immune components involved. Specific disorders are grouped according to the component of the immune system that is affected (B cell, T cell, B lymphocytes, and combined). Children with immune system disorders are at risk for infection not only from outside pathogens, but also from their own normal flora.

B-CELL DISORDERS

In B-cell disorders, inadequate or a nearly absent number of immunoglobulins may be present. Maternal antibodies naturally protect newborns during the first few months of life; thus B-cell disorders do not become apparent until the third month of life. Most of the congenital immunodeficiency disorders (for example, selective IgA deficiency and common variable immunodeficiency) are genetically X-linked and are more likely in male children.

In B-cell disorders, the child usually has recurrent infections, beginning with respiratory infections. Infections of the skin and mucous membranes, typically seen in B-cell disorders, are generally more severe, and complications are frequent. Many children develop weight loss and fail to meet developmental milestones.

Specific treatment of B-cell disorders depends on the actual disorder. General treatment principles include supporting immune function through maintenance of barriers, providing good nutrition, preventing infection, administering prophylaxis antibiotics or antiviral agents, and administering selected vaccinations. Stem cell transplants are indicated for selected disorders.

T-CELL DISORDERS

Disorders affecting T lymphocytes are infections that begin in infants younger than 6 months of age. It is rare for a disorder of T lymphocytes to occur in isolation; generally abnormalities of T lymphocytes are either a component of a combined immune disorder or associated with a syndrome of congenital anomalies. For example, with DiGeorge syndrome, there is a constellation of congenital anomalies, including heart defects, absence of the parathyroid gland, abnormal facial characteristics, and an absent or underdeveloped thymus. These infants have a variety of clinical problems shortly after birth related to cardiac defects and disturbances in calcium regulation secondary to the parathyroid absence. The alteration in immune function is highly variable depending on whether there is a functioning thymus. Those without a functioning thymus have decreased counts of T lymphocytes and therefore have a limited ability to fight infection. These infants have both fungal and viral infections early in infancy. They are treated symptomatically and with antibiotic prophylaxis to prevent *Pneumocystis carinii* infection. Definitive treatment of the immunodeficiency includes thymus transplant and stem cell or histocompatibility antigen HLA-identical bone marrow transplant.

B-LYMPHOCYTE DISORDERS

Disorders affecting B lymphocytes and antibody production tend to occur in older infants and children. Specific B-lymphocyte disorders result in a failure to produce adequate numbers of antibodies. Passive protection from maternal antibodies masks these disorders during the first few months of life. Children with B-lymphocyte disorders have multiple bacterial infections and failure to thrive. Treatment consists of the administration of specific immunoglobulins to replace missing factors and antibiotics that aggressively treat bacterial infections.

A specific B-lymphocyte disorder in children is transient hypogammaglobulinemia of infancy, in which the infant immune system is delayed in production of antibodies, sometimes until the child is 12 to 36 months of age. Support with immunoglobulin administration and antibiotics is needed until the child begins to produce antibodies. The condition is more common in premature infants and is self-limiting, resolving as the immune system matures and begins to produce antibodies.

COMBINED IMMUNODEFICIENCY DISORDERS

Combined immunodeficiency disorders affect multiple components of the immune system. They are more severe, occur in early infancy, and are often fatal during childhood. Severe combined immunodeficiency disease (SCID) is the most severe form of combined immunodeficiency. It is a congenital condition and results in absence or abnormal function of the B lymphocytes, T lymphocytes, and natural killer cells. The child with this disorder often has recurrent infections by the age of 3 months. Typical infections for SCIDs include otitis media, thrush, and pneumonia. The children often have diarrhea that contributes to failure to thrive. The infections are difficult to eliminate, tend to recur, and may be caused by unusual organisms such as *Pneumocystis carinii* or cytomegalovirus. Medical management includes antibiotics and immune globulin administration to control infections. A stem cell or bone marrow transplant is generally attempted. Without aggressive treatment, these children die before 2 years of age.

 ***Nursing Insight*—** *Wiskott–Aldrich syndrome*

Wiskott–Aldrich syndrome is an example of a combined immunodeficiency syndrome. It results in thrombocytopenia, abnormal levels of B lymphocytes, and alteration in T-lymphocyte function. Wiskott–Aldrich syndrome is an X-linked congenital disorder, occurring only in boys. Typically, children have bloody diarrhea during infancy secondary to the platelet dysfunction. Other typical symptoms include eczema, recurrent infections, and failure to thrive. Children with Wiskott–Aldrich syndrome are at greater risk for lymphoma and leukemia. Medical management includes antibiotics, replacement of specific immunoglobulins, and eventual stem cell transplant.

Immunodeficiency Disorders

HUMAN IMMUNODEFICIENCY VIRUS

Human immunodeficiency virus (HIV) is caused by HIV-1 and is the primary cause of acquired immunodeficiency syndrome (AIDS) in infants and children. The HIV virus selectively targets and destroys T cells, thereby destroying cellular immunity. The child is virtually unprotected against a number of opportunistic infections and bacterial, fungal, and viral diseases. Every system is affected (Feeney, 2004).

Nursing Care Plan The Child with Immunosuppression

Nursing Diagnosis: Risk for infection related to immunosuppression

Measurable Short-term Goal: Child remains free from symptoms of infection.

Measurable Long-term Goal: Child regains natural resistance to infection.

NOC Outcomes:
Immune Status (0702) Natural and acquired appropriately targeted resistance to internal and external antigens
Infection Severity (0703) Severity of infection and associated symptoms

NIC Interventions:
Infection Protection (6550)
Infection Control (6540)

Nursing Interventions:

1. Institute universal precautions and designated isolation precautions as appropriate.

   RATIONALE: Precautions protect the nurse, child, and family members from the transfer of microorganisms.

2. Demonstrate and instruct visitors to wash hands on entering and leaving the patient's room and to use protective equipment properly.

   RATIONALE: Hand washing and proper use of gloves, masks, or cover gowns eliminate major transmission routes for many organisms.

3. Monitor for systemic and localized signs of infection every 2–4 hours when the child is hospitalized and at each interaction in providing community-based health care. Assess temperature, lung sounds, and condition of skin, as well as mucous membranes for pain, redness, and edema.

   RATIONALE: Fever or respiratory symptoms may be the only overt signs of infection in an immunosuppressed child. Systematic monitoring allows early recognition and treatment of infection.

4. Monitor laboratory values as obtained: absolute granulocyte count, WBC count, and differential results.

   RATIONALE: Changes in lab values alert the caregiver to developing infection. The immunosuppressed patient may not exhibit overt signs of an inflammatory response.

5. Promote a balanced diet of favorite foods, prepared and presented attractively. Allow only cooked fruits and vegetables if the child is neutropenic.

   RATIONALE: Deficient intake of protein; vitamins A, C, or E; iron; or zinc may have a detrimental effect on the immune system and place the child at increased risk for infection. Cooking fruits and vegetables helps to eliminate harmful organisms.

6. Encourage rest and sleep by providing a quiet environment.

   RATIONALE: Sufficient rest and sleep will help bolster the body's immune system.

7. Administer antibiotics and immunizations as prescribed, following CDC and AAP recommendations.

   RATIONALE: Antibiotics may be prescribed prophylactically or to treat identified infections. Most children who are able to produce antibodies are given killed vaccines.

Centers for Disease Control and Prevention (CDC) data indicate that the route of infection for the majority of children with AIDS younger than 15 years of age is prenatal transmission. Other sources of exposure are hemophilia/coagulation disorders, receipt of contaminated blood or tissue, and unidentified risk.

Prenatal transmission, also known as vertical transmission, occurs when an HIV-infected mother passes the virus on to her child. Vertical transmission may occur in utero, during birth via blood, from amniotic fluid and exposure to genital tract secretions, or after birth through the breast milk. Maternal factors, such as the stage of the illness and amount of virus in her system, affect the risk of transmission of the virus to the child. An example of an antiretroviral medication, zidovudine (AZT), given during pregnancy has demonstrated that the transmission of the virus can be prevented. This information has prompted CDC to make recommendations for pregnant women to

have voluntary prenatal testing. When a pregnant woman is HIV-positive, the infant is delivered by cesarean section and administered antiretroviral drug therapy soon after birth, which significantly reduce the risk of HIV infection in the neonate.

Before mandatory screening of blood and blood products in 1985, HIV was transmitted to children through blood transfusions. Most of the children infected with the virus were being treated for hemophilia. In the adolescent population, HIV infection occurs as a result of unprotected sexual activities and intravenous drug abuse. Prevention strategies in this age group focus on education about transmission and reduction in high-risk sexual practices.

The nurse understands that HIV selectively attacks a subset of T lymphocytes, the helper T cells. As the virus invades the helper T cells and takes over the cell for viral replication, the T cell becomes nonfunctional. A specific function of helper T cells is recognition of foreign cells; in their absence, infection is more likely. HIV also affects B-lymphocyte function, adding to the difficulty in fighting infection.

When the HIV virus is present, there is an immediate drop in CD_4^+ (helper T cell) levels. The drop is followed by an immune response, which then raises the levels and marks the beginning of a latent period that may last 10 years or longer. At some point the CD_4^+ levels again decrease and when they reach critical levels the symptoms begin to appear, heralding the onset of AIDS. In children with prenatally acquired HIV, the latency period may be very short. In children who have visible symptoms during infancy an accelerated course of disease is typical and most of these children develop manifestations of AIDS by their first year of life. Their prognosis is very poor. The majority of HIV-infected children develop symptoms more slowly, initially developing clinically recognizable AIDS at 18 to 24 months of age.

Signs and Symptoms

Common clinical manifestations of HIV infection in children are lymphadenopathy, hepatosplenomegaly, chronic diarrhea, failure to thrive, oral thrush, skin infections, fevers, and recurrent infections. Chronic diarrhea with malabsorption of nutrients contributes to a failure to grow. A variety of chronic infections further complicate normal growth and development.

Diarrhea and poor nutritional status set the stage for skin breakdown that provides a portal of entry for opportunistic and bacterial infections. Infections of the mucous membranes also provide a site of entry for infection, and pain from mucosal lesions further complicates nutritional status. Lymphadenopathy and hepatosplenomegaly are seen secondary to immune system involvement.

In addition, early onset of recurrent respiratory infections and progressive neurological involvement are common in children. The cumulative results of many serious infections are multiple developmental delays, with progressive impairment of motor skills and intellectual function.

Diagnosis

Diagnosis of HIV infection in children is necessary whenever there is a suspicion that the child may have the virus. Diagnosis of HIV infection in children requires a multipronged approach using appropriate testing and clinical observation. In infants, the diagnosis can be complicated by the transmission of maternal antibodies.

Diagnostic testing for infants with suspected or unknown prenatal exposure to the HIV virus should include a PCR test as soon as possible after birth. If the results of the test are positive, a repeat PCR test should be performed as soon as possible. Two positive PCR tests confirm the diagnosis. If there is still enough suspicion that the infant may have HIV and the initial results are negative, the PCR test needs to be repeated again at 1 to 2 months of age, 3 to 6 months of age, and 15 to 18 months of age. Children with more than two negative tests results performed after the age of 6 months (and completed more than 1 month apart) may be considered HIV negative. For initial screening in children over the age of 18 months of age, the ELISA test may be used. Again, positive results should be confirmed by repeat testing.

Nursing Care

The primary concern for early and accurate identification of children with HIV infection is beginning treatment. The goals of treatment for HIV-positive children are to slow progression to AIDS, prevent further infections, promote normal growth and development, prevent complications including cancers, and prolong and improve quality of life.

Caring for children with HIV/AIDS is a multifaceted process and includes both psychological and physiological care. Because the diagnosis and treatment for HIV can be devastating, it is important for the nurse to provide psychological care. First, the nurse must assess the family's support systems and coping mechanisms. The nurse must also assess the family's ability, desire, and skills needed to care for the child. The nurse can ask about extended family or other avenues for support such as church groups, community agencies, and friends. If the mother is also infected with HIV, the nurse must determine the best way to care for both patients. It is critical to help the family access available resources such as social workers, pastors, insurance companies, and community health clinics. Often, the acute care setting nurse can initiate the coordination of ongoing care by contacting a case manager. The case manager can then assist the family through the complexities of the health care system.

Physiological nursing care for HIV is supportive, as there is no cure for infection with the virus. Priority nursing care focuses on decreasing the potential for opportunistic infection. The nurse must be ready to manage the infections that the child acquires. Often prompt and vigorous antimicrobial therapy for treatment of infections is needed. *Pneumocystis carinii* is a common infection that occurs in early infancy before absolute confirmation of HIV status. For this reason, according to current CDC guidelines, all infants born to HIV-infected mothers are routinely started on a prophylactic antibiotic regimen for this organism. Trimethoprim-sulfamethoxazole (TMP-SMZ) (Bactrim or Septra) is the agent of choice for this treatment. Intravenous immune globulin has also been used to prevent bacterial infections in children younger than the age of 2. In addition, the nurse can teach the family signs and symptoms of infection and encourage them to limit the child's exposure to large crowds of people and those with notable infections.

Labs: HIV Testing

There are two primary methods for confirming the diagnosis of HIV:

Enzyme-linked immunosorbent assay (ELISA) is a test that identifies the presence of HIV antibodies and is performed within 48 hours after birth. ELISA is fairly inexpensive, but is not as sensitive as polymerase chain reaction and sometimes produces some false-negative results. The use of ELISA is also ineffective in children younger than 18 months owing to the presence of maternal antibodies.

Polymerase chain reaction (PCR) is a test that identifies the proviral DNA specific to HIV. The PCR is more expensive but has greater sensitivity. However, the PCR has a greater number of false-positive results.

Labs: Blood Culture

Blood does not normally contain any bacteria or fungi. A simple blood culture can detect bacteria or fungi in the blood. Children with weakened immune systems (e.g., as a result of AIDS, cancer, chemotherapy, or medications such as corticosteroids) are more susceptible to an infection in the blood. To test for an infection in the blood, a phlebotomist draws a sample of blood from a vein. In the laboratory, the blood sample is mixed with substances that promote the growth of bacteria or fungus. In most cases, bacteria can be detected in the blood culture within 2–3 days. Some types of blood infections can take 10 days or longer to detect and results of tests for fungal infections in the blood can take up to 30 days. A normal blood culture (negative) result indicates that no bacteria or fungus has been found in the blood. An abnormal (positive) result indicates that bacteria or fungus has been found in the blood.

A significant concern in children with HIV is the risk of rapidly progressive disease with commensurate high mortality in infancy. There is no reliable indicator for which children will develop rapidly progressive disease and which children will have a slower course of disease progression. For children with the HIV virus, there are several recommendations for antiviral treatment that are in a constant state of revision and controversy. Following are the most recent recommendations from the National Guideline Clearinghouse (2008).

- Antiviral treatment is *initiated* for children under 1 year with known or suspected HIV and who have clinical symptoms
- Antiviral treatment is *considered* for children under 1 year who are asymptomatic
- Antiviral treatment is *initiated* in children older than 1 year with known or suspected HIV and who have clinical symptoms
- Antiviral treatment is *strongly recommended* for children with overt AIDS or severe depression of immune response, characterized by rapidly declining CD_4^+ levels
- Antiviral treatment is *considered* in children with mild–moderate clinical symptoms with depressed but not rapidly declining CD_4^+ levels
- Antiviral treatment *may be* postponed for those children who are asymptomatic

ANTIVIRAL THERAPY. Antiviral therapy includes nucleoside analogs or nucleoside reverse transcriptase inhibitors (NRTIs) such as zidovudine (AZT), didanosine (Videx), zalcitabine (Hivid), stavudine (Zerit), or lamivudine (Epivir) that inhibit the action of viral reverse transcriptase, an enzyme in the conversion for RNA to DNA. Common side effects of these medications include fever, headache, insomnia, myalgia, nausea, vomiting, diarrhea, anorexia, and bone marrow suppression. The nurse can help the family understand the importance of antiretroviral therapy and teach parents the common side effects. Other considerations for antiretroviral therapy include actual delivery of the medication to the child in a safe and effective manner, using the five rights of medication administration. It is important for the nurse to note that many antiretroviral medications are not well tolerated by children due to taste. In addition, the medication regimen can be quite complex, requiring the family to adhere to a complicated schedule of medication administration and

---

medication: Trimethoprim-Sulfamethoxazole (TMP-SMZ; Bactrim or Septra)

Trimethoprim-sulfamethoxazole (trye-**meth**-oh-prim/sul-fa-meth-**ox**-a-zole)

Indications: Prevention of *Pneumocystis carinii* pneumonia (PCP). Prevention of bacterial infections in an immunosuppressed child.

Actions: Combination inhibits the metabolism of folic acid in bacteria at two different points.

Therapeutic Effects: Bactericidal action against susceptible bacteria.

Pharmacokinetics:
ABSORPTION: Well absorbed from the GI tract.

Contraindications and Precautions:
CONTRAINDICATED IN: Hypersensitivity to sulfonamides or trimethoprim, megaloblastic anemia secondary to folate deficiency, severe renal impairment, and children younger than 2 months of age.

Adverse Reactions and Side Effects: Hepatic necrosis, nausea, vomiting, diarrhea, toxic epidermal necrolysis, Stevens–Johnson syndrome, erythema multiforme, rashes, agranulocytosis, aplastic anemia, and phlebitis with IV insertion.

Route and Dosage for PCP Prevention:
PO (CHILDREN): 75 mg/m^3 TMP/325 mg/m^3 SMZ q12h on 3 consecutive days/week. Not to exceed 320 mg TMP/1600 mg/SMZ per day.

Nursing Implications:
1. Assess child for infection. Advise the family to notify the health care provider for any signs of infection.
2. Assess for allergy to sulfonamides.
3. Monitor lab values periodically throughout therapy. May produce elevated serum bilirubin, creatinine, and alkaline phosphatase.

Data from Deglin, J.H., & Vallerand, A. (2009). *Davis's drug guide for nurses* (11th ed., pp. 1205–1207). Philadelphia: F.A. Davis.

---

monitoring. The nurse can assist the family about how to understand the prescribed medicine routine by creating a written schedule of medications, common side effects, and when to call the physician.

SYMPTOMATIC AND SUPPORTIVE CARE. Symptomatic and supportive care of children with AIDS is similar to that for children with immunodeficiency conditions (see Nursing Care Plan: The Child with Immunosuppression). Essential in the child's care are palliative and comfort care measures. Proper hygiene, comfortable clothing, good nutrition, play, rest, and social interaction are all important aspects of care for the child. The nurse should ensure good communication between the family and health care professionals to facilitate a realistic ongoing treatment plan.

Adolescents present their own specific challenges when infected with HIV. Based on their desire to be independent, an adherence to complicated treatment regimens may be a struggle. The nurse must work closely with the adolescent to identify strategies for managing a complex medical illness with the need to be independent and socialize with peers. Often, referral to an adolescent support group is helpful for children in this age group.

Another aspect when caring for the HIV-positive child is immunizations. Immunization is usually not a controversial treatment component. In general, children should receive all immunizations including pneumococcal and influenza vaccines. Live vaccines, such as varicella and measles–mumps–rubella (MMR), can be administered if the immunocompromise is not severe. Additional boosters may be needed for children with HIV due to decreased ability to produce antibodies.

PAIN MANAGEMENT. Pain management is a significant care concern for children with HIV. Pain in children can be multfactorial, resulting from inflammation, systemic manifestation of AIDS such as cardiomyopathy, drug toxicities, invasive secondary infections, and medical procedures used to monitor and treat the HIV infection. The majority of HIV-infected children report pain as a factor affecting their daily lives. Successful management of pain is based on the same principles of pain management found in other illnesses. Diligence in identification of pain, goals, and strategies to manage pain, implementation of nonpharmacological and pharmacological pain management strategies, and ongoing pain assessments are all-important in the plan of care. Pain control is a major factor in quality of life and hence a primary goal for the nurse.

 Complementary Care: *Nonpharmacological adjuncts to pain management*

Pain management in children with HIV can be challenging. Proper pain management involves both pharmacological and nonpharmacological strategies. Nonpharmacological techniques are based on the child's own experiences and preferences. Some examples of nonpharmacological techniques include guided imagery, hypnosis, prayer, meditation, music or aromatherapy. Nonpharmacological techniques also promote *preparation, distraction*, and *relaxation* for the child.

Developmentally appropriate *preparation* before painful procedures has been shown to decrease the anticipation of pain, thus decreasing the pain experience. Child life specialists may assist the nurse to prepare the child for procedures. Preparation may include diagrams, pictures, handling equipment, meeting personnel, or visiting special rooms, such as recovery or the intensive care units.

Distraction can be useful, particularly for younger children. Techniques such as blowing bubbles, singing songs, blowing pinwheels, or reading a favorite book may turn their attention away from the procedure. Family members can be encouraged to participate in distraction by providing a favorite toy.

Relaxation can be effective in pain control and actually decreases pain in the child. Nurses can teach relaxation skills to parents early in the course of HIV. A deep sense of relaxation can be obtained through guided imagery or hypnosis. The nurse can encourage parents to purchase or borrow easy-to-read relaxation books that will help them direct the relaxation with their child.

TREATING MALNUTRITION. Malnutrition, associated with either weight loss or obesity, is a common problem in children with HIV and a contributing factor to immune dysfunction. AIDS-induced diarrhea, coupled with the common symptom of anorexia, may lead to deficiencies of micro- and macro-nutrients as well as an overall deficit in caloric intake. A new problem that has surfaced is children who have become obese. Obesity occurs secondary to the side effects of some of the medications commonly used to treat HIV coupled with decreased physical activity. Malnutrition in the form of either weight loss or obesity leads to poor nutrition in HIV-infected children, underscoring the need for continuous assessment and attention. The nurse understands that early involvement of a nutritional expert to provide consultation with the family is beneficial. The nutritionist can address specific nutritional needs and provide education about healthy dietary choices. In addition, the nutritionist can perform a nutritional assessment that includes monitoring heights and weights, evaluating laboratory values, and screening for dietary difficulties.

The nurse must understand that early use of oral supplementation is recommended to proactively meet nutritional goals. The overall goal of oral supplementation is prevention of malnutrition. In addition, aggressive oral care is emphasized as important to prevent oral lesions that may add to decreased intake. Another way to ensure adequate nutrition is the initiation of parenteral (tube) feedings. Parenteral feeding is used for the most severe cases in which all attempts at normal oral nutrition have failed. The inherent risks of invasive oral or nasal catheters can negatively affect the already immunocompromised child, making this a high-risk course of treatment. However, parenteral nutrition may correct the nutritional deficiencies and therefore is a consideration when other routes have failed.

THE TEAM APPROACH. Care of the child with HIV/AIDS is complex and best managed through collaboration with the family and others (nurse, physician, pain specialist, psychologist, nutritionist, social worker, child life specialist, and schoolteacher). The family is encouraged to view the team members as a collaborative team of professionals and then see themselves as equal participants in their child's care.

 Collaboration in Caring— *Collaboration between the family and others*

Nurse: Provides coordination of team and acts as the bridge between the family and others, assists family and child to assume an active role in the care, identifies conditions requiring intervention, provides treatments or referrals as needed, helps the family create a livable plan for their unique situation

Physician: Provides and directs all medical care and monitors infections/complications, and growth and development

Pharmacist: Provides the medication and acts as a resource to help the family understand drug actions, interactions, dosing parameters, and adverse side effects

Pain specialist: Provides management for acute and chronic pain

Psychologist: Assists the child and family to identify positive coping strategies for life with HIV/AIDS.

Nutritionist: Provides early and ongoing support for nutritional needs

Social worker: Provides support, community resources, and possible ways to manage finances

Child life specialist: Provides support for normal development and coping strategies

Schoolteacher: Assists family with a realistic educational plan through episodes of illness

Now Can You—Discuss human immunodeficiency virus (HIV)?

1. Describe the pathophysiology of HIV?
2. Differentiate between tests used to diagnose HIV infection?
3. Describe symptomatic and supportive care measures for chidren with HIV/AIDS?
4. Discuss the importance of treating malnutrition in children with HIV/AIDS?

Transplantation

Stem cell transplantation is the surgical removal of tissue from one part of the body (or individual) and its implantation into another part of the body (or individual). There are three types of stem cell transplants: autologous, isogeneic, and allogenic. In **autologous** transplant, the child's own cells are taken, stored, and reinfused after the child has received chemotherapy. In **isogeneic** transplantation, the cells are taken from an identical twin, and in **allogeneic** transplantation the cells are from a donor (family member) who has a compatible human leukocyte antigen. The National Marrow Donor Program is used when no relative is found to match the child.

NURSING CARE

After the surgery, post-transplant immunosuppression is critical. Children are placed in a medically induced state of immunosuppression to maintain sufficient immune system function to resist infection while at the same time suppressing the immune system just enough to decrease the possibility of tissue rejection.

Nursing Insight— Monoclonal antibody

A monoclonal antibody is a type of antibody that is highly specific to a single antigen. These antibodies are generated in a laboratory setting. They identify and target microorganisms, white blood cells, hormones, and tumor antigens. Monoclonal antibody is used to treat transplant rejection, autoimmune diseases, and certain cancers.

Medically induced post-transplant immunosuppression is accomplished in three phases; induction, maintenance, and rejection. In the *induction phase*, the child is given medications to suppress immune function. In the *maintenance phase* a combination of medications is often given to provide the correct amount of immunosuppression that allows the graft to flourish but does not leave the child vulnerable to infections. In an acute *rejection phase*, episodes are treated with increased immunosuppression medications to stop immune system attack on the graft site.

Corticosteroids are the drug of choice for medically induced immunosuppression because they are potent anti-inflammatory agents and act to inhibit T-lymphocyte activation and cytokine (proteins produced primarily by white blood cells) production (Copenhaver et al., 2004). However, corticosteroids are nonspecific in their action, producing a generally less responsive state of immune function. This presents a delicate balance for any child

undergoing corticosteroid treatment. Although these medications are used primarily in post-transplant scenarios, it is important to recognize that children with other conditions are treated with corticosteroids, such as children with asthma or an autoimmune disorder such as systemic lupus erythematosus. It is important for the nurse to remember that any child taking corticosteroids to prevent post-transplant rejection or other illnesses is at higher risk for infections secondary to a slow and inefficient immune response.

Nursing care for children taking immunosuppressive medications includes prevention of infection by limiting exposure to overcrowded areas and infected individuals, promotion of good nutrition and general health, and maintenance of barriers, including skin and mucous membranes. Early identification and aggressive treatment for any infection is paramount.

 clinical alert

Administration of steroids

The nurse or parents must *never* stop the administration of any steroids abruptly due to adrenal insufficiency. Although adrenal insufficiency is a risk at any time with systemic administration of steroids, the greatest risk comes with sudden withdraw of the medication. Clinical manifestations of adrenal insufficiency include hypotension, weight loss, weakness, nausea, vomiting, anorexia, lethargy, confusion, and restlessness. Nursing implications include assessing for signs and symptoms of adrenal insufficiency. In addition, educating parents about taking steroids as ordered is essential. Steroids come in a dose package that specifically gives correct dosage and the exact number of pills that are taken each day. Steroids must be tapered slowly when it is time to discontinue the medication.

Autoimmune Disorders

An **autoimmune disorder** is the immune response against one of the body's own tissues or cells. Autoimmunity results from the body's inability to distinguish self from nonself, wherein the immune system carries out immune responses against normal cells and tissues. The disorders can be organ specific or systemic, as in systemic lupus erythematosus, juvenile rheumatoid arthritis, immune-complex diseases, and anaphylaxis.

SYSTEMIC LUPUS ERYTHEMATOSUS

Systemic lupus erythematosus (SLE) is a multisystem chronic autoimmune disorder of the blood vessels and connective tissue. The exact cause of SLE is unknown, although it is tied to genetic predisposition coupled with unidentified trigger(s) that cause the disease to activate. Suspected triggers include estrogen, infections, ultraviolet light, pregnancy, and certain drugs. The signs, symptoms, and course of disease are variable and dependent on the exact body systems that are affected, ranging from mild to life threatening. SLE has unpredictable periods of exacerbation (flares-ups) and remissions (lessening in intensity or degree). SLE is most common in adolescent and young adult females, African Americans, and Hispanics.

medication: Methylprednisolone (A-Methapred)

Methylprednisolone (meth-ill-pred-**niss**-oh-lone)

Indications: Anti-inflammatory or immunosuppressant agent

Actions: Suppress inflammation and the normal immune response.

Therapeutic Effects: Suppression of inflammation and modification of the normal immune response.

Pharmacokinetics:
ABSORPTION: Well absorbed after oral administration.

Contraindications and Precautions:
CONTRAINDICATED IN: Acute untreated infections.
CAUTIONS: Chronic use in children will result in decreased growth. During stress (surgery, infections) supplemental doses may be needed.

Adverse Reactions and Side Effects: Peptic ulceration, anorexia, nausea, acne, decreased wound healing, hirsutism, petechiae and bruising, muscle wasting, osteoporosis, cushingoid appearance, and thromboembolism.

Route and Dosage:
PO (CHILDREN): 0.417 mg/kg–1.67 mg/kg (12.5–50 mg/m^2)/day in 3–4 divided doses.
RECT (CHILDREN): 0.5–1 mg/kg (15–30 mg/m^2) daily or every other day for at least 1 week.
IV, IM (CHILDREN): 139–835 mcg/kg (4.16–25 mg/m^2) every 12–24 hours.

Nursing Implications:
1. Assess for signs and symptoms of adrenal insufficiency (hypotension, weight loss, weakness, nausea, vomiting, anorexia, lethargy, confusion, restlessness).
2. Monitor fluid status, daily weights.
3. Monitor electrolytes and glucose levels.
4. Administer oral medications with food.
5. Instruct family regarding need to take medications as ordered due to risk of adrenal insufficiency with sudden withdraw of medication.
6. Instruct family regarding possibility of immunosuppression, need to avoid ill contacts and report possible infections to health care provider immediately.
7. Instruct family to inform health care provider promptly for severe abdominal pain, tarry stools, increased bruising, nonhealing sores, sudden weight gain, or behavioral changes.
8. Immunizations should be discussed with the health care provider on an individual basis.

Data from Deglin, J.H., & Vallerand, A. (2009). *Davis's drug guide for nurses* (11th ed., pp. 350–357). Philadelphia: F.A. Davis.

SLE may have either an acute or a vague onset. The basic pathophysiology of SLE includes autoantibodies that attach to the body proteins, creating antigen–antibody complexes. These antigen–antibody complexes are then deposited throughout the body, causing widespread tissue damage. Systems affected vary widely, but the kidneys, spleen, joints, and heart are the most frequently involved.

Signs and Symptoms

The symptoms are highly variable in both presentation and severity. Typical symptoms may include a fever, malaise, chills, fatigue, and weight loss. As the disease progresses symptoms may include a characteristic malar photosensitive rash (butterfly rash on the face); arthritis; photosensitivity; serositis; proteinuria; immunological and hematological disorders, such as hemolytic anemia, lymphocytopenia, thrombocytopenia, and vasculitis; and an abnormal antinuclear antibody (ANA).

Diagnosis

Definitive medical diagnosis is based on the presence of four or more of the aforementioned symptoms. Laboratory tests include a complete blood cell count with differential, metabolic chemistry panel, urinalysis, antinuclear antibody, anti-DNA antibody, complement 3 (C3), complement 4 (C4), quantitative immunoglobulins, rapid plasma reagin (RPR), lupus anticoagulant, and antiphospholipid antibodies (Lehman, 2002).

Nursing Care

Nursing care is based on managing pain and inflammation, treating symptoms, and preventing complications. Treatment of pain and inflammation in mild SLE is generally accomplished with nonsteroidal anti-inflammatory medications (NSAIDs). Antimalarial medications are also used in mild SLE to control symptoms of arthritis, skin rashes, mouth ulcers, fever, and fatigue. The nurse needs to tell parents that it sometimes takes a long time before the therapeutic effects of antimalarial medications are evident.

Nursing care for severe (increased inflammation) SLE requires the addition of corticosteroids. Corticosteroids are given to the child when the child does not respond to NSAIDs or antimalarial medications. Corticosteroids are highly effective in reducing inflammation and symptoms, although they also have the serious side effect of immunosuppression. During an exacerbation period, corticosteroids may be initiated in high doses. After symptoms are under control, the dose is tapered down to the lowest therapeutic level. It is important to tell the parents that steroids must be tapered slowly when it is time to discontinue the medication.

The most potent type of medication used to treat severe SLE includes immunosuppressive agents. These medications are used when the disease has reached a serious state in which severe signs and symptoms are present. Immunosuppressive agents may also be prescribed if there is a need to avoid corticosteroids. The decision to use immunosuppressives requires serious consideration due to significant side effects, primarily related to general immunosuppression. Examples of immunosuppressive agents used in treatment of SLE include azathioprine (Imuran), cyclophosphamide (Cytoxan), and methotrexate (Rheumatrex). Each medication has unique and serious risks such as bone marrow depression and hepatotoxicity. The nurse must reinforce information on the action of the medication as well as the side effects with the parents before administration of this medication.

In addition to medication, nursing care also focuses on palliative care and providing psychosocial support. It is important that the child maintain good nutrition, rest and exercise, avoid the sun, and encourage the expression of feelings about the condition. Although there is no specific diet for SLE, a balanced diet, low in salt (if the child becomes hypertensive or nephrotic), is encouraged. Rest and exercise include periods where the child is active during remissions and is resting during exacerbation. Avoidance of sun exposure is stressed because of the photosensitive rash that occurs with SLE. Use of sunscreen is important, and planning outdoor activities in the shade or staying indoors may be necessary. Because this condition may be difficult for the child and family to cope with and understand, encouraging the expression of feelings or joining a support group is encouraged. Parents should notify teachers, coaches, and others about their child's condition so they can help monitor the child and obtain necessary treatment if needed. It is also the nurse's responsibility to help the child and family identify possible triggers, such as sunlight and emotional stress, and assist the family to find ways to avoid them.

clinical alert

Systemic lupus erythematosus

SLE is a condition with varying signs and symptoms and requires continued careful assessment to ensure prompt recognition of an exacerbation. Prevention of exacerbations is the most important component of nursing care for children with SLE. It is important for the family to understand the importance of rest and adequate nutrition to help maximize immune system function. This disease often affects adolescents, so the facial rash, fatigue, and arthritic changes may put the child at risk for depression and altered body image. Referral to support groups helps the child to adjust to life with SLE.

Nursing Insight— *SLE resources*

The nurse can encourage an adolescent recently diagnosed with SLE to contact a local support group. In addition, several good resources are available online through the organizations located at the following Web sites:

- Lupus Foundation of America
  http://www.lupus.org/
- National Institute of Arthritis and Musculoskeletal and Skin Disorders
  http://www.niams.nih.gov
- SLE Foundation, Inc.
  http://www.lupusny.org/
- Association of Rheumatology Health Professionals, American College of Rheumatology
  http://www.rheumatology.org/
- Arthritis Foundation
  http://www.arthritis.org/

JUVENILE RHEUMATOID ARTHRITIS

Juvenile rheumatoid arthritis (JRA) is a chronic autoimmune inflammatory disease and is the most common type of arthritis in children. There are three types of JRA:

- Pauciarticular: Affects the knees, ankles, and elbows; more frequent in females
- Systemic: Characterized by high fever, polyarthritis, rheumatoid rash, involves joints and internal organs: affects males and females equally
- Polyarticular: Involves five or more joints (usually small joints in the fingers and hands); may also involve ankles, knees, feet, hips, and neck

The cause of JRA is unknown, and it occurs in early (2 to 5 years of age) or later (9 to 12 years of age) childhood. If JRA has an early onset, there is better chance of complete recovery. This condition has typical cycles of remission and exacerbation. Remission can last for months or years. During the active disease state, children experience decreased mobility, swelling, and pain due to joint inflammation. Scar tissue eventually develops, resulting in limited range of motion and interference with normal growth and development. Other organs such as the heart, lungs, liver, and eyes can eventually be affected.

Signs and Symptoms

Symptoms of JRA can be limited to a few joints or multiple joints. Initially, parents may notice the child limping, favoring a particular joint, complaining of pain, uneven growth in a limb, swelling in large joints (knees), loss of motion, and stiffness. Other symptoms include fever, rash, lymphadenopathy, hepatomegaly, and splenomegaly. The main complication for children with JRA is interference with growth and development.

Diagnosis

The physician bases diagnosis on the assessment findings, reported history, and laboratory tests such as rheumatoid factor, antinuclear antibody, and human leukocyte antigen (HLA).

Nursing Care

The priority nursing goal is to relieve pain and prevent contractures. Nursing care for the child with JRA includes guiding the family through medical appointments, drug therapy, physical therapy, other important care aspects, and surgery if necessary. The child with JRA can spend significant time in a physician's office. The nurse can provide parental support, answer questions, and communicate concerns and complications to the physician. Drug therapy includes the use of salicylates (aspirin) or nonsteroidal anti-inflammatory drugs such as naproxen (Aleve), sulfasalazine (Salazopyrin), and methotrexate (Rheumatrex) may be prescribed if the child does not respond to salicylates. If the disease moves into a more severe state, steroids may be used.

A common treatment for JRA is ongoing physical therapy. The use of therapeutic exercise can restore or facilitate normal function or development in the child with JRA. Children should also be encouraged to perform activities of daily living. During bouts of pain and inflammation, warm compresses can be applied.

Other important care aspects include providing good nutrition, teaching the child and family how to manage the disease, offering support, devising proper school accommodations, and expressing the importance of routine medical visits. Some states offer summer camps for children with JRA. The camp environment gives the child a chance to have fun and the parent a needed respite. The web site: http://www.arthritis.org/ offers essential information for children and families. In children with contractures, surgery may help relieve pain or improve joint function.

Nursing Insight— *Immune-complex diseases*

Immune-complex diseases occur when antibodies attach to antigens and destroy them. These complexes circulate in the blood and attach to the walls of blood vessels, producing a local inflammatory response. Examples of immune-complex diseases include glomerulonephritis, serum sickness, arthritis, and vasculitis (Venes, 2009).

Allergic Reaction

ANAPHYLAXIS

The body reacts to a foreign substance called an antigen (such as allergens, foods, animals, chemical agents, or fungal spores) that set off an allergic reaction (Venes, 2009). The most severe allergic reactions are associated with insect bites, latex products, penicillin medications, immunizations, blood, or radiological contrast media. A severe allergic reaction is called anaphylaxis. **Anaphylaxis** is the immediate hypersensitivity reaction to an excessive release of chemical mediators affecting the entire body. Anaphylaxis is a medical emergency.

Signs and Symptoms

Signs and symptoms of anaphylaxis develop suddenly and require prompt recognition and treatment.

 Nursing Insight— *Signs and symptoms of anaphylaxis*

Wheezing
Tachycardia
Hypotension
Cyanosis
Alteration in level of consciousness
Nasal congestion
Facial edema
Anxiety
Hives
Urticaria
Nausea and vomiting
Abdominal pain
Laryngospasm
A sense of impending doom
Vascular collapse and cardiac arrest

Diagnosis

Diagnosis of anaphylaxis is based on the exposure to the antigen and the signs and symptoms.

Nursing Care

 Critical Nursing Action Anaphylaxis

Immediate nursing care for anaphylaxis includes the following actions:

- Perform cardiopulmonary resuscitation.
- Activate the emergency system.
- Ensure adequate airway—endotracheal intubation or oxygen.
- Administer epinephrine (adrenaline).
- Place a tourniquet proximal to the site of injection or insect sting.
- Keep the child lying flat, warm, and with feet slightly elevated.
- Administer corticosteroids and antihistamines.
- Determine the cause of the attack.

Basic life support must be initiated with support of airway, breathing, and circulation (ABCs). Administration of oxygen and initiation of an intravenous (IV) therapy with an isotonic crystalloid solution as soon as possible are

 medication: Epinephrine (Adrenaline)

Epinephrine (e-pi-**nef**-rin)

Indications:
IV: Management of severe allergic reactions

Actions: Inhibits the release of mediators of immediate hypersensitivity reactions from mast cells.

Therapeutic Effects: Maintenance of heart rate and blood pressure.

Pharmacokinetics:

Absorption: Well absorbed.

Contraindications and Precautions:
CONTRAINDICATED IN: Hypersensitivity.

Adverse Reactions and Side Effects:
CNS: Nervousness, restlessness, tremor.
CV: Arrhythmias, hypertension, tachycardia.

Route and Dosage:
IV (SEVERE ANAPHYLAXIS): 0.1–0.25 mg q5–15min; may be followed by a 1–4 mcg/min continuous infusion (may be increased up to 1.5 mcg/kg per minute).

Nursing Implications:
1. Assess volume status. Hypovolemia should be corrected before administration of IV epinephrine.
2. Monitor blood pressure, perfusion, ECG, respiratory rate, and urine output during administration.
3. Assess for hypersensitivity reaction: rash, urticaria, swelling of face, lips, eyelids.
4. IV administration: Administer at a dilution of 1:10,000. This may be prepared through dilution of 1 mg of 1:1000 solution in at least 10 mL of 0.9% NaCl.
5. Administer each 1 mg of 1:10,000 solution over at least 1 minute.

Data from Deglin, J.H., & Vallerand, A. (2009). *Davis's drug guide for nurses* (11th ed.). Philadelphia: F.A. Davis.

standard treatment. Epinephrine (adrenaline) injection is administered intramuscularly or intravenously to provide reversal of pulmonary bronchospasm and constriction of blood vessels, thereby improving respiratory status and blood pressure. Ongoing assessment for shock is necessary and can be treated via IV fluid bolus. Occasionally antihistamines and corticosteroids may be added to further control symptoms after the initial stabilization. The majority of children respond positively to the treatment, with a full recovery.

For children who have experienced an anaphylaxis reaction the nurse must provide follow-up care to families to prevent recurrences. If the child has allergies that cannot be completely eliminated, a follow-up referral to an allergist for desensitization treatments or a self-administration epinephrine prescription, such as an EpiPen, is warranted. It is important that parents are taught to recognize early indicators of anaphylaxis and are confident in their ability to act quickly on this assessment.

 Collaboration in Caring— *Peanut allergies in school*

According to data from the National Institute of Allergy and Infectious Disease, approximately 3% of school-age children in the United States are affected by peanut allergies.

Exposure to peanuts for a sensitive child may result in symptoms ranging from simple hives and itching to anaphylaxis. For children with severe allergies a seemingly insignificant exposure, such as coming in contact with a cafeteria table that has been brought in contact with a peanut or oils from a peanut, may result in a rapidly progressive life-threatening reaction. The pediatric nurse plays a critical role in collaboration with the family and school personnel to create an environment for a child with peanut allergy to safely attend school. The nurse assists the family in establishing a coordinated plan including the following key components:

- Education of the school staff regarding peanut allergies. Include all staff who may be supervising this student and who may be in a position to recognize and intervene in an emergency.
- Outline an emergency plan specific for this student to include:
  - Specific instructions for staff in the event of a reaction
  - Location of emergency medications
  - Identification and elimination of risks
  - Emergency phone numbers
  - Establish a "peanut-free" zone in the cafeteria.
  - Send a letter to parents who may provide snacks to the child, such as parents of children in the same class, from a sports team, or a club, informing them of the presence of a child with a severe peanut allergy.

---

 medication: Diphenhydramine (Benadryl)

Diphenhydramine (dye-fen-**hye**-dra-meen)

Indications: Relief of allergic symptoms caused by histamine release, including anaphylaxis, allergic rhinitis, allergic dermatoses. Relief of pruritus.

Actions: Antagonizes the effects of histamine at H_1-receptor sites. Significant CNS depressant and anticholinergic properties.

Therapeutic Effects: Decreased symptoms of histamine excess (sneezing, rhinorrhea, nasal and ocular pruritus, ocular tearing and redness, urticaria).

Pharmacokinetics:
ABSORPTION: Well absorbed after oral or IM administration.

Contraindications and Precautions:
CONTRAINDICATED IN: Hypersensitivity.

Adverse Reactions and Side Effects: Drowsiness, paradoxical excitation (more common in children), anorexia, dry mouth.

Route and Dosage:
PO (CHILDREN 6–12 YEARS): 12.5–25 mg q4–6h.
PO (CHILDREN 2–6 YEARS): 6.25–12.5 mg q4–6h.
IM/IV (CHILDREN): 1.25 mg/kg 4 times/day. Not to exceed 300 mg/day.

Nursing Implications:
1. Provide child and family education regarding medication, caution not to exceed recommended dose.
2. Inform parents that medication may cause drowsiness or excitability in child.
3. Provide education regarding common side effect of dry mouth. Management strategies include frequent mouth care and oral rinses.

Data from Deglin, J.H., & Vallerand, A. (2009). *Davis's drug guide for nurses* (11th ed.). Philadelphia: F. A. Davis.

 Now Can You— Recognize and intervene in anaphylaxis?

1. Identify the life-threatening symptoms of an anaphylaxis reaction?
2. Prioritize interventions in treatment of an anaphylaxis reaction?

Infectious Diseases of Childhood

INFECTION

The occurrence of infectious disease in children is the result of an interaction between several factors including the child, the environment, and the agent causing the illness (Table 26-1). There are two main models used to illustrate this relationship, the most common being the epidemiological triangle (Fig. 26-2).

In the epidemiological triangle the host, environment, and agent make up the three sides of an equilateral triangle. The *host* is the organism from which a parasite obtains its nourishment, the *environment* is the surroundings or conditions that influence the organism, and the *agent* causes the actual effect (disease) (Venes, 2009). This model illustrates the codependence that these three factors have on one another and recognizes that change in any one of the three factors will influence the risk or probability of a child contracting the disease.

Many factors unique to the pediatric population such as age, sex, physical, and psychosocial factors all play a role in the susceptibility of the host to an infectious disease. The normal development of the child's immune system is also a major factor in many infectious diseases especially during the early childhood years.

The final element in the triangle, the agent contains specific information, including infectivity, pathogenicity, and virulence, that assists the nurse in developing the appropriate plan of care. Infectivity is the mode of transmission, incubation period, and communicable period. The mode of transmission is how the pathogen actually gains access to the body. With this knowledge, the nurse can plan care to eliminate unnecessary portals of entry (multiple IV sites) and thoroughly inspect the skin on a routine basis. Knowledge about the incubation period (onset of symptoms) to the actual illness or the

Text continued on page 839

Host

Agent   Environment

Figure 26-2 Epidemiological triangle.

Table 26-1 Communicable Diseases in Childhood

Disease	Clinical	Treatment	Complications
Chickenpox (Viral) *Causative Agent* Varicella-zoster virus, a herpes virus. *Epidemiology* Highly contagious disease. Peak incidence in spring. *Mode of Transmission* Airborne and spread through contact with respiratory secretions and contact with lesions. *Infection Control* Incubation period from 13 to 17 days. Children are considered contagious 1 day before the eruption of lesions to the time when all lesions have crusted, or up to 6 days after appearance of the rash. The period of communicability may be prolonged in children who are immunocompromised. Airborne and contact precautions are needed for hospitalized children during the period of communicability.	Manifestations. Acute onset of malaise, fever, and irritability followed by rash. Rash described as a "tear drop on a rose petal." Begins with a macule on a red base, this progresses to a clear vesicle, later forms a crust. The lesions are severely pruritic and eruptions may continue to occur for up to 5 days. Generally first appears on the face and trunk, but may spread anywhere on the body.	Supportive. Varicella-zoster immune globulin (VZIG) may be given to within 72 hours of exposure to immunocompromised children following exposure with the goal of preventing the disease. VZIG provides only temporary immunity so is reserved only for high-risk individuals who are unable to receive vaccine. Acyclovir used for immunocompromised child presenting with chickenpox. Must be used within 24 hours of onset to be effective. Oral antihistamines, baking soda, oatmeal baths, and calamine lotion to manage itching.	10% of the children with chickenpox develop a complication. Immunocompromised children have high risk for complications (including those on steroids for treatment of asthma). Most common complications are bacterial superinfections of lesions, encephalitis, varicella pneumonia, and thrombocytopenia. Use of aspirin-containing medications has been linked with Reye syndrome in children with chickenpox.
Diphtheria (Bacterial) *Causative Agent* *Corynebacterium diphtheriae* bacillus *Epidemiology* Occurs mostly in fall and winter and in unimmunized or partially immunized persons.	Gradual onset of symptoms with a low-grade fever, anorexia, malaise, rhinorrhea, cough, hoarseness, stridor, cervical lymphadenitis, and pharyngitis. Hallmark sign is fuzzy gray or black covering over the tonsils, hard and soft palates, and posterior pharynx. May produce profound difficulty breathing due to narrowing of the upper airway.	IV antitoxin and antibiotics within 3 days of onset of symptoms (IV sensitivity testing must be done before administration). Oral antihistamines, baking soda or oatmeal baths, and calamine lotion to help control itching. All contacts are given prophylactic antibiotic treatment and immunization boosters.	Respiratory compromise secondary to the endotoxin produced membrane covering much of the upper airway. Membrane may require removal, but bleeding may result in the endotoxin spreading beyond the respiratory tract to cause myocarditis, peripheral neuropathy, or an ascending paralysis similar to Gullian-Barré.

Table 26-1 Communicable Diseases in Childhood—cont'd

Disease	Clinical	Treatment	Complications
Mode of Transmission: Transmitted through airborne droplets, contact with respiratory secretions, contact with contaminated household articles, close personal contact with infected persons. *Infection Control* 2–7 days incubation period (may be longer). If not treated may remain contagious for up to 4 weeks. Contagious for 4 days after antibiotic treatment instituted. Droplet and contact precautions used for hospitalized children.			
Infectious Mononucleosis (Viral) *Causative Agent* Epstein–Barr virus (EBV). *Epidemiology* Most persons become infected with EBV sometime during their life (usually adolescence or young adulthood). Infection with EBV during this time of life causes symptoms of infectious mononucleosis 35%–50% of the time. *Mode of Transmission* Transmitted via intimate contact with the saliva of an infected individual. *Infection Control* Incubation period is 4–6 weeks. Infected persons may shed virus intermittently and without symptoms throughout life. No isolation beyond standard precautions needed.	Fever, pharyngitis, and lymphadenopathy lasting from 1 to 4 weeks. Fatigue and some degree of hepatosplenomegaly.	Steroids may be considered in the case of respiratory difficulty secondary to swelling of the upper airways.	Respiratory compromise secondary to airway swelling and exudative pharyngitis, aseptic meningitis, encephalitis. Rarely splenic rupture. Possible thrombocytopenia and agranulocytosis.
Fifth Disease (Erythema Infectiosum) (Viral) *Causative Agent* Human parvovirus B19. *Epidemiology* Children 5–14 years of age, most often during spring. *Mode of Transmission* Transmission via contact with respiratory secretions. *Infection Control* Incubation period for 4–14 days. Contagious before onset of rash. No isolation required.	Stage 1: 2–3 days, mild systemic symptoms that mimic flu. Stage 2: deep red rash appears on cheeks, circumoral pallor; 1–4 days later a symmetric, lacy red rash appears on the trunk and limb. Stage 3: lasts 1–3 weeks, the rash disappears, but may reappear after exposure to sunlight or heat.	Treatment is symptomatic.	Arthralgia and arthritis are the most common complications in otherwise healthy children. Children with underlying hemolytic conditions may experience transient aplastic crisis requiring hospitalization. Fetal death may occur if mother is infected during pregnancy. Exposure to sunlight and heat may exacerbate the rash.

Continued

Table 26-1 Communicable Diseases in Childhood—cont'd

Disease	Clinical	Treatment	Complications
Haemophilus Influenzae Type B (Bacterial) *Causative Agent* *Haemophilus influenzae* type B. *Epidemiology* Occurs most often in spring and summer with infants and children in daycare. *Mode of Transmission* Spreads via direct contact or inhalation of droplets from infected persons. *Infection Control* Incubation period is unknown and the disease is likely contagious for up to 3 days following onset of symptoms. Agent may colonize in respiratory tract of an asymptomatic person. Preventable with vaccine.	Begins as an upper respiratory infection. Bacteria subsequently pass into the blood and may be spread to sites throughout the body. Symptoms of infection are dependent on the site and may include sinusitis, otitis media, upper and lower airway infections, septic arthritis, and cellulites. In infants this organism is an important cause of sepsis.	Antibiotic administration for persons. Prophylactic treatment with Rifampin for unimmunized household contacts.	Death may occur secondary to serious infections with *Haemophilus influenzae* type B if not treated.
Influenza (Viral) *Causative Agent* The flu is caused by influenza viruses A and B. *Epidemiology* Occurs more often in the winter months. *Mode of Transmission* Transmitted via droplets from person to person. *Infection Control* Incubation period is typically 1–4 days (young children may be infectious for up to 10 days before the onset of symptoms). Preventable with vaccine.	Rapid onset of fever, myalgia, headache, sore throat, rhinitis, and nonproductive cough. Otitis media and nausea and vomiting are common in younger children with influenza.	Supportive.	Febrile seizures in young children. Secondary bacterial pneumonia and exacerbation of underlying chronic illness.
Mumps (Parotitis) (Viral) *Causative Agent* Paramyxovirus. *Epidemiology* Occurs most often in winter and spring. Most often seen in unvaccinated adolescents (may be prevented with vaccine).	Mild systemic symptoms including malaise, low-grade fever, anorexia, ear pain and headache, and pain with chewing. As the disease advances, bilateral or unilateral parotid gland swelling appears; swelling generally peaks around the third day and lasts up to 6 days.	Control symptoms. Supportive with hydration and nutrition.	Aseptic meningitis (occurs in 50%–60% of children). Symptomatic meningitis, headache, stiff neck, and photophobia (occurs in approximately 15% of the cases). Orchitis is the most common complication in post-pubertal males (50%). Sterility secondary to this complication is rare. Less common complications are oophoritis, pancreatitis, myocarditis, and deafness.

Table 26-1 Communicable Diseases in Childhood—cont'd

Disease	Clinical	Treatment	Complications

Mode of Transmission

Transmission spreads via droplets directly from an infected person (saliva and respiratory secretions). Virus may be airborne through infected droplets.

Infection Control

The most contagious period is from 2 days before symptoms begin to 6 days after they end.

Hospitalized children require droplet precautions.

Pertussis (Bacterial)

Causative Agent

Bordetella pertussis bacteria.

Epidemiology

Occurs in unimmunized or partially immunized persons.

Immunity gained through immunizations in infancy wane, generally by adolescence.

Adults and adolescents who are no longer immune provide a major reservoir for pertussis.

Can spread to incompletely immunized infants and children.

Mode of Transmission

Transmission takes place through direct contact with respiratory secretions.

Infection Control

Incubation period 3–21 days.

Communicable for 5–7 days after the initiation of antibiotic therapy.

Hospitalized children should be placed on droplet precautions until the period of communicability has passed.

This is a reportable disease.

Clinical	Treatment	Complications
Onset of symptoms is insidious. First mimics a mild upper respiratory illness with a nonproductive cough (most contagious stage). After 1–2 weeks the cough becomes more severe at night and productive of thick, stringy mucus. Eventually paroxysmal coughing episodes begin, which end in the classic "whoop" of inspiratory stridor. Severe coughing episodes may lead to vomiting and decreased intake of food and liquids, may last up to 4 weeks, then gradually subsides, but may last for months.	Antibiotics to eliminate the *Bordetella pertussis* infection and supportive care. Infants younger than 6 months of age and those with severe disease are hospitalized for close observation of respiratory status. Maintain open airway. Monitor oxygen saturation. Provide gentle suction if needed.	Apnea is common in children younger than 6 months of age. Seizures. Pneumonia. Encephalopathy. Death.

Pneumococcal Disease (Bacterial)

Causative Agent

Streptococcus pneumoniae.

Epidemiology

Occurs in colder months when persons spend more time in close quarters.

Clinical	Treatment	Complications
Symptoms related to site of infection. Upper respiratory infection, sinusitis, otitis media, and pneumonia.	Penicillin. Penicillin-sensitive strains.	Causes bacteremia in children. Septic arthritis. Osteomyelitis. Endocarditis. Meningitis. Brain abscess.

Continued

Table 26-1 Communicable Diseases in Childhood—cont'd

Disease	Clinical	Treatment	Complications
Mode of Transmission Spreads through contact with infected respiratory secretions. Multiple strains. *Infection Control* Incubation 1–3 days. Many types may be prevented by use of vaccine. The vaccine is offered to children at high risk of pneumococcal disease. Concern about development of antibiotic-resistant strains.			
Poliomyelitis (Viral) *Causative Agent* Enterovirus. *Epidemiology* Most common in infants and young children. Virus lives in the throat and gastrointestinal tract. *Mode of Transmission* Transmitted via fecal–oral route primarily, but may also be respiratory. Most cases in the United States in recent years due to the administration of live vaccine (inactivated IPV now given). *Infection Control* Incubation period 7–10 days, may last as long as 20 days. Children contagious from 7 to 10 days before symptoms develop until 7–10 days after symptoms appear. Standard and droplet precautions are used for children hospitalized to control infection.	Affects central nervous system. Initially presents with nonspecific symptoms such as low-grade fever and sore throat. May start mild and progress to transient pain and stiffness in the child's neck, back, and legs or it may be severe, progressing to meningeal signs and respiratory compromise. Paralytic polio the most severe manifestation (severe muscle pain followed by paralysis most often affecting the legs but sometimes affecting other muscles, including those used in respiration).	No treatment. Supportive during the rehabilitation phase. Physical therapy to maximize function.	Permanent paralysis. Respiratory arrest. Aseptic meningitis.

Table 26-1 Communicable Diseases in Childhood—cont'd

Disease	Clinical	Treatment	Complications
Roseola (Exanthem Subitum) (Viral) *Causative Agent* Human herpesvirus 6. *Epidemiology* Occurs primarily in children ages 6–24 months. Occurs any time of the year. *Mode of Transmission* Transmitted through contact with infected respiratory secretions. *Infection Control Incubation* Between 5 and 15 days. Infectious during the febrile period. Transmission prevented through standard precautions and good hand washing.	Sudden high fever (up to 104.4°F [40.2°C]), lasts 3–5 days. As fever begins to decrease, a discrete, red, maculopapular rash appears on the trunk and spreads to head and extremities (may last several days).	Supportive. Relieve fever. Monitor for febrile seizures.	Very high fevers, raising concern for febrile seizures in susceptible children.
Rubeola: Measles (Viral) *Causative Agent* Morbillivirus. *Epidemiology* Peaks in winter and spring. Occurs in outbreaks among unimmunized populations. *Mode of Transmission* Via the respiratory tract through droplets, direct contact with infectious secretions or occasionally airborne. *Infection Control* Incubation is 8–12 days. Airborne precautions until 5 days after appearance of the rash. Measles is a reportable disease.	Prodromal phase: 3–5 days, high fever, cough, coryza, and conjunctivitis; Koplik's spots appear on the buccal mucosa 2 days before the onset of the rash. Deep red rash, maculopapular rash begins at the hairline and spreads to face, trunk, upper and then lower extremities. After 4–7 days rash begins to fade, temperature begins to fall, other symptoms begin to subside. Other common symptoms during the acute phase includes anorexia, malaise, fatigue, and generalized lymphadenopathy.	Manage fever, itching, photophobia, cough, anorexia.	Pneumonia. Otitis media. Encephalitis. Younger children, medically fragile children, and children with underlying immunosuppression are at greater risk for complications.

Continued

Table 26-1 Communicable Diseases in Childhood—cont'd

Disease	Clinical	Treatment	Complications
Scarlet Fever (Bacterial) *Causative Agent* Group A beta-hemolytic streptococci (GAS). *Epidemiology* Occurs secondary to a pharyngeal infection with GAS. This is seen most frequently in late fall through spring. *Mode of Transmission* Spread through direct contact with infectious respiratory secretions. *Infection Control* Incubation period is 2–5 days. Children with untreated infections remain contagious for weeks with the highest risk of transmission during the acute phase of the illness. Children should remain home from school until they have been on antibiotics for at least 24 hours and are also afebrile.	Acute onset of fever, sore throat, rhinitis, headache, and tender cervical nodes. Sandpaper-like rash appears 12–48 hours after onset of symptoms, rash is most prominent in creases and blanches to touch. In 3–4 days, the rash begins to fade and the tips of toes and fingers begin to peel. On day 4–5 bright red strawberry tongue develops.	Antibiotics Supportive care for throat pain and fever.	Untreated strep infections may lead to retropharyngeal abscess, acute rheumatic fever, acute glomerulonephritis, toxic shock syndrome, bacteremia, and necrotizing fascitis.
Tetanus (Bacterial) *Causative Agent* *Clostridium tetani.* *Epidemiology* Not transmitted person to person. *Mode of Transmission* Occurs in humans through wounds which come in contact with soil contaminated with the *Clostridium tetani* bacillus. Most common in children. This is secondary to a cut or deep puncture wound. Neonatal tetanus occurs in newborns delivered in unsanitary conditions. *Infection Control* The incubation period for tetanus is 2–14 days. Prevention is immunization and postexposure prophylaxis. Neonatal tetanus prevented through improved sanitation of delivery condition.	*Clostridium tetani* produces a neurotoxin that affects the muscles and nerves. Early signs are headache and restlessness, followed by stiffness of the neck and jaw. This stiffness progresses to painful spasms of the masticatory muscles accompanied by difficulty opening the mouth and dysphagia. Localized painful muscle spasm may begin to occur at the site of the wound. This eventually progresses up the trunk to the point of opisthotonos, a severe spasm of back muscles, causing the back to arch acutely. As the neurotoxin spreads widely throughout the body, seizures are possible.	Administer tetanus immune globulin (TIG) to neutralize the neurotoxin. Antibiotics eliminate the bacillus from the body. Surgical débridement of the wound to control infection. Antispasmodic agents, such as diazepam (Valium), to reduce spasms.	Potential for spasms in all muscle groups. Laryngospasm. Respiratory muscle spasms (may compromise breathing and lead to death).

time that the child is able to transmit the pathogen to others (communicable period or portal of exit) allows the nurse to alert others that the child is infectious and isolate the child for a certain period.

Pathogenicity is the percentage of those children exposed to the pathogen that will eventually develop the disease. This information is helpful to the nurse in the community when assessing citywide outbreaks. The nurse can notify schools, community centers, churches, shopping malls, and other public places that an outbreak exists and that it is best to avoid these areas, especially for high-risk children. **Virulence** is the severity of the health problems caused by the agent. The more virulent the disease the more necessary it is to curtail its spread. For example, in winter, during an influenza outbreak, a number of schools close so they can be thoroughly cleaned and sanitized. Pathogenicity and virulence are often key considerations in development and implementation of public health programs.

Although the epidemiological triangle is useful in understanding the interdependence of factors involved in infection, understanding the Chain of Infection Model is also important (Fig. 26-3). The model illustrates the steps that must occur for transmission as well as demonstrating possible ways to stop transmission of the disease. For instance, a pathogenic microorganism or a disease-causing agent is present. The agent must have a reservoir where the pathogen can grow. Reservoirs may be human hosts, animals, and the soil. With knowledge about the reservoir, the nurse can eliminate it to break the chain. A mosquito abatement program to control West Nile virus is an example of an attempt to alter the chain of infection via reservoir elimination.

Public health immunization campaigns are another example of a way to decrease the reservoir for diseases. The next three links in the chain involve the escape of the pathogen from the reservoir into the host. Knowledge about the routes of transmission (contact, droplet, airborne) enables the nurse to initiate appropriate isolation precautions. The final link involves a susceptible host. Susceptibility is decreased mainly via good general health practices such as good hygiene, nutrition, and decrease in stress.

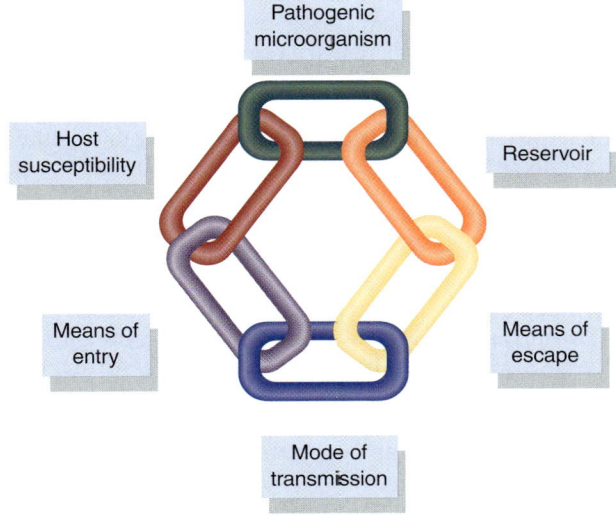

Figure 26-3 Chain of infection model.

 Nursing Insight— *Infections*

There are three types of infections: bacterial, viral, and fungal.

- Bacterial infections are caused by single-celled living microorganisms and include *Streptococcus*, *Staphylococcus*, and *Escherichia coli*. Common bacterial infections are described in Chapter 24.
- Viruses (e.g., influenza, HIV) are not living organisms and require living hosts (such as people, plants, or animals) to multiply. Some viral infections are contagious while others are not.
- Fungal infections are pathological invasions of the body by yeast or other fungi (e.g., athlete's foot, yeast infections). Fungal infections are most likely to occur in children with a compromised immune system (Venes, 2009).

It is important to understand the differentiation between bacterial, viral, and fungal infections so the proper medication is given. Antibacterial antibiotics treat bacterial infections, antiviral antibiotics are available to treat some types of viral infections, and antifungal agents are used to treat fungal infections.

Signs and Symptoms

Although each infectious condition has unique signs and symptoms, several symptoms are common in varying degrees among several illnesses. Common signs and symptoms can include fever, malaise, anorexia, and pruritus (itching) from rashes.

Diagnosis

Diagnosis of an infectious disease is confirmed by type of infection, signs and symptoms, along with various diagnostic means.

 diagnostic tools Identification of an Infectious Disease

- Complete blood count (CBC) with differential
- Urinalysis (UA)
- Spinal fluid analysis
- Cultures from fluids, secretions, drainage
- Pulse oximetry
- Chest radiograph
- Computerized tomography

Nursing Care

Building on the scientific foundation of immunology, the pediatric nurse can provide specific care measures to promote immune function and to provide education to families.

 critical nursing action Skin Care and Nutritional Support

Simple nursing actions such as good skin care and nutrition help maintain the barriers and the natural immune response. The skin can be maintained by good hygiene measures such as hand washing and paying attention to any breaks or openings on the skin surface. Through good nutrition, the innate physical, chemical, and mechanical barriers are preserved and the risk for infection is decreased. Adequate nutrition also promotes prompt healing and decreases the potential for skin breakdown. Maintaining barriers and the immune response is particularly important in children whose immune system is not yet fully mature and for children who are at risk for immunosuppression.

An important topic in education is promoting stress reduction in children. Stress in children may also negatively affect the immune system and is associated with increased risk for infections. Recent advances in science support the connection between daily life stress and immune function in children. Although the exact mechanism is unknown, more than one negative life event positively correlated with a significant drop in helper T cells in children with AIDS (Howland et al., 2000). This kind of information can help the nurse promote optimal immune function through minimizing negative life events for children.

Nursing care for the child with an infectious disease also centers on accurate assessment, prevention of disease transmission, treating the signs and symptoms, teaching families about universal precautions, and preventing complications.

assessment tools Key Components of Physical Assessment for the Child with an Infectious Disease

Vital Signs

- Temperature
- Heart rate
- Respiratory rate
- Blood pressure
- Pain

Respiratory Assessment

- Upper respiratory infection symptoms
- Breath sounds
- Work of breathing
- Pulse oximeter reading
- Skin/mucous membrane color
- Secretions; color, character, amount

Neurological Assessment

- Febrile seizures
- Early identification of neurological complications
- Level of consciousness

Gastrointestinal Assessment

- Fluid intake
- Presence of vomiting or diarrhea

Skin

- Presence of rash, pruritus, lesions

Across Care Settings: Caring for the child with an infectious disease

The majority of children with an infectious disease are cared for in the home or by a child-care provider.

Nursing care for the children and their families includes prevention of common illnesses along with their complications. Prevention of disease transmission within the family or community is essential. Key points to prevent transmission include:

- Good hand washing practices
- Covering the mouth and nose when coughing or sneezing
- Disposal or cleansing of articles contaminated with respiratory or gastric secretions such as tissues, blankets, and toys
- Early identification of illness, with isolation from other children during infectious stages

The nurse can assist families in managing the signs and symptoms. Fever is common. The nurse can teach parents about the use of acetaminophen (Children's Tylenol) or ibuprofen (Children's Advil) for treatment of fevers. It is essential that parents follow the directions on the medication label. Cool moist compresses to the head, as well as sponging or tepid baths, can reduce the fever.

Nursing Insight— *Pathophysiology of a fever*

The hypothalamus is the thermostat of the body. As blood circulates through the hypothalamus, it directs the various body organs to either conserve or dissipate the heat, (depending on the blood's temperature). If the body temperature is lower than normal, vasoconstriction is initiated to conserve heat, or shivering/chills occur that increase heat production. When a child has a fever (excess heat), the body's temperature, heart, and respiration rates increase. Vasodilatation occurs and the skin becomes flushed and warm to the touch. When the fever "breaks" the child may start to perspire and the heart and respiration rates return to normal.

clinical alert

Reye syndrome risk with use of aspirin

The administration of salicylates (aspirin) to children with acute viral illness is linked to Reye syndrome. It is critical that nurses teach parents about Reye syndrome and provide education regarding use of aspirin-free medications for control of fever in children (National Reye Syndrome Foundation: www.reyessyndrome.org/).

Common medications that contain salicylates (aspirin) are:

- Alka-Seltzer
- Anacin
- Ascriptin
- Bayer Arthritis Pain and Aspirin preparations
- Bufferin
- Doan's
- Dristan
- Ecotrin
- Excedrin
- Kaopectate
- Pamprin
- Pepto-Bismol
- Sine-Off Sinus Medicaine
- St. Joseph Adult Aspirin
- Vanquish

Malaise (weakness) tends to correlate with fevers and providing a quiet, restful environment during the acute phase of illness may assist in the management of this symptom. If the child is anorexic, offering small amounts of fluids frequently helps keep the child hydrated. Sometimes a room-temperature lemon-lime soft drink or ice-pop will taste good to the child. Also offering small amounts of favorite foods, soft foods, or bland foods may help with the anorexia. If the anorexia becomes worrisome to parents, the nurse can encourage them to contact their health care provider.

Pruritus is associated with many of the common infectious diseases and can be a source of distress for the child and a potential site for secondary infection due to skin breakdown. Educating the family about how to effectively control the itching is an important part of the nursing care plan. Parents may be advised to keep the child's fingernails short and place soft mittens on younger children to prevent scratching. Oatmeal or Aveeno baths may provide some relief, as does Caladryl lotion. Parents are advised to change bed linens frequently and avoid use of harsh soaps during the time of illness to avoid further irritation. Light clothing often helps keep perspiration and heat rashes to a minimum. An oral antihistamine such as diphenhydramine (Benedryl) may be useful in cases of severe pruritus.

The pediatric nurse can educate families and day care providers about universal precautions. Emphasize hand washing, cleaning of toys and surfaces, and proper disposal of diapers. The pediatric nurse also provides education to families about the importance of excluding the child from school and other activities during the illness. Sound knowledge about the routes of transmission assists the nurse in developing a plan of care for the hospitalized child that includes environmental precautions that minimize the risk of transmission.

 Optimizing Outcomes— **Children with infectious diseases**

The best outcome for the child with an infectious disease is the prevention and early identification of complications. The nurse must pay careful attention to fluid deficit, upper respiratory tract infection, and neurological difficulties.

Although potential complications are specific to each illness, there are general symptoms that are associated with many of the infectious diseases. Children with infectious disease often are at risk for developing a fluid deficit due to a combination of anorexia, nausea, vomiting, and sore throat. The nurse can assist families in managing fluid deficit by offering the child small amounts of liquids frequently and offering favorite fluids to the child such as juice, soda, or water. Respiratory infections are also common. A cool steamer, decongestants, or gentle nasal suctioning with a bulb syringe may help diminish respiratory difficulty. Neurological symptoms include general lethargy (sluggishness or tiredness) that may progress to decreased responsiveness. Generalized irritability that progresses to inconsolable crying, seizures, or meningeal symptoms, including stiff neck and photophobia, may be present. Parents must be instructed to call the health care provider if these neurological symptoms occur or the child is unresponsive.

critical nursing action Seeking Immediate Help

Respiratory symptoms are a major component of many of the common infectious illnesses of childhood. Respiratory symptoms of concern include increased work of breathing; inability to swallow, including drooling; muffled voice; or very rapid or slow respirations. The nurse must instruct the family to seek help immediately if the child exhibits any of these signs of respiratory deterioration.

Common Viral Infections

There are more that 400 types of viruses, which are the smallest infectious agents known today. When a virus enters a cell, it can trigger a disease process immediately or remain dormant for many years. The virus can enter any organ of the body by attaching to the cell membrane,

assembling the cells into a more mature form that is then capable of affecting other cells and taking over cellular function. Viruses are responsible for such diseases as cytomegalovirus (CMV), herpes zoster, small pox (variola), and infectious mononucleosis.

CYTOMEGALOVIRUS INFECTIONS

Cytomegalovirus (CMV) is a member of the herpes family, infecting up to 85% of the population of the United States by the age of 40. CMV is transmitted via close contact with body fluids of an infected person. The disease is not highly contagious and transmission is easily prevented with good hand washing. Young children in daycare are a major reservoir for this disease. For non-immunocompromised children who acquire CMV after birth there are few symptoms and no long-term health consequences.

Signs and Symptoms

A few children will have symptoms similar to those of mononucleosis with a prolonged fever and mild hepatitis. Disease in a non-compromised host is self-limiting and requires no more than symptomatic support. After the initial infection with CMV the virus remains dormant in body cells. The virus may be reactivated with impairment in the body's immune system.

A very small percentage of pregnant women acquiring a primary CMV infection during their pregnancy will give birth to an infant suffering from congenital CMV disease. These infants are at risk for long-term hearing or vision deficits and varying degrees of mental retardation.

CMV infection is a significant risk for unborn and immunocompromised children. Common manifestations of CMV infection in this population are pneumonia, retinitis, and symptoms of gastrointestinal dysfunction.

Diagnosis

Urine, saliva, blood, and biopsy samples can be used for virus isolation to make a diagnosis. CMV pneumonia is suggested by radiograph and lung CT scan.

Nursing Care

CMV is a major cause of morbidity and mortality in immunocompromised children. Whenever possible, exposure to the CMV virus via blood products should be avoided. Ganciclovir (Cytovene), an antiviral agent, is used in the treatment of life-threatening CMV in this population. The most common symptom after resolution of the acute phase of the infection is fatigue, which may be present for as long as 18 months after the primary infection. The nurse teaches the patient that the average time to recovery from fatigue is 1 to 2 months. Patients should resume activity as tolerated.

 clinical alert

Preventing CMV infection in immunocompromised children

CMV infection is a source of significant morbidity and mortality in immunocompromised children. Good handwashing is the best preventive measure. Disposable gloves should be worn when handling linen or underclothes soiled with feces or urine. CMV-negative blood should be provided to immunocompromised children.

medication: Ganciclovir (Cytovene)

Ganciclovir (gan-**sye**-kloe-vir)

Indications:
Treatment of CMV retinitis in immunocompromised children.
Prevention of CMV infection in transplant children at risk.

Actions: CMV converts ganciclovir to its active form inside the host cell, where it inhibits viral DNA polymerase.

Therapeutic Effects: Antiviral effect directed against CMV-infected cells.

Pharmacokinetics:
ABSORPTION: 5–9% absorbed with oral administration. IV administration results in complete bioavailability.

Contraindications and Precautions:
CONTRAINDICATED IN: Hypersensitivity to ganciclovir or acyclovir.

Adverse Reactions and Side Effects:
Seizures, headache, malaise, drowsiness, ataxia,
GI bleeding, nausea, vomiting, increased liver enzymes
Neutropenia, thrombocytopenia, anemia
Hypotension, hypertension
Renal toxicity

Route and Dosage:
Pediatric doses not established.
IV (ADULTS): Induction 5 mg/kg q12h for 14–21 days
MAINTENANCE: 5 mg/kg/day or 6 mg/kg for 5 days/week; may increase to q12h.
PO (ADULTS): Maintenance: 1000 mg 3 times/day or 500 mg 6 times/day

Nursing Implications:
1. Pediatric dose not established.
2. Increased risk of bone marrow depression when used with antineoplastics or zidovudine.
3. Assess child during treatment of signs of infection, bleeding, or development of CMV retinitis.
4. Administer IV at slow rate, using in-line filter.
5. Advise child/family to notify health care provider for any signs of bleeding.

Data from Deglin, J.H., & Vallerand, A. (2009). *Davis's drug guide for nurses* (11th ed., pp. 594–596). Philadelphia: F. A. Davis.

HERPES ZOSTER

The varicella-zoster virus (the same virus that causes chickenpox) causes herpes zoster. This virus is seen in older children and young adults. The first time the child is exposed to this virus, he or she contracts chickenpox. On a subsequent exposure, due to reactivation of the virus, herpes zoster occurs.

Signs and Symptoms

Initial signs and symptoms include cutaneous vesicular lesions that follow the nerve pattern on the face, trunk, and upper back area. It is important to note that the child will experience pain from the nerve involvement.

Diagnosis

Diagnosis of herpes zoster is based on patient history and physical examination findings.

Nursing Care

Nursing care includes measures to decrease the itching and pain. Acetaminophen (Children's Tylenol) may be given for pain. Acyclovir (Zovirax) is administered because it inhibits viral DNA synthesis, thus limiting the disease. Cool water compresses, cool baths, and calamine lotion can relieve the itching.

SMALLPOX

Smallpox (variola) has been eradicated since 1995 but is stored in laboratories worldwide and has a mortality rate of 50%. It is spread easily from one person to another via direct or indirect contact. The period of communicability is from the time of rash onset until all the lesions have been crusted over and shed.

Signs and Symptoms

Similar to chickenpox, smallpox has lesions, but can be differentiated as the smallpox lesions produce pus. Other signs and symptoms are chills, fever, headache, and vomiting.

Diagnosis

Smallpox is diagnosed based on the patient's history and clinical signs and symptoms. The disease can be definitively diagnosed by isolation of the virus from the blood or lesions, or by identification of antibodies in the blood made in response to the virus. Smallpox is diagnosed in specialized laboratories with appropriate testing techniques and measures to protect the laboratory workers.

Nursing Care

Nursing care includes isolation until all lesions have been shed, treating the signs and symptoms, and possibly administering an antibiotic to prevent a secondary condition. Passive immunity includes the administration of vaccinia immune globulin (VIG). Active artificial immunity is not recommended.

INFECTIOUS MONONUCLEOSIS

The Epstein–Barr virus is responsible for infectious mononucleosis, which is communicable during the actual phase of the illness (7 to 10 days). Historically, infectious mononucleosis was first discovered as a disease that was transmitted through kissing. Although it can occur at any age, the disease is most commonly found in adolescents and young adults.

Signs and Symptoms

The cervical lymph nodes become swollen, firm, and tender. Other symptoms are chills, fever (103.3°F [39.6°C]), headache, anorexia, and malaise. Also during the initial disease phase, the spleen may become enlarged. Because rupture is possible, the nurse must not palpate the spleen or place any pressure over the area.

Diagnosis

The monospot test was designed to detect the disease. A positive test result confirms the disease. If necessary, a blood test can be drawn to confirm the presence of Epstein–Barr virus.

Nursing Care

The nurse must communicate to the parents the importance of bedrest, maintaining hydration, decreasing fever, and isolation during the acute phase. Sharing drinking cups with family members and peers is not advisable. Children can experience general fatigue or weakness for up to 6 weeks after the acute phase. It is important that they continue to include rest periods and fluids during their normal daily routine.

Common Fungal Infections

Any disease introduced by a fungus is called a mycosis. Fungi are either unicellular (yeasts) or multicellular (molds) and larger than bacteria. Fungal diseases are categorized according to the particular body tissue they affect. Most infections in children are superficial subcutaneous infections of the skin, hair, nails, or mucous membranes associated with either overgrowth of fungi normally present or introduced through breaks in the skin. Superficial findings include slight itching, red or gray patches, dryness, and brittle hair. Transmission is by the inhalation of spores. There are four superficial fungal infections seen in children: tinae capitis, pedis, cruris, and corporis (Table 26-2).

CANDIDA ALBICANS (ORAL THRUSH)

Most infants have natural yeast in their mouths called *Candida albicans*. Owing to the immature immune system in infants, the yeast in their mouths can overgrow and lead to an infection called oral thrush.

Signs and Symptoms

Signs and symptoms of oral thrush include white plaques on the surface of the tongue and the buccal (cheek) membranes.

Diagnosis

C. albicans is diagnosed via a microscopic examination of the plaques (Venes, 2009).

Nursing Care

Maintaining nutrition is a priority nursing care measure of the child. This fungal infection is painful and the child may not eat well. Nystatin (Mycostatin) is the medication that effectively treats thrush. It is administered with a gloved finger using a swab placed on the buccal membranes. The medication must be administered after feedings so it will remain in contact with the fungi rather than being washed away immediately during the feeding.

The nurse can also educate the parents about the prevention of oral thrush. If the infant is bottle-fed oral thrush can be prevented by thoroughly cleaning the bottle nipples in hot water. If the infant is breastfed and the mother's nipples are sore and reddened the nurse can encourage the mother to contact the physician about possible use of an antifungal ointment on the nipples while the infant is also treated with Nystatin (Mycostatin). Pacifiers can be thoroughly cleaned in hot water also.

 Nursing Insight— *Candidal organisms in the diaper area*

Candida can also grow in the diaper area, causing a bright red diaper rash. Changing diapers frequently, exposing the area to air, and applying Nystatin (Mycostatin) ointment is prescribed. The nurse must be aware that candidiaisis can be a generalized infection, especially in newborns. It must be treated immediately to prevent it from becoming systemic.

Table 26-2 Fungal Infections			
Fungal Infection	**Location**	**Treatment**	**Parent Information**
Tinea Capitis (Ringworm)	Begins as an infection of a single hair follicle but spreads rapidly in a circular pattern and produces a one-inch-in-diameter lesion. The circular pattern becomes filled with dirty-appearing scales and the hairs involved break off.	Oral griseofulvin (Fulvicin)	Adolescents warned not to use alcohol due to tachycardia Children do not need to be kept home from school Family members must not share towels or combs
Tinea Pedis (Athlete's Foot)	Skin lesions between the toes and on the plantar surface of the foot	Liquid preparations of clotrimazole (Lotrimin)	Antiseptic foot baths Do not let others share personal items such as footwear, towels, clothes, or sports equipment Wear thongs or swim shoes in public showers and stockings/shoes in locker rooms
Tinea Cruris (Jock Itch)	Found on the inner aspects of thighs and scrotum	Liquid or powder preparations of clotrimazole (Lotrimin)	Shower or bathe frequently if necessary Dry scrotal area thoroughly when damp Wear cotton underwear Do not let others share personal items such as footwear, towels, clothes, or sports equipment
Tinea Corporis (Epidermal Layer of the Skin)	Fungal infection of the epidermal layer of the skin that has a circular lesion with a clear center and scaly inflammation	Topical clotrimazole (Lotrimin)	Do not let others share personal items such as footwear, towels, clothes, or sports equipment

Nursing Insight— Systemic fungal infection

A systemic fungal infection, known as systemic mycosis, occurs primarily through inhalation of fungal spores. The specific fungal agent determines the course and severity of the infection. Systemic mycosis is not transmitted from person to person. One type of systemic mycotic infection is aspergillosis, which is found in airborne dust particles, compost heaps, or air vents. The condition usually manifests in children who already have a weakened immune system. Aspergillosis usually affects open spaces in the body, such as cavities that have formed in the lungs from preexisting lung diseases. It is characterized by a slow-progression chronic illness and spreads rapidly through the bloodstream to the brain and kidneys. This infection is very serious and difficult to treat. The main medical treatment for aspergillosis is the administration of intravenous amphotericin B (Amphocin) and supportive management for complications from either the active disease or subsequent treatment.

---

 medication: Amphotericin B (Amphocin)

Amphotericin (am-foe-**ter**-i-sin)

Indications: Treatment of active, progressive, potentially fatal fungal infections.

Actions: Binds to fungal cell membrane, allowing leakage of cellular contents.

Therapeutic Effects: Fungistatic action.

Pharmacokinetics:
ABSORPTION: Not absorbed orally.

Contraindications and Precautions:
CONTRAINDICATED IN: Hypersensitivity.

Adverse Reactions and Side Effects: Headache, hypotension, diarrhea, nausea, vomiting, nephrotoxicity, hypokalemia, chills, fever, and hypersensitivity reactions.

Route and Dosage: Specific dosage and duration of therapy depend on infection being treated.
  Amphotericin deoxycholate:
IV (CHILDREN): 0.25 mg/kg infused initially; increase by 0.25 mg/kg every other day to a maximum of 1 mg/kg per day.
  Amphotericin B cholesteryl sulfate:
IV (CHILDREN): 3–4 mg/kg per day
  Amphotericin B lipid complex:
IV (CHILDREN): 5 mg/kg per day
  Amphotericin B liposome:
IV (CHILDREN): 3–5 mg/kg q24h

Nursing Implications:
1. Premedication with antipyretics, corticosteroids, antihistamines, and anitemetics may reduce incidence of fever, chills, headache, nausea, or vomiting.
2. Monitor VS and above-noted symptoms every 15–30 minutes during test dose and every 30 minutes for 2–4 hours after the test dose.
3. Monitor VS and the aforementioned symptoms closely for the first 1–2 hours of each subsequent dose.
4. Monitor for thrombophlebitis as drug is highly irritating to tissues.
5. Monitor CBC and platelet counts weekly, BUN and serum creatinine every other day while increasing dose then twice weekly. Monitor potassium and magnesium levels biweekly.
6. Ensure resuscitation equipment readily available before administration.

Data from Deglin, J.H., & Vallerand, A. (2009). *Davis's drug guide for nurses* (11th ed.). Philadelphia: F.A. Davis.

---

 nursing diagnoses The Child with an Infectious Disease

- Hyperthermia related to disease process
- Risk for Fluid Volume Deficit, related to decreased intake
- Impaired Skin Integrity, related to pruritis
- Deficient Knowledge, related to disease process and self-care

 case study Infant with Pertussis

A 3-month-old infant is admitted with a history of "cold" symptoms for the last 2 weeks. The parents report the symptoms of fever, malaise, and a hacking cough that seems much worse at night. The cough tends to come in clusters and has been increasing in intensity over the past 3 days. The parents have brought the infant into the emergency room because he is now vomiting during the coughing spells and then turns blue around his mouth. An initial diagnosis of pertussis is made.

Critical Thinking Questions

1. The parents ask about transmission of pertussis for themselves and for the other children. How would the nurse best respond?

2. What preparations should the nurse take now to prevent the spread of this disease?

3. What actions should the nurse take during a coughing spell?

4. The family asks about the length of the illnesses. What is the nurse's response?

◆ See Suggested Answers to Case Studies in the text on the Electronic Study Guide or DavisPlus.

Immunizations

The cornerstone of infectious disease prevention in pediatrics is an immunization program in which the child receives the necessary vaccines. Vaccines are produced by using weakened or killed microbes, inactivated toxins, or subunits of disease-causing microbes. The goal of an immunization program is to bring about active immunity to guard against the onset of a specific antigen. The immune system response occurs through an exposure to a naturally occurring antigen or artificially through a vaccine-mediated exposure.

 Nursing Insight— Vaccine

The general requirements for development and implementation of a vaccine are:

- There must be a risk of the disease for the individual or population.
- The risk of the vaccine itself must be minimal and outweighed by the risk of the disease.
- The vaccine must be given at a time when it is effective.
- The immunization itself must be effective in promoting an immune response (National Institutes of Health, 2003). Understanding Vaccines: What They Are and How They Work. http://niaid.nih.gov/ NIH publication No. 03-4219.

An understanding about the different types of vaccines can assist the nurse in planning care that maximizes the effectiveness of vaccine and anticipates possible complications that can occur. Traditional vaccines include inactivated vaccines, live attenuated vaccines (weakened), and toxoids. *Inactivated vaccines* are produced when the disease-causing microbe is killed but is still capable of inducing the human body to produce antibodies (e.g., inactivated poliovirus vaccine). They are very safe and require little special handling. These types of vaccines stimulate a relatively weak immune response. For this reason, repeated boosters are required. The *live virus (attenuated) vaccine* is made by using a disease-causing organism that is not killed, but is grown under special conditions designed to decrease virulence (e.g., measles vaccine). Vaccines made with live organisms require special care, such as refrigeration. Live vaccines have the potential for mutation, allowing the organism to revert to a more virulent form. Due to the increased risk of mutation, live vaccines are not recommended for children (or adults who have close proximity to the child) with compromised immune systems. A *toxoid vaccine* is used in an inactivated form and is effective in producing an immune response geared toward a toxin-producing organism. The toxoid has been treated with either heat or a chemical to weaken its toxic effect but retains it antigenicity (e.g., tetanus toxoid).

More recent vaccine development has produced subunit vaccines, polysaccharide vaccines, conjugate vaccines, and recombinant vaccines. *Subunit vaccines* use only a portion of the virus or bacterium to produce the desired immunological response without the undesirable effects that occur with some of the other surface antigens (e.g., *Bordetella pertussis* vaccine included in the acellular DPT). This subunit vaccine produces immunity to *B. pertussis* with less risk so it may be more safely given to infants and young children.

Some bacteria possess a polysaccharide outer capsule that protects them from recognition and phagocytosis by the immune system. Organisms with this coating include *Haemophilus influenzae* B (HiB), *Streptococcus pneumoniae*, and *Neisseria meningitides*, each of which may produce a very serious case of pneumonia or meningitis in an infant or young children. *Polysaccharide vaccines* (Pneumovax), made from portions of the polysaccharides making up the protective capsule of these organisms, have long been available and are effective in producing immunity in children older than the age of 2 years. At exposure the polysaccharide capsule does not elicit a T-cell response, the duration of immunity is variable and not life long. In addition, these antigenic components are not recognized by the immune system of children younger than 2 years of age and it is children in this age group who are at highest risk for serious pulmonary or neurological infection resulting from these bacteria.

The development of *conjugate vaccines* has provided an option for protecting infants and young children. The conjugate vaccine links a recognizable antigen with the "hidden" bacterial antigen, thereby enabling the immature immune system to identify the bacteria as nonself and respond. In this way, the infant's T cells may identify the otherwise unrecognizable antigen, providing both an improved primary response and conferring immunological memory. An example of a conjugate vaccine used in children younger than 2 years of age is the *H. influenzae* type b (Hib) vaccine. Before the advent of this vaccination, pediatric meningitis resulting from Hib infection was a common cause of morbidity in infants.

Production of the *recombinant vaccine* uses genetic engineering to insert the genes for production of the antigens desired into a low virulent vector. The vector then can be used to easily produce quantities of the antigen for further purification into a subunit vaccine. The only recombinant vaccine currently used is hepatitis B virus (HBV). The HBV surface antigen is injected into yeast cells that produce quantities of the antigen for use in vaccination against hepatitis B.

 Nursing Insight— *The role of the nurse with immunizations*

The primary nursing goal is up-to-date immunizations for all children based on their particular health status. The pediatric nurse has several roles in the area of immunization. Addressing family concerns regarding immunizations is an important role of the nurse. The nurse also plays a key role in organizing and carrying out vaccination programs and distributing accurate and timely information regarding childhood immunizations. In addition, the nurse must use the current immunization schedule (www.cdc.gov/vaccines/recs/schedules) and recognize that the complicated schedule may pose some challenges for parents. The nurse can ensure that the parent has a vaccine information sheet (VIS) that records the immunizations. The nurse must also remind parents when the next immunizations are due. The nurse must recognize that explosion of information about immunizations available via the World Wide Web has both benefits and disadvantages. Through the Web, parents are bombarded with information regarding the types and safety of immunizations. The nurse must stay abreast of current information and discuss the parents' concerns. The nurse must also attempt to contact and immunize high-risk un-immunized children such as children who are homeless, immigrant, refugee, home schooled, frequently mobile, or who have a chronic or life-threatening illnesses. The pediatric nurse is also actively involved in statewide reporting of adverse effects of the vaccine.

Be sure to— **Be aware of legal considerations in immunization education**

The National Childhood Vaccine Injury Act of 1986 provides that parents or legal representatives of children receiving immunizations must be given a VIS developed by the Centers for Disease Control and Prevention (CDC) before immunization. The purpose of the VIS is to ensure uniform education regarding vaccines. The VIS must be used with the following vaccinations: DTaP, Td, MMR, polio, hepatitis B, Hib, varicella, and pneumococcal conjugate.

Full compliance with this law requires the nurse to:

- Provide the parent or legal guardian with the appropriate VIS before immunization.
- Record on the medical record the date that the VIS was given, the date of publication for the VIS, the name, address, and title of the person giving the vaccine, the date of administration of the vaccine, the manufacturer of the vaccine, and the vaccine lot number.
- The VIS must not be altered in any way.
- VIS forms (in many languages) may be accessed at www.cdc.gov/nip or www.immunize.org

• Hardcopies may be ordered through the CDC Web site: www.cdc.gov/nip/publications
• Individual state health departments with camera-ready copies can be obtained.
• Additional resources and additional education provided to the parent must also be recorded.

Note: Additional VISs are available for use with other common childhood vaccines, although use with other vaccines is strongly encouraged.

NURSING CARE

Nursing care for the child receiving immunizations requires the integration of several nursing roles. The nurse must be diligent in maintaining current knowledge about the medication's action and potential side effects and any contraindications to immunizations. In addition, the pediatric nurse must remain abreast about the current immunization schedule as well as being skilled in the actual administration of the vaccine. Setting up immunization clinics and long-term tracking of children who have and have not received immunizations are important, as well as accurate documentation and follow-up care. The pediatric nurse who works in the infectious disease area must cultivate specific channels for keeping up to date. The Department of Health and Human Services: Centers for Disease Control and Prevention http://www.cdc.gov/vaccines/ has updated information. The pediatric nurse uses current information to discuss the immunization plan and concerns with the family, prior to immunization (Diekeman, 2005).

Family Teaching Guidelines...
Immunizations

How To: Increasing immunization administration and compliance requires that the nurse work with the family to address the administration of the vaccine as well as their educational concerns.

Essential Information: When working with families the nurse can:

1. Discuss the actual administration and potential side effects of the vaccine with the parents.
2. Develop programs and materials that educate parents about immunizations.
3. Identify opportunities for administering immunizations by providing immunization clinics in nontraditional settings such as churches, synagogues, mosques, community centers, or shopping malls.
4. Provide opportunities and encourage parents to communicate their concerns about immunizations.
5. Encourage parents to investigate immunizations using reputable Web sites and other resources.
6. Assist the parents in understanding how to keep track of immunizations and when the next immunizations are due.
7. Assist parents in investigating funding resources for immunizations (this is a possible barrier to immunization for many families).

critical nursing action   Identifying Contraindications to Immunizations

A contraindication to vaccine administration indicates that the child has an increased risk of serious side effects from the vaccine and therefore should not receive that vaccine. There are very few real contraindications to vaccinations. Only one universal contraindication exists to all vaccines:

• Previous severe allergic reaction (anaphylaxis) to the vaccine or its component of vaccine.

Individual vaccines carry additional contraindications:

• Diphtheria, Tetanus, and Pertussis (DTaP) vaccine: Progressive neurological disease, i.e., infantile spasms, encephalopathy
• Measles, Mumps, and Rubella (MMR) vaccine: Pregnancy, severe immunodeficiency
• Varicella: Severe immunosuppression

Circumstances requiring postponement of vaccine administration include:

• Moderate to severe illness
• Administration of immunoglobulin within the last 3–11 months (precise period depends on specific immunoglobulin)

Note: Individual vaccines may have additional contraindications and precautions. Safe administration of vaccines requires the nurse to screen for contraindications and precautions prior to administration.

clinical alert

Adverse effects of immunizations

• Local effects are mild and occur most frequently (soreness, redness, and pain at the site of injection). These effects can be managed through local application of heat or ice to the site.
• Systemic effects are less frequent and include fever and mild irritability. These are managed with acetaminiophen (Children's Tylenol) administration before immunization, continuing every 4 hours as needed for 24 hours.
• An allergic reaction is rare but serious. The pediatric nurse and parents should watch for signs of an allergic response and seek medical assistance immediately should their child exhibit any of the following symptoms: high fever; altered mental status, including excessive irritability, lethargy, nonresponsiveness, or seizures; increased work to breathe; hoarseness or wheezing when breathing; hives; or pale or cool skin.

The immunizations are administered according to manufacturers' recommendations. During the immunization process, the nurse takes the time to address the unique concerns of each family. The parent's role after immunization is to understand and treat side effects. It is important for the nurse to communicate to parents when to call the physician. Once parental concerns have been addressed, the child can be released from the clinic when there are no signs of adverse reaction and the family understands when to notify the care provider (an allergic reaction).

 Now Can You— Safely give immunizations?

1. Identify contraindications to immunizations?
2. Discuss three strategies for increasing the administration of immunizations in children?
3. Identify key points of family education regarding immunization?

Animal-Borne Infectious Diseases

Animals serve as a reservoir for certain infectious diseases, including rabies, West Nile virus, and avian influenza. Nurses participate in prevention of these diseases through education for families about strategies that minimize exposure to infected animals, mosquitos, and infected birds.

Teaching children about animal safety is also important. The nurse can proactively talk to families and children about the risk of approaching unknown animals. Typically, rabies is not readily noticed through behavior of infected animals; for this reason children should be warned to be wary of unfamiliar animals.

Nurses can strategize with families about ways to avoid mosquito bites in areas where these insect diseases are common. Protection from exposure includes protective clothing, minimizing exposure of the skin, and use of insect repellents such as diethyltoluamide (DEET) sprayed on the clothing of children older than 1 year of age. It is important to emphasize to parents the potential for anything applied directly to the skin to be absorbed systemically in young children. Due to the risk of systemic absorption, safe use of insect repellents requires application to clothing rather than the child directly.

RABIES

Rabies is an acute viral infection of the nervous system caused by rhabdoviridae lyssavirus. The primary agent for this virus is carnivorous wild animals. Transmission of this disease occurs through direct contact with the brain tissue or the saliva from infected animals. The nurse must remember that untreated or inadequately treated rabies is fatal in humans (Hanlon, Niezgoda, Morrill, & Rupprecht, 2000).

The typical incubation period for rabies is 3 to 8 weeks but may extend for several months. The highest incidence of this disease occurs in children younger than 15 years of age. Only a small percentage, 10% to 15%, of persons with exposure to rabies goes on to develop the disease. However, the disease carries 100% mortality once symptoms are present. Treatment must be initiated as soon as possible after exposure and before the onset of symptoms.

Signs and Symptoms

Typical signs and symptoms of rabies include an initial period of generalized flu symptoms, including malaise, fever, and sore throat. The disease then progresses to alterations in mental status including seizures and hyperexcitability. The respiratory tract is then affected, leading to spasms that cause severe impairment of respiratory function, including respiratory arrest.

Diagnosis

Tests are performed on samples of saliva, serum, spinal fluid, and skin biopsies of hair follicles at the nape of the neck for rabies antigen.

Nursing Care

The nurse knows that postexposure treatment for rabies includes wound cleansing with a virucidal agent, administration of human rabies immune globulin (HRIG), and administration of a rabies vaccine series. HRIG is typically given in a total dose of 20 IU/kg body weight. A portion of the total dose is given into the tissue surrounding the wound through a series of injections given all around the wound boarders. Depending on the volume of medication to be given and the size of the wound, there may be medication remaining after the wound has been encircled with the HRIG. Any remaining medication is given IM at a site distant from the wound. For example, if the child is being treated for a small bite wound on the right forearm, the prescribed volume and dose of HRIG would be given in small injections all around the wound. If on completion of this process there remained 0.5 mL of HRIG it could be given IM in the left vastis lateralis. As with other types of immune globulins, the primary goal of administration of the HRIG is to provide a rapid, short-term passive immunity.

Active immunity is provided postexposure through completion of a rabies vaccine series using human diploid cell rabies vaccine (HDCV). This medication is given IM at the same time as HRIG (day 0) and again on days 3, 7, 14, and 28. Some sources recommend another dose on day 90. The HIG and HDCV are well tolerated in children. Support is needed due to the frightening nature of the disease, the urgency of the treatment, and the need for multiple injections (Jackson, Warrell, & Rupprecht, 2003).

 clinical alert

Postexposure treatment for rabies

Owing to the traumatic nature of treatment postexposure, seriousness of rabies, and poor prognosis, exercising caution with unknown animals is essential. Most exposures to rabies occur through bites of wild animals, which allow contaminated saliva to enter the bite wound. If an animal has injured a child, the parents must contact their health care provider immediately!

WEST NILE VIRUS

West Nile virus causes an infection that is spread by mosquitoes that become infected when they bite infected birds (Morse, 2003). Infected mosquitoes then may spread the virus to children. West Nile virus infection has been documented in children as young as 1 month of age. The incidence of severe disease in children is rare (O'Leary et al., 2004). The incubation period for West Nile virus is from 3 to 14 days.

Signs and Symptoms

Most of the time West Nile virus causes few symptoms lasting 3 to 6 days, or the symptoms are so mild children do not realize they have been infected. Typical symptoms include headache, malaise, anorexia, nausea, vomiting, myalgia, eye pain, generalized lymphadenopathy, and a maculopapular rash found on the trunk, neck, and extremities. In rare cases, the virus can lead to encephalitis or meningitis.

Diagnosis

Diagnosis of West Nile virus is confirmed by specific IgM antibody in cerebrospinal fluid. Because IgM antibody does not readily cross the blood–brain barrier, IgM antibody in CSF strongly suggests acute CNS infection (Campbell, Marfin, Lanciotti, & Gubler, 2002).

Nursing Care

Nursing care of children with West Nile virus includes education about the disease itself and its prevention. Treatment is supportive based on the signs and symptoms. Nurses can also provide information about the relative infrequency of severe disease in children. Responding to parental concerns, nurses can help them plan strategies for minimizing exposure to mosquito bites. Of particular concern is also minimizing possible side effects related to systemic absorption of insect repellents.

" What to say " — *Use of insect repellents*

Concerned about exposure to insect bites and the possibility of infectious disease transmitted through this route, parents at times apply insect repellents such as diethyltoluamide (DEET) directly on their children. Although the nurse must provide education to change this behavior, it is important to support the parents' intent of decreasing the risk of infection in their child. The nurse can appraise the parents about the intent of the action while providing them with the correct information that the insect repellent must be applied to the child's clothing. Applying the insect repellant to the clothing decreases the chance of systemic absorption (through the skin) of a potentially harmful substance.

AVIAN INFLUENZA

Influenza pandemics are recurring events. In this past century influenza pandemics occurred in 1918, 1957, and 1968. Recently, one particular strain of the Avian Influenza, H5N1, has been identified by the World Health Organization (WHO) as a strain with this potential (WHO, 2006a).

Avian influenza, known commonly as bird flu, refers to an influenza virus that occurs naturally in birds worldwide. Although occurring chiefly in birds, certain subtypes of the virus may mutate and transfer to humans. Because this strain of virus has not been previously circulated in the human population, the potential for an influenza pandemic is present. This particular influenza virus is transmitted via the respiratory route and the resulting infection is likely to be more severe than typical influenza, as the human immune system currently lacks the ability to respond swiftly to this new threat.

Currently transmission is thought to occur primarily through direct contact with infected birds or the secretions or excretions of the infected animals. Confirmed cases of avian influenza in humans have occurred in those with contact with domestic birds, primarily poultry, infected with the virus. Known cases have been confined to Asia and Europe.

Person-to-person spread has been reported very rarely and is limited to one direct, close contact. In 2006, the WHO reported 228 confirmed human cases of the H5N1 strain of avian influenza, and documented with 130 deaths (World Health Organization, 2006a). As of Wednesday, May 16, 2007, in Indonesia, WHO confirmed 15 additional cases, including 13 deaths, of human infection with H5N1 avian influenza (WHO, 2007).

clinical alert

Clusters of human H5N1 cases

As reported on the CDC Web site (http://www.cdc.gov/flu/avian/outbreaks/current.htm), "Clusters of human H5N1 cases ranging from 2–8 cases per cluster have been identified in most countries that have reported H5N1 cases. Nearly all of the cluster cases have occurred among blood-related family members living in the same household. Whether such clusters are related to genetic or other factors is unknown. While most people in these clusters have been infected with H5N1 virus through direct contact with sick or dead poultry or wild birds, limited human-to-human transmission of H5N1 virus cannot be excluded in some clusters."

The WHO is working closely with heath departments worldwide to coordinate surveillance and pandemic preparation in an attempt to avert or lessen the expected impact of the threatening pandemic. Avain influenza should be considered in a child with moderate to severe respiratory symptoms who meets one of the following criteria: has traveled to an area with known outbreaks of avian influenza in the domestic poultry, has had contact with infected birds, or has had close contact with a person infected with avian influenza.

Signs and Symptoms

Symptoms of avian influenza in humans have ranged from typical symptoms of influenza, such as cough, sore throat, fever, and myalgia to severe pneumonia and acute respiratory distress.

Diagnosis

Avian influenza cannot be diagnosed on the basis of symptoms alone. It is usually diagnosed by collecting a swab from the nose or throat during the first few days of illness to test for avian influenza virus.

Nursing Care

Treatment includes supportive and symptomatic care, including aggressive treatment of complications such as pneumonia. Antiviral medications may also be used. There are four antiviral medications: amantadine (Symmetrel), rimantadine (Flumadine), osteltamivir (Tamiflu), and zanamivir (Relenza) currently approved for use in treatment of influenza in humans. Effectiveness varies with the particular strain of virus.

The H5N1 virus seen in human cases in Asia has proven to be resistant to amantadine (Symmetrel) and rimantadine (Flumadine). CDC does not recommend use of these agents. The latest (2006b) WHO guidelines suggest the use of osteltamivir (Tamiflu) as the first-line antiviral treatment if it is available but note this recommendation is based on very few cases and lacks strong evidence. WHO and CDC continue to monitor the cases of avian influenza in humans and provide updates on recommendations for specific treatment. Research focused on development of a vaccine to protect against H5N1 virus has been underway since April 2005 and clinical trials are ongoing.

Family Teaching Guidelines...
Preparing for an Influenza Pandemic

How To: Actions taken by individuals and communities help to decrease the impact of an influenza pandemic. Nurses can work with families to provide them the information needed to prepare adequately.

Essential Information: When working with families the nurse can:

1. Discuss the differences between seasonal flu and pandemic flu.
2. Describe actions being taken by the health care community to monitor and prepare for the pandemic and encourage families to take an active role.
3. Assist families to establish their own plan for care in the event of a pandemic including:
   • Storage of a 2-week supply of food and water for the family.
   • Maintenance of a supply of needed medications.
   • Maintenance of a supply of over-the-counter medications needed to treat symptoms of flu.
   • Establish a plan for family members living alone.
4. Encourage families to become involved with community groups to help prepare and plan for the pandemic.
5. Reinforce basic infection control techniques to limit spread of influenza.
6. Provide families with links to CDC resources with preparation checklists. Encourage them to utilize the checklists to assist in preparation.

Source: http://www.pandemicflu.gov/plan/checklists.html

An Emerging Issue in Infectious Disease: Resistant Organisms

In recent years, there has been a steady increase in the incidence of infections with antibiotic-resistant organisms in the United States and in many countries around the world. Several factors have been associated with the genesis and spread of these organisms. On a global scale, bacterial resistance, due to misuse. is an escalating problem in many countries providing an ever-increasing reservoir for resistant organisms to thrive.

 Ethnocultural Considerations— Antibiotic Use Around the World

Further increasing the likelihood of inadequate treatment is the common cultural practice in many countries of taking an incomplete course of treatment. Conditions for the development of antibiotic-resistant organisms include overcrowded living conditions and lack of potable water and basic sanitation. In many developing countries, the likelihood of transmission of resistant organisms from person to person is high. Inadequate equipment or surveillance furthers the problem of antibiotic resistance around the world. In the era of global travel, the increase in community-acquired antibiotic-resistant organisms in any part of the world becomes a necessary component of the discussion of infection control policies worldwide.

Overuse of antibiotics is the primary factor for the development of antibiotic resistance as well as noncompliance with a prescribed course of treatment. Person-to-person transmission of antibiotic-resistant organisms occurs primarily through nosocomial transmission in hospitalized children and now also may be occurring in the community at large.

The costs, both human and monetary, of antimicrobial resistance are large (McGowan, 2001). Specific strategies directed at control of antibiotic-resistant organisms are development of new antimicrobial agents and surveillance programs to identify incidence of current misuse. Isolation measures to prevent the spread of infection in both the hospital and broader community, education of health care professionals about the increased incidence of resistant organisms, and improving correct use and compliance of antibiotics are necessary.

Within both the acute care environment and in the community nurses can promote public awareness and develop strategies to decrease the transmission of antibiotic resistant organisms. Specifically, nurses can spread the word about overuse and provide family education about completing a prescribed course of treatment. Measures that help nurses provide effective antibiotic therapy are knowledge about exact dosing, medications that decrease efficacy, and duration of treatment. The nurse must also maintain updated knowledge of current practices in infection control. Consult an infection control specialist and decrease the spread of nosocomial transmission in the hospital. Nurses are the bridge between the actual infection and public health awareness.

 Now Can You— Describe the role of the nurse in antibiotic-resistant organisms?

1. Identify conditions for the development of antibiotic-resistant organisms?
2. Discuss ways that nurses can promote public awareness about antibiotic overuse?

ANTIBIOTIC ALTERNATIVES

As concerns about antibiotic-resistant organisms increase, alternatives for prevention of disease are being pursued with increased vigor. Monoclonal and probiotics antibodies are now considered for the future in the control of infectious disease in children. Monoclonal antibiotics are based on the same premise as passive immunity and have demonstrated effectiveness in passive immunity for a large number of infectious diseases acquired in childhood. Monoclonal antibodies are applied to mucosal surfaces to prevent disease transmission at the site of entry. The main drawback of this type of protection is the cost and time associated with production of sufficient amounts of antibodies. However, advances in technology will soon shorten the availability time and resources needed to manufacture new monoclonal antibody preparations. Since monoclonal antibodies produce only passive immunity, much more emphasis has gone into development of vaccines for stimulating active immunity.

Probiotics are another new area of research. Probiotics are bacteria that colonize in the intestine and participate in the intestinal microenvironment in such a way as to improve immune function. To be effective, probiotics must be able to survive the trip through the digestive tract and colonize primarily in the colon. It is believed that once in the colon, the probiotics act to reinforce the mucosal barrier through reducing gut permeability and enhancing local immune response, such as IgA release. It is unclear about the role that probiotics will play in the prevention of illness.

 Nursing Insight— *Probiotics*

Children with rotaviral gastroenteritis who received the probiotic *Lactobacillus* had reduced severity and duration of acute diarrhea.

"What to say" — *Home care instructions*

The nurse is providing home care instructions to the parents of a 2-year-old child presenting with symptoms of a viral illness. The parents tell the nurse they are unhappy with the physician's decision not to prescribe antibiotics. The nurse responds by asking:

- Tell me more. What has been your past experience with treating similar illnesses?

- What are your concerns with this illness? What do you believe will happen if antibiotics are prescribed to treat your child at this time?

- What are your plans to care for your child? Under what circumstances will you contact your health care provider to discuss a change in treatment plan?

summary points

- Infectious and immune diseases represent a significant pediatric health concern for the child, family, and public.

- The body's first line of defense is the skin and the second is the immune response.

- Congenital immunodeficiency disorders are rare but include more than 70 specific types of disorders. These conditions result in life-long impairment of immune system function. This impairment then results in an increase in incidence, severity, and recurrence of infections.

- The goals of treatment for HIV-positive children are to slow progression of AIDS, prevent further infections, promote normal growth and development, prevent complications including cancers, and prolong and improve quality of life.

- After surgery, post-transplant immunosuppression is critical and children are placed in a medically induced state of immunosuppression.

- An autoimmune disorder is the immune response against one of the body's own tissues or cells. Examples of autoimmune disorders are systemic lupus erythematosus, juvenile rheumatoid arthritis, and anaphylaxis.

- There are three types of infections (bacterial, viral, and fungal). Although each infectious condition has unique signs and symptoms, several symptoms are common in varying degrees among several illnesses. Common signs and symptoms include fever, malaise, anorexia, and pruritus from rashes.

- The cornerstone of infectious disease prevention in pediatrics is an immunization program where the child receives necessary vaccines.

- Animals serve as a reservoir for certain infectious diseases, including rabies, West Nile virus, and avian influenza. Nurses participate in prevention of these diseases by educating families about strategies that minimize exposure to infected animals, mosquitoes, and infected birds.

- There has been a steady increase in the incidence of infections with antibiotic-resistant organisms in the United States and in many countries around the world.

review questions

Multiple Choice

1. The pediatric nurse provides health prevention teaching to a group of parents in a community clinic regarding communicable diseases. Teaching should include:
   A. Administering salicylates (aspirin) for fever
   B. Bathing the child with harsh soap to prevent the spread of the disease
   C. The application of soft mittens to prevent scratching
   D. Providing layers of clothing to keep the child warm

2. A 13-year-old girl is admitted to the pediatric unit with a diagnosis of infectious mononucleosis. Upon assessment, the nurse records a history of swollen lymph nodes, fever of 103.5°F, headache, anorexia and malaise. The nursing plan of care includes:
   A. Bedrest, maintaining hydration, decreasing fever and isolation
   B. Assessing bowel sounds and administering Nystatin (Mycostatin)
   C. Collecting a urine sample and administering antiviral therapy
   D. Maintaining NPO, inserting a nasogastric tube and cool baths

3. The pediatric nurse provides patient education to the parents of a child with chickenpox. The teaching should include the potential complications that may come about secondary to this illness. All of the following are common complications EXCEPT:
   A. Febrile seizures
   B. Encephalitis
   C. Reye syndrome
   D. Thrombocytopenia

True/False

4. Prevention and control of infections and communicable diseases is a primary goal of national, state, and local health agencies, addressed largely through surveillance, public education, and immunization programs.

5. The pediatric nurse correctly teaches parents that disorders of the immune system are always acquired.

6. When caring for a child with an immune disorder the nurse correctly explains to parents that antibiotics reinforce the mucosal barrier by reducing gut permeability and enhancing local immune response.

7. When conducting patient teaching, the nurse will communicate that the child who is infected with the HIV virus will have a decreased CD4 or helper T-cell count.

Fill-in-the-Blank

8. When teaching parents about the immune system, the nurse stresses that the main purpose of the immune response is to _____ the body against microorganisms, parasites, and foreign cells like cancer cells.

9. An HIV-infected mother has been admitted to the hospital in labor. The nurse bases the plan of care upon the understanding that initiation of _____ _____ and delivery via _____ _____ reduce the risk of HIV infection in the neonate.

10. The pediatric nurse administers _____ (_____), the medication of choice in treating Candida Albicans (Oral Thrush).

Case Study

11. A 2-year-old boy is admitted with Systemic lupus erythematosus (SLE) with a history of fever, malaise, chills, fatigue and weight loss. Nursing care is based on managing:
   A. Offering support, administering antiviral medication and forcing fluids
   B. Administering salicylates (Aspirin), applying warm compresses and bedrest
   C. Maintaining nutrition, assessing bowel sounds and providing diversional activities
   D. Managing pain and inflammation, treating symptoms and preventing complications

12. The nurse is preparing to administer *Lactobacillus* (*L. acidophilus*) to a 4-year-old patient. The parent asks the nurse why the child is receiving this medication. The nurse's best reply is:
   A. "I'm not sure but I'll ask the doctor to come and speak with you."
   B. "It's an antibiotic to help clear up the infection."
   C. "It's an electrolyte to help treat the dehydration."
   D. "It's a medication that helps reduce the severity and duration of the diarrhea."

See Answers to End of Chapter Review Questions on the Electronic Study Guide or DavisPlus.

REFERENCES

Bulechek, G., Butcher, H.M., & Dochterman, J. (2008). *Nursing interventions classification (NIC)* (5th ed.). St. Louis, MO: C.V. Mosby.

Campbell, G.L., Marfin, A.M., Lanciotti, R.S., & Gubler, D.G. (2002). West Nile virus. *Lancet Infectious Diseases, 2*, 519–529.

Centers for Disease Control and Prevention (CDC). (2005). West Nile Virus (WNV) Infection: Information for Clinicians. Retrieved from http://www.cdc.gov/ncidod/dvbid/westnile/resources/fact_sheet_clinician.htm (Accessed July 3, 2008).

Centers for Disease Control and Prevention (CDC). (2006). Key facts about avian influenza (flu) and avian influenza A (H5N1) virus. Retrieved from http://www.cdc.gov/flu/avian/gen-info/facts.htm (Accessed July 3, 2008).

Centers for Disease Control and Prevention (CDC). (2008). Avian influenza: current H5N1 situation. Retrieved from http://www.cdc.gov/flu/avian/outbreaks/current.htm (Accessed July 3, 2008).

Copenhaver, C.C., Gern, J.E., Li, Z., Shult, P.A., Rosenthal, L.A., Mikus, L.D., Kirk, C.J., Roberg, K.A., Anderson, E.L., Tisler, C.J., DaSilva, D.F., Hiemke, H.J., Gentile, K., Gangnon, R.E., & Lemanske, R.F. Jr. (2004). Cytokine response patterns, exposure to viruses, and respiratory infections in the first year of life. *American Journal of Respiratory Critical Care Medicine, 170*(2), 175–180.

Deglin, J., & Vallerand, A. (2009). *Davis's drug guide for nurses* (11th ed.). Philadelphia: F.A. Davis.

Diekeman, D.S. (2005). Responding to parental refusal of immunization of children. *Pediatrics, 115*(5), 1428–1431.

Feeney, M.E. (2004). HIV and children: The developing immune system fights back. *West Indian Medical Journal, 53*(5), 359–362.

Hanlon, C.A., Niezgoda, M., Morrill, P.A., & Rupprecht, C.E. (2000). The incurable wound revisited: Progress in human rabies prevention? *Vaccine, 19*, 2273–2279.

Hoffjan, S., Nicolae, D., Ostrovnaya, I., Roberg, K., Evans, M., D., L., Walker, K., P., & R.(2005). Gene-environment interaction effects on the development of immune responses in the 1st year of life. *American Journal of Human Genetics, 76*, 696–704.

Howland, L.C., Gortmaker, S.L., Mofenson, L.M., Spino, C., Gardner, J.D., Gorski, H., Fowler, M.G., & Oleske, J. (2000). Effects of negative life events on immune suppression in children and youth infected with human immunodeficiency virus type 1. *Pediatrics, 106*(3), 540–546.

Jackson, A.C., Warrell, M.J., & Rupprecht, C.E. (2003). Management of rabies in humans. *Clinical Infectious Disease, 36*, 60–63.

Johnson, M., Bulechek, G., Butcher, H., McCloskey Dochterman, J., Maas, M., Moorehead, S., & Swanson, E. (2006). *NANDA, NOC, and NIC linkages: Nursing diagnoses, outcomes, & interventions* (2nd ed.). St. Louis, MO: Mosby Elsevier.

Lehman, T.J.A. (2002). Early diagnosis of SLE in childhood. *Lupus News, 22*(3).

Lupus: A Child Care Guide for Nurses and Other Health Professionals. (2001). Cygnus Corporation, Rockville, MD, and Johnson, Bassin, & Shaw, Inc., Silver Spring, MD, under contract NOI-AR-4-2213

McGowan, J.E., Jr. (2001). Economic impact of antimicrobial resistance. *Emerging Infectious Diseases. 7*(2), 286–292.

Moorehead, S., Johnson, M., Maas, M., & Swanson, E. (2008). *Nursing outcomes classification (NOC)* (4th ed.). St. Louis, MO: C.V. Mosby.

Morse, D.L. (2003). West Nile virus—Not a passing phenomenon. *The New England Journal of Medicine, 348*, 2173–2174.

NANDA International (2007). *NANDA-I nursing diagnoses: Definitions and classifications 2007–2008*. Philadelphia: NANDA-I.

National Guideline Clearinghouse (2008). Retrieved from http://www.guideline.gov/summary/summary.aspx?doc_id=12248&nbr=6332&ss=6&xl=999 (Accessed July 3, 2008).

National Institutes of Health (NIH). (2003). Understanding vaccines: What they are and how they work. Retrieved from http: //niaid.nih.gov/. NIH publication No. 03-4219 (Accessed July 3, 2008).

National Institutes of Health (NIH). (2005a). Guidelines for use of anti-retroviral medications in pediatric HIV infection. Retrieved from http://aidsinfo.nih.gov/ (Accessed July 3, 2008).

National Institutes of Health (NIH). (2005b). Supplement II: Pediatric: Managing complications of HIV infection. Retrieved from http://aidsinfo.nih.gov/ (Accessed July 3, 2008).

O'Leary, D.R., Marfin, A.A., Montgomery, S.P., Kipp, A.M., Lehman, J.A., Biggerstaff, B.J., Elko, V.L., Collins, P.D., Jones, J.E., & Campbell, G.L. (2004). The epidemic of West Nile virus in the United States, 2002. *Vector-Borne and Zoonotic Diseases, 4* (1), 61–70.

Venes, D. (Ed.). (2009). *Taber's cyclopedic medical dictionary* (21st ed.). Philadelphia: F.A. Davis

Weerkamp, F., de Haas, E.F.E, Naber, B.A.E., Comans-Bitter, W.M., Gogers, A.J.J., van Dongen, J.J.M., & Staal, F.J.T. (2005). Age-related changes in the cellular composition of the thymus in children. *Journal of Allergy and Clinical Immunology, 115* (4), 834–839.

World Health Organization (WHO). (2006a). Ten things you need to know about pandemic influenza. Retrieved from http://www.who.int/csr/disease/influenza/pandemic10things/en/ (Accessed July 3, 2008).

World Health Organization (WHO). (2006b). Rapid advice guidelines on pharmacolgocal management of humans infected with avian Influenza A (H5N1) Virus. Retrieved from http:www.who.int/medicines/publications/WHO_PSM_PAR_2006.6.pdf. (Accessed June 27, 2006).

World Health Organization (WHO). (2007). Avian influenza update information. Retrieved from http://www.medicalecology.org/diseases/influenza/influenza_update.htm (Accessed July 3, 2008)

CONCEPT MAP

Immunodeficiency Disorders
Congenital: B-cell disorders; T-cell disorders; B-lymphocyte disorders; Wiskott-Aldrich syndrome
Acquired: Pediatric HIV

Transplantation

Autoimmune Disorders
- SLE
- JRA

Allergic Reaction
- Anaphylaxis

Communicable Diseases/Childhood:
- Chickenpox, diphtheria, mononucleosis, Fifth disease, influenza, mumps, pertussis, pneumococcal disease, polio, roseola, rubella, rubeola, scarlet fever, tetanus, bacterial, viral and fungal infections, rabies, west Nile

Common Viral Infections
- CMV
- Herpes zoster
- Small pox
- Infectious mononucleosis

Common Fungal Infections
- Candidiasis
- Systemic fungal infections

Animal Borne
- Rabies
- West Nile
- Avian flu

The Immune System
The body's defense:
- Skin
  – Mechanical and chemical barriers
- Immune response

Caring for the Child with Immunologic or Infectious Conditions

Pathological Concepts:
Epidemiological Triangle
Host: susceptibility
Environment: transmission
Agent: characteristics

Across Care Settings:
- Prevent transmission of infections within the family and/or community

Clinical Alert:
- Diaper rash = portal of entry
- Never stop steroids abruptly
- Lupus: prevent infections; immediate treatment for rabies
- No ASA with viral illness; educate re: dehydration symptoms
- Only CMV negative blood to immunocompromised children
- Check for adverse reactions/ allergic reactions to immunizations
- Exercising caution with unknown animals
- Clusters of Human H5NI cases

Critical Nursing Action:
- Skin care/nutrition
- Identify contraindications to immunizations
- Teach significance of respiratory symptoms
- Immediate nursing care for anaphylaxis
- Have solid knowledge of IVIG

Where Research And Practice Meet:
- IV assessment form
- Improper use of antibiotics
- Research focuses on development of vaccine to protect against H5NI virus

Family Teaching Guidelines:
- Identify barriers to compliance with immunizations
- Immunization schedules, funding

Nursing Insight:
- Understand immunoglobulins
- Children are more vulnerable to infections
- SLE support groups
- Know s/s of anaphylaxis
- Understand physiology of a fever
- Primary nursing role is up-to-date immunizations
- DEET can be absorbed systemically
- Teach patients how to evaluate internet information

General Nursing Care:
Child With An Infection
- Manage fever
- Quiet environment
- Control itching
- Frequent, small amounts of favorite liquids
- Infant: bulb suction congested nares
- Teach significance of:
  – Complications/secondary infections
  – Transmission prevention

Promoting a Healthy Immune System:
- Minimize/decrease stress related to negative life events
- Promote immunizations
- Promote integrity of body's defense to infections

Resistant Organisms:
- Antibiotic alternatives

General Nursing Care:
Child Immunologic Disorder:
- Prevent infection
- Promote adequate nutrition
- Attend to alterations in comfort
- Monitor mucous membranes
- Prevent alterations in skin integrity
- Encourage parents to take an active role in care of the child
- Assess child for attainment of developmental milestones

Now Can You:
- Identify nursing actions that support immune functioning
- Identify three strategies for decreasing transmission of infections
- Identify two important teaching points for families related to antibiotic treatment
- Identify major nursing considerations in the care of the child with HIV

Caring for the Child with a Cardiovascular Condition

 I dedicate this chapter to the children with cardiac disease who I have cared for over the last 25 years in the Pediatric ICU, Cardiology, and Cardiovascular surgery. There are so many children, who have had immediate and lasting results from treatment (those are the ones I rarely see in follow-up) and then there are those I see chronically, year after year, perhaps since infancy, who have grown to college age. These children have the strength to survive and to live day to day with the constant reminder of their illness. They live with tachycardia, cyanosis, shortness of breath and poor growth patterns and low exercise tolerance. Year after year, month after month, or even week after week these children return for blood tests, electrocardiograms, echocardiograms, and invasive procedures such as cardiac catheterizations and multiple surgeries. They give me strength.

—Judy Marshall

LEARNING TARGETS *At the completion of this chapter, the student will be able to:*

◆ Understand the anatomy and physiology of the heart.

◆ Discuss congenital heart disease (heart defects) and the effect on children.

◆ Recognize major cardiac diseases and conditions together with related nursing care measures.

◆ Identify the importance of interventional cardiac catheterization procedures in the care of children with cardiac conditions.

◆ Describe important surgical interventions and postoperative management used for children with a cardiac condition.

◆ Develop a nursing care plan for caring for a child with cardiac conditions.

◆ Explain nursing care for the child in the Pediatric Intensive Care Unit (PICU) and surgical/ medical unit.

◆ Describe how to care for children with cardiac conditions across care settings.

---

 moving toward evidence-based practice Development risks in participants with Hypoplastic Left Heart Syndrome and Transposition of the Great Arteries

Brosig, C.L., Mussatto, K.A., Kuhn, E.M., & Tweddell, J.S. (2007). Neurodevelopmental outcome in preschool survivors of complex congenital heart disease: implications for clinical practice. *Journal of Pediatric Health Care, 21*(1), 3–12.

The purpose of this study was to compare the neurodevelopmental outcome of preschool children who had surgical repair for hypoplastic left heart syndrome (HLHS) with those who had surgical repair for transposition of the great arteries (TGA).

Past research has suggested that neurodevelopmental delays in individuals with congenital heart disease (CHD) are related to chronic hypoxia, inadequate cerebral perfusion, and decreased systematic oxygen delivery, which may be experienced during the preoperative, perioperative, and postoperative periods.

The researchers of this investigation contend that diagnostic and surgical advances in the past 10 years have improved the neurodevelopmental outcomes of persons undergoing HLHS and TGA repair procedures. Surgical repair for HLHS is associated with multiple risks due to "deep hypothermic circulatory

(continued)

moving toward evidence-based practice (continued)

arrest (DHCA), the prolonged effects of hypoxia at a time of critical brain growth, and the stress of multiple surgical procedures spaced over a 2- to 4-year interval" (p. 4).

Persons with TGA generally undergo one surgical procedure, the arterial switch operation (ASO), which provides complete repair of the defect and maintains normal anatomy and oxygen saturation.

The study sample was selected from two cohort groups: one group included children ages 3–6 "who survived the Norwood procedure for HLHS" or other forms of congenital heart disease that produced "significant obstruction to the systemic circulation" (p. 4). The second group was selected from children ages 3–6, who survived the arterial switch operation for transposition of the great arteries.

All participants received surgical care between 1996 and 1999 at a Midwestern hospital. All procedures were performed by the same cardiac surgeons. Study eligibility requirements included meeting the age and diagnostic criteria and coming from a primarily English-speaking family. Children who had other major congenital anomalies, medical conditions, or treatments deemed to exert an adverse impact on development were excluded.

The final sample included 13 participants in each group. All chart reviews were completed by one investigator. The neurodevelopmental assessment was performed by a pediatric psychologist who was unaware of the child's cardiac diagnosis and surgical history.

Several instruments, including McCarthy Scales of Participant's Abilities, Woodcock Johnson III Tests of Achievement, Developmental Test of Visual–Motor Integration, Receptive Once-Word Vocabulary Test, Expressive One-Word Vocabulary Test, and Child Behavior Checklists were used. The tools were selected based on findings from previous studies.

Analysis of demographic data revealed the following:

- The mean age of the participants was 4.7 years.
- The mean age of the TGA group was 4.6 years; the mean age of the HLHS group was 3.9 years.

- Ninety-six percent of the participants were Caucasian; 73% were male.
- All participants were considered to be from middle-class families.
- Twelve percent of the participants were enrolled in special education services.

Analysis of surgical data revealed the following:

- Participants in the HLHS cohort experienced longer hospital stays after surgery (mean = 26 days) vs. 16.5 days for the participants in the TGA cohort.
- Participants in the HLHS cohort experienced a longer duration of time (mean = 282 minutes) on cardiopulmonary bypass than did the TGA cohort (mean = 200 minutes).
- Participants in the HLHS group experienced an average of 65 minutes on deep hypothermic circulatory arrest; the TGA cohort experienced an average of 14 minutes on deep hypothermic circulatory arrest. Hypothermic circulatory arrest involves an induced state of hypothermia combined with use of extracorporeal circulation and anesthesia management, the purpose of which is to rest the heart and decrease myocardial oxygen requirements while surgical repair is completed.
- Participants in the HLHS group had an average of three surgeries; those in the TGA cohort had an average of one surgery.

Analysis of cohort scores on the various testing instruments revealed that, in general, the HLHS cohort demonstrated more difficulties with visual–motor skills, expressive language, attention, and externalizing behavior than did the TGA group.

1. What might be considered as limitations to this study?
2. How is this information useful to clinical nursing practice?

See Suggested Responses for Moving Toward Evidence-Based Practice on the Electronic Study Guide or DavisPlus.

Introduction

Children with cardiac problems are a complex population of patients. The heart is integral to all other bodily systems. Whereas a child can survive on one kidney or one lung, heart disease is not self limited and affects most other bodily systems. The nurse must understand various cardiac diseases and problems; treatment of cardiac disease; and care measures for an infant, child, or adolescent with cardiac conditions. Cardiac defects are often associated with other syndromes (Table 27-1).

A & P review Understanding the Heart

Anatomy

A child's heart contracts 60–180 times per minute depending on his or her age. The heart never stops beating although it decelerates during rest and sleep and accelerates during excitement, exercise, or illness.

Chambers

The heart consists of four chambers, two of which act as reservoirs (atria) and two as pumping chambers (ventricles) (Fig. 27-1).

The right atrium is a reservoir or collecting chamber for the peripheral venous return. The right atrium receives deoxygenated blood from the entire body (except lungs) through the superior and inferior venae cavae and coronary sinus with an approximate oxygen saturation of 70%.

The left atrium receives fully oxygenated blood from the lungs through the pulmonary veins, with an approximate oxygen saturation of 100% (Venes, 2009). The ventricles are the remaining two chambers in the heart. From the atria, blood empties into the ventricles through atrioventricular valves. The right ventricle has smaller muscle mass with trabeculated surfaces. The right ventricle receives blood from the right atrium and pumps it into the lungs via the pulmonary artery.

Table 27-1 Syndromes Associated with Cardiac Disease

Syndrome/Disease/ Chromosomal Aberrations	Cardiac Defect/Condition	Other Physical Findings
Down Syndrome	AV canal, VSD	Down's facies, developmental delay
Noonan Syndrome	Fulmonic valve stenosis, LVH	Elfin facies, pectus deformity, joint laxity, undescended testes, spine abnormalities, hypotonia, seizures
Williams Syndrome	Supravalvular aortic stenosis, PA stenosis	Williams' facies: include a small upturned nose, long philtrum (upper lip length), wide mouth, full lips, small chin, and puffiness around the eyes; hypercalcemia, dental abnormalities, renal problems, sensitive hearing, hypotonia, joint laxity, overly friendly personality
DiGeorge or Velo–cardio–facial Chromosome	Interrupted aortic arch, truncus arteriosus, VSD, PDA, TOF	Decreased immune response, low set ears, palate problems, hypoparathyroidism and hypocalcemia
Duchenne's Muscular Dystrophy	Cardiomyopathy	Generalized weakness and muscle wasting first affecting the muscles of the hips, pelvic area, thighs, and shoulders; calves are often enlarged
Marfan Syndrome	Aortic aneurism, aortic and/or mitral regurgitation	Arms disproportionately long, tall thin with laxity of joints, dislocation of lenses, spinal problems, stretch marks, hernia, pectus abnormalities, restrictive lung disease
Trisomy 18	VSD, PDA, PS	Multiple joint contractures, spina bifida, hearing loss, radial aplasia (underdevelopment or missing radial bone of forearm), cleft lip, birth defects of the eye
Trisomy 13	VSD, PDA, dextrocardia	Omphalocele, holoprosencephaly (an anatomic defect of the brain involving failure of the forebrain to divide properly), kidney defects, skin defects of the scalp
CHARGE	TOF, truncus arteriosus, vascular ring, interrupted aortic arch	Coloboma of the eye, Heart defects, Atresia of the choanae, Retardation of Growth and development, and Ear abnormalities and deafness
Fetal Alcohol Syndrome	VSD, PDA, ASD, TOF	Growth deficiencies, skeletal deformities, facial abnormalities, organ deformities: genital malformations; kidney and urinary defects, central nervous system handicaps
VATER (VACTERLS)	VSD and others	Vertebral anomalies, vascular anomalies, Anal atresia, Cardiac anomalies, Tracheo–esophageal (T–E) fistula, Esophageal atresia, Renal anomalies, radial dysplasia, Limb anomalies, Single umbilical artery
Turner Syndrome	CoA, ASD, AS	Kidney problems, high blood pressure, overweight, hearing difficulties, diabetes, cataracts, and thyroid problems, lack of sexual development, a "webbed" neck, a low hairline at the back of the neck, drooping of the eyelids, dysmorphic, low set ears, abnormal bone development, multiple moles

The left ventricle typically is thicker with a smooth interior. The left ventricle receives blood from the left atrium and pumps it into the systemic circulation via the aorta (Venes, 2009).

Valves

There are four valves in the heart. Two are atrioventricular (AV) valves connecting the atria and ventricles (Fig. 27-2). The tricuspid valve connects the right atrium to the right ventricle and is so named because it consists of three cusps or "doors" that open to allow blood flow into the adjoining chamber and shut to prevent backflow. The mitral valve, called a bicuspid valve for its two cusps, connects the left atrium to the left ventricle. The aortic and pulmonary valves are both tricuspid and are called semilunar valves because each cusp looks like a half-moon. The pulmonary valve is located at the junction of the right ventricle and pulmonary artery. It prevents regurgitation of blood from the pulmonary artery to the right ventricle. The aortic valve, located at the junction of the left ventricle and the ascending aorta, also prevents regurgitation into the left ventricle (Venes, 2009).

Vessels

Aside from the chambers and the valves in the heart, there are major vessels that lead to and from the heart. The vena cava carries the blood from body tissues to the right atrium. The superior vena cava enters from above the heart and carries blood from the head, arms, and upper body. The inferior vena cava enters from below the heart and carries blood from the legs, abdominal organs, and lower part of the body. The pulmonary artery is the only named artery in the body that carries deoxygenated blood. It is called an artery because it carries blood away from the heart, but since it arises from the right ventricle, it carries deoxygenated blood. It carries this blood to the pulmonary capillary bed, where it interfaces with the alveoli in the lungs and "picks up" oxygen. From the lungs, the blood returns to the heart through the pulmonary veins into the left atrium (the only veins that carry oxygenated blood). The blood leaves the left ventricle through the aortic valve, through the aorta and out to the body (Fig. 27-3).

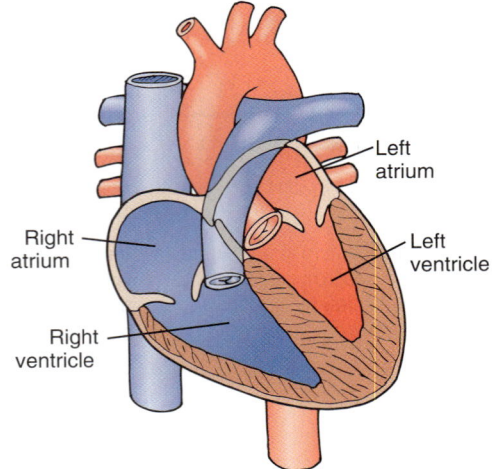

Figure 27-1 Chambers of the heart.

Figure 27-3 Vessels of the heart.

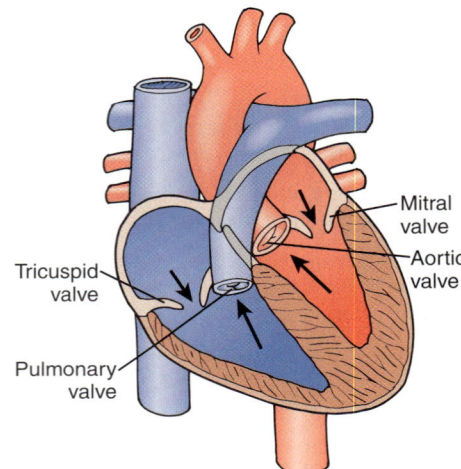

Figure 27-2 Valves of the heart.

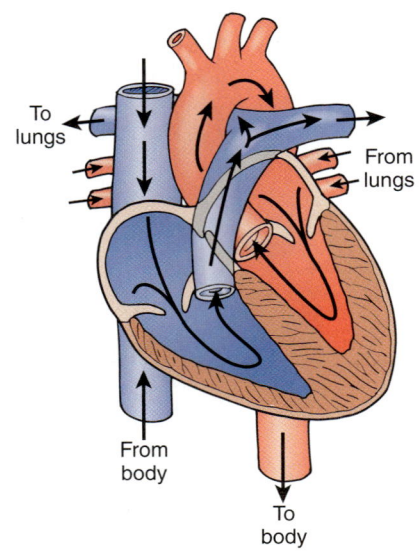

Figure 27-4 Normal blood flow.

Normal Flow

It is important to understand the flow of blood through the cardiovascular system because an interruption in any one of the vessels, valves, or chambers causes a disruption in the cardiac output. (Fig. 27-4) shows a schematic representation of normal blood flow through the heart.

Physiology

The simplest way to understand the physiology of the heart is to comprehend that the purpose of the heart is to pump blood. This vital pumping function provides a means to carry oxygen via the hemoglobin to the tissues. Without oxygen delivery, cells die and ultimately body systems fail. The heart must maintain a cardiac output at all times.

Cardiac output is the amount of blood discharged from the left or right ventricle per minute (Venes, 2009). Cardiac output is the product of stroke volume (SV) and heart rate (HR) (CO = SV × HR).

Stroke volume is the amount of blood ejected by the left ventricle with each heartbeat (Venes, 2009). Stroke volume is the product of preload, after-load,

and contractility (inotropy) (SV = Preload × afterload × contractibility).

An altered cardiac output limits the blood's ability to provide oxygen to the tissues. Since heart rate and the size of the heart vary with the size of the child, the volume of cardiac output will vary accordingly. A variety of methods measure cardiac output with varying degrees of accuracy. The Fick calculation is the most accurate way to measure cardiac output (Fig. 27-5). ◆

$$\text{Pulmonary flow } (Q_p) = \frac{\text{V}_{O_2}}{C_{PV} - C_{PA}}$$

$$\text{Systemic flow } (Q_s) = \frac{\text{V}_{O_2}}{C_{AO} - C_{MV}}$$

Figure 27-5 Fick calculation.

Nursing Insight— *Congestive heart failure*

Many congenital and acquired cardiac conditions result in congestive heart failure (CHF). Much of the basic nursing care of a patient with a cardiac condition is dependent on the degree of the CHF.

Cardiac failure occurs when the heart can no longer fully accomplish its intended purpose. CHF, or called simply heart failure, is characterized by the inability of the cardiac muscle to perform its proper function of moving blood forward. Blood is "congested" in a backward direction. The heart's pumping action is lost so the blood backs up into other areas of the body such as the lungs or the liver. This backward congestion of fluid eventually fills into the periphery.

Signs and Symptoms

The signs and symptoms of CHF vary with age and whether the fluid is more congested on the right or left side. Infants present with poor feeding, poor growth, irritability, shortness of breath (SOB), or excessive sweating. In advanced stages an enlarged liver or edema develops. Older children show poor growth, shortness of breath, and exercise intolerance. Peripheral edema in children does not present in the same way as in adults. Ascites rarely occurs in children except in the most dramatic cases and more often in teenagers. Babies and toddlers exhibit puffy eyelids, swelling of hands and feet, and the fontanel may be bulging. Congenital heart disease (CHD), arrhythmias, or other cardiac diseases such as cardiomyopathy (CM) or Kawasaki disease can lead to CHF.

Diagnosis

Diagnosis includes patient history and physical examination findings including vital signs (blood pressure and pulses may be diminished), weight gain, or changes in breath sounds. Diagnostic measures include B-natriuretic peptide, chest x-ray exam, exercise test, echocardiogram, magnetic resonance imaging (MRI), and cardiac catheterization.

Nursing Care

CHF is treated with medications or, if due to some congential defects, surgery. Positive inotropes such as digoxin (Lanoxin) or even the stronger dopamine drugs are used when poor contractility is the cause of CHF. If increased preload is the cause, then diuretics such as furosemide (Lasix) or hydrochlorothiazide (Aquazide) may be used. Vasodilators such as captopril (Capoten) or enalapril (Vasotec) are prescribed if increased afterload is the causative factor. Often all three are used in conjunction. Because of the risk of dehydration, fluid restriction is not often used in pediatrics except in the worst cases.

Congenital Heart Disease

Congenital heart disease is a defect in the heart, great vessels, or a noted disease pattern after birth. Congenital heart defects occur in approximately 1% of all pregnancies and 1 in 170 live births (Neilson & Robin, 2002). There are various ways by which the nurse can recognize a congenital heart defect, including recognizing the shunting pattern and recognizing cyanotic versus acyanotic congenital heart defects.

CYANOTIC VERSUS ACYANOTIC CONGENITAL HEART DEFECTS

Congenital heart defects are sometimes classified as cyanotic versus acyanotic: many, but not all, cardiac defects involve mixing of blood. If the deoxygenated or venous blood from the right side of the heart is forced into the left side of the heart (called right to left shunting) as in cyanotic defects, the overall oxygen saturation of the blood will drop. The range may be normal (96-100%) to as low as 70%. In acyanotic defects the oxygenated blood shunts from the left to the right. This type of mixing will not affect the overall oxygenation status.

In the presence of normal hemoglobin, a decrease in the oxygen saturation to 85% will cause an outward sign of cyanosis (bluish coloration) that appears around the lips, nose, and mouth of babies and toddlers and in the nail beds of older children. If the decreased oxygen state is chronic, the child eventually will develop clubbing of the fingernails. The longer and lower the oxygen saturation the more evident the clubbing. The physiological explanation for this change is that the capillaries enlarge to accommodate the low saturation in an attempt to deliver more blood to the periphery.

Another long-term effect of low oxygenation is polycythemia. Polycythemia is the increase in the red blood cell production in response to the low oxygen output. The patient has hemoglobin (Hgb) levels greater than 15 (g/dL). The condition also causes thickening of the blood and predisposes the child to thrombi and stroke.

Nursing care entails monitoring and maintaining the child's oxygen and nutritional status. The nurse educates the family regarding rest periods and managing the child's fatigue.

 Now Can You— **Understand the heart?**

1. Discuss the anatomy and physiology of the heart?
2. Identify signs and symptoms in a child with congenital heart disease?

Segmental Classification of Congenital Heart Defects

In the United States, cardiac defects occur in 8 to 12 per 1000 (1%) live births (Park, 2003). There are several approaches to classifying heart lesions. Table 27-2 shows the traditional approach. The nurse may best understand the cardiac defects via a segmental approach organized by the type of defective physical structure. This segmental approach includes of the septum or septae [pl] (chamber walls), vessels and valves, conal– truncal defects, and combination defects. Nichols. D.G., et al, (2006) critical heart disease in infants and children, 2nd ed., Pg. 3.

DEFECTS IN THE SEPTUM

Atrial Septal Defect

Atrial septal defect (ASD) is a simple defect of the atria. During fetal development, the septal wall forms between the 4th and 8th week of life when two septae, the primum and secundum, stretch across the center of the common atrium (Fig. 27-6). Eventually these septae overlap, but not completely and form area small opening called the foramen ovale. The foramen ovale is a necessary structure during

Table 27-2 Classification of Cardiac Defects

Class	Name	Prevalence (% of all defects)	Types or Forms	Associated Defects
L–R Shunt	Atrial–septal defect	5–10 (50–100)	Secundum or primum or sinus venosus	PAPVR or MVP
	Ventricular septal defect	20–25 (200–250)	Perimembranous, muscular, multiple	PDA, CoA, AV prolapse
	Patent ductus arteriosus	5–10 (50–100)	Large shunt or small	
	AV canal	0.02 (0.20)	Complete or partial; balanced or unbalanced	AV regurgitation. 30% of cases occur with Down syndrome
	Partial anomalous pulmonary venous return	<1 (10)	TAPVR	ASD
Obstructive Lesions	Pulmonary stenosis	5–8 (50–80)	Valvular, subvalvular, supravalvular (PA)	VSD, Noonan syndrome
	Aortic stenosis	0.05 (0.50)	Valvular, subvalvular, supravalvular	Bicuspid aortic valve, Williams syndrome, IHSS
	Coarctation of the aorta	5–10 (50–100)	Preductal, postductal, ascending aorta, descending aorta	Bicuspid AV, aortic hypoplasia, VSD, PDA, abnormal MV
	Interrupted aortic arch	0.01 (0.10)	Type of coarctation, types A, B, C	PDA, VSD, bicuspid AV, MV deformity, truncus arteriosus, subaortic stenosis
Cyanotic Defects	Transposition of the great arteries	0.05 (0.50)	D-type, L-type	ASD, VSD, PDA, PS
	Tetralogy of Fallot	0.10 (1.00)	PS or PA or absent PV with PS	May be cyanotic or acyanotic if PS is mild
	Total anomalous pulmonary venous return	0.01 (0.10)	Supracardiac, cardiac draining into RA, cardiac draining into the coronary sinus, infracardiac; obstructive	ASD or PFO
	Tricuspid atresia	1–2 (10–20)		ASD, VSD, PDA, CoA, TGA
	Pulmonary atresia	<1 (10)	Variable RV sizes	ASD, PFO, or PDA
	Epstein's anomaly	<1 (10)	Variable degrees of displacement	WPW, RA hypertrophy, ASD
	Truncus arteriosus	<1 (10)	Types I-IV showing various placements of PA arising from the aorta	Large VSD, right Ao arch, DiGeorge syndrome
	Single ventricle	<1 (10)	DILV or RV	ASD, PS, PA, CoA, VSD, asplenia, polysplenia, TGV
	Double outlet right ventricle	<1 (10)	Types are by the position of the VSD: subaortic VSD, subpulmonary VSD, remote VSD, subaortic VSD with PS, doubly committed VSD	VSD, PS
	Splenic syndromes	<1 (10)	Asplenia and polysplenia	Various redundant cardiac structures or absence of structures

The numbers in parentheses indicate the number of infants born with defects out of 100,000 live births.
© Judith M. Marshall, 2006.

fetal life, but should close within hours after birth. Sometimes the foramen ovale may persist until 1 year of life. An ASD results when the two septae fail to overlap properly. There are two variations of the defect: primum (high on the septal wall) and secumdum (low on the wall).

SIGNS AND SYMPTOMS. A murmur may or may not be present and the child may or may not have a right ventricle (RV) heave or a thrill (abnormal tremor accompanying a vascular or cardiac murmur felt on palpation) (Venes, 2009). At worst case, the ASD in the child is the source of right atrial enlargement caused by fluid overload from left to right shunting through the opening in the atrial wall. This fluid overload can extend to the right ventricle, which is the source of the RV heave, and show an axis deviation (evidence of ventricular enlargement) on an ECG. This defect also produces a fixed split second heart sound. The liver becomes engorged as result of this fluid overload. Other signs and symptoms of cardiac failure such as shortness of breath, respiratory distress, periorbital edema, failure to thrive, and increased respiratory infections may be noted. These signs gradually worsen with time unless the defect is repaired. An ASD, along with atrial fibrillation, may predispose the child to stroke due to the tendency of blood pooling and risk of thrombus formation.

DIAGNOSIS. The ASD is confirmed by chest x-ray exam, echocardiography, cardiac catheterization, and ECG.

Figure 27-6 Atrial septal defect.

NURSING CARE. Without treatment, certain types of ASDs may close spontaneously in the first year of life and the child typically shows no outward signs of a malformation. The ASD, if not closed spontaneously, may be closed with a surgical procedure or interventional cardiology where a closure device is inserted. Nursing care focuses on postoperative management of the child.

> **critical nursing action** Postoperative management
>
> Provide immediate postoperative care in the intensive care unit:
>
> - Record the vital signs frequently until the child is stable.
> - Maintain vascular access systems (there may be several):
>   - A peripheral IV is used to administer fluid and medications.
>   - A central venous pressure (CVP) line inserted in a large vessel in the neck or groin is used to measure pressure in the right atrium.
>   - Intracardiac catheters are inserted in the right atrium, left atrium, and pulmonary artery and are used to measure the pressures inside the cardiac chambers that provide essential information about cardiac output, blood volume, pulmonary pressures, ventricular function, and drug therapy response.
>   - Assess for complications such as cardiac, neurological, pulmonary, or hematologic changes; infection; and delayed growth and development.
>   - Assess and maintain respiratory status. Respiratory assessment is performed frequently and oxygen is delivered via mechanical ventilation.
>   - Suction secretions.
>   - Monitor fluid status. Accurately measure the intake and output of all fluids.
>   - Monitor blood lab values for postoperative bleeding and post-pump electrolyte imbalances.
>   - Maintain chest tubes that remove secretions and re-expand the lungs. Check drainage for quantity and color.
>   - Manage pain via comfort measures and the administration of medication.
>   - Consider the child's level of development in order to provide developmentally appropriate care.
>   - Ensure rest, which is essential to promote healing and decrease the work load of the heart.
>   - Group nursing care to avoid imposing unnecessary fatigue and weakness.
>   - Provide emotional support and information about home care.

Ventricular Septal Defect

A ventricular septal defect (VSD) is the most common congenital heart defect. Fortunately, it is one of the mildest. A VSD forms much the same way as an ASD. In fetal development at the approximate gestational age of 4 to 8 weeks, the wall is formed when a superior and inferior limb (like a divider) of tissue come together to create a wall between the two chambers. A defect in the formation of this wall can be a single opening or be fraught with multiple defects, sometimes called a Swiss cheese VSD (Fig. 27-7).

The defect may be located anywhere on the ventricular septal wall. Usually those in the muscular septum close spontaneously. If left alone, individuals can live a long normal life. At the worst case, the child suffers from right ventricular overload from left-to-right (acyanotic) shunting of blood due to the high-pressure gradient from the left to the right side. Generally, a VSD is repaired surgically. However, in the future, the use of a transcatheter closer device may be more common.

SIGNS AND SYMPTOMS. Most patients with VSDs are asymptomatic. If the VSD is large and there is a significant left to right shunt, the patient develops signs of right ventricular failure, such as shortness of breath, feeding

Figure 27-7 Ventricular septal defect.

difficulties, poor growth, easy fatigability, and recurrent pulmonary infections. Typically, a harsh murmur (along with a thrill at the lower left sternal border) is detected at the well-baby checkups.

DIAGNOSIS. Diagnosis is based on an audible heart murmur along with other signs and symptoms. A chest radiograph, ECG, echocardiogram, or cardiac catheterization may help confirm the diagnosis.

NURSING CARE. Care of the child with VSD is similar to that of the child with ASD. Nursing care focuses on postoperative management of the child.

Atrioventricular Canal Defect

An atrioventricular canal defect (AVC) is also known as complete AVC or endocardial cushion defect (ECD). This defect is somewhat of a combination of an ASD and VSD. However, it is much more than that, as it involves the valves. In its simplest definition, an AVC is a large hole in the center of the heart. The endocardial cushion fails to form properly. There are openings on the atrial wall and the ventricular wall, and the tricuspid and mitral valve come together to form one large valve (Fig. 27-8). These defects are often seen in children with Down syndrome, although 70% of AV canal defects are seen in children who have no other anomalies. This defect must be repaired surgically if the child is to live a normal life span. Although the blood is mixed through this large open space, the shunt is left to right and the child is not cyanotic.

SIGNS AND SYMPTOMS. Signs and symptoms of cardiac failure such as shortness of breath, respiratory distress, periorbital edema, failure to thrive, increased respiratory infections, and distended liver may be noted. These signs will gradually worsen with time unless the defect is repaired. There are many variations of this defect including partial ECD.

DIAGNOSIS. A complete physical examination, including listening to the heart and lungs, helps in the diagnosis. A heart murmur is verified. Additional tests such as chest x-ray and ECG support the diagnosis. An echocardiogram, cardiac catheterization, and cardiac magnetic resonance imaging (MRI) confirm the diagnosis.

NURSING CARE. Care of the child with AVC more complex than that of the child with ASD and VSD. Prior to surgery, nursing care is geared toward optimizing the cardiac output and ensuring adequate weight gain. Nursing care focuses on postoperative management of the child.

 Nursing Insight— *Care of the child with congenital heart defects*

The hospital nurse most often cares for a child with a congenital heart defect when the child is admitted for surgery. Occasionally, a child with a defect may be admitted for reasons not related to the heart. The child should always be monitored for signs of CHF and measures taken to prevent fatigue, fluid overload, or infections.

The school nurse may also have students with congenital heart defects. Typically, the cardiologist or cardiology nurse practitioner submits letters to the school that outline the plan of care and any physical or activity restrictions. Anyone caring for a child who is taking cardiac medications must understand the effects, side effects, and proper dosing.

DEFECTS OF THE VESSELS AND VALVES

Patent Ductus Arteriosus

A patent ductus arteriosus is the simplest form of vessel defect (Fig. 27-9). Remember that the ductus arteriosus is a normal structure during fetal life. In utero, the pulmonary resistance is high because the lungs are filled with fluid rather than air. The blood is oxygenated through the placenta by the umbilical vein. Instead of the blood flowing from the pulmonary artery (PA) to the lungs, the ductus is a pop-off valve for the large volume of fluid. As the blood flow follows the "path of least resistance," the blood moves through the ductus, into the aorta, and out to the body tissues. Directly after birth and the baby's first breaths, the pulmonary resistance drops and the blood flows from the PA into the lungs. Since there is decreased flow through the PDA, the duct starts to close. Changes in prostaglandin level assist the closure as well. In 8 to 10% of the population, the PDA remains open (Park, 2003). It can take as long as 1 year for the PDA to close completely. The pediatric cardiologist monitors the asymptomatic child up to 1 year for spontaneous closure of the PDA.

Figure 27-8 Atrioventricular canal defect.

Figure 27-9 Patent ductus arteriosus.

If a large PDA is not closed, severe long-term sequelae may ensue. At birth, the pulmonary resistance is higher than the left-sided pressures. As this gradient reverses, the left-sided pressure forces blood toward the right side through the PDA. Eventually, the fluid congests the right side of the heart and the pulmonary bed. The right ventricle hypertrophies in an attempt to mobilize fluid forward. The defect occurs alone or in combination with coarctation of the aorta.

SIGNS AND SYMPTOMS. The PDA murmur is distinctive in sound and location. This murmur is heard best at the left subclavicular margin and is described as machine-like, to and fro or continuous. Other symptoms include frequent colds and susceptibility to RSV, fatigue, poor feeding, and poor growth pattern. The blood pressure reveals a wide pulse pressure.

DIAGNOSIS. The presence of the characteristic machine-like murmur under the left clavicle along with symptoms of heart failure leads to the diagnosis of patent ductus arteriosus. Chest radiograph shows an enlarged heart and evidence of an excessive blood flow to the lungs. An echocardiogram confirms the diagnosis, demonstrating the size of the ductus arteriosus and enlargement of heart chambers due to the extra blood flow.

NURSING CARE. A PDA may be closed surgically or with a transcatheter device. The PDA may also be "forced" closed using the medication indomethacin (Indocin). Nursing care focuses on postsurgical measures, such as care of the wound, monitoring vital signs, and ensuring adequate hydration and nutrition.

 Nursing Insight— *Subacute bacterial endocarditis prophylaxis (SBE)*

If the child has a high risk for bacterial endocarditis, the physician will prescribe antibiotics before dental work and surgery. The child may require this for only 6 months after the defect is repaired. Each case is treated individually according to published American Heart Association guidelines.

Pulmonic Stenosis

Pulmonic stenosis or pulmonic valve stenosis (PS or PVS) is a malformation of the pulmonary artery or pulmonic valve. The narrowing of the valve causes an increased workload on the right ventricle (Fig. 27-10), which in turn leads to congestive heart failure (CHF) with symptoms such as hepatomegaly. This condition is frequently associated with Noonan syndrome and is part of the combination condition called tetralogy of Fallot.

 Nursing Insight— *An insufficient valve*

Valves may be congenitally malformed, or become physically altered because of disease. If the valve does not close properly, there may be leakage called regurgitation or insufficiency when the valve is stiff or stenotic. When the valve is insufficient, the ventricle must pump with greater force to push blood through a stiff or "sticky" door. Because of the backflow of blood, the ventricle pumps with a greater force of contraction because there is more volume and thus more stretch (Starling's law). This constant added force eventually wears on the cardiac muscle.

Figure 27-10 Pulmonary stenosis.

SIGNS AND SYMPTOMS. A heart murmur is the most common sign of pulmonic stenosis. During periods of increased blood pressure, such as with excitement, exercise, crying or fever the child may experience dyspnea (breathlessness) or in the most severe cases, brief moments of cyanosis when the blood flow does not reach the pulmonary bed.

DIAGNOSIS. Diagnosis is confirmed by the presence of a heart murmur, electrocardiogram, and echocardiogram. Cardiac catheterization measures the degree of pulmonary stenosis.

NURSING CARE. Depending on the gradient (difference in the pressure measurements), the cardiologist may choose to observe the child closely over time before recommending interventions. Interventions include balloon angioplasty or valvuloplasty (a procedure that reopens narrowed blood vessels and restores forward blood flow) or open heart surgery. Since this valve is in an area of low flow and low pressure, these children often do well with one intervention, but should be monitored periodically for restenosis. Care measures help the patient to reduce stressful situations that may cause high blood pressure.

 Nursing Insight— *Pulmonary atresia*

Pulmonary atresia is a fatal defect if not corrected or palliated (treated to reduce effect) early in life. Pulmonary atresia is absence of the pulmonary valve, pulmonary artery, or both (Fig. 27-11). The child must have an ASD or patent foramen ovale (PFO) (the opening present in utero and at birth which closes spontaneously) and/or a PDA in order to survive. If these are not present, emergency procedures are performed to save the child's life. Initially prostaglandin (PGE$_1$) is infused to maintain patency (free flow) of the PDA. A balloon atrial septostomy (formation of an opening in a septum) is performed to create an ASD (Venes, 2009). Primary surgical repair includes a shunt (diversion) or a conduit (channel). Later, a Fontan procedure (a procedure used to repair complex single ventricle type congenital heart defects) may be needed.

Figure 27-11 Pulmonary atresia.

Aortic Stenosis

Aortic stenosis or aortic valve stenosis (AS or AVS) is a malformation and narrowing in the aorta or around the aortic valve (Fig. 27-12). A narrowing in this area causes an increased workload on the left ventricle which eventually leads to hypertrophy (increase in size) and heart failure. This condition may also be acquired after birth.

SIGNS AND SYMPTOMS. In children with aortic stenosis, a murmur may be audible during the systolic phase of the cardiac cycle. A click may be heard and a thrill may be noted. The child may have chest pain or fatigue and syncope on exertion. Critical AS causes heart failure in neonates. Variations of this defect are supra- and subvalvar stenosis and an association with bicuspid aortic valve.

DIAGNOSIS. Diagnosis is based on the clinical findings, chest x-ray exam, and echocardiogram. An ECG may show left ventricular hypertrophy. Cardiac catheterization is the definitive test, also measuring the exact gradient.

NURSING CARE. In critical situations with very narrow valves, preload and afterload reduction medication is indicated. Since this valve is in a high-flow high-pressure area,

it is more critical to correct. A balloon angioplasty or valvuloplasty is performed to open the narrow area. Another treatment mode is surgical intervention to repair or replace the valve. Nursing care is based on medical and/or postoperative management. Aortic stenosis requires lifelong monitoring.

Coarctation of the Aorta

Coarctation of the aorta (CoA) is a narrowing or stricture of the descending aorta distal to the carotid arteries. The coarctation is classified by its location: preductal, ductal, or postductal (Fig. 27-13).

SIGNS AND SYMPTOMS. Normally, blood pressure in the legs should be higher or equal to that in the arms. When a BP in the lower extremities measures >10 mm Hg less than that in the upper extremities, the practitioner suspects a CoA (Park, 2003). Occasionally, the BP in the right arm is higher than in the left. This usually occurs with a preductal coarctation in which the blood flow to the left arm is supplied by the flow of blood through the ductus, which is a lower pressure system. For this reason, if only one upper extremity is used as comparison to the lower extremities, it should be the right arm. If a child is hypertensive, the nurse should suspect CoA. The child may shows signs of CHF. The child may have pain in the legs or cyanotic lower extremities.

DIAGNOSIS. The classic diagnostic feature of this defect is a high gradient, which is the difference in the pressure measurements between the arms and legs.

NURSING CARE. Surgery is always indicated for this condition. Nonsurgical treatment for older infants and adolescents involves a balloon angioplasty and stent placement. Nursing care focuses on postoperative management of the child. The child is seen in follow-up for evidence of restenosis.

Tricuspid Atresia

Tricuspid atresia (TA) is caused by an error in the formation of the tricuspid valve. As a single defect, this condition is incompatible with life, since no blood from the RA reaches the RV and thus the right ventricular outflow tract

Figure 27-12 Aortic stenosis.

Figure 27-13 Coarctation of the aorta.

Figure 27-14 Tricuspid atresia.

Figure 27-15 Epstein's malformation.

(RVOT) leading to the PA and the lungs. For this reason, most children born with TA also have co-morbidity with a septal defect such as ASD or VSD as well as a PDA. The deoxygenated blood must reach the pulmonary bed to sustain life (Fig. 27-14).

SIGNS AND SYMPTOMS. The initial signs are dramatic; as the PDA starts to close in the hours after birth, the child becomes severely cyanotic, tachycardic, and dyspneic. A heart murmur is generally present.

DIAGNOSIS. Tricuspid atresia may be discovered during a routine prenatal ultrasound imaging or at birth based on the signs and symptoms. Diagnostic testing includes ECG, echocardiogram, chest radiograph, and cardiac catheterization.

NURSING CARE. Tricuspid atresia requires emergency intervention. Initially, the neonate is given PGE_1 to keep the PDA from closing. In addition, if there is no ASD or PFO, an emergent balloon atrial septostomy is performed to ensure survival. The next step is to perform a systemic–pulmonary (SP) shunt if the pulmonary blood flow is deficient or a PA band if the pulmonary blood flow is excessive. Eventually a Glenn procedure may be done and Fontan procedure is the definitive surgery. Nursing care focuses on postoperative management of the child.

 clinical alert

Survival

With any congenital defect, as long as there is mixing of oxygenated and deoxygenated blood, the child survives. A more definitive surgery such as a Fontan procedure is performed at a later date to correct the condition (Table 27-4).

 Nursing Insight— Epstein's malformation

Epstein's malformation occurs when the tricuspid valve is displaced into the right ventricle (Fig. 27-15). Typically, in this condition, an ASD is present. The ventricle and the atria may become hypertrophied and this condition is often associated with supraventricular arrhythmias, particularly Wolff–Parkinson–White syndrome. With Epstein's malformation the child may live normally or require treatment. Surgical intervention is the treatment of choice.

Total Anomalous Pulmonary Venous Return

Total anomalous pulmonary venous return (TAPVR) is a condition in which the pulmonary blood flow returns to the heart through the right atrium rather than the left (Fig. 27-16). The child usually has an ASD, allowing the blood to flow back to the left ventricle and out to the body tissues. As a consequence of ASD, mixing of venous blood with arterial blood may occur, causing a cyanotic condition. One problem for a child with TAPVR is that a high volume of blood returns to the right side of the heart, causing right-sided hypertrophy and enlargement. If an ASD is not present, one is created with a balloon septostomy. A variation of this condition is partial anomalous pulmonary venous return (PAPVR), in which two of the veins return blood to the left side and two of the veins return blood to the right side. Other variations are simply in routing of the blood flow back to the heart.

Figure 27-16 Total anomalous venous return.

SIGNS AND SYMPTOMS. The child has cyanosis, respiratory distress, lethargy, poor and rapid breathing, poor feeding, frequent respiratory infections, and signs of heart failure.

DIAGNOSIS. Diagnosis is based on signs and symptoms and diagnostic testing including ECG, echocardiogram, chest x-ray exam, and cardiac catheterization.

NURSING CARE. The treatment for TAPVR is complete surgical repair. Post-surgery, the child can live a full normal life, but should be followed routinely (every 1 to 2 years) for any reoccurring stenosis. Nursing care focuses on postoperative management of the child.

CONAL–TRUNCAL DEFECTS

Conal–truncal defects develop during the formation of the trunk dissection. Embryologically, the pulmonary artery and the aorta begin as a large "trunk." The ventricles then fold on over, the atria rise into position, and the great vessels form when the trunk twists around and septates (having a dividing wall). Transposition of the great vessels and truncus arteriosus occur in children when there is a disruption in this process.

Transposition of the Great Arteries or Vessels

Transposition of the great arteries or vessels (TGA or TGV) occurs in utero when the signals cross and instead of twisting there is simply a septation and the aorta arises from the right side of the heart and the pulmonary artery arises from the left (Fig. 27-17).

SIGNS AND SYMPTOMS. Symptoms appear at birth or soon afterwards and include cyanosis, shortness of breath, poor feeding, and eventually clubbing of the fingers and toes.

DIAGNOSIS. Diagnosis is based on signs and diagnostic testing includes pulse oximetry, ECG, echocardiogram, chest x-ray exam, and cardiac catheterization. If an echocardiogram is done before birth, it is called a fetal echocardiogram.

NURSING CARE. The severity of the signs and symptoms direct the timing of treatment. TGA in all cases must be surgically corrected, typically with an arterial switch

where research and practice meet:
Repair of Transposition of the Great Vessels or Arteries

Until approximately 1975, TGV or TGA was corrected through a palliative procedure called a Mustard or Senning in which a tunnel or baffle was created in the right atria shunting blood to the left atria, then the left ventricle and therefore out the aorta. This was not a definitive repair and the children were often cyanotic and many times did not survive into adulthood. In 1975 a surgical procedure called arterial switch was first performed. By 1985, this procedure had replaced the Mustard and Senning as the treatment of choice (Park, 2003). In surgery the position of the aorta and the PA are permanently switched. Arterial switch is not without long-term side effects, but after surgery the child can lead a full, normal acyanotic life.

operation (ASO) (Table 27-4). This is considered a definitive repair and the prognosis is good. Nursing care focuses on postoperative management of the child.

Truncus Arteriosus

Truncus arteriosus is a complicated cyanotic lesion with a poor prognosis if not treated surgically. In truncus arteriosus, the trunk has neither twisted or septated. There are multiple variations of the condition, classed I to IV, but the general physiology is that the aorta and pulmonary arteries (PAs) are combined, with full mixing of blood (Fig. 27-18). Sometimes the PAs arise from the aorta, either ascending or descending.

SIGNS AND SYMPTOMS. Clinical signs and symptoms of truncus arteriosus include cyanosis, congestive heart failure, and low cardiac output.

DIAGNOSIS. Diagnosis is based on signs and diagnostic testing that include pulse oximetry, ECG, echocardiogram, chest radiograph, and cardiac catheterization.

NURSING CARE. This condition requires palliative and complete surgical repair. Treatment for children includes aggressive medical regimen with inotropic medications along with preload and afterload reduction. Nursing care focuses on postoperative management of the child.

Figure 27-17 Transposition of the great vessels.

Figure 27-18 Truncus arteriosus.

COMBINATION DEFECTS

Tetralogy of Fallot

Tetralogy of Fallot (TOF) is a combination defect. *Tetra* is from the Latin root "four" and Fallot is the name of the physician who defined it as a syndrome or common grouping. There are four associated conditions: VSD, overriding aorta, hypertrophic RV, and pulmonary stenosis or atresia. With advanced technology and early screening, this condition is diagnosed at an early age. As recently as the 1980s TOF was undetected for many years, and in developing countries remains so even today.

SIGNS AND SYMPTOMS. In TOF, a stenotic vessel and high pulmonary vascular resistance (PVR) cause the right ventricle to hypertrophy (Fig. 27-19).

clinical alert

Tetralogy of Fallot

The hallmark sign of TOF is cyanosis with crying or playing, which is relieved by squatting or drawing up the legs. These episodes (called "TET" spells)—are cyanotic events exacerbated by excitement and crying, then relieved by a decrease in pulmonary vascular resistance.

DIAGNOSIS. Diagnosis of TOF is based on signs and symptoms such as cyanosis, breathing difficulties, fainting, fatigue and weakness, slow growth, or developmental delay. Tests, including ECG, echocardiogram, chest x-ray exam, and cardiac catheterization, confirm the diagnosis.

NURSING CARE. Nursing care focuses on postoperative management of the child because the treatment for TOF is surgical repair. Presurgical care involves preventing or minimizing symptoms associated with the defect.

 Nursing Insight— *A way to remember cyanotic defects*

The nurse can remember that all defects starting with a "T" are cyanotic defects. There is no special reason why; it is just a convenient way to remember which defects are cyanotic.

Complex Single Ventricle Type Defects

Complex single ventricle defects are cyanotic conditions with full mixing of oxygenated and deoxygenated blood. The main concern is that there is only one physiological pumping chamber or ventricle. A VSD may be present. In these conditions, palliative procedures allow the child to grow until a definitive repair may be performed. Hypoplastic left heart syndrome is a condition in this category.

 Nursing Insight— *Hypoplastic left heart syndrome*

Hypoplastic left heart syndrome is a life-threatening defect that must be treated shortly after birth in order to sustain life. The left ventricle is extremely small or hypoplastic and unable to maintain an adequate cardiac output. The right ventricle

must act quickly as the primary pumping mechanism of the cardiac system (Fig. 27-20). This is possible only if there is a left-to-right connection. If there is no ASD an artificial shunt or pathway must be created shortly after birth. Prostaglandin (PGE_1) is given to keep the PDA open. A Norwood procedure is the first stage in the process along with a Blalock-Taussig (BT) shunt. Eventually a Glenn procedure provides more blood flow and ultimately a Fontan procedure is performed. The only other option for treatment is a cardiac transplantation. Occasionally, in the most severe cases, palliative care measures are discussed with the family.

 nursing diagnoses Congenital Heart Defects

- Decreased cardiac output related to structural factors of congenital heart defect and ineffective contraction of the cardiac muscle
- Ineffective breathing pattern related to pulmonary congestion and decreased cardiac output
- Activity intolerance related to decreased cardiac output
- Risk for infection related to debilitated state, decreased oxygenation, decreased cardiac output

Figure 27-19 Tetralogy of Fallot.

Figure 27-20 Hypoplastic left heart syndrome.

case study Infant with a Heart Murmur

Abby, a 1-month-old infant, is seen in the community clinic for a heart murmur first noted at birth. The clinic nurse obtains a history from the mother about the infant's weight gain, feeding patterns, and behavior. The mother reports that the baby has "gained some weight, tires when feeding, and sleeps most of the time." The nurse then performs a nursing assessment and hears an aortic murmur. This type of murmur is detected as an abnormal, soft blowing sound heard during the systolic phase of the cardiac cycle. The nurse understands the murmur may be a sign of aortic valvular disease such as aortic stenosis.

critical thinking questions

1. What suggestions can the nurse give Abby's mother about feeding the baby?

2. Discuss important aspects about oral medication administration.

◆ See Suggested Answers to Case Studies in text on the Electronic Study Guide or DavisPlus.

Cardiac Diseases

Children with cardiac diseases are at risk for alterations in growth and development, nutrition, psychosocial functioning, and schooling. Other risks include infection, acquiring other diseases, and even cardiopulmonary arrest. Sometimes these children have significantly altered life styles and undergo constant medical treatment.

SUBACUTE BACTERIAL ENDOCARDITIS

Subacute bacterial endocarditis (SBE) occurs subsequent to a bacterial infection or introduction of an infective agent into the child's blood stream. SBE is most commonly seen in patients with an unrepaired congenital heart defect or valve disease, but can also occur in normal hearts. The infection may be caused by an invasive procedure such as surgery, urological procedures, or most often dental cleaning. The bacterium in the blood stream adheres to a rough area in the heart such as a stenotic valve or an area of turbulent flow. The bacterium colonizes and causes tissue destruction.

SIGNS AND SYMPTOMS. Initially, vague symptoms may include a low-grade fever, malaise, loss of appetite, and muscle aches. A high fever, chills, sweating, stiff joints, or back pain can indicate that acute illness has occurred. As the condition worsens, symptoms of heart failure occur (Venes, 2009).

DIAGNOSIS. A thorough medical history and a physical exam are essential to diagnosis. The history includes symptoms, questions about a heart murmur or valve replacement, surgery, as well as any recent risk factors for a bacterial or fungal infection (dental procedures or catheter for dialysis), recent fever, chills, or flulike symptoms lasting more than 2 weeks. A physical exam may reveal eye hemorrhage petechiae, fluid in the lungs, or signs of a stroke. Blood cultures to identify bacteria or fungi in the bloodstream may detect endocarditis.

NURSING CARE. SBE is treated with antibiotics, but the most effective approach is prevention. The guidelines for administration and dosage of prophylactic antibiotics are determined by the American Dental Association (ADA) and the American Heart Association (AHA). Guidelines for prescribing prophylaxis treatment were updated in April 2007:

- Patients with prosthetic cardiac valve
- Patients who previously had endocarditis
- Patients with congenital heart disease only in the following categories:
  - Unrepaired cyanotic congenital heart disease, including those with palliative shunts and conduits
  - Completely repaired congenital heart disease with prosthetic material or device, whether placed by surgery or catheter intervention, during the first 6 months after the procedure
  - Repaired congenital heart disease with residual defects at the site or adjacent to the site of a prosthetic patch or prosthetic device (which inhibit endothelialization)
- Cardiac transplantation recipients with cardiac valvular disease or in the first 6 months post transplant.

If valve destruction occurs, the valve may need to be repaired or replaced.

KAWASAKI DISEASE

Kawasaki disease, also known as mucocutaneous lymph node syndrome, is a multisystem disease affecting the cardiovascular system. The cause is unknown, but a defective immune response to an infectious process is thought to be responsible. Kawasaki disease is not congenital or contagious. During the acute phase, diffuse vasculitis leads to long-term cardiovascular problems in one out of every five patients affected. One long-term sequelae of Kawasaki disease is aneurysm formation in arterial vessels (all aneurysms are concerning but most worrisome are those of the coronary arteries). Other sequelae are myocarditis or rhythm disturbances.

SIGNS AND SYMPTOMS. Signs and symptoms of Kawasaki disease are the result of vasculitis affecting all organ systems.

clinical alert

Kawasaki disease

There is no specific test to detect Kawasaki disease. The diagnosis is based on symptoms. Together with persistent fever (5 days or more spiking to 104°F [40°C]), if the patient has four of the five signs listed below a Kawasaki diagnosis may be made:

- Skin rash
- Cervical lymphadenopathy, typically unilateral, greater than 1.5 mm in diameter
- Edema and erythema of hands and feet with eventual peeling of skin
- Irritation and inflammation of the mouth with "strawberry tongue," erythema, and cracking lips
- Conjunctivitis without exudate

DIAGNOSIS. Children with fever and fewer than four signs in the presence of vessel aneurysm can also be diagnosed with Kawasaki disease. Other inflammatory diseases such as Rocky Mountain spotted fever, scarlet fever, or toxoplasmosis should be ruled out. Complete blood count (CBC), erythrocyte sedimentation rate (ESR), electrocardiogram, and echocardiogram help to confirm diagnosis.

NURSING CARE. Nursing care begins with the administration of IV immunoglobulin (IVIG) and aspirin (ASA), which are used primarily for their anti-inflammatory effects. Other treatments such as steroids, plasma exchange, or cytotoxic agents may be used if this initial therapy is ineffective (AHA, 2006).

clinical alert

Thrombus formation

Children with aneurysm formation as a result of Kawasaki disease also require long-term follow-up for continued assessment related to other vascular changes such as stenosis or tortuosity (twisting) (AHA, 2006; Park, 2003). Occasionally, cardiac catheterization is indicated to diagnose aneurysm formation. In the event of thrombus (blood clot) formation, the nurse understands that the treatment is the same as any patient who is at risk for a myocardial infarction. Thrombotic agents, such as streptokinase (Streptase), urokinase (Abbokinase), and alteplase (Activase), have been used with some success in thrombus formation. Long-term use of anti-coagulants such as warfarin (Coumadin) or clopidogrel (Plavix) may be used to prevent thrombus formation in the engorged or aneurysmal vessels.

 Across Care Settings: **American Heart Association**

The American Heart Association has complete up-to-date information about diagnosis and treatment of Kawasaki disease (http://www.americanheart.org).

The nurse can communicate to the family that the frequency of follow-up visits to the physician is usually determined by the initial episode and how fast initial treatment was delivered. Often these children undergo a dobutamine (Dobutrex) or exercise stress test to assess the vascular response to exercise. Coronary bypass surgery is rarely needed and a very small number of children with Kawasaki disease-related complications require a cardiac transplantation.

CARDIOMYOPATHY

Cardiomyopathy (CM) is a condition in which the cardiac muscle becomes dilated, hypertrophied, stiff, or inflamed. There are various classifications and causes, but the end result is the same. The cardiac muscle no longer functions adequately and treatment must ensue to sustain life.

SIGNS AND SYMPTOMS. Ocassionally, the child with CM has a variety of vague symptoms such as weakness,

excessive tiredness, shortness of breath, exercise intolerance, heart palpitations, chest pain, poor feeding, and slow weight gain. The child may also experience fainting or lightheadedness.

 Nursing Insight— *Three classes of cardiomyopathy*

Dilated (DCM) or congestive cardiomyopathy is the most common form and is due to weakened contractions leading to dilation of all four chambers of the heart. The weakened contractions are thought to be caused by myocardial damage, as a result of toxic agents. Dilated cardiomyopathy is caused by myocardial damage from chemotherapy, microbes, bacteria, viruses, immunological defects, or nutritional disorders.

Hypertrophic cardiomyopathy (HCM) is usually a familial disorder. It is a condition in which the ventricle is hypertrophied, swollen, or thickened in the absence of other cardiac conditions. The pumping mechanism of the ventricle is usually hyperdynamic, but the filling is hindered because of thickening of the ventricle.

Restrictive (RCM) is the least occurring type of cardiomyopathy and is characterized by unusually noncompliant ventricular walls that fail to relax. The size of the ventricle is normal, but the atria are enlarged because of the impaired diastolic filling due to stiffness in the ventricle (Park, 2003).

DIAGNOSIS. Diagnosis includes a complete physical examination that may reveal a murmur, gallop, and venous congestion as demonstrated by hepatomegaly or distended neck veins. An electrocardiogram may show right- or left-sided enlargement and possible Q waves. Tachycardia, cardiac rhythm disturbances, or ventricular ectopy is often seen. An echocardiogram provides the exact diagnosis. A family history of cardiomyopathy or sudden death of unknown causes in a family member may also alert the practitioner to seek a definitive diagnosis for CM.

NURSING CARE. Nursing care includes a medication regimen that is aimed at improving function of the cardiac muscle. Angiotensin-converting enzyme (ACE) inhibitors or angiotensin receptor blockers have positive inotropic properties influencing the force of muscular contractility (Venes, 2009) and must be continued until the muscle becomes stronger; the need for them may be life long. Other treatment includes beta-blocker therapy and nutritional supplementation particularly with carnitine (Carnitor or L-carnitine). Diuretic and inotropic therapy is also recommended, except in the case of hypertrophic CM.

After the diagnosis, the child with CM must be followed closely for further complications, preferably in a recognized cardiomyopathy program. The nurse can communicate to the family that frequent echocardiograms are warranted to assess the size and function of the ventricular wall as well as to note improvement or deterioration of the condition. The family must also understand that the child is placed on activity restrictions to prevent overstimulation of the heart muscle (Park, 2003). The ultimate treatment quite often is cardiac transplantation.

> ### medication: Carvedilol
>
> Carvedilol (kar-**ve**-dil-ole)
>
> Beta (β)-Adrenoreceptor blocker, α-adrenergic
>
> **Pregnancy Category:** C
>
> **Indications:** Carvedilol is indicated for the treatment of mild-to-severe heart failure of ischemic or cardiomyopathic origin.
>
> **Actions:** Beta blockers slow tachycardia and vasodilation; Carvedilol decreases peripheral vascular resistance, decreases renal vascular resistance, reduces plasma renin levels, and increases atrial natriuretic peptide levels.
>
> **Therapeutic Effects:** Increases stroke volume, decreases blood pressure and improves renal flow, decreases heart rate.
>
> **Pharmacokinetics:**
> Bioavailability 25–35%
> Onset of effect: 1–2 hours
> Half-life: 7–10 hours
>
> **Contraindications and Precautions:** Monitor for possible deterioration of CHF, liver injury, bronchospastic disease, thyrotoxicosis.
>
> **Adverse Reactions and Side Effects:** Chest pain, dizziness, hyperglycemia, bradycardia, nausea
>
> **Route and Dosage:**
> Oral: 0.07 mg/kg per dose
> Maximum dose: 0.5 mg/kg
> Once or twice daily dosing
> Reduce dose for bradycardia <55 beats per minute
>
> **Nursing Implications:**
> 1. Initiate with low dose and titrate up as tolerated.
> 2. Monitor blood pressure for 1 hour after initial dosing.
> 3. Monitor blood pressure, pulse, and ECG frequently.
> 4. Take with food.
>
> Data from Deglin, J.H., & Vallerand, A. (2009). *Davis's drug guide for nurses* (11th ed., pp. 271–273). Philadelphia: F.A. Davis.

Nursing Insight— *Rheumatic fever*

Rheumatic fever (RF) is a group-A hemolytic streptococcal infection affecting multiple bodily systems such as the heart, the joints, subcutaneous tissue, and at times the nervous system. During the acute phase of rheumatic fever, the entire heart may suffer due to vegetations or deposits of the offending organism that grow on the valves of the heart causing permanent damage. The aortic and mitral valves are most often valves involved. The mitral damage may result in mitral stenosis (MS) or mitral regurgitation (MR). Aortic regurgitation (AR) also results from rheumatic fever (AHA, 2006; Parillo, 2006).

Often individuals who have had rheumatic fever as children require a valve replacement at some time in their lives. The nurse understands that when a valve is replaced in infancy or childhood, it must be replaced every 5 years to accommodate the child's growth. Valves replaced during adolescence can last up to 10 years.

Additional Cardiac Conditions

CARDIAC TRAUMA

Cardiac trauma can result from a variety of injuries such as a motor vehicle crash or sports activity. Even a child wearing a seat belt in a car can sustain cardiac trauma. Damage to the heart muscle also occurs as the result of a direct blow to the thorax overlying the heart (e.g., a baseball or steering wheel). Electrocution (injury from electricity) can also cause damage to the cardiac muscle. In cardiac trauma, the particular damage to the heart can be a ventricular rupture, a great vessel tear, damage to the pericardial sac or coronary arteries, cardiac tamponade, myocardial infarction, or arrhythmias.

SIGNS AND SYMPTOMS. The signs and symptoms are related to the type of cardiac trauma sustained and can range from minor reports of pain to severe cardiac shock. The diagnosis is made based on a thorough history of including type of trauma, force of trauma, associated injuries and loss of consciousness.

DIAGNOSIS. The diagnosis of cardiac trauma is made with electrocardiogram (ECG), echocardiogram, cardiac enzymes–specifically troponin I, and chest x-ray exam. All of these tests will indicate cardiac muscle damage. A CT or MUGA scan may be helpful in determining other injuries, but does not correlate to outcome.

NURSING CARE. Nursing care is based on the extent and exact type of the injury. The nurse understands that essential nursing care includes bedrest. Activity restrictions must also be enforced until the cardiac muscle heals. In addition, antiarrhythmics, inotropic agents, and pericardiocentesis (aspiration of fluid from the pericardiac sac) may be required. A cardiac rehabilitation program can be recommended.

Nursing Insight— *Cardiac tumors*

Cardiac tumors are rare in children and are almost exclusively rhabdomyomas (Park, 2003). There is actually a newer edition, but I do not have it so I do not know what it says and if anything is different. Other tumors are teratomas, fibromas, and myxomas. Most of the tumors are benign but significant because they occupy space and may restrict the normal filling and flow of blood. Surgical removal is the treatment of choice for cardiac tumors. At times, rhabdomyomas may regress; therefore intervention may be delayed. At times, it is surgically unsafe to remove the tumor and a cardiac transplant is needed. A long-term consequence of cardiac tumors includes scar tissue formation, which in turn may lead to arrhythmias.

Nursing Insight— *Hypercholesterolemia–hyperlipidemia*

The etiology for hypercholesterolemia–hyperlipidemia in children is classified as primary and secondary. A primary cause is hereditary predisposition (Park, 2003) and children may develop atherosclerotic lesions as early as infancy.

Hypercholesterolemia is more often due to secondary causes. Secondary causes are exogenous (originating outside an organ), endocrine, or metabolic disorders; liver diseases; renal diseases; or other miscellaneous reasons such as anorexia nervosa or collagen diseases. Children with cardiac transplant have a high incidence of hyperlipidemia because of the immunosuppressant drug cyclosporine-A (Neoral). In addition, children with cardiac transplant form atherosclerotic lesions at a very rapid rate and the child risks facing coronary artery bypass graft (CABG), or worse, a second transplant surgery. The nurse can communicate to the family that treatment of hyperlipidemia for children with a transplanted heart is more aggressive than for the general population.

Family Teaching Guidelines...
Hypercholesterolemia–Hyperlipidemia

ESSENTIAL INFORMATION

There are two types of primary hypercholesterolemia–hyperlipidemia: familial hypercholesterolemia and familial combined hyperlipidemia. The standards for childhood cholesterol levels are different from those for adults (Table 27-3).

Although the standard levels are different, the treatment goals are similar to those for adults and include diet modification, exercise, and medication. A recommended balanced nutrition is one that provides less than 10% of total calories from saturated fatty acids, 30% or less of total calories from fat, and less than 300 mg of cholesterol each day. The nurse can help the family decrease the fat and cholesterol intake to 7% of fatty acids, 25% or less total calories from fat, and less than 200 mg of cholesterol per day. Pharmacological treatment is recommended for children older than 8 years whose LDL cholesterol is high.

Recommendations for screening children after age 2 and no later than 10 years old are:

◆ At least one parent with high cholesterol

◆ A family history of early heart disease such as a male parent or grandparent with CHD before age 55 or a female parent or grandparent with CHD before age 65

◆ Family History of Diabetes, Hypertension -or Obesity

◆ Child with Obesity (≥ 85th percentile)

◆ Immunosuppressant drug use (AHA, 2005)

Table 27-3 Cholesterol Levels in Children

	Desirable	Borderline	Associated with Higher Risk
Total cholesterol	Less than 170	170–199	200 or more
LDL cholesterol	Less than 110	110–129	130 or more

Source: American Heart Association, www.americanheart.org

HYPERTENSION

High blood pressure or hypertension (HTN) is an elevated blood pressure and is uncommon in children.

SIGNS AND SYMPTOMS. Signs and symptoms depend on the underlying causes. Elevated blood pressure (not in the recommended range) is a key sign (see Table 21-2). A young child may be irritable where an older child may complain of changes in vision, dizziness, or headaches.

DIAGNOSIS. Taking a detailed medical and thorough family history is important in the diagnosis of hypertension. A child is hypertensive if the blood pressure is above the 95th percentile for age, height, and gender. As a screening tool, the nurse should consider any reading greater than 20 mm Hg above normal blood pressure for

the child's age as high. A teenager is considered an adult for treatment purposes and follows the same guidelines as adults. The extent of further testing is based on the degree of blood pressure elevation. The nurse knows that high blood pressure or hypertension may indicate a coarctation of the aorta, kidney disease, left ventricular hypertrophy (LVH), or early-onset familial hypertension. Some cardiology centers conduct hypertension follow-up for families with a strong history.

NURSING CARE. Nursing care for the child with hypertension is based on education about the condition, diet, exercise, lifestyle modification, and medication. Medications for high blood pressure or hypertension include beta-blockers and ACE inhibitors.

 Ethnocultural Considerations— **Hypertension**

Based on familial predisposition, hypertension has a higher incidence among African American children than in other ethnic groups. Nursing care for this group of children includes educating the child and family about the condition, promoting a reasonable sodium intake, and teaching the family how to reduce the saturated fat and cholesterol in their diet.

IDIOPATHIC PULMONARY ARTERIAL HYPERTENSION

Pulmonary arterial hypertension (IPAH) is a condition of high blood pressure in the lungs. It may result from cardiac defects or may be idiopathic (without recognizable cause). It is a severe disease resulting in death if not treated. Normally, the desired pulmonary blood pressure is low, allowing blood to flow easily from the right side of the heart. The pressure in the right side of the heart is lower than in the left (the left reflecting the systemic blood pressure). If the pressure in the lungs is high, as with IPAH, the right ventricle must pump harder to force the blood to the lungs. Over time, this wears on the ventricle and causes right ventricular hypertrophy (RVH). Eventually, the heart fails and congestive symptoms develop.

SIGNS AND SYMPTOMS. Symptoms of IPAH include shortness of breath (dyspnea), especially during exercise, chest pain, weakness, fatigue, dizziness, leg swelling, and fainting episodes.

DIAGNOSIS. In the early stages of the disease, a physical exam may be normal because diagnosis of IPAH may take several months. However, as the condition progresses, a physical exam shows a heart murmur, enlargement of the neck veins, liver and spleen enlargement, leg swelling, parasternal heave, ascites, and clubbing.

Diagnostic tests such a pulmonary arteriogram, echocardiogram, chest radiograph, cardiac catheterization, and pulmonary function tests may help confirm the diagnosis.

NURSING CARE. Until recently, treatment for idiopathic pulmonary arterial hypertension included oxygen, which relaxes the arteries of the lungs, calcium channel blockers that relax the blood vessels, and diuretics which decrease the volume in the vessels. However, these treatments may also have an untoward effect of lowering the overall blood pressure.

where research and practice meet:
Innovative Treatment Strategies for Idiopathic Pulmonary Arterial Hypertension

Innovative treatment strategies that are producing promising results for idiopathic pulmonary arterial hypertension include:

- Prostacyclin (Flolan) dilates blood vessels and decreases pulmonary vascular resistance.
- Inhaled nitric oxide relaxes pulmonary, but not systemic, blood vessels.
- Sildenafil (Revatio) decreases pulmonary artery pressures and bosentan (Tracleer) blocks endothelin-1 (hormone that causes vasoconstriction). (http://www.revatio.com/; www.tracleer.com)

The nurse must remember that the treatment for IPAH is complicated, ongoing, and the condition has no cure. The only definitive treatment is a lung or heart–lung transplant, the latter because there is already heart damage to the right ventricle. Treatment for IPAH caused by cardiac defects is aimed at the cause of the defect.

NEURALLY MEDIATED SYNCOPE

Neurally mediated syncope (NMS) is a condition caused by an exaggerated response to a normal bodily function. It is also called vasovagal syncope. The baroreceptors in the carotid artery act as a regulator of blood pressure during certain situations. If the system is stressed such as during extreme heat, pain, fright, or prolonged standing, the initial response is a release of epinephrine, stimulating the sympathetic nervous system. This stimulation in turn raises the blood pressure. The baroreceptors send messages to control the blood pressure. In neurally mediated syncope (NMS), the baroreceptor response is exaggerated causing the blood pressure and the heart rate to drop significantly and suddenly.

SIGNS AND SYMPTOMS. The main sign is a temporary loss of consciousness (a fainting spell). Occasionally, the response is so dramatic that the child may experience a seizure.

DIAGNOSIS. A thorough history and other tests rule out other diagnosis such as seizures or Long QT syndrome. The definitive diagnosis of neurally mediated syncope is made via the tilt test but can be made on history alone.

diagnostic tools Tilt Test

Neurally mediated syncope (NMS) is diagnosed with a tilt table test. The nurse assists by placing the child in a supine position on a table equipped with a foot board. The table may be tilted to an position anywhere between 45 and 90 degrees. After a short time, the table is tilted to a full 90 degree angle so that the child stands upright. This maneuver may or may not reproduce fainting or symptoms. If the tilt test is positive, the nurse will see a remarkable drop in blood pressure or heart rate and the child will experience syncope or presyncope (dizziness or lightheadedness). If the child does not exhibit any symptoms, such as syncope or lightheadedness, the table is laid flat again and isoproterenol (Isuprel) is administered to stimulate a fast heart rate. This chemical mimics the fight or flight (fear, pain, anxiety) response that may occur before episodes of syncope. The table is then tilted again to elicit a syncopal response or a drop in the blood pressure. If there is no response or change in vital signs, the test is considered negative and other causative factors are evaluated.

NURSING CARE. Treatment for NMS may be as simple as increasing the child's sodium and water intake. An adrenocorticosteroid such as fludrocortisone (Florinef) may be given to retain fluid. The next level of treatment is a beta-blocker, which regulates the exaggerated response. The nurse monitors for frequency, severity, and precipitating factors of syncope.

"What to say" — *Neurally mediated syncope (NMS)*

It is important that the nurse communicate to the family that NMS is concerning based on the potential for injury if the child loses consciousness. If a teen with syncope is of driving age, he or she must be syncope free for 6 months in some states before the teen may drive again.

LONG Q-T SYNDROME

Long Q-T syndrome (LQTS) is an electrophysiological condition predisposing the child to fatal arrhythmias such as ventricular tachycardia (VT), torsade de pointes, and ventricular fibrillation (VF) (Fig. 27-21). LQTS is a familial disorder, and if one child is affected, all siblings and parents should be tested. If parents are positive then the siblings of the positive parent and first cousins should be evaluated. There are a variety of known factors and genetic chromosomal markers in a person with LQTS. Long QT syndrome is among a group of defects of the ion channels (channelopathies) on the cardiac cell membrane. Currently genetic researchers are studying this phenomenon in hopes of better treatment or developing a cure. A prolonged QT interval can also be acquired from medications and various toxins (www.azcert.org/medical-pros/drug-lists/drug-lists.cfm).

SIGNS AND SYMPTOMS. A nursing assessment includes a history of fainting triggered by intense emotions, vigorous physical activity, swimming, auditory stimuli (such as a school bell), and upon awakening. Other signs and symptoms of LQTS are palpitations, seizure, or sudden death. The child and family most likely are unaware that they have this problem. Because sudden death is one of the symptoms, the child's first episode may be the last.

DIAGNOSIS. An ECG should be performed in all children with seizures of sudden onset, fainting, or near drowning episodes. The child may be asymptomatic and may present at routine exam with a prolonged QT on ECG.

Figure 27-21 Long QT syndrome.

NURSING CARE. The nurse understands that the primary treatment is medication. The most frequently used medications are beta-blockers. Treatment also includes pacemaker-defibrillator (insertion) or left cardiac sympathetic denervation. It is important that the nurse communicates to the family that the most common cause of treatment failure is noncompliance with medication (Moss & Robinson, 2002).

Rhythm Disturbances

 Nursing Insight— *Electrocardiogram*

The abbreviations ECG/EKG are used interchangeably. (The K is the abbreviation for the German *kardio* [cardiac].) An ECG is a graphic display of electrical activity produced by changes in the intracellular charge of the cardiac muscles. The components of an ECG are marked with the letters PQRST (Fig. 27-22).

 Collaboration in Caring: *Nurses caring for children with heart arrhythmias*

The nurse working in a cardiac area with children who experience arrhythmias and require cardiac telemetry can acquire specific knowledge about the ECG and learn about basic arrhythmia interpretation. The nurse who cares for children on a cardiac floor or in the intensive care unit (ICU) can acquire more advanced information through a course on 12-lead ECG. Pediatric Advanced Life Support (PALS) and a pediatric emergency course are essential.

 Optimizing Outcomes— **Rhythm disturbances**

The nurse who can determine the baseline rhythm and recognize changes will facilitate the best outcome for a child with an arrhythmia. The nurse must know the ramifications of these changes. Important questions the nurse can ask about rhythm disturbances are:

Is the rhythm potentially fatal?
Will it alter the cardiac output?

 Nursing Insight— *Rhythm disturbances and the effect on cardiac output*

Tachycardia is the name for a fast heart rate. It describes any condition in which the heart beats faster than the standard pediatric heart rate values and includes sinus tachycardia, supraventricular tachycardia, atrial tachycardia, atrial flutter, atrial fibrillation, junctional tachycardia, and ventricular tachycardia (see Table 21–2). If the heart rate is too fast, the diastolic phase shortens in relation to the length of the full cardiac cycle. The ventricle is not allowed enough filling time; therefore the stroke volume is less, decreasing the cardiac output.

Bradycardia is the name for a slow heart rate. This is any condition where the heart beats slower than the standard pediatric heart rate values. This type of arrhythmia includes sinus bradycardia, junctional and idioventricular rhythms, and the slow phase of sick sinus syndrome. In a bradycardic child, the cardiac output is affected because the heart rate is slow. Initially, the body tries to compensate by increasing the contractile force, thus increasing the stroke volume (SV). Eventually, this will plateau or the cardiac muscle may not be strong enough to compensate as in congestive heart failure (CHF) or cardiomyopathy.

Blocks are disruptions in the flow of electrical current throughout the heart. They include bundle branch block (BBB) and first-, second-, and third-degree blocks. First- and second-degree type I blocks may incur no interference in the cardiac output, whereas second- and third-degree blocks are more severe and require intervention in order to maintain adequate circulation.

Lethal rhythms are those producing little or no cardiac output and include ventricular tachycardia, ventricular fibrillation, torsades de pointes, pulseless electrical activity (PEA; formerly known as electromechanical dissociation [EMD]), or asystole.

 Nursing Insight— *Sinus arrhythmias*

A normal irregular rhythm in which the rhythm varies with respiration is called sinus arrhythmia. Sinus arrhythmia has no adverse effect on the cardiac output.

* The heart rate increases with inspiration. (Remember: "Inspiration" and "Increase" both start with an "I".)
* The heart rate decreases with expiration.

Invasive Tests

CARDIAC CATHETERIZATION

Cardiac catheterization is an invasive test performed for a number of reasons. The purpose of the cardiac catheterization is to determine the pressures within the child's heart vessels and to provide a radiographic picture of the anatomy by measuring the size and shape of vessels, valves, and ventricles. A cardiac catheterization is necessary to perform a myocardial biopsy. Corrective procedures, called interventional catheterizations, may be performed in the cardiac catheterization lab.

 diagnostic tools Cardiac Catheterization

The cardiac catheterization procedure takes place in a cardiac catheterization lab where the child is sedated or anesthetized. First, an introducing sheath is placed in a major vessel such as the femoral vein or artery. Next, a long hollow tube or catheter is threaded through this sheath and into the heart. The physician uses real-time radiographic study or fluoroscopy to monitor the movement of the catheter and to prevent perforation. During a cardiac catheterization, pressure is measured in the ventricles and the vessels. The normal pressure of the left ventricle correlates with the normal blood pressure for age. The normal pressures in the right ventricle and right and left atrium are similar to those of an adult patient. Elevated pressures can indicate a variety of illnesses and will usually support or refute the suspicions of the diagnostician. For example, high pressure in the right ventricle may indicate a ventricular septal defect (VSD) with left-to-right shunting or pulmonary artery

Definition	ECG Diagram	Myocardial Conduction Pathways
The components of the ECG were labeled PQRST by Einthoven in 1895.		**Complete cycle**
P wave = depolarization of the atria		**P wave**
PR interval = time it takes for the impulse to get to the AV node. *Repolarization of atria is "buried" in the QRS complex*		
QRS complex = depolarization of the ventricle		**QRS interval**

Continued

Definition	ECG Diagram	Myocardial Conduction Pathways
QT interval = time from start of depolarization to end of repolarization of the ventricle. Also represents relative refractory period.		
ST segment represents early ventricular repolarization		
T wave is the repolarization of the ventricle		

Figure 27-22 Components of electrocardiogram.

stenosis or pulmonary hypertension. Radio-opaque dye is injected through the catheter and the flow of the dye is observed on fluoroscopy. The "shape" the dye is the shape of the inside of the heart, giving a picture of the anatomy of the ventricle, valves, vessels, and any defects that may be present.

The overall risks for the child undergoing a cardiac catheterization are minimal. Because this is an invasive procedure, the nurse must know the risks of bleeding, infection, thrombus, arrhythmia, perforation, stroke, or even death (resulting from previous named risks).

 clinical alert

Postcatheterization

The nurse must monitor pressure dressing in the groin, heart rate, respirations and blood pressure.

ANGIOGRAPHY

Angiography not only depicts the structure and function of the ventricles, the vessels, and the valves. It is also useful to determine size and location of septal defects. After placement of the catheter in the heart, radio-opaque contrast medium is injected into the chambers and vessels of the heart. If there is a defect, the contrast highlights septal openings, narrow vessels, and extra vessels. An angiogram provides the physicians important information to direct the medical and surgical treatment.

BIOPSY

Biopsy of the myocardium is performed routinely for children who have had a cardiac transplant or determining the cause of Myocarditis or cardiomyopathy. Children with cardiac transplant undergo routine biopsies to assess for rejection. Several small pieces of myocardial tissue are removed and then analyzed by a laboratory specialist for cellular changes. The sample may also contain microbial organisms responsible for the cellular changes seen in cardiomyopathy.

CLOSURE DEVICES

It is possible to close simple congenital intracardiac communications or shunts in the cardiac catheterization laboratory rather than with major surgery. Atrial septal defects and an opening called a patent foramen ovale are closed with transseptal closure devices. The cardiologist places these transseptal closure devices across the septum, through the defect, and deploys the device to form a seal around the opening. In the case of a PDA closure, a plug type device is used.

By approximately 6 weeks after the closure device is placed, the child's own tissue grows over the device (endothelialization) and by 6 months, a permanent seal is created. In addition, yearly follow-up visits to the cardiologist are recommended along with an ECG, an echocardiogram, and possibly a chest radiograph. The provider will explain the risk of embolization of the device. Embolization occurs when the device becomes dislodged from its intended location, migrating to the atria, pulmonary artery, the ventricle, or aorta. The nurse will support this with education.

OPENING DEVICES

Angioplasty or Valvuloplasty

Narrow vessels or valves may be opened or dilated with a balloon angioplasty or valvuloplasty as an initial treatment or a stent may be placed in a vessel as a long-term treatment (Fig. 27-23). This treatment is performed during a cardiac catheterization procedure. A special catheter with a balloon (similar to a Foley catheter) is passed into the heart and into the narrow vessel. The balloon is then inflated, causing the stenotic area to expand. Sometimes the stenosis recoils days, months, or years after the balloon procedure. The procedure may then be repeated but this time a stent (a wire mesh tube) is placed over the balloon. The balloon is again inflated and the stent is left in place. This repair is permanent and requires surgical extraction if removal is necessary.

Balloon Atrial Septostomy

Balloon atrial septostomy is an emergent palliative procedure necessary to keep the child alive when the heart has no means of blood flow to the pulmonary system or body such as in tricuspid atresia or hypoplastic left heart. A catheter with a balloon is passed into the right atrium, pushed across the foramen ovale (PFO), entering the left atrium. The balloon is inflated and then pulled forcefully across to the right atrium, creating an opening large enough to accommodate blood flow. Infusion of prostaglandin is a palliative treatment prior to the septostomy to keep the PDA open and allow blood flow to the pulmonary bed or body.

NURSING CARE

The nurse must be aware of specific aspects of caring for a child in the post-cardiac catheterization period (Box 27-1). The child has a pressure dressing in the inguinal area of the leg at the insertion site. If an internal jugular vein is used, a small bandage covers the site on the neck.

The nurse monitors the heart rate, respirations, and blood pressure and makes note that it is in the same range as measured precatheterization. If tachycardia is identified postcatheterization, the nurse should suspect pain or dehydration. Acetaminophen is given for the pain. If the child is dehydrated, the nurse can administer fluid boluses. Signs of infection are rare in the first few hours postcatheterization.

The nurse must remember that children with cardiac disease may be cyanotic. It is important to obtain a baseline oxygen saturation and monitor the child with that number in mind. Some children normally have a value as low as 85%. The nurse should confirm the range of normal oximeter readings with the practitioner.

Figure 27-23 Balloon angioplasty with stent.

Box 27-1 Typical Post Cardiac Catheterization Medical Orders

Admit to postsurgical observation unit.

VS q15min × 4, then q1hr × 2, then q2hr × 2, then q4hr

Check pulses with vital signs, especially on affected extremity.

Check pressure dressing with vital signs for bleeding

Keep O$_2$ saturation above_____.

Call house officer for heart rate > _____, blood pressure > _____ (age and baseline dependent) and temperature >_____ .

Call house officer for complaints of abdominal pain or no urine output

Give acetaminophen for pain.

Give anti-emetics for nausea Keep flat in bed for 6 hours.

The child may be placed on cardiac telemetry if arrhythmias were induced during the catheterization. Normally, if the child has a non-electrophysiological diagnosis, any arrhythmias seen during the procedure disappear when the catheters are removed, but subsequent monitoring may be required.

There are specific growth and development issues to consider postcatheterization. After a cardiac catheterization, a child is required to lie flat for up to 6 hours depending on the insertion site of the catheter. The supine position minimizes the risk of bleeding through the insertion site. A younger child may need to be restrained with leg immobilization devices to keep the leg straight. Older children or adolescents are usually cooperative unless they are developmentally delayed. Sometimes the nurse may administer sedation to keep the child still, but this may delay the discharge and holds certain risks. Generally, an infant or child does well if the mother is allowed to stay at the bedside or hold the child. Allowing the infant to feed is also calming.

The nurse can communicate to the family that after a cardiac catheterization, the child will be on the same medications as before. Specifically, if any devices remain in the body such as closure devices or stents, the child will take a baby aspirin (ASA) for 6 months after the procedure. The aspirin prevents clot formation while endothelialization (growth of new tissue) occurs around the artificial device. Subacute bacterial endocarditis prophylaxis (SBE) precautions should be followed for 6 months for device placement patients. The nurse can tell the family that after 6 months of placement of the device, no special precautions are needed.

clinical alert

Blood pressure postinterventional catheterization

The child's blood pressure should remain within normal limits. One specific measurement the nurse must watch is the pulse pressure; which is the difference between the systolic and diastolic blood pressure. A normal pulse pressure range is <40 mm Hg.

Children with PDA have a wide pulse pressure (>40 mm Hg). After the closure of a PDA, the pulse pressure should be within normal range. A sudden widening of the pulse pressure postprocedure may indicate a dislodged or embolized device. This event requires urgent measures by the physician or resident in house, who must be contacted immediately. Embolization of the device can cause stroke, thromboembolic events, or death.

The nurse can communicate to the family that the child's growth must be considered before placing a stent. Some stents are expandable and must be redilated at a later date to accommodate for the growth of the child. If it is known that a child must have a more definitive surgery, a stent may be placed, knowing that it will be extracted at a later date. Risks include vascular tear or embolization of the device. Absorbable stents are in the experimental phase.

Surgical Interventions

Surgical repair may be palliative repair or complete anatomical repair. Palliative repair is usually considered when the child is very young and the complete anatomical repair is too complex for him or her to tolerate. The surgeons perform a temporary, palliative repair to allow the child time to grow and develop to a point when the more definitive procedure may be tolerated. The child may be cyanotic after a palliative repair, but less cyanotic than if the surgery were delayed. These children are followed closely by the cardiologist until the time when a complete repair may be done. A complete repair is considered a cure or definitive treatment. However, as the child grows or hemodynamic requirements change, a complete repair may have to be revised (Table 27-4).

PACEMAKERS

Pacemakers are used to treat cardiac conditions such as heart block or severe bradycardia, sick sinus syndrome, some junctional or idioventricular rhythms and lethal arrhythmias. Pacemaker therapy may be internal or external, temporary or permanent. The nurse understands that external pacing is always temporary. The surgeon may elect to place temporary pacing wires if the child has complications of heart block during surgery, or if the surgical area is near or on the conduction tissue.

❝ What to say ❞ — *Pacemakers*

The nurse communicates to parents that permanent pacemakers may be placed in the abdomen in younger children and in the subclavicular area in older children. Consideration is taken for children who are athletic, as the pacemaker generator must be protected. Care is taken when deciding to place a permanent pacemaker.

Pacemaker generators must be replaced every 5–10 years. When a pacemaker is placed in an infant, a replacement may be necessary 15 times in his or her lifetime. Pacemaker insertion for neurally mediated (AKA vasovagal) syncope is controversial. Currently the AHA and American College of Cardiology (ACC) do not recommend pacemaker placement for neurally mediated syncope.

NURSING CARE. Nursing care of the pacemaker postoperative patient is the same as for any surgical procedure, including watching for signs of infection and ensuring the incision remains intact. The nurse communicates to the family that follow-up care requires routine pacemaker testing as recommended by the pacemaker center placing the device. Essential information for the family is to understand that after initial follow-up procedures, evaluation of the pacemaker is usually performed every 6 months to 1 year, but can be as often as every 3 months.

CARDIAC TRANSPLANTATION

Cardiac transplantation requires complex multidisciplinary management and is used as a treatment for severe, life-threatening cardiac conditions. Although still rare, there were 5767 reported pediatric cardiac transplants performed across the nation between 1982 and 2003 (Boucek et al., 2006). Transplantation is performed only under the most grave of circumstances, in situations in which the child would otherwise die.

A progressive heart transplantation program includes a cardiomyopathy treatment program to prevent the need for transplantation. The transplantation team

Table 27-4 Surgical Repairs of Cardiac Defects

Repair and Intended Effect	Defects	Potential Long-term Implications and Sequelae
Palliative Repairs		
PA banding: • A restrictive band is placed around the main pulmonary artery to decrease uncontrolled pulmonary blood flow and prevent the development of pulmonary hypertension and eventual right heart failure.	VSD, single ventricle, tricuspid atresia.	Eventual decreased O_2 saturations with growth/aging, right ventricular hypertrophy, if the band becomes too tight with growth of the child. Excessive flow to left pulmonary artery and left pulmonary HTN r/t stenosis of the right pulmonary artery, related to possible migration of an encroachment on the right PA. Possible revision of banding.
Blalock–Taussig shunt (modified): • A Gore-Tex graft conduit is placed between the right or left subclavian artery and the ipsilateral pulmonary artery to provide controlled pulmonary blood flow.	Cyanotic heart defects such as HLHS, TOF, pulmonary atresia, tricuspid atresia.	Mild pulmonary artery distortion at site of anastomosis, inability of shunt size to increase with growth/aging, thrombus formation on graft site, potential coronary ischemia r/t pulmonary "steal" of blood flow during diastole.
• Sano shunt. • A Gore-Tex graft conduit is placed between the single ventricle and the pulmonary artery to provide controlled pulmonary blood flow.	Cyanotic heart defects such as HLHS, pulmonary atresia, tricuspid atresia, single ventricle defects.	Mild pulmonary artery distortion at site of anastomosis, thrombus formation on graft site, inability of shunt size to increase with growth/aging.
• Atrial septectomy. • A communication is surgically created by tearing a hole or incision in between the left and right atria. This encourages mixing of blood flow at the atrial level and encourages pulmonary blood flow. More invasive than ballooning of septum as seen in Rashkind procedure. Considered to be a palliative procedure prior to complete repair.	Single ventricle physiology with intact atrial septum, unrepaired TGA.	Eventual development of heart failure if further palliation/repair is not sought.
Definitive (or Complete) Repairs		
Patch closures: • Native cardiac tissue (pericardium) or a prosthetic patch is sutured in place over a septal defect to effectively close the communication between the atria or ventricles.	ASD, VSD, AV canal.	Incomplete closure of defect, arrhythmia, potential for patch dehiscence, AV block (VSD closures).
• Ductal ligation. • A tie or clip is placed around the patent ductus arteriosus and tightened to prevent excessive pulmonary blood flow from the aorta.	PDA.	Incomplete closure of ductus and associated residual pulmonary shunting, mobilization of device.
• COA repair. • Narrowing in the proximal, distal, or arch of the aorta is reduced or eliminated via surgical resection of stenosed area, patch placement to increase aortic diameter, subclavian flap aortoplasty or bypass grafting.	Coarctation of aorta.	Restenosis or recoarctation of affected portion of aorta, transient spinal ischemia and associated paraplegia, paradoxical hypertension, possible need for re-repair or angioplasty.
Valvuloplasty: • A malformed, damaged, or stenotic valve is surgically revised to correct the associated malfunction.	Destructive endocarditis, valvular stenosis.	Incomplete or unsuccessful revision of affected valve; thromboemboli formation, additional valvular damage and possible need for valve replacement.
• Artificial valve replacement. • A faulty or damaged native valve is replaced with a valve made of either human or animal tissue or a mechanical valve.	Endocarditis, failed Ross, valvular stenosis.	Need for a lifetime of replacement prosthetic valve procedures; need for long-term oral anticoagulation; thromboemboli formation, aortic or pulmonary insufficiency.
Ross procedure: • A damaged or dysfunctional aortic valve is removed and replaced with the patient's pulmonic valve, which is then replaced with a donor homograft valve.	Destructive endocarditis, valvular aortic stenosis.	Aortic/pulmonary valve stenosis, gross valvular dysfunction, aortic or pulmonary insufficiency, potential for a lifetime of possible prosthetic valve replacements, risk for heart block.

Table 27-4 Surgical Repairs of Cardiac Defects—cont'd

Repair and Intended Effect	Defects	Potential Long-term Implications and Sequelae
Konno procedure: • A faulty aortic valve is replaced with a prosthetic valve while the narrowed aortic root is enlarged via patch placement to increase systemic blood flow. Ross-Konno procedure combines replacement of aortic valve with native pulmonary valve and aortic root enlargement.	Any left ventricular outflow tract obstruction such as aortic valve hypoplasia, sub-aortic stenosis.	Potential failure of aortic valve graft and persistent aortic stenosis, Thromboemboli formation on grafted valves, Potential need for life-long oral anticoagulation, potential for development of heart block, aortic insufficiency.
Damus–Kaye–Stansel: • Prosthetic conduits are placed between the proximal main pulmonary artery and the aorta and between the right ventricle and the distal pulmonary artery. Existing VSD is closed and the existing aortic valve may be closed or left unclosed. This procedure attempts to reroute in appropriate pulmonary and systemic blood flow.	TGA with VSD; DORV with VSD.	Aortic insufficiency, thromboemboli formation in cases of complete aortic valve closure, need for periodic surgical conduit replacements, coronary ischemia.
Rastelli: • The main pulmonary artery is divided from its incorrect origin on the LV and is re-attached to the RV using a prosthetic conduit. A tunnel is then created between the existent VSD and aorta, effectively re-routing blood from the LV to systemic outflow.	DORV, TGA + VSD + sub-aortic stenosis/pulmonic stenosis truncus arteriosus type I.	Conduit obstruction and resultant heart failure, arrhythmia, thromboemboli formation, failure of prosthetic conduits to allow increased flow with growth/aging, implicit need for eventual RV-PA conduit replacements.
Arterial switch (ASO): • The great arteries (main pulmonary artery and aorta) are divided from the LV and RV respectively and reattached to their appropriate locations on the RV (MPA) and LV (aorta). The coronary arteries are also divided from the MPA and transplanted to the neo-aorta.	TGA.	Arrhythmia, coronary artery obstruction, LV ischemia and dysfunction, aortic insufficiency, supravalvular pulmonic stenosis, branch pulmonary artery stenosis.
Staged Repairs Modified Norwood: • The main pulmonary artery is divided from the branch pulmonary arteries and patched to the hypoplastic aortic arch, creating a hybrid systemic arterial outflow from the RV. An atrial septectomy is created via catheterization or surgical incision to allow for left to right shunting, so that oxygenated pulmonary venous blood is directed toward systemic outflow. A systemic–pulmonary shunt (Sano or Blalock–Taussig) is created to allow pulmonary arterial blood flow, as the creation of single ventricle physiology only has a direct connection to systemic outflow. This stage creates a single ventricle that is responsible for pulmonary and systemic circulation.	Stage 1 repair for HLHS.	Coronary ischemia due to diastolic "steal" of aortopulmonary shunt if BT shunt is used, pulmonary artery distortion, cyanosis, aortic outflow obstruction, tricuspid insufficiency, potential stenosis of systemic-pulmonary shunt, FTT, feeding difficulties, arrhythmia.
Glenn: • The systemic–pulmonary (BT or Sano) is taken down or ligated with clips. The SVC is connected to the branch pulmonary arteries. The existent ASD is enlarged if necessary to allow for continued left to right shunting of oxygenated blood into the systemic outflow. This stage attempts to reduce the workload of the heart so that the single ventricle is only pumping to the systemic circulation.	Stage 2 repair for HLHS, tricuspid atresia.	Elevated upper body venous pressures related to increased PVR, hypoxemia, upper body swelling, headache, arrhythmia, stenosis at area of SVC-PA anastomosis, development of aortopulmonary collateral vessels.
Fontan: • The procedure attempts to establish separate pulmonary and systemic circulations by attaching the IVC directly to the RPA-SVC anastomosis with a Gore-Tex extracardiac conduit. This allows for passive flow of systemic venous return directly to the pulmonary arteries and completely bypasses the RA. The existent single ventricle continues to receive pulmonary arterial flow and pump to the systemic circulation via the neo-aorta constructed in Stage 1 repair.	Stage 3 repair for HLHS, tricuspid atresia.	Obstruction of conduit leading to systemic venous pooling, thromboemboli formation, arrhythmia, systemic venous hypertension, protein-losing enteropathy, right heart failure leading to hepatosplenomegaly.

Other Fontan techniques route caval flow through a conduit partly routed through the RA, which may lead to complications. Newer techniques bypass the RA completely. Occasionally, fenestrations or holes are created between the IVC-RPA conduit and the RA to allow for a "pop-off" of extra fluid, which is thought to prevent some postoperative complications.

Continued

Table 27-4 Surgical Repairs of Cardiac Defects—cont'd		
Repair and Intended Effect	**Defects**	**Potential Long-term Implications and Sequelae**
Infrequently Used Repairs Blalock-Taussig shunt (classic): • The right or left subclavian artery is divided from the aorta and attached to the ipsilateral (same side) pulmonary artery to provide controlled pulmonary blood flow.	Cyanotic heart defects such as HLHS, TOF, pulmonary atresia, tricuspid atresia.	Mild pulmonary artery distortion at site of anastomosis, resultant ischemia to hand or arm on ipsilateral side of anastomosis with associated limb length discrepancy and perfusion, potential coronary ischemia related to pulmonary "steal" of blood flow during diastole.
Waterston-Cooley shunt: • A connection is created between the ascending aorta to right pulmonary artery to increase pulmonary blood flow; now considered obsolete as a result of development of superior shunts. This procedure is RARELY performed today.	Cyanotic heart defects.	Right pulmonary artery distortion at site of anastomosis, inadequate pulmonary blood flow and persistent cyanosis, excessive pulmonary blood flow and development of pulmonary hypertension, right pulmonary artery stenosis and possible need for major reconstructive surgery.
Potts shunt: • A connection is created between the descending aorta to the left pulmonary artery to increase pulmonary blood flow; now considered obsolete as a result of development of superior shunts. This procedure is RARELY performed today.	Cyanotic heart defects.	Left pulmonary artery distortion at site of anastomosis, inadequate pulmonary blood flow and persistent cyanosis, excessive pulmonary blood flow and development of pulmonary hypertension, difficulty of shunt take-down.
Senning: • Conduits or baffles made from pericardium or synthetic material are placed between the RA and the LV pulmonic outflow and between the LA and the RV aortic outflow. These conduits allow appropriate pulmonary and systemic circulation without switching placement of the great arteries.	TGA.	Atrial dysrhythmias, baffle obstructions or leaks, right heart failure related to use of right ventricle as systemic pump. Tricuspid or mitral insufficiency, thromboemboli.
Mustard: • Conduits or tunnels are created between the RA and the LV pulmonic outflow and between the LA and the RV aortic outflow using atrial tissue. These conduits allow appropriate pulmonary and systemic circulation without switching placement of the great arteries.	TGA.	Atrial dysrhythmias, conduit obstructions or leaks, right heart failure related to use of right ventricle as systemic pump. Tricuspid or mitral insufficiency, thromboemboli.

Source: © Judith M. Marshall, Ellen Reyerson 2006 (From Mavroudis & Backer, 2003).

attempts to correct the condition early on and to prevent the child's condition from progressing to the point of no return. It is certainly more desirable to perform a transplant long before the child is gravely ill, but it is also difficult to justify the need for transplantation to a family whose child is playful and seems "normal" to them. Although survival rates continue to improve, there are limitations.

clinical alert

Complications of cardiac transplantation

The four main complications of cardiac transplantation are:

• Rejection
• Infection
• Posttransplant lymphoproliferative disorder (PTLD)
• Transplant coronary artery disease (TCAD)

Although transplantation saves lives and greatly improves the quality of life, it is often said that transplantation is exchanging one disease for another. Living with a transplanted heart is considered a chronic condition, but it is manageable. The child and his or her family must follow a strict regimen of medication, diagnostic tests, blood tests, and clinic follow-up.

 Across Care Settings: **The transplantation team**

The cardiac transplantation team consists of nurse practitioners, physicians, surgeons, nurses, social workers, medical psychologists, religious leaders, school nurses, and school officials. Most important, the child and his or her parents, and extended family are involved in the caretaking decisions. The child and his or her family must be hypercompliant with the regimen in order to prevent rejection of the cardiac muscle.

NURSING CARE. The priority nursing intervention is to help the family understand the importance of medication compliance. There is no room for a less than rigorous approach when administering the medications. This is a difficult endeavor, but the positive aspect is that the child will live. The medication regimen includes as many as three anti-rejection medications (immunosuppressants), antihypertensive drugs, electrolyte supplements, diuretics, anticoagulants, and antihyperlipidemics. These medications must be given every day. The immunosuppressants prevent the body's immune system from rejecting the transplanted heart muscle and must be given within a 1 hour window of time.

Another important nursing intervention is communicating to the family about the frequent follow-up visits to the clinic, which will help ensure close monitoring by the cardiac transplantation team. Sometimes the child will come to the hospital as frequently as every week for follow-up care.

Following the transplant, the nurse can educate the family about cardiac catheterization with myocardial biopsy that is performed as often as every 2 weeks in the initial postoperative phase and during times of rejection. The family also must understand that every year coronary angiography is performed with cardiac catheterization to assess for coronary atherosclerosis, a side effect of the immunosuppressant drugs. The nurse must understand the principles of myocardial rejection. Myocardial rejection is the most severe consequence of cardiac transplant. Rejection can lead to systemic failure, and depending on the grade, usually requires hospitalization. This necessitates frequent follow-up and biopsies.

Children who have received a transplanted heart are subject to many emotional and psychological issues. As it is difficult to live one's life with any heart defect or other chronic defects, imagine a life of a child locked into this intensive medical regimen. Children who received their transplant as infants or toddlers may be more adjusted psychologically (because it is the only life they know), but may suffer more developmental delays. These children may have suffered brain anoxia, or are delayed because of frequent hospitalizations. Most children do well, attending school and continuing on to college. Psychosocial adjustment depends on the coping skills and support systems of the child and the family. In addition, physical growth can be stunted because of frequent prednisone dosing. Alterations in growth and development also have an emotional impact on the child's life.

Nursing Care for the Child with a Cardiac Condition

The nursing plan of care for the child with a cardiac condition consists of assessment, outcomes, intervention, and evaluation.

CARING FOR THE CHILD IN THE PEDIATRIC INTENSIVE CARE UNIT

Postcardiac surgical patients generally require admission to a pediatric intensive care unit (PICU) for recovery. PICU admission requires specific care by highly trained nurses. The child generally stays on the unit for approximately 2 to 3 days for simple repairs and 5 to 10 days for more complicated repairs. The child is then transferred to a cardiac step-down or cardiac care unit. If the child has other body system failures or does not respond well to the surgery, very lengthy postoperative PICU admissions may ensue. The PICU stay is also influenced by the child's condition before surgery or any perioperative complications. The patient in the PICU most likely is intubated, has chest tubes, a nasogastric tube, and Foley catheter. There are multiple peripheral and central intravenous lines. The nurse may care for a patient with temporary pacer wires. Postsurgical patients have a large dressing on the surgical site (mid-sternum or lateral). When this dressing is removed, there are usually steri-strips or Dermabond™ on the skin.

Nursing care for the child in the PICU integrates important concepts such as assessment, nutrition, hygiene, activity and psychosocial care. Emphasis for care also includes taking vital signs, maintaining growth and development, administering medications, performing lab tests, and interpreting an ECG.

 clinical alert

Postoperative Vital Signs

The routine for vital signs (VS) in the PICU is much more rigorous than on a general or telemetry floor. Typically, recovery of cardiac surgical patients takes place in the ICU rather than in the postanesthesia unit. These patients may be very sick and require close monitoring and a one-on-one patient assignment. The VS should be taken every (q) 15 minutes for the first few hours then q30min, then q1hr until the child is stable. The nurse can adjust the frequency depending on the stability of the patient. All changes in VS, no matter how subtle, should be documented and reported to the physician or practitioner.

Growth and development is a consideration for any hospital admission. Often PICU patients post-cardiac surgery are heavily sedated or chemically paralyzed to maintain stability. When caring for a sick child, the nurse should consider the child's level of development. Soft music can be played for any child, and older children should be talked to and explanations given for any touching or procedures. The nurse should encourage the parents to talk to the child as well. It has been documented that after sedated or chemically paralyzed patients are brought to consciousness, they can tell their caretakers about events and conversations heard throughout the day. Never assume that your patient cannot hear what is said (The Joint Commission, 2004).

Be sure to— Administer medication properly

It is crucial for the nurse to understand the desired and undesired effects of the child's medication. Before giving any medication, the nurse must check the proper dosage (with calculations) and route. At times, medications are given in very small amounts and an error in decimal placement can mean a fatal overdose or other detrimental effects. Be sure to use the 7 rights of medication administration.

Nursing Care Plan   The Child with a Cardiac Condition

Nursing Diagnosis: Decreased cardiac output related to alterations in preload, afterload and inotropic function of the heart

Measurable Short-term Goal: The child will maintain heart rate, respirations, and blood pressure within acceptable limits (specify).

Measurable Long-term Goal: The child will tolerate daily activity without signs of cardiac decompensation.

NOC Outcomes:

Cardiac Pump Effectiveness (0400) Adequacy of blood volume ejected from the left ventricle to support systemic perfusion pressure.

Vital Signs (0802) Extent to which temperature, pulse, respiration, and blood pressure are within normal range

NIC Interventions:

Cardiac Care: Acute (4044)
Fluid/Electrolyte Management (2080)
Medication Administration (2300)
Vital Signs Monitoring (6680)

Nursing Interventions:

1. Assess vital signs: blood pressure, respirations, lung sounds, and apical and peripheral heart rate for a full minute (specify frequency). Monitor temperature every 4 hours.

   RATIONALE: Changes in cardiac output will be reflected in changes in blood pressure, respiratory status, and heart rate. Fever and infectious processes increase cardiac workload.

2. Provide continuous cardio-respiratory monitoring and evaluation of oxygen saturation levels as ordered.

   RATIONALE: Continuous cardiac monitoring provides objective data about cardiac functioning. Oxygen saturation above 95% indicates adequate respiratory status.

3. Weigh the child daily at the same time, on the same scale, and dressed in the same manner.

   RATIONALE: Congestive heart failure results in fluid accumulation reflected by weight gain. Decreased weight may indicate therapeutic effects of treatment.

4. Administer supplemental humidified oxygen as ordered.

   RATIONALE: Adequate oxygenation enhances tissue perfusion and decreases tachypnea and metabolic demands. Humidification moistens secretions to keep the airway clear.

4. Administer cardiac, diuretic, and other medications as ordered by care giver (specify drug, dose, route, and times).

   RATIONALE: (Specify the action of the particular drug related to cardiac output.)

5. Promote adequate rest and uninterrupted sleep by clustering nursing care. Collaborate with parents to reduce stress for child.

   RATIONALE: Rest and stress reduction reduce the work of the heart.

6. Position the child upright at a 30- or 60-degree angle (semi-Fowler's position).

   RATIONALE: Elevating the head of the bed enhances lung expansion, decreases venous return to the heart, redistributes blood to dependent areas, and relieves pressure on the diaphragm.

7. Monitor fluid and electrolytes as obtained. Maintain fluid restrictions if ordered (specify).

   RATIONALE: Excess fluid volume increases the work of the heart, while electrolyte alterations interfere with the electrophysiology and function of the cardiac muscle.

8. Provide ongoing education and support to the family. Encourage verbalization of concerns, feelings and questions.

   RATIONALE: Adequate knowledge and emotional support lessens the family and child's anxiety levels.

Labs: Laboratory Values

Laboratory values are unstable and close monitoring is necessary. Electrolyte measurement, particularly potassium, is perhaps the most critical lab test in the initial postoperative period because the cardiac bypass machine hemolyzes the cells, thus creating a high concentration of extracellular potassium. Hemoglobin and hematocrit tests check for possible bleeding and coagulation factors can be affected by pump time. The child will probably be on a ventilator and arterial blood gases must be assessed frequently to determine the concentration of the gases like carbon dioxide and oxygen.

The patient is on a cardiac monitor and the nurse should observe for both subtle and obvious changes. Postoperative arrhythmias may be caused by electrolyte disturbances or trauma caused by surgery.

TRANSFERRING THE STABLE CHILD TO A SURGICAL OR MEDICAL UNIT

When the postsurgical child becomes more stable, he is transferred to the surgical or cardiac floor. Commonly, a pediatric patient with a newly diagnosed cardiac condition is transferred to a tertiary care center for more definitive treatment. The nurses on this type of unit are trained in caring for cardiac patients. These units are usually equipped with telemetry monitoring.

On most telemetry units, vital signs are taken frequently, but not as often as in the PICU. The stable child requires less frequent vital signs monitoring. Typically, most telemetry units require measurement of vital signs every 4 hours.

Optimizing Outcomes— Waking the child during the night for vital signs

The best outcome for a child with a cardiac condition is proper healing along with adequate growth and development. Studies show that sleep is necessary for proper healing and that a full sleep cycle allows certain hormones (cortisol and growth hormone) and chemicals necessary for healing and growth. Copstead, L. C., and Banasik, J. L., 2009. Pathophysiology, 4th ed., page 914. Also; http://cme.medscape.com/viewarticle/502825. And; http://www.ncbi.nlm.nih.gov/pmc/articles/PMC1188300/. The nurse should assess if the child needs to be awakened during the night for vital signs or can be allowed to sleep. Many necessary VS can be taken from the monitor.

Medications given to patients on the medical/surgical unit usually do not require constant monitoring or adjusting. Some children are admitted to a medical/surgical unit for the sole purpose of starting a new medication and monitoring its effects. These children are not "sick" per se, but the medications can cause such adverse effects that close monitoring is necessary.

Although it is important to draw blood for laboratory analysis at specific times, it is not always possible on the medical/surgical unit where the phlebotomist may make rounds only at certain times of the day. Often it may be necessary for the nurse to draw the blood. The nurse understands that lab tests on the surgical/medical unit are necessary to follow up on certain conditions that may affect the cardiac system such as anemia or coagulopathies. Nurses caring for children on ECG monitoring should understand the basics of the ECG recording.

CARING FOR CHILDREN WITH CARDIAC CONDITIONS ACROSS CARE SETTINGS

The homebound child or one who visits the cardiac clinic requires specific nursing care. Often, his parents or other primary caregivers extend care into the home or community. One philosophy of family-centered care is that the parent or primary care taker always knows the child best and the nurse should rely on their judgment if they call with changes or concerns.

 Across Care Settings: **The clinic**

Caring for the child with a cardiac condition in a clinic includes:
- Monitor HR, BP, RR and pulse oximeter. Compare these vital signs values to previous visits or values from the parents or home health nurse.
- Review medications and changes noted by the caregiver. The clinic nurse verifies medications and provides proper teaching. Ensure that the family has enough refills and of the proper dosage. Occasionally medications are adjusted during a phone triage visit. Proper documentation is essential. Medications are frequently altered at clinic visits related to growth of the child.
- Laboratory tests may be performed in conjunction with the clinic visit. Ordering of these tests may be dependant to the previous lab values and the medications taken. Many children require warfarin (Coumadin) to prevent thrombus. The prothrombin time (PT) and international normalized ratio (INR) should be checked on a routine basis. The nurse must also note if any changes have been made to the warfarin (Coumadin) dosage. The clinic nurse must remember that shortly after initiation of warfarin (Coumadin) the PT/INR is checked frequently until stabilized. After stabilization, the follow-up is usually 4 weeks to 3 months. The nurse must communicate to the family that the response to Coumadin (warfarin) is affected by diet. The present recommendations are to adjust the Coumadin (warfarin) dosage rather than the diet, as families will be more compliant (Ansell et al., 2004; http://chestjournal.org/cgi/content/abstract/126/3_suppl/204S). There is a commercially available home monitoring device for these patients, which is a good option for those with unstable values.
- Electrogram monitoring usually includes a 12-lead ECG that provides a snapshot view of potential or existing arrhythmias and estimated chamber size or strain on the heart muscle. Often Holter monitors or event recorders are applied in the clinic setting. Parents may be given other recording devices for home use such as an apnea monitor or pulse oximeter. Parents should be advised not to become too preoccupied with these devices and learn to rely on their own instincts or assessment skills. An echocardiogram is frequently performed to assess for changes in chamber size or valve disease. The nurse can explain to the parents that this test often takes one hour, but is easily on the same day as the clinic visit.

Inevitably, the cardiac pediatric patient will attend school. Frequently, the school nurse or other school official will be called upon to provide care for this child. At the minimum, schools should have an automatic external defibrillator device installed. Personnel with direct contact with the child should complete a CPR course. Often it is the school nurse who first identifies a cardiac problem, hearing a murmur on a routine visit to the office or the child has a syncopal or palpitation episode. A child with long QT syndrome may have a first event while participating in school activities such as physical education, swimming, or even when the school bell is sounded. The school nurse should be prepared.

The school nurse also has other responsibilities. Typically vital signs in the school setting will coincide with administration of medication or an untoward event. If there is an event, the school nurse is responsible for stabilization until EMS arrives on the scene. Children may be taking medication frequently during the day, which necessitates administration by the school nurse. The nurse

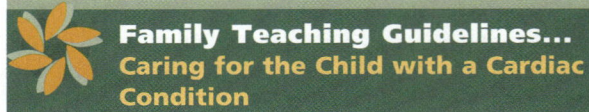

Family Teaching Guidelines...
Caring for the Child with a Cardiac Condition

HOW TO:

Teaching the child and family about the cardiac condition is essential to ensure proper growth and development as well as helping the child achieve his or her highest level of health. Essential information includes cardiopulmonary resuscitation, vital signs, medications, the disease entity, and resources.

ESSENTIAL INFORMATION

Vital Signs: Often it is noted that a parent is waking during the night to take VS, as is done in the hospital setting. One philosophy is that the child at home should lead as normal a life as possible and not become a cardiac cripple. There is rarely a need for a full-time nurse for cardiac reasons alone, but a home health nurse may evaluate the child at intervals to see if help at home is needed.

Medication: Often, children with cardiac disease require lifelong medication administration. Some require medication only until the surgery is completed and within the initial postoperative period. As in the case with the cardiac transplant child, the family must receive crucial information related to the timing and the routine of medication administration. In other cases, the cardiac drugs may be given safely with basic instruction. The nurse can also teach the family that one of the most important aspects of medication administration is proper dosing. Many of the medications are given in a liquid form. The medication dosing should always be in milliliters (mL) or cubic centimeters (cc) and not tsp or other household measures, as the family may use a kitchen teaspoon instead of 5 mL.

Disease Entity: It is important to educate the family about the disease entity itself. Because there are many resources in print and on the Internet, it is important to ensure that the child and family are receiving and reading the most up-to-date and accurate information possible. An informed family and child will be less anxious and perhaps more compliant. Educating families also builds a relationship necessary for a team approach in treating the cardiac disease.

Cardiopulmonary Resuscitation: CPR training provided by a certified instructor or fire department personnel is essential because many cardiac disease predispose to arrhythmias.

The following are resources for families and children:

American Heart Association: www.americanheart.org
Cardiomyopathy: www.cardiomyopathy.org
Children's Heart Society: www.childrensheart.org
Congenital Heart Information Network: www.tchin.org
Heart Rhythm Society: www.hrsonline.org
Heart Transplant: www.cota.org, www.a-s-t.org, www.
    ishlt.org
Kawasaki Disease: www.kdfoundation.org
Long QT Syndrome: www.long-qt-syndrome.com
March of Dimes: www.marchofdimes.com
Pectus: www.pectusinfo.com
Sudden Arrhythmia Death Syndrome (SADS)
    Foundation: www.sads.org

should understand the actions, interactions, and side effects of medications the students are taking even if not given in school.

Typically the school nurse does not perform lab tests in the school setting. In addition, there will be no electrogram equipment in the school, although if the child has a Holter monitor or event recorder in place, the school nurse may be responsible for reapplying electrodes or helping to fill out the diary. The school nurse should understand the purpose of these recordings and must be familiar with the location and use of any defibrillation equipment placed in the school.

summary points

◆ Congenital heart disease describes a congenital defect in the heart, valves or great vessels. Congenital heart defects occur in about 1% of all pregnancies and in 1 in 170 live births.

◆ Children with cardiac diseases are at risk for alterations in health such as growth and development, nutrition, psychosocial implications, and schooling, as well as being at an increased risk for infection, acquiring other diseases, and even cardiopulmonary arrest. Sometimes these children have significantly altered lifestyles and undergo constant medical treatment. The nurse must have a good understanding of common cardiac diseases in children and be able to provide essential nursing care measures.

◆ The nurse provides nursing care to the child who has undergone procedural treatments with closure devices or surgery.

◆ The nursing plan of care for the child with a cardiac condition consists of assessment, outcomes, intervention, and evaluation.

◆ Postcardiac surgical patients generally require admission to a pediatric intensive care unit for recovery. Pediatric intensive care unit (PICU) admission requires specific care by highly trained nurses.

◆ When the postsurgical child becomes more stable, he or she is then transferred to the surgical or cardiac floor.

◆ The parents or other primary caregivers extend care into the home or community.

◆ Teaching the child and family about the cardiac condition is essential to ensure proper growth and development as well as helping the child achieve their highest level of health. Essential information includes cardiopulmonary resuscitation, vital signs, medications, the disease entity, and resources.

review questions

Multiple Choice

1. When the heart condition coarctation of the aorta is suspected, the pediatric nurse will include which of

the following in the nursing assessment? *(Select all that apply.)*
   A. Take the child's blood pressures in all four extremities.
   B. Have the child lie down while taking the blood pressure.
   C. Encourage the child to play with a toy during the blood pressure assessment.
   D. Encourage the pediatrician to order acetaminophen to sedate the child.

2. The pediatric nurse recognizes that a possible long-term condition associated with Kawasaki disease is:
   A. Cervical lymphadenopathy
   B. Aneurysm formation
   C. Shortness of breath
   D. Mitral valve damage

3. The cardiac condition tetralogy of Fallot includes which of the following defects? *(Select all that apply.)*
   A. Pulmonary stenosis or atresia
   B. Ventricular septal defect
   C. Overriding aorta
   D. Hypertrophic right ventricle

4. A 14-year-old child with a history of rheumatic fever is being discharged to home after a heart valve replacement. What information would be important for the pediatric nurse to communicate to the family during discharge teaching?
   A. "The heart valve will last the child's entire lifetime."
   B. "The child will be on thrombotic agents for life."
   C. "The child may be at risk for frequent fainting episodes."
   D. "Approximately every 10 years the heart valve may need to be replaced."

5. What is a priority nursing intervention for the child who has undergone an interventional cardiac catheterization procedure?
   A. Administer morphine sulfate (Astramorph) for pain.
   B. Compare preintervention saturation levels with postintervention saturation levels.
   C. Ensure that the head of the bed is elevated to a 30-degree angle at all times.
   D. Remove the pressure dressing 1 to 2 hours post-cardiac catheterization.

True/False

6. The nurse understands that at this time there is no cure for idiopathic pulmonary arterial hypertension.

7. The pediatric nurse understands that a blood pressure greater than 20 mm Hg above the normal blood pressure for the child's age is considered as a high blood pressure reading.

8. The pediatric nurse recognizes that a lung or heart–lung transplant is the only definitive treatment for primary pulmonary hypertension.

9. The pediatric nurse must teach the parents of any child with an unrepaired cyanotic heart defect about the need for subacute bacterial endocarditis prophylaxis (SBE) therapy.

Fill-in-the-Blank

10. The child with an atrial septal defect has _____ to _____ shunting because the pressure is _____ on the _____ side of the heart.

11. In the cardiac condition transposition of the great vessels, the _____ arises from the _____ ventricle of the heart and the _____ _____ arises from the _____ ventricle of the heart.

See Answers to End of Chapter Review Questions on the Electronic Study Guide or DavisPlus.

REFERENCES

American Heart Association. (2004). Scientific statement: Diagnosis, treatment, and long-term management of Kawasaki disease. *Circulation, 110,* 2747–2771

American Heart Association (AHA). (2005). Scientific statement: Dietary recommendations for children and adolescents. *Circulation, 112,* 2061–2075.

Ansell, J., Hirsh, J., Poller, L., Bussey, H., Jacobson, A., & Hylek, E. (2004). The Pharmacology and Management of the Vitamin K Antagonists: The Seventh ACCP Conference on Antithrombotic and Thrombolytic Therapy. *Chest, 126*(3), 204S–233S.

Boucek, M.M., Edwards, L.B., Keck, B.M., Trulock, E.P., Taylor, D.O., & Hertz, M.I. (2006). Registry of the International Society for Heart and Lung Transplantation: Eighth Official Pediatric. *J Heart Lung Transplant,* 968.

Bulechek, G., Butcher, H.M., & Dochterman, J. (2008). *Nursing interventions classification (NIC)* (5th ed.). St. Louis, MO: C.V. Mosby.

Deglin, J., & Vallerand, A. (2009). *Davis's drug guide for nurses* (11th ed.). Philadelphia: F.A. Davis.

Johnson, M., Bulechek, G., Butcher, H., McCloskey Dochterman, J., Maas, M., Moorehead, S., & Swanson, E. (2006). *NANDA, NOC, and NIC linkages: Nursing diagnoses, outcomes, & interventions* (2nd ed.). St. Louis, MO: Mosby Elsevier.

Mavroudis, C., & Backer, C.L. (2003). *Pediatric cardiac surgery* (3rd ed.). St. Louis, MO: C.V. Mosby.

Moorehead, S., Johnson, M., Maas, M., & Swanson, E. (2008). *Nursing outcomes classification (NOC)* (4th ed.). St. Louis, MO: C.V. Mosby.

Moss, A.J., & Robinson, J.L. (2002). The long-QT syndrome. *Circulation, 105,* 784

NANDA International (2007). *NANDA-I nursing diagnoses: Definitions and classifications 2007–2008.* Philadelphia: NANDA-I.

Neilson, D., & Robin, N. (2002). Advances in the genetics of pediatric heart disease. *Contemporary Pediatrics, 19*(1), 85–100.

Park, M. (2003). *The pediatric cardiology handbook* (3rd ed.). St. Louis, MO: C.V. Mosby

Parrillo, S.J. (2006). Rheumatic fever. *eMedicine* http://www.emedicine.com/emerg/topic509.htm

Pophal, S. (2006). Evaluation of heart murmurs in primary care. *The child's doctor.* http://www.childrensmemorial.org/cme/online/article.asp?articleID=154

The Joint Commission (2004). Retrieved from http://www.jointcommission.org/SentinelEvents/SentinelEventAlert/sea_32.htm (Accessed July 5, 2008).

Venes, D. (Ed.). (2009). *Taber's cyclopedic medical dictionary* (21st ed.). Philadelphia: F.A. Davis.

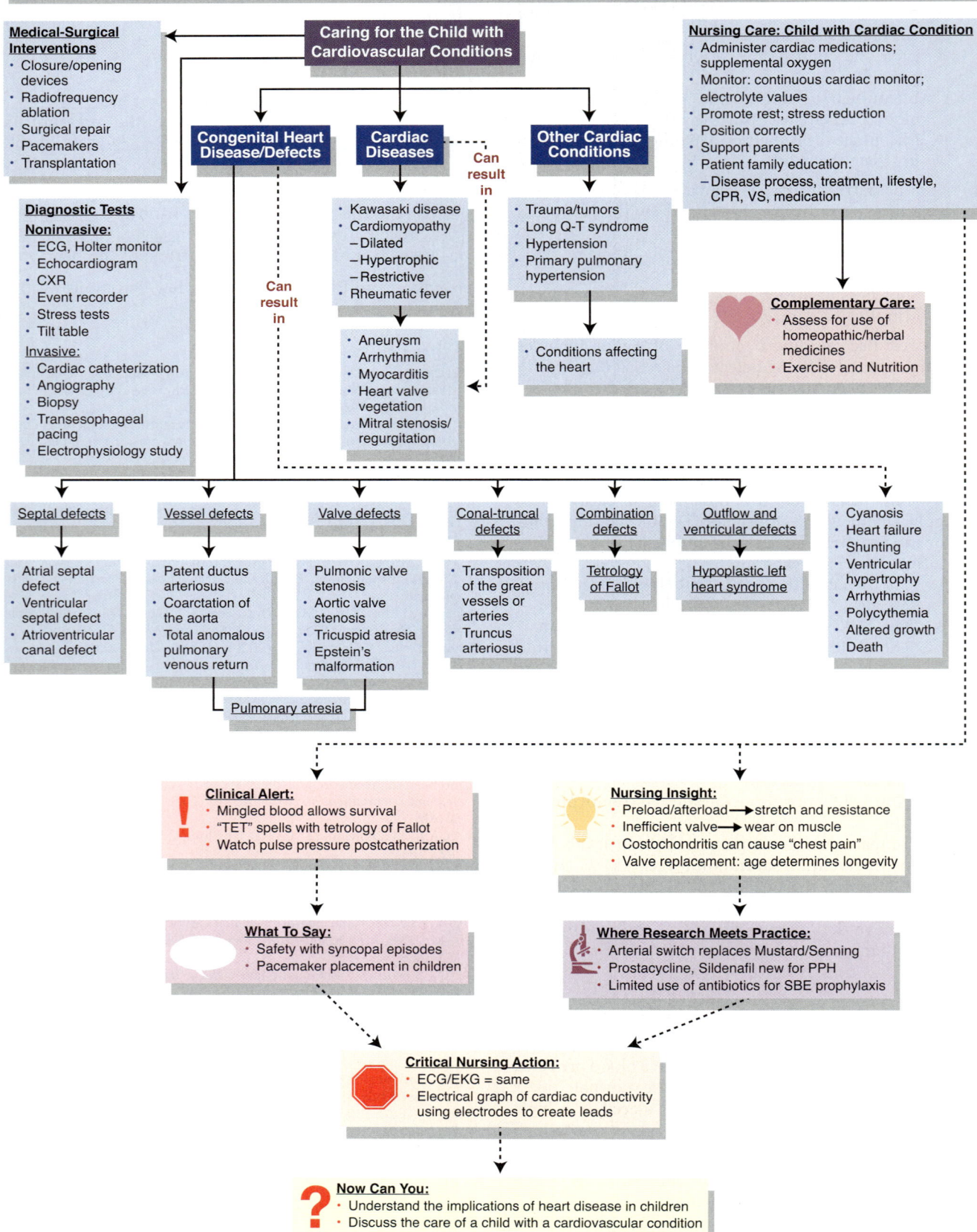

CONCEPT MAP

Caring for the Child with Cardiovascular Conditions

Medical-Surgical Interventions
- Closure/opening devices
- Radiofrequency ablation
- Surgical repair
- Pacemakers
- Transplantation

Nursing Care: Child with Cardiac Condition
- Administer cardiac medications; supplemental oxygen
- Monitor: continuous cardiac monitor; electrolyte values
- Promote rest; stress reduction
- Position correctly
- Support parents
- Patient family education:
  - Disease process, treatment, lifestyle, CPR, VS, medication

Congenital Heart Disease/Defects

Cardiac Diseases

Can result in

Other Cardiac Conditions

Diagnostic Tests
Noninvasive:
- ECG, Holter monitor
- Echocardiogram
- CXR
- Event recorder
- Stress tests
- Tilt table

Invasive:
- Cardiac catheterization
- Angiography
- Biopsy
- Transesophageal pacing
- Electrophysiology study

Can result in

- Kawasaki disease
- Cardiomyopathy
  - Dilated
  - Hypertrophic
  - Restrictive
- Rheumatic fever

- Aneurysm
- Arrhythmia
- Myocarditis
- Heart valve vegetation
- Mitral stenosis/regurgitation

- Trauma/tumors
- Long Q-T syndrome
- Hypertension
- Primary pulmonary hypertension

- Conditions affecting the heart

Complementary Care:
- Assess for use of homeopathic/herbal medicines
- Exercise and Nutrition

Septal defects
- Atrial septal defect
- Ventricular septal defect
- Atrioventricular canal defect

Vessel defects
- Patent ductus arteriosus
- Coarctation of the aorta
- Total anomalous pulmonary venous return

Pulmonary atresia

Valve defects
- Pulmonic valve stenosis
- Aortic valve stenosis
- Tricuspid atresia
- Epstein's malformation

Conal-truncal defects
- Transposition of the great vessels or arteries
- Truncus arteriosus

Combination defects
Tetrology of Fallot

Outflow and ventricular defects
Hypoplastic left heart syndrome

- Cyanosis
- Heart failure
- Shunting
- Ventricular hypertrophy
- Arrhythmias
- Polycythemia
- Altered growth
- Death

Clinical Alert:
- Mingled blood allows survival
- "TET" spells with tetrology of Fallot
- Watch pulse pressure postcatherization

Nursing Insight:
- Preload/afterload → stretch and resistance
- Inefficient valve → wear on muscle
- Costochondritis can cause "chest pain"
- Valve replacement: age determines longevity

What To Say:
- Safety with syncopal episodes
- Pacemaker placement in children

Where Research Meets Practice:
- Arterial switch replaces Mustard/Senning
- Prostacycline, Sildenafil new for PPH
- Limited use of antibiotics for SBE prophylaxis

Critical Nursing Action:
- ECG/EKG = same
- Electrical graph of cardiac conductivity using electrodes to create leads

Now Can You:
- Understand the implications of heart disease in children
- Discuss the care of a child with a cardiovascular condition

Caring for the Child with an Endocrinological or Metabolic Condition

No More Sweets for Me

No more sweets for me
today, I must abstain; not to overindulge.
Tomorrow I can have some more
If I have one I'm still ok,
If I choose two I should be all right
If I take three I better be careful
I don't want to over due it

I don't like Halloween, too much candy for me
I want, but can't have dessert, and birthday cake
I don't want to complain, but some days it just doesn't seem fair
But in the end I'll be happier,
at least that's what you keep telling me.

—Nicholas Zahara-Such

LEARNING TARGETS *At the completion of this chapter, the student will be able to:*

◆ Describe the anatomy and normal function of the endocrine system.

◆ Recognize pathophysiological conditions of the endocrine system.

◆ Identify nursing insights necessary for the holistic care of a child with an endocrine or metabolic condition.

◆ Plan collaborative care for a child with an endocrine or metabolic condition.

◆ Identify complementary measures to provide alternatives to care within the child's culture.

◆ Define pharmacological and therapeutic measures to treat a child with an endocrine condition.

◆ Develop family teaching plans to optimize outcomes in a child with a chronic endocrine or metabolic condition.

◆ Use critical thinking measures to evaluate care of a child with an endocrine or metabolic condition.

 moving toward evidence-based practice Glycemic Control of Children with Diabetes

Stallwood, L. (2005). Influence of caregiver stress and coping on glycemic control of young children with diabetes. *Journal of Pediatric Health Care, 19*(5), 293–300.

The purpose of this study was to examine the influence of caregiver stress, perceived stress and coping during the management and glycemic control of young diabetic children.

Current literature stresses the importance of maintaining acceptable glucose levels to avoid diabetic complications. Control is accomplished through adherence to a prescribed

management regimen. Previous research supports the notion that diabetes-related stress is a major contributor to decreased success in the home management of diabetes.

This investigation was part of a larger project that focused on the "relationships of the caregiver's diabetes-related stress, perceived stress, and coping with home management and

(continued)

moving toward evidence-based practice (continued)

glycemic control" (p. 295). Measures of stress, perception of stress, coping, and adaptation, as described in the Double ABCX Model of Family Adaptation, provided the framework for the study.

A cross-sectional correlational design was used. The convenience sample consisted of 73 primary caregivers of children younger than 9 years who were present in a children's hospital diabetes clinic waiting room.

To be eligible for inclusion in the study, the primary caregiver was required to meet the following criteria:

- Function as "the primary caregiver of diabetes-related home management for a child younger than 9 years of age, and
- Able to speak and understand English" (p. 295).

The children of the caregivers were required to meet the following criteria:

- A diagnosis of "Type-1 diabetes for a minimum of 3 months
- Taking a combination of short-acting and long-acting insulin in 2–4 daily injections, and
- Free of a major co-morbid chronic illness" (p. 295).

Data collection took place before the primary caregiver was seen by the diabetes health care team.

Level of stress, defined as "pressures that accompany the stress of home management," was measured by the Problem Areas in Diabetes (PAID) scale. The tool used a 5-point Likert-type scale where 1 was "not a problem" and 5 was "a serious problem."

The Appraisal of Diabetes Scale (ADS) was used to measure the perception of stress, defined as "the meaning the caregiver assigns to the situation." This instrument used a 5-point Likert-type scale and included questions such as: "How upsetting is your child's diabetes for you?" and "How much control over your child's diabetes do you have?" Higher scores were indicative of higher levels of perceived stress.

The Coping Health Inventory for Parents (CHIP) scale was used to measure coping. This instrument consisted of 45 self-report items to evaluate the caregiver's perceptions of methods currently used to manage the child with a chronic condition. Three types of coping patterns were examined: family life, external relationships, and relationships with health care providers and other persons who provide care to children with chronic illnesses.

Hemoglobin A_{1c} (Hgb A_{1c}) was used to assess level of glycemic control. Target ranges of the A_{1c} (Hgb A_{1c}) for the diabetic clinic were >7 mg/dL to <9 mg/dL. Increased levels of Hgb A_{1c} are associated with increased blood sugar levels: with each 1.0 increase in the Hgb A_{1c}, there is an average mean blood glucose change of 30 mg/dL.

The Diabetes Self-Management Profile (DSMP) was used to assess home diabetes management. This instrument assessed the following five domains over the previous 3 months: exercise frequency, hypoglycemia awareness and preparedness, food measurement and diet alterations based on activity and insulin administration, frequency of blood glucose testing, and timing and technique of insulin administration. Higher scores on the DSMP were indicative of better home diabetes management.

Analysis of the data revealed the following findings:

- The caregivers' ages ranged from 19 to 66 years; mean age 35 years.
- The caregivers' levels of education ranged from 10 to >16 years.
- Of those who reported income, 43 had an annual income of <$50,000.
- The average length of time since receiving a diagnosis of diabetes was 2.5 years, with a range of 3 months to 7 years.
- Thirty-seven of the caregivers were Caucasian and 29 African American. Sixty-two of the primary caregivers identified themselves as the child's mother; 8 identified themselves as the child's father.

Results from the Hgb A_{1c} reports revealed that 33 children scored within an acceptable range, 35 scored outside of the acceptable range, and no data were available for 5 children.

The researcher concluded that increased levels of caregiver stress as indicated by the Problem Areas in Diabetes (PAID) scale were associated with higher levels of perceived stress as measured by the Appraisal of Diabetes Scale (ADS). This finding may point to a direct relationship between stress and the perception of diabetes-related stress.

A negative relationship was found between received stress on the appraisal of Diabetes Scale (ADS) and the HgBA$_{1c}$ levels, which may be interpreted as showing that the role of stress was being a motivator for attaining glycemic control.

A negative relationship was also found between home management and Hgb A_{1c} levels, suggesting that children of caregivers with a higher level of home management were better able to attain acceptable Hgb A_{1c} levels.

A negative relationship was also noted in relation to the child's age and the PAID score, which might suggest the presence of higher levels of stress in families with younger diabetic children.

The researcher reported that no significant relationship was found between data from the Diabetes Self-Management Profile (DSMP) and the Coping Health Inventory for Parents (CHIP) scale.

1. What might be considered as limitations to this study?
2. How is this information useful to clinical nursing practice?

See Suggested Responses for Moving Toward Evidence-Based Practice on the Electronic Study Guide or DavisPlus.

Introduction

The endocrine system consists of multiple organs throughout the body. One of the main purposes of these organs is to secrete hormones that regulate various bodily functions. Hormones are chemicals that the body creates, such as proteins consisting of amino acid chains or steroids derived from fatty (cholesterol derived) substances. Although their derivations can vary, hormones act solely as "messengers," moving from system to system coordinating the functions of many parts of the body.

In the care of children, it is important to remember that the endocrine system controls growth and development as well as energy use and energy stores; it also controls levels of sugar, salt, and fluids in the bloodstream. While hormones regulate a child's response to stress or physical trauma, they play a vital role in sexual development as well.

This chapter provides a review about the anatomy and physiology of the endocrine system as well as the hormones it produces and the conditions that are commonly seen in children with endocrine or metabolic conditions. Current treatments and nursing strategies to augment the treatment and care of the child are discussed. Complementary care measures are included for the nurse to gain a repertoire of care modalities.

A & P review **Organs of the Endocrine System**

The hypothalamus is located in the center of the brain and is one of the main control centers of the body. Its main function is to communicate the messages of the central autonomic nervous system to the organs/glands of the endocrine system, thus working to create and maintain homeostasis throughout the body.

The pineal body is a photosensitive gland that receives light through the optic nerve. The pituitary gland is connected to the hypothalamus by a stem-like structure. It has two parts: the anterior and the posterior pituitary. It is said that the pituitary gland is the "master" because of its effect on growth and the functions of other glands in the body. The thyroid gland is located in the front of the neck just below the larynx. The two lobes of the thyroid are connected by an isthmus, which is a small band of tissue. The thyroid produces two hormones called thyroxin (T_4) and triiodothyronine (T_3).

There are four parathyroid glands, two embedded on the posterior side of each lobe of the thyroid gland. The parathyroid glands produce parathyroid hormone (PTH). The adrenal glands are located on the top of each kidney. Each gland has an outer (cortex) portion and an inner (medulla) portion. The hypothalamus has control on the adrenal glands by causing the anterior pituitary to release adrenocorticotropic hormone (ACTH) releasing hormone. Each part of the adrenal cortex produces different hormones. The pancreas is located in the abdomen, just behind the stomach near the duodenum. It functions as both an endocrine (without ducts) gland by secreting hormones and also as an exocrine (with ducts) gland. As an exocrine gland, it produces and secretes digestive enzymes directly into the small intestine through ducts. As an endocrine gland, it produces both insulin and glucagon which in turn are carried to the body through the bloodstream. These hormones are antagonistic and have opposite effects on metabolism.

The gonads, namely the ovaries in females and the testes in males, produce several steroidal sex hormones. Generally, these sex hormones produce and regulate changes in the male and female body at puberty. ◆

Pathophysiological Conditions of the Endocrine System

CONDITIONS OF THE ANTERIOR PITUITARY

Since the anterior pituitary gland is responsible for the production of many hormones that influence and regulate growth, metabolic activity, and eventually sexual development, conditions of the anterior pituitary are a result of either an over or underproduction of their essential hormones. These conditions include growth hormone deficiency, precocious puberty, and acromegaly.

Hypopituitary

Hypopituitary or growth hormone deficiency (GHD) is an endocrine condition that is generally due to a decreased production of GH by the anterior pituitary gland. It is seen in children who present with short stature (below the 3rd or 5th percentile) and is characterized by delayed skeletal growth.

The incidence of GHD has not yet been established with 100% certainty, but generally, its prevalence has been reported to be about 1 out of every 3500 children. Boys are referred more often than girls for short stature because it is believed that small females are more accepted in our society. Incidence among boys and girls is about equal.

Recent studies have tried to isolate the cause of hypopituitarism. Some cases, which have been spontaneous in nature, have led to the identification and characterization of numerous genes and factors as the causes. Generally, the majority of the cases are still considered to have no known cause and idiopathic in nature. In addition there are many other causes including genetic, congenital, acquired (due to trauma or CNS infections), tumors in the region of the hypothalamus or pituitary, as well as secondary causes such as cranial irradiation and transient causes such as psychosocial deprivation.

SIGNS AND SYMPTOMS. Usually in the neonatal period, infants with GHD are of normal birth weight and length. The delayed or absent growth begins to be assessed in the first 2 years of life. Delayed growth of less than 2 inches (4 to 5 centimeters) in a year should be evaluated further. Assessment must be done carefully and consistently at each visit to the pediatrician. The rate of growth can be measured using the metric system to increase the preciseness of the measurement. If a child is seen to have "fallen off" the growth chart, height or weight plateaus, stays the same, or dramatically is less than last visit, further evaluation is warranted.

critical nursing action Proper Growth Assessment

It is imperative that the nurse plot the child's height and weight accurately at each outpatient visit on the appropriate growth chart (Fig. 28-1). If the child is of short stature (below the 3rd or 5th percentile) and is not chartable on the usual chart or has Down syndrome, the pediatric nurse should go to the Center of Disease Control Web site for the most appropriate chart, located at http://www.cdc.gov/nchs/about/major/nhanes/growthcharts/charts.htm. It is important to use the same growth chart at each visit. The nurse must remember to weigh an infant completely undressed (including diaper) and young child in underwear with socks only.

Other signs and symptoms include delayed closure of the anterior fontanel; delayed dental eruption; greater weight to height ratio with increased abdominal (truncal) fat; decreased muscle mass; poor development of bridge of nose giving a child-like appearance; protrusion of the frontal skull bones; delayed puberty, including a high-pitch voice and a small penis or testes in boys; and hypoglycemia.

It is important to also note and alert the physician about episodes of frequent or recurrent hypoglycemia, prolonged jaundice, or micropenis in the neonatal period, as these may indicate the possibility of congenital hypopituitarism (Allen, 2006).

DIAGNOSIS. A diagnostic work-up begins with a review of all previous growth charts to determine the rate of growth. Special attention is given to children in the less than 3rd or 5th percentile or to any child whose growth has ceased. Bone age determination by radiograph of the wrist, knee, or hand is usually less than the child's chronological age, thus indicating a delayed skeletal maturation. Magnetic resonance imaging (MRI) of the brain is also performed. Baseline blood tests and pituitary function tests are needed to confirm the diagnosis. Various pituitary function tests are given to stimulate growth hormone (GH) release. The GH stimulants are medications that include insulin, glucagon, clonidine, arginine, or L-dopa. One or more of these may be administered during testing

to stimulate a rapid release of GH. Small percentages of children do not respond to these pituitary tests and must be retested. When peak GH levels are less than 10 nanograms per liter (ng/L) the diagnosis is confirmed.

NURSING CARE. The nurse assists the child in reaching the goals of treatment, which are that the child achieves a normal growth rate and eventually reaches a normal adult height. Treatment is considered simple with the administration of human recombinant GH (replacement therapy with daily subcutaneous injections).

Although significant side effects of GH are rare, it is important to know that they may include increased intracranial pressure (ICP), gynecomastia, arthralgia, and edema. Children who complain of a headache must be carefully monitored because this may be the only sign of ICP. Managing these side effects may mean that the GH dose is temporarily reduced or stopped. GH therapy can also decrease a child's sensitivity to insulin, but there are few reported cases of diabetes mellitus while the child is on GH treatment. Recombinant human GH is a safe treatment for children with idiopathic short stature. Studies that assess the frequency of rare side effects and long-term follow-up are necessary (Quigley et al., 2005).

When a child is diagnosed with GHD, careful and consistent growth measurements are as essential as plotting the measurements on the appropriate growth chart. Children should be measured and weighed no less than once every 6 months on an outpatient basis.

 critical nursing action Daily Weights to Ensure Accurate Medication Doses

When the child is hospitalized, the nurse must be conscientious and recalculate medication dosages with every weight variance. Physicians must be notified if the dose ordered is now inaccurate based on the most current weight. Daily weight measures using kilograms ensures that accurate medication dosages are calculated and given.

Parents need to be given as many supportive resources as possible. Specific foundations have Web sites that will link the family with other families going through the same treatment. Some reliable resources that parents could be referred to include: the Human Growth Foundation http://www.hgfound.org/, the Short Stature Foundation http://www.kumc.edu/gec/support/dwarfism.html, or the Magic Foundation http://www.magicfoundation.org/www.

These Web sites may also help parents find financial support as the GH treatments can be expensive and sometimes insurance does not cover the condition. The drug companies that produce GH also have programs that can assist families who cannot pay for the treatments.

Children with GHD can be small framed and of short stature. It is important to stress to the families to treat the child for their age, not their size. Frequently, teachers or other adults treat a child with GHD differently than a child of the same age and normal size. Children with GHD should be encouraged to play sports that do not involve size, such as swimming, ice skating, dancing, and gymnastics. They should also be encouraged to dress age-appropriately. Supporting the family to help the child attain a positive self-image is of the utmost importance. The nurse should help

Figure 28-1 The nurse is measuring the child's height to ensure growth and development are on target.

the child realize that self-determination and confidence, not height, achieve goals. Classmates can be insensitive to the child's feelings and can even tease the untreated short child. Adolescence, with the focus on body image, can be an especially difficult time. It is best to begin treatment as early as possible when a near normal height can be reached and before the psychological effects of short stature harm the child.

Another important aspect of nursing care includes patient and family teaching about the condition, its treatment, and providing as much support as possible. Parents need to be taught about GH replacement therapy, its preparation, and administration of the subcutaneous injections. Just as with other daily subcutaneous injections, rotating sites, potential side effects, and actions to take if necessary must be taught to the parents. Parents should be prompted to think of ideas that would decrease the child's stress regarding the daily injections.

The nurse can also remember to encourage the parents to take the child with GHD to the dentist regularly because the GH treatments cause the child's teeth to be softer and much more susceptible to cavities.

 ❝ What to say❞ — *Helping children express themselves*

Children can be apprehensive about daily injections of any kind. It is important for the nurse to be as honest as possible regarding the GH treatments. The nurse can refer the family to the Magic Foundation Web site for on-line videos that address this topic. The nurse can help the child express answers to the following questions:

"How do you feel?"

"What do you tell your friends about your condition and the GH medication?"

"How have you changed since the GH treatments began?"

"What advice do you have for other children beginning GH treatment?"

❈ Complementary Care: *Therapeutic touch*

Therapeutic touch (TT) or massage is a form of energy therapy that helps the body release endorphins. Endorphins (or more correctly endomorphines) are *endogenous opioid* biochemical compounds. Endorphins are peptides produced by the pituitary gland and the hypothalamus and resemble the opiates in their abilities to produce analgesia and a sense of well-being. In other words, endorphins work as "natural pain killers." Using drugs may increase the effects of the endorphins (A.D.A.M., 2006). Energy therapy does not promote GH release and therefore would not replace conventional GH treatments, but it certainly can be used to adjunct the GH therapy.

The nurse should constantly be aware of individual patient goals and the progress made toward achievement, that is, to know and accurately communicate the growth status of the child and the child's psychological acceptance of his body image. The nurse must ascertain the status of these vital outcomes. The pediatric nurse should be alert to facial expressions of uncertainty. Sometimes families are afraid to ask or fear that the question is unintelligent.

❈ Collaboration in Caring— *A team approach*

The nurse can make referrals for psychological counseling for the child or family if warranted. Even when the pediatric nurse is not certain about the child's psyche, the referral should be made and the decision left to the specialist.

Pituitary Hyperfunction

Pituitary hyperfunction or precocious puberty (early or premature) is a condition that occurs with hyperfunction of the pituitary gland. Generally, puberty occurs between 8 and 13 years of age in girls and between 9 1/2 and 14 in boys. In girls, precocious puberty is when any of the following secondary sexual characteristics develop before 8 years of age: breasts, armpit or pubic hair, mature external genitalia, and the first menstruation. In boys, precocious puberty is when any of the following secondary sexual characteristics such as mature external genitalia; growth of body hair, including facial, underarm, abdominal, chest, and pubic hair; increase in size of and mass of muscles; deepening of the voice; and change in the shape of the face and skeleton before 9 years of age.

Most often precocious puberty is idiopathic in girls and the incidence is about five times higher than in boys (Traggiai & Stanhope, 2003). In males, it is usually due to central nervous system (CNS) abnormalities, or lesions such as a benign hypothalamic tumor, brain injury, or another type of brain tumor. Other known causes include postinfections (encephalitis or meningitis), congenital adrenal hyperplasia, tumors of the ovary, adrenal gland or testicle, exogenous sources or androgens.

SIGNS AND SYMPTOMS. Similar characteristics of precocious puberty appear in boys and girls, as well as ones specific to each sex. In boys, the following signs and symptoms may be seen: facial hair, penile growth, increased masculinity, testicular enlargement, and voice changes. In girls these characteristic signs and symptoms are likely: breast development, onset of menarche, ovary enlargement, and cysts on ovaries. Commonly seen in both boys and girls are the following: armpit hair, pubic hair, body odor, acne, emotional lability and mood swings, and growth spurts in height. Advanced bone age equals increased skeletal growth which in turn equals increased height initially. If untreated, epiphyseal plates (growth plates) close early and growth stops.

DIAGNOSIS. The nurse understands that blood tests include measurement of luteinizing hormone (LH), follicle-stimulating hormone (FSH), testosterone, or estradiol. Testing to stimulate the release of gonadotropins confirm the diagnosis. In addition, radiological studies should be done to calculate the child's bone age. Because of the high incidence of CNS involvement in males, skull CT and/or MRI is usually indicated.

The pediatric nurse must perform a complete history and assessment of the child's pubertal status including a Tanner staging of sexual maturation. Growth charts should also be completed to determine the exact age that linear growth spiked. Breast, genital, pubic hair, and testicular development should be documented. The nursing history should include exposure to hormones, CNS infection or trauma, and the family history of the age at puberty onset.

clinical alert

Exogenous hormones

Many commercially purchased female products contain estrogen. Facial creams, hair products, and other "beauty" aids can contain hormones or placenta extracts. Some shampoos specifically marketed to African Americans have been found to contain hormones. Children can readily absorb enough of these exogenous hormones to present with precocious puberty. The nurse can refer parents to the Web site on Organic Parenting http://www.primalspirit.com/ps3_1lyn-piluso.htm

The nurse must alert parents of the dangers of hidden toxins in everyday products that can harm their children. They must also be cognizant of "endocrine disruptors," and can refer families to http://www.mindfully.org/Pesticide/EDs-PWG-16jun01.htm

NURSING CARE. The nurse assists in providing treatment for precocious puberty. Treatment includes gonadotropin-releasing hormone (GnRH) agonists (Kaplowitz, 2006) which can be given via subcutaneous injection daily or as a depot injection once every 3 to 4 weeks or has been given intranasally two to three times daily. Initially the treatments stimulate gonadotropin release, but when given over the long term, they suppress the release of gonadotropins by acting on the pituitary gland.

Treatments cause a decrease in growth rate and a stabilization or regression in development of secondary sexual characteristics. Sizes of the breasts, ovaries, uterus, and testes, as well as erection frequency, all decrease. The success of the treatment is measured via growth charts and blood levels of gonadotropins and sex steroids. When treatments are stopped, puberty promptly begins.

Consistent, accurate record keeping of the child's growth rate must be documented because while on treatment the child's growth rate declines. The nurse must continue to assess and document the progression or regression of the child's secondary sex characteristics. Nursing care must also focus on the accuracy of medication delivery. The pediatric nurse should provide accurate information to both the child and the family about medication preparation, action, and administration techniques.

It is important to approach the child in a manner appropriate to his or her level of emotional and cognitive development. Information provided to both the child and family should include the physical changes that the child is experiencing as well as on the child's disturbed body image. The nurse understands that help should be given to the child and family regarding manner of dress. Loosely fitting clothing may help to conceal the abruptly changing body image. The nurse can also make referrals to counseling.

Depending on the age of the child, the child should be included in the teaching as much as appropriate. Providing information about normal development during puberty helps the caregivers and the child understand the physical and emotional changes that occur with the early onset of puberty. In addition, the nurse understands that decreased stress and low-fat diets are some of the latest discoveries related to decrease premature sexual maturation. In other words, obesity, especially in females, and stress are the newest suspected causes of early puberty. Pediatric nurses must stay critically aware of the child's feelings and help the parents develop ways to stay "connected" to their child with precocious puberty.

Optimizing Outcomes— **Financial Resources**

Helping the parents identify financial resources for assistance if necessary ensures the best outcomes of the care and treatments given. GnRH analog depot treatments are very costly and can range from $700 to $1000 per injection. These treatments are usually covered by the insurance companies, but some require the injection to be given in the physician's office. For those with limited insurance resources, some pharmaceutical companies provide assistance and give treatments at limited or no cost.

Across Care Settings: A team approach

Precocious puberty has its greatest effect on the child and family both psychologically and psychosocially. It is to the child's and family's best interest for the primary care pediatrician to make referrals to an endocrinologist and psychologist as soon as possible. Especially in very young children, early referrals can help to prevent serious psychological trauma and help the child begin to adjust to his or her changing body. Communication among members of the entire team is essential for ongoing collaboration and the best possible outcomes.

Acromegaly and Gigantism

The term "acromegaly" comes from the Greek words *acro* (extremities) and *megaly* (enlargement). Acromegaly can be recognized by abnormal or overgrowth of the hands and feet, as well as other signs such as enlargement of the facial features in an adult. Although both acromegaly and gigantism have a similar cause, they are different. Acromegaly occurs in adulthood, when the long bones of the legs and arms have stopped growing (Understanding Acromegaly http://www.acromegalyinfo.com/info/understanding/home.jsp).

In children, before closure of the bone growth plates, the condition is known as gigantism. Gigantism caused by large amounts of GH results in excessive growth of the long bones in a child. Children affected by gigantism can grow to extraordinary heights. It also affects the child's muscle and organ growth, making the child look very large for his or her age. It may be noted as early as the sixth to ninth month of life. Whether acromegaly or gigantism, these conditions involve changes in the way the body functions and can delay puberty. Over time, these changes can cause complications (such as cardiomegaly or diabetes) that can be life threatening. It is imperative to obtain an early diagnosis and initiate a treatment plan as soon as the condition has been discovered. Early treatment can prevent irreversible changes that can ultimately lead to a premature death. Mortality rates can be two to fourfold higher in these patients because of the strain this excessive growth has on the vital organs such as the heart and pancreas.

Acromegaly/gigantism is a rare disease that affects about three to six out of every million people in the United States. Acromegaly/gigantism is caused by the uncontrolled hypersecretion of GH by the pituitary. In most cases, the cause of this excessive production of GH is a noncancerous tumor on the pituitary. Gigantism may also be caused by multiple endocrine neoplasms, McCune Albright syndrome (MAS), neurofibromatosis, or Carney complex.

 Nursing Insight— *Understanding acromegaly/ gigantism*

To understand the causes and treatment of acromegaly/ gigantism, the nurse needs to understand the three important hormones that circulate throughout the body to regulate many of the body's most basic activities:

- Growth hormone (GH)
  - The pituitary releases GH in short spurts throughout the day and night, resulting in constantly varying GH levels.
  - When a person has acromegaly/gigantism, abnormally high levels of GH are released by the pituitary. Too much GH causes changes in physical characteristics and other aspects of the body.
- Insulin-like growth factor (IGF-1): IGF-1 levels rise whenever GH levels rise, but IGF-1 is released more evenly than GH, and IGF-1 levels remain higher longer. Researchers believe that elevated IGF-1 levels probably cause most of the changes to one's body that are associated with acromegaly.
- Somatostatin: One of the main effects of somatostatin is its ability to control the amount of GH in the body. Researchers have taken advantage of this knowledge in developing treatments for acromegaly. Natural somatostatin is broken down by the body in a matter of minutes, whereas treatments based on somatostatin remain active much longer.

SIGNS AND SYMPTOMS. The signs and symptoms of acromegaly/gigantism may include gradual enlargement of the hands and feet in adults (may be indicated by increased ring or shoe size), and rapid growth during childhood (giantism in children). There may be swelling of soft tissue, skin tags, thyroid disorders, muscle weakness, and fatigue. Skin changes (thickening, oiliness, and acne, hirsutism) and coarsening of facial features, including forehead, nose, lips, tongue, and jaw, are common.

These changes do not appear in adults until 30 or 40 years of age, whereas in children, a rapid increase in skeletal growth would be seen each time the child is plotted on the appropriate growth chart.

Beside the changes in appearance, acromegaly/gigantism produces body function changes. These symptoms are listed in the order of most frequent to least frequent and become more pronounced as the child becomes older: arthralgia (arthritis-like joint pain), delayed onset of puberty or amenorrhea or irregular menstruation in women, excessive perspiration, sleep apnea, headaches, paresthesia or carpal tunnel syndrome, loss of libido or impotence, hypertension, goiter, and visual field defects.

DIAGNOSIS. The best way to diagnose acromegaly is to measure serum GH levels after an overnight fast and then again after giving a glucose drink (oral glucose tolerance test). A glucose ingestion of 75 grams would lower a healthy person's GH level to less than 2 ng/mL. In a child with gigantism and an overproduction of GH, this reduction would not be seen.

As a response to increases in GH, insulin-like growth factor (IGF-1), produced in the liver, also increases. IGF-1 levels are much more stable over time than GH, therefore, it provides a more reliable test than GH levels.

Since more than 90% of children with acromegaly/ gigantism suffer from benign tumors of the pituitary gland (an adenoma), other tests, such as head scans by MRI or by computed tomography (CT), look specifically for a pituitary growths or tumors. These tumors are usually the source of the excessive GH secretion.

NURSING CARE. Nursing care includes assisting in providing treatments that are aimed toward curing the cause. If there is a tumor, surgical removal is warranted. It has been found that surgery is the curative treatment of choice in 80% of the cases. Unfortunately, there are cases in which the surgical procedures cannot completely remove the tumor.

In these instances, medications are the treatments of choice. Somatostatin analogs or dopamine agonists are effective in reducing the release of GH secretion. The dopamine agonists are usually less effective medications but are usually the first drug of choice because they are easy to administer orally. Somatostatin analogs must be administered by a subcutaneous injection every 8 hours and can be difficult to administer.

In 2003, pegvisomant (Somavert) (a new drug class, GH receptor antagonist) became available. Traditionally, reducing pituitary tumor secretion of GH has been the treatment of choice, thus lowering serum IGF-I levels. Pegvisomant (Somavert) blocks the actions of circulating GH excess, but does not lower serum GH levels (Freda, 2006). Although dosages are not clearly identified for children (Schwartz, 2007), this medication is easy to administer and can be given once every 24 hours by subcutaneous injection.

Another attempt to slow GH release has been with radiation therapy. This is the slowest course of treatment in that it can take 5 to 10 years to see the full effects and almost always affects the proper excretion of other hormones as well. Many other hormones can be affected resulting in hypothyroidism, adrenal insufficiency, hypogonadism, and rarely diabetes insipidus. Radiation therapy has many side effects in children, such as learning disabilities, obesity, and emotional changes. Most experts use radiation only when all other treatments fail.

Nursing care should focus on the initial aspects of accurate assessment of growth by using the correct growth chart and by meticulously documenting height and weight at each outpatient visit. When a child is affected with gigantism, the patterns of abnormal growth are quite recognizable. Rather than just unusual tallness, there is a characteristic body build consisting of heavy thick bones, especially jaw, and unusually large hands and feet. Careful physical assessment is important to observe and document, as is the cognizance of laboratory values. Clinically an accurate assessment is one of the most important aspects of care.

In addition to assessment, the pediatric nurse should focus on the medication that the child receives. Medication regimens should be followed thoroughly and patient family teaching is of utmost importance. Medication regimens, including the administration of subcutaneous injections, and regular physician visits are extremely important. Follow-up home care may be needed in some cases depending on the status of the child's health and the resources available to the family. In the first few weeks of treatment, home health nursing visits would benefit the family by reinforcing the discharge teaching and by giving them a sense of confidence regarding the medication delivery and care of the child.

Postsurgical care after pituitary tumor excision requires precise critical neurosurgical care. Neurological and vital signs must be taken frequently. Depending on the surgical site (sometimes it is removed through the nose), care must include observations and documentation of dressing, wound, and drainage. Usually the first dressing is changed by the surgeon or advanced practice nurse. It is necessary to follow hospital protocols and physician's orders with regard to the appropriate care to give postoperatively.

Complications of this condition are numerous, and the focus of care should be measured to intervene and prevent them. The nurse must remember that lifelong monitoring and evaluation are vital in order to maintain optimal health. This is a very rare disorder, with little clinical experience in children. Multi-team efforts can help to extend and normalize life as much as possible. The earliest interventions can help prevent many serious complications that can lead to a premature death. Progressive, untreated disease can cause serious complications, such as hypertension, cardiomyopathy, and subsequent cardiovascular disease, osteoarthritis, diabetes mellitus, polyps of colon, sleep apnea, carpal tunnel syndrome, hypopituitarism, uterine fibroid tumors, spinal cord compression, and vision loss.

CONDITIONS OF THE POSTERIOR PITUITARY

Diabetes Insipidus

Diabetes insipidus is caused when there is an insufficient production of antidiuretic hormone (ADH). ADH acts on the kidneys to conserve water by controlling the kidneys' urine output. ADH is secreted by the hypothalamus and stored in the posterior pituitary gland before it is released into the bloodstream. When sufficient ADH is secreted, the amount of urine output is decreased to avoid dehydration. When a child has diabetes insipidus, there is insufficient ADH resulting in excessive production of extremely dilute urine. This causes the child to be excessively thirsty. In simple terms, diabetes insipidus can be called a disease of water regulation, causing the child to exhibit polydipsia (extreme thirst) and polyuria (excessive urination). Diabetes insipidus is categorized into two groups:

Central diabetes insipidus (or neurogenic), the production or secretion of ADH is insufficient. It can be caused by damage directly to the pituitary gland, such as head injury, neurosurgery, a genetic disorder, and other diseases.

Nephrogenic diabetes insipidus, the lack of the kidney's appropriate response to normal levels of ADH. It can be caused by drugs or chronic disorders, such as kidney failure, sickle cell disease, or polycystic kidney disease.

Generally occurring *suddenly*, diabetes insipidus can be due to many medical or surgical conditions:

Surgical (most common causes):

- Damage due to neurosurgery (i.e., hypothalamus or pituitary gland)
- Brain injury or tumor excision

Medical:

- Hypothalamus malfunction (insufficient ADH production)
- Pituitary gland malfunction (ADH is not released into the bloodstream)
- Vascular abnormalities or cerebral vascular accident (CVA) or "stroke"
- Infection
  - Encephalitis—brain inflammation
  - Meningitis—inflammation of meninges
  - Sarcoidosis—inflammation of the lymph nodes and other tissues throughout the body
  - Tuberculosis—infectious disease
- Family heredity—genetic defect (Chan & Roth, 2006)

SIGNS AND SYMPTOMS. Children experience and verbalize symptoms of the disease very differently. Infants are very difficult to assess because verbalization is through crying no matter what the problem is. It is helpful to separate signs and symptoms of diabetes insipidus into infant and child categories to accurately ascertain which symptom the pediatric patient is manifesting.

 assessment tools Signs and Symptoms of Diabetes Insipidus

Infant can manifest the following:	Child may experience these symptoms:
Irritability	Excessive thirst (polydipsia)
Poor feeding *(despite vigorous suck)*	Excessive urine production (polyuria)
Failure to grow/thrive	Enuresis (nocturnal bed wetting)
Vomiting	
Constipation	
High fevers	

 clinical alert

Dehydration

Dehydration can be seen in all cases, causing the infant/child to be irritable with many other manifestations, including dry mucous membranes, decreased skin turgor, decreased tears when crying, sunken fontanel and tachycardia. If dehydration is severe, the child's pulse may be thready and very rapid. Hypotension may also be present and could lead to hypovolemic shock. If dehydration occurs, it is important to administer IV fluids.

DIAGNOSIS. After a complete history, physical examination, and daily log of fluid and dietary intake and output patterns, the first morning urine is usually collected and subsequently tested for specific gravity, osmolarity, and sodium. Ideally, the morning urine would be collected after an overnight fast. If the urine is dilute (specific gravity of 1.005 or less) and the osmolarity (greater than 300 Osmol/kg) and sodium (as high as 170 mEq/L) are elevated, the diagnosis can be effectively confirmed. Diagnosis can be difficult in infants because they excrete dilute urine naturally.

 diagnostic tools Diagnosis of Diabetes Insipidus

The diagnosis of diabetes insipidus, including type (neurogenic central or nephrogenic) can be given definitively after a water deprivation test. This test is done under close supervision of the patient's vital signs. Urine and blood are collected early in the day and tested for osmolarity and electrolytes. The child is then deprived of water until significant dehydration occurs. The child is weighed every 2 hours until 2%–5% of body weight is lost. Urine specific gravity is monitored hourly; this test can be stopped if the specific gravity is 1.014 or higher. Urine and blood specimens can be sent for osmolarity midway through the deprivation test, i.e., 2 hours in an infant and 4 hours in a child. This water deprivation test should never be longer than a total of 4 hours in an infant and 7 hours in a child. During this test, the child may become febrile and develop hypotension. Vital signs should be watched very closely and taken every hour if necessary. A 24-hour urine collection may also be ordered to determine total daily urine output.

NURSING CARE. It is essential to differentiate between central (neurogenic) and nephrogenic diabetes insipidus before decisions are made regarding treatments and nursing care. For central diabetes insipidus, when polyuria is persistent, intranasal, parenteral, or oral doses of desmopressin (DDAVP) are the treatments of choice. Desmopressin (DDAVP) is a synthetic vasopressin analogue (Children's Hospitals and Clinics of Minnesota, 2007b). The diuretic chlorothiazide (Diuril) is given to decrease urine volume by up to 75%.

Nephrogenic diabetes insipidus cannot be effectively treated with DDAVP because of the lack of effective receptor sites, thus making the kidney unresponsive. Diuretics, amiloride (Midamor) (potassium-sparing diuretic) and indomethacin (Indocin) (nonsteroidal prostaglandin) or aspirin are all useful to help treat the child.

 Nursing Insight— *Action of diuretics on the kidney*

Diuretics impede the sodium chloride reabsorption that occurs in the distal tubule of the kidney. This reduces the loss of free water and increases the concentration of the child's urine. Reduction in urine volume derives from a concomitant action on the proximal tubule, which causes reabsorption of sodium chloride from the glomerular filtrate, thus drawing additional water along. This results in both a smaller volume and a higher concentration of the urine (Chan & Roth, 2006).

It is important for the nurse to remember that a diet low in solutes helps this condition. Generally, infants should be given breast milk because it is naturally low in solutes. Protein content in diets should be about 6% of an infant's diet and only 8% of a young child's diet. This should be enough to allow normal growth but not cause a solute excess.

The nurse should observe the child and closely monitor urine output. In addition, the nurse must keep very close track of fluid balance. The best way to measure fluid balance is by weighing the patient daily. Daily weights should be done using exact conditions (i.e., same scale, infants completely undressed including diaper, young child in underwear with socks only). Output measurements must also be exact and include weighing diapers in grams for infants. All output voided into the toilet or into a urinal

should be caught in a container to enable precise measurement of urine in milliliters. Record keeping and communication to the rest of the health care team should emphasize exact amounts taken in and excreted. The pediatric nurse should closely monitor the child for subtle signs of impending dehydration or fluid imbalance.

Caring for a child with diabetes insipidus can be difficult during the water deprivation test. The child becomes very irritable due to thirst and it may be difficult for the child to understand why he or she cannot drink. The child becomes more and more irritable, which is frustrating for the parents to deal with as well. Extreme patience is necessary to help the child and parents during this time. The nurse and parents can alternate holding and comforting the child as well as using distraction methods.

Accurate administration of medications is also a key factor when providing nursing care. The intranasal form of desmopressin (DDAVP) may be difficult to give and special care should be taken to give the medication accurately and also teach the parents proper administration.

Patient and parent teaching, as with most conditions, is of utmost importance. Parents must be taught to replace fluids in the very young child or infant because these patients cannot be relied on to accurately express thirst nor can these patients obtain a drink on their own without help from an adult. Also, common gastrointestinal illnesses that either increase fluid needs or decrease intake must be identified and the nurse must alert parents to the seriousness of these conditions that can lead to life-threatening fluid and electrolyte imbalances (Chan & Roth, 2006). Early discovery and care of the child with diabetes insipidus is important. This condition demands close monitoring of the fluid and electrolyte balance to prevent complications (Hudson, 2007). Family involvement is the key to successful home management. Helping the family by beginning a log of accurate intake, output, and daily weight while the child is hospitalized can be the greatest asset and optimize outcomes to this very challenging care situation.

 clinical alert

Critical thinking question

Will you always see poor skin turgor or tenting of abdominal skin? The answer is *no*. When the child has hypernatremic dehydration, skin turgor is not decreased despite the state of dehydration (Chan & Roth, 2006).

This state of hypernatremia places the child at an increased risk for seizures. If left untreated, diabetes insipidus can cause a child to have brain damage and impaired mental function or attention-deficit/hyperactive disorder (ADHD), short attention span, or restlessness (Children's Hospital Boston, 2007).

 medication: Accurate Administration of Intranasal Medication Doses

Intranasal DDAVP is administered through a rhinal tube. Ensure the child blows his or her nose before the medication is given. Positioning the child on the side the medication is given enhances the absorption of the medication. Instructions to parents should be as clear as possible. Refer to the Family Resource Center Library at www.childrensmn.org for explicit patient family education materials.

where research and practice meet:
Alternative Measures for Diabetes Insipidus

Alternative measures could be significant in treating the common childhood illnesses such as the vomiting and diarrhea that can be fatal in a child with diabetes insipidus. In all instances, it is crucial to prevent dehydration. There are many homeopathic therapies that treat diarrhea that have been proven to be more effective than some conventional treatments. Homeopathy is defined as stimulating the natural healing abilities of the body to cure the disease.

In a recent study of children with acute diarrhea, those who received individualized homeopathic treatment for 5 days had a significantly shorter duration of diarrhea than children who received placebo. Some of the most effective homeopathic remedies are listed below. An experienced homeopath assesses the physical, emotional, and intellectual make-up when determining the most appropriate remedy for a particular individual (A.D.A.M., 2004).

Arsenicum album—used for foul-smelling diarrhea from food poisoning or traveler's diarrhea with burning sensation in the abdomen and around the anus. This remedy is most appropriate for individuals who feel exhausted yet restless and whose symptoms tend to worsen in the cold and improve with warmth. Vomiting may also occur. *Arsenicum* may also be used to prevent diarrhea when traveling

Chamomilla—used for greenish, frothy stool that smells like rotten eggs; used primarily for children, especially those who are irritable, argumentative, and difficult to console; commonly recommended for colicky or teething infants

Calcarea carbonica—used for children who fear being in the dark or alone and who perspire heavily while sleeping; stools have a sour odor

Mercurius—used for foul-smelling diarrhea that may have streaks of blood accompanied by a sensation of incomplete emptying; this remedy is most appropriate for individuals who tend to feel exhausted after bowel movements, experience extreme changes in body temperatures, perspire heavily, and have a thirst for cold fluids

Podophyllum—used for explosive, gushing, painless diarrhea that becomes worse after eating or drinking; exhaustion often follows bowel movements and the individual for whom this remedy is appropriate may experience painful cramps in lower extremities; often used in infants for diarrhea experienced from teething

Pulsatilla—used for diarrhea that occurs after consuming too much fruit or rich, greasy food; stools are greenish in infants and of changing consistencies in older children

Sulfur—used for irritable and crying children; may have a red ring around the anus and diarrhea with the odor of rotten eggs

Veratrum album—used for profuse, watery diarrhea accompanied by stomach cramps, bloated abdomen, vomiting, exhaustion, and chills; the diarrhea is worsened by fruit, and the individual craves cold liquids (A.D.A.M., 2006).

Therapies such as acupuncture (used with children in China but not used for diarrhea in the United States), hypnosis, relaxation therapy as well as conditioning have been used and found to be useful in the treatment of vomiting.

Collaboration in Caring— *Collaboration with parents*

Collaboration with the parents helps to manage the child's care at home. It is important to also keep the physician alerted to any dehydration states the child may acquire. Early recognition of the disease in addition to recognizing excessive fluid losses, as well as the ability to replace excessive losses, is the key to long-term survival. A dietician or pediatric endocrinologist may also work closely with the primary pediatrician and the family to care for this child.

Syndrome of Inappropriate Antidiuretic Hormone

Although syndrome of inappropriate antidiuretic hormone (SIADH) is rare in children, it can be caused when excessive levels of antidiuretic hormones (ADH) are produced. Without ADH the kidneys and body cannot conserve the correct amount of water. The syndrome causes the body to retain water and causes levels of certain electrolytes (sodium) in the blood to decrease. Despite this decrease in osmolarity and electrolytes, the kidneys respond to the excessive ADH by causing more water reabsorption. Eventually this results in water intoxication, which is a large amount of water to a decreased amount of sodium in the extracellular fluid. Hyponatremia results with cellular edema.

SIADH occurs most frequently in children with CNS infections, intrathoracic disease, and can occur in postoperative patients. Among premature neonates, the syndrome most often accompanies brain injury and is closely associated with intracranial hemorrhage (Ferry, 2006). It can also be caused by hypoxia and positive pressure ventilation. In other cases, some medications (diuretics) and chemotherapy may produce the antidiuretic hormone. Other causes may include the following: meningitis, encephalitis, brain tumors, psychosis, lung diseases, head trauma, Guillain-Barré syndrome (GBS), certain medications such as diuretics or chemotherapy, damage to the hypothalamus or pituitary gland during surgery, as well as positive pressure ventilation.

SIGNS AND SYMPTOMS. Every child experiences and expresses symptoms quite differently. Symptoms in more severe cases of SIADH may include nausea and vomiting, seizures, personality changes such as irritability, combativeness, confusion, and hallucinations as well as stupor and coma (Lucile Packard Children's Hospital at Stanford, 2007).

Other signs and symptoms may include increased blood pressure, weight gain with no externally visible edema, decreased urine output despite a high specific gravity, and fluid and electrolyte imbalance. As the electrolyte (especially sodium) levels decrease the child becomes lethargic and confused. Often, if the child is old enough, complaints of a headache are also common. Eventually, altered levels consciousness followed by seizures and coma can be seen.

DIAGNOSIS. SIADH is diagnosed through serum level tests.

 diagnostic tools Serum Levels

Laboratory serum levels are monitored. Diagnosis is confirmed when the following values are found:
- High urine osmolarity (greater than 1200 Osmol/kg)
- High urine specific gravity (greater than 1.030)
- Low serum osmolarity (less than 275 mOsmol/kg)
- Low serum sodium (less than 125 mEq/L)
- Decreased BUN (less than 10 mg/dL)
- Decreased hematocrit

NURSING CARE. Fluid restriction is the cornerstone of care for a child with SIADH. The fluid restriction is begun at 75% of maintenance and decreased further to half of maintenance only if there is no improvement within 4 to 6 hours. Hypertonic sodium chloride solution is given if severe hyponatremia and severe neurological disease are present. Corticosteroids are given only when adrenal insufficiency is present. Vasopressin analogs are still experimental treatments.

Fluid restriction is the most difficult aspect of nursing care. This restriction can be challenging to maintain, especially if the child is old enough to reach the sink or water fountain. Fluid intake by all routes must be recorded as intake. The pediatric nurse must meticulously monitor and record all intake and output. Sometimes, the placement of a Foley catheter is necessary or weighing soiled diapers in grams is needed to ensure accurate measurements of output. The nurse must remember to obtain the weight of a clean diaper so that it can be subtracted from that of the soiled diaper weight before recording the output.

Medications should be given with meals to prevent any unnecessary fluid intake. If the child is thirsty, he or she can be offered hard candy to suck, providing the child's medical condition does not contraindicate the sugar. To prevent water reabsorption in the intestines, tap water and saline enemas should be avoided. Irrigate all oral tubes with normal saline rather than with water to prevent pulling of sodium thus creating an even greater electrolyte imbalance. Oral mucous membranes can be kept moist by providing frequent mouth care. Avoid alcohol-based mouth washes as these dry out the mucous membranes. The nurse must also monitor the child's nutritional status. A diet high in sodium and protein should be encouraged as this increases urine excretion.

The nurse understands that neurological assessments are also imperative. Assessing level of consciousness, headache (if child can verbalize), and seizure activity can be indications of *severe* electrolyte imbalance. Seizure precautions must be set up and implemented at the bedside.

Finally, the pediatric nurse should evaluate for fluid retention. When fluid retention is suspected, monitoring of input and output (I & O), baseline weight, and daily weight is essential. The nurse evaluates patients for edema in dependent areas and assesses the child's lungs to detect overhydration and monitor skin turgor carefully. Each of these assessments must be clearly communicated to subsequent physicians and nurses who will assume care for the child.

Educating parents about the importance of fluid balance is a significant aspect of teaching the care of a child with SIADH. The family must also be taught that a daily weight of the child is the most important indicator of fluid balance. Maintaining fluid balance and avoiding excessive fluid intake should also be emphasized. The pediatric nurse should be sure to include hidden sources of water in foods to optimize the outcomes of this child's care. Family members should be taught to measure the urine output accurately, using whatever is appropriate for the child (i.e., diaper weights, urinal use, or toilet "hats"). In addition to teaching all of the care aspects for the child with SIADH, the pediatric nurse should be sure to include basic information about SIADH and its causes, signs, and symptoms.

Along with the primary care physician, an endocrinologist, often a nephrologist, a neurologist, and possibly a pediatric intensive care specialist may need to be consulted if the child manifests severe clinical, neurological symptoms.

 Now Can You— Describe conditions of the anterior and posterior pituitary?

1. Describe conditions of the anterior pituitary?
2. Discuss nursing care for conditions of the anterior pituitary?
3. Describe conditions of the posterior pituitary?
4. Discuss nursing care for conditions of the posterior pituitary?

CONDITIONS OF THE THYROID

Hypothyroidism

Congenital hypothyroidism affects about one in every 4000 newborns in North America. In hypothyroidism the thyroid gland is underactive, secreting too little thyroid hormone for the body to function normally. If left untreated hypothyroidism can lead to a goiter. The thyroid gland secretes thyroid hormones, which control the speed of metabolism. Brain development, as well as the normal growth of the child, depends on normal levels of thyroid hormone. Hypothyroidism was once referred to as cretinism and was thought to be a major cause of severe mental retardation, but this view is not held today. In older children and young adults, hypothyroidism can also cause diverse symptoms including slowed heart rate, chronic tiredness, and inability to tolerate cold. The child may feel physically tired, mentally fatigued, and thus learning may be impaired. Infants can be born with congenital hypothyroidism, and hypothyroidism can develop in children of any age. Iodine is needed to produce thyroid hormones and is contained in many foods.

SIGNS AND SYMPTOMS. Hypothyroidism has varying levels of manifestations from subtle in infancy to overt as the child matures. In an infant the signs and symptoms are prolonged newborn jaundice, poor feeding and constipation, cool, mottled skin, increased sleepiness, decreased crying, larger-than-normal soft spots on the skull, umbilical hernia (a soft protrusion around the navel), and a large tongue.

As the child begins to grow and mature, hypothyroidism manifests in these ways: short stature for age and delayed eruption of baby teeth, delays in major developmental milestones, puffy facial features, severe mental retardation, protruding abdomen and umbilical hernia, dry skin and sparse hair.

The older child has the most overt symptoms, much like those found in the adult. These include slow heart rate, tiredness, inability to tolerate cold, dry, flaky skin, puffiness in the face (especially around the eyes), impaired memory and difficulty in thinking (appears as a learning disability), emotional depression, drowsiness, even after sleeping through the night, heavy or irregular menstrual periods (in girls at the age of puberty), and constipation.

DIAGNOSIS. Congenital hypothyroidism is usually detected during the routine newborn screening. Blood samples taken reveal abnormally low levels of T3 and T4.

 clinical alert

Hyponatremia

It is critical to remember that the hyponatremia (low serum sodium of less than 125 mEq/L) may cause seizures in the child with SIADH. Keeping the serum sodium level as near as normal is the goal of treatment. The pediatric nurse must be thorough and accurately track intake, output, and daily weights of the child.

Sometimes seen as an inborn error of thyroid hormone synthesis, the ill child's thyroid cannot produce T3 and T4 despite increasing levels of thyroid-stimulating hormone (TSH) produced by the pituitary (Cleary & Green, 2005). Further diagnosis may include a scan of the thyroid gland to check for abnormalities. Diagnosis is relatively simple, requiring one blood test once hypothyroidism is suspected.

NURSING CARE. Early diagnosis of hypothyroidism is of the utmost importance. One study suggests that the optimal care would include early diagnosis as soon after birth as possible and normalization of blood levels of thyroid hormone with low-dose levothyroxine (Synthroid) for one month (Yang et al., 2005). Daily treatment involves giving the child a prescription thyroid replacement hormone. The initial dose for an infant is between 25 and 50 mcg per day. Iodine supplementation is also appropriate in some cases. The easiest supplements are given in the diet. The goal of treatment is normal hormone levels within the infant's first 4 weeks of life. Frequent (usually weekly) visits to the treating physician for follow-up blood tests and adjustments of the dose are necessary. Once the baby's hormone levels are properly adjusted, return outpatient visits are needed every 2 to 3 months for the first 3 years of life. Thyroid hormone treatment may be needed for life, but fortunately, treatment is simple, inexpensive, and easily monitored.

 Nursing Insight— Formula

Soy-based formula may cause a decrease in the absorption of levothyroxine (Synthroid). Switching an infant from a milk-based formula to a soy-based formula may increase the dose of thyroid hormone needed to maintain a euthyroid status (having a normally functioning thyroid gland) (Postellon, 2006).

Parents are taught proper administration of the medication. The pills can be crushed in a spoon, dissolved with a small amount of water or other liquid immediately before administration, and administered to the child with a syringe, dropper, or nipple. Toddlers can be allowed to readily chew the tablets (Postellon, 2006).

Parents need to be informed that careful and regular monitoring of the child's growth, weight gain, and developmental milestone progression helps to validate that the dosing and medication administration are sufficiently accurate to achieve positive results. Laboratory blood tests

 medication: Accurate Administration of Hormone Tablets

Hormone tablets (or any pills) should never be mixed in a full bottle of formula. It is best to avoid ruining the taste of the infant's sole source of nutrition. Second, placing the medication in a full bottle will require the baby to drink the entire bottle to obtain the entire dose. Leaving even a small amount of formula on the bottom of the bottle could mean that the child will be under dosed. Most drug references state that hormone tablets mix very unevenly in solution and it is difficult for them to stay in suspension. It is best to crush and mix it in a small amount of fluid immediately before administration. The solution is then drawn up into an oral syringe and given before the feeding.

of T4 and TSH every 4 to 6 months during the first year of life and every 2 to 4 months afterward also keep close track of the child's hormone levels. Parents should also be encouraged to seek early evaluation and intervention to any problems that become readily recognizable. Educating the parents completely at the very beginning regarding the diagnosis, its signs and symptoms, care, treatment, and outcomes of care ensures that they know what to watch for and are astute as to the most effective care possible.

It is essential that the nurse is aware that congenital hypothyroidism is an important cause of mental retardation and that it is definitely preventable with the earliest identification and subsequent treatment. Educating parents regarding the signs and symptoms helps to identify the condition early so treatment can be started as soon as possible. Alerting the families with infants with this condition that life-time treatment prevents mental retardation is an important component of teaching. Newborn lab results must be assessed and follow-up for any abnormal results is mandatory.

For children whose condition is not rapidly diagnosed or treated, the return of normal thyroid function may take a long time. The child may exhibit dramatic changes in behavior. Continued care by the primary physician, the endocrinologist, and a psychotherapist may be necessary. It should be brought to the teacher's attention as well as any ongoing recommendations to help the child achieve his or her optimum potential.

Graves' Disease

Graves' disease (hyperthyroidism) is the most common cause of hyperthyroidism in children (Ferry, 2006). Many researchers believe that Graves' disease is caused by an antibody that overstimulates the thyroid, causing an excess production of thyroid hormone. It is categorized as an autoimmune disorder.

Graves' disease is most common in young to middle-aged women and tends to run in families. Incidence increases with age, reaching a peak during adolescence. It is rare in children younger than 5 years of age (Ferry, 2006).

SIGNS AND SYMPTOMS. Excessive thyroid hormone affects all organ systems of the body. Symptoms of Graves' disease are identical to those of hyperthyroidism, with the addition of three other symptoms. Although these symptoms present somewhat differently in each child, they are: (1) goiter (enlarged thyroid gland which may cause a bulge in the neck and dysphagia); (2) raised, thickened skin over the shins, back of feet, back, hands, or face; and (3) swollen, reddened eyes that bulge (exophthalmos).

Other signs and symptoms can include fast heart rate with palpitations, high blood pressure, moist skin and increased perspiration, shakiness and tremor, nervousness and confusion, increased appetite accompanied by weight loss, difficulty sleeping, constant stare, sensitivity of eyes to light, and changes in menstrual periods.

DIAGNOSIS. As with other thyroid conditions, blood levels of thyroid hormones confirm the diagnosis. These hormones are elevated. TSH levels are decreased because the high levels of T3 and T4 inhibit the anterior pituitary's production of TSH (Amer, 2005).

NURSING CARE. Physical assessment is first and foremost in the care of the child with Graves' disease. The astute nurse may identify these children when they are referred for evaluation of symptoms of attention deficit/ hyperactivity disorder (ADHD). A complete history including school performance and how distracted the child has been, together with sleep patterns, will aid in the ongoing care of the child. Once the child is diagnosed, treatment regimens must be taught to the child and family and strictly followed. The nurse knows that treatment for hyperthyroidism is specifically individualized for each patient. Ultimately, the goal of treatment is to restore the thyroid gland to normal function in which the production of thyroid hormone is at normal levels.

Treatment may include:

- Antithyroid medications (PTU-propylthiouracil or MTZ—methimazole) to help lower the level of thyroid hormones by blocking the synthesis of T3 and T4. Pharmacotherapy has been used the longest, but has toxic side effects (Table 28-1).
- Radioactive iodine therapy (in the form of a pill or liquid), which damages thyroid cells (destruction can take 6 to 18 weeks) to decrease the production of thyroid hormones
- Surgery to remove the overactive nodule of the thyroid (subtotal thyroidectomy)
- Beta-blocking agents (Inderal) to block the action of thyroid hormone on the body (these drugs do not change the levels of thyroid hormone in the blood, but make the patient feel better by relieving tachycardia, restlessness, and tremors).

Children with Graves' disease are treated on an outpatient basis for the most part. The parents need to know the significance of continuing the medication regimen even after the symptoms of hyperthyroidism have resolved. Parents must also be taught to watch for medication side effects. The importance of routine blood tests must also be emphasized as well as following through with all return visits to the physician. If referrals are made, the importance of keeping these appointments must also be stressed.

Even though the child is being treated for hyperthyroidism, the signs and symptoms of hypothyroidism must also be taught to the family so that if treatments become toxic they would know what symptoms to observe in the child. Emergency numbers and referrals must be provided to the family in the event that any of the severe reactions occur.

The importance of a low-stress, low-pressure environment should also be reinforced because increased tension could exacerbate the symptoms. The child may also exhibit sudden bursts of emotion such as crying, excitement, or irritability. The family should be taught to expect these feelings and that the ill child is not able to control them. The importance of discussing feelings with the child should be stressed in order to minimize these outbursts. Parents should be instructed to notify the child's school nurse and teacher about these feelings. The school nurse may need to be involved in the medication regime during school operational hours. In this case, a note from the child's physician is required. The teachers must also be alerted to the child's illness and the potential lack of focus in class. It may even be necessary to have the child tutored so that the child is able to catch up to the lessons.

The surgical option is used as a last resort when treatments have not resulted in permanent remission or when the parents cannot comply with the medication regimen. Although the treatment choice is a very delicate matter that should be thoroughly discussed between the physician and family, some physicians feel that total thyroidectomy is the preferred treatment for patients with Graves' disease (Lee, Grumbach, & Clark, 2007).

It is essential for the pediatric nurse to be very astute and know all of the many signs and symptoms of hyper- and hypothyroidism, because when the child begins to deteriorate it happens very quickly and there is not enough time to wait for lab results. The only indication for care in the hospital as an inpatient is if the child with hyperthyroidism experiences a thyroid storm.

 clinical alert

Thyroid storm

A thyroid storm is a rare and potentially fatal complication of hyperthyroidism. It typically occurs in patients who experience a precipitating event such as surgery, infection, or trauma. A thyroid storm must be recognized and treated on signs and symptoms alone, as laboratory confirmation often cannot be obtained in a timely manner. Patients typically appear markedly *hypermetabolic* with high fevers, tachycardia, nausea and vomiting, tremulousness, agitation, and psychosis if untreated. Patients may also become stuporous or comatose with hypotension.

CONDITIONS OF THE PARATHYROID

Hypoparathyroidism

Hypoparathyroidism is a rare condition in which there is inadequate production of parathyroid hormone. It can also occur when the parathyroid hormone that is produced cannot be used by the body or the kidneys and bones cannot respond to the production of parathyroid hormone. This deficiency of parathyroid hormone decreases the calcium level in the blood and increases the phosphate levels.

Hypoparathyroidism may be either inherited or acquired. It can result from a variety of causes:

- Underdeveloped parathyroid glands at birth (inherited)
- Medical treatment (radiation to thyroid gland, drug treatment, thyroid or parathyroid surgery) (acquired)
- An underlying medical condition such as cancer, neck trauma, Wilson's disease (high level of copper in tissues), an excess of iron in tissues, and low levels of magnesium (acquired)

Table 28-1 Side Effects of Antithyroid Medications	
Mild Effects	**Severe Effects (can be *Fatal*)**
Skin rash	Agranulocytosis (sore throat, high fever)
Mild leukopenia	Lupus-like syndrome
Loss of taste	Hepatitis
Arthralgia	Hepatic failure
Loss/abnormal hair pigmentation	Glomerulonephritis

The cause of hypoparathyroidism may also be idiopathic in that the parathyroid suddenly stops functioning for no known reason. It has also been associated with other conditions, especially cardiac defects, such as DiGeorge syndrome.

Nursing Insight— *DiGeorge syndrome*

DiGeorge syndrome is an example of a defect in parathyroid gland development. DiGeorge syndrome is comprised of hypoparathyroidism, T-cell abnormalities and cardiac anomalies.

SIGNS AND SYMPTOMS. The following signs and symptoms often appear in children with hypoparathyroidism: poor tooth development, vomiting, headaches, mental deficiency, seizures and uncontrollable, painful spasms of the face, hands, arms, and feet. Infants with hypoparathyroidism may be extremely irritable and have rigid muscles. They may also have abdominal distention and episodes of apnea causing irregular cyanosis.

DIAGNOSIS. A thorough history and physical, including muscle spasms, twitches, or seizure activity, is noted. Any vomiting with abdominal distention should be noted. Apnea episodes with or without cyanosis should be noted. Blood work including calcium (low), phosphate (high), magnesium (low), and low parathyroid hormone confirms the diagnosis. Bone or soft tissue abnormalities (increased bone density) are evaluated with radiographs and CT scans. A 12-lead EKG may reveal a prolonged QT interval.

NURSING CARE. Teaching the families about the disease, its signs and symptoms, as well as the importance of lifelong treatment optimizes the outcomes of the child's care. A lifelong regimen of dietary or supplemental calcium and vitamin D is usually required to restore calcium and mineral balance. In the acute phase of hypoparathyroidism, calcium is administered intravenously; diuretics may be prescribed in that circumstance as well to prevent overexcretion of calcium in the urine and to reduce the amount of calcium and vitamin D needed. The active form of vitamin D, 1, 25-dihydroxyvitamin D, is preferred in the treatment of hypoparathyroidism.

Hypocalcemia that produces the symptoms of hypoparathyroidism, such as seizures, tetany, and laryngospasms, requires intravenous calcium. The pediatric nurse must continuously monitor the child with telemetry for cardiac arrhythmias and blood pressure for life-threatening hypotension. Seizure precautions should be maintained until calcium levels approach a normal level. Once serum calcium levels are greater than 7.5 mg/dL the intravenous calcium can be stopped.

critical nursing action Accurate Administration of Intravenous Calcium

It is important for the pediatric nurse to scrupulously check the IV site for accurate placement as infiltration of the intravenous calcium supplements causes extravasation and sloughing of the tissue around the site. Intravenous calcium supplements must be properly calculated, diluted, and administered strictly according to hospital's standards of care and protocols.

Oral calcium and vitamin D are administered as soon as possible. The nurse must monitor the success of the oral forms of calcium and vitamin D for at least 24 hours after intravenous calcium is stopped because "rebound" hypocalcemia can occur. The pediatric nurse must be alert for subtle changes in the child's status.

Nursing Insight— *Assessing for Hyperreflexia of Muscles*

The nurse can assess for hyperreflexia (increased action of the reflexes) by tapping on the facial nerve. If there is a spasm of the facial muscles, this is a positive Chvostek sign (facial muscle spasm) and confirms the fact that the child has muscle pain, cramps, and probably twitches. These muscle manifestations may progress to numbness and tingling of the hands and feet as well as stiffness. Remember infants and small children cannot express these manifestations, and therefore just cry to communicate pain.

The prognosis for hypoparathyroidism is fairly good, especially with an early diagnosis. No special diet is needed, but adequate calcium and vitamin D intake is recommended. If phosphorus levels are extremely elevated, a diet may be given that excludes high-phosphorus foods such as eggs and dairy products.

Nursing Insight— *Proper nutrition for hypoparathyroidism*

The following supplements have been used clinically and, therefore, may be valuable adjuncts in the treatment of hypoparathyroidism:
* Calcium, if dietary intake is not adequate.
* Magnesium, which aids in the absorption of calcium; also, often low levels of magnesium are present in the case of hypoparathyroidism.
* Boron, which enhances the absorption of calcium.
* Vitamin K, produced by bacteria in the intestines or obtained through the diet (e.g., dark leafy greens) is important for the uptake of calcium by cells throughout the body.
* Foods rich in calcium include almonds, legumes, dark leafy greens, blackstrap molasses, oats, sardines, tahini, prunes, apricots, and sea vegetables.
* Calcium and vitamin D are thought to be best absorbed in an acidic environment (e.g., lemon juice may be added to salad to facilitate calcium absorption).
* Limit carbonated beverages, as they are high in phosphates and may reduce calcium absorption; dairy may diminish calcium absorption for similar reasons.
* Avoid caffeine (such as in coffee, black tea, colas, and chocolate); it can lead to calcium loss through the urine (A.D.A.M., 2006).

Children with hypoparathyroidism may be asymptomatic and often report vague symptoms. Therefore, it is vital to report any new onset of seizure or movement disorder to the physician immediately. Further evaluation should include serum calcium levels being checked.

The nurse can tell the family that the primary care provider will consult with an endocrinologist but will continue to manage the care of the child. Careful monitoring of calcium levels and doses of the medications ensures that the levels of calcium stay in the low to normal range. Close assessment helps to alleviate complications such as nephrocalcinosis. The nurse can also communicate that annual renal ultrasounds will ensure that this renal condition is not present.

Hyperparathyroidism

Hyperparathyroidism is rare in children. Primary hyperparathyroidism is more common in females and in adolescents. It is caused by overactive parathyroid glands that produce high levels of parathyroid hormone (PTH), which results in increased levels of serum calcium. The excess calcium leads to osteoporosis and osteomalacia (both bone-weakening diseases). Remember that high levels of parathyroid hormone cause the bones to demineralize, which increases the serum calcium levels. PTH also acts on the kidney to conserve calcium and excrete phosphate. Another result of the increased serum calcium is the development of kidney stones. Kidney stones form because of the high levels of calcium excreted into the urine by the kidneys. Primary hyperparathyroidism may develop as a result of one of the following conditions:

- Single or multiple benign tumors in the parathyroid glands
- Parathyroid hyperplasia (excessive growth of normal parathyroid cells)
- Parathyroid malignancies (rare)
- Certain endocrine disorders, such as type I and II multiple endocrine neoplasia (MEN) syndromes

SIGNS AND SYMPTOMS. At least 50% of patients with primary hyperparathyroidism have no symptoms, and approximately 1% of cases go undiagnosed. When symptoms do occur, they are generally attributed to persistently high levels of calcium. Symptoms include bone and joint pain, bone loss leading to osteoporosis with possible bone fractures, muscle weakness, abdominal discomfort due to pancreatitis, heartburn, nausea and vomiting, constipation, lack of appetite, peptic ulcers, kidney stones, excessive thirst, excessive urination, depression, anxiety, memory loss, and excessive drowsiness or fatigue.

DIAGNOSIS. Although this diagnosis is frequently delayed in children, it is usually diagnosed when the child becomes symptomatic. Evaluation of elevated blood calcium and parathyroid hormone levels is diagnostic in 100% of the children (Kollars et al., 2005). If radiographs are performed, the child's bones may show signs of rickets (Fig. 28-2).

NURSING CARE. Parathyroidectomy is effective and restores the normal blood calcium levels. This surgery has few complications and is the treatment of choice in children with primary hyperparathyroidism (Kollars et al., 2005). Unfortunately, if diagnosis is late, this surgical procedure cannot reverse the late effects of hyperparathyroidism on other organs, like the kidneys.

Postoperative care of the child after removal of the parathyroid is focused on airway management and frequent assessments for respiratory distress or airway obstruction due to edema at the surgical site. As with all surgical procedures, continual monitoring for signs of infection and hematoma should be done. Additional nursing care should focus on fluid management and

Figure 28-2 A radiograph taken to diagnose rickets.

consistent monitoring of the child's intake, output, and electrolyte balance.

The child and her family must be taught to consistently observe for signs and symptoms of hypocalcemia. Learning to administer calcium supplements is invaluable in that this treatment may need to be done for life.

Family members should also be taught to realize that frequent blood draws may be necessary initially to monitor calcium and phosphorus levels. The nurse can explain to the family that eventually the lab work can be done less frequently, but it needs be stressed that these blood tests are an important part of the continued health care of the child. The primary health care provider may recommend that the child take particular nutritional supplements because a child with primary hyperparathyroidism may develop deficiencies. Vitamins C and K as well as manganese are necessary for normal bone formation.

CONDITIONS OF THE ADRENALS

Acute Adrenocortical Insufficiency

 Nursing Insight— *An adrenal crisis is a life-threatening condition*

Adrenal crisis is a life-threatening condition in which the anterior pituitary gland does not make enough adrenocorticotropic hormone (ACTH). ACTH is responsible for regulating the adrenal gland (a gland near the kidneys that makes hormones that regulate bodily functions). Adrenal crisis is very serious, and children with adrenal crisis require *immediate* treatment. Parents need to seek emergency medical care immediately if they suspect an adrenal crisis.

Adrenal crisis may be caused by any of the following: rapid withdrawal from steroid therapy, sepsis, surgical stress, bleeding into the adrenal glands, pituitary necrosis, or thyroid hormone replacement in someone with adrenal insufficiency. The following factors increase the chance of developing adrenal crisis: septic shock, adrenal insufficiency, or use of steroid medications. If the child has any of these risk factors, the physician must be notified.

> ### critical nursing action Steroid Administration
>
> Steroid administration is never stopped abruptly. Steroids must be slowly weaned according to the physician's orders. An abrupt withdrawal can cause an adrenal crisis.

SIGNS AND SYMPTOMS. The child in adrenal crisis may exhibit any of these symptoms. Yet, it is important for the pediatric nurse to remember that these symptoms may also be caused by other, less serious health conditions. However, it is vital to report any of the following signs and symptoms to the physician: weakness, feeling tired all the time, nausea, vomiting, loss of appetite, weight loss, low blood pressure, abdominal pain, fever, confusion or coma, diarrhea, cyanosis, and dehydration.

DIAGNOSIS. Tests to diagnose adrenal crisis may include chest radiograph, computed tomography (CT) scan of the abdomen, and blood tests that detect ACTH and electrolytes levels, red blood cells, and other autoimmune or endocrine disorders.

NURSING CARE. Initially, steroid IV hydrocortisone (A-Hydrocort) and antibiotic drugs are needed to treat an adrenal crisis. If the child is vomiting or unconscious, the nurse gives these medications by injection or intravenously (IV). Owing to fluid loss, the child is given IV fluids to reverse dehydration, electrolyte imbalances, and hypovolemia. Whole blood may be given if the child has hemorrhaged. If the child is in severe crisis and has a decreased blood pressure, vasopressor may be used to raise the child's blood pressure quickly by vasoconstriction.

When all of these conditions are corrected and the child is stable, the cortisone medications and sodium chloride (NaCl) may be given orally. Retention of sodium is maintained by replacing aldosterone with synthetic steroids that retain salt.

The pediatric nurse must be cognizant of the fact that this crisis can be fatal and may quickly appear. The nurse must use constant assessment, and recognition of the signs and symptoms is essential. It may be necessary to take the child's vital signs every 15 minutes, always carefully watching for the most subtle signs of the onset of shock. These subtle signs of shock can include a slight cooling of the hands and feet along with a decrease in skin color. For instance, the infant's periphery goes from pink to extreme pallor.

 Ethnocultural Considerations— **Shock in dark-complexioned children**

When assessing for shock in children with a dark complexion remember to look at the palms of the hands, soles of the feet and lips to ascertain color changes.

The nurse recognizes that fluid shifts may also occur quickly, so lab values must be reviewed often. Cortisone and sodium chloride treatments are often given rapidly to

> ### Labs: Potassium Depletion
>
> Since treatments for adrenal crisis cause potassium depletion, it is crucial to keep a close watch on the child's lab values. Nursing assessments should always be mindful of the warning signs of hyperkalemia and hypokalemia (apnea, cardiac arrhythmias, paralysis, poor muscle control, and weakness).

rectify ominous situations. A consequence of this rapid treatment is an abnormally low potassium level such that the child can now be at risk for flaccid paralysis or seizures. It is good practice to keep the child in constant observation and to perform frequent assessments.

The nurse must monitor IV fluid rates and remain in constant communication with the physician so that responses to the treatments are known and counteracted if necessary. The pediatric nurse should be prepared to act quickly.

Medication administration is also a significant part of nursing care. Medications and doses should be given as prescribed by physician. Once the child has stabilized, clear, oral fluids can be initiated slowly. It would defeat the purpose if, in the child's eagerness to drink, he or she began to vomit again. For this reason, encourage the child to drink slowly. If the child refuses to drink, other forms of liquid such as ice pops, frozen ice, gelatin, or broth may give the child incentive to take fluids orally.

In this situation, parents are often in a state of confusion and shock because the treatments and changes in their child's condition occur so rapidly. The nurse should calmly explain the treatment and the child's response often. To decrease the parents' fear, noting slight improvements in the child's status helps them remain positive. Since neurological symptoms can be so devastating, remind the parents that these are only temporary and that paralysis will be reversed once the child is stabilized.

Discharge preparation should be started as soon after the crisis as possible. Keep in mind the readiness of the parents to learn. Be sure that the parents are ready to listen and learn about the care of the child at home. In some cases, it may be necessary to wait a day until the parents feel secure about the fact that their child will be going home under their care.

Parents need to know that some teens do not take prescribed medication doses because of the side effects. The nurse can reassure parents that this may happen and to call the primary pediatrician if it does.

Chronic Adrenocortical Insufficiency

Chronic adrenocortical insufficiency, or Addison's disease, is the result of an underactive adrenal gland. An underactive adrenal gland produces insufficient amounts of cortisol and aldosterone.

 Nursing Insight— *Cortisol and aldosterone*

Cortisol is a steroid hormone that helps to control the body's metabolism of fats, proteins, and carbohydrates; suppresses inflammatory reactions in the body; and affects immune system functions.

Aldosterone is a steroid hormone that controls sodium and potassium in the blood.

The onset of this disease may occur at any age. Most of the time, the cause of the disease is unknown. About one-third of Addison's disease cases are caused by the actual destruction of the adrenal glands through cancer, infection, an autoimmune process, or other diseases. Other causes may include the following:

- Use of corticosteroids as a treatment (such as prednisone) may cause a slowdown in production of natural corticosteroids by the adrenal glands and mimic Addison's disease.
- Certain medications used to treat fungal infections may block production of corticosteroids in the adrenal glands, causing signs and symptoms similar to those of Addison's disease.
- Rarely, Addison's disease is inherited as an X-linked, recessive trait, where the gene responsible for the condition is located on the X chromosome and passed down from a healthy female carrier to her sons who are affected. In this form, symptoms typically begin in childhood or adolescence.

Failure to produce adequate levels of cortisol can occur for different reasons. Corticosteroids play an important role in helping the body fight infection and promote health during physical stress. The problem may be due to a disorder of the adrenal glands themselves or to inadequate secretion of ACTH by the pituitary gland. The lack of adrenal hormones may cause:

- Elevated levels of potassium.
- Extreme sensitivity to the hormone insulin, which normally is present in the bloodstream. This sensitivity may lead to low blood sugar levels.
- Increased risk during stressful periods, such as surgery, infection, or injury.

PRIMARY ADRENAL INSUFFICIENCY. Most cases of primary adrenal insufficiency are caused by the gradual destruction of the adrenal cortex, the outer layer of the adrenal glands, by the body's own immune system. About 70% of reported cases of Addison's disease are caused by autoimmune disorders, in which the immune system makes antibodies that attack the body's own tissues or organs and slowly destroy them. Adrenal insufficiency occurs when at least 90% of the adrenal cortex has been destroyed. As a result, often both glucocorticoid (cortisol) and mineralocorticoid (aldosterone) hormones are lacking. Sometimes only the adrenal gland is affected, as in idiopathic adrenal insufficiency. In other cases, additional endocrine glands are also affected, as in the polyendocrine deficiency syndrome.

POLYENDOCRINE DEFICIENCY SYNDROME. The polyendocrine deficiency syndrome is classified into two separate forms:

- Type I occurs in children, and adrenal insufficiency may be accompanied by underactive parathyroid glands, slow sexual development, pernicious anemia, chronic *Candida* infections, chronic active hepatitis, and hair loss.
- Type II, often called *Schmidt's syndrome*, usually affects young adults. Features of type II may include an underactive thyroid gland, slow sexual development, diabetes, vitiligo, and loss of pigment on areas of the skin.

Scientists think that the polyendocrine deficiency syndrome is inherited because frequently more than one family member tends to have one or more endocrine deficiencies.

SIGNS AND SYMPTOMS. It is important to note that mild symptoms of Addison's disease may manifest only when the child is under physical stress. The most common symptoms of Addison's disease may often be seen individually or in any combination. Remember that each child experiences symptoms very differently. The astute pediatric nurse consistently observes for any of the following symptoms: weakness; fatigue; dizziness; rapid pulse; dark skin that is first noted on hands and face; black freckles; bluish-black discoloration around the nipples, mouth, rectum, scrotum, or vagina; weight loss; dehydration; loss of appetite; intense salt craving; muscle aches; nausea; vomiting; diarrhea; and an intolerance to the cold.

If left untreated, Addison's disease can lead to severe abdominal pain, extreme weakness, low blood pressure, kidney failure, and shock, especially when the child experiences physical stress. Although the symptoms of Addison's disease may resemble other problems or medical conditions, it is best for the pediatric nurse to encourage the parents to always consult the child's physician for a diagnosis confirmation.

The symptoms progress slowly and are usually ignored until a stressful event such as an illness or an accident causes the child's condition to worsen. This is called an addisonian crisis, or acute adrenal insufficiency. In most cases, symptoms are severe enough that patients seek medical treatment before a crisis occurs. However, in a few children, symptoms first become readily apparent during an addisonian crisis.

 clinical alert

Symptoms of an Addisonian crisis

Symptoms of an addisonian crisis include sudden penetrating pain in the lower back, abdomen, or legs, severe vomiting and diarrhea, dehydration, low blood pressure, and a loss of consciousness. If left untreated, a child with Addison's disease in crisis can die (NIH Publication No. 04–3054 June 2004).

DIAGNOSIS. Aside from the clinical symptoms and the signs found on physical examination, including low blood pressure, a diagnosis of Addison's disease is usually confirmed by laboratory tests. Typically, a patient has low blood sodium, high potassium, and low blood sugar. The initial test for adrenal insufficiency is the measurement of serum cortisol levels. The serum cortisol level is drawn in the morning between 6:00 A.M. and 8:00 A.M. because the levels are the highest at this time owing to circadian rhythm. Cortisol levels greater than 19 mg/dL are considered normal, whereas levels less than 3 mg/dL are diagnostic of Addison's disease (Liotta, 2007). Levels between 3 and 19 mg/dL are considered indeterminate and further testing is necessary.

NURSING CARE. Addison's disease is treatable with oral forms of the missing hormones. Cortisol (Solu-Cortef) is available in tablet form, and it is given two to three times a day. This medication helps maintain the child's blood glucose levels (Children's Hospital and Clinics of Minnesota, 2006).

If the patient has an illness that is accompanied by vomiting, an intramuscular injection of cortisol (Solu-Cortef) must be given at home. Then the patient must be taken to an emergency room for further treatment. All patients or their parents must have a dose of Cortisol (Solu-Cortef) available at home and be instructed on the proper technique to administer it during a crisis.

When a child is hospitalized in an adrenal crisis, the focus of nursing care is on fluid and electrolyte replacement. The pediatric nurse must monitor closely for signs of hypovolemic shock. The nurse understands that peripheral circulation must be checked often. Frequently, hourly assessments help the nurse detect subtle changes that can be the earliest indicators of potential imbalances not yet detected by laboratory tests.

 Optimizing Outcomes— **Hormone treatment**

The best outcome of care for the child is optimized with adequate hormonal treatment. Hormone treatment helps maintain a normal growth pattern. Even though a child with Addison's disease rarely grows beyond the fifth percentile, development during puberty is normal (Liotta, 2007).

Parents need to be aware of the diligent commitment that is necessary to giving the child medications routinely and regularly. They must plan medication delivery into their day so that it is never forgotten. The morning rush to school, the bus, or carpool may not be the best time to plan the cortisol replacements. Parents must also know that the drug cannot be stopped suddenly and that if the child is unable to ingest it due to vomiting, the injectable hydrocortisone must be given intramuscularly. Teaching IM injections is also necessary. Another important aspect of parent teaching involves providing information on the side effects of the drug as well as the signs and symptoms of adrenal crisis. A home free of stress is the best environment for a child with Addison's disease because the body needs increased cortical hormones during times of stress and this child's body is unable to produce the hormone. During times of emotional stress or physical stress, the parents may have to give additional hormone replacements. Since dehydration and stress situations are the likely triggers of a crisis, instructing parents to keep the child well hydrated in situations such as extreme heat, exercise, or influenza is warranted. These conditions should be discussed before discharge so that the parents feel in control when at home.

One of the best recommendations to make to parents when caring for a child with Addison's disease is to purchase a medical alert bracelet or tag for the child to wear. This would ensure that the treatment of a child in crisis would not be delayed. It is also important to teach the family and the child about electrolyte loss (especially sodium) during vigorous exercise or on extremely hot days when the child would perspire. Eating more salty food and drinking more water in the hot weather helps the child maintain a mineral balance in his or her body that will ward off a crisis.

 clinical alert

Cortisone insufficiency

When caring for this child, whether in the hospital or clinic, the pediatric nurse must be aware of the signs and symptoms observed before an adrenal crisis: headache, dizziness, and nausea or vomiting (stomach ache) or "wobbly knees." By the time the child exhibits extreme weakness and mental confusion the adrenal crisis is imminent.

Parents also need much support to manage the care and the medications of a child with Addison's disease. This is often very frightening for parents. A well thought through plan can help the parents be ready for any emergency.

Collaboration in Caring— *The child with Addison's disease*

Along with the primary care pediatrician or family physician, the endocrinologist is an important member of the team. Including the parents as members of this team will ensure that they will feel in better control of potential crisis situations. As the child matures and becomes a teenager, it is essential to include him or her as well so that the child is educated and understands the consequences of skipping doses of medication or of stress. The child also needs to be competent to administer emergency, injectable doses of the cortisone.

Cushing's Syndrome

Cushing's syndrome is a rare disorder that seldom is seen in young people younger than 20 years of age. It is hormonal in nature and presents when a person has been exposed to increased levels of cortisone for an extended period of time. When seen in young children it is often caused by an adrenal tumor or prolonged steroid therapy.

About 10 to 15 million new cases are diagnosed annually. It is estimated that only 10% of all individuals affected in a year are children (Keil, 2007). Although the true etiology of Cushing's syndrome is not clear, it can be due to several causes including the oversecretion of the pituitary, causing an excessive amount of serum ACTH and of the adrenal gland, causing an overload of glucocorticoids, usually tumor related. Long-term administration or large amounts of corticosteroids are also known to cause a child to present with Cushing's syndrome. If a child's adrenal glands are insensitive to normal levels of cortisone then levels can become dramatically abnormal (Keil, Batista, & Stratakis, 2003).

SIGNS AND SYMPTOMS. The signs and symptoms of Cushing's syndrome develop gradually, so insidiously in fact that it may be years before the child shows clearly visible signs of Cushing's syndrome. Often children are hypokalemic, causing alkalosis due to potassium excretion and hypercalcemic due to excessive amounts of urinary calcium.

 Nursing Insight— *Signs and symptoms of Cushing's syndrome*

Common signs and symptoms of Cushing's syndrome include weight gain, especially pendulous abdomen; fatigue; muscle wasting and weakness, thin extremities; round "moon"

face; facial flushing; fatty pad between shoulders (buffalo hump); pink or purple stretch marks (striae) on abdominal skin, thighs, breasts, and arms.

The child's skin is also thin and fragile with little subcutaneous tissue causing easy bruising; slow healing of cuts. There may also be insect bites, and infections due to a lessened inflammatory response.

The child may exhibit depression; anxiety and irritability; euphoria and frank psychoses; irregular or absent menstrual periods in females; and erectile dysfunction in males.

Hyperglycemia may eventually lead to latent or overt diabetes, high blood pressure, or arteriosclerosis.

Owing to the excess production of androgens, signs and symptoms related to secondary sexual characteristics can also be seen.

DIAGNOSIS. Children who are being evaluated for Cushing's syndrome must be seen by a pediatric endocrinologist because test result adjustments must be considered before the diagnosis is confirmed. Levels of cortisone are recorded so that escalating levels are clearly seen.

A 24-hour urine collection is a valuable tool to determine if the child's urine is clear of free cortisol. Because 24-hour urine collections can be very difficult to obtain in an infant and child, sometimes the test must be duplicated to obtain reliable results. It is important to remember that in order to correctly interpret the results of the 24-hour urinary free cortisol (UFC), the result must be "corrected" for the child's body surface area. Since cortisone is released by the child's body in response to stress, several other conditions could cause high UFC levels, for instance, physical stress, such as overexertion or obesity, and emotional stress such as depression.

Cortisol levels can also be measured in a child's saliva by taking both a midnight and morning sample. Levels are usually at the lowest point at midnight and the highest in the morning. This normal pattern is lost in children with Cushing's syndrome and the midnight levels are not very different from the morning levels.

Diagnosis is based on the results of not only urine and saliva screening but also on serum blood levels, including fasting blood glucose, and electrolyte levels as well as a bone scan for osteoporosis and a radiograph of the skull for an enlarged sella turcica. An MRI of the pituitary as well as a CT scan of the child's adrenal glands may also be performed. The medical history of the child may also hold the key to the diagnosis. A complete physical exam including the review of several growth charts may indicate that there is a decline in linear growth with a simultaneous dramatic increase in weight gain. Testing does not stop with a diagnosis confirmation. Additional results need to be investigated to determine the cause of the syndrome.

NURSING CARE. As with many diseases, the best treatment is based on the exact cause. Tumors in either the pituitary or in the adrenal glands must often be excised. Referrals to a neurosurgeon are necessary. If it is determined that surgery is not possible radiation therapy is used. Treatments can also include pharmaceuticals that inhibit the production of cortisol. Nursing care depends on the cause and the treatment of the illness. If the child has a surgical intervention, nursing care involves preoperative assessments and fluid hydration as well as postoperative assessments, pain control, and medication regimens. When a child's adrenal glands have been removed, cortisol replacement is necessary. This medication is best given early in the morning or every other day to decrease the side effects. This regime closely mimics the body's normal diurnal pattern of cortisone secretion.

The nurse needs to teach the child and family about the disease, its cause, and subsequent treatments. If a surgical intervention is indicated, thorough preoperative and postoperative teaching must be done. Often the operating room is a very frightening place for children. Many pediatric hospitals perform this teaching well before the procedure and have children tour and touch equipment when they are in a relaxed state of mind, which enables the day of the procedure to go much more smoothly.

Teaching the parents how to give the medication, including the injectable form that is given during an emergency situation, helps gain the confidence necessary to manage a child recovering from Cushing's syndrome. It is important to inform the parents that the "Cushing-like" appearance will decrease as the child recovers.

Finally, it is very important to alert the parents to watch for signs of adrenal insufficiency. If corticosteroid treatments are stopped, the child will exhibit signs of adrenal insufficiency. Encourage the family to have the child wear medical alert identification at all times.

Congenital Adrenal Hyperplasia

Children born with congenital adrenal hyperplasia (CAH) lack the ability to produce cortisol. The condition begins early during the fetal gestational period and the infant is born with the disease. With this deficiency, or lack of cortisol, the negative feedback system fails, causing an excessive amount of corticosteroid-releasing hormone to be secreted from the hypothalamus as well as ACTH from the anterior pituitary. Overproduction of ACTH in turn causes the adrenal glands to become hyperplastic, causing an excessive amount of androgens to be secreted.

The most common cause of CAH is due to a deficiency of 21-hydroxylase (an enzyme, steroid), which is seen in about 1 out of every 15,000 live births (Glatt, Garzon, & Popovic, 2005). This deficiency leads to two major problems: deficient production of both cortisol and aldosterone as well as shunting of steroid precursors that form androgens (Bowen, 2003). The abnormal production of androgens causes an abnormal development of sexual organs in male infants and virilization in females. It results in the masculinization of females, which makes the sex of the baby unclear due to ambiguous genitalia (*pseudohermaphroditism*) or more male-like features.

SIGNS AND SYMPTOMS. Generally, the male infant has no physical differences until later in childhood when the early development of pubic hair, penal enlargement, or both are accompanied by accelerated linear growth and advancement of skeletal maturation (Wilson, 2006c). At birth, it is the female who has malformed external genitalia. The clitoris is enlarged and there can be a fusion of the labial folds; this can give the female a male appearance externally. Internally, the uterus, fallopian tubes, and ovaries are normal.

DIAGNOSIS. Despite the fact that prenatal screening is used to diagnosis CAH as early as possible, false positives indicate that the physician needs to be cognizant of the clinical signs and symptoms postnatally, because milder cases may be missed by the newborn screening programs (Kaye, 2006). Elevated serum levels of 17-hydroxyprogesterone (17-OHP) may indicate the disease. It is important to note that these levels are highest in preterm infants. The levels decrease as infants mature, except in an infant with CAH, in whom the levels continue to escalate.

Although considered a "social emergency," care must be taken to determine the actual diagnosis of the child with ambiguous genitalia. Chromosomes can be studied microscopically to determine the child's gender.

NURSING CARE. Health care professionals must maintain a positive atmosphere from the moment the baby is born. In the delivery room, a positive emotional tone has a lasting effect on the parents' understanding of this disease.

Nearly all children diagnosed with CAH are treated with replacement of glucocorticoids. By alleviating the deficiency of cortisol, the negative feedback loop suppresses ACTH secretion and thus prevents adrenal stimulation.

The mineralocorticoid fludrocortisone (Florinef) or hydrocortisone (A-Hydrocort) is also given. Neither of these drugs has significant side effects at replacement doses. Side effects are seen only when doses exceed those necessary for replacement. If the levels are above normal, the child can acquire acne, an elevated blood pressure, or even growth retardation.

Since these medications need to be given throughout the child's life, parents need to be instructed to give the medication regularly. Often, making the administration part of the family's routine will ensure that the medication is not forgotten. The alternative route to the oral medication, namely the intramuscular medication, must also be taught in the event that the child has an illness in which oral doses are contraindicated. Emergency procedures, including IM injection of hydrocortisone, must be taught to the parents. It is essential for the family to know that if the medication cannot be given at all, the child must be taken to the emergency department of the closest hospital for treatment. It is always good advice to recommend that the child wear a medical alert tag.

Since all females with CAH are fertile, surgical repair can be performed once the replacement of hormones has begun. Usually it is done before the girl's first birthday, and if necessary, may be further corrected before menarche.

 Nursing Insight— *Congenital adrenal hyperplasia*

It is important to address congenital adrenal hyperplasia (CAH) and the decision about whether to wait to perform surgical correction until the child can participate in the discussions. Questions to consider include: Since the surgery is usually cosmetic in nature, what harm would there be to wait? What are the consequences of early surgical repair? Will the nerve endings to the female's clitoris be damaged? What impact will the early surgery have on the child's sexuality in later life and on the sexual identity of the child? Obviously, the decision is very complex and requires careful thought. The nurse can also examine personal thoughts about what makes up a child's sexuality.

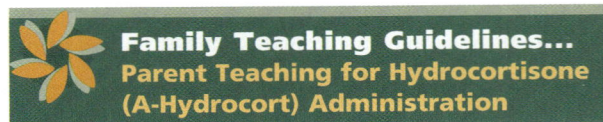

Family Teaching Guidelines...
Parent Teaching for Hydrocortisone (A-Hydrocort) Administration

ESSENTIAL INFORMATION

◆ Medication must be used as prescribed.

◆ Parents must know to always have the injectable hydrocortisone available at home, school and wherever the child travels.

◆ An emergency kit should be on hand at all times with a cortisol supply to administer to the child during acute illness, vomiting, diarrhea or during stressful circumstances. When oral doses cannot be tolerated, the injectable dose should be readily available.

◆ Administer the medication *on time* because this follows the child's body's normal cortisol release patterns (Wilson, 2006c).

Much parental teaching is needed not only regarding the medication and its various route/administration methods, but also about this chronic illness and its treatment, as well as pre- and postoperative teaching if genital reconstruction will be done. Emotional support of the parents is also essential for this lengthy process.

Family education, including siblings and grandparents, must be provided and the pediatric nurse can best help the parents address these family members. Referring to the infant as a "beautiful baby" will help the parents accept the baby as early as possible.

As with any lifelong illness, it is important for the parents to acknowledge the importance of regular checkups. The primary pediatrician, as well as the endocrinologist, pharmacist, dietician, and nurse, should work together to support the entire family to reach their maximum potential.

 nursing diagnoses Congenital Adrenal Hyperplasia

• Risk for Deficit Fluid Volume related to the excess salt excretion of the kidneys and the failure of the negative feedback system.
• Risk for Disproportionate Growth related to initial accelerated growth and early fusion of the epiphyseal plates of the long bone.
• Risk for Impaired Parenting related to the fact that the sex of the child will be uncertain until the karyotype result is determined.
• Caregiver Role Strain related to a chronic, life-threatening illness that can cause strain on the entire family.

Hyperaldosteronism

Hyperaldosteronism produces excessive secretion of aldosterone, which may be caused by an adrenal tumor or syndrome that is due to an enzyme deficiency. Similar to other endocrine disorders, hyperaldosteronism becomes symptomatic with excessive sodium levels and deficient potassium levels as well as fluid retention. (A.D.A.M., 2004).

SIGNS AND SYMPTOMS. With fluid retention, the child becomes hypervolemic and presents with a headache and hypertension. The hypokalemia causes the child to have muscle weakness, paresthesia, and may cause episodic paralysis and tetany. The low potassium levels can lead to polydipsia and polyuria.

DIAGNOSIS. When a young child presents with hypertension, the physician must rule out adrenal tumors. In addition to the hypertension, the child presents with hypokalemia and polyuria; if these conditions fail to respond to ADH administration, the clinical diagnosis of hyperaldosteronism is suspected.

NURSING CARE. Nursing care and treatment are similar to those for chronic adrenocortical insufficiency. Initially, the potassium depletion is replaced and the diuretic spironolactone (Aldactone) causes diuresis and thus blocks the aldosterone effects by preserving potassium and promoting sodium and water excretion.

Surgical excision of the affected adrenal gland or tumor is always recommended. Once the gland or tumor is excised, it is common for the child to experience hypoaldosteronism postoperatively. Hyperkalemia is also seen in this period due to the potassium replacements. Children may need mineralocorticoid supplementation for several months after the removal of the adrenal gland or tumor. Although postoperatively the blood pressure declines, it may not be sustained and may also need to be controlled with sodium restriction diet, or antihypertensive medications.

Any child admitted with hypertension should be observed closely for the signs and symptoms of hyponatremia and hyperkalemia. Excessive thirst, bed wetting or unexplained weakness should begin to raise suspicions in the nurse that the child has a serious illness. When vital sign assessments do reveal hypertension, it is important to notify the physician immediately and to continue frequent vital signs until a physician performs a thorough physical.

Once the diagnosis is confirmed, the nursing care focuses on preoperative care and teaching. The treatment plan must be followed, but more importantly taught to the family because often the child will need medication that must be adjusted for growth for the duration of the condition.

Postoperative care again focuses on the child's immediate status and care on continual assessments of fluid balance, incision site, as well as adherence to the medication regime. If diuretics are ordered, it is best to administer as early in the day as possible to avoid bed wetting at night. Since the potassium supplements can be difficult to swallow, mixing with strong flavored juice helps make the medication more palatable.

The medication regimens are the focus of parent teaching (i.e., give diuretics early in the day). Alerting the parents to subtle signs of electrolyte imbalances is the best weapon against serious consequences. Parents should know the signs and symptoms of hypo- and hyperkalemia. The parents can also meet with a dietician to discuss foods that are high in potassium so that they can be included in the child's diet. Being open and available to answer questions or to help the parents in any way is the best support that can be given to the family.

Pheochromocytoma

Pheochromocytoma is a condition in which there is an adrenal gland tumor. Unlike other tumors, it may not be physically connected to the adrenal gland. In this case, it is called *extra*-adrenal. The tumor intermittently releases excessive catecholamines (i.e., epinephrine and norepinephrine), making the child hypertensive at times.

Although pheochromocytoma is rare in childhood, it generally occurs between 6 and 14 years of age (Baykan et al., 2005). Children have a higher incidence of bilateral tumors than adults do and a lower incidence of malignancy (Vuguin, 2007).

SIGNS AND SYMPTOMS. Hypertension is the most common symptom of pheochromocytoma. It is sometimes very extreme, with the systolic reading reaching as high as 250 mm Hg. Each child may experience symptoms differently. Typical symptoms are tachycardia, arrhythmias, heart palpitations, headache, dizziness, poor weight gain, growth failure, nausea, vomiting, abdominal pain, pale skin, clammy skin, profuse sweating, cool extremities, polydipsia, and polyuria. Pheochromocytoma can mimic the signs and symptoms of diseases such as hyperthyroidism or diabetes mellitus.

DIAGNOSIS. Thorough assessments begin with a complete medical history and physical examination. Additional studies to diagnosis pheochromocytoma may include blood chemistry and urinalysis to measure hormone levels, CT scan to locate tumor, and an MRI scan to create an image of the functioning adrenal gland.

NURSING CARE. Nursing management includes caring for the child undergoing surgery to remove the tumor. If the tumor is bilateral and both adrenal glands must be removed, the child will be placed on lifelong treatment with mineralocorticoids and glucocorticoids. Tumor removal causes an excessive release of catecholamines, causing severe hypertension and tachyarrhythmias. Other complications include hypovolemic shock, and catecholamine withdrawal can cause a dramatic shift in blood pressure now leading to hypotension.

To avoid these challenging and life-threatening surgical complications, preoperative treatment with medication to inhibit the effects of the catecholamines is begun 1 to 3 weeks before surgery. The drug used most often is an α-adrenergic blocking agent, phenoxybenzamine (Dibenzyline). This medication is long acting, can be given by mouth every 12 hours, and is suitable for long-term use. This blocking agent may be combined with β-adrenergic blocking agents to increase the efficacy of the treatment.

Treatment is continued to keep blood pressure within a normal range and to decrease or eliminate hypertensive attacks that include facial flushing, headaches, tachycardia, nausea and vomiting, as well as hyperglycemia.

As with any of these disorders, it is imperative that the pediatric nurse be alert during assessments for the most subtle signs of the impending disorder. Hypertension or hypertensive attacks are sometimes the first sign that should be acted upon. The nurse must thoroughly document history of the symptoms and precipitating factors.

> **Labs: Hyperaldosteronism**
>
> Lab results indicate decreased potassium level, increased aldosterone level, and decreased renin activity. Urinalysis reveals an elevated aldosterone level. A CAT scan of the child's abdomen reveals an adrenal mass and an EKG shows abnormalities that can occur with low potassium levels.

Frequent assessment of vital signs is essential preoperatively. The preoperative nurse should note any hypertensive states or signs of congestive heart failure (CHF). Blood glucose levels should also be taken at least daily. Prompt reporting of any hyperglycemic readings is important.

Postoperatively, the nurse should continue close observation and assess for signs and symptoms of shock that could be caused from the removal of excess catecholamines. Just as preoperatively, the hospital environment should be calm. Undue physical or emotional stress should be avoided for the child's best possible recovery. Parents should be allowed to room in and stay with the child. This helps to alleviate the stress that leaving the child can cause. Distractive play should be encouraged as long as it does not exceed the child's energy level.

Parent teaching about the diagnosis should focus on the signs and symptoms of the condition. Careful observation of the precipitating factors that cause stress can be helpful to keep the child's metabolic needs at a minimum. Anxiety can cause stress, exaggerate the symptoms, and increase metabolism, which causes more catecholamines to be secreted and stimulates a severe hypertensive crisis with possible tachyarrhythmias as well. The parents need to know that touching or palpating the mass can further harm the child in the same manner as stress.

---

 critical nursing action Pheochromocytoma

The child with pheochromocytoma can potentially be very ill. The nurse should remember to perform assessments frequently. Since the adrenal tumor may sometimes be visible abdominally, it is critical to remember *not* to touch or manipulate it in any way. Palpation can cause a further release of catecholamines increasing the likelihood of a severe hypertensive crisis that could cause potentially harmful tachyarrhythmias.

Metabolic Conditions

Metabolic conditions of the pancreas most often involve the destruction of the islets of Langerhans (beta [β cells]), which causes a failure to produce and secrete enough insulin to digest the carbohydrates, proteins, and fats eaten by the child. Most commonly called "diabetes," it is one of the leading causes of chronic illness in the United States. As American society unknowingly increases carbohydrate intake the incidence of diabetes is on the rise. It is important to note that previously, diabetes was merely classified as child (type 1—insulin dependent) or adult (type 2—*non*-insulin dependent) depending at the time of onset and insulin dependency. Today classification is much more complex because either type can affect a person of any age and can be either insulin dependent or non–insulin-dependent.

- Type 1 diabetes mellitus: due to β-cell destruction resulting in definite insulin dependency
- Type 2 diabetes mellitus: due to insulin resistance in which the body fails to recognize and use insulin properly

DIABETES MELLITUS TYPE 1

Type 1 diabetes is an autoimmune disease that arises when a child with a particular genetic makeup is exposed to any precipitating event, such as infection, particularly a virus or other environmental factors such as diet. This is the most common form of diabetes in persons younger than 40 years of age. Children with type 1 diabetes make up about 10% to 15% of all people with diabetes. In the United States it is about 127,000 cases (ADA, 2007b).

SIGNS AND SYMPTOMS. Even though the production of insulin decreases very gradually over many years, the manifestations of type 1 diabetes seem to appear abruptly, and the pancreatic cells can no longer make insulin. There are several signs and symptoms a child could exhibit. There may be excessive urination, in volume and frequency (polyuria), and loss of bladder control in children after they had already been trained, especially at night. Excessive intake of water and/or food (polydipsia and/or polyphagia), unintended weight loss over several days and tendency to be thin is common. Glucose levels in the blood and urine (hyperglycemia and glycosuria) are high. Nausea and vomiting, abdominal pain or discomfort; weakness and excessive fatigue; increased susceptibility to infection, especially urinary tract, respiratory, and skin infections; dehydration; blurred vision; irritability; restlessness; and/or apathy are also common.

DIAGNOSIS. Primarily, elevated blood glucose levels (usually in excess of 200 mg/dL) and elevated hemoglobin (A_{1C}) (greater than 7.0) level are indicative of diabetes mellitus. There are also changes in the child's urine where both sugar and ketones may also be increased. The child usually presents with the complaint of the usual triad of symptoms (polyuria, polydipsia, and polyphagia). Repeat fasting blood glucose and at least two random elevated blood glucose studies make the final determination of the diagnosis.

NURSING CARE. Type 1 diabetes affects mostly children. There are five major components of management and care: insulin types, diet and nutrition, exercise, stress management, and blood glucose and ketone monitoring. Long-term treatments focus on reducing symptoms and preventing complications. Each of these therapies is a vital part of effective metabolic control. Although children and

---

 where research and practice meet:
Type 1 Diabetes is not Purely Genetic

Most recently published from the University of Philadelphia and McGill University in Montreal, a fifth gene variant has been identified that increases a child's risk for type 1 diabetes. With hopes to isolate the genes and determine their function researchers will be better able to treat type 1 diabetes early, perhaps even before the child's entire islet cells are destroyed (*Science Daily*, 2007). Research has indicated that the cause of type 1 diabetes is not purely genetic. Studies of identical twins have shown that identical twins do not always both acquire the disease. This indicates that environmental factors may play a significant role as well. Environmental factors include viral infections, congenital rubella, excessive nitrates in foods, and early cow's milk introduction into the child's diet, although there is no conclusive evidence at this time (Chase & Eisenbarth, 2005).

adolescents can be taught to perform the components, family management has proven to afford the diabetic child an improved glycemic control (Wysocki, Buckloh, Lochrie, & Antal, 2005).

Because high glucose levels and ketoacidosis are critical situations, a child initially diagnosed with type 1 diabetes usually is hospitalized to control the blood glucose level and to determine what type, dose, and frequency of insulin works best for the child.

Insulin Types. Many factors influence the child's insulin requirements. Insulin needs are affected by the child's nutritional intake and physical energy expended, as well as the child's emotional and stress level that accompany normal activities like growth spurts, puberty, and illness. Despite these variables that make insulin regulation extremely difficult, it is the foundation of treatment for a child with type 1 diabetes.

Many types of insulin are available today. Generally, the type of insulin used for each individual patient is based on the child's blood glucose levels and the child's lifestyle (Children With Diabetes, 2006). Combinations of long-, intermediate-, and short-acting insulin ("insulin cocktails") are given subcutaneously throughout the day in an attempt to simulate the body's natural release of the hormone (Tables 28-2 and 28-3).

- Humalog/NovoLog insulin is clear and usually taken immediately before meals. This regular insulin works so quickly that it can even be taken after meals. It is usually used for children who are picky eaters or toddlers who do not always eat the same amount of food and thus can take the insulin right after they eat.
- Regular insulin is also clear and begins to act quickly; it merely takes slightly longer to reach its peak than Humalog or NovoLog.
- NPH insulin is cloudy and absorbs more slowly. It is made with a protein enabling its slow release. Even though the peak and the duration can vary from child to child, generally when this insulin is taken in the morning it does not take effect until the afternoon.
- Ultralente insulin peaks somewhat more slowly than the previous NPH. It can be given at dinner and its effects can help maintain a normal blood glucose level until morning.
- Lantus insulin is a clear insulin that lasts 24 hours with steady levels giving it nearly no peaking action. It is like NPH in that it is consistent and predictable in its action, but can vary within the same child in the time it takes to peak from one day to the next. Lantus, like all types of insulin, is given subcutaneously but since it cannot be mixed with any other insulin, it must be given as a separate injection.
- Lente, 70/30, and 75/25 "cocktail" insulin is premixed to allow the child the benefit of several types of insulin with the benefit of one injection. As many as three types of insulin can be mixed together. The premixed varieties are usually used by families who do not want to have to draw from several bottles.

Insulin must be given by subcutaneous injection. Parents should be lead to expect that their child may need one to four injections per day and that generally the more injections, the greater the blood glucose control. Children are very fearful of injections. Parents need time, patience, and encouragement. Help them practice giving injections away from the child to alleviate the child's fears and to boost their confidence. Audio and visual injection techniques can be viewed on the BD Diabetes Web site: http://www.bddiabetes.com/us/main.aspx?cat=1&id=258 (see Procedure 28-1).

With some children and adolescents, the use of the insulin pump is increasing because the delivery of insulin is steady throughout the day, which most closely resembles the body's natural response. Recent research has shown that with proper training and follow-up, insulin pump therapy provides a lasting and effective treatment modality (Joslin Diabetes Center, 2006). Since pumps can be easily mistaken for a cell phone, pager, or iPod, communication with school teachers regarding the use and occasional beep is essential (Fig. 28-3).

Table 28-2 Insulin Types and Peak Affects

Insulin Name	Insulin Type	Begins to Work	Peak Effect	Used Up
Humalog/ NovoLog	Short-acting	10–15 minutes	30–90 minutes	4 hours
Regular	Short-acting	30–60 minutes	2–4 hours	6–9 hours
NPH	Intermediate acting	1–2 hours	3–8 hours	12–15 hours
Ultralente	Intermediate acting	2–4 hours	6–14 hours	18–20 hours
Lantus	Long-acting	1–2 hours	2–22 hours	24 hours

Table 28-3 Insulin "Cocktails"

Insulin Name	Insulin Type	Begins to Work	Peak Effect	Used Up
Lente	Premixed	1–2 hours	3–14 hours	18–20 hours
70/30 NPH/Regular	Pre-mixed	30–60 minutes	3–8 hours	12–15 hours
75/25 NPH/Humalog	Pre-mixed	10–15 minutes	30 minutes– 8 hours	12–15 hours

medication: Insulin Dosage and Frequency

Although the dosage of insulin is based on the individual needs of the child or adolescent, the precise dose needed for each individual child cannot be predicted. Common insulin dosage for a child is generally 0.75–1.0 unit per kilogram per day.

Common insulin dosage for an adolescent is usually 1.0–1.7 units per kilogram per day. If two doses of insulin are the goal of treatment, then usually 60%–75% of the insulin is given before breakfast, with the remainder given with the dinner meal.

Procedure 28-1 Teaching Parents How to Inject Insulin

Purpose

To teach parents how to inject insulin

Equipment

Insulin bottle from refrigerator (remove up to 1 hour before injection to allow it to warm to room temperature)

Appropriate syringe (U-30, U-50, or U-100)

Alcohol wipes

Container for the dirty, used syringe

Steps

1. Check the expiration date on the insulin bottle.

   RATIONALE: *Ensures that the insulin has not expired.*

2. Wash hands.

   RATIONALE: *Prevents the spread of bacteria.*

3. Clean rubber stopper on insulin bottle with alcohol wipe.

   RATIONALE: *Promotes asepsis.*

4. Remove syringe cap and pull air into the syringe line up the end of the black plunger to the exact amount the insulin dose will be.

   RATIONALE: *Ensures accurate dosage of insulin to be drawn up.*

5. Put the syringe needle through the bottle rubber top and push syringe plunger so that all the air goes from the syringe into the bottle.

6. Turn the insulin bottle upside down and pull the syringe plunger so that the insulin enters the syringe until the top of the black plunger exactly lines up with the dose of insulin to be given.

7. Remove every air bubble, always checking that the dose is exact.

   RATIONALE: *Exact dosing is essential in managing the child's condition.*

8. Choose (or let the child choose) the site of the injection.

   RATIONALE: *Allowing the child to participate may help them feel more in control of his condition.*

9. Clean the injection site with an alcohol swab.

   RATIONALE: *Alcohol will decrease the presence of microorganisms.*

10. Pinch up the skin slightly and gently, with the syringe at a 90-degree angle (perpendicular) to the skin, with a dart-like motion, insert the needle into the skin, release the skin.

    RATIONALE: *Ensures proper medication administration.*

11. Slowly inject the dose of insulin.

12. Discard the used syringe in a hard, rigid container with a tight-fitting lid.

Clinical Alert The nurse teaches the parents to evaluate the child for the signs and symptoms of either hypo- or hyperglycemia. In understandable terms, explain these signs and symptoms to the parents so they can watch for them at home.

Hypoglycemia (*LOW* Blood Sugar)

Cold, pale skin (cold sweat)

Shakiness/hand tremors

Sudden hunger (crave salt/sweet)

Emotional outbursts (personality changes)

Drowsiness/extremely tired

Pounding heartbeat/palpitations

Nervousness/dizziness

Anxiety/irritability

Headache, mental confusion, difficulty concentrating

Numbness or tingling of lips/mouth

Poor coordination/staggering unable to walk

Slurred or slow speech

Dilated, enlarged pupils

Fainting (needs emergency treatment *NOW*)

Hyperglycemia (*HIGH* Blood Sugar)

Increased thirst, even if consuming a large amount of liquids

Loss of appetite, nausea/vomiting

Weakness, stomach pains/aches

Heavy, labored breathing

Fatigue, tired often sleepy

Large amounts of sugar in urine

Ketones in urine

Frequent urination

Blurred/double vision

Teach Parents

If the child expresses that the injection is painful, the following measures can be taken to decrease the pain:

- Inject room temperature insulin.
- Clear even the tiniest air bubbles from the syringe.
- Let the alcohol dry completely before injection.
- Tell the child to relax muscles in area of injection (the more tense the muscles during injection, the more painful the procedure).
- Use syringelike dart to pierce skin quickly.
- Do not change the needle direction during insertion or withdrawal.
- Never reuse syringes.
- Rotate sites with *each* injection (giving the insulin in the *same* place twice in one day can cause unnecessary discomfort for the child and undue stress on the tissue).

- Document exactly where each injection was given so as to avoid the same place more than once a day.
- Create and keep a Diabetes Management Notebook with the plan and a place to record daily blood sugar values as well as doses of insulin administered including injection site.

Procedure 28-1 Teaching Parents How to Inject Insulin—cont'd

For example:

Date	Blood Glucose AM	Blood Glucose PM	Insulin Dose Given and Time	Injection Site	Given by
8/9/07	124		4 units Regular at 0700	right mid-arm	Mom
8/9/07		144	4 units Regular 4 units NPH 1230	left mid-thigh	Dad

Documentation

Mother gave 4 units of Regular at 0700 in right mid-arm, noted by R. Such, RN

Father gave 4 units of Regular and 4 units NPH at 1230 in left mid-thigh, noted by R. Such, RN

Diet and Nutrition

According to the American Diabetes Association, Medical Nutrition Therapy (MNT) is important in preventing and managing diabetes as well as preventing the development of diabetic complications. These nutritional recommendations and interventions for diabetes are intended to help those with diabetes and their health care providers (ADA, 2007a). Contrary to past belief, there are no forbidden foods in the diabetic child's diet. This is considered a unique time in the life cycle and even though some foods are more nutritious than others, no food is automatically eliminated. The goal for a dietary plan should balance various foods and include the caloric intake from:

- Carbohydrates (50–60%)—milk, fruits, vegetables, grains (wheat, rice, corn, oats, barley)
- Fats (20–30%)—mayonnaise, butter, margarine, oils (corn, olive, canola, peanut, etc.)
- Proteins (10–20%)—meats, eggs, cheese, beans, legumes (lentils)

It is also recommended that diet plans be revised at least annually. The goal of treatment for children with type 1 diabetes is that the blood glucose levels are maintained at a relatively normal level or as close to normal as possible. A_{1C} levels are indicative of the average blood glucose levels over the past several (2 to 3) months (Table 28-4).

Table 28-4 Equivalent of A_{1C} Level and Blood Glucose Level

Hemoglobin A_{1C} Levels (mean %)	Mean Blood Glucose Level (mg/dL)
Normal 4	60
4.5	
5	90
5.5	
6	120
Slightly Elevated 6.5	
7	150
7.5	
8	180
Elevated 8.5	
9	210
9.5	
10	240
Severely Elevated 10.5	
11	270
11.5	
12	300
12.5	
13	330
13.5	
14	360

Figure 28-3 Wearing an insulin pump is a good way for children to regulate glucose levels.

Modified from the American Diabetes Association (2005). Standards of medical care in diabetes: clinical practice recommendations. *Diabetes Care 28* (Supplement), S4–S36.

Nursing Insight— *Equivalent of A_{1C} level and blood glucose level*

Although a child with type 1 diabetes does not need any special foods, it is imperative that his or her food intake is coordinated with the peak action of the insulin injected subcutaneously. Normally, the child with type 1 diabetes needs as many calories and variety of foods that are necessary for the normal growth and development of any child. Timing is the key to success. Specific parameters have been set by the ADA regarding the type 1 diabetes A_{1C} goals for each specific age group (Table 28-5).

Exercise

Exercise and extracurricular activities should never be restricted unless the child with type 1 diabetes has health issues that warrant activity restriction. Children are much more likely to have a hypoglycemic crisis and must be reminded that calorie intake and insulin dosage may need adjustment with increased activity. Exercise is an excellent way to increase the cells' sensitivity to insulin and actually helps insulin to be better utilized by the body.

The spontaneity of childhood activity does not leave much time for parents to plan appropriate meals and snacks. Often it is difficult to encourage snacks before the activity. Remind parents that snacking during an activity may ward off a hypoglycemic crisis later.

Stress Management

Normal childhood milestones create varying times of stress in a child's life. From report cards to college preparation, growing young people experience anxiety, adjustments, and depression. It has been found that A_{1C} levels increase with depression. It is important to consult with mental health professionals for patient screening and also to become a part of the team in order to create a network of referrals for each particular family.

Blood Glucose and Ketone Monitoring

The ADA has recommended that the health care provider weigh the benefits of lowering the child's blood glucose levels against the unique risk of hypoglycemia. Children

Figure 28-4 Home monitoring requires parents to perform glucose checks on the child with diabetes.

with type 1 diabetes may lack the capacity to recognize and respond to hypoglycemic symptoms. Hypoglycemic unawareness is a unique challenge for all pediatric health care professionals and parents. Home glucose monitoring occurs 3 to 6 times per day (Fig. 28-4). With home testing, glucose control is more exact than in the past. The importance of home monitoring is a vital aspect of care. Parents can be reassured that the glucose monitor is generally covered under most insurance plans.

Urine testing for ketones should be performed at least every 3 hours during a child's illness. It should also be checked whenever blood glucose readings exceed 240 mg/dL or when the child experiences unexplained weight loss even if he or she is well. Ketones in the urine are indicative of insulin deficiency.

Long-term Treatments

Long-term treatments focus on reducing symptoms and preventing complications such as blindness, kidney-failure, and limb amputation. The goal of care is to prolong life while enabling the child to grow into adulthood.

The focus of nursing care for a child with type 1 diabetes should be based on the cornerstones of nursing care

Table 28-5 Plasma Blood Glucose and A_{1C} Goals for Type 1 Diabetes by Age Group

Age Group (years)	Plasma Blood Glucose Goal Range (mg/dL)		Hemoglobin A_{1C} %	Rationale
	MORNING BEFORE MEALS	BEDTIME/ OVERNIGHT		
Toddlers and preschoolers (0–6 years)	100–180	110–200	<8.5% (but >7.5%)	High risk/vulnerability to hypoglycemia
School age (6–12 years)	90–180	100–180	<8%	Risk of hypoglycemia and low risk of complications prior to puberty
Adolescents and young adults (13–19 years)	90–130	90–150	<7.5%	• Risk for severe hypoglycemia • Developmental and psychological issues Lower goal < 7.0% is reasonable if it can be achieved without excessive hypoglycemia

Modified from the American Diabetes Association (2007). Standards of medical care in diabetes – 2007. *Diabetes Care 30* (Supplement), S4–S41.

with great emphasis placed on teaching the child and family about the chronic illness and its management. The nurse must continually assess the child's blood glucose, as well as observe for signs of complications or complex management issues. Most importantly, the nurse must assess the child and family's readiness to learn. Once the family is ready, the nurse must take every opportunity to teach the family about the illness or the child's care. By expanding the understanding and knowledge of the child and his or her caregivers, the nurse is creating the skills necessary for the home management of this chronic illness.

 nursing diagnoses The Child with Type 1 Diabetes

• Risk for injury related to hypoglycemia or hyperglycemia
• Knowledge deficit related to management of type 1 diabetes
• Interrupted family processes related to management of the chronic illness
• Disturbed body image related to management of type 1 diabetes

Once the plan is complete, the nurse may begin to implement it. Education of the child and family can begin once the child is stable and ready to learn. It is an ongoing process and continues whether the child is in the hospital, or at home, just going for an outpatient visit. Outcomes can then be evaluated to determine if the child's glucose levels are normalized, if there are adequate insulin levels, and to determine if the child has a positive body image and is capable of managing the diabetes in the home with the support and guidance of others. Finally, the nurse evaluates that the child does not manifest the signs and symptoms of either hypo- or hyperglycemia.

Patient/Family Teaching that Optimizes Outcomes

Higher caregiver knowledge was associated with better glucose control/outcomes in young children with diabetes (Stallwood, 2006). Education is the main route by which a family achieves the best glucose control for the child with type 1 diabetes. The better the blood glucose is controlled, the less frequent the child experiences complications. Education must focus on insulin types; use; administration and schedule; meal planning including the balance of carbohydrates, proteins, and fats; physical exercise; blood glucose monitoring; and extremity care.

Children with diabetes could use alternative therapies to help manage blood glucose levels and to prevent any of the complications associated with the condition:

• Lifestyle changes, particularly diet and exercise
• Medications, namely insulin for individuals with type 1 diabetes
• Stress reduction and relaxation techniques
• Acupuncture for pain from nerve damage

Stressful life events can worsen diabetes in several ways. For example, stress stimulates the nervous and endocrine systems in ways that increase blood glucose levels and disrupt healthy behaviors (eating habits, etc.). Stress management is an integral part of the treatment of diabetes. Studies have shown that diabetics who participate in biofeedback sessions are more likely to reach normal blood glucose levels. Although other studies have produced results that contradict this, researchers and clinicians generally agree that long-term stress is likely to worsen diabetes and that biofeedback, tai chi, yoga, and

 Family Teaching Guidelines...
Dealing with a Hypoglycemic Crisis

How To: Recognize the signs of hypoglycemia (child is pale, sweaty, dizzy, "shaky" [tremors], confused, irritable, numb on lips or mouth and can have an altered mental status)

ESSENTIAL INFORMATION

◆ Check blood glucose level.

◆ If blood glucose is below 70 mg/dL, rapidly give one of the following sources of carbohydrates (about 10–15 grams each), the right amount to treat hypoglycemia:
  • 1/2 to 3/4 cup of orange or grape juice (a juice box is good when one is away from home)
  • 2 glucose tablets or 2 doses of glucose gel
  • 2–4 pieces of hard candy
  • 5 gumdrops
  • 1–2 tablespoons of honey
  • 1 small box of raisins
  • 6 oz. regular (not diet) soda (about half a can)
  • 2 tablespoons of cake icing

◆ Recheck blood glucose in 15 minutes, if reading is still below 70 mg/dL, then

◆ Give another glass of juice, etc.

◆ Recheck blood glucose again after another 15 minutes.

◆ When blood glucose returns to at least 80 mg/dL a more substantial snack (nonconcentrated sugar) may be given, i.e., cheese and crackers, bread and peanut butter, etc. if the next meal is more than 30 minutes away or if a physical activity/exercise is planned.

◆ If the child is unconscious, glucagon should be given either subcutaneously or intramuscularly (ADA, 2007a).

other forms of relaxation may help motivate people with diabetes to change their habits in order to manage their condition.

 Nursing Insight— *Differentiation between hypo- and hyperglycemia*

The nurse can help the family understand the differentiation between hypo- and hyperglycemia, a difference that is critical for the nurse to be able to easily recognize (Table 28-6, p. 911).

 Across Care Settings: A team approach

The care of a child with type 1 diabetes is very complex. A team approach with the family at the core of the team is paramount. The child should be included in the plan and the care as much as possible (whenever appropriate). The most effective team consists of several members across the specialties within the hospital, including primary pediatrician, pediatric endocrinologist, diabetes nutritionist and nurse educator, exercise physiologist, as well as mental health professionals for psychological support as needed.

Nursing Care Plan The Child with Type 1 Diabetes

Nursing Diagnosis: Imbalanced Nutrition: Less than Body Requirements related to inability to metabolize carbohydrates

Measurable Short-term Goal: The child will exhibit blood glucose levels between (specify range for age).

Measurable Long-term Goal: The child will not experience hypoglycemia or diabetic ketoacidosis.

NOC Outcomes:
Nutritional Status: Biochemical Measures (1005)
   Body fluid components and chemical indices of nutritional status
Nutritional Status: Food and Fluid Intake (1008)
   Amount of food and fluid taken into the body over a 24-hour period

NIC Interventions:
Hyperglycemia Management (2120)
Hypoglycemia Management (2130)
Teaching: Prescribed Diet (5614)

Interventions:

1. Identify when the child and family are ready and motivated to learn all aspects of diabetic care.

   RATIONALE: Children and families need time to accept this chronic illness and will not be able to learn until ready.

2. Explain clearly signs and symptoms of hypoglycemia, hyperglycemia, and diabetic ketoacidosis with appropriate treatment options.

   RATIONALE: Children are highly susceptible to hypoglycemia and cannot always verbalize exactly how they feel.

3. Provide multiple opportunities to practice blood glucose testing and insulin preparation and administration.

   RATIONALE: Children and families learn best with multiple demonstrations and return demonstrations. Various scenarios will enhance their problem-solving and critical thinking skills.

4. Include the parents and child in the development of the diabetic management plan including diet and exercise.

   RATIONALE: Plans that include the input from the child and the family are more likely to be successful.

Lines of communication must be kept open to best serve the family and the child. It is also vital to include other significant adults (living in the home) into the diabetic child's plan of care.

The glucose balance of a child with type 1 diabetes is daunting. Because glucose control highly depends on monitoring and regulating the child's diet, exercise, and insulin dose and administration, those significant people in the child's daily life must know the plan. That is, the child's teachers, coach, school nurse, counselor, principal, or assistant and even the "lunch mom" must know those appropriate parts of the plan in order to help actualize it. A child should not be left unsupported at any time. Whether in Sunday school or at the school play, those responsible adults must know the appropriate care of the diabetic child.

DIABETES MELLITUS TYPE 2

Unlike type 1 diabetes, type 2 diabetes is caused by the body's resistance to recognize and utilize insulin rather than a deficient production of insulin as in type 1. For years, type 2 diabetes was labeled as "adult-onset," but in the past several decades there has been an alarming increase in type 2 diabetes in young people.

It is estimated that over one-third of all people with type 2 diabetes are undiagnosed. The increase of type 2 diabetes in the adolescent population has been dramatic over the past decade (ADA, 2007b). It is estimated that more than 2.7 million teens in the United States have impaired fasting blood glucose levels (Duncan, 2006).

where research and practice meet:
Alternatives to Injectable Insulin

Alternatives to injectable insulin are in development. Several variant routes are being studied in an attempt to change the method of delivery of insulin doses. Currently the inhaled method is approved only for use with adults, but with more research, it will be seen in the pediatric population soon. Other methods of delivery under investigation include transdermal, buccal (sprayed into the back of the mouth to be absorbed by the oral mucosa), and oral methods. As with any new technology, stringent criteria must be met in order to be prescribed the alternate medication. Children need to reap the benefits of these advanced scientific/medical breakthroughs. Islet cell transplants or pancreatic transplantation may offer a cure to patients in the future (Juvenile Diabetes Research Foundation International, 2006).

 ***Ethnocultural Considerations*— People from some ethnic backgrounds are more prone to type 2 diabetes**

Type 2 diabetes in children is often associated with ethnic background (African American, Hispanic, Asian, or American Indian), obesity (85% at diagnosis), and a family history of type 2 diabetes (74–100%) as well as with insulin resistance.

Insulin resistance is when the individual cells do not recognize the insulin molecule and resist its influence. The

Table 28-6 Clinical Comparison of Hypoglycemia and Hyperglycemia

Clinical Condition	Manifestations	Critical Nursing Actions
Hypoglycemia		
Too much insulin for amount of food eaten	Rapid onset	• Give 15 grams of carbohydrates (½ glass orange juice)
	Irritable	
	Nervous	
Injected insulin into muscle	Shaky feeling, tremors	• Recheck blood glucose in 15 minutes
Too much activity for insulin dose	Difficult to concentrate	• If blood glucose is <70 mg/dl give another 15 grams of carbohydrates
	Difficult to speak	
Too much time between meals	Behavior change	• Recheck again in another 15 minutes
	Confused	
	Repeats over and over	
Too few carbohydrates eaten	Unconscious	• If unconscious, give IM glucagon
	Seizure	
Illness or stress	Tachycardia	
	Shallow breathing	
	Pale, sweaty	
	Hungry	
	Headache	
	Dizzy	
	Vision blurry or double	
	Photophobic	
	Numbness of mouth or lips	
Hyperglycemia		
Too little insulin for the food eaten	Gradual onset	• Give additional insulin at usual injection time
	Lethargic	
	Sleepy	
Illness or stress	Slow response	• Use sliding scale doses for specific level of blood glucose
	Confused	
Too many carbohydrates eaten	Breaths deeply and rapidly	• Increase fluids
	Skin flushed and dry	
Meals too close together	Mucous membranes dry	• If ketones are elevated, give an extra insulin injection
Too many snacks	Thirsty, hungry, dehydrated	
Insulin given just under skin	Weak, tired, headache	
Too little activity	Abdomen hurts	
	Nausea and vomiting	
	Vision blurry	
	Shock	

cell membrane does not allow the insulin to initiate the normal enzymatic reactions that cause metabolism. The glucose cannot be utilized by the cells, the cells begin to be "starved," and the blood glucose levels slowly but steadily rise.

SIGNS AND SYMPTOMS. Children with type 2 diabetes often have no symptoms, and their condition is detected only when a routine exam reveals high blood glucose levels or complications appear. Occasionally, a child with type 2 diabetes may experience some of the following symptoms which tend to appear gradually over time: numbness or burning sensation of the feet, ankles, and legs, blurred or poor vision, impotence, fatigue, and poor wound healing. In some cases, symptoms may mimic type 1 diabetes and appear more abruptly. These symptoms include excessive urination and thirst, yeast infections, whole body itching, and even coma.

DIAGNOSIS. In the 2007 ADA position statement, specific criteria were established for type 2 diabetes testing in children:

- Overweight defined as a BMI greater than 85th percentile for age and sex, weight greater than 85th percentile for height, or weight greater than 120% of ideal weight for height

  Plus *two* of the following risk factors:

- Family history of type 2 diabetes in a first- or second-degree relative
- Race/ethnicity (Native American, African American, Latino, Asian American, Pacific Islander)
- Signs of insulin resistance or a condition associated with insulin resistance such as acanthosis nigricans (black-brown velvety skin condition on the back of the neck, axilla, arms, caused by too much insulin in the blood), hypertension, dyslipidemia, or polycystic ovary syndrome (PCOS)
- Maternal history of diabetes or gestational diabetes mellitus (GDM)

Blood glucose testing should begin at age 10 years or at the onset of puberty if younger. The frequency of this testing should be every 2 years. The preferred test is the fasting blood glucose level (ADA, 2007b). Diagnosis is confirmed with two fasting blood glucose results that exceed 125 mg/dL or two random blood glucose readings over 200 mg/dL.

NURSING CARE. The management of type 2 diabetes can vary depending on the severity of the disease. With normal or near normal A_{1C} levels, nutritional teaching, such as decreasing calories, and behavioral changes, especially increasing activity, are pivotal to successful therapy. Teaching lifestyle modification must include the entire family to ensure compliance (McKnight-Menci, Sababu, & Kelly, 2005).

With a mildly elevated A_{1C} level (6.2% to 9.0%) an oral hypoglycemic agent such as metformin (Actoplus MET) may be given (Ibanez et al., 2006). The medication, in combination with lifestyle modification, usually successfully lowers the blood glucose level. With severe presentation (>9.0%) treatment is similar to that of type 1 diabetes. Insulin is given either intravenously or subcutaneously until the child is stabilized. Oral hypoglycemic agents can be given, particularly if the child has lost weight (Chase & Eisenbarth, 2005).

Increased awareness of the escalating type 2 diabetes crisis in the pediatric population can give the nurse the necessary tools to begin to fight this problem. Nurses, no matter what their care setting or work environment, should teach the public about the value of weight control, active lifestyles, and role model a healthy example for teachers, families, and most importantly the children.

Teaching the child, parents, teachers, counselors, coaches, and clergy should be his primary focus of care. Healthy eating habits and increasing activity in a sedentary lifestyle are very difficult. All of this must be done without compromising normal growth and development while improving the quality of life.

The nurse must provide diabetes education for the entire household (Table 28-7). For instance, if a grandmother resides in the patient's home, but was not included in the teaching, she may unknowingly sabotage the efforts to change eating habits and lifestyle. The pediatric nurse must be cognizant of any factors that may make compliance difficult and talk to the parents and the child about home routines, especially those around mealtime and activities.

Consistent monitoring for complications of diabetes is a critical component of the care of a diabetic child. The pediatric nurse must be alert to the signs and symptoms of eminent complications. The signs of acute complications include hypoglycemia, weight loss, and diabetic ketoacidosis. Long-term complications involve the degradation of vital bodily systems, including cardiopathy, nephropathy, neuropathy, and retinopathy. Many complications can have devastating effects, including growth failure, delayed puberty, menstrual disturbances, emotional disturbances, cataracts, impaired cognitive function, hyperlipidemia, and breakdown or buildup of subcutaneous tissue at injection sites.

The nurse must communicate not only with the primary pediatrician but with the endocrinologist, the nutritionist, the diabetic nurse educator, the pharmacist, the social worker, the school nurse, and the home health nurse, so that everyone is knowledgeable about the individual needs of each particular child and his family.

DIABETIC KETOACIDOSIS

Diabetic ketoacidosis (DKA) is the presenting complaint in nearly one fourth of all newly diagnosed pediatric patients with type 1 diabetes mellitus (Young, 2007). It is a very complex combination of hyperglycemia, ketosis, and acidosis resulting from severely deficient insulin in either type 1 or type 2 diabetes. The abnormal metabolism of carbohydrates, protein, and fat that leads to very high glucose levels that cause DKA. It is important to know that DKA is the leading cause of death in children with type 1 diabetes.

Although the exact incidence is unknown, it is estimated that about 4 to 8 children per 1000 present with DKA at the time of diagnosis. In many cases, this is a common occurrence with young children who have difficulty verbalizing the classic signs and symptoms.

SIGNS AND SYMPTOMS. It is important to note that in the toddler age group, the classic manifestations of DKA are often absent. Many times the child is not known to be diabetic because the onset can be often insidious, but if it is known, a complete history, especially noting the compliance with insulin regimens and the name of the endocrinologist, is essential.

Some of the following signs and symptoms may be difficult for the young child to verbalize: fatigue and malaise, nausea/vomiting, abdominal pain, polydipsia, polyuria, polyphagia, weight loss, and fever.

The physical manifestations include altered mental status (the child may be alert or in a coma), tachycardia, tachypnea or hyperventilation (Kussmaul respirations), normal or low blood pressure, increased capillary refill time, poor perfusion, lethargy and weakness, and fever; acetone (fruity) odor of breath indicates metabolic acidosis.

Table 28-7 Educating Different Groups on Diabetes			
Content Topics	**Parent**	**Child**	**Adolescent**
Disease Process	• Include type of diabetes. • Treatment options • Benefits of healthy lifestyle	• Explain disease simply. • Begin to teach self-care. • Include in treatment plan.	• Talk to as an adult. • Expect self-care, but also expect limitations.
Nutritional Guidelines	• Address breastfeeding. • Erratic eating habits • How to read labels • Family grocery shopping • Controversy of artificial sweeteners	• How to make appropriate food choices (restaurant) • How to change food behavior habits (fast food) • Guidelines for meal and snack planning • After school and "party" eating habits • Coordination of school, activities, and meals • Meal swapping/sharing	
Activities	• Explain how activity and glucose level interact. • Younger children have high energy level. • Incorporate walking into family outings.	• Limit sitting in front of TV or computer. • Play outside. • Join a sport or activity. • Walk to friend's house if possible.	• Explain how exercise increases glucose use. • Decrease sedentary (computer) time. • Exercise every day, not just on weekends. • Increase time, amount, and frequency of activity.
Medications	• Understand medication to be given. • Discuss dose, frequency, action, adverse reactions. • Insulin storage, dose, administration technique if appropriate • Choose med schedule to fit family's lifestyle.	• Needs supervision at all times. • Plans meds around normal schedule. • Provide for lunch time dose if needed (talk to school RN, teacher).	• Self-treatment • Adapting to hectic high school schedule • Treat to target blood glucose. • Monitor patterns in blood glucose to improve control.
Complications	• Discuss signs/symptoms of hypo/hyperglycemia.	• Begins to understand hyper/hypoglycemia.	• Identify cause and effect of hyper/hypoglycemia.
Acute	• Discuss DKA. • Emergency procedures • When to come to the ER	• Recognizes patterns. • Links causes to high and low blood sugar. • Understands consequences of actions.	• How to prevent high and low blood sugars • Driving precautions
Chronic	• Explain risk of long term uncontrolled diabetes and effect on neurological and vascular systems.	• Explain effect of long-term, uncontrolled diabetes on neurological and vascular systems.	• Explain effect of long-term, uncontrolled diabetes on neurological and vascular systems.
Outcome Criteria	• Family lifestyle changes • Discuss goals that can be met. • Boost confidence in technical skills. • Management of child during illness • Understand blood glucose readings and A_{1C} results.	• Work toward independence. • Learn technical skills; expect frustrations. • Emotional immaturity	• Goals should be realistic and attainable. • Problem solving each day • How to manage heat, sun, dehydration

Continued

Table 28-7	Educating Different Groups on Diabetes—cont'd		
Content Topics	**Parent**	**Child**	**Adolescent**
Psychosocial Adjustments	• Avoid giving too much responsibility too soon. • Identify friends where child could spend the night (friends know child's care routine). • Notify teachers and principal of child's health needs. • Adaptation of family life to incorporate care without stress • Stress reduction • Parental relief (who could stay overnight with family so parents can "get away")?	• Blood glucose testing before meals at friends, in restaurant, at school (in public) • Learn weight control. • Manage overnight stays. • Healthy habits amidst unhealthy environments	• Body image and weight concerns • Puberty and effect of hormonal changes • Learn to prevent complications. • Prevent DKA. • Modify high-risk behaviors. • Diabetes and dating, sex and conception • Peer pressure • Alcohol, tobacco, drugs

Source: Atkinson, A., & Radjenovic, D. (2006). Meeting quality standards for self-management education in pediatric type 2 diabetes. *Diabetes Care, 40–46*.

DIAGNOSIS. Diagnosis is confirmed with a blood glucose of greater than 200 mg/dL, ketonuria, or ketonemia with a serum bicarbonate level of less than 15 mEq/L. The pH of the blood will indicate the degree of the acidosis, that is,

• Mild DKA—venous blood pH equals 7.2 to 7.3
• Moderate DKA—venous blood pH equals 7.10 to 7.19
• Severe DKA—venous blood pH below 7.10

clinical alert

Diabetic ketoacidosis

Infection is the most frequent cause of DKA, particularly in known diabetics. Aggressive evaluation for infection always is necessary. Antibiotic therapy should strongly be considered until the culture results are known. The following patient-related issues can also be considered:

• Patient has poor compliance with existing insulin regimens.
• Patient exhibits underlying endocrine changes of adolescence.
• Thelarche—before puberty, just at the beginning of rapid growth.
• Adrenarche—activity of the adrenal cortex intensifies and hormones increase (at about 8 years of age).
• Menarche—the first menstruation usually occurs between 9 and 17 years of age.
• The caregiver's lack of competence.
• Insulin pump failure may occur.

NURSING CARE. Care of the patient with DKA is based on four essential physiologic principles (Chase & Eisenbarth, 2005):

• Restore fluid volume.
• Return child to a glucose utilization state by inhibiting lipolysis.
• Replace the child's body electrolytes.
• Correct acidosis, restore acid–base balance.

Children in DKA are unstable. Fluids and electrolytes can shift rapidly. The acid–base balance can fluctuate.

Therefore, do not expect exact treatment protocols with precise steps to follow because treatment ensues based on the signs and symptoms presented by the child and by the lab results. The nurse can expect to rapidly change intravenous solutions and to adjust the plan before one therapy is completed. The outcome of care is to restore hemodynamic and acid–base balance slowly, reducing the acidosis and restoring the child to a normal stabilized state.

The diabetic child in DKA is usually in the intensive care unit. The pediatric intensive care unit nurse must assess the child rapidly, frequently, and thoroughly. The focus of nursing care is to replenish the intravascular volume. Fluid status can be determined by the child's weight, skin turgor, pulse rate, level of consciousness, and blood pressure. As fluid and electrolyte deficits are replaced carefully and the child slowly returns to an acid–base balance status. Ongoing maintenance fluids are then given.

Nursing assessment of acidosis can be ascertained by the presence of Kussmaul breathing, flushed cheeks, acetone (fruity) breath, and complaints of back and abdominal pain. The bedside nurse is responsible to observe and document the child's response to each of the interventions. This requires a skilled nurse who understands and is comfortable with the care of a child in DKA.

With a child in DKA possibly comatose and in the intensive care unit, stress levels of the parents and caregivers are increased. The nurse must stay calm and think clearly. Performing assessments every 15 minutes is not too often. One aspect of assessment that is essential to know is the sound of Kussmaul breathing. **Kussmaul breaths** are very deep and laborious. In an attempt to correct the metabolic acidosis, the respiratory system works hard to "blow off" excess carbon dioxide. When a child breathes this way, some say it sounds like a locomotive.

Blood glucose is monitored every hour with the blood glucose goal results at approximately 100 to 180 mg/dL. When the child's blood glucose returns to a value below 300 mg/dL, 5% dextrose may be added back to the maintenance IV. Some physicians prefer a two-bag system hanging at the bedside, one IV bag with and one without glucose. Given through a Y-port, the nurse is able to infuse either one fluid or the other or both if the child needs them.

Serum potassium levels must also be checked regularly. Initially the DKA causes the child to be hyperkalemic. As the acidosis improves, and insulin and glucose are given, the child becomes hypokalemic. When the child's urinary output is adequate, potassium may be added to the IV fluids. With normal potassium levels, the child in DKA may need potassium. With abnormally low potassium levels, the ill child may need as much as 40 to 80 mEq/L. Placing the child on telemetry and obtaining an EKG may be needed to monitor for lethal arrhythmias.

Insulin infusions are begun at 0.1U/kg per hour. As the hyperglycemia and acidosis are corrected, the insulin rate is decreased. The insulin infusion is continued until the pH and the acidosis are corrected.

The child's electrolytes are carefully monitored and the acid–base balance is checked and documented every 2 to 4 hours. As the DKA is resolved, usually in 24 to 48 hours, and the child tolerates oral fluids, the insulin administration is switched to a subcutaneous regimen.

 case study A 3-Year-Old Child with Type 1 Diabetes Who is Vomiting

It is the middle of December and this young family is busy with holiday preparations, the children only have a week left of school before the holiday break, and Johnny, the first-grader, has had "a runny nose." It is craft day and the children are excited. The 3-year-old sister begins to cry. She is flushed and seems feverish and will not drink her favorite juice. The mother calls the clinic and states, "My daughter has vomited twice and is a newly diagnosed type 1 diabetic, I cannot get her to drink, what should I do, I think she may have the flu?"

critical thinking questions

1. What is the most important concept to relay to this mother?
2. How can she get the child to drink?
3. What should she do for the fever?
4. Should the mother call 911 or take the child to the Emergency Department?

◆ See Suggested Answers to Case Studies in text on the Electronic Study Guide or DavisPlus.

With the diabetic child in the intensive care unit, there are many members of the health care team working together in collaboration to prevent future episodes. In some cases, it was unknown that the child had diabetes and the DKA is the first time the parents realize that their child is ill. Whatever the scenario, working together, keeping lines of communication open, and realizing that the plan is ever-evolving keep everyone focused on the best possible outcomes for each child.

To prevent DKA, families must be taught to check and recheck blood glucose levels or urine ketone levels any time the child is sick (vomiting) or if a blood glucose result is greater than 240 mg/dL. Ideally, the parents should be taught and become comfortable with the child's management plan before discharge. Meals and insulin administration should be planned to give the child the most normal blood glucose level on average

(A_{1C}). Parents need to know that long-term complications occur when blood glucose is abnormally high and that keeping the blood glucose at as normal a level as possible will be the best protection their child can receive.

 Now Can You— Discuss Diabetes Mellitus?

1. Examine the difference between type 1 diabetes mellitus and type 2 diabetes mellitus?
2. Discuss the nursing care for the child with type 1 diabetes?
3. Discuss the nursing care for the child with type 2 diabetes?
4. Discuss the nursing care for the child with diabetic ketoacidosis (DKA)?

summary points

◆ The endocrine system controls a child's growth and development.

◆ Hormones regulate a child's response to stress and physical trauma.

◆ The nurse must document consistent, accurate record-keeping of child's growth rate because while he or she is on most treatments, these measurements are essential parameters of goal attainment.

◆ Complementary care could be significant in treating the common childhood illnesses but should be verified with a physician before all treatments.

◆ Dehydration is a severe problem, causing the infant/child to be irritable with many other manifestations, including dry mucous membranes, decreased skin turgor (tenting of abdominal skin in infant), decreased tears when crying, sunken fontanel, and tachycardia. The nurse must act quickly to avoid serious consequences of hypotension and shock.

◆ Pharmaceutical treatments are successful only with proper administration, the nurse must ensure that the medications are given accurately and that parents are taught techniques correctly.

◆ The nurse must educate parents regarding the signs and symptoms of endocrine conditions for the condition to be recognized early and treated as soon as possible.

◆ Insufficient amounts of cortisol and aldosterone cause Addison's disease.

◆ Children with aldosterone deficiencies may also present with hyponatremia, dehydration, and hyperkalemia. If not diagnosed early after birth, this salt wasting may become life-threatening with the infant in adrenal crisis.

◆ Diabetes is one of the leading causes of chronic illness in the United States.

◆ Type 2 diabetes is caused by the body's inability to recognize and utilize insulin rather than a deficient production of insulin as in type 1 diabetes and has become an epidemic in the pediatric population.

◆ Diabetic ketoacidosis (DKA) is a potentially fatal condition marked by an accumulation of ketones and increased acidity of the blood.

review questions

Multiple Choice

1. The pediatric nurse is providing discharge teaching to the family of a child who has been newly diagnosed with acromegaly. Included in the teaching should be the discussion of possible signs and symptoms that may occur. Which of the following signs and symptoms should be included?
   A. Hypotension
   B. Arthralgia
   C. Early onset of menarche
   D. Small fingers and toes

Select All that Apply

2. A parent of a child with growth hormone deficiency is interviewed in the public health clinic. Which of the following signs and symptoms must be included in the discussion?
   A. Short stature below the 3rd or 5th percentile
   B. Early closure of the anterior fontanel
   C. Delayed dental eruption
   D. High-pitched voice

3. The mother of a 7-year-old African American girl brings her daughter to the pediatrician's office for an annual examination. On assessment, the pediatric nurse notes which of the following signs or symptoms, which may suggest a diagnosis of precocious puberty?
   A. Breast development
   B. Some pubic hair
   C. Brittle hair
   D. Beginning of menstruation

4. A 9-year-old who has recently had surgery that involved the pituitary gland is now exhibiting signs and symptoms of diabetes insipidus. Which of the following signs and symptoms help confirm the nurse's suspicions?
   A. Vomiting
   B. Enuresis
   C. Polyuria
   D. Polydipsia

True/False

5. If the child receiving human recombinant growth hormone therapy begins complaining of a headache, the pediatric nurse should suspect that this symptom may be indicative of increasing intracranial pressure.

6. The child who is on strict intake and output must be evaluated for fluid retention. As a component of the nursing assessment, the pediatric nurse should auscultate the child's lung sounds to detect over-hydration.

7. To ensure that the infant receives the full dosage of the ordered hormone tablet, the prudent pediatric nurse should dilute the medication in the infant's bottle of formula.

8. The pediatric nurse would not be surprised to see a child with acromegaly exhibit a rapid increase in skeletal growth each time the child's height and weight is plotted on the growth chart.

Fill-in-the-Blank

9. The child with growth hormone deficiency will have studies done to evaluate his/her bone age. It would not be unrealistic to expect to find the child's _____, _____, or _____ size to be less than the child's chronological age.

10. It is important to note that in the _____ age group, the classic manifestations of DKA are often absent.

See Answers to End of Chapter Review Questions on the Electronic Study Guide or DavisPlus.

REFERENCES

A.D.A.M. (2004). *Alternative Medicine*. From http://www.adam.com/ (Accessed July 15, 2008).

A.D.A.M. (2006). *Alternative Medicine*. From http://www.adam.com/ (Accessed July 15, 2008).

Allen, D.B. (2006). Growth hormone therapy for short stature: Is the benefit worth the burden? *Pediatrics, 118,* 343–348. Retrieved from www.aapublications.org (Accessed February 21, 2007).

Amer, K.S. (2005). Advances in assessment, diagnosis, and treatment of hyperthyroidism in children. *Journal of Pediatric Nursing, 20,* 119–126.

American Diabetes Association (ADA). (2007a). Nutrition recommendations and interventions for diabetes. *Diabetes Care,* S48-S65.

American Diabetes Association (ADA). (2007b). Standards of medical care in diabetes—2007. *Diabetes Care,* S4–S41.

Atkinson, A., & Radjenovic, D. (2006). Meeting quality standards for self-management education in pediatric type 2 diabetes. *Diabetes Care,* 40–46.

Baykan, A., Narin, N., Kendirci, M., Akcakus, M., Kucukaydin, M., & Patiroglu, T. (2005). Pheochromocytoma presenting with polydipsia and polyuria in a child. *Erciyes Medical Journal, 27,* 128–131.

Bowen, R. (2003, August 28). Congenital adrenal hyperplasia. Retrieved from http://www.vivo.coxlostate.edu/hbooks/pathphys/endocrine/adrenal (Accessed November 20, 2008).

Bulechek, G., Butcher, H.M., & Dochterman, J. (2008). *Nursing interventions classification (NIC)* (5th ed.). St. Louis, MO: C.V. Mosby.

Chan, J.C., & Roth, K.S. (2006, July 26). Diabetes insipidus. Retrieved from http://www.emedicine.com/ped/topic580.htm (Accessed July 14, 2008).

Chase, H.P., & Eisenbarth, G.S. (2005). Diabetes mellitus. In W.W. Hay (Ed.). *Current Pediatric Diagnosis & Treatment* (pp. 1006–1013). New York: Lange Medical Books/McGraw-Hill.

Children's Hospital Boston. (2007). Diabetes insipidus. Retrieved from www.childrenshospital.org (Accessed July, 14, 2008).

Children's Hospital Boston. (2007). Hypoparathyroidism. Retrieved from www.childrenshospital.org/az/Site1132/printerfriendlypageS1132PO.html (Accessed November 20, 2008).

Children's Hospital and Clinics of Minnesota. (2007a). Adrenal insufficiency: Hormone replacement therapy. Retrieved from www.childrensmn.org (Accessed July 15, 2008).

Children's Hospitals and Clinics of Minnesota. (2007b). Desmopressin (DDAVP) for diabetes insipidus. Retrieved from www.childrensmn.org (Accessed July 15, 2008).

Children With Diabetes. (2006). What is insulin? Retrieved from http://www.childrenwithdiabetes.com/ (Accessed July 15, 2008).

Cleary, M.A., & Green, A. (2005). Developmental delay: When to suspect and how to investigate for an inborn error of metabolism. *Archives of Disease in Childhood, 90,* 1128–1132.

Demirel, F., Özer, T., Gurel, A., Acun, C., Ozdemir, H., Tomac, N., et al. (2004). Effect of iodine supplementation on goiter prevalence among the pediatric population in a severely iodine deficient area. *Journal of Pediatric Endocrinology Metabolism, 17,* 73–76.

Duncan, G.E. (2006). Prevalence of diabetes and impaired fasting glucose levels among US adolescents: National Health and Nutrition Examination Survey, 1999-2002. *Archives of Pediatrics & Adolescent Medicine.* 160 (5), 523–528.

Ferry, R.J. (2006). EMedicine: Graves' disease. Retrieved from http://www.emedicine.com/ped/topic899.html (Accessed November 20, 2008).

Freda, P.U. (2006). Pegvisomant therapy for acromegaly. *Expert Review of Endocrinology & Metabolism, 1,* 489–498.

Glatt, K., Garzon, D.L., & Popovic, J. (2005). Congenital adrenal hyperplasia due to 21-hydroxylase deficiency. *Journal for Specialists in Pediatric Nursing, 10,* 104.

Hudson, M.J. (2007). Complications of diabetes insipidus: The significance of headache. *Pediatric Nursing*, 1–4.

Ibanez, L., Ong, K., Valls, C., Marcos, M.V., Dunger, D.B., & De Zegher, F. (2006). Metformin treatment to prevent early puberty in girls with precocious pubarche. *Journal of Clinical Endocrinology and Metabolism, 91*, 2888–2891.

Johnson, M., Bulechek, G., Butcher, H., McCloskey Dochterman, J., Maas, M., Moorehead, S., & Swanson, E. (2006). *NANDA, NOC, and NIC linkages: Nursing diagnoses, outcomes, & interventions* (2nd ed.). St. Louis, MO: Mosby Elsevier.

Joslin Diabetes Center. (2006, November 2). Science Daily: Study shows durability of insulin pump therapy for adolescents. Retrieved from http://www.sciencedaily.com/release/2006/10/061031191125.html (Accessed November 20, 2008).

Juvenile Diabetes Research Foundation International. (2006, November). Paths to a cure. Retrieved from http://www.jdrf.org/index.cfm?page_id101979 (Accessed July 15, 2008).

Kaplowitz, P.B. (2006, June 16). EMedicine—Precocious puberty. Retrieved from http://www.emedicine.com/ped/topic1882.html (Accessed August 7, 2007).

Kaye, C.I., & The Committee on Genetics. (2006). Newborn Screening Fact Sheets. *Pediatrics, 118*, E934–e963.

Keil, M., Batista, D., & Stratakis, C.A. (2003). *The National Institutes of Health, Bethesda, MD. Early identification of Cushing's's syndrome in children*. Retrieved from http://www.csrf.net/index.htm (Accessed July 15, 2008).

Kollars, J., Zarroug, A.E., Van Heerden, J., Lteif, A., Stavlo, P., Suarez, L., Moir, C., Ishitani, M., & Rodeberg, D. (2005). Primary hyperparathyroidism in pediatric patients. *Pediatrics, 115*, 974–980.

Lee, J.A., Grumbach, M.M., & Clark, O.H. (2007). Controversy in clinical endocrinology: The optimal treatment for pediatric Graves' disease is surgery. *Journal of Clinical Endocrinology and Metabolism, 92*(3), 801–803.

Lee, M.M. (2006). Idiopathic short stature. *The New England Journal of Medicine, 354*, 2576–2582.

Liotta, E.A. (2007, February 21). EMedicine: Addison disease. Retrieved from http://emedicine.com/derm/topic761.html (Accessed March 18, 2007).

Lucile Packard Children's Hospital at Stanford (2007). Retrieved from http://www.lpch.org/HealthLibrary/ChildrensHealthAZ/index.html (Accessed November 20, 2008).

McKnight-Menci, H., Sababu, S., & Kelly, S.D. (2005). The care of children and adolescents with type 2 diabetes. *Journal of Pediatric Nursing, 20*, 96–106.

Moorehead, S., Johnson, M., Maas, M., & Swanson, E. (2008). *Nursing outcomes classification (NOC)* (4th ed.). St. Louis, MO: C.V. Mosby.

NANDA International (2007). *NANDA-I nursing diagnoses: Definitions and classifications 2007–2008*. Philadelphia: NANDA-I.

NIH Publication No. 04-3054 (2004, June). Addison's disease. Retrieved from http://www.endocrine.niddlc.nih.gov/pubs/addison/addison.htm (Accessed November 20, 2008).

Postellon, D. (2006, August 23). EMedicine: Congenital hypothyroidism.

Quigley, A.C., Gill, M.A., Crowe, J.B., Robling, K., Chipman, J.J., Rose, R.S., et al. (2005). Safety and growth hormone treatment in pediatric patients with idiopathic short stature. *The Journal of Clinical Endocrinology & Metabolism, 90*, 5188–5196.

Schwartz, R.A. (2007, June 12). Emedicine—Acromegaly. Retrieved from http://www.emedicine.com/derm/topic593.html (Accessed August 9, 2007).

Science Daily (2007). Gene's role in type 1 diabetes discovered. Retrieved from http://www.sciencedaily.com/ (Accessed July 14, 2008).

Stallwood, L. (2006). Relationship between caregiver knowledge and socioeconomic factors on glycemic outcomes of young children with diabetes. *Journal for Specialists in Pediatric Nursing, 11*, 158.

Traggiai, C., & Stanhope, R. (2003). Disorders of pubertal development. *Best Practice and Research Clinical Obstetrics and Gynecology, 17*, 41–56.

Vuguin, P. (2007). EMedicine: Pheochromocytoma. Retrieved from http://www.emedicine.com/ped/topic1788.html (Accessed July 15, 2008).

Wilson, T.A. (2006a, April 7). EMedicine: Adrenal Insufficiency. Retrieved from http://www.emedicine.com/ (Accessed July 15, 2008).

Wilson, T.A. (2006b, June 16). EMedicine: Adrenal hypoplasia. Retrieved from http://www.emedicine.com/ (Accessed July 15, 2008).

Wilson, T.A. (2006c, November 17). EMedicine: Congenital adrenal hyperplasia. Retrieved from http://www.emedicine.com/ (Accessed July 15, 2008).

Wysocki, T., Buckloh, L.M., Lochrie, A.S., & Antal, H. (2005). The psychologic context of pediatric diabetes. *Pediatric Clinics of North America, 52*, 1755–1778.

Young, G.M. (2007, January 4). EMedicine: Pediatrics, diabetic ketoacidosis. Retrieved from http://www.emedicine.comEMERG/topic373.html (Accessed November 20, 2008).

 For more information, go to http://davisplus.fadavis.com/

CONCEPT MAP

Organs
- Hypothalamus
- Pituitary gland
- Thyroid and parathyroid
- Adrenal gland
- Pancreas
- Pineal body
- Ovary or testes

Hormones
- ADH
- Growth hormone
- TSH; PTH
- ACTH-Releasing
- Aldosterone
- Insulin

Caring for the Child with an Endocrinologic or Metabolic Condition

General Potential Nursing Care
Assessments: thorough nursing history; school performance; sleep patterns; growth measurements, including skeletal; presence of abnormal physical characteristics for age and body build; vital signs; heart rate/rhythm/perfusion; urine output; daily weight, I&O; fluid/electrolyte balance; neurological assessment
Interventions: approach child using correct emotional and cognitive developmental level; address body image issues; manage stress; encourage exercise/activity/adjust diet; provide emergency treatments for acute conditions; care of the post-surgical child; care of the child with chronic illness; includes collaborative and interdisciplinary care
Teaching: about condition itself; treatments; resources/ foundations; administration of, compliance with and side effects of medications; treatments for home care (i.e., wts, I&O); follow up appointments; S & S of complications

Adrenal Conditions
- Adrenocortical insufficiency
  – Acute: life threatening < ACTH
  – Chronic: Addison;
  – Cushing's syndrome
- CAH: congenital adrenal hyperplasia
- Hyperaldosteronism
- Pheochromocytoma

Metabolic Conditions
Pancreatic
- Type I diabetes
  – autoimmune
- Type II diabetes
  → With all, failure to produce sufficient insulin
  → DKA: prevalent in Type I

Thyroid Conditions
- Hypothyroid sm: untreated = Goiter
- Hyperthyroidism: Graves disease

Parathyroid Conditions
- Hypoparathyroidism: inherited or acquired
- Hyperparathyroidism: leads to osteoporosis; osteomalacia

Pituitary Conditions
Anterior →
- Hypopituitary: GHD
- Hyperpituitary
  – Precocious puberty: sex characteristics < age 8-9
  – Acromegaly/gigantism: abnormal/overgrowth hands/feet/facial features

Posterior →
- Diabetes insipidus: < ADH production, gross water loss
- SIADH: > ADH, gross water retention

Clinical Alert:
- Exogenous hormones in OTC female products
- Dehydration can lead to hypovolemic shock
- Tenting not always seen in dehydration
- Hyponatremia can precipitate seizures
- Thyroid storm: potentially fatal
- Signs/symptoms of impending adrenal crisis
- Assess ABCs first in impending shock
- Infection is a major cause of DKA

Critical Nursing Action:
- Assess ht and wt. accurately
- Thoroughly assess IV site when infusing IV Ca^{2+}
- Never stop steroids suddenly
- Never touch/manipulate visible pheochromocytoma

Optimizing Outcomes:
- Help parents to access financial resources for tx.
- Use hormones to treat Addison

Nursing Insight:
- Accurate medication doses are based on daily weights
- GH, IGF-I, somatostatin are involved in acromegaly
- Action of diuretics on the kidney
- Soy-based formula may decrease absorption of levothyroxine
- DiGeorge syndrome = defect in parathyroid development
- How to assess for hyperreflexia Ca^{2+}/Mg^{2+} used to tx hypoparathyroidism

Ethnocultural Considerations:
- Assess palms/lips for color
- Changes in dark complexions
- Necessary for tx of CAH in Type II DM

Where Research Meets Practice:
- Type 1 diabetes is not purely genetic; environmental factors
- Use of homeopathy in acute diarrhea
- Inhaled insulin

Complementary Care:
- Therapeutic touch or massage
- Nutrition & herbs that help thyroid function

What To Say:
- Help child express anxiety about daily injections
- Differentiate between hypo/hyperglycemia

Collaboration In Caring:
- Psychological counseling is part of the team approach
- Nuclear medicine studies and surgery often part of tx

Now Can You:
- Describe conditions of the anterior/posterior pituitary
- Examine nursing care for conditions of the thyroid
- Discuss diabetes mellitus type 1 and 2 and associated nursing care

Across Care Settings:
- Refer to endocrinologist and psychologist for precocious puberty
- Team approach for DM type I treatment

Be Sure To:
- Teach parents re: f/u appointments
- Treat adrenal crisis STAT

Caring for the Child with a Neurological or Sensory Condition

"The brain is wider than the sky,
For, put them side by side,
The one the other will include
With ease, and you beside.
The brain is deeper than the sea,
For, behold them, blue to blue
The one the other will absorb
As sponges, buckets do."

—Emily Dickinson

LEARNING TARGETS *At the completion of this chapter, the student will be able to:*

◆ Discuss the physiology and normal function of the nervous system.

◆ Discuss the neurological assessment of a pediatric patient.

◆ Examine the altered states of consciousness along with the nursing care for a pediatric patient.

◆ Explore increased intracranial pressure (ICP) and the impact on the child's life.

◆ Identify conditions that cause a dysfunction of the nervous system.

◆ Recognize signs and symptoms of life-threatening complications of neurological disorders and sensory disorders.

◆ Discuss nursing care for various conditions affecting a child's nervous system and senses.

◆ Identify agencies and organizations available to provide support for a child and his or her family.

◆ Formulate a plan of care for a child with a neurological and/or sensory disorder.

◆ Prioritize nursing interventions when planning care for a patient with an alteration in neurological or sensory function.

---

 moving toward evidence-based practice Connection Between Epilepsy and Migraine Headache

Stevenson, S.B. (2006). Epilepsy and migraine headache: Is there a connection? *Journal of Pediatric Nursing Care, 20*(3), 167–171.

The purpose of this study was to investigate the prevalence of migraine headache in children with epilepsy and the presence of both migraine and epilepsy in the family history.

A sample of 470 pediatric participants was selected from a retrospective chart review of children with a primary diagnosis of epilepsy that were evaluated for follow-up in a neurology clinic between January 2003 and June 2004.

• The diagnosis of epilepsy was based on the International Classification of Diseases, Ninth Revision, Clinical Modification (ICD-9-CM) epilepsy codes.

• The definition for migraine headache included one or more of the following: phonophobia, photophobia, or other visual changes, and headache with nausea and/or vomiting.

• Descriptions for migraine headache or symptoms in participants too young to describe specific symptoms were based on parental reports. Information about family history included reports about close relatives with complaints of migraine headache, other types of headaches, epilepsy, or both (any type of headache and epilepsy).

(continued)

Data from the participants' charts was obtained through interviews conducted by physicians, residents, nurses, and medical students. Analysis of demographic data revealed that:

- The participants' mean age was 10.6 years: 29% were ages 1–7 years; 62% were ages 8–17 years; and 9% were age 18 years or older.
- Fifty-five percent were males.
- Headaches (any type of headache) were reported by 22.1% of females and 18.3% of males.
  - Participants younger than 7 years of age reported headaches 10% of the time.
  - Participants between 8 and 17 years of age reported headaches 23.5% of the time.
  - Participants between the ages of 18 and 26 years of age reported headaches 24% of the time.
- Sixty-nine participants reported both epilepsy and migraine headaches.
- Fourteen participants reported a family history of migraine, 97 had a positive family history of epilepsy,

and 11 reported a family history of both migraine headache and epilepsy.

Twenty percent of the participants reported headaches. This figure is consistent with headache incidence reported in other national studies. Occurrence of migraine headache in the general pediatric population ranges from 2.7% to 11%.

The increased presence of a family history of epilepsy and the prevalence of comorbid conditions, i.e., epilepsy and migraine, were also supported in the literature.

The researcher concluded that a higher incidence of migraine headaches occurs among the pediatric population diagnosed with epilepsy than in the general population.

1. What might be considered as limitations to this study?
2. How is this information useful to clinical nursing practice?

See Suggested Responses for Moving Toward Evidence-Based Practice on the Electronic Study Guide or DavisPlus.

Introduction

The nervous system is a complex system of structures that initiate, coordinate, and control all major functions of the body. A dysfunction of the nervous system resulting from internal and/or external factors may occur throughout the life span. The nervous system of a fetus is fragile. Injury to the nervous system may result in a life-altering or life-threatening disorder. In addition to congenital disorders, infants and children may be exposed to microbes that result in illnesses with short- and/or long-term effects. Traumatic events such as near drowning and head trauma sometimes have devastating neurological consequences. Congenital disorders, illnesses, and accidents affect not only the infant or child, but also the entire family. This chapter provides a review of the alterations related to congenital anomalies, illness, traumatic events, and sensory disorders.

A & P review **The Nervous System**

The nervous system is made up of the central nervous system (CNS) that consists of the brain and spinal cord and the peripheral nervous system. The peripheral nervous system (PNS) consists of the cranial nerves, the spinal nerves, and peripheral nerves. The peripheral nervous system is subdivided into the sensory-somatic nervous system and the autonomic nervous system. The brain is a network of nerve cells called neurons, which consist of axons and dendrites. Axons take information away from the cell body and dendrites bring information to the cell body. Brain tissue may be white or gray. White matter consists of axons that are coated with myelin, which allow nerve impulses to travel rapidly, and gray matter is made of neuronal cell bodies and surrounds the cerebral hemispheres, thus forming the cerebral cortex. Areas of gray matter are also found deep in the brain and include the

basal ganglia (affects movement), the hypothalamus (maintains homeostasis and regulates blood pressure, heart rate, and temperature), and the thalamus (processes sensory impulses and sends them to the cerebral cortex). Another important structure of the nervous system is the spinal cord.

The spinal cord is a mass of nerve tissue encased in a vertebral column, and the cord contains sensory and motor pathways. The spinal cord does not extend the length of the vertebral canal. A disruption in the pathway from the brain to the peripheral nervous system and spinal cord results in altered neurological function (Bickley & Szilagyi, 2003). ◆

Altered States of Consciousness

A child who is fully conscious is aware of the environment and self. The child is able to react to internal and external stimuli in an appropriate manner. A decrease in this awareness may result in a decrease or alteration in consciousness. Consciousness comprises two components: arousal and thought content. Arousal or level of consciousness (awareness of the environment) is a child's level of alertness or responsiveness to stimuli. Level of consciousness is controlled by the reticular activating system and the cerebral hemispheres of the brain. Cognitive cerebral function cannot occur without an active reticular activating system.

Content of thought includes all cognitive functions that ensure awareness of affective states, self, and environment. Content of thought is controlled by language and attention, concept and reasoning, memory, and the executive system (the cognitive processes involving logic, planning, analysis, and reasoning). An alteration in content of thought may be caused by internal or external factors including structural, metabolic, and psychogenic. Structural factors are abnormalities of the anatomy of the brain. Metabolic factors include infections, trauma, congenital anomalies, vascular anomalies, and toxins (McCance & Huether, 2002). Psychogenic factors are influenced by psychological disturbances within a child.

When determining the etiology of an altered state of consciousness, organic and functional causes must be evaluated. Whatever the etiology of the alteration, there are degrees of consciousness. Abnormal responses and nursing actions to assess the state of consciousness are identified in Table 29-1.

THE UNCONSCIOUS CHILD

Unconsciousness is a state in which a child's cerebral function is depressed. Unconsciousness ranges from a stupor (aroused only with vigorous or unpleasant stimulation) to a coma (state of unconsciousness when the child cannot be aroused) (Venes, 2009). A child may be in an unconscious state for many reasons. The more common etiologies for unconsciousness in a pediatric patient are infection, trauma, and hypoxemia. The unconscious child requires astute and continuous monitoring by the nurse. The nurse carefully monitors vital signs, level of consciousness, reflexes, and pupil reaction. The nurse carefully and meticulously documents the objective data obtained to determine any deterioration that may alter therapy. The cause of the patient's unconscious state guides the nursing care and medical management. Unconsciousness caused by trauma requires a different plan of care than unconsciousness caused by an infection. The child may be in this state for a short time or for an extended time depending on the etiology, the effectiveness of treatment, and the ability to return to a normal

state of consciousness. The nurse also assesses the child for any seizure activity that may occur as a result of cerebral ischemia and edema.

Caring for the Unconscious Child

EVALUATING NEUROLOGICAL STATUS. The nurse carefully monitors the child's neurological status by assessing his or her level of consciousness (LOC) with the use of a pediatric Glasgow Coma Scale (GCS). The pediatric Glasgow Coma Scale consists of three components of assessment: eye opening, verbal response, and motor response (Fig. 29-1).

 Nursing Insight— *Assigning a numeric value for level of response*

When performing an assessment using the Pediatric Glasgow Coma Scale, the nurse assigns a numeric value to each of the levels of response (1–15).

- Score of 9–15 (unaltered state of consciousness)
- Score of 8–4 (state of coma)
- Score of 3 or below (deep coma)

Coma scale scores may fluctuate if a change in neurological state occurs, including cerebral ischemia, the administration of medications, including paralytics and sedatives, and a regaining of consciousness.

Table 29-1	States of Consciousness Technique and Patient Response	
State	**Technique**	**Abnormal Response**
Alertness	Speak in a normal tone of voice	An alert patient answers appropriately while opening his eyes and responding fully
Lethargy	Speak in a loud voice	A lethargic patient opens his eyes but appears drowsy; answers questions appropriately but falls asleep easily
Obtundation	Shake gently to arouse	An obtunded patient opens his eyes and looks at the stimuli; appears slightly confused; alertness and interest in surroundings are decreased
Stupor	Use a painful stimuli	A stuporous patient only responds to painful stimuli; verbal responses are absent or slow; responsiveness to a painful stimuli ceases
Coma	Apply repeated painful stimuli	A comatose patient does not respond to internal or external stimuli; he remains in an un-arousal state with eyes closed

Source: Bickley, L. & Szilagyi, P. (2003). *Bate's guide to physical examination and history taking* (8th ed.). Philadelphia: Lippincott Williams & Wilkins.

Figure 29-1 The pediatric Glasgow Coma Scale.

MONITORING VITAL SIGNS. The nurse carefully monitors, measures, and documents vital signs, level of consciousness, reflexes, and pupil reaction as prescribed by the health care provider or as dictated by facility policy. The frequency of vital sign measurement is dependent on the etiology, neurological status, and cerebral involvement. Any change in vital signs needs to be evaluated because the child's condition can deteriorate rapidly. The child's vital signs may need to be assessed every 15 minutes or more often if the neurological state or physical state is unstable. If the child's condition is stable, vital signs may be measured every 2 hours.

Cerebral infections can cause elevated temperatures, so the child's temperature must be measured every 2 to 4 hours. Intracranial bleeding may cause hyperthermia (body temperature elevated above the normal range). Administering antipyretics, applying a hypothermic blanket, providing a tepid bath, and maintaining a cool environment are used to decrease temperature.

MANAGING THE AIRWAY. A priority for any unconscious child is obtaining and maintaining a patent airway. Cardiopulmonary resuscitation may be the initial treatment. If a child is unconscious because of trauma or a neck injury, the respiratory structures may be damaged. If the structures are damaged or if edema is present, the airway may be compromised. A child with a fractured cervical spine injury may also be unable to breathe independently. The nurse needs to maintain adequate positioning and deliver oxygen by using various devices or mechanical assistance to maintain adequate respiratory function.

When caring for an unconscious child, the nurse meticulously monitors respiratory status including respiratory rate and rhythm, use of accessory muscles, apnea, level of consciousness, breath sounds, and level of oxygenation. A child in a light coma still may be able to cough and swallow and maintain adequate respiratory function. A child in a deep coma may be unable to swallow and adequately handle oral secretions. It is important to note that the gag reflex of an unconscious child may be impaired. The nurse suctions the airway to remove secretions that may obstruct the airway or that may be aspirated. The nurse must be careful when suctioning the child's airway because intracranial pressure may increase.

A child who cannot maintain respiratory function needs to be mechanically ventilated. The child may need ventilator assistance for only a short time or may be dependent on the ventilator indefinitely. When caring for a mechanically ventilated child, the nurse monitors the arterial blood gases. The nurse may administer medications to sedate or relax the child to prevent injury related to manipulation of the endotracheal tube or accidental extubation.

The unconscious child who is intubated for an extended period of time requires a tracheostomy. The nurse performs tracheostomy care for these patients. The nurse changes the child's position at least every 2 hours and performs chest physiotherapy to prevent respiratory complications of atelectasis and pneumonia.

MANAGING BLADDER AND BOWEL ELIMINATION. A child who has been continent may become incontinent during an unconscious state. The child may also experience urinary retention (incomplete emptying of the bladder) or a bladder infection. An indwelling catheter may be necessary if urinary function is lost and accurate output measurement is required.

Meticulous catheter care is imperative to prevent a urinary tract infection, which may further compromise the child's condition. If the child is in an extended state of unconsciousness, the indwelling catheter may be removed and the nurse may perform intermittent catheterizations. If the child regains consciousness and has no physical dysfunctions preventing bladder control, the nurse initiates bladder retraining. If a catheter is not inserted, a diaper may be used, and the nurse weighs the diaper to obtain accurate urine output measurement.

Bowel elimination in an unconscious child may also be affected. The child may experience constipation because of immobility. The child may also lack dietary fiber and experience medication side effects that can alter bowel elimination. The nurse monitors the child's bowel habits to assess for constipation and impactions. Stool softeners, suppositories, or enemas may be necessary to promote bowel elimination.

MAINTAINING HYDRATION AND NUTRITION. The hydration and nutritional needs of an unconscious child must be met based on the specific condition and progress of the child. The fluid needs of the child are based on weight, age, and illness or injury. The nurse administers intravenous fluids to promote fluid and electrolyte balance, prevent dehydration, and maintain urine output. The nurse carefully monitors intravenous fluid therapy and assesses for fluid overload.

If the child remains in an unconscious state, fluid and enteral feedings are administered through a nasogastric or gastrostomy tube. Feedings may be continuous or bolus. Before administering fluid or feeding, the nurse verifies placement of the tube in order to prevent aspiration. Gastric residuals must be measured before feedings are administered. If the residual is excessive (determined by the physician), the nurse replaces the gastric contents and delays the feeding as prescribed by the physician. If the residuals are consistently too great, the composition, frequency, and amount of enteral formula may need to be changed. When enteral feedings are first initiated, the child may experience diarrhea. The nurse must assess the child frequently for diarrheal stools. Also, in order to prevent dehydration, constipation, and renal complications, the nurse administers water through the nasogastric or gastrostomy tube.

PROVIDING PROPER HYGIENE. Skin care is imperative when caring for an unconscious child. The child's skin is fragile and prone to breakdown. The nurse can bathe the child every other day or as needed. The perineal area is cleansed often, sometimes several times a day. The child who is unable to move may develop pressure ulcers. The nurse assesses areas on the child's body that are prone to breakdown such as the shoulder, ankle, elbow, and trochanter. The child's position is changed every 2 hours, and pressure-relieving devices are used to prevent pressure ulcer formation. The nurse assesses skin folds for maceration due to moisture and keeps the child's skin dry and clean of body secretions and excretions.

Providing mouth care is an important nursing action because the child may have dry mucous membranes. The nurse cleans and moistens the child's mouth at least twice daily and assesses for any mouth ulcers or irritation, and lip emollients are applied to the mouth to prevent dryness (Fig. 29-2).

An unconscious child may not close his or her eyes or may keep the eyes open for long periods of time, and corneal irritation may develop. The nurse assesses the child's eyes for irritation and inflammation and may administer artificial tears at least every 2 hours to lubricate the eyes.

POSITIONING AND EXERCISE. The unconscious child is placed in a position that prevents aspiration and is anatomically correct. The nurse elevates the head of the bed 30 degrees and maintains the child's head in a midline position to prevent jugular compression and facilitate venous drainage. This position prevents increased intracranial pressure (ICP) due to jugular vein compression. The nurse performs passive range-of-motion exercises at least every 2 hours to prevent the development of contractures.

 Complementary Care: *The benefits of massage*

The oldest and simplest form of nursing care may be massage. Massage was used in ancient Egypt, China, and India to treat disease and injuries. Therapeutic massage has been performed to promote a sense of well-being and enhance self-esteem while benefiting the immune and circulatory systems. The resulting sense of well-being has been found to decrease the amount of circulating stress hormones cortisol and norepinephrine that may weaken the immune system. The decreased anxiety and tension allow people to feel more serene and enhances their ability to cope with life stressors. As a result of the many benefits of massage, different massage techniques have been integrated into various complementary therapies.

All forms of touch are perceived through the body's largest organ, the skin. Thousands of specialized receptors found in the dermis react to external stimuli, including touch, by

Figure 29-2 The nurse cleans and moistens the child's mouth at least twice daily.

sending messages to the brain through the nervous system. Gentle massage or stroking releases endorphins (the body's natural pain killers) and a feeling of comfort is experienced. Stronger, more vigorous massage helps to stretch tense and uncomfortable muscles, leading to improved mobility and flexibility. Also, massage aids in relaxation by affecting the body system that controls blood pressure, digestion, and respiration. The stimulation of circulation improves the supply of oxygen and nutrients to the body's tissues and enhances skin tone. Stimulation of the lymphatic system improves the body's ability to eliminate lactic acid and other chemical wastes that cause muscle stiffness and pain (Woodham & Peters, 2006).

When caring for an unconscious child, the nurse can incorporate therapeutic massage. The child may benefit from the many positive results of massage (e.g., decreased blood pressure, increased circulation, increased skin tone, improved peristalsis). Benefits of massage may also include decreased anxiety, decreased skin breakdown, and decreased constipation.

PERSISTENT VEGETATIVE STATE

A persistent vegetative state is a complete unawareness of the environment accompanied by sleep–wake cycles. The diagnosis of this condition is established if it is present for 1 month after acute or nontraumatic brain injury or has lasted for 1 month in children with degenerative or metabolic disorders or developmental malformations (Venes, 2009).

The primary causes of a persistent vegetative state are developmental malformations, metabolic and degenerative disorders affecting the nervous system, and acute traumatic and nontraumatic brain injuries. The most common cause of acute brain injury associated with a persistent vegetative state is a hypoxic–ischemic **encephalopathy** (generalized brain dysfunction marked by varying degrees of impairment of speech, cognition, orientation, and arousal) and trauma (Venes, 2009).

A child in a persistent vegetative state remains unconscious but has irregular episodes of wakefulness alternating with sleeping. The child exhibits nonpurposeful movements and sounds. Most children in this state have adequate respiratory function although they may have previously required a tracheotomy or mechanical ventilation. A child's persistent vegetative state may be for a short period of time or lifelong. A child's recovery from a persistent vegetative state is dependent on the etiology. A child who is in a persistent vegetative state because of trauma may recover some function even though complete recovery of function is rare. If a metabolic or degenerative disorder is the cause of the persistent vegetative state, the child does not recover any function because of the progressive nature of the disease. A child with a congenital malformation severe enough to cause a persistent vegetative state does not acquire any awareness of self or environment. The life expectancy of a child in a persistent vegetative state is shortened due to respiratory complications (Ashwal, 2004). The nursing care provided for a pediatric patient in a persistent vegetative state is similar to care provided for an unconscious child.

nursing diagnoses The Unconscious Child

- Impaired Mobility related to altered neurological functioning
- Impaired Gas Exchange related to increased intracranial pressure
- Risk for Impaired Skin Integrity related to decreased mobility and incontinence
- Risk for Infection related to invasive hospital procedures
- Risk for Aspiration related to enteral feeding
- Risk for Altered Bowel Elimination related to decreased peristalsis

Family Support

The outcome for a child in a state of unconsciousness is uncertain. The family of a child who is in a persistent vegetative state experiences many emotions including fear, guilt, anxiety, anger, and depression. The nurse helps them cope with this difficult situation and plays a major role in providing support to the family members.

The intensive care unit can be a frightening environment because of the equipment, monitors, procedures, and invasive lines. The nurse helps the parents face this new environment and difficult experiences by being supportive and honest. The nurse facilitates family members' acceptance and healing by allowing them to express their feelings and to participate in the child's care. The nurse encourages the family to touch and talk to the child, which offers comfort and stimulation. Parents are asked to bring familiar toys. After the child's condition has stabilized, parents may decide to care for the child in the home or place the child in an extended care facility. Sometimes parents must make the difficult decision to end measures that are sustaining the child's life.

"What to say" — *Parental education*

The nurse must provide the family with specific instructions if the child is going to be cared for at home. Skills required to care for the child at home are determined by the condition of the child. The nurse communicates information about bathing, feeding, medication administration, medical equipment, tracheostomy suctioning, gastrostomy tubes, urinary catheterization, positioning, and range-of-motion exercises. The importance of performing these procedures correctly is also stressed. To validate parental understanding, the nurse asks the parents to demonstrate the tasks. Parents may appear reluctant and fearful. The nurse must remain supportive and patient as parents learn new skills.

The nurse also discusses signs and symptoms of complications with the parents that may need further medical evaluation. The parents must also be able to identify nonverbal indicators of illness or distress because the child is unable to communicate pain or discomfort. The nurse may suggest that the parents ask family and friends to care for the child occasionally. Some communities have respite care centers for parents with medically fragile children.

The community health nurse can assist the parents with the child's care and be a resource to answer questions, address concerns, and find other community resources.

INCREASED INTRACRANIAL PRESSURE

A delicate balance exists between the volume of the intracranial vault and the contents including the brain, blood, and cerebrospinal fluid (CSF). The CSF is the fluid of the brain and spinal cord that supplies nutrients and removes waste products and also serves as a watery cushion that absorbs shock to the central nervous system (Venes, 2009). The **intracranial pressure** (ICP) is the pressure of the CSF in the subarachnoid space between the skull and the brain.

clinical alert

Monroe–Kellie hypothesis

The pressure–volume relationship among the blood, intracranial pressure (ICP), volume of cerebrospinal fluid (CSF), and brain tissue and cerebral perfusion pressure is known as the Monroe–Kellie hypothesis or Monroe–Kellie Doctrine. The hypothesis states that if one of the components increases, the other components must compress (LeJune & Howard-Fain, 2002). The body tries to compensate by an increase in CSF absorption, a decrease in CSF production, a reduction in blood volume, or a decrease in brain mass. When compression is exhausted, the ICP rises. As a result of increased ICP, blood flow and oxygen delivery may be compromised. When blood flow and oxygen decrease, secondary brain injury occurs (Marcoux, 2005).

Nursing Insight— *Increased intracranial pressure*

Increased intracranial pressure (ICP) can have devastating and long-term consequences for the child and family. Infants and children whose fontanels have not closed are able to compensate for increased ICP for a short time. The child's fontanels bulge and skull sutures may separate to accommodate the increased volume.

A child can have increased ICP as a result of many internal or external factors. If the child has suffered a primary brain injury, the child is at risk for developing increased ICP and secondary brain injuries. Primary brain injury is irreversible, immediate, and can result from traumatic injuries (e.g., a blow to the head) or nontraumatic injuries (a tumor or infection). Secondary brain injuries include hypoxia, hypercapnia (increased serum CO_2), hypotension, acidosis, and reduced oxygen delivery (LeJune & Howard-Fain, 2002). The etiologies of increased ICP can be classified by the mechanism through which the ICP is increased. Many disorders increase brain mass or volume, including contusions (bruises), a brain tumor, a subdural or epidural hematoma (swelling composed of blood), or an abscess (a collection of pus).

Generalized brain swelling can be caused by ischemic–anoxic states, hypertensive encephalopathy, acute liver failure, hypercapnia, or Reye syndrome that may result in a decrease in cerebral perfusion with minimal brain shifts. An increase in venous pressure can result from venous sinus thrombosis, obstruction of superior mediastinal or jugular veins, or cardiac failure. If an obstruction to CSF flow or absorption is present, ICP increases. Some disorders in which CSF is obstructed are hydrocephalus, extensive meningeal disease, or obstruction in superior sagittal sinus and cerebral convexities. Meningitis, choroid plexus tumor, and subarachnoid hemorrhage can increase CSF production, resulting in increased ICP (Dennis & Mayer, 2001).

The cranium and vertebral body form a rigid container, and if any of its contents increase, an increase in ICP occurs. Small increases in brain volume do not result in an immediate increase in ICP because the CSF is able to be displaced into the spinal cord. The tentorium between the hemispheres and cerebellum and the falx cerebri between the hemispheres are slightly flexible, allowing for some stretching. An infant's normal ICP values are 2 to 6 mm Hg, young children's values are 3 to 7 mm Hg, and older children's values are 0 to 10 mm Hg. Once the ICP reaches approximately 20 mm Hg, small increases in blood volume can result in extreme elevations in ICP.

 Nursing Insight— *Cerebral perfusion pressure (CPP)*

The difference between the mean arterial pressure within the cerebral vessels and ICP is termed cerebral perfusion pressure (CPP). The CPP is calculated by subtracting the ICP from the mean arterial pressure: (CPP = MAP − ICP).

One of the primary dangers of increased ICP is that decreasing cerebral perfusion can cause ischemia (Dennis & Mayer, 2001). As the ICP nears the level of the mean systemic pressure, it is more difficult for blood to enter the intracranial space. The body's natural response to a decrease in CPP is to increase blood pressure and dilate the blood vessels in the brain. The vasodilation results in increased cerebral blood volume that increases ICP and lowers CPP further. This vicious cycle results in widespread reduction in cerebral blood flow and perfusion leading to ischemia and brain infarction. CPP should be maintained at greater than 50 to 70 mm Hg with increased ICP because a lower level may result in secondary hypoxic–ischemic injury (Marcoux, 2005). An increase in blood pressure may also make intracranial hemorrhages bleed more quickly, which increases ICP. If brainstem compression is involved, the respiratory center is affected and respiratory depression and arrest may occur.

SIGNS AND SYMPTOMS. The signs and symptoms of a child with increased ICP demonstrate are related to cerebral edema and ischemia (Table 29-2).

 Nursing Insight— *Cushing's triad*

A child with significantly increased intracranial pressure may exhibit Cushing's triad. Symptoms of Cushing's triad are hypertension (with widening pulse pressure), bradycardia, and an irregular respiratory pattern. Cushing's triad is usually indicative of impending herniation (the displacement of the foramen magnum; Venes, 2009).

DIAGNOSIS. The diagnosis of increased ICP is based on signs and symptoms exhibited by the child and diagnostic tests results. **Papilledema** (a mass of blown-out

Table 29-2	Signs and Symptoms of Increased Intracranial Pressure in Infants	
Early Signs and Symptoms	**Late Signs and Symptoms**	
Headache	Further decrease in LOC	
Emesis	Bulging fontanels (infant)	
Change in LOC	Decreasing spontaneous movements	
Decrease in GCS score	Posturing	
Irritability	Papilledema	
Sunsetting eyes	Pupil dilation with decreased or no response to light	
Decreased eye contact (infant)	Increased blood pressure	
Pupil dysfunction	Irregular respirations	
Cranial nerve dysfunction	Cushing's triad (late, ominous sign)	
Seizures		

Adapted from Marcoux, K. (2005). Management of increased intracranial pressure in the ill child with an acute neurological injury. *AACN Advanced Critical Care*, 16(2), 212-231.

blood vessels located around the optic nerve) is an important sign of increased ICP. This finding can be observed when the nurse assesses the child's eyes with an ophthalmoscope.

 diagnostic tools Determining Increased Intracranial Pressure (ICP)

Magnetic resonance imaging (MRI) or computed tomography (CT) is used to determine the etiology and severity of increased ICP. As a rule, CT contrast should be avoided in the presence of intracranial bleeding. The child's ICP can also be monitored by inserting an intracranial catheter.

NURSING CARE. The nurse closely monitors the pediatric patient with increased ICP because changes in the neurological status can occur very quickly and may have life-threatening consequences. The nurse's initial assessment provides a baseline by which the child's progress is evaluated. The goals of the child's care are to provide general supportive care and prevent secondary injury.

A priority nursing intervention is maintenance of a patent airway. Inadequate oxygenation or excess carbon dioxide causes cerebral blood vessels to dilate, resulting in an increase in ICP. The child should be intubated if the Glasgow Coma Score is less than 8 (Marcoux, 2005). If the child is intubated, the nurse monitors the ventilator equipment too. It is important to maintain normal ventilation with a P_{O_2} of 120 to 140 mm Hg and a P_{CO_2} of 30 to 35 mm Hg. Sometimes positive end expiratory pressure (PEEP) is necessary to maintain oxygenation saturations above 95%.

If the child's condition deteriorates, hyperventilation, with an Ambu-bag, may be performed until the ICP decreases. Hyperventilation is aimed at keeping a low level of serum P_{CO_2} so that cerebral blood flow decreases and reduces cerebral blood volume, thereby reducing ICP. Prolonged hyperventilation is avoided because it may cause hypotension due to decreased venous return (Marcoux, 2005). Mild hyperventilation may be prescribed by some health care providers. If the child is not intubated, supplemental oxygenation will be necessary. If possible, the nurse positions the child on the side in order to decrease possible airway obstruction.

The child's vital signs are monitored very closely. Intracranial bleeding is often accompanied by an increase in body temperature which is usually resistant to antipyretic agents. Hyperthermia is to be avoided because brain metabolic needs will be greatly increased. The nurse may use a hypothermic blanket if the child's temperature is higher than 102°F (39°C).

 critical nursing action Assessing for Hypothermia

When using a hypothermic blanket, the nurse must monitor the patient's temperature continuously to prevent hypothermia (a body temperature below 95°F [35°C]). Hypothermia causes shivering and an increase in ICP.

Acetaminophen (Children's Tylenol) or ibuprofen (Children's Advil) may be administered by the nurse to lower the child's temperature. Cooling the environment may help as well.

The head of the bed can be elevated 15 to 30 degrees to promote venous blood return, but a side effect of elevating the head is that the pressure of blood being delivered to the brain decreases, resulting in inadequate blood supply and perfusion. Another simple way to decrease ICP (particularly in trauma patients) is to loosen clothing around the neck.

 clinical alert

Patient safety

Never place the patient's head lower than the body. This position significantly increases the patient's ICP.

Administer intravenous fluid cautiously because hypertonic IV solutions have an osmotic effect. Normal saline, lactated Ringer's solution, and albumin are primarily used.

 Nursing Insight— *Intravenous fluids*

Hypotonic intravenous fluids (a combination of dextrose [5% or 10%] and sodium chloride [0.22% or 0.3%]) are avoided because they cross the blood–brain barrier resulting in increased cerebral edema and ICP.

If a child has increased ICP and has inadequate circulation, fluid administration takes priority over concern about cerebral edema. Fluid restriction is contraindicated in children who are poorly perfused with brain pathology or hypovolemic (an insufficient amount of fluid in the circulatory system) because hypovolemia results in decreased cerebral perfusion. To closely monitor fluid balance, the nurse accurately measures and records intake and output.

Another responsibility of the nurse is to protect the child from injury. The child with increased ICP may be predis-

posed to seizures. The nurse administers antiseizure medications as prescribed. Phenytoin (Dilantin) or a similar medication may be used. The nurse also places the child under seizure precautions. The nurse monitors seizures for such factors as frequency, severity, and type of seizure.

 clinical alert

Seizure precautions

- Maintain airway patency—Ensure nothing is placed in the child's mouth during a seizure. A loose tooth may be aspirated or knocked out.
- Monitor oxygenation—The child's color should remain pink. The pulse oximeter should read 95% or greater and the heart rate should be normal or slightly raised.
- Administering medications—When administering intravenous medications during a seizure, give the medication slowly to reduce the risk of side effects such as respiratory or circulatory failure.
- Raise and pad the side rails when the child is in bed or crib— The child needs to be protected from self harm (Fig. 29-3).
- Helmet—If the child has frequent seizures, a helmet can be worn to protect his head in case of a fall.
- Medical alert bracelet—The child who has seizures should wear a medical identification bracelet at all times.

The nurse must provide emotional support to the child and family. The nurse allows the child and family to express their feelings, can offer a support group, and reminds the family to treat the child as normally as possible.

 Nursing Insight— *Phenytoin (Dilantin)*

Phenytoin (Dilantin) may cause gingival hyperplasia. The nurse observes for swelling and bleeding of the child's gums and provides good dental hygiene. Parents need to be taught the necessity of performing proper hygiene.

Figure 29-3 An important care measure is padding the side rails.

medication: Mannitol (Osmitrol)

Mannitol (**man**-i-tol)

Classifications: Osmotic diuretic, diagnostic agent

Indications: Reduction of intracranial pressure and treatment of cerebral edema

Action: Increases the osmolarity of the glomerular filtrate, preventing the reabsorption of water and resulting in a loss of sodium chloride and water.

Contraindications: Use cautiously with hypersensitivity, anuria, and active intracranial bleeding.

Incompatibilities: Do not add to blood products.

Adverse Reactions and Side Effects: Confusion, headache, blurred vision, rhinitis, chest pain, pulmonary edema, tachycardia, nausea, thirst, vomiting, renal failure, urinary retention, dehydration, hyperkalemia, hypernatremia, hypokalemia, hyponatremia and phlebitis at the IV site.

Route and Dosage: Reduction of intracranial/intraocular pressure: 1–2 g/kg as a 15–20% solution over 30–60 minutes

Nursing Implications:
1. Do not administer electrolyte-free mannitol with blood products. If blood is administered, add at least 20 mEq of NaCl to each liter of mannitol.
2. Confer with physician regarding placement of an indwelling Foley catheter (except when used to decrease intraocular pressure).
3. Administer by IV infusion undiluted.

Evaluation/Desired Outcomes:
1. Urine output of at least 30–50 mL/hr or an increase in urine output in accordance with patient parameters set by physician
2. Reduction in intracranial pressure
3. Reduction in intraocular pressure
4. Excretion of certain toxic substances

Data from Deglin, J.H., & Vallerand, A. (2009). *Davis's drug guide for nurses* (11th ed., pp. 770–771). Philadelphia: F.A. Davis.

The nurse may also administer medications to decrease cerebral edema. A drug frequently prescribed is mannitol (Osmitrol).

Barbiturates may be administered to reduce ICP. Barbiturates cause the blood vessels in the brain to constrict but the blood vessels in the rest of the body to dilate. The nurse must carefully monitor volume status and blood pressure. The use of steroids with increased ICP is controversial. Corticosteroids reduce vasogenic edema surrounding brain abscesses and tumors and after neurosurgical manipulation such as with tumor resection. Corticosteroids have no effect on cytotoxic brain edema resulting from metabolic, infectious, or hypoxic–ischemic disorders (Dennis & Mayer, 2001).

The child with increased ICP may require analgesia and sedation. The child who is hospitalized for increased ICP is usually in an intensive care unit or in an area where he or she is closely monitored. Overstimulation from the child's environment, in addition to fear and pain, may increase the ICP. Pain and agitation should be treated aggressively if increased ICP is present. Nursing actions that may increase ICP include endotracheal suctioning, bathing, and positioning. If the child's ICP becomes dangerously high, the child should be sedated and, if necessary, paralyzed. Narcotics such as morphine (Astramorph) or fentanyl (Sublimaze) and benzodiazepines such as lorazepam (Ativan) are titrated to the desired effect.

 Optimizing Outcomes— Intracranial pressure monitoring

A pressure line may be inserted to accurately monitor ICP. Several types of monitoring devices are available, including intracranial bolts, intraventricular catheters, and intraparenchymal fiberoptic catheters. Intracranial pressure monitoring is indicated for the child who has a GCS score <8, exhibits signs of increasing ICP, who is post major neurosurgical procedures, or has a high probability of having increased ICP. The best outcome for ICP monitoring is to maintain cerebral perfusion pressure between 50 and 70 mm Hg, maintain ICP <20, and detect occurrences such as herniation or bleeding (Marcoux, 2005).

A craniotomy (an incision through the cranium) is recommended only when all other measures have been unsuccessful. A complication of a craniotomy is herniation of the brain through the defect, leading to further edema and an increase in ICP. After a craniotomy, the nurse assesses the child for signs and symptoms of infection and increased ICP postoperatively.

SEIZURE DISORDERS

A seizure is an electrical disturbance within the brain, resulting in changes of motor function, sensation, or cognitive ability. Seizure activity is classified according to the area of the brain experiencing the abnormal electrical activity and the neuromuscular sensory and psychogenic alteration from the electrical conduction disturbance. The incidence and onset of seizure disorders varies by age and underlying physical or pathological condition. Seizures may be genetically linked in susceptible children or the etiology may be unknown. Seizures can result from a traumatic brain injury, an infection in the central nervous system, toxic ingestion, endocrine dysfunction, atrial–venous malformation, or an anoxic episode. Neonates may develop seizures due to intrapartum or postpartum anoxic episodes, maternal ingestions or exposure to teratogens, and prenatal infections. Hypoglycemia and congenital malformations can also cause neonatal seizures in the first month of life. The prevalence of seizures is approximately 4 to 6 cases per 1000 children but the type of seizure incidence varies according to genetic predispositions in families (Richardson, 2006).

 Nursing Insight— Febrile seizures

Febrile seizures occur in less than 5% of the population and typically are seen in children younger than 3 years of age. Children may experience a febrile seizure between the ages of 6 months to 5 years but the most common occurrence is in the first 1 to 2 years of life. The exact etiology of febrile seizures has not been clearly identified. There may be a family history of seizure activity or febrile seizures. The child has a normal EEG without epileptiform (having the appearance of epilepsy) activity. In the emergency room, the nurse notes that the child with a febrile illness has a generalized tonic–clonic seizure lasting less than 15 minutes with a loss of consciousness. This pathological process can be controlled with antipyretics and anticonvulsant therapy, but this treatment is controversial and prescribed mainly in the case of anxious parents and/or prolonged febrile seizures (O'Dell et al., 2005; Robertson and Shilkofski, 2005). There is no preceding aura and the child may be postictal (confused) for a short time after the seizure is over. There is a slightly increased incidence of epilepsy in children with febrile seizures over the general population, especially if other types of seizures or abnormal CNS development are present in the child or the family (Robertson & Shilkofski, 2005).

SIGNS AND SYMPTOMS. Although seizures in children may be a direct result of a known disease process or injury, most seizures have unknown causes. Head injuries, infection, brain tumors, anoxic or hypoxic events such as a near drowning or intrauterine fetal compromise, or metabolic imbalance events can precipitate seizures in infants and children. Because seizures can indicate a disease process rather than be a disease entity alone, all pediatric seizures are thoroughly investigated (Table 29-3).

DIAGNOSIS. Seizures are diagnosed clinically with the use of neurological testing. Neurological testing procedures are used to determine the etiological epileptic focal center in the brain causing the abnormal electrical activity. In-depth testing of the neurological system helps to classify the type of seizure and determine appropriate anticonvulsant therapy. The neurological exam consists of a cranial nerve assessment, deep tendon reflex, sensory and motor response, level of consciousness, and hearing and pupil checks. A computed tomography (CT) scan or an MRI may be performed to look for CNS malformation, lesions, neoplasms, hemorrhage, trauma, foreign body, or edema. An angiography is done to assess for arteriovenous malformations that may be hereditary. New-onset seizures may suggest malignant neoplasms and warrant emergent neuroimaging.

Electroencephalogram (EEG) is the accepted standard test for diagnosing a seizure disorder. The EEG evaluates the electrical activity of the brain while the brain is in a sleepy or drowsy state and also when stimulated (Fig. 29-4). Loud noises, bright lights, and rapid flashing images are presented during the procedure and the resulting electrical brain wave response is graphed. This information is useful to the neurologist in diagnosing the type of seizure activity, especially if the history and exam do not support a clear diagnosis. Video EEG can also be done if the EEG is inconclusive or if the child experiences sleep and waking onset seizures. Positron emission tomography (PET) is performed if brain structures require outlining or mapping before a surgical procedure, but is not routinely indicated for seizure evaluations.

NURSING CARE. Seizure management is a collaborative effort among the nurse, the medical team, the primary care provider, and the family. Specific nursing care for a child with seizures is determined by the type of seizure. If the etiologic agent for the seizure is pathological in origin, seizures are managed medically until the cause can be resolved. If the cause is a brain tumor, the mass is excised.

Table 29-3   Types of Seizures and Signs and Symptoms

Type of Seizures	Brain Location/Cause	Signs and Symptoms
Partial (Focal)	Localized to one area	One area affected: hands, lips, wrist, arms, face. Impaired loss of consciousness at onset.
Partial complex (psychomotor)	Temporal lobe	Loss of consciousness and loss of awareness or surrounding. Change in behavior: lip smacking, picking, inappropriate mannerisms, confusion follows the seizure.
Partial simple		Lasts 5 minutes, child only remembers the aura. Automatisms are noted. No loss of consciousness or awareness. Motor signs are isolated to one area of the body and then spread to the rest of the body. May experience senses such as buzzing sounds, tingling, flashing lights, anxiety, fear, or anger.
Generalized		
Tonic clonic	Genetic predisposition or brain injury secondary to anoxia	Partial simple and complex seizures evolve to generalized seizures. Aura is experienced followed by loss of consciousness and tone. Patient falls to the floor with tonic–clonic muscle contractions. Patient is postictal and confused after the seizure is over. Loss of urine may occur.
Atonic: loss of muscle tone, drop attacks. Absence (petit mal)		Sudden drop to the floor due to loss of motor muscle tone. Seen in children 2–4 years of age.
		No loss of consciousness but experiences loss of awareness. Non-convulsive. Periods of staring or minor movements lasting seconds. May occur several times a day, interferes with learning and schoolwork.
Tonic		Stiffening of the body that is sustained, involving all four extremities.
Myoclonic	Metabolic etiology	Single or multiple jerks or flexion of limbs.
Clonic		Intermittent rhythmic jerking, 1–3 per second, may start in one body location and move or migrate to another location.
Myoclonic and Akinetic		Complete or total lack of movement.

Source: Fox, J.A. (2002). *Primary health care of infants, children and adolescents.* St. Louis, MO: C.V. Mosby.

Figure 29-4 The EEG evaluates the electrical activity of the brain while the brain is in a sleepy or drowsy state and when stimulated.

If the cause is endocrine dysfunction, it is resolved. If infection is present, appropriate antibiotic therapy is initiated. If the cause of the seizure is unknown and a structural abnormality is not present, the child is placed on an anticonvulsant therapy specific for the type of seizures being experienced.

The nurse completes a detailed history of the seizure event, an in-depth review of the child's prenatal and postnatal history, and review of systems. The event history must include antecedent events that may have precipitated the seizure such as dehydration, video gaming, exercise, or any ingestion of substances that may cause seizures. Information regarding the type of activity during the seizure, any loss of consciousness, loss of urine, noises made, cyanosis, and history of present illness is also retrieved from the persons who witnessed the event. Due to the genetic predisposition of some types of seizures, a family history of and type of seizure activity must obtained. The neurological exam is completed by the physician or a neurological specialist. Pseudoseizures (false) seizures are evaluated as neurological episodes until determined to be psychological or not pathological in nature and etiology.

 critical nursing action Nursing Care for the Child Having a Seizure

1. Call for help. In a hospital, use the designated emergency number. In the community setting call 911.
2. Maintain a patent airway. If the airway is occluded, open the airway with a jaw thrust maneuver. Administer oxygen if needed and available. Do not put anything in the mouth. If the situation warrants emergency medical care, qualified health care personnel can insert an appropriate sized oral airway.
3. Loosen restrictive clothing to ensure adequate circulation to essential body organs.
4. Administer medications such as diazepam (Valium), lorazepam (Ativan), or fosphenytoin (Cerebyx) as ordered by the physician. **Do not do this with a neonate.** These medications become toxic due to immature liver function.
5. Monitor respiratory status and circulatory status throughout the seizure.
6. If the child has a seizure (convulsion), the nurse positions the child in a lateral position to prevent aspiration (entry of secretions into tracheobronchial passages) (Fig. 29-5).
7. Inform the child that they have just had a seizure. Tell the family that the child may still be confused and disoriented for a short time.
8. Stay with the child. Support is essential because a seizure is frightening to both the child and family.
9. Document all important details about the seizure, care provided, and notification to physician, and condition of child after the seizure.

Airway management is the priority nursing intervention for the child experiencing a seizure. Oxygenation, supportive ventilation and removal of obstructing secretions or foreign bodies with proper body positioning to prevent injury are required for a successful outcome. The child who has experienced a seizure needs continuous monitoring of respiratory status because seizure medications that are administered intravenously during a seizure can cause a decreased level of consciousness, apnea, and hypotension. The seizure either arrests independently or after medication administration.

Anticonvulsant therapy is the mainstay for seizure management in children. Many medications are available and have varying therapeutic effects on the brain (Table 29-4). The correct medication must be selected to treat the specific electrical abnormality or clinical symptomatology. The child who has seizures may require daily medication such as fosphenytoin (Cerebyx) or phenytoin (Dilantin) to control the seizure activity and to prevent further seizures. During a seizure, intravenous medications such as diazepam (Valium) or lorazepam (Ativan) are administered to stop the seizure activity and to prevent respiratory compromise.

Phenobarbital (luminal sodium) may be given intravenously (usually a loading dose of 20 to 40 mg/kg given one time is ordered to treat status epilepticus followed by

Figure 29-5 When the seizure is over, place the child in the recovery position on the left lateral recumbent position.

Table 29-4 Seizure Medications

Type of Seizure	Medication	Dose Range	Adverse Reactions	Nursing Care
Partial Complex (Psychomotor)	Carbamazepine (Tegretol)	10–30 mg/kg per day in divided doses. Increase until best response is achieved.	Drowsiness, nausea, liver changes, increased appetite.	Give with food but not with milk.
	Valproic acid (Depakene)	0.1–0.2 mg/kg/day in two or three divided doses per day.	Confusion, ataxia, nystagmus, nausea, gingival hyperplasia, bleeding disorders.	Always give with food and monitor serum drug levels. Teach parents about oral hygiene and wear a medical alert tag. Teach parents to watch for adverse effects indicating toxicity.
	Phenytoin (Dilantin)	5 mg/kg per day in two to three divided doses.	May cause dizziness, drowsiness, or physical incoordination. Avoid abrupt discontinuation of use. Daily multivitamin is recommended while on this medication.	Give with water, juice or milk.
	Phenobarbital (Luminal)	Infants 5–6 mg/kg per day in one or two divided doses		
	Fosphenytoin (Cerebyx)	Children 1–6 years, 6–8 mg/kg per day in one or two divided doses. Loading dose of 10–20 mg/kg. Then 4–6 mg/kg per day.		
Generalized Tonic–clonic	Valproic acid (Depakene) and carbamazepine (Tegretol). Phenytoin (Dilantin). Phenobarbital	May be an inexpensive medication.	Monitor for sleepiness, hyperactivity, drowsiness and school performance changes.	
	Ketogenic diet high in fat and low in protein and carbohydrates.	Causes a high level of ketones which decrease myoclonic or tonic–clonic seizure activity.	Nausea, vomiting, headache, drowsiness, dizziness	This diet is hard to maintain for a long period of time due to the lack of food variety and difficulty of food preparation and parental involvement.
Absence (Petit Mal)	Ethosuximide (Zarontin) or Valproic Acid	3–8 mg/kg per day		Avoid antacids.
Partial Simple	Topiramate (Topamax)	1–3 mg/kg per day	Weight loss, dizziness, diarrhea, cognitive dysfunction.	Avoid antidepressants and antacids.

a maintenance dosing regimen). However, the onset is less rapid and there may be cardiac arrhythmias associated with this medication.

Many anticonvulsant medications can become toxic when taken on a daily basis. Baseline liver function, renal function, and hematological values should be assessed before initiation of pharmacotherapy and retained for future reference. Anticonvulsant drug serum levels are also monitored to maintain therapeutic levels. Children outgrow the dosage and begin having seizures due to lowered serum levels. Drug serum levels should be assessed every 3 to 6 months.

Nursing care also includes seizure precautions according to hospital protocol, which includes padded side rails or bed rails, oxygen, and suction equipment readily available, IV access, and anticonvulsant medications at the bedside according to physician prescription.

The hospitalized child should receive continuous cardiac, respiratory, and oxygen monitoring. Centrally located monitoring on the nursing unit for ease of observation in case of seizure activity is necessary. Baseline seizure activity for some children may be several seizures a day without compromise. The child must be continually monitored while an inpatient. Do not allow the child to bathe independently until the seizures have been arrested and controlled.

All caregivers of children with seizures should be instructed in CPR techniques. Medication information such as type of medication, dose, route, and frequency of dosing must be explained to the parents. The regimen must also be adhered to in the day care setting. The child should not be left alone until the seizures have been controlled and he or she is seizure free for several months. Adolescents may drive (depending on State Laws) and participate in sports with therapeutic serum anticonvulsant drug levels and a seizure-free duration of at least 6 months.

School nurses and teachers should be informed about the child's seizure condition and follow institutional procedures if the child experiences a seizure in school or day care. Medical alert identification bracelets should be worn by younger children and may be worn by older children and adolescents.

 Now Can You— Discuss seizures and related nursing care?

1. Identify the difference between tonic and clonic seizures.
2. Identify absence seizures from complex or partial seizures.
3. Identify the medications for the different types of seizures.
4. Identify the nursing care for a patient experiencing a seizure.

Inflammatory Neurological Conditions

MENINGITIS

Meningitis is an inflammation of the structures in the central nervous system caused by an infectious process. The meninges are composed of three membranes that cover the brain, protecting it from injury and infection: the dura mater, arachnoid mater, and pia mater. These structures house arterioles, venules, and cerebrospinal fluid to protect, bathe, and provide chemical functional support for the brain and its contents. Meningitis is either septic or aseptic. Septic or pyogenic meningitis is caused by a bacterial pathogen such as *S. pneumoniae*, *N. meningitides*, *Escherichia coli*, or *Haemophilus influenzae* type B. Aseptic meningitis is caused by a known or unknown viral agent typically presenting at peak seasonal viral illness intervals in the fall and winter.

Meningitis can develop at any time during childhood. During the neonatal period, meningitis results from a pathogen transmitted during the labor and delivery process or while in utero. The most common types of neonatal meningococcal infections are caused by herpes simplex, Group B beta-hemolytic *Streptococcus*, and *E. coli*. In older infants and children, a peak incidence of *S. pneumoniae* is noted in the winter months. In summer months, bacterial organisms such as *N. meningitides* and non-bacterial agents such as rhinoviruses and adenoviruses are more prevalent. *Haemophilus influenzae* type B, once a deadly pathogen, has almost been eradicated now with scheduled routine childhood immunizations (Centers for Disease Control and Prevention [CDC], 2007).

Bacterial meningitis is the result of bacterial dissemination from a nasopharyngeal or a hematological inoculation. The pathogen migrates into the cerebrospinal fluid and imbeds in the subarachnoid space. The body reacts to the infiltration with a severe inflammatory response and white blood cell proliferation. Systemic septicemia, surgical procedures involving the central nervous system, a penetrating wound, otitis media, sinusitis, cellulitis of the scalp or facial structure, dental caries, pharyngitis, and orthopedic diseases and procedures are also antecedent events leading to bacterial meningitis.

SIGNS AND SYMPTOMS. A child with meningitis may initially appear to be mildly ill with general vague or subtle symptoms such as lethargy, malaise, irritability, vomiting, fever, and diarrhea. If left unrecognized and untreated, meningitis may progress rapidly to a critical state depending on the age of the patient and the etiological pathogen. Younger infants and children succumb rapidly to meningitis and children with meningococcemia, *H. influenzae* type B, and *E. coli* become quite toxic and deteriorate quickly if untreated.

Infants generally present with nuchal rigidity, a bulging fontanel, fever, and poor feeding. Other symptoms may include seizures, photophobia, anorexia, and emesis.

---

 assessment tools Kernig's or Brudzinski Sign

Classic finding on examination for a child suspected of meningitis include a positive Kernig's or Brudzinski sign (Behrman, Kleigman, & Jenson, 2004). These exams indicate meningeal irritation resulting in hyperreactive reflexes (Fig. 29-6*A*). The test for Kernig's sign is conducted with the child lying supine with the hips flexed. As the nurse raises the lower leg to straighten the leg the child either cries out or resists the leg extension. If the child experiences pain behind the knee as the knee is fully extended, this is an abnormal finding. Bilateral increased resistance and pain upon extension of the knee is a positive Kernig sign and may indicate meningeal irritation.

Brudzinski's sign (Fig. 29-6*B*) is conducted with the child lying flat. The nurse attempts to raise the head toward the child's chest and place the chin on the chest. If there is pain or resistance, the child immediately flexes the hip and knee. If the child exhibits flexion of the hips and knees when the nurse performs the maneuver, meningeal inflammation may be present (Bickley & Szilagyi, 2003).

Nursing Insight— Viral or aseptic meningitis

The etiological pathogen in viral or aseptic meningitis is a viral agent. The most common pathogens are herpes and adenovirus; in most cases the etiologic agent is unknown. Some cases are the result of partially treated bacterial meningitis (Behrman et al., 2004). Clinically the child with viral meningitis presents with the same vague or subtle symptoms; however, the child does not become toxic or as acutely ill as the

A

B

Figure 29-6 Classic finding on examination for a child suspected of meningitis include a positive Kernig's or Brudzinski sign.

patient with bacterial meningitis. Diagnosis is based on CSF analysis, CSF gram stain, and culture; results are typically negative unless a viral agent is identified.

DIAGNOSIS. The nurse conducts a review of the current illness with specific information obtained regarding duration of symptoms, ill contacts in the family or school settings, seizures, loss of sleep or weight, anorexia, emesis, behavioral changes and immunization status. A complete blood count (CBC) reveals an elevated white blood cell (WBC) count and any clotting deficiencies. A disseminated intravascular coagulation (DIC) panel is collected to rule out a coagulation disorder when the child presents with petechial hemorrhage, shock, and meningococcemia. Blood cultures are obtained to identify the potential hematological origin. A lumbar puncture is also performed for CSF analysis including chemistry and cell counts as well as culture and gram stain for bacterial or viral diagnosis. Meningitis is diagnosed based on the results of the lumbar puncture.

NURSING CARE. Essential nursing care includes assessing neurological status at least every 2 to 4 hours. The child's level of consciousness and the use of a pediatric Glasgow coma scale, pupil response, and overall activity provide clues to the child's neurological status (e.g., increase in ICP or response to antibiotic and fluid therapy). In small infants ICP can be subjectively monitored by palpating the anterior fontanel while the patient is lying supine. If the fontanel is tense and bulging, this may suggest increased ICP, particularly when combined with photophobia, irritability, a high-pitched cry, anorexia, and emesis. Infants with open fontanels and an enlarging head circumference during or post meningitis infection may indicate hydrocephalus and must be monitored. The child with an increasing head size and symptoms of increased ICP requires radiological evaluation such as a CT scan or MRI (Fig. 29-7). To prevent additional increased ICP the child's

Figure 29-7 The child with an increasing head size and symptoms of increased ICP requires radiological evaluation such as a CT scan.

room is kept quiet, dim, and without loud or noxious visual, auditory, or olfactory stimuli.

The onset of seizure activity associated with meningitis is managed medically and seizure precautions are maintained at all times. The child with meningitis may develop new-onset seizures and is treated with anticonvulsant therapy. The child is also kept NPO until nausea and vomiting has been resolved.

Comfort care includes a dim room, antipyretic therapy for fever management, nutrition as tolerated, and emotional and social support. Care for malaise with massage, nonsteroidal anti-inflammatory drugs (NSAIDs), warm baths, and rest.

Infections of the central nervous system can upset the family. The nurse can educate the family and the child about the disease and treatment options. The nurse also explains that long-term parenteral access may be maintained with a peripherally inserted central catheter (PICC) and intravenous antibiotics can be continued at home with the assistance of a home health nurse.

ENCEPHALITIS

Encephalitis is usually viral in origin and occurs with an acute febrile illness that is characterized by cerebral edema and infection of surrounding meninges. Less common etiologies are fungal, bacterial, and parasitic infections, exposure to toxins or drugs, and cancer (Wisniewski, 2003). The most common types of viral encephalitis are caused by arthropod-borne viruses (mosquito-borne) and the herpes simplex type I. Systemic viral illnesses such as rabies, mononucleosis, and poliomyelitis may also result in encephalitis. When obtaining a history and physical, the nurse must ask the parent about exposure to possible sources of encephalitis (McCance & Huether, 2002).

All types of encephalitides cause meningeal involvement. Widespread nerve cell degeneration is caused by arthropod-borne viral encephalitides. Acute viral encephalitis is the result of direct viral infection of the neural cells accompanied by associated perivascular inflammation and destruction of brain gray matter.

SIGNS AND SYMPTOMS. The symptoms experienced by children vary from mild to life-threatening. The severity of the illness depends on the child's age, immune system stability, underlying cause, and duration of illness. The child who has a compromised immune system is at greater risk. Primary encephalitis occurs when a toxin or pathogen directly attacks the spinal cord and brain. The most common causes of primary encephalitis are mosquito-borne viruses and herpes simplex. Secondary encephalitis is the result of an immune response to a foreign object or toxin within the body or an infection in another part of the body. Depending on the source of the encephalitis and the severity of the illness, signs and symptoms of the virus develop within hours to weeks after exposure. Encephalitis caused by bacteria usually results in a more serious illness state.

Signs and symptoms of encephalitis include disorientation, confusion, headache, high fever, photophobia, lethargy, aphasia, hallucinations, seizures, nuchal rigidity, and coma (Wisniewski, 2003).

Nursing Care Plan The Child with Meningitis

Nursing Diagnosis: Decreased Intracranial Adaptive Capacity related to inflammatory process secondary to microbial invasion of the central nervous system

Measurable Short-term Goal: The child will not experience complications from increased intracranial pressure (ICP).

Measurable Long-term Goal: The child will recover completely with no residual neurological deficits.

NOC Outcomes:

Neurological Status: Autonomic (0910) Ability of the autonomic nervous system to coordinate visceral and homeostatic function

Tissue Perfusion: Cerebral (0406) Adequacy of blood flow through the cerebral vasculature to maintain brain function

NIC Interventions:

Intravenous Therapy (4200)
Neurologic Monitoring (2620)
Cerebral Edema Management (2540)
Seizure Precautions (2690)

Nursing Interventions:

1. Implement universal precautions. Initiate respiratory isolation for first 24 hours of antibiotic administration for bacterial meningitis (specify). Instruct family in correct procedures.

   RATIONALE: Universal precautions help prevent transmission of infection. Respiratory isolation prevents droplet transmission of bacteria to family and caregivers until the prescribed antibiotic has been implemented for 24 hours.

2. Initiate and maintain intravenous access (specify fluids and rate) as ordered. Monitor hourly intake and output, notifying the caregiver if urine output is less than 0.5–1 mL/kg per hour.

   RATIONALE: Intravenous access is required for optimal medication administration; fluids promote adequate hydration; decreased output may signal impending syndrome of inappropriate antidiuretic hormone (SIADH).

3. Administer prescribed IV antibiotic, antiviral, steroid, and antipyretic medications as prescribed (specify drug, dose, route, and times).

   RATIONALE: Antimicrobial medications should be administered as soon as possible. Drugs that are specific for the cultured microorganism will be most effective in combating infection. Steroids reduce cerebral edema, decreasing meningeal irritation to help prevent complications such as hearing loss, hydrocephalus, and learning disorders.

4. Monitor vital signs every 1–4 hours (specify, depending on severity of symptoms). Place on cardiac monitor as indicated (specify).

   RATIONALE: Changes in vital signs such as tachycardia, tachypnea, and hypotension signal increasing intracranial pressure and possible septicemia.

5. Monitor neurological status and symptoms closely; compare with baseline for child.

   RATIONALE: Decreased consciousness and changes in reflexes may signal increasing ICP.

6. Maintain the child in a quiet darkened environment with padded side rails up when in bed.

   RATIONALE: Promotes comfort by reducing noise, light, and activity. Padded side rails may help prevent injury in the event of seizure activity.

DIAGNOSIS. The clinical symptoms of encephalitis mimic those of other neurological disorders. When obtaining a history and physical, the nurse assesses the child's skin for any lesions that might be vector bites. The nurse asks the child and family about possible exposure to mosquitoes, bats, or other sources of encephalitis. The family needs to be questioned about outdoor play, camping trips, unvaccinated pets, wild animals, medication, and recent illnesses. MRI or CT may be used to determine any cerebral edema, shifts within the brain, or focal lesions. The health care provider may also order cerebral fluid analysis, an electroencephalogram, and lab work. Brain biopsy is the test for a definitive diagnosis (Wisniewski, 2003).

Across Care Settings: Complications from encephalitis

The complications resulting from encephalitis may include motor or cognitive deficits, seizure disorders, hearing or vision loss, memory loss, and paralysis (Wisniewski, 2003). If a child has permanent or lingering problems, the treatment plan for them may be multidisciplinary. This multidisciplinary approach optimizes the child's recovery and maximizes skills necessary for life.

NURSING CARE. Treatment for encephalitis is determined by the etiology. Viral encephalitis is treated with an antiviral medication such as acyclovir (Zovirax) (McCance & Huether, 2002). Encephalitis of a bacterial origin is treated with a narrow-spectrum antibiotic. Other medications that may be prescribed are antipyretics, anticonvulsants, analgesics, and anti-inflammatory agents (Wisniewski, 2003).

The nurse must be astute when caring for a child with encephalitis because of the rapid neurological changes that may occur with the illness. The nurse provides care and support for the child and the family during the acute and convalescent phases of the disease process. During the acute phase of the disease, the nurse administers intravenous fluids, medications, and nutrition. Seizure precautions must be initiated because of cerebral edema and increased ICP. To decrease ICP, the nurse performs interventions such as ongoing neurological assessments, ensuring the child is afebrile and seizure free, maintaining homodynamic stability, and positioning the child to avoid neck vein compression. The nurse also carefully monitors the child's fluid and electrolyte balance and watches for syndrome of inappropriate antidiuretic hormone (SIADH) (Wisniewski, 2003). Suctioning and percussion are not recommended unless the child has a current respiratory condition.

 Across Care Settings: Community education about DEET (N, N-diethyl-m-toluamide)

The nurse can educate others in the community about DEET. "Insect repellents containing DEET (N,N-diethyl-m-toluamide, also known as N,N-diethyl-3-methylbenzamide) with a concentration of 10% appear to be as safe as products with a concentration of 30% when used according to the directions on the product labels." The American Academy of Pediatrics recommends that repellents with DEET should not be used on infants younger than 2 months old. (American Academy of Pediatrics: http://www.bt.cdc.gov/cdclinkdisclaimer.asp?a_gotolink=http://www.aap.org/family/wnv-jun03.htm)

BRAIN ABSCESS

A brain abscess is an uncommon but life-threatening infection that occurs when infectious material collects in brain tissue. Brain abscesses affect more males in the first 2 decades of life and comprise approximately 1% of all space-occupying lesions in the United States (Bader & Littlejohns, 2004). Brain abscess may result from an infection of contiguous structures (e.g., otitis media, dental infection, mastoiditis, and sinusitis), after penetrating head trauma or surgery, hematogenous spread from a distal location (endoscopy, lung infections), and after meningitis. The child with congenital cyanotic heart disease is more predisposed to developing a brain abscess because he or she has frequent and recurrent episodes of otitis media and sinusitis (Brook, 2004).

The infection can enter the brain by several routes, such as necrotic areas of bone, if sinusitis is present. If a child has otitis media, the infection can enter directly through the ear. Trauma causing an open fracture of the skull may also result in an abscess. Infection in another

> **Labs: Brain Abscess**
>
> Serum laboratory studies, including complete blood count, blood cultures, and C-reactive protein, may be ordered. With a brain abscess, the child usually demonstrates moderate leukocytosis, and an elevated erythrocyte rate and C-reactive protein level. If the abscess is aspirated, the specimen should be cultured to identify the causative microorganism (Brook, 2004).

part of the body can travel through the vascular system to the brain and result in an abscess (Brook, 2004).

SIGNS AND SYMPTOMS. The signs and symptoms exhibited by a child with a brain abscess may be minor or life-threatening. Symptoms may occur for up to 2 weeks before a definitive diagnosis is made. The signs and symptoms include a localized headache, fever, drowsiness, stupor, confusion, general or focal seizures, focal motor or sensory impairments, ataxia, nausea and vomiting, papilledema, and hemiparesis. General seizures and mental changes can also occur. A brain abscess may present as encephalitis accompanied by symptoms of increased ICP. If a brain abscess ruptures, meningitis can occur (Brook, 2004). Residual deficits including hydrocephalus may exist after a rupture.

DIAGNOSIS. Diagnosis is made based on the clinical presentation and MRI or CT. The MRI differentiates between an abscess, tumor, and stroke.

NURSING CARE. Nursing care focuses on assessment of the neurological status, response to treatment, medication administration, and supportive care. The nurse continually monitors the neurological status to identify any changes in ICP that may require more aggressive intervention and documents the child's condition.

The nurse monitors serum labs, especially blood glucose and potassium levels, because of the effects that corticosteroid therapy has on body systems. Based on the laboratory results, the nurse may need to administer insulin or electrolytes (Smeltzer, 2008). The course of the medical treatment may be short or long, depending on the causative agent, area of brain affected, and size of the abscess. Most brain abscesses require a lengthy course of antimicrobial therapy (4 to 8 weeks) because the brain tissue takes time to heal (Brook, 2004) (Table 29-5).

If the child does not respond to antimicrobial therapy or does not meet the criteria for medical therapy alone, surgery may be required. The abscess can either be aspirated or excised (Brook, 2004). If surgery is performed, the nurse must assess the child postoperatively for possible neurological complications such as meningitis or cerebral edema. The child's safety becomes a priority so the nurse must implement fall and seizure precautions (Smeltzer, Bare, Hinkle, & Cheever, 2008).

REYE SYNDROME

For many years, childhood illnesses and discomforts were managed with the administration of aspirin (acetylsalicylic acid). Acetylsalicylic acid is a component found in many over-the-counter medications to relieve fever, muscle aches, and nausea (Table 29-6). Reye syndrome was first identified in 1963 and reached a peak in the 1970s

Table 29-5	Antimicrobial Therapy Used in Brain Abscesses
Cause of Brain Abscess	**Therapy**
Meningitis	Neonates: Cefotaxime + ampicillin
	Infants and children: Ceftriaxone or cefotaxime + vancomycin
Cyanotic congenital heart disease	Ampicillin + chloramphenicol, or ceftriaxone + metronidazole, or ampicillin-sulbactam
Otitis or sinusitis	Ampicillin + chloramphenicol, or ceftriaxone + metronidazole, or ampicillin-sulbactam
Ventriculoperitoneal shunt or trauma	Vancomycin + antipseudomonal

and early 1980s. The syndrome can affect persons of all ages but it usually affects children. Reye syndrome is primarily associated with the administration of aspirin during viral illnesses (Bhutta, Savell, & Schexnayder, 2003). A decline in the incidence of Reye syndrome has been evident in the recent past, primarily due to the decreased administration of acetylsalicylic acid and parental education about the disease.

Reye syndrome affects all organs of a child's body but causes the most damage to the brain and liver. The brain is affected by an increase in ICP and other organs are affected by an accumulation of fat. The disorder is considered to be a two-phase illness because it usually occurs in conjunction with a viral infection, especially varicella (chickenpox) or influenza (flu). The child develops the disorder during the recovery phase of the viral infection. Reye syndrome may be misdiagnosed because the symptoms mimic those of other neurological illnesses such as meningitis, encephalitis, diabetes, poisoning, drug overdose, and sudden infant death syndrome.

SIGNS AND SYMPTOMS. The signs and symptoms of the illness are a result of hyperammonemia, hypoglycemia

Table 29-6	Medications Containing Acetylsalicylic Acid
Nonprescription Products	**Prescription Products**
Alka-Seltzer	Darvon
Excedrin	Norgesic
Pepto-Bismol	Robaxisal
Anacin	Talwin
Kaopectate	Butalbital
BC	Percodan
Pamprin	Roxiprin
	Lortab
	Propoxyphene
	Soma

and an increase in short-chain fatty acids found in the serum after the liver becomes involved. The liver has diffuse deposits of lipids with an absence of necrosis or inflammatory reaction. Azotemia (excess urea in the serum) also occurs as a result of fatty degeneration of the kidneys (McCance & Huether, 2002).

There are several stages of Reye syndrome. The child may progress through all of the stages or stop at any stage if treatment is effective (McCance & Huether, 2002).

 Nursing Insight— *The stages of Reye syndrome*

Stage   I: Lethargy, vomiting, drowsiness, liver dysfunction
Stage II: Disorientation, combativeness, aggressiveness, delirium, hyperactive reflexes, hyperventilation, shallow breathing, stupor, liver dysfunction
Stage III: Obtundation, coma, decorticate posturing hyperventilation
Stage IV: Deepening coma, large fixed pupils, decerebrate posturing, loss of ocular reflexes, liver dysfunction
Stage V: Loss of deep tendon reflexes, seizures, flaccidity, respiratory arrest, usually no liver function

DIAGNOSIS. Because a number of inherited metabolic diseases present with many of the same symptoms as Reye syndrome, these illnesses need to be excluded before a diagnosis of Reye syndrome can be made. When obtaining a history and physical, the nurse must ask about recent viral illnesses and the use of any medications containing acetylsalicylic acid. The nurse performs a complete neurological assessment. A definitive diagnosis of this syndrome is established with a liver biopsy obtained during the illness or at autopsy. Other diagnostic tests that may be ordered are serum tests including liver enzymes, blood glucose, ammonia level, coagulation studies, and others to exclude metabolic inherited disorders. The child may have a lumbar puncture to rule out infections, including meningitis and encephalitis.

If a liver biopsy is to be performed, the nurse prepares the child and family by explaining that the child may be given a sedative to help calm him or her. If the child is old enough, the nurse can allow the child to practice the position that is needed for the procedure (lying on the back with the right hand under the head). The nurse tells the family that during the procedure an ultrasound is used to guide the needle. The child will have a small incision where the biopsy needle was inserted and a bandage over the insertion site.

 critical nursing action Liver Biopsy

After a liver biopsy, the nurse must monitor for bleeding. The child is predisposed to bleeding after the procedure because the liver is highly vascular and Reye syndrome causes hepatomegaly and liver dysfunction. After the biopsy, the physician places a dressing to splint the puncture site and positions the child to lie on the right side for 2 hours (Lewis, Heitkemper, Dirksen, O'Brien, & Bucher, 2007).

The anticipated results of a liver biopsy would include elevated liver enzymes (aspartate aminotransferase and alanine aminotransferase), low blood glucose, elevated serum creatinine and blood urea nitrogen, prolonged prothrombin and partial thromboplastin times, and elevated serum ammonia.

NURSING CARE. Reye syndrome is an illness that progresses quickly and may not have a favorable outcome. The nurse performs astute neurological assessments because of the high incidence of increased ICP and brain injury. The child's level of consciousness, seizure activity, and reflex function are assessed to determine the stage of the illness. To reduce the risk of increased ICP, the nurse carefully administers intravenous fluids. The intravenous fluids may include glucose to correct hypoglycemia and potassium, chloride, and sodium to correct electrolyte imbalances. Corticosteroids may be prescribed to decrease cerebral edema and inflammation, and insulin may be administered to increase glucose metabolism. Diuretics may be prescribed to enhance fluid elimination, resulting in decreased ICP. If the child is experiencing respiratory difficulty, the nurse monitors the oxygen saturation concentration with the use of pulse oximetry. Supplemental oxygen may be administered via nasal cannula. If the child's condition worsens, the child may need intubation and mechanical ventilation. The health care provider may insert an arterial line to monitor blood pressure and obtain arterial blood gases. The nurse then assesses the insertion site for complications of infection and leaking. The nurse initiates seizure precautions if the child demonstrates signs of increased ICP. Invasive procedures are limited and handled carefully because of the risk of bleeding due to liver involvement. Emotional support is provided to the child and parents.

 ### *Across Care Settings:* Reye syndrome

The child may have residual physical and psychological conditions because of brain injury. The nurse can provide information about resources available to support survivors and their caregivers. These resources include Crippled Children's Services, child developmental clinics, State Developmental Disabilities Agencies, local school systems, and health departments. Caregivers should familiarize themselves with legal acts that protect patient rights including Equal Opportunities for Individuals with Disabilities Act, Americans with Disabilities Act of 1990, Title 42, Chapter 126, Sec. 12101-12213 (National Reye Syndrome Foundation, 2008).

 ### **"What to say"** — *Can I give my child aspirin?*

If a parent asks, "Can I give my child aspirin?" the nurse should respond:

"No product containing acetylsalicylic acid should be given to any person younger than 19 years of age because of the risk of Reye syndrome."

GUILLAIN-BARRÉ SYNDROME

Guillain-Barré syndrome (GBS) is a rare self-limiting disease characterized by clinical manifestations of ascending muscle weakness or paralysis. GBS is a rare and potentially debilitating self-limiting autoimmune disease. If it is effectively and supportively managed, full recovery can be anticipated.

GBS is the most common form of acquired acute paralysis in children. Loss of function can range from fatigue and lethargy to complete paralysis of the lower limbs extending upward and affecting upper motor and sensory neuron pathways.

The incidence of GBS is about 0.5 to 1 cases per 100,000 children younger than 18 years of age. School-age children are most susceptible and more males than females are affected (Sladky, 2004). The syndrome is an acute autoimmune inflammatory response resulting in one of two subtypes: acute inflammatory demyelinating neuropathy (AIDP), causing transient ascending paralysis of both sensory and motor neuropathy (Hughes & Cornblath, 2005), or acute motor axonal neuropathy (AMAN), or a combination of the two subtypes (Lu et al., 2000). The child loses motor function and in some cases sensation in peripheral, spinal, sensory, and motor neurons. Infrequently cranial nerve function is also involved (Sladky, 2004).

The exact cause of GBS is unknown. The syndrome may follow an antecedent gastrointestinal or respiratory illness. Commonly occurring etiologic pathogens are *Mycoplasma pneumoniae*, the Epstein–Barr virus, cytomegalovirus, *Varicella*, and *Campylobacter jejuni*. Inflammatory mediators penetrate the Schwann cells in the nerve axons, causing demyelinization (removal of the myelin sheath of nerve tissue) and denuding (loss of nerve covering) of the neuronal pathways, resulting in decreased conduction of sensory and motor peripheral and spinal pathways. Areas of nerve involvement are assessed and monitored as nerve function and sensation is blocked or slowed. Some cases of GBS have been linked to several vaccines such as meningococcal, influenza, swine vaccine, and rabies vaccine, but the evidence is weak and anecdotal (Aschenbrenner, 2006; Schessl, Luther, Kirshner, Mauff, & Korinthenberg, 2004).

SIGNS AND SYMPTOMS. The initial diagnosis of GBS may be missed owing to the wide variety of presenting signs and symptoms that can be attributed to other disease causes. GBS becomes clinically apparent as the child progresses through three phases. Each phase is marked by a leveling of symptoms. The acute phase is preceded by a febrile viral illness, ataxia, lethargy, motor and sensory nerve weakness, and pain in the lower extremities that continues to progress up the body starting in the lower extremities. This phase may take several days or weeks and seems to plateau at around 2 to 3 weeks. During this time, the level of functional and sensory loss may necessitate ventilatory and or oxygen support if respiratory function is compromised. The second phase is the plateau phase, which is characterized by arrested progression in the degree of involvement or loss of sensation and function. This phase has no specific duration and lasts for varying intervals. The recovery phase begins with the return of motor and sensory function. The degree of disability is assessed and rehabilitation services are begun. Physical and occupational therapy are necessary to aid the child's return to normal function; recovery occurs over time, most cases resolving in 4 to 8 weeks.

DIAGNOSIS. Diagnosis of GBS is based on clinical and laboratory procedures. The child presents with muscle weakness, sensory disturbances, loss of deep tendon reflex responses, and muscle paralysis. Elevated CSF protein levels in the absence of infection support the clinical diagnosis. Sensory and motor nerve conduction studies such as electromyography (EMG) define the subtype classification and degree of inflammatory involvement; results will demonstrate blocked impulses or conduction slowing along the peripheral motor and sensory nerve endings (Sladky, 2004).

NURSING CARE. Supportive measures are the hallmark of care for the patient with GBS. Plasma exchange and intravenous immunoglobulin therapies shorten the disease duration, support the recovery phase, and reduce the duration of disability. Corticosteroid use may be initiated to slow the inflammatory response. The use of high-dose steroid therapy alone remains poorly established as single regimen therapy for GBS in children (Kuwabara, 2004; van Doorn, 2005).

Vigilant clinical monitoring related to the progression of motor, sensory, and functional losses, as well as the degree of respiratory compromise, are the priority nursing assessments. As GBS progresses, the nurse monitors pulse oximetry, respiratory function, ease of breathing, and lung sounds for potential atelectasis leading to pneumonia. Respiratory support is provided with intermittent positive pressure breathing, cough assist, and incentive spirometry. Frequent repositioning is also required every 2 hours. To maintain urinary output it may be necessary to use an indwelling urinary catheter or intermittent clean catheterization. Parenteral or enteral nutrition is maintained if the child is unable to meet nutritional intake needs or is experiencing dysphagia.

The nurse must assess the pain level in the child. GBS is painful and requires opioid analgesia that is administered on a scheduled basis to treat the severe neuralgia. Children with GBS may underreport the pain associated with the neuritis and expect the nurse to understand their discomfort. The nurse must have a high index of suspicion and proactively manage the pain in GBS.

Immobilization and loss of function can lead to muscular contracture and loss of function after the inflammation has subsided. Passive range-of-motion exercises, frequent position changes, and hand and foot orthotics or splints may be used temporarily to preserve function and prevent contractures. Skin integrity over bony prominences or pressure areas must be monitored and managed aggressively with padding, massaging, close inspection, and frequent repositioning. Age-appropriate developmental activities are provided daily as the child is able. Offer visual and auditory stimulation frequently to meet the child's cognitive, social, and emotional needs. School work, crafts, and books provide respite from the boredom and may prevent behavioral and emotional disorders related to the debilitation and limitations of the disease.

🌼⚙️ **nursing diagnoses** Guillain-Barré syndrome

- Ineffective Breathing Patterns related to ascending loss of nerve function
- High Risk for Alteration in Airway Clearance related to muscle weakness and/or paralysis
- Alterations in Comfort related to neuralgia
- Social Isolation related to debilitation and limitations imposed by the child's disease
- Powerlessness related to loss of function and sensation

Developmental Neurological Conditions

SPINA BIFIDA

Neural tube defects (NTDs) are a group of birth defects in which malformations of the brain and spinal cord occur and the structures lack protection of soft tissue and bone. NTDs develop when the neural tube fails to close during fetal development. Usually, the nerves below the defect are impaired, although some sparing of nerves with subsequent partial functioning may occur (Brown, 2001).

Spina bifida is the most frequently occurring and permanently disabling birth defect in the United States. No two people affected by this disorder are alike. It accounts for approximately two-thirds of all NTDs. Spina bifida is derived from the Latin words that mean "cloven backbone." It is a congenital spinal deformity occurring early during gestation (18 to 28 days). The etiology of the disorder can be multifaceted, including environmental and genetic risks. Environmental predisposing factors include exposure to prolonged hyperthermia, diabetes mellitus, and the consumption of seizure medications during early pregnancy. Poor nutrition is an environmental risk factor. Presumptive genetic predisposing factors include hereditary defects in not only the absorption of folic acid but also in its utilization. Usually, the nerves below the defect are impaired, although some sparing of nerves with subsequent partial functioning may occur (Brown, 2001).

SIGNS AND SYMPTOMS. The signs and symptoms demonstrated by children with spina bifida vary depending on the level of the lesion and the type of defect. Spina bifida occulta is the least severe form of spina bifida. There is a localized defect of the vertebral arch and no spinal cord or meningeal involvement. A dimple or tuft of hair may be seen on the infant's back. If the child has a **meningocele,** a protruding sac is located on the cervical, thoracic, or lumbar spine at the level of the defect and a thin layer of muscle and skin usually covers the lesion. Meninges (membranes) protrude through the defect in the spine but no involvement of neural elements is present. Neurological functioning is usually not affected.

A myelomeningocele is the most severe form of spina bifida and is evident on delivery. The meninges protrude through the defect and the meninges contain spinal cord elements. It appears as a very pronounced skin defect usually covered by a transparent membrane and may even have neural tissue attached to the inner surface. The higher the defect is located on the spine, the greater the loss of spinal cord function because usually no neurological function is found below the defect. The bony prominences of the unfused neural arches can be felt at the defect's lateral border. When the child is born, the membrane covering the defect may be intact or may leak CSF. If the membrane is not intact, the risk for infection and neuronal damage is increased. Until the defect is surgically closed, CSF may accumulate, which results in further dilation and enlargement of the sac and further neuronal damage may occur. The involvement of the spinal cord has greater implications for the function of the child during childhood.

DIAGNOSIS. After 12 to 14 weeks of pregnancy, prenatal diagnosis can be made if the defect is visible through ultrasound examination. During pregnancy, maternal serum testing of alpha-fetoprotein is performed to determine the presence of a neural tube defect. An elevated alpha-fetoprotein level may be indicative of a neural tube defect because open neural defects leak this substance into surrounding amniotic fluid, and a small portion is absorbed into the mother's blood. On delivery, the defect is usually visible, and a diagnosis is made. The defect is examined to determine the type and severity of the defect, and contents of the sac are assessed for meninges, CSF, and spinal cord. An MRI or a CT scan identifies the neurological structures contained in the sac.

NURSING CARE. On delivery, the nurse assesses the defect for the type of contents in the sac and measures the defect. A priority nursing concern is prevention of injury and infection of the sac. The nurse assesses the sac for indications of infection including redness, purulent drainage, bleeding, and necrosis. If the sac ruptures and leaks CSF, the patient is at risk of developing meningitis.

 critical nursing action Preventing Injury of the Sac

As quickly as possible and using sterile technique, the nurse covers the defect with a sterile nonadherent dressing moistened with sterile saline to maintain moisture and to prevent drying. The dressing is changed every 2 to 4 hours as prescribed and when soiled.

The nurse positions the newborn in a prone position and does not place a diaper over the defect in order to prevent pressure on the sac, rupture, and infection of the sac. A laminectomy (the excision of a vertebral posterior arch, usually to remove a lesion or herniated disk) and closure of the defect is performed as soon after birth as possible to preserve the neurological function present, prevent infection or rupture, improve the appearance, and allow easier handling of the baby (Venes, 2009). Intravenous antibiotics are administered to prevent infection preoperatively and postoperatively.

The nurse evaluates the orthopedic function of the newborn. A low thoracic lesion may cause total flaccid paralysis of the lower body. A small sacral lesion may cause only patchy areas of decreased sensation in the feet. Movement or lack of movement of the extremities is assessed and documented. The child may have contractures of the hips, knees, and ankles, and the hips may be dislocated. The nurse prevents joint contractures or prevents further joint contractures by performing passive range-of-motion exercises but does not perform range-of-motion exercises of the hips because hip displacement is common. Clubfeet are a common orthopedic complication of spina bifida because the fetus cannot move the lower extremities in utero. As the child gets older, locomotion may be facilitated with the use of braces, wheelchairs, and walkers.

The bladder and bowel function of children with spina bifida may be affected to varying degrees. During the neonatal period, the nurse assesses the voiding and defecation patterns of the newborn. The newborn who constantly dribbles urine may have a neurogenic bladder and may experience urinary retention and overflow with a risk of urinary tract infections. A newborn who voids at spaced intervals may be able to achieve some level of urinary continence later in life because there is some innervation of the bladder. Anticholinergics may be administered to improve urinary continence and antispasmodics to control bladder spasms.

Constipation and impaction are a common complaint associated with spina bifida. The child's diet needs to include fiber and fluid. If constipation occurs, stool softeners and laxatives may be administered. A child with spina bifida may not be able to feel the urge to defecate and bowel incontinence may result. The child may need to wear diapers, and as he or she gets older, psychosocial disturbances, including depression, embarrassment, and shame, may be experienced. If adequate innervation of the bowel exists, bowel training may be attempted.

 critical nursing action Do Not Obtain a Rectal Temperature

Do not obtain a rectal temperature of a child with spina bifida because rectal irritation and rectal prolapse may occur.

Preserving skin integrity is an important nursing responsibility. Preoperatively, the nurse ensures no pressure is placed on the vulnerable defect. Postoperatively, the surgical incision is protected by not applying pressure on the area. Perineal irritation and skin breakdown may occur if incontinence is a problem. The nurse checks the perineum for stool and urine and changes the diaper as needed. The patient who is in a wheelchair for the majority of the day is prone to skin breakdown of the coccyx due to pressure. Areas where orthopedic devices apply pressure need to be padded well and assessed frequently.

The child with spina bifida is at risk for neurological complications, including meningitis, because of the possibility of infection of the CSF and meninges and the possibility of hydrocephalus because an obstruction to CSF absorption may occur. Early signs of infection include irritability, elevated temperature, and lethargy. Antibiotics are administered postoperatively to prevent or treat infection. The infant's vital signs and neurological function are monitored closely to identify changes that may indicate infection. The nurse performs dressing changes using sterile technique and assesses the surgical site for redness, purulent drainage, and odor. The site is assessed for CSF leakage.

Because hydrocephalus may develop after surgical repair, the nurse measures the infant's head circumference as prescribed. The nurse assesses the fontanels for bulging and cranial sutures for separation. The infant is maintained in a position that does not place pressure on the surgical site. The nurse provides postoperative pain management because when the infant cries, ICP increases. Pain management must be administered carefully so neurological impairment does not occur.

Spina bifida may be prevented by controlling environmental factors which increase the risk of a woman having a child with the disorder. It is imperative the pregnant women receive education on these risk factors. Women who are pregnant should decrease exposure to hyperther-

where research and practice meet:
Latex Allergy

Research has shown that 18%–73% of people with spina bifida demonstrate sensitivity to latex. The proposed theory is that these individuals become sensitized after repeated exposure to latex early in life. Nurses caring for children with spina bifida should provide a latex-free environment.

Referrals can be made so that families can obtain information regarding latex allergy. Organizations include Spina Bifida Association of America, Allergy to Latex Education and Resource Team and Education for Latex Allergy/Support Team & Information Coalition (National Association of Neonatal Nurses, 2003).

mia (e.g., saunas, hot tubs). A pregnant patient with diabetes mellitus must be closely monitored. The patient must understand the importance of maintaining blood glucose levels within a normal range by adherence to an appropriate diet, exercise regimen, and medication therapy. Some antiseizure medications may result in spina bifida. A woman receiving these medications needs to notify the physician immediately if she becomes pregnant so the medication therapy can be altered. Every woman of childbearing age should ingest 400 mcg of folic acid per day to prevent neural tube birth defects. Sources of folic acid include green leafy vegetables, liver, legumes, orange juice, fortified breakfast cereals, and multivitamins.

HYDROCEPHALUS

Hydrocephalus occurs in approximately 1 to 2 of every 1000 live births. The term hydrocephalus is derived from the Greek, *hydor* (water) and *kephale* (head). Many functions are served by the CSF, including buffering of the brain, helping maintain normal chemical balances, and assisting in the maintenance of the very important blood–brain barrier (Chiafery, 2006).

CSF is formed and secreted by the choroid plexus (the ventricle's highly vascular lining). Newborns produce approximately 25 mL of CSF per day and children produce between 25 and 500 mL per day (Greenberg, 2001). After it is secreted, the CSF circulates through the intracranial vault and the spinal cord. With hydrocephaly, there is an increase of CSF production, an impedance to CSF absorption, or an obstruction of flow. As the fluid volume increases in the ventricles, pressure increases within the intracranial vault.

Congenital anomalies, including Chiari I and II malformations, Dandy–Walker malformation, and aqueductal stenosis, are the most common causes of hydrocephaly during the neonatal and early infancy periods. Acquired hydrocephaly occurs after birth and in infancy, usually resulting from intraventricular hemorrhage due to prematurity (Greenberg, 2001). Other causes of acquired hydrocephaly include tumors, head injury, bleeding, and infections.

There are two categories of hydrocephalus. Communicating hydrocephalus occurs when there is full communication between the subarachnoid space and ventricles. The causes of communicating hydrocephalus are defective absorption of CSF (most often), overproduction of CSF

(rarely), and venous drainage insufficiency (occasionally). Noncommunicating hydrocephalus occurs when CSF flow within the ventricular system or the ventricular outlets to the arachnoid space is prevented. Noncommunicating hydrocephalus occurs when there is obstruction of the flow of CSF (extraventricular or intraventricular) and includes tumors, anatomic malformations, or cerebral edema. Most cases of hydrocephalus are obstructive.

SIGNS AND SYMPTOMS. The signs and symptoms of hydrocephalus vary based on the child's age and cause and rate of hydrocephalus development. The child may demonstrate signs and symptoms of increased ICP, if the disorder is severe enough. On tapping of the skull, a resonant sound termed Macewen's sign or "cracked pot" sound is heard after cranial suture separation occurs. The infant may have difficulty holding the head upright. The face and cranial vault may be disproportionate and an unusually prominent forehead may be present. Dramatic head growth and enlargement, optic chiasm, and compression of optic nerves occur in untreated hydrocephalus (McCance & Huether, 2002).

DIAGNOSIS. Congenital hydrocephalus can be diagnosed with ultrasound during a prenatal examination or discovered during infancy or even early childhood. Hydrocephalus may be suggested by symptoms exhibited by the patient such as increasing head circumference inconsistent with normal growth.

 diagnostic tools Hydrocephalus

The primary means of diagnosis is through imaging studies (CT, MRI, ultrasound), which usually reveal enlargement of ventricles. A cisternogram (radiographic evaluation) may be used to evaluate CSF flow dynamics in the child's brain and spinal cord. During the procedure, dye is injected into the subarachnoid area around the brain. Once the dye has circulated through the CSF path, a series of pictures is taken. The procedure is performed to reveal CSF concentration, leakage, obstruction, and pressure.

Lumbar puncture may be used to examine CSF and measure pressure. The nurse may perform transillumination to show abnormalities of the various areas of the child's head. Thinning or separation of the bones of the skull may be identified with radiographs of the skull. An ultrasound of the brain possibly may show ventricular dilation, hydrocephalus, or intraventricular bleeding.

 Nursing Insight— Ventricular shunts

A shunt may be placed in a child to drain excessive intracranial CSF. Ventricular shunts have greatly improved the quality of life for children with hydrocephalus. A ventricular shunt consists of several parts including a proximal catheter that enters the lateral ventricle, a one-way valve that is set at a desired pressure to prevent CSF being drained too fast due to gravity, a small reservoir, and a distal catheter that terminates in the peritoneal cavity or alternate drainage site. The peritoneal cavity is the preferred site for placement of the distal catheter because of easy accessibility and decreased risk of complications. When the catheter is placed in the peritoneum, the shunt is called a ventriculoperitoneal shunt (Fig. 29-8).

Figure 29-8 A child may have a shunt placed to drain excessive intracranial CSF.

NURSING CARE. It is important for the nurse to understand the function of shunts and nursing care of the child with a shunt. Other sites for shunt placement other than the head are the right atrium of the heart and the pleural space of the lungs. The alternate sites pose the risks of pleural effusion, emboli, pneumothorax, respiratory distress, and endocarditis. The child with a shunt is at risk for complications related to surgery to place the shunt and the shunt itself. Complications related to shunts and shunt placement include infection, abdominal complications (i.e., bowel perforation, abscesses, and ileus), and shunt failure (Chiafery, 2006). The child may also be at risk for meningitis and encephalitis postoperatively because the shunt is placed in the ventricles of the brain and any introduction of infectious agents causes a potentially life-threatening illness. Infective complications occur in approximately 5% to 10% of shunt operations. Most shunt infections occur within the first 3 months after the surgical procedure and are more frequent in children younger than 6 months of age (Spyros, 2004). Common signs and symptoms demonstrated by a child with a shunt infection include decreased LOC, irritability, increased ICP, seizures, poor feeding, and an alteration in vital signs. Antibiotic-impregnated catheters are available and can be used for patients at high risk for infection and those who have had prior shunt infections (Chiafery, 2006).

Another complication of shunts is overdrainage. The child complains of postural headaches when sitting up, but the headache resolves when lying down. On rare occasions, a subdural hematoma develops when there is rapid decompression of the ventricles. If drainage of CSF occurs too quickly, intracranial bleeding may occur because the brain shifts into the area occupied by the ventricles (McLone, 2001).

A frequent complication is shunt malfunction (e.g., kinking, blockage, infection, and incorrect positioning due to the child's growth). A child with shunt malfunction needs surgery to replace the defective shunt. The nurse needs to make caregivers aware of the frequent rate of shunt malfunction and provide them with information regarding signs and symptoms of failure as manifested by increased ICP.

Another procedure performed to relieve increased ICP is called endoscopic third ventriculostomy. This procedure also presents complications. Children who are candidates for this procedure are those with obstructive hydrocephalus such as with a tumor or aqueductal stenosis. An endoscope is introduced and used to visualize the floor of the ventricle and a fenestration is made, which allows the CSF to flow around the obstruction (Greenberg, 2001). A child may experience life-threatening complications related to this procedure including hemorrhage, subdural hematoma, CSF leakage, bradycardia, and injury to structures located in the area of surgery. The injury to the hypothalamus may result in diabetes insipidus, loss of thirst, loss of appetite, and amenorrhea (Walker, 2004). The child needs to be monitored because the fenestration may close or narrow resulting in enlarged ventricles and increased ICP (Chiafery, 2006).

When obtaining a history and physical, the nurse must question the caregiver about predisposing factors to hydrocephalus. The nurse carefully examines the child to identify the presence of any immediate life-threatening symptoms. These symptoms exhibited by the child may be indicative of increased ICP or infection. If necessary, the nurse implements emergent measures to save the child's life. The child with hydrocephaly may need only pharmacological therapy to decrease CSF and ICP or a surgical procedure may be necessary to decrease them. The nurse performs nursing actions related to increased ICP and the proposed course of treatment. The child's head circumference is obtained and documented to identify any major changes that need to be evaluated.

 assessment tools Head Circumference Measurement

Birth to 3 months Note the average head size at birth is 33–38 cm (12–14 inches)	Head circumference increases 2 cm/month (0.75 inch)
4–6 months Note the average head size at 6 months is 43 cm (17 inches)	Head circumference increases 1 cm/month (0.4 inch)
6 months to a year Note the average head size at 1 year is 46 cm (18 inches) By 1 year of age the child's head size has increased by 33% http://pediatrics.about.com/cs/weeklyquestion/a/032002_ask.htm	Head circumference increases 0.5 cm/month (0.2 inch)

Ethnocultural Considerations— Head circumference and infants of Asian heritage

The standard head circumference charts used today were developed in Denver, Colorado in the 1960s and were based on Caucasian American samples. This assessment tool does not allow for any difference in standards with reference to ethnicity. Infants of Asian heritage generally have smaller head circumferences in comparison to Caucasian infants. When Asian infants are measured using the current tool, the measurement obtained may indicate the infant is small for gestational age (SGA). However, this may not be true. The infant may be considered to be at risk for medical diseases and

Procedure 29-1 Measuring Head Circumference

Purpose

Measuring head circumference is an important component of evaluation of a child's growth as well as his or her health status.

Equipment

Flexible nonstretchable tape measure
Child's chart

Steps

1. Obtain a flexible nonstretchable tape measure (preferably one in which one end inserts into the other end).

2. Allow the parent to hold the child in his or her arms or lap.

   RATIONALE: *Parents holding the child may help decrease the child's anxiety.*

3. Remove braids, barrettes, or other hair decorations.

   RATIONALE: *The hair must lie flat in order to obtain an accurate measurement of head circumference.*

4. Place the tape measure over the most prominent part of the occiput (back of the head) and just above the supraorbital ridges (above the eyebrows).

   RATIONALE: *The landmarks ensure accurate measurement.*

5. Pull the tape measure snugly to compress the hair and underlying tissues.

   RATIONALE: *Ensures accurate measurement.*

6. Read the measurement to the nearest 0.1 cm or 1/8 inch.

7. Document the measurement on the chart.

   Clinical Alert If an abnormal circumference is found based on the child's age, reposition the tape and measure the head circumference again. The new measurement should agree with the first measurement within 0.2 cm or 1/4 inch.

Teach Parents

To help ensure an accurate head circumference measurement, teach the parents how to hold the child firmly while offering verbal comfort and encouragement.

Documentation
9/10/10 1200 Head Circumference 43 cm (17 inches).
—M. Cannon, RN

complications based on data that may not be accurate. When using the current tool to obtain a head circumference measurement of an Asian infant, the nurse must recognize that the data obtained may not be accurate with regard to ethnicity. The nurse should determine if the infant exhibits other physical findings associated with SGA.

The child who is to receive a ventricular shunt receives a preoperative intravenous antibiotic to help prevent development of infection. During the preoperative period, medications including acetazolamide (Diamox) and furosemide (Lasix) may be prescribed to decrease the production of CSF. These medications are sometimes used to postpone the need for shunt insertion. Preoperatively, the nurse ensures support of the child's head. The child requires frequent position changes of the head because hydrocephalus causes the skin of the scalp to thin, and prolonged pressure may result in impaired skin integrity.

Postoperatively, the child receives intravenous antibiotics and is monitored for infection. The nurse observes for redness along the shunt tract in addition to palpating for warmth to assess for infection. Other signs of shunt infection are fever, irritability, lethargy, abdominal discomfort, and apnea (Greenberg, 2001). The most common organisms that cause CSF infections in infants and children are *Staphylococcus aureus* and *Staphylococcus epidermis*. Adolescents are more likely to experience an infection resulting from *Propionibacter acne*, which is a slow growing infection of the CSF.

 critical nursing action Intravenous Therapy

If shunt surgery is anticipated, the nurse should not use scalp veins for intravenous therapy as the IV may be located near the surgical site.

Neurological assessment is paramount in the postoperative period after shunt insertion. Irritability, lethargy, or other alterations in neurological function may be indicative of meningitis or increased ICP. The nurse assesses and documents the child's vital signs and neurological assessments every 15 minutes or as prescribed by the surgeon. The child's head circumference is measured daily, and the fontanels are assessed for bulging and the sutures for separation. The nurse examines the child's eyes regularly because shunt malfunction may result in pressure on the optic nerve, and if not treated promptly, irreversible damage occurs.

If peritonitis develops, the child may complain of diffuse abdominal pain and tenderness along with nausea and vomiting. When taking vital signs, the nurse pays particular attention to an elevated temperature and rapid pulse. Peritonitis results in leukocytosis (an increase in white blood cells); therefore, lab results are closely monitored. The nurse observes for signs of hypovolemia and shock resulting from loss of electrolytes and fluids into the abdominal cavity and assesses for rebound tenderness and muscle rigidity. When assessing the abdomen, the nurse auscultates for hypoactive or absent bowel sounds to identify a paralytic ileus. The nurse obtains an abdominal circumference measurement to assess for distention. To promote accuracy, the nurse puts a mark on the abdomen so the tape measure is placed in the same spot every time. Safety precautions are implemented as pain and fever may cause the child to become disoriented.

When positioning the child, the nurse elevates the head no higher than 30 degrees in order to prevent ventricular decompression and places the child on the unoperated side to prevent pressure on the shunt. If increased CSF occurs, the physician may prescribe for the child to be elevated higher than 30 degrees. The shunt may be manually purged but only in extreme cases due to the risk of a subdural hematoma.

❝What to say❞ — *Parental education about ventricular shunts*

The nurse can communicate to the parents that a child with hydrocephalus needs continuous monitoring and assessment because hydrocephalus is a lifelong disorder. Educate parents so they can recognize complications of hydrocephalus, including increased ICP and shunt malfunction (kinking, plugging within the ventricle from tissue or exudate or obstruction at the distal end from thrombosis or displacement of the tubing due to growth). Shunt infection can happen any time but most often occurs 1–3 months after placement. Instruct parents to assess for common signs and symptoms (nausea and vomiting, headache, change in customary behavior, lethargy, unresponsiveness, elevated temperature). Explain that the child will not be able to participate in contact sports because of the possibility of shunt damage. The importance of safe transport and positioning (a reclining car seat) is also emphasized.

❝What to say❞ — *Growth and development concerns*

The nurse assesses the child's growth and development and compares the findings to established normal parameters so any delays and issues can be addressed and appropriate referrals made if necessary. Explain to caregivers that the child may experience delays in achieving developmental milestones. The child with hydrocephalus usually has a larger than normal head and may find it difficult to support the head. Rolling over and sitting up for the child may be delayed or difficult. The nurse informs the parents that as the child grows, the body grows more in proportion to the head size (Chiafery, 2006). Alert parents that they need to implement safety measures relevant to an enlarged head, including support while in a car seat or high chair.

CEREBRAL PALSY

Cerebral palsy (CP), the most common permanent physical disability of childhood, is characterized by physical impairment and mild to severe physical and mental dysfunction (Fig. 29-9). The United Cerebral Palsy Foundation estimated

Figure 29-9 The child with cerebral palsy has physical impairment and has mild to severe physical and mental dysfunction.

that approximately 764,000 adults and children in the United States in 2001 were diagnosed with cerebral palsy (Krigger, 2006). Cerebral palsy is a nonprogressive neurological disorder that results from brain injury occurring before cerebral development is complete. Since brain development continues for the first 2 years of life, the disorder can be a result of brain injury occurring not only during the prenatal period but also during the perinatal and postnatal periods. Prenatal risk factors include asphyxia, infections (i.e., rubella, cytomegalovirus, and toxoplasmosis), intracranial hemorrhage, blood incompatibility, and trauma. The perinatal risk factors for CP are low birth weight, birth at less than 32 weeks of gestation, and intracranial hemorrhage. Postnatal risk factors include viral encephalitis, bacterial meningitis, falls, child abuse, and motor vehicle accidents.

SIGNS AND SYMPTOMS. The signs and symptoms vary depending on the area of the brain involved and the extent of damage. Some children with CP may only have some awkwardness and can lead relatively normal lives while others are severely disabled and require extensive assistance. There are four types of CP. Spastic CP is the most common type. A child with spastic CP has stiff muscles because of increased muscle tone, and the muscles are predisposed to contracture. Children with this type of CP have poor control of posture, coordinated movement, and balance. Spastic CP is often classified according to the limbs affected (i.e., diplegia, hemiplegia, quadriplegia, monoplegia, and triplegia). Children with spastic diplegia (both legs are involved) have difficulty walking because of tight muscles in the hips and legs and may have scissoring (legs turn inward and cross at the knees) (Sankar & Mundkur, 2005).

Children with ataxic cerebral palsy have difficulties with balance and depth perception. They walk with an unsteady gait, demonstrate poor coordination, and often have fine motor control problems. Athetoid CP or dyskinetic CP is characterized by uncontrolled involuntary writhing movement of extremities. In severe cases, the facial muscles may be affected and drooling, speech difficulties, and grimacing may occur. In mixed CP, a child has two or more types of CP. Some of the common symptoms of mixed CP are difficulty or inability to walk, speech difficulty, swallowing problems, breathing difficulties, bowel or bladder incontinence, seizures, vision problems, learning disabilities, hearing deficits, attention or behavioral problems, and impaired senses (Sankar & Mundkur, 2005).

? case study Infant Amy Moore

Infant Amy Moore, 9 months old, has been referred to a neurologist by a pediatrician for evaluation. The neurologist questions the infant's mother about her pregnancy, the birth, and Amy's physical and psychosocial development. The mother stated Amy is her first child, and she had a complicated pregnancy. She was diagnosed with cytomegalovirus at 26 weeks of gestation and pregnancy-induced hypertension at 28 weeks. She delivered Amy at 32 weeks because of rapid progression of the hypertension. At birth, Amy weighed 2 pounds and 9 ounces, and her Apgar scores at birth were 3 and 6. Based on her initial assessment, Amy was transferred to the NICU and remained there for 65 days Amy was mechanically ventilated for 26 days and received enteral feedings. While in the NICU, Amy had a small intraventricular hemorrhage. Amy weighed 4 pounds and 10 ounces when discharged. The mother states that she is concerned about Amy's physical and psychosocial development. Physical assessment findings are as follows: poor eye contact, anterior fontanel soft, slight drooling of oral secretions, mild head lag, few facial expressions, hypotonic extremity muscles, and right handedness noted.

critical thinking questions

1. What risk factors predisposed Amy to CP?

2. What physical assessment findings demonstrated by Amy are indicative of CP?

◆ See Suggested Answers to Case Studies in text on the Electronic Study Guide or DavisPlus.

DIAGNOSIS. Diagnosis is primarily based on clinical symptoms demonstrated by the child. The child may exhibit muscular hypotonia (low tension) or hypertonia (high tension). A child with CP may demonstrate hand preference by 6 months of age instead of 12 months. An important sign of CP is persistence of some primitive infant reflexes (i.e., Moro and crossed extensor reflexes) because these reflexes normally disappear between 6 months and 12 months of age. CT, MRI, and cerebral ultrasound are tests used to diagnose CP.

NURSING CARE. The child with CP has some degree of muscular dysfunction. Splints and braces may be necessary to facilitate muscle control and improve body functioning. The nurse encourages the child to perform self-care tasks. Assistive devices may be necessary to allow the child to perform these tasks, including large handled brushes and toothbrushes. Clothing should be easy to manipulate. To reduce muscle spasms and prevent fatigue, allow frequent rest periods.

The nurse administers medications that reduce muscle spasms. Skeletal muscle relaxants may be used for short-term control with older children and adolescents. Dantrolene (Dantrium) is administered to decrease spasticity, but the child must be monitored for hepatic impairment. The use of baclofen (Lioresal) has increased. Baclofen (Lioresal) can be administered intrathecally via an infusion pump to provide continuous and controlled relief (Krigger, 2006). Neurolytic agent nerve blocks provide a temporary decrease in spasticity. Paralysis of specific muscles can be achieved by the injection of botulinum (Botox), but the long-term effects have not been determined. Antianxiety medications such as diazepam (Valium) may be administered to older children and adolescents to reduce excessive motion and tension. Also, children with CP are predisposed to seizures. Medications including phenobarbital (Luminal) and phenytoin (Dilantin) may be administered to control seizures.

The child who does not respond to conservative management may need surgical intervention. Surgical procedures provide joint stability and balanced muscle power and may include tendon lengthening, release of spastic wrist flexor muscles, and correction of spastic hip adduction. Selective dorsal rhizotomy (severing of dorsal sensory fibers that have an abnormal response resulting in spasticity) may be performed to improve the child's ability to sit, stand, and walk.

Feeding problems may be experienced by the child due to impaired muscle control and strength. If the child can feed independently, she is encouraged to do so. Utensils with large handles may be used for easier manipulation. The child must be fed in an upright position and not hurried while eating because of the danger of aspiration. Assistance may be provided by standing behind the child and guiding the hand to the mouth. The nurse can stabilize the mandible in a child with poor facial muscle control by placing a hand on the child's mandible.

Children with CP may or may not demonstrate intellectual deficits. The degree of deficit depends on the severity of brain injury. Children with CP need intellectual stimulation. If possible, the child with CP should be enrolled in school to foster relationships, self-esteem, and normalcy. Participating in activity programs helps incorporate play into exercise. Toys are chosen based on cognitive, not chronological age. The environment needs to be safe because the child may not comprehend the concept of danger.

Neurological Injuries

NEAR DROWNING

Near drowning or submersion injuries (SIs) are a major cause of death and disability in children. Children are at risk for a SI because of the inability to swim, fatigue, inadequate muscle strength, and lack of knowledge of water safety. A child who has a SI may have only short-term complications or may have long-term life-altering disabilities. Early and aggressive medical treatment is paramount in the care of the child, and the child's prognosis depends on the treatment provided.

Near drowning involving children is usually preventable, yet more than 1500 children in the United States die every year from submersion injuries. Males are approximately four times more likely to experience a SI as females. Children younger than 3 years of age and adolescents 15 to 19 years of age are at the highest risk. SI in a child may have various causes (e.g., trauma, seizure, abuse).

A submersion injury occurs when a child who is submerged in water tries to breathe and aspirates water (wet drowning) or has a laryngospasm without aspiration (dry drowning). The most significant contributing factors to morbidity and mortality are hypoxemia with decreasing oxygen delivery to vital tissues. CNS damage may occur during the incident (primary injury) or may result from ongoing pulmonary injury, injury due to reperfusion, or multiorgan dysfunction (secondary injury). Early resuscitation is associated with an improved prognosis. Clinicians use an Orlowski scale to predict the likelihood of neurologically intact survival (Verive, 2006).

 assessment tools Orlowski Scale

Clinical Application
Each item is assigned one point. If a child has a score of 2 or less, there is a 90% likelihood of a complete recovery. If a child has a score of 3 or more, there is a 5% chance of survival (Verive, 2006).

- Three years of age or older
- Submersion time greater than 5 minutes
- No resuscitation efforts for more than 10 minutes after rescue
- Comatose on admission to the emergency room
- Arterial pH <7.10

SIGNS AND SYMPTOMS. Near drowning affects many organ systems. The child may experience cerebral edema if prolonged submersion exists. Varying degrees of alterations in level of consciousness may be present. The child may have altered surfactant volume or function or both, resulting in atelectasis and severe injury to the pulmonary capillary bed with resulting pulmonary edema. The child experiences respiratory distress with cyanosis, hypoxia, wheezing, and rales. Acute respiratory distress syndrome (ARDS) is a common complication of SI because of altered surfactant function and pulmonary edema (Verive, 2006). Pneumonia may develop if the water contains bacteria or other microbes. If the immersion occurs in water containing chemicals, such as household cleaning substances, the child may develop chemical pneumonitis. Cardiovascular complications are common.

The child may be hypovolemic due to increased capillary permeability. Vasodilation may occur if rewarming is performed and hypotension may result. The child may experience myocardial dysfunction including ventricular dysrhythmias, pulseless electrical activity (PEA), and asystole as a result of hypoxemia, acidosis, hypothermia, and electrolyte abnormalities (Verive, 2006).

DIAGNOSIS. Arterial blood gas analysis, which detects carboxyhemoglobin and methemoglobinemia; continuous pulse oximetry; and chest radiography help assess the respiratory system. CT and cervical spine imaging are used to evaluate the neurological system. The cardiovascular system is evaluated with echocardiography and electrocardiography. Laboratory tests usually include complete blood count, blood coagulation studies, liver enzymes, renal function tests (BUN and creatinine), serum electrolytes, and serum glucose (Verive, 2006).

NURSING CARE. When caring for a patient admitted because of near drowning, a priority nursing responsibility is assessing and maintaining the airway (Orlowski & Szpilman, 2001). If respiratory or cardiac arrest occurs, life support measures are implemented. Suctioning is performed to remove debris, secretions, or emesis that may obstruct the airway (Orlowski & Szpilman, 2001). The nurse inserts a nasogastric tube to remove gastric contents and relieve abdominal distention in order to reduce the risk of vomiting and aspiration. Oxygenation is a primary concern. A nonrebreather mask may be used if the child is not intubated but oxygen saturation and respiratory status must be closely monitored in case respiratory deterioration occurs (Ross, 2005). The nurse understands that the child who is in respiratory compromise (hypoxic or apneic) or unconscious needs immediate intubation. The nurse evaluates the child for symptoms that may indicate other injuries including head or spinal trauma.

 clinical alert

Cricoid pressure
To avoid vomiting during intubation, apply cricoid pressure or empty the stomach contents with a nasogastric tube (Orlowski & Szpilman, 2001).

HEAD INJURY

Traumatic brain injury (TBI) occurs when a jolt or blow to the head disrupts the normal function of the brain. The effects of a TBI may be as mild as a brief loss of consciousness or as severe as a vegetative state or death.

Each year in the United States, approximately 1.5 million people experience a TBI. 50,000 die (2685 are children), and as many as 5.3 million persons are currently living with a long-term disability. Each year many children from 0 to 14 years of age experience varying degrees of brain injury. Approximately 435,000 children are seen in emergency departments for accidents involving a head injury and 37,000 of those evaluated are hospitalized (National Center for Injury Prevention and Control, 2008). The primary causes of pediatric TBIs are motor vehicle crashes, bicycle accidents, sports trauma, violence, and falls. Any child with a TBI must be evaluated for child abuse.

A TBI can be classified as penetrating (e.g., bullet entering the brain) or nonpenetrating (e.g., fall from a tree). A TBI is further classified as primary or secondary. Primary injury occurs directly from the trauma and secondary injury is a result of complications (e.g., cerebral ischemia, hemorrhage). Children are predisposed to head injury because their heads are larger in relation to their body sizes, an unsteady gait, and thinner, softer cerebral tissue. Direct brain injury occurs when the skull vault is impended. A skull fracture may or may not be present. Indirect brain injury results when structural deformation occurs. Rotational acceleration and deceleration forces are usually present in motor vehicle accidents and they produce tearing and shearing injuries of the brain (Benham & Chavda, 2002).

SIGNS AND SYMPTOMS. The child may exhibit obvious signs including bleeding from the scalp, depression of the skull, or a visible penetrating wound. Other typical signs and symptoms are loss of consciousness, an alteration in consciousness, seizures, and combativeness. These are primarily the result of cerebral ischemia and necrosis and increased ICP.

DIAGNOSIS. A CT or an MRI identifies intracranial bleeding, compression of cerebral tissue, the presence of penetrating foreign objects, and skull fractures. An electroencephalogram (EEG) may be prescribed to determine if the child has brain activity abnormalities. ICP monitoring, cerebral blood flow, and CPP are measured if increased ICP is present. Cerebral oxygenation is monitored with the use of jugular venous bulb saturation and concentration or near infrared spectroscopy (Woodrow, 2000).

NURSING CARE. The child with a TBI needs immediate care to prevent life-threatening complications or death. Airway patency is a priority. The nurse delivers supplemental oxygen via a bag-valve-mask device until the airway is established. The child may need to be intubated and mechanically ventilated if a patent airway is not possible due to injury to the neck or pharynx, if level of consciousness is depressed, or if the neurological state is expected to deteriorate.

The nurse inserts two large-bore IV needles and administers hypertonic fluid to maintain adequate circulation. Intravenous fluids are warmed if hypothermia is a concern. If blood loss is greater than 30% of the child's total blood volume, blood products are administered (Brettler, 2004).

Assessment of the child's neurological status is imperative. The nurse uses the Pediatric Glasgow Coma scale to evaluate neurological status. The child's pupil size and reactivity are assessed and a difference or change is reported. Reflexes are assessed to determine brainstem involvement, and if the brainstem is injured, the child's prognosis is poor. The nurse palpates the skull to identify any fractures or depressions. Signs of a basal skull fracture include leakage of CSF from the ears or nose, hemotympanum (blood in the middle ear), mastoid ecchymosis (Battle's sign), and periorbital ecchymosis (raccoon eyes) (Bergsneider & Kelly, 2003). The nurse assesses the patient for increased ICP. If increased ICP is present, appropriate measures are implemented.

 critical nursing action Basal skull fracture

Do not insert an NG tube if a basal skull fracture is suspected because the tube may enter the brain through the fracture. Insert an orogastric tube if needed instead (Brettler, 2004).

SHAKEN BABY SYNDROME

Shaken baby syndrome results from major rotational forces and angular deceleration encountered when an infant is shaken forcefully. The injury may be intentional or unintentional. Most victims of shaken baby syndrome are younger than 6 months of age and the source of the abuse is usually the father or a male acquaintance of the mother. The prognosis for an infant depends on the severity of the injury and response to medical therapy. Complications a child may experience are neuromotor impairment, visual impairment, and developmental delays.

SIGNS AND SYMPTOMS. Symptoms of severe injury include seizure activity, apnea, bulging or full fontanels, coma, hemorrhage, bradycardia, and complete cardiovascular collapse. Symptoms exhibited in less severe cases include vomiting, hypothermia, poor feeding or failure to thrive, increased sleeping, lethargy, or irritability and difficulty arousing.

DIAGNOSIS. CT scan or MRI is used to determine if a subdural or subarachnoid hemorrhage is present. Radiographs of the skull determine if any skull fractures are evident and an ocular funduscopic exam is used to assess for retinal hemorrhage, a classic sign of shaken baby syndrome.

 Nursing Insight— Shaken baby syndrome

The hallmark of shaken baby syndrome is an absence of external trauma to the head, face, and neck of an infant along with massive intracranial or intraocular bleeding.

NURSING CARE. Nursing care involves initiation and maintenance of respiratory and cardiovascular support if necessary. The nurse needs to assess for increased ICP, insert a nasogastric or orogastric tube, assess for seizure activity, implement seizure precautions, maintain adequate fluid and nutritional intake, and assess and document any visible injuries.

The child may have either short-term or long-term impairment. Long-term impairment requires therapy consisting of gastrostomy tube feedings, a tracheostomy, pressure ulcer prevention, and other measures for children in a vegetative state. An important measure to prevent this abuse is educating parents and other caregivers (Smith, 2003).

The long-term outcome for a child with shaken baby syndrome or a TBI may be uncertain. The child's prognosis is affected by many variables including the degree of cerebral involvement, areas of the brain affected, severity of intracranial hemorrhaging, and medical management provided. The child may have minimal deficits or complications or she may experience severe and life-altering complications. The nurse must honestly address parental concerns and questions and provide information about agencies that can provide assistance and support them. The parents need to realize the child may never return to the prior level of cognitive and physical functioning.

 Be sure to— Legal and ethical responsibility related to shaken baby syndrome

Nurses are legally and ethically required to report any incidences of probable abuse to the proper authorities. The health care facility should have relevant policy and procedure guidelines available.

SPINAL CORD INJURY

Spinal cord injury without radiographic abnormality (SCIWORA) is a closed spinal cord injury resulting in stretching of the spinal cord without bony involvement or radiographic abnormalities. SCIWORA occurs in more than 50% to 70% of spinal cord injuries in children. SCWIORA usually occurs in children younger than 8 years of age because they are at risk for high cervical injuries because of their disproportionately larger head in relation to their body. As the child grows the spinal cord becomes less elastic but is covered by strengthened bony prominences; this added protection accounts for better resistance to injury as the child ages. The long-term outcome for children with SCIWORA is related to the etiology of the injury and the degree of functional loss.

The incidence of spinal cord injury (SCI) is based on pediatric demographics, gender, and age of the child. SCIs are seen more in the summer with bike riding, swimming and diving activities, football playing, and motor vehicle collisions. Spinal cord injuries have been associated with traumatic births and child abuse in children younger than 1 year of age. SCIs are also associated with fighting with guns and knives and other forms of violence.

Spinal cord injury involves injury to the spinal cord in any or all of the following regions: cervical, thoracic, lumbar, or sacral. SCIs are due to direct or indirect force causing a contusion or bruising, compression, hemorrhage, or significant vascular damage resulting in paresthesia (loss of sensation) or paralysis (loss of function) below the level of injury. There are four types of SCIs: (1) cord resection, when the spinal cord is completely severed; (2) cord laceration caused by a blunt instrument such as a knife; (3) cord contusion caused by swelling and edema; and (4) cord injury in which there is no necrosis or obvious injury.

There are three phases of injury: acute, secondary, and chronic. The acute phase is the immediate time of injury to a few days later in which there is damage to the tissues resulting in cell necrosis. Immediately after the insult there is hemorrhage and edema combined with electrolyte and fluid shifts. The cord then experiences a spinal shock that lasts for 24 hours (Hulsebosch, 2002). The secondary phase occurs at the time of injury and continues over several weeks. The child's neurological status at this phase determines recovery outcomes. The chronic phase is marked with scarring and progression or regression of function. The nurse understands that complete resection of the spinal cord results in complete loss of motor function and sensation below the area of injury (Hulsebosch, 2002). Regardless of the mechanism of injury, the result is either temporary or permanent loss or alteration of autonomic, motor, and sensory function.

SIGNS AND SYMPTOMS. Clinically, the child has injury to the back, neck, thoracic, or lumbar area followed by numbness, tingling, or loss of function. Loss of anal tone and the ability to urinate independently, combined with an abnormal neurological examination of any of the four extremities, are present. There may be neck or back pain or tenderness. The child may or may not have an obvious deformity of a bony prominence.

DIAGNOSIS. The International Standards for Neurological and Functional Classification of Spinal Cord Injury identify two levels of spinal cord loss and function. Tetraplegia, currently replacing the term quadriplegia, is due to a spinal cord injury at the cervical level that involves all four extremities. Paraplegia is the result of thoracic, lumbar, or sacral injury loss of function and sensation in the lower extremities (Dawodu, 2007).

The clinical diagnosis of SCIWORA and SCI is made both clinically and radiologically. Loss of motor function, sensation, and anal tone on exam clinically define the level of injury and degree of involvement. Radiological examination with spine series, CT scan, or MRI identifies the type of injury, the presence of hemorrhage or inflammation, and the degree of bony involvement, if any.

clinical alert

Autonomic dysreflexia

Autonomic dysreflexia is a stress syndrome caused by massive amounts of stimuli overloading the autonomic system resulting in hyperactive sympathetic stimulation. This leads to a myriad of symptoms such as extreme anxiety, headache, visual and auditory sensation changes, nausea, seizures, hypertension, peripheral vascular dilation or flushing, and bradycardia. This situation is an emergent condition requiring immediate management of hypertension, cardiac, and neurological complications.

NURSING CARE. The priorities of trauma care are attention to airway management, breathing or ventilatory support, circulation support, disability identification, and exposure of known and unknown physical limitations. Immediate cervical (c-spine) immobilization is maintained continuously. Treat a SCI with full body immobilization and maintain with lumbar–thoracic–sacral orthotics (TLSOs), which are rigid body casts that maintain neuromuscular alignment until the injury is resolved.

If a child has a high cervical injury or if an open airway cannot be maintained, a temporary or permanent tracheostomy is necessary for the child to breathe. Mechanical ventilation may be a lifelong need for patients with a high C-4 injury. Cardiovascular and circulatory support is maintained with adequate fluid resuscitation, inotropic medications, and blood products to maintain circulation, cardiac output, and renal function during the immediate posttraumatic event. Large doses of steroid therapy may be used after the initial injury for up to 6 days to reduce spinal cord inflammation.

After the child is stabilized, there are several facets of ongoing care. Maintaining adequate respiratory function is necessary. The nurse works to maintain a patent airway with frequent suctioning. Tracheotomy care and proper neck and body alignment to prevent potential aspiration complications is required twice daily. Continuous mechanical ventilation or oxygen support monitoring is a priority in nursing care.

The nurse also monitors appropriate daily fluid intake and output measurements and ensures adequate daily fluid requirement needs are met. Renal function is evaluated with daily monitoring of serum chemistry values and urine specific gravity measurements.

A child immobilized by a spinal cord injury may have slowed peristaltic function and may require medications such as metoclopramide (Reglan), laxatives, or stool softeners to prevent constipation, gastric overdistention, and fecal impaction. Bowel training may be a chronic issue for most children with SCI. Stool bulking with high-fiber foods may promote stool formation. Lower intestinal evacuation may be necessary with enemas, suppositories, and colonic irrigations. Exercise and abdominal massage promote peristaltic activity, and planned colonic irrigations may be used if the child experiences unplanned fecal soiling.

Nutritional support is a collaborative issue among the physician, the nurse, and the dietician. Enteral feedings may be needed until the child is able to chew and swallow without threat of aspiration. A child with altered oral pharyngeal motility or dysphagia may require an oral pharyngeal motility (OPM) study before oral feedings. Nasogastric or gastrostomy devices for enteral feedings can be implemented if the child's swallowing is impaired or if there is a threat of aspiration.

The nurse should provide emotional and social support, as the child with a spinal cord injury and his family have unique collective and individual needs. The younger child does not understand the loss of function immediately and is more concerned with parental presence and fear issues. The older child understands the loss of function and sensation and is more cooperative and eager to return to normal living as much as possible. Encourage older children and adolescents to participate in their own care as much as possible. All daily activities such as bathing, dressing, eating, grooming, and bowel and bladder care should be performed by the older child as he is able.

The adolescent presents a unique developmental challenge. The realization about the loss of friends, athletic participation, and social disruption may place the teen at risk for depression, withdrawal, isolation, and suicide. The nurse must look for these changes and recommend antidepressant medication in order to promote optimal function and return to a healthy emotional status.

The child with SCI requires lifelong care and support. This places a financial, mental, physical, and emotional strain on the family. The nurse must recognize caregiver role strain and offer or encourage respite care for the caregivers as needed.

 Collaboration in Caring— *Spinal Cord Injury*

Nursing care of the child with spinal cord injury is an interdisciplinary approach. The child works together with the family; medical team; physical, speech, occupational, and respiratory therapists; and social workers to coordinate the services needed for individualized care.

 nursing diagnoses Spinal Cord Injury

- Impaired Urinary Elimination related to neuromuscular alteration.
- Constipation related to sensory and motor impairment
- Ineffective Individual Coping related to traumatic spinal cord injury and potential loss of function.
- Impaired Physical Mobility related to neuromuscular functional loss.
- Risk for Injury related to loss of sensation and motor function.
- Risk for Impaired Skin Integrity related to loss of sensation.
- Situational Alteration in Self-Esteem related to change in lifestyle.

Nontraumatic Neurological Conditions

HEADACHES

Headaches are a common occurrence in the pediatric population. Headaches are classified as primary or secondary and further classified into subtypes according to International Classification of Headache Disorders (ICHD-II) (Silberstein et al., 2005). The International Classification of Headache Disorders is a useful tool in classifying acute and chronic headaches in school-age children and adolescents but lacks sensitivity in diagnosing benign headaches in preschool and younger children (Balottin et al., 2005; Bigal, Rapoport, Tepper, Sheftell, & Lipton, 2005).

Headaches can occur in 90% of children. Most causes of a childhood headache are based on a simple etiology such as minor trauma, emotions, genetic predisposition, illness, environmental factors, or certain food and beverages (Mayoclinic.com, 2008).

SIGNS AND SYMPTOMS. Primary headaches are headaches caused by tight muscles with no etiological agent. Triggers of primary headaches have been identified as lack of sleep, stress, exercise, hunger, loud noise or persistently loud noises, weather changes, and hormonal changes due to menstrual cycles in females. Secondary headaches are associated with an organic disorder such as trauma, vascular changes, infectious processes, substance use, brain neoplasms, or psychogenic issues.

Headaches are further classified into subtypes based on descriptive symptoms and frequency of disturbances. Tension headaches are common among school-age children and are associated with stress. The tension headache is located in the back of the head at the base of the skull and feels like a dull moderate pain. This pain may radiate bilaterally and may be located just above the neck and shoulders. Loss of vision, nausea, photophobia, and auditory sensitivity are not associated with tension headaches. Sleep may be affected for children with these headaches.

Migraines are another type of headache and can be present in the preschool or school-aged child. Most often, there is a family history of migraines. Migraine headache pain is located on one side of the head with a throbbing or pulsating quality that radiates. An aura may precede the migraine headache and is accompanied by nausea, vomiting, diaphoresis, pallor, photophobia, and auditory sensitivity. The aura may be sensed by a noxious smell, bright lights, or a change in vision. Migraines are not easily remedied with rest alone and typically require prophylactic and acute management.

Cluster headaches are a series of headaches over a period of weeks or months that vary in intensity and can be very debilitating. The pain is usually unilateral, behind one eye, and results in ptosis (drooping), pupil constriction, erythema, and edema of the affected eye. Rhinorrhea is also present with clear drainage in the absence of an upper respiratory illness.

DIAGNOSIS. Headache diagnoses are based on clinical symptoms according to the ICHD-II criteria. Diagnosis is based on inclusion and exclusion clinical criteria. Clinical diagnosis is difficult with a young child because of cognitive and communication barriers. A history of headache signs are difficult to piece together as the symptoms may mimic those of other minor pediatric illnesses. Neuro-imaging studies are warranted with sudden severe onset of headaches, history of trauma, family history of brain neoplasms or vascular malformations, change in neurological function, signs of increased intracranial pressure or visual disturbances, new seizure onset, unexplained ataxia, or alterations in level of consciousness (Lewis et al., 2002).

Diagnostic assessment begins with a full neurological examination, history of present illness, family headache history, review of symptoms, and headache history including patterns, antecedent events, and symptom management. Decisions for diagnostic neuroimaging, lumbar puncture, or EEG testing are based on patient data obtained at the time of the neurological evaluation. Routine neuroimaging is not indicated in the presence of a normal neurological exam (Lewis et al., 2002).

NURSING CARE. Combined pharmacological and non-pharmacological therapies along with child and family education can successfully manage the child with primary headaches.

Prophylactic medication such as beta-blockers, calcium channel blockers, antidepressants, and anticonvulsants or a combination of these can help the child cope with primary headaches. Acute episodes are treated with acetaminophen (Children's Tylenol) and ibuprofen (Children's Advil). Intranasal sumatriptan (Imitrex) or dihydroergotamine mesylate (DHE) is administered subcutaneously.

Child and family education must target migraine prophylaxis, identification, and management of headache triggers and symptom management with analgesia. Migraine prophylaxis includes medications such as topiramate (Topamax), sumatriptan (Imitrex), ergotamine (Cafergot), NSAIDs, antiemetics, and sedative analgesics. Pharmacology therapy is titrated to individual child needs and desired function.

Intramuscular or intranasal dihydroergotamine can be also used for moderate to severe migraines in adolescents (Hamalainen, 2006; Robertson & Shilkofski, 2005; Saper & Silberstein, 2006).

The nurse educates the family on recognition of headache aura, prophylaxis strategies, and management intervention, including medication, relaxation strategies, and environmental modifications (e.g., noise reduction, dim or dark room). The nurse evaluates the effectiveness of the medication and monitors for adverse reactions. Treatment also involves rest and stress reduction strategies such as soothing baths, music, guided imagery or massage therapy.

Sensory Conditions

EYE DISORDERS

Children may experience a myriad of common eye disorders. The parent may notice an abrupt change or changes in vision function. Children are not acutely aware of changes in vision or eye disturbances and may not voice complaints of vision difficulty unless there is an injury. Common childhood eye disorders are classified as refractive disorders, astigmatism, amblyopia, strabismus, or organic diseases (Watkinson & Graham, 2005) (Table 29-7).

 Nursing Insight— *Vision*

Vision occurs as a result of light reflection from an object passing through the cornea, aqueous humor, pupil, lenses, and vitreous humor and finally absorbed by the retina. The retina then converts the light to an electrical impulse that travels from the optic nerve to the visual cortex of the brain. The retina is composed of rods and cones that are used in night, color, daylight, and eye movement functions. The rods and cones communicate electrical energy to the retina, which then sends an impulse to the optic nerve. The majority of the blood vessels radiate from the optic nerve and the retina. The fovea centralis, which is located in the center of the macula about 2.5 disc diameters from the optic nerve, is responsible for color perception.

Refractive Disorders

The most common category of vision disorders in children is refractive errors (Simon & Kaw, 2001). Light refraction is the bending of light as it passes through a lens. As light passes through an opening in the pupil, the lens directs the light to the retina to initiate vision. In very young infants, the light rays fall behind the retina due to the shallowness of the eye. Most children are hyperopic (farsightedness). The amount of hyperopia diminishes as the child ages. In hyperopia, vision is unclear at a close range and is clearer at a far range. Young children with hyperopia may have trouble focusing on projects requiring close range visions and may lose interest. Hyperopia usually diminishes by age 5 but in some cases may persist. These children require convex lenses to correct the refractive disorder. If a child reports headaches, dizziness, or eye strain after doing school work, hyperopia is suspected and a referral is made for vision assessment (Simon & Kaw, 2001).

Some children develop myopia (nearsightedness) in the school years, particularly if there is a familial history of myopia. In myopia, light rays do not reach the retina causing blurred vision at a far range and clear vision at a close range. Children who have myopia may squint, complain of nearsightedness, and are unable to see the blackboard, television, or street signs but can clearly read a book or a computer screen at close range. About 10% of school-aged children have myopia. This condition continues to progress in severity until puberty when progression plateaus (Watkinson & Graham, 2005).

Correction of myopia includes concave lenses in eye glasses or contact lenses. Laser assisted surgery keratomileusis (LASIK) is available for the adolescents if desired. The age for LASIK surgery is controversial. If the procedure is performed before full eye growth maturity has been reached, additional surgery may be needed (U.S. Food and Drug Administration, 2007).

Astigmatism

Astigmatism is an irregular curvature or uneven contour of the eye resulting in impaired light refraction. The cause is unknown. Astigmatism may be present at birth or acquired. Light rays are unevenly distributed in the eyes, causing blurred vision at all distances. This condition is associated with birth hyperopia and myopia.

Table 29-7 Common Acute Eye Disorders

Eye Disorder	Cause/Organism	Signs and Symptoms	Treatment
Conjunctivitis	An inflammation of the conjunctiva caused by bacterial, viral or allergic agents.	Excessive tearing, erythema, and edema with clear, watery discharge, yellow or green drainage, and eyelid crusting. Bacterial and viral agents are difficult to discriminate clinically without a culture. Viral usually seen in children older than age 6 years with a clear watery drainage. Allergic: cobble stoning and pallor of the conjunctiva, pruritus, watery clear drainage.	Apply warm soaks to remove crusting, use good hand hygiene and apply cool compresses to edematous eyes. Antibiotic ointment or solutions are used for bacterial infections. Family education includes good hand hygiene before and after touching the eye, non-sharing of personal items such as pillow cases and washcloths and careful disposal of used tissues and wipes. Older children who wear contact lenses or use cosmetics should discard used materials and begin use of new materials after the infection has resolved. School attendance is permissible after the discomfort and drainage has subsided, usually after 24 hours of treatment. If symptoms are not improved in 24–48 hours the family should seek additional follow-up medical care. Conjunctivitis associated with herpes may be treated with oral or parenteral antiviral agents. Herpetic ophthalmicus is one of the leading causes of vision loss in children (Shaikh and Ta, 2002). Allergic conjunctivitis treated with allergen avoidance and antihistamines.
Neonatal Conjunctivitis– Ophthalmia Neonatorium	Chemical irritation caused by maternal sexually transmitted diseases acquired at birth. *Chlamydia, gonorrhea, herpes.*	Purulent drainage either white or yellowish.	Prophylactic antibiotic ointment is used in all neonates. Lack of treatment can cause eye damage.
Stye	A localized inflammatory swelling of one or more of the glands of the eyelid. They are mildly tender, and may discharge some purulent fluid (Venes, 2009).	Painful, erythematous lesion on the lid margin. Slight edema, some lymph node tenderness or induration.	Apply warm moist compresses with an antibiotic ointment. Good hand hygiene is necessary.
Chalazion	Granuloma of the meibomian gland on the eyelid. Cause unknown.	Hard, small nodule on either eyelid may be painful.	Applying warm moist compresses and massage, with antibiotic ointment, may resolve the condition spontaneously. Surgical removal or steroid injections may be used to reduce size and symptoms such as ptosis.
Blepharitis Marginalis	Staphylococcal infection of the lid margin.	Erythematous eyelid margin with crusted eye drainage.	Apply an antibiotic ointment to the lower affected eyelid. Apply warm moist compresses to remove crusting drainage.
Keratitis	Inflammation and infection of the corneal layers due to bacterial, viral, fungal or foreign body infiltration.	Very painful, excessive tearing, photophobia and erythema.	An ophthalmologist must examine the cornea to monitor or treat potential scarring and prevent loss of vision.
Periorbital Cellulitis	Inflammation of the subcutaneous tissues and skin about the eye may be bacterial or viral.	Edema, pain, erythema in the skin and orbital folds of the affected eye.	Use intravenous antibiotic therapy for 7 days.
Blocked Tear Duct	Obstruction of the nasolacrimal tear duct causing inflammation or cystitis.	Tearing, yellow drainage, crusting, small bump in the inner canthus of the affected eye. Usually unilateral, may be painful.	Apply warm compresses and gentle massage of the lacrimal sac with the forefinger milking any exudates toward the nose. This condition may require probing of the duct by an ophthalmologist if no improvement is noted in 6 months (Fox, 2002).

Corrective lenses usually solve the problem. Sometimes surgery is indicated but is not usually necessary. If a child complains of headaches, blurry vision, dizziness after doing close work or difficulty reading, he or she is referred to an ophthalmologist.

Amblyopia

Amblyopia ("lazy eye") is one of the most common monocular eye disorders in children leading to loss of vision. Approximately 2% to 5% of children in the United States experience this condition. Strabismus and anisometropia are the most prevalent forms of amblyopia in children. **Strabismus,** or crossed eye appearance, results in malalignment of the eyes. The child attempts to compensate for this unequal vision by preferentially choosing to use one eye and not the other eye. When the child focuses on an object, one eye wanders off of the focused object while the other eye looks straight ahead. The child then experiences two separate images instead of one and develops a stronger eye. The brain eventually suppresses central mission in the unused eye causing amblyopia.

Anisometropia is a condition in which the refractive power of the eyes is unequal (Venes, 2009). If the refractive errors are significantly different in one eye the child becomes dependent on the eye that is more easily focused, leading to an irreversible loss of vision potential (Simon & Kaw, 2001). Amblyopia can also result from excessive patching, ptosis, or cataracts. Amblyopia is treated with corrective lenses for up to 6 months or until improvement plateaus, then surgery is indicated (Holmes & Llarke, 2006).

The goal of amblyopia treatment is to improve visual acuity of the weaker eye and prevent permanent loss of vision or visual impairment. Occlusion therapy or patching of the normal eye is done to restore strength and function to the lazy eye (Fig. 29-10). Duration of occlusion therapy is widely debated. No clear evidence exists. Patching for as little as 1 to 2 hours per day may be as effective as patching the entire day (Allison, 2005).

Child and parental compliance with occlusion therapy is complicated and stressful for both. Children may experience a stigma with patching at school or at home, making the treatment more debilitating than the vision loss. Children are too young to appreciate the significance of the therapy and attempt to remove or hide the patches.

Figure 29-10 Occlusion therapy or patching of the normal eye is done to restore strength and function to the lazy eye.

Compliance is better if patching is disguised behind eyeglasses or if patching time is shortened.

Amblyopia is treatable if detected at an early age. Treatment should be initiated during the preschool years if possible (Watkinson & Graham, 2005). The success of amblyopic therapy diminishes after age 6. Correction after age 10 is very limited. It is recommended that preschoolers be screened for visual acuity using the Snellen E chart, and most schools comply.

 Optimizing Outcomes— Early vision screening

Early screening for all children at risk for amblyopia and aggressive prompt treatment will result in the best outcome and prevention of visual impairment.

Strabismus

Strabismus is a condition of nonparallelism in the different fields of gaze causing visual lines to cross even when focused on the same object. Weakened or misaligned extraocular muscles pull the eyes in different directions resulting in a cross eyed appearance. Strabismus occurs in 2% to 7% of children, affecting males and females equally, and has an inherited pattern in about half of the cases.

assessment tools   Strabismus

Three forms of strabismus describe the eye deviation noted on an exam:
- Esotropia: Eye turns toward the midline of the face or nose
- Exotropia: Eye turns away from the midline of the face
- Hypertropia: Eye turns toward the forehead or a downward turning

SIGNS AND SYMPTOMS. Intermittent esotropia is seen in normal children younger than 3 years of age when the child is tired, ill, or with a sudden change in light or distance. Persistent squinting, head tilting, clumsiness, or decreased visual acuity may also be assessed. Pseudostrabismus is an appearance of crossed eyes but is due to physical attributes such as prominent epicanthal folds and a flattened nasal bridge. Children outgrow this condition over time. True strabismus does not change without intervention and can lead to amblyopia and loss of vision.

DIAGNOSIS. Childhood screening is begun as early as 3 to 6 months of age. The corneal light reflex test and the cover test are performed to detect strabismus, the cover test being the most reliable. The cover test is more sensitive in that eye movement is noted in response to covering and uncovering the child's eye while focusing on an object. This test requires the child's cooperation. The cover test is performed by having the child focus on a toy or favorite object and covering one eye. If the uncovered eye moves, that eye was not fixated on the object and strabismus is suspected.

 assessment tools   Hirschberg Asymmetrical Corneal Light Reflex Test

The Hirschberg asymmetrical corneal light reflex test is performed by holding a pen light or flash light in front of the child's face. The light reflection is noted on the cornea in both eyes. Symmetrical placement on both eyes at the same time and in the same location on each eye is a negative corneal light reflex exam and indicates normal muscle alignment. A positive asymmetrical corneal light reflex test is when the light falls slightly medially to the center of the pupil on the iris. The presence of an asymmetrical corneal light reflex is a positive exam and is suggestive of strabismus. A cover test is then performed.

NURSING CARE. Early identification and recognition of all children suspected for strabismus is critical in order to prevent vision loss. Treatment involves ocular patching of the stronger eye in order to force the weaker eye to work independently and "exercise" to strengthen extraocular muscles. Occlusion therapy should be conducted under the care of a pediatric ophthalmologist. Patching is most successful if implemented before age 3 to 4 years. Glasses and pharmacotherapy may be used. *Oculinum botulinum* toxin (Botox) may also be used for treatment of strabismus in children. Botox can be used in conjunction or as an alternative to surgery. The toxin is injected into the extraocular muscle, causing misalignment and produces a temporary muscle shortening that results in a parallelism of vision. The Botox effects last for up to 3 months and repeat injections may be performed. Potential complications include retrobulbar hemorrhage, ocular needle penetration, and ptosis.

The nurse provides families and children with referral sources, support groups, information, and schooling. School-based screening programs are essential for early detection, identification, and initiation of treatment of strabismus-related eye disorders. The school nurse may also be involved when treatment is needed during school hours.

Color Blindness

Color blindness is an X-linked recessive inheritable color vision deficiency that causes loss of accurate color perception. Males are more affected (8%) than females (less than 0.5%). Color blindness may be selective, partial, or complete (all colors). Complete color blindness is rare and results in perception of only shades of gray. Color blindness is a deficiency of photosensitive pigments (red, green, blue, yellow) located in the cones of the retina. Color blindness is untreatable, nonprogressive, and nondebilitating.

Color blindness is detected using colored charts called the Ishihara Test plates (Fig. 29-11). Each chart is com-

posed of colored dots with a number located in the center of the plate in a different color, usually yellow, red, green, or brown. The child is asked to identify the number or the shape in the center of the chart. A child without a color vision deficiency sees the object clearly. A child with color blindness sees only the plate of dots without an image or the image is blurred and indistinct.

Children can learn to compensate for their color deficiency with support from family members, teachers, and friends. Some alterations in daily function may be affected but they can be compensated for with minor behavioral alterations. For instance, at a traffic signal the child will need to learn to identify the signal by order rather than by color. Assistance with clothing selection may be necessary as well as labeling the clothes. The nurse can provide reassurance to parents that color blindness does not lead to loss of vision.

Nystagmus

Nystagmus is a rapid irregular involuntary eye movement caused by a disorder of the central nervous system that may be congenital or acquired. There are many types of nystagmus. The eyes may rotate in a lateral direction, clockwise or counterclockwise direction, up and down, or any combination of these movements. Eye movement is repetitive and involuntary and in some cases can be managed by gaze redirection.

Congenital nystagmus is usually mild and nonprogressive and persists into adulthood. Brain injuries are the most common cause of acquired nystagmus. Any child who develops nystagmus early in life should be evaluated for an underlying central nervous system cause. If an identifiable cause is not clear, neuroimaging, such as an MRI, is warranted to rule out the possibility of a neoplasm. Prognosis is based on the etiologic cause. Extraocular surgery may correct some forms of congenital nystagmus. Acquired nystagmus treatments are based on the existing etiology (Watkinson & Graham, 2005).

Cataracts

A cataract is a clouding or a haziness of the corneal lens. Significant irreversible vision disorders are caused by cataracts. Cataracts can be located unilaterally in one eye or bilaterally in both eyes. Cataracts can be acquired or congenital resulting in partial or complete occlusion or both. Acquired cataracts can be caused by maternal infection acquired during pregnancy, trauma to the eye, radiation, or systemic diseases. Some cataracts are due to family inheritance patterns. Congenital cataracts are present in neonates with syndrome anomalies or mothers with TORCH (toxoplasmosis, rubella, cytomegalovirus, herpes simplex or HIV) infection during pregnancy. Congenital cataracts can be autosomal dominant in genetically linked families. However, X-linked and recessive genetic situations have been reported.

SIGNS AND SYMPTOMS. During an eye exam with an ophthalmoscope, a cataract is obvious to the examiner. The direct pupil check yields an abnormal or absent red reflex. Excessive tearing and extraocular movements may be seen. Strabismus is usually present. If a child has a cataract, the cover test is abnormal or of poor fixation quality. Photophobia is always present along with

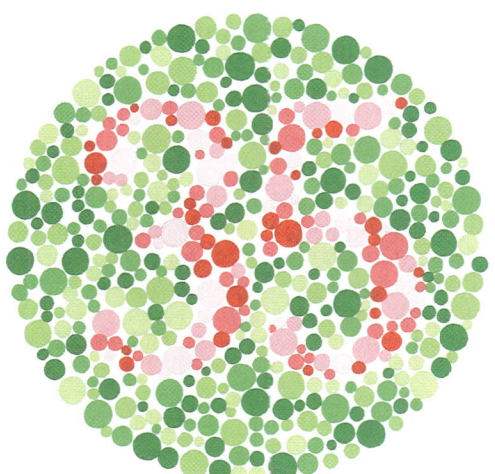

Figure 29-11 Color blindness is detected using colored charts called the Ishihara Test plates.

decreased visual acuity. The infant or child may appear inattentive or have abnormal eye movements that seem random and disorganized.

DIAGNOSIS. A pediatric ophthalmologist performs a complete eye examination. Diagnosis is made when the lens appears cloudy or there is a white or dulled red reflex.

NURSING CARE. Early detection and diagnosis of a congenital cataract prevents loss of visual acuity. Referral to a pediatric ophthalmologist is indicated. In most cases, a laser procedure is performed to remove the cataract and then a small incision is made to place the lens. The child who is undergoing a cataract removal is usually admitted to the outpatient surgery unit. Postoperative nursing care for the child includes monitoring nausea, emesis, pain, hemorrhage, and signs of infection. Keep the child free from wrenching, coughing, crying, and active play that can cause increased intraocular pressure. Postoperative eye drops include a steroid preparation to reduce inflammation and prevent adhesions. Mydriatic eye drops prevent adhesions of the pupils and topical antimicrobial eye solutions prevent infection.

Follow-up care of the child is based on loss of visual acuity. Some children need glasses for correction of refraction errors. Other children may need an antiglaucoma medication to prevent intraocular pressure development. Postoperative education for the family and child includes signs and symptoms of infection, hemorrhage, increased intraocular pressure, and activity restrictions until cleared by the physician. If amblyopia is evident, the unoperated eye is patched in order to force the operative eye to "exercise," which strengthens the extraocular muscles.

Glaucoma

Glaucoma is an increase of the intraocular pressure (IOP) in the eye due to an obstruction or impaired outflow of aqueous humor (clear fluid) that leads to retinal damage and eventual necrosis of the optic nerve. Optic nerve cupping is seen with ophthalmoscope examination. The eye enlarges due to increased IOP, causing a thinned cloudy appearing cornea. The sclera may appear bluish.

Glaucoma can be congenital or acquired. Some cases of pediatric glaucoma are due to eye trauma or from surgical procedures. Congenital or infantile glaucoma is a rare condition presenting with corneal opacification (or clouding), corneal enlargement, and eye pain. Another rare type of congenital glaucoma is when the iridocorneal (the junction of the iris and the cornea) angle of the eye at the Canal of Schlemm causes an obstruction of outflow of aqueous humor from the eye. This condition appears in the first year of life and if left untreated results in blindness.

SIGNS AND SYMPTOMS. Signs of infantile glaucoma include a triad of symptoms: buphthalmos (enlarged eye globe), epiphora (excessive tearing), and photophobia (sensitivity to light). There is also pain, excessive blinking due to the photophobia, and corneal cloudiness. Older infants experiencing light sensitivity turn away from the light, become irritable, and rub their eyes. Most infants have obvious signs of glaucoma by 4 to 5 months of age.

DIAGNOSIS. A complete eye examination is performed by a pediatric ophthalmologist. Tonometry (measurement of tension) is used to evaluate intraocular pressure. Prior to the procedure, the child is pre-medicated with a topical anesthetic in order to obtain a reliable measure. Early surgical intervention is done to remove obstructions and allow the flow of aqueous humor into the Canal of Schlemm. Rapid intervention reduces the risk of option disk necrosis and retinal ischemia.

NURSING CARE. The nurse provides pre- and postoperative family-centered care and education. Prior to surgery the nurse prevents intraocular pressure increase by maintaining a quiet, calm environment with dim lighting. Antiglaucoma medications provide temporary relief of IOP. Analgesia is given for pain as well as using anxiety reduction strategies such as distraction, massage, music, and parental presence. Favorite toys, pacifiers, and blankets are used to comfort the child. Preoperative care includes parental teaching about the condition. In the postoperative period, the nurse teaches the parents about eye dressings, medications, signs and symptoms of infection, and increased IOP, activity limitations, and follow-up care.

Retinoblastoma

Retinoblastoma is a malignant tumor of the retina seen only in children. It is a rare condition, accounting for fewer than 3% of the cases of childhood cancers. This tumor can spread to the optic nerve and invade the brain, lymph nodes, facial bones, and bone marrow.

SIGNS AND SYMPTOMS. In retinoblastoma a whitish or yellow color of the pupil called leukocoria or cat's eye reflex is noted instead of the usual red reflex. Late manifestations include visual acuity disturbances, pain, inflammation, and hyphema (blood in the anterior chamber of the eye) (Venes, 2009).

DIAGNOSIS. Diagnosis is made when either the absence or abnormality of the red reflex is noted by the examiner.

NURSING CARE. Treatment is based on unilateral or bilateral presentation and degree of cancer infiltration. Because this tumor is a rapidly progressing cancer, early detection, laser, radiation or cryotherapy (use of ice compresses), or enucleation (removal of the eye) is necessary for survival. If the eye is saved and vision is still present but altered by the tumor, other therapies such as radiation are used to shrink the tumor. Systemic chemotherapy is used to treat metastases. Once the tumor invades other organs the success of treatment is diminished.

EYE INJURIES

Foreign Bodies

When a child has a foreign body penetrating the eye, careful history of the injury and assessment dictate immediate action. An intraocular penetration injury or laceration (tear) to the corneal or eye globe requires an immediate transport to the local emergency room. An eye shield is used to prevent further trauma and all bleeding should be controlled before transport.

In foreign body penetration, vision loss is prevented by timely prompt medical treatment. The triage nurse must be able to recognize an emergent situation from a nonemergent injury. If a foreign body is visualized in the conjunctival sac, a physician can carefully remove the object using a cotton-tipped applicator or warmed normal saline irrigation. Glass particles are removed carefully using a with warm normal saline. Foreign bodies need to be removed meticulously to avoid a corneal abrasion.

Corneal Abrasion

Corneal abrasion is a nonpenetrating injury to the cornea. Common objects that cause an abrasion include contact lens, human fingers, animal nails, sticks, flying objects, pens, pencils, and glass. Corneal abrasions are painful. Treatment is necessary if purulent eye drainage is present. Medications include topical antibiotic solutions or ointments if infection is suspected. Administer analgesics for pain. An eye patch is placed to prevent the child from rubbing or scratching the eye causing further irritation and potential self-inoculation of bacteria. An ophthalmologist should reexamine in 1 to 2 days.

Hyphema

Hyphema is a hemorrhage into the anterior chamber of the eye. The eye requires rest and possible evacuation of the bleeding. Evacuation prevents globe rupture due to increased intraocular pressure (IOP). The child is hospitalized to monitor the IOP and to promote decreased activity. The head of bed is raised to 30 degrees and the room is kept dimly lit with minimal activity. Both eyes are patched to prevent excessive ocular movement and increased intraocular pressure.

Chemical Burns

Chemical burns to the eye are treated with rapid eye flushing for 15 to 30 minutes followed by pH analysis of the chemical agent. Eye patching and referral to an emergency room or an ophthalmologist is essential to evaluate for further treatment.

critical nursing action Chemical Burns

Nursing care of the patient with a chemical burn requires prompt assessment. The nurse assesses the injury and monitors the patient for signs of infection, hemorrhage, and increased IOP. Provide emotional and social support for the child and family. The nurse stresses the importance of follow-up care that involves evaluation of the cornea for scarring and IOP testing to determine post inflammatory response. Instruct the family that patching and eye medication may be required at home. School and normal activities are allowed after physician consultation.

HEARING LOSS

Hearing loss is diagnosed in approximately 12,000 children per year, resulting in speech and language difficulties, social and developmental delays, and slowed academic progress with psychological and occupational difficulties. Hearing loss can be caused by several factors. Approximately one third of all cases are due to genetic causes, one third of all cases are due to nongenetic influences, and one third of all cases are of unknown causes. Causes of nongenetic acquired hearing loss are seen in conditions such as meningitis and maternal TORCH infections during pregnancy, with cytomegalovirus being the most common. Prevention of hearing loss is important for children of all ages. Hearing loss is prevented by reducing noise levels to less than 50 dB.

A middle ear infection, otitis media, is associated with allergies and causes hearing loss in children. Seventy-five percent of children experience at least one ear infection before the age of three. Hearing loss affects approximately 17 children in 1000 under age 18 years of age. Two to three children per 1000 are born with hearing abnormalities. Of these children, 90% are born to parents who can hear (National Institute on Deafness and other Communication Disorders, 2007).

Hearing loss may be caused by conduction abnormalities associated with structural anomalies of the inner and outer ear or sensory neural hearing loss due to central nervous dysfunction. Central nervous dysfunction includes damage to the cerebral cortex, brainstem, or cranial nerve VIII. Hearing loss is also seen with severe neurological insult from trauma, anoxia, infections, or malformations.

A hearing disorder can involve a combination of both conductive and sensory-neural abnormalities. Sensory-neural hearing loss is a common sequelae of bacterial meningitis affecting approximately 10% of these children with bacterial meningitis. Rapid identification and prompt treatment can prevent post meningitis hearing loss (Klutz, Simon, Chennupati, Giannoni, & Manolidis, 2006).

SIGNS AND SYMPTOMS. Hearing loss is quantified in terms of severity and degree of functional disability and may be unilateral or bilateral (Table 29-8). Detection of hearing loss in children requires a high index of suspicion if noted developmental milestones are not observed. Any child suspicious for a hearing loss should receive a prompt referral to an audiologist. Maternal reports of infant hearing concerns should be immediately investigated and treated in order to prevent long-term consequences.

 Nursing Insight— *Risk factors*

Critical risk factors for hearing loss in neonates also include extracorporeal membrane oxygenation (ECMO), systemically administered ototoxic medications, phototherapy, and severe hypoxic ischemic encephalopathy post resuscitation or asphyxia.

Table 29-8 Classification of Hearing Loss

Level of Hearing Loss	Range	Description
Normal	0 dB–15 dB	No impairment. Able to hear all speech sounds
Slight	16 dB–25 dB	Vowel sounds are heard clearly may miss some consonant sounds
Mild	26 dB–40 dB	Hears some speech
Moderate	41 dB–55 dB	No speech heard
Moderate/severe	56 dB–70 dB	No speech heard
Severe	70 dB–90 dB	No speech heard and no other sounds heard
Profound loss	91+dB or more	No speech and no other sounds heard

Source: American Speech-Language-Hearing Association (2007).

DIAGNOSIS. Early detection and intervention for children with hearing loss has been recommended by the Joint Committee on Infant Hearing. Universal infant hearing screening before 1 month of age is recommended. Newborn readiness for discharge includes a hearing screening evaluation. If newborn hearing loss is suspected, a more extensive audiological evaluation is recommended by 3 months of age. Treatment for the hearing loss should begin by 6 months of age (Joint Committee on Infant Hearing, 2000; Walter et al., 2000). Hearing loss is determined by analyses of many kinds of hearing tests performed by a licensed audiologist.

 diagnostic tools Audiologic Testing

Audiologic testing may include one or several procedures:

The otoacoustic emissions test (OAE) or an auditory brainstem evoked response (ABER) performed by a licensed, certified audiologist further defines the degree of hearing loss. This is a very reliable test that measures acoustic responses produced by the inner ear and cochlear function. A small probe is placed in the outer ear canal and senses sounds that are reflected or echoed back out of the ear. This bounced back sound is the otoacoustic emission that may spontaneously occur or be evoked.

The automated auditory brainstem evoked response (AABER), or the ABER, records electrical activity in response to auditory stimuli received from electrodes placed on the scalp. The electrical impulse reflects cochlear, auditory brainstem and cranial nerve VIII vibration pathways. The AABER places a series of clicking sounds through ear phones placed over the infant's or child's ears. The sounds are then converted to waveforms and detected as electrical activity by the scalp sensors. The strength of the stimulus level is in the normal voice and hearing range of 35–50 dB. The AABER is useful for screening newborns with congenital hearing loss or postneonatal intensive care therapies such as mechanical ventilation.

Audiography can be performed in children older than 3 years of age who are able to cooperate and follow directions. This test requires the child to raise his hand in response to normal hearing tones. The screening is performed under the supervision of a clinically competent audiologist, speech pathologist, or appropriately supervised personnel (American Speech-Language-Hearing Association, 2007).

A routine otoscopic examination is also performed by a health care provider to evaluate the presence of a middle ear effusion or otitis media (Fig. 29-12). Part of the otoscopic examination also involves the use of the pneumoscope to assess for tympanic membrane mobility.

If the hearing loss continues to be suspected, a **tympanogram** (radiographic examination of the eustachian tubes and middle ear after introduction of a contrast medium) may be completed (Venes, 2009). The tympanogram evaluates the tympanic membrane (TM) compliance to air pressure. An ear-tight probe containing a small speaker, microphone, and air pump is placed into the external auditory canal. The probe then determines the flexibility of the TM in response to positive and negative pressure levels. The normal result is a mountain peak plotted on a graph depicting the positive and negative pressure levels. A flat or absent mountain peak suggests a conductive hearing loss due to obstruction.

NURSING CARE. Appropriate treatment for the hearing loss is based on underlying pathological conditions, presence of organic diseases, the severity of the hearing loss, the degree of frequency loss, and any CNS abnormalities.

Figure 29-12 A routine otoscopic examination of the child is also performed by a health care provider to evaluate the presence of a middle ear effusion or otitis media.

Ear infections are treated with appropriate antimicrobial therapy with close follow-up to monitor for the hearing loss or language delays as well as to monitor response to therapy. Children who have chronic ear infections may have surgery to restore inner ear function with myringotomy tubes placed in the tympanic membrane for effusion drainage and pressure equilibrium.

Simple conduction loss due to cerumen (ear wax) impaction can be treated with over-the-counter preparations, water irrigations and foreign body removal. Stapedectomy (excision of the stapes to improve the hearing) and tympanoplasty (restores function to the sound-transmitting mechanism of the middle ear) have been shown to be effective in restoring the hearing for conduction disorders. Severe to profound hearing loss is treated using cochlear implants that provide sound awareness and support speech development. Cochlear implants carry a risk of meningitis.

Amplification aids (hearing aids) are small microphones that amplify sounds. Amplification devices are fitted to infants as young as 4 weeks old. Most children with mild to moderate hearing loss require some form of amplification. The amplification frequency and ranges are predetermined.

The amplification device is placed in the child's ear, turned on, and then the volume of amplification is adjusted to the child's comfort level. In preverbal children nonverbal cues of irritability such as crying, restlessness, or agitation may signal the need to adjust the volume. Care and maintenance of the hearing aid involve keeping the unit clean and dry with a dry cloth, avoiding water immersion and replacing batteries frequently. Background noise can be distracting to infants wearing a hearing aid. Hearing aids can be removed while sleeping. High-pitched sounds called acoustic feedback can also be disrupting. This sound may not be realized by the hearing-impaired child but can be easily remedied by turning the volume down on the hearing aid, removing the aid, and inspecting the ear for cerumen impaction, cleaning the device or securing proper installation in the external ear canal.

Nurses provide emotional, educational, and collaborative support for the child with a hearing loss and his family. Sign language services may be required as well as visual aids that support nonverbal communication and lip reading. The family needs to investigate home safety measures that protect the hearing-impaired child from inadvertent injury. Supervision may be required at all times. Other assistive communication techniques that may be used include lip reading, finger spelling, and cuing. The family can use cued speech, a visual communication system that uses hand and mouth shapes along with gestures to cue a sound or a consonant. This serves as a supplement to lip reading and sign language. Adolescents should be encouraged to turn down radios, stereos, personal music devices such as iPods, MP3 players, and cell phones in order to prevent the hearing loss.

 Be sure to — **Follow rules set forth in the Individuals with Disability Education Act of 2004**

Children identified with a hearing loss should begin school at an early age in order to prevent early developmental delays in speech and language development. All levels of education should have hearing conservation and loss prevention curricula. The school nurse plays a pivotal role in initiating and monitoring these programs (Folmer, 2003). Early intervention services are implemented in the family using a multi-tiered approach. The Individuals with Disability Education Act of 2004 (IDEA) (http://idea.ed.gov/) ensures that children older than 3 years receive assistive services throughout the school years up to age 21.

The hearing-impaired child needs support services in school and elsewhere to communicate and learn. Early recognition, prevention, treatment, and support services combined with healthy family and individual coping ensures optimal growth and development for the child with a hearing disorder. The hearing-impaired children can have the same cognitive ability as children who have no hearing loss. Hearing loss accounts for most language delays seen in children.

 Nursing Insight— *Communicating with the hearing impaired child*

- Recognize behavioral cues suggestive of hearing loss.
- Obtain the child's attention before speaking.
- Face the child when talking.
- Position yourself at the child's eye level.
- Talk slowly and loudly.
- Modify the environment; unnecessary noises should be reduced.
- Offer emotional support: a child with a hearing loss may face a potential stigma associated with their communication difficulty.

Language Disorders

Communication is a process of complex interaction involving the exchange of information, feelings, ideas, and interactions. Verbal speech together with a language framework provides the basic component of communication. Nonverbal gestures, tones and body movements provide as much if not more communication than words. Language development is a process of giving and receiving of information and processing and organization of meaning in order to exchange information, thoughts and feelings. The ability to understand what is said is receptive language. The ability to clearly speak to other is expressive language. Speech impairment is an inability to make voice sounds or produce quality sounds; children may experience any combination of hearing speech and/or language disorders.

Children understand more than they can express at a very early age as language is learned last. The majority of a child's speech should be clearly understood by 3 to 4 years of age. Most communication skills are learned by age 5. Approximately 5% of all children have a language disorder.

 Nursing Insight— *A language quick reference tool*

The child's language should be understood

- 50% of the time by age 2 years
- 75% by age 3 years
- 100% by age 4 years
- There may be something wrong if the child is not talking appropriately for his age.
- Sentences should be as long as their age.

Jacobsen, C. (2007). Director Hearing and Speech Clinic, Children's Mercy Hospital, Kansas City, MO. Personal communication January 17, 2007.

SIGNS AND SYMPTOMS. Language disorders can be related to physical, emotional, environmental, social, neurological and/or cognitive influences or any combination of these. For some children, delayed competency of language milestones persist into the school age years and slows academic achievement (Dale, Price, Bishop, & Plasmin, 2003). Hearing, cognition, and oral motor ability must be present for language to develop.

DIAGNOSIS. Early detection and intervention for young children with a language disorder prevents many forms of delay in child development. A communication disorder is considered delayed when the child is not meeting predictable developmental sequencing for their age.

NURSING CARE. Speech and language difficulties have been positively correlated with occupational and academic success as well as personal, social, and emotional health.

The nurse is in a key position to recognize speech and language developmental delays. Knowledge about development milestones assist the nurse in recognizing children who are at risk or experiencing a difficulty. The overall nursing goal of early recognition is to prevent a communication, language, and literacy delay that significantly impacts the child at an early age and potentially for life.

 nursing diagnoses Language Disorders

- Social Isolation related to inability to communicate, decreased level of consciousness and/or hospitalization
- Impaired Verbal Communication related to articulation difficulties or environmental deprivation
- Parental Knowledge Deficit related to lack of understanding of normal language development

Family Teaching Guidelines
Language Disorder

How To: Tell family that a language disorder is an impairment in the child's ability to understand or use words correctly, an ability to express one's self, follow directions, understand words, or any combination of these conditions

ESSENTIAL INFORMATION

◆ Help the child learn how to say speech sounds correctly.

◆ Help the child improve language comprehension such as increasing their vocabulary.

◆ Help the child with conversational and story-telling skills.

◆ Help the child and family understand the disorders may impact the child's educational and social interactions.

◆ Advise the family about how to find a speech pathologist in the community; schools, rehabilitation, community and private clinics and home services may be utilized to meet the child's needs (American Speech-Language-Hearing Association, 2007).

summary points

◆ Unconsciousness is a state where there is a depression of a child's cerebral function. Unconsciousness ranges from a stupor (only aroused with vigorous or unpleasant stimulation) to a coma (state of unconsciousness when the child cannot be aroused).

◆ A persistent vegetative state is a complete unawareness of the environment accompanied by sleepwake cycles. The primary causes of a persistent vegetative state are developmental malformations, metabolic and degenerative disorders affecting the nervous system and acute traumatic and non-traumatic brain injuries.

◆ The pediatric patient may experience minor or major complications with increased intracranial pressure (ICP).

◆ Increased ICP can be fatal if not treated because of the effect of edema on the brain.

◆ A seizure is caused by an imbalance in the normal inhibition and excitement of neural tissue. Seizure activity is classified according to the area of the brain experiencing the abnormal electrical activity and the neuromuscular sensory and psychogenic alteration from the electrical conduction disturbance.

◆ Encephalitis is usually viral in origin and occurs with an acute febrile illness characterized by cerebral edema and infection of surrounding meninges. Signs and symptoms of encephalitis include disorientation, confusion, headache, high fever, photophobia, lethargy, aphasia, hallucinations, seizures, nuchal rigidity and coma.

◆ The child with Reye syndrome will normally be a previously healthy child and is usually recovering from a recent viral infection such as varicella (chickenpox), influenzae B, gastroenteritis or an upper respiratory infection. The child may progress through all of the stages of Reye syndrome or may stop at any stage if treatment is effective.

◆ Guillain-Barré syndrome (GBS) is a rare self-limiting disease characterized by clinical manifestations of ascending muscle weakness and/or paralysis.

◆ There are two categories of hydrocephalus. Communicating hydrocephalus occurs when there is full communication between the subarachnoid space and ventricles. Noncommunicating hydrocephalus occurs when CSF flow within the ventricular system or the ventricular outlets to the arachnoid space is prevented. Most cases of hydrocephalus are obstructive.

◆ Cerebral palsy is a nonprogressive neurological disorder that results from brain injury occurring before cerebral development is complete.

◆ When caring for a patient admitted with near drowning, a priority nursing responsibility is assessing and maintaining the airway.

◆ The primary causes of pediatric traumatic brain injuries are motor vehicular crashes, bicycle accidents, sports trauma, violence, and falls.

◆ The priorities of trauma care for a child with a spinal cord injury are initiated with primary attention to airway management, breathing and/or ventilatory support, circulation support, disability identification and exposure of known and unknown physical limitations.

◆ Headaches can occur in 90% of children. However, most causes of a childhood headache are based on a simple etiology such as minor trauma, emotions, genetic predisposition, illness, environmental factors or even food and beverages.

◆ Children may experience a myriad of common eye disorders, which may present as an abrupt change or changes in vision function; eye function may never be identified unless screened for by health care professionals.

◆ Hearing loss is diagnosed in approximately 12,000 children per year, resulting in speech and language difficulties, social and developmental delays and slowed academic progress with psychological and occupational difficulties.

◆ Early detection and intervention for young children with a language disorder prevents many forms of delay in child development.

review questions

Multiple Choice

1. The pediatric nurse is offering a health prevention lecture to the community. Included in the teaching should be:
   A. The use of DEET (*N,N*-diethyl-*meta*-toluamide) containing products is contraindicated in school-age children.
   B. Avoiding areas infested with mosquitoes can be helpful in preventing encephalitis.
   C. The incidence of Reye syndrome has increased due to the use of acetaminophen (Tylenol).
   D. The *Varicella* vaccine should not be given to children with arthritis or Kawasaki disease.

2. A 3-year-old with a history of hydrocephalus has recently undergone a ventriculo-peritoneal shunt insertion. The pediatric nurse is aware that postoperative care should include:
   A. Assessing for signs of complications such as infection and neurological function.
   B. Maintaining the head of the bed at a 90-degree angle to facilitate drainage.
   C. Encouraging the patient to lie on the operative site to decrease pressure.
   D. Encouraging the patient to lie flat in bed for the first 24 to 48 hours.

3. A 12-month-old, who was born at 28 weeks of gestation, is admitted for a neurological work-up. While obtaining the nursing history, the nurse assesses that the infant has stiff muscles, poor control of posture, coordinated movement, and balance. The nurse suspects that he has (*Select All that Apply*)
   A. Spina bifida
   B. A seizure disorder
   C. Hydrocephalus
   D. Cerebral palsy

4. The pediatric nurse is admitting a child with a history of seizure activity. The nurse is aware that seizure precautions must be assembled at the bedside, which includes:
   A. A ventilator machine
   B. Suction equipment
   C. A padded tongue blade
   D. Intubation equipment

Select All that Apply

5. A child is admitted to the intensive care unit following a motor vehicle accident. The pediatric nurse utilizes the Pediatric Glasgow Coma Scale to evaluate the child's neurological status. Which assessments does this scale include?
   A. Verbal response
   B. Vital signs
   C. Eye opening
   D. Motor response

6. A child with a history of recurrent episodes of ear infections has suffered hearing loss. The pediatric nurse is aware that children with hearing loss may also suffer from which of the following?
   A. Language difficulties
   B. Visual disturbances
   C. Social delays
   D. Developmental delays

True /False

7. The pediatric nurse is aware that the unconscious child with a neck injury may have respiratory involvement. The nurse should use caution when suctioning this child in order to prevent a rise in intracranial pressure.

8. Infants whose fontanels have closed are able to compensate for increased intracranial pressure for a longer time period than infants with open fontanels.

9. A 16-year-old is being discharged after a 4-month hospitalization due to a spinal cord injury. Included in the discharge teaching instructions to the parents, the pediatric nurse stresses that the parents should monitor the adolescent for signs of depression and feelings of isolation.

10. The use of prolonged video gaming has been found to be a high risk precipitating factor for seizures in children.

Fill-in-the–Blank

11. When a pediatric nurse is performing a neurological assessment of a child, the assessment must be tailored to the child's _____ and _____ _____.

12. _____ - _____ syndrome is the most common form of acquired acute paralysis in children.

See Answers to End of Chapter Review Questions on the Electronic Study Guide or DavisPlus.

REFERENCES

American Optometric Association. Retrieved from http://www.aoa.org/x4688.xml (Accessed January 13, 2007).

American Speech-Language-Hearing Association. Retrieved from www.asha.org/public/hearing/disorders/type.htm (Accessed January 13, 2007).

Aschenbrenner, D.S. (2006). Meningococcal vaccine and Guillain-Barre syndrome. *American Journal of Nursing, 103*(1), 34.

Ashwal, S. (2004). Pediatric vegetative state: Epidemiological and clinical issues. *NeuroRehabilitation, 19,* 349–360.

Bader, M.K., & Littlejohns, L.R. (eds.) (2004). *AANN core curriculum for neuroscience in Nursing* (4th ed.). St. Louis, MO: W.B. Saunders.

Balottin, U., Termine, C., Nicoli, F., Quadrelly, M., Ferrari-Ginevra, O., & Lanzai, G. (2005). Idiopathic headaches in children under six years of age: A follow-up study. *Headache, 45*(6), 705–715.

Behrman, R., Kleigman, R., & Jenson, H. (2004). *Nelson textbook of pediatrics* (16th ed.). Philadelphia: W.B. Saunders.

Benham, J., & Chavda, S.V. (2002). Head trauma. *Trauma, 6,* 101–110.

Bergsneider, M., & Kelly, D.F. (2003). Brain injury. In G.P. Naude, F.S. Bongard, & D. Demetriades (eds.), *Trauma secrets* (2nd ed., pp. 51–59). Philadelphia: Hanley & Belfus.

Bhutta, A., Savell, V., & Schexnayder, S. (2003). Reye's syndrome: Down but not out. *Southern Medical Journal, 96*(1), 43–45.

Bickley, L., & Szilagyi, P. (2003). *Bate's guide to physical examination and history taking* (8th ed.). Philadelphia: Lippincott Williams & Wilkins.

Bigal, M.E., Rapoport, A.M., Tepper, S.J., Sheftell, F.D., & Lipton, R.B. (2005). The classification of chronic daily headaches in adolescents—A comparison between the second edition of the international classification of headaches disorders and alternative diagnostic criteria. *Headache. Special Series: Headache Research Methodology 45*(5), 582–589.

Brettler, S. (2004). Trauma nursing: Traumatic brain injury. Retrieved from http://www.rnweb.com/rnweb/article/articleDetail.jsp?id=110100 (Accessed July 22, 2008).

Brook, I. (2004). Microbiology and management of brain abscess in children. *Journal of Pediatric Neurology, 2*(3), 125–130.

Brown, J. (2001). Orthopaedic care of children with Spina Bifida: You've come a long way, baby. *Orthopaedic Nursing, 20*(4), 51–58.

Bulechek, G., Butcher, H.M., & Dochterman, J. (2008). *Nursing interventions classification (NIC)* (5th ed.). St. Louis, MO: C.V. Mosby.

Centers for Disease Control and Prevention (2007). Meningococcal disease: Frequently asked questions. Retrieved from http://www.cdc.gov/ncidod/DBMD/diseaseinfo/meningococcal_g.htm (Accessed November 23, 2008).

Chiafery, M. (2006). Care and management of the child with shunted hydrocephalus. *Pediatric Nursing, 32*(3), 222–225.

Dale, P., Price, T., Bishop, D., & Plomin, R. (2003, June). Outcomes of early language delay: I. Predicting persistent and transient language difficulties at 3 and 4 years. *Journal of Speech, Language, and Hearing Research, 46*(3), 544–560. doi:10.1044/1092-4388(2003/044).

Dawodu, S.T. (2007). Spinal cord injury: Definition, epidemiology, pathophysiology. Retrieved from http://www.emedicine.com/pmr/topic182.htm (Accessed November 23, 2008).

Deglin, J., & Vallerand, A. (2009). *Davis's drug guide for nurses* (11th ed.). Philadelphia: F.A. Davis.

Dennis, L.J., & Mayer, S.A. (2001). Diagnosis and management of increased intracranial pressure. *Neurology India,* June. Retrieved from http://www.neurologyindia.com/oldsite/suppl-1/1508fl.shtml (Accessed February 3, 2007).

Eyemedlink.com. http://www.eyemdlink.com/EyeProcedure.asp?Eye ProcedureID=59 (Accessed November 23, 2008).

Fox, J.A. (2002). *Primary health care of infants, children and adolescents.* St. Louis, MO: C.V. Mosby.

Greenberg, M.S. (2001). *Handbook of neurosurgery* (5th ed.). New York: Thieme Medical Publishers.

Hamalainen, M.L. (2006). Migraines in children and adolescents: A guide to drug treatment therapy in practice. *CNS Drugs, 20*(10), 813–820.

Harrell, R.W. (2002). PureTone evaluation. In J. Katz (Ed.). *Handbook of clinical audiology* (5th ed., p. 82). Philadelphia: Lippincott/Williams & Wilkins.

Holmes, J.M., & Llarke, M.P. (2006). Amblyopia. *Lancet, 3647,* 1341–1351.

Hughes, R.A., & Cornblath, D.R. (2005). Guillain-Barré syndrome. *Lancet, 366,* 1653–1666.

Hulsebosch, C.E. (2002). Recent advances in pathophysiology and treatment of spinal cord injury. *Advances in Physiology Education, 26,* 238–255.

ICHD-II International classification of the headache disorders, 2nd ed. (2004). *Cephalalgia, 24* (S1), 1–22.

Individuals with Disability Education Act of 2004. Retrieved from http://idea.ed.gov (Accessed November 23, 2008).

Jacobsen, C. (2007). Director Hearing and Speech Clinic, Children's Mercy Hospital, KC, MO. Personal communication January 17, 2007.

Jafari, A., Malayeri, S., & Ashayeri, H. (2007). The ages of suspicion, diagnosis, amplification and intervention in deaf children. *International Journal of Pediatric Otorhinolaryngology, 71,* 35–40.

Johnson, M., Bulechek, G., Butcher, H., McCloskey Dochterman, J., Maas, M., Moorehead, S., & Swanson, E. (2006). *NANDA, NOC, and NIC linkages: Nursing diagnoses, outcomes, & interventions* (2nd ed.). St. Louis, MO: Mosby Elsevier.

Joint Committee on Infant Hearing Year 2000 position statement: Principles and guidelines for early detection and intervention program. *Pediatrics, 106*(4), 795–817.

Kemp, D.M. (2005). In Grose, C. (Ed). Q and A: Prophylaxis against rabies in children exposed to bats. *The Pediatric Infectious Disease Journal, 24*(12), 1109.

Klutz, J.Q., Simon, L.M., Chennupati, S.K., Giannoni, C.M., & Manolidis, S. (2006). Clinical predictors for hearing loss in children with bacterial meningitis. *Archives of Otolaryngology, Head and Neck Surgery, 132,* 941–945.

Krigger, K. (2006). Cerebral palsy: An overview. *American Academy of Family Physicians, 73*(1), 91–100.

Kuwabara, S. (2004). Guillain-Barre syndrome. *Drugs, 64*(6), 597–610.

LeJune, M., & Howard-Fain, T. (2002). Caring for patients with increased intracranial pressure. *Nursing, 32*(11), 1–5.

Lewis, D.W., Ashwal, S., Dahl, G., Dorgad, D., Hirtz, D., Prensky, A., et al. (2002). Practice parameter: Evaluation of children and adolescents with recurrent headaches: Report of the Quality Standards Subcommittee of the American Academy of Neurology and the Practice committee of Neurology Society. *Neurology, 59,* 490–498.

Lewis, S., Heitkemper, M., Dirksen, S., O'Brien, P., & Bucher, L. (2007). *Medical-surgical nursing: Assessment and management of clinical problems.* St. Louis, MO: Mosby Elsevier.

Lu, J.L., Sheikh, K.A., Wu, H.S., Zhang, J., Jiang, A., Cornblath, D.R., et al. (2000). Physiologic-pathologic correlation in Guillain-Barre syndrome in children. *Neurology, 54*(1), 33.

Marcoux, K. (2005). Management of increased intracranial pressure in the ill child with an acute neurological injury. *AACN Advanced Critical Care, 16*(2), 212–231. Retrieved from http://www.nursingcenter.com/library/JournalArticle.asp? Article_ID=594176 (Accessed November 23, 2008).

Mayoclinic.com. (2008). Retrieved from http://www.mayoclinic.com/health/headaches/HE99999. (Accessed July 22, 2008).

McCance, K., & Huether, S. (2002). *Pathophysiology: The biologic basis for disease in adults and children* (4th ed.). St. Louis: C.V. Mosby.

McLone, D.G. (Ed.). (2001). *Pediatric neurosurgery* (4th ed.). New York: W.B. Saunders.

Moore, A.J., & Shevell, M. (2004). Chronic daily headaches in pediatric neurology practice. *Journal of Child Neurology, 19*(12), 925–929.

Moorehead, S., Johnson, M., Maas, M., & Swanson, E. (2008). *Nursing outcomes classification (NOC)* (4th ed.). St. Louis, MO: C.V. Mosby.

NANDA International (2007). *NANDA-I nursing diagnoses: Definitions and classifications 2007–2008.* Philadelphia: NANDA-I.

National Association of Neonatal Nurses. (2003). Retrieved from http://www.nann.org/ (Accessed November 23, 2008).

National Center for Injury Prevention and Control. (2008). What is traumatic brain injury. Retrieved from http://www.cdc.gov/ncipc/tbi/TBI.htm (Accessed November 23, 2008).

National Institute on Deafness and other Communication Disorders. Statistics about hearing, balance, ear infections, and deafness. Retrieved from www.nidcd.nih.gov/health/statistics/hearing.asa. (Accessed November 23, 2008).

National Reye Syndrome Foundation (2008). Retrieved from http://www.reyessyndrome.org/ (Accessed November 23, 2008).

O'Dell, C., Shinnar, S., Ballaban-Gil, K., Nornick, M., Sigalova, M., Kang, H., et al. (2005). Rectal diazepam gel in the home management of seizures in children. *Pediatric Neurology, 33,* 166–172.

Orlowski, J.P., & Szpilman, D. (2001). Drowning: Rescue, resuscitation, and reanimation. *Pediatric Clinics of North America, 48*(3), 627–646.

Richardson, B. (2006). *Practice guidelines for pediatric nurse practitioners.* St. Louis, MO: Elsevier-Mosby.

Robertson, J., & Shilkofski, N. (2005). *The Harriet Lane handbook* (17th ed.). Philadelphia: Elsevier/Mosby.

Ross, J. (2005). Summer injuries: Near drowning. Retrieved from RNweb at http://www.rnweb.com/rnweb/article/articleDetail.jsp?id=168160 (Accessed December 4, 2006).

Sankar, C., & Mundkur, N. (2005). Cerebral Palsy-Definition, Classification, Etiology and Early Diagnosis. *Indian Journal of Pediatrics, 72*(10), 865–868.

Saper, J.R., & Silberstein, S. (2006). Pharmacology of dihydroergotamine and evidence for efficacy and safety in migraine. *Headache.* 46(Supplement 4), S171–S181.

Schessl, J., Luther, B., Kirshner, T., Mauff, G., & Korinthenberg, R. (2004). Infections and vaccination preceding childhood Guillain-Barré syndrome: a prospective study. *European Journal of Pediatrics, 1265,* 605–612.

Shaikh, S., & Ta, C.N. (2002). Evaluation and management of herpes zoster ophthalmicus. *American Family Physician, 66*(1), 1723–1730, 1732.

Silberstein, S.D., Olesen, J., Bousser, M.G., Diener, H.C., Dodick, D., First, M., Goadsby, P.J., Göbel, H., Lainez, M.J., Lance, J.W., Lipton, R.B., Nappi, G., Sakai, F., Schoenen, J., & Steiner, T.J. (2005). *The International Classification of Headache Disorders* (2nd ed., ICHD-II)—revision of criteria for 8.2 Medication-overuse headache. *Cephalalgia, 25*(6), 460–465.

Simon, J.W., & Kaw, P. (2001). Commonly missed diagnoses in the childhood eye examination. *American Family Physician, 62*(4), 623–628.

Sladky, J.T. (2004). Guillain-Barré syndrome in children. *Journal of Child Neurology, 19*(3), 191–200.

Smeltzer, S., Bare, B., Hinkle, J., & Cheever, K. (2008). *Brunner & Suddarth's Textbook of Medical-Surgical Nursing* (11th ed.). Philadelphia: Lippincott Williams & Wilkins.

Smith, J. (2003). Shaken baby syndrome. *Orthopaedic Nursing, 22*(3), 196–203.

Spyros, S. (2004). Management of spina bifida, hydrocephalus and shunts. Retrieved from http://www.emedicine.com/ped/topic2976.htm (Accessed November 17, 2006).

U.S. Food and Drug Administration (2007). *Lasik Eye Surgery.* Retrieved from http://www.fda.gov/CDRH/LASIK/ (Accessed July 22, 2008).

van Doorn, P.A. (2005). Treatment of Guillain-Barré syndrome and CIDP. *Journal of the Peripheral Nervous System: JPNS, 10*(2), 113–127.

Venes, D. (Ed.). (2009). *Tabers cyclopedic medical dictionary* (21st ed.). Philadelphia: F. A. Davis.

Verive, M. (2006). Near drowning. Retrieved from www.emedicine.com/ped/topic/2570.htm (Accessed November 23, 2008).

Walter, W.C., Cunningham, G.C., Davis, J.G., Morton, C.C., Elsas, L J., Finitzo, T., et al. (2000). Statement of the American College of Medical Genetics on Universal Newborn Hearing Screening. *Genetics in Medicine, 2,* 145–150.

Watkinson, S., & Graham, S. (2005). Visual impairment in children. *Nursing Standard, 19,* 51, 58–65.

Wisniewski, A. (2003). Closing in on clues to encephalitis. *Nursing, 33*(4), 70–71.

Woodham, A., & Peters, D. (2006). Healing massage. *Saturday Evening Post,* May/June, 2006.

CONCEPT MAP

Caring for the Child with a Neurological or Sensory Condition

Ethnocultural Considerations:
- Child of Asian heritage will have smaller head circumference

Neurological Injuries
- Near drowning
- Head injury
- Shaken baby syndrome
- Spinal cord injury

Non-traumatic Conditions
- Headaches

Developmental Conditions
- Spina Bifida
- Hydrocephalus
- Cerebral Palsy

Altered States of Consciousness
- Unconscious child
- Persistent Vegetative state
- Increased intracranial pressure
- Seizures

Inflammatory Conditions
- Meningitis
- Encephalitis
- Brain abcess
- Reye's Syndrome
- GBS

Sensory:
Eye disorders
- Refractive; astigmatism; amblyopia; strabismus color blindness; nystagmus; cataracts; glaucoma: retinoblastoma; eye injuries

Ear
- Hearing loss; language

General Nursing Care
- Airway management: adequate oxygenation; ventilatory support; prevent aspiration
- Neurological assessment: LOC; Glasgow; motor function; cognitive and functional ability; bowel/bladder function; assess/monitor for ICP
- Assess: Vital signs; fluid/electrolyte balance; lab results; signs/symptoms of condition complications
- Hydration: based on age, weight and illness: Tend to nutrition: possible enteral feeding
- Maintain temperature
- Maintain mobility: positioning; exercise; ROM
- Manage pharmacotherapy as ordered
- Safety: Seizure precautions/management; prevent injury; immobilization of spinal cord injury; care with head elevation
- Provide hygiene; comfort care; supportive measures; emotional support for child/family

Prevention strategies
- Kill vectors/identify organisms
- No ASA for children
- Control environmental factors associated with neural tube defects
- Encourage: helmet use; swimming safety; educate re: decrease in risk behaviors

Nursing Insight:
- Coma scale uses numeric values for LOC
- Infant skull can compensate for ICP
- Cushing's triad indicates brain herniation
- No hypotonic fluids in ICP
- Dilantin causes gingival hyperplasia
- Reye's syndrome has 4 stages
- Ventricular shunts drain excess CSF
- Shaken baby syndrome: hallmarks = external trauma with brain/eye bleed
- Autonomic dysreflexia is emergent
- Children can have febrile seizures
- Triad of symptoms for infant glaucoma
- 2 types of meningitis; SIADH can occur
- ECMO, oxytoxics, hypoxia = some risks for infant hearing loss

Be Sure To:
- Report suspected child abuse
- Provide services listed in IDEA for child with hearing loss

Complementary Care:
- Massage has many benefits: e.g.: decreases pain, anxiety, increases mobility, flexibility; stimulate circulation

Critical Nursing Action:
- Maintain elevation of head 30 degrees in ICP
- Monitor for bleeding post liver bx.
- Prevent injury to "sac" of spina bifida; no rectal temps
- No venous access in scalp veins in child with shunt
- Basilar skull fracture: no NG
- Child with chemical burns to eye needs prompt assessment

Collaboration In Caring:
- Need interdisciplinary approach in SCI
- Learn how to communicate with the hearing impaired child

Optimizing Outcomes:
- CPP should be 50–70 mm Hg. ICP < 20
- Screen early for amblyopia

Across Care Settings:
- Multiple potential deficits after encephalitis → multidisciplinary care
- Community education re: DEET
- Need community resources to deal with residual effects of Reye's

What To Say:
- Teach skills necessary to care for unconscious child at home
- No ASA to those under 19 y/o
- Educate parents re: lifelong care of child with hydrocephalus as well as growth and development issues

Clinical Alert:
- Components of seizure precautions
- Use cricoid pressure to prevent aspiration during intubation

Now Can You:
- Identify major neurological conditions that occur in children
- Discuss the nursing care of the child with a neurological condition
- Care for a child having: ICP, seizures

Caring for the Child with a Musculoskeletal Condition

 Our bodies are our gardens, to which our wills are gardeners

—William Shakespeare (1564–1616)

LEARNING TARGETS *At the completion of this chapter, the student will be able to:*

- Describe the major structural or functional anomalies of the musculoskeletal system.
- Describe the signs and symptoms for children with different musculoskeletal conditions.
- Explain diagnostic procedures for children with musculoskeletal conditions.
- Examine therapeutic communication techniques for children with musculoskeletal conditions.
- Apply the nursing process in caring for children with musculoskeletal conditions.
- Teach health promotion strategies to the family for children with musculoskeletal conditions.
- Identify community resources for the families with children who have musculoskeletal conditions.
- Apply teaching, learning principles in developing a plan for home care for children with musculoskeletal conditions.
- Identify common pharmacological treatments and side effects used in children with musculoskeletal conditions.
- Identify complementary therapies used for children with musculoskeletal conditions.
- Identify across care settings appropriate for children with musculoskeletal conditions.

---

 moving toward evidence-based practice Use of Calcium in Children with Juvenile Rheumatoid Arthritis

Stark, L.J., Davis, A.M., Janicke, D.M., Mackner, L.M., Hommel, K.A., Bean, J.A., Lovell, D., Heubi, J.E., & Kalkwarf, H.J. (2006). A randomized clinical trial of dietary calcium to improve bone accretion in children with juvenile rheumatoid arthritis. *The Journal of Pediatrics, 148,* 501–507.

The purpose of this study was to investigate the impact of behavioral intervention (BI) on the bone mass and maintenance of calcium intake at 6-month and 12-month periods in children diagnosed with juvenile rheumatoid arthritis (JRA).

Study participants were recruited from the outpatient rheumatology centers of three pediatric medical centers in the Midwest. The children who were selected ranged in age from 4 to 10 years. Children who were excluded: (1) had other conditions that affected growth, (2) had non-English speaking parents, (3) had used systemic corticosteroids within the previous 3 months, or (4) were taking calcium supplements. Of 194 eligible families, 49 families agreed to participate, met the criteria, and continued in the study until its completion.

The study design was a randomized trial that compared a group of children who received a six-session BI to a group of children who received a three-session Enhanced Standard of Care (ESC). Three-day diaries were kept to assess calcium intake. Dual energy x-ray absorptiometry (DEXA) was used to assess total bone mineral content (BMC), arm and leg BMC, and lumbar spine bone mineral density.

Separate but simultaneous baseline group sessions were held for both the BI and ESC participants. The meetings were held to instruct parents on how to record and keep a food diary. Fun activities and high-calcium snacks were provided for the children during the sessions.

(continued)

moving toward evidence-based practice (continued)

Intervention with both the ESC and BI groups was initiated with identical dietary counseling. Over an 8-week period, families in the ESC group attended three sessions; families in the BI group attended six sessions. The dietary goal of increasing calcium intake to 1500 mg/day was set for both the ESC and BI groups along with encouragement to consider achieving 400 mg at each meal and 300 mg at each snack time during the day.

Specific Group Interventions

Enhanced Standard of Care (ESC) group

Sessions for the ESC group included (1) a baseline assessment and training, (2) individual treatment session, and (3) individual posttreatment assessment and feedback. Information about optimal calcium intake and JRA was provided to parents and their children during the second session. Families received grafted feedback documenting their child's average calcium intake at each meal and a notebook with informational materials about foods high in calcium.

Behavioral Intervention (BI) group

Sessions for the BI group included (1) a baseline assessment and training, (2) four weekly treatment sessions, and (3) a posttreatment assessment during the 8th week. Information about nutrition and child behavior management strategies aimed at assisting the child in meeting daily calcium intake goals was provided.

Parents in the BI group were instructed:

- To avoid using consequences, coaxing, or commenting when the goals were not met.
- On the use of a technique termed "shaping" —the gradual introduction of a new food.

Children in the BI group received:

- Instruction about the importance of a high-calcium diet.
- A meal at each session with the goal of consuming their calcium goal for which a prize was earned.

Both groups were instructed to record food intake in a diet diary. They were also educated about behavioral management techniques such as praise and encouraged to place stickers on the child's meal chart when calcium goals were met. Calcium intake and bone mass were evaluated for both groups at 6 and 12 months after the treatment sessions.

Data Collection

Self-report questionnaires and charts were reviewed at baseline and at 12 months to compare the number and types of medications and the number of inflamed joints. Seven-day food records were reviewed in the food diaries at baseline, after treatment, and at the 6- and 12-month follow-up visits. Intake was evaluated by a dietician for daily calcium, calories, protein, carbohydrates, and fats.

Total body and lumbar spine bone mass was measured using a dual energy x-ray absorptiometer at baseline and at 6 and 12 months posttreatment. Each child's height, weight, and body-fat measurements were also taken at each of the three points of time. Vitamin D concentration was measured using a Dia Sorin 25-OH-D assay, also at baseline and 6 and 12 months posttreatment.

Results

- The groups were predominantly composed of female Caucasian children.
- The average age of the children in the ESC group was 6.8 years; in the BI group the average age was 6.1 years.
- The children in the ESC group maintained a baseline calcium intake of 1300 mg/day at both 6- and 12-month follow-up visits.
- The children in the BI group maintained an average calcium intake of 1500 mg/day at both the 6- and 12-month follow-up visits. This amount represented an increase from the 972 mg/day calculated at the baseline. The difference between groups was not significant.
- Total body bone mineral content gain of the BI group was 4% greater at the 6-month follow-up visit and 2.9% greater at the 12-month follow-up visit than the gains of the ESC group.
- The bone mineral content gain for arms and legs of the BI group was 7.1% greater at the 6-month follow-up visit and 5.3% greater at the 12-month follow-up visit than the gains of the ESC group.
- The children in the BI group grew an average of 2.91 inches (7.4 cm) between baseline and at the 12-month assessment, compared to 2.88 inches (7.3 cm) in the ESC group. This increase in growth was not significant.
- Children in the BI group gained an average of 8.14 lbs. (3.7 kg), compared to 7.7 lbs. (3.5 kg) for the ESC group. The increase in weight was not significant.
- The average serum 25-OH-D concentration did not vary between or within the groups at any assessment point.
- The study findings revealed that there was a greater total body bone mineral content increase in the children with an increased dietary calcium intake.
- The researchers concluded that use of BI is effective in increasing calcium intake in children with JRA over a 12-month period.

---

1. What might be considered as limitations to this study?
2. How is this information useful to clinical nursing practice?

See Suggested Responses for Moving Toward Evidence-Based Practice on the Electronic Study Guide or DavisPlus.

Introduction

Children are by nature very active and their musculo-skeletal system plays a major role in their growth and development. When their ability to interact with the environment is impaired, possibly through a musculoskeletal system disorder, they are at risk for impaired growth and development. Alterations in the musculoskeletal system may be related to a congenital defect such as muscular dystrophy, clubfoot, or osteogenesis imperfecta. Other alterations may be related to an acquired defect such as Legg–Calve–Perthes disease, slipped femoral capital epiphysis, fractures, soft tissue or sports injuries, Osgood–Schlatter disease, osteomyelitis, juvenile arthritis, scoliosis, tetanus, or osteoporosis.

This chapter discusses some of the more common alterations in mobility among children, the challenges they face, and the short-term and long-term goals. It also covers diagnostic analysis for the child with musculoskeletal conditions.

A & P review

Movement is made possible by the musculoskeletal system, which consists of the bones, joints, ligaments and tendons and muscles. These structures provide protection for the vital organs inside the body. Children are more likely to suffer from conditions of the musculoskeletal system because their musculoskeletal system is still growing. On the positive side, because the bones are still growing in a child, a fracture heals much faster than in an adult. Conversely, if the fracture penetrates the growth plate in a child, growth of that bone is interrupted. Some conditions involving the musculoskeletal system may have only a slight effect on the child's ability to mobilize and be short-term. Other conditions may have a significant effect, be debilitating and long term.

Bones

Bones are classified by their size and shape. Long bones are found in the extremities, including the fingers and toes. Most childhood disorders are located in the long bones. Short bones are located in the ankle and wrist. Flat bones are located in the skull, scapulae, ribs, sternum, and clavicle. Irregular bones are the vertebrae, pelvis, and facial bones. Long bones consist of the epiphysis (rounded, end portion), the diaphysis (long, central portion), and the metaphysis (thin portion between the epiphysis and the diaphysis). Long bones grow in length at the epiphyseal plate (cartilage segment) when the cartilage segment cells grow away from the shaft of the bone. The cartilage cells are replaced by bone. The diaphysis of the long bones is covered by periosteum (an outer, sensitive layer). The width of the bone is increased by pressing against the periosteum. Some disorders, such as osteomyelitis, cause damage to the periosteum and can interrupt bone growth.

Bones need nutrients in order to grow. Calcium is a main component of bones and is required for bone formation, resorption (bone breakdown), and remodeling (new bone replacing old bone). Calcitonin, parathyroid hormone, vitamin D, other minerals, and enzymes all play a role in the processes of resorption and remodeling. The central part of a long bone contains the marrow. Red marrow is responsible for production of red and white blood cells and platelets. Yellow marrow is responsible for the production of fat cells. Bones have an excellent blood supply, which enable the production of blood components for the body. Bone cells die and the necessary production of blood components is interrupted if there is no blood supply to the long bones.

Ligaments and Tendons

Ligaments are fibrous bands of connective tissue linking two or more bones or cartilages together. They provide stability to a joint during both movement and rest. The blood supply to ligaments is very small and they lack elasticity. Therefore, an injury to a ligament can take a long time to heal. Tendons are also fibrous connective tissue that attaches muscles to bones and other parts. There is also very little blood supply to the tendons and an injury to a tendon can also involve a lengthy recovery.

Muscles

Muscles consist of striated muscles and smooth muscles. Skeletal muscle is a type of *striated muscle* that attaches to tendons.

Skeletal muscles are used to create *movement* through contraction by applying *force* to *bones* and *joints*. These muscles can contract voluntarily (by somatic *nerve* stimulation) or can contract involuntarily through *reflexes*. *Smooth muscle* is a type of muscle found in the walls of all the hollow organs of the body (except the heart). Smooth muscles are involuntary muscles and are under the control of autonomic nervous system. For example, smooth muscles regulate the flow of blood in the arteries, move food through the *gastrointestinal tract* and expel urine from the bladder. ◆

Nurses play an important role in assisting the parents to find methods to help the child maintain normal growth and development as well as adapting or overcoming musculoskeletal system impairment. The nurse understands that casts, skin traction, skeletal traction, and distraction devices are ways to immobilize an extremity. The nurse evaluates the child through physical assessment. Laboratory studies and diagnostic tests can help establish the cause and nature of the musculoskeletal injury or condition. The results of these tests are then used to help the nurse develop an appropriate plan of care.

⚙ diagnostic tools Orthopedic Imaging Tests

Diagnostic Imaging Test	Benefits	Limitations
Radiograph	Easily available Visualizes fractures well No sedation needed Inexpensive	Two-dimensional Does not visualize soft tissue such as cartilage Patient must be positioned properly Radiation exposure
Fluoroscopy	Guides many orthopedic procedures Can be used with contrast Real-time radiography Inexpensive	Radiation exposure
Arthrography	Provides visualization of joints Three-dimensional view	Risk of reaction to contrast Depends on the skill of the radiographer Radiation exposure

🔧 diagnostic tools Orthopedic Imaging Tests—cont'd

Diagnostic Imaging Test	Benefits	Limitations
Computed tomography (CT scan)	Cross-sectional view of anatomy Clearer than radiographs Software programs can show reconstruction Can use contrast	Expensive May require sedation Risk of reaction to contrast
Bone scan (nuclear medicine)	Excellent at finding changes in bone as a result of infection, trauma, or tumor	Takes 4 hours Not always available on emergency basis Cannot distinguish benign from malignant tumors Radiation exposure to entire body IV access required
Ultrasound	Easily available No radiation No sedation needed Good for visualizing soft tissue masses and cysts Painless Inexpensive	Limited use Depends on the skill of the radiographer
Magnetic resonance imaging (MRI)	Visualizes hard and soft tissue and bone marrow No radiation	Not readily available No metal can be present in the vicinity Sedation may be needed Need experienced radiologist to read MRI

Immobilizing Devices

The nurse understands that casts, skin traction, skeletal traction, and distraction devices are four different methods to immobilize an extremity. Each of these methods is effective in treating musculoskeletal conditions in the child. There are benefits and risks associated with each of these methods. Specific nursing interventions need be initiated with each of these immobilization devices.

CASTS

Casts are a solid mold applied for immobilization purposes for fractures, dislocations, and other injuries. Casts are made of either a synthetic material such as fiberglass or plaster of Paris. Fiberglass is preferred because it is lighter in weight and dries within 30 minutes. Plaster of Paris casts take about 10 to 72 hours to dry.

There are four categories of casts: upper extremity, lower extremity, spinal or cervical, and total body. An upper extremity or lower extremity cast provides absolute immobility of the affected extremity (Fig. 30-1). A complex or extensive fracture may require a rigid spinal or cervical cast for a long period of time. A total body cast such as a hip spica cast (also called a spica cast) immobilizes the hips and thighs so that bones or tendons can heal properly after hip surgery. A bilateral long leg cast with an abduction bar (crossbar connects the cast together at ankle level) is also used for significant immobilization. Both the hip-spica and bilateral long leg cast with an

🔧 Labs: Blood and Body Fluid Analysis for the Child with Alterations in Musculoskeletal Conditions

Diagnostic Test	Function of the Test	Indications	Normal Values

Complete blood count (CBC)
CBC differential
	Blood sample evaluates many aspects.
	Breaks down WBC into various types (five total).
	Numbers indicate a percentage of total WBC
	Indicates the type of infection.
		Platelets indicate a bleeding disorder.
		>WBC indicates a bacterial infection or septic arthritis.
		Monocytes indicate a long-term infectious process.
		Lymphocytes indicate an increase in viral illness.
		Eosinophils indicate an allergic or parasitic condition.
		Basophils indicate a chronic inflammatory condition.
		Neutrophils (polys)
		    Bands are immature neutrophils.
		    Segs are mature neutrophils.
		    (Left-shift describes an increase in the band neutrophils.)
		Suggests a severe bacterial infection such as sepsis.
			Platelets: 150,000–400,000/μL
			WBC: 4500–10,000/μL
			0% for bands and 31–57% for segs
			Presence of bands is highly indicative of a bacterial infection

C-Reactive protein (CRP)	Measures a protein in blood that is released when an infection is present.	>0.9 indicates an infection or septic arthritis.	<1.0 mg/dL
Calcium and phosphate	Measures the amount of these minerals.	Low levels may indicate rickets.	Calcium: 8.5–11 mg Phosphorus: 3.0–4.5 mg/dL
Rheumatoid factor (Rh factor)	Measures the body's autoimmune response to an antigen.	If positive, may indicate juvenile arthritis. Not all children with juvenile arthritis have a positive Rh factor.	Negative
Erythrocyte sedimentation rate (ESR)	Measures the speed at which RBCs settle out in solution.	Elevated indicates septic arthritis. May also indicate infection.	0–10 mm/hr
Blood cultures	Measures whether microorganisms grow out in the lab.	Can identify an organism causing infection. Forty percent of children with septic arthritis have a positive blood culture.	No growth
Bone biopsies	Diagnose tumor or infection of the bone.	Osteomyelitis Bone tumor	Normal bone cells
Fluid aspiration from joints	Diagnose an infection of the joint or drain fluid from joint to relieve pressure.	Drainage is purulent. Culture of fluid is positive.	Clear fluid No growth from culture

abduction bar encase the trunk up to the nipples and both legs to the toes.

When a child is placed in a total body cast, parents have a much easier time caring for a child in a bilateral long leg cast that has an abduction bar than a child in a hip-spica cast. The nurse can teach parents that periodically, the cast needs to be changed. The two most common reasons to change a cast are when it becomes soiled or wet. Also, incision sites under a cast need to be assessed for infection. This includes checking for a foul odor, drainage from inside the cast, or staining through the cast.

Cast Complications

Complications can occur when a child is immobilized in a cast. The major complication is **compartment syndrome**. Compartment syndrome is caused by an accumulation of fluid in the fascia. This increases the pressure on the muscles, blood vessels, and nerve tissue that the fascia surrounds. Too much pressure can cause tissue ischemia, nerve damage, and necrosis. Unchecked compartment syndrome can result in the loss of the limb and possibly the loss of the child's life. A fasciotomy (surgical incision where a division of a fascia occurs) may be necessary to relieve the pressure. Pressure sores secondary to a tight cast or poor padding are another complication.

When a child is placed in a hip-spica cast, cast syndrome can occur. **Cast syndrome** occurs when a portion of the duodenum is compressed between the superior mesenteric artery and the aorta, causing vomiting, abdominal distention, and bowel obstruction.

 critical nursing action Cast Syndrome

Cast syndrome can be prevented by three nursing interventions:

Frequent repositioning
Fluids and increased fiber in the child's diet
Cutting a "belly hole" or a window in the cast to allow for abdominal expansion

Figure 30-1 A cast is applied to the affected extremity to keep it immobile while healing.

Nursing Care

Nursing care of the child in a cast begins with pre-application teaching to the child and family. For example, allow a preschool-age child to apply a cast to a doll. Then, give the child time to play with the casted doll before actually applying the cast to the child. When a child has any type of cast the nurse performs a neurovascular assessment with vital signs. An assessment is also done any time neurovascular compromise is suspected. A nursing assessment for a child with a cast includes the 5 "P"s: pain, pulse, pallor, paresthesia, and paralysis.

After the cast is applied, the nurse can facilitate drying of the cast by leaving the cast open to air. The cast has a hollow sound when it is dry. The nurse understands that it is never acceptable to use a hair dryer to facilitate drying. The heat from the hair dryer can cause a burn injury under the cast. The nurse can instruct the family that careful handling of the cast is an important intervention that prevents dents in the cast. Dents can cause pressure points on the tissue under the cast and ultimately result in a pressure sore.

Children treated with a plaster of Paris hip-spica cast are placed on a Bradford Frame, which elevates the child off the bed and facilitates drying of the plaster cast. The frame is secured to the bed and the child is secured to the frame. There is a hole in the frame to allow for elimination. Children treated with a fiberglass hip-spica cast are placed in the bed with pillows to support the lower extremities.

During the course of the drying phase and ongoing cast care, the child is turned every 2 hours. Frequent turning helps to facilitate drying and prevents cast syndrome if the child is in a hip-spica cast. At times, the cast may be bivalved meaning that it is cut down one or both sides with scissors to allow for expansion. The bivalved procedure is done to alleviate pressure, monitor for infection, or to help maintain proper hygiene. After the cast is bivalved, the affected extremity is elevated when the child is in bed, in a chair, or a wheelchair.

Elevation of the affected extremity helps with the child's pain control and prevents damage caused by pressure. If the child has a single-extremity cast, a waterproof plastic sleeve can be used to protect the cast and provide a seal with the skin proximal to the cast. It is also important for the nurse to explain to parents of a child in a cast that the child needs to be held. The nurse can help parents adjust to holding their child with a cast.

Hygiene is a major concern for a child in any type of cast but especially a hip-spica cast or bilateral long leg casts with an abduction bar. The nurse understands that protecting the proximal edges of the long leg casts and the perineal area of the hip-spica cast from soiling is a key hygienic intervention that is achieved by petaling the cast (Procedure 30-1).

 Nursing Insight— *Modifications for a child in a hip-spica cast*

Modifications need to be made for a child in a hip-spica cast. The hip-spica cast prevents the child from sitting normally; therefore, parents need a way to help their child adapt. One suggestion for modification is a toddler car seat that does not have sides. Toddler car seats are designed to help the small child with a hip-spica cast to sit fairly normal. They also have

Procedure 30-1 Petaling a Cast

Purpose

The purpose of petaling a cast is to promote good hygiene by protecting the proximal edges of the long leg casts and the perineal area of the hip-spica casts from soiling.

Equipment

Moleskin
1-inch waterproof adhesive tape
Plastic bag to place adhesive tape on
Scissors

Steps

1. Use scissors to cut 1-inch-wide by 1 1/2- to 2-inch-long strips of moleskin.

   RATIONALE: *Cutting the material ahead of time, along with the proper size of moleskin, facilitates application.*

2. Use scissors to cut 1-inch-wide strips of waterproof adhesive tape. The length of the waterproof adhesive tape should be about 1 1/2 to 2 inches long.

   RATIONALE: *Waterproof adhesive tape helps provide a protective barrier for the skin.*

3. The edge on one end of both the moleskin and waterproof adhesive tape must be rounded.

   RATIONALE: *Rounded edges keep the moleskin and waterproof adhesive tape edges from rolling.*

4. Place strips of the 1-inch waterproof adhesive tape on the plastic bags.

5. Apply the first strip of waterproof adhesive tape to any edge of the cast that is likely to become soiled by urine or stool. Place the rounded ends of the moleskin and adhesive tape over the cast edge to the outside.

6. Tuck the straight (unrounded) end inside the cast.

7. With your forefinger, gently ensure that the inside end is flat and not sticking to the child's skin.

8. Repeat the procedure, overlapping each additional strip, until all rough edges are completely covered.

9. Begin the same procedure with the moleskin to edges of the cast that are not likely to become soiled by urine and stool.

Clinical Alert It is a good idea to petal the edges of the cast that are likely to be soiled by urine and feces on the first postoperative day and preferably before the Foley catheter is removed.

Teach Parents

The nurse can teach the parents that diapering needs to be modified. To achieve this, a small diaper or peripad is placed in the perineal area with all edges of the cast outside this small diaper. Then a larger diaper is placed outside the smaller diaper and taped in the normal fashion. The nurse needs to ensure that the perineal edges of the cast remain outside of the diaper.

Documentation

1/9/10 0900 Upper edge of cast soiled and moist. Cast petaling performed. Waterproof adhesive tape to the upper edge of the cast, then moleskin applied. After petaling; the cast is noted to be clean and dry. No adverse reactions noted.

—M. O'Connor, MS, RN

a 5-point restraint system. Another suggestion is allowing a child to sit in a wagon with siderails. Feeding a child in a hip-spica cast can also be a challenge. Placing the child in the prone position on the floor is a good modification and makes it easier for the child to feed herself. Allowing the child to have supervised time while prone on a blanket helps the child to maintain developmental milestones.

Bathing the child with a cast is also an important nursing intervention. If the child has a small extremity cast a typical bath can be taken as long as the cast is protected from water. A large plastic bag can be placed over the cast during the bath. If the child is in a bilateral long-leg cast with an abduction bar, or a hip-spica cast, the nurse can teach the parent how to bathe the child by giving a sponge bath. In addition, frequent diaper changes help prevent complications such as skin breakdown and infection. Good perineal care is essential for children of all ages.

During the casting period, the child may be prone to constipation due to inactivity. The nurse can teach the family about the importance of good fluid intake and calling the health care professional about laxatives or stool softeners if needed.

Sometimes the child experiences some itching under the cast. Itching can be prevented by keeping the skin in good condition by turning the child every 2 hours and keeping the cast clean and dry. It is important for the nurse to tell parents that some children try to push items under the cast to scratch the area. The nurse can teach the parents and the child that absolutely nothing should be placed under the cast. If the itching is severe, the nurse can instruct the parent to call the health care provider about medication.

Cast care also includes taking care of the cast when it is being removed. The nurse must explain to the child that the sound of the cast saw is loud and can be frightening. It is difficult for the child to believe that the saw will not cut his or her skin. Reassure the child that she will not be injured with the cast removal. When the cast is removed, the child's skin is dry and flaky and the muscles are weak and possibly stiff. It is important to consider the child's emotions about the cast because the child may have grown used to it and think of it as a part of him or her.

Principles of Traction

The nurse recognizes that the main principle of traction is to reduce dislocations and immobilize fractures in the child. During the application of traction, one body part is pulled in one direction (traction) against a counterpull in the opposite direction (countertraction). The traction and the countertraction are the actual weights and pulleys. There are two main types of traction: skin traction and skeletal traction.

SKIN TRACTION

Skin traction is used for an extremity with a type of strapping material applied to the limb. Skin traction is used for short periods of time. Bryant's traction is one type of skin traction and is used to treat developmental dysplasia of the hip, shortened limb, and femur fractures in children

younger than 2 to 3 years of age. The child must weigh less than 26.4 lb (12 kg) to use Bryant's traction. In Bryant's traction, the child lies supine with thighs flexed and the hips slightly off the bed. Moleskin straps are applied to the child's calves and the pull is in only one direction. The nurse understands that the child's body is the countertraction. In modified Bryant's traction, the hips remain on the bed, but the legs are abducted.

Russell's traction is another type of skin traction that is used when the child weighs more than 26.4 lb (12 kg). It is most often used to stabilize femur fractures until a callus forms or with Legg–Calve–Perthes disease. With this type of traction, the child lies supine with hip flexed and abducted. There are two lines of pull in Russell's traction and the hips need to remain in alignment (Fig. 30-2). The child should have a trapeze secured on a cross-bar above the bed to assist with repositioning and maintaining upper body strength. In this type of traction a sling is placed under the knee. The placement of the sling is assessed frequently. Countertraction is increased with the foot of the bed elevated and the head of the bed flat.

Balanced suspension is used to suspend and immobilize the leg without traction to the rest of the body. Balanced suspension is achieved by attaching the Pearson attachment to the Thomas splint. This allows the leg to be "suspended" over the bed. A footplate can be attached to the end of the bed to reduce the incidence of foot drop. The nurse ensures that the bed remain flat to decrease the flexion in the hip. If the child has the bed in semi-Fowler's position, the head of the bed is lowered for 20 minutes per day.

Nursing Care

Nursing care for the child in skin traction requires a neuromuscular assessment to the affected extremity every 4 hours. Watch for web space numbness in fingers and toes. Web space numbness may indicate compartment syndrome. For any child in traction, it is necessary to assess circulation, sensation, pain, pallor, cyanosis, movement, and decreased pulse every 2 to 4 hours.

The nurse must ensure that the traction weights are checked and hanging free and that the child is in alignment with the traction. Skin traction needs to be removed and reapplied every 4 hours.

Perform skin care every 4 hours. The skin under the straps needs to be inspected and treated with rubbing alcohol to remove the body oils, which might cause the straps to slip. The nurse pays particular attention to the bony prominences that can break down easily. Do not

Figure 30-2 The child in Russell's traction (with trapeze).

massage bony prominences and ensure protective foam is in place. If the child has Ace wraps, protect the Ace wraps from urine and stool. The nurse can have two sets of Ace wraps for the child. Keep one set washed and ready to be used in case the other set becomes soiled. While the child is in traction, the nurse can initiate diversional activities to keep the child occupied while in traction (e.g., movie videos, board and video games, puzzles, blocks, and other toys that are easy for the child to handle).

SKELETAL TRACTION

Skeletal traction is used when more pulling force is needed than can be withstood by skin traction. Since the advent of newer orthopedic devices that achieve similar outcomes as skeletal traction and allow the child to be cared for at home rather than in the hospital, skeletal traction is used much less frequently. However, skeletal traction is still used when the weight of the traction needs to be more than 5 pounds.

In children, skeletal traction is used for long periods of time until the bone is ready for casting or **open reduction** (surgery to place the bones in their proper position). Many children needing skeletal traction have sustained multiple injuries. In skeletal traction, a pin is placed through the bone distal to the fracture. It is extremely important to note that with skeletal traction, the weights cannot be removed. There are three common forms of skeletal traction: Crutchfield tongs, 90/90 femoral traction, and Dunlop traction.

Crutchfield Tongs

Crutchfield tongs are used in the treatment of cervical and thoracic fractures. The tongs are placed into the child's skull (Fig. 30-3). The pull is along the axis of the spine. The traction usually hangs off the head of the bed. The counter-traction is the body. The tongs need to be assessed every 8 hours and as needed for placement and looseness. The nurse uses log rolling to turn the child in Crutchfield tongs. When this type of traction is used, pin care (gently cleansing the wound with saline-moistened gauze and applying antibiotic ointment with a cotton-tipped applicator if prescribed by the physician) needs to be done every shift. Neurovascular signs need to be assessed every 4 hours (more often if needed) due to the pressure on the spinal cord. Other important nursing care measures include pain control, meeting nutrition and elimination needs, providing proper hygiene, maintaining developmental milestones, giving emotional support and allowing for spiritual care. The family can be encouraged to express feelings of worry, helplessness, and frustration.

Figure 30-4 The 90/90 femoral traction is most commonly used to treat femur fractures and complicated femur fractures.

90/90 Femoral Traction

The 90/90 femoral traction is most commonly used to treat femur fractures and complicated femur fractures. A pin is placed in the femur, distal to the fracture. Weights are attached to a sling that supports the calf and also to the pin that causes the traction (Fig. 30-4). The body is the counter-traction. Femoral traction is more effective in children older than 6 years of age. Often femoral traction is used for the first 2 to 3 weeks after a femur fracture until enough of a callus forms. After a callus forms, a hip-spica cast is applied. The nurse needs to perform pin care every shift or according to the hospital policy. The nurse also needs to meet the holistic health needs of the child and family.

Maintaining the child in this type of alignment can be challenging. Sometimes there is a need for restraints to keep the child in proper alignment. If restraints are needed, hospital policy needs to be strictly followed and the nurse needs to obtain an order from the physician. Generally, a hospital restraint policy states that the restraints need to be removed every 2 hours for 10 minutes while the child is awake and every 4 hours for 10 minutes while the child sleeps. The restraint order also needs to be renewed by the physician every 24 hours. A better solution than restraints is constant supervision by parents, family members, friends and hospital staff. Often a hospital will have a volunteer program or a child-life specialist who can help with diversion activities.

Dunlop Traction

Dunlop traction is used in the treatment of a supracondylar fracture of the humerus. In this type of traction, a pin is placed in the humerus, distal to the fracture. Weights are attached to the forearm and to the pin that causes the traction. The body is the countertraction (Fig. 30-5).

Figure 30-3 Crutchfield Tongs are used in the treatment of cervical and thoracic fractures.

Figure 30-5 Dunlop traction is used in the treatment of a supracondylar fracture of the humerus.

Volkmann's ischemia can occur with children in Dunlop traction. The child complains of numbness, tingling, and a decreased sensation in the fingers. An important nursing intervention is to ask the child to wiggle the fingers to help relieve the discomfort.

Nursing Care

Assessment is the key nursing care measure for a child in skeletal traction. Neurovascular status must be assessed carefully and every 1 to 2 hours for the first 48 hours and then every 4 hours after that if there is no compromise in circulation. The nurse needs to know the symptoms of compartment syndrome and report them to the physician immediately.

Figure 30-6 The nurse assesses capillary refill time.

 Nursing Insight— *Performing the neurovascular assessment*

- **Pain**—Does the child complain of pain in the affected limb? Is it relieved by narcotic medication? Does it become worse when fingers or toes are flexed? If yes, notify physician *immediately* (compartment syndrome).
- **Sensation**—Can the child feel touch on the extremity? Is two-point discrimination decreased? If yes, notify the physician immediately (compartment syndrome).
- **Motion**—Can the child move fingers or toes? Lack of movement may indicate nerve damage.
- **Temperature**—Does the affected limb feel warm? Does it feel cool? A cool extremity may change to feeling warm if a blanket is placed over it and the extremity is elevated. If the extremity is still cool after these interventions, there is poor circulation.
- **Capillary refill time (CRT)**—Apply brief pressure to the nail bed and note how quickly pink color returns to the nail bed. CRT of less than 3 seconds is the norm. If CRT is greater than 3 seconds, circulation is poor (Fig. 30-6).
- **Color**—Note the color of the affected limb. Compare it to the color of the unaffected limb. Pink is the norm. If the color is paler than in the unaffected limb, circulation is poor.
- **Pulses**—Check pulses distal to the injury or cast. If the pulse is difficult to locate, assess with a Doppler. If the cast covers the foot or hand, it may not be possible to check the pulse but the other neurovascular assessment can be implemented.

The nurse also needs to understand the principles of traction and the reason why the traction has been applied. Other nursing care measures include maintaining the traction, maintaining the alignment of the traction with the child, preventing skin breakdown, providing pin site care, managing pain, maintaining good nutrition and elimination, preventing complications, and preparing the family for discharge.

Maintaining the traction involves assessing the desired line of pull with the relationship between the distal part and the proximal part. The nurse ensures that:

- The ropes are in the center part of the pulley, taut, and are intact, without knots.
- The pulleys are checked often to be sure they are in their original place and that the wheels of the pulley move freely.

- The amount of the weights is correct and that they are hanging freely.
- The bed is positioned with the head or the foot of the bed elevated as ordered so that the correct amount of pull is achieved with the traction and countertraction.
- The skeletal traction is not removed. If a child needs to be moved or if the traction needs to be adjusted, the nurse contacts the surgeon.

Maintaining the alignment of the traction with the child can be a challenge. By nature, children are unable to remain still in bed for extended periods of time. The nurse needs to realign the child in the bed often. Emphasis is on ensuring that the shoulder, hip, and leg are in a straight line with the lines of traction. Diversional activities are essential in assisting the child to maintain proper alignment. Collaboration with the child-life specialist also helps the child.

To prevent skin breakdown, place the child on an alternating-pressure mattress or a foam mattress overlay. A nursing assessment of the child's body is done to look for redness or breakdowns, especially on bony prominences receiving the greatest pressure. The nurse can wash and dry the child's skin daily or more frequently if needed. The nurse can also change the child's position every 2 hours to relieve pressure.

The nurse assesses pin sites every 8 hours for signs and symptoms of infection to prevent osteomyelitis.

Managing the child's pain is essential and the nurse can use pharmacological and nonpharmacological care measures. The nurse must use good judgment about the administration of pain medication by not waiting too long to administer pain medication and being alert for any adverse side effects. Effective pain control methods include epidural with bupivacaine (Marcaine) and a narcotic such as morphine sulfate (Astramorph) or hydromorphone (Dilaudid), patient-controlled analgesia (PCA) with morphine sulfate (Astramorph), or hydromorphone (Dilaudid). Antispasmodics such as diazepam (Valium) will give relief to the child with muscle spasms. The nurse can also ask the parents to participate in pain

where research and practice meet:
Pin Care

Pin site infection has been a problem for nursing practice. Hospital policy and procedure manuals each have a specific procedure to follow to help prevent this problem. Few multicenter studies have been done to determine which method is in fact most effective. Patterson (2005) completed a multicenter, prospective, randomized pin-care study over a 2-year period. The goal was to determine which of seven different methods is most effective in preventing pin-site infections:

1. Half-strength hydrogen peroxide cleansing and gauze wraps
2. Half-strength hydrogen peroxide cleansing and Xeroform wraps
3. Saline cleansing and gauze wraps
4. Saline cleansing and Xeroform wraps
5. Antibacterial soap and water cleansing and gauze wraps
6. Antibacterial soap and water cleansing and Xeroform wraps
7. Stable dressings with no pin cleansing

The results showed that 527 pins had an average infection rate of 20%. Ninety-eight pins had stage II infections and 12 pins had stage III infections. None had a deep infection or osteomyelitis.

The conclusion of this study suggests that there may be some factors involved in pediatric pin-site infection that were not covered in this study. It is clear that half-strength hydrogen peroxide and Xeroform wraps were superior to antibacterial soap and water cleansing. This was a pilot study and indicates a need for further research in this area.

assessment and pain management by offering comfort measures. Diversional activity also might help manage pain. The nurse can involve the child-life specialist in this aspect of care. The nurse can work collaboratively with the physical therapist to perform passive and active range-of-motion exercises to prevent weakness in uninvolved extremities. If pain is under control, the child may be able to perform minimal activities of daily living while on bedrest.

Maintaining good nutrition is essential for the child in skeletal traction. The hospital nutritionist can visit with the family to discuss healthy meals. The child may tolerate six small meals and healthy snacks instead of the traditional meal schedule. The nurse can offer the child healthy drinks and snacks. A sticker reward chart may be an effective measure to encourage good nutrition and reward healthy food choices. The child also needs to be assessed for regular elimination to ensure she does not become constipated or acquire a urinary tract infection.

The nurse must be alert to the child in skeletal traction, as serious complications can occur. Osteomyelitis (inflammation of bone and marrow, usually caused by infection) is a major, serious complication. The nurse also helps to prevent complications such as pneumonia, circulatory compromise, ischemia, and problems of disuse with uninvolved extremities. Any circumferential dressing has a potential to cause impaired circulation so dressings are assessed for tightness. Any restrictive bandages or devices are also assessed to ensure that they are neither too tight nor too loose. The nurse needs to assess for the 5 P's. Any notation of these symptoms may indicate circulatory compromise and possible ischemia. A burning sensation is associated with ischemia and can be an early indicator of neurovascular problems.

Nursing Insight— Preventing pneumonia

Respiratory care includes assessment and methods to increase lung expansion to prevent pneumonia. An incentive spirometry can be used for the school-age and adolescent child (Fig. 30-7). Younger children are not able to understand how to use the incentive spirometer, but the nurse can use creative measures to encourage expansion of the lungs (e.g., blowing a pinwheel, bubbles, a musical instrument, or a small folded paper triangle across the bedside table).

Preparing the family for discharge is essential to ongoing care of the child as the child will most likely have long-term casting or continued immobility. While the child is hospitalized, the nurse can coordinate a care conference to help plan discharge and home care. The family needs to learn about making adaptations in the home environment to ensure a safe environment and allow the child as much movement as possible. The family also needs psychosocial support in order to assist them in coping with the child's ongoing musculoskeletal condition. The nurse can help the family and the child achieve the best possible psychosocial outcome by arranging for home nursing care, physical and/or occupational therapy along with how to obtain durable medical equipment.

Nursing Insight— Distraction devices

Distraction devices are usually used to lengthen a bone. The surgeon performs an osteotomy (cuts through a bone) and places the distraction device. A distraction device can be placed in any long bone such as the femur and mandible, as well as in bones in the hand and the foot. Nursing care of the child with a distraction device is much the same as for the child in skeletal traction.

Now Can You— Discuss nursing care for musculoskeletal conditions?

1. Discuss the nursing care for a child with a cast?
2. Perform a Neurovascular Assessment?
3. Describe the principles of traction?
4. Describe the nursing care for skin and skeletal traction?

Figure 30-7 Blowing into incentive spirometer helps expand the lungs and prevent pneumonia.

Common Musculoskeletal Conditions found in Children

CLUBFOOT

Clubfoot is a foot deformity diagnosed in newborns. In children who have not had effective treatment, the most severe form of this condition resembles a "club." There are about one dozen different types of clubfoot. The most severe form and most commonly known is talipes equinovarus. The foot defect can be unilateral (more common) or bilateral. Talipes equinovarus affects boys twice as often as girls. Clubfoot deformities tend to run in families and are associated with spina bifida.

Signs and Symptoms

In clubfoot, the foot is plantar-flexed with an inverted heel and adducted forefoot The defect is rigid and cannot be manipulated into a neutral position. There is a possibility that the position of the fetus in utero influences the formation of clubfoot.

> 66 **What to say** 99 — *Talipes equinovarus (clubfoot)*

A mother has just delivered a baby with clubfoot. The parents are in the delivery room and are visibly upset. The parents are most likely in a state of shock and denial. The family does not understand what implications this has for their newborn.

The nurse can ask questions such as:
"How are you feeling at this time?"
"Do you know what this condition is called?"
"Do you know anything about clubfoot?"
"Can I stay with you to offer support while you hold the baby?"
"After you rest we can talk more about the baby's condition."

Diagnosis

Diagnosis of clubfoot is made by visualization during the newborn nursing assessment.

Nursing Care

Treatment is begun as soon as possible after birth. Clubfoot can be treated with serial casting (replacing plaster casts) on the affected extremity(s) at specified intervals to permit progressively greater ranges of joint motion so that the maximum range needed for function may be restored (Venes, 2009). While casted, the affected extremity is manipulated into a more normal position and a cast is applied to hold this position. In the beginning, the cast is changed frequently and eventually reduced to a weekly basis until overcorrection of the position is achieved. Overcorrection is the goal for serial casting because the ligaments and muscles are shortened and when the casts are finally removed, there is a tendency for these muscles and ligaments to pull the foot back into the clubfoot position. Overcorrection enables this pull to level off at a normal position. The nurse communicates to the family that exercises, splints, special shoes, or casts may be prescribed on a long-term basis.

where research and practice meet:
Clubfoot Casting Techniques

Lifelong atrophy of the calf is common for children with clubfoot, requiring long-term follow-up care. A study by Ippolito, Farsetti, Caterini, and Tudisco (2003) compared two different techniques for treatment of congenital clubfoot. The authors found that serial casting followed by an open heel–cord lengthening and a limited posterior ankle release had much better long-term results than the group of children who received serial casting followed by an extensive posteromedial casting (Venes, 2009).

Nursing care for a child undergoing nonsurgical management of clubfoot includes passive range of motion (ROM) and care of the daily cast application after manipulation. Since manipulation of the affected extremity with serial casting can cause discomfort because the muscles and ligaments are being stretched, pain medication is indicated. Neurovascular assessments must be done every 1 to 2 hours for the first 24 to 48 hours after cast application and every 4 hours thereafter, until a new cast is placed. The nurse needs to assess for swelling. The cast is left open to air to aid in the drying process, and the extremity is elevated. The nurse must teach parents important neurological assessments and cast care.

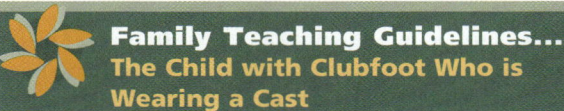

Family Teaching Guidelines…
The Child with Clubfoot Who is Wearing a Cast

HOW TO:

The nurse can teach the parents how to care for their child with a clubfoot who is wearing a cast. The nurse can instruct the parents to:

- Give the child emotional support and reassurance that she will return to her normal activities soon after the cast is removed.
- Maintain the child's normal development by playing, reading, and spending time with the child.
- Keep the cast and surrounding area clean and dry and reposition her every 2 hours.
- Elevate an extremity and use good hygiene to prevent skin breakdown.
- Notify the health care provider if she has a fever, signs and symptoms of infection, or unrelieved pain.
- Take her to the health care professional if the cast is damaged (soft, loose, or cracked) or cast syndrome is suspected.

ESSENTIAL INFORMATION

- Follow-up care is essential.
- Inform the parents that there may be a potential for reoccurrence of the clubfoot.
- Teach the parents about the importance of monitoring their child for cast complications.

Severe cases of clubfoot may require surgery when the infant is 9 to 12 months of age. An orthopedic surgeon lengthens the tendons to help ease the foot into a more normal position. Postoperative care involves assessing the neurovascular status. The nurse also needs to observe for swelling in the ankle and foot. The key to preventing swelling is to elevate the ankle and foot. The nurse must assess for drainage from the cast as well as for signs of infection, including purulent drainage, fever, and chills. The nurse is aware that pain management is important postoperatively. Pain medication is initially administered intravenously with morphine sulfate (Astramorph). When the child can tolerate fluids and food, they can be switched to oral pain medication.

In either case serial casting or surgery, the nurse needs to keep the cast clean. The young child needs to be diapered in such a way that the cast is outside of the edges of the diaper. Double diapering and changing the diaper frequently are also methods to keep the cast clean. The older child may have to change underwear frequently. It is not feasible to bathe the child in a tub of water with bilateral long leg casts with an abduction bar so a sponge bath is given. The nurse can provide the family with emotional support. Distraction techniques and age appropriate toys can help the child to handle the long recovery process.

 ### Collaboration in Caring— *Clubfoot*

Collaboration with the surgical team is required in the care of the child with clubfoot. The orthopedic surgeon directs the serial casting. In some cases, surgery is needed after the serial casting. Collaboration with physical therapy is essential since the physical therapist directs the passive range-of-motion exercises. The nurse teaches the parents about the serial casting process and how to provide home care. The nurse helps direct the family to a respite care center and parenting help line.

 ### nursing diagnoses A Child with Clubfoot

- Impaired Physical Mobility related to external devices (casts)
- Impaired Parenting related to growth and development lag
- Risk for Impaired Skin Integrity related to external devices (casts)
- Knowledge Deficit related to treatment and home care

LEGG–CALVE–PERTHES DISEASE

Legg–Calve–Perthes disease (LCPD) is a self-limiting disease that has an insidious onset and traditionally had been accepted as a disorder of growth. It affects boys five times more frequently than girls. Most cases are boys ages 4 to 8 years and are blue-eyed with very fine light-colored hair and of shorter stature. It is an aseptic necrosis (necrosis occurring without infection) of the femoral head. It can take 18 months to 4 years for this condition to resolve.
There are four stages of LCPD:

- Aseptic necrosis (flattening of the femoral head)—lasts several weeks, presents with synovitis and a decrease in ossification in the nucleus of the femoral head secondary to ischemia

- Revascularization—lasts 6 to 12 months; increased joint space, increased cartilage thickness, decrease in size and density of femoral head
- New bone formation—lasts 1 to 2 years, collapse and superolateral displaced head, avascular bone is reabsorbed
- Regenerative phase—reconstitution of femoral head with remodeling and final healing

Signs and Symptoms

The child complains of hip or knee soreness or stiffness. This pain increases with activity and decreases with rest. The child presents with a painful limp and may also have quadriceps muscle atrophy. There may also be joint dysfunction and limited ROM.

Diagnosis

A radiograph establishes the initial diagnosis LCPD. The definitive diagnosis is made by MRI, which shows osteonecrosis.

Nursing Care

The goal of treatment is to keep the femoral head in the acetabulum. There is an initial period of non–weight-bearing (NWB) for 7 to 10 days. During this time, traction, braces, or a hip-spica cast may be used. Obtaining a history is important in assessing the child with possible LCPD. This history will uncover how long the child has been limping and the severity of the pain. The nurse understands that the child will describe the pain as increasing in intensity with activity and decreasing with rest. The nurse's assessment of ROM will determine limitations on abduction and internal hip rotation. An assessment of the thigh and buttock area will reveal a wasting of the muscles. A shortening of the extremity on the affected side indicates that the femoral head has collapsed. The orthopedic surgeon directs the care and decides when surgery is needed.

When the child is receiving conservative treatment, the nurse needs to assess the skin in the brace, traction, or cast. The nurse needs to prepare the child and family for an x-ray exam and MRI. If the child is being treated with a brace, collaboration with the Orthotics team (a team of experts who teach others how to use orthopedic appliances) is required. The child needs to be maintained on bedrest to reduce the inflammation and restore motion. Pain management needs to be included in the nursing plan of care. The nurse can communicate to the family that the child will need to avoid weight-bearing activities and that mobility restrictions need to be maintained. While the child has mobility restrictions, passive and active ROM need to be implemented.

Ongoing treatment consists of conservative therapy for 1 to 3 years in NWB braces or serial casting. Neurovascular assessments need to be done while the child is in traction or a cast. If the child has undergone surgery for an osteotomy and a hip-spica cast is required, the nurse needs to implement the usual postoperative care measures in addition to the care of a child in a cast. Pain relief is achieved with the administration of nonsteroidal anti-inflammatory drugs (NSAIDs) such as ibuprofen (Children's Advil).

Since it is very difficult for a child to remain on bedrest, emotional support and diversional activities are essential. It is also important for the nurse to teach the family about home care. The nurse can discuss the importance of adaptive play. After the physician has communicated that the condition has resolved the child can return to normal activity in about 3 to 4 months.

Across Care Settings: Visiting nurse

After hospitalization, when the child with Legg–Calve–Perthes disease is dismissed to home the visiting nurse can:
- Assess the family support systems while the child and the family are in their own environment.
- Ensure that the family is able to provide the care needed.
- Ensure compliance with the use of the conservative devices.
- Ensure the NWB status of the child.
- Assess the knowledge of the parents and child about ongoing care.
- Encourage the use of creative quiet activities and hobbies.
- Ask the family about follow-up care with the physician.

nursing diagnoses A Child with Legg–Calve–Perthes Disease

Risk for Injury related to altered mobility secondary to Legg–Calve–Perthes Disease treatment
Impaired Physical Mobility related to external devices
Risk for Impaired Skin Integrity related to external devices
Body Image Disturbance related to immobility
Knowledge Deficit related to treatment and home care

SLIPPED FEMORAL CAPITAL EPIPHYSIS

Slipped femoral capital epiphysis (SFCE) affects 2 to 10 per 100,000 children. It occurs two to five times more frequently in males than in females. A higher proportion of children with SFCE are obese. SFCE occurs more frequently in the Eastern United States and in African American children. The cause is unknown, but there is a genetic component and it may be related to endocrine abnormalities.

When this condition occurs, the capital femoral epiphysis (top of the femur) slips through the epiphysis (growth plate) in a posterior direction.

assessment tools Slipped Capital Femoral Epiphysis

The nurse understands that capital femoral epiphysis is classified by stage and severity:

Stage
- Preslip—The child complains of weakness in the leg. Pain in knee or hip when standing or walking for long periods of time.
- Acute slip—The child falls and then reports hip pain.
- Chronic slip—The femoral head gradually slips off the femoral neck and then remodels for the incorrect position.
- Acute-on-chronic—Slow progressive slip that then becomes more displaced when the child falls.

Severity
- Grade I: Preslip—There is a widening of the physis without any displacement of the epiphysis.
- Grade II: Minimal slip—There is a one-third displacement of the femoral head from the femoral neck.
- Grade III: Moderate slip—There is more than one-third but less than one-half displacement of the femoral head from the femoral neck.
- Grade IV: Severe slip—There is more than one-half displacement of the femoral head from the femoral neck.

Signs and Symptoms

Symptoms appear gradually. Pain in the groin or referred pain to the thigh or knee is the child's primary presenting complaint. This occurs because the child is externally rotating the leg to relieve pressure on the hip joint. The parent usually notices that the child is limping and favoring that extremity. During examination, the child complains of pain during internal rotation of the hip. Other conditions associated with SFCE are hypothyroidism, renal osteodystrophy, and postradiation therapy.

Acute slip symptoms are present for less than 3 weeks. Chronic slip symptoms are present for more than 3 weeks or even months. Along with the expressed symptoms, the hip does not fully rotate internally and abduction is limited. The affected leg may be shorter if the child has a moderate or severe slip.

Diagnosis

A radiograph reveals a slipped epiphysis and the diagnosis is made.

Nursing Care

Once a child has been diagnosed with SFCE, no weight bearing is permitted. The goal of nursing care is to prevent further slippage. No ROM should be attempted if the child has an acute slip because it may cause further damage. The nurse can communicate to the family that the hip cannot be reduced manually as that will cause further damage to the femoral head. Forced bedrest with the child in traction decreases synovitis (inflammation of a synovial membrane) in the hip. If the child has an acute slip, split Russell's traction may be instituted for a few days before surgery.

Surgery (pinning) is the intervention of choice for a child with mild to moderate SFCE. The pinning consists of a percutaneous insertion of a large screw or pin into the femoral head to hold it in place. There is a small incision and the child stays in the hospital for less than 24 hours. After 1 week, the child may bear full weight and the pin is removed at a later date.

With severe SFCE, an osteotomy is required, which consists of a breaking and resetting of the bone. This prevents further slippage and restores hip motion to normal. It is a much more extensive surgery, requiring a longer hospitalization and prolonged immobilization.

The nurse needs to assist the family in adjusting to the sudden hospitalization, NWB status of the child, and the impending surgery. After surgery, postoperative pain management is managed with intravenous narcotics and changed to oral narcotics once the child is tolerating liquids and solid food. The nurse also monitors the neurovascular status frequently.

After surgery, the nurse collaborates with physical therapy to teach the child crutch walking. The physical therapy initiates ambulate with crutches. After that, the nurse needs to continue ambulation with the child using crutches until discharge.

The child is discharged when pain is controlled with oral narcotics and the child can ambulate safely with crutches. It may be helpful to arrange for a visiting nurse to ensure that the child can ambulate safely with crutches at home. If the child still needs assistance with ambulation at home, a physical therapist can visit the home and reinforce teaching.

FRACTURES

Fractures occur when a bone undergoes more stress than it can absorb. Skeletal fractures account for 10% to 15% of all childhood injuries. The most common causes of fractures are falls, motor vehicle accidents, and bicycle accidents. There are differences between a fracture in a child and a fracture in an adult. A child's bone heals faster because of a higher metabolic rate and because the epiphyseal plate (growth plate) is still open. However, any damage to the epiphyseal plate can result in a limb length discrepancy, joint incongruity, and a progressive angular deformity of the limb. During birth, an infant can suffer a fracture of the collarbone. Otherwise, fractures in infancy are rare because the infant has limited mobility. During the first 2 years of life, fractures may be the result of physical maltreatment.

Signs and Symptoms

Fractures are characterized as open and closed. With an open fracture, the bone has penetrated through the skin. It is designated type I, II, or III, based on the degree, severity of soft tissue damage, size of the wound, and amount of contamination. The potential for infection is greatest with an open fracture. A closed fracture involves no break in the skin. Classification of fractures involves identifying the locations and descriptive nature of the fracture. The location is where the fracture occurs along the shaft of the bone. Fractures can be described in terms of the amount of injury.

 assessment tools Classification of Fractures by Location

Epiphyseal
  Type I
    Separation of epiphysis
    May be mistaken for a sprain
    Does not usually affect growth
  Type II
    Fracture separation of the epiphysis
    Circulation remains intact
    Does not usually affect growth
  Type III
    Fracture through the epiphysis into the joint
    Does not usually affect growth f reduced properly
  Type IV
    Fracture through epiphysis into the joint and the metaphysis
    Open reduction and internal fixation necessary
    Can prevent growth disturbance
  Type V (rare occurrence)
    Crush injury to epiphyseal plate
    Results in premature closure of the epiphyseal plate
    Growth arrest occurs

Diaphysis
  Proximal
  Midshaft
  Distal

 assessment tools Classification by Type of Break

Transverse
  Line crosses the shaft at a 90-degree angle

Spiral
  A diagonal line coils around the bone
  Caused by a twisting force

Oblique
  A diagonal line across the bone

Greenstick
  Bone is bent, but not broken
  More common in children

Comminuted
  Three or more fracture fragments

Compression
  Bone becomes wider and more flat
  Usually seen in the spine

The severity of the fracture depends on the amount of force placed on the bone and the strength of the bone, the size of the bone, and the direction of the force. Once a bone is fractured, inflammation happens. Osteoblasts (bone-forming cells) activate within 24 hours to begin making new bone. A callus forms during the first few weeks. Complete callus formation and establishment of compact bone takes 4 to 12 weeks. Remodeling (rounding off angles and filling in hollows) continues for up to 1 year. In children, the ends of the bone do not need to be perfectly aligned because the bone has an enhanced ability to remodel.

Diagnosis

A fracture is suspected by presenting symptoms, trauma history, and physical examination of the child. X-ray exam is the primary method to diagnose fractures. When an x-ray film is taken, the nurse understands that there needs to be at least two views (anteroposterior and lateral). The joints above and below the suspected fracture must be included in the radiographic evaluation. CT scans, MRI, fluoroscopy, and myelograms may also be used to diagnose fractures.

Nursing Care

The nurse obtains a history from the child and family describing how the injury occurred. In cases where maltreatment may be involved, it is helpful to ask the child how the injury occurred in the absence of the caregiver. Depending on the type and location of the fracture, children generally heal without complications. Nursing care involves preventing complications such as limping, decreased ROM, and nerve deficits.

Specific treatment depends on the type and location of the fracture. If the bones are not displaced, no reduction of the fracture is needed. If the bones are displaced, a reduction of the fracture is needed, in which the ends of the bone are placed close together or aligned. A **closed reduction** aligns the fractured ends by manually manipulating the extremity or traction. This is performed by a physician under conscious sedation or general anesthesia. The goal is to reduce the fracture as soon as possible.

An **open reduction** is performed when the fracture cannot be reduced by closed methods or when torn muscles or ligaments need to be repaired. Internal fixation is used to stabilize the bone ends until healed. Internal fixation is achieved with percutaneous pins or with screws, plates, or rods. For example, an intramedullary fixation rod can be placed in the shaft of the femur. After the bone has healed, the hardware can be removed.

After closed or open reduction, the fractured bone must be immobilized to maintain the position of the fracture, prevent rotation and shearing of the fracture, and permit active muscle contraction. Immobilization is achieved with splints, braces, casts, external fixators, or traction. Immobilization relieves pain and allows for ease of movement of the unaffected areas of the body. It is important to mobilize the child as quickly as possible in order to avoid hazards of immobility.

Open fractures present additional concerns. The potential for infection from contamination is great. Antibiotics must be administered in the emergency department and continued for at least 3 days after the injury. Surgery for wound cleansing, débridement, and stabilization of the fracture needs to be performed urgently. If the wound is small, the surgeon may surgically close the wound. Most often, the wound is left open and draining until the infection is eradicated. The child may have to return to surgery later for more débridement or closure of the wound.

clinical alert

Complication of the child with a fracture

The classic sign of compartment syndrome is unrelenting pain that is unrelieved by narcotics. The nurse must notify the physician immediately. The priority intervention for compartment syndrome is prevention. Prevention is achieved by elevating the extremity to prevent excessive swelling and frequent neurovascular checks.

After open or closed reduction, the nurse needs to perform frequent checks to assess for pain, numbness, or tingling. Nursing actions that can help to prevent complications and restore function are frequent neurovascular assessments, notifying the surgeon of any changes, elevating the affected extremity above the level of the heart, and applying cold packs (15 minute intervals) for the first 24 hours after the injury. The nurse can teach the family that nutrition can be addressed by providing a well-balanced diet with protein, calcium, and iron. A child in a hip-spica cast should eat small, frequent meals to avoid abdominal distention. The child should also increase fluids and fiber in the diet to prevent constipation.

critical nursing action   Caring for a Child with a Fracture in a Cast

- Elevate the extremity with the cast on pillows for at least the first 24 hours.
- Avoid indenting the cast.
- Assess the extremity for swelling and discoloration.
- Observe the extremity for sensation and movement.
- Notify a health care professional immediately if abnormalities are noted.
- Follow activity restrictions.
- Do not allow the affected limb to hang down for any length of time.
- Prevent the child from putting anything inside the cast.
- Keep a clear path for ambulation.
- Ensure the child uses crutches appropriately.
- Encourage rest.
- Encourage good nutrition to promote healing.
- Encourage quiet activities.
- Ensure child moves joints above and below cast.

After surgery, if the child has any open wounds or pins from traction or a distraction device, the nurse assesses the wound(s) and performs pin care every 8 hours to prevent infection. For any type of fracture it is critical that the nurse assesses and treats pain frequently. Intravenous opioids are administered for the first 24 hours. Once the child is tolerating liquids and a regular diet, pain medication is switched to the oral route. Acetaminophen (Tylenol) with codeine or oxycodone (Percocet) is the preferred narcotic. The nurse may supplement the medication with regular acetaminophen (Tylenol) to reach the maximum safe dose to achieve the best pain control during hospitalization. It is important for the nurse to differentiate between pain and muscle spasms with a child who has had a fractured femur. Muscle spasms are extremely painful. Diazepam (Valium) is the best choice for an antispasmodic medication. Muscle spasms generally subside after the first week.

The child and family may experience anxiety related to the unplanned hospital admission and possible surgery. It is important for the nurse to provide emotional support to the child and the family.

 Collaboration in Caring— *Caring for a child with a fracture*

- A child-life specialist can initiate play to help reduce the anxiety of a child with a fracture. He can assist the child with working through fears and frustrations with medical play, art therapy, and distraction.
- Social services personnel may also be available to assist the family on admission to the emergency department and can continue to support the family during the child's hospitalization. At discharge, they can arrange for transportation as well as identify helpful community resources.
- A school teacher or tutor can assist a child who is hospitalized for an extended period of time.

Complications that can occur with fractures are shock, fat emboli, deep vein thrombosis, pulmonary embolism, and infection. Late complications that can occur are malunion, nonunion, refracture, joint stiffness, reflex sympathetic dystrophy, loss of reduction, posttraumatic arthritis, delayed union, and pseudoarthritis.

Discharge teaching helps parents feel more comfortable caring for their child at home. It is important to review the treatment plan, principles of bone healing, how to perform a neurovascular assessment and cast care. Parents need to be aware that adaptations to the home environment need to be in place to ensure the child's safety. The physical therapist can help the family learn methods for transfer and use of assistive devices at home.

 case study The Child with a Fracture Who Has Complications

A 12-year-old child was admitted with a femur fracture the previous night. He has a morphine sulfate (Astramorph) PCA that has a dose that is safe and effective. The leg is elevated on two pillows and ice packs are in place. The nurse performs the neurovascular assessments with the first morning vital signs. During the following hour, the child complains that on the numerical pain scale, the pain is 10 out of 10. The nurse checks the history on the PCA pump and finds that the child has requested numerous doses, but has received the maximum number of doses possible in the past hour. The neurovascular assessment reveals that the pulse is absent and the extremity is cool and pale. The capillary refill time is greater than 3 seconds.

critical thinking questions

1. Describe compartment syndrome?

2. What should the nurse do first?

3. What is the priority intervention for compartment syndrome, and how is it achieved?

◆ See Suggested Answers to Case Studies in text on the Electronic Study Guide or DavisPlus.

SOFT TISSUE INJURIES

Soft tissue injuries (sprains and strains) are unusual in young children. These injuries are more often seen in the adolescent age group. The growth plate of the epiphysis is weaker than the ligaments in younger children because of the new bone formation and is prone to fracture rather than sprains or strains. With puberty, skeletal growth declines and the growth plates begin to close. The growth plates become less susceptible to injury and the ligaments and tendons become more susceptible to injury. The ankle is the most frequently sprained or strained joint. The prognosis is good for first- and second-degree sprains. Severe sprains (third-degree) have an increased risk of recurrent injury, persistent instability, and traumatic arthritis.

Signs and Symptoms

Signs and symptoms of a sprain include pain, swelling, bruising, instability, and loss of the ability to move and use the joint. Signs and symptoms of a strain are pain, limited motion, muscle spasms, muscle weakness, swelling, cramping, and inflammation.

Diagnosis

A history needs to be obtained from the child as well as the parents. The history reveals important information about the injury, swelling and local hemorrhage at the injury site. The child's most painful area is examined last. An x-ray exam is performed if there is an obvious fracture or misalignment.

 assessment tools Sprains are Classified According to Severity

First Degree
Mild; ligament is stretched and the affected joint is stable.
Minimal pain, swelling, ecchymosis.
Full ROM and weight bearing.

Second Degree
Moderate; ligament is partially torn and joint laxity is present.
Moderate pain, swelling, and ecchymosis.
Motion is slightly limited and painful.
Mild joint laxity with tenderness over the joint.
May be unable to bear weight.

Third Degree
Severe; ligament is completely torn and joint is unstable.
Significant swelling and severe ecchymosis occurs within the first 30 minutes.
Severe pain over the joint makes examination difficult.
Cannot bear weight or otherwise use the extremity.

Nursing Care

Immediately after the initial injury, it is most important for the nurse to use the RICE acronym (Fig. 30-8):

R—Rest; resting the injured extremity prevents further injury and allows the ligament to heal

I—Ice; ice for the first 48 hours, keep ice packs in place for 15-minute intervals to decrease swelling

C—Compression; apply an Ace wrap or some other method to apply pressure to the affected joint to help reduce swelling

E—Elevation and early motion of the affected joint; elevation reduces swelling and early motion of the affected joint helps keep the full ROM

Immobilization of the joint is recommended based on the severity of the injury. Mild sprains are immobilized with external support with an elastic bandage, brace, or ankle lacer. Moderate sprains require a posterior splint or cast for 2 to 3 weeks in conjunction with crutches. Severe sprains require conservative or surgical treatment with a cast for 4 to 6 weeks and no weight-bearing activities. Early motion after the injury, with gentle stretching and a strengthening program, speeds recovery.

Collaboration with the physical therapist is necessary in caring for the child with a soft tissue injury. The physical therapist teaches the patient quadriceps and hamstring exercises, a range-of-motion program for ankle injuries, and crutch walking. To prevent nerve damage, the physical therapist ensures that the patient bears weight on his hands, not the axillae.

The nurse has an important role in teaching home care for the child with a soft tissue injury. The nurse teaches the proper technique for wrapping the affected joint and ensures that it is followed. The nurse communicates to the caregiver that it is important to start wrapping the area distally and work up to the proximal area beyond the level of the injury. The child needs a physical activity restrictions school note for the physical education teacher and coach. If the child has a mild sprain, sports activities can be resumed in 2 to 3 weeks. If the child has a moderate sprain, the child can participate in partial weight-bearing activities using crutches and return to full weight-bearing and sports activities gradually. If the child has a severe sprain, sports activities can be resumed in approximately 4 to 8 weeks.

Figure 30-8 The nurses uses the "RICE" acronym.

Sports Injuries

Sports injuries occur as a result of competitive sports in three quarters of all middle and high schools in the United States. One-half of boys and one quarter of girls ages 8 to 16 have participated in competitive sports. The increase in popularity of competitive sports, recreational sports, and cheerleading has significantly increased the number of overuse injuries, sprains, strains, and dislocations. The causes of these injuries may be a result of inadequate health physicals, hazardous practice and play areas, training and practice errors, improper safety equipment, improper nutrition, overtiredness, and a limited awareness or concern for the possible risk factors. Sports injury may involve fractures, sprains and strains as well as knee and elbow injuries.

A child who participates in sports where the legs are being used, such as skiing, soccer, football, or track, is at risk for a knee injury such as a tear in the anterior cruciate ligament (ACL). The injury occurs when the ACL is stretched or torn during a sudden twisting motion when the feet stay planted one way and the knee turns the opposite way.

A child who participates in sports where the arms are being used, such as baseball, basketball, or tennis, is at risk for an elbow injury. Each of these sports involves a repetitive forward motion of the arm and the child is not able to extend the elbow fully. This is due to injury to the muscle consisting of tiny tears and contractures.

Signs and Symptoms

A ruptured or torn ACL causes instability and pain in the knee. In an elbow injury, pain and tenderness, as well as the loss of full extension of the elbow, occur 24 to 48 hours after the injury. This injury is commonly known as "Little Leaguer's elbow."

Diagnosis

Diagnosis of a sports injury is based on an x-ray exam followed by an MRI.

Nursing Care

Treatment for a knee injury depends on whether the injury is mild or severe and whether there was a twisting action involved in the injury. A mild injury is treated with bedrest and ice. A topical anesthetic may be applied locally to minimize pain and oral pain medication can be given. After 24 hours, heat is applied, which aids in healing. If the injury is more severe and the knee joint fills with fluid a physician will aspirate the excess synovial fluid. A cast may need to be applied in order to completely immobilize the joint. It takes the same length of time for a severe ligament injury to heal as a bone, therefore the cast remains in place for about 8 weeks. Arthroscopy can be performed to see the joint and repair torn ligaments or cartilage.

If the injury involved a severe twisting motion, the kneecap may be dislocated (slips around to the posterior side of the knee). The knee appears deformed and a physician slides the kneecap back into place immediately. The child is placed in a leg immobilizer for about a week. If this type of injury occurs frequently, surgery on the ligaments is necessary. Quadriceps exercises, which consist of straight leg raising exercises, help prevent a kneecap dislocation from occurring again.

For an elbow injury, exercises to strengthen the flexor muscles help prevent further injury. Children need extra protection against injury to the epiphyseal plates until they have fused (between the ages of 14 and 17 years of age). To prevent elbow injuries, children who participate in ball sports need time to warm-up. Pitching breaking balls and curve balls should be discouraged. Pitching should also be limited to six innings per week with a 3-day rest period between games. Treatment of the "Little Leaguer's Elbow" consists of applying ice for 15 minutes three times per day. Administering an anti-inflammatory agent may help the child be comfortable. Cortisone injections into the joint can also be helpful, but only a limited number can be used. Treatment for a more severe case consists of rest and immobilization of the elbow until pain, tenderness, and limited movement disappear. Permanent damage to the epiphyseal line and an elbow deformity can be the result of inadequate treatment for this injury.

OSGOOD–SCHLATTER DISEASE

Osgood–Schlatter disease is a painful prominence of the tibial tubercle. It is a common problem in active older school-age children and adolescents. It is a self-limiting disease, which is more prevalent in boys. It occurs in boys between the ages of 10 and 15 years and in girls between the ages of 8 and 13 years. It can occur bilaterally or unilaterally.

Osgood–Schlatter disease is caused by a repetitive injury and repair to the tibial tubercle where the patellar tendon attaches. There is a strong quadriceps contraction and an immature ossification center resulting in inflammation and small avulsions (tearing away) of the bone. The cycle continues with new bone forming each time the injury and the body attempts to heal itself (Cassas & Cassettari-Wayhs, 2006). Osgood–Schlatter disease does not result in long-term complications and the prognosis is good.

Signs and Symptoms

The major symptom is pain below the kneecap that is aggravated by activity and relieved by rest. Symptoms resolve around the time skeletal growth ceases (about puberty). The child experiences pain when asked to squat or extend the knee against resistance.

Diagnosis

An x-ray exam of the knee is performed to rule out a tumor. History and the presenting symptoms assist in making this diagnosis. Pain that occurs when the child is asked to squat or extend the knee against resistance is a good indicator of Osgood–Schlatter disease.

Nursing Care

Pain control is an important nursing action for a child with Osgood–Schlatter disease. The pain medication of choice is an NSAID. The knee should be iced after exercising. An elastic wrap or neoprene sleeve over the knee during activity also helps to relieve the pain. Surgical management is rare, unless a piece of bone has completely torn free from the tibial tubercle. Surgery would consist of excision of this bone fragment. The surgery is performed after the child has reached bone maturity to avoid damage to the epiphyseal plate.

The nurse teaches the family that the child is to have limited activity. Once the symptoms improve, the child may return to normal activities. The nurse can provide support to the child by helping the child to cope with the activity restrictions and social interactions. The nurse collaborates with the physical therapist to teach the child exercises to strengthen the upper body. The physical therapist also teaches the child to perform lower extremity isometrics. These exercises help the child maintain strength while the injured knee heals.

Osteomyelitis

Osteomyelitis is an infection of the bone and the tissues around the bone.

 clinical alert

Osteomyelitis

The nurse understands that osteomyelitis needs immediate treatment.

Osteomyelitis most commonly occurs in healthy children. Osteomyelitis can cause massive destruction of bone, sepsis, and possibly death. Osteomyelitis often involves the long bones in the lower extremities in children, but it can involve any other bone in the body. Many bacteria can cause osteomyelitis, most commonly *Staphylococcus aureus*.

 Nursing Insight— *Osteomyelitis*

Acute osteomyelitis can be caused by the following:

- An open fracture
- Penetration of the skin by a contaminated object
- A septic joint
- An infected wound
- Bacterial infection from somewhere else in body, like dental caries
- Blunt trauma
- Premature babies and infants with birth complications during the 1st year of life

Osteomyelitis occurs when bacteria lodge and multiply in the middle of the bone where circulation is sluggish. The infection spreads to the ends of the bones and can destroy the epiphyseal plate in children. The inflammatory process produces pus, edema, and vascular congestion in the area of infection (Fig. 30-9). Pressure in the bone increases and eventually cuts off the blood supply, causing necrosis. The body attempts to lay down new bone over the necrotic bone. The prognosis is good if the osteomyelitis is treated promptly with intravenous antibiotics.

Signs and Symptoms

The signs and symptoms of osteomyelitis can be overt or subtle. The child comes to the clinic with pain in the affected bone. The child's history may reveal a fall or bumping of the affected extremity. History also reveals a

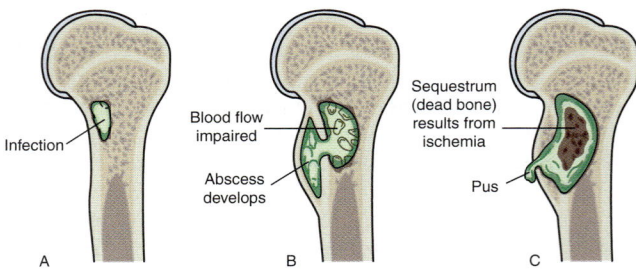

Figure 30-9 Sequence of osteomyelitis development. *A.* Infection begins. *B.* Blood flow is blocked in the arc of infection and an abscess with pus forms. *C.* Bone dies within the infection site and pus continues to form.

recent infection such as a cold or otitis media. Sometimes the child has a fever. The child is irritable and guards the affected limb. There is localized tenderness, redness, warmth, and pain on palpation. Occasionally, there is soft tissue swelling around the area.

Diagnosis

Osteomyelitis is suspected when the child presents with the clinical manifestations. X-ray exam and a bone scan confirm the diagnosis. Blood cultures help determine the causative bacteria.

Nursing Care

Treatment for osteomyelitis is a course of broad-spectrum antibiotics. Antibiotics are begun after blood cultures are drawn. The exact antibiotic prescribed will depend on the causative bacteria. The child is hospitalized on antibiotic therapy. It is important for the nurse to evaluate the child's response to the antibiotic therapy about 2 or 3 days after the initial dose. If the child demonstrates a response to the intravenous antibiotic therapy at this point, more blood cultures are drawn, intravenous antibiotics are stopped, and the child continues therapy on oral antibiotics for 4 to 8 weeks at home. If the child demonstrates poor response to the intravenous antibiotic therapy, antibiotic therapy is continued for a much longer period. The nurse monitors the erythrocyte sedimentation rate (ESR). This lab study is a good indication of whether the infection is resolving. As the infection resolves, the ESR decreases to normal. Palliative measures such as rest, oral pain medication, good nutrition and diversional activity can also help. The nurse can also teach parents about the importance of antibiotic compliance.

 clinical alert

Chronic osteomyelitis

Chronic osteomyelitis is uncommon and occurs when bone tissue dies as a result of the lost blood supply. The frequency of chronic osteomyelitis has diminished due to an increased awareness of the need for prompt, aggressive treatment. However, children with chronic osteomyelitis have had symptoms for longer than 3 weeks and there is a history of prior bone infection within weeks or months after surgery or trauma. The treatment for chronic osteomyelitis is prolonged, painful, and frustrating for the child and family. Pain control is an important nursing action for the child

with chronic osteomyelitis. The nurse understands that it is important to make the child as comfortable as possible. For the first few days of hospitalization, the affected limb is placed in a splint. Oral analgesics, including acetaminophen (Children's Tylenol), ibuprofen (Children's Motrin), or narcotic analgesics such as acetaminophen with codeine (Percocet) can be used to manage pain. The intravenous site should be monitored for infiltration because the antibiotics used to treat osteomyelitis are caustic to the veins. A peripherally inserted central catheter (PICC) or tunneled central line is placed if intravenous therapy continues for more than 2 to 3 days. Diversional activities should be employed while the child is in the hospital and at home while activity is limited.

The nurse has an important role in teaching home care for the child with osteomyelitis. The child may be discharged on a regimen of home intravenous antibiotics. This requires a sustained commitment from the family. The nurse needs to assess if a family member can maintain the child at home on intravenous therapy. Antibiotics that can be scheduled every 8 to 12 hours may have a better compliance rate than more frequently scheduled antibiotics. A parent who has to administer one or two antibiotics every 4 to 6 hours can become sleep deprived very quickly. The child may return to school if the antibiotics are on a 12-hour schedule. A home school teacher or tutor is needed if the antibiotics are scheduled more frequently.

 Now Can You— Discuss osteomyelitis?

1. Describe the symptoms of osteomyelitis?
2. Describe the critical nursing actions for a child with osteomyelitis?

JUVENILE ARTHRITIS

Juvenile arthritis is an autoimmune, inflammatory process with unknown origin, but is thought to be triggered by an infection. Peak onset occurs in two different age groups (between 1 and 3 years or age and between 8 and 12 years of age). Females are affected twice as frequently as males. Symptoms can range from very mild to very severe. Juvenile arthritis is the leading cause of blindness and disability in children. Juvenile arthritis is not a childhood version of rheumatoid arthritis. The prognosis of juvenile arthritis is considered good. Success related to how the child and family cope with the condition is based on how well the child meets developmental milestones. If juvenile arthritis occurs in a younger child, growth retardation usually occurs.

Human leukocyte antigens (HLAs) play a role in the disease. There is chronic inflammation of the synovial membrane with effusion and destruction of the articular cartilage. Immune complexes in the blood and synovial tissue initiate the inflammatory response by activating the plasma protein complement. Excessive fluid is produced that is watery, thin, and lacks mucin. The synovium swells and thickened villi and nodules protrude into the joint cavity. The nurse understands that a restriction in the joint capsule and ligaments leads to a decreased joint movement and tendonitis. Ankylosis (adhesions) also develop between joint surfaces, which can further limit joint mobility.

The prognosis for children with juvenile arthritis is that 60% to 70% will have remissions. Approximately 45% will still have active disease 10 years after diagnosis, which results in disability in adulthood.

Signs and Symptoms

The child with juvenile arthritis has joints that are swollen, tender, and warm to touch, and limited ROM. The joints are stiff and have loss of motion, especially in the morning. Intermittent joint pain that lasts longer than 6 weeks should be suspect for juvenile arthritis. The child may also present with a rash. The child may try to protect the affected joint and may even refuse to walk if the joint is a weight-bearing joint. Systemic symptoms include malaise, fatigue, and lethargy. There is a history of a late afternoon fever with a temperature spike up to 105.1°F (40.6°C). Infection, injury, and surgery may precipitate a flare-up. There are many types of juvenile arthritis. Three different types are described in Table 30-1.

Diagnosis

There is no actual test for juvenile arthritis; therefore, diagnosing juvenile arthritis may be difficult. The diagnosis is made by excluding other conditions that may cause similar symptoms or other possible causes such as viral infections. The white blood cell (WBC) and erythrocyte sedimentation rate (ESR) are important laboratory values to monitor. The character, frequency, and severity of systemic and articular (joint capsule) manifestations are critical factors in diagnosing juvenile arthritis. Radiographs or bone scans to detect changes in bones and joints may be used. Any joint swelling or pain that has lasted longer than 6 weeks should be assessed for possible juvenile arthritis. The child with juvenile arthritis has a pattern of remissions and exacerbations.

Nursing Care

Medications are a key factor in the management of the child with juvenile arthritis. The nurse can teach the child and the family about the different medications required in the treatment of juvenile arthritis.

The outcomes of the nursing interventions for JA are to prevent injuries and identify exacerbations. This requires teaching the child and family about the disease and proper care. The nurse can teach the caregiver how to assess the child for warmth, tenderness, pain, and limitations in ROM. The family must be alert for increasing irritability, guarding, and refusal to bear weight and take action by encouraging rest. The nurse can help parents learn proper positioning of the inflamed joints and the appropriate application of heat or cold. A physical therapist can design an exercise program with isometric exercises and passive ROM. Part of home care includes the need for a diet high in fiber, protein, calcium, and adequate fluid intake. The nurse also needs to develop a plan of care that aids parents in providing age-appropriate activities and reinforces independent activities. After an exacerbation the child needs to be encouraged to resume pre-exacerbation activities. The parents need to break the cycle of dependence, but this can be very difficult. It is best to involve the child in the decision-making process as much as possible. Psychosocial adjustment of the child is assessed by school performance and peer activities. Attending professional counseling sessions or support groups can be encouraged.

 nursing diagnoses A Child with Juvenile Arthritis

- Chronic pain related to joint inflammation
- Impaired physical mobility related to joint discomfort and stiffness
- Altered family processes related to a situational crisis (child with a chronic illness)

Table 30-1 Types of Juvenile Arthritis			
	Polyarticular	**Pauciarticular**	**Systemic Onset**
Number of Joints Involved	Five or more	Four or fewer	Any number
Joints Affected	Usually small joints of fingers and hands	Usually large joints, knees, ankle, elbow	Any joint
	Weight-bearing joints	Usually particular joint on one side of body	
	Same joint on both sides		
Sex Affected	Girls more than boys	Girls more than boys (most common type)	Boys and girls equally
Body Temperature	Low-grade fever	Low-grade fever	High spiking fever lasting for weeks or months
Other Symptoms	Stiffness and minimal joint swelling	Iridocyclitis (eye inflammation)	Macular rash on chest, thighs
	Rheumatoid nodules on elbow or other body area receiving pressure from chairs, shoes	Painless joint swelling with little redness	Inflammation of heart and lungs
			Anemia
	(+) Rheumatoid factor in 20% of cases	(+) ANA titer (possible)	
	(+) ANA titer is possible	(+) HLA antigen (possible in boys)	Enlarged lymph nodes, liver, and spleen
	Elevated WBC, complement and erythrocyte sedimentation rate		Rarely (+) rheumatoid factor and ANA titer
			Elevated WBC

medications: Treatments for Juvenile Arthritis

- NSAIDs (nonsteroidal anti-inflammatory drugs). Only a few NSAIDs have been approved for use with juvenile arthritis. The approved NSAIDs are ibuprofen (Children's Advil), naproxen (Aleve), tolmetin (Tolectin), and choline magnesium trisalicylate (Trilisate). Other NSAIDs commonly used are indomethacin (Indocin) and diclofenac (Cataflam). If an NSAID is selected, it is usually chosen based on dosing schedule, patient preference, or medication taste because there is a lack of agreement on the best NSAID for patients with juvenile arthritis.
- Disease-modifying antirheumatic drugs (DMARDs) are agents that prevent or relieve rheumatism. Some of the more commonly used DMARDs are methotrexate (Rheumatrex), cyclophosphamide (Cytoxan), sulfasalazine (Azulfidine), and infliximab (Remicade). Methotrexate (Rheumatrex) is most frequently prescribed for juvenile arthritis patients. It is effective in polyarticular JA and has been used for the past 10 years. The most common side effect of methotrexate (Rheumatrex) is gastrointestinal symptoms.
- New drugs potentially available for use with juvenile arthritis are leflunomide (Arava) and etanercept (Enbrel). Leflunomide is an immunosuppressant. The side effects of these drugs are diarrhea, elevated liver enzymes, alopecia, and rash. They have been approved for use in adult patients with adult RA, but have not yet been approved for use with children. There is a teratogenic potential that would be of concern with children, particularly adolescent girls. The other new drug, etanercept (Enbrel), has been found to reduce the signs and symptoms of moderately severe to severe polyarticular juvenile arthritis. It is a potent inhibitor of tumor necrosis factor (TNF), which is a key proinflammatory cytokine found in the synovial tissue of patients with juvenile arthritis (Ilowite, 2002).
- Infliximab (Remicade) is another TNF-neutralizing agent. Efficacy data are limited for use of this medication. There needs to be a large-scale evaluation of the effectiveness of this drug (Ilowite, 2002).
- Prednisone (Deltasone) and other corticosteroids are very potent and should be administered at the lowest possible dose and for the shortest possible period of time. Side effects, such as Cushing syndrome, osteoporosis, increased risk of infection, glucose intolerance, cataracts, and growth retardation, can occur.

MUSCULAR DYSTROPHIES

Muscular dystrophies (MDs) are a group of muscle disorders that cause the gradual wasting of symmetrical groups of skeletal muscle. It is the most common group of muscle disorders in childhood. All muscular dystrophies are a result of a genetic defect that causes the degeneration of muscle fibers. Most muscular dystrophies are identified in early childhood. Thirty percent of the time, muscular dystrophy is caused by a spontaneous mutation and 65% of muscular dystrophy cases are sex-linked recessive disorders. Muscular dystrophies are divided into three types: pseudohypertrophic muscular dystrophy (Duchenne's muscular dystrophy), congenital myotonic dystrophy and facioscapulohumeral muscular dystrophy.

Duchenne's is the most common and serious type of muscular dystrophy. Duchenne's muscular dystrophy is a sex-linked recessive disease, so it generally only affects males. Duchenne's muscular dystrophy affects 1 in 3600 males. Females are usually carriers. In a case such as a female child with Turner's syndrome, where the child

receives only one X-gene from the mother, the female child could have Duchenne's muscular dystrophy.

Congenital myotonic dystrophy is an autosomal dominant inherited disease. The disease process begins while the fetus is in utero. The infant usually dies before 1 year of age due to the inability to maintain respiratory function. Facioscapulohumeral muscular dystrophy is an autosomal dominant trait carried on chromosome 4. Symptoms progress slowly, making a normal life span possible.

Signs and Symptoms

There is a belief that a protein is absent from the muscle. The muscle fibers degenerate and are replaced by fat and connective tissue. Muscle wasting and contractures of the calf muscle are replaced by fat. There is a progressive symmetrical muscle wasting and weakness without loss of sensation.

In Duchenne's muscular dystrophy, the symptoms first appear after the child is able to walk, usually about 3 to 7 years of age. Duchenne's muscular dystrophy most often affects the pelvis and shoulders. The child develops a waddling, wide-based gait. The calf muscles become weak and hypertrophied.

With congenital myotonic dystrophy, the newborn may already have severe muscle weakness at birth. Muscle degeneration continues until there is inadequate respiration. Symptoms of facioscapulohumeral muscular dystrophy occur after the child is 10 years old. The main symptom is facial weakness. The child becomes unable to wrinkle the forehead and cannot whistle.

assessment tools   Gower Maneuver

A child with muscular dystropy uses the Gower maneuver to rise from the floor. The Gower maneuver is when the child must move to a kneeling position with hands also on the floor to stabilize. Then the child, while keeping hands on the floor, rises to feet. The child comes to a standing position by using the hands to walk up the legs until in a standing position.

Diagnosis

Children with a positive family history are at risk for Duchenne's muscular dystrophy. These children should be monitored for clinical symptoms that do not usually appear until preschool years. Serum creatinine kinase (CK) levels should be monitored. CK levels are elevated in the early stages of the disease. As muscle bulk decreases, the CK levels also decrease. Definitive diagnosis is made by muscle biopsy (the removal of muscle tissue for microscopic examination and chemical analysis) and electromyelogram (EMG, a graphic record of resting and voluntary muscle activity as a result of electrical stimulation) (Venes, 2009). Diagnosis of congenital myotonic dystrophy is based on serum enzyme analysis and muscle biopsy. Muscle biopsy and serum enzyme analysis are used for diagnosing facioscapulohumeral muscular dystrophy.

Nursing Care

Treatment for muscular dystrophy is aimed at maintaining independant living for the child as long as possible. These children rarely live beyond 20 years of age. Since death is usually a result of respiratory complications, the key is to prevent respiratory infections. Monitoring the respiratory status is critical. Any respiratory infection must to be treated quickly and aggressively with antibiotics, postural drainage, and chest physiotherapy (CPT).

The nurse also needs to monitor the child's skin. As the child's mobility decreases, the skin can deteriorate quickly. It may be necessary to arrange for a special bed with an air cushion that can assist the caregiver in turning the child frequently. The nurse can teach the family to provide meticulous skin care.

Transferring the child in and out of bed and into a chair may eventually need to be performed with a Hoyer lift. Toileting can become an issue when the child is no longer able to ambulate and is required to wear diapers. Safety factors are essential in the care of the child with MD.

Nutrition is another focus for the nurse. The nurse should monitor the child's weight gain. A diet that is low in calories and high in protein helps prevent obesity. A high-fiber diet and adequate fluid intake help prevent constipation. The nurse can teach the caregiver to begin a regimen of stool softeners and laxatives to help prevent constipation.

Assessment of the child's mobility is an important nursing action to help the child maintain ambulation for as long as possible. Active and passive ROM is also performed. Splinting and bracing may be recommended by the physician to prevent contractures.

The nurse can help foster independence and self-care. It is important to teach the child how to achieve an optimal level of functioning. The nurse can teach the child how to make adaptations so he can participate in self-care measures. Encouraging the child to be involved in activities that will maintain independence is important. For example, swimming is a good activity to achieve independence because when he is in the water, exercises can be done without the child feeling the weight of his body.

The nurse recognizes that the child and family need emotional support. The nurse should encourage the child and family to participate in support groups. The Muscular Dystrophy Association is an excellent resource for these families and children (http://www.mda.org/). Parents should be referred for genetic counseling. With muscular dystrophy, the parents must watch their child pass away gradually.

Collaboration in Caring— *A child with muscular dystrophy*

Coordination of the child's health care requires collaboration with physicians, physical therapists, nutritionists, social workers, medical equipment companies, faith communities and the family. The nurse should assess the family's ability to cope with their child's chronic illness and poor prognosis. The nurse assesses the support and resources available to the family. The nurse can help the family find proper community and online resources because the child will eventually need an electric wheelchair, Hoyer lift, and modifications to the home environment.

Complementary Care: *Muscular dystrophy*

Children who suffer from muscular dystrophy often turn to alternative or complementary therapies since there is no cure. Wenneberg, Gunnarsson, and Ahlstrom (2004) performed a quantitative and qualitative study using a qigong. The conclusion from this two-part study was that qigong was accepted as a new, innovative exercise program. Qigong may lower the rate of decline in general health.

nursing diagnoses A Child with Muscular Dystrophy

- Impaired Physical Mobility related to chronic degenerative disease process
- Self-care Deficits; Bathing/Hygiene, Dressing, and Grooming related to chronic degenerative disease process
- Risk for Injury related to decreasing mobility secondary to chronic degenerative disease process
- Fatigue related to increased energy expenditure
- Altered Grieving related to chronic and terminal illness
- Altered Family Processes related to chronic and terminal illness
- Impaired Gas Exchange related to diminishing muscle function secondary to muscular dystrophy
- Altered Nutrition related to chronic and debilitating disease process

SCOLIOSIS

Scoliosis is a nonpainful lateral curvature of the spine and is the most common spinal deformity in children. The spine either curves laterally in only one direction ("C" curve) or in two opposite directions ("S" curve). There is a lateral deviation and rotation of each vertebra, which accentuates the deformity. Idiopathic scoliosis is common in female children and in families in which another member has been affected by scoliosis. Idiopathic scoliosis is the predominant form and there is no recognizable cause. Unequal leg lengths, such as untreated developmental dysplasia of the hip (DDH), can cause scoliosis. Congenital scoliosis is related to vertebral anomalies. It can also be associated with other congenital anomalies, such as myelomeningocele (spina bifida), osteogenesis imperfecta, or muscular dystrophy. Paralytic scoliosis occurs in association with neuromuscular diseases such as cerebral palsy, paraplegia, and quadriplegia.

Signs and Symptoms

Scoliosis may first be suspected by the child's parents or the school nurse. The school nurse performs scoliosis checks on all children between 9 and 15 years age. The primary care practitioner also assesses the child for alignment of the midline of the neck, shoulders, and hips. The child is asked to bend at the waist with arms hanging loosely. This is called the Adam's position or the bend over test (Fig. 30-10). The nurse practitioner assesses for unequal shoulder heights, scapulae prominences and heights, waist angles, rib prominences, chest asymmetry, and leg length discrepancy. It is also necessary to assess the skin for hairy patches, nevi, café au lait, lipomas, and dimples. A neurological and cardiac exam may be performed to rule out Marfan syndrome.

Nursing Care Plan The Child with a Musculoskeletal Disorder

Nursing Diagnosis: Impaired Physical Mobility related to physical disability or mechanical restrictions.

Measurable Short-term Goal: The child will engage in activities appropriate to current physical limitations.

Measurable Long-term Goal: The child will regain maximum mobility.

NOC Outcomes:
Mobility (0208) Ability to move purposefully in own environment independently with or without assistive device
Transfer Performance (0210) Ability to change body location independently with or without assistive device

NIC Interventions:
Activity Therapy (4310)
Environmental Management (6480)
Self-Care Assistance: Transfer (1806)

Nursing Interventions:

1. Monitor the child for complications of immobility (specify, e.g., peripheral pulses, capillary refill, skin integrity, muscle weakness).

   RATIONALE: Provides prevention or early recognition of complications to decrease their severity.

2. Allow the child to make as many realistic choices as possible and encourage independence in activities of daily living.

   RATIONALE: Empowers the child by allowing him or her to exercise as much control as possible over self and the environment.

3. Select appropriate transport for the child and promote as much mobility as possible (specify, such as a wheelchair, crutches, stretcher, go-cart, or stroller).

   RATIONALE: Mobility promotes normality and helps prevent feelings of isolation.

4. Encourage the child to go to the playroom if possible or arrange for the child-life therapist to visit the child.

   RATIONALE: Increases child's mobility and decreases isolation. The child-life specialist promotes normal growth and development.

5. If the child is immobile for a long period of time, plan periodic rearrangement and redecoration of the room with input from the child as appropriate.

   RATIONALE: Change breaks up the monotony of the immobilization and provides an opportunity for engagement and creativity.

Figure 30-10 The child is asked to bend at the waist with arms hanging loosely. This is called the Adam's position or the bend-over test. Scoliosis is obvious in this adolescent.

Diagnosis

Diagnosis is confirmed by radiography. The physician looks at the Cobb angle (a measure of the curvature of the spine in degrees). The number of degrees helps the physician decide what type of treatment is necessary. A scoliosis curve of 10 degrees is normal and the child will continue to be assessed for scoliosis at regular checkups until pubertal maturation and growth are complete. The primary health care provider monitors the number of degrees; a curve between 10 and 40 degrees (mild) will generally suggest a back brace. A curve of more than 40 degrees (severe) revealed by x-ray exam requires treatment and the child is referred to an orthopedic surgeon.

Severe scoliosis can lead to respiratory compromise, as the lung under the shortened side of the body will not be able to fully expand. Severe scoliosis can also have a negative effect on the hips and knees.

Nursing Care

Scoliosis screening is a critical nursing action. Bracing and exercise are the usual treatments for mild cases of scoliosis. Bracing stops the progression of scoliosis. The molded brace is worn 23 hours per day. The patient may only remove the brace to shower. The adolescent wears a special T-shirt under the brace to prevent skin irritation. The nurse can communicate to the child and family that compliance with bracing improves the outcome for this condition. The major problem with bracing is body image. Many adolescents do not want to wear the brace at school or while they are with their friends. The nurse can communicate to the family that the best way to increase compliance is to include the adolescent in decisions. Exercises recommended by a physical therapist help the muscles in the back gain strength.

 Complementary Care: *Exercise and bracing*

Thompson (2004) revealed outcomes from exercises alone and chiropractic therapy are rarely therapeutic in managing scoliosis. Transcutaneous electrical stimulation has also proved ineffective. Exercises are of benefit when used in conjunction with bracing to maintain and strengthen the muscles of the back and abdomen.

Surgical treatment is necessary when pulmonary function becomes compromised, sitting or walking becomes difficult because of poor balance, pain, curves are noted as severe by x-ray exam, and for cosmetic reasons. The surgical method is reserved for the most severe cases of scoliosis. The surgeon can approach either anteriorly, posteriorly, or both. When both approaches are used, the anterior approach is done first and then 1 week later, the posterior approach is done. In severe cases, halo traction may be used before surgery to better align the vertebrae. Surgery should be delayed as long as possible because the fusion of the vertebrae will stop spinal growth.

When surgery is scheduled, the nurse should explain to the child and parents what to expect. Prior to surgery, a tour of the ICU can help alleviate the child's anxiety. It is also important to stress that after surgery the child will have an indwelling urinary catheter in place. The nurse can also teach range-of-motion exercises before surgery.

In the postoperative phase, the child remains in the ICU overnight. The nurse assesses vital signs and neurological status every 1 to 2 hours after surgery. Once the child is stable she is transferred to the inpatient area where vital signs and neurological assessments continue to be preformed every 4 hours. The nurse also understands the importance of monitoring fluid balance. Renal function is monitored because the kidneys are hypoperfused during surgery. The child may also have had blood transfusions.

Pain is controlled with narcotic analgesics and the child should not wait too long to communicate that he or she is in pain. Pain is controlled with a PCA. While the child is receiving narcotics, the nurse monitors oxygen saturation (Fig. 30-11). The child will also have a nasogastric tube hooked up to low suction. When the child's bowel sounds return, the nurse discontinues the nasogastric tube. The child's diet then advances from clear liquids to a regular diet.

Figure 30-11 While the child is receiving narcotics, the nurse monitors oxygen saturation.

The child may have a chest tube in place. The chest tube will be hooked up to suction at first and then placed on water seal. When drainage has ceased, the chest tube is removed. Radiography is usually performed the day after chest tube removal to ensure that no pneumothorax is developing. Incentive spirometry, chest physiotherapy (CPT), and coughing and deep breathing exercises are used to prevent atelectasis and pneumonia. The nurse must also assess for signs of symptoms of infection every 4 hours, such as fevers, chills, redness and pain at the incision site, and drainage from the incision site.

 critical nursing action Logrolling

Positioning of the patient is also an important nursing action. The patient must be turned using the logrolling technique. Logrolling involves two or more nurses turning the patient in complete unison. The head, shoulders, hips, and legs are turned as one unit, thereby keeping the back in a straight line as the patient is turned (Fig. 30-12).

Figure 30-12 The patient must be turned using the logrolling technique.

The surgeon may require the patient to wear an orthotic brace. Collaboration with the orthotist is necessary to ensure that the brace fits properly. The nurse checks for pressure points under the brace for the first couple of days after implementation of the brace. Range-of-motion exercises are also performed to keep the uninvolved extremities from becoming weak.

A nutritionist helps prevent constipation by suggesting adding fiber and fluids to the diet. Foods high in iron, folate, and vitamin C should be added to the patient's diet. Psychosocial aspects of care for this child include nursing actions that maintain or build his or her self-esteem. Because some musculoskeletal conditions have visible deformities, the nurse should address body image concerns and anxiety. Certain situations may create an inability for the child to interact physically or socially, or may cause the child to feel alienated from the peer group. Other psychosocial concerns related to the family are daily living routines and family functions, continued care of other siblings and financial burdens. Compliance with the treatment regime is important to ensure the best outcome for the child.

Discharge teaching is done after assessing the level of knowledge by the patient and the family. Discharge teaching should include a variety of topics. The physical therapist will continue to be involved with this child on an outpatient basis for rehabilitation. The school nurse should be notified about the patient's activity restrictions as the adolescent will have activity restrictions for 6 to 9 months postoperatively. Activities such as bike riding, roller blading, skiing, mowing the lawn, shoveling snow, or any lifting of more than 10 pounds is not allowed until the activity restriction is lifted.

The nurse can teach the parents to be alert for unfavorable signs such as pain, infection and difficulty breathing. Teaching the family about the brace including the signs and symptoms of skin breakdown is important. Be sure to instruct that the patient's head should not be raised more than 30 degrees without the jacket brace. Provide the family with information on community resources available to them and arrange for counseling for the adolescent, particularly if compliance with wearing the brace is an issue. The nurse can encourage the adolescent to be as active as possible and keep follow-up appointments.

? case study Scoliosis

An 11-year-old girl has a history of idiopathic scoliosis. She is otherwise healthy. She has just arrived from the PACU after a posterior spinal fusion with instrumentation. The child had a blood loss of 1200 mL and received PRBCs (packed red blood cells) and 450 mL of cell saver in the operating room. She also received 2 L of lactated Ringer's solution in the PACU. She has a central line for intravenous access. Her vital signs are: heart rate, 120–130 beats/min; blood pressure, 92/48; temperature 97.2°F (36.2°C). Her face, hands, and feet are edematous. She denies discomfort and appears relaxed.

critical thinking questions

1. After attaching the patient to the apenic and bradycardia monitor (A & B monitor) and obtaining report, what would the nurse's initial assessment include?

2. What assessments place the child at risk?

3. What additional information should the nurse consider?

4. What other problem might the nurse anticipate?

5. Taking into consideration the characteristics of the middle childhood stage of growth and development, what can the nurse do to optimize the plan of care?

6. What are important home care instructions?

◆ See Suggested Answers to Case Studies in text on the Electronic Study Guide or DavisPlus.

KYPHOSIS

Kyphosis is a nonpainful spinal curvature in the sagittal plane. It is commonly described as "hunchback." Slight kyphosis is found in the normal spine. Families usually seek treatment when the kyphosis becomes noticeable. In children, kyphosis is caused by a congenital or acquired condition. Some congenital causes of kyphosis are ankylosing spondylitis, metabolic disorders, osteogenesis imperfecta, spina bifida, Paget's disease, and Scheuermann's disease, which causes juvenile or adolescent kyphosis because there are wedge-shaped vertebrae in the thoracic region. In acquired kyphosis, the child can voluntarily bend the spine to correct the curvature. In addition, there is no underlying evidence of structural changes seen with acquired kyphosis. Kyphosis is potentially serious because of the risk of progressive deformity.

Signs and Symptoms

Parents may first notice uneven shoulder height in their child. The adolescent may also have complaints of pain in the thoracic region.

Diagnosis

Kyphosis is most commonly diagnosed in early adolescence during routine back screening for scoliosis. If kyphosis is suspected, a complete examination should include a complete orthopedic and neurological exam. Radiographs confirm the diagnosis and are used to follow progression of the disease. If the curve exceeds 50 degrees; it is considered abnormal (kyphotic).

Nursing Care

Nonsurgical treatment is recommended for acquired kyphosis when it is between 50 and 70 degrees. It may be possible to treat the child with continued observation and thoracic hyperextension exercises, or a brace may be needed. Surgical treatment is recommended when the curve is greater than 70 degrees. Anterior–posterior spinal fusion is the surgery of choice. The child with congenital kyphosis does not respond well to bracing, so surgery is necessary. The nursing care for the child with a surgical repair for kyphosis is the same as for the child with scoliosis.

LORDOSIS

Lordosis is a spinal curvature in the sagittal plane (Fig. 30-13). It is seen in conjunction with flexion contractures of the hip, scoliosis, obesity, developmental dysplasia of the hip (DDH), and slipped femoral capital

Figure 30-13 Lordosis is present in the normal spine and is not considered a major deformity.

epiphysis (SFCE). Lordosis is present in the normal spine and is not considered a major deformity.

Signs and Symptoms

Lordosis is commonly described as "swayback," an excessive backward cavity of the spine.

Diagnosis

The parents may first notice that the child's clothing is not fitting properly. This may precipitate a visit to the primary care provider. If lordosis is suspected, the full diagnostic exam includes a full orthopedic and neurological examination. Radiographs confirm the diagnosis and are used for follow-up progression of the disease.

Nursing Care

Treatment involves reducing the predisposing factors such as obesity. Reducing the predisposing factors can also be temporarily achieved with postural exercises and support garments.

SPINAL FUSION

In spinal fusion the vertebrae are fused together to maintain alignment. This is usually the surgical procedure used to correct scoliosis. Instrumentation (an application of metal screws, bolts, wires to straighten the spine) is usually performed with the spinal fusion. The instrumentation holds the vertebrae in place until the fusion has healed.

Nursing Care

Important nursing interventions for a child who has had a spinal fusion are similar to those for a child who has had a surgical repair of scoliosis. The usual postoperative routines are followed. Vital signs are monitored hourly while the child is in the ICU. Once on the inpatient unit, the vital signs are monitored at least every 4 hours (more frequently if needed). Encourage the child to use the incentive spirometer every hour, or an alternative method if they are not developmentally capable, to expand the lungs.

The nurse also monitors fluid balance. Syndrome of inappropriate antidiuretic hormone (SIADH) is very common in the child who has had a spinal fusion because of change in the fluid volume. Anesthetic medications as well as the physical and emotional stress of the surgery can lead to SIADH.

The nurse must assess circulation in the child's lower extremities, the incision, the bowel sounds in all four quadrants along with the softness of the abdomen each time vital signs are assessed. Any changes in the neurovascular status and signs of redness, swelling, drainage, or dehiscence (separation of the suture line) must be reported to the physician.

Pain from a spinal fusion surgery can be severe. Various methods are used to control pain in the postoperative patient. Continuous infusion of an opioid can be used for nonverbal patients. PCA is effective and commonly used for those patients who are able. In some cases, an epidural with bupivacaine (Marcaine) anesthetic alone or combined with an opioid such as morphine sulfate (Astramorph) or hydromorphone (Dilaudid) is used with success. Pain management is usually switched to the oral route by postoperative day three. The oral analgesic of choice is acetaminophen (Tylenol) with codeine. Acetaminophen (Tylenol) with codeine can be administered to children who are too young for oxycodone (Percocet) and is available in a liquid form, if needed. For older children, oxycodone (Percocet) can be used as the oral drug of choice.

Ambulation is permitted (usually about five days postoperatively). Early mobilization is important in the care of the child who has had a spinal fusion to prevent atelectasis, pneumonia, pulmonary emboli, phlebitis, and skin breakdown. The nurse should also perform passive ROM to all extremities. To turn the patient, the nurse needs to use the logrolling technique.

Nutrition is important for wound and bone healing. A regular diet with added calcium, fiber, and fluids is maintained. Encourage the child who has had a spinal fusion to increase fluid intake and consume foods high in fiber to help to relieve constipation. Docusate (Colace) can be administered to soften the stools. Vitamin C and protein help the healing process and should be added to the child's diet. Calcium supplements should be considered if the child's diet is not well balanced. The child may need iron supplementation to augment anemia caused by the surgery.

Collaboration with physical therapy is necessary to assist with ambulation training in addition to ROM exercises. The physical therapist also teaches strengthening and isometrics exercises. The wheelchair may need to be adjusted if the child is wheelchair-bound. The orthotist fabricates the orthotic brace and makes any necessary adjustments.

The nurse arranges for home care for the child. A caregiver needs to be home with the child at all times. The child will need durable medical equipment for the home environment, such as an elevated toilet seat and shower chair. A hospital bed may also be needed in some circumstances. The nurse can explain activity restrictions to the child and caregivers (no twisting or bending, no lifting of heavy objects, no contact or high-impact sports for 2 years). The child may return to school about 4 to 6 weeks after surgery.

Tetanus

Tetanus (lockjaw) is a preventable, acute, and potentially fatal disease. Tetanus occurs when an exotoxin, which is produced by an anaerobic, gram-positive bacillus

(*Clostridium tetani*) forms spores. The spores are found in soil, dust, and human gastrointestinal tracts. These spores enter the body through wounds such as burns; stabs; minor, unnoticed breaks in the skin; and the umbilical cord of a newborn.

 Ethnocultural Considerations— **Tetanus**

Spores entering through the umbilical cord of the newborn are seen more often in developing countries, where women are not immunized against tetanus, contaminated instruments are used to cut the umbilical cord, or poultices are made from cow dung or fermented milk and used for cord care. The greatest incidence of tetanus is during warmer months when people are outdoors more frequently.

Prevention of tetanus is the best defense. For the organism to grow in the human, four requirements must be fulfilled: a presence of tetanus spores, an injury to the tissues, wound conditions that enable multiplication of the spores, and a susceptible host. When the natural defense mechanisms fail, the organism proliferates and forms exotoxins known as tetanospasmin. Tetanospasmin affects the central nervous system through the neuron axons and the vascular system.

 Across Care Settings: **Tetanus prophylaxis**

Tetanus prophylaxis through immunization is the key to preventing tetanus. The nurse plays a key role in ensuring that the immunization is complete. The school nurse and the nurse in the primary care provider's office are in the best position to ensure that complete tetanus immunization occurs.

Signs and Symptoms

Symptoms of tetanus can develop between 5 and 15 days after the initial wound. The child initially presents with a progressive stiffness and tenderness of the muscles in the neck and jaw and has trismus (difficulty opening the mouth). Risus sardonicus (a peculiar grin) is also present due to facial muscle spasms.

As the disease progresses, there is more involvement of the muscles in the body. Opisthotonus posturing occurs when there is a rigid and severe arching of the back, with the head thrown backwards. There is also a board-like rigidity of the abdomen and limb muscles. The child develops difficulty swallowing. The child becomes hypersensitive to stimuli such as a slight noise, bright lights, and gentle touch. These stimuli trigger paroxysmal muscular contractions lasting from seconds to minutes. As the disease progresses further, the contractions recur with increasing frequency until they are almost continuous. Laryngospasm and tetany of the respiratory muscles develop. As a result, secretions accumulate, atelectasis and pneumonia develop, and finally respiratory arrest occurs. During all of these phases of symptomology, the child remains alert. Pain and distress can be determined through the child becoming tachycardic, sweating, and an anxious expression. Generally, the child remains afebrile. If a fever occurs, it is only a mild fever.

Diagnosis

Diagnosis is based on patient history and physical examination findings.

Nursing Care

Prophylactic therapy is administered after trauma. Tetanus antitoxin (TAT) is no longer available in the United States. An unprotected or inadequately immunized child who has sustained an injury that is prone to tetanus needs to be given tetanus immune globulin (TIG). Tetanus toxoid (tetanus toxin modified so that its toxicity is reduced, while retaining its capacity to promote active immunity) is administered (Venes, 2009). The child continues to receive the complete immunization for tetanus at the correct intervals. The nurse communicates to the family that antibiotics will be prescribed to control the proliferation of exotoxin. Antibiotics of choice are penicillin G (Pfizerpen) or erythromycin (Erythrocin). Tetracycline (Sumycin) may be used in older children whose dentition is complete.

If prophylaxis is not used, treatment in the acute phase of the disease is through aggressive support in the ICU. The child is closely monitored and given respiratory support in a quiet environment. Fluids and electrolytes, as well as caloric intake, are monitored closely. The nurse initiates nasogastric (NG) enteral feedings for the child. In the case of severe laryngospasm, total parenteral nutrition or enteral feedings through a gastrostomy tube (GT) may need to be initiated. Recurrent laryngospasm may necessitate endotracheal intubation and mechanical ventilation.

One key to providing nursing care for the child with tetanus is to control or eliminate stimulation from light, sound, and touch. The nurse understands the importance of avoiding unnecessary handling and sudden or loud noises. The nurse must perform frequent neurological and vital sign assessments. Assess oxygen saturation and arterial blood gases regularly. Emergency equipment must be placed close to the child's bed. Oropharyngeal suctioning is done when there is an accumulation of secretions. The nurse assesses for excessive central nervous system depression and for muscle spasms. Medication administration is an important nursing action to keep the child as comfortable as possible. If a neuromuscular blocking agent is being used, the nurse needs to pay close attention to the effects of those agents (see Medication box).

 Nursing Insight— *Neuromuscular blocking agent*

Important ideas to remember when caring for a child treated with a neuromuscular blocking agent:

- The child has total paralysis, including respiratory function.
- The child is not able to communicate.
- The child is anxious.
- The child is aware of all activity around him or her.
- The child is terrified.
- The nurse needs to anticipate the child's needs.
- The nurse needs to explain all procedures.
- The nurse should never leave the child alone.
- The nurse should reduce anxiety in the child by
  - Using a calm, reassuring manner
  - Support and understand the child's fear
  - Encourage the parents to stay with the child
- The nurse needs to medicate the child with an anxiolytic (antianxiety agent).

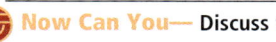

medications: Pharmaceuticals Used for Tetanus

Medications are used to alleviate the muscle spasms and seizures.

- Diazepam (Valium) is the drug of choice to control seizures. It is a benzodiazepine, anxiolytic and an anticonvulsant (Robertson and Shilkofski, 2005).
- Lorazepam (Ativan) may also be used. It is also a benzodiazepine anticonvulsant. It may cause respiratory depression especially when used in combination with other sedatives. Onset of action is 1–5 minutes intravenously, 30–60 minutes intramuscularly, and 20–30 minutes orally with a duration of action of 6 to 8 hours. Flumazenil (Romazicon) is the antidote (Robertson and Shilkofski, 2005).
- Intrathecal baclofen (Lioresal) is a centrally reacting skeletal muscle relaxant and can be effective in treating these children. Abrupt withdrawal of the medication should be avoided. Oral doses should be administered with food or milk and should be used with caution in children with a seizure disorder or impaired renal function (Robertson and Shilkofski, 2005).
- Dantrolene sodium (Dantrium) is a skeletal muscle relaxant and can be effective. Caution should be used when administering to a child with cardiac or pulmonary impairment. Unnecessary exposure to light should be avoided. This medication should not be allowed to extravasate into the surrounding tissue. Discontinue if benefits are not evident in 45 days (Robertson and Shilkofski, 2005).
- Midazolam (Versed) is a benzodiazepine and can also be effective. Contraindicated in patients with narrow angle glaucoma and shock. It causes respiratory depression, hypotension, and bradycardia. Cardiovascular monitoring is necessary. Doses should be reduced when given in combination with narcotics or in patients with respiratory compromise. Serum concentrations may be increased by cimetidine (Tagamet), erythromycin, itraconazole, ketoconazole, and protease inhibitors. Sedative effects may be antagonized by theophylline. The effects of the medication can be reversed with flumazenil (Romazicon) (Robertson and Shilkofski, 2005).
- Neuromuscular blocking agents are used when the child is suffering severe unresponsive tetanus. These two are nondepolarizing neuromuscular blocking agents.
- Rocuronium (Zemuron) may cause hypertension, hypotension, tachycardia, and bronchospasm. There is a risk of increased neuromuscular blockade when administered in conjunction with aminoglycosides, clindamycin, tetracycline, magnesium sulfate, quinine, quinidine, succinylcholine, and inhalation anesthetics. There is a risk of a reduction in neuromuscular blocking effects when used in conjunction with carbamazepine, phenytoin, azathioprine, and theophylline. Peak effects occur in 0.5–1 minute. Duration is 30–40 minutes (Robertson and Shilkofski, 2005).
- Vecuronium bromide (Norcuron) may cause arrhythmias, rash, and bronchospasm. It should be used with caution in patients with renal or hepatic failure and neuromuscular disease. Infants from 7 weeks to 1 year of age are more sensitive to the medication and may have a longer recovery period. Children from 1 to 10 years may need higher and more frequent doses. Potency can be increased with administration of enflurane, isoflurane, aminoglycosides, magnesium salts, tetracyclines, bacitracin, and clindamycin. Neostigmine, pyridostigmine, and edrophonium are antidotes. Onset is 1–3 minutes. Duration is 30–90 minutes (Robertson and Shilkofski, 2005).

The nurse assesses hydration and nutrition. The child must be maintained on total parenteral nutrition (TPN) or enteral feeds through a NG tube or gastrostomy tube.

The nurse collaborates with the respiratory therapist and physician to ensure that the child receives adequate respiratory support and that seizures are kept under control. The nurse needs to collaborate with the pharmacist regarding the administration of the medications to eradicate the exotoxin from the child. Nursing care should be clustered so that the child has a chance to rest and recover from the stress of the intervention.

Now Can You— Discuss tetanus?

1. Describe the prophylaxis treatment for a child at risk of tetanus?
2. Describe the symptoms of tetanus?
3. Describe the critical nursing actions needed to care for a child with tetanus?
4. Describe the medications and the important facts regarding the medications for a child with tetanus?

OSTEOGENESIS IMPERFECTA

Osteogenesis imperfecta (OI), or brittle bone disease, is the most common genetic disorder of the bone. Osteogenesis imperfecta is a group of autosomal dominant diseases characterized by excessive fragility of the bones causing a high rate of fracture. It occurs equally in all races and is equally prevalent between males and females. It is a biochemical defect that causes a decrease in the synthesis of collagen. It affects all connective tissue in the body. Children may become disabled as a result of the severe deformities.

Signs and Symptoms

In OI, the joints are lax and the muscles are small and weak. Any undue stress on the bone causes a fracture (e.g., changing the infant's diaper can cause a femur fracture). The fracture heals within the normal period, but the bone lacks the normal strength. Bone deformities such as bowing and growth pattern disturbances occur. Some newborns die of complications caused by the extreme fragility of the bones.

Diagnosis

Reliable prenatal diagnosis about OI is not currently available. Diagnosis is based on the severity of clinical symptoms and the level of disability. There are five major types of OI that are based on severity and the mode of genetic transmission (Table 30-2).

A unique feature of this disease is that there is very little bruising or swelling, only tenderness at the fracture site. Laboratory studies are not useful in the diagnosis of osteogenesis imperfecta. Radiographic studies show multiple normal callus formations at new fracture sites, evidence of previous fractures, and skeletal deformities. In addition, radiographs will reveal generalized osteopenia, which is an insufficiency of bone. A collagen biopsy will confirm the diagnosis.

Nursing Care

Treatment can include surgery to reduce fractures, correct spinal deformities, and straighten long bones. Intramedullary rodding of the femur is not a perfect solution, but can provide stability to a deformed bone. A solid intramedullary rod is easier to insert, but does not grow with the child and needs to be replaced every 2 to 4 years. A telescoping intramedullary rod is more complicated to insert, but can be adjusted as the child grows.

Table 30-2 Major Types of Osteogenesis Imperfecta

Type I	Type II	Type III	Type IV	Type V
Autosomal dominant	Autosomal recessive	Most autosomal recessive	Autosomal dominant	Autosomal dominant
Subtypes A, B, and C		Few autosomal dominant	Subtypes A and B	
Blue sclerae present	Lethal	Blue sclerae at birth	Normal sclerae in both subtypes	Normal sclerae
	Stillbirth at 50%	Less blue with age		
Subtypes A and B have severe bone fragility with spontaneous decrease in fractures during adolescence	Thin, fragile skin	Severe bone fragility	Subtype A has mild to moderate bone fragility, short stature, variable deformity	Clinically similar to type IV
	Multiple rib fractures	Fractures present at birth		Hyperplastic callus
Subtype C has no bone fragility	Diffuse osteopenia in face and skull	Death in childhood	Subtype B has mild to moderate bone fragility, short stature, variable deformity PLUS dentinogenesis imperfecta instead of normal teeth	Collagen mutation is negative
Subtype B and C have dentinogenesis imperfecta instead of normal teeth				
			Subtype B is about 6% of all cases	
Hearing loss between 20 and 30 years of age	Beak-like nose	Development of kyphoscoliosis	Bowing of lower limbs	Bowing of lower limbs
Flat feet	Short, bent, and deformed limbs	Skull deformity	Generalized osteopenia	Generalized osteopenia
Kyphosis as an adult	10% of cases classified as type II	Short stature		
Excessive hyperlaxity of ligaments		Generalized osteopenia		
Mild short stature		Diaphoresis		
Two-thirds of cases classified as type I				

In an article by Rauch and Gilorieux (2004, p. 1377) the most important therapeutic advance is the introduction of bisphosphonate (Reclast). Bisphosphonate (Reclast) is an inhibitor of osteoclastic bone resorption and is used in treatment for moderate to severe forms of OI. The best treatment regimen and the long-term outcomes of bisphosphonate (Reclast) therapy are unknown. Treatment with bisphosphonate (Reclast) is an adjunct therapy for children with OI and should be used in conjunction with physical therapy, rehabilitation, and orthopedic care.

When caring for an infant who presents with a fracture, it is important to rule out OI as well as child abuse. In many instances, the diagnosis of OI is made after the family has been evaluated for possible child abuse or neglect. This can be a very difficult time for the family.

> ### 🌀 where research and practice meet:
> **Osteogenesis imperfecta**
>
> Nonsurgical treatment with olpadronate (a bone-resorption inhibitor) therapy has been studied in a blinded placebo-controlled trial with a 2-year follow-up in the Netherlands. The study concluded that fracture risk was decreased. Patients who were treated with olpadronate had greater increases in spinal bone mineral content and bone mineral density (Sakkers et al., 2004).

❝ What to say ❞ — *Osteogenesis imperfecta*

An important nursing intervention for the nurse is to teach the parents of an infant just diagnosed with osteogenesis imperfecta to watch for signs of a fracture. The nurse can communicate that the signs of fracture include irritability, fever, and refusal to eat. The nurse should tell parents of an older child that signs to watch for are pain, swelling, and possible deformity at the site.

If the child is going for surgery to reduce and immobilize a fracture, ensure that the child is adequately hydrated with intravenous fluids. Postoperative care involves frequent vital sign and neurovascular assessments. Pain management is also an important critical nursing action. Intravenous narcotics are administered as indicated. If the child is old enough to use a patient-controlled analgesia (PCA), it should be used to keep pain control at a more constant, therapeutic level. When the child is able to tolerate solid food, pain medication is changed to an oral narcotic such as acetaminophen (Children's Tylenol) with codeine. Children with OI have excessive fluid loss through their skin, so they have a much greater need for hydration. The nurse assesses hydration status with every vital sign assessment.

Social development may be delayed in a child with OI because of increased dependence on parents and decreased social interactions. Play and physical therapy should be used with these children. Family can play with the child. The physical therapist directs range-of-motion exercises and muscle-strengthening exercises. The physical therapist also helps the child regain mobility after surgery or a fracture and ensures that the child can use the ambulatory devices safely. If deformities are present, ambulatory devices such as a walker or wheelchair may be necessary.

Most families are unaware of the different types of OI and the prognosis for each type. Encourage parents to receive genetic counseling. Causing a fracture is the biggest fear of these parents. Focus information toward the specific type of OI. Specific instructions about how to hold their infant, change the infant's diaper, and position their infant to reduce the possibility of fracture should be reviewed to help parents feel comfortable caring for their infant. The goal is to achieve a balance between protecting the child from fractures and allowing the child to live as normal a life as possible.

Osteoporosis

Osteoporosis is a condition that develops in postmenopausal women. The bones lose density and calcium and become brittle. Fractures of the hip and vertebrae are common in women with osteoporosis. Adequate intake of calcium and vitamin D are very important during the adolescent years when bone formation is maximized. This helps prevent osteoporosis in later years. Many adolescents do not ingest the necessary requirements of calcium and vitamin D, which puts them at risk for osteoporosis later in life. Some lifestyle choices also put adolescents at risk for osteoporosis (e.g., smoking, using alcohol, drinking excessive amounts of soda, keeping their weight very low).

A study by Lypaczewski, Lappe, and Stubby (2002) showed that the intake of calcium in school-age and adolescent girls plays an important role in preventing the development of osteoporosis. It is important for nurses to educate parents and children about the need to have adequate calcium intake in childhood as a means to prevent osteoporosis in adulthood.

Children can develop osteoporosis related to imbalanced nutrition or some pathological conditions. Osteopenia or low bone mass, between 1 and 2.5 standard deviations below the norm, precedes osteoporosis. Premature, very low birth weight infants often suffer from osteopenia of prematurity because bone mass is acquired in the last weeks of gestation. These infants may have an inability to ingest sufficient nutrients due to their prematurity or other health problems related to their prematurity. Physical activity helps increase bone mass. Activity is often less in premature infants so there is a decreased amount of mechanical loading on their bones.

Older children can also present with osteoporosis as a result of decreased mechanical loading. Children who have a health condition that results in decreased ambulation or minimal pressure on the long bones are at risk for osteoporosis. Children with any of the following diseases are at risk for osteoporosis: spina bifida, cerebral palsy, juvenile arthritis, osteogenesis imperfecta, diabetes, growth hormone deficiency, and Turner syndrome. Immobilization can also lead to osteoporosis, so children who are immobilized in traction or children who are wearing a cast are at risk.

Signs and Symptoms

The precursor to osteoporosis is osteopenia. Osteoporosis is a disease that strikes silently. Signs or symptoms may not become apparent for years. It may become apparent when an infant or child suffers a fracture and the x-ray exam confirms this diagnosis.

Diagnosis

Diagnosis includes complete blood count (CBC), sedimentation rate, urinalysis, chemistry panel, arthritis panel, serum protein electrophoresis, and x-ray of the involved bones. A skeletal survey may be necessary. Bone scans are often useful.

Nursing Care

Nursing care includes encouraging dietary intake of calcium and vitamin D and physical activity to promote bone strength.

 Ethnocultural Considerations— **Caring for a Hispanic child**

Families of Hispanic background believe in *mal ojo* or "the evil eye." They believe that the *mal ojo* is an illness that affects children and occurs when someone with special powers looks at or admires a child, but does not touch the child. For this reason, it is very important for a nurse to touch the child when making an admiring statement about him or her. The parents may call a *curandera* or *curandero* to treat the child through touch and prayer. They may have the child wear special amulets or charms to protect him or her from the *mal ojo*. Hispanic families believe that the saints help their sick child recover. They may place holy pictures of saints on or near their child. It is very important for the nurse to respect this practice and not replace the pictures, amulets, or charms on or near the child in the absence of the parents. (Information retrieved from personal communications with R. Spector, PhD [2006], who has performed extensive research on cultural competence and with a Hispanic student from the Dominican Republic.)

summary points

- Growth and development of the musculoskeletal system play a major role in the normal growth and development of the child.

- The nurse understands that casts, skin traction, skeletal traction, and distraction devices are effective methods in treating musculoskeletal conditions in the child.

- Complications can occur when a child is immobilized in a cast. The major complication that can occur is compartment syndrome, which is caused by an accumulation of fluid in the fascia.

- A nursing assessment of a child in a cast includes the 5 P's: pain and point to tenderness, pulse present at the distal site, pallor, paresthesia, and paralysis.

- The nurse recognizes that the main principle of traction is to reduce dislocations and immobilize fractures in the child.

◆ When caring for a child with a musculoskeletal condition a neurovascular status must be assessed carefully and every 1 to 2 hours for the first 48 hours. A thorough neurovascular status consists of pain, sensation, motion, temperature, capillary refill time, color, and pulses.

◆ The nurse understands that symptoms of compartment syndrome include a burning sensation, pain, pallor, pulselessness, paresthesia, and paralysis.

◆ Distraction devices are usually used to lengthen a bone where the surgeon cuts through a bone and places the distraction device.

◆ Clubfoot is a term used to describe a foot deformity diagnosed in newborn infants. The most severe form of this condition resembles a "club" and is called talipes equinovarus. It requires long-term follow-up since there is a residual lifelong atrophy of the calf muscle.

◆ There are four stages of Legg–Calve–Perthes disease (LCPD); aseptic necrosis, revascularization, new bone formation and the regenerative phase. It is a self-limiting disease that can take between 18 months to 4 years for the child to emerge from it. The child needs to participate in non–weight-bearing activities during the course of the disease.

◆ Nursing care of the child with slipped femoral capital epiphysis (SFCE) includes bedrest, assisting the family in adjusting to the sudden hospitalization, non–weight-bearing status of the child, and the impending surgery. After surgery, the nurse also needs to monitor the neurovascular status frequently and manage pain.

◆ Nursing diagnoses for a child with a fracture include risk for injury related to external devices, impaired physical mobility related to external devices, and risk for impaired skin integrity related to external devices.

◆ Soft tissue injuries are sprains and strains and are unusual in young children. Sprains and strains are often seen in the adolescent age group.

◆ The increase in popularity of competitive sports, recreational sports, and cheerleading has significantly increased the number of overuse injuries, sprains, strains, and dislocations.

◆ The nurse understands that all types of osteomyelitis require immediate treatment.

◆ The child with juvenile arthritis will have joints that are swollen, tender, and warm to touch and limited ROM. The joints will have a loss of motion and will be stiff, especially in the morning. Intermittent joint pain that lasts longer than 6 weeks should be suspect for juvenile arthritis.

◆ In Duchenne's muscular dystrophy, the symptoms first appear after the child is able to walk, usually about 3 to 7 years of age. The child develops a waddling, wide-based gait and uses the Gower maneuver to rise from the floor.

◆ Positioning of the child after surgery for scoliosis is an important nursing action. The child must be turned using the logrolling technique.

◆ Early mobilization is important in the care of the child who has had a spinal fusion. Early mobilization prevents atelectasis, pneumonia, pulmonary emboli, phlebitis, and skin breakdown.

◆ Prevention of tetanus is the best defense; tetanus prophylaxis through immunization is the key to preventing this condition.

◆ Reliable prenatal diagnosis about osteogenesis imperfecta (OI) is not currently available. Diagnosis is based on the severity of clinical symptoms and the level of disability.

◆ Research shows that an intake of calcium in school age and adolescent girls plays an important role in preventing the development of osteoporosis.

review questions

Multiple Choice

1. The pediatric nurse is caring for a 5-year-old child in traction related to a broken femur. The nurse understands the importance of performing a neurovascular assessment every 4 hours. Select all of the following nursing interventions that apply to a neurovascular assessment.
   A. Assess the child's respiratory rate.
   B. Assess the child's ability to move his toes.
   C. Assess the child's color of the affected leg.
   D. Assess the child's pedal pulse.
   E. Assess the child's abdominal pain.

2. The nurse is experiencing some difficulty when caring for a child who is immobilized due to traction. The nurse consults the child-life specialist and a plan is developed to decrease this child's anxiety as well as provide stimulation. The priority intervention is:
   A. Providing diversional activities
   B. Allowing tutoring once a day
   C. Consulting the social worker
   D. Administering pain medication

3. The nurse is preparing a 7-year-old child to have a cast removed from his leg. The nurse can prepare the child for cast removal with which statement?
   A. "As soon as the cast comes off, you can get up and move around."
   B. "The sound of the cast removal instrument will be very loud."
   C. "You must sit very still so we don't accidentally hurt your leg."
   D. "Don't worry, you will be asleep during the cast removal."

Select All that Apply

4. An 8-year-old boy is admitted to the hospital to rule out Legg–Calve–Perthes disease. During the admission interview, the parent tells the nurse that her son has been complaining of hip pain for the past 2 weeks. Which of the following assessment findings helps the nurse confirm the diagnosis of Legg–Calve–Perthes disease?
   A. The pain increases with activity and decreases with rest.

B. The nurse notices that the child has a painful limp.

C. There is quadriceps muscle atrophy.

D. The parent reports that the child currently has a fever.

5. A 10-year-old child is being discharged home with a diagnosis of juvenile arthritis. The pediatric nurse is aware that the family will need discharge teaching. Which of the following care measures should the nurse include in the discharge teaching plan?

A. Teach the family about passive range-of-motion exercises.

B. Teach the family that most children develop other disabilities.

C. Teach the family about corticosteroid medication therapy.

D. Teach the family that the prognosis for remissions is 100%.

True/False

6. The pediatric nurse is aware that a fracture in a child will occur when the bone undergoes more stress than it can absorb.

7. When a child falls and damages the epiphyseal plate, the affected limb can suffer length discrepancy and deformity.

8. The pediatric nurse is aware that the best treatment for compartment syndrome is prevention.

9. Based on the bone structure of an infant who has osteogenic imperfecta, the nurse knows that changing the infant's diaper usually results in a femur fracture.

Fill-in-the-Blank

10. When caring for a child with a broken leg, it is important for the nurse to perform pin care in an effort to prevent _____.

11. The child with a slipped femoral capital epiphysis will complain of pain in the _____ or referred pain to the _____ of the affected _____.

12. A compression fracture usually occurs in the _____.

See Answers to End of Chapter Review Questions on the Electronic Study Guide or DavisPlus.

REFERENCES

Bulechek, G., Butcher, H.M., & Dochterman, J. (2008). *Nursing interventions classification (NIC)* (5th ed.). St. Louis, MO: C.V. Mosby.

Cassas, K.J., & Cassettari-Wayhs, A. (2006). Childhood and adolescent sports-related overuse injuries. *American Family Physician, 73*, 6.

Fallath, S., & Letts, M. (2004). Slipped capital femoral epiphysis: an analysis of treatment outcome according to physeal stability. *Canadian Journal of Surgery, 47*(4), 284–289. Retrieved from the CINAHL Plus with Full Text database (Accessed October 27, 2006).

Ilowite, N. (2002). Current treatment of juvenile rheumatoid arthritis. *Pediatrics, 109*, 109–115.

Ippolito, E., Farsetti, P., Caterini, R., & Tudisco, C. (2003). Long-term comparative results in patients with congenital clubfoot treated with two different protocols. *Journal of Bone and Joint Surgery, 85-A*(7), 1286–1294.

Johnson, M., Bulechek, G., Butcher, H., McCloskey Dochterman, J., Maas, M., Moorehead, S., & Swanson, E. (2006). *NANDA, NOC, and NIC linkages: Nursing diagnoses, outcomes, & interventions* (2nd ed.). St. Louis, MO: Mosby Elsevier.

Lypaczewski, G., Lappe, J., & Stubby, J. (2002). 'Mom & me' and healthy bones: An innovative approach to teaching bone health. *Orthopedic Nursing, 21*(2), 35–42. Retrieved from the CINAHL Plus with Full Text database (Accessed July 23, 2008).

Moorehead, S., Johnson, M., Maas, M., & Swanson, E. (2008) *Nursing outcomes classification (NOC)* (4th ed.). St. Louis, MO: C.V. Mosby.

NANDA International (2007). *NANDA-I nursing diagnoses: Definitions and classifications 2007–2008.* Philadelphia: NANDA-I.

Patterson, M. (2005). Multicenter pin care study. *Orthopedic Nursing, 24*(5), 349–360. Retrieved from the CINAHL Plus with Full Text database (Accessed December 29, 2006).

Rauch, F., & Gilorieux, F. (2004). Osteogenesis imperfecta. *Lancet, 363*(9418), 1377–1385. Retrieved from the CINAHL Plus with Full Text database (Accessed October 27, 2006).

Robertson, J., & Shilkofski, N. (2005). *Harriet Lane handbook: A manual for pediatric house officers* (17th ed.) St. Louis, MO: C.V. Mosby.

Saakers, R., Kok, E., Engelbert, R., van Dongen, A., Jansen, M., Pruiis, H. Verbout, A., Schweitzer, D., & Uiterwaal, C. (2004). Skeletal effects and functional outcome with olpadronate in children with osteogenesis imperfecta: A 2-year randomised placebo-controlled study. *The Lancet, 1:363*, 1427–1431. Retrieved from the CINAHL Plus with Full Text database (Accessed July 23, 2008).

Thompson, G.H. (2004). The spine. In R.E. Behrman, R.M. Kliegman, & H.B. Jenson (Eds.). *Nelson textbook of pediatrics* (17th ed.). Philadelphia: W.B. Saunders.

Venes, D. (Ed.). (2009). *Taber's cyclopedic medical dictionary* (21st ed.). Philadelphia: F.A. Davis.

Wennerberg, S., Gunnarsson, L., & Ahlstrom, G. (2004a). Using a novel exercise programme for patients with muscular dystrophy, Part I: A qualitative study. *Disability and Rehabilitation, 26*(10), 586–594.

Wennerberg, S., Gunnarsson, L., & Ahlstrom, G. (2004b) Using a novel exercise programme for patients with muscular dystrophy, Part II: A quantitative study. *Disability and Rehabilitation, 26*(10), 595–602.

 For more information, go to http://davisplus.fadavis.com/

CONCEPT MAP

Diagnostics → **Caring for the Child with a Musculoskeletal Condition**

Imaging Tests
- Radiography
- Fluoroscopy
- Arthrography
- CT/bone scan
- Ultrasound
- MRI

Lab Tests
- CBC, ESR, RF
- C-reactive protein
- Calcium/phosphorus
- Bone biopsy
- Fluid aspirations

Orthopedic Injuries
- Fractures
  - Open/closed
  - Classified by location/type
- Soft tissue: sprains/strains
- Sports-related
- Osgood-Schlatter disease
- Knee, elbow injuries
- Dislocations
- Overuse injuries

Congenital/Genetic Link
- Club foot
- Muscular Dystrophy
- Osteogenesis imperfecta
- Slipped femoral capital epiphysis

Immobilization Devices

Casts
- Made of fiberglass or plaster-of-Paris
- Four categories

Traction
- Skin: Bryant's; Russell's
- Skeletal: Crutchfield tongs; 90/90 femoral; Dunlop

Distraction Devices
- To lengthen a bone e.g., Ilizarov fixator

General Nursing Care
- Assessments: hx. of musculoskeletal injuries; mobility impairments/physical restrictions; pain/pain patterns; symmetry; muscle tone; skin; neurovascular
- Care: pain/spasm management; control swelling (RICE); maintain appropriate mobility status; passive ROM; cast care; pin care; well-balanced diet/adequate fluids; prevent further injury by preventing complications; ID exacerbations of chronic conditions; collaborate with orthopedic team
- Support family: help family to → provide age-appropriate diversions, foster independence/self-care; find community resources. Teach correct home care techniques; discuss continuance of education at home; help child cope with activity restrictions.

Growth Disorder
- Legg-Calve-Perthes disease

"Injuries" related to Infection
- Tetanus (lockjaw)
- Osteomyelitis

Other Disorders
- Osteoporosis
- Juvenile arthritis

Spinal Issues
- Scoliosis
- Kyphosis
- Lordosis
- Spinal fusion

Where Research And Practice Meet:
- Pin care: ½ H_2O_2 and Xeroform wraps
- Olpdronate increases mineral content/density of spinal bone

Clinical Alert:
- Alterations in 5 P's
- Classic sign of compartment syndrome: unrelenting pain/unrelieved by narcotics
- Osteomyelitis needs immediate treatment
- Hip-spica cast—be alert for cast syndrome

Nursing Insight:
- Performing neurovascular assessment
  - use of the 5 P's
- LCPD stages: aseptic necrosis, revascularization, new bone formation regeneration
- Neuromuscular blocking agents are used when child is suffering severe tetanus
- Prevent pneumonia by assessing lungs and increasing lung expansion

Ethnocultural Considerations:
- Tetanus: increased during warmer months/in developing nations; in substance abusers
- Hispanic belief in "mal ojo"

What To Say:
- Encourage attachment; allow for verbalization of grief in talipes equiovarus
- Parents → watch for fractures in osteogenesis imperfecta

Critical Nursing Action:
- Use positioning, fiber, fluids to prevent cast syndrome
- Child with casted fracture: prevent complications/attend to safety
- Know when to use log-rolling

Optimizing Outcomes:
- Neurovascular assessment: Pain <5; strong pulse; + sensation distally; + strong distal movement; CRT, 3 sec. pink distal extremity

Collaboration In Caring:
- Child with a fracture; child-life, social services, school teacher
- Coordinate a care conference to help plan discharge and home care
- Modifications in the home environment (physical therapist)
- Child with MO → multifaceted team of HCP

Now Can You:
- Discuss care concerns for the child in a cast or traction
- Describe signs/symptoms and important nursing actions for children with musculoskeletal disorders

Caring for the Child with an Integumentary Condition

 In almost all diseases, the function of the skin is, more or less, disordered; and in many most important diseases, nature relieves herself almost entirely by the skin. This is particularly the case with children. However, the excretion, which comes from the skin, is left, unless removed by washing or by the clothes. Every nurse should keep this fact constantly in mind: if the nurse allows the sick to remain unwashed, or their clothing to remain on them after being saturated with perspiration or other excretion, the nurse is interfering injuriously with the natural processes of health just as effectually as if the nurse were to give the patient a dose of slow poison by the mouth. Poisoning by the skin is no less certain than poisoning by the mouth—only it is slower in its operation.

—Florence Nightingale

LEARNING TARGETS: *At the completion of this chapter, the student will be able to:*

- Discuss the pathophysiology and normal function of the skin.
- Identify common pediatric skin diseases and conditions.
- Explore nursing care for various skin conditions and diseases.
- Plan care for a child with skin diseases and conditions.
- Identify types of wounds and wound healing.
- Identify common pharmacological treatments for skin disorders.
- Plan care for a pediatric client with a burn injury.
- Discuss pressure formation and treatment in children.

---

 moving toward evidence-based practice Nonchemical Head Lice Treatment

Goates, B.M., Atkin, J.S., Wilding, K.G., Birch, K.G., Cottam, M.R., Bush, S.E., & Clayton, D.H. (2006). An effective nonchemical treatment for head lice: A lot of hot air. *Pediatrics, 118,* 1962–1970.

The purpose of this study was to examine the effectiveness of various methods that use hot air to kill head lice infestation and the nits (the egg of a louse or another parasitic insect). The literature review identified that the incidence of head lice infestation is on the increase.

There are three common approaches for treating head lice infestations: chemical shampoos, specialized louse combs, and home remedies. However, each approach has its limitations. The researchers asserted that treatment with hot air provides a fast, safe effective method for killing both the lice and the nits.

Infested children were solicited from area elementary schools. Children younger than 6 years of age and individuals who had

used head lice shampoos or home remedies within the preceding 2 weeks were excluded from the study. One hundred and sixty-nine children who demonstrated evidence of infestation were interviewed. Confirmation of infestation was determined by the researchers through carefully combing the subjects' hair and noting the presence of one or more living, moving lice.

In addition, the parent/guardian of children in area elementary schools was asked to participate in a telephone interview that elicited information regarding a past history of treatment for head lice infestation.

Study participants received one of six hot air treatment methods. Treatments were conducted by the researchers in the home and

(continued)

---

moving toward evidence-based practice (continued)

each required approximately 1 hour. The hot air treatment methods included the following: a bonnet-style hair dryer; a handheld blow-dryer with a diffuser; a handheld blow-dryer with directed heating; a wall-mounted dryer (similar to those found in public restrooms for drying hands), a "LouseBuster" with sections; and a "LouseBuster" with hand piece.

The "LouseBuster" was described as a "custom-built, high-volume, hot-air blower" developed for the study. The "Louse-Buster" with sections was compared to a wall-mounted dryer with a long flexible hose that could be aimed at the participant's scalp. The "LouseBuster" with sections was designed to deliver twice the volume (of hot air) of a handheld blow dryer. The "LouseBuster" with hand piece included a comb-like attachment with coarse teeth that could be pulled through the hair during the treatment. Before implementation of the hot air treatment, each participant's hair was carefully combed with a LiceMeister comb until infestation was confirmed by the presence of one or more living, moving lice. Next, the hair on one side of the scalp was thoroughly combed to remove all lice and eggs. The retrieved nits were placed in an incubator. When no additional lice or nits were found, the child's entire scalp was treated via one of the six hot-air methods. After the hot air treatment was completed, the other side of the scalp was combed for the same length of time spent on the first side. Lice and nits obtained from the second hair combing were collected and incubated for later comparison.

A tally was made of the number of live versus dead lice retrieved from each side of the scalp. The retrieved lice were reexamined periodically for 18 hours to check for the "resurrection effect," in which lice appearing to be killed are not actually dead. The effectiveness of the treatment method was determined "by comparing the percentage of dead lice and non-hatching eggs on the pretreatment and post treatment sides of the scalp (p. 1964)."

The median age of the participants was 10 years; 94.1% were female. The total duration of treatment for each method ranged from 30 to 35 minutes. The mean recorded temperature for the six hot air devices ranged from 130.6°F to 141.4°F (54.8°C to 60.8°C); the mean temperature delivered with all six treatment methods was 131°F (55°C), which has been reported to effectively kill hatched lice.

Treatment method and louse and egg mortality were as follows:

Treatment method	Louse mortality (%)	Louse egg mortality (%)
• Bonnet-style hair dryer	10.1	88.8
• Handheld blow-dryer with a diffuser	20.8	96.7
• Handheld blow-dryer with directed heating	55.3	97.9
• Wall-mounted dryer	62.1	96.5
• "LouseBuster" with sections	76.1	94.0
• "LouseBuster" with hand piece	80.1	98.0

All six hot air methods had an effect on the presence of lice and/or nits. The percentage of killed lice (louse mortality) varied considerably with the percentage of unhatched eggs (egg mortality). The hot air method was effective regardless of hair length or hair thickness and worked equally well for children from diverse ethnic backgrounds, though no data were available regarding participants' hair length or ethnicity. The researchers concluded that one 30-minute application of hot air could effectively and safely eradicate head lice.

---

1. What additional information would you want to consider before recommending the LouseBuster hot air treatment for children with head lice infestation?
2. How is this information useful to clinical nursing practice?

See Suggested Responses for Moving Toward Evidence-Based Practice on the Electronic Study Guide or DavisPlus.

Introduction

The skin is the largest organ in the body; its main purpose is to protect the deeper issues from injury and from foreign matter invasion. The skin also protects the body from exposure to a variety of environmental, pest, tactile, and chemical irritants on a daily basis that can disrupt the effectiveness of the skin as a protective barrier.

Other functions of the skin include synthesis of vitamin D from ultraviolet light, aiding in water retention, and ridding the body of toxins. The skin also helps regulate temperature and initiates the sensations of touch, pain, heat, and cold in the body. While most skin conditions are common across the age span, children are often at a higher risk for certain skin conditions based on their large body surface area and still maturing immune system.

This chapter provides an overview of skin conditions that are common during infancy, childhood, and adolescence. Varieties of treatment regimens with appropriate nursing actions for treating a child with a skin condition are discussed. Complementary regimens and other insights for the nurse are also included.

A & P review   **The Skin**

The skin has three layers: the epidermis, the dermis, and the subcutaneous fatty layer (Fig. 31-1). These three layers act to provide the body with a barrier against external invaders. Each layer of the skin contains specific properties. The epidermis is the outlet for the sweat glands and the hair follicles protrude through this layer. The dermis contains the nerves, muscles, connective tissue, sebaceous and sweat glands, blood vessels, and lymph channels. The subcutaneous fatty layer separates the skin from the underlying tissue as well. While all the accessory structures of the skin—the hair, sebaceous glands, exocrine glands, and apocrine glands—are present at birth, most are immature and cannot function to their full potential until middle childhood (Jarvis, 2005) (Table 31-1). ◆

Figure 31-1 The skin has three layers: the epidermis, the dermis, and the subcutaneous fatty layer.

Table 31-1	Integumentary Changes as Children Grow	
Newborn	**Child**	**Adolescent**
Skin is thin.	Skin thickens with age.	Skin reaches adult thickness.
Friction can cause blistering easily.	Friction and shear are not as destructive to the child's skin, but skin is still developing the bond between epidermis and dermis.	The epidermis and dermis are bound together and firm.
Eccrine sweat glands are functional.	Eccrine sweat glands are functional.	Eccrine sweat glands are fully functional and testosterone increases sweating in the male.
Apocrine sweat glands are not functional.	Apocrine sweat glands grow larger preparing for pubescence.	Apocrine sweat glands are mature at puberty.
Color is lighter than normal for race/ethnicity. Newborns/infants should avoid direct exposure to the sun.	Color is normal for race/ethnicity. Skin is easily sunburned, especially in fair-haired, fair-skinned children.	Color is normal for race/ethnicity functional at adult levels. Melanin is normal and provides some UV protection; however, protection from direct sun is still important.

✿ Nursing Insight— *Infant skin and temperature*

An infant's skin is very thin and contains very little subcutaneous fat. For this reason, temperature regulation becomes an important issue, as the infant tends to lose heat rapidly. Take care not to leave an infant uncovered and exposed for a prolonged time. Owing to their immature neurological system and large body surface area, infants have more difficulty in regulating their body temperature.

Skin Lesions

A skin lesion is a circumscribed area of altered tissue (Venes, 2009). When assessing the skin for a skin lesion, it is important to note the size, shape, color, and texture. The two main types of lesions are primary and secondary. Primary lesions include macules, papules, patches, nodules, tumors, vesicles, pustules, bullae, and wheals. Macules, papules, and nodules are found in children and adolescents with acne. Vesicles and pustules are seen in the child with chickenpox and impetigo. Wheals are often seen in the child with an allergic reaction. Secondary lesions are those that happen as a result of changes from the primary lesions. They include crusts, scales, lichenification, scars, keloids, fissures, erosions, and ulcers (Table 31-2).

Notably visible lichenification or the thickening of the skin with hyperpigmentation is often found on children who have atopic dermatitis. Ulcers may be associated with cancer. Scars are the result of a wound. Keloids, seen mainly in persons of color, result from hypertrophy of the scar tissue that extends beyond the wound edges (Venes, 2009).

Nursing Care Plan   The Child with Eczema

Nursing Diagnosis: Impaired Skin Integrity related to inflammatory processes

Measurable Short-term Goal: The child will regain skin integrity.

Measurable Long-term Goal: The child will not experience secondary infection.

NOC Outcomes:
Tissue Integrity: Skin and Mucous Membranes (1101) Structural intactness and normal physiological function of skin and mucous membranes.
Allergic Response: Localized (0705) Severity of localized hypersensitive immune response to a specific environmental (exogenous) antigen

NIC Interventions:
Infection Protection (6550)
Skin Care: Topical Treatments (3584)
Pruritis Management (3550)

Nursing Interventions:

1. Review family history for allergies or eczema.

   RATIONALE: Assists with diagnosis of lesions as infantile eczema is often associated with familial tendencies.

2. Assess child's skin lesions for location, size, type, drainage, signs of secondary infection, and any precipitating factors.

   RATIONALE: Provides baseline data from which to evaluate improvement or worsening of the condition. Intense itching and scratching may disrupt skin integrity further and lead to secondary infections.

3. Administer cool compresses or medications as ordered to relieve itching and treat secondary infection (specify drug, dose, route, and times).

   RATIONALE: Cold helps reduce irritation. Antihistamines and/or topical steroids may be prescribed to reduce inflammation and pruritis and antibiotics may be required for secondary infection.

4. Teach the family to promote skin hydration by bathing child in a lukewarm bath without harsh soaps and to apply emollient lotions to damp skin.

   RATIONALE: Hot water and harsh soaps may exacerbate the skin irritation. Emollient lotions help trap moisture next to the skin to reduce irritation and itching.

5. Teach the family to dress child in light, soft, nonirritating clothing and to keep the child's fingernails short, smooth, and clean.

   RATIONALE: Overheating and irritating fabrics may increase pruritis and inflammation. Nail care may help prevent secondary infection from itching.

6. Assist the family to identify and remove potential irritants from the child's environment, including harsh detergents, perfumes, rough fabrics, and animal dander.

   RATIONALE: A nonirritating environment helps reduce flare-ups of the condition.

Wounds and Wound Healing

Typical wounds found in the child are a result from cuts, scrapes, and burns, and can be secondary to surgical intervention. When an injury has occurred, skin healing has three phases and these often overlap. The first stage, inflammation, reflects the skin's initial healing response and lasts about 2 to 5 days. This is a preparatory stage for repair. Under normal circumstances, the wound seals itself with blood coagulation, followed by vasodilatation that allows the leukocytes to ingest the bacteria and debris at the site of the injury (Fishman, 2006). In the second phase, proliferation, the blood flow is reestablished to the site and natural débridement occurs. In this phase, lasting 2 days to 3 weeks, the wound contracts and a fine layer of epithelial cells cover the site of new collagen (Fishman, 2006). Finally, during remodeling, the third phase, collagen production occurs that allows for scar formation. This phase, lasting 3 weeks to 2 years, allows the collagen to increase the tensile strength of the newly mended tissue. Scar strength is only 80% as strong as the original tissue (Fishman, 2006) (Fig. 31-2).

 Nursing Insight— Superficial wound management

As a pediatric nurse, it is important to note that in the area of superficial wound management wounds are often closed with tissue adhesives (DERMABOND) that work like glue. While the adhesive is effective in wound closure, the cosmetic outcome is not statistically different from suturing (Ong, Jacobson, & Joseph, 2002). Tending to wounds in this way has decreased both child and parent anxiety.

Skin Infections

A number of invaders can affect the skin and these can be bacterial, viral, or fungal in nature. While most of the skin conditions resulting from these invaders respond quickly to treatment, others require an extended time for healing. The specific pathogens that are responsible for the infection, as well as the treatment and sequelae of the infection, affect

Text continued on page 1002

Table 31-2 Common Skin Lesions and Associated Conditions

Lesion Name	Description	Associated Condition (example)
Primary Lesions		
Macules	Flat, circumscribed area that has color change: <1 cm in diameter	Freckles, flat moles, petechiae, measles, scarlet fever
Papules	Raised, circumscribed area: <1 cm diameter	Warts, moles, lichen planus, scabies
Patches	Macule that is flat and nonpalpable, irregular shape: <1 cm diameter	Port-wine stains, café-au-lait spots, capillary hemangios
Nodules	Raised, firm, circumscribed (deeper than a papule), 1–2 cm diameter	Lipomas, erythema nodosum
Tumors	Raised and solid; may be clear, deep in the dermis, >2 cm in diameter	Lipoma, hemangiomas, neoplasms, benign tumors

Continued

Table 31-2 Common Skin Lesions and Associated Conditions—cont'd

Lesion Name	Description	Associated Condition (example)
Vesicles	Raised, circumscribed, superficial, filled with serous fluid, <1 cm in diameter	Varicella, herpes zoster (shingles)
Pustules	Raised, superficial, like vesicle, but fluid is purulent	Impetigo, acne
Bullae	Vesicle >1 cm in diameter	Blister
Wheals	Raised, irregular shaped, cutaneous swelling, solid; diameter is variable (usually transient)	Urticaria, insect bites, allergic reaction
Secondary Lesions Crusts	Dried body fluid on the skin surface: serum, pus, or blood	Disease where the skin weeps: eczema, impetigo, seborrhea

Table 31-2 Common Skin Lesions and Associated Conditions—cont'd

Lesion Name	Description	Associated Condition (example)
Scales	Raised cluster of keratinized cells, irregular, diameter is variable, can be thick or thin, dry or oily	Seborrheic dermatitis, dry skin, skin flaking after allergic reaction
Lichenification	Rough, thickened epidermal area often in the flexor surface of extremity	Chronic dermatitis
Scars	Fibrous tissue, thin or thick, coloration may be lighter or darker than surrounding skin	Healing wound of any etiology
Keloids	Fibrous tissue (scar) of irregular shape, raised and grown beyond the boundary of the original wound	Postoperative wound healing (more common in persons of color)
Fissures	Linear crack in the epidermis may be deeper; moist or dry	Athlete's foot; cracks at the corner of the mouth or anus

Continued

Table 31-2	Common Skin Lesions and Associated Conditions—cont'd	
Lesion Name	**Description**	**Associated Condition (example)**
Erosions	Depressed, moist, loss of part of the epidermis	After rupture of vesicle or bulla, e.g., Varicella
Ulcers	Concave, moist, loss of epidermis and dermis	Ulceration: stasis, decubitus

Source: Potter & Perry (2004).

both the treatment regimen and the healing response. Three specific pathogens are identified as the most frequent causes of bacterial skin infections: *Staphylococcus aureus, Streptococcus,* and *Pseudomonas*. Viral infections can be caused by any number of viruses but those encountered the most often include a member of the poxvirus group, herpes simplex I or II, and the human papilloma virus (HPV). Fungal infections are also caused by a wide variety of pathogens, the most common being *Candida albicans*.

BACTERIAL INFECTIONS

Acne

Acne vulgaris is the most common bacterial skin disorder (Fig. 31-3). Although acne generally begins in the teen years, it can begin earlier in some children. The onset of adrenal androgenic hormones in the prepubertal child is the primary reason for the occurrence of acne.

SIGNS AND SYMPTOMS. With increase in the androgenic hormones, there is an increase in the size of the sebaceous glands and consequently more sebum secreted. With the increase in sebum secretion, the follicle (a small secretory sac) enlarges, placing the person at risk for a keratin plug. These plugs result in the presence of a comedo that is called a "whitehead." At times, the comedo becomes inflamed and creates enough pressure to rupture. If a follicle is dilated enough to reach the skin surface, a comedo may form what is often called a "blackhead." Hyperpigmentation (increase in color) in the area of insult will remain for weeks to months. If the area is aggravated by mechanical means, such as scratching, squeezing, or harsh chemical cleansers, a scar may form. When inflammation deepens into the dermis, there is a potential for scarring. Often, adolescents who have excessive sebum have more acne present, as sebum is a growth medium for *Propionibacterium acnes* (*P. acnes*) (Lehman, 2001).

DIAGNOSIS. A thorough skin assessment is the method of diagnosis for acne along with a complete history. For an assessment, the nurse can prepare the teen by making sure

Figure 31-2 Three phases of wound healing.
A. Inflammation. *B.* Proliferation. *C.* Remodeling.

- Blood cells fibrin
- Macrophages
- Collagen
- Fibroblasts
- Collagen
- Fibroblasts

Figure 31-3 Acne generally begins in the teen years.

her face, scalp, chest, and back are exposed. Laboratory tests may be ordered when an underlying endocrine disorder is suspected.

NURSING CARE. Adolescents may suffer a psychological burden related to their acne. The nurse must realize that it is important to elicit information from the adolescent about his or her feelings and relationships and if acne is affecting these relationships. If necessary, the nurse can refer the adolescent for further support and intervention.

❝ What to say ❞ — *Assessing acne in an adolescent*

When assessing acne in an adolescent the nurse can ask specific questions that may help guide the acne treatment regimen.

- "When did your acne begin?"
- "What types of cleaning products, makeup, or moisturizers and hair care products are you currently using?"
- "What medications you are taking, including over-the-counter and natural products?"
- "What type of foods do you eat?"
- "Have you noticed certain foods, activities, or environmental factors that affect your acne?"
- "Do you notice a change in your acne related to your menses?"
- "What other dermatologic problems have you had recently or in the past?"
- "Can you tell me how you feel having acne?"

Acne treatment can be as simple as decreasing the use of abrasive cleansers and harsh products or as involved as minor surgery. Most adolescent acne improves with cleansing and proper moisturizing with a water-soluble moisturizer.

 critical nursing action   Cleansing the Adolescent's Face

The nurse can follow these steps when cleansing the adolescent's face:

1. Use a warm moist cloth with antibacterial soap to soak away some of the crusting and then gently wipe away as much crusting as possible before applying the antibiotic topical ointment.
2. Apply the prescribed antibiotic topical ointment with a cotton swab or the finger of a gloved hand.
3. Apply a water-soluble moisturizer.
4. Encourage good hand washing techniques before and after the cleansing.

Note: If the teen is cooperative, allow her as much autonomy in cleansing and treating the area as possible.

If the cleansing approach is not successful, acne washes with benzoyl peroxide may be used. If over-the-counter preparations have not been effective, the adolescent may seek advice from a physician. The physician may then prescribe topical antibiotics such as erythromycin (E-Mycin), clindamycin (Cleocin), and tetracycline (Sumycin). The next line of treatment includes topical retinoids,

including tretinoin (Retin-A), adapalene (Differin), or tazarotene (Tazorac). These treatments tend to be very drying and must not be covered with moisturizers or makeup. Teaching the teen to use these medications at bedtime may increase adherence (Table 31-3).

 Nursing Insight— *Tetracycline (Sumycin)*

Tetracycline (Sumycin) will autofluorescence in the presence of ultraviolet light, thus making the person noticeably "glow" in environments that are lit by black lights. Tetracycline (Sumycin) can also darken the teeth in children younger than the age of 8 years and should not be used in this age group.

When cleansing and topical treatments are ineffective, systemic oral antibiotic therapy may be necessary for teens with especially difficult to resolve acne. The primary systemic medications used are antibiotics, including tetracycline (Sumycin), minocycline (Minocin), doxycycline (Vibramycin), and erythromycin (Erythrocin). If the acne is excessively inflammatory, the incidence of scarring increases and a more potent oral medication may be used. The primary acne medication for inflammatory acne is isotretinoin (Accutane) (Cullen & Lucky, 2001). Follow up, teaching, and monthly visits to the dermatologist are imperative for the adolescent and family when this medication is prescribed.

 Be sure to— **Isotretinoin (Accutane)**

Isotretinoin (Accutane) has been shown to cause severe birth defects. Therefore, women must not take this medication if there is any chance of becoming pregnant. Be sure to discuss this with any adolescent where pregnancy is a possibility. Pregnancy tests must be performed before treatment with this medication, monthly during treatment, and 1 month after the cessation of treatment. Women considering this treatment must use two forms of birth control. Visit iPLEDGE: Committed to Pregnancy Prevention program at http://www.ipledgeprogram.com/ to view the information appropriate for clients undergoing isotretinoin (Accutane) treatment. Other side effects include hypercholesteremia, drying of the mucous membranes, decreased night vision, headaches, depression, and liver damage.

Give adolescents strict instructions not to share this medication with peers and to report any change in mood. Suicidal tendencies have been linked to isotretinoin (Accutane) therapy. If a teen is under the legal age limit, the parents or guardians must read, complete, and sign a designated form that proves they have been informed

Labs: **Liver Enzymes**

Liver enzymes must be drawn once a month to ensure that liver damage is not occurring from the isotretinoin (Accutane). Medication refills are not authorized unless the individual submits to the pregnancy testing guidelines and has blood testing of the liver enzymes. Teens are particularly difficult to manage because they often feel invincible and because they are not as likely to be compliant with this treatment unless a direct effect is seen quickly in their acne improvement.

Table 31-3 Medications for Acne

Name	Indications	Actions	Therapeutic Effect	Contraindications and Precautions
Erythromycin (E-Mycin)	Treatment of acne	Inhibits protein synthesis of bacterial ribosome	Anti-infective	Hypersensitivity, known alcohol intolerance
Clindamycin (Cleocin)	Treatment of skin infections: acne	Inhibits protein synthesis of bacterial ribosome	Anti-infective	Hypersensitivity, previous pseudomembranous colitis, severe liver impairment
Tetracycline (Sumycin)	Treatment of various infections: acne	Inhibits protein synthesis of bacterial ribosome	Anti-infective	Hypersensitivity, known alcohol intolerance, pregnancy, lactation
Tretinoin (Retin-A)	Acne, acute promyelocytic leukemia, wrinkles	By stimulating the transcription process, it increases epidermal cell mitosis and epidermal cell turnover	Anti-acne, antineoplastic, retinoid	Hypersensitivity
Adapalene (Differin)	Acne, chloasma, keratosis	Thought to normalize epithelial cells	Retinoid-like effect	Hypersensitivity
Tazarotene (Tazorac)	Acne, psoriasis, wrinkles	Studies suggest: inhibits growth of human keratocyte	Retinoid	Hypersensitivity, pregnancy
Minocycline (Minocin)	Treatment of various infections: acne	Inhibits protein synthesis of bacterial ribosome	Anti-infective	Hypersensitivity, known alcohol intolerance, pregnancy, lactation
Doxycycline (Vibramycin)	Treatment of various infections: acne Treatment of anthrax	Inhibits protein synthesis of bacterial ribosome	Anti-infective	Hypersensitivity, known alcohol intolerance, pregnancy, lactation
Isotretinoin (Accutane)	Acne	Reduces sebaceous gland size and inhibits sebaceous gland activity	Anti-acne, retinoid	Hypersensitivity, pregnancy

Adverse Reactions and Side Effects	Route and Dosage	Nursing Implications
Nausea/vomiting, rashes	Topical and systemic	Assess child for infection. Obtain specimen for culture and sensitivity before dosing. Assess for improvement in the child's condition.
Diarrhea, rashes, pseudomembranous colitis	Topical and systemic	Assess child for infection. Obtain specimen for culture and sensitivity before dosing. Monitor bowel elimination. Assess for improvement in the child's condition.
Nausea/vomiting, diarrhea, photosensitivity	Systemic	Assess patient for infection. Obtain specimen for culture and sensitivity before dosing. Monitor liver and kidney functions. Assess for improvement in the child's condition.
Oral: Dysrhythmia Topical: Erythema, scaling, dryness, itching, photosensitivity	Systemic and topical Oral: capsule, liquid filled: 10 mg Topical cream: 0.02%, 0.025%, 0.05%, 0.1% Topical gel/jelly: 0.01%, 0.025%, 0.04%, 0.1% Topical solution: 0.05% Usually used one time a day before bed	Assess patient for sensitivity. Assess for superinfection. Assess for improvement in the child's condition.
Erythema, scaling, dryness, itching, photosensitivity	Topical Gel 0.1% Solution 0.1% Usually used one time a day before bed	Assess patient for sensitivity. Assess for superinfection. Assess for improvement in the child's condition.
Topical: Erythema, scaling, dryness, itching, photosensitivity	Safety not established in children <12 years old Topical cream: 0.05%, 0.1% Topical gel/jelly: 0.05%, 0.1%	Assess patient for sensitivity. Assess for superinfection. Assess for improvement in the child's condition.
Nausea/vomiting, diarrhea, photosensitivity	Systemic	Assess patient for infection. Obtain specimen for culture and sensitivity before dosing. Observe for change in skin pigmentation. Monitor liver and kidney functions. Assess for improvement in the child's condition.
Nausea/vomiting, diarrhea, photosensitivity	Systemic	Assess patient for infection. Obtain specimen for culture and sensitivity before dosing. Monitor liver and kidney functions. Assess for improvement in the child's condition.
Dermatologic: Cheilitis, dry skin, itching. Endocrine metabolic: Serum triglycerides raised Hepatic: Hepatotoxicity Psychiatric: Aggressive behavior, depression, violent behavior	Systemic Safety and effectiveness in children less than 12 years not established 1 mg/kg/day ORALLY in 2 divided doses	Obtain a pregnancy test, two tests at baseline, followed by tests monthly during therapy, at the completion of therapy and 1 month after the discontinuation of therapy. Assess for depression, psychosis, suicidal ideation, or aggressive behavior. Monitor hepatic function by obtaining a lipid panel; weekly or biweekly intervals. Register for iPLEDGE Program: www.ipledgeprogram.com. Assess for improvement in the child's condition.

about the risks associated with isotretinoin (Accutane). The iPLEDGE Program is designed to ensure safe administration, prescription, and consumption of this medication. There are exact guidelines that must be followed when filling the prescription. The physician informs parents or guardians about the specific rules and regulations associated with this medication (iPLEDGE, 2005).

Impetigo

Impetigo is a highly contagious bacterial infection. The child is predisposed to the infection via dry or cracked skin where bacteria may invade. Impetigo may be caused by *Staphylococcus aureus* (*S. aureus*) and *Streptococcus pyogenes* (*S. pyogenes*) or both (Watkins, 2005). On rare occasions, other bacteria may be responsible for the skin infection. Infants and children who have a less developed immune system are more prone to this condition as well as children who are in close contact with other children through daycare and school associations (Hill, 2003).

SIGNS AND SYMPTOMS. Impetigo is a bacterial infection of the skin often found on and around the mouth of the child or elsewhere on the face (Fig. 31-4). It can also appear on the hands, neck, trunk, buttocks, or extremities. The lesions begin as a vesicle or pustule surrounded by edema (swelling) and erythema (redness) a common sign of inflammation (Watkins, 2005). Later these lesions erupt, leaving honey-colored exudate. This exudate becomes crusty in appearance and sticky to the touch. The child may experience pruritus (itching) that is not usually painful. Over time, impetigo clears leaving no residual scarring (Watkins, 2005).

DIAGNOSIS. Impetigo is diagnosed through assessment. Rarely does the diagnosis require laboratory testing by culture. A diagnostic culture may be needed if the health care provider is unsure of the exact diagnosis, and is investigating a differential diagnosis such as contact dermatitis or herpes virus (Watkins, 2005).

NURSING CARE. Impetigo is very contagious and passed by touch from the infected child to others. Treatment options vary. Some practitioners may allow for spontaneous resolution by encouraging strict hygiene measures if the child is home and not requiring day care or school involvement. Mupirocin (Bactroban), a topical antibiotic, may be used if the skin lesions are limited (Watkins, 2005). If the skin infection is widespread, the child is required to stay home from school for 24 hours after the induction of the oral antibiotic. Dicloxacillin (Dynapen) is most commonly used for a 7-day regimen. If the child is allergic to this medication, a cephalosporin or Macrolide antibiotics may be used.

Figure 31-4 Impetigo is a highly contagious bacterial infection.

"What to say" — *Teaching about impetigo*

When the nurse is caring for the child with impetigo, it is important to teach the child and caregiver:

- "Do not be embarrassed."
- "It is very important to wash your hands."
- "Try not to scratch the lesions."
- "It is not nice to make fun of other children."

Cellulitis

Cellulitis is a spreading bacterial infection that enters via existent openings in the skin caused by dermatological conditions or trauma that then spreads into the interstitial space. The most common bacteria causing cellulitis are *S. pyogenes* and *S. aureus* (Venes, 2009), particularly *S. pyogenes*. The most frequent location of cellulitis is the face and extremities, particularly the lower legs, but cellulitis can occur anywhere on the body (Venes, 2009).

SIGNS AND SYMPTOMS. The infected area is edematous (swollen), erythematosus (red), and hot to the touch. It is likely that the child will experience discomfort on palpation of the indurated area. Often the child experiences malaise, fever, and chills. Lymphadenitis (inflammation of the lymph nodes) may or may not be present in the region.

DIAGNOSIS. A complete history and physical is the usual method of diagnosis. Lab tests, radiological testing, or

---

Family Teaching Guidelines...
Cellulitis

HOW TO TEACH THE CAREGIVER TO:

- Administer all antibiotics as ordered. Stress to the caregiver not to stop the antibiotics when the skin appears to have improved. The caregiver must realize that failure to finish the antibiotics may result in recurrence of the infection.

- Use warm moist packs to relieve discomfort as needed. If cool moist packs relieve discomfort, this is acceptable.

- Use analgesics such as ibuprofen (Children's Advil) or acetaminophen (Children's Tylenol) if necessary for comfort. If the skin infection is in a limb, elevate the limb to provide comfort and decrease swelling.

- Contact the physician if the redness or edema appears to be worsening, if the child's pain is increasing, or if the temperature remains above 101.5°F (38.6°C) 48 hours after the beginning of antibiotic administration.

ESSENTIAL INFORMATION

Cellulitis is an infection of the skin caused by a bacterium. Cellulitis does not spread from person to person. The bacterium enters the skin and infects the soft tissue through a sore or a cut. If the cellulitis is around the eye, the original infection may have begun in the nose or sinuses. The infected area may look red or purple and be swollen; it will also be tender to pressure. The child may have a fever.

surgical biopsy is used only in the presence of severe infection. Complete blood counts and blood cultures are ordered to rule out septicemia (infection of the blood).

 clinical alert

Group A Streptococcus

Group A *Streptococcus* can cause necrotizing fasciitis (flesh-eating bacteria). Be alert to the following clinical manifestations of necrotizing fasciitis: bruising, crepitus, or bullae filled with bluish/purple colored fluid over the induration (an area of hardened tissue). (Venes, 2009).

NURSING CARE. Benzathine penicillin G (Pfizerpen) orally is usually the antibiotic of choice. Children allergic to penicillin may be given first-generation cephalosporins, then Macrolide antibiotics. One-time intramuscular benzathine penicillin G (Bicillin L-A) may be given in the practitioner's office.

 Optimizing Outcomes— **Family compliance**

The best outcome for a child receiving an antibiotic is for the family to be adherent and administer the entire medication as prescribed. If the family has a history of nonadherence to a medical plan, or if the child cannot take the medication as prescribed, the nurse must notify the health care provider immediately. The health care provider may then choose to order a single dose of intramuscular penicillin instead of the oral medication. Using a topical anesthetic such as EMLA (lidocaine/prilocaine) at the injection site at least an hour before the injection can help decrease the pain.

If a child has a severe case of cellulitis, hospitalization and intravenous antibiotics may be necessary. In addition, steroids to decrease inflammation such as prednisolone (Pediapred) may be ordered but are not routine. Another nursing intervention for symptom control is the administration of an anti-inflammatory medication such as ibuprofen (Children's Advil).

 nursing diagnoses Cellulitis

- Impaired skin integrity related to inflammatory process damaging skin
- Pain related to inflammatory changes in tissues from infection
- Ineffective tissue perfusion: peripheral related to edema.

VIRAL INFECTIONS

Human Papillomavirus

Human papillomavirus infections (warts) are common among children. The human papillomavirus can cause warts by invading the epithelial cells in the skin. The wart is transmitted by direct skin-to-skin or mucous membrane contact as well as from hard surface areas such as plantar warts from gymnasium floors. The usual incubation period is 2 to 6 months but in some cases there is a latency period. Three types of warts occur in children: common wart (verruca vulgaris) the plantar wart (verruca plantaris) and the flat wart (verruca plana).

 medication: Benzathine Penicillin G (Bicillin L-A)

Benzathine penicillin G (ben-za-theen, pen-i-**sill**-in, gee) Bicillin L-A

Pregnancy Category: B

Indications: Treatment of a wide variety of infections: pharyngeal/tonsil/skin as well as prophylaxis for rheumatic fever.

Actions: Binds to bacterial cell wall, resulting in cell death.

Therapeutic Effects: Bacteriostatic action against susceptible bacteria spectrum: *Streptococci, Staphylococci,* and some gram-negative organisms

Pharmacokinetics:
ABSORPTION: IM delayed and prolonged to sustain therapeutic blood levels.

Contraindications and Precautions:
CONTRAINDICATED IN: Hypersensitivity

Adverse Reactions and Side Effects:
Pain at injection site
GASTROINTESTINAL: Diarrhea, epigastric distress, nausea/vomiting
ENDOCRINE: Rash
RESPIRATORY: Anaphylaxis

Route and Dosage:
IM: Children >27 kg, 900–1.2 million units (single dose)
IM: Children <27 kg, 300,000–600,000 units (single dose)

Nursing Implications:
Assess for history of hypersensitivity.
Observe patient for signs of anaphylaxis for a minimum of 15 minutes after injection.
Reconstitute with D5W or 0.9% NaCl.
Administer deeply in a well-developed muscle mass.

Data from Deglin, J.H., & Vallerand, A.H. (2009). *Davis's drug guide for nurses* (11th ed., pp. 958–961). Philadelphia: F.A. Davis.

SIGNS AND SYMPTOMS. Warts are a cutaneous elevation of the skin (Venes, 2009). The warts are rough, raised, and flesh-colored and can occur anywhere on the body (Fig. 31-5). Flat warts generally occur on the face or legs and are sometimes flesh-colored and rarely rough. Plantar warts are found on the soles of the feet on weight-bearing surfaces. They are difficult to differentiate from corns and calluses but usually have a small dark dot near the center secondary to thrombosed vessels. Warts are usually not painful, nor do they itch unless other skin irritation is present. Occasionally, plantar warts cause foot pain if they grow large, and can be surgically removed if painful and not responding to other treatments.

Figure 31-5 Warts are a cutaneous elevation of the skin.

DIAGNOSIS. Diagnosis is based on presenting signs, symptoms, and visual inspection. Often the family makes a diagnosis at home and treats the wart with over-the-counter medications before seeking medical advice. Physician advice is usually sought after a long period of failed resolution, or an increase in the number or size of the warts.

NURSING CARE. The nurse can communicate to the caregiver that most of the time no intervention is needed for warts because 75% of warts resolve on their own within 2 years. Several medications, both over-the-counter and prescription, are available for wart treatment (Table 31-4).

Figure 31-6 Herpes simplex virus 1. Cold sore.

 Now Can You— Discuss bacterial, viral, and fungal skin infections?

1. Name one condition in each category of skin infection?
2. Discuss the priority nursing interventions for the named condition?

 Complementary Care: *Topical agents*

Topical agents that promote healing are frequently used for rashes: cow udder balm (bag balm), green tea extract, vitamin E preparations, aloe vera, milk, calamine, and colloidal oatmeal (Beltrani, 2002).

Herpes Simplex

The herpes simplex virus causes herpes infections. There are two types of herpes virus. Herpes simplex virus 1 (HSV-1) is the common cold sore (Fig. 31-6). HSV-1 can cause painful blisters on mucosal surfaces of the skin, and the most common location for HSV-1 is on the face, usually on the lips and in or near the mouth and nose. HSV-1 can also affect the sclera or the eyelid (Hurtado, 2005; Venes, 2009). Herpes simplex virus 2 (HSV-2) is genital herpes (Fig. 31-7).

Figure 31-7 Herpes simplex virus 2. Genital warts.

Table 31-4 Human Papillomavirus			
Type of Wart	**Common warts (verruca vulgaris)**	**Flat Warts (verruca plana)**	**Plantar Wart (verruca plantaris)**
Treatment and Description	Topical: keratolytic acids (OTC)	Topical tretinoin cream (Prescription)	Topical keratolytic acids
	This topical treatment is applied by dropper or cotton swab. Place the thick liquid directly on the top of the wart taking care to keep this highly acidic fluid off the surrounding skin. The wart will peel away in layers as the acid kills the superficial layers, one at a time.	This topical treatment is applied by using a gloved hand/finger in a thin coating.	This topical treatment is applied by dropper or cotton swab. Place the thick liquid directly on the top of the wart taking care to keep this highly acidic fluid off the surrounding skin. The wart will peel away in layers as the acid kills the superficial layers, one at a time.
	Liquid Nitrogen Cryosurgery		**Liquid Nitrogen Cryosurgery**
	The application of liquid nitrogen to the wart by the practitioner is a common method, which often expedites the wart's demise. The practitioner will direct a narrow flow of the liquid nitrogen to the wart directly, causing it to freeze and therefore killing the warty tissue. This is mildly painful, but efficient.		(with paring and topical chemodestruction to enhance its effectiveness)
			The application of liquid nitrogen to the wart'd by the practitioner is a common method, which often expedites the wart's demise. The practitioner will direct a narrow flow of the liquid nitrogen to the wart directly, causing it to freeze and therefore killing the warty tissue. This is mildly painful, but efficient.

Source: Krusinski, P.A., & Flowers, F.P. (2000, March). Common viral infection of the skin. Retrieved from http://merck.micromedex.com/index.asp?page=bpm_brief&article_id=CPM02DE404&hilight=herpesvirus.

SIGNS AND SYMPTOMS. An infection by a herpes simplex virus is evident by watery blisters in the skin or mucous membranes of the mouth, lips, or genitals. After the virus has been introduced into the body, it establishes a latent infection. Based on a variety of stimuli such as a febrile illness, emotional stress, sexual contact, or ultraviolet light exposure, a lesion appears. The lesions are tender, burn, tingle, or itch before the sore actually appears. The sore usually begins as a red rash progressing on to blisters (vesicles) that open up, leaving a painful ulceration. These ulcerations are virulent and highly contagious (Hurtado, 2005).

DIAGNOSIS. When the child and family arrive at the clinic, the nurse can communicate to them that no specific diagnostic testing is required and that visualization of the lesion is often the only procedure required to diagnose the condition. A family history may reveal that the virus has recently affected other family members. If a differential diagnosis is needed, the practitioner may perform a viral culture of an open area to determine if the lesions are the herpesvirus or a different virus such as the varicella virus (chickenpox) which is similar in appearance.

NURSING CARE. Even though there are no treatments that can cure this viral infection, there are medications that decrease the length of the outbreak and/or increase the intervals between outbreaks. Acyclovir (Avirix) is a prescribed oral medication that can be prescribed for a child older than the age of 2, for their first outbreak or for outbreak suppression. Over-the-counter topical preparations such as docosanol (Abreva) can be used by children older than the age of 12 for local relief of symptoms and potentially to limit the length of the outbreak.

Family Teaching Guidelines...
Herpes Simplex Virus (HSV-1)

HOW TO:

The child and family need to understand how to decrease transmission of this virus and prevent subsequent outbreaks.

ESSENTIAL INFORMATION

◆ Teach the child to keep his or her hands away from the face.

◆ Teach the child good hand washing techniques. To wash the proper amount of time, young children can be taught to sing the alphabet song while rubbing their hands together.

◆ Decrease stressful situations.

◆ Avoid prolonged sun exposure.

◆ Moisturize the lips and use a moisturizing sunscreen on the lips during the summer months (Hurtado, 2005).

 Across Care Settings: Supporting the child during treatment

• The community nurse has an important role in supporting the child and family during treatment. Tell the child and family the origin, signs, and symptoms of the virus in age-appropriate language.

• Create an environment of trust; allowing the child to keep a parent close may help the child cope with the clinic visit better.

• Monitor pain response throughout the visit to determine if the parent will need information about adequate pain control such as acetaminophen (Children's Tylenol).

FUNGAL INFECTIONS

Cutaneous Candidiasis

Candida albicans is the most common of the *Candida* fungi (yeast). It lives naturally in the gut and oral mucosa but is not a threat to intact skin. *Candida* overgrowth can occur in newborns who acquire this fungal infection during the birth process from the vaginal canal of an infected mother. Children who have an immune disorder are at risk for developing oral (thrush) or diaper area candidiasis. Children who use corticosteroid inhalers for allergy and asthma prophylaxis and treatment may develop oral candidiasis as well. Rinsing the mouth after each inhaler dose decreases the likelihood of developing oral candidiasis. Immunocompromised children may develop candidiasis more easily than healthy children.

SIGNS AND SYMPTOMS. The fungal rash appears in the infant's mouth or diaper area and occasionally in the folds of the axillae or the groin. In the mouth, the lesions appear as white or gray plaque that cannot be removed. The plaque can be on the tongue, buccal (cheek) area, or gingival (gums). On the skin, the rash is a fine red and slightly raised with a scallop-like border. A few stray papules may be present near the border of this moist rash area.

DIAGNOSIS. A thorough history of the mother and child's existing conditions, as well as a current visualization of the lesions, helps diagnose this condition. If there is a need for a differential diagnosis, a fungal culture can be obtained (Procedure 31-1).

NURSING CARE. Oral candidiasis is treated with kinesthetic nystatin (Mycostatin) orally after each feeding or two or three times per day. The nurse has a gloved hand and uses a swab to apply the medication to the insides of both cheeks. Remember to use a separate swab for each cheek. Topical treatment for skin infections includes nystatin (Mycostatin), clotrimazole (Lotrimin), miconazole (Monistat), or ketoconazole (Nizoral) ointment applied with a gloved finger applied in a thin layer on the infected area two or three times per day.

 Nursing Insight— How to tell oral thrush from formula or breast milk on the tongue of an infant

Sometimes after an infant drinks formula or breastfeeds, a white film is noted on the tongue. To differentiate the formula or breast milk from oral thrush the nurse can use a tongue

Procedure 31-1 Obtaining a Fungal Culture

Purpose

The purpose of obtaining a fungal culture is to test for the presence of fungi, and, if found, identify the type.

Equipment

Gloves
Tongue blade
Sterile cotton swab
Sterile test tube

Steps

1. Explain the procedure to the child in age-appropriate terms.

   RATIONALE: *A simplified explanation may help decrease anxiety.*

2. Gather all supplies.

3. Aseptically place a sterile cotton swab against a plaque.

   RATIONALE: *Using a tongue blade to keep the child's mouth open and the tongue out of the way.*

4. Vigorously rub the plaque with the cotton swab.

   RATIONALE: *Twirling the swab so that all sides of the swab are exposed to the plaque.*

5. Place the swab into a covered, sterile test tube provided by the laboratory and place in a biohazard bag.

   RATIONALE: *Maintains universal precautions.*

6. Have the specimen transported to the lab within 15–30 minutes.

   RATIONALE: *Timely delivery will help ensure accuracy of test results.*

Clinical Alert The nurse must remember that attempting to remove the oral thrush can cause the lining of the oral mucosa to bleed.

Teach Parents

The final culture is not available for 48–72 hours; preliminary culture results may be available sooner.

Note

The specimen must have a label with the child's name, identification numbers, date/time of collection and the nurse's name or initials.

Caution: Monitor the child's mucosa for bleeding.

Documentation
9/25/10 1500 An oral culture was obtained. Child tolerated the collection without difficulty; no pain or bleeding noted.
—C. Kildare, RN

---

blade to gently scrape the white film. If the nurse can remove the film, it is formula or breast milk. If the nurse cannot remove the film, it is thrush.

Ringworm

Ringworm (dermatophytoses) is a fungal infection that affects the skin, hair, or nails (Fig. 31-8). Children of all ages are affected. It may be spread from person to person or from animal to person. Ringworm may also be spread by contact with inanimate objects such as clothing, furniture, or bed linen of another infected person. Some children may be colonized but remain asymptomatic.

Figure 31-8 Ringworm is a fungal infection that affects the skin, hair, or nails.

The most common ringworm infections are as follows:

Tinea capitis—involves the hair of the scalp, usually seen in pre-pubertal children between the ages of 1 and 10 years.

Tinea corporis—involves the skin of the body, except the scalp, groin, hands and feet; seen in children and adolescents

Tinea cruris—known as "jock itch"; involves the inner thighs, inguinal creases, or perineal area (rare before adolescence)

Tinea pedi—athlete's foot; involves the kinesthetic webbed areas of the toes and feet, seen in children and adolescents

SIGNS AND SYMPTOMS. Symptoms include round, scaly lesions. These areas may be red or inflamed. The patient may have areas that appear bald, due to hair that has broken off. There may be small black dots on the scalp. The child may experience slight itching.

DIAGNOSIS. Ringworm diagnosis is made by visual inspection using a Wood lamp that discloses yellowish gold fluorescent coloration. A potassium hydroxide (KOH) preparation of scrapings is also diagnostic, demonstrating groups of thick-walled spores and myriad short thick angular hyphae resembling spaghetti (Behrman et al., 2004).

NURSING CARE. For most types of ringworm treatment with antifungal drugs in the form of skin creams, lotions or ointments is adequate. If the infection is widespread or affects the hair or nails, griseofulvin (Fulvicin, or Grasactin) in tablet form is prescribed for the child. The medication must be taken for at least 6 weeks to be effective. Absorption of the medication is enhanced if it is given with a high-fat meal. Other drugs such as miconazole (Monistat), fluconazole (Diflucan), and terbinafine (Lamisil) are not yet approved for children (American Academy of Pediatrics [AAP], 2003). Antifungal shampoo is often recommended. The child is checked periodically throughout treatment to be sure a proper response is noted. The nurse must stress that everyone in the family needs to be treated and it is essential not to share hair brushes or bath towels. Specifically, with tinea capitis the effected area of hair growth may take 6 to 12 months to grow or it may not grow back at all. The nurse can provide emotional support and suggest hairstyles to help conceal tinea capitis.

Dermatitis

Dermatitis is an inflammatory rash marked by itching and redness that occurs due to numerous conditions. There are three common classifications of dermatitis in children: contact, atopic, and seborrheic.

CONTACT DERMATITIS

Contact dermatitis can occur if an allergen or skin irritant is encountered (Venes, 2009). In children, the irritative agents that cause this type of skin sensitivity are often soaps or detergents. For infants, the diaper area is especially prone and could be the result of diaper perfumes, cloth diaper detergents, or diaper wipes (Fig. 31-9) (American Academy of Family Physicians [AAFP], 2005). Children playing out of doors may encounter varying plant life that can cause contact dermatitis, specifically poisonous oaks, ivies, or sumacs.

Signs and Symptoms

In the case of contact dermatitis, the skin becomes irritated, inflamed, and pruritic within 48 hours of contact with the offending agent. Vesicles and bullae may be present in this area as well. Vesicles may rupture and weep a serous fluid. The presence of urticaria (hives) is expected (Beltrani, 2002).

Figure 31-9 Contact dermatitis can occur if an allergen or skin irritant is encountered.

Diagnosis

A complete history of contacts both in and out of doors for a child appearing in the community health clinic helps determine the diagnosis. If a differential diagnosis is required because there are atypical lesions, a biopsy may be performed (Beltrani, 2002). If the offending agent is not easily determined, an allergist may be the next appropriate referral to determine if allergic contact dermatitis is the diagnosis. One method of determining an allergy is by completing patch testing. The allergist prepares the proper concentration of allergens in a paraffin base and places this on the child's skin, usually the back, holding it in place with hypoallergenic tape. The patch is left in place for varying times based on the type of allergy being assessed (48 hours of wear is a standard). After the time has passed, the skin is assessed for reaction that is measured by redness and edema.

Nursing Care

On diagnosis, if the nurse notices that there are weepy lesions, a drying agent such as an over-the-counter product such as Domeboro powder (active ingredient, aluminum sulfate) may bring relief. For pruritic relief cool baths are effective. For a longer effect, a low dose of over-the-counter hydrocortisone (A-Hydrocort) cream can be applied with a gloved finger. Oral steroids such as prednisone (Deltasone) are used only if more than 10% of the child's body surface area is involved (Beltrani, 2002). If discomfort from agents such as poison ivy or oak is the concern, a topical anesthetic such as Dermoplast may bring relief. The nurse must remember that children suffering from severe pruritus may require a sedative for sleeping purposes.

 Collaboration in Caring— *A severe allergic reaction*

The parents and community nurse must notify the school nurse, day care providers, coaches, and other adult leaders who spend time with the child about the diagnosed allergy. Everyone must be informed on how to use an EpiPen or EpiPen Jr. (epinephrine). EpiPens are usually kept in the school nurse's office. During sports activities, a second EpiPen may be given to the coach or the assistant. Along with documentation of the allergy, contact information, and the EpiPen that is on-hand, ready access to a phone for emergency medical assistance is a necessity.

nursing diagnoses Contact Dermatitis

- Impaired Skin Integrity related to allergic reaction
- Acute Discomfort related to inflammation of the skin
- Alteration in Sleep Pattern related to pruritus

ATOPIC DERMATITIS

Atopic dermatitis is a chronic skin condition with no known etiology. This condition is found in children with allergies and in children whose family has a history of allergies, asthma, and rhinitis. Approximately 50% of persons with atopic dermatitis present in the first year of life and an additional 30% in the years between ages 1 and 5. Although the etiology may be genetic, the child may also have immunological impairment. It is also possible for the etiology to be environmental in nature (e.g., pollution, indoor allergens such as cigarette smoke, or infections).

Signs and Symptoms

The child with atopic dermatitis has a red, raised rash that is both pruritic and painful with red papules that may have a serous exudate (clear fluid) during an acute phase. The rash is dry and easily cracks and excoriates in the subacute phase. As the disease progresses and the rash become chronic, the skin thickens, lichenification is present, and the papules become fibrotic. In the infant, the rash usually presents on the head, face, and lateral arms and legs. In the older child, the rash presents in the folds of the arms and legs, occasionally on the eyelids and neck.

Diagnosis

A complete family history and visual assessment of the child reveals the common signs of this condition. Blood tests reveal an increase in circulating IgE antibodies.

Nursing Care

critical nursing action Preventing Atopic Dermatitis Secondary Infection

When a child has atopic dermatitis, prevention of secondary infection is very important. Prevention of a secondary infection requires good hygiene processes, following prescribed treatment protocols, and maintaining skin hydration. Close and frequent monitoring and assessment of the rash is an important nursing measure.

SEBORRHEIC DERMATITIS

Chronic seborrheic dermatitis affects 2% to 5% of the population. Although it can affect young children, the peak incidence occurs in persons aged 18 to 40 years. There are many theories about the etiology of seborrheic dermatitis. This condition may have a genetic predisposition. In immunosuppressed individuals, *Pityrosporum ovale* may be the offending fungus.

Signs and Symptoms

The child who comes to the community health clinic with red to pink patches with loose, yellow, greasy scaling has seborrheic dermatitis. This skin rash is found on the face, across the cheekbones, in the fold around the nostrils, and behind the ears. It is also found on the scalp and eyebrows and may be found on the chest and back as well.

Diagnosis

The child who is diagnosed with seborrheic dermatitis has the defined rash. The nurse must understand that it may be necessary to differentiate between other conditions such as lupus, rosacea, and atopic or contact dermatitis.

Nursing Care

The nurse is aware that antifungal therapy is used if the etiology is *Pityrosporum ovale*. If the condition is not fungal in nature, topical corticosteroids may be used intermittently. It is important for the nurse to remember that low-dose corticosteroid topical applications are to be used on the face and other thinner skin surfaces. For the hair, antiseborrheic

shampoos that contain one of the following active ingredients can be used: coal tar, ketoconazole (Nizoral), selenium sulfide (Exsel), or zinc pyrithione (Denorex). It is more efficacious if the child or adolescent rotates types of shampoos. The nurse can communicate to the family that some of these shampoos with these active ingredients are marketed as "anti-dandruff" shampoos.

CUTANEOUS SKIN REACTIONS

Cutaneous skin reactions are a manifestation of an allergic response. The offending allergen can be introduced into the system in a variety of ways such as ingestion, inhalation, or coming into direct contact.

Signs and Symptoms

There are four basic types of skin reactions in an allergic response: exanthema (eruption), urticarial (itching), blistering (swelling), or pustular (a small elevated skin lesion filled with white blood cells) (Venes, 2009). It is paramount that the nurse look beyond the outer surface of the skin and assess for the root of the problem that may be a life-threatening condition associated with a systemic allergic response. An allergic reaction can be mild or a severe immediate hypersensitivity to an excessive release of chemical mediators affecting the entire body from medications, insects, foods, immunizations, diagnostic contrast media, or the administration of blood products. During the assessment phase, the nurse must appraise the face for swelling, especially around the lips, and including the tongue. It is essential that the nurse check the throat, using a light, but avoid using a tongue blade. Use of a tongue blade may stimulate more oral/pharyngeal swelling. Check nasal passages for edema (swelling) and erythema (redness) to ensure a patent airway. Airway compromise is a medical emergency.

critical nursing action Assessing for a Systemic Allergic Response

The nurse must recognize the key assessments in a systemic allergic response. Any edema or laryngospasms in the airway has the potential to cause blockage. If airway obstruction is noted, the Emergency Medical System must be initiated and airway, breathing, and circulation (ABCs) are begun. The nurse must assess for cyanosis as well as listening for audible sounds of upper airway respiratory distress such as wheezing or stridor. Assessing the vital signs, specifically, hypotension, which may lead to vascular collapse and cardiac arrest, is a critical indication that the allergic response may be systemic. Other important treatment measures include administering epinephrine (Adrenalin), keeping the child lying flat and warm with the feet slightly elevated, and administering oxygen if available. Immediate transport to an emergency medical facility is essential.

Once the possibility of compromised airway is dismissed, the nurse needs to assess whether the reaction is systemic. The nurse can then evaluate the skin lesions thoroughly determining the exact type of skin reaction.

Diagnosis

Visual assessment along with a complete history may help the nurse determine the cause. The nurse can find out specific details such as time and place of onset, ingested prescription medications, over-the-counter medications, bug bites, use of herbal/cultural remedies, and their relationship to the cutaneous eruptions. A nonjudgmental approach helps the nurse obtain the essential information that is necessary to determine which agent is the cause of the reaction. It is important to note that medication reactions can occur with the first dose of medication or even with a medication that the child has taken for months or years.

clinical alert

Stevens Johnson syndrome (erythema multiforme)

Stevens Johnson syndrome (erythema multiforme) or toxic epidermal necrolysis is a serious reaction that may result in death (Venes, 2009). The condition may be triggered by infections or certain medications such as anticonvulsants, nonsteroidal anti-inflammatory medications, or antibiotics. The leading cause of Stevens Johnson syndrome is severe allergic response to a medication. The syndrome often begins with a nonspecific upper respiratory system infection. The defining signs of this condition are bullae that appear on the lips, mouth, eyes, and genitalia, often in a target-like pattern. Purulent conjunctivitis is common as well as skin lesions that may rupture. Fever, neutropenia, chills, malaise, weakness, and anemia may occur. Once this condition has been diagnosed, it is essential to eliminate the causative agent, and treat the skin lesions using aseptic technique along with an air/fluid-filled bed, nutritional support, IV fluids, and pain management. Antibiotics can be given for secondary infections. An ophthalmologist should be contacted to assess for lesions in the eyes. These fluid-filled lesions begin to erupt and then slough off. This sloughing can occur internally as well as externally. It is vital to ensure a patent airway. This may progress to the necessity of intubation and mechanical ventilation. As these lesions rupture, large amounts of body surface area may become exposed. The child may experience large fluid losses and must be treated similar to a burn patient.

Nursing Care

Nursing care of a nonsystemic allergic reaction must also begin immediately. The nurse can emphasize the immediate discontinuation and avoidance of the offending agent. Administering oral antihistamines and topical corticosteroids decreases the symptoms of rash and pruritis. The nurse can also communicate to the parents that children returning to school after diagnosis may benefit from non-sedating antihistamines. See Family Teaching Guidelines (Lice) Pediculosis page 1014.

 Across Care Settings: **Prevention**

The pediatric community health nurse can create a detailed record for each child including a history and a list of all allergies. Asking specific questions about medications, insects, foods, immunizations, diagnostic contrast media, or the administration of blood products may help decrease the chance of serious reactions in the future. When a certain allergy is identified, the nurse can teach the child and parent about the allergy and ways to avoid contact with the offending agent. The information can also be passed along to the school nurse or other adults such as coaches or group leaders who are in contact with the child.

Infestations

LICE

Lice (pediculosis) is a common childhood condition that can be passed among friends and family. Approximately 10 to 12 million people are infested yearly; one fourth of them are children in elementary school. Females are at higher risk because they are more likely to share combs, brushes, and hair accessories (Wiederkehr & Schwartz, 2003). There are three kinds of lice: scalp (pediculosis capitis), body (pediculosis corporis), and pubic area (pediculosis pubis). The louse pierces the skin and sucks blood. The bites can cause severe itching and can predispose the child to a secondary infection.

Signs and Symptoms

Lice (pediculosis) and their eggs (nits) can infest the body in any of the aforementioned locations but primarily choose areas that have longer hair. In children, one is most likely to find lice on the head and the live bugs tend to live near the nape of the neck and behind the ears. They lay their eggs at the base of the hair shaft, where they can be seen as pearlescent tear drops.

Diagnosis

For lice, the clinical presentation and identification of the louse and/or its eggs is important. Persistent itching of the head is the classic sign.

Nursing Care

The nurse can instruct the parents that visual inspection of the home, including clothes and bedding, is important but it is often difficult to see lice because of their small size.

MITE INFESTATION

Mite infestation (scabies) results from an infestation with *Sarcoptes scabiei* and is typically seen in children with a weakened immune system. Scabies is transmitted by close personal contact with an infected person and is more common in persons who live in crowded conditions or share a bed. The scabies mite cannot survive for more than 3 days away from the skin. Although scabies mites are found in the United States, there are significantly more documented cases in South America and Central America and infestation is endemic in some developing countries (Wiederkehr & Schwartz, 2003). This condition is highly contagious and while children of all ages are affected, it is most commonly seen in children younger than 2 years of age.

Signs and Symptoms

In this condition, the female arachnid scabie burrows into the outer layer of the epidermis and lays her eggs, leaving a trail of debris and feces. The larvae hatch in approximately 2 to 5 days and proceed to the surface of the skin. This cycle repeats every 7 to 14 days. The original mite dies in the burrow after 4 to 5 weeks. The scabies rash is red streaked and appears linear from the burrowing. The mites, eggs, and their excrement cause intense itching, especially at night. There are also signs of papules that are a result of inflammation secondary to infestation (Wiederkehr & Schwartz, 2003).

Family Teaching Guidelines...
Lice (Pediculosis)

HOW TO TREAT LICE (PEDICULOSIS)

◆ Assess for lice using good lighting and examining the child's head to identify both live lice (very small and brown or black) and nits.

◆ Separate sections of the hair to go through. Particularly pay attention to the area behind the ears and the nape of the neck.

◆ Teach the family member that this dandruff-like appearance cannot be easily removed by combing because of the sticky adherence of the nit.

If the family member is unsure of what to do, they can call their primary care provider. The primary care provider instructs them to purchase an over-the-counter pediculicide shampoo in which the active ingredient is either permethrin, for an infant/young child, or malathion or lindane, for older children.

The nurse can instruct the family to wash the hair according to the product's instructions. If a child is unable to tolerate these shampoos, former remedies including the use of asphyxiants like petrolatum and food oils (e.g., olive oil may be used) (Wiederkehr & Schwartz, 2003). Once the shampoo is rinsed from the hair, remove nits by backcombing with a fine-tooth comb (nits are easier to remove when the hair is damp).

The nurse can also instruct the family member to remove nits from eyelashes by applying petrolatum jelly to the eyelashes twice a day for 8 days. (Nits on the eyelashes of a child are sometimes a sign of sexual abuse. The nurse must report any suspicious findings.)

The nurse can stress to the family member to implement house cleaning (dust, vacuum, scrub); wash clothing and bedding; and wipe off hats, bicycle helmet, and toys. If a soft or cloth toy like stuffed animals is not washable, it must be bagged in a sealed plastic bag and away from family members' rooms for 14 days.

Launder all bed linens in hot water and then placed in the dryer. Pillows should be thrown away if used by the child to avoid reinfestation. Anti-lice sprays can be used for furniture and other environmental objects that are not disposable.

Hair care items can be boiled (hot water above 140°F) or soaked in anti-lice shampoo and **never** shared.

The family member can check the school's anti-lice policy; children must remain home from school until lice-free. The child may be required to be checked by the school nurse or day care provider before returning.

Instruct the family member that the child should be rechecked for infestation in 7–10 days if the itching resumes, interferes with the child's sleep, or if the condition does not clear after 1 week of treatment

ESSENTIAL INFORMATION

To prevent the spread of acquired head lice (pediculosis) the nurse can have the mother:

◆ Ask other family members if there is a recent history of another family member with infestation.

◆ Remind family members and friends that because they may acquire head lice (pediculosis) from the affected child, they should take the same actions (listed above) if they are in close contact with or sleep in the same bed with the child (The National Pediculosis Association, Inc., 2008).

Diagnosis

In assessing for scabies, it is essential to check all pruritic areas for the primary burrows and secondary inflammatory papules (raised, circumscribed lesions) (Wiederkehr & Schwartz, 2003). A skin scraping may be viewed under the microscope for evidence of the mite, eggs, or feces. As an alternate assessment tool, the nurse can use a fountain pen and place the tip at the opening of a suspected burrow. "If the ink seeps into the skin, the burrow will look different than the surrounding skin, thus identifying a burrow" (Wiederkehr & Schwartz, 2003). If scabies are not identifiable by visual inspection, skin scrapings, or other clinical testing, and an IgE blood level may be drawn. Eosinophilia (large number of eosinophils) may be present with scabies infestation (Wiederkehr & Schwartz, 2003).

Nursing Care

Treatment of scabies is similar to pediculosis and requires a scabacide that is applied only to the scalp and forehead of infants. First a warm soap and water bath is given, then 5% permethrin cream (Elimite) or lotion is applied. Treatment is repeated in 1 week. All persons in close contact with the child should be treated concurrently (Wiederkehr & Schwartz, 2003). The nurse can suggest to the parents that a dishwasher with no other contents works well for cleaning washable toys and hair items. Treating all clothing, bedding, towels, and cloth toys by washing them in hot water and then placing them in the dryer is necessary to kill all scabies.

 nursing diagnoses Lice and Mite Infestation

- Altered Comfort related to pruritis secondary to infestation
- Potential Altered Health Maintenance related to nonadherence of cleaning regimen
- Potential for Social Isolation related to isolation from peers during treatment
- Pain related to secondary infection
- Risk for Infection related to impaired skin integrity, primary infestation, secondary pruritus

Bites and Stings

INSECTS

The most common insect bite comes from the mosquito. Spider and tick bites are also prevalent among children. The stings experienced most frequently are from bees, wasps, and hornets, and in some parts of the United States, scorpions. Other insects are also likely to bite, such as some types of flies, fleas and fire ants.

Signs and Symptoms

The mosquito bite causes discrete, red papules and edema at the site that produces itching, burning, and minimal discomfort. A spider's bite can cause local reaction (e.g., erythema, itching, and pain at the site that is usually self-limiting).

 Nursing Insight— *The brown recluse and black widow spiders' bite*

The bite of the brown recluse spider begins with itching, pain, and erythema and then due to the venomous sting advances into a purple lesion that signals the beginning of necrosis. The site becomes red with blisters, has a white ring and is surrounded by irregular erythematosus.

Black widow spider's bite leaves a stinging sensation at the time of the bite along with two fang bite marks, edema, petechiae, and erythema. The neurotoxin is usually self-limiting, but can result in more severe anaphylactic reaction. A systemic reaction from the neurotoxic venom can occur in 1 to 3 hours, with symptoms peaking in 3 hours and then diminishing in 72 hours. A systemic reaction includes muscle rigidity of the abdomen and torso, muscle cramps near the bite, malaise, sweating, dizziness, restlessness, insomnia, nausea and vomiting, hypertension, arrhythmias, and oliguria (low urine output).

A tick bite produces a reddened area of the skin that can be raised and itchy. A tick bite may cause a general sick feeling with fever, headache and nausea. The tick can stay on the skin and carry a risk of Rocky Mountain spotted fever or Lyme disease (Table 31-5).

Bee or wasp/hornet stings cause a mild local reaction that includes pain, erythema, and edema. If the reaction is systemic generalized urticaria (hives), flushing, and angioedema occur. Wheezing can be seen in some children but anaphylaxis is rare.

Diagnosis

Diagnosis of insect bites and stings are based on the child's history and physical findings.

Nursing Care

To protect against insect bites and stings the nurse can stress that children and adolescents adhere to the following directives when out of doors: wear light-colored clothing with minimal patterns, wear minimal perfumes or colognes, and cover the skin whenever possible to decrease the chance of insect bites and stings.

 clinical alert

A severe reaction to a bite

A child who has had a severe reaction to a bee or wasp sting should wear a medical alert bracelet or necklace and carry an EpiPen (epinephrine) or EpiPen Junior.

Specific care measures for mosquito bites and therefore, mosquito-borne illnesses are the use of bug sprays applied sparingly to the child's clothing to help decrease bites and therefore lower the risk for contracting West Nile virus, a significant mosquito-borne illness in the United States today. The CDC (CDC, 2005b) is now recommending two new repellants that do not contain N-diethyl-*m*-toluamide (DEET), a common ingredient in most bug sprays. The two new repellants are oil of lemon eucalyptus (Repel) and picaridin (KBR3023) (Cutter Advanced Insect Repellant), easily found in local stores that carry brand name bug repellant sprays (CDC, 2005b).

 Now Can You— **Identify the types of insect bites**

1. Identify the local symptoms of insect bites and stings?
2. Identify which spider bite may produce an anaphylactic reaction?
3. Discuss specific care measures for mosquito bites?

ANIMAL BITES

Dog bites account for the majority of animal bites to children. In fact, in the United States, approximately 800,000 dog bites are reported each year and 50% of them involve children. Boys are bitten more often than girls and children between the ages of 5 and 9 are most at risk (National Center for Injury Prevention and Control 2008). Oftentimes the child knows the animal and may have been bitten due to improper behavior such as interfering with feeding, playing, or taunting. Dog bites are sharp lacerations whereas cat bites cause deep puncture wounds.

Signs and Symptoms

When assessing animal bites it is important that the nurse consider the location, redness and swelling, number of puncture wounds, abrasions, and lacerations. Remember that any drainage or redness or swelling that extends beyond the primary site of the bite may be a sign of a complication such as cellulitis. The nurse must also assess for damage in the nervous, muscular, and vascular systems.

Diagnosis

Diagnosis of animal bites is based on patient history and physical findings. To diagnose a more severe problem, a radiographic evaluation or CT scan may be required.

Nursing Care

The nurse must take an accurate history about the incident and gather information about the exact injury, circumstances surrounding the attack, and location of the animal if known. The animal bite requires a good cleaning with soap and water and thorough rinsing. The nurse can then cover the wound with a topical antibiotic and clean dry dressing that helps to protect it from infection. Small wounds can be closed with adhesive strips (Band-Aid) and larger wounds may need suturing. Wounds over the joints must be elevated and immobilized.

If the wound was a crushing injury from a larger or stronger animal, an evaluation in the provider's office or an emergency department is required to rule out damage to deeper structures. A tetanus booster is required if the child has not had one in the last 5 years (Stump, 2006). Rarely do animal bites require oral antibiotics, but the wound should be assessed daily for signs of infection.

Table 31-5 Insect Bites

Bite	Local Reaction	Treatment for Local Reactions
Mosquitoes and Fleas Systemic reaction is possible: Allergic reaction; wheezing, urticaria, laryngeal edema, shock.	Red papules Itching, sometimes burning Local swelling (from foreign proteins) Minimal pain	Cleanse Cold compresses to the site Antihistamines, oral or topical
Bees, Wasps, and Hornets Systemic reaction is possible: Urticaria, flushing, angioedema, pruritis, wheezing	Redness and swelling (from venomous enzymes) Mild pain	Remove stinger quickly by scraping, not pinching Cleanse Cold compresses to the site Elevate the extremity Antihistamines A dash of meat tenderizer with a drop of water on the sting, massaged in for approximately five minutes will decrease pain
Fire Ants Systemic and anaphylactic reaction is possible.	Redness, swelling, and induration (from neurotoxin, creates a histamine response) Red, itchy wheal that turns into a cloudy vesicle within 24 hours	Cleanse Cold compresses Antihistamines, oral or topical Elevate extremity
Ticks Systemic allergic reaction is possible. Lyme disease is possible: Bull's-eye rash with erythema migrans, followed by fatigue, malaise, and joint pain	Tick is usually found with head burrowed into the skin The tick must be removed Area is generally reddened, and occasionally itchy	Remove tick Cleanse Cold compresses Monitor for rash over the next month
Brown Recluse Spider Systemic reaction is possible in 12–72 hours: Fever, chills, malaise, arthralgia, nausea, and vomiting. Intravascular hemolysis resulting in anemia.	Red swollen "bull's eye" wound that turns purplish with an outer area of white induration Skin necrosis occurs (the venom is proteolytic and cytoxic) Painful	Cleanse Ice to the site Apply topical antibiotic cream or lotion Seek emergency assistance
Black Widow Spider Systemic reaction possible in 1–3 hours, diminishing within 72 hours: Muscle rigidity, malaise, sweating, nausea and vomiting, hypertension, arrhythmia, oliguria, restlessness, insomnia	Redness and swelling Fang marks Petechiae branching out from site Stinging sensation	Cleanse Ice Antihistamine, orally Hydrocortisone topically Seek emergency assistance to manage any neurotoxic symptoms

Source: CDC (2005).

It is essential that the nurse find out if the animal is rabid. Human rabies immune globulin (HRIG) or human diploid cell rabies vaccine (HDCV) should be given to all children who have been bitten by an unknown wild or domestic animal that is positive for rabies or bitten by an animal in which rabies cannot be excluded (Merlin & Bertolini, 2005). Unknown dogs or other mostly domesticated animals may not require rabies prophylaxis. The local health department has information regarding best practice based on reported rabies cases in the local area (Stump, 2006).

" What to say " — *Animal bite prevention*

The nurse can teach the following safety tips to children and parents when encountering dogs or other unfamiliar animals:

- Never leave a child alone with an animal.
- Never put your face close to an animal.
- Spay or neuter the pet to reduce aggression.
- Avoid dogs and animals that you do not know.
- Seek permission to touch or pet an animal.

- Avoid any contact with wild animals.
- Do not run away from aggressive animals. Lie down in a ball, protecting the face, and remain quiet.
- Never overexcite or tease an animal.
- Play with animals only when an adult is present.
- Report any strange behavior from an animal, even if it is a familiar animal
- Do not disturb animals that are eating, sleeping, or nursing their young.

(National Center for Injury Prevention and Control 2008).

HUMAN BITES

Human bites can be quite common and usually occur in toddlers and young children. Human bites carry a higher risk for infection than do animal bites. Further, human bites may carry blood-borne diseases such as hepatitis B or C and human immunodeficiency virus (HIV).

Signs and Symptoms

A human bite displays as redness, swelling, a break in the skin, fever, and signs of infection.

Diagnosis

Diagnosis of a human bite is based on patient history and physical findings.

Nursing Care

The nurse must take an accurate history about the incident and gather information about the exact injury. After the bite, if the skin is broken, the nurse communicates to the family that both the biter and the bitten are at risk for blood-borne diseases. Both children need to be tested according to blood-borne pathogen exposure precautions. The nurse irrigates the wound with Ringer's solution or with soapy water. Vigorously scrubbing of the wound is not recommended. After irrigation, a topical antibiotic is gently applied to the wound followed by a clean dry dressing. The extremity is elevated and the area must be monitored daily for an infection. If any infection is noted, the primary health care provider must be notified. The child's immunization record needs to be evaluated by the nurse for status of tetanus coverage. The child can be cared for at home, alerting the parents to signs and symptoms of infection and proper wound care.

Diseases from Bites

LYME DISEASE

Lyme disease is a tick-borne infection with multiple system involvement. It is an inflammatory response to the spirochete *Borrelia burgdorferi* and is the most common vector-borne disease in the United States. Lyme disease has been found in 49 of the 50 states. Eighty percent of the Lyme disease cases occur in the Northeastern, Mid-Atlantic, and North Central states (CDC, 2005d). Deer ticks, which carry this disease are located in the Midwestern, Northwestern, and Southwestern states.

 Nursing Insight— *Lyme disease in California*

Western black-legged ticks are the vector ticks responsible for Lyme disease in California (CDC, 2005d).

Exposure occurs in any outdoor setting where ticks are endemic. Animals such as dogs and cats can also have the disease. Lyme disease occurs year round, with the highest incidence of infection in the summer. Children between 5 and 14 years of age are at highest risk because of outdoor activities. Infection does not induce immunity. Nymph (young) ticks feed on mammals in the spring, summer, and fall. The tick must feed for 36 hours to transmit the disease. It takes 48 hours after contact with a human to introduce the spirochete into the feeding site where the tick has buried its head. Any rash that appears before 48 hours is an allergic reaction or infection, not Lyme disease. The infection is not contagious from person to person.

Signs and Symptoms

During the history and physical, the nurse must always ask the family member if there has been an occurrence of a tick bite. The bite is often found in the groin, axilla or thigh.

 assessment tools Lyme Disease Presents in Three Stages

In the first stage, days to weeks after the tick bite, the child has a mild local rash. The rash from Lyme disease may occur as a bull's-eye rash or as disseminated erythematous (red) rash and erythema migrans (bull's-eye rash) (CDC, 2005d). Erythema migrans occurs in up to 90% of cases within a month of the bite. Other symptoms include headache, nuchal rigidity (stiff neck), and joint and muscle pain.

In the second stage, the disease may last from a few days to up to 10 months after the tick bite. During stage 2, the infection spreads through the blood and the child may exhibit signs of arthritis (especially in the knees), arthralgia (muscle pain), cardiac dysrhythmias, lymphadenopathy, pericarditis, or meningoencephalitis.

In the third stage, lasting from weeks to years after the tick bite (chronic stage), the child develops mild to severe arthritis. Neurological symptoms that occur in stage 3 include cranial nerve palsy, depression, meningitis, neuropathy, radiculopathy, and encephalopathy.

Diagnosis

After a tick bite, the nurse assesses the bite area for the distinguishing bull's-eye rash. Assessing joints for inflammation is necessary. A child's knees are the primary site for sudden onset arthritis, and it occurs without prior arthralgia (muscle pain), as in the case of chronic arthritis. Differentially, small joints are rarely inflamed in Lyme disease as they are in rheumatoid arthritis.

Lab testing may be performed to determine if the condition is present. The enzyme-linked immunosorbent assay (ELISA) is performed with follow-up of positive results with the Western blot for confirmation of Lyme disease, if seroconversion has occurred. The ELISA methods may sometimes provide a false-positive result because of cross-reactive antibodies to other spirochetal infections (Behrman et al., 2004). Seroconversion takes at least 6 weeks in Lyme disease, so the child is treated symptomatically while waiting for lab confirmation. The child will have specific IgM antibodies that will appear first at 3 to 4 weeks and peak at 6 to 8 weeks, then usually decline. The IgG antibodies appear at 6 to 8 weeks, peak after 4 to 6 months and may remain elevated indefinitely (Behrman et al., 2004).

Nursing Care

The first step is to remove all ticks immediately and properly. The nurse must remember to tell parents to remove a tick, grasping it gently but firmly with fine-point tweezers where the mouth part is attached. Pulling gently to avoid squeezing of the tick's body (to avoid leaving any tick parts in the host) until it releases is important. Then the nurse can teach the family to clean the area with soap and water (AAP, 2003). The nurse explains to the parents to save the intact tick in a sealable bag in the freezer with the date of the bite recorded (in case the tick needs to be tested for disease).

A 2-week course of oral antibiotics is given if infection is suspected. Amoxicillin (Amoxil) or cefuroxime (Ceftin) are the most often used antibiotics in children 8 years of age or younger. Doxycycline (Vibramycin) or tetracycline (Sumycin) is given to children older than the age of 8 years. If recurrent arthritis, central nervous system complications, or carditis occurs, treatment lasts for 4 weeks with intravenous ceftriaxone (Rocephin), cefotaxime (Claforan) or penicillin G (Pfizerpen). With early detection and treatment, the prognosis is good; however, relapse can occur.

ROCKY MOUNTAIN SPOTTED FEVER

Some ticks, the dog tick and the Rocky Mountain wood tick, harbor the organism *Rickettsia rickettsii* that can be transmitted to the human host after a tick bite. Rocky Mountain spotted fever (RMSF) has been found in 38 of the 50 states, with a highest incidence in Oklahoma and North Carolina (CDC, 2005c). Between 250 and 1200 cases of RMSF are confirmed in the United States each year, with 90% diagnosed between April and September (CDC, 2005c). The peak age for RMSF is 5 to 9 years of age, with more than two-thirds of the cases occurring in children younger than 15 years (CDC, 2005c). The incubation period lasts 2 to 12 days after the bite of an infected tick.

Signs and Symptoms

RMSF is a multisystem disease that can be mild, moderate, or severe. The onset can be either gradual or sudden. Sudden onset is characterized by nausea, vomiting, lack of appetite, abdominal pain, malaise, deep muscle pain, and severe headache along with a diffuse red macular (flat, circumscribed) rash that blanches with pressure, occurring 3 to 5 days after the onset of fever (CDC, 2005c).

The rash starts on the extremities, including the palms of the hands and soles of the feet and moves to the trunk. The classic petechial spotted rash does not occur until approximately 6 or more days after the initial symptoms. Along with the rash, diarrhea and joint pain also occur (CDC, 2005c). The child may have splenomegaly, hepatomegaly, and jaundice.

Diagnosis

Diagnosis is based on the classic triad of presenting symptoms, which include rash, fever, and history of a tick bite (CDC, 2005c). Often symptoms are vague and particularly difficult to diagnose if the child or parents do not recall a tick bite. Laboratory testing may prove useful.

 Labs: Results and Rocky Mountain Spotted Fever (RMSF)

The nurse can expect elevations in white blood cell (WBC) count, thrombocytopenia (low platelets), hyponatremia (a decreased concentration of sodium in the blood), and elevated liver enzymes (CDC, 2005c). The child's WBCs will likely remain low in the early stage and rise to slightly abnormal in later stages.

WBCs: 5000–10,000/mm³. Later stage: 10,000–12,000/mm³
Platelets: 150,000–400,000/mm³. Thrombocytopenia <150,000/mm³
Na: 136–145 mEq/L. Hyponatremia <136 mEq/L
Bilirubin (total): 0.3–1.0 mg/dL. Hyperbilirubinemia >1.0 mg/dL.
Urine testing may reveal red cells and protein (Gandhi, 2005).

Nursing Care

Treatment should begin based on clinical symptoms and epidemiology. An indirect immunofluorescence assay specific for RMSF antibodies or a skin biopsy using immunostaining procedure is conducted (CDC, 2005c). Tetracycline (Sumycin) is effective against RMSF. The earlier it is administered, the quicker the patient responds to antibiotics and experiences fewer sequelae (CDC, 2005c; Gandhi, 2005). Tetracycline (Sumycin) therapy is continued for 3 days after the fever subsides. If tetracycline (Sumycin) cannot be used (in the case of children younger than the age of 8 years), doxycycline (Vibramycin) can be used and chloramphenicol (Chloromycetin) is the next alternative (CDC, 2005c; Gandhi, 2005). Supportive therapy for other symptoms may include antipyretics, anti-inflammatory medication, and IV fluids.

CAT SCRATCH DISEASE

Cat scratch disease (CSD) is a self-limiting illness lasting 6 to 12 weeks that begins with a scratch or bite from a cat (CDC, 2006). Domestic cats are reservoirs for the bacillus *Rochalimaea henselae*, which causes the disease response in humans (CDC, 2006).

Signs and Symptoms

The symptoms of cat scratch disease include tender lymphadenopathy (swollen lymph nodes) in the region of the scratch or bite that begins 1 to 3 weeks after the initial inoculation (CDC, 2006). Most children experience general malaise and low-grade fever. Some children experience nausea, vomiting, and weight loss. Others may experience sore throat and anorexia. Generalized rashes and thrombocytopenia purpura have been noted in some children. Some children may experience all of these symptoms (CDC, 2006).

Diagnosis

During the assessment, the nurse asks the parent or child about a recent history related to a cat scratch or bite. A positive response to CSD specific antigen, a confirming lymph node biopsy, and other lab findings that conclude another etiology for lymphadenopathy are used to confirm or refute the diagnosis (CDC, 2006).

Nursing Care

Antibiotics are used to treat CSD. Other treatments and care are not typically indicated.

Burns

The skin is the most important organ system to protect the body from infection, regulate body temperature, and serve as a barrier to prevent body fluid loss. Damage from burns causes major alterations in the skin. Burns occur every day in the United States; more than 1 million persons seek care for burns each year (American Burn Association, 2006). Burns that affect children can be accidental or the result of intention to harm and are the third leading cause of death (after motor vehicle crashes and drowning). Boys between the ages of 1 and 4 are twice as likely as girls to be burned, and the average of pediatric burn patients is 32 months of age (Perry, 2003). Thirty-three percent of all burns affect children younger than the age of 19 years (American Burn Association, 2006). Some children are at higher risk for burns due to their environment, their behavior, and their age. Burns are a result of either chemical, electrical, radiation, or thermal insult. The most common burns affecting children are thermal. Infants and children younger than 5 years are most likely to suffer burns from scalding. The risk of injury from fire is highest in the 5- to 20-year-old population (American Burn Association, 2006).

 Nursing Insight— *Development*

Children at different developmental stages are at risk for different types of burns:

Infants—incur burns by scalding liquids and house fires
Toddlers—incur burns by spilling hot liquids on themselves
Preschool children—incur burns by appliances (irons, curling irons) or scalding liquids
School-age children—incur burns by playing with matches, climbing trees or high-voltage towers and chemical burns from curious experimentation
Adolescents—incur burns by thermal, chemical, and electrical means, but primarily fire

THERMAL BURNS

Thermal burns are the most common type of burn in childhood. Thermal burns occur as a result of flame, flash, scalds, or contact with hot objects, or radiation. In the toddler age group, scald burns from hot liquid or hot grease is common and account for 80% of all thermal injuries. This type of burn accounts for a majority of childhood burn hospitalizations in this age group (Reed & Pomerantz, 2005).

 Nursing Insight— *Common Causes of Burns*

- Flame   Ignition of combustible materials and contact with fire, fireworks, candles, campfires
- Flash   Caused by explosions, especially with combustible fuels like gasoline, kerosene, and charcoal lighter; fireworks; hairspray
- Scald   Occur when hot liquid is spilled on a child (oil, grease, coffee, hot tea, soup) or from hot tap water in sinks and bathtubs or from steam
- Contact   Exposure to a hot object like an oven, hot iron, radiator, hot light bulb, or heating device.

Four out of five U.S. fire deaths occur in the home (Karter, 2001). This accounts for 82% of all civilian fire deaths (National Fire Protection Agency, 2007). Cooking is the most common cause of residential fires, with the leading cause of fire related deaths linked to smoking (Ahrens, 2001).

 Ethnocultural Considerations— **Vulnerable populations**

African and Native Americans (CDC, 2006) and persons living in rural areas (Ahrens, 2001) are most vulnerable to fire-related injuries and death.

Nearly one half of all home fire deaths are in homes without smoke detectors (Ahrens, 2001). Smoke detectors have a major impact on decreasing the likelihood of death from a house fire, and all homes should be equipped with at least one smoke detector per floor (U.S. Fire Administration, 2005). Thermal injuries from campfires occur when children fall into the fire or by touching the embers around an already extinguished fire. A lack of adult supervision is usually responsible for this type of injury (Klein, Heimbach, Honari, Engrav, & Gibran, 2005).

 Across Care Settings: **Burn prevention**

Nurses can remind parents to be sure to check that their home hot water heater is set at no higher than 120°F to prevent scald injuries. Nurses should also remind parents to turn the pot handles inward when cooking and to make sure all cords from cooking appliances are not dangling and are away from children's reach (American Burn Association, 2007).

 where research and practice meet:
Pediatric Scald Burns

A study by Greenhalgh et al. (2006) looked at the design flaws in instant cup of soup containers. With scald injuries being the most common type of burn injury in children, heating prepackaged soups are a frequent cause. All pediatric scald burns caused by soup between June 1997 and August 2004 were examined. Safety statements and recommendations as to use of the microwave oven were documented but were inconsistent. During the study period, 99 admitted patients and 80 outpatients who were treated for burns caused by soup were examined. Of the 13 different types of soups, 11 required the addition of hot water and 2 were prepackaged to eat out of the container. Twelve containers had round bases and were tall and narrow and one was short and rectangular. Their height/base area ratio was measured. The most significant contributor to the ease of tipping over was the height of the container. Instant soups are packaged in containers that are tall with a narrow base that predisposes them to being knocked over and spilled. Simple redesigning of the instant soup packages with a wider base and shorter height, along with the requirements for warnings about the risk of burns, would reduce the frequency of soup burns.

CHEMICAL BURNS

Between 25,000 and 100,000 chemical burns are reported in the United States each year. Collectively burns have a morbidity and mortality rate of less than 1%. Children and adults are reported to have similar rates of exposure. More than 25,000 different chemicals can produce either acid or alkali burns. The burn usually results from a direct chemical injury, but there may also be components of a thermal burn caused by an exothermic reaction (Reed & Pomerantz, 2005).

Chemical burns can be divided into the following categories: acid, alkali, oxidants, and other. Children are likely to be burned as they explore the environment. Acids tend to cause self-limiting tissue damage by denaturing protein, whereas alkalis cause fat saponification and the burning continues into deeper tissue (Cox, 2005). In any chemical burn, immediate flushing of the skin can significantly decrease the burn injury (Cox, 2005). Chemical burns require a visit to the emergency department for full decontamination, for the chemical to be neutralized, and for a complete evaluation (Cox, 2005).

Household chemicals that are available to children are the most frequent cause of chemical burns (Whetstone, 2005). Acid burns result in coagulation necrosis, which usually limits the depth and penetration of the burn. Some common household examples that contain acid include drain cleaners (sulfuric acid or hydrochloric acid), toilet cleaners (hydrochloric acid or phosphoric acid), and car batteries (sulfuric acid). Sometimes burns involving bases with high pHs are worse than those from acid because they actually produce a type of necrosis called liquefactive, which causes a deeper penetrating and more significant burn. Some common alkalis include lye (sodium hydroxide), cement (calcium, potassium, and sodium hydroxide), oven and drain cleaner (sodium or potassium hydroxide), and various detergents (Reed & Pomerantz, 2005). All household chemicals should be out of the reach of children by placing them on high shelves for children who cannot climb, or locking them in cabinets. Parents who do not understand these basic principles put their children at risk for a chemical burn.

clinical alert

Material safety data sheets

To protect personal and patient safety the nurse must know where to find the material safety data sheets (MSDS) in a health care setting. Many organizations have a special telephone hot line for MSDS information when you encounter chemical exposures. The nurse must also know the phone number of the local poison control center. The poison center provides accurate telephone advice and faxes important information regarding the management of chemicals spilled on or ingested by your patients.

ELECTRICAL

Electrical burns result in more than 1500 deaths per year and more than 4000 emergency department visits. Electric burns also account for 2% to 3% of all admissions to hospital burns centers. Up to one-third of electrical burns are household burns that are seen most often in children. Electrical burns result from thermal energy that is produced as an electrical current passes through the body. The amount of thermal energy is directly related to the degree of electrical current. The longer the individual is in contact with the electrical source, the more severe the injury. Electrical outlets and loose or frayed cords are dangerous for small children and are directly responsible for the majority of electrocutions in children younger than 12 years.

Parents should childproof their homes by keeping all cords away from children, taking appliances with frayed cords out of service and covering all exposed outlets with childproof covers (at least in the first 5 years of a child's life) (Reed & Pomerantz, 2005).

If a child suffers any type of electrical burn, he or she must be treated in the emergency department and monitored for a minimum of 4 hours (O'Conner & Besner, 2004). If a low-voltage burn was encountered, the child will not likely have cardiac involvement. Cardiac monitoring should take place in the emergency department while the child is being observed for any other sequelae. If the wound is small and manageable in an outpatient setting, and the child did not have any adverse cardiac events, did not lose consciousness, and did not suffer the injury while the skin was wet, the child can be discharged after observation (O'Conner & Bessner, 2004). Typically, low-voltage electrical injuries do not cause a significant internal burn effect (Selvaggi, Monstrey, van Landuyt, Hamdi, & Blondeel, 2005). If the child has any of the aforementioned adverse reactions, he or she must be hospitalized for more intensive monitoring and treatment.

If the child suffers a high-voltage electrical assault he or she is at high risk for a cardiac arrest, and must be monitored. Blood vessels, nerves, and muscles readily conduct electricity and are also destroyed as the electrical current makes its way through the child's body (Selvaggi et al., 2005).

 Nursing Insight— Alternating current

The nurse can remember that alternating current is more damaging than direct current, as it causes a "lock-on" effect that does not allow the child to release and stay released from the source (Selvaggi et al., 2005).

RADIATION

The nurse must educate parents how to protect children from the sun by applying a sunscreen of SPF 15 or above. Ultraviolet rays from the sun are most intense between the hours of 10:00 A.M. and 4:00 P.M. Children should be strongly encouraged to play indoors or in shaded areas during these times. Further, infants younger than the age of 6 months should not wear sunscreen and should never be in direct sunlight. Exposure to sun occurs on cloudy days too, so children can protect their skin by covering up with clothing or applying sunscreen on these days as well. Special attention to sunscreen around water is encouraged, as even waterproof sunscreen requires reapplication approximately every hour. Sunscreen should be reapplied per package directions and must completely cover all exposed skin.

CLASSIFICATION OF BURNS (FIG. 31-10)

First Degree

First-degree burns (superficial thickness) are usually erythematous (reddened) and painful (e.g., sunburn from ultraviolet exposure). These burns involve the intact epidermis without blistering. This type involves only the outer layer of the epidermis, and fluid loss is not a problem. Several days after the initial burn, peeling of the skin begins because of superficial cell death. This type of burn heals without scarring in 4 to 5 days (Reed & Pomerantz, 2005).

Second Degree

Second-degree burns (superficial partial thickness, or deep partial thickness) involve partial destruction of the dermis and appear red and painful with blister formation. They have a weeping or moist appearance, and usually heal with minimal scarring in 7 to 10 days. Dark-skinned individuals may lose melanin and develop hypopigmentation on healing (Reed & Pomerantz, 2005).

Second-degree burns involve greater than 50% of the dermis. They destroy nerve fibers and as a result are less painful. These burns have a white pale appearance and usually take 2 to 3 weeks or longer to heal. It can be difficult to distinguish between this type of burn and third-degree burns. Frequently severe scarring develops and patients are at risk for contractures. These patients are at risk for fluid volume loss. Surgical consultation is necessary because skin grafting is usually required (Reed & Pomerantz, 2005).

Third Degree

This is the most severe burn (full thickness). It appears white, waxy, or leathery and does not bleed or blanch. The skin may also be black in color, called eschar. Typically, these burns are less painful because the nerve fibers in the dermis were completely destroyed. Patients with these burns are at high risk for infections and severe fluid volume loss. Patients with this type of burn are immediately referred to a burn center and a surgeon because of risk of significant scarring on healing and they frequently require grafting. This type of burn takes several weeks to heal.

Fourth Degree

Although this terminology is not commonly used, fourth degree burns involve the destruction of the underlying structures such as tendons, muscles, bone, and deep fascia. Most commonly these are seen with severe electrical injuries and in severe thermal injury (Reed & Pomerantz, 2005). This type of burn injury requires immediate transfer to a burn center. Survival of the child depends of several factors such as fluid resuscitation, decreasing the risk of infection, and restoration of function.

Classifying Burns

It is also important to determine the extent of the burn by calculating the total body surface area (TBSA). TBSA can be determined by using several methods. The Lund and Browder Chart or the Burn Calculations Rule of 9's is frequently used and gives a reasonably accurate TBSA when a quick assessment is needed (Uliasz, 2002). The Rule of 9's (modified) calculates the child's body proportions differently than the adult. After 2 years of age, as the child's proportions change, percentages are deducted from the head (1%) and added to the legs (0.5% to each leg). For example, an infant's head and neck make up 18% of the TBSA and each lower extremity accounts for 14% of the TBSA (Fig. 31-11). Burns are also categorized according to severity (Table 31-6).

Figure 31-10 Classification of burns. *A.* Partial thickness (superficial). *B.* Partial thickness (deep). *C.* Full thickness.

PERCENTAGES IN A CHILD

Figure 31-11 Rule of nines.

Table 31-6 Classification of Burn Severity

Mild	Moderate	Severe
First or second degree <10% TBSA	Second degree, 10–20% burn	Second-degree burn >20% TBSA
Third degree <2% TBSA	Third degree but <10% TBSA	Third-degree burn >10% TBSA
No area of the face, feet, hands, genitalia burned		• Burn on face, hands, feet, genitalia that may lead to functional impairment
		• Smoke inhalation present
Treated in outpatient clinic	Treated in a burn unit or hospital	Treated in a specialized burn center

 critical nursing action Criteria for Transfer to a Burn Center

- Partial thickness burns >10% total body surface area (TBSA)
- Burns that involve the face, hands, feet, or genitalia
- Third-degree burns in any group or category
- Electrical burns including lightening injury
- Chemical burns
- Inhalation burns
- Burn injuries in patients with preexisting chronic conditions that could prolong the burn recovery
- Any patient with coexisting trauma (such as fractures) where burn injury poses a greater risk of morbidity and mortality than the trauma
- Burned children in hospitals without qualified personnel or equipment to care for the care of children
- Burn injury in patients who require special emotional, social, or long-term burn rehabilitation

(American Burn Association, 2006)

NURSING CARE

Minor Burns

Minor burns are usually treated in clinics or outpatient setting unless there is suspicion of child abuse or neglect.

 critical nursing action Managing Minor Burns

In a clinic or outpatient setting the nurse can use the concept of the six "C's" to manage minor burns. The nurse can teach this method to parents and other caregivers.

- Clothing—Remove any clothing that is hot or has been in contact with the offending chemical.
- Cooling—Burns need to be cooled immediately with cool (54°F) saline soaked gauze or any available clean cloth soaked in cool water. Caution: Do not use ice!
- Cleaning—Wash wound with mild soap and rinse well with water.
- Chemoprophylaxis—Bacitracin (AK-tracin) may be used topically to prevent infection. Other types of anti-infective agents are used in moderate and major burns. A tetanus booster (Td) is also given.
- Covering—Cover the burn with gauze to prevent infection, to decrease pain, and to absorb drainage.
- Comfort—Give acetaminophen (Children's Tylenol) or ibuprofen (Children's Advil) to decrease the pain. Pain medications should be on a schedule to decrease pain in the child who has sleep, play, or mood alterations.

Source: Morgan, E.D., Bledsoe, S.C., & Barker, J. (2000). Ambulatory management of burns [Electronic Version]. *American Family Physician, 62*(9), 2015–2026.

Moderate and Major Burns

Moderate and major burns require hospitalization and some major burns require hospitalization in specialty burn-trauma units. At the site of a moderate or major burn, there is coagulative destruction of the skin and necrosis if the burn is deep. Interstitial fluids are lost secondary to increased capillary permeability. With the shift of fluids to the site of the burn, there is a hypovolemia (decrease in circulating plasma volume), which increases plasma viscosity. Increased plasma viscosity decreases cardiac output. With a decrease in cardiac output, there is a decrease in blood pressure. Breakdown of the muscle tissue in full thickness burns results in an increase in myoglobin, which decreases kidney perfusion. Increases in myoglobin are most likely in partial to full-thickness burns and when the burn is a result of electrical shock. If chemicals are swallowed, the internal burn presents as dyspnea, stridor, wheezing, and drooling (Cox, 2005). Immediate attention to the child's airway is critical. These critical burns assault the entire body system and create a stress that demands increased energy metabolism to compensate, putting the child at risk for shock.

 Optimizing Outcomes— **Overall goals of burn treatment**

The best outcomes for a burned child include interventions from the following categories:
- Burn assessment
- Fluid resuscitation
- Adequate nutrition
- Pain management
- Meticulous wound care
- Burn recovery

ASSESSMENT. Assessment of the burn history is vital. The initial nursing assessment includes emergency care related to airway, breathing, and circulation (ABCs). After the ABCs are addressed and the child is being safely transported to an emergency room, the nurse or emergency medical technician (EMT) removes all clothing and jewelry to decrease continued burning at any site.

Once the child is in a hospital, burn wounds are decontaminated and assessed for depth, surface area, and severity. Depth of the wounds is measured in millimeters or centimeters. Circumference measurements are also necessary to provide a full clinical picture. The surface of the burn wound is assessed for color, blanching, desiccation (dryness), turgor/elasticity, blisters, or sloughed blisters. TBSA and all other skin assessments are taken into consideration to help classify the burn. For some burn assessments, wounds are photographed with a camera that has a measurement graphing lens. If the burn injuries are severe and encompass large areas of the TBSA, some burn or emergency departments use video charting to record the clinical assessment.

" What to say " — *Gathering important information*

The nurse can ask these questions to gather important information:

- "What was the offending agent?"
- "When did this burn occur?"
- "Who was present or witnessed the injury?"
- "What first aid was given?"
- "How did the burn feel when it first occurred?"
- "How does the burn feel now?"
- "Has the child had any like accidents or injuries before?"
- "What other medical history is important?"

FLUID RESUSCITATION. Children with burns greater than 15% of TBSA require intravenous fluid resuscitation to maintain adequate perfusion. The IV fluid of choice is lactated Ringer's solution (Behrman et al., 2004). Fluid resuscitation is necessary to increase the patient's plasma volume and maintain blood pressure. The Parkland Formula is one means of determining the fluid needs of the child with a burn injury (Box 31-1) (Bollero, Stella, Calcagni, Guglielmotti, & Magliacani, 2000). Effectiveness of fluid resuscitation is monitored by adequate urine output. Normal urine output for children is 1 to 2 mL/kg per hour. If adequate urine output is not achieved, additional fluid resuscitation may be required.

NUTRITION. When a child has a burn, it is essential that adequate nutrition be maintained. Burn injuries place a child in a hypermetabolic state. The caloric requirement for a patient with a >30% burn is 2000 to 2200 calories/day. In major burns enteral nutrition (fed by a tube passed into the stomach) is necessary to keep up with the increased energy demand of the body, secondary to the stress response (Rimdeika et al., 2006). Enteral feeding is often initiated within 6 hours of the burn injury to support the child's increased needs. These children often need nearly twice the basal metabolic caloric requirement and nearly 2 g/kg of protein. Adequate caloric intake in the acute phase of the burn and burn treatment decreases complications, treatment length, and mortality rates (Rimdeika et al., 2006).

PAIN MANAGEMENT. Pain management is an important nursing care issue for children with burns. Pain is usually mild to moderate in children with superficial burns. As the burn depth increases to full thickness, the pain is diminished as the nerve endings are burned and no longer conduct pain messages back to the brain. The areas surrounding full-thickness burns where the tissue is viable are hypersensitive to pain reception (Selvaggi et al., 2005). It is important to provide adequate analgesia and anti-anxiety medication along with proper psychological support to reduce early metabolic stress and decrease the potential for posttraumatic stress disorder. Children with burn injuries show wide fluctuations in pain intensity. Appreciation of pain depends on the depth of the burn, stage of healing, age and stage of emotional development, cognition, experience and efficiency of the treating team, use of analgesics and other drugs, pain threshold, and interpersonal and cultural factors. From the onset of treatment, preemptive pain control during dressing changes is of utmost importance. Initially morphine sulfate (Duramorph) is most commonly used for pain. The use of anxiolytics such as midazolam (Versed) or lorazepam (Ativan) is usually very helpful and can have a synergistic effect (the interaction of elements that when combined produce a total effect that is greater than the sum of the individual elements) (Dictionary.com, 2008).

The problem of undermedication most often occurs with adolescents who fear the development of drug dependency. This may affect treatment and adequate pain relief (Behrman et al., 2004). It is important to explain to the child and the parent that withholding medications because of the fear of dependency is not a valid concern. Reassurance and education are needed for families in the area of pain management. The use of nonpharmacological interventions as well as pharmacological agents need to be used (Behrman et al., 2004).

Complementary Care: *Distraction*

The nurse can use distraction as a good technique when changing the dressings for a child with burns. The type of distraction used is based on age and developmental stage (e.g., singing, counting, watching television, focusing on picture, talking about familiar events or places, playing games or blowing pin-wheels or bubbles). If the child is anxious or has severe pain, medication may be required before and during distraction. The nurse must remember to praise the child when the dressing change is complete, with the focus on all of the positive behaviors that the child displayed.

WOUND CARE. Prevention of infection is the priority outcome when providing meticulous wound care. Wounds are initially decontaminated. Subsequent burn wound care includes cleansing the wound with a special solution or débridement (cutting away dead tissues). Escharotomy (incision into a burn in order to lessen its pull on the surrounding tissue) if a burn is circumferential may be required if circulation or perfusion is impeded. If escharotomy is required, the child is provided with conscious sedation or general anesthesia if not already sedated.

The nurse can assess the child's wound and if no eschar or devitalized tissue is present, the wound can be treated

---

Box 31-1 The Parkland Formula

4 mL of IVF × weight in kg × %TBSA

Give ½ of the total IVF volume over the 1st 8 hours.

Give the second ½ at an even rate over the next 16 hours.

Example: A child weighing 110 lb. (50 kg) with a 20%, TBSA burn requires:

4 mL × 50 kg × 20% TBSA = 4,000 mL

1st 8 hours IVF = 2000/8 hours = 250 mL/hr

next 16 hours IVF = 2000/16 hours = 125 mL/hr

Source: Behrman, R.E., Kliegman, R.M., & Jenson, H.B. (2004). *Nelson textbook of pediatrics* (17th ed.). Philadelphia: W.B. Saunders.

with antibiotic cream and re-dressed. If the wound needs to be cleansed, the nurse cleans it at the bedside with antibacterial products. The wound is softened by soaking the site with saline-soaked gauze for 15 minutes. Antibiotic ointment is applied and the wound is then re-dressed. Wounds can also be cleansed in a tub or a whirlpool, allowing the movement of the water to soften skin, and gently removing some loose dead skin. Some of the dead skin needs to be scrubbed and cut away to create clean vitalized margins.

Other methods of débriding include the use of the enzyme collagenase. This enzyme speeds débridement, resulting in earlier wound closure and a decrease in scarring (Frye & Luterman, 2005). Collagenase has been used only in wounds that do not require grafting (Frye & Luterman, 2005).

Some dressings have occlusive ability (a thin sheet of plastic that prevents air entry and retains moisture, heat, body fluids, and medication). These are used for a longer period of time than gauze-type dressings. These dressings are often transparent, so the wound can be assessed easily for signs of infection, but can remain in place if the wound is healing adequately.

IMPREGNATED DRESSINGS. Acticoat™ is an antimicrobial nanocrystalling film of pure silver. Its surface is nonadherent and nonabrasive. Acticoat™ provides a sustained release of ionic silver, which maintains the antimicrobial properties, which is effective against more than 150 pathogens. This silver-coated polyethylene mesh can be used over débrided burns, grafts, and donor sites. It is applied to the cleansed wound and sometimes wrapped in to place with sterile water-soaked gauze or sometimes placed on dry depending on the facility's standard protocol (Ülkür, Oncul, Karagoz, Yeniz, & Celikoz, 2005).

Sterile saline cannot be used to moisten Acticoat™ because the saline reacts with the silver and may precipitate the salt out of the dressing. Do not to use any topical antimicrobials with Acticoat™ as it may alter its antimicrobial properties. Acticoat™ is also available in a moisture absorbent dressing (Smith & Nephew, 2006).

Silvadene™ is a sulfonamide with broad-spectrum coverage. Silvadene™ is the most commonly used burn cream to both prevent and treat burn infection. This medication comes in tubes and in impregnated gauze wraps as well. Silvadene™ is usually applied one to two times a day and then the wound is wrapped in a gauze dressing. The nurse can instruct the family that residue is washed off with each dressing change. This cream is contraindicated for a child with a sulfa allergy (Deglin & Vallerand, 2009).

TEMPORARY SKIN REPLACEMENT. Biobrane™ is a semipermeable temporary skin substitute that is a nylon fabric with an outer silicone film, which is saturated with porcine collagen. The collagen peptides on the nylon bind to wound surface fibrin and collagen resulting in the initial adherence. Small pores in the structure allow for drainage of exudates and provide permeability for topical antibiotics. Biobrane™ is clinically indicated in superficial to mid- to partial-thickness burns but can be used on excised wound beds with or without mesh autografts. This temporary skin substitute can also be used on donor sites and in partial thickness slough disorders (Demling, DeSanti, Dennis, & Orgill, 2000).

Transcyte™ is a human fibroblast-derived temporary skin substitute that is made of silicone. It consists of a polymer membrane and neonatal human fibroblast cells cultured under aseptic conditions in vitro on a nylon mesh. The membrane provides a transparent epidermis when applied. As the fibroblasts proliferate within the nylon mesh, they secrete human dermal collagen, matrix proteins, and growth factors. It can be used on primary mid-dermal to intermediate depth wounds that may heal without grafting (second degree burns). Transcyte™ may be used as a temporary barrier before grafting. It also can be used safely with or without additional dressings (Smith and Nephew Acticoat™ Antimicrobial Barrier Dressing; Silcryst, 2008).

PERMANENT SKIN REPLACEMENT. There are three main types of grafting or permanent skin replacement. An allograft is cadaver skin. Cadaver skin is skin taken from a skin bank that can be used as a grafting host when auto grafting is not possible of a full thickness wound. Allografts are bilayer skin (both epidermis and dermis) that aids in revascularization, which makes it a favorable choice (Demling, DeSanti, Dennis, & Orgill, 2000). Allografting has the disadvantages of potential disease transmission, rejection, and difficulty in obtaining and storing it (Demling, DeSanti, Dennis, & Orgill, 2000).

Autografting is using the child's own healthy skin taken from an area not burned. Autografting harvests the child's own skin and then grafts into a new position on the child's body. The skin can be used as is or, if necessary, it is processed in a meshing machine that enlarges the surface area of the harvested skin and creates small slits for the passage of fluid and for better adherence (O'Conner & Besner, 2004). Autografting does cause permanent scarring along the slits made by the meshing machine, so it should be limited to areas of the body that clothing will cover (O'Conner & Besner, 2004).

Xenografting is the use of nonhuman skin. Xenografting is necessary for full-thickness skin loss. This type of grafting may be used in partial-thickness wounds also. Since 1965, xenograft has been limited to pigskin (Demling et al., 2000). Pigskin has a dermal layer that adheres to a partial thickness wound, providing collagen to the cleaned wound surface. Its disadvantages include potential for disease transmission and it does not always revascularize, resulting in sloughing (Demling et al., 2000).

Integra™ is a bioactive bilayer manmade permanent skin replacement. Integra™ is lined with a collagen–glycosaminoglycan matrix that biodegrades. It has a thin silicone second layer that acts as a barrier to control fluid movement in and out much like normal skin (Demling et al., 2000). Integra™ is limited, as it is only a temporary measure that allows some epithelialization and then the silicone layer is removed and autograft or cultured epithelial cells are placed (Demling et al., 2000).

For severe burn treatment, there are now cultured epithelial autografts (CEAs). This is the child's own skin cells that are grown in a laboratory. A 2×6 full-thickness biopsy is extracted from the child's own viable skin. The skin biopsy is sent to the genetics laboratory and grown for about 2 weeks. During the 2-week period, the child is covered with a synthetic dressing to enhance wound bed growth. The synthetic dressing autologous keratinocytes is co-cultured with irradiated murine cells to form epidermal autographs. The delivery of these sheets is coordinated with the burn surgeon and placed as an autograph.

where research and practice meet:
Growth Hormone
Studies have shown that intramuscular injection of growth hormone allows for rapid regeneration of the donor sites and thus more rapid reharvesting (O'Conner & Besner, 2004).

This treatment is used for patients with full-thickness burns extending over 30% of TBSA or larger. The treatment can be very expensive because these epidermal autografts are grown from the patient's own skin cells. The advantage is that they are usually not rejected by the patient's immune system. Genzyme is just one company that develops this product (Epicel) (Genzyme, 2006).

In large burns, it is difficult to find enough autodonor tissue, so the alternate methods of temporary and permanent skin replacement must be used. Postoperative orders include the appropriate dressing change for graft site and graft donor site.

BURN RECOVERY. Burn injuries for children are managed by phases of recuperation as well as by the type and severity of burns. The acute, or early phase, is from the time of the initial assault until wound closure. The second phase, recovery, is from the time of wound closure until scar maturation, which could be as long as 16 months (Selvaggi et al., 2005). It is important to remember that for some children burn recovery may last a lifetime.

Caring for a hospitalized child with burns involves the family and the health care team. The health care team can typically comprise a nurse, a pediatrician, and a physician with a specialty in burn treatment and/or surgery. Plastic surgeons often have this role. As part of discharge planning, the nurse can contact a social worker for parental and child support to help manage home care issues.

During the long-term recovery phase as the child reenters the world, there remains a need for the integrated burn team. The child may have compression garments and splints that need to be altered with growth. The child continues to need to be seen by a physical and occupational therapist to continue the work of range of motion and decrease any possibility of contracture. Scar revision may be necessary, especially if contracture occurs. When this happens, the child needs to be admitted to the hospital and treated by the plastic surgeon. Optimal functioning with minimal scarring and minimal negative psychological impact are the goals of care.

Collaboration in Caring— *A team approach*

The care of a burned child requires a team approach. During hospitalization, the nurse provides essential nursing care and acts as the advocate for the child and her family. The nurse can also coordinate care of other health care professionals such as a physical therapist who helps the child maintain or regain physical function. A dietician plans appropriate nutrition for immediate and long-term nutritional intervention. An occupational therapist helps the child adapt to activities of daily living. As the child becomes more able to return to activities including school, the case manager, either a social worker or nurse, helps bridge the information gap between agencies. Other long-term therapy,

sometimes upwards of 2 years, with rehospitalization and scar revisions, is another reason for an integrative team approach where health care professionals provide optimal care and share their knowledge of the child and family with one another over time (Hubbuck, 2003).

Hypothermia

Hypothermia is secondary to cold air exposure, wet clothes, and immersion in water. Hypothermia is also present in victims of burns, where large amounts of skin are no longer present or the child no longer has the capacity to hold heat. Hypothermia is a condition in which the child's core body temperature falls below 95°F (35°C). Hypothermia is a life-threatening emergency. The body loses heat in one of five ways: radiation, conduction, convection, evaporation, and respiration (McCullough & Arora, 2004) (Table 31-7).

Different developmental stages predispose the child to different types of exposure. Infants and young children are at higher risk due to their immature thermoregulatory system, thinner skin, and lack of subcutaneous fat. Older children are at high risk for hypothermia, as they may lack the cognitive ability to evaluate risky situations. Adolescents are at risk for hypothermia due to risk-taking behaviors such as participating in outdoor activities without proper clothing and potentially the ingestion of alcohol or other illicit drugs. In children of any age, a trauma, brain disorder, or severe sepsis can also cause hypothermia because these conditions interfere with the thermoregulation system.

 Nursing Insight— *Protecting Children from Hypothermia*

Monitoring children closely so they do not leave the house in inclement weather without adequate protection is essential information to pass along to parents. Teaching children to avoid walking on frozen lakes and ponds unless they are sure they are adequately frozen is very important. Emphasize to

Table 31-7	Types of Heat Loss
Radiation	Heat loss from the head and areas with less subcutaneous fat and thin skin; e.g., prematurity of the newborn
	This is the most rapid method of heat loss and accounts for at least 50% of heat loss
Conduction	The transfer of heat away from the body by direct contact with a cooler surface; e.g., wet clothing or immersion
Convection	The transfer of heat away from the body by the movement of air over the skin surface; e.g., wind and drafts
Evaporation	The transfer of heat away from the body; e.g., skin moisture turned to vapor as it is dried by the movement of air
Respiration	Expiration of heat from the lungs; e.g., cold and windy weather

parents the need to protect the child from all bodies of water, especially in the cooler temperatures, to avoid both the incidence of accidental drowning and immersion hypothermia.

clinical alert

Other etiologies of hypothermia

The nurse must understand that metabolic or neurological etiologies may be the cause of hypothermia in children. The cause of hypothermia is investigated when no environmental explanation for hypothermia exists.

Nursing Insight— Hypothermia

Hypothermia is also associated with near drowning. When the child's body is immersed in water, heat is lost quickly. During a near drowning, the body tries to maintain core body temperature at the expense of losing heat in the extremities. Shivering is the body's way to rewarm the blood. Increased muscle tone and increased metabolism also occur.

Signs and Symptoms

Hypothermia is classified as minor, moderate, or severe (McCullough & Arora, 2004) (Table 31-8).

Table 31-8 Hypothermia		
Classification	**Body Temperature**	**Clinical Symptoms**
Mild	93.2°–96.8°F (34°–36°C) (Venes, 2009)	Shivering
		Rapid heart rate
		Rapid respiratory rate
		Vasoconstriction
		Increased urine output
		As temperature decreases child becomes apathetic rather than excited, lethargic, and has impaired judgment
Moderate	86°–93°F (30°–34°C) (Venes, 2009)	Decreased heart rate
		Decreased respiratory rate
		Hypotension
		Loss of consciousness
		Decreased pupillary response
Severe	<86°F (30°C) (Venes, 2009)	Apnea
		Asystole
		Coma
		It may not be possible to readily differentiate between severe hypothermia and death

Diagnosis

A diagnosis of hypothermia in children is based on body temperature. Other signs of hypothermia include slurred speech, poor coordination, poor judgment, and inappropriate behavior. If no etiology of prolonged exposure to the cold, the child will need differential diagnostics to determine if the etiology is neurological or metabolic.

clinical alert

Wet clothing

Wet clothes increase the risk of hypothermia. The nurse or parents must remove wet clothing as soon as possible and replace with dry clothing.

Nursing Care

The nurse initiates emergency medical care by calling the emergency response team and by conducting a complete assessment of airway, breathing, and circulation. Cardiopulmonary resuscitation is initiated if the child's condition warrants. The nurse must record core body temperature. Rectal temperatures are most accurate and are used during the rewarming process (McCullough & Arora, 2004). Important nursing care measures include removing all cold and wet clothing, wrapping the child in warmed blankets, and administering warmed oxygen and warmed intravenous fluids to promote cardiac output. Vital signs and urine output are also monitored during the rewarming process. Electrocardiograms are used to give essential information about the heart. The nurse must remember that ventricular or atrial dysrhythmias are possible in hypothermia. After these critical measures are implemented, the nurse raises the body temperature by using a forced air warming system (e.g., the Bair Hugger™). This type of system uses convection to heat the trunk area first (McCullough & Arora, 2004).

case study Hypothermia

Eight-year-old Billy and his friends are planning to ice fish on a small farm pond about 100 yards from his back yard. Billy and his friends are cutting a small hole in the ice, about 10 feet from the shore of the pond when a cracking sound sends Billy's friends running to shore. Billy has always been braver and he continues his work to open an ice hole. In a little while, Billy's friends return to see his progress. As his friends watch from shore, they see Billy fall into the water near the edge of the pond. Billy's friends run to the house to tell Billy's mother. Billy's mother calls 911, then runs down to the pond, and pulls him out. Her cold limp son lies on the ground while she waits for the emergency medical team to arrive. While she waits, she remembers that it is best to remove any wet clothing and begins to frantically undress Billy. She then covers him in the blankets that the friends have brought down to the pond. When the medical team arrives, they find him not breathing and nonresponsive. Billy has no signs of respirations or heartbeat and his body temperature is very cold. The team begins CPR and Billy is transported to the local emergency room.

Frostbite

Frostbite in children is an injury that results from prolonged exposure (more than an hour) to severe cold and usually affects the outer extremities (ears, cheeks, nose, hands, and feet). Crystal formations occur in the tissue and blood cells, which result in dehydration of the cells and ischemic damage.

Signs and Symptoms

Symptoms of frostbite depend on the severity and depth of the cellular damage. Signs of frostbite include red, blue, or pale (waxy) skin. There is a prickling or painful sensation with superficial frostbite and painless rigid skin with deep frostbite.

Diagnosis

Frostbite can be identified by the hard, pale, and cold quality of skin that has been exposed to the cold. As the exposed skin warms and thaws, the flesh becomes red and painful.

Nursing Care

Treatment for frostbite is much like core hypothermia treatment. Place the child in a warm area, remove all wet and cold clothing, and replace with warm ones. If frostbite is in the hands or feet, they are immersed in warm tap water (100°F) for up to one half hour (McCullough & Arora, 2004). The nurse must check the water temperature frequently, as the body part cools the tub of water. Do not run warm water directly from the tap over the area, as tap water can change in temperature rapidly based on use by other household members. The water must also be monitored closely so a secondary burn does not occur in the process of rewarming. Do not rewarm the frozen part with massage or dry heat (McCullough & Arora, 2004). Massage causes the crystals that have formed in the capillaries to break through causing damage in the area. After rewarming is complete, the extremity is wrapped in a soft cloth and the child can be encourage to rest. If no subsequent problems arise, the child can remove the soft cloth and return to inside activities. If parents suspect continued problems the heath care provider is called.

🌼 nursing diagnoses Frostbite

- Impaired Skin Integrity related to freezing of the skin
- Ineffective Thermoregulation related to extended exposure to a cold environment
- Pain related to decreased circulation from prolonged exposure to cold

Pressure Ulcers

Pressure ulcers are the result of compression on one or more areas of the body for an extended period. This subsequently injures both the capillary bed and the soft tissues, allowing for decreased perfusion and subsequent breakdown. Owing to this compression, the skin cells are deprived of nutrients and needed oxygen. Metabolic waste products then accumulate, causing the injury. Any delay in intervention may cause a deep sore to form.

Pressure ulcers occur in children with decreased mobility. Premature infants, infants who have motor delays and cannot easily move their head or extremities, and children with paralysis or other forms of limited mobility are at risk. Children who use mobility devices (e.g., crutches, walkers, and wheelchairs) are at risk for developing pressure ulcers in the weight-bearing tissue used while navigating with these devices. Children and adolescents in casts or body braces are also at risk if the apparatus is ill fitting, or if the areas of pressure are not properly padded. Infants, children, and adolescents who are malnourished or have infections or anemia are at higher risk for ulceration. Children who are bed bound for any period of time, such as children with low cardiac output, are also at risk for ulceration. Children with decreased sensation to pressure or pain may also be at risk of developing skin breakdown and pressure ulcers. Friction and shear from caregivers moving the immobile child is yet another way to injure the skin and decrease local perfusion.

Signs and Symptoms

The four stages of ulcer formation can assist the nurse in thorough skin assessment (Fig. 31-12). The earliest sign of skin damage is a reddened area on the skin that does not disappear within 30 minutes of removing the cause of the pressure or irritant. The skin can appear to have an abrasion and look raw or rubbed. Further damage extends through the dermis forming the ulcer.

✳ Ethnocultural Considerations— Pressure ulcers

In children with dark pigmented skin, the area can look red or purple upon blanching.

Figure 31-12 Stages of pressure ulcer. *A.* Stage 1. *B.* Stage 2. *C.* Stage 3. *D.* Stage 4.

Diagnosis

Diagnosis is based on a good nursing assessment using reliable tools. The Braden Scale (bradenscale.com) is used to assess pressure ulcer risk every 3 to 4 days. The major components assessed in the scale are sensory perception, skin moisture, physical activity, mobility ability, nutrition, and friction and shear (Braden & Bergstrom, 1988). A standardized assessment tool such as the Neonatal Skin Condition Score for neonates may also be used as an assessment tool for at-risk neonates (Lund & Osborn, 2004).

Nursing Care

Careful inspection of a child's skin at least three times a day is essential. The nurse can note the color of the affected area, signs of infection, character of the skin lesion, wound edges, drainage, measure the diameter, and determine the depth of the pressure ulcer. The nurse proactively addresses anemia. A diet high in iron may help prevent pressure ulcers. Keep bed clothing straight and wrinkle-free to decrease areas of pressure. Air, water, or gel mattresses and pads decrease pressure areas. The nurse must keep the child's skin both clean and dry. The nurse also addresses the exact condition affecting the skin before a pressure sore actually develops. A variety of topical treatments are available (Table 31-9).

Stage one and two pressure ulcers are cleansed and allowed to dry. The nurse must also keep the child off the affected area as much as possible. With time and protective management, the wound resolves. Stage three ulcers may heal spontaneously as well. Some hydrophilic gels or hydrocolloidal dressings may be used. In stage 4 ulcers, surgical débridement and closure may be the treatment of choice.

Prevention of pressure ulcers is essential and begins by routinely moving and shifting the weight of the child off bony prominences on a regular basis. Movement must occur at least every 2 hours for the child who is confined to bed. A child in a sitting position (e.g., in a wheelchair) should shift his or her weight every 15 minutes, independently, or with assistance. If the child wears braces, the skin is

Table 31-9 Topical Treatments		
Classification	**Names**	**Precautions**
Anesthetics	Benzocaine (Americaine)	Allergy
	Lidocaine and prilocaine	Do not use over wounds
	(EMLA)	Do not use over large areas: avoid the eyes
Antibacterial	Bacitracin and polymyxin B (AK-Poly-Bac)	Allergy
	Neomycin (Myciguent)	Existing infection (for prevention of infection)
	Mupirocin (Bactroban)	Antibiotic resistance
		Use for only minor cuts/scrapes/burns
Antifungal	Clotrimazole (Lotrimin)	Cautious use in nail and scalp infections
	Ketoconazole (Nizoral)	
	Miconazole	
	(Aloe Vesta)	
	Nystatin (Mycostatin)	
Anti-itch	Diphenhydramine (Benadryl)	Allergy
		Photosensitivity
Emollients	White petrolatum jelly	Allergy
	Mineral oil	Choose fragrance free products
	Lanolin	
	Glycerin	
Steroids	Varying strengths	Allergy
	Strongest group I: betamethasone (Diprolene)	Repeated use in the same area of the skin will cause thinning of the skin
	Group II: dexamethasone (Decadron)	
	Group III: triamcinolone 0.5% (Kenalog)	May inhibit the skin's ability to fight infection
	Group IV: fluocinolone (Lidex)	
	Group V: hydrocortisone 0.2% (A-Hydrocort)	Should be used in lowest strength on the thin skin of the face and genitalia
	Group VI: desonide (Tridesilon)	Avoid the eye area: places the client at risk for glaucoma or cataract formation
	Group VII: hydrocortisone 1% (A-Hydrocort)	

Source: Data from Deglin, J., & Vallerand, A.H. (2009). *Davis's drug guide for nurses* (11th ed.). Philadelphia: F.A. Davis.

inspected for redness or irritation at least once a day. If any redness is noted, the nurse must not reapply the brace and notify the physician immediately.

summary points

◆ Children are often at risk for certain skin conditions based on their large body surface area and maturing immune system.

◆ The specific pathogen that is responsible for a bacterial, viral, or fungal infection affects both the treatment regimen and the healing response.

◆ Contact, atopic, and seborrheic dermatitis is an inflammatory rash on the skin marked by itching and redness that occurs due to numerous conditions.

◆ The offending allergen in a cutaneous skin reaction, causing an allergic response, can be introduced into the system in a variety of ways such as ingestion, inhalation, or coming in direct contact with the allergic child.

◆ Burns that affect children can be accidental or the result of intention to harm and are the third leading cause of death. Some children are at higher risk for burns due to their environment, behavior, or age.

◆ Hypothermia is a life-threatening emergency and the body loses heat in one of five ways: radiation, conduction, convection, evaporation, and respiration.

◆ Pressure ulcers are the result of compression on one or more areas of the body for an extended period; this subsequently injures both the capillary bed and the soft tissues, allowing for decreased perfusion and subsequent breakdown. A pediatric prevention plan for skin breakdown provides a simple tool to assist with pressure ulcer management.

review questions

Multiple Choice

1. A 5-year-old child is being treated for asthma and is using a corticosteroid inhaler. The mother is concerned when she notes white, patchy spots in the child's buccal area and tongue. She tries to rub them off, but is unsuccessful. The pediatric nurse recognizes these lesions as:
   A. *Candida* fungi
   B. Cellulitis
   C. Herpes simplex virus
   D. Varicella

2. A 6-year-old child is admitted from the emergency department to the pediatric unit. The pediatric nurse assesses the child and finds a rash over the abdominal area. The mother states that the child has recently complained of pain in her knees. The nurse notes that the child lives in a rural area and likes to play outdoors in the woods. Based on this information, the nurse suspects that this child has:
   A. Rocky Mountain spotted fever
   B. Cat scratch disease
   C. Lyme disease
   D. Diphtheria

True/False

3. The pediatric nurse recognizes that impetigo is usually found on the child's lips and around the face.

4. The child with atopic dermatitis has a red, raised nonpruritic rash on the face and arms.

5. Females are more likely than males to develop lice infestations because of shared combs and hair accessories.

6. Lice and their nits can infest only a child's scalp or hair.

7. Human bites carry a greater risk for infection than the bites of animals.

Fill-in-the-Blank

8. The most frequent location of cellulitis can be found on a child's_____ and _____. The area infected will be red, _____ and ____ _____to the touch.

9. Before the eruption of the herpes simplex virus, burning, _____ or an _____ _____usually occurs on the _____ or near the mouth.

Case Study

10. Beth, a 17-year-old girl, is diagnosed with acne on her face, chest, and back. She tells the pediatric nurse that she is very unhappy with "all of these ugly pimples all over my body. It's getting to the point that I don't even want to go out with my friends anymore!" What is the most therapeutic response by the nurse?
    A. "Don't worry about the acne. It will go away soon."
    B. "I'll speak with the doctor to order some medication to treat the acne."
    C. "Tell me what bothers you the most about your acne."
    D. "Let's discuss what you can do to prevent more acne from erupting."

11. What is the priority diagnosis for a 17-year-old girl with acne?
    A. Impaired skin integrity
    B. Body image disturbance
    C. Anxiety
    D. Social isolation

12. The pediatric nurse provides health promotion teaching to Beth, a 17-year-old girl with acne who is given a prescription for isotretinoin (Accutane) to treat the acne. The nurse teaches her:
    A. That she must drink two full glasses of water with this medication.
    B. That she must refrain from sexual relationships while on this medication.
    C. That she must use two forms of reliable birth control while on this treatment if sexually active.
    D. That she must eat a high-protein diet while on this medication.

See Answers to End of Chapter Review Questions on the Electronic Study Guide or DavisPlus.

REFERENCES

Ahrens, M. (2001). The U.S. fire problem overview report: Leading causes and other patterns and trends [Electronic Version]. Quincy, MA: National Fire Protection Association.

American Academy of Family Physicians (AAFP). (2004, May). Diaper rash: Tips on prevention and treatment. Retrieved from http://familydoctor.org/051.xml (Accessed July 27, 2008).

American Academy of Pediatrics (AAP) Committee on Infectious Disease (2003). *Red book: Report of the committee on infectious disease* (26th ed.) Elk Grove Village, IL.

American Burn Association (2006). National Burn Repository: 2005 Report. Retrieved from http://www.ameriburn.org/NBR2005.pdf (Accessed July 27, 2008).

American Burn Association. (2007). Burn incidence and treatment in the US: 2007 Fact Sheet. Retrieved from http://www.ameriburn.org/resources_factsheet.php (Accessed July 27, 2008).

Behrman, R.E., Kliegman, R.M., & Jenson, H.B. (2004). *Nelson textbook of pediatrics* (17th ed.). Philadelphia: W.B. Saunders.

Beltrani, V.S. (2002). An overview of chronic urticaria. *Clinical Reviews in Allergy and Immunology, 23,* 147–170.

Bollero, D., Stella, M., Calcagni, M., Guglielmotti, E., & Magliacani, G. (2000). Does inhalation injury really change fluid resuscitation needs? A retrospective analysis. *Annals of Burns and Fire Disasters, 13,* 198-200.

Braden, B., & Bergstrom, N. (1988). The Braden scale for predicting pressure sore risk. Copyright Barbara Braden and Nancy Bergstrom, 1988 All rights reserved. Retrieved from http://www.bradenscale.com/braden.PDF (Accessed July 27, 2008).

Bulechek, G., Butcher, H.M., & Dochterman, J. (2008). *Nursing interventions classification (NIC)* (5th ed.). St. Louis, MO: C.V. Mosby.

Centers for Disease Control and Prevention (CDC). (2002). Lyme disease—United States, 2000. *Morbidity and Mortality Weekly Report, 51*(2), 29–31.

Centers for Disease Control and Prevention (CDC). (2005a, September 27). Cat scratch disease. Retrieved from http://www.cdc.gov/healthypets/diseases/catscratch.htm (Accessed July 27, 2008).

Centers for Disease Control and Prevention (CDC). (2005b, July). CDC recommends two new repellents [Electronic Version]. *Physician and Sports Medicine 33*(6).

Centers for Disease Control and Prevention (CDC). (2005c, May). Rocky Mountain spotted fever. Retrieved from http://www.cdc.gov/ncidod/dvrd/rmsf/Epidemiology.htm (Accessed July 27, 2008).

Centers for Disease Control and Prevention (CDC). (2005d, October 7). Lyme disease prevention and control. Retrieved from http://www.cdc.gov/ncidod/dvbid/lyme/ld_prevent.htm (Accessed July 27, 2008).

Centers for Disease Control and Prevention (CDC). (2006, July 6). Mass casualties: Burns. Retrieved from http://www.bt.cdc.gov/masscasualties/burns.asp (Accessed July 27, 2008).

Cox, R. (2005, November). Burns, chemical. Retrieved from http://www.emedicine.com/emerg/topic73.htm (Accessed July 27, 2008).

Deglin, J.H., & Vallerand, A.H. (2009). *Davis's drug guide for nurses.* (11th ed.). Philadelphia: F.A. Davis.

Demling, R.H., DeSanti, L., & Orgill, D.P. (2000). Biosynthetic skin substitutes: Purpose, properties and clinical indications. Retrieved from http://www.burnsurgery.com/Modules/skinsubstitutes/sec4.htm (Accessed July 27, 2008).

Dictionary.com (2008). Retrieved from http://dictionary.reference.com/browse/synergistic (Accessed July 27, 2008).

Fishman, T.D. (2006). Wound care information network. Retrieved from http://www.medicaledu.com/phases.htm (Accessed July 27, 2008).

Frye, K.E., & Luterman, A. (2005). Decreased incidence of hypertrophic burn scar formation with the use of collagenase, and enzymatic debriding agent [Electronic Version]. *Wounds, 17*(2), 332–336.

Gandhi, M. (2005, June). Rocky Mountain spotted fever. Retrieved from http://www.nlm.nih.gov/medlineplus/ency/article/000654.htm (Accessed July 27, 2008).

Genzyme Biosurgery (2006). Epicel: Cultured epithelial autografts. Retrieved from http://www.genzymebiosurgery.com/ (Accessed July 27, 2008).

Greenhalgh, D.G., Bridges, P., Coombs, E., Chapyak, D., Doyle, W., O'Mara, M.S., & Palmieri, T. (2006). Instant cup of soup: Design flaws increase risk of burn. *Journal of Burn Care & Research, 27*(4), 476–481.

Hill, M. (Ed.). (2003). Dermatologic nursing essentials: A core curriculum [Electronic Version]. Dermatology Nurses Association, Mt. Laurel, NJ.

Hubbuck, C. (2003). Treatment of children with severe burns [Electronic Version]. *Lancet, 362,* 44–45.

Hurtado, R. (2005). Herpes simplex. Retrieved from http://www.nlm.nih.gov/medlineplus/ency/article/001324.htm (Accessed July 28, 2008).

iPLEDGE. (2005). iPLEDGE: Committed to pregnancy prevention. Retrieved from https://www.ipledgeprogram.com/ (Accessed July 28, 2008).

Istre G.R., McCoy, M.A., Osbom, L., Bamard, J.J., Bolton, A. (2001). Deaths and injuries from house fires [Electronic Version]. *New England Journal of Medicine, 344,* 1911–1916.

Johnson, M., Bulechek, G., Butcher, H., McCloskey Dochterman, J., Maas, M., Moorehead, S., & Swanson, E. (2006). *NANDA, NOC, and NIC linkages: Nursing diagnoses, outcomes, & interventions* (2nd ed.). St. Louis, MO: Mosby Elsevier.

Karter, M.J. (2001). Fire loss in the United States during 2000 [Electronic Version]. Quincy, MA: National Fire Protection Association, Fire Analysis and Research Division.

Klein, M.B., Heimbach, D.M., Honari, S., Engrav, L.H., & Gibran, N.S. (2005). Campfire burns: Two avenues for prevention. *Journal of Burn Care & Rehabilitation, 26*(5), 440–442.

Krusinski, P.A., & Flowers, F.P. (2000, March). Common viral infection of the skin. Retrieved from http://merck.micromedex.com/index.asp?page=bpm_brief&article_id=CPM02DE404&hilight=herpesvirus (Accessed July 29, 2008).

Lund, D., & Osborne, J. (2004). Validity and reliability of the neonatal skin condition score. *Journal of Obstetric, Gynecological and Neonatal Nursing, 33*(3), 320–327.

McCullough, L., & Arora, S. (2004). Diagnosis and treatment of hypothermia [Electronic Version]. *American Family Physicians, 70*(12).

Merlin, M., & Bertolini, J. (2005). Rabies. Retrieved from http://www.emedicine.com/emerg/topic493.htm (Accessed July 28, 2008).

Morgan, E.D., Bledsoe, S.C., & Barker, J. (2000). Ambulatory management of burns [Electronic Version]. *American Family Physician, 62*(9), 2015–2026.

Moorehead, S., Johnson, M., Maas, M., & Swanson, E. (2008) *Nursing outcomes classification (NOC)* (4th ed.). St. Louis, MO: C.V. Mosby.

NANDA International (2007). *NANDA-I nursing diagnoses: Definitions and classifications 2007–2008.* Philadelphia: NANDA-I.

National Center for Injury Prevention and Control. (2008). National dog biteprevention week. Retrieved from http://www.cdc.gov/ncipc/duip/biteprevention.htm (Accessed July 27, 2008).

National Fire Protection Association. (2007). The U.S. fire problem. Retrieved from http://www.nfpa.org/itemDetail.asp?categoryID=953&itemID=23071&URL=Research%20&%20Reports/Fire%20statistics/The%20U.S.%20fire%20problem (Accessed July 28, 2008).

National Pediculosis Association, Inc. (2008). Retrieved from http://www.headlice.org/ (Retrieved July 27, 2008).

O'Conner, A., & Besner, G.E. (2004). Burns: Surgical perspective. Retrieved from http://www.emedicine.com/PED/topic2929.htm (Accessed July 28, 2008).

Ong, C.C., Jacobsen, A.S., & Joseph, V.T. (2002). Tissue glue [Electronic Version]. *Pediatric Surgical International 18*(5-6), 552–555.

Pagana, K.D., & Pagana, T.J. (2002). *Mosby's manual of diagnostic and laboratory tests.* St. Louis, MO: C.V. Mosby.

Perry, C. (2003). Thermal injuries. In P.A. Maloney-Harmon & S.J. Czerwinski (Eds), *Nursing care of the pediatric trauma patient* (pp. 277–294). St. Louis, MO: W.B. Saunders.

Potter, P.A., & Perry, A.G. (2004). *Fundamentals of nursing: sixth edition.* St. Louis, MO: C.V. Mosby.

Reed, J.L., & Pomerantz, W.J. (2005). Emergency management of pediatric burns. *Pediatric Emergency Care, 21*(2), 118–129.

Rimdeika, R., Gudaviciene, D., Adamonis, K., Barauskas, G., Pavalkis, D., & Endzinas, Z. (2006). The effectiveness of caloric value of enteral nutrition in patients with major burns. *Burns: Journal of the International Society for Burn Injuries, 32* (1), 83-6.

Selvaggi, G., Monstrey, S., Van Landuyt, K., Hamdi, M., & Blondeel, P. (2005). Rehabilitation of burn injured patients following lightning and electrical trauma [Electronic Version]. *NeuroRehabilitation, 20,* 35–42.

Smith & Nephew Acticoat™ Antimocrobial Barrier Dressing Silcryst (2008). Acticoat antimicrobial dressing. Retrieved from http://www.acticoat.com (Accessed July 27, 2008).

Smith & Nephew. (2006). Transcyte: Human fibroblast derived temporary skin substitute. Retrieved from http://www.wound.smith-nephew.com (Accessed July 28, 2008).

Stump, J.L. (2006, February). Bites, animal. Retrieved from http://www.emedicine.com/emerg/topic60.htm National Center for Injury Section 1.01 (Accessed July 28, 2008).

Uliasz, A, (2002, July). Chapter XXI.4. Burns. Retrieved from http://www.hawaii.edu/medicine/pediatrics/pedtext/s21c04.html (Accessed July 28, 2008).

Ülkür, E., Oncul, O., Karagoz, H., Yeniz, E., & Celikoz, B. (2005). Comparison of silver-coated dressing (acticoat), chlorhexidine acetate 0.5% (Bactigrass), and fusidic acid 2% (Fucidin) for topical antibacterial effect in methicillin-resistant Staphylococci-contaminated wounds [Electronic Version]. *Burns, 31*(7), 874–877.

U.S. Fire Administration. (2005, June). Residential smoking fires and casualties. Retrieved from http://www.usfa.fema.gov/downloads/pdf/tfrs/v5i5.pdf. (Accessed July 28, 2008).

Venes, D. (Ed.). (2009). *Taber's cyclopedic medical dictionary* (21st ed.). Philadelphia: F.A. Davis.

Watkins, P. (2005). Impetigo: Aetiology, complication and treatment options [Electronic Version]. *Nursing Standard, 19*(36), 51–54.

Whetstone, W.D. (2005). Chemical burn or reaction. Retrieved from http://www.nlm.nih.gov/medlineplus/ency/article/000059.htm (Accessed July 28, 2008).

 For more information, go to http://davisplus.fadavis.com/

CONCEPT MAP

Care of the Child with an Integumentary Condition

Bites/Stings
- Insect
- Animals
- Human

- Lyme disease
- Rocky Mtn Spotted Fever
- Cat scratch fever

General Nursing Care
- Assess bitten area
- Assess for systemic reaction → necrosis, anaphylaxis
- Treat local symptoms
- Cover area
- Prevent complications: cellulitis, rabies, tetanus, other infections
- Teach: repellants, approaches

Infestations
- Lice
- Mites

General Nursing Care
- ID risk factors → close quarters, socioeconomic status
- Total body assessment
- Complete treatment of:
  - Family
  - Environment
  - Community
- Non-judgmental attitude

Skin Assessment
- A visual assessment along with a complete history is important
- Temp/texture
- Signs of trauma
- Birthmarks

Nursing Insight:
- Use proper terms for skin conditions
- Wound bond vs. sutures
- How to control and remove ticks
- Developmental stage is related to type of burn risk

Burns
- Thermal
  - Fire, scalding
- Chemical
  - Household chemicals
- Electric
  - Outlets, frayed cords
- Radiation
  - Sun

Lesions
- Primary
  - Macules, papules, tumors, pustules, wheals
- Secondary
  - Crusts, scars, keloids, ulcers

Dermatitis
- Contact
- Atopic
- Seborrheic

Critical Nursing Action:
- Proper environment for assessing skin
- Age-appropriate HSV-2 teaching; establish trust
- Prevent secondary infections in atopic dermatitis
- Assess for systemic allergic reaction

Categories
- Depth: thickness → superficial, partial, full
- Body surface area: Lund and Browder chart, Rule of 9's
- Severity: mild, moderate, major

Skin Infections
- Bacterial
  - Acne
  - Impetigo
  - Cellulitis
- Viral
  - HPV
  - HSV-1 and -2
- Fungal
  - Cutaneous candidiasis
  - Ringworm

General Nursing Care
- ID allergen/irritant
  - Use drying agent/cool baths
  - Topical or oral meds
  - Maintain skin integrity
  - Attend to self-image

Clinical Alert:
- Strep A can cause necrotizing fasciitis
- Severe med allergy can result in Stevens Johnson syndrome: can be fatal
- Core body temperature falls below 95°F (35°C) is a life-threatening emergency

Nursing: Mod → Major Burns
- Emergent care: ABC's
- Assess burn characteristics/category
- Fluid resuscitation: Parkland formula
- Nutrition: child = 2× normal requirements
- Pain management: IV opioids
- Wound care: débridement, escharotomy, cleansing
- Grafting

General Nursing Care
- Correctly identify lesion, organism
- Maintain clean, intact skin
- Monitor exudate
- Use good handwashing
- Control itching
- Thoroughly cleanse environmental transmission items
- Prevent spread; prevent self-inoculation
- Treat sequella
- Teach regarding sexual spread of HSV-2. No cure
- Instruct about mouth rinse for users of inhaled steroids
- Instruct about need for frequent diaper changes

Family Teaching Guidelines:
- Completion and correct dosing of antibiotics
- Decreasing transmission and preventing outbreaks of HSV-1 and -2
- How to assess for and treat lice

Across Care Settings:
- Six C's of minor burn management

Collaboration In Caring:
- Teach community use of Epi-pen; allergy contact information
- A team approach to care for the severely burned child

What To Say:
- Assessing acne in adolescents
- Teach child and caregiver about impetigo
- Prevent animal bites
- Gathering important burn information

Complementary Care:
- Topical agents for rashes: bag balm, aloe vera, vitamin E preparations
- Distraction: a good technique when changing burn dressings

Now Can You:
- Name one infectious condition of the skin and state priority nursing interventions
- Identify the various types of insect bites and which requires emergency treatment

Caring for the Child with a Renal, Urinary Tract, or Reproductive Condition

chapter
32

 Children are one-third of our population and all of our future.

—Select Panel for the Promotion of Child Health, 1981

LEARNING TARGETS *At the completion of this chapter, the student will be able to:*

◆ Examine fluid and electrolyte balance in children.

◆ Discuss the four signs and symptoms of a urinary tract infection.

◆ Compare the differences between acute and chronic glomerulonephritis.

◆ Examine the most common cause and spread of bacterial infection that can lead to hemolytic–uremic syndrome.

◆ Describe the nursing care and nursing diagnoses associated with renal transplant and dialysis in children.

◆ State the pathophysiology and clinical symptoms of vesicoureteral reflux.

◆ Describe how testicular torsion is considered a medical emergency.

◆ Explain the diagnosis and risks of cryptorchidism.

◆ Describe a variety of genitourinary abnormalities in male and female children.

◆ Examine the most common causes of amenorrhea in female adolescents.

---

 moving toward evidence-based practice Compliance with Care for Urinary Tract Infection

Cohen, A.L., Rivara, F.P., Davis, R., & Christakis, D.A. (2005). Compliance with guidelines for the medical care of first urinary tract infections in infants: A population-based study. *Pediatrics, 115*(6), 1474–1478.

The purpose of this study was to describe the medical care received by children enrolled in a state Medicaid program after their first urinary tract infection. The study also aimed to determine predictors for prescribed care during the child's first year of life. It is estimated that 6.5% of girls and 3.3% of boys experience a urinary tract infection (UTI) during their first year of life, with vesicoureteral reflux present in 30% to 40% of these children. The long-term impact of UTI may include a variety of conditions such as risk for recurrent urinary tract infections as well as renal scarring, disease, and hypertension. These conditions may be prevented by effective evaluation and treatment. This study was based on the American Academy of Pediatrics (1999), practice guidelines that which include "timely anatomic

imaging, timely imaging for reflux, and adequate antimicrobial prophylaxis."

- Anatomical imaging was defined as "urinary tract ultrasonography or renal scan within 3 months of initial diagnosis" (p. 1475).
- Imaging for reflux was defined as "voiding cystourethrography or renal scan within 3 months of initial diagnosis" (p. 1475).
- Antimicrobial prophylaxis was defined as "antibiotic therapy after diagnosis until imaging for reflux was performed" (p. 1475).

The retrospective cohort study used statistics obtained from a state Medicaid program database. Medicaid insurance is

(continued)

---

moving toward evidence-based practice (continued)

offered "to all children living within the state whose families earn <200% of the federal poverty level" (p. 1471).

The following inclusion criteria were used for each child:

- Born between January 1, 1999, and September 30, 2000.
- Continuously enrolled in the Medicaid program from birth through age 15 months.
- Diagnosed with a UTI during the first 12 months of life as determined by either provider-billed diagnosis (for inpatient) or provider-billed diagnosis and an antibiotic prescription filled within 1 week of diagnosis (for outpatient).
- In the case of multiple diagnoses, only children with UTI listed as the primary diagnosis or secondary diagnosis were included.
- When UTI was listed as a secondary diagnosis, the primary diagnosis was reviewed. If conditions predisposing to urinary catheterizations were present, those children were excluded.

Analysis of data examined medical management, age, gender, race, primary language of the parent, Medicaid program plan (managed care or fee-for-service), and location of household (rural or urban).

The findings were as follows:

- Of a potential 38,793 Medicaid-eligible children, 780 met the criteria for the study based on the diagnosis of a UTI during the first year of life.
- Of the 708 eligible children:
  38.7% (302) were hospitalized for the UTI.
  59.7% were female.
  17.7% were ≤90 days old.
  29.7% lived in a rural area.
  64.6% were participants in a managed care plan.
- The sample was representative of the following racial mix:
  Caucasian 43.5%
  Hispanic 27.8%
  African American 3.3%

Asian American 3.0%
American Indian 2.3%
Other 8.2%
11.9% not specified

- English was the primary language for all but 29% of the participants.
- UTI was the primary diagnosis for 83% of the participants.
- Febrile seizures, fever, and bronchiolitis were the most common primary diagnoses for those with UTI as the secondary diagnosis.
- Forty-four percent received timely anatomical imaging and 39.5% received imaging for reflux during the first year of life, as prescribed by AAP guidelines.
- Both anatomical imaging and imaging for reflux were performed in 28.2% (220) of children diagnosed with UTI.
- Anatomical imaging was performed in only 15.8% (123) and imaging for reflux only was performed in 11.3% (88).
- Fifty-one percent received an adequate course of antibiotics, according to AAP guidelines.

Children who were hospitalized for UTI were more likely to receive anatomical imaging and imaging for reflux. Children 90 days of age or younger were less likely to receive antimicrobial prophylaxis. Females were more likely to receive imaging for reflux. Children were less likely to receive appropriate imaging after the first UTI if they came from families in which English was not the primary language and if they lived in rural locations.

The overall conclusion was that there was poor compliance with AAP guidelines for children enrolled in the Medicaid program whose first UTI occurred during the first year of life.

---

1. What might be considered as limitations to this study?
2. How is this information useful to clinical nursing practice?

See Suggested Responses for Moving Toward Evidence-Based Practice on the Electronic Study Guide or DavisPlus.

Introduction

Renal and reproductive conditions in children are attributable to a variety of causes: a genetic predisposition, a condition that may have occurred during fetal development, infection, trauma, or a neurological problem. No matter what the cause, pediatric nurses must be knowledgeable about the pathophysiology of the renal system, common and uncommon renal disorders, as well as associated reproductive anomalies that can occur in children. This chapter provides a short review of the anatomy and physiology of the renal system followed by a discussion of fluid and electrolyte balance. An examination of the acute and chronic renal diseases and reproductive system problems common in children is presented. Information on diagnostic tests, medications prescribed, and developmentally appropriate nursing interventions is provided together with information about patient/family education. Preventive measures taught by nurses are provided because they can be influential in reducing the incidence of fluid and electrolyte imbalance and renal and reproductive disease.

A & P review The Kidneys

The kidney is divided into an outer cortex and inner medulla. The outer cortex is composed of the glomeruli and convoluted tubules of the nephron and blood vessels. The medulla is composed of the renal pyramid. Urine leaves the papilla of a pyramid to collect in a minor calyx. The minor calyxes come together to make the major calyces and then the renal pelvis (Hansen & Koeppen, 2002).

Each kidney is surrounded by adipose tissue to protect it from trauma, although kidneys can be injured by blows to the abdomen and such trauma as motor vehicle accidents.

Kidneys receive their blood supply through a single renal artery that comes from each side of the aorta, one to each kidney. The renal artery subdivides into five segmental arteries that feed each kidney. Each segmental artery further subdivides into multiple branches several times; the smallest of these are the afferent arterioles, which feed the glomeruli (Porth, 2004).

The glomerulus is a tuft of capillaries in a thin-walled capsule termed Bowman's capsule. While blood flows into the glomerulus through the afferent arteriole, it leaves through the efferent arterial. Fluid and blood particles are filtered through capillary membranes into a fluid-filled space in Bowman's capsule. The filtered blood is termed the filtrate.

The tubular components of the nephron are divided into four parts. The first part is a very coiled portion termed the proximal convoluted tubule, and this drains Bowman's capsule. The second part is a thin loop termed the loop of Henle, while the third part is the distal convoluted tubule. The fourth and final part is the collecting tubule, which joins several tubules together to collect filtrate. About 85% of the nephrons are cortical nephrons, so termed because they are on the superficial portion of the cortex. The remaining 15% of the nephrons penetrate deeper into the medulla and are involved with urine concentration (Porth, 2004) (Fig. 32-1). ◆

Fluid and Electrolyte Balance

Fluid balance means that the liquid in the body is regulated in such a way to maintain homeostasis (a state of equilibrium). The body's intake and output of fluid in a 24-hour period is approximately the same. A fluid deficit occurs when fluids are lost by diaphoresis, vomiting, diarrhea, or hemorrhage. A fluid overload occurs from conditions that create impaired fluid excretion, such as kidney disease or congestive heart failure. Fluid overload also can occur due to excessive administration of intravenous fluids (Venes, 2005). Fluid balance is measured by daily discrepancies in body weight and by monitoring fluid intake and output.

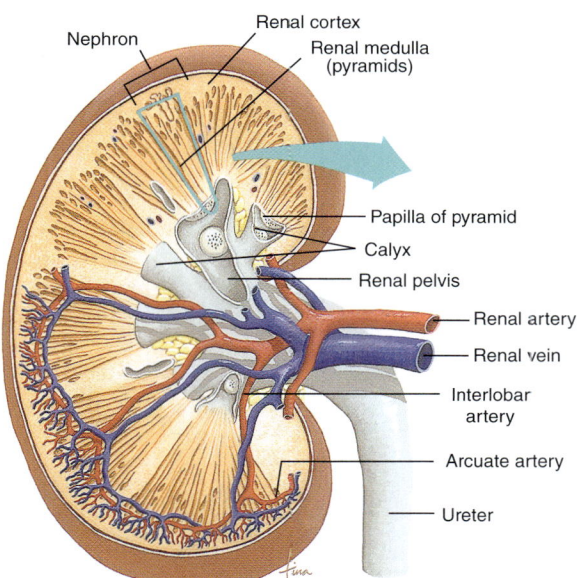

Figure 32-1 Anatomy of the kidney.

clinical alert

Calculation of daily maintenance fluid requirements

There are two methods of fluid maintenance:

The surface area method is the most common and used for children >22 lbs. (10 kg): 1500–2000 mL/m^2 per day.

Child's Weight	Daily Maintenance Fluid Requirement
0–10 kg (0–22 lbs.)	100 mL/kg of body weight
11–20 kg (24.2–44 lbs.)	1000 mL + 50 mL/kg for each kg >10
>20 kg (>44 lbs.)	1500 mL + 20 mL/kg for each kg >20

Note: The method used to measure normal urinary output is 1–2 mL/kg per hour.

Children are at a greater risk for fluid and electrolyte imbalance than adults because they have a proportionately greater amount of body water, require more fluid intake and subsequently excrete more fluid.

Nursing Insight— *Compared to adults, children are at a greater risk for fluid and electrolyte imbalance*

Children have:
- A greater body surface area
- A higher percentage of total body water (the volume of total body water decreases with increasing age)
- A greater potential for fluid loss via the gastrointestinal tract and skin
- An increased incidence of fever, upper respiratory infections and gastroenteritis
- A greater metabolic rate
- Immature kidneys that are inefficient at excreting waste products
- Kidneys that have a decreased ability to concentrate urine
- Increased risk for developing hypernatremia based on their inability to verbalize thirst

The body is continually losing water in the urine, stool, and by evaporation from the skin and lungs. If the child is not taking in enough fluids to make up for the amount lost, they can become dehydrated. Dehydration occurs when the amount of fluids leaving the body is greater than the amount of fluids being taken into the body.

clinical alert

Types of dehydration

Depending on the cause of the fluid loss, a child will lose water and electrolytes.

Dehydration is classified as isotonic, hypotonic, or hypertonic.

Isotonic dehydration occurs when electrolyte and water deficits are present in balanced proportions (sodium and water are lost in equal amounts). Serum sodium remains in normal limits 130–150 mEq/L. This is the most common type of dehydration. Hypovolemic shock is the greatest concern.

Hypotonic dehydration occurs when the electrolyte deficit exceeds the water deficit. Serum sodium concentration is <130 mEq/L. Physical signs are more severe with smaller fluid losses.

Hypertonic dehydration is the most dangerous type and occurs when water loss is in excess of electrolyte loss. Sodium serum concentration is >150 mEq/L. Seizures are likely to occur.

Assessment is a priority nursing action when caring for the child with a fluid and/or electrolyte imbalance. The astute nurse must recognize fluid deficit and excess as well as electrolyte imbalance and then provide the proper care. Sometimes emergent care is required where IV replacement of fluids and electrolytes is essential.

 ### Nursing Insight— *Fluid deficit and excess*

Fluid deficit (to determine normal values use calculation of daily maintenance fluid requirements)

Causes	Signs and symptoms	Nursing care
Diminished fluid intake	Dry skin	Determine underlying cause
Diaphoresis	Sticky mucous membranes	Replace fluids
Vomiting	Poor skin turgor	Replace electrolytes
Diarrhea	Thirst	Oral hydration
Nasogastric suction	Poor perfusion	IV hydration
Fever	Decreased urinary output	Measure intake and output
Hemorrhage	Weight loss	Monitor vital signs
	Fatigue	Monitor laboratory values (electrolytes)
	Tachycardia	
	Tachypnea	
	Decreased blood pressure	
	High urine specific gravity	
	High hematocrit	

Fluid excess (to determine normal values use calculation of daily maintenance fluid requirements)

Causes	Signs and symptoms	Nursing care
Excessive oral intake	Pulmonary edema (crackles)	Determine underlying cause
Hypotonic fluid overload	Weight gain (fluid retention)	Decrease fluid intake
Kidney disease	Lethargy	Administer diuretics
	Decreased level of consciousness	Monitor vital signs
	Slow, bounding pulse	Monitor laboratory values (electrolytes)
	Low urine specific gravity	
	Decreased hematocrit	

In the early phases of dehydration, extracellular fluids with some electrolytes are lost. If the fluid loss continues, loss of intracellular fluids can occur. Hypovolemic shock occurs when there is an insufficient amount of fluid in the circulatory system and subsequent death can result.

 ### clinical alert

Pathophysiology of dehydration

Reasons for dehydration:

- Fever
- Vomiting
- Diarrhea
- Diaphoresis
- Hemorrhage
- Burns
- Trauma
- Diminished fluid intake
- Rapid and sudden extracellular fluid loss
  - Electrolyte imbalance
  - Intracellular fluid loss
  - Cellular dysfunction

Signs of hypovolemic shock:

- Tachycardia
- Tachypnea
- Hypotension
- Cool, clammy, or cyanotic skin
- Decreased urine output
- Death

The main electrolytes are sodium (the primary electrolyte of the extracellular fluid) and potassium (the primary electrolyte of intracellular fluid). These electrolytes keep the body in balance by maintaining muscle contraction, heart rhythm and brain function. Normal values for sodium is 130 to 150 mEq/L and potassium 3.5 to 5.5 mEq/L. An imbalance in one or both of these electrolytes can cause illness in children. Calcium imbalance can also pose problems for children. The normal value for calcium is 8.8 to 10.8 mEq/L.

 ### Nursing Insight— *Electrolyte Imbalance*

Sodium (Na^+) deficit (hyponatremia; serum sodium concentration <130 mEq/L)

Causes	Signs and symptoms	Nursing care
Decreased sodium intake	Dehydration	Determine underlying cause
Excessive sweating	Nausea	
Fever	Weakness	Administer IV fluids with the appropriate amount of sodium added
Malnutrition	Lethargy	Monitor laboratory values (electrolytes)
Vomiting	Abdominal cramping	
Diarrhea	Dizziness	
Nasogastric suction	Weak pulse	
Diabetic ketoacidosis	Decreased blood pressure	
Kidney disease		

Sodium (Na⁺) excess (hypernatremia; serum sodium concentration ≥150 mEq/L)

Causes	Signs and symptoms	Nursing care
Excessive salt intake	Oliguria	Determine underlying cause
Fever	Nausea	Monitor neurological status
High insensible water loss	Vomiting	Monitor laboratory values (electrolytes)
Diabetes insipidus	Muscle twitching	
Hyper glycemia	Lethargy	
Kidney disease		

Potassium (N⁺) deficit (hypokalemia; serum potassium concentration ≤3.5 mEq/L)

Causes	Signs and symptoms	Nursing care
Diuresis	Muscle weakness	Determine underlying cause
Starvation	Muscle cramping and stiffness	Monitor vital signs
IV fluid without potassium added	Hypotension	Offer high-potassium foods
Diarrhea	Hyporeflexia	Administer oral potassium supplements (assess for adequate output before administration)
Vomiting	Cardiac arrhythmias (tachycardia or bradycardia)	Administer IV potassium slowly
Nasogastric suction	Fatigue	Obtain ECG (for IV potassium bolus)
Administration of diuretics or corticosteroids	Drowsiness	Monitor laboratory values (electrolytes)
Burns that are healing		Evaluate acid-base status
Alkalosis		

Potassium (N⁺) excess (hyperkalemia; serum potassium concentration ≥5.5 mEq/L)

Causes	Signs and symptoms	Nursing care
Increased intake of potassium	Muscle twitching	Determine underlying cause
Severe dehydration	Muscle weakness	Monitor vital signs
	Flaccid paralysis	Obtain ECG
Rapid administration of IV potassium chloride	Hyperreflexia	Administer IV fluids as ordered
Potassium sparing diuretics	Oliguria	Administer IV insulin to facilitate potassium moving into cells (if ordered)
Burns	Apnea (respiratory arrest)	Monitor laboratory values (electrolytes)

Kidney disease (failure)	Bradycardia	Evaluate acid–base status
Adrenal insufficiency (Addison disease)	Ventricular fibrillation (cardiac arrest)	
Metabolic acidosis		

Calcium (Ca²⁺) deficit (hypocalcemia; serum calcium concentration <8.8 mEq/L)

Causes	Signs and symptoms	Nursing care
Inadequate dietary intake	Tetany	Determine underlying cause
Vitamin D deficiency	Convulsions	Administer oral calcium supplement as prescribed
Feeding cow's milk to infants	Neuromuscular irritability	Administer IV calcium slowly and monitor IV site (irritation)
Advanced adrenal insufficiency	Hypotension	Monitor laboratory values (electrolytes)
	Tingling (nose, ears, toes, and fingertips)	
	Cardiac arrest	

Calcium (Ca²⁺) excess (hypercalcemia; serum calcium concentration >10.8 mEq/L)

Causes	Signs and symptoms	Nursing care
Excessive vitamin D intake	Weakness	Determine underlying cause
Acidosis	Fatigue	Obtain ECG
Immobilization (prolonged periods of time)	Constipation	Monitor laboratory values (electrolytes)
Increased bone catabolism	Anorexia	
Hyperthyroidism	Nausea	
Kidney disease	Vomiting	
	Thirst	
	Bradycardia (cardiac arrest)	

Nursing care centers on recognizing the underlying cause and then replacing water loss and electrolytes. Another nursing care measure is education. The nurse explains to parents the signs and symptoms of dehydration, the importance of offering clear liquids as ordered and home care.

🌼 **Nursing Insight**— *Fluid and electrolyte balance nursing interventions*

- Obtain daily weights (same scale, same time, and wearing the same clothing) (infants are weighed naked and often older children are weighed only in their underwear).
- Measure intake and output (weigh diapers to assess output).

- Assess hydration status which includes assessing for presence of tears, skin turgor, anterior fontanel (up to 18 months), sticky mucous membranes, sunken eyeballs, urine and stool output, weight loss, tachycardia, tachypnea, decreased blood pressure, temperature and thirst.
- Laboratory tests include specific gravity, hematocrit, blood urea nitrogen (BUN), creatinine, Na^+, K^+, and Ca^{2+}.
- Assess the type of acid–base disturbance (metabolic acidosis, metabolic alkalosis, or respiratory acidosis) (see Chapter 24).
- Administer oral clear liquids as ordered (1–2 oz. every hour).
- Start an IV for fluid and electrolyte replacement as ordered.
- Before administering intravenous potassium (K^+), ensure the child has voided (to prevent tubular necrosis).
- Cleanse perineal area and apply protective topical ointment.
- Encourage the parents to be involved in the care of child.
- Educate the parents about signs and symptoms of dehydration, rehydration and when to call the doctor.
- Encourage parents to be compliant with follow-up appointment(s).

Disorders of the Renal and Urinary Systems

URINARY TRACT INFECTIONS

An acquired infection of the urinary system caused by a bacterium, virus, or fungus is referred to as a **urinary tract infection** (UTI). Often the infection is acquired in association with newborn bacteremia seeding into the renal circulation or by the ascending route via the urinary system (Lebel, 2004). Urinary tract infection is the second most common form of bacterial infection in children, ranking only behind upper respiratory problems (Snyder, 2002). It is thought that 8% of girls and 2% of boys will have a UTI during childhood. UTIs are a serious threat to the health of any newborn, infant, preschooler, school-age child, or adolescent.

Gender, age, race, renal tissue, poor hygiene, constipation, nutritional status, adaptive and resistant qualities of the causative agents, as well as structural abnormalities, catheterization, urinary tract instrumentation, and sexual activity all contribute to the incidence and etiology of this disease (Lum, 2007; Wise & Cardinal-Busse, 2007).

During the first year of life, boys are at a greater risk for a UTI. The higher incidence in boys is partially attributed to the higher rate of congenital abnormalities in the male newborn (Lippincott Williams & Wilkins, 2004). Starting at 6 months, girls are at greater risk until school age and then again when they enter adolescence, owing to their proximity of the anus with fecal flora available to colonize easily within the urethra. Sexually active adolescent girls have a higher incidence of UTIs than do boys, as well as a greater incidence than any age group. The causative agent is *Chlamydia*.

UTIs are also more common in uncircumcised males (Elder, 2004). Circumcision reduces the risk of UTIs in boys (Lum, 2007). Breastfeeding is also correlated with a decreased incidence of infection of the urinary tract (Lebel, 2004).

 Nursing Insight— Renal scarring

"Once bacteria gain entrance into the renal medulla, an immune response is stimulated. A substance called superoxide is released and eliminates the bacteria. In the process of killing the bacteria, however, damage occurs to the tubular cell wall that produces renal scarring. Scarring causes decreased usable space in the renal parenchyma and loss of function. End-stage renal disease can occur due to scarring" (Bernstein & Shelov, 2003, p. 605).

The most common invading bacterium responsible for UTIs is *Escherichia coli*; *Klebsiella, Proteus,* enterococci, and *Staphylococcus saprophyticus* (Stead, Matthews, & Kaufman, 2004). *Pseudomonas aeruginosa* and *Staphylococcus epidermidis* also commonly cause UTI in children (Snyder, 2002).

Any alteration that interferes with elimination creates a risk for UTI. Conditions associated with chronic perineal irritation such as poor hygiene, bubble baths, soaps, pinworms, or perineal trauma that experienced cyclists, dirt bikers, or equestrians may experience are important associations to consider in predisposing the individual to UTIs. Conditions such as constipation, neurogenic bladder, and voiding dysfunction, or a history of abnormal voiding patterns are potential underlying etiological factors. It is important to consider anatomical abnormalities such as posterior urethral valves and ureterocele (Kennedy, 2003).

A child with a UTI may also have an anatomical abnormality called vesicoureteral reflux (VUR). In this condition, there is a backward (retrograde) flow of urine from the bladder intro the ureters and nephron components. It is a common underlying cause of febrile UTI in infants and very young children.

 Nursing Insight— Urinary tract infections

- The higher the infection in the urinary system, the greater the risk for morbidity and significant long-term deteriorating health alterations.
- Within the first 2 years of life, infections that progress into the renal parenchyma frequently cause scarring, resulting in hypertension leading to chronic renal failure (inability of the kidneys to function adequately) (Elder, 2004).
- There is a high occurrence of UTIs in the newborn period followed closely by ages 1 to 3 months; the most frequent pathogen is *E. coli*.
- Children with indwelling Foley catheters or on continuous antibiotics frequently can contract a UTI.

SIGNS AND SYMPTOMS. Unique age-related signs and symptoms in the neonate are failure to thrive, jaundice, fever or hypothermia, poor feeding, or vomiting. The infant usually is a poor feeder, has fever, strong-smelling urine, vomiting, and diarrhea. The preschooler often presents with anorexia and sleepiness along with vomiting, diarrhea, abdominal pain, fever, strong-smelling urine, enuresis, dysuria, urgency, or frequency. The school-age child has new enuresis, strong-smelling urine, urgency, or flank pain and some changes of personality. Adolescents often experience fatigue and flank pain. Visual inspection of external genitalia for irritation, pinworms, sexual abuse, trauma, or vaginitis is important (Egland & Egland, 2006).

Nursing Insight— *Urinary tract infections*

Adolescents are more likely to have classic adult symptoms of cystitis that is concurrent with vaginitis (35%) rather than only a UTI (17%) (Egland & Egland, 2006; Luxner, 2005). Dull flank pain and costovertebral angle are associated with renal involvement (Newberry, 2003).

DIAGNOSIS. Owing to the long-term consequences of a UTI in childhood, early accurate diagnosis and treatment are of paramount importance. Early diagnosis is essential and is based on signs and symptoms as well as urine collection to obtain the culture (Kennedy, 2003; Schwartz, 2005). A complete blood count (CBC) with differential is done, as well as a test for blood urea nitrogen (BUN) and creatinine.

To localize the actual infection, imaging studies are delayed for 3 to 6 weeks after an infection for follow-up. If, however, obstruction is suspected, imaging studies are done.

diagnostic tools Determining Problems with the Urinary Tract

- The renal ultrasound depicts the ureters but does not discern if there is an infection.
- A voiding cystourethrogram (VCUG) depicts urethral and bladder anatomy.
- An intravenous pyelogram assists with identifying the size, shape, and position of the urinary system as well as elimination function by noting length of time for passage of contrast material through the kidneys.
- Nuclear cystography visualizes the bladder and is good for detecting VUR.
- Nuclear cortical scanning detects tubular damage and scarring (Egland & Egland, 2006; Pagana & Pagana, 2003).

NURSING CARE. The goals of nursing care are to collaborate with the patient, family, and other health care providers along the continuum of care needed to diagnose and treat the urinary tract infection. Concurrent with every diagnostic test, medications prescribed, and developmentally appropriate nursing intervention provided is the underlying goal of patient/family education that explains each step of the treatment process.

The nurse obtains a history that identifies risk factors, clinical manifestations, medications given, nutritional and fluid intake needed, and output parameters required for healing to occur.

Typically, patients who require IV fluids or IV antibiotics, neonates, and infants identified as high risk are admitted to the hospital. All infants younger than 1 month with suspected UTI, even if not febrile, are admitted. There

where research and practice meet: Urinalysis

Since approximately 20% of patients with UTIs have a normal urinalysis, a urine culture and sensitivity should be obtained and sent to the lab (Cincinnati Children's Hospital Medical Center, 2005; Egland & Egland, 2006).

may be other reasons for admission based on the health care provider and/or family's collaborative decision (Cincinnati Children's Hospital Medical Center, 2005; Egland & Egland, 2006).

Parenteral antibiotics are used to treat UTIs. The most common anti-infective agents are listed in Table 32-1.

It is important to keep track of intake and output, as well as any odors associated with the urine. A fishy malodorous aroma without other clinical manifestations may still indicate a UTI and a health care provider should be consulted.

Nursing Insight— *Broad-spectrum antibiotics*

It is important that nurses emphasize the importance and rationale for taking all antibiotics for the entire designated time along with adequate intake of fluids. For children on low-dose antibiotics prophylactically, medication taken at night allows the drug more time in the bladder.

Children who receive broad-spectrum antibiotics that are likely to alter GI and periurethral flora are at increased risk for UTI because these drugs disturb the natural defense against colonization by pathogenic bacteria (Hellerstein, 2007, p. 4).

Nursing Insight— *Urinary tract infections*

The most significant risk factor for UTIs is the presence of a urinary tract abnormality that causes urinary stasis, obstruction, reflux, or dysfunctional voiding. **Pyelonephritis** (an infection in the renal pelvis) causes renal scarring and, with repeated infections, hypertension or end-stage renal disease.

VESICOURETERAL REFLUX

Normally, urine should flow downward from the kidneys through the ureters into the bladder and urethra. In vesicoureteral reflux (VUR) the urine backflows from the bladder to the ureters and back to the kidneys. The disorder occurs at the vesicoureteral junction, which normally creates a one-way valve for the urine to enter the bladder without being refluxed back into the ureters or kidneys. VUR is found as a common cause of children with UTI, and it is most frequently diagnosed between ages 2 and 3. VUR is more common in girls, is familial and is more common in Caucasians. It is a cause of UTI in infants and children, and is more commonly diagnosed after the first or second UTI episode.

Primary Vesicoureteral Reflux

A child may be born with a valvular defect at the ureter and bladder junction, due to insufficient fetal growth of the ureter. The resultant valvular defect allows urine to backflow from the bladder to the ureters. As a child grows and the ureters lengthen, this type of VUR may resolve spontaneously (National Kidney and Urologic Diseases Information Clearinghouse, 2007).

Secondary Vesicoureteral Reflux

In this category of reflux, there may be an obstruction within the urinary system, possibly related to UTI, which causes ureteral inflammation. The edema itself causes a

Table 32-1 Common Anti-infective Agents, Side Effects, and Nursing Interventions

Anti-infective	Side Effects	Nursing Intervention
Cefotaxime (IV) Claforan	Mild diarrhea, mild abdominal cramping	Monitor fluid intake.
Ampicillin (IV) Marcillin	Nausea, vomiting, diarrhea, rash	Hold and notify MD if rash or diarrhea develops. With prolonged therapy periodically monitor renal, hepatic, and hematology lab work.
Gentamicin (IV) Garamycin	Serious side effect: Ototoxicity and nephrotoxicity	Monitor urinalysis. Therapeutic peak 5–10 mcg/mL and trough 2 mcg/mL. The family needs to notify physician of any balance, hearing, urinary, or vision problems even after drug is completed.
Ceftriaxome (IV) Rocephin	Serious side effect: Antibiotic-associated colitis manifested as severe abdominal pain, tenderness, fever, and diarrhea that is severe and watery	Assess bowel pattern or pain. Monitor I & O.
Cefixime (PO) Suprax	Serious side effects: Stevens-Johnson syndrome, nephrotoxicity, blood dyscrasias Superinfections (can occur with any antibiotic)	Monitor BUN and serum creatinine, I & O. Teach how to recognize superinfection (e.g., furry tongue, perineal itching). Take with yogurt/buttermilk to decrease superinfection by maintaining intestinal flora.
Cephalexin (PO) Biocef, Keflex	Serious side effects: Antibiotic-associated colitis and other superinfections; nephrotoxicity with preexisting renal disease, angioedema, bronchospasm, and anaphylaxis especially if allergies to penicillin or cephalosporins	Monitor I & O for nephrotoxicity. Assess bowel activity and stool consistency and increasing GI effects. Take with food or milk if mild GI upset occurs. Assess mucous membranes and tongue for white patches.
Sulfamethoxazole-trimethoprim (PO) Bactrim, Septra, *Generic*	Serious side effects: Fatalities secondary to Stevens-Johnson syndrome, toxic epidermal necrolysis, fulminant hepatic necrosis, and other blood dyscrasias such as agranulocytosis, aplastic anemia	Contraindicated in children younger than 2 months of age; kernicterus may result if used with newborns. Monitor I & O; assess skin for pallor, purpura, and rash or overt signs of bleeding, swelling. Monitor hematology, liver and renal function lab results. Family needs to report new symptoms (e.g., bruising, fever, sore throat, or other skin reactions).
Nitrofurantoin (PO) Macrodantin, Furadantin	Serious side effects: Stevens-Johnson syndrome, liver toxicity, peripheral neuropathy, impairment of pulmonary function	Monitor for peripheral neuropathy (e.g., numbness and/or tingling of extremities). Monitor for liver toxicity signs and symptoms. Monitor respiratory system and chest pain, cough, or difficulty with respirations.
Ciprofloxacin (PO) Cipro	Many IV incompatibilities Serious side effects: Superinfection, nephrotoxicity, cardiac arrest, cerebral thrombosis Arthropathy may occur in children younger than 18 years	Monitor I & O; ensure that appropriate fluid intake maintained. Caution regarding sun exposure affecting eyes, skin. If contact lenses, remove if taking ophthalmic solution or ointment.

reflux of urine back to the kidneys. When urine refluxes backwards into the kidneys, it can cause hydronephrosis (distension of the kidney) and risk for pyelonephritis (kidney infection, as opposed to bladder infection).

Gradations of VUR are provided in the International Reflux Grading System, with a range from Grade I to Grade V (Fig. 32-2). These gradations were created based on the appearance of the renal pelvis and calyces on voiding cystourethrograms (VCUG; radiography of the bladder and urethra by use of a radiopaque contrast medium).

I   II   III   IV   V

Figure 32-2 Gradations of VUR are found in the International Reflux Grading System, ranging from Grade I to Grade V.

Nursing Care Plan The Child with a Urinary Tract Infection

Nursing Diagnosis: Impaired Urinary Elimination related to tissue inflammation

Measurable Short-term Goal: The child will be able to void adequate amounts of clear urine without burning, frequency, or urgency.

Measurable Long-term Goal: The child will not experience complications such as pyelonephritis.

NOC Outcome:
Urinary Elimination (0503) Collection and discharge of urine

NIC Interventions:
Medication Administration (2300)
Pain Management (1400)
Specimen Management (7820)

Nursing Interventions:

1. Assess history of urinary tract problems, family dynamics, and understanding about urinary elimination and hygiene.

   RATIONALE: Recurrent urinary tract infections may indicate lack of knowledge about urinary hygiene or may be an indication of sexual abuse.

2. Collaborate with the physician regarding the collection of a urine specimen for culture and sensitivity and follow-up culture after antibiotic administration is completed.

   RATIONALE: A urine culture will help determine the causative organism and the antibiotic that will be the most effective against the organism. Follow-up will help determine if the causative organism has been eliminated by the antibiotic.

3. Instruct family to administer medications as prescribed including antipyretics, analgesics, and the full course of antibiotics (specify drugs, doses, routes, and times).

   RATIONALE: An antipyretic is an agent that reduces a fever associated with a urinary tract infection. Urinary tract analgesics provide symptomatic relief from burning pain, frequency, and urgency. Antibiotics must be maintained at a consistent blood level for 7–10 days to kill the causative organism.

4. Assist the caregiver to plan for optimal nutrition and fluid intake that is individualized for the child (specify for age).

   RATIONALE: Good nutrition and adequate hydration is required for healthy immune response and optimal renal function.

5. Teach the child and/or family about good genital hygiene practices such as wiping from front to back and washing hands before and after elimination.

   RATIONALE: Prevents fecal–urinary contamination and the spread of infection.

6. Provide the child and family with education about urinary tract infections, including prevention by obtaining adequate fluids, voiding frequently, UTI signs and symptoms, and the necessity of completing the full course of antibiotics.

   RATIONALE: Provides new knowledge for child and family and empowers them to prevent recurrent infections.

---

 diagnostic tools Voiding Cystourethrogram (VCUG) to determine VUR

- Grade I: Urine backs up into the ureter only, and the renal pelvis appears healthy, with sharp calyces.
- Grade II: Urine backs up into the ureter, renal pelvis, and calyces. The renal pelvis appears healthy and has sharp calyces.
- Grade III: Urine backs up into the ureter and collecting system. The ureter and pelvis appear mildly dilated, and the calyces are mildly blunted.
- Grade IV: Urine backs up into the ureter and collecting system. The ureter and pelvis appear moderately dilated, and the calyces are moderately blunted.
- Grade V: Urine backs up into the ureter and collecting system. The pelvis severely dilates, the ureter appears tortuous, and the calyces are severely blunted

(Cendron & Benedict, 2006, p.1)

Grades I, II, and III reflux are considered lower grade and tend to resolve more spontaneously with cautious monitoring. Grades IV and V VUR need to be managed medically and surgically by a pediatric urologist and/or pediatric nephrologist. Candidates for surgery include children with recurrent breakthrough pyelonephritis (Gaylord & Starr, 2004), severe anatomical deformity at the ureterovesicular junction, antibiotic intolerance, medication noncompliance, and VUR in females after puberty (Montagnino & Currier, 2005).

SIGNS AND SYMPTOMS. The most common presentation for VUR is recurrent UTI. Flank pain, abdominal pain, and enuresis may coexist, although toddlers are seldom capable of describing these symptoms.

The major risk of VUR is the development of acute pyelonephritis, due to the backflow of urine toward the kidney. These children usually have a fever, nausea/vomiting, and possibly, but not always, UTI symptoms. Even one episode of febrile acute pyelonephritis can cause renal scarring in children (Montagnino & Currier, 2005).

Nursing Insight— *Children younger than 2 years old*

The risks of persistent VUR, especially in children younger than 2 years old, are significant, as the most common cause of UTI and renal scarring. Children with UTI who are younger than 2 years of age may more easily develop sepsis and become gravely ill. Infants with VUR and renal pelvis dilatation were found to usually have low-grade reflux that resolved by age two, as shown on ultrasound (Ismaili et al., 2006). Infants with high-grade reflux do not tend to resolve as spontaneously.

DIAGNOSIS. Diagnosis of VUR is most consistently based on the voiding cystourethrogram (VCUG) radiograph, which identifies the bladder, urethra, and ureters during micturition. Radiographic contrast material is observed as it refluxes back into the ureters and kidneys from the bladder.(See Diagnostic tools Voiding Cystourethrogram (VCUG) to determine VUR)

NURSING CARE.

Nursing care and treatment vary according to the grading of the reflux. In Grades I and II, the mildest types of reflux, the VUR may resolve spontaneously as the child grows. In children with more severe grades of reflux, surgical intervention may be required. This ranges from abdominal surgery to less invasive endoscopic surgery. Typical surgery involves reimplanting the ureter on the top of the bladder, so that the ureter length is long enough to prevent reflux.

Medical management for nonsurgical VUR includes vigilance in preventing and treating UTIs, especially because there is significant risk for the more dangerous pyelonephritis. Renal scarring and damage are hazards of VUR. Many children who are managed medically take prophylactic long-term antibiotics in addition to anticholinergic agents, such as oxybutynin chloride (Ditropan), to reduce bladder pressure.

Nurses have a vital role in educating the parents and family members about signs and symptoms of UTI and the importance of medication in this chronic disorder. Nurses caring for the postsurgical patient must be vigilant in monitoring intake and output as well as maintaining the patient's pain control. All tubing and drainage apparatus must be carefully labeled and monitored for any breaks in the system that could introduce infection (Kenner, Moran, Zebold, Keating, & Amlung, 2007).

 where research and practice meet:
Prophylactic Antibiotics

Many children with VUR are treated with prophylactic antibiotics, such as a daily low dose of an antibiotic. This is followed by urine culture periodically (every 2 or 3 months). Prophylactic antibiotics are often recommended until the child has been free of infection for a 12-month period (Gaylord & Starr, 2004). However, other researchers disagree and say it may not be necessary for children with VUR to take urinary antibiotic prophylaxis after an episode of acute pyelonephritis (Garin et al., 2006).

 Optimizing Outcomes— **Children with VUR and UTI**

A thorough nursing assessment promotes the best outcome for a child with VUR and UTI. Since infants and small children cannot express urinary discomfort easily, nurses can observe for discomfort during voiding or straining to void, dribbling of urine, and starting and stopping of the stream. Fever of unknown origin and irritability may be suspicious for UTI in nonverbal children especially. Nurses must take extreme care to obtain a reliable clean-catch urine specimen through assisting older children in the collection of the sample and through proper handling of a bagged specimen in younger children. It is useful to explain the urinary system to children old enough to understand it through the use of drawings, models, or dolls (Montagnino & Currier, 2005).

UNEXPLAINED PROTEINURIA

Routine office urinalysis may discover proteinuria (loss of proteins, such as albumin or globulins, in the urine). Proteinuria ranges from simple and reversible etiologies to complex, life-threatening causes.

More benign etiologies of proteinuria include orthostatic (from supine to seated or standing) or postural (affected by posture) proteinuria. This commonly asymptomatic disorder tends to occur after age 8, and is associated with upright activities during the daytime hours. It is necessary to obtain supine urine collections (normally the first morning void if the patient has not arisen during the night), which reveal a lessening or absence of protein in the case of purely orthostatic proteinuria.

Other reversible causes of proteinuria include that occurring after fever or hardy exercise. When the patient temperature subsides or the patient has not exercised heavily for 48 hours, the proteinuria subsides as well.

 Nursing Insight— *Pathological etiologies for proteinuria*

More pathological etiologies for proteinuria include glomerulonephritis, polycystic kidney disease, renal trauma, chronic pyelonephritis, acute tubular necrosis, obstructive uropathy, Henoch–Schönlein purpura, and congestive heart failure. Pregnancy and certain medications can cause proteinuria as well. Associated signs and symptoms for more pathological proteinuria include the potential presence of hematuria, edema, hypertension, fatigue, impaired growth and failure to thrive, dysuria (painful), frequency, oliguria (diminished urine), costovertebral angle (CVA) tenderness or flank pain, and joint pain (King, 2006).

SIGNS AND SYMPTOMS. The incidence of positive proteinuria by dipstick screening is seen in 10% of all children between 8 and 15 years of age. The dipstick must show 1+ (30 mg/dL) or higher level of proteinuria to be considered significant. False-positive readings for proteinuria are possible with highly concentrated urine, with specific gravity >1.015, and in this case, the proteinuria must be 2+ or higher to be considered significant. Proteinuria may also be noted in infected urine, often along with leukocytes, hematuria, and positive nitrates (King, 2006).

The nurse should note potential signs of renal disease, such as periorbital (around the eye orbit) edema and peripheral edema. The nurse also assesses blood pressure, pulse, and growth, which may be impaired with renal disease, in addition to performing an abdominal examination to assess for CVA tenderness and renal masses (Gaylord & Starr, 2004).

DIAGNOSIS. Obtain serial first-voided (the first urine of the morning) specimens for urinalysis at least three times over a 2-week span if orthostatic proteinuria is suspected. It is advisable to send urine for culture and sensitivity to rule out UTI. Any urinalysis containing proteinuria, especially higher than 1+, along with possible hematuria, white blood cells (WBCs), casts, crystals, and bacteria, is more suspicious for urological or renal disease. Additional renal serum tests that should be ordered include BUN and creatinine. A 12- or 24-hour urine test for creatinine (a chemical waste product of muscle metabolism) and protein may suggest pathology.

Further diagnostic testing may include renal ultrasound, voiding cystourethrogram (VCUG), and testing for anti-streptolysin titer (ASO) to rule out poststreptococcal glomerulonephritis. Referral to an urologist or nephrologist is necessary when proteinuria is persistent, of a high level, or is associated with other urinary abnormalities.

NURSING CARE. In the outpatient setting, the nurse can instruct the parent or child on how to obtain a first-voided morning specimen to test for orthostatic or postural proteinuria. Make certain the parent understands whether the specimen is to be returned to the office or to a laboratory. Nurses should be able to perform an accurate urine dipstick test by obtaining proper quantities of urine to dip the sticks into, and then by waiting the appropriate amount of time to test each specimen (Fig. 32-3).

Figure 32-3 Nurses should be able to perform an accurate dipstick test.

If patients require further testing in the inpatient or outpatient settings, nurses can be instrumental in educating the parents or caretakers about what each test entails. Sometimes it is possible to obtain educational handouts geared for the lay public to help patients understand what urinary disorders mean and how various urological tests are performed. In this case, the nurse's role is largely that of an educator. Nurses should also make certain that patients receive the proper follow-up after proteinuria is discovered. This may infer return visits to an outpatient setting and the establishment of appointments with a pediatric urologist or nephrologist.

HEMATURIA

Asymptomatic gross (visible) and microscopic hematuria is considered fairly common in children.

Although rare, microscopic hematuria can be the first sign of renal disease. Conversely, gross hematuria in children is more serious. The most common etiologies are poststreptococcal glomerulonephritis, hypercalciuria (with or without calculi), and IgA nephropathy. It is especially important for children with gross hematuria to undergo a significant urological work-up (Bergstein et al., 2005).

Other less common causes of hematuria include renal trauma, coagulopathy (a disorder of blood coagulation), hydronephrosis, epididymitis (inflammation of the epididymis, usually associated with a sexually transmitted infection), and tumor. UTI may cause microscopic or gross (macroscopic) hematuria. It is also important to note that exercise may induce hematuria, as well as viral and bacterial illness. Occasionally, external irritation may cause hematuria (e.g., from bubble baths, soaps, and scratching) (Gaylord & Starr, 2004).

SIGNS AND SYMPTOMS The main sign of hematuria is blood in the urine.

DIAGNOSIS. The color of the urine may be significant; tea-colored or brownish urine, especially if it contains protein and casts, signifies a nephrological disorder. Pink or red urine with or without blood clots, but without protein, usually originates in the lower urinary tract. If higher than 1+ hematuria is present on dipstick, then it is necessary to obtain a microscopic urinalysis to check for red blood cells (RBCs). Pseudohematuria is a condition that shows a false-positive dipstick but no RBCs on microscopic lab examination (Gaylord & Starr, 2004).

where research and practice meet:
Hematuria

In a study reported by Bergstein, Leiser, and Andreoli (2005), the most common etiologies for microscopic hematuria were hypercalcuria (calcium deposits in the urine) with or without renal calculi, poststreptococcal glomerulonephritis, and structural abnormalities, including a single kidney. It was significant to note that asymptomatic microhematuria had no identifiable cause in the majority of patients. It was surprising that urinary tract infection (UTI) was not the cause in any of the patients studied. Occasional low-grade vesicoureteral reflux was found in microscopic hematuria.

Urinalysis that reveals hematuria along with casts and proteinuria is highly suspicious for renal disease. UTI may show hematuria along with mild proteinuria, but without casts. Urine culture is suggested to rule out urinary tract infection in cases of hematuria. Further diagnostic work-up may include renal ultrasound, intravenous pyelography (IVP), and voiding cystourethrogram (VCUG). Referral to a pediatric urologist or nephrologist is necessary in cases of hematuria suggesting the potential for renal disease.

NURSING CARE. Depending on the cause of the hematuria, the nurse is called on to educate the child and parent or caregiver about necessary laboratory and procedural tests, in addition to giving understandable explanation of the cause of the hematuria. In the case of UTI, the nurse must educate the child or parent in the proper techniques of collecting a urine specimen (Procedure 32-1).

If the child cannot voluntarily give a urine specimen, the nurse must use appropriate bagging techniques to obtain the specimen, including clean-catch collection in all cases. The nurse is able to obtain urine specimens by collecting urine from a bag that fits over the perineum in females or over the penis in males (Fig 32-4). The skin must be dry for the bags to adhere. It is ideal to cleanse the perineum in girls or penis in boys before placing the plastic collecting bag. The bag must be removed as soon as the child voids to avoid fecal contamination. Transfer the urine to a sterile collection container and send it to the laboratory immediately.

The nurse is also responsible for accurately testing the urine with a dipstick, ensuring that there is an adequate sample and allowing the proper time limits for testing.

GLOMERULAR DISEASE

Glomerular disease (glomerulonephritis) can be due to primary kidney disease or secondary multisystem diseases that cause damage to the glomerulus. Both primary and secondary diseases are accompanied with histological evidence that captures the glomerular damage and resultant

---

Procedure 32-1 Collecting a Urine Specimen

Purpose

The purpose of collecting a urine specimen is to screen for early signs of disease.

Equipment

Packaged urine culture set (usually contains three antiseptic towelettes and a sterile urine collection plastic container)

Steps

1. Wipe (or have the child wipe) the labia or penis with the three provided iodine or antiseptic solution towelettes. In occasional situations, it is considered appropriate to use just soap and water to wash these areas. The customary procedure is to wipe the areas three times. In males, wipe the urethral tip three times in a circular fashion, once with each wipe. In a female, holding the labia open to expose the urethra, wipe the right side top to bottom and discard the wipe. Then repeat this on the left side, discarding the wipe. Wipe top to bottom over the central area where the urethral meatus is and discard that wipe.

    RATIONALE: *Cleansing removes normal flora that may contaminate a urine culture and make it impossible to tell which organisms are pathogens.*

2. Ask the child to begin to urinate into the toilet, bedpan, or urinal, and then stop urinating.

    RATIONALE: *This action flushes away urine in the distal urethra, which may be contaminated with normal flora from the skin.*

3. Position the sterile urine container so that it catches the "mid-stream" urine, which needs to be about 3 to 4 ounces of urine.

4. Remove the container and cap it, taking care not to contaminate the inner container with your gloved hands.

    RATIONALE: *Removing the container keeps the specimen sterile.*

5. Allow the child to finish voiding into the toilet, bedpan, or urinal.

    Clinical Alert Do not keep a urine culture at room temperature any longer than 10 minutes. If the specimen cannot be sent to the laboratory immediately, it is necessary to refrigerate it in a plastic specimen bag to prevent the overgrowth of organisms that interfere with the interpretation of the culture and sensitivity to specific antibiotics. The specimen is plated on a nutrient medium and bacteria that are present are allowed to grow and then are counted. Usually, different antibiotic discs are placed on the inoculated medium to show which ones decrease the colony counts (sensitivity).

Teach Parents

Parents may be responsible for collecting urine cultures from their children at home or in the medical office, so they must be instructed on the sterile techniques of handling the specimen. If the specimen is collected at home, it may need to be refrigerated before bringing it to the laboratory.

Documentation

4/20/10 0800 Specimen collected.

—M. Helming, RN

Note: Time and date of the urine collection must appear on the label and in the chart. The label should also contain the patient's name and other identifying information, such as identification number.

Figure 32-4 The nurse must be able to collect urine specimens in a bag that fits over the perineum in females or over the penis in males.

clinical manifestations and needed treatment. Acquired causes, including genetic, immunological abnormalities, disturbances of coagulation, chemical toxic events, or biochemical defects, interrupt and do varying degrees of damage to the physiological functions of the glomerulus. Acquired immunological abnormalities are the major pathophysiological mechanisms in glomerular disease (Fig. 32-5).

 Nursing Insight— *Three classic syndromes*

There are three classic syndromes that characterize the sequence of events with glomerular renal insult:

- Acute glomerulonephritis
- Nephrotic syndrome
- Hemolytic uremic syndrome

Figure 32-5 The nephron showing glomerular filtration and tubular reabsorption.

The etiology of the renal glomerular insult determines the specific condition, progression, whether acute or chronic, and its prognosis. Regardless of which classical disease or syndrome the patient has, a major concern is the prevention of or early detection and intervention for renal glomerular dysfunction before the condition worsens (Bernstein & Shelov, 2003).

Acute Glomerulonephritis

Inflammation of the glomeruli (tubules of the kidney) is called glomerulonephritis. Interference with the glomeruli filtering waste products from the blood gives rise to acute and chronic clinical manifestations. If the inflammation follows the course of an infection it is called postinfectious glomerulonephritis. If it can be directly attributed to the streptococcus organisms it is called poststreptococcal glomerulonephritis.

Post Streptococcal Glomerulonephritis

Although it is not common, it is possible for children to develop an acute glomerulonephritis within 7 to 14 days following an acute Group A beta-hemolytic streptococcal infection. Antigen–antibody complexes with the streptococcal bacteria form and are deposited in the glomeruli, causing damage. Infections that were missed or not cultured may cause patients to develop this sequela. The nurse must consider not only Group A beta-hemolytic streptococcal pharyngitis, but also other potential sources of this bacteria, such as impetigo.

SIGNS AND SYMPTOMS. Gross hematuria, either tea or coffee-colored urine, develops, accompanied at times by edema, which may be seen in the periorbital region (around the eye orbits). The process of kidney dysfunction causes disturbances in sodium and water retention, which in turn cause edema. If the symptoms become more severe, the child may develop hypertension and headache. Severe disease causes significant proteinuria and possibly even ascites, due to fluid shifting (Lum, 2007).

DIAGNOSIS. If the child has not had a diagnosed streptococcal infection in the previous 2 weeks, it is possible that the physician will order a serum antistreptolysin titer (ASO titer) that will indicate exposure to the bacteria. Serum complement (C3) is another blood test that may be positive. Urine microscopic hematuria may still be noted up to 1 year after this disease resolves. Laboratory tests such as BUN and creatinine are used to assess renal function. If children do not fully recover, they may develop nephrotic syndrome and require a renal biopsy (Lum, 2007).

NURSING CARE. Children with post streptococcal glomerulonephritis require antibiotic therapy if an infection is still found. Fluid imbalances require monitoring of fluid intake and output, as well as possible treatment with diuretic medications and antihypertension drugs. Children with severe glomerulonephritis may require peritoneal dialysis or hemodialysis. Corticosteroids may be useful to manage the acute process. In most cases, the disorder begins to resolve within 2 or 3 weeks. Nurses need to support family members through this frightening and uncommon disorder.

Nurses should assess the child's pharynx and upper respiratory tract for signs of acute infection, and a streptococcal culture is obtained. In addition to a rapid-streptococcal test, it is wise to send a full streptococcal culture swab to the laboratory for a confirmatory exam. Nurses should monitor children for hypertension and urinary output. Children who develop significant oliguria, gross hematuria, and hypertension are hospitalized due to the risk of associated acute renal failure. Nurses may need to educate patients and family members about dietary restrictions such as sodium, potassium, and fluid intake (Kenner et al., 2007).

case study   Post Streptococcal Glomerulonephritis

Sara is a 4-year-old girl who is taken to the pediatric emergency department with edematous eyelids and swollen abdomen. Sara's mother reports that along with her daughter's swollen eyelids, her daughter has a decreased appetite and has been very fatigued for the past several days.

Sara's vital signs are normal except for her blood pressure, which is 140/90. The systems review and physical exam are negative except for lesions on her ankles and a "doughy" or "dense" feeling to her abdomen, which is slightly firm to touch. The lesions are circular, crusted with sticky yellow drainage, which Sara scratches during the exam. Sara's mother reports that her daughter is allergic to amoxicillin (Amoxil) and develops a rash.

critical thinking questions

1. What is your assessment?

2. What other questions do you want to ask?

The pediatric nurse practitioner orders a flat abdominal radiograph including the kidneys, ureters, and bladder, which comes back negative. There are no abdominal masses. She then asks Sara for a urine specimen. There is hematuria and proteinuria.

3. What other laboratory test(s) should you anticipate will be needed?

4. What are two tests that would confirm a diagnosis of post-streptococcal glomerulonephritis?

5. What diet do you anticipate will be ordered for Sara?

6. What antibiotic could be given since she is allergic to amoxicillin?

7. What patient teaching would you want to provide before they go home?

◆ See Suggested Answers to Case Studies in text on the Electronic Study Guide or DavisPlus.

HEMOLYTIC UREMIC SYNDROME

Hemolytic uremic syndrome (HUS) is the most common cause of acute renal failure (ARF) in children. HUS is most commonly associated with children ingesting beef contaminated with *Escherichia coli* (*E. coli*), although other organisms, such as shigella, coxsackievirus, adenovirus, salmonella, ECHO virus, pneumococci, and rickettsia have been implicated. This potentially lethal outcome is most commonly seen in young children between 6 months and 3 years of age, but can occur in all age groups.

clinical alert

E. coli O157:H7

Undercooked ground beef has been one of the primary sources of *E. coli* O157:H7 that can cause HUS. Meat should be cooked until it reaches a temperature of 160°F and is no longer pink. *E. coli* outbreaks have occurred in fast-food and other restaurants, and have been found in unpasteurized cider, milk, juice, alfalfa sprouts, strawberries, and most recently, raw spinach.

It is believed that an endotoxin is produced from the dangerous bacteria in the gastrointestinal tract, and results in inflammation causing capillary wall destruction. This occurs also within the glomerular arterioles, and as the endothelium of the glomerulus becomes more edematous, platelets aggregate at the site of injury. A clot then forms that impedes renal circulation. This stimulates increased rennin production, which results in hypertension. These platelets are damaged and this results in thrombocytopenia, or a drop in the platelet count to less than 100,000/μL for a period of 1 to 2 weeks. The overall effect damages the glomerular blood vessels, resulting in a lesser glomerular filtration rate, lowered urine output, acute renal failure, and hypertension. The clotting and inflammatory process may also affect the respiratory system and any other body system.

SIGNS AND SYMPTOMS. Signs and symptoms of HUS include, first, gastroenteritis (inflammation of the intestines due to infection) with diarrhea and vomiting, as well as a potential upper respiratory infection. The hemolytic uremic syndrome that may result can endure from several days to two weeks. Classically, HUS must include this triad: thrombocytopenia, anemia, and acute renal failure. Pallor, lethargy, anorexia, anemia, and irritability are included in the presentation. Urine output decreases, and blood chemistries may be altered. Hepatosplenomegaly, dehydration, and bloody diarrhea are possible. The child may suffer from seizures, consciousness alteration, and may require dialysis. Thrombocytopenia (low platelet count) may cause petechiae and purpura formation, as well as ecchymosis.

DIAGNOSIS. Diagnosis of HUS includes critical analysis of laboratory results. In HUS there may be an elevation in BUN and creatinine levels. Hyperkalemia (elevated potassium level) also may occur due to decreased urinary excretion. Serum glucose levels may drop due to increased metabolic needs, but may also rise if the pancreas is affected, and some children require insulin. Other affected electrolytes include calcium, which decreases, and phosphorus, which rises.

NURSING CARE. Many of those suffering from HUS are ill enough to be in intensive care. Nurses must monitor level of consciousness, signs of increased intracranial pressure, congestive heart failure, bleeding, and hypertension (Kenner, Moran, Zebold, Keating, & Amlung, 2007). Fluid intake and output is measured every 4 hours, and up to every hour if the child is critically ill. Daily weights are essential and the nurse needs to assess electrolyte balances (sodium, potassium, chloride, and bicarbonate), as well as arterial blood gas measurements. The BUN and creatinine are important to measure to determine if renal status is worsening and the child may be at risk of needing dialysis. The lungs should be assessed for signs of congestive heart failure, such as rales. Assess for peripheral and periorbital edema, as these are indicators of worsening renal and cardiac status.

The nurse monitors the child's vital signs frequently for hypertension and tachycardia. It is recommended that children with HUS have electrocardiographic monitoring to assess for possible changes such as widened QRS complexes, heart block, and peaked T waves due to hyperkalemia (Kenner et al., 2007).

 assessment tools Hemolytic Uremic Syndrome (HUS)

Nurses should be observant for all of these risks of hemolytic uremic syndrome:
- Signs of bleeding, associated with thrombocytopenia, petechiae, epistaxis (nosebleed), prolonged bleeding at venipuncture sites, and ecchymoses.
- Signs of increased intracranial pressure, including change in level of consciousness and risk of seizure.
- Abdominal symptoms are the primary presenting complaints for children, and may occur in the form of diffuse abdominal pain, intussusception (telescoping of the bowel), nausea and vomiting, diarrhea, and fever. These abdominal symptoms may present up to 1 week after exposure to the *E. coli* O157:H7 toxin (Razzaq, 2006).

Antibiotics are contraindicated in treating HUS as they may worsen the situation. Because very young and very old patients are at highest risk for developing HUS from *E. coli* O157:H7, it is prudent to investigate whether any patient with diarrheal illness has eaten a risky food. Stool culture for *E. coli* O157:H7 is available at many laboratories, and should be ordered if there is a suspicion of contaminated food.

 Be sure to— Investigate Legal Concerns

Children who have been exposed to undercooked beef or other products containing *E. coli* O157:H7 may seek legal remedies for their suffering. Severe illness, possibly chronic renal problems, and death have been outcomes of pediatric HUS. Restaurants and food producers who are responsible for contaminated products have legal liability for personal injury. Some years ago, many outbreaks of HUS forced the fast-food industry to cook all beef sufficiently so that no redness persisted and the internal temperature of the thickest portion of the beef reaches 160°F.

HENOCH–SCHÖNLEIN PURPURA

Henoch–Schönlein purpura (HSP) includes a range of mild to severe glomerulonephritis and renal insufficiency. This disease is classified as a vasculitis (inflammation of blood vessels) because there is a component of inflammation in the arteries. HSP typically follows an upper respiratory tract infection during the ages from 4 years old to 10 years old (Olson, 2002).

SIGNS AND SYMPTOMS. Hematuria and hypertension are common features of this disorder. Other symptoms include bloody diarrhea, crampy abdominal pain, and a rash with palpable purpura (raised purpura), features found especially on the lower extremities and buttocks (Lum, 2007).

There may also be joint pain and swelling and scrotal swelling. The glomerulonephritis that develops may not occur until 2 months after the onset of symptoms. About 5% of all affected children may have a gradual progression to renal failure (Olson, 2002).

DIAGNOSIS. Diagnosis is not difficult if the classic symptoms of rash, gastrointestinal complaints or hematuria, and arthritis are present. The diagnosis of Henoch–Schönlein purpura depends on clinical findings and history. There is not a specific laboratory test for the disorder, although an elevated serum IgA level, elevated sedimentation rate, elevated platelet count, and elevated white blood cell count may be present. Urinalysis may show hematuria. A stool guaiac test (a test for unseen blood in stool) may be positive.

NURSING CARE. Although most children recover spontaneously, some can relapse and some can recover very slowly, continuing to show hematuria for up to 2 years later. Corticosteroids seem to assist the abdominal and joint pain as well as the edema, but do nothing to assist the renal compromise. Some children may require immunosuppressant medications and renal transplant.

Children with HSP are at risk of complications of intussusception (telescoping of the bowel), intestinal hemorrhage, intestinal perforation, and central nervous system and severe renal complications (Marino & Devivio, 2002). Nurses must monitor these children for signs of bleeding, pallor, vital sign alterations, abdominal pain, oliguria, and urine abnormalities.

CHRONIC GLOMERULONEPHRITIS

Chronic glomerulonephritis involves several glomerular diseases that, unlike acute poststreptococcal glomerulonephritis, do not have a tendency toward spontaneous recovery but rather are undulant (moving like waves) with primary cause difficult to establish. Advanced pathological damage to the glomeruli silently occurs.

Damage to the glomerular membrane causes permeability and electrical charge changes that permit passage rather than filtering of protein molecules. A persistent abnormal sediment is found in the urine as progressive loss of renal function occurs over time. Proteinuria and hematuria finally surface with a urinalysis obtained during a clinic visit. Renal failure can be an outcome depending on the degree of damage done to the glomerular membrane (Bernstein & Shelov, 2006).

Most often, chronic glomerulonephritis is due to acquired immunological assaults that occur to the kidney directly. Complement C3, IgG, or IgA is often found embedded in the glomeruli if a renal biopsy is performed.

Other times, chronic glomerulonephritis can be attributed to systemic disease, such as systemic lupus erythematosus, or human immunodeficiency virus infection. Nephrogenic exposure to organic solvents, mercury, and certain nonsteroidal anti-inflammatory agents can also be the etiological finding.

Because chronic glomerulonephritis has been silently undulating over several years, it is common to diagnose this during adolescence during a health care visit. Early childhood years pass without the disease being diagnosed. As the National Kidney Foundation calls for more frequent routine monitoring of glomerular filtration rate (GFR), there may be a change in how early the chronic glomerulonephritis is discovered.

SIGNS AND SYMPTOMS. A decrease in the adolescent's urine output; the presence of high blood pressure, headaches, and other signs of fluid overload such as periorbital edema; increased abdominal girth; and swelling of the labia or scrotum bring the patient to the attention of the physician. These symptoms are serious enough to warrant hospitalization and aggressive treatment.

DIAGNOSIS. Diagnosing chronic glomerulonephritis includes the use of diagnostic laboratory tests similar to that of acute or chronic renal failure: urinalysis, blood chemistry, blood urea nitrogen, serum creatinine, and pH.

NURSING CARE. Treatment depends on the degree of renal insufficiency or failure (refer to section on Acute and Chronic Renal Failure). The overall management principles for treating chronic glomerulonephritis are related to treating the etiology of primary disease or secondary disease that affects the glomerulus, preventing immune responses (or limiting them) and correcting problems of edema, hyperkalemia, or hyperlipidemia if present. If hyperlipidemia is present, nystatins cannot be given because renal damage prevents proper clearance of the drugs. Dietary management may include restriction of salt and fluid along with instituting low-potassium foods.

The use of plasma exchange may be instituted in severe cases to decrease the amount of circulating immunoglobulin that are damaging the kidney. When hypertension is present, it is generally related to fluid overload, and loop diuretics (e.g., furosemide [Lasix]) may be given to reduce the circulating intravascular fluid volume. Careful monitoring of urine output, along with weight and abdominal girth, is necessary.

The patient must be monitored vigilantly for nephrotic syndrome, chronic renal failure, end-stage renal disease, chronic or malignant hypertension, heart failure, pulmonary edema, chronic or recurrent UTIs, and infection.

Trusting, supportive, developmentally appropriate relationships are established through the caring interventions of the nurse and other health care providers. Long-term follow-up, possible renal biopsies every 2 to 5 years, and vigilant observations for possible renal failure become part of the patient and her family's everyday life. Refer to the section on acute and chronic renal failure for more specificity related to monitoring weight, abdominal girth, electrolytes (e.g., hyperkalemia with potential ECG changes) as well as acidosis and inadequate renal perfusion. If renal failure does eventually occur, the patient and family is prepared for the possibility of dialysis and renal transplant.

Now Can You—— Discuss common disorders of the urinary system?

1. Explain why the early diagnosis of urinary tract infections (UTIs) is critical?
2. Describe gradations of vesicoureteral reflux?
3. Discuss hemolytic uremic syndrome and related nursing care measures?

Structural Defects of the Urinary System

Although theoretically the urinary tract system, composed of two ureters, one bladder, and one urethra, appears independent of the kidneys, the two systems are intertwined. Abnormalities with the urinary tract system ultimately affect the other system. The abnormalities may be anatomical, infectious, cellular, inflammatory, functional, or maturational.

Bladder exstrophy, hypospadias and epispadias, and vesicoureteral reflux (VUR) are primarily urinary tract system abnormalities that damage the kidney. For instance, a kidney disease known as hydronephrosis is an accumulation of urine in the renal pelvis that results from an obstruction. These structural defects also compromise kidney function, resulting in hypertension, metabolic acidosis, inability to concentrate urine, urinary stasis and infection, and chronic renal failure. "Pyelonephritis is considered more severe than a urinary tract infection" (Potts & Mandleco, 2002, p. 617).

Other structural defects of the urinary system are referred to as obstructive uropathy, which are structural or functional abnormalities that also result in retrograde flow of urine back into the renal pelvis. The most common of these obstructive uropathies are ureteropelvic junction obstruction (an obstruction or stenosis of the ureteropelvic valve between the renal pelvis and ureters). The outcome of untreated obstructive uropathy is chronic renal failure due to the damage to the renal parenchyma from hydronephrosis.

RENAL TRAUMA

Injury to the kidney accounts for greater than 47% of the genitourinary injuries. Up to 90% of these injuries are due to blunt trauma. The most common causes of renal trauma are motor vehicle accidents, direct blows, and sports injuries or falls. Due to the larger size of the kidney in children and the greater amount of space it has in the abdomen, children are more likely to sustain renal injury.

SIGNS AND SYMPTOMS. With critical injuries, the children have localized flank tenderness, hematoma, and a palpable mass. There also can be other symptoms related to abdominal injury such as tenderness, peritonitis, paralytic ileus, and resulting hypovolemic shock.

 clinical alert

Hematuria

Hematuria is most often considered the cardinal marker of renal injury. The presence of any degree of hematuria should be regarded as a potential indication of underlying renal injury or anomaly. Hematuria out of proportion to the mechanisms of injury should suggest a congenital anomaly or neoplasm.

DIAGNOSIS. Diagnosis of renal trauma is confirmed by history and clinical findings.

NURSING CARE. Because renal trauma is a critical injury, advanced trauma life-support guidelines are followed. The goal is prevention of renal morbidity and mortality. Blunt trauma, such as bruising without any urinary extravasation (grades I, II, and III), is treated conservatively. Treatment includes bedrest, analgesia, and prophylactic antibiotics. Grades of IV and V renal trauma require referral to an urologist.

Nursing care centers on recognizing a renal injury and the potential urgency. Hematuria is the primary sign of renal injury. The nurse must gather a detailed history of the problem. Sometimes a lengthy admission process is not possible due to the impending surgery. Performing a nursing assessment, including vital signs, growth and development, nutritional and immunization status, along with a thorough physical examination, is essential. The nurse also gains crucial information such as the precipitating event, allergies, medications, general state of health, and previous hospitalizations or surgeries.

Surgery may be required if abdominal exploration is needed. The nurse must prepare both the child and family for the surgery and immediate postoperative care. Essential abbreviated information is communicated because the family may not understand the full situation. Serious injury to the urinary system often requires astute observation in the critical care unit. Nursing care must be tailored to the identified problems, in order of importance, and the nurse must develop a care plan that deals with the multifaceted problems. The nurse understands that the child will be placed on bedrest for initial observation and remain on bedrest for 3 days after internal bleeding has subsided. Monitoring vital signs, urinary, respiratory, cardiac, and gastrointestinal status as well as the surgical incision is essential. Priority actions also include monitoring intake and output, measuring weight and abdominal girth, administering intravenous fluids, and pain management. The nurse must report signs of inadequate renal perfusion (hypotension), acidosis, and observe for edema, oliguria, or anuria.

Psychosocial care of the family is also important and includes encouraging the parents to remain at the bedside, relaying appropriate developmental information, and minimizing stressors experienced by the child. The nurse may have to remind the family to avoid discussions at the bedside that may upset the child. The nurse must respect and support family's decision about medical care but can intervene if the best interest of the child is in question. Notify a hospital chaplain for spiritual care if the family desires.

ACUTE RENAL FAILURE

Acute renal failure (ARF) is a life-threatening syndrome in which there is a sudden decreased capacity of the kidneys to eliminate waste products, resulting in an inability to maintain fluid and electrolyte or acid–base balance (Kline & Milonovich, 2006). Glomerular filtration is reduced or tubular function is decreased, resulting in oliguric renal failure (less than 1 mL/kg per hour in neonates and infants, less than 5 mL/kg per hour in older children) and nonoliguric renal failure, which is more easily missed on diagnosis (Kliegman, Marcdante, Jenson, & Behrman, 2006). There are a variety of causes of ARF (Table 32-2).

In the newborn, the major causes of oliguria are congenital heart disease, respiratory distress syndrome, congenital hydronephrosis, acute tubular necrosis, and renal vein thrombosis. For children younger than age 5, the most common cause of oliguria is hemolytic uremic syndrome and poststreptococcal glomerular nephritis. Beyond 5 years of age, the pathophysiology and management is similar to that provided for adults.

Table 32-2 Causes of Acute Renal Failure		
Prerenal, Hypovolemic, Hypotension	**Intrinsic, Intrarenal, Parenchymal**	**Postrenal (Obstruction)**
Dehydration	Acute tubular necrosis	Urethral obstruction
	• Nephrotoxins (drugs) (reversible if caught early)	• Stricture
		• Posterior urethral valves
		• Diverticulum
Septic shock	Acute cortical necrosis (not reversible)	Ureterocele
Heart failure	Glomerulonephritis	Extrinsic tumor compressing bladder outlet
Hemorrhage	Interstitial nephritis	Extrinsic urinary tract tumors
Burns	Vascular	Tumor lysis syndrome
	• Renal vein thrombosis	
	• Arterial thromboembolus (umbilical artery catheter)	
	• Disseminated intravascular coagulation	
	• Immune-mediated (scleroderma)	
Peritonitis, ascites, cirrhosis	Pigmented	
	• Hemoglobinuria	
	• Myoglobinuria	

Nursing Insight— *Renal failure*

Any condition that reduces blood flow to the kidneys is prerenal failure. Intrarenal failure also referred to as intrinsic or parenchymal renal failure, is a result of destruction to the renal filtering components.

Obstruction of the outflow of urine from the bladder, ureters, or urethra is the underlying etiology of postrenal failure.

Regardless of type of acute renal failure, the clinical manifestations usually can be seen through three distinct phases: oliguric, diuretic, and recovery.

Nursing Insight— *Hemolytic uremic syndrome*

The most common cause of acute renal failure is hemolytic uremic syndrome (HUS) in North America due to hemorrhagic colitis from *E. coli*.

SIGNS AND SYMPTOMS. Signs and symptoms of acute renal failure include fever, rash, bloody diarrhea, pallor, vomiting, diarrhea, abdominal pain, hemorrhage, shock, anuria, or polyuria. Other life-threatening signs and symptoms include gastrointestinal bleeding, hypertension, anemia, neurological symptoms, as well as the skin becoming ecchymotic. Signs and symptoms of electrolyte imbalances are also seen in ARF (Table 32-3).

DIAGNOSIS. Determining if the cause of the acute renal failure is prerenal, intrarenal, or postrenal requires a very careful history, analysis of symptoms, and physical examination. A previous medical history helps to determine any previous infections such as acute glomerulonephritis or neurogenic bladder. Genetic problems such as a horseshoe-shaped kidney or one kidney can be uncovered.

Laboratory data routinely obtained are a urinalysis, blood chemistry, blood urea nitrogen, serum creatinine, and pH (Table 32-4). Common urinalysis associated findings with acute renal failure include a urinary sediment, color ranging from dirty brown, reddish brown, to bilious tinge, proteinuria, and casts (Kline & Milonovich, 2006) (Table 32-5).

Sometimes a renal biopsy is ordered if the cause of the ARF cannot be ascertained. Renal ultrasound may also be used. Renal ultrasound can assist with pinpointing obstructive uropathy. A CBC can help determine if there is thrombocytopenia due to hemolytic uremic syndrome or eosinophilia due to acute interstitial nephritis.

Acute renal failure can also be diagnosed by finding toxins in the blood. Toxins can be found if there has been exposure to heavy metals or organic solvents, which causes acute tubular necrosis. Other epidemiological

Table 32-3 Signs and Symptoms of Electrolyte Imbalances in Acute Renal Failure		
Electrolyte Imbalance	**Clinical Manifestations**	**Clinical Treatment**
Hyperkalemia (>6.0 mEq/L)	Peaked T waves, widening of QRS on ECG	Eliminate all intake of potassium (dietary, parenteral, or TPN)
Results from inability to adequately excrete potassium derived from diet and catabolized cells. In metabolic acidosis, there is also movement of potassium from intracellular fluid to extracellular fluid.	Dysrhythmias: ventricular dysrhythmias, heart block, ventricular fibrillation, cardiac arrest Diarrhea Muscle weakness	Administration of alkalinizing agents Kayexalate orally or in retention enema when K^+ >7.0 mEq/L (Other drugs may be ordered by physician including calcium gluconate 10% solution, sodium bicarbonate, and regular insulin when K^+ >7.0 mEq/L) Dialysis if other methods to reduce the potassium level are ineffective
Hyponatremia In the acute oliguric phase, hyponatremia is related to the accumulation of fluid in excess of solute.	Change in level of consciousness Muscle cramps Anorexia Abdominal reflexes, depressed deep tendon reflexes Cheyne–Stokes respirations Seizures	Electrolyte replacement, sodium bicarbonate Dialysis to correct severe electrolyte disturbance
Hypocalcemia Phosphate retention (hyperphosphatemia) depresses the serum calcium concentration. Calcium is deposited in injured cells. Hyperkalemia and metabolic acidosis may mask the common clinical manifestations of severe hypocalcemia.	Muscle tingling Changes in muscle tone Seizures Muscle cramps and twitching Positive Chvostek sign (contraction of facial muscles after tapping facial nerve just anterior to parotid gland)	Calcium gluconate Low phosphorus diet Phosphate binders, e.g., Tums tablets, calcium acetate and sevelamer (Aluminum-based binders not utilized to prevent possible aluminum toxicity.) Calcium IV not given (except for tetany to prevent calcium salt deposition into tissues) Dialysis to correct severe electrolyte disturbance

Table 32-4 Normal Urinalysis

Urinalysis	Normal Values
Appearance	Clear
Color	Amber yellow
Odor	Aromatic
pH	4.6–8.0 (average 6.0)
Osmolarity	50–1400 mOsm/L
Protein	None or up to 8 mg/dL
	50–80 mg/24 hr (at rest)
	<250 mg/24 hr (exercise)
Specific gravity	Adult: 1.005–1.030 (usually 1.010–1.025)
	Elderly: values decrease with age
	Newborn: 1.001–1.020
Leukocyte esterase	Negative
Nitrites	Negative
Ketones	Negative
Crystals	Negative
Casts	None present
Glucose	Brand new specimen: negative
	24-hour specimen: 50–300 mg/day or 0.3–1.7 mmol/day (SI units)
White blood cells (WBCs)	0–4 per low-power field
WBC casts	Negative
Red blood cells (RBCs)	Up to 2
RBC casts	None

Table 32-5 Common Urinalysis Findings of Acute Renal Failure

Urinalysis Findings	Interpretation
Urinary sediment	Intrinsic kidney failure
Color	+"Dirty" brown: Intrinsic renal failure
	+Reddish brown: Acute glomerulonephritis
	+Bilious tinge: Mixed hepatic & renal failure
Proteinuria	+Glomerulonephritis
	+Interstitial nephritis
	+Toxic and infectious causes
Casts	+Red blood cell (RBC) casts:
	Glomerulonephritis or vasculitis
	+White blood cells (WBC) casts:
	Interstitial nephritis
	+Granular casts: Glomerulonephritis
	+Uric acid crystals: Tumor lysis syndrome
	+Calcium oxalate crystals: Ethylene glycols
	Ingestion:
	+Acetaminophen (Tylenol) crystals: Acetaminophen (Tylenol)

nephrotoxic agents include treatment with aminoglycosides, amphotericin B, contrast, or chemotherapeutic agents (Schwartz, 2005).

 Nursing Insight— *Renal tubular function*

- "The fractional excretion of sodium (FENa) is an index of renal tubular function.
- FENa = ([UNA/PNA]/Ucreat/Pcreat]) × 100
- An FENa greater than 2 is correlated with acute interstitial nephritis or acute tubular necrosis.
- An FENa less than 1 is correlated with hemolytic uremic syndrome, acute glomerulonephritis, or prerenal causes."

  (Schwartz, 2005, p. 711)

Laboratory differential diagnosis of acute renal failure is also important (Table 32-6).

NURSING CARE. The nursing responsibilities for care of a patient with acute renal failure are multiple and require significant patience for a child who has a changing level of consciousness and irritability. Parents need sup-

port, particularly if they are feeling guilty that a postinfectious glomerulonephritis was not prevented by earlier treatment. Administration of medications, monitoring nutritional intake, and meticulous fluid intake and output assessment are critical to help the physician make treatment decisions.

The complications of acute renal failure are variable depending on the underlying etiology (Table 32-7). Renal-limited diseases, such as postinfectious glomerulonephritis, have a mortality rate of less than 1%. Other etiologies such as HUS, tumor lysis syndrome, and acute tubercular necrosis, all have severe multiorgan effects that increase the mortality rate to greater than 90%. Many medications are prescribed to control multisystem complications (Table 32-8).

Collaboration with the health care team is critical so that acute renal failure complications are reduced or prevented from occurring depending on whether the etiology is prerenal, intrarenal, or postrenal. Appropriate key nursing diagnoses are suggested (Bruck & Mayer, 2005; Kline & Milonovich 2006; Schwartz, 2005).

nursing diagnoses Acute Renal Failure

- Fluid Volume Excess related to fluid retention
- Risk for Injury related to accumulation of electrolytes and nitrogenous waste
- Risk for Infection related to lowered body defenses, fluid overload
- Interrupted Family Processes related to a child with a serious disease
- Knowledge Deficit related to long-term follow-up to monitor the patient's kidney status

Table 32-6 Laboratory Differential Diagnosis of Acute Renal Failure

| | Prerenal | | Intrarenal | | |
	CHILD	NEONATE	CHILD	NEONATE	POSTRENAL
Urine Na+ (mEq/L)	<20	<20–30	>40	>40	Variable, may be >40
FENa* (%) Should not be obtained after a diuretic is given as renders the test inaccurate	<1	<2–5	>2	>2.5	Variable, may be >2
Urine osmolality (mOsm/L)	>500	>300–500	>300	>300	Variable, may be <300
Serum BUN-to-creatinine ratio	>20	> or equal to 10	>10	>10	Variable, may be >20
Urinalysis	Normal		RBCs, WBCs, casts, proteinuria		Variable to normal, possible crystals
Comments	History: diarrhea, vomiting, hemorrhage, diuretics Physical: volume depletion		History: hypotension, anoxia, exposure to nephrotoxins Physical: hypertension, edema		History: poor urine stream and output Physical: flank mass, distended bladder

*FENa Fractional excretion of sodium (%) = [(urine sodium/plasma sodium) + (urine creatinine/plasma creatinine)] × 100.

RBCs, red blood cells; WBCs, white blood cells.

Table 32-7 Complications of Acute Renal Failure

Metabolic	Cardiovascular	Gastro-intestinal	Neurological	Hematological	Infection	Other
Hyperkalemia	Pulmonary edema	Nausea	Neuromuscular irritability	Anemia	Pneumonia	Hiccups
Metabolic acidosis	Arrhythmias	Vomiting		Bleeding	Septicemia	Increased parathyroid hormone
Hyponatremia	Pericarditis	Malnutrition	Asterixis (flapping tremor)		Urinary tract infection	
Hypocalcemia	Pericardial effusion	Gastrointestinal hemorrhage	Seizures			Low total triiodothyronine
Hyperphosphatemia	Pulmonary embolism		Mental status change			Low thyroxine
Hypermagnesemia	Hypertension					Normal free thyroxine
Hyperuricemia	Myocardial infarction					

Table 32-8 Medications Used to Treat Complications of Acute Renal Failure

Medication	Action/Indication	Nursing Implications
Hyperkalemia • Kayexalate	Exchanges sodium for potassium	May require up to 4 hours to take effect.
• Calcium gluconate 10%	Counteracts potassium-induced increased myocardial irritability	Monitor for ECG changes. Intravenous infiltration may result in tissue necrosis.
• Albuterol	Shifts potassium to the cells	Give by inhalation.
Metabolic Acidosis • Sodium bicarbonate or sodium citrate	Helps correct metabolic acidosis by exchanging hydrogen for potassium	Do not mix with calcium. Complications include fluid overload, hypertension, and tetany.
Hypocalcemia • Calcium gluconate 10%	Used in the presence of tetany; provides ionized calcium to restore nervous tissue function to control serum phosphorus	Administer slowly to prevent bradycardia. Monitor for ECG changes.
Malignant Hypertension (B/P > 95% for age) • Sodium nitroprusside, nitroglycerin	Relaxes smooth muscle in peripheral arterioles	Administer by continuous intravenous infusion; fall in blood pressure is seen within 10–20 minutes.

Be sure to— Record accurate weight measurement

An inaccurate weight recorded in a computer charting system can cause life-threatening harm for the patient. It is critical that when delegating to nursing assistants the nurse carefully monitor that the weight measures are being done properly. Obtain weights: same scale, same time, and wearing the same clothing (infants are weighed naked and oftentimes older children only have on their underwear). The weights are ordered once a day, before feedings, and every 12 hours for critical children.

CHRONIC RENAL FAILURE

Chronic renal failure refers to an insidious process of irreversible, progressive deterioration of the glomerular filtration rate that goes through a deteriorating continuum of four stages at variable rates for each individual patient (Table 32-9). Sometimes the process is sudden, as there can be an acute renal failure occurring secondarily in someone who already has chronic renal failure.

 Nursing Insight— Recommendation from the National Kidney Foundation

The National Kidney Foundation (2007) recommends patients and families with a background of diabetes, hypertension, or renal disease follow their glomerular filtration rate with their physician to ensure early intervention to slow the process. Reduction of the glomerular filtration results in fluid and electrolyte and acid–base imbalances causing damage and abnormalities of all organ systems.

 Ethnocultural Considerations— Kidney failure

"African Americans constitute about 32 percent of all patients treated for kidney failure in the US, but only about 13 percent of the overall US population." Furthermore, "anyone with high blood pressure, diabetes, or a family history of kidney disease is at risk and should have his or her kidney function tested."
—Former US Surgeon General Dr. Joycelyn Elders

The etiology of chronic renal failure in children is age related and dependent on the organs that are affected. For children younger than 2 years old, obstructive urop-athy or renal hypodysplasia is the common underlying problem. For children between 2 and 5 years of age, neonatal vascular accidents, renal hypodysplasia, and obstructive uropathy are factors. For older children and adolescents, glomerulonephritis, lupus nephritis, or reflux nephropathy are the underlying etiologies. Genetic considerations include polycystic kidney disease, congenital nephritic syndrome, and sickle cell disease (Schwartz, 2005, p. 712). The course of the disease is eventually fatal unless dialyses followed by kidney transplantation can be done for the patient.

SIGNS AND SYMPTOMS. Signs and symptoms of chronic renal failure are similar to those of acute renal failure. They include fever, rash, bloody diarrhea, pallor, vomiting, abdominal pain, hemorrhage, shock, anuria, or polyuria.

DIAGNOSIS. The major challenge in diagnosis and treatment is to discern whether the condition is acute or chronic renal failure and in what stage the signs and symptoms are manifesting. Acute renal failure is normally sudden, and chronic renal failure has insidious features characteristic of the system affected.

A carefully elicited history shows that all organ systems are affected to varying degrees (Table 32-10). Ultrasound shows the size of the renal organ. Although renal biopsies are important, they are not always done if the cause and treatment can be outlined without having to do the needle biopsy. The major advantage of a biopsy is that it can also assist with identifying the cause of the chronic failure and provide a map for treatment and counseling (Schwartz, 2005).

Diagnostic tests include serum chemistries, CBCs, urinalysis, parathyroid hormone, chest radiograph, bone films, renal ultrasound, and ECG if the patient is hyperkalemic. Consider the laboratory tests and results that correlate with renal failure.

❝ **What to say** ❞ — *Gathering information from the parents*

- "Does your child have any of the following symptoms?"
  - Malaise
  - Poor appetite
  - Vomiting
  - Bone pain
  - Headache (if hypertensive)
  - Polyuria

Table 32-9 Four Stages of Chronic Renal Failure According to Glomerular Filtration Rate (GFR)		
Percentage of Reduction of GFR	**Stage of Renal Failure**	**Glomerular Filtration Rate as Applied to Children Age 2 and Older***
35%–55% of normal	1. Reduced renal reserve	≥90
25%–35% of normal	2. Renal insufficiency	60–89
20%–25% of normal	3. Renal failure	30–59
Less than 20% of normal	4. End-stage renal disease (ESRD)	15–29*

*If GFR <15, dialysis is needed.

Table 32-10 Physical Examination Findings Correlated with Underlying Pathophysiological Mechanisms for Chronic Renal Failure

Organ System	Physical Findings	Correlation with Pathophysiological Mechanisms
Skeletal	Osteitis fibrosa (bone inflammation with fibrous degeneration)	Bone resorption associated with hyperparathyroidism, vitamin D deficiency, and demineralization
	Bone demineralization (principally subperiosteal loss of cortical bone in the fibers, lateral ends of the clavicles, and lamina dura of the teeth)	Lowered calcium and raised phosphate levels
	Spontaneous fractures, bone pain; osteomalacia (rickets or rachitic changes) with end-stage renal failure	
	Edema	
	Absent patella	
Cardiopulmonary	Hypertension, pericarditis with fever, chest pain, and pericardial friction rub, pulmonary edema, Kussmaul respirations	Extracellular volume expansion as cause of hypertension
	Flow murmur	Hypersecretion of renin also associated with hypertension
	Gallop	Fluid overload associated with pulmonary edema and acidosis leading to Kussmaul respirations
	Rub	
Neurological	Encephalopathy (fatigue, loss of attention, difficulty problem solving)	Uremic toxins associated with end-stage renal disease
	Peripheral neuropathy (pain and burning in the legs and feet, loss of vibration sense and deep tendon reflexes)	
	Loss of motor coordination, twitching, fasciculations, stupor, and coma with advanced uremia	
	Hypotonia	
	Irritability	
Endocrine and Reproductive	Retarded growth in children (short stature)	Decreased growth hormone
	Osteomalacia	Elevated parathyroid hormone
	High incidence of goiter	Decreased thyroid hormone
	Sexual dysfunction: menorrhagia, amenorrhea, infertility, and decreased libido in women; decreased testosterone levels, infertility, and decreased libido in men	Elevated hormones: luteinizing hormone (LH), follicle-stimulating hormone (FSH), prolactin, and LH-releasing hormone; decreased testosterone, estrogen, and progesterone
Hematological	Anemia, usually normochromic, normocytic; platelet disorders with prolonged bleeding times (increase in bleeding gums)	Reduced erythropoietin secretion associated with loss of renal mass, leading to reduced red cell production in the bone marrow; uremic toxins associated with shortened red cell survival
Gastrointestinal	Anorexia, nausea, vomiting	Retention of urea, metabolic acids, and other metabolic waste products, including methylguanidine
	Mouth ulcers, stomatitis, bad breath (uremic fetor), hiccups, peptic ulcers, gastrointestinal bleeding, and pancreatitis associated with end-stage renal failure	
Integumentary	Abnormal pigmentation and pruritus	Retention of urochromes, contributing to sallow, yellow color
		High plasma calcium levels associated with pruritus
Immunological	Increased risk of infection that can cause death; decreased response to vaccination	Suppression of cell-mediated immunity
		Reduction in number and function of lymphocytes
		Diminished phagocytosis
HEENT	Retinal changes	Uremic toxins
	Preauricular pits	
	Hearing deficit	
Abdomen	Palpable kidneys	
	Suprapubic mass	

- "Has your child had any of the following in the past?"
  - Perinatal complications
  - Oligohydramnios
  - Recurrent urinary tract infections
  - Enuresis
- "Is there any family history of renal disease? Hearing impairment?"

NURSING CARE. Once diagnosis is made from a well-taken history and there are laboratory results, patient medications are ordered (Table 32-11). The goals of nursing care for a patient with chronic renal failure are mutually established with the patient and family. Collaboration with the health care team is essential so that the quality of life can be extended as long as possible as the renal capacity diminishes and affects all organ systems. Nutritionists assist with the plan of providing meals that counteract the growth retardation. Pastoral care is helpful for the spiritual input as this chronic disease takes its toll, and end-stage renal disease occurs and hopes for transplant rise as dialysis sees the patient through kidney compensation. Meticulous nursing care is required to administer care as the multisystem organ failure begins to take place. Patient teaching along with referral to group support organizations such as the National Kidney Foundation help the patient and family cope more effectively with the renal failure.

Dialysis in Pediatric Nursing

Dialysis is a life-extending procedure for children with severe renal compromise. Dialysis may be done through the peritoneal wall (peritoneal dialysis) or through cleansing the blood by using a dialysis machine (hemodialysis). It is important to note that while dialysis is usually reserved for children in end-stage renal disease as a result of chronic renal failure, it may also be needed in acute renal failure if BUN and creatinine levels elevate.

PERITONEAL DIALYSIS

This process of dialysis utilizes the peritoneal membrane (abdominal lining) to filter blood and purify it. Using a dialysis solution composed of dextrose sugar and other minerals in water, it is inserted into the child's abdomen through an abdominal catheter. Through an osmotic process, the dialysis solution draws toxins, excess water, and waste chemicals from the blood into the dialysis solution. From there, it is drained through an abdominal tube out of the abdomen. The amount of time the dialysis solution is in the abdomen is termed the dwell time, and the entire process of filling and emptying the abdomen is termed an exchange, which normally lasts 30 to 40 minutes.

There are two essential types of peritoneal dialysis: continuous ambulatory peritoneal dialysis (CAPD) and continuous cycling peritoneal dialysis (CCPD). CCPD uses a machine termed a cycler to provide numerous exchanges during a child's sleep time. In the morning, the child has one exchange with a dwell time that lasts for the whole day, with a potential of adding a mid-afternoon treatment. In contrast, CAPD does not require a cycler machine. Instead, the dialysis solution is run from a plastic bag through the catheter, and it remains in the abdomen for several hours with a sealed catheter. After this dwell time has passed, the patient's dialysis solution with the waste products must be drained into a special disposal bag. Then another cycle of dialysis solution is begun. Each

Table 32-11 Medications Commonly Used for Children with Chronic Renal Failure		
Medication	**Action or Indication**	**Nursing Considerations**
Vitamin and mineral supplement (Nephrocaps)	Add vitamins and minerals missing from heavily restricted diet	Only prescribed vitamins should be used; over-the-counter brands may contain elements that are harmful.
Phosphate binding agents: Calcium carbonate (Tums), calcium acetate (PhosLo), or sevelamer hydrochloride (Renagel)	Reduce absorption of phosphorus from the intestines	Ensure that phosphate binding agent is aluminum free.
Calcitriol (Rocaltrol)	Replace the calcitriol that kidneys are no longer producing to keep calcium balance normal	Monitor serum calcium level. Ensure that calcium supplement is provided.
Epoetin alfa (Epogen, Procrit)	Stimulates bone marrow to produce red blood cells, treats anemia due to CRF	Given by IV or subcutaneous injection. Monitor blood pressure as hypertension is an adverse effect. Monitor hematocrit and serum ferritin level according to facility guidelines.
Iron supplementation	Treat iron deficiency when epotin alfa is prescribed	May be administered orally or IV during hemodialysis.
Growth hormone (rhGH)	Used to stimulate growth in children with CRF	Record accurate height measurements at regular intervals.
Antihypertensive agents: Angiotensin-converting enzyme (ACE) inhibitor (enalapril, lisinopril)	Used with proteinuric kidney disease as it slows the progression to ESRD	Monitor renal function and electrolyte balance.
Loop diuretics	Used when volume overload is present	

cycle lasts at least 4 to 6 hours. Most children have four cycles during the day, but sleep with the solution in their abdomen at night, unlike in CCPD.

NURSING CARE. Community nurses can assist parents and older children in learning peritoneal dialysis. The riskiest problem with peritoneal dialysis is the chance of peritonitis, an infection of the abdominal peritoneum. This is extremely serious and requires urgent antibiotic therapy, hospitalization, and follow-up with the child's nephrologist (National Kidney and Urologic Diseases Information Clearinghouse, 2007). Currently, peritoneal dialysis is considered the best choice in dialysis therapy for children, especially small children (Lum, 2007). Nurses monitor the abdominal catheter sites for signs of infection or malfunctioning equipment and make certain that the returning dialysate solution remains clear. If it is cloudy, it indicates a potential infection or problem. The nurse must notify the physician immediately (Montagnino & Currier, 2005).

HEMODIALYSIS

Children can also receive dialysis through the blood, using a special machine. This is a more complex form of dialysis that may require several months of adjustment for the child. The child's blood is moved through a filter called a dialyzer, which is part of a complex machine (Fig. 32-6). Extra water, extra salt, and toxic waste products are removed, while the blood pressure and electrolytes such as potassium, calcium, sodium, and bicarbonate are kept in balance. A special port is placed in the child, usually in the wrist, for vascular access. Through this port, the blood is removed through tubing into the dialyzer, cleansed, and then returned through a different set of tubes back to the child's body. Three types of ports are used: arteriovenous (AV) fistulas, arteriovenous (AV) grafts, and venous catheters.

The preferred type is the AV fistula, which needs to be placed weeks before starting dialysis, and it may last for a long period. In the AV fistula type, a surgeon connects an artery directly to a vein, commonly in the forearm and around the wrist. This process makes more blood flow into the vein, so it grows stronger and larger. Eventually, the vein can support repeated hemodialysis connections. A bruit is a noise heard on auscultation that can be heard over an AV fistula to make certain it is patent.

The AV graft is reserved for children with small veins that do not properly form a fistula over time. It requires a synthetic tube to be implanted under the skin of the forearm.

The venous catheter becomes an artificial vein for needle placement with hemodialysis and serves as temporary access for more urgent need to start hemodialysis because there is no time to wait for a fistula to develop. A catheter is inserted into the chest, groin, or neck, with two chambers permitting a two-way blood flow. These catheters are intended to be temporary because they clog easily, become infected frequently, and can cause vein narrowing, but they can be used until an AV fistula begins to form within the months often required (National Kidney and Urologic Diseases Information Clearinghouse, 2007).

Many children must be hemodialyzed three times a week at an outpatient dialysis center. It is possible to arrange for home hemodialysis. Since each treatment can last 3 to 4 hours, it is disruptive to the child's time, although it is possible for the child to read, write, complete homework, play video games, and watch television during this process.

SIGNS AND SYMPTOMS. At the onset of hemodialysis, a child may experience several side effects related to quick alterations in the body's chemical and water balance. Hypotension (low blood pressure) can cause weakness, dizziness, and nausea, while muscle cramps may be caused by electrolyte imbalances (National Kidney and Urologic Diseases Clearinghouse, 2007).

NURSING CARE. It is imperative for pediatric nurses to teach the patient and parents or guardians how to keep the AV fistula, AV graft, or venous catheter clean and safe. First, the access site must be kept clean and used only for

Figure 32-6 The hemodialysis process.

hemodialysis (e.g., no drawing blood from the site). Children must learn they cannot wear jewelry near the access site, cannot have a blood pressure taken on that arm, and cannot bruise the site. Nurses must instruct patients and families to avoid carrying heavy objects on that arm, to avoid sleeping with that arm under the head or body, and to check the pulse at the site daily.

This is a highly specialized form of nursing that requires additional training. The children best suited for hemodialysis have either no one at home that can assist them with peritoneal dialysis, or they live close to a dialysis center. Children on hemodialysis often are faced with missing school and social activities, leading to further isolation and emotional problems. Fluid and dietary restrictions are necessary between dialysis sessions. Hemodialysis has the benefit of rapidly improving uremic children, somewhat normalizing their growth rates, skeletal maturation, and sexual development, which may all be impaired in end-stage renal disease (Montagnino & Currier, 2005).

 critical nursing action Arteriovenous Fistulas (AV)

The pediatric nurse provides health promotion teaching to a child and family related to the care of a newly acquired arteriovenous fistula for hemodialysis treatment:

- Wash the access with soap and warm water each day, and always before dialysis.
- Instruct the child to not scratch the area or try to remove scabs.
- Check the area daily for signs of infection, including warmth and redness.
- Check that there is blood flow in the access daily. There should be a vibration (called a thrill) over the access. If this is absent or changes, a health care provider at the dialysis center should be notified.
- Take care to avoid traumatizing the arm where the access is located; do not wear tight clothes, jewelry, carry heavy items, or sleep on the arm.
- Remind health care providers not to take blood or measure blood pressure on the access arm.
- Rotate needle sites on the access. Use gentle pressure to stop bleeding when the needle is removed. If bleeding occurs later, apply gentle pressure; call a health care provider if bleeding does not stop within 30 minutes or if bleeding is excessive.

 nursing diagnoses Peritoneal Dialysis

- Acute Pain related to instillation of dialysate, temperature of dialysate
- Chronic Sorrow related to chronic disability
- Risk for Infection, Peritoneal, related to invasive procedure, presence of catheter, dialysate
- Risk for Fluid Volume Excess related to retention of dialysate
- Risk for Ineffective Coping related to disability requiring change in lifestyle

 nursing diagnoses Hemodialysis

- Excess Fluid Volume related to renal disease with minimal urine output
- Noncompliance with dietary restrictions related to denial of chronic illness
- Ineffective Health Maintenance related to deficient knowledge regarding hemodialysis procedure, restrictions, blood access care
- Powerlessness related to treatment regimen
- Risk for Infection related to exposure to blood products, risk of developing hepatitis B or C

Renal Transplantation

Children who receive renal transplants receive them from either unrelated donors who have died or from living donors. The living donors may be relatives who have ideal tissue matches or close friends. A person can live with just one full-functioning kidney, so there are healthy living donors who give up one of their kidneys to an ill child. About half of all children who receive kidney transplants obtain them from a living donor, often a parent (National Kidney and Urologic Diseases Information Clearinghouse, 2007). Children usually are maintained on peritoneal or hemodialysis until a donor kidney is available. Children in need of a renal transplant are placed on a waiting list and are registered with the United Network of Organ Sharing (UNOS), which keeps a computer network to link all organ donation centers and transplant centers. A preemptive transplant implies that a child has received a donated kidney before needing dialysis. This is associated with less chance of rejection (destruction of transplanted material at the cellular level) of the new kidney and longer duration of the transplanted kidney.

Children who are eligible for renal transplants are in end-stage renal disease (ESRD) and they include children who have been surviving on peritoneal dialysis or hemodialysis. Children with maple syrup urine disease, a disorder that causes sweet-smelling urine, are now being considered for renal transplant also. With this disease, there is a defect that causes amino acids from proteins to build up to a toxic level in the body, causing cerebral edema, neurological damage, and even death (Children's Hospital of Pittsburgh, 2005). Children must avoid proteins such as eggs, milk, and meat.

Chronic renal failure implies that only 50% or less of normal renal function is present and the renal failure has lasted several months. When chronic renal failure is considered to be permanent and irreversible, the child moves into the category of end-stage renal failure (ESRF). Children with ESRF become transplant candidates if there will be better quality of life for the child, and if the child can withstand the significant surgical risks of transplantation. The child must not be significantly immunocompromised. There is a higher mortality rate for children undergoing renal transplant than for adults (Kenner et al., 2007).

NURSING CARE. Children who receive renal transplants are on long-term medications to prevent rejection of the transplant. These medications are considered immunosuppressive. Medications include such drugs as cyclosporine and steroids. These drugs increase the child's risk for infection and can cause Cushing syndrome by affecting glucocorticosteroids. Steroids can also raise serum glucose level, giving the potential for diabetes mellitus to develop. In addition, steroids affect bone mineralization and strength, which can cause impairments in a growing child. Growth hormone has been used to counteract this problem, but it is controversial. Children receiving transplants frequently are also on antihypertensive and diuretic medications due to the common problem of hypertension causing renal disease because constricted blood vessels impair renal flow. Hypertension may be caused by renal disease related to volume overload, obstruction of the urinary tract, or congenital anomalies of the kidney (Lum, 2007). Diabetic children may also develop ESRF due to the damage that diabetes inflicts upon the renal system. Children who receive transplants may need to remain on protein-restricted diets to avoid overloading the kidneys.

clinical alert

Signs of kidney transplant rejection

Signs of kidney transplant rejection in children include hypertension, decreased urinary output, fever, weight gain, edema, graft site pain, and increasing BUN and creatinine levels (Kenner et al., 2007).

 Across Care Settings: **Children who receive renal transplants**

Children who receive renal transplants need the services of many members of the health care team: the pediatrician; the nephrologist; dialysis nurses with special training; a transplant coordinator; a social worker for information on financial assistance, transportation, and counseling; a psychologist, psychiatrist, or other counselor to handle the emotional upset children and their families go through with chronic end-stage renal disease, dialysis, and plans for transplant; and a dietitian to help the child avoid foods that can cause more toxic waste buildup and to help maintain proper nutrition, as these children are often underweight (National Kidney and Urologic Diseases Information Clearinghouse, 2007).

 Now Can You— Describe structural defects of the urinary system?

1. Discuss emergency care that involves crisis nursing management for renal trauma?
2. Examine clinical manifestations of electrolyte imbalances in acute renal failure?
3. Explain nursing care measures for a patient with acute and chronic renal failure?
4. Discuss peritoneal dialysis and hemodialysis along with nursing care?

Functional Disorders of the Urinary Tract

DYSFUNCTIONAL ELIMINATION SYNDROME/ VOIDING DYSFUNCTION

Dysfunctional elimination syndrome (DES), also called voiding dysfunction, is an abnormal but common pediatric elimination pattern associated with bladder and bowel withholding and incontinence. It has been found that UTI and VUR before age 2 is not a cause of DES (Shaikh et al., 2003). There may not be an association between DES and toilet training, but there does appear to be an association between children with encopresis (involuntary loss of bowel contents) and vulnerable children at risk.

 Nursing Insight— *Voiding disorders*

There are numerous types of voiding disorders. Urge incontinence is the most frequently seen type of voiding dysfunction. Urodynamic studies show bladder storage problems and persistent bladder contractions that cause urgency and excess voiding with holding, such as crouching, leg crossing, squatting, or dancing.

Lazy bladder syndrome occurs when children delay voiding, and the detrusor muscle of the bladder weakens, while the bladder itself enlarges. This causes incomplete voiding, minimal urge to void, and voiding infrequently, associated with increased bladder capacity.

Giggle incontinence is the leakage of urine when children are laughing and there may be some bladder instability. Anticholinergic drugs can assist with this, as well as the attention-deficit/hyperactivity (ADHD) drug methylphenidate (Ritalin).

Bladder-sphincter dyssynergia refers to a bladder disorder with elevated bladder pressure but a decrease in urine flow, leaving residual urine. The child may return quickly to the restroom after just leaving it.

Vaginal voiding is associated with dribbling after voiding, due to some urine flowing into the vaginal vault. This urine then dribbles out with standing or activity. This problem may be remedied by weight loss in overweight girls, having the girl sit backwards or straddle a toilet seat so urine is directed downward.

SIGNS AND SYMPTOMS. Symptoms of dysfunctional voiding or DES include frequency in voiding, urinary incontinence, and urgency.

 Nursing Insight— *Dysfunctional voiding and enuresis*

There is a distinction between dysfunctional voiding and enuresis. In enuresis, the child voids normally and fully but not at the socially acceptable time. In voiding dysfunction or DES, there is an abnormal emptying or storage in the bladder.

DIAGNOSIS. Physical examination includes examining the back for sacral hairy tufts and gluteal asymmetry that may be associated with neurogenic bladder issues such as spina bifida. The rectum and abdomen should be examined for evidence of constipation. The genitalia should be examined for physical abnormalities.

Diagnostic tests include VCUG, flat plate of the abdomen to assess for constipation, uroflowmetry to assess voiding flow and velocity, and the addition of electromyography to assess the pelvic floor musculature.

NURSING CARE. Nurses can assist in helping children with voiding dysfunction by identifying issues, asking the child at various times of day if he or she has voided, and asking the child if she can hold her urine if a bathroom is not always available. Monitoring stool elimination is also essential. Nurses should assess for any emotional or social problems resulting from a child's embarrassment or shame associated with voiding dysfunction.

Management includes maintaining a normal bowel regimen, with or without the use of enemas and stool softeners, such as polyethylene glycol (MiraLax) or lactulose syrup. Children need to sit on the toilet for 1 minute for each year of age after eating, to let the gastrocolic reflex relax to induce bowel elimination. Girls with an inflamed perineum from leaking urine may be soothed with baking soda sitz baths and use of barrier creams. Nurses should promote an adequate water intake in a child to maintain dilute and less acidic urine. If a child suffers from recurrent UTI, he or she may need antibiotic treatment and prophylaxis. Trimethoprim-sulfamethoxazole (Bactrim or Septra) and nitrofurantoin (Macrodantin) are the most common antibiotics used to treat prophylaxis of UTI.

 Complementary Care: *Behavioral management and biofeedback*

Complementary measures may be useful for treating voiding dysfunction. These include behavioral management and biofeedback. Nurses can promote adequate hydration by ensuring that children are hydrated with 8 ounces of water with each meal, and the child should attempt to void every 2 hours. Voiding charts and diaries may assist in behavioral tracking and recording of successes. Biofeedback training assists with gaining control over the bladder muscles and relaxing the external sphincter. Children wear electromyogram (EMG) patches near the perineum or abdomen to assist with biofeedback training. Psychological counseling is vital. Associated psychological and educational problems include learning disabilities, attention deficit hyperactivity disorder (ADHD), low motivation, sensory problems, and family issues. Parents and other family members need much assistance in dealing with these issues.

ENURESIS

One of the most distressing childhood issues is enuresis (bedwetting). The definition of enuresis is the "involuntary or unintentional urination at any age when voluntary control should be present" (Dunn, 2004, p. 293). Some sources discuss enuresis as occurring at age 5 or older (von Gontard, Freitag, Seifen, Pukrop, & Rohling, 2006; El-Radhi & Board, 2003) and other sources put the limit at age 6 and older (Dunn, 2004). This condition may be due to the neuromotor (neurological and musculoskeletal) development in children varying substantially, so that some children achieve bladder control earlier than others. The incidence is approximately 1% of the population internationally, and it is more common in boys than in girls.

 Nursing Insight— *Other issues associated with enuresis*

Enuresis may carry a genetic etiology. If one or both parents have suffered from enuresis, there is a higher likelihood their offspring may suffer too. Developmental delays in other areas, such as speech, motor, and growth, may accompany enuresis issues. One study found that the brainstem may be immature in children with enuresis problems (von Gontard et al., 2006).

There are different types of enuresis; primary nocturnal enuresis (PNE) as well as primary and secondary enuresis. PNE is bedwetting during the night. Primary enuresis occurs when children have never been able to gain urinary control. Robson, Leung, & Van Howe, (2005) found that constipation can be a major issue in primary enuresis. Secondary enuresis refers to the presence of enuresis after a child has achieved dryness for 6 to 12 months. Children who experience secondary enuresis may be the victims of sexual abuse or have other issues such as school phobias, parental divorce, or other medical problems requiring significant care. Family neglect may have also diminished a positive toileting experience. ADHD is associated with an increased incidence of secondary enuresis possibly because children with attention deficits ignore nocturnal bladder warnings and cannot sit still long enough while toileting to void.

 Ethnocultural Considerations— Enuresis

Toileting patterns and expectations vary among different cultural and ethnic groups. Enuresis may be considered more problematic for some cultures than for others, and expectations of bladder and bowel control vary among parents, teachers, health care professionals, and daycare providers as well.

SIGNS AND SYMPTOMS. Children who have nocturnal enuresis are thought to suffer from problems awakening at night in response to a full bladder, smaller nocturnal bladder capacity, or an abundance of nocturnal urine production. Children with secondary enuresis are thought to suffer more from UTIs, constipation, diabetes mellitus, obstructive sleep apnea, psychological stress, and urge syndrome with dysfunctional voiding.

DIAGNOSIS. Diagnosis is based on patient history and physical examination to rule out other medical conditions as the cause of enuresis.

NURSING CARE. The nurse understands that medication administration is the most effective care measure. Many children are embarrassed by this problem, and school functions, camp, and sleepovers become problematic. Some parents use medication only as needed for these special occasions.

The most commonly prescribed medication to treat enuresis is desmopressin (DDAVP), a synthetic analogue of the antidiuretic hormone (ADH). This medication, administered orally or via a nasal spray, acts to lower nocturnal urinary production. The spray is given intranasally at doses of 1 to 40 mcg (1 to 4 sprays) each night, beginning with the lowest effective dose. If given orally, desmopressin (DDAVP) is available in 0.2 mg tablets given in dosages of 0.2 mg to 0.6 mg per night. Success rates range from 10% to 65%, but unfortunately, relapse rates are high, at 80%, when the drug is discontinued. Although there is a slight risk of water intoxication, the drug overall appears safe and efficacious (National Guidelines Clearinghouse, 2004).

Another medication, imipramine (Tofranil), has been used for enuresis, although its significant side effect profile makes it considerably less desirable than desmopressin (DDAVP). Imipramine (Tofranil) may be used in a bedtime doses of 1 to 2.5 mg/kg with up to 60% effectiveness. As imipramine (Tofranil) is a tricyclic antidepressant, it is subject to risk of cardiac arrhythmia and therefore pretreatment EKG is required (National Guidelines Clearinghouse, 2004).

medication: Imipramine

Imipramine (im-**ip**-pra-mean)

Tofranil (brand name)

Pregnancy category: D

Indications: Depression, enuresis, bulimia, attention deficit disorder in children, obsessive–compulsive disorder, panic disorder

Actions: Tricyclic antidepressant known to increase the effect of nor-epinephrine and serotonin in the body. It also possesses anticholinergic side effects.

Contraindications and Precautions:
- Cardiovascular disease
- Seizure disorder
- Children younger than age 6
- Concomitant use of MAO inhibitors, such as Nardil and Parnate; cannot take Tofranil within 2 weeks of taking an MAO inhibitor drug.
- Recent myocardial infarction

Adverse Reactions and Side Effects:
- Nervousness, anxiety, emotional instability
- Fainting; convulsions
- Constipation, nausea, vomiting
- Fatigue; sleep disorders
- Dry mouth
- Gynecomastia
- Confusion; hallucinations
- High or low blood pressure
- Tremor; numbness

Route and Dosage: Pediatric: short-term only, not for children younger than age 6

Dosing: maximum 2.5 mg for each 2.2 pounds (or 1 kg) of body weight. Usually begins at 25 mg per day, taken 1 hour before bedtime. If necessary, increase this dose after 1 week to 50 mg per day (ages 6–11) or 75 mg per day (ages 12 and up), taken in one dose at bedtime or divided into two doses, one at mid-afternoon and one at bedtime (PDRhealth, 2007).

Nursing Implications:
- Risk of potential suicidal ideation during initiation of upward titration of this medication, especially in children and adolescents.
- Toxic and possibly fatal drug interactions can occur with concomitant use of MAO inhibitors (e.g., Nardil, Parnate), SSRI drugs (e.g., Prozac, Paxil), and clonidine (antihypertensive drug also used for ADHD).
- Blood pressure and heart rate should be assessed before treatment, and an initial EKG should be taken. Serial EKGs may be needed with dose adjustments, in order to monitor for prolonged PR and QT intervals and flattened T waves.
- Nurses must assess patients for mood alterations, hallucinations, confusion, and laboratory abnormalities (leukocytes, blood glucose, and renal and hepatic status).
- There is a significant risk of agitation, arrhythmias, hallucinations, fever, dyspnea, seizures, and vomiting in acute overdosage. Treatment consists of gastric lavage, use of charcoal, and a stimulant cathartic. Additional supportive measures are heart monitoring, respiratory status monitoring, and possibly use of antiarrhythmic and anticonvulsant agents.

Data from Deglin, J.H., and Vallerand, A. (2009). *Davis's drug guide for nurses* (11th ed., pp. 666–669). Philadelphia: F.A. Davis.

Another nursing care measure is education. The nurse can explain to the parents that sometimes enuresis is due to developmental stage of the child or the child is a deep sleeper who does not feel the urge to void. In some cases, this may improve as the child grows, but it should be monitored. Avoidance of fluids close to bedtime, avoidance of diuretic beverages or substances (coffee, tea, chocolate, colas), and use of reward charts are other techniques useful to parents. Many commercial items are available to assist

parents. These include mattress pads with alarms, watches with reminders to void, books on staying dry, and absorbent underwear.

Other complementary care modalities have been developed to assist in the management of enuresis. Nurses should familiarize themselves with these in order to instruct parents and children with this problem. One behavioral treatment that has proven very useful involves conditioning through the use of a battery-operated bed wetting alarm, a device that wakens the child if the bedding becomes wet.

 Complementary Care: *Enuresis*

- Four to six sessions of hypnotherapy can train a child to awaken when his or her bladder feels full.
- Not every child with enuresis is suffering psychological problems, but there is an increased incidence of psychological issues in secondary enuresis, including parental divorce, school trauma, hospitalization, and sexual abuse. Acupressure or massage therapy can be useful in some cases of psychological induced enuresis.
- Citrus foods, carbonated or caffeinated drinks, red dyes, and artificially colored candy may contribute to enuresis. Elimination trials can be advised by nurses.

 case study   Enuresis

Tommy is an 8-year-old boy who is brought in for a medical evaluation of enuresis. He lives with his divorced mother and a 4-year-old sister in a suburban community. Tommy is in second grade at the local public school and his grades are mostly Bs. The nurse in the pediatrician's office is responsible for taking Tommy's medical history.

critical thinking questions

1. What questions do you need to ask Tommy?

2. What questions do you need to ask Tommy's mother?

   The pediatrician is now ready to see Tommy.

3. What laboratory test(s) should you anticipate will be needed?

   The pediatrician does a well-child exam on Tommy. He is in the 50th percentile for height and the 40th percentile for weight. He has a normal exam except for a mild, excoriated pink rash in his antecubital fossae bilaterally. He is at Tanner stage I. The in-office urinalysis is normal.

   Tommy's mother is distressed that her son is still wetting the bed at age 8. This happens almost every night, and she is washing linens continuously.

4. What education can you give to Tommy's mother about enuresis?

5. What advice can you give her about tools available to help enuresis?

   The pediatrician decides to give Tommy medication for enuresis. You are the office nurse who needs to instruct Tommy and his parents in the medication.

6. What is the likely medication given?

7. What instructions do you need to give Tommy's mother about this medication?

- See Suggested Answers to Case Studies in text on the Electronic Study Guide or DavisPlus.

EXSTROPHY OF THE BLADDER

Exstrophy of the bladder is a congenital defect in which the abdominal and anterior bladder walls do not fuse during fetal development. This results in the anterior surface of the bladder being open on the abdominal wall. The defect has a variety of degrees of severity. There are a number of associated congenital anomalies or other structural alterations (epispadias, cryptorchidism, chordee (downward penis), cleft scrotum or bifid (split in two parts) clitoris, inguinal hernia, rectal prolapse, widely split symphysis pubis, and rotated hips (Stein, 2007).

SIGNS AND SYMPTOMS. The visualization that the bladder is open on the abdominal wall is the main determinant of this condition.

DIAGNOSIS. Ultrasound is the tool used to diagnose exstrophy of the bladder.

NURSING CARE. Surgery is usually necessary within the first 48 hours of the infant's life in this rare disorder. It may need to be delayed due to infant stability or other associated problems. Surgical teams work to preserve the bladder and abdominal wall and to maintain support for the bladder. The bladder may need to be augmented to improve its size and urinary diversion is sometimes required (Kenner et al., 2007).

Nurses must focus on presurgical, psychological, and medical preparation, as well as postsurgical care. The area must be kept clean because urine on the skin can cause irritation. Diapers should be loose-fitted and changed frequently. The exposed bladder may be covered with Vaseline gauze (Stein, 2007).

 Across Care Settings: **Bladder exstrophy**

Nurses must prepare daycare providers and school nurses to care for infants and children with bladder exstrophy. This may involve proper diapering and hygiene maintenance, education about the congenital anomaly and other associated anomalies and preparation for psychosexual problems that may arise as the child reaches adolescence. Hospital pediatric nurses may need to educate community nurses, who may play a role in educating daycare providers and school nurses.

 Now Can You— Discuss functional disorders of the urinary tract?

1. Describe care measures for children who experience enuresis?
2. Explain the importance of the nurse's role in community care for children with exstrophy of the bladder?

Reproductive Disorders Affecting Girls

VULVOVAGINITIS

There are various etiologies of vulvovaginitis (inflammation of the vulva and vagina) in prepubertal girls. Candidiasis, a yeast organism, is the most common source of this disorder. Vulvitis (vulvar inflammation) may be isolated or occur with vaginitis, which is vaginal inflammation. The prepubertal girl is sensitive to lack of estrogen, lack of protective hair, and lack of labial fat pads, as well as the influence of poor hygiene and proximity of the anus to the vulva. Clothing, soaps, and other chemicals may be irritating to vulvar skin. Tight jeans, ballet leotards, nylon tights, underwear, and bathing suits may all contribute to maceration and vulvar infection, especially if the weather is warm and there is associated sweating. It is common for young girls to void with their legs together, which increases the risk of urine refluxing into the vagina. Candidiasis is often associated with bubble baths in young girls, and this may also lead to UTI as well.

Nonspecific vulvovaginitis, without a clear etiology, is found in 25% to 75% of all cases in prepubertal girls. Fecal organisms have been found, and so may be a cause of vulvovaginitis in some cases, due to poor hygiene and possibly wiping back to front, spreading anal organisms. Candida, bacteroides, and some other streptococcal species have also been noted. Gram-negative *E. coli* organisms have been cultured from girls with vulvovaginitis, and these may be fecal in origin. Normal flora, including lactobacilli, diphtheroids, and *S. epidermidis*, have been noted on vaginal cultures of vulvovaginitis.

If infections that are sexually transmitted, such as those due to *Neisseria gonorrhea*, *Chlamydia trachomatis*, *Trichomonas*, herpes simplex, and human papillomavirus are found, there is high suspicion of sexual contact, either voluntary or due to sexual assault.

SIGNS AND SYMPTOMS. Vulvar itching may be the only presenting complaint without a defined etiology. Vaginal candidiasis has notable thick, curdy white discharge and is typically very pruritic. The discharge may also be foul-smelling and brown or green.

DIAGNOSIS. Diagnosis is based on patient history, clinical findings, and pH testing. Pseudohyphae (branching yeast organisms) may be found on microscopy where the pH is < 4.5.

NURSING CARE. If no etiology for vulvovaginitis is determined, the child should be instructed to avoid predisposing factors.

 Nursing Insight— *Vaginal candidiasis and diabetes mellitus*

Recurrent vaginal candidiasis should raise the suspicions of diabetes mellitus.

Treatment of vaginal candidiasis in prepubertal girls is best accomplished with over-the-counter antifungal remedies, such as miconazole (Monistat) and chlortrimazole (Gyne-Lotrimin) creams applied topically, avoiding internal insertion. Nurses should instruct young girls to wipe from the front to the back after voiding in order to avoid contaminating the perineum with stool. Educate patients in the complementary treatments.

 Complementary Care: *Vaginal candidiasis*

- Wear cotton underwear to allow better ventilation.
- Avoid wearing wet clothing, such as bathing suits, for long periods.
- Avoid bubble baths, as well as perfumes or powder near the vaginal area.

Family Teaching Guidelines...
Vulvovaginitis

HOW TO:

It may be useful for the nurse to suggest tub baths with clear, warm water one to two times daily for 10 to 15 minutes, followed by washing with a bland soap such as unscented Dove, Basis, Aveeno, or Neutrogena. The soap should not be applied to the vulvar area, and the vulva should never be scrubbed. Avoid shampooing the hair in the bathtub, so the vulva is not exposed to shampoo chemicals. Showering is an option.

After bathing, the nurse should instruct the patient to gently pat dry the vulvar area. Sleeper pajamas are not recommended due to their occlusive nature. Underwear should be all cotton for greater ventilation. They should be washed in mild, unscented detergent without bleach.

Some health care providers recommend a small amount of A+D ointment, Vaseline, or Desitin ointment to be applied to protect the vulvar skin. Loose-fitting clothing is ideal, especially in warm weather.

ESSENTIAL INFORMATION

Persistent discharge is occasionally treated with certain antibiotics in oral form or topical form. Pinworms can be a cause of recurrent vulvovaginitis. Nurses can instruct parents to inspect the anal area of their child at night with a flashlight, or apply a small piece of cellophane tape over the anal area to catch the pinworms (Emans, 2005).

medication: Medications for Candida Vulvovaginalis

Miconazole (Monistat Products)—Antifungal Agent Used Topically in the Vaginal Area

Pregnancy Category: C
- Mechanism: damages fungal cell wall membrane that causes leakage of nutrients
- Absorption: small amount through vagina
- Apply topically to external vagina very sparingly once or twice daily in adolescents; can be applied through vaginal applicator in adolescents Nystatin (Mycostatin Products)—Antifungal Agent Used Topically in the Vaginal Area

Pregnancy Category: B

Mechanism: Bonds to sterols in fungal cell membrane, causing wall permeability changes

Absorption: Not absorbed through mucous membranes; therefore safer for children and infants
- Gently massage cream or ointment onto skin two to four times per day Chlortrimazole (Lotrimin, Mycelex products): Antifungal Agent Used Topically in Vaginal Area

Pregnancy Category: B (topical)

Mechanism of Action: Binds to phospholipids in cell membrane causing cell wall permeability and loss of intracellular contents

Absorption: Negligible through intact skin topically; 3%–10% absorption through intravaginal preparations
- Vaginal cream (Mycelex) 2% bid application external vagina in children older than age 3; vaginal applicator of cream usable in children older than age 12 and adults (Taketomo, Hodding, & Kraus, 2007).

- In menstruating females, avoid using scented sanitary pads or tampons.
- Avoid excessive sugars and simple carbohydrates in the diet.
- Eat yogurt. The natural lactobacilli appears to maintain normal bacterial balance in the GI tract, keeping yeast in check.

 Nursing Insight— Vaginal foreign bodies

Insertion of a foreign object, normally by the young girl herself, usually from ages 2 to 9, has been noted to cause vaginal bleeding and/or odiferous and blood-stained vaginal discharge. The problem normally was remedied through removal and a simple Betadine irrigation (Stricker, Navratil, & Sennhauser, 2004). Sexual abuse must be ruled out.

LABIAL ADHESIONS

Labial adhesions are most common in girls from 3 months to 6 years old. This disorder is defined as the fusion of the labia minora, due to inflammation, infection, trauma, and estrogen deficit.

SIGNS AND SYMPTOMS. A thin film develops over the labia, from the posterior aspect to the anterior aspect, and if severe, even the vaginal introitus and urethral meatus are not visible. Any scarring that is not midline or seems very severe and dense should raise the suspicion of child sexual abuse or trauma. Also, intersexed (female and male physical sexual characteristics in the same individual) females may have anatomy that resembles that of labial adhesions.

DIAGNOSIS. Diagnosis is based on signs and symptoms and common associated problems such as dysuria and incontinence if urine is trapped, or dribbling after voiding in toilet-trained girls.

NURSING CARE. The nurse can communicate to the family that the condition may be a spontaneous resolution over time, lysis of adhesions, or treatment with hormone cream, such as Premarin cream 0.625 mg bid for 10 to 14 days. It is also important to inform the family that complications may include UTI due to obstruction of urine flow.

AMENORRHEA

Amenorrhea refers to the absence of menses. Primary amenorrhea is when no menses occur by the age of 17. Secondary amenorrhea implies that menses have been established, but have ceased for a minimum of 3 months. There are several possible causes: corpus luteum cyst, lactation, menopause (premature or normal), hypothyroidism or hyperthyroidism, chemotherapy, polycystic ovarian syndrome (PCOS), diabetes mellitus, stress, excessive exercise, weight loss, and pregnancy (Herban Hill & Sullivan, 2004). Pregnancy must always be considered as a cause of secondary amenorrhea, even if the patient denies sexual contact.

The etiologies of primary amenorrhea include agenesis (no formation) of the uterus, Turner's syndrome (genetic disorder with pectus excavatus, heart murmur, and short stature), imperforate hymen, and constitutional delay.

Certain medications can cause amenorrhea, including chemotherapy and medroxyprogesterone acetate (Depo Provera), which is given as a contraceptive injection.

SIGNS AND SYMPTOMS. In primary amenorrhea, the patient may exhibit abnormalities in body habitus, suggestive of delayed puberty. The Tanner stages of sexual characteristic development may show delays. In cases of secondary amenorrhea, signs and symptoms of pregnancy include mastalgia (breast tenderness); breast enlargement; nausea and possibly vomiting, especially in the early morning; gastrointestinal upset; and urinary frequency. On examination, the uterus may be enlarged and Chadwick's sign (blue or violaceous cervix) may be present, a probable sign of pregnancy that becomes evident about the fourth week of gestation.

In hypothyroidism, the patient may have dry skin, dry hair, fatigue, hoarseness, constipation, and an enlarged thyroid gland. In hyperthyroidism, the patient may exhibit oily skin and hair, diaphoresis, tachycardia, diarrhea, and a goiter (enlarged thyroid gland).

Patients with polycystic ovarian syndrome may have hirsuitism (excessive facial and bodily hair) and obesity. Corpus luteum cysts tend to cause pain in the lower quadrants that may be intermittent in nature, as some cysts resolve spontaneously. Other cysts grow and may rupture, causing significant lower quadrant abdominal pain and even peritoneal signs of rebound, guarding, and rigidity.

DIAGNOSIS. In the absence of menses, a number of laboratory tests and other diagnostic tests are often necessary in the diagnostic evaluation of amenorrhea.

---

 diagnostic tools Determining Reason for Amenorrhea

- Genetic testing may be required to determine disorders such as Turner's syndrome.
- Pelvic ultrasound or transvaginal (ultrasound wand in the vaginal canal) is used to test for pregnancy, ovarian cysts, and other gynecological abnormalities. Patients normally are required to drink four 8-ounce glasses of water 1 hour before a pelvic ultrasound to elevate the bladder in order to view the pelvic organs.

Labs: Tests for Amenorrhea

- Urine pregnancy test (urinary HCG) these tests are widely available over the counter but more sensitive tests are available in clinical facilities.
- Serum pregnancy test (qualitative or quantitative tests show positive pregnancy and approximate duration of pregnancy, respectively). Considered more accurate than urine pregnancy tests and identify pregnancy earlier.
- Thyroid stimulating hormone (TSH) is a general test for hypothyroidism and hyperthyroidism. This may be accompanied by a free thyroxine (T4) test to specify the disorder more clearly.
- Prolactin level: elevated in hyperprolactinemia, which may be seen with hypothyroidism or with a benign pituitary adenoma. Prolactin is a hormone produced in the pituitary gland and is associated with breastfeeding.
- Levels of follicle stimulating hormone (FSH) may be low in PCOS.
- Levels of luteinizing hormone (LH) may be elevated in PCOS.
- Testosterone levels may be high in PCOS, in addition to dehydroepiandrosterone (DHEA) levels.

NURSING CARE. The nurse must realize that some adolescent girls are unaware that pregnancy is possible with just genital contact. Often pregnant adolescents may be in a state of denial. The nurse should evaluate the patient with amenorrhea for signs and symptoms of pregnancy first, including weight gain, unprotected coitus, fatigue, nausea and vomiting, and mastalgia (tender breasts). A urinary human chorionic gonadotropin (hCG) test may be run and may turn positive within days after a missed menses. In cases of possibly false-negative urine pregnancy tests, it is necessary to administer the serum HCG test to determine pregnancy status. If a parent is present with a girl who may be pregnant, the nurse should attempt to have the parent wait outside in order to speak confidentially to the adolescent girl, by suggesting that at this age, it is common to interview young women alone. Invite the parent or guardian back at the conclusion of the discussion. This sometimes allows the opportunity for a young woman to discuss the possibility of pregnancy or her concerns about contraception and sexually transmitted diseases (STDs).

The nurse can also assist the patient in constructing a calendar depicting her abnormal menstrual pattern. Young girls often need to be educated about variations in menstrual cycles, and why it is essential that they keep track of their cycle days, intervals, and duration. Girls who have eating disorders such as anorexia nervosa or bulimia may incur secondary amenorrhea due to weight loss and associated alterations in estrogen. When body fat significantly decreases, amenorrhea or oligomenorrhea (infrequent menses) may occur. Young girls who exercise heavily (gymnasts or distance runners) may develop menstrual disorders, as well as young girls with eating disorders.

In the circumstance of adolescent females, those with primary amenorrhea may have family members who have experienced the same issue.

 Nursing Insight— *Imperforate hymen*

In cases of imperforate hymen (without opening), a surgical intervention is required. If laboratory testing is normal, many amenorrheic patients are given a trial of medroxyprogesterone acetate (Depo Provera), 5 or 10 mg daily for 5 or 10 days in 1 month, in an attempt to elicit the menses by causing a progesterone withdrawal bleed. Some patients are placed on oral contraceptive agents to regulate the menses and cause a monthly withdrawal bleed (Herban Hill & Sullivan, 2004).

Reproductive Disorders Affecting Boys

VARICOCELE

Varicoceles are defined as abnormal dilations in the testicular veins, normally unilateral and affecting the left testicle. Most arise after age 9, and 16% of adolescents and 15% to 20% of adult males have varicoceles. The etiology of this disorder remains unknown, but it is now considered the most common cause of male infertility that is correctable.

SIGNS AND SYMPTOMS. Frequently, varicoles are said to feel like a "bag of worms," although while still in the smaller stages, they may only feel like thickened spermatic cords.

assessment tools Valsalva Maneuver

Assessment is made by noting distended veins in the scrotum on standing, accentuation of the veins with the Valsalva maneuver, and decrease in visibility of the varicocele on taking the supine position. The testes are often smaller in varicocele.

DIAGNOSIS. Doppler ultrasonography may help to definitively determine the presence of varicocele.

NURSING CARE. Surgical ligation (binding or tying) of the spermatic veins is the curative approach to preserve fertility. This must be considered in adolescent males (Elmore & Kirsch, 2006). Nursing care centers on caring for the postsurgical patient.

CRYPTORCHIDISM

Cryptorchidism is defined as absent, undescended, or ectopic testicles. This is the most common male congenital anomaly, noted in 1% of all newborns. It may result from hormonal, anatomical, or chromosomal variations. Prematurity increases the risk of cryptorchidism. Intersex conditions such as congenital adrenal hyperplasia may be associated. In 80% of the cases, the testicles are palpable but undescended, and the scrotal sac is empty, as well as potentially flat or small. This must be distinguished from retractile testes, which are descended testicles that rise up into the groin area, but can be pushed down into the scrotum. Retractile testes are very common in young males. The remaining 20% of cases are nonpalpable testes, which may actually be in the abdomen or inguinal area, or may not be present at all.

The major risk associated with cryptorchidism is testicular cancer, which remains a lifetime risk even if the child has surgical repair. There is also risk of decreased fertility, testicular torsion, and increased trauma. If the testis does not descend permanently by age 6 months, surgical intervention is needed. All patients with a history of cryptorchidism must be vigilant with testicular self-exam and have annual testicular exams by a health care provider.

SIGNS AND SYMPTOMS. A retractile testis has descended but retracts with exam and physical stimulation. An ectopic testis is outside of the normal pathway (e.g., in the groin, abdominal wall, or perineum). After 1 year of age, it is uncommon for the testes to spontaneously descend. In 85% of affected males, the undescended testicle is unilateral and on the right.

DIAGNOSIS. Diagnosis is based on patient history, physical examination findings, and imaging tests.

NURSING CARE. The surgical repair is termed orchiopexy and is usually done between ages 1 and 2. Gentle compression of the inguinal canals should reveal a palpable nodule in undescended testicles (Fig. 32-7).

 Nursing Insight— Cryptorchidism

Observation and occasional use of hCG to stimulate testosterone production may be suggested. The nurse understands that deficient knowledge of the caregiver may exist. It is important to communicate to the caregiver that use of hCG may be alarming, in that penile growth, augmented pigmentation, and pubic hair may result. The nurse also recognizes that the caregiver may have anxiety due to the risk of testicular cancer and decreased fertility.

Figure 32-7 An undescended testis is palpable in various areas and needs to be surgically corrected.

Surgical treatment may involve use of dissolving sutures with a Tegaderm dressing (transparent dressing) over the wound. The nurse should instruct the caregiver to have the child wear loose clothing to increase comfort; use appropriate analgesics as ordered, including acetaminophen (Children's Tylenol); and observe for erythema, purulent discharge, fever, and increased pain at the incision site as potentially indicative of infection. The nurse should instruct the caregiver to change diapers more frequently and to avoid having the older child engage in any sports or straddle riding toys that might injure the surgical site (Kenner et al., 2007).

 Nursing Insight— Hydrocele

A hydrocele is a collection of fluid in the scrotal sac, related to a patent processus vaginalis, which is the channel that gives fluid the ability to move from abdomen to groin. Peritoneal abdominal fluid can pass into this patent canal, enlarging the scrotal sack. This canal is patent in up to 80% of all newborns at birth, but by the first month of life, the incidence decreases to 60% and by the age of 18 to 24 months, the incidence decreases to 20% to 30%. While this condition can rarely occur in females, primarily in intersex conditions, it is common enough in males that it must be repaired if it has not resolved by 1 year. If a hernia is found with it, earlier surgical repair is necessary.

HYPOSPADIAS AND EPISPADIAS

Hypospadias and epispadias are possibly genetic congenital conditions that imply an abnormal positioning of the urethral meatus in boys. In hypospadias, the meatus is inferior to its usual position. In epispadias, the meatus is superior to its usual position and a surgical correction with possible penile urethral lengthening may be necessary (Montagnino & Currier, 2005). Hypospadias may cause chordee, which is a bending of the penis that may later present problems with intercourse. Young males with hypospadias may not be able to urinate standing and there may be associated cryptorchidism. Patients need to be referred early to pediatric urologists for surgical repair.

SIGNS AND SYMPTOMS. Signs and symptoms of hypospadias include opening of the urethra below the tip on the bottom side of the penis, incomplete foreskin, curvature of the penis during erection, and abnormal position of the scrotum in relation to the penis. Signs and symptoms of epispadias are opening of the urethra above the tip of the penis, curvature of the penis, and urinary incontinence.

DIAGNOSIS. Diagnosis is based on patient history, physical examination findings, radiography, and ultrasound.

NURSING CARE. Surgery is usually performed before the child is 18 months old and before toilet training. Techniques reconstruct the penis to lengthen the urethra and bring it to the distal penis shaft. The chordee is straightened and often foreskin is used as a graft, so children born with hypospadias cannot be circumcised. The child may have a urethral stent or Foley catheter in place to allow urine drainage due to potential obstruction of voiding from surgical edema. A compression dressing termed a penile wrap may be used. The nurse may need to instruct the caregiver to have the child soak in warm water for 20 minutes before the surgical follow-up appointment in order to loosen the dressing. Potential surgical complications include urethral fistula (an opening that allows urine to leak to the surface), return of the meatus to its original site postsurgically, and strictures at the site of the anastomosis (Kenner et al., 2007).

In patients with hypospadias and epispadias surgical repairs are at risk of acute infection. The penile incision must be monitored for signs of infection (e.g., purulent discharge, fever, erythema). Also watch for evidence of UTI (fever; cloudy, foul urine; and hematuria). These pediatric patients also often suffer acute pain related to bladder spasm, incisional pain, and pain related to infection. Oxybutynin chloride (Ditropan) is an anticholinergic medicine that may relieve bladder spasm. Adverse effects of Ditropan include dry mouth and flushed facies.

Nurses must recognize that parents of these children may be deficient in knowledge about the defects and their repair. The nurse should assess the parent's feelings about having a child with a congenital defect (Kenner et al., 2007).

 Nursing Insight*— *Gynecomastia

Sixty percent of males may have temporary gynecomastia (breast enlargement) during puberty. This often coincides with one side of the scrotum growing faster than the other (Kenner et al., 2007).

Gynecomastia may be one of four types:

- Type I is considered benign and self-limited. It occurs during Tanner stages II and III, and most cases are unilateral. The problem may persist for 2 years.
- Type II is painful gynecomastia without any associated disease.
- Type III is gynecomastia that results from obesity.
- Type IV is related to hypertrophy of the pectoral muscles.

Type I gynecomastia has an uncertain etiology, but is thought to be related to an imbalance in estrogen and testosterone levels, or to increased prolactin levels, or possibly to abnormal serum-binding protein levels. The incidence is between 50% to 60% of all males, normally between the ages of 12 and 14. Commonly, a 1 cm to 3 cm mobile, firm, and round mass is palpable proximal to and beneath the areola. An enlarging mass or a mass that persists more than 2 years requires a diagnostic work-up to consider the differential diagnoses of breast tumor, Klinefelter's syndrome (decreased facial hair, eunuch body, normal or borderline low IQ, and micro-orchidism), drug-induced gynecomastia, and thyroid disease (Herban Hill & Sullivan, 2004).

66 What to say 99 — *Gynecomastia*

- Teach the patient and parents that gynecomastia is usually a temporary condition.
- If obesity is an issue, the nurse should work with the patient and family members to establish an age-appropriate dietary plan. Referral to a nutritionist may be useful.
- Explain to the family and patient that it may be necessary to have certain blood tests to eliminate any risk of pathological causes of the gynecomastia.
- The nurse can discuss ways the child can respond to hurtful comments from other children.

TESTICULAR TORSION

Testicular torsion is considered an emergency and surgical intervention must occur within a 4- to 8-hour time frame from the onset of symptoms, or the patient risks the need for orchiectomy (testes resection). Loss of one testis through orchiectomy has been documented to decrease sperm counts and reduce fertility. This emergency condition is most common in growing males between the ages of 10 and 19 (Mansback, Forbes, & Peters, 2005).

During the neonatal period, testicular torsion can occur because the processus vaginalis about the spermatic cord and testis can twist, causing partial or complete vascular compromise. In ages above the neonatal period, the etiology of testicular torsion is distinct; the testicle normally is attached to the tunica vaginalis, but periodically, the testicle is not attached and it hangs free to twist around the spermatic cord. This can cause torsion with painful ischemia and loss of the testis. Testicular torsion is the cause of 16% to 27% of all cases of acute scrotal pain, and thus it must be ruled out in all cases (Cole & Vogler, 2004).

SIGNS AND SYMPTOMS. Neonates present distinctly from older males with testicular torsion. In the neonate, the scrotum appears dusky colored, a solid mass is palpated, scrotal edema prevents transillumination (inspect the testis by passing a light through the scrotum), and there is minimal or no pain from testicular motion. Older males normally have severe and persistent pain, although it may begin gradually. Trauma and physical exertion may promote the development of torsion, but it may occur without any etiology. The pain may be severe enough to awaken patients at night and prevent ambulation. It is possible to have intermittent torsion, which resolves itself, but eventually a patient may develop full, emergency torsion. Fever, anorexia, nausea, and vomiting may accompany the condition (Cole & Vogler, 2004).

 critical nursing action Testicular Torsion

Essential clinical signs and symptoms the nurse should look for:

- The torsed testicle may be lying horizontally or appear higher in the scrotal sack than the opposite testicle.
- Although most commonly, the situation is unilateral, it may be bilateral. Scrotal edema is usually present within 12 hours.
- Especially in the neonate, the testicle may feel quite hard.

- One way to differentiate the diagnosis of testicular torsion is to attempt to elicit the cremasteric reflex, which is normally absent on the torsion side.
- Prehn's sign, which is relief of pain from elevating the testicle, is also usually absent in torsion (Cole & Vogler, 2004).

DIAGNOSIS. Diagnosis is based on patient history, physical examination findings, and Doppler ultrasonography.

 diagnostic tools Testicular Torsion

Doppler ultrasonography is the preferred diagnostic test, and it should be ordered immediately. In testicular torsion, the testicle may be enlarged and may reveal decreased or absent blood flow. The Doppler test can also differentiate between ischemia and inflammation, such as that seen in orchitis (inflammation of a testis) and epididymitis (inflammation of the epididymis) often associated with gonorrhea. In the case of possible false-negative results on Doppler ultrasound, a technetium scintigraphy test shows definitive testicular torsion (Ringdahl & Teague, 2006).

NURSING CARE. Manual detorsion (surgery for torsion of a testicle) by the urologist can be done with sedation and local anesthesia to provide immediate mitigation of pain (Ringdahl & Teague, 2006). Surgical consultation is always necessary and if the surgery is not performed within the 4- to 8-hour window, orchiectomy may be required. According to Gaylord and Starr (2004), the rate of saving the testicle drops steadily after 3 hours, and testicular atrophy, abscess, total loss of the testicle from necrosis, and loss of fertility may occur particularly if torsion is present for 24 hours or longer.

Reproductive Disorders Affecting Both Girls and Boys

AMBIGUOUS GENITALIA

Approximately 1 out of 2000 newborns are born in the United States with ambiguous genitalia, which cannot be properly identified as either male or female genitalia. In males, it is more typical to have underdeveloped genitalia and in females, overdeveloped genitalia are more common (Fig. 32-8). The etiology may be related to fetal or maternal hormonal imbalances.

SIGNS AND SYMPTOMS. Signs and symptoms include external reproductive organs that are not easily identified as male or female (Venes, 2009).

DIAGNOSIS. Diagnosis can include a family history of congenital adrenal cortical hyperplasia, amenorrhea and infertility in aunts, or maternal history of prostaglandin, androgen, or danazol (Danocrine, a synthetic androgen used for endometriosis) use. Diagnosis is also based on the fact that the infant has both ovaries and testes. The external genitalia may vary from fully masculine to nearly fully feminine.

NURSING CARE. The nurse may assist the patient's family by suggesting endocrinology and genetic referrals. Some patients with ambiguous genitalia become surgical candidates (Gray & Campbell, 2002).

Figure 32-8 Ambiguous genitalia.

Now Can You— Discuss reproductive disorders in girls and boys?

1. Explain family teaching measures for vulvovaginitis?
2. Describe causes of secondary amenorrhea?
3. Examine care measures for hypospadias and epispadias?
4. Discuss ambiguous genitalia?

summary points

- Pediatric nurses must be aware of the pathophysiology of the renal system, common and uncommon renal disorders, and also associated reproductive anomalies that can occur in children.

- Assessment is a priority nursing action when caring for the child with a fluid and/or electrolyte imbalance. The astute nurse must recognize fluid deficit and excess as well as electrolyte imbalance and then provide the proper care.

- Urinary tract infection is the second most common form of bacterial infection in children, ranking only behind upper respiratory problems. It is thought that 8% of girls and 2% of boys will have a UTI during childhood.

- The major risk of vesicoureteral reflux (VUR) is the development of acute pyelonephritis, due to the backflow of urine toward the kidney.

- The most common etiologies for gross hematuria include hypercalciuria with or without stones, hypertension, and glomerulonephritis. However, it is significant to note that asymptomatic microhematuria had no identifiable cause in the majority of patients.

- Glomerular disease can be due to primary kidney disease or secondary multisystem diseases that cause damage to the glomerulus. Both primary and secondary diseases are accompanied with histological evidence that captures the glomerular damage and resultant clinical manifestations and needed treatment.

- Hemolytic uremic syndrome (HUS) is considered the most common cause of acute renal failure (ARF) in children. Hemolytic uremic syndrome (HUS) is most commonly associated with children ingesting beef contaminated with *Escherichia coli* (*E. coli*).

◆ Abnormalities of the urinary tract system ultimately affect the kidneys. The abnormalities may be anatomical, infectious, cellular, inflammatory, functional, or maturational.

◆ The most common causes of renal trauma are motor vehicle accidents.

◆ Collaboration with the health care team is critical so that acute renal failure complications are reduced or prevented from occurring depending on whether the etiology is prerenal, intrarenal, or postrenal.

◆ The goals of nursing care for a patient with chronic renal disease are mutually established with the patient and family. Collaboration with the health care team is essential so that the quality of life can be extended as long as possible as the renal capacity diminishes and affects all organ systems.

◆ Children in need of a renal transplant are placed on a waiting list and are registered with the United Network of Organ Sharing (UNOS), which keeps a computer network to link all organ donation centers and transplant centers.

◆ Nurses can assist a child with dysfunctional elimination syndrome (DES) by identifying issues, asking the child at various times of day if he or she has voided, and asking if he or she can hold his or her urine if a bathroom is not always available. Nurses should assess for any emotional or social problems resulting from a child's embarrassment or shame associated with voiding dysfunction.

◆ There are a variety of reproductive disorders in girls such as vulvovaginitis, vaginal foreign bodies, labial adhesions, and amenorrhea.

◆ There are a variety of reproductive disorders in both girls and boys such as ambiguous genitalia.

◆ There are a variety of reproductive disorders in boys such as varicocele, cryptorchidism, hydrocele, hypospadias and epispadias, gynecomastia, and testicular torsion.

review questions

Select All that Apply

1. The pediatric nurse is providing critical information about a 3-year-old who was admitted to the unit with a urinary tract infection to a group of nursing students. Which of the following classic clinical signs and symptoms of urinary tract infection would be discussed?
   A. Dysuria
   B. Frequency
   C. Urgency
   D. Abdominal pain

2. The pediatric nurse is writing a comprehensive nursing care plan about chronic renal failure. Which of the following nursing diagnosis(es) would be essential for the nurse to include in the nursing care plan?
   A. Fluid Volume Deficit related to compromised regulatory mechanism.
   B. Imbalanced Nutrition Less than Body Requirements related to anorexia.
   C. Risk for Infection related to lowered body defenses.
   D. Disturbed Body Image related to growth delays.

3. The pediatric nurse is providing health promotion teaching to a child and family related to the care of a newly acquired arteriovenous fistula for hemodialysis treatment. Which of the following should be included in the teaching?
   A. Wash the access with soap and warm water each day, and always before dialysis.
   B. Check the area daily for signs of infection, including warmth and redness.
   C. Take care to avoid traumatizing the arm; no tight clothes or jewelry on the arm.
   D. Remind health care providers not to take blood pressure on the access arm.

Case Study

4. A 2-year-old child who weighs 33 lbs. (15 kg) is admitted with a kidney infection and is receiving intravenous fluids based on her weight. Which of these infusion rates based on the fluid maintenance calculation would the pediatric nurse follow?
   A. IV fluids infusing at 47 mL/hr
   B. IV fluids infusing at 52 mL/hr
   C. IV fluids infusing at 58 mL/hr
   D. IV fluids infusing at 73 mL/hr

5. The nurse assesses a 7-year-old and notes gastroenteritis with diarrhea and vomiting along with an upper respiratory infection. The nurse also notes that laboratory results of the stool culture are positive for *E. coli*. The nurse suspects that the child has:
   A. Hemolytic uremic syndrome
   B. Poststreptococcal glomerulonephritis
   C. Henoch–Schönlein purpura
   D. Urinary tract infection

Fill in the Blank

6. The child who is in acute renal failure will have signs and symptoms that include fever, rash, _____ _____, pallor, vomiting, _____ _____, hemorrhage, shock, anuria, or _____.

7. _____ _____ _____ is the most common cause of acute renal failure in children due to the pathogen, _____ _____.

8. _____ is a cause of recurrent vulvovaginitis. Treatment is best accomplished with over-the-counter _____ _____.

True or False

9. The pediatric nurse is aware that urinary tract infections are the second most common form of bacterial infection in children.

10. Circumcision increases the risk of urinary tract infections in boys.

11. Hematuria is considered the cardinal marker of renal injury in children.

12. When acute renal failure is considered to be permanent and fatal, it is called chronic renal failure.

13. Children whose status is postrenal transplant receive immunosuppressive medications to help prevent them from developing infections.

14. In most cases, children who receive kidney transplants can be on a regular diet once the transplant is accepted.

REFERENCES

American Academy of Pediatrics, Committee on Quality Improvement, Subcommittee on Urinary Tract Infections. (1999). Practice parameters: the diagnosis, treatment and evaluation of the initial urinary tract infection in febrile infants and young children. *Pediatrics*, 103(4), 843–853.

Bergstein, J., Leiser, J., & Andreoli, S. (2005). The clinical significance of asymptomatic gross and microscopic hematuria in children. *Archives of Pediatric and Adolescent Medicine, 159,* 353–355.

Bernstein, D., & Shelov, S. (2003). *Pediatrics for medical students.* Philadelphia: Lippincott Williams & Wilkins.

Berry, A. (2005, June). Helping children with dysfunctional voiding. *Urologic Nursing*, 25(3), 193–200.

Bruck, L., & Mayer, B. (2005). *Pediatric nursing made incredibly easy.* Philadelphia: Lippincott Williams & Wilkins.

Bulechek, G., Butcher, H.M., & Dochterman, J. (2008). *Nursing interventions classification (NIC)* (5th ed.). St. Louis, MO: C.V. Mosby.

Cendron, M., & Benedict, J. (2006). Vesicoureteral reflux. Retrieved from http://www.emedicine.com/med/topic2838 (Accessed January 20, 2007).

Children's Hospital of Pittsburgh. (2005). Children with Maple Syrup Urine Disease celebrate one-year post-transplant—Kids no longer have life-threatening disease. Retrieved from http: //www.sciencedaily.com/releases/2005/06/050624102658.htm (Accessed March 6, 2007).

Cincinnati Children's Hospital Medical Center (2005). Evidence-based clinical practice guidelines: ED Algorithm for medical management of uncomplicated urinary tract infections in children age 12 or less.

Cincinnati Children's Hospital Medical Center Formulary (2005). Evidence-based Clinical practice guidelines.

Cole, F. L., & Vogler, R. (2004). The acute, nontraumatic scrotum: Assessment, diagnosis, and management. *Journal of the American Academy of Nurse Practitioners*, 16(2), 50–56.

Davis's Drug Guide for Nurses (2007). Imipramine. Retrieved from http://www.drugguide.com/monograph_library/psychotropic_drugs/imipramine.htm (Accessed February 17, 2007).

Deglin, J.H., and Vallerand, A. (2009). *Davis's drug guide for nurses* (11th ed.). Philadelphia: F.A. Davis.

Dunn, A.M. (2004). Elimination patterns. In C.E. Burns, A.M. Dunn, M.A. Brady, N.B. Starr, & C.G. Blosser. (Eds.). *Pediatric primary care: A handbook for nurse practitioners* (3rd ed., pp. 285–299). St. Louis: W.B. Saunders.

Egland, A., & Egland T. (2006). Pediatrics, urinary tract infections and pyelonephritis. Retrieved from http://www.emedicine.com/emer/topic 769.htm (Accessed February 25, 2007).

Elder, J. (2004). Urinary tract infections. In R.E. Behrman, R.M. Kleigman, & H.B. Jenson (Eds.). *Nelson's textbook of pediatrics* (17th ed. pp. 1785–1789). Philadelphia: W.B. Saunders.

Elmore, J.M., & Kirsch, A.J. (2006, December). Varicocele in adolescents. Retrieved from http://www.emedicine.com/ped/topic2806.htm (Accessed January 17, 2007).

Emans, S.J. (2005) Vulvovaginal problems in the prepubertal child. In S.J. Emans, M.R. Laufer, & D.P. Goldstein, *Pediatric & adolescent gynecology* (5th ed.). Philadelphia: Lippincott Willliams & Wilkins.

Garin, E., Olavarria, F., Nieto, V., Valenciano, B., Campos, A., & Young, L. (2006, March). Clinical significance of primary vesicoureteral reflux and urinary antibiotic prophylaxis after acute pyelonephritis: a multicenter, randomized, controlled study. *Pediatrics*, 117(3), 626–632.

Gaylord, N., & Starr, N. B. (2004). Genitourinary disorders. In C.E. Burns, A.M. Dunn, M.A. Brady, N.B. Starr, & C.G. Blosser. (Eds.). *Pediatric primary care: A handbook for nurse Practitioners* (3rd ed., pp. 911–953). St. Louis: W.B. Saunders.

Gray, M., & Campbell, F. (2002). Urinary system. In J.A. Fox. *Primary health care of infants, children, & adolescents* (2nd ed., pp. 670–693). St. Louis: C.V. Mosby.

Hansen, J. T., & Koeppen, B. M. (2002). *Netter's atlas of human physiology.* Teterboro, NJ: Icon Learning Systems.

Hellerstein, S. (2007). Urinary tract infection. Retrieved from http://www.emedicine.com/ped/topic2366.htm (Accessed February 24, 2007).

Herban Hill, N., & Sullivan, L. M. (2004). *Management guidelines for nurse practitioners working with children and adolescents* (2nd ed.). Philadelphia: F. A. Davis.

Hogan, M. & White, J. (2003). Child health nursing: reviews & rationales. Upper

Ismaili, K., Hall, M., Piepsz, A., Wissing, K.M., Collier, F., Schulman, C., Avni, F.E. (2006). Primary vesicoureteral reflux detected in neonates with a history of fetal renal pelvis dilatation: A prospective clinical and imaging study. *Journal of Pediatrics, 148,* 222–227.

Johnson, M., Bulechek, G., Butcher, H., McCloskey Dochterman, J., Maas, M., Moorehead, S., & Swanson, E. (2006). *NANDA, NOC, and NIC linkages: Nursing diagnoses, outcomes, & interventions* (2nd ed.). St. Louis, MO: Mosby Elsevier.

Kennedy, T. (2003). Urinary tract infection. In C. Rudolph & A. Rudolph (Eds.). *Rudolph's Pediatrics* (21st ed., pp. 1667–1671). Chicago: McGraw-Hill.

Kenner, C., Moran, M., Zebold, K. F., Keating, B. J., & Amlung, S. R. (2007). Genitourinary alterations. In N.L. Potts & B.L. Mandleco (Eds.). *Pediatric nursing: Caring for children and their families* (2nd ed., pp. 623-659). Clifton Park, NY: Thompson Delmar.

Kliegman, R., Marcdante, K., Jenson, J. & Behrman, R.(2006). *Nelson essentials of pediatrics* Philadelphia: Elsevier Saunders.

Kline, A.M., and Milonovich, L. (2006). Renal Critical Care. In P. Slota. *Pediatric critical care core curriculum* (2nd ed., pp. 408–445). Philadelphia: Elsevier.

King, S.J. (2006). Genitourinary disorders. In B. Richardson. (Ed.). *Practice guidelines for pediatric nurse practitioners*. St. Louis: Elsevier Mosby.

Lebel, M. (2004).Urinary tract infections. In M. Crocetti & M Barone *Oski's essential pediatrics* (2nd ed., p. 76). Philadelphia: Lippincott, Williams, & Wilkins.

Lippincott Williams & Wilkins. (2004). *Straight A's in pediatric nursing.* Philadelphia: Lippincott Williams & Wilkins.

Lum, G.M. (2007). Kidney & urinary tract. In W.W. Hay, Jr., M.J. Levin, J.M. Sondheimer, & R.R. Deterding. (Eds.). *Current pediatric diagnosis & treatment* (18th ed). New York: Lange Medical Books/McGraw-Hill.

Luxner, K. (2005). Delmar's pediatric nursing care plans. Clifton Park, New Jersey: Thompson Delmar Learning.

Mansback, J.M., Forbes, P., & Peters, C. (2005, December). Testicular torsion and risk factors for orchiectomy. *Archives of Pediatric and Adolescent Medicine, 159,* 1167–1171.

Montagnino, B., & Currier, H. (2005). The child with genitourinary dysfunction. In M.J. Hockenberry, D. Wilson, & M.L. Winkelstein (Eds.). *Wong's essentials of pediatric nursing* (7th ed., pp. 984–1010). St. Louis: C.V. Mosby.

Moorehead, S., Johnson, M., Maas, M., & Swanson, E. (2008) *Nursing outcomes classification (NOC)* (4th ed.). St. Louis, MO: C.V. Mosby.

NANDA International (2007). *NANDA-I nursing diagnoses: Definitions and classifications 2007–2008.* Philadelphia: NANDA-I.

National Guideline Clearinghouse. (2004). Practice parameter for the assessment and treatment of children and adolescents with enuresis. Retrieved from http://www.guideline.gov (Accessed January 20, 2007).

National Kidney and Urologic Diseases Information Clearinghouse. Retrieved from html:// www. kidney.nnik.nih.gov (Accessed January 20, 2007).

National Kidney Foundation: Newsroom. Retrieved from http://www.kidney.org/news/newsroomnewsitem.cfm?id=378 (Accessed March 10, 2007).

Newberry, L. (2003). *Sheey's emergency nursing: Principles and practice.* St. Louis: C.V. Mosby.

Nurse's Drug Handbook (2003). Blu Bell, PA: Blanchard & Loeb, LLC.

Olson, J.C. (2002). Rheumatic diseases of childhood. In R.E. Behrman & R.M. Kliegman.

Nelson Essentials of Pediatrics. (4th ed., p. 341-358). Philadelphia: Saunders.

Pagana, K., & Pagana, T. (2003). *Mosby's diagnostic and laboratory test reference*. Philadelphia: C.V. Mosby.

PDRhealth.(2007). Tofranil. Retrieved from http://www.pdrhealth.com/drug_info/rxdrugprofiles/drugs/tof1448.shtml (Accessed April 11, 2007).

Porth, C. M. (2004). *Essentials of pathophysiology: Concepts of altered health states*. Philadelphia: Lippincott Williams & Wilkins.

Potts, N. L., & Mandleco, B. H. (2002). *Pediatric nursing: caring for children and their families*. Clifton Park, NY: Delmar.

Razzaq, S. (2006). Hemolytic uremic syndrome: An emerging risk. *American Family Physician, 74*(6), 991–996.

Ringdahl, E., & Teague, L. (2006). Testicular torsion. *American Family Physician, 74*(10), 1739–1744.

Robson, W.L.M., Leung, A.K.C., & Van Howe, R. (2005, April). Primary and secondary nocturnal enuresis: Similarities in presentation. *Pediatrics, 115*(4), 956–959. 744–750.

Schwartz, M.W. (2005).*The 5 minute pediatric consult*. Philadelphia: Lippincott, Williams & Wilkins.

Shaikh, N., Hoberman, A., Wise, B., Kurs-Lasky, M., Kearney, D., Naylor, S., Haralam, M.A., Colborn, D.K., & Docimo, S.G. (2003). Dysfunctional elimination syndrome: Is it related to urinary tract infection or vesicoureteral reflux diagnosed early in life? *Pediatrics, 112*(5), 1134–1137.

Snyder, H. (2002), Urinary Tract Infections. In G. Fleisher & S. Ludwig (Eds.). *Synopsis of pediatric emergency medicine* (4th ed. pp. 585–586). Philadelphia: Lippincott Williams & Wilkins.

Stead, L.G., Stead, S.M,, & Kaufman, M.S. (2004). *First aid for the pediatric clerkship: A student to student guide*. Chicago: McGraw-Hill.

Stein, A.M. (Ed.). (2007). *Nursing review series: Pediatric nursing*. Clifton Park, NY: Thomson Delmar Learning

Stricker, T., Navratil, F., & Sennhaurer, F.H. (2004). Vaginal foreign bodies. *Journal of Pediatrics and Child Health, 40*(4), 205–207.

The Bedwetting Store (2007). Retrieved from http://www.bedwettingstore.com

Taketomo, C. K., Hodding, J. H., & Kraus, D. M. (2007). *Pediatric dosage handbook: with international trade names index : including neonatal dosing, drug administration & extemporaneous preparations*. Lexi-Comp's drug reference handbooks. Hudson, Ohio: Lexi-Comp.

The surgical management of congenital adrenal hyperplasia. Retrieved from http://www.cornellurology.com/pediatrics/genitoplasty/shtml (Accessed January 17, 2007).

Venes, D. (Ed.). *Taber's cyclopedic medical dictionary* (20th ed) . (2005). Philadelphia: F.A. Davis.

von Gontard, A. (2003). Psychological and psychiatric aspects of nocturnal enuresis. *Monatsschrift Kinderheilkunde, 151*, 945–951.

Von Gontard, A., Freitag, C. M., Seifen, S., Pukrop, R., & Rohling, D. (2006). Neuromotor development in nocturnal enuresis. *Developmental Medicine & Child Neurology, 48*

WebMD.Urinary tract infections in teens and adults. Retrieved from http://www.webmd.com/a-to-a guides/Urinary_Tract_Infections_in_Teens-and_Adults (Accessed February 25, 2007).

Wise, B., & Cardinal-Busse, B. (2007) Common illness of the reproductive and urologic systems. In N. Ryan-Wenger *Core curriculum for primary care pediatric nurse practitioners*. St. Louis: Mosby.

 For more information, go to http://davisplus.fadavis.com/

CONCEPT MAP

Caring for the Child with a Renal Urinary Tract or Reproductive Disorder

Fluid and Electrolyte Balance
- Calculate daily maintenance fluid balance
- Children at greater risk for F/E imbalance
- Dehydration → hypervolemic shock

Where Research And Practice Meet:
- Urinalysis
- Prophylactic antibiotics for VUR
- Hematuria

Renal, Urinary Tract Reproductive Disorders

Reproductive Disorders
Boys: varicocele; cryptorchidism; hydrocele; hypo/epispadias; gynecomastia; testicular torsion
Girls: vulvovaginitis; vaginal foreign body; labial adhesions; amenorrhea
Both: ambiguous genitalia; hernias

Structural Disorders
Urinary Tract
- Bladder exostrophy
- Vesicoureteral reflux
Obstructive Uropathies
- Ureteropelvic junction
- Ureterovesicular junction
- Posterior urethral valve
Renal Trauma
- Caused by MVA, direct blows, sports injuries, falls

Renal/Urinary System Disorders
UTI
- *E.coli* most common organism
- Related to structural abnormalities, urinary stasis, poor hygiene
Vesicoureteral Reflux
- Backflow of urine to ureters; primary or secondary
Unexplained Proteinuria
- 30 mg/dl or higher; simple to life-threatening etiologies
Hematuria
- Gross/microscopic; can also have serious cause
Glomerular disease
- → Acute /Chronic/Post-streptococcal glomerulonephritis
- – Inflammation of glomeruli due to deposits of antigen/antibody complexes
- → Hemolytic uremic syndrome
- – Cascade of events affecting filtration; clotting and inflammation; affects other systems
- → Henoch-Schonlein Purpura
- – Type of vasculitis: follows URIs

General Nursing Care Assessments
- Detailed history of injury; stressors/ sexual abuse; vital signs, EKG, UA, VCUG, labs (BUN, creatinine, potassium, sodium, etc.); urine color, odor, amount (I&O); acid–base imbalances; signs of ARF; other systems for signs of infection

Care of the Postoperative Patient
- Manage wounds/dressings; ambulation; I&O; pain management

Teaching
- Prevention through proper hygiene signs/symptoms of disease; etiology of the disorder; medication compliance; collection of urine samples; diagnostic tests; dietary restrictions; home care for dialysis patients (access care, signs of peritonitis)

Other
- Disorder-related medication administration; supporting the family; emotional issues with dialysis; collaborating with family and other health care team members; care of the child in ICU

Functional Disorders
Dysfunctional voiding
- Urge incontinence; lazy bladder syndrome; giggle incontinence; bladder-sphincter dyssynergia; vaginal voiding
Enuresis
- Involuntary/unintentional voiding
Bladder exstrophy
- Congenital defect; anterior surface of bladder open on abdominal wall
- Associated with other congenital anomalies

Acute Renal Failure
- Sudden cessation of renal function
- Oliguric or nonoliguric
- Pre-, intra-, and postrenal causes
- Oliguric, diuretic, and recovery phases
Vesicoureteral Reflux
- Backflow of urine to ureters; primary or secondary
Chronic Renal Failure
- Progressive, irreversible deterioration of kidney function
- → four stages
- Etiology related to age of child and organs affected
- End stage renal disease (ESRD)

Dialysis
Peritoneal: (CAPD; CCPD)
- Peritoneal membrane filters blood
- Uses concept of exchanges
Hemodialysis
- Mechanical filtration/dialyzer
- Requires vascular access

Renal Transplant
- From cadaver or living donor
- Long term pharmacotherapy:
  – Immunosuppressants
  – Antihypertensives
  – Diuretics
- Potential for organ rejection
  – Signs/symptoms

Complementary Care:
- Behavioral management/ biofeedback for voiding dysfunction
- Enuresis: hydrotherapy; acupressure, massage
- Tx for vaginal candidiasis

Optimizing Outcomes:
- Look for objective cues for UTI in small child
- Growth and development considerations

Ethnocultural Considerations:
- Toileting practices
- African Americans constitute 32% of all patients treated for kidney failure

What To Say:
- History info for CRF
- Causes of secondary amenorrhea
- Teaching about gynecomastia
- Consequences of adolescence high risk behaviors

Critical Nursing Action:
- Clinical signs/symptoms of testicular torsion

Clinical Alert:
- UTI can be caused by adenovirus
- Proper calculation of fluid requirement
- Uncooked meat
- Hematuria cardinal marker of renal injury
- Physical findings for ARF
- Kidneys secrete erythrogenin/renin
- Kidneys activate Vitamin D which controls calcium metabolism
- Stages of transplant rejection
- Repair of hypospadias before preschool (G&D)

Now Can You:
- Name common disorders of the renal and urinary systems
- Describe structural defects of the urinary system
- Discuss functional disorders of the urinary tract
- Discuss reproductive disorders for girls and boys
- Discuss nutritional components of the renal diet

Be Sure To:
- Legal ramifications of *E.coli* 0147.H7 infection

Nursing Insight:
- How to calculate the GFR
- ESRD can occur due to scarring
- Antibiotics: compliance and UTI risk
- Risk factors for UTI
- HUS common cause of ARF
- FEna index of tubular function
- Teaching about cryptorchidism

Across Care Settings:
- Child with kidney transplant needs multidisciplinary care
- Daycare/school nurses need teaching re: caring for bladder exostrophy
- Identifying/caring for strep infection
- Proper hygiene practices

Caring for the Child with a Hematological Condition

 A Nurse's Wish

To be a nurse requires dedication,
With years of study and preparation.
I pray for guidance and humbly ask,
That I will do well with this chosen task.

When illness strikes or pain demands,
And a life is placed within my hands,
Give me compassion, knowledge and skill
To do the things that comfort and heal.

Suffering makes patients' fear grow worse
And they seek reassurance from their nurse.
Help me see things from their point of view
And always to know what is best to do.

May I have a part, in some small way,
In restoring good health to a child today.
Let my work be all that I want it to be—
I ask the great healer to work through me.

—Author Unknown

LEARNING TARGETS *At the completion of this chapter, the student will be able to:*

- Describe the hematopoietic system.
- Explain the basic components and functions of the blood.
- Discuss factors that cause deviations in normal laboratory values.
- Identify common hematological conditions in children.
- State the common signs and symptoms associated with hematological conditions, as well as diagnostic criteria.
- Discuss the nursing care of children with hematological conditions.
- Review the treatment options for children with hematological illnesses.
- Discuss blood transfusion therapy, apheresis, and thrombosis.

moving toward evidence-based practice Sickle Cell Patients with Acute Chest Syndrome and the Incidence of Asthma

Bryant, R. (2005). Asthma in the pediatric sickle cell patient with acute chest syndrome. *Journal of Pediatric Health Care, 19*(3), 157–162.

The purpose of this study was to determine whether there was an increased frequency of asthma in children who experienced acute chest syndrome (ACS) as a complication of sickle cell disease (SCD). Previous studies cited in the literature found that ACS accounts for 25% of premature deaths in children with SCD and that ACS is four times more likely to develop in children who also have asthma. ACS can be precipitated by cell sickling, which in turn may be a response to the pathogenesis associated with asthma.

The retrospective study included a descriptive chart review to identify the frequency of asthma in SCD patients admitted with ACS over a 5-year period. The diagnosis of ACS was determined using records from emergency room visits and hospitalizations at a children's hospital and a children's sickle cell clinic. All charts were reviewed for the variables of age, gender, race, length of hospital stay, type of sickle hemoglobinopathy, hemoglobin level, pulmonary function test results, and history of asthma. Children diagnosed with asthma that occurred after the ACS episode were not included. Records from a total of 60 children were included in the study.

Study participant data:

- Ninety-two percent of the children were diagnosed with Hgb SS.
- Five percent of the children were diagnosed with Hgb SC.
- Three percent of the children were diagnosed with Hgb SB thalassemia.
- The vast majority (58) of the children were of African American descent; two were described as being of Hispanic descent.

- The children's ages ranged from 1.5 to 17 years, with a mean age of 8.4 years.
- Fifty-five percent of the participants were females.
- The children's hemoglobin levels ranged from 4.4 to 12.1 g/dL, with a mean of 7.7 g/dL.
- Fifty-three percent of the children with SCD had a diagnosis of asthma or abnormal pulmonary function tests before the diagnosis of ACS.
- Children with a previous diagnosis of asthma had a mean Hgb of 7.7 g/dL.
- Children with no prior diagnosis of asthma had a mean Hgb of 7.6 g/dL.
- The mean length of hospital stay for children admitted with ACS with a prior diagnosis of asthma was 6.4 days; for children with no prior diagnosis of asthma, it was 8.6 days.

There were no significant differences in the children's age, gender, Hgb levels, or length of stay. There was no significance difference between male and female children with SCD with or without a prior diagnosis of asthma before the development of ACS.

1. What might be considered as limitations to this study?
2. How is this information useful to clinical nursing practice?

See Suggested Responses for Moving Toward Evidence-Based Practice on the Electronic Study Guide or DavisPlus.

Introduction

A hematological disorder in a child can have various causes, including injury, nutritional deficit, genetic disorder, infection, congenital problem, or any number of blood-related conditions. A thorough history and physical examination are essential in the diagnosis and care of the child with a hematological disorder, as the condition can be insidious in nature. A variety of tests can be performed to determine the functional status of the hematological system and proper care can then be provided for the child. To understand the disorders affecting children that involve the hematological system, it is imperative to comprehend the normal function of the blood and formed elements.

A & P review Hematopoietic System

Blood is composed of two parts: the fluid portion called plasma and the cellular portion. The solutes in the plasma include albumin, electrolytes, proteins, clotting factors, fibrinogen, globulins, and circulating antibodies.

The cellular portion consists of the formed elements (red blood cells [RBCs], white blood cells [WBCs], and platelets).

The primary function of the RBCs (erythrocytes) is to transport hemoglobin that carries oxygen from the lungs to the tissues. The life span of a normal RBC is approximately 120 days (Hermiston & Mentzer, 2002).

Leukocytes (WBCs) are mobile units of the body's protective system. Most leukocytes migrate to areas of serious inflammation and provide a rapid defense against any foreign agent. WBCs are also important in immune system mediation. The life span of a leukocyte is specific to the cell type.

Megakaryocytes are cells that give rise to platelets. Platelets are small fragments of megakaryocytes. Platelets are the smallest of all formed blood elements and are not really cells because they do not possess a cellular structure. The primary function of platelets is hemostasis and vascular repair after injury to a vessel wall. Platelets aggregate to form a plug. Their life span is approximately 7–10 days (Nathan, Orkin, Ginsburg, & Look, 2003). Almost a third of all circulatory platelets can be found normally in the spleen. In normal circumstances, platelets are removed by the liver and spleen in 10 days if not utilized in a clotting reaction (Turgeon, 2005). ◆

Common Hematological Conditions

Several common hematological conditions can occur in children. Some of these are acute in nature and with proper care can be easily managed. Others can be life-threatening or cause a chronic illness that can permanently impact the lifestyle of the child and his or her family. It is essential that the nurse understand the necessary care and important teaching aspects associated with these conditions.

ANEMIA

One of the most common hematological conditions of infancy and childhood is anemia (a decrease in the number of red blood cells [RBCs]). The reduction in circulating RBCs, decreases the oxygen-carrying capacity of the blood. For the majority of patients, anemia is not a disease, but rather a symptom of other diseases.

 Nursing Insight— *Causes of anemia*

- Decreased production of RBCs such as in bone marrow failure and myelodysplastic syndromes
- Increased destruction of RBCs such as sickle cell anemia or hereditary spherocytosis
- Acute or chronic blood loss
  Note: It is important to identify the cause of anemia so that the treatment plan can be tailored to the child's specific needs.

Signs and Symptoms

Anemia may be insidious and the child may be asymptomatic due to compensatory mechanisms. The child with mild anemia may be asymptomatic and not diagnosed until blood work is obtained. The initial signs of anemia vary: fatigue, shortness of breath, headache, difficulty concentrating, dizziness, and pale skin. The child with moderate to severe anemia will have overt signs and symptoms: irritability, fatigue, delayed motor development, tachycardia, shortness of breath, decreased activity level, pale skin, listlessness, systolic heart murmur, hepatomegaly, and/or congestive heart failure (Nathan et al., 2003).

 clinical alert

Screening guidelines

According to the recommendations in the American Academy of Pediatrics screening guidelines, hemoglobin and hematocrit should be evaluated once during infancy (6–9 months of age), early childhood (1–5 years of age), late childhood (5–12 years of age), and adolescence (14–20 years of age). This screening schedule should identify children who may benefit from treatment for anemia.

Diagnosis

For the child diagnosed with anemia, a thorough history and physical examination are essential to establish a possible etiology. Complete blood count (CBC) and reticulocyte count are obtained to evaluate the hemoglobin and hematocrit. Anemia exists when the hemoglobin content is less than required to meet the oxygen demands of the body.

 Nursing Insight— *Hemoglobin and hematocrit*

Hemoglobin is the iron-containing pigment of the RBC that carries oxygen from the lungs to the tissues. The hemoglobin level is measured as the amount of hemoglobin per deciliter of whole blood. The average hemoglobin in the blood varies based on the age and gender of the individual.

Normal hemoglobin (Hgb) (g/dL) lab values for children are:
   Newborn: 12.7–18.6
   2 Months: 9.0–14.0
   2 Years: 10.5–12.7
   6–12 Years: 11.2–14.8
   12–18 Years: 10.7–15.7

The hematocrit is the percent of whole blood that is composed of RBCs. The hematocrit measures both the number and size of the RBCs and is approximately three times greater than the hemoglobin value. The hematocrit indirectly measures the hemoglobin. The average hematocrit value is between 35% and 45% (Gilbert-Barness & Barness, 2003).

A child's CBC measures the formed elements in the blood, including RBCs, WBCs, and platelets, providing valuable information with regard to illnesses and disease processes that may be occurring. In addition to the quantitative analysis, the blood cells of the CBC can also be evaluated for shape, size, and color.

 Labs: Blood Values According to Age

The nurse needs to be knowledgeable about the age-specific norms for the child. Based on the child's age, there may be variations in expected ranges (Tables 33-1, 33-2, and 33-3). It is unacceptable to use generic adult values.

Labs: Complete Blood Count, Reticulocyte, and Peripheral Smear Lab Values for Children

When evaluating the presence of anemia, initial laboratory tests should include complete blood count (CBC) and a reticulocyte count. The CBC includes hemoglobin, hematocrit, RBC indices, platelet count, WBC count with a differential, and a peripheral smear to examine the morphology of the RBCs. For the patient with suspected anemia, the peripheral blood smear is imperative to confirm the appropriate diagnosis (Gilbert-Barness & Barness, 2003).

Nursing Care

Nursing care for a child with anemia varies based on the etiology. To effectively replenish the RBCs, the underlying cause must be identified. For children with mild anemia, the nurse can provide supportive care through diet or

Table 33-1 Lab Blood Values According to Age

Age/Blood Component	Newborn	2 Months	2 Years	6–12 Years	12–18 Years	Comments
Red blood cells (RBCs)	4.1–5.74	2.7–4.9	3.9–5.03	4.93–5.3	3.7–5.5	Measure of bone marrow function
Hemoglobin (Hgb) (g/dL)	12.7–18.6	9.0–14.0	10.5–12.7	11.2–14.8	10.7–15.7	Amount of hemoglobin/dL of whole blood
Hematocrit (Hct) (%)	37.4–56.1	28.0–42.0	31.7–37.7	34.0–43.9	33.0–46.2	Percentage of packed RBC to whole blood, approximately three times the Hgb content
White blood cells (WBCs)	6.8–14.3	5.0–19.5	5.3–11.5	4.5–10.1	4.4–10.2	Differential count is more important than the total number of WBCs
Platelets (x 10^3/mm^3 [μl])	164–586	164–586	206–459	189–403	175–345	Platelets contribute to blood clotting

Table 33-2 Normal White Blood Cell Differential Count According to Age

Age/White Blood Cell Component	Function	Newborn	2 Months	2 Years	6–12 Years	12–18 Years
Neutrophils (%)	Phagocytosis	19–49	15–35	13–33	32–54	34–64
Eosinophils (%)	Allergic reactions	0–4	0–3	0–3	0–3	0–3
Basophils (%)	Inflammatory reactions	0–1	0–1	0	0–1	0–1
Lymphocytes (%) (B cells and T cells)	Humoral immunity (B cell) and cellular immunity (T cell)	38–46	42–72	46–76	27–57	25–45
Monocytes (%) (macrophages)	Phagocytosis and antigen processing	0–9	0–6	0–5	0–5	0–5

Table 33-3 Red Cell Lab Values for Children

Test	Reference Range	Comments
Mean corpuscular volume (MCV)	79–95 μm^3	Average size of a single RBC, expressed as cubic microns (μm^3)
Mean corpuscular hemoglobin (MCH)	25–33 pg/cell	Average weight of the Hgb within a RBC, expressed in picograms (pg)
Mean cell hemoglobin concentration (MCHC)	31%–37% Hgb [g]/dl RBC	Average concentration of Hgb in each RBC
Reticulocyte count	0.5%–1.5%	Measure of the production of mature RBCs by the bone marrow
Peripheral smear	Size, shape and structure of the RBCs, as well as an estimate of the amount of Hgb in the RBCs	Can indicate variations in size and shape of RBCs, microcytic, macrocytic, or normocytic

vitamin supplement. Children with moderate to severe anemia may need a RBC transfusion to restore blood volume. For specific types of anemia such as decreased production of RBCs, the nurse can administer hematopoietic growth factors that may prove beneficial in decreasing the need for blood transfusions.

Proper instructions from the nurse are necessary for children with anemia. The teaching required for a child with a chronic illness is more extensive than for the child who has an acute self-limiting episode of anemia. The family must be made aware of the clinical signs and symptoms that may indicate anemia. The nurse can teach the family that alterations in daily activities may be necessary such as quiet play, allowing for periods of rest, and a diet high in iron. The child with anemia may also need to have laboratory tests and medical exams periodically to evaluate the status of the anemia.

Nursing Insight— *Evaluating a CBC*

Blood Elements	Increase	Decrease
RBC (Hgb/Hct)	Polycythemia	Anemia
WBC	Leukocytosis	Leukopenia
Platelets	Thrombocytosis	Thrombocytopenia

IRON-DEFICIENCY ANEMIA

The most prevalent nutritional disorder worldwide is iron-deficiency anemia. Iron-deficiency anemia is defined as a microcytic, hypochromic anemia caused by an inadequate supply of iron (Nathan et al., 2003). Iron is essential for the production of hemoglobin. When iron stores are inadequate, the production of hemoglobin is diminished. As a result of the decrease in hemoglobin, there is a decreased oxygen-carrying capacity of the blood. Iron-deficiency anemia is more common in infants. Premature infants are at high risk due to their decreased fetal iron supply (Nathan et al., 2003). Approximately 10% to 20% of infants and toddlers have some type of iron-deficiency anemia, with a greater incidence in children at or below poverty level.

 Across Care Settings: Women Infants and Children (WIC) program

Since the implementation of the Women Infants and Children (WIC) program, the incidence of iron-deficiency anemia has decreased. WIC serves 45% of all infants born in the United States.

The target populations for WIC participants who need nutritional counseling are low-income women with nutritionally at-risk children:

- Pregnant women (through pregnancy and up to 6 weeks after birth or after pregnancy ends)
- Breastfeeding women (up to infant's 1st birthday)
- Non-breastfeeding postpartum women (up to 6 months after the birth of an infant or after pregnancy ends)
- Infants (up to 1st birthday) and children up to their 5th birthday

It is important for the nurse to recognize the presence of iron-deficiency anemia. Because it has been associated with abnormal infant behavior, growth, and development, it needs to be corrected. Adolescents are also vulnerable to iron-deficiency anemia because of rapid growth and sometimes poor eating habits. The pathophysiology of iron-deficiency anemia can be related to various factors such as a decreased supply of iron, impaired absorption of iron, increased demand for iron, or blood loss (Box 33-1).

Signs and Symptoms

The nurse understands that the signs and symptoms of iron-deficiency anemia vary with the severity of the disorder. If a child has a mild iron-deficiency anemia, he or she may be asymptomatic. This deficiency may not be apparent until laboratory tests are performed (decreased hemoglobin/hematocrit). For children with moderate to severe iron-deficiency anemia, clinical manifestations that may be present include irritability, fatigue, delayed motor

---

Box 33-1 Common Causes of Iron-Deficiency Anemia

DECREASED IRON SUPPLY

Inadequate iron supply at birth

Nutrition

- Deficient iron intake
- Excessive milk
- Limited solid foods
- Poor eating habits, vegetarian diet, increased fast foods

INCREASED IRON DEMANDS

Growth

- Low birth weight, twins or multiple births
- Prematurity/infants
- Adolescents
- Pregnancy
- Cyanotic congenital heart diseases (i.e., tetralogy of Fallot)

BLOOD LOSS

Acute

Chronic

Parasite infection

GI tract is the most common site

INABILITY TO FORM HEMOGLOBIN

Lack of vitamin B_{12} (pernicious anemia)

Folic acid deficiency

IMPAIRED ABSORPTION

Presence of iron inhibitors

- Phytates, phosphates, or oxalates
- Gastric alkalinity
- Malabsorption syndrome (celiac disease, severe prolonged diarrhea, postgastrectomy, inflammatory bowel disease)

---

development, tachycardia, shortness of breath, decreased activity level, pale, conjunctival pallor, listless, systolic heart murmur, hepatomegaly, and congestive heart failure. Pica, the eating of items of non-nutritive value such as starch, clay, ice, or paper (Nathan et al., 2003), may also be associated with iron-deficiency anemia. Iron deficiency, alone or with anemia, may result in impairment of cognitive skills that may not be reversible.

Diagnosis

Diagnosis of iron-deficiency anemia is based on patient history and physical examination findings. Laboratory tests that are frequently performed include those that quantify or describe hemoglobin, iron concentration, and morphological changes in the RBC.

Nursing Care

The nurse understands that early identification and recognition of iron-deficiency anemia is essential. The nurse can stress to the parents that the primary goal of iron deficiency anemia is prevention. Many instances of iron-deficiency anemia can be avoided with the appropriate food selections. The nurse or dietitian can provide nutritional counseling and assist with obtaining recommended iron-fortified formula and cereal.

"What to say" — *Nutritional counseling*

- "Feed your infant breast milk or commercial infant formula recommended for the first 12 months of life."

- "Be sure to use iron-fortified cereal from 6 to 12 months of age."

- "Do not feed your infant cow's milk before 12 months of age. After 12 months of age limit the amount of cow's milk to 18 to 24 ounces per day."

- "Offering solids before bottle once solids are introduced helps prevent iron deficiency."

- "To meet recommended dietary allowances and to avoid iron-deficiency anemia, it is important for adolescents on a vegetarian diet or weight reduction diet to understand proper dietary alternatives."

- "Red meats, beans, whole grains, nuts, and iron-fortified cereals are good sources of iron."

The nurse can teach the parents how to administer oral iron supplements. The recommended dosage of elemental iron is 3 mg/kg per day based on body weight in one to two divided doses. The severity of the anemia dictates the monitoring frequency of laboratory testing and follow-up with the health care provider. Several days after initiating iron replacement therapy, the family can expect a rise in the reticulocyte count, which is an indicator of RBC production. Adequate iron replacement therapy should result in a peak reticulocyte count in 7 to 10 days (Gilbert-Barness & Barness, 2003). It is important for the nurse to communicate to the parents that this time frame is a good opportunity for the child to return to the health care provider for follow-up.

 critical nursing action Education About Oral Iron

Educating parents on the proper administration of oral iron is a vital nursing responsibility. The iron supplement needs to be taken between meals because absorption is improved in an acidic environment. Administering this medication with a glass of orange juice may also enhance absorption. Iron supplements should not be taken with tea because it may adversely affect the absorption process.

- Inform parents that liquid iron preparations may stain teeth so it is important to administer the medication with a dropper or drink it through a straw. Encourage the child to rinse his or her mouth after taking this liquid medication.
- Make parents aware that iron can be constipating and it is necessary to increase the fiber and water intake to prevent this possible complication.
- Possible side effects of iron therapy include gastric upset, nausea, vomiting, and constipation. Black tarry stools are a common finding and are normal for children taking iron supplements. Encourage parents to keep no more than a 1-month supply in the home and to store it out of reach of small children because ingestion of excessive quantities may be toxic or even fatal.

 case study Iron-Deficiency Anemia

Johnny is a 7-month-old infant visiting the Head Start clinic for a check-up. During the child's initial history, the 18-year-old mother reports that she missed her last few appointments to the clinic because she does not have any transportation. The nursing assessment reveals that the infant is pale and listless. Johnny's weight is plotted at 110% on the growth chart. The mother reports that Johnny "drinks lots of milk." "I give him milk whenever he cries." She also informs you that she has had "no money for formula but that he likes whole milk just as well." After a blood draw the nurse notes that his laboratory results are: hemoglobin = 8.8 hematocrit, 26.3. Johnny's vital signs include: axillary temperature, 97.6°F (36.4°C); heart rate, 166 beats per minute; respiratory rate, 32 breaths per minute; blood pressure, 92/45.

critical thinking questions

1. From a nursing perspective what is your primary concern?

2. What community resource can you suggest to Johnny's mother?

◆ See Suggested Answers to Case Studies in text on the Electronic Study Guide or DavisPlus.

 clinical alert

An overweight child diagnosed with iron-deficiency anemia

The clinic nurse can be vigilant for overweight infants who may have iron-deficiency anemia. While most infants diagnosed with iron-deficiency anemia are underweight, do not be misled. Infants who are overweight may also have this disorder. Many of these infants are overweight because of excessive milk ingestion, known as "milk baby." These infants are chunky, pale, and have a "porcelain-like" appearance. Other clinical features of these "milk babies" include poor muscle development and they are susceptible to infections. It is essential to obtain a comprehensive nutritional history from the parents.

EPISTAXIS

Epistaxis (nosebleeds) are common in children. Most cases are clinically benign events. The greatest concern occurs when family members or caretakers become upset at the site of blood, which may appear excessive even from a small nosebleed. Nosebleeds are related to the increased vascularity of nasal mucosa.

Signs and Symptoms

The septum of the child's nose is especially vulnerable to bleeding as a result of direct trauma, foreign body insertion, nasal gastric tube insertion, nasal intubation, nose picking, violent sneezing, inhaled drug use (e.g., cocaine) and related effects (nasal crusting), and chronic infections of the nasal tissue. Other external factors or disease states such as alterations in platelet count, hypertension, or prolonged use of acetylsalicylic acid (Children's Aspirin) or aspirin-containing products may precipitate epistaxis.

Diagnosis

To determine the cause of bleeding from the nares, the nurse can perform a thorough history and physical. The majority of the time, bleeding is an independent occurrence. If bleeding is controlled and infrequent, the nurse can identify the causative factor. The nurse should ask the parents about nose picking or foreign body aspiration. In children with reoccurring and prolonged epistaxis, a further diagnostic workup is warranted.

Nursing Care

Nursing care for a child with epistaxis focuses mainly on prevention. The nurse can tell children not to pick the nose, vigorously blow the nose, or engage in strenuous activity that is known to cause a nosebleed. Teach children to sneeze with the mouth open and gently blow the nose if needed. Inform parents to avoid giving the child acetylsalicylic acid (Children's Aspirin) or nonsteroidal anti-inflammatory drugs (NSAIDs). Cool mist humidification may also be recommended as a preventive measure. When a nosebleed occurs, the nurse can provide simple first aid measures that may assist in stopping the bleeding (Fig. 33-1).

 critical nursing action Controlling Epistaxis (Nosebleeds)

Don gloves and place the child in a sitting position, leaning forward. Apply direct pressure to the anterior nasal septum for 10–15 minutes. Remind the child to breathe through the mouth, so he or she does not become anxious. Applying ice to the nose area is beneficial. If a large amount of blood loss occurs, the nurse must monitor vital signs. In cases with severe nose bleeding that persists beyond 10–15 minutes, nasal packing may be required, as well as topical epinephrine. When an infection is present, antibiotics may be ordered (Kucik & Clenney, 2005). It is essential that the nurse keep the child and family quiet and calm by providing support and reassurance. It is important that families are able to demonstrate first aid measures necessary to control an occurrence of epistaxis.

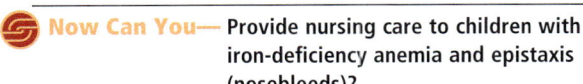 **Labs:** Epistaxis Diagnostic Workup

Laboratory tests can potentially diagnose an underlying bleeding disorder. Recommended blood tests include a CBC with differential, prothrombin time, partial thromboplastin time, and coagulation profile, if a bleeding disorder is suspected (Table 33-4).

Now Can You— **Provide nursing care to children with iron-deficiency anemia and epistaxis (nosebleeds)?**

1. Discuss the cause of iron-deficiency anemia?
2. List nursing interventions for children experiencing iron-deficiency anemia?
3. Discuss the cause of epistaxis (nosebleeds)?
4. List nursing interventions for children experiencing epistaxis (nosebleeds)?

Figure 33-1 When a nosebleed occurs, the nurse can provide simple first aid measures that may assist in stopping the bleeding.

SICKLE CELL DISEASE

One of the most common genetic hematological conditions present in children is sickle cell disease (SCD). This disorder is transmitted via an autosomal recessive pattern of inheritance. Both parents of the child must have the sickle cell gene in order for the child to have sickle cell disease (Fig. 33-2).

 Ethnocultural Considerations— Sickle cell disease

Approximately 8% of the African American population in the United States is a carrier of sickle cell trait (Turgeon, 2005). Children affected by this condition are usually of African American or Mediterranean descent. Although rare, this genetic disorder may be seen in other populations such as Hispanic, Caucasians, and Italians due to the intermarriages that have occurred throughout the world.

Patients with sickle cell *trait* have the heterozygous form of the disease. They usually are asymptomatic since they possess one sickle and one normal gene. The child with trait

Test	Range	Significance
Prothrombin time (PT)	11–14 seconds	Measures the extrinsic pathway for bleeding, requires fibrinogen, prothrombin, and factors V, VII, and X. Prolonged times may indicate deficiencies of vitamin K liver factors, malabsorption, and liver disease.
Partial thromboplastin time (PTT)	25–38 seconds	Measures the intrinsic pathway for bleeding, requires factors V, VIII, IX, X, XI, and XII and fibrinogen and prothrombin. Prolonged times may indicate a bleeding disorder.

Table 33-4 Laboratory Tests to Diagnosis Bleeding Disorder

Source: Hillman, R.S., Ault, K.A., & Rinder, H.M. (2005). *Hematology in clinical practice: A guide to diagnosis and management*. New York: McGraw-Hill.

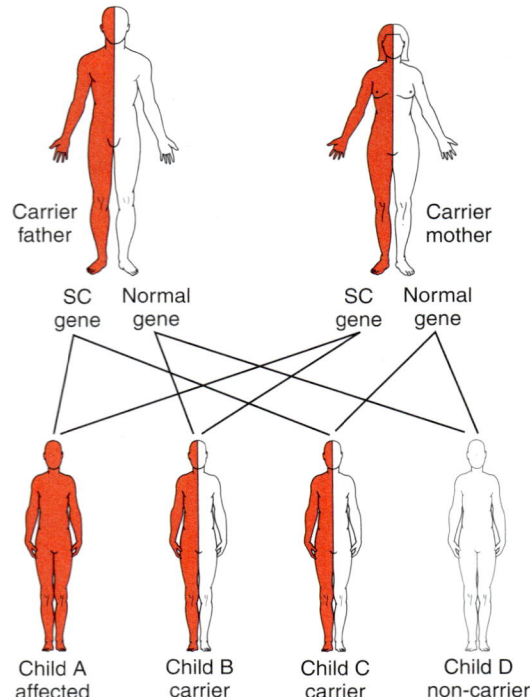

Carrier father

Carrier mother

SC gene   Normal gene

SC gene   Normal gene

Child A affected

Child B carrier

Child C carrier

Child D non-carrier

Figure 33-2 Pattern of inheritance of sickle cell disease.

may be affected only in certain situations such as high altitudes, periods of extreme stress such as dehydration, and females later in life during pregnancy. Children with sickle cell *disease*, have the homozygous form of the disorder, indicating that both genes are abnormal (Turgeon, 2005).

 Nursing Insight— *Inheritance*

Consistent with the genetic pattern of inheritance, hemoglobin genes come from both parents. If one parent has sickle cell disease and the other parent does not, the child has only the sickle cell trait. If one parent has sickle cell disease and the other has sickle cell trait, there is a 50% probability (1 out of 2) that the child will have either the sickle cell disease or the sickle cell trait. When both parents have sickle cell trait, they have a 25% probability (1 out of 4) of having a child with sickle cell disease or who will become a carrier of the disease.

The primary defect in this type of genetic disease is that the globin chain in normal hemoglobin A (HbA) is partially or completely replaced by hemoglobin S (HbS). Hemoglobin S has a substitution of the amino acid valine for glutamine which is more sensitive to the changes in the oxygen concentration in the blood. When a patient has a large amount of hemoglobin S and a decrease in oxygen levels, these abnormal hemoglobins clump together within the cell and change the shape from donut-like to a sickled shape (Fixler & Styles, 2002) (Fig. 33-3). The two most significant pathophysiological features of this disease include tissue ischemia as a result of the occlusions and the inherited fragility of the sickled cells. Once RBCs sickle, they are more fragile and easily destroyed. The surfaces of these sickled cells are also sticky and adhere to the blood

vessel walls. The shape of the sickled cell does not promote good oxygenation or movement throughout the circulatory system and hence clinical symptomatology results. If the RBCs cannot circulate through the vascular system and there are occlusions, hypoxemia may result that could lead to ischemia, infarcts, and possible tissue death (Gilbert-Barness & Barness, 2003). The average life span of a sickled RBC is approximate 30 to 45 days (Nathan et al., 2003). Owing to the shortened life span of the RBCs, children with sickle cell disease have an increased amount of hemolysis, as evidenced by their chronic anemia.

Signs and Symptoms

Because sickle cell disease is a blood disorder, all organs of the body may be affected. The signs and symptoms that may be evident in a child with sickle cell anemia are largely the result of the vaso-occlusion of the blood vessels from the sickled red blood cells and hemolysis. Other symptoms seen in children with sickle cell disease may include weakness, pallor, fatigue, tissue hypoxia, and jaundice as result of RBC hemolysis.

The most common presenting clinical manifestation is the child with pain (vaso-occlusive crisis). The pain can present anywhere in the body and is the result of the occlusion of the blood vessels.

Diagnosis

Accurate assessment and diagnosis are essential for appropriate treatment. Newborn screening is a standard in all 50 states. Infants can be identified early to elicit the appropriate diagnosis. For toddlers and preschool children who present to the health care provider with nonspecific symptoms with the presence of anemia, a thorough history and physical must be performed. If the etiology of the anemia is undetermined, a screening for sickle cell disease may be indicated. The definitive test for diagnosis of sickle cell disease or trait is hemoglobin electrophoresis (Gilbert-Barness & Barness, 2003). This assay separates the various types of hemoglobin and quantifies the percentage of various hemoglobins present. Laboratory tests including a CBC and reticulocyte count are necessary. Expected laboratory findings for sickle cell disease are decreased hemoglobin and hematocrit and an elevated reticulocyte count.

Figure 33-3 In sickle cell disease, the shape of the cell changes from a donut shape to a sickled shape.

diagnostic tools Further Testing for Infants Suspected of Having Sickle Cell Disease

If sickle cell disease is suspected, infants require further testing, such as a hemoglobin electrophoresis (Fixler & Styles, 2002). A hemoglobin electrophoresis is a more specific blood test that identifies sickle cell disease versus sickle cell trait in a child (Gilbert-Barness & Barness, 2003).

Nursing Care

The most important nursing care measure in the treatment of sickle cell disease is the early identification and treatment of hypoxic episodes. The nurse can provide supportive and specific care based on the type of crisis present. Nursing care should focus on encouraging rest, hydration, pain control, and adequate oxygenation. When providing nursing care to patients with suspected sickle cell crisis, attempts should be made to coordinate nursing care to allow adequate rest periods and to minimize unnecessary interruptions. Nursing care always includes adequate hydration (oral or intravenous). The fluid requirement recommendations are one and a half times above the child's normal calculated requirements. The nurse understands that adequate hydration promotes dilution and diminishes the possibility of hypoxic episodes. In addition to hydration, pain control is essential to adequately treat painful crisis. Pain control can be pharmacological or nonpharmacological. A combination of both is preferred. A complete nursing history should be obtained to determine what pain measures have worked in the past. Another critical assessment factor is monitoring respiratory status and oxygenation of sickle cell patients. The child with sickle cell crisis may be at risk for an acute pulmonary event that may be a result of the disease itself or the use of opiates. A complete respiratory assessment should include signs and symptoms of respiratory distress, including auscultation of lung sounds to detect decreased and abnormal breath sounds, respiratory effort and quality, continuous monitoring of oxygen saturations, color and perfusion, and any necessary laboratory or radiographic studies. If abnormal findings are present, the nurse must immediately inform the medical team so treatment can begin. For example, if the patient's oxygen saturation consistently is less than 90% on room air, supplemental oxygen may be indicated. The nurse must remember that pneumonia and pulmonary infarcts occur more often in this patient population.

 Complementary Care: *Nonpharmacological pain interventions*

In addition to administering medications for pain control, the use of nonpharmacological interventions has proven to be beneficial for many patients experiencing painful episodes from a sickle cell crisis. This may include distraction, guided imagery, relaxation techniques, music therapy, comfort care, cutaneous stimulation, and play therapy. If available at your institution, a child life specialist or other interdisciplinary team member can be consulted to assist in providing nonpharmacological interventions.

 clinical alert

When a child is asplenic

A child with a temperature greater than 101.5°F (38.6°C) requires immediate medical attention, as most children with sickle cell disease are "functionally asplenic". When a child is asplenic, he or she does not have the ability to filter certain encapsulated bacteria. This allows the bacteria to multiply within the bloodstream, causing a low-grade bacterial infection or serious sepsis. Children with sickle cell disease generally are asplenic by the age of 3–5 years. The major cause of death in children with sickle cell disease who are less than 5 years old is overwhelming infection due to *Streptococcus pneumoniae, Haemophilus influenzae* type b, and *Neisseria meningitidis* (Nathan et al., 2003). If a child with sickle cell disease has a fever, immediate treatment involves blood cultures and the implementation of parenteral broad-spectrum antibiotics. Children with sickle cell disease often receive prophylactic oral penicillin at home to prevent overwhelming sepsis. The nurse knows that this critical information is necessary for parents to ensure the child receives the pneumococcal and *H. influenzae* type B vaccine and other routine vaccinations.

For the family that seeks medical attention for the child with mild pain, the initial management consists of oral pain medication at home. Oral pain medication may consist of acetaminophen (Children's Tylenol), ibuprofen (Children's Advil), or acetaminophen with codeine (Children's Tylenol-Codeine) for mild to moderate pain. If the child continues to have pain, hospitalization may be required. For the hospitalized child with vaso-occlusive crisis, opioids such as immediate and sustained release morphine (Duramorph), oxycodone (OxyContin), hydromorphone (Dilaudid), or methadone (Methadol) may be administered around the clock. Morphine (Duramorph) is often considered the drug of choice. Morphine (Duramorph) may be administered around the clock or by patient-controlled analgesia (PCA) (Fixler & Styles, 2002). PCA is an appropriate method of pain management for children who are able to manage their own pain relief. Another medication that may be used for painful crises and does not have the common side effects of the opiate drugs is ketorolac (Toradol). Toradol is a parenteral anti-inflammatory drug that has been found to be effective in reducing pain associated with a vaso-occlusive crisis. The recommended duration of ketorolac should not exceed 5 days owing to the increased risk of gastritis and gastrointestinal bleeding.

 assessment tools Pain Assessment

Pain assessment must be documented for all patients. The use of a standardized pain assessment tool provides a more accurate assessment data. A developmentally appropriate pain assessment tool also must be used for all patients in health care settings. Pain assessment tools should be used to assess the pain on admission, reassess pain, and determine treatment effectiveness. The Joint Commission national patient safety goals recommended pain assessment as the 5th vital sign (for developmentally appropriate pain assessment tools see Chapter 21).

Children who have experienced numerous hospitalizations, cerebral vascular accident (CVA), or acute chest syndromes may be candidates for hypertransfusion therapy. These patients receive blood transfusions every 3 to 4 weeks to increase their amount of hemoglobin A. This

medication: Toradol (Ketorolac)

Toradol (tor-ah-dal)

Generic name: Ketorolac (Kee-**toe**-role-ak)

Pregnancy Category: C (D if used in the 3rd trimester)

Indications: Short term (<5 days) management of moderate to severe pain, including postoperative pain.

Actions: Inhibits prostaglandin synthesis by decreasing activity of the enzyme cyclooxygenase, which results in a decrease of prostaglandin precursors.
THERAPEUTIC EFFECTS: pain relief

Pharmacokinetics:
ORAL: Well absorbed; 100%
IM/IV: Rapid and complete

Contraindications and Precautions:
Contraindicated in: Hypersensitivity to Toradol, acetylsalicylic acid (Children's Aspirin), or other NSAIDs; patients with peptic ulcer disease or anyone with bleeding tendencies

Adverse Reactions and Side Effects: Dizziness, headache, rash, diarrhea, GI pain, bleeding, prolonged bleeding times, anaphylaxis, hypersensitivity reactions.

Route and Dosage: Ketorolac injection is approved for use in pediatric patients only as a single I.M. or I.V. dose in children 2–16 years of age; the use of ketorolac injection in children <2 years of age, the use of multiple doses of the injection in children <16 years of age, and the use of the tablets in children <16 years of age are outside of the manufacturer's recommendations; ophthalmic solutions are approved for use in children ≥3 years of age.
SINGLE-DOSE TREATMENT: Manufacturer's recommendations:
I.M.: 1 mg/kg as a single dose; maximum dose: 30 mg
I.V.: 0.5 mg/kg as a single dose; maximum dose: 15 mg

Nursing Implications:
Instruct the patient and parents on medication administration.
Do not exceed 5 days of total use.
May cause drowsiness and impair ability to perform activities requiring mental alertness.
Additional Information: 30 mg of Toradol (Ketorolac) provides analgesia comparable to 12 mg of morphine or 100 mg of meperidine.

Data from Deglin, J.H., & Vallerand, A.H. (2009). *Davis's drug guide for nurses* (11th ed.). Philadelphia: F.A. Davis.

treatment regimen is not without potential risks, which may include the transmission of various infectious diseases, an acute transfusion reaction, or iron overload from multiple blood transfusions. Chelation therapy must be initiated to prevent organ damage from iron accumulation (Fixler & Styles, 2002). An experimental treatment modality for sickle cell patients with numerous complications is a bone marrow transplant.

 Across Care Settings: **Education about sickle cell disease**

Children and families affected by sickle cell disease must learn to cope with a lifelong chronic illness. Families must be knowledgeable of the signs and symptoms of sickle cell crisis so they can report them to their primary health care provider. The community-based nurse can educate the family about the goals of ongoing care including the prevention of complications associated with infections, hypoxemia, and vaso-occlusive crisis. Ensure that parents understand that strenuous activities that

may precipitate hypoxia should be avoided. Nurses must teach parents how to avoid a sickle cell crisis by providing rest and adequate hydration. Patients with sickle cell disease are on prophylactic penicillin to prevent overwhelming sepsis and supplemental folic acid to assist with red blood cell production. Adherence to these medications is critical in preventing complications associated with this disease. The nurse can inform the parents about genetic screening and counseling.

In the event a patient experiences a mild sickle cell crisis at home, instruct him or her to stop what he or she is doing, rest, drink fluids, and take the prescribed pain medication. If improvement is not observed, notify the physician and anticipate the need for the patient to see a health care provider or to go to the nearest emergency facility for additional treatment.

Complications related to occlusion of blood vessels include splenic sequestration, functional asplenia, avascular necrosis of the femoral head, leg ulcers, hand–foot syndrome (dactylitis), and chronic organ damage. Additional complications secondary to hemolysis include anemia, cholelithiasis (gallstones), jaundice, retarded growth, and sexual maturation. The most severe complications are the occurrence of acute chest syndrome, priapism (painful and continuous erection of the penis), splenic sequestration (separation), and a CVA. These conditions are medical emergencies and treatment must be obtained immediately to prevent permanent disability or a life-threatening event (Fixler & Styles, 2002).

 nursing diagnoses Sickle Cell Disease

- Knowledge Deficit related to home care
- Pain related to tissue hypoxia secondary to vaso-occlusive crisis
- Alteration in Tissue Perfusion related to anemia
- Activity Intolerance related to anemia
- Risk for Injury related to anemia
- Altered Family Process related to hospitalization
- Ineffective Coping related to chronic illness
- Fluid Volume Deficit related to decreased fluid intake and the kidney's ability to concentrate urine
- Risk for Infection related to limited splenic filtering abilities

 case study Sickle Cell Disease

Sammy is a 16-year-old boy with a history of sickle cell disease. He also has a history of numerous admissions to the hospital for pain crisis and blood transfusions. Today, in the emergency room, Sammy complains of pain in his chest and fever. During the physical assessment the nurse notes that his lungs are congested and that he has a moist cough. His oxygen saturation is 87% on room air. Sammy's vital signs are: heart rate, 121 beats per minute; respiratory rate, 28 breaths per minute; temperature, 101.5°F (38.6°C) orally; and blood pressure on the left upper extremity, 139/96.

critical thinking questions

1. In addition to respiratory status, what are the other concerns?

2. What are the priority nursing interventions?

3. What information will the nurse teach the parents?

◆ See Suggested Answers to Case Studies in text on the Electronic Study Guide or DavisPlus.

THALASSEMIA

Beta-thalassemia is the most common inherited genetic disorder in the world (Sapountzi-Krepia et al., 2006). This condition involves a deficiency in the globin chains of the hemoglobin. It is also classified according to which specific globin chains are affected. For example, if the beta-chain is affected, the child is diagnosed as having beta-thalassemia. Beta-thalassemia also has an autosomal recessive pattern of inheritance, which is similar to the pattern of inheritance as sickle cell disease. There are three forms of beta-thalassemia:

- Thalassemia minor (or thalassemia trait) is asymptomatic, or a mild microcytic anemia is present.
- Thalassemia intermedia has signs and symptoms similar to those of splenomegaly (enlarged spleen) with severe anemia.
- Thalassemia major (the most severe form), also known as Cooley's anemia (Turgeon, 2005). Cooley's anemia was first described by Dr. Thomas Cooley in 1925 (Nathan et al., 2003). Children with thalassemia major are usually dependent on blood products in order to maintain their hemoglobin, support growth, and prevent extramedullary hematopoiesis (the production of blood cell in tissues other than bone marrow).

In addition to beta-thalassemia, there is alpha–thalassemia, which occurs when the alpha-chain is affected. These patients are sometimes mistakenly diagnosed with iron-deficiency anemia. The severity of alpha-thalassemia is based on the number of alpha genes affected. If the patient has one or two missing alpha genes, he or she is most likely asymptomatic or has a mild anemia. A patient missing three alpha genes is classified as having Hgb H disease (Turgeon, 2005), which is characterized by an excess of beta-chains, resulting from minimal production of alpha-chains in the bone marrow and development of hemoglobin H as a result (Turgeon, 2005). Although hemoglobin H has oxygen-carrying capacity, its effectiveness is somewhat decreased and these patients often present with anemia and splenomegaly (enlarged spleen).

Signs and Symptoms

Children with beta-thalassemia who are symptomatic have an enlarged liver and spleen, mild jaundice, growth retardation, and a moderate to severe anemia. Due to the rapid destruction of red blood cells, the body attempts to increase more RBC production to compensate for the anemia that is present (Turgeon, 2005). When the hemoglobin level declines and severe anemia is present, bones that normally do not produce RBCs take on this function. As a result, there may be bony deformities such as frontal bossing or maxillary prominence from the excess cell production. These children also have an increased susceptibility to infection secondary to their nonfunctioning spleen.

Diagnosis

A thorough history and physical examination are necessary for diagnosis. Frequently performed laboratory tests include those that quantify or describe hemoglobin such as a CBC with red cell indices. Laboratory studies often reveal decreased hemoglobin and hematocrit, hypochromia, microcytosis, low mean corpuscular volume (MCV), and increased reticulocyte count (Turgeon, 2005).

Labs: Hemoglobin Electrophoresis

The nurse understands that hemoglobin electrophoresis can distinguish the type and severity of the thalassemia. Electrophoresis separates hemoglobin variants based on molecular charge. Hemoglobins are then described in order of relative abundance, detecting the homozygous and heterozygous forms of the disorder (Gilbert-Barness & Barness, 2003). Based on the results of the hemoglobin electrophoresis, a referral to a hematologist may be warranted for further evaluation.

Nursing Care

The goal of nursing care for children with beta-thalassemia major (Cooley's anemia) is to prevent hypoxia by providing blood transfusion therapy usually every 3–4 weeks for the child's lifetime (Lo & Singer, 2002). These children are dependent on transfusion therapy to maintain their hemoglobin, improve the quality of their lives, prevent extramedullary hematopoiesis, promote growth and development, and reduce infections.

Children with beta-thalassemia may experience numerous complications related to their disease and/or the treatment of their disease. As a result of chronic transfusion therapy, these children are at high risk for developing hemosiderosis.

clinical alert

Accumulation of iron (hemosiderosis)

As a result of the chronic blood transfusion therapy, in which each unit contains approximately 200 mg of iron, iron may accumulate in the body. The body does not have a mechanism to remove the iron. Excess iron is stored in the tissues and organs (hemosiderosis). Hemosiderosis must be treated to prevent toxic levels of iron in the body and possible death. Iron may be removed from the body by using drugs called chelating agents that bind with the iron and allow for excretion through the urine and stool. The main chelating agent is deferoxamine B (Desferal) (Lo & Singer, 2002). This drug is rapidly excreted in the urine. It must be administered intravenously or subcutaneously over 8–10 hours, usually at bedtime, at least 5 days a week. Most parents can be taught how to insert the butterfly catheter and administer the drug via an infusion pump at home without difficulties. The treatment process with deferoxamine B (Desferal) may become burdensome, expensive, and the issue of adherence is quite often a concern for health care professionals. Routine monitoring of iron levels is indicated for patients on chelation therapy to evaluate compliance and effectiveness of treatment. Patients at risk for hemosiderosis should be evaluated for long-term complications. Complications that may occur are a result of iron deposits that may damage vital organs causing hearing loss, diabetes, organ failure, and ultimately death.

Children with beta-thalassemia (Cooley's anemia) may be cured of their disorder with a bone marrow transplant (Martin, Foote, & Carson, 2004). Finding a suitable match is often difficult. Younger children often fare significantly better than older children who are treated with bone marrow transplant, primarily because their organs have not sustained substantial damage from the chronic transfusion therapy that may have caused iron overload.

Patients with this chronic disorder and their families require supportive care by the nurse. The nurse must address the importance of blood transfusion therapy and chelation to ensure compliance with the treatment regimen. The nurse teaches the family the appropriate technique for administration of the chelation therapy. Other nursing interventions include good hand washing because these children are often asplenic, which increases their susceptibility to infection. The nurse can alert parents to seek medical attention if the child develops a temperature of 101.5°F (38.6°C). If the child has a fever, the nurse can inform the parents that antibiotic prophylaxis may be indicated. Genetic counseling is needed to guide a family on making decisions about having additional children who possibly can be affected with this inherited disorder.

HEREDITARY SPHEROCYTOSIS

Hereditary spherocytosis (HS) is a hemolytic anemia acquired via autosomal-dominant inheritance and is caused by an abnormal RBC membrane. In most cases, there is a defect of the red cell skeletal protein called spectrin or it may also include the proteins involved in the attachment of the spectrin to the membrane (Hillman, Ault, & Rinder, 2005). The severity of the disease is directly contingent on the amount of the spectrin deficiency.

The cellular defect results in an abnormal RBC membrane. The malformed cell membrane has a smaller surface area in relationship to a normal RBC and an alteration in the actual shape of the cell from donut like to that of a spherocyte. The new shape makes it difficult for the RBCs to circulate through the body, particularly to the spleen, which leads to sequestered cells and early destruction (Turgeon, 2005). HS does not involve an abnormality of the hemoglobin. Rather it is an inherited disorder, which actually transforms the configuration of the red cell membrane (Turgeon, 2005).

Signs and Symptoms

Clinical manifestations may include hyperbilirubinemia, anemia, splenomegaly, and a negative Comb's test. In many cases, there is a strong family history. Some children can present later in life with anemia, jaundice, splenomegaly, or with an aplastic crisis often linked to a viral infection. The anemia may range from mild to severe based on the extent of compensation by the body.

Diagnosis

The diagnostic workup for HS includes a thorough history and physical examination. A CBC is frequently performed. Laboratory tests often reveal a low hemoglobin level between 7 and 10 grams per deciliter. The peripheral smear reveals small, dense, round, spherical red cells. The MCV is usually normal and there is increased red cell osmotic fragility, which is a measure of the lysis of spherocytes.

Nursing Care

The nurse understands that mild to moderate cases of HS include folic acid supplementation recommended at 1 mg/day. Children who have less than 80% of normal spectrin content are candidates for a splenectomy. The splenectomy eliminates the anemia and is reserved for children with moderate to severe cases of HS. After a splenectomy, the spherocytosis of the RBCs continues, although the cells no longer become sequestered in the spleen. The red cell survival improves to near normal.

 critical nursing action Pneumococcal and *Haemophilus influenzae* Type b (Hib) Vaccine

Children with hereditary spherocytosis (HS) should receive the pneumococcal and *Haemophilus influenzae* type b (Hib) vaccine before the splenectomy to prevent life-threatening bacterial infections. Children should also be given prophylactic penicillin to prevent fatal infections.

The nurse can provide supportive care measures for all children with HS. It is essential to teach parents of children with the milder form of HS about the folic acid supplementation regimen. The nurse must pay careful attention to infection control principles for a child who has undergone a splenectomy. The nurse needs to encourage parents to adhere to a prescribed antibiotic regimen. Promote good hand washing by all care providers because these children have increased susceptibility to infection. Instruct parents on the proper method for taking a temperature. Inform parents to seek medical attention if the child develops a temperature of 101.5°F (38.6°C). The nurse can remind parents that routine visits to their health care provider must be scheduled to evaluate blood counts and the need for immunizations. Provide support to the child and family to help them cope with this lifelong illness.

HEMOPHILIA

Hemophilia is a group of bleeding disorders caused by a congenital X-linked deficiency of either clotting factor VIII or IX (Sevier, 2005).

 ***Ethnocultural Considerations*—** The royal disease

Hemophilia has been present for centuries throughout the world. Often, members of the royal English family married into royalty of other countries. Hemophilia has been referred to as "the royal disease." The marriage of England's Queen Victoria and Prince Albert hallmarked the beginning of hemophilia in the British royal line. Queen Victoria, who had nine children, was a carrier of the hemophilia gene. As a result, hemophilia was transmitted to most of the royal houses of Europe (Stevens, 1999). A specific example of the royal disease is the case of the Czar and Czarina of Russia, Nicholas II and his wife, Alexandra. As a granddaughter of Queen Victoria of England, Alexandra was a carrier of the same genetic mutation that afflicted several of the major European royal houses and passed the disease to her only son, Alexei. Because the family was killed by the Bolsheviks in 1918, it is not known whether any of the couple's four daughters (Olga, Tatiana, Maria and Anastasia) inherited the gene as carriers as their mother had before them.

Hemophilia is found in all races and is present throughout the world. This disorder is an X-linked recessive disease, males are predominately affected, and females are "carriers" of this genetic illness. In rare instances, a female may be affected with the disease when a man with hemophilia produces an offspring with a woman who is a carrier of this disorder.

In children with hemophilia, the coagulation process cannot be completed, so bleeding is prolonged. A common misconception is that bleeding is faster in these patients, but this is not the case. The prolonged bleeding is what causes the clinical manifestations to be evident. There are two basic types of hemophilia. In hemophilia A (classic hemophilia), there is a deficiency of factor VIII. In hemophilia B (Christmas disease), there is a deficiency of factor IX (Sevier, 2005). The symptoms of these bleeding disorders are clinically similar, but hemophilia A is more common (Sevier, 2005). The severity of these bleeding disorders is directly related to the degree of factor deficiency. The child with a greater degree of factor deficiency experiences more bleeding episodes than the child with mild deficiency. Hemophilia A is classified as mild, moderate, or severe based on the degree of deficiency present.

Signs and Symptoms

Often a child with hemophilia is diagnosed after presenting with bleeding or there is a known family history of bleeding disorders. Children with bleeding disorders often experience **hemarthrosis** (a bloody effusion within a joint) and soft tissue bleeding (Sevier, 2005). Children who have hemarthrosis often seek medical attention after a minor injury in which there is swelling, stiffness, tingling, decreased range of motion, or pain in the affected joint.

Most children are free of symptoms until they crawl or walk. In infancy, a bleeding disorder may be discovered at the time of circumcision. In older children, excessive bleeding may occur with a tooth extraction or tooth loss. For the child with hemophilia who experiences frequent bleeds in the joints, there may be long-term consequences including mobility limitations, bony changes, and crippling deformities.

Diagnosis

For the child who experiences moderate to severe bleeding from minor procedures or bleeding into large joints, diagnostic testing is warranted. Common diagnostic tests may include a prothrombin time (PT) and a partial thromboplastin time (PTT) (see Table 33-4). The most important test is the direct assay of plasma factor activity level for hemophilia A and B (Hillman et al., 2005). Based on the type of factor deficiency and the percentage of factor level in the plasma, the diagnosis of the type and the classification of hemophilia is confirmed.

Nursing Care

A collaborative interdisciplinary approach is essential to manage children with hemophilia. The nurse must initiate prompt treatment of bleeding episodes. The identification of the deficient factor is imperative in order to administer the proper replacement factors.

 Nursing Insight— *Proper replacement factors*

Years ago, most factor products were derived from human plasma. This treatment posed severe risks to hemophilia children due to the transmission of viral illnesses. Children who were treated with human factor products may have contracted human immunodeficiency virus (HIV) or hepatitis (Sevier, 2005). Now recombinant factor products are the main treatment of hemophilia patients (Sevier, 2005). After years of receiving replacement factor products, children may develop inhibitors to the specific coagulation proteins. The development of inhibitors poses a unique treatment challenge to manage these patients. Changes or additions to the treatment regimen may be necessary to provide adequate replacement factors.

The number one nursing priority for all patients with bleeding disorders is always patient safety, prevention of additional complications, and promoting wellness. Depending on the severity of the bleed, patients may require close observation and inpatient hospitalization. The majority of patients with hemophilia can be managed at home by informed and educated family members. Inpatient nursing care focuses on preventing additional bleeding episodes, monitoring laboratory values as indicated, and administering replacement factor products.

For children with severe hemophilia, prophylactic doses of recombinant factor products may be administered in the home setting by caretakers in order to prevent bleeding episodes. The nurse instructs family members how to administer these factor products by intravenous access. Older mature children may assume the responsibility of self-administering factor products at home after teaching has been completed. Proper administration of factor products at home improves the quality of life, decreases hospitalizations, reduces missed days in school, and prevents long-term complications for children with this chronic illness.

 nursing diagnoses Bleeding Disorders

- Risk for Injury related to bleeding tendencies
- Pain related to bleeding episodes in joints and muscles
- Knowledge Deficit related to home care
- Potential for Impaired Physical Mobility related to bleeding in the joints and muscles

VON WILLEBRAND'S DISEASE

One of the most common inherited bleeding disorders is von Willebrand's disease (vWD) (Allan & Glader, 2002), first described in 1926 by Eric von Willebrand (Turgeon, 2005). It is transmitted via an autosomal dominant pattern of inheritance, affecting males and females equally (Allan & Glader, 2002). vWD is characterized by a deficiency of von Willebrand factor (vWF) and has variable clinical manifestations. vWF plays an important role in the early phase of hemostasis by enhancing platelet aggregation and adhesion. The vWF assists in forming the "platelet plug" to the damaged endothelium and also acts as a carrier protein for coagulation factor VIII (Allan & Glader, 2002).

Signs and Symptoms

When there is a deficiency of vWF, signs and symptoms of prolonged bleeding times may be present. The most common presenting clinical manifestation is epistaxis, followed by bleeding from the oral cavity (Allan & Glader, 2002). In addition, these children may experience menorrhagia (excessive menstrual bleeding) and easy bruising.

Family Teaching Guidelines...
The Child with Hemophilia

HOW TO: Teach the Family How to Care for the Child with Hemophilia

◆ Instruct families on what signs and symptoms require prompt medical attention. Most importantly, any trauma to the head or a change in the level of consciousness is a medical emergency.

◆ Teach the family about the factor replacement products, including how to obtain the product. Often parents are instructed on how to administer prophylactic doses of factor replacement at home.

◆ Ensure that the family is aware that safety is of utmost importance. Injury prevention should be reviewed at all stages of development as risk factors change based on the child's age. Contact sports are highly discouraged. The child should be fitted for a safety helmet to prevent head injury when bike riding.

◆ The nurse communicates to the family that an interdisciplinary team meeting reviews home environmental factors that can affect the treatment plan, such as safety concerns (e.g., bunk beds, difficulty in obtaining or paying for medications, mobility issues).

◆ The nurse also informs the family that for children who have experienced bleeding into the joints, physical therapy may be necessary to preserve and maintain functional status. The physical therapist is a key member in the collaboration with the family to provide comprehensive care.

◆ The child should wear a medical alert bracelet in the event that a medical emergency occurs outside the home when his or her caretaker or parent is not present.

◆ The nurse can reinforce to the family that genetic counseling is recommended since this is an inherited disorder (Lea & Williams, 2002).

◆ Collaboration with the social worker is essential to assist with insurance issues, obtaining medications and supplies, rehabilitation services, home nursing, and other concerns. The social worker is also available for emotional and psychosocial support.

◆ Numerous resources are available at comprehensive hemophilia centers and also online by the National Hemophilia Foundation at www.hemophilia.org.

ESSENTIAL INFORMATION

As there is no known cure for hemophilia, the interdisciplinary team members, including physicians, nurses, rehabilitative services, social workers, child life specialists, and school personnel, are instrumental in teaching the family about how to care for their child with hemophilia.

Recommendations are to seek health care at a facility with a comprehensive hemophilia care center. If the treatment regimen is followed, these children can live long and productive lives. It is essential that the health care team members teach the family about the prevention of bleeding to avoid complications. If a bleeding episode occurs, the family should be instructed on the proper interventions to take. In the instance that the child has a soft tissue injury or bleeding into a joint, before seeking medical attention, the family should initiate supportive measures (i.e., application of pressure to bleeding site, ice, elevation, and rest) (Sevier, 2005).

Diagnosis

Often children are diagnosed with von Willebrand disease when excessive bleeding is present with a simple tooth loss or a minor procedure such as circumcision. A comprehensive family history is essential. The family history reveals similar bleeding manifestations in other family members since vWD is an inherited bleeding disorder. A complete physical examination is essential to detect clinical abnormalities for bleeding tendencies such as multiple sites of bruising. For a child who is experiencing moderate to severe bleeding, a thorough diagnostic evaluation is warranted. The nurse obtains blood samples for PT, PTT, fibrinogen, thrombin time, platelet function assay, CBC, vWF, and vWF antigen.

Nursing Care

Treatment for this disorder includes the administration of desmopressin (DDAVP), a synthetic analog of the antidiuretic hormone vasopressin. This hormone increases the plasma vWF and factor VIII after the administration by releasing vWF from its endothelial cell storage to produce an immediate increase in the plasma levels. This improves the platelet function and shortens the bleeding time. This treatment method may be effective in correcting the bleeding defect of vWD. In addition to the primary function of desmopressin (DDAVP), there may be secondary stabilization of additional factor VIII. Other treatment modalities of vWD include the intravenous administration of Humate-P and/or the administration of cryoprecipitate or fresh frozen plasma (FFP) (Hillman et al., 2005).

For the child identified with an inherited bleeding disorder such as hemophilia or vWD, the nurse should recommend that a medical alert bracelet be worn to appropriately alert health care personnel of the condition. Nursing care includes instructing parents about common sites of bleeding such as nosebleeds, gums, and internal bleeding. Even the smallest nosebleed can be upsetting to a child and parent. Education can also be focused on controlling the bleeding by applying pressure, applying ice, and seeking medical attention. Educate adolescent females on what constitutes excessively heavy menses. The nurse's teaching should also include tips to avoid an embarrassing moment during periods of heavy menstrual flow, such as wearing two maxi pads and not wearing light-colored pants or skirts. Small children can be instructed to avoid nose picking, vigorous nose blowing, and strenuous activity that may cause a nosebleed. Teach children to sneeze with their mouth open and gently blow nose if needed. Avoid the use of acetylsalicylic acid (Children's Aspirin) or NSAIDs, which may promote bleeding episodes. For the child prone to epistaxis, cool mist humidification may also be recommended as a preventive measure.

IDIOPATHIC THROMBOCYTOPENIA PURPURA

Idiopathic (immune) thrombocytopenia purpura (ITP) is the most frequently occurring thrombocytopenia of childhood. The cause of this hemorrhagic disorder is unknown although it may be an autoimmune response to a disease-related antigen (Di Paola & Buchanan, 2002). The characteristic features include thrombocytopenia (an excessive destruction of platelets) and purpura (discoloration caused by petechia beneath the skin). The peak incidence occurs in children 2 to 10 years of age.

There are two types of ITP: acute and chronic. The more common type is acute. Acute ITP is often benign, self-limiting, and often occurs in children younger than 10 years after an upper respiratory infection; after childhood diseases such as measles, rubella, mumps, and chickenpox; and it may also occur after an infection with parvovirus B19 (Turgeon, 2005). Acute ITP is characterized by a normal platelet count within 6 months of diagnosis with no evidence of relapse. Approximately 80% to 90% of children diagnosed with acute ITP achieve complete remission; the remaining 10% to 20% continue with symptoms and are classified as having chronic ITP (Turgeon, 2005). Chronic ITP is most common in adults. A small percentage of children have this chronic condition. Chronic ITP is defined as the persistence of thrombocytopenia (usually less than 150,000) that lasts longer than 6 months (Nathan et al., 2003). In some chronic ITP cases there seems to be a strong correlation with the development of systemic erythematosus lupus.

ITP is a disorder of increased platelet destruction caused by antiplatelet antibodies. These antiplatelet antibodies attach to the child's own platelets and the body's immune system eliminates the platelets, erroneously identifying them as bacteria. The antibodies usually responsible for this response are glycoprotein anti-IIb and IIIa. Antibodies can be identified in many children diagnosed with ITP (Di Paola & Buchanan, 2002).

Signs and Symptoms

The clinical presentation of ITP is generally a previously healthy child who may have had a recent viral infection and then presents with petechiae, bruising, mucocutaneous bleeding, and epistaxis (Sevier & Houston, 2005). Rarely does internal bleeding, such as intracranial hemorrhage, occur (Sevier & Houston, 2005). An adolescent female's chief complaint may be menorrhagia.

Diagnosis

A thorough history and physical examination are essential. Most of these patients appear healthy, with the exception of bruising and bleeding.

66 What to say 99 — *Diagnosing idiopathic (immune) thrombocytopenia purpura*

The nurse can communicate to the family about how ITP is diagnosed. It is essential that the nurse tell the family that there are no definitive tests to establish the diagnosis. Explain that other disorders such as lupus, leukemia, and lymphoma must be ruled out (Sevier & Houston, 2005). Numerous tests are required to confirm the diagnosis of ITP, including CBC and peripheral

smear examination, coagulation analysis, and possible bone marrow aspirate if steroid therapy is implemented. A bone marrow aspirate may be performed to rule out an underlying malignancy. The CBC often shows isolated and usually severe thrombocytopenia, usually a platelet count of less than 20,000 (normal platelet count is 150,000 to 400,000). The peripheral smear is often normal with the exception of thrombocytopenia with normal size to large platelets (Di Paola & Buchanan, 2002).

Nursing Insight— *Accurately diagnosing idiopathic (immune) thrombocytopenia purpura*

Often the child who presents to the emergency department with ITP may be erroneously identified as a child abuse victim. An accurate history and physical and evaluation of CBC should assist the health care team in determining the actual cause of the observed bruising/bleeding. ITP and child abuse may be easily confused. An accurate history is essential to elicit the appropriate diagnosis.

Nursing Care

The majority of patients with acute ITP may have spontaneous resolution of the disorder with no treatment (Sevier & Houston, 2005). The treatment for ITP among pediatric hematologists is not consistent, although recommendations from the American Society of Hematology have been established. General guidelines recommend that children who have a platelet count greater than 20,000 and are asymptomatic do not require treatment, and platelet counts should be monitored. Small toddlers and active children with bruising and petechia with platelet counts less than 20,000 are treated aggressively to avoid the most serious complication of a life-threatening intracranial bleed. Unless severe life-threatening bleeding is present, transfusion of platelets is not recommended to treat acute ITP because the antibodies attach the infused platelets and destroy the new platelets in a similar fashion as the destruction of the patient's own platelets.

The nurse must recognize that first-line treatment strategies may include steroid administration, intravenous immune gamma globulin (IVIG) administration, or Anti-D antibody (WhinRho) administration. Children with exceptionally low platelet counts and acute bleeding require inpatient hospitalization with close observation. These children may also receive a 2- to 3-day course of IVIG intravenously. The mechanism of action of IVIG is to prevent antibody attachment to the platelets, thereby preventing platelet destruction in the spleen. A vast majority of patients who receive IVIG experience a substantial rise in platelet count within 48 hours.

clinical alert

The administration of intravenous anti-D antibody

The newest treatment modality for acute ITP patients with an Rh + blood type is the administration of intravenous anti-D antibody. The mechanism of action of anti-D antibody is to bind to the RBCs, which are selectively destroyed in the spleen instead of platelets. The anti-D antibody coats the Rh+ RBCs with antibody, only for Rh+ patients. The anti-D–coated cells saturate the capacity of the spleen receptors, and the platelets are spared. A common side effect of anti-D antibody is a transient hemolytic anemia that often resolves as the IgG disperses. It is important that the nurse communicate to the family the other possible side effects of anti-D antibody (e.g., fever, chills, or headache after infusion). A paramount nursing action is close observation and monitoring of the child's vital signs.

 ### Nursing Insight— *Splenectomy*

In selected children in whom medical treatment has failed and there have been acute life-threatening bleeding episodes, a treatment modality may include a splenectomy. These patients must be older than 5 years of age and have low platelet counts that impact their activities of daily living (Sevier & Houston, 2005). However, advancements in medical treatment for ITP have diminished the need for the major surgical procedure of a splenectomy.

 Be sure to— Understand institutional guidelines related to intravenous immune gamma globulin (IVIG)

The nurse must understand that intravenous immune gamma globulin (IVIG) is a blood product and that blood product consent may be necessary based on institutional guidelines. Administration of this product requires frequent measurement of vital signs to monitor for possible side effects, which may include fever, chills, hypotension, nausea, and headache. It is important for the nurse to check product specific information for administration guidelines (Di Paola & Buchanan, 2002).

The nurse must teach the family the most important information related to this condition: safety. Advise parents to restrict activities such as contact sports and high-risk activities such as bicycle riding, roller skating, and riding motor scooters. Parents must be instructed on how to manage a bleeding episode in the home. Most common sites of bleeding would be minor cuts and scrapes and nosebleeds. Instruct parents to apply pressure to the injury site. If the bleeding is from the nose, the nurse can instruct the caretaker to have the child lean down and forward, pinch the bridge of the nose, and if possible apply ice. For severe bleeding that does not stop with manual pressure, the caregiver must seek medical attention. Other important teaching strategies include avoiding the use of acetylsalicylic acid (Children's Aspirin) or other aspirin-containing products, injections, the use of straight-edge razors, the use of tampons, or inserting a thermometer or suppository into the rectum. The nurse should instruct caregivers to report signs or symptoms of bleeding immediately, provide a safe environment to prevent trauma such as padding a crib and using a nail file as opposed to clippers for nail grooming. It is essential that the nurse recommends to parents of a child with chronic ITP that a medical alert bracelet be worn (Fig. 33-4).

Figure 33-4 Any child who has idiopathic (immune) thrombocytopenia purpura (ITP) should wear a medical alert bracelet.

 ### clinical alert

Intracranial bleeding

The nurse must ensure that caretakers are knowledgeable about identifying the most serious complication of ITP, an intracranial bleed. Parents must report any changes in level of consciousness or behavior, severe headaches, vision changes, ataxia, slurred speech, complaints of weakness or numbness, and severe vomiting not associated with nausea.

 ### case study Idiopathic (Immune) Thrombocytopenia Purpura

Kelly is a 4-year-old child who has just had a respiratory infection last week. When she woke up this morning to go to daycare she had bruises and petechia. She did not have a fever. The parents immediately phoned the pediatrician and were told to bring the child to the emergency department. Her physical examination was unremarkable except for her bruising, petechia, and a platelet count of 6000. All of Kelly's other labs were within normal limits. She was admitted to the hematology oncology unit.

critical thinking questions

1. What is the goal of Kelly's treatment?

2. What would you expect Kelly's treatment to consist of?

◆ See Suggested Answers to Case Studies in text on the Electronic Study Guide or DavisPlus.

DISSEMINATED INTRAVASCULAR COAGULATION

Disseminated intravascular coagulation (DIC) is a hematological illness that is secondary to an underlying disease (Turgeon, 2005). Some disease states in which children may develop DIC include sepsis (usually gram-negative bacteria), hypoxemia, major trauma with severe tissue injury, malignancy, thrombotic thrombocytopenic purpura (TTP), hemolytic uremic syndrome (HUS), extensive burns, and severe viral infections (Hillman et al., 2005).

In children with DIC, there is an abnormal coagulation process. This process is characterized by an excessive stimulation of normal coagulation that results in microthrombi. These microthrombi are released and as a result more coagulation factors and platelets are consumed and produced. When the process occurs, there is a destruction of platelets and coagulation factors resulting in hemorrhaging and thrombosis. When this clinical diagnosis of DIC is evident, there is accompanying decreased platelet count, increased prothrombin, decreased fibrinogen, and a buildup of fibrin degradation products that may develop into DIC and tissue ischemia.

Signs and Symptoms

The clinical symptomatology of excessive bleeding from orifices or due to minor procedures may lead the clinician to suspect the patient has DIC. Other pertinent assessment findings include the presence of an underlying primary illness that may place the child at high risk for developing DIC. A nursing assessment may also include the presence of petechia; purpura; hypotension; and, as the child's condition progresses, the possibility of multiorgan failure due to numerous infarctions and ischemia.

Diagnosis

There is no single test that confirms the diagnosis of DIC. The diagnosis is based on the combination of the child's clinical condition and laboratory tests pertinent to coagulopathies (Turgeon, 2005). For a child with DIC, suspicious findings include thrombocytopenia, prolonged prothrombin time (PT), prolonged partial thromboplastin (PTT), decreased fibrinogen, and increased D-dimer.

Nursing Care

When caring for a child with DIC, the nurse's primary intervention is to assess the child and provide supportive care for the symptomatology. Children with DIC are critically ill and may require management in the intensive care unit. The administration of blood and factor products is often necessary. More importantly, the underlying cause must be identified and treated. Important nursing responsibilities include early identification of risk factors that predispose patients to develop DIC. The nurse must monitor for signs of hemorrhage, bleeding, petechiae, cutaneous oozing, dyspnea, lethargy, pallor, increased heart rate, decreased blood pressure, headache, dizziness, muscle weakness, and restlessness. If the child is bleeding, it is important that the nurse does not disturb clots, uses pressure, and applies ice to control bleeding, and measures blood loss. The nurse must monitor for internal bleeding by checking both the urine and stool for occult blood (Procedure 33-1). The nurse can also obtain necessary laboratory tests and administer supportive treatments such as blood and factor products per physician orders (Hillman et al., 2005). Prognosis for DIC has improved significantly over the last two decades due to advances in supportive care such as improved antibiotics, antifibrinolytic therapy, and improvement in transfusion therapy.

When a child is critically ill and has the diagnosis of DIC, parents must be informed about the plan of care and the course of treatment. In the intensive care unit the nurse can orient families to the unit procedures, equipment, and treatments. The possibility of excessive bleeding from multiple sites may occur and could be upsetting to family members. The nurse must communicate to families about the occurrence of excessive bleeding to help decrease anxiety. Identifying areas of knowledge deficits and ensuring consistent caregivers during this time of crisis are important nursing interventions. Provide families with honest answers in clear and concise terms (see Chapters 11, 14, and 16 for further discussion).

APLASTIC ANEMIA

Aplastic anemia is rare but is one of the most serious hematological conditions that generally afflicts adolescents and young adults. It is characterized by **pancytopenia** (a reduction in all cellular elements of the blood) caused by bone marrow hematopoiesis failure (Hillman et al., 2005). Patchy brown melanin-like pigmentation of the skin (café-au-lait spots), short stature, microcephaly, mental retardation, strabismus, and other musculoskeletal and genitourinary anomalies are also associated with aplastic anemia (Turgeon, 2005).

 Nursing Insight— *Pancytopenia*

Pancytopenia is a common finding in aplastic anemia. In pancytopenia all formed elements of the blood are depressed at the same time. A patient with pancytopenia has neutropenia, decreased white blood cell count, anemia, decreased hemoglobin count and thrombocytopenia.

The body's cells arise from a universal/pluripotent "mother" cell called the stem cell (Nathan et al., 2003). In aplastic anemia, hematopoietic precursor cells are absent in the bone marrow, with the resultant space replaced by fat. This effect results in a decrease in all cell lines. Aplastic anemia can be congenital or an acquired illness.

Hereditary aplastic anemia is a congenital disorder that is relatively rare but it can occur with diseases such as Fanconi's anemia. Fanconi's anemia is inherited as an autosomal recessive trait. Fanconi's anemia accounts for 25–30% of all cases of childhood aplastic anemia (Turgeon, 2005). Children with congenital aplastic anemia have chromosomal breakages and structural abnormalities that increase the incidence of various malignancies such as leukemia.

The majority of aplastic anemia cases are considered to be idiopathic and the specific cause is never determined (Box 33-2, p. 1089). Other forms of aplastic anemia are considered secondary to etiological agents that are usually associated with various environmental factors and physical conditions.

Signs and Symptoms

The presenting signs and symptoms of a child with aplastic anemia vary by severity of bone marrow suppression. The clinical course may be acute and may progress to severe bone marrow suppression with the possibility of rapid deterioration leading to death. The condition could also have an insidious onset and chronic course (Turgeon, 2005). Classification can range from moderate aplastic anemia to very severe aplastic anemia.

Procedure 33-1 Obtaining a Fecal Occult Blood Test Sample

Purpose

A fecal occult blood test (FOBT) is performed to detect hidden (occult) blood in the stool.

Equipment

Hematest cards
Gloves
Sterile tongue blade
Chemical reagent

Steps

1. Wash hands and don gloves.

   RATIONALE: *Prevents the spread of bacteria.*

2. Verify the identity of the patient.

   RATIONALE: *Accurate patient identification is necessary in the delivery of safe care.*

3. Check the manufacturer's instructions for specific Hematest cards.

   RATIONALE: *Following the correct instructions ensures proper administration of the test as well as accurate results.*

4. Keep the Hematest cards at room temperature.

   RATIONALE: *Extreme temperatures may damage the Hematest cards.*

5. Use a sterile tongue blade to remove a sample of stool from the diaper.

   RATIONALE: *A sterile tongue blade helps to prevent contamination of the collected specimen.*

6. Place a smear of stool on both windows of the Hematest card as indicated on the instructions.

   RATIONALE: *Collecting an adequate amount of stool is necessary to complete the test.*

7. Cover the windows with the paper flaps and wait the correct amount of time before reading the results.

   RATIONALE: *It is important to follow the manufacturer's instructions.*

8. Apply the recommended drops of developing solution to the Hematest card.

   RATIONALE: *It is important to follow the manufacturer's instructions.*

9. Read the back flap of the sample card within the recommended time of application of developing solution.

   RATIONALE: *Reading the card within the recommended time is essential to performing the test accurately.*

10. The Hematest card should change color to indicate the test results.

    RATIONALE: *A change in color may indicate occult blood in the stool.*

Clinical Alert When the nurse records results, it is important to notify the health care provider of any abnormal findings. In addition, the nurse should check the expiration date on the developing solution.

Teach Parents

It is important to teach the parents the rationale for the test.

Documentation
5/20/10 1300 Stool Hematest negative.
—D. Salani, RN

Nursing Insight— *Signs and symptoms of aplastic anemia*

The child's symptoms are related to the degree of pancytopenia. Anemia, pallor, dizziness, and fatigue may be present because of a decreased RBC count. Increased bleeding and bruising, petechia, and epistaxis may be attributed to a low platelet count. Increased susceptibility to infections and oral ulcerations that do not respond well to antibiotics are related to a low WBC count. The most common presenting symptom is bleeding, usually from the nose, mouth, and gastrointestinal tract. The nurse must be aware that the child with aplastic anemia characteristically does not have the clinical finding of hepatosplenomegaly or lymphadenopathy. The child with this clinical finding is usually diagnosed with leukemia.

Diagnosis

To confirm the diagnosis of aplastic anemia and rule out other hematopoietic diseases, a bone marrow aspirate and biopsy must be performed. Children who are suspected to have aplastic anemia require a thorough history and physical and laboratory tests, including a CBC with differential. The findings of the CBC usually are consistent with all cell lines depressed. To confirm a diagnosis of aplastic anemia, a bone marrow aspiration must be performed. The results of the bone marrow aspiration generally reveal a fatty marrow with few developing blood cells.

Nursing Care

Nursing care for children with aplastic anemia varies based on the severity of illness and determination of causative factors. If the causative factor of the aplastic anemia has been identified, immediate removal of the agent is necessary. Some patients may respond to medical treatment and support. In these cases, a hematopoietic stem cell transplant may not be warranted. If there is no identified cause of the severe aplastic anemia and a suitable stem cell donor is identified, the treatment of choice is a hematopoietic stem cell transplant (HSCT). For best outcomes and long-term survival, every effort must be made to proceed to transplant as soon as possible. Following the stem cell transplant, nursing care consists of supportive care, immunosuppressive therapy, or the administration of hematopoietic growth factors.

Box 33-2 Causative Factors of Acquired Aplastic Anemia

- High dose radiation
- Autoimmune disorders
- Pregnancy
- Infectious processes
  - Hepatitis
  - Epstein–Barr virus
  - HIV
  - CMV
  - Infectious mononucleosis
- Nonpharmacological agents
  - Benzene
  - Lindane (insecticide)
  - Kerosene
  - Heavy metals
- Pharmacological agents
  - Chemotherapy
  - Chloramphenicol
  - Selected antiepileptics (carbamazepine)
  - Sulfonamides
  - Penicillamine
  - Nonsteroidal anti-inflammatory drugs (NSAIDs)
  - Antithyroid drugs
  - Psychotropics (clozapine)
  - Certain cardiovascular drugs
  - Penicillamine
  - Antithyroid drugs
  - Psychotropics (Clozapine)
  - Certain cardiovascular drugs

The nurse understands that drug therapy may be the first line of therapy while searching for a potential bone marrow donor. The two most common immunosuppressive drugs used in treating aplastic anemia include antithymocyte globulin (ATG) and high-dose cyclosporine (Neoral, Gengraf). Antithymocyte globulin (ATG) is a horse serum containing polyclonal antibodies against human T cells, and cyclosporine is also a T-cell-suppressing agent. Immunosuppressive therapies work with the child's immune system. The mechanism of action is to stimulate the bone marrow to produce cells or to reduce the patient's immune response, thereby allowing the bone marrow to work. Combined ATG and cyclosporine is the gold standard for first-line immunosuppressive therapy. There is usually a 75% to 85% response rate (Turgeon, 2005).

Another treatment modality includes the administration of hematopoietic growth factors. These growth factors are copies of substances that occur naturally in the body and attempt to stimulate the bone. Sometimes combinations of these growth factors are used to treat aplastic anemia.

 clinical alert

Anaphylactic reaction in children who receive antithymocyte globulin (ATG)

Children with aplastic anemia who receive antithymocyte globulin (ATG) require specific nursing care related to the administration of this medication. Although rare, a severe anaphylactic reaction may occur (hypotension, tachycardia, shortness of breath, chest pain). Since there is a potential risk for anaphylaxis, an antithymocyte globulin (ATG) test dose is often administered to determine if there is a potential for an adverse reaction to this medication. The child may have no adverse reaction to the test dose, but still may have a reaction to antithymocyte globulin (ATG). If the child has been identified as being "allergic" to antithymocyte globulin (ATG), administration of this medication can still take place after a desensitization process or administration of premedications such as antihistamine and steroids.

All patients diagnosed with aplastic anemia are extremely susceptible to infectious agents. These patients may not exhibit the "classic signs of infection."

 critical nursing action Supportive Care

For all patients with aplastic anemia, and especially those who are preparing for hematopoietic stem cell transplant (HSCT), the nursing care plan often consists of supportive care including transfusions of RBCs and platelets. Transfusions are used cautiously to prevent development of antibodies (alloimmunization) and possible graft versus host disease (GVHD) if this patient proceeds on to transplant. Antibiotics are often given to treat infections but are generally not recommended prophylactically.

This special population of pediatric hematology patients requires diligent nursing assessments secondary to their pancytopenia. These children may experience numerous complications from neutropenia, anemia, or thrombocytopenia. When caring for children who are neutropenic, the nurse does not traditionally see the hallmark signs of infections such as redness, swelling, and pus, since these patients do not have the neutrophils to provoke such a response. The nursing care plan can be used to monitor the subjective responses of the child.

 where research and practice meet:
Single Stem Cell Research

The first theory about a single pluripotent stem cell to repopulate was first documented in the early 1960s by Till and McCulloch. Their early research involved injecting bone marrow cells into mice. Till and McCulloch observed "small raised lumps" that grew on the spleen of the mice related to the amount of marrow cells injected. Through this experiment, the theory of a "single stem cell" was discovered (Becker, McCulloch, & Till, 1963).

medication: Hematopoietic Growth Factors

Granulocyte colony-stimulating factors (GCSF), also known as Neupogen, are one example of a hematopoietic growth factor. GCSF stimulates the WBC lines. Growth factors for the WBCs are given to prevent profound neutropenia and decrease susceptibility to life-threatening infections. In the home setting, this medication is given by subcutaneous injection once daily by the child's caregiver. Possible side effects include fever, bone pain, headache, and local reaction at the injection site.

Nursing Care Plan   The Child with Aplastic Anemia

Nursing Diagnosis: Risk for Infection related to decreased white blood cell count

Measurable Short-term Goal: Patient will be afebrile within 24 hours of initiation of antibiotic therapy.

Measurable Long-term Goal: Patient will have a decrease in the incidence of infections.

NOC Outcome:
Immune Status (0702) Natural and acquired appropriately targeted resistance to internal and external antigens

NIC Interventions:
Infection Protection (6550)
Medication Administration (2300)

Nursing Interventions:

1. Monitor temperature, blood pressure, pulse, and respirations (specify frequency).

   RATIONALE: Allows recognition of fever, tachycardia, tachypnea, or hypotension or other signs of sepsis and allows early intervention.

2. Administer antibiotics and acetaminophen per physician orders (specify drug, dose, route, and times).

   RATIONALE: Antibiotics are used promptly to treat suspected infections in the neutropenic patient. Acetaminophen is the preferred antipyretic because acetylsalicylic acid (Children's Aspirin) or NSAIDs may increase bleeding.

3. Reinforce strict hand washing and the use of antimicrobial hand gels/foams.

   RATIONALE: Hand washing is the number one method to reduce the spread of infections

4. Maintain protective isolation as per institution guidelines (specify).

   RATIONALE: Individualized isolation precautions avoid contact with infectious agents.

5. Provide or assist family member to provide meticulous oral and skin hygiene.

   RATIONALE: Reduce the portals of entry for infections.

6. Instruct family and visitors that no fresh fruits, vegetables, flowers, or plants are allowed in the child's room.

   RATIONALE: Some fresh fruits, vegetables, flowers, and plants may harbor bacteria or viruses.

Owing to the variations in severity of aplastic anemia, the nurse's teaching plan must correlate with the child's clinical condition. The nurse can provide reassurance and support to families, including basic explanations of the disease process and recommended treatment plan. It is important for the nurse to review the child's prescribed drugs and discuss possible adverse reactions. Children who do not require hospitalizations can continue a normal lifestyle with some restrictions. The nurse can communicate to the family that monitoring the child's CBC is imperative so changes in condition from mild to moderate aplastic anemia are noted. Children and their families must be aware of signs and symptoms of pancytopenia. Patients with moderate to severe aplastic anemia should be encouraged to schedule regular rest periods, avoid contacts with crowds, and avoid sources of infections (sick contacts, soil, standing water). Injury prevention may include using a soft toothbrush for oral hygiene, ensuring a safe play environment, and avoiding the use of tampons for adolescent girls. The nurse can stress the importance of meticulous oral hygiene and diligent hand washing. For additional education materials and resources for family teaching, the nurse can refer families to the Aplastic Anemia and MDS International Foundation at www.aamds.org. New therapies are being tested and developed with the hope of developing a cure of this chronic disease.

NEUTROPENIA

Neutropenia occurs when an absolute neutrophil count is less than 1000/μL in infants younger than 1 year of age and 1500/μL for those older than 1 year of age.

> ### Nursing Insight— Absolute neutrophil count (ANC)
>
> The absolute neutrophil count (ANC) is the total number of white blood cells multiplied by the percentage of neutrophils (segs and bands) to determine the ANC.

The National Cancer Institute neutropenia grading system classifies slight neutropenia as grade 1 with ANC of less than 2000, minimal neutropenia grade 2 with ANC of less than 1500, and moderate neutropenia grade 3 with ANC less than 1000. The most severe neutropenia is grade 4 with an ANC of less than 500. When caring for children with neutropenia, the nursing plan of care is based on the severity of neutropenia present.

Neutropenia is further classified as an acquired or congenital illness. Acquired neutropenia is more common than the congenital form. Viral infections (e.g., HIV, EBV, hepatitis A and B, RSV) are often a common cause of acquired neutropenia (Turgeon, 2005). Acquired neutropenia is often referred to as secondary neutropenia due to the fact that it occurs as a result of an illness or of treatment of the illness (e.g., chemotherapy, radiation therapy, immunosuppressive agents, specific medications, and malignancies). It can also result as part of the normal aging process. Congenital neutropenia (also known as primary neutropenia) is usually caused by a genetic abnormality that results in profound neutropenia. Some examples include severe combined immunodeficiency syndrome (SCIDs), Wiskott–Aldrich syndrome, and Kostmann's syndrome. Often these congenital neutropenia disorders are associated with the future development of more serious illnesses such as myelodysplastic syndromes or acute myelogenous leukemia.

Signs and Symptoms

Signs and symptoms of neutropenia include lymphadenopathy, organomegaly, pallor, bruising, petechia, and other abnormalities in appearance. The nurse observes the child for any underlying infection, especially the mouth, skin, ears, and perianal area. A fever may be the only clinical sign that an infection is present. Often the child with neutropenia may not have the classic signs of an underlying infection, so the nurse must pay close attention to the subtle signs that may be present. The reason these children do not display the classic signs and symptoms is that they do not possess the cells (i.e., neutrophils) to evoke such a response, such as redness, swelling, or pus.

Diagnosis

The child diagnosed with neutropenia requires a meticulous history and physical examination. The child's height and weight can be plotted on the growth chart to evaluate for any underlying genetic illness or deviations from the norm. The child's laboratory work-up is based on the findings from the history and physical. In most cases a CBC with differential and a peripheral smear will be performed. It is important to focus on the absolute neutrophil count (ANC) as opposed to the total WBC count. If the child has other clinical findings such as anemia, thrombocytopenia, or high MCV with normal B_{12}, a bone marrow aspirate may be indicated. The bone marrow aspirate is helpful in ascertaining the cause and treatment regimen for the neutropenia. Usually the child with congenital neutropenia has a normal cellularity with absence of mature neutrophils in the bone marrow sample. If a bone marrow aspirate cannot be obtained, a bone marrow biopsy may be required. Additional diagnostic tests may include cytogenetics (identification of chromosomes), including flow cytometry (laser device is used for the counting and measuring cells in specialized laboratories).

Nursing Care

The initial determination of the cause of the neutropenia is relevant to the plan of care. For the patient with acquired neutropenia, the etiology must be evaluated. For patients with congenital neutropenia, the nursing plan of care is based on the degree of neutropenia and physical findings. Treatment may range from supportive measures to the administration of colony-stimulating factors and in most severe cases to bone marrow transplant if necessary.

The administration of granulocyte colony-stimulating factor such as GCSF (Neupogen) stimulates the bone marrow to produce more neutrophils.

One of the most important aspects of nursing care for neutropenic patients includes monitoring for infections such as fever, absolute neutrophil count evaluation, and physical exam. In the event an infection is suspected, treatment of a documented infection in the neutropenic patient is dependent on the organism that is isolated. Empiric therapy, usually with a broad-spectrum antibiotic, is usually implemented during the period of time in which culture results are pending. Once culture results are obtained, antibiotic therapy should be evaluated for sensitivities and adjusted accordingly. The child who has neutropenia, whether it is congenital or acquired, needs specific teaching on management. Families must be instructed on when and how to appropriately wash their hands. Hands should be washed with soap and water for at least 10 to 15 seconds using a circular motion. Friction (rubbing) is the most important aspect of hand washing as it assists in removing germs from the hands. The nurse can teach parents how to appropriately check the child's temperature. Remind them to never check a temperature rectally because this route may cause a tear in the rectal mucosa, promoting an entrance for bacteria. Parents need to seek medical attention if the child develops a temperature of 101.5°F (38.6°C). Teaching the family about meticulous oral hygiene is also important. To prevent bacteria in the mouth, the child can use a soft toothbrush and rinse well after brushing. Good skin care is essential to prevent infections or breaks in the skin. The nurse can instruct caregivers to keep the neutropenic child away from anyone who is sick or recently received live vaccines. Instruct parents of a child who has had an exposure to chickenpox (i.e., any type of varicella illness) to immediately contact a health care provider. Administering the varicella-zoster vaccine may be helpful to the neutropenic child who might be exposed to an outbreak of chickenpox.

 critical nursing action The Neutropenic Child

Families and children with neutropenia can be taught the following measures to reduce the incidence of infection:

- Always keep routine visits.
- Be aware of the signs and symptoms of infections such as fever (greater than 101.5°F [38.6°C]).
- Avoid large crowds, or anyone who may be sick with a cold, flu, etc.
- Keep the child's body clean by bathing every day, and brush teeth after meals and before bedtime.
- Avoid hot tubs.
- Always be sure to wash the child's hands before eating or touching her face, eyes, nose, and mouth.
- Avoid constipation and straining to have a bowel movement by drinking two quarts of fluids each day such as water and use a stool softener.
- Avoid putting anything in the child's rectum, including thermometers and suppositories.
- Avoid exposure to fresh flowers or live plants.
- Avoid exposure to stool droppings from pets and cleaning bird cages, as well as cleaning cat litter boxes.

- Do not share bath towels or drinking glasses with others, including family members.
- Avoid eating the following items:
  - Raw milk or milk products; any milk product that has not been pasteurized, including cheese and yogurt made from unpasteurized milk
  - Raw or uncooked meat, fish, chicken, eggs, tofu
  - Foods that contain mold (e.g., blue cheese)
  - Raw honey (honey that has not been pasteurized)
  - Uncooked fresh fruit or vegetables
  - Outdated foods or foods left at room temperature for more than 2 hours
- Adolescents should not use tampons, vaginal suppositories, or douche.
- Adolescents should avoid manicures, pedicures, acrylic nails, or nail tips.
- Adolescents should use an electric shaver instead of a razor.

Blood Transfusion Therapy

With recent advances in health care and more children living with chronic illnesses, blood transfusion therapy may be required as part of the nursing care plan. Illnesses such as hematological, oncological, and other chronic conditions often necessitate the use of blood products. Nurses must be knowledgeable about blood transfusion products and specific indications for each blood product (Table 33-5). Administration of blood may vary based on institution policy and procedures and the actual product being administered.

BLOOD PRODUCT ADMINISTRATION

Most blood transfusions are delivered in the hospital. The first responsibility of the nurse who is administering a blood transfusion to a child is to review the plan of care with the family and explain in detail the indications and process of a blood transfusion. The nurse must obtain signed consent from the parent or guardian to administer blood to the child.

 Be sure to— Obtain transfusion consent

Transfusion consent must be obtained before the transfusion of all blood products. Transfusion consent must include the description of procedure for transfusion, risks and benefits, treatment alternatives, and appropriate signatures including those of the health care provider, the patient if 18 years or older, the parent or other legal representative and witness (American Association of Blood Banks [AABB], 2004). Provide the opportunity for the family to ask questions. The family has the right to revoke the consent if they wish.

After the consent process is complete, obtain the required blood samples from the patient. For example, if a child requires a packed red blood cell transfusion, a type and crossmatch is indicated in order to determine the ABO and Rh factor and to reserve the donated red blood cells for this specific child.

 clinical alert

Blood transfusion safety measure

During the collection of a blood sample for crossmatch, a blood bracelet with the specific identifying numbers is placed on the child's extremity. This safety measure is to ensure that the child receives the correct blood product crossmatched specifically for his or her blood type in order to prevent a fatality. Fatalities have occurred when these safety steps are not adhered to.

The only instance in which the nurse may transfuse a blood product in which a type and crossmatch are not obtained is in a severe emergency situation. In this situation, O negative blood (the universal donor for all blood products) is rapidly infused in order to save the child's life. In most emergency departments that treat trauma patients, a "rapid infuser" is the best method to warm and infuse the blood in a more efficient manner.

Optimizing Outcomes— **Type and screen and type and crossmatch**

The best outcome exists for the child when the nurse understand the difference between the type and screen and type and crossmatch

Type and Screen
- Obtained in anticipation that a child may need blood
- ABO group and Rh type of patient identified
- Does not remove blood from inventory

Type and Crossmatch
- Obtained if almost certain child will require blood
- ABO/Rh compatible donor red cells combined
- Cross match is good for 72 hours. (Hillman et al., 2005)

Blood is administered to the child after verifying that the correct blood product is available and that the child's clinical condition is stable (i.e., vital signs within parameters to safely administer blood). The nurse must complete the pre-assessment process for blood administration. The nurse must be aware that there are several clinical conditions that may delay the administration of a blood product:

- Fever greater than 101°F (38.3°C)
- Lack of intravenous access
- Child is unable to be closely monitored by nursing staff

Nursing Insight— *Understanding blood type*

When the clinical criterion is met, the nurse may proceed and obtain the product to be infused from the institution's blood bank or pharmacy. Understand that blood type is essential information for the nurse (Box 33-3, page 1095).

Table 33-5 Transfusion Products

Transfusion Product	Indications	Critical Nursing Actions
Red Blood Cells	Hemoglobin <8 grams on a stable patient with a chronic anemia Hypovolemia due to acute blood loss Evidence of impending heart failure secondary to severe anemia Patients on hyper transfusion regimen for sickle cell disease and history of: • Cerebral vascular accident • Splenic sequestration • Acute chest syndrome • Recurrent priapism • Preoperative preparation for surgery with general anesthesia • Hypoxia Children requiring increased oxygen-carrying capacity (i.e., complex congenital heart, intracardiac shunting, severe pulmonary disease—ARDS): • Shock states (decrease B.P., increased peripheral vasoconstriction pallor, cyanosis, diaphoretic, clamminess, mottled skin, increased oxygen requirement, decreased urinary output) • Cardiac failure • Respiratory failure requiring significant ventilatory support • Postoperative anemia	Observe for clinical signs and symptoms of anemia: • Fatigue • Syncope • Pallor • Tachycardia • Diaphoretic • Shortness of breath • Inability to perform activities of daily living Don appropriate PPE (personal protective equipment) for all blood product transfusions. Monitor vital signs per hospital policy and procedure. Monitor hemoglobin and hematocrit. During blood product infusions, observe for adverse reactions. Blood can be stored only in a designated blood refrigerator. Generally 10–15 mL/kg of packed red blood cells are transfused (Khilnani, 2005).
Autologous Blood (self-donated blood product)	For general scheduled surgical procedures in which there are clinical indications that a blood transfusion may be necessary during the intraoperative or postoperative period the patient may elect to self-donate. Check with blood bank facilities for time criteria for this type of donation. For general surgical procedures, the recommended hemoglobin is 10 grams or greater and for orthopedic surgery the recommendation is hemoglobin of 11.5 or greater.	Verify with parents that self-donation has occurred. Patient identification and administration process is the same as for all other blood products.
Whole Blood or Packed Red Blood Cells (PRBC) Reconstituted with Fresh Frozen Plasma (FFP)	Hypovolemia due to acute blood loss non-responsive to crystalloids • Hct <35% • Hypovolemia due to acute massive blood loss (i.e., major trauma) • History of blood loss at delivery or large amount of blood drawn for lab studies (10% blood volume) • Cardiac patients Hct <40% (structural heart disease, cyanosis, or congestive heart failure) • Drop in Hgb to below 10 grams intraoperatively • Exchange transfusion	Same nursing actions applicable to red blood cell infusions. In major trauma situations, patient may be transfused with O negative blood, the universal donor. Use blood warmer and rapid infuser if available.

Continued

Table 33-5 Transfusion Products—cont'd

Transfusion Product	Indications	Critical Nursing Actions
Platelets	Platelet count <20,000	Know normal platelet count (150,000 to 400,000).
	Active bleeding with symptoms of DIC or other significant coagulopathies	Obtain CBC.
		Assess bruising, petechiae, and bleeding.
	Platelet count <50,000 with planned invasive procedure (i.e., surgical procedure, central line insertion, does not include drawing blood or intramuscular injection of intravenous catheter insertion)	
	Prevention or treatment of bleeding due to thrombocytopenia (secondary to chemotherapy, radiation, or bone marrow failure)	
	Treatment of patients with severe thrombocytopenia secondary to increased platelet destruction or immune thrombocytopenia associated with complication of severe trauma	
	Massive transfusion with platelet dilution	
Fresh Frozen Plasma (FFP)	Replacement for deficiency of factors II, V, VII, IX, X, XII; protein C or protein S	Notify blood bank to thaw FFP; product must be used within 6 hours of thawing.
	Bleeding, invasive procedure, or surgery with documented plasma clotting protein deficiency (i.e., liver failure, DIC, or septic shock)	Don appropriate PPE for all blood product transfusions.
		Monitor vital signs per hospital policy and procedure.
	Prolonged PT and/or PTT without bleeding	Monitor coagulation studies.
	Significant intraoperative bleeding (>10% blood volume/hr) in excess of normally anticipated blood loss that is at high risk of clotting-factor deficiency	During FFP infusions, observe for adverse reactions.
	Massive transfusion	
	Therapeutic plasma exchanges	
	Warfarin anticoagulant overdose	
Cryoprecipitate (CRYO)	Fibrinogen levels below 150 mg/dL with active bleeding	Assess for signs and symptoms of bleeding.
	Bleeding or prophylaxis in von Willebrand's disease or in factor VIII (hemophilia A) deficiency unresponsive to or unsuitable for DDAVP or factor VII concentrates	Don appropriate PPE for all blood product transfusions.
		Monitor vital signs per hospital policy and procedure.
	Replacement therapy, bleeding or invasive procedure in patients with factor XIII deficiency	Monitor coagulation studies.
	Patients with active intraoperative hemorrhage in excess of normally anticipated blood loss who are at risk of clotting factor deficiency	During cryoprecipitate infusions, observe for adverse reactions.
Granulocytes (white blood cell transfusion)	Bacterial or fungal sepsis (proven or strongly suspected) unresponsive to antimicrobial therapy	Type and crossmatch required for all WBC transfusions.
	Infection (proven or strongly suspected) unresponsive to antimicrobial therapy	Pre-medications may be ordered, such as antihistamines or acetaminophen.
Factor VII	Treatment of factor VII deficiency	Assess for signs and symptoms of bleeding.
	Treatment of factor VIII inhibitors	Don appropriate PPE for all blood products, even recombinant.
	Treatment of factor IX inhibitors	Monitor coagulation studies.
	Idiopathic uncontrolled bleeding	If undiluted, dilute vial with indicated amount of sterile water and administer intravenously as per manufacturer's guidelines.

Table 33-5 Transfusion Products—cont'd

Transfusion Product	Indications	Critical Nursing Actions
Factor VIII Concentrate	Hemophilia A (factor VIII deficiency)	Assess for signs and symptoms of bleeding.
	Patient with factor VIII inhibitors	Don appropriate PPE for all blood products.
	Patients with von Willebrand's disease	Monitor coagulation studies.
		Check product to see if refrigeration necessary.
		Record expiration date and lot number of product.
Factor IX Concentrate (prothrombin complex)	Treatment of hemophilia B	Assess for signs and symptoms of bleeding.
	Hemophilia A with factor VIII inhibitors	Don appropriate PPE for all blood products.
	Patients with congenital deficiency of prothrombin, factor VII, and factor X	Monitor coagulation studies.
		Record expiration date and lot number of product.
Intravenous Immunoglobulin (IVIG)	Congenital or acquired antibody deficiency	Don appropriate PPE for all IVIG infusions.
	Immunological disorders such as idiopathic thrombocytopenia (ITP), Kawasaki disease	Monitor vital signs per hospital policy and procedure.
	Posttransplant patients used prophylactically, newborns with severe bacterial infections	Start infusion slowly and increase rate/titrate per physician orders. During IVIG infusion, observe for adverse reactions such as fever, chills, and headache.
		Product is obtained from pharmacy.
		Record expiration date and lot number of product.

Box 33-3 Understanding Blood Types

BLOOD TYPE	CAN GIVE TO:	TAKE FROM:
A+	A+	A+, A–, O–
A–	A+, A–	A–, O–
B+	B+	B+, B–, O+, O–
B–	B+, B–	B–, O–
AB+	AB+	All types
AB–	AB–	A–, B–, AB–, O–
O+	A+, B+, AB+, O+	O+, O–
O–	All types	O–

 clinical alert

The administration process for blood products

The nurse must understand the administration process for blood products.

Pretransfusion

- Do not call for the blood product until it is needed.
- Verify the physician's orders, including the appropriate product and volume to be infused. For packed red blood cell infusions, the appropriate volume is 10–13 cc/kg. Check with institution policies and procedures. The transfusion must be started within 30 minutes after the blood has left the blood bank.
- The maximum time for the infusion is 4 hours. Transfusion needs to start immediately due to the risk of bacterial contamination and cell lysis. Most blood banks do not accept blood back after 30 minutes.

- Follow institutional policy for obtaining, verifying, and transporting blood products obtained from the blood bank.
- Complete appropriate forms and ensure accurate patient identification.
- Indicate product type and check for any special orders such as CMV safe, irradiated.
- Always check to see if any premedications were ordered before administration.
- Use personal protective equipment. Be sure to wear goggles and gloves.
- All blood products must be checked at the patient's bedside by two appropriate health care team members as per the institution's policy.
- Remember the two patient identifiers: matching the number on the blood product and the wrist band.

Initiation of the Transfusion

- Obtain baseline vital signs.
- Start the infusion slowly for the first 15 minutes.
- Designate a nurse to remain with the patient for the first 15 minutes of transfusion in the event of an adverse reaction.

During the Transfusion

- Do not infuse any other solutions simultaneously with blood through the same intravenous line. The only exception to this is normal saline (AABB guidelines, 2004).
- Never add any medications to blood.
- Monitor vital signs per the institution's policy and procedures.
- All identification information that is attached to the blood product must remain attached until the transfusion is completed.

- Monitor for signs and symptoms of adverse reactions (see section on adverse reactions).

Posttransfusion

- Save the transfusion bag for at least 1 hour after the transfusion has ended.
- The blood slip must be completely filled out with the institution's required information.
- As per the American Association of Blood Bank (AABB) guidelines, information to be included in the child's medical record must include the transfusion order, the type of blood product, the donor unit number, date and time of transfusion, pre- and post-vital signs, the volume infused, required signatures, and if applicable any transfusion adverse events (2004).
- Place the chart copy and blood bank copy of blood slip in an appropriate area to be kept on file as per policy and procedure.

SENSITIVITY TO CULTURAL AND RELIGIOUS BELIEFS

The nurse must be sensitive to cultural and religious beliefs in order to provide the most culturally competent care to patients and their families. In most cases, the nurse is the primary health care provider at the bedside and may experience some personal conflict when providing the necessary medical care. The nurse must be knowledgeable about various belief systems that impact care and be aware of what resources are available to assist in these situations.

 Ethnocultural Considerations— Jehovah Witness

People of the Jehovah Witness faith are adamantly opposed to receiving blood and blood products. This belief is based on the literal interpretation of the Bible that states that to be transfused with blood is equivalent to eating it and therefore prohibited by scripture as cited in Leviticus 17:10-14; Acts 15:19, 20, 28, 29 and Genesis 9:3, 4. Although the Jehovah Witnesses believe it necessary to "abstain from … blood," they have the high standards of receiving all medical treatment including advanced technology. Jehovah Witnesses feel strongly that if blood is removed from the body, it cannot be reinfused (e.g., cell saver technology that could be used in the operating room). Self-donation is also prohibited based on this premise.

When caring for a child from a Jehovah Witness family, there may be an ethical and medical dilemma to provide quality medical care. The health care team should explore all alternative methods of treatment in order to respect the family's beliefs. In some circumstances when the child's life is severely threatened, the courts may be called upon. A court order may be required to proceed with the necessary medical treatment. The involvement of the court system relinquishes the family from making the decision for their child to have a blood transfusion. This transfer of responsibility may diminish the disgrace that the family might experience from other members of this religious group when this medical treatment is necessary to save the child's life (Linnard-Palmar & Kools, 2004).

TRANSFUSION REACTIONS

Most transfusion reactions occur during the initiation of a transfusion, but a reaction can occur at any time during this process (AABB, 2004). These reactions can vary from a mild reaction, such as mild fever, to the most severe complication of death. Children who have received multiple transfusions are at higher risk for developing a transfusion reaction (Knippen, 2006).

 critical nursing action The Administration of Blood

Strict observance to the institutional policy regarding the administration of blood products cannot be stressed enough. The accuracy of patient verification is a critical nursing action that can help prevent a transfusion reaction.

FEBRILE REACTION

The most common blood transfusion reaction is a nonhemolytic **febrile reaction** in which the child develops a fever greater than 1.8°F from the baseline temperature. These reactions generally occur on initiation of the transfusion, but have been known to occur up to 12 hours posttransfusion.

Signs and Symptoms

Signs and symptoms that may be present during a transfusion reaction include fever and chills, which then may progress to more serious complications such as tachycardia, tachypnea, and hypotension.

Nursing Care

With the increased use of leukocyte-depleted blood products, this type of reaction has diminished. Premedication with acetaminophen (Children's Tylenol) sometimes can prevent this type of adverse reaction. An important nursing care measure includes monitoring the child's temperature to recognize febrile reactions early and prevent progression. If the child is having a febrile response, the nurse must immediately stop the transfusion, monitor vital signs closely, and notify the physician.

ALLERGIC REACTION

Another type of nonhemolytic reaction is an allergic reaction. This reaction occurs during a transfusion in which the child has had a previous exposure to a particular allergen in the blood product. The exposure to this allergen stimulates an antibody response and an allergic transfusion reaction is then evident. An allergic reaction may occur on the second or subsequent transfusions.

Signs and Symptoms

Signs and symptoms may include rash, hives, pruritus, swelling of the lips, wheezing, and anxiety.

Nursing Care

If the nurse suspects an allergic reaction, stop the transfusion immediately, monitor vital signs closely, and notify the physician. In most cases, the administration of an antihistamine such as diphenhydramine (Benadryl) resolves an allergic response. An histamine blocker such as raniti-dine (Zantac) may be administered to aid in relieving the symptoms of a reaction. In severe allergic reactions, the child may require the administration of steroids such as hydrocortisone (Solu-Cortef) and possibly adrenaline (epinephrine). For future transfusions for this child, pro-phylaxis care may be required with diphenhydramine (Benadryl) and hydrocortisone (Solu-Cortef).

BACTERIAL CONTAMINATION

Bacterial contamination is a rare nonhemolytic reaction that generally occurs during the initiation of the infusion. The actual contamination of the blood product can occur anywhere during the process of collection, storage, and administration. Guidelines from the AABB (2004) require strict adherence to the completion of all transfusions in 4 hours or less to prevent this from happening. There are strict guidelines for blood collection centers on screening of potential donors, collection, and storage of blood products.

Signs and Symptoms

Signs and symptoms that may occur during a transfusion of blood that is contaminated are shaking chills, fever, vomiting, diffuse erythema, and the onset of hypotension that may progress to shock. In severe cases hemoglobin-uria, actual renal failure, and DIC may develop.

Nursing Care

If any of the signs and symptoms are identified the nurse must stop the transfusion immediately, monitor vital signs closely, start a normal saline infusion, notify the physician, and prepare emergency care (support oxygen-ation and ventilation, antibiotics, and vasopressors may be ordered). Nursing responsibilities include obtaining blood samples for culture and sensitivity and sending the blood product with tubing to the blood bank also to be cultured.

CIRCULATORY OVERLOAD

Circulatory overload is a rare occurrence. This reaction occurs when the infusion is given too rapidly or an exces-sive quantity of blood is given.

Signs and Symptoms

Signs and symptoms may include dry cough, dyspnea, rales, distended neck veins, hypertension/hypotension, bradycardia/tachycardia, clammy skin, and cyanosis of the extremities.

Nursing Care

The nurse understands the importance of accurate verifi-cation of physician orders, double-checking the volume to be infused, and the use of an intravenous pump. The nurse must be aware of children on fluid restriction and the accuracy of intake and output. If any of the signs and symptoms are identified, the nurse must immediately stop the transfusion, monitor vital signs closely, place the child upright with feet in a dependent position to increase venous resistance, notify physician, and prepare emer-gency care (support oxygenation and ventilation as well as diuretics may be ordered).

ACUTE HEMOLYTIC TRANSFUSION REACTION

Acute hemolytic transfusion reaction is rare but it is the most severe type of reaction. It occurs when the donor RBCs and the recipient plasma are incompatible, and there is an ABO mismatch. Acute hemolytic transfusion reactions occur upon initiation after exposure to a small amount of blood (Hillman et al., 2005).

Signs and Symptoms

Symptoms may include fever, shaking chills, pain at the intravenous site, tightness of the chest, difficulties breath-ing, impending sense of doom, pallor, jaundice, nausea/vomiting, red or black urine, flank pain, and progressive signs of shock such as tachycardia and hypotension.

Nursing Care

If any of the signs and symptoms are identified, the nurse must immediately stop the transfusion, monitor vital signs closely, start a normal saline infusion, verify patient iden-tification, notify the physician, and prepare emergency care (support oxygenation and ventilation, antihistamines, fluids, diuretics, and vasopressors may be ordered). Other nursing responsibilities include obtaining blood and urine samples and sending them to the laboratory to analyze for the presence of hemoglobin, which indicates intravascular hemolysis. Insert a urinary catheter to monitor the child's output more accurately.

 Nursing Insight— *Teaching parents*

For children receiving blood transfusions, thorough teach-ing by the nurse to the child and parents is essential to ease anxiety. The first transfusion of a blood product may be fright-ening for the child. If available, the use of a child life therapist to provide developmentally appropriate medical play could assist the child in understanding this required treatment. The nurse must alert parents to be aware of the signs and symptoms of an adverse reaction and to report any possible reaction signs and symptoms immediately. Teaching by the nurse is tailored specifically to the type of blood product being administered.

 Be sure to— Transfusion reaction procedure and documentation

For any transfusion reaction, the nurse must be aware of the appropriate procedure and documentation required by the institution when an adverse reaction occurs. The nurse can check specific institutional policies and procedures about transfusion reactions. Documentation may include completing a blood transfusion reaction form and submit-ting an incident report.

 clinical alert

Transfusion-related acute lung injury

A 2001 letter from the Food and Drug Administration (FDA) issued an alert to clinicians about transfusion-related acute lung injury (TRALI) (U.S. Food and Drug Administration, 2002). In 2003, TRALI was the most frequent cause of transfusion-related deaths

(FDA Patient Safety, 2004). This complication occurs when there is an antigen–antibody reaction. This is not characterized as the typical allergic reaction. The causes of TRALI reactions are the antibodies that are found in the donated blood. These are antibodies to human leukocytes. The donor antibodies are infused to the patient and begin to attach to the patient's white blood cells and form microaggregates. These microaggregates often end up in the lungs, which may result in a vascular permeability, pulmonary edema, and life-threatening events (Knippen, 2006).

The child who is experiencing TRALI may develop respiratory distress such as shortness of breath, hypoxia, hypotension, fever, and abnormal breath sounds. The reaction typically occurs within 1–2 hours after the transfusion has started and full-blown acute respiratory distress may occur within 6 hours (Knippen, 2006).

Based on the severity of symptoms, respiratory support with a ventilator may be indicated. For mild cases of TRALI, supportive care is indicated. If this complication is suspected, it is reportable to the FDA (U.S. Food and Drug Administration, 2002).

Bone Marrow Transplantation

Hematopoietic stem cell transplant (HSCT) is the treatment for some types of oncological illnesses and hematological diseases. There are several types of hematological diseases in which hematopoietic stem cell transplant (HSCT) may be a treatment option. For instance, a child newly diagnosed with severe aplastic anemia who has an HLA-matched sibling donor may proceed immediately to transplant as curative treatment. Children with other hematological disorders who have severe sequela, such as sickle cell disease with multiple complications such as cerebral vascular accidents (CVA) and acute chest syndromes, may also be candidates to undergo a HSCT. Children who require chronic transfusion therapy may also have the indications for HSCT such as beta-thalassemia and Diamond Blackfan anemia. Some genetic and autoimmune diseases are now being treated with hematopoietic stem cell transplant.

In these conditions, a large volume of actual bone marrow is harvested and bone marrow transplantation (BMT) is performed. The preparative BMT regimen consists of the administration of "near lethal" doses of chemotherapy and/or radiation to ablate the diseased bone marrow. This preparative regimen results in severe myelosuppression and places the child at grave risk for infection.

After the preparative regimen the bone marrow is surgically obtained and then infused through a central line. On the day of the transplant, also known as day "0," the child is given an intravenous infusion of stem cells as a "rescue" and the waiting for engraftment (when the donated cells start to grow and make new blood cells). This treatment is not without potential risks, including death. Proceeding with this type of therapy may have lifelong consequences for the patient and his or her family.

 Nursing Insight— *Hematopoietic stem cell transplants (HSCT)*

There are three types of hematopoietic stem cell transplants.

In an **autologous transplant,** the ill child is his or her own donor of stem cells. These donor stem cells are obtained by harvesting the child's cells through peripheral access or directly from the bone marrow cavity. This method is not used in hematological diseases because hematological illnesses originate in the bone marrow.

In an **allogeneic transplant,** the recipient's human leukocyte antigens (HLAs) are matched to a compatible donor, usually a sibling. The sibling must be tested by a thorough genetic investigation to determine if he or she is a carrier of the same hematological illness as the patient or is a compatible match before the transplant can occur. In other cases, the allogeneic donor is an unrelated donor but is someone who has been identified from the National Marrow Donor Program. Umbilical cord blood stem cell transplant is another allogeneic type of transplant. These rich stem cells are obtained from the childbirth process immediately after delivery of the infant. The ability to obtain stem cells in this manner is a viable alternative that recently became available.

In a **syngeneic transplant,** the donor of the bone marrow is an identical sibling.

 Nursing Insight— *Hematological diseases cured by hematopoietic stem cell transplant (HSCT)*

Severe aplastic anemia
Beta-thalassemia
Sickle cell disease
Fanconi anemia
Kostmann's disease
Diamond Blackfan anemia

The child with a hematological illness who receives a HSCT must be prepared to live with potential complications. The majority of these children receive the HSCT from an unrelated donor. This carries a greater risk of long-term complications such as acute and chronic graft versus host disease (GVHD). Other complications that may occur can be a result of the preparative regimen from the chemotherapy or radiation. Additional complications may result from infections, immunosuppression, organ dysfunction, and psychosocial impact.

Apheresis

Some children with hematological diseases may require apheresis as part of their treatment plan. The name of the apheresis procedure is identified according to a specific blood component that is extracted. This process usually takes place in the hospital setting with specially trained staff. In most institutions, children must be greater than 11 lbs. (5 kg).

The process of apheresis is the selective removal of a specific blood component from a donor or child while retransfusing the remaining components. The ultimate goal in using apheresis therapy is to deplete or collect a circulating cell or substance. Blood is removed from the child, pumped through a special cell separator in the apheresis machine that removes the specific desired component by centrifugal force, and then is returned to the patient. The mechanics of the apheresis machine are comparable to those of a dialysis machine and require two large-bore lines, one line to draw from and another to return the blood.

Nursing Insight— Pheresis

There are three types of pheresis.

Plasmapheresis is removal of plasma containing harmful components such as circulating complexes, antibodies (IgM, IgG), cholesterol, and toxins. Plasma alone is depleted from the child's blood and replaced by donor plasma or a plasma substitute that is reinfused along with the child's own RBCs, WBCs, and platelets. Critically ill patients who have conditions such as thrombotic thrombocytopenic purpura (TTP), meningococcemia, toxic ingestion, hemolytic uremic syndrome, Guillain–Barré syndrome, and systemic lupus erythematosus may require a plasmapheresis.

Erythrocytapheresis (Red Cell Exchange)

In erythrocytapheresis (red cell exchange), RBCs are removed from the patient's blood and replaced by leukocyte depleted donor red blood cells which are reinfused to the patient along with the patient's own plasma, WBCs, and platelets. Sickle cell anemia with acute chest syndrome, CVA, or severe priapism may require red cell exchange.

Leukapheresis (Stem Cell Collection or Leukodepletion)

The purpose of stem cell collection is to harvest an adequate amount of stem cells/mononuclear cells as noted by a countable marker on the white cell called a CD34 antigen. Based on the disease or reason for collecting, there may be multiple sessions in order to collect sufficient targeted cells. These mononuclear cells (monocytes) are involved in the body's immune responses. The collected stem cells are processed by the blood service and are cryopreserved in liquid nitrogen for future use. These stem cells are reinfused at a later specific date after the preparative regimen has ablated the bone marrow. Patients with solid tumors are the usual candidates to have their own stem cells removed, treated, and reinfused. Another procedure that may be used to remove excess white blood cells is leukodepletion. Leukodepletion is primarily used for patients with high white blood cell counts such as patients newly diagnosed with acute or chronic leukemia, or at risk for acute tumor lysis syndrome. Complications may develop during the apheresis process (Table 33-6).

Table 33-6 Complications of Apheresis	
Complication	**Critical Nursing Actions**
Hypocalcemia	Obtain ionized calcium levels before treatment. Correct all abnormal levels before initiating treatment.
	For apheresis lasting longer than one hour, ionized calcium levels should be monitored every hour until the end of the procedure.
	Consider calcium drip if needed:
	• Calcium chloride: 20–25 mg/kg per dose used for acute hypocalcemia
	• Calcium gluconate: 100–500 mg/kg per day
	(Robertson & Shilkofski, 2005)
Hypotension	Hypotension may occur with onset of treatment. Be sure to have fluid readily available at the bedside. Patients receiving inotropic support may need an increase in the rate of administration.
Risk for Bleeding	Prothrombin time (PT), partial thromboplastin time (PTT), fibrinogen level, platelet count, Hct, and activated clotting time (ACT) are measured before and after apheresis.
	ACT should be measured at the bedside at regular intervals, and citrate and/or heparin doses adjusted accordingly.
	Platelet or other blood products such as clotting factors may be required during the procedure.
Hypothermia	Hypothermia may result from the blood being circulated in the extracorporeal circuit outside the body.
	• Utilize blood warmer on pheresis machine.
	• Monitor frequent temperatures to avoid hypothermia.
	• Assess patient for other signs of hypothermia such as bradycardia and shivering.
	• Keep child warm with blankets and/or external warmer.
	• Increase ambient room temperature.
Transfusion Reaction	Utilize leukodepleted blood.
	Monitor for transfusion reactions from the replacement products. Follow the transfusion reaction protocol if this occurs.
	Consider administration of an antihistamine for patients receiving multiple treatments.
Infection	Maintain strict sterile technique with all intravenous lines.
Air Embolism	Monitor tubing and connection sites. Check that all are secured properly.
Thrombus	Obtain platelet count before catheter placement and be aware when possible transfusion of platelets are necessary.
	Flush vigorously with adequate volumes of normal saline as per institutional policy.

Thrombosis

A possible hematological complication for patients with chronic illness includes the development of a thrombosis (blood clot). A thrombosis is an abnormal formation of blood constituents within the vascular system. Thrombi can be caused by a variety of factors such as prolonged immobility, disease states, major surgery or trauma, hypercoagulability, venous access devices, obesity, medications, and hereditary factors. Additional complications of thrombi include stroke, deep vein thrombosis, and pulmonary emboli. Certain disease states promote a higher incidence of thrombi, such as sickle cell anemia, malignancies, and diseases of coagulation.

Signs and Symptoms

A blood clot in the lungs causes a sudden pain in the side of the chest, shortness of breath, lightheadedness, or increased heart rate. If blood appears in the urine there may be a blood clot in the kidneys. In the skin, small hemorrhagic spots may appear. If there is a blood clot in a large artery of an extremity (arm or leg), an obstruction occurs and the extremity becomes cold, pale, blue, and the pulse disappears below the obstructed site (Venes, 2009).

Diagnosis

Diagnosis is based on a nursing assessment of the lungs, urine, and skin or red, swollen, or tender extremity. A venogram (an x-ray test that shows the blood flow through the veins) is used as well as a Doppler ultrasound exam of a limb. A D-dimer blood test is also drawn.

Nursing Care

Nursing care for children with hematological diseases includes obtaining a thorough assessment of the child's risk factors for developing a thrombus. When caring for a child at risk for thrombosis a prophylactic plan of care should be individualized for each child's condition and interventions should be reviewed daily for effectiveness. All children on prolonged bedrest and those at high risk should have prophylaxis care which may include compression stockings, intermittent pneumatic compression devices, and passive range of motion. Compression stockings and intermittent pneumatic compression devices are usually used on the lower extremities. These assistive devices may promote increased venous flow and decreased venous pooling and stasis. These devices can be discontinued when the patient is ambulatory. Nursing assessment must also include a thorough skin assessment under the stocking and compression device to evaluate for redness or skin breakdown. Implementing early ambulation when appropriate is an additional preventive measure. Some children may benefit from the administration of low molecular weight heparin therapy (Vedantham, 2006).

The most serious complication associated with thrombi is the possibility of developing pulmonary emboli (sudden blockage) that can result in a life-threatening event. Deep venous thrombosis (DVT) occurs less often in children than in adults, but when it does, it has the same potential for pulmonary embolization and death (Koschel, 2004). Institutions should implement formal protocols to identify children at risk for thrombolytic events and implement preventive measures.

summary points

◆ Blood is composed of two parts, the fluid portion called plasma and the cellular portion. The solutes include albumin, electrolytes, proteins, clotting factors, fibrinogen, globulins, and circulating antibodies. The cellular portion consists of the formed elements: red blood cells, white blood cells, and platelets.

◆ Several common hematological conditions occur in children. Some of these conditions can be acute in nature and with proper care can be easily eliminated. However, others can be life-threatening or cause a chronic illness that can permanently impact the lifestyle of the child and his or her family.

◆ The nurse can stress to the parents that the primary goal with regard to iron-deficiency anemia is prevention. Nursing care consists of nutritional counseling, assistance with obtaining recommended iron-fortified formula/ cereal, and the administration of oral iron supplements.

◆ Children and families affected by sickle cell disease must learn to cope with lifelong chronic illness. The community-based nurse can educate the family about the goals of ongoing care including the prevention of complications associated with infections, hypoxemia, and vaso-occlusive crisis.

◆ Since there is no known cure for hemophilia the nurse can teach the family about how to care for the child with hemophilia. If the treatment regimen is followed, these children can live long and productive lives.

◆ Aplastic anemia is rare but one of the most serious hematological conditions that generally afflicts adolescents and young adults. This clinical syndrome is characterized by pancytopenia (a reduction in all cellular elements of the blood) caused by bone marrow hematopoiesis failure.

◆ The child who has neutropenia, whether it is congenital or acquired, will need specific teaching on management. First and foremost, the nurse can teach the importance of hand washing.

◆ The first responsibility of the nurse who is administering a blood transfusion to a child is to review the plan of care with the family, explain in detail the indications and process of a blood transfusion, and then obtain blood consent from the appropriate individual.

◆ During every transfusion the importance of strict observance to the institutional policy regarding the administration of blood products cannot be stressed enough. In addition, the accuracy of patient verification is a critical nursing action that prevents this type of acute hemolytic transfusion reaction.

◆ Some children with hematological diseases may require apheresis as part of their treatment plan. The process of apheresis is the selective removal of a specific blood component from a donor or child while retransfusing the remaining components.

◆ A possible hematological complication for patients with chronic illness includes the development of a thrombosis. A thrombosis is an abnormal formation of blood constituents within the vascular system.

review questions

Multiple Choice

1. During an assessment, the pediatric nurse finds the child to be short of breath, tachycardic, pale, and irritable. The mother reports the child also has been easily fatigued. When examining the child's complete blood count, the nurse notes:
   A. An increase in red blood cells
   B. An increase in platelets
   C. A decrease in red blood cells
   D. A decrease in white blood cells

2. After a sickle cell crisis, the family requires health promotion teaching before discharge. The pediatric nurse should include which of the following in the teaching plan about sickle cell crisis? (*Select all that apply.*)
   A. Call the pediatrician when the child has a fever above 101.5°F (38.6°C).
   B. Increase the child's fluid intake during a sickle cell crisis.
   C. Administer acetaminophen (Children's Tylenol) for pain.
   D. Encourage the child to rest during a sickle cell crisis.

3. The pediatric nurse teaches the parents of a newly diagnosed child with hemophilia important health promotion aspects. (*Select all that apply.*)
   A. Apply pressure to a bleeding injury.
   B. Administer acetylsalicylic acid (Children's Aspirin) for pain and swelling.
   C. Apply ice to the injury and elevate an extremity.
   D. Encourage the child to return to normal activities.

4. The pediatric nurse who works in a clinic with adolescents realizes that there is knowledge deficit when a 16-year-girl old says:
   A. "I take my iron supplements every night with a cup of hot tea."
   B. "Since I have become a vegetarian, I must eat whole grains and nuts."
   C. "I take my iron pill with a glass of orange juice every morning."
   D. "Since I have been taking iron pills, I've noticed that my stools are dark in color."

5. When planning care for a child with aplastic anemia, the pediatric nurse is aware of which of the following? (*Select all that apply.*)
   A. The child is at risk for bleeding due to thrombocytopenia.
   B. Invasive procedures such as taking a rectal temperature should be avoided.
   C. When the child is feeling well, it is important for the child to play.
   D. Anaphylactic precautions are set up before the administration of antithymocyte globulin.

True/False

6. The symptoms associated with idiopathic or immune thrombocytopenia purpura can be mistaken for signs of child abuse.

7. Children with sickle cell anemia have increased hemoglobin S.

8. Children with hereditary spherocytosis should receive the Hib vaccine (*Haemophilus influenzae* type b) and the pneumococcal vaccine following a splenectomy in order to prevent life-threatening bacterial infections.

9. When a child has a blood disorder, a signed consent from parents is not necessary before administering blood products.

Fill-in-the-Blank

10. A rise in the _____ _____ is an indicator of red blood cell production.

11. An accumulation of iron, termed _____, can be treated with a _____ agent.

Matching

Match the term with the correct definition.

12. Purpura
13. Thrombocytopenia
14. Hemarthrosis
15. Splenomegaly
16. Priapism
17. Dactylitis
18. Pluripotent stem cell

   a. Bloody effusion within a joint
   b. Painful and continuous penile erection
   c. "Mother cell" which gives rise to all other cell lines
   d. Hand–foot syndrome
   e. Discoloration beneath the skin caused by petechiae
   f. Decrease in the number of the platelets
   g. Enlarged spleen

See Answers to End of Chapter Review Questions on the Electronic Study Guide or DavisPlus.

REFERENCES

American Association of Blood Banks (AABB) Guidelines. (2004). Bethesda, MD: AABB Press.

Allan, G., & Glader, B. (2002). Approach to the bleeding child. *Pediatric Clinics of North America, 49*, 1239–1256.

Becker, A.J., McCulloch, E.A., & Till, J.E. (1963). Cytological demonstration of the clonal nature of spleen colonies derived from transplanted mouse marrow cells. *Nature, 197*, 452–454.

Bulechek, G., Butcher, H.M., & Dochterman, J. (2008). *Nursing interventions classification (NIC)* (5th ed.). St. Louis, MO: C.V. Mosby.

Deglin, J.H. & Vallerand, A.H. (2009). *Davis's drug guide for nures* (11th ed.). Philadelphia: F.A. Davis.

Di Paola, J., & Buchanan, G.R. (2002). Immune thrombocytopenic purpura. *Pediatric Clinics of North America, 49*, 911–928.

FDA Patient safety news October 2004.

Fixler, J., & Styles, L. (2002). Sickle cell disease. *Pediatric Clinics of North America, 49*, 1193–1210.

Geerts, W., Cook, D., Selby, R., & Etchells, E. (2002). Venous thromboembolism and its preventions in critical care. *Journal of Critical Care, 17*(2), 95–104.

Gilbert-Barness, E., & Barness, L. (2003). *Clinical use of pediatric diagnostic tests.* Philadelphia: Lippincott Williams & Wilkins.

Hermiston, M., & Mentzer, W. (2002). A practical approach to the evaluation of the anemic child. *Pediatric Clinics of North of America, 49*, 877–891.

Hillman, R.S., Ault, K.A., & Rinder, H.M. (2005). *Hematology in clinical practice: A guide to diagnosis and management.* New York: McGraw-Hill.

Johnson, M., Bulechek, G., Butcher, H., McCloskey Dochterman, J., Maas, M., Moorehead, S., & Swanson, E. (2006). *NANDA, NOC, and*

NIC linkages: Nursing diagnoses, outcomes, & interventions (2nd ed.). St. Louis, MO: Mosby Elsevier.

Khilnani, P. (2005). *Practical approach to pediatric intensive care.* Oxford University Press: New York.

Knippen, M. (2006). Transfusion-related acute lung injury. *AJN, 106*(6), 61–64.

Koschel, M. (2004). Pulmonary embolism: Quick diagnosis can save a patient's life. *AJN, 104*(6), 46–50.

Kucik, C.J., & Clenney, T. (2005). Management of epistaxis. *American Family Physician, 71*(2), 305–311.

Lea, D., & Williams, J. (2002). Genetic testing and screening, use them as part of routine nursing practice. *American Journal of Nursing, 102*(7), 36–43.

Linnard-Palmar, L., & Kools, S. (2004). Parents' refusal of medical treatment based on religious and/or cultural beliefs: The law, ethical principles and clinical implications. *Journal of Pediatric Nursing, 19*(5), 351–356.

Lo, L., & Singer, S. (2002). Thalassemia: current approach to an old disease. *Pediatric Clinics of North America, 49,* 1165–1191.

Martin, M., Foote, D., & Carson, S. (2004). Help your patient meet the challenges of beta thalassemia major. *Nursing 2004, 34*(10), 32–34.

Moorehead, S., Johnson, M., Maas, M., & Swanson, E. (2008). *Nursing outcomes classification (NOC)* (4th ed.). St. Louis, MO: C.V. Mosby.

NANDA International (2007). *NANDA-I nursing diagnoses: Definitions and classifications 2007–2008.* Philadelphia: NANDA-I.

Nathan, D.G., Orkin, S.H., Ginsburg, D., & Look, A.T. (2003). *Nathan and Oski's hematology of infancy and childhood* (6th ed.). Philadelphia: W.B. Saunders.

Robertson, J., & Shilkofski, N. (2005). *The Harriet Lane handbook* (17th ed.). Philadelphia: Elsevier Mosby.

Sapountzi-Krepia, D., Roupa, Z., Gourni, M., Mastorakou, F., Vojiatzi, E., Kouyioumtzi, A., & Van Shell, S. (2006). A qualitative study on the experiences of mothers caring for their children with Thalassemia in Athens, Greece. *Journal of Pediatric Nursing, 21*(2), 142–152.

Sevier, N. (2005). Inherited coagulation factor abnormalities: A pediatric review. *Journal of Pediatric Oncology Nursing, 22*(3), 137–144.

Sevier, N., & Houston, M. (2005). Chronic refractory ITP in children; Beyond splenectomy. *Journal of Pediatric Oncology Nursing, 22*(3), 145–151.

Sickle Cell Disease Association of America. Retrieved from www.sicklecelldisease.org (Accessed November 26, 2008).

Stevens, R. (1999). The history of haemophilia in the royal families of Europe. *British Journal of Haematology, 105*(1), 25–32.

Turgeon, M.L. (2005). *Clinical hematology: Theory and procedures* (4th ed.). Philadelphia: Lippincott Williams & Wilkins.

US Food and Drug Administration (2002). Current good manufacturing practice for blood and blood components: Adverse reaction file. Title 21 part 606.170(b).

Vedantham, S. (2006). Fending off the risky complications of DVT. *The Clinical Advisor* (May), 26–33.

Venes, D. (Ed.). (2009). *Taber's cyclopedic medical dictionary* (21st ed.). Philadelphia: F.A. Davis.

DavisPlus
DavisPlus.fadavis.com **For more information, go to http://davisplus.fadavis.com/**

CONCEPT MAP

Caring for the Child with a Hematological Condition

Anemias

Types of Anemias
- Iron deficiency
  - Microcytic or hypochromic
- Sickle cell
  - Autosomal recessive linked
  - HbA replaced by HbS
- Beta-thalassemia
  - Deficiency in globin chain
  - Most commonly inherited genetic condition
- Hereditary spherocytosis
  - Inherited hemolytic anemia
  - Deficiency of spectrin

Aplastic Anemia
- Bone marrow hematopoiesis failure
- Leads to pancytopenia

Child with Anemia: General Nursing Care
- Identify underlying cause
- Prevention, early ID and treatment of any related hypoxic episodes
- Supportive care: diet; vitamins/supplements; hydration; transfusions
- Family teaching: signs and symptoms; activity management/prevention

Critical Nursing Action:
- Educate family re: oral iron
- Several ways to manage epistaxis depending on degree
- Pneumococcal and Hib vaccines critical in HS
- Teaching family how to prevent infection in neutropenic child
- Strictly adhere to transfusion policies

What To Say:
- Nutrition counseling important in iron deficiency anemia
- Teach family how ITP is diagnosed

Neutropenia
- ANC less than 1000 < 1 yr
- ANC less than 1500 < 1 yr
- Acquired or congenital

Child with Neutropenia: Potential Nursing Care
- Determine the cause: guides care
- Implement supportive measures
- Possible use of colony-stimulating factors
- Possible bone marrow transplant

Nursing Insight:
- There are several causes of anemia and children can be asymptomatic
- Inheritance of sickle cell anemia depends on parental genotypes
- There are 3 forms of beta-thalassemia
- The degree of neutropenia is measured by the ANC
- Symptoms of aplastic anemia depend on degree of pancytopenia

Clinical Alert:
- Overweight infants can have iron deficiency anemia
- Asplenic child is at risk for sepsis
- Multiple RBC transfusions increase risk for hemosiderosis
- Special considerations for IV Anti-D antibody
- The most severe complication of ITP is a possible intracranial bleed
- Know nursing responsibilities during transfusions

Across Care Settings:
- WIC program has decreased the incidence of iron deficiency anemia
- Education about SCD: ongoing chronic lifetime disease

Now Can You:
- Correctly evaluate a CBC
- Provide care to a child with a nosebleed
- Identify the nursing responsibilities related to blood transfusion therapy
- Discuss the nursing care of a child with a hematologic condition

Bleeding Disorders

Types
- Epistaxis: nosebleed
- Hemophilia
  - Congenital deficiency of factor VIII (A): factor IX (B)
- von Willebrand's disease
- ITP
  - most frequently seen thrombocytopenia in childhood
  - possibly disease-mediated autoimmune process
- ITP
  - secondary to an underlying disease → i.e., sepsis, trauma

Child with Bleeding Disorder: Potential Nursing Care
- Prevent bleeding when possible
- Promote prompt treatment of bleeding episode
- Potential administration of:
  - Replacement factors
  - IVIG; Anti-D antibody
  - Desmopressin
- Splenectomy → treatment for life-threatening bleeding episodes
- Family teaching: safety, management of bleeding
- Potential transfusions: blood, platelets

Where Research And Practice Meet:
- Single stem cell research

Ethnocultural Considerations:
- 8% of African Americans carry Sickle cell trait
- Historically, hemophilia was prominent in European royalty
- Jehovah Witness opposed to receiving blood

chapter 34

Caring for the Child with Cancer

 Once you choose hope, anything is possible.

—Christopher Reeve

LEARNING TARGETS *At the completion of this chapter, the student will be able to:*

◆ Identify the common pediatric cancers.

◆ Understand the incidence and etiology of pediatric cancers.

◆ Describe the signs and symptoms of pediatric cancers.

◆ Explain diagnostic criteria for pediatric cancers.

◆ Explore nursing care for the pediatric cancer patient.

◆ Discuss the negative and long-term effects of chemotherapy for the pediatric cancer patient.

◆ Describe medical emergencies for the pediatric cancer patient.

◆ Examine the psychological impact of pediatric cancer.

---

 moving toward evidence-based practice Quality of Life in Children with Cancer

Yeh, C.H., Chang, C.W., & Chang, P.C. (2005). Evaluating the quality of life in children with cancer using children's self-reports and parent-proxy reports. *Nursing Research, 54*(5), 354–362.

Major advances in cancer treatment outcomes and improved survival rates make the assessment of quality of life an important concern for parents and nurses. Literature cited in this study supports the belief that proxy reports tend to have greater validity with measures of objective assessments (i.e., physical findings) than with subjective assessments such as depression and anxiety.

The purpose of the study was to explore the level of agreement about quality of life measures as self-reported by children and parent-proxy reports at two specified points in time: initially and at a 6-month follow-up.

The longitudinal study included 126 children ages 7–18 (75 children; 51 adolescents) previously diagnosed with cancer and at least one parent. The Quality of Life for Children with Cancer (QOLCC), an instrument that consists of 34 items, measures the following constructs: (1) disease state and physical symptoms; (2) physical function; (3) psychological function; (4) social function; (5) cognitive function; and (6) communication and understanding.

According to the study findings, a better quality of life for the child was reported by parents more often than by the children at both the initial and the 6-month measurement.

The investigators concluded that the parent-proxy report is not a valid tool for determining the child's perceived quality of life when the child is unable to self-report.

---

1. Based on the above synopsis, what additional data could be collected to expand the scope of this study?
2. How is this information useful to clinical nursing practice?

See Suggested Responses for Moving Toward Evidence-Based Practice on the Electronic Study Guide or DavisPlus.

Introduction

Cancer is a group of diseases in which there is out of control growth and spread of abnormal cells (anaplasia). Anaplastic cells resist normal growth controls. This abnormal cellular growth is also known as a neoplasm and is caused by one or a combination of three factors: (1) external stimuli or environment, (2) viruses that can alter the immune system and let the cancer grow, and (3) chromosomal and gene abnormalities.

 Nursing Insight— *Cell division*

Normal cells divide in an orderly fashion through the four phases of cell division. Normal cells have a control mechanism that stops division when it is complete. Cancer cells have no control mechanism as they keep dividing and replicating unchecked without stopping.

 Nursing Insight— *Oncogenes*

An oncogene is a gene found in a virus that has the ability to encourage a cell to become malignant (Venes, 2009).

A tumor is a mass of abnormally growing cells that is either benign (not cancerous), with slow and limited noninvasive growth, or malignant (cancerous), a progressively virulent growth. Cancerous growths are divided further into solid tumors (i.e., a brain tumor) and systemic cancers such as leukemia. Cancer is second only to accidents as the leading cause of death among children. It is important for the nurse to understand the terms associated with cancer (Box 34-1).

Box 34-1 Terms Associated with the Cancer Patient

Roadmap—protocol or treatment plan that is "mapped out" to guide staff and families through the treatment course.

Protocol—complete explanation of a treatment plan, includes background, drug dosages and timing, protocol requirements like tests and laboratory specimens.

Clinical trials—medical research studies conducted with volunteers. Each study is designed to answer scientific questions and to find new ways to treat cancer.

Remission—the partial or complete disappearance of signs and symptoms of disease. This does not mean "cancer free." There could still be cancer cells that are undetectable in the body. Treatment will continue during this time.

Extravasation—leaking of potentially tissue damaging medications surrounding the injection site. May cause blistering, blanching, or excoriation that may lead to ulcer and deep skin sloughing.

Induction—chemotherapy given to achieve remission.

Consolidation—chemotherapy given after induction to control microscopic disease.

Maintenance—chemotherapy given on a long-term basis to maintain remission.

Palliative care—treatment given to relieve rather than cure symptoms caused by cancer. Supportive care services are usually involved. The patient may still receive chemotherapy or radiation.

 A & P review Pattern of Tumor Progression

A tumor originates as a single transformed cell somewhere in the body. That cell must undergo a long process of growth and development before it can form a tumor. The cell also undergoes countless divisions to form a mass that may be made up of a billion cells at the time of diagnosis. Tumor cells have very stringent constraints placed upon them as they grow. Each of the newly created cells must have a steady supply of nutrients to keep growing. While the tumor may not be directly next to a capillary, it may be close enough so that oxygen and nutrients can diffuse through tissue to tumor cells. If the tumor receives a continuous supply of nutrients and blood, it grows and invades surrounding tissue. Once a tumor grows past its critical phase it induces growth of new blood vessels into the tumor mass. It can then grow much more rapidly and produce a clinically detectable tumor. If a tumor does not receive adequate blood supply and nutrients it can die. A tumor lacking a sufficient blood supply can also remain dormant for years and not grow beyond a certain size. ◆

 Nursing Insight— *Gene therapy*

The use of gene therapy is complex and in the early stages of usage for cancer patients. Gene therapy is used to understand and treat the genetic mutations that cause disease. The goal of gene therapy is to correct a genetic defect by inserting healthy copies of missing or altered genes into the defective gene (Alcoster & Rodgers, 2003). Exploring the potential benefits of gene therapy for cancer patients is proceeding cautiously.

Differences Between Childhood and Adult Cancers

Anatomically and physiologically, cancers in children differ greatly from the types of cancer occurring in adults. In children many common malignancies arise from primitive embryonic tissue where there has been a strong environmental link related to the development of cancer.

---

where research and practice meet:
Epstein–Barr Virus and Nasopharyngeal Carcinoma

Nasopharyngeal carcinoma primarily involves the lining of the nasal cavity and pharynx. It is an infrequent cause of childhood cancer. In the United States, the incidence of this tumor is approximately one in 100,000 persons younger than the age of 20, but there is a higher frequency of the tumor in North Africa and Southeast Asia. Nasopharyngeal carcinoma occurs in association with Epstein–Barr virus (EBV) infection. The virus can be detected in biopsy specimens of nasopharyngeal carcinoma, and tumor cells may have EBV antigens on their cell surface. Research is ongoing. A study by Ozyar et al. in 2004 examined 166 patients. The researchers were unable to prove a prognostically significant role of the presence of the EBV latent protein-1 and interleukin-10 expression in patients with nasopharyngeal carcinoma.

The cure rate for childhood cancers is better than for adults. The 5-year survival rate for children is 79% for those diagnosed from 1995 to 2000 as compared to 56% for children diagnosed in 1974 to 1976. The 5-year survival rate for adults has increased to 64% for all types of cancer (Jemel et al., 2005). Children tend to get cancers that affect stem cells. Adults primarily get cancers of epithelial cells, highly differentiated cells that line body cavities or cover the body surface. Pediatric cancers tend to be more aggressive and faster growing than adult cancers. They also respond more readily to chemotherapy and radiation, which target dividing cells. In comparison with adults, sometimes children with cancer are not treated locally but are referred to major cancer centers in the United States that are more familiar with research study protocols and treatment regimens. Children are also generally more resilient than adults and can tolerate more aggressive therapy. Many adults have other physiological problems that can complicate treatment.

 Now Can You— **Discuss cancer in children?**

1. Describe the pattern of tumor progression?
2. Differentiate the differences between childhood and adult cancers?

Common Childhood Cancers

LEUKEMIA

The term leukemia refers to the cancers of the blood-forming cells or hematopoiesis. There are two types of blood-forming cells: myeloid and lymphoid. Myeloid cells differentiate and form into red blood cells, monocytes, granulocytes, and platelets (Fig. 34-1). Lymphoid cells differentiate and form into B cells and T cells. In leukemia, normal hematopoiesis (production and development of blood cells) is altered. Immature blood cells multiply at the expense of normal blood cells. These immature blood cells also have a growth advantage over normal cellular elements because of an increased rate of proliferation, a decreased rate of spontaneous apoptosis (cell death), or both (Behrman, Kliegman, &

Jenson, 2004). The immature cells are known as blast cells. Normal bone marrow elements are replaced by large amounts of these immature lymphocytes (blast cells), which causes a "crowding out" of normal red blood cells, platelets, and white blood cells, resulting in pancytopenia (a marked reduction in the number of red blood cells [RBCs], white blood cells [WBCs], and platelets) and immunosuppression. Leukemia can develop at any point during the stages of normal lymphoid or myeloid differentiation in the bone marrow and can spread to the blood, lymph nodes, spleen, liver, central nervous system, or other organs (Colby-Graham & Chordas, 2003).

Classification of leukemia is based on the predominant cell line affected and the level of cellular differentiation. The terms myeloid and lymphoid denote the cell line involved. Both myeloid and lymphoid cell lines can proliferate into acute or chronic forms of leukemia. Acute leukemia is a rapidly progressing disease that affects mostly immature, undifferentiated cells that are not able to perform their normal functions. Chronic leukemia is a less rapidly progressing disease allowing for the production of mature, more differentiated cells. These cells can maintain some of their normal function. The three major classifications of childhood leukemia are acute lymphocytic leukemia, acute myelogenous leukemia, and chronic lymphocytic leukemia (Figs. 34-2 and 34-3). Chronic lymphocytic leukemia is rarely reported in children (Colby-Graham & Chordas, 2003). Juvenile chronic myelogenous leukemia (JCML) is also rare.

Figure 34-2 Dark-stained lymphoblast cells seen in acute lymphocytic leukemia (ALL), the most common type of childhood leukemia.

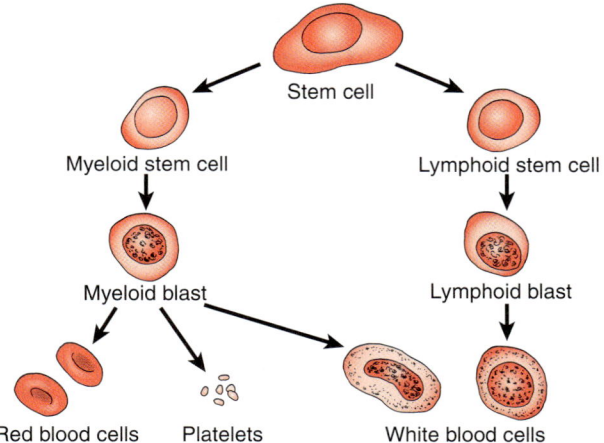

Figure 34-1 Myeloid cells differentiate and form into red blood cells, monocytes, granulocytes, and platelets.

Figure 34-3 Acute myelocytic leukemic cells (AML).

Acute Lymphocytic Leukemia

Acute lymphocytic leukemia (ALL) is the most common type of cancer in children. ALL accounts for 75% to 80% of all childhood leukemias and for approximately one-third of all childhood cancers. Approximately 2800 children are diagnosed with ALL in the United States annually (Behrman et al., 2004). The peak incidence is between 2 and 5 years of age. During infancy, boys are more likely than girls to develop ALL. The leukemic cells usually are acquired versus inherited. However, there is an increased risk among children with certain genetic disorders such as Down syndrome. A variety of factors have been implicated that might predispose children to developing leukemia (Table 34-1).

SIGNS AND SYMPTOMS. The presenting symptoms of ALL vary widely, depending on the degree of infiltration of the bone marrow and other organs by leukemic cells. Most cases have an acute onset, while in others symptoms appear slowly. Fever occurs in approximately 50% of the cases. Fatigue and lethargy are also present. ALL patients have anemia and are therefore pale. Anorexia is usually present. In more than one-third of children with ALL, especially the younger ones, bone or joint pain is present. Parents may notice a limp or the child may refuse to walk. Less common symptoms include headache, vomiting, difficulty in breathing, and low urine output. Bleeding under the skin, in the mouth, or sometimes in the eyes may be present. Petechiae can also be noted. Abdominal distention caused by an enlarged spleen as well as enlarged lymph nodes are present in more than half of the patients. Hepatomegaly may also be present.

DIAGNOSIS. A bone marrow aspirate is required to make the diagnosis of ALL. A finding of more than 25% abnormal lymphoblasts in the bone marrow is diagnostic. Other samples in the bone marrow are sent for further testing that can show chromosomal changes and better identify the specifics of the leukemia. The child's WBC count and age at diagnosis are the most important prognostic signs in ALL. The best prognosis is associated with a WBC count less than 5000/mm³ and an age of 2 to 9 years. The worst prognosis is associated with an initial WBC count of 50,000/mm³ and an age older than 10 years. Infants younger than 1 year of age at the time of diagnosis also have a very poor prognosis.

Table 34-1 Factors Predisposing to Childhood Leukemia	
Genetic Conditions	**Environmental Factors**
Down syndrome	Ionizing radiation
Fanconi syndrome	Drugs
Bloom syndrome	Alkylating agents
Shwachman syndrome	Nitrosourea
Klinefelter syndrome	Epipodophyllotoxin
Turner syndrome	Benzene exposure
Neurofibromatosis	Advanced maternal age
Li–Fraumeni syndrome	
Severe combined immune deficiency	

Infants and patients who present with specific chromosomal abnormalities have a higher risk of relapse despite intensive therapy (Behrman et al., 2004). Lumbar puncture is performed to assess for the presence of central nervous system (CNS) disease and staging of leukemia. A chest radiograph is obtained to detect a mediastinal mass. Laboratory findings show liver or kidney involvement.

 Nursing Insight— *Staging*

Staging describes the severity of the patient's *cancer*. It is the process of classifying tumors in relation to the degree of differentiation, possibility of responding to therapy, and prognosis (Venes, 2009).

Stage 0 indicates early cancer that is present only in the layer of cells in which it began.

Stage I, Stage II, and Stage III indicate more extensive disease, greater tumor size, and/or spread of the cancer to nearby lymph nodes or adjacent organs.

Stage IV indicates that the cancer has spread to another organ(s).

NURSING CARE. Without effective therapy and nursing care, ALL is fatal. Leukemia is treated with chemotherapy and includes three phases: remission-induction, consolidation, and maintenance. In the remission-induction phase, the tumor burden is reduced to an undetectable level. Ninety-five percent of children with ALL achieve remission during induction, which usually lasts 4 weeks. Once remission is achieved, most children relapse within a few months if treatment is stopped.

Chemotherapy agents used for remission-induction are vincristine (Oncovorin), L-asparaginase (Elspar), and prednisone (Deltasone) or dexamethasone (Decadron). Children who have a poorer prognosis are also given an anthracycline drug (chemotherapy drug that is known to affect and damage the heart, such as doxorubicin [Adriamycin]). Children with ALL also receive CNS prophylaxis. The prophylactic chemotherapy agent is injected intrathecally (in the spinal canal) into the cerebrospinal fluid (CSF) space during a lumbar puncture. Once the child is stable, the chemotherapy can be given in an outpatient setting.

 diagnostic tools Lumbar Puncture

A lumbar puncture (LP), also known as a "spinal tap," is the introduction of a needle into the subarachnoid space of the lumbar spinal cord. The needle is inserted with a stylet into the interspace between the third and fourth lumbar vertebrae under strict sterile technique (Fig. 34-4). This test is usually done to remove a sample of CSF to test it for infection. For cancer patients this procedure is also used to introduce chemotherapeutic agents into the CSF space. Since some medications cannot cross the blood–brain barrier without difficulty, physicians have obtained better results by introducing chemotherapeutic agents into the CSF space to kill cancer cells so they cannot "hide" behind the blood–brain barrier.

 Complementary Care: *Visualization and distraction*

The child may experience anticipatory anxiety before a procedure. The use of visualization and distraction can be helpful in these situations.

Figure 34-4 Lumbar puncture.

When using visualization, be creative. Help the child imagine a trip to his or her favorite place. Have the child close his or her eyes while the nurse plays tour guide. Ask the child questions about the favorite place and encourage the child to be part of the story or trip.

The nurse can also use distraction depending on the child's developmental level. Blowing bubbles, performing a magical light show, or simply reading a story can distract the child from the procedure.

The goal of the second phase, consolidation, is to destroy any residual leukemic cells. This phase starts immediately after remission is achieved and lasts about 6 months. Chemotherapy in this phase is frequently administered in high doses. Children are not usually hospitalized for this phase unless a complication arises. This phase may also require radiation.

The maintenance phase controls the leukemia. It can last for 2 to 3 years after diagnosis. Today, remission can be induced in 95% of children, and 5-year survival rates are nearly 80%.

 Nursing Insight— *Philadelphia chromosome*

A small number of patients with particularly poor prognostic features, principally those with a translocation known as the Philadelphia chromosome, may undergo bone marrow transplantation during the first remission. In ALL, this chromosome is similar, but not identical to, the Philadelphia chromosome of chronic myelogenous leukemia (CML) (Behrman et al., 2004).

Once the maintenance phase is completed, the caregivers and the children look forward to the return of a "normal life." Unfortunately, a number of the children do relapse. Relapse occurs in 15% to 20% of children with ALL (Behrman et al., 2004). Children who relapse while on therapy or within 6 months have a poor prognosis. This is especially true if relapse occurs shortly after completion of therapy.

 Nursing Insight— *Bone Marrow Transplant*

Bone marrow transplant is the treatment option for children who have a second remission after relapse. This treatment involves giving the child high doses of chemotherapy and/or radiation to eradicate disease or cancer and then rescuing the patient with a source of stem cells that allows for recovery of healthy bone marrow.

There are two basic types of bone marrow transplants: autologous and allogeneic. In an autologous transplant, the patient's own peripheral blood or bone marrow is given back. An allogeneic transplant can be from a matched sibling, a relative, or an unrelated donor accessed through the National Marrow Donor Program.

Acute Myelogenous Leukemia

Acute myelogenous leukemia (AML) is the second most common type of leukemia seen in children. In the United States, it comprises 11% of the cases of childhood leukemia, with approximately 380 children diagnosed annually (Behrman et al., 2004). AML is equally distributed among ethnic groups. Males and females are affected equally. Unlike ALL, the incidence of AML is constant from birth to 10 years of age, with a slight peak in adolescence. However, a neonate is more likely to have AML than ALL. The principal defect in AML appears to be an arrest in the differentiation pathway of myeloid progenitors or precursors rather than abnormal growth kinetics. The molecular mechanism that leads to a block in differentiation is mostly unknown (Colby-Graham & Chordas, 2003). AML can affect all three types of blood cells. Accordingly, a standard classification system called the French–American–British (FAB) system is used that differentiates AML into eight main types.

SIGNS AND SYMPTOMS. Children with AML may present with vague symptoms resembling the flu. Since blast cells replace the normal blood cells in the bone marrow, children with AML often present with abnormal blood counts. A decreased number of RBCs may result in anemia that may lead to decreased oxygen delivery to the blood cells and tissue. Pallor, fatigue, headache, or dizziness may result. As a result of a decreased number of platelets, thrombocytopenia, petechiae, easy bruising, nosebleeds, or bleeding gums may be present. Fever and infection may be present as a result of decreased WBCs. Bone pain and arthralgias are less common complaints in childhood. Massive hepatosplenomegaly is uncommon except in infants with AML (Colby-Graham & Chordas, 2003). Patients with AML present with signs and symptoms that infrequently occur with ALL, including subcutaneous nodules or "blueberry muffin" lesions, infiltration of the gingiva, signs and laboratory findings of disseminated intravascular coagulation (DIC), and discrete masses known as chloromas or granulocytic sarcomas that may occur in the absence of apparent bone marrow involvement (Behrman et al., 2004).

DIAGNOSIS. A bone marrow aspiration and analysis is required for a diagnosis of AML. The biopsy typically reveals a hypercellular marrow consisting of a pattern of cells with features that permit a subclassification of disease (Behrman et al., 2004). The diagnosis is typically made when there are more than 25% malignant myeloid blast cells.

NURSING CARE. Once diagnosis is made, treatment begins promptly, especially to control any copresenting symptomatology. Induction treatment includes the combination of cytarabine (Ara-C) and daunorubicin (Daunomycin). Commonly used pediatric induction therapy regimens use

Nursing Care Plan Child with Acute Lymphocytic Leukemia

Nursing Diagnosis: Risk for Infection related to neutropenia from the disease process and treatment regimen

Measurable Short-term Goal: The child will be afebrile.

Measurable Long-term Goal: The child will not experience an infection during a neutropenic episode.

NOC Outcome:
Immune Status (0702) Natural and acquired appropriately targeted resistance to internal and external antigens

NIC Interventions:
Infection Protection (6550)
Laboratory Data Interpretation (7690)
Surveillance (6650)

Nursing Interventions:

1. Monitor vital signs (specify frequency). Report a temperature 101.2°F (38.5°C) in a 24-hour period or 100.4°F (38.0°C) three times in a 24-hour period, or decrease in blood pressure to the physician.

   RATIONALE: Increased temperature, heart rate, and respiratory rate are signs of infection. A drop in blood pressure may be a late sign of septic shock.

2. Assess the child for signs of potential infection, such as mucosal ulcerations, breaks in the skin, or localized signs of infection such as pain, redness, or swelling.

   RATIONALE: The skin and mucous membranes are the first line of defense against infection, and openings in this protective barrier could be a portal for microbial entry. The child with neutropenia has diminished defense against infection, and sepsis may develop quickly.

3. Monitor laboratory values as obtained and report abnormal values to the physician.

   RATIONALE: Neutropenia from the disease process and chemotherapy increase the risk for infection. An elevated WBC count indicates an infectious process.

4. Wash hands thoroughly before and after providing care and teach the child and family when and how to wash their hands. Implement isolation precautions as ordered (specify).

   RATIONALE: Good hand hygiene is an effective and simple way to prevent transmission of infective microorganisms. Isolation precautions help protect the child from microorganisms in the hospital environment.

5. Instruct the family and visitors that no flowers, plants, fresh fruits, or vegetables should be brought into the child's room.

   RATIONALE: Promotes a safe environment for the child. Fresh plants and foods may carry infectious microorganisms that could be dangerous for the neutropenic child.

6. Flag the child's chart and alert all caregivers that the child should not use a drinking straw, have a rectal temperature taken, or receive rectal suppositories.

   RATIONALE: Protects the fragile mucous membranes of the mouth and rectum from mechanical injury, which could lead to infection.

7. Administer antibiotic and antifungal medications as ordered in a timely fashion (specify drug, dose, route, and times), and monitor for expected and adverse effects (specify).

   RATIONALE: Antibiotic therapy may be started in a child with a fever and who is neutropenic with an absolute neutrophil count (ANC) of less than 500.

---

cytarabine (Ara-C) and anthracyclines in combination with other agents such as etoposide (VP-16) and/or thioguanine (6-TG). The anthracycline that has been used most often in induction regimens for children with AML is daunorubicin (Daunomycin). Idarubicin (Idamycin) has also been used. Studies show no difference in efficaciousness between the drugs (Colby-Graham & Chordas, 2003).

Treatment has improved significantly since the first effective therapies were introduced in the 1970's. Five-year survival rates have increased from less than 5% in 1970 to 43% today as a result of treatment intensification, the incorporation of hematopoietic stem cell transplant into primary therapy, and enhanced supportive care. Aggressive multiagent chemotherapy is successful in inducing remission in about 80% of patients. Up to 10% of patients

die of either infection or bleeding before a remission can be achieved (Behrman et al., 2004). Matched-sibling bone marrow or stem cell transplantation after remission has been shown to achieve long-term disease-free survival in 60% to 70% of patients (Behrman et al., 2004).

 Now Can You— Discuss leukemia?

1. Describe the two main types of leukemia?
2. Describe the signs and symptoms of acute lymphocytic leukemia?
3. Describe three phases of acute lymphocytic leukemia chemotherapy treatment (remission-induction, consolidation, and maintenance)?
4. Discuss the purpose of a lumbar puncture?

Chronic Myelogenous Leukemia

Chronic myelogenous leukemia (CML) is a clonal disorder of the hematopoietic tissue (formation of blood cells) that accounts for 2% to 3% of all cases of childhood leukemia. About 99% of the cases are characterized by a specific translocation known as the Philadelphia chromosome. This disease has been associated with exposure to ionizing radiation, but very few children have a history of such exposure.

SIGNS AND SYMPTOMS. The presenting signs and symptoms of CML are nonspecific. They may include fever, fatigue, weight loss, and anorexia (Behrman et al., 2004).

CML is also characterized clinically by an initial chronic phase in which the malignant clone (cancerous alteration) produces an elevated leukocyte (WBC) count with increased numbers of immature granulocytes. In addition to leukocytosis, the blood counts may reveal mild anemia and thrombocytosis (increased number of platelets) (Behrman et al., 2004). The spleen is often greatly enlarged, resulting in pain in the left upper quadrant of the abdomen.

The chronic phase typically ends 3 to 4 years after onset when the CML moves into an accelerated or "blast crisis" phase. At this point, the blood counts rise dramatically and cannot be controlled with drugs. Additional manifestations may occur, including hyperuricemia and neurological symptoms, which are related to increased blood viscosity with decreased CNS perfusion (Behrman et al., 2004).

DIAGNOSIS. A diagnosis is suggested by increased numbers of myeloid cells with differentiation to mature forms in the peripheral blood smear and bone marrow. Cytogenetic studies yield the presence of the characteristic Philadelphia chromosome (Behrman et al., 2004).

NURSING CARE. Treatment of the signs and symptoms in the chronic phase can be controlled with hydroxyurea (Droxia, Hydrea), which gradually returns the leukocyte count to normal. This treatment is not definitive and does not eliminate the abnormal clone or prevent the progression of the disease. Therapy with interferon-α can produce a hematological remission in up to 70% of patients and cytogenetic remission in about 20% of patients. Combination chemotherapy has been successful in achieving remission in a small proportion of patients with CML. The optimum therapy is allogenic bone marrow or stem cell transplantation from a matched sibling, which is curative in up to 80% of children (Behrman et al., 2004).

 Nursing Insight— *Juvenile chronic myelogenous leukemia (JCML)*

Juvenile chronic myelogenous leukemia (JCML), also known as juvenile myelomonocytic leukemia, is a clonal proliferation of hematopoietic stem cells that typically affects children younger than 2 years of age. Patients with this disease do not have the Philadelphia chromosome that is characteristic of CML. JCML is rare and accounts for fewer than 2% of all cases of childhood leukemia (Behrman et al., 2004).

SOLID TUMORS

Solid tumors in children differ significantly from those in adults. There are some solid tumors that children acquire that never develop in adults, or if they do, are quite rare such as neuroblastoma, Wilms' tumor, rhabdosarcoma, and osteosarcoma (Kline & Sevier, 2003). The most common types of solid tumors found in children are discussed here. Solid tumors are named for the type of cells of which they are composed:

- Sarcoma is a cancer arising from connective or supporting tissues (e.g., bone or muscle).
- Carcinoma is cancer arising from the body's glandular cells and epithelial cells
- Lymphomas are cancers of the lymphoid organs such as the lymph nodes, spleen, and thymus that produce and store infection-fighting cells. These cells also occur in almost all tissues of the body; therefore, lymphomas may develop in a wide variety of organs.

Brain Tumors

Tumors of the brain or CNS are the second most common cancer in children after leukemia. Brain tumors in children differ greatly from those seen in adults. Virtually all childhood brain tumors are primary tumors, meaning that they originate in the brain. In contrast, in adults brain tumors are primarily metastatic, originating from another site and then spreading to the brain. The mortality rate among children and adolescents with brain tumors approaches 45% (Behrman et al., 2004).

 Nursing Insight— *Glial tumors*

Glial cells are the major supportive and structural cells of the CNS, as they form a framework supporting and nourishing nerve cells. The most common type of primary brain tumors in children are glial tumors. An example of this tumor comprises the primitive neuroectodermal tumors (PNETs), which arise almost exclusively in children. This tumor often resembles the early and undeveloped cells in an embryo and may be referred to as embryonal tumors. The most common site for this tumor is in the cerebellum.

Brain tumors are also divided into two types: supratentorial and intratentorial. Supratentorial tumors occur in the anterior two-thirds of the brain above the tentorium (dura matter located between the cerebrum and cerebellum, supporting the occipital lobes), primarily in the cerebrum. Infratentorial tumors are located in the posterior third of the brain, primarily in the cerebellum and brain stem and below the tentorium.

 Nursing Insight— *Age-related differences in primary location of the tumor*

There are age-related differences in primary location of the tumor:

Within the first year of life, supratentorial tumors predominate and include, most commonly, choroid plexus complex tumors and teratomas.

From 1 to 10 years of age, infratentorial tumors predominate, owing to the high incidence of juvenile pilocytic astrocytoma (tumor of the brain or spinal cord composed of astrocytes) and medulloblastoma (an infiltrating malignant tumor of the roof of the fourth ventricle and cerebellum) (Venes, 2009).

After 10 years of age, supratentorial tumors predominate (Behrman et al., 2004).

SIGNS AND SYMPTOMS. Clinical manifestations of patients with brain tumors depend on the tumor location, tumor type, and the age of the child. Classic signs and symptoms are related to the tumor causing obstruction of CSF drainage paths, leading to increased intracranial pressure (ICP).

Because their cranial sutures are open, infants may exhibit lethargy, irritability, and macrocephaly. They may also have a raised or tense fontanel. Projectile vomiting is often seen in the morning with little warning, or a headache may be noted.

In young children, the diagnosis of a brain tumor may be delayed because the symptoms are often similar to those of a typical gastrointestinal illness (Behrman et al., 2004). Subtle changes in personality, mentation, and/or speech may precede the classic signs and symptoms of brain tumors. Brain stem tumors are associated with cranial nerve abnormalities such as hemiparesis, a weakness on one side of the body, or a spastic gait. Older children may fall or stumble.

DIAGNOSIS. Any child who displays signs of increased ICP or other neurological signs such as ataxia, visual disturbances (if able to ascertain), or hemiparesis needs to be referred for a complete neurological exam. The diagnostic workup may include magnetic resonance imaging (MRI) or a computerized tomography (CT) scan. CT takes less time (5 to 10 minutes) and may be more appropriate if the child is able to lie still without sedation. An endocrine workup may be required for tumors that occur in the pituitary area.

✳ Nursing Insight— *Performing the neurological exam*

The main focus of a physical assessment of a child with a brain tumor should be the neurological exam. A patient's baseline assessment is important to detect any subtle changes. This exam includes vital signs; pupil size, equality, and response to light; level of consciousness; strength and equality of grip of hands; and movement of the legs. Head circumference and the assessment of the anterior fontanel is extremely important in assessing an infant's intracranial pressure. Parents may first notice behavioral changes. The nurse should perform frequent neurological exams to determine early changes in a child's condition. Detecting subtle changes in the neurological exam can be of great value in managing a child's condition and eventual prognosis. It is important for the nurse to remember that the neurological exam can change rapidly. Timely responses to neurological changes are of vital importance for the child with a brain tumor.

NURSING CARE. First the tumor is staged. Tumor tissue is needed for the pathologist to determine the histologic

diagnosis so that proper treatment can be determined. Treatment may include surgical resection, radiation therapy, chemotherapy, and or a combination of these. In addition good communication is essential because children diagnosed with a brain tumor may die.

! clinical alert

Surgical resection

The extent of surgical resection (cutting off) of the tumor correlates with the prognosis. Radical resections are particularly important in children younger than 2 years of age because cranial radiation can be deferred in these patients. Because many of the brain tumors infiltrate into surrounding normal brain, often complete resection is not possible.

After resection, postoperative care includes intravenous steroids such as dexamethasone (Decadron) to prevent edema within the brain. Anticonvulsants are indicated for the child with a supratentorial tumor where seizures are possible. Other nursing care measures include frequent neurological assessments, airway and fluid maintenance, prevention of infection, pain management, adequate nutrition and promotion of normal growth and development.

The goal of radiation therapy is to destroy the tumor while sparing normal brain tissue in the developing brain. Early use of radiation is used sparingly, related to the desire to preserve intellectual growth and decrease the possibility of growth impairment. When radiation must be used, the dose is usually high and the toxicity (poisonous) can be severe. Radiation therapy to large areas of the brain can sometimes cause changes in brain function (Venes, 2009).

In the last decade, chemotherapy has emerged as the standard care in the treatment of certain pediatric brain tumors, especially for children younger than 3 years of age. Several rounds of high-dose chemotherapy with stem cell rescue are now being offered for metastatic medulloblastoma as well as for some other incurable brain tumors.

Good communication with the care delivery team is vital. Parents and the child need much emotional support and accurate information. Nurses are the pivotal coordinators of the care in this difficult situation. The nurse needs to demonstrate a positive attitude and be reassuring to parents during difficult treatments in order to build a trusting relationship with the family.

❝ What to say❞ — *When a child is diagnosed with a brain tumor*

A 4-year-old child has just been diagnosed with a brain tumor. The pediatric nurse must realize that the family is probably in a state of shock. The family or the child does not understand the exact nature or future implications of a brain tumor. While caring for the child, the nurse must treat him or her as normally as possible. It is acceptable to communicate with the child and family while the child plays. It is also important that the nurse support the parents or caregivers and allow them time to "absorb" the diagnosis.

What would the pediatric nurse say to the family?

- "It is important for you to verbalize and express your feelings."
- "You may find it helpful to talk with others who have had the same experience as you. I have contact information for a support group. Would you like me to make a call for you?"
- "I know this is a very difficult time for you. Let's take this a day at a time and make your child's daily routine as normal as possible."

Neuroblastoma

Neuroblastoma is the third most common pediatric cancer after leukemia and brain tumors (Behrman et al., 2004). Neuroblastoma is a tumor originating from neural crest cells, which are embryological precursors of the adrenal medulla and sympathetic nervous system. These cells are present in tissues of the brain, adrenal medulla, pelvis, mediastinum, and sympathetic ganglia. A neuroblastoma tumor may occur at any of these sites.

Neuroblastoma accounts for about 8% of all childhood cancers (Behrman et al., 2004). Neuroblastoma is the most common diagnosed neoplasm in infants. The median age at diagnosis is 2 years. Ninety percent of all cases are diagnosed in children younger than 5 years. The incidence is slightly higher in males and in Caucasian non-Hispanic children (Kline & Sevier, 2003).

The etiology of neuroblastoma remains unknown. The most common site of a primary tumor is the abdomen. In about 25% of patients, the tumor arises in the adrenal gland. The next most common site is the chest, followed by the neck. Sometimes a primary tumor site cannot be identified.

Neuroblastoma is staged into low, average, and high-risk groups, as well as into a I through IV classification using the International Neuroblastoma Staging System (INSS) (Kline & Sevier, 2003). The prognosis can be determined by the age of the child, the stage of the tumor, and the histology of the tumor. The prognosis for children who have abdominal masses is poorer than for those with cervical, mediastinal, or pelvic tumors.

SIGNS AND SYMPTOMS. Children with neuroblastoma can present with a wide variety of initial symptoms depending on the primary site of the tumor. Most commonly the tumor is detected by palpation. On palpation the nurse notes that neuroblastoma crosses the midline. The tumor is noted as a hard, painless mass in the neck or abdomen. Masses of the thorax can be seen on radiographs and are usually an incidental finding on a film done to rule out pneumonia. If large enough, the tumor can produce edema of the lower extremities related to vascular compression. Unfortunately, at the time of diagnosis, 75% of patients with neuroblastoma have a tumor that has already spread or metastasized to another site. Nearly one-half of the patients have widespread metastasis to the bone that causes bone pain. The bones of the skull and orbit are also frequently affected, so swelling and bruising around the eyes are common.

DIAGNOSIS. Imaging studies such as MRI and CT scan may indicate the presence of a mass. A clear diagnosis of neuroblastoma can be made only by biopsy. Bone marrow aspiration may also be performed. Laboratory studies may be ordered, as 95% of neuroblastomas secrete catecholamines. These are secreted in the urine, so vanillylmandelic acid (VMA) and homovanillic acid (HVA) tests are used to measure the level of catecholamines or catecholamine metabolites (breakdown products) in the urine.

NURSING CARE. Treatment for neuroblastoma is determined by the stage of the disease and the age of the child. Initially surgical reaction is preformed followed by chemotherapy. In advanced stage disease, a complete surgical resection is sometimes not possible and chemotherapy is initiated. Neuroblastoma is radiosensitive, but radiation alone is not curative. Radiation is used for tumor control in conjunction with chemotherapy and autologous or allogeneic bone marrow transplant.

During the treatment phase a complete nursing assessment is vital to ensure that the child does not have an infection and their condition remains stable. Place emphasis on the child's comfort and alleviating pain. Supporting the child and the family during the diagnosis and treatment phase is most important. Encourage both the child and caregivers to share their feelings about the disease process and related treatments. Providing accurate information and education for the family is also important.

Wilms' Tumor

Wilms' tumor (nephroblastoma) is a tumor that originates in the kidney. It is named after the German doctor, Max Wilms, who first described it in 1899. Ninety percent of all kidney tumors are Wilms' tumors. Wilms' tumor is the fourth most common cancer in children.

Wilms' tumor accounts for 6% of all childhood cancers. The average age at diagnosis is between 2 and 5 years (Behrman et al., 2004). The disease occasionally affects older children and adults. Girls and boys are equally affected. The majority of Wilms' tumor cases are sporadic, although 1% to 2% of patients have a family history. One Wilms' tumor gene has been located at 11p13, but only 20% of all Wilms' tumors carry that mutation (Behrman et al., 2004). The actual cause of Wilms' tumor is unknown.

SIGNS AND SYMPTOMS. Children with Wilms' tumor present with an abdominal mass that is usually painless. Hematuria, hypertension, and pain occur infrequently. The tumor is usually discovered on a routine physical exam, or is felt or seen by a family member during bathing or routine care. Unlike neuroblastoma, the mass frequently presents on one side and seldom crosses the midline as does a neuroblastoma. Other symptoms may be aniridia (absence of the iris, the colored part of the eye), hemihypertrophy (an increased size of one half of the body), or urinary defects such as cryptorchidism and hypospadia. The tumor may be in one kidney or both kidneys (Behrman et al., 2004).

DIAGNOSIS. A child presenting with an abdominal mass needs a timely diagnostic workup. An abdominal ultrasound is often the first test ordered. An abdominal CT scan or MRI may more definitively identify other structural involvement. A complete blood count (CBC), urinalysis, and electrolyte analysis should also be ordered.

NURSING CARE. Nursing care for Wilms' tumor consists of a thorough health and history and nursing assessment. The nurse can explain to the parents that laboratory and diagnostic testing may include urinalysis, drawing blood for a complete blood count, a renal or abdominal ultrasound or CT scan, or MRI of the abdomen. If metastasis is suspected a chest x-ray exam may also be ordered. A surgical removal of the mass, which usually involves taking the entire kidney, and biopsy are performed.

Nursing care also centers on the administration of chemotherapy and post-radiation care. The first-line chemotherapeutic agents for Wilms' tumor are vincristine (Oncovorin), dactinomycin (Cosmegen), doxorubicin (Adriamycin), and cyclophosphamide (Cytoxan). More than 85% of children diagnosed with Wilms' tumor are cured with current treatment (Kline & Servier, 2003).

After surgical resection for a Wilms' tumor postoperative care is similar to care for children undergoing other abdominal surgeries. A critical postoperative assessment of the remaining kidney is necessary to ensure its function.

Foods high in calories and protein are important. If a child is unable to eat or meet basic caloric requirements for growth and development, dietary supplements, allowing the child food choices, and ensuring that food textures can facilitate eating might help. Enteral or parental feeding may be provided if necessary.

critical nursing action Palpitation of the Abdomen in a Child with Wilms' Tumor

Once a child has been diagnosed with Wilms' tumor, never palpate the abdomen or allow anyone else to do so. Palpating this kind of encapsulated tumor can cause it to rupture or lead to further metastasis.

Place a warning sign on the child's hospital room door that says, "No abdominal palpation."

case study Wilms' Tumor

A mother brings her 3-year-old to the pediatrician's office. She states that while giving her daughter a bath, she noticed a "lump" on her abdomen. The mother also says the child shows no abnormal behavior. She is sleeping and playing normally. However, the mother does state she is a picky eater, but assumes that is normal for a preschooler. The mother is concerned about a "hernia or something." On physical examination by the pediatrician, a small mass in the abdominal cavity is discovered. The pediatrician sends the child for an abdominal CT scan. The CT confirms there is a mass on the left kidney. It is classified as a stage II Wilms' tumor.

critical thinking questions

1. What is the course of treatment for this child?

2. What information does the parent need to know about nutrition?

◆ See Suggested Answers to Case Studies in text on the Electronic Study Guide or DavisPlus.

Rhabdomyosarcoma

Rhabdosarcoma is the most common pediatric soft-tissue sarcoma (Behrman et al., 2004) and accounts for 5% to 8% of all childhood cancers. Overall, two-thirds of children diagnosed with rhabdomyosarcoma will become long-term survivors. Children with distant metastatic disease at diagnosis have a poor prognosis, with only 30% surviving 5 years.

Rhabdosarcoma arises from mesenchymal cells that are normally committed to skeletal muscle formation, but can also arise from smooth muscle cells (Kline & Sevier, 2003). These tumors occur at virtually any anatomical site but are most often found in the head and neck, genitourinary tract, extremities, and trunk.

Rhabdomyosarcoma occurs with an increased frequency of patients with neurofibromatosis (Behrman et al., 2004). There are four recognizable types of rhabdomyosarcoma based on subtypes.

 Nursing Insight— *Rhabdomyosarcoma subtypes*

The embryonal type (resembling an embryo) accounts for about 60% of all cases and has an intermediate prognosis. The botryoid type resembles a "bunch of grapes" and accounts for 6% of cases. It is most often found in the vagina, uterus, bladder, nasopharynx, and middle ear. The alveolar type accounts for about 15% of cases. The tumor cells in this type tend to grow in cores that often have cleft-like spaces resembling alveoli. Alveolar tumors occur most often in the trunk and extremities and carry the poorest prognosis. The pleomorphic type (having many shapes) is rare in childhood (1% of cases).

Note: About 20% of rhabdomyosarcomas are considered to be undifferentiated (an alteration in cell character toward a malignant state) sarcomas (Venes, 2009).

SIGNS AND SYMPTOMS. Signs and symptoms of rhabdosarcoma depend on the location of the primary tumor and metastasis. In the head and neck, orbital or eyelid tumors may cause proptosis (a downward displacement of the eyeball) and may impair vision (Venes, 2009). Tumors in the nasopharynx may cause sinus obstruction or result in continual sinus drainage. If the tumor erodes through the bone to the brain, signs and symptoms of increased intracranial pressure (headache, vomiting, etc.) may be present. In the genitourinary tract, the bladder and prostate are the most common sites, and hematuria or urinary obstruction may result. Extremity sarcomas are diagnosed as the affected area begins to swell. Erythema and tenderness may occur. Other sites can be any skeletal or smooth muscle and the intrathoracic, retroperitoneal, perineal, and perianal regions (Kline & Sevier, 2003).

DIAGNOSIS. Definitive diagnosis is established by biopsy. Investigating a lesion may help with diagnosis. Paratesticular lesions may be ignored for a long time by adolescents (Behrman et al., 2004). A lesion in an extremity may be mistaken for a hematoma or hemangioma. Physical examination should also include attention to the lymph nodes. Radiographic studies should include x-ray exams, CT scan, and MRI.

NURSING CARE. Treatment is based on the primary tumor and disease stage (Behrman et al., 2004). Patients with complete surgical resected tumors have the best prognosis. Unfortunately, most rhabdomyosarcomas are not completely resectable. Chemotherapy is the standard treatment. Radiation may also be added (Kline & Sevier, 2003).

Retinoblastoma

Retinoblastoma is a malignant tumor that arises from the retina at the back of the eye during fetal life or early childhood. A retinoblastoma can grow rapidly or slowly. It may produce multiple tumors that can affect one or both eyes. It is sometimes recognized at birth. It affects mainly very young children. There is no racial or gender predominance, but there is a familial predisposition in about a third of patients. Retinoblastoma can often be seen by looking at a young person's eyes or by observing a photograph taken of the individual.

Overall, 60% of cases are unilateral and nonhereditary. Bilateral involvement is found in 42% of those presenting when younger than 1 year of age and is even less common at older ages. Close to 95% of retinoblastomas are cured (Behrman et al., 2004).

SIGNS AND SYMPTOMS. Usually retinoblastoma is detected by the caregiver, who notices a whitish glow in the pupil known as leukocoria (cat's eye reflex). This is seen instead of the red eye reflex typically seen in photographs and is the most common manifestation. Other signs include strabismus, red painful eyes, and blindness (late sign). Other less common evidence of tumor is an inward or outward turning of the eye, visual impairment, or an abnormal appearance of the eye. This abnormal appearance consists of a change in color of the iris, pupils of unequal size, or increased pressure inside the eye.

DIAGNOSIS. Retinoblastoma is usually diagnosed via an examination under anesthesia using an ophthalmoscope. Orbital ultrasound and CT or MRI may be used to evaluate the extent of intraocular disease and extraocular spread.

NURSING CARE. Treatment depends on the size and location of the tumor (or tumors), with the primary goal being cure and a secondary goal of preserving vision. Primary enucleation (removal of the eye) is usually preformed if there is no potential for useful vision (Behrman et al., 2004).

An important care measure before surgery includes showing parents a photograph of another child who has had this type of surgery. Parents will then understand that the child's facial appearance will be near normal. It is also important to inform parents that after surgery the eyelid is usually closed and their child will be wearing a patch over the operative eye. It is important to keep the operative site clean and dry. Postoperative medical orders may include eye socket irrigation and the application of an antibiotic ointment. Traditional postoperative measures such as airway and fluid maintenance, vital signs, pain management, and nutrition are also important.

The child is usually discharged in 3–4 days after the surgery. The nurse can teach parents about care of the eye socket by showing them gentle irrigation of the area (with the prescribed solution) and then applying a thin coating of the prescribed antibiotic ointment. Eye gauze pads are applied until the wound has completely healed. Enforce good hand washing for the entire family. In about 3 weeks the child is fitted for a prosthetic eye and the child's facial appearance appears near normal. Through the entire process the nurse can offer support to the child and family and encourage follow-up care.

 Nursing Insight— *Additional treatment modalities*

Cryotherapy (freezing of the tumor) and photocoagulation (laser light treatment of the tumor) is used to treat small primary tumors.

BONE TUMORS

Malignant bone tumors account for approximately 5% of all childhood cancers. The two most common bone tumors are osteogenic sarcoma and Ewing's sarcoma.

Osteosarcoma

Osteogenic sarcoma or osteosarcoma is a tumor of bone that usually occurs in the metaphysis (the growing portion of a bone) (Fig. 34-5). The long bones are more frequently affected than the flat bones such as the pelvis or skull. The leg is the most common site, with the femur (upper leg) being the most commonly affected bone, followed by the tibia (lower leg) and the humerus (upper arm). The high-risk period of developing osteosarcoma is during adolescent growth spurts. Often a traumatic event leads to the discovery of osteosarcoma as a secondary finding.

Osteosarcoma can also occur as a complication of treatment for another tumor, especially at a site of prior radiation for a tumor such as retinoblastoma. These secondary radiation-associated osteosarcomas can occur 7 to 15 years after successful treatment of the primary tumor.

 Nursing Insight— *Osteosarcoma*

The cause of osteosarcoma is unknown. Certain genetic or acquired conditions may predispose children to the development of osteosarcoma. Children with hereditary retinoblastoma have a significantly increased risk of developing osteosarcoma (Behrman et al., 2004). The annual incidence of

Figure 34-5 Osteosarcoma.

osteosarcoma in the United States is 5.6 cases per million children younger than 15 years of age. There is a slightly lower incidence in African American children. Boys are usually more often affected than are girls.

 Nursing Insight— *Osteosarcoma prognosis*

Patients with nonmetastatic extremity osteosarcoma are cured with current multiagent treatment protocols 75% of the time. Patients with pelvic tumors do not have as good a prognosis as those with extremity tumors. From 20% to 30% of patients who have limited numbers of pulmonary metastases can also be cured with aggressive chemotherapy and resection of lung nodules. Patients with bone metastasis and those with widespread lung metastasis have an extremely poor prognosis (Behrman et al., 2004).

SIGNS AND SYMPTOMS. Pain and swelling are the most common presenting symptoms. The pain increases with activity and weight bearing and may cause the child to limp. It is common for a child to have a dull aching pain for several months before diagnosis. Palpation at the site of disease often reveals tenderness, swelling, warmth, and erythema (Kline & Sevier, 2003).

DIAGNOSIS. An x-ray film may include a sunburst pattern of the affected bone. An accompanying chest x-ray exam should be performed to check for metastasis. A MRI of the entire bone should be performed to evaluate the extent of the tumor.

A nuclear medicine scan or bone scan may also be done to determine the extent of involvement in the bone (Behrman et al., 2004). Nuclear tracer isotopes such as technetium-99m or thallium-201, which are radioactive materials, show an increased uptake of radioactive material in the areas of primary tumor as well as any area of metastasis. The most common site of distant metastatic spread of osteosarcoma is to the lung.

Certain laboratory tests, such as elevated blood serum levels of serum alkaline phosphatase or lactic acid dehydrogenase, can help make the diagnosis of osteosarcoma. Although the diagnosis of osteosarcoma may be very strongly suspected after diagnostic studies, only a biopsy with microscopic examination provides final confirmation of osteosarcoma.

NURSING CARE. The primary treatment goal is total eradication of the tumor. Children with osteosarcoma receive chemotherapy first to shrink the size of the tumor. Surgical resection of the affected bone is then performed.

 Nursing Insight— *Amputation*

Amputation was the surgical treatment used almost exclusively in the past. Today a limb-saving procedure is available. Limb-sparing surgery uses cadaver bone, grafted into place to replace the section of bone that must be resected with tumor (or where the affected part of the bone is removed) and then replaced with a metal prosthesis. In the most severe cases, total limb amputation must be used. Various types of amputation can be done, including removal of the joint (disarticulation) or across-the-bone (transosseous) amputation. The decision as to which type is chosen must take into consideration the patient's lifestyle.

Ewing's Sarcoma

Ewing's sarcoma is the second most common type of bone tumor in children and young adults. Ewing's sarcoma is a highly malignant bone tumor with a histologic appearance that is different from that of osteosarcoma. Ewing's sarcoma tumors can occur anywhere in the body but is typically found in bones other than the long bones of the arms and legs. The most common sites are the pelvis, the arms and legs, and the ribs (Fig. 34-6). In the United States, the incidence of Ewing's sarcoma is 2.1 cases per million children. It is extremely rare among African American children (Behrman et al., 2004) and in Asian Americans. It is more often seen in young males than in females. Ewing's sarcoma commonly affects patients between 10 and 20 years of age.

There are two different types of tumors. The first type, Ewing's sarcoma family of tumors, refers to a group of small round cell undifferentiated tumors thought to be of neural crest origin that generally carry the same chromosomal translocation. The second type is called peripheral primitive neuroectodermal tumor (PPNET). Both of these tumor types can arise in long bone or in soft tissue (Behrman et al., 2004).

SIGNS AND SYMPTOMS. Clinical symptoms of Ewing's sarcoma are similar to those of osteosarcoma. Pain or tenderness and swelling at the site of the tumor are the usual presenting symptoms. The bone pain or swelling may be attributed to a sports injury and caregivers may delay seeking care (Behrman et al., 2004).

When the tumor is present in the chest wall, Askin tumor, the child may present with respiratory distress. The child with paraspinal or vertebrospinal tumors may present with symptoms of spinal cord compression. There may be systemic manifestations such as fever, or weight loss.

Figure 34-6 Ewing's sarcoma.

DIAGNOSIS. Diagnosis is made via biopsy of the bone lesion. A complete staging procedure must be performed. A CT scan, MRI, or radionucleotide bone scan is helpful in determining the primary site. Location of the primary tumor is important, especially with pelvic and sacral lesions, since those tumors are not resectable.

 Nursing Insight— *Metastasis*

Ten to thirty percent of patients have metastatic disease at the time of diagnosis. The lung, other bones, and the bone marrow are the most common sites of metastasis. Widespread metastasis to other bones and the bone marrow may have a poor prognosis.

NURSING CARE. Multiagent chemotherapy is important because it can rapidly shrink the tumor. Surgical resection is preferred if possible. Radiation treatment is also performed but it is associated with the risk of radiation-induced secondary tumors, especially osteosarcoma, as well as failure of bone growth in skeletally immature patients.

Patients with small, nonmetastatic, distally located extremity tumors have the best prognosis, with up to a 75% cure rate. Long-term follow-up is needed related to the chance of developing secondary malignancies. Late relapses even 10 years after initial diagnosis have been reported (Behrman et al., 2004).

LYMPHOMAS

Lymphatic tissue is present throughout the entire body. A lymphoma is a malignancy that arises from the lymphatic system.

Hodgkin's Disease

Two types of lymphomas are seen in children: Hodgkin's disease (HD) and non-Hodgkin's lymphoma (NHL). Hodgkin's disease was first described in 1832 by the English physician Thomas Hodgkin. The major difference between the two is that HD tends to involve the lymph nodes (those near the surface of the body) and NHD is frequently a disease of the tissues, especially the bowel, particularly in the region adjacent to the appendix, and in the upper mid-section of the chest (National Cancer Institute, 2008).

In the United States, HD accounts for about 5% of childhood malignancies. HD is rare in children younger than 5 years of age. There are three main age groups affected by Hodgkin's disease:

Childhood form (younger than 14 years of age)
Young adult form (15 to 34 years of age)
Older adult form (55 to 74 years of age)

There is a male predominance in patients younger than 10 years of age, with an equal gender distribution in adolescence. People with a preexisting immunodeficiency, either congenital or acquired, have an increased risk of developing HD. The role of the Epstein–Barr virus is being studied in relation to HD. The Reed–Sternberg cell, a large cell with multiple or multilobulated nuclei, is considered the hallmark of HD, although similar cells are seen in mononucleosis (Behrman et al., 2004).

SIGNS AND SYMPTOMS. The onset of HD is commonly not acute in nature. The child may have symptoms for a long time before telling anyone or seeking care. The disease is usually localized when patients present at the time of diagnosis.

Painless, firm, cervical, or supraclavicular lymphadenopathy is the most common presenting sign. Inguinal or axillary sites are uncommon areas of presentation of lymphadenopathy. These lymph nodes are different than those associated with infection in that they are hard and not painful since they are filled with cancer cells. An anterior mediastinal mass is often present and can rapidly disappear with therapy. Systemic symptoms considered important in staging are unexplained fever, weight loss, or drenching night sweats. Less common symptoms are lethargy, anorexia, pruritus, and hepatomegaly or splenomegaly (Behrman et al., 2004).

DIAGNOSIS. The only way to confirm HD is with a biopsy or removal of the enlarged lymph node. After biopsy confirms HD, several tests and scans are performed to determine the extent of spread: chest x-ray exam, CT scan, lymphangiogram to show abnormal nodes, MRI, bone scan, bone marrow biopsy, and blood tests.

NURSING CARE. Chemotherapy and/or radiation therapy may be used depending on the clinical stage at the time of diagnosis (Fig. 34-7).

Non-Hodgkin's Lymphoma

Malignant lymphoma is a cancer of lymphoid tissue. NHL is different from HD in that there is no single focal origin (the malignant cells are rarely localized). NHL has a rapid onset and presents with widespread involvement. NHL results from malignant clonal proliferation of lymphocytes of T or B or indeterminate cell origin. There are three histologic types of NHL:

- Small noncleaved cell lymphoma, with Burkitt and non-Burkitt subtypes, is a malignancy of B-cells.
- Lymphoblastic lymphoma is a malignancy of T cells.
- Large B-cell lymphoma with diffuse and anaplastic subtypes is a heterogeneous group of tumors characterized by cells that tend to be larger than cells seen in the other two subtypes of NHL.

Figure 34-7 A child receiving chemotherapy.

Among children younger than 15 years of age, 60% of lymphomas are NHL. NHL is seen from infancy through adolescence, with a peak between the ages of 7 and 11. Boys are affected more than girls. The cause is unknown, although viral, genetic, immunological, and environmental factors have been implicated.

SIGNS AND SYMPTOMS. The presenting symptom of NHL is usually pain or swelling dependent on the initial site of involvement and the extent of disease spread. The most frequent sites of involvement are the abdomen, chest, and the head or neck region. These lymphomas grow rapidly, and most children present with advanced-stage disease. Spread into the CNS may result in weakness of the facial muscles. Spread to the bone marrow may be associated with pale skin or bruising.

DIAGNOSIS. Prompt tissue diagnosis and staging is important because of the rapid growth of lymphomas. Elevated levels of serum lactic dehydrogenase (greater than 500 U/L) correlate with tumor mass and are useful in deciding on therapy intensity. Other laboratory findings vary with the site or organs involved. A CT scan or MRI of the chest or abdomen or both may assist in determining disease extent.

NURSING CARE. Aggressive multi-agent chemotherapy is started as soon as possible once the diagnosis is made and tumor staging is complete. Intrathecal chemotherapy is given for CNS prophylaxis. Children with limited disease have a good prognosis (90% cure rate). Seventy to ninety percent of those with extensive disease who receive good supportive care can expect to be cured.

 clinical alert

Discarding chemotherapy drugs

When handling equipment or material that has contained chemotherapy drugs, discard it in a designated container that is properly labeled (Fig. 34-8). Chemotherapy drugs are considered hazardous waste material.

Figure 34-8 Chemotherapy waste receptacle.

OTHER CANCERS

Liver Cancer

In the United States, primary malignant liver tumors are the tenth most frequent pediatric malignancy. However, many other kinds of cancers can spread or metastasize to the liver. The two primary types of liver cancer are hepatoblastoma and hepatocellular carcinoma.

SIGNS AND SYMPTOMS. The first sign of liver cancer is a mass in the abdomen discovered by a family member or physician during a routine exam. It is usually located in the upper right side of the abdomen. Other symptoms the child might experience are a vague feeling of abdominal fullness, pain, vomiting, diarrhea, fever, abnormal weight loss, jaundice (yellow appearance of skin or sclera), or general itching. It is not uncommon for these symptoms to be present for months before a diagnosis is made. Occasionally the liver may produce hormones that cause platelets to increase and the child has a very high platelet count.

DIAGNOSIS. X-ray, ultrasound, CT scan, and MRI are used to diagnose liver cancer. These tests enable the physician to determine the severity and metastasis. The most common areas of metastasis are to other parts of the liver, the lungs, lymph nodes in the abdomen, and rarely to the brain or bones. Biopsy of the liver cells confirms the diagnosis.

NURSING CARE. Chemotherapy may be used first to shrink the size of the tumor. The best chance of curing liver cancer is surgical removal of the tumor. More than three-fourths of the liver can be removed without any problems because the liver can regenerate or regrow. Hepatoblastoma responds very well to chemotherapy, but hepatocellular carcinoma does not respond well to any known chemotherapy. It is important to remember that new drugs are being investigated all the time.

 Nursing Insight— *Alpha-fetoprotein (AFP)*

An interesting note is that both hepatoblastoma and hepatocellular carcinoma can produce a protein called alpha-fetoprotein (AFP), which can be detected in the blood via a simple blood test. If AFP levels fall, it indicates that treatment is working. If AFP levels rise, it means the tumor is not responding.

 Nursing Insight— *Extragonadal germ cell cancer (EGC)*

Extragonadal germ cell cancer (EGC) are tumors that originate in the sperm-forming cells in the testicles (male gonads) or egg-producing cells in the ovary (female gonads). This this type of cancer is located on the midline from the pineal gland to the coccyx. EGC can be either benign or malignant. Most of the benign tumors occur in children. Surgical treatment can result in high rates of long-term survival and cure. Note: Undescended testes are associated with an increased risk of testicular cancer (Behrman et al., 2004).

Nursing Care of the Child with Cancer

Tailored nursing care of the child with cancer is important. After diagnosis/staging and during the ongoing treatment a thorough nursing assessment is crucial in order to maintain realistic optimal health and prevent complications. The nurse assesses for signs and symptoms of infection and bleeding. Additionally, the nurse monitors skin integrity (including mucous membranes), heart, kidney, bowel, lung, musculoskeletal and sensory function. Assessing the child's nutritional and pain status, as well as evaluating the child's ability to meet normal growth and developmental milestones, is also important.

There are several areas of nursing care for the child with cancer: maintaining nutrition, preventing infection, administering chemotherapy, addressing radiation side effects, understanding the use of surgery and related nursing diagnosis, pain control, offering psychosocial support, managing negative and long-term effects of cancer treatments and preventing medical emergencies. Understanding the psychological impact of pediatric cancer is also an important element of care.

NUTRITION

Good nutrition is essential for the child with cancer to promote realistic optimal health as well as maintain normal growth and development (Fig. 34-9). For the child with cancer, the demands of the illness and subsequent treatment can cause certain challenges. Malnutrition has been reported to occur in 8% to 32% of pediatric oncology patients (Bryant, 2003).

Parents frequently have anxiety about proper nutrition because the child can respond differently to treatment(s) and their desire and ability to eat and drink often times changes. Some children are able to eat enough food to have strength and energy to enjoy a normal level of activity; others are not. Poor nutrition can lead to tiredness or irritability, greater susceptibility to infections, and reduction of growth and developmental patterns.

The side effects of cancer therapy (nausea and vomiting, mouth sores, diarrhea, or constipation) can also make achieving adequate nutrition a challenge too. Chemotherapy

Figure 34-9 Good nutrition is essential for the growing child to maintain normal growth and development.

and radiation may interfere with the ability to chew and swallow. The child's sense of taste may change and their appetite may be poor.

A healthy immune system is a critical foundation of treatment. The immune system needs good nutrition for proper function. Proper immune function is possible only if the child obtains enough fluid intake and a high-calorie balanced diet, emphasizing proteins, fatty acids, vitamins, and minerals. The nurse can offer suggestions to maintain good nutrition (Box 34-2). Encourage a diet that includes foods from all four food groups.

The nurse tries simple care measures first, such as offering small frequent feedings, allowing the child food choices, choosing food textures that are appealing and providing the child adequate time to eat. If the patient is unable to maintain good nutritional status, the nurse considers enteral tube feedings. If the gastrointestinal tract is not functioning well, total parenteral nutrition (TPN) via the intravenous route may be the only option. Communicate to the child and his or her parents that tube feedings or (TPN) may be temporary and that he or she may be able to eat independently again.

 Collaboration in Caring— *The role of a nutritionist*

Consultation with the dietitian is essential to achieve the child's best nutritional outcome. If a child is unable to eat or meet basic caloric requirements for growth and development, the dietitian can recommend protein shakes and nutritional supplements. The dietitian can also teach the child and family what foods would be best tolerated for certain conditions such as oral ulcerations or difficulty in swallowing.

INFECTION

A priority nursing action is preventing infection. It is essential that the nurse monitor for systemic and localized signs of infection every 2–4 hours (take the child's temperature every 4 hours). Report a single temperature greater than 101.2°F (38.5°C) in a 24-hour period or 100.4°F (38.0°C) three times in a 24-hour period.

The nurse provides meticulous skin care and uses good hand washing. Instruct visitors to wash hands on entering and leaving the patient's room. Universal precautions and designated isolation precautions are instituted. Monitor and report laboratory values as ordered, such as absolute granulocyte count, WBC count, complete blood count (CBC) with differential, serum protein, serum albumin, and cultures. Encourage rest and sleep by providing a quiet environment.

Teaching the child and parents about the principles of prophylactic antibiotics as well as on the signs and symptoms of infection in order to promote the best possible health for the child is important.

CHEMOTHERAPY

Chemotherapy is the primary treatment modality for many pediatric cancers. The nurse administers chemotherapy using a variety of drugs to destroy or kill cancer cells. The goal of chemotherapy is to reduce the primary size of the tumor by destroying cancer cells and to prevent

Box 34-2 Suggestions for Nutrition

NAUSEA/VOMITING

- Offer plain, bland foods such as cereal, canned or fresh fruit, rice, pasta, toast, mashed potatoes, soup, crackers, or plain meat.
- Avoid spicy, heavy, or fatty foods.
- If food smells bother the child, choose cold or room-temperature foods; use a cup with a lid.
- Do not offer solid food and liquid at the same time, as this can induce nausea by making the child feel too full; give liquids 30–60 minutes after solid food.

DIARRHEA

- Offer plenty of liquids.
- Try bananas, rice, applesauce, toast, and tea.
- Cut back on fiber in the diet.

CONSTIPATION

- Provide extra liquids; offer beverages that contain caffeine, like coffee, tea, and cola.
- Increase fiber in the diet.
- Encourage the child to increase activity level.

POOR APPETITE

- Offer small amounts of food four or more times a day.
- Offer liquids between meals.
- Make every bite count by offering "power packed foods."
- Start with small portions, then gradually increase them.
- Allow the child to have foods and beverages that he or she especially likes.

SORE THROAT AND MOUTH

- Offer soft foods such as pudding, Jell-o®, macaroni and cheese, applesauce, bananas, ice cream, Italian ice, popsicles.
- Avoid acidic foods like oranges and tomatoes, spicy foods, or foods that require a lot of chewing.
- Encourage good oral hygiene.

HEARTBURN OR REFLUX

- Do not give the child high-fat, spicy foods, caffeine, citrus juices, cinnamon, peppermint, or pepper.
- Keep the child upright for at least 1 hour after eating.

DIFFICULTY CHEWING OR SWALLOWING/DRY MOUTH

- Give the child soft, moist foods.
- Encourage sips of liquids while eating.
- Avoid hard foods that require a lot of chewing.
- Cut the food into small pieces.
- Use extra butter, sauces, or gravies.
- Offer hard candy to suck on.

BELCHING, INTESTINAL GAS, OR CRAMPS

- Avoid gas-forming foods such as cabbage, broccoli, cauliflower, cucumbers, beans, and carbonated beverages.
- Encourage the child to eat or drink slowly.
- Do not allow the child to chew gum.

Source: Steen, G., & Mirro, M. (2000). *Childhood cancer: A handbook from St. Jude Children's Research Hospital.* Cambridge, MA: Perseus.

Family Teaching Guidelines...
Signs and Symptoms of Infection

HOW TO: Teach the Family How to Recognize Signs and Symptoms of Infection

The family needs to understand that any of these signs and symptoms, or a combination of them, must be reported to the physician immediately.

Fever
Decrease in temperature
Runny nose (or other respiratory illness)
Sore throat
Childhood disease such as chickenpox
Lethargy
Pale or ashen color
Chills
Diaphoresis
Poor appetite
Poor fluid intake
Nausea, vomiting, or diarrhea
Decreased urination
Foul smelling urine, or pain or burning upon urination

ESSENTIAL INFORMATION

The rectal mucosa is very vascular and an area of potential injury or a source of infection. Never take a rectal temperature, administer any rectal suppository or an enema.

those cells from spreading or metastasizing (Alcoser & Rodgers, 2003).

Chemotherapy destroys these rapidly dividing and mutating cancer cells by interfering with cell division (Alcoser & Rodgers, 2003) (Table 34-2). A variety of venous access devices are available to administer chemotherapy (Table 34-3).

RADIATION

Radiation therapy is using ionizing radiation to break apart the bonds within a cell, damaging it and causing it to die. This treatment has evolved over the years with respect to children. Today with the use of CT scan and MRI scans, it is possible to more precisely deliver radiation therapy to very specific targeted areas. External beam accounts for the majority of radiation treatments in children. The amount of radiation used is determined by the patient's age, tumor site, tumor size, tumor radiosensitivity, coexisting disease, and the use of other treatment modalities. The lowest effective dose of radiation is calculated and then delivered over a 3- to 6-week period. Treatment lasts just a few minutes. It is very important for the child to remain still and not move during treatment. Sometimes it may be necessary to sedate the child (Alcoser & Rodgers, 2003). Radiation is used with some hesitancy in children younger than 3 years of age because it can cause severe damage to healthy cells and restrict growth and fertility in the future. Nursing care includes measures that address the radiation side effects.

Table 34-2 Chemotherapeutic Agents and Common Cancer Drugs

Agent	Indications	Route	Side Effects
Asparaginase (Elspar, Kidrolase) Classification: Antineoplastic Pharmacological action: Enzyme	Acute lymphoblastic leukemia (ALL)	IM and IV	Seizures, hyperglycemia Nausea/vomiting, rashes, coagulation abnormalities, hepatotoxic, pancreatitis, anaphylaxis (have emergency medications available)
Bleomycin (Blenoxane) Classification: Antineoplastic Pharmacological: Antitumor antibiotics	Hodgkin's disease (HD) Osteosarcoma Testicular embryonal cell carcinoma	IM, IV, and SQ	Pulmonary fibrosis Pneumonitis, hypotension, nausea/vomiting, anorexia, hyperpigmentation, rashes. Anaphylaxis: fever, chills
Carboplatin (Paraplatin, Paraplatin AQ) Classification: Antineoplastic Pharmacological: Alkylating agent	Brain tumors Soft tissue sarcoma Osteosarcoma Retinoblastoma Neuroblastoma	IV	Ototoxicity, nausea/vomiting, constipation, diarrhea, stomatitis, renal and liver toxicity, hypocalcemia, hypokalemia, hyponatremia, hypomagnesemia Anaphylactic-like reactions
Corticosteroid (Dexamethasone, Decadron, Hydrocortisone, Prednisone) Classification: Corticosteroid Pharmacological: Systemic corticosteroids, anti-inflammatory	ALL Non-Hodgkin's lymphoma (NHL) HD Cerebral edema	PO, IV, and IT	Immunosuppression Weight gain, hypertension, anorexia, nausea/vomiting, acne, delayed wound healing, hirsutism, petechiae, osteoporosis, growth delay Cushingoid appearance
Cyclophosphamide (Cytoxan, Neosar, Procytox) Classification: Antineoplastic, immunosuppressant Pharmacological: Alkylating agent	NHL HD ALL Neuroblastoma Wilms' tumor Bone and soft tissue sarcoma Retinoblastoma	PO and IV	Myelosuppression Nausea, vomiting, anorexia, diarrhea, pulmonary & myocardial fibrosis, hemorrhagic cystitis, leukopenia, hematuria, alopecia, sterility, SIADH May cause second neoplasm
Daunorubicin (Daunomycin, Cerubidine) Classification: Antineoplastic Pharmacological: Anthracyclines	ALL AML Osteosarcoma Soft tissue sarcoma	IV	Blistering, myelosuppression, Cardiotoxic: arrhythmias, acute cardiac myopathy-delayed Nausea/vomiting, stomatitis, potentiation of radiation, alopecia, rash, hyperpigmentation of nails
Doxorubicin (Adriamycin, Adria, DOX, Rubex) Classification: Antineoplastic Pharmacological: Anthracyclines	ALL AML Osteosarcoma Soft tissue sarcoma Neuroblastoma	IV	Blistering, nausea/vomiting, stomatitis, esophagitis, diarrhea, red urine, anemia, hypersensitivity reaction, sterility. Cardiotoxic: arrhythmias, acute cardiomyopathy—delayed, potentiation of radiation hyperpigmentation of nails, seizures, hypertension, edema, nausea/vomiting, diarrhea, cough, shortness of breath, rash, thrombotic events
Epoetin/Erythropoietin (Epogen, EPO, Procrit) Classification: Biological Response Modifier Pharmacological: Hormone	Anemia	IV and SQ	Pulmonary edema, CHF, MI, hypotension, nausea/vomiting, anaphylaxis

Table 34-2 Chemotherapeutic Agents and Common Cancer Drugs—cont'd

Agent	Indications	Route	Side Effects
Etoposide (VP-16, VePesid) Classification: Antineoplastic Pharmacological: Podophyllotoxin derivative	AML, ALL NHL HD Bone and soft tissue sarcoma Wilms' tumor Brain tumor Neuroblastoma Retinoblastoma	IV	Excessive leukocytosis, pain, and redness at subcutaneous site
Filgrastim (GCSF—granulocyte colony stimulating factor) (Neupogen) Classification: Colony-stimulating factor Pharmacological: Hematopoietic progenitor mobilizer	Recovery drug for neutropenia	IV and SQ	Medullary bone pain
Fluorouracil (5-FU, Adrucil) Classification: Antineoplastic Pharmacological: Antimetabolite	Brain tumors Germ cell tumors Osteosarcoma Soft tissue sarcoma NHL ALL	IV	Myelosuppression, nausea/vomiting (mild), mucositis (severe), hyperpigmentation of nails, nail loss, dermatitis, phototoxicity, myelosuppression, nausea/vomiting, diarrhea, neurotoxicity (encephalopathy, hallucinations), hepatotoxicity, hemorrhagic cystitis, alopecia, sterility, may cause second neoplasm
Ifosfamide (Ifex) Classification: Antineoplastic Pharmacological: Alkylating agent	Stops methotrexate from harming the cells when given in high doses	IV	Allergic reactions: rash, urticaria, wheezing
Leucovorin (Citrovorum factor, folinic acid, Wellcovorin) Classification: Antidote (for methotrexate), vitamins Pharmacological: Folic acid analog	Recovery drug to prevent hemorrhagic cystitis from ifosfamide and cyclophosphamide	IV PO	*Dose dependent on methotrexate level *Given 24 hours after first methotrexate level has begun
Mesna (Mesnex, Uromitexan) Classification: Antidote Pharmacological: Ifosfamide detoxifying agent	Prevention of ifosfamide-induced hemorrhagic cystitis	IV, PO, IM, and IT	Dizziness, drowsiness, headache, anorexia, diarrhea, nausea/vomiting, unpleasant taste, flushing, flu-like symptoms
Methotrexate (MTX, Amethopterin) Classification: Antineoplastic Immunosuppressant Pharmacological: Antimetabolite	All Osteosarcoma NHL	IV	Myelosuppression, nausea/vomiting/stomatitis, alopecia, hepatotoxicity, neurotoxicity, photosensitivity, rash, pulmonary fibrosis, aplastic anemia
Ondansetron (Zofran) Classification: Antiemetic Pharmacological: 5-HT$_3$ antagonist	Prevention of nausea/vomiting associated with chemotherapy	IV and PO	Headache, diarrhea, constipation, dry mouth, extrapyramidal reactions
PEG-L-asparaginase (pegasparagase) (Oncospar) Classification: Antineoplastic Pharmacological: Enzymes	ALL HD	IM and IV	Seizures, pancreatitis, lip edema, headache, nausea/vomiting, diarrhea, DIC, hemolytic anemia, pancytopenia, chills, night sweats
Vincristine (Oncovorin, Vincasar PFS) Classification: Antineoplastic Pharmacological: Vinca alkaloids	Wilms' tumor Ewing's sarcoma Brain tumor	IV	Altered LOC, blistering, peripheral neuropathy, alopecia, constipation, SIADH, seizure, nausea/vomiting

IV = intravenous; IM = intramuscular; SQ = subcutaneous; PO = by mouth; IT = intrathecal.
Data from Deglin, J.H., & Vallerand, A.H. (2009). *Davis's drug guide for nurses* (11th ed.). Philadelphia: F.A. Davis.

Table 34-3 Venous Access Devices

Name	Description	Advantage	Nursing Care
Central Implanted Ports such as Infus-a-port, Mediport, port-a-cath, or Norport	A saucer-shaped plastic device with a self-sealing injection port that can be accessed from the top or side; requires placement in operating room	Decreased risk of infection Placed under the skin; reducing the chance of becoming dislodged or pulled out Limited noticeably (small bump under the skin) Patency is maintained by administering heparin after access Little maintenance or care: child can participate in regular activities	Cleanse skin with warm water and soap prior to use Administer topical anesthetic such as EMLA (lidocaine and prilocaine) before accessing the port Use a Huber needle to access the port Observe child during medication administration for dislodgment of needle When treatment complete the port must be surgically removed
Central Groshong catheter	A silicone, flexible and clear catheter; at the proximal end, there is a closed-tip two-way valve; requires placement in operating room	Easy for self-administered medications and fluids No heparin required No clamping needed due to two-way valve Minimal backflow Decreases possibility of air embolism	Weekly irrigation with normal saline Parents can learn catheter care (site must be kept clean and dry) Teaching includes; (1) strenuous activity and water sports are restricted (2) safety as the catheter protrudes from body and may be pulled out Offer support based on body image disturbance
Central tunneled catheter such as Broviac or Hickman	An open-ended silicone, flexible, radiopaque catheter. Requires placement in operating room	Easy for self-administered medications and fluids Decreases risk of infection	Daily heparin flushes Parents can learn catheter care (site must be kept clean and dry) When not in use must be clamped Teaching includes; (1) strenuous activity and water sports are restricted (2) safety as the catheter protrudes from body and may be pulled out
Peripherally inserted central catheters	Catheter made of silastic or polyurethane material Single or double lumen available Inserted into antecubital fossa passing through the cephalic or basilica vein entering the superior vena cava	Does not require placement in operating room Pediatric nurse practitioners can insert the line using a small lumen needle Decreases risk of infection	Flushed with saline using 5- to 10-mL syringe Not suitable for rapid fluid replacement (small lumen needle) Sometimes can be difficult to remove because of resistance

 clinical alert

Radiation side effects
- Nausea
- Alopecia
- Fatigue and malaise
- Low WBC
- Skin desquamation
- Mucous membrane inflammation and irritation

SURGERY

Before the development of chemotherapy and radiation, surgery was the principle treatment of children with solid tumors. Now surgery is used as an adjunct to both chemo-therapy and radiation. Tumors are usually treated with chemotherapy and radiation first to reduce the size before surgical resection. The use of surgery varies widely depending on the child's diagnosis. Surgery is also an important role in the diagnosis of a tumor via biopsy. The biopsy sample may be obtained through a fine-needle aspiration or an open biopsy procedure.

 Nursing Insight— Insertion of central venous catheters

The insertion of central venous catheters is one of the most frequent surgical procedures performed (Fig. 34-10). These long-term central venous access devices make it safer to administer chemotherapy and total parenteral nutrition, and are also used in administering of antibiotics and obtaining blood specimens (Alcoser & Rodgers, 2003).

Figure 34-10 The insertion of a central venous catheter helps in administering chemotherapy and is one of the most frequent surgical procedures performed on children with cancer.

The child may have cancer-related medical conditions before surgery; therefore the nurse understands that care measures are tailored to the child's pre- and postoperative nursing diagnoses.

 nursing diagnoses Children with Cancer

- Ineffective Airway Clearance
- Risk of Injury (bleeding) related to thrombocytopenia
- Risk for Fluid Volume Deficit related to vomiting and decreased oral intake
- Risk for Infection related to neutropenia
- Pain related to diagnosis, disease process, and treatment
- Fatigue related to anemia
- Impaired Oral Mucosa related to oral ulcerations from cancer treatment
- Imbalanced Nutrition: Less than Body Requirements related to loss of appetite, nausea, vomiting, and mucositis
- Caregiver Role Strain related to disease process and frequent hospitalizations
- Ineffective Coping related to diagnosis
- Altered Family Process related to hospitalization

PAIN CONTROL

Controlling the child's pain is an essential nursing intervention. Pain associated with cancer can be acute or chronic. Four common types of pain found in children with cancer are tumor-related pain, impingement of tumor on nervous tissue, treatment-related pain, and post-lumbar puncture headaches. Postoperative pain is also a concern after tumor resection, biopsy, amputation, or central line placement. The most effective pain management strategies reported by children with cancer are use of effective pain medications combined with adequate rest and sleep, massage, heat, distraction, and social support.

 Nursing Insight— Topical anesthetics

Use topical anesthetics when possible for procedure-related pain such as EMLA (Astra Zeneca) cream, which is a lidocaine/prilocaine 1:1 mixture. The nurse applies a thin coating of ointment to the projected insertion site(s) and covers the site(s) with a hydrocolloid dressing (such as DuoDERM). It is important to keep the cream on for at least 1 hour (sometimes longer) prior to the procedure (Bryant, 2003).

Ethnocultural Considerations— Caring for a Hispanic child with cancer

People in the Hispanic culture may approach pain with stoicism. The lack of verbal or other expression of pain does not necessarily mean that the child is pain free. Hispanics have a belief in folk health care practices and nondrug interventions. Some Hispanics do not understand the instructions for pain management. When caring for the Hispanic patient, it is important to respect his or her values and incorporate Hispanic folk practices when possible. More importantly, the nurse must provide written instruction for the child and parents in Spanish so that they understand the treatment plan. Do a thorough pain assessment and do not rely on verbal or observational cues. Explore the parents' or caregivers' and child's beliefs to achieve optimal pain control (Juarez, Ferrell, & Borneman, 1998).

PSYCHOSOCIAL SUPPORT

Psychosocial support is essential in providing holistic nursing care. Encourage 24-hour stay with parents and other family members or friends. Involve the child life specialist who can use therapeutic play or encourage arts and crafts. Video games, computers, hand-held devices or other technological equipment can be helpful when offering psychosocial support. Encourage visits to the playroom (if appropriate for the child's condition) while the child is in the hospital. Being present or simply listening can be powerful in the care of children with cancer. The nurse can also provide the family with community resources, reliable internet sources or information about support groups.

 Nursing Insight— Taking care of children with cancer

The pediatric nurse understands that children with cancer still want to be loved and treated like other children. Be sure to encourage these children to play and be involved in self-care activities as their condition allows. Encourage them to talk about their dreams, feelings, and fears. The pediatric nurse realizes that it is a privilege to share in the lives of these brave children.

Negative Effects of Chemotherapy

Chemotherapy has several associated negative effects. The nurse must recognize and provide proper nursing care to promote the best health for the child during his or her treatment.

critical nursing action Recognizing Negative Effects of Chemotherapy

Chemotherapy is toxic to the body because it kills not only cancer cells but healthy cells as well. It is important that as soon as chemotherapy is administered the nurse ensures that the child is also well hydrated so that the chemotherapeutic agent (or toxin) is flushed out of the system. A way to ensure proper hydration is to measure the specific gravity of the urine. The urine specific gravity should be 1.012 or below. If it rises above this, IV fluid boluses are required.

NAUSEA AND VOMITING

Nausea and vomiting is a major negative effect of chemotherapy and the nurse understands that the nausea may persist for weeks. Acute nausea begins 2 to 3 hours after chemotherapy starts, peaks at 4 to 10 hours, and lasts for 12 to 24 hours. Delayed nausea begins 1 to 5 days after chemotherapy, peaks 48 to 72 hours, and is less severe than acute nausea. Anticipatory nausea is psychological and the nurse understands that it is important to medicate the child if he or she complains about nausea.

It is also important for the nurse to be knowledgeable about medications (antiemetics) that can prevent or lessen nausea and vomiting in children (Fig. 34-11).

ALOPECIA

Hair loss (alopecia) is another negative effect associated with cancer treatment (Fig. 34-12). Not all children undergoing chemotherapy lose their hair. When it does occur, it may be devastating to the child and the family. Providing a wig or a hat and helping the child present a positive body image and peer acceptance is crucial. There are agencies (i.e., http://www.locksoflove.org/) that assist with providing the child with a wig.

medication: Common Antiemetics

Odansetron (Zofran)
0.15 mg/kg every 8 hours
Duration:
IV: 24 hours
PO: 8 hours
Not as effective as a prn
Not as effective if vomiting has begun
While the child is receiving chemotherapy, give 30 minutes before chemotherapy, then every 6–8 hours for 24 hours

Diphenhydramine (Benadryl)
1 mg/kg per dose every 6 hours
PO/IV immediate onset
Duration 4–7 hours
SIDE EFFECTS: sedation, dry mouth, blurred vision

Lorazepam (Ativan)
IV: 0.4 mg/kg/dose every 6 hours
IV duration: 4–6 hours
Often used for anticipatory nausea/vomiting
Side effects: sedation, euphoria

"What to say" — *If I lose my hair will it grow back?*

Many children who start chemotherapy have many questions, especially wanting to know "if my hair falls out, will it grow back"? Children worry about their appearance to an extent that depends on their age. The nurse should explain that the hair will probably start to fall out 10 days to 2 weeks after chemotherapy begins and that it may fall out in sections. The nurse can assure the child that once the chemotherapy has been completed, their hair will grow back. Try to make this experience as positive as possible by emphasizing there are wigs available as well as scarfs, and "cool" hats and

Figure 34-11 It is important for the nurse to be knowledgeable of medications (antiemetics) that can prevent or lessen nausea and vomiting in children receiving chemotherapy.

Figure 34-12 Alopecia is a negative effect associated with cancer treatment that can make the child feel very self-conscious.

caps to cover the child's head. Encourage the child to speak with others his or her age who have been through this experience. It is important for the nurse to emphasize the fact that just because his or her hair falls out, it does not change the person the child is inside. The child is the same person, who just looks a little different for a little while. The nurse can make this a special event by arranging for a first "cool hat" purchase before the child leaves the hospital.

EXTRAVASATION

Chemotherapeutic drugs must be handled carefully to avoid extravasation (accidental leakage of drug into the subcutaneous tissues surrounding the injection site/IV site). This is caused by known vesicants or a chemotherapy agent that can produce a blister or tissue destruction (Box 34-3). It is also important to handle chemotherapy agents safely (Box 34-4). For central lines it is important to make sure there is a blood return in the line to ensure patency before administering any chemotherapeutic agents by this route.

 clinical alert

Monitor closely the intravenous (IV) site

Before administering a known "vesicant," a chemotherapy agent that can result in tissue necroses and even potentially the loss of a limb, make sure the peripheral IV or central line is patent. This involves more than flushing the IV site. Some institutions require a return blood flow, which is important to ensure the peripheral line is patent because the infiltration of a known vesicant can result in blistering, tissue sloughing, and severe cellulites. In rare cases, this can cause cellulitis that turns into a more severe infection. It is important that the nurse infusing these agents be specially trained and certified in the administration of chemotherapy agents. Through this training, the nurse learns that vigilant monitoring is paramount.

Box 34-3 Agents Known to Cause Extravasation

TPN and other hyperosmolar fluids

Dilantin

Chemotherapeutic agents Doxorubicin, Daunorubicin, Mitomycin C, Vincristine, Vinblastine, VP-16, Dacarbazine

---

Box 34-4 Safe Handling of Chemotherapeutic Agents

- Use disposable gloves and gowns when handling or preparing chemotherapy medications to prevent contact with medication.
- Use aseptic technique when administering medications.
- Prepare drugs in a well ventilated room.
- Dispose of all medications, contaminated needles, syringes, intravenous tubing, gloves, and gowns in an appropriate leakproof, puncture-resistant container.

Source: Alcoser, P., & Rodgers, C. (2003). Treatment strategies in childhood cancer. *Journal of Pediatric Nursing*, 18(2), 103–112.

MUCOSITIS

Mucositis is a diffuse inflammation of the mucosa of the mouth, a change in the integrity of the mucous membranes characterized by soreness, redness, and swelling. Lesions on the mucous membranes allow bacteria to attach themselves to the affected areas and are a source of localized and systemic infection. Mucositis is caused by chemotherapy and radiation to the head and neck. It is essential to keep the oral cavity clean by rinsing the mouth with a solution (e.g., Peridex, sodium bicarbonate swish and spit, Nystatin swish and swallow, a "magic mouthwash" consisting of milk of magnesia and Carafate).

DIARRHEA AND CONSTIPATION

Diarrhea may occur with chemotherapy. The nurse must assess the rectal mucosa to prevent infection. Gently cleaning the skin around the anus with a soft cloth and warm water is important. Applying a barrier cream (such as Desitin) and allowing the irritated skin to be exposed to open air as much as possible may be necessary. Have the child drink plenty of clear fluids (based on 24-hour intake) and eat small amounts of soft bland low fiber foods such as bananas, rice, noodles, white bread, or skinned chicken. Avoiding greasy, fatty, spicy, or fried foods, as well as raw vegetables/fruits and whole-grain breads (cereals, nuts, and popcorn), can help. It is also important to discourage gas-forming foods (beans, cabbage, and carbonated beverages) and limiting beverages with caffeine. The nurse communicates to parents that they can contact the health care provider about an over-the-counter medication for diarrhea such as Loperamide (Imodium) or a prescription medication like Diphenoxylate (Lomotil).

If the child becomes constipated, the nurse can suggest foods high in fiber (fruits and vegetables) and drink plenty of fluid such as water and juices. Normal activity and playing if approved by the health care provider can help. The nurse can instruct parents to ask their health care provider for medications that will help with the constipation. The health care provider may prescribe medications such as Docusate sodium (Colace) or Bisacodyl (Dulcolax).

ANEMIA

Anemia can also be acquired during chemotherapy. Bone marrow suppression, nutritional deficiencies, and blood loss may all lead to anemia below 8 g/dL. While the cancerous cells are being killed, sometimes healthy cells such as RBCs are killed also.

Some signs of anemia are severe fatigue, headache, irritability, or tachycardia (Bryant, 2003). For children with mild anemia, the nurse can provide supportive care guidelines for improving the anemia through diet or vitamin supplementation. Children with moderate to severe anemia may need a RBC transfusion to restore blood volume. For specific types of anemia such as decreased production of RBCs, the nurse can administer hematopoietic growth factors (filgrastim [Neupogen]) that may prove beneficial in decreasing the need for blood transfusions.

THROMBOCYTOPENIA

Like RBCs, platelets can also be destroyed. Platelets are important for the clotting of the blood. Thrombocytopenia is a decreased number of platelets (less than 100,000 μL) (Bryant, 2003). Thrombocytopenia develops as a result of increased destruction, decreased production, or loss of platelets. A platelet transfusion should be given if platelet counts drop to less than 50,000 μL, if the patient has spontaneous bleeding, or if an invasive procedure is scheduled (Behrman et al., 2004).

NEUTROPENIA

Neutropenic children have few WBCs and often do not show signs of infection, such as swelling, redness, or drainage. The only sign may be fever. A fever in an oncology patient is 101.2°F (38.5°C) in a 24-hour period or 100.4°F (38.0°C) three times in a 24-hour period. Take only axillary or oral temperature.

A severe neutropenic patient has an absolute neutrophil count (ANC) of <500/mm³. An ANC of ≥500 to <1000/mm³ is considered moderately neutropenic, and an ANC of ≥1000 to <1500/mm³ is considered mildly neutropenic. When a child undergoing chemotherapy develops a fever, it is considered an emergency.

---

 diagnostic tools Calculating the Absolute Neutrophil Count (ANC)

Formula: (WBC × 10) × (Bands + Neutrophils)
Example: WBC = 8.8, Neutrophils = 82, Bands = 5
    ANC = (8.8 × 10) × (82 + 5)
    ANC = (88) × (87)
    ANC = 7656

Two sets of blood cultures are required for the neutropenic patient before the start of antibiotics. Antibiotics should be started as soon as possible, no later than 1 hour after admission. The nurse must monitor vital signs very closely when administering antibiotics due to the release of endotoxin that may occur. Left unchecked, this condition may lead to septic shock.

Optimizing Outcomes— **Neutropenic patient admitted to a pediatric unit**

A 2-year-old neutropenic oncology patient is admitted to the in-patient pediatric unit. The unit is full and bed space is limited. It is the middle of winter and there are several patients with respiratory syncytial virus and rotavirus on the floor. In what type of room should the child be placed?

Best Outcome: To ensure the best outcome, place the child in a private room by him- or herself. If a private room is not available, assigning the child to a room with someone noninfectious, such as a child with a fractured femur, is acceptable.

LONG-TERM EFFECTS OF CANCER TREATMENTS

Now that children with cancer are surviving longer, researchers are just beginning to understand the long-term effects of cancer treatments. Children undergoing cancer treatments are assessed for acute effects at the time but also need follow-up care in adulthood to assess for potential long-term effects. A long-term survivor of any cancer is considered a child who has been in remission for 5 years or who has been off cancer therapy for 2 years.

For example, high-tone hearing loss may be a side effect of cisplatin (Platinol). Other chemotherapeutic agents can cause loss of speech, impairment in depth perception, and increased response time can be a problem for the adolescent who wishes to drive. Lung problems can be caused by scarring of lung tissue or a reduction in lung elasticity during breathing. Shortness of breath and a reduced capacity to exercise can significantly impact the child. Kidney problems include bleeding, damage to the tubules that affects electrolyte exchange and salt balance, and protein wasting. Musculoskeletal defects involving the bones or soft tissue and teeth have been reported. Functional and/or mobility deficits may persist if an amputation was performed. Hormonal abnormalities that are often treatable may also exist. Cancer treatment can sometimes produce sterility. Hearing, skin problems and cardiac dysfunction are some of the late side effects that children are left to deal with later in life.

Children who had radiation to the brain may show growth retardation, cognitive impairment, and/or learning disabilities. Damage to the hypothalamus may cause an irreversible disorder called diabetes insipidus (DI). A type of nerve damage called peripheral neuropathy can lead to decreased reflexes and weakness. The thyroid gland is also sensitive to radiation and may pose problems later in life.

Medical Emergencies

Due to his or her altered state of health, a child with cancer is prone to various conditions that may constitute a medical emergency, including accidents, infections, allergic reactions, or common childhood diseases. If one or more of these conditions is negatively affecting the child, the pediatric nurse must act quickly and notify the physician or oncologist caring for the child in order to prevent a life-threatening condition or further complications.

HEMORRHAGIC CYSTITIS

When caring for an oncology patient who is undergoing chemotherapy, using certain chemotherapy agents, such as cyclophosphamide (Cytoxan) or ifosfamide (Ifex), can cause hemorrhagic cystitis (bloody or painful urination). Radiation may also cause hemorrhagic cystitis. This condition can range from mild dysuria (painful urination) with urinary frequency to severe hemorrhage significant enough to damage the epithelial lining of the bladder. Patients also have leukocytes, erythrocytes, and clots in the urine. The best way to treat hemorrhagic cystitis is to prevent it with adequate hydration before and during the administration of chemotherapy. Be sure to test the urine for blood, pH and specific gravity. The specific gravity should be less than 1.010. If it is not, a bolus of IV fluid is required (Box 34-5 and Procedure 34-1). If the urine is positive for blood, send an immediate urinalysis sample to the lab and notify the physician immediately. Monitoring of intake and output is vital as well as a daily blood urea nitrogen (BUN) and creatinine. Mesna (Mesnex, Uromitexan) is a drug given to prevent hemorrhagic cystitis by helping to protect the lining of the bladder.

Procedure 34-1 Checking Urine Specific Gravity

Purpose

The purpose of checking the specific gravity of urine is to measure the concentration of the particles in the urine.

Equipment
- Refractometer
- 3- or 5-mL syringe (needleless)

Steps

1. Have the child urinate into a urine collection receptacle.

   RATIONALE: *The urine collection receptacle is not a sterile container.*

2. Using a 3- or 5-mL syringe, draw up 0.5 mL of urine into the syringe.

3. Place the syringe into a universal precaution container.

   RATIONALE: *Promotes a safe environment.*

4. Take the urine specimen to the testing area.

   RATIONALE: *A specific testing area promotes a safe environment.*

5. Open the refractometer.

6. Place one drop of urine in the center of the square opening.

7. Close the lid.

8. Look through the focused eyepiece to see the horizontal line clearly.

   RATIONALE: *Ensures accurate measurement of specific gravity.*

9. Note where the blue horizontal line crosses the markings (see picture below).

   RATIONALE: *The blue horizontal line that crosses the markings is the specific gravity reading.*

Clinical Alert If the institution does not have a refractometer, it is acceptable to use a urine dipstick, with the realization that this is not as detailed. The specific gravity markings on a urine dipstick are in increments of 0.005. On a refractometer, the markings are in increments of 0.001.

Teach Parents

The nurse can teach the parents about the purpose of a specific gravity measurement.

Documentation
Specific gravity done at 1300 h. Specific gravity = 1.010.
—M. Godshall, RN

Box 34-5 Checking Urine Specific Gravity

SPECIFIC GRAVITY
- Check urine specific gravity for patients receiving Cytoxan, ifosfamide, cisplatin, high-dose carboplatin, high-dose methotrexate.
- Specific gravity must be less than or equal to 1.010 before the start of chemotherapy and then for at least 24 hours after its completion.
- If at any time the specific gravity rises above 1.010, the patient should receive a fluid bolus (extra fluid). DO NOT turn off the main IV. The bolus is in addition to the main IVF.
- If giving more than two or three fluid boluses, notify the oncologist on call.

URINE pH
- Monitor when the patient is receiving methotrexate.
- Urine pH must be higher than 7.0 before starting methotrexate, and must be maintained at that level until the methotrexate serum blood level is <0.1 mg/dl.
- Before receiving high-dose methotrexate, patients are hydrated with IVF of D5¼ with 40 mEq/L of $NaHCO_3$. The $NaHCO_3$ is needed to keep the urine alkalinized.

TUMOR LYSIS SYNDROME

Tumor lysis syndrome is a life-threatening condition that may develop in children with cancer. Tumors with high growth rates, large volume, or that are widely disseminated such as Burkitt's lymphoma, lymphoblastic lymphoma, T-cell, and ALL are associated with this disorder. Tumor lysis syndrome may result from cell death related to a chemotherapy agent or the malignancy itself.

SIGNS AND SYMPTOMS. Children develop lethargy, nausea and vomiting, oliguria, flank pain, pruritus, tetany, and altered level of consciousness. Renal failure can also occur.

DIAGNOSIS. After the cell dies, there is a rapid (12 to 72 hours after treatment starts) release of intracellular contents (metabolites) that leads to hyperuricemia, hypocalcemia, hyperphosphatemia, and hyperkalemia. An astute nursing assessment and immediate laboratory results can help diagnose this condition.

NURSING CARE. It is important to keep the urine alkalinized and maintain a low-phosphate diet. Administration of allopurinol (Aloprim) to reduce uric acid formation and promote excretion of byproducts of purine metabolism is essential. Maintaining adequate hydration is also paramount. Monitoring electrolytes such as calcium, magnesium, phosphorus, potassium, as well as kidney function with measurements such as BUN and creatinine, is very important. Sometimes dialysis or exchange transfusions are necessary to decrease the metabolic consequence that causes an even more severe effect on the child.

SEPTIC SHOCK

The patient who is neutropenic and has a fever is at great risk for septic shock. Septic shock happens in a child who is undergoing or has just finished chemotherapy and/or radiation. The level of the WBCs that fight infection and invading organisms is extremely low (neutropenia).

When the child is admitted to the hospital with a fever, he or she is given an antibiotic regimen to cover both gram-positive and gram-negative bacteria within a 1-hour window of the patient arriving on the inpatient unit. As the antibiotic destroys the cell wall of the bacteria, endotoxin is released from the cell wall. This endotoxin starts a cascade and overwhelms the compromised body's ability to deal with the endotoxin.

SIGNS AND SYMPTOMS. Signs can include confusion, fever, increased respirations (tachypnea), decreased urinary output, and cold, clammy skin. The patient becomes pale and the heart rate increases in an attempt to compensate, and then suddenly the patient's blood pressure plummets (late sign). Laboratory studies reveal acidosis and sometimes renal failure (Venes, 2009).

 Nursing Insight— **Hypotension**

Pediatric patients compensate for shock by increasing the heart rate. When that is no longer effective, the blood pressure falls rapidly.

DIAGNOSIS. Vigilant monitoring of signs and symptoms by the nurse who is giving antibiotics to a neutropenic patient is crucial in diagnosing this condition.

 clinical alert

Septic shock

It is important to remember that this septic shock response can occur immediately or up to 48 to 72 hours later.

NURSING CARE. By the time the blood pressure drops, the situation is ominous.

 critical nursing action Nursing Care for Septic Shock

For a child who is neutropenic and is admitted for a fever, and is being given antibiotics, the nurse must take vital signs every 10 to 15 minutes during the antibiotic administration to recognize signs of septic shock. Recognizing the other signs is also crucial. Remember that a drop in blood pressure is a late sign. Be ready to administer large amounts (1-L bags) of an isotonic fluid, such as normal saline

(20 mL/kg) rapidly to prevent circulatory collapse and possibly death. Be sure to check peripheral pulses and capillary refill to monitor perfusion (whether the blood is reaching the extremities). In an emergency remember the ABCs and other emergent care measures:

Airway

Breathing

Circulation

Fluid resuscitation

Evaluation of etiology (CBC, electrolytes, DIC panel, blood cultures, liver and renal functions)

Blood products

Antibiotics

Vasopressors

 clinical alert

Other emergencies

- Superior vena cava syndrome—obstruction or thrombus in the superior vena cava, superior mediastinum syndrome—tracheal compression.
- Pericardial effusion—fluid in the pericardial cavity, between the visceral and the parietal pericardium. This condition may produce symptoms of cardiac tamponade, such as difficulty in breathing (Venes, 2009).
- Pleural effusion—fluid in the thoracic cavity between the visceral and parietal pleura. It may be seen on a chest radiograph if the fluid exceeds 300 mL (Venes, 2009).
- Abdominal emergencies—esophagitis, gastric hemorrhage, perirectal abscess, hemorrhagic pancreatitis, massive acute hepatomegaly, bowel obstruction.
- Neurological conditions—stroke, seizure, spinal cord compression.
- Shock—hypovolemic, cardiogenic, distributive.
- Hyperleukocytosis—WBC count greater than $100,000/mm^3$.

The Psychological Impact of Pediatric Cancer

The psychological impact that cancer has on the entire family is enormous. The feelings of shock, denial, confusion, and fear strike everyone. Families may feel someone or something is to blame for their child's illness. Adding to the stress is the feeling of having absolutely no control over any part of the situation. Feelings of any kind during this situation are normal as everyone reacts differently.

Sometimes one of the best sources of support for the parents are other parents who have gone through the experience of their child having cancer. It is important to encourage families to develop support systems whether they are family, friends, or other people who may be able to help in some way.

Many parents maintain a bedside vigil, which is understandable because they want to be there for their child. As this can be very wearing and tiring (Fig. 34-13), the nurse can communicate to the parents that it is important that they get adequate rest and nutrition to avoid becoming sick themselves.

Figure 34-13 Many parents maintain a bedside vigil to support their child during treatment for cancer.

Depending on his or her level of understanding, it is important for the parents and health care team to be honest with the child. A multidisciplinary approach is necessary and the goal of the team is to communicate enough information so that the child can make sense of the situation without becoming overwhelmed. Information must be tailored to each child's developmental stage. The nurse must keep the lines of communication open.

Families may ask questions such as, Why did this happen? Why does my child suffer? What did I do wrong? These are normal feelings for families when a child is diagnosed with cancer. Steen and Mirro (2000) stated, "faith is like a lens through which you experience all of life. During this process grief comes into play. When grief and faith meet, a crisis of faith occurs" (p. 283). The nurse understands that it is important to offer spiritual support when the child and family are ready. The child may feel a sense of spirituality through the nurse. The nurse can ask the hospital Chaplin or Faith Community Nurse to visit on a regular basis, use prayer or meditation if requested or read from a spiritual/inspirational text. Be sure to allow the child and family quiet time during the day to be alone and meditate if they choose.

Help the child and family express his or her feelings. Being present and giving reassurance that he or she is not being punished is important. Through the nurse's care the child will know that he or she is loved. Many parents tell the nurse how they were touched deeply knowing that the nurse really cared for their child (Fig. 34–14).

❝What to say❞ — *To siblings of an ill child*

While children with cancer are undergoing many stressful events, as a pediatric nurse do not forget about the sibling(s) of the children with cancer. Visiting a sick sibling is stressful for both the ill child and the sibling. The nurse can help make the sibling's day special by telling them a story, or giving them a sticker or a coloring book and crayons. Encourage the ill child to color a picture for their sibling and hang it in the room.

A sincere demeanor and common pleasantries such as saying hello or calling the sibling by their name can make the visit special and less stressful.

? case study Family Dilemma

An 18-year-old adolescent named Joe who is dying from liver cancer is admitted to your pediatric unit. His parents are divorced. He lives with his father. He has a sister who lives with the mother. The mother is remarried and therefore Joe has a stepfather as well. You are the nurse caring for this family. No one but Joe wants to talk about the fact that he is dying. The father tries to keep Joe's spirits up with jokes. The mother appears to be in denial and will not accept the possibility that Joe is dying. He is receiving antibiotic therapy and continued chemotherapy, which at this point is palliative. One day when you are caring for Joe, he says to you that he is tired of being in pain and just wants to die. He says "I know I am dying, but my family refuses to accept it." He is a mature young man, and you listen as he tells you of the dreams he had to go to a state college. He tells you that he has spoken to his oncologist who has agreed to stop chemotherapy for him. He is 18 and legally an adult. His mother now refuses to visit him because she feels everyone has given up on him. Joe is the only one who is realistic about his future and disease progression.

critical thinking question

1. As Joe's nurse, how would you help him and his family so that he can experience a peaceful death?

   Note: This is a true story and Joe died peacefully with his father and nurse at his bedside.

◆ See Suggested Answers to Case Studies in text on the Electronic Study Guide or DavisPlus.

Figure 34-14 Through the nurse's care the child will know that he or she is loved.

summary points

◆ Cancer is a group of diseases in which there is out-of-control growth and spread of abnormal cells known as anaplasia (loss of the normal pattern of growth of cells).

◆ In children many common malignancies arise from primitive embryonic tissue where there has been a strong environmental link related to the development of cancer.

◆ Acute leukemia is a rapidly progressing disease that affects mostly immature, undifferentiated cells. Chronic leukemia is a less rapidly progressing disease allowing for the production of mature, more differentiated cells.

◆ The most common types of solid tumors in children include brain tumors, neuroblastoma, rhabdosarcoma, retinoblastoma and nephroblastoma (Wilms' tumor).

◆ The two most common bone tumors are osteogenic sarcoma and Ewing's sarcoma.

◆ Lymphoma is a malignancy that arises from the lymphatic system. Two types of lymphomas are seen in children: Hodgkin's disease (HD) and non-Hodgkin's lymphoma (NHL).

◆ Liver and extragonadal germ cell cancer are other types of cancer seen in children.

◆ Nursing care for a child with cancer: maintaining nutrition, preventing infection, administering chemotherapy, addressing radiation side effects, understanding the use of surgery and related nursing diagnosis, pain control, offering psychosocial support, managing negative and long-term effects of cancer treatments and preventing medical emergencies.

◆ Understanding the psychological impact of pediatric cancer is also an important element of care.

review questions

Multiple Choice

1. A 3-year-old girl is admitted to your unit with acute lymphocytic leukemia. She received chemotherapy treatment 10 days ago and her neutrophil count is low. The nurse utilizes critical thinking and assigns her in a room with:
A. A 3-year-old admitted with bronchiolitis
B. A 5-year-old with a fractured femur
C. A 4-year-old admitted with a streptococcal infection
D. A 3-year-old with a history of diarrhea

2. The pediatric nurse provides health promotion teaching to the parents of a 6-year-old boy who has been discharged after chemotherapy. The nurse should instruct them:
A. "Do not allow your child to play with any children for a few days."
B. "Be sure to encourage your child to brush his teeth vigorously every day."
C. "If your child feels warm, be sure to take his temperature rectally."
D. "If your child has a temperature of 101.2°F (38.5°C) bring him to the emergency room immediately."

True/False

3. The pediatric nurse who is assessing a child with a decreased number of platelets (thrombocytopenia) is aware that this child may present with clinical manifestations such as bleeding gums, nosebleeds, and easy bruising.

4. The pediatric nurse recognizes that a child with acute myelogenous leukemia has "blueberry muffin" lesions.

5. Sarcomas are solid tumors that may develop in lymphoid organs such as the thymus, spleen, and lymph nodes.

6. During nursing rounds, the pediatric nurse discusses that leukemia is the first most common pediatric cancer, brain tumors are second, and neuroblastoma is the third most common pediatric cancer.

7. The pediatric nurse recognizes that children with leukemia who relapse while on chemotherapy or within 6 months after cessation of chemotherapy have a poor prognosis.

8. During the physical assessment, the pediatric nurse carefully palpates the scrotum to confirm that both testicles are present since a child with undescended testes has an increased risk of developing testicular cancer.

Fill-in-the-Blank

9. Ninety-five percent of children with acute lymphocytic leukemia will achieve remission during the _____ _____ of chemotherapy treatment. If treatment is stopped during this phase, _____ cells will reappear. This is why _____ treatment is crucial. Because leukemic cells can cross the _____ _____ _____ and most chemotherapy does not, central nervous system prophylaxis treatment is necessary. This medication is injected _____ into the cerebrospinal fluid space during a lumbar puncture.

10. The second phase of chemotherapy treatment is called the _____ phase. The goal of this phase is to eliminate any residual leukemic cells. _____ _____ is also required during this phase of treatment.

11. The _____ _____ phase maintains control of leukemia. This phase can last for _____ to _____ years after diagnosis.

12. Children with cancer should be encouraged to play in the playroom as long as their _____ _____ are within normal. Allowing the child to continue with recreational activities helps to promote a sense of normalcy.

Case Study

13. Johnny, a 5-year-old boy, is admitted to the pediatric unit to rule out a brain tumor. The nurse performs a neurological exam. Which of the following does the nurse note to be indicative of increasing intracranial pressure?
A. A bulging fontanel with irritability
B. Speech disturbance with vomiting

C. A blood pressure of 98/58 with an apical pulse of 90

D. Hyperactivity with a temperature of 101.2°F (38.5°C)

14. The diagnosis is confirmed that Johnny has a brain tumor. The parents are very upset and say to the nurse, "I can't believe my son is going to die. What am I going to do"? The most therapeutic response that the nurse can say is:

A. "Your son is not going to die. We will take good care of him."

B. "I will call the hospital minister to come and speak with you."

C. "I can understand how upset you must be feeling, but we need to take this one day at a time."

D. "I will be here every day to help your son. Would you like me to introduce you to another family with a child who has the same illness?"

See Answers to End of Chapter Review Questions on the Electronic Study Guide or DavisPlus.

REFERENCES

Alcoser, P., & Rodgers, C. (2003). Treatment strategies in childhood cancer. *Journal of Pediatric Nursing, 18*(2), 103–112.

Behrman, R., Kliegman, R., & Jenson, H. (Eds.). (2004). *Nelson textbook of pediatrics* (17th ed.). Philadelphia: W.B. Saunders.

Bryant, R. (2003). Managing side effects of childhood cancer treatments. *Journal of Pediatric Nursing, 18*(2), 113–125.

Bulechek, G., Butcher, H.M., & Dochterman, J. (2008). *Nursing interventions classification (NIC)* (5th ed.). St. Louis, MO: C.V. Mosby.

Colby-Graham, M., & Chordas, C. (2003). The childhood leukemias. *Journal of Pediatric Nursing, 18*(2), 87–94.

Deglin, J.H., & Vallerand, A.H. (2009). *Davis's drug guide for nurses* (11th ed.). Philadelphia: F.A. Davis.

Jemel, A., Murray, T., Ward, E., Samuels, A., Tiwardi, R.C., Ghafoor, A., E.J., & Thun, M.J. (2005). Cancer statistics 2005. *CA A Cancer Journal for Clinicians, 55*, 10–30. Retrieved from http://caonline.amcancersoc.org (Accessed August 15, 2008).

Johnson, M., Bulechek, G., Butcher, H., McCloskey Dochterman, J., Maas, M., Moorehead, S., & Swanson, E. (2006). *NANDA, NOC, and NIC linkages: Nursing diagnoses, outcomes, & interventions* (2nd ed.). St. Louis, MO: Mosby Elsevier.

Juarez, G., Ferrell, B., & Borneman, T. (1998). Influence of culture on cancer pain management in Hispanic patients. *Cancer Practice, 6*(5), 262–269.

Kline, N., & Sevier, N. (2003). Solid tumors in children. *Journal of Pediatric Nursing, 18*(2), 96–102.

Moorehead, S., Johnson, M., Maas, M., & Swanson, E. (2008) *Nursing outcomes classification (NOC)* (4th ed.). St. Louis, MO: C.V. Mosby.

NANDA International (2007). *NANDA-I nursing diagnoses: Definitions and classifications 2007–2008*. Philadelphia: NANDA-I.

National Cancer Institute. (2008). Solid tumors in children. Retrieved from http://www.cancer.gov/search/results.aspx (Accessed May 14, 2008).

Ozyar, E., Ayhan, A., Korcum, A., & Atahan, I. (2004). Prognostic role of Epstein-Barr virus latent membrane protein-1 and interleukin-10. Expression in patients with nasopharyngeal carcinoma. *Cancer Investigation, 22*(4), 483–491.

Steen, G., & Mirro, M. (2000). *Childhood cancer. A handbook from St. Jude Children's Research Hospital*. Cambridge, MA: Perseus.

Venes, D. (2009). *Taber's cyclopedic medical dictionary* (21st ed.) Philadelphia: F.A. Davis.

 For more information go to http://davisplus.fadavis.com/

CONCEPT MAP

Caring for the Child with Cancer

Influences: Certain Viruses; Genetics → **Cancer** → Anaplasia/neoplasm: → **Malignant: in children**
- From embryonic tissue
- Affects stem cells

→ **Metastasis**

Benign

Types of Cancers in Children
Leukemias
- Acute lymphocytic leukemia
- Acute myelogenous leukemia
- Chronic myelogenous leukemia
- Juvenile chronic myelogenous
Solid Tumors
- Brain tumors
  - Glial → astrocytomas; ependyomas
  - Primitive neuroectodermal tumor
- Neuroblastoma; nephroblastoma
- Rhabdosarcoma; retinoblastoma
Bone Tumors
- Osteosarcoma; Ewing's sarcoma
Lymphomas
- Hodgkin's/Non-Hodgkin's
Liver cancer
Extragonadal Germ Cell

Where Research And Practice Meet:
- EBV link to nasopharyngeal cancer

Treatment Options

Collaboration In Caring:
- Nutritionist

Radiation Therapy:
Use of lowest therapeutic dose over 3- to 6-wk period

Surgery:
To diagnose cancer through biopsy; removal of tumor; insert central venous catheter

HSCT: Bone Marrow Transplant:
High-dose chemotherapy followed by stem cell rescue
Autologous or allogeneic transplants

Gene Therapy:
Developing slowly; to correct genetic defects

Chemotherapy:
Primary treatment; use of drugs to kill cancer cells by interrupting cell division; toxic to some non-cancerous cell lines

General Nursing Care
- Thorough physical assessment for side effects of all treatments
- Nutritional support
- Psychological support
- Pain management

Specific Nursing Care:
Child Receiving Chemotherapy
- Nausea/vomiting: anticipate timing; give antiemetics
- Alopecia: provide wig/wig info
- Extravasation: know drugs, know facility policy
- Mucositis: mouth care; appropriate products; close inspection
- Diarrhea/constipation: NO enemas if neutropenic; increased liquids; skin care to rectal area
- Anemia: assessment, transfusion
- Neutropenia: defined by absolute neutrophil count; protect from infection; neutropenic precautions
- Thrombocytopenia: pay attention to bleeding
- Pain control

Nursing Care: Oncologic/Medical Emergencies
- Hemorrhagic cystitis: urine for specific gravity/blood; IV fluid bolus; monitor I&O, BUN and creatinine
- Tumor lysis syndrome: hydration; allopurinol; exchange transfusions
- Septic shock: intense monitoring and assessment of vital signs; triple antibiotic therapy; fluid resuscitation; possible ICU

What To Say:
- Have positive attitude; help family maintain normalcy
- Allow time to absorb dx
- Encourage verbalization; provide reassurance/support group
- Include ill child in discussions
- Encourage sibling participation

Critical Nursing Action:
- Never palpate Wilms' tumor
- Hydration critical during chemotherapy
- Recognizing septic shock

Family Teaching Guidelines:
- Recognizing signs of infection

Nursing Insight:
- Cell division
- Focused neuro exam done for child with brain tumor
- Gene therapy and staging
- Bone marrow transplant

Clinical Alert:
- Chemo drugs are biohazardous waste
- Assess for hemorrhagic cystitis
- Avoid rectal route for meds/temps
- Be aware of other medical emergencies

Ethnocultural Considerations:
- Hispanic patients and pain control issues; cultural health beliefs

Now Can You:
- List/describe the cancerous growths that affect children versus adults
- Discuss various treatment modalities used in cancer treatment

Complementary Care:
- Visualization using scenarios meaningful to children
- Distraction

Caring for the Child with a Chronic Condition or the Dying Child

 We don't have to wait until we are very sick and know this might be "it." We can get support from the day we learn something could happen.

—Mattie Stepanek

LEARNING TARGETS *At the completion of this chapter, the student will be able to:*

◆ Define what is meant by a chronic condition.

◆ Explore chronic conditions and the role of technology in their management.

◆ Discuss the impact of a chronic condition for children of all ages.

◆ Recognize the emotional responses to a chronic condition.

◆ Explain important aspects of a chronic condition such as establishing a therapeutic relationship, growth and development, education, and cultural issues.

◆ Explore the aspects of the dying process and related nursing care.

◆ Describe palliative, hospice, and end-of-life care for the dying child.

◆ Explore grief and saying good-bye.

◆ Describe additional nursing aspects related to the death of a child such as preparing a remembrance packet, organ tissue donation and funerals.

◆ Explore what it means to care as a professional caregiver.

---

 moving toward evidence-based practice Quality of Life in Chronically Ill Children

Svavarsdóttir, E.K. & Črlygsdóttir, B. (2006). Comparison of health-related quality of life among 10 to 12 year old children with chronic illnesses and healthy children: The parents' perspective. *The Journal of School Nursing, 22*(3), 178–185.

The purpose of this study was to compare mothers' and fathers' perceptions of the health-related quality of life of well children and those with chronic illness. The study was conducted as part of a larger cross-sectional study: the Health-Related Quality of Life (HRQOL) among 10- to 12-year-old school children.

Twelve randomly selected public elementary schools from one city were selected for this study. Data were collected over a 3-month period.

Participants in the study were recruited from a total population of 1079 children in the 5th and 6th grades and their parents. From the total population, 480 children (209 boys and 271 girls) and 912 parents (519 mothers and 402 fathers) agreed to participate in the study. A majority of the children (70.2%) lived in a household where both parents were present,

8.1% lived with one biological parent or a stepparent, and 21% lived with only one parent.

Information collected included:

- Demographic data (collected from parents and children) that included information about health status and the presence of chronic conditions or illnesses in the child
- Children's experiences with bullying either as a victim or a perpetrator (reported by children)
- Children's visits to the school nurse over a 1-week period and their level of involvement in after-school activities (reported by children)
- Parents' ratings of the child's complaints of various symptoms such as headaches, stomachaches, dizziness, and difficulty sleeping

(continued)

moving toward evidence-based practice (continued)

- Parents' reports of the child's chronic physical conditions or illnesses including allergies/eczema, migraines, asthma, seizures/epilepsy, diabetes and "other"
- Parents' reports of the child's chronic psychiatric conditions or illnesses including learning disabilities, hyperactivity/ attention-deficit disorder, dyslexia, developmental delay, autism, and "other."

Study Tools

The Health Promotion Scale-Parents' Proxy Report was used to measure the parents' perception of the children's level of health promotion. This tool contained 21 items and 5 subscales: social-support, life-appreciation, health-responsibility, stress-management, and nutrition behavior. The tool was a modification of a previously tested measure. Parents were asked to rate items on a 5-point Likert-type scale with 1 = never to 5 = always. The total score could range from 0 to 84.

A 23-item Pediatric Quality of Life Inventory scale was also used. This tool contained four subscales: physical functioning, emotional functioning, social functioning, and school functioning. Parents were asked to rate each item based on how they perceived problems in each area over the previous month from "never a problem" to "almost always a problem."

Data analysis revealed the following findings:

- 84.8% of the mothers had technical-school institution or university-level education.
- 88% of the fathers had technical-level institution or university-level education.
- 81.5% of mothers were married or cohabiting with their partner.

- 95.2% of fathers were married or cohabiting with their partner.
- 87.4% of the mothers were working outside the home.
- 98.9% of the fathers were working outside the home.
- 27% of the children were diagnosed with chronic health conditions or illnesses (56% of those were physical conditions or illnesses; 47% were considered psychiatric conditions or learning disabilities, hyperactivity, or dyslexia).
- 299 students were involved in after-school activities.
- 21 children identified being bullied by other children.
- 48 children engaged in school nurse visits during the past month.

Overall Findings

- The fathers' evaluation of the girl's quality of life (77.91) was significantly higher than the evaluation of the boy's quality of life (74.87).
- There was no significant difference between the mothers' and fathers' quality-of-life scores.
- Parents of children with chronic health conditions perceive their child to have a low quality of life, as compared with parents of children without chronic health conditions.

1. Given the synopsis provided above, what additional information might help the reader to gain a better understanding about the variations between the fathers' and mothers' perception of their children's quality of life and school functioning?

2. How is this information useful to clinical nursing practice?

See Suggested Responses for Moving Toward Evidence-Based Practice on the Electronic Study Guide or DavisPlus.

Introduction

A chronic condition is a health situation that persists over time, usually longer than 3 months, or one in which recovery progresses slowly. A chronic condition is a physical, psychological, or cognitive impairment that places limitations on the child's daily activities and requires ongoing care. The condition may require that the child and family rely on another individual's assistance in carrying out the activities of daily living. A chronic condition can be a congenital defect or a problem that occurs during fetal development. At birth, a chronic condition can arise from sepsis, prematurity, or intraventricular hemorrhage. It can also develop from a genetic predisposition. The chronic condition can be acquired sometime during the child's life as a result of an illness, accident, or injury. Either a chronic (or acute) condition can lead to a child's death.

 Nursing Insight— Chronic Conditions

Brain: Cerebral palsy (CP) or a seizure disorder
Heart: Congenital or acquired heart disease
Lungs: Cystic fibrosis, bronchopulmonary dysplasia (BPD), or asthma

Muscular or skeletal: Muscular dystrophy or skeletal malformations
Abdominal organs: Kidneys (renal failure), liver (cirrhosis), or intestine (short bowel syndrome)
Skin: Eczema, dermatitis, or conditions such as Lyme disease that can cause chronic arthritis
Psychological: Depression, bipolar disorder, or autism
Cognitive: Down syndrome, developmental or learning disabilities

Conditions such as diabetes, cancer, and human immunodeficiency virus (HIV) are considered chronic. The condition may also have been acquired through an acute medical condition such as an infection or from a trauma such as near drowning, motor vehicle crash, head injury, or shaken baby syndrome (SBS). Whatever the reason for the chronic condition, it becomes a lifelong situation for the child and family. The impact and adaptation to the condition depend on its severity, the age at which the insult occurred, the overall effect on the growth and developmental aspects, and the child's and family's responses to the condition.

The child with the chronic condition may require the use of adaptive devices (e.g., wheelchairs, walkers, braces, crutches) that help to overcome environmental barriers (Schmitke & Scholmann, 2002) (Fig. 35-1). The nurse must remember that when caring for the child with a chronic condition, the child may feel more like his or her unaffected peers than different from them.

 Nursing Insight*— *Other terms associated with a chronic condition

There are other terms used to describe a child who is unable to actively participate in daily activities and needs ongoing care.

Disability is similar to a chronic condition in that it also refers to the limitations that prevent or interfere with a child's ability to perform daily activities.

Handicap is the inability to carry out tasks or access certain aspects of the environment due to one or more impairments. The terms "activity limitation" or "participation restriction" are preferred by many specialists in physical, occupational, and speech therapy as well as those in related fields (Venes, 2009).

A Chronic Condition and Its Relationship to Technology

In the United States today, the increase in chronic conditions may be partially attributed to technological life-saving and life-sustaining measures or technological devices that can now diagnose and treat diseases that previously were either undiagnosed or untreatable. For instance, the use of a refined diagnostic tool such as a level 2 ultrasound has enabled health care providers to find

Figure 35-1 Some children who have a chronic condition require an adaptive device to help with mobility.

 where research and practice meet:
Where Do Children with a Chronic Condition Die?

Feudtner, Silveira, and Christakis (2002) researched where children with chronic conditions die. Their study found 52% of deaths occurred in the hospital, 17.2% occurred at home, 8.5% occurred in the emergency department, and 21.7% were classified as other. Infants (younger than 1 year of age) with chronic illness died predominantly in the hospital (88.4%–99.6%). Beyond the first year of life, the incidence of children with a chronic condition who died at home increased from 21% in 1980 to 43% by 1998.

developmental problems while the infant is still in the mother's womb. Once the condition is diagnosed, health care professionals can begin to develop a plan of care. The child who is born prematurely benefits from medical technology such as a ventilator that enables the infant to live. While technology has many benefits and has enabled some children to live, it has also caused them to be dependent on technology for survival. **Technology dependent** means the child is reliant on some type of medical device to compensate for the loss of normal use of a vital body function. The Technology Related Assistance for Individuals with Disabilities Act Amendments of 1994 provide for programs that support the development, acquisition, or application of assistive technology devices or equipment to assist the child living with limitations (Venes, 2009). The child may also require substantial skilled nursing care to avert death and further disability.

Be sure to — Understand the type of technological equipment required

Technology dependent children are grouped according to the type of equipment required. According to a United States Congress report, the groups are designated from the most complex equipment to the least complex equipment required:

- Group 1—Children who require a ventilator
- Group 2—Children who require devices for total parenteral nutrition
- Group 3—Children who have a daily dependence on some other device for respiratory or nutritional support (e.g., tracheostomy, oxygen support, tube feeding)
- Group 4—Children who require an apnea monitor, peritoneal dialysis or hemodialysis or other devices, such as catheters and colostomy bags
- The infants and children who fall into groups 1 and 3 are further defined as needing high-technology care; medically fragile (Judson, 2004).

Impact of a Chronic Condition

A chronic condition affects the child and family differently depending on the age at diagnosis. It can create a threat of the unknown, loss of control, and long-term effects yet to be discovered. Depending on the degree of illness, frequent hospitalizations or clinic visits may be needed. Frequent visits to the hospital can create stress because normal home routines are disrupted and more demands are placed on the caregivers, who now must balance time between the sick child in the hospital and other responsibilities at home and work. This lack of control and sense of powerlessness may lead some parents to become controlling and overprotective (Melnyk, Feinstein, Moldenhouer, & Small, 2001).

The child may also have to cope with unfamiliar people, places, and medical treatments. The family, depending on the coping mechanisms, may become overwhelmed and unable to deal or cope with the condition and related treatments. Because the condition is life long, the family may experience social, financial, and psychological strain as a result.

The nurse can assist the family in developing an ongoing plan of care to meet the child's physical, emotional, and spiritual needs. The nurse can offer ongoing support and supply resources to help ensure successful coping. The nurse caring for the family must remember that uncertainty and fear about the future is a constant worry for the parents of a chronically ill child (Melnyk et al., 2001).

IMPACT OF A CHRONIC CONDITION ON THE INFANT

In infancy, the developmental task is to achieve an emotional attachment or a bond with the primary caregiver. The need for necessary treatments or hospitalizations may require a separation from the caregiver that can interfere with the bonding process. Pain due to invasive procedures and forced changes in diet and sleep may alter normal growth and developmental milestones (Armstrong-Dailey & Zarbock, 2001).

Nursing Care

Priority nursing interventions include rocking, holding, comforting, and using a soothing voice. It is also important to provide visual and auditory stimulation. Brightly colored mobiles, calming music, low lighting, grouping nursing cares, and protecting nap time can assist in the healing process. The crib or nursery area must be maintained as a safe place where invasive procedures are not performed. The nurse must also encourage parents to hold the infant whenever possible, regardless of the amount of wires and equipment to which the infant is attached (Fig. 35-2). Siblings can be encouraged to visit and participate in simple care-taking measures or create pictures to hang up in the room (Armstrong-Dailey & Zarbock, 2001).

 case study An Infant with a Chronic Condition

Cindy, a mother at 24 weeks' gestation with twins, developed HELLP syndrome (a condition characterized by *h*emolysis, *e*levated *l*iver enzymes, and *l*ow *p*latelets; a serious complication of preeclampsia) and went into premature labor. The birth was further complicated when the first baby died from a heart defect and the second baby experienced significant medical conditions. The living infant was placed on a ventilator and subsequently developed the chronic lung condition bronchopulmonary dysplasia (BPD). After 3 months in the intensive care unit, the infant was transferred to a rehabilitation facility closer to the parents'

Figure 35-2 It is important for parents to hold and care for their chronically ill child.

home. As the days turned into months, the infant developed sepsis, pneumonia, and had one episode of cardiopulmonary arrest. With the decline in health, one nurse at the rehabilitation faculty felt that the nursing care was no longer helpful and was actually causing pain. However, another nurse believed that the infant could eventually go home. As time progressed, the infant's condition continued to deteriorate, and during this time the infant received extreme care that included oscillatory ventilation, numerous medications and other painfully invasive procedures. The parents voiced that everything possible be done for the infant. Later, the infant died at the rehabilitation facility at the age of 14 months.

critical thinking questions

1. The infant had several chronic conditions. How can the care given to the infant be viewed by the nurse?

2. What are extreme care measures?

3. What happens when the nurse feels that the treatments have become more of a burden than a benefit?

4. Does the nurse suffer?

5. What if the nurse's beliefs about care differ from those of the institution?

◆ See Suggested Answers to Case Studies in text on the Electronic Study Guide or DavisPlus.

IMPACT OF A CHRONIC CONDITION ON THE TODDLER

For the toddler, the major developmental task is initiating autonomy or self-control. When the child has a chronic condition, accomplishing this task is in jeopardy. The most frightening aspects of illness and hospitalization for the toddler are pain, anxiety, and separation from parents. The toddler is also sensitive to bodily harm (Armstrong-Dailey & Zarbock, 2001).

The child's chronic condition can hinder both gross and fine motor development. Frequent or repeated hospitalizations cause the toddler stress. The toddler has a tremendous capacity to withstand the stress provided that the relationship (attachment) to the parents is maintained. It is important for the nurse to encourage parents to stay with the child by giving 24-hour unlimited visitation and proper sleeping accommodations.

The most common coping method employed by the chronically ill toddler is regression.

 Nursing Insight— *Regression*

Regression is an abnormal return to an earlier reaction, characterized by emotions or behaviors that are inappropriate for the current age and may include the loss of recently acquired skills (Venes, 2009). Regression can be both physical and emotional. For example physical regression occurs when a toddler refuses to continue bowel or bladder training. Regression can be considered emotional when a child refuses to talk, withdraws, or becomes easily irritated.

Nursing Care

Priority nursing interventions for the toddler with a chronic condition include maintaining the bond between the parents and child, promoting realistic developmental skills, and not reacting negatively to regression. Praise the child for all attempts at self-care. The nurse can also give parents instructions about realistic methods of discipline. Parents may be reluctant to enforce rules for the chronically ill child based on feelings and concerns about the child's condition. In turn, the child may react emotionally (naughtily) to inconsistent discipline patterns. Without consistent limitations, the toddler may feel insecure and unable to complete developmental tasks essential to the promotion of autonomy.

Pain management includes medication and other traditional nursing comfort measures such as clean sheets, good hygiene measures, oral care, and skin care.

Because the toddler needs a set routine, the nurse can also encourage parents to maintain the child's normal home schedule as much as possible. The nurse can allow the child to express feelings through play and artwork. Sometimes the toddler uses a toy to project personal feelings (Armstrong-Dailey & Zarbock, 2001).

IMPACT OF A CHRONIC CONDITION ON THE PRESCHOOLER

The developmental task of a preschooler is to create a sense of initiative. A painful treatment, isolation, separation from a parent, or loss of autonomy or mobility can be associated with chronic illness and the preschooler is likely to interpret this experience as punishment for real or imagined wrongdoing (Armstrong-Daley & Zarbock, 2001).

The preschooler with a chronic condition may react aggressively to the impact of illness by throwing toys, biting, and hitting other people. The preschooler may also regress, withdraw from others, wet the bed, have difficulty sleeping, or refuse to cooperate (Armstrong-Dailey & Zarbock, 2001). The nurse must remember that young children accept the literal meanings of words. If death is associated with "going to sleep" the child may fear going to sleep. The child also may have nightmares that symbolize fears.

Nursing Care

Priority nursing interventions include providing the preschooler with the opportunity to express fears and frustrations. At this age, storytelling and reading books about the illness may be helpful in providing a nonthreatening approach to the topic. The preschooler can express concerns through dramatic play. The nurse can ask the child life specialist for assistance with methods of expression. It is essential that the nurse communicate to the parents that the preschooler's sense of security is derived from schedules and rules. Parents can be encouraged to maintain as normal a home schedule as possible and enforce consistent limits. The nurse can also teach the parents that the child needs constant reassurance that nothing the child has done has caused the illness. The nurse caring for the preschooler must remember that honesty is important when explaining and preparing for procedures. The preschooler has a limited concept of time, so general terms like after lunch, after your nap, or at bedtime when describing time-related events is important (Armstrong-Dailey & Zarbock, 2001).

IMPACT OF A CHRONIC CONDITION ON THE SCHOOL-AGE CHILD

During the school-age period, the child who had achieved a certain degree of autonomy and independence strives to develop a sense of industry. The school-age child takes pride in the ability to assume some new responsibility. Peer relationships become extremely important at this age. Separation from the peer group is often a difficult consequence of a chronic condition. The school-age child who experiences interrupted independence coupled with little peer interaction may show anger by refusing to comply with treatments or compliance with a special diet. The school-age child can listen attentively but sometimes does not completely comprehend all of the information. He or she may be reluctant to ask questions or admit that she does not know the answer. It is easy for the child to misinterpret medical information (Armstrong-Dailey & Zarbock, 2001). The nurse must remember that the school-age child has an increased awareness about the significance of illness and may understand the lifelong consequences of the chronic condition.

Nursing Care

Priority nursing interventions for the school-age child include pain assessment. The nurse can use the FLACC pain scale (see Table 21-8), the Wong-Baker FACES pain scale, or the numeric pain scale (see Fig. 21-14). The child needs to be reassured that his or her personal behavior has not caused the illness. It is important for the nurse to answer questions about treatment, procedures, and medications honestly and at a level the school-age child can understand. Play can be used as an outlet or a temporary escape from the illness. Allowing for unstructured play may enhance feelings of control and predictability during hospitalization or clinic visits (Armstrong-Dailey & Zarbock, 2001). Include peers as much as possible. The nurse can teach parents how to help the child attain realistic independence by allowing him or her to play with friends, attend school, choose activities, and enjoy private time. The nurse can communicate to the family that the school-age child is acutely aware of nonverbal cues and often understands more information than parents and caregivers realize. For this reason, it is important to encourage the child to maintain open and honest dialog with family and caregivers (Armstrong-Dailey & Zarbock, 2001).

 Collaboration in Caring— *Child life specialist*

Whenever a child is diagnosed with a chronic condition, it is important to involve the child life specialist. Because the child with a chronic condition often spends significant amounts of time in the hospital, the days can be long and boring. The child life specialist is an expert in child development and therapeutic play. She can assist in diversion activities during procedures, arrange for therapeutic play, or simply let the child take time to play (Fig. 35-3).

IMPACT OF A CHRONIC CONDITION ON THE ADOLESCENT

Adolescence is a time of increasing independence, autonomy, and vulnerability. It is a time to ask, "who am I?" and a time when self-esteem is closely related with peer acceptance. To complicate matters, during a chronic illness the adolescent may be placed on a pediatric ward or on an adult floor. Neither situation seems to be the right fit (Armstrong-Dailey & Zarbock, 2001). Previously independent, the adolescent is now faced with a chronic condition

Figure 35-3 The child life specialist is called upon to work with a child who has been diagnosed with a chronic condition.

and may be required to accept help from others. Dependence on caregivers and family for physical care, coupled with a lack of privacy, can crush the adolescent's sense of autonomy. Based on this loss of independence, the adolescent may exhibit maladaptive coping behaviors such as hostility, aggression, and even refusal of treatment. Sometimes when presented with frequent medications, tests, appointments, and other procedures, the adolescent is easily overwhelmed and may show regression in behavior. Besides worrying about the condition, self-esteem, and identity, the adolescent may show concern about the burdens and strains the family may now face.

Nursing Care

Priority nursing interventions for the adolescent with a chronic condition include providing solitary time to help the adolescent regain control. The nurse understands that it is important to give the adolescent realistic choices to enhance control when possible. Realistic choices include when to bathe, sleep, eat, and visit with friends. They should be included in medical-related matters when possible. The nurse must remember that peers can be a strong source of support for each other, so peer interaction is important. The adolescent can be encouraged to expand networks of social support through peer groups and other community programs when possible. A support group may help normalize the adolescent's crisis and give him or her a new source of strength and hope (Armstrong-Dailey & Zarbock, 2001).

IMPACT OF A CHRONIC CONDITION ON THE SIBLING

It is important for the nurse to understand that a chronic condition also has an effect on siblings. The sibling may be affected in ways such as experiencing decreased self-esteem, receiving less support from parents, exhibiting mood swings, lacking an understanding about the condition, and displaying a negative attitude toward the ill sibling's condition (Williams et al., 2002). The sibling may also have feelings of jealousy, embarrassment, resentment, loneliness, and isolation (Beckman, 2002). For some siblings the chronic condition means the loss of a playmate. A young child, who has a vivid imagination, may believe he or she caused the condition or may fear that he or she might acquire the same condition as the sibling (Beckman, 2002).

Nursing Care

Priority nursing interventions include instructing the parents to maintain familiar home routines as much as possible for the sibling. In addition, the nurse can help the parents include the sibling in simple care. Remind the parents that providing information about the ill child may decrease stress reactions in the sibling.

Optimizing Outcomes— **The sibling**

How does the nurse handle "acting out" in the sibling?

Best outcome: The sibling has time to regain control and can express feelings. To convey genuine understanding the nurse might say, "You seem very angry today (reflection). It is all right to be angry about your sister's condition and about the situation (validating the sibling's feelings). It must be difficult for you to have your sister in the hospital (empathizing and understanding)." The nurse can then help the sibling find a positive outlet for the anger such as art therapy (channeling). The nurse can encourage the sibling to tell an adult when the anger returns (providing an outlet).

The Child Living with a Chronic Condition

Judson (2004) suggests that 15% to 18% of children in the United States have a chronic health condition. Each year about 50,000 children acquire a permanent disability as a result of injury or illness. Asthma is the leading chronic condition in the United States, affecting about 6 million children. Other chronic conditions are sickle cell disease (SDS), bronchopulmonary dysplasia (BPD), congenital heart disease (CHD), cystic fibrosis (CF), type 1 and type 2 diabetes mellitus, epilepsy, and chronic renal failure.

 Nursing Insight— *Children living with chronic conditions*

According to Judson (2004), children living with a chronic condition experience one or more of these symptoms:

* Limitation in bodily functions appropriate for age and development
* Disfigurement
* Dependence on medical technology
* Dependence on medication or special diet to ensure normal functioning or control of the condition
* Ongoing need for medical care or related services compared to other children of the same age
* Special ongoing treatments at home or at school

A child living with a chronic condition requires day-to-day care and can become a source of stress for parents and other caregivers. Melnyk et al. (2001) describes day-to-day care as "chronic burden of care."

 Nursing Insight— *Caregiver burden*

Caregiver burden, as described by Kuster, Badr, Chang, Wuerker, and Benjamin (2004), is the unrelenting pressure and anxiety in providing daily care to a child with disabilities while meeting other family needs and can be a major source of stress.

Balancing the demands of the child's chronic condition and the parent's personal and family responsibilities can be challenging and exhausting. Many daily health care regimens for the ill child are time consuming, rigorous, and unrelenting, which prove taxing to both the parents and child. The complex schedule of care for the ill child, combined with family responsibilities such as shopping, preparing meals, doing laundry, cleaning, spending time with the other children and getting them to school, paying bills, and finding personal time for self and marriage, can be overwhelming even with the best of support

systems and help in place. Parents of a child living with a chronic condition frequently experience role and marital strain as well as higher levels of psychological distress such as depression and anxiety compared to parents of healthy children (Melnyk et al., 2001).

The financial burden of ongoing care is also a concern. Continuous health care is expensive. Other costs related to housing, lifestyle modifications, special equipment, and special services for the child are also expensive. Some of these costs may not be reimbursed by private health care insurance plans (Melnyk et al., 2001).

Nursing Care

The nurse must communicate to the family that overwhelming feelings can be discussed with a health care professional and that respite care is available.

 Across Care Settings: **Respite care**

Respite care is short-term care offered to families living with a child who has a chronic condition. The main goal of respite care is to provide relief for family members of the burden and stress of sustained care giving (Venes, 2009). Parents can also use respite care in situations in which someone besides them can accompany the child to a doctor's appointment. The availability of respite care varies in every community (Orloff, Quance, Perszyk, Flowers, & Veale, 2004). It is important to note that respite care is not always paid for by private insurance. Sometimes state agencies or national programs can reimburse the family for respite care.

 case study The Frequently Hospitalized Child and His Family

Jack is a 7-year-old boy who is admitted to the inpatient unit at the local children's hospital with a diagnosis of cerebral palsy, apnea, and seizure disorder. He has been admitted to the hospital numerous times in the past. Soon after he was admitted, Jack's mother leaves the hospital and goes home to tend to another child who is 4 years old. When Jack is at home, the mother has difficulty getting anyone to watch Jack because of his apnea spells that can happen several times a day. The father refuses to stay alone with Jack for fear that "something might happen to Jack when he is alone with him." Some of the nurses on the unit talk despairingly about the mother because they think that the mother does not care about Jack, as evidenced by "dropping him off and leaving him alone." A few of the nurses fail to understand the complexity of the total situation. However, one nurse notices that the mother visits Jack every day at lunchtime, staying at Jack's bedside for about 1 hour.

critical thinking questions

1. As a nurse supervisor, what can be said to the staff nurses when making judgments about the mother?

2. What kind of support systems does Jack's mother have in place at home? What can be done to increase support in the home?

3. Do you think this mother is suffering from "caregiver burden" and may be in need of respite care?

◆ See Suggested Answers to Case Studies in text on the Electronic Study Guide or DavisPlus.

Emotional Responses to a Chronic Condition

When a child is diagnosed with a chronic condition, the family equilibrium is disrupted and emotional responses follow. The family is faced with multiple, powerful stresses related to the medical diagnosis, treatment, and the course of the disease that may include a fatal outcome. At the time of initial diagnosis, it is not possible for the family to comprehend the diagnosis and the impact it may have on family life. Initially, the emotional response is shock and chaos. Family members may experience anger, fear, disbelief, anxiety, pain, stress, and feelings described as an "emotional roller coaster" (Gibbons, 2001).

The nurse must understand that there is no typical response and must be prepared to expect a wide range of responses from the family. The nurse must also remember that the emotional reaction may also differ depending on the specific diagnosis and whether there is a chance for the child to be cured. If a child has been ill for a long period, some parents may express relief at finally having an answer to the child's illness. The parental reaction to the diagnosis of asthma will be different than the reaction to a diagnosis of cancer in their child.

Nursing Care

The priority nursing intervention for the family's emotional responses to a chronic condition is communication. The nurse can communicate to the family that the child can continue to live a good life and not just merely exist. The nurse can help the family understand that the child needs to participate in normal childhood activities (when possible) such as remaining involved in the family's typical lifestyle, going to school, playing with friends as well as expecting to be disciplined and acting in a responsible manner. Sometimes simple childhood activities sustain the foundation for the child to embrace life. It is important to remember that regular daily activities must not be lost in the frantic endeavor to treat the condition. The family can be taught that the child needs to incorporate the condition and treatment into a new daily routine (Gibbons, 2001).

The nurse can also communicate important information to the family related to treatment, procedures, medicine, and visits to the hospital or clinic. Potts and Mandleco (2002) found that children who do not focus on the positive aspects of the condition may blame themselves or others and display negativity and irritability.

Because parents are grieving, they may have difficulty in understanding how their family life can return to normal. Parents may blame themselves for not having been able to prevent the condition, especially if the condition is a congenital defect. Based on a myriad of emotions, one parent may blame the other parent. In addition, a parent may not be able to bond with the child. Sometimes, as a defense mechanism, a parent may be fearful of bonding with the child in case the child dies. The nurse can listen carefully to the family's concerns and communicate the importance of bonding, spending quality time with the ill child and promoting as normal a life as possible.

Parents of a child with a chronic condition may also report episodes of recurrent sorrow, particularly at times of important transitions in the child's life that remind them that the child is not the same as other healthy children. The period of episodic grieving interspersed with periods of denial is called **chronic sorrow.** Episodic grieving is a coping mechanism allowing parents to adjust to the situation while permitting them to carry on with daily life and other responsibilities (Melnyk et al., 2001). The nurse can discuss the importance of the parent's continued involvement in the care of the child through these recurrent sorrowful periods. The nurse can also give parents information about community resources and help them sort through the details of medical care.

" What to say " — *Talking about the chronic condition*

When talking about the child's chronic condition with the family, the nurse must be sure to use the child's name and personalize the discussion. It is important that the nurse avoid labeling the child by, for example, saying "CF kids." Instead, the nurse can say, "Timmy will need ongoing care for his cystic fibrosis." This kind of communication places the emphasis on the child and not on the condition. It is also important to listen to the family so that home routines can be continued during hospitalization.

Important Aspects When Caring for a Child with a Chronic Condition

ESTABLISHING A THERAPEUTIC RELATIONSHIP

The nurse understands the importance of establishing a therapeutic relationship with the child and his or her family who are living with a chronic condition. This therapeutic relationship is vital when providing family-centered care because the family has a tremendous amount of responsibility in the care of the child.

Nursing Care

Care may be technical as well as emotional in nature. For the nurse to build a successful therapeutic relationship with the family, the nurse must first establish trust.

---

 critical nursing action Establishing Trust with the Family

Godshall (2003) suggests that the nurse take the following actions when establishing trust:

- Consider the needs of the entire family; do not forget the siblings.
- Familiarize yourself with the child's condition and know about the disease process.
- Be open and honest.
- Show the family that the burden of care is understood. Burden of care includes the combination of physical, psychological, social, and financial burdens the family may face.
- Take time to listen to the child and to the caregiver.
- Include parents in the plan of care. Some parents like to participate in the child's care while the child is hospitalized. It is also important to maintain home rituals as much as possible while the child is hospitalized.

- Treat each child as an individual. It is essential that the nurse not label the child according to the disease process.
- Allow the child to make decisions about the care when possible. Decision making is especially important for the adolescent.
- Maintain confidentiality.
- Do not prematurely judge the parents. Some parents cannot stay with the child in the hospital based on personal needs and responsibilities.
- Arrange for continuity of nursing care.
- Assess the family's support systems and resources.

GROWTH AND DEVELOPMENT

The child with a chronic condition may experience negative physical growth (growth failure) and developmental aspects. **General growth failure** means that the child grows more slowly and that the height and weight is in a lower percentile on the growth charts than for children of the same age. It may result from the condition itself or from related treatments and medications. Conditions such as cystic fibrosis or end-stage renal disease may significantly alter the growth process.

The pathophysiology of the condition may affect the child's growth. For example, if the child has a severe hypoxia problem, the tissues may simply not receive the needed oxygen required to promote normal growth. Treatment protocols associated with chemotherapeutic agents may hinder growth or damage usual organ functioning.

The child with altered growth may be delayed developmentally as well. The child may achieve developmental milestones much later than do peers or not at all. The nurse must be aware that the parents may positively or negatively affect the child's development. For instance, a parent, teacher, or guardian who is fearful of consequences of a child's condition may unduly restrict a child's opportunity for interaction and subsequently hinder development (e.g., parents of a child with autism do not allow him or her to play with peers). Conversely, some parents can embrace the child's condition and help the child attain the most realistic potential. The child's personality, temperament, and motivation may help or hinder developmental attainment.

Nursing Care

An important nursing care measure related to growth is carefully plotting their growth using charts from the National Center for Health Statistics (NCHS) http://www.cdc.gov/nchs/about/major/nhanes/growthcharts/charts.htm. When a child is unable to take adequate nutrition by mouth, an alternate feeding method is used to maintain and promote growth in the child. The type of feeding method selected depends on the child's medical condition.

The nurse can encourage parents to maintain realistic developmental milestones. Helping the child interact with children of his or her own age (when possible) and creating a social network consisting of family, friends and others in the community can help maintain development. Finding appropriate social activities also positively affects the child's development.

EDUCATION

By federal law, all children, including those with a chronic condition, are entitled to a free education that is matched to the developmental and functional capabilities of the child. School personnel must be informed about any chronic condition. Today's educators need to receive special training to prepare them for ongoing monitoring and care of the child. Along with adequate training, resource allocation is needed to support the child and can help make entry into the school less challenging (Kliebenstein & Broome, 2000).

Nursing Care

The nurse can discuss home schooling as an educational alternative. Helping the family understand laws about educational services is important.

> **Be sure to—** Observe federal laws providing educational services for children
>
> *Education for All Handicapped Children Amendments,* PL 99-457 of 1986 expanded the scope of PL 94-142 to include appropriate services for infants and toddlers with disabilities and the families.
>
> *Individuals with Disabilities Education Act* (IDEA), PL 105-17 of 1997 ensures that all children with disabilities have available to them a free appropriate public education that emphasizes special education and related services designed to meet their unique needs and prepare them for employment and independent living. Every child with a disability must have a written individualized education plan (IEP), and parents have the right to question placement decisions and due process when settling differences.
>
> *Rehabilitation Act,* PL 93-112 of 1973, prohibits discrimination against people with a disability. Section 504 specifies that each student who has a disability be entitled to accommodations needed to attend school and participate as fully as possible in school activities.
>
> *The Education for All Handicapped Children Act,* PL 94-142 of 1975, mandated that all children, even those with handicaps, be provided with public education and related services.

CULTURAL ISSUES

Understanding ethnocultural aspects of the child who has a chronic condition is paramount. Ethnocultural considerations emphasize cultural sensitivity in both the hospital and community settings.

Nursing Care

Field and Berman (2003) state that the nurse should assess the language and nonverbal cues being used by the child and family. The nurse must also try to determine the locus of control and where the decision–making process lies (with the parents exclusively or if it involves a larger social unit of the family). The nurse must consider the relevance of religious beliefs and spiritual practices, particularly about death, the existence of an afterlife, and the belief in miracles. The nurse can evaluate whether expressions of pain and related aspects are allowable in the culture or looked at as signs of weakness. Assessing how hope for future recovery is negotiated within the family is also important.

In working with a family dealing with a chronic condition, the nurse must assess how the members express grief. Some families feel that grief is a private matter and tend to suppress feelings until they are alone. Other families outwardly express sorrow by crying or moaning. It is important to recognize those beliefs and culture influence the family's reactions to grief and death.

The Dying Child

Dying is the total cessation of life. Death is difficulty to comprehend and might be considered mysterious, ambiguous or confusing for the child and family. The dying process is unique and the exact time or date of death is unpredictable. When the child enters the dying process the body begins to shut down physically as well as emotionally and spiritually. This failure might happen slowly or rapidly depending on the circumstance.

 critical nursing action Do Not Resuscitate

The Do Not Resuscitate (DNR) request means withholding life-sustaining treatment and requires that no attempt be made to revive a child who has clinically died. Withholding life-sustaining medical treatment includes decisions to withhold, withdraw, or limit medical treatment. Some medical ethicists feel that there is no difference between withholding and withdrawing treatment if the treatment is no longer beneficial to the child.

When making recommendations to withhold, withdraw, or limit medical treatment, the benefits of treatment must be weighed against the burden of continuing treatment for the child. The nurse understands that a do-not-resuscitate (DNR) order means that no lifesaving measures will be initiated in the event of cardiac or respiratory arrest. This decision also can mean removing medical equipment such as a ventilator or monitor, dialysis machine, feeding tube used for artificial nutrition, and intravenous fluids for hydration. Aggressive treatments such chemotherapy or radiation therapy are also terminated.

Wiegand (2006) states that the child and family participating in the process of withdrawal of life-sustaining therapy need consistency among health care providers and the delivery of consistent messages. All members of the interdisciplinary team need to communicate effectively with each other so that families receive ongoing and reliable information.

PERCEPTIONS OF DEATH

Perceptions of death vary across the age continuum. The nurse needs to prioritize nursing actions and assist the child according to the appropriate developmental level to help make the transition to death fearless, peaceful, and painless.

Death for the infant is undefined yet related to the level of cognitive development. The infant's perception of death is based on the degree of discomfort and the reactions of the parent and others in the environment. The nurse can ensure that the infant's basic physiological needs are met and that the child is able to build trust with caregivers.

Toddlers have a more developed perception of death and can sense by the way that the parents react that something is wrong. The toddler is unable to distinguish fact from fantasy, which inhibits a true comprehension of death. Death for the toddler may mean separation from parents or disruption in routine. The dying toddler responds with fear and sadness. It is important for the nurse to encourage parents to stay with the child by giving 24-hour unlimited visitation, ensure their needs are met and comfort is maintained.

The preschool child seems to comprehend death more than can be verbalized. The preschooler is able see the body changing and can understand that something is wrong. Fear of death may be present as early as 3 years of age and nurses can discuss death simply and honestly in response to the child's questions. It is important for the nurse to keep answers short. The nurse remembers that the preschooler is a magical thinker and may view illness or injury as punishment for bad behavior. Reinforce that their condition is not caused by bad behavior. Because preschoolers are concrete thinkers, death should not be described as "going to sleep." A child of this age takes this response literally and fears going to sleep so the nurse must never equate sleep with death.

The school-age child often has a realistic understanding about the seriousness of the condition, but the understanding of death is not precise until he or she can understand the concept of time. Kübler-Ross (1983) found that after the age of 8 or 9 children understand the permanence of death. The school-age child is aware of nonverbal cues and often understands more of what is overheard than parents and nurses realize. Attempts to shield the school-age child from death can be perceived as distrust. The nurse must include children of this age in discussions about their care, condition, treatment or non-treatment, prognosis, and death.

The adolescent has the capacity to understand death at the adult level, but has difficulty accepting it as reality and often thinks that death can be defied. The adolescent thinks that the body is invincible, hence some of the risk-taking behaviors among this group. Adolescence is a difficult time to deal with death because establishing identity and independence is important. The adolescent has a fear of becoming dependent on parents. The nurse can help the family realize that even though the cognitive ability to understand death is present the emotional maturity to face death is absent.

The nurse and family can include the adolescent in decision making. The adolescent might wish to write a final poem or message as well as say good-bye to friends. It is important to allow the adolescent to talk about feelings and disappointments about goals and experiences never to be attained.

 where research and practice meet:
Causes of Death

Anderson and Smith (2005) studied the various causes of death among children ages birth to 19. Currently, in infants, the main cause of death is prematurity, congenital defects and infections. Death in toddlers and children is a result of accidents and injuries. School-age children die from cancers and unintentional injuries. The leading causes of death in adolescents are homicide, suicide, and cancer.

BEFORE THE CHILD DIES

Before the child dies the nurse completes the institution's checklist to ensure that all of the necessary institutional policies and procedures are followed. The nurse can contact the bereavement team before the death so they are ready to offer support when the death occurs. The nurse can also create a file that includes community resources that the family may need after the death to receive ongoing support.

A ledger may be created as a follow-up for acknowledging important times in the child's life (e.g., on the child's birthday or another special day). Later on, the nurse can send a "thinking of you" card to let the family know that the child is still remembered on these occasions. The nurse can also make note of the child's death date in order to make a follow-up phone call that can allow parents to ask unanswered questions or express feelings.

Signs and Symptoms

The nurse recognizes physical signs of impending death. Knowing the normal physical processes may help the family through the experience.

 assessment tools Recognition of Physical Signs of Impending Death

- Loss of sensation
- Loss of the body's ability to maintain thermoregulation: skin may feel cool
- Loss of bowel and bladder function
- Loss of awareness, consciousness and slurring of speech
- Alteration in respiratory status
- Cheyne–Stokes respirations (a waxing and waning of respiration in the depth of breathing with regular periods of apnea)
- Noisy chest or respirations with the accumulation of fluid in the lungs or in the posterior pharynx
- Decreased, weak, or slow pulse rate and drop in blood pressure

Nursing Care

Once medical treatment is halted and the family has determined that death is inevitable, the focus of nursing care is about allowing the child to die. Ward (2006) finds that the nurse can shift from the curative technological approach to providing care that enables the child to move toward death by accessing his or her own inner resources.

To help the child have a peaceful death comfort measures are essential which can help create a positive outcome at the time of the child's death as well as later on for the family. The nurse must be aware of family needs and communicate genuine feelings of kindness and sympathy to the family.

 Nursing Insight— *Presence*

The nurse may wonder how to respond to the family at the time of the child's death. The death of a child is a sorrowful time for the family. One primary intervention for the nurse is to be present. Presence includes a receptive, nonverbal posture that signals to the family that the nurse is willing to sit quietly and listen. Being present may reduce the family's feelings of isolation. It is important to remember that the family may not need the nurse to say profound words. They may simply want the nurse's support and willingness to remain in the room.

 where research and practice meet:
Facilitators and Barriers to Providing a "Good Death" Experience in the ICU

A study by Beckstrund, Callister, and Kirchoff (2006) listed facilitators and barriers to providing a "good death" experience in the ICU.

Facilitators
- Make environmental changes to facilitate dying with dignity.
- Communicate challenges.
- Manage pain and discomfort.
- Follow child and family wishes for end-of-life care.
- Promote early cessation of treatments if requested.
- Eliminate aggressive treatments, especially when they would be futile.
- Ensure effective communication among the total health care team.

Barriers
- Staffing patterns and nursing shortage.
- Treatments based on medical regimens rather than on child and family needs.

Mays (2005) noted that relationships are extremely important during the dying process and that physical contact is a major source of comfort to both the child and family. A simple touch from the nurse's hand, gently stroking the child's head, or the placement of a favorite toy next to the child shows the family that the nurse truly cares about the child. When a nurse offers touch, the family members may lean in toward the nurse and respond positively. The nurse must also be sensitive to a family who is not comfortable with being touched, who may respond with stiffening or drawing back. In this situation, the nurse can quietly remove the hand and perhaps take a step back. The nurse must also have the insight to realize that this is not the time to share personal stories about loss. It is important for the nurse to keep the focus on the family.

It is important that the nurse give the family choices about what is possible during the dying process. The nurse can ask the family members if holding the child is desired. If death is imminent, the nurse must be sure to tell the family that death could occur while holding the child. Sometimes parents request to get into the bed with the child. This behavior is acceptable during the death of a child.

The nurse must assess the situation and accurately determine the proper environment. Sometimes it is appropriate for the nurse to give the family short periods to be alone with the child or the family may want a health care professional in the room at all times. When the nurse presents these choices, if the family does not respond, ask the family again, a few moments later, as sometimes the family member cannot absorb everything that is occurring.

 Across Care Settings: Care of the dying child

Heller and Solomon (2005) found that slightly more than half of the parents recalled that their child was cared for in more than one setting near the end of life (either one or more hospital units or in different hospitals, or moved between the hospital, home, or long-term care setting).

Most parents felt that care was well coordinated. Parents who felt differently stated that there was inadequate discharge planning and poor preparation related to home care, disjointed outpatient care, inadequate staffing levels to provide sufficient care, poor organization of care, and staff who were unprepared to care for gravely ill children, as well as the staff not knowing the child and family. These factors were frustrating for parents. When a gravely ill child will be cared for in the home it is essential to begin discharge planning early and have a discharge family meeting to ensure that all aspects related to the child's care are covered before the parents are expected to provide the care independently (Fig. 35-4).

PALLIATIVE CARE, HOSPICE CARE AND END-OF-LIFE CARE

Care of the dying child also includes holistic nursing interventions that address the physical, emotional, and spiritual aspects of the child and family. Care of the dying child can be addressed in three ways: palliative care, hospice care and end-of-life care. These three ways are similar yet different from one another.

Palliative Care. With technological advances, nurses and other health care professionals are faced with decisions as to when to stop treatment once it is initiated. **Palliative care** is a term that has drawn much attention in health care today.

 Nursing Insight— *Palliative care*

The American Academy of Pediatrics (AAP, 2002) describes palliative care in a policy statement entitled Palliative Care for Children. In this policy statement palliative care is described as enhancing quality of life in the face of an ultimately terminal condition.

In 2008, The World Health Organization discussed palliative care as providing physical, emotional, and spiritual care of the child and family. Palliative care refers to the type of care that the child receives at the end of life after it becomes obvious that no cure is possible.

Figure 35-4 The health care team is of tremendous support to parents and family of a chronically ill or dying child.

The main aspect of palliative care is that it follows a medical model of care through the hospital and follows the hospital's rules. Hain, Weinsten, Oleske, Orloff, & Cohen (2004) state that sound scientific principles should govern care. Important nursing interventions of palliative care include relief from pain, dyspnea, and other distressing symptoms. Emotional and spiritual aspects are essential care measures that help the child and family function as actively as possible until the child's death. Palliative care addresses conditions such as loneliness that cause distress and detract from the child's enjoyment of life. In addition, the nurse can provide a support system to help the child and family members cope during the illness and bereavement process.

Palliative care measures neither hasten nor postpone death. For a child receiving sometimes rigorous medical treatments, the nurse must consider that the benefit of the treatment outweighs the burden of care. For example, a child who has already been diagnosed with metastatic bone cancer should not have to undergo further painful and invasive procedures like injection of radioisotopes to prove something that is already known. This type of care is considered an unnecessary burden to the child.

With palliative care measures, dying at home care is not always possible. Some institutions have implemented Palliative Care Units (PCUs). In some institutions, a PCU works well; in others a PCU may not be a good choice for the child because the environment has a medical focus.

 Complementary Care: *Complementary and alternative medicine*

Complementary and alternative medicine (CAM) therapy has become increasingly popular in palliative care. Neuhouser, Patterson, Schwartz, Hedderson, Bowen, & Standish (2001) state that 66% of children with cancer use some form of CAM. This includes self-care practices such as relaxation, aromatherapy, acupuncture, or other therapies performed by a licensed practitioner. Other therapies, including dietary supplements and herbal remedies, are unregulated. A study by Pitetti, Singh, Hornyak, Garcia, & Herr (2001) found that CAM therapies are frequently used to treat children. Many of the parents of children using CAM therapy use it themselves. A large proportion of children taking herbal medications are also taking over-the-counter medications. Sanders et al. (2003) found that the use of CAM therapy in children with special needs is common. The frequency and type of CAM are dependent on the child's condition and prognosis. This study also found that the use of spiritual blessings and prayers was beneficial to various types of chronic conditions.

Advantages of CAM

- Easy to understand.
- Familiar methods.
- Many are noninvasive.
- Many have fewer side effects compared to medical treatments.
- Help improve the overall quality of life.
- Help maintain current state of health.
- More holistic and in balance with nature (Suzuki, 2004).

Disadvantages of CAM

- Some treatments are complex.
- They have not undergone adequate testing of effectiveness.
- Many herbal preparations and remedies lack FDA approval.
- Many not covered by third-party reimbursement.

What makes CAM controversial?

One of the main controversies is that many of the therapies have not been tested through research. CAM therapies have not been proven effective 100% of the time. Some health care providers find that it is through pure belief that these measures work, similar to a placebo effect and that people who are drawn to CAM are desperate and "will try anything." In addition, some health care providers are concerned that some patients may refuse traditional medicine based on belief in CAM.

Hospice Care. **Hospice care** refers to a program that focuses on quality of life for dying persons. It is a method of treating a serious illness when cure or meaningful improvement is no longer possible, and end-of-life care describes a certain time frame wherein care is given during the final 6 months of life (AAP, 2000). According to Children's Hospice International (2005), the focus of hospice care for the child is on life and living, improving the quality of the life for the child and the ongoing lives of the family. In 1967, Dr. Cicely Saunders established the first hospice, St. Christopher's Hospice in London.

The main aspect of hospice care is that it uses a variety of services (medical equipment, diagnostics, and therapeutic interventions) provided by a multidisciplinary group consisting of physicians; nurses; and other personnel, such as chaplains, health aides, and bereavement counselors

 critical nursing action The hospice approach

- Family-centered care is essential.
- A comprehensive, holistic approach can meet the child's physical, emotional, social, and spiritual needs.
- Effective symptom control and pain management is paramount.
- Care is provided by an interdisciplinary team.
- The child can be cared for at home or in a homelike environment.
- Coordination and continuity of care is a priority.
- In addition to regularly scheduled home care visits, services are available on a 24-hour, 7-day-a-week, on-call basis.
- The focus of care is on improving the quality of remaining life; that is, on palliative, not curative, measures.
- Bereavement follow-up services are offered to family members in the year after the death of the loved one (Lattanzi-Licht & Connor, 1995).

Once hospice care is initiated, the nurse can help the family determine the best place for the child to spend the final days. Most children prefer to die at home surrounded by family. The concept of children's home hospice care is a growing alternative to in-patient hospital care for the dying child. Holistic care measures can be implemented easily in the home. The child who is cared for in the home receives nursing care that includes visits, treatments, medications, supplies, and equipment offered by the home care agency. At home, the child is exposed to normal daily activities and surrounded by family members as death draws near. When the child is at home, he or she may be able to continue to play with other children and "feel normal" for as long as possible.

The nurse understands that remaining in the home environment may not always be possible. Assuming care for a dying child can be an overwhelming duty. Some parents simply have too much grief to care for the dying child and other children along with household responsibilities.

Hospice care also provides respite care that allows family members to "take a break" or "time off" to reenergize before returning to the role of primary caregiver. In addition to the actual care of the dying child, hospice care also offers professional support after the death of the child.

❝What to say❞ — *Children's Hospice International, 2005*

Children's Hospice International, 2005 states that it is important to give clear answers to children who are dying. Evasive answers may confuse the child. The nurse must remember that the child may be at a developmental level at which he or she may take conversations literally. When the nurse is talking to the child, it is important to remember:

- Do not tell the child that death is sleeping peacefully. The child may fear going to sleep.
- Do not tell the child abstract concepts like, "It is God's will" or "you are such a good boy that God wants you to be with him." He or she may start to misbehave so as not to die.
- Approach the child with compassion, honesty, support, and love.

(Adapted from Children's Hospice International, 2005).

End-of-Life Care. After it has been determined that the end of life is near (about 6 months) for the child, care measures can be initiated to help the child die peacefully and without pain. End-of-life care recognizes that each child and family has unique needs at this time.

End-of-life care should be accessible to the child and the family in their desired setting (the home, inpatient hospice, or intensive care unit). The home is usually the preferred site (Children's International Project on Palliative/Hospice Services [ChIPPS]. Compendium of Pediatric Palliative Care. Alexandria, VA: National Hospice and Palliative Care Organization, 2003).

The main aspect of end-of-life nursing care is to provide the best quality of life possible for the child and family. End-of-life care is a holistic approach to care that includes physical, emotional, social, spiritual interventions, and complementary care. Quality of life can be enhanced by offering support to the bereaving child and family, relieving distressing symptoms, and providing respite.

 critical nursing action Holistic Care for the Dying Child

Comfort Measures	Emotional Support	Spiritual Interventions	Complementary Care
Pain management	Active listening and showing empathy	Offering presence	Art therapy
Good hygiene		Meditation	Energy-based therapy (healing touch, therapeutic touch, Reiki)
Repositioning	Distraction	Music	
Nutrition and diet management	Encourage positive coping	Prayer	Relaxation
	Encourage verbalization and ventilation of feelings		Guided imagery

Physical or occupational therapy	Psychotherapy referral	Read from spiritual text or poetry	Acupuncture
Help the family create new rituals when the old ones no longer work due to the disease process	Suggest support groups	Allow for sacrament	Reasonable exercise
	Discuss topics about grief, loss, isolation, fear, guilt, and relationships	Contact the family's religious or spiritual community	Aromatherapy
	Discuss concerns about life after the child's death that relate to family, friends, and others	Discuss God/ Higher Power, or spiritual source	

Providing end-of-life nursing care means addressing pain in the dying child. This can be difficult, as pain is a subjective experience. Some children can clearly describe the pain while others cannot. Dying children who are nonverbal have the most difficulty in conveying pain. The nurse can communicate to the family the necessity of pain management.

clinical alert

Principles of pain medication administration

- Give pain medications orally for as long as possible.
- Alternate routes for pain medication administration include intravenous, subcutaneous, transcutaneous, transmucosal, rectal, nasal, epidural, and intrathecal. The enteral route (or through a gastrostomy tube) is the preferred route for children in the dying process.
- Consider using an appropriate adjuvant (a drug added to a prescription to hasten or increase the action of a principal ingredient in the medication).
- Adjuvants offer analgesia in certain situations, and include anticonvulsants, antidepressants, or muscle relaxants.

(Hain et al., 2004).

Questions and concerns raised about the end of life can be discussed with the nurse as they arise. When a child is dying, parents tend to want to protect him or her from death by avoiding the subject or not talking about death. Some parents feel that if they discuss death with the child, the child may lose hope (Mazanec & Tyler, 2003). The nurse can help the family understand that the child may want to talk about death. The nurse can communicate to the family that the child does not want to be left alone. The child may be more afraid of being abandoned. The nurse can also inform the family about other good resources.

Across Care Settings: National Cancer Institute

The National Cancer Institute (NCI) has resources available by calling the Cancer Information Service (CIS) Toll-free: 1–800–4–CANCER (1–800–422–6237) TTY (for deaf and hard of hearing callers): 1–800–332–8615.

The NCI's Web sites are located at http://www.cancer.gov or http://www.cancer.gov/cancer_information/coping/ (click on the title under "End-of-Life Issues.") Cancer information specialists offer online assistance through the *LiveHelp* link on the NCI's Web site.

Fact Sheets
- The NCI fact sheet about hospice care includes contact information for hospice organizations.
- The NCI Advance Directives fact sheet discusses a patient's rights regarding medical treatment.
- The NCI fact sheet on Home Care for Cancer Patients provides information and resources related to home care services.
- The NCI booklet Advanced Cancer: Living Each Day provides support to cancer patients, families, and friends.

Ethnocultural Considerations— Cultural practices

The nurse must be knowledgeable of cultural practices of the child and family. It is important for the nurse to include the right support person to facilitate the cultural care of the dying child. By including cultural rituals or customs, nursing care can ease the death process for the child and family. Special ceremonies or rites may be requested by the family and should be accommodated whenever possible. Other cultural care measures may include use of spiritual texts and symbols, prayer or meditation, chanting, offering music, lighting a candle, listening in silence, being present in the moment, or including other methods of care as deemed appropriate by the culture.

AFTER THE CHILD DIES

If the family arrives at the unit after the child has died, the nurse must take the time to prepare the family about the child's appearance and description of the death. The nurse can describe the child's dress, hairstyle, if the child's eyes are open or closed, any noticeable injuries, positioning of the child, and what occurred at the moment of death. It is essential that the nurse give the family the choice of seeing the child alone or having the nurse accompany them into the room. If the family chooses to be alone, the nurse must stay close by in case the family has questions or needs.

Nursing Insight— *Handling the child's belongings*

When handling the belongings of a child who has died, the nurse must treat them gently and with respect. The nurse can give the belongings to the family in a special container or package, not simply placing them in a plastic bag, as this action may appear insensitive. The nurse must remember that these items are the final possessions of the child.

Collaboration in Caring— *A father's story*

One father tells about a personal precious moment after the death of a child. The father said that as he held his adolescent daughter as she was dying, he felt her heart stop beating next to his chest. This was the actual moment when the daughter's heart took its last beat. The father treasures this moment. The nurse caring for the child was privileged to hear this father's story and collaborate with him in caring for his child during her death. The compassionate nurse is honored to be present for these moments in time, holding dear, and striving to make the tragedy of the death of a child special, positive, and memorable for the family.

 nursing diagnoses The Dying Child

- Pain related to frequent invasive procedures
- Alteration in Family Process related to frequent hospitalization
- Anxiety related to separation from caregivers
- Alteration in Nutrition: Less than Body Requirements related to decreased appetite from disease process
- Anticipatory Grieving by family related to prognosis of disease process and imminent death of child
- Social Isolation related to frequent hospitalizations
- Depression related to the potential for death
- Fear related to the child's understanding of the disease process and the unknown
- Altered Coping Mechanism related to parental anxiety and stress from imminent death of the child
- Knowledge Deficit related to the disease process, unknown outcome, and possible experimental treatment

Grieving

From the moment that a family has been informed about the child's fatal condition the family's life changes direction and grieving begins (Fig. 35-5).

 Nursing Insight— *Grief*

Grief is a normal and appropriate emotional response to loss. Grief is unique to every individual and there is no timetable in which grief is complete. The stages of grief may come and go. Feelings of grief can return when least expected. Parents may not realize that grief begins the moment the child's diagnosis is communicated (Steen & Mirro, 2000).

Figure 35-5 The hospital chaplain or another religious figure can offer spiritual support to the child and his or her family.

Signs and Symptoms

Grief can be an emotional response as well as a physical response to death.

 Nursing Insight— *Somatic Grief Response*

Somatic grief response can be described as:

- Somatic distress that includes feelings of tightness in the throat or chest, sighing
- Weakness or shortness of breath
- Preoccupation with the image of the deceased (e.g., hearing or seeing the person who died)
- Inability to focus on anything other than the loved one who died
- Emotionally distancing self from others
- Feelings of guilt
- Feeling responsible for the loved one's death.
- Searching for what could have been done differently, thinking in terms of "if I only had done…"
- Hostile reactions that include feelings and expressions of anger
- Inability to complete daily tasks

Nursing Care

A nursing plan of care is essential when caring for the grieving family.

The nurse can also offer ongoing emotional support to help the family understand the situation.

 What to say — *Helping the family understand the situation*

After the child's initial diagnosis, the family may ask the nurse questions such as, What did I do to deserve this? Did I do something wrong? Am I being punished? The nurse can listen empathetically to the family and encourage them to "take it one day and sometimes one moment at a time". The nurse can help the family understand that there may be "good days" and that inevitably there will be "bad days." The nurse can give the family hope that over time the emotional pain may dissipate and that they can better understand the experience of their child's death.

GRIEF THEORIES

It is important for the nurse to understand grieving from well known theories in order to provide proper support (Steen & Mirro, 2000).

Kübler-Ross's Stages of Grief

Elisabeth Kübler-Ross (1983) described five stages of grieving.

DENIAL AND ISOLATION. This stage includes feelings of numbness, disbelief, and shock. Denial is a way of protecting the family and child from the emotional pain that may be too severe to handle all at once. The numbness can also help the family or the child by creating emotional distance from the pain, thereby allowing continuation of daily responsibilities.

Nursing Care Plan The Grieving Family

Nursing Diagnosis: Anticipatory grieving related to poor medical prognosis for child

Measurable Short-term Goal: Family will explore their beliefs and feelings about the medical prognosis.

Measurable Long-term Goal: Family will begin the grieving process, using resources and positive coping mechanisms.

NOC Outcomes:
Family Coping (2600) Family actions to manage stressors that tax family reserves
Grief Resolution (1304) Adjustment to actual or impending loss

NIC Interventions:
Anticipatory Guidance (5210)
Family Integrity Promotion (7100)
Grief Work Facilitation (5290)
Sibling Support (7280)

Nursing Interventions:

1. Develop a trusting relationship with child and family by spending time with them, using active listening techniques, and providing consistency in assignment of nurses to care for the child.

   RATIONALE: Enhances family comfort and enables the family to build trust with the nursing staff.

2. Assess the family's understanding, beliefs, and feelings about the child's prognosis.

   RATIONALE: Assists the family to organize and verbalize their concerns while allowing for correction of misunderstandings.

3. Provide ongoing information about the child's condition and what to expect next. Allow time for questions and reassurance.

   RATIONALE: Allows the family to understand what is happening and to prepare themselves for the next stage in a supportive environment.

4. Provide the child and family with a quiet space and protect their private time together from unnecessary interruptions.

   RATIONALE: Ensures privacy for family to freely experience and show feelings without worrying about strangers and interruptions.

5. Encourage the family to participate in the child's care as much as possible, if desired.

   RATIONALE: Care provided by a familiar person may ease the child's anxiety and allows the family to demonstrate their love for the child.

6. Refer the family and child for spiritual care and/or professional support as needed (specify, e.g., pastoral care, family spiritual advisor, social services, grief counseling, or grief support groups).

   RATIONALE: Support systems can offer the family and child a constant source of support during the dying process and after the death of the child.

 Nursing Insight— Denial and isolation

The nurse can acknowledge these feelings of numbness and remind the family to slow down, "take it easy," and pay attention to safety measures and retain healthy habits.

ANGER. Anger can be one of the most difficult stages. At this point, the family and child have developed awareness about the reality of the diagnosis. The feelings of anger, fear, and guilt can be an overwhelming but a normal response to the impending death. Both the family and child may become angry with God or experience a spiritual crisis.

 Nursing Insight— Anger

The nurse can give spiritual care by calling upon a hospital chaplain or the family's personal clergy to provide support. The nurse can use prayer, meditation, reading from a spiritual text or just being present with the family. The nurse can also encourage the family to find a positive outlet for the emotions. Positive outlets can include talking with other family members or friends, nurses, and families at the hospital, or expressing feelings in a support group. Physical exercise is another positive way to release anger. Family members can be encouraged to write in a journal or draw to express emotions. The child can express anger through therapeutic play or art therapy.

BARGAINING. It is common for the family members to ask, "What did I do to make this happen?" It is normal for the family to try to bargain with either self or with "God" in hopes that the child's life will be spared. The family may express guilt at times for disciplining the child on occasion. The family may also feel punishment for personal life circumstances. Specifically, a mother might wonder if she caused the illness or injury during pregnancy. During this stage, it is natural for the family to make vows of personal improvement if the child is cured.

Nursing Insight— *Bargaining*

It is important for the nurse to talk to the family about bargaining and reinforce that the child's illness is not anyone's fault.

DEPRESSION. When the illness can no longer be denied or bargained away, the family and child may begin to feel a profound sadness.

 ### Nursing Insight— *Depression*

The nurse understands that this sadness or depression is to be expected.

There are some warning signs that the nurse must be aware of that indicate extra help is needed during this period of depression (e.g., insomnia or excessive sleeping, nightmares, weight gain or weight loss, loss of concentration that interferes with the ability to function normally, overwhelming anger, and constant fear or worry about the physical wellness of other family members). If the nurse assesses that any of these signs are present, it is imperative to talk to the hospital social worker, physician or a professional counselor to obtain help.

ACCEPTANCE. Accepting a child's illness and possible death means that the family or child has made an emotional adjustment to the illness. Although the family and child may still feel as if they are on an emotional roller coaster, the difficulties will become more predictable and manageable. At this phase, many family members find strength and joy in everyday living. Family members begin looking for meaning and a reason about why this happened to the child and what impact this experience may have on the future.

 ### Nursing Insight— *Acceptance*

The nurse can remain present with the family and continue to offer support and encouragement. The nurse can provide community resources for the family to help them continue in the grieving process.

 ### Nursing Insight— *Miles and Perry's Stages of Grief*

Miles and Perry (1985), two other well known grief theorists, identify three phases of parental grief.

Phase 1
Phase 1 is a state of numbness and shock. The parents may seem to be in a trance and display no emotion. Some parents may try to comfort others, yet show no emotion themselves.

Phase 2
Phase 2 is a period of intense grief. The parents may cry. Some parents express grief loudly with outbursts, while others cry quietly. Some parents display inappropriate silliness or euphoria. It is a mistake for the nurse to judge a parent as unaffected or uncaring because of the type of emotional reactions at the time of death.

Phase 3
Phase 3 is a period of reorganization. Initially the parents are in a state of emotional shock and forget important information. Later parents can remember verbatim the information that was given at the time of the child's death.

Epperson's Theory of Grieving

It is important for the nurse to remember that no two families go through the grieving process at the same time or at the same pace. A family who experiences a sudden or catastrophic loss appears to go through a slightly altered grief process. Epperson's theory about catastrophic grief may be helpful in the emergency department setting. With the absolute loss of a child already evident, bargaining is absent and depression is replaced with remorse. According to Morroni-Leash (1994), Epperson's theory of the grieving process includes six phases.

HIGH ANXIETY. High anxiety is described as a time of great stress, with many physical manifestations of emotional upheaval.

 ### Nursing Insight— *High anxiety*

A nursing assessment of the family member finds agitation, rapid respiration and increased heart rate, irritability, muscular tension, and fainting, along with digestive or bowel changes that may result in nausea and diarrhea. It is important to refer the family member to a health care provider.

DENIAL. Denial is a protective emotional reaction to postpone the realization of the loss until sufficient psychological preparation has been made.

 ### Nursing Insight— *Denial*

The nurse understands that this phase should not be hurried and a period of acute denial is normal. However, the denial should not persist beyond the viewing of the child's body and after the family has departed the hospital. If denial continues the nurse needs to refer the family member to a health care provider or a professional counselor.

ANGER. Anger is a common emotional response and can be directed inwardly, toward another family member, or toward others. Usually the anger is a diffuse kind that lashes out at society or life in general, with the feeling that the loss was somehow "allowed" to occur. Many times, the anger may be an attempt to affix blame. The anger is usually brief.

 ### Nursing Insight— *Anger*

During an assessment, if the nurse sees that the anger persists, a complex underlying cause such as fear needs to be addressed further by a mental health specialist.

REMORSE. Remorse includes feelings of both guilt and sorrow. The family regrets that the accident or illness occurred and feels responsible that it could not be prevented.

Nursing Insight— *Remorse*

The nurse understands that this is the "if only....." stage. Nursing care includes giving the family repeated reassurance that personal actions were reasonable. In situations of true culpability, the responsible family member needs intensive support and counseling in order to come to terms with personal liability.

GRIEF. Grief is an intense period of overwhelming sadness. The duration and intensity of the grief depend on factors such as the medical condition of the child, existing support systems, and culpability in the disease or injury scenario.

Nursing Insight— *Grief*

The nurse can provide emotional support and genuine caring during this phase.

RECONCILIATION. Reconciliation is described as the final phase to be experienced and may be an end point to the acute family crisis.

Nursing Insight— *Reconciliation*

The nurse can tell the family that reconciliation is a time when the family begins to adapt to the existing circumstances and begins to move on with life (see Chapter 3 for further discussion).

Ethnocultural Considerations— **The Hispanic culture and grief**

Hispanics (Latinos) are persons of Mexican, Cuban, Puerto Rican, Central or South American, or other Spanish origins. As a result of this diversity, grieving behaviors surrounding the death of a child might take different forms. One example is a Hispanic family who is of the Catholic faith and who has a close extended family network within the social structure. Based on their culture and way of grieving, their infant child who has died is viewed as an angel who has returned to heaven. This belief brings comfort to the parents and the extended family, particularly the grandparents, and allows them to move on through the grieving process. To honor the deceased child, pictures are displayed in the home as a tribute, keeping the memory alive. There is a specified grieving time called *luto*. When this family is in *luto*, few celebratory activities takes place, and usually no parties are attended and music is not played in the home. Outward expressions of happiness are discouraged for usually a year. In some instances, the relatives may wear black clothing to signify that they remember the loved one. If these traditions are not observed, there may be criticism from others. Any criticism is of the utmost concern to the family.

Coping Patterns

Grief reactions can differ. Certain behaviors by the family directly after a notification of illness or impending death tend to be magnifications of their predominant stress-coping behaviors in times of duress. In times of stress, the child and parents may revert backwards to familiar ways of coping. It is important to note that if there is too much damage to a familiar lifestyle or family structure, the child or parents may become unable to cope.

NURSING CARE. The nurse must recognize the exhibited coping patterns and find ways to support the family directly or indirectly. The nurse can listen, sit silently, refer a pastoral care person, offer spiritual care such as prayer, or encourage journal writing or reading from a spiritual text. If the nurse notices that the behavior is destructive to self or others it is necessary to call in a physician or a professional counselor. The nurse should not alter the coping pattern completely because alteration could strip the child and family completely of protective buffers and leave them exposed to more pain than bearable.

Pathological Grief

On occasion, personal support systems do not adequately allow the individual to cope and the family members may experience dysfunction or pathological grief. Intense grief feelings or a dysfunctional personality may easily bring on **pathological grief** (deviation from a healthy or normal grief) such as violence, addictions, or poor decision making.

Nursing Insight— *Subtle indicators of grief*

These subtle signs are warning signs and may not necessarily indicate a severe problem. It is the intensity and duration of these behaviors that are the deciding factors indicating the need for professional help.

* Absence of grief such as showing little or no emotion
* Persistent blame or guilt
* Anxiety
* Aggressive and destructive outbursts
* Depression and suicidal thoughts or actions
* Unwillingness to speak about the deceased
* Expressing only positive or only negative feelings about the deceased
* Prolonged dysfunction in school
* Always assuming a caregiver role
* Stealing or other illegal acts
* Signs of addictive behavior; drugs, food, certain activities

TYPES OF PATHOLOGICAL GRIEF. Another type of pathological condition is suicidal ideation and can occur when an individual is notified about the death of a child. The individual may feel intense hopelessness, helplessness, and loss of love. It is very important that the nurse recognize these feelings and listen carefully to the individual who may be expressing suicidal ideas. The nurse must immediately obtain professional psychiatric help for the individual.

The sudden loss of a child may be perceived like an emotional assault and an assertion of vulnerability. Therefore, sometimes an individual becomes violent when experiencing this significant loss in control. When the behavior of the individual escalates beyond the realm of verbal interchange, pathology is present. The nurse must try to understand the cause of the violent behavior. If the nurse notices that a family member displays a violent reaction, steps must be taken for other family members to avoid any confrontation with the individual. The nurse can attempt to quietly remove the person to a private area away from others. It is essential that the nurse not be placed in a situation of personal risk. If the violent individual threatens the nurse or others, it is important to obtain help quickly and activate the facility's security personnel.

Homicidal ideation must never be ignored. The nurse understands that homicidal threats can occur when a child dies due to negligence (whether real or perceived, such as drunken driving or intentional violence). Sometimes after a cooling-down period, the individual regains a calm demeanor and the potential for the violence may diminish. Most often, the violent individual is able to regain self-control and stabilize him- or herself. If this is not the case, the nurse must call for the hospital security guard or the local police to deal with the individual.

Grief that is influenced by drugs and alcohol dramatically alters the individual's ability to work through the grieving process. Illegal narcotic or alcoholic substances cause emotional responses to be exaggerated and uncontrolled. The ability of family members to unite in support of each other can be greatly reduced in this situation. An important nursing management strategy is to call in other family members, friends, or professional counselors to provide immediate help and extended support for the individual under the influence of drugs or alcohol.

Extreme denial is another abnormal response to grief. Most often grief reaches its peak within 3 or 4 months after the bereavement. However, when this does not happen, psychosomatic, psychoneurotic, and psychotic reactions can occur with increased frequency. If an individual is unable to start accepting what has happened beyond the viewing of the child's body or extends grieving into months after the child's death, the nurse needs to be aware of a pathological denial response. The nurse can help the family member find an appropriate community resource or support group.

Now Can You— Discuss the dying child?

1. Discuss nursing care for the dying child?
2. List three nursing diagnoses related to the dying child?
3. Assist the child and family through the grieving process?
4. Recognize pathological grief?

Saying Good-bye

At the time of death, the parents of a dying child can be in extreme grief, and saying good-bye to the child is an important process.

Nursing Care

The nurse can facilitate the saying good-bye process in several ways. It is important for the nurse to remember that the process of saying good-bye should not be rushed. It is paramount that throughout the process the nurse calls the child by name, which helps parents and family members feel that the nurse genuinely cares and that the child is special.

❝ What to say ❞ — *Comforting a family*

The nurse understands that it is important to avoid platitudes such as "time heals all wounds," "you wouldn't want him to live like that," "you're lucky; it could have been much worse," "you can always have another child." These phrases minimize the loss and have little comforting effect. They may be upsetting to the family and make them feel that somehow this child's life has limited value. It is better to say nothing if you do not know what to say. Some appropriate responses are:
"I'm sorry."
"This must be terribly hard for you."
"Is there anyone I can call for you?"
"Would you like me to stay with you for a while?"

During the good-bye, the nurse keeps the child covered up and as warm as possible. The parents may want to assist in the immediate postmortem care as a way of saying good-bye. Parents can give the child their last bath, comb the hair, wash the face, or dress the child in a clean set of clothing. Allowing parents to hold the child one more time as the final good-bye is said is an act of compassion. Extended family members, friends, and others may come to say good-bye as well. The nurse can encourage the parents and others to talk about memories of the child. Crying is common for the parents, family, friends, and the nurse. If the nurse cannot keep personal emotional control, another nurse should offer relief.

The nurse's role after the child's death is to be supportive and allow the family to dictate the "good-bye" time line. If an extended time frame is needed to say good-bye, the nurse can contact pastoral care services to coordinate a private viewing time in the chapel. After the good-bye, it is important that the nurse ensure that the parents and others have departed from the hospital before transporting the child to the morgue.

THE SIBLING SAYS GOOD-BYE

The sibling relationship is sometimes one of the most consistent and ongoing relationships for a child. It can involve many feelings and experiences, including disharmony. In a sibling relationship, the child may experience love, caring, sharing, comforting, playing, jealousy, envy, fighting, and blaming. To the child, the sibling is not only a brother or sister, but also many times a playmate, friend, or support system. The child and sibling have learned and grown with each other and now the relationship is lost.

When a child dies, the surviving sibling may be mistakenly overlooked. Sometimes overlooking another child is unintentional as the focus is placed on the child who died or on the parents. Sometimes there is a perception that the sibling will "be all right." The child may have been sent away to a grandparent or neighbor while the brother or sister was dying in the hospital. Sending the sibling away must not be viewed as negative behavior by the parent because the parent may be too overcome with personal emotions to care properly for the other child. When a child dies, the surviving sibling loses not only a brother or sister but sometimes also the grieving parents because they may be unable to attend to his or her needs. It is also important to remember that the sibling may experience guilt feelings, thinking he or she may have done "something" to make the child sick, or has done something wrong and is now being punished.

Nursing Care

The nurse must encourage the family to include the sibling when saying good-bye.

critical nursing action The Sibling

The nurse's role in relation to the sibling consists of a variety of nursing interventions:

- Listen and help the sibling express his or her feelings.
- Model to the family about how to acknowledge the sibling's presence during this difficult time (initiate a simple conversation, turn on cartoons, offer a drink or snack, or show the sibling how to touch the dying child).
- Explain the situation to the sibling and relate appropriate information in terms understandable for the sibling's age.
- Allow visitation during appropriate times.
- Help the sibling understand that he or she is not responsible for the death.
- Contact a child life specialist who can assist the sibling with art therapy.
- Encourage simple ways to be involved in the care such as making a final gift for the sibling to keep at the bedside.
- Remind the family that the sibling is also experiencing a loss.
- Give siblings the chance to say good-bye.

REMEMBRANCE PACKET

After the death of a child, ongoing nursing care includes creating a remembrance packet to give to the family. When creating this memory packet, the nurse must gain permission from the parents to include personal aspects. If a camera is available, the nurse can take pictures of the

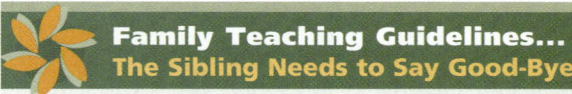

Family Teaching Guidelines...
The Sibling Needs to Say Good-Bye

HOW TO: Teach the Family to Help the Sibling say good-bye:

- Teach the family that it is important that the sibling be included in the grieving process and have the opportunity to say good-bye.
- Instruct families to bring the sibling for short visits when possible.
- During visitation encourage the family to have another support person with the sibling such as a friend or grandparent.
- Tell the family that the sibling can write letters or draw pictures for the child as a way of saying good-bye.

ESSENTIAL INFORMATION

Kübler-Ross (1983) states that the child who has been included in the death and mourning process with the family is able to let go in a healthy way.

child. Taking pictures can be especially important in the death of an infant if parents have not yet taken pictures. Sometimes the nurse may want to make a plaster impression of the child's hand or footprints. A lock of hair from the back of the child's head can be included in the remembrance packet. The nurse can suggest to the parents that baptismal certificates or candles can also be incorporated into the remembrance packet.

The nurse understands that in the death of a young infant and, especially with young parents, the gathered items may be refused. If permission is granted to collect the items, it is important to place them in an envelope or box and keep them for a later date. Some parents are in a state of shock but may ask for them later. After the child's death, the nurse can mail a sympathy card to the parents that may also become a part of the remembrance packet.

ORGAN TISSUE DONATION

In many states, a discussion soon after death about organ tissue donation is required by law. Organ tissue donation may be a sensitive issue for the nurse. The bereavement team or nurse must understand when it is appropriate to approach the family. The bereavement team is a group of trained professionals who know how to approach the topic of organ tissue donation while maintaining dignity and respect for the deceased child. In some circumstances, the family may approach the nurse about organ tissue donation. Sometimes, the physician provides information about organ tissue donation.

Certain criteria must be met for the child to be an organ or tissue donor. Depending on the type of illness, criteria may not be met for organ tissue donation. Nurses should be aware of common questions that the family may ask about organ tissue donation in order to help the family make an informed decision. Sometimes after the organ tissue donation, the family of the child gains comfort in knowing that the death of the child enabled another child to live.

FUNERALS

The nurse may be asked by families to attend the funeral of the child. The presence of the nurse at the funeral is meaningful to the child's family and may bring the family comfort and convey a sense of caring for the deceased child. Attending the funeral is a personal decision for the nurse. While attending the funeral, the service may be difficult and bring up emotions for the nurse or it may assist the nurse in the grieving process and promote closure. Attending the service may be a meaningful way for the nurse to express feelings for the child and the family. If the nurse cannot attend the funeral, sending a card is a sign of caring about the child and family.

Caring for the Professional Caregiver

Caring for the dying child and family can be one of the greatest challenges presented to the nurse. A nurse caring for the dying child can experience personal emotions. One emotion is attachment and it can vary from close contact with the child and family to distancing him- or herself from the situation. The nurse may also feel a sense of helplessness about not being able to alter the outcome of death, especially in an acute death situation. In caring for a child with a chronic condition, the nurse has time to prepare for the child's death. Either way, the death of a child may not be easy for the nurse.

Caring for the child who is dying requires specialized knowledge and skill, sustaining an ongoing and special relationship with families, and at times advocacy. In addition, caring for a seriously ill or dying child requires compassion, sympathy, and empathy. This type of care can require enormous physical, emotional, and spiritual energy. Often the nurse is able to do this effortlessly. However, it is important to realize that the nurse can become depleted based on constant demands from the dying child and family. When the demands of care exceed personal energy, the nurse's personal energy may be threatened. The nurse may begin to wonder what personal threshold can be endured. Health care professionals are not expected to deliver high-quality care when personal emotions have been shattered (Rushton, 2004).

 Nursing Insight— *Burnout, compassion fatigue syndrome, and moral distress*

The nurse must understand the concepts of burnout, compassion fatigue syndrome, and moral distress.

- Burnout is a state of physical, emotional, and mental exhaustion caused by long-term involvement in emotionally demanding situations. It emerges gradually and is a result of emotional exhaustion and job stress.
- Compassion fatigue syndrome is characterized by a sense of helplessness, confusion, and isolation from supporters and can have a more rapid onset and resolution than burnout.
- Moral distress occurs when the nurse is unable to translate personal moral choices into action. The nurse acts in a manner contrary to personal or professional values which undermines integrity. During moral distress, the nurse experiences feelings of frustration, anger and anxiety.

It is important for the nurse to recognize that simple actions can help relieve burnout, compassion fatigue syndrome, and moral distress. Sharing grief with the child's family after death can help both the nurse and family deal with feelings about the loss of the child. Most institutions have grief counselors and support services available to the nurse. Debriefing sessions with professional grief counselors after the child's death have proven to be helpful. Journal writing is an avenue many nurses explore. The nurse must remember to ask for personal support as well as to be supportive to other nurses. The nurse can also consider organized support sessions after the death of a child. It may be helpful for the nurse to talk with the physician or professional counselor for reassurance that a change in the nursing care would not have changed the outcome.

Another aspect is personal suffering. Suffering is multifaceted. Suffering happens when the nurse feels little control over the practice environment. Even though caring for the dying child and family is a privilege that offers personal rewards, the nurse must recognize that personal suffering is possible (Rushton, 2004). A good way to address the nurse's suffering is to attend a forum specifically for discussion, reflection, and shared understandings about suffering. During the forum, the nurse can express personal feelings, frustrations, and disappointments. The nurse can also use strategies in the work setting such as journal writing, quiet time, prayer, or meditation that acknowledges and allows the nurse to process the grief and loss. The nurse should accept compassion and care from others. Self-care practices away from the workplace such as exercise, leisure activities with friends and family, and solitary time for reflection and renewal have great value. It is important for the nurse to create healthy boundaries, setting proper limits for compassion and self-sacrifice with the child and his family as well as oneself.

 Nursing Insight— *Paying attention to personal needs*

The nurse can pay attention to personal needs by asking:

- How do I feel?
- Am I comfortable caring for a child who is dying?
- Can I cope with the needs of the family as well?
- Am I becoming overwhelmed or attached when caring for this child and family?

If the nurse feels uncomfortable with any of these questions, it is time for reflection and self-care. The nurse understands that these feelings are normal and are a part of the human experience. The nurse must know when the situation becomes too great to bear. It is difficult to help the patient and the family if the nurse is not coping. Remember there are employee assistance programs or forums at most institutions to assist the nurse with coping.

summary points

- A chronic condition is a physical, psychological, or cognitive condition that places limitations on daily activities or functions usually for longer than 3 months and may require relying on another individual to assist in daily care.

- A chronic condition may affect each developmental phase and the family's social, financial, and psychological resources.

- Technological advances now save premature infants, as well as infants and children who are very ill, leading to an increase in the number of children who are dependent on technology.

- Chronic sorrow is a coping mechanism that permits parents to carry on with life and daily responsibilities.

- The nurse caring for the child and family with a chronic condition must establish a therapeutic relationship.

- Death is difficult to comprehend and might be considered mysterious, ambiguous or confusing for the child and family. The dying process is unique and the exact time or date of death is unpredictable.

- Perceptions of death vary across the age continuum.

- To help the child have a peaceful death comfort measures are essential which can help create a positive outcome at the time of the child's death as well as later on for the family.

◆ Care of the dying child also includes holistic nursing interventions that address the physical, emotional, and spiritual care of the child and family.

◆ A nursing plan of care is essential when caring for the grieving family as well as recognizing pathological grief.

◆ At the time of death, the parents and siblings of a dying child can be in extreme grief, and saying good-bye to the child is an important process.

◆ There are additional nursing aspects related to the death of a child such as a remembrance packet, organ tissue donation and funerals.

◆ Caring for the dying child and family can be one of the greatest challenges presented to the nurse.

review questions

Multiple Choice

1. The pediatric nurse enters the room of an infant newly diagnosed with cerebral palsy and finds the mother tearful, looking over her baby's crib. The nurse places her hand on the mother's shoulder and the mother cries, "I wish my son was normal!" The nurse's best therapeutic response is:
   A. "I know what you mean. This is very difficult".
   B. "Sit down and let's talk about how you're feeling."
   C. "I am here to help you." "I will come back later?"
   D. "Where is your husband? Can he help you now?'

2. The pediatric nurse working in an acute inpatient unit understands that a Do Not Resuscitate order includes which of the following measures?
   A. Administering radiation therapy in an attempt to eradicate the disease.
   B. Administering antibiotic therapy as scheduled by the physician.
   C. Administering no lifesaving measures in the event of a respiratory arrest.
   D. Administering feeding via an orogastric tube for artificial nutrition.

3. A chronic illness can have a direct effect on the family as a whole. The pediatric nurse is aware that the impact of the chronic illness depends on the: (*Select all that apply.*)
   A. Severity of the illness
   B. Growth and developmental age when the insult occurred
   C. Hospital and community resources available to the family
   D. Family's coping mechanisms
   E. Child's response to the condition

4. When assessing the chronically ill toddler, the pediatric nurse notes signs of impending death. The nurse recognizes the importance of supporting this family through this difficult experience and reviews which of the following as signs of impending death with the family members? (*Select all that apply.*)
   A. Skin is cool to the touch
   B. Quiet, easy respirations
   C. Rapid regular pulse
   D. Noisy, irregular respirations
   E. Sleeping for long periods of time
   F. Difficult to arouse

True/False

5. The child who is chronically ill always has physical involvement.

6. A priority nursing intervention for the adolescent with a chronic condition includes providing group therapy to help the adolescent to regain control.

7. During the time of death, the nurse should leave the family alone to grieve privately.

8. Palliative nursing care can provide relief of pain and other distressing symptoms but cannot postpone death.

9. According to developmental specialists, the preschool age group is a period of concrete thinking and so, death should be described as "going to sleep".

Fill-in-the-Blank

10. The pediatric nurse is aware that the leading cause of death in the school age group is _____.

11. It is important for the pediatric nurse to understand that according to normal growth and development the preschooler is a _____ _____ and may view illness as a punishment for bad behavior.

12. The _____ is unable to distinguish fear from fantasy which inhibits a true comprehension of death.

13. The _____ seems to comprehend death more than can be verbalized.

14. The _____ has difficulty accepting death as a reality and therefore thinks the body is invincible and engages in _____ _____ behaviors.

15. According to Kübler Ross, children after the ages of ____to____ understand the permanence of death. This age group understands more of what is overheard than parents and nurses realize. Attempts to shield this age group from death can often be perceived as _____.

Short Answer

16. The parent of the dying child asks the nurse if he/she can hold the child. What action is appropriate for the nurse to take?

See Answers to End of Chapter Review Questions on the Electronic Study Guide or DavisPlus.

REFERENCES

American Academy of Pediatrics (AAP) (2002). Palliative care for children, *Pediatrics, 106*(2), 351–357.

Anderson, R., & Smith, B. (2005). Deaths: Leading causes for 2002. *National Vital Statistics Report, 53*(17), 1–89.

Armstrong-Dailey, A., & Zarbock, S. (2001). *Hospice care for children*, 2nd ed. New York: Oxford University Press.

Beckman, P.J. (2002). Providing family centered services. In M.L. Batshaw (Ed.), *Children with disabilities*, 5th ed. (pp. 683–691). Baltimore: Brooks.

Beckstrand, R.L., Callister, L.C., & Kirchhoff, K.T. (2006). Providing a "good death": Critical care nurses suggestions for improving end-life-care. *American Journal of Critical Care, 15*(1), 38–45.

Bulechek, G., Butcher, H.M., & Dochterman, J. (2008). *Nursing interventions classification (NIC)* (5th ed.). St. Louis, MO: C.V. Mosby.

Caring Connections (2005). Differences between palliative care and hospice. Retrieved from http://www.caringinfo.org (Accessed August 22, 2008).

Children's Hospice International (2005). Retrieved from http://www.chionline.org/resources (Accessed August 22, 2008).

Children's International Project on Palliative/Hospice Services (ChIPPS). Compendium of Pediatric Palliative Care. Alexandria, VA: National Hospice and Palliative Care Organization, 2003.

Feudtner, C., Silveira, M.J., & Christakis, D.A. (2002). Where do children with complex chronic conditions die? Patterns in Washington State, 1980–1998. *Pediatrics – Springfield, 109*, 656–660.

Field, M.J., & Behrman, R.F. (2003). *When children die: Improving palliative and end-of-life care for children and their families.* Washington, DC: National Academic Press.

Gibbons, M. (2001). Psychosocial aspects of serious illness in childhood and adolescence. In A. Armstrong-Dailey & S. Zarbock (Eds.), *Hospice care for children,* 2nd ed. (pp. 49–67). New York: Oxford.

Godshall, M. (2003). Caring for the families of chronically ill kids. *RN, 66*(2), 30–35.

Hain, R., Weinsten, S., Oleske, J., Orloff, S.F., & Cohen, S. (2004). Holistic management of symptoms. In B.S. Carter & M. Levetown, (Eds.), *Palliative care for infants, children, and adolescents: A practical handbook* (pp. 163–195). Baltimore: The Johns Hopkins University Press.

Heller, K.S., & Solomon, M.Z. (2005). Continuity of care and caring: What matters to parents of children with life-threatening conditions. *Journal of Pediatric Nursing, 20*(5), 335–346.

Johnson, M., Bulechek, G., Butcher, H., McCloskey Dochterman, J., Maas, M., Moorehead, S., & Swanson, E. (2006). *NANDA, NOC, and NIC linkages: Nursing diagnoses, outcomes, & interventions* (2nd ed.). St. Louis, MO: Mosby Elsevier.

Judson, L. (2004). Protective care: Mothering a child dependent on parenteral nutrition. *Journal of Family Nursing, 10*(1), 93–120.

Kliebenstein, M.A., & Broome, M.E. (2000). School re-entry for the child with chronic illness: Parent and school personnel perceptions. *Pediatric Nursing, 26*(6), 579–582.

Kübler-Ross, E. (1983). *On children death.* New York: Macmillan.

Kuster, P.A., Badr, L.K., Chang, B.L., Wuerker, A.K., & Benjamin, A.E. (2004). Factors influencing health promoting activities of mothers caring for ventilator assisted children. *Journal of Pediatric Nursing, 19*(4), 276–287.

Lattanzi-Licht, M., & Connor, S. (1995). Care of the dying: The hospice approach. In H. Wass & R.A. Neimeyer (Eds), *Dying: Facing the facts.* Washington, DC: Taylor and Francis.

Mays, M. (2005). Comfort care as experienced by oncology nurses. Unpublished master's thesis, Nebraska Methodist College, Omaha.

Mazanec, P., & Tyler, M. (2003). Cultural considerations in end-of-life care: How ethnicity, age, and spirituality affect decisions when death is imminent. *American Journal of Nursing, 103*(3), 50–58.

Meleski, D.D. (2002). Families with chronically ill children. *American Journal of Nursing, 102*(5), 47–54.

Melnyk, B.M., Feinstein, N.F., Moldenhouer, Z., & Small, L. (2001). Coping in parents of children who are chronically ill: Strategies for assessment and intervention. *Pediatric Nursing, 27*, 548–558.

Miles, M., & Perry, K. (1985). In M.C. Slota (Ed.), *Core curriculum for critical care nurses* (pp. 28-29). Philadelphia: W.B. Saunders,

Moorehead, S., Johnson, M., Maas, M., & Swanson, E. (2008). *Nursing outcomes classification (NOC)* (4th ed.). St. Louis, MO: C.V. Mosby.

Morroni-Leash, R. (1994). *Death notification: A practical guide to the process.* Vermont: Upper Access.

NANDA International (2007). *NANDA-I nursing diagnoses: Definitions and classifications 2007–2008.* Philadelphia: NANDA-I.

National Cancer Institute (2006). Retrieved from http://www.cancer.gov (Accessed August 22, 2008).

Neuhouser, M.L., Patterson, R.E., Schwartz, S.M., Hedderson, M.M., Bowen, D.J., & Standish, L.J. (2001). Use of alternative medicine by children with cancer in Washington state. *Preventive Medicine, 33*(5), 347–354.

Orloff, S., Quance, K., Perszyk, S., Flowers, W., & Veale, E. (2004). Psychosocial and spiritual needs of the child and family. In K.M. Foley, B.S. Carter, & M. Levetown (Eds.), *Palliative care for infants, children, and adolescents* (pp. 141–162). Baltimore: Johns Hopkins University Press.

Pitetti, R., Singh, S., Hornyak, D., Garcia, S.F., & Herr, S. (2001). Complementary and alternative medicine use in children. *Pediatric Emergency Care, 17*(3), 165–169.

Potts, N., & Mandleco, B. (2002). *Pediatric nursing: Caring for children and their families.* Clifton Park, NY: Delmar.

Rushton, C.H. (2004). Ethics and palliative care in pediatrics. *American Journal of Nursing, 104*, 54–64.

Sanders, H., Davis, M., Duncan, B., Meany, J., Hayes, J., & Barton, L. (2003). Use of complementary and alternative medical therapies among children with special health care needs in Southern Arizona. *Pediatrics, 111*(3), 584–587.

Schmitke, J., & Scholmann, P. (2002). Chronic conditions. In N. Potts & B. Mandleco (Eds.), *Pediatric nursing: Care for children and their families* (pp. 493–515). Clifton Park, NY: Delmar.

Steen, G., & Mirro, M. (2000). *Childhood cancer. A handbook from St. Jude Children's Research Hospital.* Cambridge, MA: Perseus.

Suzuki, N. (2004). Complementary and alternative medicine: A Japanese perspective. *Evidenced-based Complementary and Alternative Care, 1*(2), 113–118.

Venes, D. (Ed.). (2009). *Taber's cyclopedic medical dictionary* (21st ed.). Philadelphia: F.A. Davis.

Ward, S. (2006). What healing means to nursing students: A phenomenological study. *Health Ministry Journal, 2*(1), 15–27.

Wiegand, D. (2006). Withdrawal of life-sustaining therapy after sudden, unexpected life-threatening illness or injury: Interactions between patients' families, healthcare providers, and the healthcare system. *Journal of Critical Care, 15*(2), 178–187.

Williams, P., Williams, A.R., Graff, J., Hanson, S., Stanton, A., Hafeman, C., Liebergen, A., Leuenber, K., Setter, R., Ridder, L., Curry, H., Barnard, M., & Sanders, S. (2002). Interrelationships among variables affecting well siblings and mothers in families of children with a chronic condition or disability. *Journal of Behavior Medicine, 25*(5), 411–424.

 For more information, go to http://davisplus.fadavis.com/

CONCEPT MAP

Nursing Insight:
- Know examples of chronic conditions/AKA: handicap/disability
- Understand symptoms for chronic conditions
- Caregiver burden
- Grief normal/appropriate
- Somatic grief response
- Use care with belongings of child who has died
- Take care of yourself/self-insight

Be Sure To:
- [✓] Understand type of technological equipment
- Know laws: educational services

Where Research And Practice Meet:
- 52% of children with chronic conditions die in hospitals
- There are facilitators and barriers to good death

Collaboration In Caring:
- Child life specialist

Complementary Care:
- Acupuncture; herbs; relaxation; prayers

Infant
- Separation: disrupts bonding
- Alteration in growth & development

Toddler
- Interruption of development: autonomy/self control
- Hinders fine/gross motor
- Anxiety; Regression

Preschool Child
- Interrupts initiative
- Perceives treatment as punishment
- Aggression; withdrawal; regression

School-aged Child
- Interrupts industry; peer interactions; independence
- Anger; refusal to comply with treatment

Adolescent
- Loss of peer interaction negative self-esteem/sexual identity
- Loss of autonomy/control
- Maladaptive coping; Worry about family

Sibling
- Decreased self-esteem; less parental support; mood swings
- Loneliness/isolation

Nursing: Infant
- Hold; rock; comfort
- Encourage parent–child bonding/holding
- Visual/auditory stimulation

Nursing: Toddler
- Promote parent–child bond; realistic developmental skills
- Teach realistic methods of discipline
- Maintain normal schedule

Nursing: Preschool Child
- Allow expression of fears/frustration
- Storytelling/books/dramatic play
- Normal schedule = security
- Use honesty; explain all procedures

Nursing: School-aged Child
- Clarify their understanding of information
- Reassure: behavior doesn't cause illness
- Unstructured play
- Allow choices when possible

Nursing: Adolescent
- Base care on "stage" of adolescence
- Allow choices to enhance control
- Peer/social support

Nursing: Sibling
- Maintain familiar routines
- Include sibling in simple aspects of care
- Provide information about ill child

- Frequent hospitalization
- Chronic burden of care
- Threat of unknown
- Social, financial, psychological strain
- Stress/increased demands/role strain
- Interruption of normal routine
- Loss of control/powerlessness
- Balancing care with other responsibilities

Impact on family

Impact on child

Chronic Condition

Caring for the Child with a Chronic Condition or the Dying Child

Emotional Responses
- Will differ depending on illness/prognosis
- Shock, fear, anger, disbelief anxiety, "roller coaster" of feelings, chronic sorrow

General Nursing Interventions: Dying Child
- Therapeutic communication relay sympathy, kindness
- Demonstrate caring: touch, placing toys
- Give family realistic choices in the process
- Provide information re: actual death of child
- Facilitate "saying good-bye" no time limit; include sibling(s)
- Provide ongoing care for family after child's death
- Provide community resources

Palliative Care
- End of life when cure not possible
- Enhances quality of life
- Alleviate/control distressing symptoms
- Medical model; hospital care
- Also addresses emotional/spiritual needs

Hospice Care
- Comprehensive, holistic care
- Patient/family is unit of care
- Quality of life not cure
- Respite care/follow-up bereavement care for family

Nursing Interventions
- Communication is KEY
- Topics
  – Continue regular daily activities: incorporate disease into routine; help child to live life
- Treatments; procedures; meds
- Handling self-blame/chronic sorrow
- Participation in child's care

Grief

End of Life Care
- Facilitate discussions about death
- Continue palliative care: control pain
- Take proactive approach to impending death
- Create remembrance packet for family
- Provide care for the caregiver

- Nursing care based on theory:
  – Kübler-Ross; Lindemann
  – Miles and Perry; Epperson
- Accept family in whatever stage of grief they are in
- Help families to retain healthy habits/find positive outlet for emotions
- Reinforce: illness is no one's fault
- Recognize coping patterns used
- Identify pathological grief:
  – "Competition of drama"
  – Suicidal/homicidal ideation
  – Drug and alcohol use
  – Extreme denial
- Collaborate with licensed professionals
- Provide community resources

Critical Nursing Action:
- Establish trust with family
- Help the sibling
- Hospice approach
- Holistic care for dying child

Other Important Aspects of Care
- Establish a therapeutic relationship
- Assess for alterations/delays in growth and development
- Promote/advocate for child's right to education
- Assess cultural aspects that affect response to illness

Optimizing Outcomes:
- Handle acting out with use of reflection/validation

What To Say:
- Use child's name in discussions on disease
- Practice "presence" at time of death
- Listen empathetically to family questions avoid using platitudes
- Give clear answers to dying child

Across Care Settings:
- Respite care
- Early and comprehensive discharge planning key to coordination

Ethnocultural Considerations:
- Culturally appropriated spiritual care
- Special needs of the Latino culture related to grief

? Now Can You:
- Define chronic conditions
- List 3 nursing diagnoses related to the dying process
- Differentiate between hospice and palliative care
- Assist the child and family through the grieving process

Centigrade to Fahrenheit Temperature Conversions

Conversion Formulas

°F = (°C × 9/5) + 32, or (°C × 1.8) + 32

°C = (°F − 32) × 5/9, or (°F − 32) × 0.55

°C	°F
35.0	95.0
35.2	95.4
35.4	95.7
35.6	96.1
35.8	96.4
36.0	96.8
36.2	97.2
36.4	97.5
36.6	97.9
36.8	98.2
37.0	98.6
37.2	99.0
37.4	99.3
37.6	99.7
37.8	100.0
38.0	100.4
38.2	100.8
38.4	101.1
38.6	101.5
38.8	101.8
39.0	102.2
39.2	102.6
39.4	102.9
39.6	103.3
39.8	103.6
40.0	104.0
40.2	104.4
40.4	104.7
40.6	105.1
40.8	105.4

Appendix B

Expected Temperatures in Children

Age	Fahrenheit (°F)	Centigrade (°C)
2 months	99.4	37.5
4 months	99.5	37.5
1 years	99.7	37.7
2 years	99.0	37.2
4 years	98.6	37.0
6 years	98.3	36.8
8 years	98.1	36.7
10 years	98.0	36.7
12 years	97.8	36.6

Photo and Illustration Credits

NURSING CARE PLANS

NIC and NOC information by permission of Elsevier.

CHAPTER 2

Figure 2-1 Courtesy of Public Health Practice, St. Cloud, Minnesota.

CHAPTER 3

Figure 3-1 Courtesy of Family Ties Project, Washington, DC. Life Planning for Families Affected by HIV/AIDS.

CHAPTER 4

Figure 4-1 U.S. Department of Agriculture, Food and Nutrition Service, September 2005.

Figure 4-2 Centers for Disease Control and Prevention, 2008.

Figure 4-3 Dillon, P. (2007). *Nursing health assessment: A critical thinking, case studies approach* (2nd ed., p. 612). Philadelphia: F.A. Davis.

Figure 4-4 Dillon, P. (2007). *Nursing health assessment: A critical thinking, case studies approach* (2nd ed., p. 631). Philadelphia: F.A. Davis.

Figure 4-5 Dillon, P. (2007). *Nursing health assessment: A critical thinking, case studies approach* (2nd ed., p. 634). Philadelphia: F.A. Davis.

Figure 4-6 Dillon, P. (2007). *Nursing health assessment: A critical thinking, case studies approach* (2nd ed., p. 635). Philadelphia: F.A. Davis.

Figure 4-7 Dillon, P. (2007). *Nursing health assessment: A critical thinking, case studies approach* (2nd ed., p. 640). Philadelphia: F.A. Davis.

Figure 4-8 Dillon, P. (2007). *Nursing health assessment: A critical thinking, case studies approach* (2nd ed., p. 641). Philadelphia: F.A. Davis.

Figure 4-9 Dillon, P. (2007). *Nursing health assessment: A critical thinking, case studies approach* (2nd ed., p. 641). Philadelphia: F.A. Davis.

Figure 4-10 Dillon, P. (2007). *Nursing health assessment: A critical thinking, case studies approach* (2nd ed., p. 642). Philadelphia: F.A. Davis.

Figure 4-11 Dillon, P. (2007). *Nursing health assessment: A critical thinking, case studies approach* (2nd ed., p. 642). Philadelphia: F.A. Davis.

Figure 4-12 Dillon, P. (2007). *Nursing health assessment: A critical thinking, case studies approach* (2nd ed., p. 642). Philadelphia: F.A. Davis.

Figure 4-13 Williams L., & Hopper P. (2007). *Understanding medical surgical nursing* (3rd ed., p. 896). Philadelphia: F.A. Davis.

Visual breast inspection. Dillon, P. (2007) *Nursing health assessment: A critical thinking, case studies approach* (2nd ed., p. 544). Philadelphia: F.A. Davis.

Arms raised overhead. Dillon, P. (2007). *Nursing health assessment: A critical thinking, case studies approach* (2nd ed., p. 544). Philadelphia: F.A. Davis.

Nipple assessment. Dillon, P. (2007). *Nursing health assessment: A critical thinking, case studies approach* (2nd ed., p. 550). Philadelphia: F.A. Davis.

Breast palpation. Dillon, P. (2007). *Nursing health assessment: A critical thinking, case studies approach* (2nd ed., p. 550). Philadelphia: F.A. Davis.

CHAPTER 5

Figure 5-1 Dillon, P. (2007). *Nursing health assessment: A critical thinking, case studies approach* (2nd ed., p. 612). Philadelphia: F.A. Davis.

Figure 5-3 Dillon, P. (2007). *Nursing health assessment: A critical thinking, case studies approach* (2nd ed., p. 612). Philadelphia: F.A. Davis.

Figure 5-4 Dillon, P. (2007). *Nursing health assessment: A critical thinking, case studies approach* (2nd ed., p. 613). Philadelphia: F.A. Davis.

Figure 5-5 Scanlon V., & Sanders T. (2007). *Essentials of anatomy and physiology* (5th ed., p. 458). Philadelphia: F.A. Davis.

Figure 5-7 Scanlon V., & Sanders T. (2007). *Essentials of anatomy and physiology* (5th ed., p. 463). Philadelphia: F.A. Davis.

Figure 5-8 Scanlon V., & Sanders T. (2007). *Essentials of anatomy and physiology* (5th ed., p. 464). Philadelphia: F.A. Davis.

Figure 5-13 Scanlon V., & Sanders T. (2007). *Essentials of anatomy and physiology* (5th ed., p. 467). Philadelphia: F.A. Davis.

Figure 5-14 Dillon, P. (2007). *Nursing health assessment: A critical thinking, case studies approach* (2nd ed., p. 613). Philadelphia: F.A. Davis.

Figure 5-16 Dillon, P. (2007). *Nursing health assessment: A critical thinking, case studies approach* (2nd ed., p. 617). Philadelphia: F.A. Davis.

Figure 5-19 Scanlon V., & Sanders T. (2007). *Essentials of anatomy and physiology* (5th ed., p. 459). Philadelphia: F.A. Davis.

Figure 5-20 Scanlon V., & Sanders T. (2007). *Essentials of anatomy and physiology* (5th ed., p. 460). Philadelphia: F.A. Davis.

Figure 5-21 Scanlon V., & Sanders T. (2007). *Essentials of anatomy and physiology* (5th ed., p. 457). Philadelphia: F.A. Davis.

CHAPTER 6

Figure 6-2 Hatcher R.A., et al. (2005). A pocket guide to managing contraception. Tiger, Georgia: Bridging the Gap Foundation.

CHAPTER 7

Figure 7-1 Courtesy of National Human Genome Research Institute, Bethesda, Maryland.

Figure 7-2 Scanlon V., & Sanders T. (2007). *Essentials of anatomy and physiology* (5th ed., p. 488). Philadelphia: F.A. Davis.

Figure 7-3 Scanlon V., & Sanders T. (2007). *Essentials of anatomy and physiology* (5th ed., p. 477). Philadelphia: F.A. Davis.

Figure 7-5 Scanlon V., & Sanders T. (2007). *Essentials of anatomy and physiology* (5th ed., p. 489). Philadelphia: F.A. Davis.

Figure 7-7 Scanlon V., & Sanders T. (2007). *Essentials of anatomy and physiology* (5th ed., p. 491). Philadelphia: F.A. Davis.

Figure 7-8 Scanlon V., & Sanders T. (2007). *Essentials of anatomy and physiology* (5th ed., p. 478). Philadelphia: F.A. Davis.

Figure 7-9 Scanlon V., & Sanders T. (2007). *Essentials of anatomy and physiology* (5th ed., p. 484). Philadelphia: F.A. Davis.

Figure 7-10 Scanlon V., & Sanders T. (2007). *Essentials of anatomy and physiology* (5th ed., p. 479). Philadelphia: F.A. Davis.

Figure 7-12 Polan, E.U., & Taylor, D.R. (2007). *Journey across the life span: Human development and health promotion* (3rd ed., p. 77). Philadelphia: F.A. Davis.

Figure 7-13 Polan, E.U., & Taylor, D.R. (2007). *Journey across the life span: Human development and health promotion* (3rd ed., p. 77). Philadelphia: F.A. Davis.

Figure 7-14 Courtesy of National Human Genome Research Institute, National Institutes of Health, Bethesda, Maryland.

Figure 7-15 Courtesy of National Human Genome Research Institute, National Institutes of Health, Bethesda, Maryland.

Figure 7-16 Courtesy of National Human Genome Research Institute, National Institutes of Health, Bethesda, Maryland.

Figure 7-18 Venes, D. (2005). *Taber's cyclopedic medical dictionary* (20th ed., p. 1165). Philadelphia: F.A. Davis.

CHAPTER 8

Figure 8-3 Dillon, P. (2007). *Nursing health assessment: A critical thinking, case studies approach* (2nd ed., p. 840). Philadelphia: F.A. Davis.

Figure 8-5 Dillon, P. (2007). *Nursing health assessment: A critical thinking, case studies approach* (2nd ed., p. 834). Philadelphia: F.A. Davis.

Figure 8-6 Dillon, P. (2007). *Nursing health assessment: A critical thinking, case studies approach* (2nd ed., p. 834). Philadelphia: F.A. Davis.

Figure 8-9 Dillon, P. (2007). *Nursing health assessment: A critical thinking, case studies approach* (2nd ed., p. 834). Philadelphia: F.A. Davis.

Figure 8-11 Dillon, P. (2007). *Nursing health assessment: A critical thinking, case studies approach* (2nd ed., p. 841). Philadelphia: F.A. Davis.

CHAPTER 9

Figure 9-4 Dillon, P. (2007). *Nursing health assessment: A critical thinking, case studies approach* (2nd ed., p. 833). Philadelphia: F.A. Davis.

Figure 9-5 Dillon, P. (2007). *Nursing health assessment: A critical thinking, case studies approach* (2nd ed., p. 836). Philadelphia: F.A. Davis.

Figure 9-6 Dillon, P. (2007). *Nursing health assessment: A critical thinking, case studies approach* (2nd ed., p. 836). Philadelphia: F.A. Davis.

Figure 9-7 Dillon, P. (2007). *Nursing health assessment: A critical thinking, case studies approach* (2nd ed., p. 838). Philadelphia: F.A. Davis.

Figure 9-8 Dillon, P. (2007). *Nursing health assessment: A critical thinking, case studies approach* (2nd ed., p. 838). Philadelphia: F.A. Davis.

Figure 9-9 Dillon, P. (2007). *Nursing health assessment: A critical thinking, case studies approach* (2nd ed., p. 838). Philadelphia: F.A. Davis.

Figure 9-10 Dillon, P. (2007). *Nursing health assessment: A critical thinking, case studies approach* (2nd ed., p. 838). Philadelphia: F.A. Davis.

Figure 9-11 Dillon, P. (2007). *Nursing health assessment: A critical thinking, case studies approach* (2nd ed., p. 838). Philadelphia: F.A. Davis.

Figure 9-12 Dillon, P. (2007). *Nursing health assessment: A critical thinking, case studies approach* (2nd ed., p. 837). Philadelphia: F.A. Davis.

Figure 9-13 Dillon, P. (2007). *Nursing health assessment: A critical thinking, case studies approach* (2nd ed., p. 837). Philadelphia: F.A. Davis.

Figure 9-14 Dillon, P. (2007). *Nursing health assessment: A critical thinking, case studies approach* (2nd ed., p. 837). Philadelphia: F.A. Davis.

Figure 9-15 Dillon, P. (2007). *Nursing health assessment: A critical thinking, case studies approach* (2nd ed., p. 631). Philadelphia: F.A. Davis.

Figure 9-16 Dillon, P. (2007). *Nursing health assessment: A critical thinking, case studies approach* (2nd ed., p. 635). Philadelphia: F.A. Davis.

Figure 9-17 Dillon, P. (2007). *Nursing health assessment: A critical thinking, case studies approach* (2nd ed., p. 840). Philadelphia: F.A. Davis.

Figure 9-18 Dillon, P. (2007). *Nursing health assessment: A critical thinking, case studies approach* (2nd ed., p. 641). Philadelphia: F.A. Davis.

CHAPTER 10

Figure 10-2 Copyright 2001, The Dr. Spock Company.

Figure 10-8 Courtesy of Indiana Perinatal Network.

CHAPTER 11

Figure 11-1 Venes, D. (2005). *Taber's cyclopedic medical dictionary* (20th ed., p. 1757). Philadelphia: F.A. Davis.

Figure 11.3 Wedding, M.S.. & Toenjes, S.A. (1998). *Medical laboratory procedures* (2nd ed., p. 57). Philadelphia: F.A. Davis.

Figure 11-4 Holloway, B., Moredich, C., & Aduddell, K. (2006). *OB peds women's health notes: Nurse's clinical pocket guide*, p. 43, Philadelphia: F.A. Davis.

Figure 11-5 Holloway, B., Moredich, C., & Aduddell, K. (2006). *OB peds women's health notes: Nurse's clinical pocket guide*, p. 45, Philadelphia: F.A. Davis.

Figure 11-6 Gilbert, E.S., & Harmon, J.S. (2003). *Manual of high risk pregnancy and delivery* (3rd ed., p. 562). St. Louis: Mosby.

Figure 11-7 Dillon, P. (2007). *Nursing health assessment: A critical thinking, case studies approach* (2nd ed., p. 785). Philadelphia: F.A. Davis.

Figure 11-8 Scanlon V., & Sanders T. (2007). *Essentials of anatomy and physiology* (5th ed., p. 59). Philadelphia: F.A. Davis.

Figure 11-9 Compiled by Patricia M. Sauer. High-risk pregnancy: Chronic medical conditions. Copyright March of Dimes Birth Defects Foundation, 1998.

Figure 11-11 Kendrick, J. (2004). *Diabetes in pregnancy* (3rd ed., p. 54). March of Dimes.

CHAPTER 12

Figure 12-1 Holloway, B., Moredich, C., & Aduddell, K. (2006). *OB peds women's health notes: Nurse's clinical pocket guide*, p. 63. Philadelphia: F.A. Davis.

Figure 12-9 Holloway, B., Moredich, C., & Aduddell, K. (2006). *OB peds women's health notes: Nurse's clinical pocket guide*, p. 53. Philadelphia: F.A. Davis.

Figure 12-13 Dillon, P. (2007). *Nursing health assessment: A critical thinking, case studies approach* (2nd ed., p. 837). Philadelphia: F.A. Davis.

Figure 12-14 Holloway, B., Moredich, C., & Aduddell, K. (2006). *OB peds women's health notes: Nurse's clinical pocket guide*, p. 55. Philadelphia: F.A. Davis.

Figure 12-15 Holloway, B., Moredich, C., & Aduddell, K. (2006). *OB peds women's health notes: Nurse's clinical pocket guide*, p. 56. Philadelphia: F.A. Davis.

Figure 12-16 Holloway, B., Moredich, C., & Aduddell, K. (2006). *OB peds women's health notes: Nurse's clinical pocket guide*, p. 57. Philadelphia: F.A. Davis.

Figure 12-17 Holloway, B., Moredich, C., & Aduddell, K. (2006). *OB peds women's health notes: Nurse's clinical pocket guide*, p. 59. Philadelphia: F.A. Davis.

Figure 12-18 Holloway, B., Moredich, C., & Aduddell, K. (2006). *OB peds women's health notes: Nurse's clinical pocket guide*, p. 60. Philadelphia: F.A. Davis.

Figure 12-19 Holloway, B., Moredich, C., & Aduddell, K. (2006). *OB peds women's health notes: Nurse's clinical pocket guide*, p. 61. Philadelphia: F.A. Davis.

Figure 12-20 Holloway, B., Moredich, C., & Aduddell, K. (2006). *OB peds women's health notes: Nurse's clinical pocket guide*, p. 60. Philadelphia: F.A. Davis.

CHAPTER 15

Figure 15-1 Holloway, B., Moredich, C., & Aduddell, K. (2006). *OB peds women's health notes: Nurse's clinical pocket guide*, p. 83. Philadelphia: F.A. Davis.

Figure 15-2 Dillon, P. (2007). *Nursing health assessment: A critical thinking, case studies approach* (2nd ed., p. 844). Philadelphia: F.A. Davis.

Figure 15-4 Dillon, P. (2007). *Nursing health assessment: A critical thinking, case studies approach* (2nd ed., p. 514). Philadelphia: F.A. Davis.

Figure 15-8 Holloway, B., Moredich, C., & Aduddell, K. (2006). *OB peds women's health notes: Nurse's clinical pocket guide*, p. 79. Philadelphia: F.A. Davis.

Figure 15-9 Courtesy of Medela Corporation, McHenry, Illinois.

Figure 15-10 Courtesy of Medela Corporation, McHenry, Illinois.

Figure 15-11 Courtesy of Medela Corporation, McHenry, Illinois.

CHAPTER 16

Figure in Procedure 16-1. Holloway, B., Moredich, C., & Aduddell, K. (2006). *OB peds women's health notes: Nurse's clinical pocket guide*, p. 83. Philadelphia: F.A. Davis.

CHAPTER 18

Figure 18-2 Dillon, P. (2007). *Nursing health assessment: A critical thinking, case studies approach* (2nd ed., p. 857). Philadelphia: F.A. Davis.

Figure 18-3 Dillon, P. (2007). *Nursing health assessment: A critical thinking, case studies approach* (2nd ed., p. 857). Philadelphia: F.A. Davis.

Figure 18-4 Dillon, P. (2007). *Nursing health assessment: A critical thinking, case studies approach* (2nd ed., p. 856). Philadelphia: F.A. Davis.

Figure 18-5 Dillon, P. (2007). *Nursing health assessment: A critical thinking, case studies approach* (2nd ed., p. 856). Philadelphia: F.A. Davis.

Figure 18-6 Dillon, P. (2007). *Nursing health assessment: A critical thinking, case studies approach* (2nd ed., p. 857). Philadelphia: F.A. Davis.

Figure 18-7 Courtesy of Mead Johnson Nutritionals.

Figure 18-8 Courtesy of Mead Johnson Nutritionals.

Figure 18-9 Dillon, P. (2007). *Nursing health assessment: A critical thinking, case studies approach* (2nd ed., p. 859). Philadelphia: F.A. Davis.

Figure 18-11 Dillon, P. (2007). *Nursing health assessment: A critical thinking, case studies approach* (2nd ed., p. 859). Philadelphia: F.A. Davis.

Figure 18-12 Dillon, P. (2007). *Nursing health assessment: A critical thinking, case studies approach* (2nd ed., p. 861). Philadelphia: F.A. Davis.

Figure 18-13 Dillon, P. (2007). *Nursing health assessment: A critical thinking, case studies approach* (2nd ed., p. 860). Philadelphia: F.A. Davis.

Figure 18-14 Dillon, P. (2007). *Nursing health assessment: A critical thinking, case studies approach* (2nd ed., p. 860). Philadelphia: F.A. Davis.

Figure 18-16 Dillon, P. (2007). *Nursing health assessment: A critical thinking, case studies approach* (2nd ed., p. 861). Philadelphia: F.A. Davis.

Figure 18-17 Dillon, P. (2007). *Nursing health assessment: A critical thinking, case studies approach* (2nd ed., p. 862). Philadelphia: F.A. Davis.

Figure 18-18 Dillon, P. (2007). *Nursing health assessment: A critical thinking, case studies approach* (2nd ed., p. 863). Philadelphia: F.A. Davis.

Figure 18-19 Dillon, P. (2007). *Nursing health assessment: A critical thinking, case studies approach* (2nd ed., p. 864). Philadelphia: F.A. Davis.

Figure 18-20 Dillon, P. (2007). *Nursing health assessment: A critical thinking, case studies approach* (2nd ed., p. 864). Philadelphia: F.A. Davis.

Figure 18-21 Dillon, P. (2007). *Nursing health assessment: A critical thinking, case studies approach* (2nd ed., p. 864). Philadelphia: F.A. Davis.

Figure 18-22 Dillon, P. (2007). *Nursing health assessment: A critical thinking, case studies approach* (2nd ed., p. 865). Philadelphia: F.A. Davis.

Figure 18-23 Dillon, P. (2007). *Nursing health assessment: A critical thinking, case studies approach* (2nd ed., p. 873). Philadelphia: F.A. Davis.

Figure 18-24 Dillon, P. (2007). *Nursing health assessment: A critical thinking, case studies approach* (2nd ed., p. 866). Philadelphia: F.A. Davis.

Procedure 18-3, first photo Dillon, P. (2007). *Nursing health assessment: A critical thinking, case studies approach* (2nd ed., p. 866). Philadelphia: F.A. Davis.

Procedure 18-3, second photo Dillon, P. (2007). *Nursing health assessment: A critical thinking, case studies approach* (2nd ed., p. 866). Philadelphia: F.A. Davis.

Procedure 18-3, third photo Dillon, P. (2007). *Nursing health assessment: A critical thinking, case studies approach* (2nd ed., p. 866). Philadelphia: F.A. Davis.

Table 18-2 Palmar grasp. Dillon, P. (2007). *Nursing health assessment: A critical thinking, case studies approach* (2nd ed., p. 869). Philadelphia: F.A. Davis.

Table 18-2 Toe or plantar grasp. Dillon, P. (2007). *Nursing health assessment: A critical thinking, case studies approach* (2nd ed., p. 869). Philadelphia: F.A. Davis.

Table 18-2 Rooting and sucking reflex. Dillon, P. (2007). *Nursing health assessment: A critical thinking, case studies approach* (2nd ed., p. 871). Philadelphia: F.A. Davis.

Table 18-2 Extrusion reflex. Dillon, P. (2007). *Nursing health assessment: A critical thinking, case studies approach* (2nd ed., p. 871). Philadelphia: F.A. Davis.

Table 18-2 Stepping reflex. Dillon, P. (2007). *Nursing health assessment: A critical thinking, case studies approach* (2nd ed., p. 870). Philadelphia: F.A. Davis.

Table 18-2 Tonic neck or fencing reflex. Dillon, P. (2007). *Nursing health assessment: A critical thinking, case studies approach* (2nd ed., p. 868). Philadelphia: F.A. Davis.

Table 18-2 Glabellar reflex. Dillon, P. (2007). *Nursing health assessment: A critical thinking, case studies approach* (2nd ed., p. 872). Philadelphia: F.A. Davis.

Table 18-2 Babinski reflex. Dillon, P. (2007). *Nursing health assessment: A critical thinking, case studies approach* (2nd ed., p. 869). Philadelphia: F.A. Davis.

Table 18-2 Moro reflex. Dillon, P. (2007). *Nursing health assessment: A critical thinking, case studies approach* (2nd ed., p. 868). Philadelphia: F.A. Davis.

Table 18-2 Magnet reflex. Dillon, P. (2007). *Nursing health assessment: A critical thinking, case studies approach* (2nd ed., p. 873). Philadelphia: F.A. Davis.

Table 18-2 Galant reflex or trunk incurvation reflex. Dillon, P. (2007). *Nursing health assessment: A critical thinking, case studies approach* (2nd ed., p. 873). Philadelphia: F.A. Davis.

Table 18-2 Crawling reflex. Dillon, P. (2007). *Nursing health assessment: A critical thinking, case studies approach* (2nd ed., p. 872). Philadelphia: F.A. Davis.

Table 18-2 Crossed extension. Dillon, P. (2007). *Nursing health assessment: A critical thinking, case studies approach* (2nd ed., p. 872). Philadelphia: F.A. Davis.

CHAPTER 19

Figure 19-3 Stevens, B., Johnston, C., Petryshen, P., & Taddio, A. (1996). Premature infant pain profile: Development and initial validation. *Clinical Journal of Pain, 12*(1), 13–22.

Figure 19-6 Courtesy of William A. Silverman, MD.

CHAPTER 21

Figure 21-1 Dillon, P. (2007). *Nursing health assessment: A critical thinking, case studies approach* (2nd ed., p. 856). Philadelphia: F.A. Davis.

Figure 21-14B *Wong's essentials of pediatric nursing* (6th ed). St. Louis: Mosby. Copyright by Mosby, Inc. Reprinted with permission.

Preliterate eye chart. Wilkinson, J.M., & Van Leuven, K. (2007). *Fundamentals of nursing: Theory, concepts & applications*, Vol. 2, p. 254. Philadelphia: F.A. Davis.

Snellen standard eye chart. Wilkinson, J.M., & Van Leuven, K. (2007). *Fundamentals of nursing: Theory, concepts & applications*, Vol. 2, p. 254. Philadelphia: F.A. Davis.

CHAPTER 24

Heimlich maneuver, back blows. Hopkins, T., & Myers, E. (2007). *Medical surgical notes* (2nd ed., p. 168). Philadelphia: F.A. Davis.

Heimlich maneuver, chest thrusts. Hopkins, T., & Myers, E. (2007). *Medical surgical notes* (2nd ed., p. 168). Philadelphia: F.A. Davis.

CHAPTER 26

Table 26-1 Chickenpox. Courtesy of the Centers for Disease Control and Prevention.

Table 26-1 Diphtheria. Courtesy of the Centers for Disease Control and Prevention.

Table 26-1 Fifth disease. Courtesy of the Centers for Disease Control and Prevention.

Table 26-1 Mumps. Courtesy of the Centers for Disease Control and Prevention.

Table 26-1 Pertussis. Courtesy of the Centers for Disease Control and Prevention.

Table 26-1 Poliomyelitis. Courtesy of the Centers for Disease Control and Prevention.

Table 26-1 Measles. Courtesy of the Centers for Disease Control and Prevention.

Table 26-1 Scarlet fever. Courtesy of the Centers for Disease Control and Prevention.

Table 26-1 Tetanus. Courtesy of the Centers for Disease Control and Prevention.

CHAPTER 29

Figure 29-1 Teasdale, G., & Jennett, B. (1974). Assessment of coma and impaired consciousness. A practical scale. *The Lancet, 13*;2(7872), 81-84.

Figure 29-6 Dillon, P. (2007). *Nursing health assessment: A critical thinking, case studies approach* (2nd ed., p. 784). Philadelphia: F.A. Davis.

Figure 29-11 Scanlon, V., & Sanders T. (2007). *Essentials of anatomy and physiology* (5th ed., p. 209). Philadelphia: F.A. Davis.

CHAPTER 30

Figure 30-9 Williams, L.S., & Hopper, P.D. (2007). *Understanding medical surgical nursing* (3rd ed., p. 1006). Philadelphia: F.A. Davis.

Figure 30-10 Dillon, P. (2007). *Nursing health assessment: A critical thinking, case studies approach* (2nd ed., p. 708). Philadelphia: F.A. Davis.

Figure 30-13 Dillon, P. (2007). *Nursing health assessment: A critical thinking, case studies approach* (2nd ed., p. 708). Philadelphia: F.A. Davis.

Assessment Tools: Transverse break. Williams, L.S., & Hopper, P.D. (2007). *Understanding medical surgical nursing* (3rd ed., p. 995). Philadelphia: F.A. Davis.

Assessment Tools: Spiral break. Williams, L.S., & Hopper, P.D. (2007). *Understanding medical surgical nursing* (3rd ed., p. 995). Philadelphia: F.A. Davis.

Assessment Tools: Oblique break. Williams, L.S., & Hopper, P.D. (2007). *Understanding medical surgical nursing* (3rd ed., p. 995). Philadelphia: F.A. Davis.

Assessment Tools: Greenstick break. Williams, L.S., & Hopper, P.D. (2007). *Understanding medical surgical nursing* (3rd ed., p. 995). Philadelphia: F.A. Davis.

Assessment Tools: Comminuted break. Williams, L.S., & Hopper, P.D. (2007). *Understanding medical surgical nursing* (3rd ed., p. 995). Philadelphia: F.A. Davis.

CHAPTER 31

Figure 31-1 Scanlon, V., & Sanders, T. (2007). *Essentials of anatomy and physiology* (5th ed., p. 91). Philadelphia: F.A. Davis.

Figure 31-3 Goldsmith, L.A., Lazarus, G.S., & Tharp, M.D. (1997). *Adult and pediatric dermatology*, p. 351. Philadelphia: F.A. Davis.

Figure 31-4 Williams, L.S., & Hopper, P.D. (2007). *Understanding medical surgical nursing* (3rd ed., p. 1226). Philadelphia: F.A. Davis.

Figure 31-5 Williams, L.S., & Hopper, P.D. (2007). *Understanding medical surgical nursing* (3rd ed., p. 1237). Philadelphia: F.A. Davis.

Figure 31-6 Dillon, P. (2007). *Nursing health assessment: A critical thinking, case studies approach* (2nd ed., p. 297). Philadelphia: F.A. Davis.

Figure 31-7 Dillon, P. (2007). *Nursing health assessment: A critical thinking, case studies approach* (2nd ed., p. 246). Philadelphia: F.A. Davis.

Figure 31-8 Dillon, P. (2007). *Nursing health assessment: A critical thinking, case studies approach* (2nd ed., p. 241). Philadelphia: F.A. Davis.

Figure 31-9 Dillon, P. (2007). *Nursing health assessment: A critical thinking, case studies approach* (2nd ed., p. 246). Philadelphia: F.A. Davis.

Figure 31-10A Trofino, R.B. (1991). *Nursing care of the burn-injured patient*, plate 1. Philadelphia: F.A. Davis.

Figure 31-10B Trofino, R.B. (1991). *Nursing care of the burn-injured patient*, plate 2. Philadelphia: F.A. Davis.

Figure 31-10C Trofino, R.B. (1991). *Nursing care of the burn-injured patient*, plate 3. Philadelphia: F.A. Davis.

Figure 31-11 Venes, D. (2005). *Taber's cyclopedic medical dictionary* (20th ed., p. 1931). Philadelphia: F.A. Davis.

Figure 31-12 Dillon, P. (2007). *Nursing health assessment: A critical thinking, case studies approach* (2nd ed., p. 239). Philadelphia: F.A. Davis.

Table 31-2 Macules. Dillon, P. (2007). *Nursing health assessment: A critical thinking, case studies approach* (2nd ed., p. 231). Philadelphia: F.A. Davis.

Table 31-2 Papule. Dillon, P. (2007). *Nursing health assessment: A critical thinking, case studies approach* (2nd ed., p. 233). Philadelphia: F.A. Davis.

Table 31-2 Patches. Dillon, P. (2007). *Nursing health assessment: A critical thinking, case studies approach* (2nd ed., p. 233). Philadelphia: F.A. Davis.

Table 31-2 Tumors. Dillon, P. (2007). *Nursing health assessment: A critical thinking, case studies approach* (2nd ed., p. 234). Philadelphia: F.A. Davis.

Table 31-2 Vesicles. Courtesy of Centers for Disease Control and Prevention.

Table 31-2 Pustules. Courtesy of Centers for Disease Control and Prevention.

Table 31-2 Bullae. Courtesy of Centers for Disease Control and Prevention.

Table 31-2 Wheals. Courtesy of Centers for Disease Control and Prevention.

Table 31-2 Crust. Courtesy of Centers for Disease Control and Prevention.

Table 31-2 Scales. Courtesy of Centers for Disease Control and Prevention.

Table 31-2 Licherification. Courtesy of Centers for Disease Control and Prevention.

Table 31-2 Keloids. Dillon, P. (2007). *Nursing health assessment: A critical thinking, case studies approach* (2nd ed., p. 237). Philadelphia: F.A. Davis.

Table 31-2 Fissure. Dillon, P. (2007). *Nursing health assessment: A critical thinking, case studies approach* (2nd ed., p. 238). Philadelphia: F.A. Davis.

Table 31-2 Ulcer. Dillon, P. (2007). *Nursing health assessment: A critical thinking, case studies approach* (2nd ed., p. 238). Philadelphia: F.A. Davis.

CHAPTER 32

Figure 32-1 Scanlon V., & Sanders T. (2007). *Essentials of anatomy and physiology* (5th ed., p. 422). Philadelphia: F.A. Davis.

CHAPTER 33

Figure 33-3 Harmening, D.M. (1997). *Clinical hematology and fundamentals of hemostasis* (3rd ed., p. 176). Philadelphia: F.A. Davis.

CHAPTER 34

Figure 34-2 Harmening, D.M. (1997). *Clinical hematology and fundamentals of hemostasis* (3rd ed., p. 176). Philadelphia: F.A. Davis.

Figure 34-3 Harmening, D.M. (1997). *Clinical hematology and fundamentals of hemostasis* (3rd ed., p. 176). Philadelphia: F.A. Davis.

Figure 34-5 McKinnis, L.N. (2005). *Fundamentals of musculoskeletal imaging* (2nd ed., p. 56). Philadelphia: F.A. Davis.

Figure 34-6 McKinnis, L.N. (2005). *Fundamentals of musculoskeletal imaging* (2nd ed., p. 76). Philadelphia: F.A. Davis.

APPENDICES ON ELECTRONIC STUDY GUIDE AND DAVISPLUS

The Pregnant Patient's Bill of Rights. With permission from Alliance for the Improvement of Maternity Services.

Clinical Position Statement: The Role of the Registered Nurse (RN) in the Care of Pregnant Women Receiving Analgesia/Anesthesia by Catheter Techniques (Epidural, Intrathecal, Spinal, Patient-Controlled Epidural Analgesia [PCEA] Catheters). With permission from Association of Women's Health, Obstetric and Neonatal Nurses.

Clinical Position Statement: The Role of the Nurse in the Promotion of Breastfeeding. With permission from Association of Women's Health, Obstetric and Neonatal Nurses.

Core Competencies for Health Professionals. With permission from National Coalition for Health Professional Education in Genetics.

Index

Note: Page numbers followed by f refer to figures; page numbers followed by t refer to tables; page numbers followed by b refer to boxes.

A

A & P (anatomy and physiology) review
  blood components, 1072–1073
  endocrine system, 887
  epidural space, 419–420, 419f
  fetal circulation, 604–605
  fetal lungs, 604
  fetal skull, 359, 361, 361b, 361f
  gastrointestinal system, 786
  heart, 854–856, 856f
  immune system, 820–821
  kidneys, 1034–1035, 1035f
  lactation-related breast changes, 473
  menstrual cycle, 125, 125f
  musculoskeletal system, 964
  nervous system, 922
  oogenesis, 117, 117f
  placental hormone, 194–195
  primary germ layers, 176
  respiratory function, 542
  respiratory system, 751
  skin, 996, 997f
  spermatogenesis, 132, 133f
  tumor progression, 1105
Abarelix, in infertility, 157t
Abdomen
  auscultation of, in child assessment, 679
  in child assessment, 679–680, 679f
  distention of, in neonate, 584
  examination of, in prenatal assessment, 236
  pain in. See Abdominal pain
  palpation of
    in child assessment, 680
    contraindication to, 1113
    in neonate, 583–584
  quadrants of, 679, 679f
  trauma to, 814, 815t
Abdominal pain
  in children, 787
  in constipation, 804
  in intussusception, 791, 791f
  in malrotation, 791–792
  during pregnancy, 279–280
ABO isoimmunization, 328
Abortion
  clinical, 153–154
    complications of, 145, 154
    dilation and evacuation for, 145
    elective, 153
    methotrexate for, 154
    mifepristone for, 154
    therapeutic, 153
    vacuum aspiration for, 153–154
  spontaneous, 280, 295–296
    alcohol use and, 261
    history of, 225
Abruptio placentae, 280, 299–300, 299b, 299f, 300b, 450, 452
Abscess, brain, 936, 937t
Absolute neutrophil count, 1090, 1126
Abstinence, 144, 246
Acceptance, in grieving, 1149
Accidents. See also Trauma
  in adolescent, 85
  in young children, 31
Acculturation, 66
Accutane, 275
Acetaminophen
  in fever, 684
  in otitis media, 768

Acetazolamide, with ventricular shunt, 943
Acetylsalicylic acid. See Aspirin
ACHES signs, 148
Achondroplasia, 586
Acidosis, 752t
  in acute renal failure, 1052t
  neonatal, 611, 612t
Acne, 1002–1006
  diagnosis of, 1002–1003
  neonatal, 575
  signs and symptoms of, 1002, 1002f
  treatment of, 1003–1004, 1004t–1005t
Acoustic stimulation, in fetal assessment, 342
Acquired immunodeficiency syndrome (AIDS). See Human immunodeficiency virus (HIV) infection
Acrocyanosis, in newborn, 393, 545
Acromegaly, 890–892
Across care settings. See Care settings
Acticoat, for burn wound, 1024
Acupressure
  in labor-related pain, 410
  in pregnancy-related nausea and vomiting, 297
Acupuncture, in labor-related pain, 410
Acute chest syndrome, in sickle-cell disease, 1072
Acute hemolytic transfusion reaction, 1097–1098
Acute lung injury, transfusion-related, 1097–1098
Acute lymphocytic leukemia, 1106, 1106f, 1107–1108, 1107t, 1109
Acute myelocytic/myelogenous leukemia, 1106, 1106f, 1108–1109
Acyclovir
  in chickenpox, 832t
  in herpes simplex virus infection, 627, 1009
Adam's position, 983, 984f
Adapalene, in acne, 1004t–1005t
Adaptive devices, in chronic conditions, 1135, 1135f
Addisonian crisis, 901
Addison's disease, 900–902
Adhesive, tissue, 998
Admission procedures, for childbirth, 369–372, 370t
Adnexa, 116, 117f
Adolescent. See also Children; Young adulthood
  accidents in, 85
  acne in, 1002–1006, 1002f, 1004t–1005t
  amenorrhea in, 1062–1063
  anorexia nervosa in, 84, 737–738
  bicycle safety for, 86
  bimanual pelvic palpation for, 89–90, 91f
  body piercing by, 87
  bone mineral density in, 151
  bulimia nervosa in, 84
  cervical cancer screening for, 89
  chronic condition in, 1138
  cognitive development of, 660
  communication with
    about acne, 1003
    about adolescent mother discharge, 506
    for decision-making, 660
    about discharge, 506
    about sex, 245
    about weight loss, 83–84

death perceptions of, 1142
definition of, 642
dental care for, 84
Depo-Provera effects in, 151
depression in, 723, 727t
  alcohol and, 717–718
  nursing care plan for, 724
  obesity and, 83
development of, 660–661
  concept map for, 663
  hospitalization and, 707t
  milestones in, 670t
  pregnancy and, 247
  tasks of, 80, 82, 82b
developmental disabilities in, 740–743
diabetes mellitus in, 64, 83
discipline for, 660–661
driving safety for, 85–86
eating and activity habits of, 71–72
eating disorders in, 84, 737–738
emotional development of, 660
firearm safety for, 86
gynecological examination for, 88–91, 88f, 89f, 91f
gynecomastia in, 659, 1065
health promotion for, 73, 87–91
health status of, 32
helmet use by, 86
HIV infection in, 825
homicide and, 85
human papillomavirus infection in, 90t, 1007–1008, 1007f
informed consent from, 660
insulin resistance in, 83
intimate partner violence in, 346–347
irritable bowel syndrome in, 792–793
learning disorders in, 743
menstrual disorders in, 91–92
moral development of, 660
mother's pregnancy and, 210
nutrition for, 71–72, 82–84, 249
obesity in, 83, 738–739
oral contraceptives for, 148
osteoporosis prevention for, 88
pain management for, 695t
Pap smear for, 89
pelvic examination for, 88–91, 88f, 89f, 91f
physical development of, 660
play for, 82t
posttraumatic stress disorder in, 722
pregnancy in, 243, 245–249
  assessment of, 248
  case study of, 450, 501
  complications with, 344
  cultural influences on, 246, 246b
  decline in, 215
  denial of, 247
  developmental impact of, 209, 247
  father and, 249
  infant bonding and, 500, 501
  labor and, 377
  nursing interventions for, 248–249, 377
  nutrition in, 249
  postpartum period after, 506–507
  prevention of, 243, 245–246, 245t
  risk for, 247
procedure preparation for, 686
rectovaginal palpation in, 90–91, 91f
reproductive health safety for, 86
risk-taking behavior by, 85

The Women's Health Companion to Maternal-Child Nursing Care

Optimizing Outcomes for Mothers, Children, & Families

The Women's Health Companion to Maternal-Child Nursing Care

Optimizing Outcomes for Mothers, Children, & Families

Shelton M. Hisley, PhD, RNC, WHNP-BC

Assistant Professor of Nursing (Retired)
University of North Carolina at Wilmington
Wilmington, North Carolina

 F.A. Davis Company · Philadelphia

F.A. Davis Company
1915 Arch Street
Philadelphia, PA 19103
www.fadavis.com

Printed in the United States of America

Last digit indicates print number: 10 9 8 7 6 5 4 3 2

Publisher: Lisa B. Deitch
Director of Content Development: Darlene D. Pedersen
Project Editor: Jamie Elfrank
Design & Illustration Coordinator: Carolyn O'Brien

As new scientific information becomes available through basic and clinical research, recommended treatments and drug therapies undergo changes. The author(s) and publisher have done everything possible to make this book accurate, up to date, and in accord with accepted standards at the time of publication. The author(s), editors, and publisher are not responsible for errors or omissions or for consequences from application of the book, and make no warranty, expressed or implied, in regard to the contents of the book. Any practice described in this book should be applied by the reader in accordance with professional standards of care used in regard to the unique circumstances that may apply in each situation. The reader is advised always to check product information (package inserts) for changes and new information regarding dose and contraindications before administering any drug. Caution is especially urged when using new or infrequently ordered drugs.

Library of Congress Cataloging-in-Publication Data
Hisley, Shelton M.
The women's health companion to maternal-child nursing care: optimizing outcomes for mothers, children, and families/Shelton M. Hisley.
  p. ; cm.
Includes bibliographical references and index.
ISBN-13: 978-0-8036-2814-4
1. Maternity nursing--Textbooks. I. Hisley, Shelton M. II. Title.
  [DNLM: 1. Maternal-Child Nursing--methods. 2. Cultural Diversity. 3. Evidence-Based Nursing--methods. 4. Holistic Nursing--methods. WY 157.3
  W263m 2009]
RG951.W37 2009
618.2'0231--dc22

                                        2008051815

Health Promotion Approach to the Women's Health Content

The broad directives set forth in the Healthy People 2010 national initiative are central in the development and delivery of contemporary medical and nursing education. Today's emphasis on health care has shifted from an illness-focused model to a preventive model grounded in the shared goals of health promotion, health protection, and preventive services for all individuals. Consistent with this model, nursing education today embraces a wellness-centered approach that emphasizes health promotion and maintenance. The women's health information offered in the *Women's Health Companion to* *Maternal-Child Nursing Care: Optimizing Outcomes for Mothers, Children, & Families* is framed in a health promotion context designed to appeal to nursing educators and students alike. Constructed to compliment and enhance the parent text *Maternal-Child Nursing Care: Optimizing Outcomes for Mothers, Children, & Families, the Women's Health Companion* is presented in a similar style with special features that parallel those found in the basic book and emphasize the nurse's role in health promotion and community-based care. This information is designed to allow students to increase their understanding about strategies for promoting women's health and enhance their expertise in caring for women of all ages in a variety of settings.

Table of Contents

Promoting Reproductive Health Through an Understanding of Sexually Transmitted Diseases   73

Promoting Reproductive Health Through an Understanding of Cervical Cytology Screening, Human Papillomavirus, and Cervical Cancer   90

Promoting Menopausal Health   113

Promoting Mental Health and Physical Safety Through an Understanding of Intimate Partner Violence

Shelton M. Hisley, PhD, RNC, WHNP-BC

 I Got Flowers Today

I got flowers today.
It wasn't my birthday or any other special day.
We had our first argument last night, and he said a lot of cruel things that really hurt me.
I know he is sorry and didn't mean the things he said.
Because he sent me flowers today.

I got flowers today.
It wasn't our anniversary or any other special day.
Last night he threw me into a wall and started to choke me.
It seemed like a nightmare.
I couldn't believe it was real.
I woke up this morning sore and bruised all over.
I know he must be sorry.
Because he sent me flowers today.

I got flowers today,
And it wasn't Mother's Day or any other special day.
Last night he beat me up again.
And it was much worse than all the other times.
If I leave him, what will I do?
What about money?
I'm afraid of him and scared to leave.
But I know he must be sorry.
Because he sent me flowers today.

I got flowers today.
Today was a very special day.
It was the day of my funeral.
Last night he finally killed me.
He beat me to death.
If only I had gathered enough courage and strength to leave him,
I would not have gotten flowers…today.

—Paulette Kelly

LEARNING TARGETS *At the completion of this chapter the student will be able to:*

◆ Define the term *intimate partner violence.*

◆ Describe the different types of intimate partner violence.

◆ Identify a national health goal related to intimate partner violence and discuss how nurses may be instrumental in helping the nation to achieve this goal.

◆ Discuss characteristics of the three phases typically included in a cycle of violence and describe how partners generally react during each phase.

◆ Explain how to conduct intimate partner violence screening and assessments.

◆ Describe the nurse's role in planning and providing care for victims of intimate partner violence.

Introduction

This chapter focuses on violence against women and the nurse's role in promoting mental health and physical safety for victims of intimate partner violence. Formerly termed *domestic violence* (DV), *intimate partner violence* (IPV) is considered a more modern term that recognizes that in contemporary society, intimate partners do not always share the same household. IPV is a significant public health problem that causes physical and emotional trauma for women, men, and children and leads to a myriad of health problems for the victims. Individuals who have been abused may be subjected to unnecessary diagnostic testing for various chronic problems that may be related to physical and emotional abuse. Although the physical manifestations of abuse may be treated by the health-care professional, it is incumbent upon the nurse to also address the underlying causes of the injuries and empower the victim with safety information and other appropriate resources (Krieger, 2008; Mahoney, 2006).

Nurses have long been at the forefront of research in the area of violence against women. Early investigations by Campbell (1986), Parker and McFarlane (1991), and McFarlane and colleagues (1991) helped to raise awareness about this significant public health problem (Williams, Brackley, Hibler, & Prater, 2008). Nurses who care for women and are advocates for the prevention of abuse are perfectly situated to screen patients and educate others on the importance of screening (Moran, 2008).

An important *Healthy People 2010* national goal clearly underscores the magnitude of intimate partner violence: *Reduce physical abuse directed at women by male partners to no more than 27 per 1,000 couples from a current baseline of 30 per 1,000 couples.* Nurses can be instrumental in helping the nation to achieve this goal by routinely assessing women and their families to identify those at risk, assisting with counseling or initiating referrals for professional care, and maintaining contact to ensure that appropriate follow-up mechanisms are in place (Family Violence Prevention Fund, 2008a; U.S. Department of Health and Human Services [USDHHS], 2000).

Definition, Incidence, and Impact on Individuals and Society

Intimate partner violence (IPV) is defined as physical, sexual, or psychological harm or social isolation perpetrated by a current or former partner (adult or adolescent), in an intimate or dating relationship. The violence can occur between members of heterosexual or homosexual couples and does not require sexual intimacy. The abuser's actions are intended to instill fear and to intimidate and control the victim (Davila, 2006; Family Violence Prevention Fund, 2008a; Stinson & Robinson, 2006; Ward & Wood, 2009; Yonaka, Yoder, Darrow, & Sherck, 2007).

Viewed as a potentially preventable public health problem, IPV affected more than 32 million individuals in the United States between 1993 and 2005. Around the world, at least one in every three women has been beaten, coerced into sex, or otherwise abused during her lifetime. Intimate partner violence is the most common form of violence directed against women, and according to the World Health Organization (WHO), one out of every six women has been a victim of IPV. In many situations, women are victimized more than once by the same partner. In this country, it is estimated that approximately 5.3 million women experience IPV each year, and women have a one in four chance of becoming a victim of IPV at some point during their lifetime. During 2001, more than half a million American women (588,490 women) were victims of nonfatal violence at the hands of an intimate partner. In 2005, IPV resulted in 1,510 deaths; of these deaths, 22% were males and 78% were females (Centers for Disease Control and Prevention [CDC], 2009; Moran, 2008; Tjaden & Thoennes, 2000a; WHO, 2005; Williams et al., 2008).

✸ *Nursing Insight*— *IPV: Appreciating the scope of the problem*

In 2007, the Bureau of Justice Statistics of the U.S. Department of Justice published "Intimate Partner Violence in the United States," a report that showed that, sadly, statistics on IPV have not changed much over the past few years. "Domestic homicides against women rose from 1,155 murders in 2004 to 1,181 in 2005. That means that, on average, in 2005 more than three women a day were murdered by their husbands or boyfriends in the United States" (Family Violence Prevention Fund, 2007). Findings from a study conducted by the CDC (2003) showed that there are approximately 2 million injuries to women from IPV each year, and nearly one in four women report experiencing violence by a current or former spouse or boyfriend during some time in her life (Family Violence Prevention Fund, 2008b).

A man with a history of violence often brings violence into the family. The abuser's expressions of violent behavior usually erupt early in the courtship and grow progressively worse. Violence is used to handle conflicts, and the abuser exerts power to elicit a pervasive feeling of powerlessness in those around him. Male abusers frequently have a history of early and prolonged exposure to family violence as children, and alcohol is often associated with the violent behavior (Blereau, 2009; Bull, 2009; Krieger, 2008).

According to the U.S. Department of Justice (2007), female victims are substantially more likely than male victims to be killed by an intimate partner. In fact, male abusers kill their female partners four times more often than female abusers kill males involved in IPV. From 1976 to 2004, most homicides involved spouses, although in recent years the number of deaths by boyfriends and girlfriends has increased. More than two-thirds of spouse and ex-spouse victims of IPV were killed by firearms between 1976 and 2004. Interestingly, during this time period, female abusers were more likely to kill their partners with knives than were any other group of intimates (Krieger, 2008; Rennison, 2003).

Intimate partner violence reaches across all strata of society and affects persons regardless of economic status, ethnic background, educational level, or religious status. The economic toll of the violence is substantial. It is estimated that the costs of IPV, physical assault, and stalking exceed $5.8 billion per year. Of this amount, $4.1 billion is directly related to physical and mental health services (CDC, 2003; Moran, 2008; Tjaden & Thoennes, 2000a; U.S. Department of Justice, 2007; Ward & Wood, 2009; Yonaka et al, 2007). Individuals affected by IPV experience a productivity loss of 8 million days of paid work (the equivalent of 32,000 full-time jobs) and approximately 5.6 million days of unpaid household work each year (CDC, 2003).

Ethnocultural Considerations— *Intimate partner violence*

According to Tjaden and Thoennes (2000b), in the United States, the groups found to have the highest prevalence of IPV are American Indian and Alaskan Native women and men, African American women, and Hispanic women. Glass (2005) reported that Latinas are known to under-use traditional intervention services such as domestic violence shelters, health-care services, and law enforcement agencies because of a lack of health insurance, language and cultural barriers, and a general distrust of formal systems. Caucasian women report less IPV than do non-Caucasians, and Asian women report significantly less IPV than do other racial groups. Peedicayil and colleagues (2004) conducted a study of 9,938 women in India and reported a 13% prevalence rate of moderate to severe violence—including slapping, beating, kicking, and use of a weapon—during pregnancy. It is important for nurses to remember that violence may be underreported as a result of cultural norms. Although cultures may differ in their perceptions and definitions of abuse, the act of inflicting harm to another is against the law.

Those who perpetrate the abuse may refuse to allow their victims to work or attend school. Women who are abused are more likely to be unemployed, suffer from health problems, and receive public assistance than are women who are not victims of abuse. Those with severe and persistent mental illness are more likely to be involved in controlling and violent relationships. In the workplace, an additional burden is frequently placed on coworkers to compensate for the IPV victim's repeated absenteeism. Another indicator of the substantial economic burden of abuse is reflected in the millions of tax dollars channeled into supporting programs created to assist IPV victims (Krieger, 2008; Moracco et al., 2004).

Nursing Insight— *Accuracy issues with reported IPV statistics*

Accuracy in regard to IPV statistics is difficult to determine. It is estimated that only 20% to 50% of the assaults are actually reported to the police (National Domestic Violence Hotline, 2008). According to Tjaden and Thoennes (2000a), only 25% of all physical assaults against women, and fewer assaults against men, are reported to police. Coker and colleagues (2002) estimated that 29% of all women and 22% of all men will experience physical, sexual, or psychological abuse at some point in their lifetime. Victims of abuse may be reluctant to report personal violence because of fear or embarrassment or because those from whom they sought help did not directly ask about abuse.

According to Johnson and Leone (2005), victims of repeated violence over time sustain more serious injuries than do victims of one-time abuse incidents. Young women and economically challenged individuals are affected more often by IPV than any other population (Heise & Garcia-Moreno, 2002). Economic hardship is known to exacerbate IPV. Financial stress may lead to more frequent and violent abuse: Out-of-work husbands and boyfriends spend more time at home and thus have more opportunities to abuse their partners, and women are less likely to leave abusive situations for fear that they will not be able to support themselves (Blereau, 2009; Johnson & Leone, 2005).

Approximately 50% of children living in homes of intimate partner violence are also victimized. Children living in households affected by maternal abuse are 57 times more likely to suffer personal harm and are at greater risk for psychiatric disorders, developmental problems, school failure, violence against others, and low self-esteem. Those who perpetrate IPV create instability within their families while causing untold physical and psychological damage (Bull, 2009; Krieger, 2008; Parkinson, Adams, & Emerling, 2001).

Nursing Insight— *Recognizing social factors in violent behavior*

Violent behavior in intimate relationships is often rooted in multiple social factors. For example, the perpetrators and victims of family violence may learn about violent behavior by either witnessing or experiencing it firsthand. Other social factors include poverty and oppression, low income, unemployment, difficulty in maintaining interpersonal ties, marital instability and disruption, and single-parent families (Hamolia, 2005).

The CDC National Center for Injury Prevention and Control (2003) and other researchers list multiple factors that place an individual at risk for committing intimate partner abuse and for being a victim of intimate partner abuse (Tables 1-1 and 1-2).

 Now Can You— Discuss certain facts about IPV?

1. Define the term *intimate partner violence*?
2. Identify a national goal related to IPV and discuss how nurses can be instrumental in helping the nation to achieve this goal?
3. Explain why it is difficult to obtain accurate statistics about the prevalence of IPV?
4. List 10 risk factors for committing IPV and 10 risk factors for being a victim of IPV?

Types of Abuse

Abuse may occur in many forms, and victims may be repeatedly subjected to more than one type of abuse. Physical abuse is only one manifestation of intimate partner violence. Other types of abuse include sexual abuse, mental (emotional) abuse, social abuse, and economic abuse.

PHYSICAL ABUSE

Physical abuse may include spitting, kicking, punching, grabbing, slapping, or strangulation. The abused woman may be seen in the health clinic, doctor's office, or emergency department with vague, chronic, nonspecific complaints, and often there is a history of overuse of health services or unexplainable injuries such as bruises and fractures. Nurses should be alert to the patient's chronic issues as possible symptoms of abuse. For example, the woman may seek treatment for headaches, anxiety, stress, insomnia, or fatigue. The IPV victim's appearance may vary: She may be disheveled, dirty, and distressed or neat, well groomed, and calm. Oftentimes, abused women are

Table 1-2 Risk Factors for Being a Victim of Intimate Partner Violence

Individual Factors	Relationship Factors
History of child abuse	Marital conflict
History of physical abuse	Marital instability
History of sexual abuse	Male dominance in the family
Prior injury from the same partner	Poor family functioning
Having a verbally abusive partner	Partner history of alcohol or drug abuse
Economic stress, low income	
Tobacco, alcohol, and illicit drug use	
Depression or suicide attempts	
History of sexually transmitted infections	
Young age (less than 24 years, especially adolescents)	
Lack of high school diploma	
Unplanned pregnancies (often as a result of birth control sabotage)	

subjected to unnecessary diagnostic testing to determine the cause of the chronic conditions (Krieger, 2008; Mahoney, 2006; Ward & Wood, 2009).

 Optimizing Outcomes— Recognizing signs of intimate partner violence

By recognizing signs of IPV, nurses can be instrumental in helping to make an accurate diagnosis and in securing appropriate assistance for the abused woman. Specifically, the nurse should remain alert to the following indicators, which may be signs of IPV:

- Overuse of health services
- Vague, nonspecific complaints
- Repeated missed appointments
- Unexplained injuries
- Untreated serious injuries
- Significant delay between the injury and the presentation for care
- Injuries that do not match the patient's description of how they were incurred
- Evidence or a history of previous injuries
- Bilateral or multiple injuries in various stages of healing
- Intimate partner who refuses to leave the patient's side
- Intimate partner who insists on explaining how the injury was incurred (Blereau, 2009; Krieger, 2008)

Certain behavioral clues may point to abuse. For example, the intimate partner may refuse to leave the victim during the interview and physical assessment. The abuser may display extreme attentiveness toward the victim and attempt to describe to the care provider exactly how the injuries were sustained. The abuser may hover,

Table 1-1 Risk Factors for Committing Intimate Partner Violence

Individual Factors	Relationship Factors
Young age	Marital conflict
Low self-esteem	Marital instability
Low income	Male dominance in the family
Low academic achievement	Poor family functioning
Aggressive or delinquent behavior as a child	Emotional dependence and insecurity
Alcohol or drug use	Belief in strict gender roles
Witnessing or experiencing childhood violence	Desire for power and control in relationships
Social isolation	Angry or hostile behavior toward a partner
Unemployment	

dominate, and control the information given. The abuser may refuse to allow the victim to share private time with the health professional. The information about the circumstances surrounding the injury may not match the actual injuries. Frequently, victims suffer repeated injuries and delay medical treatment for serious injuries. Research conducted by Crandall and associates (2004) revealed that 93% of female IPV victims had made at least one previous injury visit to a health-care facility, and 44% of women murdered during an IPV episode had visited an emergency department within 2 years of being murdered (Krieger, 2008; Ward & Wood, 2009).

 Optimizing Outcomes— Recognizing physical patterns of IPV injury

Nurses should be aware that physical injuries inflicted during intimate partner violence are likely to appear in a central pattern on the face, chest, breasts, abdomen, and neck. The patient may complain of abdominal pain upon palpation, chest pain related to rib trauma, or musculoskeletal pain accompanied by redness and swelling. Bruises may be noted on the inner aspect of the arms and/or legs, along with injuries suggestive of a defensive-type posture, such as an injury to the ulnar aspect of the forearm (Ward & Wood, 2009).

Intimate partner violence frequently results in head, neck, and facial injuries. It is estimated that up to 90% of abused victims sustain head and neck injuries, and IPV is believed to account for between 34% and 73% of all facial injuries in women (Blereau, 2009).

Arosena and colleagues (2009) discovered that specific patterns of facial injury are more likely to be associated with IPV than with other sources of injury, such as motor vehicle crashes or even with assault by a stranger. The researchers reviewed the medical and dental records of 326 women with facial trauma treated by specialists at a university hospital. Their findings revealed that injuries around the eye or upper face were more likely to be associated with IPV, while mandible fractures were more likely to be caused by assault by an unknown assailant. Victims of IPV more often sustained zygomatic complex fractures, orbital blow-out fractures, and intracranial injuries than did other patients with facial trauma (Arosarena, Fritsch, Hsueh, Aynehchi, & Haug, 2009; Blereau, 2009).

 Nursing Insight— *IPV and patterns of facial trauma*

A woman's face is the most meaningful area on her person. According to an otolaryngologist who has extensively studied injuries inflicted during IPV, the pattern of facial trauma sustained is reflective of this fact. Thus, hitting in the face figures prominently in IPV. This particular pattern may be contrasted with that typically seen in the assault of a robber, for example, whose ultimate goal is primarily to disable the victim (Blereau, 2009; Lite, 2009).

Women who are strangled during IPV may or may not demonstrate physical evidence of an injury to the neck. Strack and McClane (1999) reported that visible evidence

such as red marks, scratches, scrapes, bruises, or rope burns may be apparent in only 15% of strangulation cases. Nurses should be alert to patient complaints such as persistent throat pain, voice changes, or difficulty swallowing, which may be indicators of neck trauma sustained during an act of violence. Chin abrasions may be present—as the victim lowers the chin in an instinctive effort to protect the neck, the skin is scraped against the abuser's hands. Victims of strangulation attempts should be evaluated for possible damage (e.g., fracture) to the hyoid bone, a small horseshoe-shaped bone in the neck that supports the tongue. Although breathing difficulty may initially appear to be mild, damage to the hyoid bone or other underlying structures may result in fatal asphyxiation up to 36 or more hours after the assault (Krieger, 2008; Strack & McClane, 1999).

 Nursing Insight— *Recognizing the unique problems of older women subjected to IPV*

Women of all ages are at risk for IPV. When trying to leave an abuser, older women may face challenges such as feelings of shame and worries about money. However, abused women who are 55 years and older are confronted with still another challenge. Having grown up and gotten married during a time when IPV was often ignored, older women have suffered many years of abuse and, like other victims of IPV, frequently have problems with poor self-image and guilt. Older women who have been abused are also less likely to confide in anyone about the abuse, they may have health problems that keep them dependent on their abusive partner, feel committed to caring for their abusive and aging partners, and are fearful of being alone (American College of Obstetricians and Gynecologists [ACOG], 2008; USDHHS, 2009).

 Now Can You— Discuss physical injury associated with IPV?

1. Identify eight clinical red flags that may be indicative of IPV?
2. Describe behavioral characteristics of the abuser that may be indicative of IPV?
3. Explain what is meant by a "central pattern" of injury and why this is often observed in victims of IPV?

SEXUAL ABUSE

Sexual abuse may include the abuser's use of force to carry out sexual intercourse or other sexual activities against the victim's will. It may include forced participation in an early initiation of sexual activity; forced participation in sexual activity viewed to be humiliating or degrading; decreased condom use or otherwise unprotected sexual intercourse; having multiple sexual partners; and trading sex for food, money, drugs, or other items. Sexual abuse may increase the likelihood of exposure to sexually transmitted diseases (STDs), including HIV and AIDS. Recurrent vaginal infections and/or an unusually high number of STDs or frequent miscarriages can be warning signs of sexual abuse. Interestingly, sexual assaults committed by strangers are more likely to be reported than are rapes and sexual assaults committed by an intimate partner (CDC, 2003;

Family Violence Prevention Fund, 2008b; Krieger, 2008; Rennison, 2003; Ward & Wood, 2009).

Another manifestation of sexual abuse involves forcing undesired pregnancy or forcing pregnancies to rapidly occur after one another. Pregnancy constitutes an especially dangerous time for abused women. Physical violence during pregnancy has far-reaching effects for the infant as well as the mother. Battery during pregnancy is associated with a greater incidence of low-birth-weight neonates, preterm birth, and neonatal death. According to the Family Violence Prevention Fund (2008b), IPV accounts for 31% of the homicides among pregnant women and is the leading cause of traumatic death for pregnant and postpartum women in the United States (Krieger, 2008; Yost, Bloom, McIntire, & Leveno, 2005).

 ### Nursing Insight— *Maternal intimate partner violence: The sobering statistics*

Women who experience abuse in the year prior to and/or during a recent pregnancy are 40% to 60% more likely than nonabused women to suffer from high blood pressure, vaginal bleeding, severe nausea, and kidney or urinary tract infections during pregnancy. They are also more likely to require hospitalization during pregnancy and are 37% more likely to give birth to preterm infants. Neonates born to abused mothers are 17% more likely to be underweight at birth and are 30% more likely than other infants to require neonatal intensive care (Silverman, Decker, Reed, & Raj, 2006).

MENTAL (EMOTIONAL) ABUSE

Mental or emotional abuse includes acts such as coercion, making threats, and stalking. The abuser may verbally abuse the victim with criticism, insults, put-downs, or name calling. The perpetrator may use facial expressions or gestures to intimidate and instill fear. Other forms of emotional abuse include the perpetrator's use of threats of harm to children, family members, or pets. Not uncommonly, abusers destroy the victim's property, abuse their pets, or display weapons to force the victim into submission. The abuser may mislead children into viewing the victim as having "earned" the abuse by causing the perpetrator to become angry—in this situation, the children often blame the victim for the resulting violence. The perpetrator frequently places the blame on the victim—denying fault and instead claiming that any physical injury resulted from the victim's "clumsiness." Often, the victim's injuries are minimized and the abuser creates excuses for the abusive behavior. The perpetrator may also attempt to convince others that the victim is incompetent or guilty of fabrication and not to be believed or taken seriously (Krieger, 2008).

 Now Can You— Discuss aspects of sexual and mental abuse?

1. Identify four examples of sexual abuse?
2. Describe maternal and neonatal problems that may stem from abuse during pregnancy?
3. Identify three characteristics of mental abuse?

SOCIAL ABUSE

Social abuse may include the abuser isolating or limiting the victim's contact and time spent with family and friends; the abuser may also require the victim to obtain permission to leave the house. The victim may be forbidden from seeking outside employment or from attending school. The perpetrator may conduct "odometer checks" on the victim's car to confirm that the victim has not left home and in some situations, the victim is required to provide a detailed account of any time spent away from the abuser. The victim may be denied access to medical services. The abuser may prevent the victim from keeping medical or other appointments, thereby creating strain on relationships with health-care providers, employers, friends, and family members (Krieger, 2008; Plichta, 2004).

The abuser may harm the victim's reputation and intimidate the victim's family and friends. Not infrequently, a breakdown in the victim's interpersonal relationships occurs, removing an important source of emotional support for the victim. Social abuse may include the perpetrator stalking the victim. According to the CDC (2003), 1 million women and 371,000 men are stalked by IPV abusers. It has been estimated that only 50% of stalking activity against women is actually reported to the police. Stalking constitutes a serious threat, and the victim should be encouraged to report this behavior to the police (CDC, 2003; Krieger, 2008; Tjaden & Thoennes, 2002a).

ECONOMIC ABUSE

Economic abuse may include the abuser's controlling all aspects of the victim's finances, refusing to share money, forcing the victim to account for any money spent, and forbidding the victim from working outside of the home. For the perpetrator, these actions help to bring about the victim's emotional and financial dependency on the abuser. The abuser may force the victim to repeatedly miss work, place frequent telephone calls to the victim at the workplace, or show up at the workplace unannounced in an attempt to jeopardize the victim's work ethic and job security. According to the American Bar Association (2008), 70% of IPV victims are employed, and greater than 70% of them admit that their abusers harass them at work, either over the telephone or in person. Also, abusers cause more than 60% of their victims to be late or absent from work or both (American Bar Association, 2008; Krieger, 2008).

 ### Nursing Insight— *Use of the power and control wheel to enhance understanding*

The Power and Control Wheel (Figure 1-1) was developed by battered women in Duluth, Minnesota. The women, all victims of IPV, were attending women's education groups sponsored by the women's shelter. The Power and Control Wheel is meant to graphically illustrate the scope of men's abusive behaviors toward women.

The Equality Wheel (Figure 1-2), also developed by the Minnesota Domestic Abuse Intervention Project, was created to describe the changes needed for men who batter to move from being abusive to being part of a nonviolent partnership. Used together, the wheels provide a mechanism for identifying and exploring abuse and then making behavioral changes toward nonviolent behavior.

Figure 1-1 The Power and Control Wheel: A model of power and control issues that perpetuate battering. (Developed by the Duluth Domestic Abuse Intervention Project, Duluth, Minnesota.)

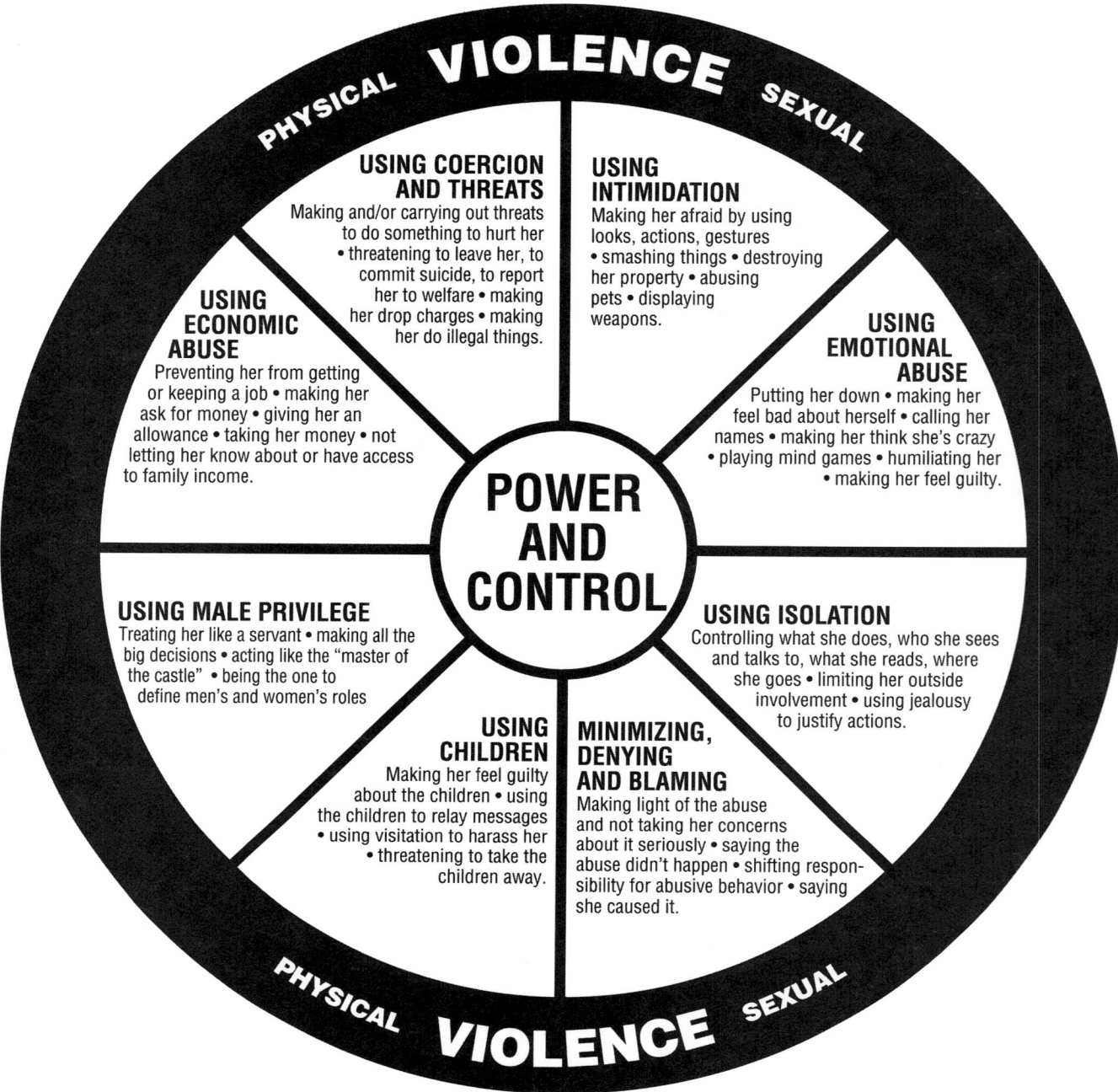

DOMESTIC ABUSE INTERVENTION PROJECT

202 East Superior Street
Duluth, Minnesota 55802
218-722-2781
www.duluth-model.org

Figure 1-2 The Equality Wheel: May be used in concert with the Power and Control Wheel to help individuals see alternate ways of being in relationships with women that are free of violence and controlling behavior. (Developed by the Duluth Domestic Abuse Intervention Project, Duluth, Minnesota.)

Optimizing Outcomes— Recognizing vulnerable victims of abuse

Nurses should be aware that certain vulnerable individuals might be more likely to be affected by IPV. Women with disabilities are vulnerable to physical, sexual, and mental abuse, neglect, and exploitation. The abuse may include withholding necessary assistive devices, care, or treatment. Immigrant and refugee women are at risk for violence and abuse because of isolation and manipulation by their partners, language and cultural differences, and a prevailing lack of awareness of their rights and legal and social resources (ACOG, 2007).

Now Can You— Discuss aspects of social and economic abuse?

1. Describe three characteristics of social abuse?
2. Describe three characteristics of economic abuse?
3. Explain how the Power and Control Wheel and the Equality Wheel may be used to enhance understanding about male-directed abusive behavior toward women and offer behavioral strategies for the transition into a nonviolent, noncontrolling relationship?

Phases of Abuse

Three phases of abuse have been identified: (1) tension building; (2) acute violence; and (3) a tranquil, loving period of calm and remorse, sometimes termed the "honeymoon period." Although not all abusive relationships follow this cycle, many victims can readily recognize this pattern (Walker, 1979, 1984).

TENSION-BUILDING PHASE

The first phase is characterized as a period of increasing tension. During this time, the abuser demonstrates hostility and anger without culminating into violent outbursts. The victim senses the escalating behavior and attempts to placate the abuser. In many situations, the victim's behavior postpones rather than prevents the abuse. At some point, the victim realizes that she cannot control the violent behavior and withdraws to cope. This action only heightens the abuser's anger (Krieger, 2008; Walker, 1979, 1984).

VIOLENCE PHASE

In the second phase, the abuser discharges the pent-up tension. This phase may be triggered by an internal response in the abuser or by an external crisis. Over a period of hours or days, the abuser may engage in a number of violent acts, such as biting, slapping, punching, stomping, choking, pushing, burning, or mutilation. Most injuries are directed at the face, neck, chest, breasts, buttocks, and abdomen; the hands and forearms are often damaged as the victim attempts to protect herself. The abuser often makes the victim feel that she has angered the abuser and thus is responsible for the abuse. Frequently, the woman minimizes the extent of injury and is reluctant to seek medical care (Krieger, 2008; Walker, 1979, 1984).

THE HONEYMOON PHASE

During the third phase, the abuser feels remorse and apologizes profusely. He promises that the abuse will never happen again and may even believe that it will not. The abuser showers his victim with love and kindness, lulling her into forgiveness and a desire to continue the relationship. The victim desperately wants to believe her abuser and is renewed in her hope that he really will change. This phase provides the positive reinforcement for remaining in the relationship. The victim denies the reality that the abuse will recur. Unless there is some intervention at this point, this phase will end and the cycle of violence will be repeated (Krieger, 2008; Varcolis, Carson, & Shoemaker, 2006; Walker, 1979, 1984).

VICTIMS' REACTIONS TO THE PHASES OF ABUSE

Victims react in various ways to each of the three phases of abuse. During the first, or tension-building, phase, the woman uses denial as a defense mechanism. If the relationship is not terminated at this point, the abuse continues to escalate in frequency and violence, and the victim indirectly "gives permission" for the abuse to continue. During the second (violence) phase, the woman can no longer deny that the violence is occurring. Unfortunately, she is unable to stop the violence because she is fearful of provoking further violence. She resorts to the use of various coping mechanisms such as dutiful obedience and cooperation as she conforms to the abuser's wishes in a desperate effort to reduce the violence. This behavior has been termed "learned helplessness." Not surprisingly, the victim feels hopeless, powerless, and depressed and may have difficulty seeking help at this point because she is immobilized by a sense of guilt and does not believe that others may wish to help her.

 Nursing Insight— *Gaining an understanding of the IPV victims' behavior/recovery phases*

Kearney's (2001) seminal research was designed to gain insight into why IPV victims remain with or return to their abusers. Four phases of IPV victim recovery were identified:
Enduring love/relationship obligation: Characterized by a desire to love/be loved; belief that the relationship is "forever"; fearfulness of disclosure to family and friends; personal feelings of shame and guilt and self-blame for the abuse
The more I do, the worse I am: Characterized by attempts to meet the abuser's needs despite the fact that the abuse now occurs routinely; feelings of self-doubt, loss of personal identity; displaying of harmful behaviors (e.g., substance abuse, alcoholism, suicide attempts) to cope with the emotional strain or coping behaviors (e.g., extreme dieting or overeating) to gain some semblance of control over their lives (CDC, 2003)
I've had enough: Characterized by the realization that the relationship is abusive and will not be tolerated, but fear of the unknown and a lack of information about how to seek safe shelter—this point in the relationship is an opportune time for nurses to advocate for victims by providing support, education, and information about community resources

I was finding me: Characterized by the ability to live a life separate from the abuser; may need tools (e.g., economic resources) to remain independent; requires continued support and encouragement; ongoing self-discovery/recovery; moving from the role of "victim" to one of "survivor"

 Now Can You— **Discuss the phases of abuse?**

1. Identify the three phases of abuse and describe characteristics of each phase?
2. Explain how victims often react to each of the three phases of abuse?
3. Describe how Kearney's (2001) research provides insights into IPV victims' behavior and how this information is useful to nurses?

Intimate Partner Violence Screening, Documenting, and Reporting

SCREENING FOR IPV

In 2000, the American Nurses Association (ANA) published a position statement on violence against women. This important document advocates universal screening, routine assessment, and documentation of abuse for all victims in any health-care setting. Universal screening means that *all* patients are assessed for IPV, regardless of the presence or absence of any abuse indicators. Routine screening can facilitate early identification of IPV when signs and symptoms may not be readily apparent and timely referral for appropriate services that may prevent further injury (Ward & Wood, 2009; Wilson, Lane, & Gillespie, 2006). If the screening tool suggests that the patient may be at high risk for abuse, a more detailed assessment should be performed (Krieger, 2008).

 Nursing Insight— *Recognizing potential barriers to IPV screening*

Nurses must be aware of potential barriers to routine IPV screening in the clinical setting. Time constraints, a lack of awareness of IPV, a lack of instructions on how to inquire about abuse, language and cultural differences, and a practitioner's personal history of abuse are factors that may prevent health-care professionals from performing routine IPV screening (Yonaka et al., 2007). Chang and colleagues (2003) explored positive and negative consequences of IPV screening. Positive consequences included the following: a feeling that the practitioners cared, growing awareness that IPV is a problem, and a reduction in the victims' sense of social isolation. Negative consequences included feelings of being judged and being intruded upon, increasing anxiety, and disappointment in the practitioner's response (Williams et al., 2008).

In 2004, the U.S. Preventive Services Task Force (USPSTF) found insufficient evidence to recommend for or against routine screening of women for IPV. The Task Force noted that the potential harms (e.g., anxiety, fear of being stigmatized) of screening for IPV need to be documented in more rigorous studies. In addition, the USPSTF reported that no studies have determined the validity

 where research and practice meet: **Routine Screening for IPV**

Williams and colleagues (2008) conducted a pilot study designed to assess the IPV screening practices of advanced practice nurses and physicians. The participants completed a survey about routine IPV screening of female patients and whether they had received IPV-related education. Based on the findings, the researchers suggested that professional educational programs routinely include content on IPV screening, beliefs, practices, and barriers to screening and concluded that despite the USPSTF position against routine screening, practitioners should routinely screen for IPV to err on the side of patient safety.

---

of the screening tools designed to identify IPV. Although current evidence to support routine screening is insufficient, health-care settings may still provide a unique opportunity for IPV victims to confide in their care providers and to seek help. Despite a lack of confirmed efficacy, national consensus guidelines still recommend routine screening (Family Violence Prevention Fund, 2008b; Klevens & Saltzman, 2009; Williams et al., 2008).

" What to say " — *Conducting the IPV interview*

After ensuring privacy, the nurse should maintain eye contact and begin with a statement such as "In this office, a part of our routine care is to ask about intimate partner violence." Then, proceed with open-ended questions such as, "How are things at home? Do you feel safe at home? Do you feel safe in your community?" If injuries are present, it is important to acknowledge them and ask how they occurred. If the patient's responses do not seem to match the mechanism of the injury, voice concern about the inconsistency, but don't push for details. Always promote trust and convey caring and let the patient know that violence is wrong and that no one deserves to be hurt. Demonstrating a nonjudgmental attitude and creating trust is an essential strategy in facilitating the patient's disclosure of abuse, especially in a busy clinical setting. Research suggests that IPV screening does not necessarily add significant time to a patient visit (Bull, 2009; Du Plat-Jones, 2006; Rhodes et al., 2007; Ward & Wood, 2009).

Once a patient discloses abuse, the nurse should facilitate an assessment to determine urgent safety needs and to guide the plan of care. If the patient is in immediate danger, an assessment for suicide and/or homicide may be indicated as well (Ward & Wood, 2009).

 Nursing Insight— *Finding the right words to facilitate understanding and disclosure of abuse*

Patients may not always use the word *abuse* when describing their intimate relationships. It is important to be aware of words that suggest that abuse is occurring. For example, the patient may confide that her partner "has a temper" or "gets angry easily." Using the same terms expressed by the patient may enhance her comfort in confiding about the full extent of the abuse (Krieger, 2008; Valente, 2002).

Across Care Settings: Community resources share in supporting the victim of IPV

When IPV is identified, nurses and other health-care professionals share the responsibility of offering referrals to confidential victim and social support resources within the community. Referrals should be made regardless of whether the woman chooses to report the abuse to law enforcement. In the ideal situation, all health-care providers should be a part of a coordinated community response to reduce domestic violence, a response in which shelters, hospitals, health-care providers, legal advocates, and law enforcement work together to improve safety and save lives (Association of Women's Health, Obstetric, and Neonatal Nurses, 2007; Krieger, 2008).

A number of screening tools have been developed to assess for intimate partner violence. These include the Woman Abuse Screening Tool (WAST) (Brown, Lent, Schmidt, & Sas, 2000), Abuse Risk Inventory, Conflict Tactics Scale (Yegadis, 1989), and the Danger Assessment Scale (Campbell, 1989). The Abuse Assessment Screen (Family Violence Prevention Fund, 2004) is a brief, easy-to-use validated tool that contains five simple questions along with a body map to provide visual reference for physical injury (see Figure 1-3). If the woman has disclosed IPV, the nurse must document that a risk assessment was completed (Family Violence Prevention Fund, 2004; Ward & Wood, 2009).

DOCUMENTING IPV

Accurate documentation is essential, as it provides a record of the abuse, facilitates communication among the various professionals who are dealing with the case, and provides a record of previous episodes of abuse. Since documentation provides evidence of abuse escalation, it can be beneficial in helping the patient to recognize and acknowledge the abuse (Ward & Wood, 2009).

 Be sure to— Obtain patient consent before IPV information disclosure

Nurses are aware that careful documentation of IPV-related information is essential in supporting the victim's assertions and charges. Proper documentation enables the woman to obtain protection and assistance, which may range from obtaining a restraining order to receiving victim compensation. However, nurses must remember that disclosure of confidential information may take place only with the explicit consent of the patient (Griffith, 2008; Rhodes et al., 2007; Ward & Woods, 2009).

In addition to obtaining the past health history, social history, and sexual history, the nurse documents subjective data related to the current IPV incident. Information recorded includes a description of the incident in the patient's own words. If the victim names the abuser, the name should be documented as well. All subjective information provided by the patient is recorded in quotation marks to indicate that the statements represent exactly what the patient said. It is important to record

the time that the patient reports that the incident occurred, as well as the time that the patient's descriptive statements were made. The nurse also notes the date and location of the incident (Family Violence Prevention Fund, 2004; Ward & Wood, 2009).

The patient's general appearance and demeanor is recorded, and additional subjective information, such as reported threats and psychological abuse perpetrated by the abuser, is documented as well. Findings from the physical examination are carefully documented. Body maps are useful in accurately pinpointing the areas of injury, including the location, size, and age. Once the patient's signed consent has been obtained, photographs may be taken. Photographs provide an excellent visual record of the injuries. Additional information including the results of laboratory and diagnostic tests, radiography, and all referrals (e.g., other health-care professionals, local shelters) are recorded on the patient's health record (Ward & Wood, 2009).

 Optimizing Outcomes— With photographs of the injuries

A minimum of three photographs should be taken of each injury: a full body photograph of the victim to establish identity, an injury photo taken a medium distance from the body, and a close-up photo of each individual injury. All photographs are clearly labeled with the patient's name, date, time that they were taken, and the photographer's name. Ideally, a blue background, which shows the depth and defines the clarity of an injury, is used. Additional photographs can be taken at the follow-up visit (2 to 4 days) to provide additional documentation of the progression of the injuries (Family Violence Prevention Fund, 2004; Hamme, Moynihan, & Pagliaro, 2005; Pyrek, 2006; Ward & Wood, 2009).

REPORTING IPV

It is important for nurses to be knowledgeable about IPV reporting guidelines for their particular practice state. Proponents of mandatory IPV reporting describe the following benefits associated with mandatory IPV reporting:

Facilitates the prosecution of perpetrators
Helps to identify victims; promotes interventions
Improves data collection (Lewis-O'Connor, 2004; Ward & Wood, 2009)

 Be sure to— Be knowledgeable of state law regarding reporting of IPV

Nurses must be familiar with laws on the mandatory reporting of IPV; requirements vary from state to state. Currently, six states (California, Kentucky, New Mexico, Rhode Island, New Hampshire, and Colorado) have laws requiring comprehensive reporting of IPV obtained by either victim disclosure or suspicion of IPV. A synopsis of current state statutes and reporting guidelines is available at http://www.endabuse.org/userfiles/file/Consensus.pdf. The Association of Women's Health, Obstetric and Neonatal Nurses

1) Have you ever been emotionally or physically abused by your partner or someone important to you?

    Yes ☐   No ☐

    If yes by whom? _____

    Total number of times _____

2) Within the last year, have you been hit, slapped, kicked or otherwise physically hurt by someone?

    Yes ☐   No ☐

    If yes by whom? _____

    Total number of times _____

3) Since you've been pregnant, have you been hit, slapped, kicked, or otherwise physically hurt by someone?

    Yes ☐   No ☐

    If yes by whom? _____

    Total number of times _____

4. Within the last year, has anyone forced you to have sexual activities?

    Yes ☐   No ☐

    If yes by whom? _____

    Total number of times _____

5. Are you afraid of your partner or anyone you listed above?

    Yes ☐   No ☐

MARK THE AREA OF INJURY ON A BODY MAP AND SCORE EACH INCIDENT ACCORDING TO THE FOLLOWING SCALE.

If any of the descriptions for the higher number apply, use the higher number.

1 = Threats of abuse including use of a weapon
2 = Slapping, pushing; no injuries and/or lasting pain
3 = Punching, kicking, bruises, cuts, and/or continuing pain
4 = Beating up, severe contusions, burns, broken bones
5 = Head injury, internal injury, permanent injury
6 = Use of weapon; wound from weapon

Figure 1-3 Abuse Assessment Screen. (Produced by the Family Violence Prevention Fund, 383 Rhode Island St., Ste. 304, San Francisco, CA, 94103-5133, (415) 252-8900, TTY: (800) 595-4889, www.endabuse.org.)

(AWHONN) supports health-care professionals reporting IPV with the informed consent of the abused woman. However, the organization recognizes that health-care providers must abide by state law (AWHONN, 2007).

However, it must be pointed out that mandatory reporting violates the framework on which the ethical codes of nursing are based. The ANA Code of Ethics for Nurses, provision 3, states, "the nurse promotes, advocates for, and strives to protect the health, safety, and rights of the patient" (ANA, 2005). Mandatory reporting of IPV may place victims in danger and violates the victim's right to make personal choices. Furthermore, mandatory reporting laws place the responsibility of the victim's safety on health-care professionals, who, in turn, must rely on law enforcement and the courts to provide safety for the victim. This process may not necessarily be a desirable alternative, considering that in many situations, the abuser is incarcerated for only a brief period of time (Smith, Rainey, Smith, Alamares, & Grogg, 2008; Ward & Wood, 2009).

 Now Can You— Discuss IPV screening, documenting, and reporting?

1. Explain the nurse's role in conducting screening for IPV?
2. Describe how to document IPV and identify when the patient's informed consent must be obtained?
3. Identify the IPV reporting requirements of your practice state?

Nursing Interventions

EDUCATION AND COUNSELING

Education and counseling constitutes an essential nursing role in IPV care. The nurse should inquire about violence and family conflict, listen to the woman's story, and provide information and referrals. Nurses should reassure their patients that they will provide help regardless of whether they choose to remain in the relationship. Nurses must assist victims of violence by informing them of available options and by providing support in making decisions. Allowing the woman to break the cycle of abuse restores her power and enables her to regain control of her life (Burge, Schneider, Ivy, & Catala, 2005; Coker et al., 2007; Ward & Wood, 2009). Nursing diagnoses may be related to physical injuries, emotional trauma, and the need for seeking help (see Box 1-1). In addition, abused women may be formally diagnosed as having posttraumatic stress disorder (PTSD) if their symptoms meet the explicit criteria outlined in the *Diagnostic and Statistical Manual of Mental Disorders* (American Psychiatric Association, 2000).

Nurses can educate their patients about strategies to protect themselves from harm in their home environment. When physical abuse appears to be imminent, women should be taught to remove themselves from the kitchen where there are weapons such as knives that may be used to inflict harm. Victims should also be taught to stay out of bathrooms, closets, or small spaces where the abuser can trap the victim. If possible, the woman should leave the home or go to a room with a door or window to escape or lock the abuser outside. Women should be encouraged to call 911 in an emergency and go to their health-care

Box 1-1 Examples of Nursing Diagnoses for Victims of IPV

- Powerlessness related to perception that it is impossible to leave the abusing partner
- Fear related to the ongoing threat of violence
- Social Isolation related to the need to conceal evidence of the abuse
- Ineffective Denial related to an inability to acknowledge that the partner is abusive
- Compromised Family Coping related to the dysfunctional relationship between self and the abusive partner
- Chronic, Situational Low Self-esteem related to the continuing physical and mental abuse
- Helplessness related to the ongoing exposure to physical, mental, sexual, social, and economic abuse
- Injury related to physical and emotional abuse
- Knowledge Deficit related to the cycle of violence
- Knowledge Deficit related to available resources

provider or nearest emergency room for care when their injuries require medical attention. Victims may go to a local women's shelter or crisis center for housing and counseling. It has been estimated that 50% of all homeless women and children in the United States are fleeing IPV. They may also call the National Domestic Violence Hotline (1-800-799-SAFE [7233]) for additional information and assistance. Women should also be encouraged to learn self-defense skills through enrollment in a course, if possible, and to seek education from an IPV program (American Bar Association, 2008; Family Violence Prevention Fund, 2008b; Krieger, 2008; National Domestic Violence Hotline, 2008).

The woman may also be encouraged to prepare a packed bag with essential items that will be needed if she needs to make a hasty escape from her abuser. Hiding the bag in a handy, safe place or leaving it with a neighbor helps to ensure that the "ready escape bag" will be available if needed. Necessary items include certain documents that will be needed to establish stability, such as housing and financial assistance (Krieger, 2008).

 Optimizing Outcomes— With a ready escape bag containing important items

Nurses can teach IPV victims how to assemble a ready escape bag to facilitate a hasty departure from an unsafe home situation. The bag should contain money, an extra set of car keys, birth certificates, lists of medications and doses, medical records (for self and children), passports, court papers, Social Security card, car title, insurance card, and immigration papers (Krieger, 2008; Ward & Wood, 2009).

It is important to ensure that the woman keeps all information about her safety plan stored in a safe place away from her abuser. Danger to the victim is heightened if the abuser believes that the victim may leave or report the abuse to the police (Family Violence Prevention Fund, 2004; Ward & Wood, 2009).

If the abuser has moved out of the home, the woman should be advised to change the locks on the doors and secure locks for the windows. She may ask neighbors to call the police if they observe the abuser at the victim's house, and the victim and neighbor(s) may develop a system of signals to alert the neighbor when to call the police. The nurse should counsel the woman to obtain an unlisted phone number, block caller ID, and use an answering machine to screen phone calls. Rather than use a personal home computer, it may be wise to use a friend's or library computer, as the abuser may be able to monitor the woman's computer activities or have access to the e-mail addresses of the victim's family members and friends. The woman should also be encouraged to change her online passwords and create a new e-mail account to avoid the abuser's harassment (Krieger, 2008). Additional safety strategies are listed in Box 1-2.

⊛ **Optimizing Outcomes— Using the ABCDEs to provide sensitive care for the IPV victim**

Nurses should remember the "ABCDEs of Caring" (Campbell & Furniss, 2002) to provide appropriate, sensitive care for victims of IPV:

A – Reassuring the woman that she is not **alone**

B – Expressing the **belief** that violence directed against the woman is unacceptable and not her fault

C – **Confidentiality** of the shared information will be maintained (explain the mandatory reporting laws of the practice state, when applicable)

D – **Documentation** – descriptive documentation includes quoted statements, accurate descriptions of all injuries, and photographs (with the woman's written consent)

E – **Education** about the cycle of violence and community and national resources

S – **Safety**—always the most important component of the intervention, especially since one of the most dangerous times for the victim is when she decides to leave her abuser

---

TREATMENT AND FOLLOW-UP

In the clinic, office, or hospital setting, nurses should carefully document all injuries in great detail and use body maps to enhance clarification. Terms such as *strangulation* should be used in place of *choked,* which implies that a foreign object has been lodged in the patient's trachea or esophagus. By definition, strangulation is an assault with malicious intent that causes harm to the victim. Treatment interventions and discharge information must be clearly noted on the chart, along with a description of all referrals and follow-up options that were provided to the patient. Nurses can offer immediate contact with an IPV counselor either in person or by phone, and referral to a mental health provider may also be appropriate (Krieger, 2008; Ward & Wood, 2009).

Nurses must ensure that an adequate referral system is in place for victims of IPV. A number of resources are available to assist nurses in providing appropriate, sensitive care in a timely manner and to take action against IPV perpetrators (Box 1-3). Establishing a professional relationship with the local domestic violence center empowers the nurse with a variety of resources to better help the victim of abuse (Ward & Wood, 2009).

IPV centers offer services that frequently include a 24-hour hotline, advocacy with community systems, and temporary shelter for victims who cannot return home because of safety concerns for themselves and their children. Advocacy with community systems includes referral for services such as legal aid, housing, mental health, substance abuse, and dental referral resources. In most situations, IPV centers also assist victims in accessing local and state government programs (Ward & Wood, 2009).

Nurses who deal with victims of IPV should also be familiar with the local sexual assault center. Women who have been sexually assaulted can benefit from the specialized services (e.g., individualized counseling, support

---

Box 1-2 Safety Strategies for Victims of IPV

Nurses can teach women to do the following:
- Remain aware of surroundings at all times.
- Shop and bank at different places, especially if being stalked.
- Use different routes for driving to work, or try to receive rides from different persons.
- Obtain a protection order.
- Refrain from lunching alone.
- Cancel all joint credit card and bank accounts.
- Ask for workplace escorts to the car or public transportation.
- Determine whether an immediate danger exists; if so, go to a safe place and call 911 (Krieger, 2008).

Box 1-3 Additional IPV Resources

Centers for Disease Control and Prevention
http://www.cdc.gov/ncipc/dvp/IPV/default.htm
DomesticViolence.org
http://www.domesticviolence.org/
Family Violence Prevention Fund
http://www.endabuse.org/
Medline Plus
http://www.nim.nih.gov/medlineplus/domesticviolence.html
National Center for Victims of Crime, Stalking Resource Center
1-800-394-2255
National Coalition Against Domestic Violence
http://www.ncadv.org/
National Domestic Violence Hotline
1-800-799-SAFE (1-800-787-3224 (TTY))
http://www.ndvh.org
National Teen Dating Abuse Helpline
1-866-331-9474
Rape, Abuse, and Incest National Network (RAINN)
1-800-656-HOPE (4673)
U.S. Department of Justice
http://www.ovw.usdoj.gov/domesticviolence.htm
WomensHealth.gov
http://www.4women.gov/violence/types/domestic.cfm
World Health Organization
http://www.who.int/entity/violence_injury-prevention/violence/world-report/factsheets/en/ipvfacts.pdf

groups) provided by these centers. Nurses can also advocate for IPV awareness and assistance by placing information about local resources in various public and private locations throughout the clinic or office (e.g., waiting area, bathroom, examination room) where patients can have ready access to them. Many clinics distribute business-size IPV cards that contain essential information such as strategies for self-protection and protection of children and the National Domestic Violence Hotline phone number. The business-size card is particularly useful as it can be easily concealed (Ward & Wood, 2009).

Nurses must also recognize the victim's need for legal information. For those with access to a computer, the Web site WomensLaw.org (http://www.womenslaw.org) contains an abundance of easy-to-understand information for women living with or escaping IPV. The Web site offers suggestions for obtaining restraining orders, court forms and other legal documents, and provides locations for various law enforcement offices (Ward & Wood, 2009). Women who have no access to a computer may receive assistance by dialing the toll-free phone number for the National Domestic Violence Hotline (1-800-799-SAFE).

Excellent IPV resources are available for nurses and other health-care professionals. The Minnesota Center Against Violence and Abuse (http://www.mincava.umn.edu) offers educational resources for training on violence of any type, including IPV, teen violence, and dating violence.

 Optimizing Outcomes— With an IPV tool designed especially for health-care professionals

The Minnesota Center Against Violence and Abuse Web site offers "A Medical Provider's Guide to Managing the Care of Domestic Violence Patients Within a Cultural Context," a training and reference guide for health-care professionals. This tool is designed to help reduce cultural, linguistic, and systemic barriers that keep IPV victims, particularly immigrant women and women of color, from reporting abuse to their care providers (Ward & Wood, 2009).

Once a patient leaves the health-care setting, a lack of personal contact does not mean that interventions cannot occur. McFarland and colleagues (2004) used telephone interviews to conduct a longitudinal study on abused women. After an initial personal contact with abused women to ask about inclusion in the study and to obtain informed consent, researchers contacted the women with either six intervention and four follow-up calls (experimental group) or four follow-up calls only (control group). During the phone calls, the interviewers asked women in the experimental group to answer yes or no to a series of safety-promoting behaviors. These behaviors included such actions as hiding money, hiding house and car keys, removing weapons from the house, asking neighbors to call police if violence begins, establishing a code with family and friends, and obtaining items such as birth certificates, important phone numbers, identification cards, and rent and utility receipts. The research findings indicated that women in the intervention group (those who received six additional phone calls) practiced more safety-promoting behaviors than did those in the

control group and that the required nursing time was minimal. Such research findings are significant in supporting the important role that nurses and other members of the health-care team can have in helping victims of domestic violence take control of their environments and practice positive behaviors that can break the cycle of abuse.

Now Can You— Discuss the nurse's role when caring for victims of IPV?

1. Formulate five nursing diagnoses that may be appropriate for victims of IPV?
2. Describe three ways that IPV victims can enhance personal safety at home and items that they should include in a "ready escape bag"?

summary points

- *Intimate partner violence* (IPV) is defined as physical, sexual, or psychological harm or social isolation perpetrated by a current or former partner in an intimate or dating relationship.
- The abuser's actions are intended to instill fear and to intimidate and control the victim.
- Intimate partner violence reaches across all strata of society and affects persons regardless of economic status, ethnic background, educational level, or religious status.
- Women who are abused are more likely to be unemployed, suffer from health problems, and receive public assistance than are women who are not victims of abuse.
- Routine screening can facilitate early identification of IPV when signs and symptoms may not be readily apparent.
- Accurate documentation of abuse is essential, and nurses must be knowledgeable about IPV reporting guidelines for their particular practice state.
- Nurses must assist victims of violence by informing them of available options and by providing support in making decisions.

review questions

Multiple Choice

1. Nurses should be alert to signs of IPV, which may include
   A. Overuse of health services
   B. Injuries consistent with the patient's explanation as to cause
   C. Consistency in keeping health-care appointments
   D. Reporting specific, descriptive complaints

2. Potential barriers to routine IPV screening in the clinical setting may include
   A. Having an awareness of IPV
   B. Sharing the patient's language and cultural values
   C. Understanding how to inquire about abuse
   D. Having a personal history of abuse

3. When physical abuse is imminent, a home safety strategy that the nurse can teach the patient is to
  A. Hide in the bathroom
  B. Seek shelter in a closet
  C. Remove herself from the kitchen
  D. Confront the abuser in an assertive way

4. The nurse can encourage the woman to develop a plan to facilitate safety from the abuser. A safety strategy is to
  A. Pack a ready escape bag containing essential items
  B. Leave a "good-bye" note for the abuser
  C. Maintain usual habits for banking and shopping
  D. Keep computer e-mail accounts and online passwords as originally set up

5. IPV is an abusive relationship characterized by the abuser's desire to have
  A. The victim's sympathy
  B. Power and control in the relationship
  C. A sense of intimacy
  D. Financial security

REFERENCES

American Bar Association. (2008). *Survey of recent statistics.* Commission on Domestic Violence. Retrieved January 31, 2010, from http://www.abanet.org/domviol/statistics.html

American College of Obstetricians and Gynecologists (ACOG). (2008). *Guidelines for women's health care. A resource manual* (3rd ed.). Washington, DC: Author.

American Nurses Association. (2000). *Violence against women* (Position statement). Retrieved January 30, 2010, from http://www.nursingworld.org/MainMenuCategories/HealthcareandPolicyIssues/ANAPositionStatements/social.aspx

American Nurses Association (ANA). (2005). *Code of ethics for nurses with interpretive statements.* Retrieved February 2, 2010, from http://nursingworld.org/MainMenuCategories/ThePracticeofProfessionalNursing/EthicsStandards/CodeofEthics.aspx

American Psychiatric Association. (2000). *Diagnostic and statistic manual of mental disorders* (4th ed., text revision). Washington, DC: American Psychiatric Association Press.

Arosarena, O. A., Fritsch, T. A., Hsueh, Y., Aynehchi, B., & Haug, R. (2009). Maxillofacial injuries and violence against women. *Archives of Facial Plastic Surgery, 11*(1), 48–52.

Association of Women's Health, Obstetric and Neonatal Nurses. (2007). *Mandatory reporting of intimate partner violence* (Position paper). Washington, DC: Author. Retrieved January 30, 2010, from https://www.awhonn.org/awhonn/content.do?name=05_HealthPolicyLegislation/5H_PositionSta tements.htm

Blereau, R. P. (2009). Woman with multiple head and neck injuries. *Consultant, 49*(9), 565–568.

Brown, J., Lent, B., Schmidt, G., & Sas, G. (2000). Application of the Women Abuse Screening Tool (WAST) and WAST-Short in the family practice setting. *Journal of Family Practice, 49*(10), 896–903.

Bull, A. (2009). Screening for intimate partner violence: Offering the tissue box. *Journal for Nurse Practitioners, 5*(8), 620–621.

Burge, S. K., Schneider, F. D., Ivy, L., & Catala, S. (2005). Patients' advice to physicians about intervening in family conflict. *Annals of Family Medicine, 3*(3), 248–254.

Campbell, J. (1986). Nursing assessment for risk of homicide with battered women. *Advances in Nursing Science, 8*(4), 36–51.

Campbell, J. (1989). Women's responses to sexual abuse in intimate relationships. *Health Care for Women International, 10*(1), 335–340.

Campbell, J., & Furniss, K. (2002). *Violence against women: Identification, screening, and management of intimate partner violence.* Washington, DC: Association of Women's Health, Obstetric, and Neonatal Nurses.

Centers for Disease Control and Prevention (CDC), National Center for Injury Prevention and Control. (2003). *Costs of intimate partner violence against women in the United States.* Retrieved January 29, 2010, from http://www.cdc.gov/violenceprevention/pub/IPV_cost.html

Centers for Disease Control and Prevention (CDC). (2009). *Intimate partner violence: Fact sheet.* Retrieved January 29, 2010, from http://www.cdc.gov/violenceprevention/pdf/IPV_factsheet-a.pdf

Chang, J. C., Decker, M., Moracco, K. E., Martin, S. L., Petersen, R., & Frasier, P. Y. (2003). What happens when health care providers ask about intimate partner violence? A description of consequences from the perspectives of female survivors. *Journal of the American Medical Women's Association, 58*(2), 76–81.

Coker, A., Davis, K., Arias, Il, Desai, S., Sanderson, M., Brandt, H., & Smith, P. H. (2002). Physical and mental health effects of intimate partner violence for men and women. *American Journal of Preventive Medicine, 23*(4), 260–268.

Coker, A. L., Flerx, V. C., Smith, P. H., Whitaker, D. J., Fadden, M. K., & Williams, M. (2007). Partner violence screening in rural health care clinics. *American Journal of Public Health, 97*(7), 1319–1325.

Crandall, M., Nathens, A., Kernic, M., Holt, V., & Rivara, F. (2004). Predicting future injury among women in abusive relationships. *Journal of Trauma—Injury Infection and Critical Care, 56*(8), 906–912.

Davila, Y. (2006). Increasing nurses' knowledge and skills for enhanced response to intimate partner violence. *Journal of Continuing Education in Nursing, 37*(4), 171–177.

Du Plat-Jones, J. (2006). Domestic violence: The role of health professionals. *Nursing Standard, 21*(10), 44–48.

Family Violence Prevention Fund. (2004). *National consensus guidelines on identifying and responding to domestic violence victimization in health care settings.* Updated February 2004. Retrieved February 2, 2010, from http://www.endabuse.org/userfiles/file/Consensus.pdf

Family Violence Prevention Fund. (2007). *Justice Department releases '05 intimate partner violence data.* Retrieved January 29, 2010, from http://www.endabuse.org/content/features/detail/919/

Family Violence Prevention Fund. (2008a). *Intimate partner violence and Healthy People 2010 fact sheet.* Retrieved January 29, 2010, from http://www.endabuse.org/userfiles/file/Children_and_Families/ipv.pdf

Family Violence Prevention Fund. (2008b). *Survey finds health problems more common for victims of violence.* Retrieved January 29, 2010, from http://www.endabuse.org/content/news/detail/1070

Griffith, R. (2008). Patient confidentiality: Rights and duties of nurse prescribers. *Nurse Prescribing, 6*(3), 116–120.

Hamme, R., Moynihan, B., & Pagliaro, E. (2005). *Forensic nursing.* Sudbury, MA: Jones and Bartlett.

Hamolia, C. (2005). Preventing and managing aggressive behavior. In G. Stuart & M. Laraia (Eds.), *Principles and practice of psychiatric nursing* (8th ed.). St. Louis, MO: Mosby.

Heise, L., & Garcia-Moreno, C. (2002). Violence by intimate partners. In E. Krug, L. Dahlberg, & J. Mercy (Eds.), *World report on violence and health* (pp. 87–121). Geneva, Switzerland: World Health Organization.

Johnson, M., & Leone, J. (2005). The differential effects of intimate terrorism and situational couple violence. *Journal of Family Issues, 26*(8), 322–349.

Kearney, M. (2001). Enduring love: A formal theory of women's experience of domestic violence. *Research in Nursing and Health, 24*(3), 270–282.

Klevens, J., & Saltzman, L. E. (2009). The controversy on screening for intimate partner violence: A question of semantics? *Journal of Women's Health, 18*(2), 143–145.

Krieger, C. L. (2008). Intimate partner violence: A review for nurses. *Nursing for Women's Health, 12*(3), 226–234.

Lewis-O'Connor, A. (2004). Policy perspectives. "Dying to tell?" Do mandatory reporting laws benefit victims of domestic violence? *American Journal of Nursing, 104*(10), 75–76.

Lite, J. (2009). Domestic violence victims have distinct facial injuries, study says. *Scientific American 60-second science blog.* Retrieved January 29, 2010, from http://www.scientificamerican.com/blog/post.cfm?id=domestic-violence-victims-have-dist-2009-01-19

Mahoney, B. (2006). Reducing barriers against routine screening for intimate partner violence. *American Journal for Nurse Practitioners, 10*(10), 45–58.

McFarlane, J., Christoffel, K., Bateman, L., Miller, V., & Bullock, L. (1991). Assessing for abuse: Self-report versus nurse interview. *Public Health Nursing, 8*(4), 245–250.

McFarland, J., Malecha, A., Gist, J., Watson, K., Batten, E., Hall, I., & Smith, S. (2004). Original research: Increasing the safety promoting behaviors of abused women. *American Journal of Nursing, 104*(3), 40–51.

Moran, B. A. (2008). Intimate partner violence: The difference nurses can make. *Nursing for Women's Health, 12*(3), 194–196.

Moracco, K., Brown, C., Martin, S., Chang, J., Dulli, L., Loucks-Sorrell, M., Turner, T., Bou-Saada, I., & Starsoneck, L. (2005). Mental health issues among female clients of domestic violence programs in North Carolina. *Psychiatric Services, 55*(9), 1036–1040.

National Domestic Violence Hotline. (2008). *National domestic violence hotline*. Retrieved January 29, 2010, from: http://www.ndvh.org

Parker, B., & McFarlane, J. (1991). Nursing assessment of the battered pregnant woman. *American Journal of Maternal Child Nursing, 16*(6), 161–164.

Parkinson, G., Adams, R., & Emerling, F. (2001). Maternal domestic violence screening in an office-based pediatric practice. *Pediatrics, 108*(6), E43.

Peedicayil, A., Sadowski, L. S., Jeyaseelan, L., Shankar, V., Jain, D., Suresh, S., & Bangdiwala, S. I. (2004). Spousal physical violence against women during pregnancy. *British Journal of Obstetrics and Gynaecology, 111*(7), 682–687.

Plichta, S. (2004). Intimate partner violence and physical health consequences: Policy and practice implication. *Journal of Interpersonal Violence, 19*(6), 1296–1323.

Pyrek, K. (2006). *Forensic nursing*. New York: CRC Press.

Rennison, C. (2003). *Intimate partner violence, 1993–2001*. Washington, DC: U.S. Department of Justice, Bureau of Justice Statistics (Publication No. NCJ197838).

Rhodes, K. V., Frankel, R. M., Levinthal, N., Prenoveau, N., Bailey, J., & Levinson, W. (2007). "You're not a victim of domestic violence, are you?" Provider–patient communication about domestic violence. *Annals of Internal Medicine, 147*(9), 620–627.

Silverman, J. G., Decker, M. R., Reed, E., & Raj, A. (2006). Intimate partner violence victimization prior to and during pregnancy among women residing in 26 U.S. states: Associations with maternal and neonatal health. *American Journal of Obstetrics and Gynecology, 195*(1), 140–148.

Smith, J., Rainey, S., Smith, K., Alamares, C., & Grogg, D. (2008). Barriers to the mandatory reporting of domestic violence encountered by nursing professionals. *Journal of Trauma Nursing, 15*(1), 9–11.

Stinson, C., & Robinson, R. (2006). Intimate partner violence: Continuing education for registered nurses. *Journal of Continuing Education in Nursing, 37*(2), 58–64.

Strack, G. B., & McClane, G. (1999). *How to improve your investigation and prosecution of strangulation cases*. Austin, TX: National Center of Domestic and Sexual Violence. Retrieved January 30, 2010, from http://www.ncdsv.org/images/strangulation_article.pdf

Tjaden, P., & Thoennes, N. (2000a). *Full report of the prevalence, incidence, and consequences of violence against women: Findings from the National Violence Against Women Survey, 2000*. Retrieved January 29, 2010, from http://www.ncjrs.gov/pdffiles1/nij/183781.pdf

Tjaden, P., & Thoennes, N. (2000b). *Extent, nature and consequences of intimate partner violence: Findings from the National Violence Against Women Survey*. Washington, DC: National Institute of Justice and the Centers for Disease Control and Prevention.

U.S. Department of Health and Human Services. (2000). *Healthy People 2010*. Washington, DC: Author.

U.S. Department of Health and Human Services. National Women's Health Information Center. (2009). *Violence against women. Domestic and intimate partner violence*. Retrieved January 29, 2010, from http://www.womenshealth.gov/violence/types/domestic.cfm

U.S. Department of Justice, Bureau of Justice Statistics. (2007). *Criminal victimization*. Retrieved January 29, 2010, from http://bjs.ojp.usdoj.gov/index.cfm?ty=pbdetail&iid=1000

U.S. Preventive Services Task Force. (2004). Screening for family and intimate partner violence. *Annals of Internal Medicine, 140*(8), 382–386.

Valente, S. (2002). Evaluating intimate partner violence. *Journal of the American Academy of Nurse Practitioners, 14*(6), 505–516.

Varcolis, E., Carson, V., & Shoemaker, N. (2006). *Foundations of psychiatric mental health nursing: A clinical approach*. St. Louis, MO: Saunders Elsevier.

Walker, L. (1979). *The battered woman*. New York: Harper & Row.

Walker, L. (1984). *The battered woman syndrome* (Vol. 6). New York: Springer.

Ward, C., & Wood, A. (2009). Intimate partner violence: NP role in assessment. *American Journal for Nurse Practitioners, 13*(10), 9–15.

Williams, G. B., Brackley, M. H., Hibler, T. R., & Prater, S. J. (2008). Screening for intimate partner violence. *Women's Health Care: A Practical Journal for Nurse Practitioners, 7*(8), 10–26.

Wilson, J., Lane, E., & Gillespie, T. (2006). Identifying and responding to intimate partner violence in the health care setting. *Oklahoma Nurse, 51*(2), 28–33.

World Health Organization. (2005). *WHO multi-country study on women's health and domestic violence against women. Summary report of initial results on prevalence, health outcomes, and women's responses*. Geneva, Switzerland: Author.

Yonaka, L., Yoder, M., Darrow, J., & Sherck, J. (2007). Barriers to screening for domestic violence in the emergency department. *Journal of Continuing Education in Nursing, 38*(1), 37–45.

Yegadis, K. (1989). *Women's mental health in primary care*. Philadelphia: W. B. Saunders.

Yost, N., Bloom, S., McIntier, G., & Leveno, K. (2005). A prospective observational study of domestic violence during pregnancy. *Obstetrics and Gynecology, 106*(1), 61–65.

 For more information, go to http://davisplus.fadavis.com/

Promoting Reproductive Health Through an Understanding of Premenstrual Syndrome

Shelton M. Hisley, PhD, RNC, WHNP-BC

Live your life while you have it.
Life is a splendid gift—there is nothing small about it.

—Florence Nightingale

LEARNING TARGETS *At the completion of this chapter, the student will be able to:*

◆ Identify diagnostic criteria for premenstrual syndrome.

◆ Discuss the unique characteristics of symptoms that accompany premenstrual syndrome.

◆ Describe nonpharmacological and pharmacological approaches to care for women who experience premenstrual syndrome.

◆ Discuss the nurse's role when caring for a patient with a premenstrual disorder.

Introduction

This chapter explores premenstrual syndrome (PMS), a common women's health problem during the childbearing years. In the past, many in the medical profession viewed symptoms of PMS to be wholly attributable to the woman's emotional state and without any physiological basis. PMS-related research was infrequently conducted and consisted mostly of anecdotal experiences. As the women's movement grew in strength and the public's awareness about women's health issues increased, views began to shift. At the same time, a growing body of medical information began to identify various physiological imbalances and theories were proposed to explain the causes of PMS. Today, PMS is viewed as a complex interplay of genetic influences and various hormonal imbalances that can adversely affect a woman's physical, mental, and emotional health (Dickerson, 2007). Various nonpharmacological and pharmacological therapies have been shown to be effective in reducing PMS symptoms. Nurses have traditionally played an important role in promoting women's reproductive health. They can be instrumental in helping women to deal with premenstrual disorders by offering ongoing education and support. These interventions empower women to seek and embrace strategies to help them gain control over their lives and, ideally, to enjoy life more fully.

Scope of the Problem

Premenstrual disorders affect many women during the reproductive years. *Premenstrual syndrome* (PMS) is defined as the presence of emotional and physical symptoms and behavioral changes that occur during the second half, or luteal phase, of the menstrual cycle and cease at or within a few days after the onset of menses. The timing of the symptoms in relation to the menstrual cycle, rather than the symptoms themselves, constitutes the unique element in this disorder.

 A & P Review **Phases of the Uterine (Endometrial) Cycle**

Following menstruation (the "menstrual phase"), follicle-stimulating hormone (FSH) stimulates the growth and development of the ovarian graafian follicle, which secretes estrogen. The first phase of the menstrual cycle is termed the "follicular" or "proliferative" phase; this phase lasts from the end of menses through ovulation (approximately days 7–14). When estrogen production reaches a peak, the pituitary gland releases luteinizing hormone (LH), which triggers ovulation. The "luteal phase" of the ovarian cycle begins at ovulation and ends with the onset of menses. The corpus luteum produces some estrogen but mainly produces progesterone. Eighty percent of all the progesterone secreted during the entire menstrual cycle is secreted during the first 8 days after ovulation. In the absence of fertilization, the life span of the corpus luteum is 14 days. Thus, the luteal phase of the uterine cycle is 14 days in length. As the end of the luteal phase nears, low levels of FSH and LH cause degeneration of the corpus luteum, which is associated with declining levels of estrogen and progesterone. The decreased hormonal levels trigger degeneration of the endometrium and the onset of menses (the "menstrual phase"). ◆

Criteria for Diagnosis

The diagnosis of PMS depends on the determination of the following three criteria:

- The woman's symptoms occur in a cyclic pattern.
- The symptoms are not caused by any underlying physical or mental condition.
- The symptoms greatly disrupt one or more areas of the woman's life.

Since 1987, PMS has been recognized as a mental disorder. More than 150 symptoms, which can affect almost every organ system in various combinations and intensity, have been identified (American College of Obstetricians & Gynecologists [ACOG], 2000, 2007; American Psychiatric Association [APA], 2000; Association of Women's Health, Obstetrical and Neonatal Nurses [AWHONN], 2003; Dickerson, 2007; Polaneczky, 2007).

 Nursing Insight— *PMS and PMT*

Premenstrual syndrome is sometimes referred to as "premenstrual tension syndrome" (PMT). When first described in 1931, premenstrual tension centered on women's symptoms of tension, self-deprecation, and severe depression during the 7 to 10 days preceding menstruation. By the 1950s, the spectrum of reported symptoms had dramatically increased, and there was a growing realization that the previously described "tension" was just one aspect of the problem. A medical report published in 1953 introduced the term "premenstrual syndrome" to encompass the extensive list of symptoms, and this is the name most often used today.

Prevalence and Economic Impact

Sources vary in estimates of the number of women who experience symptoms of PMS. It has been estimated that over 80% of childbearing-age women experience various emotional and physical changes during the premenstrual period. However, according to experts, most patients who self-diagnose do not actually have PMS (ACOG, 2000, 2007). Of the women with premenstrual symptoms, approximately 20% to 40% regard the emotional and physical changes as difficult, although only 5% to 10%

report a significant degree of impact on their work or lifestyle (ACOG, 2007; Arrowsmith, 2007).

Nevertheless, the disability associated with premenstrual disorders is quite substantial. Women who suffer from PMS reportedly have higher absenteeism from work and make more visits to ambulatory health-care facilities than those who do not experience PMS. On average, women with premenstrual disorders have an increase of $59 in direct annual health-care costs and $4,333 in indirect costs (Borenstein et al., 2003; Whyte & Peraud, 2009).

Symptoms of PMS

Over 100 physical and behavioral symptoms have been experienced by women during the premenstrual period (see Box 2-1). It is important to remember that to meet the criteria for a premenstrual disorder, the symptoms must be confined to the luteal phase of the menstrual cycle and they must resolve after the onset of menstruation.

Clinical criteria from the U.S. National Institute of Mental Health for the diagnosis of PMS include a significant change in the intensity of symptoms between the follicular and late luteal phases. These changes must occur for at least two consecutive cycles (Dickerson, 2007; Whyte & Peraud, 2009). Other definitions, such as symptom intensity, have been developed for research purposes. According to ACOG, at least one of the affective and/or somatic symptoms associated with PMS must be present—and appropriately timed with the menstrual cycle—to meet the diagnostic criteria. Speroff and Fritz (2005) proposed a simple, commonsense definition of PMS: "The cyclic appearance of one or more of a large constellation of symptoms just prior to menses, occurring to such as degree that lifestyle or work is affected,

Box 2-1 Selected Premenstrual Symptoms Reported by Women	
• Irritability	• Joint pain
• Anxiety	• Sore throat
• Mood swings	• Cramps
• Depression	• Nausea
• Hostility	• Insomnia
• Headaches	• Water retention
• Dizziness	• Fatigue
• Fainting	• Increased appetite
• Shakiness	• Cold sweats
• Bloating	• Hot flashes
• Weight gain	• Lack of coordination
• Sugar cravings	• Easy bruising
• Constipation	• Palpitations
• Diarrhea	• Hives
• Backache	• Joint swelling
• Asthma	• Hay fever
• Migraine	• Breast tenderness
• Breast swelling	

followed by a period of time entirely free of symptoms" (p. 247).

It has been noted that PMS symptoms commonly occur in clusters, with some women reporting as many as 10 symptoms at one time. Those who experience severe symptoms may be prone to extremes of behavior, with an increased likelihood of accidents, alcohol abuse, and suicide attempts. For others, PMS symptoms may be described as annoying but mild (Dickerson, 2007).

 Now Can You— Discuss certain broad aspects of PMS?

1. Explain why the timing of symptoms is an essential component of premenstrual syndrome?
2. Identify three criteria necessary for a diagnosis of PMS?
3. Identify at least 20 symptoms that may be associated with PMS?

Premenstrual Dysphoric Disorder (PMDD)

Premenstrual dysphoric disorder (PMDD) is a diagnostic term for the most severe form of PMS as defined by the APA's *Diagnostic and Statistical Manual of Mental Disorders* (4th edition, text revision) (*DSM-IV-TR*). It is estimated that nearly 5 million American women have PMDD (Whyte & Peraud, 2009). PMDD pertains to women with PMS who suffer from more severe and disabling emotional symptoms. PMS and PMDD may be viewed as a spectrum of premenstrual disorders that begins with mild emotional and/or physical symptoms that are cyclic but not debilitating and proceeds through PMS to PMDD (Dickerson, 2007; Whyte & Peraud, 2009). Women with PMDD most frequently report the following symptoms: abdominal bloating, anxiety, tension, breast tenderness, crying episodes, depression, fatigue and a lack of energy, irritability, difficulty concentrating, appetite changes, thirst, and swelling of the extremities (Speroff & Fritz, 2005).

 Optimizing Outcomes— When evaluating a patient for PMS/PMDD symptoms

When evaluating a patient with PMS/PMDD symptoms, the nurse must always take any report of suicidal thoughts or other indicators of extreme mood change most seriously. The woman will need appropriate medications, close follow-up, and referral to a qualified mental health professional. In the ideal situation, mental examinations are timed to occur during both the luteal and follicular phases of the menstrual cycle. If the patient experiences significant mood symptoms (e.g., suicidal ideation) during both the luteal and follicular phases, referral to a psychiatrist is indicated. Once she is stable, various interventions such as lifestyle changes, dietary alterations, and conventional and complementary care approaches can be initiated that will become an important part of her long-term health promotion and maintenance (Dickerson, 2007; Whyte & Peraud, 2009).

Women who seek care for symptoms associated with premenstrual disorders should be given a complete physical examination and thorough clinical evaluation to rule out illness that may be the source of the symptoms. A detailed health history is the cornerstone in the accurate diagnosis of PMS/PMDD. It is crucial that careful attention be paid to the cyclic timing of symptoms. For most women with PMS, symptoms develop from 2 to 12 days prior to menstruation and resolve within 24 hours following the onset of menses. Women who have symptoms that primarily occur during the menstrual flow or during the first 2 weeks of the menstrual cycle do not have PMS as defined in the literature (Dickerson, 2007; Speroff & Fritz, 2005; Whyte & Peraud, 2009).

 Nursing Insight— *Identifying populations most likely to experience PMS*

Although all age groups are affected, women in their 20s and 30s most frequently report symptoms of premenstrual disorders. It is important to note that premenstrual disorders:
- Occur only in ovulatory women
- Occur only during the luteal phase of the menstrual cycle
- Resolve within 4 days following the onset of menses

The occurrence of premenstrual disorders is not dependent on the presence of monthly menses. Interestingly, women who have had a hysterectomy without bilateral salpingo-oophorectomy (removal of both ovaries) can still have cyclic PMS symptoms (Andolsek & Rapkin, 2006).

Causes of Premenstrual Disorders

Clinical research has not yet determined the exact cause of premenstrual disorders. Variations in the cyclical fluctuation of estrogen and progesterone may well account for symptoms in certain individuals. However, the cause is believed to be multifactorial—that is, a genetic predisposition and multiple biological, psychosocial, and sociocultural factors most likely play a role in the development of premenstrual disorders (Nelson & Baldwin, 2007; Taylor, Schuiling, & Sharp, 2006; Whyte & Peraud, 2009).

Although it was once believed that low levels of progesterone were the primary cause of PMS, research has failed to find a significant difference between PMS sufferers and non-PMS sufferers in levels of various hormones, including progesterone, estradiol, FSH, LH, prolactin, sex hormone binding-globulin (SHBG), and testosterone. It has been proposed, however, that women with PMS may have a greater biological vulnerability to the normal fluctuations in hormone levels than do women without PMS (Nelson & Baldwin, 2008). There appears to be a genetic component to the development of PMS. Women who have a genetic predisposition to the development of PMS are believed to have a heightened sensitivity to various cyclic hormonal changes or a varied response to naturally occurring neurotransmitters (e.g., serotonin). Interestingly, a genetic predisposition to PMS is also known to be associated with a predisposition to other psychiatric disorders (Halbreich, 2003; Whyte & Peraud, 2009).

It has been demonstrated that levels of the gonadal steroids (i.e., androgens, estrogens, progestogens) are the same in patients with and without PMS. However, the responses to fluctuating levels of the hormones are different in women with PMS. Another area of research has explored the role of the neurotransmitters serotonin and gamma-aminobutyric acid (GABA) in the etiology of premenstrual disorders. It has been suggested that a dysregulation in serotonin in particular is linked to many of the psychological symptoms in PMS, such as tension, irritability, and dysphoria (an emotional state characterized by anxiety, depression, or unease) (Clayton, Keller, Leslie, & Evans, 2006; Nelson & Baldwin, 2008; Whyte & Peraud, 2009).

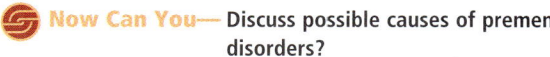 **Optimizing Outcomes**— Teaching women about the serotonin–stress relationship

Nurses can empower women with information about the normal workings of their bodies and how certain lifestyle changes may promote an enhanced sense of well-being and diminish PMS symptoms. For example, explaining the relationship between cyclic estrogen fluctuation and changes in serotonin levels may be beneficial in promoting an understanding about serotonin, one of the natural brain chemicals that assists one in coping with life's normal stressors.

Other clinical investigations have focused on the renin–angiotensin–aldosterone system. It has long been noted that many premenstrual symptoms, such as bloating, breast swelling, and weight gain, are caused by fluid retention. Estrogen increases the production of the serum globulin angiotensinogen (a precursor for angiotensin), which leads to increased aldosterone and fluid levels. Under normal circumstances, progesterone competes with aldosterone and prevents excessive fluid retention. However, in the late luteal phase of the menstrual cycle, declining progesterone levels give rise to an increase in the effect of estrogen (Nelson & Baldwin, 2008; Whyte & Peraud, 2009).

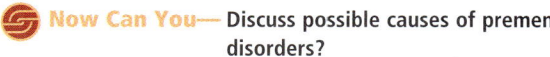 **Now Can You**— Discuss possible causes of premenstrual disorders?

1. Describe premenstrual dysphoric disorder?
2. List three characteristics common to premenstrual disorders?
3. Describe three possible causes of premenstrual disorders?

Diagnosis

In general, the diagnostic workup for PMS/PMDD consists of four components:

1. A detailed history with a focus on the medical, psychosocial, psychosexual, and substance abuse histories (the gynecological history must include the timing of the symptoms and the regularity of the menstrual cycle)
2. A complete physical examination
3. Laboratory tests (as appropriate to rule out other disorders such as hypothyroidism)
4. A record of the woman's symptoms over a 2- or 3-month period

 Nursing Insight— *Hormonal testing unnecessary in PMS diagnosis*

Laboratory testing of the sex steroid hormonal levels is not necessary for the diagnosis of PMS. Depending on the history and clinical findings, appropriate serum testing may include a chemistry profile, a complete blood cell count, or measurement of the thyroid-stimulating hormone level (Whyte & Peraud, 2009).

 Optimizing Outcomes— Recognizing other conditions that may masquerade as premenstrual disorder

When interviewing patients with premenstrual disorder symptomatology, it is essential to obtain a detailed history. Dysmenorrhea, hypothyroidism, depressive disorders, pain disorders, and generalized anxiety disorders are other conditions that may produce similar symptoms. Hypothyroidism, for example, may be associated with fatigue, bloating, irritability, and depression. Breast disease (breast tenderness) or anemia (fatigue) may be responsible for other common symptoms. Various gynecological disorders such as polycystic ovary syndrome or endometriosis may also cause symptoms that can be confused with PMS (Whyte & Peraud, 2009).

THE SYMPTOM DIARY

The patient must be instructed to record her symptom types, timing, and severity each day. Maintaining a prospective symptom diary for at least two to three consecutive menstrual cycles is an essential element in the diagnostic workup for premenstrual disorders. Because many medical disorders are exacerbated during the luteal phase, the symptom diary is instrumental in determining the severity and the timing of the symptoms (Nelson & Baldwin, 2008; Whyte & Peraud, 2009).

Several symptom inventories are available. The use of a standardized form such as the Daily Record of Severity of Problems (DRSP) was designed to diagnose PMDD. This tool has shown high test/retest reliability and is available on the Internet from the Madison Institute of Medicine at http://www.pmdd.factsforhealth.org (Endicott, Nee, & Harrison, 2006). Other symptom diaries designed to track premenstrual symptoms include the Calendar of Premenstrual Experiences (COPE), the Penn Daily Symptom Report (DSR), and the Premenstrual Symptoms Screening Tool (PSST) (Freeman, DeRubeis, & Rickels, 1996; Steiner, Macdougall, & Brown, 2003).

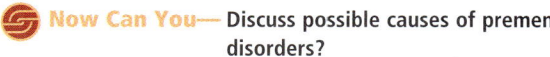 **Optimizing Outcomes**— A daily calendar alternative for tracking PMS symptoms

As an alternative method to using a commercially available symptom inventory form, the nurse may teach the patient how to record her symptoms by taking notes on a regular calendar each day. The woman is taught to write down the symptoms experienced each day, note their severity, and record the dates of her menstrual period. If the number of symptoms is excessive or overwhelming, the patient may record only the three to five symptoms that most profoundly bother her. Under ideal circumstances, the patient's weight, basal body temperature, or home ovulation test results are also documented (Nelson & Baldwin, 2008).

The daily symptom records are useful in that they often heighten the patient's awareness of her symptoms, allow her to gain insights into her problem, and empower her to become more involved in her diagnostic workup and treatment plan. A discussion of cyclic hormonal changes and PMS may be of benefit in heightening an understanding of premenstrual disorders and in promoting a greater sense of control over the situation. If the woman is reluctant to track her daily symptoms, her partner or a family member can be taught to assist with the data collection. It is helpful to ask the patient to continue her charting after therapy has been initiated so that she can identify which interventions improve her symptoms (Nelson & Baldwin, 2008; Whyte & Peraud, 2009).

After the patient has been instructed in the use of a daily symptom diary, she should return in 2 or 3 months for an evaluation of her symptom pattern. Symptoms do not need to recur with equal intensity in each cycle. In fact, the patient may experience different symptoms during different cycles. It is important to recognize, however, that the diagnosis of PMS/PMDD hinges on the timing of symptoms: They must peak in the luteal phase and disappear with the onset of menses (Nelson & Baldwin, 2008).

DIAGNOSTIC CRITERIA FOR PMS AND PMDD

According to ACOG (2000), to meet the diagnostic criteria for premenstrual syndrome, at least one of the following symptoms must be present; occur during the luteal phase of the menstrual cycle, and resolve within 4 days of the onset of menses. Also, the symptoms must not represent an exacerbation of another disorder, and the symptoms should be bothersome but not necessarily debilitating.

PMS Affective Symptoms

- Angry outbursts
- Irritability
- Mild psychological discomfort
- Confusion
- Poor concentration
- Depression
- Sleep disturbances
- Social withdrawal

PMS Somatic Symptoms

- Abdominal bloating
- Headache
- Aches and pains
- Swelling of the extremities
- Breast tenderness
- Weight gain
- Change in appetite

Diagnostic criteria for premenstrual dysphoric disorder defined by the APA include four major symptom categories and seven additional symptoms. To meet the criteria, the woman must report that her symptoms interfere with her usual activities; the symptoms must not represent an exacerbation of another disorder; at least five symptoms must be present for 1 to 2 weeks premenstrually, with relief by the fourth day of menses; and the criteria must be confirmed by prospective daily ratings for at least two cycles (APA, 2000; Dickerson, 2007; Nelson & Baldwin, 2008).

PMDD Major Symptom Categories (at least one must be present)

- Anger or irritability
- Anxiety, edginess, nervousness
- Depressed mood
- Moodiness

Other, Additional PMDD Symptoms (at least five must be present)

- Appetite changes or cravings
- Decreased interest in usual activities
- Difficulty concentrating
- Fatigue
- Feelings of being overwhelmed or out of control
- Insomnia or hypersomnia
- Physical symptoms (listed in the PMS diagnostic criteria)

 Now Can You— **Discuss aspects of the PMS/PMDD diagnostic workup?**

1. Discuss four components of a diagnostic workup for premenstrual disorders?
2. Teach a patient how to keep a symptom diary?
3. Identify the three components of diagnostic criteria for premenstrual disorders as defined by ACOG?

Patient Care and Management of PMS Symptoms

Women with mild to moderate symptoms of PMS often respond well to reassurance, emotional support, and simple health promotion strategies. Education constitutes a central component in the care of women with PMS. Nurses can teach women about self-help modalities intended to reduce symptoms and enhance coping with various discomforts.

Nonpharmacological therapies are often initiated during the initial visit; patients can then implement them as they complete their daily symptom charting and discuss helpful and non-helpful approaches at the follow-up visit. The first step in treatment centers on validating the woman's experience and acknowledging that the symptoms are real and have a physiological base. For many women, the simple act of validation brings relief and opens the door to healing. Nursing diagnoses, such as Cyclic Pelvic Pain and Related Discomforts (Collins Sharp, Taylor, Thomas, Killeen, & Dawood, 2002) are developed to address the patient's specific symptoms:

- Anxiety related to anticipation of cyclical discomfort
- Depression related to cyclical hormonal changes
- Excess Fluid Volume related to cyclical hormonal changes
- Pain related to cyclical breast changes

"What to say" — *Teaching patients about strategies to cope with PMS symptoms*

Nurses can suggest strategies to help women cope with specific PMS symptoms. For example, a fitted support or sports bra may ease the discomfort associated with breast tenderness. Abdominal pain and backache are often relieved with the local application of heat; some women benefit from performing stretching exercises, and NSAIDs are useful in reducing the production of pain-producing prostaglandins. Others may be interested in exploring the possibility of using extended cycle hormonal contraceptives to prevent ovulation. The nurse can also encourage the patient to engage in relaxation techniques and, if available, participate in a PMS support group to help reduce premenstrual tension and anxiety. Support groups provide a forum for the sharing of feelings and concerns and offer an opportunity for learning new strategies for self-care.

PHYSICAL ACTIVITY

Various lifestyle changes have been shown to improve PMS symptoms for many women. These include physical activity, aerobic exercise, stress reduction, and relaxation techniques such as yoga and meditation. Nurses should encourage patients with PMS, as well as all women, to regularly engage in physical activity. Vigorous aerobic exercise may lift the mood, reduce stress, and diminish certain physical symptoms in PMS. The 2008 Physical Activity Guidelines for Americans recommend that adults engage in at least 150 minutes per week of moderate-intensity, or 75 minutes a week of vigorous-intensity, aerobic physical activity or an equivalent combination of moderate- and vigorous-intensity aerobic activity (U.S. Department of Health and Human Services, 2008).

DIETARY ALTERATIONS, VITAMINS, AND MINERALS

Dietary alterations may play a role in reducing certain premenstrual disorder symptoms, although various clinical investigations have not conclusively determined that modification of specific substances, including caffeine, sugar, fat, soy, and complex carbohydrates, ameliorates premenstrual symptoms. Drinking an increased amount of water beginning around 7 to 10 days before menstruation may help to decrease fluid retention.

Complementary Care: *Enhancing comfort with water and other natural diuretics*

Nurses can encourage women with PMS symptoms related to excessive fluid retention to reduce their sodium intake and consume increased amounts of water during the days preceding the expected menses. The water may serve as a natural diuretic and help reduce edema. Foods that may promote a natural diuresis include peaches, parsley, watermelon, asparagus, and cranberry juice.

Vitamins and minerals have also been prescribed to reduce PMS symptoms. Pyridoxine (vitamin B_6), which plays a role in the biosynthesis of neurotransmitters, may be useful in diminishing premenstrual breast pain and depression. Supplementation with vitamin E (alpha-tocopherol) or magnesium may be beneficial in reducing certain PMS symptoms, although stronger evidence exists for the supplementation of calcium and vitamin D. Calcium may be of benefit in reducing PMS symptoms through its interaction with estrogen and parathyroid hormone (Nelson & Baldwin, 2008; Whyte & Peraud, 2009).

 critical nursing action Counseling About Vitamin Supplements

When counseling about vitamin supplements for premenstrual disorders, the nurse must ensure that women understand the dangers of vitamin overdose. Dosages of vitamin B_6 must remain lower than 100 mg/day, as excessive amounts may lead to peripheral neuropathy. Vitamin E supplements should never exceed 400 IU per day; higher amounts are associated with a number of side effects, including diarrhea, flatulence, bloating, weakness, headache, fatigue, abdominal pain, blurred vision, and an increased risk of bleeding.

HERBAL SUPPLEMENTS AND OTHER COMPLEMENTARY AND ALTERNATIVE MEDICINE MODALITIES

Chasteberry (*Vitex agnus-castus*) has been used throughout the ages to treat a variety of conditions. The fruit of the chaste tree, chasteberry is also known as "monk's pepper." Today this herb is used widely in Europe for a variety of gynecological disorders, including PMS, dysfunctional uterine bleeding, and menstrual cycle irregularities. The German Commission E approved the use of chasteberry for irregularities of the menstrual cycle, cyclical breast discomfort, and PMS (Blumenthal, 2000). Native to western Asia and southwestern Europe, chasteberry is now grown in the southeastern United States. It can be prepared as a medicinal tea and is also available as a tincture and in capsule form. Chasteberry is well tolerated; reported adverse effects are infrequent and include gastrointestinal complaints, dizziness, and dry mouth (Roemheld-Hamm, 2005).

Evening primrose oil (*Oenothera biennis*) has been recommended for relief of PMS-related breast tenderness; but to date, clinical trials of this omega-6 essential fatty acid–rich supplement have failed to demonstrate statistically or clinically significant results.

For many women, various nonpharmacological approaches may diminish PMS symptoms. Trials of cognitive behavioral therapy, group therapy, and relaxation therapy have demonstrated improvement in physical and/or psychological symptoms of PMS, although few studies have randomized patients. For some women, other modalities such as massage, yoga, aromatherapy, biofeedback, acupuncture, hypnosis, reflexology, chiropractic, and light therapy may have a beneficial effect on

PMS symptoms (Andolsek & Rapkin, 2006; Nelson & Baldwin, 2008; Whyte & Peraud, 2009).

 ### *Nursing Insight*— *Asian medicine and PMS*

Nurses should recognize that the fundamental healing approach offered in Asian medicine may well be of benefit in diminishing symptoms of PMS. With the Asian perspective, premenstrual syndrome is viewed as an energetic imbalance, a blockage and stagnation of vital energy, or "chi," which normally flows through the body and enlivens it. When an individual's vital energy is blocked in the pelvic region, it can be manifest in many of the symptoms associated with PMS. Asian healing approaches are designed to restore and balance the body energies, thereby allowing the hormonal and nervous systems to return to a harmonious equilibrium.

PHARMACOLOGICAL INTERVENTIONS

If the nonpharmacological approaches fail to provide satisfactory symptom relief in 2 to 3 months, medication is often initiated. There are two major pharmacological strategies to treatment. One targets the central nervous system processes that are believed to contribute to premenstrual mood symptoms; the other approach centers on eliminating the hormonal cyclicity by suppressing ovulation. Pharmacological therapy is reserved for women who qualify as having PMDD or severe manifestations of PMS. The U.S. Food and Drug Administration (FDA) has approved two categories of medications for premenstrual disorders: selective serotonin reuptake inhibitors (SSRIs) and an oral contraceptive that contains the progestin drospirenone (Nelson & Baldwin, 2008; Whyte & Peraud, 2009).

The SSRIs that have received FDA approval for the treatment of PMDD are fluoxetine (Prozac, Sarafem), sertraline (Zoloft), and controlled-release paroxetine (Paxil CR). Currently, these medications constitute the mainstay of medical treatment. They have been studied extensively for the treatment of PMS symptoms, and dosing may be administered on a continuous or intermittent schedule. Luteal-phase dosing should be initiated about 14 days before menses and continued until the onset of menstruation. Use of any of the central nervous system agents for treatment of PMS/PMDD does not contraindicate the use of any hormonal or nonhormonal contraceptive method to prevent pregnancy (Nelson & Baldwin, 2008; Whyte & Peraud, 2009).

 ### Be Sure to— Teach about potential adverse effects associated with SSRIs

Although most patients tolerate SSRIs without difficulty, nurses must make certain that the patient is aware of the following side effects associated with these medications: nausea, nervousness, anxiety, headache, drowsiness, dizziness, impaired concentration, decreased libido, and insomnia. The risk of side effects is dose related—lower doses, which often suffice for the symptoms of PMS—are associated with fewer side effects. Also, limiting dosing days to the luteal phase of the cycle has also been shown

to be effective in PMS/PMDD. Teaching women about their specific medications is an important step in helping them to understand their diagnosis and the rationale for the prescribed pharmacological treatment (Deglin & Vallerand, 2009; Nelson & Baldwin, 2008; Whyte & Peraud, 2009).

Spironolactone (Aldactone), a potassium-sparing diuretic, is another nonhormonal medication that has been shown to be beneficial in the treatment of PMS. Administered in a dosage of 25 mg two to four times a day during the luteal phase, this agent reduces bloating and improves mood in many patients. However, it should be noted that use in PMS management is considered to be off-label (Nelson & Baldwin, 2008).

Ovulation suppressants may be beneficial in the treatment of PMS. Although oral contraceptive pills (OCPs) have been used to treat premenstrual symptoms, most clinical trials have not demonstrated any efficacy in this approach. For some women, however, extended-cycle dosing of continuous OCPs or regular administration of Depo-Provera may be useful in providing symptom relief—these agents suppress ovulation and reduce the number of withdrawal bleeding episodes (and associated symptoms) experienced each year (Nelson & Baldwin, 2008).

The FDA has approved one oral contraceptive for the treatment of PMDD in women who desire contraception. Marketed under the trade name Yasmin, this medication contains ethinyl estradiol and drospirenone, a novel progestin. Yasmin is administered for 24 days and followed by a 4-day hormone-free interval. Clinical trials with this medication demonstrated significant improvement in physical, psychological, and behavioral symptoms of PMS/PMDD (Pearlstein, Bachmann, Zacur, & Yonkers, 2005; Yonkers et al., 2005).

 ### case study Patient with Premenstrual Syndrome

Cassandra Burney is a 29-year-old primigravida who visits the women's health clinic for an evaluation of bothersome premenstrual symptoms. Presently, Cassandra is not sexually active, but she has a diaphragm for birth control and is pleased with her contraceptive method. Her menstrual periods are regular, occur every 28 to 30 days, are moderate in flow, and last 6 to 7 days. Cassandra tells the nurse that each month beginning approximately 1 week before the onset of menstrual flow, she experiences painful, tender, swollen breasts; bloating; weight gain; and feelings of "being down" and irritable.

critical thinking questions

1. What additional information is needed to help confirm the diagnosis of PMS?

2. What can the nurse teach Cassandra about PMS and self-care strategies that may help to minimize her symptoms?

◆ See Suggested Answers to Case Study at the end of this chapter.

Now Can You— Discuss nursing care for patients with premenstrual disorders?

1. Describe the nurse's major role when caring for a patient with a premenstrual disorder?
2. Discuss various nonpharmacological therapies for premenstrual disorders?
3. Discuss various pharmacological therapies for premenstrual disorders?

summary points

◆ Premenstrual syndrome may be viewed as a complex constellation of genetic influences and hormonal imbalances that adversely affects a woman's physical, mental, and emotional health.

◆ Women have reported over 100 different physical and behavioral symptoms during the premenstrual period.

◆ The cause of PMS is believed to be multifactorial.

◆ To meet the criteria for PMS, the woman's symptoms must occur cyclically, be unrelated to any physical or mental condition, and greatly disrupt one or more areas of the woman's life

◆ The diagnostic workup for a premenstrual disorder includes the patient history, a physical examination, appropriate laboratory tests, and review of the daily symptom diary.

◆ Management of premenstrual syndrome may include nonpharmacological and pharmacological approaches.

◆ Nurses are instrumental in helping women to deal with premenstrual disorders by offering ongoing education and support.

review questions

Multiple Choice

1. In earlier times, premenstrual syndrome was thought to be related to:
   A. The patient's emotional makeup
   B. Pregnancy
   C. Insanity
   D. Tobacco use

2. One of the criteria for the diagnosis of premenstrual syndrome is that the symptoms:
   A. Occur during the menstrual phase of the uterine cycle
   B. Persist for 25 or more days
   C. Are not caused by any underlying physical or mental condition
   D. Occur during the proliferative phase of the uterine cycle

3. Most women with PMS experience relief of symptoms:
   A. During the luteal phase of the uterine cycle
   B. Within 24 hours following the onset of menstrual flow
   C. Around the time of ovulation
   D. Following removal of the uterus (hysterectomy)

4. An important component in the diagnostic workup for PMS involves:
   A. Obtaining serum levels of iron and prolactin
   B. Evaluating the basal body temperature
   C. Assessing the urine for glucose, protein, and ketones
   D. Evaluating the daily symptom diary

5. The nurse teaches the woman with PMS about self-help strategies to help diminish symptoms. For example, the nurse may suggest:
   A. Decreasing physical activity approximately 1 week before expected menses
   B. Decreasing the intake of water approximately 5 to 7 days before menstruation
   C. Taking evening primrose oil during the menstrual period
   D. Engaging in relaxation techniques and stress-relief therapies such as massage and yoga

REFERENCES

American College of Obstetricians and Gynecologists (ACOG). (2000). *Premenstrual syndrome* (ACOG Practice Bulletin No. 15). Washington, DC: Author

American College of Obstetricians and Gynecologists (ACOG). (2007). *Women's health care: A resource manual* (3rd ed.). Washington, DC: Author.

American Psychiatric Association (APA). (2000). *Diagnostic and statistical manual of mental disorders* (4th ed., text revision). Washington, DC: American Psychiatric Association Press.

Andolsek, K. M., & Rapkin, A. J. (2006). Contraceptive use in women with premenstrual disorders. *Dialogues in Contraception, 10*(4), 4–7.

Arrowsmith, F. M. (2007). Preventing the cycle of migraine: A review of patient issues for NPs. *American Journal for Nurse Practitioners, 11*(8), 42–54.

Association of Women's Health, Obstetrical and Neonatal Nurses. (2003). *Evidence-based practice guideline: Nursing management for cyclic perimenstrual pain and discomfort.* Washington, DC: Author.

Blumenthal, M. (2000). *German Federal Institute for Drugs and Medical Devices. Commission E Herbal Medicine: Expanded commission E monographs.* Newton, MA: Integrative Medicine Communications.

Borenstein, J. E., Dean, B. B., Endicott, J., Wong, J., Brown, C., Dickerson, V., & Yonkers, K. A. (2003). Health and economic impact of the premenstrual syndrome. *Journal of Reproductive Medicine, 48*(7), 515–24.

Clayton, A. H., Keller, A. E., Leslie, C., & Evans, W. (2006). Exploratory study of premenstrual symptoms and serotonin variability. *Archives of Women's Mental Health, 9*(1), 51–57.

Collins Sharp, B. A., Taylor, D. L., Thomas, K. K., Killeen, M. B., & Dawood, M. Y. (2002). Perimenstrual pain and discomfort: The scientific basis for practice. *Journal of Obstetric, Gynecologic, and Neonatal Nursing, 31*(6), 637–649.

Deglin, J. H., & Vallerand, A. H. (2009). *Davis's drug guide for nurses* (11th ed.). Philadelphia: F. A. Davis.

Dickerson, V. M. (2007). Premenstrual syndrome and premenstrual dysphoric disorder: Individualizing therapy. *Female Patient, 32*(1), 38–46.

Endicott, J., Nee, J., & Harrison, W. (2006). Daily record of severity of problems (DRSP): Reliability and validity. *Archives of Women's Mental Health, 9*(1), 41–49.

Freeman, E. W., DeRubeis, R. J., & Rickels, K. (1996). Reliability and validity of a daily diary for premenstrual syndrome. *Psychiatry Research, 65*(2), 97–106.

Halbreich, U. (2003). The etiology, biology, and evolving pathology of premenstrual syndromes. *Psychoneuroendocrinology, 28*(suppl. 3), 55–99.

Nelson, A. L., & Baldwin, S. (2008). Menstrual disorders and related concerns. In R. Hatcher, J. Trussell, A. Nelson, W. Cates Jr., F. Stewart, & D. Kowal (Eds.), *Contraceptive technology* (19th ed., pp. 469–476). New York: Thomson Reuters.

Pearlstein, T. B., Bachmann, G. A., Zacur, H. A., & Yonkers, K.A. (2005). Treatment of premenstrual dysphoric disorder with a new drospirenone-containing oral contraceptive formulation. *Contraception, 72*(5), 414–421.

Polaneczky, M. (2007). Premenstrual syndrome/premenstrual dysphoric disorder. *Female Patient, 32*(9), 40–45.

Roemheld-Hamm, B. (2005). Chasteberry. *American Family Physician, 72*(5), 821–824.

Speroff, L., & Fritz, M. A. (2005). *Clinical gynecologic endocrinology and infertility* (7th ed.). Philadelphia: Lippincott Williams & Wilkins.

Steiner, M., Macdougall, M., & Brown, E. (2003). The premenstrual symptoms screening tool (PSST) for clinicians. *Archives of Women's Mental Health, 6*(3), 203–209.

Taylor, D., Schuiling, K. D., & Sharp, B. A. (2005). Menstrual cycle pain and discomforts. In K. D. Schuiling & F. Liskis (Eds.), *Women's gynecologic health* (pp. 474–500). Sudbury, MA: Jones & Bartlett.

U.S. Department of Health and Human Services. (2008). *Physical activity guidelines for Americans: 2008 activity guidelines for Americans summary.* Retrieved September 1, 2009, from http://www.health.gov/paguidelines/guidelines/summary.aspx

Whyte, J., & Peraud, P. (2009). Premenstrual disorders: A primary care primer. *Consultant, 49*(1), 15–24.

Yonkers, K. A., Brown, C., Pearlstein, T. B., Foegh, M., Sampson-Landers, C., & Rapkin, A. (2005). Efficacy of a new low-dose contraceptive with drospirenone in premenstrual dysphoric disorder. *Obstetrics & Gynecology, 106*(3), 492–501.

suggested answers to case study

1. It is important that the nurse determine the timing and duration of Cassandra's symptoms in order to establish that they are consistent with premenstrual syndrome. To meet the criteria for PMS, the symptoms must occur during the luteal phase of the menstrual cycle and resolve within 4 days after the onset of menstrual flow. Although the patient states that her symptoms occur cyclically, it is important to document this information. The nurse teaches Cassandra how to use a symptom diary to record her premenstrual symptoms each day, note their severity, and record the dates of her menstrual period. Cassandra is asked to bring the diary with her when she returns to the clinic for an evaluation in 3 months.

2. The nurse teaches Cassandra about the relationship between normal cyclic hormonal variations and accompanying physiological changes. This information serves to validate the patient's experience with her monthly discomforts and acknowledges that the symptoms are real and have a physiological base. The information also increases Cassandra's understanding about premenstrual disorders and promotes a greater sense of control over her situation. The nurse counsels Cassandra to wear a supportive bra to minimize breast tenderness. Other self-care strategies are centered on facilitating fluid excretion: limiting the intake of salt- and sodium-containing foods and increasing the consumption of water and other natural diuretic foods such as watermelon, cranberry juice, peaches, asparagus, and parsley approximately 7–10 days before the menstrual period is expected. The nurse can also suggest that Cassandra engage in stress-reduction techniques (e.g., exercise, yoga, meditation, massage therapy) in anticipation of the cyclical hormonal changes each month and participate in a PMS support group, if available.

 For more information, go to http://davisplus.fadavis.com/

Promoting Breast Health

Shelton M. Hisley, PhD, RNC, WHNP-BC

3

 Life begins each morning . . .
Each morning is the open door to a new world—new vistas, new aims, new tryings.

—Leigh Hodges

LEARNING TARGETS *At the completion of this chapter, the student will be able to:*

◆ Describe normal breast anatomy.

◆ Teach a patient how to perform breast self-examination.

◆ Differentiate among various breast abnormalities.

◆ Discuss diagnostic modalities and treatment options for breast cancer.

◆ Describe the nurse's role in promoting breast health.

Introduction

This chapter discusses the promotion of breast health in women. Most concerns about breast care and problems are first voiced in the primary care setting. Nurses who work with women are in an ideal position to educate about the importance of breast health awareness and suggest strategies to promote the early identification of benign and malignant breast disease. As is true with other types of cancers, early detection is key in the successful treatment of breast cancer. Most experts agree that breast cancer is not a singular disease. Instead, it is believed that malignancies of the breast stem from many types of disease, each with distinct histological, biological, and immunological characteristics. A myriad of dietary, socioeconomic, and environmental factors most likely serve as causative or contributing influences in the development of breast cancer. Breast health is an important issue for women; maintaining breast health is an essential strategy for maintaining optimal physical and psychological health.

⬡ Optimizing Outcomes— A holistic approach to breast care

Owing to the likelihood that multiple factors play a role in the development of breast cancer, nurses can embrace a holistic approach to women's health care that is centered on health promotion. This strategy focuses on individualized patient education and counseling concerning diet, lifestyle habits, and environmental exposure—all aspects of health over which individuals have control. The general health benefits of these types of changes have been proven in terms of improved quality of life. Prevention strategies such as these, when combined with early detection, empower women with knowledge and heightened awareness of the normal workings of their bodies and equips them with tools for self-care. The nurse's involvement in patient education and awareness of breast health constitutes an essential action for helping the nation to achieve an extremely important Healthy People 2010 goal: Reduce breast cancer deaths to no more than 20.6 per 100,000 women from a baseline of 23 per 100,000 (USDHHS, 2000).

Benign and Malignant Breast Diseases: The Scope of the Problem

Fibrocystic breast changes, also known as benign breast disease (BBD), are believed to occur in over 50% of women. Benign breast conditions include cysts, tumors, masses, nipple discharge, infection, and inflammation of the ducts. Although not malignant, the discovery of a benign breast mass may evoke feelings of fear, anxiety, and vulnerability and trigger worry about the future. And women have cause for concern, as research has shown that some types of BBD are an important risk factor for the later development of breast cancer (Hartman, Sellers, & Frost et al., 2005; Lee, 2009).

Breast cancer is the most common cancer in women in the United States, except for skin cancer, and it is the second leading cause of cancer deaths in women (American

Cancer Society [ACS], 2009a; Smith, 2007). The American Cancer Society predicts that in 2009, an estimated 192,370 new cases of invasive breast cancer will be diagnosed, and there will be 40,170 deaths from breast cancer. Presently, the chance of a woman developing invasive breast cancer at some time during her life is approximately 1 in 8 (12%). The chance of dying from breast cancer is around 1 in 35 (3%). Women who live in North America have the highest rate of breast cancer in the world. To gain a perspective on the magnitude of the problem, nurses can reflect on the fact that approximately 2.5 million breast cancer survivors are living in the United States today (ACS, 2009a).

 Nursing Insight— Breast cancer among American women

Besides skin cancer, breast cancer is the most commonly diagnosed cancer among women in the United States. More than 1 in 4 cancers are breast cancer. From 2001 to 2004, the incidence of breast cancer in this country decreased by 3.5% per year. One theory regarding this decrease centers on the reduced use of hormone therapy by women after the results of the Women's Health Initiative were published in 2002. These results suggest a correlation between hormone therapy and increased breast cancer risk (ACS, 2009a; BreastCancer.org, 2008). Women of different ages have different risks of breast cancer. A woman's risk increases with age until she reaches menopause; breast cancer risk then increases more slowly with the advancing years.

Anatomy of the Breast

To enhance an understanding of the breast, it is helpful to review normal breast anatomy. The female breasts, or mammary glands, are considered to be accessory organs of the reproductive system. The two breasts lie over the pectoral and anterior serratus muscles. Breast tissue, which consists primarily of glandular, fibrous, and adipose tissue suspended within the conical-shaped breasts by Cooper's ligaments, is richly supplied with a dense network of blood vessels and lymph vessels (Fig. 3-1).

A & P review **Components of the Breast**

The glandular tissue contains 15 to 24 lobes that are separated by fibrous and adipose tissue. Each lobe contains several lobules composed of numerous alveoli clustered around tiny ducts that are layered with secretory cuboidal epithelium called alveoli or acini (Fig. 3-2).

The epithelial lining of the ducts secretes various components of milk. The ducts from several lobules come together to form the lactiferous ducts, which are larger ducts that open on the surface of the nipple. The lymphatic vessels carry lymph, an alkaline, clear, colorless tissue fluid, away from the breast. Most of the lymph vessels of the breast lead to the nodes in the axillae. The lymph nodes are small, kidney-shaped organs of lymphoid tissue (Fig. 3-3). An increase in the size of the node (lymphadenopathy) indicates a high level of activity (e.g., infection or cancer).

Outer parts of the breasts include the nipples, areolae, and Montgomery tubercles. The nipples contain several pores that secrete colostrum (breast fluid that precedes breast milk) and breast milk during lactation. The nipples consist primarily of erectile tissue to assist with infant

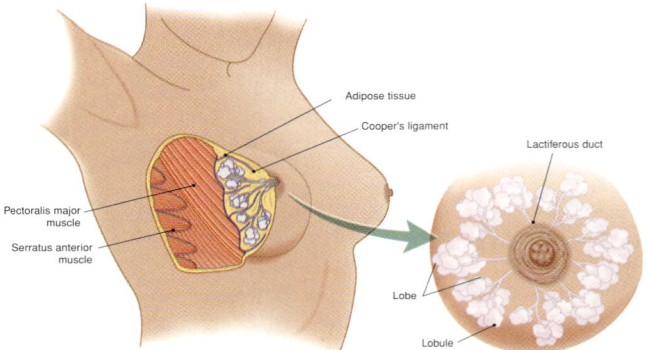

Figure 3-2 Cross section of breast; note lobe and lobule shown in detailed area

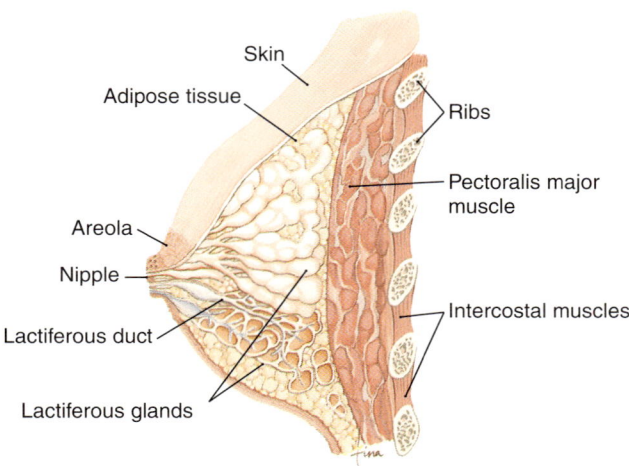

Figure 3-1 Mammary gland shown in a midsagittal section

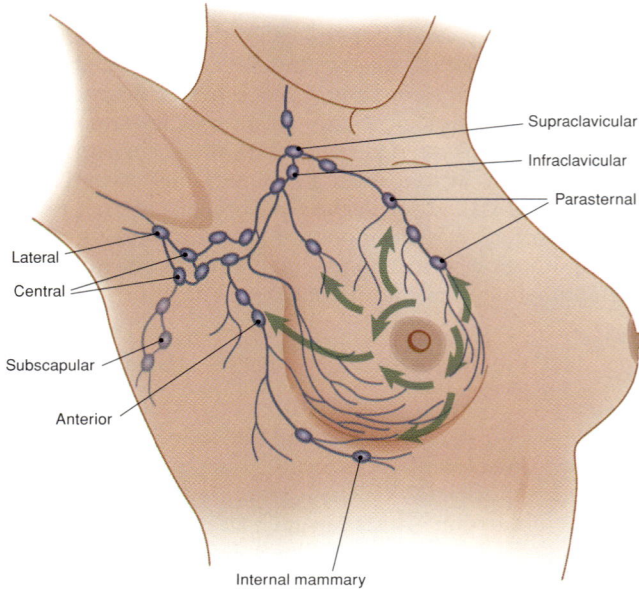

Figure 3-3 Lymph nodes

latch-on during suckling. The areola is a more deeply pigmented area that surrounds the nipple. Its diameter ranges from 1 to 3.9 inches (2.5 to 10 cm). The Montgomery tubercles are papillae located on the surface of the nipple and the areola; they secrete a fatty substance that lubricates and protects the nipple and areola during breastfeeding.

The primary function of the breasts is to provide nutrition to offspring through the process known as lactation. In American culture, the breasts are also closely linked with "womanhood." Many equate large breasts with increased sexiness and eroticism. Because the breasts serve as a source of sensual pleasure for both men and women, injury to or the loss of a breast can trigger major psychological distress for both genders.

The Nurse's Role in Teaching About Breast Health

The promotion of breast health encompasses several areas, including cancer screening, optimal nutrition, and physical activity. It is important for nurses to educate women throughout the life span about strategies for promoting breast health. Personal awareness of the normal appearance and feel of the breasts constitutes an essential first step in promoting and maintaining breast health. Nurses working with women in a variety of settings are perfectly situated to offer information about strategies for promoting breast health and for performing self-examinations. By providing information in a nonthreatening, therapeutic environment, nurses can help to allay women's fears and present self-examination as a positive, empowering experience.

"What to say" — *Teaching about breast health*

During a discussion about breast health, the nurse may wish to include the following information:

- As you age, your breasts experience loss of milk glands and shrinkage of collagen. This causes an increase in the fat tissue and loosening of the breast tissue. Instead of getting larger with the increase in fat tissue, however, the breast tissue begins to sag, causing the breasts to drop.
- Breast tissue weighs less than most people think: an A-cup weighs ¼ lb, a B-cup weighs ½ lb, a C-cup weighs ¾ lb, and a D-cup weighs about 1 lb.
- The skin covering the breasts stretches as you grow, causing the skin to become thinner than the skin on other parts of the body.
- It is not uncommon for women to have some degree of hair surrounding their nipples. The darker the skin, the more hair there is likely to be.
- A woman's nipples may be different sizes and may be placed in slightly different locations on each breast. This may cause the nipples to point in different directions, which is considered a normal finding.
- Fluctuating hormone levels during the monthly cycle cause changes in breast tissue. Following menstruation, when hormone levels are at their lowest, the breast tissue is smooth and nontender.

As estrogen levels increase at mid-cycle, the breasts may become more sensitive. Also, just before menstruation, when progesterone is elevated, many women's breasts become swollen and tender, with palpable nodules.

- Ideally, your health-care provider should perform your clinical breast examination 1 week following menstruation, when the breast tissue is nontender and smooth.
- Breast implants still pose health risks, including deflation, leakage, and wrinkling. In addition, capsular contraction can occur, causing the scar tissue surrounding the implant to tighten and the breast to become hard.
- The area between the breasts has several oil and sweat glands, creating an atmosphere conducive to the growth of bacteria.
- Sleeping on your side, with a pillow to support your breasts, provides the best position for maintaining breast shape and contour over time.
- Regular exercise can strengthen the pectoral muscles, reducing sagging over time and creating a natural lift.
- It is not uncommon to have a third nipple, stemming from breast buds that form during early fetal development. These extra nipples, however, rarely contain milk glands.
- Pregnancy darkens the color of the nipple, which is an enhancement for the breastfeeding baby. This darker color does not disappear after pregnancy.
- The left breast is usually larger then the right breast.
- Breasts do not reach their full size until the early 20s.

LIFESTYLE CHOICES AND BREAST HEALTH

Lifestyle choices, including moderate alcohol consumption, weight maintenance, and avoidance of smoking can affect breast health as well. Alcohol consumption is known to be associated with an increased risk of breast cancer. The American Cancer Society (2009b) recommends limiting alcohol intake to one drink per day. The risk of breast cancer is increased 1.5 times in women who consume two to five drinks per day.

Routine exercise, which helps to maintain a healthy weight, is associated with a decreased risk of breast cancer. Maintenance of a healthy weight is recommended for optimum breast health. Obesity is associated with an increased risk of breast cancer, particularly in postmenopausal women. Following menopause, estrogen is produced in the fat cells. In combination with dietary fat, estrogen significantly increases the likelihood of breast cancer development. Smoking is associated with an increased risk of breast cancer, lung cancer and heart disease in women.

 Now Can You— **Discuss breast health promotion?**

1. Describe normal breast anatomy?
2. Discuss the nurse's role in teaching about breast health?
3. Develop an educational program that includes essential information about the breasts?

Breast Awareness and Cancer Screening

Breast self-examination (BSE), clinical breast exams, and mammography (x-ray filming of the breasts) can assist in early detection and early treatment (Fig. 3-4). The initiation and frequency of mammography depends on the woman's age and risk factors. Magnetic resonance imaging (MRI) (a noninvasive nuclear procedure for imaging tissues with high fat and water content) appears to be especially useful in detecting tumors in women with an inherited susceptibility to breast cancer, and recent findings suggest that this diagnostic method can detect cancer in the contralateral breast that was missed by mammography in women with recently diagnosed breast cancer (Lehman, Gastonis, Kuhl, Hendrick, Pisano, Hanna, Peacock, et al., 2007). As a screening tool, MRI may be useful for women with breast implants in whom mammography is difficult or to determine the integrity of the implants. It has been demonstrated that breast MRI is most effective for identifying tissue with increased blood flow, such as neoplastic tumors. However, breast MRI is not a substitute for a mammogram and it should not be used for routine screening of the average-risk woman. Limitations associated with this diagnostic modality include the expense, the limited specificity, and false-positive results (Aliotta & Schaeffer, 2006; Bleicher, Ciocca, Egleston, Sesa, Evers, Sigurdson, & Morrow, 2009; Smith, 2007).

 Optimizing Outcomes— Screening for breast cancer

Best outcome: Monthly breast-self examination, annual clinical breast examinations, and routine mammography allow women and their health-care providers to detect potentially cancerous tumors at the earliest stage possible. This multi-pronged screening approach facilitates early diagnosis and early treatment, providing the best outcome possible.

Ethnocultural Considerations . . . Breast Cancer Screening

There are notable differences in breast cancer screening practices among women of different ethnic backgrounds. Although African American women are at a lower risk for developing breast cancer than Caucasian women, they are more likely to die from breast cancer due to late diagnosis. According to Husaini and associates (2001), African American women are more likely to have mammogram screening if they are older, married, have a higher level of education, and believe that early detection could lead to a cure. A positive family history of breast cancer and church affiliation have no influence on the incidence of detection.

Asian American and Pacific Islander women have very low rates of breast cancer screening. Factors responsible for the low screening rates include lack of health insurance, low income, and lack of a primary-care provider (Kagawa-Singer & Pourat, 2000).

Breast cancer causes a significant number of deaths in Filipino women. In a study by Wu and Bancroft (2006), researchers found that women were more likely to follow recommended screenings if there is support from physicians and family members, and if they had insurance. In addition, the presence of physical symptoms, family history of breast cancer, and health literacy promote adherence to recommendations.

BREAST SELF-EXAMINATION

Familiarization with one's breasts facilitates the early detection of problems and allows for prompt evaluation. Breast self-examination is a way for women to learn how their breasts normally feel. Routinely performing BSE is an approach that focuses on the importance of self-awareness and helps women to notice changes in breast tissue (ACS, 2009a). When teaching women about breast self-examination, the nurse can display pictures of breast tissue and discuss the normal irregular contours of breasts. Breast models are also helpful and allow women to feel normal and abnormal masses; these teaching aides may be beneficial in diminishing women's fears about checking their own breasts. Since menstruating women often experience increased discomfort and lumpiness in their breasts during the second half of the menstrual cycle, the ideal time to perform BSE is during the week after menstruation.

Routinely performing BSE helps women to perfect their technique and become familiar with the contours and tissue characteristics unique to their own breasts. Then, if they detect changes that are worrisome to them or that persist, they can schedule an evaluation (Smith, 2007). Nurses can be instrumental in facilitating women's awareness of and comfort with detecting changes in their breasts (Ruhl, 2007).

Breast self-examination is a simple yet powerful self-help behavior that can save lives. Over 75% of breast cancers are discovered by women themselves. The current procedure for performing BSE differs from previous recommendations endorsed by the American Cancer Society. The changes in technique represent an extensive review of the medical literature and input from an expert medical advisory group (ACS, 2008). Despite the advantages of performing BSE, it should be noted that according to the latest (2009) statement from the U.S. Preventive Services Task Force (USPSTF), insufficient evidence was found to recommend for or against teaching or performing routine breast self-examination (http://www.ahrq.gov/clinic/pocketgd09/gcp09s2.htm).

Figure 3-4 Mammogram

Family Teaching Guidelines...
Breast Self-Examination

1. Visually inspect the breasts in front of a mirror. Assess for color, contour, shape, and size. Assess for dimpling or puckering of the skin; change in nipple direction; and redness, rash, or swelling (Fig. 3-5).

2. Repeat first step with the arms slightly raised above the head (Fig. 3-6).

3. Inspect and palpate the nipple. Gently squeeze the nipple between the thumb and forefinger, looking for discharge. Many women, especially those who have had children, are able to express some discharge by squeezing the nipples. Discharge that is of concern is most often spontaneous (ACS, 2008) (Fig. 3-7).

4. Palpate the breast and axillae. Recline on the bed and place a pillow under each shoulder during palpation. Use the left hand to palpate the right breast, and the right hand to palpate the left breast. Using the finger pads of the three middle fingers, palpate the entire surface of the breast. Use overlapping dime-sized

circular motions and apply three different levels of pressure: *light pressure* is best to feel the tissue closest to the skin; *medium pressure* is best to feel a little deeper; and *firm pressure* is used to feel the tissue closest to the chest and ribs (Fig. 3-8).

5. Move around the breast in an up and down pattern, checking the entire breast area until only the ribs are felt; repeat the entire technique on the opposite breast (ACS, 2008)./ftgnl.

The American Cancer Society endorses "breast awareness." Breast awareness, or being aware of how the breasts normally look and feel, may be achieved by feeling the breasts for changes or by using a step-by-step approach (BSE) on a specific schedule (e.g., after menses when the breasts are not tender or swollen) (ACS, 2009a). According to the American College of Obstetricians and Gynecologists (ACOG), despite a lack of definitive data for or against BSE, the technique has the potential to detect palpable breast cancer and can be recommended (ACOG, 2007).

🌼 *Nursing Insight*— *Breast implants and BSE*

If they choose to do so, women with breast implants may perform BSE. Following surgery, it may be helpful for the surgeon to guide BSE teaching by identifying the edges of the implant to enhance the patient's understanding of the new contours of her breasts. For some, the increased prominence of the breast tissue following implant surgery may make it easier to perform the examination. Women who are pregnant or breastfeeding may also choose to examine their breasts regularly (ACS, 2009b).

CLINICAL BREAST EXAMINATIONS

Annual clinical breast examinations (CBE) performed by a trained health-care professional are an important tool in the early detection of breast cancer. Inflammatory breast cancer, a rare and aggressive type that may cause swelling and redness, often does not show up on mammography. Also, the clinical breast examination provides an opportunity for the clinician to reinforce a woman's self-examination technique, discuss concerns, and emphasize the value in becoming intimately familiar with the contour of one's own breasts.

All women should have a clinical breast examination performed at recommended intervals by a skilled health-care provider. The clinical breast examination should be performed at least every 3 years for women aged 18 to 39, and every year after age 40. According to the American Cancer Society (2009c), the clinical breast examination serves as a complement to mammography, and there may be some benefit in having the CBE performed shortly before the mammogram. It is important for nurses to provide information about the benefits and limitations of the CBE, as well as BSE (ACOG, 2007; ACS, 2009c).

MAMMOGRAPHY

A mammography examination is used to aid in the early diagnosis of breast cancer (Fig. 3-9). The examination, which requires exposure to small doses of ionizing radiation, allows for identification of small breast tissue abnormalities that may require further investigation. In recent times, two enhancements have been made to traditional mammography techniques: digital mammography and computer-aided detection (CAD). Digital mammography, also called full-field digital mammography (FFDM), converts the x-rays to electrical signals, similar to those found in digital cameras. These signals produce images that can be viewed on a computer screen or printed on special film. The images are stored for future comparison. Digital mammography provides improved screening for women determined to be at high risk for developing breast cancer (Pisano et al., 2005). This latest technology is enhanced with the use of computer software that highlights areas of increased density, masses, and calcifications.

 Nursing Insight— *Calcium deposits within breast tissue*

Calcifications (calcium deposits) detected on mammography may be identified as *macrocalcifications* or as *microcalcifications*. Macrocalcifications, degenerative changes resulting from old trauma, inflammation, or aging of the breast arteries, occur in approximately one-half of women in the United States who are over age 50 and are usually not related to malignancy. Microcalcifications are small specks of calcium that may be present as "residue" in areas of rapidly dividing cells (e.g., a neoplasm). A cluster of microcalcifications may be indicative of a small cancer.

Figure 3-9 Mammography showing breast cancer

Screening mammography is beneficial as routine breast surveillance for the asymptomatic woman. Clinical detection through the use of breast self-examination generally does not occur until the tumor approximates the size of a walnut. By the time a palpable mass or lump is detected, the tumor most likely has been growing for some time. Hence, routine screening mammograms provide a much earlier, high-sensitivity study of developing tumors at the lowest possible cost. In addition, a screening mammogram enables the radiologist to identify changes such as calcifications that may point to malignancy (Smith, 2007).

 Nursing Insight— *Differentiating between screening mammography and diagnostic mammography*

Screening mammograms are performed to check for breast cancer in women who have no signs or symptoms of the disease. They usually involve two x-rays of each breast. *Diagnostic* mammograms are performed to check for breast cancer after a lump or other sign or symptom of breast cancer has been detected. They may also be used to evaluate changes discovered during a screening mammogram or to view breast tissue when it is difficult to obtain a screening mammogram because of special circumstances, such as the presence of breast implants. Diagnostic mammography takes longer to perform because more x-rays are taken to obtain views of the breast from several angles (National Cancer Institute [NCI], 2009a).

The value of routine screening mammography for women age 50 and older has been well established. Recommendations for mammography screening in women ages 40 to 49 have been met with some controversy. Analysis of the major studies of women in this age group has shown a marginal benefit in decreasing the death rate from breast cancer. However, it should be noted that:

- Findings from older studies may be flawed because mammography was much cruder 30 years ago.
- Breast cancer in women ages 40 to 49 occurs with less frequency.
- Mammography in premenopausal women historically has not been as accurate owing to the density of breast tissue in women in this age group, as compared with breast tissue in postmenopausal women. Mammography may miss as many as 25% of invasive cancers in women ages 40 to 49 years, as compared with 10% in women age 50 years and older.
- Certain tumors, even when detected early, are not curable. In general, younger women tend to have more rapidly growing tumors than do older women. This finding may be related to the higher levels of estrogen in the blood and tissues of premenopausal women that can stimulate tumor growth or a genetic predisposition that becomes expressed in this age group (Smith, 2007).

In 2002, the U.S. Preventive Services Task Force (USPSTF) issued a recommendation that women undergo screening mammography every 1 to 2 years, beginning at age 40. Guidelines from the American College of

Obstetricians and Gynecologists, the American Medical Association, and the American Academy of Family Physicians are similar, with annual mammography recommended after age 50 (Smith, 2007). Presently, the American Cancer Society recommends that women age 40 and older receive yearly mammograms in addition to clinical breast examinations, and they should continue to perform breast self-examination monthly (ACS, 2009d).

In November 2009, the USPSTF issued new breast cancer screening recommendations for the general population. Based on evidence review, the updated guidelines recommend against routine mammography screening for women before age 50 years, suggest that screening end at age 74 years, and recommend changing the screening interval from 1 year to 2 years. Several professional organizations have voiced their objections to the new recommendations. The American Cancer Society, the American College of Radiology, the American College of Obstetricians and Gynecologists, and several other expert groups recommend that clinicians and patients continue to follow the earlier guidelines (Barclay, 2009; USPSTF, 2009).

Since mammography is considered a less useful screening and diagnostic tool in women younger than age 40, the health-care provider must determine the use of mammography in this patient population on an individual basis. When compared with film mammography, full-field digital mammography has been determined to be more accurate, especially for women younger than age 50, those with dense breast tissue, and those who are premenopausal or perimenopausal (Pisano et al., 2005; Smith, 2007).

Optimizing Outcomes— **Recognizing mammography barriers to enhance counseling and empower women**

Women may be reluctant to obtain a mammogram for a number of reasons, including a fear of pain associated with the test and a fear of the test findings. Other barriers to breast cancer screening include older age, cultural patterns and health beliefs, lack of knowledge and information, lack of motivation, expense, lack of availability of mammography services, lack of physician referral, lack of health-related social support, cancer fatalism, and the presence of disabilities (Barr, Giannotti, Van Hoof, Mongoven, & Curry, 2008; Farmer, Reddick, D'Agostino, & Jackson, 2007; Kang, Thomas, Kwon, Hyun, & Jun, 2008; Kim & Kim, 2008; Makuc, Breen, Meissner, Vernon, & Cohen, 2007; Wang, Mandelblatt, Liang, Ma, & Schwartz, 2009; Young & Severson, 2005). Nurses can empower women by providing factual information, by addressing specific concerns, and by working with other professionals to help remove barriers to screening. Compliance with mammography guidelines may be improved by strategies such as reminder postcards or telephone calls and direct health-care provider referrals.

"What to say" — *Preparing for a mammogram*

Nurses can counsel women about strategies to enhance mammography results and minimize discomfort associated with the procedure. For example, the nurse can provide the following information:

- Choose a mammography facility that is accredited by the American College of Radiology; ensure that the mammogram is performed by a registered technologist and that the radiologist is trained specifically to interpret mammography.
- Remove powder, deodorant, and perfume prior to the mammogram (these substances may create shadows).
- Schedule the mammogram when the breasts are less tender (e.g., after the menstrual period).
- Ask for the use of a soft pad to cushion the breasts during mammography compression.
- Take acetaminophen, ibuprofen, or aspirin as needed for relief of discomfort.

BREAST TOMOSYNTHESIS: A NEW TOOL FOR BREAST CANCER SCREENING

Mammography, which produces a two-dimensional x-ray image of the breast, is the traditional first-choice modality for the early detection of breast cancer. However, mammography interpretation, especially in women with dense, fibroglandular breasts, has inherent limitations. With a standard mammogram, normal breast structures are superimposed on each other, creating an overlapping image that may mimic or mask a lesion and lead to false-positive or false-negative findings. Tomosynthesis, available in some research settings, is a new advancement in breast imaging. This modality produces breast views in numerous thin slices, providing a three-dimensional image (and better visualization) of breast tissue. Similar to mammography, the breast is compressed with the tomosynthesis technique and the total radiation dose is comparable to the dose of a single-view mammogram. Research is presently underway to determine the clinical utility, guidelines, applications, and cost-effectiveness of this innovative, new diagnostic tool (Buzek, 2009; Diekmann & Bick, 2007; Rafferty, 2004; Rafferty, 2007).

where research and practice meet: **Cultural Barriers Toward Mammography Screening**

Kang and associates (2008) explored Korean women's attitudes toward and barriers to mammography screening. The women's beliefs that an absence of symptoms meant there was no need for a breast examination constituted a major finding of the study. Other variables that were identified as barriers to screening included a lack of information and fear about x-rays and test results and fear of discomfort and pain. Other researchers (Wang et al., 2009) investigated the role of knowledge, culture, and attitude as barriers to mammography screening among immigrant Chinese women. Study findings revealed that women who were least likely to obtain mammography were recent immigrants and those with a low income, limited English ability, and lacking regular sources of health care. Findings from both studies underscore the importance of culturally sensitive education and counseling to improve the use of mammography screening services among women of varying ethnic backgrounds.

Now Can You— Discuss methods of breast awareness
and cancer screening?

1. Explain what is meant by the term "breast awareness" and
   identify the recommended guidelines for clinical breast
   examinations and screening mammography?

2. Teach a patient the proper procedure for breast self-
   examination?

3. Explain how to prepare for a mammogram?

Benign Breast Masses

It has been estimated that at some time during adulthood, 50% of women will experience a breast problem.
Fortunately, most breast tumors are benign. Breast cysts
are a common finding; they may be fluid-filled or solid.
Fluid-filled cysts, also termed "**fibrocystic changes**," are
often tender and fluctuate in size with the menstrual
cycle. These changes are the most common benign breast
condition and occur most often during the childbearing
years. Although the cause is unknown, an imbalance of
estrogen and progesterone may play a role in the development of fluid-filled breast masses. It is believed that
fibrocystic changes in the breasts are exacerbated by caffeine intake. Therapeutic interventions involve differentiating between fibrocystic changes and breast cancer.
Screening methods include clinical breast examinations,
mammography, and ultrasonography. The physician may
choose to aspirate fluid-filled cysts for evaluation to
determine if malignant cells are present. Patients should
be advised that although aspiration may eliminate the
cysts, they frequently re-form.

 Optimizing Outcomes— Teaching about fibrocystic
breast changes

When teaching women about breast health and BSE,
nurses can include information about fibrocystic changes,
palpable thickening in the breasts often associated with
pain and tenderness that fluctuates with the menstrual
cycle. Fibrocystic changes are common, benign, and tend
to appear during the second and third decades of life.
Treatment for the condition centers on relief of symptoms
and may include analgesics, nonsteroidal anti-inflammatory drugs (e.g., ibuprofen), diuretics, use of a supportive
bra, avoidance of caffeine and other stimulants (called
methylxanthines), tobacco, and alcohol, and the application
of heat to the breasts.

Fibroadenomas are solid cysts composed of stromal
(connective) and glandular tissue. They are usually moveable and nontender. Fibroadenomas are the second most
common benign breast condition (fibrocystic changes are
the most common) and are usually located in the upper
outer quadrant of the breast. This tumor occurs most
often in women who are in their 20s and 30s. The use of
oral contraceptives before age 20 has been linked to the
risk of fibroadenomas (ACS, 2009b).

Lipomas are mobile, nontender fat tumors that are
soft with discrete borders. Lipomas may develop anywhere in the body, including the breasts. **Intraductal**
papillomas are small, wartlike growths in the lining of
the milk ducts near the nipple. These rare, benign tumors
usually produce a clear or bloody nipple discharge. They
may be felt as a small lump behind or next to the
nipple.

Mammary duct ectasia is an inflammation of the
ducts located behind the nipple. Occurring most often
in peri- and postmenopausal women, this condition
produces a thick, sticky nipple discharge that may be
purple, brown, or white in color. Upon inspection, the
nipple and adjacent breast tissue may be tender and red
and the nipple may be pulled inward. Duct ectasia
may resolve spontaneously, or it may require treatment
with warm compresses and antibiotics. In some situations, surgical removal of the abnormal duct is necessary. This lesion does not increase the risk of breast
cancer.

 Nursing Insight— *Nonproliferative and*
proliferative breast lesions

The presence of cysts in the breasts does not necessarily
increase a woman's risk for breast cancer. It has been estimated that approximately 70% of fibrocystic changes are *non-*
proliferative lesions; 26% of changes are *proliferative lesions*
without atypical or unusual growing cells (termed "atypia"),
and *proliferative lesions with atypical hyperplasia* represent the
remainder of fluid-filled breast lesions. Nonproliferative (multiplying) lesions do not affect breast cancer risk. Proliferative
lesions without atypia may slightly increase cancer risk, and
proliferative lesions with atypical hyperplasia raise the risk of
cancer (ACS, 2009c).

Mastitis is an infection of the breast that occurs when
bacteria enter the mammary ducts through a nipple. Most
often, bacteria are introduced during breastfeeding. Localized pockets of infection produce tender, warm lumps and
the adjacent axillary lymph nodes are frequently enlarged
and painful. Mastitis is usually treated with antibiotics
and warm compresses. If there is no improvement in
symptoms following antibiotic therapy, further screening
is indicated to rule out inflammatory carcinoma, a rare
form of breast cancer that may cause redness, warmth,
swelling, and skin texture changes in the affected breast.

Breast trauma or injury may produce an accumulation of blood at the site (hematoma) or destruction of the
mammary fatty tissue ("fat necrosis"), which can appear
as a lump. A biopsy may be performed to rule out malignancy. There is no evidence that breast injury causes
cancer.

Evaluating Breast Abnormalities

Over the past decade, breast cancer screening methods,
especially mammography, have become more precise,
allowing for earlier diagnosis. Improved screening and
increased public awareness have accounted for the dramatic increase in the detection of breast cancer. Earlier
diagnosis has resulted in a decrease in mortality rates.

If an area of abnormal breast tissue is detected during
the clinical breast examination, unless there is a high

index of suspicion, the woman is usually asked to return for a second evaluation after her next menstrual period. In many situations, she is also referred for a mammography. A limitation of mammography is the inability of this modality to differentiate between solid and cystic masses. An ultrasound examination (ultrasonography; sonography) may be performed at the time of the mammography to determine whether the lump is solid or fluid-filled.

Further testing is indicated if the breast mass persists after the next menstrual period, or if any abnormality is identified on mammography or sonography. If the ultrasound examination reveals that the lump is solid, the suspicious tissue is biopsied for further analysis. If the mass is fluid-filled, a needle aspiration is performed, and the woman is monitored for the development of additional cysts. Ultrasound may be used to guide the needle aspiration. If a distinct, palpable lump persists despite normal findings on mammography, immediate follow-up and evaluation are indicated.

A biopsy of any suspicious area is needed to provide a tissue sample for analysis so that a definitive diagnosis can be made. Although mammography is considered to be the best detection method for early breast cancer, it is often unable to distinguish between benign and malignant tumors. The American Cancer Society estimates that four out of every five biopsy results are not cancer (ACS, 2009c).

Breast MRI is used with increasing frequency to evaluate abnormal breast findings and to screen women at high risk for breast cancer. This screening modality is especially beneficial for breast masses that are not visualized mammographically, for lobular cancers, and for patients at risk for bilateral disease. MRI of the breast has shown an overall sensitivity to breast cancer of 95% (Esserman, Lane, Ewing, & Hwang, 2005; Knutson & Steiner, 2007; Smith, 2007). Recent evidence suggests that this diagnostic method can detect cancer in the contralateral breast that was missed by mammography in women with recently diagnosed breast cancer (Lehman et al., 2007; Pomeranz, 2007).

The American Cancer Society recommends both MRI scans and mammograms once per year for women considered as high risk—those whose chance of developing breast cancer during their lifetime is greater than 20%—beginning at age 30. Younger women frequently develop more aggressive cancers and they tend to have more dense breasts, a factor that makes it more difficult to detect cancerous changes via mammography alone (ACS, 2009c; Pomeranz, 2007).

BIOPSY

Most often, the diagnosis and treatment of breast abnormalities is a two-step process: A biopsy is obtained and evaluated and then based on this information, decisions are made regarding the treatment. Palpation alone cannot determine whether or not a suspicious mass or lump is cancer. Likewise, neither the clinical breast examination nor available technology can provide definitive proof that a suspicious lesion is cancerous. All that can be concluded from these modalities is that "no evidence of cancer is found." Confirmation of cancer can be made only by examining the suspicious tissue (Smith, 2007). A number of different biopsy procedures may be used to

obtain a sample of breast tissue or fluid within the breast tissue for evaluation. These include fine needle aspiration, core needle aspiration, and surgical or open biopsy.

Fine Needle Aspiration (FNA)

The FNA technique involves the use of a fine needle that is carefully guided into the suspicious area while the practitioner palpates the lump. It is usually conducted in the office setting. If the abnormality is too small to feel, ultrasound or a stereotactic biopsy can be used to help locate and ensure an adequate sampling of the suspicious tissue. In the latter technique, the biopsy is conducted with the aid of mammography. The needle is guided to the area by computer-assisted x-ray, which can help the examiner precisely control the needle placement. Then suction is applied to the needle. FNA is used to determine whether the lump is a fluid-filled cyst or a solid tumor (Smith, 2007) (Fig. 3-10).

 clinical alert

Indications for breast biopsy

A biopsy obtained by FNA with a stereotactic core needle or by surgical excision is usually recommended for any breast mass that does not resolve spontaneously within one or two menstrual cycles and for all postmenopausal women. It is important to note that negative results from mammography and ultrasonography are not always accurate enough to rule out cancer (Venes, 2009).

If fluid is aspirated, the FNA procedure may eliminate the lump altogether and provide a preliminary diagnosis. In some situations it is necessary to perform further testing. Additional evaluation may be indicated if the fluid is dark in color, or if the fluid-filled cyst has recurred several times, or if the sample has been obtained from a postmenopausal woman, who would not be expected to have breast cysts because of low estrogen levels. Clear fluid is usually indicative of a benign cyst; cloudy or bloody fluid may be present in benign or malignant tumors (Smith, 2007).

If no fluid is aspirated or if a residual thickened area remains after aspiration of the fluid, a core needle biopsy is performed. The false-positive rate for needle aspiration is almost zero. False-negative results occur more frequently because the needle may have missed the abnormal tissue. If no abnormalities are found with aspiration, follow-up mammography or sonography is recommended in

Figure 3-10 Fine needle breast biopsy

approximately 2 to 4 months to assess for recurrence of the cyst (Smith, 2007).

Core Needle Biopsy

In this technique a large-bore needle is used to remove a small cylinder of tissue. The needle placement is often guided as with the fine needle aspiration procedure. Core needle biopsy may be performed with the use of a local anesthetic in the office setting. The procedure may be painful, but there is usually little or no scarring. Core biopsy samples can identify invasive cancer and they can also provide prognostic biomarkers to help direct the course of treatment (Smith, 2007).

Optimizing Outcomes— With stereotactic biopsy

The Mammotome and the Advanced Breast Biopsy Instrument (ABBI) are stereotactic biopsy methods that remove more tissue than a core needle biopsy. The Mammotome is a type of vacuum-assisted biopsy that uses a hollow probe instrument to remove about twice as much tissue as a core biopsy. Performed in the outpatient setting under local anesthesia, this procedure requires no stitches and leaves minimal scarring. The ABBI method uses a rotating circular knife equipped with a thin heated electrical wire to remove a large cylinder of abnormal tissue. This procedure requires sutures and is more likely to leave a minimal scar. In some centers, the biopsy is guided by an MRI, which locates the tumor, plots its coordinates, and precisely aims the stereotactic biopsy instrument into the tumor. Automated Tissue Excision and Collection (ATEC) is a biopsy technique that combines vacuum-assisted breast biopsy with MRI-assisted guidance. This method, which allows many samples to be taken through one small cut in the skin, requires only a local anesthetic. It is being studied in women who have had a personal or family history of breast cancer, in those who have had previous breast surgery, and in women with dense breast tissue who cannot be accurately screened with tests such as mammography or sonography (ACS, 2009d).

Surgical or Open Biopsy

In many instances, removal of all or a portion of the tissue for microscopic analysis may be indicated. When this is the case, a number of decisions must be made concerning the amount of tissue needed, since the goal is to obtain surgical margins that are free of possible malignant tissue. If possible, the incision is made near the areola of the nipple to minimize scarring and disfigurement. The surgical or open biopsy is considered the most accurate biopsy technique for large masses or for large areas of suspicion and may involve removal of the entire tumor (excisional biopsy) or a small part of a large tumor (incisional biopsy) (ACS, 2009d; Smith, 2007). Depending on the situation, the procedure may be performed using local anesthesia or regional anesthesia; if the tumor is deep inside the chest, general anesthesia may be required.

Skin ("Punch") Biopsy

A punch biopsy may be used to confirm a diagnosis of inflammatory breast cancer or Paget's disease (carcinoma of the mammary ducts) of the nipple.

Testing for Estrogen and Progesterone Receptors

Normal breast tissue contains hormone receptors that respond to the stimulatory effects of estrogen and progesterone. An estrogen receptor is a cellular protein that binds the female sex steroid hormones. When circulating estrogens attach to it, they stimulate the cells to transcribe DNA and manufacture proteins. This process typically leads to cellular growth and proliferation. Many types of breast cancers retain estrogen receptors, and for these particular tumors, estrogen enhances proliferation of the malignant cells. The same situation occurs with tumors having progesterone receptors.

An important component in the evaluation of a woman with early breast cancer is to test for the presence of hormone receptors. The estrogen and progesterone receptor proteins are present in the cell cytoplasm and may be located on the surface of some of the breast cancer cells. When present, the receptors bind to the estrogen or progesterone, and the binding promotes growth of the malignant cells. A malignant breast tumor may have estrogen receptors, progesterone receptors, or both types. Determining the patient's hormone receptor status through biologic testing of the tumor type provides valuable information concerning the predicted response to hormone manipulation therapy. Tumors that lack hormone receptors will not respond to hormone therapy. In general, postmenopausal women tend to be estrogen receptor positive; premenopausal women tend to be estrogen receptor negative (Venes, 2009).

Evaluating Breast Symptoms

Breast symptoms may occur in benign and malignant conditions. For example, the woman may experience nipple discharge, skin changes, or breast pain. It is important that each symptom be evaluated to determine its significance and the need for further testing or treatment.

NIPPLE DISCHARGE

Any spontaneous nipple discharge should be promptly evaluated. In most cases, nipple discharge results from a physiological event (e.g., infection) or hormonal imbalance. However, a small percentage of women who experience this symptom are diagnosed with a serious pituitary disorder or malignancy.

 Optimizing Outcomes— Use of the ductogram to evaluate nipple discharge

A ductogram is sometimes performed to determine the cause of nipple discharge. Also called a "galactogram," this test involves the placement of radiopaque dye (instilled via a tiny plastic tube) into the nipple. An x-ray is then taken to determine the presence of a ductal mass.

Galactorrhea (the continuation of milk secretion after breastfeeding has ceased) is characterized by a spontaneous bilateral, milky, sticky discharge. Galactorrhea normally occurs during pregnancy due to increased circulating levels of prolactin. Elevated prolactin levels may also be associated with a thyroid disorder, a pituitary tumor, chest wall surgery, or trauma. Some women develop galactorrhea during therapy with certain neuroleptic drugs or oral contraceptives. In addition to evaluation of serum prolactin levels, diagnostic testing may also include a ductogram, microscopic analysis of the nipple discharge, a thyroid profile, pregnancy testing, and mammography.

Serous or bloody nipple discharge may be caused by an intraductal papilloma, a rare, benign condition of unknown etiology that develops in the terminal nipple ducts. Purulent nipple discharge is typically associated with breast infection. Occasionally, breast cancer produces a spontaneous unilateral discharge that may be bloody, serous, or watery. The bloody discharge associated with breast cancer ranges from bright red to black and the serous discharge is thin, sticky, and yellow to light orange in color (Smith, 2007).

False discharge is a term that refers to fluid that appears on the nipple or areola but is not secreted by breast tissue. False discharge may be bloody, clear, colored, purulent, serous, or viscous. Various conditions such as eczema, dermatitis, nipple trauma, and Paget's disease may be associated with false nipple discharge.

 Nursing Insight— Recognizing symptoms that may point to Paget's disease

Paget's disease is an inflammatory, malignant neoplasm that originates in the nipple. This rare tumor accounts for only 1% of all cases of breast cancer. It usually occurs with invasive ductal carcinoma and can cause scaling, bleeding, oozing, and crusting of the nipple. The woman may complain of burning or itching in the affected area. Nurses should remind women that an important component of breast awareness and self-examination involves visualization and inspection of the nipples and that any changes should be promptly reported.

SKIN CHANGES

Erythema, or reddening of the skin, may be related to benign or malignant conditions. Infection, the most common cause of breast erythema in young women, is usually accompanied by increased tenderness and localized warmth. Infection is treated with a course of antibiotic therapy. Reddening that occurs at the end of the nipple may be associated with Paget's disease, and a biopsy is required for diagnosis. Changes in the breast skin color and texture that resemble orange peel (*peau d'orange*) may result from inflammatory breast cancer and require immediate evaluation. Other skin changes associated with inflammatory breast cancer include the presence of pink, purplish, or bruised skin; a pitting or ridging of the skin; and a nipple newly turning inward (Ruhl, 2007). **Mondor disease** of the breast is a rare, self-limiting condition characterized by thrombophlebitis of the superficial veins. Symptoms include skin redness, edema, and pain in the affected area. The condition may occur after trauma or appear without apparent cause. Although Mondor disease is usually benign, it may be associated with breast cancer and hypercoagulability (Marcovici, 2007; Venes, 2009).

BREAST PAIN

The most common type of breast pain occurs cyclically and is associated with the period of time that immediately precedes the onset of menses. While the exact etiology is unknown, cyclical breast pain has been linked to hormonal imbalances. The pain may be experienced in one or both breasts. An association between methylxantines (a group of chemicals present in tea, colas, coffee, and chocolate) and premenstrual breast pain has been established. In general, breast pain is not associated with breast cancer, although women with breast cancer may complain of a localized tightening or pulling sensation or a localized burning or itching.

 Now Can You— Discuss breast abnormalities?

1. Describe the following types of breast masses: fibrocystic changes, fibroadenomas, intraductal papillomas, mammary duct ectasia?
2. Identify and describe four methods for evaluating breast abnormalities?
3. Explain the significance of testing for estrogen and progesterone receptors?

Breast Cancer

RISK FACTORS

Risk factors for breast cancer may be related to demographics, personal health history, lifestyle choices, and defects in certain genes. As is the case with many other diseases, the greater the number of risk factors that are present, the greater the likelihood of developing breast cancer. A listing of specific risk factors is presented in Box 3-1. It is important to note, however, that approximately 70% to 80% of women who develop breast cancer have none of the known risk factors (ACS, 2009b; Smith, 2007). Nurses may assist women in assessing their personal risk for breast cancer with the Breast Cancer Risk Assessment Tool.

 Optimizing Outcomes— The Breast Cancer Risk Assessment Tool

The National Cancer Institute (NCI) and the National Surgical Adjuvant Breast and Bowel Project (NSABP) have developed an interactive computer tool to estimate a woman's risk of developing invasive breast cancer. The tool, designed for use by health professionals, has recently been updated for African American women. The tool predicts a woman's risk of breast cancer in 5 years and over the lifetime (to age 90 years). Various risk factors, including present age, number of first-degree relatives affected, age at menarche, age at first live birth, the number of breast biopsies, and a history of abnormal hyperplasia in breast biopsy specimens, are assessed. The tool is available at the Web site http://www.cancer.gov/bcrisktool/ (NCI, 2009b).

Demographics and Personal Health History

Advancing age constitutes the single most important risk factor for breast cancer. A woman's risk increases as her age increases. According to the American Cancer Society,

Box 3-1 Risk Factors Associated with Breast Cancer

- Defects in breast cancer gene 1 (*BRCA1*) or breast cancer gene 2 (*BRCA2*)
- Gender: 100 times more likely to occur in females than in males
- Age: Increasing age—2 out of 3 invasive breast cancers occur in women age 55 and older
- Personal history of breast cancer in at least one breast
- Family history of breast cancer
- Exposure to chest radiation
- Excess weight
- Exposure to estrogen: early onset of menarche, late menopause, or use of hormonal therapy
- Race: Caucasians more likely to develop breast cancer than Hispanics or African Americans
- Smoking
- Exposure to carcinogens
- Excessive use of alcohol
- Diagnosis of precancerous breast changes
- Increased breast density revealed on mammography
- Exposure to diethylstilbestrol (DES)—mothers and female offspring

Source: American Cancer Society (2009b).

approximately 1 out of 8 invasive breast cancer diagnoses are among women younger than age 45; approximately 2 out of 3 women with invasive breast cancer are age 55 or older when they are diagnosed (ACS, 2009b). Breast cancer is more prevalent in women than in men. In males, breast cancer accounts for only 0.7% of all breast cancer diagnoses (ACS, 2009b; Smith, 2007).

Caucasian women are more likely to develop breast cancer than are African American women. Statistically, however, African American women are more likely to die from their disease than are Caucasian women, and they are also more likely to be diagnosed with higher-grade tumors associated with a poorer prognosis. Reasons for this finding may include an inability to obtain health care or screening mammography, not following up after receiving abnormal test results, distrust of the health-care system, and the belief that mammograms are not needed (U.S. Department of Health and Human Services [USDHHS], 2008). Also, higher-grade tumors may occur more frequently in African American women, even those who receive regular screening (Smith-Bindman, Miglioretti, Lurie, Abraham, Barbash, Strzelczyk, et al., 2006). Asian, Hispanic, and Native American women have an overall lower risk of developing and dying from breast cancer (ACS, 2009b; Centers for Disease Control and Prevention [CDC], 2009).

Women who currently have or have been previously diagnosed with cancer in one breast have three to four times the risk of developing new cancer in the same or other breast than do their counterparts who have never had breast cancer (ACS, 2009b). A history of a family member, especially a mother or sister, who received a diagnosis of breast cancer also increases the risk, especially if the cancer occurred prior to menopause. Interestingly, however, approximately 70% to 80% of women who develop breast cancer do not have a family history of this disease.

Lifestyle-Related Factors

Women who have had no children or who had their first child after age 30 have a slightly increased risk of breast cancer, owing to increased exposure to estrogen. Also, women who use oral contraceptives (OC) have a slightly greater risk of breast cancer than women who never used them. However, after discontinuation of OC use, the risk decreases; approximately 10 years after discontinuing the OC, there is no increased risk of breast cancer. Postmenopausal combined hormone therapy (i.e., estrogen + progestin) is associated with an increased risk of breast cancer; the use of estrogen alone for less than 10 years does not appear to increase the risk. Breastfeeding, especially for 1 to 2 years, appears to slightly reduce the risk for breast cancer (ACS, 2009b).

Being overweight or obese increases breast cancer risk, especially for postmenopausal women, and especially if the extra weight has been gained in adulthood and is accumulated at the waist. Following menopause, adipose tissue becomes the primary source of estrogen. Postmenopausal weight loss lowers circulating estrogen levels, and since estrogens are directly related to the risk of breast cancer, it is believed that weight loss may decrease the risk. Regular exercise also appears to reduce breast cancer risk; the American Cancer Society recommends 45 to 60 minutes of intentional physical activity 5 or more days a week (ACS, 2009b; Eliassen, Colditz, Rosner, et al., 2006; Hellwig, 2007; Theroux, 2007).

Alcohol use increases breast cancer risk, especially for women who drink more than 1 alcoholic beverage per day. Women who consume 2 to 5 alcoholic drinks daily have about 1½ times the risk of women who consume no alcohol. According to the American Cancer Society (2009b), women should limit their alcohol consumption to no more than 1 drink a day. Smoking or secondhand

Family Teaching Guidelines...
Tips for Reducing Breast Cancer Risk

Nurses can teach families about simple at-home strategies that may reduce breast cancer risk:

Diet and exercise: Reducing calories and engaging in regular exercise may slow tumor growth and lower the amount of circulating leptin, a fat-released protein that has been linked to breast cancer.

Extra-virgin olive oil: Contains polyphenol compounds that suppress a breast cancer-promoting gene.

Apples: Phenols found in apples may combat malignant tumors.

Vitamin D: Prevents the division of cancer cells and activates a tumor-suppressing protein.

Folate: Consuming foods that contain the B-vitamin folate (e.g., leafy green vegetables, beans, and fortified cereals) may help to mitigate the increased breast cancer risk associated with drinking alcohol.

Soy supplements: Soy contains isoflavones, substances that act like estrogen and may stimulate the growth of certain types of breast cancer. Supplements that contain concentrated amounts of isoflavones should be avoided. However, healthy soy foods such as edamame, soy milk, and tofu are not considered harmful.

exposure to tobacco smoke as a risk factor for breast cancer is controversial; all women should be counseled to stop smoking and avoid secondhand smoke as a health-promoting strategy (ACS, 2009b).

Nursing Insight— *Controversial breast cancer risk factors*

It has been suggested that various factors, including dietary fat, antiperspirants, bras, breast implants, environmental chemicals, abortions, and night work, increase the risk for breast cancer. It is important for nurses to know about these claims so that they can address their patients' concerns and provide appropriate counseling. The dietary intake of fat has not been clearly linked with an increased risk for breast cancer. However, high-fat diets can lead to obesity, which is a breast cancer risk factor. Although one postulate is that the absorption of chemicals in underarm antiperspirants may lead to cancer, there is no evidence to support this theory. Bras, purported to obstruct lymph flow, have also been implicated in the development of breast cancer. However, there is no scientific evidence to support this claim. Although breast implants do not increase breast cancer risk, scar tissue associated with the silicone implants may make mammography interpretation more difficult. Presently, there are no data supporting a definite link between breast cancer and environmental chemicals (e.g., DDE [a pesticide]; polychlorinated biphenyls [PCBs]). Neither induced nor spontaneous abortions are related to an increased risk for breast cancer. Some researchers have proposed that, owing to a disruption in the hormone melatonin, there is a link between working at night and breast cancer; this theory is currently undergoing investigation (ACS, 2009b).

Gene Defects

Approximately 5% to 10% of breast cancer cases are hereditary, resulting from gene defects, or mutations, passed on from a parent. The identification of the *BRCA1* and *BRCA2* genes was a pivotal discovery that clearly demonstrated the role of heredity and genetic mutations in the development of breast and ovarian cancer. It is estimated that approximately 10% of ovarian cancer cases and 3% to 5% of breast cancer cases are due to genetic mutations in *BRCA1* and *BRCA2*. Hereditary breast and ovarian cancer syndrome is an inherited cancer-susceptibility syndrome (ACOG, 2009; ACS, 2009b; Lessick, 2007).

Clinical Alert

Recognizing Hallmarks of Hereditary Breast and Ovarian Cancer Syndrome

When taking the patient history, nurses must be aware of the following indicators of hereditary breast and ovarian cancer syndrome: multiple family members with breast cancer or ovarian cancer or both; the presence of both breast cancer and ovarian cancer in a single individual; and early age of breast cancer onset. Women with these risk factors can be referred for clinical genetic testing for gene mutations. Information gained from the testing allows for the identification of individuals who are at substantial risk of breast cancer and ovarian cancer and the timely institution of screening and prevention strategies to reduce the woman's personal risk (ACOG, 2009).

Approximately 1 in 300 to 1 in 800 individuals in the general population are estimated to carry a mutation in *BRCA1* or *BRCA2*. Normally, *BRCA1*, located on chromosome 17, and *BRCA2*, located on chromosome 13, help to prevent cancer by manufacturing proteins that halt the abnormal growth of cells. However, individuals who inherited a mutated copy of either gene from a parent have an increased risk of developing breast and/or ovarian cancer. For a woman with a *BRCA1* mutation, the risk of ovarian cancer is 39% to 46%. For a woman with a *BRCA2* mutation, the risk of ovarian cancer is 12% to 20%. The estimated lifetime risk of breast cancer with a *BRCA1* or *BRCA2* mutation is 65% to 74%. For women with breast cancer, the 10-year actuarial risk of developing subsequent ovarian cancer is 12.7% for *BRCA1* mutation carriers and 6.8% for *BRCA2* mutation carriers. In the United States, *BRCA* mutations occur most often in Jewish women of Ashkenazi (Eastern European) origin. In fact, an estimated 1 in 40 Ashkenazi Jews carries a specific "founder mutation" in *BRCA1* or *BRCA2*. Other rare gene mutations, such as ATM, p53, CHEK2, PTEN and CDH1, are less common causes of inherited breast cancer. Genetic testing to identify mutations in the *BRCA* and other genes is available; women who seek this testing should be offered counseling to help them make an informed decision (ACOG, 2009; ACS, 2009b; Hughes & Ravnikar, 2009).

TUMOR TYPES

There are several types of breast cancer. The majority of breast cancers represent a type of adenocarcinoma, which arises from the glandular tissue (i.e., ducts and lobules of the breast). Four subtypes account for most breast cancers. Occasionally, a single breast tumor can have a combination of these types or a mixture of invasive and in situ cancer. The term *in situ* indicates that the cancer cells remain confined to the ducts (ductal carcinoma in situ) or lobules (lobular carcinoma in situ); they have not penetrated into deeper breast tissues or spread to other organs in the body. Invasive carcinomas have grown beyond the layer of cells where the cancer originated. Most breast cancers are invasive carcinomas—either invasive ductal carcinoma or invasive lobular carcinoma (ACS, 2009e).

Ductal Carcinoma In Situ (DCIS) and Lobular Carcinoma In Situ (LCIS)

The most common type of noninvasive breast cancer, ductal carcinoma in situ, is confined within the ducts and has not spread into the surrounding breast tissue. DCIS accounts for approximately 1 in 5 new breast cancer cases. It is most often detected by mammography and has an excellent cure rate (ACS, 2009e).

Lobular carcinoma in situ (LCIS) (sometimes termed "lobular neoplasia") begins in the milk-producing glands and does not penetrate the wall of the lobules. LCIS is not considered a true cancer, although this neoplasm is sometimes classified as a type of noninvasive breast cancer. LCIS is rarely an invasive cancer, but women with this type have a higher risk of developing an invasive breast cancer in the same breast or in the opposite breast (ACS, 2009e).

Figure 3-11 Invasive ductal carcinoma

Invasive (Infiltrating) Ductal Carcinoma (IDC)

The most common type of breast cancer, invasive ductal carcinoma (IDC), originates in a mammary duct, penetrates through the ductal wall, and grows into the fatty tissue of the breast. (Fig. 3-11) Metastasis (spread) to other parts of the body may occur through the lymphatic system and bloodstream. Approximately 8 out of 10 invasive breast cancers are infiltrating ductal carcinomas. Women with this type of tumor usually present with a discrete, solitary breast mass (ACS, 2009e; Smith, 2007).

Invasive (Infiltrating) Lobular Carcinoma (ILC)

Invasive (infiltrating) lobular carcinoma (ILC) originates in the lobules (milk-producing glands). Like invasive ductal carcinoma, this neoplasm has spread into the fatty tissue and can metastasize to other parts of the body. Approximately 1 out of 10 invasive breast cancers is an ILC, and women with this type are more likely than those with other cancers to have bilateral disease. ILC may be harder to detect by mammography; breast MRI is often helpful in the diagnosis (ACS, 2009e; Capobianco, Spaliviero, Dessole, Rocca, Cherchi, Ambrosini et al., 2007; Smith, 2007).

Inflammatory Breast Cancer (IBC)

Inflammatory breast cancer (IBC) is a rare neoplasm that tends to grow more quickly and aggressively than the more common types of breast cancer. There is usually no lump or tumor, and the skin often exhibits changes similar to an infectious process such as mastitis. The affected breast may appear inflamed: red, thickened, tender, itchy, or larger than the unaffected breast. Because metastasis has usually occurred by the time of diagnosis, the cure rate is lower with IBC than with other types of breast cancer (Smith, 2007).

 Optimizing Outcomes— **Teaching about inflammatory breast cancer**

Although inflammatory breast cancer is rare, nurses should educate women about the signs and symptoms (ACS, 2009f):

- Breast swelling, which is usually sudden with one breast much larger than the other
- Itching
- A pink, red, or dark-colored area, sometimes with a texture like the skin of an orange (*peau d'orange*)
- Ridges and thickened areas of the skin

- Breast feeling warm to the touch
- Nipple retraction
- Breast pain

In the early stages, IBC may be mistaken for infection, resulting in a delay in diagnosis. Also, because there is no defined lump, this neoplasm may not be detected by mammography. MRI, which allows for precise measurement of the associated skin changes, is the most sensitive imaging test for IBC. Positron emission tomography (PET) scanning combined with computed tomography (CT) may be used to detect areas of metastasis (lymph nodes and organs) (ACS, 2009f).

 Ethnocultural Considerations... African American Women and Inflammatory Breast Cancer

Inflammatory breast cancer accounts for approximately 1% to 3% of all breast cancers diagnosed in the United States. Symptoms (e.g., redness, increased warmth, changes in the skin texture termed *peau d'orange* ["orange peel"]) that occur with this rare type of breast cancer are related to interference with lymph drainage by the malignant cells. Inflammatory breast cancer tends to occur more often in younger women; African American women appear to be at a higher risk than Caucasian women (ACS, 2009f).

INDICATORS OF DISEASE PROGNOSIS

A number of variables, such as the cancer stage, type, and tumor size, the presence of lymph node involvement (Fig. 3-12), and the presence of hormone receptor levels and HER2/neu (human epidermal growth factor receptor 2) in the tumor tissue, are associated with the likelihood of breast cancer recurrence.

 Nursing Insight— *Understanding about human epidermal growth factor receptor 2 (HER2/neu)*

Human epidermal growth factor receptor 2, a protein involved in normal cell growth, is found on some types of cancer cells, including breast and ovarian. Approximately 20% of breast cancers have an amplification (or overexpression) of the *HER2/neu* gene. Overexpression of this receptor in breast cancer is associated with increased disease recurrence and a worse prognosis. All newly diagnosed breast cancers should be tested for HER2/neu because HER2-positive cancers are more likely to benefit from treatment with medications that specifically target the HER2/neu protein, such as trastuzumab (Herceptin) and lapatinib (Tykerb) (ACS, 2009e; NCI, 2009c).

Identification of these factors allows for development of an individualized plan of treatment. The majority of women with negative lymph nodes (approximately 60% of women diagnosed with breast cancer today) will be cured by surgery alone. Approximately 30% of women with breast cancer will develop recurrent disease within 10 years of the initial treatment. In addition to identifying hormone receptor status and the histological tumor type,

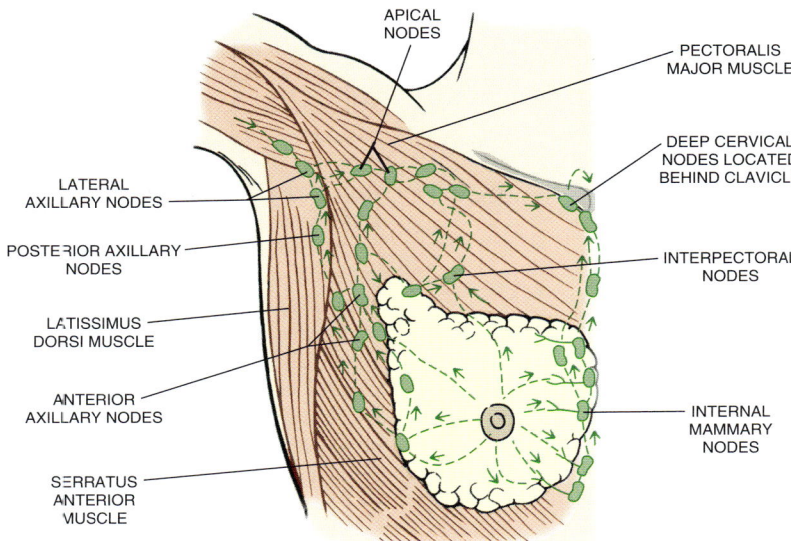

APICAL
NODES

PECTORALIS
MAJOR MUSCLE

DEEP CERVICAL
NODES LOCATED
BEHIND CLAVICLE

LATERAL
AXILLARY NODES

POSTERIOR AXILLARY
NODES

INTERPECTORAL
NODES

LATISSIMUS
DORSI MUSCLE

ANTERIOR
AXILLARY NODES

INTERNAL
MAMMARY
NODES

SERRATUS
ANTERIOR
MUSCLE

Figure 3-12 Breast cancer: possible paths of lymphatic spread

information concerning the status of the axillary lymph nodes and the overall tumor size is useful in determining the disease prognosis (ACS, 2009e).

Axillary Nodes

It has long been recognized that tumor involvement of the axillary nodes is an important indicator for breast cancer prognosis. Clinical assessment of the axillary nodes is associated with a 30% false-positive and false-negative rate. Thus, pathological staging of the patient's lymph nodes is an essential step in the development of the treatment plan. Seventy percent of women with negative nodes survive 10 years following their breast cancer treatment. The disease prognosis worsens as the number of positive lymph nodes increases. Recurrence of breast cancer occurs in approximately 75% of women who have multiple positive nodes (Smith, 2007).

Sentinel node biopsy is a technique that targets selected lymph nodes during biopsy. A radioactive tracer (dye) injected into the region of the tumor travels through the lymphatic system to a lymph node. This node, termed the "sentinel node," is the first node that receives lymphatic drainage from the tumor. If no cancer is detected in this node, the patient is able to avoid more extensive lymph node surgery with its accompanying side effects, such as lymphedema (swelling of the arm) (ACS, 2009e).

Tumor Size

There is a direct relationship between the size of the tumor and the risk of recurrence. Prior to the widespread use of mammography, fewer than 8% of women with node-negative breast cancer had tumors that were less than 1 cm in diameter. Tumors of this size are associated with a relative 5-year survival that approaches 99%. Women with tumors that measure 1–3 cm have a relative 5-year survival rate of approximately 91%, and those with tumors that measure greater than 3 cm have a 5-year survival of approximately 85%. Women whose tumors are

greater than 3 cm have a breast cancer recurrence rate that exceeds 50% (Smith, 2007).

CANCER STAGING SYSTEM

The stage of cancer is based on the size of the tumor, the number of lymph nodes involved, and whether the cancer has spread. The American Joint Committee on Cancer TNM system is the most commonly used system to describe the stages of breast cancer. The *clinical stage* is based on findings from the physical examination, biopsy, and imaging tests; the *pathologic* stage combines these three diagnostic modalities with the results of surgery. Pathologic staging, which includes detailed information about the breast mass and adjacent lymph nodes, provides a more accurate description of the tumor.

Optimizing Outcomes— Staging cancer to guide development of a treatment plan

The TNM staging system classifies cancers based on their T, N, and M stages:

- **T** = Tumor: size and spread within the breast and to nearby organs
- **N** = Nodes: spread to the lymph nodes
- **M** = Metastasis: spread to distant organs

Additional letters or numbers are added after the T, N, and M to provide further details about the tumor, lymph nodes, and metastasis to distant organs, such as the bones, lungs, brain, and liver. Breast cancer stage grouping is a process that combines the T, N, M information to allow for the identification of cancers with similar stages, which are usually treated in a similar way. Stage is delineated in Roman numerals and progresses from Stage I (least advanced) to Stage IV (most advanced); Stage 0 identifies noninvasive cancer (ACS, 2009g) (Box 3-2).

Box 3-2 The Breast Cancer Staging System

Stage 0: Ductal carcinoma in situ (DCIS), the earliest form of breast cancer.

Stage I: The tumor measures 2 cm in diameter or less and there is no involvement of the lymph nodes and no distant metastasis.

Stage II: The tumor measures 2.0 cm in diameter (or less) to 5.0 cm. Depending on the specific findings, the cancer may have spread to the axillary or internal mammary lymph nodes but has not spread to distant sites.

Stage IIIA: One of the following applies:

1. The tumor is not more than 5 cm across and has spread to 4–9 axillary lymph nodes, or it has enlarged the internal mammary lymph nodes; no distant metastasis.
2. The tumor is larger than 5 cm across and does not grow into the chest wall or skin. It has spread to 1–9 axillary nodes or to internal mammary nodes; no distant metastasis.

Stage IIIB: The tumor has grown into the chest wall or skin and one of the following applies:

1. No spread to the lymph nodes; no distant metastasis.
2. Spread to 1–3 axillary lymph nodes and/or small amounts of cancer are found in the internal mammary lymph nodes (per sentinel lymph node biopsy); no distant metastasis.
3. Spread to 4–9 axillary lymph nodes, or enlargement of the internal mammary lymph nodes; no distant metastasis.

Stage IIIC: The tumor is any size, and one of the following applies:

1. Cancer has spread to 10 or more axillary lymph nodes; no distant metastasis.
2. Cancer has spread to the lymph nodes beneath the clavicle; no distant metastasis.
3. Cancer has spread to the lymph nodes above the clavicle; no distant metastasis.
4. Cancer involves the axillary lymph nodes and there is enlargement of the internal mammary lymph nodes; no distant metastasis.
5. Cancer has spread to 4 or more axillary lymph nodes, small amounts of cancer are present in the internal mammary lymph nodes (per sentinel lymph node biopsy); no distant metastasis.

Stage IV: The cancer can be any size (any "T"), may or may not have spread to nearby lymph nodes (any "N"). It has metastasized ("M") to distant organs or to distant lymph nodes.

Source: ACS (2009g).

 Now Can You— Discuss aspects of breast cancer diagnosis and staging?

1. Identify and describe at least 12 risk factors associated with breast cancer?
2. Describe at least 6 signs and symptoms associated with inflammatory breast cancer?
3. Explain why the hormone receptor status, tumor type and size, and presence of positive axillary lymph nodes are important indicators for the overall breast cancer prognosis?
4. Explain what is meant by the TNM cancer staging system and why this information is useful?

BREAST CANCER TREATMENT

Medical management of breast cancer is complicated and may require a multitreatment approach, including surgery and adjunctive treatment, such as radiation, chemotherapy, and hormone therapy. The simplest surgical treatment option is a lumpectomy: The lump and an area of surrounding normal tissue are removed. The lumpectomy is usually followed by radiation treatment to remove any remaining cancerous cells. A partial or segmental mastectomy involves removal of the tumor, the surrounding breast tissue, a portion of the lining of the chest wall, and some of the axillary lymph nodes. This procedure is usually followed with radiation therapy as well. A simple mastectomy involves the removal of all the breast tissue along with the area surrounding the nipple and areola. Radiation, chemotherapy, or hormone therapy may follow this surgical procedure. In a modified radical mastectomy, the entire breast and several axillary lymph nodes are removed, leaving the chest wall intact. While this procedure makes breast reconstruction easier for the patient, complications including lymphadenopathy and paresthesia are more likely to occur (ACS, 2009c).

 Optimizing Outcomes— Counseling women about chemotherapy side effects

When counseling patients about expected side effects from chemotherapy, nurses can reassure them that there are medications available now that are highly effective in reducing nausea and vomiting, the major symptoms traditionally associated with chemotherapy. Other side effects include a change in appetite, loss of hair, mouth or vaginal sores, suppression of the immune system that leads to an increased chance of infection, anemia, fatigue, menstrual cycle changes, and infertility. With the exception of infertility, most of the side effects are temporary (Smith, 2007).

Many women choose to undergo breast reconstruction after a mastectomy. This surgical option, performed by a plastic surgeon, is a personal decision that requires considerable individualized counseling and education. Since the reconstruction can be performed at the same time as the mastectomy, it is important to consider the options early. Breast reconstruction methods include use of a synthetic breast implant or reconstruction using one's own tissue. Synthetic implants typically are composed of a silicone shell filled with a saline solution. A tissue expander may be needed to cover the implant. To accomplish tissue expansion, an empty implant shell is placed under the skin and muscles and is gradually filled with the saline solution over several months. Once the skin is stretched sufficiently, the expander is removed and replaced with a permanent implant. Recovery usually takes several weeks.

Women who choose to undergo breast reconstruction using their own tissue may have a transverse rectus abdominis myocutaneous (TRAM) flap procedure. The breast is reconstructed using fat and muscle tissue taken from the abdomen, back, and buttocks. Recovery following the procedure usually takes 6 to 8 weeks, and there is an increased risk of infection and tissue necrosis. Deep inferior epigastric perforator (DIEP) reconstruction is a slightly less complicated surgical procedure. This method is similar to the TRAM flap procedure, but the abdominal muscles are left intact. The DIEP procedure is associated with fewer complications and less postoperative pain. Following reconstruction of the breast tissue, the surgeon can reconstruct the nipple and areola using tissue from other areas of the body. A small mound is constructed to resemble a nipple, and tattooing may be used to create an areola. In this situation, the surgeon applies a skin graft to the areolar region, slightly raises the skin, and then tattoos the skin graft.

Adjuvant therapies may include radiation therapy, chemotherapy, or hormone therapy. Radiation is usually begun 3 to 4 weeks after surgery, and treatments are given 5 days per week for 5 to 6 weeks. Chemotherapy that includes a combination two or more drugs may also be prescribed. Chemotherapeutics may be administered orally or intravenously and usually require four to eight treatments over 3 to 6 months. Hormone therapy is most commonly used to treat advanced metastatic cancer or as an adjuvant treatment to prevent recurrence of cancer. Normally, estrogen and progesterone bind to receptor sites in the breast tissue and encourage growth of cancerous cells. Prescribed hormone medications bind to the sites instead and prevent estrogen from reaching them. Medications used in hormone treatment include tamoxifen (Nolvadex), a selective estrogen receptor modulator (SERM), and aromatase inhibitors, which block the conversion of androgens into estrogen.

Nursing Insight— *Anti-angiogenesis therapy for cancer treatment*

Angiogenesis, which comes from the Greek words *angio* ("making new blood vessels") and *genesis* ("beginning"), is the process of making new blood vessels. Anti-angiogenesis is a targeted therapy that uses drugs or other substances to halt the tumor's production of new blood vessels. New anti-angiogenesis drugs that may prove useful in the treatment of breast cancer are currently under development and investigation (ACS, 2009h).

Optimizing Outcomes— Using genomics to guide breast cancer care

Genomic medicine encompasses the disciplines of gene mapping and sequencing and the study of the functions and interactions of all genes in the genome (a complete copy of the genetic material in an organism). Genomics focuses on developing tests that are both prognostic (i.e., based on factors such as tumor size, lymph node involvement, hormone receptor status) and predictive. *Prognostic* testing identifies the likelihood of cancer recurrence; *predictive* testing identifies the relative resistance of a cancer to specific treatments. Breast cancer specialists use information from genomics-driven specialized tests (e.g., Mammoprint; Oncotype DX; HOXB13/IL17BR) to develop an individualized treatment approach based on recurrence risk and predicted benefits of specific therapies (Moeller, 2008).

NURSING CARE FOR WOMEN DEALING WITH BREAST CANCER

Nurses must be sensitive to the fact that once a woman has received a diagnosis of breast cancer, her life is forever changed. Compassionate care during this difficult time

where research and practice meet:
Enhancing patient follow-up after breast cancer surgery

After surgery, women diagnosed with early stage breast cancer often benefit from treatment with chemotherapy, radiation, or hormonal therapy. For this reason, surgeons typically refer these patients to oncologists and assume that the cancer specialist is following up on them appropriately. Unfortunately, some women, especially African Americans and Hispanics, never see an oncologist. To keep these patients from being lost to follow-up, researchers developed a tracking system to determine if patients visited an oncologist and alert the surgeon to those who did not so that they could provide timely follow-up.

Bickell and colleagues (2008) compared the treatment of 639 women with early stage breast cancer who were seen at six city hospitals between January 1999 and December 2000 to 300 women who were seen between September 2004 and March 2006, the time period in which the tracking system was used. The rates of oncology consultations, chemotherapy, and hormonal therapy were higher for all women after the tracking system was in place. According to the investigators, the tracking system eliminated the racial disparity for African American and Hispanic women regarding the underuse of radiation, chemotherapy, and hormonal therapy. For example, after the tracking system was implemented, underuse of radiotherapy declined from 23% to 10%, underuse of chemotherapy decreased from 26% to 6%, and underuse of hormonal therapy diminished from 27% to 11% for African American and Hispanic women.

The researchers suggest two strategies to ensure that patients receive proper care for early stage breast cancer: Ensure that the tumor registry personnel follow up with patients to determine if they have visited an oncologist; and mandate that insurers require an oncology consultation for all patients diagnosed with invasive breast cancer to ensure that the women receive appropriate treatment. Nurses can be instrumental in ensuring proper oncology follow-up by counseling women about the importance of continued specialized cancer care after surgery and by participating in tracking efforts to prevent loss of patient contact after surgical intervention.

includes providing emotional support; empowering the patient and her family with current, evidence-based information; assisting them with immediate needs; and directing them to available resources. Personal and professional resources are essential as the woman works her way through the diagnostic process, the necessary decision-making concerning treatment and possible breast reconstruction, the surgery and adjuvant therapies, and the future with its uncertainties. Women who are confronted with breast cancer frequently discover an inner strength that they did not know existed. Examples of appropriate nursing diagnoses for women who have received a diagnosis of breast cancer are listed in Box 3-3.

Nurses can be a tremendous source of support and advocacy for women who are diagnosed with breast cancer. It is important to encourage patients to carefully consider all options and seek other opinions or other providers if they do not feel comfortable with recommendations. Nurses can direct women to the wealth of reliable information about breast cancer treatment and recovery available in books and on Internet sites and to the opportunities for personal sharing through local and national support groups.

Box 3-3 Examples of Nursing Diagnoses for Women Diagnosed With Breast Cancer

- Anticipatory grieving
- Anxiety
- Body image disturbance
- Denial
- Dysfunctional grieving
- Fear
- Grief
- Hopelessness
- Impaired skin integrity
- Ineffective individual or family coping
- Knowledge deficit
- Low self-esteem
- Pain
- Powerlessness
- Spiritual distress

 Collaboration in Caring— *Resources for women with cancer*

An important nursing role in the care of women with cancer centers on sharing information about the various resources that are available to them. These include:

- National Breast and Cervical Cancer Early Detection Program, NCCDPHP, CDC
- National Cancer Institute, NIH, HHS
- Office of Minority Health, OPHS, OS, HHS
- American Cancer Society
- Cancer.net
- BreastCancerTrials.org
- Celebrating Life Foundation
- Sisters Network® Inc.
- Susan G. Komen Breast Cancer Foundation
- Lance Armstrong Foundation and University of Pennsylvania
- NCI Community Cancer Centers Program
- National Coalition for Cancer Survivorship

For many, holistic medicine offers an additional healing approach to assist the body, mind, and spirit through the rigors of cancer diagnosis and treatment and to foster healing throughout the recovery process. The woman's immune system can be supported and enhanced naturally through dietary and safe herbal remedies, along with practices that reduce stress and help restore physical and emotional harmony and balance. For example, patients may benefit from imagery, aromatherapy, meditation, music therapy, dance therapy, journal writing, humor, art therapy, and hypnosis. Other modalities such as acupuncture, Ayurveda, Qigong, yoga, and tai chi may provide relief from unpleasant symptoms and be instrumental in lifting the body and spirit during the journey to recovery.

 Optimizing Outcomes— **Complementary and alternative therapies for cancer patients**

Many women find that various complementary and alternative therapies help to relieve cancer side effects and discomforts and enhance and enrich their lives during treatment and into recovery. Nurses can empower women with specific information and direct them to available resources. The American Cancer Society provides an up-to-date Internet source for complementary and alternative therapies. It is available at http://www.cancer.org/docroot/ETO/ETO_5.asp?sitearea5ETO.

Today there are an estimated 11 million cancer survivors living in the United States. Nurses who care for women across the life span are likely to see patients who are dealing with the psychosocial and physical effects of cancer treatments, which may occur for months or years after the treatment has ended. Development of a cancer survivorship care plan can help to ensure coordination of care and appropriate follow-up and empower the woman to understand and participate in her continuing care (Ruhl, 2009). Cancer survivorship care plans have been recommended by a variety of groups, including the Institute of Medicine (IOM), which, along with the National Research Council, produced a major report on cancer survivorship in 2005 (Greenwood & Stovall, 2005).

Optimizing Outcomes— **With a cancer survivorship care plan**

First introduced for survivors of childhood cancers, cancer survivorship care plans have recently been recommended for adult survivors. Components of the survivorship plan, which should be provided to the patient's primary care physician, include a summary of treatment, the possible short- and long-term effects of treatment, late toxicity monitoring, monitoring for primary cancer recurrence or a second cancer, identification of the provider responsible for survivor care, psychological and vocational needs, community support resources, and recommendations for preventive care and practices. For women, additional information should include genetic issues, the effects of treatment on future pregnancy and fertility, and menopausal issues (Cox, 2009; Ganz & Hahn, 2008; Ruhl, 2009; Ruhl & Moran, 2008).

Nurses are perfectly situated to provide cancer survivor care. With a holistic and family-centered approach that emphasizes patient education, health promotion, and preventive care practices, nursing can fully embrace the cancer survivorship movement to empower women and their providers with a comprehensive, holistic plan for continuing care in the aftermath of cancer. Owing to the dynamic nature of the survivorship plan, evolving scientific evidence about the specific cancer type, management of short- and long-term treatment sequelae, and the need for screening for recurrence and other cancers can be readily incorporated into the plan. This information can help to inform the woman's decision-making and allow her and her care provider to be proactive in both the planning and management of her health after cancer (Ruhl, 2009).

case study: Midlife Woman Treated for Breast Cancer

Dorothy is a 56-year-old postmenopausal Caucasian woman who received a diagnosis of early stage breast cancer approximately 6 months ago. Dorothy's treatment, which included a lumpectomy followed by radiation therapy, was uncomplicated and her physician has told her that her chance for a cure is "excellent."

Today, during an interview at the woman's health clinic, Dorothy confides in the nurse that she is concerned about herself because she feels "down and out." She admits that physically, she feels just fine and is very relieved to have the treatment behind her. Lately, however, she has been concerned about "the way my body looks." As a result of the surgery and radiation therapy, Dorothy has experienced a decrease in breast size in the affected breast. Although she acknowledges that "in the grand scheme of things, this change is a minor thing," the alteration in breast appearance is concerning to her.

critical thinking questions

1. What is a priority nursing intervention for Dorothy?

2. What information should the nurse provide to Dorothy?

3. What other actions should the nurse take?

♦ See suggested answers to case studies on DavisPlus.

 Now Can You— **Discuss aspects of breast cancer treatment?**

1. Identify four treatment modalities for breast cancer?
2. Describe the nurse's role in breast cancer treatment care?
3. Identify the components of a cancer survivorship care plan and explain why this information is useful?

summary points

♦ Maintaining breast health is an essential strategy for maintaining optimal physical and psychological health.

♦ Nurses are in an ideal position to educate women about breast health and strategies for the identification of benign and malignant breast disease.

♦ Breast cancer is the most common cancer in women in the United States, except for skin cancer, and it is the second leading cause of cancer deaths in women.

♦ Dietary, socioeconomic, and environmental factors most likely contribute to the development of breast cancer.

♦ A number of screening and diagnostic methods, including mammography, ultrasonography, magnetic resonance imaging, and biopsy, may be used in the clinical evaluation of the breasts.

• Risk factors for breast cancer may be related to demographics, personal health history, lifestyle choices, and defects in certain genes.

• The cancer staging system, based on the size of the tumor, the number of lymph nodes involved, and the presence of metastasis, is used to guide the development of a treatment plan for breast cancer.

• Breast cancer treatment may include surgery, radiation, chemotherapy, hormone therapy, and complementary and alternative therapies.

• The nursing role in caring for women with breast cancer includes providing emotional support, empowering the patient and her family with current information, assisting them with immediate needs, and directing them to available resources.

review questions

Multiple Choice

1. When teaching women how to perform proper breast self-examination (BSE), the nurse advises:
   a. Avoid the axillary area
   b. Refrain from squeezing the nipples
   c. Place the arm adjacent to the breast being examined in a relaxed position alongside the thigh
   d. Use the finger pads to apply light, medium, and firm pressure

2. Breast magnetic resonance imaging (MRI) is useful in screening:
   a. Women with recently diagnosed breast cancer
   b. Postmenopausal women
   c. All women
   d. Women whose screening mammograms are satisfactory

3. Ultrasound can reveal whether a breast mass is:
   a. Malignant
   b. Benign
   c. Fluid-filled or solid
   d. Potentially malignant

4. Known risk factors for breast cancer include:
   a. Slender body type
   b. Pregnancy before the age of 20
   c. Age greater than 50
   d. Menopause before the age of 50

5. Treatment for breast cancer may include:
   a. Estrogen therapy
   b. Anti-angiogenesis drugs
   c. Lactation suppressants
   d. Oral contraceptives

REFERENCES

Aliotta, H.M., & Schaeffer, N.J. (2006). Breast conditions. In K.D. Schuiling & F. E. Likis (Eds.), *Women's gynecologic health.* Sudbury, MA: Jones & Bartlett Publishers.

American Cancer Society (ACS). (2008). *How to perform a breast self-exam.* Retrieved from http://www.cancer.org/docroot/CRI/content/CRI_2_6x_How_to_perform_a_breast_self_exam_5.asp (Accessed October 1, 2009).

American Cancer Society (ACS). (2009a). *How many women get breast cancer?* May 6, 2009. Retrieved from http://www.cancer.org/docroot/CRI/content/CRI_2_2_1X_How_many_people_get_breast_cancer_5.asp (Accessed September 13, 2009).

American Cancer Society (ACS). (2009b). *What are the risk factors for breast cancer?* Retrieved from http://www.cancer.org/docroot/CRI/content/CRI_2_4_2X_What_are_the_risk_factors_for_breast_cancer_5.asp?sitearea= (Accessed October 29, 2009).

American Cancer Society (ACS). (2009c). *Cancer reference information.* Retrieved from http://www.cancer.org/docroot/CRI/content/CRI_2_4_6x_For_Women_Facing_a_Breast_Biopsy.asp (Accessed October 5, 2009).

American Cancer Society (ACS). (2009d). *Mammograms and other breast imaging procedures.* Retrieved from http://www.cancer.org/docroot/CRI/content/CRI_2_6X_Mammography_and_other_Breast_Imaging_Procedures_5.asp?sitearea= (Accessed October 6, 2009).

American Cancer Society (ACS). (2009e). *What is breast cancer?* Retrieved from http://www.cancer.org/docroot/CRI/content/CRI_2_4_1X_What_is_breast_cancer_5.asp?sitearea= (Accessed October 15, 2009).

American Cancer Society (ACS). (2009f). *Inflammatory breast cancer.* Retrieved from http://www.cancer.org/docroot/CRI/content/CRI_2_6X_Inflammatory_Breast_Cancer.asp (Accessed October 16, 2009).

American Cancer Society (ACS). (2009g). *How is breast cancer staged?* Retrieved from http://www.cancer.org/docroot/CRI/content/CRI_2_4_3X_How_is_breast_cancer_staged_5.asp?rnav=cri (Accessed October 16, 2009).

American Cancer Society (ACS). (2009h). *Anti-angiogenesis treatment.* Retrieved from http://www.cancer.org/docroot/ETO/eto_1_3_Antiangiogenesis_Therapy.asp (Accessed October 17, 2009).

American College of Obstetricians and Gynecologists (ACOG). (2007). *Guidelines for women's health care: A resource manual.* (3rd ed.). Washington, DC: Author.

American College of Obstetricians and Gynecologists (ACOG). (2009). *Hereditary breast and ovarian cancer syndrome* (Practice Bulletin No. 103). *Obstetrics and Gynecology, 113*(4), 957–966.

Barclay, L. (2009). *New breast cancer screening guidelines opposed.* Retrieved from http://www.medscape.com/viewarticle/712720?src (Accessed January 5, 2010).

Barr, J.K., Giannotti, T.E., Van Hoof, T.J., Mongoven, J., & Curry, M. (2008). Understanding barriers to participation in mammography by women with disabilities. *American Journal of Health Promotion, 22*(6), 381–385.

Bickell, N.A., Shastri, K., Fei, K., Oluwole, S., Godfrey, H., Fiotis, K., Srinivasan, A., & Guth, A.A. (2008). A tracking and feedback registry to reduce racial disparities in breast cancer care. *Journal of the National Cancer Institute, 100*(23), 1717–1723.

Bleicher, R.J., Ciocca, R.M., Egleston, B.L., Sesa, L., Evers, K., Sigudson, E.R., & Morrow, M. (2009). Association of routine pretreatment magnetic resonance imaging with time to surgery, mastectomy rate and margin status. *Journal of the American College of Surgeons, 209*(2), 180–187.

BreastCancer.org. (2008). *Breast cancer statistics.* Retrieved from http://www.breastcancer.org/symptoms/understand_bc/statistics.jsp (Accessed October 11, 2009).

Buzek, N. (2009). Breast tomosynthesis: The future of breast imaging? *Advance for Nurse Practitioners, 17*(10), 25–28.

Capobianco, G., Spaliviero, B., Dessole, S., Rocca, P.C., Cherchi, P.L., Ambrosini, G., Meloni F., & Meloni, G.B. (2007). Lymph node axillary metastasis from occult contralateral infiltrating lobular carcinoma arising in accessory breast: MRI diagnosis. *Breast Journal, 13*(3), 305–307.

Centers for Disease Control and Prevention (CDC). (2009). *Breast cancer rates by race and ethnicity.* Retrieved from http://www.cdc.gov/cancer/breast/statistics/race.htm (Accessed October 12, 2009).

Cox, T. (2009). *Breast cancer survivorship.* Oncology Nursing Society Special Interest Group Newsletter, 7:1. Retrieved from http://onsop-content.ons.org/Publications/SIGNewsletters/sur/sur7.1.html (Accessed October 29, 2009).

Diekmann, F., & Bick, U. (2007). Tomosynthesis and contrast-enhanced digital mammography: Recent advances in digital mammography. *European Journal of Radiology, 17*(12), 3086–3092.

Eliassen, A.H., Colditz, G.A., Rosner, B., Willet, W.C., & Hankinson, S. C. (2006). Adult weight change and risk of postmenopausal breast cancer. *Journal of the American Medical Association, 296*(2), 193–201.

Farmer, D., Reddick, B., D'Agostino Jr., R., & Jackson, S.A. (2007). Correlates of mammography screening in older African American women. *Oncology Nursing Forum, 34*(1), 117–123.

Ganz, P.A., & Hahn, E.E. (2008). Implementing a survivorship care plan for patients with breast cancer. *Journal of Clinical Oncology, 26*(8), 659–767.

Hartman, L.C., Sellers, T.A., Frost, M.H, Lingle, W.L., Degnim, A.C., Ghosh, K., Vierkant, R.A., Maloney, S.D., Pankratz, S., Hillman, D. W., Suman, V.J., Johnson, J., Blake, C., Tlsty, T., Vachon, C.M., Melton, L.J., & Visscher, D.W. (2005). Benign breast disease and the risk of breast cancer. *New England Journal of Medicine, 353*(3), 229–237.

Hellwig, J.P. (2007). Breast cancer: Lower fat intake may reduce recurrence. *Nursing for Women's Health, 11*(2), 121–122; 124–128.

Hughes, K.S., & Ravnikar, V. (2009 Suppl). Risk assessment and management of women with BRCA mutations. *The Female Patient, 34*(11), 1–4.

Kang, H.S., Thomas, E., Kwon, B.E., Hyun, M.S., & Jun, E.M. (2008). Stages of change: Korean women's attitudes and barriers toward mammography screening. *Health Care for Women International, 29*(2), 151–164.

Kim, J.H., & Kim, O. (2008). Predictors of perceived barriers to mammography in Korean women. *Asian Nursing Research, 2*(2), 74–81.

Knutson, D., & Steiner, E. (2007). Screening for breast cancer. Current recommendations and future directions. *American Family Physician, 75*(11), 1660–1666.

Lee, E. (2009). Evidence-based management of benign breast diseases. *The American Journal for Nurse Practitioners, 13*(7/8), 22–31.

Lehman, C.D., Gastonis, C., Kuhl, C., Hendrick, R.E., Pisano, E.D., Hanna, L., Peacock, S., et al. (2007). MRI Evaluation of the contralateral breast in women with recently diagnosed breast cancer. *The New England Journal of Medicine, 356*(13), 1295–1303.

Lessick, M. (2007). Genetic testing for breast and ovarian cancer: Ethical, legal, and psychosocial considerations. *Nursing for Women's Health, 11*(4), 390–401.

Makuc, D.M., Breen, N., Meissner, H.I., Vernon, S.W., & Cohen, A. (2007). Financial barriers to mammography: Who pays out-of-pocket? *Journal of Women's Health, 16*(3), 349–360.

Marcovici, I. (2007). Mondor disease of the breast. *Female Patient, 32*(10), 53–58.

Moeller, M. (2008). Genomics in breast cancer care. *Women's Health Care: A Practical Journal for Nurse Practitioners, 7*(9), 19–24.

National Cancer Institute (2009a). *Fact sheet: Mammograms.* Retrieved from http://www.nci.nih.gov/cancertopics/factsheet/Detection/screening-mammograms (Accessed October 11, 2009).

National Cancer Institute (2009b). *Breast Cancer Risk Assessment Tool.* Retrieved from http://www.cancer.gov/bcrisktool/Default.aspx (Accessed October 15, 2009).

National Cancer Institute. (2009c). *General information about breast cancer.* Retrieved from http://www.cancer.gov/cancertopics/pdq/treatment/breast/HealthProfessional/page2 (Accessed October 16, 2009).

Pisano, E., Gastonis, C., Hendrick, E., Yaffe, M., Braum, J., Acharyya, S., et al. (2005). Diagnostic performance of digital versus film mammography for breast cancer screening: The results of the American College of Radiology Imaging Network (ACRIN) digital mammographic imaging screening trial (DMIST). *The New England Journal of Medicine, 353*(17), 1773–1783.

Pomeranz, S.J. (2007). Breast MRI scans: What women need to know. *Radiology Today, 8*(10), 8–10.

Rafferty, E.A. (2004). Tomosynthesis: New weapon in breast cancer fight. *Imaging Economics.* Retrieved from http://www.imagingeconomics.com/issues/articles/2004-04_12.asp (Accessed October 11, 2009).

Rafferty, E.A. (2007). Digital mammography: Novel applications. *Radiologic Clinics of North America, 45*(1), 831–843.

Ruhl, C. (2007). Breast health screening: What all women should know. *Nursing for Women's Health, 11*(3), 326–330.

Ruhl, C. (2009). Cancer survivor care planning: A dynamic approach to cancer survivors' futures. *Nursing for Women's Health, 13*(5), 427–431.

Ruhl, C., & Moran, B. (2008). The clinical content of preconception care; preconception care for special populations. *American Journal of Obstetrics and Gynecology, 199*(6), (Suppl. B), S384–S388.

Smith, E.C. (2007). Breast cancer fundamentals. *Clinician Reviews, 17*(10), 32–40.

Smith-Bindman, R., Miglioretti, D.L., Lurie, N., Abraham, L., Barbash, R.B., Strzelczyk, J., et al. (2006). Does utilization of screening mammography explain racial and ethnic differences in breast cancer? *Annals of Internal Medicine, 144*(3), 541–553.

Theroux, R. (2007). Breast cancer after menopause: Do weight and exercise affect risk? *Nursing for Women's Health, 11*(3), 319–321.

U.S. Department of Health & Human Services (USDHHS). (2000). *Healthy People 2010*. Washington, DC: Author.

U.S. Department of Health & Human Services (USDHHS). (2008). *Minority women's health: Breast cancer*. Retrieved from http://64.94.16.210/minority/africanamerican/bc.cfm (Accessed October 12, 2009).

U.S. Preventive Services Task Force. (2009a). *Screening for breast cancer. Guide to preventive services, 2009, Section 2. Recommendations for adults*. Retrieved from http://www.ahrq.gov/clinic/pocketgd09/gcp09s2.htm (Accessed October 1, 2009).

U.S. Preventive Services Task Force. (2009b). Screening for breast cancer: U.S. Preventive Services Task Force recommendation statement. *Annals of Internal Medicine, 151*(10), 716–726.

Venes, D (Ed.). (2009). *Taber's cyclopedic medical dictionary* (21st ed.). Philadelphia: F.A. Davis.

Wang, J.H., Mandelblatt, J.S., Liang, W., Yi, B., Ma, I-Jung, & Schwartz, M.D. (2009). Knowledge, cultural, and attitudinal barriers to mammography screening among nonadherent immigrant Chinese women. *Cancer, 15*(20), 4828–4838.

Young, R.F., & Severson, R.K. (2005). Breast cancer screening barriers and mammography completion in older minority women. *Breast Cancer Research and Treatment, 89*(2), 1573–1577.

 For more information, go to http://davisplus.fadavis.com/

Promoting Reproductive Health Through an Understanding of Various Gynecological Disorders

Shelton Hisley, PhD, RNC, WHNP-BC

Both within the family and without,
our sisters hold up our mirrors,
our images of who we are and of
who we can dare to become.

—Elizabeth Fishel

LEARNING TARGETS *A the completion of this chapter, the student will be able to:*

- Describe various gynecological disorders and discuss implications for patient counseling and teaching.
- Describe various causes of abnormal uterine bleeding.
- Develop a nursing plan of care for a patient with a diagnosis of endometriosis.
- Develop a nursing plan of care for a patient with a diagnosis of polycystic ovary syndrome.
- Identify signs and symptoms that may be associated with vaginal, ovarian, endometrial, and vulvar carcinoma.
- Describe a strategy for increasing women's awareness of potential ovarian cancer symptoms.
- Teach a woman how to perform vulvar self-examination.

Introduction

This chapter explores several gynecological disorders in women. To deliver safe, effective care, nurses who care for women should be familiar with the special aspects of various gynecological conditions. It is important to remember that the human body functions as a whole system. Although a gynecological problem may initially appear to be confined to the pelvis, it could actually result from a host of other influences, activities, and imbalances. For example, amenorrhea, or absence of menses, may be related to excessive exercise, eating disorders, obesity, weight loss, stress, chronic illness, or endocrine disorders that adversely affect the normal functioning of the menstrual cycle (American College of Obstetricians and Gynecologists [ACOG], 2007).

Mutual trust and respect in the nurse–patient relationship help to facilitate appropriate discussion of questions and concerns about various health issues. Women's emotional responses to certain gynecological disorders may profoundly affect their quality of life and ability to function. The nurse must always remain sensitive to women's unique problems related to the functioning of their reproductive systems and offer holistic, individualized care that empowers them to seek and embrace strategies to restore balance and control over their lives.

Menstrual Disorders

Menstrual disorders, specifically amenorrhea, irregular bleeding, and dysmenorrhea, constitute some of the most common reproductive problems in women. Premenstrual syndrome, another problem frequently encountered in the clinical setting, is discussed in Chapter 2. Potential

<table>
<tr><td>

Box 4-1 Potential Nursing Diagnoses for Women with Menstrual Disorders

• Ineffective Coping related to emotional and physical effects that stem from the disorder
• Knowledge Deficit related to the cause, treatment, and self-care strategies of the disorder
• Disturbed Body Image related to sexual dysfunction associated with the disorder
• Situational Low Self-esteem related to an inability to conceive
• Acute Pain related to the menstrual disorder

</td></tr>
</table>

nursing diagnoses for women with various menstrual disorders are presented in Box 4-1.

AMENORRHEA

Under normal circumstances, the menstrual cycle is dependent on the integrated functioning of the hypothalamus, pituitary gland, ovaries, uterus, cervix, and vagina. Amenorrhea, or a lack of menstruation, may result from abnormalities of the structure or function of any of these organs.

The term *amenorrhea* is rooted from the Greek "a" = no + "men" = month + "rhoia" = flow = "no monthly flow." Amenorrhea may be classified as "primary" or "secondary." With primary amenorrhea, menstruation never takes place. With secondary amenorrhea, menstruation starts but then stops. The nurse should refer the patient for an evaluation for amenorrhea when the following circumstances are present.

Primary

• Lack of secondary sex characteristics by age 14–15
• Lack of menarche (the initial menstrual period) by age 15
• Lack of menses within 3 years after breast development (thelarche) or the appearance of pubic or axillary hair (pubarche or adrenarche) (ACOG, 2007)

Primary amenorrhea may be caused by a number of conditions, including pregnancy, lactation, missed abortion, eating disorders (e.g., anorexia nervosa, bulimia), obesity, hyperthyroidism, hypoglycemia, cystic fibrosis, Crohn's disease, genetic abnormalities, congenital absence of the cervix and/or vagina, and polycystic ovary syndrome.

Secondary

Secondary amenorrhea is defined as an absence of menses for at least 3 months in a woman who has previously had regular monthly menses, or a lack of menses for at least 6 to 12 months in a woman who normally experiences irregular menses. The term *delayed menses* is used in situations where the amenorrhea is for a shorter period of time (ACOG, 2007; Hatcher et al., 2008). Pregnancy, lactation, premature ovarian failure (menopause before age 40), weight loss, eating disorders, and obesity are conditions that may cause secondary amenorrhea. Other causes include hormonal contraceptive effects and post–oral contraceptive pill amenorrhea, pituitary gland dysfunction (e.g., hyperprolactinemia), polycystic ovary syndrome,

emotional or physical stress, frequent strenuous exercise, chronic illness (e.g., colitis, kidney failure, cystic fibrosis), cancer chemotherapy, ovarian cysts or tumors, and certain endocrine disorders such as Cushing's syndrome and thyroid dysfunction (ACOG, 2007).

When evaluating a patient for amenorrhea, the first step is to test for pregnancy. Once pregnancy has been ruled out, the patient undergoes a thorough physical examination and, depending on the findings, additional testing that may include laboratory and diagnostic testing (e.g., ultrasonography). In many situations, a careful review of the woman's health history can provide clues as to the cause(s) of the amenorrhea (ACOG, 2007; Hatcher et al., 2008).

 Nursing Insight— *Perspectives on amenorrhea*

Amenorrhea is a symptom, not a condition. In the United States, approximately 2% to 5% of all women of childbearing age are affected by amenorrhea. Although the cause is generally not a life-threatening condition, amenorrhea can be associated with significant potential morbidity. In most situations, amenorrhea is reversible with treatment for the underlying condition (ACOG, 2007).

ABNORMAL GENITAL BLEEDING

Any bleeding other than what is expected in a normal ovulatory cycle is considered abnormal genital bleeding. This condition constitutes one of the most frequent reasons for patient visits to the clinic or private office and accounts for approximately 19% of all gynecological complaints. The source of the bleeding may be the rectum, urinary tract, vulva, vagina, cervix, or uterus. Conditions that may cause abnormal bleeding include pregnancy and pregnancy-related complications, trauma, infection, endocrine abnormalities, lesions, or tumors (ACOG, 2007; Nelson & Baldwin, 2008).

 Nursing Insight— *Understanding correct terminology for abnormal genital bleeding*

Nurses who care for women should be familiar with terminology for abnormal genital bleeding, which is classified by the timing of the bleeding and the duration of the flow. The use of accurate terminology helps to promote effective communication and justifies appropriate work-ups and therapies. Patient-recorded menstrual calendars are beneficial in facilitating the accurate documentation of bleeding patterns.

Metrorrhagia is bleeding that occurs at abnormal times during an ovulatory cycle—that is, the woman experiences bleeding more frequently than every 21 days.

Menorrhagia is excess bleeding (80 mL or more, or bleeding that lasts longer than 7 days) during the expected time of menstrual flow.

Menometrorrhagia is a combination of the above two bleeding abnormalities—the woman experiences excessive bleeding and frequent bleeding at abnormal times during the cycle.

Polymenorrhea is bleeding that occurs at short intervals (less than 21 days).

Intermenstrual bleeding is bleeding of variable amounts that occur between regular menses.

Postcoital bleeding is bleeding that occurs after sexual intercourse (ACOG, 2007; Nelson & Baldwin, 2008; Stern, 2009).

A number of possible diagnoses are associated with bleeding disorders. Although many factors influence a woman's menstrual patterns, one of the first considerations is the patient's age. In an adolescent female, approximately 20 hormonal cycles occur before ovulation takes place on a regular basis. Bleeding that is irregular in both timing and amount tends to be the rule rather than the exception during early adolescence. Similarly, perimenopausal women commonly experience an increased variation in their menstrual intervals and in the quantity of flow during the 5 years that precede menopause. The cause of abnormal genital bleeding can range from simple to complex. Evaluation requires a careful and thorough history and work-up, including a physical examination, laboratory tests, and appropriate diagnostic tests such as ultrasonography (Nelson & Baldwin, 2008; Speroff & Fritz, 2005).

 Optimizing Outcomes— Using patient age to guide the work-up for abnormal genital bleeding

The patient's age is an important consideration in the evaluation of abnormal genital bleeding. For example during *adolescence*, a common cause is persistent anovulation, or failure to ovulate, which may be related to contraception, pregnancy, polycystic ovary syndrome, or coagulopathies.

During *mid-life* (30s–40s), women most often develop abnormal genital bleeding from pregnancy, structural lesions (e.g., leiomyomata [fibroid tumors], polyps), and anovulation, including that caused by polycystic ovary syndrome, hormone therapy, and endometrial hyperplasia.

During *menopause*, bleeding most often results from hormone therapy, endometrial atrophy, leiomyomata, endometrial hyperplasia, and malignancy (ACOG, 2007; Nelson & Baldwin, 2008).

DYSMENORRHEA

Dysmenorrhea, defined as painful menstruation, is one of the most common gynecological problems occurring in women of all ages. For most, the pain develops during or shortly before the onset of menstruation and is most intense in the suprapubic region or in the lower abdomen. Symptoms including nausea, vomiting, diarrhea, headaches, and lightheadedness may accompany the pain. Dysmenorrhea can cause significant disruption with daily activities each month, resulting in absence from school and missed time from work. Dysmenorrhea may be classified as primary (intrinsic and usually early onset) or secondary (results from some other physical cause and usually has a later onset) (Nelson & Baldwin, 2008).

Primary dysmenorrhea usually begins within 1 to 3 years following menarche and results from physiological causes—no pathology is present. In general, women with primary dysmenorrhea are ovulatory and thus produce progesterone in the luteal phase. Progesterone stimulates the production of prostaglandins in the base of the endometrium. Found in various tissues throughout the body, prostaglandins are substances that control local functions such as vasodilation and vasoconstriction. Women with primary dysmenorrhea produce excessive amounts of prostaglandin F2-alpha, which increases the force of the uterine contractions. Uterine contractions reduce blood flow to the uterus, causing ischemia and pain. The pain usually begins at the onset of menstrual flow and persists for 8 to 48 hours. During menstruation, the highest levels of prostaglandins are released during the first 48 hours. When the prostaglandins are introduced into the general circulation by uterine contractions, they can produce symptoms of headache, nausea, vomiting, and diarrhea (ACOG, 2007; Nelson & Baldwin, 2008).

Secondary dysmenorrhea is due to some other physical cause and usually is of a later onset. Women with secondary dysmenorrhea also complain of painful uterine cramping with menstruation but frequently have other accompanying complaints, such as dyspareunia or nonmenstrual pelvic pain. By definition, pain that occurs with secondary dysmenorrhea is related to uterine or pelvic pathology. The treatment for secondary dysmenorrhea should be targeted to the underlying cause and should be reflective of the patient's desire for fertility. When surgical intervention is not required, the treatments helpful for primary dysmenorrhea are often successful in reducing the symptoms of secondary dysmenorrhea (ACOG, 2007; Nelson & Baldwin, 2008).

The most common causes of secondary dysmenorrhea are adenomyosis, endometriosis, pelvic adhesions, and neoplasia. Adenomyosis is a condition characterized by the presence of endometrial glands and stoma that are embedded in the myometrium (the deep muscle layer of the uterus). Adenomyosis most commonly occurs in parous women. Each month, normal ovarian hormonal changes cause stimulation of the ectopic (abnormally located) endometrial tissue and produce sloughing within the myometrium. In addition to dysmenorrhea, women with adenomyosis may also experience heavy menses and perimenstrual pain. The uterus is enlarged, boggy, and tender immediately before and during menses (ACOG, 2007; Nelson & Baldwin, 2008).

Endometriosis is a condition characterized by implantation of endometrial tissue outside the uterus. Women with endometriosis experience painful menses due to the cyclic shedding of the ectopic endometriotic implants and the local inflammatory response triggered by the shedding. The pain associated with endometriosis often occurs just prior to the onset of menses. (See later discussion of endometriosis.) Pelvic adhesions may also cause secondary dysmenorrhea. Pelvic adhesions are fibrous bands that may result from previous pelvic inflammatory disease, appendicitis, and pelvic or abdominal surgery. *Neoplasia* is a term that refers to the abnormal proliferation of benign or malignant cells (ACOG, 2007; Bloski & Pierson, 2008; Nelson & Baldwin, 2008). (See later discussion about various neoplastic processes.)

Health-care teaching for women experiencing dysmenorrhea should be holistic in nature and include relaxation and breathing techniques, the use of heat to reduce uterine contractions and increase blood flow to the uterine tissues, exercise or rest, and the use of NSAIDs to inhibit the synthesis of prostaglandin. These drugs not only improve the cramping pain but also reduce backache, headaches, and gastrointestinal symptoms. When taken at the onset of menses, NSAIDs reduce the release of prostaglandins and considerably decrease menstrual blood loss. Other therapeutic interventions for dysmenorrhea include hormonal contraceptives (e.g., combined oral contraceptive pills, depo medroxyprogesterone acetate [Depo-Provera], the levonorgestrel-releasing intrauterine system [LNG-IUS]), which reduce menstrual blood loss and decrease the production of prostaglandins (Nelson & Baldwin, 2008).

Complementary Care: *Measures for Relief From Dysmenorrhea*

Throughout the ages, women have resorted to the use of various herbal remedies such as cramp bark, wild yam, black haw, ginger, and raspberry leaf to ease the pain of menstrual cramps. The nurse should counsel patients that because herbal preparations may be toxic and also interact with other medications, only preparations obtained from reputable companies should be used. Other strategies for relief from menstrual pain include the application of heat or cold, massage, meditation, and progressive relaxation. Exercise is beneficial for some women. Physical activity enhances blood flow to the pelvis and reduces pelvic congestion. Dietary strategies include the use of natural diuretics such as peaches, parsley, and cranberry juice to reduce edema and limiting the intake of meat.

Now Can You— Discuss abnormal genital bleeding, dysmenorrhea, and vaginal infections?

1. Define the terms *metrorrhagia, menorrhagia, menometrorrhagia, and polymenorrhea*?
2. Differentiate primary dysmenorrhea from secondary dysmenorrhea and identify three possible causes of secondary dysmenorrhea?
3. Develop a holistic teaching plan for women who experience dysmenorrhea?

Common Vaginal Infections

Under normal circumstances, the vaginal environment functions as an ecosystem that maintains a steady state as it interacts with the environment outside the vagina. Many organisms, including certain bacteria and yeast, normally reside in the vagina. In fact, at any given time, from 5 to 10 different types of microorganisms are normally present in the vaginal flora. *Lactobacillus* is the dominant bacterial genus. It plays an essential role in helping to maintain the vaginal balance by producing byproducts such as lactic acid and hydrogen peroxide. These byproducts allow the vagina to maintain a healthy acidic pH of less than 4.5, which prevents the overgrowth of less desirable vaginal microorganisms. If the delicate balance of microorganisms is upset, the potentially pathogenic minor bacteria can proliferate to a concentration that causes symptoms (ACOG, 2007; Hatcher et al., 2008; Nyirjesy & Sobel, 2005).

Nursing Insight— *Understanding vaginal infections*

During the reproductive years, the normal vaginal pH range is between 3.8 and 4.2, which falls within the acidic spectrum of the pH scale. Anaerobic bacteria are unable to colonize and thrive in the normally acidic vaginal environment, and lactobacilli become the predominant bacteria. When anaerobic bacteria are able to colonize, they eradicate the lactobacilli, creating an alkaline environment that allows continued colonization. Vaginal infections primarily occur in two ways: An imbalance and overgrowth of organisms that normally inhabit the vagina proliferate and cause symptoms, or organisms are introduced into the vagina, usually from intimate sexual contact. Factors that may cause an alteration in the normal vaginal environment include stress, douching, feminine hygiene products, harsh soaps, dietary changes (e.g., sugar, caffeine), sexual intercourse, barrier contraceptive methods (e.g., condoms, diaphragms), spermicides, synthetic underwear or tight-fitting pants, illness, chronic metabolic conditions (e.g., diabetes), immunosuppression, certain medications, and pregnancy (Coughlin & Secor, 2010; Hatcher et al., 2008).

Optimizing Outcomes— Teaching women strategies for promoting vaginal health

Nurses can be instrumental in promoting vaginal health by teaching women about the normal functioning of their bodies. Women can be taught that leukorrhea is a normal vaginal discharge that undergoes hormonally mediated changes throughout the menstrual cycle. In the early (proliferative) phase, estrogen promotes a clear, thin, stretchy vaginal discharge. Later, the discharge becomes thick and tacky in response to the effects of progesterone, the dominant hormone during the second half of the cycle. The normal vaginal discharge varies in quantity from woman to woman, and often from cycle to cycle. Nurses can help patients explore ways to promote a balanced vaginal environment through alterations in lifestyle and choice of birth control method. Women should be taught that douching is discouraged, as it has a drying effect on the vagina and disrupts the normal vaginal flora. Douching can also cause an increase in the amount of vaginal discharge normally present and has been shown to contribute to serious infection of the upper reproductive tract (ACOG, 2007; Hatcher et al., 2008; Vermund & Allen, 2009).

A number of infections and conditions that involve the vaginal environment are commonly seen in women with gynecological disorders. These include bacterial vaginosis, candidiasis, sexually transmitted diseases (STDs), cervicitis, and pelvic inflammatory disease (PID). Cervicitis may be accompanied by a purulent discharge, which may be a symptom of infection with gonorrhea or chlamydia. Less commonly encountered conditions include vaginal carcinoma (primary, which is rare, or secondary, which results from the spread of cancer to the vagina from another site), cancer associated with in utero exposure to diethylstilbestrol (DES), and toxic shock syndrome (TSS). STDs and PID are discussed in a separate chapter.

BACTERIAL VAGINOSIS

Bacterial vaginosis (BV) was previously called "nonspecific vaginitis," *Haemophilus vaginitis*, or *Gardnerella*. BV is the most common vaginal infection in women, and although it is a sexually associated condition, it is not usually considered to be a specific STD. This vaginal infection is related to a lack of hydrogen peroxide–producing lactobacilli (microorganisms that normally maintain a low vaginal pH) and a dramatic overgrowth of the vaginal resident bacterium *Gardnerella vaginalis* and anaerobic bacteria (e.g., *Mycoplasma hominis, Mobiluncus, Bacteroides, Prevotella, Peptostreptococcus, Eubacterium, Escherichia coli*, and group B streptococci). Anaerobic bacteria thrive in a low-oxygen environment (ACOG, 2007; Coughlin & Secor, 2010; Hatcher et al., 2008).

 Ethnocultural Considerations— Prevalence of bacterial vaginosis

Bacterial vaginosis affects approximately 30% of reproductive-age women. In the United States, African American women are infected with BV at three times the rate of Caucasian women. The prevalence rate of BV is highest in African American women without Hispanic heritage (50.3%) and Mexican American women (28.8%) when compared with non-Hispanic Caucasian women (22.4%) (Coughlin & Secor, 2010; Koumans et al., 2007).

Women with BV may be asymptomatic. When present, symptoms include a thin white or gray adherent vaginal discharge with a "fishy" amine odor, and women often report that the odor is worse after intercourse and following menses. The diagnosis is made on the basis of a positive finding on the "whiff" test—the characteristic amine odor is produced when a sample of the discharge is combined with a 10% solution of potassium hydroxide (KOH). Microscopic examination of the vaginal fluid (i.e., a wet mount) reveals the presence of clue cells, which are sloughed vaginal epithelial cells coated with bacteria that cling to the edges of the cells. Clue cells have a granular appearance with indistinct, blurry borders (Fig. 4-1).

 Nursing Insight— The vaginal wet mount

A wet mount, also known as a "wet-prep" or "wet smear," is frequently used in the clinical setting to diagnose three of the most common vaginal infections: bacterial vaginosis, trichomoniasis, and yeast (candidiasis). To perform this test, the clinician inserts a speculum and uses a moist cotton swab to take a sample of the discharge from the posterior vaginal fornix. The discharge is then placed on a glass slide and viewed under a microscope. Alternately, a dry swab may be used: The sample is placed in 1 mL of saline, mixed, and placed on a slide or a drop of saline is placed on a slide and the sample is added to it. A cover slip is then applied and the slide is promptly viewed.

Typically, when BV is present, the vaginal pH is above the normal value of 4.5. Because BV may occur concurrently with other STDs (e.g., chlamydia, gonorrhea, genital herpes), it is important to screen for STDs as well (ACOG, 2007; Coughlin & Secor, 2010; Elkins & Mayeaux, 2010; Hatcher et al., 2008).

 Optimizing Outcomes— With vaginal pH testing kits for home and clinical use

Self-diagnosis of vaginal infections based on symptoms alone is inaccurate approximately 50% of the time. Over-the-counter vaginal pH screening tests (e.g., Vagisil Screening Kit for vaginal infections, VI-SENSE) can help distinguish vaginal symptoms that require attention from a health-care provider. The Vagisil Screening Kit contains plastic wands with attached pH paper; the woman touches the wand to the vaginal wall to moisten the pH paper and withdraws the device. The vaginal pH level is then compared to the color on the pH guide. A pH value of 4.5 suggests that the vaginal symptoms are due to candidiasis (yeast); a pH reading of 5.0 or higher indicates that the vaginal symptoms are likely due to BV, trichomoniasis, or a mixed infection, and office follow-up is necessary (Dunican, 2008; Scolaro, Lloyd, & Helms, 2008; Wysocki, 2009).

The VS-SENSE is a swab-based test to detect vaginitis in the clinical setting. The VS-SENSE indicates by color change the elevated vaginal acidity levels associated with bacterial vaginosis and trichomonas. This new screening test offers immediate results and assists in detecting BV and trichomonas even when *Candida* (yeast) symptoms mask the more serious infections.

When BV is detected in an asymptomatic woman, it is usually not treated unless the patient will be undergoing an invasive surgical procedure, such as abortion, hysterectomy, or insertion of an intrauterine device. These procedures increase the risk of pelvic infection in the presence of BV. Bacterial vaginosis has also been shown to be associated with various pregnancy complications, such as spontaneous abortion, preterm birth, and infection following cesarean birth (ACOG, 2007; Coughlin & Secor, 2010; Hatcher et al., 2008).

Symptomatic women are typically treated with metronidazole (Flagyl), which is given either orally (500 mg twice a day for 7 days) or vaginally (metronidazole gel, 0.75% [Metro-Gel], 5 grams intravaginally for 5 days). Flagyl should not be used in women with a history of seizures. No alcohol should be ingested 24 hours before or after taking this medication, since the combination of metronidazole and alcohol causes abdominal discomfort, nausea, vomiting, and headache. Since nausea is the most common side effect, nurses should advise women to always take the medication with food. Metronidazole

Figure 4-1 Clue cell (Venes, D. (Ed.). (2009). *Taber's cyclopedic medical dictionary* (p. 397, 21st ed.). Philadelphia: F. A. Davis)

readily crosses the placenta and should not be taken during the first trimester of pregnancy; it is also contraindicated in breastfeeding women. Clindamycin (Cleocin) given orally (300 mg twice a day for 7 days) or in a 2% vaginal cream (5 grams intravaginally for 7 days) or in a vaginal ovule (100 mg at bedtime for 3 days) is also used to treat bacterial vaginosis. This medication is especially useful in individuals with an allergy or intolerance to metronidazole. Tinidazole (Tindamax), an oral medication, may also be used to treat BV in non-pregnant, adult women. The recommended dose is 2 grams once daily for 2 days, or 1 gram once daily for 5 days, and this medication should be taken with food. The half-life of this medication is twice as long as that of metronidazole, and it has fewer side effects. Alcohol should be avoided during the 3 days after taking tinidazole because of its longer half-life. Because treatment of male sexual partners has no effect on the recurrence rate in female partners, male treatment is not indicated (ACOG, 2007; Centers for Disease Control and Prevention [CDC] 2006a; Coughlin & Secor, 2010; Elkins & Mayeaux, 2010; Hatcher et al., 2008). Health professionals should consult the CDC Web site (http://www.cdc.gov/std/treatment/2006/vaginal-discharge.htm#vagdis2) for the most current guidelines on BV treatment.

CANDIDIASIS

Commonly known as a yeast infection, candidiasis is generally caused by *Candida albicans* (Fig. 4-2). Other related yeast species (e.g., *C. tropicalis, C. glabrata, C. parapsilosis, C. krusei, C. lusitaniae*), however, can also be causative agents as well. Infection with candidiasis is usually characterized by intense vulvar pruritus (itching) and irritation and a thick, white, cottage cheese–like vaginal discharge that may have a sour odor. The discharge may be observed on the vaginal walls, cervix, and labia, and the vulva and labial folds are red and edematous. The patient may complain of dyspareunia and dysuria, although symptoms are subtler in some women. The diagnosis of candidiasis is made on the basis of microscopic examination of the vaginal discharge. A saline and KOH wet smear reveals budding yeast or pseudohyphae. The vaginal pH is usually unaltered, although it may be slightly more acidic than normal. During the examination, it is important to rule out STDs (Watson & Ng, 2008).

Figure 4-2 Gram's stain of *Candida albicans* (purple) in blood (× 640) (Venes, D. (Ed.). (2009). *Taber's cyclopedic medical dictionary* (p. 354, 21st ed.). Philadelphia: F. A. Davis)

Optimizing Outcomes— Recognizing factors that are associated with vulvovaginal candidiasis

Certain factors are associated with vulvovaginal candidiasis, such as the use of broad-spectrum antibiotics and systemic corticosteroids, which can cause a reduction in the normal protective vaginal flora (Pirotta & Garland, 2006; Sheary & Dayan, 2005); high-dose oral contraceptives; and uncontrolled diabetes and allergies, especially allergic rhinitis (White, Vanthuyne, Wood, & Ayres, 2004). Spermicidal creams have also been associated with vaginal yeast infections. Nurses can advise women who use these medications or products about strategies to enhance the normal vaginal environment and reduce the likelihood of vulvovaginal candidiasis (Watson & Ng, 2008).

Candidiasis is treated with antifungal medications, and many over-the-counter agents such as miconazole (Monistat) and clotrimazole (Gyne-Lotrimin) are available. Most of the commercial products are fungistats that inhibit the organisms from reproducing, so the woman's immune system can suppress the yeast. Patients can apply a topical antifungal cream to the vulva as well as the intravaginal cream or suppositories. It is important to remind women that creams and vaginal suppositories are oil based and may weaken latex condoms or diaphragms (CDC, 2006a). Although these medications are available without prescription, the nurse should advise patients to avoid self-treatment without first undergoing a clinical evaluation to confirm the diagnosis of vulvovaginal candidiasis. Treatment of asymptomatic sexual partners is not generally necessary (ACOG, 2007; Watson & Ng, 2008).

Complementary Care: *Measures for Vaginal Candidiasis*

Nurses can educate women about strategies to relieve symptoms of candidiasis and help prevent recurrent yeast infections. For example, women can be advised to take sitz baths for comfort and add Aveeno powder to the bath. Boric acid, 600 mg in size 0 gelatin capsules inserted in the vagina each night for 14 days, has been reported to be effective against resistant infections. Vaginal suppositories containing acidophilic bacteria, as well as long-term (6 months) daily ingestion of dairy products or powders, capsules, or tablets that contain *Lactobacillus acidophilus* are other strategies that anecdotally have been associated with prevention and relief of symptoms, although the evidence supporting this intervention is conflicting (Falagas, Betsil, & Athansion, 2006; Goodman, Herman, Murdaugh, Moneyham, & Phillips, 2007). Nurses can also teach women to wear cotton underwear to enhance ventilation of the genital area, avoid wearing tight-fitting pants or wet clothing (e.g., bathing suits) for prolonged periods of time, and avoid potential irritants such as perfumed soaps; bubble baths; hot tubs; and the application of perfumes, sprays, or powder near the vaginal area.

Stronger antifungal prescription medications are available in creams or suppositories, along with oral preparations, including fluconazole (Diflucan), itraconazole (Sporanox), and ketoconazole (Nizoral). Although the oral medications are associated with various side effects (e.g., nausea, vomiting, diarrhea, abdominal pain, head-ache), they tend to be well tolerated by most women. Ketoconazole is associated with hepatotoxicity, and base-line and ongoing liver function monitoring is recom-mended. Oral antifungals and boric acid suppositories should not be used during pregnancy. Topical antifun-gals have limited systemic absorption and are considered safe for maternal use. Women who have recurrent yeast infections should be evaluated for diabetes and infection with HIV (CDC, 2006a; Hatcher et al., 2008; Watson & Ng, 2008).

 Now Can You— Discuss various aspects of vaginitis?

1. Develop an educational tool for teaching women about promoting healthy vaginal environment.
2. Compare and contrast bacterial vaginosis and vaginal candidiasis.
3. Describe strategies intended to relieve symptoms and help prevent recurrence of vaginal candidiasis.

Vaginal Carcinoma

Vaginal carcinoma is any type of cancer that forms in the tissues of the vagina. Vaginal carcinomas can be primary or secondary or related to in utero diethylstilbestrol (DES) exposure. Vaginal cancer is extremely rare, occurs primarily in women over age 50, and accounts for only 1% to 2% of gynecological malignancies. It is frequently asymptomatic and first detected during a routine gyneco-logical examination. Abnormal vaginal bleeding consti-tutes the most common symptom of this type of cancer, and the bleeding may be postcoital, intermenstrual, pre-pubertal, or postmenopausal. Other symptoms include foul-smelling vaginal discharge, dysuria, dyspareunia, and pelvic pain.

There are two primary types of vaginal cancer: squa-mous cell carcinoma and adenocarcinoma. Most lesions (85% of cases) are squamous cell carcinomas that arise from the thin, flat, squamous cells that line the vagina. These kinds of cancers develop over a period of many years and are usually found in women between the ages of 60 and 80. Vaginal squamous cell carcinoma occurs most often in women with a history of infection with human papillomavirus (HPV) (genital warts) or cervical or vulvar cancer. The time from HPV infection to the development of invasive cancer is believed to be from 5 to 10 years. In most cases, the cancer initially spreads super-ficially within the vaginal wall and later invades the para-vaginal tissues and the parametria (the connective tissue and fat adjacent to the uterus). Distant metastases occur most commonly in the lungs and liver (National Cancer Institute [NCI], 2009).

Vaginal adenocarcinoma (occurring in approximately 15% of cases) arises from the glandular or secretory cells that line the vagina and produce some vaginal fluids. Adenocarcinoma is more likely than squamous cell can-cer to spread to the lungs and lymph nodes. The most common type of vaginal adenocarcinoma usually devel-ops in women over the age of 50. Clear cell adenocarci-noma is another type of vaginal cancer that usually occurs in women who were exposed to diethylstilbestrol (DES) in utero.

 Nursing Insight— *Understanding diethylstilbestrol (DES)*

Diethylstilbestrol (DES) is a nonsteroidal, synthetic estro-gen that is several times more potent than natural estrogens. In the United States, DES was prescribed to approximately 5 to 10 million mothers during the late 1930s until the early 1970s as a preventative treatment to reduce the likelihood of spontaneous abortion or preterm birth (Smith, 1948). It was taken off the market when study results revealed that DES was linked to abnormalities in both male and female offspring of women who received this drug during pregnancy. Structural alterations, changes in the tissue of the vagina and cervix, and infertility have been linked to in utero DES exposure. The incidence of DES-related clear cell adenocarcinoma is highest for those women who were exposed during the first 3 months of their mother's pregnancy. The highest incidence of occur-rence is between ages 17 and 21. The incidence of vaginal clear cell adenocarcinoma peaked in the early 1970s and is now rare, since DES use during pregnancy diminished during the early 1960s and was banned in the early 1970s (Helming, 2009; Stern, 2007).

Other less common forms of vaginal cancer include germ cell tumors (e.g., teratoma, endodermal sinus tumors), which are rare and found most often in infants and children; malignant melanoma; and sarcoma botryoi-des, a rhabdomyosarcoma that is also found most often in infants and children. Screening for malignancies of the vagina is similar to screening for cervical cancer. In addi-tion to a history and physical examination, diagnostic testing for vaginal carcinoma includes a pelvic exam, Pap smear, biopsy, and colposcopy (an examination of the cervix, using a lighted instrument that magnifies the tis-sues). Other diagnostic modalities may include laboratory testing and imaging studies (ACOG, 2007; NCI, 2009; Stern, 2007).

The prognosis for vaginal carcinoma depends primarily on the type and stage of the condition at the time of diag-nosis, but survival is reduced in women who are older than 60 years of age, are symptomatic at the time of diag-nosis, have lesions of the middle and lower third of the vagina, or have poorly differentiated tumors. Treatment modalities depend on the stage of the condition; surgery or radiation therapy is highly effective in the early stages, while radiation therapy is the primary treatment for the more advanced stages. Chemotherapy has not been shown to be curative for advanced vaginal cancer (ACOG, 2007; NCI, 2009; Stern, 2007).

Toxic Shock Syndrome

Toxic shock syndrome (TSS) is a rare, sometimes fatal condition that affects many body systems. Although this disorder is not well understood, TSS is believed to be asso-ciated with tampon use during menses. However, TSS can also occur in children, men, and non-menstruating women. Non-menstrual TSS risk is increased for women who use vaginal barrier contraceptives. The incidence of TSS peaked during the late 1970s and 1980s, most likely because of the widespread availability of superabsorbent tampons. A few specific tampon designs and high-absorbency tampon materials were found to have some association with an increased risk of TSS; these products are no longer sold in the United States. Today, the overall rate of TSS is 1 to 3 cases per 100,000 people per year, and only 55% of current cases are associated with menstruation (Hatcher et al., 2008).

⟳ Be sure to— Teach about toxic shock syndrome

Women who use a diaphragm, cervical cap, or contraceptive sponge should be aware of the possible association between these devices and toxic shock syndrome. Common signs of TSS include fever of sudden onset greater than 102.2°F (38.9°C), diffuse rash, vomiting, diarrhea, malaise, muscle aches, and hypotension with a systolic blood pressure less than 90 mm Hg. Patients who experience these symptoms should seek medical care immediately; left untreated, TSS can be fatal within hours (CDC, 2005).

Toxic shock syndrome is caused almost exclusively by toxins produced by some strains of the colonized bacterium *Staphylococcus aureus*. Toxins produced from the bacterium *Streptococcus pyogenes* may also cause TSS (sometimes referred to as "Toxic Shock–Like Syndrome" [TSLS] or "Streptococcal Toxic Shock Syndrome" [STSS]). Although the exact mechanism of cause is unknown, several conditions are believed to contribute to the development of menstrual TSS. These include alterations in the normal vaginal flora, a neutral vaginal pH, mechanical blockage of menstrual flow, contamination of tampons by the bacteria *S. aureus*, absorption of bacteria-resistant cervical fluids, the superabsorbent or synthetic materials found in some tampons, and damaged cervical or vaginal tissue. The toxin implicated in menstrual TSS is capable of entering the bloodstream by crossing the vaginal wall in the absence of ulcerations (Hatcher et al., 2008).

⟳ Optimizing Outcomes— Strategies to reduce risk for menstrual TSS

Nurses can teach women about strategies to minimize the risk of contracting menstrual TSS. For example, menstruating women may use sanitary pads or choose a tampon with the minimum absorbency needed to manage the menstrual flow and use the tampons only during active menstruation. Women can be taught to change tampons frequently (at least every 6 hours) and alternate sanitary pads with tampons, especially during the night. Nurses should emphasize that if symptoms suggestive of TSS occur, the tampon should be removed and medical attention sought immediately.

The diagnosis of TSS is made on the basis of physical examination findings and symptoms, along with results of a complete blood count, which often shows an elevated white blood cell count indicative of an acute infectious process. Treatment of this potentially life-threatening condition involves immediate hospitalization with fluid replacement and aggressive antibiotic therapy. Antibiotics should cover both *S. aureus* and *S. pyogenes* and may include a combination of cephalosporins, penicillins, and vancomycin, along with clindamycin or gentamicin. With appropriate care and prompt treatment, patients usually recover within 2 to 3 weeks (Hatcher et al., 2008).

 Nursing Insight— Formulating appropriate nursing diagnoses for patients with TSS

Nursing diagnoses for patients with TSS may focus on Hyperthermia (related to the inflammatory process/hypermetabolic state and dehydration), Deficient Fluid Volume (related to increased gastric losses, fever, and decreased intake), Acute Pain (related to the inflammatory process, effects of circulating toxins, and skin disruptions), and Impaired Skin/Tissue Integrity (related to the effects of circulating toxins and dehydration).

Urinary Tract Infections

Because of the widespread prevalence of urinary tract infections in women, a brief description of the problem is included in this discussion of gynecological disorders. Urinary tract infection (UTI) is defined as significant bacteriuria in the presence of symptoms. UTIs occur more frequently in women than in men because of the shorter route from the external environment to the bladder in women, along with the close proximity of the urethra to the vaginal and anal areas. UTIs account for a significant number (>6 million) of physician/health clinic visits each year, and it is estimated that 20% of women will be affected by a UTI at some time during their lifetime (ACOG, 2008a).

Under normal circumstances, the flow of urine keeps bacteria flushed from the urinary tract, and the entire urinary system remains sterile. The bladder wall possesses antibacterial properties, and the urine is usually acidic, which inhibits growth of bacteria.

A & P review The Female Urinary Tract and Bacterial Exposure

The female and male urinary tracts are relatively the same except for the length of the urethra. Owing to this difference, women are 30 times more likely to develop UTIs than are men. The female urethra is approximately 1.5 inches long; the male urethra is approximately 8 inches long. In women, bacteria from fecal matter can be easily transferred to the vagina or the urethra (Figs. 4-3 and 4-4). Most UTIs arise from one type of bacteria, *Escherichia coli*, which normally lives in the colon. Other common culprits include *Enterococcus faecalis*, *Staphylococcus saprophyticus*, *Klebsiella pneumoniae*, and *Proteus mirabilis*. Chlamydia and mycoplasma may also cause UTIs in both women and men, but these infections tend to remain limited to the urethra and reproductive system. Unlike *E. coli*, chlamydia and mycoplasma may be sexually transmitted (Sadovsky, 2007). ◆

Risk factors for UTIs include extremes of age, altered immunity, diabetes, urinary tract obstructions, pregnancy, sexual activity, and diaphragm use. Irritation of the urethra during sexual activity can cause bacteria to migrate upward

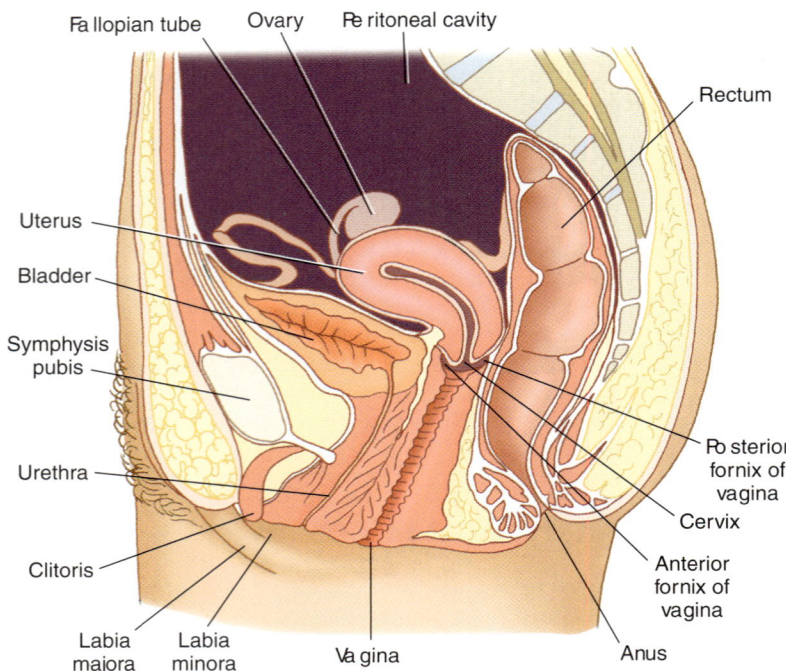

Figure 4-3 Internal female genitalia (Dillon, P. M. (2007). *Nursing health assessment: A critical thinking approach* (2nd ed., p. 612). Philadelphia, F. A. Davis)

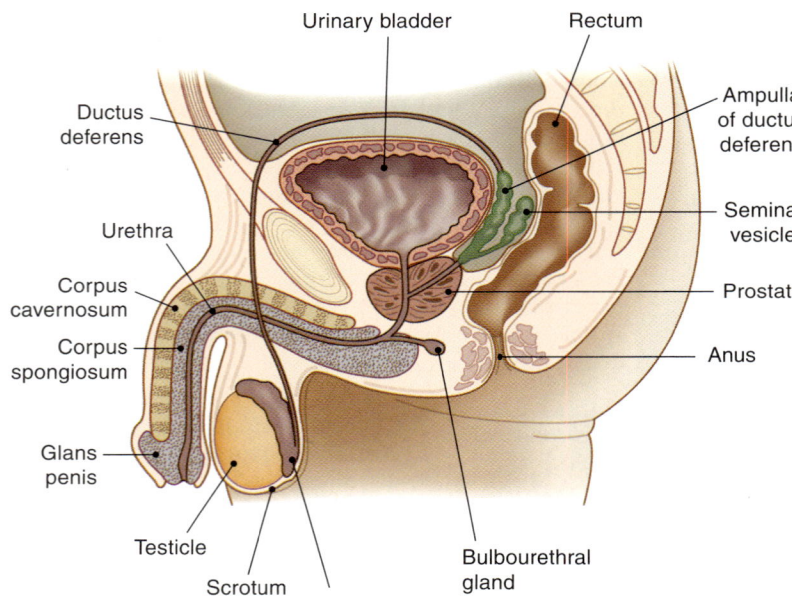

Figure 4-4 Male genitourinary system (Dillon, P. M. (2007). *Nursing health assessment: A critical thinking approach* (2nd ed., p. 651). Philadelphia, F. A. Davis)

into the urinary tract. Spermicides may alter the vaginal pH and decrease levels of normal protective bacteria, allowing harmful bacteria to grow in the vagina, which can then migrate to the bladder. Allergy to certain ingredients in soaps, vaginal creams, bubble baths, or other chemicals used in the genital area may cause tissue injury that can allow for the introduction of bacteria.

✿ Nursing Insight— *Recognizing signs and symptoms of a UTI*

Nurses should be alert to certain patient symptoms that may be indicative of a UTI. Dysuria (pain with urination),

urinary frequency, urgency, a sensation of bladder fullness, suprapubic tenderness, and cloudy, foul-smelling urine are classic symptoms associated with a UTI. If the infection has ascended to the kidneys, the woman may experience pain in the lower back region where the vertebrae and ribs meet (costovertebral angle tenderness), and fever may be present.

Diagnosis for a UTI varies according to the location and extent of the infection. For uncomplicated infection of the lower urinary tract, the diagnosis is made on the basis of symptoms and urinalysis, including the microscopic examination of a clean-catch urine sample (Procedure 1) for the presence of white or red blood cells and

Procedure 1 Obtaining a Midstream Urine Sample

Preparation

1. Complete the information requested on the container label. Include the patient's full name and the date and time of collection of the specimen. If a requisition is needed, note the date and time on the requisition.

2. Explain the procedure to the woman to ensure she understands why a urine sample is requested, the purpose of any tests to be performed, and directions on how to obtain a midstream urine sample.

Equipment

Approved empty sterile container for collection
Towelette for cleaning in between the labia
Tissue

Procedural Steps

Instruct the patient to do the following:

1. Wash and dry your hands thoroughly or use an alcohol-based hand rub

   RATIONALE: *To reduce the risk of specimen contamination. Alcohol-based hand rubs are fast acting, reduce the number of microorganisms on the skin, and may cause less skin irritation or dryness.*

2. Remove the container cap and set it on a clean, even surface with the inner surface pointing up. Do not touch the inner surface of the lid or the container.

   RATIONALE: *To reduce the risk of specimen contamination.*

3. Sit on the toilet seat and separate the labia (vaginal lips) using your nondominant hand. Clean the urogenital area from the front to back with the towelette provided. Wipe for only one stroke and then discard the towelette.

   RATIONALE: *To reduce the risk of specimen contamination and to reduce the number of microorganisms on the skin. Cleansing from front to back prevents bringing rectal contamination forward.*

4. Holding the labia apart, begin to pass urine. Allow the beginning urine go directly into the toilet.

   RATIONALE: *The initial stream of urine washes urethral microorganisms and other debris away from the urethral meatus. The midstream collection ensures that a sterile specimen is obtained.*

5. Continue to urinate and hold the container under the urine stream. Avoid touching the inside of the container. Remove the container when it is approximately half full.

6. Carefully replace the cap and secure tightly.

   RATIONALE: *Placing the cap on the container prevents inadvertent spilling and possible contamination of the urine specimen.*

7. Wash your hands again after the specimen collection.

   Clinical Alert Pregnant women are at an increased risk for developing urinary tract infections, especially if they are diabetic or have gestational diabetes. Urinary tract infections may also predispose to the onset of preterm labor.

bacteria. Complicated cases require a urine culture and sensitivity. In some practice settings, a leukocyte esterase or nitrite urine dipstick screening test to detect bacteriuria in women with suspected uncomplicated urinary tract infections is used (ACOG, 2008a).

Teach the patient to recognize common signs of a UTI:

- Dysuria—pain (burning sensation) on urination
- Urinary frequency associated with small amounts of urine
- Hematuria—blood or red blood cells in the urine

Treatment for uncomplicated lower urinary tract infections may be initiated in non-pregnant women with antibiotic therapy given over a 3-day course. Medications commonly used include co-trimoxazole (e.g., Bactrim, Septra), nitrofurantoin macrocrystals (e.g., Macrodantin), and amoxicillin/clavulanate (e.g., Augmentin). If the woman complains of intense dysuria, a bladder analgesic such as phenazopyridine (Pyridium), given for 1 to 2 days, is beneficial in alleviating the bladder discomfort (ACOG, 2008a).

 Optimizing Outcomes— Strategies to promote bladder health and decrease the incidence of UTI

Nurses can teach women about strategies to promote bladder health and decrease the likelihood of developing a UTI. For example, the nurse may advise the patient to:

- Void frequently (every 2–4 hours); avoid postponing urination (allowing urine to remain in the bladder allows bacteria to multiply).
- Empty the bladder before and after intercourse; drink liquids before and after intercourse.
- Remain hydrated to keep bacteria flushed out of the urinary tract system.
- Drink fruit juices to acidify the urine; take vitamin C regularly to inhibit bacterial growth.
- Wipe the urethral meatus and perineum from front to back after voiding.
- Avoid harsh soaps, powders, sprays; avoid bubble baths and bath oils.
- Wear cotton underwear; avoid tight-fitting underwear and pants.

Now Can You— Discuss various aspects of vaginal carcinoma, toxic shock syndrome, and urinary tract infections?

1. Identify risk factors for vaginal carcinoma?
2. Develop an educational program to teach women about toxic shock syndrome?
3. Discuss urinary tract infections and describe five strategies to reduce risk for a UTI?

Endometriosis

First described by Dr. John Sampson in the 1920s, endometriosis is defined as the growth, adhesion, and progression of endometrial glands and tissue outside of the uterine cavity with cellular activity evident in lesions, nodules, and cysts. Women ages 30 to 40 are most likely to develop endometriosis, and the condition is found in 20% to 40% of infertile women and in up to 33% of women with chronic pelvic pain. Endometrial lesions have been discovered on the ovaries, fallopian tubes, lining of the inside of the pelvic cavity, cervix, bladder, bowel, brain, nostrils, liver, and lungs (Fig. 4-5) (Audebert et al., 1992; Bloski & Pierson, 2008; Sampson, 1940).

Each month, the misplaced endometrial tissue responds to cyclic hormonal stimulation during the secretory and proliferative stages of the menstrual cycle, growing and thickening in a similar fashion to the endometrial tissue normally lining the uterus. During the ischemic and menstrual phases of the cycle, however, the misplaced endometrial tissue breaks down and bleeds into the surrounding tissue, causing inflammation. The released blood becomes trapped in the surrounding tissues, causing the development of blood-containing cysts. The recurrence of inflammation in the areas outside of the uterus eventually results in scarring, fibrosis, and the development of adhesions, scar tissue that binds the organs together, causing increased abdominal pain and a risk of infertility (Guo & Wang, 2006; Bloski & Pierson, 2008; Speroff & Fritz, 2005; Woodson, 2007).

 Nursing Insight— *Understanding terms associated with endometriosis*

Endometriosis is the presence of endometrial glands and tissue outside the uterus. An *endometrioma* is a solitary, non-neoplastic mass that contains endometrial tissue. An endometrioma is also referred to as an *endometrioid cyst*. Endometrioid cysts, often filled with dark, reddish-brown blood, may range in size from 0.75 to 8 inches (19.05 mm–20.32 cm). An endometrioid cyst is sometimes called a "chocolate cyst" because it is filled with old blood.

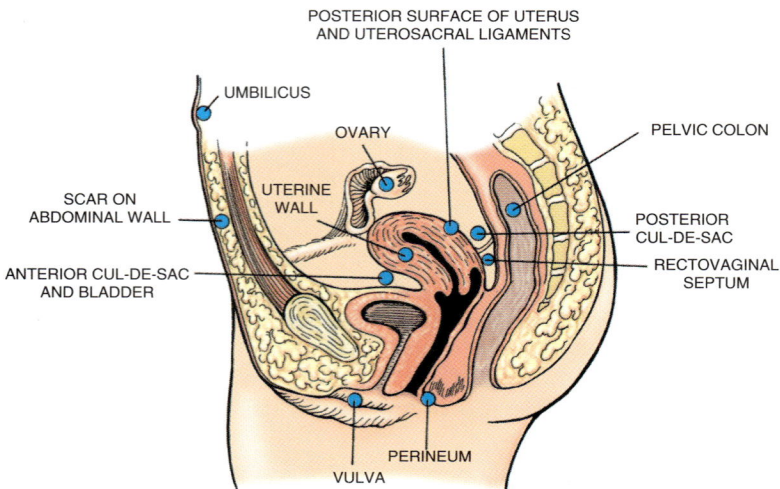

Figure 4-5 Possible sites of occurrence of endometriosis (Venes, D. (Ed.). (2009). *Taber's cyclopedic medical dictionary* (p. 768, 21st ed.). Philadelphia: F. A. Davis)

ETIOLOGY AND PATHOGENESIS

The exact cause and pathogenesis of endometriosis is not known. One of the most widely accepted theories is Sampson's theory, or "retrograde menstruation." This theory postulates that during menstruation, endometrial tissue is transported through the fallopian tubes into the peritoneal cavity, where it implants on the ovaries and other structures. Although retrograde menstruation occurs in most women, it is not clear why some develop endometriosis and others do not. The level of functioning of the immune system is thought to be a factor in the development of endometriosis, although the exact mechanism is unknown. Interestingly, women with endometriosis tend to develop additional symptoms such as allergies, fibromyalgia, asthma, eczema, autoimmune inflammatory disease, chronic fatigue syndrome, and hypothyroidism. Also, there is a higher risk of breast cancer in women diagnosed with endometriosis after age 40 because of their prolonged exposure to elevated endogenous estrogen (Bertelsen et al., 2007; Bloski & Pierson, 2008; Sinaii, Cleary, Ballweg, Nieman, & Stratton, 2002).

SIGNS AND SYMPTOMS

The signs and symptoms of endometriosis vary from woman to woman, and the severity of symptoms may increase over time. However, the most common symptom is pelvic pain. The pain, which usually begins 1 or 2 days before the expected menses, may be unilateral or bilateral and frequently lasts until the end of menstruation. Some patients experience a constant, debilitating pain that interferes with their normal daily activities. Bowel symptoms such as diarrhea, pain with defecation, constipation, and rectal bleeding with significant bowel involvement may also occur. Other symptoms include dyspareunia, dysuria, various gastrointestinal symptoms, low back pain, infertility, and menstrual dysfunction. Interestingly, the severity of pain does not correlate well with the extent of the condition. Thus, severe disease may go undetected (Bloski & Pierson, 2008; Chopin et al., 2006; Denny & Mann, 2007; Ninia, 2007).

DIAGNOSIS

The diagnosis of endometriosis can be difficult to confirm owing to the wide variation in symptoms. Diagnostic laparoscopy to allow for visualization and biopsy of the lesions remains the gold standard for diagnosis, after other causes of pelvic pain (e.g., upper genital tract infection, pelvic inflammatory disease) have been ruled out. A vaginal ultrasound may also be performed to provide imaging of the displaced endometrial tissue or cyst(s), although it may be difficult to differentiate between other pathological entities such as tubal cysts, abscesses, and ectopic pregnancy (Bazot et al., 2003; Bloski & Pierson, 2008).

Optimizing Outcomes— **Endometriosis staging to guide care**

The American Society for Reproductive Medicine (ASRM) has developed classification and staging guidelines to assist with endometriosis diagnosis, prognosis, treatment, and progress and communication among health professionals.

Staging is based on the extent of the spread of the lesions, the density of pelvic adhesions, involvement of pelvic organs, and the degree of fallopian tube occlusion. In the standardized schema, endometriosis is classified into four stages: Stage 1—minimal, Stage 2—mild, Stage 3—moderate, and Stage 4—severe. Interestingly, women with minimal or mild endometriosis have been shown to have high degrees of pain and infertility while women with Stage 4 disease have been asymptomatic and diagnosed during laparoscopy for various procedures such as tubal ligation (ASRM, 2006; Bloski & Pierson, 2008).

TREATMENT OPTIONS

Because endometriosis can persist during a woman's entire reproductive life, her treatment plan should be individualized and holistic. When determining the best approach for therapy, many factors must be taken into account, such as the woman's desire for future pregnancy, the size of her current family, and general lifestyle patterns. Although there are no ideal treatments for endometriosis, the planned course of therapy is based on the severity of symptoms and the woman's or couple's goals. Treatment plans generally begin with the least invasive approach and progress to more invasive therapies. Regardless of the treatment, however, approximately 10% to 20% of women with endometriosis experience a recurrence of the condition.

Medical Therapy

The goal of medical treatment is to reduce the amount of estrogen in the body so that menstruation and the subsequent growth of endometrial tissue are suppressed. To accomplish the suppression of endogenous estrogen, two main classes of drugs are used: GnRH-agonists and gonadotropin inhibitors. GnRH-agonists such as leuprolide (Lupron), goserelin (Zoladex), and nafarelin (Synarel) suppress the secretion of pituitary gonadotropins. This action causes anovulation and amenorrhea, which result in shrinkage of the endometrial tissue. The patient experiences significant pain relief and an interruption in the further development of endometrial lesions. Common side effects are similar to those associated with natural menopause and include hot flashes; vaginal dryness; loss of libido; emotional lability; and mild, reversible bone loss. Treatment is limited to 5 months due to the decrease in bone mineral density associated with these medications (Bloski & Pierson, 2008; Crosignani, Olive, Bergqvist, & Luciano, 2006; Deglin & Vallerand, 2009).

Danazol (Danocrine, Cyclomen) is a synthetic androgen that acts as a pituitary gonadotropin inhibitor. This medication causes anovulation by suppressing the secretion of follicle-stimulating hormone (FSH) and luteinizing hormone (LH). Pain relief results from the hypoestrogenic environment, endometrial atrophy, and regression of the endometrial lesions. Because this medication is an androgenic synthetic steroid, masculinizing side effects such as acne, hirsutism, deepening of the voice, weight gain, decreased breast size, and oily skin are common. Other side effects include headaches, flushing, sweating, atrophic vaginitis, and edema. The duration of treatment is approximately 6 months, due to the multitude of adverse side effects (Blosky & Pierson, 2008; Deglin & Vallerand, 2009).

Contraceptive medications are also used to treat endometriosis. Combination oral contraceptives contain progestins and estrogen—hormones that suppress gonadotropins, prevent ovulation, and cause endometrial atrophy. Pain relief, related to a thinning of the endometrial lining and regression of the endometriotic implants, is achieved in approximately 75% of patients. Side effects include irregular bleeding, weight gain, headache, thrombophlebitis, benign liver tumors, and gallbladder disease. Medroxyprogesterone (Depo-Provera) is an injectable progesterone that also suppresses gonadotropins and thins endometrial tissue. Potential adverse side effects associated with this medication include weight gain, headache, abdominal discomfort, and irregular bleeding. Treatment outcomes are similar to those achieved with oral contraceptives (ASRM, 2006; Bloski & Pierson, 2008; Brankin & Cackovic, 2010; Deglin & Vallerand, 2009).

Anastrozole (Arimidex) and letrozole (Femara) are aromatase inhibitors that decrease levels of circulating estrogen by inhibiting the peripheral conversion of androgens. Potential adverse effects include headache, nausea, diarrhea, hot flashes, and an increased risk of osteoporosis with long-term use. Treatment is limited to 6 months due to the decrease in bone mineral density. Up to 90% of patients experience alleviation of symptoms during and up to 15 months post-treatment (Ailawadi, Jobanpufra, Kataria, Gurates, & Bulun, 2004; Bloski & Pierson, 2008; Deglin & Vallerand, 2009; Shippen & West, 2004).

Surgical Treatment

Laparoscopy with biopsy of the lesions is the only accurate method to diagnose and determine the severity of endometriosis. During the laparoscopy, surgical removal of the lesions, adhesions, and cysts may be conducted via excision, electrocautery, or laser vaporization. The recurrence rate of endometriotic lesions after 5 years is 19% with laparoscopic removal of the lesions and 10% with hysterectomy (removal of the uterus) and bilateral oophorectomy (removal of the ovaries). Women who undergo a bilateral oophorectomy are usually treated with hormone therapy, as the benefits outweigh the risk of endometriosis recurrence (ASRM, 2006; Bloski & Pierson, 2008).

IMPLICATIONS FOR NURSES

Counseling and support constitute the cornerstone of nursing care for women diagnosed with endometriosis. It is incumbent upon nurses who care for women with this chronic condition to remain knowledgeable about endometriosis so that they can provide factual information about treatment options, including the risks and benefits of each. Therapeutic listening reflects respect and encourages patients to share intimate details about sensitive issues, such as dyspareunia. Teaching patients about endometriosis empowers them to participate in their treatment plan and explore approaches such as alternative methods of pain control and lifestyle and diet modifications that may enhance well-being and improve functionality (Bloski & Pierson, 2008; Huntington & Gilmour, 2005). Potential nursing diagnoses for women with endometriosis are presented in Box 4-2.

 Collaboration in Caring— *Assisting women with endometriosis*

Women with endometriosis can benefit from a multidisciplinary approach to treatment. The health-care team, composed of professionals with skills to address the many difficulties associated with this chronic condition, may include dietitians, physiotherapists, psychologists, and chronic pain specialists. Also, nurses may suggest referral to local support groups and national organizations such as Resolve (http://www.resolve.org), an organization for infertile couples, or the Endometriosis Association (http://www.endometriosisassn.org). Nurses can remain up-to-date on evidence-based guidelines for the treatment of endometriosis through the European Society for Human Reproduction & Embryology (SHRE) Web site (http://www.guidelines.endometriosis.org) or the National Guideline Clearinghouse Web site (http://www.guideline.gov) (Bloski & Pierson, 2008).

 Now Can You— **Discuss various aspects of endometriosis?**

1. Describe the chronic condition of endometriosis, and define the term *endometrioma*?
2. Discuss the modalities and goals of medical and surgical treatment for endometriosis?
3. Develop a nursing plan of care for a patient with endometriosis?

Leiomyomas (Fibroids)

Uterine leiomyomas (also called fibroids) are the most common solid pelvic tumors in women and the leading indication for hysterectomy. Fibroids arise from a singular neoplastic smooth muscle cell in the uterus and grow slowly. Although the exact cause is unknown, the growth of leiomyomas is dependent on estrogen. They are almost always benign (ACOG, 2008b).

 Nursing Insight— *Understanding terminology for uterine fibroid tumors*

A leiomyoma, or fibroid, is a benign tumor composed of nonstriated muscular tissue. The plural form of leiomyoma is either *leiomyomas* or *leiomyomata*.

Leiomyomas may be located in various places in and around the uterus. The most common fibroids form within the uterine wall. They can vary greatly in size and may protrude into the uterine cavity, bulge outward through the uterine wall and into the pelvic cavity, or grow on a stalk called a "pedicle" that can become twisted and cause pain. Leiomyomas are more common in African American women, and some studies report the presence of fibroids in 70% of Caucasian women and more than 80% of African American women by age 50 years. Stimulated by estrogen and progesterone, the tumors occur more frequently with increasing age and regress after menopause (ACOG, 2008b; Day Baird, Dunson, Hill, Cousins, & Schectman, 2003).

SIGNS, SYMPTOMS, AND DIAGNOSIS

The two most common symptoms of uterine leiomyomas for which women seek medical treatment are abnormal uterine bleeding and pelvic pressure. Frequently, however, fibroids cause no symptoms and are first discovered during a routine bimanual pelvic examination. When abnormal bleeding is present, it is usually reported as heavy or prolonged menstrual bleeding, which may result in iron-deficiency anemia. In some situations, the bleeding significantly disrupts the woman's normal daily activities. The pelvic and abdominal discomfort is often described as "pressure." Depending on the location of the leiomyoma, pressure may be experienced in the bladder or rectal regions, leading to difficulty with urination or defecation or dyspareunia. Also, depending on their size and location, leiomyomas can interfere with fertility (ACOG, 2008b; Fraser, Critchley, Munro, & Broder, 2007).

On examination, the uterus is nontender and may feel enlarged, irregularly shaped, or both. Pregnancy must always be ruled out. An ultrasound examination can confirm the presence of the leiomyoma and provide baseline measurements. Sometimes a hysteroscopy, an office procedure that uses an instrument to view the uterine cavity, or a laparoscopy, an outpatient hospital procedure that uses an instrument to view the uterus and surrounding structures, is performed to aid the diagnosis (ACOG, 2008b).

TREATMENT

In general, patients with leiomyomas are seen in the office every 3 to 6 months as long as they are experiencing mild symptoms. If heavy and prolonged bleeding or severe pain occurs, however, referral to a specialist for further evaluation is indicated. Interventions may include drug therapy, uterine artery embolization, myomectomy, hysterectomy, and laser surgery, electrocauterization, or magnetic resonance imaging (MRI)–guided focused ultrasound surgery.

Drug Therapy

Contraceptive steroids (estrogen and progestin combination and progestin alone) may be prescribed to control heavy periods and dysmenorrhea. Gonadotropin-releasing hormone (GnRH) agonists including leuprolide acetate (Lupron, Synarel) suppress the production of estrogen and progesterone and shrink the tumors, although the effects of these agents is temporary, with gradual recurrent growth of leiomyomas within several months following the cessation of treatment. Also, the significant menopausal symptoms such as vaginal dryness, hot flashes, and mood changes along with decreased bone mineral density limit use of these medications to no more than 6 months. Antiprogesterone agents such as mifepristone (Mifeprex) may also be useful in controlling leiomyoma symptoms. Recurrence of tumor growth following cessation of treatment tends to be slower than with other medications; however, further study is needed. Potential side effects include endometrial hyperplasia and alterations in liver functioning (ACOG, 2008b).

Uterine Artery Embolization (UAE)

Performed by interventional radiologists, this treatment involves the injection of polyvinyl alcohol pellets into selected blood vessels to block the blood supply to the fibroid and cause shrinkage and resolution of symptoms. UAE is performed under local anesthesia and conscious sedation. An incision is made into the groin, a catheter is threaded from the femoral artery into the uterine artery, and an arteriogram identifies the major blood vessels that supply the leiomyoma. Most tumors shrink in size by 50% within 3 months following treatment. Women who wish to undergo this procedure should be advised that data are lacking about the long-term effects on fertility and future pregnancies (ACOG, 2008b; Society of Obstetricians and Gynaecologists of Canada, 2005; Spies et al., 2005).

Myomectomy and Hysterectomy

For women who desire uterine preservation, myomectomy (removal of the leiomyoma) may be an option. Depending on the size and number of tumors, this surgical procedure may be accomplished during a laparotomy, a laparoscopy, or a hysteroscopy. Myomectomy can be performed through a laparoscopic or abdominal incision approach or a vaginal (hysteroscopic) approach. The uterus (and therefore childbearing potential) is preserved, although most myomectomy patients will require a cesarean birth. Hysterectomy (removal of the uterus) may be the treatment of choice if heavy, persistent bleeding cannot be controlled by any other means (ACOG, 2008b).

Laser Surgery, Electrocauterization, and MRI-Guided Focused Ultrasound Surgery

Laser surgery and electrocauterization may be used to destroy small leiomyomas with a vaginal (hysteroscopic) or abdominal (laparoscopic) approach. Laser coagulation vaporizes the fibroids and produces necrosis. However, although the uterus remains intact, endometrial scarring may diminish future fertility (ACOG, 2008b).

In 2004, the U.S. Federal and Drug Administration (FDA) granted approval for the use of an MRI-guided system for the localization and treatment of uterine leiomyomas with focused ultrasound therapy. This treatment is a noninvasive approach that uses high-intensity ultrasound waves directed into the leiomyoma. The ultrasound energy penetrates soft tissue and causes necrosis. Adverse effects include heavy menses and persistent pain; further studies regarding the long-term efficacy of this treatment modality are indicated (ACOG, 2008b).

Optimizing Outcomes— Following surgical intervention for leiomyomas

Nurses can educate women undergoing surgical interventions for leiomyomas about strategies to enhance comfort and promote healing. Nurses can teach women to:

- Take all prescribed medications.
- Contact the physician for symptoms including bleeding, cramping, fever of 39°C (102.2°F) or greater, gastrointestinal changes, signs of wound infection (redness, swelling, heat, or pain at the incision site), urinary retention, abnormal vaginal discharge.
- Consume foods high in protein, iron, and vitamin C to facilitate tissue healing; drink plenty of fluids.
- Avoid straining during bowel movements.
- Follow the physician's recommendations regarding physical activity and driving.
- Follow the physician's orders regarding tub baths and the resumption of intercourse.

Abnormal Uterine Bleeding

Abnormal uterine bleeding, a common problem for women, may be associated with major disruptions in daily functioning. Typically, the abnormal uterine bleeding is categorized as either *structural* or *dysfunctional*. Dysfunctional uterine bleeding is a diagnosis that is made only after all pathological causes of bleeding, such as leiomyomata, polyps, endometrial hyperplasia, and cancer, have been excluded. An accurate diagnosis for the cause of the bleeding should be established. Based on age alone, endometrial assessment to exclude cancer should be performed on any woman older than 35 years. In addition to a physical examination, diagnostic tests used to evaluate women with abnormal uterine bleeding may include a pregnancy test to rule out ectopic pregnancy, Pap smear, complete blood count, evaluation for endocrine dysfunction, endometrial biopsy, transvaginal ultrasound, hysteroscopy, and dilatation and curettage (D & C) (ACOG, 2007).

ABNORMAL BLEEDING RELATED TO STRUCTURAL CAUSES

Structural causes of uterine bleeding include leiomyomata, polyps, and infection. Uterine fibroid tumors are often asymptomatic and first detected during a bimanual pelvic examination. Precancerous or cancerous conditions of the uterus or cervix can also cause abnormal bleeding (ACOG, 2007).

ABNORMAL BLEEDING RELATED TO DYSFUNCTIONAL CAUSES

Dysfunctional uterine bleeding is defined as noncyclic menstrual blood flow that is derived from the endometrium. The bleeding may range from spotty to excessive and may be prolonged. It is most commonly caused by hormonal imbalances, which account for approximately 75% of cases of irregular bleeding. Heavy bleeding is a common problem for women during the perimenopausal period between the ages of 40 and 50. As ovulation becomes more erratic, levels of progesterone decrease. An important function of progesterone is to stabilize the uterine endometrial lining. In the absence of progesterone, the bleeding may become unpredictable, excessive, or prolonged. Abnormal uterine bleeding may also occur during adolescence, before a pattern of regular ovulatory cycles has been established. Other conditions that may cause abnormal bleeding include thyroid or adrenal gland disorders, polycystic ovary syndrome, clotting disorders, liver or kidney disease, leukemia, herbal preparations such as ginseng, or medications such as anticoagulants (ACOG, 2000, 2007; Keehbauch & Nystrom, 2007; Speroff & Mishell, 2007; Wolfe, 2006).

 Nursing Insight— *Clotting disorders may cause abnormal uterine bleeding*

Nurses should be aware that abnormal uterine bleeding may be related to an undiagnosed coagulopathy such as defects in primary hemostasis, platelet deficiency (e.g., leukemia, idiopathic thrombocytopenia), platelet dysfunction (e.g., von Willebrand disease), and abnormalities of secondary homeostasis (congenital factor deficiencies). von Willebrand disease is a genetic bleeding disorder caused by a defect or deficiency of a blood-clotting factor (von Willebrand factor). This condition occurs in approximately 1% of all women and is the most common medical disorder associated with menarche (ACOG, 2007).

TREATMENT

Depending on the cause, treatment for abnormal uterine bleeding may include drug therapy and/or surgery. Medical management is the preferred method of therapy for anovulatory uterine bleeding. The goals of medical treatment are to alleviate the acute bleeding, prevent future episodes of noncyclic bleeding, decrease the woman's risk of long-term complications from anovulation, and improve her overall quality of life. It is important for nurses to counsel patients that the treatment may initially cause heavy menstrual bleeding related to buildup of the endometrium. However, the bleeding should diminish over the course of 3 to 4 months.

Depending on the patient's age and physical findings, medications used include conjugated equine estrogens, low-dose combination oral contraceptives, cyclic progestogens, iron supplementation, prostaglandin synthetase inhibitors (e.g., indomethacin [Indocin]), and NSAIDs (e.g., aspirin, ibuprofen, naproxen). The FDA recently approved an oral nonhormonal product to treat heavy menstrual bleeding. Tranexamic acid (Lysteda) works by stabilizing a protein that helps blood to clot. Because the use of this medication while taking hormonal contraceptives may increase the risk of blood clots, stroke, or heart attack, women using hormonal contraception should take tranexamic acid only if there is a strong medical need and the benefits outweigh the potential risks (ACOG, 2007; FDA, 2009).

Surgical procedures to treat abnormal uterine bleeding include dilation and curettage (D & C), hysteroscopic-assisted endometrial ablation, thermal balloon ablation, and hysterectomy. These interventions are indicated for patients who fail to improve with medical therapy and who desire no future fertility. Women with significant acute bleeding may need a D & C for the immediate control of bleeding as well as for diagnosis. However, the beneficial effects associated with this surgical intervention are only temporary, and the D & C procedure is no longer the mainstay of treatment (ACOG, 2007; Nelson & Baldwin, 2008).

A surgical alternative to hysterectomy is endometrial ablation, a procedure that uses a lighted viewing instrument (hysteroscope) and other instruments to destroy (ablate) the uterine lining. Endometrial ablation is generally performed in an outpatient facility or hospital. The procedure may be done using a local or spinal anesthesia, although general anesthesia is sometimes used. Recovery following endometrial ablation generally ranges from a few days to a couple of weeks.

 Nursing Insight— *Understanding endometrial ablation*

Endometrial ablation is used to control heavy, prolonged vaginal bleeding for the following circumstances: The bleeding has not responded to other treatments; childbearing is completed; the patient prefers not to have a hysterectomy to control the bleeding; or other medical problems prevent a hysterectomy. The five FDA-approved methods use a variety of energy sources to achieve endometrial destruction, and each is designed to ablate down to the basal layer to prevent regeneration and subsequent menstrual flow. Endometrial ablation may be accomplished by laser beam (laser thermal ablation), electricity, freezing, microwave, or heat (thermal ablation, using radiofrequency or a balloon filled with heated saline solution). With thermal balloon ablation, a flexible balloon attached to a thin probe is inserted through the cervix and inflated in the uterus with sterile saline. The saline, heated to approximately 85°C, destroys the uterine lining. With all ablation techniques, the endometrium heals by scarring, which usually reduces or prevents uterine bleeding. Fertility is not preserved, although there is a remote possibility of pregnancy if a portion of the endometrium is left intact. Contraception is recommended for women who have not completed menopause (ACOG, 2000; Fothergill & Sulak, 2010; Song, 2007).

Hysterectomy

A hysterectomy is a surgery to remove the uterus. After cesarean section, hysterectomy is the second most frequently performed major surgical procedure for women of reproductive age in the United States. Each year in this country, approximately 600,000 hysterectomies are performed, and an estimated 20 million women have had a hysterectomy. The three conditions most commonly associated with hysterectomy are uterine leiomyomata, endometriosis, and uterine prolapse. Other indications include cancer (i.e., uterine, ovarian, cervical, endometrial), adenomyosis (a condition in which endometrial tissue grows into the myometrium), chronic pelvic pain, and abnormal vaginal bleeding (ACOG, 2007, 2009a; CDC, 2006b).

During the surgery, the whole uterus or a part of it may be removed. A *partial*, *subtotal*, or *supracervical* hysterectomy involves removal of the upper part of the uterus, leaving the cervix in place. A *total* hysterectomy removes the whole uterus and cervix, and a *radical* hysterectomy removes the whole uterus, along with the tissue on both sides of the cervix and the upper part of the vagina. This particular surgery is done mostly when there is cancer present.

❝What to say❞ — *"What to say" — When explaining surgical approaches for hysterectomy*

Several different surgical approaches are used to perform removal of the uterus. To determine the most appropriate method, the physician assesses a number of factors, including the patient's health history, reason for the surgery, and personal preference. The nurse can explain the various procedures:

Abdominal hysterectomy: A 5- to 7-inch incision is made in the low abdomen, just above the pubic hairline. The incision may be in a vertical or horizontal direction. The uterus is removed through the incision. Recovery time varies from 4 to 6 weeks.

Vaginal hysterectomy: An incision is made in the vagina, and the uterus is removed through the vagina.

Laparoscopic hysterectomy: An instrument with a thin, lighted tube and small camera (laparoscope) is inserted into the abdomen to allow for visualization of the pelvic organs. Three or four small cuts are made in the abdomen for insertion of the laparoscope and other instruments. The uterus is divided into small segments and removed through the incisions.

Laparoscopically assisted vaginal hysterectomy (LAVH): The uterus is removed through the vagina, and the laparoscope is used to guide the procedure.

Robotic surgery: The doctor uses a special machine to perform the surgery like laparoscopic surgery. This method is most often used when a patient has cancer or is very obese and vaginal surgery is considered unsafe.

Recovery from vaginal or laparoscopic surgery generally takes from 3 to 4 weeks.

Prior to the surgery, a psychological assessment is an essential component of care. The nurse should ensure that the woman has an opportunity to consider the personal significance of the loss of her uterus, discuss misconceptions about the effects of the surgery, and ensure that she has an adequate support system for postoperative care and concerns. Recovery from a hysterectomy is a very personal experience that is shaped by a myriad of factors, such as the woman's age, her physical and emotional health, reason for the surgery, and type of surgery performed. The nurse can help to empower women facing uterine surgery by creating a therapeutic environment where the patient feels safe in sharing feelings and expressing concerns. Other nursing actions to help prepare the woman for the surgery and promote a healthy recovery include providing information, engaging the assistance of other health professionals, and making referrals when appropriate.

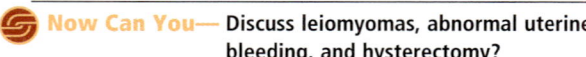

Now Can You— **Discuss leiomyomas, abnormal uterine bleeding, and hysterectomy?**

1. Identify common treatment modalities for leiomyomas, and develop a postoperative teaching plan for the woman undergoing a surgical intervention?
2. Differentiate between structural and dysfunctional abnormal uterine bleeding?
3. Discuss the nurse's role when caring for the patient who will undergo a hysterectomy?

Ovarian Tumors

Because the ovary is composed of many different tissue types, growths or tumors involving the ovary may be of various types. Interestingly, more than 50 different types of ovarian tumors have been identified. Two of the most common types of ovarian tumors are follicular cysts and corpus luteum cysts, which are included in this discussion.

Nursing Insight— *Understanding about ovarian cysts*

Ovarian cysts affect women of all ages; the vast majority of them are considered functional, or physiologic. Most disappear within a few weeks without treatment. Ovarian cysts occur most often during the childbearing years and typically represent a normal process. A dermoid cyst is an abnormal cyst that usually affects younger women; it may range in size from 1 cm (less than a half inch) up to 45 cm (17 inches) in diameter. A dermoid cyst is usually a benign tumor (2% are malignant) sometimes referred to as a mature cystic teratoma. Originating from a totipotential germ cell, the cyst is similar to those present on skin tissue and can contain fat and occasionally bone, hair, and cartilage. A dermoid cyst can cause the ovary to twist ("torsion") and produce severe abdominal pain.

FOLLICULAR CYSTS

A follicular cyst is the most common growth that occurs on the ovary. It develops during the first half of the menstrual cycle, called the "follicular phase." This type of ovarian cyst, termed a "functional" or "simple" cyst, forms when ovulation does not occur. Instead, the developing dominant follicle continues to grow and evolves into a large, fluid-filled cyst that contains a high concentration of estrogen. The follicular cyst can also form from one of the smaller follicles that failed to regress after another ovarian follicle gained dominance. Follicular cysts usually produce no symptoms and disappear spontaneously within a few months. However, approximately one-fourth of women with follicular cysts report symptoms such as pain or the sensation of a heavy, achy feeling in the pelvis.

The diagnosis is generally made on the basis of symptoms and bimanual examination. Ultrasonography may be used to confirm the findings and rule out pregnancy. Expectant management ("watch and wait") and a repeat examination in 6 to 10 weeks is the treatment of choice unless symptoms worsen. The majority of follicular cysts resolve after two to three menstrual cycles without intervention. On occasion, oral contraceptive pills are prescribed to hasten cyst resolution (ACOG, 2007).

CORPUS LUTEUM CYSTS

A corpus luteum cyst forms from the corpus luteum during the second half, or luteal phase, of the menstrual cycle. The woman with a corpus luteum cyst may experience menstrual irregularity (e.g., delayed menses), although most often, the cyst regresses and disappears spontaneously within one or two menstrual cycles. The cyst may, however, fill with fluid or blood and persist on the ovary. Less commonly, the cysts rupture and can cause severe abdominal pain from the associated bleeding. When this occurs, surgical removal of the cyst may be necessary.

Polycystic Ovary Syndrome

Polycystic ovary syndrome (PCOS), also called Stein-Leventhal syndrome, is one of the most common endocrine disorders in reproductive-age women, affecting 1 in 15 women of childbearing age (Speroff & Mishell, 2007). The disorder occurs when an endocrine imbalance results in elevated levels of estrogen, testosterone, and luteinizing hormone (LH) and a decreased secretion of follicle-stimulating hormone (FSH). Multiple follicular cysts develop on one or both ovaries and produce excessive amounts of estrogen. Clinical findings associated with PCOS include obesity, hirsutism, acne, and infertility. Menstrual irregularity, which occurs in approximately 75% of women with PCOS, may be the first presenting symptom suggestive of the disorder. Women with this condition often have insulin resistance and are at an increased risk for developing type 2 diabetes mellitus (Speroff & Mishell, 2007). There is also an increased risk for coronary artery disease, hypertension, cancer (e.g., endometrial, ovarian, breast), and dyslipidemia. PCOS is often diagnosed during adolescence, and the prevalence of the disorder in Mexican Americans is twice that of other ethnic groups (ACOG, 2009b; DuRant, Leslie, & Critch, 2009; Lindenbaum, 2010).

Optimizing Outcomes— **With lifestyle modifications to improve PCOS**

Diet, exercise, and weight loss are considered the best first-line interventions to improve PCOS. An increase in exercise combined with dietary change has been shown to reduce diabetes risk comparable to or better than medication. Weight control improves many aspects of the condition, leading to more regular menstrual cycles, reduced androgen levels, lowered lipid levels, and better glucose metabolism. To achieve weight loss, a low-fat, high-fiber diet with low-glycemic-index carbohydrates is recommended. Typically, women with PCOS have unique challenges achieving and maintaining healthy weights. Because they consume less energy metabolizing their food, they often require a lower-calorie diet than other women to lose weight. Obese women with PCOS should follow a hypocaloric diet (500 kcal/d deficit) that reduces the glycemic load. Reducing alcohol consumption is another way to decrease caloric intake. Moderate physical activity combined with muscle-strengthening exercises improves insulin sensitivity and helps to limit the loss of lean muscle mass. Cognitive behavior therapy, which involves teaching problem-solving skills and enhancing and reframing perceptions, may be useful in helping women with PCOS to overcome the barriers to adopting lifestyle changes needed to improve health (ACOG, 2009b; DuRant, Leslie, & Critch, 2009; Fan et al., 2008; Hoeger, 2007; Lindenbaum, 2010; Nelson, 2009).

Medical treatment of patients with PCOS usually depends on the presenting signs and symptoms. For women who are not attempting to conceive, combination low-dose hormonal contraceptives are the usual treatment because they inhibit LH and decrease testosterone levels. Oral contraceptives may also lessen acne and hirsutism. If pregnancy is desired, medications to induce ovulation, such as clomiphene citrate (Clomid) are usually prescribed. Insulin medications for type 2 diabetes such as metformin hydrochloride (Glucophage) are used to lower insulin, testosterone, and glucose levels, which, in turn, can reduce symptoms of acne, hirsutism, abdominal obesity, and other symptoms associated with PCOS (ACOG, 2007, 2009b; Lindenbaum, 2010; Neal, Formyduval, & Taylor, 2009; Speroff & Mishell, 2007).

Nurses can counsel women with PCOS about their chronic disorder and the potential long-term effects on their health. A holistic approach to care encompasses a variety of lifestyle strategies, such as diet, exercise, and weight loss along with prescribed medications, when

needed, to achieve good clinical outcomes and a better quality of life. Referrals for resources including cognitive behavior therapy, counseling for issues concerning body image and self-esteem, and support groups and nutritional information may be appropriate as well (DuRant, Leslie, & Critch, 2009; Lindenbaum, 2010).

Ovarian Cancer

Ovarian cancer is the leading cause of gynecological deaths and the fourth most common cause of cancer deaths in women, resulting in 16,000 deaths annually. Ovarian cancer accounts for about 3% of all cancers in women, and a woman's risk of getting invasive ovarian cancer during her lifetime is approximately 1 in 71. About two-thirds of women with ovarian cancer are 60 or older, and it is slightly more common in Caucasian women than in African American women (American Cancer Society [ACS], 2009a).

Although the cause is unknown, there are identified risk factors, including nulliparity, pregnancy later in life, obesity (body mass index of at least 30), the presence of *BRCA1* and *BRCA2* genes, a personal history of breast cancer, and a family history of breast, ovarian, or colorectal cancer. Associative causes include the use of fertility medications, exposure to asbestos, genital exposure to talcum powder, a high-fat diet, and childhood mumps infection. Pregnancy and oral contraceptive use provide some protection against ovarian cancer, and the use of postmenopausal estrogen may increase the risk (ACS, 2009a).

Unfortunately, the signs and symptoms of ovarian cancer are often vague until late in development. Ovarian cancer should be considered in any woman over age 40 who has complaints of vague abdominal or pelvic discomfort or enlargement, back pain, indigestion, inability to eat normally, feeling full after eating only a small amount, a sense of bloating, constipation, urinary incontinence of recent onset, or unexplained weight loss. Enlargement of the abdomen due to accumulation of fluid (ascites) is the most common sign. Since ovarian cancer is a rapidly growing neoplasm, the diagnosis is often not made until the cancer has metastasized (ACOG, 2002; ACS, 2009a; Goff, Mandel, et al., 2007).

Ovarian cancer is rarely diagnosed early. In fact, nearly 70% of women with ovarian cancer have already experienced metastatic spread outside of the pelvis by the time of the initial diagnosis. Methods for mass screening and early detection have not been successful, and currently an annual bimanual examination is recommended. Tests that are used most frequently to screen for ovarian cancer include transvaginal sonography, which can be used to determine the size, location, and quality (e.g., fluid filled, solid) of the mass and serum CA-125 antigen levels (ACOG, 2002; ACS, 2009a).

 Optimizing Outcomes— **Biomarkers for epithelial ovarian cancer**

CA-125 is a serum protein that is higher in many women with epithelial ovarian cancer. In premenopausal women with symptoms, a CA-125 measurement is frequently not useful because elevated levels of the protein are associated

---

where research and practice meet:
HER LIFESTYLE Mneumonic for Recognizing PCOS

Neal, Formyduval, and Taylor (2010) developed HER LIFESTYLE, a tool designed to aid health-care providers in recognizing and managing PCOS in their adolescent patients. The mnemonic can be incorporated into clinical practice to assist with educational efforts about lifestyle modification and its positive effects on PCOS. Specifically, the mnemonic includes the following:

H—Hirsutism (discuss treatment options for this sensitive issue)
E—Education (educate about potential complications of PCOS, treatment options, lifestyle modifications)
R—Reassure (reassure that options are available to help manage PCOS)
L—Lose weight (to decrease symptoms and risk factors associated with PCOS)
I—Irregular periods (consider PCOS as a possible cause of irregular periods)
F—Fertility (impaired fertility, a complication of PCOS, can be devastating)
E—Exercise (include regular exercise in lifestyle changes)
S—Skin (assess for skin changes [e.g., acne, acanthosis nigricans]), consider treatment options
T—Talk (take time to talk with adolescent patients with PCOS; changes now can affect future health)
Y—Youth (consider the patient's developmental stage and present concerns)
L—Long-term consequences (stress what may happen without treatment; assess personal perception of risk)
E—Eating plan (encourage a high-fiber, low-fat diet; assess progress with each visit)

with a variety of common benign conditions (e.g., uterine leiomyomata, PID, endometriosis, pregnancy). In postmenopausal women with a pelvic mass, a CA-125 measurement may be helpful in predicting a higher likelihood of a malignant tumor than a benign tumor, although a normal CA-125 measurement alone does not rule out ovarian cancer. Human epididymis protein 4 (HE4) is a secreted glycoprotein expressed in normal glandular epithelium of the reproductive tract. HE4 has been validated as a serum tumor marker for epithelial ovarian cancer (EOC), and it has recently been cleared by the FDA as a monitoring tool for patients diagnosed with EOC. A new ovarian cancer blood test, called OVA1, has also recently gained FDA approval. The OVA1 biomarker panel can help assess the likelihood of malignancy of an ovarian tumor before surgery and facilitate decisions about referral to a gynecological oncologist (ACOG, 2002; ACS, 2009a; Moore & MacLaughlan, 2009).

A strong family history of breast cancer may be caused by an inherited mutation in the *BRCA-1* or *BRCA-2* gene. Since alterations in these genes have been detected in women with ovarian cancer, screening women with the BRCA mutations can be performed to determine whether they carry these genes. Interestingly, these mutations also increase the risks for primary peritoneal carcinoma and fallopian tube carcinoma (ACOG, 2002; ACS, 2009a).

Laparotomy is performed for surgical confirmation and clinical staging, which provides direction to the treatment and prognosis of the cancer. The preferred treatment for ovarian cancer is surgical removal and usually requires a hysterectomy with bilateral salpingo-oophorectomy. After surgery, chemotherapy (administered intravenously and intraperitoneally), sometimes combined with immunotherapy, is used to treat any remaining cancer. Radiation therapy may be used as a palliative measure, although it is not typically used as a treatment option for ovarian cancer (ACOG, 2008c; Goff, Matthews, et al., 2007; Hordern, 2007).

Optimizing Outcomes— Enhancing ovarian cancer awareness

Nurses can help promote women's awareness and understanding of their bodies by empowering them with information about specific symptoms that may be associated with ovarian cancer. The Geoff Symptom Index was developed to aid in the early identification of women with potential ovarian cancer. The tool focuses on symptoms most often seen among women who were later diagnosed with ovarian cancer. The easy-to-administer symptom index includes the following symptoms: bloating, pelvic or abdominal pain, difficulty eating or feeling full quickly, and urinary urgency or frequency. Scientists note that the frequency and/or number of symptoms are correlated with the diagnosis of ovarian cancer, and women who experience any of these symptoms on a daily basis for more than a few weeks should be counseled to contact their women's health-care specialist. Recently, the Ovarian Cancer National Alliance issued Interim Practice Guidance for the diagnosis of ovarian cancer. Posted online, these guidelines represent the first time that ovarian cancer diagnostic protocols have been made available to the public. In conjunction with the Gynecologic Cancer Foundation, a Symptom Diary, designed to help women measure the persistency and severity of their symptoms, is also available at http://www.ovariancancer.org/diary (Fife, 2007; Goff, Mandel, et al., 2007; Hellwig, 2007).

Endometrial Cancer

In the United States, cancer of the endometrium is the most common gynecological malignancy. According to estimates from the ACS (2009b), for the year 2009, approximately 42,000 new cases of cancer of the uterine corpus (body) were diagnosed. The estimates include both endometrial cancers and uterine sarcomas (which are rare and represent 2% of uterine body cancers). Most uterine malignancies arise within the inner lining of the uterus and are adenocarcinomas that develop from overgrowth (hyperplasia) of the endometrium. Uterine cancer is rarely found in women under age 40; approximately 70% of all cases are found in women in the 50–69 age group. The average chance of a woman being diagnosed with endometrial cancer during her lifetime is about 1 in 40. Currently, there are over 500,000 survivors of endometrial cancer living in this country. Interestingly, this cancer is more common in Caucasian women, but African American women are more likely to die from it (ACOG, 2005, 2007; ACS, 2009b).

 Nursing Insight— *Estrogen and endometrial cancer*

There is an established relationship between unopposed (i.e., absence of progesterone) exogenous estrogen and uterine cancer. Progesterone inhibits the growth of cells stimulated by estrogen and causes them to enter a more mature secretory state. Postmenopausal women who receive estrogen therapy without progesterone have much higher rates of uterine cancer.

 Ethnocultural Considerations— Endometrial cancer in African American women

The lifetime mortality risk for Caucasian women with uterine cancer is 2.8% (risk for disease) and 0.48% (risk for death), as compared with African American women, whose risk for developing this condition is 1.7% and whose risk for dying from the condition is 0.73%. The 5-year survival rate for Caucasian women older than 65 years is 80.8%; for African American women in the same age group, the 5-year survival rate is 53.3%. It is unclear whether the high mortality in African American women is a result of delayed treatment, lack of access to care, or a higher likelihood of cancers with more serious prognostic characteristics. It is known, however, that of women with endometrial cancer, only 52% of African American women older than 50 years have the condition confined to the uterus at the time of the original surgery, as compared with 73% of Caucasian women older than 50 years (ACOG, 2008c; Ries et al., 2004).

The exact cause of uterine cancer is not known. However, risk factors have been established. These include unopposed estrogen therapy, nulliparity or low parity, early menarche (before age 12), late menopause (after age 55), therapy with tamoxifen (an anti-estrogen medication used in the prevention and treatment of breast cancer), infertility, diabetes, gallbladder disease, PCOS, a history of ovarian granulosa-theca cell tumors, hypertension, diabetes mellitus, a high-fat diet (which increases the levels of circulating estrogen), and obesity. Factors associated with a lower risk for endometrial cancer include multiparity, use of combination oral contraceptives, use of an intrauterine device, and menopausal estrogen therapy combined with progesterone therapy for women who have a uterus. A genetic syndrome known as hereditary nonpolyposis colon cancer has also been associated with both endometrial and ovarian cancer (ACOG, 2005, 2007; ACS, 2009b).

Endometrial cancer is slow growing, and over 75% of the neoplasms are adenocarcinomas that develop from endometrial hyperplasia. Most women are symptomatic in the early stages of this cancer, a factor that leads to early diagnosis and, frequently, successful treatment. There are no effective screening methods to detect endometrial cancer. Instead, women and their health-care providers must rely on signs and symptoms of the condition. For postmenopausal women, the cardinal symptom is vaginal bleeding; perimenopausal women may experience heavy or prolonged menstruation or spotting or bleeding between menses. Other symptoms for women in all age groups include pelvic pain, dyspareunia, and weight loss (ACOG, 2005, 2009a; ACS, 2009b).

Pelvic examination may reveal a uterine enlargement or mass. A patient who has abnormal vaginal bleeding should have an endometrial biopsy. Fractional curettage, a procedure that involves a scraping of the endocervix and the endometrium to obtain tissue for histological evaluation, may also be performed. Other diagnostic tests that may be conducted include hysteroscopy (examination of the uterus through an endoscope) and transvaginal ultrasound. If invasive endometrial cancer is present, systematic surgical staging is performed. The workup may also include chest radiography, abdominal computed tomography (CT) scan, MRI, cystoscopy, proctoscopy, liver function tests, renal function tests, bone scans, and serum testing for the presence of cancer antigen 125 (CA-125, released by some endometrial and ovarian cancers) to determine the extent of metastasis (ACOG, 2005, 2009a; ACS, 2009b).

Endometrial cancer is staged based on its location and extension into surrounding tissue and distant metastases. Treatment involves total abdominal hysterectomy along with removal of the ovaries, fallopian tubes, and local lymph nodes. Following the surgery, radiation therapy, chemotherapy, or hormone therapy may be prescribed, depending on the clinical findings. When diagnosed and treated early, survival rates are good. For all cases of endometrial cancer, the relative 5-year survival rate is approximately 83%; for cancers treated at an earlier stage, the 5-year survival rate exceeds 92% (ACOG, 2007; ACS, 2009b).

🔄 **Now Can You—** **Discuss ovarian tumors and endometrial cancer?**

1. Differentiate between ovarian follicular cysts and corpus luteum cysts?
2. Develop a holistic nursing plan of care for a woman with a diagnosis of polycystic ovary syndrome?
3. Develop an ovarian cancer awareness educational program for women?
4. Discuss the major risk factors for endometrial cancer, and identify the primary presenting symptom?

Diseases of the Vulva

The external female genital organs, or vulva, include all visible structures that extend externally from the mons pubis to the perineum. The vulvar tissue is richly supplied with sweat and sebaceous glands, and some areas contain hair follicles as well. The vulvar region supports a moist environment that contains increased concentrations of skin bacteria.

Symptoms of vulvovaginal disorders are common, often chronic, and can significantly interfere with a woman's sexual function and sense of well-being. Obtaining a detailed health history is an essential tool in the patient assessment, and it is important to remember that systemic conditions such as Crohn's disease can cause vulvar symptoms. Vulvar pruritus, or itching, is the most frequent symptom, and women often delay evaluation because they self-treat with readily available vaginal preparations. Other commonly reported symptoms in the vulvar region include a sensation of burning, the presence of a lump or sore, vaginal discharge, a rash, and pain. Frequently encountered vulvar conditions include vaginal infections, Bartholin's gland abscess, parasites, molluscum contagiosum, and vulvar warts (ACOG, 2008d).

VAGINAL INFECTIONS

Vaginal infections can produce vulvar symptoms. Candidiasis (yeast infection) often is associated with intense itching and tissue irritation. Women who are immunocompromised, diabetic, overweight, or receiving long-term antibiotic therapy are especially susceptible to vulvar yeast infections that may be resistant to treatment. Because the infection may stem from multiple types of yeast or include bacterial organisms, it is important to perform an appropriate diagnostic evaluation (ACOG, 2008d).

BARTHOLIN'S GLAND ABSCESS

The Bartholin's glands, also known as the greater vestibular or vulvovaginal glands, are located deep within the posterior portion of the vestibule near the posterior vaginal introitus (Fig. 4-6).

A & P review **The Bartholin's Glands**

The vestibule is essentially an oval-shaped space enclosed by the labia minora. It contains openings to the urethra and vagina, the Skene's glands, and the Bartholin's glands. This area of a woman's anatomy is extremely sensitive to chemical irritants. The Bartholin's glands secrete a clear mucus that moistens and lubricates the vagina during sexual arousal. ◆

Bartholin's cysts are the most common benign lesions of the vulva. Obstruction of the Bartholin duct leads to enlargement and formation of a cyst. The cyst may cause

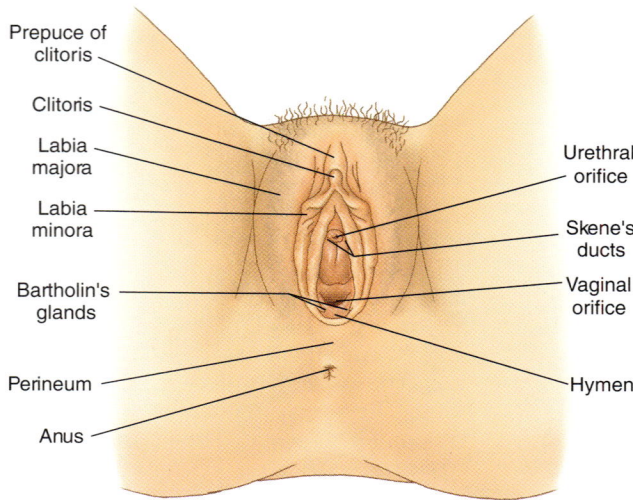

Figure 4-6 labels:
- Prepuce of clitoris
- Clitoris
- Labia majora
- Labia minora
- Bartholin's glands
- Perineum
- Anus
- Urethral orifice
- Skene's ducts
- Vaginal orifice
- Hymen

Figure 4-6 Female external genitalia (Dillon, P. M. (2007). *Nursing health assessment: A critical thinking approach* (2nd ed., p. 612). Philadelphia, F. A. Davis)

Figure 4-7 Molluscum contagiosum (Venes, D. (Ed.). (2009). *Taber's cyclopedic medical dictionary* (p. 1498, 21st ed.). Philadelphia: F. A. Davis)

no symptoms, but if it enlarges or becomes infected, the woman frequently experiences pain, dyspareunia, and an awareness of a tender mass in the area. When symptomatic, incision and drainage provides temporary relief. Because Bartholin's cysts tend to recur, a permanent opening for drainage may be recommended. Rarely, the abscess is caused by gonorrhea. Bartholin's abscesses are highly unusual in postmenopausal women and should be evaluated to rule out malignancy (ACOG, 2008d).

PARASITES

Lice or mites may infect the vulva. Intense itching of the skin that contains hair follicles is characteristic of infestation. Scabies, a dermatitis caused by the itch mite *Sarcoptes scabiei,* produces areas of excoriation composed of scaly papules and insect burrows. Scabies is transmitted by person-to-person contact or through infested bedding and clothing. The itching tends to worsen at night. Scabies spreads on the skin by fingernail contamination. Diagnosis is made by microscopic examination of skin scrapings to detect the presence of the mite, its eggs, or its excretions (Venes, 2009).

 Nursing Insight— *Formulating appropriate nursing diagnoses for patients with scabies*

Nursing diagnoses for patients with scabies usually focus on Impaired Skin Integrity related to the presence of invasive parasites and the development of pruritus and Deficient Knowledge regarding the communicable nature of the infestation, possible complications, therapy, and self-care needs related to a lack of information or misinterpretation.

MOLLUSCUM CONTAGIOSUM (SEED WART)

Molluscum contagiosum is a rash composed of small, dome-shaped papules with a central crater filled with a cheesy (caseous) material (Fig. 4-7). The lesions of molluscum

contagiosum are caused by a pox virus. In adults, transmission is primarily sexual; in children, transmission is non-sexual and via fomites, substances that adhere to and transmit infection (Venes, 2009).

VULVAR CONDYLOMATA

A condyloma (plural: *condylomas, condylomata*) is a growth that resembles a wart on the skin or mucous membrane, usually of the genitals or anus. Vulvar condylomata, also known as "warts," "genital warts," and "venereal warts," are caused by certain strains of the human papillomavirus, different from those that produce cervical lesions. Condylomata can appear as small, thickened growths or large cauliflower-like masses on the vulva, along the perineum, or in and around the anus. The benign growths can be treated with chemicals, cryosurgery, electrosurgery, or laser vaporization. None of the treatments are fully successful, however, and recurrence is common. Despite removal of the lesions, surrounding tissues continue to harbor the human papillomavirus. Condylomata may be spread by physical contact with an area containing a wart, and the spread of a wart from one labium to the other by autoinoculation is possible (ACOG, 2008d; Venes, 2009). (See further discussion about human papillomavirus in Chapter 5.)

 Nursing Insight— *Premalignant and malignant vulvar lesions*

Most vulvar cancer is squamous in origin. Because the vulva is covered with skin, any malignancy that appears elsewhere on the skin can also occur on the vulva. *Vulvar intraepithelial neoplasia* (VIN) is a cancer precursor often associated with human papillomavirus. The most common symptom of VIN is persistent itching; localized burning and/or skin thickening or discoloration (e.g., red, pink, lighter, or darker) in the affected area may also be present. Biopsy is needed for diagnosis. Women who have a history of genital warts and who smoke have an increased risk of developing vulvar cancer. *Invasive vulvar cancer* is the presence of a malignant lesion that breaks through the cellular basement membrane. This type of cancer occurs most often in older (70+ years) women, and in the United States it is responsible for 5% of all female genital malignancies. Treatment involves surgical excision (vulvectomy) and inguinal lymphadenectomy (ACOG, 2008d; ACS, 2009c).

Melanoma is the second most common type of invasive vulvar malignancy, but it is extremely rare, accounting for less than 5% of all vulvar cancers. Most melanomas are located on the labia minora or clitoris and are blue-black in color. They have a jagged or fuzzy border, and the lesions may be raised or ulcerated. Although the condition may affect women of all ages, vulvar melanoma is more common in older (70+ years) women, and over 90% occur in Caucasian women. Biopsy is needed for diagnosis, and treatment involves surgical excision and in some situations inguinal lymphadenectomy (ACOG, 2008d; ACS, 2009c).

Paget disease is another rare neoplasm of the vulva. It also occurs more commonly in older (70+ years) women. Symptoms include intense vulvar itching and soreness, usually of long duration. Lesions of Paget disease are thick, often leading to an impression of leukoplakia. The affected area may also be red, moist, and elevated; biopsy is necessary for diagnosis. Treatment consists of surgical excision (ACOG, 2008d; ACS, 2009c).

THE NURSE'S ROLE IN PROMOTING VULVAR HEALTH

Nurses should be aware of common vulvar irritants and allergens (see Box 4-3) so that they can provide appropriate patient counseling and offer strategies for promoting and maintaining a healthy vulvar environment to reduce the risk of irritation and infection. Nurses can also teach women to wear cotton underwear, keep the vulvar area clean and dry, avoid douching, and perform monthly vulvar self-examination.

Box 4-3 **Common Vulvar Irritants and Allergens**

Adult or baby wipes
Antiseptics (e.g., povidone iodine, hexachlorophene)
Body fluids (e.g., semen, saliva)
Colored or scented toilet paper
Condoms (lubricant or spermicide containing)
Contraceptive creams, jellies, foams, nonoxynol-9, and lubricants
Dyes
Emollients (e.g., lanolin, jojoba oil, glycerin)
Laundry detergents, fabric softeners, and dryer sheets
Rubber products (including latex)
Sanitary products, including tampons and pads
Soaps, bubble bath and salts, shampoos, and conditioners
Tea tree oil
Topical anesthetics (e.g., benzocaine, lidocaine, dibucaine)
Topical antibacterials (e.g., neomycin, bacitracin, polymyxin)
Topical antimycotics (e.g., imidazoles, nystatin)
Topical corticosteroids
Topical medications, including trichloroacetic acid, 5-fluorouracil, and podofilox or podophyllin
Vaginal hygiene products, including perfumes and deodorants

Source: ACOG, 2008d.

Family Teaching Guidelines...
Performing Vulvar Self-examination

To prepare for vulvar self-examination, the woman places a flashlight and mirror within easy reach. She washes her hands, removes clothing from the waist down, and sits comfortably on the floor or bed, with a pillow support behind her back. The following steps should then be performed:

1. While bending her knees, she leans backward and allows her knees to fall slightly apart to expose the genital area. The mirror and flashlight should be positioned for optimal visualization.
2. External inspection of the genital area includes visualizing the labia, the clitoris, the urethral meatus, the vaginal opening, and the anal opening.
3. Using her fingers, the woman should gently spread the labia and inspect the vaginal vault. The vaginal walls should be pink and contain small folds or ridges called rugae.
4. The vaginal discharge should be evaluated at this time as well. Normal vaginal discharge is clear to cloudy and white, with a slightly acidic odor; it may be thick or thin, depending on the timing of the examination with regard to the menstrual cycle.
5. Findings that need to be reported to the health-care provider include the presence of sores or growths on the labia or vaginal walls, an unpleasant odor to the vaginal discharge, and tissue redness. Sores, redness, abnormal growths, malodorous or excessive vaginal discharge, and itching may indicate irritation or infection.

Source: Vulval Pain Society, 2008.

Now Can You— **Discuss conditions of the vulva?**

1. Describe signs, symptoms, and treatment modalities for a Bartholin gland cyst?
2. Discuss signs and symptoms of vulvar carcinoma, and identify populations at greatest risk for development of this type of cancer?
3. Teach a patient how to perform vulvar self-examination?

summary points

◆ Menstrual disorders, such as amenorrhea, irregular bleeding, and dysmenorrheal, constitute some of the most common reproductive problems in women.

◆ Endometriosis is a chronic condition characterized by the presence of endometrial glands and tissue outside the uterus.

◆ Uterine leiomyomas are the most common solid pelvic tumors in women and the leading indication for hysterectomy.

◆ Dysfunctional uterine bleeding is defined as noncyclic menstrual blood flow that is derived from the endometrium.

◆ Ovarian cysts affect women of all ages, although they occur most often during the childbearing years and typically represent a normal process.

◆ Polycystic ovary syndrome occurs when an endocrine imbalance results in elevated levels of estrogen, testosterone, and luteinizing hormone and a decreased secretion of follicle-stimulating hormone.

◆ Ovarian cancer is the leading cause of gynecological deaths and the fourth most common cause of cancer deaths in women.

◆ In the United States, cancer of the endometrium is the most common gynecological malignancy, and approximately 70% of all cases are found in women in the 50–69 age group.

◆ Nurses can promote vulvar health by teaching women about strategies such as the avoidance of common vulvar irritants and how perform vulvar self-examination.

review questions

Multiple Choice

1. The nurse is aware that secondary amenorrhea may be caused by:
A. Lactation
B. Crohn's disease
C. Congenital absence of the vagina
D. Polycystic ovary syndrome

2. During patient teaching, the nurse explains that primary dysmenorrhea is related to:
A. Pregnancy
B. Leiomyoma
C. Perimenopause
D. Prostaglandins

3. When providing counseling for a patient with a diagnosis of endometriosis, the nurse explains that:
A. Consuming a high-fat diet may help to minimize symptoms.
B. Medical treatment is designed to reduce the amount of estrogen in the body.
C. Laparoscopic surgical removal of the lesions results in a permanent cure.
D. Infertility is a rare complication of the condition.

4. The nurse explains to a patient with a diagnosis of abnormal uterine bleeding that thermal balloon ablation is a technique developed to:
A. Restore fertility
B. Destroy the uterine lining
C. Treat uterine cancer
D. Open blocked fallopian tubes

5. Nurses can teach women about strategies to promote vulvar health, such as:
A. Performing monthly vulvar self-examination
B. Using scented toilet paper
C. Douching once a week
D. Wearing synthetic underwear

REFERENCES

Ailawadi, R. K., Jobranpufra, S., Kataria, M., Gurates, B., & Bulun, S. E. (2004). Treatment of endometriosis and chronic pelvic pain with letrozole and norethindrone acetate: A pilot study. *Fertility and Sterility, 81*(2), 290–296.

American Cancer Society (ACS). (2009a). *What are key statistics about ovarian cancer?* Retrieved March 10, 2010, from http://www.cancer.org/docroot/cri/content/cri_2_4_1x_what_are_the_key_statistics_for_ovarian_cancer_33.asp

American Cancer Society (ACS). (2009b). *Detailed guide: Endometrial cancer.* Retrieved March 11, 2010, from http://www.cancer.org/docroot/CRI/content/CRI_2_4_1x_What_is_Endometrial_Cancer.asp?sitearea=

American Cancer Society (ACS). (2009c). *Detailed guide: Vulvar cancer.* Retrieved March 11, 2010, from http://www.cancer.org/docroot/CRI/content/CRI_2_4_1X_What_is_vulvar_cancer_45.asp?sitearea=

American College of Obstetricians and Gynecologists (ACOG). (2000). *Management of anovulatory bleeding* (Practice Bulletin No. 14, pp. 1049–1056). Washington, DC: Author.

American College of Obstetricians and Gynecologists (ACOG). (2002, December). The role of the generalist obstetrician–gynecologist in the early detection of ovarian cancer (ACOG Committee Opinion No. 280). *Obstetrics and Gynecology, 100*(6), 1413–1416.

American College of Obstetricians and Gynecologists (ACOG). (2005). *Management of endometrial cancer* (Practice Bulletin No. 65, pp. 1258–1269). Washington, DC: Author.

American College of Obstetricians and Gynecologists (ACOG>. (2007). *Women's health care: A resource manual.* (3rd ed.). Washington, DC: Author.

American College of Obstetricians and Gynecologists (ACOG). (2008a). *Treatment of urinary tract infections in non-pregnant women* (Practice Bulletin No. 91, pp. 10–12). Washington, DC: Author.

American College of Obstetricians and Gynecologists (ACOG). (2008b). *Alternatives to hysterectomy in the management of leiomyomas* (Practice Bulletin No. 96, pp. 388–397). Washington, DC: Author.

American College of Obstetricians and Gynecologists (ACOG). (2008c). Intraperitoneal chemotherapy for ovarian cancer (ACOG Committee Opinion No. 396). *Obstetrics and Gynecology, 111*(3), 249–251.

American College of Obstetricians and Gynecologists (ACOG). (2008d). *Diagnosis and management of vulvar skin disorders* (Practice Bulletin No. 93, pp. 370–379). Washington, DC: Author.

American College of Obstetricians and Gynecologists (ACOG). (2009a). Choosing the route of hysterectomy for benign disease (ACOG Committee Opinion No. 444). *Obstetrics and Gynecology, 114*(5), 1156–1158.

American College of Obstetricians and Gynecologists (ACOG). (2009b). *Polycystic ovary syndrome* (Practice Bulletin No. 108, pp. 936–948). Washington, DC: Author.

American Society for Reproductive Medicine (ASRM). (2006). Endometriosis and infertility. *Fertility and Sterility, 86*(4), 156–160.

Audebert, A., Backstrom, T., Barlow, D.H., Benagiano, G., Brosens, I., Buhler, K., Donnez, J., Evers, J., Pellicer, A., & Mettler, L. (1992). Endometriosis 1991: A discussion document. *Human Reproduction, 7*(3), 432–435.

Bazot, M., Detchev, R., Cortez, A., Amouyal, P., Uzan, S., & Darai, E. (2003). Transvaginal sonography for the prediction of location of deep pelvic endometriosis. *Human Reproduction, 18*(8), 1686–1692.

Bertelsen, L., Mellemkjaer, L., Frederiksen, K., Kjaer, S. K., Brinton, L. A., Sakoda, L. C., van Valkengoed, I., & Olsen, J. H. (2007). Risk for breast cancer among women with endometriosis. *International Journal of Cancer, 120*(6), 1372–1375.

Bloski, T., & Pierson, R. (2008). Endometriosis and chronic pelvic pain: Unveiling the mystery behind this complex condition. *Nursing for Women's Health, 12*(5), 382–395.

Brankin, C. A., & Cackovic, M. (2010). Oral contraceptives for the treatment of pain associated with endometriosis. *Contemporary OB-GYN, 55*(3), 42–43.

Centers for Disease Control and Prevention (CDC). (2005). *Toxic shock syndrome.* Retrieved February 20, 2010, from http://www.cdc.gov/ncidod/dbmd/diseaseinfo/toxicshock_t.htm

Centers for Disease Control and Prevention (CDC). (2006a). *Sexually transmitted diseases treatment guidelines.* Retrieved February 15, 2010, from http://www.cdc.gov/std/treatment/2006/vaginal-discharge.htm#vagdis2

Centers for Disease Control and Prevention (CDC). (2006b). *Women's reproductive health: Hysterectomy.* Retrieved March 1, 2010, from http://www.cdc.gov/reproductivehealth/WomensRH/Hysterectomy.htm

Chopin, N., Ballester, M., Borghese, B., Fauconnier, A., Foulot, H., Marlartic, C., & Chapron, C. (2006). Relation between severity of dysmenorrhea and endometriosis. *Acta Obstetricia et Gynecologica Scandinavica, 85*(11), 1375–1380.

Coughlin, G., & Secor, M. (2010). Bacterial vaginosis: Update on evidence-based care. *Advance for Nurse Practitioners, 18*(1), 41–45.

Crosignani, P., Olive, D., Bergqvist, A., & Luciano, A. (2006). Advances in the management of endometriosis: An update for clinicians. *Human Reproduction Update, 12*(2), 179–189.

Day Baird, D., Dunson, D. B., Hill, M. C., Cousins, D., & Schectman, J. M. (2003). High cumulative incidence of uterine leiomyoma in African American and Caucasian women: Ultrasound evidence. *American Journal of Obstetrics & Gynecology, 188*(7), 100–107.

Deglin, J., & Vallerand, A. (2009). *Davis's drug guide for nurses* (11th ed.). Philadelphia: F. A. Davis.

Denny, E., & Mann, C. H. (2007). Endometriosis-associated dyspareunia: The impact on women's lives. *Journal of Family Planning and Reproductive Health Care, 33*(3), 189–193.

Dunican, K. (2008). OTC product: Vagisil Screening Kit for vaginal infections. *Journal of the American Pharmacists Association, 48*(2), e33.

DuRant, M. E., Leslie, N. S., & Critch, E. A. (2009). Managing polycystic ovary syndrome: A cognitive behavioral strategy. *Nursing for Women's Health, 13*(4), 293–300.

Elkins, B. L., & Mayeaux Jr., E. J. (2010). Bacterial vaginosis: Diagnosis and therapy. *Female Patient, 35*(3), 42–46.

Falagas, M. F., Betsil, G. I., & Athansion, S. (2006). Probiotics for prevention of recurrent vulvovaginal candidiasis: A review. *Journal of Antimicrobial Chemotherapy, 58*(9), 266–272.

Fan, A. Z., Russell, M., Naimi, T., Li, Y., Liao, Y., Jiles, R., & Mokdad, A. H. (2008). Patterns of alcohol consumption and the metabolic syndrome. *Journal of Clinical Endocrinology & Metabolism, 93*(10), 3833–3838.

Fife, A. (2007). Ovarian cancer: This "silent killer" does make noise. *Clinician Reviews, 17*(9), 10–16.

Fothergill, R., & Sulak, P. J. (2010). Ovulatory heavy menstrual bleeding. *Female Patient, 35*(3), 15–19.

Fraser, I. S., Critchley, H. O., Munro, M. G., & Broder, M. (2007). A process designed to lead to international agreement on terminologies and definitions used to describe abnormalities of menstrual bleeding. *Fertility & Sterility, 87*(3), 466–476.

Goff, B. A., Mandel, L. S., Drescher, C. W., Urban, N., Gough, S., Schurman, K. M., Patras, J., Mahony, B.S., & Andersen, M. R. (2007). Development of an ovarian cancer symptom index: Possibilities for earlier detection. *Cancer, 109*(2), 2031–2042.

Goff, B. A., Matthews, B. J., Larson, E. H., Andrilla, C. H., Wynn, M., Lishner, D. M., & Baldwin, L. M. (2007). Predictors of comprehensive surgical treatment in patients with ovarian cancer. *Cancer, 109*(10), 2031–2042.

Goodman, P., Herman, J., Murdaugh, C. L., Moneyham, L. D., & Phillips, K. D. (2007). Role of decision-making in women's self-diagnosis and management of vaginitis. *Women's Health Care, 6*(2), 57–63.

Guo, S. W., & Wang, Y. (2006). The prevalence of endometriosis in women with chronic pelvic pain. *Gynecologic & Obstetric Investigation, 62*(3), 54–58.

Hatcher, R. A., Trussell, J., Nelson, A., Cates, F., Stewart, F., & Kowal, D. (Eds.). (2008). *Contraceptive technology* (19th ed.). New York: Ardent Media.

Hellwig, J. P. (2007). Ovarian cancer: Considering symptoms. *Nursing for Women's Health, 11*(2), 123.

Helming, M. B. (2009). Three generations and counting: The many health threats of DES. *Advance for Nurse Practitioners, 17*(8), 27–30.

Hoeger, K. M. (2007). Obesity and lifestyle management in polycystic ovary syndrome. *Clinical Obstetrics and Gynecology, 50*(1), 277–294.

Hordern, B. (2007). Finding ovarian cancer early: What to look for. *Clinical Advisor, 10*(5), 99–103.

Huntington, A., & Gilmour, J. A. (2005). A life shaped by pain: Women and endometriosis. *Journal of Clinical Nursing, 14*(9), 1124–1132.

Keehbauch, J. A., & Nystrom, J. (2007). Diagnosis and management of abnormal uterine bleeding. *Female Patient, 32*(7), 38–40.

Koumans, E. H., Sternberg, M., Vruce, C., McQuillan, G., Kendrick, J., Sutton, M., & Markowitz, L. E. (2007). The prevalence of bacterial vaginosis in the United States, 2001–2004; Associations with symptoms, sexual behaviors, and reproductive health. *Sexually Transmitted Diseases, 34*(11), 864–869.

Lindenbaum, C. (2010). Polycystic ovarian syndrome: Where genetics and environment collide. *Advance for Nurse Practitioners, 18*(2), 20–27.

Moore, R. G., & MacLaughlan, S. (2009). A novel approach for the risk assessment of a pelvic mass for ovarian cancer. *Female Patient, 34*(9), 31–37.

National Cancer Institute (NCI). (2009). *Vaginal cancer.* Retrieved February 16, 2010, from http://www.cancer.gov/cancertopics/pdq/treatment/vaginal/HealthProfessional/

Nelson, A. L. (2009). Metabolic syndrome in women with polycystic ovary syndrome. *Female Patient, 32*(8), 15–22.

Nelson, A. L., & Baldwin, S. (2008). Menstrual disorders and related concerns. In R. Hatcher et al. (Eds.), *Contraceptive technology* (19th ed., pp. 451–469). New York: Ardent Media.

Neal, D. D., Formyduval, A. M., & Taylor, J. S. (2010). HER LIFESTYLE: A mneumonic for addressing polycystic ovary syndrome in adolescents. *Nursing for Women's Health, 13*(6), 473–478.

Ninia, J. G. (2007). Pelvic congestion syndrome. *Female Patient, 32*(8), 41–49.

Nyirjesy, P., & Sobel, J. D. (2005). Advances in diagnosing vaginitis: Development of a new algorithm. *Current Infectious Disease Reports, 7*(16), 458–462.

Pirotta, M. V., & Garland, S. M. (2006). Genital *Candida* species detected in samples from women in Melbourne, Australia, before and after treatment with antibiotics. *Journal of Clinical Microbiology, 44*(6), 3213–3217.

Ries, L. A. G., Eisner, M. P., Kosary, C. L., Hankey, B. F., Miller, B. A., Clegg, L., Mariotto, A., Feuer, E.J., & Edwards, B. K. (Eds.). *SEER cancer statistics review, 1975–2001.* Bethesda, MD: National Cancer Institute. Retrieved March 9, 1010, from http://seer.cancer.gov/csr/1975_2001/

Sadovsky, R. (2007). Managing first-time and recurrent UTIs. *Clinical Advisor, 9*(5), 46–51.

Sampson, J. A. (1940). The development of the implantation theory for the origin of peritoneal endometriosis. *American Journal of Obstetrics and Gynecology, 40*(6), 549–557.

Scolaro, K. L., Lloyd, K. B., & Helms, K. L. (2008). Devices for home evaluation of women's health concerns. *American Journal of Health-System Pharmacists, 65*(4), 299–314.

Sheary, B., & Dayan, L. (2005). Clinical practice. Recurrent vulvovaginal candidiasis. *Australian Family Physician, 34*(9), 147–150.

Shippen, E. R., & West, W. J. (2004). Successful treatment of severe endometriosis in two premenopausal women with an aromatase inhibitor. *Fertility and Sterility, 81*(5), 1395–1398.

Sinaii, N., Cleary, S. D., Younes, N., Ballweg, M., & Stratton, P. (2002). High rates of autoimmune and endocrine disorders, fibromyalgia, chronic fatigue syndrome and atopic diseases among women with endometriosis: A survey analysis. *HumanReproduction, 17*(10), 2715–2724.

Smith, O. W. (1948). Diethylstilbestrol in the prevention and treatment of complications of pregnancy. *American Journal of Obstetrics and Gynecology, 56*(3), 821–834.

Society of Obstetricians and Gynaecologists of Canada. (2005). SOGC clinical guidelines: Uterine fibroid embolization (UFE). *International Journal of Gynaecology and Obstetrics, 89*(3), 305–318.

Song, A. H. (2007). Global endometrial ablation devices: Minimally invasive surgical alternatives to hysterectomy. *Female Patient, 32*(7), 46–50.

Speroff, L., & Fritz, M. A. (2005). *Clinical gynecologic endocrinology and infertility* (7th ed.). Philadelphia: Lippincott Williams & Wilkins.

Speroff, L., & Mishell Jr., D. R. (2007). Polycystic ovary syndrome: Management and contraception. *Dialogues in Contraception, 11*(1), 5–7.

Spies, J. B., Myers, E. R., Worthington-Kirsch, R., Mulgund, J., Goodwin, S., & Mauro, M. (2005). The FIBROID registry: Symptom and quality-of-life status 1 year after therapy. *Obstetrics and Gynecology, 106*(6), 1309–1318.

Stern, J. L. (2007). *Cancers and treatments: Vagina.* Retrieved February 18, 2010, from http://womenscancercenter.com/info/types/typehome.html

Stern, L. (2009). Assessing excessive menstrual bleeding. *Clinical Advisor, 12*(1), 25–37.

U.S. Food and Drug Administration (FDA). (2009). *FDA approves Lysteda to treat heavy menstrual bleeding.* Retrieved March 5, 2010, from http://www.fda.gov/NewsEvents/Newsroom/PressAnnouncements/2009/ucm190551.htm

Venes, D. (2009). *Taber's cyclopedic medical dictionary* (21st ed.). Philadelphia: F. A. Davis.

Vermund, S. H., & Allen, K. L. (2009). Douching is a remediable risk factor for sexually transmitted infections. *The Female Patient, 34*(7), 37–39.

Vulval Pain Society. (2008). *How to perform a vulval self-exam.* Retrieved March 9, 2010, from http://vulvalpainsociety.org/index.php?page=self-examination

Watson, C., & Ng, G. (2008). Not that itch again: Dealing with recurrent vulvovaginal candidiasis. *Nursing for Women's Health, 12*(3), 215–223.

White, D., Vanthuyne, P., Wood, M., & Ayres, J. (2004). Zafirlukast for severe recurrent vulvovaginal candidiasis: An open label pilot study. *Sexually Transmitted Infections, 80*(2), 219–222.

Wolfe, J. (2006). Polycystic ovary syndrome: Case study decision tree. *Women's Health Care, 5*(7), 19–31.

Woodson, S. A. (2007). Chronic pelvic pain: Can you guess the cause? *Nursing for Women's Health, 11*(2), 200–204.

Wysocki, S. (2008). Vaginal pH as an OTC screening tool for vaginitis. *Advance for Nurse Practitioners, 17*(20), 29–35.

 For more information, go to http://davisplus.fadavis.com/

Promoting Reproductive Health Through an Understanding of Sexually Transmitted Diseases

Shelton M. Hisley, PhD, RNC, WHNP-BC

 We may run, walk, stumble, drive, or fly, but let us never lose sight of the reason for the journey, or miss a chance to see a rainbow on the way.

—Gloria Gaither

LEARNING TARGETS *At the completion of this chapter, the student will be able to:*

◆ Discuss signs and symptoms, modes of transmission, and treatment options for the most common sexually transmitted diseases (STDs).

◆ Identify various safer sex strategies.

◆ Describe the nurse's role in STD counseling and education.

Introduction

This chapter focuses on sexually transmitted diseases (STDs). Information regarding signs, symptoms, modes of transmission, and treatment options for various STDs is presented, along with a discussion of the nurse's role in promoting reproductive health. STDs encompass more than 25 infectious organisms that cause reproductive tract infections that are primarily transmitted by close, intimate contact. Nurses are perfectly situated to provide evidence-based, culturally sensitive STD counseling and education that facilitates understanding of these potentially lethal health threats and empowers women to make informed choices in their intimate relationships.

In many clinical settings, the terms *sexually transmitted disease* and *sexually transmitted infection* are used interchangeably. "Sexually transmitted disease" is the accepted subject heading in the PubMed database, and *STD* is also the term used by the Centers for Disease Control and Prevention (CDC) (Royer & Cerf, 2009). According to the CDC (2006b), an important component of STD health care is that providers use language that is understandable to patients. Owing to the fact that stigma associated with an STD can be a barrier to appropriate diagnosis and treatment (Royer & Zahner, 2009), some clinicians use the term STI instead of STD because discussing an infection with a patient may be less embarrassing than discussing a disease (Marrazzo et al., 2007).

In addition to the short-term emotional and physical distress usually associated with a reproductive tract infection, many serious long-term effects may also result from many of the STDs. Potential complications include fallopian tube blockage with resultant infertility, an increased risk of ectopic pregnancy, chronic pelvic pain, an increased risk of liver cancer and serious liver disease, and death. Women suffer more long-term reproductive consequences from STDs than do men, and women are more likely than men to acquire an infection from any single sexual encounter. Unfortunately, owing to the asymptomatic nature of many STDs, treatment is often delayed, and this factor increases the likelihood of more serious long-term consequences (Adler, 2007; Johnson-Mallard & Lengacher, 2007).

The incidence of several STDs has increased over the past few years. In late 2009, the CDC released STD Surveillance Data for the year 2008. According to the findings, Chlamydia remains the most commonly reported infectious disease in the United States. The rate of this infection has increased by 9.2% as compared to the 2007 data; however, it is important to note that the increase could be related to factors such as improved screening

where research and practice meet:
Exploring young women's beliefs about the terms *sexually transmitted disease* **and** *sexually transmitted infection*

It is unknown whether patients understand what their health-care provider means when using the terms *sexually transmitted disease* and *sexually transmitted infection*, and recent research (Royer, 2008) suggests that some female patients may be more familiar with the terms *sexually transmitted disease* or *STD*.

Royer and Cerf (2009) conducted a survey to determine whether young women differentiate between the terms *sexually transmitted disease* and *sexually transmitted infection* and, if so, whether their reasons were consistent with those of health-care providers. A total of 302 women aged 18 to 24 completed a survey that measured beliefs about STDs and whether they considered the terms *sexually transmitted disease* and *sexually transmitted infection* to be interchangeable. Fifty-seven percent responded that *sexually transmitted disease* and *sexually transmitted infection* do *not* mean the same thing; 28% believed that *STD* and *STI do* mean the same thing; and 15% responded that they did not know. The investigators concluded that while a majority of the young women do differentiate between the two terms, their rationale for doing so is not consistent with the rationale used by health-care providers. Based on the findings, the researchers suggested that professionals clarify their use of the terms *sexually transmitted disease* and *sexually transmitted infection* when talking with patients as a strategy to improve health communication and to improve STD health care.

methods and testing. Rates of gonorrhea have dropped from the 2007 data, with approximately 111 cases per 100,000 individuals. Similarly to Chlamydia, gonorrhea continues to be under-diagnosed and under-reported. Syphilis is on the comeback, with an increase of 18%, as compared to the 2007 data. Interestingly, at one point, this disease was once on the verge of elimination, but there have been increasing numbers of reported cases since 2001. Much of the increase has occurred among men who have sex with men and is attributed to increased rates of unsafe sexual practices (CDC, 2009a).

Nursing Insight— *The National Health Initiative addresses sexually transmitted diseases*

Several *Healthy People 2010* National Health Goals specifically focus on STDs:

- Reduce the proportion of adolescents and young adults with *Chlamydia trachomatis* infections from baselines of 12% (females) and 15% (males) to a target of 3%.
- Reduce new cases of gonorrhea to an incidence of no more than 19 new cases/100,000 people from a baseline of 123/100,000.
- Reduce primary and secondary syphilis to an incidence of no more than 0.2 cases/100,000 people from a baseline of 3.2 per 100,000.
- Reduce genital herpes to an incidence of no more than 14% from a baseline of 17%.
- Reduce pelvic inflammatory disease to an incidence of no more than 5% of women aged 15 through 44 from a baseline of 8% (U.S. Department of Health and Human Services [USDHHS], 2000).

Nurses can help the nation to meet these goals by providing education about methods of preventing STDs and information about how to recognize the signs and symptoms of these illnesses. Nurses can design studies and engage in research to provide evidence-based practice strategies for issues such as teaching women about safer sex practices, teaching youth about the methods of transmission of infection and the long-term consequences of the diseases, and ways that health professionals can increase STD awareness in their practice settings.

HIV/AIDS

In the years since acute HIV infection was first described, research has identified the cellular mechanisms that accompany its clinical presentation. HIV most commonly enters the host through percutaneous or genital routes. Once the virus has penetrated the mucosal epithelium, it infects macrophages, CD4+ T cells, and dendritic cells and spreads to the systemic lymph nodes within 2 days after infection. Within 3 days, it is detectable in the plasma. Plasma viremia then results in dissemination to various body organs, including the brain and spleen (Kahn & Walker, 1998; Swan, 2009).

Infection with HIV leads to a progressive disease that results in AIDS. The AIDS epidemic has in some way touched everyone's life, and the health profession has been affected profoundly. Many individuals living in the United States remain ignorant of the fact that AIDS affects men, women, and children and has reached epidemic proportions in many areas. Because HIV infection can remain asymptomatic for years, infected women can unknowingly harbor and transmit the virus. Women who are infected with HIV have special gynecological health needs that must be assessed and addressed (Marrazzo et al., 2007).

In this country, more and more young people, especially women, are contracting HIV. Most women are infected during sex with an HIV-infected man or while using HIV-contaminated syringes for the injection of drugs such as heroin, cocaine, and amphetamines. According to the CDC (2009b), approximately 56,300 individuals were newly infected with HIV in 2006. In 2007, the estimated number of persons diagnosed with AIDS was 37, 041. This is a higher estimate than those made in previous years and underscores the need to keep HIV prevention at the top of the public health agenda. In the United States, women ages 15 to 44 years represent one of the fastest growing segments of the epidemic. It is important to note that women are more likely than men to acquire HIV at any one contact (CDC, 2009b; Swan, 2009).

Ethnocultural Considerations— HIV disparities in the United States

According to the CDC, African American females are severely and disproportionately affected by HIV infection. In 2006, the HIV diagnosis rate for African American females (56.2) was more than 19 times the rate for Caucasian females (2.9). The rate for Hispanic women was 15.1, more than 5 times that for Caucasian females. Among American Indians/Alaska Natives, the rate for females (4.6) was nearly twice the rate for Caucasian females (CDC, 2008a).

Today, AIDS is the leading cause of death among young women in most of the world. The majority of women contracted the disease by exposure to infected men. The ratio of infected men and women worldwide approaches 1:1. Both sexual activity and IV drug use play major roles in current transmission statistics.

RISK FACTORS

Lifestyle behaviors that place a woman at risk for contracting HIV are listed in Box 5-1. When obtaining the patient history, it is important to routinely inquire about symptoms that may be associated with HIV. Although primary HIV infection is typically asymptomatic, women may describe nonspecific flulike discomforts such as fever, headache, night sweats, malaise, muscle aches, nausea, diarrhea, weight loss, sore throat, skin rash, and lymphadenopathy (Marrazzo et al., 2007).

 Nursing Insight— *Current investigations in HIV prevention*

In early 2009, the National Institutes of Health (NIH) published promising findings from a multisite clinical trial of topical products designed to reduce the risk of HIV. One product, a vaginal microbicide known as PRO 2000/5, is a vaginal gel applied before sex. The trial sites were in four African countries and also in the United States. When women used the PRO 2000/5 gel plus condoms, they had 30% fewer HIV infections than those offered only condoms or condoms plus a placebo gel. Reported adherence to the gel was very high, at 81%.

DETECTION, TESTING, AND DOCUMENTATION

Detecting HIV is a primary step in prevention of the virus. The CDC (2006a) recommends opt-out HIV testing for all patients in all health-care settings, including pregnant women. (*Opt-out testing* is defined as performing HIV screening after notifying the patient that the test will be performed and that the patient may elect to decline or defer testing. Assent is inferred unless the patient declines testing. *Opt-in testing* means that testing is offered and the patient is required to actively give permission before it can occur.) This latest guideline represents a major change from previous recommendations, which encouraged opt-in testing and suggested that providers consider HIV prevalence and individual risk factors when making recommendations for HIV testing to patients. The American College of Obstetricians and Gynecologists (ACOG) supports routine screening for women aged 19 to 64 years and recommends screening for patients at high risk, including adolescents who are, or ever have been, sexually active. The latest guidelines are aimed at improving access to HIV testing across the country and increasing the number of individuals who are tested each year. It is estimated that up to 25% of persons infected with HIV are unaware of their status, and universal testing may identify more of them (ACOG, 2007; CDC, 2006a; Glynn & Rhodes, 2005; Swan, 2009).

 Optimizing Outcomes— **With CDC-endorsed HIV testing**

The CDC (2006) has published the following recommendations for HIV testing:
Patients in all health care settings:
- Perform HIV screening on every patient after informing the patient that testing will be performed unless the patient declines (opt-out testing).
- Screen patients at highest risk for HIV at least annually.
- General consent for medical care should be sufficient to encompass consent for HIV testing; no separate written consent should be required.
- Prevention counseling should not be required with HIV testing.

Pregnant women:
- Include HIV screen in routine prenatal testing for all pregnant women.
- Screening should be on an opt-out basis.
- General consent for medical care should be sufficient to encompass consent for HIV testing; no separate written consent should be required.
- Repeat HIV testing in the third trimester is recommended.

It is important for the nurse to assess the patient's level of understanding to ensure that she is aware of the legal, emotional, and medical implications of a positive or negative HIV test before she takes the test. Pregnancy is not encouraged for women who are HIV-positive; contraceptive counseling should be offered to HIV-positive women who do not desire pregnancy. Post-test counseling centers on telling the patient her test results, explaining the meaning of the results, and reinforcing infection prevention measures. Women should be advised that if they have been exposed in the past 6 months, they should be retested. All pre-and post-test counseling should be documented on the patient's chart.

 Be sure to— **Conform to HIPAA regulations**

If the HIV test results are to be placed on the patient's medical record, they are then available to everyone who accesses the chart. The patient must be advised of this policy before testing. Health-care facilities must have policies in place to safeguard patient information from inadvertent or inappropriate breaches of confidentiality. In some clinical settings, HIV-related information is maintained in a separate chart and a code is assigned for HIV test results. In other facilities, HIV-related information is removed from the medical record before it is released. Federal regulations set forth in the Health Insurance Portability and Accountability

---

Box 5-1 Risk Factors for HIV Infection

- Current or past history of drug use, especially IV drug use
- History of prostitution
- Frequent sexual intercourse with multiple partners
- Engaging in sexual intercourse under the influence of drugs
- Engaging in sexual intercourse with men who also have sex with men
- Residing in an area with a high prevalence of HIV infection (e.g., rural South and Northeast U.S.)
- Having received a blood transfusion or blood products before 1985

Source: CDC, 2009c.

Act (HIPAA) also provide specific rules for what information may be shared with other practitioners and agencies with and without an individual's permission. Results of HIV testing may need to be recorded and stored in a certain way. It is incumbent upon nurses to be familiar with the legal requirements that exist in the particular practice setting (ACOG, 2007; Marrazzo et al., 2007).

HIV infection is usually diagnosed via the HIV-1 and HIV-2 antibody tests. A schema for HIV screening in women is presented in Figure 5-1. Antibody testing is first performed with a sensitive screening test such as the enzyme-linked immunoassay (ELISA) (also called enzyme immunoassay [EIA]), which detects serum antibodies to HIV. Reactive screening tests are then confirmed by an additional test such as the Western blot or, less commonly, an immunofluorescence assay (IFA). If a positive antibody test is confirmed by a supplemental test, the woman is infected with HIV and is capable of infecting others. These diagnostic tests are very reliable; false-positive and false-negative results are rare. In general, seroconversion for HIV in adolescents and adults occurs from 6 to 12 weeks after transmission of the virus; HIV antibodies are detectable in at least 95% of patients within 3 months after infection (CDC, 2006a).

 Nursing Insight— *Home testing for HIV*

Patients who are reluctant to visit a care provider for testing can purchase a home collection kit at a pharmacy and collect their own finger-prick blood sample. The sample is then mailed to a lab and the patient may call for anonymous results and telephone counseling a few days later (Marrazzo et al., 2007).

Methods of rapid testing for HIV antibodies use a blood sample obtained by finger stick, venipuncture, or an oral fluid sample. The rapid tests can help to reduce unrecognized infections by improving access to testing in both clinical and nonclinical settings and increase the proportion of those tested who learn their results. Rapid testing facilitates patients receiving their test results the same day, usually at the encounter where the test specimen was collected. Like the conventional HIV EIAs, the rapid HIV tests are screening tests that require confirmation if reactive. Although false negatives are rare, they may occur in an individual who has been acutely infected but who has not yet developed HIV antibodies. All of the rapid tests are interpreted visually and require no instrumentation (Greenwald, Burstein, Pincus, & Branson, 2006; Swan, 2009).

Currently, no cure is available for HIV. Current standard of care for HIV is highly active antiretroviral therapy (HAART), a combination of oral antiretroviral agents that inhibit different targets of the virus (Marrazzo et al., 2007). The use of antiretroviral agents has been demonstrated to be effective in maintaining the health of HIV-positive women and in reducing or preventing the perinatal transmission of the virus. A number of opportunistic infections often accompany HIV infection. Information and current guidelines about management are available at the CDC AIDS Prevention hotline (1-800-CDC-INFO [232-4636]) and at their Web site, http://www.cdc.gov/hiv/.

SPECIAL CONCERNS FOR HIV-POSITIVE WOMEN

Women who are HIV positive may experience a number of psychosocial issues. They are often primary caregivers who bear the burden of responsibility for the care of their children. The illness presents major challenges in keeping appointments, receiving adequate rest, and complying with medication regimens. Other immediate needs may involve housing and financial difficulties, and in many situations, other family members are infected as well.

Gynecological problems are also a major concern. Owing to the immunocompromised state, vulvovaginal candidiasis, genital warts caused by human papillomavirus (HPV), and genital herpes lesions are more common and more severe in HIV-infected women. Menstrual problems such as heavy bleeding may require hormonal intervention to address the anemia and lessen the discomfort. However, because the relationship between HIV and menstrual disruption is unclear, all menstrual irregularities should be investigated (ACOG, 2007; Marrazzo et al., 2007).

 Across Clinical Settings: Reducing HIV-related occupational risks for health-care providers

There are three routes of transmission for HIV: direct sexual contact, perinatal transmission from the HIV-infected mother to her fetus or newborn, and direct inoculation with contaminated blood products, needles, or syringes. All health-care providers who may come in contact with

Figure 5-1 Screening for HIV in Women

contaminated blood products, needles, or syringes in any acute care, long-term care, or home care settings are at risk for occupational exposure to HIV. To address this risk, the CDC developed standard precautions, a set of principles to be used in the care of all patients at all times. To minimize personal risk, all health-care workers should consistently comply with the precautions.

 Now Can You— Discuss aspects of HIV infection?

1. Identify six risk factors for HIV infection?
2. Describe what is meant by "opt-out" HIV testing recommended by the CDC?
3. Discuss special concerns for HIV-positive women?

Chlamydia Trachomatis

Chlamydia trachomatis infection is the most common bacterial sexually transmitted disease in the United States and the leading cause of preventable infertility and ectopic pregnancy. Other potential complications include pelvic inflammatory disease (PID) and Fitz-Hugh-Curtis syndrome (infection of the liver capsule). Approximately 1.1 million cases were reported to the CDC (2009d) in 2007, and more than half occurred in women 15 to 25 years old. The reported rate of Chlamydia infection for women substantially exceeds the rate for men, primarily due to increased detection of asymptomatic infection in women through screening. It is estimated that 1 in 10 adolescent girls tested for Chlamydia is infected. Teenage girls tend to have the highest rates of Chlamydial infection. *C. trachomatis* is widespread geographically and is highly prevalent among economically disadvantaged young women (CDC, 2009d; Hackett, 2010; Hoover, Tao, & Kent, 2008; Ravin, 2007).

 Optimizing Outcomes— Teaching patients about STD prevention

Nurses can teach patients about strategies to prevent or decrease the transmission of Chlamydia and other STDs: practicing abstinence from sexual intercourse or sharing a mutually monogamous relationship with a partner who has been tested and is known to be uninfected and correctly and consistently using latex condoms, and avoiding condoms lubricated with the spermicide Nonoxynol-9 (N-9), an agent that has been associated with disruption of the genital epithelium, which may increase the risk for the transmission of infection.

The majority (75%) of Chlamydial infections are asymptomatic, especially in women. Only about 30% of those infected have a mucopurulent cervical discharge; other symptoms include spotting or postcoital bleeding and dysuria. Infected women who use oral contraceptives may report breakthrough bleeding. Chlamydia infection of the cervix causes inflammation that produces microscopic ulcerations, which may increase the risk for contracting HIV (Marrazzo et al., 2007; Weber-LaShore & Biro, 2009).

The CDC and the U.S. Preventive Services Task Force (USPSTF) recommend annual screening for Chlamydia in all sexually active women aged 25 years and younger. Chlamydia infection can be diagnosed using several different testing methods, such as culture, direct immunofluorescence, nucleic acid hybridization, and EIA, all of which require a pelvic examination to collect cervical epithelial cells. The nucleic acid amplification test (NAAT), which can detect Chlamydia from a cervical or vaginal swab (self- or clinician-collected) or urine sample (first few drops of the stream), is considered to be the most sensitive and specific test (CDC, 2009d; Hoover & Tao, 2008; USPSTF, 2001; Weber-La-Shore & Biro, 2009).

 Optimizing Outcomes— Recognizing and addressing barriers to screening for Chlamydia

Although Chlamydia screening is considered a priority preventive service, it remains underutilized by health-care providers. Barriers to screening include a lack of awareness that patients are sexually active and at risk for STDs, a lack of reimbursement for the time required to conduct patient testing and counseling, and a lack of knowledge that screening can be performed without a pelvic examination. Strategies to change provider behavior include the use of computerized reminders, placement of Chlamydia collection swabs alongside Pap test collection materials, and the practice of performing routine Chlamydia screening with other laboratory testing (CDC, 2009d; Christiansen-Lindquist, Tao, Hoover, Frank, & Kent, 2009; Hackett, 2010).

Unlike viruses, the Chlamydia bacterium is susceptible to antibiotics. The recommended antibiotic options for treatment of *C. trachomatis* include doxycycline 100 mg orally twice a day for 7 days or azithromycin 1 gm orally, given in a single dose. Alternatives are ofloxacin 300 mg orally two times a day for 7 days or erythromycin ethylsuccinate 800 mg orally four times a day for 7 days. In general, the erythromycin-based regimens are inferior to the other medications and should be used as a second-line therapy (CDC, Workowski, & Berman, 2006b; CDC, 2009d; Marrazzo et al., 2007).

Gonorrhea

Gonorrhea is caused by the gram-negative intracellular diplococcal bacterium *Neisseria gonorrhoeae*. Approximately 650,000 new cases of gonorrhea occur each year, making it the second most commonly reported STD in the United States. Similar to Chlamydia, gonorrhea is prevalent in the adolescent population and disproportionately affects minority groups. The rate of gonorrheal infections in African American women is 18 times higher than in Caucasian women (CDC, 2006b; Marrazzo et al., 2007; Weber-LaShore & Biro, 2009).

 Nursing Insight— *The magnitude of Chlamydial and gonorrheal infections in young women*

In 2008, there were more than 1.5 million total cases of Chlamydia and gonorrhea reported to the CDC, making them the two most commonly reported infectious diseases in the United States. Adolescent girls and young women are especially hard hit by these two diseases. The largest number of reported cases of both Chlamydia and gonorrhea in 2008 was among girls between 15 and 19 years of age, followed closely by young women 20 to 24 years of age. Because patients with gonorrhea are often co-infected with Chlamydia, dual treatment may be indicated (CDC, 2009a; Weber-LaShore & Biro, 2009).

In men, symptoms usually consist of dysuria and penile discharge. Women, however, are commonly asymptomatic. When present, symptoms are frequently less specific than in males but may include abnormal vaginal discharge, irregular menses, postcoital bleeding, low backache, and urinary frequency and dysuria.

The USPSTF recommends annual screening of all sexually active women 25 years old and younger; the CDC supports these recommendations. Gonorrhea is most often tested through government screening programs (CDC, 2009a; USPSTF, 2005). Testing methods include culture, nucleic acid hybridization, and NAAT. Either cervical swab or urine can be used as the specimen for NAAT.

The recommended therapies for gonorrhea include cefixime 400 mg orally single dose or ceftriaxone 125 mg IM single dose. Other treatment options include the following three synthetic broad-spectrum antibiotics known as "quinolones": ciprofloxacin 500 mg orally single dose, ofloxacin 400 mg orally single dose, or levofloxacin 250 mg orally single dose. However, these medications should be avoided in persons who may have acquired their infection outside the United States or in California or Hawaii, where rates of quinolone resistance are considerable (CDC, 2006b; Marrazzo et al., 2007). Sex partners also require treatment. Health professionals should consult the CDC's Web site (http://www.cdc.gov/std/treatment) for frequent updates regarding treatment recommendations.

Optimizing Outcomes— With home screening for *C. trachomatis* and *N. gonorrhoeae*

Graseck, Secura, Allsworth, Madden, and Peipert (2010) recently conducted a study to compare the acceptability of home screening with clinic-based screening for two STDs (*C. trachomatis* and *N. gonorrhoeae*). In a telephone interview, women (ages 14–45 years) were given a choice of no-cost screening with vaginal swabs for self-collection mailed to their home (detailed instructions and a pre-addressed and stamped specimen mailer were included in the kit) or screening that was available without an appointment at area family planning clinics. The participants were much more likely to choose to screen for STDs at home than at a clinic or with their own medical provider. The researchers concluded that future interventions to increase screening rates in young women should consider alternative screening strategies such as home-based or patient-controlled testing.

Pelvic inflammatory disease (PID) develops in up to 40% of untreated women with cervical gonorrhea and may progress to a systemic infection. Patients with gonorrhea who have oral sex should be evaluated and treated for pharyngeal gonorrhea as necessary. Rectal testing for Chlamydia and gonorrhea may improve case-finding for both STDs; recent research (Barry, Kent, Philip, & Klausner, 2010) revealed that among women, rectal infections were as common as genital infections. Maternal transfer of both gonorrhea and Chlamydia may occur during childbirth, causing neonatal eye infection (ophthalmia neonatorum), scalp abscess at the site of fetal monitors, rhinitis, or anorectal infection (Marrazzo et al., 2007).

Trichomoniasis

Caused by the protozoan *Trichomonas vaginalis*, trichomoniasis is the most common curable STD in the United States. An estimated 5 million new cases occur in this country each year. Infection with trichomoniasis has been shown to increase the risk of HIV transmission. Although infection with *T. vaginalis* may be asymptomatic, it often produces a profuse frothy gray or yellow-green vaginal discharge with a foul odor. Erythema, edema, and pruritus of the external genitalia may be present, and the patient may report dysuria and dyspareunia. Upon examination, small red ulcerations in the vagina or on the cervix ("strawberry cervix") may be observed. The pH of the vaginal discharge is usually higher (more alkaline) than normal (CDC et al., 2006b; Marrazzo et al., 2007; Sorvillo, Smith, Kerndt, & Ash, 2001; Weber-LaShore & Biro, 2009).

Microscopic evaluation is used to confirm trichomoniasis. Microscopic examination of the vaginal secretions on a wet prep reveals the motile trichomonad parasites. *T. vaginalis* can also be detected by performing the rapid trichomoniasis test (results available in 10 minutes) or by performing the Affirm VP III test (results available in 45 minutes). The most sensitive and specific method of diagnosis of trichomoniasis is by performing a vaginal culture (CDC et al., 2006b; Weber-LaShore & Biro, 2009).

 ***Nursing Insight*—** *The vaginal wet mount*

A wet mount, also known as a "wet-prep" or "wet smear," is frequently used in the clinical setting to diagnose three of the most common vaginal infections: bacterial vaginosis, trichomoniasis, and yeast (candidiasis). To perform this test, the clinician inserts a speculum and uses a moist cotton swab to take a sample of the discharge from the posterior vaginal fornix. The discharge is then placed on a glass slide and viewed under a microscope. Alternately, a dry swab may be used: The sample is placed in 1 mL of saline, mixed, and placed on a slide, or a drop of saline is placed on a slide and the sample is added to it.

The slide may be warmed briefly (to increase motility of the trichomonads). A cover slip is then applied and the slide is promptly viewed.

Metronidazole (Flagyl), the medication of choice for trichomoniasis, is associated with a 95% cure rate. Metronidazole may be administered as a single dose—2 g orally—or 500 mg orally twice daily for 7 days. Alternately, tinidazole (Tindamax) 2 g orally single dose may be used, and this medication is recommended for the treatment of metronidazole-resistant *T. vaginalis* infections. Partners should be simultaneously treated, and patients should be counseled to use condoms to prevent future infections and to avoid drinking alcohol until 24 hours after completing metronidazole therapy and 72 hours

(3 days) after completing tinidazole therapy. Combining these medications with alcohol ingestion may produce a reaction characterized by flushing, nausea, vomiting, headache, and abdominal cramps (CDC et al., 2006b; Deglin & Vallerand, 2009; Marrazzo et al., 2007; Weber-LaShore & Biro, 2009).

 Now can you— **Discuss Chlamydia, gonorrhea, and trichomoniasis?**

1. Explain why infection with *Chlamydia trachomatis* poses such a danger to young women?
2. Identify the U.S. population that is at highest risk for infection with gonorrhea?
3. Describe patient education that should accompany metronidazole therapy?

Pelvic Inflammatory Disease (PID)

Pelvic inflammatory disease (PID) is an acute infection of the uterus and fallopian tubes, which, if left untreated or unresolved, results in scarring, adhesions, or blockage of the fallopian tubes. A number of different organisms (e.g., *Escherichia coli*, *Mycoplasma hominis*) are usually involved, but the most common causative agents are *Chlamydia trachomatis* (> 50%) and *Neisseria gonorrhoeae*. In the United States, PID accounts for nearly 180,000 hospitalizations every year, and 1 in 7 reproductive-aged American women reports having received treatment for PID. Since PID may be caused by many organisms and encompasses a wide spectrum of pathological processes, the infection may be acute, subacute, or chronic. The two greatest reproductive consequences of acute PID are infertility and tubal pregnancy resulting from scarring of the fallopian tubes (Marrazzo et al., 2007).

 Nursing Insight— *Recognizing risk factors for pelvic inflammatory disease*

When taking a sexual history, nurses should be aware of certain factors—such as a history of multiple sexual partners, a new partner in the last 6 months, lower age at first intercourse, and lower economic status—that place women at increased risk for PID. Age constitutes another risk factor: Adolescents have the highest incidence of PID of any age group, and 70% of all cases of PID occur in women under age 25. Women who use intrauterine devices (IUDs) are also at increased risk if they have more than one sexual partner or if their partner has other sexual partners, because they are at higher risk for an STD (Marrazzo et al., 2007).

Symptoms of PID can range from none to severe abdominal, uterine, and ovarian pain and tenderness; abnormal bleeding; nausea; and vomiting. The infected individual may also experience extreme tenderness when the cervix is moved on examination ("cervical motion tenderness"; the "chandelier sign"). Fever, chills, and an elevated white blood cell (WBC) count and erythrocyte sedimentation rate (ESR) may also be present.

PID can be treated on an outpatient basis, but hospitalization may be necessary, depending on the individual case. For patients treated on an outpatient basis,

reexamination within 48 to 72 hours is a crucial part of therapy. Combined drug therapy is advised, especially at the initiation of treatment, because the full spectrum of all organisms involved is often unknown. The CDC provides specific guidelines for PID treatment (http://www.cdc.gov/std/treatment/2006/pid.htm). Also, a PID Teaching Module for physicians, advanced practice nurses, and physician assistants is available at http://www2a.cdc.gov/STDTraining/Ready-To-Use/Manuals/PID/pid-notes-2009.pdf.

Human Papillomavirus (HPV)

Human papillomavirus (HPV), which causes genital warts (also called condylomata acuminata), is a DNA virus transmitted by skin-to-skin contact. There are more than 100 viral types currently identified, and of these, more than 30 types can infect the genital area. Approximately one-half of all HPV genital infections occur in young women and men between the ages of 15 and 24 years. The majority of HPV infections are asymptomatic, unrecognized, or subclinical. Genital HPV infection can cause warty growths in the vagina or on the vulva, perineum, or anal area. The growths can be single or multiple, and they are soft and fleshy and usually painless. Other strains of HPV infect the cervix and remain unnoticed until findings from a routine Pap smear reveal the presence of the virus. Certain viral types are associated with the growth of abnormal cervical cells, which can lead to cancer of the cervix (CDC et al., 2006b; Mayeaux, 2007; Schmidt, 2007).

 Optimizing Outcomes— **HPV prevention and testing**

Strategies for prevention of HPV include sexual abstinence, confining sexual intimacy to a long-term monogamous relationship, and prophylactic vaccination. A vaccine against HPV types 6, 11, 16, and 18 first became available in 2006 and is recommended for all females, ages 9 to 26 years (Advisory Committee on Immunization Practices, 2009; ACOG, 2006). Although testing is available based on HPV-DNA in cervical cells, routine screening is not recommended except in specific circumstances following an abnormal Pap test (CDC et al., 2006b; Nelson, 2007).

Several topical chemical agents are available for the treatment of external genital warts. These include trichloroacetic acid (TCA) and podophyllin (provider administered) and podofilox 0.5% (Condylox) and imiquimod (Aldara), both of which are patient administered. Cryotherapy (freezing), CO_2 laser surgery, electrosurgery, and surgical removal are other treatment options, depending on the severity of the lesions and resistance to treatment (CDC et al., 2006b; Marrazzo et al., 2007).

When clinician-administered agents are used, the nurse should stress the importance of returning for regular treatment until the lesions have resolved. Once the warts have responded to therapy, no special follow-up is necessary. Owing to the risk of sequelae from cervical cancer, regular Pap smears are crucial for all women with documented HIV infection. Nurses should also encourage tobacco cessation to reduce the risk of HPV and neoplasia (Marrazzo et al., 2007).

Herpes Simplex Virus (HSV) 1 and 2

Herpes simplex virus 1 and 2 (HSV-1 and HSV-2), also known as human herpes virus 1 and 2 (HHV-1 and HHV-2), are members of the herpes virus family *Herpesviridae* that infect humans. Both HSV-1 and HSV-2 are transmitted horizontally during close contact with an infected person who is shedding virus from the skin, often in saliva or in genital secretions. Although transmission occurs most often when lesions are present, viral shedding and transmission can also occur in the absence of visible sores. HSV-1 is usually transmitted during childhood via nonsexual contacts. It is most commonly associated with cold sores or fever blisters on the mouth or face. Genital HSV-1 may result from oral–genital sexual contact with a person infected with oral HSV-1. Genital HSV-1 is unlikely to recur, and treatment may only be needed in persons with initial symptoms (Xu et al., 2006).

HSV-2 is primarily a sexually transmitted disease. HSV-2 is associated with genital lesions, although, depending on sexual practices, HSV-1 and HSV-2 are not exclusively associated with the respective sites. HSV-2 occurs more frequently in women than in men, which most likely results from the greater incidence of male-to-female transmission. HSV-infection rates are significantly higher among African Americans (46%) than among Caucasians (18%). Although HSV infection is not a reportable disease, it is estimated that 50 million Americans are infected with genital herpes (CDC et al., 2006b; Winer & Richwald, 2007).

Most infected persons have no or only minimal signs or symptoms from HSV-1 or HSV-2 infection. If symptoms develop during the first HSV-2 outbreak, they usually appear within 2 weeks after exposure and can be very pronounced. Owing to the fact that the body has not had an opportunity to develop antibodies, symptoms that result from a primary HSV infection are usually much more severe than with subsequent outbreaks (CDC et al., 2006b; Gardner, 2006).

 ### Nursing Insight— *Recognizing signs and symptoms of HSV infection*

Symptoms of HSV-2 infection are similar to those that occur with the flu—malaise, muscle aches, and headache. Other symptoms include dysuria and the development of multiple fluid-filled, blister-like lesions, which can be extremely tender and persist for 2 to 3 weeks (Fig. 5-2). Before the appearance of the lesions, the patient may experience a period of prodromal symptoms characterized by skin sensitivity and nerve pain in the area where the lesions will appear. Reddening of the skin frequently follows these symptoms. The lesions form pustules and ulcers that dry up, crust over, and then heal without scarring. The woman may also experience itching, inguinal tenderness, vulvar edema, and a heavy watery or purulent vaginal discharge. In some instances, women with "chronic yeast infections" are actually experiencing herpes outbreaks that go undiagnosed because the typical herpetic lesions are not present (CDC et al., 2006b; Gardner, 2006).

Typically, recurrent outbreaks are less severe than the primary infection and usually involve localized symptoms with less severe lesions that last 5 to 7 days. The prodromal characteristic genital tingling sensation is common

Figure 5-2 Herpes Vulvovaginitis

with recurrence. The virus then enters a latent stage in the nerves at the base of the spine, only to reactivate when the patient's immune system is weakened. The lesions may occur along any skin surface supplied by that particular distribution (e.g., vulva, vagina, cervix, urethral meatus, buttocks). Because transmission of the virus is most likely during an active outbreak, patients should abstain from sexual contact during this time. However, viral transmission may occur at any time when the infected individual is producing and releasing ("shedding") the virus, and some individuals shed virus between active outbreaks (Gardner, 2006).

In most situations, a diagnosis of HSV is suspected based on the patient history and physical examination. HSV can be confirmed by obtaining a viral culture from the exudate swabbed from the vesicular (blister) lesion. Testing for the presence of HSV-2 antibodies in capillary blood or serum (i.e., HSV glycoprotein G-specific antibodies, IgG by immunoblot [HerpeSelect]) is also available for clinical use. However, screening of the general population is not indicated (CDC et al., 2006b; Nelson, 2007).

The goal of treatment for herpes is to hasten healing and reduce symptoms. Several oral antiviral medications (e.g., acyclovir [Zovirax], valacyclovir [Valtrex], famciclovir (Famvir]) are available and may be used for primary or recurrent episodes or as daily suppressive therapy. The medications do not eradicate the infection, nor do they alter subsequent risk, frequency, or recurrences once the medication has been stopped. When indicated, acyclovir may be administered intravenously for 5 to 7 days for severe symptoms (CDC et al., 2006b; Nelson, 2007).

 ### Optimizing Outcomes— **Teaching women about HSV infection**

Providing counseling and education are essential components of holistic care for women with herpes infections. Nurses should offer information about the etiology, signs, symptoms, modes of transmission, treatment options, and the possibility of suppression therapy to prevent partner transmission. It is important to advise women about the times when transmission is most likely and the need to avoid sexual contact beginning with the onset of prodromal symptoms until all lesions have healed. Some experts recommend the consistent use of condoms for all individuals with genital herpes. Nurses can help women explore potential precipitating factors in the reactivation of the latent herpes virus. Triggers may include stress, menstruation, febrile illnesses, chronic illnesses, and ultraviolet light. Some patients find that keeping a personal diary provides insights about precipitating events for their herpetic outbreaks.

 Complementary Care— *Measures to reduce HSV discomforts and outbreaks*

For many women, certain comfort measures and dietary changes are useful in decreasing HSV symptoms and the frequency and severity of HSV outbreaks. Comfort measures may include warm sitz baths with baking soda or oatmeal, the use of cotton underwear, the use of a hair dryer (on the cool setting) to enhance drying of the lesions, the application of compresses containing peppermint oil and clove oil to the lesions, and the application of cool, wet, black tea bags or tea tree oil applied to the lesions. Oral analgesics including aspirin or ibuprofen may help relieve pain. Dietary strategies center on consumption of a diet rich in vitamin C, B-complex vitamins, zinc, and calcium and the daily use of kelp powder and sunflower seed oil as well as the amino acid l-lysine, which is thought to suppress the herpes simplex virus (Gardner, 2006; Stonehouse & Studdiford, 2007).

Syphilis

One of the oldest known sexually transmitted diseases, syphilis is caused by the spirochetal bacterium *Treponema pallidum*. It is believed that the organism is transmitted through microscopic abrasions that can occur during sexual intercourse. Kissing, biting, and oral–genital sex may also be modes of transmission. Congenital syphilis occurs via maternal–fetal transmission. Syphilis cannot be contracted through toilet seats, daily activities, hot tubs, or sharing eating utensils or clothing. Left untreated, syphilis can cause severe systemic disease and death. In 2008, there were 13,500 reported cases of primary and secondary syphilis, and this figure represents the highest number of cases since 1995 and an increase over 2007, when there were 11,466 reported cases. Less than a decade ago, syphilis was on the verge of elimination. However, syphilis reemerged as a public health threat in 2001, and rates of infection have steadily increased since then (CDC, 2009a).

Although the majority of reported syphilis cases in the United States occur among men who have sex with men, rates among women have increased each year since 2004. In 2008, the syphilis rate among women increased 36% from the previous year (1.1 cases per 100,000 females in 2007, as compared with 1.5 cases in 2008). The syphilis rate among African American women increased to 7.6 cases per 100,000 in 2008, up from 5.5 reported cases in 2007. Also, the rate of reported syphilis cases among Hispanics (4.7 per 100,000) was double that of Caucasian (2.2 per 100,000) (CDC, 2009a).

 Optimizing Outcomes— **Through targeted syphilis screening efforts**

The CDC (2009a) and the USPSTF (2009) recommend that persons at increased risk for syphilis infection (i.e., all men who have sex with men) be tested at least annually for syphilis and that all pregnant women be screened for syphilis at the first prenatal visit to avoid transmission to their infants.

Syphilis is a complex disease with several stages. Different manifestations occur depending on the stage of the disease. In the primary stage, approximately 10 to 90 days after the initial exposure, a painless ulcer (chancre) appears at the point of contact, which is usually the genitalia. Lymphadenopathy may also be present. The lesion may persist for 4 to 6 weeks and usually resolves on its own without treatment (CDC, 2009a).

Secondary syphilis occurs 6 weeks to 6 months after the appearance of the chancre. During this stage, patients may have fever, a sore throat, weight loss, skin rash on the trunk and extremities (Fig. 5-3), headache, generalized malaise, mucous patches on the genitals or in the mouth, lymphadenopathy, alopecia, and the appearance of moist, flat warts in the genital and anal areas (condylomata lata). If left untreated, the symptoms resolve within 2 to 10 weeks. Approximately one-third of infected individuals will then develop tertiary syphilis (CDC, 2009a; Marrazzo et al., 2007).

Tertiary syphilis usually occurs 1 to 10 years after the initial infection, although in some cases systemic symptoms may not appear until 30 to 50 years later. This stage is characterized by the formation of gummas (soft, tumorlike

Figure 5-3 Secondary Syphilitic Rash on Chest and Palms

balls of inflammation). Other manifestations of tertiary syphilis include neuropathic joint disease (degeneration of joint surfaces), neurosyphilis, and cardiovascular syphilis. It is estimated that approximately 20% to 30% of untreated individuals with syphilis develop tertiary syphilis (CDC, 2009a).

 Nursing Insight— *Understanding the entity termed "latent syphilis"*

Latent syphilis is defined as having serological proof of infection without signs or symptoms of the disease. Latent syphilis may be "early" or "late." By definition, early latent syphilis is having the infection for greater than 2 years but without clinical evidence of the disease. This stage is treated with a single intramuscular injection of a long-acting penicillin. Late latent syphilis requires 3 weekly intramuscular injections of a long-acting penicillin (CDC, 2009a).

Effective tests and treatments for syphilis were developed during the 20th century. Microscopy of fluid from the primary or secondary lesion using darkfield illumination is highly accurate in detecting *T. pallidum*. Screening tests include the Rapid Plasma Reagin (RPR) and Venereal Disease Research Laboratory (VDRL). When positive, the tests should be followed up by a more specific treponemal test. Tests based on monoclonal antibodies and immunofluorescence, including treponema pallidum hemagglutination assay (TPHA) and fluorescent treponemal antibody absorption (FTA-ABS) are more specific tests. Tests based on ELISAs are also used to confirm results of the simpler screening tests for syphilis. Neurosyphilis is diagnosed via analysis of the cerebrospinal fluid. Because there is some evidence that the incidence of neurosyphilis is higher in HIV patients, some experts recommend that all HIV-positive individuals have a lumbar puncture to assess for asymptomatic neurosyphilis (CDC, 2009a).

Penicillin, in the form of penicillin G, is the treatment of choice for syphilis, and the specific regimen and duration depends on the length of infection. Doxycycline and tetracycline may be used as alternative treatments for individuals who are allergic to penicillin (CDC, 2009a). For the most current treatment guidelines, health professionals may visit the CDC Web site at http://www.cdc.gov/mmwr/preview/mmwrhtml/rr5511a1.htm.

 Be sure to— **Teach patients about the possibility of a Jarisch-Herxheimer reaction**

The Jarisch-Herxheimer reaction occurs when large quantities of toxins are released into the body as bacteria, typically spirochetal bacteria, die during treatment with antibiotics. Death of the bacteria and the associated release of endotoxins occur more quickly than the liver and kidneys can remove the toxins. Fever, chills, headache, myalgia, and exacerbation of skin lesions are the hallmarks of this acute reaction. In syphilis, the duration is usually only a few hours but can persist for much longer with other diseases. Treatment, aimed at reducing symptoms, centers on the use of analgesics and antipyretics.

 Now Can You— **Discuss PID, HPV, HSV, and syphilis?**

1. Identify six risk factors for PID?
2. Describe strategies for HPV prevention?
3. Discuss the nurse's role in teaching women about HSV infection?
4. Differentiate among the primary, secondary, and tertiary stages of syphilis?

Hepatitis

Hepatitis is the leading cause of liver cancer and the most common reason for liver transplantation. In the United States, an estimated 1.2 million individuals are living with chronic hepatitis B virus (HBV) and 3.2 million persons are living with chronic hepatitis C virus (HCV). Many are unaware that they are infected. Each year, an estimated 25,000 persons become infected with the hepatitis A virus (HAV), 43,000 with hepatitis B, and 17,000 with hepatitis C (CDC, 2010).

 Nursing Insight— *Hepatitis A virus*

Formerly known as "infectious hepatitis," hepatitis A is an acute infectious disease of the liver caused by HAV. Every year, approximately 10 million people worldwide are infected with the virus, and the incidence of infection is highest in developing countries and in regions with poor hygiene standards. HAV causes no clinical signs and symptoms in over 90% of infected children, and since the infection confers lifelong immunity, the disease is of no special significance to the indigenous population. In the United States, HAV is primarily contracted by susceptible young adults, the majority of whom are infected with the virus during trips to countries with a high incidence of the disease. There is no specific treatment for HAV. Hepatitis A can be prevented by vaccination, good hygiene, and sanitation (Connor, 2005; Ryan & Ray, 2005; Steffen, 2005; Thiel, 1998).

HEPATITIS B VIRUS (HBV)

In 2007, an estimated 43,000 persons in the United States were newly infected with HBV. The highest incidence of HBV occurs in persons aged 20 to 49 years, and the virus is 50 to 100 times more contagious than HIV. It causes liver disease and can be fatal. Each year, approximately 6,000 Americans die from complications resulting from HBV infection (CDC, 2009e).

Hepatitis B virus is a species of the genus *Orthohepadnavirus*, which is a part of the *Hepadnaviridae* family of viruses. This virus causes the disease hepatitis B. The incubation period from the time of exposure to the onset of symptoms is 6 weeks to 6 months. HBV is found in highest concentrations in blood and in lower concentrations in other body fluids such as semen, vaginal secretions, and wound exudates. Although heterosexual intercourse is the predominant mode of transmission, HBV may also be spread through blood-to-blood contact. Blood-to-blood contact can occur through the sharing of razors, toothbrushes, and manicure tools, as well as through contaminated instruments used for dental procedures, tattooing, and body piercing. Vertical transmission occurs when a pregnant woman passes the virus to her fetus. HBV is not spread through food or water, sharing eating utensils, breastfeeding, hugging, kissing, hand holding, coughing, or sneezing (CDC, 2009e; Holloway & D'Acunto, 2006).

 Optimizing Outcomes— Identifying populations at increased risk for HBV

Nurses should be aware of certain factors that place men, women, children, and intimate partners at increased risk for HBV. Taking a detailed patient history can help nurses to identify these individuals, who include (CDC 2009e):

- Infants born to infected mothers
- Sex partners of infected persons
- Sexually active persons who are not in a long-term (> 6 months) mutually monogamous relationship
- Men who have sex with men
- Injection drug users
- Household contacts of persons with chronic HBV infection
- Health-care and public safety workers at risk for occupational exposure to blood or blood-contaminated body fluids
- Hemodialysis patients
- Residents and staff of facilities for developmentally disabled persons
- Travelers to countries with intermediate or high prevalence of HBV infection

Signs and symptoms of infection with HBV are often absent, especially in children under age 5 years and in newly infected immunosuppressed adults. However, it is estimated that up to 50% of persons older than 5 years have initial signs and symptoms of the infection, such as fever, fatigue, loss of appetite, nausea, vomiting, abdominal pain, dark-colored urine, clay-colored stools, joint pain, and jaundice. On average, symptoms appear from 60 to 150 days after exposure to HBV and last for several weeks (CDC, 2009e).

 Nursing Insight— *Acute and chronic HBV infection*

Acute HBV infection ranges from asymptomatic or mild disease to fulminate hepatitis (rare). The disease is more severe among older adults (> 60 years). The risk for chronic infection varies according to the age at infection and is greatest among young children: Approximately 90% of infants and 25% to 50% of children (ages 1–5 years) will remain chronically infected with HBV. The vast majority (> 95%) of adults with HBV infection recover completely and do not become chronically infected. Approximately 25% of those who become chronically infected during childhood and 15% of those who become chronically infected after childhood die prematurely from cirrhosis or liver cancer, and the majority remain asymptomatic until the onset of cirrhosis or end-stage liver disease. In the United States, chronic HBV infection results in an estimated 2,000 to 4,000 deaths each year (CDC, 2009e).

Individuals at high risk for contracting HBV should be screened on a regular basis. The USPSTF (2004) recommends that all women should be screened for HBV at the first prenatal visit, regardless of whether they have been tested previously, and screening should be repeated later in the pregnancy for women with high-risk behaviors. No routine screening is recommended for the general population. Testing for HBV is complex. There are a number of different markers identified in a blood test, some of which indicate active infection, chronic carrier state, or past infection (American Academy of Pediatrics & ACOG, 2007; CDC, 2009e; USPSTF, 2004).

 Optimizing Outcomes— With vaccines for hepatitis B prevention

Two single-antigen vaccines (Engerix-B and Recombivax HB) and three combination vaccines are licensed in the United States. The combination vaccines include the following: Comvax (combined hepatitis B-*Haemophilus influenzae* type b [Hib])—cannot be administered before age 6 weeks or after age 71 months); Pediarix (combined hepatitis B, diphtheria, tetanus, acellular pertussis [DtaP], and inactivated poliovirus [IPV] vaccine)—cannot be administered before age 6 weeks or after age 7 years; and Twinrix (combined hepatitis A and hepatitis B vaccine—recommended for persons age 18+ years who are at risk for both HAV and HBV). The vaccination schedule most often used for children and adults is three intramuscular injections; the second and third doses administered 1 and 6 months after the first dose. After a person has been exposed to HBV, appropriate prophylaxis (i.e., hepatitis B vaccine), given as soon as possible but preferably within 24 hours, can effectively prevent infection. Although persons who have already been infected with HBV will receive no benefit from vaccination, there is no risk to a previously infected person who receives the vaccination (CDC, 2009e).

The CDC (2009e) Advisory Committee on Immunization Practices has published recommendations for hepatitis B vaccination. At-risk individuals who should receive HBV vaccination are presented in Box 5-2. The Advisory Committee has also determined that adults who receive care in health-care, evaluation, and treatment settings should also receive HBV vaccination. Specific settings are presented in Box 5-3.

There is no specific therapy for acute hepatitis B infection; treatment is supportive. Several antiviral drugs (adefovir dipivoxil [Preveon, Hepsera], interferon alfa-2b [Peg-Intron], pegylated interferon alpha 2-a [Pegasys], lamivudine [Epivir], entecavir [Baraclude], telbivudine [Tyzeka]) are used for treatment of chronic infection. Individuals with chronic HBV infection require medical evaluation and regular monitoring to determine whether the disease is progressing and to identify liver damage or hepatocellular carcinoma (cancer of the liver) (CDC, 2009e).

HEPATITIS C VIRUS (HCV)

Largely unknown to the American public, hepatitis C virus (HCV) infection is the most common chronic bloodborne infection in the United States. According to the CDC (2009f), approximately 3.2 million persons are chronically infected. Previously known as "non-A, non-B hepatitis," up to 85% of individuals infected with HCV will progress to chronic viral hepatitis.

Box 5-2 Individuals Who Should Be Vaccinated Against Hepatitis B

- All infants, beginning at birth
- All children aged <19 years who have not been vaccinated previously
- Susceptible sex partners of hepatitis B surface antigen (HbsAg)–positive persons
- Sexually active persons who are not in a long-term, mutually monogamous relationship (e.g., >1 sex partner during the previous 6 months)
- Persons seeking evaluation or treatment for an STD
- Men who have sex with men
- Injection drug users
- Susceptible household contacts of HbsAg-positive persons
- Health-care and public safety workers at risk for exposure to blood or blood-contaminated body fluids
- Persons with end-stage renal disease, including predialysis, hemodialysis, peritoneal dialysis, and home dialysis patients
- Residents and staff of facilities for developmentally disabled persons
- Travelers to regions with intermediate or high rates of endemic HBV infection
- Persons with chronic liver disease
- Persons with HIV infection
- All other persons seeking protection from HBV infection—acknowledgment of a specific risk factor is not a requirement for vaccination

Source: CDC, 2009e.

Box 5-3 Settings Where Hepatitis B Vaccination Should Be Administered to All Adults Who Receive Care

- STD treatment facilities
- HIV testing and treatment facilities
- Facilities providing drug-abuse treatment and prevention services
- Health-care settings targeting services to injection drug users
- Correctional facilities
- Health-care settings targeting services to men who have sex with men
- Chronic hemodialysis facilities and end-stage renal disease programs
- Institutions and nonresidential day-care facilities for developmentally disabled persons

Source: CDC, 2009e.

HCV is primarily spread through blood-to-blood contact and less efficiently through semen, saliva, or urine. As with HBV, transmission of HCV can potentially occur through blood contact with shared needles, razors, and toothbrushes. Persons at risk for HCV include those with STDs such as hepatitis B and HIV and those with multiple sex partners, a history of blood transfusions, or a history of IV drug use. Currently, no vaccine for HCV infection is available (CDC, 2009f).

Newly acquired HCV infection is often asymptomatic. When symptoms occur, however, they may include fever, fatigue, dark-colored urine, clay-colored stools, abdominal pain, anorexia, nausea, vomiting, joint pain, and jaundice. Approximately 20% to 30% of individuals newly infected with HCV experience fatigue, abdominal pain, poor appetite, or jaundice. The average time period from exposure to symptom onset (if any) is 4 to 12 weeks (CDC, 2009f).

 Nursing Insight— Progression of acute HCV infection to chronic HCV infection to death

Of every 100 persons infected with HCV, approximately 75 to 85 will develop chronic infection; 60 to 70 will develop chronic liver disease; 5 to 20 will develop cirrhosis over a period of 20 to 30 years; and 1 to 5 will die from the consequences of chronic infection (e.g., liver cancer or cirrhosis). Chronic HCV infection, the leading indication for liver transplantation in this country, accounts for an estimated 8,000 to 10,000 deaths in the United States each year (CDC, 2009f).

According to the CDC (2009f), certain individuals and populations should be tested for HCV infection (Box 5-4). Blood tests that may be performed to test for HCV infection include screening tests for antibody to HCV (e.g., EIA, enhanced chemiluminescence immunoassay [CIA]), recombinant immunoblot assay [RIBA]), qualitative tests to detect presence or absence of the virus, and quantitative tests to detect the amount of virus. The CDC provides a table on interpretation of HCV test results for health professionals, available at http://www.cdc.gov/hepatitis/HCV/PDFs/hcv_graph.pdf.

Following diagnosis, HCV-infected patients should be evaluated for the presence of chronic liver disease and determination of the need for hepatitis B vaccination. Combination therapy with pegylated interferon and ribavirin is the treatment of choice for individuals with chronic hepatitis C. According to the CDC (2009f), success rates are improved with the addition of polymerase and protease inhibitors to standard pegylated interferon/ribavirin combination therapy.

 Optimizing Outcomes— With holistic nursing care for women with chronic hepatitis

Nurses can empower women with chronic hepatitis infection by providing education and counseling about strategies to optimize health, reduce the transmission of infection, and communicate concerns with intimate sexual partners. Referrals to local resources such as professional

Box 5-4 Testing for HCV Infection

The CDC (2009f) recommends that the following individuals are at increased risk for HCV infection and should undergo testing:

- Persons who have ever injected illegal drugs, including those who injected only once many years ago
- Recipients of clotting factor concentrates made before 1987
- Recipients of blood transfusions or solid organ transplants before July 1992
- Patients who have ever received long-term hemodialysis treatment
- Persons with known exposures to HCV (e.g., health-care workers after needle sticks involving HCV-positive blood, recipients of blood or organs from a donor who later tested HCV-positive)
- All persons with HIV infection
- Patients with signs or symptoms of liver disease (e.g., abnormal liver enzyme tests)
- Children born to HCV-positive mothers (to avoid detecting maternal antibody, testing should not be performed prior to 18 months of age)

counselors and peer support groups may also be of benefit. Nurses can teach women about the importance of maintaining a high level of personal hygiene with measures such as performing strict hand washing after toileting and ensuring the careful disposal of all tampons, sanitary pads, and bandages. Patients can also be taught to avoid sharing razor blades, toothbrushes, needles, and manicure implements and to promptly clean blood spills with soap and water. Non-HBV-vaccinated male sexual partners should consistently use latex condoms. Nutritional strategies may include the consumption of a low-protein, low-fat diet; avoidance of protein or amino acid supplements; the use of an antioxidant formula vitamin supplement; and the avoidance of alcohol and tobacco. Patients are also advised to avoid medications that are hepatotoxic (e.g., Tylenol) (Holloway & D'Acunto, 2006).

HEPATITIS D VIRUS (HDV)

Hepatitis D virus (HDV) is a single-stranded circular RNA molecule with some double-stranded attachments. HDV infection can only occur in a person already infected with HBV; a person can be infected by HBV and HDV simultaneously or by HBV first. Infection with HDV is clinically indistinguishable from other forms of hepatitis. After exposure, the incubation period is 21 to 45 days. Up to 90% of cases of HDV are asymptomatic, but when present, symptoms include jaundice, fatigue, abdominal pain, confusion, pruritus, anorexia, nausea, vomiting, and joint pain (Kellogg-Spadt, 2009).

Serum testing is complex and includes assays for serum HDAg, serum HDV RNA, anti-HDV antibody, and tissue markers for HDV infection. Transmission of HDV occurs through body fluids, including blood, semen, vaginal fluids, and saliva. Perinatal transmission is rare. Nurses can teach women to reduce their risk of contracting HDV through the avoidance of illicit IV drugs and the consistent practice of safer-sex strategies (e.g., latex condoms during vaginal, anal, and oral sex). Women may also wish to consider vaccination against hepatitis B (Kellogg-Spadt, 2009).

Now Can You— Discuss aspects of viral hepatitis?

1. Identify populations at greatest risk for infection with HBV?
2. Identify seven settings where hepatitis B vaccination should be administered to adults who receive care?
3. Explain how the hepatitis virus may be transmitted?

Chancroid, Lymphogranuloma Venereum, Granuloma Inguinale, and Pthirus Pubis (Pubic Louse)

Although they occur less commonly, STDs including chancroid, lymphogranuloma venereum, granuloma inguinale, and pubic lice may be identified in the clinical setting.

CHANCROID

Caused by the gram-negative streptobacillus *Haemophilus ducreyi*, infection with chancroid begins with a small bump (usually on the labia majora) that quickly develops into a painful ulcer with a base that is covered with a gray or yellow-gray material. Symptoms include dysuria and dyspareunia. Inguinal adenopathy is present in approximately one-third of infected individuals. The diagnosis is made via special culture media. Treatment consists of a single oral dose (1 g) of azithromycin (Zithromax), a single intramuscular dose (250 mg) of ceftriaxone (Rocephin), oral ciprofloxacin (Cipro) (500 mg bid) for 3 days, or oral erythromycin (E-Mycin, E.E.S.) (500 mg tid) for 7 days (CDC et al., 2006b).

LYMPHOGRANULOMA VENEREUM

Lymphogranuloma venereum (LGV) is caused by the bacterium *Chlamydia trachomatis*. Primarily an infection of the lymphatics and lymph nodes, LGV gains entrance through breaks in the skin or via the mucous membranes. The primary infection produces a self-limited, painless genital ulcer at the contact site approximately 3 to 12 days after exposure. Owing to its hidden location, women frequently are unaware of its presence. The second stage, which usually occurs from 10 to 30 days later, involves the lymph nodes and lymphatic drainage pathways. Localized symptoms include cervicitis, perimetritis, salpingitis, and lymphadenitis; systemic symptoms include fever, decreased appetite, and malaise. The diagnosis is based on clinical suspicion, epidemiological information, and the exclusion of other causes, along with *C. trachomatis* testing. Serological testing is also available. LGV is treated with doxycycline (Vibramycin) 100 mg orally bid for 21 days or erythromycin base (E-base, Robimycin) 500 mg orally qid for 21 days (CDC et al., 2006b).

GRANULOMA INGUINALE

Granuloma inguinale (also known as "donovanosis") is a genital ulcerative disease caused by the intracellular gram-negative bacterium *Klebsiella granulomatis*. The disease commonly produces painless, progressive, beefy-red ulcerative lesions; regional lymphadenopathy is absent. The lesions most commonly occur on the labia or perineum. The diagnosis is made based on the patient's sexual history, absence of inguinal lymphadenopathy, and identification of the lesions. Tissue biopsy may be used to aid in diagnosis. Granuloma inguinale is treated with doxycycline (Vibramycin) 100 mg orally bid for at least 3 weeks and until all lesions have completely healed. Alternative regimens include azithromycin (Zithromax) (1 g orally once per week × 3 weeks, ciprofloxacin (Cipro) (750 mg orally bid × 3 weeks) or trimethoprim-sulfamethoxazole (Bactrim) (one double-strength [160 mg/800 mg] tablet orally bid × 3 weeks) (CDC et al., 2006b).

PTHIRUS PUBIS

Lice are parasitic insects that can be found on the head and body, including the pubic area. Human lice survive by feeding on human blood. Lice infestations are primarily spread by close person-to-person contact. Lice move by crawling—they are unable to hop or fly. The Pthirus pubis (pubic louse, "crab" louse) is very short (1.1 to 1.8 mm in length) and crablike in appearance (Fig. 5-4). Pubic lice are typically found attached to hair in the pubic area but can sometimes be found on coarse hair in the eyebrows, eyelashes, beard, mustache, chest, or armpits. Pubic lice are usually spread through sexual contact and are most common in adults. Although they do not transmit disease, secondary bacterial infection can occur from scratching of the skin. Pubic lice and nits (eggs) may be large enough to be seen with the naked eye, although a magnifying lens may be necessary to find them (CDC, 2008b).

🅢 Optimizing Outcomes— Through prevention and control of pubic lice

The nurse counsels infected women about strategies to help prevent and control the spread of pubic lice. Patients are taught to (CDC, 2008b):

- Ensure that all sexual contacts are examined and all infested persons are treated.
- Avoid sexual contact until treatment and reevaluation have been completed.
- Machine wash all clothing and bedding in hot (at least 130°F) water and machine dry on the high heat drying cycle. Clothing and items that are not washable can be dry-cleaned or sealed in a plastic bag and stored for 2 weeks.
- Avoid the sharing of clothing, bedding, and towels.
- Avoid the use of fumigant sprays or fogs—these products can be toxic if inhaled or absorbed through the skin.

A lice-killing lotion containing 1% permethrin or a mousse containing pyrethrins and piperonyl butoxide can be used to treat pubic lice. These products are readily available over-the-counter without a prescription at a local drugstore. When used exactly according to the instructions listed on the package, these medications are safe and effective (CDC, 2008b).

The Nurse's Role in Fostering Reproductive Health Through STD Education and Counseling

When educating women about STDs, nurses should include basic information along with sexual decision-making skills. When dealing with adolescents, it is often helpful to discuss basic communication skills needed to negotiate in a relationship and how to operate from an internal value system rather than submit to peer pressure. Educating women about the workings of their bodies and encouraging them to be active participants in their own

health care enhances their personal control over their reproductive health. Nurses can empower women of all ages by providing them with specific strategies for making safe choices in their intimate relationships. When appropriate, teaching about strategies for "safer sex" provides guidance and serves to foster wellness and promote reproductive health (Box 5-5). During STD counseling, the nurse can emphasize that condoms offer the best protection against the transmission of disease and stress that intimate sexual contact should be avoided if the person or partner has any sore areas or visible lesions (Marrazzo et al., 2007).

During private counseling sessions, it is important to inquire about substance use and other high-risk behaviors that may increase the likelihood of exposure to an STD.

Box 5-5 Safer Sex Strategies for Sexual Intimacy and HIV and STD Prevention

STRATEGIES CONSIDERED TO BE SAFE

- Sexual fantasies
- Massage
- Hugging
- Body rubbing
- Dry kissing
- Masturbation without contact with the partner's semen or vaginal secretions
- Erotic conversation, books, movies, videos, or DVDs
- Eroticizing feet, fingers, buttocks, abdomen, ears, or other body parts
- All sexual activities when both partners are monogamous and known by testing to be free of HIV and other STDs

STRATEGIES WITH A LOW RISK, CONSIDERED TO BE POSSIBLY SAFE

- Wet kissing with no broken skin, cracked lips, or damaged mouth tissue
- Hand-to-genital touching or mutual masturbation
- Vaginal or anal intercourse using latex or plastic condom
- Oral sex on a woman using a latex or plastic barrier, such as a female condom, dental dam, or modified male condom (especially if the woman does not have a vaginal infection with discharge and is not menstruating)
- Oral sex on a man using a latex or plastic condom
- All sexual activities, when both partners agree to a monogamous relationship and trust each other

STRATEGIES CONSIDERED UNSAFE IN THE ABSENCE OF HIV TESTING AND TRUST AND MONOGAMY

- Blood contact of any kind, including menstrual blood
- Any vaginal or anal intercourse without a latex or plastic condom
- Oral sex on a woman without a latex or plastic barrier, such as a female condom, dental dam, or modified male condom, especially if she has a vaginal infection with discharge or is menstruating
- Semen in the mouth
- Oral–anal contact
- Sharing sex toys or douching equipment
- Any sex that causes tissue damage or bleeding (e.g., rough vaginal or anal intercourse, rape, fisting)

Source: Marrazzo et al., 2007.

Figure 5-4 Pubic Louse

A woman who drinks heavily or who practices binge drinking may not remember the details of sexual encounters that took place while intoxicated. A history of injected drug use increases the risk for infection with hepatitis and HIV; women who smoke have a higher rate of cervical cancer (Marrazzo et al., 2007; Ravin, 2007).

 ### Nursing Insight— *Contraceptive choice and safer sex*

Nurses should recognize that women who use nonbarrier contraceptive methods (e.g., oral contraceptive pills [OCPs], IUDs, subdermal hormonal implants) usually choose these methods for the freedom involved. Thus it is important to inform oral contraceptive users that the "pill" may cause changes in the cervix and in the immune system that increase susceptibility to HIV infection. Women who are in new or nonmonogamous relationships should be encouraged to use a barrier method along with the OCP, IUD, or subdermal hormonal implant.

The nurse should approach the counseling sessions with sensitivity and awareness that the individual may feel uncomfortable with sharing personal information about the sexual history or STD infection in the past. When possible, partners should be included in discussions concerning reproductive health issues.

 ### Optimizing Outcomes— **Reducing the likelihood of STD transmission and progression of disease**

To promote health maintenance and safety and reduce the likelihood of STD transmission, nurses can teach women:

- How to use condoms (male and female, if appropriate) properly
- How to perform a genital self-examination
- To avoid the sharing of personal care items, such as toothbrushes and razors
- To take all prescribed antibiotics, even if symptoms resolve
- To abstain from sexual intercourse until both partners have completed treatment (to prevent reinfection)
- To return for evaluation, as indicated, after treatment has been completed

Nurses should also inquire about vaginal douching, a common practice among women in the United States. Findings from a 2001 survey (Sutton, Bruce, & Sternberg, 2006) showed that approximately 22% of women douche, with the prevalence highest among African American women (50%). To date, no study has shown that douching is in any way beneficial to a woman's reproductive health or that it decreases the risk for contracting an STD. In fact, women who douche are at increased risk for STDs, especially if they are less educated, are economically disadvantaged, have more sexual partners, have higher-risk sexual partners, or have a past history of pelvic inflammatory disease. Owing to their biological and behavioral vulnerability to STDs, at-risk adolescents may experience even greater risks associated with douching (Martino & Vermund, 2002; Vermund & Allen, 2009).

 ### Nursing Insight— *Douching and STIs*

Douching increases the risk for STDs by washing away the resident lactobacilli, which increase vaginal acidity, thereby creating an inhospitable environment for pathogens. The lactobacilli also adhere to epithelial cells that prevent pathogen adherence. Without a preponderance of beneficial lactobacilli, the vaginal acidity decreases and pathogens can more readily adhere to the vagina (Schwebke, 2000). Younger women who douche and are more sexually active may be at an especially high risk for contracting an STD; the risk with douching may not be as great for older women (Vermund & Allen, 2009).

Nurses who work with women of all ages can provide counseling about the harmful effects of douching. The information should be presented in a patient-centered, nonjudgmental manner that is appropriately attuned to the patient's age, culture, sexual orientation, and developmental level. When appropriate, engaging the support of influential family members (e.g., mothers, sisters, mothers-in-law) may also be of benefit in effecting the desired behavioral change (Vermund & Allen, 2009).

Nursing diagnoses for women with STDs are developed after careful consideration of all patient assessment data, the plan of treatment, and specific directives from the health-care provider. One appropriate diagnosis, for example, may focus on the threat to physiological functioning: "Acute Pain/Impaired Tissue Integrity related to effects of the infection process/excoriation of pruritic areas/hygiene practices." Another may address the emotional dimensions of the diagnosis: "Anxiety/Situational Low Self-Esteem/Disturbed Body Image related to perceived effects on intimate relationships and long-term sequelae of infection," or "Social Isolation and Impaired Social Interaction related to perceived effects on relationships with others if the STD status is not known." A nursing diagnosis that addresses educational needs is "Deficient Knowledge related to transmission/prevention/reinfection/management of infection or safer sex behaviors."

Nursing interventions center on the use of therapeutic communication to foster nonjudgmental, culturally appropriate discussion to facilitate learning and understanding. Providing emotional support is an essential component of care. The nurse assesses the patient's (and partner's, if appropriate) level of knowledge about the infection and uses this information to develop an individualized teaching plan. Emphasis is placed on the use and importance of safe sexual practices and, depending on the treatment regimen, the need to complete all prescribed medication and return for further evaluation. Referral to support groups may be appropriate.

In some situations, the patient may confide that she is too embarrassed to reveal information about the STD to her intimate partner and ask for guidance. The nurse can assist her by offering strategies, such as role-playing, for approaching the partner and sharing the information. It is important to emphasize that although this is a difficult topic for discussion, most individuals would rather know about the possibility that they are infected rather than not know. Exploring ways of communicating sensitive information is an important nursing intervention that can strengthen the therapeutic relationship, enhance adherence with the treatment plan, and improve STD case finding.

❝**What to say**❞ — *Exploring strategies for communicating STD infection information*

When counseling the patient about how she may approach her intimate partner about her STD, the nurse may suggest that she use statements such as "I care about you and I want you to know that I am concerned about your health. I want you to know that I am undergoing treatment for an STD—and you need to be evaluated as well."

Now Can You— **Describe the nurse's role in promoting reproductive health?**

1. Identify eight "safer sex" strategies?
2. Explain patient teaching about the practice of douching?
3. Formulate three potential nursing diagnoses for a woman with an STD?
4. Discuss aspects of patient education and counseling about STDs?

summary points

◆ STDs encompass more than 25 infectious organisms that cause reproductive tract infections.

◆ Potential complications of STDs include infertility, ectopic pregnancy, chronic pelvic pain, liver disease, liver cancer, and death.

◆ Chlamydia, the most commonly reported infectious disease in the United States, is the leading cause of preventable infertility and ectopic pregnancy.

◆ Once on the verge of elimination, syphilis has reemerged as a common STD.

◆ In the United States, women represent one of the fastest growing segments of the HIV epidemic.

◆ Gonorrhea and Chlamydia are prevalent in the adolescent population and disproportionately prevalent in minority groups.

◆ Infection with *Trichomonas vaginalis* increases the risk of HIV transmission.

◆ Pelvic inflammatory disease is most often caused by the organisms *Chlamydia trachomatis* and *Neisseria gonorrhoeae*.

◆ Hepatitis is the leading cause of liver cancer and the most common reason for liver transplantation.

◆ In the area of reproductive health promotion, an important nursing role centers on education about STDs, safer sex strategies, and actions to reduce the likelihood of STD transmission.

review questions

Multiple Choice

1. Self-care measures that reduce the transmission of STDs include:
A. Withdrawal of the penis before ejaculation
B. Douching immediately after sexual intercourse
C. Use of barrier methods of contraception
D. Mutual masturbation

2. Strategies for safer sex that avoid contact with bodily fluids include:
A. Erotic massage
B. Oral–genital stimulation
C. Careful anal intercourse
D. Consensual sharing of sex toys

3. Factors that place women at increased risk for HIV infection include:
A. History of premenstrual syndrome
B. History of prostitution
C. History of a seizure disorder
D. History of an ectopic pregnancy

4. The most common STD that frequently produces no signs or symptoms in women is:
A. Chancroid
B. Herpes
C. Chlamydia
D. Syphilis

5. The first sign of syphilis is a sore that is:
A. Painful
B. Filled with clear fluid
C. Itchy and scaly
D. Painless

REFERENCES

Adler, S. (2007). The importance of routine STD screening. *Clinical Advisor, 10*(6), 35–40.

Advisory Committee on Immunization Practices, Vaccines for Children Program. (2009). *ACIP provisional recommendations for HPV vaccine.* Retrieved March 20, 2010, from http://www.cdc.gov/vaccines/recs/provisional/downloads/hpv-vac-dec2009-508.pdf

American Academy of Pediatrics and the American College of Obstetricians and Gynecologists. (2007). *Guidelines for perinatal care* (6th ed.). Washington, DC: Author.

American College of Obstetricians and Gynecologists (ACOG). (2006, September). ACOG Committee Opinion No. 344: Human papillomavirus vaccination. *Obstetrics and Gynecology, 108*(4), 699–705.

American College of Obstetricians and Gynecologists (ACOG). (2007). *Women's health care: A resource manual* (3rd ed.). Washington, DC: Author.

Barry, P. M., Kent, C. K., Philip, S. S., & Klausner, J. D. (2010). Results of a program to test women for rectal Chlamydia and gonorrhea. *Obstetrics and Gynecology, 115*(4), 753–759.

Centers for Disease Control and Prevention (CDC). (2006a). Revised recommendations for HIV testing of adults, adolescents, and pregnant women in health-care settings. *MMWR Recommendations and Reports, 55*(RR14), 1–17.

Centers for Disease Control and Prevention (CDC), Workowski, A., & Berman, S. M. (2006b). *Sexually transmitted diseases treatment guidelines, 2006. Morbidity and Mortality Weekly Report, 55*(RR-11), 1–94.

Centers for Disease Control and Prevention (CDC). (2008a). *HIV and AIDS in the United States: A picture of today's epidemic.* Retrieved March 20, 2010, from http://www.cdc.gov/hiv/topics/surveillance/pdf/us_media.pdf

Centers for Disease Control and Prevention (CDC). (2008b). *Pubic "crab" lice.* Retrieved April 2, 2010, from http://www.cdc.gov/lice/pubic/index.html

Centers for Disease Control and Prevention (CDC). (2009a). *Sexually transmitted diseases surveillance, 2008.* Retrieved March 18, 2010, from http://www.cdc.gov/std/stats08/main.htm

Centers for Disease Control and Prevention (CDC). (2009b). *Basic statistics.* Retrieved March 20, 2010, from http://www.cdc.gov/hiv/topics/surveillance/basic.htm

Centers for Disease Control and Prevention (CDC). (2009c). *AIDS in the United States by geographic distribution.* Retrieved March 20, 2010, from http://www.cdc.gov/hiv/resources/Factsheets/geographic.htm

Centers for Disease Control and Prevention (CDC). (2009d). Chlamydia screening among sexually active young female enrollees of health plans—United States, 2000–2007. *MMWR Morbidity and Mortality Weekly Report, 58*(14), 362–365

Centers for Disease Control and Prevention (CDC). (2009e). *Hepatitis B information for health professionals.* Retrieved March 24, 2010, from http://www.cdc.gov/hepatitis/HBV/HBVfaq.htm#treatment

Centers for Disease Control and Prevention (CDC). (2009f). *Hepatitis C information for health professionals.* Retrieved April 4, 2010, from http://www.cdc.gov/hepatitis/HCV/index.htm

Centers for Disease Control and Prevention (CDC). (2010). *Viral hepatitis.* Retrieved March 22, 2010, from http://www.cdc.gov/hepatitis/

Christiansen-Lindquist, L., Tao, G., Hoover, K., Frank, R., & Kent, C. (2009). Chlamydia screening of young sexually active, Medicaid-insured women by race and ethnicity, 2002–2005. *Sexually Transmitted Diseases, 36*(10), 642–646.

Connor, B. A. (2005). Hepatitis A vaccine in the last-minute traveler. *American Journal of Medicine, 118*(Suppl. 10A), 58S–62S.

Deglin, J. H., & Vallerand, A. H. (2009). *Davis's drug guide for nurses* (11th ed.). Philadelphia: F. A. Davis.

Gardner, J. (2006). What you need to know about genital herpes. *Nursing 2006, 36*(10), 26–27.

Glynn, M., & Rhodes, P. (2005). *Estimated HIV prevalence in the United States at the end of 2003.* Abstract presented at the National HIV Prevention Conference, 2005, Atlanta.

Graseck, A. S., Secura, G. M., Allsworth, J. E., Madden, T., & Peipert, J. F. (2010). Home screening compared with clinic-based screening for sexually transmitted infections. *Obstetrics and Gynecology, 115*(4), 745–752.

Greenwald, J. L., Burstein, G. R., Pincus, J., & Branson, B. (2006). A rapid review of rapid HIV antibody tests. *Current Infectious Disease Reports, 8*(11), 125–131.

Hackett, K. M. (2010). Chlamydia screening. *Advance for Nurse Practitioners, 18*(2), 16.

Holloway, M., & D'Acunto, K. (2006). An update on the ABCs of viral hepatitis. *Clinical Advisor, 9*(6), 26–40.

Hoover, K., & Tao, G. (2008). Missed opportunities for Chlamydia screening of young women in the United States. *Obstetrics & Gynecology, 11*(5), 1097–1102.

Hoover, K., Tao, G., & Kent, C. (2008). Low rates of both asymptomatic Chlamydia screening and diagnostic testing of women in U.S. outpatient clinics. *Obstetrics & Gynecology, 112*(4), 891–898.

Johnson-Mallard, V., & Lengacher, C. A. (2007). STD health communication intervention. *Women's Health Care, 6*(8), 27–31.

Kahn, J. O., & Walker, B. D. (1998). Acute human immunodeficiency virus type 1 infection. *New England Journal of Medicine, 339*(1), 33–39.

Kellogg-Spadt, S. (2009). Hepatitis D: Implications for sexuality. *American Journal for Nurse Practitioners, 13*(10), 39–40.

Marrazzo, J. A., Guest, F., & Cates, Jr., W. (2007). Reproductive tract infections, including HIV and other sexually transmitted infections. In R. Hatcher, J. Trussell, A. Nelson. W. Cates Jr., F. Stewart, & D. Kowal (Eds.), *Contraceptive technology* (19th ed., pp. 499–557). New York: Thomson Reuters.

Martino, J. L., & Vermund, S. H. (2002). Vaginal douching: Evidence for risks or benefits to women's health. *Epidemiologic Review, 24*(2), 109–124.

Mayeaux, E. J., Jr. (2007). External genital warts: An update. *Female Patient, 32*(12), 33–35.

National Institutes of Health (NIH). (2009). *BufferGel and PRO 2000/5: Vaginal gels to prevent HIV infection in women.* Retrieved April 5, 2010, from http://clinicaltrials.gov/ct2/show/NCT00074425

Nelson, A. L. (2007). Sexually transmitted treatment guidelines, 2006: An update. *Forum, 5*(1), 2–5.

Ravin, C. R. (2007). Preventing STDs: Ask the questions. *Nursing for Women's Health, 11*(1), 88–91.

Royer, H. R., & Cerf, C. (2009). Young women's beliefs about the terms sexually transmitted disease and sexually transmitted infection. *Journal of Obstetric, Gynecologic, & Neonatal Nursing, 38*(6), 686–692.

Royer, H. R., & Zahner, S. (2009). Providers' experiences with young people's cognitive representations and emotions related to prevention and treatment of sexually transmitted infections. *Public Health Nursing, 26*(2), 161–172.

Ryan, K. J., & Ray, C. G. (Eds.). (2004). *Sherris medical microbiology* (4th ed., pp. 541–544). New York: McGraw-Hill

Schmidt, J. V. (2007). HPV vaccine: Implications for nurses and patients. *Nursing for Women's Health, 11*(1), 83–87.

Schwebke, J. R. (2000). Vaginal infections. In M. B Goldman & M. C. Hatch (Eds.), *Women and health.* San Diego: Academic Press.

Sorvillo, F., Smith, L., Kerndt, P., & Ash, L. (2001). *Trichomonas vaginalis, HIV, and African-Americans. Emerging Infectious Diseases, 7*(6), 38–49.

Steffen, R. (2005). Changing travel-related global epidemiology of hepatitis A. *American Journal of Medicine, 118*(10), 46–49.

Stonehouse, A., & Studdiford, J. (2007). Allergic contact dermatitis from tee tree oil. *Consultant, 47*(8), 781.

Sutton, M. Y., Bruce, C., & Sternberg, M. R. (2006). *Prevalence and correlates of vaginal douching among women in the United States, 2001–2002.* Paper presented at the National STD Prevention Conference, May 2006, Jacksonville, FL.

Swan, A. M. (2009). Acute HIV infection in primary care. *Advance for Nurse Practitioners, 17*(9), 49–54.

Thiel, T. K. (1998). Hepatitis A vaccination. *American Family Physician, 57*(7), 1500–1501.

U.S. Department of Health and Human Services (USDHHS). (2000). *Healthy People 2010: Understanding and improving health.* Washington, DC: U.S. Government Printing Office.

U.S. Preventive Services Task Force (USPSTF). (2001). Screening for Chlamydial infection: Recommendations and rationale. *American Journal of Preventive Medicine, 20*(3 Suppl.), 90–94.

U.S. Preventive Services Task Force (USPSTF). (2004). *Screening for hepatitis B virus infection.* Retrieved March 25, 2010, from http://www.ahrq.gov/clinic/uspstf/uspshepb.htm

U.S. Preventive Services Task Force (USPSTF). (2005). Screening for gonorrhea: Recommendation statement. *Annals of Family Medicine, 3*(3), 263–267.

U.S. Preventive Services Task Force. (2009). U.S. Preventive Services Task Force Reaffirmation Recommendation Statement: Screening for syphilis infection in pregnancy: *Annals of Family Medicine, 150*(5), 705–709.

Vermund, S. H., & Allen, K. L. (2009). Douching is a remediable risk factor for sexually transmitted infections. *Female Patient, 34*(7), 37–39.

Weber-LaShore, A., & Biro, F. M. (2009). Cervicitis and sexually transmitted infections in the adolescent population. *Female Patient, 34*(6), 34–36.

Winer, S., & Richwald, G. A. (2007). Genital HSV update. *Forum, 5*(2), 18–22.

Xu, F., Sternberg, M. R., Kottiri, B. J., McQuillan, G. M., Lee, F. K., Nahmias, A. J., et al. (2006). Trends in herpes simplex virus type 1 and type 2 seroprevalence in the United States. *Journal of the American Medical Association, 296*(8), 964–973.

Promoting Reproductive Health Through an Understanding of Cervical Cytology Screening, Human Papillomavirus, and Cervical Cancer

Shelton M. Hisley, PhD, RNC, WHNP-BC

Life is what happens to you
When you're making other plans

—Betty Talmadge

LEARNING TARGETS *At the completion of this chapter, the student will be able to:*

- Describe the cervical epithelium and the process of metaplasia
- Discuss methods of cervical cytology screening
- Identify treatment options for various preinvasive conditions of the cervix
- Identify risk factors for human papillomavirus (HPV)
- Discuss the HPV–cervical cancer link
- Identify risk factors for cervical cancer
- Develop materials for patient education and counseling regarding cervical cytology screening, human papillomavirus, and cervical cancer

Introduction

This chapter, which explores cervical cytology screening, focuses on human papillomavirus (HPV) and its association with premalignant and malignant cervical disease. HPV is a nonenveloped, double-stranded DNA virus. It is the most common sexually transmitted disease in the United States. More than 40 HPV types that can infect the genital areas of males and females exist, and these HPV types can also infect the mouth and throat.

According to the Centers for Disease Control and Prevention (CDC) (2009a), approximately 20 million Americans are currently infected with HPV, and another 6 million people become newly infected each year. HPV is so common that at least 50% of all sexually active men and women get it at some point in their lives. Around 1% of sexually active adults in the United States have genital warts at any one time, and each year approximately 12,000 American women get cervical cancer. HPV infection is known to be the primary cause of cervical cancer. Other cancers that may be caused by HPV include pharyngeal, vulvar, vaginal, penile, and anal (CDC, 2009a).

Although HPV has been recognized since 1907, it has only been within the past three decades that an understanding of the virus has evolved and its link to cervical and other cancers has been clearly established. The past 10 years have brought major advances in cervical screening technologies with the advent of liquid-based Pap tests and HPV testing. Most recently, two HPV vaccines have become available. The vaccines are indicated for the prevention of cervical cancer, genital warts, and dysplastic or precancerous cervical lesions caused by several of the HPV viruses types (American Cancer Society [ACS], 2010; CDC, 2009b; Howley, Yang, Spalholz, & Rabson, 1986; Moore & Seybold, 2007; National Association of Nurse Practitioners in Women's Health [NPWH], 2007; Wysocki, Reiter, & Berman, 2007).

The Cervix and the Cervical Transformation Zone

To enhance understanding about the uterine cervix and the cervical Pap test, it is important for the nurse to be knowledgeable about cervical cytology and the normal cellular changes that occur throughout a woman's life. The surface of the cervix and the canal that leads into the uterus—termed the "endocervical canal"—is composed of two types of cells: squamous epithelium and columnar epithelium.

A & P review Cervical Cell Types, the Squamocolumnar Junction, and the Transformation Zone

The cervix, which is typically 2.5 cm long, communicates with the endometrial cavity of the corpus uteri (uterine body) through the internal os and with the vagina through the external os. The vaginal portion (also called the exocervix, ectocervix, or portio vaginalis) is covered by stratified *squamous epithelium.* The squamous epithelium is smooth and light pink in appearance. The cervical canal is covered by *columnar epithelium,* which also forms endocervical glands, more correctly called "clefts." In young women, columnar epithelium can also be noted on the outer surface of the cervix around the external cervical os. The glandular tissue has a rough texture and is dark pink in color.

The area in which the squamous epithelium and the columnar epithelium come together on the cervix is called the *squamocolumnar junction (SCJ).* The SCJ is located where the more delicate, darker pink columnar cells that line the uterus meet the sturdier, lighter pink squamous epithelium of the vagina. Throughout the reproductive years, some columnar cells at the SCJ are replaced by squamous epithelium through a process termed squamous metaplasia. The area between the old and new SCJ is called the *transformation zone.* The size of the transformation zone varies from 2 to 15 mm. In most adult women, the squamocolumnar junction is not an abrupt meeting point but a zone containing irregular areas of glandular and squamous epithelium. This site undergoes continuous cell growth and replacement. The squamous type of cell replaces the columnar type of cell in a constant cycle of cell turnover, which is influenced by the female hormones. Metaplasia, which is a normal process of cell turnover, occurs most rapidly during adolescence and pregnancy. Cervical cancer usually develops in this area of rapid cell division. The immature cells undergoing the transformation from columnar to squamous tissue are especially vulnerable to events that can change the genetic material of the cells. These changes, or mutations, may result in the development of premalignant or malignant

cells (Teitelman, Stringer, Averbuch, & Witkoski, 2009; Wysocki et al., 2007). ◆

 Nursing Insight— *Natural migration of the transformation zone*

In infants and postmenopausal women, the transformation zone is located deep within the endocervical canal. In women of childbearing age, beginning at puberty, the transformation zone moves out of the endocervical canal and lies primarily on the ectocervix; this movement is termed *cervical ectopy.* Elevated hormone states that occur, for example, during pregnancy and with the use of hormonal contraception, may cause the transformation zone to become enlarged or more greatly exposed (Woodson, 2008).

Cervical Cancer Screening

DEVELOPMENT OF THE PAP TEST

Prior to the 1940s when the Pap test for cervical cytological screening became widely available, cervical cancer was the most common cause of cancer death in women in the United States. Over the last 30 years, the incidence of invasive cervical cancer has decreased by 50 percent. The ACS (2010) estimated that in 2009 around 11,270 new cases of invasive cervical cancer would be diagnosed, and around 4,070 American women would die from cervical cancer.

 Nursing Insight— *Origins of the Pap test*

The Pap test is named for Dr. George Papanicolaou, the physician who, along with Dr. Herbert Traut, developed the procedure in the 1930s. The Pap test is a cytological study used to detect cancer in cells that an organ has shed. Although used most often in the diagnosis and prevention of cervical cancers, the Pap test is also of value in detecting pleural or peritoneal malignancies and in the evaluation of cellular changes caused by radiation, infection, or atrophy. In women's health, the Pap test is a screening technique used to detect cervical cancer or cervical abnormalities that may progress to cancer. The test can detect 95% of all cervical cancers and precancerous abnormalities. In the years since World War II, the Pap test has become the most widely used cancer screening method in the world, and it is the most successful cancer screening technique in medical history. Pap screening reduced cervical cancer death rates by 74% between 1955 and 1992, and the rate continues to decline by about 2% each year (Venes, 2009).

 Nursing Insight— *Screening and early detection for cervical cancer*

The goal of screening for cervical cancer is to detect cervical cell changes and early cervical cancers before any symptoms develop. *Screening* refers to the use of tests (e.g., the Pap test) and exams to find a disease, such as cancer, in individuals who have no symptoms. *Early detection* means applying a strategy that results in an earlier diagnosis of cervical cancer than otherwise might have occurred. Screening tests offer the best chance to detect cervical cancer at an early stage when successful treatment is likely. Screening for cervical cancer is especially beneficial because it affords an opportunity to detect abnormal cell changes (precancers) so that they can be treated before they progress to cervical cancer (ACS, 2009a).

PAP TEST TECHNIQUES

The Pap test is usually a part of a routine pelvic examination. A sample of cervical epithelium is gathered from the squamocolumnar junction, which can often be visualized on the cervix. An adequate Pap test should contain both columnar cells and squamous cells, which indicates that the squamocolumnar junction was sampled. The Pap test is obtained before any digital examination of the vagina is performed and before any endocervical bacteriological specimens are collected. Prior to insertion, the vaginal speculum may be moistened with water or saline if necessary; no other lubricants are recommended. The examiner may use a large cotton-tipped applicator to remove excess cervical discharge before the cytological specimen is obtained (Teitelman et al., 2009).

Various sampling devices (e.g., spatula [paddle], cervix brush, plastic "broom") may be used (Fig. 6-1). When conventional Pap tests are performed, a single microscope slide, combining both the endocervical and ectocervical samples, or two separate glass slides can be used. The exocervix (outer area) is first sampled with the spatula (Fig. 6-2). This is done first to minimize the possibility of obscuring the cells with blood. The endocervix (inner area) is then sampled with the brush placed into the cervical os. The plastic "broom-like" brush is designed to simultaneously sample the endocervix and the exocervix. This device is inserted and rotated 360 degrees for a total of three to five times. If the patient has had a hysterectomy, the vaginal cuff (the portion of the vagina that remains open to the peritoneum following removal of the uterus) is sampled. The vaginal wall is usually not sampled unless the woman is approaching menopause, and in that case, a second sample may be obtained to evaluate the hormonal effects on vaginal tissue (ACOG, 2007; Policar, 2008).

The cytology sample is promptly transferred onto one or two thin glass slides and the sampling device is discarded. With this method of Pap testing, the most important consideration is rapid fixation. The slide should be

Figure 6-2 Taking a Cervical Smear (Source: From *Nursing Health Assessment: A Critical Thinking, Case Studies Approach,* 2nd ed., by P. M. Dillon, 2007, Philadelphia: F. A. Davis, p. 637.)

sprayed with a preservative within 5 seconds to prevent drying of the specimen (Bickley & Szilagyi, 2007; Dillon, 2007) (Fig. 6-3). Drawbacks of the conventional "slide method" of Pap test collection include the possibility of inadequate cellular sampling, the presence of artifacts (e.g., blood, discharge, lubricant) that obscure the cervical cells, the clinician's failure to properly "fix" the specimen in a timely manner, and inaccurate interpretation by the laboratory cytologist (ACOG, 2009a; Wysocki et al., 2007).

Today, the majority of cervical cytology screening performed in the United States uses a liquid-based process (e.g., ThinPrep Pap Test, BD SurePath Pap Test). With the liquid-based technique, exfoliated cells are collected from

Figure 6-3 A Cytology Brush and Spatula are Used for Specimens Obtained During a Conventional Pap Test. The Specimen Is Placed onto a Thin Glass Side and Immediately Sprayed with a Preservative (Fixative) (Source: From *Nursing Health Assessment: A Critical Thinking, Case Studies Approach,* 2nd ed., by P. M. Dillon, 2007, Philadelphia: F. A. Davis, p. 65.)

Figure 6-1 Tools for Pap Test (top to bottom): Cytobrush, Cervical Cytobroom, and Wooden Spatula (Source: From *Taber's Cycolpedic Medical Dictionary,* 21st ed., by D. Venes, 2009, Philadelphia: F. A. Davis, p. 1697.)

the transformation zone of the cervix and transferred to a vial of liquid alcohol-based preservative. The sample is then processed in the laboratory and a slide is produced for interpretation. With this method, almost all of the sample cells are transferred to the liquid preservative, and most of the contaminating blood, inflammatory cells, and debris are filtered out. However, heavy menstrual blood may limit the number of squamous cells available for interpretation. Prompt suspension of the cells in the liquid preservative eliminates the problem of air-drying artifact, a factor that can limit the interpretation of conventional cervical cytology (American College of Obstetricians and Gynecologists [ACOG], 2009a).

 Nursing Insight— *Comparing the conventional Pap test with the liquid-based Pap test*

In the conventional Pap test, cell samples are obtained from the vagina, cervix, and cervical canal and spread on a glass slide. In liquid-based Pap testing, cell samples are collected using a special brush that is immediately washed in an alcohol-based fluid. In the laboratory, a special machine filters out the cells from the solution and deposits them in a thin, uniform monolayer (a single layer of cells) on a glass slide. Analysis usually includes initial computer screening followed by slide review by a cytotechnologist. The liquid-based Pap test method removes contaminants such as blood and mucus, which frequently obscure cells in the conventional Pap test. The monolayer of cells is also easier to examine under the microscope, resulting in an increased rate of detection of abnormal cells. The disadvantage of the liquid-based method primarily centers on the increased cost incurred by the collection fluid and the continuing operation of the laboratory filtering machine.

With the liquid-based technology, between 50,000 and 70,000 diagnostic cells are available for screening; with the conventional process, approximately 4,000 to 300,000 cells are "smeared" onto a slide, where they often overlap or are obscured by non-cervical material. In addition, according to the laboratory-based cytotechnologists, the liquid-based tests are easier to read. Although the liquid-based cytology is more expensive than conventional cytology, it provides the added ability to test for HPV, gonorrhea, and Chlamydia from the same sample (ACOG, 2009a; Gupta, 2007).

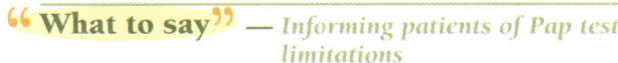 **"What to say"** — *Informing patients of Pap test limitations*

Counseling patients about Pap test limitations constitutes a central role for nurses in women's health care. Nurses can advise about the limits of Pap test accuracy while reassuring them that the Pap test is the single most reliable method to detect preinvasive cancer of the cervix. However, there is no guarantee that any single Pap test will identify abnormal cells that may be present. Rescreening, when necessary, carries the burden of an additional expense, which may or may not be covered by insurance, whether funded by private, state, or federal sources (ACOG, 2009a; Gupton, 2007).

 Now Can You— Describe normal cervical epithelium and the cervical Pap test?

1. Identify the types of cells normally found in the cervix?
2. Define the terms *squamous metaplasia, squamocolumnar junction, and transformation zone?*
3. Describe the proper technique for obtaining a Pap test, and compare the liquid-based method with the conventional slide method?

INITIATION AND RECOMMENDED FREQUENCY OF CERVICAL CANCER SCREENING

Cancer of the cervix is usually a slow-growing neoplasm that is almost always caused by infection with the sexually transmitted disease human papillomavirus (HPV). (See later discussion of HPV in this chapter.) Screening for cervical cancer should begin at age 21 years, regardless of the woman's sexual history. Cervical neoplasia develops in susceptible individuals in response to infection with a high-risk type of HPV (i.e., types 12–14, 20, and 21). HPV causes carcinogenesis in the transformation zone of the cervix, where the process of squamous metaplasia replaces columnar epithelium with squamous epithelium. Squamous metaplasia is particularly active in the cervix during adolescence and early adulthood. HPV is commonly acquired by young women shortly after the initiation of vaginal intercourse, but in most situations the HPV is cleared by the immune system within 1 to 2 years without producing neoplastic changes. The risk of neoplastic transformation increases in women whose HPV infections persist. The recommendation to initiate cervical cancer screening at age 21 years regardless of the age of onset of sexual intercourse is based in part on the very low incidence of cancer in younger women. It is also based on the potential for adverse effects associated with follow-up of young women with abnormal cytology screening results (ACOG, 2009a).

 Nursing Insight— *Potential adverse effects associated with cervical cancer screening in adolescents*

Initiating cervical cancer screening in the adolescent population may result in increased anxiety, morbidity, and expense from the testing and overuse of follow-up procedures. The emotional impact of labeling an adolescent with both a sexually transmitted disease (i.e., HPV) and a potential precancer must be considered in light of the fact that the adolescent period is characterized by emerging sexuality and a heightened concern for self-image. Sexually active adolescents (i.e., females younger than 21 years) should be counseled and tested for STDs and educated about safer sex and contraception. These measures may be carried out without cervical cytology screening and, in the asymptomatic patient, without the use of a speculum (ACOG, 2009b; Wright et al., 2007).

Cervical cytology screening is recommended every 2 years for women aged 21 to 29 years, with either conventional or liquid-based cytology. Women aged 30 years and older who have had three consecutive cervical cytology test results that are negative for intraepithelial (potentially precancer) lesions and malignancy may be screened every 3 years. Women with the following risk factors may require more frequent cervical cytological screening (ACOG, 2009a):

- Women who are infected with HIV
- Women who are immunosuppressed (e.g., those who have received renal transplants)
- Women who were exposed to diethylstilbestrol (DES) in utero
- Women previously treated for cervical intraepithelial neoplasia (CIN) 2, CIN 3, or cancer

⊛ Be sure to— Educate patients about strategies to optimize cervical cancer screening

Nurses can teach patients about strategies to optimize cervical cancer screening. In the ideal situation, the Pap test should be collected at midcycle. Patients should avoid intercourse, douching, or the use of vaginal medications for 24 to 48 hours prior to the test. The presence of infection (e.g., yeast) can cause vaginal inflammation and interfere with the test results. Over-the-counter vaginal creams, gels, foams, or suppositories used within 24 to 48 hours before the Pap test is obtained may interfere with the collection of an adequate cytological specimen.

CERVICAL CANCER SCREENING IN THE OLDER WOMAN

Cervical cancer tends to occur in midlife. It rarely develops in women younger than age 20. Most cases of cervical cancer and related deaths occur in women older than age 50. Almost 20% of women with cervical cancer are diagnosed over age 65. In fact, many older women do not realize that the risk of developing cervical cancer is still present as they age. Sadly, up to two-thirds of older women with cervical cancer have not received adequate Pap screening prior to their cancer diagnosis. Thus, all women with a cervix should continue to receive Pap test screening according to standard guidelines and their care provider's recommendations (ACS, 2010; Chase & Tewari, 2010; Gupton, 2007; Olbrys, 2010).

Currently, the ACS suggests that cervical cancer screening may be stopped in women aged 70 years or older if they have had three or more recent consecutive negative test findings and no abnormal test findings in the previous 10 years (ACS, 2009). The U.S. Preventive Services Task Force (USPSTF) (2007) recommends screening cessation in women older than 65 years with negative test results who are not otherwise considered to be high risk for cancer. ACOG has determined that it is reasonable to discontinue cervical cancer screening at either 65 years of age or 70 years of age in women who have three or more negative cytology test results in a row and no abnormal test results in the past 10 years (ACOG, 2009a). A summary of the current ACOG recommendations concerning cervical cancer screening is presented in Box 6-1. All expert groups are in agreement that cervical cancer screening can be discontinued in women who have had a hysterectomy if the surgery was performed for benign reasons and there is no past history of high-grade cervical lesions.

Box 6-1 Cervical Cancer Screening: ACOG Recommendations

The following ACOG recommendations for cervical cancer screening (2009) are based on good and consistent scientific evidence (Level A):

- Cervical cancer screening should begin at age 21 years. Screening before age 21 should be avoided because it may lead to unnecessary and harmful evaluation and treatment in women at very low risk of cancer.
- Cervical cytology screening is recommended every 2 years for women between the ages of 21 years and 29 years.
- Women aged 30 years and older who have had three consecutive negative cervical cytology screening test results and who have no history of CIN 2 or CIN 3, are not HIV infected, are not immunocompromised, and were not exposed to diethylstilbestrol (DES) in utero may extend the interval between cervical cytology examinations to every 3 years.
- Both liquid-based and conventional methods of cervical cytology are acceptable for screening.
- In women who have had a total hysterectomy for benign indications and have no prior history of high-grade CIN, routine cytology testing should be discontinued.
- Co-testing using the combination of cytology plus HPV DNA testing is an appropriate screening test for women older than 30 years. Any low-risk woman aged 30 years or older who receives negative test results on both cervical cytology screening and HPV DNA testing should be rescreened no sooner than 3 years subsequently.

⊛ Be sure to— Document all communications concerning Pap tests

When Pap test results are received, it is essential that patients be promptly notified of abnormal results. Neglect to do so may result from a breakdown in communication between the care provider and the office staff or from poor follow-up efforts to contact patients. Documentation of test results and patient follow-up efforts is equally important. It is essential that information regarding efforts to report results, make treatment recommendations, and order appropriate follow-up, as well as efforts to obtain patient history and informed consent or informed refusal, be documented in the chart (Duffy, 2009).

Across Care Setting: Ensuring cervical cancer screening for medically underserved women

In this country, all states are making cervical cancer screening more available to medically underserved women through the National Breast and Cervical Cancer Early Detection Program (NBCCEDP). The program provides free or low-cost breast and cervical cancer screening to women with no health insurance. The goal of NBCCEDP is to reach as many women in medically underserved communities as possible, including older women, women without health insurance, and women who are members of racial and ethnic minorities. Nurses can contact the Department of Health in their practice state for specific information regarding program location and eligibility requirements, or they may contact the CDC at 1-800-CDC-INFO, or visit the CDC Web site at www.cdc.gov/cancer/nbccedp.

INTERPRETING CERVICAL CYTOLOGY FINDINGS: THE BETHESDA SYSTEM TERMINOLOGY

The Bethesda System is the classification for abnormal cervical cytology and histology that is most commonly used today. First developed in 1988 under sponsorship of the National Institutes of Health (NIH), the updated 2001 Bethesda System terminology is used to describe the categories of epithelial cell abnormalities, including atypical squamous cells (ASC), low-grade or high-grade squamous intraepithelial lesions (LSIL or HSIL), and glandular cell abnormalities, including atypical glandular cells (AGC) and adenocarcinoma in situ (AIS). Histology diagnoses of abnormalities are reported as CIN Grades 1–3 (ACOG, 2008). The 2001 Bethesda System terminology is presented in Box 6-2.

 Optimizing Outcomes— With the Bethesda System: A standardized approach for cytology/histology findings and interpretation to guide patient care

Over the years, the Bethesda System has undergone a number of major changes in approach and terminology in attempts to standardize reporting systems worldwide and provide more information about what was actually identified in the cellular sample. Developed by major medical groups including the ACOG, the ACS, the Association of Reproductive Health Professionals (ARHP), and the American Society for Colposcopy and Cervical Pathology (ASCCP), the original guidelines have undergone review several times in past years in response to emerging data on the role of HPV in cervical cancer. The latest (2007) ASCCP consensus guidelines reflect evidence-based advances in the understanding of the natural history of HPV, its influence on the development of cervical dysplasia and cancer, and the role of Pap tests with a

liquid-based sample (ACOG, 2008; Wright et al., 2007; Wysocki et al., 2007).

 Now Can You— Discuss cervical cytology screening?

1. Identify the appropriate time for initiation and recommended frequency for cervical cancer screening according to guidelines established by ACOG?
2. Explain why cervical cancer screening in the adolescent population is discouraged?
3. Teach a patient how to prepare for her Pap test and include three strategies intended to optimize the test results?

FOLLOW-UP FOR ABNORMAL CERVICAL CYTOLOGY SCREENING RESULTS

Depending on the result of the Pap test, further evaluation or treatment or both may be indicated. Reflex HPV DNA testing is an option for the management of an ASCUS Pap test result. Reflex HPV DNA testing is performed to determine whether HPV is present and if referral for colposcopy is indicated. Women of all ages with ASCUS Pap test results should be tested for HPV. The liquid-based Pap samples can be immediately tested for HPV if there is an ASCUS result. Women with an ASCUS Pap result who test positive for HPV should be referred for colposcopy with directed biopsy and endocervical sampling (ACOG, 2008; Wysocki et al., 2007).

Colposcopy

Colposcopy is a medical diagnostic procedure that uses a colposcope to provide an illuminated, magnified view of the cervix and the tissues of the vagina and vulva. The colposcope is a low-powered binocular microscope with a powerful light source mounted to allow visualization of the vagina and cervix during a pelvic examination. This instrument allows for a close-up view of the cervix and surrounding tissue for evaluation. The main goal of colposcopy is to prevent cervical cancer by the early detection and treatment of precancerous lesions.

❝What to say❞ — *Preparing the patient for colposcopy*

The nurse can do much to allay a patient's anxiety about colposcopy. The nurse may offer the following description of the procedure to help the patient understand what to expect:

Once you have emptied your bladder, I will assist you into position (dorsal lithotomy) for a pelvic examination. The clinician (colposcopist) will insert a vaginal speculum and most likely use cotton swabs to apply an acetic acid (vinegar) solution to the cervix. Abnormal areas turn white (acetowhite) and become more prominent in response to the acetic acid, allowing for improved visualization. Areas that turn white after the application of acetic acid or have an abnormal vascular pattern are often considered for biopsy. If no lesions are visible, an iodine solution (Schiller's or Lugol's solution) may be applied to the cervix and vagina to help highlight areas of abnormality. The colposcopist determines the

---

Box 6-2 The 2001 Bethesda System Terminology

SQUAMOUS CELL
* ASC
* Of undetermined significance (ASC-US) (the most minor form of cytological abnormality detected on the Pap test)
* Cannot exclude high-grade SIL*
* LSIL (encompasses HPV, mild dysplasia, and CIN1)**
* HSIL (encompasses HPV, moderate and severe dysplasia, CIS, and CIN 2 and CIN 3)
* Squamous cell carcinoma

GLANDULAR CELL
* AGC (a cytological abnormality of the glandular cells that line the endocervix or uterus)
* Atypical glandular cells, favors neoplasia
* Endocervical adenocarcinoma in situ
* Adenocarcinoma

* SIL: cytological abnormalities identified on the Pap test, classified as low-grade (LSIL) or high-grade (HSIL).
** CIN: cervical cancer precursor (confirmed by biopsy), divided into low-grade (CIN1) and high-grade (CIN2/3) (ACOG, 2008; Wysocki et al., 2007).

areas with the highest degree of visible abnormality and may obtain biopsies from these areas. A numbing medication (lidocaine) is used to diminish discomfort, especially if many biopsy samples are taken. Although not common, potential complications include bleeding and infection. To minimize the risk of infection, you should use a panty liner or sanitary napkin and avoid sexual intercourse until all vaginal bleeding or discharge has stopped. Your health-care provider may advise you to take a mild pain reliever such as ibuprofen approximately 30 minutes to 1 hour before the procedure and afterward as needed for cramping and discomfort. Be sure to promptly notify your health-care provider if you develop any signs of infection, such as fever, continued pain, bleeding, foul-smelling vaginal discharge, or painful urination (dysuria), or have any concerns. Also, it is a good idea to bring a support person with you.

Endocervical Sampling

Endocervical sampling is performed if the colposcopy is unsatisfactory (e.g., no lesions are identified, or the endocervical canal cannot be fully visualized) and in women who have follow-up colposcopy after treatment for CIN 2 or 3 with a positive endocervical margin. Endocervical sampling may be conducted either with vigorous endocervical brushing or by the traditional endocervical curettage (ECC), a procedure that uses a sharp, spoon-shaped instrument (curette). A small tissue sample is obtained and sent to a pathology lab for evaluation. Examination of the tissue allows for determination of whether abnormal lesions are located inside the endocervical canal; this information is an important determinant in the treatment plan (ACOG, 2008; ACOG, 2009a).

During the endocervical sampling procedure, which usually only takes a few minutes, the patient will most likely experience abdominal pain and menstrual-like uterine cramps. Endocervical sampling is not indicated in the pregnant patient. Monsel's Solution (Basic Ferric Sulfate Solution, a hemostatic agent) is applied with large cotton swabs to the surface of the cervix to control bleeding. This solution, which is mustard colored, turns black when exposed to blood. After the procedure, the Monsel's Solution is expelled naturally. The nurse can explain to the patient that she may experience a thin, coffee-ground-like vaginal discharge for several days after the procedure (ACOG, 2009a).

🔴 Optimizing Outcomes— Addressing abnormal Pap test results during pregnancy

The management of abnormal Pap test results during pregnancy takes into consideration the duration of the pregnancy, the woman's desire to maintain the pregnancy, and the degree of cellular abnormality. Colposcopy is used for diagnosis, and the primary goal of both cytology and colposcopy is to identify invasive cancer that requires treatment before or at the time of delivery. Cervical biopsies are safe and should be performed for suspected high-grade disease or cancer. Biopsy during pregnancy has not been linked to fetal loss or preterm birth. Endocervical sampling should not be performed. Unless invasive cancer is identified, treatment is postponed until after the pregnancy has ended (ACOG, 2008).

MANAGEMENT OF ABNORMAL CERVICAL CYTOLOGY/COLPOSCOPY FINDINGS

There are a number of ways to treat the lesions identified in a colposcopic examination; the treatment depends on the location and severity of the lesions. Four types of interventional techniques are available: cryosurgery, laser ablation, conization, and the loop electrosurgical excision procedure.

Cryosurgery

Cryosurgery (cryotherapy), a gynecological treatment that involves the freezing of cervical tissue, is performed in the office setting. The patient is assisted into a dorsal lithotomy position and a vaginal speculum is inserted. Cryo probes are placed over the abnormal areas on the cervix. Liquid nitrogen flows through the cryo probes at a temperature of approximately –50°C, making the metal cold enough to freeze and destroy the tissue. Cryosurgery is relatively painless and produces very little scarring. An "ice ball" forms on the cervix, killing the superficial abnormal cells. The most effective treatment result is obtained by a process of freezing for 3 minutes, allowing the area to thaw, and then refreezing for 3 more minutes. Throughout the procedure, the patient may experience slight cramping and/or a sensation of cold or heat. Cryosurgery effectively destroys all of the abnormal cervical tissue in over 85% of cases (ACOG, 2008).

66 What to say 99 — Teaching patients about aftercare following cryosurgery

Offering explanations about what to expect following cryosurgery and alerting patients to danger signs constitutes an important nursing role. The nurse can counsel the patient that she:

- may return to most normal activities the day following the cryosurgery;
- will experience a foul-smelling watery vaginal discharge, caused by sloughing of the necrotic cervical tissue, for a few weeks;
- should avoid inserting anything (tampons, douches) into the vagina and refrain from intercourse for at least 2 to 3 weeks;
- should promptly call her health-care provider if she experiences any symptoms of infection (fever, vaginal bleeding heavier than a normal menstrual cycle, severe or increasing pelvic pain, foul-smelling or yellow-green vaginal discharge); and
- should be sure to return for her follow-up appointment and comply with her health-care provider's recommendations for repeat Pap testing.

A long-term complication of cryosurgery concerns the migration of the squamocolumnar junction (the transformation zone—the area on the cervix where the outer squamous cells meet the inner glandular columnar cells). Following the procedure, the squamocolumnar junction migrates upward into the cervical canal. The relocation of the transformation zone may create the need for a more invasive procedure in the future if abnormal lesions occur that are not visible with the colposcope (i.e., the abnormal cells are located inside the endocervical canal). Although rare, cryosurgery may cause scarring of the cervix and lead to stenosis (narrowing) of the cervical opening, making future cervical cytology screening (Pap testing) and evaluation (colposcopy) difficult (ACOG, 2008).

Laser Ablation

Laser ablation (destruction) involves the use of a thin, high-energy beam of light precisely directed at the abnormal tissue to cause cell destruction through vaporization. Depending on the circumstances, the procedure may be performed in the office, or outpatient setting of the clinic or hospital. The technique uses a laser (mounted on a colposcope) to vaporize the transformation zone, where the abnormal cells are located. Advantages of laser ablation include rapid healing (3–4 weeks), minimal scarring, and no retraction of the transformation zone. Following laser ablation, patients may experience less vaginal discharge than with cryosurgery, but they may experience more discomfort immediately after the procedure. Vaginal spotting or bleeding may occur for several days after the surgery.

66 What to say 99 — *Preparing the patient for cervical laser ablation*

Prior to the procedure, the nurse provides information, answers questions, and asks the patient to empty her bladder. The nurse may offer the following description of the procedure to help the patient understand what to expect:

- Medication will be given to decrease cramping and to numb the area to be treated.
- Everyone in the room will wear special glasses and surgical masks.
- Because laser burns or vaporizes cells, there will be a small amount of smoke present, and a smoke evacuator is used to remove the smoke from the air.

- The entire procedure (when done in the office or clinic) will take approximately 5 to 20 minutes, depending on the size of the abnormal area.
- Recovery time is minimal; most women leave within 20 minutes following the procedure.
- Some vaginal discharge is normal, but immediately report bleeding heavier than a menstrual period or yellow-green, foul-smelling discharge.
- A mild analgesic such as acetaminophen or ibuprofen may be taken as needed for pain, but severe abdominal pain should be reported immediately.
- Intercourse, douching, or the use of tampons should be avoided for 3 weeks.
- A fever above 100°F (38°C) should be reported immediately.
- Tub baths and showers may be taken, and you may return to work the day after the treatment.
- It is a good idea to ask a support person to accompany you to the appointment.
- Be sure to keep your follow-up appointment and follow your health-care provider's recommendations for repeat Pap testing.

Conization: Cold Knife Cone; Laser Conization; Loop Electrosurgical Excision Procedure (LEEP)

Conization of the cervix is defined as excision of a cone-shaped or cylindrical wedge from the uterine cervix that includes the transformation zone and all or a portion of the endocervical canal (Fig. 6-4). This procedure may be done when the lesion found on colposcopy extends into the endocervical canal and cannot be fully seen. Cold knife conization (CKC; also known as "cone biopsy") involves the use a scalpel without electrosurgical current; laser conization employs use of a laser for the excision of

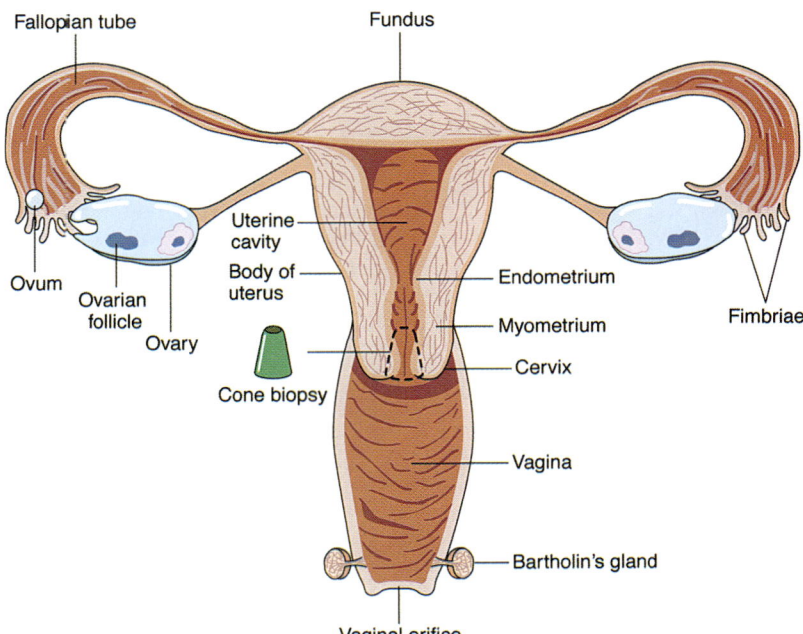

Figure 6-4 Cervical Conization (Source: From *Understanding Medical-Surgical Nursing,* 3rd ed., by L. S. Williams and P. D. Hopper, 2007, Philadelphia, F. A. Davis, p. 928.)

tissue. Cold knife and laser conization, which are usually performed in the hospital outpatient surgical center, may be done for diagnostic purposes, or for therapeutic purposes, to remove precancerous cells. Techniques for diagnostic and therapeutic conization are virtually identical. Depending on the circumstances and setting, patients may receive a local anesthetic with IV sedation, regional anesthesia, or general anesthesia. Potential complications of cervical conization include infection, bleeding, and cervical scarring or stenosis (narrowing); the procedure may also increase the risk of cervical incompetence and preterm birth (ACOG, 2008; Burkman, 2010; Shanbhag, Clark, Timmaraju, Bhattacharya, & Cruickshank, 2009).

Conization performed with electrosurgical loop is called the loop electrosurgical excision procedure (LEEP), or large loop excision of the transformation zone (LLETZ). LEEP uses a low-voltage electrical current to remove abnormal cervical tissue. With this procedure, the cervix is anesthetized with a local anesthetic, and a fine wire loop electrode is used to simultaneously remove and cauterize a portion of the cervix. The advantage of the electrosurgical loop procedure and other excisional techniques (e.g., CKC) over the ablative therapies (e.g., cryosurgery, laser vaporization) is that the tissue is removed, not destroyed. Thus, the tissue is available for evaluation by a pathologist. Also, the LEEP procedure is fast (20–30 minutes), virtually bloodless, and may be performed in the office. Following the procedure, healing is rapid, and there is only a mild vaginal discharge afterward. Patients may experience mild pain and cramping for the first few hours after the LEEP; the discomfort can be relieved by oral medications. Possible short- and long-term complications include bleeding, cervical stenosis, preterm birth, infertility, and loss of cervical mucus (ACOG, 2008; Burkman, 2010).

6️⃣ **What to say** — *Preparing the patient for cervical conization*

An important nursing role in caring for the patient who will undergo cervical conization centers on education and support. Prior to the conization, the nurse answers questions and addresses concerns. The nurse may offer the following description of the procedure to help the patient understand what to expect:

- The procedure will take less than 1 hour.

- Some form of anesthesia will be used to control pain.

- Depending on the type of anesthesia to be used, nothing should be taken by mouth for 8 hours prior to the procedure (when IV sedation or general anesthesia is planned).

- The physician will first insert a vaginal speculum and then use a knife (CKC), laser, or heated loop (LEEP) to remove a cone-shaped section of tissue (containing any abnormal cells) from the cervix.

- Self-absorbable sutures may be placed in the cervix to control bleeding.

- Analgesics may be taken as needed for pain control after the conization.

- If the conization is performed in an outpatient surgery center, and depending on the type of anesthesia used,

you may leave after you are fully awake, but someone must be with you to drive you home.

- If the conization is planned as an office procedure (LEEP), an electrosurgical dispersive pad (a gel-covered adhesive electrode that provides a safe return path for the electrosurgical current) will be placed on your thigh and removed after the procedure.

- Vaginal bleeding or discharge may be present for several days after the conization; a panty liner or sanitary napkin should be worn to protect clothing.

- Tampons, douches, and sexual intercourse should be avoided for 4 to 6 weeks.

- You should avoid lifting items heavier than 25 pounds for at least 1 week.

- Tub baths and showers may be taken as desired.

- Any signs of infection or other complications (e.g., fever, chills, foul-smelling discharge from the vagina, worsening abdominal pain, heavy vaginal bleeding [may not occur until about 1 week after the procedure, when the healing scar is shed from the cervix]) should be promptly reported to your health-care provider.

- It is important to return for the postoperative examination and to follow your health-care provider's recommendations for repeat Pap testing.

 Now Can You— Discuss diagnostic/treatment modalities for abnormal cervical cytological screening results?

1. Describe colposcopy, and explain how to prepare a patient for a colposcopic examination?
2. Discuss the importance of endocervical sampling?
3. Compare and contrast cervical cryosurgery, laser ablation, and conization, and provide patient teaching for each of these treatment modalities?

Human Papillomavirus

The human papillomavirus (HPV) is a DNA tumor virus that can infect cutaneous and mucosal surfaces, including the anogenital epithelium. Anogenital and cutaneous HPV infections are very common, but only a small fraction of genital infections actually progress to cancer. Cervical cancer, rarely found among women in celibate religious orders, has long been associated with intimate sexual activity. Owing to the rising epidemic of the sexually transmitted HPV infection, the average age of women with abnormal Pap test findings is declining steadily. HPV is most prevalent among the younger population of women, although it does occur with the same frequency in older women as well (Teitelman et al., 2009; Wysocki et al., 2007).

 Nursing Insight— *The papillomavirus–cancer link*

Many of the papilloma viruses cause papillomas. Papillomas are not cancers and are more commonly called warts. The most important risk factor in the development of cervical cancer is infection with a high-risk strain of HPV. The virus–cancer connection occurs as a result of alterations in the cervical cells that can lead to the development of CIN, which can then lead to cancer. HPV is passed from one individual to another during skin-to-skin contact. Although the virus is frequently transmitted during vaginal intercourse, anal intercourse, or oral sex, intercourse does not have to take place for HPV to be spread from one person to another. Skin-to-skin contact with an area of the body infected with HPV is the only requirement for transmission (ACS, 2010).

where research and practice meet:
Incidence of HPV infection in new sexual relationships

According to a recent study, more than half (56%) of young adults who reported that they were involved in a new sexual relationship were infected with HPV; of those, nearly half (44%) were infected with an HPV type that causes cancer. The results also indicated a high probability of HPV transmission between partners. When one partner had HPV, the researchers observed that in 42% of couples, the other partner also had the infection. If one partner was infected with HPV, the other partner's chance of also being infected with the same HPV type increased more than 50 times. The researchers concluded that the study findings support the belief that HPV infection is very common among young adults and underscore the importance of prevention programs for HPV-associated diseases such as cervical cancer screening and HPV vaccination (Burchell, Tellier, Hanley, Coutlee, & Franco, 2010).

HPVs are a family of more than 100 virus types with a multitude of manifestations that include common warts, plantar warts, skin cancers, anal and genital warts, recurrent respiratory papillomatosis (a rare, benign infection of type HPV 6 or 11—it passes from mothers to neonates during vaginal childbirth), head and neck cancers, genital cancers, and cervical cancer (Hellwig, 2006; Moore & Seybold, 2007; Schmidt, 2007). Young men and women between the ages of 15 and 24 account for approximately half of all new HPV infections (Cates, Brewer, Fazekas, Mitchell, & Smith, 2006).

Nursing Insight— *Maternal HPV and neonatal laryngeal papillomatosis*

Transmission to the infant of HPV type 6 or 11 is known to be possible during vaginal childbirth, but it is rare. Most experts believe that the risk of cesarean birth to both the mother and her infant exceeds the risk of neonatal genital warts or laryngeal papillomatosis (the presence of HPV 6– or 11–induced warts in the larynx or upper airway). However, cesarean birth may be indicated for women with genital warts if the pelvic outlet is obstructed or if vaginal birth would result in excessive bleeding. Once the maternal warts are no longer present, especially if the woman has had no detectable HPV lesions for 6 months or more, transmission of HPV to the infant during a vaginal birth becomes increasingly unlikely (ASCCP, 2010; CDC, 2006).

Of more than 100 known types of HPV, approximately 40 strains are believed to be capable of infecting the genital

tract. HPV types 6 and 11 have been identified as "low risk." These are the types most likely to be associated with condylomata acuminata (genital warts), benign cervical changes, and low-grade cervical intraepithelial lesions. Important associations have been identified between HPV type 16 and squamous cell carcinoma and between type 18 and cervical adenocarcinoma. In fact, these two HPV strains together are responsible for approximately 70% of all cervical cancers. Many other HPV types (i.e., types 31, 33, 35, 39, 45, 51, 56, 58, 59, 68, 73) are considered to be "high risk" (they carry the potential to cause cervical cancer), and one or more of these particular types is detected in nearly every patient diagnosed with cervical cancer (Moore & Seybold, 2007). High-risk HPV produces no visible symptoms; instead, it is detected by DNA testing for the virus, or on the basis of abnormal Pap test results. HPV is the primary cause of cervical neoplasia, and persistent infection with high-risk types of HPV constitutes the most significant risk factor for cervical cancer (ACS, 2010; Moore & Seybold, 2007; Teitelman et al., 2009; Woodson, 2008).

HPV DNA TESTING

Most HPV infections produce no symptoms, and frequently a woman learns that she has been exposed to the virus only after undergoing a routine Pap test. Reflex HPV DNA testing, performed on a sample of vaginal or cervical cells collected during a pelvic examination, is most commonly performed on cells collected from residual preservative when liquid-based cytology is used. The HPV DNA test can often be performed on the same sample collected for the Pap test. HPV DNA testing assesses exfoliated cervical cells for the presence of 1 or more of 13 or 14 of the 15 to 18 potentially cancer-causing HPV types (ACOG, 2009a; Gupton, 2007).

Optimizing Outcomes— Through co-testing: A combination of cytology + HPV DNA testing

Although the Pap test can detect cellular changes caused by high-risk types of HPV, it is not as sensitive as the HPV test, which specifically detects the viral DNA. DNA testing for HPV has gained widespread acceptance as an additional cervical cancer screening tool and as follow-up to abnormal changes detected with a Pap test. Today, there are several DNA HPV tests that can detect either the majority of the high-risk types of HPV or specific subtypes, such as HPV-16 and HPV-18. The tests are performed on cervical or vaginal cells collected through self-sampling or obtained by a health-care provider during a pelvic examination. Co-testing using the combination of cytology plus HPV DNA testing is an appropriate screening test for women older than 30 years. ACOG recommends that women 30 years or older be offered an HPV DNA test in addition to their Pap test and pelvic exam, and this recommendation is supported by various organizations, including the ACS, the National Institutes of Health (NIH), the ASCCP, the NPWH, and the American Medical Women's Association (AMWA). The HPV DNA test is not recommended for screening adolescents because infections with HPV are relatively common in this age group and often resolve without treatment or complications (ACOG, 2008; Duffy, 2008; Garfield, Gavaghan, Poret, & Ilika, 2010).

POTENTIAL MANIFESTATIONS OF HPV INFECTION

In women with HPV infection, abnormal findings on Pap screening are common. Of persons infected with HPV, only about 1% develop external genital warts, while approximately 10% develop cervical lesions. When present, HPV lesions most often occur on the posterior part of the vaginal introitus. Other locations include the buttocks, vulva, vagina, urethra, anus, and cervix. Four different types of genital warts have been identified (Box 6-3). It is possible to be infected with several different genotypes of HPV; some may be associated with a low risk, while others are associated with a high risk for the development of cervical cancer (ACOG, 2008; ACS, 2010; Moore & Seybold, 2007).

> **"What to say"** — *Counseling patients about abnormal Pap test results and HPV*

It is incumbent upon the nurse to listen generously to patient concerns about HPV and cervical cancer and offer support in coping with abnormal or positive results. Nurses should be sensitive to the fact that sharing the results of an abnormal Pap test with a patient can evoke feelings of anxiety, fear, and difficulty assimilating the implications of the results. In this situation, the nurse may wish to include the following information:

Your abnormal Pap test result is not a diagnosis of a disease; it merely alerts us to the fact that there is a need for closer surveillance (e.g., more frequent testing) or further evaluation (e.g., colposcopy). Because it takes so long for cervical changes caused by HPV to develop into cancer, women who obtain Pap tests regularly are very unlikely ever to develop cervical cancer because there is plenty of opportunity to identify and treat the problem at an early stage (ASCCP, 2010; Woodson, 2008).

HPV is an elusive virus with a clinical course that is characterized by spontaneous regressions and recurrences. Once a woman contracts genital HPV, she may develop a latent HPV infection, a subclinical HPV infection, a clinical HPV infection (manifested by the appearance of warts and/or cervical changes), or regression of the HPV lesions (Box 6-4). For most women, HPV infection resolves without intervention. It is estimated that up to 70% of HPV infections clear in 1 year and 91% of infected women do not have detectable levels of cervical

---

Box 6-4   Potential Manifestations of HPV Infection

Following exposure to HPV, one or more of the following may occur (ASCCP, 2010):

Latent HPV infection: No detectable warts are present (i.e., undetectable by visual inspection, cytology, or HPV testing) and the person is non-contagious. However, because the virus can move from latency to "expressed" HPV disease (e.g., warts, cervical cell changes), there is no guarantee that the person will remain noncontagious indefinitely.

Subclinical HPV infection: Applies to changes in the skin cells of the lower genital tract that cannot be seen with the naked eye. The most common subclinical change is intraepithelial neoplasia of the cervix (cervical "precancerous change," dysplasia, CIN 1, 2, or 3) that can be seen following the application of vinegar (acetic acid) to the skin, followed by close examination (e.g., colposcopy magnification) of areas that turn white (acetowhitening). Although subclinical HPV may appear anywhere in the lower genital tract, acetowhitening is very nonspecific and often unrelated to HPV. Tissue biopsy must be used to confirm the diagnosis of HPV infection.

Clinical HPV: The presence of warts and precancerous changes on the external genitalia (vulvar and perianal intraepithelial neoplasia; cervical and other lower genital tract cancers) that can be seen with the naked eye. Common clinical manifestations of HPV are:

- Condyloma acuminata: Raised, cauliflower-appearing (papillary) warts. Most are caused by the low-risk HPV 6 or 11 and are generally found on the external vulva, although they may also appear in the vagina, cervix, and anus.
- Condyloma planum: "Flat" warts; although most are caused by HPV 16 or other high-risk types, they should be treated as genital warts and not as a true precancerous condition.
- High-grade intraepithelial neoplasia: "Precancerous" flat HPV lesions that may appear on the vulva and the perianal and anal canal area. They can be very white (due to thick layers of keratin) or red (due to an increased blood supply) or various shades of brown to dark gray (due to increased pigment).
- Cancer: HPV is the cause of virtually all cancers of the cervix, as well as about 80% of vaginal cancers and 90% of anal cancers. In any of these areas, the cancer may appear as a nodule, erosion, ulcer, or thickening.

Immune mediated regression:

- Most HPV lesions eventually resolve because of a host immune response to the virus. This is especially true for genital warts and CIN 1 because neither is truly precancer. Approximately 40%–50% of CIN 2 will resolve spontaneously; CIN 3 is considered a true cancer precursor, although some CIN 3 may resolve spontaneously to an immune-mediated regression.
- It is not known whether an immune-mediated regression clears that particular HPV type from the body completely or just suppresses it to the point where it is not likely to be contagious or cause HPV-induced disease in the future.

Box 6-3   Types of Genital Warts

Condyloma acuminata are soft, moist, pink, red, or gray lesions that may occur singularly or in multiples. The warts occur on moist surfaces and often cluster to form a cauliflower shape.

Smooth papular warts are small dome-shaped papules that are usually skin colored. They occur on hair-bearing or non-hair-bearing skin and do not occur on mucosal tissue.

Keratotic genital warts have a thick layer and often look like "common" warts. They develop on hair-bearing or on non-hair-bearing skin and other non-skin tissues.

Flat warts are generally flat or slightly raised with flat tops. These lesions can occur on moist or on dry tissue (Wysocki et al., 2007).

HPV infection after 2 years. It is unknown whether the virus is truly absent or is simply reduced to undetectable levels. For the remaining 10% of women, persistent infection with certain types of HPV constitutes the major risk factor for cervical cancer (Dunne & Markowitz, 2006; Frazer et al., 2006; Schmidt, 2007).

> *Nursing Insight*— *HPV and chronological age*

HPV infections are most common in teenagers and women in their early 20s, with prevalence decreasing as women age. Most women will come in contact with HPV shortly after they become sexually active; by age 50, more than 80% of women will have had HPV at some time in their lives. In adolescents and young women, HPV infections and dysplasia (precancerous changes) are likely to resolve spontaneously. This finding suggests that HPV infections detected in older women are more likely to reflect persistent infections acquired in the past (ACOG, 2009a; ASCCP, 2010; Lara-Torre & Murchison, 2009).

The triggers that activate HPV and cause abnormal cell growth, as well as why some lesions heal on their own and others become precancerous, are not known. Cervical infections are caused by a group of about 15 oncogenic (cancer causing) types of HPV. Persistent infection with these viruses can lead to a precancerous condition. While the vast majority of cervical HPV infections (including those caused by the oncogenic types) heal through the body's natural immune response, some of them persist and can eventually progress to invasive cervical cancer. The strains most strongly associated with cervical cancer are types 16, 18, 31, and 45, and a few others, to a lesser degree. However, in most women with high-risk types of cervical HPV, cervical cancer will not develop (Kiviat, Hawes, & Feng, 2008; NPWH, 2007).

 Nursing Insight— *Routine clinical examinations for HPV are not performed with STD screening*

Couples who are contemplating a sexual relationship should always be encouraged to undergo STD testing prior to initiating intercourse. However, because HPV is so very common and most often undetectable, neither the CDC nor the American Medical Association recommends clinical examinations for HPV as a component of STD screening.

 Now Can You— **Discuss certain aspects of HPV?**

1. Identify the population at highest risk for contracting HPV?
2. Briefly discuss the link between HPV and cervical cancer?
3. Explain the process of "co-testing" and identify patients for whom this procedure is most appropriate?

THE NURSING ROLE IN REDUCING PATIENT RISK FOR CERVICAL CANCER

Currently, researchers continue to investigate factors that may promote the development of cervical cancer. The role and the progression of HPV-induced lesions into cancer have recently become clearer. Research has demonstrated that cigarette smoking interferes with women's ability to clear an HPV infection and is associated with an increased risk of new HPV infection, persistent HPV infection, and cervical cancer. Also, a dose–response relationship with the amount of tobacco consumed has been noted (Lindstrom et al., 2008; Oh, Ju, Franceschi, Quint, & Shin, 2008). Other potential factors that link HPV with cervical cancer include long-term oral contraceptive use, young age, nutritional deficiency, presence of other genital tract infections, and immunodeficiency, such as occurs with HIV infection. For women with a healthy immune system, it may take decades for cervical cancer to develop from an initial exposure to high-risk viral types (Moore & Seybold, 2007; NPWH, 2007; Wysocki et al., 2007).

 Optimizing Outcomes— **Identifying risk factors associated with HPV infection and HPV-related cervical disease**

To guide clinical HPV screening and educational efforts, nurses who work with women of all ages should be aware of certain risk factors that are associated with HPV infection and/or HPV-related cervical disease (Escobar & Orr, 2008), including the following:

- A sex partner more than 2 years older
- More than three lifetime sex partners
- A new sex partner in the last 12 months
- Illegal drug use in the last 12 months
- Engaging in intercourse while impaired by alcohol
- Never having been married

A recent review of the literature revealed that several studies have linked HPV and cervical cancer to intimate partner violence in women, likely because women victims are less able to successfully negotiate strategies for safer sex, such as condom usage and monogamy, with an abusive partner. Women who have sex with women (WSW) are also at risk of contracting HPV. Although less common than heterosexual transmission, woman-to-woman HPV transmission is possible. Many WSW also report a history of sexual encounters with men. WSW may be less likely to seek regular pelvic examinations and Pap tests, although these health-promoting practices are recommended for women regardless of their sexual partners' gender (Coker, 2007; Hutchinson, Thompson, & Cederbaum, 2006; Marazzo, Koutski, Kiviat, Kuypers, & Stine, 2001; Teitelman et al., 2009).

An important role for nurses in reproductive health promotion centers on counseling and education about strategies to enhance the immune system and reduce the risk for contracting HPV and other STDs. For example, the nurse can teach patients that refraining from smoking; limiting the use of alcohol; consuming a healthy, nutritious diet; and avoiding exposure to chemical and environmental hazards are health practices that enhance the strength of the immune system. Observing sexual abstinence or, if sexually active, consistently using condoms or receiving prophylactic HPV vaccination are other preventive strategies to reduce the risk for infection. The nurse can counsel women that they can lower their chance of getting HPV by remaining in a faithful relationship with one partner, by limiting the number of sex partners, and by choosing a partner who has had no or few prior sex partners (ASCCP, 2010; CDC, 2009).

 Optimizing Outcomes— **Heightening HPV awareness: The AWHONN "Be Confident!" campaign**

In January 2010, the Association of Women's Health, Obstetric and Neonatal Nurses (AWHONN) launched the "Be Confident!" campaign for adolescents and parents. The grant-funded program features brochures, posters, articles, and a public service announcement to educate adolescents and young women about HPV and encourage informed decisions about cervical health issues. Available in English and Spanish, the comic book–style posters and brochures are intended to encourage open discussions between young women and their parents and health-care providers. According to the organization, outreach to the Hispanic community constitutes a heavy emphasis of the campaign. Hispanic females have the highest incidence of cervical cancer among all groups of women and often experience disparities in access to cervical cancer screening and access to information related to cervical cancer screening and prevention (AWHONN, 2010). AWHONN is distributing the educational materials to health-care providers and community health settings; additional copies may be downloaded at www.awhonn.org/HPV.

The patient with genital warts may benefit from HPV counseling sessions that include her intimate partner. Meeting with both partners provides an opportunity for the couple to learn that HPV infection is common and probably shared between partners and affords the possibility for other STD evaluation and screening along with Pap screening. The nurse can again emphasize the importance of routine cytological screening for cervical cancer (CDC, 2006).

Optimizing Outcomes— **With condoms to reduce the risk of contracting HPV**

Latex condoms offer some protection against HPV, and consistent condom use appears to reduce the risk of HPV transmission by about 70%. However, condoms protect only those areas of skin that they cover—and many infected individuals have HPV in non-covered areas of their skin that come into contact with their partner's skin. Secretions may also be a source of HPV-infected skin cells that could come into contact with a partner's uncovered skin areas. Spermicides and condoms coated with spermicide are not effective in preventing HPV and may cause microscopic abrasions that facilitate transmission of HPV and other STDs. Because female condoms cover more of the female introital epithelium at risk for HPV, they may provide a more protective barrier for both partners. However, the female condom may also be more easily dislodged during intercourse (ASCCP, 2010).

"What to say" — *When discussing HPV with patients*

When discussing HPV, the nurse can be instrumental in dispelling various myths and misconceptions about genital HPV. Providing current, evidence-based information empowers the woman to make informed choices and decisions about her reproductive health. Depending on the situation, sharing the following information may be appropriate:

Genital HPV is very common. It is primarily transmitted through sexual contact involving genital skin, and penetrative intercourse is not required. The only way to entirely eliminate the possibility of being exposed to HPV is abstinence from any form of genital–genital or oral–genital contact. The lifetime likelihood of getting genital HPV is estimated at 75 to 90%, and the risk of exposure to HPV is estimated to be approximately 15 to 25% per partner. That is, for every sexual partner one has, there is up to a 25% chance of being exposed to some type of HPV. Because HPV rarely causes symptoms, most people who get HPV never know they have it—they do not develop genital warts, receive an abnormal Pap test result, or develop any other manifestations of HPV that they can identify. An HPV diagnosis does not necessarily mean that your partner has not been monogamous; it means only that the infection was contracted at some point in that person's life. HPV testing is not indicated for partners of persons with genital warts. An abnormal Pap test result does not necessarily mean that a woman is at high risk for cervical cancer. The abnormal result can be related to infection, local irritation, a low-risk HPV type, or a higher risk HPV type. Depending on the degree of abnormality, further evaluation or a follow-up Pap test obtained 3 months later may be rec ommended. Reflex HPV DNA testing may obviate the need for repeated Pap tests—and if no high-risk HPV types are identified, the Pap test may be repeated in 1 year. Only one in four cases of cervical lesions, if left untreated, will progress to cancer, and treatment is almost always successful in preventing cancer if the cells are discovered early. Undergoing routine Pap testing according to the recommendations of your health-care provider is an important preventive strategy (ASCCP, 2010; CDC, 2006).

HPV VACCINES

A vaccine (Gardasil) against HPV types 6, 11, 16, and 18 became available in 2006. Gardasil is the first HPV vaccine in the United States. The quadrivalent recombinant (non-live virus) vaccine is recommended for females ages 9 to 26 years. (The quadrivalent HPV vaccine may also be given to males ages 9 through 26 years to reduce their likelihood of acquiring genital warts; ideally the vaccine should be administered before potential exposure to HPV through sexual contact.) Vaccination consists of three intramuscular injections given over 6 months, with the second dose to be given 2 months after the first dose and the third dose given 6 months after the first dose. If the HPV vaccine schedule is interrupted, the vaccine series does not need to be restarted (ASCCP, 2010; CDC, 2009; Moore & Seybold, 2007; Wysocki et al., 2007).

The HPV vaccine is supplied in prefilled syringes for single use only and in single-use vials; the vials must be stored under refrigeration and protected from light. The vaccine is highly protective, especially when the vaccination occurs before sexual activity. Although the vaccine does not prevent infection with all types of HPV, it provides protection against the HPV types associated with 70% of cervical cancers (16, 18), and 90% of external genital warts (6, 11). However, if a woman has already been infected with HPV 16, 18, 6, or 11, the vaccine offers no protection, and only limited or no protection against the other HPV types. Hence, the protection afforded by the vaccine is lower in women who have had sex prior to vaccination. The quadrivalent vaccine has also been demonstrated to protect against vulvar and vaginal cancers (ASCCP, 2010; CDC, 2009; Moore & Seybold, 2007; Wysocki et al., 2007).

Cervarix is a bivalent vaccine that protects against HPV 16 and 18. Approved by the FDA in 2009, Cervarix also consists of three intramuscular injections given over 6 months; the second dose is given 1 month after the first dose and the third dose is given 6 months after the first dose (ASCCP, 2010; CDC, 2009; Moore & Seybold, 2007; Wysocki et al., 2007).

 ### Be sure to— Offer HPV vaccines to appropriate patients

It is important that an HPV vaccine be administered before people become sexually active. The CDC's Advisory Committee on Immunization Practices (CDC ACIP, 2009) recommends that Gardasil and Cervarix be routinely given to girls when they are 11 or 12 years old. However, Gardasil can be started as early as age 9 and can also be given to women 13 to 26 years old. Cervarix is approved for use in females 10 through 25 years of age. Although the vaccine series should begin before the initiation of sexual intercourse, a "catch-up" series is recommended for young women in the older age group who are already sexually active. HPV vaccines are not recommended for use in pregnant women, but pregnancy testing is not needed before vaccination. Completion of the HPV vaccine series should occur before pregnancy or after a pregnancy is complete. The HPV vaccines are contraindicated for persons with a history of immediate hypersensitivity to any vaccine component. The quadrivalent HPV vaccine (Gardasil) is contraindicated for persons with a history of immediate hypersensitivity to yeast. The bivalent HPV vaccine (Cervarix) in prefilled syringes is contraindicated for persons with an anaphylactic latex allergy. Because the HPV vaccines are not live vaccines, they may be administered either simultaneously or at any time before or after an inactivated or live vaccine. Syncope may occur after vaccination; to avoid patient injury related to a syncopal episode, the nurse should consider observing the patient for 15 minutes after the vaccination is administered. The most commonly reported adverse reactions to the vaccinations include pain, redness, and swelling at the injection site and fatigue, headache, muscle and joint aches, and gastrointestinal distress. Since the vaccines do not cover all of the HPV types that can cause cervical cancer, routine Pap test screening is still recommended for those who have been vaccinated against HPV (CDC, 2009; Markowitz et al., 2007; Rome & Hicks, 2009).

 ### Be sure to— Be knowledgeable about immunization laws in your practice state

Federal law does not explicitly require parental consent for immunizations such as the HPV vaccine. However, it does require that prior to administration the parent or guardian receive federally mandated vaccine information statements on any immunizations their children will receive. State law is the authority on whether parental consent is required. Minor consent laws are based on status (e.g., emancipated, married, in armed services, "mature" minor, pregnant, incarcerated) and services they are seeking (e.g., pregnancy-related care, family planning, and sexual health services) (Burns, Walsh, & Popovich, 2010; English, Shaw, McCauley, & Fishbein, 2008). It is essential that the health-care provider have an understanding of the laws in the particular practice state; this information is available at www.cahl.org.

 ### Be sure to— Comply with federal mandates regarding HPV vaccination for immigrant women

Although compulsory HPV vaccination is not currently mandated for any U.S. population, immigrant women aged 11–26 years are now required to receive the first injection (of the three doses) of the vaccine as a result of the 1996 Illegal Immigration Reform and Immigrant Responsibility Act. According to this law, immigrants applying for visas to enter the United States or to adjust their immigration status must receive the inoculations that the CDC ACIP recommends for U.S. residents (Hachey, Allen, Nothnagle, & Boardman, 2009).

 ### where research and practice meet: Identifying disparities in attitudes, acceptability, and beliefs about the HPV vaccine

Several epidemiological and behavioral studies have identified disparities in attitudes, acceptability, and beliefs about the HPV vaccine (Burns et al., 2010). Watts and colleagues (2009) found that acceptance of the HPV vaccine was high among Latina women for themselves and their daughters, and this was primarily motivated by concern for cancer prevention. An investigation by Cates and colleagues (2009) discovered racial differences between African American and Caucasian in HPV knowledge in a rural Southern U.S. sample; Caucasian were significantly more informed about the HPV vaccine. African American were significantly less likely to perceive cervical cancer as a threat to their daughters' health and had lower intentions to vaccinate their daughters against HPV than whites. Based on their research, Gottlieb and Brewer (2009) concluded that the demographic factors of race and educational level were found to influence the use of information sources to learn about the HPV vaccine; this finding may be used to guide communication-based interventions for future research and practice. Other investigators (Brewer & Fazekas, 2007; Fazekas, Brewer, & Smith, 2008; Kahn et al., 2008; Marshall, Phillip, Don, & Peter, 2007) reported factors (i.e., lack of insurance or resources to pay for the vaccine, perception that the vaccine is unsafe, fear that receipt of the vaccine would encourage sexual behavior, and personal perception of being at low risk for HPV and cervical cancer) that may inhibit patients' intention to receive the HPV vaccine or parents' intention to have their child receive the HPV vaccine. These studies highlight the importance of the nurse's role in developing culturally appropriate health promotion programs that target vaccination education and outreach. To successfully accomplish this goal, nurses must seek the latest evidence-based information about vaccines, remain knowledgeable about current vaccination guidelines, and possess an awareness of various behavioral disparities that place some populations at greater risk than others (Burns et al., 2010; Theroux, 2008).

 ### Collaboration in Caring— *Securing funding resources for HPV vaccination*

Most health insurance plans cover the recommended HPV vaccines, although some plans may not cover any or all vaccines. The Vaccines for Children (VFC) program helps families of eligible children who may not otherwise have access to vaccines. The program provides vaccines at no cost to physicians who serve eligible children. Children younger than 19 years of age are eligible for VFC vaccines if they are Medicaid eligible, American Indian, Alaska Native, or have no health insurance. "Underinsured children" who have health insurance that does not cover vaccination can receive VFC vaccines through Federally Qualified Health Centers or Rural Health Centers (CDC, 2009). For more information about the program, nurses may visit the CDC Web site at www.cdc.gov/vaccines/programs/vfc/.

AWHONN supports HPV vaccination for the prevention of cervical cancer along with regular cervical cancer screening with Papanicolaou and HPV tests, as recommended. The organization also supports policies that ensure universal access to HPV vaccination and cervical cancer screening and treatment. In the revised and reaffirmed "HPV Vaccination for the Prevention of Cervical Cancer" Position Statement (November, 2009), AWHONN endorsed the establishment of adolescent health visits (to include health counseling, physical assessment, and vaccinations) and called for the establishment of programs specifically designed to educate young women and men, parents, and providers about HPV and the importance of HPV vaccination.

In an effort to increase public awareness of the need for vaccination, Merck (manufacturer of Gardasil) launched a multimedia campaign about HPV and cervical cancer prevention using their vaccine. Other organizations including the CDC and the National Federation of Planned Parenthood have created consumer education Web sites. And recently, the Society for Adolescent Medicine, the National Basketball Association, the Women's National Basketball Association, and Sanofi Pasteur (a vaccine manufacturer) have collaborated in launching a national program designed to heighten public awareness of the importance of vaccinations for teens.

 Collaboration in Caring— *A team approach to a teen-targeted immunization campaign*

The NBA and the WNBA have collaborated with the Society for Adolescent Medicine and Sanofi Pasteur (a vaccine manufacturer) to create "Vaccines for Teens," a national program designed to educate parents and their teens about the need to get vaccinated. The campaign Web site (www.vaccinesforteens.net/) is one component of the larger effort to make parents and teens aware of the dangers of four serious diseases (meningococcal disease/meningococcal meningitis, pertussis, influenza, and HPV) that can easily be spread from person to person. The Web site, which includes a brief athlete-narrated video, describes each disease and provides links for additional resources.

HPV EDUCATION AND COUNSELING FOR TEENS AND THEIR PARENTS

An essential area for nurses in HPV awareness and prevention centers on education and counseling for adolescents and teens and their parents. Because both males and females may be at risk for acquiring HPV, educational efforts should target both genders (Pollack, Balkin, Edouard, Cutts, & Broutet, 2007). It is important that reproductive health counseling provide developmentally appropriate information. Preteens tend to be concrete thinkers, and teenagers are more likely to engage in risky health behaviors. Understanding the tasks associated with normal adolescent development is an essential element that guides the nurse in establishing and directing a therapeutic dialogue. Communicating with young patients about HPV, the HPV vaccine, and other health issues may be enhanced by listening attentively, using terms the adolescent understands, remaining focused, and avoiding lectures and writing during the course of the conversation (Neinstein, 2008).

 Nursing Insight— *Understanding normal adolescent development*

The period of adolescence is characterized by rapid physical, emotional, and intellectual changes and development. Developmental tasks of adolescence center on establishing autonomy and identity, integrating physical changes into a new body image, and operating within the peer group. Adolescents experience feelings of invulnerability that may lead to an increased willingness to expose them to risk. Adolescents often tend to underestimate the personal risk of health hazards and unhealthful behaviors (Kahn, 2008; Woodson, 2008).

During the course of the conversation, it is helpful to focus on strategies to minimize HPV risk (e.g., minimizing sexual partners, using condoms, avoiding smoking) and discuss the HPV vaccination in terms of its value for the prevention of genital warts and cervical dysplasia. The nurse should emphasize the importance of completing the HPV vaccine series, once initiated. The nurse can encourage the teen to take responsibility for her health by discussing how a healthy lifestyle can contribute to disease prevention. Teens should also be reminded of the importance of cervical cancer screening beginning at age 21 (Taylor & Smith, 2009; Woodson, 2008).

 Optimizing Outcomes— NASPAG: A resource for health professionals who provide gynecologic care for adolescents

The North American Society for Pediatric and Adolescent Gynecology (NASPAG) is a nonprofit organization dedicated to educating health-care professionals in pediatric and adolescent gynecology. NASPAG's mission is to provide a forum for education, research and communication among health professionals who provide gynecological care to children and adolescents. The Web address for NASPAG is www.naspag.org.

Nurses can also teach parents about strategies to enhance effective HPV communication with their daughters. Some parents may believe that giving their daughters the HPV vaccine somehow implies that they are encouraging sexual activity. In this situation, it may be beneficial to use a seat belt analogy: Just as the seat belt does not give someone permission to drive recklessly, the HPV vaccination does not imply that it is okay to have sex (Woodson, 2008). Nurses should encourage frequent, age-appropriate dialogue between parents and their children. For younger girls, ongoing parent–adolescent communication about issues such as personal sexual risk and partner relationship dynamics is an important strategy in STD prevention (Teitelman et al., 2009). The nurse can model for parents how to have honest, open communications about HPV information and use discussion about HPV and the vaccine as a basis for future discussions about sexuality and reproductive health as their daughters grow older (Woodson, 2008). Parent–daughter communication about partner sexual pressure has been associated with increased condom use (Teitelman, Ratcliffe, & Cederbaum, 2008).

TREATMENT FOR HPV

The risk of developing genital warts after sexual intercourse with someone who has warts is greater than 65%. Once exposed to genital warts, most individuals will develop them within 4 weeks to 8 months. Genital warts are usually not painful, but they can interfere with normal bodily functions, such as urination and defecation, making these actions painful and uncomfortable. Although no treatment has been developed for latent HPV infection, several therapies are available to manage external genital warts and clearly identifiable subclinical HPV lesions on the vulva, cervix, and vagina. The goal of all therapies is to destroy the visible lesions and reduce patient symptoms. In the majority of patients, treatment produces wart-free periods. Treatment, however, does not eliminate HPV infection. Eradication of the virus is not considered to be conclusive even after there is no visible evidence of wart tissue because of the high incidence of recurrence (Woodson, 2008).

 Optimizing Outcomes— With treatment for HPV

Treatment options for HPV include the provider-administered medications podophyllin resin, trichloroacetic acid (TCA), or bichloracetic acid (BCA), which are carefully applied to each wart and allowed to air-dry. Patient-applied medications include podofilox solution or gel (Condylox) and imiquimod cream (Aldara). Podophyllin, podofilox, and imiquimod should not be used during pregnancy. No one treatment is ideal for all warts. Surgical therapies used to eliminate the lesions include cryosurgery, manual excision, electrosurgical excision, and laser vaporization. Injection of interferon is another treatment but one that is usually reserved for recurrent lesions unresponsive to standard treatments such as cryosurgery with liquid nitrogen or cryoprobe, electrocautery, and laser vaporization. Interferon is a naturally occurring substance that boosts the immune system and interferes with the ability of viruses to reproduce (CDC, 2006).

One's degree of contagiousness following treatment depends on how successful the treatment was in destroying the HPV lesions (where potentially infectious HPV particles are known to be present) and how successful the individual's immunity is in suppressing any HPV that might still be present in apparently normal skin. Most people treated for external warts do not experience a complete resolution even after several treatments. This is because most treatments destroy the HPV lesions but cannot eliminate any HPV in surrounding apparently normal skin. Until the individual's immune system responds and suppresses the remaining HPV, new lesions may appear (ASCCP, 2010).

Once no further HPV lesions are detectable by clinical exam, and no new lesions have appeared over several subsequent months, the chance of shedding enough HPV to be contagious dramatically falls. Although it is impossible to advise anyone exactly when they have little to no chance of passing HPV to a partner, as months pass with no new lesions found by a clinician, the possibility of being contagious becomes increasingly remote (ASCCP, 2010).

Now Can You— Discuss HPV education, vaccination, and treatment?

1. Develop HPV educational programs specifically suited for adolescents, parents of adolescents, reproductive-age women, and older women?
2. Identify six risk factors associated with HPV infection and HPV-related cervical disease?
3. Discuss HPV vaccination: identify who should receive the vaccines, how and when the vaccines should be given, nursing implications for administration, and patient education concerning vaccination?
4. Identify medical and surgical treatment modalities for HPV-related genital warts?

Cervical Cancer

Cervical cancer is a malignant neoplasm that forms in the tissues of the cervix. Worldwide, cervical cancer is the second most common type of cancer in women. It is much less common in the United States because of the routine use of cervical cytological screening. Cervical cancers originate in the cells on the surface of the cervix, which are composed of squamous and columnar epithelium.

Nursing Insight— The uterine cervix and cervical cancers

Approximately 80% to 90% of cervical cancers are squamous cell carcinomas—neoplasms that originate in the squamous cells that cover the surface of the exocervix. Most of the remaining cervical cancers are adenocarcinomas, which are becoming increasingly more common in women born in the last 20 to 30 years. Cervical adenocarcinoma develops from the mucus-producing gland cells of the endocervix. Less commonly, cervical cancers have features of both squamous cell carcinomas and adenocarcinomas and are called adenosquamous carcinomas or mixed carcinomas (ACS, 2009).

The development of cervical cancer, which is typically a very slow process, begins as dysplasia, a precancerous condition. Dysplasia, which can be detected by a Pap test, is 100% treatable. Most women who are diagnosed with cervical cancer today have not had regular Pap tests or they have not followed up on abnormal results. Undetected, precancerous changes can develop into cervical cancer and spread to the bladder, intestines, lungs, and liver (ACS, 2009).

 ### Collaboration in Caring— *The Pearl of Wisdom Campaign to Prevent Cervical Cancer*

The Pearl of Wisdom Campaign to Prevent Cervical Cancer is a united, global effort to raise awareness of the opportunities now available to prevent cervical cancer. The campaign reaches women, health-care providers, policy makers, health advocates, and the media in an effort to increase awareness of the new means of preventing cervical cancer, encourage women to take full advantage of these methods, and advocate for the implementation of these tools for girls and women everywhere. The Pearl of Wisdom Campaign was started by the European Cervical Cancer Association, which includes 100 organizations from across Europe, including cancer charities, cancer treatment centers, medical associations, university teaching hospitals, and health education organizations. The campaign promotes the "Pearl of Wisdom" as the global symbol for cervical cancer prevention in the same way as the pink ribbon serves the breast cancer campaign. Launched in the United States in 2009, the campaign is led by the national nonprofit organization Tamika and Friends, Inc. All profits from purchases of the Pearl of Wisdom pin go to the U.S. Pearl of Wisdom Campaign Fund to support cervical cancer prevention activities. Campaign partners, which include more than 24 national as well as local women's health and advocacy organizations, distribute simple, consistent key messages about cervical cancer to ensure that their collective voices effectively reach women. Additional information about the Pearl of Wisdom Campaign to Prevent Cervical Cancer may be found at the organization Web site: www.pearlofwisdom.us/about_us.

RISK FACTORS

Although the exact mechanism for the progression of cervical cancer is unknown, several key contributing factors have been identified (Box 6-5). Nurses must remain up-to-date about cancer risk factors so that they can appropriately identify and screen individuals at risk and provide accurate, culturally centered patient counseling and education. As is true in other areas of health promotion, it is useful to focus teaching efforts on risk factors such as lifestyle choices (e.g., tobacco and alcohol use, diet, sexual practices, HPV exposure) over which the woman has some control.

 ### *Ethnocultural Considerations*— Cervical cancer

Cervical cancer disproportionately affects low-income women and women of color. The CDC (2008) estimates that cervical cancer treatment costs $160 million each year. In this country, cervical cancer occurs most often in Hispanic women, at a rate that is more than twice what is seen in non-Hispanic Caucasian women. African American women develop this cancer about 50% more often than non-Hispanic Caucasian women and have the highest mortality (ACS, 2010). In Caucasian women in the United States, the rate of new-onset cer-

---

Box 6-5 Cervical Cancer Risk Factors

- HPV infection (the most important risk factor)
- Cigarette smoking (doubles the risk for cervical cancer)
- Immunosuppression (HIV increases the likelihood for infection with HPV, which increases the risk for cervical cancer. Also, the immune system normally destroys/slows the growth of cancer cells)
- Co-infection with other STDs (e.g., Chlamydia, herpes simplex virus)
- Diet (low in fruits and vegetables increases the risk; obesity increases the risk of cervical adenocarcinoma)
- Early onset of sexual activity (before age 16)
- Inadequate cervical screening
- Male sexual partner who has had other partners, especially if a previous partner had cervical cancer
- Multiple sexual partners (three or more in a lifetime)
- An uncircumcised sexual partner
- Oral contraceptives (long-term use increases the risk; however, the risk returns to normal after discontinuation)
- Multiple full-term pregnancies (three or more full-term pregnancies are associated with an increased risk; reasons unknown)
- Young age at first full-term pregnancy (women younger than 17 years with first full-term pregnancy are almost two times more likely to get cervical cancer later in life than those who postpone pregnancy until 25 years or older)
- Poverty (most likely related to lack of cervical cancer screening)
- In utero exposure to diethylstilbestrol (DES) (increased risk for clear-cell adenocarcinoma of the vagina or cervix; risk is greatest if DES exposure occurred during the first 16 weeks of pregnancy; there may also be an increased risk of squamous cell cancers and precancers of the cervix linked to HPV)
- Family history of cervical cancer (if the mother or a sister had cervical cancer, the woman's chances of developing the condition are two to three times higher)
- Alcoholism

Sources: ACS (2009); Moore & Seybold (2007); Wysocki et al. (2007).

---

vical cancer peaks in the middle of the fifth decade of life and then decreases. The peak incidence in Hispanics is in the early 70s, and for women of Asian or Pacific Island ethnicity, the incidence peaks in the late 70s. The incidence of cervical cancer continues to increase throughout life in African American women in the United States (Ries et al., 2009). Factors that may influence cervical screening behaviors for these populations of women include a lack of a health promotion/disease prevention perspective, a lack of knowledge about Pap tests, financial barriers, and failure of health-care providers to recommend screening (Giarratano, Bustamante-Forest, & Carter; Wysocki et al., 2007).

SYMPTOMS

Most of the time, early cervical cancer produces no symptoms. In fact, patients with cervical cancer usually do not experience any problems until the cancer is advanced and has spread. An important nursing role in cervical cancer education centers on emphasizing the importance of routine cervical cancer screening and teaching women about symptoms that may be associated with cancer of the cervix.

Optimizing Outcomes— Teaching about symptoms of cervical cancer

Nurses should emphasize that although early cervical cancer usually produces no symptoms, patients should remain alert to the following signs and symptoms that may be associated with the disease:

- Continuous vaginal discharge, which may be pale, watery, pink, brown, bloody, or foul smelling
- Abnormal vaginal bleeding between menstrual periods, after intercourse, or after menopause
- Menstrual periods that become heavier and last longer than usual
- Any vaginal bleeding after menopause

Signs and symptoms that may be associated with *advanced* cervical cancer include:

- Loss of appetite
- Weight loss
- Fatigue
- Pelvic pain
- Back pain
- Leg pain
- Single swollen leg
- Heavy vaginal bleeding
- Leaking of urine or feces from the vagina
- Bone fractures

 Optimizing Outcomes— With a new tool to predict cervical cancer risk

A new tool for assessing cervical cancer risk may offer health-care professionals a simpler method for making treatment decisions. Katki and colleagues (2009) at the National Cancer Institute are developing a tool that uses cervical precancer (i.e., CIN Grade 3 or higher) as a common treatment threshold. The tool, which is based on the established predictability of cervical precancer, will allow clinicians to use their personal digital assistants or computers to accurately calculate a patient's current, 1-year, 3-year, and 5-year risk of developing cervical precancer based on the woman's age, current test results, and available past test results. This information can then be used to guide development of an appropriate plan of care.

DIAGNOSTIC WORKUP AND TREATMENT OF CERVICAL CANCER

Once a diagnosis of cervical cancer has been made, the physician orders additional tests to determine if the cancer is confined to the local area or has spread to distant organs. This process is termed *staging*. Tests that may be appropriate include x-ray computed tomography (CT scan), magnetic resonance imaging (MRI), positron emission tomography (PET scan), cystoscopy, chest x-ray, and intravenous pyelogram (IVP). The cancer stage is based on where the cancer is found (Box 6-6).

Treatment for cervical cancer depends on the stage of the cancer—whether it is localized or has spread to surrounding tissues or distant organs. A high-grade, preinvasive lesion (i.e., carcinoma in situ [CIS]) is removed to

---

Box 6-6 Stages of Invasive Cervical Cancer

STAGE I
The tumor has invaded the cervix beneath the top layer of cells. Cancer cells are located only in the cervix.

STAGE II
The tumor extends to the upper part of the vagina. It may extend beyond the cervix into nearby tissues toward the pelvic wall. The tumor does not invade the lower third of the vagina or the pelvic wall.

STAGE III
The tumor extends to the lower part of the vagina. It may also have invaded the pelvic wall. If the tumor blocks the flow of urine, one or both kidneys may not be working well.

STAGE IV
The tumor invades the bladder or rectum, or the cancer has spread to other parts of the body.

RECURRENT CANCER
The cancer was treated but has returned after a time during which it could not be detected. The cancer may show up again in the cervix or in other parts of the body.

Source: NCI (2009).

---

prevent progression to invasive disease. A conization procedure is usually recommended, although hysterectomy may be advised, depending on the individual situation (ACOG, 2009a).

 Nursing Insight— *Factors that influence cervical cancer prognosis*

A number of factors influence the prognosis for a woman who has received a diagnosis of cervical cancer. These factors include the type of cancer, the stage of the disease, and the woman's age and general physical condition. Precancerous conditions are completely curable when followed up and treated properly. The 5-year survival rate for cancer that has not spread beyond the cervical area is 92%. However, the 5-year survival rate falls steadily as the cancer extends to other areas in the body (NCI, 2009).

 Collaboration in Caring— *Using a team approach to facilitate treatment of cervical cancer*

Depending on the cervical cancer stage, the health-care provider may wish to refer the woman to the care of a gynecological oncologist, a surgeon who specializes in treating gynecological cancers. Other members of the health-care team who may be involved in the patient's treatment plan include medical oncologists, radiation oncologists, oncology nurses, mental health professionals, and registered dieticians.

Surgery

For invasive cancer, radiation can be used alone or in combination with some form of surgery. Surgery options range from cervical conization to radical hysterectomy. A radical trachelectomy involves removal of the cervix, part of the vagina, and the lymph nodes in the pelvis. This surgery is reserved for a small number of women with small tumors who desire pregnancy in the future. Total hysterectomy involves removal of the cervix and the uterus. Radical hysterectomy involves removal of the uterus, cervix, parametrium (tissue surrounding the uterus), ovaries, fallopian tubes, upper vagina, and some or all of the local lymph nodes (NCI, 2009).

Nursing Insight— *Understanding pelvic exenteration*

Pelvic exenteration is a rare, extreme procedure that is used to treat recurrent cervical cancer that has spread to surrounding organs. This surgery, which involves removal of the same organs and tissues as radical hysterectomy, may also include removal of the bladder, rectum, part of the colon, and/or the vagina.

Radiation Therapy

Radiation therapy (RT) uses high-energy x-rays to destroy cancer cells. Cancers that extend beyond the cervix into the pelvis, lower vagina, and urinary tract typically receive radiation. RT may be combined with surgery or chemotherapy to treat early cervical cancers and more invasive stages of the disease; it can also be used to relieve symptoms caused by advanced cancer. Radiation may be delivered by external beam, by radioactive implants placed directly at the cancerous site ("internal therapy"), or by a combination of these two therapies.

External Therapy

External beam radiation, administered the same way as a diagnostic x-ray, is usually given five times a week for 5 or 6 weeks, with an extra boost of radiation at the end of that time. With this treatment modality, the entire pelvic area is irradiated, including the rectum, large intestine, small intestine, bone, and skin. Providing education and emotional support are key components of nursing care for women receiving external beam radiation. The nurse can encourage the patient to remain as active as possible throughout the course of therapy. Patients should be counseled that they might experience certain side effects in the treatment target area, such as hair loss, dry or irritated skin, or permanent darkening of the skin. While undergoing external RT, patients are cautioned not to remove any skin markings made by the radiologist (NCI, 2009).

Optimizing Outcomes— With strategies to promote comfort during external radiation therapy

Nurses can teach women who are undergoing external beam RT about strategies to promote comfort and healing. For example, the nurse can suggest that the patient:

- Practice good personal hygiene
- Use lotions or creams only with the physician's approval, and remain vigilant about skin care and the condition of the treatment area
- Wear loose clothing over the treatment area
- Wear cotton underwear

- Expose the treatment area to air whenever possible
- Avoid exposing the treatment area to temperature extremes
- Avoid the use of adhesive tape in the treatment area

After completion of the external RT, patients are taught about self-care strategies to promote comfort and healing, and they are advised that side effects from the therapy may persist for weeks after the therapy has ended.

"What to say" — *Teaching about self-care strategies after external radiation therapy*

Nurses can empower women with self-care strategies to promote comfort and healing after the completion of external RT. For example, the nurse may tell the patient to:

- Be sure to consume a nutritious diet
- Drink plenty of fluids
- Obtain adequate rest, and take naps as needed
- Take medications as prescribed; check with your health-care provider before taking any non-prescribed medications
- Maintain good oral and skin care
- Anticipate that the effects from the radiation may persist for 10 days to 2 weeks after the last treatment
- Anticipate that signs of healing will occur in about 3 weeks after the last treatment
- Avoid infection; report any symptoms of infection to your health-care provider
- Promptly report symptoms of complications, such as gastrointestinal symptoms (e.g., continued nausea, vomiting, anorexia, diarrhea) or skin symptoms (e.g., redness, swelling, pain, pruritus at the radiation site) to your health-care provider.

Internal Therapy

Implant radiation, also known as brachytherapy ("slow therapy"), involves placement of the radioactive material as close to the tumor as possible while sparing the adjacent healthy tissue. The radioactive material is either placed in a capsule and inserted into the cervix or placed in thin needles that are inserted directly into the tumor. This method of treatment takes place in the hospital setting. The patient stays in the hospital for 1 to 3 days while the implants remain in place; during this time, the patient is considered radioactive. The device is removed before discharge. Brachytherapy is then repeated several times over a period of 1 to 2 weeks. Once the radioactive material has been removed, no radioactivity remains in the body. In some situations, the internal radiation therapy is delivered during a brief treatment session, and the patient is able to go home afterward. In premenopausal women, sterility and cessation of menstruation usually occur after brachytherapy. Patients should be advised to promptly report signs of infection (i.e., vaginal or rectal bleeding, hematuria, foul-smelling vaginal discharge, fever, abdominal distention or pain) to their health-care provider (NCI, 2009).

ⓢ Be sure to— Monitor and limit personal radiation exposure

Nurses and other health-care providers who come in direct contact with patients receiving internal radiation therapy should monitor their personal radiation exposure by wearing a film badge or other device to determine the amount of exposure received. When providing direct patient care, isolation techniques (i.e., good hand-washing technique, wearing gloves when handling bodily fluids) are observed, and time spent in close proximity to the patient is limited to 30 minutes or less per 8 hours to avoid exposure to gamma rays. It is important to use the principles of time, distance, and shielding to protect from personal radiation exposure and to explain to the patient and her family why nursing care is focused on providing only essential care during the course of internal radiation therapy. Also, the nurse explains that pregnant women and children younger than 16 should not visit the patient. If the radiation source becomes dislodged, a radiation specialist uses special long-handled tongs to remove the device and place it in a lead container. All linens and dressings are considered contaminated (Venes, 2009).

Along with physical care, education and emotional support remain central in the nursing care for all patients undergoing radiation therapy. Understandably, patients experience considerable emotional distress related to their diagnosis, fear of the anticipated treatment (e.g., pain, perceived personal radioactivity, adverse effects on bodily functions), and concerns about the impact of their treatment on family members. Potential nursing diagnoses for patients undergoing radiation therapy for the treatment of cervical cancer are presented in Box 6-7.

Nurses can advise patients undergoing external RT that although the affected area may look and feel sunburned, the treated tissues usually regain their normal appearance within 6 to 12 months. It is also important that all patients

be counseled about common RT side effects, such as fatigue, diarrhea, frequent or uncomfortable urination, loss of hair in the genital area, and vaginal dryness, itching, and burning. Patients should also be advised to abstain from intercourse until a few weeks following completion of the RT. In general, patients who are treated with internal RT may resume intercourse in 7 to 10 days. Altered patterns of sexuality related to RT side effects are not unusual. Patients may experience a decrease in vaginal secretions and sensation, as well as vaginal stenosis (narrowing). These aftereffects can cause coital pain and discomfort and can contribute to diminished sexual desire. Depending on the specific problem, the nurse may offer suggestions such as applying water-based lubricants for vaginal dryness and/or the regular use of a vaginal dilator for vaginal stenosis; patient/partner referral to other resources may be appropriate (NCI, 2009). Other complications of external beam radiation and brachytherapy are listed in Box 6-8.

Chemotherapy

Chemotherapy may be used for cervical cancer that has either metastasized too far from its origin to be treated by surgery or radiation or that has recurred. It may also be used to relieve pain associated with advanced cervical cancer or to shrink cancer to an operable size before surgery is performed. This treatment modality is termed *neo-adjuvant chemotherapy,* and it can help to prevent cervical cancer from spreading. Chemotherapeutic agents most often used to treat advanced or recurrent cervical cancer include cisplatin (Cisplatinum, Platinol), ifosfamide (Ifex), paclitaxel (Taxol), cyclophosphamide (Cytoxan), and 5-fluorouracil (5-FU). The medications are either administered by mouth or via IV infusion. Chemotherapy treatments are usually alternated with "recovery periods" that allow the patient a rest time before beginning a new cycle of therapy (NCI, 2009).

Combination chemotherapy, which involves the combination of two or more chemotherapy medications, may be more effective than any single agent. When used in association with surgery or radiation, chemotherapy can help to prevent the spread or recurrence of cervical cancer. Nurses

---

Box 6-7 **Potential Nursing Diagnoses for Patients Undergoing Radiation Therapy for Cervical Cancer**

Knowledge Deficit related to planned treatment procedures

Fear and Anxiety related to
- diagnosis
- pain
- interference with sexual functioning
- concerns about personal radioactivity
- responses of family members and significant others

Disturbed Sensory Perception related to
- internal radiation therapy
- restricted contact with visitors and health-care professionals

Risk for Skin Integrity Impairment related to
- external radiation exposure
- immobility and bedrest (with internal radiation therapy)

Risk for Physical Injury related to dislodgment of the radiation source (with internal RT)

Acute Pain related to internal radiation applicators

Box 6-8 **Complications of External Beam Radiation and Brachytherapy**

Proctitis (inflammation of the rectum)

Cystitis (inflammation of the bladder)

Vaginal scarring and stenosis

Anemia and/or bruising

Thrombophlebitis, pulmonary embolism, pneumonia (related to immobility associated with internal radiation therapy)

Increased risk of infection

Skin rash, inflammation, pruritus

Sexual difficulties

Premature menopause

Vesicovaginal fistula (development of an abnormal connection between the vagina and the bladder or rectum)

Source: NCI (2009).

can counsel patients undergoing chemotherapy about common side effects associated with these medications, which include nausea and vomiting, change in appetite, oral lesions, vaginal sores, temporary hair loss, fatigue, bruising and bleeding, skin rash, joint pain, swelling in the legs and feet, susceptibility to infection, anemia, menstrual cycle changes, onset of early menopause, and infertility. In most situations, women who undergo chemotherapy for cervical cancer are already infertile as a result of surgery or RT. Physicians may prescribe hormones to help offset the symptoms associated with premature menopause (NCI, 2009).

 Optimizing Outcomes— Biological therapy to boost cervical cancer treatment

Biological therapy may be used to treat cancer that has metastasized to other body organs. Interferon, a cell protein that provides immunity to viral infections, is the type of biological therapy most often used. Biological therapy is usually administered on an outpatient basis and is sometimes combined with chemotherapy. Nurses can counsel women about possible side effects associated this treatment modality, including:

- Flulike symptoms: fever and/or chills; muscle aches; weakness; diarrhea, nausea, or vomiting
- Rash
- Loss of appetite
- Easy bleeding or bruising (NCI, 2009)

 Optimizing Outcomes— Supportive care for cancer patients

Nurses can inform women who have received a diagnosis of cancer about supportive care that is available at any stage of the disease. Patients may find information about relief from the side effects of treatment, tips to help to control pain and other symptoms, and emotional support to help them cope with the feelings associated with a diagnosis of cancer. Resources for coping are available on the NCI Web site at www.cancer.gov/cancertopics/coping and from NCI's Cancer Information Service at 1-800-4-CANCER or LiveHelp (www.cancer.gov/help).

Nurses are perfectly situated to provide women with factual information about cervical cancer screening, HPV, and cervical cancer. For example, nurses can explain that while HPV is the cause of cervical cancer, most HPV infections resolve without treatment and do not progress to cervical cancer, especially when regular screening is performed. Most new HPV infections occur in women in their 20s, but the most common decades of life for cervical cancer to be diagnosed is in the 40s and 50s, and 25% of new diagnoses occur in women over age 60. Sharing this information empowers patients with the essential knowledge they need to make informed choices about seeking continued screening at the recommended intervals (Ruhl, 2008; Saslow, 2008).

Teaching women about risk factors for cervical cancer may motivate them to stop smoking or seek regular cervical cancer screening, if they have not done so in the past.

Sharing information about strategies to reduce exposure to HPV (e.g., using condoms, limiting sexual partners, practicing monogamy) may assist in making decisions about intimate relationships. Women of all ages should be educated about the HPV vaccine—although the upper age limit for the vaccine is 26, they may be mothers, grandmothers, aunts, or sisters of preteen or teen girls. Because one concern about the HPV vaccine centers on a potential for patient and care provider complacency about cervical cancer screening, it is imperative that nurses continue to emphasize the importance of routine screening according to current early-detection guidelines (Ruhl, 2008; Saslow, 2008).

Nurses who care for pregnant women can use prenatal visits as an opportunity to counsel patients about the HPV vaccine and cervical cancer prevention and encourage them to begin the series during the postpartum visit. Nurses can support funding for programs that increase access to Pap testing and HPV vaccination for economically disadvantaged women. Finally, through age-appropriate, culturally sensitive educational efforts, nurses can empower patients to make informed choices about the HPV vaccine and, if they do choose to initiate the vaccine, encourage completion of the series (Teitelman et al., 2009).

 Now Can You— Discuss aspects of cervical cancer?

1. Identify at least 15 risk factors for cervical cancer?
2. Teach a woman how to recognize symptoms of cervical cancer?
3. Describe the various treatment modalities for cervical cancer?
4. Discuss the nursing role in caring for patients undergoing treatment for cervical cancer?

summary points

- Cervical cancers originate in the cells on the surface of the cervix, which are composed of squamous and columnar epithelium.

- Cytological screening for cervical cancer should begin at age 21 years, regardless of the woman's sexual history.

- An important nursing role in cervical cancer education centers on emphasizing the importance of routine cervical cancer screening and teaching women about symptoms that may be associated with cancer of the cervix.

- Infection with human papillomavirus (HPV) is known to be the primary cause of cervical cancer.

- An essential area for nurses in HPV awareness and prevention centers on education and counseling for adolescents and teens and their parents.

- The HPV vaccines are indicated for the prevention of cervical cancer, genital warts, and dysplastic or precancerous cervical lesions caused by several of the HPV viruses types.

- Routine Pap test screening is recommended for women regardless of whether they have received the HPV vaccine.

◆ Nurses are perfectly situated to provide women with factual information about cervical cancer screening, HPV, and cervical cancer.

review questions

Multiple Choice

1. The squamocolumnar junction of the cervix:
   A. Is shed during menstruation
   B. Is devoid of cellular growth and replacement
   C. Is the area where the squamous epithelium and the columnar epithelium come together
   D. Surrounds the vaginal introitus

2. The nurse teaches the patient that she can enhance the accuracy of her Pap test screening by:
   A. Avoiding intercourse for 48 hours before the test
   B. Douching 24 hours before the test
   C. Scheduling the appointment to occur during menstruation
   D. Using lubricants with intercourse 24 hours before the test

3. The liquid-based process for cervical cytology screening can also be used to test for:
   A. HIV
   B. Syphilis
   C. Bacterial vaginosis
   D. Chlamydia trachomatis

4. If an abnormal Pap test result requires further evaluation, a procedure that allows for a close-up visualization of the vagina and cervix is:
   A. Colposcopy
   B. Cryosurgery
   C. Endocervical curettage
   D. Conization

5. The nurse teaches about risk factors for cervical cancer, which include:
   A. Initiation of sexual activity after age 26
   B. A history of three or more sexual partners
   C. A history of infection with the varicella virus
   D. Nulliparity

REFERENCES

American Cancer Society (ACS). (2009). *Cervical cancer: Prevention and early detection*. Retrieved April 10, 2010, from http://www.cancer.org/docroot/CRI/content/CRI_2_6x_cervical_cancer_prevention_and_early_detection_8.asp?sitearea=FED

American Cancer Society (ACS). (2010). *Detailed guide: Cervical cancer*. Retrieved April 10, 2010, from http://www.cancer.org/docroot/CRI/content/CRI_2_4_2X_What_are_the_risk_factors_for_cervical_cancer_8.asp

American College of Obstetricians and Gynecologists (ACOG). (2007). *Guidelines for women's health care: A resource manual*. Washington, DC: Author.

American College of Obstetricians and Gynecologists (ACOG). (2008, December). *ACOG Practice Bulletin No. 99, Management of abnormal cervical cytology and histology* (pp. 402–427). Washington, DC: Author.

American College of Obstetricians and Gynecologists (ACOG). (2009a, December). *ACOG Practice Bulletin No. 109, Cervical cytology screening* (pp. 1409–1420). Washington, DC: Author.

American College of Obstetricians and Gynecologists (ACOG). (2009b, June). *ACOG Committee Opinion No. 436, Evaluation and management of abnormal cervical cytology and histology in adolescents*. *Obstetrics and Gynecology, 113*(6), 1422–1425.

American Society for Colposcopy and Cervical Pathology. (2010). *Human papillomavirus (HPV)*. Retrieved April 13, 2010, from http://www.asccp.org/hpv_history.shtml

Association of Women's Health, Obstetric, and Neonatal Nurses. (2009). AWHONN Position Statement: HPV vaccination for the prevention of cervical cancer. *Journal of Obstetric, Gynecologic, & Neonatal Nursing, 39*(11), 129–130.

Association of Women's Health, Obstetric, and Neonatal Nurses. (2010). *Nursing association launches HPV awareness & education campaign*. Retrieved April 20, 2010, from https://www.awhonn.org/awhonn/content.do?name=07_PressRoom/7B7_Jan06_HPVBeConfident.htm

Bickley, L. S., & Szilagyi, P. G. (2007). *Bates' guide to physical examination and history taking* (9th ed.). Philadelphia: Lippincott Williams and Wilkins.

Brewer, N. T., & Fazekas, K. I. (2007). Predictors of HPV vaccine acceptability: A theory-informed, systematic review. *Preventive Medicine, 45*(2-3), 107–114.

Burchell, A. N., Tellier, P. P., Hanley, J., Coutlee, F., & Franco, E. L. (2010). Human Papillomavirus infections among couples in new sexual relationships. *Epidemiology, 21*(1), 31–37.

Burkman, R. T. (2010). New screening recommendations: Benefits and harms are in the eye of the beholder. *Female Patient, 35*(3), 12–13.

Burns, J. L., Walsh, L. J., & Popovich, J. M. (2010). Practical pediatric and adolescent immunization update. *Journal for Nurse Practitioners, 6*(4), 254–266.

Cates, J. R., Brewer, N. T., Fazekas, K. I., Mitchell, C. E., & Smith, J. S. (2009). Racial differences in HPV knowledge, HPV vaccine acceptability, and related beliefs among rural Southern women. *Journal of Rural Health, 25*(1), 93–97.

Centers for Disease Control and Prevention (CDC). (2006). *Sexually transmitted diseases treatment guidelines 2006*. Retrieved April 20, 2010, from http://www.cdc.gov/std/treatment/2006/genital-warts.htm

Centers for Disease Control and Prevention (CDC). (2009a). *Genital HPV infection—CDC fact sheet*. Retrieved April 20, 2010, from http://www.cdc.gov/STD/HPV/STDFact-HPV.htm

Centers for Disease Control and Prevention (CDC). (2009b). *HPV vaccine—questions & answers*. Retrieved April 20, 2010, from http://www.cdc.gov/vaccines/vpd-vac/hpv/vac-faqs.htm

Centers for Disease Control and Prevention, Advisory Committee on Immunization Practices (CDC ACIP). (2009). *Provisional recommendations for HPV vaccine*. Retrieved April 18, 2010, from http://www.cdc.gov/vaccines/recs/provisional/downloads/hpv-vac-dec2009-508.pdf

Chase, D. M., & Tewari, K. S. (2010). Update on cervical cancer screening. *Female Patient, 35*(1), 16–21.

Coker, A. L. (2007). Does physical intimate partner violence affect sexual health? A systematic review. *Trauma Violence and Abuse, 8*(2), 149–77.

Dillon, P. M. (2007). *Nursing health assessment: A critical thinking, case studies approach* (2nd ed.). Philadelphia: F. A. Davis.

Duffy, P. J. (2009). Cervical cancer risk management: A legal perspective. *Female Patient (Suppl.), 34*(1), S1–12.

Dunne, E. F., & Markowitz, L. E. (2006). Genital human papillomavirus infection. Emerging Infections. *Clinical Infectious Diseases, 43*(1), 624–629.

Escobar, P. F., & Orr, J. W. (2008). The human papillomavirus vaccine: Current status. *Female Patient, 33*(11), 18–22.

English, A., Shaw, F. E., McCauley, M. M., & Fishbein, D. B. (2008). Legal basis of consent for health care and vaccination for adolescents. *Pediatrics, 121*, S85–87.

Fazekas, K., Brewer, N. T., & Smith, J. (2008). HPV acceptability in a rural Southern area. *Journal of Women's Health, 17*(6), 539–547.

Frazer, I. H., Cox, J. T., Mayeaux, E. J., Jr., Franco, E. L., Moscicki, A. B., & Palefsky, J. M., et al. (2006). Advances in prevention of cervical cancer and other human papillomavirus-related diseases. *Pediatric Infectious Disease Journal, 25*(2 Suppl.), S65–S81.

Garfield, S., Gavaghan, M., Poret, A., & Ilika, K. (2010). HPV DNA co-testing adoption and its effect on patient annual visits. *Female Patient, 35*(4), 53–56.

Giarratano, G., Bustamante-Forest, R., & Carter, C. (2005). A multicultural and multilingual outreach program for cervical and breast cancer screening. *Journal of Obstetric, Gynecologic, and Neonatal Nursing, 34*(4), 395–402.

Gottlieb, S. L., & Brewer, N. T. (2009). Disparities in how parents are learning about the human papillomavirus vaccine. *Cancer Epidemiology, Biomarkers & Prevention, 18*(2), 363–372.

Gupton, N. E. (2007). Are Pap tests in danger of being phased out? *Clinical Advisor, 10*(4), 89–92.

Hachey, K. J., Allen, R. H., Nothnagle, M., & Boardman, L.A. (2009). Requiring human papillomavirus vaccine for immigrant women. *Obstetrics & Gynecology, 114*(5), 1135–1138.

Hellwig, J. P. (2006). HPV linked to common skin cancer. *AWHONN Lifelines, 10*(4), 289–294.

Howley, P. M., Yang, Y. C., Spalholz, B. A., & Rabson, M. S. (1986). Papillomavirus transforming functions. *Ciba Foundation Symposium, 120,* 39–52.

Hutchinson, M. K., Thompson, A. C., & Cederbaum, J. A. (2006). Multisystem factors contributing to disparities in preventive health care among lesbian women. *Journal of Obstetric, Gynecologic & Neonatal Nursing, 35*(3), 393–402.

Kahn, J. A. (2008). Human papillomavirus infections and anogenital warts. In L. Neinstein, C. M. Gordon, D. K. Katzman, D. S. Rosen, & E. R. Woods (Eds.), *Adolescent health care* (5th ed., pp. 842–849). Philadelphia: Lippincott Williams & Wilkins.

Kahn, J., Rosenthal, S., Jin, Y., Huang, B., Namakydoust, A., & Zimet, G. (2008). Rates of Human papillomavirus vaccination, attitudes about vaccination, and human papilloma-virus prevalence in young women. *Obstetrics and Gynecology, 111*(4), 1103–1110.

Katki, H. A., Wacholder, S., Solomon, D., Castle, P. E., & Schiffman, M. (2009). Risk estimation for the next generation of prevention programmes for cervical cancer. *Lancet Oncology, 10*(11), 1022–1023.

Kiviat, N. B., Hawes, S. E., & Feng, Q. (2008). Screening for cervical cancer in the era of the HPV vaccine: The urgent need for both new screening guidelines and new biomarkers. *Journal of the National Cancer Institute, 100*(5), 290–291.

Lara-Torre, E., & Murchison, A. B. (2009). Case management of cervical cytology and histology in the adolescent patient. *Female Patient, 34*(11), 34–37.

Lindstrom, A. K., Ekman, K., Stendahl, U., Tot, T., Henriksson, R., Hedman, H., & Hellberg, D. (2008). LRIG1 and squamous epithelial uterine cervical cancer: Correlation to prognosis, other tumor markers, sex steroid hormones, and smoking. *International Journal of Gynecological Cancer, 18*(2), 312–317.

Markowitz, L. E., Dunne, E. F., Saraiya, M., Lawson, H. W., Chesson, H., & Unger, E. R. (2007). Quadrivalent human papillomavirus vaccine: Recommendations of the advisory committee on immunization practices (ACIP). *Morbidity and Mortality Weekly Report, Recommendations and Reports, 56*(RR-2), 1–24.

Marrazzo, J. M., Koutsky, L. A., Kiviat, N. B., Kuypers, J. M., & Stine, K. (2001). Papanicolaou test screening and prevalence of genital human papillomavirus among women who have sex with women. *American Journal of Public Health, 91*(6), 947–952.

Marshall, H., Phillip, R., Don, R., & Peter, B. (2007). A cross-sectional survey to assess community attitudes to introduction of human papillomavirus vaccine. *Australian and New Zealand Journal of Public Health, 31*(3), 235–242.

Moore, S. L., & Seybold, V. K. (2007). HPV vaccine. *Clinician Reviews, 17*(1), 36–42.

National Association of Nurse Practitioners in Women's Health. (2007). Guidelines for screening and management of cervical disease. *Women's Health Care: A Practical Journal for Nurse Practitioners, 6*(1), 24–32.

National Cancer Institute (NCI). (2009). *Cervical cancer treatment.* Retrieved April 27, 2010, from http://www.cancer.gov/cancertopics/pdq/treatment/cervical/healthprofessional

Neinstein, L. S. (2008). Office visit and interviewing. In L. Neinstein, C. M. Gordon, D. K. Katzman, D. S. Rosen, & E. R. Woods (Eds.), *Adolescent health care* (5th ed., pp. 25–41). Philadelphia: Lippincott Williams & Wilkins.

Oh, J. K., Ju, Y. H., Franceschi, S., Quint, W., & Shin, H. R. (2008). Acquisition of new infection and clearance of type-specific human papillomavirus infection in female students in Busan, South Korea: A follow-up study [Electronic version]. *BMC Infection Diseases,* 8(13). Retrieved April 30, 2010, from http://www.biomedcentral.com/content/pdf/1471-2334-8-13.pdf

Olbrys, K. (2010). Cervical screening: Assessment and referral. *Journal for Nurse Practitioners, 6*(2), 151–152.

Policar, M. S. (2008). Female genital tract cancer screening. In R. A. Hatcher, J. Trussell, A. Nelson, F. Cates, F. Stewart, & D. Kowal. (Eds.). *Contraceptive technology* (19th ed., pp. 559–581). New York: Ardent Media.

Pollack, A. E., Balkin, M., Edouard, L., Cutts, F., & Broutet, N. (2007). Ensuring access to HPV vaccines through integrated services: A reproductive health perspective. *Bulletin of the World Health Organization, 85*(1), 57–63.

Ries, L. A., Melbert, D., Krapcho, M., Stinchcomb, D. G., Howlader, N., Horner, M. J., et al. (Eds.). (2009). *SEER cancer statistics review, 1975-2006.* Bethesda, MD: National Cancer Institute. Retrieved April 22, 2010, from http://seer.cancer.gov/csr/1975_2006/

Rome, E. S., & Hicks, C. W. (2009). Human papillomavirus vaccine: The current picture. *Female Patient, 34*(10), 34–39.

Ruhl, C. (2008). The future of the Pap: Where is cervical cancer screening headed? *Nursing for Women's Health, 12*(5), 427–431.

Saslow, D. (2008). Current issues in cervical cancer screening. *Female Patient, 33*(7), 20–23.

Schmidt, J. V. (2007). HPV vaccine: Implications for nurses and patients. *Nursing for Women's Health, 11*(1), 83–87.

Shanbhag, S., Clark, H., Timmaraju, V., Bhattacharya, S., & Cruickshank, M. (2009). Pregnancy outcome after treatment for cervical intraepithelial neoplasia. *Obstetrics & Gynecology, 114*(4), 727–735.

Taylor, J. S., & Smith, J. (2009). Concurrent STIs in adolescents with abnormal cervical cytologic findings. *Women's Health Care: A Practical Journal for Nurse Practitioners, 8*(12), 17–23.

Teitelman, A. M., Ratcliffe, S. J., & Cederbaum, J. A. (2008). Parent–adolescent communication about sexual pressure, maternal gender norms about relationship power and HIV protective behaviors of minority urban girls. *Journal of the American Psychiatric Nurses Association, 14,* 50–60.

Teitelman, A.M., Stringer, M., Averbuch, T., & Witkoski, A. (2009). Human papillomavirus, current vaccines, and cervical cancer prevention. *Journal of Obstetric, Gynecologic, and Neonatal Nursing, 38*(1), 69–80.

Theroux, R. (2008). The HPV vaccine: Rates, attitudes and acceptability. *Nursing for Women's Health, 12*(5), 423–426.

U.S. Preventive Services Task Force. (2007). *Guide to clinical preventive services 2007: Recommendations of the U.S. Preventive Services Task Force* (AHRQ Publication No. 07-05100). Available at http://www.ahrq.gov

Venes, D. (2009). *Taber's cyclopedic medical dictionary* (21st ed.). Philadelphia: F. A. Davis.

Watts, L. A., Joseph, N., Wallace, M., Rauh-Hain, J. A., Muzikansky, A., Growdon, W. B., & del Carmen, M. G. (2009). HPV vaccine: a comparison of attitudes and behavioralperspectives between Latino and non-Latino women. *Gynecologic Oncology, 112*(3), 577–582.

Woodson, S.A. (2008). *HPV counseling: A clinician resource.* Washington, DC: Association of Women's Health, Obstetric and Neonatal Nurses (AWHONN).

Wright, T. C., Massad, L. S., Dunton, C. J., Spitzer, M., Wilkinson, E. J., & Solomon, D. (2007). 2006 consensus guidelines for the management of women with abnormal cervical cancer screening tests. *American Journal of Obstetrics and Gynecology, 197*(4), 346–355.

Wysocki, S., Reiter, S., & Berman, N.R. (2007). Strategies for preventing cervical cancer and HPV-related disease: The role of vaccination. *Women's Health Care, 6*(1), 6–22.

Promoting Menopausal Health

Shelton M. Hisley, PhD, RNC, WHNP-BC

You can't turn back the clock.
But you can wind it up again.

—Bonnie Pruden

LEARNING TARGETS *At the completion of this chapter, the student will be able to:*

◆ Identify physiological changes that occur during the menopausal period.

◆ Identify self-care strategies to promote health during midlife and the later years.

◆ Recognize various risk factors for cardiovascular disease and osteoporosis.

◆ Develop an educational program for perimenopausal women that focuses on potential health threats and empowers women with strategies to optimize physical and emotional well-being.

Introduction

This chapter explores the years surrounding the menopausal transition. By 2025, 1.1 billion women worldwide will be postmenopausal. In 1900, the average age of menopause was 46 years and the average life expectancy was 51 years, although many women lived well beyond this age. In contemporary times, American women, on average, can expect to live to be 80 years old and spend close to one-third of their lives as postmenopausal women. For the modern woman, menopause does not mark the end of life. Instead, it represents a transition into another phase, with a potential life span of another 30 to 50 years (Burdette, Moore, Speroff, & Wysocki, 2009; Edelman, 2010).

A healthy lifestyle that balances optimal nutrition and regular exercise with mental and social stimulation helps women to lead productive, enriched lives well into the ninth decade. The period surrounding the menopause offers a unique time for women to evaluate their physical and emotional health, make plans for the future, and prepare for many, many healthy years ahead. With evidence-based information about menopause and the normal aging process, as well as various health issues such as cardiovascular disease and osteoporosis, nurses can empower women with the tools they need to prepare for and embrace the coming years with energy, enthusiasm, and strategies for optimizing their health and well-being. Armed with factual information, women can actively partner with their health-care provider in the decision-making process. Nurses are perfectly positioned to provide ongoing menopausal education and counseling to assist women in making fully informed choices.

While menopause is a natural, inevitable process, women do have control over how they pass through this special time of life. They can engage in strategies to ease uncomfortable symptoms and minimize their risks of chronic disease. For example, refraining from smoking, maintaining appropriate weight through exercise and diet, limiting alcohol intake, reducing stress, remaining socially active, and recognizing that happiness and long-term health come about through a personalized approach are tools that help women to enjoy good health during the later years of life. As a noted author observed, "the wise woman achieves menopause, it does not overcome her" (Weed, 2002). During this special time in their lives, many women describe an enhanced sense of well-being, hard-won individuality, and a positive attitude for living life to its fullest.

The Climacteric, Premenopause, Menopause, Perimenopause, and Postmenopause

The *climacteric* is a transitional time in a woman's life marked by declining ovarian function and decreased hormone production. The climacteric begins at the onset of ovarian decline and ends with the cessation of postmenopausal symptoms. *Menopause*, a term derived from Latin *mensis* for "month" and Greek *pausis*, meaning "to cease," refers to the last menstrual period and can be dated with certainty only 1 year after menstruation ceases. Menopause is defined as the permanent cessation of menses resulting from reduced ovarian hormone secretion that occurs naturally or is induced by surgery, chemotherapy, or radiation. The average age at menopause in the United States is 51.4 years; the normal age at menopause ranges from 40 to 58 years (Nelson, Haney, Humphrey, Miller, Nedrow, Nicolaidis, Vesco, Walker, Bougatsos, & Nygren, 2005).

Premenopause is the time up to the beginning of perimenopause, but the term is also used to define the time up to the last menstrual period. *Perimenopause* is the period of time preceding menopause, usually between 2 and 8 years before menopause. The age at onset of perimenopause ranges from 39 to 51 years. Although perimenopause may last as few as 2 or as many as 10 years; on average, it lasts 4 years. During this time of transition, levels of estrogen and progesterone increase and decrease at uneven intervals, causing the menstrual cycle to become longer, shorter, and eventually absent. Ovulation is sporadic. Symptoms of perimenopause, including irregular menses, hot flashes, vaginal dryness, dyspareunia, and mood changes are associated with the fluctuation and decline in hormone levels. *Postmenopause* begins when ovarian estrogen terminates, ovulation ceases, and menstrual periods have stopped for 12 consecutive months. During postmenopause, estrogen is produced solely by the adrenal glands. Women typically enter postmenopause between the ages of 40 and 58; the average age is 51 (Edelman, 2010; Nelson et al., 2005).

 Nursing Insight— *Perspectives on the perimenopausal period*

Every woman travels her own unique course through perimenopause. Interestingly, the term *perimenopause* is a relatively new concept—the word was not even listed in a medical dictionary until after 1989. The term *menopausal transition* describes the years from the onset of the loss of ovarian cycling to the last menstrual period. Menopause occurs regardless of a woman's age when the number of remaining ovarian follicles falls below a critical level of about 1000. The health habits established during the perimenopausal and early postmenopausal years can determine the woman's health status and quality of life for her critical elderly years after age 75, when serious health problems are greatest (Nelson & Stewart, 2008).

Throughout the menopausal transition, changes take place in both the physiological and emotional domains. Hormone levels shift, readjust, and reach new balances, and the tissues and organs whose function is influenced by these hormones also change structurally and functionally. At the same time, mental and emotional alterations occur as well. While some of the changes are physiological in nature, others involve various dimensions of self-perception and self-concept as women are challenged to deal with this natural passage into a new phase of life.

 Ethnocultural Considerations— Views on menopause

Cross-cultural studies have revealed that the menopausal experience is greatly influenced by the attitudes of the culture and community in which women reside. In the United States, owing in part to the present-day graying of the baby-boom generation, attitudes toward menopause and aging are undergoing change. For many traditional cultures throughout the world, menopause represents a time for women to assume leadership roles in the community and a time for honor and recognition as one of the tribal members with an accumulation of wisdom. American women are embracing this broad cultural perspective as an opportunity to shift self-perception and create a positive cultural image of women during this stage of life. Today, the majority of American women do not believe that menopause interferes with their quality of life (National Institutes of Health [NIH], 2005).

Signs and Symptoms of Menopause

A number of signs and symptoms typically herald the physical changes that take place during the menopausal transition. During this time, nurses can empower women with various strategies to promote mental and physical well-being. Potential nursing diagnoses for women experiencing the perimenopausal period are presented in Box 7-1.

 Nursing Insight— *Body systems affected by the natural decline in estrogen*

Estrogen secretion naturally declines as women age. Estrogen receptors are plentiful throughout the female body. During the childbearing years, estrogen is a dominant hormone that regulates the menstrual cycle and exerts important effects on the reproductive and urinary tracts, the heart and blood vessels, bones, breasts, skin, hair follicles, mucous membranes, pelvic muscles, and the brain. Loss of estrogen is associated with a multitude of acute symptoms, including hot flashes, sleep disruptions, and mood changes. For many women, menopause-related estrogen depletion is also associated with longer-term manifestations such as urogenital symptoms (Allmen & Moore, 2010).

MENSTRUAL CYCLE CHANGES

It is rare for a woman to cease menstruation all at once. Most often, the menstrual periods become progressively more irregular. The volume of blood flow is variable as well and may be accompanied by midcycle spotting. Changes in bleeding patterns largely result from a lack of ovulation. The absence of ovulation interrupts the production of progesterone, the hormone that stabilizes the endometrium, or uterine lining. Under the influence of prolonged, continuous estrogen, the endometrium continues to proliferate and may only be irregularly sloughed off. When bleeding does occur, it may be heavier or more prolonged. The endometrial lining may also develop irregular or thickened areas; it may not slough off evenly or in its entirety, and these events cause the menses to stop and start again.

Box 7-1 **Potential Nursing Diagnoses for Perimenopausal Women**

- Knowledge deficit related to menopause and its management
- Risk for injury related to osteoporosis and coronary heart disease
- Sexual dysfunction related to physiological changes associated with declining estrogen levels
- Readiness for enhanced family coping related to the menopausal transition
- Risk for situational low self-esteem related to the physical and emotional changes during the menopausal transition

Although irregular menses is usually a normal part of the perimenopausal process, any heavy bleeding should be investigated. Uterine fibroids, a frequent cause of increased bleeding, are common in perimenopausal women. Cervical or uterine cancer should also be considered as a possible cause of this symptom. If heavy bleeding is an ongoing problem and cancer has been ruled out, hormonal intervention in the form of low-dose oral contraceptives, progesterone alone, or another form of hormone therapy (HT) may be suggested. If fibroids are the cause of heavy bleeding, medical or surgical intervention may be advised. (See Bonus Chapter 4 for a discussion of uterine cancer and fibroid tumors and Bonus Chapter 6 for a discussion of cervical cancer.) It is important to remember that although fertility declines during this transitional period, it does not disappear until menopause is complete. Menopause is signaled by the passage of one full year without menstruation. For most women, birth control remains an important consideration during the perimenopausal period (Alexander, 2007; Nelson & Stewart, 2008; Secor & Simon, 2006).

HORMONAL CHANGES

During the perimenopausal period, hormone levels are frequently erratic, with highs and lows occurring without the usual synchronicity. A common hormonal pattern that occurs when ovulation becomes unpredictable is an elevated estrogen level throughout the cycle with low progesterone levels during the second half of the cycle, when progesterone is normally at its peak. Some women develop very low levels of estrogen as well. At this time, ovarian function declines and the ovaries lose their ability to manufacture large amounts of sex hormones. The physiological feedback loops between the ovaries, the hypothalamus, and the pituitary glands also lose their synchronized pattern. Progesterone undergoes the most dramatic drop during menopause because its production depends upon ovulation and the development of the corpus luteum.

Small amounts of estrogen continue to be produced by the ovaries for up to 10 years following cessation of menses. The body has other means of estrogen production, however. The woman's fat cells convert androgens produced by the adrenal glands to estrogens. Androgens are female forms of "male-type" hormones that are produced by the ovaries and the adrenal glands. Androgens are responsible for the maintenance of muscle strength and the sex drive. As estrogen and progesterone levels fall, the effects of the androgens often become relatively more pronounced. For example, these hormones can produce an increase in facial hair often noted after menopause. For some women, androgen levels (including testosterone) fall as well, producing symptoms of low libido or decrease in muscle mass with a relative increase in the amount of adipose (fat) tissue (Wysocki, 2009a).

SKIN AND HAIR CHANGES

Declining levels of estrogen affect many tissues throughout the body. The skin and mucous membranes become dry. The fatty layer beneath the skin tends to shrink, and this change is associated with an overall decrease in elasticity and moisture. The skin feels rougher to the touch, and the outer skin may be looser than the deeper layers, which results in wrinkling. The skin produces less melanin, and it can burn more easily. The increasing predominance of androgens often causes a darker, thicker, more wiry hair to appear on the symphysis pubis, underarm area, chest, lower abdomen, and back. Some women experience an increase in facial hair, and the hair on the head may become dry. Pubic and axillary hair often thins. Genetically susceptible women may experience female pattern (scalp) hair loss, a condition most likely related to the altered estrogen-to-androgen ratio that accompanies menopause (Bergfeld & Harrison, 2009; Freeman, 2009).

BREAST CHANGES

Glandular tissues in the breasts shrink during the menopausal period. The breasts may lose their fullness and flatten and drop. The nipples may become smaller and flatter.

UROGENITAL CHANGES

Vaginal changes may accompany the perimenopausal period, or they may not occur for several years after menopause. The mucous membranes, previously supported by estrogen stimulation, become thin, dry, and fragile. The vagina loses its rough texture and dark pink coloration and becomes smooth and pale. The vagina also shortens and narrows. Women may experience vaginal itching, burning, bleeding, or soreness. The vagina lubricates more slowly, and there is a diminished amount of cervical mucus produced. Owing to these changes, intercourse often becomes painful. Bleeding and/or pain may occur following minimal trauma, such as that occurring during intercourse or a pelvic examination. Vulvar changes may also make activities such as riding a bicycle uncomfortable. There is also an alteration in the normal vaginal flora, which results in a decrease in the normal protective mechanisms of the vagina. Declining estrogen secretion is accompanied by a corresponding reduction in the lactobacilli needed to maintain a healthy acidic vaginal environment. With these changes in pH, normally harmless pathogens may colonize the more alkaline vagina, potentially leading to infection. When the vaginal mucosa becomes inflamed, the condition is termed "atrophic vaginitis," a condition characterized by burning, leukorrhea and malodorous yellow discharge (Greenblum, Greenblum, & Neff, 2009; Mehta & Bachmann, 2008; North American Menopause Society [NAMS], 2007; Wysocki, 2009a).

A & P review **Estrogen Deficiency and Urogenital Atrophy**

Estrogen plays a critical role in maintaining the structure and function of the vagina. The layers of the vaginal mucosa, which is estrogen sensitive, are composed of *parabasal* (the least mature), *intermediate* or *basal* (larger and polygon-shaped), and *superficial* squamous cells (the most mature). Prior to menopause, the matured vaginal epithelium has more superficial cells than parabasal cells, indicating the presence of estrogenic stimulation. In menopausal women, systemic declines in estrogen levels correspond to decreased cellular maturation. The proportion of superficial cells present on cytological examination is expressed as the *vaginal maturation index* (VMI). The VMI is a ratio of parabasal, intermediate, and superficial squamous cells found on a cytological smear of cells taken from the upper one-third of the vagina. Although infrequently used in clinical practice today, the maturation index of vaginal cells is useful in evaluating the qualitative response of the vaginal tissue to estrogen. Under the influence of estrogen, mature superficial cells predominate; when estrogen levels are low, parabasal cell numbers fall, leading to gradual atrophic changes in the tissues of the vagina, vulva, urethra, and trigone area of the bladder. Some menopausal women experience urinary problems, including increased urinary tract infections (Allmen & Moore, 2010; Greenblum, Greenblum, & Neff, 2009; Mehta & Bachmann, 2008; NAMS, 2007; Wysocki, 2008, 2009a). ◆

Menopause-induced changes in the genitourinary tract can produce symptoms that include urinary urgency, increased frequency, stress or urge incontinence, and recurrent urinary tract infections. Unlike other symptoms associated with menopause, such as hot flashes, those of urogenital atrophy often worsen with advancing age. Vulvovaginal or urinary atrophic symptoms in postmenopausal women can cause significant reductions in quality of life, avoidance of sexual intercourse, and emotional distress (Burdette, 2009; Goldstein & Alexander, 2005). More than one-third of women over the age of 60 in the United States have some form of urinary incontinence (Alexander, 2007). The prevalence of incontinence appears to increase gradually during young adult life, peak around middle age, and then steadily increase during the later years. The estimated annual direct cost of urinary incontinence in women in this country is around $12.43 billion (ACOG, 2007).

A & P review Estrogen Deficiency and Urogenital Changes

In the urinary tract, estrogen deficiency causes urethral and bladder mucosal thinning, urethral shortening, weakening of the sphincter, decreased bladder capacity, increased postvoid residual urine volume, and uninhibited detrusor muscle contractions. After menopause, the urethral mucosa atrophies, and the collagen content in the connective tissue surrounding the urethra decreases; blood flow in the urethra is also reduced. These changes may cause dysuria, urinary frequency, and stress incontinence; estrogen-deficient women may also be susceptible to recurrent urinary tract infections. Owing to a decrease in collagen and elastin, declining estrogen levels also contribute to loss of mechanical support of the pelvic diaphragm (Goldstein & Alexander, 2005; Palacios, 2009; Wysocki, 2008). ◆

Nursing Insight— *Menopause and pelvic floor dysfunction*

Pelvic organ support is provided by the physiologically complex interactions between the vagina, the levator ani muscles and their fascial coverings, the connective tissue attachments to the bony pelvis (including the uterosacral ligaments), the arcus tendineus fascia pelvis, and the perineal body and perineal membrane. The pelvic floor muscles atrophy after menopause, becoming weak and unable to adequately support the pelvic structures and organs. As the pelvic organs shift position, they begin to press against the vagina, resulting in prolapse, usually of the vagina or bladder. A prolapse can result in pain during intercourse and urinary incontinence. Exercises can strengthen the muscles; however,

muscle damage cannot be reversed. Surgery is the primary treatment for pelvic prolapse; the timing of the surgery depends on the woman's symptoms and their effect on her daily activities. Some symptoms can be medically managed until surgery is appropriate. Many treatment options are available for urinary incontinence, especially if it is not accompanied by a cystocele, which results when the bladder herniates into the vagina (Jones, Bryson, & Harmanli, 2010).

Urinary incontinence has been shown to affect women's social, clinical, and psychological well-being. It is estimated that fewer than one-half of all incontinent women seek medical assistance for this problem, even though urinary incontinence can often be treated (ACOG, 2007). Loss of estrogen supply to the estrogen-dependent tissues of the genitourinary tract results in a decrease in muscle tone and control in the bladder and urethra. Stress urinary incontinence (SUI) is a disturbance in urinary control (e.g., loss of urine) due to sudden increases in intra-abdominal pressure that often occurs during sneezing, coughing, or laughing. SUI is more likely to occur in women who have given birth. For most women, pelvic muscle exercises, known as Kegel exercises, can be very effective in strengthening the pelvic floor and in improving symptoms associated with SUI. Some practitioners provide patients with "Kegel beads" to encourage and remind them to perform the exercises. Patients are instructed to slide the beads from one side of the chain to the other until all sets (10) are performed for the day (Jones, Bryson, & Harmanli, 2010).

❝What to say❞ — *Teaching patients how to perform Kegel exercises*

To teach patients about Kegel exercises, the nurse may provide the following information:

Kegel exercises strengthen the pelvic floor and should help decrease your urinary symptoms. To perform the Kegel exercise:

- First, contract the vaginal opening as if you are trying to stop the flow of urine.
- Now hold to a count of 6.
- Relax to a count of 10, then repeat these steps 10 more times.
- Perform 5 to 10 sets of Kegel exercises each day.

For patients who are unable to isolate the levator ani, electrical stimulation and/or muscle biofeedback may be helpful. Electrical stimulation during Kegel exercises stimulates and contracts the pelvic muscles in a manner similar to the Kegels. This approach, conducted in the health-care practitioner's office, may be helpful for women who have difficulty contracting the pelvic muscles voluntarily. It involves the use of a device that delivers current to the pudendal nerve through a vaginally placed probe (Jones, Bryson, & Harmanli, 2010).

Biofeedback therapy has been used to assist the re-education of patients with pelvic floor spasms and has been shown to result in significant symptomatic improvement after several months of therapy. Biofeedback utilizes a vaginal sensor that measures the level of muscle activity generated by voluntary pelvic floor contraction. With biofeedback, the patient is taught to voluntarily control the pelvic muscles and bladder. With an electrode attached to the skin, biofeedback machines measure the electrical signals elicited when the pelvic muscles and urinary sphincter are contracted. Through the visual cues from the graph shown on the monitor, patients can learn to control these muscles voluntarily (Jones, Bryson, & Harmanli, 2010).

Vaginal cones, which may also be vaginal weights, can be used to strengthen the vaginal muscles as well. The woman is instructed to insert the tampon-shaped cone into the vagina while in a standing position, beginning with the lightest weight. Once inserted, the patient should contract the levator ani muscles in an effort to keep the cone in place for 15 to 20 minutes. As the muscles strengthen, the patient then transitions, one at a time, to the next heaviest cone. It is helpful to use the cone while doing Kegel exercises as well. As the pelvic muscles strengthen, patients can use the cones while engaging in exercise (Jones, Bryson, & Harmanli, 2010).

Some women choose to use a pessary, which is a device inserted into the vagina to support the prolapsed bladder or uterus. This device must be fitted by a health-care practitioner and needs to be removed and cleaned regularly with soap and water to reduce the risk of infection. Surgical intervention for a prolapsed bladder usually involves an anterior repair (colporrhaphy). This procedure involves shortening of the pelvic muscles to provide better support for the bladder.

Urinary urgency and/or frequency combined with an involuntary loss of urine are common signs of an overactive bladder. Pharmacologic management of incontinence is aimed at relaxing the involuntary contractions that occur at the bladder. For overactive bladder, common medications include tolterodine (Detrol), oxybutynin (Ditropan), and imipramine (Tofranil). Common side effects associated with these medications include dry mouth, nausea, dizziness, drowsiness, and constipation. Low-dose vaginal estrogen creams, tablets, or rings may also be prescribed to provide relief of urinary symptoms (Alexander, 2007).

Promoting Sexual Health During the Menopausal Years

Years ago, researchers Masters and Johnson studied sexuality in menopausal women and found that there is a general reduction in the four phases of the sexual response cycle with increasing years after menopause. However, they also discovered that women who maintained regular sexual activity experienced vaginal lubrication similar to levels expected in women who were premenopausal, and these women continued to be capable of full sexual response and enjoyment. Sexual activity is also beneficial in improving tone and blood flow to the pelvic floor.

Nursing Insight— *Sexual responsiveness in older women*

Sexual responsiveness reaches a peak for women in their late 30s and can remain on a high plateau into the 60s. Some women report an increased sexual desire after menopause. The fear of unwanted pregnancy often frees women to be much more sexually expressive and responsive than they were in their premenopausal years.

The two most important influences on older women's sexual activity are the strength of the relationship and the health status of each partner. The lack of an available partner can have a negative effect on sexual intimacy for many midlife and older women. Older widowed, divorced, and lesbian women may have fewer opportunities to develop close relationships because they are less sought after. When discussing sexuality issues with older women, it is important for nurses to provide accurate information and offer support and nonjudgmental guidance. The nurse can reassure the woman that the desire for sex into old age is a natural one and the body continues to have the capacity for sexual satisfaction (ACOG, 2007).

Many women do, however, experience changes in libido (sex drive), reduction in vaginal lubrication, discomfort during intercourse, and changes in orgasmic response in the years after menopause. The use of various oils (e.g., vegetable, vitamin E, olive) or vaginal lubricants that are specifically formulated for menopausal vaginal discomfort allows many older women to continue to enjoy sexual intercourse. Lengthening the foreplay time may promote enhanced vaginal lubrication as well.

"What to say" — *Initiating dialogue about menopausal sexual difficulties*

When discussing menopause-related problems, it is important to use patient-friendly terms such as *vaginal dryness, discomfort,* or *irritation,* rather than *sexual dysfunction.* Owing to the fact that the patient may be reluctant to initiate dialogue about sexual or urinary problems, the nurse may enhance the woman's comfort level with questions such as

- "Many women come to our office with various complaints such as vaginal dryness, itching, and pain with sex. Have you experienced any of these problems?"

- "Have you had any problems with frequent urination, leaking urine, or burning during urination?"

- "Have you tried any vaginal lubricants or other products to enhance comfort during intercourse?" (Allmen & Moore, 2010; Reiter, 2009).

Nurses can empower perimenopausal women with strategies to help combat vaginal dryness. Depending on the situation, the nurse may offer the following suggestions:

- Remain sexually active—sexual activity increases blood flow to the vagina, increases elasticity and lubrication of the vaginal tissues, and maintains muscle tone. Orgasm, achieved by any means, helps to decrease vaginal atrophy.

- Consume phytoestrogen-containing foods and herbs.

- Consider vitamin E, which has an estrogenic effect—apply vitamin E oil to the vagina; take vitamin E supplements (contraindicated in women with hypertension) (Constantino & Guaraldi, 2008).

- Consider the use of vegetable or olive oil, which is more soothing to the genital tissue than the commercially available alcohol-based products, but be aware that the oils can degrade latex condoms (Allmen & Moore, 2010).

- Consider vitamin C and bioflavonoids, substances that increase estrogen levels.

If natural remedies and interventions do not alleviate the discomfort associated with vaginal dryness, a number of nonprescription, nonhormonal products are available. For example, Replens, Me Again, Astroglide, Good Clean Love, and KY Liquibeads assist with moisture, lubrication, coital comfort, and normalization of vaginal pH. The duration of effectiveness is generally 24 to 48 hours. However, nonhormonal lubricants and moisturizers do not restore the integrity of the vagina. Nurses should caution women to avoid the use of Vaseline and other petroleum-based products, which can increase the chance for infection. Also, some over-the-counter products have an alcohol base and can have an undesirable drying effect (Alexander, 2007; Allmen & Moore, 2010; Kellogg-Spadt, 2010).

For women who experience a significant decrease in sex drive along with intolerable vaginal symptoms, the use of estrogen therapy, delivered in the form of a vaginal cream, tablet, or a silastic device may be helpful (ACOG, 2007). Presently, U.S. Food and Drug Administration (FDA) guidelines recommend the use of a vaginal hormonal preparation for menopausal women whose only symptom is vaginal atrophy (Alexander, 2007; Nelson & Stewart, 2008; NAMS, 2007, 2010a).

⑤ Optimizing Outcomes— With the therapeutic effects of vaginal estrogen therapy

Vaginal estrogen therapy promotes a healthy vaginal ecology by restoring vaginal pH to premenopausal levels and normalizing vaginal cytology. Treatment also leads to substantial subjective relief and marked improvement of vulvovaginal atrophy manifestations. Restoration of the vaginal mucosa with subsequent improvement in symptoms associated with vaginal atrophy is likely to improve sexual function by facilitating intercourse. Vaginally delivered estrogen therapy may also reduce urinary urge incontinence and diminish the recurrence of urinary tract infections (Allmen & Moore, 2010).

Low-dose vaginal estrogen cream (e.g., Premarin, Estrace) has been shown to significantly improve symptoms associated with vaginal dryness and reduce the incidence of urinary tract infections. Because systemic absorption of estrogen is minimal, most experts do not recommend the concomitant use of progestins to prevent endometrial hyperplasia in women who have a uterus. Typically, the woman is instructed to insert the estrogen cream into her vagina every day for the first 3 weeks, and then twice a week or as needed. Nurses need to instruct patients to discontinue local estrogen therapy for several days before a Pap screening so as not to obscure the cytology slide. A tablet that contains a low dose of estradiol (i.e., Vagifem) is also available; it is inserted in the vagina twice a week. Nurses should counsel all women who use estrogen therapy to promptly report any vaginal bleeding or breast pain (Alexander, 2007; Greenblum, Greenblum, & Neff, 2009; Secor & Simon, 2006; Wysocki, 2008).

Hormonal vaginal rings, which are silastic devices impregnated with estrogen (estradiol) offer another option. The vaginal rings Estring and Femring are designed to deliver a slow release of estrogen (estradiol) locally to the vagina. The vaginal ring is inserted for a period of 3 months and then replaced by the patient or physician. The Estring is formulated with an ultralow dose of estradiol (7.5 micrograms released per day) and is associated with minimal systemic absorption. No concomitant progestin therapy (to prevent endometrial hyperplasia in women who have a uterus) is necessary. The Femring is formulated with a higher dose of estradiol (available to deliver 0.05 mg per day or 0.1 mg per day) and women with an intact uterus who use this product should almost always receive a progestin to avoid endometrial hyperplasia. Some older women with limited dexterity may experience difficulty positioning the vaginal ring, and the ring may become dislodged with intercourse, douching, or defecation (Greenblum, Greenblum, & Neff, 2009; Secor & Simon, 2006; Wysocki, 2008).

⑤ Be sure to— Consider Lichen sclerosus et atrophicus as another cause of vulvovaginal symptoms

Lichen sclerosus et atrophicus (LS&A) is a rare, benign, chronic, and progressive skin condition that usually affects the vulva in postmenopausal women. Lesions of vulvar LS&A appear as thin, white, glistening scaly patches with diffuse borders affecting the labia majora and minora. Diagnosis is made by the histological examination of a vulvar punch biopsy. Hormonal factors, genetics, immunological abnormalities, and local factors such as infection have been suggested as possible causes, although the actual etiology of LS&A is unknown. Most patients complain of nonspecific vulvar irritation or discomfort of variable intensity. Interestingly, some women are completely asymptomatic; others with severe disease and related symptoms (e.g., intense pruritus, pain, ulceration) may develop dysuria, dyspareunia, and vaginal or meatal stenosis. Treatment usually consists of the nightly application of a topical corticosteroid such as clobetasol (Temovate, Clobex) or halobetasol propionate (Ultravate). Because patients with genital LS&A are at an increased risk for the development of squamous cell cancer, routine follow-up is essential (Patel & Nunley, 2010; Pugliese, Morey, & Peterson, 2007).

HOT FLUSHES, HOT FLASHES, NIGHT SWEATS, AND SLEEP DISTURBANCES

One of the hallmarks of menopause is the occurrence of the vasomotor symptoms hot flushes, hot flashes, and night sweats. A *hot flush* is a visible red flush of skin and perspiration. A *hot flash* is a sudden warm sensation in the neck, head, and chest; heat may be radiated from all parts of the body. During a hot flash, skin temperatures rise as a result of peripheral vasodilation and sweating begins primarily on the upper body. Most women describe a sudden sweeping wave of heat sensation that spreads over the body. An increase in the heart rate of about 7 to 15 beats per minute occurs at approximately the same time as the peripheral vasodilation and sweating. It may take up to 30 minutes or longer for skin temperatures to return to normal. Hot flashes can occur infrequently (e.g., monthly; weekly) or frequently (hourly), although there is usually an individual pattern. A circadian rhythm has been observed, with hot flash frequency peaking in the early evening hours—about 3 hours after the peak in core body temperature (NAMS, 2007).

Night sweats are characterized by profuse perspiration and heat radiating from the body during the night. The woman's sleep may be interrupted each night because her nightclothes and bed linens become soaked with perspiration. Hot flashes constitute the most common symptom reported by women experiencing menopause and are present in 68% to 90% of women. They can occur often throughout the day and create anxiety, distress, and a significantly decreased quality of life (Edelman, 2010; Nelson & Stewart, 2008).

 Nursing Insight— *Vasomotor symptoms and NAMS terminology*

The terms *vasomotor symptoms*, *hot flash*, and *hot flush* are often used to describe the same phenomenon. The North American Menopause Society (NAMS) defines vasomotor symptoms as a global term that encompasses both hot flashes and night sweats. NAMS prefers the term *hot flash* rather than *hot flush* (NAMS, 2007).

For some women, hot flashes are only a significant problem for 1 to 2 years; others experience vasomotor symptoms that can persist for up to 15 years. Approximately 10% to 15% of women characterize their hot flashes as "debilitating." In many non-Westernized cultures, hot flashes either do not occur or are so minimal they are barely noticed. In this country, hot flashes cause women to seek medical advice more than any other symptom of menopause (Alexander, 2007; Secor & Simon, 2006).

The cause of the alternating vasodilation and vasoconstriction associated with hot flashes is not well understood, but it is known that this symptom is related to hormonal changes that affect the temperature-regulating centers in the hypothalamus. Low levels of estrogen alone are not responsible. It is believed that the presence of estrogen, followed by its withdrawal, triggers an imbalance in the body's temperature control center, which subsequently decreases the core body temperature. The body then attempts to activate heat centers to readjust the body's thermostat (Alexander, 2007). Other problems that may be associated with vasomotor instability include dizziness, numbness, or tingling in the fingers and toes and headaches. Environmental and lifestyle factors such as being in a crowded or warm room, consuming hot drinks, alcohol, or spicy foods, and stress can precipitate or aggravate an episode of vasomotor symptoms.

 Be sure to— **Consider alternate causes for various vasomotor symptoms**

The nurse should be aware of other conditions that may cause vasomotor symptoms in women. These include thyroid disease, epilepsy, infection, pheochromocytoma (a rare tumor of the adrenal gland), leukemia, pancreatic tumors, autoimmune disorders, new-onset hypertension, and mast-cell disorders. Also, some medications, such as tamoxifen (Nolvadex) and raloxifene (Evista) can cause hot flashes. Night sweats may be associated with more serious diseases, such as tuberculosis and lymphoma (NAMS, 2007).

Sleep disturbance is a more prevalent complaint for women than men. It is associated with menopausal symptoms (e.g., hot flashes, night sweats) and most importantly, with comorbidities (e.g., obesity, diabetes, depression, esophageal reflux) and stress. Sleep disorders in midlife women should not be attributed solely to the menopausal symptom experience. Referral for clinical evaluation to assess for primary sleep disorders such as restless legs, insomnia, or sleep-disordered breathing may be appropriate (Minarik, 2009; Reeve & Bailes, 2010; Valerio, 2009).

 Now Can You— **Discuss certain aspects of menopause?**

1. Differentiate among the terms *climacteric, premenopause, perimenopause,* and *postmenopause*?
2. Identify menstrual cycle changes, hormonal changes, skin and hair changes, and urogenital changes that typically accompany menopause?
3. Describe four strategies for maintaining and promoting sexual health and enjoyment during the menopausal transition and later years?
4. Identify and describe various vasomotor symptoms that frequently accompany menopause?

Promoting Comfort During the Menopausal Transition

COMPLEMENTARY AND ALTERNATIVE MEDICINE

Complementary and alternative medicine (CAM) includes a broad base of healing philosophies, approaches, and therapies that conventional medicine has not commonly understood or used. In general, a therapy is termed "complementary" when it is used *in addition to* conventional treatment, and it is called "alternative" when it is used *instead of* conventional treatment (NAMS, 2007).

Many women use CAM approaches such as stress management, guided imagery, biofeedback, massage therapy, yoga, chiropractic care, acupuncture, and dietary supplements to relieve various menopausal symptoms. Other nonmedicinal interventions for the relief of mild vasomotor symptoms include engaging in regular exercise; consuming cool, refreshing foods such as cabbage, cucumbers, and pineapple; minimizing the intake of alcohol, fatty foods, sugar and caffeine; avoiding "triggers" such as hot drinks, alcohol, or spicy foods; and dressing in layers to keep cool. Wearing clothing made of cotton, washable linen, or fabrics that wick perspiration away from the skin and increase air movement can increase comfort. Synthetic fabrics such as polyester should be avoided, as they can trap body heat and trigger hot flashes. Nurses can also counsel women to drink 8 to 10 glasses of water each day and perform deep-breathing or paced-respiration exercises at the beginning of a hot flash to diminish its effects (Alexander, 2009; Burdette

Box 7-2 Alternative Medical Systems, Mind–Body Medicine, Manipulative and Body-Based Methods, and Energy Medicine

ALTERNATIVE MEDICAL SYSTEMS

Traditional Chinese Medicine (TCM)

Traditional Chinese medicine (TCHM) is a system of healing that in written form dates back to 200 BC. TCM emphasizes the proper balance of two opposing and inseparable forces: yin and yang. Yin represents the cold, slow, or passive principle, and yang represents the hot, excited, or active principle. An imbalance of these two forces is thought to lead to blockage in the flow of qi (pronounced "chee" and meaning vital energy) and of blood along pathways known as meridians. TCM consists of a group of techniques and methods, including acupuncture, herbal medicine, oriental massage, and qi gong, to bring the body back into harmony and balance (NAMS, 2007).

Ayurveda

Ayurveda is India's traditional system of medicine. Meaning "science of life," Ayurvedic medicine is a comprehensive system that places equal emphasis on body, mind, and spirit and strives to restore the innate harmony of the individual. Some of the primary Ayurvedic treatments include diet, exercise, meditation, herbs, massage, exposure to sunlight, and controlled breathing (NAMS, 2007).

Homeopathic Medicine

Homeopathy is an unconventional Western system that is based on the principle that "like cures like" (i.e., large doses of a particular substance may produce symptoms of an illness; very small doses will cure it). Very small doses of specially prepared plant extracts and minerals are used to stimulate the body's defense mechanisms and healing processes to treat illness. The homeopathic approach focuses on the links among an individual's physical, emotional, and mental symptoms (NAMS, 2007).

Naturopathic Medicine

In naturopathic medicine, disease is viewed as a manifestation of alterations in the processes by which the body naturally heals itself, and emphasis is placed on health restoration rather than on disease treatment. Practitioners of naturopathic medicine employ a variety of healing practices, including diet and clinical nutrition, homeopathy, acupuncture, herbal medicine, hydrotherapy, spinal and soft-tissue manipulation, physical therapies involving electric currents, ultrasound and light therapy, therapeutic counseling, and pharmacology (NAMS, 2007).

MIND–BODY MEDICINE

Mind–body medicine focuses on the interactions among the brain, mind, body, and behavior and the powerful ways in which emotional, mental, social, spiritual, and behavioral factors can directly affect health. Mind–body medicine is an approach that respects and enhances each person's capacity for self-knowledge and self-care and emphasizes techniques that are grounded in this approach. Hypnosis, dance, music, and art therapy, prayer and mental healing, relaxation and visual imagery, meditation, and yoga are typical techniques used with this approach (NAMS, 2007).

MANIPULATIVE AND BODY-BASED METHODS

These methods are based on manipulation and/or movement of structures and systems of the body, including bones and joints, the soft tissues, and the circulatory and lymphatic systems. While there is considerable variation in the training and approaches of manipulative and body-based providers, they all share certain principles, such as the belief that the human body is self-regulating and has the ability to heal itself. Practitioners of manipulative and body-based methods include osteopathic physicians (DOs), massage therapists, and reflexologists (NAMS, 2007).

ENERGY MEDICINE

Energy therapies focus on either energy fields originating within the body (putative energy fields [biofields], which cannot be measured) or those from other sources (veritable energy fields that involve the use of measurable wavelengths and frequencies, also called electromagnetic fields). Examples of putative energy medicine include qi gong, reiki, intercessory prayer, and healing touch (NAMS, 2007).

---

et al., 2009; Kupferer, Dormire, & Becker, 2009; Nachtigall et al., 2006; Nelson et al., 2006).

Daily aerobic exercise helps to reduce the frequency and severity of hot flashes by assisting in body temperature regulation. Exercise is also beneficial in reducing cardiovascular disease and osteoporosis risk and helps to maintain normal glucose levels and weight. Midlife women who engage in regular exercise report a higher quality of life, and routine exercise can help to improve depression, muscular soreness or stiffness, palpitations, memory, and sleep quality (Alexander, 2009).

In 1998, the U.S. Congress established The National Center for Complementary and Alternative Medicine (NCCAM) at the National Institutes of Health to stimulate, develop, and support research on CAM for the benefit of the public. NCCAM was charged with providing the American public with reliable information about the safety and effectiveness of CAM practices. NCCAM groups CAM therapies into the following five major domains: Alternative Medical Systems, Mind-body Medicine, Manipulative and Body-based Methods, Energy Medicine, and Biologically-based Treatment (NAMS, 2007).

Alternative Medical Systems

Alternative medical systems include complete systems of theory and practice that have evolved independently of and often prior to the conventional biomedical approach. Many are traditional systems of medicine practiced by individual cultures throughout the world. Alternative medical systems, mind–body medicine, manipulative and body-based methods, and energy medicine are briefly described in Box 7-2.

 Nursing Insight— *Traditional Chinese medicine and menopause*

Traditional Chinese medicine (TCM) includes menopause as part of a phenomenon that involves an imbalance of body energy. The TCM practitioner may use herbs, meditative or breathing exercises, massage, or diet to help a woman restore and balance the energy and therefore reduce menopausal symptoms. TCM practitioners may also use acupuncture for treating symptoms associated with menopause (NAMS, 2007).

Biologically Based Treatments

Biologically based complementary and alternative medicines include biologically based practices, interventions, and products, many of which overlap with conventional medicine's use of dietary supplements. Botanical therapies are complex mixtures of preparations made from the whole plant or plant part, such as root, leaves, gum, resin, or essential oil. Most botanical therapies are medicinal herbs. A medicinal herb is a plant or plant part that produces and contains chemical substances that act upon the body (NAMS, 2007).

 Complementary Care: *Herbal therapies: Modes of administration*

Herbal therapies intended for ingestion may be administered in a variety of ways, such as:

- Tea infusions (soft, aromatic parts of the plant are steeped, not boiled, in water)

- Tea decoctions (barks and roots, boiled in water)
- Essential oils (highly concentrated)
- Tinctures and fluid extracts (herbs macerated into water-alcohol mixtures)
- Dried standardized extract (these typically contain part of a plant but can contain the whole plant; extracts are standardized to one ingredient only)
- Homeopathic preparations (extremely diluted) (NAMS, 2007)

The most studied of the botanicals for menopause-related conditions are compounds often termed *phytoestrogens* (sometimes called "dietary estrogens"). Phytoestrogens are a diverse group of naturally occurring nonsteroidal plant compounds that have a structural similarity with estradiol and are able to exert estrogenic and/or antiestrogenic effects. There are three principal groups of phytoestrogens: isoflavones, coumestans, and lignans. Because herbal compounds containing phytoestrogens are not FDA regulated, there is no proof of the efficacy, safety, or overall quality of the products. Until such information becomes available, these remedies should be considered to have the same issues as traditional menopausal hormone therapy (discussed later in this chapter) (Alexander, 2006; Alexander, 2007; Lake, 2007; McKee & Warber, 2005; NAMS, 2007).

Be sure to— Advise women to use isoflavones with caution

Isoflavones (e.g., red clover, soy) are the most widely used phytoestrogens for menopause. Isoflavones comprise a class of organic compounds, often naturally occurring, related to the isoflavonoids. Some isoflavones and isoflavone-rich foods possess activity against cancer, including certain types of breast and prostate cancer. Isoflavones are produced almost exclusively by members of the bean family, and soybeans are the most common source of isoflavones in human food. Soy and other iso-flavone supplements are regulated in the United States as dietary supplements; their effectiveness has not been well established, and they are not monitored for purity, amount of active ingredient, or health claims (Alexander, 2009; Geller & Studee, 2008; NAMS, 2007).

Phytoestrogens interact with estrogen receptors in the body. Foods that contain phytoestrogens include wild yams, cashews, peanuts and almonds, dandelion greens, apples, cherries, alfalfa sprouts, sage, black beans, and soy products (e.g., beans, flour, milk, sauce). The use of soy-rich foods has also been investigated as an alternative to hormone therapy for menopausal symptoms. According to the Natural Standard database, there is good evidence for sage and soy for menopause symptom management (http://www.naturalstandard.com/). NAMS concedes that soy products may have small benefits in the treatment of vasomotor symptoms in the short term (12 weeks), but not for longer periods (6 to 12 months). According to NAMS (2007), there is strong evidence that soy is non beneficial in the prevention of postmenopausal bone loss, but may be useful in maintaining cognitive function; however, additional studies are needed (Albertazzi, 2005; NAMS, 2007).

An important role for nurses centers on counseling women to become informed about any herbal preparations they are considering and to consult with their health-care providers before using any of them. Nurses should explain that before using any substance, it is important to understand the mechanisms of action, contraindications, and potential adverse effects. Herbs may be beneficial in resolving physical symptoms as well as mood swings and depression. To obtain current information about various dietary supplements, health professionals and consumers may consult various Internet sites such as those offered by the U.S. National Library of Medicine and the National Institutes of Health (http://www.nlm.nih.gov/medlineplus/dietarysupplements.html and http://www.nlm.nih.gov/medlineplus/druginformation.html) and the U.S. Department of Agriculture National Agricultural Library (http://fnic.nal.usda.gov/nal_display/index.php?info_center=4&tax_level=2&tax_subject=274&topic_id=1331). Nurses may also inform patients who wish to use soy, herbs, or other dietary supplements about ConsumerLab (http://www.consumerlab.com), an independent company that tests and provides objective reviews of many over-the-counter consumer supplements; there is an annual subscription fee to access the information (Alexander, 2009).

Oriental herbal teas composed of licorice, ginseng, sage, coptis, red raspberry leaf, and Chinese rhubarb may provide some relief for hot flashes. Dong quai and black cohosh have been used for various menopausal discomforts. Dong quai, the most commonly prescribed Chinese herbal medicine for "female problems," purportedly regulates and balances the menstrual cycle and is said to "strengthen the uterus." It is also purported to exert estrogenic activity. However, Dong quai has not been found to be useful in reducing hot flashes and is not recommended for this symptom. Also, Dong quai can trigger heavy uterine bleeding and should never be used by women who have fibroids, hemophilia, or other blood-clotting problems; it is contraindicated for use with anticoagulants (ACOG, 2001; Alexander, 2009; NAMS, 2007).

Black cohosh (*Cimicifuga racemosa*) may be helpful in the short-term (less than 2 years) treatment of menopausal symptoms, including hot flashes, sleep disorders, anxiety, and depression. Black cohosh is not recommended for women with a history of liver problems or for those using hepatotoxic medications. Both Dong quai and black cohosh have been investigated for effectiveness, with varying results. According to NCCAM (http://nccam.nih.gov/), there is very little high-quality scientific evidence about the effectiveness and long-term safety of complementary and alternative medicine for menopausal symptoms (ACOG, 2001; Alexander, 2009; Geller & Studee, 2008; NAMS, 2007).

Complementary Care: *St. John's wort, valerian, chasteberry, and ginseng*

St. John's wort and valerian root have been used for mood disturbances during menopause. The flower *hypericum perforatum*, known as St. John's wort, has been used for centuries to treat mild to moderate depression. Commercial preparations typically contain the generally recommended doses and one capsule is taken three times a day. Side effects are similar to, but much less than, those associated with standard antidepressant medications and include fatigue, dry mouth, dizziness, and constipation. St. John's wort should not be used concomitantly with psychotropic medications. Valerian root (*Valeriana officinalis*), has traditionally been used as a tranquilizer and soporific. Valerian improves subjective experiences of sleep when taken nightly for 1 to 2 weeks. Although it has no demonstrable toxicity, there have been reports of adverse reactions and visual disturbances. Little is known about the actions, effects, or potential interactions of valerian with other medications (ACOG, 2001; NAMS, 2007).

Some practitioners have recommended chasteberry and ginseng for menopausal loss of libido. Chasteberry, or vitex, is also known as Chaste tree, Monk's pepper, agnus castus, Indian spice, sage tree hemp, and tree wild pepper. It has been used for vaginal dryness at menopause and also for depression and to enhance libido in menopausal women. Asian ginseng (*Panax ginseng*) is promoted as an "adaptogen" that helps one cope with stress and boost immunity. Ginseng is also reputed to be an aphrodisiac, although this claim has not been substantiated by medical evidence (ACOG, 2001; NAMS, 2007). According to the Natural Standard database, there is poor evidence for ginseng and chasteberry in the treatment of menopausal symptoms. However, there is good evidence for both sage and soy in menopause symptom management.

 Now Can You— Discuss various CAM therapies for menopausal symptoms?

1. Identify and briefly describe three alternative medical systems?
2. Describe the major focus of mind–body medicine and identify six examples of typical techniques used with this approach?
3. Briefly explain the techniques of *intercessory prayer* and *healing touch*?
4. Provide appropriate counseling to a woman who wishes to use herbal products?

HORMONAL THERAPIES

Estrogen is the only pharmacologic therapy that is government approved in the United States and Canada for treating menopause-related symptoms. Estrogen-containing drugs for menopausal use are divided into two categories: estrogen therapy (ET) and combined estrogen-progestogen therapy (EPT) (NAMS, 2010a).

 Nursing Insight— *NAMS menopausal hormone therapy terminology*

Estrogen therapy (ET)—unopposed estrogen prescribed for postmenopausal women who have had a hysterectomy.
Estrogen plus progestogen (EPT)—a combination of estrogen and progestogen (either progesterone or progestin, synthetic forms of progesterone). Although the available data suggest that the benefits of EPT are almost exclusively due to the estrogen, progestogen reduces the risk of endometrial adenocarcinoma in women with a uterus—and this risk is significantly increased in women who use unopposed estrogen.

Hormone therapy (HT)—encompasses both ET and EPT. The FDA refers to EPT as HT.
Local therapy—vaginal ET administration that does not result in clinically significant systemic absorption.
Progestogen—encompasses both progesterone and progestin.
Systemic therapy—HT administration that results in absorption in the blood high enough to provide clinically significant results.
Timing of HT initiation—length of time after menopause when HT is initiated. (NAMS, 2010a)

Previously, the terms *estrogen replacement therapy* and *hormone replacement therapy* were used. However, according to NAMS, the term *replacement* is a misnomer because postmenopausal levels of HT provide only a small fraction of the estrogen the ovaries once produced. The FDA declared that "replacement" can no longer be used by marketers of products available in the United States. The FDA uses "ET" to describe unopposed estrogen therapy and "HT" to describe EPT. NAMS, however, prefers using "HT" to encompass all hormone therapy used for menopause and "EPT" to more clearly describe combined therapy (Bachmann, 2009; NAMS, 2007; Theroux, 2008).

Menopause hormone therapy (HT) is a controversial issue. A brief review of the historical background, recent research, and current guidelines for use of HT can assist women and their health-care providers in making the appropriate decisions concerning this treatment option.

Historical Background

The widespread practice of prescribing estrogen began in the 1960s. Estrogen was touted as a wonder drug that offered women the opportunity to age more slowly. By 1975, conjugated equine estrogen, marketed under the name of Premarin, was one of the most frequently prescribed drugs in the United States. Premarin is derived from the urine of pregnant mares. For many years, animal rights activists have promoted public awareness of cruelty to these animals and their offspring involved in the production of Premarin (National Women's Health Network, 2000).

In 1975, two studies were published that showed a 2- to 8-fold increase in the rate of uterine cancer among non-hysterectomized women receiving estrogen therapy. The risk was linked to estrogen dosage and the duration of treatment. In response to this finding, a number of women's organizations sought to heighten public awareness of the risks associated with estrogen use, claiming that women were not given adequate information to make informed choices. As this information became more widespread, use of estrogen in this country declined. Later studies were conducted to investigate combinations of estrogen and a progestin (a synthetic form of progesterone). Results of these studies revealed that the estrogen-progestin combination protected against precancerous changes of the uterine lining. Based on these findings, there was a shift to the use of estrogen-progestin combinations (National Women's Health Network, 2000).

By the late 1980s, results of several studies had shown that women who received estrogen were less likely to suffer heart attacks than those who did not receive estrogen. Although the FDA refused to grant the manufacturer approval for promoting estrogen as a heart disease preventive, many clinicians were recommending estrogen for this purpose. The combination of estrogen along with a progestin also began to be prescribed for this same purpose, even though the combination had not been in use long enough to evaluate its effect on heart disease. The Postmenopausal Estrogen/Progestin Interventions (PEPI) study, published in 1995, showed that the most commonly used progestin, medroxyprogesterone acetate (Provera), greatly interfered with the positive effect of estrogen alone on high-density lipoprotein (HDL) levels. Natural progesterone (i.e., oral micronized progesterone), also used in the study, did not negate the positive effects of estrogen on HDL levels (National Women's Health Network, 2000). Major findings from more recent studies, including the Heart and Estrogen/Progestin Replacement Study (HERS I and II), the Nurse's Health Study, and the Women's Health Initiative (WHI) are summarized in Box 7-3.

Menopausal Hormone Therapy: Considerations and Choices

Owing to the findings from large-scale prospective clinical trials such as the WHI, which demonstrated that hormone therapy is not without risks, the FDA and several professional organizations recommend prescribing the lowest effective dose for the shortest duration of time consistent with treatment goals for the individual patient. Growing evidence indicates that the benefits and risks vary with the type of estrogen and progestogen prescribed, as well as the route of administration, timing of therapy, baseline risk of disease, chronological age, age at menopause, cause of menopause, time since menopause, and previous use of

where research and practice meet:
Considerations of the WHI Research Results

Findings from the WHI research may be used to guide patient education and counseling. Nurses should consider the following points (ACOG, 2007; Burdette et al., 2009; Secor & Simon, 2006; Theroux, 2008; Utian, 2008):

The HT arm of the WHI trial was stopped because the rate of breast cancer crossed a predetermined boundary set at the initiation of the trial. However, breast cancer rates had not reached statistical significance when the trial was halted.

The fact that that the slight increase in invasive breast cancer was noted during the fourth year of the study, along with the trend toward a later decrease in the total number of breast cancer cases, suggests that HT promotes the growth of existing breast cancer, rather than causes breast cancer. No increased risk in breast cancer was seen among women on estrogen therapy for an average of 7.1 years. Estrogen-progestin therapy, and to a lesser extent, estrogen therapy, increases breast cell proliferation, breast pain, and mammographic density. Hormone therapy may impede the diagnostic interpretation of mammograms. Women with risk factors for breast cancer (e.g., positive family history, early puberty, late parity) should be individually assessed before initiating HT for the relief of moderate to severe vasomotor symptoms.

For the first time in terms of any therapy, findings from the WHI study indicated that HT reduces hip fractures and colon cancer.

Box 7-3 Major Findings From The HERS and WHI Studies

THE HEART AND ESTROGEN/PROGESTIN REPLACEMENT STUDY (HERS), THE HEART AND ESTROGEN/PROGESTIN REPLACEMENT STUDY FOLLOW-UP (HERS II), AND THE NURSE'S HEALTH STUDY

- Designed to assess the relationship between hormone therapy (HT) and coronary artery disease events among postmenopausal women.
- Although findings from the HERS II study showed that HT did not provide cardiac protection in women who had previously been diagnosed with heart disease, re-analysis of data indicated that certain women (e.g., women on statin medications to lower cholesterol) experienced fewer problems associated with thromboembolic events (Alexander, 2007).

THE WOMEN'S HEALTH INITIATIVE (WHI)

- A long-term primary prevention trial conducted with 25,000 healthy postmenopausal women.
- Purpose: To evaluate the safety and effectiveness of estrogen as well as an estrogen/progestin combination given to healthy women over a 9-year period beginning in 1993, with final analysis planned for 2005.
- Designed to assess the major benefits and risks of hormone therapy with regard to coronary heart disease, venous thrombotic events, breast cancer, colon cancer, and fractures.
- Quality of life issues, such as a reduction in hot flashes and vaginal dryness, were not included (Secor & Simon, 2006).
- In July, 2002, after approximately 5 years of follow-up, the estrogen and progestin arm of the WHI trial was halted because the predetermined boundary for invasive breast cancer was exceeded. At this time, it was concluded that the risks outweighed the benefits for the indicators that were being studied.
- The risk of cardiovascular disease, coronary heart disease, stroke, and venous thromboembolism was increased as well (Theroux, 2008; Writing Group for the Women's Health Initiative Investigators, 2002).
- There was a 37% and a 24% decrease in colorectal cancer and total fractures, respectively.
- Of importance, there was no difference in rates of mortality between the two groups (i.e., those who did receive HT and those who did not receive HT).
- In 2004, the estrogen-only trial was also halted because the risk with the conjugated equine estrogen (Premarin) for stroke was elevated and the other endpoints were unlikely to change with continuation of the trial (Burdette et al., 2009; Hsia et al., 2006; Secor & Simon, 2006).
- Later analysis of the findings suggested that timing of hormone therapy use has an effect: In the age 50 to 59 cohort, coronary heart disease was decreased. Based on this information, it is believed to be safest to begin hormone therapy within 10 years of menopause.
- Another follow-up study of the WHI participants demonstrated that women ages 50 to 59 who were on estrogen therapy had lower amounts of calcium deposits in their coronary arteries.

Sources: Alexander, 2007; Dranov, 2007; Secor & Simon, 2006; Williams & Brownlee, 2010; Writing Group for the Women's Health Initiative Investigators, 2002.

---

any hormone (Altman, 2008, 2009; Bachmann, 2009; Berga, 2009; Sherman, 2009a; Gersh, 2009; Nachtigall, 2009). A summary of NAMS (2010a) recommendations concerning HT for the treatment of various menopausal symptoms is presented in Box 7-4.

Today, clinicians have a wide variety of estrogen products from which to choose, including oral tablets; transdermal patches; and topical sprays, gels, and lotions, as well

Box 7-4   Summary of NAMS 2010 Recommendations for HT Use

Vasomotor symptoms: Moderate to severe vasomotor symptoms (e.g., hot flashes, night sweats) remain the primary indication for HT; it is also the best treatment for moderate to severe vulvar and vaginal atrophy; local vaginal ET is recommended for treating urogenital atrophy alone; systemic or local ET can relieve dyspareunia.

Osteoporosis: Extended HT is an option for women with decreased bone mass; benefits decrease quickly once therapy has ended.

Coronary heart disease (CHD): HT is not recommended as a sole or primary indication for coronary protection at any age; starting ET alone soon after menopause may slow development of calcified atherosclerotic plaque and lower CHD risk.

Stroke: HT is not recommended for primary or secondary prevention of stroke.

Venous thromboembolism (VTE): Most likely an increased risk of VTE with oral HT, especially in women with a history of VTE or factor V Leiden (a hypercoagulability disorder).

Diabetes mellitus: Inadequate evidence to recommend HT as the sole or primary indication for preventing diabetes in perimenopausal or post-menopausal women.

Endometrial cancer: Women with an intact uterus taking systemic ET should take concomitant progestogen to counteract the risk of endometrial cancer; HT is not recommended for women with a history of endometrial cancer.

Breast cancer: Diagnosis of breast cancer increases with EPT use longer than 3 to 5 years; women who start EPT shortly after menopause may have a greater risk than women who start more than 5 years afterward; ET use in breast cancer survivors has not been proven to be safe and may be associated with an increased risk of recurrence.

Ovarian cancer: Data on HT and ovarian cancer conflict; the association between ovarian cancer and HT beyond 5 years is rare.

Cognitive aging and dementia: HT is not recommended for the sole or primary indication of preventing cognitive aging or dementia or to enhance cognitive function in younger postmenopausal patients with intact ovaries.

Mood and depression: Although HT might have a positive effect on mood and behavior, HT is not an antidepressant and should not be considered as such; evidence is insufficient to support HT use for the treatment of depression.

Sources: Altman, 2009; Bachmann, 2009; Burdette, Moore, Speroff, & Wysocki, 2009; Freeman, 2009; Helmrich, 2010; Hess, London, Moore, & Simon, 2009; Henderson, 2009; Margolis, 2010; NAMS, 2010a; Utian, 2008.

Box 7-5   Examples of Estrogen and Progestogen Products for Menopause-Related Symptoms

ESTROGEN ONLY
Estrace (oral tablet, vaginal cream)
Femtrace (oral tablet)
Ogen (oral tablet)
Premarin (oral tablet, vaginal cream)
Estraderm, Vivelle, Climara (transdermal patch)
Divigel, EstroGel (transdermal gel)
Femring, Estring (vaginal ring)
Vagifem (vaginal tablet)
Evamist (topical spray)

PROGESTOGEN ONLY
Provera (oral tablet)
Prometrium (oral tablet)

ESTROGEN-PROGESTOGEN COMBINATIONS
CombiPatch (transdermal patch)
Climara Pro (transdermal patch)
Femhrt (oral tablet)
Prempro (oral tablet)

protection, osteoporosis prevention, short- and long-term hormone use, and alternatives to HT. Women who are taking or considering HT only for the prevention of cardiovascular disease should be counseled about other strategies to lower their risks of heart disease.

 Nursing Insight— *Hormone therapy and heart disease*

According to the American College of Obstetricians and Gynecologists (ACOG) (2008) and the North American Menopause Society (NAMS) (2010a), menopausal HT should not at present be used for the primary or secondary prevention of coronary heart disease. Recent analyses suggest that HT may not increase CHD (coronary heart disease) risk for select populations of women who have experienced menopause recently. Hormone therapy should be limited to the treatment of menopausal symptoms at the lowest effective dosage over the shortest duration possible and continued use should be reevaluated on a periodic basis.

as vaginal creams, tablets, and rings. The choice of therapy is often based on patient preference. Examples of estrogen and progestogen products for menopause-related symptoms are presented in Box 7-5; NAMS has prepared charts for health-care providers that include information about all estrogen and progestogen products that are currently available in the United States and Canada. The charts may be viewed at http://www.menopause.org/edumaterials/hormoneprimer.aspx (Bachmann, 2009; Margolis, 2010; NAMS, 2010a; Theroux, 2008; Utian, 2008; Utian, Archer, Bachmann, et al., 2008).

The Nursing Role in Menopausal Hormone Therapy Counseling

When counseling women about HT benefits and risks, it is helpful to consider a number of factors, such as cardiac

Women who are taking HT only for the prevention of osteoporosis should be assessed for their personal osteoporosis risk and should be advised to consult with their health-care provider about continuing HT for this purpose. There are many alternatives (i.e., bisphosphonates, calcitonin) that should be considered for women whose only need for HT is the prevention of osteoporosis (ACOG, 2004; Alexander, 2007; Bachmann, 2009; Dranov, 2007; National Osteoporosis Foundation [NOF], 2008; Secor & Simon, 2006). (See discussion of osteoporosis later in this chapter.)

For women who seek short-term (1 to 4 years) relief of menopausal symptoms, the benefits of HT most likely outweigh the risks. Although certain symptoms such as hot flashes and night sweats tend to be of short duration for most women, other menopausal symptoms such as vaginal dryness generally continue throughout the post-menopausal period. Also, many women believe that estrogen helps them to feel, think, and sleep better. These women may conclude that for them, the added benefits of fracture prevention and colon cancer reduction associated with HT outweigh the risks. Nurses may share information about alternatives to HT, such as the use of vaginal lubricants, and strategies for relief from sleep disturbances (Ruhl, 2010). However, the decision to continue with long-term HT is one that must be made on an individual basis following consideration of each woman's benefits and risks, including those benefits and risks that were not addressed in the WHI study.

Large randomized controlled trials, including the WHI, have suggested that hormone therapy reduces the incidence of diabetes among postmenopausal women. The reason for this benefit is unknown, although it may be related to lower weight gain or reduced insulin resistance among women using HT. However, there is inadequate evidence to recommend hormone therapy solely for diabetes prevention in perimenopausal women. Also, it is important to bear in mind that the WHI studied only one preparation of HT. Hence, data generated from the WHI study cannot be applied to all HT therapies. An important role for nurses who care for midlife women involves providing them with current evidence-based information about HT along with culturally appropriate resources for promoting menopausal health (Alexander, 2007; Dranov, 2007; NAMS, 2010a; Secor & Simon, 2006).

Estrogens do not cause endometrial cancer, as long as an appropriate dosage of progestogen (either as progestin or progesterone) is added to the hormonal regimen. Individual regimens and formulations differ and include both synthetic and natural formulations, and each route and type of progestogen carries different effects, risks, and benefits. Evidence shows that women who use combined HT are no more likely than those who have never used HT to develop overgrowth (hyperplasia) of the endometrium or endometrial cancer (LaCroix, 2005; Liu, 2007; NAMS, 2010a; Secor & Simon, 2006).

"What to say" — *Counseling patients about bleeding symptoms when systemic HT is first initiated*

Nurses should educate women who plan to initiate HT about certain symptoms, such as vaginal spotting and unscheduled bleeding, that often occur as the body adapts to a new hormonal milieu. Nurses may offer the following information:

- Vaginal bleeding and spotting are most likely to occur in the first 3 months after initiation of therapy.
- Follow-up visits should be scheduled at 1 and 3 months—and improvement in symptoms should be noted at that time.
- It is important to promptly report the following symptoms: persistent bleeding, bleeding that stops but then starts again, or the presence of blood clots in the vaginal discharge (Liu, 2007).

Evidence that the risk of depression is higher in early menopause is mixed. Although two small randomly controlled trials found that short-term estrogen therapy is effective for the treatment of affected perimenopausal women, another trial found no such benefit for depressed older postmenopausal women. Presently, there is insufficient evidence for using hormone therapy to treat depression in general (Dranov, 2007). Also, despite earlier findings, no evidence has been generated to support the use of hormone therapy to prevent dementia or cognitive decline. Beginning estrogen-progestogen therapy after age 65 for these reasons may actually increase the risk of dementia within the subsequent 5 years. Studies that investigated whether dementia can be prevented in women who begin hormone therapy during the menopause transition or early postmenopause period provided insufficient evidence of help or harm. Estrogen therapy does not appear to have any effect on Alzheimer's disease (Gies & Lessick, 2009; Dranov, 2007). The U.S. Preventive Services Task Force (USPSTF) and ACOG advise against the use of HT to improve cognition or to prevent or treat dementia (ACOG, 2004b; Alexander, 2007; USPSTF, 2009).

Educating Patients About Hormone Therapy Options

In general, transdermal estrogen (estradiol) provides the same relief of menopausal symptoms as do the oral preparations but without the side effects of breast tenderness or fluid retention. Transdermal estradiol delivery systems have been shown to be safer than oral administration in reducing certain markers of cardiovascular risk. Since the hormones bypass the liver and are directly absorbed into the bloodstream, transdermal administration is more effective in maintaining stable blood levels of estrogen. Also, because the transdermal estradiol is absorbed directly into the body, first-pass metabolism by the gastrointestinal tract and liver is avoided. When given orally, larger doses of estrogen are required to achieve therapeutic levels and to offset metabolism by the liver and inactivation by the gut wall. In addition, when compared with the transdermal formulations, oral estrogen therapy has been shown to increase the risk of venous thromboembolic disease (Altman, 2009; Dranov, 2007; Secor & Simon, 2006; Shulman, 2008).

No large studies have compared the advantages and disadvantages of the different transdermal formulations. The patch, applied one or two times a week to a hairless area of the skin, is considerably more irritating to the skin than either the gel or emulsion. Also, the gel and the emulsion are more discrete than the patch. To use the gel or emulsion, the patient applies the product to clean, dry, intact skin at the same time each day. The emulsion is applied to the complete surface of both legs once a day; the gel is applied to one upper arm and shoulder once a day. An estradiol transdermal spray, now available, is applied to a small area on the inner forearm once daily; the dose can be increased to two or three sprays as needed for symptom control. The application site should be allowed to dry for 2 minutes before it is covered with clothing and the site should not be washed for 30 minutes after application. When applying two or three sprays, the applicator cone should be placed adjacent to, but not overlapping, the area of the previous administration. All of these products should be used for the shortest possible period of time and require 4 to 12 weeks before relief of symptoms is obtained (Altman, 2009; Minkin, 2010; Secor & Simon, 2006; Shulman, 2008).

Nurses can empower women with current evidence-based information about contraindications, risks, and side effects of various hormone therapies. Providing this information helps guide patients to make appropriate, informed decisions. The risks and side effects of estrogen and progestogen are presented in Box 7-6.

 Be sure to— Be knowledgeable of the contraindications to estrogen

Nurses who care for patients who use estrogen therapy must be knowledgeable of the absolute contraindications to estrogen. These include the following:
- Known or suspected estrogen-dependent cancer
- Known, suspected, or history of breast cancer except in appropriately selected patients being treated for metastatic disease
- Undiagnosed abnormal genital bleeding
- Active or history of deep venous thrombosis, pulmonary embolism
- Active or recent (within the past year) arterial thromboembolic disease (e.g., stroke, myocardial infarction)
- Liver dysfunction or disease
- Known or suspected pregnancy
- Known hypersensitivity to ET/EPT (NAMS, 2007; Reiter, 2009)

 Optimizing Outcomes— Using the NAMS 2010 position statement to guide care

The North American Menopause Society's evidenced-based 2010 Position Statement emphasizes recent data on breast cancer, cognitive aging/decline and dementia, coronary heart disease, stroke, and discontinuation of therapy. It also includes new sections on ovarian and lung cancer. The full text is available on the NAMS Web site at http://www.menopause.org/PSHT10.pdf.

Bioidentical Compounds

The term *bioidentical hormones* was introduced by Jonathan Wright, MD, a practitioner who used the term to communicate his still unsubstantiated claim that plant-derived hormones are "identical" in molecular structure to human hormones. When used to describe hormones, "bioidentical" simply means chemically indistinguishable from the hormones produced in a woman's body (e.g., estradiol-17β and progesterone) during her reproductive years. Numerous FDA-approved drugs contain these hormones and therefore are also "bioidentical" (Box 7-7) (ACOG, 2005; Alexander, 2006, 2007; Altman, 2008, 2009; Burkman, 2009; Dranov, 2007; NAMS, 2010a; Rosenthal, 2008, 2009; Secor & Simon, 2006).

Compounded bioidentical hormones are plant-derived hormones (e.g., from wild yam or soy) that are prepared by a pharmacist and can be custom-made for a patient according to a physician's specifications. Bioidentical compounds have been promoted as a natural approach; the claim is that

---

Box 7-6   **Risks and Side Effects of Estrogen and Progestogen**

RISKS OF ESTROGEN
Breast cancer
Endometrial cancer
Increased risk of stroke
Small increase in the risk of venous thromboembolism
Possible small increase in the risk of coronary events
Worsening of hypertriglyceridemia
Possible worsening of gallbladder disease
Deterioration of liver function in women with severe liver disease
Worsening of edema in women with severe cardiac disease
Worsening of pain from benign breast disease
Increased risk of gallbladder disease

SIDE EFFECTS OF ESTROGEN
Worsening of estrogen-dependent conditions, such as uterine fibroids and endometriosis
Increase in fibrocystic breast problems
Vaginal bleeding
Hypertension
Nausea and vomiting
Headaches, jaundice, and fluid retention
Impaired glucose tolerance
Changes in the shape of the cornea (sometimes leading to contact lens intolerance)

SIDE EFFECTS OF PROGESTOGEN
Fluid retention
Breast tenderness
Jaundice
Nausea
Insomnia
Depression
Menstrual bleeding

Sources: Altman, 2009; NAMS, 2007; Reiter, 2009.

Box 7-7   **FDA-Approved Pharmaceutical Bioidentical Hormone Preparations**

- Oral estradiol (Estrace, Femtrace)
- Estradiol transdermal patches (Alora, Climara, Esclim, Estraderm, Menostar, Vivelle, Vivelle-dot)
- Estradiol transdermal gel (Divigel, Elestrin, EstroGel)
- Estradiol spray (Evamist)
- Estradiol topical emulsion (Estrasorb)
- Vaginal estradiol cream (Estrace) and ring (Estring, Femring)
- Progesterone as oral micronized progesterone (Prometrium) and vaginal gel (Crinone)
- Estradiol patches are available in combination with a synthetically produced progestin; no combination bioidentical preparations are on the market.

Sources: Minkin, 2010; Moore, 2010; Weil, 2009.

they replace specific hormones that are naturally present in a woman's body. Because the only truly natural source of human estradiol is the human ovary, all plant sources must be processed to synthesize estradiol. Therefore, all bioidentical products are, in actuality, synthetic (ACOG, 2005; Alexander, 2006, 2007; Altman, 2008, 2009; Burkman, 2009; Dranov, 2007; Moore, 2010; NAMS, 2010a; Secor & Simon, 2006; Weil, 2009).

Many bioidentical replacement hormones are compounded in private laboratories or pharmacies as individualized made-to-order products. The hormones prepared by a compounding pharmacist are not regulated and FDA approved. Women need to be made aware of the limitations and poor results that may be associated with this therapy (ACOG, 2005; Alexander, 2006, 2007; Altman, 2008, 2009; Dranov, 2007; Minkin, 2010; NAMS, 2010a; Secor & Simon, 2006). However, certain bioidentical preparations of estrogen or progestin are approved by the FDA for oral, intravaginal, transdermal, or percutaneous applications. These particular medications have undergone strenuous testing for safety, efficacy, and quality control. *Compounded* bioidentical formulations are not FDA-regulated in the same way. These products are not subject to rigorous testing or quality control standards. Also, the compounded products do not include a package insert that lists important contraindications, warnings, and precautions—which may make them appear to be safer than traditional therapy medications. These products lack standardization and in many cases, the specific active ingredients and minimally effective dosages are not known (ACOG, 2005; Alexander, 2006, 2007; Altman, 2008, 2009; Altman, Moore, Speroff, & Wysocki, 2009; Moore, 2010; NAMS, 2010a).

 Nursing Insight— *Being wary of compounded bioidentical hormone formulations is warranted*

Custom-made HT formulations, called *bioidentical hormone therapy,* or BHT, are compounded for an individual according to a health-care provider's prescription. Often touted as "natural," in actuality, bioidentical hormones are all synthesized, making terms such as *natural* and *nonsynthetic* inaccurate and meaningless. The American College of Obstetricians and Gynecologists (ACOG) and the North American Menopause Society (NAMS) consider the bioidentical hormone preparations to have the same safety risks as traditional hormone therapy and assert that they may carry additional risks associated with the compounding process. In addition, evidence-based data supporting the efficacy of bioidentical compounded preparations are lacking. The risks, benefits, and quality of these products have not been evaluated through rigorous testing, a standard requirement for traditional hormone therapy medications (ACOG, 2005; Alexander, 2007; Altman, 2008, 2009; NAMS, 2010a; Secor & Simon, 2006).

These products are custom compounded to "normalize" a woman's hormone levels. However, natural levels of estrone, estradiol, and other hormones are in constant flux, so they are impossible to normalize. Procedures such as having personal hormone levels measured via blood tests or saliva tests as a basis for compounding "individualized" HT products are expensive and useless; no scientific data exist to indicate what these levels should be (Altman, 2008, 2009; Altman, Moore, Speroff, & Wysocki, 2009; NAMS, 2010a).

 Across Care Settings: ETIQ, an estrogen therapy awareness campaign

In late 2010, the National Association of Nurse Practitioners in Women's Health (NPWH) launched ETIQ, a Web site, http://www.ETIQ.info, created to empower women with credible information about menopause and advances in estrogen therapy. The campaign was inspired by findings from a recent (2010) survey that revealed women were unaware of the differences between FDA-approved estrogen therapies and those that are compounded at the pharmacy level. The goal of the ETIQ campaign is to heighten awareness of bioidentical estrogen options that are FDA approved so that women can make more informed choices about how best to manage the symptoms of menopause. NPWH hopes to enhance awareness of the advances in new delivery methods of estrogen, such as transdermals, in the form of gels, sprays, and creams, which may be preferred options for some women. The organization also hopes to help women become aware that FDA-approved estrogen therapies are tightly monitored for safety and efficacy whereas compounded estrogen formulations are not.

NONHORMONAL PRESCRIPTION MEDICATIONS

Women who experience debilitating vasomotor symptoms and wish to avoid traditional hormone therapy (HT) may be willing to try certain prescription medications, including antidepressants, belladonna alkaloid preparations, anticonvulsants, or antihypertensive agents.

 Nursing Insight— *Nonhormonal medications for vasomotor symptoms*

Various nonhormonal medications have been prescribed for the relief of severe vasomotor symptoms. Antidepressant agents known as selective serotonin reuptake inhibitors (SSRIs), including fluoxetine (Prozac), paroxetine (Paxil), citalopram (Celexa), escitalopram (Lexapro), and sertraline (Zoloft), and serotonin/norepinephrine reuptake inhibitors (SNRIs), including venlafaxine (Effexor), and desvelafaxine (Pristiq), may reduce hot flashes (Kupferer, Dormire, & Becker, 2009). However, studies that compared the efficacy of venlafaxine with that of medroxyprogesterone acetate (MPA, a progestational agent) found that a single dose of MPA alleviated hot flashes more effectively than did daily use of the antidepressant (Alexander, 2007; Hess, London, Moore, & Simon, 2009; Loprinzi et al., 2006).

Belladona alkaloid preparation is a combination of phenobarbital, caffeine, and belladonna. This medication may be useful for certain women with sleep-related vasomotor symptoms. However, this agent is contraindicated with a number of other medications and may interact with many other substances, including acetaminophen, alcohol, antacids, certain antibiotics, digoxin, metronidazole, and warfarin (Alexander, 2007).

In some women, clonidine (Catapres), an antihypertensive medication, and gabapentin (Neurontin), an anticonvulsant, have been useful in controlling hot flashes (Hess, London, Moore, & Simon, 2009; Minarik, 2010).

Now Can You— Discuss certain aspects of menopausal hormone therapy?

1. Identify the NAMS recommendations for HT use for the following conditions: vasomotor symptoms, osteoporosis, coronary heart disease, diabetes mellitus, and cognitive functioning?
2. Explain why a progestogen may be appropriate for a patient who wishes to use HT?
3. Counsel a patient about the proper use of various transdermal formulations?
4. Explain what is meant by the term *bioidentical hormones?*

Cardiovascular Disease

Cardiovascular disease (CVD) is the number-one killer of older American women; the diagnosis of heart disease presents a greater challenge in women than in men. This disease includes coronary heart disease (CHD), stroke, congestive heart failure (CHF), hypertension, and other diseases of the heart and vascular system. Over the past few decades, improved prevention and treatment have reduced the annual number of CVD deaths in men, but not in women. Cardiovascular disease is a particularly important problem among minority women. The death rate due to CVD is substantially higher in African American women than in Caucasian women. Despite the heightened public awareness of cardiovascular disease in women, the majority of women in this country continue to underestimate their risk of dying as a result of CVD (American Heart Association [AHA], 2010).

 Nursing Insight— *Women and cardiovascular disease*

Compared to men, many women before the age of menopause appear to be partly protected from coronary heart disease, heart attack, and stroke. As women age, their risk of heart disease and stroke begins to rise and keeps rising. The reasons for the lower incidence of coronary heart disease and stroke in younger women are not clear. Results from clinical trials have shown that estrogen therapy alone or in combination with progestin does not protect from heart disease or stroke. The American Heart Association does not advise women to undertake postmenopausal hormone therapy to reduce the risk of coronary heart disease or stroke (AHA, 2010).

Cardiovascular disease is a chronic, degenerative disease. While the exact mechanisms are not well understood, it is known that there is deterioration in arterial wall elasticity due to the deposition of plaque containing cholesterol and other compounds. The plaque formation may result from attempts by the body to repair damage to the lining of blood vessels. Blood flow is slowed through the narrowed areas, and clots tend to form around the deposits, causing further occlusion of the vessels (AHA, 2010).

According to the American Heart Association, the risk of heart disease and stroke increases with age. CVD ranks first among all disease categories in hospital discharges for women, and nearly 38% of all female deaths in this country occur from coronary heart disease, hypertension, stroke, congestive heart failure, and other cardiovascular diseases.

The risk of heart disease and stroke increases with age, and in the year 2006, more than 36 million American women were 55 and older. More women than men die of stroke. Interestingly, low blood levels of "good" cholesterol (high density lipoprotein or HDL) appear to be a stronger predictor of heart disease death in women than in men in the over-65 age group. High blood levels of triglycerides (another type of fat) may be a particularly important risk factor in women and the elderly (AHA, 2010).

THE AMERICAN HEART ASSOCIATION GUIDELINES FOR WOMEN

The AHA 2007 Guidelines for Preventing Cardiovascular Disease in Women emphasize that health-care professionals should focus on women's lifetime heart disease risk, rather than just the short-term risk. This approach underscores the importance of healthy lifestyles in women of all ages to reduce the long-term risk of heart and blood vessel diseases. The new guidelines for risk assessment include personal risk factors and family history, as well as the Framingham Risk Score, which estimates the risk of developing CHD within 10 years. The guidelines include expanded recommendations on lifestyle factors such as physical activity, nutrition, and smoking cessation, as well as specific recommendations on drug treatments for blood pressure and cholesterol control (AHA, 2010; McNeal & Birchem, 2009a; Mosca et al., 2007; Wenger, 2007).

 Nursing Insight— *The Framingham Risk Score (FRS) and the Reynolds Risk Score (RRS)*

Some experts have expressed concerns about the utility of the Framingham Risk Score (FRS) for women, pointing out that it does not reflect the risk of developing "soft" endpoints that are more common in women, such as stroke, angina, or need for coronary revascularization. Furthermore, the 10-year risk projection in the FRS may underestimate a woman's risk for developing CHD because women tend to live longer than men, resulting in an increased lifetime risk even if one risk factor is left untreated. To address these concerns, the Reynolds Risk Score (RRS) has recently been introduced, and it may be a superior indicator of CVD risk, especially in postmenopausal women. The Reynolds Score measures the same risk factors as the FRS but also includes family history, glycosylated hemoglobin value, and high sensitivity C-Reactive Protein (hs-CRP) levels (a biomarker associated with subclinical inflammation). Patients and health-care providers may learn more about the RRS by visiting http://www.reyoldsriskscore.org/ or http://www.hearthealthywomen.org/index.php?view=article&id=90&Itemid=1&option=com_content (Blumenthal, Michos, & Nasir, 2007; McNeal & Birchem, 2009a; Ridker, Buring, Rifai, & Cook, 2007).

The new guidelines state that the use of unregulated dietary supplements is not a proven method of preventing heart disease. Research that has become available since the last guidelines were developed suggests that health-care providers should consider recommending aspirin to women over age 65 to prevent stroke. For women younger than age 65, routine use of aspirin is not recommended to prevent myocardial infarction (MI), owing to an increased risk of cerebral and gastrointestinal bleeding. In addition, health-care providers should avoid the use of menopausal therapies such as hormone therapy or selective estrogen receptor modulators (SERMs) (e.g., raloxifene, tamoxifen) to prevent heart disease because they have been shown to be ineffective in protecting the heart and may, in fact, increase the risk of a stroke. Estrogen plus progestin can increase the risk of MI, breast cancer, venous thromboembolism, stroke, dementia, and ovarian cancer. In women who have undergone hysterectomy, estrogen alone confers a risk of stroke and dementia/memory loss. Likewise, no cardiovascular benefit has been shown for SERMs (AHA, 2010; Flores & Taylor, 2010; McNeal & Birchem, 2009b; Manson, 2009; Mosca et al., 2007; Wenger, 2007).

 Optimizing Outcomes— With AHA Guidelines for women's heart health

The AHA Guidelines for women include the following:

- Recommended lifestyle changes to help manage blood pressure include weight control; increased physical activity; alcohol moderation; sodium restriction; and an emphasis on eating fresh fruits, vegetables, and low-fat dairy products.
- Besides advising women to stop smoking, the 2007 guidelines recommend counseling, nicotine replacement, or other forms of smoking cessation therapy.
- Physical activity recommendations for women who need to lose weight or sustain weight loss include a minimum of 60 to 90 minutes of moderate-intensity activity (e.g., brisk walking) on most, and preferably all, days of the week.
- All women should be encouraged to reduce the intake of saturated fats to less than 7% of calories.
- All women should be encouraged to consume oily fish at least twice a week, and women with heart disease should consider taking a capsule supplement of 850 to 1000 mg of EPA (eicosapentaenoic acid) and DHA (docosahexaenoic acid) (2 to 4 grams for women with high triglycerides).
- Women at high risk for CVD should consider taking 325 mg of aspirin per day.
- Antioxidant supplements such as vitamins E, C, and beta-carotene should not be used for primary or secondary prevention of CVD.
- Folic acid should not be used to prevent CVD.

(AHA, 2010; Manson, 2009)

where research and practice meet: Women's Awareness of Heart Disease and Stroke

Christian, Rosamond, White, and Mosca (2007) conducted a study to evaluate trends in women's awareness, knowledge, and perceptions related to cardiovascular disease since 1997, when the American Heart Association initiated a national campaign for women. An interviewer-assisted questionnaire was used to assess CVD awareness, knowledge, and perceptions among a nationally representative sample of 1005 women. Their findings indicated that while CVD awareness has increased significantly among women since 1997, the racial/ethnic gap in awareness has not narrowed. Based on their research, the investigators call for educational efforts to increase heart disease and stroke awareness that target racial/ethnic minorities, especially Hispanics.

Across Care Settings: The AHA Go Red For Women movement

In 2004, the American Heart Association launched its multitiered marketing campaign, the "Go Red for Women" movement, to raise women's awareness of their risk for heart disease and empower them to take charge of their heart health. In 2010, the AHA set a strategic goal of reducing death and disability from cardiovascular disease and strokes by 20% while improving the cardiovascular health of all Americans by 20% by the year 2020. Nurses and patients can obtain accurate, up-to-date information about heart disease and stroke and the "Go Red for Women" movement by calling 1-888-MY-HEART or by visiting http://www.goredforwomen.org/.

Be sure to— Teach women about heart attack warning signs

As with men, women's most common heart attack symptom is chest pain or discomfort. But women are somewhat more likely than men to experience some of the other common symptoms, particularly shortness of breath, nausea and vomiting, and back, neck, tooth, or jaw pain. Atypical symptoms that have been reported include fatigue, weakness of the arms or shoulders, dizziness, gaslike pain, indigestion, pain between the shoulder blades, restlessness, and a feeling of impending doom (AHA, 2010; Vassar, 2009).

RISK FACTORS FOR CVD

Women are considered to be at high risk for cardiovascular disease if they have established CVD or CHD, peripheral artery disease, cerebrovascular disease, chronic renal disease, or diabetes mellitus. Other risk factors for coronary disease are listed in Box 7-8.

Fortunately, many of the major CVD risk factors can be significantly modified through therapeutic lifestyle changes

---

Box 7-8 Risk Factors for Cardiovascular Disease

Increasing age (about 83% of people who die of CHD are 65 or older)

Heredity (including race). Children of parents with heart disease are more likely to develop it themselves. African Americans have more severe high blood pressure than do Caucasians and a higher risk of heart disease. Heart disease is also higher among Mexican Americans, Native Americans, native Hawaiians and some Asian Americans—and this is partly due to higher rates of obesity and diabetes in these populations.

Cigarette smoking

Obesity

Elevated serum cholesterol levels

Metabolic syndrome

Hypertension (often related to the use of alcohol, cigarettes, excessive sodium, and obesity)

Other modifiable factors such as a high-fat diet, sedentary lifestyle, stressful lifestyle

Sources: Mosca et al., 2007; Ruhl, 2009; Vassar, 2009.

and pharmacotherapy. Modifiable risk factors include smoking, hyperlipidemia, diabetes mellitus (DM), hypertension (HTN), and obesity. Educating women about strategies to control these five risk factors can empower them to make the changes that can greatly reduce their lifetime risk for CVD.

Smoking has been associated with early CVD events and doubles the risk of developing CVD by age 70. Nurses can encourage women to avoid both cigarette smoking and secondhand exposure to environmental tobacco smoke. When discussing smoking cessation strategies, it may be useful to identify and address barriers to smoking cessation, such as a fear of weight gain, a lack of support, a lack of interest, and a long-standing use of smoking as a stress reliever (Vassar, 2009).

 Optimizing Outcomes— Medications to treat tobacco dependence

Patients may benefit from medications to treat tobacco dependence. These include bupropion (Wellbutrin, Zyban), supplemental nicotine (Nicoderm CQ, Nicorette), varenicline (Chantix), clonidine (Catapres), and nortriptyline (Sensoval, Aventyl). All of these agents significantly increase the rate of long-term smoking abstinence, especially varenicline and nicotine nasal spray (Nicotrol NS) (McNeal & Birchem, 2009b).

Abnormal lipid levels—including elevated low-density lipoprotein cholesterol (LDL-C), low high-density lipoprotein cholesterol (HDL-C), elevated total cholesterol, and elevated triglycerides (TG)—are associated with an increased long-term likelihood of CVD. A fasting lipid profile should be obtained for women beginning at age 20 and then every 5 years thereafter. If a dyslipidemia is identified, secondary causes such as diabetes mellitus (DM), hypothyroidism, obstructive liver disease, chronic renal failure, and medication-induced changes should be considered (McNeal & Birchem, 2009b; Vassar, 2009).

DM is a significant risk factor for CVD. In women, having DM confers a myocardial infarction (MI) risk equal to that in someone who has established coronary artery disease (CAD). Women with DM have a 57.3% risk for CVD by age 75, compared with a 16.3% risk in women without DM (Vassar, 2009).

Hypertension (HTN) is also a significant risk factor for CVD, although the relative risk is closely correlated to how well women can control their blood pressure. Among U.S. women age 20 years and older, 15.5% have been diagnosed with HTN. Sadly, most of these women remain unaware that HTN constitutes a major risk factor for CVD (Vassar, 2009).

As of 2004, 61.9% of women in the United States were classified as overweight or obese. Obesity is more prevalent in women, especially minorities and those with a lower socioeconomic status. Overweight and obesity are independent and contributory risk factors to CVD. Body mass index (BMI) greater than 25 kg/m² is independently associated with an increased risk of CVD, with an even larger risk in persons with a BMI equal to or greater than 30. Those with a BMI of 40 kg/m² or greater tend to experience MI 12 years earlier than those with a normal BMI (Madala, Franklin, & Chen et al., 2008). Moreover, overweight and obesity are known contributors to other risk factors, such as DM, HTN, and dyslipidemia (McNeal & Birchem, 2009b; Vassar, 2009).

 Nursing Insight— *Understanding the term cardiometabolic health*

The term *cardiometabolic health*, promoted by the American Diabetes Association (ADA) since 2006, describes an individual's level of risk for developing diabetes and CVD; it's based on an assessment of all the factors, called "cardiometabolic risk factors," that contribute to risk for these conditions. In 2006, the ADA launched its Cardiometabolic Risk Initiative, which is a national campaign to encourage health-care providers to focus on the prevention, recognition, and treatment of all risk factors (e.g., smoking, obesity, physical inactivity, psychological stress) for CVD and type 2 diabetes (ADA, 2006; Ruhl, 2009).

THE NURSING ROLE IN PROMOTING CARDIOVASCULAR HEALTH

Nurses have a central role in promoting cardiovascular health through education and counseling about heart disease. Nurses can empower women with strategies to make lifestyle modifications to address the five major risk factors (smoking, dyslipidemia, DM, HTN, and obesity) for cardiovascular disease. Diets high in saturated fat, trans-fatty acids, cholesterol, calories, alcohol, and salt and low in fiber, fruits, and vegetables have been shown to contribute to HTN, DM, dyslipidemia, and obesity. Dietary changes to reduce blood pressure may include incorporation of the Dietary Approaches to Stop Hypertension (DASH) diet. The DASH diet emphasizes low sodium intake (2.3 g/day or less) and the consumption of fruits, vegetables, low-fat/nonfat dairy foods, whole grains, lean meat, fish, poultry, nuts, and beans (McNeal & Birchem, 2009b; Vassar, 2009). Nurses and patients may learn more about the DASH Diet Eating Plan by visiting the Web site at http://www.dashdiet.org/.

Complementary Care: *Olive oil to promote cardiovascular health*

When counseling women about dietary modifications to promote CV health, nurses can encourage them to use olive oil in their cooking. In 2004, the U.S. Food and Drug Administration approved labeling olive oil as a nonpharmaceutical product that reduces the risk of coronary heart disease. Olive oil has been shown to reduce after-meal lipemia and to promote more rapid metabolism of the damaging, oxidative chylomicrons formed after eating fats (Covas, 2007; Ruano, Lopez-Miranda, & de la Torre et al., 2007; Sego, 2009). A botanical product, olive oil may produce allergic reactions in sensitive individuals, so skin patch testing for patients with significant sensitivity histories is advised. While there are no known drug interactions, highly antioxidant compounds can increase the potency of warfarin (Coumadin); nurses should advise patients who use this anticoagulant to proceed with caution. Most studies are conducted with extra virgin olive oil using a daily intake of 1 to 2 ounces (30 to 60 mL), the amount typically found in salad dressings, cooking, and spreads (Sego, 2009).

A lack of physical activity is also known to contribute to CVD. Exercise inhibits atherosclerosis (Fig. 7-1); reduces inflammatory responses; improves endothelial function; and reduces obesity, HTN, dyslipidemia, and insulin resistance (AHA, 2002; Lichtenstein, Appel, Brands, & Carnethon et al., 2006; Perry & Bennett, 2006; Slentz, Duscha, & Johnson et al., 2004; Vassar, 2009).

 Optimizing Outcomes— With exercise to decrease CHD and DM risk

Exercise has been documented to decrease the risk of CHD by 40%, stroke by 30%, and type 2 diabetes mellitus by 30%. Nurses can encourage patients to exercise for a total of at least 30 minutes over the course of a day; 60 minutes is optimal, and 90 minutes is recommended for weight loss (AHA, 2002; McNeal & Birchem, 2009b). Evidence indicates that community-based physical activity programs are effective in reducing new cases of cancer (i.e., breast, colon), type 2 diabetes, and heart disease. Community-based interventions may include mass communication efforts, social support networks, individualized physical activity goal-setting and monitoring, and enhanced access to services such as fitness centers, bike paths, and walking trails (Hellwig, 2009; Kapustin, 2010). "Choose To Move," offered by the AHA, is a free 12-week physical activity program for women that provides step-by-step instructions for simple exercises, motivational tips, and information about nutrition, heart disease and stroke. Women may register by visiting the Web site at http://www.choosetomove.org/.

Nurses can also explore and address barriers to prevention and treatment of CVD. Barriers may be perceived or actual; mental or physical; or economic, geographic, or cultural. Exploring these barriers in a nonthreatening, culturally sensitive, therapeutic environment empowers women to identify and overcome them so that they may take action to improve their cardiovascular health (Ruhl, 2009; Vassar, 2009). It is well established that women who have limited access to health care have more adverse health outcomes, including CVD (Ruhl, 2009; Zhang, Geiss, Cheng, Beckles, Gregg, & Kahn, 2008).

 Nursing Insight— Barriers to CVD prevention and treatment

Nurses can help women identify barriers to actions that promote their cardiovascular health. Barriers may include:

- Confusion concerning information in the media
- The belief that a supreme being ultimately determines one's health
- The perception that one is not at risk for CVD
- A reluctance to make a change in lifestyle
- The belief that nothing can be done to prevent CVD
- A lack of time, energy, support, willpower
- An overwhelming feeling of stress that prevents participation in CVD prevention or treatment activities
- A lack of resources (financial, access to healthy foods, access to exercise space, family obligations) (Christian, Rosamond, White, & Mosca, 2007; Mosca, Mochari, & Christian et al., 2006; Mosca, Ferris, Fabunmi, & Robertson, 2004; Thanavaro, 2005; Vassar, 2009).

When counseling women about personal risk for CVD, nurses can inform them about the Reynolds Risk Score, developed by experts at Brigham and Women's Hospital in Boston. The interactive tool calculates the risk of having a heart attack, stroke, or other form of heart disease in the next 10 years. Nurses can also inform women about HeartHub (http://www.hearthub.org/), the AHA's patient portal for information, tools, and resources about CVD and stroke. This Internet resource offers a wealth of current information about various cardiovascular-related topics, such as warning signs for heart attack, stroke, and cardiac arrest, and provides self-assessment activities for personal risk of diabetes, heart attack, and high blood pressure. The HeartHub Internet site offers information in Spanish, Vietnamese, and simplified and traditional Chinese.

Across Care Settings: The National Coalition for Women with Heart Disease

For more than a decade, WomenHeart Champions have been educating, supporting, and advocating in communities nationwide for prevention, early detection, timely and accurate diagnosis and treatment, and effective health-care policy to help women better understand about heart

Normal artery

Atherosclerotic artery

Figure 7-1 A. Cross-section of normal coronary artery. **B.** Coronary artery with atherosclerosis narrowing the lumen. (Scanlon V.C., & Sanders T.: *Essentials of anatomy and physiology*, 5th ed., Philadelphia, F. A. Davis Company, 2007, p. 280.)

A

B

disease. Often misdiagnosed and undertreated, more than 41 million American women are living with or at risk for developing heart disease. WomenHeart, the National Coalition for Women with Heart Disease, is the only national organization dedicated to promoting women's heart health. To learn more about this organization, women may visit the organization's Web site at http://www.womenheart.org.

Remaining up-to-date about current, evidence-based CVD information empowers nurses to offer care that promotes and optimizes women's cardiovascular health. Nurses can appropriately counsel patients about interventions that have been found harmful or are ineffective in preventing CVD in women. For example, both folic acid and antioxidant supplementation have been found ineffective in the primary and secondary prevention of CVD. Also, women younger than age 65 should not routinely use aspirin to prevent myocardial infarction. Finally, hormone therapy and estrogen-receptor modulators are no longer recommended for primary or secondary prevention of CVD in women (Manson, 2009; Mosca, Banka, & Benjamin et al., 2007; Smith, Allen, & Blair et al., 2006; Vassar, 2009).

 Optimizing Outcomes— **Resources for health-care providers**

The American Heart Association (AHA) and American College of Cardiology (ACC) have published guidelines to assist practitioners in the prevention of CVD. The AHA has published *Evidence-Based Guidelines for Cardiovascular Disease Prevention in Women: 2007 Update*, and the AHA and ACC have jointly published AHA/ACC *Guidelines for Secondary Prevention for Patients With Coronary and Other Atherosclerotic Vascular Disease: 2006 Update: Endorsed by the National Heart, Lung, and Blood Institute*. This publication summarizes the highlights of these guidelines and is a rich resource for health-care professionals. Both sets of guidelines focus on major CVD risk factor reduction and the use of pharmacotherapy in patients with established CVD (Mosca, Banka, Benjamin, & Berra et al., 2007; Smith, Allen, & Blair et al., 2006; Vassar, 2009).

 Now Can You— **Discuss certain aspects of cardiovascular disease?**

1. Discuss the utility of two tools specifically developed to determine risk for cardiovascular disease?
2. Identify at least five AHA guidelines for promoting heart health in women?
3. Develop a patient teaching program that focuses on five modifiable risk factors for cardiovascular disease?

Osteoporosis

As individuals age, their bone density progressively decreases. Osteoporosis is a generalized, metabolic disease characterized by decreased bone mass and an increased incidence of bone fractures (Fig. 7-2). Osteopenia is a condition where bone mineral density is lower than normal, and many clinicians consider it to be a precursor to osteoporosis. Osteoporosis is a largely preventable complication of menopause. Screening strategies and pharmacological interventions are available to prevent and treat osteoporosis.

Nursing Insight— *Appreciating the full impact of osteoporosis-related fractures*

Hip fractures, which occur on average at age 82, elicit a particularly devastating toll, resulting in higher cost, disability, and mortality than all other osteoporotic fracture types combined. Hip fractures cause up to a 25% increase in mortality within 1 year of the incident. Approximately 25% of women require long-term care after a hip fracture, and 50% will experience some long-term loss of mobility. Vertebral fractures may cause substantial pain as well as loss of height and exaggerated thoracic kyphosis (abnormal curvature of the thoracic spine). Spinal pain and deformity can greatly restrict normal movement, including bending and reaching. Thoracic fractures may restrict lung function and cause digestive problems. Osteoporotic fractures exert a psychological toll as well. Pain, loss of mobility, change in body image, and loss of independence can exert a strong negative impact on self-esteem and mood (NAMS, 2010b).

Normal Bone

Osteoporosis

A

B

Figure 7-2 **A.** Normal spongy bone, as in the body of a vertebra. **B.** Spongy bone thinned by osteopososis. (Scanlon V.C., & Sanders T.: *Essentials of anatomy and physiology,* 5th ed., Philadephia, F. A. Davis Company, 2007, p. 113.)

NORMAL BONE PHYSIOLOGY

Bone is a living tissue. It is involved in a wide range of biochemical processes, which result in the constant break-down and reformation of new bone replacing weakened areas with new, well-formed tissue. Bone is composed of two types of cells, osteoblasts and osteoclasts (Fig. 7-3), as well as an intercellular matrix. The intercellular matrix is composed of organic compounds, such as collagen and other proteins, and inorganic components responsible for bone rigidity, including minerals such as calcium phosphate, calcium carbonate, magnesium, fluoride, sulfate, and other trace elements that form crystalline structures called *hydroxyapatites* (NAMS, 2010b).

A & P review **The Bone Remodeling Unit**

The bone-remodeling unit is the site on the surface of the bone where osteoblasts and osteoclasts act to form and resorb bone. Bone is constantly being remodeled to provide optimal support and to repair damage occurring from daily activities. An osteoblast (from the Greek words for "bone" and "germ," or embryonic) is a mononucleate cell that is responsible for bone formation. Osteoblasts produce osteoid, which is composed mainly of collagen. Osteoblasts are also responsible for mineralization of the osteoid matrix. Bone is a dynamic tissue that is constantly being reshaped by osteoblasts, which build bone, and osteoclasts, which resorb bone. An osteoclast (from the Greek words for "bone" and "broken") is a type of bone cell that removes bone tissue by removing its mineralized matrix and breaking up the organic bone, a process termed *bone resorption*. Osteoclasts and osteoblasts are instrumental in controlling the amount of bone tissue: osteoblasts form bone; osteoclasts resorb bone. Osteoblast cells tend to decrease as individuals age, thus decreasing the natural renovation of bone tissue (Fig. 7-4) (ACOG, 2004; NAMS, 2010b). ◆

 Nursing Insight— *Gonadal hormones and bone metabolism*

Estrogen inhibits bone resorption by binding to estrogen receptors in bone tissue and also by blocking the production of cytokines, substances that increase the number of osteoclasts. Estrogen, however, is not the only hormone that has an important influence on the health of bone. Two other hormones produced by the ovaries, progesterone and dehydroepiandrosterone (DHEA), influence bone metabolism as well. Testosterone (one of the male hormones also produced by women) may also play a role in bone health (ACOG, 2008, NOF, 2008).

There are two major types of bone: cortical and trabecular. Cortical bone forms the outer shell of all bones and accounts for 75% of total bone mass. Trabecular bone is the spongy, interlacing network of struts that forms the internal support within the cortical bone. Trabecular bone is concentrated in the vertebral bodies and pelvis and at the ends of the long bones. Trabecular bone accounts for only 25% of total bone mass, but because of its spongy, open architectural structure, it accounts for most of the bone volume. Bone remodeling units are limited to the bone surface. Because trabecular bone has a larger surface area, it has a higher turnover rate than cortical bone. Trabecular bone is most likely to show early bone loss, but it also is the first bone type to show response to therapy (ACOG, 2004).

Bone formation and resorption are ongoing processes that are usually "in balance" in young adults who have adequate nutrition and exercise and experience normal puberty. Bone mass peaks at approximately 30 years in both men and women. After reaching peak bone mass, approximately 0.4% of bone is lost per year in both genders. Bone strength is determined by the total bone mass and the integrity of its protein and crystal matrix. Bone strength is also related to the efficiency of bone repair in response to mild trauma, which produces microfractures. Remodeling tends to occur along lines of stress, increasing the strength in those weakened areas (NOF, 2008).

 Nursing Insight— *The menopause–bone loss link*

In addition to the bone loss with aging that naturally occurs in both genders, women lose approximately 2% of cortical bone and 5% of trabecular bone per year for the first 5 to 8 years after menopause. With menopause and aging, the coordinated "balance" between osteoclasts and osteoblasts may be disturbed, resulting in excessive bone resorption and loss of both bone density and structure. In women who are recently menopausal, excess bone loss commonly is caused by excessive osteoclast-mediated resorption. In later postmenopausal years, suppressed osteoblast activity and inadequate formation of bone may play a major role in the progression of osteoporosis, providing an opportunity for new therapeutic approaches, such as stimulating bone formation. Osteoporosis is more common in women than in men in part because of the accelerated loss of bone that occurs after menopause (ACOG, 2004).

Bone health promotion typically centers on methods of ensuring adequate intake of calcium. However, bone health maintenance and the prevention of fractures should encompass other strategies, such as preventing the loss of calcium and other minerals from the bone, maintaining the soft tissue components around the bone, and promoting the efficiency of bone repair (NOF, 2008; Speroff & Fritz, 2005).

Figure 7-3 Osteoclast. (Venes, D.: *Taber's cyclopedic medical dictionary*, 21st ed., Philadelphia, F. A. Davis Company, 2009, p 1655.)

Figure 7-4 The ossification process in a long bone. **A.** Progression of ossification from the cartilage model of the embryo to the bone of a young adult. **B.** Microscopic view of an epiphyseal disc showing cartilage production and bone replacement. (Scanlon V.C., & Sanders T.: *Essentials of anatomy and physiology*, 5th ed., Philadelphia, F. A. Davis Company, 2007, p. 110.)

Nursing Insight— *Fractures commonly associated with osteoporosis*

Three major types of fractures may occur as a result of osteoporosis:

Spontaneous vertebral crush fracture—the vertebrae become so weak that one vertebra collapses under the minimal stress of lifting or due to the weight of the woman's body. This action causes a loss of height and kyphosis, or dowager's hump, the curvature of the upper back often present in older people.

Colle's fracture—a transverse fracture of the distal radial metaphysis with displacement of the hand posteriorly and outward. This fracture occurs when a person breaks a fall by landing on a hand, causing fracture of the radius (Venes, 2009).

Osteoporotic hip fracture—The hip fracture related to the osteoporotic process is the most severe form of these three types of fractures.

Tooth loss and periodontal disease represent other aspects of osteoporosis.

In the United States, it is estimated that 10 million individuals have osteoporosis and almost 34 million more are estimated to have osteopenia, or low bone mass, placing them at increased risk for osteoporosis. Of the 10 million Americans estimated to have osteoporosis, 8 million are women and 2 million are men. Although osteoporosis is often considered to be an older person's disease, it can strike at any age. Both osteopenia and osteoporosis increase the risk of fracture (ACOG, 2007; NOF, 2008b).

 Ethnocultural Considerations—
Osteoporosis

Osteoporosis varies among ethnic groups. Asian Americans and Caucasians are more often affected by osteopenia/osteoporosis than are African Americans. African American women have approximately a 6% higher bone mineral density than Caucasian women. Among non-Hispanic African American women who are older than age 50, 5% have osteoporosis and 35% have osteopenia. Among Hispanic women over age 50, 10% have osteoporosis and 49% have osteopenia. When compared with other ethnic/racial groups, the risk of osteoporosis is increasing most rapidly among Hispanic women. And among non-Hispanic Caucasian women and Asian American women who are 50 and older, approximately 20% have osteoporosis, while 52% have osteopenia. (ACOG, 2004; NOF, 2008b; Speroff & Fritz, 2005)

Osteoporosis constitutes a major health threat for women. In this country, the incidence of osteoporosis-related fractures has increased over the past 20 years. Most fractures occur at the femoral neck, the vertebrae, and the distal radius. Postmenopausal women who experience a hip or symptomatic vertebral fracture have a 6- to 8-fold increased risk of death in the year following their fracture. On an annual basis, the associated costs of osteoporosis-related fractures exceed $14 billion, and this figure is expected to increase as life expectancy increases and the population ages (Alexander, 2007; Nelson & Stewart, 2008).

 Nursing Insight— *Heredity and bone mass*

The single largest factor that influences a woman's peak bone mass (i.e., the maximal bone mineral density [BMD] gained during the skeletal development and maturation phase) is genetics. Up to 80% of the variability in peak bone mass is attributable to genetic factors alone. Female children of women with osteoporotic fractures have lower bone mass than would be expected for their age when compared with unrelated individuals. First-degree relatives of women with osteoporosis have lower bone mass than those with no family history of osteoporosis. (ACOG, 2004; NAMS, 2007; NAMS, 2010b)

CAUSES

Stated in simple terms, osteoporosis occurs when the normal balance of bone formation and bone resorption is disrupted. In women and young adults, bone growth and calcium deposition take place continuously throughout young adulthood. Bone mass generally reaches a peak around age 30. As women grow older, net bone loss gradually occurs due to an imbalance in bone tissue and metabolism. A deficiency of estrogen worsens the situation, as does the inefficiency in calcium and vitamin D assimilation that naturally occur as women age (Nelson & Stewart, 2008; NOF, 2008; Speroff & Fritz, 2005).

During the first five to six years following menopause, women lose bone density six times more rapidly than men. By the age of 65, one-third of women have experienced a vertebral fracture; by the age of 80, women have lost approximately 47% of the trabecular bone, which is concentrated in the vertebrae, pelvis, and other flat bones, and the epiphyses. The most well-defined risk factor for the development of osteoporosis is the loss of the protective effects of estrogen, which occurs with declining ovarian function during perimenopause (NOF, 2008).

Osteoporosis may result from other causes, including rheumatoid arthritis, chronic lung disease, anorexia nervosa, and endocrine diseases such as diabetes, hypogonadism, overactive thyroid, and hyperparathyroidism. Also, certain prescription drugs, including glucocorticoids (e.g., prednisone), anticoagulants (e.g., heparin), chemotherapeutic agents, anticonvulsants (e.g., phenytoin), and some diuretics (e.g., furosemide), as well as some over-the-counter aluminum-containing antacids (e.g., Maalox), can contribute to bone loss. An excessive caffeine intake increases calcium excretion, and excessive alcohol use (i.e., three or more drinks per day) interferes with calcium absorption and depresses bone formation (NOF, 2008).

 Optimizing Outcomes— **With routine postmenopausal osteoporosis risk assessment**

All postmenopausal women should be assessed for risk factors associated with osteoporosis and fracture. This assessment requires a history, physical examination, and any necessary diagnostic tests. The goals of this evaluation are to evaluate fracture risk, to rule out secondary causes of osteoporosis, to identify modifiable risk factors, and to determine appropriate candidates for pharmacologic therapy (NAMS, 2010b).

RISK FACTORS

There are a number of risk factors for osteoporosis. Non-modifiable factors include genetic background and medical conditions (presented in Box 7-9). Modifiable risk factors related to lifestyle include smoking (active or passive); alcohol use; low dietary calcium; vitamin D insufficiency; high dietary intake of sodium, protein, caffeine, phosphates, sugar, and refined flour products; lack of sun exposure or a deficiency of vitamin D; and lack of exercise (NOF, 2008).

 Nursing Insight— Tobacco use and osteoporosis risk

Compared with nonsmokers, women smokers tend to lose bone more rapidly, have lower bone mass, and reach menopause 2 years earlier, on average. The mechanisms by which smoking might adversely affect bone mass are not known, although some experts suggest that cigarette smokers may have impaired calcium absorption and lower estradiol levels (NAMS, 2010b).

DIAGNOSING OSTEOPOROSIS

A *clinical* diagnosis of osteoporosis is made when a postmenopausal woman suffers a nontraumatic, nonpathological fracture of the spine. A *radiological* diagnosis is based on the T score, which is obtained from bone densitometry

---

analysis. The first-line technique for assessing BMD (bone densitometry) is the central dual-energy x-ray absorptiometry, or C-DEXA (or DEXA). This test assesses BMD in the spine, hip, and waist.

 diagnostic tools Bone Density Scan (DEXA)

Bone density scanning, also called dual-energy x-ray absorptiometry (DEXA) or bone densitometry, is an enhanced form of x-ray technology that is used to measure bone loss. Central DEXA is today's established standard for measuring BMD and is most often performed on the lower spine and hips. Central DXA devices, consisting of a large, flat table and an "arm" suspended overhead, are usually located in hospitals and medical offices. Peripheral devices (pDEXA) that use x-ray or ultrasound are sometimes used to screen for low bone mass. Peripheral devices measure bone density in the wrist, heel, or finger and are often available in drugstores and mobile health vans in the community. The pDEXA device, much smaller than the central DEXA device, is a portable box-like structure with a space for the foot or forearm to be placed for imaging. Although bone tests at peripheral sites can identify women at risk of fracture, they are not useful for the diagnosis of osteoporosis and have limited or no value in the follow-up of patients. In some communities, a computed tomography (CT) scan with special software can also be used to diagnose or monitor low bone mass. This is accurate but less commonly used than DEXA scanning. DEXA is effective in tracking the effects of treatment for osteoporosis and other conditions that cause bone loss; the DEXA test can also assess an individual's risk for developing fractures (NAMS, 2010b).

DEXA works by measuring a specific bone or bones (e.g., spine, hip, waist). The density of these bones is then compared with an average index based on age, sex, and size to determine risk for fractures and the stage of an individual's osteoporosis. Results are generally scored by two measures, the T-score and the Z-score. The T-score refers to the extent of bone loss and is reflective of the number of standard deviations by which a patient's BMD falls below the expected BMD score for healthy young women. Every decrease of 1 standard deviation represents approximately a 12% reduction in BMD, which translates into a 1.5- to 3.0-fold increase in fracture risk (NOF, 2008).

 Nursing Insight— Understanding the BMD Z-score and T-score

The Z-score is the number of standard deviations above or below the mean for the patient's age, sex, and ethnicity. The Z-score is used in premenopausal women, men under the age of 50, and in children. The T-score, which is also the number of standard deviations above or below the mean, is a comparison of a patient's BMD to that of a healthy 30-year-old of the same sex and ethnicity. This value is used in postmenopausal women and men over age 50 because it better predicts risk of future fracture. The World Health Organization T-score criteria are as follows:

- Normal: a T-score of –1.0 or higher
- Osteopenia: a T-score less than –1.0 and greater than –2.5
- Osteoporosis: a T-score equal to or less than –2.5 (i.e., the bone density is 2.5 standard deviations below the mean of a 30-year-old healthy woman)

Scores indicate the amount one's bone mineral density varies from the mean. Negative scores indicate lower bone density; positive scores indicate higher bone density.

Box 7-9 Nonmodifiable Risk Factors for Osteoporosis

Gender: Eighty percent of the 10 million Americans who have osteoporosis are women.

Race: Caucasian, Asian, and Latina women are at the highest risk; African American women have a lower risk.

Advanced age

History of:
- Previous fractures that occurred without any major trauma, or fracture after the age of 50
- Poor absorption of calcium and other minerals or nutrients due to celiac disease, chronic diarrhea, low stomach acid (common in older individuals), surgical removal of part of the stomach or intestines

Family history of female osteoporosis or fractures or both

Body build: Women who are small-boned and slim and have small muscle mass are at greater risk than women with other body builds

Current osteopenia

Early menopause (before age 40 years, or if surgically induced); amenorrhea; never having gone through a pregnancy

Diabetes; liver disease; kidney disease with dialysis; daily use of thyroid replacement medication (greater than 2 grains); hyperthyroidism; hyperparathyroidism

Lactose intolerance: Present in 60% of women with osteoporosis and in only 15% of the general population

Use of phenytoin sodium (Dilantin), a medication that interferes with the body's ability to absorb calcium; aluminum-containing antacids; steroid medications

Sources: ACOG, 2004; NAMS, 2007; NAMS, 2010b; NOF, 2008.

"What to say" — *Preparing patients for a C-DXA examination*

The nurse can do much to allay the patient's anxiety about a scheduled bone densitometry test. The nurse explains why the test is performed, how the test is performed, and what information will be gained from the test results. The nurse may also counsel the patient about how to prepare for the test. For example, the nurse may say:

- The bone density test is a quick, noninvasive, painless procedure.
- The amount of radiation used is extremely small—less than one-tenth the dose of a standard chest x-ray and less than a day's exposure to natural radiation.
- DXA bone density testing is the most accurate method available for the diagnosis of osteoporosis and is also considered an accurate estimator of fracture risk.
- No radiation remains in your body after an x-ray examination.
- On the day of the exam, you may eat normally. You should not take calcium supplements for at least 24 hours before your exam.
- You should wear loose, comfortable clothing and avoid garments that have zippers, belts, or buttons made of metal. Objects such as keys or wallets that would be in the area being scanned should be removed.
- You may be asked to remove some or all of your clothes and to wear a gown during the exam. You may also be asked to remove jewelry, dentures, eyeglasses, and any metal objects or clothing that might interfere with the x-ray images.
- You will be positioned on a padded table and your legs will be supported on a padded box (to flatten the pelvis and lumbar spine). You must hold very still and you may be asked to hold your breath for a few seconds while the x-ray picture is being taken.
- The DEXA bone density test is usually completed within 10 to 30 minutes, depending on the equipment used and the parts of the body being examined.
- You should inform your health-care provider if you recently had a barium examination or have been injected with a contrast material for a CT scan or radioisotope scan. In this event, you may have to wait 10 to 14 days before undergoing the DEXA test.
- You should inform your health-care provider and the x-ray technologist if there is any possibility that you may be pregnant.

Optimizing Outcomes— Routine height assessments to detect asymptomatic osteoporosis

As women grow older, routine height assessments should become standard practice during annual examinations. Loss of height may indicate bone loss in asymptomatic women. Height loss in women who are in their 40s or early 50s should signal a need for further testing to determine the cause. After achieving maximal height, women can lose up to 1.0 to 1.5 inches (2.0 to 3.8 cm) of height as part of the normal aging process, primarily as a result of degenerative arthritis and shrinkage of intervertebral disks. Height loss greater than 1.5 inches increases the likelihood that a vertebral fracture is present. The nurse should measure height using an accurate method such as a wall-mounted ruler or a stadiometer (an instrument used to measure both sitting and standing height) (NAMS, 2010b; NOF, 2008).

According to recommendations established by the ACOG, the USPSTF, NAMS, and NOF, health-care providers should routinely screen all women older than 65 for osteoporosis, regardless of risk factors. Women with risk factors should be screened beginning at age 60.

Be sure to— Teach women about osteoporosis early warning signs

Teaching women about the early warning signs of osteoporosis constitutes an important nursing role in the promotion of bone health. Nurses should alert women to the following signs and symptoms that may signal bone loss and advise them to promptly contact their health-care provider if they experience them:

- Sudden onset of insomnia and restlessness
- Leg and foot cramps that occur frequently during the night
- Persistent low back pain
- Gradual loss of height
- Development of gum disease or loose teeth

In this country, women typically reach menopause around age 51, and most bone loss occurs during the first 5 to 7 years after cessation of menses. Thus, it may be prudent to begin screening at an earlier age. It is generally recommended that the BMD be reassessed every 3 to 5 years. For certain women, including those who are undergoing treatment for osteoporosis and those who are immobilized, the BMD may need to be measured beginning at an earlier age and more often, such as every 6 to 24 months (ACOG, 2008b; Goldstein, 2008; NAMS, 2010b; NOF, 2008, USPSTF, 2002).

Nursing Insight— ACOG recommendations for bone mineral density (BMD) testing

ACOG (2008b) has published the following recommendations for BMD testing:

- Bone mineral density testing should be recommended to all postmenopausal women aged 65 years or older regardless of risk factors.
- Bone mineral density testing may be recommended for postmenopausal women younger than 65 years who have one or more risk factors for osteoporosis. According to current risk factors, all Caucasian postmenopausal women younger than 65 years would be candidates for BMD testing.
- Bone mineral density testing should be performed on all postmenopausal women with fractures to confirm the diagnosis of osteoporosis and determine disease severity.

Optimizing Outcomes— With the FRAX Assessment Tool

The launch of the World Health Organization (WHO) technical report *Assessment of Osteoporosis at the Primary Health Care Level* and the related Fracture Risk Assessment Tool (FRAX) are major milestones toward helping health professionals worldwide to improve identification of patients at high risk of fracture. The practical Web-based tool FRAX assesses the 10-year risk of osteoporosis fracture. An individual's risk factors such as age, sex, weight, height, and femoral neck BMD (if available) are entered into the tool, followed by clinical risk factors, which include a prior fragility fracture, parental history of hip fracture, tobacco smoking, long-term use of glucocorticoids, rheumatoid arthritis, other causes of secondary osteoporosis, and daily alcohol consumption. The FRAX tool then provides a figure indicating a 10-year fracture probability as a percentage, which, together with a clinical assessment, provides guidance for determining access to treatment in health-care systems. Estimates are available for U.S. Caucasian, African American, Hispanics, and Asian Americans. It is expected that the software needed to provide the FRAX model calculations will be loaded into most DEXA machines by 2011. The FRAX algorithm is intended for use with postmenopausal women and men age 50 and older and applies only to previously untreated patients. The FRAX model is available on the NOF Web site (http://www.nof.org) or at the FRAX Web site (http://www.shef.ac.uk/FRAX/) (Ettinger & Ettinger, 2009; Goldstein, 2008; Kessenich, 2009; Nelson, 2009; Watts, Ettinger, & LeBoff, 2009).

PROMOTING BONE HEALTH THROUGH OPTIMAL NUTRITION

Although it is impossible to determine the precise effect of diet on bone health, there is at least circumstantial evidence that the standard American diet, which frequently contains excessive sugar, refined grains, and caffeine, promotes the development of osteoporosis. Other dietary factors that adversely affect bone health include alcohol and protein, phosphorus, and sodium. The relationship between these substances and their impact on bone loss is presented in Box 7-10.

Nurses can empower women with information about the value of optimal nutrition in reducing osteoporosis risk. Consuming a diet that is composed primarily of plant-based, unprocessed whole foods is an important strategy in the promotion of bone health and the prevention of osteoporosis. Examples of plant-based nutritious substances include legumes, fresh fruits and vegetables, whole grains, nuts, and seeds. These foods provide a rich supply of nutrients in the right proportions to enhance their absorption and use. In addition to calcium, many vitamins, such as vitamins K, B_6, C, and D, and minerals, such as manganese, magnesium, boron, and zinc, play an important role in maintaining bone mass and in preventing bone loss (Box 7-11) (NAMS, 2010b; NOF, 2008c).

Calcium

Calcium deficiency is only one of the predisposing factors for the development of osteoporosis in women,

---

Box 7-10 Selected Dietary Substances and Their Association With Bone Loss

Sugar: The average American ingests 139 pounds of refined sugar each year. Sugar intake may be associated with large increases in urinary calcium excretion. Owing to the fact that 99% of the body's calcium is stored in bone, and the blood maintains a very narrow concentration range of calcium, when the body loses calcium, it is likely to be from bone.

Refined grains: The nutrient-rich portions of grains have been removed through refinement, including vitamin B complex, calcium, magnesium, and zinc.

Caffeine: Caffeine in coffee, tea, and soft drinks, as well as similar substances in chocolate and some drugs, causes calcium to be excreted in the urine. Increased calcium excretion causes a systemic acidosis that stimulates bone resorption.

Alcohol: Excessive alcohol intake interferes with calcium absorption and depresses bone formation.

Protein, phosphorus, and sodium: The typical American diet contains excessive amounts of protein, phosphorus, and sodium. Calcium is mobilized to neutralize the acidic by-products and is then excreted in the urine, causing a loss of calcium from the body. Phosphorus is an ingredient in many soft drinks, and excess protein results from the high consumption of meat and dairy products in the average American diet.

Oxalate and phytate sodium: Foods with high amounts of oxalate and phytate reduce the absorption of calcium contained in those foods. Examples of foods high in oxalate include spinach, rhubarb, and beet greens. Legumes (e.g., pinto beans, navy beans, peas) are high in phytate. To reduce the phytate level, soak the legumes in water for several hours; discard the water, then cook them in fresh water. Wheat bran is also high in phytate; take calcium supplements 2 or more hours before eating any foods with 100% wheat bran.

---

and not everyone with osteoporosis is deficient in calcium. Calcium balance and metabolism in the body are complex and involve a number of factors, including ingestion, absorption, use, and excretion. In addition, calcium balance is modulated by various hormonal systems. Adequate calcium intake for osteoporosis prevention should begin early in life when bone mass is reaching its peak. This important period for bone health occurs during the late teens to early 20s (Speroff & Fritz, 2005).

 Optimizing Outcomes— With skeletal health promotion in children and adolescents

An important role for nurses who work with men, women, and families centers on promoting bone health and preventing osteoporosis. Ideally, protection against osteoporosis should begin in childhood and adolescence, with efforts focused on building bone mass. Children should be encouraged to eat calcium-rich foods, and nurses should teach parents to encourage regular exercise, including participation in school gym classes and sports programs, to build strong bones and establish healthy lifestyle habits. Parents also should be informed about the negative effects that eating disorders, excessive dieting, excessive exercise, alcohol consumption, and smoking exert on bone density. From the mid-20s through age 35, focus should continue to be placed on building and maintaining bone mass

Box 7-11 Selected Vitamins and Minerals and Their Role in Promoting Bone Health

Vitamin K: Along with calcium, vitamin K is involved in bone metabolism. This important vitamin attracts calcium into the matrix to form bone—the process of bone mineralization and fracture healing. The current adequate intake value for vitamin K is 90µ/day. Vitamin K is found in several forms: vitamin K_1 (Phylloquinone), the form occurring naturally in plants; vitamin K_2 (Menaquinone), the form produced by intestinal bacteria and also derived from putrefied fish meal; and synthetic vitamin K (Menadione). Humans are unable to synthesize vitamin K. It must either be acquired from dietary sources or as metabolic by-products of intestinal bacteria. Sources of vitamin K include dark green leafy vegetables (e.g., cabbage, broccoli, lettuce, spinach, cauliflower); soybeans; strawberries; and certain dairy products such as egg yolks, butter, and cheese. Vitamin K supplements are contraindicated in women taking warfarin (Coumadin) (NAMS, 2010).

Vitamin B_6: Vitamin B_6 (pyridoxine) is believed to be involved in bone matrix formation. Sources of this vitamin include whole grains, fish, chicken, organ meats, nuts, watermelon, and tomatoes.

Vitamin C: It has been known from the days of widespread scurvy that vitamin C (ascorbic acid) is necessary for normal bone formation. This vitamin promotes the formation and cross-linking of some of the structural proteins found in bone. Vitamin C is present in citrus fruits, strawberries, melons, broccoli, tomatoes, potatoes, and raw deep green leafy vegetables.

Vitamin D: Calcium metabolism and absorption depend upon the presence of vitamin D. Vitamin D is made from either of two inert precursors: vitamin D_2 (ergocalciferol) or D_3 (choecalciferol). D_2 is plant derived and obtained through diet; D_3 is produced in the skin with exposure to sunlight. Exposing the skin to ultraviolet rays from the sun causes the cholesterol beneath the skin's surface to be converted to vitamin D, which is then stored in the liver until needed. Vitamin D increases the absorption of calcium by the intestines and promotes calcium uptake into the bone. With aging, there is a decrease in the synthesis of vitamin D by the skin. This problem is exacerbated by the common tendency for older individuals to decrease their exposure to the sun. Sun exposure consisting of as little as 10 to 15 minutes each day can have a positive impact on bone health by improving calcium absorption and use. Vitamin D deficiency that stems from reduced sun exposure increases the risk of other conditions, including colorectal, breast, and pancreatic cancer (Giovannucci, 2009; Rutecki, 2009). Wearing a sunscreen with a sun protection factor of 8 or more blocks the skin's ability to produce vitamin D by 95%. Dietary sources of vitamin D include saltwater fish, egg yolks, butter, cod liver oil, fortified milk, margarine, cereals and bread products, liver, and supplements. Fortified substances usually provide 100 IU per serving (Dawson-Hughes et al., 2005; Jockers, 2007; Mayhew, 2009; Syroney & Franjesevic, 2010). Certain medications (e.g., anticonvulsants, thiazide diuretics, corticosteroids, cimetidine [Tagamet], heparin, and some cholesterol-lowering agents) can prevent vitamin D absorption, and in some individuals, malabsorption may be related to loss of gastrointestinal acidity or malfunction of the proximal small bowel (Malone & Kessenich, 2008). The National Osteoporosis Foundation (NOF, 2008) recommends that adults under age 50 obtain 400 to 800 IU/day and that adults age 50 and over obtain 800 to 1000 IU/day. Vitamin D_3, also called cholecalciferol, is the form of vitamin D that best supports bone health (NAMS, 2007; NAMS, 2010b; NOF, 2008c).

through a calcium-rich diet. After age 35, bone resorption exceeds bone formation. At that time, emphasis should be placed on preventing bone loss through a healthy diet, use of calcium supplements, and engaging in weight-bearing exercises such as weight-lifting, walking, jogging, dancing, and climbing stairs (Venes, 2009).

The National Institutes of Health Office of Dietary Supplements (2009) recommends the following calcium dietary allowances for women, which represent the amounts of calcium required to maintain adequate rates of calcium retention and bone health in healthy individuals:

- 9 to 13 years: 1300 mg/day
- 14 to 18 years: 1300 mg/day (same amount for pregnant and lactating individuals)
- 19 to 50 years: 1000 mg/day (same amount for pregnant and lactating individuals)
- 50+ years: 1200 mg/day

When considering dietary sources of calcium, most people are aware that dairy products are rich in calcium, but many do not realize that the animal protein in these products can interfere with the body's ability to absorb the calcium. Other substances that can inhibit calcium absorption are found in wheat bran, raw spinach, salt, caffeine, alcohol and tobacco, and fructose (present in many soft drinks). An important nursing role in promoting bone health centers on teaching women about good nutritional sources of calcium.

"What to say" — *Educating women about dietary calcium*

Nurses can teach women about calcium-rich dietary sources. The nurse may offer the following information:

- Dietary sources are the preferred means of obtaining adequate calcium intake because there are other essential nutrients in high-calcium foods.
- Milk, yogurt, ice cream, and cheese are rich sources of calcium.
- Nondairy calcium sources include vegetables such as Chinese cabbage, kale, and broccoli.
- Most grains do not have high amounts of calcium unless they are fortified; however, they contribute calcium to the diet because they do have small amounts and people consume them frequently.
- Seafood, including sardines and salmon, are good sources of calcium.
- Puddings, instant breakfast drinks, cottage cheese, and sour cream are good sources of calcium.
- Many products, such as soy milk, rice, yogurt, cereals, and orange juice, are now available with extra calcium added.
- Reduced-fat or low-fat products contain at least as much calcium per serving as high-fat dairy products, and they offer an alternative for women concerned about body weight and lipid profiles.
  (Dawson-Hughes et al., 2008; NAMS, 2007)

Some individuals are lactose intolerant and have difficulty digesting dairy products because they lack the enzyme lactase, which is needed to break down the milk sugar lactose. Lactose intolerance is fairly common in adults, particularly African Americans, Asians, Native Americans, and Inuits (Alaska natives). Persons with lactose intolerance experience abdominal cramping, bloating, and diarrhea following milk consumption, although many can tolerate small amounts of milk without symptoms. Calcium sources such as yogurt, sweet acidophilus milk (fermented with certain bacteria), buttermilk, cheese, chocolate milk, and cocoa may be tolerated even when fresh milk is not. Lactase supplements such as Lactaid are available to consume with milk, and lactase-treated milk is also available in many markets. The lactase in these products digests the lactose in the milk so that lactose-intolerant persons can drink milk without experiencing unpleasant intestinal symptoms (NOF, 2008c).

Optimizing Outcomes— Teaching women about strategies to enhance calcium absorption

The absorption of calcium depends upon adequate acidity in the stomach. Low stomach acid is a common problem that becomes more prevalent with increasing age. When counseling women about strategies to optimize the absorption of calcium, the nurse can offer the following advice:

* Eat slowly and chew well.
* Limit fluid intake with meals.
* Consider the use of digestive enzymes.

Most women will need an additional 600 to 900 mg of calcium per day over their usual daily dietary intake to reach recommended levels. Among the many calcium supplements are various formulations available in oral tablets, chewable tablets, dissolvable oral tablets, and liquids. Patients should be advised that the "best" supplement for them is the one that best meets their needs, based on tolerance, convenience, cost, and availability. Nurses can teach women that when choosing a calcium supplement, special consideration should be given to the product's purity, absorbability, tolerance, and possibility of interactions with other drugs. Although vitamin D is necessary for the absorption of calcium, it is not necessary that it be included in the calcium supplement. Calcium citrate tends to be better tolerated than calcium carbonate; however, it is a more expensive form of calcium supplement. Most individuals adequately absorb calcium carbonate, a less expensive calcium source, unless there is a problem with insufficient stomach acid. Antacids are not the best sources of calcium, as they can cause other problems, such as kidney stones, and they may aggravate other medical conditions as well. Furthermore, some antacids also contain aluminum, which can cause the body to lose calcium. Nurses can reassure women that total calcium intakes of up to 1500 mg/day do not appear to increase the risk of developing renal calculi and may actually reduce it. Also, women should not exceed the recommended daily requirement for calcium, as there appears to be no benefit to consumption of amounts in excess of 1500 mg/day (NAMS, 2007, 2010b; NOF, 2008c).

"What to say" — Providing guidance to assist women in choosing calcium supplements

When discussing calcium supplements, the nurse may offer the following advice:

* *Purity:* Choose only those supplements that are known brand names that have proven reliability. The product label should include the term *purified* or have the USP (U.S. Pharmacopeia) symbol, although the USP label is voluntary and not all products display this symbol. Avoid calcium extracted from unrefined oyster shell, bone meal, or dolomite without the USP—these products historically have contained higher lead levels or other toxic materials (NOF, 2008).

* *Absorbability:* Most brand-name calcium products are readily absorbed by the body. If the product label does not state that it is absorbable, it is easy to determine absorbability by doing this: place the tablet in a small amount of warm water for 30 minutes and stir occasionally. If the tablet has not dissolved within this time period, it probably will not dissolve in the stomach. Calcium supplements in chewable and liquid form dissolve well because they are broken down before they enter the stomach. Calcium, whether in the diet or from supplements, is best absorbed when it is taken several times a day in amounts of 500 mg or less. Calcium carbonate is absorbed best when taken with food; calcium citrate can be taken any time (NOF, 2008).

* *Tolerance:* Although calcium supplements are well tolerated by most people, certain preparations can cause side effects such as gas or constipation in some individuals. If simple strategies such as increased fluids and fiber intake do not resolve the symptoms, try another calcium source. A combined calcium-magnesium product may be helpful if constipation is a problem. It is best to increase the intake of any calcium supplement gradually, beginning with 500 mg a day for several days, and add additional calcium slowly (NOF, 2008).

* *Interactions with other drugs:* Before taking any calcium supplement, it is important to talk with your health-care provider or pharmacist about possible interactions between prescription or over-the-counter medications and the calcium supplements. For example, calcium supplements may interfere with the absorption of the antibiotic tetracycline. Calcium also interferes with iron absorption and should not be taken at the same time as the iron supplement unless the iron supplement is taken with vitamin C or calcium citrate. Any medication that is to be taken on an empty stomach should not be taken with a calcium supplement (NOF, 2008c).

* *Dietary factors that limit calcium absorption:* Consumption of certain foods, including those that contain oxalic acid (found in spinach, rhubarb, and some other green vegetables), large amounts of grains that contain phytates (e.g., wheat bran, soy protein isolates), and, possibly, tannins (found in tea) are known to limit calcium absorption from the intestines (NAMS, 2007)

Optimizing Outcomes— With NOF resources for patients and health-care professionals

Boning Up on Osteoporosis is a 100+ patient-care handbook that offers current information on the prevention, diagnosis, and treatment of osteoporosis. The handbook also includes detailed nutrition information and exercises for individuals with low bone density and osteoporosis. It may be purchased from the NOF online store at http://www.nofstore.org/.

The *Clinician's Guide to Prevention and Treatment of Osteoporosis* was published in 2008, and an online updated version became available in January 2010. This resource was developed to inform clinical decision making for the management of men and women at high fracture risk. It integrates the expression of a patient's fracture risk as a 10-year probability with current clinical recommendations for the management of osteoporosis. Health-care professionals may obtain a single print copy of the 2008 *Clinician's Guide* at no charge; additional quantities may be purchased from the NOF online store.

PROMOTING BONE HEALTH THROUGH PHYSICAL ACTIVITY

Immobilization and bedrest are associated with an increase in bone loss. During travel in space, astronauts have experienced accelerated rates of bone loss. It is known that overall bone mass is directly related to weight-bearing physical exercise. Women who regularly engage in exercise programs that include weight-bearing and muscle-strengthening elements can help prevent postmenopausal bone loss and reduce their risk of falling. The bone-building effect of exercise results mainly from the repetitive physical stress applied to the bones. With weight-bearing exercise, pressure is placed on the bones either by the weight of the body or by the force of muscular contractions. Effective exercises for menopausal women that are generally safe and contribute to cardiovascular health and bone mass are walking, stair climbing, gardening, weight lifting, and low-impact aerobics. An effective program involves regular exercise for at least 30 minutes, every day of the week. Also, the 30 minutes do not need to be done all at once—physical activity may be divided into 10-minute segments, if desired (NOF, 2008d).

 Optimizing Outcomes— With exercises to promote balance, posture, and function

Nonimpact exercises improve balance, posture, and movement and help to increase muscle strength and decrease the risk of falls and fractures. Balance exercises such as Tai Chi strengthen the legs and enhance the balance. Posture exercises that improve one's posture and help reduce rounded shoulders decrease the risk of fractures, especially in the spine. Functional exercises enhance the performance of daily activities and decrease the risk of falls and fractures. Yoga and Pilates can also improve strength, balance, and flexibility. Individuals with osteopenia or osteoporosis should avoid certain positions such as forward-bending exercises to prevent fractures (NOF, 2008d).

When counseling older women, it is helpful to include information about safety and prevention of falls. Many factors, such as frailty, altered balance, poor vision, and use of certain medications can contribute to falls (Box 7-12). Strategies to minimize falls include lowering the bed, removing throw rugs, illuminating dark areas with night lights, using safety treads and safety rails in the bathroom, ensuring ready access to a telephone, eliminating exposed electrical cords, ensuring stair safety (handrails, good condition, nonslip surfaces), and removing all clutter from the floors. Also, older women should be advised to avoid

Box 7-12 Medical Risk Factors for Falls

- Age
- Anxiety and agitation
- Arthritis of the lower extremities
- Arrhythmias
- Dehydration
- Depression
- Female gender
- Impaired transfer and mobility
- Malnutrition
- Medications that cause oversedation (e.g., narcotic analgesics, anticonvulsants, psychotropics)
- Orthostatic hypotension
- Poor vision and use of bifocals
- Previous fall
- Reduced problem solving or mental acuity and diminished cognitive skills
- Urgent urinary incontinence
- Vitamin D insufficiency
- Kyphosis
- Poor balance
- Reduced proprioception
- Muscle weakness

Sources: Dawson-Hughes et al., 2008; NAMS, 2010b.

wearing slippery-soled shoes or slippers, since they provide insufficient support, traction, and stability (Kaunitz, 2008; Nelson & Stewart, 2008).

 Optimizing Outcomes— Potential nursing diagnoses for women with osteoporosis

Nursing diagnoses for women with osteoporosis may focus on potential or real problems such as trauma, pain, or impaired mobility:

Risk for Trauma (related to loss of bone density/integrity; increasing risk of fracture with minimal or no stress)

Acute/Chronic Pain (related to vertebral compression on spinal nerves/muscles/ligaments, spontaneous fractures, possibly evidenced by verbal reports, guarding/distraction behaviors, self-focus, and changes in sleep pattern)

Impaired Physical Mobility (related to pain and musculoskeletal impairment, possibly evidenced by limited range of motion, reluctance to attempt movement/expressed fear of re-injury, and imposed restrictions/limitations) (Venes, 2009)

MEDICATIONS FOR THE PREVENTION AND/OR TREATMENT OF OSTEOPOROSIS

A number of medications are effective in preserving bone mineral density. FDA-approved osteoporosis treatments have been shown to decrease fracture risk in patients who have had fragility fractures and/or osteoporosis as diagnosed by DEXA. NOF treatment guidelines state that treatment should be recommended to anyone who faces at least a 3% risk of suffering hip fracture in the next 10 years and to anyone who has at least a 20% risk of sustaining any major bone fractures in that time frame; this is based on a cost-effectiveness model. Pharmacotherapy may also reduce fractures in patients with osteopenia without fractures. There is no consensus about when to initiate therapy to prevent fractures; the health-care provider should assess the potential benefits and risks of therapy in each patient on an individual basis (Cadarette, Katz, Brookhart, Levin, Stedman, Choudhry, & Solomon, 2008; Nelson, 2009; NOF, 2008a).

 Nursing Insight— *ACOG and NAMS recommendations for osteoporosis pharmacotherapy*

ACOG (2008b) recommends osteoporosis pharmacotherapy for the following women:
- Postmenopausal women who have experienced a fragility or low-impact fracture
- Postmenopausal women with no risk factors who have a BMD T-score determined by central dual energy x-ray absorptiometry (C-DEXA) of less than –2
- Postmenopausal women with risk factors for fracture who have a BMD T-score by C-DEXA of less than –1.5

NAMS (2010) recommends osteoporosis pharmacotherapy for:
- All postmenopausal women who have had an osteoporotic vertebral or hip fracture
- All postmenopausal women who have BMD values consistent with osteoporosis (i.e., T-scores equal to or worse than –2.5 at the lumbar spine, femoral neck, or total hip region)
- All postmenopausal women who have T-scores from –1.0 to –2.5 and a 10-year risk, based on the FRAX calculator, of major osteoporotic fracture (spine, hip, shoulder, or wrist) of at least 20% or hip fracture of at least 3%

The FDA has approved a number of medications for the prevention and/or treatment of postmenopausal osteoporosis. These include, in alphabetical order, bisphosphonates (alendronate, alendronate plus D, ibandronate, resedronate, risedronate with 500 mg of calcium carbonate and zoledronic acid), calcitonin, estrogens (estrogen and/or hormone therapy), estrogen agonist/antagonists (raloxifene), and parathyroid hormone (PTH). Certain medications are available in oral and intravenous forms; specific information about each medication is presented in Box 7-13. Combination therapy (usually a bisphosphonate with a nonbisphosphonate) can provide additional small increases in BMD when compared with monotherapy. However, the impact of combination therapy on fracture rates is unknown. Presently, combination therapy is reserved for treatment failures when compliance has been assured (Dawson-Hughes, Lindsay, Khosla, Melton, Tosteson, Favus, & Baim, 2008; NAMS, 2010b; Pinkerton & Dalkin, 2007).

 Nursing Insight— *Empowering women with information about medication options*

An intravenous bisphosphonate may be an appropriate choice when a patient prefers less frequent dosing. Because an IV formulation must be administered by a health-care professional (in an infusion center or infusion-equipped office setting), use of an IV bisphosphonate ensures adherence for the indicated treatment period. Prior to the initiation of any therapy, it is important to inform the patient of various medication dosing and delivery options so that she may participate in the decision-making process, when possible (Bachmann, 2008; Sunyecz & Derman, 2007).

 Nursing Insight— *FDA-approved expanded use of Forteo*

In late 2009, the FDA approved a new use for the osteoporosis medication Forteo (teriparatide) to treat osteoporosis associated with sustained, systemic glucocorticoid therapy in men and women who have a high risk of fracture. Glucocorticoid therapy is the most common cause of secondary osteoporosis—approximately 50% of individuals who are prescribed chronic glucocorticoid therapy will eventually have an osteoporotic fracture. Glucocorticoid medication can lead to a reduction in bone formation, and Forteo has been shown to counter this effect by stimulating bone formation (Scott, 2009).

The Nurse's Role in Fostering Safe Use of Osteoporosis Medications

Nurses have an essential education and counseling role in caring for women who take prescribed osteoporosis medications in terms of advising them about potential risks and side effects as well as the importance of adhering to specific dosing recommendations for the bisphosphonates. The oral bisphosphonates share a common risk profile in terms of their potential to cause gastrointestinal problems, including difficulty swallowing, gastroesophageal reflux, inflammation of the esophagus, and gastric ulcer. Oral bisphosphonates are contraindicated in individuals with reflux, gastroesophageal reflux disease, and other esophageal abnormalities. Neither IV ibandronate nor IV zoledronic acid has been associated with adverse upper gastrointestinal events. Side effects for all of the bisphosphonates may include abdominal, bone, joint, or muscle pain. The nurse should emphasize that deviating from the dosing instructions increases the likelihood of experiencing gastrointestinal symptoms (ACOG, 2004; Cole, 2009; Dawson-Hughes et al., 2008; Kaunitz, 2008; NAMS, 2010b; Pinkerton & Dalton, 2009; Wysowski, 2009).

It is essential that the oral bisphosphonates be taken on an empty stomach first thing in the morning with 8 ounces of plain water, with no additional food or drink consumption for at least 30 minutes, and that the patient remain upright during this time. Not following the instruction to take the medication with only plain water can substantially reduce bisphosphonate absorption; substituting coffee or juice for water can reduce drug absorption by as much as 60%. Oral bisphosphonates are contraindicated in women with uncorrected hypocalcemia, an inability to sit or stand for 30 to 60 minutes, esophageal stricture, or severe renal impairment. Side effects associated with the IV administration of bisphosphonates include flu-like symptoms: fever, pain in the muscles or joints, and headache. Eye inflammation (uveitis) is a rare side effect (ACOG, 2004; Cole, 2009; Dawson-Hughes et al., 2008; Gertz, Holland, Kline,

Box 7-13 FDA-Approved Medications for the Prevention and/or Treatment of Postmenopausal Osteoporosis

BISPHOSPHONATES

Bisphosphonates are synthetic forms of a class of compounds found in the body. These compounds bind to the crystals in the bone matrix and inhibit bone resorption. Women who cannot or who choose not to take estrogen are good candidates for bisphosphonate therapy. Bisphosphonates inhibit normal physiological bone resorption as well as abnormal bone resorption, thereby halting bone loss, increasing bone mineral density, and reducing the risk of fractures (Dawson-Hughes et al., 2008; Kagan, 2009; Miller, 2009).

Alendronate (Fosamax, Fosamax Plus D) is FDA approved for the prevention (5 mg PO daily or 35 mg PO weekly) and treatment (10 mg PO daily or 70 mg PO weekly) of postmenopausal osteoporosis. A liquid formulation is available, as well as a formulation that contains 5600 IU of vitamin D. This medication is now available as a generic preparation in the United States. Alendronate reduces the incidence of spine and hip fractures by about 50% over 3 years in patients with a prior vertebral fracture, and it reduces the incidence of vertebral fractures by about 48% over 3 years in patients without a prior vertebral fracture (Dawson-Hughes et al., 2008; Pinkerton & Dalkin, 2009).

Etidronate (Didrocal) is approved in Canada for osteoporosis prevention and treatment in postmenopausal women (400 mg/day for 14 days every 3 months, with calcium taken between cycles). In the United States, etidronate is approved only for treatment of Paget's disease, not for osteoporosis therapy (NAMS, 2010b).

Ibandronate (Boniva) is FDA approved for the treatment of postmenopausal osteoporosis (2.5 mg daily tablet, 150 mg monthly tablet, and 3 mg every 3 months by intravenous injection). The oral preparations are also approved for the prevention of postmenopausal osteoporosis. Ibandronate reduces the incidence of vertebral fractures by about 50% over 3 years (Dawson-Hughes et al., 2008; Pinkerton & Dalkin, 2009).

Risedronate (Actonel, Actonel with Calcium) is approved by the FDA for the prevention and treatment of postmenopausal osteoporosis (5 mg daily tablet or 35 mg weekly tablet, packaged with 5 tablets of 500 mg calcium carbonate or 75 mg tablets on 2 consecutive days every month, or 150 mg monthly tablet). This medication reduces the incidence of vertebral fractures by about 41% to 49% and nonvertebral fractures by about 36% over 3 years, with significant risk reduction occurring after 1 year of treatment in patients with a prior vertebral fracture (Dawson-Hughes et al., 2008; Pinkerton & Dalkin, 2009).

Zoledronic acid (Reclast—USA; Aclasta—Canada) is approved by the FDA for the treatment (5 mg by intravenous infusion over at least 15 minutes once yearly) and prevention (an infusion administered every 2 years is now approved in the United States) of osteoporosis in postmenopausal women. Zoledronic acid reduces the incidence of vertebral fractures by about 70%, hip fractures by about 41%, and nonvertebral fractures by about 25% over 3 years. Zoledronic acid is also indicated for the prevention of new clinical fractures in patients who have recently had a hip fracture. Prior to administration, patients must have two blood tests: One is for creatinine to confirm that kidney function is normal; the other test is for calcium to confirm that the serum calcium level is within normal limits (Dawson-Hughes et al., 2008; NAMS, 2010b; Pinkerton & Dalkin, 2009).

CALCITONIN

Salmon calcitonin (Miacalcin, Fortical) is FDA approved for the treatment of osteoporosis in women who are at least 5 years postmenopausal. It is delivered as a single daily intranasal spray that provides 200 IU of the drug. Subcutaneous administration by injection also is available; side effects associated with this administration route include local inflammation and flushing of the face or hands. Intranasal calcitonin is generally considered safe although some patients experience rhinitis and, rarely, epistaxis. Oral calcitonin has been approved by the FDA for the treatment of osteoporosis. However, because calcitonin is a less effective agent than other pharmacological therapies for osteoporosis, it is reserved as an alternative for women who cannot or choose not to take one of the other osteoporosis agents (ACOG, 2004; Dawson-Hughes et al., 2008; NAMS, 2010b; Sherman, 2009b).

ESTROGEN/HORMONE THERAPY (ET/HT)

Estrogen therapy (Climara, Estrace, Estraderm, Estratab, Ogen, Ortho-Est, Premarin, Vivelle) and hormone therapy (Activella, Femhrt, Premphase, Prempro, etc.) are approved by the FDA for the prevention of osteoporosis and relief of vasomotor symptoms and vulvovaginal atrophy associated with menopause. Women who have not had a hysterectomy require HT, which contains a progestin to protect the uterine lining. The Woman's Health Initiative (WHI) found that 5 years of HT (Prempro) reduced the risk of clinical vertebral fractures and hip fractures by 34% and other osteoporotic fractures by 23% (Dawson-Hughes et al., 2008).

The WHI reported increased risks of myocardial infarction, stroke, invasive breast cancer, pulmonary emboli, and deep vein phlebitis during 5 years of treatment with conjugated equine estrogen and medroxyprogesterone (Prempro). Subsequent analysis of these data showed no increase in cardiovascular disease in women who started treatment within 10 years of menopause. In the estrogen-only arm of WHI, no increase in breast cancer incidence was noted over 7.1 years of treatment. Other doses and combinations of estrogen and progestins were not studied. Because of the risks, ET/HT should be used in the lowest effective doses for the shortest duration to meet treatment goals. When ET/HT use is considered solely for the prevention of osteoporosis, the FDA recommends that approved nonestrogen treatments should first be carefully considered (Dawson-Hughes et al., 2008).

ESTROGEN AGONIST/ANTAGONIST

Formerly known as a selective estrogen-receptor modulator (SERM), the drug raloxifene (Evista) is approved by the FDA for both prevention and treatment of osteoporosis in postmenopausal women. Raloxifene reduces the risk of vertebral fractures by about 30% in patients with a prior vertebral fracture and by about 55% in patients without a prior vertebral fracture over 3 years. Bone loss often resumes when raloxifene therapy is stopped. Raloxifene is indicated for the reduction in risk of invasive breast cancer in postmenopausal women with osteoporosis. This medication increases the risk of deep vein thrombosis to a degree similar to that observed with estrogen, and it also increases the frequency of night sweats and hot flashes (ACOG, 2004; Dawson-Hughes et al., 2008; NAMS, 2010b).

PARATHYROID HORMONE (PTH)

Teriparatide (recombinant human PTH 1-34, marketed as Forteo) is approved by the FDA for the treatment of osteoporosis in postmenopausal women at high risk for fracture. It is a bone-building (anabolic) agent that directly stimulates osteoblastic bone formation, resulting in substantial increases in trabecular bone density and connectivity. This mechanism of action is very different from that of antiresorptive agents such as estrogen and bisphosphonates, which reduce bone resorption. It is administered by daily subcutaneous injection. Teriparatide in a dose of 20 mcg daily has been shown to decrease the risk of vertebral fractures by 65% and nonvertebral fractures by 53% in patients with osteoporosis, after an average of 18 months of therapy. This medication should only be used for a maximum of 2 years, and it is contraindicated in patients with an increased risk of osteosarcoma and those having prior radiation of the skeleton, bone metastases, hypercalcemia, or a history of skeletal malignancy. Teriparatide is also indicated for the treatment of glucocorticoid-induced osteoporosis and male osteoporosis (Dawson-Hughes et al., 2008; NAMS, 2010b).

Matuszewski, Freeman, Quan, Lasseter, Mucklow, & Porras, 1995; Kaunitz, 2008; Pinkerton & Dalton, 2009; Sunyecz & Derman, 2007; Wysowski, 2009).

There have been rare reports of osteonecrosis (death of the bone cells or tissue) of the jaw with bisphosphonate medications. Nearly all of these cases occurred in cancer patients receiving an intravenous bisphosphonate. Although unusual, there are also reports of osteonecrosis of the jaw in patients being treated with the bisphosphonate tablets alendronate (Fosamax), ibandronate (Boniva), and risedronate (Actonel) for osteoporosis prevention or treatment. Although the risk for this complication in healthy women is estimated as less than 1 in 100,000 treatment years, dental evaluation is recommended prior to the initiation of bisphosphonate therapy. Also, there have been rare reports of esophageal cancer in women taking oral bisphosphonates. Owing to this potential complication, patients with Barrett's esophagus (a premalignant condition caused by an abnormal change in the cells of the distal portion of the esophagus) should not use oral bisphosphonates. An essential component of health teaching for all women who take oral bisphosphonate tablets includes the warning that side effects such as chest pain, new or worsening heartburn, or difficult or painful swallowing must be immediately reported to the health-care provider (ACOG, 2004; Cole, 2009; Dawson-Hughes et al., 2008; Pinkerton & Dalton, 2009; Wysowski, 2009).

Because bisphosphonates are associated with esophageal irritation, it is important to provide detailed dosing information when counseling women about the use of these medications. Alendronate and risedronate tablets should be taken first thing in the morning with 8 ounces of plain water. Patients using the liquid formulation of alendronate should swallow one bottle (75 mL) and follow with at least 2 ounces of plain water. After taking these medications, patients must wait at least 30 minutes before eating, drinking, or taking any other medication. Patients should remain upright (sitting or standing) during this interval (Dawson-Hughes et al., 2008).

Oral ibandronate tablets should be taken on an empty stomach, the first thing in the morning, with 8 ounces of plain water (no other liquid). After taking this medication, patients should be instructed to wait at least 60 minutes before eating, drinking, or taking any other medication. Patients must remain upright for at least 1 hour after taking the medication. Ibandronate, 3 mg per 3 mL prefilled syringe, is given by intravenous injection over 15 to 30 seconds, once every 3 months. Patients should be advised that serum calcium and creatinine levels will be checked before each injection (Bachmann, 2009; Dawson-Hughes et al., 2008; Pinkerton & Dalton, 2009).

❝ **What to say** ❞ — *Preparing patients for zoledronic acid infusion*

Nurses can help prepare patients who will be treated with an intravenous infusion of zoledronic acid (Reclast) by offering the following information:

- Eat normally and drink at least 2 glasses of fluids before the treatment.
- Your treatment will take at least 15 minutes.

- You may resume your normal activities immediately after the treatment.
- After the first treatment, common side effects may include flu-like symptoms such as fever, muscle or joint pain, and headache.
- You may receive acetaminophen (Tylenol) prior to the infusion to reduce the risk of developing these symptoms; after the treatment, you may continue to use a mild pain reliever as needed for discomfort.
- Side effects are much less common after successive treatments.

  (Bachmann, 2008; Dawson-Hughes et al., 2008).

NOF recommends BMD testing every 2 years. For women undergoing pharmacological therapy for osteoporosis, a repeat C-DEXA scan should be performed 2 years after the initiation of treatment and at subsequent 2-year intervals (Dawson-Hughes, 2008; Simon, 2008).

🄢 **Optimizing Outcomes**— Educating women about osteoporosis resources for consumers

- *Know My Bones* is a new educational program for women diagnosed with postmenopausal osteoporosis. The program, available at http://www.knowmybones.com, offers women new insights in understanding the science of bone health, healthful high-calcium recipes, helpful lifestyle tips, and more. The Know My Bones Council, formed to enhance educational efforts about postmenopausal osteoporosis, includes members such as Amgen, Inc. (an international biotechnology company), the National Osteoporosis Foundation, the National Association of Nurse Practitioners in Women's Health, and the Society for Women's Health Research.
- The U.S. Department of Health & Human Services (DHHS) Agency for Healthcare Research and Quality (AHRQ)'s Effective Health Care summary guides have produced *Osteoporosis Treatments That Help Prevent Broken Bones: A Guide for Women After Menopause*, a resource for consumers. The guide is based on a government-funded review of research reports about osteoporosis treatments to prevent broken bones and is available at http://effectivehealthcare.ahrq.gov/index.cfm/search-for-guides-reviews-and-reports/?pageaction=displayproduct&productID=92&returnpage=.

🄢 **Optimizing Outcomes**— With professional resources to guide clinical care

Several clinical and governmental organizations have published guidelines to assist clinicians in informing and guiding women toward appropriate treatments that will help to relieve their menopausal symptoms without placing their health in undue jeopardy. These organizations include the American College of Obstetricians and Gynecologists (ACOG); the North American Menopause Society (NAMS); the National Association of Nurse Practitioners in Women's Health (NPWH); the National Osteoporosis Foundation (NOF); the International Osteoporosis Foundation (IOF); the Association of Women's Health, Obstetric, and

Neonatal Nurses (AWHONN); the U.S. Food and Drug Administration (FDA), and the U.S. Preventive Services Task Force (USPSTF). Nurses can use these recommendations to discuss options with their patients and provide current, evidence-based care (Alexander, 2007).

Now Can You— Discuss certain aspects of osteoporosis?

1. Explain why menopausal women are at increased risk for osteoporosis and how to conduct a risk assessment for the condition?
2. Counsel a woman about preparing for a C-DEXA examination?
3. Develop an osteoporosis educational program that includes strategies for reducing risk and tips for optimizing bone health?
4. Counsel a woman about the safe use of medications for the prevention and/or treatment of osteoporosis?

---

summary points

◆ Today, American women can expect to live to be 80 years old and spend close to one-third of their lives as menopausal women.

◆ Nurses can empower midlife women with factual, evidence-based information about menopause, the normal aging process, and strategies to optimize cardiovascular and skeletal health.

◆ Complementary and alternative medicine approaches such as stress management, guided imagery, biofeedback, yoga, and massage therapy may be useful in minimizing various menopausal symptoms.

◆ An important role for nurses centers on counseling women to become informed about any herbal preparations they are considering and to consult with their health-care providers before using any of them.

◆ Estrogen-containing drugs for menopausal use are divided into two categories: estrogen therapy (ET) and combined estrogen-progestogen therapy (EPT).

◆ The number-one killer of older American women is cardiovascular disease, which includes coronary heart disease, stroke, congestive heart failure, hypertension, and other diseases of the heart and vascular system.

◆ Educating women about strategies to control the five cardiovascular risk factors (smoking, hyperlipidemia, diabetes mellitus, hypertension, obesity) can empower them to make changes that can greatly reduce their lifetime risk for cardiovascular disease.

◆ Bone health promotion includes strategies such as optimizing calcium intake, preventing the loss of calcium and other minerals from the bone, maintaining the soft tissue components around the bone, and promoting the efficiency of bone repair.

◆ An essential role for nurses who care for women who take prescribed osteoporosis medications centers on education and counseling about potential risks and side effects as well as the importance of adhering to specific dosing recommendations for the bisphosphonates.

review questions

Multiple Choice

1. Normal physiological changes that accompany menopause include:
   a. Vaginal lengthening with an increased production of cervical mucus
   b. An increase in muscle mass
   c. Less elastic skin with decreased melanin
   d. Increased levels of estrogen and progesterone

2. Nurses can teach women about self-care strategies to help reduce menopausal symptoms, such as:
   a. Dressing in layers
   b. Consuming foods and beverages that contain caffeine
   c. Reducing physical activity
   d. Consuming foods that are highly seasoned

3. According to recommendations from the North American Menopause Society, recommendations for hormone therapy use include:
   a. Prevention of diabetes mellitus
   b. Short-term treatment for severe vasomotor symptoms
   c. Prevention of coronary heart disease
   d. Prevention of dementia

4. Risk factors for cardiovascular disease include:
   a. Normal body weight
   b. Parkinson's disease
   c. Psychological stress
   d. Regular dietary consumption of fiber, fruits, and vegetables

5. Risk factors for osteoporosis include:
   a. Excessive sun exposure
   b. Large body build
   c. Late menopause
   d. Caucasian ethnicity

REFERENCES

Alexander, I.M.(2006). Bioidentical hormones for menopause therapy: Separating the myths from the reality. *Women's Health Care,* 5(1), 7–17.

Alexander, I.M. (2007). Overview of current HT recommendations using evidence-based decision making. *American Journal for Nurse Practitioners,* 11(10), 29–41.

Alexander, I.M. (2009). Harnessing the hot flash: More choices for midlife women. *Advance for Nurse Practitioners,* 17(7), 31–34.

Allmen, T., & Moore, A. (2010). Attention and intervention: Responding to vaginal changes of menopause. *Women's Health Care: A Practical Journal for Nurse Practitioners,* 9(5), 38–51.

Altman, A.M. (2008). Postmenopausal hormone therapy—updates. *Women's Health Care,* 7(10), 7–15.

Altman, A. (2009). Transdermal hormone therapy compared to oral hormone therapy: The impact of the first-pass effect. *Contemporary OB/GYN (Supplement),* 22(1), S8–S12.

Altman, A.M., Moore, A., Speroff, L., & Wysocki, S. (2009). Tackling the tricky issue of bioidentical hormones. *Women's Health Care: A Practical Journal for Nurse Practitioners,* 8(7), 7–15.

American College of Obstetricians and Gynecologists (ACOG). (2001). *Use of botanicals for management of menopausal symptoms.* (Practice Bulletin Number 28), 1–10. Washington, DC: Author.

American College of Obstetricians and Gynecologists (ACOG). (2004a). *Osteoporosis.* (Practice Bulletin Number 50), 1170–1183. Washington, DC: Author.

American College of Obstetricians and Gynecologists (ACOG). (2004b). Hormone therapy: Cognition and dementia. *Obstetrics and Gynecology,* 104(Suppl), 25S–40S.

American College of Obstetricians and Gynecologists (ACOG). (2005). *Compounded bioidentical hormones.* (Committee Opinion Number 322), 298–299. Washington, DC: Author.

American College of Obstetricians and Gynecologists (ACOG). (2007). *Women's health care: A Resource manual* (3rd ed.). Washington, DC: Author.

American College of Obstetricians and Gynecologists (ACOG). (2008a). *Hormone therapy and heart disease.* (Committee Opinion Number 420), 115–118. Washington, DC: Author.

American College of Obstetricians and Gynecologists (ACOG). (2008b). *Low bone mass (osteopenia) and fracture risk.* (Committee Opinion Number 407), 102–104. Washington, DC: Author.

American Diabetes Association (ADA). (2006). *The cardiometabolic risk initiative: Moving beyond the metabolic syndrome.* Retrieved June 5, 2010, from http://professional.diabetes.org/ResourcesForProfessionals.aspx?cid=60379

American Heart Association (AHA). (2002). National Cholesterol Education Program (NCEP) Expert Panel on Detection, Evaluation, and Treatment of High Blood Cholesterol in Adults (Adult Treatment Panel III). Third report of the National Cholesterol Education Program (NCEP) Expert Panel on Detection, Evaluation, and Treatment of High Blood Cholesterol in Adults (Adult Treatment Panel III) Final Report. *Circulation, 106*(25), 3143–3421.

American Heart Association (AHA). (2010). *Heart disease & stroke statistics: 2010 update.* Retrieved May 18, 2010, from http://www.americanheart.org/downloadable/heart/1265665152970DS-3241HeartStrokeUpdate_2010.pdf

American Heart Association (AHA). (2010). *Facts about women and cardiovascular diseases.* Retrieved May 18, 2010, from http://www.americanheart.org/presenter.jhtml?identifier=1200011

Bachmann, G.A. (2008). A menopausal hormone therapy update. *The Female Patient, 34*(3), 24–25.

Bachmann, G.A. (2008). The utilization of intravenous bisphosphonates. *The Female Patient (Supplement), 33*(11), S9–12.

Berga, S.L. (2009). Putting hormones and aging into perspective: State of hormone therapy for vasomotor symptoms. *Contemporary OB/GYN (Supplement), 22*(1), S3–S7.

Bergfeld, W.F., & Harrison, S. (2009). Treating osteoporosis and postmenopausal hair loss. *Contemporary OB/GYN, 54*(5), 32–33.

Blumenthal, R.S., Michos, E.D., & Nasir, K. (2007). Further improvements in CHD risk prediction for Women. *Journal of the American Medical Association, 297*(6), 641–643.

Burdette, L. (2009). Managing the vaginal and urinary symptoms of postmenopausal urogenital atrophy: A case-based approach. *Women's Health Care: A Practical Journal for Nurse Practitioners, 8*(9), 12–21.

Burdette, L., Moore, A., Speroff, L., & Wysocki, S. (2009). Hormone therapy in menopause: Applying research findings to optimal patient care and education. *Women's Health Care: A Practical Journal for Nurse Practitioners, 8*(5), 10–21.

Burkman, R.T. (2009). Are your patients asking for bioidentical hormones? *The Female Patient, 34*(6), 15–16.

Cadarette, S.M., Katz, J.N., Brookhart, M.A., Levin, R., Stedman, M.R., Choudhry, N.K., & Solomon, D.H. (2008). Trends in drug prescribing for osteoporosis after hip fracture, 1995–2004. *Journal of Rheumatology, 35*(2), 319–326.

Christian, A.H., Rosamond, W., White, A.R., & Mosca, L. (2007). Nine-year trends and racial and ethnic disparities in women's awareness of heart disease and stroke: An American Heart Association national study. *Journal of Women's Health, 16*(1), 68–81.

Cole, R.E. (2009). A new drug in a new class for postmenopausal osteoporosis. *The Female Patient, 34*(11), 20–24.

Costantino, D., & Guaraldi, C. (2008). Effectiveness and safety of vaginal suppositories for the treatment of the vaginal atrophy in postmenopausal women: An open, non-controlled clinical trial. *European Review for Medical and Pharmacological Sciences, 12*(6), 411–416.

Dawson-Hughes, B., Lindsay, R., Khosla, S., Melton, L.J., III, Tosteson, A.N.A., Favus, M., & Baim, S. (2008). *Clinician's guide to prevention and treatment of osteoporosis.* National Osteoporosis Foundation: Washington, DC.

Dranov, P. (2007). Homone therapy is making a comeback. *The Clinical Advisor, 10*(5), 72–83.

Edelman, J. (2010). Managing the menopausal patient. *The Clinical Advisor, 55*(1), 84.

Ettinger, B., & Ettinger, K.M. (2009). FRAX: Using the new fracture risk assessment tool. *Contemporary OB/GYN, 54*(7), 22–28.

Flores, V., & Taylor, H.S. (2010). Current and future SERMs: An update. *The Female Patient, 35*(5), 21–24.

Freeman, R. (2009). Changes in hair growth patterns in postmenopausal women. *The Female Patient, 34*(10), 47–48.

Freeman, S.B. (2009). Micronized progesterone: An important option for oral hormone therapy. *Women's Health Care: A Practical Journal for Nurse Practitioners, 8*(12), 7–13.

Geller, S.E., & Studee, L. (2008). Botanical and dietary supplements for menopause. *The Female Patient, 33*(6), 19–24.

Gersh, F.L. (2009).Estradiol gel 0.1% clinical data. *Contemporary OB/GYN (Supplement).* 22(1), S16–S19.

Gertz, B.J., Holland, S.D., Kline, W.F., Matuszewski, B.K., Freeman, A., Quan, H., Lasseter, K.C., Mucklow, J.C., & Porras, A.G. (1995). Studies of the oral bioavailability of aldendronate. *Clinical Pharmacology & Therapeutics, 58*(3), 288–298.

Gies, C., & Lessick, M. (2009). Alzheimer disease in women: A clinical and genetics perspective. *Nursing for Women's Health, 13*(4), 314–324.

Giovannucci, E. (2009).Vitamin D and cancer incidence in the Harvard cohorts. *Annals of Epidemiology, 19*(4), 84–88.

Goldstein, S.R. (2008). Osteoporosis: Screening and diagnosis in clinical practice. *The Female Patient (Supplement), 33*(11), S1–4.

Goldstein, L., & Alexander, J.L. (2005). Practical aspects in the management of vaginal atrophy and sexual dysfunction in perimenopausal and postmenopausal women. *Journal of Sexual Medicine, 2*(Suppl. 3), 154–165.

Greenblum, C., Greenblum, J., & Neff, D. (2009). Vaginal estrogen use in menopause: Is it safe? *The American Journal for Nurse Practitioners, 13*(9), 26–35.

Hellwig, J.P. (2009). Economics of exercise: Community-based physical activity programs are cost effective. *Nursing for Women's Health, 13*(1), 16.

Helmrich, G. (2010). NAMS position on hormone therapy. *Menopause, 19*(4), 34–36.

Henderson, V.W. (2009). Estrogen-containing hormone therapy and cognition: Consensus and controversy. *The Female Patient, 34*(5), 25–27.

Hess, H., London, A., Moore, A., & Simon, J. (2009). Pharmacologic treatment options for menopausal symptoms. *The Female Patient (Supplement), 34*(5), S1–58.

Hsia, J., Langer, R.D., Manson, J.E., Kuller, J., Johnson, K.C., & Hendrix, S.L., et al. (2006). Conjugated equine estrogens and coronary heart disease: The Women's Health Initiative. *Archives of Internal Medicine, 166*(3), 357–365.

Jones, K.A., Bryson, E., & Harmanli, O. (2010). Successful pelvic floor rehabilitation practice for the obstetrician/gynecologist. *The Female Patient, 35*(5), 41–43.

Kagan, R. (2009). Charting a course for postmenopausal women after hormone therapy. *Contemporary OB/GYN, 54*(11), 22–24.

Kapustin, J. (2010). Chronic disease prevention across the lifespan. *The Journal for Nurse Practitioners, 6*(1), 16–24.

Kaunitz, A.M. (2008). Counseling patients on the management of osteoporosis. *The Female Patient (Supplement), 33*(11), S13–16.

Kellogg-Spadt, S. (2010). Vulvovaginal atrophy: Who benefits most from estrogen therapy? *Advance for Nurse Practitioners, 18*(4), 31–36.

Kessenich, C.R. (2009). Fracture risk assessment in osteoporosis management. *The American Journal for Nurse Practitioners, 13*(9), 36–42.

Kupferer, E.M., Dormire, S.L., & Becker, H. (2009). Complementary and alternative medicine use for vasomotor symptoms among women who have discontinued hormone therapy. *Journal of Obstetric, Gynecologic, and Neonatal Nurses, 38*(1), 50–59.

LaCroix, A.Z. (2005). Estrogen with and without progestin: Benefits and risks of short-term use. *American Journal of Medicine, 118*(12 Suppl. 2), 79–87.

Lake, K. (2007). Beware of bioidentical hormones! *The Clinical Advisor, 10*(9), 121.

Lichtenstein, A.H., Appel, L.J., Brands, M., et al. (2006). Diet and lifestyle recommendations revision 2006: A scientific statement from the American Heart Association nutrition committee. *Circulation, 114*(1), 82–96.

Liu, J.H. (2007). Progestins in hormone therapy: What are the options? *Female Patient, 32*(2), 33–39.

Loprinzi, C.L., Levitt, R., Barton, D., Sloan, J.A., Dakhil, S.R., Nikcevich, D.A., et al. (2006). Phase III comparison of depomedroxyprogesterone acetate to vanlafaxine for managing hot flashes: North Central

Cancer Treatment Group Trial N99C7. *Journal of Clinical Oncology*, 24(9), 1409–1414.

Madala, M.C., Franklin, B.A., Chen, A.Y., & Berman, A.D., et al. (2008). Obesity and age of first non-ST segment elevation myocardial infarction. *Journal of the American College of Cardiology*, 52(12), 979–985.

Malone, R.W., & Kessenich, C. (2008). Vitamin D deficiency: Implications across the lifespan. *The Journal for Nurse Practitioners*, 4(6), 448–454.

Manson, J.E. (2009). Expert advice on aspirin, MI, and stroke. *Contemporary OB-GYN*, 54(9), 66–67.

Margolis, M. (2010). How drug delivery and pharmacokinetics impact estrogen therapy. *The Female Patient (Supplement)*, 35(5), S1–S8.

Mayhew, M.S. (2009). Vitamin D deficiency and treatment. *The Journal for Nurse Practitioners*, 5(10), 773–774.

McKee, J., & Warber, S.L. (2005). Integrative therapies for menopause. *Southern Medical Journal*, 98(3), 319–326.

McNeal, C.J., & Birchem, J. (2009a). Cardiovascular disease in women, part 1: Identification of women at risk. *The Female Patient*, 34(6), 43–48.

McNeal, C.J., & Birchem, J. (2009b). Cardiovascular disease in women, part 2: The therapeutic spectrum. *The Female Patient*, 34(7), 44–50.

Mehta, A., & Bachmann, G. (2008). Vulvovaginal complaints. *Clinical Obstetrics and Gynecology*, 51(3), 549–555.

Miller, P.D. (2009). Treating osteoporosis and postmenopausal hair loss. *Contemporary OB/GYN*, 54(5), 31–32.

Minarik, P.A. (2009). Sleep disturbance in midlife women. *Journal of Obstetric, Gynecologic, and Neonatal Nurses*, 38(3), 333–343.

Minkin, M.J. (2010). Transdermal estrogen therapy: Personalized treatment approaches. *The Female Patient*, 35(6), 16–18.

Moore, A. (2010). Bioidentical hormone therapy: What practitioners need to know now. *Women's Health care: A Practical Journal for Nurse Practitioners*, 9(5), 10–18.

Mosca, L., Banka, C.L., Benjamin, E.J., Berra, K., Bushnell, C., Dolor, R.J., et al. (2007). Evidence-based guidelines for cardiovascular disease prevention in women: 2007 update. *Circulation*, 115(11), 1481–1501.

Mosca, L., Ferris, A., Fabunmi, R., & Robertson, R.M. (2004).Tracking women's awareness of heart disease: An American Heart Association national study. *Circulation*, 109(5), 573–579.

Mosca, L., Mochari, H., Christian, A., Berra, K., Taubert, K., Mills, T., Burdick, K.A., & Simpson, S.L. (2006). National study of women's awareness, preventive action, and barriers to cardiovascular health. *Circulation*, 113(4), 525–534.

Nachtigall, L.E. (2009). Understanding the pathophysiology of estrogen clotting issues: Oral vs transdermal routes. *Contemporary OB/GYN (Supplement)*, 22(10), S12–S16.

Nachtigall, L.E., Baber, R.J., Barentsen, R., Durand, N., Panay, N., & Pitkin, J., et al. (2006). Complementary and hormonal therapy for vasomotor symptom relief: A conservative clinical approach. *Journal of Obstetrics and Gynaecology Canada*, 28(4), 279–289.

National Institutes of Health. (2005). National Institutes of Health state-of-the science conference statement: Management of menopause-related symptoms. *Annals of Internal Medicine*, 142(12 Part 1), 1003–1013.

National Institutes of Health. (2009). *Dietary supplement fact sheet: Calcium*. Retrieved May 30, 2010, from http://ods.od.nih.gov/factsheets/calcium.asp

National Osteoporosis Foundation (NOF). (2008a). *Medications to prevent & treat osteoporosis*. Retrieved May 18, 2010, from http://www.nof.org/patientinfo/medications.htm

National Osteoporosis Foundation (NOF). (2008b). *Fast facts on osteoporosis*. Retrieved May 25, 2010, from http://www.nof.org/osteoporosis/diseasefacts.htm

National Osteoporosis Foundation (NOF). (2008c). *Prevention: Calcium*. Retrieved May 30, 2010, from http://www.nof.org/prevention/calcium2.htm

National Osteoporosis Foundation (NOF). (2008d).*Prevention: Exercise for healthy bones*. Retrieved May 28, 2010, from http://www.nof.org/prevention/exercise.htm

National Women's Health Network. (2000). *Taking hormones and women's health: Choices, Risks, and benefits* (5th ed.). Washington, DC: Author.

Nelson, A.L. (2009). Fracture risk reduction: How to use FRAX in your practice. *The Female Patient*, 34(2), 22–24.

Nelson, A.L., & Stewart, F.H. (2003). Menopause and perimenopausal health. In R. Hatcher, J. Trussell, A. Nelson, W. Cates, Jr., F. Stewart, & D. Kowal (Eds.), *Contraceptive technology*, (19th ed., pp. 699–745). New York: Thomson Reuters.

Nelson, H.D., Haney, E., Humphrey, L., Miller, J., Nedrow, A., Nicolaidis, C., Vesco, K., Walker, M., Bougatsos, C., & Nygren, P. (2005). Management of menopause-related symptoms. Summary, Evidence Report/Technology Assessment: Number 120. *AHRQ Publication No. 05-E016-1*. Retrieved June 8, 2010, from http://www.ahrq.gov/clinic/epcsums/menosum.htm

Nelson, H.D., Vesco, K.K., Haney, E., Fu, R., Nedrow, A., & Miller, J., et al. (2006). Non-hormonal therapies for menopausal hot flashes: Systematic review and meta-analysis. *Journal of the American Medical Association*, 295(17), 2057–2071.

Palacios, S. (2009). Managing urogenital atrophy. *Maturitas*, 63(4), 315–318.

Patel, P., & Nunley, J.R. (2010). Lichen sclerosis et atrophicus. *The Clinical Advisor*, 35(2), 59–60.

Pinkerton, J.V., & Dalkin, A.C. (2007). Combination therapy for treatment of osteoporosis: A review. *American Journal of Obstetrics and Gynecology*, 197(6), 559–565.

Pinkerton J.V., & Dalkin, A.C. (2009). Approaches to the treatment of osteoporosis. *The Female Patient*, 34(6), 30–33.

Pugliese, J.M., Morey, A.F., & Peterson, A.C. (2007). Lichen sclerosus: Review of the literature and current recommendations for management. *The Journal of Urology*, 178(6), 2268–2276.

Reeve, K., & Bailes, B. (2010). Insomnia in adults: Etiology and management. *The Journal for Nurse Practitioners*, 6(1), 53–60.

Reiter, S. (2009). Sexual dysfunction and vaginal atrophy in menopausal women: An approach to effective communication and management. *Women's Health Care: A Practical Journal for Nurse Practitioners*, 8(9), 22–33.

Ridker, P.M., Buring, J.E., Rifai, N., & Cook, N.R. (2007). Development and validation of improved algorithms for the assessment of global cardiovascular risk in women: The Reynolds Risk Score. *Journal of the American Medical Association*, 297(6), 611–619.

Rosenthal, M.S. (2008). Ethical problems with bioidentical hormones. *International Journal of Impotence Research*, 20(1), 45–52.

Rosenthal, M.S. (2009). Bioidentical hormones: Ethics and misinformed consent. *The Female Patient*, 34(8), 28–31.

Ruhl, C. (2009). Cardiometabolic health: Connecting the dots. *Nursing for Women's Health*, 13(1), 78–82.

Ruhl, C. (2010). Sleep is a vital sign: Why assessing sleep is an important part of women's health care. *Nursing for Women's Health*, 14(3), 243–247.

Rutecki, G.W. (2009). May the sun shine half day long: Balancing the risks and benefits of sun exposure. *Consultant*, 49(8), 509.

Scott, A. (2009). FDA approves new drug indication for Forteo. *Drug Topics E-News*. Retrieved May 30, 2010, from http://drugtopics.modernmedicine.com/drugtopics/Community+Practice/FDA-approves-new-drug-indication-for-Forteo/ArticleStandard/Article/detail/614527

Secor, R.M., & Simon, J.A. (2006). New options for treating the symptoms of menopause. *Women's Health in Primary Care*, 6(4), 44–52.

Sego, S. (2009). Olive oil. *The Clinical Advisor*, 12(9), 71–72.

Sherman, C. (2009a). Hormone therapy following menopause. *The Clinical Advisor*, 12(11), 29–35.

Sherman, C. (2009b). Osteoporosis: No gender gap for therapy. *The Clinical Advisor*, 12(6), 16–20.

Shulman, L.P. (2008). Advances in treating vasomotor symptoms in postmenopausal women. *The Female Patient (Supplement)*, 33(6), S27–31.

Simon, J.A. (2008). Pharmacologic prevention and treatment of osteoporosis. *The Female Patient (Supplement)*, 33(11), S5–8.

Slentz, C.A., Duscha, B.D., & Johnson, J.L., et al. (2004). Effects of the amount of exercise on body weight, body composition, and measures of central obesity: STRRIDE—a randomized controlled study. *Archives of Internal Medicine*, 164(1), 31–39.

Smith, S.C., Jr., Allen, J., Blair, S.N., & Bonow, R.O., et al. (2006). ACC guidelines for secondary prevention for patients with coronary and other atherosclerotic vascular disease: 2006 update: Endorsed by the National Heart, Lung, and Blood Institute. *Circulation*, 113(19), 2363–2372.

Speroff, L., & Fritz, M.A. (2005). *Clinical gynecologic endocrinology and infertility* (7th ed.). Philadelphia: Lippincott Williams & Wilkins.

Syroney, L., & Franjesevic, A. (2010). Vitamin D deficiency: Screening and treatment in primary care. *Advance for Nurse Practitioners*, 18(5), 37–40.

Thanavaro, J.L. (2005). Barriers to coronary heart disease risk modification in women without prior history of coronary heart disease. *Journal of the American Academy of Nurse Practitioners*, 17(11), 487–493.

Theroux, R. (2008). Postmenopausal hormone use: What does the latest evidence show? *Nursing for Women's Health, 12*(1), 56–61.

The North American Menopause Society (NAMS). (2007). *Menopause practice: A clinician's guide* (3rd ed.). Cleveland, OH: Author.

The North American Menopause Society (NAMS). (2010a). *Estrogen and progestogen use in postmenopausal women: 2010 position statement of The North American Menopause Society, 17*(2), 242–255.

The North American Menopause Society (NAMS). (2010b). *Osteoporosis in postmenopausal women: 2010 position statement.* Retrieved June 1, 2010, from http://www.medscape.com/viewarticle/714984_2

U.S. Preventive Services Task Force (USPSTF). (2002). *Osteoporosis screening.* Retrieved May 25, 2010, from http://www.ahrq.gov/clinic/3rduspstf/osteoporosis/

U.S. Preventive Services Task Force (USPSTF). (2009). *Guide to clinical preventive health services, 2009: Recommendations of the U.S. Preventive Services Task Force* (AHRQ Publication No. 09-IP006). Available from http://www.ahrq.gov

Utian, W.H. (2008). The practical clinical application of the NAMS 2008 position statement on estrogen and progestogen use in postmenopausal women. *Women's Health Care: A Practical Journal for Nurse Practitioners, 7*(8), 50–59.

Utian, W.H., Archer, D.F., Bachmann, G.A., et al; North American Menopause Society. (2008). Estrogen andprogestogen use in postmenopausal women: July 2008 position statement of The North American Menopause Society. *Menopause, 15*(4, pt 1), 584–602.

Valerio, T.D. (2009). Much more than a nuisance: Health consequences of sleep disorders. *Advance for Nurse Practitioners, 17*(9), 57–60.

Vassar, K.A. (2009). Promoting cardiovascular health in women. *Women's Health Care: A Practical Journal for Nurse Practitioners, 8*(12), 28–33.

Venes, D. (2010). *Taber's cyclopedic medical dictionary* (21st ed.). Philadelphia: F.A. Davis Company.

Watts, N.B., Ettinger, B., & LeBoff, M.S. (2009). FRAX facts. *Journal of Bone and Mineral Research, 24*(3), 975–979.

Weed, S. (2002). *New menopausal years, the wise woman way: Alternative approaches for Women.* Woodstock, NY: Ash Tree.

Weil, E. (2009). Bioidentical hormones: Examining the debate. *Advance for Nurse Practitioners, 17*(9), 37–41.

Wenger, N.K. (2007). Cardiovascular risk assessment and intervention strategies in women. *Women's Health in Primary Care, Supplement,* September, 2007, S1–S11.

Williams, J. K., & Brownlee, J. (2010). The dietary clinical trials of the Women's Health Initiative: Part 2. *The Female Patient, 35*(4), 39–41.

Writing Group for the Women's Health Initiative Investigators. (2002). Risks and benefits of estrogen plus progestin in healthy postmenopausal women. *Journal of the American Medical Association, 288* (7), 321–333.

Wysocki, S. (2008). Etiology, consequences, and management of vaginal atrophy. *The American Journal for Nurse Practitioners, 12*(11/12), 36–46.

Wysocki, S. (2009a). Local estrogen therapy—Preferred treatment for symptoms of menopausal vulvovaginal atrophy. *Women's Health Care: A Practical Journal for Nurse Practitioners, 8*(11), 8–16.

Wysocki, S. (2009b). Targeting the urogenital health of postmenopausal women: A spotlight on vaginal atrophy. *Women's Health Care: A Practical Journal for Nurse Practitioners, 9*(9), 10–11.

Wysowski, D.K. (2009). Reports of esophageal cancer with oral bisphosphonate use. *New England Journal of Medicine, 360*(1), 89–90.

 For more information, go to http://davisplus.fadavis.com/

Index